FUNDAMENTAL VIROLOGY

Fourth Edition

FUNDAMENTAL VIROLOGY

Fourth Edition

Editors-in-Chief

David M. Knipe, Ph.D.
Higgins Professor of Microbiology and Molecular Genetics
Harvard Medical School
Boston, Massachusetts

Peter M. Howley, M.D.
George Fabyan Professor of Comparative Pathology
Department of Pathology
Harvard Medical School
Boston, Massachusetts

Associate Editors

Diane E. Griffin, M.D., Ph.D.
Department of Molecular Biology and Immunology
Johns Hopkins School of Public Health
Baltimore, Maryland

Robert A. Lamb, Ph.D., Sc.D.
Howard Hughes Medical Institute
Department of Biochemistry, Molecular Biology, and Cell Biology
Northwestern University
Evanston, Illinois

Malcolm A. Martin, M.D.
Laboratory of Molecular Microbiology
National Institute of Allergy and Infectious Diseases
National Institutes of Health
Bethesda, Maryland

Bernard Roizman, Sc.D.
Departments of Molecular Genetics and Cell Biology and Molecular Biology and Biochemistry
University of Chicago
Chicago, Illinois

Stephen E. Straus, M.D.
Chief, Laboratory of Clinical Investigation
National Institute of Allergy and Infectious Diseases
Director, National Center for Complementary and Alternative Medicine
National Institutes of Health
Bethesda, Maryland

LIPPINCOTT WILLIAMS & WILKINS
A **Wolters Kluwer** Company
Philadelphia • Baltimore • New York • London
Buenos Aires • Hong Kong • Sydney • Tokyo

Acquisitions Editor: Jonathan Pine
Developmental Editor: Anne Snyder
Production Editor: Robin E. Cook
Manufacturing Manager: Tim Reynolds
Cover Designer: Patricia Gast
Compositor: Lippincott Williams & Wilkins Desktop Division
Printer: Courier Westford

530 Walnut Street
Philadelphia, PA 19106 USA
LWW.com

Printed in the USA

Library of Congress Cataloging-in-Publication Data

Fundamental virology / editors-in-chief, David M. Knipe, Peter M. Howley ; associate editors, Diane E. Griffin ... [et al.].–4th ed.
p. ; cm.
Consists of selected chapters reprinted from: Fields virology. 4th ed. c2001.
Includes bibliographical references and index.
ISBN 0-7817-1833-3
1. Viruses. 2. Virology. I. Knipe, David M. (David Mahan), 1950–
II. Howley, Peter M. III. Griffin, Diane E. IV. Fields virology.
[dNLM: 1. Viruses. 2. Virus Replication. QW 160 F981 2001]
QR360 .F847 2001
616'.0194–dc21

2001029482

Care has been taken to confirm the accuracy of the information presented and to describe generally accepted practices. However, the authors, editors, and publisher are not responsible for errors or omissions or for any consequences from application of the information in this book and make no warranty, expressed or implied, with respect to the currency, completeness, or accuracy of the contents of the publication. Application of this information in a particular situation remains the professional responsibility of the practitioner.

The authors, editors, and publisher have exerted every effort to ensure that drug selection and dosage set forth in this text are in accordance with current recommendations and practice at the time of publication. However, in view of ongoing research, changes in government regulations, and the constant flow of information relating to drug therapy and drug reactions, the reader is urged to check the package insert for each drug for any change in indications and dosage and for added warnings and precautions. This is particularly important when the recommended agent is a new or infrequently employed drug.

Some drugs and medical devices presented in this publication have Food and Drug Administration (FDA) clearance for limited use in restricted research settings. It is the responsibility of the health care provider to ascertain the FDA status of each drug or device planned for use in their clinical practice.

10 9 8 7 6 5 4 3 2 1

Contents

Part II. Specific Virus Families

Contributing Authors

L. Andrew Ball, *Professor, Microbiology Department, University of Alabama at Birmingham, Birmingham, Alabama*

Kenneth I. Berns, M.D., Ph.D., *Vice-President of Health Affairs, Dean, College of Medicine, Professor, Department of Molecular Genetics and Microbiology, Powell Gene Therapy Center, University of Florida, Gainesville, Gainesville, Florida*

Christine A. Biron, M.D., *Esther Elizabeth Brintzenhoff Professor of Medical Science and Chair, Department of Molecular Microbiology and Immunology, Brown University, Providence, Rhode Island*

Allan M. Campbell, Ph.D., *Professor, Department of Biological Sciences, Stanford University, Stanford, California*

Donald M. Coen, Ph.D., *Professor, Department of Biological Chemistry and Molecular Pharmacology, Harvard Medical School, Boston, Massachusetts*

Charles N. Cole, Ph.D., *Professor, Department of Biochemistry, Dartmouth Medical School, Hanover, New Hampshire*

Richard C. Condit, Ph.D., *Professor, Department of Molecular Genetics and Microbiology, University of Florida College of Medicine, Gainesville, Florida*

Suzanne D. Conzen, M.D., *Assistant Professor, Hematology/Oncology Section, Department of Medicine, University of Chicago School of Medicine, Chicago, Illinois*

Daniel DiMaio, M.D., *Professor, Department of Genetics, Yale University School of Medicine, New Haven, Connecticut*

Eric O. Freed, Ph.D., *Principal Investigator, Laboratory of Molecular Microbiology, National Institute of Allergy and Infectious Diseases, National Institutes of Health, Bethesda, Maryland*

Paul D. Friesen, Ph.D., *Professor, Institute for Molecular Virology, University of Wisconsin, Madison, Madison, Wisconsin*

Donald Ganem, M.D., *Professor and Vice Chair, Department of Microbiology, University of California, San Francisco, San Francisco, California*

Stephen P. Goff, Ph.D., *Higgins Professor of Biochemistry, Department of Biochemistry and Molecular Biophysics, Columbia University College of Physicians and Surgeons, New York, New York*

Stephen C. Harrison, Ph.D., *Higgins Professor of Biochemistry, Investigator, Howard Hughes Medical Institute, Department of Molecular and Cellular Biology, Harvard University, Boston, Massachusetts*

Kathryn V. Holmes, Ph.D., *Department of Microbiology, University of Colorado Health Sciences Center, Denver, Colorado*

Jay W. Hooper, Ph.D., *Staff Scientist, Virology Division, United States Army Medical Research Institute of Infectious Diseases, Frederick, Maryland*

Peter M. Howley, M.D., *George Fabyan Professor of Comparative Pathology, Chairman, Department of Pathology, Harvard Medical School, Boston, Massachusetts*

Eric Hunter, Ph.D., *Professor of Microbiology, Director, UAB Center for AIDS Research, University of Alabama at Birmingham, Birmingham, Alabama*

Elliott Kieff, M.D., Ph.D., *Harriet Ryan Albee Professor, Departments of Medicine/Microbiology and Molecular Genetics, Harvard Medical School, Boston, Massachusetts*

David M. Knipe, Ph.D., *Higgins Professor of Microbiology and Molecular Genetics, Department of Microbiology and Molecular Genetics, Harvard Medical School, Boston, Massachusetts*

Daniel Kolakofsky, Ph.D., *Department of Genetics and Microbiology, University of Geneva Medical School, Geneva, Switzerland*

Robert M. Krug, Ph.D., *Institute for Cellular and Molecular Biology, University of Texas at Austin, Austin, Texas*

Michael M. C. Lai, M.D., Ph.D., *Professor, Department of Molecular Microbiology and Immunology, University of Southern California, Los Angeles, California*

Robert A. Lamb, Ph.D., Sc.D., *John Evans Professor of Molecular and Cellular Biology, Department of Biochemistry, Molecular Biology and Cell Biology, Investigator, Howard Hughes Medical Institute, Northwestern University, Chicago, Illinois*

Sondra G. Lazarowitz, Ph.D., *Professor, Department of Plant Pathology, College of Agriculture and Life Sciences, Cornell University, Ithaca, New York*

Arnold J. Levine, Ph.D., *Professor, Department of Cancer Biology, The Rockefeller University, New York, New York*

Brett D. Lindenbach, *Howard Hughes Medical Institute, Institute for Molecular Virology, University of Wisconsin, Madison, Wisconsin*

Douglas R. Lowy, *Chief, Laboratory of Cellular Oncology, Division of Basic Sciences, National Cancer Institute, National Institutes of Health, Bethesda, Maryland*

Malcolm A. Martin, M.D., *Chief, Laboratory of Molecular Microbiology, National Institute of Allergy and Infectious Diseases, National Institutes of Health, Bethesda, Maryland*

Lois K. Miller, Ph.D. (deceased), *Departments of Genetics and Entomology, University of Georgia, Athens, Georgia*

Bernard Moss, M.D., Ph.D., *Laboratory Chief, Laboratory of Viral Diseases, National Institute of Allergy and Infectious Diseases, National Institutes of Health, Bethesda, Maryland*

Nicholas Muzyczka, Ph.D., *Professor, Department of Molecular Genetics and Microbiology, Director, Powell Gene Therapy Center, University of Florida College of Medicine, Gainesville, Florida*

Neal Nathanson, M.D., *Director, Office of AIDS Research, National Institutes of Health, Bethesda, Maryland, and Professor and Chair Emeritus, University of Pennsylvania School of Medicine, Philadelphia, Pennsylvania*

Joseph R. Nevins, Ph.D., *James B. Duke Professor and Chairman, Department of Genetics, Duke University Medical Center, and Investigator, Howard Hughes Medical Institute, Durham, North Carolina*

Max L. Nibert, Ph.D., *Department of Microbiology and Molecular Genetics, Harvard Medical School, Boston, Massachusetts*

Michael B. A. Oldstone, M.D., *Division of Virology, Department of Neuropharmacology, The Scripps Research Institute, La Jolla, California*

Peter Palese, M.D., *Professor and Chair, Department of Microbiology, Mount Sinai School of Medicine, New York, New York*

Alexander Pfeifer, M.D., *Postdoctoral Research Associate, Laboratory of Genetics, The Salk Institute for Biological Studies, La Jolla, California*

Stanley B. Prusiner, M.D., *Professor of Neurology, Institute for Neurodegenerative Diseases, University of California, San Francisco, San Francisco, California*

Vincent R. Racaniello, Ph.D., *Higgins Professor, Department of Microbiology, Columbia University College of Physicians & Surgeons, New York, New York*

Charles M. Rice, Ph.D., *Center for the Study of Hepatitis C, Laboratory for Virology and Infectious Disease, The Rockefeller University, New York, New York*

Alan B. Rickinson, M.D., *Cancer Research Campaign for Cancer Studies, University of Birmingham, Birmingham, United Kingdom*

Bernard Roizman, Sc.D., *Departments of Molecular Genetics and Cell Biology, and Molecular Biology, The Marjorie B. Kovler Viral Oncology Laboratories, University of Chicago, Chicago, Illinois*

John K. Rose, Ph.D., *Professor, Departments of Pathology and Cell Biology, Yale University School of Medicine, New Haven, Connecticut*

Charles E. Samuel, Ph.D., *Professor, Department of Molecular, Cellular, and Developmental Biology, University of California, Santa Barbara, Santa Barbara, California*

Leslie A. Schiff, M.D., *Department of Microbiology, University of Minnesota Medical School, Minneapolis, Minnesota*

Milton J Schlesinger, Ph.D., *Professor Emeritus, Department of Molecular Microbiology, Washington University School of Medicine, St. Louis, Missouri*

Sondra Schlesinger, Ph.D., *Professor, Department of Molecular Microbiology, Washington University School of Medicine, St. Louis, Missouri*

Connie S. Schmaljohn, Ph.D., *Chief, Department of Molecular Virology, United States Army Medical Research Institute of Infectious Diseases, Frederick, Maryland*

Robert Schneider, M.D., *Professor, Department of Microbiology, New York University Medical Center, New York, New York*

Ganes C. Sen, Ph.D., *Professor, Department of Molecular Biology, Lerner Research Institute, The Cleveland Clinic Foundation, Cleveland, Ohio*

Thomas E. Shenk, Ph.D., *Elkins Professor, Department of Molecular Biology, Princeton University, Princeton, New Jersey*

Kenneth L. Tyler, M.D., *Professor of Neurology, Medicine, Microbiology, and Immunology, University of Colorado Health Sciences Center, Denver, Colorado*

Inder M. Verma, Ph.D., *American Cancer Society Professor of Molecular Biology, Laboratory of Genetics, The Salk Institute for Biological Studies, La Jolla, California*

Michael A. Whitt, M.D., *Associate Professor, Department of Molecular Sciences, University of Tennessee Health Science Center, Memphis, Tennessee*

J. Lindsay Whitton, M.D., Ph.D., *Professor, Department of Neuropharmacology, The Scripps Research Institute, La Jolla, California*

Reed B. Wickner, M.D., *Chief, Laboratory of Biochemistry and Genetics, National Institute of Diabetes, Digestive and Kidney Diseases, National Institutes of Health, Bethesda, Maryland*

John A. T. Young, Ph.D., *The Howard M. Temin Professor in Cancer Research, McCardle Laboratory for Cancer Research, University of Wisconsin, Madison, Madison, Wisconsin*

Preface

The field of virology includes a broad range of subjects, ranging from the study of macromolecular structures of viruses to the molecular biology of viral replication, and from the interaction of the virus with the host cell to viral pathogenesis and the mechanisms of clinical disease in humans. Despite significant advances in medicine over the past half century, viruses remain as major pathogens in humans. Nevertheless, viruses have provided simple systems for scientific studies that continue to yield major insights into molecular genetics and eukaryotic molecular biology. The goal of *Fields Virology*, from which the present volume is derived, is to bring together basic and medical aspects of virology in a unified, comprehensive presentation. Thus, *Fields Virology* serves as an up-to-date reference and textbook for medical and graduate students as well as for scientists, physicians, and investigators interested in viruses as they are represented in the biological sciences.

This book, the fourth edition of *Fundamental Virology*, consists of a set of chapters reprinted from *Fields Virology*, Fourth Edition. Its purpose to provide a text for graduate and upper-level undergraduate students, researchers, scientists, and investigators whose primary interests are directed toward basic aspects of virology rather than its more clinical or applied areas. Like previous editions, the fourth edition is divided into two parts. The first part (Chapters 1 through 17) presents the basic concepts of general virology; the second part (Chapters 18 through 37) describes the biochemistry, molecular biology and cellular aspects of replication of selected individual viruses from the various virus families.

There have been many major advances in basic virology since the last edition, and all of the chapters have been updated to reflect these advances. In addition, we have added new chapters on principles of virology, virus entry and uncoating, replication of RNA viruses, replication of DNA viruses, virus assembly, and virus vectors and their applications to enhance the use of this book as a textbook for courses in general or molecular virology. We anticipate that course instructors may wish to further supplement the material in this book with material on pathogenesis and medical aspects of other viruses from *Fields Virology* that have not been included in *Fundamental Virology*.

We wish to thank Anne Snyder, Robin Cook, and Jonathan Pine at Lippincott Williams and Wilkins and Lisa Holik at Harvard Medical School for all of their many important contributions to the preparation of this book.

David M. Knipe, Ph.D.
Peter M. Howley, M.D.

Preface

SECTION I

General Virology

CHAPTER 1

The Origins of Virology

Arnold J. Levine

Virology, as a subject matter, has had a remarkable history. Viruses, because of their predatory nature, have shaped the history and evolution of their hosts. Virtually all living organisms, when studied carefully, have viral parasites, and so these smallest of living entities exert significant forces on all life forms, including themselves. The medical consequences of viral infections of humans have altered our history and have resulted in extraordinary efforts on the part of virologists to study, understand, and eradicate these agents. These virologists have elucidated new principles of life processes and taken major new directions in science. Many of the concepts and tools of molecular biology have been derived from the study of viruses and their host cells. This chapter is an attempt to review selected portions of this history as it relates to the development of new concepts in virology (50,51).

THE DEVELOPMENT OF THE CONCEPT OF VIRUSES

The Early Period: The 19th Century

By the last half of the 19th century, the existence of a diverse microbial world of bacteria, fungi, and protozoa was well established. As early as 1840, the noted German anatomist Jacob Henle of Gottingen (the discoverer of Henle's loop and the grandfather of 20th-century virologist Werner Henle) hypothesized the existence of infectious agents that were too small to be observed with the light microscope and that were able to cause specific diseases. In the absence of any direct evidence for such entities, however, his ideas failed to be accepted. It was at this time that three major advances in microbiology came together to set the stage for the development of the concept of a submicroscopic agent that would come to be called a virus.

The first of these ideas was the demonstration that the spontaneous generation of organisms did not occur. This notion had a long history, with experiments both supporting and refuting it. The credit, however, for finally disproving this hypothesis is commonly given to Louis Pasteur (1822–1895), who employed his swan-neck flasks to strike a mortal blow to the concept of spontaneous generation. Pasteur went on to study fermentation by different microbial agents. During these studies, he made it clear that "different kinds of microbes are associated with different kinds of fermentations" and he extended this concept to disease processes. Building on this, Robert Koch (1843–1910), a student of Jacob Henle and a country doctor in a small German village, demonstrated that the anthrax bacillus was the cause of this disease (1876) and that the tubercle bacillus was the cause of tuberculosis in humans (1882). Little of this would have been possible without the third major contribution by Joseph Lister (1827–1912). Once it was clear that organisms reproduce new organisms, the importance of a sterile field, whether in surgery or for the isolation of new organisms, became clear. Lister contributed the technique of limiting dilution to obtain pure cultures of organisms, and Koch developed solid media, the isolation of separate individual colonies of bacteria to obtain pure cultures, and the use of stains to visualize these microorganisms. Although many scientists of that day contributed to these tools and concepts, it was principally Pasteur, Lister, and Koch who put together a new experimental approach for medical science.

These studies formalized some of Jacob Henle's original ideas in what are now termed Koch's postulates for defining whether an organism was indeed the causative agent of a disease. These postulates state that (a) the organism must be regularly found in the lesions of the disease, (b) the organism must be isolated in pure culture, (c) inoculation of such a pure culture of organisms into a host should initiate the disease, and (d) the organism must be recovered once again from the lesions of the host. By the end of the 19th century, these concepts became the dominant paradigm of medical microbiology. They outlined an experimental method to be used in all situations. It was only when these rules broke down and failed to yield a causative agent that the concept of a virus was born.

The Discovery Period: 1886–1903

Adolf Mayer (1843–1942), a German scientist trained in the field of chemical technology (who had studied fermentation and plant nutrition), became the director of the Agricultural Experiment Station at Wageningen, Holland, in 1876. A few years later (1879), he began his research on diseases of tobacco and, although he was not the first to describe such diseases, he named the disease tobacco mosaic disease after the dark and light spots on infected leaves. In one of Mayer's experiments, he inoculated healthy plants with the juice extracted from diseased plants by grinding up the infected leaves in water. This was the first experimental transmission of a viral disease of plants, and Mayer reported that, "in nine cases out of ten (of inoculated plants), one will be successful in making the healthy plant . . . heavily diseased" (109). Although these studies established the infectious nature of the disease, neither a bacterial nor a fungal agent could be consistently cultured or detected in these extracts, so Koch's postulates could not be satisfied. In a preliminary communication in 1882 (108), he speculated that the cause could be a "soluble, possibly enzyme-like contagium, although almost any analogy for such a supposition is failing in science." However, 4 years later, in his definitive paper on this subject, Mayer concluded that the mosaic disease "is bacterial, but that the infectious forms have not yet been isolated, nor are their forms and mode of life known" (109).

The next step was taken by Dimitri Ivanofsky (1864–1920), a Russian scientist working in St. Petersburg. In 1887 and again in 1890, Ivanofsky was commissioned by the Russian Department of Agriculture to investigate the cause of a tobacco disease on plantations in Bassarabia, Ukraine, and the Crimea. Ivanofsky rapidly repeated Mayer's observations, demonstrating that the sap of infected plants contained an agent able to transmit the disease to healthy plants, and he added one additional step. He passed the infected sap through a filter that blocked the passage of bacteria—the Chamberland filter, made of unglazed porcelain. The Chamberland filter, perfected to purify water by Charles Chamberland, one of Pasteur's collaborators, contained pores small enough to retard most bacteria. On February 12, 1892, Ivanofsky reported to the Academy of Sciences of St. Petersburg that "the sap of leaves infected with tobacco mosaic disease retains its infectious properties even after filtration through Chamberland filter candles" (79). The importance of this experiment is that it provided an operational definition of viruses, an experimental technique by which an agent could qualify as a virus.

Ivanofsky, like Mayer before him, failed to culture an organism from the filtered sap and failed to satisfy Koch's postulates. He, too, was bound by the paradigm of the times suggesting that the filter might be defective or something might be wrong with his methods. He even suggested the possibility that a toxin (not a living/reproducing substance) might pass through the filter and cause the disease. As late as 1903, when Ivanofsky published his thesis (80), he could not depart from the possibility that bacteria caused this disease and that he and others had somehow failed to culture them. The dogma of the times and the obvious success of Koch's postulates kept most scientists from interpreting their data in a different way. It is equally curious that, at this time (1885), Pasteur was working with viruses and developing the rabies vaccine (117) but never investigated the unique nature of that infectious agent.

The third scientist to play a key role in the development of the concept of viruses was Martinus Beijerinck (1851–1931), a Dutch soil microbiologist who collaborated with Adolf Mayer at Wageningen. Beijerinck also showed that the sap of infected tobacco plants could retain its infectivity after filtration through a Chamberland candle filter. [He was unaware of Ivanofsky's work at the time (1898).] He then extended these studies by showing that the filtered sap could be diluted and then regain its "strength" after replication in living, growing tissue of the plant. The agent could reproduce itself (which meant that it was not a toxin) but only in living tissue, not in the cell-free sap of the plant. This explained the failure to culture the pathogen outside its host, and it set the stage for discovery of an organism smaller than bacteria (a filterable agent), not observable in the light microscope, and able to reproduce itself only in living cells or tissue. Beijerinck called this agent a "*contagium vivum fluidum*" (9), or a contagious living liquid. This concept began a 25-year debate about the nature of viruses; were they liquids or particles? This conflict was laid to rest when d'Herelle developed the plaque assay in

1917 (33) and when the first electron micrographs were taken of tobacco mosaic virus (TMV) in 1939 (88).

Thus, Mayer, Ivanofsky, and Beijerinck each contributed to the development of a new concept: a filterable agent too small to observe in the light microscope but able to cause disease by multiplying in living cells. Loeffler and Frosch (101) rapidly described and isolated the first filterable agent from animals, the foot-and-mouth disease virus, and Walter Reed and his team in Cuba (1901) recognized the first human filterable virus, yellow fever virus (122). The term *virus* [from the Latin for slimy liquid or poison (76)] was at that time used interchangeably for any infectious agent and so was applied to TMV. The literature of the first decades of the 20th century most often referred to these infectious entities as filterable agents, and this was indeed the operational definition of viruses. Sometime later, the term *virus* became restricted in use to those agents that fulfilled the criteria developed by Mayer, Ivanofsky, and Beijerinck and that were the first agents to cause a disease that could not be proven by using Koch's postulates.

The Plant Viruses and the Chemical Period: 1929–1956

Tobacco mosaic virus (TMV) continued to play a central role in exploring the nature and properties of viruses. The early decades of the 20th century saw the development of techniques to purify enzymes (proteins). The notion that viruses were proteins and so could be purified in the same way was first appreciated and applied by Vinson and Petre (1927–1931) at the Boyce Thompson Institute in Philadelphia. They precipitated the infectious TMV agent [using an infectivity assay developed by Holmes (75)] from the crude sap of infected plants using selected salts, acetone, or ethyl alcohol (144). They showed that the infectious virus could move in an electric field, just as proteins did. At the same time, H. A. Purdy-Beale, also at the Boyce Thompson Institute, produced in rabbits antibodies directed against TMV that could neutralize the infectivity of this agent (121). At the time, this was taken as further proof of the protein nature of viruses. With the advent of purification procedures for viruses, both physical and chemical measurements of the virus became possible. The strong flow birefringence of purified preparations of TMV was interpreted (correctly) to show an asymmetric particle or rod-shaped particle (136). Max Schlesinger (129), working on purified preparations of bacteriophages in Frankfurt, Germany, showed that they were composed of proteins and contained phosphorus and deoxyribonucleic acid. This led to the first suggestion that viruses were composed of nucleoproteins. The crystallization of TMV in 1935 by Wendell Stanley (132), working at the Rockefeller Institute branch in Princeton, New Jersey, brought this infectious agent into the world of the chemists. Within a year, Bawden and Pirie (7,8) had demonstrated that crystals of TMV contained 0.5% phosphorus and 5% RNA. The first "view" of a virus came from x-ray crystallography using these crystals to show rods of a constant diameter aligned in hexagonal arrays containing RNA and protein (14). The first electron micrographs of any virus, those of TMV, were taken with a microscope built in Germany, and they confirmed the rod shape of the virus particle (88).

The x-ray diffraction patterns (14) suggested that TMV was built up from repeating subunits. These data and other considerations led Crick and Watson (29) to realize that most simple viruses had to consist of one or a few species of identical protein subunits. By 1954–1955, several techniques had been developed to dissociate TMV protein subunits, and TMV could be reconstituted from its RNA and protein subunits (57) to produce infectious virus. The principles of virus self-assembly (20) were appreciated using TMV, and in 1962 Caspar and Klug (23) elegantly described the geometric principles of icosahedral virus structure for many of the isometric viruses. Thus, from 1929 to 1962, both the structures and the chemical compositions of viruses were elucidated.

As early as 1926, H. H. McKinney (110) reported the isolation of "variants" of TMV with a different plaque morphology that bred true and could be isolated from several geographic locations (111). In 1933, Jensen (85) confirmed McKinney's observations and demonstrated reversion mutations for this phenotype. Thus, viruses, like all living and replicating entities, could mutate and therefore had genetic information. That the genetic information resides in the RNA of TMV was shown 30 years later by an infectious RNA assay (56,65). This was the first demonstration that RNA could be a genetic material. This followed Avery's DNA transformation experiments with pneumococcus (4) and the Hershey-Chase experiment with bacteriophages (73), both of which demonstrated that DNA was the more common genetic material. TMV RNA and its nucleotide sequence helped to confirm codon assignments for the genetic code, added clear evidence for the universality of the genetic code, and helped to elucidate the mechanisms of mutation by several diverse mutagens (55). TMV and its related plant viruses have contributed significantly to both the origins and the development of virology.

THE BACTERIOPHAGES

The Early Period: 1915–1940

In 1915, Frederick W. Twort was the superintendent of the Brown Institution in London. In his research, Twort was looking for variants of vaccinia virus, used in the smallpox vaccine, that would replicate in simple defined media outside living cells. In one of his experiments, he inoculated a culture dish of nutrient agar with an aliquot of the smallpox vaccine and, although the virus failed to replicate, bacterial contaminants grew in the agar dish very readily. As Twort continued to incubate his cultures, he noticed that some bacterial colonies underwent a visible change and became "watery looking" (i.e., more transparent). Such colonies were no longer able to replicate when subcultured (i.e., the bacteria had been killed). Twort called this phenomenon glassy transformation, and he went on to show that infecting a normal colony of bacteria with the glassy transforming principle would kill the bacteria. The glassy entity readily passed through a porcelain filter, could be diluted a million-fold, and when placed upon fresh bacteria would regain its strength, or titer (140–142).

Twort (140) published a short note describing all this and suggested that one explanation of his observation was a virus of bacteria. Twort's research was interrupted by World War I, in which he served. When he returned to London, he did not continue this line of research and made no further contributions in this area.

At the same time, Felix d'Herelle, a Canadian medical bacteriologist, was working at the Pasteur Institute in Paris. In August 1915, a cavalry squadron of French soldiers were quartered in Maisons-Lafitte, just outside Paris, and a rampant *Shigella* dysentery infection was devastating the entire outfit. D'Herelle readily isolated the dysentery bacillus from filtered emulsions of the feces of sick men and cultured them. As the bacteria grew and covered the surface of the Petri dish, d'Herelle occasionally observed clear circular spots where no bacteria grew, and he called these *taches vierges*, or plaques. D'Herelle (33,34) was able to follow the course of an infection in a single patient, noting when the bacteria were most plentiful and when the plaques appeared. He was able to demonstrate that the plaques appeared on the fourth day after infection and killed the bacteria in the culture dish; interestingly, the patient began to improve on the fourth day after infection.

D'Herelle named these viruses bacteriophages, and he went on to develop techniques utilized to this day in virology. He developed the use of limiting dilutions with the plaque assay to titer the virus preparation. He reasoned that the appearance of plaques showed that the virus was particulate, or "corpuscular." D'Herelle also demonstrated that the first step of a virus infection was for the agent to attach (adsorb) to the host cell, which he showed by the co-sedimentation of virus and host after mixing the two. (He showed that the virus was lost from the supernatant fluid.) The attachment of a virus occurred only when bacteria sensitive to the virus were mixed with it, demonstrating the host range specificity of a virus at the adsorption step. He described cell lysis and the release of infectious virus in clear and modern terms. D'Herelle (34,35) was in many ways one of the founders of the principles of modern virology.

By 1921, an increasing number of lysogenic bacterial strains had been isolated, and it became impossible to separate the virus from its host in some experiments. This led Jules Bordet (18) of the Pasteur Institute in Brussels to suggest that the transmissible agent described by d'Herelle was nothing more than a bacterial enzyme that stimulates its own production. Although that was an incorrect conclusion, it is remarkably close to the present ideas of prion structure and replication (see Chapter 37).

Throughout the decades of the 1920s and 1930s, d'Herelle focused his efforts on the potential medical applications of his research, but it never bore fruit. What basic research was being carried out at that time was often confused by the interpretations that resulted from the strong personalities of individual scientists in the field. Although it was clear that there were many diverse bacteriophages and that some were lytic while some were lysogenic, their interrelationships remained ill-defined. The highlight of this period was the demonstration by Max Schlesinger (128,130) that purified phages had a maximum linear dimension of 0.1 micron and a mass of about 4×10^{-16} grams and that they were composed of protein and DNA in roughly equal proportions. In 1936, no one quite knew what to make of that observation, but it would begin to make a great deal of sense over the next 20 years.

The Modern Period: 1938–1970

Max Delbrück was trained as a physicist at the University of Gïttingen, and his first position was at the Kaiser Wilhelm Institute for Chemistry in Berlin. There he joined a diverse group of individuals actively discussing how quantum physics related to an understanding of heredity. Delbrück's interest in this area led him to develop a quantum mechanical model of the gene, and in 1937 he applied for and obtained a fellowship to study at the California Institute of Technology. Once at Caltech, he teamed up with another research fellow, Emory Ellis (44), who was working with a group of bacteriophages, T2, T4, T6 (the T-even phages). Delbrück soon appreciated that these viruses were ideal for the study of virus replication. These phages represented a way to probe how genetic information could determine the structure and function of an organism. From the beginning, these viruses were viewed as model systems for understanding cancer viruses or even for understanding how a sperm fertilizes an egg and a new organism develops. Ellis and Delbrück (45) designed the one-step growth curve experiment, in which an infected bacterium liberates hundreds of phages synchronously after a one-half hour latent or eclipse period. This experiment defined the latent period, when viral infectivity was lost. This became the experimental paradigm of the phage group.

At the outbreak of World War II, Delbrück remained in the United States (at Vanderbilt University) and met an Italian refugee, Salvador E. Luria, who had fled to America and was working at Columbia University in New York (with phages T1 and T2). They met at a meeting in Philadelphia on December 28, 1940, and spent the next 2 days planning experiments at Columbia. These two scientists were to recruit and lead a growing group of researchers focused on using bacterial viruses as a model for understanding life processes. Central to their success was an invitation to spend the summer of 1941 at Cold Spring Harbor Laboratory doing experiments. The result was that a German physicist and an Italian geneticist joined forces throughout the years of World War II to travel throughout the United States and recruit a new generation of biologists who came to be known as the phage group.

Shortly thereafter, Tom Anderson, an electron microscopist at the RCA Laboratories in Princeton, New Jersey, met Delbrück, and by March 1942 the first clear pictures of bacteriophages had been obtained (104). About the same time, the first mutants of these phages were isolated and characterized (102). By 1946, the first phage course was being taught at Cold Spring Harbor, and in March 1947, the first phage meeting attracted eight people. From these humble beginnings grew the field of molecular biology, which focused on the bacterial host and its viruses.

The next 25 years (1950–1975) was an intensely productive period of virus research with bacteriophages. Hundreds of virologists produced thousands of publications that covered three major areas: (a) lytic infection of *E. coli* with the T-even phages; (b) the nature of lysogeny, using lambda phage; and (c) the replication and properties of several unique phages such as ϕX174 (single-stranded circular DNA), the RNA phages, T7, and so forth. It is simply not possible here to review all this literature, which laid the foundations for modern molecular virology and biology, so only selected highlights of this era will be mentioned.

By 1947–1948, the idea of examining, at the biochemical level, the events occurring in phage-infected cells during the latent period had come into its own. Seymour Cohen [who had trained first with Erwin Chargaff at Columbia University, studying lipids and nucleic acids, and then with Wendell Stanley working on TMV RNA, and who had taken Delbrück's phage course (1946) at Cold Spring Harbor] examined the effects of phage infection on DNA and RNA levels in infected cells using a colorimetric analysis (26,27). These studies showed a dramatic alteration of macromolecular synthesis in phage-infected cells: (a) The net accumulation of RNA stopped in these cells. [Later this would be the basis for detecting a rapidly turning over species of RNA and the first demonstration of messenger RNA (3)]. (b) There was a cessation of DNA synthesis for 7 minutes, followed by a resumption of DNA synthesis at a 5- to 10-fold increased rate. (c) At the same time, Monod and Wollman (112) showed that the synthesis of a cellular enzyme, the inducible β-galactosidase, was inhibited after phage infection. These experiments divided the viral latent period into early (prior to DNA synthesis) and late times. These results, more importantly, made the clear point that a virus could redirect cellular macromolecular synthetic processes in infected cells (28).

By the end of 1952, two experiments had a critical effect on this field. First, Hershey and Chase (73) utilized differentially labeled viral proteins ($^{35}SO_4$) and nucleic acids ($^{32}PO_4$) to follow phage attachment to bacteria. They were able to shear the viral protein coats from the bacteria using a Waring blender and thus leave only the DNA associated with the infected cells. This enabled them to prove that the DNA had all the information needed to reproduce 100 new viruses. The Hershey-Chase experiment came at the right time to be appreciated in light of the novel structure of DNA elucidated by Watson and Crick 1 year later (145). Together, these experiments formed a cornerstone of the molecular biology revolution (21).

The second experiment in virology carried out in 1953, which was to have an important influence, was done by G. R. Wyatt and S. S. Cohen (155). They identified a new base, hydroxymethylcytosine, in T-even phage DNA; this new base took the place of cytosine, which was present in bacterial DNA. This began a 10-year study of how deoxyribonucleotides were synthesized in bacteria and phage-infected cells, and it led to the critical observation that the virus introduces genetic information for a new enzyme into the infected cell (53). By 1964, Mathews et al. (28) had proved that hydroxymethylase does not exist in uninfected cells and must be encoded for by the virus. These experiments introduced the concept of early enzymes, utilized in deoxypyrimidine biosynthesis and DNA replication (90), and provided clear biochemical proof that the virus encoded new information expressed as proteins in an infected cell. A detailed genetic analysis of these phages identified and mapped the genes encoding these phage proteins and added to this concept. Indeed, the genetic analysis of the rII A and B cistrons of T-even phages became one of the best-studied examples of "genetic fine structure" (10,11). The replication of viral DNA using phage mutants and extracts to complement and purify enzyme activities *in vitro* contributed a great deal to our modern understanding of how DNA duplicates itself (1). Finally, a detailed genetic analysis of phage assembly, utilizing the complementation of phage assembly mutants *in vitro*, is a lucid example of how complex structures are built by living organisms using the principles of self-assembly (41). The genetic and biochemical analysis of phage lysozyme helped to elucidate the molecular nature of mutations (135), and phage (amber) mutations provided a clear way to study second-site suppressor mutations at the molecular level (12). The circular genetic map of the T-even phages (134) was explained by the circularly permuted, terminally redundant (giving rise to phage heterozygotes) conformation of these DNAs (139).

The remarkable reprogramming of viral and cellular protein synthesis in phage-infected cells was dramatically revealed by an early use of sodium dodecyl sulfate (SDS)-polyacrylamide gels (93), showing that viral proteins are made in a specific sequence of events ever subdividing the early and late proteins. The underlying mechanism of this temporal regulation led to the discovery of sigma factors modifying RNA polymerase and conferring gene specificity (67). The study of gene regulation at almost every level (transcription, RNA stability, protein synthesis, protein processing) was revealed from a set of original contributions derived from an analysis of phage infections.

Although this remarkable progress had begun with the lytic phages, no one knew quite what to make of the lysogenic phages. This changed in 1949 when André Lwoff at the Pasteur Institute began his studies with *Bacillus megaterium* and its lysogenic phages. By use of a micromanipulator, single bacteria were shown to divide up to 19 times, never liberating a virus. When lysogenic bacteria were lysed from without, no virus was detected. But from time to time a bacterium spontaneously lysed and produced many viruses (106). The influence of ultraviolet light in inducing the release of these viruses was a key observation that began to outline this curious relationship between a virus and its host (107). By 1954, Jacob and Wollman (82,83) at the Pasteur Institute had made the important observation that a genetic cross between a lysogenic bacterial strain (Hfr, lambda) and a nonlysogenic recipient resulted in the induction of the virus after conjugation, a process they called zygotic induction. In fact, the position of the lysogenic phage or prophage in the chromosome of its host *E. coli* could be mapped by the standard interrupted mating experiment after a genetic cross (83). This was one of the most critical experiments in the conceptual understanding of lysogenic viruses for several reasons: (a) It showed that a virus behaved like a bacterial gene on a chromosome in a bacteria; (b) it was one of the first experimental results to suggest that the viral genetic material was kept quiescent in bacteria by negative regulation, which was lost as the chromosome passed from the lysogenic donor bacteria to the nonlysogenic recipient host; and (c) this helped Jacob and Monod to realize as early as 1954 that the "induction of enzyme synthesis and of phage development are the expression of one and the same phenomenon" (106). These experiments laid the foundation for the operon model and the nature of coordinate gene regulation.

Although the structure of DNA was elucidated in 1953 (145) and zygotic induction was described in 1954, the relationship between the bacterial chromosome and the viral chromosome in lysogeny was still referred to as the attachment site and literally thought of in those terms. It was not until Campbell (22) proposed the model for lambda integration of DNA into the bacterial chromosome, based on the fact that the sequence of phage markers was different in the integrated state than in the replicative or vegetative state, that the truly close relationship between a virus and its host was appreciated. This led to the isolation of the negative regulator or repressor of lambda, a clear understanding of immunity in lysogens, and one of the early examples of how genes are regulated coordinately (120). The genetic analysis of the lambda bacteriophage life cycle is one of the great intellectual adventures in microbial genetics (72). It deserves to be reviewed in detail by all students of molecular virology and biology.

The lysogenic phages such as P22 of *Salmonella typhimurium* provided the first example of generalized transduction (157), whereas lambda provided the first example of specialized transduction (114). That viruses could carry within them cellular genes and transfer such genes from one cell to another provided not only a method for fine genetic mapping but also a new concept in virology. As the genetic elements of bacteria were studied in more detail, it became clear that there was a remarkable continuum from lysogenic phages to episomes, transposons and retrotransposons, insertion elements, retroviruses, hepadnoviruses, viroids, virosoids (in plants), and prions. Genetic information moves between viruses and their hosts to the point where definitions and classifications begin to blur.

The genetic and biochemical concepts that derive from the study of bacteriophages made the next phase of virology possible. The lessons of the lytic and lysogenic phages were often relearned and modified as the animal viruses were studied.

ANIMAL VIRUSES

The Early Period (1898–1965): Discovery and Cell Culture

Some of the highlights of the early period of animal virology are summarized in Table 1. Once the concept of a filterable virus took hold, this experimental procedure was applied to many diseased tissues. Filterable agents, unable to be seen in a light microscope, that replicate only in living animal tissue were found. There were truly some surprises, such as a virus—yellow fever virus—transmitted by a mosquito vector (122), specific visible pathologic inclusion bodies (viruses) in infected tissue (80,116), and even viral agents that can "cause cancer" (43,123). Throughout this early time period (1900–1930), a wide variety of viruses were found (see Table 1) and characterized with regard to their size (using the different pore sizes of filters), resistance to chemical or physical agents (e.g., alcohol, ether), and pathogenic effects. Just based on these properties, it became clear that viruses were a very diverse group of agents. Some were even observable in the light microscope (vaccinia in dark-field optics). Some were inactivated by ether, whereas others

TABLE 1. *Landmarks in animal virus research: The early period (1898–1965)*

Date	Virologist	Discovery
1898	F. Loeffler, P. Frosch	First demonstration of a filterable animal virus (foot-and-mouth disease virus)
1898	G. Sanarelli	Myxomatous virus
1901	W. Reed et al.	First human virus (yellow fever virus)
1901	A. Lode, J Gruber	Fowl plague virus
1903	P. Remlinger, Riffat-Bay	Rabies virus
1903	A. Negri	The inclusion bodies of rabies virus
1908	V. Ellerman, O. Bang	First demonstration of a leukemia-causing virus
1909	K. Landsteiner, E. Popper	Poliovirus
1911	P. Rous	First demonstration of a solid tumor virus; Rous sarcoma virus
1912	A. Carrel	Tissue culture of chick embryo explant
1913	E. Steinhardt et al.	An early example of virus propagation in tissue culture
1931	J. Furth	Use of mice as a host for viruses
1931	A. Woodruff, E. Goodpasture	Use of the embryonated chicken egg as a host for viruses
1931	R. Shope	Swine influenza virus
1933	W. Smith et al.	Human influenza virus
1933	R. Shope	Rabbit papilloma virus (first DNA tumor virus)
1933	Staff of the Jackson Memorial Laboratory	Mouse mammary tumors
1936	P. Rous, J. Beard	Rabbit papilloma virus induces carcinomas in a different species.
1941–50	G. Hirst	Influenza virus hemagglutination (HA), HA inhibition by antibody, receptor-destroying enzyme (neuraminidase—the first virus-associated enzyme)
1948–55	Sanford et al.	Culture of single animal cells
	J. Enders et al.	Nonneural tissue (human) supports poliovirus replication in culture
	G. Gey et al.	Single cell cultures, HeLa cervical carcinoma
	H. Eagle	The optimal medium for growing cells
1952–65	Dulbecco, Darnell, Baltimore, et al.	Poliovirus—plaque assay and origins of the molecular biology of animal viruses using poliovirus

were not. The range of viral diseases affected every tissue type. Viruses gave rise to chronic or acute disease; they were persistent agents or recurred in a periodic fashion. Viruses might cause cellular destruction or induce cellular proliferation. For the early virologists, unable to see their agents in a light microscope and often confused by this great diversity, there had to be an element of faith in their studies. In 1912, S. B. Wolbach, an American pathologist, remarked, "It is quite possible that when our knowledge of filterable viruses is more complete, our conception of living matter will change considerably, and that we shall cease to attempt to classify the filterable viruses as animal or plant" (151).

The way out of this early confusion was led by the plant virologists and the development of techniques to purify viruses and characterize both the chemical and physical properties of these agents (see previous section, The Plant Viruses and the Chemical Period: 1929–1956). The second path out of this problem came from the studies with bacteriophages, where single cells infected with viruses in culture were much more amenable to experimental manipulation and clear answers than were virus infections of whole animals. Whereas the plant virologists of that day were tethered to their greenhouses and the animal virologists were bound to their animal facilities, the viruses of bacteria were studied in Petri dishes and test tubes. Progress in simplifying the experimental system under study came one step at a time; from studying animals in the wild, to laboratory animals, such as the mouse (59) or the embryonated chicken eggs (152), to the culture of tissue, and then to single cells in culture. Between 1948 and 1955, a critical transition converting animal virology into a laboratory science came in four important steps: (a) Sanford et al. (126) at the National Institutes of Health (NIH) overcame the difficulty of culturing single cells, (b) George Gey (64) and his colleagues at Johns Hopkins Medical School cultured and passaged human cells for the first time and developed a line of cells (HeLa) from a cervical carcinoma, (c) Harry Eagle (40) at the NIH developed an optimal medium for the culture of single cells, and (d) in a demonstration of the utility of all this, Enders and his colleagues (46) showed that poliovirus could replicate in a nonneuronal human explant of embryonic tissues.

These ideas, technical achievements, and experimental materials had two immediate effects in virology. First, they led to the development of the polio vaccine as the first vaccine produced in cell culture. From 1798 to 1949, all the vaccines in use (smallpox, rabies, yellow fever, influenza) had been grown in animals or embryonated chicken eggs. Poliovirus was grow in monkey kidney cells (74,98) incubated in flasks. Second, the exploitation of cell culture for the study of viruses began the modern era of molecular virology. The first plaque assay for an animal virus in culture was with poliovirus (36), and it led to an analysis of poliovirus every bit as detailed and important as the contemporary work with bacteriophages. The simplest way to document this statement is for the reader to compare the first edition of General Virology by S. E. Luria in 1953 (103) to the second edition by Luria and J. E. Darnell in 1967 (105) and to examine the experimental descriptions of poliovirus infection of cells. The present era of virology had arrived, and it would continue to be full of surprises.

The Modern Period: 1960 to the Present

In this chapter, information has been presented chronologically or in separate virus groups (plant viruses, bacteriophages, and animal viruses), which reflects the historical separation of these fields. In this section, the format changes because the motivation for studying viruses began to change during this period. Virologists began to use viruses to probe questions central to understanding all life processes. Because viruses replicate in and are dependent on their host cells, they must use the rules, signals, and regulatory pathways of the host. Virologists began to make contributions to all facets of biology. These ideas began with the phage group and were continued by the animal virologists. Second, during this period (1970 to the present), the recombinant DNA revolution began, and both bacteriophages and animal viruses played a critical and central role in this revolution. Viruses were used to probe many diverse questions in biology. For these reasons, the organization of this section focuses on the accomplishments of cellular and molecular biology, where viruses were used. Some of the landmarks in virology since 1970 are listed in Table 2.

The Role of Animal Viruses in Understanding the Basic Outlines of Eukaryotic Gene Regulation

The closed circular and superhelical nature of polyoma virus DNA was first elucidated by Dulbecco and Vogt (37) and Weil and Vinograd (147). The underlying reason for this structure of DNA was first shown to be the packaging of the DNA of simian vacuolating virus 40 (SV40), wound around nucleosomes (63), which produced a superhelix when the histones were removed. These observations proved to be excellent models for the *E. coli* genome (153) and the mammalian chromosome (94). The unique genomes of viruses, with single-stranded DNA (131), plus or minus strand RNA, or double-stranded RNA, are the only life forms that have adopted these modes of information storage.

Important elements of the eukaryotic transcription machinery have been elucidated with viruses. The first transcriptional enhancer element (acts in an orientation- and distance-independent fashion) was described in the SV40 genome (68), as was a distance- and orientation-dependent promoter element observed with the same virus. The transcription factors that bind to the promoter, SP-1 (38), or to the enhancer element, such as AP-1, AP-2 (96), and which are essential to promote transcription along with the basal factors, were first described with SV40. AP-1 is composed of fos and jun family member proteins, demonstrating the role of transcription factors as oncogenes (17). Indeed, the great majority of experimental data obtained for basal and accessory transcription factors come from *in vitro* transcription systems using the adenovirus major late promoter or the SV40 early enhancer–promoter (146). Our present-day understanding of RNA polymerase III promoter recognition comes, in part, from an analysis of the adenovirus VA gene transcribed by this polymerase (54).

Almost everything we know about the steps of messenger RNA (mRNA) processing began with observations made with viruses. RNA splicing of new transcripts was first described with the adenoviruses (13,25). Polyadenylation of mRNA was first observed with poxviruses (86) using a system where the first DNA-dependent RNA polymerase in a virion was discovered (87). The signal for polyadenylation in the mRNA was first found using SV40 (52). The cap and methylation of bases at the 5′ end of mRNA was first detected using reoviruses (60). What little is known about the process of RNA transport out of the nucleus has shown a remarkable discrimination of viral and cellular mRNAs by the adenovirus E1B-55Kd protein (118).

Translational regulation has been profitably studied using poliovirus RNA (or TMV RNA), where internally regulated initiation entry sites (IRES) have been described (84). The discovery of the role of interferon in inducing a set of gene products that act on translational regulatory events owes its origins to virology (77,78). Similarly, the viral defenses against interferon by the adenovirus VA RNA has provided unique insight to the role of eIF-2 phosphorylation events (89). Posttranslational processing of proteins by proteases, carbohydrate addition to proteins in the Golgi apparatus, phosphorylation by a wide variety of important cellular protein kinases, or the addition of fatty acids to membrane-associated proteins have all been profitably studied using viruses. Indeed, a good deal of our present-day knowledge in cell biology of how protein trafficking occurs and is regulated in cells comes from the use of virus-infected cell systems. Clearly, the field of gene regulation has relied on virology for many of its central tenets.

The Role of Animal Viruses in the Recombinant DNA Revolution

The discovery of the enzyme reverse transcriptase in retroviruses (5,138) not only helped to prove how retroviruses replicate but also provided an essential tool to produce complementary DNAs (cDNAs). The first restriction enzyme map of a chromosome, *Hin*dII plus III, was with SV40 DNA (30,31), and the first DNA to show the speci-

TABLE 2. *Landmarks in virology: 1970 to present*

Regulation of gene expression
- Elucidation of DNA structure and chromosome organization (37,63,83,139,147)
- Transcriptional signals identified:
  - SV40-enhancer elements (68)
  - Adenovirus—major late promoter (146)
  - SV40-poly A signals (52) and pox viruses poly A polymerase (86)
- Reoviruses—cap and methylation structure on m-RNA
  - Poliovirus—internal ribosomal initiation entry sites (84)
  - Interferon regulates translational efficiency (77,78).
- Adenovirus—mRNA splicing (13,25)
  - Adenovirus, HIV, HTLV-1-RNA transport from the nucleus (EIB 55k, Rev, Rex) (118)

Recombinant DNA revolution
- Reverse transcriptase discovered (5,138)
- SV40 restriction enzyme map (30,31)
- DNA cloning: hemoglobin into SV40 (81)
- Gene therapy-cloning with SV40 (66), retroviruses (148), adenoviruses (62,70), adeno-associated viruses (125)
- Lambda virus vectors for gene cloning used in the isolation of hepatitis C virus (24)

Oncology
- Viruses isolated that cause human cancers:
  - Epstein-Barr virus (19,47,71)
  - Hepatitis B virus (92,16)
  - Hepatitis C virus (24)
  - Human papilloma viruses (158)
  - Karposi sarcoma virus
  - Human T-cell leukemia virus (137,143,156,119)
- Discovery of oncogenes in Rous sarcoma virus (133)
- Insertional activation of oncogenes by retroviruses (69)
- Description of tumor suppressor gene products SV40 T-antigen-p53 (95,100) and the retinoblastoma susceptibility protein and adenovirus E1A; the papilloma virus E6/E7 proteins—p53/Rb interactions (32,39,95,100,127,149,150)

Vaccines
- Salk and Sabin vaccines for poliovirus (98)
- Hepatitis B vaccine—recombinant subunit vaccine, prevents virus infections and cancers
- Smallpox vaccine used to eliminate a disease for the first time (154)

Drug development
- Acyclovir, HSV-2, selected herpesviruses
- Protease inhibitors, reverse transcriptase inhibitors—HIV, triple drug therapy
- Interferons—hepatitis B, C, multiple sclerosis

Epidemological advances
- Understanding genetic shifts and drifts in influenza A virus
- AIDS first described (1981) and the human immunodeficiency virus discovered in 1983 (6), 1984 (61)
- Prion diseases recognized and the mechanisms elucidated
- High-volume nucleotide sequencing uncovers evolutionary relationships between viruses and genes involved in virulence.

Viral pathogenesis
- Role of viral and host genes in pathogenesis
- Role of the immune system and its response to viral infections in pathogenesis
- Understanding of host cell or tissue preferences by viruses
- Emergence of hemorrhagic fever viruses and episodic infections
- Elucidation of the mechanisms involved in viral persistence and chronic infections
- Understanding cellular apoptosis and viral countermeasures to this process

The future, 2000–2050
- A human population growth to 8–10 billion people on earth
- A dramatic increase in cities with large urban populations (10–20 million people)
- For the first time, more people over the age of 60 than under the age of 3–4 years
- Enhanced population mobility
- Decline in the number of rural spaces
- These conditions describe the need for an excellent worldwide microbial surveillance system and rapid responses to ever-evolving agents.

HIV, human immunodeficiency virus; HTLV, human T-cell leukemia virus; SV, simian virus; AIDS, acquired immunodeficiency syndrome.

ficity of a restriction enzyme was SV40 DNA with *Eco*RI (113,115). Some of the earliest DNA cloning experiments used SV40 DNA into lambda, or human β-hemoglobin genes into SV40 DNA, to construct the first mammalian expression vectors (81). Indeed, a debate about these very experiments led to a temporary moratorium on all such recombinant experiments. From the beginning, several animal viruses had been developed into expression vectors for foreign genes, including SV40 (66), the retroviruses (148), the adenoviruses (62,70), and adeno-associated virus (125), which has the remarkable property of site preferential integration (91). Modern day strategies of gene therapy will surely rely on some of these recombinant viruses. The first cDNA cloning of hemoglobin sequences utilized lambda vectors for the cloning and replication of these mRNA copies. In a nice twist of events, the long-elusive hepatitis virus C (non-A, non-B) was cloned from serum using recombinant DNA techniques, reverse transcriptase, and lambda phage vectors (24).

The Role of Animal Virology in Oncology

It is not too strong a statement to say that we owe a great proportion of our present understanding of the origins of human cancers to two major groups of animal viruses, the retroviruses and DNA tumor viruses. The oncogenes were first discovered and proven to exist in a virus and then in the host cell genome using Rous sarcoma virus (133). A wide variety of retroviruses have captured, altered, and delivered oncogenes to the virologists (see Chapter 10). The insertion of retroviruses into the genomes of cancerous cells also helped to locate additional oncogenes (69). The second group of genes that contribute to the origins of human cancers, the tumor suppressor genes (97), has been shown to be intimately associated with the DNA tumor viruses. Genetic alterations at the p53 locus are the single most common mutations known to occur in human cancers (60% to 65% of the time) (99). The p53 protein was first discovered in association with the SV40 large T-antigen (95,100). SV40, the human adenoviruses, and the human papillomaviruses all encode oncogenes that produce proteins that interact with and inactivate the functions of two tumor suppressor gene products, the retinoblastoma susceptibility gene product (Rb) and p53 (32,39,95,100,127, 149,150). The cellular oncogenes and the tumor suppressor genes in human cancers have been studied and understood most profitably using these viruses.

The viruses that cause cancers have provided some of the most extraordinary episodes in modern animal virology. The recognition of a new disease and the unique geographic distribution of Burkitt's lymphomas in Africa (19) set off a search for viral agents that cause cancers in humans. From D. Burkitt (19) to Epstein, Achong, and Barr (47) to W. Henle and G. Henle (71), the story of the Epstein-Barr virus and its role in several cancers, as well as in infectious mononucleosis, provides us with the best in detective story science. The story is not yet complete and many mysteries remain. Similarly, the identification of a new pathologic disease, adult T-cell leukemia, in Japan by K. Takatsuki (137,143) led to the isolation of a virus that causes the disease by I. Miyoshi and Y. Hinuma (156) and the realization that this virus [human T-cell leukemia virus (HTLV-1)] had been found previously (119) by Gallo and his colleagues. Although this discovery provided the virus, there is yet to be a satisfactory explanation of how this virus contributes to adult T-cell leukemia.

Equally interesting is the road to the hepatitis B virus and hepatocellular carcinomas. By 1967, S. Krugman and his colleagues (92) had good evidence distinguishing between hepatitis A and B viruses, and in the same year B. Blumberg et al. (16) detected the Australia antigen. Through a tortuous path, it eventually became clear that the Australia antigen was a diagnostic marker (a coat protein) for hepatitis B. Although this freed the blood supply of this dangerous virus, Hilleman at Merck, Sharp and Dohme and the Chiron Corporation (which later isolated the hepatitis C virus) went on to produce the first human vaccine that prevents hepatitis B infections and very likely hepatocellular carcinomas associated with chronic virus infections (see Chapter 87 in *Fields Virology*, 4th ed.). The idea of a vaccine that can prevent cancer [first proven with the Mareck's disease virus and T-cell lymphomas in chickens (15,42)] comes some 82 to 85 years after the first discoveries of tumor viruses by Ellerman, Bang, and Rous. At present, an experiment is under way in Taiwan, where 63,500 newborn infants have been inoculated to prevent hepatitis B infections. Based on the epidemiologic predictions, this vaccination program should result in 8,300 fewer cases of liver cancer in that population some 40 to 50 years from now.

Vaccines

The Salk and then Sabin poliovirus vaccines were the first beneficial products of the cell culture revolution. In the early 1950s in the United States, just before the introduction of the Salk vaccine, about 21,000 cases of poliomyelitis were reported annually. Today, the number is fewer than 10 (see Chapter 16) (98).

Among the most remarkable achievements of our century is the complete eradication of smallpox, a disease with a history of over 2,000 years (154). In 1966, the World Health Organization began a program to immunize all individuals who had come into contact with an infected person. This strategy, as opposed to trying to immunize an entire population (which simply was not possible), worked and, in October 1977, Ali Maolin of Somalia was the last person in the world to have a naturally occurring case of smallpox (barring laboratory accidents). Because smallpox has no animal reservoir and requires person-to-person contact for its spread, most scientists agree that we are free of this disease (154). What most scientists do not agree on is whether we should store smallpox virus samples as a reference for the future (2).

The viral vaccines used in the past have included live attenuated vaccines, killed virus vaccines, and subunit vaccines. Both the killed virus vaccine (Salk) and the recombinant subunit vaccine (hepatitis B, S antigen) were new to the modern era of virology. In the future, we will see one virus (e.g., vaccinia virus) presenting the antigens of a different virus, the injection of DNA-encoding viral antigens, and the use of specific interleukins or hormones with vaccines to stimulate immunity at specific locations in the host and to elucidate specific immunoglobulin classes. Considering that the first vaccines (for smallpox) were reported in the Chinese literature of the 10th century (48), these ideas can be traced back in time to the origins of virology.

Although vaccines have been extraordinarily successful in preventing specific diseases, there had been very few natural products or chemotherapeutic agents that cured or reduced the symptoms of virus infections. That changed dramatically with the development of acyclovir by Burrows-Wellcome, which requires both a viral enzyme (thymidine kinase) to activate it (by phosphorylation) and a second enzyme to incorporate it into viral DNA, employing its specificity for the viral encoded DNA polymerase. This drug blocks HSV-2 reactivation from latency and stopped a growing epidemic in the 1970s and 1980s (Chapter 15 in *Fields Virology*, 4th ed.). Similarly, the interferons (Chapter 12) have come into use clinically for hepatitis B and C infections, cancer therapy, and multiple sclerosis. The interferons, found in the course of studying virus interference (77,78), will modulate the immune response and have an increasing role to play in treatments of many clinical syndromes.

An overview of the modern period of animal virology would not be complete without mentioning the appearance of an apparently new virus during the decades of the 1970s and 1980s, the human immunodeficiency virus. It was first recognized as a new disease entity by clinicians and epidemiologists, and they rapidly tracked down the venereal mode of virus transmission. Blood products and transplants provided the fluid and tissue samples for virologists to detect this virus. The first published report of acquired immunodeficiency syndrome (AIDS) was in June 1981. The first publications describing a candidate virus for this disease were in 1983 (6) and then 1984 (61). Had this virus and disease begun in 1961 instead of 1981, neither the nature of retroviruses nor the existence of its host cell (CD-4 helper T-cell) would have been understood. The rapid development of a diagnostic test has helped to remove the virus from the blood supply and to test individuals for the virus.

The development of the first drugs to treat human immunodeficiency virus (HIV) infections (e.g., zidovudine) proved disappointing because of the rapid development of resistance to the drug via mutations in the reverse transcriptase gene. The mutation rates by retroviruses (1 in 10^4 to 10^5 nucleotides polymerized) are very high and the solution to this problem is to give multiple drugs simultaneously, requiring mutations at different loci to develop resistance. The use of two different drugs directed against reverse transcriptase and a third drug that is an HIV protease inhibitor provides a cocktail that can reduce the viral load to a nondetectable level in a patient. Eliminating the integrated and silent copies of the viral DNA from the host cell does not look promising. The highest priority will be the development of an HIV vaccine. This is clearly a major challenge for the future.

Epidemiologic Adventures in Virology

The field of the epidemiology of viruses (see Chapter 14 in *Fields Virology,* 4th ed.) got a terrific boost in the last half of the 20th century with the advent of specific molecular tools [antibodies, polymerase chain reaction (PCR), rapid diagnostic tests] to detect viruses in body fluids or tissue samples, to compare and classify these agents rapidly, and to determine the relationships between virus strains. The marriage of behavioral, geographic, and molecular epidemiology made this a most powerful science. The previous section reviewing advances in oncology pays tribute to this strategy by D. Burkitt and K. Takatsuki, leading to the identification of Epstein-Barr virus (EBV) and HTLV-1. Similarly, the recombinant DNA revolution overcame the problems of propagating the human papillomaviruses, permitting the isolation of new virus serotypes and setting off epidemiologic correlations for high- or low-risk cancer viruses (158). The human papillomaviruses (see Chapter 30 as well as Chapter 66 of *Fields Virology,* 4th ed.) differ in transmission, location on the body, their nature of pathogenesis, persistence, and so forth. Similarly, the first recognition of the so-called slow viruses, which cause spongiform encephalopathies (Chapter 37), came from epidemiologic studies with humans and animals.

With the evolutionary development of a sophisticated immune system in vertebrates, the viruses of these hosts faced a new challenge in that they could no longer productively infect their hosts more than once. For their part, these viruses responded with the establishment of latency (herpesviruses), attacking directly the cells involved in the immune response (HIV), setting up persistent or chronic infections, or devising rapid methods for antigenic changes (influenza A virus). This ability of influenza A to undergo antigenic drift and shift resulted in the development of a lifestyle that uses Darwinian principles in a time frame shorter than that of any other organism. G. Hirst and his colleagues (1941–1950) developed the diagnostic tools to follow this. This permitted both the typing of the hemagglutinin of influenza A strains and the monitoring of the antibody response to it in patients (see Chapter 24 and Chapter 47 of *Fields Virology,* 4th ed.). This has been used, with more and more sophisticated molecular approaches, to prove the presence of animal reservoirs for this virus, the reassortment of chromosomes between human and animal virus strains (antigenic shift), and a high rate of mutation (antigenic drift) caused by RNA-dependent RNA synthesis with no known RNA editing or corrective mechanisms. How these molecular events led to episodic local epidemics and worldwide pandemics has now been explained in broad outline. Although most viruses tend to come to equilibrium with their hosts and become endemic [see, for example, the introduction of the North American myxoma–fibroma virus into the wild European rabbit population in Australia (49)], influenza A virus remains epidemic, changing from local to pandemic via an antigenic shift of its HA subunit gene. These studies (Chapter 24 and Chapter 47 of *Fields Virology,* 4th ed.) have revealed an extraordinary lifestyle. Similarly, the study of the mechanisms of viral pathogenesis and the role of the immune system in this process have led to new insights in the virus–host relationship.

The field of viral epidemiology is changing rapidly with the advent of a new branch termed molecular epidemiology. The PCR technologies permit rapid sampling of viruses without growth in culture or plaque purification. Rapid genome sequencing has revealed sequence relationships between viruses, and sequence heterogeneity within a virus population. Mutation rates are documented and localized in the genome, and their biologic consequences are tested. Just two mutations altered the feline panleukopenia virus into a canine parvovirus, for the first time highly pathogenic and transmissible in dogs. Similarly, the earliest isolates of HIV (ZR 1959) suggest an HIV origin in the 1940s to 1950s derived from a chimpanzee lentivirus in Africa. Rapid mutation forming a population of viruses or clades followed.

Molecular epidemiology will now be required to detect and follow emerging viruses. Whether the next emerging epidemic will result from a novel variant of Ebola virus, Hantan virus, or Norwalk virus, or the more common possibility of a new pandemic variant of influenza virus remains to be seen. What is much clearer, however, is that the demographics of the human population on earth have begun to change. Even as birth rates slow, earth will house 8 to 10 billion people by 2050 to 2100. For the first time, there will be three to four times more people above the age of 60 than below 3 to 4 years of age. We will become an increasingly urban population, with more than 20 to 30 cities containing more than 10 million people. Clearly, human behavioral patterns (increased population density, increased travel, increased ages of the population) will provide the environment for the selection of emerging viruses and the challenges to the new field of molecular epidemiology.

Host–Virus Interactions and Viral Pathogenesis

The modern era of virology (1960 to present), which was developed largely with studies in cell culture, described in great detail the replicative cycles of viruses. Virologists demonstrated the elaborate interactions between viral genomes or viral proteins and host cell proteins. As indicated previously, this resulted in an extraordinary inquiry into the functions of infected or uninfected host cells using the tools of both molecular and cell biology. As this approach matured, the questions became more detailed and of less general interest, and so virologists turned back to the natural host animal, or a related animal model, to address new sets of questions. Chief among these questions was, how does a virus cause disease processes in the animal? How do we quantitate viral virulence and what is the genetic basis of an attenuated virus? These studies have identified, in selected viruses, a set of genes and functions that broadly impact on viral virulence.

Six categories of such factors have been explored to date. First, mutations in genes that impair virus replication in the host reduce the number of viruses produced below a level required to produce disease. These are essential genes (essential for life) *in vivo*. A second class of mutations has been identified in viral genes: These mutations impair virulence but do not alter normal virus replication at least in some cell or tissue types. Here, host or tissue range mutations are most common. Mutations can change the pattern of virus adsorption to a particular cell type and so prevent viral entry into a cell. Mutations in viral enhancer elements can alter the ability of a virus to transcribe its genes in selected cell types. All three strains of the Sabin poliovirus attenuated vaccine contain mutations in the viral RNA 5′ untranslated region, which reduce translation of these RNAs in selected cells (i.e., neurons) but still allow replication in other cells and immunization of the host. A third class of genes critical to regulating viral virulence produce gene products that modify the host defenses. HIV infection kills CD-4 T-cells and eliminates an immune response. Some viruses encode genes that produce virokines that are secreted from infected cells and modify the immune response to infection. Other viruses produce proteins that alter the human leukocyte antigen (HLA) presentation of viral antigens in infected cells, whereas some viruses produce superantigens that stimulate or eliminate lymphoid cells of a selected specificity or with a class of receptors. Many viruses produce proteins that block infected cells from undergoing apoptosis in response to a virus infection. Some viruses, such as African swine fever virus, secrete a pro-apoptotic factor that kills lymphocytes and enhances its virulence. A fourth class of genes and products produced by viruses that impacts on virulence enhances the spread of a virus in the host organism. Some viruses contain signals that permit the virus to bud from an infected cell specifically at the apical or basolateral surfaces of a tissue, permitting selected spread *in vivo*. Some of the RNA viruses acquire infectivity by budding out of a cell using specific proteolytic cleavage of their glycoproteins. This is done in some cases by a viral protease and in others by a cellular protease, each requiring a specific amino acid sequence in the glycoprotein for proper cleavage and spread of the virus. Altering this sequence alters the host cell, which can then give rise to infectious virus, and it can also impact on virulence.

A wide variety of polymorphisms or mutations in the host animal can modulate resistance or virulence of a virus. These mutations can even be selected for during viral epidemics, thus changing the hosts' gene pool. In humans, polymorphisms in a cytokine or cytokine receptor gene imparts resistance to HIV infection at the level of viral absorption. Variations in the immune responses of diverse hosts in a population will result in large variations in the virulence of a virus. The mechanisms used by the host to minimize viral diseases after infection will be a major subject for study in the future.

Finally, changes in population density, life styles, cultural traditions, and economic factors have all played a major role in virus virulence. Poliovirus was a minor endemic virus infection for 3,000 years prior to the introduction of improved sanitation in the last century. This created a population that was infected with this virus for the first time at a later age and resulted in poliovirus epidemics that included tens of thousands of cases. It may not have been a coincidence that the worst influenza epidemic in the century, killing 40 million people, started about 1918 toward the end of World War I, with so many people dislocated and moving about the world in very poor conditions. Cultural and environmental changes will surely play a role in the virulence of viruses.

AFTERWORD: D'HERELLE'S DREAM AND KOCH'S POSTULATES

It was d'Herelle's dream to use bacteriophages as a "magic bullet" to kill bacteria and cure diseases caused by these agents. The ultimate historical irony of that dream was played out by some of the participants described in this chapter over the same time frame.

The story begins in 1884, when Friedrich Johannes Loeffler in Germany used Koch's postulates to isolate and identify the bacterium that causes diphtheria. [Fourteen years later, he and Paul Frosch (both had been trained by R. Koch) would isolate the foot-and-mouth disease virus, the first animal virus to be isolated.] Loeffler was surprised to note, however, that when he inoculated the bacteria into an animal, the bacilli were detected only at the site of the local injection, whereas the abnormalities responsible for the disease were visible in the heart, liver, kidneys, and so forth. Loeffler hypothesized that the bacilli produced a toxin that caused the disease at remote sites in the body with no detectable bacteria. In the next step (in 1888), Emile Roux and A. Yersin (at the Pasteur Institute) demonstrated a heat-labile soluble toxin in the fluid phase above the diphtheria bacillus cultures. An injection of the toxin (which could be filtered through a Chamberland filter) into animals reproduced the symptoms. Emile Roux was a student of Pasteur's who worked with Chamberland on his filters. When Ivanofsky suggested that the filterable agent in his TMV preparations was a toxin, he credited Roux for this idea and his work on diphtheria toxin as precedence (76). In 1898, E. I. E. Nocard and Roux isolated from cows a pleuropneumonia organism that could pass through a Chamberland filter, could be seen as microscopic dots in the light microscope, and could be replicated in collodion sacs in a cell-free meat infusion in the peritoneal cavity of a rabbit. In this way they discovered mycoplasma, a bacteria that violated the "filterable agent" concept of a virus or a liquid that could replicate only in an intracellular environment. In fact, in 1903, Roux challenged Beijerinck's idea of a fluid contagium by calling it "very original" but not distinguishable from his tiny mycoplasma spores, which were microorganisms. In 1903, Roux (124) wrote the first review article on viruses, entitled "Sur les microbes dits 'invisible.' "

By 1890 in Germany, von Behring and Kitasato treated the diphtheria toxin with chemical agents to inactivate it and then immunized animals with it. They demonstrated that serum from immunized animals protected other animals from the toxin and, on Christmas night in 1891 in Berlin, this antitoxin was first given to a child with diphtheria. Shibasaburo Kitasato had also developed a microorganism filter with somewhat finer pores than the Chamberland filter, and he even sold it commercially. Loeffler, in 1898, used both the Chamberland and the Kitasato filters to test whether foot-and-mouth disease virus was retained by or passed through these two filters. This virus readily passed through the Chamberland filter but lost virulence by repeated filtration through a Kitasato filter. Loeffler used these data to claim that the virus was particulate, or corpuscular, partly stopped by the Kitasato filter, and he thus challenged Beijerinck's concept of a fluid contagium (a liquid virus). Beijerinck responded that he felt that the foot-and-mouth disease virus was adsorbed to the Kitasato filter and was not stopped by its smaller pore size. The scientific arguments concerning the nature of viruses continued.

In 1923, G. Ramon introduced a formalin-treated diphtheria toxin as an immunizing agent, and an effective vaccine was in hand that all but eliminated this disease from countries that had an active vaccination program. Although that should have been the end of a good story, it was not. In 1951, V. J. Freeman (58) made the unexpected observation that all virulent strains of *Corynebacterium diphtheriae* are lysogenic with a phage called beta. If the bacteria are cured of this prophage, they fail to produce toxin and are avirulent. Indeed, the gene for this toxin is encoded by the phage genome and is regulated by the metabolic state of the bacteria. The lysogenic virus causes this disease. Koch's postulates had been circumvented by the intimate association of a virus and its host as first described by Lwoff and his colleagues. D'Herelle's dream of a phage curing a disease was given a cruel twist of fate in this case. These filterable agents, be they toxins, viruses, or even viruses that produce toxins when lysogenic in their host and so cannot pass a filter, all have the power to present a most confusing or at the very least a complex picture to the observer.

It is a tribute to the scientists of those times that they came so close to describing reality, while inferring the existence of organisms that could not be seen except by their effect on a host. These 100 years of virology have forged new concepts and provided novel insights into the processes of life.

REFERENCES

1. Alberts BM, Bedinger BP, Formosa T, et al. Studies on DNA replication in the bacteriophage T4 in vitro systems. *Cold Spring Harb Symp Quant Biol* 1982;47:655–668.
2. Altman LK. Smallpox virus, frozen in 2 labs, escapes a scalding end for now. *New York Times*, Natl Ed. 1993, Dec 25:1,8.
3. Astrachan L, Volkin E. Properties of ribonucleic acid turnover in T2-infected *Escherichia coli*. *Biochem Biophys Acta* 1958;29:536–539.
4. Avery OT, MacLeod CM, McCarty M. Studies on the chemical nature of the substance inducing transformation of pneumococcal types: Induction of transformation by a deoxyribonucleic acid fraction isolated from pneumococcus type III. *J Exp Med* 1944;79:137–158.
5. Baltimore C. RNA-dependent DNA polymerase in virions of RNA tumour viruses. *Nature* 1970;226:1209–1222.
6. Barre-Sinoussi F, Chermann JC, Rey F, et al. Isolation of a T-lymphotropic retrovirus from a patient at risk for acquired immune deficiency syndrome (AIDS). *Science* 1983;110:868–871.
7. Bawden FC, Pirie NW. The isolation and some properties of liquid crystalline substances from solanaceous plants infected with three strains of tobacco mosaic virus. *Proc R Soc Med* 1937;123:274–320.
8. Bawden FC, Pirie NW, Bernal JD, Fankuchen I. Liquid crystalline substances from virus infected plants. *Nature* 1936;138:1051–1052.
9. Beijerinck MW. Concerning a contagium vivum fluidum as a cause of the spot-disease of tobacco leaves. *Verh Akad Wetensch*, Amsterdam, II 1898;6:3–21.
10. Benzer S. Fine structure of a genetic region in bacteriophage. *Proc Natl Acad Sci U S A* 1955;41:344–354.
11. Benzer S. Genetic fine structure. In: *Harvey Lectures,* vol 56. New York: Academic Press, 1961:1.
12. Benzer S, Champe SP. Ambivalent rII mutants of phage T4. *Proc Natl Acad Sci U S A* 1961;47:1025–1038.
13. Berget SM, Moore C, Sharp PA. Spliced segments at the 5′ terminus of adenovirus 2 late mRNA. *Proc Natl Acad Sci U S A* 1977;74: 3171–3175.
14. Bernal JD, Fankuchen I. X-ray and crystallographic studies of plant virus preparations. *J Gen Physiol* 1941;25:111–165.
15. Biggs PM, Payne LN, Milne BS, et al. Field trials with an attenuated cell-associated vaccine for Mareck's disease. *Vet Rec* 1970;87: 704–709.
16. Blumberg BS, Gerstley BJS, Hungerford DA, et al. A serum antigen (Australia antigen) in Down's syndrome, leukemia and hepatitis. *Ann Intern Med* 1967;66:924–931.
17. Bohmann D, Bos TJ, Admon A, et al. Human proto-oncogene c-*jun* encodes a DNA binding protein with structural and functional properties of transcription factor AP-1. *Science* 1987;328:1386–1392.
18. Bordet J. Concerning the theories of the so-called "bacteriophage." *Br Med J* 1922;2:296.
19. Burkitt D. A children's cancer dependent on climatic factors. *Nature* 1962;194:232–234.
20. Butler PJG, Klug A. Assembly of the particle of TMV from RNA and disk of protein. *Nature New Biol* 1971;229:47.
21. Cairns J. The autoradiography. In: Cairns J, Stent GS, Watson JD, eds. *Phage and the Origins of Molecular Biology.* Cold Spring Harbor, NY: Cold Spring Harbor Laboratory Press, 1966:252–257.
22. Campbell AM. Episomes. *Adv Genet* 1962;11:101–145.
23. Caspar DLD, Klug A. Physical principles in the construction of regular viruses. *Cold Spring Harb Symp Quant Biol* 1962;27:1–32.
24. Chov Q-L, Kuo G, Weiner AJ, et al. Isolation of a cDNA clone derived from a blood-borne non-A, non-B viral hepatitis genome. *Science* 1989;88:359–362.
25. Chow LT, Gelinas RE, Broker TR, Roberts RJ. An amazing sequence arrangement at the 5′ ends of adenovirus 2 messenger RNAs. *Cell* 1977;12:1–8.
26. Cohen SS. The synthesis of bacterial viruses in infected cells. *Cold Spring Harb Symp Quant Biol* 1947;12:35–49.
27. Cohen SS. Synthesis of bacterial viruses; synthesis of nucleic acid and proteins in *Escherichia coli* infected with T2r+ bacteriophage. *J Biol Chem* 1948;174:281–295.
28. Cohen SS. *Virus-induced Enzymes.* New York: Columbia University Press, 1968.
29. Crick FHC, Watson JD. The structure of small viruses. *Nature* 1956; 177:473–475.
30. Danna K, Nathans D. Specific cleavage of SV40 DNA by restriction endoculease of *H. influenzae. Proc Natl Acad Sci U S A* 1971;68: 2913–2918.
31. Danna KJ, Sack GH Jr, Nathans D. Studies of simian virus 40 DNA. VII. A cleavage map of the SV40 genome. *J Mol Biol* 1973;78: 363–376.
32. DeCaprio JA, Ludlow JW, Figge J, et al. SV40 large tumor antigen forms a specific complex with the product of the retinoblastoma susceptibility gene. *Cell* 1988;54:275–283.
33. d'Herelle FH. Sur un microbe invisible antagoniste des bacilles dysentériques. *C R Hebd Seances Acad Sci Paris* 1917;165:373–390.
34. d'Herelle F. Le microbe bactériophage, agent d'immunité dans la peste et le barbone. *C R Hebd Seances Acad Sci Paris* 1921;172:99.
35. d'Herelle F. *The Bacteriophage and Its Behavior.* Baltimore: Williams & Wilkins, 1926.
36. Dulbecco R, Vogt M. Some problems of animal virology as studied by the plaque technique. *Cold Spring Harb Symp Quant Biol* 1953;18: 273–279.
37. Dulbecco R, Vogt M. Evidence for a ring structure of polyoma virus DNA. *Proc Natl Acad Sci U S A* 1963;50:236–243.
38. Dynan WS, Tjian R. The promoter specific transcription factor Sp1 binds to upstream sequences in the SV40 early promoter. *Cell* 1983; 35:79–87.
39. Dyson N, Howley PM, Munger K, Harlow E. The human papillomavirus-16 E7 oncoprotein is able to bind to the retinoblastoma gene product. *Science* 1989;243:934–937.
40. Eagle H. The specific amino acid requirements of a human carcinoma cell strain HeLa in tissue culture. *J Exp Med* 1955;102:37–48.
41. Edgar RS, Wood WB. Morphogenesis of bacteriophage T4 in extracts of mutant-infected cells. *Proc Natl Acad Sci U S A* 1966;55:498–505.
42. Eidson CS, Kleven SH, Anderson DP. Vaccination against Marek's disease. In: *Oncogenesis and Herpesvirus.* Lyon: International Ongeny Research on Cancer, 1972:147.
43. Ellermann V, Bang O. Experimentelle Leukamie bei Huhnern. *Zentralbl Bakteriol Alet I* 1908;46:595–597.
44. Ellis EL. Bacteriophage: One-step growth. In: Cairns J, Stent GS, Watson JD, eds. *Phage and the Origins of Molecular Biology.* Cold Spring Harbor, NY: Cold Spring Harbor Laboratory Press, 1966: 53–62.
45. Ellis EL, Delbrück M. The growth of bacteriophage. *J Gen Physiol* 1939;22:365–384.
46. Enders JF, Weller TH, Robbins FC. Cultivation of the Lansing strain of poliomyelitis virus in cultures of various human embryonic tissues. *Science* 1949;109:85–87.
47. Epstein MA, Achong BG, Barr YM. Virus particles in cultured lymphoblasts from Burkitt's lymphoma. *Lancet* 1964;1:702–703.
48. Fenner F, Nakano JH. Poxviridae: The poxviruses. In: Lennette EH, Halonen P, Murphy FA, eds. *The Laboratory Diagnosis of Infectious Diseases: Principles and Practice*, vol. 2: *Viral, Rickettsial and Chlamydial Diseases.* New York: Springer-Verlag, 1988:177–210.
49. Fenner F, Woodroofe GM. Changes in the virulence and antigenic structure of strains of myxomavirus recovered from Australian wild rabbits between 1950 and 1964. *Aust J Exp Biol Med Sci* 1965;43: 359–374.
50. Fields BN, Knipe DM, Chanock RM, et al., eds. *Fields Virology*, 1st ed. New York: Raven Press, 1985.

51. Fields BN, Knipe DM, Chanock RM, et al., eds. *Fields Virology,* 2nd ed. New York: Raven Press, 1990.
52. Fitzgerald M, Shenk T. The sequence 5′-AAUAAA-3′ forms part of the recognition site for polyadenylation of late SV40 mRNAs. *Cell* 1981;24:251–260.
53. Flaks JG, Cohen SS. Virus-induced acquisition of metabolic function. I. Enzymatic formation of 5′-hydroxymethyldeoxycytidylate. *J Biol Chem* 1959;234:1501–1506.
54. Fowlkes DM, Shenk T. Transcriptional control regions of the adenovirus VAI RAN gene. *Cell* 1980;22:405–413.
55. Fraenkel-Conrat H, Singer B. The chemical basis for the mutagenicity of hydroxylamine and methoxyamine. *Biochim Biophys Acta* 1972; 262:264.
56. Fraenkel-Conrat H, Singer B, Williams RC. Infectivity of viral nucleic acid. *Biochim Biophys Acta* 1957;25:87–96.
57. Fraenkel-Conrat H, Williams RC. Reconstitution of active tobacco mosaic virus from its inactive protein and nucleic acid components. *Proc Natl Acad Sci U S A* 1955;41:690–698.
58. Freeman VJ. Studies on the virulence of bacteriophage-infected strains of *Corynebacterium diphtheriae. J Bacteriol* 1951;61: 675–688.
59. Furth J, Strumia M. Studies on transmissible lymphoid leukemia of mice. *J Exp Med* 1931;53:715–726.
60. Furuichi Y, Morgan M, Muthukrishnan S, Shatkin AJ. Reovirus mRNA contains a methylated, blocked 5′-terminal structure: m5G(5′) ppp(5′)GmpCp. *Proc Natl Acad Sci U S A* 1975;72:362–366.
61. Gallo RC, Salahuddin SZ, Popovic M, et al. Frequent detection and isolation of cytopathic retroviruses (HTLV-III) from patients with AIDS and at risk for AIDS. *Science* 1984;224:497–500.
62. Gaynor RB, Hillman D, Berk AJ. Adenovirus early region 1A protein activates transcription of a nonviral gene introduced into mammalian cells by infection or transfection. *Proc Natl Acad Sci U S A* 1984;81: 1193–1197.
63. Germond JE, Hirt B, Oudet P, et al. Folding of the DNA double helix in chromatin-like structures from simian virus 40. *Proc Natl Acad Sci U S A* 1975;72:1843–1847.
64. Gey GO, Coffman WD, Kubicek MT. Tissue culture studies of the proliferative capacity of cervical carcinoma and normal epithelium. *Cancer Res* 1952;12:264–265.
65. Gierer A, Schramm G. Infectivity of ribonucleic acid from tobacco mosaic virus. *Nature* 1956;177:702–703.
66. Goff SP, Berg P. Construction of hybrid viruses containing SV40 and lambda phage DNA segments and their propagation in cultured monkey cells. *Cell* 1976;9:695–705.
67. Gribskov M, Burgess RR. Sigma factors from *E. coli, B. subtilis,* phage SP01 and phage T4 are homologous proteins. *Nucleic Acids Res* 1986;14:6745–6763.
68. Gruss P, Dhar R, Khoury G. Simian virus 40 tandem repeated sequences as an element of the early promoter. *Proc Natl Acad Sci U S A* 1981;78:943–947.
69. Hayward WS, Neel BG, Astrin SM. Activation of a cellular *onc* gene by promoter insertion in ALV-induced lymphoid leukosis. *Nature* 1981;290:475–480.
70. Hearing P, Shenk T. Sequence-independent autoregulation of the adenovirus type 5 E1A transcription unit. *Mol Cell Biol* 1985;5: 3214–3221.
71. Henle G, Henle W, Diehl V. Relation of Burkitt's tumor-associated herpes-type virus to infectious mononucleosis. *Proc Natl Acad Sci U S A* 1968;59:94–101.
72. Hershey AD, ed. *The Bacteriophage Lambda.* New York: Cold Spring Harbor Laboratory Press, 1971.
73. Hershey AD, Chase M. Independent functions of viral protein and nucleic acid in growth of bacteriophage. *J Gen Physiol* 1952;36:39–56.
74. Hilleman MR. Historical and contemporary perspectives in vaccine developments: From the vantage of cancer. In: Melnick JL, ed. *Progress in Medical Virology*, vol 39. Switzerland: S Karger, 1992:1–18.
75. Holmes FA. Local lesions in tobacco mosaic. *Bot Gaz* 1929;87:39–55.
76. Hughes SS. *The Virus: A History of the Concept.* London: Heinemann Education Books, 1977.
77. Isaacs A, Lindenmann J. Virus interference I. *Proc R Soc Lond* 1957;147B:258–267.
78. Isaacs A, Lindenmann J. The interferon II. Some properties of interferon. *Proc R Soc Lond* 1957;147B:268–273.
79. Ivanofsky D. Concerning the mosaic disease of the tobacco plant. *St Petersburg Acad Imp Sci Bul* 1892;35:67–70.
80. Ivanofsky D. On the mosaic disease of tobacco. *Z Pfanzenkr* 1903;13: 1–41.
81. Jackson DA, Symons RH, Berg P. Biochemical method for inserting new genetic information into DNA of simian virus 40: Circular SV40 DNA molecules containing lambda phage genes and the galactose operon of *Escherichia coli. Proc Natl Acad Sci U S A* 1972;69: 2904–2909.
82. Jacob F, Wollman EL. Etude génétique d'un bactériophage tempéré d'*Escherichia coli.* I. Le système génétique du bactériophage l. *Ann Inst Pasteur* 1954;87:653–673.
83. Jacob F, Wollman EL. *Sexuality and the Genetics of Bacteria.* New York: Academic Press, 1961.
84. Jan SK, Davies MV, Kaufman RJ, Wimmer E. Initiation of protein synthesis by internal entry of ribosomes into the 5′ nontranslated region of encephalomyocarditis virus RNA in vivo. *J Virol* 1989;63: 1651–1660.
85. Jensen JH. Isolation of yellow-mosaic virus from plants infected with tobacco mosaic. *Phytopathology* 1933;23:964–974.
86. Kates J, Beeson J. Ribonucleic acid synthesis in vaccinia virus. II. Synthesis of polyriboadenylic acid. *J Mol Biol* 1970;50:19–23.
87. Kates JR, McAuslan BR. Poxvirus DNA-dependent RNA polymerase. *Proc Natl Acad Sci U S A* 1967;58:134–141.
88. Kausche GA, Ankuch PF, Ruska H. Die Sichtbarmachung von PF lanzlichem Virus in Ubermikroskop. *Naturwissenschaften* 1939;27: 292–299.
89. Kitajewski J, Schneider RJ, Safer B, Shenk T. An adenovirus mutant unable to express VAI RNA displays different growth responses and sensitivity to interferon in various host cell lines. *Mol Cell Biol* 1986; 6:4493–4498.
90. Kornberg A. Biological synthesis of deoxyribonucleic acid. *Science* 1960;131:1503–1508.
91. Kotin RM, Siniscalco RJ, Samulski RJ, et al. Site-specific integration by adenovirus-associated virus. *Proc Natl Acad Sci U S A* 1990;87: 2211–2215.
92. Krugman S, Giles JP, Hammond J. Infectious hepatitis: Evidence for two distinctive clinical, epidemiological and immunological types of infection. *JAMA* 1967;200:365–373.
93. Laemmli UK. Cleavage of structural proteins during the assembly of the head of bacteriophage T4. *Nature* 1970;227:680–685.
94. Laemmli UK, Cheng SM, Adolph KW, et al. Metaphase chromosome structure: The role of nonhistone proteins. *Cold Spring Harb Symp Quant Biol* 1978;42:351–360.
95. Lane DP, Crawford LV. T antigen is bound to a host protein in SV40-transformed cells. *Nature* 1979;278:261–263.
96. Lee W, Haslinger A, Karin M, Tjian R. Activation of transcription by two factors that bind promoter and enhancer sequences of the human metallothionein gene and SV40. *Nature* 1987;325:368–372.
97. Levine AJ. The tumor suppressor genes. *Ann Rev Biochem* 1993;62: 623–651.
98. Levine AJ. The origins of the small DNA tumor viruses. *Adv Cancer Res* 1994;65:141–168.
99. Levine AJ, Momand J, Finlay CA. The p53 tumor suppressor gene. *Nature* 1991;351:453–456.
100. Linzer DIH, Levine AJ. Characterization of a 54K dalton cellular SV40 tumor antigen in SV40 transformed cells. *Cell* 1979;17:43–52.
101. Loeffler F, Frosch P. *Zentralbl Bakteriol 1 Orig* 1898;28:371.
102. Luria SE. Mutations of bacterial viruses affecting their host range. *Genetics* 1945;30:84–99.
103. Luria SE, ed. *General Virology*, 1st ed. New York: Wiley, 1953.
104. Luria SE, Anderson TF. Identification and characterization of bacteriophages with the electron microscope. *Proc Natl Acad Sci U S A* 1942;28:127–130.
105. Luria SE, Darnell JE, eds. *General Virology*, 2nd ed. New York: J Wiley and Sons, 1967.
106. Lwoff A. The prophage and I. In: Cairns J, Stent GS, Watson JD, eds. *Phage and the Origins of Molecular Biology.* Cold Spring Harbor, NY: Cold Spring Harbor Laboratory Press, 1961:88–99.
107. Lwoff A, Siminovitch L, Kjeldgaard N. Induction de la lyse bactériophagique de la totalité d'une population microbienne lysogène. *C R Acad Sci Paris* 1950;231:190–191.
108. Mayer A. On the mosaic disease of tobacco: Preliminary communication. *Tijdschr Landbouwk* 1882;2:359–364.

109. Mayer A. On the mosaic disease of tobacco. *Landwn VerSStnen* 1886; 32:451–467.
110. McKinney HH. Factors affecting the properties of a virus. *Phytopathology* 1926;16:753–758.
111. McKinney HH. Mosaic diseases in the Canary Islands, West Africa, and Gibraltar. *J Agric Res* 1929;39:557–578.
112. Monod J, Wollman EL. L'inhibition de la croissance et de l'adaption enzymatique chez les bactéries infectées par le bactériophage. *Ann Inst Pasteur* 1047;73:937–957.
113. Morrow JF, Berg P. Cleavage of simian virus 40 DNA at a unique site by a bacterial restriction enzyme. *Proc Natl Acad Sci U S A* 1972;69: 3365–3369.
114. Morse ML, Lederberg EM, Lederberg J. Transduction in *Escherichia coli* K12. *Genetics* 1956;41:142–156.
115. Mulder C, Delius H. Specificity of the break produced by restricting endonuclease R1 in SV40 DNA as revealed by partial denaturation. *Proc Natl Acad Sci U S A* 1972;69:3215.
116. Negri A. Beitrag zum Stadium der Aetiologie der Tollwuth. *Z Hyg Infektkrankh* 1903;43:507–528.
117. Pasteur L. Méthode pour prévenir la rage après morsure. *C R Acad Sci* 1885;101:765–772.
118. Pilder S, Moore M, Logan J, Shenk T. The adenovirus E1B-55Kd transforming polypeptide modulates transport or cytoplasmic stabilization of viral and host cell mRNA. *Mol Cell Biol* 1986;6:470–476.
119. Poiesz BJ, Ruscetti FW, Gazdar AF, et al. Detection and isolation of type C retrovirus particles from fresh and cultured lymphocytes of a patient with cutaneous T-cell lymphoma. *Proc Natl Acad Sci U S A* 1980;77:7415–7419.
120. Ptashne M. *A Genetic Switch, Gene Control and Phage Lambda.* Palo Alto, CA: Blackwell Science, 1987.
121. Purdy-Beale HA. Immunologic reactions with tobacco mosaic virus. *J Exp Med* 1929;49:919–935.
122. Reed W, Carroll J, Agramonte A, Lazear J. *Senate Documents* 1901; 66(822):156.
123. Rous P. A sarcoma of the fowl transmissible by an agent separable from the tumor cells. *J Exp Med* 1911;13:397–399.
124. Roux E. Sur les microbes dits invisible. *Bull Inst Pasteur Paris* 1903; 1:7–12,49–56.
125. Samulski RJ, Chang L-S, Shenk T. Helper-free stocks of recombinant adeno-associated viruses: Normal integration does not require viral gene expression. *J Virol* 1989;63:3822–3828.
126. Sanford KK, Earle WR, Likely GD. The growth in vitro of single isolated tissue cells. *J Natl Cancer Inst* 1948;23:1035–1069.
127. Sarnow P, Ho YS, Williams J, Levine AJ. Adenovirus E1B-58Kd tumor antigen and SV40 large tumor antigen are physically associated with the same 54Kd cellular protein in transformed cells. *Cell* 1982;28:387–394.
128. Schlesinger M. Die Bestimmung von Teilchengrïsse und Spezifischem gewicht des Bakteriophagen durch Zentrifugierversuche. *Z Hyg Infektionskrankh* 1932;114:161.
129. Schlesinger M. Zur Frage der chemischen Zusammensetzung des Bakteriophagen. *Biochem Z* 1934;273:306–311.
130. Schlesinger M. The fuelgen reaction of the bacteriophage substance. *Nature* 1936;138:508–509.
131. Sinsheimer RL. A single-stranded DNA from bacteriophage Ø174. *Brookhaven Symp Biol* 1959;12:27–34.
132. Stanley W. Isolation of a crystaline protein possessing the properties of tobacco-mosaic virus. *Science* 1935;81:644–645.
133. Stehelin D, Varmus HE, Bishop JM, Vogt PK. DNA related to transforming gene(s) of avian sarcoma viruses is present in normal avian DNA. *Nature* 1976;260:170–173.
134. Streisinger G, Edgar RS, Denhardt GH. Chromosome structure in phage T4. I. Circularity of the linkage map. *Proc Natl Acad Sci U S A* 1964;51:775–779.
135. Streisinger G, Mukai F, Dreyer WJ, et al. Mutations affecting the lysozyme of phage T4. *Cold Spring Harb Symp Quant Biol* 1961;26: 25–30.
136. Takahashi WN, Rawlins RE. Method for determining shape of colloidal particles: Application in study of tobacco mosaic virus. *Proc Natl Acad Sci U S A* 1932;30:155–157.
137. Takatsuki K, Uchuyama T, Ueshima Y, et al. Adult T-cell leukemia: Proposal as a new disease and cytogenetic, phenotypic and function studies of leukemic cells. *Gann Monogr* 1982;28:13–21.
138. Temin HM, Mizutani S. RNA-dependent DNA polymerase in virions of Rous sarcoma virus. *Nature* 1970;226:1211–1213.
139. Thomas CA Jr. The arrangement of information in DNA molecules. *J Gen Physiol* 1966;49:143–169.
140. Twort FW. An investigation on the nature of the ultramicroscopic viruses. *Lancet* 1915;189:1241–1243.
141. Twort FW. The bacteriophage: The breaking down of bacteria by associated filter-passing lysins. *Br Med J* 1922;2:293.
142. Twort FW. The discovery of the bacteriophage. *Sci News* 1949;14:33.
143. Uchiyama T, Yodoi J, Sagawa K, et al. Adult T-cell leukemia: Clinical and hematologic features of 16 cases. *Blood* 1977;50:481–492.
144. Vinson CG, Petre AW. Mosaic disease of tobacco. *Botan Gaz* 1929;87: 14–38.
145. Watson JD, Crick FHC. A structure for deoxyribonucleic acid. *Nature* 1953;171:737–738.
146. Weil PA, Luse DS, Segall J, Roeder RG. Selective and accurate initiation of transcription at the Ad2 major late promoter in a soluble system dependent on purified RNA polymerase II and DNA. *Cell* 1979; 18:469–484.
147. Weil R, Vinograd J. The cyclic helix and cyclic coil forms of polyoma viral DNA. *Proc Natl Acad Sci U S A* 1963;50:730–736.
148. Weiss R, Teich N, Varmus H, Coffin J, eds. RNA tumor viruses. New York: Cold Spring Harbor Laboratory Press, 1982.
149. Werness BA, Levine AJ, Howley PM. Association of human papillomavirus types 16 and 18 E6 proteins with p53. *Science* 1990;248: 76–79.
150. Whyte P, Buchkovich KJ, Horowitz JM, et al. Association between an oncogene and an anti-oncogene: The adenovirus E1a proteins bind to the retinoblastoma gene product. *Nature* 1988;334:124–129.
151. Wolbach SB. The filterable viruses: A summary. *J Med Res* 1912;27: 1–25.
152. Woodruff AM, Goodpasture EW. The susceptibility of the chorio-allantoic membrane of chick embryos to infection with the fowl-pox virus. *Am J Pathol* 1931;7:209–222.
153. Worcel A, Burgi E. On the structure of the folded chromosome of *E. coli. J Mol Biol* 1972;71:127–139.
154. World Health Organization. The global eradication of smallpox. Final report of the Global Commission for the Certification of Smallpox Eradication (History of International Public Health, no 4). Geneva: World Health Organization, 1980.
155. Wyatt GR, Cohen SS. The basis of the nucleic acids of some bacterial and animal viruses: the occurence of 5-hydroxymethylcytosine. *Biochem J* 1952;55:774–782.
156. Yoshida M, Miyoshi I, Hinuma Y. Isolation and characterization of retrovirus from cell lines of human adult T-cell leukemia and its implications in the disease. *Proc Natl Acad Sci U S A* 1982;79:2031–2035.
157. Zinder ND, Lederberg J. Genetic exchange in *Salmonella. J Bacteriol* 1952;64:679–699.
158. zur Hausen H. Viruses in human cancers. *Science* 1991;254: 1167–1172.

CHAPTER 2

Principles of Virology

Richard C. Condit

Viruses are unique in nature. They are the smallest of all self-replicating organisms, historically characterized by their ability to pass through filters that retain even the smallest bacteria. In their most basic form, viruses consist solely of a small segment of nucleic acid encased in a simple protein shell. They have no metabolism of their own but rather are obliged to invade cells and parasitize subcellular machinery, subverting it to their own purposes. Many have argued that viruses are not even living, although to a seasoned virologist they exhibit a life as robust as any other creature.

The apparent simplicity of viruses is deceptive. As a group, viruses infect virtually every organism in nature, they display a dizzying diversity of structures and lifestyles, and they embody a profound complexity of function.

The study of viruses, virology, must accommodate both the uniqueness and the complexity of these organisms. The singular nature of viruses has spawned novel methods of classification and experimentation entirely peculiar to the discipline of virology. The complexity of viruses is constantly challenging scientists to adjust their thinking and their research to describe and understand some new twist in the central dogma revealed in a "simple" virus infection.

This chapter explores several concepts fundamental to virology as a whole, including virus taxonomy, virus cultivation and assay, and virus genetics. The chapter is not intended as a comprehensive or encyclopedic treatment of these topics but rather as a relatively concise overview with sufficient documentation for more in-depth study. In addition to primary resources and practical experience, the presentation draws heavily on previous editions of *Fields Virology* (29–31) for both the taxonomy and the genetics material, plus several excellent texts for material on virus cultivation and assay (16,28,35,50,57,60,65). It is hoped that this chapter will be of value to anyone learning virology at any stage: a novice trying to understand basic principles for the first time, an intermediate student of virology trying to understand the technical subtleties of virologic protocols in the literature, or a bewildered scientist in the laboratory wondering why the temperature-sensitive mutant sent by a colleague does not seem to be temperature sensitive.

VIRUS TAXONOMY

A coherent and workable system of classification, a taxonomy, is a critical component of the discipline of virology. However, the unique nature of viruses has defied the strict application of many of the traditional tools of taxonomy used in other disciplines of biology. Thus, scientists who concern themselves with global taxonomy of organisms have traditionally left the viruses scattered throughout the major kingdoms, reasoning that viruses have more in common with their individual hosts than they do with each other (66). By contrast, for practical reasons at least, virologists agree that viruses should be considered together as a separate group of organisms regardless of host, be it plant, animal, fungus, protist, or bacterium, a philosophy borne out by the observation that in several cases viruses now classified in the same family, for example family *Rhabdoviridae*, infect hosts from different kingdoms. Interestingly, the discipline of virus taxonomy brings out the most erudite and thought-provoking, virtually philosophical discussions about the nature of viruses, probably because the decisions that must be made to distinguish one virus from another require the deepest thought about the nature of viruses and virus evolution. In the end, all of nature is a continuum, and the business of taxonomy has the unfortunate obligation of drawing boundaries within this continuum, an artificial and illogical task but necessary nevertheless. The execution of this obligation results today in a free-standing virus taxonomy, overseen by the International Committee on Taxonomy of Viruses (ICTV), with rules and tools unique to the discipline of virology. The process of virus taxonomy that has evolved uses some of the hierarchical nomenclature of traditional taxonomy, identifying virus species and grouping them into genera, genera into families, and families into orders, but at the same time, to cope with both the uniqueness and diversity of viruses as a group, the classification process has been deliberately nonsystematic and thus is "based upon the opinionated usage of data" (73).

Most important, the virus taxonomy that has been developed works well. For the trained virologist, the mention of a virus family or genus name, such as family *Herpesviridae* or genus *Rotavirus*, immediately conjures forth a set of characteristics that form the basis for further discussion or description. Virus taxonomy serves an important practical purpose as well, in that the identification of a limited number of biologic characteristics, such as virion morphology, genome structure, or antigenic properties, quickly provides a focus for identification of an unknown agent for the clinician or epidemiologist and can significantly impact further investigation into treatment or prevention of a virus disease. Virus taxonomy is an evolving field, and what follows is a summary of the state of the art, including important historical landmarks that influenced the present system of virus taxonomy, a description of the system used for virus taxonomy and the means for implementation of that system, and a very brief overview of the taxonomy of viruses that infect humans and animals.

History and Rationale

Virology as a discipline is scarcely 100 years old, and thus the discipline of virus taxonomy is relatively young. In the early 1900s, viruses were initially classified as distinct from other organisms simply by virtue of their ability to pass through unglazed porcelain filters known to retain the smallest of bacteria. As increasing numbers of filterable agents became recognized, they were distinguished from each other by the only measurable properties available, namely the disease or symptoms caused in an infected organism. Thus animal viruses that caused liver pathology were grouped together as hepatitis viruses, and viruses that caused mottling in plants were grouped together as mosaic viruses. In the 1930s, an explosion of technology spawned a description of the physical properties of many viruses, providing numerous new characteristics for distinguishing viruses one from another. The technologies included procedures for purification of viruses, biochemical characterization of purified virions, serology, and, perhaps most important, electron microscopy, in particular negative staining, which permitted detailed descriptions of virion morphology, even in relatively crude preparations of infected tissue. In the 1950s, these characterizations led to the distinction of three major animal virus groups, the myxoviruses, the herpesviruses, and the poxviruses. By the 1960s, because of the profusion of data describing numerous different viruses, it became clear that an organized effort was required to classify and name viruses, and thus the ICTV (originally the International Committee on the Nomenclature of Viruses, ICNV) was established in 1966. The ICTV functions today as a large, international group of virologists organized into appropriate study groups, whose charge it is to develop rules for the classification and naming of viruses, and to coordinate the activities of study groups in the implementation of these rules.

Early in its history, the ICTV wrestled with the fundamental problem of developing a taxonomic system for classification and naming of viruses that would accommodate the unique properties of viruses as a group, and that could also anticipate advancements in the identification and characterization of viruses. Perhaps the most critical issue was whether the classification of viruses should consider virus properties in a monothetical, hierarchical fashion, or in a polythetical, hierarchical fashion (definition to follow). A monothetical, hierarchical classification, modeled after the Linnean system used for classification of plants and animals, would effectively rank individual virus properties, such as genome structure or virion symmetry, as being more or less important relative to each other, and use these individual characteristics to sort viruses into subphyla, classes, orders, suborders, and families (63). Whereas the hierarchical ordering of viruses into groups and subgroups is desirable, a strictly monothetical approach to using virus properties in making assignments to groups was problematic because both the identification of individual properties to be used in the hierarchy, and the assignment of a hierarchy to individual properties seemed too arbitrary.

A polythetic approach to classification would group viruses by comparing simultaneously numerous properties of individual viruses, without assigning a universal priority to any one property. Thus, using the polythetic approach, a given virus grouping is defined by a collection of properties rather than a single property, and virus groups in different branches of the taxonomy may be characterized by different collections of properties. One argument against the polythetic approach is that a truly systematic and comprehensive comparison of dozens of individual properties would be at least forbidding if not impossible. However, this problem could be avoided by the adoption of a nonsystematic approach, namely, using study groups of virologists within the ICTV to consider together numerous characteristics of a virus and make as rational an assignment to a group as possible. Therefore, the system that is currently being used is a nonsystematic, polythetical, hierarchical system. This system differs from any other taxonomic system in use for bacteria or other organisms, but it is effective and useful, and it has withstood the test of time (72). As our understanding of viruses increases, and as new techniques for characterization are developed, notably comparison of gene and genome sequences, the methods used for taxonomy will undoubtedly continue to evolve.

As a consequence of the polythetic approach to classification, the virus taxonomy that exists today has been filled initially from the middle of the hierarchy by assigning viruses to genera, and then elaborating the taxonomy upward by grouping genera into families and to a limited extent families into orders. By 1970, the ICTV had established two virus families, each containing two genera, 24 floating genera, and 16 plant "groups" (106). A rigorous species definition (100), discussed later, was not approved by the ICTV until 1991, but it has now been applied to the entire taxonomy and has become the primary level of classification for viruses. As of this writing, the complete virus taxonomy comprises 3 orders, 69 families, 9 subfamilies, 243 genera, 1550 species, and 2404 tentative species (101). The complete virus taxonomy is far too extensive to relate here, but examples of the results of the taxonomy are offered in Tables 1 and 2. Table 1 lists the distinguishing

TABLE 1. *Summary of characteristics of major animal virus families*

Family	Nucleocapsid morphology	Envelope	Virion morphology	Genome[a]	Host[b]
dsDNA viruses					
Adenoviridae	Icosahedral	No	Icosahedral	1 linear, 30–42 kb	V
Herpesviridae	Icosahedral	Yes	Spherical, tegument	1 linear, 120–220 kb	V
Papillomaviridae	Icosahedral	No	Icosahedral	1 circular, 8 kb	V
Polyomaviridae	Icosahedral	No	Icosahedral	1 circular, 5 kb	V
Poxviridae	Ovoid	Yes	Ovoid	1 linear, 130–375 kb	V, I
ssDNA viruses					
Parvoviridae	Icosahedral	No	Icosahedral	1 linear–sense, 5 kb	V, I
RNA and DNA reverse-transcribing viruses					
Hepadnaviridae	Icosahedral	Yes	Spherical	1 circular DNA, 3 kb	V
Retroviridae	Spherical or rod-shaped	Yes	Spherical	1 linear RNA dimer, 7–11 kb	V
dsRNA viruses					
Reoviridae	Icosahedral	No	Icosahedral, layered	10–12 linear, 18–30 kb	V, I, P
Negative-sense ssRNA viruses					
Arenaviridae	Helical filaments	Yes	Spherical	2 linear, 5–7 kb	V
Bornaviridae	ND	Yes	Spherical	1 linear, 9 kb	V
Bunyaviridae	Helical filaments	Yes	Spherical	3 linear, 10–23 kb	V, I, P
Filoviridae	Helical filaments	Yes	Pleomorphic, filamentous	1 linear, 19 kb	V
Orthomyxoviridae	Helical filaments	Yes	Pleomorphic, spherical	8 linear, 12–15 kb	V
Paramyxoviridae	Helical filaments	Yes	Pleomorphic, spherical, filamentous	1 linear, 15–16 kb	V
Rhabdoviridae	Coiled helical filaments	Yes	Bullet-shaped	1 linear, 11–15 kb	V, I, P
Positive-sense ssRNA viruses					
Arteriviridae	Icosahedral	Yes	Spherical	1 linear, 13 kb	V
Astroviridae	Icosahedral	No	Icosahedral	1 linear, 7–8 kb	V
Caliciviridae	Icosahedral	No	Icosahedral	1 linear, 8 kb	V
Coronaviridae	Helical rod	Yes	Pleomorphic, spherical, rod-shaped	1 linear, 20–33 kb	V
Flaviviridae	Polyhedral	Yes	Spherical	1 linear, 10–12 kb	V, I
"Hepatitis E-like viruses"	Spherical	No	Spherical	1 linear, 7 kb	V
Picornaviridae	Icosahedral	No	Icosahedral	1 linear, 7–8 kb	V, I
Togaviridae	Icosahedral	Yes	Spherical	1 linear, 10–12 kb	V, I
Subviral agents					
Prions	—	—	—	—	V, F

[a]Number of segments, conformation, size.
[b]V, vertebrate; P, plant; I, insect; F, fungus.
ND, not determined.

TABLE 2. *Taxonomy of the order* Mononegavirales

Order Family	Subfamily	Genus	Type species	Host
Mononegavirales				
Bornaviridae		*Bornavirus*	*Borna disease virus*	Vertebrates
Filoviridae		Marburg-like viruses	*Marburg virus*	Vertebrates
		Ebola-like viruses	*Zaire Ebola virus*	Vetebrates
Paramyxoviridae	*Paramyxovirinae*	*Respirovirus*	*Sendai virus*	Vertebrates
		Rubulavirus	*Mumps virus*	Vertebrates
		Morbillivirus	*Measles virus*	Vertebrates
	Pneumovirinae	*Pneumovirus*	*Human respiratory syncytial virus*	Vertebrates
		Metapneumovirus	*Turkey rhinotracheitis virus*	Vertebrates
Rhabdoviridae		*Vesiculovirus*	*Vesicular stomatitis Indiana virus*	Vertebrates
		Lyssavirus	*Rabies virus*	Vertebrates
		Ephemerovirus	*Bovine ephemeral fever virus*	Vertebrates
		Novirhabdovirus	*Infectious hematopoietic necrosis virus*	Vertebrates
		Cytorhabdovirus	*Lettuce necrotic yellow virus*	Plants
		Nucleorhabdovirus	*Potato yellow dwarf virus*	Plants

Source: From ref. 101, with permission.

characteristics of the major animal virus families detailed in this edition of *Fields Virology,* and Table 2 provides an example of the entire taxonomic classification of one virus order, the order *Mononegavirales.*

The ICTV Universal System of Virus Taxonomy

Structure and Function of the ICTV

The ICTV is a committee of the Virology Division of the International Union of Microbiological Societies. The objectives of the ICTV are to develop an internationally agreed-upon taxonomy and nomenclature for viruses, to maintain an index of virus names, and to communicate the proceedings of the committee to the international community of virologists. The ICTV publishes an update of the taxonomy at approximately 3-year intervals (27,33, 68,69,73,106). At the time of this writing, the most recent report is the seventh (101). The ICTV also supports a web site (http://www.ncbi.nlm.nih.gov/ICTV/), which contains all its published information in a conveniently interactive format, plus links to additional sites of interest, including the universal virus database of the ICTV (ICTVdB), described later.

Virus Properties and Their Use in Taxonomy

As introduced previously, the taxonomic method adopted for use in virology is polythetic, meaning that any given virus group is described using a collection of individual properties. The description of a virus group is nonsystematic in that there exists no fixed list of properties that must be considered for all viruses, and no strict formula for the ordered consideration of properties. Instead, a set of properties describing a given virus is simply compared with other viruses described in a similar fashion to formulate rational groupings. Dozens of properties can be listed for description of a virus, but they break down generally into virion morphology, including size, shape, capsid symmetry, and presence or absence of an envelope, virion physical properties, including genome structure, sensitivity to physical or chemical insults; specific features of viral lipids, carbohydrates, and structural and nonstructural proteins; antigenic properties; and biologic properties including replication strategy, host range, mode of transmission, and pathogenicity (72,73).

The Hierarchy

The ICTV has adopted a universal classification scheme that employs the hierarchical levels of order, family, subfamily, genus, and species. Because the polythetic approach to classification introduces viruses into the middle of the hierarchy, and because the ICTV has taken a relatively conservative approach to grouping taxa, levels higher than order are not currently used. Levels lower than species, such as strains and variants, are not officially considered by the ICTV but are left to specialty groups.

A virus species is defined as "a polythetic class of viruses that constitutes a replicating lineage and occupies a particular ecological niche" (100). The formal definition of a polythetic class is "a class whose members always have several properties in common although no single common attribute is present in all of its members" (101). Thus, no single property can be used to define a given species, and application of this formal definition of a polythetic class to species accounts nicely for the inherent variability found among members of a species. The qualification of a replicating lineage implies that members of a species experience evolution over time with consequent variation, but that members share a common ancestor. The qualification of occupation of an ecologic niche acknowledges that the biology of a virus, including such properties as host range, pathogenesis, transmission, and habitat, are fundamental components of the characterization of a virus. In the most recent report of the ICTV, study group members have listed the criteria that identify each species, then listed species according to the criteria. In addition, some viruses are listed as tentative species because their taxonomic status cannot currently be unambiguously determined. Last, a type species, the species used to define the taxon, has been identified for each genus.

Taxonomic levels higher than species are formally defined by the ICTV only in a relative sense—namely, a genus is a group of species sharing certain common characters, a subfamily is a group of genera sharing certain common characters, a family is a group of genera or subfamilies sharing certain common characters, and an order is a group of families sharing certain common characters. As the virus taxonomy has evolved, these higher taxa have acquired some monothetic character. They remain polythetic in that they may be characterized by more than one virus property, but they violate the formal definition of a polythetic class in that one or more defining properties may be required of all candidate viruses for membership in the taxon. Not all taxonomic levels need be used for a given grouping of viruses, thus whereas most species are grouped into genera and genera into families, not all families contain subfamilies, and only a few families have been grouped into orders. Consequently, the family is the highest consistently used taxonomic grouping, it therefore carries the most generalized description of a given virus group, and as a result it has become the benchmark of the taxonomic system. Most families have distinct virion morphology, genome structure, and/or replication strategy (Table 1).

Nomenclature

The ICTV has adopted a formal nomenclature for viruses, specifying suffixes for the various taxa, and rules for written descriptions of viruses. Names for genera, subfamilies, families, and orders must all be single words, ending with the suffixes -virus, -virinae, -viridae, and -virales, respectively. Species names may contain more than one word and have no specific ending. In written usage, the formal virus taxonomic names are capitalized and written in italics, and they are preceded by the name of the taxon, which is neither capitalized nor italicized. For species names that contain more than one word, the first word plus any proper nouns are capitalized. As an example, the full formal written description of human respiratory syncytial virus is order *Mononegavirales*, family *Paramyxoviridae*, subfamily *Pneumovirinae*, genus *Pneumovirus*, species *Human respiratory syncytial virus*.

Order of Presentation of the Viruses

For convenience in presenting or tabulating the virus taxonomy, informal categorical groupings of taxa have been created and together are called an order of presentation. Although superficially the order of presentation appears to function as a higher taxonomic level, it is important to understand that no hierarchy or official taxonomic classification is intended. Currently, the criteria used to specify the order of presentation are nature of the viral genome, strandedness of the viral genome, polarity of the genome, and reverse transcription. In addition, two categories have been created for subviral agents, one for viroids and another for satellites and prions. Finally, a category exists for unassigned viruses. These criteria give rise to nine groupings in the order of presentation, specifically dsDNA viruses, ssDNA viruses, dsRNA viruses, negative-sense ssRNA viruses, positive-sense ssRNA viruses, DNA and RNA reverse transcribing viruses, subviral agents (viroids), subviral agents (satellites and prions), and unassigned viruses. Table 1 provides an example of the usage of the order of presentation.

Universal Virus Database of the ICTV

To facilitate the management and distribution of virologic data, the ICTV has established the universal virus database of the ICTV (ICTVdB). The ICTVdB is accessible on the worldwide web at http://life.anu.edu.au/viruses/welcome.htm, with mirror sites in Europe (http://www.res.bbsrc.ac.uk/mirror/auz/welcome.htm) and North America (http://www.ncbi.nlm.nih.gov/ICTVdB/welcome.htm). The ICTVdB, constructed from virus descriptions in the published reports of the ICTV, comprises searchable descriptions of all virus families, genera, and type species, including microscopic images of many viruses. The ICTVdB is a powerful resource for management of and access to virologic data, and it promises to considerably extend the reach and capability of the ICTV.

VIRUS CULTIVATION AND ASSAY

Different branches of science are defined in large part by their techniques, and virology is no exception. Although the study of viruses uses some general methods that are common to other disciplines, the unique nature of viruses and virus infections requires a unique set of technical tools designed specifically for their investigation. Conversely, what we know and can know about viruses is delimited by the techniques used, and therefore a genuine understanding of virology requires a clear understanding of virologic methods. What follows therefore is a summary of the major techniques essential and unique to all of virology, presented as fundamental background for understanding the discipline.

Initial Detection and Isolation

The presence of a virus is evidenced initially by effects on a host organism, or, in the case of a few animal viruses, by effects on cultured cells. Effects on animal hosts include a broad spectrum of symptoms, including skin and mucous membrane lesions; digestive, respiratory, or neurologic disorders; immune dysfunction; or specific organ failure such as hepatitis or myocarditis. Effects on cultured cells include a variety of morphologic changes in infected cells, termed cytopathic effects and described in detail later in this chapter and in Chapter 18 in *Fields Virology*, 4th ed. Both adenovirus (87) and the polyomavirus SV40 (98) were discovered as cell culture contaminants before they were detected in their natural hosts.

Viruses can be isolated from an affected host by harvesting excreted or secreted material, blood, or tissue and testing for induction of the original symptoms in the identical host, or for induction of some abnormal pathology in a substitute host or in cell culture. Historically, dogs, cats, rabbits, rats, guinea pigs, hamsters, mice, and chickens have all been found to be useful in laboratory investigations (57), although most animal methods have now been replaced by cell culture methods (65). Once the presence of a virus has been established, it is often desirable to prepare a genetically pure clone, either by limiting serial dilution or by plaque purification.

Viruses that are cultivated in anything other than the natural host may adapt to the novel situation through acquisition of genetic alterations that provide a replication advantage in the new host. Such adaptive changes may be accompanied by a loss of fitness in the original host, most notably by a loss of virulence or pathogenicity. Although this adaptation and attenuation may present problems to the basic scientist interested in understanding the replication of the virus in its natural state, it also forms the basis of construction of attenuated viral vaccines.

Hosts for Virus Cultivation

Laboratory Animals and Embryonated Chicken Eggs

Prior to the advent of cell culture, animal viruses could be propagated only on whole animals or embryonated chicken eggs. Whole animals could include the natural host—laboratory animals such as rabbits, mice, rats, and hamsters. In the case of laboratory animals, newborn or suckling rodents often provide the best hosts. Today, laboratory animals are seldom used for routine cultivation of virus, but they still play an essential role in studies of viral pathogenesis.

The use of embryonated chicken eggs was introduced to virology by Goodpasture et al. in 1932 (38) and developed subsequently by Beveridge and Burnet (3). The developing chick embryo, 10 to 14 days after fertilization, provides a variety of differentiated tissues, including the amnion, allantois, chorion, and yolk sac, which serve as substrates for growth of a wide variety of viruses, including orthomyxoviruses, paramyxoviruses, rhabdoviruses, togaviruses, herpesviruses, and poxviruses (57). Members of each of these virus families may replicate in several tissues of the developing egg, or replication may be confined to a single tissue. Several viruses from each of the groups just mentioned cause discrete and characteristic foci when introduced onto the chorioallantoic membrane (CAM) of embryonated eggs, thus providing a method for identification of virus types, or for quantifying virus stocks or assessing virus pathogenicity (Fig. 1). Although the embryonated eggs have been almost wholly replaced by cell culture techniques, they are still the most convenient method for growing high-

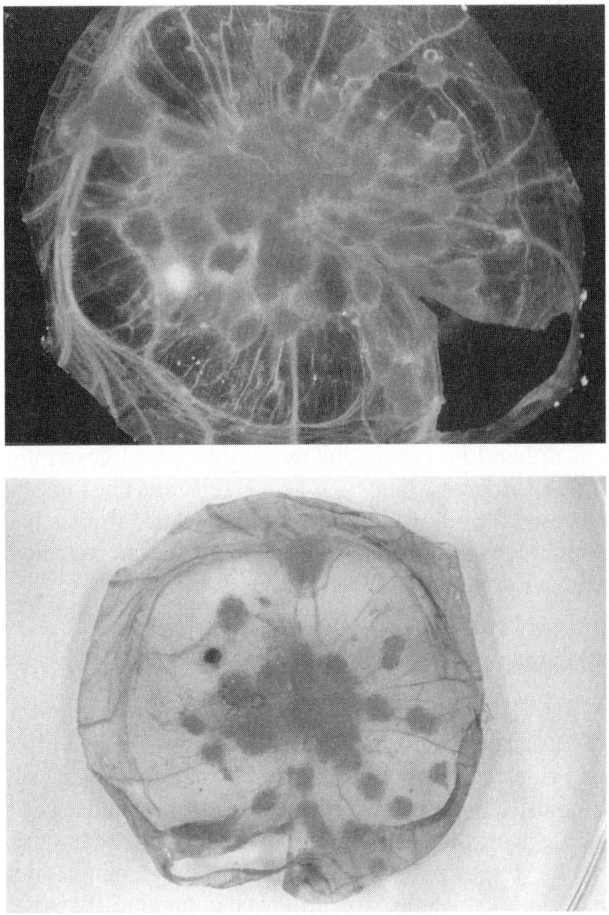

FIG. 1. Cowpox-induced pock formation on the chorioallantoic membrane of chick embryos. The CAMs of intact chicken embryos, 11 days old, were inoculated with cowpox and the eggs were incubated for an additional 3 days at 37.5°C. CAMs were then dissected from the eggs and photographed. The membrane shown at the *top* was untreated, and the membrane at the *bottom* was stained with nitroblue tetrazolium (NBT), an indicator of activated heterophils (34). Wild-type cowpox forms hemorrhagic pocks on the membrane (*top and bottom*). Spontaneous deletion mutants of cowpox virulence genes occur at a high frequency, resulting in infiltration of inflammatory cells into the pock. This infiltration of inflammatory cells causes the pocks to appear white in unstained membrane preparations or dark on NBT-stained membranes. The unstained membrane preparation contains a single white pock; the NBT-stained preparation contains a single dark pock. (Courtesy of Dr. R. Moyer.)

titer stocks of some viruses, and they thus continue to be used both in research laboratories and for vaccine production. In addition, pock formation on the CAM still provides a specialized method for assay of variants of poxviruses: wild type rabbitpox and cowpox viruses cause red hemorrhagic pocks on the CAM, whereas viruses deficient in specific virulence genes cause white pocks as a result of the infiltration of the lesions with inflammatory cells (34,77) (Fig. 1).

Cell Culture

The maintenance of animal cells *in vitro*, described generally (albeit incorrectly) as tissue culture, can be formally divided into three different techniques: organ culture, primary explant culture, and cell culture. In organ culture, the original three-dimensional architecture of a tissue is preserved under culture conditions that provide a gas–liquid interface. In primary explant culture, minced pieces of tissue placed in liquid medium in a culture vessel provide a source for outgrowth of individual cells. In cell culture, tissue is disaggregated into individual cells prior to culturing. Only cell culture will be discussed in detail here, as it is the most commonly used tissue culture technique in virology.

Cultured cells currently provide the most widely used and most powerful hosts for cultivation and assay of viruses. Cell cultures are of three basic types: primary cell cultures, cell strains, and cell lines, which may be derived from many animal species, and which differ substantially in their characteristics. Viruses often behave differently on different types of cultured cells, and in addition each of the culture types possesses technical advantages and disadvantages. For these reasons, an appreciation of the use of cultured cells in animal virology requires an understanding of several fundamentals of cell culture itself. A detailed description of the theory and practice of cell and tissue culture is provided by Freshney (35), and several additional texts provide excellent summaries of cell culture as it specifically applies to virology (16,28,50).

Primary Cell Culture

A primary cell culture is defined as a culture of cells obtained from the original tissue that have been cultivated *in vitro* for the first time, and that have not been subcultured. Primary cell cultures can be established from whole animal embryos, or from selected tissues from embryos, newborn animals, or adult animals of almost any species. The most commonly used cell cultures in virology derive from primates, including humans and monkeys; rodents, including hamsters, rats, and mice; and birds, most notably chickens. Cells to be cultured are obtained by mincing tissue, and dispersing individual cells by treatment with proteases and/or collagenase to disrupt cell–cell interactions and interactions of cells with the extracellular matrix. With the exception of cells from the hemopoietic system, normal vertebrate cells will grow and divide only when attached to a solid surface. Dispersed cells are therefore placed in a plastic flask or dish, the surface of which has been treated to promote cell attachment. The cells are incubated in a buffered nutrient medium in the presence of blood serum, which contains a complex mixture of hormones and factors required for the growth of normal cells. The blood serum may come from a variety or sources, but bovine serum is most commonly used. Under these conditions, cells will attach to the surface of the dish, and they will divide and migrate until the surface of the dish is covered with a single layer of cells, a monolayer, whereupon they will remain viable but cease to divide. If the cell monolayer is "wounded" by scraping cells from an isolated area, cells on the border of the wound will resume division and migration until the monolayer is reformed, whereupon cell division again ceases. These and other observations led to the conclusion that the arrest of division observed when cells reach confluency results from cell–cell contact, and it is therefore called contact inhibition. Primary cultures may contain a mixture of cell types, and they retain the closest resemblance to the tissue of origin.

Subcultivation

Cells from a primary culture may be subcultured to obtain larger numbers of cells. Cells are removed from the culture dish and disaggregated by treating the primary cell monolayer with a chelating agent, usually ethylenediamine tetra-acetic acid (EDTA), or a protease, usually trypsin, or both, giving rise to a single-cell suspension. This suspension is then diluted to a fraction of the original monolayer cell density and placed in a culture dish with fresh growth medium, whereupon the cells attach to the surface of the dish and resume cell division until once again a monolayer is formed and cell division ceases. Cultures established in this fashion from primary cell cultures may be called secondary cultures. Subsequently, cells may be repeatedly subcultured in the same fashion. Each subculturing event is called a passage, and each passage may comprise a number of cell generations, depending on the dilution used during the passage. Most vertebrate cells divide at the rate of approximately one doubling every 24 hours at 37°C. Thus, a passage performed with an eightfold dilution will require three cell doublings over 3 days before the cells regain confluency.

Cell Strains

Normal vertebrate cells cannot be passaged indefinitely in culture. Instead, after a limited number of cell generations, usually 20 to 100 depending on the age and species of the original animal, cultured normal cells cease to divide and they degenerate and die, a phenomenon called crisis or senescence (Fig. 2) (45). Starting with the establishment of a secondary culture and until cells either senesce or become transformed (as will be described later), the culture is termed a cell strain, to distinguish it from a primary culture on the one hand, or a transformed, immortal cell line, on the other hand. During culture, cells in a strain retain their original karyotype and are thus called euploid; however, culturing induces profound changes in the composition and characteristics of the cell strain, and these changes are manifested early during the passage history and may continue during passage. Whereas primary cell cultures may contain a mixture of cell types that survive the original plating of cells, only a few cell types survive subculturing, so that by the second or third passage typically only one cell type remains in the cell strain.

Cell strains are usually composed of one of two basic cell types, fibroblast-like or epithelial-like, characterized based on their morphology and growth characteristics (Fig. 3). Fibroblasts have an elongated, spindle shape, whereas epithelial cells have a polygonal shape. Although after only a few passages only one cell type may remain in a cell strain, continued passage may select for faster-growing variants, such that the characteristics of a cell strain may change with increasing passage number. Despite the fact that normal cell strains experience senescence in culture, they may be maintained for many years by expanding the culture to a large number of cells early during the passage history and storing numerous small samples of low-passage cells by freezing. Thus, as a given strain approaches high passage number and senescence, low-passage cells of the same strain may be thawed and cultured.

Cell Lines

At any time during the culture of a cell strain, cells in the culture may become transformed, meaning that they are no longer subject to crisis and senescence but can be passaged indefinitely. Transformation is a complex phenomenon, discussed in more detail later and in Chapter 10, but in the context of cell culture, the most important characteristic of transformation is that the transformed cells become immortalized. Immortal cell cultures are called cell lines, or sometimes continuous cell lines, to distinguish them from primary cultures and cell strains. Immortalization can occur spontaneously during passage of a cell strain, or it can be induced by treatment with chemical mutagens, infection with tumorigenic viruses, or transfection with oncogenes. In addition, cells cultured from tumor tissue frequently readily establish immortal cell lines in culture. Spontaneous immortalization does not occur in cultured cells from all animal species. Thus, immortalization occurs frequently during culture of rodent cells, for example in mouse and hamster cell strains, and it has been observed in monkey kidney cells, but it occurs rarely if at all during the culture of chicken or human cells. Immortalization is typically accompanied by genetic changes—such cells become aneuploid, containing abnormalities in the number and structure of chromosomes relative to the parent species, and not all cells in a culture of a continuous cell line necessarily display the same karyotype. Like cell strains, cell lines are usually composed of cells that are either fibroblast-like or epithelial-like in morphology.

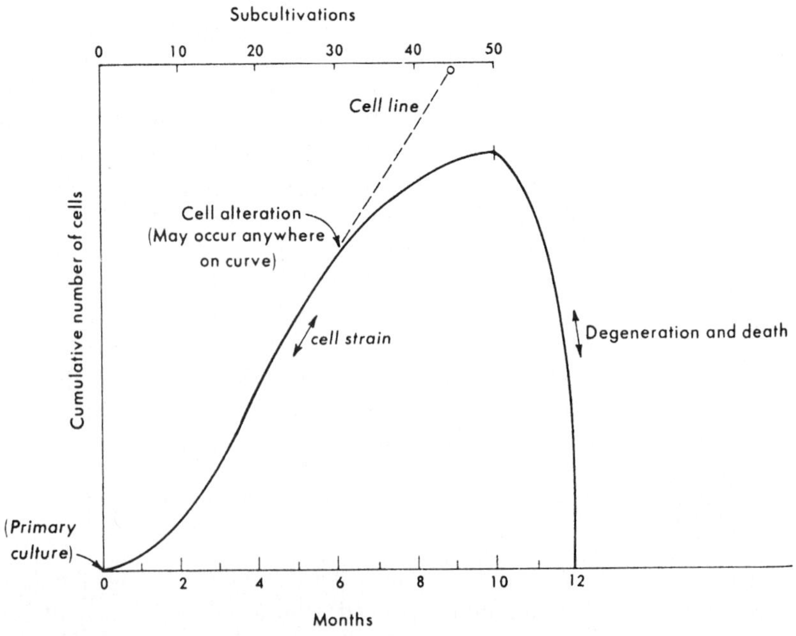

FIG. 2. Growth of cells in culture. A primary culture is defined as the original plating of cells from a tissue, grown to a confluent monolayer, without subculturing. A cell strain (*solid line*) is defined as a euploid population of cells subcultivated more than once *in vitro*, lacking the property of indefinite serial passage. Cell strains ultimately undergo degeneration and death, also called crisis or senescence. A cell line (*dashed line*) is an aneuploid population of cells that can be grown in culture indefinitely. Spontaneous transformation or alteration of a cell strain to an immortal cell line can occur at any time during cultivation of the cell strain. The time in culture and corresponding number of subcultivations or passages are shown on the abscissas. The ordinate shows the total number of cells that would accumulate if all were retained in culture. (From ref. 16 and adapted from ref. 45, with permission.)

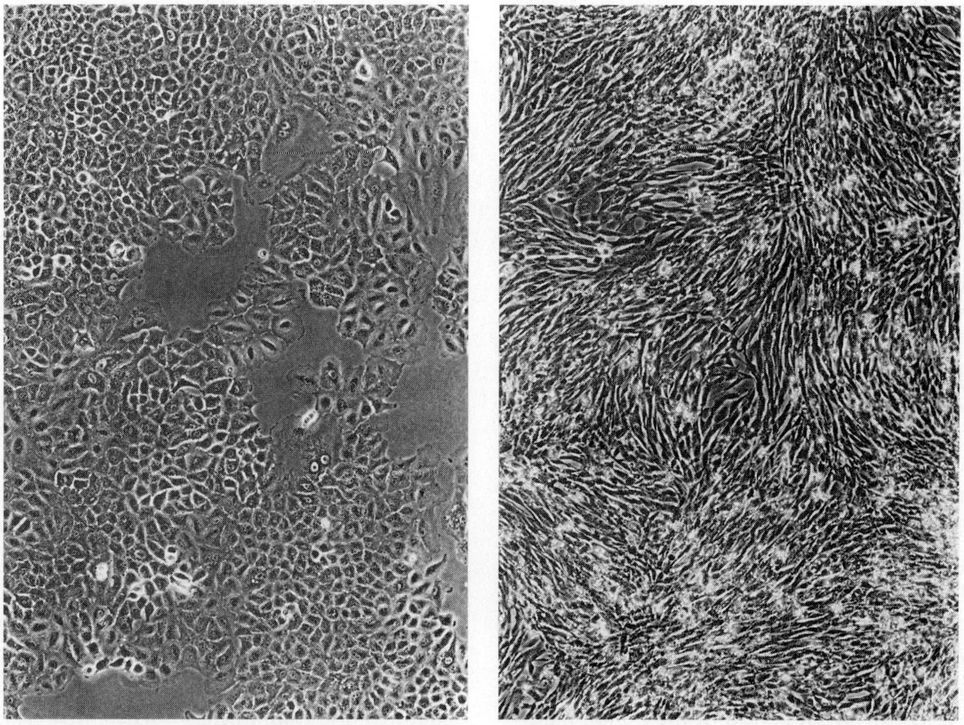

FIG. 3. Cultured cell types. Phase-contrast photomicrographs are shown. *Left*: Epithelial-like cells, A549, a human lung carcinoma cell line, a slightly subconfluent monolayer. *Right*: Fibroblast-like cells, BHK, a baby hamster kidney cell line. (A549 cell culture, courtesy of J. I. Lewis. BHK cell culture, courtesy of D. Holmes and S. Moyer.)

As with the propagation of cell strains, continued culture of a cell line may result in selection of specific variants that outgrow other cells in the culture over time, and thus with passage the character of a cell line may change substantially, and cell lines of the same origin cultured in different laboratories over a period of years may have significantly different characteristics. It is prudent, therefore, to freeze stocks of cell lines having specific desirable properties so that these cells can be recovered if the properties disappear during culture. Likewise, it makes sense to obtain a cell line showing certain desired characteristics directly from the laboratory that described those characteristics, because cells from alternative sources may differ in character.

Transformation

Transformed cells are distinguished from normal cells by a myriad of properties, which can be grouped into three fundamental types of changes: immortalization, aberrant growth control, and malignancy. Immortalization refers simply to the ability to be cultured indefinitely, as described in the preceding section. Aberrant growth control comprises a number of properties, several of which have relevance to experimental virology, including loss of contact inhibition, anchorage independence, and tumorigenicity. Loss of contact inhibition means that cells no longer cease to grow as soon as a monolayer is formed and will now grow on top of one another. Anchorage independence means that the cells no longer need to attach to a solid surface to grow. Anchorage independence is often assayed as the ability to form colonies suspended in a semisolid medium such as agar, and a practical consequence of anchorage independence is the ability to grow in liquid suspension. Tumorigenicity refers to the ability of cells to form a tumor in an experimental animal, and malignancy refers to the ability to form an invasive tumor *in vivo*. Of course, malignancy is of vital importance as a phenomenon in its own right, but it has limited application in virology except within the specific discipline of tumor virology (Chapter 10).

It is important to note that the many properties of transformed cells are not necessarily interdependent, and no one property is an absolute prerequisite for another. Thus, transformation is thought to be a multistep genetic phenomenon, and varying degrees of transformation are measurable. Tumorigenicity is often regarded as the most stringent assay for a fully transformed cell, and it is most closely correlated with anchorage independence.

The fact that the various characteristics of transformed cells are not interdependent has important consequences for experimental virology, especially in the assay of tumor viruses. Specifically, a transformed cell line that is immortalized but still contact-inhibited may be used in a viral transformation assay that measures the further transformation to loss of contact inhibition. When cells in a monolayer are transformed by a tumor virus and lose contact inhibition, they grow on top of a confluent monolayer forming a *focus*, or a pile of cells, which is readily distinguishable from the rest of the monolayer. This property forms the basis for quantitative biologic assay of tumor viruses (102), described in more detail later.

Advantages and Disadvantages of Different Cultured Cell Types

The various types of cultured cells just described have specific application to different problems encountered in experimental virology. For most applications, an adherent cell line provides the most useful host cell. Cell lines are relatively easy to maintain because they can be passaged indefinitely, and adherence is a prerequisite for a plaque assay (described later). A distinct technical advantage of adherent cells is that the culture medium can easily be changed for the purposes of infection or metabolic labeling by simply aspirating and replacing fluid from a monolayer, a process that requires repeated centrifugations with suspension cells. By contrast, relative to adherent cell lines, suspension cell lines are easier to sample than adherent cells, and they produce large numbers of cells from a relatively small volume of medium in a single culture vessel, which has significant advantages for some high-volume applications in virology. Unfortunately, not all viruses will grow on a cell line, and often under these circumstances, a primary cell culture will suffice. This may reflect a requirement for a particular cell type found only under conditions of primary cell culture, or it may reflect a requirement for a state of metabolism or differentiation closely resembling the *in vivo* situation, which is more likely to exist in a primary culture than it is in a cell line.

Last, some viruses do not grow in cell culture at all, and in these cases investigators are reliant either on the old expedients of natural hosts, laboratory animals, or embryonated eggs, or on some more modern advances in tissue culture and recombinant DNA technology. The papilloma viruses, which cause warts, provide an enlightening example of this situation (Chapter 30). Although the viral nature of papillomatosis was demonstrated over 90 years ago, progress on the study of papilloma viruses was seriously hampered in the virology heyday of the mid-20th century because the viruses grow well only on the natural host; they do not grow in culture. The inability to grow in culture is now reasonably well understood: It results from a tight coupling of the regulation of viral gene expression with the differentiation state of the target epithelial cell, which in turn is tightly coupled to the three-dimensional architecture of the epidermis, which is lost in culture. Specialized tissue culture techniques have now been developed that result in the faithful reconstruction of an epidermis by seeding primary keratinocytes on a *feeder* layer composed of an appropriate cell line, and incubating these cells on a *raft*, or grid, at a liquid–air interface. On these raft cultures the entire replication cycle of a papilloma virus can be reproduced *in vitro*, albeit with difficulty (6). In the meantime, it is significant that a large fraction of the genetics and biology of papillomaviruses was determined primarily through the use of recombinant DNA technology, without ever growing virus in culture. Thus, the genetic structure of both the model bovine papillomavirus and many human papillomaviruses has been determined by cloning genomic DNA from natural infections, and regulation and function of many genes can be gleaned from sequence alone, from *in vitro* assays on individual gene products expressed *in vitro*, and from cell transformation assays that use all or parts of a papillomavirus genome. In summary, the inability to grow a virus in culture, while it increases the challenge, no longer presents an insurmountable impediment to understanding a virus.

Recognition of Viral Growth in Culture

Three principal methods exist for the recognition of a virus infection in culture: cytopathic effect, formation of inclusion bodies, and hemadsorption. Cytopathic effect refers to pronounced morphologic changes induced in individual cells or groups of cells by virus infection, which are easily recognizable under a light microscope. Inclusion bodies are more subtle alterations to the intracellular architecture of individual cells. Hemadsorption refers to indirect measurement of viral protein synthesis in infected cells, detected by adsorption of erythrocytes to the surface of infected cells. Cytopathic effect is the simplest and most widely used criterion for infection, but not all viruses cause a cytopathic effect, and in these cases other methods must suffice.

Cytopathic effects, or CPE, comprise a number of cell phenomena, including rounding, shrinkage, increased refractility, fusion, aggregation, loss of adherence, or lysis. CPE caused by a given virus may include several of these phenomena in various combinations, and the character of the CPE may change reproducibly during the course of infection. CPE caused by a given virus are very reproducible and can be so precisely characteristic of the virus type that significant clues to the identity of a virus can be gleaned from the CPE alone (Chapter 18 in *Fields Virology*, 4th ed.). Fig. 4 depicts different CPE caused by two viruses, measles and vaccinia. Most important to the trained virologist, a simple microscopic examination of a cell culture can reveal whether an infection is present, what fraction of cells are infected, and how advanced the infection is. In addition, because cytopathology results directly from the action of virus gene products, virus mutants can be obtained that are altered in cytopathology, yielding either a conveniently marked virus or a tool to study cytopathology per se.

The term *inclusion bodies* refers generally to intracellular abnormalities specific to an infected cell and discernible by light microscopy. The effects are highly specific for a particular virus type, so that, as is the case with CPE, the presence of a specific type of inclusion body can be diagnostic of a specific virus infection. Electron microscopy, combined with a more detailed understanding of the biology of many viruses, reveals that inclusion bodies usually represent focal points of virus replication and assembly, which differ in appearance depending on the virus. For example, Negri bodies formed during a rabies virus infection represent collections of virus nucleocapsids (67).

Hemadsorption refers to the ability of red blood cells to attach specifically to virus-infected cells (90). Many viruses synthesize cell attachment proteins, which carry out their function wholly or in part by binding substituents such as sialic acid that are abundant on a wide variety of cell types, including erythrocytes. Often, these viral proteins are expressed on the surface of the infected cell, for example in preparation for maturation of an enveloped virus through a budding process. Thus, a cluster of infected cells may be easily detectable to the naked eye as areas that stain red after exposure to an appropriate preparation of red blood cells. Hemadsorption can be a particularly useful assay for detecting infections by viruses that cause little or no CPE.

Virus Cultivation

From the discussion just presented, it should be clear that ultimately the exact method chosen for growing virus on any particular occasion will depend on a variety of factors, including (a) the goals of the experiment—namely, whether large amounts of one virus variant or small amounts of several variants are to be grown, (b) limitations in the in vitro host range of the virus—namely, whether it will grow on embryonated eggs, primary cell cultures, continuous adherent cell lines, or suspension cell lines, and (c) the relative technical ease of alternative possible procedures. Furthermore, the precise method for harvesting a virus culture will depend on the biology of the virus—for example, whether it buds from the infected cell, lyses the infected cell, or leaves the cell intact and stays tightly cell associated. As a simple example, consider cultivation of a budding, cytopathic virus on an adherent cell line. Confluent monolayers of an appropriate cell line are exposed to virus diluted to infect a fraction of the cells, and the progress of the infection is monitored by observing the development of the CPE until the infection is judged complete based on experience with the relationship between CPE and maximal virus yield. A crude preparation of virus can be harvested simply by collecting the culture fluid; it may not even be necessary to remove cells or cell debris. Most viruses can be stored frozen indefinitely either as crude or purified, concentrated preparations.

Quantitative Assay of Viruses

Two major types of quantitative assays for viruses exist, physical and biologic. Physical assays, such as hemagglutination, electron microscopic particle counts, optical density measurements, and immunologic methods, quantify only the presence of virus particles, whether or not the particles are infectious. Biologic assays, such as the plaque assay or various endpoint methods that have in common the assay of infectivity in cultured cells or *in vivo*, measure only the presence of infectivity, and they may not count all particles present in a preparation, even many that are in fact infectious. Thus a clear understanding of the nature and efficiency of both physical and biologic quantitative virus assays is required to make effective use of the data obtained from any assay.

Biologic Assays

The Plaque Assay

The plaque assay is the most elegant, the most quantitative, and most useful biologic assay for viruses. Developed originally for the study of bacteriophage by d'Herelle in the early 1900s (15), the plaque assay was adapted to animal viruses by Dulbecco and Vogt in 1953 (22), an advance that revolutionized animal virology by introducing a methodology that was relatively simple and precisely quantitative, that enabled the cloning of individual genetic variants of a virus, and that permitted a qualitative assay for individual virus variants that differ in growth properties or cytopathology.

The plaque assay is based simply on the ability of a single infectious virus particle to give rise to a macroscopic area of cytopathology on an otherwise normal monolayer of cultured cells. Specifically, if a single cell in a monolayer is infected with a single virus particle, new viruses resulting from the initial infection can infect surrounding cells, which in turn produce viruses that infect additional surrounding cells. Over a period of days, the exact length of time depending on the particular virus, the initial infection thus gives rise through multiple rounds of infection to an area of infection called a plaque. Photomicrographs of plaques are shown in Fig. 4, and stained monolayers containing plaques are shown in Fig. 5.

The plaque assay can be used to quantify virus in the following manner (Fig. 5). A sample of virus of unknown concentration is serially diluted in an appropri-

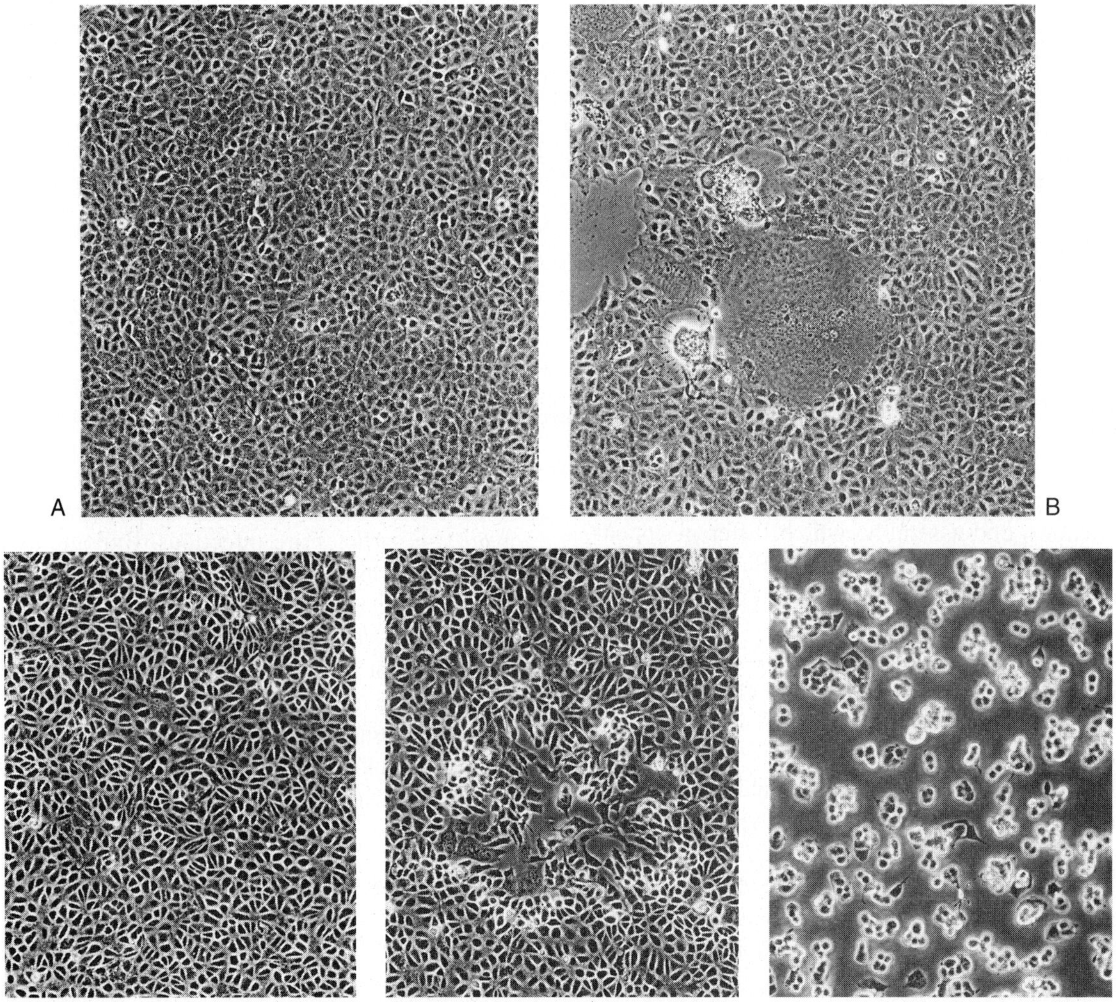

A B C,D E

FIG. 4. Virus-induced cytopathic effects (CPE). Phase-contrast photomicrographs are shown. **A:** Uninfected A549 cells, a human lung carcinoma cell line. **B:** A549 cells infected with measles virus at a multiplicity of infection (moi) of less than 0.01 pfu/cell. Individual plaques can be discerned. Measles fuses cells, causing formation of syncytia. In mid field is a large syncytium containing multiple nuclei. Surrounding this area are additional syncytia, including two that have rounded and are separating from the dish. **C:** Uninfected BSC40 cells, an African green monkey cell line. **D:** BSC40 cells infected with vaccinia virus at an moi of less than 0.01 pfu/cell. A single plaque is shown in the middle of the field. **E:** BSC40 cells infected with vaccinia virus at an moi of 10 pfu/cell, 48 hours after infection. All cells are infected and display complete CPE. (Cultures of vaccinia infections courtesy of J. I. Lewis. Cultures of measles infections courtesy of S. Smallwood and S. Moyer.)

FIG. 5. Plaque assay. Monolayers of the African green monkey kidney cell line BSC40 were infected with 0.5-ml portions of 10-fold serial dilutions of wild-type vaccinia virus or the temperature-sensitive vaccinia mutant, *ts*56, as indicated. Infected monolayers were overlaid with semisolid medium and incubated at 31°C or 40°C, the permissive and nonpermissive temperatures for *ts*56, in the presence of 45 μM isatin-β-thiosemicarbasone (IBT) or in the absence of drug as indicated, for 1 week. Agar overlays were removed and monolayers were stained with crystal violet. Wild-type vaccinia virus forms plaques at both 31°C and 40°C, but plaque formation is inhibited by IBT. Spontaneous IBT-resistant mutants in the wild-type virus stock are revealed as plaques forming at 10^{-3} and 10^{-4} dilutions in the presence of IBT. The *ts*56 mutant carries a single-base missense mutation in the vaccinia gene G2R (70). G2R is an essential gene that when completely inactivated renders the virus dependent on IBT, hence *ts*56 is not only temperature sensitive, forming plaques at 31°C but not at 40°C in the absence of IBT, but it is also IBT dependent at 40°C, forming plaques in the presence but not the absence of IBT. The *ts*56 mutant is slightly defective at 31°C: It forms smaller-than-wild-type plaques, and it is IBT resistant, forming plaques both in the presence and in the absence of drug, a phenotype intermediate between the wild-type IBT-sensitive phenotype and the null G2R mutant IBT-dependent phenotype. Wild-type, temperature-insensitive revertants present in the *ts*56 stock are revealed as plaques growing on the 10^{-3} plate at 40°C. Based on this assay, the titer of the wild-type stock is 1.6×10^9 pfu/ml, and the titer of the *ts*56 stock is 2.0×10^8 pfu/ml. (Plaque assays courtesy of J. I. Lewis.)

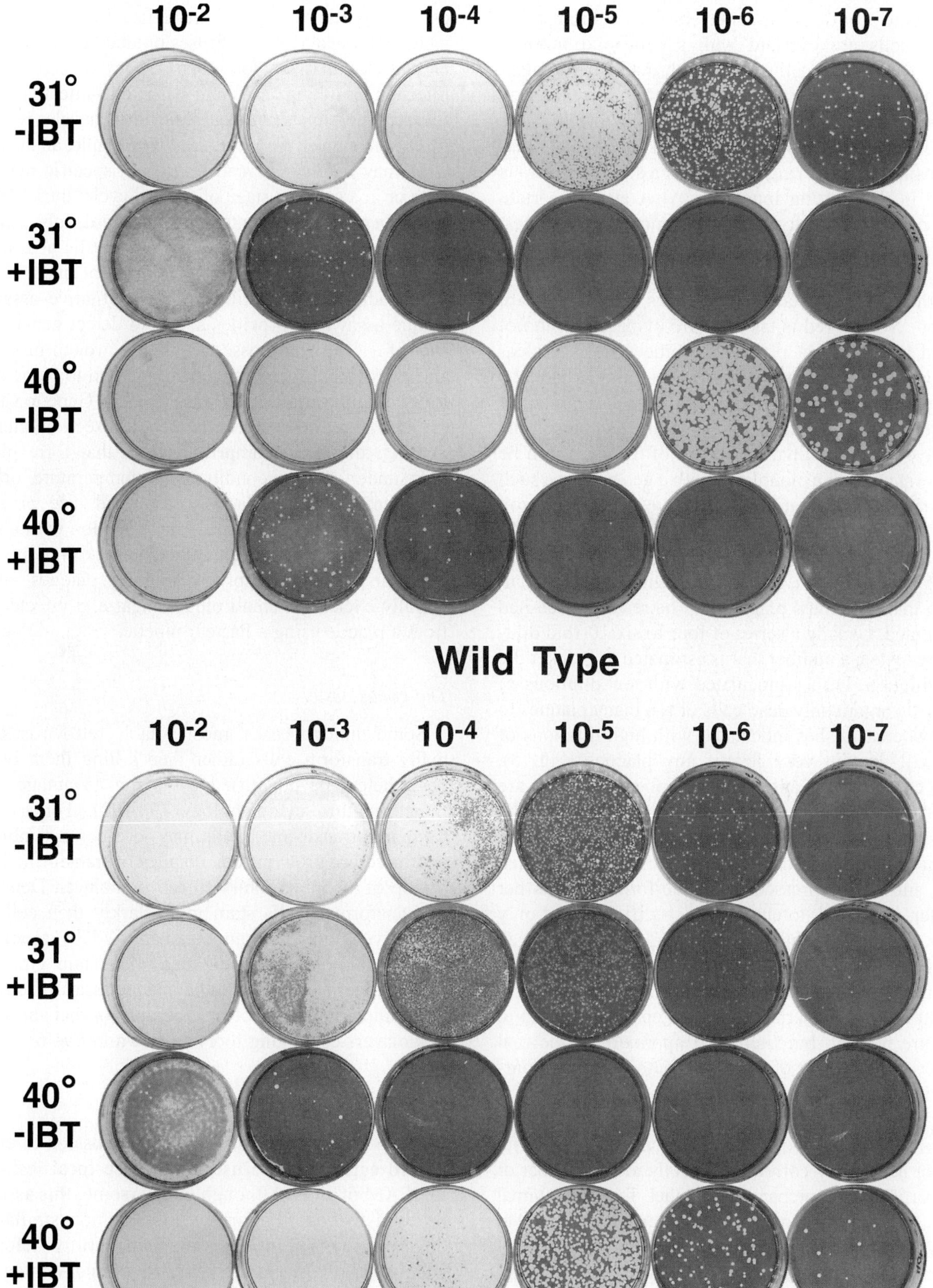
10-2
10-3
10-4
10-5
10-6
10-7
31°
-IBT
31°
+IBT
40°
-IBT
40°
+IBT
Wild Type
10-2
10-3
10-4
10-5
10-6
10-7
31°
-IBT
31°
+IBT
40°
-IBT
40°
+IBT
ts56

ate medium, and measured aliquots of each dilution are seeded onto confluent monolayers of cultured cells. Infected cells are overlaid with a semisolid nutrient medium usually consisting of growth medium and agar. The semisolid medium prevents formation of secondary plaques through diffusion of virus from the original site of infection to new sites, ensuring that each plaque that develops in the assay originated from a single infectious particle in the starting inoculum. After an appropriate period of incubation to allow development of plaques, the monolayer is stained so that the plaques can be visualized. The staining technique depends on the cytopathology, but vital dyes such as neutral red are common. Neutral red is taken up by living cells but not by dead cells, so that plaques become visible as clear areas on a red monolayer of cells. In cases where the virus cytopathology results in cell lysis or detachment of cells from the dish, plaques exist literally as holes in the monolayer, and a permanent record of the assay can be made by staining the monolayer with a general stain such as crystal violet, prepared in a fixative such as ethanol. The goal of the assay is to identify a dilution of virus that yields 20 to 100 plaques on a single dish—that is, a number large enough to be statistically significant yet small enough that individual plaques can be readily discerned and counted. Usually a series of four to six 10-fold dilutions are tested, a number that is estimated to bracket the target dilution. Dishes inoculated with low dilutions of virus will contain only dead cells or too many plaques to count, whereas dishes inoculated with high dilutions of virus will contain very few if any plaques (Fig. 5). Dishes containing an appropriate number of plaques are counted, and the concentration of infectious virus in the original sample can then be calculated by taking into account the serial dilution. The resulting value is called a titer, and it is expressed in plaque-forming units per milliliter, or pfu/ml, to emphasize specifically that only viruses that are capable of forming plaques have been quantified. Titers derived by serial dilution are unavoidably error prone simply because of the additive error inherent in multiple serial pipetting steps; errors of up to 100% are normal, but titers that approximate the real titer to within a factor of 2 are satisfactory for most purposes.

A critical benefit of the plaque assay is that it measures infectivity, but it is important to understand that infectivity does not necessarily correspond exactly to the number of virus particles in a preparation. In fact, for most animal viruses, only a fraction of the particles, as few as 1 in 10 to 1 in 10,000, may be infections as judged by comparison of a direct particle count (described later) with a plaque assay. This low efficiency of plating, or high particle-to-infectivity ratio, may have several causes. First, to determine a particle to infectivity ratio, virus must be purified to determine the concentration of physical particles, and then it must be subjected to plaque assay. If the purification itself damages particles, the particle-to-infectivity ratio will be increased. Second, some viruses produce empty particles, or particles that are for other reasons defective during infection, resulting in a high particle-to-infectivity ratio. Last, it is possible that not all infectious particles will form plaques in a given plaque assay. For example, an infectious virus may require that cells exist in a specific metabolic state or in a specific stage of the cell cycle; thus, if not all cells in a culture are identical in this regard, only a fraction of the potentially infectious virions may be able to successfully launch an infection and form a plaque.

In addition to its utility as a quantitative assay, the plaque assay also provides a way to detect genetic variants of a virus that possesses altered growth properties, and it provides a very convenient method to clone genetically unique variants of a virus (Fig. 5). Genetic variants are considered in detail in the genetics section later, but, in brief, they may comprise viruses that form plaques only under certain conditions of temperature or drug treatment, or form plaques of altered size or shape. Because each plaque results from infection with a single infectious virus particle, unique genetic variants of a virus can be cloned simply by "picking" plaques—that is, literally excising a small plug of agar and infected cells from a plaque using a Pasteur pipette.

The Focus Assay

Some tumor viruses, most notably retroviruses, normally transform cells rather then killing them but can nevertheless be quantified by taking advantage of the transformation cytopathology (94,102). For example, retrovirus-transformed cells may lose contact inhibition and therefore grow in foci, or piles of transformed cells, on top of a contact-inhibited cell monolayer. Dense foci of transformed cells stain more darkly than cells in a monolayer and thus can be quantified by treating an infected monolayer with an appropriate stain. Otherwise, the focus assay is similar to the plaque assay in both technique and function. Photomicrographs of foci and stained monolayers containing foci are shown in Fig. 6.

Pock Formation

As mentioned previously in the discussion of embryonated eggs, many viruses will cause focal lesions on the CAM of eggs. Although cumbersome, this assay can be used to quantify viruses in a fashion similar to a plaque assay. The pock assay found utility before the adaptation of the plaque assay to animal virology, but now it has largely been replaced by other assays utilizing cultured cells and is used only for specialized purposes as noted previously. An example of a pock assay is shown in Fig. 1.

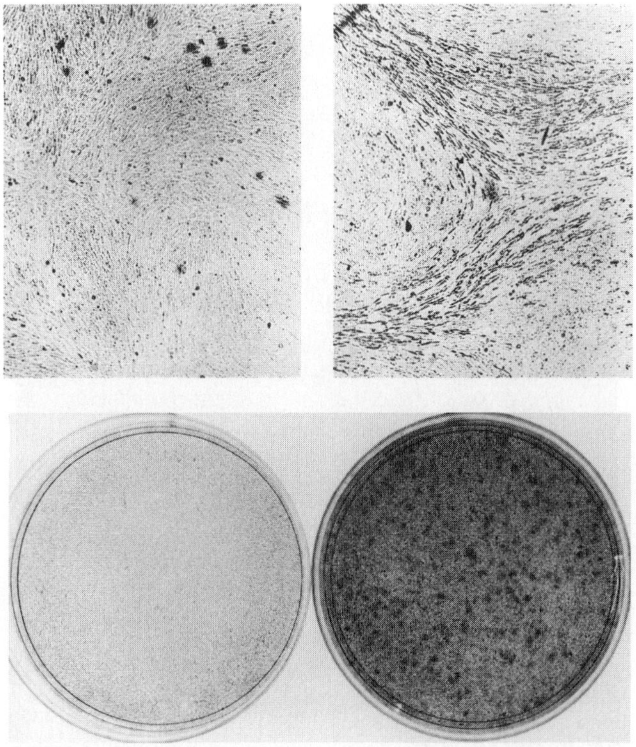

FIG. 6. Focus assay. Monolayers of the NIH3T3 mouse fibroblast cell line were infected with Maloney murine sarcoma virus. The *top two panels* show photomicrographs of uninfected cells (*left*) and a single virus-induced focus (*right*). The *bottom two panels* show stained dishes of uninfected (*left*) and infected (*right*) cells. Foci are clearly visible as darker areas on the infected dish. (Courtesy of D. Blair.)

Endpoint Method

Viruses that cannot be adapted to either a plaque or a focus assay, but that nevertheless cause some detectable pathology in cultured cells, embryonated eggs, or animals, can be quantified using an endpoint method. Briefly, virus is serially diluted and multiple replicate samples of each dilution are inoculated into an appropriate assay system. After a suitable incubation period, an absolute judgment is made as to whether or not an infection has taken place. The dilution series is constructed so that low dilutions show infection in all replicate inoculations, high dilutions show infection in none of the inoculations, but some dilutions result in infection in some but not all inoculations. Statistical methods, described in more detail later, have been devised to calculate the dilution of virus that results in infection in 50% of replicate inoculations, and titers are expressed as the infectious dose 50, or ID_{50}. Assay systems are various and include, for example, observation of CPE in cultured cells, yielding tissue culture infective dose 50 (or $TCID_{50}$); cytopathology or embryonic death in inoculated embryonated chicken eggs, yielding egg infectious dose 50 (or EID_{50}); or death of an experimental laboratory animal, yielding lethal dose 50 (or LD_{50}). Like the plaque assay, the focus assay, and the pock assay, the endpoint method has the advantage of measuring infectivity, but it is important to note that the unit of infectivity measured by the endpoint method may require more than one infectious particle.

A sample determination of a $TCID_{50}$ (65) is shown in Table 3. The data for this experiment would be collected by infecting replicate cell monolayers in a multiwell dish with serial dilutions of virus, and after an appropriate incubation period inspecting the wells for the presence of CPE. Inspection of the data reveals that a 10^{-6} dilution of virus results in infection in more than 50% of replicate wells, whereas a 10^{-7} dilution of virus results in infection in fewer than 50% of replicate wells. Thus, the dilution that would yield infection in exactly 50% of samples lies between 10^{-6} and 10^{-7}. The precise dilution required for infection of 50% of the wells can be calculated by either of two methods, the Spearman Karver method (53,92) (not shown) or the Reed-Muench method (83).

The Reed-Muench method is carried out as follows. First, the cumulative number of infected (column A in Table 3) or uninfected (column B in Table 3) samples is determined by progressively summing the infected samples from the highest dilution to the lowest dilution, and the uninfected samples from the lowest dilution to the highest dilution. Using these numbers, a ratio or percent of infection is calculated for each dilution. The dilution that would yield 50% infected samples is then estimated by determining the proportionate distance between the 10^{-6} and 10^{-7} dilutions that would correspond to 50%

TABLE 3. *Data for calculation of $TCID_{50}$*

Log of virus dilution	Infected test units	Cumulative infected (A)	Cumulative uninfected (B)	Ratio of A/(A + B)	Percent infected
–5	5/5	9	0	9/9	100.0
–6	3/5	4	2	4/6	66.7
–7	1/5	1	6	1/7	14.3
–8	0/5	0	11	0/11	00.0

TCID, tissue culture infective dose.
Source: From ref. 65, with permission.

infection. This distance is the ratio of the distance between 50% infection and the percent positive above 50%, divided by the total distance between the percent positive above 50% and the percent positive below 50%:

$$\frac{(\text{\% positive above 50\%}) - 50\%}{(\text{\% positive above 50\%}) - (\text{\% positive below 50\%})} = \text{proportionate distance,}$$

or

$$\frac{66.7\% - 50\%}{66.7\% - 14.3\%} = 0.3.$$

Knowing the proportionate distance between dilutions, the endpoint is calculated taking into consideration the exact dilutions used:

$$(\text{log dilution above 50\%}) + (\text{proportionate distance} \times \text{log dilution factor}) = \log TCID_{50},$$

or

$$(-6) + (0.3 \times 1.0) = -6.3.$$

Therefore the $TCID_{50} = 10^{-6.3}$. The reciprocal of this number is used to express the titer in infectious units per unit volume. Thus, if 0.1 ml had been used for inoculation of each test well in the assay, the final titer would be $10^{7.3}$ $TCID_{50}$/ml.

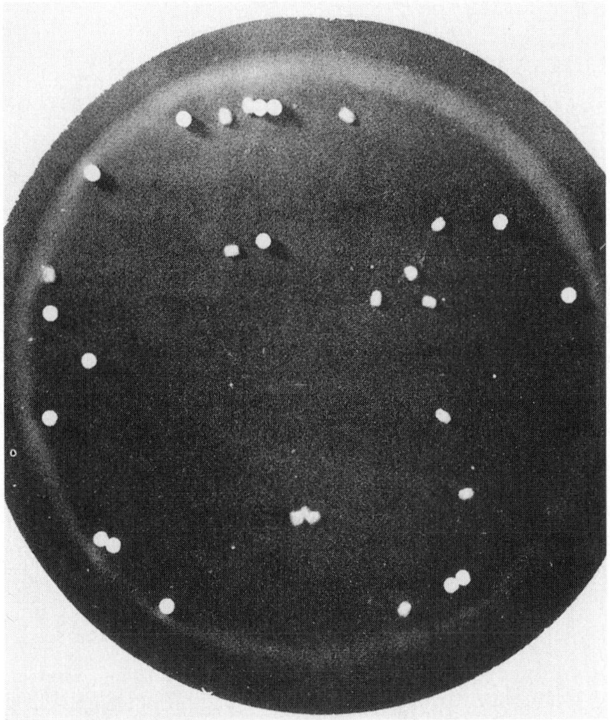

FIG. 7. Direct electron microscopic particle count. An electron micrograph of a spray droplet containing 15 latex beads (*spheres*) and 14 vaccinia virus particles (*slightly smaller, brick-shaped particles*). (From ref. 23, with permission.)

Physical Assays

Direct Particle Count

The concentration of virus particles in a sample of purified virus can be counted directly using an electron microscope (62,104). Briefly, a purified preparation of virus is mixed with a known concentration of microscopic marker particles such as latex beads, which can be easily distinguished from virus particles with the electron microscope. Samples of the solution containing virus and beads are then applied to an electron microscope grid and visualized after shadowing or staining. The volume of liquid applied to a given area of the grid can be determined by counting the beads. The virus particles in the same area can then be counted, resulting in an accurate determination of the concentration of virus particles in the original solution. An example of an electron microscopic count of vaccinia virus is shown in Fig. 7. Given a solution of virus with a known concentration determined by microscopic particle count, the same solution can be subjected to any number of chemical or spectophotometric analyses to yield a conversion from protein content, nucleic acid content, or simply absorbance at a fixed wavelength to a concentration of virus in particles per unit volume. Thus, once a microscopic particle count has been performed, future quantitative assays of purified virus are greatly simplified. It is important to note that the direct particle count does not distinguish infectious from noninfectious particles.

Hemagglutination

As noted previously in the discussion of hemadsorption, many viruses synthesize cell attachment proteins, which carry out their function wholly or in part by binding substituents such as sialic acid that are abundant on a wide variety of cell types, including erythrocytes. Because these cell attachment proteins decorate the surface of the virion, virions may bind directly to erythrocytes. Because both the virions and the erythrocytes contain multiple binding sites for each other, erythrocytes will agglutinate, or form a network of cells and virus, when mixed with virus particles in sufficiently high concentration. Agglutinated erythrocytes can be easily distinguished from cells that are not agglutinated, and thus hemagglutination can be used as a simple quantitative assay for the presence of a hemagglutinating virus.

In practice, a hemagglutination assay is carried out as follows (Fig. 8). Virus is serially diluted and mixed with a fixed concentration of erythrocytes. The mixture is allowed to settle in a specially designed hemagglutination tray containing wells with rounded bottoms. Erythrocytes that are not agglutinated are free to roll to the bottom of the well, forming a dense, easily recognizable button, or cluster of cells. Erythrocytes that are agglutinated are not free to roll to the bottom of the well, but

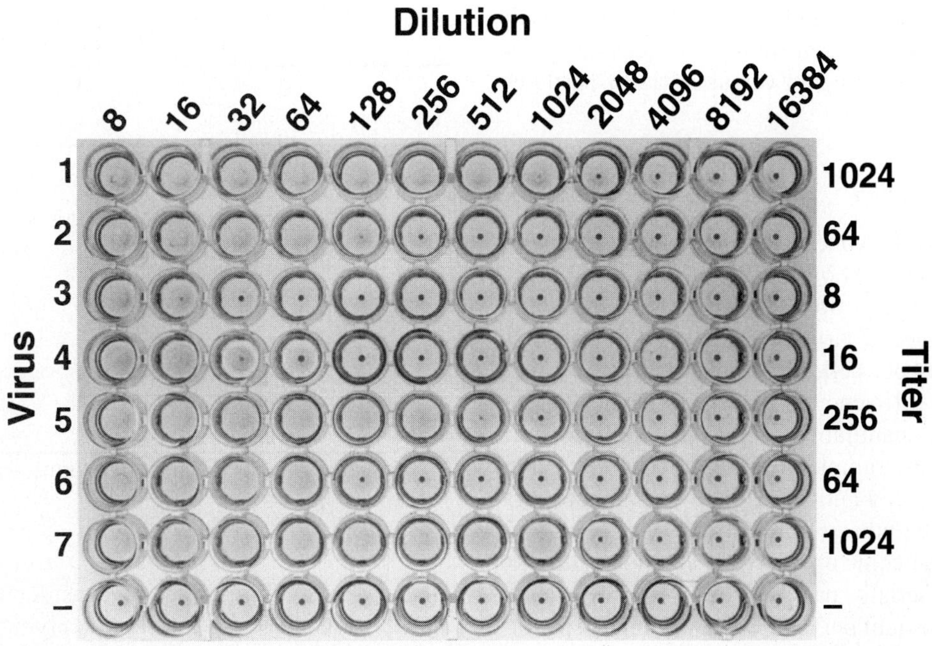

FIG. 8. Hemagglutination assay. Seven different samples of influenza virus, numbered 1 through 7 at the left, were serially diluted as indicated at the *top*, mixed with chicken red blood cells (RBC), and incubated on ice for 1 to 2 hours. Wells in the bottom row contain no virus. Agglutinated RBCs coat wells evenly, in contrast to nonagglutinated cells, which form a distinct button at the bottom of the well. The HA titer, shown at the right, is the last dilution that shows complete hemagglutination activity. (Courtesy of J. Talon and P. Palese.)

instead evenly coat the bottom surface of the well. One hemagglutination (HA) unit is defined as the minimum amount of virus required to cause agglutination, and the titer of the virus solution, expressed as HA units/ml, can be calculated taking into account the serial dilution. It is noteworthy that, like the direct particle count assay, the hemagglutination assay does not distinguish infectious from noninfectious particles. In addition, since it may require many particles to cause a detectable hemagglutination, one HA unit may represent many physical particles.

Quantitative Considerations in Virus Assay, Cultivation, and Experimentation

Dose Response in Plaque and Focus Assays

With few exceptions, the number of infectious units observed on a given plate in a plaque assay is a linear function of the dilution of the virus, thus the development of plaques follows single-hit kinetics, proving that each plaque results from infection with a single virus particle. Exceptions include the murine sarcoma viruses, assayed in a focus assay, which require co-infection with both a defective transforming virus and a nondefective helper virus, in which case the number of foci observed relative to the dilution used follows two-hit kinetics (40).

Comparison of Quantitative Assays

As noted in the individual descriptions, the various quantitative assays of viruses measure different physical and biologic properties, and a one-to-one correlation between assays cannot be assumed. Table 4 summarizes the titers of an influenza virus preparation as measured by several different assays, providing an example of the magnitude of differences that might be expected between the various assays. Hence, relative to a direct particle count, the efficiency of plating the influenza sample shown in Table 4 is 10^{-1} as assayed in eggs, 10^{-2} as assayed in a plaque assay, and 10^{-7} as assayed in a hemagglutination assay. As indicated in the forgoing discussion, some of the differences result from different properties being measured—for example, physical par-

TABLE 4. *Comparison of quantitative assay efficiency*

Method	Amount (per ml)
Direct electron microscope (EM) count particles	10^{10} EM
Quantal infectivity assay in eggs	10^9 egg ID_{50}
Quantal infectivity assay by plaque formation	10^8 pfu
Hemagglutination (HA) assay	10^3 HA units

ID, infectious dose; pfu, plaque-forming units.
Source: From ref. 28, with permission.

ticles versus infectivity—and some differences result from differences in the sensitivity of the assay—for example, direct particle count versus assay of particles by hemagglutination.

Multiplicity of Infection

Multiplicity of infection, often abbreviated moi, measures the average amount of virus added per cell in an infection. Multiplicity of infection can be expressed using any quantitative measure of virus titer, for example particles per cell, HA units per cell, $TCID_{50}$ per cell, or pfu per cell. Because the efficiency of plating varies depending on the method of quantitation used, some knowledge of the infectivity of the sample or the efficiency of plating is required to correctly anticipate the consequences of a particular moi. The moi used in different protocols can have a profound outcome on the procedure. For example, some viruses, if serially passaged at an moi of greater than one infectious unit per cell, will accumulate spontaneously deleted defective particles, which are maintained during passage by the presence of complementing wild-type helper virus (103). Passage of the same virus at very low moi, for example 0.01 infectious units per cell, discourages the accumulation of defective particles because few cells will be co-infected with an infectious and a defective particle, and defective particles cannot replicate in the absence of a wild-type helper. On the other hand, most metabolic labeling experiments are done at a high moi, for example 10 infectious units per cell, to ensure that all cells in the culture are infected and that the infection is as synchronous as possible. For such experiments, use of too low an moi may result in an apparently asynchronous infection and a high background because of the presence of uninfected cells in the culture.

The Poisson distribution can be used to predict the fraction of cells in a population infected with a given number of particles at different mois. As applied to virus infections, the Poisson distribution can be written as follows:

$$P(k) = e^{-m}m^{k}/k!,$$

where $P(k)$ = the probability that any cell is infected with k particles, m = moi, and k = number of particles in a given cell.

Note that to determine the fraction of uninfected cells in any experiment, that is when $k = 0$, the equation simplifies to

$$P(0) = e^{-m}$$

For practical purposes, solution of this equation for given values of m and k (other than 0) is most easily accomplished using published tables (109). Sample solutions are shown in Table 5 for commonly used mois.

TABLE 5. *The Poisson distribution: values of* P(k) *for various values of* m *and* k

	moi (m)			
#/cell (k)	1	3	5	10
0	0.37	0.05	0.01	0.00
1	0.37	0.15	0.03	0.00
2	0.18	0.22	0.08	0.00
3	0.06	0.22	0.14	0.01
4	0.02	0.17	0.18	0.02
5	0.00	0.10	0.18	0.04
6	0.00	0.05	0.15	0.06
7	0.00	0.02	0.10	0.09
8	0.00	0.00	0.07	0.11
9	0.00	0.00	0.04	0.13
10	0.00	0.00	0.02	0.13

Note: See text for definitions of terms and equations.

Inspection of this table and consideration of the error inherent in any virus titration involving a serial dilution leads to some significant practical guides in experimental design. Note first that in a culture infected at an moi of 1 pfu/cell, 37% of cells remain uninfected, an unacceptably high number for an experiment designed to measure a single round of synchronous infection. An moi of at least 3 is required to infect 95% of the cells in culture. Given that titers can easily be inaccurate by a factor of 2, use of a calculated moi of 10 ensures that 99% of the cells in a culture will be synchronously infected even if the measured titer is twofold higher than the actual titer.

One-Step Growth Experiment

A classic experiment developed initially for bacteriophage (24) and still frequently used to determine the essential growth properties of a virus is the one-step growth experiment. The goal of the one-step growth experiment is to measure the time course of virus replication and the yield of virus per cell during a single round of infection. The experiment is carried out as follows. Several dishes containing confluent monolayers or an appropriate culture cell are infected simultaneously with virus at a high moi, for example 10 pfu/cell. After an adsorption period, monolayers are washed to remove unabsorbed virus and then incubated in culture medium. At various times after infection, virus from individual dishes is harvested, and at the completion of the experiment, the virus titer in samples representing each time point is determined. The virus yield at each point can be converted to pfu/cell by dividing the total amount of virus present in the sample by the number of cells originally infected in the sample.

The results from one example of a one-step growth experiment, in this case comparing growth of wild-type vaccinia virus and a temperature-sensitive (*ts*) mutant at permissive and nonpermissive temperatures, are shown in Fig. 9. Several features of the growth curve are noteworthy. First, during the first several hours of the wild-type infection or the *ts*56 infection at the permissive temperature, the titer in the cultures decreases and then increases. This dip in the growth curve, called *eclipse*, results from the following sequence: Early during the experiment, the virus that attaches to the cell surface but is not yet uncoated remains infectious. Then, infectivity is lost during the first few hours of infection (the eclipse phase), when the virus is uncoated. Infectivity is then recovered only after new virus is produced. The infection then enters a rapid growth phase, followed by a plateau. The plateau results from the fact that all infected cells have reached the maximal yield of virus, or they have died or

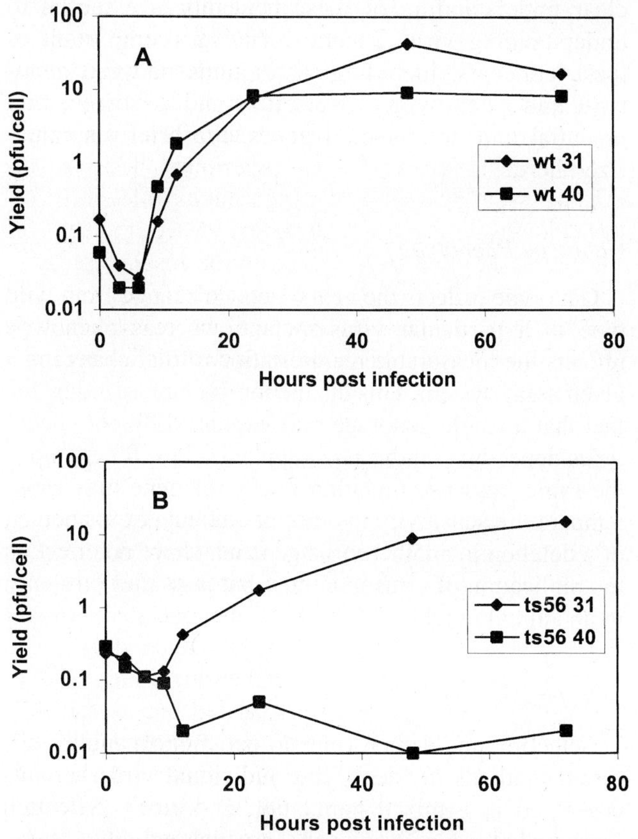

FIG. 9. One-step growth experiment. Monolayers of the African green monkey kidney cell line BSC40 were infected at an moi of 6 pfu/cell with wild-type vaccinia virus (*top panel*) or the temperature-sensitive vaccinia mutant, *ts*56 (*bottom panel*), and incubated at the permissive temperature, 31°C, or the nonpermissive temperature, 40°C, as indicated. Samples were harvested at various times and the titer determined by plaque titration on BSC40 cells at 31°C. The wild-type virus grows equally well at 31°C and 40°C. The *ts*56 grows more slowly than the wild type at 31°C but ultimately produces a yield of virus comparable to wild type. The *ts*56 does not grow at 40°C. (From ref. 41, with permission.)

lysed, depending on the type of virus infection. The time interval from infection to plateau represents the time required for a single cycle of growth, and the yield of virus at plateau shows the amount of virus produced per cell.

The experiment in Fig. 9 demonstrates the utility of the one-step growth experiment. As judged by this experiment, wild-type virus grows with identical kinetics and to the identical yields at both 31°C and 40°C, permissive and nonpermissive temperatures for the temperature-sensitive mutant, respectively. The temperature-sensitive mutant, *ts*56 (70), grows more slowly than wild-type virus at 31°C, indicating some defective character even at the permissive temperature, although at plateau the yields of mutant virus at 31°C are equivalent to those of the wild-type virus. The experiment demonstrates conclusively that the mutant does not grow at all at the nonpermissive temperature, 40°C.

Multiplicity of infection is a critical factor in the design of a virus growth experiment. A true one-step growth experiment can be done only at high moi. If the moi is too low and a large fraction of cells are left uninfected, then virus produced during the first round of infection will replicate on previously uninfected cells, and thus multiple rounds of infection rather than one round will be measured. A growth experiment done at low moi has utility in that it measures both growth and spread of a virus in culture, but the time from infection to plateau does not accurately reflect the time required for a single cycle of infection. It is also noteworthy that some mutant phenotypes are multiplicity dependent (5).

VIRUS GENETICS

Viruses are subject to the same genetic principles at work in other living systems, namely mutation, selection, complementation, and recombination. Genetics impacts all aspects of virology, including the natural evolution of viruses, clinical management of virus infections, and experimental virology. For example, antigenic variation, a direct result of mutation and selection, plays a prominent role in the epidemiology of influenza virus and human immunodeficiency virus (HIV) in the human population, and mutation to drug resistance offers a significant challenge to the clinical management of virus infections with antiviral drugs. This section deals primarily with the application of experimental genetic techniques to basic virology.

The ultimate goal of experimental virology is to understand completely the functional organization of a virus genome. In a modern context, this means determination of the structure of a virus genome at the nucleotide sequence level, coupled with isolation of mutational variants of the virus altered in each gene or control sequence, followed by analysis of the effects of each mutation on the replication and/or pathogenesis of the virus. Thus, genetic analysis of viruses is of fundamental importance to experimental virology.

Before the advent of modern nucleic acid technology, that is during a "classical" period of "forward" genetics, genetic analysis of viruses consisted of the random, brute-force isolation of large numbers of individual virus mutants, followed first by complementation analysis to determine groupings of individual mutants into genes, then recombination analysis to determine the physical order of genes on the virus genome, and finally the phenotypic analysis of mutants to determine gene function. This approach, pioneered in the 1940s, 1950s, and 1960s in elegant studies of several bacteriophage, notably lambda, T4, and T7 (Chapter 17), was the primary method for identifying, mapping, and characterizing virus genes. The application of cell culture techniques to animal virology opened the door to classical genetic analysis of animal viruses, resulting in a flurry of activity in the 1950s through the 1970s, during which time hundreds of mutants were isolated and analyzed in prototypical members of most of the major animal virus families (32). Modern nucleic acid technology introduced in the 1970s brought with it a variety of techniques for physical mapping of genomes and mutants, including restriction enzyme mapping, marker rescue, and DNA sequence analysis, which together replaced recombination analysis as an analytic tool. Mutants and techniques from that classical period continue to be of enormous utility today, but recombinant DNA technology has brought with it reverse (or "punk") genetics, in which the structure of the genome is determined first, using entirely physical methods, and then the function of individual genetic elements is determined by analyzing mutants constructed in a highly targeted fashion.

The genetic approach to experimental virology, or any field of biology for that matter, has the profound advantage of asking of the organism under study only the most basic question, "What genes do you need to survive, and why do you need them?" without imposing any further bias or assumptions on the system. And organisms often respond with surprises that the most ingenious biochemist or molecular biologist would never have imagined. What follows is a summary of the critical elements of both the classical and modern approaches to virus genetics as applied to experimental virology.

Mutants

Wild-Type Virus

It is important to understand that in the context of experimental virus genetics, a virus designated as wild type can differ significantly from the virus that actually occurs in nature. For example, virus genetics often relies heavily on growth and assay of viruses in cell culture, and, as noted previously, natural isolates of viruses may undergo significant genetic change during adaptation to cell culture. In addition, viruses to be designated wild type should be plaque purified before initiating a genetic study, to ensure a unique genetic background for mutational analysis. Last, viruses may be specifically adapted for use in genetic analysis, for example by passage under conditions that are to be restrictive for conditionally lethal mutants so that the analysis can be initiated with a preparation free of spontaneous mutants.

Fundamental Genetic Concepts

Concepts fundamental to genetic analysis of other organisms apply to genetic analysis of viruses, and a clear understanding of these concepts is essential to understanding virus genetics. The most important of these concepts, including distinctions between genotype and phenotype, a selection and a screen, and essential and nonessential genes, are briefly summarized here.

Genotype/Phenotype

Genotype reflects the actual genetic change from wild type in a particular virus mutant, whereas phenotype reflects the measurable manifestation of that change in a given assay system. This distinction is emphasized by the fact that a single genotype may express different phenotypes depending on the assay applied. Thus, for example, the same missense mutation in a virus gene may cause temperature sensitivity in one cell line but not in another, or a deletion in another virus gene may have no effect on the replication of virus in culture but may alter virulence in an animal model.

Selection/Screen

Selection and screen refer to two fundamentally different methods of identifying individual virus variants contained in a mixed population of viruses. Selection implies that a condition exists in which only the desired virus will grow, while growth of unwanted viruses is suppressed. Thus, a drug-resistant virus can be identified by plating a mixture of wild-type, drug-sensitive viruses, and mutant, drug-resistant viruses together on the same cell monolayer in the presence of the inhibitory drug, thereby selecting for drug-resistant viruses, which grow, and selecting against wild-type viruses, which do not grow (Fig. 5). A screen implies that both the desired virus variant and one or several other unwanted virus types grow under a given condition, so that many viruses must be analyzed individually to identify the desired variant. For example, in searching for a temperature-sensitive mutant—that is, a virus whose growth is inhibited relative to wild-type virus at an elevated temperature—no condition exists under which the mutant alone will grow. Therefore, virus must be plated at a low temperature at which both wild-type and mutant virus will grow, and plaques must be tested individually for temperature sensitivity.

Sometimes, a screen can be streamlined by introducing a phenotypic marker into the variant of choice. For example, a knockout virus might be constructed by inserting the beta-galactosidase gene into the virus gene to be inactivated. In the presence of an appropriate indicator dye, viruses containing the insertional knockout produce blue plaques and can therefore be distinguished from unmodified viruses, which form clear plaques, growing on the same plate (107). This example is still a screen, because both wild-type and mutant viruses grow under the conditions used, but the screen is simplified because mutant viruses can be readily identified by their color, obviating the need to pick and test individual plaques. Selections have considerable advantages over screens but are not always possible.

Essential/Nonessential

The terms *essential* and *nonessential* describe phenotypes, specifically whether a given gene is required for growth under a specific condition. Most viruses are finely tuned through selection to fit a specific niche. Not all viral genes are absolutely required for virus replication in that niche; some may simply confer a subtle selective advantage. Furthermore, if the niche is changed, for example from a natural animal host to a cell line in a laboratory, some genes that may have been essential for productive infection in the animal may not be required for replication in cell culture. Genes that are required for growth under a specific condition are termed essential, and those that are not required are termed nonessential. Because as a phenotype, essentiality may be a function of the specific test conditions, the test conditions need to be specified in describing the mutation; for example, the herpesvirus thymidine kinase gene is nonessential for virus replication in cell culture. A genes that is essential or nonessential under a given condition presents unique characteristics for analysis. Thus, mutants in nonessential genes may be easy to isolate because the gene can be deleted, but the function of the gene may be difficult to determine because, by definition, nonessential genes have no phenotype. On the other hand, genes that are essential can be used to study gene function by characterizing the precise replication defect caused by a mutation in the gene, but acquiring the appropriate mutant is confounded by the necessity for identifying a condition that will permit growth of the virus for study.

Mutation

Spontaneous Mutation

Spontaneous mutation rates in viruses are measured by fluctuation analysis (51), a technique pioneered by Luria and Delbruck (61) for analysis of mutation in bacteria, and later adapted to viruses by Luria (59). Fluctuation analysis consists of measuring the proportion of spontaneous mutants with a particular phenotype in many replicate cultures of virus, and applying the Poisson distribution to these data to calculate a mutation rate. It is important to note that, because spontaneous mutations occur at random and may occur only rarely, the raw data in a fluctuation analysis display enormous scatter, with some cultures containing a high proportion of mutants and some containing no mutants. Thus, from a practical perspective, although the proportion of mutants in a single culture of virus may reflect the mutation rate, it does not necessarily provide an accurate measure of mutation rate.

Both DNA and RNA viruses undergo spontaneous mutation, but the spontaneous mutation rate in RNA viruses is usually much higher than in DNA viruses. In general, the mutation rate at a specific site in different DNA viruses ranges from 10^{-8} to 10^{-11} per replication, whereas in RNA viruses it is at least 100-fold higher, between 10^{-3} and 10^{-6} per replication. The difference in mutation rate observed between RNA and DNA viruses is thought to result primarily from differences in the replication enzymes. Specifically, the DNA-dependent DNA polymerases used by DNA viruses contain a proofreading function, whereas the reverse transcriptases used by retroviruses and the RNA-dependent RNA polymerases used by RNA viruses lack a proofreading function. The difference in spontaneous mutation rate has profound consequences for both the biology of the viruses and for laboratory genetic analysis of viruses. Specifically, RNA viruses exist in nature as "quasi-species" (19)—that is, populations of virus variants in relative equilibrium with the environment but capable of swift adaptation because of their high spontaneous mutation rate (Chapter 13 in *Fields Virology*, 4th ed.). On the other hand, DNA viruses are genetically more stable but less adaptable. In the laboratory, the high mutation rate in RNA viruses presents difficulties in routine genetic analysis because mutants easily revert to a wild-type virus that can outgrow the mutant virus.

It is noteworthy that whereas the actual mutation rate at a single locus is probably relatively constant for a given virus, the apparent mutation rate to a given phenotype depends on the nature of the mutation(s) that can give rise to that phenotype. For example, spontaneous mutation to bromodeoxyuridine (BUdR) resistance in vaccinia virus may occur at least 10 to 100 times more frequently than spontaneous reversions of temperature-sensitive mutations to a wild-type, temperature-insensitive phenotype. In the case of BUdR resistance, any mutation that inactivates the thymidine kinase causes resistance to BUdR, and thus there are literally hundreds of different ways in which spontaneous mutation can give rise to BUdR resistance. By contrast, a temperature-sensitive mutation is usually a single-base missense mutation: There may exist only one possible mutational event that could cause reversion to the wild-type phenotype, and thus the apparent spontaneous mutation rate for the revertant phenotype is lower than the apparent spontaneous mutation rate to the BUdR resistance phenotype.

From a practical perspective, the apparent spontaneous mutation rate for specific selectable phenotypes may be sufficiently high that induction of mutants is unnecessary for their isolation. Note, for example, that the wild-type vaccinia virus culture titered in Fig. 5 contains numerous spontaneous isatin-beta-thiosemicarbasone (IBT)-resistant viruses that could easily be plaque-purified from assays done in the presence of IBT. However, for most mutants (e.g., temperature-sensitive mutants), in which the desired mutational events are rare and a screen must be used rather than a selection, induced mutation is required for efficient isolation of mutants.

Induced Mutation

Under most circumstances, the incidence of spontaneous mutations is low enough that induction of mutation is a practical prerequisite for isolation of virus mutants. It is usually desirable to induce limited, normally single-base changes, and for this purpose, chemical mutagens are most appropriate. Commonly used chemical mutagens are of two types, *in vitro* mutagens and *in vivo* mutagens (20). *In vitro* mutagens work by chemically altering nucleic acid and can be applied by treating virions in the absence of replication. Examples of *in vitro* mutagens include hydroxylamine, nitrous acid, and alkylating agents, which through chemical modification of specific bases cause mispairing leading to missense mutations. *In vivo* chemical mutagens comprise compounds such as nucleoside analogs, which must be incorporated during viral replication and thus must be applied to an infected cell. One of the most effective mutagens is an alkylating agent, nitrosoguanidine, which, although it is capable of alkylating nucleic acid *in vitro*, is most effective when used *in vivo*, where it works by alkylating guanine residues at the replication fork, ultimately causing mispairing.

The effectiveness of a mutagenesis is often assayed by observing the killing effect of the mutagen on the virus, the assumption being that many mutational events will be lethal, and thus an effective mutagenesis will decrease a virus titer relative to an untreated control. However, killing does not always correlate precisely with mutagenesis, especially with an *in vitro* mutagen that can damage virion structure without necessarily causing mutation. An alternative method for assessing mutagenesis is to monitor an increase in the mutation frequency to a selectable phenotype where possible. For example, in vaccinia virus, mutagenesis causes a dose-dependent increase in resistance to phosphonoacetic acid, a drug that prevents poxvirus replication by inhibiting the viral DNA polymerase (11). In summary, use of mutagens can increase the mutation frequency several hundred fold, such that desired mutants may comprise as much as 0.5% of the total virus population.

Double Mutants/Siblings

The existence of double mutants and siblings can theoretically complicate genetic analysis of a virus. Double (or multiple) mutants may contain more than one mutation contributing to a phenotype. Theoretically, because the probability that a double mutant will be created increases as the dose of a mutagen is increased, there is a practical limit to the amount of induced mutation that is desirable. Double mutants are usually revealed as mutants that are noncomplementing with more than one mutant, or that are impossible to map by recombination or physical methods. Siblings result from replication of mutant virus either through amplification of a mutagenized stock, or during an *in vivo* mutagenesis. The only completely reliable method to avoid isolation of sibling mutants is to isolate each mutant from an independently plaque-purified stock of wild-type virus. In practice, siblings seldom present a problem serious enough to justify the effort required to avoid them.

Mutant Genotypes

There exist two basic categories of mutation, base substitution and deletion/insertion mutations. Both mutation types can occur with consequence in either a protein coding sequence or in a control sequence, such as a transcriptional promoter, a replication origin, or a packaging sequence. Base substitution mutations consist of the precise replacement of one nucleotide with a different nucleotide in a nucleic acid sequence. In coding sequences, base substitution mutations can be silent, causing no change in amino acid sequence of a protein; they can be missense, causing replacement of the wild-type amino acid with a different residue; or they can be nonsense, causing premature translation termination during protein synthesis. Deletion and insertion mutations comprise deletion or insertion of one or more nucleotides in a nucleic acid sequence. In a coding sequence, deletion or insertion of multiples of three nucleotides can result in precise deletion or insertion of one or more amino acids in a protein sequence. In a coding sequence, deletions or insertions that do *not* involve multiples of three nucleotides result in a shift in the translational reading frame, which almost invariably results in premature termination at some distance downstream of the mutation. In general, nonsense mutations, frameshift mutations, or large in-frame insertions or deletions are expected to inactivate a gene, whereas missense mutations may cause much more subtle phenotypes such as drug resistance or temperature sensitivity.

Mutant Phenotypes

In the context of experimental virology, where the goal is to understand the function of individual virus genes, the most useful mutants are those that inhibit virus replication by inactivating a virus gene. The nonproductive infections with these lethal mutants can be studied in detail to determine the precise aspect of virus replication that has been affected, thus providing information about the normal function of the affected gene. However, one must be able to grow the mutant to conduct experiments, so a condition must be found in which the mutation in question is not lethal, hence the general class of mutant phenotypes called conditional lethal. Conditional lethal mutants comprise by far the largest and most useful class of mutant phenotypes; they consist of host-range, nonsense, temperature-sensitive, and drug-dependent phenotypes, and they will be described individually later. Two additional classes of mutant phenotypes, resistance and plaque morphology, which have very specific application to genetic analysis of viruses, will also be described.

Host-Range

A host-range virus mutant is broadly defined as a mutant that grows on one cell type and not on another, in contrast to the wild-type virus, which grows on both cell types. Two general subcategories of host-range mutants exist, natural and engineered. Natural host-range virus mutants are relatively rare, primarily because they must be identified by brute-force screen or serendipity, in many cases in the absence of a viable rationale for the targeted host range. The existence of a host-range phenotype implies that a specific virus–host interaction is compromised, which also implies that for any specific host-range phenotype, only one virus gene (or a limited number) will be targeted. A classic example of a natural host-range mutants are the *hrt* mutants of mouse polyoma virus, which affect both small and middle T antigens, and which grow on primary mouse cells but not continuous mouse 3T3 cell lines (2). Engineered host-range mutants are constructed by deleting an essential gene of interest in the virus while at the same time creating a cell line that expresses the gene. The engineered cell line provides a permissive host for growth of the mutant virus because it complements the missing virus function, whereas the normal host lacking the gene of interest provides a nonpermissive host for study of the phenotype of the virus. This technology has been useful for studying a variety of viruses, notably herpes simplex virus, where it has facilitated study of several essential virus genes (17,107).

Nonsense Mutants

Nonsense mutants are those that contain a premature translation termination mutation in the coding region of the mutant gene. Nonsense mutants are formally a specific class of conditionally lethal, host-range mutants. Specifically, the permissive host is one that expresses a tRNA containing an anticodon mutation that results in insertion of an amino acid in response to a nonsense codon, thus restoring synthesis of a full-length polypeptide and suppressing the effects of the virus nonsense mutation. The nonpermissive host is a normal cell in which a truncated, nonfunctional polypeptide is made. In practice, most nonsense mutants in existence have been isolated by random mutagenesis followed by a brute-force screen for host range. Nonsense mutants have three distinct advantages for the conduct of virus genetics: (a) Mutants can be isolated in virtually any essential virus gene using one set of permissive and nonpermissive hosts and one set of techniques, (b) the mutations result in synthesis of a truncated polypeptide, thereby facilitating identification of the affected gene, and (c) virus mutants can be relatively easily engineered, as the exact sequence of the desired mutation is predictable.

Nonsense mutants have provided the single most powerful genetic tool in the study of bacteriophage, where efficient, viable nonsense-suppressing bacteria are readily available. Unfortunately, attempts to isolate nonsense-suppressing mammalian cells have met with only limited success, probably because the nonsense-suppressing tRNAs are lethal in the eucaryotic host (89).

Temperature Sensitivity

Temperature sensitivity is a type of conditional lethality in which mutants can grow at a low temperature but not at a high temperature, in contrast to wild-type virus, which grows at both temperatures. Genotypically, temperature-sensitive mutants are usually relatively subtle, single amino acid substitutions that render the target protein unstable and hence nonfunctional at an elevated or nonpermissive temperature, while leaving the protein stable and functional at a low, permissive temperature. In practice, temperature-sensitive mutants are usually isolated by random mutagenesis followed by brute-force screening for growth at two temperatures. Screening can be streamlined by a plaque enlargement technique in which mutagenized virus is first plated at a permissive temperature, then stained and shifted to a nonpermissive temperature after marking the size of plaques, to screen for plaques that do not increase in size at the nonpermissive temperature (91). Replica plating techniques that permit relatively straightforward screening of thousands of mutant candidates in yeast and bacteria have not been successfully adapted to virology, and thus a screen for temperature sensitivity, even when streamlined with plaque enlargement, ultimately depends on the laborious but reliable process of picking and testing individual plaques.

Temperature-sensitive mutants have the profound advantage of theoretically accessing any essential virus gene using a single set of protocols. Temperature-sensitive mutants have proved enormously useful in all branches of virology, but they have been particularly useful for the study of animal viruses, where nonsense suppression has not been a viable option. Cold-sensitive mutants—that is, mutants that grow at a high but not a low temperature—comprise a relatively rare but nevertheless useful alternative type of temperature-sensitive mutants.

Temperature-sensitive mutants can actually be divided into two subclasses, thermolabile and temperature-sensitive-for-synthesis mutants (108). Thermolabile mutants are those in which the gene product can be inactivated following synthesis by a shift from the permissive to the nonpermissive temperature. Mutants that are temperature sensitive for synthesis display gene dysfunction only if the infection is held at the nonpermissive temperature during synthesis of the mutant gene product; if the gene product is made at the permissive temperature, it cannot be inactivated by raising the temperature. Clearly, the two mutant types can be distinguished by performing appropriate temperature-shift experiments. Thermolability obviously implies that a protein preformed at the permissive temperature is directly destabilized by raising the temperature. Temperature-sensitive-for-synthesis mutations commonly involve multisubunit structures or complex organelles: Theoretically, the quaternary structure of a complex formed correctly at the permissive temperature stabilizes the mutant protein, making the mutation resistant to temperature shift. If a temperature-sensitive-for-synthesis mutant protein is synthesized at the nonpermissive temperature, it may be degraded before assembly or may not assemble properly because of misfolding. For most purposes, the thermolabile and temperature-sensitive-for-synthesis mutant types are equally useful.

Drug Resistance/Dependence

A number of antiviral compounds have now been identified, and virus mutants that are resistant to or that depend on these compounds have found utility in genetic analysis of viruses. A few compounds have been identified that target similar enzymes in different viruses, including phosphonoacetic acid, which inhibits DNA polymerases (44,93), and BUdR, which targets thymidine kinases (21,97). More often, however, antiviral drugs are highly specific for a gene product of one particular virus—for example, guanidine, which targets the polio 2C NTPase (78,79); acyclovir, which targets the herpes simplex virus thymidine kinase and DNA polymerase (8,88); amantidine, which targets the influenza virus M2 virion integral membrane ion channel protein (43); and IBT, which is highly specific for poxviruses and targets at least two genes involved in viral transcription (10,70). Drugs that are most useful are those that inhibit wild-type virus growth in a plaque assay without killing cells in a monolayer, so that resistant or dependent viruses can be selected by virtue of their ability to form plaques on a drug-treated monolayer. Examples of both drug resistance and drug dependence are shown in Fig. 5.

Drug-resistant or -dependent virus mutants have two general uses in virus genetics. First, they can be useful for identifying the target or mechanism of action of an antiviral drug. For example, studies of influenza virus mutants resistant to amantidine were of importance in characterizing both the M2 gene and the mechanism of action of amantidine (80). Second, resistant or dependent mutants provide selectable markers for use in recombination mapping, for the assessment of specific genetic protocols, or for selection of recombinant viruses in reverse genetic protocols. For example, guanidine resistance has been used as a marker for use in three-factor crosses in recombination mapping of poliovirus temperature-sensitive mutants (14); phosphonoacetic acid resistance and IBT dependence have been used in vaccinia virus to assess the efficiency of marker rescue protocols (26,41); and acyclovir resistance and BUdR resistance, resulting from mutation of the herpesvirus or poxvirus thymidine kinase genes, have been used both in herpes viruses and in poxviruses to select for insertion of engineered genes into the viral genome (9,64,74).

Plaque Morphology

Plaque morphology mutants are those in which the appearance of mutant plaques is readily distinguishable from that of wild-type plaques. Most commonly, the morphologic distinction is plaque size—that is, mutant plaques may be larger or smaller than wild-type plaques. However, other morphologic distinctions are possible—for example, formation of clear versus turbid bacteriophage plaques. Most plaque morphology mutants affect very specific virus functions, which in turn affect the virus–host relationship in a fashion that impacts on the appearance of a plaque. Notable examples from bacteriophage research include clear plaque mutants of bacteriophage lambda and rapid lysis mutants of the T-even bacteriophage. Wild-type lambda forms turbid plaques because some percentage of cells are lysogenized and thus survive the infection, leaving intact bacteria within a plaque. Clear mutants of lambda typically affect the lambda repressor so that lysogeny is prevented and all infected bacteria lyse, resulting in a clear plaque (52). Wild-type T-even phages produce small plaques with a turbid halo because only a fraction of infected bacteria lyse during a normal infection, a phenomenon called lysis inhibition. Rapid lysis mutants, which affect a phage membrane protein, do not display lysis inhibition and as a result form large, clear plaques (46). Examples from animal virus research include large plaque mutants of adenovirus and syncytial mutants of herpes simplex virus. The large plaque phenotype in adenovirus results from faster-than-normal release of virus from infected cells (56). Syncytial mutants of herpes virus affect virus surface glycoproteins and result in fusion of infected cells, whereas wild-type virus causes cells to round and clump without significant fusion. Thus, *syn* mutants form large clear plaques readily distinguishable from the smaller dense foci caused by wild-type virus (86). All of these specific plaque morphology mutants have value either in the study of the actual functions affected, or as specific phenotypic markers for use in recombination studies, where they can be used in the same fashion as drug-resistance markers, described previously.

In addition to the existence of specific plaque morphology loci in several viruses, it is noteworthy that any mutation that effects virus yield or growth rate may result in the production of a smaller-than-wild-type plaque, which can be useful in genetic experiments. Thus, many temperature-sensitive mutants form smaller-than-wild-type plaques even at the permissive temperature because the mutant gene may not be fully functional even under permissive conditions, and this property is often useful in mutant isolation or for distinguishing wild-type from mutant virus in plaque assays involving several virus variants. Note, for example, in Fig. 5 that the vaccinia virus temperature-sensitive mutant *ts*56 forms smaller-than-wild-type plaques at the permissive temperature, 31°C. Last, intragenic or extragenic suppressors of conditional lethal virus mutants may grow poorly relative to the wild-type virus and form small plaques as a result, facilitating their isolation from a mixture containing true wild-type revertant viruses (13).

Neutralization Escape

Neutralization escape mutants are a specific class of mutants selected as variant viruses that form plaques in the presence of neutralizing antibodies. Such mutants affect the structure or modification of viral surface proteins. They have been of value in studies of virus structure, antigenic variation, and virus–cell interactions (37,47).

Reversion

Reversion may be defined as mutation that results in a change from a mutant genotype to the original wild-type genotype. Accordingly, revertants in a stock of mutant virus are revealed as viruses that have acquired a wild-type phenotype. For example, Fig. 5 shows that when the vaccinia virus temperature-sensitive mutant *ts*56 is plated at the nonpermissive temperature, a number of plaques with wild-type morphology, probably revertants, are detectable at low dilutions of virus. Spontaneous reversion of missense mutations probably results from misincorporation during replication, as the reversion frequency of different viruses often reflects the error rate of the replication enzyme. Spontaneous reversion of significant deletion mutations occurs rarely if at all, as reversion would require replacement of missing nucleotides with the correct sequence.

Reversion impacts on viral genetics in two ways. First, in any genetic experiment involving mixed infections with two genetically different viruses, wild-type viruses can arise either through reversion or recombination, and in most cases it is important to be able to distinguish between these two processes. This is discussed in more detail later in the sections describing complementation and recombination. Second, as described previously in the description of spontaneous mutation, if the spontaneous reversion rate is extremely high, revertants can easily come to dominate a mutant virus stock, thus obscuring the mutant phenotype and causing serious difficulties in both genetic and biochemical analysis of mutants.

Leakiness

Not all conditionally lethal mutants are completely defective in replication under nonpermissive conditions, and leakiness is a quantitative measure of the ability of a mutant virus to grow under nonpermissive conditions. Leakiness can be quantified with a one-step growth experiment. To quantify leakiness of a temperature-sensitive mutant, for example, cells are infected at a high moi with wild-type or mutant virus, infected cells are incubated at either permissive or nonpermissive temperatures, and maximal virus yields are then determined by plaque titration under permissive conditions so that the growth of mutant and wild-type virus can be quantitatively compared. Ideally, for wild-type virus the ratio of the yield for infections done at the nonpermissive temperature relative to the permissive temperature should be 1—that is, the virus should grow equally well at both temperatures. For mutant viruses, the ratio of the yield for infections done at the nonpermissive temperature relative to the permissive temperature may range from less than 10% to as much as 100%, even for mutants that are clearly defective in plaque formation under nonpermissive conditions. Mutants that are "tight" (i.e., that grow poorly under nonpermissive conditions) are desirable for phenotypic characterization relative to leaky mutants, because leaky mutants will logically display considerable wild-type phenotypic behavior.

In special cases, extreme leakiness is an expected and desirable trait. Specifically, virus mutants that are wild type for replication and production of infectious virions but defective in cell-to-cell spread have a phenotype characterized by defective plaque formation, which requires spread, but 100% leakiness, which does not require spread if assayed in a high moi, one-step growth protocol (4).

Genetic Analysis of Mutants

Complementation

Complementation analysis provides a general method for determining whether two different virus mutants affect the same or different genes. The quantitative test to determine complementation is a two-step procedure in which co-infections are first done to induce an interaction between two mutants, then the results of those infections are quantitatively assessed by plaque titration. The test compares the ability of two mutants to grow in mixed, relative to single, infections under nonpermissive conditions. Specifically, cells are first infected with two different virus mutants at high moi so that all cells are co-infected with both mutants, and infected cells are incubated under nonpermissive conditions where neither mutant alone can replicate, for an interval sufficient to achieve maximal virus yield. Single high-moi infections under nonpermissive conditions are performed as controls. Virus is then harvested, yields are quantified by plaque titration under both permissive and nonpermissive conditions, and a complementation index (CI) is calculated according to the following formula:

$$\frac{\text{yield } (A + B)_p - \text{yield } (A + B)_{np}}{\text{yield } (A)_p + \text{yield } (B)_p} = \text{CI},$$

where A and B represent individual virus mutants and the subscripts p and np represent the conditions, permissive or nonpermissive, under which the virus yields were plaque-titrated. Because both mutant and wild-type viruses will be counted in plaque titrations done at the permissive temperature, the first term in the numerator, yield $(A + B)_p$, measures the yield of all viruses, both mutant and wild type, from the initial high-moi mixed infections done under nonpermissive conditions. The second term in the numerator, yield $(A + B)_{np}$, measures the yield of wild-type viruses, mostly recombinants, from the high-moi mixed infections done under nonpermissive conditions, because only wild-type viruses will be counted in plaque titrations done at the nonpermissive temperature. Subtraction of the wild-type viruses from the total viruses leaves a count of only the mutant viruses in the numerator. The denominator measures the ability of each of the mutants to grow in single high-moi infections done initially under nonpermissive conditions.

If the two mutants, A and B, are in different virus genes, then in the mixed infection done under nonpermissive conditions mutant A can contribute wild-type B gene product and mutant B can contribute wild-type A gene product. Thus, the mutants can help or complement each other, resulting in a high yield of mutant virus in the mixed infection compared to the single infections, and a CI significantly greater than 1. If the two mutants A and B affect the same gene, then the wild-type gene product will be lacking in the mixed infection. In this case, the

TABLE 6. *Complementation between* ts *mutants of Sindbis virus*

Complementation Group	Mutant	Complementation level in mixed infection with *ts*21	*ts*19	*ts*17	*ts*4	*ts*24	*ts*11	*ts*6	*ts*2	*ts*5	*ts*10	*ts*23	*ts*20
A	*ts*21	—	0.2	0.1	0.1	1.5	17.6	200	43	27	24	ND	ND
A	*ts*19		—	0.4	0.5	3.2	120	485	ND	16	19	43	12
A	*ts*17			—	ND	4.5	30	393	25	31	17	19	23
A	*ts*4				—	0.36	9.0	127	19	ND	27	ND	8
A	*ts*24					—	4.2	364	22	29	18	16	5
A′	*ts*11						—	280	1.8	50	43	ND	12
B	*ts*6							—	62	93	64	68	21
C	*ts*2								—	1.0	36	27	5.2
C	*ts*5									—	345	61	8.0
D	*ts*10										—	0.7	16.7
D	*ts*23											—	8.5
E	*ts*20												—

ND, not determined.
Source: From ref. 76, with permission.

yield from the mixed infection will be equivalent to the yield from the single infections, and the CI should not exceed 1. In practice, because of error in plaque assays and from other sources, mixed infections with mutants in the same viral gene will often yield complementation indices of slightly greater than 1, and the practical cutoff must be determined empirically for a given viral system.

An example of complementation analysis for several mutants of Sindbis virus is shown in Table 6. Close examination of these data demonstrates both the utility and the vagaries of complementation analysis. For example, *ts*21, *ts*19, and *ts*17 clearly form a complementation group, as they are all noncomplementing with each other, and they complement all other mutants with the exception of *ts*24. The *ts*24 mutant is retained in group A because it is clearly noncomplementing with two other group A mutants, despite relatively high complementation indices with *ts*19 and *ts*17. The *ts*6 mutant is unusual in that it yields, for unknown reasons, relatively high complementation indices with all other mutants. The complementation pattern observed with *ts*11 is erratic; it was originally assigned to an independent group, then to group A, and finally to an independent group called A′ to indicate uncertainty in the assignment (76).

Qualitative complementation tests have also been devised for use with both bacterial and mammalian viruses (7,11,96). These qualitative tests are much easier to perform than quantitative tests and in practice just as reliable. In general, these tests are designed so that bacterial lawns or eukaryotic cell monolayers are infected either singly or with two viruses under nonpermissive conditions and at relatively low moi. The moi must be high enough so that numerous cells are doubly infected in the mixed infection, but low enough so that most cells are uninfected and a lawn or monolayer is maintained. Complementing mutant pairs produce plaques or cleared areas under nonpermissive conditions, whereas noncomplementing mutant pairs do not. An example of a qualitative complementation test is shown in Fig. 10. A disadvantage of the qualitative test is that it theoretically does not discriminate between complementation and recombination, but in practice this deficiency has not been a problem.

Complementation analysis has been of tremendous benefit in sorting mutants in most but not all viral systems. A notable exception is poliovirus, where complementation between temperature-sensitive mutants *in vivo* is not observed. The lack of complementation in picornaviruses may be related to the unique mechanism of viral gene expression, in which all protein products are produced from a polyprotein precursor by proteolytic cleavage. If individual temperature-sensitive mutants affect structure, synthesis, or cleavage of the polyprotein precursor, they may behave as if they all belong to a single complementation group, even though they may map to different protein end products.

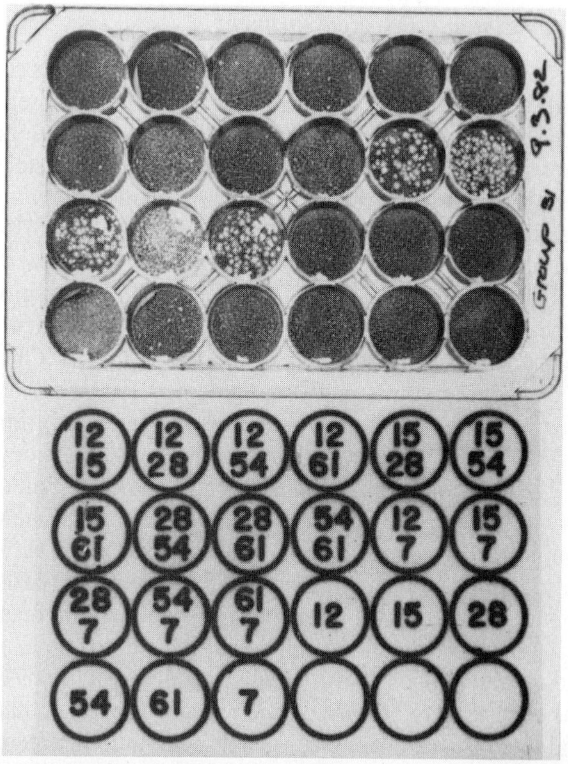

FIG. 10. Qualitative complementation test. This test was done to confirm that five different vaccinia virus temperature-sensitive mutants, *ts*12, *ts*15, *ts*28, *ts*54, and *ts*61, all reside in the same complementation group. Monolayers of the African green monkey kidney cell line BSC40 grown in a 24-well dish were infected at very low moi (0.03 pfu/cell) with individual mutants or mutant pairs. The dish was incubated at a nonpermissive temperature (40°C) for 3 days and stained with crystal violet. The stained dish is shown at the *top*, and a key to the infections is shown at the *bottom*. Mixed infections in the first 10 wells represent all possible pairwise combinations of the five candidate temperature-sensitive mutants, and the absence of plaques in these wells confirms that they all reside in a single complementation group. As a control, each mutant was also tested with another temperature-sensitive mutant, *ts*7, which was known to be in a different complementation group. The presence of plaques in each of the mixed infections containing *ts*7 represents positive complementation and confirms the validity of the test. Each mutant was tested in a single infection as an additional control. (From ref. 12, with permission.)

As a concept, complementation impacts broadly on virology and is not limited simply to the grouping of conditionally lethal mutants into genes. For example, the growth of engineered host-range deletion mutants in essential virus genes, discussed previously, relies on complementation of the missing viral function by an engineered cell line that expresses the wild-type viral gene product. In addition, the accumulation of defective virus genomes at high-multiplicity passage, also discussed previously, results from a complementing helper function provided by wild-type virus.

Recombination and Reassortment

Recombination describes a process by which nucleic acid sequences from two genotypically different parental viruses are exchanged so that the progeny contain sequences derived from both parents. In viral systems, there exist three distinct mechanisms of recombination, dictated by the structures of the viral genomes. For DNA viruses, recombination occurs by the physical breakage and rejoining of parental DNA molecules through regions of sequence homology, in a fashion similar or identical to the same process in bacteria or higher organisms. Of the RNA viruses containing nonsegmented genomes, only picornaviruses, coronaviruses, togaviruses, and retroviruses display efficient recombination, which is thought to occur during replication via "copy choice"—namely, switching templates during replication so that the newly synthesized genome contains sequences from two different parental molecules (39,48,54,55). For RNA viruses containing segmented genomes, recombination occurs through reassortment of individual parental genome segments into progeny viruses. Historically, recombination has been used to construct genetic maps of virus mutants and to construct novel virus genotypes. Although recombination mapping has been largely replaced by physical mapping techniques such as marker rescue, a technical knowledge of recombination mapping can contribute to an appreciation of the complexity of genetic interactions between viruses.

The methods used to determine recombination frequencies are the same regardless of genome structure or mechanism of recombination. Like complementation, the quantitative test to determine recombination frequency between two mutants, called a two-factor cross, is a two-step procedure, but in this case co-infections are first done under conditions permissive to recombination, and then the fraction of recombinants relative to the total virus yield is quantitatively assessed by plaque titration. Specifically, cells are first infected with two different virus mutants at high moi so that all cells are co-infected with both mutants, and infected cells are incubated under permissive conditions so that both mutants have maximal opportunity for interaction, for an interval sufficient to achieve maximal virus yield. Single high-moi infections under permissive conditions are performed as controls. Virus is then harvested, yields are quantified by plaque titration under both permissive and nonpermissive conditions, and a recombination frequency is calculated according to the followng formula:

$$\frac{\text{yield }(A + B)_{np} - \text{yield }(A)_{np} - \text{yield }(B)_{np}}{\text{yield }(A + B)_{p}} \times 2 \times 100\% = \text{RF},$$

where A and B represent individual virus mutants and the subscripts p and np represent the conditions, permissive or nonpermissive, under which the virus yields were plaque-titrated. The first term in the numerator, yield $(A + B)_{np}$, quantifies wild-type virus emerging from the mixed infection, including both recombinants and revertants, because only wild-type virus will grow in the plaque assay done under nonpermissive conditions. The second and third terms in the numerator, yield $(A)_{np}$ and yield $(B)_{np}$, quantify wild-type virus emerging from the control single infections, providing a measure of reversion in each of the two mutants. Subtraction of the revertants from the total yield of wild-type virus leaves a measure of recombinants only in the numerator. The denominator, yield $(A + B)_{p}$, quantifies the total virus yield from the mixed infection including both wild-type and mutant virus, as all input virus types will grow in the plaque assay done under permissive conditions. The quotient is multiplied by a factor of 2 to account for unscored progeny representing the reciprocal of the wild-type recombinants, namely double mutants, and converted to a percent.

Recombination mapping in DNA viruses relies on the assumption that the frequency of recombination between two genetic markers is proportional to the distance between the two markers. For several DNA viruses, observed recombination frequencies comprise a continuous range from less than 1% up to a theoretical maximum of 50%, allowing the construction of linear genetic maps (32).

In viruses with segmented genomes, recombination between markers on the same segment is extremely rare, but reassortment of segments is extremely efficient, so that recombination is an all-or-none phenomenon, with markers on the same segment displaying no recombination, and markers on different segments displaying very high levels of recombination (82). For these reasons, genetic exchange in segmented RNA viruses is commonly called reassortment rather than recombination. Reassortment analysis for segmented viruses is useful for determining whether two mutants map to the same genome segment, but it cannot be used to determine the order of markers on a given segment. Mutants can be mapped to individual RNA segments by performing intertypic crosses between virus types that differ in the electrophoretic mobility of each RNA segment. Specifically, if crosses are performed between a wild-type virus of one type and a mutant virus of another type and numerous wild-type progeny analyzed, one segment bearing the wild-type allele will be conserved among all the progeny, while all other segments will display reassortment (82).

Marker Rescue

Marker rescue is a physical mapping technique that measures directly whether a given virus mutation maps within a specific subfragment of a virus genome. Use of marker rescue is confined to DNA viruses in which homologous recombination takes place, but it has been of enormous value in these systems. The application of the technique varies somewhat depending on the virus system under study, but the general principles are the same. Specifically, full-length mutant viral genomic DNA plus a wild-type DNA genomic subfragment, usually a cloned DNA molecule, are introduced into cells under conditions permissive for recombination and for wild-type virus replication. For viruses that contain infectious DNA—for example, herpesviruses (95), adenoviruses (36), and polyomaviruses (58,71)—the mutant genomic DNA and the wild-type genomic subfragment may be cotransfected into cells. For viruses containing noninfectious genomic DNA—for example, poxviruses (99)—the mutant DNA must be introduced into cells by infection with the mutant virus, and this is followed by transfection with the wild-type DNA subfragment. In either case, the protocol allows for homologous recombination between the mutant genome and the wild-type DNA subfragment. If the wild-type DNA subfragment contains the wild-type allele for the mutation, the recombination can exchange the wild type for the mutant sequence in the mutant genome, creating wild-type virus. Conversely, if the wild-type fragment does not contain the wild-type allele for the mutation, no wild-type virus, above a background of revertants, will be created in the experiment.

The presence of wild-type virus can be assayed using either a two-step or a one-step protocol. In the two-step protocol, depending on the nature of the mutation being rescued, infected and/or transfected cells are incubated under permissive conditions to facilitate recombination and replication, or under nonpermissive conditions to select for wild-type recombinants; then wild-type virus yields are quantified by plaque titration under nonpermissive conditions. In the one-step protocol, the infection and/or transfection is done so that only a small fraction of the cells in a monolayer are infected, and cells are then incubated under nonpermissive conditions so that wild-type virus formed during a successful rescue will form plaques on the monolayer (99). In short, regardless of the precise method used, conversion, or rescue, of mutant virus to wild type with a given wild-type DNA fragment means that the mutation maps within that fragment. Initial marker rescue mapping experiments may be facilitated by the use of a few large but overlapping wild-type DNA fragments, and fine mapping may be accomplished with fragments as small as a few hundred nucleotides. Marker rescue mapping has completely replaced recombination mapping as a method for mapping DNA virus mutants, and precise genetic maps of several DNA viruses have now been constructed.

Reverse Genetics

Prior to the advent of recombinant DNA and DNA sequencing technologies, classical genetic analysis, namely random isolation and characterization of virus mutants, was one of the few effective methods for identifying, mapping, and characterizing virus genes, and it was the only method for obtaining virus mutants. With the current ready availability of genomic sequences for virtually all the prototypical members of each virus family and a versatile package of genetic engineering tools, the experimental landscape has changed completely. One can now conduct a genetic analysis with a reasonably complete foreknowledge of the genetic structure of the virus, focus attention on individual genes of interest, and deliberately engineer mutations in genes to study their function. Termed reverse genetics, this process has come to dominate the genetic analysis of viruses.

Reverse genetic analysis involves two distinct considerations: strategies for construction of cloned mutations and strategies for incorporation of mutations into viral genomes. The principles governing these strategies are highly dependent on the structure of a given viral genome and the strategy of virus replication, and thus they vary in the extreme. However, a few general principles can be identified and are discussed later.

Incorporation of Mutations into Viral Genomes

The methods used for incorporation of mutations into viral genomes depend on several features of the individual virus under consideration, including genome size, whether the nucleic acid is infectious, and whether the genome is RNA or DNA. For DNA or RNA viruses with relatively small genomes and for which the nucleic acid is infectious, incorporation of a given mutation into the viral genome is a relatively straightforward matter of cloning the desired mutation in a full-length genomic clone in a prokaryotic vector, then transfecting cells with the mutant nucleic acid. For examples, engineered mutations have been constructed in both picornaviruses (18) and polyomaviruses (1) using full-length genomes.

For DNA viruses that are either too large or too complex to be easily manipulated as a full-length genomic clone, or that contain genomes that are not infectious as nucleic acids, incorporation of mutations into the viral genome requires homologous recombination catalyzed in infected and/or transfected cells, in a fashion virtually identical to marker rescue protocols described previously. For example, *in vivo* recombination has been used very successfully to construct numerous engineered mutations in both vaccinia virus (75) and herpes simplex virus (107).

For RNA viruses whose genomic nucleic acid is not infectious and for which homologous recombination is not an option, the protocols for incorporation of mutations into the genome become more complex and tailored to the particulars of replication of individual viruses. For example, construction of engineered mutations in rhabdoviruses requires construction of a full-length genomic clone which contains the mutation, and which can be transcribed from a bacteriophage T7 promoter. The mutant viral genome is activated by cotransferation with T7 promoter-driven plasmids encoding all required rhabdovirus replication proteins into cells infected with a recombinant vaccinia virus expressing T7 RNA polymerase (84). Similarly, construction of influenza virus recombinants requires co-transfection of multiple plasmids encoding the mutant RNA segment and several influenza replication proteins, and co-infection with a helper virus (81).

The methods used for isolation of the desired mutant virus depend on the nature of the mutation being constructed, and on the method of incorporation into the virus genome. In situations not requiring *in vivo* homologous recombination between cloned mutant DNA and wild-type virus, only the mutant allele of the target gene is present in the construction, all virus recovered from the construction will be mutant, and no selection or screen for mutants is required. This situation applies, for example, to construction of mutations in papovaviruses, picornaviruses, or rhabdoviruses, as described previously. In situations when *in vivo* homologous recombination is used to incorporate the cloned mutation into a wild-type genome, for example in poxviruses or herpesviruses, both mutant and wild-type viruses emerge from the mutant construction protocol, and thus a screen or selection is required to identify the mutant of interest. For mutations in nonessential genes, this may be a relatively straightforward matter of inserting into the target gene a color marker such as beta-galactosidase to facilitate a screen (107), or inserting a dominant selectable marker such as *E. coli* guanine phosphoribosyltransferase (25), to facilitate a selection. For conditionally lethal phenotypes such as temperature sensitivity, although techniques exist that enrich for recombinant viruses, mutant isolation ultimately relies on a screen of individual mutants for differential growth under permissive and nonpermissive conditions.

Construction of Cloned Mutations

Construction of cloned mutations for use in virology is problematic only if the gene in question is essential, necessitating isolation of a conditionally lethal mutation. For genes that are nonessential, construction of a cloned mutation is a simple matter of engineering a null mutation, for example a deletion, insertion, or nonsense mutation, into the cloned gene sequence. Three basic types of engineered conditionally lethal mutations are currently in use: host-range deletion mutants that rely on the availability of a complementing host cell, temperature-sensitive mutants constructed by clustered charge-to-alanine scanning, and artificially induced gene regulation. For host-range deletion mutants, the primary problem is construction of a host cell that expresses the target gene in a fashion appropriate for complementation of a null mutant in the virus. Once a cell line has been isolated, construction of the cloned mutation in the virus gene follows the same principles governing construction of a null mutation in a nonessential gene. The fundamental problem in creating temperature-sensitive mutations is that it is currently impossible to predict from primary amino acid sequence or even from three-dimensional protein structure what type of mutation will render a protein temperature sensitive. This difficulty has been partially overcome with the use of clustered charge-to-alanine scanning mutagenesis, in which clusters of three or more charged residues in the primary amino acid sequence of a protein are all changed to alanine (105). In theory, charge clusters are likely to reside on the surface of the protein, where they may facilitate protein–protein interactions, and neutralization of the charge by replacement with alanine may weaken such interactions without seriously disrupting the three-dimensional conformation of the protein. In practice, as much as 30% of clustered charge-to-alanine scanning mutants prove to be temperature sensitive *in vivo*, and this mutagenesis technique has been successfully used to construct temperature-sensitive mutants of both picornaviruses and poxviruses (18,42). Last, conditionally lethal mutants have been constructed in poxviruses by placing essential genes under lactose operator–repressor control in the viral genome (85).

Viral Interference, Defective Interfering Particles

Interference refers generally to a phenomenon whereby infection by one virus results in inhibition of replication of another virus. Several distinct types of interference have been described (28), including direct heterologous interference, interferon-mediated heterologous interference, and defective interfering (DI) particle–mediated homologous interference. Direct heterologous interference describes a negative interaction between viruses of two different types, even different families, wherein viral gene products or alterations in the intracellular environment induced by one virus disrupt replication of another virus. The incompatibility of heterologous virus infections is not surprising, given the intricate interplay of virus and host functions in an infection, and the enormous variety of intracellular changes induced by different viruses. In interferon-mediated heterologous interference, discussed in detail in Chapter 12, infection by one virus induces interferon synthesis by the infected cell, and the interferon in turn induces an antiviral state in neighboring uninfected cells. DI particle–mediated homologous interference has been of particular interest to geneticists because of insights into the mechanisms of virus replication provided by defective interfering particles.

Defective interfering particle–mediated homologous interference was first described by von Magnus (103), who noted that serial undiluted passage of influenza virus resulted in a dramatic decrease in infectious titer, whereas the number of particles remained constant. Essentially the same phenomenon was subsequently observed in a wide variety of RNA and DNA animal viruses, and in both plant and bacterial viruses (49). The mechanism of interference in each case is similar: Virus stocks accumulate DI particles, which are virus particles that contain genomes that are grossly altered genetically, usually by significant deletion of essential functions, but that nevertheless retain critical replication origins and packaging signals, allowing for amplification and packaging in co-infections with complementing wild-type "helper" virus. DI particles usually display a replication advantage relative to wild-type virus, resulting from increases in the copy number or efficiency of replication origins. DI particles actively inhibit replication of wild-type virus, presumably by competing for limiting essential replication factors. Study of DI particles has provided significant insight into the viral replication, in particular structure and function of replication origins.

REFERENCES

1. Barkan A, Welch RC, Mertz JE. Missense mutations in the VP1 gene of simian virus 40 that compensate for defects caused by deletions in the viral agnogene. *J Virol* 1987;61:3190–3198.
2. Benjamin TL. Host-range mutants of polyoma virus. *Proc Natl Acad Sci U S A* 1970;67:394–401.
3. Beveridge WIB, Burnet FM. The cultivation of viruses and Rickettsiae in chick embryo. *Med Res Counc Spec Rep Ser (Lond)* 1946;256.
4. Blasco R, Moss B. Extracellular vaccinia virus formation and cell-to-cell virus transmission are prevented by deletion of the gene encoding the 37,000-dalton outer envelope protein. *J Virol* 1991;65: 5910–5920.
5. Cai W, Schaffer PA. Herpes simplex virus type 1 ICP0 regulates expression of immediate-early, early, and late genes in productively infected cells. *J Virol* 1992;66:2904–2915.
6. Chow LT, Broker TR. In vitro experimental systems for HPV: Epithelial raft cultures for investigations of viral reproduction and pathogenesis and for genetic analyses of viral proteins and regulatory sequences. *Clin Dermatol* 1997;15:217–227.
7. Chu CT, Schaffer PA. Qualitative complementation test for temperature-sensitive mutants of herpes simplex virus. *J Virol* 1975;16: 1131–1136.
8. Coen DM, Schaffer PA. Two distinct loci confer resistance to acycloguanosine in herpes simplex virus type 1. *Proc Natl Acad Sci U S A* 1980;77:2265–2269.
9. Coen DM, Weinheimer SP, McKnight SL. A genetic approach to promoter recognition during trans induction of viral gene expression. *Science* 1986;234:53–59.
10. Condit RC, Easterly R, Pacha RF, et al. A vaccinia virus isatin-beta-thiosemicarbazone resistance mutation maps in the viral gene encoding the 132-kDa subunit of RNA polymerase. *Virology* 1991;185: 857–861.
11. Condit RC, Motyczka A. Isolation and preliminary characterization of temperature-sensitive mutants of vaccinia virus. *Virology* 1981;113: 224–241.
12. Condit RC, Motyczka A, Spizz G. Isolation, characterization, and physical mapping of temperature-sensitive mutants of vaccinia virus. *Virology* 1983;128:429–443.
13. Condit RC, Xiang Y, Lewis JI. Mutation of vaccinia virus gene G2R causes suppression of gene A18R *ts* mutants: Implications for control of transcription. *Virology* 1996;220:10–19.
14. Cooper PD. Genetics of picornaviruses. In: Fraenkel-Conrat H, Wagner RR, eds. *Comprehensive Virology.* New York: Plenum Press, 1977: 133–207.
15. d'Herelle F. *The Bacteriophage and Its Behavior.* Baltimore: Williams & Wilkins, 1926.
16. Davis BD, Dulbecco R, Eisen HN, Ginsberg HS. *Microbiology*, 4th ed. Philadelphia: JB Lippincott, 1990.
17. DeLuca NA, McCarthy AM, Schaffer PA. Isolation and characterization of deletion mutants of herpes simplex virus type 1 in the gene encoding immediate-early regulatory protein ICP4. *J Virol* 1985;56:558–570.
18. Diamond SE, Kirkegaard K. Clustered charged-to-alanine mutagenesis of poliovirus RNA-dependent RNA polymerase yields multiple temperature-sensitive mutants defective in RNA synthesis. *J Virol* 1994;68:863–876.
19. Domingo E, Holland JJ, Biebricher C, Eigen M. Quasi-species: The concept and the word. In: Gibbs A, Calisher CH, Garcia-Arenal F, eds. *Molecular Basis of Virus Evolution.* Cambridge: Cambridge University Press, 1995:181–191.
20. Drake JW, Baltz RH. The biochemistry of mutagenesis. *Annu Rev Biochem* 1976;45:11–37.
21. Dubbs DR, Kit S. Isolation and properties of vaccinia mutants deficient in thymidine kinase inducing activity. *Virology* 1964;22: 214–225.
22. Dulbecco R, Vogt M. Some problems of animal virology as studied by the plaque technique. *Cold Spring Harb Symp Quant Biol* 1953;18: 273–279.
23. Dumbell KR, Downie AW, Valentine RC. The ratio of the number of virus particles to infective titer of cowpox and vaccinia virus suspensions. *Virology* 1957;4:467–482.
24. Ellis EL, Delbruck M. The growth of bacteriophage. *J Gen Physiol* 1939;22:365–384.
25. Falkner FG, Moss B. *Escherichia coli gpt* gene provides dominant selection for vaccinia virus open reading frame expression vectors. *J Virol* 1988;62:1849–1854.
26. Fathi Z, Sridhar P, Pacha RF, Condit RC. Efficient targeted insertion of an unselected marker into the vaccinia virus genome. *Virology* 1986;155:97–105.
27. Fenner F. The classification and nomenclature of viruses: Second report of the International Committee on Taxonomy of Viruses. *Intervirology* 1976;7:1–115.
28. Fenner F, McAuslan BR, Mims CA, et al. *The Biology of Animal Viruses.* New York: Academic Press, 1974.
29. Fields BN, Knipe DM, Chanock RM, et al. *Fields Virology*, 2nd ed. New York: Raven Press, 1990.
30. Fields BN, Knipe DM, Chanock RM, et al. *Fields Virology*, 1st ed. New York: Raven Press, 1985.
31. Fields BN, Knipe DM, Howley PM, et al. *Fields Virology*, 3rd ed. Philadelphia: Lippincott-Raven, 1996.
32. Fraenkel-Conrat H, Wagner RR. *Comprehensive Virology.* New York: Plenum Press, 1977.
33. Francki RIB, Fauquet CM, Knudson DL, Brown F. *The Classification and Nomenclature of Viruses: Fifth Report of the International Committee on Taxonomy of Viruses.* Vienna: Springer-Verlag, 1991.
34. Fredrickson TN, Sechler JM, Palumbo GJ, et al. Acute inflammatory response to cowpox virus infection of the chorioallantoic membrane of the chick embryo. *Virology* 1992;187:693–704.
35. Freshney RI. *Culture of Animal Cells*, 3rd ed. New York: Wiley-Liss, 1994.
36. Frost E, Williams J. Mapping temperature-sensitive and host-range mutations of adenovirus type 5 by marker rescue. *Virology* 1978;91: 39–50.
37. Gerhard W, Webster RG. Antigenic drift in influenza A viruses. I. Selection and characterization of antigenic variants of A/PR/8/34 (HON1) influenza virus with monoclonal antibodies. *J Exp Med* 1978;148:383–392.
38. Goodpasture EW, Woodruff AM, Buddingh GJ. Vaccinal infection of the chorio-allantoic membrane of the chick embryo. *Am J Pathol* 1932;8:271–281.
39. Hahn CS, Lustig S, Strauss EG, Strauss JH. Western equine encephalitis virus is a recombinant virus. *Proc Natl Acad Sci U S A* 1988;85:5997–6001.
40. Hartley JW, Rowe WP. Production of altered cell foci in tissue culture by defective Maloney sarcoma virus particles. *Proc Natl Acad Sci U S A* 1966;55:780–786.
41. Hassett DE, Condit RC. Targeted construction of temperature-sensitive mutations in vaccinia virus by replacing clustered charged residues with alanine. *Proc Natl Acad Sci U S A* 1994;91:4554–4558.
42. Hassett DE, Lewis JI, Xing X, et al. Analysis of a temperature-sensitive vaccinia virus mutant in the viral mRNA capping enzyme isolated

by clustered charge-to-alanine mutagenesis and transient dominant selection. *Virology* 1997;238:391–409.
43. Hay AJ, Wolstenholme AJ, Skehel JJ, Smith MH. The molecular basis of the specific anti-influenza action of amantadine. *EMBO J* 1985;4: 3021–3024.
44. Hay J, Subak-Sharpe JH. Mutants of herpes simplex virus types 1 and 2 that are resistant to phosphonoacetic acid induce altered DNA polymerase activities in infected cells. *J Gen Virol* 1976;31: 145–148.
45. Hayflick L, Moorhead PS. The serial cultivation of human diploid cell strains. *Exp Cell Res* 1961;25:585–621.
46. Hershey AD. Spontaneous mutations in bacterial viruses. *Cold Spring Harb Symp Quant Biol* 1946;11:67.
47. Holland TC, Sandri-Goldin RM, Holland LE, et al. Physical mapping of the mutation in an antigenic variant of herpes simplex virus type 1 by use of an immunoreactive plaque assay. *J Virol* 1983;46:649–652.
48. Hu WS, Temin HM. Effect of gamma radiation on retroviral recombination. *J Virol* 1992;66:4457–4463.
49. Huang AS, Baltimore D. Defective interfering animal viruses. In: Fraenkel-Conrat H, Wagner RR, eds. *Comprehensive Virology.* New York: Plenum Press, 1977:73–116.
50. Joklik WK, Willett HP, Amos DB, Wilfret CM. *Zinsser Microbiology*, 20th ed. Norwalk, CT: Appleton & Lange, 1992.
51. Jones ME, Thomas SM, Rogers A. Luria-Delbruck fluctuation experiments: Design and analysis. *Genetics* 1994;136:1209–1216.
52. Kaiser AD. Mutations in a temperate bacteriophage affecting its ability to lysogenize *E. coli. Virology* 1957;3:42.
53. Karber G. Beitrag zur kollektiven Behandlung pharmakologischer Reihenversuche. *Arch Exp Path Pharmak* 1931;162:480–483.
54. Keck JG, Stohlman SA, Soe LH, et al. Multiple recombination sites at the 5′-end of murine coronavirus RNA. *Virology* 1987;156:331–341.
55. Kirkegaard K, Baltimore D. The mechanism of RNA recombination in poliovirus. *Cell* 1986;47:433–443.
56. Kjellen LE. A variant of adenovirus type 5. *Arch Ges Virusforsch* 1963;13:482–488.
57. Kuchler RJ. *Biochemical Methods in Cell Culture and Virology.* Stroudsburg, PA: Dowden, Hutchingon & Ross, 1977.
58. Lai CJ, Nathans D. Mapping temperature-sensitive mutants of simian virus 40: Rescue of mutants by fragments of viral DNA. *Virology* 1974;60:466–475.
59. Luria SE. The frequency distribution of spontaneous bacteripohage mutants as evidence for the exponential rate of phage reproduction. *Cold Spring Harb Symp Quant Biol* 1951;16:463–470.
60. Luria SE, Darnell JE, Baltimore D, Campbell A. *General Virology*, 3rd ed. New York: John Wiley & Sons, 1978.
61. Luria SE, Delbruck M. Mutations of bacteria from virus sensitivity to virus resistance. *Genetics* 1943;28:491–511.
62. Luria SE, Williams RC, Backus RC. Electron micrographic counts of bacteriophage particles. *J Bacteriol* 1951;61:179–188.
63. Lwoff A, Horne R, Tournier P. A system of viruses. *Cold Spring Harb Symp Quant Biol* 1962;27:51–55.
64. Mackett M, Smith GL, Moss B. Vaccinia virus: A selectable eukaryotic cloning and expression vector. *Proc Natl Acad Sci U S A* 1982;79: 7415–7419.
65. Mahy BWJ, Kangro HO. *Virology Methods Manual.* San Diego: Academic Press, 1996.
66. Margulis L. *Five Kingdoms: An Illustrated Guide to the Phyla of Life on Earth*, 3rd ed. New York: WH Freeman, 1998.
67. Matsumoto S. Rabies virus. *Adv Virus Res* 1970;16:257–302.
68. Matthews REF. Classification and nomenclature of viruses: Third report of the International Committee on Taxonomy of Viruses. *Intervirology* 1979;12:132–296.
69. Matthews REF. Classification and nomenclature of viruses: Fourth report of the International Committee on Taxonomy of Viruses. *Intervirology* 1982;17:1–199.
70. Meis RJ, Condit RC. Genetic and molecular biological characterization of a vaccinia virus gene which renders the virus dependent on isatin-beta-thiosemicarbazone (IBT). *Virology* 1991;182:442–454.
71. Miller LK, Fried M. Construction of the genetic map of the polyoma genome. *J Virol* 1976;18:824–832.
72. Murphy FA. Virus taxonomy. In: Fields BN, Knipe DM, Howley PM, et al., eds. *Fields Virology*, 3rd ed. Philadelphia: Lippincott-Raven, 1996:15–57.
73. Murphy FA, Fauquet CM, Bishop DHL, et al. *Virus Taxonomy: The Classification and Nomenclature of Viruses. The Sixth Report of the International Committee on Taxonomy of Viruses.* Vienna: Springer-Verlag, 1995.
74. Panicali D, Paoletti E. Construction of poxviruses as cloning vectors: Insertion of the thymidine kinase gene from herpes simplex virus into the DNA of infectious vaccinia virus. *Proc Natl Acad Sci U S A* 1982;79:4927–4931.
75. Perkus ME, Goebel SJ, Davis SW, et al. Deletion of 55 open reading frames from the termini of vaccinia virus. *Virology* 1991;180: 406–410.
76. Pfefferkorn ER. Genetics of togaviruses. In: Fraenkel-Conrat H, Wagner RR, eds. *Comprehensive Virology.* New York: Plenum Press, 1977: 209–238.
77. Pickup DJ, Ink BS, Hu W, et al. Hemorrhage in lesions caused by cowpox virus is induced by a viral protein that is related to plasma protein inhibitors of serine proteases. *Proc Natl Acad Sci U S A* 1986;83: 7698–7702.
78. Pincus SE, Diamond DC, Emini EA, Wimmer E. Guanidine-selected mutants of poliovirus: Mapping of point mutations to polypeptide 2C. *J Virol* 1986;57:638–646.
79. Pincus SE, Rohl H, Wimmer E. Guanidine-dependent mutants of poliovirus: Identification of three classes with different growth requirements. *Virology* 1987;157:83–88.
80. Pinto LH, Holsinger LJ, Lamb RA. Influenza virus M2 protein has ion channel activity. *Cell* 1992;69:517–528.
81. Pleschka S, Jaskunas R, Engelhardt OG, et al. A plasmid-based reverse genetics system for influenza A virus. *J Virol* 1996;70: 4188–4192.
82. Ramig RF, Fields BN. Genetics of reoviruses. In: Joklik WK, ed. *The Reoviridae.* New York: Plenum Press, 1983:197–228.
83. Reed LJ, Muench H. A simple method for estimating 50% endpoints. *Am J Hyg* 1932;27:493–497.
84. Roberts A, Rose JK. Recovery of negative-strand RNA viruses from plasmid DNAs: A positive approach revitalizes a negative field. *Virology* 1998;247:1–6.
85. Rodriguez JF, Smith GL. Inducible gene expression from vaccinia virus vectors. *Virology* 1990;177:239–250.
86. Roizman B. Polykaryosis: Results from fusion of nononucleated cells. *Cold Spring Harb Symp Quant Biol* 1962;27:327–342.
87. Rowe WP, Huebner RJ, Gilmore LK, et al. Isolation of a cytopathogenic agent from human adenoids undergoing spontaneous degeneration in tissue culture. *Proc Soc Exp Biol Med* 1953;84:570–573.
88. Schnipper LE, Crumpacker CS. Resistance of herpes simplex virus to acycloguanosine: Role of viral thymidine kinase and DNA polymerase loci. *Proc Natl Acad Sci U S A* 1980;77:2270–2273.
89. Sedivy JM, Capone JP, RajBhandary UL, Sharp PA. An inducible mammalian amber suppressor: Propagation of a poliovirus mutant. *Cell* 1987;50:379–389.
90. Shelokov A, Vogel JE, Chi L. Hemadsorbtion (adsorbtion-hemagglutination) test for viral agents in tissue culture with special reference to influenza. *Proc Soc Exp Biol Med* 1958;97:802–809.
91. Simpson RW, Hirst GK. Temperature-sensitive mutants of influenza A virus: Isolation of mutants and preliminary observations on genetic recombination and complementation. *Virology* 1968;35:41–49.
92. Spearman C. The method of right and wrong cases (constant stimuli) without Gauss's formulae. *Br J Psychol* 1908;2:227–242.
93. Sridhar P, Condit RC. Selection for temperature-sensitive mutations in specific vaccinia virus genes: Isolation and characterization of a virus mutant which encodes a phosphonoacetic acid-resistant, temperature-sensitive DNA polymerase. *Virology* 1983;128:444–457.
94. Stoker MGP, Macpherson I. Transformation assays. In: Maramorosch K, Koprowski H, eds. *Methods in Virology.* New York: Academic Press, 1967:313–336.
95. Stow ND, Subak-Sharpe JH, Wilkie NM. Physical mapping of herpes simplex virus type 1 mutations by marker rescue. *J Virol* 1978;28: 182–192.
96. Studier FW. The genetics and physiology of bacteriophage T7. *Virology* 1969;39:562–574.

97. Summers WP, Wagner M, Summers WC. Possible peptide chain termination mutants in thymide kinase gene of a mammalian virus, herpes simplex virus. *Proc Natl Acad Sci U S A* 1975;72:4081–4084.
98. Sweet BH, Hilleman MR. The vacuolating virus SV40. *Proc Soc Exp Biol Med* 1960;105:420–427.
99. Thompson CL, Condit RC. Marker rescue mapping of vaccinia virus temperature-sensitive mutants using overlapping cosmid clones representing the entire virus genome. *Virology* 1986;150:10–20.
100. Van-Regenmortel MH. Virus species, a much overlooked but essential concept in virus classification. *Intervirology* 1990;31:241–254.
101. Van-Regenmortel MH, Fauquet CM, Bishop CM, et al. *Virus Taxonomy: The Seventh Report of the International Committee on Taxonomy of Viruses.* San Diego: Academic Press, 2000.
102. Vogt PK. Focus assay of Rous sarcoma virus. In: Habel K, Salzman NP, eds. *Fundamental Techniques in Virology.* New York: Academic Press, 1969:198–211.
103. Von Magnus P. Incomplete forms of influenza virus. *Adv Virus Res* 1954;2:59–78.
104. Watson DH, Russell WC, Wildy P. Electron microscopic particle counts on herpes virus using phosphotungstate staining technique. *Virology* 1963;19:250–260.
105. Wertman KF, Drubin DG, Botstein D. Systematic mutational analysis of the yeast ACT1 gene. *Genetics* 1992;132:337–350.
106. Wildy P. Classification and nomenclature of viruses: First report of the International Committee on Taxonomy of Viruses. *Monogr Virol* 1971;5:1–181.
107. Yu D, Sheaffer AK, Tenney DJ, Weller SK. Characterization of ICP6::lacZ insertion mutants of the UL15 gene of herpes simplex virus type 1 reveals the translation of two proteins. *J Virol* 1997;71:2656–2665.
108. Yu MH, King J. Surface amino acids as sites of temperature-sensitive folding mutations in the P22 tailspike protein. *J Biol Chem* 1988;263:1424–1431.
109. Zwillinger D. *CRC Standard Mathematical Tables and Formulae*, 30th ed. Boca Raton: CRC Press, 1996.

CHAPTER 3

Principles of Virus Structure

Stephen C. Harrison

Virus particles have evolved to transfer genetic material between cells and to encode information sufficient to ensure their own continued propagation. They are, in effect, extracellular organelles. They contain most or all of the molecular machinery necessary for efficient and specific packaging of viral genomes, escape from an infected cell, survival of transfer to a new host cell, attachment, penetration, and initiation of a new replication cycle. In many cases, the molecular machinery works in part by subverting more elaborate elements of the host cell apparatus for carrying out related processes. The principles of virus structure thus arise from the requirements imposed by the functions just outlined on the evolution of viral molecular architecture.

What are these requirements? One of the simplest and most general is the formation of a closed shell to protect viral nucleic acid during its passage from one cell to another. A second is one of genetic economy: the information necessary to specify the structural proteins must not exhaust the coding capacity of the viral genome. A third is the embodiment of specific strategies for exit and entry. The principles of protein folding and assembly, the sources of specificity in protein–protein interactions, and the possibilities for triggered conformational changes have determined what sorts of structures are observed. Indeed, much of our appreciation of these principles and possibilities has come from the study of viruses because they are among the simplest and most accessible of macromolecular machines.

Viruses come in many shapes and sizes. The broadest distinction is between the so-called enveloped and nonenveloped viruses, that is, those that contain or do not contain, respectively, a lipid-bilayer membrane. Most enveloped viruses acquire their envelope by budding through a membrane of the host cell into some extracytoplasmic compartment—either through the plasma membrane itself or through a membrane of the endoplasmic reticulum (ER) or Golgi apparatus. This last step in viral assembly is thus also an important part of the mechanism by which the virus escapes from an infected cell. Enveloped viruses then enter another host cell by fusion of their membrane with a membrane of the cell being infected. Again, this can be either the plasma membrane or the membrane of an internal compartment, such as an endosome. Nonenveloped viruses generally escape by lysis of the cell in which they have propagated, and their mechanism of entry is still incompletely understood.

Further categorization of virus structures depends on details of their molecular organization. The progress made recently in understanding viral architecture in atomic detail now allows us a glimpse of underlying similarities across various families of viruses, and the final section of this chapter attempts to develop some of those categories. We need first, however, to outline how virus structures are studied and to introduce the language needed to describe them. Integrated into this introduction is a synopsis of the principles of virus assembly and a discussion of how observed structural similarities relate to functional homologies in viral entry.

HOW VIRUS STRUCTURES ARE STUDIED

Electron microscopy is the most useful way to determine the general morphology of a virus particle. For examining infected cells and larger, isolated particles, the traditional thin-sectioning methods are used. The thickness of a section and the coarseness of staining methods limit resolution to about 50 to 75 Å, even in the best cases. (*Resolution* means the approximate minimal size of a substructure that can be detected or separated in an image from its neighbor. Recall that one atomic diameter is 2–3 Å; an α-helix, 10 Å; and a DNA double helix, 20 Å.) Negative staining, with uranyl acetate, potassium phosphotungstate, or related electron-dense compounds, gives somewhat more detailed images of isolated and purified virus particles. Viruses embedded in negative stain are often relatively well preserved. The electron beam destroys the particle itself very rapidly, but it leaves the dense "cast" of stain undamaged for much longer. If the particle is fully covered by the negative stain, the image contains contrast from both the upper and the lower surface of the particle, and visual interpretation of finer aspects of the image can be difficult (34).

Recently, methods for preserving viruses and other macromolecular assemblies by rapid freezing to liquid nitrogen or liquid helium temperatures have permitted visualization of electron-scattering contrast from the structures in the particle itself and not just from the cast created by a surrounding of negative stain (3). Moreover, quantitative methods for image analysis, originally developed for studying negatively stained particles, have been applied effectively to such images (3,34). Thus, a three-dimensional reconstruction of the electron-scattering density in a hepatitis B virus capsid has been computed to 7 Å resolution, permitting a tracing of the polypeptide chain later verified by x-ray crystallography at much higher resolution (14,115). An advantage of such cryoelectron microscopy is that regular images can be selected from a heterogeneous field, allowing study of unstable or relatively impure preparations. A gallery of cryoelectron microscopy images is shown in Figure 1.

The detail obtained from even the most elegant of electron microscopy methods still falls short of what is required to understand molecular interactions. A higher-resolution picture can be obtained by x-ray diffraction methods, if single crystals of the relevant structure can be prepared. It has been known since the 1930s that simple plant viruses, such as tomato bushy stunt virus (TBSV), can be crystallized (8), and the first x-ray studies of such crystals were carried out as early as 1938 (11). Crystallization of poliovirus and other important animal viruses showed that the approach could be extended to human pathogens (95). The first complete high-resolution structure of a crystalline virus was obtained from TBSV in 1978 (61), and since then, the structures of a number of animal, plant, and insect pathogens have been determined. Only very regular structures can form single crystals; to study the molecular details of larger and more complex virus particles, it is necessary to dissect them into well-defined subunits or substructures. This dissection was originally done with proteases, by disassembly, or by isolation of substructures from infected cells. For example, the structure of the influenza virus hemagglutinin (114)—the first viral glycoprotein for which atomic details were visualized—was obtained from crystals of protein cleaved from the surface of purified virions (113); the structure of the adenovirus hexon was obtained from excess unassembled protein derived from adenovirus-infected cells (86). Recently, this dissection has more commonly been carried out using recombinant expression (e.g., of a fragment of gp120 from human immunodeficiency virus type 1 [HIV-1]) (65).

VIRUSES AS MOLECULAR PACKAGES

The simplest sort of package is a shell that can assemble spontaneously from a single component. The observation that certain viruses, particularly tobacco mosaic virus (TMV), assemble *in vitro* from dissociated components led Crick and Watson (33) to propose that virus shells would be highly symmetric objects. The arguments behind this proposal were simple: genetic efficiency requires that the viral coat be composed of many identical subunits, and experimentally observed self-assembly requires that the interactions among these subunits be specific and well defined. Identical subunits with specific interactions in general produce symmetric structures.

What is meant by *symmetric*? The rigorous definition of symmetry involves an operation, such as a rotation, that brings an object into self-coincidence. For example, if the ring of three commas in Figure 2 is rotated by 120 or 240 degrees, it will not be possible to recognize that a rotation has occurred (assuming that the commas are truly indistinguishable). The full symmetry of an object is defined by the collection of such operations that apply to it. In the case of protein assemblies, these operations can be rotations, translations, or combinations of the two. A symmetry axis that includes rotation by 180 degrees is called a *twofold axis* or a *dyad*; one with a 120-degree rotation (and, of course, a 240-degree rotation as well) is called a *threefold axis*; and so forth. Note the distinction between shape and symmetry: the *shape* of an object refers to the geometry of its outline, whereas its *symmetry* refers to the operations that describe it. The set of commas in Figure 2 has threefold symmetry; so does an

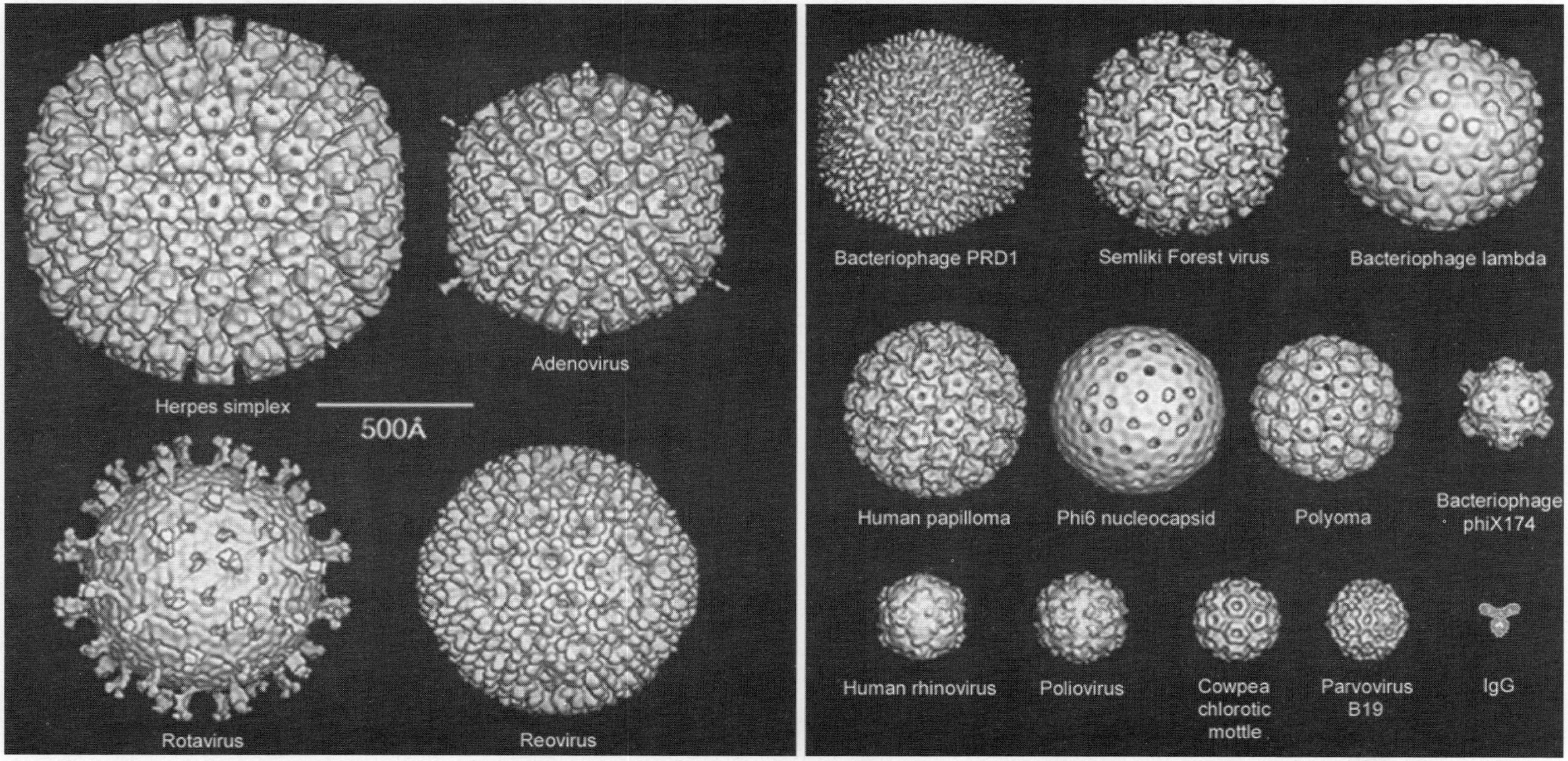

FIG. 1. A gallery of image reconstructions from cryoelectron microscopy of icosahedrally symmetric virus particles. The images illustrate the variety of sizes and specializations, even in these highly regular structures. The particles are labeled; the herpes simplex image is the nucleocapsid only. The image of an immunoglobulin molecule (IgG) is included on the same scale as the virus images, for direct comparison. The scale bar corresponds to 500 Å. (Modified from ref. 3, with permission.)

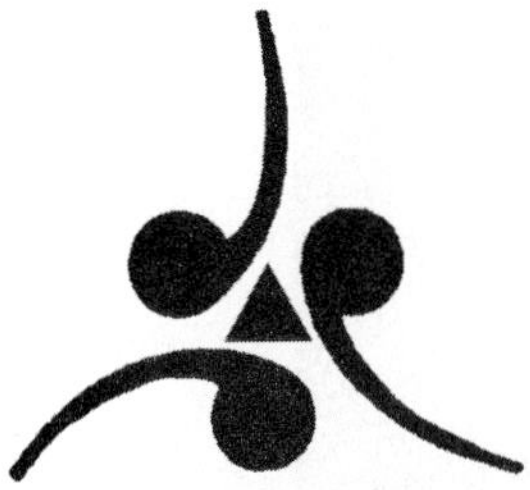

FIG. 2. Three commas, arranged with threefold symmetry. The threefold rotation axis passes through the solid triangle in the center of the diagram.

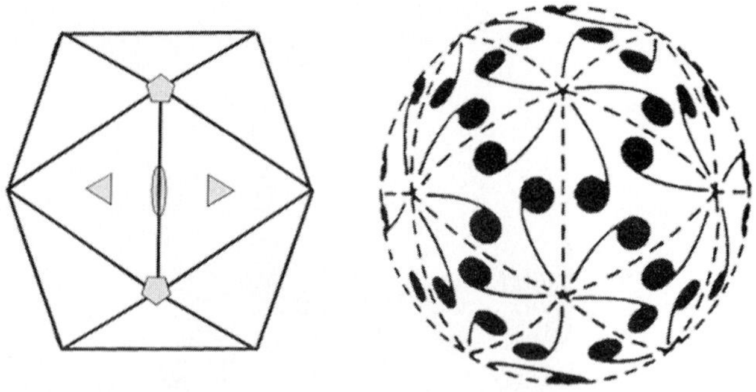

FIG. 3. *Left:* Outline of an icosahedron, showing some of the symmetry axes. Fivefold axes (*vertices*) are represented by pentagons; threefold axes (*faces*) by triangles; twofold axes (*edges*) by ovals. *Right:* 60 commas, distributed with icosahedral symmetry on the surface of a sphere. The *dashed lines* correspond to the edges of an icosahedron, projected onto the spherical surface.

equilateral triangle, the beer-company symbol with interlocked rings, and countless other objects with unrelated shapes.

Closed shells composed of identical subunits that interact through conserved, specific interfaces and that have a more or less spherical outline can have one of only three symmetries: the symmetry of the regular tetrahedron, the cube, or the regular icosahedron. These shells accommodate 12, 24, or 60 subunits, respectively. The icosahedral shells are obviously the most efficient of the three designs: they use the largest number of subunits to make a container of a given size, and hence they use subunits of the smallest size and the smallest coding requirement. Indeed, many of the viruses of interest to medical virologists contain at least some element with an icosahedrally symmetric shell, and the tetrahedral and cubic symmetries have not appeared in any normal virus assembly. We therefore describe icosahedral symmetry in some detail. Again, note the distinction between icosahedral symmetry and icosahedral shape. Not all objects with icosahedral symmetry have even the vague outline of an icosahedron; conversely, painting a single asymmetric object, like a comma, on each face of an icosahedron, rather than three such objects related by a threefold axis, would destroy the symmetry of the decorated object but would not affect its shape.

Icosahedral Shells

Icosahedral Symmetry

The diagram in Figure 3 shows the operations that belong to an icosahedrally symmetric object. They are a collection of twofold, threefold, and fivefold rotation axes. Placement of a single, asymmetric object on a surface governed by this symmetry leads to the generation of 59 others, when the various rotations are applied. One such object, one sixtieth of the total shell, can therefore be designated as an *icosahedral asymmetric unit,* the fundamental piece of structure from which all the rest can be produced by the operations of icosahedral symmetry. With a typical, compact protein domain of 250 to 300 amino acid residues, close to the upper limit for most single protein domains, what sort of container can we construct? Suppose that the protein is so constructed that 60 copies fit together into a 30 Å thick shell with no significant gaps. The cavity within that shell will then have a radius of about 80 Å, which can contain a 3-kb piece of single-stranded DNA or RNA (ssDNA or ssRNA, respectively), tightly condensed. A few, very simple virus particles indeed conform to this description. The parvoviruses (see Chapter 32) contain a 5.3-kb ssDNA genome, and their shells contain 60 copies of a protein of about 520 residues (Fig. 4). The capsid protein therefore uses up about one third of the genome. (*Capsid,* from the Latin *capsa,* for box, is used to describe the protein shell that directly packages DNA or RNA; *nucleocapsid* is sometimes used to refer to the shell plus its nucleic acid contents.) Likewise, the satellite of tobacco necrosis virus (STNV) contains 60 copies of a 195-residue subunit and a 1120 ssRNA genome, of which over half is used for the coat protein (68). As the name implies, however, STNV is actually a defective virus, and it requires tobacco necrosis virus co-infection to propagate.

There are various ways in which viruses have evolved to produce larger icosahedral shells and thus to package larger genomes. The simplest is just to use several different subunits, each of "garden-variety" size, to make up one icosahedral asymmetric unit. The picornaviruses (e.g., polioviruses, rhinoviruses) have 60 copies of three distinct proteins, VP1, VP2, and VP3, each of between 230 and 300 amino acid residues, as well as 60 copies of a small internal peptide, VP4 (Fig. 5; see Chapter 18). The shell has a cavity about 95 Å in diameter, which contains an RNA genome of 7.5 to 8 kb. The picornaviruses thus expend about one third of their genome to encode the structural proteins of the virion. (*Virion* is used interchangeably with *complete virus particle.*) We note here two other important features of picornavirus molecular

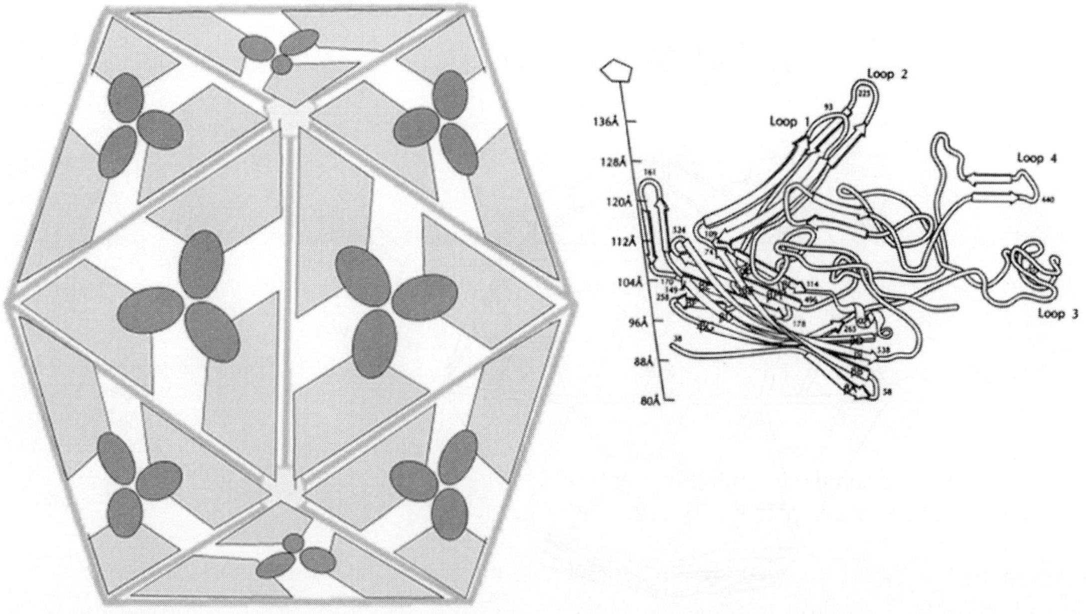

FIG. 4. *Left:* Diagram of the packing of 60 protein subunits in the shell of a parvovirus. The *trapezoids* represent a jelly-roll β-barrel domain (see Fig. 5) that forms the core of each subunit, and the *ovals* represent loops, emanating from the jelly-roll domain, which form contacts about the threefold axes. *Right:* Ribbon diagram of the folded subunit of canine parvovirus, viewed perpendicular to the fivefold and twofold axes, that is, as if viewing from the "southeast" the subunit that is just to the lower right of center in the larger packing diagram. The position and orientation of a fivefold axis, with respect to the subunit, are shown by the line with a fivefold symbol at its end. The jelly-roll β-barrel is at the *lower left* of this ribbon diagram, and the loops extend into the page toward the *upper right.* (From ref. 101, with permission.)

architecture. First, the folded structures of VP1, VP2, and VP3 are all based on the same kernel—a domain known as a *jelly-roll β-barrel* (see Fig. 5). This is the same fold that is found in the single subunits of the parvoviruses and of STNV. It is a module particularly well suited to the formation of closed, spherical shells, because of its blocklike, trapezoidal outline, but its prevalence among viral subunits may be evidence of a deeper evolutionary relationship. A second noteworthy feature of picornavirus design is the use of armlike extensions of the subunits for tying together the assembled particle (see Fig. 5). The importance of scaffold-like intertwining of subunit arms was first discovered in the simple plant viruses (61). In effect, folding of part of the subunit and assembly of the shell are concerted processes.

Quasi-Equivalence

A conceptually more complex, but evolutionarily simpler and more economical, way to build a shell of more than 60 average-sized subunits was described by Caspar and Klug in 1961 (23). It is illustrated by the diagram of 180 commas in Figure 6. The commas have similar interactions (head to head in pairs; neck to neck in rings of three; tail to tail in rings of five or six), but they fall into three sets, designated *A, B,* and *C.* If the commas are taken to represent proteins, the conformational differences between A and B positions, for example, involve the differences between rings of five and rings of six, for contacts involving the parts of the proteins symbolized by the tails. Caspar and Klug (23) postulated that protein subunits might have the sort of flexibility or capacity for conformational switching needed to accommodate in this way, and that viruses with more than 60 chemically and genetically identical subunits might exhibit the sort of near equivalence seen in the A, B, and C conformers in the comma illustration. Caspar and King (23) called this sort of local distortability, which might conserve the specificity and character of protein contacts, "quasi-equivalence."

Quasi-equivalent designs are exemplified by a number of plant and animal viruses, such as TBSV (61) and Norwalk virus (78), as illustrated in Figures 7 to 9. In TBSV and Norwalk virus, there are 180 genetically and chemically identical subunits that compose the capsid. The subunits are actually larger than those of the picornaviruses, but most of the extra size comes from a second, projecting domain that serves functions other than the construction of a closed shell. The size of the *shell domain* (S domain) in both cases is just about 200 residues, and the folded structure of the domain is again a jelly-roll β-barrel. The important feature of the packing of these 180 S domains is illustrated by the TBSV diagram in Figure 8. The contents of an icosahedral asymmetric unit can be

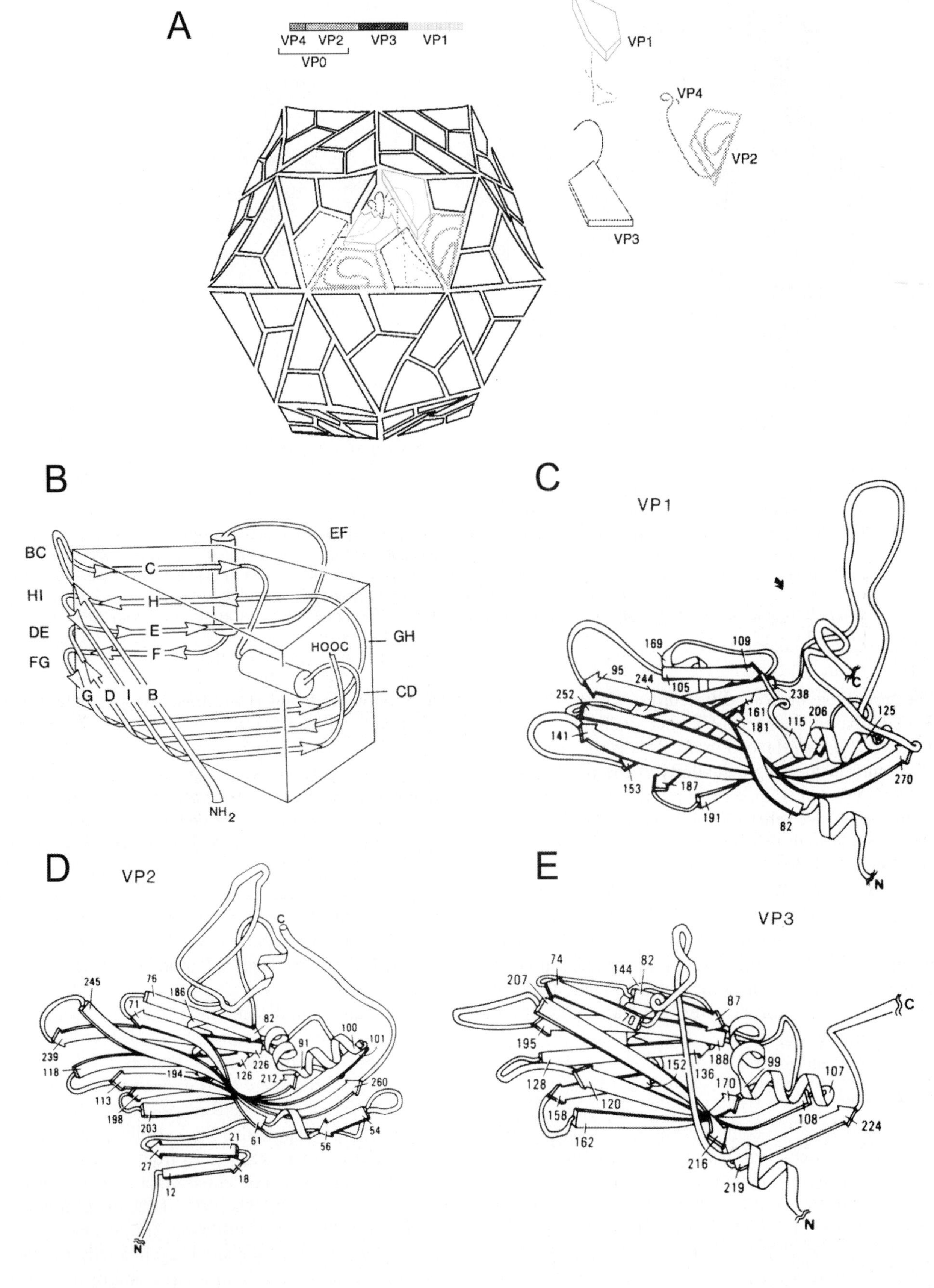
A
VP4 VP2
VP3
VP1
VP0
VP1
VP4
VP2
VP3
B
BC
HI
DE
FG
C
H
E
F
G D I B
EF
GH
HOOC
CD
NH2
C
VP1
169
109
95
244
105
252
238
161
181
115
206
125
141
153
187
191
82
270
C
N
D
VP2
245
76
186
71
82
100
101
91
239
118
226
126
212
194
260
113
198
203
61
56
54
21
27
18
12
C
N
E
VP3
74
82
144
207
87
70
C
195
152
188
99
136
170
107
128
120
158
162
108
224
216
219
N

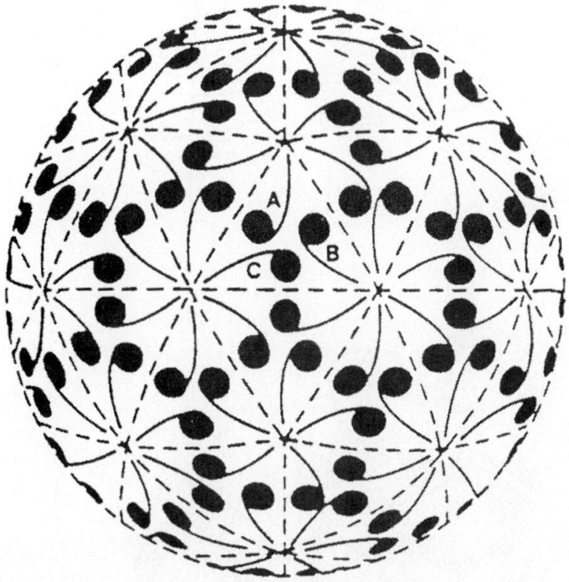

FIG. 6. Quasi-equivalent arrangement of 180 commas, in a T=3 icosahedral surface lattice on a sphere. Compare Figure 3 (*right*), a T=1 arrangement of 60 commas with icosahedral axes oriented similarly.

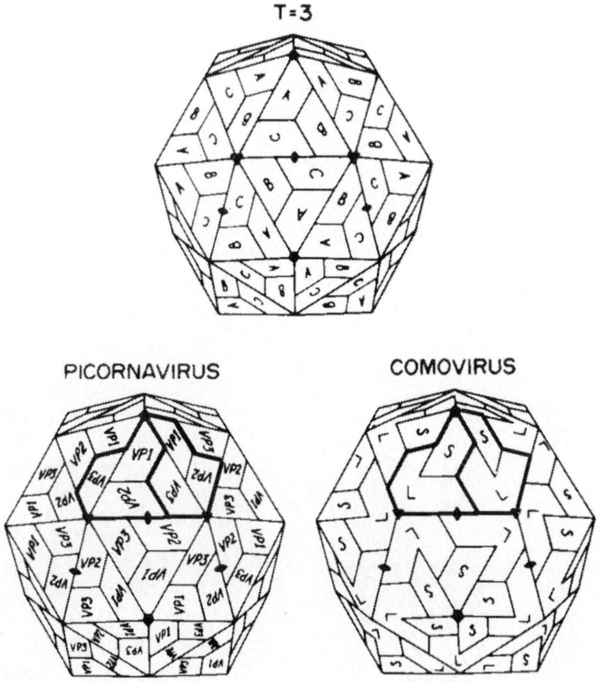

FIG. 7. Comparison of the packing of the jelly-roll β-barrel domains in T=3 plant and insect viruses; vertebrate picornaviruses; and plant comoviruses. In T=3 structures, the A, B and C subunits are chemically identical. In picornaviruses, VP1, VP2, and VP3 are different, but similar in the way the polypeptide chains folds (see Fig. 5). In comoviruses, the large subunit contains two β-barrel domains, in positions corresponding respectively to C and B in T=3 structures or to VP2 and VP3 in picornaviruses, and the small subunit contains one such domain, in a position corresponding to A or VP1. The diagrams are oriented (with respect to the icosahedral axes) like in Figs. 3 and 5**A**, but tilted slightly upward. The trapezoidal outlines represent subunits; the lettering or numbering on the subunits is oriented to show the rotational relationships among them. The small, solid symbols represent symmetry axes as defined in Figure 3. The heavy outlines in the lower two diagrams surround two protomers, related to each other by the fivefold axes toward the top of the diagrams. In Figure 5**A**, these are the protomers for which the N-terminal extensions of the subunits and VP4 are shown. The protomer on the right in the picornavirus diagram is the one shown in the "exploded" view on the upper right of Figure 5**A**. (Courtesy of J. Johnson.)

described as three chemically identical subunits, with somewhat different conformations. These conformers are denoted A, B, and C, echoing the designation of commas in Figure 6. The differences among the conformers reside principally in an ordered or disordered conformation for part of the N-terminal arm and in the angle of the hinge between the S domain and the *projecting domain* (P domain). The A and B conformations are nearly identical, with disordered arms and similar hinge angles. The C conformation has an ordered arm and a different hinge angle from A and B. The ordered arms extend along the base of the S domain and intertwine with two others around the icosahedral threefold axis. Thus, the whole collection of 60 C-subunit arms forms a coherent inner scaffold.

FIG. 5. Organization of the protein shell of picornaviruses. **A:** Subunit packing. *Upper left:* The order of domains in the precursor polypeptide chain. The cleavages between VP0 and VP3 and between VPP3 and VP1 are performed by a viral protease; the cleavage of VP0 to VP2 and VP4 is autolytic. Each subunit contains a jelly-roll β-barrel (*trapezoidal solid*), with highly variable loops and long N- and C-terminal extensions (*curved lines*). Two protomers (VP1, VP2, VP3, and V4) are shown in more detail in the center of the diagram. Distinct line qualities are used for each type of subunit. The diagram on the right is an "exploded view" of the right-hand protomer in the packing diagram. **B:** Schematic diagram of the folding of a polypeptide chain into a jelly-roll β-barrel. The strands are lettered in the order of their sequence in the chain. Strands B, I, D, and G form one sheet; C, H, E, and F, the other. The interstrand loops are designated BC, CD, etc. In picornaviruses and T=3 plant viruses, there are usually α-helices in the positions, shown as a cylinders. **C** to **E:** Ribbon diagrams of the jelly-roll cores of VP1 to VP3 of poliovirus. The numerals show residue numbers in each chain. Note how the loops give each subunit distinct characteristics. There is no evident sequence similarity, despite the similarity of fold. The small, curved arrow in C points to the entrance of a hydrophobic channel in the β-barrel, where various antipicornaviral drugs bind, blocking one or more steps in viral entry.

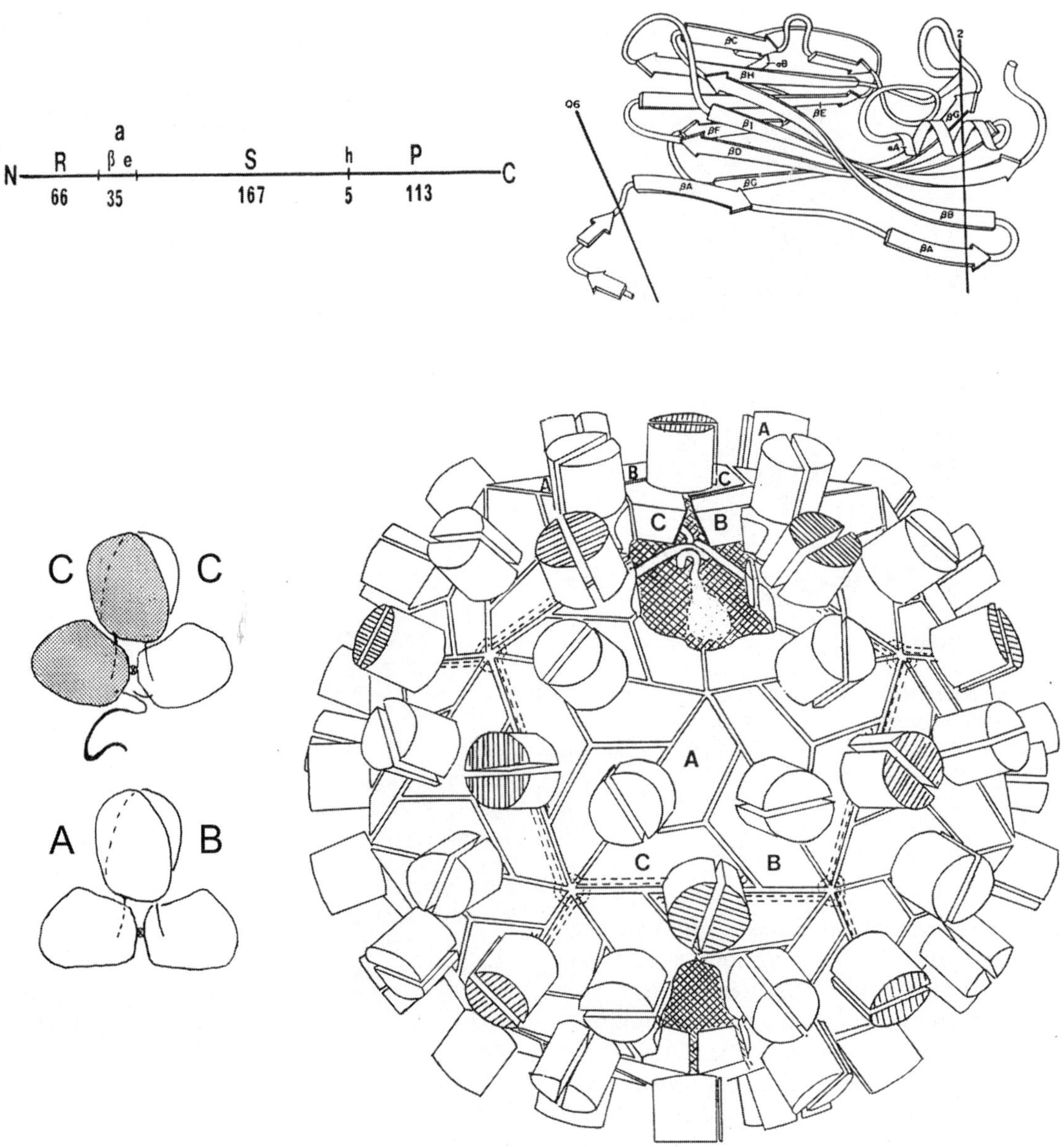

FIG. 8. Molecular architecture of tomato bushy stunt virus (TBSV), illustrating some of the principles of domain organization and quasi-equivalent interaction described in the text. TBSV is an icosahedrally symmetric, RNA-containing particle with 180 identical subunits. The 40-kd coat protein is organized into four regions: a positively charged, N-terminal R-segment; a connecting arm (*a*), and two compactly folded domains—*S* (shell) and *P* (projecting). There is a hinge (*h*) between the S and P domains. The relationship of the domains and connecting segments to the sequence (N- to C-terminus) is shown at the *upper left.* A ribbon diagram of the S domain is shown in the *upper right,* in an orientation corresponding to the similar diagrams in Figures 4 and 5. Note how closely related are the folds of the β-barrels in all the subunits illustrated in these figures. The R segment of TBSV is probably irregularly folded in the particle interior; it interacts with viral RNA. By analogy with work on alfalfa mosaic virus (see text), a short piece of the R segment might be recognized by the RNA packaging signal, but this interaction has not been defined for TBSV. The arm is folded against the S domain on 60 of the subunits (those in positions symmetrically related to *C*), but it extends inward in a more disordered way on the remaining 120 (positions equivalent to *A* and *B*). The folded arms form an internal framework (*dashed lines* in full-particle diagram), with three arms meeting and interdigitating at each of the icosahedral threefold positions (cutaway in full-particle diagram). The shell can be considered an assembly of 90 dimers—30 C/C dimers, with ordered arms and rather little local curvature and 60 A/B dimers, with disordered arms and significant local curvature (*lower left*). The ordered framework of arms forces the bases of the S domains apart, whereas along the line that bisects an A/B dimer (the line that joins a fivefold to an icosahedral threefold), the bases of the S domains come together. The detailed side-chain interactions along the fulcrum of this contact remain essentially unchanged, however. Note that the interdomain hinges are essentially passive followers, so that the pair-wise clustered P domains simply project out along the strict and local twofold axes, and the weak interdomain contacts within a subunit do not significantly influence their orientation.

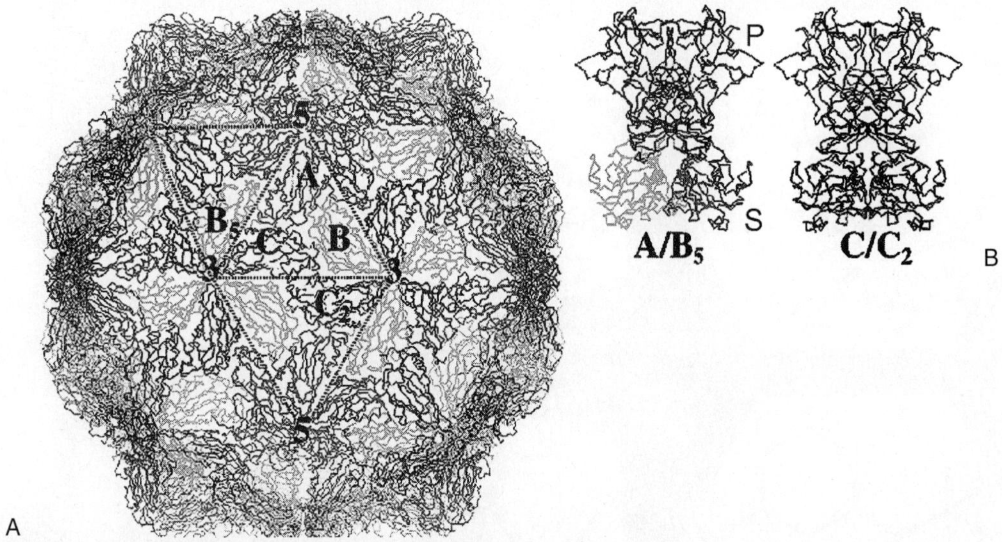

FIG. 9. Molecular architecture of the capsid of Norwalk virus, a human pathogen with a T=3 structure. The subunit arrangement resembles that in TBSV (see Fig. 8). There is a shell (*S*) domain with a jelly-roll β-barrel fold and a protruding (*P*) domain. The packing of S domains is shown in **A**. The P domain in Norwalk virus does not resemble the P domain in TBSV—it is larger, and it has two distinct subdomains—but it also forms strong dimer contacts. By comparing the side-view images of A/B and C/C dimers in part **B** of this figure with those in the lower left of Figure 8, the reader can see that the basic packing principle is similar in the two particles: the A/B contact generates curvature, whereas the C/C contact is relatively flat. The fulcrum around which the S-domain contact rotates in Norwalk virus is somewhat closer to the inward-facing margin of the domain than it is in TBSV. (From ref. 78, with permission.)

How equivalent or nonequivalent are the actual intersubunit contacts in TBSV or in other examples of quasi-equivalent designs? Most of the interfaces are quite conserved, with very modest local distortions that do not significantly change the way individual amino acid side chains contact each other. The interfaces between conformers that do exhibit noteworthy differences are those that include the ordered C-conformer arms in one of their quasi-equivalent locations. Even at these interfaces, however, where a clear switching mechanism takes place, many side-chain contacts are conserved around the "fulcrum" of the differences created by C-arm insertion (see Fig. 8).

The ways of subdividing an icosahedral shell, to create quasi-equivalent subunit packing as in TBSV and Norwalk virus, were enumerated by Caspar and Klug (23). Only certain multiples of 60 subunits can be accommodated in this way; they are given by the formula $T=h^2 + hk + k^2$, where *h* and *k* are any integer or zero. The multiple T is known as the *triangulation number* because, as illustrated by comparison of the 60- and 180-comma structures in Figures 3 and 6, it corresponds to subtriangulations of an icosahedral net on the surface of a sphere. Such nets are known as *surface lattices,* and they are another way of describing the symmetry of a closed-shell arrangement of building blocks. If an icosahedrally symmetric structure is imagined as a folded-up hexagonal net (Fig. 10), 12 uniformly spaced sixfold vertices are transformed into fivefold vertices. The intervening twofold, threefold, and sixfold symmetry axes of the flat net are transformed either into quasi-twofold, quasi-threefold, and quasi-sixfold axes of the icosahedral net (i.e., approximate symmetry axes that apply only locally to the subunits in the immediate neighborhood) or, in some cases, into strict icosahedral twofolds or threefold axes (see Fig. 10). A number of the designs predicted by the Caspar and Klug concepts have been found among various viruses of vertebrates, insects, and plants (see Fig. 1; see also ref. 3).

The external appearance of the virus particles in Figure 1 do not in all cases immediately reveal the underlying quasi-equivalent design. At high enough resolution, they will do so, of course, but as seen in the electron microscope at moderate resolution, they reveal variously disposed "bumps" rather than individual protein subunits. The bumps usually correspond to projecting parts of subunits, clustered around local symmetry axes. The 90 bumps in a three-dimensional reconstruction from electron micrographs of negatively stained TBSV, for example, correspond to pair-wise clustered P domains of the protein subunit, projecting at the 30 strict twofold and 60 quasi-twofold positions. In a frequently found arrangement, the intersubunit contacts are particularly tight and prominent around fivefold and quasi-sixfold axes in the surface lattice, as in the images of the herpesvirus capsid, bacteriophage P2, and cowpea chlorotic mottle virus (CCMV) in Figure 1 (*hexamer-pentamer clustering*). In low-resolution electron micrographs, such as those taken of negatively stained particles, the struc-

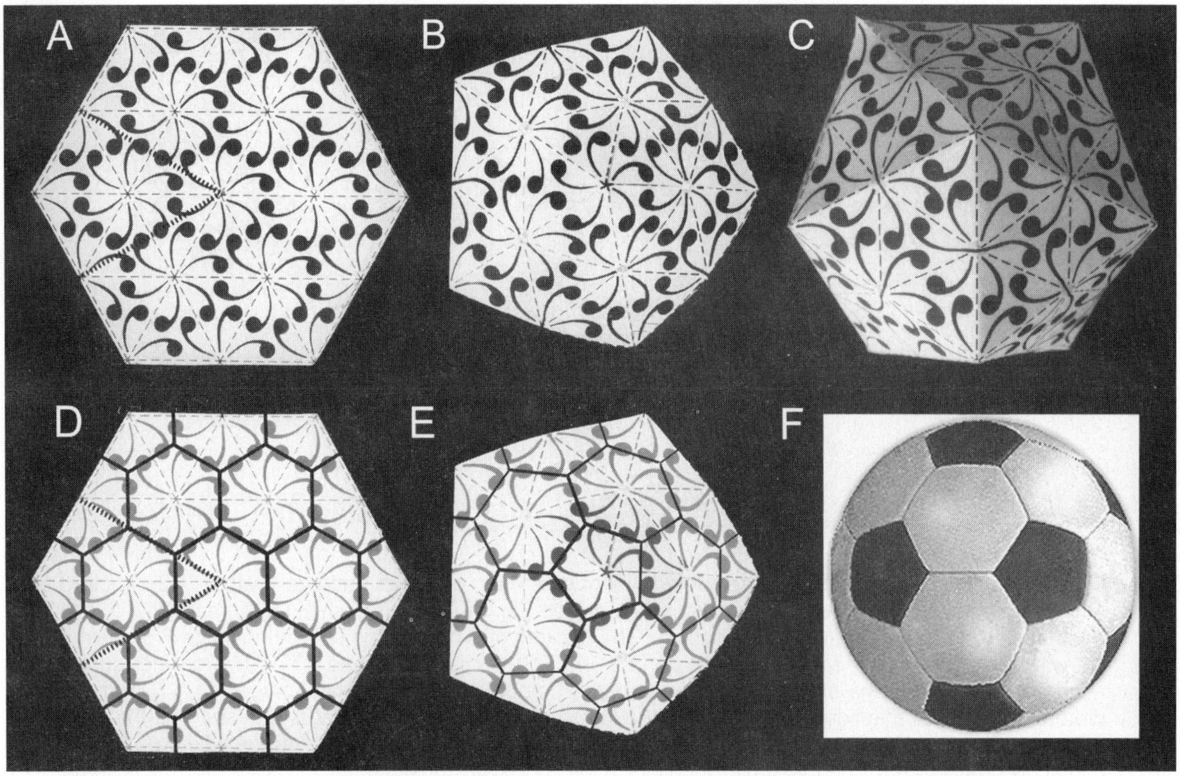

FIG. 10. **A:** Portion of a hexagonal lattice. Six triangular cells of the lattice meet at each lattice point, and each triangular cell contains three "subunits" (*commas*). Thus, there is a sixfold symmetry axis at each lattice point, a threefold symmetry axis at the center of each triangle, and a twofold axis at the midpoint of each edge. Imagine that the lattice extends indefinitely in all directions. **B:** Curvature can be introduced by transforming one of the sixfold positions into a fivefold (*center*). A 60-degree "pie slice" has been removed from the object in **A** by cutting along the heavy dotted lines, and the cut edges have been joined to generate the curved lattice shown here. **C:** If further cuts are made at regular intervals in an extended lattice, such as the one in **A**, and the edges joined as in **B**, a closed solid can be produced. In the case of the icosahedral solid shown here, vertices of the lattice separated by two cell edges have been transformed into fivefold axes, whereas the intervening lattice points have been left as local sixfold axes, producing a T=4 (h=2, k=0) structure. Notice that the local sixfold axes are actually only approximately sixfold in character; they correspond strictly to the twofold axes of the icosahedral object. **D:** Lines joining the centers of the triangular cells in **A** create a pattern of hexagons. **E:** When a sixfold is transformed into a fivefold, a hexagon becomes a pentagon. **F:** If second nearest-neighbor lattice points are all transformed into pentagons, a "soccer ball" figure results. This is a T=3 structure. A description of the lattice as a network of hexagons and pentagons is complementary to its description as a network of triangles. The representations in Figures 3 and 6 use triangles. The representations in Figures 11 and 12 use hexagons and pentagons. One representation for a given structure can easily be derived from the other.

ture of CCMV (see Fig. 1) would simply have 32 smooth bumps, rather than obviously subdivided hexamers and pentamers. In general, hexamer-pentamer clustering produces $10(T-1)+12$ bumps in an icosahedral lattice with triangulation number T. Before the molecular principles of virus structure were fully understood, these bumps were called *capsomeres* (meaning the structural units of the capsid). This word is sometimes still used when referring to apparent morphologic units on the surface of a virus shell, but it is best reserved for cases in which all capsomeres are the same and hence represent a defined oligomer, as in the pentameric units of papovaviruses (see later).

Some noteworthy variations on subtriangulated icosahedral designs are nonetheless in keeping with the basic Caspar-Klug notion of quasi-equivalence, namely, that once a stable and specific protein interface has evolved, structures requiring deviations from simple designs generally make use of the possibility for flexing the contact, rather than developing a completely different specificity within the same surface of the folded subunit. One such variation is found in elongated structures with hemi-icosahedral caps (Fig. 11). Near the poles of these caps, the shell looks like a normal icosahedral design. As the lattice approaches the equator, however, the regular interspersion of fivefold and quasi-sixfold axes gives way to sixfold axes only, so that

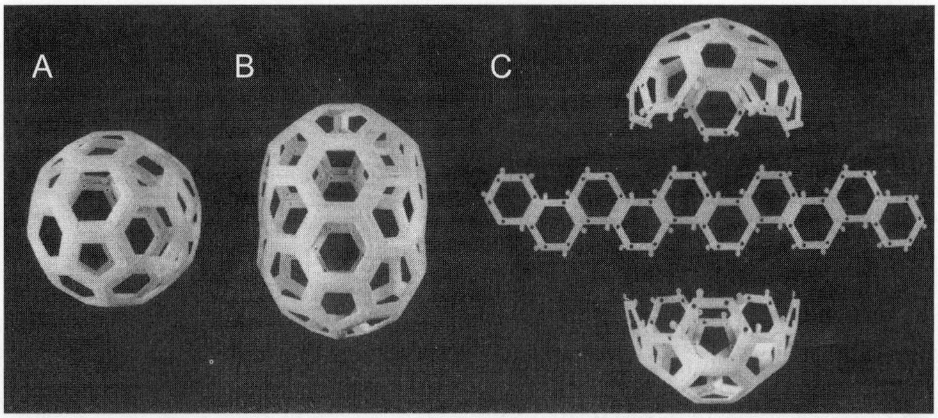

FIG. 11. A: Schematic representation of a T=3 lattice. Compare the soccer ball in Figure 10**F**. In this figure, the lattice is oriented so that there are pentagons at the north and south poles. Altogether, there are 12 pentagons and 20 hexagons (180 subunits) in a T=3 assembly. **B:** Schematic representation of the lattice describing phage ϕ29. There are 12 pentagons and 30 hexagons (240 subunits). Again, there are pentagons at the poles of the structure. **C:** The ϕ29 lattice can be derived by cutting the T=3 structure into two hemispheres, each with a pentagon at its pole, and adding a band of 10 hexagons around the equator. (From ref. 112, with permission.)

there is a tubular region around the middle of the particle. The tubular region can be of varying extent; in extreme cases, it can be much longer than the caps themselves. A further variation on this theme is found in the shells formed by the CA fragment of the lentivirus Gag protein. Conical structures seen within HIV-1 particles have been shown to be based on the sort of arrangement shown in Figure 12, where one cap has more than six fivefold axes and the other has less, so that the diameters of the two caps are different (50). (Note that if there are only sixfold and fivefold vertices in a closed surface lattice, there will always be exactly 12 of the latter.)

A key issue in assemblies with quasi-equivalent contacts, like those just illustrated, is positional regulation. Of the different quasi-equivalent interactions, what determines, for any given site, which state is actually present? Consider for definiteness the T=3 design exemplified by TBSV (see Fig. 8). Structures like this one are known to assemble from dimers of the protein subunit. We can think of the dimer as having two states: the A-B state, characterized by unfolded arms and one position for the interdomain hinge, and the C-C state, characterized by folded arms and another position for the interdomain hinge. Experiments show that assembly proceeds by addition of dimers to a growing shell and that the curvature of the growing shell is always nearly correct (94) (Fig. 13). That is, when a dimer adds to a shell, it adopts the correct state, and the characteristics of the site at which the dimer adds determine that state. Assembly mechanisms of this kind depend on getting started correctly—having a correct initial nucleus—and on addition of defined "assembly units." In the case of TBSV, the initial nucleus probably includes an RNA packaging signal, and the assembly unit is the subunit dimer.

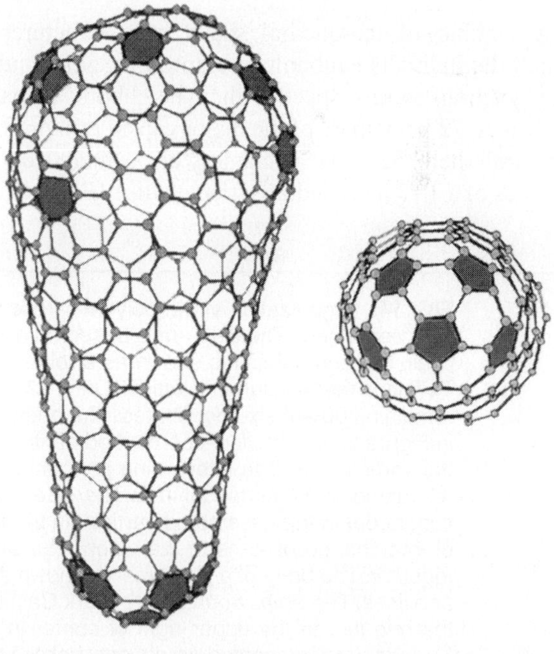

FIG. 12. *Left:* a conelike lattice of hexagons and pentagons, representing the rearranged ("mature") capsid of human immunodeficiency virus type 1. There are seven pentagons in the upper curved surface and five in the lower one. Thus, the upper surface contains a bit more than a full hemisphere and the lower surface, a bit less. *Right:* View from below, showing the five-pentagon surface. Addition of one more pentagon would turn it into a T=3 hemisphere. (From ref. 50, with permission.)

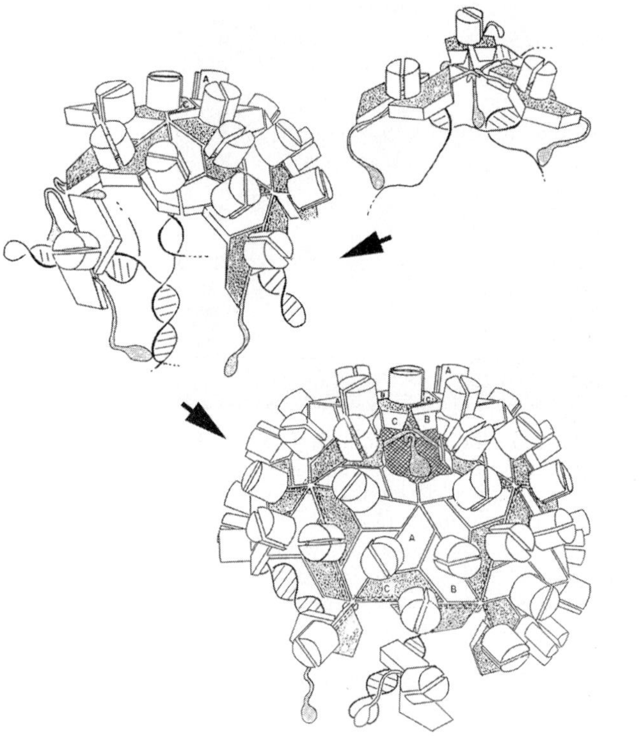

FIG. 13. Model for assembly of a T=3 virus shell (derived from work on turnip crinkle virus; see ref. 94). The key steps are: specific initiation, propagation by addition of a defined assembly unit, and closure. In the case of most T=3 structures that have been studied, the assembly unit is a dimer of the subunit. The initiation structure is shown as a trimer of dimers, nucleated by interaction with a packaging signal on the RNA. All the dimers adopt the C/C (ordered arm) conformation (see Fig. 8). An alternative model, probably not ruled out by the data, would be a pentamer of dimers, all in the A/B conformation (disordered arms), also nucleated by the packaging signal. In either case, the key characteristic of each addition step is that the conformation of the assembly unit that associates with the growing shell is uniquely determined by the nature of the site at which it adds. In the model shown here, the first addition to the trimer of C/C dimers is necessarily an A/B dimer because the interdigitated arms prevent further ordered arms around that threefold, and the assembly unit that slips in must necessarily leave its arms in a disordered state.

More Complex Icosahedral Shells

Pentameric Assembly Units in Papovaviruses

A number of icosahedral shells have structures in which the individual subunits are not in roughly equivalent positions with respect to their neighbors. In papovaviruses, 72 pentamers of the major capsid protein form the viral shell (82). The pentamers are centered on the vertices of a T=7 icosahedral surface lattice (Fig. 14), but of these, only 12 can be on fivefold positions, and the remainder are six-coordinated. That is, 60 of the 72 pentamers are "fivefold pegs in sixfold holes." In the case of the polyomaviruses (such as SV40 and murine polyoma), each subunit has an extended, C-terminal arm that issues from the body of the pentamer and invades a subunit in a neighboring pentamer (67). Thus, each subunit donates and accepts an arm. The interactions made by the arms are essentially invariant: they fit the same way into every

FIG. 14. Organization of the polyomaviruses (67). **A:** Overview of the particle, showing the packing of VP1 pentamers. The diagram is based on a molecular graphics representation in which the polypeptide chain of each subunit is shown as a folded line. The pentamers are all centered on lattice points of a T=7 icosahedral surface lattice. Only 12 of those lattice points are five-coordinated, however; the remaining 60 are six-coordinated. The orientation of the particle corresponds to that of the icosahedron in Figure 3; note the five-coordinated pentamers toward the top and bottom of the image, along the central vertical axis. The intervening pentamers are six-coordinated. **B:** A six-coordinated VP1 pentamer, "extracted" from the model in **A.** The extended carboxyl-terminal arms are shown in the conformations they adopt in the assembled particle; in the free pentamer, they are disordered and flexible. **C:** Pattern of interchange of arms in the virion. The arms "invade" neighboring pentamers, to link the structure together. The body of a pentamer is shown as a five-petalled flower; the arms are cylinders (α-helices) and lines. The *small open circles* mark Ca^{2+} sites. The central pentamer in this diagram corresponds to the one just to the upper right of center in **A. D:** The subunit, viewed normal to the pentamer axis. Strands are represented as *ribbons;* helices, as *cylinders;* loops as *narrow tubes.* The two sheets of the β-barrel domain are in different *dark shades;* the carboxyl-terminal arms are pale; the amino-terminal arms are somewhat darker. The complete carboxyl-terminal arm seen here actually emanates from a subunit in another pentamer; only the initial, α-helical segment of the arm from this subunit is shown because it then extends out of the page. Note how the amino-terminal segment clamps the invading arm in place. The small ball represents the site of a Ca^{2+} ion. **E:** Interaction of VP2 (or VP3) with VP1. The VP1 pentamer is shown in cross-sectional "side" view, with the outside of the virion at the top and the inside at the bottom. The C-terminal part of VP2 (identical with the C-terminal part of VP3) inserts from within the virion, into the conical hollow in the pentamer (4,25).

target subunit. The essential variability lies in the way an arm bridges from one pentamer to the next, in other words, in the flexibility of the arm as it passes across the boundary between the pentamer from which it emanates and the pentamer into which it inserts. The folded part of the subunit is a jelly-roll β-barrel, just as in the RNA viruses with quasi-equivalent designs, but the long axis of the domain is oriented essentially radially, rather than tangentially, in the shell.

The assembly unit of the papovavirus shell is a pentamer (91), and just as the assembly mechanism for a T=3 shell described previously involves a unique nucleation event, followed by successive addition of individual dimers, so the likely mechanism for assembly of the papovavirus shell involves a specific initiation step followed by successive addition of pentamers. A scheme can be drawn by which the nature of a site for pentamer addition, at the growing edge of the shell, determines where

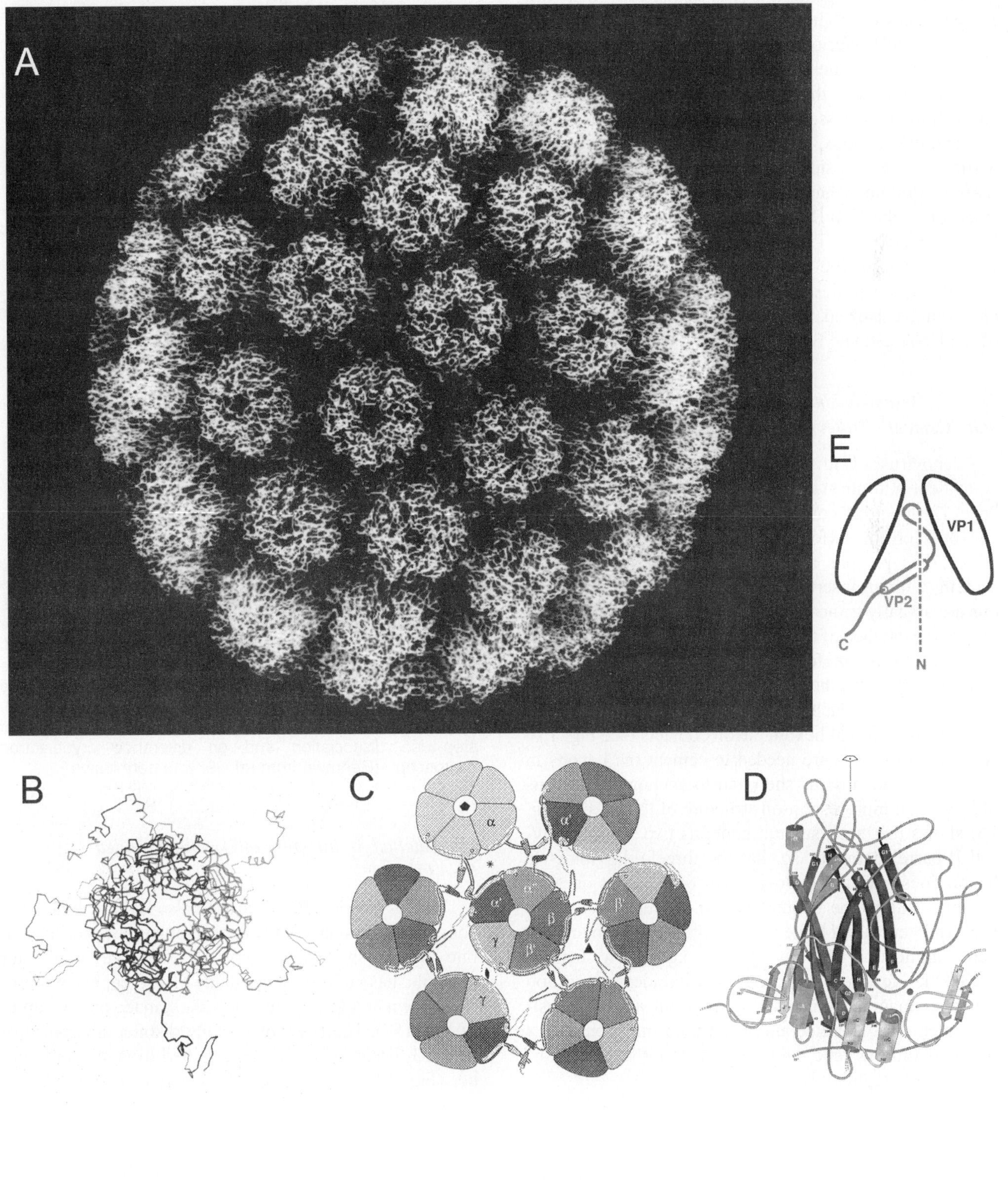

the C-terminal arms of the new pentamer will insert (96). A clear advantage of the papovavirus design is that there is a single type of preformed assembly unit: the pentamer.

Scaffold Proteins in Phage and Herpesvirus Capsid Assembly

Structures with hexamers and pentamers of the same protein species cannot assemble by simple addition of a single kind of assembly unit, and they consequently require a substantially more intricate assembly mechanism. For example, genuine T=7 structures do exist, with 12 pentamers and 60 hexamers made of the same subunit. The heads of bacteriophages, such as lambda and P22, are examples of such designs (79). Unlike the papovaviruses, however, they cannot be put together from a unique kind of subassembly. Indeed, their assembly pathway is quite complex, involving formation of a precursor particle (the procapsid) with participation of an internal scaffold protein, which is degraded or recycled before insertion of the viral DNA (22). Herpesvirus capsids (see Fig. 1), which have T=16 shells with 12 pentamers and 150 hexamers of the major capsid protein (VP5 in the case of herpes simplex virus type 1 [HSV-1]), also assemble around a scaffold, which is degraded before insertion of the DNA genome (see Chapter 33).

Trimeric Assembly Units, Chemically Distinct Pentons, and "Cement" Proteins in Adenoviruses

Adenoviruses (Fig. 15) exhibit a combination of nonequivalent and quasi-equivalent interactions (98). They have 12 "pentons" on the fivefold positions, and 240 "hexons" on the sixfold positions of a T=25 icoshedral lattice. The pentons are pentamers of the penton-base protein, with an inserted, trimeric fiber (105). The hexons are actually trimers, not hexamers, of the hexon protein, and each face of the icosahedron is triangulated into a net with local threefold (rather than sixfold) symmetry. Within a face, the hexons make essentially equivalent interactions with each other, but at the edges, there are completely different hexon–hexon contacts (see Fig. 15). Additional proteins are needed to cement the hexons in place in the adenovirus shell and to anchor the pentons (47,99). The high-resolution structure of the hexon (Fig. 16) shows that each subunit contains two similar jelly-roll β-barrel domains, so that the threefold symmetric hexon does have a pseudo-sixfold (86). Just as one can imagine taking one subunit of a T=3 quasi-equivalent shell and generating three related but distinct subunits by gene duplication and divergence (e.g., going from a TBSV-like design to a picornavirus-like design), so too can one imagine taking a subunit from a true, quasi-equivalent, T=25 lattice and generating the adenovirus-like structure by gene duplication without separation of the two polypeptide chains.

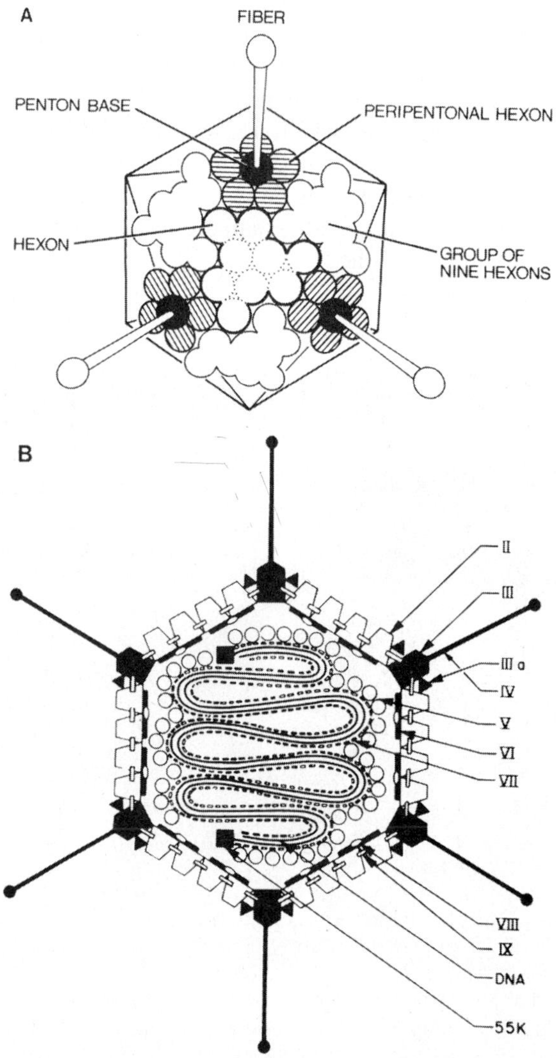

FIG. 15. A: Diagram of the adenovirus particle, showing the location of major protein subassemblies. The nine hexons drawn as a group and the "peripentonal" hexons are trimers of the same polypeptide; they are distinguished only by their location in the structure. (Illustration by John Mack. From ref. 16, with permission.) **B:** Cross-section showing the probable location of the principal polypeptide components and the viral DNA. The assignment for proteins other than II (hexon), III (penton base), and IV (penton fiber) is based on studies of step-wise dissociation and on difference cryoelectron microscopy. (Redrawn from ref. 39, with permission.)

Multishelled Architecture of Double-Stranded RNA Viruses

Double-stranded RNA viruses also exhibit both nonequivalent and quasi-equivalent interactions, but in separate protein shells. The core of bluetongue virus, for example, has an inner shell, made of 120 copies of a protein known as VP3, and an outer shell, made of 780 copies of VP7 (57). There are two totally distinct environments for VP3, because 2 is not a permitted triangulation number (Fig. 17). The amino acid side chains on the lateral

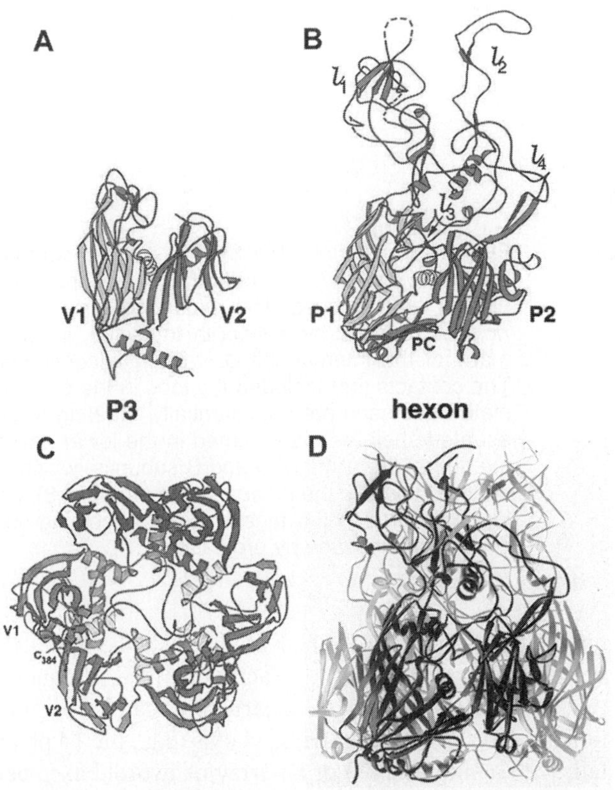

FIG. 16. Comparison of the adenovirus hexon structure and the P3 outer-shell protein from bacteriophage PRD1. **A** and **B:** The polypeptide chains of P3 and adenovirus hexon. The direction of view is perpendicular to the threefold axis. The two β-barrel domains are shown in *gray;* the loops between strands in each domain and between domains are shown in a *lighter shade.* Note that these domains are oriented so that their β-strands would run radially in the virus particle, as in the polyomaviruses, rather than tangentially, as in the picornaviruses. Except for the much more restricted loops of the "tower," P3 closely resembles hexon. **C:** Top view of the PRD1 P3 trimer, showing its pseudo-hexagonal outline. The adenovirus hexon would have, near its base, a very similar outline; this is the part of the trimer that interacts with others in the lattice of the virion shell (compare Fig. 15A). **D:** Side view of the adenovirus hexon trimer. The black subunit, in the foreground, is in the same orientation as the single subunit in **A.** The loops of the individual chains fold extensively with each other. These loops would probably not be ordered in a monomeric subunit, and it is likely that subunit folding and trimer assembly occur coordinately. (**A** to **C** redrawn from ref. 10, with permission; **D** courtesy of R. Burnett.)

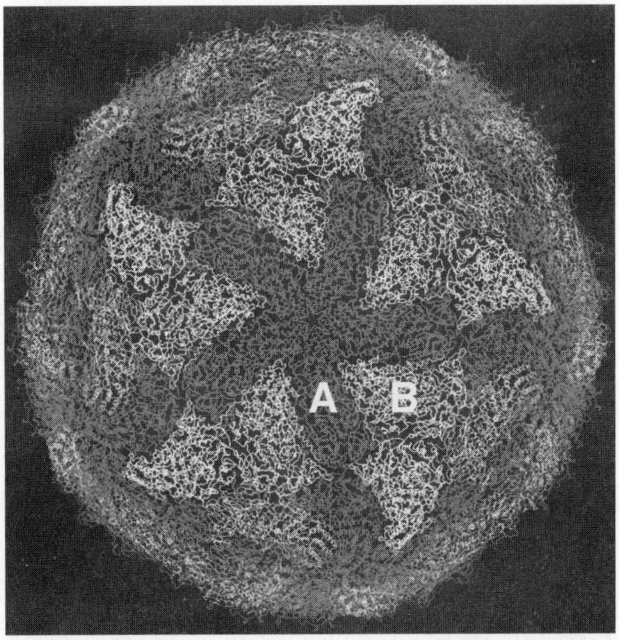

FIG. 17. A structure with 120 identical subunits: the principal shell of the inner capsid particle (core) from reovirus (83). The 60 dark copies of the protein λ1 (one of which is labeled *A*) and the 60 lighter copies (*B*) have different interactions within the shell. For example, the "tips" of five A subunits contact each other around a fivefold axis, whereas the corresponding surfaces of B subunits touch different parts of A subunits. Thus, the same molecular surface makes two quite different, yet specific, interactions. A similar arrangement of the protein VP3 is found in the core of bluetongue virus (57).

surfaces of VP3 have different partners, depending on the interface in which they lie. The distortion of the subunit itself, when the two environments are compared, is quite small. By contrast, the VP7 shell has a classic, T=13, quasi-equivalent design. The contacts between VP7 trimers resemble each other closely. Intershell contacts are obviously highly variable because there is no match between the triangulation of the two shells. It is likely that addition of VP7 nucleates at threefold positions, where there is a match in symmetry of the two layers; these strong intershell contacts can then initiate lateral propagation of the VP7 lattice by addition of further trimers.

Rearrangements in Icosahedral Lattices

Icosahedral surface lattices can undergo rearrangements, which preserve the overall symmetry of the structure but change the pattern of specific intersubunit contacts. There is often an accompanying change in the diameter of the shell. The T=3 plant viruses expand, in most cases reversibly, when the calcium cations that stabilize a particular set of subunit interfaces are removed (87) (Fig. 18). This swelling is believed to be the first step in disassembly. Plant viruses are injected by their vectors directly into the cytoplasm of the recipient cell, where they are exposed to a low Ca^{2+} environment. A similar, but transient, expansion occurs when poliovirus binds its receptor (9). The double-stranded DNA (dsDNA) bacteriophages insert their genomic DNA into a preformed "prohead," and the outer shell of the prohead generally expands as its subunits shift around to form the mature structure (22). Herpesviruses likewise package DNA into a procapsid, which undergoes structural changes in the process, but without a change in diameter (100).

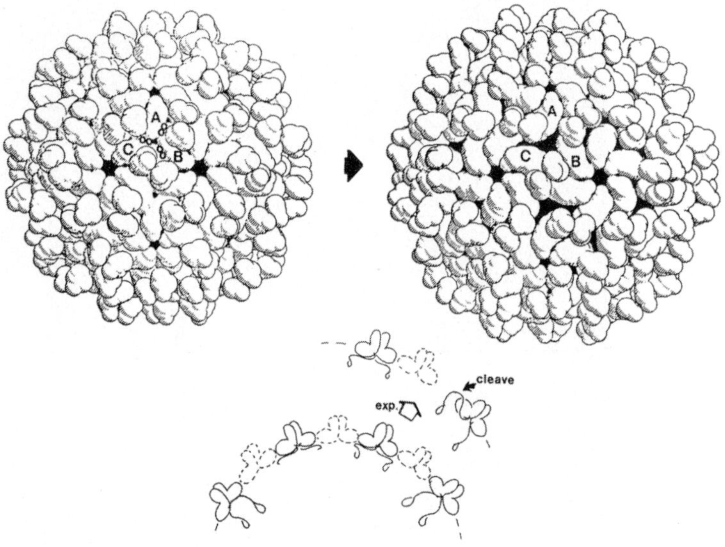

FIG. 18. Expansion of TBSV. The mature, compact particle (*upper left*) expands when Ca^{2+} ions (*small circles*) are removed. The expanded form (*upper right*) is reached by a smooth transition, in which many of the intersubunit contacts are conserved. The contacts that included the ions in the compact state have separated substantially, creating a fenestrated shell. As diagrammed in the lower part of the figure, the arms of A and B subunits, which do not participate in the inner scaffold (see Fig. 8), can loop out through the fenestrations, becoming susceptible to cleavage by proteases.

Symmetry Mismatches

The papovavirus structures have already provided us with one example of mismatched symmetry—what we called a "fivefold peg in a sixfold hole." A somewhat different example is the way these same pentamers bind the internal proteins, VP2 and VP3 (4,25). These proteins are the same, except for an about 100-residue N-terminal extension unique to VP2. Each VP1 pentamer binds one internal protein, through interaction with residues near the common C-terminus (see Fig. 14**E**). In the virus particle, all five symmetry-related registers of the VP1-VP2/3 interaction occur, so that the internal protein projecting inward from a given VP1 pentamer adopts one of five equally likely orientations. A similar rotational randomness is likely to characterize the adenovirus fiber, which is a trimeric molecule anchored in a pentameric base (see Fig. 15). Symmetry mismatch appears to be used in rotary motors, such as those that package DNA or RNA in phage heads, to subdivide a full rotation into discrete steps.

Helical Tubes

Isometric virus structures occur much more frequently than tubular ones, perhaps because of the inherently greater efficiency of nucleic acid packaging within a quasi-spherical cavity. There are, however, a number of well-known and widely studied helical and filamentous viruses, and the nucleocapsids (protein-coated nucleic acid) of many enveloped, negative-strand RNA viruses are helical arrays, which coil within the virion and uncoil when released.

Helical structures are organized around a single axis (the *helix axis*). They can be described by the number of units per turn, u (not necessarily integral), and the axial rise per unit, p. (Axial rise is the increment in "height" along the helix axis between one unit and the next.) The pitch of the helix, P, defined as the distance along the helix axis corresponding to exactly one turn, is equal to the product of u and p. Helical structures can have a rotation axis coincident with the helix axis (e.g., the T4 phage tail, with a sixfold axis) or an array of twofold axes per-

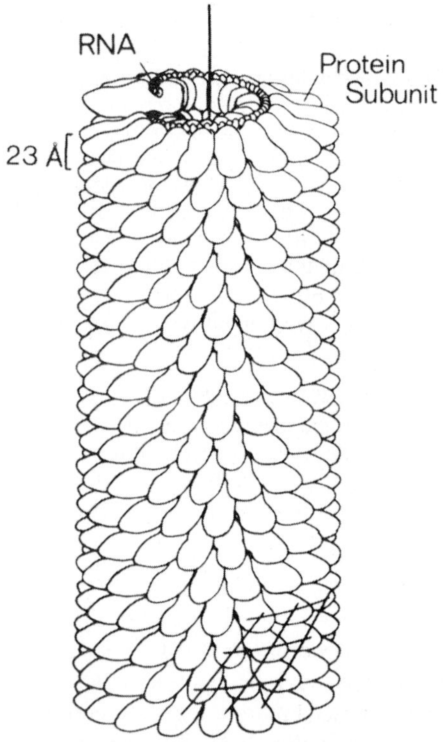

FIG. 19. The helical structure of tobacco mosaic virus (TMV). There are 161/3 subunits per turn of the helix, which has a 23 Å pitch. Three RNA nucleotides fit into a groove on each subunit. There is an about 30 Å diameter hollow along the axis. The surface lattice (four "unit cells") is indicated in the lower part of the figure.

pendicular to the helix axis (as in DNA). The diagram of TMV in Figure 19 illustrates that a structure with helical symmetry (in this case, having $u = 16^1/_3$, $p = 1.4$ Å, and $P = 23$ Å) can also be described by reference to a surface lattice—the network connecting equivalent units in the curved surface. The lattice lines correspond to different helical paths, as shown in the figure and described in more detail in the caption.

In TMV, and probably in the nucleocapsids of negative-stranded RNA viruses like influenza and vesicular stomatitis virus (VSV), the RNA winds in a helical path that follows the protein. That is, the tubular package does not simply contain the RNA, it co-incorporates it. There are exactly three nucleotides per subunit in TMV, and they fit into a defined groove between the helically arrayed proteins. By contrast, the protein coat of a filamentous, ssDNA phage, such as M13, forms a sleeve that surrounds and constrains the closed, circular genome, without there being a specific way in which each subunit "sees" one or more nucleotides (51). Thus, there can be a non-integral ratio of nucleotides to protein monomers.

Genome Packaging

Incorporation of viral nucleic acid must be specific but independent of most of its base sequence. Therefore, viral genomes often contain a *packaging signal*—a short sequence or set of sequences that directs encapsidation. Recognition of the packaging signal depends on the nature of the genome and on the complexity of the assembly mechanism. The coats of simple viruses usually assemble around the genomes, and in these cases, there is likely to be a direct interaction between genome and capsid protein. More complex viruses sometimes insert nucleic acid into a preformed shell, and genome recognition is a property of the packaging system. If replication and packaging are closely coupled in some way, there may be no requirement for a specific packaging signal at all, as may be true of the picornaviruses.

In positive-stranded RNA viruses, no definite overall secondary or tertiary fold is needed for the genomic RNA, aside from the restriction that it fit within the shell. This restriction is actually quite severe, and the RNA is generally packed very tightly, approximating the density of RNA in crystals (e.g., of tRNA). Even random-sequence ssRNA contains about 60% to 70% of its nucleotides in base-paired stems (55), and to fit efficiently within the interior of a capsid, these RNA stems must pack tangentially, many in contact with the inward-facing surface of the shell. Such packing can be achieved by assembly around the RNA, without defined capsid–RNA interactions. In some viruses, segments of partially ordered RNA appear, packing into shallow grooves on the inner capsid surface (27,42). The ordered structures of these segments may result simply from the shape of the groove and the possible structures that a tightly packed polynucleotide chain can adopt. There do not appear to be any base-specific contacts in these ordered segments.

Recognition of RNA packaging signals has been analyzed in detail in a few cases. In RNA phage such as MS2 and R17, the packaging signal folds into a stem-loop structure (Fig. 20**A**), recognized by a dimer of the coat protein (the assembly unit for this T=3 particle) (20,103,104). Bases of the loop in the packaging signal and a looped-out base in the stem fit into a groove on the inward-facing surface of the subunit dimer, and conserved bases make defined protein contacts. The MS2 subunit has a structure unrelated to those of nonenveloped positive-stranded RNA viruses of eukaryotes, many of which recognize their genomic RNA, not through a groove-like site on the protein, but rather through a flexibly extended, positively charged protein arm, often at the N-terminus. In the case of alfalfa mosaic virus, the arm may fit against a recognition structure formed by the folded RNA packaging signal (2). In a sense, the RNA "recognizes" the packaging signal, rather than the other way around. A similar recognition principle determines the specificity of interactions between the Tat protein of HIV-1 and its cognate site, TAR, on the HIV-1 RNA (80), as well as of those between HIV-1 Rev and its cognate site, the RRE (6). It may also apply to the way the positively charged, N-terminal arm of alphavirus capsid proteins direct specific RNA packaging.

Retroviral packaging signals, known as *psi* sequences, are recognized by the nucleocapsid (NC) domain of the Gag protein. The HIV-1 psi element has a stem-loop structure that associates with two "zinc-knuckle" modules in HIV-1 NC (35) (see Fig. 20**B**). The two zinc modules are flexibly linked in unbound NC, but they adopt a defined, three-dimensional organization in complex with the RNA. Thus, the structure of the RNA imparts additional order to the protein element with which it binds.

Helical structures must unwind any base-paired stems of an RNA genome in order to package it. For example, TMV assembly begins at an internal origin sequence, about 1 kb from the 3′ end of the genome (102,117). A 75-base sequence containing a presumptive stem-loop structure is sufficient to initiate specific encapsidation (see Fig. 20**C**), which proceeds by a mechanism that requires the 5′ end of the RNA to be drawn through a channel along the axis of the assembling particle (17). This process may be described as an assembly-driven helicase. In negative-stranded RNA viruses such as influenza, the sequences that determine encapsidation by the nucleocapsid protein are probably in the conserved termini of the genome segments (see Chapter 24).

The mechanism of overall condensation of a viral genome may be distinct from the specific recognition just discussed. If there is no regular, repeated interaction between coat protein and nucleic acid, there are various strategies for neutralizing the net negative charge on the nucleic acid. Those icosahedral viruses with inwardly

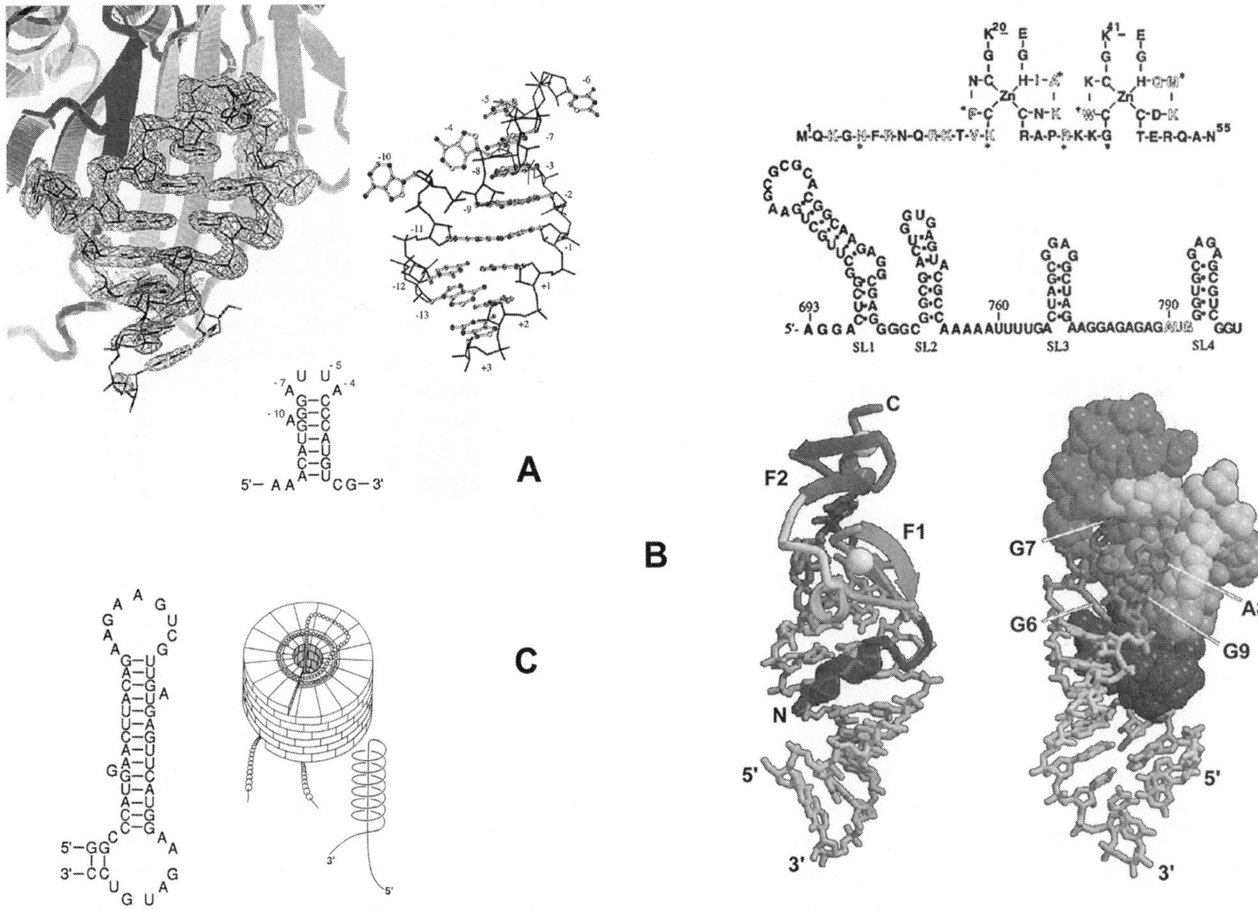

FIG. 20. RNA virus packaging signals. **A:** Recognition of the bacteriophage MS2 packaging sequence (a stem-loop structure, with a sequence shown in the lower part of the figure) by a dimer of the coat protein. The stem-loop fits into a hollow on the inward-facing surface of the protein (*upper left*); three bases in the loop and a looped-out base in the stem are critical for specific recognition; the stem structure presents them to the protein in correct spatial orientation (*upper right*). (Redrawn from ref. 104, with permission.) **B:** Recognition of the human immunodeficiency virus type 1 packaging sequence by the dual "zinc knuckle" element in the NC protein. The amino acid sequence of this 55-residue element is shown at the *top,* using single-letter notation. The nucleotide sequence of the packaging signal ("psi sequence") in the genomic RNA is shown in the *middle.* Note that it contains four distinct stem-loops. The two zinc knuckles (F1 and F2) fold around the loop at the tip of stem-loop 3 (SL3), and a segment N-terminal to the first Zn knuckle forms an α-helix in the widened major groove of the RNA. The NC peptide itself is ordered only within each Zn-liganding fold (about 16 residues each), and the two knuckles are flexibly linked. The structure of SL3 thus imposes additional structure on the peptide, including the N-terminal helix. (Redrawn from ref. 35, with permission). **C:** Assembly of TMV from an assembly origin that lies just upstream of the coat-protein coding sequence at the 3′ end of the genome (17,117). The sequence and likely secondary structure of the assembly origin are shown on the left. The location of this origin, roughly 500 nucleotides from the 3′ end of the RNA, implies that the 5′ end of the RNA runs back along the axis of the assembling particle, as shown on the right.

projecting, positively charged arms use most of these arms for nonspecific interactions with RNA and only one or a few for specific recognition. In the picornaviruses, polyamines are incorporated to achieve charge neutralization. Double-stranded DNA viruses use either cellular histone to condense the viral chromosome (polyomaviruses) or basic, virally encoded proteins (adenoviruses). The dsDNA bacteriophages and the herpesviruses "pump" DNA into a capsid precursor, using adenosine triphosphate hydrolysis to drive condensation. The most efficient packing of a double-stranded genome within a hollow shell can be achieved by uniform coiling of the dsDNA or dsRNA, such that in cross-section, adjacent segments are hexagonally arrayed (37,54). DNA is packed this way in herpesviruses and in phage heads (Fig. 21**A**), as is dsRNA in reoviruses and their relatives (83). Reoviruses have segmented genomes, and each segment may form an independent coil (see Fig. 21**B**).

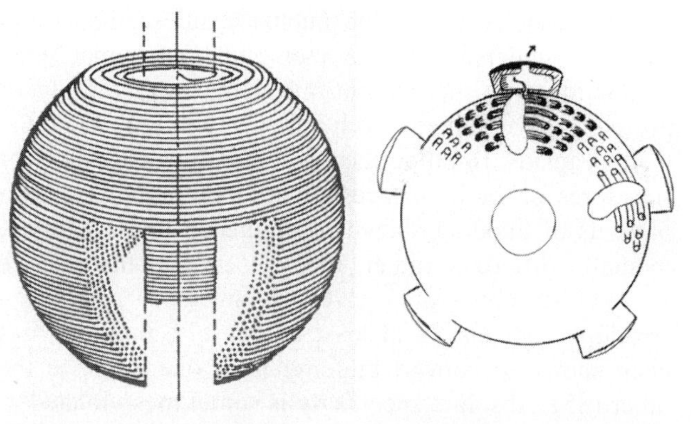

FIG. 21. Packing of double-stranded nucleic acid in virions. **A:** Uniform coiling of DNA within the head of bacteriophage lambda and its relatives (37). The DNA is introduced into a prohead by the action of an adenosine triphosphate–driven rotary motor. In the filled, mature phage head, adjacent, parallel segments of DNA form a local hexagonal packing (*cutaway view toward the bottom of the drawing.*) **B:** Model for coiling of double-stranded RNA (dsRNA) genomic segments within the core of reovirus and other dsRNA viruses (54,83). The negative strand for each segment is generated by the polymerase (*oval outline*), after core assembly in which are packaged one each of the positive-stranded segments. Each genomic segment must be transcribed multiple times, probably by the polymerase around which it is coiled. The transcript exits through a pore along the fivefold axis; in the case of orthoreoviruses, it passes through the chamber of a capping-enzyme complex (*hollow turrets*).

Viral Membranes

Budding

Most enveloped viruses (except for the large and very complex poxviruses) acquire their membrane, a lipid bilayer with associated proteins, by budding through an appropriate cellular membrane—the plasma membrane in many cases, the ER, Golgi apparatus, or nuclear membrane in others (Fig. 22). Using the cell's compartmentalization mechanisms, these viruses direct the insertion of their surface glycoproteins into the relevant membrane of the cell. Budding is driven either by interactions between cytoplasmic tails of the glycoproteins and assembling or preassembled internal structures, by lateral interactions between glycoprotein subunits, or by a combination of both. In some cases, assembly of an internal structure on the cytoplasmic face of the membrane is sufficient to drive budding, even if glycoproteins are lacking. Pinching off from the cell surface, or into the lumen of the ER or Golgi apparatus, appears not to need a cellular activity; assembly of viral components provides the force needed to distort the membrane bilayer. The lipids in the resulting bilayer derive from the cell, whereas the proteins are virally encoded. To a first approximation, the incorporated lipids represent a sample of those in the membrane through which the virus budded, but the significance of potential detailed specificities in lipid incorporation are still poorly understood. Viruses that emerge through the plasma membrane contain phospholipid and cholesterol in characteristic proportions, whereas those that emerge into the lumen of the ER contain almost no cholesterol. Cholesterol tends to increase the thickness of a bilayer, by restricting free rotation around single bonds in the fatty acid chains of adjacent phospholipids (81). The lengths of α-helical transmembrane segments in viral glycoproteins vary accordingly: from about 26 residues in influenza (which buds at the cell surface) to 18 to 20 residues in yellow fever (which buds into the ER).

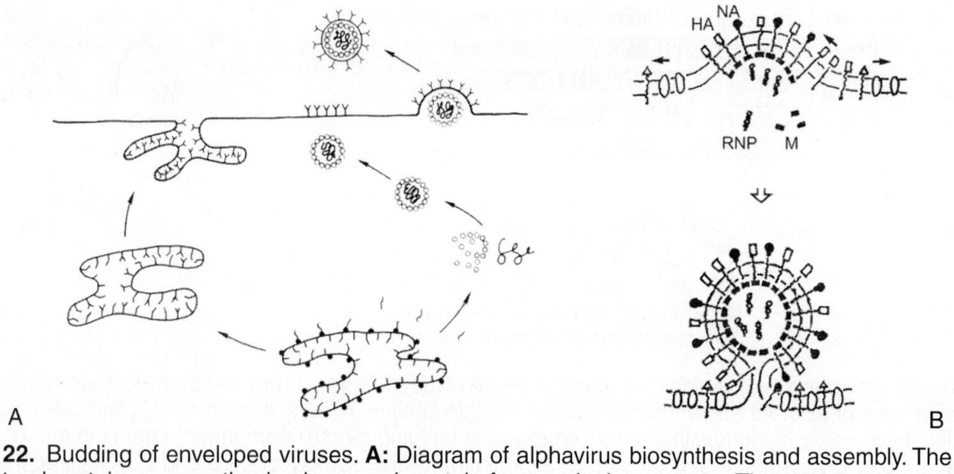

FIG. 22. Budding of enveloped viruses. **A:** Diagram of alphavirus biosynthesis and assembly. The viral structural proteins are synthesized as a polyprotein from a single message. The core protein, a serine protease that acts only on its own polypeptide chain, cleaves itself from the precursor at an early stage. The ribosomes and nascent viral polyprotein then associate with endoplasmic reticulum membranes to complete synthesis of the glycoproteins, which are exported to the cell surface by the standard constitutive route through the Golgi compartments. Core protein and RNA assemble to form nucleocapsids, which associate with glycoprotein patches and initiate budding. **B:** Influenza virus budding. Nucleocapsid protein (N), matrix protein (M), and glycoproteins (HA, NA) are synthesized from independent messages. Glycoproteins arrive at the cell surface by the usual route. Budding is a coassembly at the cell surface of the glycoproteins with M and with RNP segments. Host cell proteins are excluded (*arrows*).

Figure 22 illustrates features of the budding process in two examples—an alphavirus (Sindbis) and an orthomyxovirus (influenza). The structure of the nucleocapsid varies with virus type. It is a compact, spherical particle in the alphavirus; a filamentous, helical nucleocapsid in paramyxoviruses and rhabdoviruses; and a multisegmented helical nucleocapsid in the orthomyxoviruses. The viral glycoproteins are anchored in the cellular membrane by a transmembrane hydrophobic segment (in some cases, a hydrophobic hairpin), and there is a small cytoplasmic domain. In alphaviruses (see Fig. 22**A**), a core particle (nucleocapsid) assembles independently in the cytoplasm. Interactions between the core and the cytoplasmic tail of the glycoproteins then determine the location of budding. Lateral interactions of the glycoproteins also appear to assist the budding process. In orthomyxoviruses such as influenza (see Fig. 22**B**), an M (matrix) protein associates with the nucleocapsid segments and with the underside of the membrane, presumably by interaction with the cytoplasmic domains of the glycoproteins. M organizes both the glycoproteins and the nucleocapsids. Budding then proceeds by coassembly of structures on both surfaces of the membrane. The two patterns of budding shown in Figure 22 are not fundamentally different; rather, they depend on the relative strength of core–core, envelope–envelope, and core–envelope contacts. In at least one case, a mutation has been shown to convert budding from one mode to the other (85). Absolute specificity is sometimes violated in viral budding, leading to cases of phenotypic mixing, in which, for example, SV5 glycoproteins can be found in the membrane of VSV. In retroviruses (Fig. 23), cleavage of core proteins after budding leads to major internal rearrangements.

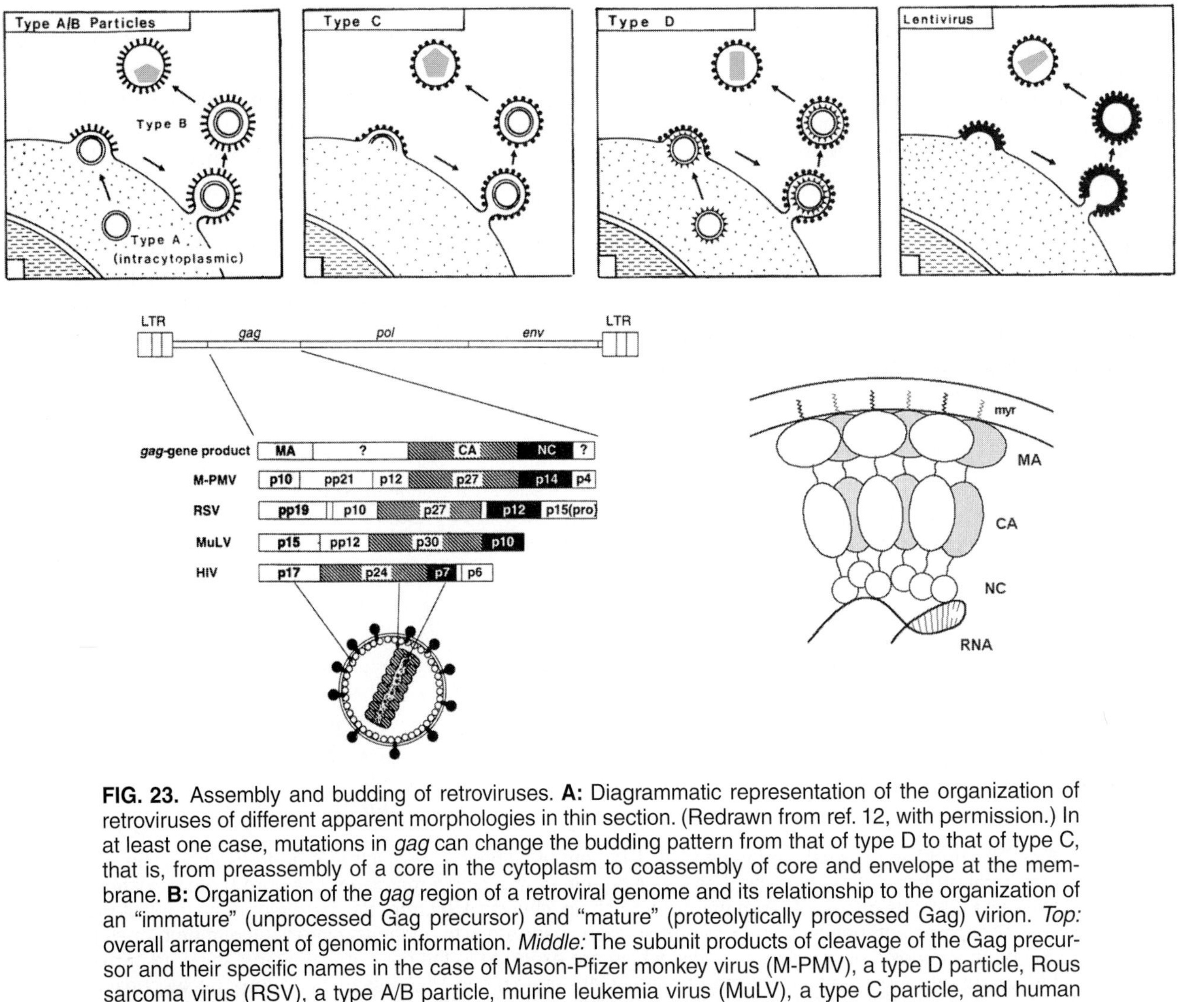

FIG. 23. Assembly and budding of retroviruses. **A:** Diagrammatic representation of the organization of retroviruses of different apparent morphologies in thin section. (Redrawn from ref. 12, with permission.) In at least one case, mutations in *gag* can change the budding pattern from that of type D to that of type C, that is, from preassembly of a core in the cytoplasm to coassembly of core and envelope at the membrane. **B:** Organization of the *gag* region of a retroviral genome and its relationship to the organization of an "immature" (unprocessed Gag precursor) and "mature" (proteolytically processed Gag) virion. *Top:* overall arrangement of genomic information. *Middle:* The subunit products of cleavage of the Gag precursor and their specific names in the case of Mason-Pfizer monkey virus (M-PMV), a type D particle, Rous sarcoma virus (RSV), a type A/B particle, murine leukemia virus (MuLV), a type C particle, and human immunodeficiency virus (HIV), a lentivirus. *Bottom:* Representation of an HIV particle, showing locations of MA, CA, and NC proteins (Redrawn from ref. 64, with permission). **C:** Diagram of the organization of the HIV Gag precursor. The MA domain is myristoylated at its N-terminus, facilitating its association with the membrane. It forms a trimer. The CA domain dimerizes, through its carboxyl-terminal subdomain. This combination of trimer and dimer formation may help drive extended lateral association and budding.

The simplest enveloped virus particles—those of the alphaviruses and the flaviviruses—are icosahedrally symmetric. In these positive-stranded RNA viruses, one-to-one interactions between the envelope glycoprotein and the nucleocapsid subunit appear to ensure coherence between external and internal structures (28,106) (Fig. 24; see Fig. 22**A**). The larger, negative-stranded RNA bunyaviruses also have an icosahedrally symmetric envelope (a T=12 lattice), but their internal structures are probably not icosahedrally organized (108), and the outer lattice is the major determinant of symmetry and stability. The rhabdoviruses have a helically organized shaft with a (probably hemi-icosahedral) cap at one end. The orthomyxoviruses, like influenza A, bud out as variable elongated structures with no overall symmetry, although there is probably considerable local order. Retrovirus particles also do not appear to have a global symmetry. The fluid character of a lipid bilayer means that the virus can form a closed structure without a perfect surface lattice. Defects in a protein layer that would produce unacceptable holes in a nonenveloped virus are tolerable if the barrier protecting the genome is a lipid membrane rather than a protein shell.

Internal Structures

As Figures 22 to 24 suggest, the proteins on the internal side of viral envelopes are significantly more varied in design than those in the outer shells of nonenveloped viruses, where most of the known outershell protein structures contain jelly-roll β-barrel domains. The alphaviruses have subverted a serine protease to serve as the principal domain of the capsid subunit (C) (29). The protease is functional in the single step required to cleave C from the nascent polyprotein of these positive-stranded RNA viruses. The core, sealed within the bilayer, can afford to be fenestrated. The hexamer and pentamer clusters of the protease domains do not contact each other, and coherence of the T=4 icosahedral lattice is maintained by interacting N-terminal arms. Thus, these positively charged arms, like those of TBSV (see Fig. 8), appear to knit the core together as well as to recognize and neutralize RNA. The hepatitis B capsid is also an open, almost lattice-like, structure, formed by a largely α-helical subunit that can assemble into either T=3 or T=4 shells (14). The retroviral Gag precursor is usually anchored by an N-terminal myristoyl group to the membrane bilayer, and successive domains are separated by cleavage into radially organized layers (see Fig. 23 and Chapter 27). The structures of the various domains from HIV-1 Gag have been determined (44), as have those of certain domains from a few other retroviruses.

Most viral envelope proteins are so-called type I membrane proteins, with a single transmembrane α-helix linking the ectodomain and the cytoplasmic tail. The transmembrane helices have been resolved in a recent cryoelectron microscopy study of Semliki Forest virus (69). In some positive-stranded RNA viruses, like the flaviviruses, where structural proteins are derived from a polyprotein precursor, the anchor may be an α-helical hairpin that traverses the membrane twice (24). Contacts between the cytoplasmic tails of viral envelope glycoproteins and target sites on the underlying core of matrix subunits generally determine specificity of envelope protein incorporation. These interactions usually involve a short segment of envelope polypeptide, fitting against a site on the internal protein (13,66,75). Individual interactions are weak, and bilayer disruption by nonionic detergents readily dissociates them. But the cooperativity imparted by lateral contacts, both within the core or matrix and within the outersurface layer, is strong, and the ensemble of cooperative, weak interactions drives budding.

Surface Proteins

The proteins on the surface of an enveloped virus must carry out at least two functions: receptor (and co-receptor) binding and fusion. In addition, there may be a receptor-destroying enzyme (e.g., the influenza-virus neuraminidase or the coronavirus esterase), to promote viral release. The membrane of influenza A contains a fourth activity: a proton channel that assists uncoating and transcriptase activation (M2). In some cases (e.g., rhabdoviruses and retroviruses), the receptor-binding and fusion activities are combined in a single protein; in others (e.g., paramyxoviruses), there are two distinct proteins to carry out these functions. A trimeric, coiled-coil fusion-protein structure, found in a wide range of enveloped viruses, is described later under Membrane Fusion.

Viral Entry into Cells

Receptor Binding

There are no simple generalizations about virus receptors and how they bind with viral surfaces (see Fig. 24). We note two broad issues here. The first is that most viruses have evolved a mechanism to avoid "getting stuck" at the cell surface when emerging from an infected cell. Many viruses simply bind weakly to their receptors and thus can dissociate in a reasonable time. The virulence of polyomavirus in mice is inversely related to viral affinity for its sialoglycoconjugate receptor (Fig. 25**A**), demonstrating that spread in the animal host, rather than entry into cells, is the principal correlate of pathogenesis (7). Like polyoma, influenza virus recognizes a sialic acid–containing carbohydrate for cell attachment (77) (see Fig. 25**B**). A receptor-destroying enzyme (neuraminidase) is present on the surface of the virion; its activity allows release of newly assembled virions from the cell surface through which they have budded (76). The neuraminidase is thus required for effective spread of the virus, and the enzyme is the target of antiinfluenza drugs, developed in part by exploiting knowledge of the neuraminidase structure (109). HIV-1 has several mecha-

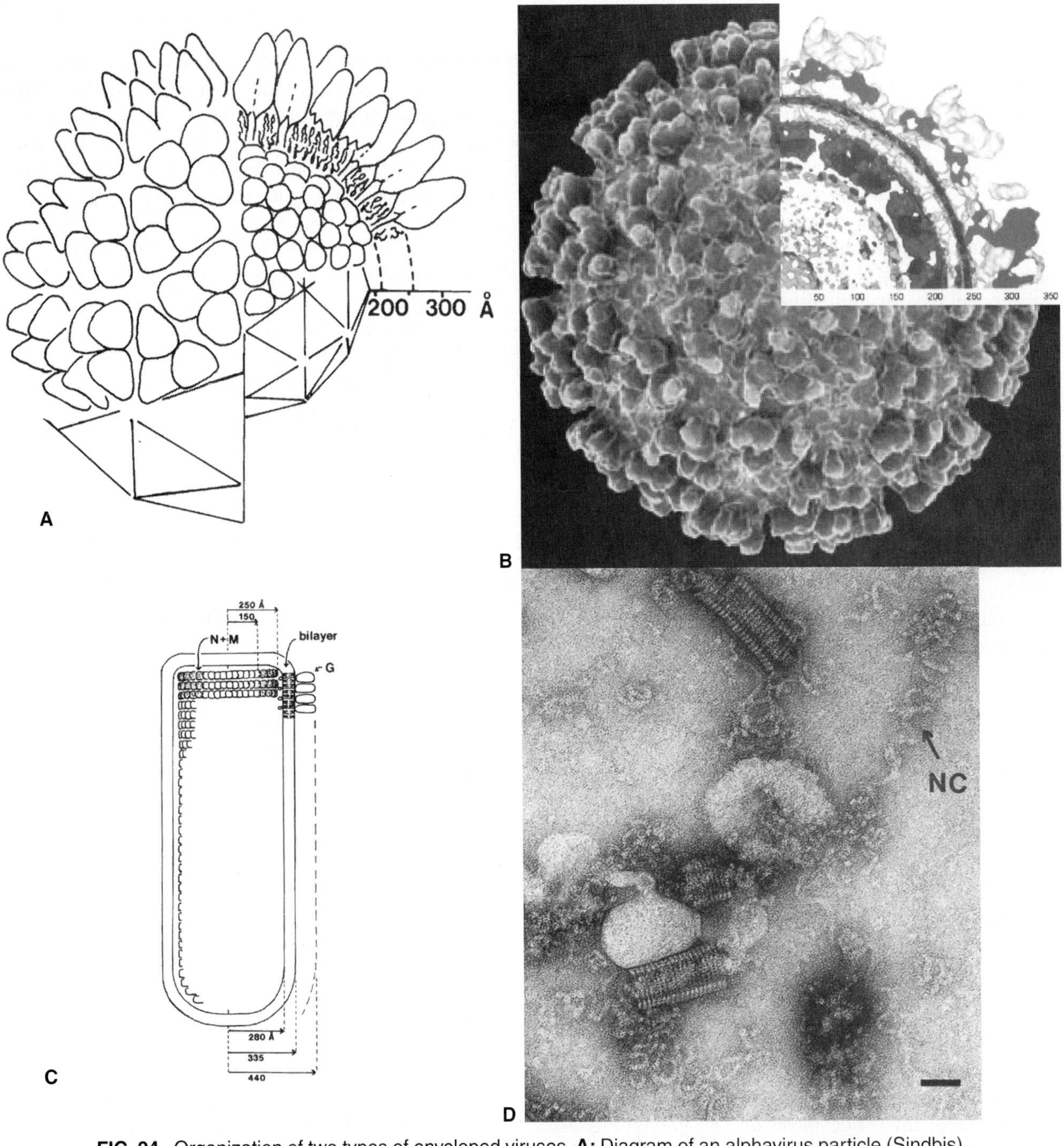

FIG. 24. Organization of two types of enveloped viruses. **A:** Diagram of an alphavirus particle (Sindbis). The pear-shaped objects represent the ectodomains of E1 and E2, closely associated as heterodimers and further clustered into trimers in the T=4 icosahedral lattice that describes the surface organization (107). There are 240 E1:E2 heterdimers in the complete particle. Hydrophobic transmembrane segments of E1 and E2 penetrate the lipid bilayer. A 33-residue internal domain on E1 mediates interactions with the core. The core also has a T=4 icosahedral structure (28). **B:** Reconstruction of the closely related Semliki Forest virus particle from cryoelectron microscopy at 10 Å resolution. Most of the figure shows a surface rendering; the *upper right-hand quadrant* shows a thin cross-section, with a scale to show radius (in angstoms), for comparison with the diagram in **A**. (Redrawn from ref. 69, with permission.) **C:** Diagram of the vesicular stomatitis virus (VSV) particle, showing the relationship of nucleocapsid (N), matrix protein (M), and glycoprotein (G) to the lipid bilayer. The scale of this diagram is about half that of the diagram in **A**, but the VSV genome is only slightly larger than that of Sindbis. The Sindbis RNA, which collapses into stem-loop structures in the interior of the core, is therefore markedly more condensed than the VSV RNA, which winds as an extended strand along the helical nucleocapsid. **D:** Electron micrograph of disrupted VSV, showing partially disassembled "cores." The hollow tubes are helically coiled nucleocapsid (*NC*), fixed into a rigid structure by interaction with M, which has probably dissociated from the more loosely coiled NC (e.g., *upper right*). Paramyxovirus nucleocapsids have a rather similar appearance, after release from disrupted particles.

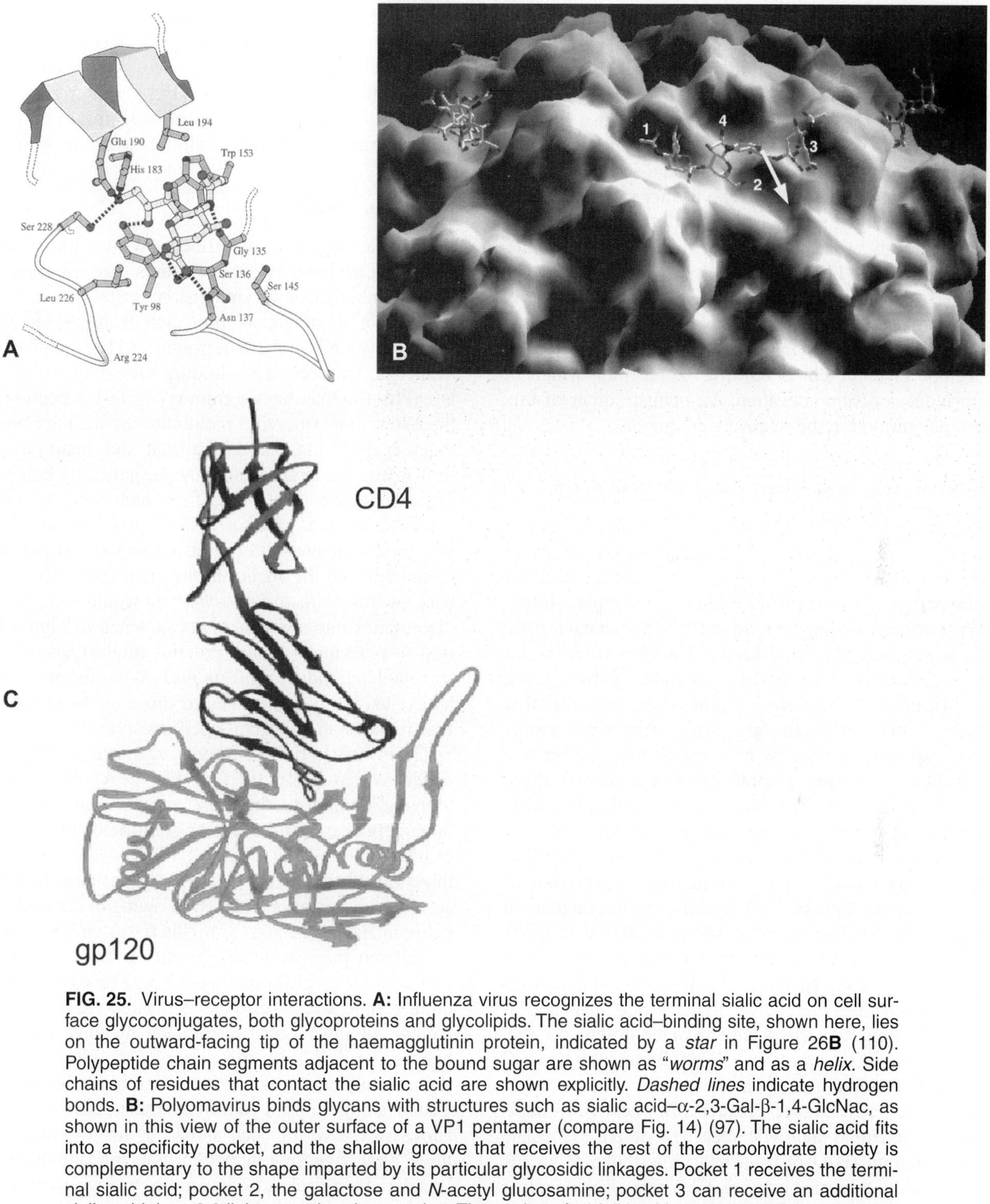

FIG. 25. Virus–receptor interactions. **A:** Influenza virus recognizes the terminal sialic acid on cell surface glycoconjugates, both glycoproteins and glycolipids. The sialic acid–binding site, shown here, lies on the outward-facing tip of the haemagglutinin protein, indicated by a *star* in Figure 26**B** (110). Polypeptide chain segments adjacent to the bound sugar are shown as "*worms*" and as a *helix.* Side chains of residues that contact the sialic acid are shown explicitly. *Dashed lines* indicate hydrogen bonds. **B:** Polyomavirus binds glycans with structures such as sialic acid–α-2,3-Gal-β-1,4-GlcNac, as shown in this view of the outer surface of a VP1 pentamer (compare Fig. 14) (97). The sialic acid fits into a specificity pocket, and the shallow groove that receives the rest of the carbohydrate moiety is complementary to the shape imparted by its particular glycosidic linkages. Pocket 1 receives the terminal sialic acid; pocket 2, the galactose and *N*-acetyl glucosamine; pocket 3 can receive an additional sialic acid, in α-2,6 linkage to the glucosamine. The pockets for sialic acid are structurally unrelated to the influenza sialic acid site. The affinity for an individual receptor group is very low (about 1 mmolar). The virus can probably bind glycan that is attached to any cell surface glycoprotein; the position and direction of the protein linkage is shown by the arrow. **C:** The complex of the core of the human immunodeficiency virus type 1 receptor–binding domain, gp120, with the receptor, CD4 (65). A key phenylalanine on CD4 fits into a hydrophobic pocket on gp120 (*center*).

nisms for down-regulating its receptor (CD4) after infection, both to avoid envelope–receptor interactions within the secretory pathway and to facilitate viral release after budding (see Chapter 28). The second broad issue is that some viruses require a cascade of at least two distinct receptors, in order to enter efficiently. One receptor is required for initial cell attachment and a second for triggering fusion or penetration. The former may be a quite broadly distributed molecule, like sialic acid or other glycans (heparan sulfate for HSV-1), or it may be a quite specific protein, like the adenovirus receptor, CAR, or the HIV-1 receptor, CD4 (see Fig. 25**C**). The latter is often called a *co-receptor,* for example, the chemokine receptors for HIV-1. In the case of HIV-1, CD4 primes the envelope glycoprotein to bind the co-receptor, which in turn induces fusion activation. An obligate order of this sort may turn out to be relatively common.

An Irreversible Step Between Assembly and Entry

Assembly of TMV protein and RNA into infectious particles was among the key observations that triggered thinking about viral symmetry. *In vitro* self-assembly of components from the mature virion into complete infectious particles is, however, an exceptional characteristic of the simplest plant and bacterial RNA viruses. A far more general property of virus assembly pathways is a modification, often a simple proteolytic cleavage, that "primes" the particle for large-scale, irreversible events accompanying entry. Loss of a scaffolding protein is a particularly extreme example of such a modification. Picornaviruses such as polio assemble from VP0, VP1, and VP3, but autolytic cleavage of VP0 into VP4 (an internal peptide) and VP2 accompanies assembly (see Chapter 18). When receptor binding triggers expansion of the viral shell, exit of VP4 renders the rearrangement irreversible (9). The receptor acts as a catalyst to lower the energy barrier to an irreversible reorganization. The function of this reorganization is viral entry, and the triggering mechanism has evolved to occur only in an appropriate location. Reoviruses have an outer protein, $\sigma 3$, that caps the penetration protein, $\mu 1$ (36). Proteolytic removal of $\sigma 3$ is required to render the particle competent to attach and penetrate (see Chapter 26). There is, in addition, an essential autolytic cleavage of $\mu 1$ (73). The hemagglutinin (HA) of influenza virus folds in the ER into a stable, trimeric structure. Cleavage of one peptide bond in HA by the protease, furin, in a compartment late in the secretory pathway, primes the protein to undergo a dramatic, low-pH triggered rearrangement (Fig. 26), which mediates fusion of viral and target cell membranes. In effect, cleavage renders the virion form of HA metastable, but the barrier to rearrangement is so great at neutral pH that no conformational change occurs. Proton binding in the low pH environment of the endosome removes this barrier and triggers a refolding of the HA protein. Protons have the role taken in other cases by a second receptor (e.g., the chemokine receptors for HIV-1). The expression "spring loaded" has been used to describe the state of HA at neutral pH after cleavage to HA1 and HA2 (21). "Jack-in-the-box" might be a comparable image for poliovirus after cleavage of VP0.

Membrane Fusion

The rearrangement of influenza virus HA, shown in Figure 26, has two essential features that also characterize a number of other viral fusion proteins. The first is ejection of a previously protected hydrophobic *fusion peptide,* which is at the N-terminus of HA2 in the case of influenza. The second is a folding back of the fusion protein (HA_2) so that the N-terminus (the fusion peptide) and the C-terminus (the viral membrane anchor) are brought together (92,111). Assuming that the fusion peptide inserts into the target membrane, as generally believed, a possible intermediate state, for which there is indirect evidence in the case of HIV-1 gp41, would be an extended structure with the fusion peptide buried in one membrane and the anchor in the other (Fig. 27). Folding back of this *prefusion intermediate* would bring the two membranes into apposition. As sketched in Figure 27, a ring of rearranged fusion proteins might be required to surround and induce a *fusion pore.* What further molecular events, if any, are needed to cause the two bilayers to fuse remains an important open question.

The influenza HA is a trimer, organized by a central α-helical coiled-coil (114) (see Fig. 25**A**). HA_1 forms a globular domain at the "top" of the molecule, with a binding pocket for the receptor, sialic acid (110). Binding of protons at low pH leads initially to dissociation of the three HA_1 "heads" from their docked positions (but not to complete dissociation from HA_2, owing to disulfide links between HA_1 and HA_2) (52). This first step liberates HA_2 to undergo the rearrangement shown in Figure 26. The product of this conformational change (see Fig. 25**B**) is a quite simple structure: there is a three-chain, α-helical, coiled-coil inner core, surrounded by three outer-layer helices, derived from the part of each HA_2 chain that immediately precedes the transmembrane anchor (15). The fusion proteins of paramyxoviruses, retroviruses, and filoviruses have all been shown to form similar structures, after triggering by fusion-inducing signals (93).

Are rodlike structures the only way in which molecular fold-back can bring about close approach of two membranes? Apparently not, because the flaviviruses have quite a different structure for their fusion protein, as exemplified by the E protein from tick-borne encephalitis virus (84). In that case, the fusion peptide is an internal loop, and the protein is a platelike rather than a rodlike molecule. Moreover, the E protein itself does not undergo cleavage; rather, proteolytic processing of a second protein, PrM, is the step that primes the virion for a

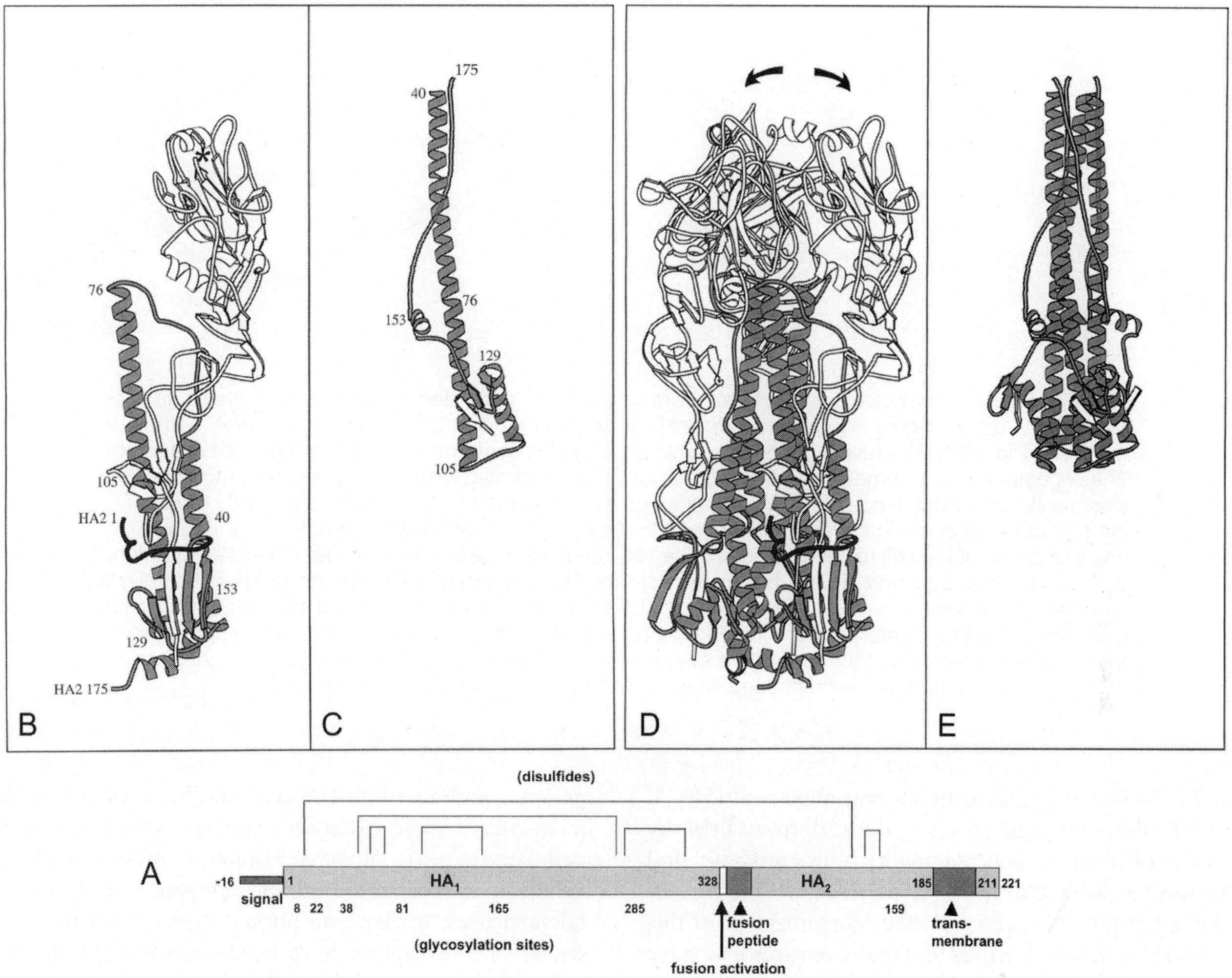

FIG. 26. Influenza-virus haemagglutinin (*HA*). **A:** Schematic representation of the primary structure of the 1968 Hong Kong virus HA, showing the ectodomain, HA_1 + HA_2(1–185), the transmembrane anchor (HA_2 185–211), and the cytoplasmic domain (HA_2 212–221). The cleavage site between HA_1 and HA_2 is labeled *fusion activation.* The secretion signal sequence (removed by signalase), S-S bridges, carbohydrate (CHO) attachment sites, and fusion peptide (N-terminus of HA_2) are shown. The uncleaved precursor is known as HA_0. **B** to **E:** The folded structure of HA and its rearrangement when exposed to low pH. **B:** The HA monomer: HA_1 is *light;* HA_2 is *dark;* the fusion peptide is *black.* Residue numbers in HA_2 are shown at several key positions to assist in visualizing the conformational change that occurs on fusion activation. The receptor-binding pocket in the β-barrel "top" domain of HA_1 is indicated with a *star* (compare Fig. 25**A**). The viral membrane would be at the bottom of this part of the figure. The transmembrane and cytoplasmic segments are not shown. **C:** The HA_2 monomer in the fusion-active form. A short segment of HA_1 (*white*) remains bound to the rearranged HA_2 in this structure. Note the dramatic conformational change, in which residues 40 to 105 become a continuous α-helix. The introduction of a kink at residue 105 also causes the "bottom" part of the molecule to turn upward, so that the N- and C-termini of the fragment are next to each other. Thus, the fusion peptide, extending from the N-terminus, and the transmembrane segment, extending from the C-terminus, would be spatially adjacent after the full conformational change. **D:** The HA trimer. The subunit toward the right in this illustration is viewed in essentially the same orientation as the monomer in **B.** HA_2 is shaded. Exposure to low pH initiates a conformational change, causing the "top" domains of HA_1 to move apart (*arrows at top of diagram*). **E:** The rearranged $\mathbf{HA_2}$ trimer. Imagine the tops of HA_1 to have spread to either side, and the three HA_2 monomers to have undergone rearrangement to the conformation shown in **C**. (Courtesy of F. Hughson, modified.)

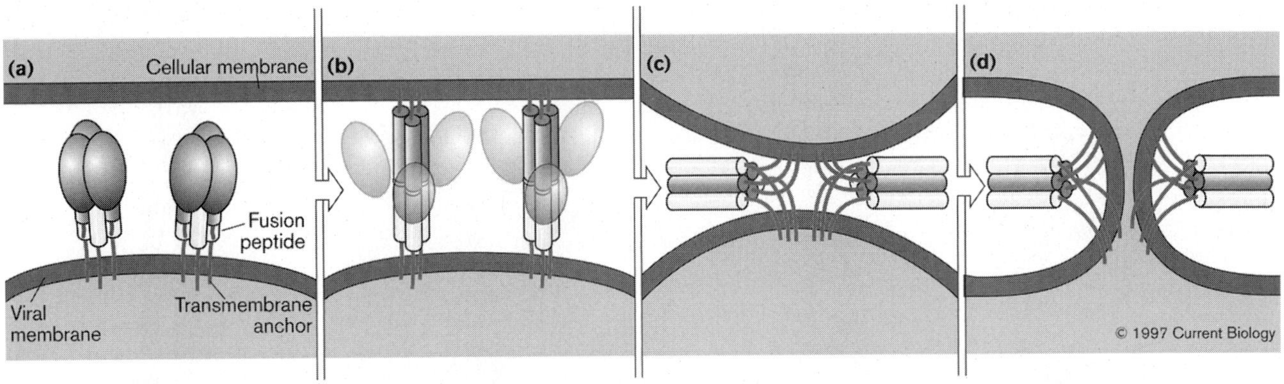

FIG. 27. Fusion. Schematic diagram of membrane fusion, as catalyzed by viral fusion proteins such as influenza virus hemagglutinin (HA). **A:** Neutral pH conformation of HA trimers in the viral membrane (compare Fig. 25D). The fusion peptides are buried. **B:** Initial conformation change triggered by low pH. The receptor-binding domains of HA_1 (ellipsoids) have separated from each other and from the HA_2 stems (although in influenza, they remain attached by a disulfide bond; in retroviruses, the corresponding SU fragment dissociates). The fusion peptides have been thrust by the conformational change into the membrane of the cell to be infected. **C:** The HA_2 stem folds back to form a chain-reversed structure, as seen in Figs. 26**C** and **E**. The fusion peptide and the transmembrane anchor of HA are brought together by the folding back. Because the former lies in the cell membrane and the latter in the viral membrane, the two membranes are forced to approach each other. As suggested by the diagram, more than one HA trimer is needed to form an effective fusion structure. **D:** Putative fusion pore, formed by local rearrangement of the two apposed bilayers. (Adapted from ref. 63, with permission).

low-pH triggered conformational rearrangement (58). E and M (the truncated product, derived from PrM by removal of most of its ectodomain) form an icosahedral array on the surface of the virus particle, and the fusion-inducing step involves a concerted reorganization of this array (41). The alphaviruses and rhabdoviruses also have fusion proteins with internal loops as their putative fusion peptides (see Chapters 19 and 22).

Penetration of Nonenveloped Viruses

Nonenveloped viruses must breach a membrane to access the cytoplasm or nucleus of a cell, but unlike their enveloped cousins, they cannot do so by membrane fusion. The molecular mechanism by which a nonenveloped virus particle, bound at the surface of a cell or taken up into an endosome, translocates itself (or its genome) across the intervening lipid bilayer is not fully understood. In general, it appears that binding of a receptor or co-receptor induces a conformational change in the virion and that a consequent exposure of previously buried hydrophobic elements is important for penetration. In several cases, at least one of the exposed hydrophobic elements is an N-terminal myristoyl group: on VP4 in picornaviruses (30), on VP2 in polyomaviruses (90), and on μ1 in reoviruses (74). Myristoyl groups target proteins to membranes, and it is logical to suppose that exposure of the myristoylated protein leads it to associate with membranes and ultimately to contribute to penetration.

One class of models for nonenveloped virus penetration invokes formation of a pore, through which the viral genome is drawn into the cell; another class of models postulates a more extensive, transient disruption of the cell membrane (or of the endosome) in order to admit the virion (in altered form) into the cytoplasm. In the case of adenoviruses, uptake into an endosome and subsequent endosomal disruption have been reported (43,56). The subviral particle admitted to the cytoplasm lacks pentons, as a result of events triggered by receptor and co-receptor binding; this partially stripped virion subsequently disassembles in association with a nuclear pore. The dsRNA viruses must likewise insert an intact, roughly 700 Å diameter inner capsid particle (the *core* in the case of reoviruses; the *double-layered particle* in the case of rotaviruses) into the cytoplasm. Indeed, this particle never uncoats because it contains the enzymes necessary for mRNA synthesis and modification (see Chapter 26 and Chapter 54, *Fields Virology*, 4th ed.). In the case of picornaviruses, receptor binding triggers a rearrangement or destabilization of the virion, exposing the myristoylated VP4 as well as a hydrophobic N-terminal segment of VP1 (45,53,59,60,71). Formation of a pore in the endosomal membrane, through which the RNA passes, has been proposed. Such a model requires a mechanism by which secondary structural elements in the RNA are melted out to make translocation possible but for which candidate helicases have not been demonstrated. One possibility would be a ribosome, by analogy with an uncoating mechanism established (*in vitro*) for certain positive-stranded RNA plant viruses. With those viruses, exposure of the 5′ end of the RNA (e.g., through expansion of the virion induced by intracellular ionic conditions) leads to association of ribosomes with the still largely packaged RNA genome, and progress of the ribosome along the message-sense genome appears to generate uncoating (114). A similar mechanism could, in principle, draw RNA through a membrane pore as well as through an opening in the viral shell. An alternative picture for picornavirus penetration involves membrane disruption (a "large" pore), either by the altered particle plus VP4 or by the dissociated components; RNA unwinding is not required in this model.

STRUCTURE-BASED CATEGORIES OF VIRAL DESIGNS

A particularly noteworthy consequence of the proliferation of high-resolution structural information about viruses is the frequent discovery of totally unexpected relationships. This sort of surprise came early, when the determination of the structure of southern bean mosaic virus (SBMV) revealed that it closely resembled TBSV (1). Equally striking was the relationship between the picornaviruses and the T=3 plant viruses (62,89). Even the development of sensitive sequence alignment methods has failed to predict structural homologies that are obvious once high-resolution three-dimensional images are available. Thus, the number of strategies that evolution has found, for carrying out the functions that are embodied in virions, is smaller than one might have imagined. In the sections that follow, we attempt to group certain viruses or viral substructures, not by replication strategy or host range, but rather by three-dimensional organization and its functional consequences. The available structural information is by no means sufficient to make a full catalog, but there is reason to believe that in the future, newly determined structures are quite likely to look like something we have already seen in another, perhaps superficially unrelated, virus particle.

Simple, Icosahedrally Symmetric Capsids with Jelly-Roll β-Barrel Subunits

Small, Nonenveloped, Positive-Stranded RNA Viruses

The comparison in Figure 7 shows that picornaviruses and T=3 plant viruses have closely related architectural features, based on 180 jelly-roll β-barrels. Variant packing of the same sort of domain yield T=1 and T=4 structures, such as those found in STNV and in nodaviruses, respectively. Common features in addition to the shell domains themselves are the formation of an internal network of amino-terminal arms and (in the T=3 and T=4 structures) a specific switching mechanism to ensure accurate assembly. When this switching mechanism is disturbed (e.g., through cleavage of the amino-terminal arms), the same subunit that makes a T=3 structure can instead make a T=1 structure (94). Although the shells have a similar basic architecture, the loops between framework elements of the jelly-roll β-barrel vary enormously from one virus to another. These variations give rise to differences in receptor interactions, antigenic characteristics, and particle stability. The RNA bacteriophages have a T=3 icosahedral shell, but with a very different subunit architecture (104).

Parvoviruses

Parvoviruses have T=1 icoshedral shells (101). The subunit has a standard jelly-roll framework, but substantial insertions into the interstrand loops increase the volume of the capsid it forms. The jelly-roll cores pack neatly around the fivefold and twofold axes, roughly as in the T=1 variants of T=3 structures, but a very large (more than 200-residue) segment between strands G and H makes expanded contacts between threefold related monomers (see Fig. 4). The ssDNA phage ϕX174 has a shell in which subunits with a jelly-roll framework (protein F) interact very roughly, as in parvoviruses (70). Twelve pentamers of a distinct, jelly-roll subunit (protein G) decorate the surface: the protein G pentamers resemble the polyomavirus VP1 capsomeres in the packing of their subunits. Because there may be a restricted number of ways to organize jelly-roll structures into icosahedral shells, these similarities may not imply close evolutionary relationships.

Double-Stranded DNA Viruses

Papovaviruses

As described earlier (see Fig. 14), the assembly unit of the polyomaviruses and papillomaviruses is a pentamer of the major capsid protein (VP1 in polyomaviruses; L1 in papillomaviruses). The axes of the 72 pentamers that form the viral shell align with the vertices of a T=7 icosahedral lattice, but they do not conform to its symmetry because even the six-coordinated vertices have pentamers of the protein (82). The subunits have jelly-roll β-barrels as a framework, with relatively elaborate loops facing outward (26,67). Both the polyomaviruses and papillomaviruses have an internal protein (VP2/VP3 and L2, respectively). VP2 is probably required for penetration; L2 may have a similar function.

Adenoviruses

The architecture of adenoviruses is based on a shell of hexons, centered at the six-coordinated vertices of a T=25 icosahedral surface lattice. The hexons are trimers with an approximate internal repeat, making them pseudohexamers (see Fig. 16). The same fold has been discovered in the principal outershell subunit, P3, of bacteriophage PRD1 (10). The phage protein looks like a "stripped-down" version of the hexon: it lacks the elaborate projecting loops that form the principal antigenic structures in the adenovirus protein. This striking relationship between an animal-virus structural protein and a phage structural protein is evidently more than a simple convergence, but how viruses have made the presumed evolutionary jump is not clear. Phage PRD1 has a separate penton-base subunit and a penton fiber, just like adenoviruses, but it also has a lipid membrane just beneath the outer, adenovirus-like, pseudo T=25 lattice (10). Thus, the common shell can clearly be combined with different internal structures, depending on strategies for assembly, entry, and uncoating.

Herpesvirus Capsids

Herpesviruses are enveloped particles, but the capsid is an independently assembling entity that has many of the characteristics of a nonenveloped particle (100,116). The high-resolution structure of the principal herpesvirus capsid protein has yet to be determined. Moderate-resolution studies of capsid structure and assembly, using electron cryomicroscopy, show that the hexamers and pentamers of the major capsid protein are held together at local threefold positions by a heterotrimeric "triplex" complex, which may serve a function analogous to the cement proteins in adenoviruses. Assembly of the herpesvirus capsid by way of a scaffold-containing procapsid regulates morphogenesis at a different level (72).

Double-Stranded RNA Viruses

All dsRNA viruses of the *Reoviridae* family have a common design for the 120-subunit shell that serves as the major framework of the particle (57,83). The 120- to 140-kd protein that forms this shell—known as $\lambda1$ in reoviruses, VP2 in rotaviruses, VP3 in orbiviruses, and so forth—has the shape of a flattened teardrop. Five copies radiate from a fivefold axis, like petals of a gently cupped flower, and five further copies insert between them. This decamer may also be the assembly unit. Certain other components (an RNA polymerase or helicase; capping enzymes) are associated with each fivefold, and it is logical to suppose that they are incorporated as part of a 12-decamer assembly mechanism (see Chapter 26). The outer layers of protein, which surround the common framework, differ significantly from one genus of this family to another. Of the nine genera, four have pentameric "turrets" that project outward from each fivefold axis of the framework shell. The structure of the reovirus core (83) shows that the turrets are hollow cylinders, with the active sites of the capping enzymes facing their inner cavity. The mRNA is capped as it is exported through these structures. Members of the other five genera contain a protein with the various capping activities inside the framework shell; it is likely that the capping protein is associated directly with the polymerase. The outermost layers of the dsRNA viruses are specialized for their specific routes of assembly and entry, and the proteins in this layer appear to be the least conserved from one genus to another.

There are three other families of dsRNA viruses, including ones that infect lower eukaryotes as well as the enveloped $\phi6$ phage of *Pseudomonas syringae*. Image reconstructions from electron cryomicroscopy of exemplars of each of these families demonstrate structural features in common with *Reoviridae* (3). The fungal and bacterial viruses both have a principal shell with 120 subunits. Thus, it is possible that the designs of all dsRNA viruses, even those of bacteria, are based on a similar framework.

Enveloped Positive-Stranded RNA Viruses

The alphaviruses and flaviviruses are T=4 and (probably) T=3 icosahedral assemblies, respectively (41,107). There is at present no structural information for pestiviruses or for hepatitis C. The various proteins derive from a single polyprotein; in the alphaviruses, the core and the envelope have the same T=4 surface lattice, as expected from a uniform stoichiometry. Parallels between alphaviruses and flaviviruses are only hinted at by structures currently known. The flavivirus envelope proteins are PrM and E, found in that order in the polyprotein. PrM is a "chaperone" subunit: cleavage of PrM exposes E for low-pH triggered rearrangement. The corresponding envelope proteins in alphaviruses are PE2 and E1; cleavage of PE2 to E2 and E3 (E3 is lost in some cases, not in others) primes E1 for a fusion transition. Appreciation of detailed structural parallels, if any, between flavivirus E and alphavirus E1 must await the crystal structure of the latter (F. Rey, in progress). The flavivirus receptor-binding domain is on E; the alphavirus receptor-binding protein is E2. Transfer of this function from the fusion subunit to the chaperone subunit may parallel the association of receptor binding and fusion on one protein in orthomyxoviruses and the separation of these functions in paramyxoviruses.

Enveloped Viruses with Trimeric, α-Helical, Coiled-Coil Fusion Proteins

A Fundamental Fusion Module

The envelopes of orthomyxoviruses, paramyxoviruses, filoviruses and retroviruses all contain a glycoprotein with a fundamental fusion module, into which may be inserted domains that carry out other functions. Using the HA of influenza virus A as a model (see Fig. 26), the fusion module comprises HA_2 plus the very beginning and the very end of HA_1. The HA_1 N- and C-terminal segments are part of the folded structure of the fusion module in its precursor state; they do not contribute to the rearranged structure that forms after triggering by exposure to low pH. The organization of the hemagglutinin-esterase-fusion (HEF) protein of influenza C (and of

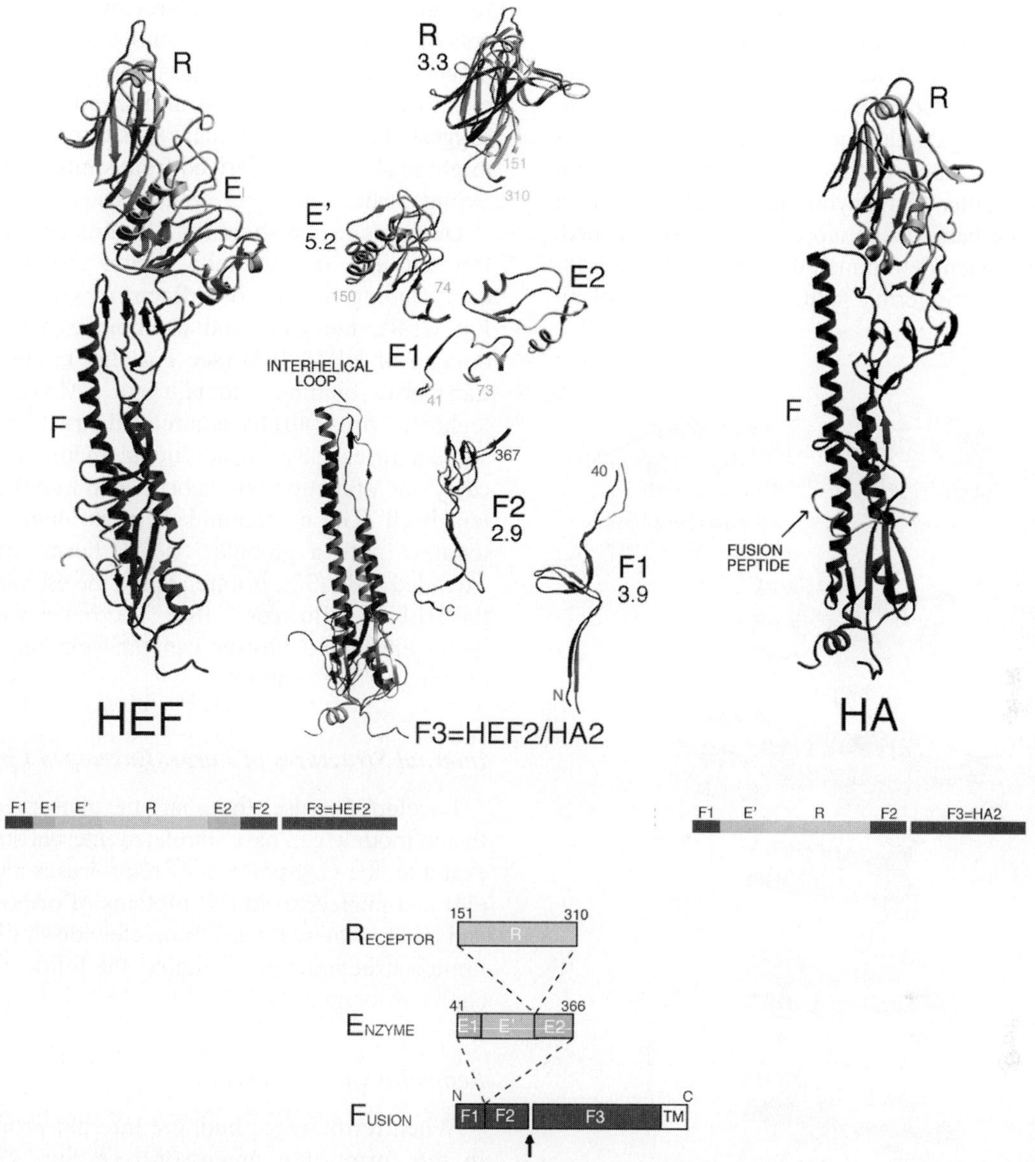

FIG. 28. Comparison of the fusion proteins from influenza C (*HEF*—haemagglutinin-esterase-fusion protein) and influenza A (*HA*) reveals a common core fusion module (*F*), into which evolution appears to have inserted the enzymatic domain (*E*) that catalyzes cleavage of the receptor (in influenza C) and then a receptor-binding domain (*R*). Parts of the E domain have been deleted in the HA of influenza A, leaving R as the only functional part of the insert. (Influenza A has a separate receptor-destroying enzyme, the neuraminidase.) The pattern of insertions is shown in the diagram at the *bottom* of the figure. The core F module thus comprises a segment F1, N-terminal to the insertion point for E (and R), and a segment F2-F3, C-terminal to this point. The fusion-activating cleavage separates F2 from F3 (*arrow in bottom diagram*). F3 is thus known as HEF_2 or HA_2 in influenza C and A, respectively. After triggering by low pH, F3 rearranges. *Top left: Ribbon diagram of one subunit of the HEF trimer from influenza C.* Top right: Similar diagram of a subunit of the HA trimer from influenza A. Compare the view of the HA subunit in Figure 26**B**. Beneath each ribbon diagram is a *bar,* showing the arrangement of segments in the polypeptide chain, *shaded* to correspond to the shading in the ribbon diagram. In the *top center* are ribbon diagrams of the various segments, with their conformations in HEF and HA superimposed. (From ref. 92, with permission; see also ref. 87).

coronaviruses) is particularly revealing (88) (Fig. 28). This protein has three activities: receptor (9-*O*-acetyl-sialic acid) binding (H), receptor hydrolysis (E), and fusion (F). The receptor-binding domain (homologous to the receptor-binding domain in HA from influenza A) is inserted into a surface loop on the esterase domain (homologous to other acetyl hydrolases), which is in turn inserted into the basic fusion apparatus as just defined. Structures have been determined of fusion-module fragments (in the posttriggering state) from members of all four groups of viruses listed previously. They reveal variants of a conserved, trimeric unit (Fig. 29). Although the precursor state (before triggering) is known only for HA of influenza A and HEF of influenza C, it is plausible to suggest that similar final (posttriggering) structures might in all cases be derived from similar initial (pretriggering) structures.

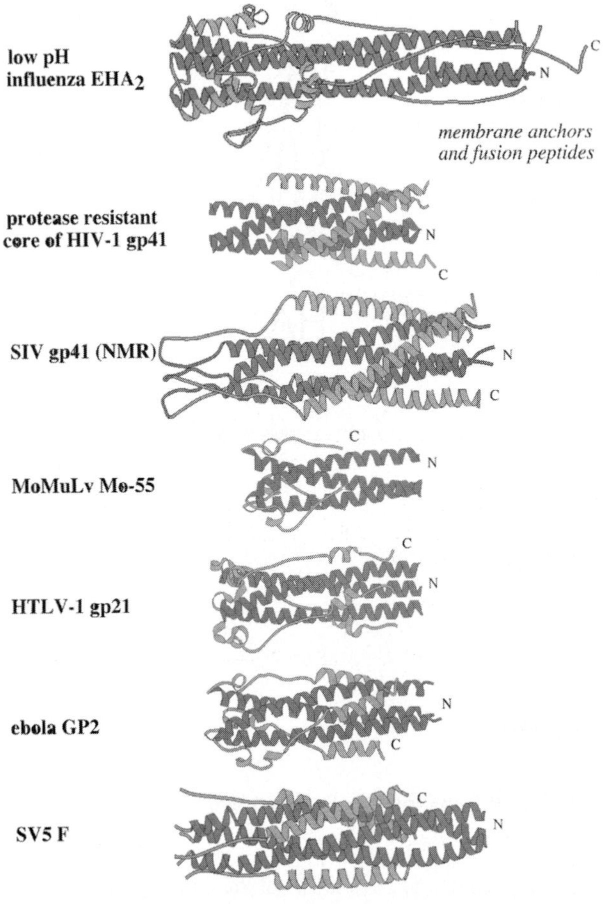

FIG. 29. The core fusion modules from influenza virus (HA_2), human immunodeficiency virus type 1 (HIV-1) and simian immunodeficiency virus (SIV; gp41), Moloney murine leukemia virus (TM), human T-cell lymphotropic virus type 1 (HTLV-1; gp21), Ebola virus (GP2), and SV5 (F), all rearrange after triggering to form related structures. There is a central coiled-coil, formed by three copies of the polypeptide chain segment that immediately follows the fusion peptide, and an outer layer of three helices, formed by the polypeptide chain segments that immediately precede the transmembrane anchor. The fusion peptides and membrane anchors are thus brought together (on the right-hand side of the figure). The fold-back regions on the left have various sizes and characteristics, and they have been deleted in most of the structures actually determined. Note that in all cases, the structures shown here correspond to the "F3" segment of a fusion protein, as defined in Figure 28. (From ref. 92), with permission.)

Diverse receptor-binding domains can evidently be inserted into the common fusion module. The sialic acid–binding domain of influenza virus HA (110) (see Fig. 25**B**), the CD4 and chemokine receptor–binding domain of HIV-1 (65) (see Fig. 25**C**), and the arginine transporter–binding domain of Moloney murine-leukemia virus (40) have unrelated structures. Moreover, some viruses have an additional membrane protein to carry out a function not incorporated into the fusion protein itself. The neuraminidase of influenza A and B, a tetramer with a globular "head" borne on a flexible, extended stalk (32), is unrelated to the esterase domain in the HEF of influenza C (88). The outer surfaces of the larger enveloped viruses can thus exhibit considerable combinatorial variability.

Internal Structures of Large, Enveloped Viruses

Enveloped viruses that share the conserved coiled-coil fusion module can have unrelated internal structures. For example, the Gag proteins of retroviruses and the matrix (M) and nucleocapsid (N) proteins of orthomyxoviruses and paramyxoviruses are completely dissimilar. From the limited structural data available, the following groupings can be discerned.

Retroviral Gag Proteins

When retroviruses bud, the internal protein (Gag) is in the form of a precursor (see Fig. 23). The key domains of this precursor are MA (matrix), CA (capsid), and NC (nucleocapsid); some retroviruses have additional fragments. MA, which trimerizes (probably already before cleavage of the precursor), associates with the inner face of the bilayer. Except in avian retroviruses, it bears an N-terminal myristoyl group, which helps anchor it to the membrane. MA from HIV-1 and from human T-cell lymphotropic virus type II (HTLV-II) have similar structures (31). In HIV-1, MA forms regions of hexagonal lattice, but it does not appear to make a regular icosahedral shell (46). Cleavage of the Gag precursor, subsequent to budding, leads to significant internal rearrangements. In this process, CA assembles into a defined, internal capsid that encloses the two packaged copies of the RNA genome and the associated NC domains. The morphology of the capsid, as seen in the electron microscope, appears to differ from one type of retrovirus to another; a detailed picture is available only for HIV-1 (48–50). Nonetheless, clear structural similarities among CA proteins from HIV-1, HTLV-I, and Rocus sarcoma virus (19) suggest that the fundamental assembly scheme is likely to be similar in all cases. The NC domain contains one or two (depending on the virus) zinc knuckle domains—small, folded modules stabilized by a Zn^{2+} ion (see Chapter 27). These structures recognize the specific viral packaging signal (see Fig. 20**B**), but they also interact nonspecifically with other segments of genomic RNA (35).

Nucleocapsids and Matrix Proteins of Negative-Stranded RNA Viruses

The genomes of negative-stranded RNA viruses are associated with the viral nucleocapsid protein (N), which remains bound even during transcription. The N proteins of myxoviruses, paramyxoviruses, filoviruses, and rhabdoviruses have similar molecular masses (about 50 kd), and apparent N-protein sequence similarities have been reported among members of the last three of these viral families (5). The ribonucleoprotein complex of Sendai virus has been analyzed by electron microscopy (38). Its most condensed form is a stiff, helical rod, with a pitch of 53 Å and about 13.1 NP subunits per left-handed turn. RNA and protein are wound together, and there appear to be exactly six nucleotides per subunit (18,38). The total length of the rod is 1.1 μm (11,000 ÅÅ); its outer diameter is about 200 Å, and there is a 50 Å diameter hollow core. This form is clearly too stiff and too long to fit into the roughly spherical virions, of about 1000 Å diameter, and indeed much more flexible rods can be seen, corresponding to various degrees of uncoiling of the helix just described (38). The stiff rod could, in principle, represent a transcriptionally active state, if the polymerase were to wind its way down the central hollow and if the bases of the encapsidated RNA were to face inward. Alternatively, it may simply be an intermediate between initial assembly and viral budding.

The VSV ribonucleoprotein complex (RNP) contains eight to nine nucleotides per N-protein subunit. Association with the matrix protein (M) imparts a fixed, tightly coiled structure to the RNP, and this assembly also gives the virion its elongated, bullet-like shape. The dimensions of the viral core are shown in Figure 24**C**. It has a much larger diameter than the paramyxovirus RNP rod just described. The rigid form of the VSV RNP–M complex can be produced either by recombinant coexpression of N and M (which presumably leads to assembly on cellular RNA) or by disassembly of virions. Removal of M produces a far more loosely and flexibly coiled form of the RNP: images from electron microscopy resemble a released spring (Fig. 24**D**). M also mediates incorporation of the envelope glycoprotein (G). Its location with respect to the RNP coil has not, however, been determined unambiguously. Thus, although the structural information currently available hints strongly at parallels between paramyxoviruses and rhabdoviruses, the details remain to be determined.

REFERENCES

1. Abad-Zapatero C, Abdel-Meguid SS, Johnson JE, et al. Structure of southern bean mosaic virus at 2.8 Å resolution. *Nature* 1980;286: 33–39.
2. Ansel-McKinney P, Gehrke L. RNA determinants of a specific RNA-coat protein peptide interaction in alfalfa mosaic virus: Conservation of homologous features in ilarvirus RNAs. *J Mol Biol* 1998;278: 767–85.
3. Baker TS, Olson NH, Fuller SD. Adding the third dimension to virus life cycles: Three-dimensional reconstruction of icosahedral viruses. *Microbiol Mol Biol Rev* 1999;63:862–922.
4. Barouch DH, Harrison SC. The interaction between the major and minor coat proteins of polyomavirus. *J Virol* 1994;68:3982–3989.
5. Barr J, Chambers P, Pringle CR, Easton AJ. Sequence of the major nucleocapsid protein gene of pneumonia virus of mice: Sequence comparisons suggest structural homology between nucleocapsid proteins of pneumoviruses, paramyxoviruses, rhabdoviruses, and filoviruses. *J Gen Virol* 1991;72:677–685.
6. Battiste JL, Mao H, Rao NS, et al. Alpha helix-RNA major groove recognition in an HIV-1 rev peptide-RRE RNA complex. *Science* 1996;273:1547–1551.
7. Bauer PH, Cui C, Stehle T, et al. Discrimination between sialic acid-containing receptors and pseudoreceptors regulates polyomavirus spread in the mouse. *J Virol* 1999;73:5826–5832.
8. Bawden FC, Pirie NW. Crystalline preparations of tomato bushy stunt virus. *Br J Exp Pathol* 1938;29:251–263.
9. Belnap DM, Filman DJ, Trus BL, et al. Molecular tectonic model of virus structural transitions: The putative cell entry states of poliovirus. *J Virol* 2000;74:1342–1354.
10. Benson SD, Bamford JK, Bamford DH, Burnett RM. Viral evolution revealed by bacteriophages PRD1 and human adenovirus coat protein structures. *Cell* 1999;98:825–833.
11. Bernal JD, Fankuchen I. Structure types of protein "crystals" from virus-infected plants. *Nature* (London) 1939;139:923–924.
12. Bernhard W. Electron microscopy of tumor cells and tumor viruses: A review. *Cancer Res* 1958;18:491–509.
13. Bottcher B, Tsuji N, Takahashi H, et al. Peptides that block hepatitis B virus assembly: Analysis by cryomicroscopy, mutagenesis and transfection. *EMBO J* 1998;1998:23.
14. Bottcher B, Wynne SA, Crowther RA. Determination of the fold of the core protein of hepatitis B virus by electron cryomicroscopy. *Nature* 1997;386:88–91.
15. Bullough PA, Hughson FM, Skehel JJ, Wiley DC. The structure of influenza haemagglutinin at the pH of membrane fusion. *Nature* 1994; 371:37–43.
16. Burnett RM. Structural investigations on hexon, the major coat protein of adenovirus. In: McPherson A, Jurnak FA, eds. *Biological macromolecules and assemblies*. New York: Wiley, 1984:337–385.
17. Butler PJ, Finch JT, Zimmern D. Configuration of tobacco mosaic virus, RNA during virus assembly. *Nature* 1977;265:217–219.
18. Calain P, Roux L. The rule of six, a basic feature for efficient replication of Sendai virus defective interfering RNA. *J Virol* 1993;67: 4822–4830.
19. Campos-Olivas R, Newman JL, Summers MF. Solution structure and dynamics of the Rous sarcoma virus capsid protein and comparison with capsid proteins of other retroviruses. *J Mol Biol* 2000;296:633–649.
20. Carey J, Cameron V, de Haseth PL, Uhlenbeck OC. Sequence-specific interaction of R17 coat protein with its ribonucleic acid binding site. *Biochemistry* 1983;22:2601–2610.
21. Carr CM, Kim PS. A spring-loaded mechanism for the conformational change of influenza hemagglutinin. *Cell* 1993;73:823–832.
22. Casjens S, King J. Virus assembly. *Annu Rev Biochem* 1975;44: 555–611.
23. Caspar DLD, Klug A. Physical principles in the construction of regular viruses. *Cold Spr Harb Symp Quant Biol* 1962;27:1–24.
24. Chambers TJ, Hanh CS, Galler R, Rice CM. Flavivirus genome organization, expression, and replication. *Annu Rev Microbiol* 1990;44: 649–688.

25. Chen X, Stehle T, Harrison SC. Crystal structure of a C-terminal fragment of polyomavirus internal protein VP2 and its interaction with VP1. *EMBO J* 1998;17:3233–3240.
26. Chen XS, Garcea R, Goldberg I, Harrison SC. Structure of small virus-like particles assembled from the L1 protein of human papillomavirus 16. *Mol Cell* 2000;5:557–567.
27. Chen ZG, Stauffacher C, Li T, et al. Protein-RNA interactions in an icosahedral virus at 3.0 A resolution. *Science* 1989;245:154–159.
28. Cheng RH, Kuhn RJ, Olson NH, et al. Nucleocapsid and glycoprotein organization in an enveloped virus. *Cell* 1995;80:621–630.
29. Choi H-K, Tong L, Minor W, et al. Structure of sindbis virus core protein reveals a chymotrypsin-like serine proteinase and the organization of the virion. *Nature* 1991;354:37–43.
30. Chow M, Newman JF, Filman D, et al. Myristylation of picornavirus capsid protein VP4 and its structural significance. *Nature* 1987;327:482–486.
31. Christensen AM, Massiah MA, Turner BG, et al. Three-dimensional structure of the HTLV-II matrix protein and comparative analysis of matrix proteins from the different classes of pathogenic human retroviruses. *J Mol Biol* 1996;264:1117–1131.
32. Colman PM, Varghese JN, Laver WG. Structure of the catalytic and antigenic sites in influenza virus neuraminidase. *Nature* (London) 1983;303:41–47.
33. Crick FHC, Watson JD. Structure of small viruses. *Nature* (London) 1956;177:473–375.
34. Crowther RA, Klug A. Structural analysis of macromolecular assemblies by image reconstruction from electron micrographs. *Annu Rev Biochem* 1975;44:161–182.
35. De Guzman RN, Wu ZR, Stalling CC, et al. Structure of the HIV-1 nucleocapsid protein bound to the SL3 psi-RNA recognition element. *Science* 1998;279:384–388.
36. Dryden KA, Wang G, Yeager M, et al. Early steps in reovirus infection are associated with dramatic changes in supramolecular structure and protein conformation: Analysis of virions and subviral particles by cryoelectron microscopy and image reconstruction. *J Cell Biol* 1993;122:1023–1041.
37. Earnshaw WC, Harrison SC. DNA arrangement in isometric phage heads. *Nature* 1977;268:598–602.
38. Egelman EH, Wu SS, Amrein M, et al. The Sendai virus nucleocapsid exists in at least four different helical states. *J Virol* 1989;63:2233–2243.
39. Everitt E, Lutter L, Philipson L. Structural proteins of adenovirus, XII. Location and neighbor relationship among proteins of adenovirion type 2 as revealed by enzymatic iodination, immunoprecipitation and chemical cross-linking. *Virology* 1975;67:197–208.
40. Fass D, Davey RA, Hamson CA, et al. Structure of a murine leukemia virus receptor-binding glycoprotein at 2.0 angstrom resolution. *Science* 1997;277:1662–1666.
41. Ferlenghi I, Thomas D, Rey F, et al. Molecular organization of a recombinant subviral particle from tick-borne encephalitis virus. *Mol Cell* (in press).
42. Fisher AJ, Johnson JE. Ordered duplex RNA controls capsid architecture in an icosahedral animal virus. *Nature* 1993;361:176–179.
43. FitzGerald DJ, Padmanabhan R, Pastan I, Willingham MC. Adenovirus-induced release of epidermal growth factor and Pseudomonas toxin into the cytosol of KB cells during receptor-mediated endocytosis. *Cell* 1983;32:607–617.
44. Frankel AD, Young JA. HIV-1: Fifteen proteins and an RNA. *Annu Rev Biochem* 1998;67:1–25.
45. Fricks CE, Hogle JM. Cell-induced conformational change in poliovirus: Externalization of the amino terminus of VP1 is responsible for liposome binding. *J Virol* 1990;64:1934–1945.
46. Fuller SD, Wilk T, Gowen BE, et al. Cryo-electron microscopy reveals ordered domains in the immature HIV-1 particle. *Curr Biol* 1997;7:729–738.
47. Furciniti PS, Van Oostrum J, Burnett RM. Adenovirus polypeptide IX revealed as capsid cement by difference images from electron microscopy and crystallography. *EMBO J* 1989;8:3563–3570.
48. Gamble TR, Vajdos FF, Yoo S, et al Crystal structure of human cyclophilin A bound to the amino-terminal domain of HIV-1 capsid. *Cell* 1996;87:1285–1294.
49. Gamble TR, Yoo S, Vajdos FF, et al. Structure of the carboxyl-terminal dimerization domain of the HIV-1 capsid protein. *Science* 1997;278:849–853.
50. Ganser BK, Li S, Klishko VY, et al. Assembly and analysis of conical models for the HIV-1 core. *Science* 1999;283:80–83.
51. Glucksman MJ, Bhattacharjee S, Makowski L. Three-dimensional structure of a cloning vector: X-ray diffraction studies of filamentous bacteriophage M13 at 7 Å resolution. *J Mol Biol* 1992;226:455–470.
52. Godley L, Pfeifer J, Steinhauer D, et al. Introduction of intersubunit disulfide bonds in the membrane-distal region of the influenza hemagglutinin abolishes membrane fusion activity. *Cell* 1992;68:635–645.
53. Gomez Yatal A, Kaplan G, Racaniello VR, Hogle JM. Characterization of poliovirus conformational alteration mediated by soluble cell receptors. *Virology* 1993;197:501–505.
54. Gouet P, Diprose JM, Grimes JM, et al. The highly ordered double-stranded RNA genome of bluetongue virus revealed by crystallography. *Cell* 1999;97:481–490.
55. Gralla J, DeLisi C. mRNA is expected to form stable secondary structures. *Nature* 1974;248:330–332.
56. Greber UF, Willetts M, Webster P, Helenius A. Stepwise dismantling of adenovirus 2 during entry into cells. *Cell* 1993;75:477–486.
57. Grimes JM, Burroughs JM, Gouet P, et al. The atomic structure of the bluetongue virus core. *Nature* 1998;395:470–478.
58. Guirakhoo F, Heinz FX, Mandl CW, et al. Fusion activity of flaviviruses: Comparison of mature and immature (prM-containing) tick-borne encephalitis virions. *J Gen Virol* 1991;72:1323–1329.
59. Guttman N, Baltimore D. A plasma membrane component able to bind and alter virions of poliovirus type 1: Studies on cell-free alteration using a simplified assay. *Virology* 1977;82:25–36.
60. Hall L, Rueckert RR. Infection of mouse fibroblasts by cardioviruses: Premature uncoating and its prevention by elevated pH and magnesium chloride. *Virology* 1971;43:152–165.
61. Harrison SC, Olson A, Schutt CE, et al. Tomato bushy stunt virus at 2.9 Å resolution. *Nature* (London) 1978;276:368–373.
62. Hogle JM, Chow M, Filman DJ. Three-dimensional structure of poliovirus at 2.9 Å resolution. *Science* 1985;229:1358–1365.
63. Hughson FM. Enveloped viruses: A common mode of membrane fusion. *Curr Biol* 1997;7:R565–569.
64. Hunter E. Macromolecular interactions in the assembly of HIV and other retroviruses. *Semin Virol* 1994;5:71–83.
65. Kwong PD, Wyatt R, Robinson J, et al. Structure of an HIV gp120 envelope glycoprotein in complex with the CD4 receptor and a neutralizing human antibody. *Nature* 1998;393:648–659.
66. Lee S, Owen KE, Choi HK, et al. Identification of a protein binding site on the surface of the alphavirus nucleocapsid and its implication in virus assembly. *Structure* 1996;4:531–541.
67. Liddington RC, Yan Y, Zhao HC, et al. Structure of simian virus 40 at 3.8 Å resolution. *Nature* 1991;354:278–284.
68. Liljas L, Unge T, Jones TA, et al. Structure of satellite tobacco necrosis virus at 3.0 Å resolution. *J Mol Biol* 1982;159:93–108.
69. Mancini EJ, Clarke M, Gowen BE, et al. Cryo-electron microscopy reveals the functional organization of an enveloped virus, Semliki Forest virus. *Mol Cell* 2000;5:255.
70. McKenna R, Xia D, Willingman P, et al. Atomic structure of single-stranded DNA bacteriophage FX174 and its functional implications. *Nature* 1992;355:137–143.
71. Moscufo N, Yafal AG, Rogove A, et al. A mutation in VP4 defines a new step in the late stages of cell entry by poliovirus. *J Virol* 1993;67:5075–5078.
72. Newcomb WW, Homa FL, Thomsen DR, et al. Assembly of the herpes simplex virus capsid: characterization of intermediates observed during cell-free capsid formation. *J Mol Biol* 1996;263:432–446.
73. Nibert ML, Fields BN. A carboxy-terminal fragment of protein ml/m1C is present in infectious subvirion particles of mammalian reoviruses and is proposed to have a role in penetration. *J Virol* 1992;66:6408–6418.
74. Nibert ML, Schiff LA, Fields BN. Mammalian reoviruses contain a myristoylated structural protein. *J Virol* 1991;65:1960–1967.
75. Owen KE, Kuhn RJ. Alphavirus budding is dependent on the interaction between the nucleocapsid and hydrophobic amino acids on the cytoplasmic domain of the E2 envelope glycoprotein. *Virology* 1997;230:187–196.
76. Palese P, Tobita K, Ueda M, Compans RW. Characterization of temperature sensitive influenza virus mutants defective in neuraminidase. *Virology* 1974;61:397–410.

77. Paulson JC, Sadler JE, Hill RL. Restoration of specific myxovirus receptors to asialoerythrocytes by incorporation of sialic acid with pure sialyltransferases. *J Biol Chem* 1979;254:2120–2124.
78. Prasad BV, Hardy ME, Dokland T, et al. X-ray crystallographic structure of the Norwalk virus capsid. *Science* 1999;286:287–290.
79. Prasad BV, Prevelige PE, Marietta E, et al. Three-dimensional transformation of capsids associated with genome packaging in a bacterial virus. *J Mol Biol* 1993;231:65–74.
80. Puglisi JD, Tan R, Calnan BJ, et al. Conformation of the TAR RNA-arginine complex by NMR spectroscopy. *Science* 1992;257:76–80.
81. Rand RP, Luzzati V. X-ray diffraction study in water of lipids extracted from human erythrocytes: The position of cholesterol in the lipid lamellae. *Biophys J* 1968;8:125–137.
82. Rayment I, Baker TS, Caspar DLD, Murakami WT. Polyomavirus capsid structure at 22.5 Å resolution. *Nature* 1982;295:110–115.
83. Reinisch K, Nibert M, Harrison SC. The reovirus core: structure of a complex molecular machine. *Nature* 2000;404:960–967.
84. Rey FA, Heinz FX, Mandl C, et al. The envelope glycoprotein from tick-borne encephalitis virus at 2 Å resolution. *Nature* 1995;375:291–298.
85. Rhee SS, Hunter E. A single amino-acid substitution within the matrix protein of a type D retrovirus converts its morphogenesis to that of a type C retrovirus. *Cell* 1990;63:77–86.
86. Roberts MM, White JL, Grütter MG, Burnett RM. Three-dimensional structure of the adenovirus major coat protein hexon. *Science* 1986;232:1148–1151.
87. Robinson IK, Harrison SC. Structure of the expanded state of tomato bushy stunt virus. *Nature* (London) 1982;297:563–568.
88. Rosenthal PB, Zhang X, Formanowski F, et al. Structure of the haemaggluntinin-esterase-fusion glycoprotein of influenza C virus. *Nature* 1998;396:92–96.
89. Rossmann MG, Arnold E, Erickson JW, et al. Structure of a human common cold virus and functional relationship to other picornaviruses. *Nature* 1985;317:145–153.
90. Sahli R, Freund R, Dubensky T, et al. Defect in entry and altered pathogenicity of a polyoma virus mutant blocked in VP2 myristylation. *Virology* 1993;192:142–153.
91. Salunke DM, Caspar DLD, Garcea RL. Self-assembly of purified polyomavirus capsid protein VP1. *Cell* 1986;46:895–904.
92. Skehel JJ, Wiley DC. Coiled coils in both intracellular vesicle and viral membrane fusion. *Cell* 1998;95:871–874.
93. Skehel JJ, Wiley DC. Receptor binding and membrane fusion in virus entry: The influenza hemagglutinin. *Annu Rev Biochem* 2000;69:531–569.
94. Sorger PK, Stockley PG, Harrison SC. Structure and assembly of turnip crinkle virus. II. Mechanism of reassembly in vitro. *J Mol Biol* 1986;191:639–658.
95. Steere RL, Schaffer FL. The structure of crystals of purified mahoney poliovirus. *Acta Biochem Biophys* 1958;28:241.
96. Stehle T, Gamblin SJ, Yan Y, Harrison SC. The structure of simian virus 40 refined at 3.1 Å resolution. *Structure* 1996;4:165–182.
97. Stehle T, Yan Y, Benjamin TL, Harrison SC. Structure of murine polyomavirus complexed with an oligosaccharide receptor fragment. *Nature* 1994;369:160–163.
98. Stewart PL, Burnett RM, Cyrklaff M, Fuller SD. Image reconstruction reveals the complex molecular organization of adenovirus. *Cell* 1991;67:145–154.
99. Stewart PL, Fuller SD, Burnett RM. Difference imaging of adenovirus: Bridging the resolution gap between x-ray crystallography and electron microscopy. *EMBO J* 1993;12:2589–2599.
100. Trus BL, Booy FP, Newcomb WW, et al. The herpes simplex virus procapsid: Structure, conformational changes upon maturation, and roles of the triplex proteins VP19c and VP23 in assembly. *J Mol Biol* 1996;263:447–446.
101. Tsao J, Chapman MS, Agbandge M, et al. The three-dimensional structure of canine parvovirus and its functional implications. *Science* 1991;251:1456–1464.
102. Turner DR, Joyce LE, Butler PJG. The tobacco mosaic virus assembly origin RNA. *J Mol Biol* 1988;203:531–547.
103. Valegard K, Murray JB, Stockley PG, et al. Crystal structure of an RNA bacteriophage coat protein-operator complex. *Nature* 1994;371:623–626.
104. Valegard K, Murray JB, Stonehouse NJ, et al. The three-dimensional structures of two complexes between recombinant MS2 capsids and RNA operator fragments reveal sequence-specific protein-RNA interactions. *J Mol Biol* 1997;270:724–738.
105. van Raaij MJ, Mitraki A, Lavigne G, Cusack S. A triple beta-spiral in the adenovirus fibre shaft reveals a new structural motif for a fibrous protein. *Nature* 1999;401:935–938.
106. Vogel RH, Provencher SW, von Bonsdorff CH. Envelope structure of Semliki Forest virus reconstructed from cryo-electron micrographs. *Nature* 1986;320:533–535.
107. Von Bonsdorff CH, Harrison SC. Sindbis virus glycoproteins form a regular icosahedral surface lattice. *J Virol* 1975;16:141–145.
108. Von Bonsdorff CH, Pettersson RF. Surface structure of Uukuniemi virus. *J Virol* 1975;16:1296–1307.
109. von Itzstein M, Wu W-Y, Kok GB, et al. Rational design of potent sialidase-based inhibitors of influenza virus replication. *Nature* 1993;363:418–423.
110. Weis W, Brown J, Cusack S, et al. The structure of the influenza virus haemagglutinin complexed with its receptor, sialic acid. *Nature* (London) 1988;333:426–431.
111. Weissenhorn W, Dessen A, Calder LJ, et al. Structural basis for membrane fusion by enveloped viruses. *Mol Membr Biol* 1999;16:3–9.
112. Wikoff WR, Johnson JE. Virus assembly: Imaging a molecular machine. *Curr Biol* 1999;9:R296–300.
113. Wiley DC, Skehel JJ. Crystallization and x-ray diffraction studies on the haemagglutinin glycoprotein from the membrane of influenza virus. *J Mol Biol* 1977;112:343–347.
114. Wilson IA, Skehel JJ, Wiley DC. Structure of the haemagglutinin membrane glycoprotein of influenza virus at 3 Å resolution. *Nature* (London) 1981;289:366–373.
115. Wynne SA, Crowther RA, Leslie AG. The crystal structure of the human hepatitis B virus capsid. *Mol Cell* 1999;3:771–780.
116. Zhou ZH, Dougherty M, Jakana J, et al. Seeing the herpesvirus capsid at 8.5 Å. *Science* 2000;2888:877–880.
117. Zimmern D, Wilson TMA. Location of the origin for viral reassembly on tobacco mosaic virus RNA and its relation to stable fragment. *FEBS Lett* 1976;71:294–298.

CHAPTER 4

Virus Entry and Uncoating

John A. T. Young

IDENTIFICATION AND CHARACTERIZATION OF VIRAL RECEPTORS AND CORECEPTORS

The first step of viral infection requires the binding of viral attachment proteins to specific cell surface receptors and, in some cases, also to coreceptors. Following binding, viruses penetrate a cellular membrane, delivering the viral genome into the host cell cytoplasm. Viral genomes enter cells either as naked nucleic acid molecules, as is seen with a number of plus-strand RNA viruses, or instead as nucleoprotein complexes as with minus-strand RNA viruses, retroviruses, and DNA viruses. Coincident with, or immediately following, their entry into the cell, virions undergo *uncoating* events involving the step-wise disassembly of viral components, leading to genome replication.

This chapter will review some aspects of our current understanding of viral entry and uncoating mechanisms.

Viral Receptors and Coreceptors

Because of their critical involvement in the early steps of infection, viral receptors and coreceptors are major determinants of viral tropism. Viral receptors are defined as cell surface factors that bind directly to native virions and include proteins such as the CD4 receptor for the human and simian immunodeficiency viruses (HIV and SIV, respectively) (130) and polio virus receptor (PVR) for polioviruses (141). In addition to primary binding receptors, some viruses also interact with secondary receptors (coreceptors) that can bind either to native virions or instead to altered forms of virions that are produced as a result of the primary binding step. Viral coreceptors include a variety of CC and CXC chemokine receptors for different strains of HIV and SIV (19), the HveA, HveB, and HveC mediators of herpesvirus entry (82,143,213), and specific integrins used by adenoviruses (222).

Genetic and Receptor-Interference Approaches to Understand Viral Receptors

Genetic and viral receptor-interference studies have been used widely to characterize the nature of virus–receptor interactions. A classical genetic approach is to mate together two parental individuals, one that expresses candidate receptors and the other that does not. The individual progeny of these crosses are then analyzed for their susceptibility to viral infection. These studies can establish the existence of one or more putative viral receptor genes, can determine whether such genes are autosomal or sex-linked, may reveal functionally distinct alleles of these genes, and will establish whether susceptibility to infection is a dominant or a recessive trait.

A second genetic approach involves mapping a putative receptor gene to a specific chromosomal location by analyzing panels of somatic cell hybrids formed between donor cells that express receptors and recipient cells that do not. The chromosomal location of a putative receptor gene can then be deduced by identifying donor cell–derived genomic DNA fragments that are shared between independent somatic cell hybrids that display the appropriate receptor activity. This approach led to the mapping of the putative receptor genes for polytropic and xenotropic murine leukemia viruses (MLVs) and for measles virus, to specific portions of chromosomes 1 from mice and humans, respectively (63,101).

Receptor-interference studies can classify viruses into different receptor usage groups and can indicate whether virus infection abrogates expression of a putative receptor. One approach is based on the principle that cells infected by a given virus are often resistant to superinfection by other viruses that use the same receptor. By contrast, the infected cells remain fully susceptible to infection by viruses that use distinct cellular receptors (Fig. 1A). This technique led to the classification of retroviruses into several distinct receptor usage groups (190).

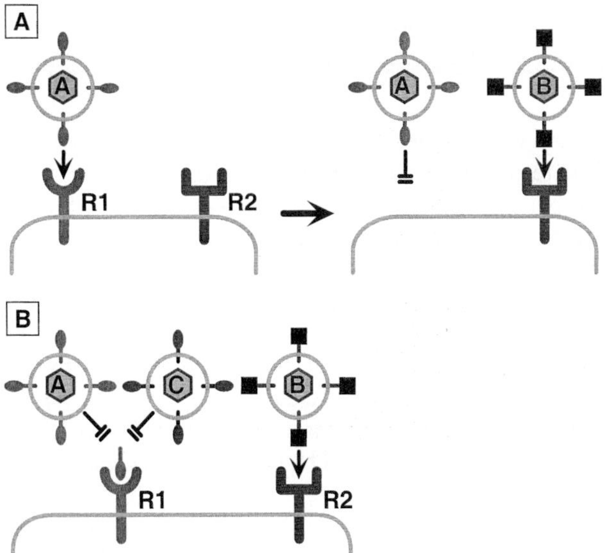

FIG. 1. Viral receptor interference. **Panel A:** Following infection. The cellular receptors for virus type A and virus type B are designated as R1 and R2, respectively. Following infection, expression of the type A viral attachment protein may interfere with the function of R1, leading to a specific block to superinfection by other type A viruses. **Panel B:** Mediated by a soluble viral attachment protein. In this example, type A viruses and type C viruses share the R1 receptor. A soluble form of the type A viral attachment protein may block infection by types A and C viruses, but it will have no effect on the type B virus–R2 interaction.

Although most viruses that establish receptor-interference are thought to do so by forming a complex between newly synthesized viral attachment proteins and the cellular receptor, in most cases the cellular compartment where this occurs is not known. However, in the case of HIV-1, the viral envelope protein (Env) can form a complex with CD4 within the endoplasmic reticulum (ER) and thus interfere with the transport of the receptor to the cell surface (46). HIV-1 encodes two accessory proteins, Vpu and Nef, that also contribute to receptor down-regulation: Vpu causes the ubiquitin-dependent proteolysis of ER-retained CD4 proteins by a mechanism that involves the cellular proteins beta TrCp and Skp1p (132), and Nef seems to serve as an adaptor protein that can target cell surface CD4 for endocytic uptake through clathrin-coated pits (153). Although the Env, Vpu, and Nef proteins of HIV-1 are each capable of reducing cell surface levels of CD4, maximal receptor down-modulation occurs when all three proteins are expressed (37).

A second receptor-interference method used to define viral receptor usage groups relies on the ability of a soluble viral attachment protein to block infection by other viruses that share the same receptor (Fig. 1B). This technique was employed using soluble adenovirus-type 2 (Ad-2) fiber protein to indicate that Ad-2, Ad-5, and Coxsackie B viruses interact with a common receptor (127, 160). This notion was later confirmed when the Coxsackie and adenovirus receptor (CAR) that is shared by these viruses was identified (15,203).

Identification of Viral Receptors

Protein Receptors

Various techniques have been employed to identify viral receptors and coreceptors, including the use of specific monoclonal antibodies raised against cell surface proteins, gene and/or cDNA transfer strategies, the virus overlay protein blot assay, and screening the functions of cell surface proteins that are highly related to known viral receptors (Table 1).

Monoclonal antibodies that bind to specific cell surface proteins and block viral infection have been used extensively to identify viral receptors. Receptors identified by this approach include CD4 for HIV-1 (48,119, 130), intercellular adhesion molecule (ICAM)-1 for the major subgroups of rhinoviruses (89,192), MHVR/Bgp1(a) for mouse hepatitis virus A59 (68), $\alpha 2\beta 1$ integrin for echoviruses 1 and 8 (17), CAR for coxsackie B viruses, and adenoviruses (15,203), CD46 for measles virus (63), CR2 for Epstein-Barr virus (73,78,147), CD55 for different subtypes of echoviruses and coxsackie B viruses (14,16,212), aminopeptidase N for human coronavirus-229E and transmissible gastroenteritis virus

TABLE 1. *Protein viral receptors and coreceptors*

Virus	Family	Receptor	Function	Refs.
G-protein-coupled receptors				
HIV	*Retroviridae*	CXCR4	Chemokine receptor	71
HIV	*Retroviridae*	CCR3	Chemokine receptor	40, 62
HIV	*Retroviridae*	CCR2b	Chemokine receptor	62
HIV	*Retroviridae*	CCR8	Chemokine receptor	180
HIV/SIV	*Retroviridae*	CCR5	Chemokine receptor	4, 40, 55, 62, 65
HIV/SIV	*Retroviridae*	Bonzo/STRL-33/TYMSTR	Chemokine receptor	5, 56, 125, 126
HIV/SIV	*Retroviridae*	BOB/GPR15	Chemokine receptor	56, 69
SIV	*Retroviridae*	GPR1	Chemokine receptor	69
Proteins with multiple membrane-spanning domains				
GALV/FeLV-B/SSAV	*Retroviridae*	PiT-1	Phosphate transport	152, 201
MLV-E	*Retroviridae*	MCAT-1	Cationic amino acid transport	3
MLV-A	*Retroviridae*	PiT-2	Phosphate transport	142, 207
MLV-X/MLV-P	*Retroviridae*	XPR1/Rmc1/SYG1	Transporter	12, 199, 229
Immunoglobulin-related proteins				
Poliovirus	*Picornaviridae*	PVR	Unknown	141
PRV/BHV-1	*Herpesviridae*	PVR	Unknown	82
HSV-1/HSV-2/PRV	*Herpesviridae*	Prr2/HveB	Unknown	213
HSV-1/HSV-2/ BHV-1/PRV	*Herpesviridae*	Prr1/HveC	Unknown	82
Coxsackie B	*Picornaviridae*	CAR	Unknown	15, 203
Ad-2/Ad-5	*Adenoviridae*	CAR	Unknown	15, 203
MHV-A59	*Coronaviridae*	MHVR/Bgp1 (a)	Biliary glycoprotein	68
Major rhinoviruses	*Picornaviridae*	ICAM-1	Cell adhesion/signaling	89, 192
HIV/SIV	*Retroviridae*	CD4	T-cell signaling	130
HHV-7	*Herpesviridae*	CD4	T-cell signaling	129
Low-density lipoprotein receptor–related proteins				
ALV-A	*Retroviridae*	TVA	Unknown	11
Minor rhinoviruses	*Picornaviridae*	LDLR/α2MR/LRP	Lipoprotein receptors	97
Integrins				
Adenovirus	*Adenoviridae*	$\alpha v\beta 3$	Vitronectin binding	222
Coxsackie A9	*Picornaviridae*	$\alpha v\beta 3$	Vitronectin binding	176
Adenovirus	*Adenoviridae*	$\alpha v\beta 5$	Vitronectin binding	222
Echoviruses-1/-8	*Picornaviridae*	$\alpha 2\beta 1$	Collagen/laminin binding	17
Tumor necrosis factor receptor–related proteins				
ALV-B/D/E	*Retroviridae*	TVB	Apoptosis-inducing receptor	1, 26
HSV-1	*Herpesviridae*	HveA	LIGHT receptor	136, 146
Small consensus repeat–containing proteins				
EBV	*Herpesviridae*	CR2	C3d/C3dg/iC3b binding	73, 78, 147
Measles	*Paramyxoviridae*	CD46	Complement inhibition	63
Echoviruses	*Picornaviridae*	CD55	Complement inhibition	14, 212
Coxsackie B-1/-3/-5	*Picornaviridae*	CD55	Complement inhibition	16, 184
Miscellaneous				
BLV	*Retroviridae*	BLVRcp1	Unknown	9
Coronavirus-229E/TGEV	*Coronaviridae*	Aminopeptidase-N	Metalloproteinase	54, 231
LCMV/lassa fever virus	*Arenaviridae*	α-Dystroglycan	Laminin/agrin binding	31
Sindbis	*Togaviridae*	Laminin receptor	Laminin binding	211

Note: See text to identify abbreviations.

(54,231), and the high-affinity laminin receptor for Sindbis virus (211). Antibodies specific for the $\alpha v\beta 3$ and $\alpha v\beta 5$ integrins were also used to demonstrate that these cell surface factors can facilitate a post-binding step of adenovirus entry (222).

Gene-transfer and cDNA-transfer methods have been used to clone viral receptor and coreceptor genes. These approaches involve preparing genomic DNA libraries or cDNA libraries from donor cells that express a viral receptor and then introducing these molecules into a recipient cell type that lacks the receptor. Transduced cells that express the receptor are then identified either (a) because they become susceptible to viral infection or to virus-induced cell–cell fusion, or (b) because they acquire an ability to bind to a viral attachment protein. The viral receptor gene/cDNA can then be directly cloned from these cells.

Viral receptors and coreceptors that were identified by gene/cDNA transfer include PVR for polioviruses (141), PiT-1 for gibbon ape leukemia viruses/subgroup B feline leukemia viruses/simian sarcoma-associated viruses (152), ATRC1/MCAT-1 for ecotropic MLV (3), TVA and TVB for subgroups A, B, and D avian leukosis virus (ALV) (11,26,232), PiT-2 for amphotropic MLVs (142), CXCR4 for X4-tropic strains of HIV-1 (71), and HveA and HveB/Prr2 (poliovirus receptor-related protein 2) for herpes simplex viruses (HSV) (143,213). The use of retroviral cDNA libraries has greatly accelerated the pace of discovering new viral receptors, because putative receptor cDNA molecules can be directly isolated from transduced cells by polymerase chain reaction (PCR) amplification using oligonucleotide primers that are derived from the flanking sequences of the retroviral vector (12,56,168,199,229).

Several viral receptors, including low-density lipoprotein receptor (LDLR)-related receptor proteins for minor subgroups of rhinovirus (97) and α-dystroglycan for lymphocytic choriomeningitis virus and lassa fever virus (31), have been identified using the virus overlay protein blot assay. This assay relies on virion binding to receptors that have been immobilized on a membrane following SDS-polyacrylamide gel electrophoresis.

In some cases, receptors for specific viruses have been identified by testing the activities of either known viral receptors or highly related proteins. For example, the fact that HSV-1 and HSV-2 use Prr2/HveB as a mediator of viral entry led to the finding that these viruses can also use the highly related Prr1 protein for entry (82). Similarly, the identification of the CXCR4/fusin α-chemokine receptor for T-cell tropic strains of HIV (71), coupled with the observation that entry of macrophage-tropic (M-tropic) strains of HIV can be blocked specifically by certain β (CC)-chemokines (43), led to the remarkable discovery that a number of CXC and CC chemokine receptors can serve as coreceptors for different strains of HIV and SIV (5,39,40,55,56,62,65,69,125,126,180).

Carbohydrate Receptors

Certain viruses have evolved to use carbohydrate receptors that are expressed as components of cell surface glycoproteins or glycolipids (Table 2). Because these receptors are generally expressed on cell types from a number of different species, viruses that use carbohydrate receptors tend to have a broad host range.

Carbohydrate receptors can be identified by determining whether the treatment of cells with carbohydrate-destroying enzymes impacts virus binding and infection. Neuraminidase treatment was used to implicate sialic acid–bearing oligosaccharides as receptors for influenza A virus (158), Sendai virus (133), reovirus type 3 (7), porcine rotavirus (177), murine polyomavirus (80), and canine parvovirus (10). Furthermore, virus binding was restored by adding back sialic acid residues to asialylated membranes, confirming the role of this carbohydrate in virus attachment (18,80,93,158,177,198). Similar studies performed using heparinase- and/or heparitinase-treated cells indicated that HSV-1 and human cytomegalovirus (CMV) bind to cell surface heparan sulfate molecules, a result that was confirmed when these viruses failed to attach to cells deficient in heparan sulfate proteoglycan synthesis (45,227).

Carbohydrate-containing receptors have also been implicated using specific monoclonal antibodies that block viral attachment. An antibody that recognizes galactosyl ceramide (GalCer) specifically blocked HIV infection of certain cell types, suggesting that this glycolipid may act as an alternative viral receptor (92). Indeed, GalCer can bind with a high affinity to the HIV-1 Env protein (92,128).

Antibody-Dependent Enhancement of Viral Entry

In addition to classical receptor/coreceptor-dependent mechanisms of entry, viruses may also enter cells when they become complexed with subneutralizing amounts of virus-specific antibodies. Virus–antibody complexes can then be taken up into cells following their binding to immunoglobulin receptors expressed on the cell surface. This type of antibody-dependent enhancement (ADE) of viral infection has been observed through cellular Fc receptors with dengue virus (52), West Nile virus (32,159), influenza A viruses (202), and HIV-1 and HIV-2 (99,137,200). This effect is also seen with Epstein-Barr

TABLE 2. *Carbohydrate viral receptors*

Virus	Family	Receptor	Refs.
Influenza A	*Orthomyxoviridae*	Sialic acid–containing oligosaccharides	158
Sendai	*Paramyxoviridae*	Sialic acid–containing oligosaccharides	93, 133
Reovirus-3	*Reoviridae*	Sialic acid–containing oligosaccharides	7
Murine polyomavirus	*Papovaviridae*	Sialic acid–containing oligosaccharides	80
Canine parvovirus	*Parvoviridae*	Sialic acid–containing oligosaccharides	80
Influenza C	*Orthomyxoviridae*	9-O-acetylsialic acid	10
Human/bovine coronaviruses	*Coronaviridae*	N-acetyl-9-O-acetylsialic acid	209
HIV	*Retroviridae*	Galactosyl ceramide	92
HSV	*Herpesviridae*	Heparan sulfate	128
Human CMV	*Herpesviridae*	Heparan sulfate	45

HIV, human immunodeficiency virus; HSV, herpes simplex virus; CMV, cytomegalovirus.

virus (EBV) that is complexed with polymeric immunoglobulin A (pIgA) specific for the viral gp340 protein, raising the interesting possibility that this pathway of EBV infection may be important at mucosal surfaces of the body where this virus persists and where pIgA is produced (186). The existence of these alternative viral entry pathways indicates that in the absence of a robust immune response that generates high titers of neutralizing antibodies, viruses may be able to bypass their normal requirements for receptors and coreceptors for cell entry, potentially expanding their *in vivo* cell-type tropism.

THE ROLE OF ENDOCYTOSIS IN VIRAL ENTRY

After binding viral receptors and/or coreceptors, there are at least two major mechanisms of viral entry that can be distinguished by their requirement for a low pH environment. The pH-independent mechanism of viral entry is proposed to occur at neutral pH, involving viral entry either directly at the plasma membrane or instead from within endosomal compartments following endocytosis of virus–receptor complexes (Fig. 2) (Table 3). By contrast, the pH-dependent mechanism involves the trafficking of virus–receptor complexes to endosomes with an acidic lumenal pH, where the high concentration of protons serves to facilitate viral entry. These distinct mechanisms of viral entry have been distinguished by testing the effect on viral infectivity of treating cells with agents that act to neutralize acidic endosomal compartments such as lysosomotropic agents, carboxylic ionophores, and v-type H^+/ATPase inhibitors such as bafilomycin A1.

There are two major endocytic pathways that lead to virus uptake from the cell surface, one that is clathrin dependent and the other that is clathrin independent. Electron microscopy has proved useful for uncovering which of these pathways is used by a specific virus—for example, this approach provided strong evidence that influenza A virus enters cells through clathrin-coated pits

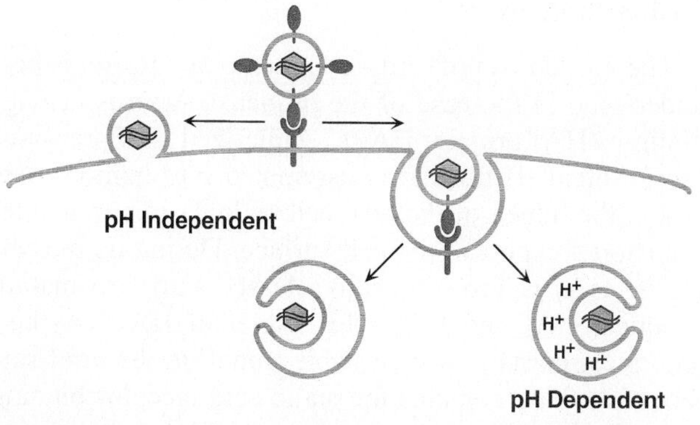

FIG. 2. The pH-independent and pH-dependent mechanisms of viral entry.

TABLE 3. *Examples of pH-Dependent and pH-Independent viruses*

pH-Dependent	pH-Independent
Influenza A virus	Retroviruses
Semliki Forest virus	Herpes simplex viruses
Vesicular stomatitis virus	Vaccinia virus
Reoviruses	Rotaviruses
Adenovirus	Paramyxoviruses

(135). However, a caveat in using this approach is that RNA viruses usually have a high particle-to-infectivity ratio, so there can be no guarantee that a virus that is imaged represents one that is truly infectious. Therefore, a more definitive approach is to assess the impact on virus infection of expressing dominant negative inhibitors that block cellular endocytic pathways.

Two such inhibitors have been tested for their impact on viral entry, dominant negative forms of the cellular guanosine triphosphatase (GTPase) dynamin and of caveolin. Dynamins constitute a large protein family with at least 27 distinct protein isoforms that are encoded by three separate cellular genes (Dyn1 to Dyn3) (138,182). These proteins are proposed to be "pinchases," or mechanoenzymes, that can constrict and sever membrane tubules into discrete membrane vesicles (138). Expression of a dominant-negative, GTPase-defective form of Dyn1 inhibits endocytosis through clathrin-coated pits as well as from caveolae, which are microdomains of the plasma membrane that are rich in cholesterol and glycosphingolipids (138,182). The dominant-negative Dyn1 protein blocks the entry of Semliki Forest virus, Sindbis virus, influenza virus, human rhinovirus 14, and adenovirus, indicating that each of these viruses uses a dynamin-dependent pathway for viral entry (58,178,210). By contrast, poliovirus and Moloney murine leukemia virus are apparently unaffected by the expression of this mutant protein, indicating that these viruses use a dynamin-independent mechanism of entry (58,121). A dominant-negative form of caveolin that prevents endocytosis through caveolae has been used to implicate these plasma membrane microdomains as the major sites of SV40 uptake into cells (100,150,157,179).

Factors That Influence Receptor Choice

A comparison of known viral receptors and coreceptors reveals that members of a given virus family have evolved to use a variety of different cell surface factors for viral entry. For example, a cell surface glycolipid, multiple membrane-spanning transporter proteins, and proteins that are members of the immunoglobulin, LDLR, and tumor necrosis factor receptor (TNFR) superfamilies are used as retroviral receptors (see Tables 1 and 2). Similarly, different picornaviral receptors include immunoglobulin-related proteins, an LDLR-related protein, integrins, and small consensus repeat–containing proteins that regulate complement activation (see Table 1).

Despite this heterogeneity of viral receptor usage, it is striking that several distinct viruses use precisely the same receptor. Two herpesviruses, pseudorabies virus and bovine herpes virus-type 1, can use the same cellular receptor as poliovirus, a picornavirus (see Table 1). Also, CD4 is a receptor used by retroviruses and by a herpesvirus, whereas CAR and $\alpha v\beta 3$ integrin are used by picornaviruses and adenoviruses (see Table 1).

This apparent convergence of receptor usage may simply be a coincidence. However, it seems much more likely that viruses have evolved to recognize receptors that have properties that are particularly well suited for mediating viral entry. Although these factors remain largely unknown, it intuitively seems that one important property would be the close proximity of the viral attachment site to the host cell membrane. Indeed, by varying the distance between the measles virus attachment site on the CD46 receptor and the host cell membrane, it has been possible to uncouple virus binding from entry (27). An additional factor that could influence receptor choice is the localization of that protein within specific microdomains of the plasma membrane and the subsequent membrane trafficking of that protein after virus binding—for example, SV40 binding leads to a clustering of the major histocompatibility complex (MHC) class I molecule receptors in caveolae, which represent the site of virus uptake into the cell (150,157).

Another factor that can influence receptor choice is the presence of receptor-associated signal transduction pathways that may facilitate steps of viral replication either during or after viral entry. Endocytosis of adenoviruses is stimulated by a signal transduction pathway linked to the integrin coreceptor that activates phosphoinositide-3-OH kinase (PI3K) and cellular Rho GTPases to stimulate the necessary rearrangements of the actin cytoskeleton (123,196). The actin cytoskeleton is also implicated as playing a critical role in the entry mechanisms used by other viruses such as HIV (103) and MLV (117). The interaction between the EBV gp350/220 protein and the CR2 receptor also activates a receptor-associated protein phosphorylation pathway that is important for the early steps of EBV replication (41,174). Similarly, the interaction of the CMV gB protein with an as yet unidentified receptor activates the interferon-responsive pathway, which may provide an optimal cellular environment for the subsequent transcription of viral genes (24).

Receptor interference, which is often observed after virus infection, may represent another selective force on viral receptor usage. For those viruses that assemble and bud at the plasma membrane, this block to cell surface receptor expression is presumably necessary to allow the efficient release of nascent viral particles. The fact that HIV-1 has evolved three separate mechanisms to interfere with cell surface CD4 expression (37) underscores the importance of receptor down-regulation for viral replication.

As discussed, receptor interference can prevent viral receptor expression on the cell surface because newly synthesized receptors and viral attachment proteins can form a complex that is retained within the cell. It therefore follows that the expression level of a given cellular factor may dictate whether it can be used as a viral receptor. Those factors that are expressed at a low level will presumably be more easily titrated out by viral attachment proteins than are factors that are expressed at a higher level.

Receptor interference may also prevent that cellular receptor from interacting with its cognate ligand and thus abrogate the normal receptor function. If the ligand–receptor pair in question plays a critical role in host defenses against virus infection, then this mechanism of interfering with receptor function may provide an additional level of selection on receptor choice. Indeed, this may explain why subgroups B, D, and E of ALV use TVB, a TNFR-related death receptor, as a viral receptor. TVB is most closely related to the human TRAIL (TNF-related apoptosis-inducing ligand) receptors, TRAIL-R1 (or DR4), and TRAIL-R2 (or DR5). TRAIL and its receptors have been implicated in the induction of apoptosis in cell populations infected with several distinct classes of viruses including HIV-1, human CMV, and adenoviruses (113,183,225). Therefore, certain subgroups of ALV may have evolved to use the TVB receptor, at least in part, because after the establishment of receptor interference, the infected cells may be protected against cell death induced by the cognate ligand (26).

ENVELOPED VIRUS ENTRY

Enveloped viruses have a lipid bilayer, or envelope, that surrounds their nucleocapsids. Therefore, the entry of these viruses into cells requires the fusion of viral and cellular membranes by a process that is driven by viral glycoproteins located on the virus surface.

The Influenza A Virus Paradigm and Related Viral Fusion Proteins

The mechanism of virus–cell membrane fusion is best understood in the case of the influenza A virus hemagglutinin (HA) protein. HA is synthesized as a precursor glycoprotein (HA_0) that is assembled into homotrimers within the lumen of the host cell endoplasmic reticulum prior to its export to the cell surface. During its biosynthesis, HA_0 is proteolytically cleaved into two mature subunits, HA_1 and HA_2. This trimer of HA_1/HA_2 heterodimers exists as a metastable trimer on the viral surface (33). HA_1 contains the sialic acid receptor binding site of the viral glycoprotein, and HA_2 contains two hydrophobic regions that are important for the complete fusion of virus and cell membranes, an N-terminal fusion peptide, and a membrane anchor located near the C-terminal end.

Following receptor binding, influenza viruses are endocytosed via clathrin-coated pits and then trafficked to acidic endosomes. The acidic lumenal environment of these endosomal compartments then activates irreversible conformational changes in HA that promote membrane fusion. These structural alterations can be detected as an increased susceptibility of the protein to cleavage by specific proteases such as trypsin and proteinase K (59,163). Also, these structural changes can be detected using conformation-specific antibodies to monitor the appearance and disappearance of certain epitopes of HA. For example, the fusion peptide region of HA_2, which is found buried at the trimer interface in the native HA structure, becomes rapidly exposed following low pH treatment, leading either to aggregation of the viral protein or to its attachment to membranes (59,115,187,219). By contrast, an epitope located at the interface between two HA_1 subunits in the native trimer is lost following this treatment, indicating that the HA_1 subunits must be dissociated from each other during the fusion reaction (115,219). Indeed, when intermonomer disulfide bonds were introduced into HA_1 subunits to prevent their dissociation from each other, this led to a specific block to the fusion activity of the viral glycoprotein (84,114).

During low pH–induced activation, the HA trimer is converted from its metastable state to one in which HA_2 adopts a highly stable trimeric structure. During this conversion, the hydrophobic fusion peptide regions of HA_2 are predicted to be displayed at the tip of a long, triple-stranded, α-helical coiled coil region that forms the core of the structurally altered viral glycoprotein (29,33,34). X-ray crystal structures of the native form of HA_2, as well as of an apparent postfusion form of this glycoprotein, are described in Chapter 3 and will not be discussed in detail here.

The exposed fusion peptide regions of HA_2 are critical for the membrane fusion reaction and have been proposed to bind directly to target membranes (Fig. 3). The importance of these regions for membrane fusion has been demonstrated using mutant viruses bearing amino acid replacements within this hydrophobic region. Although these altered viral glycoproteins can still bind to sialic acid receptors and are capable of undergoing the characteristic low pH–induced structural changes, their membrane fusion activities are abrogated (51,83,193). In addition, experiments performed with liposomes containing radiolabeled photoreactive lipids have demonstrated that the fusion peptide region is the only domain of HA_2 that becomes associated with a target lipid bilayer following the low pH activation (66).

It is thought that, following attachment of the HA_2 fusion peptides to the target membrane, this protein undergoes additional rearrangements, bringing the viral

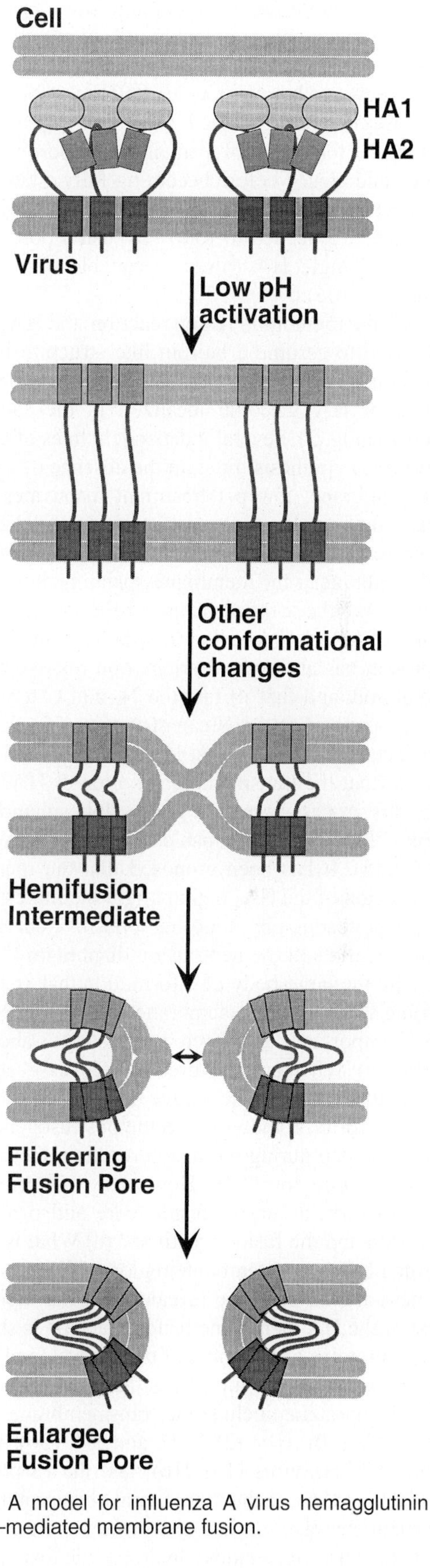

FIG. 3. A model for influenza A virus hemagglutinin (HA) protein–mediated membrane fusion.

and target lipid bilayers into close apposition (see Fig. 3). These rearrangements are thought to lead initially to mixing of lipids between the outer leaflets of membranes, a process known as hemifusion, leading to the formation of a hemifusion diaphragm (see Fig. 3). This step is then followed by the formation of a small fusion pore that flickers open and closed before becoming fully dilated (191). It has been suggested that at least three and perhaps six HA trimers are needed to form the fusion pore (22,50), although a single HA trimer is capable of perturbing membranes (106).

During the membrane fusion reaction, the HA_2 protein is proposed to assume a hairpin-like structure in which the fusion peptide domains and the transmembrane domains of HA_2 become localized in the same lipid bilayer (see Fig. 3). Several independent lines of evidence support this hypothesis. First, in the absence of a suitable target membrane, low pH treatment inactivates virions because the newly exposed fusion peptide domains become inserted in the viral membrane—that is, in the same membrane as the membrane-spanning domain (215, 218). Second, the x-ray structure of the low pH form of the core of HA_2 has revealed that the C-terminal end of this protein has an inverted orientation relative to its N-terminal end, and that in fact the N- and C-termini can combine, generating an N-cap structure (38). Whatever the precise mechanism is that leads to membrane fusion, it is clear that the transmembrane region of HA_2 is critical for this process because a glycosylphosphatidylinositol-linked form of HA is capable only of mediating hemifusion (115). It has been proposed that the membrane-anchor region of the HA_2 region might facilitate the complete fusion reaction by imposing a positive curvature on the inner leaflets of the hemifusion diaphragm (139).

Despite the large body of information that is available regarding HA-mediated membrane fusion, there are still several important unanswered questions about this process: (a) What are the precise step-wise structural changes that convert the native HA protein from its metastable form on the virion to the postfusogenic state? (b) At what step during the fusion reaction does the HA_2 hairpin structure form? (c) How many HA trimers are needed to form an active fusion pore and mediate the hemifusion and the fusion reactions? (d) What is the precise role of the transmembrane region of HA_2?

Structural analyses have revealed that the basic architecture of the HA membrane fusion machine is shared by the glycoproteins of a number of other enveloped viruses, including retroviruses, filoviruses, and paramyxoviruses. These glycoproteins include the transmembrane proteins of Mo-MLV (70), HIV (35,217), and SIV (30); the GP2 protein of Ebola virus (131,216); and the F_1 protein of SV5 (8). Like HA_2, each of these viral glycoproteins is the C-terminal cleavage product of a precursor envelope glycoprotein, and each contains a hydrophobic fusion peptide located near the N-terminal end and a single membrane-spanning anchor region located near the C-terminal end. Each of these viral glycoproteins can fold into a rodlike structure similar to that of activated HA_2, with the fusion peptide regions located at the tip of a central, triple-stranded, α-helical coiled, coil. Also, in some of these glycoproteins, three antiparallel helices are packed against the central, triple-stranded coil, coil domain, providing additional support for the idea that the fusion peptide and transmembrane regions of these glycoproteins become located in the same lipid bilayer at a late stage during membrane fusion (8,30,35,131,216,217).

In addition to the structural similarities observed between retroviral transmembrane and influenza virus HA_2 proteins, there is also biochemical evidence that, like HA, retroviral Env proteins must undergo conformational changes leading to viral entry. However, as most retroviruses are thought to enter cells by a pH-independent mechanism, it is presumed that fusion-activating conformational changes in Env are induced upon receptor/coreceptor binding. Consistent with this hypothesis, CD4-binding can induce conformational changes in the HIV-1 surface protein (SU) that, in lab-adapted viral strains, causes dissociation of the surface protein from the transmembrane protein, increases the exposure of certain antibody epitopes of Env, increases the susceptibility of the viral glycoprotein to protease cleavage, and leads to exposure of the coreceptor binding site of SU (173,181, 206,226,228). CD4 and coreceptor interactions also lead to exposure of hydrophobic determinants of HIV Env proteins as measured using a fluorescent probe that binds specifically to hydrophobic groups (108). Additional evidence for receptor-induced structural changes in retroviral glycoproteins has been obtained for a soluble ALV-A Env protein that is induced to undergo structural changes leading to fusion-peptide exposure and to stable liposome binding following its interaction with the TVA receptor (49,96).

Other Types of Viral Fusion Proteins

Although the core structural elements of the membrane fusion machinery described for the influenza HA protein are shared by many viruses, other enveloped viruses use fusion proteins with different architectures to enter cells. For example, the G protein of the rhabdovirus vesicular stomatitis virus (VSV) is a homotrimer of a single protein subunit with an internal hydrophobic fusion peptide region (79,220,233) that becomes labeled by hydrophobic photoactivatable probes under conditions that stimulate viral fusion (67). However, unlike HA, which irreversibly associates with target membranes following low pH-induced activation, VSV-G reversibly associates with these membranes, implying that it is less stably associated with target bilayers (156).

Another type of viral fusion protein is represented by the E protein of the tick-borne encephalitis virus (TBE), a flavivirus that contains two transmembrane segments and has a putative internal fusion peptide (171). The E protein of TBE exists as a dimer that is parallel to the membrane on the virus surface but is converted to a trimer that is active for membrane fusion when incubated under low pH conditions needed for membrane fusion (6,171).

Alphaviruses have yet another type of viral glycoprotein complex. Semliki Forest virus has three envelope proteins: E1 and E2, which are both type 1 membrane glycoproteins, and E3, which is an extrinsic protein. These proteins assemble as E1/E2/E3 heterotrimers. At low pH, the viral glycoprotein complex undergoes conformational changes leading to the formation of a stable E1 homotrimer that mediates membrane fusion (72,94).

More complex viral fusion machines are seen with the herpesviruses. Usually, five glycoproteins of HSV-1 are required for viral entry: gB and gC, which bind to cell surface heparan sulfate molecules; gD, which interacts with herpesvirus entry mediators such as HveA (143); and the gH/gL heterodimer, which participates in membrane fusion (166). Additionally, viral glycoproteins such as the gE/gI complex and gM can facilitate viral spread into certain cell types by interacting with receptors that are expressed at cell–cell junctions (166).

Regulating Viral Fusion Proteins

The membrane fusion activities of viral glycoproteins need to be tightly regulated to prevent their premature activation during viral protein synthesis and assembly. As described, the fusion activities of viral glycoproteins can be controlled by receptor/coreceptor interactions and by exposure to a suitable, low pH–containing environment. A number of viral glycoproteins are also regulated by proteolytic cleavage of their extracellular domains, which converts an energetically stable precursor glycoprotein to a metastable form that is then capable of being triggered for membrane fusion. This form of regulation is seen with the glycoproteins of orthomyxoviruses, paramyxoviruses, and retroviruses (95).

Amino acid residues located within the transmembrane and cytoplasmic tail domains of viral glycoproteins can also regulate their fusogenic activity. For example, the Env proteins of Mason Pfizer monkey virus and Mo-MLV become competent for fusion following viral protease-mediated cleavage at a specific site in their cytoplasmic tail domains (25,165,170). As retroviral proteases become activated at a late stage of viral replication that is coincident with, and/or occurs shortly after, virus budding, this form of regulation ensures that the viral glycoproteins are not prematurely activated within the virus producer cell. Specific mutations introduced into the transmembrane domain of VSV-G or into the transmembrane region or cytoplasmic tail domains of influenza virus HA, have also been shown to selectively block complete membrane fusion without affecting hemifusion (42,140). However, how these residues act to regulate membrane fusion remains to be determined.

Another mode of regulating viral fusion protein activity is seen with paramyxoviruses. For most of these viruses, with the exception of SV5, the fusogenic activity of the F protein is tightly regulated by its association with the homologous hemagglutinin (HN) protein that is responsible for receptor binding. Therefore, the fusion activation of paramyxoviral F proteins generally involves homotypic HN-F interactions following receptor binding (57,195,230). The coordinated action of separate viral attachment and fusion proteins presumably evolved to ensure that the fusion protein would become activated only following viral attachment to an appropriate target cell surface.

NONENVELOPED VIRUS ENTRY

Nonenveloped virus entry into cells involves either the formation of proteinaceous pores in a host cell membrane, as has been suggested for picornaviruses, or processes that disrupt the integrity of a cellular membrane, as seems to be the case for adenoviruses and reoviruses. A common feature of each of these viral entry mechanisms is the orchestrated disassembly of the virion leading to loss of specific capsid proteins and to the interaction of the viral particle with a host cell membrane.

It has been proposed that the positive-stranded RNA genome of picornaviruses enters cells through a proteinaceous core composed of viral proteins. Mature picornaviral virions contain a single copy of plus-stranded genomic RNA and 60 copies each of four viral proteins, VP1, VP2, VP3, and VP4. The VP1 proteins of poliovirus and of rhinovirus contain a deep surface depression, or canyon, located at each fivefold axis of symmetry. This canyon represents the site of receptor interaction on the viral surface (154,164).

During poliovirus entry, the viral particle undergoes a series of structural changes at the cell surface that are predicted to lead to the transfer of the viral RNA genome into the host cell cytoplasm to begin replication. The first change detected is the conversion of mature virions sedimenting as 160S particles to those that sediment at 135S (223). This alteration involves the loss of VP4, which is located within the virion interior, and the buried hydrophobic N-terminus of VP1 is translocated to the virion surface to mediate membrane binding (164,223). Thus, as for a number of enveloped viruses, exposure of hydrophobic viral protein surfaces is a critical event and required for poliovirus entry. A second similarity between polioviruses and the enveloped viruses discussed earlier is that poliovirus virions seem to exist in a metastable state and are converted to more highly stable forms during the process of viral entry (223). At physiologic temperatures, poliovirus is a conformationally dynamic entity, with VP4 and the N-terminal end of VP1 being transiently and reversibly exposed on the virus surface by a so-called breathing mechanism, even in the absence of a target cell (124). Reversible conformational changes in viral capsids have also been noted with rhinovirus (122), and with the nodavirus Flock House virus (23).

The data implicating 135S particles as obligatory intermediates during poliovirus entry are compelling. Receptor binding converts native virions to 135S particles, a result that indicates that the receptor alone may be capable of triggering the first steps of viral uncoating (164, 223). However, it is still not clear whether the 135S particles are obligatory intermediates during poliovirus entry or instead are simply dead-end products. In support of their importance, 135S particles are infectious, albeit at much reduced levels compared to mature virions (47). Arguing against their importance, cold-adapted poliovirus mutants seem to enter cells without the need to generate 135S particles (64). These disparate findings might be rationalized if 135S particles are short-lived only in the case of cold-adapted viral strains (223). Additional experimentation is needed to validate the role of the 135S particles during poliovirus entry.

The next stage in poliovirus entry is predicted to involve the conversion of the 135S particle to an 80S form that is devoid of RNA and that probably represents the empty protein capsid (91,204). Furthermore, it has been proposed that an amphipathic helix located at the exposed amino-terminus of VP1, and the N-terminal myristic acid group of the extruded VP4 protein might participate in the formation of protein channels in host cell membranes that could allow translocation of the poliovirus genomic RNA into the cytoplasm (13,91,204). However, it is not yet clear exactly how the viral RNA exits from the virion (13).

Adenovirus is predicted to enter cells by perturbing the integrity of cellular endosomal membranes, thus allowing viral nucleoprotein complexes access to the host cell cytoplasm. Adenovirus is a nonenveloped DNA virus that contains 11 different types of protein, including 12 complexes of penton base, each with an associated fiber protein. Following the binding of the viral fiber protein to the CAR receptor, the viral penton base interacts with specific host cell integrins. Following virus uptake into the host cell by receptor-mediated endocytosis, adenoviruses enter the cytoplasm after the pH-dependent lysis of endosomes, a step that is facilitated by the penton base–integrin interaction (221). Coincident with endosomal lysis, the viral nucleocapsid begins to disassemble with the fiber, penton base, and viral IIIa proteins being shed from the viral particles (88).

Reoviruses are also proposed to enter cells by perturbing a cellular membrane after being trafficked to a low-pH endosomal compartment. However, in contrast to the situation with adenoviruses where low pH is proposed to play a direct role in the membrane perturbation event, the role of low pH in the case of reoviruses is to activate cellular cysteine proteases that cleave the viral outer capsid proteins σ3 and μ1/μ1C, giving rise to infectious subviral particles (ISVPs). ISVPs are then capable of infecting cells in a pH-independent manner. It has been suggested that removal of the σ3 protein of reoviruses may lead to conformational changes in μ1/μ1C that in turn lead to membrane perturbation (105).

VIRAL UNCOATING

The events that immediately follow viral penetration into the host cell, but precede replication of the viral genome, are commonly referred to as uncoating. These events may be intrinsically coupled with those leading to cellular membrane penetration, as in the case of picornaviruses, which must simply introduce their plus-stranded RNA genome into the host cell cytoplasm for replication to proceed. Other viruses, however, introduce viral nucleoprotein complexes into the cell, and for these viruses a series of disassembly steps that occur after virus entry are required for successful uncoating.

Most RNA viruses are replicated in the host cell cytoplasm, presumably because their replication via the associated RNA-dependent RNA polymerase does not usually require activities provided by the host cell nucleus. By contrast, most DNA viruses, retroviruses, hepadnaviruses, and other RNA viruses such as the orthomyxovirus influenza A virus must access the host cell nucleus for replication to proceed. These viruses require nuclear functions involved in cellular DNA and RNA synthesis as well as in RNA processing. These viruses must traverse the physical barrier imposed by the nuclear envelope in addition to that imposed by the plasma/endosomal membrane.

The nuclear envelope consists of a double membrane, within which are embedded nuclear pore complexes (NPCs) made up of more than 50 different types of nucleoporins that regulate the transport of macromolecules into and out of the nucleus (86). Active transport of proteins and of nucleoprotein complexes through the NPC is mediated by specific transport signals designated as nuclear localization signals (NLSs). The NLS is recognized by importin-α, an NLS receptor, which in turn binds to importin-β, a transport receptor that facilitates binding to, and translocation through, the NPC (86). The importin-α and -β subunits are then exported—shuttled—back to the cytoplasm in a complex with the GTP-bound form of the cellular GTPase Ran (RanGTP) (86). The GTPase activity of Ran becomes activated in the cytoplasm by RanGAP1, giving rise to RanGDP, an event that leads to release of the importin subunits so that they can engage in a new round of nuclear import. RanGDP is then returned to the nucleus where a guanine nucleotide exchange factor (RCC1) acts to regenerate RanGTP for a new round of nuclear export. It has been proposed that the GTP hydrolysis that is associated with the establishment of the nucleocytoplasmic gradient of RanGTP is the driving force for cellular nuclear import and export pathways (86).

Influenza A viruses and lentiviruses such as HIV-1 seem to employ several distinct NLSs on viral core proteins for efficient targeting of viral nucleoprotein complexes to the host cell nucleus. Influenza A viruses contain eight single-stranded negative-sense RNA segments that encode viral proteins. Within the virion, these segments are found as viral ribonucleoprotein complexes (vRNPs) containing the nucleoprotein NP and the viral polymerase complex, and these vRNPs are associated in turn with the viral M1 protein. An essential step of influenza virus uncoating is the dissociation of M1 from the vRNPs. M1 dissociation occurs under low pH conditions when the virus is trafficked to acidic endosomal compartments, and it results from the translocation of protons through the M2 ion channel located on the virus surface (28,134,161). Thus, this critical step of viral uncoating is linked both spatially and temporally within the cell to that of HA-mediated membrane fusion. Following M1 dissociation, the viral RNPs are trafficked to the host cell nucleus to begin replication by a mechanism that presumably involves nuclear localization signals contained on each of the NP and polymerase proteins (2, 107,148,149,214). The NLS of the NP protein has been found to interact with an importin-α/β complex (155).

Lentiviral preintegration complexes (PICs) consist of viral DNA, the matrix protein (MA), nucleocapsid (NC), reverse transcriptase (RT), integrase (IN), and the Vpr accessory protein (194). These viruses differ from most other retroviruses in that they are able to infect nondividing cell types such as macrophages, and thus their entry into the host cell nucleus is not dependent on nuclear envelope breakdown. Several distinct nuclear-targeting signals have been found associated with HIV-1 core proteins. The Vpr protein, which is associated with viral PICs, is an importin-β-like protein that can bind importin-α and is proposed to target the viral core particles to nuclear pores where it interacts with nucleoporins to facilitate viral translocation into the nucleus (77,162,208). Additional nuclear localization signals have been described in the viral integrase protein that mediate interactions with importins (81), as well as in the viral MA protein, although the existence of this latter signal has been the subject of much controversy (76,169).

Posttranslational modifications of viral proteins may regulate their nuclear uptake, as has been seen with the hepatitis B virus core protein, where the NLS is exposed to interact with an importin-α/β complex after protein phosphorylation (110). It has been proposed that this phosphorylation step involves protein kinase C molecules assembled into hepatitis B viral capsids (110). Also, the nuclear transport of HIV-1 PICs can be regulated by the phosphorylation status of the viral MA protein, which is a substrate for the virion-associated mitogen-activated protein kinase (ERK/MAPK) (104).

Viruses have evolved to use components of the host cell cytoskeleton to facilitate their intracellular trafficking to sites of virus replication, as exemplified by adenovirus and by the herpesvirus HSV-1. Intracellular adenoviral complexes are translocated to the NPC through their association with the minus-end-directed microtubule motor complex of dynein and dynactin (197). Adenovirus capsids then dissociate at the NPC so that viral DNA and protein VII can enter the nucleus to begin genome replication (87).

Following HSV-1 entry at the plasma membrane and dissociation of the viral tegument proteins, the capsids associate with dynein, which is proposed to traffic these complexes toward NPCs (189). Once docked at the NPC, HSV-1 DNA is delivered into the host cell nucleus, leaving the empty capsid behind (189). Transport along microtubules probably represents an important event during HSV-1 infection of neuronal cells, where the viral capsids have to travel some distance from the site of virus entry to the nucleus.

INHIBITORS OF VIRAL ENTRY

Specific inhibitors of viral entry have been useful reagents for studying the basic mechanisms of this first step of viral replication and represent attractive antiviral agents because their action does not require that they be taken up into cells. Several different classes of viral entry inhibitor have been described, including neutralizing antibodies, soluble receptors, peptide inhibitors, small molecules, and ligand-based inhibitors that bind to target viral receptors or coreceptors (Fig. 4).

Neutralizing Antibodies

One of the ways by which the host organism can restrict viral entry into cells is to produce neutralizing antibodies that bind to and inhibit the function of viral attachment and fusion proteins. These antibodies can block infection by binding directly to the receptor-interaction site located on viral proteins, as has been seen with human rhinovirus 14 (36) and with influenza virus HA (20). Alternatively, these antibodies can block infection

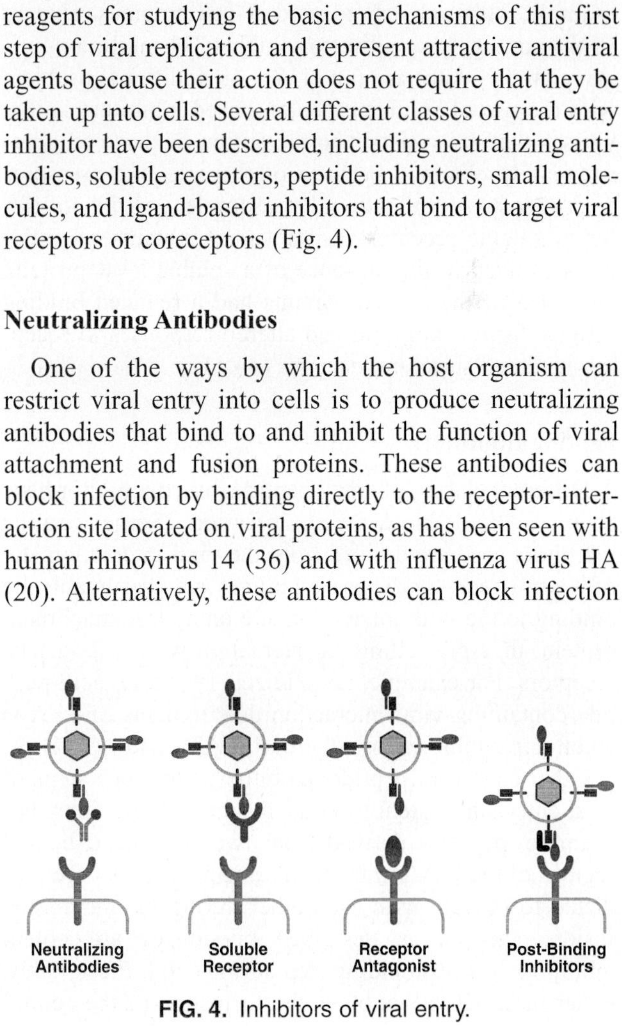

FIG. 4. Inhibitors of viral entry.

by binding to an epitope that is located outside of the receptor-binding site, where they sterically hinder the receptor association (75). Neutralizing antibodies that block viral association with coreceptors by binding to receptor-induced epitopes located on viral proteins have also been described in the case of HIV-1 (120,228).

Soluble Receptors

Soluble proteins composed of the extracellular domains of viral receptors have been used as reagents to block viral infection. Examples of such soluble receptors include PVR for polioviruses (111,112), ICAM-1 for rhinoviruses (90), and CD4 for HIV-1 (53,74,102,188,205). These agents act by binding to, and occluding, the receptor-binding site of the viral attachment protein. In addition, some soluble viral receptors are capable of triggering a series of conformational changes in virion proteins that are similar to those that occur normally during viral entry and that lead to virus inactivation (85,90).

Although soluble receptors might appear to be suitable antiviral reagents, their efficacy as viral entry inhibitors has been compromised by the fact that independent viral isolates are differentially sensitive to their action. For example, although lab-adapted, T-cell tropic strains of HIV-1 are highly sensitive to soluble CD4-inhibition, primary viral isolates are not (118). An additional problem with the use of soluble receptor–based inhibitors is that viruses that are resistant to the action of these reagents are readily obtained because of the selective pressures they impose on replication. For example, a variety of different soluble receptor–resistant (srr) mutants of poliovirus evolved in the presence of a soluble PVR protein, and most of these viral variants had a reduced binding affinity for receptor and had altered responses to receptor-mediated structural changes (44,112).

Peptide Inhibitors

Different classes of small peptide–based inhibitor have been used to block viral infection. Some peptide inhibitors used are derived from the viral interaction site of a viral receptor. These inhibitors act presumably by binding to the viral interaction site on a viral attachment protein, thus preventing its interaction with cell surface receptors. For example, an oxidized 19–amino acid peptide containing viral interaction determinants of TVA is an effective inhibitor of subgroup A ALV entry (234).

Other classes of peptide inhibitor act to block steps of viral entry subsequent to virus–receptor interactions. For example, peptides derived from two separate α-helical regions of the HIV-1 transmembrane protein that are predicted to interact with each other during the membrane fusion reaction, as described previously, are potent inhibitors of a postbinding step during entry. Presumably, either these inhibitors block the formation of the central coiled coil of the transmembrane protein trimer, or they block the contacts that are formed between this central trimer and the outer-layer α-helices of the transmembrane protein (35,217,224). Peptides corresponding to similar regions of other viral fusion proteins are also effective viral entry inhibitors—for example, in the case of paramyxovirus F_1 proteins (109,167). These inhibitors have been used to define an intermediate "lipid-mixing only" step in the viral fusion reaction, where hemifusion has apparently occurred but complete membrane fusion has not (109,145).

This class of peptide inhibitor has already shown some promise in the clinic, at least when administered at a high dose to HIV-infected individuals (116). However, as with soluble receptors, it seems that one problem that will be encountered with these reagents is the evolution of inhibitor-resistant viral strains with mutations that interfere with inhibitor binding and/or function (172).

Another class of peptide inhibitor that acts to block virus infection after receptor binding are those that antagonize the function of viral coreceptors. For example, the T22 and ALX40-4C peptides that are antagonists of CXCR4 can inhibit entry of T-cell-tropic HIV-1 (61,146).

Small-Molecule Inhibitors

Small-molecule inhibitors of viral entry include the drug amantadine hydrochloride, which was instrumental in revealing the ion channel activity of the influenza A virus M2 protein that is essential for the low pH–induced dissociation of M1 from viral RNPs during viral entry (28,161). Other small-molecule inhibitors act by binding to and inactivating viral proteins that are necessary for entry—for example, the compound WIN 52084 acts to block viral entry when located in a hydrophobic pocket that is located in the canyon floor of the VP1 protein. It does so by preventing dynamic conformational changes in the viral capsid that are necessary for infectivity (122). Also, small-molecule inhibitors of influenza A virus entry have been described that act either by blocking the necessary conformational changes in HA or by prematurely activating these changes (98). Other classes of small molecules have been described that are antagonists of viral receptors and/or coreceptors. These molecules include the bicyclam AMD3100 antagonist of CXCR4 function, which prevents entry of T-cell-tropic strains of HIV into cells (60).

Ligand-Based Inhibitors

In some cases, it has been possible to block viral entry using naturally occurring ligands or ligand derivatives that bind to viral receptors and coreceptors, thus interfering with viral entry. Examples of naturally occurring ligands used as viral inhibitors are the α-chemokine SDF-1, and the β-chemokines RANTES, MIP-1α, and MIP-1β that block viral entry by binding to the HIV coreceptors CXCR4 and CCR5, respectively (4,21,40,43,55,65,151). An example of a chemically modified form of one of these ligands that can still block viral entry without potentiating the normal function of the receptor is amino-oxypentane (AOP)-RANTES (185). However, selection of viral variants that resist inhibition may restrict the utility of this approach, in this case by selecting for viruses that use other HIV coreceptors (144).

CONCLUDING REMARKS

Over the course of the last decade, much has been learned about how virus–receptor interactions lead to viral entry. The exact mechanisms of viral entry into cells are beginning to be revealed through the combined use of biochemical, genetic, and structural analyses of specific viral proteins or whole virions. Also, a number of different cell surface proteins and carbohydrates that serve as viral receptors have been identified and their viral binding determinants defined. The challenge that lies ahead is to understand the step-wise series of events leading to viral entry that occur after virus binding to receptors/coreceptors, and in the presence of other activators such as low pH conditions.

The mechanisms of viral uncoating are also beginning to be understood. Future research in this area should provide valuable new information about this important step of viral replication. It will undoubtedly shed new insights into how viruses exploit host cell processes for their own ends, and it will, we can hope, provide a new set of targets for the development of antiviral strategies.

REFERENCES

1. Adkins HB, Brojatsch J, Naughton J, et al. Identification of a cellular receptor for subgroup E avian leukosis virus. *Proc Natl Acad Sci U S A* 1997;94:11617–11622.
2. Akkina RK, Chambers TM, Londo DR, Nayak DP. Intracellular localization of the viral polymerase proteins in cells infected with influenza virus and cells expressing PB1 protein from cloned cDNA. *J Virol* 1987;61:2217–2224.
3. Albritton LM, Tseng L, Scadden D, Cunningham JM. A putative murine ecotropic retrovirus receptor gene encodes a multiple membrane-spanning protein and confers susceptibility to virus infection. *Cell* 1989;57:659–666.
4. Alkhatib G, Combadiere C, Broder CC, et al. CC CKR5: A RANTES, MIP-1alpha, MIP-1beta receptor as a fusion cofactor for macrophage-tropic HIV-1. *Science* 1996;272:1955–1958.
5. Alkhatib G, Liao F, Berger EA, et al. A new SIV coreceptor, STRL33. *Nature* 1997;388:238.
6. Allison SL, Schalich J, Stiasny K, et al. Oligomeric rearrangement of tick-borne encephalitis virus envelope proteins induced by an acidic pH. *J Virol* 1995;69:695–700.
7. Armstrong GD, Paul RW, Lee PW. Studies on reovirus receptors of L cells: Virus binding characteristics and comparison with reovirus receptors of erythrocytes. *Virology* 1984;138:37–48.
8. Baker KA, Dutch RE, Lamb RA, Jardetzky TS. Structural basis for paramyxovirus-mediated membrane fusion. *Mol Cell* 1999;3:309–319.
9. Ban J, Portetelle D, Altaner C, et al. Isolation and characterization of a 2.3-kilobase-pair cDNA fragment encoding the binding domain of the bovine leukemia virus cell receptor. *J Virol* 1993;67:1050–1057.
10. Barbis DP, Chang SF, Parrish CR. Mutations adjacent to the dimple of the canine parvovirus capsid structure affect sialic acid binding. *Virology* 1992;191:301–308.
11. Bates P, Young JA, Varmus HE. A receptor for subgroup A Rous sarcoma virus is related to the low density lipoprotein receptor. *Cell* 1993;74:1043–1051.
12. Battini JL, Rasko JEJ, Miller AD. A human cell-surface receptor for xenotropic and polytropic murine leukemia viruses: Possible role in G protein-coupled signal transduction. *Proc Natl Acad Sci U S A* 1999;96:1385–1390.
13. Belnap DM, Filman DJ, Trus BL, et al. Molecular tectonic model of virus structural transitions: The putative cell entry states of poliovirus. *J Virol* 2000;74:1342–1354.
14. Bergelson JM, Chan M, Solomon KR, et al. Decay-accelerating factor (CD55), a glycosylphosphatidylinositol-anchored complement regulatory protein, is a receptor for several echoviruses. *Proc Natl Acad Sci U S A* 1994;91:6245–6624.
15. Bergelson JM, Cunningham JA, Droguett G, et al. Isolation of a common receptor for Coxsackie B viruses and adenoviruses 2 and 5. *Science* 1997;275:1320–1323.
16. Bergelson JM, Mohanty JG, Crowell RL, et al. Coxsackievirus B3 adapted to growth in RD cells binds to decay-accelerating factor (CD55). *J Virol* 1995;69:1903–1906.
17. Bergelson JM, Shepley MP, Chan BM, et al. Identification of the integrin VLA-2 as a receptor for echovirus 1. *Science* 1992;255:1718–1720.
18. Bergelson LD, Bukrinskaya AG, Prokazova NV, et al. Role of gangliosides in reception of influenza virus. *Eur J Biochem* 1982;128:467–474.
19. Berger EA, Murphy PM, Farber JM. Chemokine receptors as HIV-1 coreceptors: Roles in viral entry, tropism, and disease. *Ann Rev Immunol* 1999;17:657–700.
20. Bizebard T, Gigant B, Rigolet P, et al. Structure of influenza virus haemagglutinin complexed with a neutralizing antibody. *Nature* 1995;376:92–94.
21. Bleul CC, Farzan M, Choe H, et al. The lymphocyte chemoattractant SDF-1 is a ligand for LESTR/fusin and blocks HIV-1 entry. *Nature* 1996;382:829–833.
22. Blumenthal R, Sarkar DP, Durell S, et al. Dilation of the influenza hemagglutinin fusion pore revealed by the kinetics of individual cell–cell fusion events. *J Cell Biol* 1996;135:63–71.
23. Bothner B, Dong XF, Bibbs L, et al. Evidence of viral capsid dynamics using limited proteolysis and mass spectrometry. *J Biol Chem* 1998;273:673–676.
24. Boyle KA, Pietropaolo RL, Compton T. Engagement of the cellular receptor for glycoprotein B of human cytomegalovirus activates the interferon-responsive pathway. *Mol Cell Biol* 1999;19:3607–3613.
25. Brody BA, Rhee SS, Hunter E. Postassembly cleavage of a retroviral glycoprotein cytoplasmic domain removes a necessary incorporation signal and activates fusion activity. *J Virol* 1994;68:4620–4627.
26. Brojatsch J, Naughton J, Rolls MM, et al. CAR1, a TNFR-related protein, is a cellular receptor for cytopathic avian leukosis-sarcoma viruses and mediates apoptosis. *Cell* 1996;87:845–855.
27. Buchholz CJ, Schneider U, Devaux P, et al. Cell entry by measles virus: Long hybrid receptors uncouple binding from membrane fusion. *J Virol* 1996;70:3716–3723.
28. Bui M, Whittaker G, Helenius A. Effect of M1 protein and low pH on nuclear transport of influenza virus ribonucleoproteins. *J Virol* 1996;70:8391–8401.
29. Bullough PA, Hughson FM, Skehel JJ, Wiley DC. Structure of influenza haemagglutinin at the pH of membrane fusion. *Nature* 1994;371:37–43.
30. Caffrey M, Cai M, Kaufman J, et al. Three-dimensional solution structure of the 44 kDa ectodomain of SIV gp41. *EMBO J* 1998;17:4572–4584.
31. Cao W, Henry MD, Borrow P, et al. Identification of alpha-dystroglycan as a receptor for lymphocytic choriomeningitis virus and lassa fever virus. *Science* 1998;282:2079–2081.
32. Cardosa MJ, Gordon S, Hirsch S, et al. Interaction of West Nile virus with primary murine macrophages: Role of cell activation and receptors for antibody and complement. *J Virol* 1986;57:952–959.
33. Carr CM, Chaudhry C, Kim PS. Influenza hemagglutinin is spring-loaded by a metastable native conformation. *Proc Natl Acad Sci U S A* 1997;94:14306–14313.

34. Carr CM, Kim PS. A spring-loaded mechanism for the conformational change of influenza hemagglutinin. *Cell* 1993;73:823–832.
35. Chan DC, Fass D, Berger JM, Kim PS. Core structure of gp41 from the HIV envelope glycoprotein. *Cell* 1997;89:263–273.
36. Che Z, Olson NH, Leippe D, et al. Antibody-mediated neutralization of human rhinovirus 14 explored by means of cryoelectron microscopy and x-ray crystallography of virus-Fab complexes. *J Virol* 1998;72:4610–4622.
37. Chen BK, Gandhi RT, Baltimore D. CD4 down-modulation during infection of human T cells with human immunodeficiency virus type 1 involves independent activities of vpu, env, and nef. *J Virol* 1996;70: 6044–6053.
38. Chen J, Skehel JJ, Wiley DC. N- and C-terminal residues combine in the fusion-pH influenza hemagglutinin HA(2) subunit to form an N cap that terminates the triple-stranded coiled coil. *Proc Natl Acad Sci U S A* 1999;96:8967–8972.
39. Choe H, Farzan M, Konkel M, et al. The orphan seven-transmembrane receptor apj supports the entry of primary T-cell-line-tropic and dual-tropic human immunodeficiency virus type 1. *J Virol* 1998;72: 6113–6118.
40. Choe H, Farzan M, Sun Y, et al. The beta-chemokine receptors CCR3 and CCR5 facilitate infection by primary HIV-1 isolates. *Cell* 1996;85:1135–1148.
41. Cirone M, Angeloni A, Barile G, et al. Epstein-Barr virus internalization and infectivity are blocked by selective protein kinase C inhibitors. *Int J Cancer* 1990;45:490–493.
42. Cleverley DZ, Lenard J. The transmembrane domain in viral fusion: Essential role for a conserved glycine residue in vesicular stomatitis virus G protein. *Proc Natl Acad Sci U S A* 1998;95:3425–3430.
43. Cocchi F, DeVico AL, Garzino-Demo A, et al. Identification of RANTES, MIP-1 alpha, and MIP-1 beta as the major HIV-suppressive factors produced by CD8+ T cells. *Science* 1995;270:1811–1815.
44. Colston E, Racaniello VR. Soluble receptor-resistant poliovirus mutants identify surface and internal capsid residues that control interaction with the cell receptor. *EMBO J* 1994;13:5855–5862.
45. Compton T, Nowlin DM, Cooper NR. Initiation of human cytomegalovirus infection requires initial interaction with cell surface heparan sulfate. *Virology* 1993;193:834–841.
46. Crise B, Buonocore L, Rose JK. CD4 is retained in the endoplasmic reticulum by the human immunodeficiency virus type 1 glycoprotein precursor. *J Virol* 1990;64:5585–5593.
47. Curry S, Chow M, Hogle JM. The poliovirus 135S particle is infectious. *J Virol* 1996;70:7125–7131.
48. Dalgleish AG, Beverley PC, Clapham PR, et al. The CD4 (T4) antigen is an essential component of the receptor for the AIDS retrovirus. *Nature* 1984;312:763–767.
49. Damico RL, Crane J, Bates P. Receptor-triggered membrane association of a model retroviral glycoprotein *Proc Natl Acad Sci U S A* 1998;95:2580–2585.
50. Danieli T, Pelletier SL, Henis YI, White JM. Membrane fusion mediated by the influenza virus hemagglutinin requires the concerted action of at least three hemagglutinin trimers. *J Cell Biol* 1996;133: 559–569.
51. Daniels RS, Downie JC, Hay AJ, et al. Fusion mutants of the influenza virus hemagglutinin glycoprotein. *Cell* 1985;40:431–439.
52. Daughaday CC, Brandt WE, McCown JM, Russell PK. Evidence for two mechanisms of dengue virus infection of adherent human monocytes: Trypsin-sensitive virus receptors and trypsin-resistant immune complex receptors. *Infect Immun* 1981;32:469–473.
53. Deen KC, McDougal JS, Inacker R, et al. A soluble form of CD4 (T4) protein inhibits AIDS virus infection. *Nature* 1988;331:82–84.
54. Delmas B, Gelfi J, L'Haridon R, et al. Aminopeptidase N is a major receptor for the entero-pathogenic coronavirus TGEV. *Nature* 1992; 357:417–420.
55. Deng H, Liu R, Ellmeier W, et al. Identification of a major coreceptor for primary isolates of HIV-1. *Nature* 1996;381:661–666.
56. Deng HK, Unutmaz D, KewalRamani VN, Littman DR. Expression cloning of new receptors used by simian and human immunodeficiency viruses. *Nature* 1997;388:296–300.
57. Deng R, Wang Z, Mahon PJ, et al. Mutations in the Newcastle disease virus hemagglutinin-neuraminidase protein that interfere with its ability to interact with the homologous F protein in the promotion of fusion. *Virology* 1999;253:43–54.
58. DeTulleo L, Kirchhausen T. The clathrin endocytic pathway in viral infection. *EMBO J* 1998;17:4585–4593.
59. Doms RW, Helenius A, White J. Membrane fusion activity of the influenza virus hemagglutinin. The low pH-induced conformational change. *J Biol Chem* 1985;260:2973–2981.
60. Donzella GA, Schols D, Lin SW, et al. AMD3100, a small molecule inhibitor of HIV-1 entry via the CXCR4 coreceptor. *Nat Med* 1998;4: 72–77.
61. Doranz BJ, Grovit-Ferbas K, Sharron MP, et al. A small-molecule inhibitor directed against the chemokine receptor CXCR4 prevents its use as an HIV-1 coreceptor. *J Exp Med* 1997;186:1395–1400.
62. Doranz BJ, Rucker J, Yi Y, et al. A dual-tropic primary HIV-1 isolate that uses fusin and the beta-chemokine receptors CKR-5, CKR-3, and CKR-2b as fusion cofactors. *Cell* 1996;85:1149–1158.
63. Dorig RE, Marcil A, Chopra A, Richardson CD. The human CD46 molecule is a receptor for measles virus (Edmonston strain). *Cell* 1993;75:295–305.
64. Dove AW, Racaniello VR. Cold-adapted poliovirus mutants bypass a postentry replication block. *J Virol* 1997;71:4728–4735.
65. Dragic T, Litwin V, Allaway GP, et al. HIV-1 entry into CD4+ cells is mediated by the chemokine receptor CC-CKR-5. *Nature* 1996;381: 667–673.
66. Durrer P, Galli C, Hoenke S, et al. H+-induced membrane insertion of influenza virus hemagglutinin involves the HA_2 amino-terminal fusion peptide but not the coiled coil region. *J Biol Chem* 1996;271: 13417–13421.
67. Durrer P, Gaudin Y, Ruigrok RW, et al. Photolabeling identifies a putative fusion domain in the envelope glycoprotein of rabies and vesicular stomatitis viruses. *J Biol Chem* 1995;270:17575–17581.
68. Dveksler GS, Pensiero MN, Cardellichio CB, et al. Cloning of the mouse hepatitis virus (MHV) receptor: Expression in human and hamster cell lines confers susceptibility to MHV. *J Virol* 1991;65: 6881–6891.
69. Farzan M, Choe H, Martin K, et al. Two orphan seven transmembrane segment receptors which are expressed in CD4-positive cells support simian immunodeficiency virus infection. *J Exp Med* 1997;186: 405–411.
70. Fass D, Harrison SC, Kim PS. Retrovirus envelope domain at 1.7 angstrom resolution. *Nat Struct Biol* 1996;3:465–469.
71. Feng Y, Broder CC, Kennedy PE, Berger EA. HIV-1 entry cofactor: Functional cDNA cloning of a seven-transmembrane, G protein-coupled receptor. *Science* 1996;272:872–877.
72. Ferlenghi I, Gowen B, de Haas F, et al. The first step: Activation of the Semliki Forest virus spike protein precursor causes a localized conformational change in the trimeric spike. *J Mol Biol* 1998;283:71–81.
73. Fingeroth JD, Weis JJ, Tedder TF, et al. Epstein-Barr virus receptor of human B lymphocytes is the C3d receptor CR2. *Proc Natl Acad Sci U S A* 1984;81:4510–4514.
74. Fisher RA, Bertonis JM, Meier W, et al. HIV infection is blocked in vitro by recombinant soluble CD4. *Nature* 1988;331:76–78.
75. Fleury D, Barrere B, Bizebard T, et al. A complex of influenza hemagglutinin with a neutralizing antibody that binds outside the virus receptor binding site. *Nat Struct Biol* 1999;6:530–534.
76. Fouchier RA, Meyer BE, Simon JH, et al. HIV-1 infection of non-dividing cells: Evidence that the amino-terminal basic region of the viral matrix protein is important for Gag processing but not for post-entry nuclear import. *EMBO J* 1997;16:4531–4539.
77. Fouchier RA, Meyer BE, Simon JH, et al. Interaction of the human immunodeficiency virus type 1 Vpr protein with the nuclear pore complex. *J Virol* 1998;72:6004–6013.
78. Frade R, Barel M, Ehlin-Henriksson B, Klein G. Gp140, the C3d receptor of human B lymphocytes, is also the Epstein-Barr virus receptor. *Proc Natl Acad Sci U S A* 1985;82:1490–1493.
79. Fredericksen BL, Whitt MA. Vesicular stomatitis virus glycoprotein mutations that affect membrane fusion activity and abolish virus infectivity. *J Virol* 1995;69:1435–1443.
80. Fried H, Cahan LD, Paulson JC. Polyoma virus recognizes specific sialyligosaccharide receptors on host cells. *Virology* 1981;109:188–192.
81. Gallay P, Hope T, Chin D, Trono D. HIV-1 infection of nondividing cells through the recognition of integrase by the importin/karyopherin pathway. *Proc Natl Acad Sci U S A* 1997;94:9825–9830.
82. Geraghty RJ, Krummenacher C, Cohen GH, et al. Entry of alphaherpesviruses mediated by poliovirus receptor-related protein 1 and poliovirus receptor. *Science* 1998;280:1618–1620.
83. Gething MJ, Doms RW, York D, White J. Studies on the mechanism of membrane fusion: Site-specific mutagenesis of the hemagglutinin of influenza virus. *J Cell Biol* 1986;102:11–23.

84. Godley L, Pfeifer J, Steinhauer D, et al. Introduction of intersubunit disulfide bonds in the membrane-distal region of the influenza hemagglutinin abolishes membrane fusion activity. *Cell* 1992;68: 635–645.
85. Gomez Yafal A, Kaplan G, Racaniello VR, Hogle JM. Characterization of poliovirus conformational alteration mediated by soluble cell receptors. *Virology* 1993;197:501–505.
86. Gorlich D, Kutay U. Transport between the cell nucleus and the cytoplasm. *Ann Rev Cell Dev Biol* 1999;15:607–660.
87. Greber UF, Suomalainen M, Stidwill RP, et al. The role of the nuclear pore complex in adenovirus DNA entry. *EMBO J* 1997;16: 5998–6007.
88. Greber UF, Willetts M, Webster P, Helenius A. Stepwise dismantling of adenovirus 2 during entry into cells. *Cell* 1993;75:477–486.
89. Greve JM, Davis G, Meyer AM, et al. The major human rhinovirus receptor is ICAM-1. *Cell* 1989;56:839–847.
90. Greve JM, Forte CP, Marlor CW, et al. Mechanisms of receptor-mediated rhinovirus neutralization defined by two soluble forms of ICAM-1. *J Virol* 1991;65:6015–6023.
91. Hadfield AT, Lee WM, Zhao R, et al. The refined structure of human rhinovirus 16 at 2.15 A resolution: Implications for the viral life cycle. *Structure* 1997;5:427–441.
92. Harouse JM, Bhat S, Spitalnik SL, et al. Inhibition of entry of HIV-1 in neural cell lines by antibodies against galactosyl ceramide. *Science* 1991;253:320–323.
93. Haywood AM. Characteristics of Sendai virus receptors in a model membrane. *J Mol Biol* 1974;83:427–436.
94. Helenius A, Kartenbeck J, Simons K, Fries E. On the entry of Semliki Forest virus into BHK-21 cells. *J Cell Biol* 1980;84:404–420.
95. Hernandez LD, Hoffman LR, Wolfsberg TG, White JM. Virus-cell and cell-cell fusion. *Ann Rev Cell Dev Biol* 1996;12:627–661.
96. Hernandez LD, Peters RJ, Delos SE, et al. Activation of a retroviral membrane fusion protein: Soluble receptor-induced liposome binding of the ALSV envelope glycoprotein. *J Cell Biol* 1997;139:1455–1464.
97. Hofer F, Gruenberger M, Kowalski H, et al. Members of the low density lipoprotein receptor family mediate cell entry of a minor-group common cold virus. *Proc Natl Acad Sci U S A* 1994;91:1839–1842.
98. Hoffman LR, Kuntz ID, White JM. Structure-based identification of an inducer of the low-pH conformational change in the influenza virus hemagglutinin: Irreversible inhibition of infectivity. *J Virol* 1997;71: 8808–8820.
99. Homsy J, Meyer M, Tateno M, et al. The Fc and not CD4 receptor mediates antibody enhancement of HIV infection in human cells. *Science* 1989;244:1357–1360.
100. Hooper NM. Detergent-insoluble glycosphingolipid/cholesterol-rich membrane domains, lipid rafts and caveolae. *Mol Membr Biol* 1999; 16:145–156.
101. Hunter K, Housman D, Hopkins N. Isolation and characterization of irradiation fusion hybrids from mouse chromosome 1 for mapping Rmc-1, a gene encoding a cellular receptor for MCF class murine retroviruses. *Somat Cell Mol Genet* 1991;17:169–183.
102. Hussey RE, Richardson NE, Kowalski M, et al. A soluble CD4 protein selectively inhibits HIV replication and syncytium formation. *Nature* 1998;331:78–81.
103. Iyengar S, Hildreth JEK, Schwartz DH. Actin-dependent receptor colocalization required for human immunodeficiency virus entry into host cells. *J Virol* 1998;72:5251–5255.
104. Jacque JM, Mann A, Enslen H, et al. Modulation of HIV-1 infectivity by MAPK, a virion-associated kinase. *EMBO J* 1998;17:2607–2618.
105. Jane-Valbuena J, Nibert ML, Spencer SM, et a. Reovirus virion-like particles obtained by recoating infectious subvirion particles with baculovirus-expressed sigma3 protein: An approach for analyzing sigma3 functions during virus entry. *J Virol* 1999;73:2963–2973.
106. Jiricek R, Schwarz G, Stegmann T. Pores formed by influenza hemagglutinin. *Biochim Biophys Acta* 1997;1330:17–28.
107. Jones IM, Reay PA, Philpott KL. Nuclear location of all three influenza polymerase proteins and a nuclear signal in polymerase PB2. *EMBO J* 1986;5:2371–2376.
108. Jones PL, Korte T, Blumenthal R. Conformational changes in cell surface HIV-1 envelope glycoproteins are triggered by cooperation between cell surface CD4 and coreceptors. *J Biol Chem* 1998;273: 404–409.
109. Joshi SB, Dutch RE, Lamb RA. A core trimer of the paramyxovirus fusion protein: Parallels to influenza virus hemagglutinin and HIV-1 gp41. *Virology* 1998;248:20–34.
110. Kann M, Sodeik B, Vlachou A, et al. Phosphorylation-dependent binding of hepatitis B virus core particles to the nuclear pore complex. *J Cell Biol* 1999;145:45–55.
111. Kaplan G, Freistadt MS, Racaniello VR. Neutralization of poliovirus by cell receptors expressed in insect cells. *J Virol* 1990;64:4697–4702.
112. Kaplan G, Peters D, Racaniello VR. Poliovirus mutants resistant to neutralization with soluble cell receptors. *Science* 1990;250: 1596–1599.
113. Katsikis PD, Garciaojeda ME, Torresroca JF, et al. Interleukin-1-beta converting enzyme-like protease involvement in Fas-induced and activation-induced peripheral blood T cell apoptosis in HIV infection-TNF-related apoptosis inducing ligand can mediate activation-induced T cell death in HIV infection. *J Exp Med* 1997;186: 1365–1372.
114. Kemble GW, Bodian DL, Rose J, et al. Intermonomer disulfide bonds impair the fusion activity of influenza virus hemagglutinin. *J Virol* 1992;66:4940–4950.
115. Kemble GW, Danieli T, White JM. Lipid-anchored influenza hemagglutinin promotes hemifusion, not complete fusion. *Cell* 1994;76: 383–391.
116. Kilby JM, Hopkins S, Venetta TM, et al. Potent suppression of HIV-1 replication in humans by T-20, a peptide inhibitor of gp41-mediated virus entry. *Nat Med* 1998;4:1302–1307.
117. Kizhatil K, Albritton LM. Requirements for different components of the host cell cytoskeleton distinguish ecotropic murine leukemia virus entry via endocytosis from entry via surface fusion. *J Virol* 1997;71: 7145–7156.
118. Klasse PJ, Moore JP. Quantitative model of antibody- and soluble CD4-mediated neutralization of primary isolates and T-cell line-adapted strains of human immunodeficiency virus type 1. *J Virol* 1996;70:3668–3677.
119. Klatzmann D, Champagne E, Chamaret S, et al. T-lymphocyte T4 molecule behaves as the receptor for human retrovirus LAV. *Nature* 1984;312:767–768.
120. Kwong PD, Wyatt R, Robinson J, et al. Structure of an HIV gp120 envelope glycoprotein in complex with the CD4 receptor and a neutralizing human antibody. *Nature* 1998;393:648–659.
121. Lee SY, Zho Y, Anderson WF. Receptor-mediated moloney murine leukemia virus entry can occur independently of the clathrin-coated-pit-mediated endocytic pathway. *J Virol* 1999;73:5994–6005.
122. Lewis JK, Bothner B, Smith TJ, Siuzdak G. Antiviral agent blocks breathing of the common cold virus. *Proc Natl Acad Sci U S A* 1998; 95:6774–6778.
123. Li EG, Stupack D, Klemke R, et al. Adenovirus endocytosis via alpha (V) integrins requires phosphoinositide-3-OH kinase. *J Virol* 1998;72: 2055–2061.
124. Li Q, Yafal AG, Lee YM, et al. Poliovirus neutralization by antibodies to internal epitopes of VP4 and VP1 results from reversible exposure of these sequences at physiological temperature. *J Virol* 1994;68: 3965–3970.
125. Liao F, Alkhatib G, Peden KW, et al. STRL33, a novel chemokine receptor-like protein, functions as a fusion cofactor for both macrophage-tropic and T cell line-tropic HIV-1. *J Exp Med* 1997;185: 2015–2023.
126. Loetscher M, Amara A, Oberlin E, et al. TYMSTR, a putative chemokine receptor selectively expressed in activated T cells, exhibits HIV-1 coreceptor function. *Curr Biol* 1997;7:652–660.
127. Lonberg-Holm K, Crowell RL, Philipson L. Unrelated animal viruses share receptors. *Nature* 1976;259:679–681.
128. Long D, Berson JF, Cook DG, Doms RW. Characterization of human immunodeficiency virus type 1 gp120 binding to liposomes containing galactosylceramide. *J Virol* 1994;68:5890–5898.
129. Lusso P, Secchiero P, Crowley RW, et al. CD4 is a critical component of the receptor for human herpesvirus 7: Interference with human immunodeficiency virus. *Proc Natl Acad Sci U S A* 1994;91:3872–3876.
130. Maddon PJ, Dalgleish AG, McDougal JS, et al. The T4 gene encodes the AIDS virus receptor and is expressed in the immune system and the brain. *Cell* 1986;47:333–348.
131. Malashkevich VN, Schneider BJ, McNally ML, et al. Core structure of the envelope glycoprotein GP2 from Ebola virus at 1.9-A resolution. *Proc Natl Acad Sci U S A* 1999;96:2662–2667.
132. Margottin F, Bour SP, Durand H, et al. A novel human WD protein, h-beta TrCp, that interacts with HIV-1 Vpu connects CD4 to the ER degradation pathway through an F-box motif. *Mol Cell* 1998;1: 565–574.

133. Markwell MAK. New frontiers opened up by the exploration of host cell receptors. In: Kingsbury DW, ed. *The Paramyxoviruses*. New York: Plenum Press, 1991.
134. Martin K, Helenius A. Transport of incoming influenza virus nucleocapsids into the nucleus. *J Virol* 1991;65:232–244.
135. Matlin KS, Reggio H, Helenius A, Simons K. Infectious entry pathway of influenza virus in a canine kidney cell line. *J Cell Biol* 1981; 91:601–613.
136. Mauri DN, Ebner R, Montgomery RI, et al. LIGHT, a new member of the TNF superfamily, and lymphotoxin alpha are ligands for herpesvirus entry mediator. *Immunity* 1998;8:21–30.
137. McKeating JA, Griffiths PD, Weiss RA. HIV susceptibility conferred to human fibroblasts by cytomegalovirus-induced Fc receptor. *Nature* 1990;343:659–661.
138. McNiven MA, Cao H, Pitts KR, Yoon Y. The dynamin family of mechanoenzymes: Pinching in new places. *Trends Biochem Sci* 2000; 25:115–120.
139. Melikyan GB, Brener SA, Ok DC, Cohen FS. Inner but not outer membrane leaflets control the transition from glycosylphosphatidylinositol-anchored influenza hemagglutinin-induced hemifusion to full fusion. *J Cell Biol* 1997;136:995–1005.
140. Melikyan GB, Lin SS, Roth MG, Cohen FS. Amino acid sequence requirements of the transmembrane and cytoplasmic domains of influenza virus hemagglutinin for viable membrane fusion. *Mol Biol Cell* 1999;10:1821–1836.
141. Mendelsohn CL, Wimmer E, Racaniello VR. Cellular receptor for poliovirus: Molecular cloning, nucleotide sequence, and expression of a new member of the immunoglobulin superfamily. *Cell* 1989;56: 855–865.
142. Miller DG, Edwards RH, Miller AD. Cloning of the cellular receptor for amphotropic murine retroviruses reveals homology to that for gibbon ape leukemia virus. *Proc Natl Acad Sci U S A* 1994;91:78–82.
143. Montgomery RI, Warner MS, Lum BJ, Spear PG. Herpes simplex virus-1 entry into cells mediated by a novel member of the TNF/NGF receptor family. *Cell* 1996;87:427–436.
144. Mosier DE, Picchio GR, Gulizia RJ, et al. Highly potent RANTES analogues either prevent CCR5-using human immunodeficiency virus type 1 infection in vivo or rapidly select for CXCR4-using variants. *J Virol* 1999;73:3544–3550.
145. Munoz-Barroso I, Durell S, Sakaguchi K, et al. Dilation of the human immunodeficiency virus-1 envelope glycoprotein fusion pore revealed by the inhibitory action of a synthetic peptide from gp41. *J Cell Biol* 1998;140:315–323.
146. Murakami T, Nakajima T, Koyanagi Y, et al. A small molecule CXCR4 inhibitor that blocks T cell line-tropic HIV-1 infection. *J Exp Med* 1997;186:1389–1393.
147. Nemerow GR, Wolfert R, McNaughton ME, Cooper NR. Identification and characterization of the Epstein-Barr virus receptor on human B lymphocytes and its relationship to the C3d complement receptor (CR2). *J Virol* 1985;55:347–351.
148. Neumann G, Castrucci MR, Kawaoka Y. Nuclear import and export of influenza virus nucleoprotein. *J Virol* 1997;71:9690–9700.
149. Nieto A, de la Luna S, Barcena J, et al. Complex structure of the nuclear translocation signal of influenza virus polymerase PA subunit. *J Gen Virol* 1994;75:29–36.
150. Norkin LC. Simian virus 40 infection via MHC class I molecules and caveolae. *Immunol Rev* 1999;168:13–22.
151. Oberlin E, Amara A, Bachelerie F, et al. The CXC chemokine SDF-1 is the ligand for LESTR/fusin and prevents infection by T-cell-line-adapted HIV-1. *Nature* 1996;382:833–835.
152. O'Hara B, Johann SV, Klinger HP, et al. Characterization of a human gene conferring sensitivity to infection by gibbon ape leukemia virus. *Cell Growth Differ* 1990;1:119–127.
153. Oldridge J, Marsh M. Nef—An adaptor adaptor? *Trends Cell Biol* 1998;8:302–305.
154. Olson NH, Kolatkar PR, Oliveira MA, et al. Structure of a human rhinovirus complexed with its receptor molecule. *Proc Natl Acad Sci U S A* 1993;90:507–511.
155. O'Neill RE, Jaskunas R, Blobel G, et al. Nuclear import of influenza virus RNA can be mediated by viral nucleoprotein and transport factors required for protein import. *J Biol Chem* 1995;270:22701–22704.
156. Pak CC, Puri A, Blumenthal R. Conformational changes and fusion activity of vesicular stomatitis virus glycoprotein: [125I]iodonaphthyl azide photolabeling studies in biological membranes. *Biochemistry* 1997;36:8890–8896.
157. Parton RG, Lindsay M. Exploitation of major histocompatibility complex class I molecules and caveolae by simian virus 40. *Immunol Rev* 1999;168:23–31.
158. Paulson JC, Rogers GN. Resialylated erythrocytes for assessment of the specificity of sialyloligosaccharide binding proteins. *Methods Enzymol* 1987;138:162–168.
159. Peiris JS, Gordon S, Unkeless JC, Porterfield JS. Monoclonal anti-Fc receptor IgG blocks antibody enhancement of viral replication in macrophages. *Nature* 1981;289:189–191.
160. Philipson L, Lonberg-Holm K, Pettersson U. Virus-receptor interaction in an adenovirus system. *J Virol* 1968;2:1064–1075.
161. Pinto LH, Holsinger LJ, Lamb RA. Influenza virus M2 protein has ion channel activity. *Cell* 1992;69:517–528.
162. Popov S, Rexach M, Zybarth G, et al. Viral protein R regulates nuclear import of the HIV-1 pre-integration complex. *EMBO J* 1998;17: 909–917.
163. Puri A, Booy FP, Doms RW, et al. Conformational changes and fusion activity of influenza virus hemagglutinin of the H2 and H3 subtypes: Effects of acid pretreatment. *J Virol* 1990;64:3824–3832.
164. Racaniello VR. Early events in poliovirus infection: Virus-receptor interactions. *Proc Natl Acad Sci U S A* 1996;93:11378–11381.
165. Ragheb JA, Anderson WF. pH-independent murine leukemia virus ecotropic envelope-mediated cell fusion: Implications for the role of the R peptide and p12E TM in viral entry. *J Virol* 1994;68: 3220–3231.
166. Rajcani J, Vojvodova A. The role of herpes simplex virus glycoproteins in the virus replication cycle. *Acta Virol* 1998;42:103–118.
167. Rapaport D, Ovadia M, Shai Y. A synthetic peptide corresponding to a conserved heptad repeat domain is a potent inhibitor of Sendai virus-cell fusion: An emerging similarity with functional domains of other viruses. *EMBO J* 1995;14:5524–5531.
168. Rasko JEJ, Battini JL, Gottschalk RJ, et al. The RD114 simian type D retrovirus receptor is a neutral amino acid transporter *Proc Natl Acad Sci U S A* 1999;96:2129–2134.
169. Reil H, Bukovsky AA, Gelderblom HR, Gottlinger HG. Efficient HIV-1 replication can occur in the absence of the viral matrix protein. *EMBO J* 1998;17:2699–2708.
170. Rein A, Mirro J, Haynes JG, et al. Function of the cytoplasmic domain of a retroviral transmembrane protein: p15E-p2E cleavage activates the membrane fusion capability of the murine leukemia virus Env protein. *J Virol* 1994;68:1773–1781.
171. Rey FA, Heinz FX, Mandl C, et al. The envelope glycoprotein from tick-borne encephalitis virus at 2 A resolution. *Nature* 1995;375: 291–298.
172. Rimsky LT, Shugars DC, Matthews TJ. Determinants of human immunodeficiency virus type 1 resistance to gp41-derived inhibitory peptides. *J Virol* 1998;72:986–993.
173. Rizzuto CD, Wyatt R, Hernandez-Ramos N, et al. A conserved HIV gp120 glycoprotein structure involved in chemokine receptor binding. *Science* 1998;280:1949–1953.
174. Roberts ML, Luxembourg AT, Cooper NR. Epstein-Barr virus binding to CD21, the virus receptor, activates resting B cells via an intracellular pathway that is linked to B cell infection. *J Gen Virol* 1996;77: 3077–3085.
175. Rogers GN, Herrler G, Paulson JC, Klenk HD. Influenza C virus uses 9-O-acetyl-N-acetylneuraminic acid as a high affinity receptor determinant for attachment to cells. *J Biol Chem* 1986;261:5947–5951.
176. Roivainen M, Piirainen L, Hovi T, et al. Entry of coxsackievirus A9 into host cells: Specific interactions with alpha v beta 3 integrin, the vitronectin receptor. *Virology* 1994;203:357–365.
177. Rolsma MD, Kuhlenschmidt TB, Gelberg HB, Kuhlenschmidt MS. Structure and function of a ganglioside receptor for porcine rotavirus. *J Virol* 1998;72:9079–9091.
178. Roy AMM, Parker JS, Parrish CR, Whittaker GR. Early stages of influenza virus entry into MV-1 lung cells: Involvement of dynamin. *Virology* 2000;267:17–28.
179. Roy S, Luetterforst R, Harding A, et al. Dominant-negative caveolin inhibits H-ras function by disrupting cholesterol-rich plasma membrane domains. *Nat Cell Biol* 1999;1:98–105.
180. Rucker J, Edinger AL, Sharron M, et al. Utilization of chemokine receptors, orphan receptors, and herpesvirus-encoded receptors by diverse human and simian immunodeficiency viruses. *J Virol* 1997; 71:8999–9007.
181. Sattentau QJ, Moore JP. The role of CD4 in HIV binding and entry. *Philos Trans R Soc Lond B Biol Sci* 1993;342:59–66.

182. Schmid SL, Mcniven MA, Decamilli P. Dynamin and its partners—A progress report. *Curr Opin Cell Biol* 1998;10:504–512.
183. Sedger LM, Shows DM, Blanton RA, et al. IFN-gamma mediates a novel antiviral activity through dynamic modulation of TRAIL and TRAIL receptor expression. *J Immunol* 1999;163:920–926.
184. Shafren DR, Bates RC, Agrez MV, et al. Coxsackieviruses B1, B3, and B5 use decay accelerating factor as a receptor for cell attachment. *J Virol* 1995;69:3873–3877.
185. Simmons G, Clapham PR, Picard L, et al. Potent inhibition of HIV-1 infectivity in macrophages and lymphocytes by a novel CCR5 antagonist. *Science* 1997;276:276–279.
186. Sixbey JW, Yao QY. Immunoglobulin A-induced shift of Epstein-Barr virus tissue tropism. *Science* 1992;255:1578–1580.
187. Skehel JJ, Bayley PM, Brown EB, et al. Changes in the conformation of influenza virus hemagglutinin at the pH optimum of virus-mediated membrane fusion. *Proc Natl Acad Sci U S A* 1982;79:968–972.
188. Smith DH, Byrn RA, Marsters SA, et al. Blocking of HIV-1 infectivity by a soluble, secreted form of the CD4 antigen. *Science* 1987;238: 1704–1707.
189. Sodeik B, Ebersold MW, Helenius A. Microtubule-mediated transport of incoming herpes simplex virus 1 capsids to the nucleus. *J Cell Biol* 1997;136:1007–1021.
190. Sommerfelt MA, Weiss RA. Receptor interference groups of 20 retroviruses plating on human cells. *Virology* 1990;176:58–69.
191. Spruce AE, Iwata A, White JM, Almers W. Patch clamp studies of single cell-fusion events mediated by a viral fusion protein. *Nature* 1989; 342:555–558.
192. Staunton DE, Merluzzi VJ, Rothlein R, et al. A cell adhesion molecule, ICAM-1, is the major surface receptor for rhinoviruses. *Cell* 1989;56:849–853.
193. Steinhauer DA, Wharton SA, Skehel JJ, Wiley DC. Studies of the membrane fusion activities of fusion peptide mutants of influenza virus hemagglutinin. *J Virol* 1995;69:6643–6651.
194. Stevenson M. Portals of entry—Uncovering HIV nuclear transport pathways. *Trends Cell Biol* 1996;6:9–15.
195. Stone-Hulslander J, Morrison TG. Mutational analysis of heptad repeats in the membrane-proximal region of Newcastle disease virus HN protein. *J Virol* 1999;73:3630–3637.
196. Stupack ELD, Bokoch GM, Nemerow GR. Adenovirus endocytosis requires actin cytoskeleton reorganization mediated by rho family GTPases. *J Virol* 1998;72:8806–8812.
197. Suomalainen M, Nakano MY, Keller S, et al. Microtubule-dependent plus- and minus end-directed motilities are competing processes for nuclear targeting of adenovirus. *J Cell Biol* 1999;144:657–672.
198. Suzuki Y, Matsunaga M, Matsumoto M. N-Acetylneuraminyllactosylceramide, GM3-NeuAc, a new influenza A virus receptor which mediates the adsorption-fusion process of viral infection. Binding specificity of influenza virus A/Aichi/2/68 (H3N2) to membrane-associated GM3 with different molecular species of sialic acid. *J Biol Chem* 1985;260:1362–1375.
199. Tailor CS, Nouri A, Lee CG, et al. Cloning and characterization of a cell surface receptor for xenotropic and polytropic murine leukemia viruses. *Proc Natl Acad Sci U S A* 1999;96:927–932.
200. Takeda A, Tuazon CU, Ennis FA. Antibody-enhanced infection by HIV-1 via Fc receptor-mediated entry. *Science* 1988;242:580–583.
201. Takeuchi Y, Vile RG, Simpson G, et al. Feline leukemia virus subgroup B uses the same cell surface receptor as gibbon ape leukemia virus. *J Virol* 1992;66:1219–1222.
202. Tamura M, Webster RG, Ennis FA. Antibodies to HA and NA augment uptake of influenza A viruses into cells via Fc receptor entry. *Virology* 1991;182:211–219.
203. Tomko RP, Xu RL, Philipson L. HCAR and MCAR—The human and mouse cellular receptors for subgroup C adenoviruses and group B coxsackieviruses. *Proc Natl Acad Sci U S A* 1997;94:3352–3356.
204. Tosteson MT, Chow M. Characterization of the ion channels formed by poliovirus in planar lipid membranes. *J Virol* 1997;71:507–511.
205. Traunecker A, Luke W, Karjalainen K. Soluble CD4 molecules neutralize human immunodeficiency virus type 1. *Nature* 1988;331:84–86.
206. Trkola A, Dragic T, Arthos J, et al. CD4–dependent, antibody-sensitive interactions between HIV-1 and its coreceptor CCR-5 *Nature* 1996;384:184–187.
207. van Zeijl M, Johann SV, Closs E, et al. A human amphotropic retrovirus receptor is a second member of the gibbon ape leukemia virus receptor family. *Proc Natl Acad Sci U S A* 1994;91:1168–1172.
208. Vodicka MA, Koepp DM, Silver PA, Emerman M. HIV-1 Vpr interacts with the nuclear transport pathway to promote macrophage infection. *Genes Dev* 1998;12:175–185.
209. Vlasak R, Luytjes W, Spaan W, Palese P. Human and bovine coronaviruses recognize sialic acid-containing receptors similar to those of influenza C viruses. *Proc Natl Acad Sci U S A* 1994;85:4526–4529.
210. Wang K, Huang S, Kapoor-Munshi A, Nemerow G. Adenovirus internalization and infection require dynamin. *J Virol* 1998;72:3455–3458.
211. Wang KS, Kuhn RJ, Strauss EG, et al. High-affinity laminin receptor is a receptor for Sindbis virus in mammalian cells. *J Virol* 1992;66: 4992–5001.
212. Ward T, Pipkin PA, Clarkson NA, et al. Decay-accelerating factor CD55 is identified as the receptor for echovirus 7 using CELICS, a rapid immuno-focal cloning method. *EMBO J* 1994;13:5070–5074.
213. Warner MS, Geraghty RJ, Martinez WM, et al. A cell surface protein with herpesvirus entry activity (HveB) confers susceptibility to infection by mutants of herpes simplex virus type 1, herpes simplex virus type 2, and pseudorabies virus. *Virology* 1998;246:179–189.
214. Weber F, Kochs G, Gruber S, Haller O. A classical bipartite nuclear localization signal on Thogoto and influenza A virus nucleoproteins. *Virology* 1998;250:9–18.
215. Weber T, Paesold G, Galli C, et al. Evidence for H(+)-induced insertion of influenza hemagglutinin HA_2 N-terminal segment into viral membrane. *J Biol Chem* 1994;269:18353–18358.
216. Weissenhorn W, Carfi A, Lee KH, et al. Crystal structure of the Ebola virus membrane fusion subunit, GP2, from the envelope glycoprotein ectodomain. *Mol Cell* 1998;2:605–616.
217. Weissenhorn W, Dessen A, Harrison SC, et al. Atomic structure of the ectodomain from HIV-1 gp41. *Nature* 1997;387:426–430.
218. Wharton SA, Calder LJ, Ruigrok RW, et al. Electron microscopy of antibody complexes of influenza virus haemagglutinin in the fusion pH conformation. *EMBO J* 1995;14:240–246.
219. White JM, Wilson IA. Anti-peptide antibodies detect steps in a protein conformational change: Low-pH activation of the influenza virus hemagglutinin. *J Cell Biol* 1987;105:2887–2896.
220. Whitt MA, Zagouras P, Crise B, Rose JK. A fusion-defective mutant of the vesicular stomatitis virus glycoprotein. *J Virol* 1990;64:4907–4913.
221. Wickham TJ, Filardo EJ, Cheresh DA, Nemerow GR. Integrin alpha v beta 5 selectively promotes adenovirus mediated cell membrane permeabilization. *J Cell Biol* 1994;127:257–264.
222. Wickham TJ, Mathias P, Cheresh DA, Nemerow GR. Integrins alpha v beta 3 and alpha v beta 5 promote adenovirus internalization but not virus attachment. *Cell* 1993;73:309–319.
223. Wien MW, Chow M, Hogle JM. Poliovirus: New insights from an old paradigm. *Structure* 1996;4:763–767.
224. Wild CT, Shugars DC, Greenwell TK, et al. Peptides corresponding to a predictive alpha-helical domain of human immunodeficiency virus type 1 gp41 are potent inhibitors of virus infection. *Proc Natl Acad Sci U S A* 1994;91:9770–9774.
225. Wold WSM, Doronin K, Toth K, et al. Immune responses to adenoviruses: Viral evasion mechanisms and their implications for the clinic. *Curr Opin Immunol* 1999;11:380–386.
226. Wu L, Gerard NP, Wyatt R, et al. CD4-induced interaction of primary HIV-1 gp120 glycoproteins with the chemokine receptor CCR-5 *Nature* 1996;384:179–183.
227. WuDunn D, Spear PG. Initial interaction of herpes simplex virus with cells is binding to heparan sulfate. *J Virol* 1989;63:52–58.
228. Wyatt R, Kwong PD, Desjardins E, et al. The antigenic structure of the HIV gp120 envelope glycoprotein. *Nature* 1998;393:705–711.
229. Yang YL, Guo L, Xu SA, et al. Receptors for polytropic and xenotropic mouse leukemia viruses encoded by a single gene at Rmc1. *Nat Genet* 1999;21:216–219.
230. Yao Q, Hu X, Compans RW. Association of the parainfluenza virus fusion and hemagglutinin-neuraminidase glycoproteins on cell surfaces. *J Virol* 1997;71:650–656.
231. Yeager CL, Ashmun RA, Williams RK, et al. Human aminopeptidase N is a receptor for human coronavirus 229E. *Nature* 1992;357:420–422.
232. Young JA, Bates P, Varmus HE. Isolation of a chicken gene that confers susceptibility to infection by subgroup A avian leukosis and sarcoma viruses. *J Virol* 1993;67:1811–1816.
233. Zhang L, Ghosh HP. Characterization of the putative fusogenic domain in vesicular stomatitis virus glycoprotein G. *J Virol* 1994;68: 2186–2193.
234. Zingler K, Belanger CA, Peters R, et al. Identification and characterization of the viral interaction determinant of the subgroup A avian leukosis virus receptor. *J Virol* 1995;69:4261–4266.

CHAPTER 5

Replication Strategies of RNA Viruses

L. Andrew Ball

INTRODUCTION

Replication of genetic information is the single most distinctive characteristic of living organisms, and nowhere in the biosphere is this process accomplished with greater economy and apparent simplicity than among the RNA viruses. To achieve the expression, replication, and spread of their genes, different families of RNA viruses have evolved diverse genetic strategies and life cycles that exploit the biology and biochemistry of their hosts in many different ways. Because the global environments in which viruses replicate and evolve are dictated largely by their hosts, understanding virus replication also illuminates host biology at the molecular, cellular, organismal, and population levels. Each infection represents an encounter between the genetic program of a virus and that of its host, and the ensuing interplay reflects the current status of their ongoing co-evolution. The details not only enrich our understanding of the biosphere in general and virus–host relationships in particular, but also create opportunities for the rational development of antiviral drugs and for domesticating viruses as expression vectors, live attenuated vaccines, and pesticides. This chapter presents an overview of the replication strategies of the major families of RNA viruses that infect animals, attempting wherever possible to identify the general principles that guide and constrain RNA virus replication and evolution. Most of the references cite review articles where citations of the primary literature can be found.

Unique Pathways and Enzymes

RNA viruses are the only organisms known to use RNA as their genetic material. They accomplish this by replicating their genomes through one of two unique biochemical pathways: either RNA-dependent RNA synthesis (RNA replication) or, among the retroviruses, RNA-dependent DNA synthesis (reverse transcription) followed by DNA replication and transcription. Both these pathways require enzyme activities that are not usually found in uninfected host cells and must therefore be encoded in the viral genome and expressed during infection. Furthermore, in some families of RNA-containing viruses, these unique synthetic processes are required right at the start of the infectious cycle. This necessitates copackaging of the corresponding polymerase and other associated enzymes with the viral genome during the assembly of virus particles in preparation for the next round of infection.

Whatever the structure and replication strategy of their genomes, all viruses must express their genes as functional

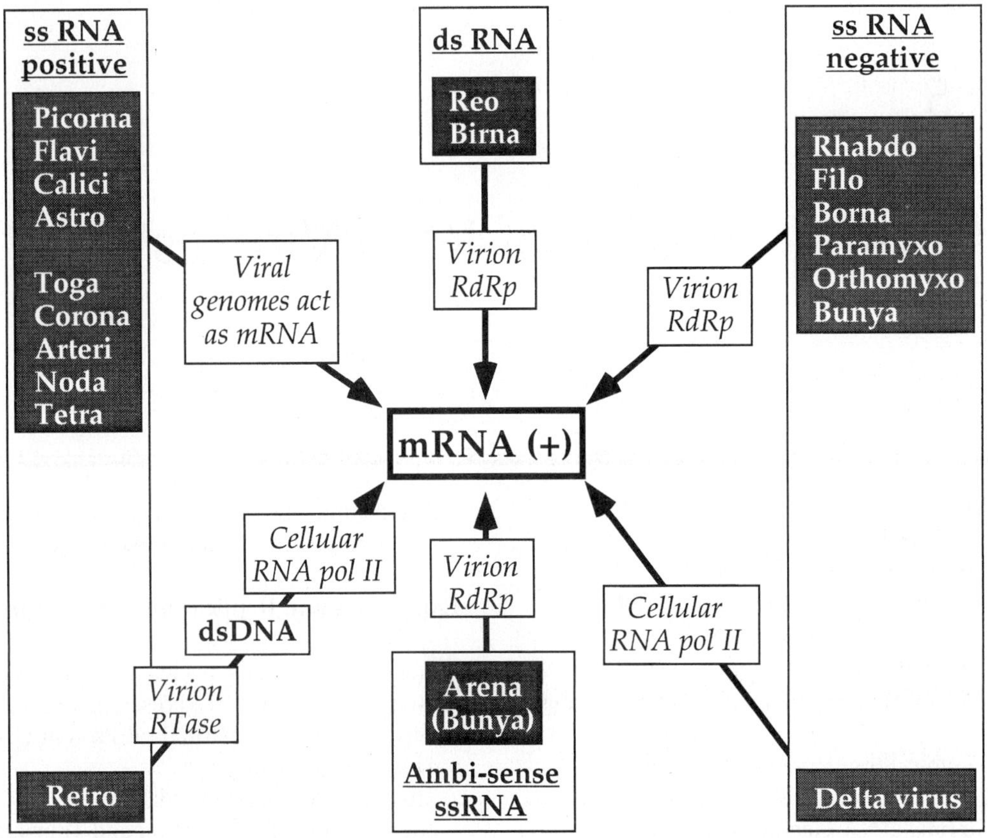

FIG. 1. Pathways of primary mRNA synthesis by RNA viruses of animals. How RNA viruses produce mRNA at the start of infection depends on the nature of the viral genome.

mRNAs early in infection to direct the cell's translational machinery to make viral proteins. The various genetic strategies used by RNA viruses can therefore be organized into a simple conceptual framework centered around viral mRNA (Fig. 1). By convention, mRNA is defined as positive sense and its complement as negative sense. The pathways leading from genome to message vary widely among the different virus families and form the basis of viral taxonomy. Their variety suggests that RNA viruses either had several different origins or that they have diverged expansively since their most recent common ancestors. Although it is generally believed that viruses originated from cellular organisms, it remains possible that some RNA virus components are descended directly from a primordial RNA or ribonucleoprotein world, which may have predated the emergence of DNA and cells.

RNA Replication is Error Prone

The polymerases that catalyze RNA replication and reverse transcription have minimal proof-reading activities. As a result, their error rates are about 10 thousand times higher than those encountered during DNA replication, and they approximate the reciprocal of the number of nucleotides in the viral genome (10,19,32). This means that the genome of any individual RNA virus particle will contain an average of one or more mutations from the consensus wild-type sequence for that virus species. This simple fact has far-reaching consequences for the biology and evolution of RNA viruses, because it means that an RNA virus population does not represent a homogenous clone—either in nature or in the laboratory—but rather a molecular swarm of related nucleotide sequences clustered in sequence space around a master consensus sequence (14). This molecular swarm or "quasi-species" provides a fertile source of phenotypic variants that can respond rapidly to changing selection pressures by shifting its composition. As a consequence, RNA viruses can evolve up to one million times faster than can DNA-based organisms (10,14).

Their rapid rates of evolution are not without cost to RNA viruses, however, because high polymerase error rates impose upper limits on genome size. The combination of replicative error rate and genome size defines an "error threshold" above which a virus cannot maintain even the sequence integrity of its quasi-species (14). As a result, few RNA virus genomes contain more than 30 kilobases (kb), and most have between 5 kb and 15 kb. RNA genomes of this size are poised just below their error thresholds, and whereas their genetic diversity inevitably wastes individual progeny that may carry lethal mutations, the cost is offset by the potential for rapid evolutionary response.

Subcellular Sites of Genome Replication

Whereas most DNA viruses of eukaryotes (apart from the poxviruses) replicate their genomes in the nucleus, most RNA viruses replicate in the cytoplasm. However, in addition to the retroviruses, which integrate DNA copies of their genomes into cellular chromosomes, other notable exceptions to this generalization are the orthomyxo- and bornaviruses whose linear negative-sense RNA genomes replicate in the nucleus. The circular RNA genome of hepatitis delta virus, like the viroids of plants, also replicates in the nucleus (Table 1). Each site of replication presents distinct opportunities and challenges in terms of which cellular components and pathways are available to be parasitized, and how the synthesis and trafficking of viral proteins, genome replication, virion assembly, and the release of progeny can be coordinated. For example, RNA splicing occurs only in the nucleus, so this way to access multiple open reading frames in a single transcript can be used only by the retro-, orthomyxo-, and bornaviruses that transcribe there. It is interesting that the paramyxoviruses, which replicate in the cytoplasm, have instead evolved a transcriptional editing mechanism that achieves the same result (8).

Levels of Segmentation: Genes, mRNAs, and Proteins

Another distinctive feature of eukaryotic cells—besides their partitioning into nuclear and cytoplasmic compartments—has a profound influence on the biology of their viruses. On most mRNAs, eukaryotic ribosomes require a methylated cap structure at the 5′ end that plays a critical role in signaling the initiation of protein synthesis. As a result, eukaryotes generally obey the rule "one mRNA, one polypeptide chain," and with very few exceptions, each message operates as a single translational unit. Similarly, viral RNA-dependent RNA polymerases (RdRp's) generally appear somewhat limited in their ability to access internal initiation sites on RNA templates, and this creates the problem of how an RNA virus can derive several separate protein products from a single genome. Through evolution, different RNA virus families have found three solutions: fragmentation at the level of proteins, mRNAs, or genes, with some viruses using more than one level. For example, RNA viruses in the picorna-, toga-, flavi-, and retrovirus families rely on extensive proteolytic processing of polyprotein precursors to derive their final protein products (13). Others (in the corona-, arteri-, rhabdo-, and paramyxovirus families, among others) depend on complex transcriptional mechanisms to produce several different monocistronic mRNAs from a single RNA template (8,26,39). Still others (in the reo-, orthomyxo-, bunya-, and arenavirus families, among others) have solved the problem by fragmenting their genomes and assembling virions that contain multiple genome segments, each often representing a single gene (see Table 1) (15,40,45). Among plant viruses, such RNA genome segments are often packaged into separate virions, necessitating co-infection by several virus particles to transmit infectivity (50), but the genome segments of animal viruses are usually copackaged. In contrast, DNA viruses seldom use either genome segmentation or polyprotein processing. This is likely due to the relative ease with which monocistronic mRNAs can be transcribed from internal promoter sites on double-stranded (ds) DNA and

TABLE 1. *Families of RNA-containing viruses that infect animals*

Virus family	Genomic RNA				RNA replication	
	ss/ds	Polarity[a]	Topology	Segments	Enzyme	Intracellular site
Picornaviridae	ss	Positive	Linear	1	Viral RdRp	Cytoplasm
Flaviviridae	ss	Positive	Linear	1	Viral RdRp	Cytoplasm
Caliciviridae	ss	Positive	Linear	1	Viral RdRp	Cytoplasm
Astroviridae	ss	Positive	Linear	1	Viral RdRp	Cytoplasm
Togaviridae	ss	Positive	Linear	1	Viral RdRp	Cytoplasm
Nodaviridae	ss	Positive	Linear	2	Viral RdRp	Cytoplasm
Tetraviridae	ss	Positive	Linear	1 or 2	Viral RdRp	Cytoplasm
Coronaviridae	ss	Positive	Linear	1	Viral RdRp	Cytoplasm
Arteriviridae	ss	Positive	Linear	1	Viral RdRp	Cytoplasm
Retroviridae	ss	Positive	Linear	2 (identical)	Virion RTase	Nucleus/Cytoplasm
Birnaviridae	ds	Both	Linear	2	Virion RdRp	Cytoplasm
Reoviridae	ds	Both	Linear	10–12	Virion RdRp	Cytoplasm
Rhabdoviridae	ss	Negative	Linear	1	Virion RdRp	Cytoplasm
Filoviridae	ss	Negative	Linear	1	Virion RdRp	Cytoplasm
Bornaviridae	ss	Negative	Linear	1	Virion RdRp	Nucleus
Paramyxoviridae	ss	Negative	Linear	1	Virion RdRp	Cytoplasm
Bunyaviridae	ss	Negative or ambisense	Linear	3	Virion RdRp	Cytoplasm
Orthomyxoviridae	ss	Negative	Linear	6–8	Virion RdRp	Nucleus
Delta virus (also viroids)	ss	Negative	Circular	1	RNA pol II	Nucleus
Arenaviridae	ss	Ambisense	Linear	2	Virion RdRp	Cytoplasm

[a]Polarity of the encapsidated RNA. By convention, mRNA is defined as having positive polarity.
ss, single-stranded; ds, double-stranded.

the use of differential splicing of nuclear transcripts to express promoter-distal open reading frames.

STRUCTURES AND ORGANIZATION OF VIRAL RNA GENOMES

Unlike cellular genomes, which uniformly consist of dsDNA, viral RNA genomes provide examples of almost every structural variation imaginable. As shown in Table 1, different families of RNA viruses have genomes that consist of either ds or single-stranded (ss) RNA; of either positive, negative, or mixed (ambi-sense) polarity; of either linear or circular topology; and of either single or multiple RNA segments. Each of these variations has consequences for the pathways of genome replication, viral gene expression, and virion assembly.

Single- and Double-Stranded RNA Genomes

Although all RNA genomes replicate through conventional Watson–Crick base-pairing between complementary template and daughter strands, different RNA virus families encapsidate and transmit different molecular stages of the RNA replication cycle. Families of ssRNA viruses outnumber families of dsRNA viruses by almost 10 to one, roughly the inverse of the ratio found among DNA viruses. In view of the greater stability of ds nucleic acids of both types, this difference calls for an explanation. Two possibilities seem plausible: first, dsRNA viruses must somehow circumvent the translational suppression resulting from the coexistence of equimolar amounts of antisense RNAs. How the dsRNA reoviruses solve this problem is described in Chapter 26. Second, dsRNA is widely recognized by the cells of higher eukaryotes as a signal for the induction of defense mechanisms that act to suppress viral replication, such as the interferon system in vertebrates (27; also see Chapter 12) and gene silencing in plants (30). These two effects probably suffice to explain the relative scarcity of dsRNA viruses.

For these same reasons, it is important even for ssRNA viruses to limit the accumulation of replicative intermediates that contain regions of dsRNA, and the strategies to ensure this differ between positive- and negative-strand viruses. All positive-strand RNA viruses synthesize disproportionately low levels of negative-sense RNA—typically 1% to 5% of the levels of positive-sense RNA—and thereby minimize the potential for dsRNA accumulation. Conversely, negative-strand viruses, which need substantial amounts of both positive- and negative-sense RNAs to use as messages and progeny genomes, respectively, usually prevent them from annealing to one another by keeping the genomic RNA covered with a viral nucleocapsid protein (7,39).

Positive- and Negative-Sense RNA Genomes

The differences between positive- and negative-strand RNA viruses extend beyond the polarity of the RNA assembled into virions. Positive-sense RNA genomes exchange their virion proteins for ribosomes and cellular RNA-binding proteins at the start of infection. Once synthesized and assembled, the virus-specified RdRp and other nonstructural proteins replace the ribosomes to accomplish RNA replication. Virion structural proteins are reacquired during the assembly of viral progeny. In contrast, negative-sense RNA genomes and their antigenomic complements remain associated with their nucleocapsid proteins both within virus particles and throughout the viral replication cycle, even during RNA replication. These fundamentally different adaptations can be attributed to the fact that whereas positive-sense genomes must satisfy criteria for translation that are dictated by the host cell, negative-sense genomes and antigenomes must satisfy only the template requirements of the virus-specified RdRp because they are replicated but never translated. Although it remains unclear how polymerases can copy protein-coated RNA templates, the mechanism was surely refined during the coevolution of negative-strand viral nucleocapsids and their RdRp's relatively free from cellular constraints. Double-stranded RNA genomes are intermediate between these extremes: the parental genome segments remain sequestered in subviral particles, whereas positive-sense precursors to the progeny dsRNAs are initially unencapsidated. These distinctions most likely reflect significant differences in the structures of the viral RdRp–template complexes and in the molecular mechanisms of replication of positive, negative, and dsRNA genomes.

Linear and Circular RNA Genomes

RNA replication not only requires an acceptable error rate, as discussed earlier, but also must avoid the systematic deletion or addition of nucleotides. Genome termini are particularly troublesome in this respect, which has been dubbed "the end problem." For DNA replication, the end problem is exacerbated by the fact that DNA polymerases cannot initiate daughter strands and must therefore depend on primers, which creates the additional complication of how to replicate the primer-binding site(s). Among several known solutions, the most economical and widespread in nature is to eliminate the ends by covalently circularizing the DNA, as in prokaryotic genomes.

Unlike DNA polymerases, most RNA polymerases do not require primers, so RNA genomes are less susceptible to the end problem. Accordingly, most RNA virus genomes are linear molecules. Covalently closed circular RNAs are found only in hepatitis delta virus in animals (see Table 1), and among the viroids and some other subviral RNA pathogens that infect plants (9,24). Nevertheless, the termini of linear RNAs are especially vulnerable to degradation, and their replication is likely to be particularly error prone. Consequently, every family of RNA viruses has features designed to preserve the termini of the genome. For example, many positive-strand RNA genomes carry the 5′-caps and 3′-poly(A) tracts that protect the termini of eukaryotic mRNAs against degradation, and similar roles are likely played by the Vpg protein that is covalently bound to the 5′ end of picornavirus RNAs (36), and by the stable RNA secondary structures found at the 3′ ends of flavivirus and other genomes. The 3′ ends of many plant virus RNAs form cloverleaf structures that resemble tRNAs so closely that they are recognized by cellular tRNA charging and modifying enzymes (12). In addition to playing protective roles, terminal modifications of positive-sense RNAs also may serve to bring their ends together by binding to interacting cellular proteins such as the poly(A)-binding protein and cap-binding complex, thereby forming noncovalent functionally circular complexes that may promote repetitive translation by ribosomes and repetitive replication by RdRp's.

Unlike the genomes of positive-sense RNA viruses, negative- and ambisense RNA genomes rarely carry covalent terminal modifications. Instead, these RNAs routinely show some degree of terminal sequence complementarity, which is thought to stabilize the viral nucleocapsid in a panhandle structure and promote RNA replication, perhaps by rendering the template functionally circular, as described for positive-strand RNAs (see Chapters 22, 23, and 24). Terminal complementarity also may enable the RNA ends to act as telomeres for one another, with the 5′ end serving as a template to restore nucleotides eroded from the 3′ end.

In other solutions to the end problem, there is evidence that some ambisense arenaviruses may be able to tolerate a substantial level of sequence variation at the termini of their genomic RNAs, presumably by locating all necessary cis-acting signals internally, well away from the RNA termini (41; also see Chapter 50 in *Fields Virology*, 4th ed.). Retroviral genomes conversely are terminally redundant, and have direct repeats of between 12 and 235 nucleotides at each end that maintain and restore the integrity of the termini during reverse transcription and virus replication (28; also see Chapter 27).

Segmented and Nonsegmented RNA Genomes

Although genome segmentation facilitates the production of multiple gene products in eukaryotic cells, it also means that the various genome segments must each contain appropriate cis-acting signals to mediate their expression, replication, and assembly into virions. In some virus families with segmented genomes (such as the orthomyxoviruses and some reoviruses), these signals comprise conserved sequences at the RNA termini, but in others (such as the bipartite noda- and tetraviruses), significant sequence conservation between the segments is undetectable. In these cases, the specificity of RNA replication and assembly is presumably determined by conserved RNA secondary or tertiary structures. However, the mechanisms that coordinate the replication and packaging of multiple genome segments remain poorly understood for any eukaryotic virus.

Evidently the evolutionary barrier between viruses with segmented and nonsegmented RNA genomes is readily traversed, because both genome types occur in members of the alphavirus-like supergroup, a taxonomic cluster based on phylogenetic comparisons of viral nonstructural protein sequences (23). Indeed, among the tetraviruses, segmented and nonsegmented genomes can be found even within the same family (31). Furthermore, the genomes of some toga- and rhabdoviruses, which are naturally nonsegmented, have been experimentally divided in two without destroying viral infectivity, thus confirming the flexibility of RNA virus genomes in this regard. Nevertheless, genome segmentation has major effects on the biology of a virus, because individual segments can often reassort between dissimilar strains in co-infected cells, enabling segmented genome viruses to make substantial evolutionary leaps by horizontal gene transfer. This mechanism underlies the antigenic shifts that produce new pandemic strains of the orthomyxovirus influenza (see Chapter 47 in *Fields Virology*, 4th ed.).

Cis-Acting Signals and Specificity

Replication and packaging of viral RNAs display striking specificity; both processes unerringly pick the correct viral molecules from among thousands of cellular RNAs that may be much more abundant. This is generally attributed to the presence of cis-acting signals that selectively channel the viral RNAs into replication and assembly complexes, but in most RNA virus genomes, these signals remain to be clearly identified. Those that have been characterized mostly comprise not linear nucleotide sequences but RNA secondary structures such as bulged stem-loops, tRNA-like cloverleaves, and pseudoknots, which are thought to create distinctive three-dimensional molecular shapes that interact specifically with viral enzymes and structural proteins (11). However, although high-resolution structures have been determined for some RdRp's, reverse transcriptases, and several viral capsids, our understanding of the molecular basis of specificity in RNA replication and virus assembly is limited by our scant knowledge of the three-dimensional structures of the viral RNA and its cis-acting signals. Not infrequently, the structural basis of RNA selectivity during replication and assembly has proved elusive, perhaps because the specificity determinants can be redundant, dispersed, or global properties of the viral genome. Furthermore, in both RNA replication and assembly, specific initiation is followed by less specific RNA–protein interactions that propagate the reactions. The transitions between these different stages are largely unexplored, and much remains to be learned concerning the recognition of cis-acting RNA signals and how they promulgate RNA replication and virus assembly.

Satellite RNAs and Defective RNA Genomes

Occasionally RNA molecules arise that are neither independently infectious nor essential for infectivity but nevertheless contain cis-acting signals that promote their own replication and/or packaging by the proteins encoded by another virus. Such satellite RNAs are parasitic on the parent virus and can modulate its replication and virulence (46). Among the RNA viruses of animals, a prime example is hepatitis delta virus, which packages its genome in virion proteins encoded by the hepadnavirus hepatitis B, and can severely exacerbate its pathogenicity (24; also see Chapter 88 in *Fields Virology*, 4th ed.). Dependence of an RNA satellite on a DNA virus parent is unusual; more commonly, satellite RNAs are replicated and encapsidated by the proteins of an RNA virus parent with which they share at least some sequence homology. In some instances, satellite RNAs encode their own distinct capsid proteins, or proteins required for RNA replication (as in the case of hepatitis delta virus), but in others, they are translationally silent. Satellite RNAs are much more common among the viruses of plants than in those of animals (see Chapter 14), perhaps because the transmission of animal viruses between hosts generally involves narrower bottlenecks, which select against the spread of satellites.

In contrast to the transmission of viral infection between hosts, the spread of infection within a single animal usually involves successive episodes of localized virus replication, which resemble the conditions of plaque formation and serial high-multiplicity passage in cell culture. These conditions favor the generation and amplification of defective viral RNAs, which can arise from simple deletions of viral genes as well as from more complex genome rearrangements that occur during RNA replication. Like satellite RNAs, defective RNAs parasitize the parent virus and usually interfere with its replication, but because they also depend on it for their own survival, they typically establish a fluctuating coexistence (46). Most families of animal RNA viruses readily generate defective interfering (DI) RNAs in cell culture, but their influence on viral disease and evolution is less well understood.

EXPRESSION AND REPLICATION OF RNA VIRUS GENOMES

Variety of RNA Virus Genome Strategies

The type of RNA genome largely determines whether the first step of macromolecular synthesis is translation, transcription, or RNA replication. Viruses with positive-sense ssRNA genomes (except the retroviruses) deliver their genomic RNAs directly to cellular ribosomes and

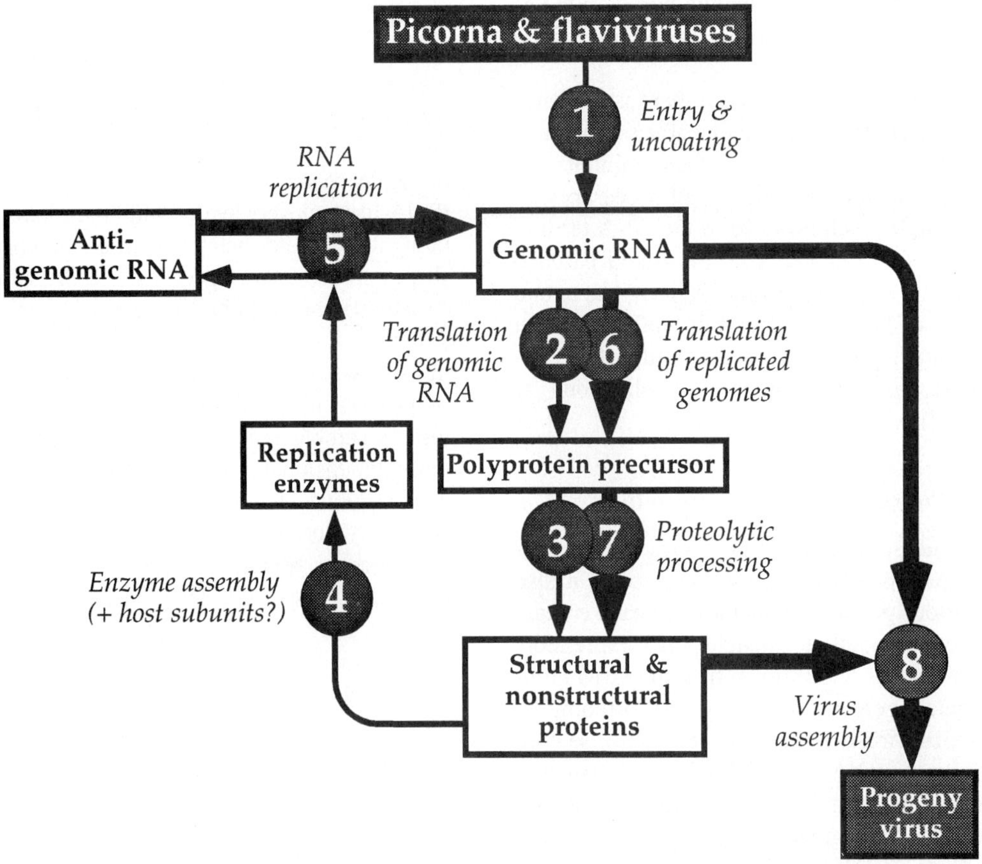

FIG. 2. Replication scheme of positive-strand RNA viruses that make no subgenomic mRNAs. After entry and uncoating (*step 1*), genomic RNA is used directly as the mRNA for both nonstructural and structural proteins (*steps 2 and 3*). The nonstructural proteins catalyze RNA replication via the synthesis of antigenomic RNA (*steps 4 and 5*). Replication produces more genomic RNA for further translation of viral proteins (*steps 6 and 7*) and for assembly with the structural proteins to produce progeny virus particles (*step 8*). For further details, see Chapters 18 and 20. In this and the figures that follow, *arrow thickness* denotes the relative magnitude of the reactions.

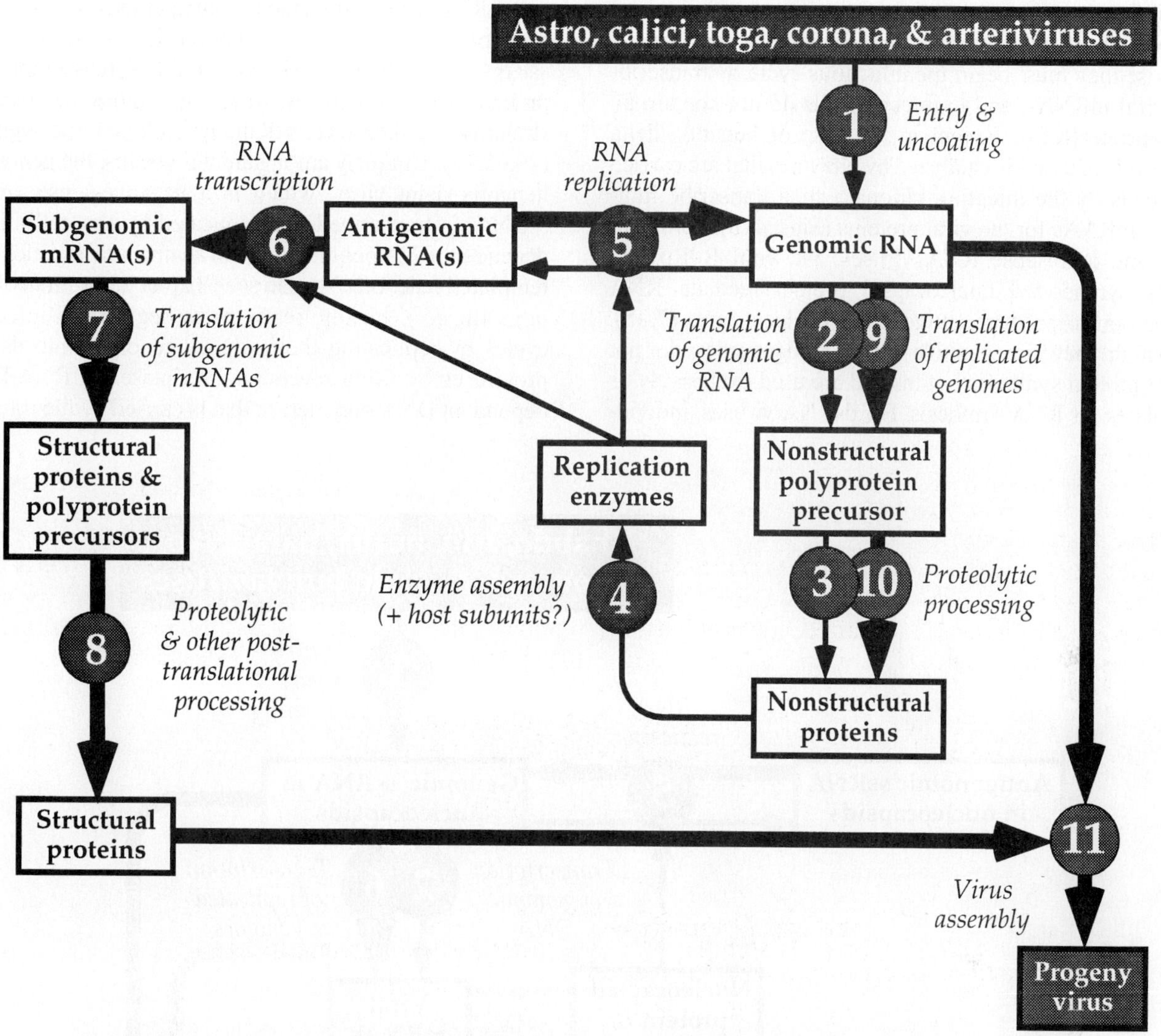

FIG. 3. Replication scheme of positive-strand RNA viruses that make one or more subgenomic mRNAs. After entry and uncoating (*step 1*), genomic RNA is used directly as the mRNA for nonstructural proteins that include the viral RNA-dependent RNA polymerases (RdRp's) (*steps 2 and 3*). The RdRp catalyzes RNA replication through the synthesis of full-length antigenomic RNA (*steps 4 and 5*). It also transcribes one or more subgenomic mRNAs (*step 6*), which direct synthesis of the viral structural proteins (*steps 7 and 8*). Replicated genomes are translated to produce more nonstructural proteins (*steps 9 and 10*), and assembled with structural proteins into progeny virus particles (*step 11*). Note that the corona- and arteriviruses (Chapter 21 as well as Chapter 37 from *Fields Virology,* 4th ed.) synthesize their subgenomic mRNAs by a very different mechanism from that used by the toga-, astro-, and caliciviruses (Chapter 19 as well as Chapter 27 from *Fields Virology,* 4th ed.).

begin the infectious cycle with translation (Figs. 2 and 3). Accordingly, these genomic RNAs are infectious even when completely deproteinized, as was first shown for tobacco mosaic virus RNA in classic work that helped to establish that genes were composed of nucleic acids rather than proteins (17). Positive-sense RNA viruses fall into two groups: those that produce subgenomic mRNAs and those that do not. For viruses in the latter group (like the picorna- and flaviviruses), genomic RNA directs the synthesis of a single polyprotein precursor to both the structural and nonstructural viral proteins, which are therefore produced in equimolar amounts (see Fig. 2). After cleavage by proteases contained within the polyprotein itself, the nonstructural proteins catalyze RNA replication to produce progeny genomes that assemble with the processed structural proteins to form progeny virus particles. For positive-sense viruses in the other group, which include the astro-, calici-, toga-, corona-, and arteriviruses (see Fig. 3), genomic RNA directs the synthesis of a precursor to only the nonstructural proteins, which include the viral RdRp. This enzyme then transcribes one or more subgenomic mRNAs that encode the structural proteins. Their greater transcriptional complexity allows these viruses to produce their proteins in dissimilar amounts.

Viral genomes that consist of negative- or ambisense ssRNA or of dsRNA are not infectious by themselves because they must begin the infectious cycle by transcribing viral mRNAs, and uninfected cells do not contain an appropriate RdRp. Except in the case of hepatitis delta virus, this reaction is catalyzed by enzymes that are carried into cells by the infecting virions, which transcribe individual mRNAs for the viral proteins (Figs. 4–6). For negative- and ambisense RNA viruses, the viral RdRp and newly synthesized nucleocapsid protein mediate RNA replication to produce antigenomic nucleocapsids (7,35). Although they are positive sense, antigenomes do not direct protein synthesis but instead are used exclusively as templates for RNA synthesis. For dsRNA viruses, individual mRNAs are transcribed from genome segments that remain enclosed in subviral particles (see Fig. 6). These ssRNAs and their translation products reassemble into progeny subviral particles, where the synthesis of negative-strand RNAs then recreates the dsRNA genome segments (40,45,47). Uniquely among animal viruses, the genome of hepatitis delta virus, which is a negative-sense circular ssRNA, is transcribed and replicated by the cell's DNA-dependent RNA polymerase II in an uncharacteristic RNA-templated reaction (24; also see Chapter 88 of *Fields Virology*, 4th ed.). Finally, retroviruses begin their infectious cycles by replicating their ssRNA genomes into dsDNA proviruses by using reverse transcriptase, an RNA/DNA-dependent DNA polymerase that is carried by the infecting

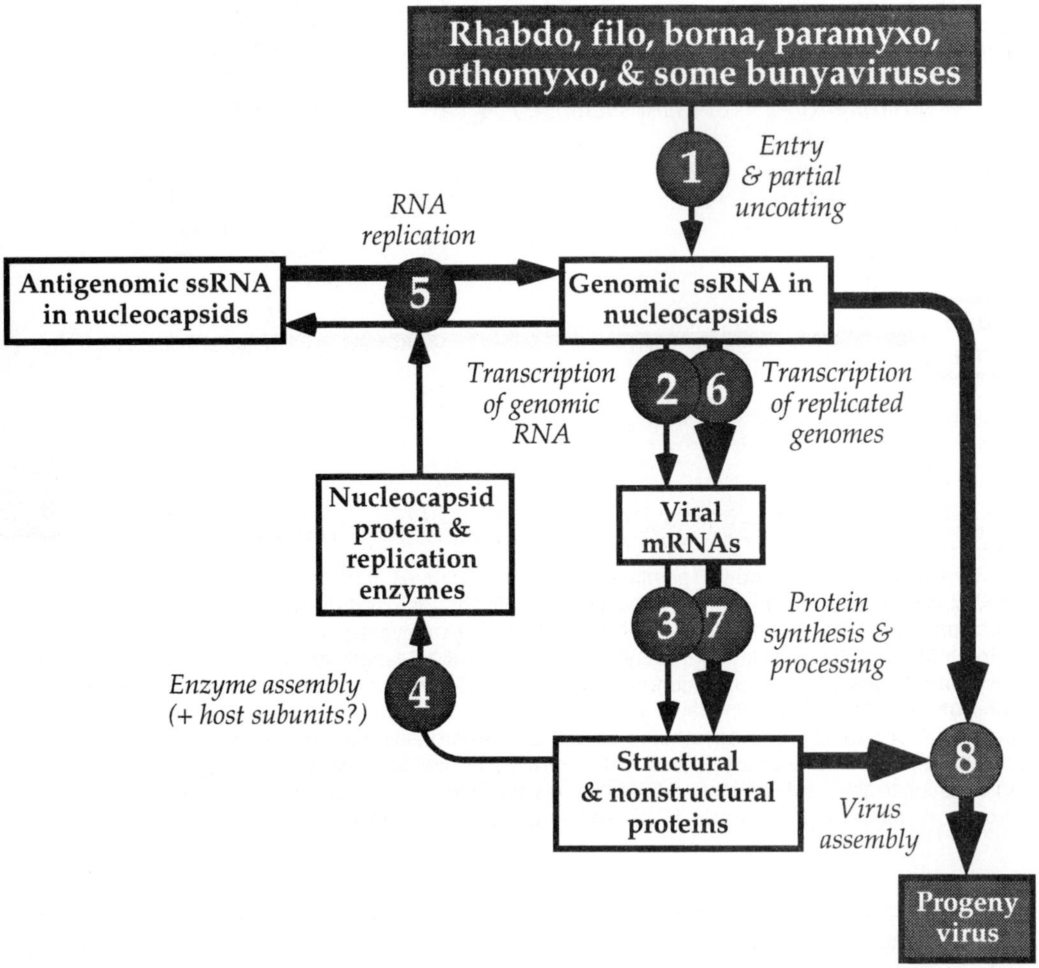

FIG. 4. Replication scheme of negative-strand RNA viruses. After entry and partial uncoating (*step 1*), encapsidated viral RNAs are transcribed by the nucleocapsid-associated RNA-dependent RNA polymerases (RdRp's) to produce mRNAs (*step 2*) for the viral proteins (*step 3*). These catalyze RNA replication through the synthesis of antigenomic nucleocapsids (*steps 4 and 5*). Replication produces more genomic nucleocapsids for further transcription (*step 6*) and translation (*step 7*) of viral genes, and for assembly with the structural proteins to produce progeny virus particles (*step 8*). Orthomyxo- and bornaviruses transcribe and replicate in the nucleus, and some of their mRNAs are spliced (Chapter 24 as well as Chapter 51 of *Fields Virology*, 4th ed.). The other virus families listed replicate in the cytoplasm and avoid splicing (Chapters 22, 23 and 25; as well as Chapter 40 of *Fields Virology*, 4th ed.). Some bunyavirus genomes are negative sense and some are ambisense (Chapter 25 and Chapter 49 of *Fields Virology*, 4th ed.; see Fig. 5).

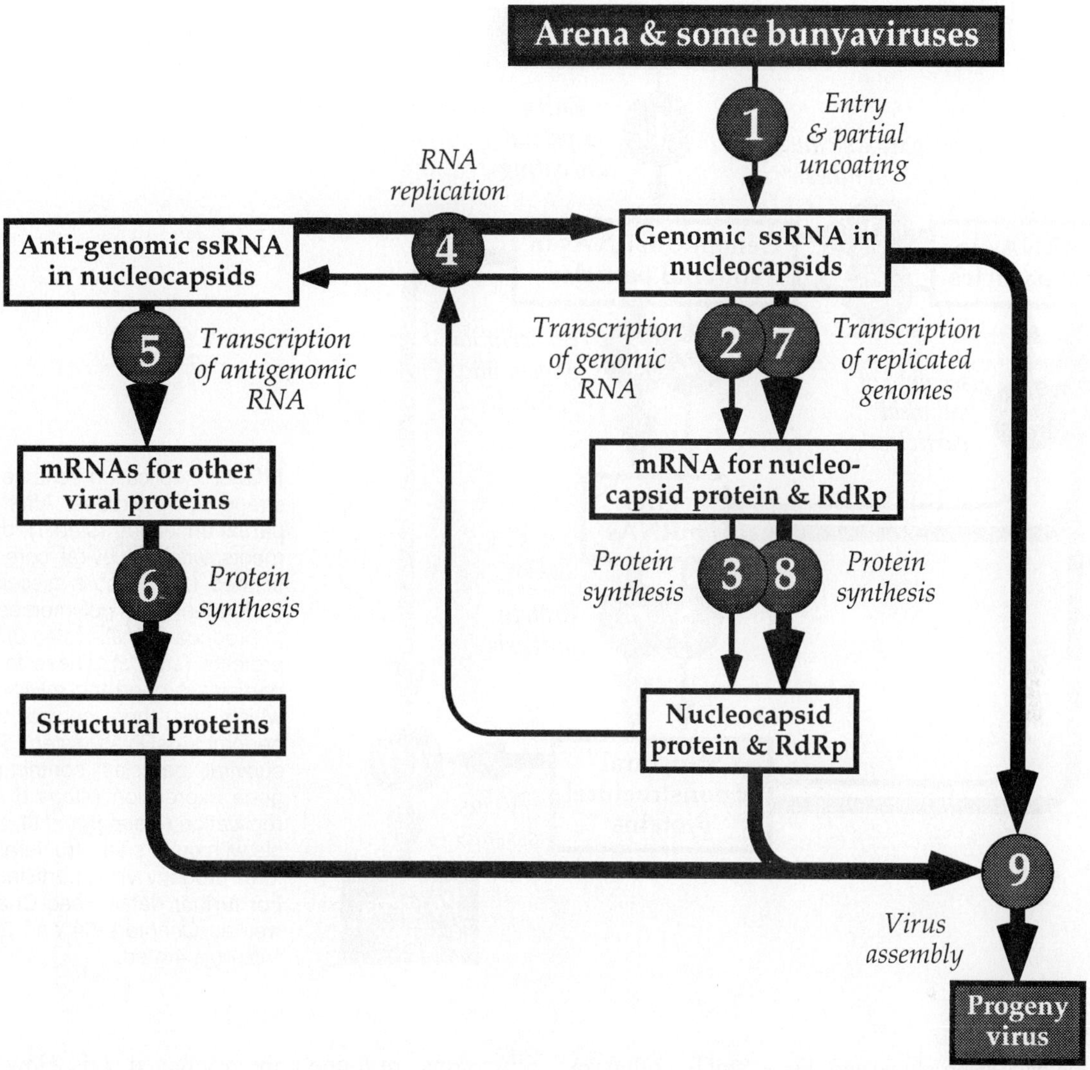

FIG. 5. Replication scheme of ambisense RNA viruses. After entry and partial uncoating (*step 1*), encapsidated viral RNAs are partially transcribed by the nucleocapsid-associated RNA-dependent RNA polymerases (RdRp's) to produce mRNAs (*step 2*) for the nucleocapsid protein and RdRp (*step 3*). These catalyze RNA replication through the synthesis of antigenomic nucleocapsids (*step 4*), which serve both as templates for transcription of mRNAs (*step 5*) for the other viral proteins (*step 6*), and for the production of more genomic nucleocapsids. Replicated genomic nucleocapsids serve as templates for transcription (*step 7*) and translation (*step 8*) of viral genes, and for assembly with the structural proteins to produce progeny virus particles (*step 9*). Some bunyavirus genomes are ambisense and some are negative sense (see Fig. 4). For further details, see Chapters 25 and 27.

virion (28). After integration into a host chromosome, proviral DNA is transcribed by cellular RNA polymerase II to produce unspliced and spliced viral mRNAs that direct viral protein synthesis (Fig. 7).

Regulation of Gene Expression

DNA viruses typically express different sets of genes before and after DNA replication, predominantly making catalytic amounts of nonstructural proteins during the prereplicative or early phase of infection, and stoichiometric amounts of structural proteins later, after DNA replication has amplified the gene copy-number. In contrast, most RNA viruses show little differentiation between the pre- and postreplicative phases of the infectious cycle, expressing their genes at roughly the same relative levels throughout infection. In cases like the toga- and influenza viruses, in which some temporal modulation of gene expression does occur, the differences are subtle and are accomplished mostly at the transcriptional level through modulation of mRNA levels.

However, posttranscriptional controls and countermeasures dominate the struggle between eukaryotic cells and viruses for the supremacy of gene expression. Apart from the retroviruses, RNA viruses generally inhibit host protein synthesis either directly or indirectly, and some specific

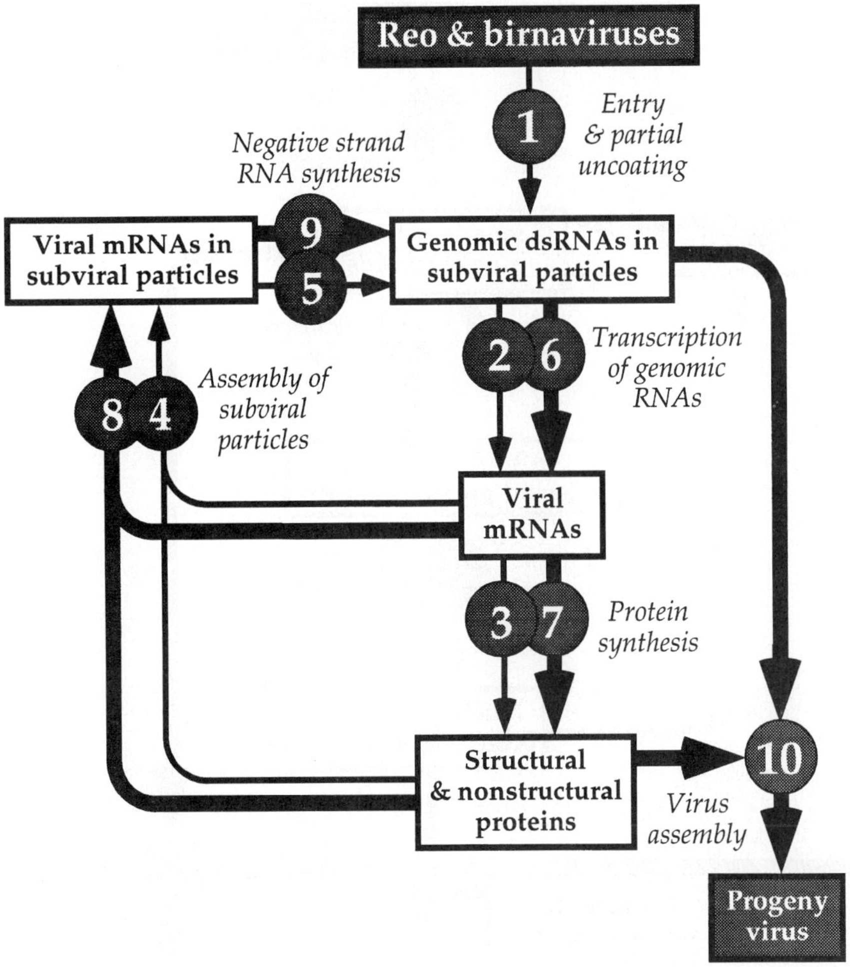

FIG. 6. Replication scheme of double-strand RNA viruses. After entry and partial uncoating (*step 1*), dsRNA segments within subviral cores are transcribed by the core-associated RNA-dependent RNA polymerases (RdRp's) to produce mRNAs (*step 2*) for the viral proteins (*step 3*). These form subviral particles around the mRNAs (*step 4*), which are then copied to produce genomic dsRNAs (*step 5*). Progeny subviral particles contribute to viral gene expression (*steps 6 and 7*) and replication (*steps 8 and 9*), and assemble with outer shell structural proteins to form progeny virus particles (*step 10*). For further details, see Chapter 26 as well as Chapters 54 and 56 of *Fields Virology*, 4th ed.

mechanisms have been elucidated. For example, influenza virus blocks the splicing and nuclear export of cellular mRNAs, whereas polio- and rhinoviruses degrade mRNA cap-binding protein, but some other viruses monopolize translation simply by flooding the cell with highly efficient mRNAs (1). To counteract virus infection, some cells have evolved antiviral defense mechanisms such as gene silencing in plants and the interferon system in vertebrates, which intervene posttranscriptionally to degrade viral mRNAs and inhibit their translation (27,30; also see Chapter 12). In response, many viruses have acquired mechanisms to neutralize or evade these cellular defenses in ways that provide valuable insights into virus–host coevolution (1). Because retroviruses integrate DNA copies of their genomes into cellular chromosomes, their replication depends on the survival and proliferation of the host cell. Many retroviruses therefore express oncogenes that override cell-cycle controls and drive infected cells to divide (28).

Structural and Nonstructural Proteins

By definition, virus-specified structural proteins are incorporated into virus particles, whereas nonstructural proteins are found only in infected cells. However, negative-, ambisense, and dsRNA viruses assemble their RdRp's and associated enzymes into progeny virions and therefore encode predominantly or exclusively structural proteins. In addition to the polymerase, virus-encoded enzymes often include one or more proteases, an RNA helicase, guanylyl- and methyl-transferases, poly(A) polymerase, sometimes a nuclease, and in the case of the retroviruses, a DNA integrase. However, for several RNA viruses, the evidence that these enzymes are virally encoded is only circumstantial or is based on inconclusive sequence homologies.

The proteases process the primary translation products of which they are a part by cleaving them at highly specific target sequences, and in some picornavirus-infected cells, they also selectively inhibit host cell protein synthesis by cleavage of the cellular cap-binding protein (13). Particularly among the larger RNA viruses, RNA helicases may be required to disrupt inter- or intramolecular base-pairing during RNA synthesis, although some RdRp's are capable of melting RNA duplexes without help (21). Guanylyl- and methyltransferases construct the 5′-caps found on the mRNAs of almost all eukaryotic

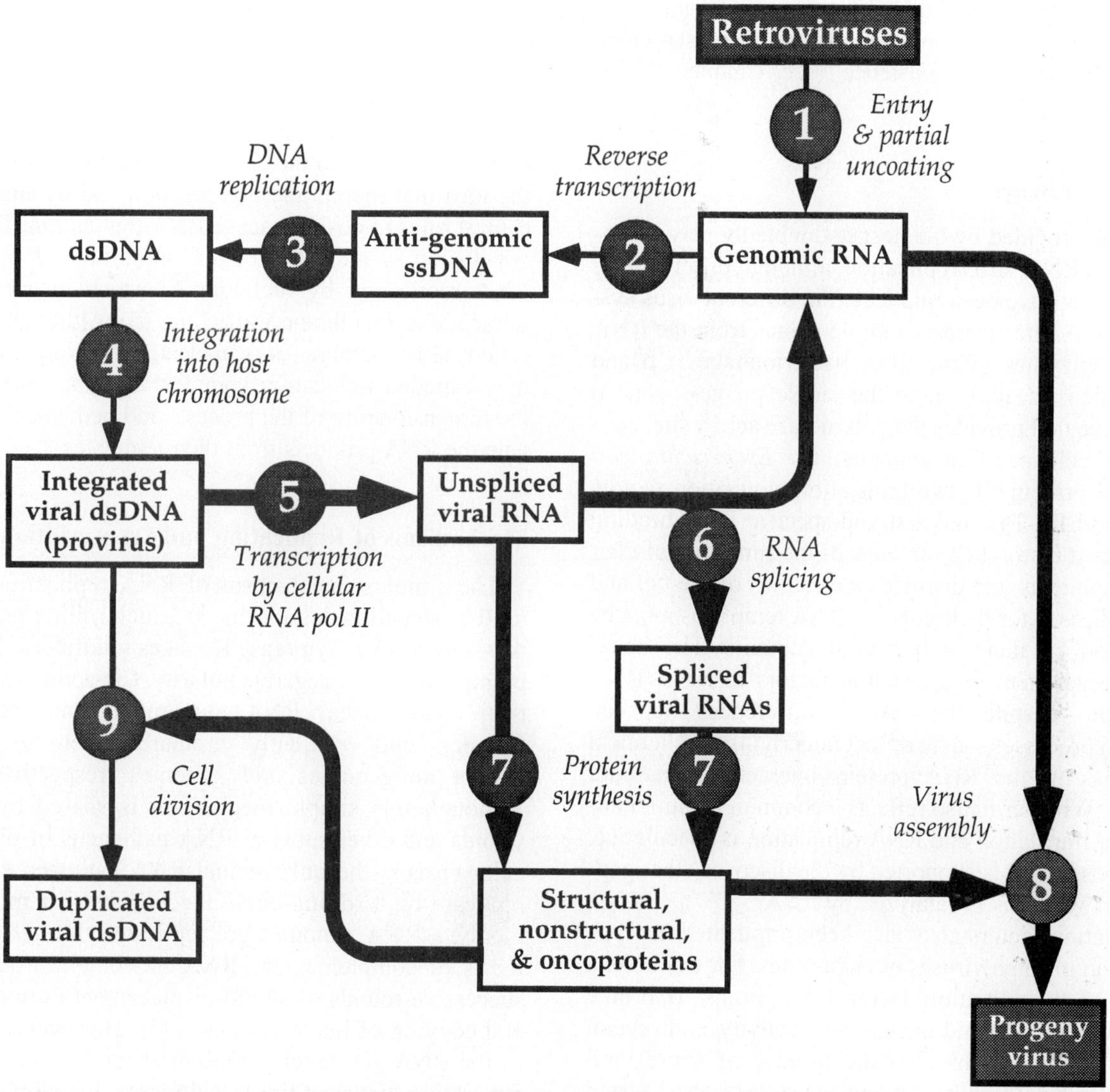

FIG. 7. Replication scheme of retroviruses. After entry and partial uncoating (*step 1*), genomic RNA is copied to dsDNA by reverse transcriptase (*steps 2 and 3*) and covalently integrated into cellular DNA in the nucleus by DNA integrase (*step 4*). Both enzymes are present in the viral core. The integrated viral genome (or provirus) is transcribed by cellular RNA polymerase II (*step 5*) to produce viral RNA transcripts that function both as precursors to mRNAs for the viral proteins (*steps 6 and 7*) and for assembly into progeny virus particles (*step 8*). For further details, see Chapter 58 of *Fields Virology*, 4th ed .

RNA viruses (42), except for the picornaviruses, which are uncapped, and the orthomyxo- and bunyaviruses, which steal the caps from cellular mRNAs by means of a cap-specific endonuclease (3,15,37). At their 3′ ends, most animal virus mRNAs carry untemplated poly(A) tails, although 3′ tRNA-like structures are common among plant RNA viruses (12,50). Polyadenylation is usually ascribed to a stuttering side-reaction of the viral RdRp rather than to a separate poly(A) polymerase, as in poxviruses, although the enzymology of the reaction remains to be clearly defined (38).

Comparisons among the amino acid sequences of viral RdRp's establish clear phylogenetic relationships that also reflect other differences in viral genome structures and strategies (23). Moreover, the x-ray crystal structures of the polio- and hepatitis C virus RdRp's (4,18) show unmistakable resemblances not only to one another but also to those of reverse transcriptases, as well as DNA-dependent RNA and DNA polymerases. Although the overall levels of amino acid sequence homology among these diverse polymerases are statistically insignificant, RdRp's share many of the characteristic polymerase motifs that occupy critical positions in the three-dimensional architecture of the polymerase active site (20,34). Taken together, the structural homologies of their RdRp's firmly anchor the RNA viruses to the rest of the biosphere, and suggest that despite their diversity, these viruses radiated from common ancestors that probably escaped from cellular origins to establish a transmissible parasitic existence (see Chapter 13 of *Fields Virology*, 4th ed.).

Host-Cell Proteins

Proteins provided by the host undoubtedly play essential roles in RNA virus replication, although different cellular proteins have been implicated in different virus systems (25,44). The clearest example comes from the RNA replicase enzymes of the RNA bacteriophages Qβ and MS2, which, in addition to the single phage-specified polypeptide that provides the polymerase active site, contain four cell-specified subunits: the *Escherichia coli* ribosomal protein S1, two translation elongation factors (EF-Tu and EF-Ts), and a strand-specific RNA-binding protein, host factor-1 (2). In view of the similarity of their host components, the distinct specificities of the Qβ and MS2 replicases for their cognate RNA templates must be determined by their unique viral subunits. The unexpected recruitment of translation factors to assist RNA replication—despite the evident differences between these two processes—may reflect underlying biochemical similarities in the RNA–protein interactions that are involved. Whether it also reflects a common evolutionary origin for translation and RNA replication is speculative, but the possibility is supported by the discovery that peptide bond synthesis is catalyzed by RNA.

Translation factors also have been implicated in RNA replication in some viruses of eukaryotes. For example, a subunit of the initiation factor eIF-3 binds to brome mosaic virus RdRp and increases its activity, and several other host proteins bind to the termini of some viral RNAs in infected cells. Among these are poly(A)- and polypyrimidine tract-binding proteins, calreticulin, and the snRNA-binding proteins Ro and La (5,29). Although it is often difficult to distinguish fortuitous interactions from those that play functional roles, the development of cell-free systems and recombinant strains of yeast that support the complete replication of certain viral RNAs promises clarification from biochemical and genetic studies, respectively (5).

Host-Cell Membranes

Unlike phage replicases, the RdRp's of eukaryotic viruses are invariably found associated with some type of supramolecular assembly: host-cell membranes for positive-sense RNA viruses, nucleocapsids for negative-sense RNA viruses, and subviral particles for dsRNA viruses. In general, the intracellular membranes of cells infected with positive-sense RNA viruses undergo proliferation and redistribution to form anchor sites for the viral RNA replication complexes. When these complexes are released from membranes during purification, they generally lose the ability to catalyze true RNA replication, although they often retain the more limited ability to copy an RNA template into its complement. In the case of the nodavirus flock house virus, true RNA replicase activity was restored to partially purified RdRp by adding glycerophospholipids to the cell-free extract (49), reinforcing the idea that membrane organization and dynamics play central roles in positive-sense RNA replication. The same conclusion is indicated by the inhibition of poliovirus RNA replication by brefeldin A, which interferes with intracellular membrane trafficking (5). Although the specific role of membranes is unclear, it is thought that they may expedite replication complex assembly by reducing the dimensionality of the process, and perhaps also segregate the RNA products from their templates.

Mechanisms of Replication and Transcription

The simplest mechanism of RNA replication is that used by hepatitis delta virus, in which rolling-circle synthesis by RNA polymerase II makes multimeric RNAs of both positive and negative polarity. Cis-acting ribozymes then cleave linear RNA monomers from these concatamers and covalently circularize them to produce mature antigenomes and genomes, respectively (24). Although this simple mechanism is shared by several viroids and other subviral RNA pathogens of plants (9), delta virus is the only animal RNA pathogen known to replicate by a rolling-circle mechanism. Far more commonly, ssRNA genomes are replicated through the synthesis of complementary RNA monomers produced by successive rounds of strand-displacement during end-to-end copying of linear templates (5). However, both ends of the RNA are generally required for template activity, suggesting that even linear RNAs may function as if they were circular, perhaps to facilitate reiterative replication and to hinder erosion of the termini.

The relative levels of genomic and antigenomic RNAs are regulated in different ways in different virus families. In the case of Qβ, negative-strand synthesis is limited by the requirement for an additional host subunit that is not needed for the synthesis of positive-sense RNA (2). In some other systems, it appears that different cis-acting RNA signals are largely responsible for determining the relative template activities of the complementary strands, although it is possible that different host factors are involved here, too. For the togavirus Sindbis, negative-sense RNA is synthesized only by a transient version of the RdRp, an intermediate in the proteolytic processing pathway of the viral nonstructural proteins (43). As infection proceeds, the increased viral protease cleaves this intermediate and thereby switches the template specificity of the RdRp to the synthesis of positive-sense RNA (see Chapter 19).

Unlike the enzymes that replicate DNA, which usually require primers, most RdRp's can initiate RNA synthesis *de novo.* However, there are exceptions: picornavirus

RdRp's use a small viral protein (Vpg), which is first covalently uridylated and then used as a primer for all viral RNA synthesis (36). In another mechanism of priming, the enzymes encoded by orthomyxo- and bunyaviruses cleave short capped oligonucleotides from host mRNAs and use them to prime transcription, although for replication, they initiate RNA synthesis *de novo* (37). Arenavirus RdRp's also initiate replication *de novo,* but they start at the penultimate nucleotide of the template and then realign the nascent strand and use it to prime replication of the entire genome, including the 3′ nucleotide (16; also see Chapter 50 of *Fields Virology*, 4th ed.). The ability of some plant virus RdRp's to restore several nucleotides to the 3′ ends of their templates suggests that additional novel mechanisms of initiation await discovery (22).

Viral RdRp's also sometimes catalyze unorthodox reactions during RNA chain elongation. For example, some paramyxovirus polymerases edit selected transcripts internally by specifically inserting one or more nontemplated nucleotides, thereby allowing ribosomes access to additional open reading frames and expanding the coding potential of the viral genome (8). Somewhat similarly, negative-strand RNA virus RdRp's generally polyadenylate their transcripts by stuttering on short runs of U residues in the template (38). Finally, almost all RdRp's occasionally switch templates during replication, thereby producing recombinant progeny molecules that, as satellite or DI RNAs, can influence both the course of infection and the evolution of the virus (6,33,48).

SUMMARY AND PERSPECTIVES

The many different genome strategies of RNA viruses furnish a wealth of unique biochemical pathways found nowhere else in the biosphere. As our understanding deepens, we can look forward to new opportunities for the development of antiviral agents that specifically target these pathways, like the successful antiretroviral protease inhibitors, for example. Furthermore, it is now possible to recover infectivity from cDNA clones of many RNA viruses and thus to manipulate their genotypes and phenotypes in systematic and deliberate ways. This technology has far-reaching potential for the creation of novel reagents, including recombinant vaccines, biopesticides, targeted cytolytic agents, and vectors for gene therapy. Both as foes and friends of mankind, RNA viruses have an interesting and exciting future.

REFERENCES

1. Ball LA. Virus-host cell interactions. In: Collier L, Balows A, Sussman M, eds. *Topley and Wilson's microbiology and microbial infections.* Vol 5. London: Arnold Publishers, 1998:115–146.
2. Blumenthal T, Carmichael GG. RNA replication: Function and structure of Qβ replicase. *Annu Rev Biochem* 1979;48:525–548.
3. Bouloy M. Bunyaviridae: Genome organization and replication strategies. *Adv Virus Res* 1991;40:235–275.
4. Bressanelli S, Tomei I, Roussel A, et al. Crystal structure of the RNA-dependent RNA polymerase of hepatitis C virus. *Proc Natl Acad Sci U S A* 1999;96:13034–13039.
5. Buck KW. Comparison of the replication of positive-stranded RNA viruses of plants and animals. *Adv Virus Res* 1996;47:159–251.
6. Bujarski JJ, ed. RNA recombination. In: *Seminars in virology*. Vol 8. London: Academic Press, 1997.
7. Conzelmann KK. Nonsegmented negative-strand RNA viruses: Genetics and manipulation of viral genomes. *Annu Rev Genet* 1998;32:123–162.
8. Curran J, Kolakofsky D. Replication of paramyxoviruses. *Adv Virus Res* 2000;54:403–422.
9. Diener TO, ed. The viroids. In: Fraenkel-Conrat H, Wagner RR, series eds. *The viruses*. New York: Plenum Press, 1987.
10. Domingo E, Holland JJ. RNA virus mutations and fitness for survival. *Annu Rev Microbiol* 1997;51:151–178.
11. Draper DE. Themes in RNA-protein recognition. *J Mol Biol* 1999; 293:255–270.
12. Dreher TW. Functions of the 3′-untranslated regions of positive-strand RNA viral genomes. *Annu Rev Phytopathol* 1999;37:151–174.
13. Dougherty WG, Semler BL. Expression of virus-encoded proteinases: Functional and structural similarities with cellular enzymes. *Microbiol Rev* 1993;57:781–822.
14. Eigen M. Viral quasispecies. *Sci Am* 1993;269:42–49.
15. Elliott RM, ed. The *Bunyaviridae.* In: Fraenkel-Conrat H, Wagner RR, series eds. *The viruses*. New York: Plenum Press, 1996.
16. Garcin D, Lezzi M, Dobbs M, et al. The 5′ end of Hantaan virus (Bunyaviridae) RNAs suggest a prime-and-realign mechanism for the initiation of RNA synthesis. *J Virol* 1995;69:5754–5762.
17. Gierer A, Schramm G. Infectivity of ribonucleic acid from tobacco mosaic virus. *Nature* 1956;177:702–703.
18. Hansen JL, Long AM, Schultz SC. Structure of an RNA-dependent RNA polymerase of poliovirus. *Structure* 1997;5:1109–1122.
19. Holland JJ, ed. Genetic diversity of RNA viruses. *Curr Top Microbiol Immunol* 1992;17.
20. Ishihama A, Barbier P. Molecular anatomy of viral RNA-directed RNA polymerases. *Arch Virol* 1994;134:235–258.
21. Kadare G, Haenni AL. Virus-encoded RNA helicases. *J Virol* 1997; 71:2583–2590.
22. Kao CC. Initiation of viral RNA synthesis: More than one way to get a good start. *Virology* (in press).
23. Koonin EV, Dolja VV. Evolution and taxonomy of positive-strand RNA viruses: Implications of comparative analysis of amino acid sequences. *Crit Rev Biochem Mol Biol* 1993;28:375–430.
24. Lai MM. The molecular biology of hepatitis delta virus. *Annu Rev Biochem* 1995;64:259–286.
25. Lai MM. Cellular factors in the transcription and replication of viral RNA genomes: A parallel to DNA-dependent RNA transcription. *Virology* 1998;244:1–12.
26. Lai MM, Cavanagh D. The molecular biology of coronaviruses. *Adv Virus Res* 1997;48:1–100.
27. Leaman DW. Mechanisms of interferon action. *Prog Mol Subcell Biol* 1998;20:101–142.
28. Levy JA, ed. The *Retroviridae* In: Fraenkel-Conrat H, Wagner RR, series eds. *The viruses*. Vol 4. New York: Plenum Press, 1995.
29. Li HP, Huang P, Park S, et al. Polypyrimidine tract-binding protein binds to the leader RNA of mouse hepatitis virus and serves as a regulator of viral transcription. *J Virol* 1999;73:772–777.
30. Meyer P, ed. Gene silencing in higher plants and related phenomena in other eukaryotes. *Curr Top Microbiol Immunol* 1995:197.
31. Miller LK, Ball LA, eds. The insect viruses. In: Fraenkel-Conrat H, Wagner RR, series eds. *The viruses.* New York: Plenum Press, 1998.
32. Moya A, Elena SF, Bracho A, et al. The evolution of RNA viruses: A population genetics view. *Proc Natl Acad Sci U S A* 2000;97: 6967–6973.
33. Nagy PD, Simon AE. New insights into the mechanisms of RNA recombination. *Virology* 1997;235:1–9.
34. O'Reilly EK, Kao CC. Analysis of RNA-dependent RNA polymerase structure and function as guided by known polymerase structures and computer predictions of secondary structure. *Virology* 1998;252: 287–303.
35. Patton JT, Davis NL, Wertz G. N protein alone satisfies the requirement for protein synthesis during RNA replication of vesicular stomatitis virus. *J Virol* 1984;49:303–309.
36. Paul A, van Boom JH, Fillippov D, et al. Protein-primed RNA synthesis by purified RNA polymerase. *Nature* 1998;393:280–284.
37. Plotch SJ, Bouloy M, Ulmanen I, et al. A unique cap ($^{m7}GpppX_m$)-depen-

dent influenza virion endonuclease cleaves capped RNA to generate the primers that initiate viral RNA transcription. *Cell* 1981;23:847–858.
38. Poon LLM, Pritlove DC, Fodor E, et al. Direct evidence that the poly(A) tail of influenza A virus mRNA is synthesized by reiterative copying of a U track in the virion RNA template. *J Virol* 1999;73:3473–3476.
39. Pringle CR, Easton AJ. Monopartite negative strand RNA genomes. *Semin Virol* 1997;8:49–57.
40. Ramig RF, ed. Rotaviruses. *Curr Top Microbiol Immunol* 1994;185.
41. Salvato MS, ed. The *Arenaviridae.* In: Fraenkel-Conrat H, Wagner RR, series eds. *The viruses.* New York: Plenum Press, 1993.
42. Shuman S, Schwer B. RNA capping enzyme and DNA ligase: A superfamily of covalent nucleotidyl transferases. *Mol Microbiol* 1995;17: 405–410.
43. Strauss JH, Strauss EG. The alphaviruses: Gene expression, replication, and evolution. *Microbiol Rev* 1994;58:491–562.
44. Strauss JH, Strauss EG. With a little help from the host. *Science* 1999;283:802–804.
45. Tyler KL, Oldstone MBA, eds. Reoviruses 1: Structure, proteins, and genetics. *Curr Top Microbiol Immunol* 1998;233.
46. Vogt PK, Jackson AO, eds. Satellites and defective viral RNAs. *Curr Top Microbiol Immunol* 1999;239.
47. Wickner RB. Double-stranded RNA viruses of *Saccharomyces cerevisiae. Microbiol Rev* 1996;60:250–265.
48. Worobey M, Holmes EC. Evolutionary aspects of recombination in RNA viruses. *J Gen Virol* 1999;80:2535–2543.
49. Wu S-X, Ahlquist P, Kaesberg P. Active complete *in vitro* replication of nodavirus RNA requires glycerophospholipid. *Proc Natl Acad Sci U S A* 1992;89:11136–11140.
50. Zaccomer B, Haenni AL, Macaya G. The remarkable variety of plant RNA virus genomes. *J Gen Virol* 1995;76:231–247.

CHAPTER 6

Replication Strategies of DNA Viruses

Daniel DiMaio and Donald M. Coen

All viruses, whether they contain RNA or DNA genomes, adsorb to cell membranes, enter cells, uncoat, express their genes, replicate their genomes, assemble new virions, and exit from cells. These activities entail interactions with the host cell that range from simple binding to cellular receptors to complex modulation of host processes. In addition, DNA viruses carry out some steps that RNA viruses do not. For most DNA viruses, these steps include transport of virion DNA into the nucleus, initiation of transcription from this DNA and induction of transcription of additional viral genes, preparation of the cell for viral DNA replication, replication of the DNA genome, resolution and packaging of DNA into virions, and egress from the nucleus. In addition, many DNA viruses have evolved interesting mechanisms to evade host defenses, and many DNA viruses can cause tumors in animals. The intimate relationship between viruses and their host cells dictates that viruses exploit key cellular regulatory systems and usurp important cellular processes to carry out successful infection. Thus, studies of various aspects of DNA virus replication have provided fundamental new insights into important cellular processes including gene expression, DNA replication, and cell-cycle control.

This chapter reviews most of the steps just listed that are specific to DNA viruses. Nuclear entry and egress (which are not employed by poxviruses) are discussed in Chapter 7, and virus assembly and packaging of DNA per se are discussed in Chapter 8. Because of space constraints, this review cannot be comprehensive. A limited—and necessarily subjective and arbitrary—set of examples from various mammalian viruses is presented to illustrate unifying themes and interesting exceptions.

TRANSCRIPTION OF VIRAL DNA

Each mammalian cell contains about 6×10^9 base pairs of DNA and $>10^4$ active promoters. This presents a considerable challenge for viral DNA to compete effectively in recruiting the cellular transcriptional machinery to viral promoters. Moreover, once recruited, the machinery must generate viral transcripts efficiently. To meet this challenge, DNA viruses have adopted strategies to permit efficient initiation of transcription at one or more specific promoters on viral DNA shortly after it enters the nucleus. These promoters drive the transcription of what are frequently termed immediate early genes.

Enhancers

To recruit the transcriptional machinery to immediate early viral promoters and activate transcription, many

DNA viruses contain enhancers—*cis*-acting regulatory sequences that, unlike promoters, can activate transcription from thousands of base pairs (bps) upstream or downstream of the transcriptional start site. This defining feature of enhancers emphasizes the competitive advantage they confer on viral promoters. Indeed, the high activity of the cytomegalovirus immediate early enhancer/promoter accounts for the popularity of its use in expression vectors. Although cellular genes frequently contain enhancers, the first enhancer to be recognized was that of the papovavirus SV40 (3,30,56). The SV40 enhancer consists of two tandem repeats of 72 bp, which contain binding sites for at least six different transcription factors, including multiple binding sites for certain factors. Although it is possible to create a synthetic enhancer by multimerizing a binding site for a single transcription factor, the multiplicity of factors and binding sites characteristic of natural enhancers appears to be required for optimal enhancer function.

Many enhancers also contain binding sites for "architectural" proteins, which do not necessarily have transcriptional activation functions on their own but rather promote the stereospecific, three-dimensional assembly of enhancer-protein complexes ("enhanceosomes") (9). These nucleoprotein complexes can then activate transcription by interactions with the RNA polymerase II transcriptional machinery with considerable potency and specificity (29,72,73). Indeed, subtle sequence changes in papovavirus enhancers can drastically affect their function in different cell types (39).

Virion Transcription Factors

In addition to enhancers, some DNA viruses encode proteins that are packaged into virions, enter the cell with the viral DNA, and then facilitate transcription of immediate early genes. An extreme example of this is provided by poxviruses, which replicate in the cytoplasm and make no use of the cellular transcription machinery. Rather, as described in Chapter 35, poxviruses encode and package in virions their own RNA polymerases, capping and polyadenylation enzymes, and transcription factors. Upon entry into the cell and uncoating, the viral transcription machinery becomes active and synthesizes viral immediate early transcripts.

A more general example is the herpes simplex virus (HSV) transactivator VP16 (also known as αTIF) (58,72,74). HSV VP16 is synthesized late in infection and is packaged into the portion of the virion known as tegument, which lies between the capsid and the envelope. Upon entry of HSV into cells, VP16 is transported to the nucleus and forms a complex with at least two cellular proteins—Oct-1, which is a transcription factor that recognizes an eight-bp DNA sequence, and HCF-1. This tripartite complex binds to specific DNA sequences with the consensus TAATGARAT (R = purine) upstream of HSV immediate early genes, with much of the DNA binding specificity and affinity provided by Oct-1. The complex then serves as a strong activator of transcription. Much of the activation is due to the C-terminal "activation domain" of VP16. This domain, when linked to virtually any sequence-specific DNA-binding domain that binds upstream of a TATA-box element of a promoter, can activate transcription in any eukaryote. Indeed, VP16 has served as a paradigmatic transcriptional activator. The VP16 activation domain can interact with many different proteins in the cellular transcriptional machinery, and it remains controversial as to whether any one protein is most important for its transcriptional activity. Indeed, the ability of VP16 to interact with more than one protein may account for the strength of its activation domain, given the evidence that this domain functions to recruit the transcriptional machinery to promoters rather than to stimulate the activity of any particular transcription protein (e.g., 41). Regardless, in the absence of an intact VP16 activation domain, the expression of HSV immediate early genes and viral replication is greatly impaired (1,64).

Stimulation of Gene Expression by Viral Immediate Early Proteins

As infection proceeds, DNA viruses typically express their genes in a highly ordered sequence. Although expression of viral genomes can be regulated posttranscriptionally, major control is exerted at the level of transcription. Viral immediate early genes generally encode proteins that stimulate expression of viral genes that are expressed subsequently during infection (the early and late genes). This enables early and late promoters, which usually lack enhancers or binding sites for transcription complexes such as those formed by virion proteins like VP16, to compete effectively with cellular promoters for the transcriptional machinery. Expression of some viral genes (e.g., papillomavirus late genes) is restricted to cells in a particular state of differentiation. Tissue-specific expression of essential cellular transcription factors may underlie this restriction. It should also be noted that several viruses also encode proteins that repress expression of certain viral genes at particular times in the virus life cycle. In addition, many viruses affect cellular gene expression. This can entail the induction and repression of specific genes, as well as a more nonspecific shut-off of cellular gene expression. The latter topic is considered in Chapter 7.

There appear to be many mechanisms by which viral immediate early proteins function. Certain of these proteins, such as the Epstein-Barr virus (EBV) BZLF1 protein (also known as Zta or Zebra), can behave like cellular transcription factors in that they bind to specific sequences upstream of genes and activate transcription (66). Other immediate early proteins increase the activity of cellular sequence-specific transcription factors. For example, the adenovirus E1A protein displaces members of the transcription factor E2F family from inhibitory retinoblastoma (Rb) family proteins. This increases transcription of adenovirus early genes that contain E2F binding sites (44) [and also has important consequences on cellular transcription and, indirectly, on viral and cellular DNA replication (see later)]. Other immediate early proteins, such as HSV ICP4, appear to stimulate transcription by direct interaction with the transcriptional machinery without binding to specific DNA sequences in the target promoter (31,36), while still others, like HSV ICP27, appear to stimulate viral gene expression by both transcriptional and posttranscriptional mechanisms (38,51,65). The net result of the activities of these viral proteins is that cells devote most of their gene expression machinery to production of viral gene products.

PREPARING THE CELL FOR VIRAL DNA REPLICATION

Viral Effects on Cell Cycle Progression

During productive viral infection, many DNA viruses carry out prodigious feats of DNA replication, in which a single viral genome gives rise to up to 100,000 or more genome copies in the course of a few days. This requires the action of many proteins, including DNA binding proteins and polymerases, as well as an abundant supply of nucleotides. Replication of some DNA viruses occurs only in cells that are naturally replicating their own DNA, thereby providing the necessary cellular environment for viral DNA replication. Many other DNA viruses also rely largely on the cellular DNA replication machinery, but these viruses encode proteins that induce cells to enter the necessary replicative state. Finally, some of the largest DNA viruses make limited use of the cellular replication machinery but rather encode viral versions of many of the necessary proteins.

The parvoviruses are among the simplest DNA viruses and contain single-stranded linear genomes. Parvoviruses can undergo DNA replication and carry out their full infectious cycle only in cells undergoing cellular DNA replication—that is, only in cells in the S-phase of the cell cycle (70,79). In fact, viral gene expression is not activated until after the cells enter S phase and the incoming DNA genome is converted into a double-stranded form suitable as a template for transcription (15). However, unlike certain other viruses that require cells to be actively replicating cellular DNA, parvoviruses are unable to induce the cells to enter S-phase, and thus they can carry out successful infection only if they encounter cells already committed to DNA synthesis. Some parvoviruses, notably adeno-associated virus (AAV), have even more stringent requirements and can replicate only if helper adenoviruses or herpesviruses provide viral gene products that permit parvovirus gene expression and DNA replication (7,62). Certain forms of cellular stress, such as DNA damage, can also induce a cellular state compatible with AAV DNA replication (62,83,84).

Many other DNA viruses induce cells to enter the replicative state required for viral DNA replication. For these viruses, viral DNA replication is the result of collaboration between cellular replication proteins and viral proteins that have direct roles in replication, such as initiator proteins that localize the replication apparatus to the viral replication origin. These DNA viruses generally induce cells to enter this essential replicative state by encoding proteins that participate in specific protein–protein interactions with key cellular regulatory molecules, and some of these viral proteins have molecular chaperone activity that enables them to assemble these protein complexes (4,8,67). Often, these interactions lead to the neutralization of cellular tumor suppressor proteins such as p53 and members of the Rb protein family, whereas in other cases, these interactions result in the activation of cellular growth-stimulatory signal transduction pathways, which may indirectly inhibit Rb activity (Table 1).

The viral proteins that induce the replicative state commonly inactivate Rb family members $p105^{Rb}$, p107, and p130 (13). Rb inactivation relieves repression and releases E2F transcription factors to stimulate expression of numerous cellular proteins required for S-phase, including DNA polymerase α, thymidine kinase, ribonucleotide reductase, and thymidylate synthase (Fig. 1) (17,20,34). Some viral proteins, such as adenovirus E1A and human papillomavirus (HPV) E7, directly bind Rb proteins and inhibit Rb function, thereby activating E2F (2,27,81). Other viral proteins regulate the activity of cyclin-dependent kinases (cdks), which catalyze the phosphorylation of Rb, resulting in release of active E2F and transcription of E2F-regulated genes. Viral proteins that indirectly influence Rb activity in this way include herpesviruses-encoded cyclins that bind and activate cdks (40) and a variety of proteins that impair the expression or activity of proteins that inhibit cdk activity. For example, adenovirus E1B 55K and E4orf6 protein and HPV E6 inhibit the activity of p53, a transcriptional activator (24,61,80). Several viral proteins target the p53 coactivator CBP/p300. Abrogation of p53 function results in decreased expression of the p53-responsive gene encoding the cdk inhibitor p21, thus stimulating cdk

TABLE 1. *Mobilization of the host cell replication machinery by DNA Viruses*

Neutralization of tumor suppressor function
Direct effects on retinoblastoma expression or activity
Stimulation of cyclin-dependent kinase activity
Activation of growth-promoting signal transduction pathways
Receptor tyrosine kinase pathways
Intracellular signal transduction pathways

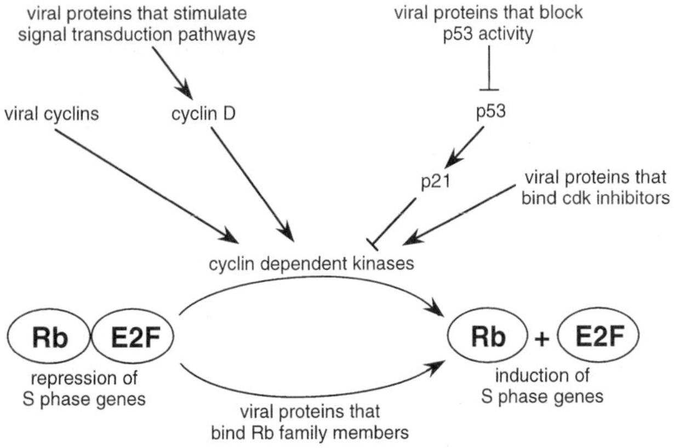

FIG. 1. Inactivation of retinoblastoma family members and activation of E2F by DNA tumor viruses. Viral proteins can cause the release of E2F family transcriptional activators from Rb-E2F repressor complexes by stimulating the activity of cyclin-dependent kinases or by binding directly to Rb family members. See text for details and examples.

activity. Similarly, adenovirus E1A binds the related cdk inhibitor p27, neutralizing its effects (50). SV40 large T antigen is a particularly versatile protein that not only binds and inactivates both Rb and p53 (19,45,49) but also carries out several functions directly required for viral DNA replication (see later) as well as essential roles in other aspects of the virus life cycle. Another mechanism is employed by polyomavirus middle T antigen and bovine papillomavirus E5 protein, which activate growth factor receptor signaling cascades and presumably induce expression of the cyclin D regulatory subunit of the cdks, thereby stimulating cdk activity and Rb phosphorylation (22,23,59). Certain herpesvirus and hepadnavirus proteins also appear to stimulate signal transduction cascades by activating intracellular signal transduction proteins such as NFκB, $p21^{ras}$, and $pp60^{c\text{-}src}$ (23). Although poxviruses encode growth factor homologs, these do not appear essential for viral DNA replication; rather, they are involved in various aspects of viral pathogenesis (6).

Not surprisingly, induction of a panel of cellular DNA replication proteins has profound consequences on the host cell, which is often induced to undergo DNA replication and proliferation as a by-product of this mobilization of the cellular replication machinery. When this proliferative signal is sustained and tolerated, for example in nonpermissive cells that are unable to support viral DNA replication, the cells may undergo stable growth transformation, a topic covered in detail in Chapter 10. Thus, not only do many DNA viruses induce quiescent cells to reenter the cell cycle, but they also transform cells in culture and cause tumors in animals. Viewed in this light, the ability of many DNA tumor viruses to induce transformation is not a feature of normal viral replication but rather an aberrant cellular response to the need of the virus to generate the proper cellular milieu for viral DNA replication. In accord with this view, the parvoviruses, which as noted previously lack the ability to stimulate cellular DNA replication, are one of the few DNA virus groups that do not transform cells. However, the relationship between the ability of viruses to stimulate cellular DNA synthesis and to transform cells is not simple. For example, some herpesviruses stimulate DNA synthesis, others do not, and still others actually inhibit cell proliferation. Such large viruses, with their large coding capacity, are able to create the proper environment for viral DNA replication without relying on mobilization of the cellular replication machinery.

The cell cycle normally is tightly regulated to prevent excess proliferation and ensure that each step in the cycle is successfully completed before the next step begins. When the cell cycle is disrupted, as is the case when unscheduled cellular DNA synthesis occurs, cells often initiate a suicidal response called *apoptosis*, or programmed cell death. Apoptosis is characterized by specific morphologic changes and biochemical events, including the activation of caspase proteases and the degradation of cellular DNA, and it is regulated by components of the cell cycle machinery. For example, E2F1 can stimulate apoptosis, and p53 appears to play a central role in mediating apoptosis in response to diverse stimuli. Because viruses often target these same cell cycle components, viral proteins can induce or inhibit apoptosis. In fact, DNA virus infection and the DNA synthesis response it elicits often induces host cell apoptosis. Because apoptosis and the resulting premature cell death can curtail virus production, viruses have evolved numerous mechanisms to inhibit apoptosis, including the neutralization of p53 function. Therefore, transformation by some viruses requires the seemingly antagonistic action of two or more viral proteins. For example, adenovirus E1A stimulates both proliferation and apoptosis, in part by inactivating Rb proteins and releasing active E2F1. Stable transformation ensues only if viral E1B gene products prevent E1A-induced apoptosis by interfering with p53 function or by acting downstream of p53 in the apoptotic pathway (18,60). By neutralizing p53, HPV E6 may block a similar apoptotic activity of E7. These relationships suggest that some viral oncogenes have evolved to thwart antiviral host defenses, such as apoptosis or interferon induction, by interfering with cellular pathways that mediate these defense mechanisms (54).

Whether viral oncogenes primarily function to generate the milieu for viral DNA replication or to counteract host defense mechanisms, the fundamental strategy is the same: The virus has evolved proteins that influence intracellular processes to allow vegetative viral replication, and the ability of these proteins to induce cell transformation and tumorigenesis is an unintended consequence of the underlying cellular biochemistry. The papillomaviruses are unusual in that benign tumor formation is an integral part of the virus life cycle. However, even for these viruses, carcinogenic progression is not a normal feature of the virus life cycle but rather a response to defective viruses with deregulated oncogene expression.

Provision of Nucleotides for DNA Replication

As described, parvoviruses require cells to be in S-phase to replicate, and papovaviruses and adenoviruses stimulate cells to enter S-phase. The requirement for S-phase is, in part, a requirement for cells to supply deoxynucleoside triphosphates (dNTPs) for DNA synthesis. Via effects on Rb and E2F family members, papovaviruses and adenoviruses induce the synthesis of enzymes such as ribonucleotide reductase that are required to generate sufficient dNTPs for viral DNA replication (Fig. 2). In contrast, herpesviruses and poxviruses are able to replicate in resting cells. One reason that these viruses can circumvent the requirement for S-phase is that they encode enzymes for dNTP synthesis, both of the *de novo* pathway (e.g., ribonucleotide reductase) and the salvage pathway (e.g., thymidine kinase) (see Fig. 2). In the case of HSV and varicella zoster virus, viral-encoded thymidine kinases provide Achilles heels for antiviral chemotherapy because these viral enzymes phosphorylate nucleoside analogs such as acyclovir more efficiently than do cellular enzymes. Following conversion by cellular enzymes to their triphosphate form, these dNTP analogs selectively impair viral DNA replication (37).

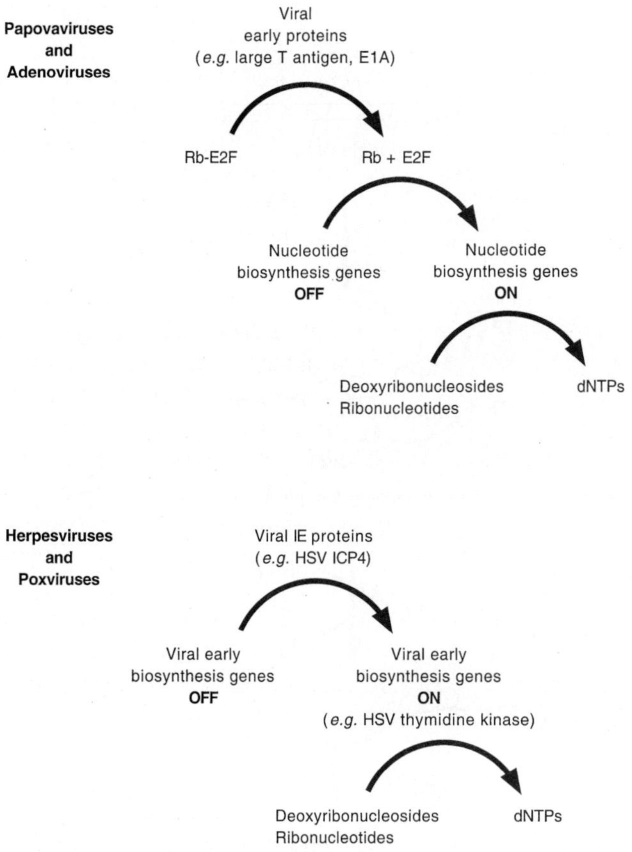

FIG. 2. Mechanisms of provision of nucleotides for DNA replication. **Top:** Papovaviruses and adenoviruses encode viral proteins such as SV40 large T antigen and the adenovirus E1A protein, which displace members of the E2F family of transcriptional activators from the retinoblastoma protein (Rb), as indicated in Fig. 1. The E2F transcription factors are then free to induce expression of numerous cellular genes required for DNA replication, including those that encode proteins that catalyze the formation of deoxyribonucleoside triphosphates (dNTPs) from deoxynucleosides or ribonucleotides. **Bottom:** Herpesviruses and poxviruses encode viral immediate early (IE) proteins such as herpes simplex virus (HSV) ICP4, which induce expression of viral enzymes involved in deoxyribonucleotide biosynthesis, such as HSV thymidine kinase.

VIRAL DNA REPLICATION

Initiation of Viral DNA Replication

Replication of DNA virus genomes generally initiates at specific sites called origins. Unlike most cellular origins, which are active once and only once per cell cycle, a viral replication origin can fire many times during a single replication cycle. Replication proceeds away from the origin either by utilizing classic replication forks with lagging and leading strand synthesis or by displacement synthesis with leading strand synthesis only. Viruses have evolved a number of strategies to assemble the replication apparatus at the origin and initiate DNA synthesis at the correct position. Most commonly, a viral early protein binds directly and specifically to the double-stranded DNA that comprises the origin and recruits the cellular replication machinery to this site. Other viral genomes have a 3′ end base-paired to a template strand that can be extended by polymerase, whereas in some cases unusual protein-priming strategies are used. Despite the diversity of initiation mechanisms, a common theme is the use of specific protein–protein interactions to recruit essential viral and cellular replication proteins to participate in replication initiation.

The role of the SV40 large T antigen in origin-dependent viral DNA replication has been particularly well studied (21,32,48). Large T antigen is the only SV40 protein required for viral DNA replication. It binds tightly and specifically to the SV40 origin, a short segment of viral DNA shown by numerous studies to be the necessary and sufficient *cis*-acting element for initiation of bidirectional viral DNA replication in permissive monkey cells. Elegant genetic studies established that the binding of large T antigen to the origin is required for replication (63). In the presence of ATP, hexameric complexes of large T antigen bind specifically to the origin and carry out several functions essential for replication initiation (Fig. 3). Large T antigen induces local DNA distortion and melting at AT-rich sequences within the origin. Large T antigen then associates with the cellular replication protein A (RPA), a single-stranded DNA binding protein, thereby permitting extensive DNA unwinding catalyzed by the intrinsic ATP-dependent helicase activity of large T antigen (52). DNA polymerase α-primase binds directly to the origin-bound large T antigen, and this replicative polymerase synthesizes short RNA sequences that serve as primers for viral DNA synthesis. The importance of the interaction between large T antigen and DNA polymerase α-primase is highlighted by the finding that the inability of viral DNA to replicate in nonpermissive cells is the result of the inability of large T antigen to recognize DNA polymerase α-primase from these cells (6,25,28,68). The molecular chaperone activity of large T antigen may play an important role in assembling the protein complexes necessary for initiation of replication.

Similar initiation strategies are used by other viruses with double-stranded origins. However, unlike SV40, in which all the required viral replication functions are contained within a single viral protein, other viruses are not so parsimonious. For example, the papillomaviruses encode two proteins, E1 and E2, required in *trans* for efficient viral DNA replication in rodent fibroblasts (75). The E1 protein appears to be the major viral replication protein, and, like large T antigen, is an ATP-dependent helicase. Both the E1 and E2 proteins bind to specific

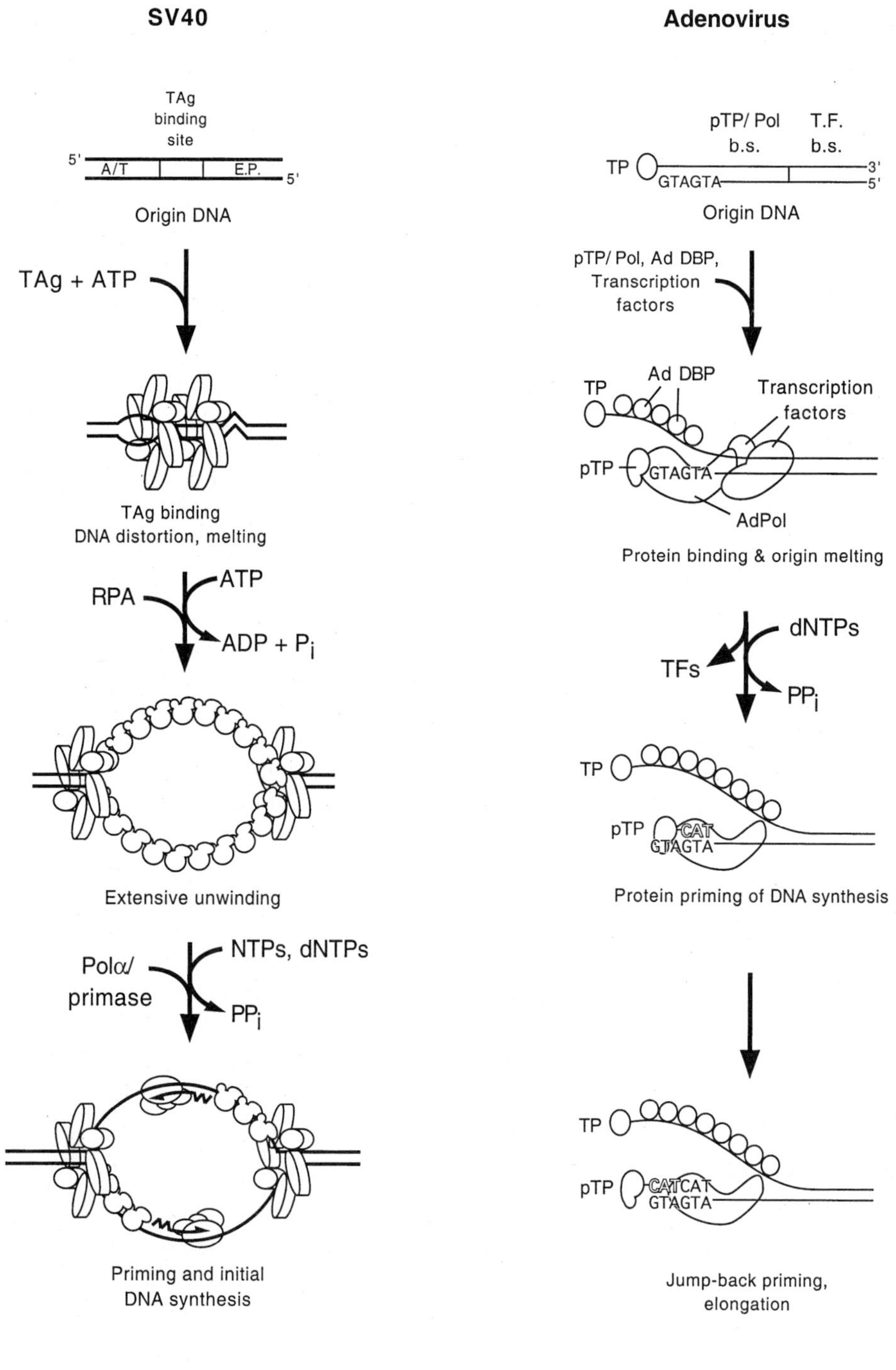

DNA sequences in the origin region, and they bind to each other (53). The presence of the E2 protein in the complex facilitates the specific, high-affinity binding of E1 to the origin. Moreover, both the E1 and E2 proteins participate in specific protein–protein interactions that localize cellular replication proteins such as DNA polymerase α-primase and RPA to the origin. The presence of more than one viral protein at the origin raises the possibility that different combinatorial multimeric protein complexes may play distinct roles in different phases of the virus life cycle, such as stable maintenance of plasmids at a low copy number during latent infection versus rapid amplification of viral DNA during vegetative DNA replication. Origins also often contain binding sites for cellular transcription factors, which may facilitate replication, perhaps by altering chromatin structure or by recruiting replication proteins. Some of the large DNA viruses, including HSV, have multiple specific origins (55,76). Unlike the case of the polyomaviruses and papillomaviruses, the detailed mechanics of origin recognition and initiation of replication have not been completely worked out for the larger DNA viruses, in part because of the lack of suitable *in vitro* DNA replication systems for these viruses. Indeed, the development and analysis of *in vitro* replication systems for small viral genomes has led to the identification of essential cellular replication proteins and to many important insights into the mechanism of cellular DNA replication (see later) (11,42,48).

The linear DNA packaged by a number of viruses has base-paired 3′ ends that are extended as the initial steps in viral DNA replication. In the case of parvoviruses, these base-paired primer-template structures are formed by complicated stem-loop structures occurring at the ends of the viral genome that is otherwise single-stranded (15). These 3′ ends are extended by cellular DNA polymerase in a reaction that does not appear to require viral proteins. The resulting double-stranded DNA replication intermediates are then nicked at specific sites by viral NS or Rep proteins to generate primers for ongoing DNA synthesis. Cellular DNA binding proteins collaborate with the viral proteins to ensure efficient nicking. These viral proteins also presumably play an important role in recruiting cellular replication proteins, including DNA polymerase, to these sites. The ends of the linear poxvirus genomes are imperfectly base-paired hairpin loops. Recent evidence indicates that these ends can serve as the sites of replication initiation in the cytoplasm, but the details of initiation of this virus group are obscure (26). Indeed, it is not known whether poxviruses encode all essential origin recognition and replication proteins, or whether the cell also makes a contribution.

The most unusual strategy for initiating viral DNA replication is the use of proteins as primers. The adenoviruses are the prototype viruses that use this strategy (33). Adenovirus DNA replication origins are located at inverted repeats at both ends of the linear double-stranded viral genome. The 5′ end of each DNA strand contained within the virus particle is covalently linked to a virally encoded protein (the terminal protein). Immediately adjacent to the terminal protein are specific DNA sequences that comprise a core origin and an auxiliary region that binds cellular transcription factors. Viral DNA synthesis is initiated when a complex of the adenovirus DNA polymerase and the precursor to the terminal protein (preter-

FIG. 3. Two mechanisms of initiation of DNA replication.
Left: A model for initiation of SV40 DNA synthesis. The *top panel* shows the SV40 origin with a binding site for SV40 large T antigen (TAg) flanked by a highly AT-rich sequence (A/T) and a modestly AT-rich sequence known as the early palindrome (E.P.). In the presence of ATP, two TAg hexamers form on the TAg binding site, leading to distortion and melting of the AT-rich sequences. Then, in the presence of the cellular heterotrimeric single-stranded DNA binding protein, replication protein A (RPA), TAg extensively unwinds origin DNA, a reaction driven by ATP hydrolysis. The four-subunit cellular DNA polymerase α/primase (Polα/primase) then binds to each single strand and catalyzes the incorporation of nucleoside triphosphates (NTPs) into RNA primers on each strand (*zigzag line*). The DNA polymerase catalyzes the incorporation of deoxynucleoside triphosphates (dNTPs), extending the RNA primers into newly synthesized strands of DNA. Polα/primase is then replaced at the primer terminus by replication factor C and subsequently the DNA polymerase δ complex (not shown; see Fig. 4 for subsequent steps).
Right: A model for initiation of adenovirus DNA synthesis. The *top panel* shows the adenovirus terminal protein TP bound to the 5′ end of an adenovirus origin of DNA synthesis at a terminus of adenovirus DNA. Near the end of the DNA is a binding site for the preterminal protein (pTP)-adenovirus DNA polymerase (Pol) complex (pTP/Pol b.s.) and an adjacent binding site for cellular transcription factors (T.F. b.s.). These transcription factors interact with Pol such that pTP/Pol binds to the template strand (sequence 5′-ATGATG-3′OH) with a serine side chain in pTP placed opposite the G, four bases from the 3′ end of the viral DNA. This interaction is abetted by the adenovirus single-stranded DNA binding protein (Ad DBP), shown coating the TP-bound strand, thereby favoring the melting of origin sequences. Pol then adds a C to the serine hydroxyl moiety in the pTP protein primer and extends that C two bases in a template-dependent fashion, synthesizing the sequence CAT. The pTP/Pol bound to the newly synthesized CAT sequence then "jumps-back" to the very end of the template strand, and the CAT serves as a primer for elongation of the rest of the daughter DNA strand (see Fig. 4).

TABLE 2. *Proteins that act at replication forks*

Replication protein	Function
DNA Polymerase	Elongate DNA chains
Polymerase-accessory proteins (e.g., PCNA)	Stimulate polymerase, increase processivity
ss DNA binding protein	Remove hairpins, etc., especially on lagging strand
Primase	Lay down RNA primers on lagging strand
RNases	Remove RNA primers
Ligase	Seal nicks, especially on lagging strand
Helicase	Unwind DNA at fork
Topoisomerase	Remove superhelicity ahead of fork

PCNA, proliferating cell nuclear antigen.

minal protein, pTP) binds to the origin and melts the origin region in conjunction with a virally encoded single-stranded DNA binding protein (see Fig. 3). The binding of viral proteins to the origin may be assisted by transcription factors bound to the auxiliary sequences and by the bound terminal protein, although these proteins are not absolutely required. The adenovirus polymerase then adds nucleotides directly to pTP by a remarkable template-dependent mechanism that entails a "jump back" so that the first bases added correspond to the sequence of the 5′ ends of the genome (12,43). The DNA 3′hydroxyl group of the pTP–oligonucleotide complex is then extended by viral DNA polymerase (see next section).

Provision and Action of Proteins That Act at the Replication Fork

Once viral DNA replication is initiated, the elongation phase of DNA synthesis proceeds via the concerted action of multiple proteins at replication forks. At replication forks in most organisms, one strand (the leading strand) is replicated by simple 5′-3′ extension in a continuous manner. Because the other strand (the lagging strand) must also be synthesized 5′-3′, it is replicated discontinuously, by repeated synthesis and joining of short Okazaki fragments. Table 2 lists proteins that act at replication forks, and their functions.

FIG. 4. Contrasting sets of proteins at the replication fork.
Top: A replication fork during SV40 DNA replication. The replication fork is shown as a branched DNA molecule, with 5′ and 3′ ends indicated. On the right, downstream of the replication fork, either a type I or a type II topoisomerase (Topo I or II) releases supercoiling generated during DNA synthesis. At the replication fork, a hexamer of SV40 large T antigen (TAg), the only viral protein present, serves as a helicase, unwinding DNA in front of the DNA synthetic machinery. The leading strand for DNA synthesis is shown as the bottom of the two branches with the two-subunit DNA polymerase δ (Polδ) bound to the processivity factor, proliferating cell nuclear antigen (PCNA; this is trimeric, but it is shown as a ring around the DNA). The heteropentameric replication factor-C (RF-C) is drawn as a large oval bound to Polδ and PCNA. RF-C loads the PCNA ring onto DNA, which is then recognized by Polδ. The Polδ complex synthesizes DNA in a continuous fashion, starting from the RNA–DNA primers laid down by DNA polymeraseα/primase at the SV40 origin (see Fig. 3). The lagging strand for DNA synthesis is shown as the top of the two branches. Closest to the replication fork is the four-subunit DNA polymerase α/primase (Polα/primase). The primase subunit lays down RNA primers (*zigzag line*) on the lagging strand, and the DNA polymerase extends the RNA into newly synthesized DNA (*straight line*). To the left of the Polα/primase is replication protein A (RPA), coating single-stranded DNA ahead of Polα/primase. To the left of the RPA is a stretch of RNA–DNA primer previously synthesized by Polα/primase. The Polδ/PCNA/RF-C complex, having assembled at the primer terminus, is drawn as extending the DNA strand. Farther to the left, a previously synthesized RNA primer is being digested by RNase H1. The nuclease FEN-1 (also known as MF-1) will remove the last ribonucleotide of the RNA primer. After the Polδ complex finishes extending the DNA strand, DNA ligase I will ligate together the two Okazaki fragments. Although events on the leading and lagging strands are shown as occurring separately, there is evidence that they are coordinated within a large macromolecular complex.
Bottom: A replication fork during adenovirus DNA synthesis. The replication fork is shown as a branched DNA molecule. On the *right*, downstream of the replication fork, supercoiling generated during DNA synthesis is released by type I or type II topoisomerase, the only cellular protein present. The top branch is a single strand of parental viral DNA displaced during DNA synthesis, coated with the adenovirus single-stranded DNA binding protein (Ad DBP) and with the 5′ end bound to terminal protein (TP). The double-stranded bottom branch is made up of a parental template strand and a newly synthesized strand whose 5′ end is bound to preterminal protein (pTP) and whose 3′ end is being extended by the adenovirus DNA polymerase. This enzyme synthesizes DNA in a continuous fashion starting from the pTP protein primer, as described in Fig. 3. Events at the adenovirus replication fork are much simpler than those at the SV40 replication fork, largely because there is no lagging strand synthesis.

DNA viruses employ different strategies to provide these proteins. For the most part, small DNA viruses use cellular proteins at the replication fork. The best understood of these viruses is SV40 where the replication proteins involved were identified following the development of a cell-free system for replicating SV40 DNA *in vitro* (48) (Fig. 4). Subsequent work led to the purification of 10 proteins that are sufficient to catalyze the replication of SV40 DNA *in vitro* (32,77,78). Nine cellular activities were purified: DNA polymerase α, which is mainly responsible for initiating DNA synthesis at the origin and during lagging strand synthesis; primase, which is associated with DNA polymerase α and primes DNA synthesis at the origin and during the synthesis of Okazaki fragments; DNA polymerase δ, which is mainly responsible for leading-strand synthesis and for completing synthesis of Okazaki fragments; proliferating cell nuclear antigen (PCNA), which binds to DNA polymerase δ and forms a ring around DNA, thereby increasing polymerase processivity; replication factor-C, which loads the PCNA ring onto DNA and stimulates polymerase δ; RPA, a single-stranded DNA binding protein; RNase H, which removes all but one ribonucleotide of the RNA primer; FEN-1 (also known as MF-1), an exonuclease that removes the remaining ribonucleotide; DNA ligase I, which ligates together Okazaki fragments; and either topoisomerase I or topoisomerase II to remove superhelicity during synthesis. Although it is difficult to demonstrate that these cellular proteins perform these functions during SV40 replication in living cells, the importance of their homologs for chromosomal DNA replication in yeast supports this idea. SV40 large T antigen, the only required viral protein, provides the requisite helicase function at the replication fork, in addition to the origin-binding and unwinding activities during initiation alluded to previously.

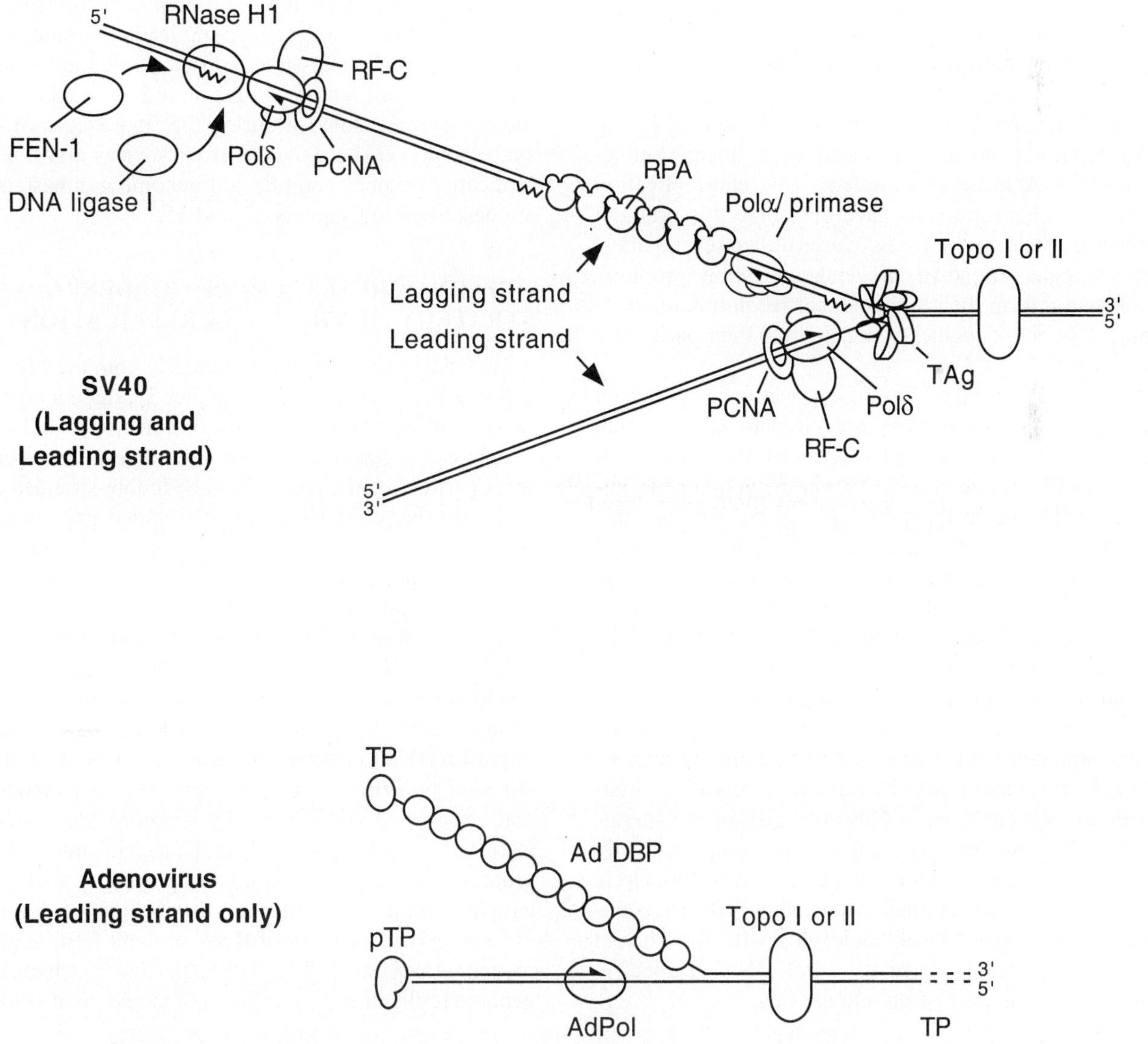

Other viruses provide almost all of the replication fork proteins. The elongation phase of adenovirus DNA replication *in vitro* requires only the single subunit adenovirus DNA polymerase; the adenovirus single-stranded DNA binding protein, which can increase the processivity of the polymerase; and either cellular topoisomerase I or II (57) (see Fig. 4). This remarkable simplicity is due in part to the unusual nature of adenovirus DNA replication, which does not entail lagging-strand synthesis (see later). Larger DNA viruses provide more activities still. For example, herpesviruses each encode a DNA polymerase, a processivity factor, a primase–helicase complex, and a single-stranded DNA binding protein (10). It is not known whether herpesviruses or poxviruses, whose full complement of virally encoded replication proteins has probably not yet been identified, require cellular proteins at all for synthesis of viral DNA.

STRATEGIES TO ENSURE COMPLETE REPLICATION, GENOME RESOLUTION, AND PACKAGING

It is critical for all organisms to replicate their entire genome. In most organisms, this problem is exacerbated by the semidiscontinuous nature of DNA replication, in which replication of the lagging strand requires laying down a primer; thus, one strand of a linear double-stranded DNA is never completed (the end-replication problem). Eukaryotic cells have overcome this problem by the use of telomeres. DNA viruses utilize several alternate strategies to solve the end-replication problem, which also inform their strategies for resolution of replicating DNA into daughter molecules and their packaging into virions.

Papovaviruses avoid the end-replication problem by being endless—that is, they are circular. Bidirectional replication generates complete circular daughter DNA molecules that are then resolved via the action of topoisomerase II (21). In the virion and in the cell nucleus, papovavirus DNA, like cellular DNA, is wound around nucleosomes, which are disrupted during replication. Daughter DNA molecules then reassemble into nucleosomes that are mixtures of "old" and "new" histones (82); thus, daughter minichromosomes are generated that are the substrates for packaging into new virions.

For other DNA viruses, virion DNA is not a simple double-stranded circle and is not wound around nucleosomes. Herpesvirus DNA is linear in the virion but circularizes when it enters cells. However, instead of generating circular daughter molecules, replication evidently generates long, concatameric molecules via rolling circle and perhaps recombinational mechanisms (10). To regenerate linear progeny DNA molecules with the correct ends, viral proteins cleave the viral DNA at specific sequences during packaging into capsids.

Adenoviruses, poxviruses, and parvoviruses, all with linear genomes, solve the end-replication problem in very different ways from papovaviruses and herpesviruses. Following initiation at one end of the adenovirus genome by protein priming (see earlier), DNA is extended from the protein primer continuously to the other end of the genome, displacing the preexisting parental strand intact (46). The displaced parental single-stranded DNA is replicated after its self-complementary inverted termini anneal, reconstructing a double-stranded origin, which is recognized by the initiation proteins (see earlier), leading to synthesis of another parental-daughter duplex. Thus, each parental duplex can be replicated semiconservatively. The linear daughter DNAs are substrates for packaging into adenovirus virions, and pTP is cleaved to generate terminal protein. Poxviruses have linear genomes with sealed hairpin ends, so they are effectively circular single-stranded DNAs. They evidently also replicate via leading-strand synthesis only, involving the generation of concatameric, double-stranded genomes that are resolved into unit-length daughter molecules by cleavage at specific DNA sequences by viral proteins. Parvoviruses utilize similar mechanisms involving leading-strand synthesis to generate double-stranded replicative intermediates, but mature unit-length, single-stranded daughter DNA molecules are displaced during the final stages of DNA synthesis (71). These stages of parvovirus and poxvirus replication require complicated genome gymnastics that are described in Chapters 32 and 35.

HEPADNAVIRUSES: A RUBE GOLDBERG STRATEGY OF VIRAL DNA REPLICATION

Hepadnaviruses have a particularly complicated replication scheme, described in Chapter 35, that incorporates several of the features already outlined here and defies simple categorization. The viral genome in extracellular virus particles is a circular, largely double-stranded DNA molecule that contains a single-stranded gap. In a step similar to that used by parvoviruses, the 3′ end of the shorter strand is extended to generate the fully double-stranded circular genome as the first step in viral DNA replication. With the aid of a viral enhancer, cellular RNA polymerase II then transcribes the nuclear double-stranded DNA genome from a specific promoter to generate a terminally redundant linear RNA pregenome that is packaged into immature virus particles. The single-stranded pregenome is later replicated to generate the mature, gapped virion DNA by virion reverse transcriptase (69), which utilizes several mechanisms including protein-priming similar to that employed by adenovirus, template jumping similar to that employed by retroviruses, and scavenging of RNA primers from degraded pregenomic viral RNA. Although this mechanism of genome replication may appear cumbersome, it evidently serves the needs of hepadnaviruses very well, as they often establish persistent infections that last for decades.

EVASION OF HOST DEFENSES AND LATENCY

Cells mount stout defenses against viral infection. Infection can induce the synthesis of interferons, which initiate a complex series of antiviral responses that inhibit virus replication. Cells can also respond to virus infection by undergoing apoptosis. If apoptosis occurs early during the virus life cycle, virus replication is terminated by the premature demise of the host cell, limiting virus yield. (Later in the life cycle, some viruses actively stimulate apoptosis, which might facilitate virus release and dissemination.) Finally, organisms can mount effective immune and inflammatory responses that prevent virus infection or lead to clearance of the virus or of virally infected cells. Spurred on by their evolutionary need to replicate and spread, viruses have evolved a number of mechanisms to overcome these defenses. The study of viral proteins that interfere with the cellular defense machinery is providing new insights into important cellular processes, such as immune recognition and apoptosis, and these viral proteins are being used as tools to identify and characterize key cellular proteins involved in these processes. Details of the interaction of host defense systems and viruses can be found in Chapters 7, 11, and 12, and in the chapters on specific viral groups.

Latent Infection

An effective mechanism of evading host defenses is for a virus to withdraw into a latent state in which the viral DNA is present at a low copy number, few viral proteins are expressed, and the cellular defenses are not mobilized. At some later time, perhaps when conditions are more conducive to virus replication, the virus can reenter the lytic, vegetative cycle. Herpesviruses commonly employ this strategy. A striking example is the latency involving varicella zoster virus, a herpesvirus that causes chicken pox during childhood but commonly sets up a latent infection in the neurons in dorsal root ganglia. When immunity has waned decades after the initial infection and acute disease, the virus can reinitiate lytic replication, resulting in lesions termed shingles in the body segment innervated by the affected dorsal root ganglion. The reactivated virus can even be transmitted to a new host.

In general, the mechanisms underlying establishment and release from latency are not well understood. EBV latency in B lymphocytes has been studied intensively (see Chapter 75 of *Fields Virology,* 4th ed.), and its regulation exemplifies many of the principles discussed in this chapter. Upon infection of B cells, latency is established via an elaborate interplay of host and viral transcription factors acting at various viral promoters to activate or repress transcription. During latency, the viral genome is present in only a few extrachromosomal copies per cell, and the virus evades the immune system by expressing very few proteins, at least some of which are poor immunogens. In latently infected nondividing cells, viral proteins are not even required for replication of EBV DNA. In latently infected dividing cells, EBV DNA is replicated using a specific viral origin sequence and cellular replication proteins, and it is segregated properly to daughter cells by the action of the viral protein EBNA-1. At a low spontaneous rate, or at a high rate in response to certain stimuli such as chemical inducers, there is a dramatic induction of viral DNA synthesis utilizing a different replication origin and viral replication proteins. The viral protein Zta (or Zebra) appears to play the primary role in induction of EBV (16). This DNA-binding transcriptional activator induces the efficient expression of a variety of virus lytic cycle genes, including those required for high-level viral DNA replication. The molecular events responsible for activation of Zta during spontaneous and induced escape from latency are not known.

Smaller DNA viruses, such as papillomaviruses and some parvoviruses, also undergo latent infections. In the case of the papillomaviruses, the basal epithelial cells in virus-induced warts are latently infected: The viral genomes are present at low copy number, late gene products are not expressed, and no virus particles are produced. In the more differentiated cells of the same lesion, latency is disrupted and active viral replication and production of infectious virions takes place. The nature of the switch between latent and vegetative replication is obscure, but it appears to be tightly linked to the state of differentiation of the host cell. In latent parvovirus infection, the viral genome is integrated into the cellular DNA. Superinfection of these latently infected cells with helper adenoviruses or herpesviruses supplies factors required for reentry into vegetative parvovirus replication.

Transmission of Latent Viral Genomes to Daughter Cells

During latent infection, viral genomes must be faithfully segregated during cell division. Some latent viral genomes are integrated into the cellular DNA and are replicated and segregated passively during the appropriate stage of the cell cycle. This is the case for the nonautonomous parvovirus AAV, which in the absence of helper function stably integrates with high efficiency into a specific site in a cellular chromosome and remains latent until helper function is provided (14). Other latent viral genomes are often maintained as relatively low copy number plasmids. For these viruses, unequal segregation would lead to the loss of the viral DNA in some daughter cells. Bovine papillomavirus, which replicates as a nuclear plasmid in transformed rodent fibroblasts, has

TABLE 3. *Strategies utilized during DNA virus replication*

Step	Strategy	Viruses
Initiation of transcription	Strong enhancer(s) Virion protein(s)	Papovaviruses, adenoviruses, hepadnaviruses Herpesviruses, poxviruses
Stimulation of subsequent viral gene expression	Viral-encoded transactivators	All
Mobilization of cell cycle	Inactivation of tumor suppressors Stimulation of signal transduction pathways	Papovaviruses, adenoviruses Some papovaviruses, some herpesviruses
Provision of deoxynucleoside triphosphates	Stimulation of cell enzymes Synthesis of viral enzymes	Papovaviruses, adenoviruses Herpesviruses, poxviruses
Initiation of DNA synthesis	Internal origin-recognition proteins Protein-primers plus sequence recognition Preexisting or newly formed primers	Papovaviruses, some herpesviruses Adenoviruses, hepadnaviruses Parvoviruses, poxviruses, hepadnaviruses, some herpesviruses (?)
Provision of replication fork proteins	Mainly cellular proteins Mainly viral proteins	Parvoviruses, papovaviruses Adenoviruses, herpesviruses, poxviruses, hepadnaviruses
Genome completion and resolution	Circles to circles Circles to linear RNAs to circles Linears to linears Linears to circles to linears Hairpins to concatamers to hairpins	Papoviruses Hepadnaviruses Adenoviruses Herpesviruses Parvoviruses, poxviruses
Evasion of host defenses	Interference with host defense systems Latent infections	Adenoviruses, papovaviruses, poxviruses, herpesviruses Some parvoviruses, some papovaviruses (including papillomaviruses), herpesviruses

devised a clever strategy to achieve proper genome distribution during cell division (35,47). The viral E2 replication protein not only binds viral DNA but also associates with mitotic cellular chromosomes. The E2 protein thus tethers the viral DNA to the cell chromosomes as they undergo migration during mitosis and cytokinesis, and the viral DNA hitchhikes a ride into the daughter cells. The EBV protein EBNA1 may carry out a similar function during viral genome segregation during latency. In this fashion, the viruses take advantage of the elaborate cellular machinery that ensures proper chromosome segregation during cell division.

SUMMARY AND PERSPECTIVES

Viruses have evolved many different strategies to effect their replication. The diverse strategies employed for each step in replication are summarized in Table 3. Despite this diversity, there are remarkable similarities in how rather different viruses execute specific steps in their replication. For example, replication of the smallest (parvovirus) and that of the largest (poxvirus) viral DNAs appear to employ similar "rolling hairpin" mechanisms. These similarities presumably reflect the ability of viruses to identify and exploit or interfere with conserved cellular processes to carry out the essential steps of the virus life cycle: viral gene expression, genome replication, evasion of host defenses, and production of progeny virions. Viruses thus continue to be unique and powerful tools to elucidate these fundamental cellular processes. Unfortunately, many intricate and interesting mechanisms utilized by DNA viruses are not outlined in this brief chapter. Some of these mechanisms are described in the chapters on the various viruses in this volume; others remain to be uncovered.

REFERENCES

1. Ace CI, McKee TA, Ryan JM, et al. Construction and characterization of a herpes simplex virus type 1 mutant unable to transinduce immediate-early gene expression. *J Virol* 1989;63:2260–2269.
2. Bandara LR, LaThangue NB. Adenovirus E1a prevents the retinoblastoma gene product from complexing with a cellular transcription factor. *Nature* 1991;351:494–497.
3. Banerji J, Rusconi S, Schaffner W. Expression of a β-globin gene is enhanced by remote SV40 DNA sequences. *Cell* 1981;27:299–308.
4. Brodsky JL, Pipas JM. Polyomavirus T antigens: Molecular chaperones for multiprotein complexes. *J Virol* 1998;72:5329–5334.
5. Brückner A, Stadlbauer F, Guarino LA, et al. The mouse DNA polymerase α-primase subunit p48 mediates species-specific replication of polyomavirus DNA in vitro. *Mol Cell Biol* 1995;15:1716–1724.
6. Buller RM, Chakrabarti S, Cooper JA, et al. Deletion of the vaccinia virus growth factor gene reduces virus virulence. *J Virol* 1988;62: 866–874.
7. Buller RML, Janik JE, Sebring ED, Rose JA. Herpes simplex virus types 1 and 2 help adeno-associated virus replication. *J Virol* 1981;40: 241.
8. Campbell KS, Mullane KP, Aksoy IA, et al. DnaJ/hsp40 chaperone

domain of SV40 large T antigen promotes efficient viral DNA replication. *Genes Dev* 1997;11:1098–1110.
9. Carey M. The enhanceosome and transcriptional synergy. *Cell* 1998;92: 5–8.
10. Challberg M. Herpesvirus DNA replication. In: DePamphilis ML, ed. *DNA Replication in Eukaryotic Cells.* Cold Spring Harbor, NY: Cold Spring Harbor Laboratory Press, 1996;721–750.
11. Challberg MD, Kelly TJ Jr. Adenovirus DNA replication in vitro. *Proc Natl Acad Sci U S A* 1979;76:655–659.
12. Challberg MD, Ostrove JM, Kelly TJ Jr. Initiation of adenovirus DNA replication: Detection of covalent complexes between nucleotide and the 80-kilodalton terminal protein. *J Virol* 1982;41:265–270.
13. Chellappan S, Kraus VB, Kroger B, et al. Adenovirus E1A, simian virus 40 tumor antigen, and human papillomavirus E7 protein share the capacity to disrupt the interaction between transcription factor E2F and the retinoblastoma gene product. *Proc Natl Acad Sci U S A* 1992;89: 4549–4553.
14. Cheung A-K, Hoggan MD, Hauswirth WW, Berns KI. Integration of the adeno-associated virus genome into cellular DNA in latently infected human Detroit 6 cells. *J Virol* 1980;33:739–748.
15. Cotmore SF, Tattersall P. DNA replication in the autonomous parvoviruses. *Semin Virol* 1995;6:271–281.
16. Countryman J, Jenson H, Seibl R, et al. Polymorphic proteins encoded within BZLF1 of defective and standard Epstein-Barr viruses disrupt latency. *J Virol* 1987;61:3672–3679.
17. Cress WD, Nevins JR. Use of the E2F transcription factor by DNA tumor virus regulatory proteins. *Curr Top Microbiol Immunol* 1996; 208:63–78.
18. Debbas M, White E. Wild-type p53 mediates apoptosis by E1A, which is inhibited by E1B. *Genes Dev* 1993;7:546–554.
19. DeCaprio JA, Ludlow JW, Figge J, et al. SV40 large tumor antigen forms a specific complex with the product of the retinoblastoma susceptibility gene. *Cell* 1988;54:275–283.
20. DeGregori J, Kowalik T, Nevins JR. Cellular targets for activation by the E2F1 transcription factor include DNA synthesis- and G1/S-regulatory genes. *Mol Cell Biol* 1995;15:4215–4224. (Erratum: 15: 5846–5871)
21. DePamphilis ML, Bradley MK. Replication of SV40 and polyomavirus. In: Salzman N, ed. *The Papovaviridae*, vol. 1. New York: Plenum Press, 1996;99–246.
22. Dilworth SM. Polyoma virus middle T antigen: Meddler or mimic? *Trends Microbiol* 1995;3:31–35.
23. DiMaio D, Lai C-C, Klein O. Virocrine transformation: The intersection between viral transforming proteins and cellular signal transduction pathways. *Ann Rev Microbiol* 1998;52:397–421.
24. Dobner T, Horikoshi N, Rubenwolf S, Shenk T. Blockage by adenovirus E4orf6 of transcriptional activation by the p53 tumor suppressor. *Science* 1996;272:1470–1473.
25. Dornreiter I, Erdile LF, Gilbert IU, et al. Interaction of DNA polymerase alpha-primase with cellular replication protein A and SV40 T antigen. *EMBO J* 1992;11:769–776.
26. Du S, Traktman P. Vaccinia virus DNA replication: Two hundred base pairs of telomeric sequence confer optimal replication efficiency on minichromosome templates. *Proc Natl Acad Sci U S A* 1996;93: 9693–9698.
27. Dyson N, Howley PM, Münger K, Harlow E. The human papilloma virus-16 E7 oncoprotein is able to bind to the retinoblastoma gene product. *Science* 1989;243:934–937.
28. Eki T, Enomoto T, Masutani C, et al. Mouse DNA primase plays the principle role in determination of permissiveness for polyomavirus DNA replication. *J Virol* 1991;65:4874–4881.
29. Grosschedl R. Higher-order nucleoprotein complexes in transcription: Analogies with site-specific recombination. *Curr Opin Cell Biol* 1995; 7:362–370.
30. Gruss P, Dhar R, Khoury G. The SV40 tandem repeats as an element of the early promoter. *Proc Natl Acad Sci U S A* 1981;78:943–947.
31. Gu B, DeLuca NA. Requirements for activation of the herpes simplex virus glycoprotein C promoter in vitro by the viral regulatory protein ICP4. *J Virol* 1994;68:7953–7965.
32. Hassell JA, Brinton BT. SV40 and polyomavirus DNA replication. In: DePamphilis ML, ed. *DNA Replication in Eukaryotic Cells.* Cold Spring Harbor, NY: Cold Spring Harbor Laboratory Press, 1996; 639–677.
33. Hay RT. Adenovirus DNA replication. In: DePamphilis ML, ed. *DNA Replication in Eukaryotic Cells.* Cold Spring Harbor, NY: Cold Spring Harbor Laboratory Press, 1996;699–719.
34. Hiebert SW, Chellappan SP, Horowitz JM, Nevins JR. The interaction of RB with E2F coincides with an inhibition of the transcriptional activity of E2F. *Genes Dev* 1992;6:177–185.
35. Ilves I, Kivi S, Ustav M. Long-term episomal maintenance of bovine papillomavirus type 1 plasmids is determined by attachment to host chromosomes, which is mediated by the viral E2 protein and its binding sites. *J Virol* 1999;73:4404–4412.
36. Imbalzano AN, Shepard AA, DeLuca NA. Functional relevance of specific interactions between herpes simplex virus type 1 ICP4 and sequences from the promoter-regulatory domain of the viral thymidine kinase gene. *J Virol* 1990;64:2620–2631.
37. Jamieson AT, Subak-Sharpe JH. Biochemical studies on the herpes simplex virus-specified deoxypyrimidine kinase activity. *J Gen Virol* 1974;4:481–492.
38. Jean S, LeVan KM, Song B, et al. Herpes simplex virus 1 ICP27 is required for transcription of two viral late genes in infected cells (submitted).
39. Jones NC, Rigby PWJ, Ziff EB. Trans-acting protein factors and the regulation of eukaryotic transcription: Lessons from studies on DNA tumor viruses. *Genes Dev* 1988;2:267–281.
40. Jung JU, Stager M, Desrosiers RC. Virus-encoded cyclin. *Mol Cell Biol* 1994;14:7235–7244.
41. Keaveney M, Struhl K. Activator-mediated recruitment of the RNA polymerase II machinery is the predominant mechanism for transcriptional activation in yeast. *Mol Cell* 1998;1:917–924.
42. Kelly TJ. DNA replication in mammalian cells: Insights from the SV40 model system. *Harvey Lect* 1989-1990;85:173–188.
43. King AJ, van der Vliet PC. A precursor terminal protein trinucleotide intermediate during initiation of adenovirus DNA-replication-regeneration of molecular ends in vitro by a jumping back mechanism. *EMBO J* 1994;13:5786–5792.
44. Kovesdi I, Reichel R, Nevins JR. Identification of a cellular factor involved in E1A transactivation. *Cell* 1986;45:219–228.
45. Lane DP, Crawford LV. T antigen is bound to a host protein in SV40-transformed cells. *Nature* 1979;278:261–263.
46. Lechner RL, Kelly TJ Jr. The structure of replicating adenovirus 2 DNA molecules. *Cell* 1977;12:1007–1020.
47. Lehman CW, Botchan MR. Segregation of viral plasmids depends on tethering to chromosomes and is regulated by phosphorylation. *Proc Natl Acad Sci U S A* 1998;95:4338–4343.
48. Li JJ, Kelly TJ. Simian virus 40 DNA replication in vitro. *Proc Natl Acad Sci U S A* 1984;81:6973–6977.
49. Linzer DI, Levine AJ. Characterization of a 54K dalton cellular SV40 tumor antigen present in SV40-transformed cells and uninfected embryonal carcinoma cells. *Cell* 1979;17:43–52.
50. Mal A, Poon RY, Howe PH, et al. Inactivation of p27Kip1 by the viral E1A oncoprotein in TGFβ-treated cells. *Nature* 1996;380:262–265.
51. Mears WE, Rice SA. The herpes simplex virus immediate-early protein ICP27 shuttles between nucleus and cytoplasm. *Virology* 1998;242: 128–137.
52. Melendy T, Stillman B. An interaction between replication protein A and SV40 T antigen appears essential for primasome assembly during SV40 DNA replication. *J Biol Chem* 1993;268:3389–3395.
53. Mohr IJ, Clark R, Sun S, et al. Targeting the E1 replication protein to the papillomavirus origin of replication by complex formation with the E2 transactivator. *Science* 1990;250:1694–1699.
54. Moore PS, Chang Y. Antiviral activity of tumor-suppressor pathways: Clues from molecular piracy by KSHV. *Trends Genet* 1998;14: 144–150.
55. Morcaski ES, Roizman B. Herpesvirus-dependent amplification and inversion of a cell-associated viral thymidine kinase gene flanked by viral a sequences and linked to an origin of viral DNA replication. *Proc Natl Acad Sci U S A* 1982;79:5626–5630.
56. Moreau P, Hen R, Wasylyk B, et al. The SV40 72 base pair repeat as a striking effect on gene expression both in SV40 and other chimeric recombinants. *Nucleic Acids Res* 1981;9:6047–6067.
57. Nagata K, Guggenheimer RA, Hurwitz J. Adenovirus DNA replication in vitro: Synthesis of full length DNA with purified proteins. *Proc Natl Acad Sci U S A* 1983;80:4266–4270.
58. O'Hare P. The virion transactivator of herpes simplex virus. *Sem Virol* 1993;4:145–155.
59. Petti L, Nilson L, DiMaio D. Activation of the platelet-derived growth

factor receptor by the bovine papillomavirus E5 protein. *EMBO J* 1991;10:845–855.
60. Rao L, Debbas M, Sabbatini P, et al. The adenovirus E1A proteins induce apoptosis, which is inhibited by the E1B 19-kDa and Bcl-2 proteins. *Proc Natl Acad Sci U S A* 1992;89:7742–7746. (Erratum, *Proc Natl Acad Sci U S A* 1992;89:9974.)
61. Sarnow P, Ho YS, Williams J, Levine AJ. Adenovirus E1b-58kd tumor antigen and SV40 large tumor antigen are physically associated with the same 54-kd cellular protein in transformed cells. *Cell* 1982;28:387–394.
62. Schlehofer JR, Ehrbar M, zur Hausen H. Vaccinia virus, herpes simplex virus, and carcinogens induce DNA amplification in a human cell line and support replication of a helpervirus dependent parvovirus. *Virology* 1986;152:110–117.
63. Shortle DR, Margolskee RF, Nathans D. Mutational analysis of the simian virus 40 replicon: Pseudorevertants of mutants with a defective replication origin. *Proc Natl Acad Sci U S A* 1979;76:6128–6131.
64. Smiley JR, Duncan J. Truncation of the C-terminal acidic transcriptional activation domain of herpes simplex virus VP16 produces a phenotype similar to that of the in1814 linker insertion mutation. *J Virol* 1997;71:6191–6193.
65. Smith IL, Hardwicke MA, Sandri-Goldin RM. Evidence that the herpes simplex virus immediate early protein ICP27 acts post-transcriptionally during infection to regulate gene expression. *Virology* 1992;186:74–86.
66. Speck SH, Chatila T, Flemington E. Reactivation of Epstein-Barr virus: Regulation and function of the BZLF1 gene. *Trends Microbiol* 1997;5: 399–405.
67. Srinivasan A, McClellan AJ, Vartikar J, et al. The amino-terminal transforming region of simian virus 40 large T and small t antigens functions as a J domain. *Mol Cell Biol* 1997;17:4761–4773.
68. Stadlbauer F, Voitenleitner C, Brückner A, et al. Species-specific replication of simian virus 40 DNA in vitro requires the p180 subunit of human DNA polymerase α-primase. *Mol Cell Biol* 1996;16:94–104.
69. Summers J, Mason WS. Replication of the genome of a hepatitis B-like virus by reverse transcription of an RNA intermediate. *Cell* 1982;29: 403–415.
70. Tattersall P. Replication of the parvovirus MVM. I. Dependence of virus multiplication and placque formation on cell growth. *J Virol* 1972;10:586–590.
71. Tattersall P, Ward DC. Rolling hairpin model for replication of parvovirus and linear chromosomal DNA. *Nature* 1976;263:106–109.
72. Thompson CC, McKnight SL. Anatomy of an enhancer. *Trends Genet* 1992;8:232–236.
73. Tjian R, Maniatis T. Transcriptional activation: A complex puzzle with few easy pieces. *Cell* 1994;77:5–8.
74. Triezenberg SJ. Structure and function of transcriptional activation domains. *Curr Opin Genet Dev* 1995;5:190–196.
75. Ustav M, Stenlund A. Transient replication of BPV-1 requires two viral polypeptides encoded by the E1 and E2 open reading frames. *EMBO J* 1991;10:449–457.
76. Vlazny DA, Frenkel N. Replication of herpes simplex virus DNA: Location of replication recognition signals within defective virus genomes. *Proc Natl Acad Sci U S A* 1981;78:742–746.
77. Waga S, Bauer G, Stillman B. Reconstitution of complete SV40 DNA replication with purified replication factors. *J Biol Chem* 1994;269: 10923–10934.
78. Waga S, Stillman B. Anatomy of a DNA replication fork revealed by reconstitution of SV40 DNA replication in vitro. *Nature* 1994;369: 207–212.
79. Walter S, Richards R, Armentrout RW. Cell cycle-dependent replication of the DNA of minute virus of mice, a parvovirus. *Biochim Biophys Acta* 1980;607:420–431.
80. Werness BA, Levine AJ, Howley PM. Association of human papillomavirus types 16 and 18 E6 proteins with p53. *Science* 1990;248:76–79.
81. Whyte P, Buchkovich KJ, Horowitz JM, et al. Association between an oncogene and an anti-oncogene: The adenovirus E1A proteins bind to the retinoblastoma gene product. *Nature* 1988;334:124–129.
82. Wolffe AP. Chromatin structure and DNA replication: Implications for transcriptional activity. In: DePamphilis ML, ed. *DNA Replication in Eukaryotic Cells*. Cold Spring Harbor, NY: Cold Spring Harbor Laboratory Press, 1996;271–293.
83. Yakinoglu AO, Heilbronn R, Burkle A, et al. DNA amplification of adeno-associated virus as a response to cellular genotoxic stress. *Cancer Res* 1988;48:3123–3129.
84. Yakobson B, Koch T, Winocour E. Replication of adeno-associated virus in synchronized cells without the addition of a helper virus. *J Virol* 1987;61:972–981.

CHAPTER 7

Virus–Host Cell Interactions

David M. Knipe, Charles E. Samuel, and Peter Palese

By definition, viruses are unable to replicate on their own but must enter a host cell and use the host-cell macromolecular machinery and energy supplies to replicate. Thus, in many ways the study of viral replication is a study of the interactions of viruses with their host cells. The study of virus–host cell interactions has impacted several areas of biology and biomedical science. First, investigation of the mechanisms by which viruses replicate in, alter, or take over their host cells has often led to insight into basic cell biologic and molecular biologic mechanisms. Viruses often target critical regulatory events in the host cell; thus, knowledge of the processes subverted by viruses has often highlighted cellular regulatory mechanisms.

Second, during their replication within cells, viruses exploit host-cell molecules and processes at the expense of the host cell, which may result in cell injury or death. These injurious effects of viral replication in cells are one of the basic causes of viral disease. Therefore, precise knowledge of the pathogenic mechanisms by which viruses replicate in specific tissues, spread, and cause disease must come, in part, from studies of the intracellular replication of the virus. Over the past 45 years, increasing understanding of the mechanisms of viral replication has emerged from biochemical and cell biologic studies of virus replication in cultured cells. Investigators of viral pathogenesis have recently attempted to define the molecular events occurring in different cell types during the series of stages that define viral pathogenesis within a host organism.

Third, the definition of antiviral strategies requires knowledge of the replicative mechanisms of viruses and the identification of replicative steps that involve virus-specific processes and not host-cell processes.

This chapter will focus on the interactions of viruses with an individual host cell. Chapter 9 discusses the events that lead to (a) spread of a virus from one cell to another within a host organism, (b) induction of disease, and (c) spread within the environment. Virus infection of a cell can lead to any of several possible outcomes. First, a nonproductive infection can occur in which viral replication is blocked, and the host cell may or may not survive. After the nonproductive infection, the viral genome may be lost from the cell. Alternatively, the viral genetic information may become integrated as DNA in the cellular genome or may persist as episomal DNA in these surviving cells. If the growth properties of the cell are altered to make it oncogenic, this would constitute an oncogenic transformation event (see Chapter 10). The virus may become dormant with limited or no viral gene expression, and a latent infection is established (see Chapter 9). Second, a productive viral infection may result in which the host cell dies and lyses. Third, the cell may survive and continue to produce virus at a low level, resulting in a chronic infection (see Chapter 9).

Which of these possible scenarios is realized is determined by the nature of the interactions between the virus and the host-cell constituents. For example, a nonproductive infection may result if a host-cell component necessary for viral replication is not present. One of the main goals of this chapter is to describe the types of interactions between virus-encoded macromolecules and the host cell, which may define the ultimate outcome of a virus infection. This chapter will examine (a) the molecular and cell biologic events that allow viral replication, (b) the ways in which viruses modify their host cells to promote their own replication, and (c) the kinds of mechanisms that may have evolved in cells to prevent virus infection. The types of experimental approaches used to obtain evidence for specific virus–host interactions will also be discussed.

The study of virus–cell interactions really started with the growth of viruses in cultured cells (83). Although infection of host organisms had given some indication of cell death resulting from viral infection, there was little clear evidence of other effects of viruses on the host cell before the infection of cultured cells and the identification of cytopathic effect (CPE) of viruses on cells (82). The elucidation of viral replication strategies in the 1950s and 1960s provided the broad outlines of virus replication. More recently, better probes for nucleic acids and proteins have allowed more precise descriptions of the molecular events of viral replication in a host cell. The techniques of molecular genetics and cell biology have begun to define the specific host-cell molecules and cellular compartments with which virus-encoded molecules interact.

In addition to classifying virus–host cell interactions in terms of the final outcome of the infection, virus–cell interactions can also be described in molecular terms with regard to individual replication events. For example, the effects of viruses on the host cell may be mediated by addition or substitution of a virus-specific macromolecule into a cellular complex or structure. Alternatively, the virus may mediate a covalent or noncovalent modification of a host-cell molecule. Virus infection may cause a disassembly or rearrangement of a host-cell complex or structure, or virus infection may lead to the assembly of a new infected cell–specific complex or structure in the infected cell. After defining these molecular interactions, the challenge for us as virologists is to relate this molecular information back to the biology of the virus in the host cell and ultimately the host organism.

CYTOPATHIC EFFECTS OF VIRUS INFECTION

One of the classic ways of detecting virus replication in cells was the observation of changes in cell structure, or CPEs, resulting from virus infection (Figs. 1–3, and see Fig. 1 in Chapter 18 of *Fields Virology*, 4th ed.). Some of the most common effects of viral infection are mor-

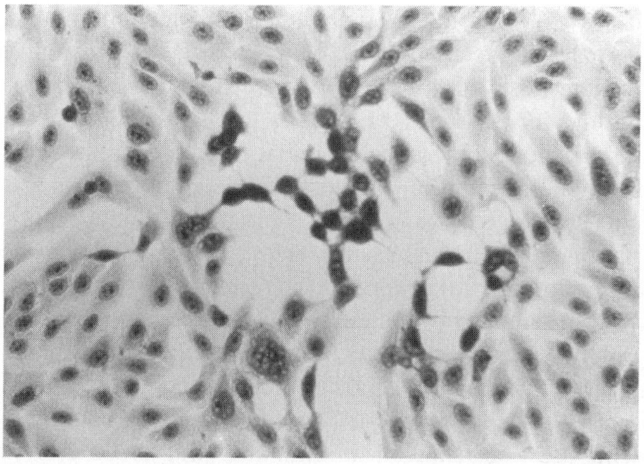

FIG. 1. Cytopathic effect (CPE) resulting from virus infection. The center portion of the figure shows monkey (Vero) cells rounding up and detaching from the substrate after infection with Herpes simplex virus 1 (HSV-1). A normal monolayer of cells is visible around the focus of CPE. The cells were fixed with methanol and stained with Giemsa stain. Micrograph courtesy of M. Kosz-Vnenchak.

phologic changes such as (a) cell rounding and detachment from the substrate (see Fig. 1), (b) cell lysis, (c) syncytium formation (see Fig. 2), and (d) inclusion body formation (see Fig. 3). The occurrence of cell morphologic changes resulting from CPE has even led to classification schemes for viruses. In 1954, Enders (1982) proposed classifying viruses into the following groups: (a) those causing cellular degeneration; (b) those causing formation of inclusion bodies and cell degeneration; and (c) those causing formation of multinucleated cells or syncytial masses and degeneration, with or without inclusion bodies. However, as described in Chapter 2, other classification schemes based on virion and genome structure and modes of replication have provided much better ways of classifying viruses.

The CPE of viruses on cells has also been called cell injury. These terms tend to emphasize the pathology of the host cell; however, from a virologist's point of view, we will see that many of the host-cell alterations by virus infection can now be explained as changes in the host cell that permit necessary steps in viral replication. Thus, many of the CPEs or cell injuries are secondary effects of the virus doing what it needs to do to replicate and are not simply toxic effects of viral gene products on the host cell. Some viral gene products cause toxic effects to the host with no apparent purpose, but as we learn more about the precise mechanisms of virus–cell interactions, many of these effects will likely be explained as aspects of essential steps in viral replication. For example, an adenovirus virion component was shown more than 30 years ago to cause monolayer cells to detach from the culture substrate (87,257), and this was later shown to be caused by the penton base protein (32,328,353). This remained an unexplained toxic effect until it was

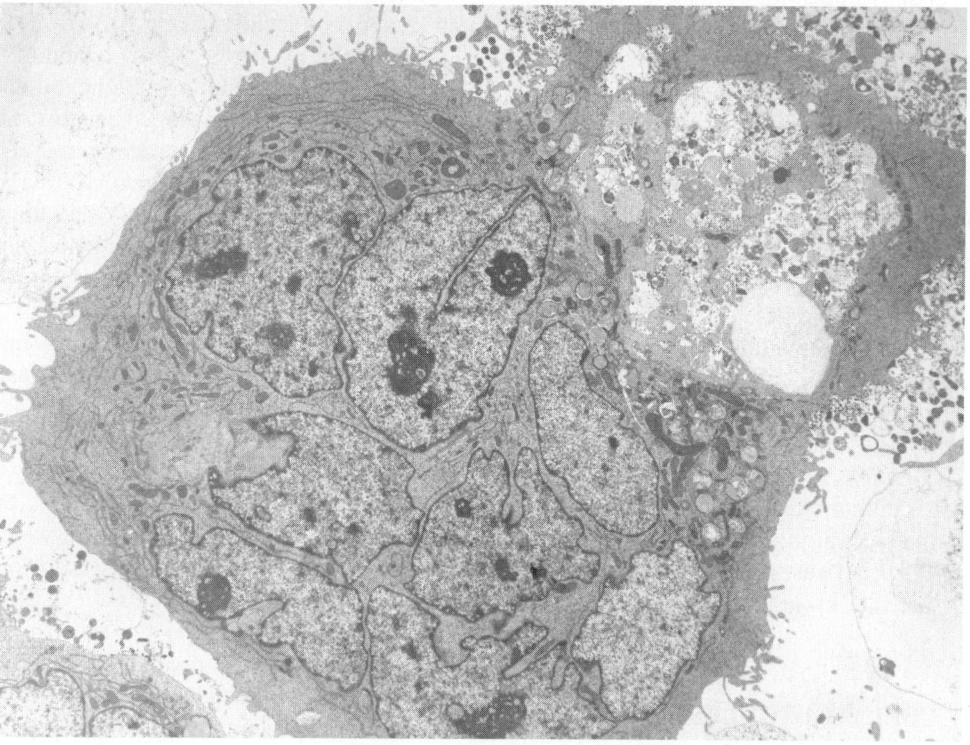

FIG. 2. A syncytium formed by human immunodeficiency virus (HIV) infection of T cells. Electron micrograph courtesy of J. Sodroski.

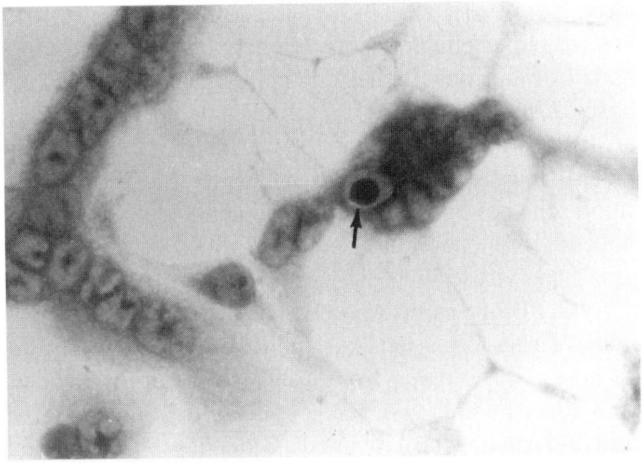

FIG. 3. Inclusion body formation in infected cells. The *arrow* indicates an intranuclear eosinophilic inclusion in a cell infected with HSV-1. The inclusion is surrounded by a clear halo. The cells were stained with hematoxylin and eosin. Micrograph courtesy of M. Kosz-Vnenchak.

observed that the penton base protein binds to α_V integrins during adenovirus internalization (368). Thus, penton base protein causes cell detachment by binding through RGD sequences to cell-surface integrins, thereby displacing vitronectin from the integrins. The interaction of vitronectin and integrins is involved in cell attachment and spreading on the culture substrate.

A number of reviews and monographs have examined the various aspects of cytopathology resulting from virus infection (96,175,304). The reader is referred to these sources for detailed discussion and references on these topics. Determining the primary cause of death of a cell resulting from viral infection can be a complex and difficult issue because of the numerous events occurring within the infected cell. It is also apparent now that there are at least two general pathways for cell death: necrosis and apoptosis (programmed cell death). Necrosis involves the death of a cell as a result of physical damage or toxic agents. During necrosis, there is disruption of the mitochondria, swelling of the cell, disruption of organized structure, and lysis. Apoptosis involves cell death in situations controlled by physiologic stimuli during development and hormonal signaling in response to DNA damage. During apoptosis, there is DNA condensation and fragmentation, cell shrinkage, and membrane blebbing. Cell death due to viral infection could result from either mechanism in that viruses may have toxic effects on the host cell, activate programmed cell death pathways, or both.

USE OF HOST CELL MOLECULES AND PROCESSES FOR VIRAL ENTRY

Viruses must enter the host cell to replicate. Therefore, they must cross the cell plasma membrane to gain access to the cellular synthetic machinery in the cytoplasm and, in some cases, the nucleus of the host cell. Virus entry into the host cell has been divided into two events: (a) binding to cell-surface receptors and (b) penetration of the plasma membrane, or entry. These processes are described in detail in Chapter 4; thus, the purpose of this discussion is only to highlight the aspects of the host cell that are utilized during virus entry. Virus particles serve to protect the viral genome during spread from cell to cell or from one host to the next. The lipid envelope and the protein capsid act to protect the genome from nucleolytic attack or chemical reaction in the extracellular environment. As the virus enters a new host cell, these components must be removed to allow the viral genome to be replicated. Thus, viruses have evolved to have a stable, protective particle that can be readily disassembled in a new host cell. For the enveloped virus, cell entry by fusion serves two functions, a means to cross the plasma membrane barrier and a means to remove its outer coat, the envelope.

Viruses utilize a wide variety of cell-surface molecules as their receptors in that they can use protein molecules, carbohydrates, or glycolipids for their initial attachment to cells. Additional molecules or coreceptors may be involved in the fusion event between the viral envelope and the cellular plasma membrane. After binding to its surface receptor, a virus must cross the plasma membrane to replicate. Two general pathways have been defined for virus entry: (a) surface fusion between the viral lipid envelope and the cell plasma membrane and (b) receptor-mediated endocytosis (Fig. 4). Enveloped viruses can gain entry to the cytoplasm by fusion of their lipid envelope with the plasma membrane or endosomal membrane, whereas nonenveloped viruses must use alternative strategies to cross the membrane.

Fusion at the surface involves the cellular plasma membrane (see Fig. 4, panel I), and uptake into the cell by endocytosis involves normal endocytotic mechanisms for uptake of molecules into vesicles within cells (see Fig. 4, panel IIA). Cellular proton pumps lower the pH in the endocytotic vesicles, activating membrane fusion between the viral and cellular membranes or activating enzymes that lyse the vesicle (see Fig. 4).

Based on these entry processes, virus–host interactions can be divided into at least seven strategies (Fig. 5). This classification depends on whether the viruses are enveloped or nonenveloped, and in which cell compartment replication and virus assembly or budding takes place. In the case of poliovirus (PV) (see Fig. 5, line 1), the native virion binds to the specific PV receptor and undergoes a receptor-mediated conformational change. The altered (A) particles, which appear to have lost an internal viral protein (VP4), form a pore in the endosome structure, thereby releasing the viral RNA into the cytoplasm. Certain members of the picornavirus group (but not PV) and other nonenveloped RNA viruses, including

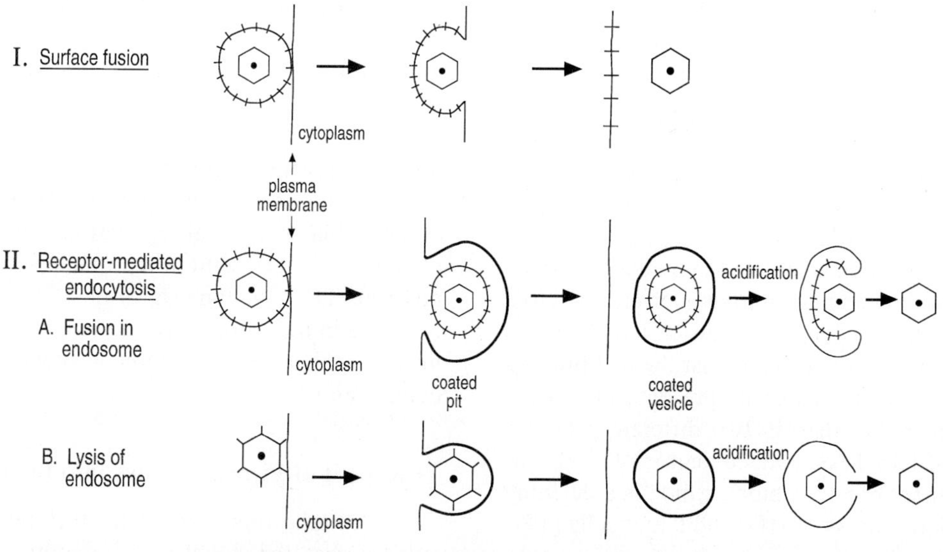

FIG. 4. Pathways for viral entry of the host cell.

reovirus, have been shown to require the acidification of endosomes (119).

Even more complex is the entry of adenovirus, another nonenveloped virus (see Fig. 5, line 6). Following attachment to the cell and internalization, the virus undergoes a series of changes in which the viral protein interactions of the capsid are broken down. The acidification of the endosome is a required step in entry as well as the activity of the viral protease (120).

Many enveloped viruses, including paramyxoviruses such as Newcastle disease virus and the Sendai and parainfluenza viruses, fuse directly with the cytoplasmic

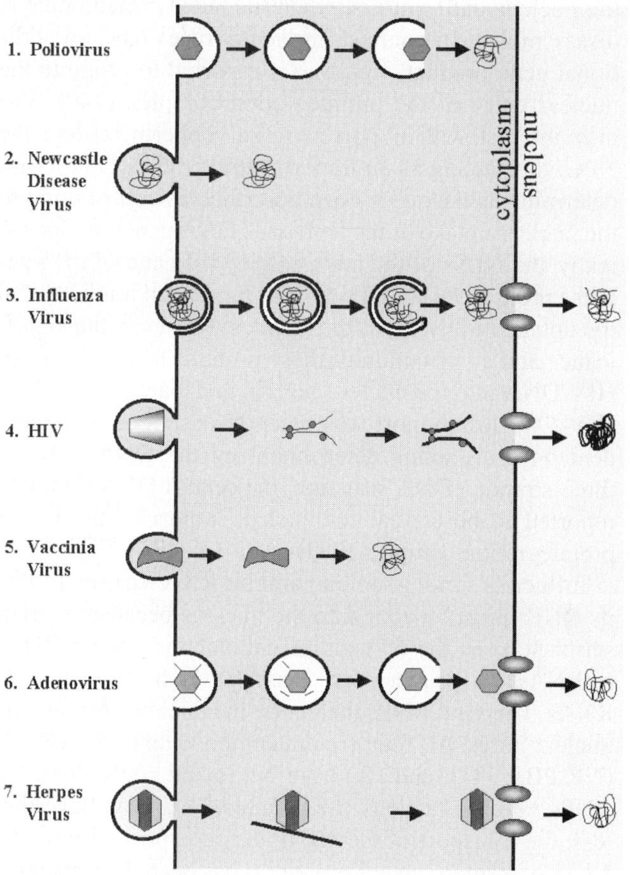

FIG. 5. Entry mechanisms for different classes of viruses. Nonenveloped RNA viruses such as poliovirus (*line 1*) and DNA viruses such as adenovirus (*line 6*) enter the cell by endocytosis at the cytoplasmic membrane. Enveloped RNA or DNA viruses can enter the cell by fusion at the cell membrane [Newcastle disease virus (*line 2*), HIV (*line 4*), vaccinia (*line 5*), and herpes (*line 7*) viruses] or by endocytosis and subsequent fusion of the viral and vesicular membranes [influenza virus (*line 3*)]. Viral replication may ensue in the cytoplasm (*lines 1, 2, 5*), or viral genomes are transported through the nuclear pore into the nucleus (*lines 3, 4, 6, and 7*), where they are replicated. For the sake of clarity, not all viral proteins implicated in entry are shown. Line 7 depicts only one of the two possible routes of HIV egress described in the text.

membrane at neutral pH (see Fig. 5, line 2). For all of these viruses, the first step involves the binding of HN to its sialic acid receptor, which may cause HN to undergo a conformational change. This in turn triggers a conformational change in the F protein, which expresses the fusion peptide and allows it to embed in and perturb the cell membrane. This ultimately leads to the fusion of the cell and viral lipid bilayer (187,363).

A similar mechanism is postulated to mediate entry of retroviruses, including human immunodeficiency virus (HIV) (see Fig. 5, line 4). One of the differences between paramyxoviruses and retroviruses is that the cell binding and fusion activities of the latter are present in the same viral glycoprotein rather than in two different proteins. Also, the entry of HIV has an added degree of complexity in its requirement of coreceptors, which is a defining factor in the fusion process of HIV and target cells (19).

In contrast to the fusion at plasma membranes observed for many enveloped viruses, influenza viruses undergo an acid pH–mediated membrane fusion and entry process (see Fig. 5, line 3). Following binding to sialic acid on the cell surface via the hemagglutinin, the virus–receptor complex is endocytosed and the acidified environment of the endosome triggers a conformational rearrangement of the viral surface protein. The fusion reaction facilitated by the influenza virus hemagglutinin is one of the best characterized processes in virology and it has helped to provide a detailed understanding of viral entry mechanisms (363).

To promote the release of the influenza viral ribonucleoprotein (vRNP) into the cytoplasm and to conclude the uncoating process, protons in the acidic endosome are pumped into the interior of the virus (see Fig. 5, line 3). The M2 protein in the influenza virion envelope serves as a proton channel (263,332) that exposes the nucleocapsid to low pH conditions, resulting in a conformational change in the M1 protein and its irreversible dissociation from the nucleocapsids (38,210). The antiviral drugs amantadine and rimantadine can block this ion channel and thereby interfere with uncoating of influenza A viruses (but not influenza B viruses).

The alphaherpesviruses make initial contact with the cell by low-affinity binding to glycosaminoglycans (i.e., heparan sulfates; see Fig. 5, line 7). Subsequent interactions with membrane coreceptors facilitate fusion of the viral membrane and the plasma membrane and subsequent entry. In the cytoplasm, the capsid structures undergo a microtubule-mediated transport to the nuclear pore complex (NPC) (322).

TARGETING OF VIRAL GENOMES TO INTRACELLULAR SITES FOR TRANSCRIPTION AND/OR REPLICATION

Once the viral nucleocapsid has gained entry to the cytoplasm, it needs to be targeted to the intracellular site where transcription and/or replication of the viral genome can take place. For most DNA viruses, the viral genome must localize into the nucleus, usually through the nuclear pores. The reverse transcription product of the retrovirus genome also must be transported into the nucleus. In general, trafficking of viral genomes into the cell nucleus involves normal cellular pathways, and, as described later, optimal replication may require targeting to specific sites within the nucleus. In contrast, the poxvirus DNA genome and most RNA virus genomes replicate in the cytoplasm. As we will see, some of these viruses replicate their genome at specific sites within the cytoplasm.

Transport of Viral Genomes into the Cell Nucleus

The cellular mechanisms for transport of macromolecules across the double membranous nuclear envelope involve the recognition of a nuclear localization signal (NLS) on the protein by cellular proteins called importins. This complex then binds to fibrils extending from the NPC and moves to the NPC. Translocation through the nuclear pore involves a complex of the Ran GTP-binding protein and p10 or NTF2.

Most viral nucleocapsids are too large to move through the nuclear pores, so alternative macromolecular complexes containing the viral genome must move through them. Retroviruses, except the lentiviruses, cannot enter the nucleus until mitosis, when the nuclear membrane is disassembled. In contrast, the lentiviruses have an additional gene product, Vpr, that is reported to promote the nuclear entry of the preintegration complex (140). Vpr may interact with importin α (karyopherin α) and the NPC, thus acting as an importin itself (357). Other viral determinants have also been described as contributing to the nuclear uptake of the lentivirus DNA genome. Specifically, the NLSs of the matrix (MA) (95) and of the integrase protein (IN) of HIV-1 (104) have been implicated in the uptake of DNA into the nucleus. However, the significance and contribution of these proteins to the import of HIV DNA into the nucleus remain in debate (98). In fact, HIV-1 nuclear import was recently described as dependent on a cis-acting determinant on the DNA itself. A three-stranded DNA structure, the central DNA flap, was reported to be crucial for nuclear import of the HIV-1 preintegration complex (383).

Influenza virus is unique among RNA viruses in that its RNPs must localize into the nucleus because its transcriptase uses the 5′ ends of cellular messenger RNAs (mRNAs) as primers for transcription of the genomic RNAs. The viral RNPs then enter the nucleus through the nuclear pores. All four protein components of the vRNPs (NP, PB1, PB2, and PA) have NLSs and could drive the RNPs into the nucleus (65,243,244,319,360). Nevertheless, the transport of the vRNP depends primarily on the NLSs present in the NP protein. It has been demonstrated that NP binds to the NPI-1 (karyopherin α protein), which then binds karyopherin β, resulting in a docking complex at the nuclear pore (Fig. 6). In studies with permeabilized cells, the influenza virus NP has been shown to be the crucial factor in allowing the import of the incoming RNP from the cytoplasm to the nucleus.

The DNA viruses uncoat their genomic DNA before it enters the nucleus through the nuclear pores. After adenovirus enters the cell by endocytosis and disruption of the endosome, it binds to microtubules that mediate movement to the nuclear membrane. The adenovirus capsids then bind to the NPC (228), and the viral DNA is transferred into the nucleus in a process that requires metabolic energy (47). The capsid is disassembled during or soon after release of the DNA. Herpesvirus nucleocapsids bind to the dynein motor protein, which transports the nucleocapsid along microtubules to the microtubule-organizing center located near the nucleus (322). These nucleocapsids also bind to the NPC, and the DNA is transferred into the nucleus, but the empty capsid remains at the nuclear pore. Simian virus 40 (SV40) and polyoma viruses are both taken into the cell in endocytotic vesicles, and delivery of the virions from the vesicles to the cytoplasm, the endoplasmic reticulum, and the nucleus has been reported (123,165,217). The precise route of entry of the papovaviruses into the nucleus remains to be defined.

Once within the nucleus, viral DNAs appear to be targeted to specific sites for transcription and possibly initiation of replication. The genomic DNAs of herpes simplex virus (HSV), adenovirus, and SV40 localize to intranuclear sites at the periphery of nuclear domain 10 (ND10) structures, where immediate-early and early gene transcription takes place (155,216). HSV DNA replication proteins localize to these same sites, at which viral DNA synthesis then initiates (216,352). As viral DNA replication progresses, these punctate structures grow into the larger replication compartments in the infected cell nucleus (66). The mechanisms of targeting viral DNA and viral proteins within the cell nucleus remain to be defined, but these viral processes provide some of the best evidence for specific structural organization of the interior of the cell nucleus.

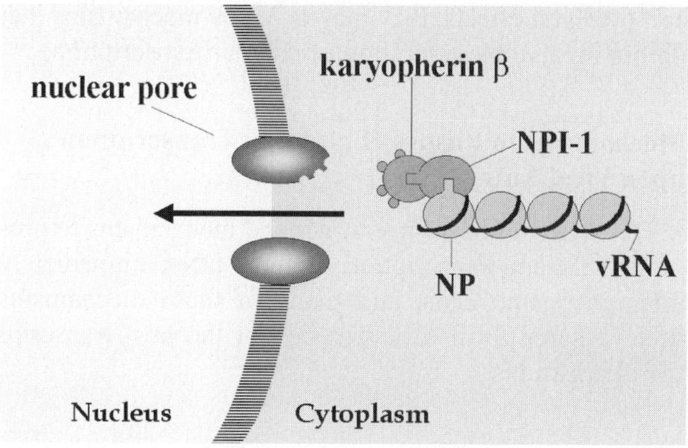

FIG. 6. Influenza viral ribonucleoprotein (RNP) import. Import of influenza viral RNPs is mediated by soluble cellular proteins NPI-1 (karyopherin α) and by karyopherin β. Interaction of the RNP complexes with these cellular factors is mediated by nuclear localization signals (NLSs) located on the viral nucleoprotein (NP). The NLS receptor consists of NPI-1, which binds to the NLS, and karyopherin β, which interacts directly with the proteins of the nuclear pore.

Targeting of Viral Genomes in the Cytoplasm

Much less is known about the localization of viral genomes to specific sites in the cytoplasm for replication. It has long been known that PV replicates on membranes in the cytoplasm (40,62), and other positive-strand RNA viruses also replicate on the cytoplasmic face of internal membranes (13,24,124,308,356,364). In contrast, other viruses such as vesicular stomatitis virus (VSV) and paramyxoviruses replicate on the cytoskeleton (128,131, 142).

TAKING OVER THE CELLULAR TRANSCRIPTION MACHINERY

Viral mRNA is needed during replication of viruses to encode viral proteins for replication of the genomic nucleic acid and for virion assembly. In the case of positive-strand RNA viruses, genomic RNA can be used as mRNA directly, so synthesis of viral RNA need not precede initial rounds of translation. However, for negative-strand RNA viruses and DNA viruses, *de novo* synthesis of viral mRNA must occur. If the virion contains an RNA polymerase, then synthesis of viral mRNA may depend on cellular factors to only a limited extent. However, if the virus uses cellular polymerases to synthesize mRNA, specific mechanisms may have evolved to promote transcription of viral DNA or to shift the host-cell RNA polymerase to the transcription of viral DNA. Viruses may even encode a new transcription factor (29).

DNA viruses often exhibit two general phases of transcription during infection of the host cell. First, they must ensure efficient transcription of at least part of their DNA genome immediately upon entry into the cell, a process known as immediate-early or early gene transcription. This has been accomplished by packaging a new polymerase in the virion (poxviruses), packaging a transcriptional adaptor molecule in the virion (HSV), or having a strong transcriptional enhancer upstream from the promoter for the immediate-early genes (e.g., adenovirus, papovaviruses, and cytomegalovirus). Second, they must be capable of efficient transcription of the later viral genes, called early, delayed-early, and late genes. The strategy used by DNA viruses to achieve this last aim is to encode a trans-activator protein as an immediate-early or early viral gene product that activates later viral gene expression after the viral DNA template has increased in number. The following sections describe how viruses inhibit host-cell transcription and ensure efficient immediate-early transcription and later viral gene transcription.

The general process of transcription in eukaryotic cells can be described as follows: Preinitiation complexes are formed by the binding of the general transcription factors, primarily transcription factors II-D (TFII-D), TFII-B, and TFII-I, to the promoter, and this complex then positions RNA polymerase II (pol II) near the start site of transcription. The pol II molecules that initiate transcription are not phosphorylated on the C-terminal domain (CTD), which consists of 52 repeats of a heptapeptide sequence (YSPTSPT). Molecules bound to the CTD also interact with activators bound to the DNA, and these interactions increase the number of initiation events. The general transcription factor TFII-E is bound to pol II and binds TFII-H, which contains DNA helicases and the CDK-activating kinase. The helicase activities open the double-stranded DNA so that it can be transcribed by pol II, and the kinase activity phosphorylates the CTD, which destabilizes the binding of the mediators and activators. Elongation factors, which include capping enzymes, splicing factors, and polyadenylation machinery, can then bind to the CTD and promote elongation. Viruses target several of these steps to inhibit pol II transcription or to divert it to their own advantage.

Inhibition of Cellular Transcription

Infection with many viruses leads to an inhibition of transcription of cellular protein-coding genes by host RNA pol II. However, little is known about how DNA viruses cause an inhibition of host-cell transcription, except for possible competition for RNA pol II and cell transcription factors. For RNA viruses, which do not use host-cell RNA polymerases for their replication, the presumed advantage conferred by this inhibition would be to provide larger pools of ribonucleoside triphosphate pools for viral RNA synthesis. Possible mechanisms for inhibition of host transcription have been formulated for cells infected with the RNA viruses VSV and PV. VSV infection causes rapid inhibition of host RNA synthesis, and this inhibition requires transcription of the viral genome (213,362). Two viral components have been implicated in the process of RNA pol II inhibition. Earlier data suggested that the leader RNA—a short (approximately 50 nucleotides long) transcript synthesized from the 3′ end of the virion genome—has this activity (125). However, Dunigan et al. (80) cast doubt on this interpretation because the kinetics of expression of the leader RNA in infected cells did not correlate with the timing of the shut off of host mRNA transcription. The second component of VSV that has been shown to inhibit host transcription is the M (matrix) protein (26). This activity of the M protein appears to be independent of that required for viral assembly at the cytoplasmic membrane (93). The inhibition of RNA pol II–dependent transcription by the VSV M protein is not cell-type specific. Although the mechanism by which the VSV M protein exerts its activity is not well defined, recent data suggest that the TFII-D is altered, resulting in an inhibition of host transcription (379). This inactivation of TFII-D is probably not mediated through a direct protein–protein interaction, but rather through indirect effects of the VSV M protein in the nucleus. Yet another mechanism of modulation of TFII-D by viruses has been observed. Infection by PV results in the proteolytic cleavage of TATA-binding protein (TBP) through the viral protease 3C (53).

Transcription factor II-D is not unique in being a target for virus-mediated inhibition of transcription. Inhibition of host mRNA transcription may involve cleavage of capped host mRNAs through a viral polymerase complex. It appears that influenza viruses inhibit the expression of host genes at least in part through the viral activity of cap snatching, which is localized to the nucleus of infected cells (182). In addition, it has been reported that the influenza A virus NS1 protein targets the poly(A)-binding protein II (PAB-II) and the cleavage and polyadenylation specificity factor (CPSF) of the cellular 3′-end processing machinery (48,235). When both host activities are inhibited by the viral NS1 protein, this should result in a severe reduction of the level of functional host mRNA transcripts. Whether the induction of a proteolytic activity (301) in influenza virus-infected cells is a third major factor contributing to the remarkable ability of influenza viruses to shut off host transcription remains to be seen.

On the other hand, many RNA viruses—including negative-strand RNA viruses such as Sendai virus—do not appear to have an appreciable effect on host transcription. Although these viruses can cause cytopathic and cytolytic effects, they may do so by mechanisms that do not involve the inhibition of cellular transcription.

Mechanisms to Ensure High-Level Transcription upon Viral Entry

DNA viruses have several general mechanisms to promote efficient transcription of their DNA immediately after entry into cells, and many of these mechanisms involve some form of subversion of the host transcriptional apparatus.

Packaging a Virally Encoded RNA Polymerase in the Virion

Poxviruses contain a double-stranded DNA genome but replicate in the cytoplasm. These viruses have evolved their own transcriptional and DNA replication machinery, allowing these processes to occur in the cytoplasm, almost completely independent of the host cell nucleus. The poxvirus particle contains a virally encoded RNA polymerase (166) capable of transcribing about one half of the viral genome (30,250). The presence of the RNA polymerase in the virion ensures efficient transcription of the viral genome upon entry into the cell.

Packaging a Transcriptional Activator in the Virion

The best-known example of a virion trans-activator is the HSV virion protein 16 (VP16). HSV VP16 (also called αTIF or Vmw65) is assembled into the virion and, when introduced into the cell, becomes a part of a transcriptional activation complex that specifically stimulates viral immediate-early (α) gene expression (41,271). VP16 binds to host-cell proteins (221,272); specifically, it is thought to bind to at least one host factor, the HCF protein complex (180), and this complex binds to the transcription factor Oct-1 bound to DNA (112). One portion of VP16 binds to HCF and Oct-1, whereas another activates transcription (346) by binding to basal transcription factors. Thus, HSV provides for adequate transcription of its immediate-early genes by carrying in its virion a viral trans-activator that binds to a cellular protein, which in turn binds to specific DNA sequences located in immediate-early gene promoters, thereby stimulating transcription and causing increased transcriptional initiation on immediate-early viral gene promoters that contain this specific sequence.

Use of an Enhancer to Ensure High-Level Immediate Transcription

An alternative mechanism by which DNA viruses promote efficient transcription of viral genes immediately after infection is to have an enhancer sequence located upstream of these genes. Enhancers are blocks of DNA sequences containing multiple binding sites for transcription factors acting in synergy to promote high-level transcription from a nearby gene. They act in a position- and orientation-independent manner. Enhancers were, in fact, first identified in viral genomes (12,17). For example, the early transcriptional units of SV40 virus (12,17), polyoma virus (351), human papilloma virus (58), the adenovirus E1A transcriptional unit (139), and the human cytomegalovirus IE1/IE2 transcriptional unit (31,343) all contain enhancers. These enhancer sequences provide for utilization of multiple cellular transcription factors in the transcription of the earliest genes of these viruses immediately after infection.

Mechanisms for Activation of Later Viral Genes

Many DNA viruses encode trans-activators among their earliest gene products. The SV40 large T-antigen stimulates late transcription, both by promoting viral DNA replication and by binding to host-cell transcription factors (127). The adenovirus E1A, the HSV ICP4, and the papilloma virus E2 proteins all serve to stimulate later viral gene transcription by altering the activity of host-cell RNA pol II. The mechanism of trans-activation has been most extensively studied with the adenovirus E1A proteins (23,160). The E1A gene encodes two mRNAs, 13S and 12S, by differential splicing, and much of the trans-activation activity is caused by the 13S gene product. The E1A proteins increase the expression of pol II–transcribed genes (121,152,237) and pol III–transcribed genes (20,109,144). The promoter requirements for E1A trans-activation coincide with basal-level promoter elements (22,238). The E1A proteins do not bind to DNA specifically or efficiently, and there is now considerable evidence that E1A stimulates transcription through various effects on cellular transcription factors (191,316,374). The numerous specific effects of E1A are described in detail in Chapter 31, but the general mechanisms are relevant here. The E1A protein activates transcription by interacting with basal transcription factors, by interacting with activating proteins that bind to upstream promoter and enhancer elements, and by interacting with other regulatory or DNA-binding proteins. E1A protein binds directly to the TBP of TFII-D to activate transcription (145,192), and it also binds to p53 and Dr1 and relieves their repressive effects on transcription (146,179). E1A can also bind to TAF subunits of TFII-D and TFII-F (110,198,218).

E1A can activate transcription of certain genes by binding to the pRb protein, releasing E2F to activate transcription at its cognate sites (8). E1A can also activate transcription by binding to ATF transcription factors, by binding to YY1 to relieve its repressive effects, and by binding to AP1 to activate transcription. E1A activates pol III transcription of the adenoviral VA genes by increasing the amount of the IIIC2a transcription factor.

Promotion of RNA Polymerase II Elongation on Viral Templates

Transcription of the HIV genome by pol II is very inefficient in the absence of prior viral gene expression. However, when the HIV Tat protein is expressed, it serves as a novel transcription activator in that it regulates elongation rather than initiation of transcription and acts by binding to the nascent transcript rather than to DNA (337). Pol II initiates transcription in the HIV long terminal repeat (LTR) promoter but synthesizes only short RNA products. Tat binds to a specific sequence called the trans-activation response (TAR) element on the nascent RNA molecule and promotes elongation of transcription. This is accomplished by Tat interacting with the cyclin subunit of the positive elongation factor b (P-TEFb) and with TAR. Tat also interacts with cyclin T1 and recruits the cyclin-dependent kinase 9, which phosphorylates the CTD of pol II. This phosphorylation activates pol II for elongation along the proviral genome. Thus, HIV Tat promotes transcription of the HIV genome by a novel mechanism, and elucidation of this mechanism has provided insight into the molecules regulating transcriptional elongation.

VIRUSES CAN REGULATE CELLULAR SIGNAL TRANSDUCTION PATHWAYS

Viruses often modify the host cell signal transduction pathways for their own benefit. The effect may be exerted by the binding of virions to a surface receptor on the cell surface, by a new protein encoded by modifying the activity of a cellular protein, or by a viral protein mimicking a cellular protein. For example, binding of human cytomegalovirus to the cell surface is believed to activate NF-κB (34), which would induce expression of cellular regulatory proteins, some of which would block the interferon response (386). Similarly, binding of Epstein-Barr virus to its receptor, CR2, activates B-cell signaling pathways (286). As a third example of this mechanism, binding of adenovirus to α_V integrins activates mitogen-activated protein (MAP) kinase signaling pathways (236). An example of a different mechanism is human herpesvirus 8, which is associated with Kaposi's sarcoma, encoding a protein, vIRF, that heterodimerizes with the host interferon regulatory factor, IRF-1, and blocks its action in interferon responses (see later).

TAKING OVER THE CELLULAR RNA PROCESSING AND TRANSPORT MACHINERY

RNA splicing and transport to the cytoplasm are cellular pathways often used by viruses for maturation of their mRNA from nucleus to cytoplasm. In fact, the first evidence for RNA splicing came when the adenovirus late mRNAs were mapped on the viral DNA by R-loop hybridization (21,51). These studies showed that adenoviral late mRNAs are encoded by noncontiguous portions of the genome. Splicing of the viral mRNA precursors is accomplished by cellular enzymes recognizing splice donor and acceptor sequences in the viral RNA. However, some viruses use the cellular splicing mechanisms but regulate the extent to which the full-length transcript is spliced. For example, influenza and retroviruses have transcripts that are infrequently spliced (see Chapters 24 and 27). In cells infected with influenza virus, the viral NS1 and M1 RNAs are spliced to yield the NS2/NEP and M2 mRNAs, respectively, at a frequency of 10% (186, 188). Although splicing of the NS1 RNA is inefficient, formation of the spliceosome complex involving the snRNPs U1, U2, U4, U5, and U6 is efficient (2). Thus, the block seems to occur after formation of the spliceosome complex. The block may be mediated by the structure of the RNA itself or by a virus-encoded protein. This appears to be a situation in which virus infection determines the extent of splicing of one of the viral RNAs, thereby regulating the levels of one of its own gene products. The NS1 gene product has been postulated to be responsible for this regulatory event (181). However, a mutant influenza virus lacking the entire NS1 open reading frame (ORF) was shown to have normal levels of splicing of the viral mRNAs (106).

Adenovirus inhibits maturation of cellular mRNA at a different stage. In adenovirus-infected cells, cell transcripts are synthesized and processed but do not accumulate in the cytoplasm (15). The adenoviral E1B-55kD and E4-34kD proteins are required for inhibition of transport of cellular mRNA as well as for promotion of cytoplasmic accumulation of viral mRNA (7,130,262). The E1B and E4 proteins have been observed to localize within and around the nuclear inclusions where viral transcription is believed to occur (245). Thus, these proteins may redistribute a cellular factor involved in mRNA transport. This system may provide important insights into the regulation and specificity of mRNA transport.

A similar observation has been made in cells infected with HSV, in which transport and processing of host-cell RNA is inhibited (359). In HSV-infected cells, small nuclear ribonucleoprotein particles become aggregated (211), and this may be related to impaired transport or splicing. The HSV IE protein ICP27 or IE63 has been reported to be necessary and sufficient for this effect (133,134,259), possibly by affecting phosphorylation of SRP proteins. Only four of the more than 70 HSV genes contain introns. Thus, inhibition of host-cell splicing should contribute to host shutoff, but the mechanisms for specific retention of viral RNA splicing, if any exist, are unknown.

The regulation of RNA maturation may also provide a mechanism for temporal regulation of viral gene expression. HIV encodes several regulatory gene products from spliced mRNAs. One of these regulatory gene products, the *rev* gene product, stimulates the cytoplasmic accumulation of unspliced viral mRNAs that encode the viral structural proteins (90,173,207,294,323,341). The Rev protein seems to promote the export of newly synthesized viral transcripts to the cytoplasm so that the splicing pathway is avoided (208). The Rev protein enters the nucleus using a classic NLS and binds to the viral RNA via a Rev-responsive element (RRE) (61). The Rev-RNA complex is then recognized by the nuclear export machinery. Specifically, it appears that the nuclear export signal (NES) of rev binds to the CRM1 exportin (94), which in turn interacts with members of the nucleoporin family. The NES-mediated interaction of Rev with CRM1 is inhibited by the drug leptomycin B (371). Lentiviruses, including HIV and human T-cell lymphoma virus (HTLV)-1, have developed this mechanism of a viral protein (Rev and Rex, respectively) that binds to viral RNAs and chaperones them through the NPC.

Other retroviruses also transport unspliced or partially spliced viral mRNAs from the nucleus into the cytoplasm. However, they do this by relying on a different mechanism. Many oncovirus RNAs possess so-called constitutive transport elements (CTEs), which interact directly with the cellular RNA export machinery without the mediation of a rev-like viral protein. Tang et al. (336) showed that a cellular RNA helicase A binds to the CTE from simian retrovirus (SRV)-1 and thus facilitates the export process. Similar CTE-like elements are found in all oncovirus RNAs, and they are thought to allow unspliced (or partially spliced) viral mRNAs to be effectively transported from the nucleus to the cytoplasm. Like the retroviruses, the hepatitis B viruses produce RNA transcripts in the nucleus that possess a cis-acting post-transcriptional regulatory element (PRE) that facilitates interactions with the nuclear export machinery (289).

Influenza viruses face yet another RNA maturation/transport problem. Not only does transcription of viral mRNAs occur in the nucleus, but also the entire genome of the virus replicates in infected cells. In fact, one incoming genome complement (consisting of eight RNA segments) may result in the amplification of up to 100,000 copies, which must then be transported out of the nucleus. The work of many groups now indicates that the newly amplified virion (v) RNAs are not in naked form in the nucleus but exist as complexes with the viral NP and the polymerase (P) proteins. In addition, the presence of the viral M1 protein appears to be necessary for the formation of mature nucleoplasmic vRNP structures destined for export into the cytoplasm (366). Finally, the influenza virus nuclear export protein (NEP) (formerly the NS2 protein), which had no previously assigned function, has been shown to facilitate the nuclear export of virion RNAs by acting as an adaptor between vRNP/M1 complexes and the nuclear export machinery of the cell. NEP interacts with cellular nucleoporins and CRM1 and can functionally replace the effector domain of the HIV-1 Rev protein. A functional domain on the NEP with characteristics of an NES was mapped: It mediates rapid nuclear export when cross-linked to a reporter protein. Microinjection of anti-NEP antibodies into infected cells inhibited nuclear export of vRNPs, suggesting that the Rev-like NEP mediates this process. In the model shown in Figure 7, NEP acts as a protein adaptor molecule bridging influenza vRNPs and the NPCs of infected cells. This novel export mechanism for genomic viral RNA differs from that mediated by Rev for HIV-1 RNA in that the influenza viral NEP does not interact directly with the virion RNA. Rather, the NEP functions as a chaperone for the newly formed influenza virus ribonucleoprotein complexes.

Influenza virus intervenes in and takes advantage of the host-cell mRNA maturation pathway in another novel way. Influenza mRNA transcription from the genomic RNA segments occurs in the host cell nucleus (141). Cellular nascent transcripts are cleaved by a virus-encoded endonuclease, and the 5′ end of the host transcript is used

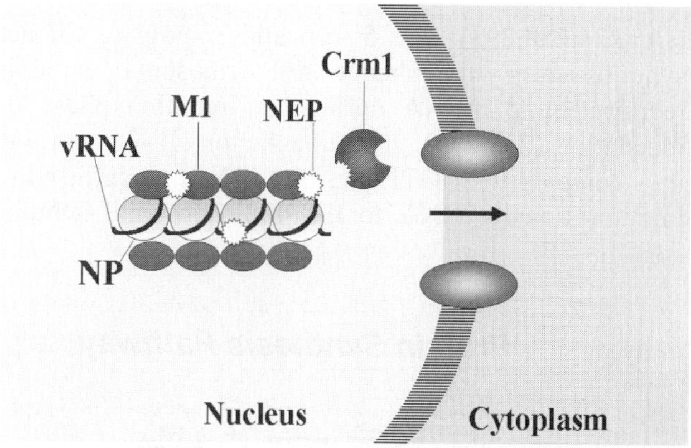

FIG. 7. Influenza viral ribonucleoprotein (RNP) nuclear export. The nuclear export of amplified influenza viral RNP complexes is mediated by the viral nuclear export protein (NEP). NEP interacts with a cellular export factor, Crm1, and with the viral RNPs via the viral matrix (M1) protein. By interacting with the cellular export machinery, NEP mediates the transport of the viral genome from the nucleus to the cytoplasm via the nuclear pore.

as a primer for synthesis of viral mRNA from the viral genome (33,266). Thus, influenza virus transcriptional complexes subvert the host mRNA maturation pathway to obtain primer molecules for the viral transcriptional process, and then the virus most likely uses the cellular mRNA export machinery to transport its viral mRNAs out of the nucleus.

TAKING OVER THE TRANSLATIONAL MACHINERY: STRATEGIES FOR OPTIMIZATION OF VIRAL PROTEIN SYNTHESIS AND ANTAGONISM OF CELLULAR PROTEIN SYNTHESIS

Animal viruses utilize the host translational machinery for production of their own proteins. The biochemical pathway of mRNA translation in animal cells is summarized in Figure 8. Several strategies are utilized by viruses to optimize their own protein synthesis, and to antagonize cellular protein synthesis, by altering the host translational machinery. For some virus–cell combinations, the efficiency of mRNA translation (that is, the amount of protein produced per unit of mRNA) varies during the infective process. Multiple biochemical mechanisms account for the translational control observed in virus-infected cells. Many, but not all, are operative at the initiation phase of mRNA translation, the phase generally believed to be rate-limiting.

Two steps of translation regulated during initiation are the recruitment of the small (40S) ribosomal subunit to mRNA, and the binding of the initiator transfer RNA (met-tRNAi) to the 40S subunit. Most cellular and viral mRNAs found in animal cells possess a 5′-terminal cap [7mG(5′)ppp(5′)N] structure and a 3′-terminal poly A tail (224,258,293). The 5′-cap and 3′-poly A tail act synergistically to enhance 40S ribosomal subunit recruitment to mRNA during the initiation phase of translation (258,293). Initiation factor eIF-2 functions in a complex with GTP and met-tRNAi to deliver the initiator transfer RNA to the 40S ribosomal subunit (224). The 40S small ribosomal subunit is recruited to the mRNA 5′-cap structure by protein synthesis initiation factor eIF-4F in a process that requires ATP. The eIF-4F is composed of three subunits: eIF-4A (which is an RNA-dependent ATPase), eIF-4E (which interacts directly with the cap structure), and eIF-4G (formerly known as p220). The eIF-4G factor appears to function as a scaffold, binding several initiation factors during the assembly of the mRNA-ribosome initiation complex including eIF-3, -4A, and -4E, as well as the poly(A)-binding protein PABP (224,227,258).

Modification of Initiation Factor Function Involved in Recruitment of the 40S Ribosomal Subunit to mRNA

For many members of the *Picornaviridae* family, infection leads to a rapid and efficient inhibition of cellular protein synthesis. One of the best-characterized examples of the selective shutoff of host cell translation in infected cells is provided by poliovirus. Cellular protein synthesis is drastically reduced within about 1 to 2 h after PV infection (256). PV and other picornavirus mRNAs lack the 5′-cap structure (14,293). Their translation initiation occurs by a cap-independent mechanism, in which the 40S subunit binds directly to an internal ribosome entry site (IRES) located in the 5′-UTR region of the picornavirus RNA (158,255,347). Translation of 5′-capped cellular mRNAs is inhibited at the initiation step in picornavirus-infected cells because of proteolytic inactivation of the eIF-4G subunit of the

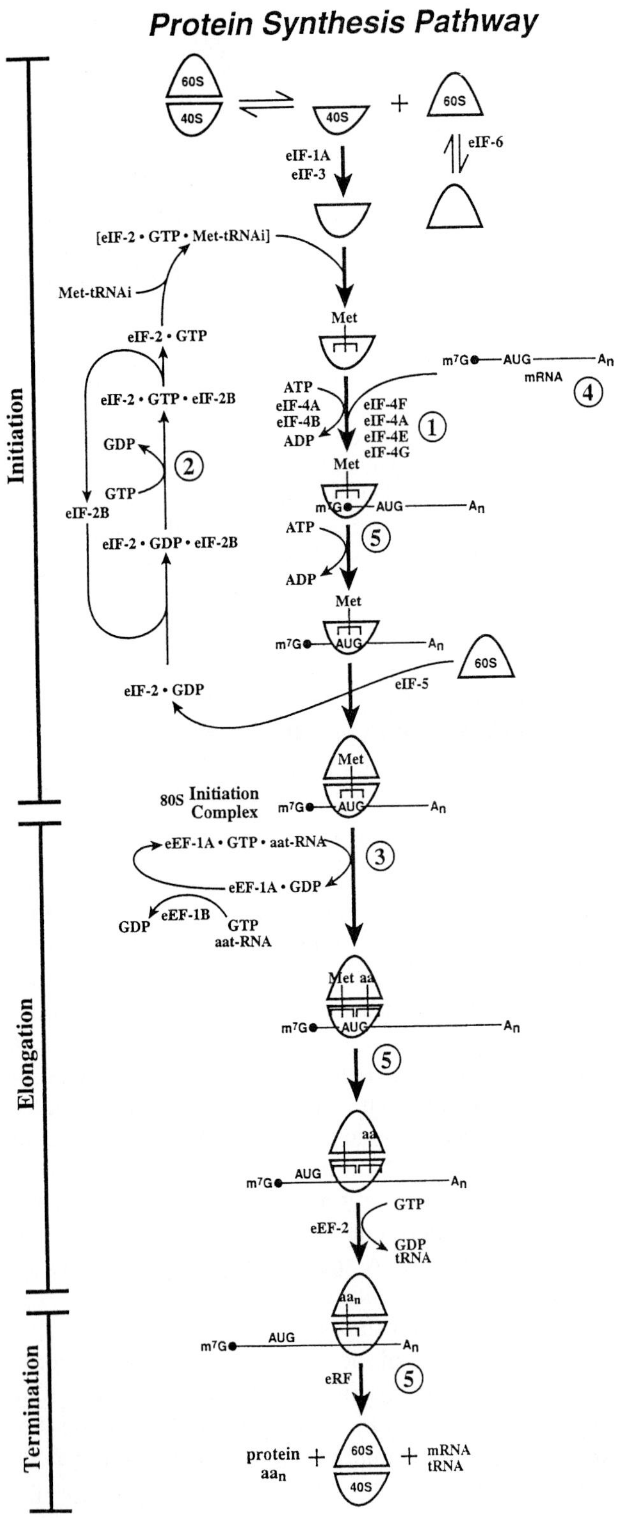

FIG. 8. The cellular protein synthesis pathway and examples of the modification of the process by viruses. **1:** Modification of eIF-4F initiation factor function involved in recruitment of the 40S subunit to mRNA. Picornaviral 2A protease catalyzes cleavage of the eIF-4G component of the eIF-4F complex and also the poly A binding protein; phosphorylation of the eIF-4E component is decreased in cells infected with adenovirus, influenza virus, and encephalomyocarditis virus. **2:** Modification of eIF-2 initiation factor function involved in binding of tRNA to the 40S subunit. Phosphorylation of the α subunit of eIF-2 is antagonized by several viral RNAs (including adenovirus VA1 and Epstein-Barr virus EBER) and proteins [including reovirus σ3, vaccinia E3L and K3L, hepatitis C virus NS5A and E2, influenza virus NS1, and Herpes simplex virus (HSV) γ34.5 and Us11]. **3:** Elongation factor function is altered in cells infected with human immunodeficiency virus, HSV, and vesicular stomatitis virus. **4:** Host-cell mRNA is degraded in cells infected with HSV, influenza virus, and poxvirus. **5:** Unconventional strategies used for viral protein synthesis include leaky scanning and ribosome shunting during initiation, frameshifting during elongation, and suppression of termination.

cap binding protein complex eIF-4F (14). Two functional homologs of the eIF-4G factor have been identified, eIF-4GI and eIF-4GII. Both eIF-4GI and -4GII are cleaved in PV-infected (117) and rhinovirus-infected (333) cells. The cleavage of eIF-4GII coincides with the shutoff of host protein synthesis and, at least for PV and HRV-14, this eIF-4GII cleavage appears to be the rate-limiting step in the shutoff process. The molecular basis for the differential susceptibility of eIF-4GI and -4GII to proteolytic degradation, and the physiologic significance of the differential sensitivity in the context of the virus–host interaction, are not yet fully resolved. In addition, whether this cleavage pattern is general for all picornavirus infections is not yet clearly established. The picornaviral 2A proteases ($2A^{pro}$) catalyze the cleavage of eIF-4GI and II (189). However, eIF-4G is not the only target of picornavirus $2A^{pro}$. For example, Coxsackie virus $2A^{pro}$ also catalyzes the cleavage of PABP (170). This may represent an additional mechanism for shutoff of host protein synthesis in picornavirus-infected cells. The eIF-4G subunit binds PABP and functions in poly(A)-dependent translation (258). Thus, the possibility of a synergistic reduction in host protein synthesis arises in picornavirus-infected cells by cleavage of two different factors by viral 2A proteases, eIF-4G and PABP, that interact during the process of initiation of translation to synergistically enhance 40S ribosomal subunit recruitment to mRNAs.

In group A rotavirus-infected cells, the nonstructural viral protein NSP3A appears to play an important role in the efficient expression of viral proteins by disruption of cellular eIF-4G factor function. NSP3A is bound to the 3′ end of viral mRNAs. NSP3A also interacts *in vivo* with the initiation factor eIF-4GI, an association that evicts the cellular PABP from eIF-4GI (264). The translation of the viral mRNA, which is not polyadenylated, thus is enhanced at the expense of the translation of the cellular polyadenylated mRNA by the action of NSP3A. Despite binding on the same site on eIF-4GI, the PABP and NSP3 do not have strong sequence similarities even in their respective eIF-4GI binding domains.

Phosphorylation of the mRNA 5′-cap binding protein eIF-4E correlates with increased translation rates (115,171). Initiation factor eIF-4G recruits MAP kinase–activated protein kinase Mnk1 to phosphorylate eIF-4E (361). The extent of eIF-4E phosphorylation is often decreased in virus-infected cells, including cells infected with adenovirus, influenza virus, PV and, encephalomyocarditis (EMC) virus, but not with Semliki Forest virus or reovirus (172). For example, in adenovirus-infected cells, the vast majority (>95%) of the eIF-4E factor is dephosphorylated. A late adenovirus gene function impairs the phosphorylation of eIF-4E, an effect that coincides with the inhibition of cell protein synthesis. Presumably, the relative amounts of eIF-4E required for efficient translation of the viral and cellular mRNAs differ, possibly because of differences in relative structures among the RNAs. The function of eIF-4E is also regulated through binding to a family of translational repressor proteins designated as 4E-BPs. Binding of 4E-BPs to eIF-4E depends on the phosphorylation status of 4E-BP; thus, the 4E-BPs act in their unphosphorylated form as inhibitors of eIF-4E function. Dephosphorylation of 4E-BP1 following infection with picornaviruses such as PV and EMC virus has been observed, and in the case of EMC virus, the time course of 4E-BP dephosphorylation generally coincides with the shutoff of host protein synthesis (115). Thus, both 4E-BP1 dephosphorylation and eIF-4GII cleavage may contribute to picornavirus-mediated shutoff of host protein synthesis.

Influenza virus infection results in a dramatic shutoff of cellular protein synthesis. This shutoff is concomitant with the selective translation of viral mRNAs, mediated in part by the cellular RNA-binding protein GRSF-1, a positive-acting translation regulatory factor that binds to specific G-rich sequences within the 5′-UTR region of influenza virus mRNA (251). Influenza virus mRNAs contain the cellular 5′-cap structure and about a dozen nucleotides from host mRNA sequences at their 5′ end and are translated by a 5′ cap-dependent mechanism. The precise mechanism by which GRSF-1 enhances viral mRNA translation is not yet known, but it may involve interaction with eIF-4G, which is known to interact with the PABP. Dephosphorylation and inactivation of eIF-4E also plays a role in the shutoff of host cell translation in influenza virus–infected cells (115,172). Influenza virus mRNAs display a decreased requirement for eIF-4F relative to host mRNAs, thus allowing them to be translated in the presence of low levels of the cap-binding complex factor.

Modification of Initiation Factor Function Involved in Binding of Initiator Transfer RNA to the 40S Ribosomal Subunit

Initiation factor eIF-2 is composed of three subunits (α, β, and γ). Phosphorylation of eIF-2α correlates with decreased translation rates and suppression of cell proliferation (55,298,334), and phosphorylation of the α subunit mediates an inhibition of translation. Among the protein kinases that phosphorylate eIF-2α is the RNA-dependent protein kinase PKR (298). PKR plays a central role in the regulation of protein synthesis in virus-infected cells (55,295,297,298). PKR possesses a double-stranded RNA binding domain that consists of two tandem copies of a conserved dsRNA-binding motif (dsRBM). Binding of structured RNAs of viral origin to the dsRBM motifs occurs in a sequence-independent fashion and leads to either activation or inhibition of kinase enzymatic activity. Following catalytic activation by an RNA-dependent intermolecular autophosphorylation,

PKR then catalyzes the phosphorylation of eIF-2α at serine residue 51. This modification of eIF-2α leads to an inhibition of protein synthesis, because it blocks the eIF-2B catalyzed guanine nucleotide exchange reaction of eIF-2:GDP (55,298).

During virus infection, PKR may become activated by viral RNA molecules and then in some cases later inhibited, thereby reversing any PKR kinase–mediated translational block that had been established. The mechanism by which PKR-catalyzed phosphorylation of eIF-2 is antagonized differs among viruses and can involve either RNA or protein modulators. The best-characterized viral RNA inhibitor of PKR is the adenovirus virus–associated VAI RNA (214). VAI RNA is produced in large amounts at late times after infection, and it subsequently impairs activation of PKR and phosphorylation of eIF-2α (214,215). Viral mutants that lack functional VAI RNA multiply poorly because of the dominant effect of virus-specific RNAs that activate PKR, thereby causing an inhibition of late viral protein synthesis. Adenovirus VAI RNA is bound by the dsRBMs of PKR, the same motifs that also bind activator RNAs (219). Modulation of eIF-2α phosphorylation is the primary function of viral VAI RNA, at least in cell culture, because substitution of serine 51 with alanine not only eliminates the phosphorylation site on the eIF-2α substrate but functionally complements the deletion of VA from the virus genome. Epstein-Barr virus–encoded RNAs (EBER), which functionally can substitute for adenovirus VAI RNA *in vivo*, also inhibit PKR activation (55).

The fundamental importance of PKR in the modulation of the translational pattern in virus-infected cells is further demonstrated by the large number of viruses that encode proteins that affect PKR function and subsequently the biochemical activity of initiation factor eIF-2 (102,215,298). The σ3 major capsid protein of reovirus was among the first animal virus proteins identified that antagonize PKR function by sequestering activator dsRNAs (299). The preferential translation of reovirus mRNAs and the inhibition of cellular protein synthesis appear to be mediated in part by a σ3-dependent mechanism that depends on both the subcellular localization of σ3 (303) and the interaction of σ3 with μ1c, the other major outer capsid protein of reovirions (380). Proteolytic cleavage of σ3 results in enhanced dsRNA binding activity (299), but the association of σ3 with μ1c eliminates dsRNA-binding activity and the ability to antagonize PKR function and stimulate protein synthesis (380). Reovirus mRNAs also can activate PKR. For example, the poorly translated S1 mRNA that encodes the minor capsid protein σ1 is an efficient activator of PKR, whereas the efficiently translated S4 mRNA that encodes σ3 is a poor PKR activator (298,299).

In influenza virus–infected cells, changes in the translational machinery mediated by down-regulation of PKR occur by two different strategies. One involves the viral nonstructural RNA-binding protein NS1 (102,137) and the other involves the activation of the stress-related cellular $P58^{IPK}$ inhibitor of PKR (223). NS1, an abundant protein in influenza virus–infected cells, performs several regulatory functions during the viral infective cycle including regulation of synthesis, transport, splicing, and translation of mRNAs. NS1 prevents activation of PKR by binding to dsRNA activators. Temperature-sensitive mutant influenza A viruses with an RNA-binding defective NS1 protein cannot block activation of PKR in infected cells. These ts mutant virus strains exhibit temperature sensitivity in virus protein synthesis at the translational level, in a manner that correlates with increased activation of PKR and phosphorylation of eIF-2α. $P58^{IPK}$, a constitutively expressed cellular protein, inhibits PKR activity through direct protein–protein interaction with PKR. Influenza virus infection activates $P58^{IPK}$ by promoting dissociation from its negative regulator, heat-shock protein 40; thus, cellular $P58^{IPK}$ is believed to be targeted with hsp70 to PKR, thereby inhibiting kinase function in influenza virus–infected cells (223). The baculovirus PK2 gene product also inhibits PKR by a dimerization mechanism. Baculovirus PK2 protein is a truncated viral kinase that forms a heteromeric complex with the cellular PKR, thereby blocking kinase autophosphorylation and eIF-2α phosphorylation. Insect cells infected with wild-type baculovirus, but not PK2-deleted virus, exhibit reduced phosphorylation and increased translational activity (72).

Hepatitis C (HCV) and vaccinia viruses provide examples of animal viruses that encode multiple proteins that act synergistically to disrupt PKR function. Two HCV-encoded proteins, the nonstructural protein NS5A (101) and the envelope protein E2 (338), have been reported to prevent activation of PKR. NS5A of HCV interacts with a region of the PKR catalytic domain that also serves as a dimerization domain, thereby disrupting PKR dimerization and PKR-mediated eIF-2α phosphorylation (101). The HCV envelope protein E2 also appears to bind to and inhibit PKR (338). Interestingly, E2 contains a sequence identical to the phosphorylation sites of the PKR kinase and the eIF-2α substrate, but the contribution of E2 as a potential pseudosubstrate to the antagonism of PKR in natural infections is unknown, given the different subcellular localizations expected for PKR and this portion of E2. Inhibition of PKR by the NS5A and E2 proteins of HCV may facilitate survival and proliferation of the infected host, ultimately leading to HCV-associated hepatocellular carcinoma (342).

Vaccinia virus also encodes two gene products, E3L and K3L, that stimulate translation through inhibition of the PKR kinase (55,298). E3L and K3L function by different mechanisms. The viral E3L protein is a dsRNA binding protein that both sequesters dsRNA activators of PKR (314) and interacts directly with the eIF-2α substrate-binding region of PKR (309), thereby down-regulating PKR autoactivation and eIF-2α phosphorylation. The vaccinia K3L protein is a virus-encoded homolog of the eIF-2α substrate. The K3L pseudo-substrate inhibits PKR-catalyzed phosphorylation of eIF-2α (167).

TAR, a highly structured RNA leader element located at the 5′ end of all HIV transcripts, activates the PKR kinase (55,206). HIV uses two proteins to counter this TAR-mediated activation of PKR. PKR function is down-regulated by the cellular TAR-RNA binding protein TRBP, which forms an inactive heterodimer with PKR (16), and by the viral trans-activating Tat protein, which inhibits autophosphorylation of PKR and competes with eIF-2 (35). HIV Tat protein also activates transcription factor NF-κB through a process that requires the function of the PKR kinase (69). The relative roles during the HIV infective process of the negative (35) and positive (69) effects of Tat protein on PKR kinase activity are not yet fully resolved.

In HSV-infected cells, the viral γ34.5 protein affects phosphatase function, thereby blocking the shutoff of protein synthesis mediated by activated PKR. In the absence of the γ34.5 gene, eIF-2α is phosphorylated and protein synthesis is impaired beginning at about 5 hours after infection; however, in the presence of γ34.5, protein synthesis continues even though PKR is activated. The γ34.5 protein binds to the protein phosphatase 1α and redirects it to dephosphorylate eIF-2αP (138). The HSV U_S11 protein can substitute for the γ34.5 protein if it is present early in infection before PKR is activated. U_S11 protein blocks the shutoff of protein synthesis by binding to PKR and blocking the subsequent phosphorylation of eIF-2α (43).

Modification of Elongation Factor Function in Virus-Infected Cells

Viral proteins also interact with the translation elongation factors eEF-1A (formerly known as EF-1α) and eEF-1B (52,64,168,169,376). Factor eEF-1A is the protein synthesis elongation factor involved in the delivery of aminoacylated transfer RNAs to the ribosome A site as an eEF-1A:GTP:aa-tRNA ternary complex during the process of polypeptide chain elongation (see Fig. 8). The matrix MA protein and the $Pr55^{gag}$ polyprotein of HIV-1 both interact with eEF-1A (52). This interaction appears selective, as eEF-1A does not associate with nonlentiviral MA proteins. RNA, possibly the eEF-1A:aminoacyl-tRNA complex, is involved in the eEF-1A interaction with MA/Gag. The interaction between eEF-1A and MA/Gag leads to an inhibition of translation (52). Elongation factor eEF-1B catalyzes the exchange of GDP for GTP on the eEF-1A factor. The second coding exon of the HIV-1 Tat protein interacts with the δ subunit of eIF-1B and specifically inhibits cellular translation, without significantly affecting the efficiency of viral translation (376). Interaction of viral proteins with eEF-1 delineates a possible mechanism for HIV-1–mediated modulation of host translation.

In addition to the functions that translation elongation factors play during the process of protein synthesis, the eEF-1B factor also is implicated as a component of the RNA replication complex of VSV (64). Purified VS virions include packaged eEF-1B, which interacts with the L protein of VSV to give an active viral RNA polymerase, in striking similarity to earlier observations made with Qβ RNA phage where the bacterial homolog of eEF-1B is involved in viral RNA replication. The eEF-1A factor has been shown to bind RNA genomes of some viruses, for example West Nile virus genomic RNA (28) and tRNA-like structures from plant viral RNAs (113), and, like eEF-1B, it may play a role in RNA replication.

Degradation of Cellular mRNA in Virus-Infected Cells

Degradation of the host mRNA following virus infection provides an additional mechanism to modulate the utilization of ribosomes and factors of the translational machinery for preferential translation of viral mRNAs and also to delay the host response to infection. For example, following infection with HSV, influenza virus, or poxvirus, inhibition of cellular translation occurs and a decrease in intact host-cell mRNA is observed (92,153, 242,282). For viruses such as these that have a lytic life cycle, an overall reduction in the level of cellular mRNAs, together with high rates of transcription of a comparatively small number of viral genes, creates an environment where highly abundant viral mRNAs can effectively out-compete relatively more scarce cellular mRNAs for the translational machinery.

An important question concerns the origin of the nuclease(s) that catalyze the degradation of cellular mRNAs in infected cells. Probably the earliest HSV gene that plays a significant role in abating or delaying the host response to infection through degradation of mRNA is U_L41, which encodes a protein that is introduced into the cell in virions at the time of infection (278). Although the HSV virion host shutoff (vhs) activity of the U_L41 protein reduces the synthesis of host proteins by causing the destruction of mRNA, it apparently does so in a nonspecific manner, as the half-lives of both host and viral mRNAs are reduced by the U_L41 protein (185,246,382). U_L41 has the biochemical properties of an RNase, but it has not been unequivocally resolved whether U_L41 alone possesses ribonucleolytic activity or whether an accessory component is required. Interestingly, the U_L41 function of HSV-2 strains generally leads to shutoff of the host more rapidly and completely than that seen with HSV-1 strains (88,91). Because there is no apparent discrimination between host and viral mRNA in the degradative process, in addition to providing a means for inhibiting host translation, it is conceivable that the U_L41 viral function promotes the shutoff of immediate-early and early gene expression in the HSV lytic cycle.

Another cellular RNA degradation pathway that can be activated by viral infection, which is also up-regulated by interferons, is the 2-5A system. Interferon treatment of cells induces a family of RNA-dependent 2′-5′ oligoadenylate synthetases (279,297,315). These enzymes synthesize novel 2′-5′-phosphodiester-linked oligoadenylates (2-5A) that function to activate an endoribonuclease, designated as RNase L. The 2-5A dependent RNase L degrades single-stranded RNAs by preferentially cleaving uridylate-rich sequences. Although RNase L is constitutively present in most types of mammalian cells, because the 2-5A effector of the nuclease is unstable, the effects of 2-5A are transient. Among the small structured viral RNAs that can activate 2-5A synthetase are the EBER-1 RNA of Epstein-Barr virus, the VAI RNA of adenovirus, and the TAR RNA of HIV-1 (71,206,310).

Unconventional Translational Strategies Used for Viral Protein Production

Most viral mRNAs found in the cytoplasm of infected cells possess the following five features: (a) a 5′-terminal cap structure; (b) a 5′-untranslated sequence; (c) an ORF that typically begins with an AUG codon and ends with an UAA, UAG, or UGA codon; (d) a 3′-untranslated sequence; and (e) a poly A tail. Following attachment of the small ribosomal subunit at or near the 5′ end of the mRNA and identification of the functional AUG initiation codon by the scanning 40S subunit, the host translational machinery reads the single ORF of the mature viral mRNA to produce a single protein product (178). In addition to this conventional strategy, viruses also utilize a number of other strategies in specific instances to optimize the production of their protein products, strategies that include leaky scanning, ribosome shunting, translational frameshifting, and suppression of termination, as well as posttranscriptional RNA editing to alter the expression of viral genetic information.

Leaky Scanning

Some animal virus families include members that encode functionally polycistronic mRNAs in which translation initiation occurs alternatively at one or more AUG initiation sites in the same mRNA (296). The efficiency of translational initiation at a given AUG codon is thought to be modulated in part by the position and context of the start codon. The leaky scanning model provides a conceptual framework for understanding the process of initiation of translation on those viral mRNAs that utilize more than one AUG codon for initiation (178). According to the model, 40S ribosomal subunits bind at or near the 5′ end of the mRNA and advance linearly until an AUG codon in a favorable context is reached, at which point assembly of complete 80S ribosomes takes place and initiation of polypeptide chain synthesis begins. If the 5′-proximal AUG codon is in an optimal context with purines in the −3 and +4 positions relative to the A of the AUG, initiation is typically unique and efficient. If the context is suboptimal, initiation at that codon is inefficient, scanning is leaky, and consequently some of the 40S subunits bypass the first suboptimal AUG and begin initiation at a downstream AUG positioned in a more favorable context. Thus, leaky scanning provides a mechanism by which multiple viral proteins may be produced from a single mRNA.

For several of the polycistronic viral mRNAs, the AUG codon of the 5′-proximal upstream cistron is present in a suboptimal context, whereas the initiation codon of the internal downstream cistron is often, but not always, present in an optimal context (178,296). Thus, some of the scanning 40S ribosomal subunits would presumably "leak" past the suboptimal initiation site and begin translation at the downstream initiation site, which may occur either in the same or different ORF (296). The relative efficiency of utilization of the upstream and downstream initiation codons may be of possible regulatory importance, as certain polycistronic mRNAs appear to be organized so that the relative abundance of the proteins encoded by the different cistrons correlates with the relative strength of the initiation codon.

A number of animal virus genes encode mRNAs in which different in-frame AUG initiation sites are alternatively utilized to generate related forms of a protein that differ in their amino terminal sequences. This is exemplified by the SV40 late 19S mRNAs encoding capsid proteins VP2 and VP3. The less abundant VP2 capsid protein is synthesized from the 5′-proximal AUG, which is in a suboptimal context, and the more abundant VP3 capsid protein is synthesized from an in-frame downstream AUG codon in a more favorable context (307). About 70% of the scanning ribosomes are estimated to bypass the VP2 initiator AUG and instead initiate translation at the downstream VP3 translation start site. Several examples of polycistronic viral mRNAs exist in which two proteins are produced from different, overlapping reading frames, as exemplified by the reovirus S1 mRNA, which encodes the minor capsid protein σ1 and the nonstructural protein σ1ns, also known as σ1S (296). The steady-state distribution of translating ribosomes on reovirus S1 mRNA is not uniform, and interactions may occur between ribosomes in different reading frames. Ribosome pausing occurs at sites of initiation and termination of translation, both for the simple S4 mRNA in which a single ORF is utilized to produce the major capsid protein σ3 and for the more complex S1 mRNA, where two overlapping ORFs are utilized. For the polycistronic S1 mRNA, the rate-limiting initiation event at the downstream favorable AUG utilized for ORF2 initiation of σ1ns synthesis leads to ribosome stacking and elongation arrest in the upstream σ1 ORF1 that encodes the minor capsid attachment protein (78).

Ribosome Shunting

Ribosome shunting refers to the process by which intervening regions of an mRNA are bypassed without scanning by ribosomes during the translation process. Examples in which ribosome shunting or jumping occurs include animal cells infected with adenovirus (381) and papilloma virus (281) and plant cells infected with cauliflower mosaic virus (76). In the case of adenovirus late mRNAs that are preferentially translated during infection, ribosomes are recruited to the 5′ end of the tripartite leader RNA and then are translocated to a downstream AUG codon without scanning the intervening sequences (381). The tripartite leader confers preferential translation by reducing the requirement for initiation factor eIF-4F, the rate-limiting cap binding complex. Adenovirus inhibits cell protein synthesis, in part, by inactivating eIF-4F. The tripartite leader directs both 5′ linear scanning and ribosome jumping when eIF-4F is abundant, but it exclusively uses the jumping mechanism at late times after infection when the level of eIF-4E phosphorylation is reduced and eIF-4F function is impaired (381).

Translational Frameshifting

In addition to the conventional process of mRNA translation where a single ORF is read by an elongating ribosome, some retroviruses, coronaviruses, toroviruses, arteriviruses, and astroviruses exploit the ability of the host cell ribosomes to shift from one reading frame to another in response to signals programmed by the mRNA (36,89). The elongating ribosome typically slips backward by one nucleotide (−1), resulting in a change in reading frame. For many retroviruses, production of the polymerase gene products occurs following a −1 frameshift during translation. The *pol* gene partially overlaps and is in the −1 reading frame with respect to the upstream *gag* gene. As exemplified by Rous sarcoma virus (157) and HIV (156), a small fraction of the ribosomes (about 5%) shift reading frames during translation to produce a Gag-Pol fusion protein, whereas the majority of ribosomes (about 95%) terminate at the end of the *gag* ORF. This provides a mechanism for viruses to synthesize, from a single mRNA, relatively large amounts of an upstream product (e.g., Gag structural proteins) compared to the downstream product (e.g., reverse transcriptase). Two cis-acting viral mRNA signals are involved in the process of −1 ribosome frameshifting: a slippery sequence where the ribosome changes reading frame, and a stimulatory structure located downstream (36,89). Pseudoknot structures involved in frameshifting of various retroviral RNAs and infectious bronchitis coronavirus RNA are believed to impose a thermodynamic barrier to elongating ribosomes, resulting in ribosome pausing, which increases the opportunity that ribosome-bound tRNAs will slip into the −1 reading frame at the slippery sequence because of specific interaction between the viral mRNA and host protein synthesizing machinery (49,233). Small amounts of HSV thymidine kinase enzyme can be produced by drug-resistant strains utilizing a translational recoding mechanism of +1 (or −2) frameshifting (147). Thus, this provides a general mechanism whereby specific viral RNA sequences cause ribosomal slippage so that small amounts of an essential viral protein can be synthesized.

Suppression of Translational Termination

The UAG, UGA, and UAA codons typically specify translation termination. However, termination can sometimes be leaky. Expression of limited amounts of a viral protein can be achieved by suppression of a stop codon, resulting in the synthesis of a carboxy-terminally extended protein. For certain retroviruses, as exemplified by murine leukemia viruses (MuLV), this is the mechanism used to express the *pol* gene as a Gag-Pol fusion protein by reading through the *gag* stop codon to produce viral reverse transcriptase (261). The amber UAG codon of MuLV is decoded as glutamine, thus allowing read-through to permit expression of downstream Pol ORF sequences at about 5% to 10% efficiency (4,261). Suppression of translational termination is also observed with some alphaviruses, as exemplified by Sindbis virus, where read-through of an opal UGA codon occurs to produce nsp4, a nonstructural protein required for viral RNA polymerase activity (195). No cases of read-through are yet known for UAA, a commonly used translation termination codon. Like frameshifting, the suppression of translational termination by ribosome read-through requires cis-acting sequences on the viral mRNA to interact with the host translational machinery to make the nonsense stop codon an inefficient terminator, and thus subject to read-through to allow the regulated expression of downstream viral ORFs (4,195).

Posttranscriptional RNA Editing

RNA editing is a posttranscriptional process by which RNA transcripts are covalently modified in a manner that potentially alters the function of the encoded product. Site-selective conversion of adenosine to inosine represents one such editing process, catalyzed by RNA-specific adenosine deaminases (ADAR). This A-to-I RNA editing modifies the expression of genetic information by changing codons, as inosine is read as guanine instead of adenine by ribosomes and polymerases. Two types of A-to-I editing processes have been described in viral RNAs. First, modifications characteristic of adenosine deamination are found at multiple sites, as exemplified by the extensive adenosine modifications present on the viral antisense RNA late in polyoma virus infection (183) and by the biased hypermutations observed in negative-stranded RNA virus genomes during lytic and persistent infections, as in the case of measles virus (44). Second, highly site-specific A-to-I modifications have also been identified at one or a few sites in certain viral and cellular RNA transcripts, as demonstrated by the editing of hepatitis delta virus (HDV) RNA (270) and pre-mRNAs encoding the glutamate GluR and 5HT-2c serotonin receptor channel subunits (200), respectively. Editing of these viral and cellular RNAs results in codon changes and thus mRNAs that encode protein products with altered functional activities. In the case of HDV infections, RNA editing plays an essential role in the production of two forms of hepatitis delta antigen (HDAg) from the same ORF. A-to-I editing at adenosine 1012 of HDV antigenomic RNA has the effect of converting an amber UAG termination codon to a UGG tryptophan codon in the mRNA (270), thereby extending the ORF. The two HDAg proteins encoded by the ORF have different functions in the viral life cycle. Small HDAg is required for RNA replication, and large HDAg, which inhibits replication, is required for packaging of viral RNA. Interestingly, the human ADAR gene is regulated by two promoters, one of which is interferon inducible and one of which is not inducible (111). The possible roles of RNA editing by ADAR in viral pathogenesis are numerous but so far have not yet been studied extensively.

NUCLEAR LOCALIZATION OF DNA REPLICATION AND ASSEMBLY PROTEINS

During viral infection, proteins encoded by certain viruses must localize from the cytoplasm into the nucleus to replicate viral genomes, to regulate viral transcription and RNA processing, and to assemble progeny viral capsids. In general, viral proteins use cellular machinery for localization through the nuclear pores into the nucleus (reviewed in ref. 366). In fact, the first NLS was identified as PKKKRKV in the SV40 large T-antigen (162). The importin α/β complex binds to this sequence and attaches to fibrils that extend to the nuclear pore. Once at the nuclear pore, the complex binds to the nucleoporins and the protein is transported into the nucleus. Some proteins, such as the SV40 large T-antigen, can localize to the nuclear compartment independently of other viral proteins and assemble into higher-order complexes after they enter the nucleus. Other proteins, such as the HSV helicase–primase complex (209) or capsid proteins (241,285), must assemble into a complex in the cytoplasm prior to localization into the nucleus.

TAKING OVER THE CELLULAR DNA REPLICATION MACHINERY

Inhibition of Host-Cell DNA Replication

Both RNA and DNA viruses cause the inhibition of host-cell DNA synthesis. There are several possible reasons for viral inhibition of cell DNA synthesis: (a) to provide precursors for viral DNA synthesis, (b) to provide host-cell structures and/or replication proteins for viral DNA synthesis, or (c) as a secondary effect of inhibiting cellular protein synthesis. The possible mechanisms by which virus infection might inhibit cellular DNA synthesis are discussed individually.

A Secondary Effect of Inhibiting Cell Protein Synthesis

There appears to be a small pool of an essential cell DNA replication protein (or proteins), as suggested by the decrease in rate of DNA chain growth seen within minutes after inhibition of protein synthesis (265,329). It has been proposed that some viruses, such as the herpesviruses, inhibit cellular DNA synthesis as a consequence of inhibiting cellular protein synthesis (164), and indeed, the two shutoff functions do map together on the HSV genome (91). HSV and adenovirus DNA synthesis do not require the limiting cellular factor, or the factor is not limiting in infected cells because their DNA synthesis continues independently of whether protein synthesis is ongoing or not (148,287).

Displacement of Cellular DNA from Its Normal Site of Replication

Herpesvirus infection has been variously reported to displace cellular DNA from the nuclear membrane (240) or to cause the displacement of cellular chromatin to the periphery of the nucleus (63,305). In either case, the cell DNA could be displaced from its normal site for replication because cell DNA synthesis has been reported to occur on the "nuclear cage" (220), or the nuclear matrix (18). The exposed sites on the nuclear matrix may provide a structural framework for viral DNA replication and late transcription (174).

Recruitment of Cell DNA Replication Proteins to Viral Structures

Several studies have shown that HSV infection leads to a redistribution of the host-cell DNA replication apparatus (66,369). This type of event could serve the dual function of providing cellular factors for viral DNA replication and inhibiting cell DNA synthesis, thereby reserving deoxynucleoside triphosphates for viral DNA synthesis.

Degradation of Cellular DNA

Infection by vaccinia virus leads rapidly to a marked inhibition of cell DNA synthesis. A virion-associated DNase enters the host cell nucleus and acts on single-stranded DNA (ssDNA) (267,268). This inhibition is mediated by the action of a virion component on the host cell.

Mechanisms by Which DNA Viruses Ensure the Availability of a DNA Replication Apparatus

DNA viruses need a replication apparatus for amplification of their genomic nucleic acid. Although the host-cell enzymes may be used for DNA replication, they may not always be available for use by the virus. Thus, several strategies have evolved to ensure the availability of DNA replication machinery. These range from encoding an entirely new replication apparatus to inducing host cell DNA synthesis to allow the virus to use the cellular machinery.

Viruses Can Encode a New Replication Apparatus

The poxviruses replicate entirely in the cytoplasm. Indeed, poxviral DNA synthesis can occur in enucleated cells. Therefore, they must encode all (or nearly all) of the proteins needed for replication of their DNA in the cytoplasm. Similarly, retrovirions contain an enzyme capable of copying the genomic RNA into DNA. This step is not possible in cells without the virion enzyme, because a cellular reverse transcriptase is not available to copy the viral RNA. For these viruses, DNA synthesis is usually not restricted in different cells, because the enzymes are virally encoded.

The herpesviruses encode several proteins that form a major part of the replication complex. For example, HSV encodes seven viral proteins required for and directly involved in viral DNA replication (46,373). In addition, HSV encodes several other enzymes involved in providing deoxynucleoside triphosphate precursors for viral DNA synthesis: thymidine kinase, ribonucleotide reductase, and dUTPase. HSV replicates in the resting neuron and has apparently evolved to encode these DNA replication proteins because they are expressed at low levels in resting neurons. Some cellular proteins may be involved in HSV DNA replication. Although the identity and role of specific cell proteins in HSV DNA replication have not been defined, the cellular DNA replication machinery is redistributed after HSV infection so as to co-localize with viral proteins in the cell nucleus (66). HSV DNA replication proteins also bind to the nuclear matrix (274), so cellular proteins may be required to anchor DNA replication complexes and thereby promote optimal HSV DNA synthesis. However, HSV blocks cells from progressing into S phase (66), so any cellular proteins required for HSV DNA synthesis may be present in non-S phase cells.

Viruses Can Induce Cellular DNA Synthesis

Some viruses, especially the DNA tumor viruses, rely on the host-cell DNA replication machinery, and to ensure its availability, they induce S phase in their host cells if they are not cycling or are in G0 phase. SV40 and polyoma viruses encode one protein, large T-antigen, which essentially inserts itself into the host-cell replication complex and directs it to replicate viral DNA. The SV40 large T-antigen (a) binds to the SV40 DNA sequences that serve as the origin of DNA replication (344), (b) interacts with the cellular α-DNA polymerase (318), and (c) acts as a helicase (324). Through these and possibly other functions, T antigen promotes replication of the SV40 chromosome. T antigen could be viewed as an origin-binding protein that substitutes for an analogous cellular protein. The specific interaction of T antigen with host proteins is apparent in other ways. SV40 DNA replication can occur in extracts prepared from only certain cell types (196), and the interaction between T antigen and the α polymerase–primase complex seems to define or play a role in defining this specificity (230). Thus, the permissivity of a cell for viral growth may be defined by the ability of a viral DNA replication protein to interact with the cellular DNA replication apparatus.

However, the levels of several critical components of the cellular DNA replication apparatus are limiting, except during S phase. Thus, the host DNA replication machinery would not be available at all stages of the cell cycle. Polyomaviruses have long been known to induce S phase in resting (G0) cells (79), and the mechanisms for this effect are now understood. SV40 T antigen forms complexes with pRb and related proteins (68), releasing transcription factors of the E2F family that are important for expression of cellular DNA replication and cell cycle proteins such as c-fos, c-myc, DNA pol α, dihydrofolate reductase, thymidine kinase, thymidylate synthetase, and cdc-2 (239). Thus, activation of E2F contributes to the preparation of the host cell for viral DNA replication.

Adenovirus encodes a DNA polymerase, a terminal protein, and an ssDNA-binding protein for viral DNA replication (see Chapter 31), but the remainder of the replication proteins and nucleotide metabolism enzymes are host-cell gene products. Thus, adenovirus also induces its host cell to enter S phase. Like SV40 T-antigen, the E1A proteins bind to pRb (367), releasing E2F and activating transcription of cell cycle genes. It is also becoming clear that adenovirus infection disrupts a number of protein complexes that are involved in regulation of the cell cycle. The adenovirus E1B-55K protein binds to the cellular p53 protein (302), inactivating the G1 cell cycle block imposed by p53. This also contributes to activation of the host-cell S phase and the optimal conditions for viral DNA synthesis.

Maintenance of Viral DNA Within the Host Cell

Viruses whose DNA genomes persist within growing cells have evolved mechanisms for their genomes to be maintained stably in these cells via association with cellular chromosomes. There are two types of mechanisms by which viral DNA is stably maintained within the host cell in association with chromosomes. First, the viral DNA can be integrated into the cellular chromosome and propagated as part of the cellular DNA. For example, retrovirus DNA is integrated into the cellular genome after its synthesis by the reverse transcriptase (see Chapter 58 of *Fields Virology*, 4th ed.). Integration is promoted by the viral integrase function, but host functions can modulate the process. For example, the mouse Fv-1 gene mediates a postpenetration block to MuLV DNA integration (135,197,330). Thus, this host gene can define the host range of MuLV in mouse cells.

Second, viral DNA can be maintained as an extrachromosomal circular molecule in the infected cell. For example, Epstein-Barr virus (EBV) DNA is maintained in latently infected B lymphocytes as an episomal molecule (1) and requires a specific sequence, oriP, for replication and maintenance in latently infected B cells (377). Epstein-Barr nuclear antigen 1, EBNA-1, is also required for EBV DNA maintenance (377). Although EBNA-1 was thought to serve as an origin-binding protein, recent studies have shown that it plays a role in maintenance of the DNA rather than in its synthesis (3). EBNA-1 binds to specific sequences on viral DNA (277) and also binds to cellular chromosomes (126). Thus, EBNA-1 is thought to maintain EBV DNA in growing B cells by linking the viral DNA to cellular chromosomes. The related gammaherpesvirus, human herpesvirus-8 or Kaposi's sarcoma-associated herpesvirus also encodes a latency-associated nuclear antigen that tethers viral DNA to cellular chromosomes (11,56). Similarly, the papillomavirus genome contains sequences (called plasmid maintenance sequences) needed to maintain and replicate the DNA as an extrachromosomal element (149,203). Long-term maintenance of these plasmid genomes depends on attachment to host chromosomes, which is mediated by the viral E2 protein (151,193,317). In addition, these extrachromosomal elements appear to be subject to the normal copy number control existing in the normal cell because there is a constant number of episomal copies of these viral DNA molecules per cell as the cells divide. In contrast, HSV DNA can apparently persist during latent infection of neurons in a nonreplicating form because the host cell is not dividing.

ASSEMBLY OF FACTORIES FOR NUCLEIC ACID REPLICATION AND VIRION ASSEMBLY

Viral replication complexes, transcriptional complexes, replicative and assembly intermediates, and nucleocapsids and virions often accumulate in specific locations within the host cell and form structures called factories or inclusion bodies. The location of these structures obviously reflects the site of replication of a given virus. They may form in the nucleus, as do the inclusion bodies or factories in cells infected with herpesviruses (Fig. 9) or adenoviruses, or in the cytoplasm, as do the factories in reovirus-infected (Fig. 10) or poxvirus-infected cells or the Negri bodies in rabies virus–infected cells. Inclusion bodies have been useful in diagnostic virology because areas of altered staining can be detected at specific locations in the cell with specific staining properties, either basophilic or acidophilic, characteristic of individual groups of viruses. Crystalline arrays of capsids or nucleocapsids may accumulate in these inclusions (see Fig. 10). The assembly of these new structures in the cell may alter or displace host-cell components and lead to one form of CPE.

Much as other viral proteins have provided probes for important cell biologic questions, HSV DNA replication proteins and their localization to intranuclear inclusions have provided a situation in which to study intranuclear localization mechanisms. Initial studies characterized the nuclear inclusions of herpesvirus-infected cells and their molecular components. Electron microscopy (EM) of herpesvirus-infected cells showed electron-translucent intranuclear inclusions surrounded by marginated and compacted cell chromatin (63) (see Fig. 9). Light microscopic observation of nuclear inclusions shows an hourglass appearance of the inclusions at early times and an eosinophilic staining at later times (232,321) (see Fig. 3). Immunofluorescence experiments using antibodies specific for HSV DNA replication proteins have shown that viral DNA replication proteins accumulate in intranuclear foci by 3 hours postinfection and that these foci enlarge into globular nuclear structures called replication compartments (Fig. 11) (66,274). The replication compartments are likely to be equivalent to (a) the translucent nuclear inclusions seen by EM (see Fig. 9) and (b) the early nuclear inclusions seen by light microscopy.

These replication compartments are located in the interior of the nucleus as shown by EM (63,306) (see Fig. 9) and by confocal microscopy (67). Bromodeoxyuridine pulse labeling followed by immunofluorescence detection of bromodeoxyuridine-substituted DNA has shown that viral DNA synthesis occurs in the replication compartments (66). This technique allows the determination of the cellular location of DNA synthesis. Similarly, *in situ* hybridization with a viral DNA probe has shown that progeny HSV DNA accumulates in replication compartments (Fig. 12). The initial sites of formation of these compartments most likely takes place at specific loca-

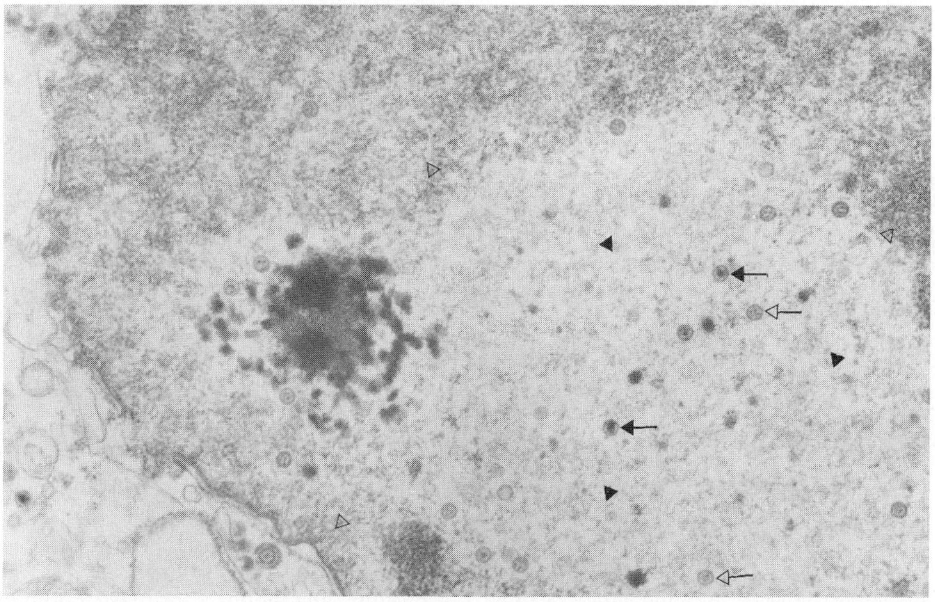

FIG. 9. Electron microscope visualization of nuclear inclusion areas. The *filled triangles* denote the electron-translucent nuclear inclusion area in a human HEp-2 cell infected with HSV-1. The *filled arrows* indicate full capsids, and the *unfilled arrows* indicate empty capsids. The *unfilled triangles* indicate host chromatin compressed to the periphery of the nucleus, apparently by the nuclear inclusion. Micrograph courtesy of D. Furlong and B. Roizman.

tions in the nucleus defined by the availability of host-cell proteins or structures (67), near ND10 sites in the nucleus (216,352). The accumulation of progeny DNA, the probable template for late gene transcription and the viral transcriptional trans-activator protein ICP4 (177, 276), pol II (283), and pulse-labeled viral RNA (260) in replication compartments argue that late gene transcription takes place in the replication compartments. Thus, late gene transcription is likely compartmentalized in infected cell–specific nuclear structures. Empty capsids appear to be assembled around dense bodies or in the inclusions within the infected cell nucleus, whereas encapsidation of viral DNA appears to occur within the inclusion body itself (see Fig. 9). Therefore, these

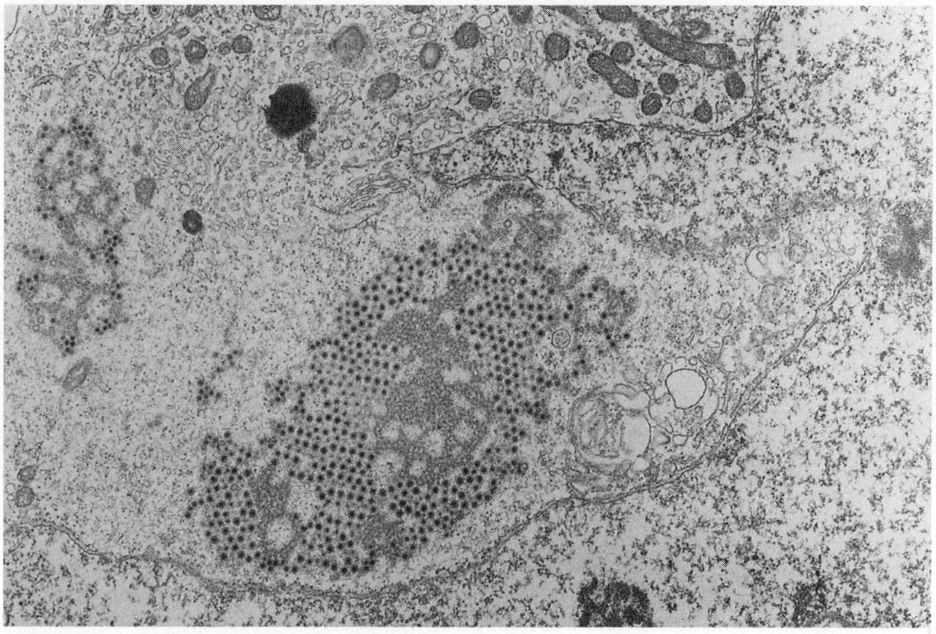

FIG. 10. Electron microscope visualization of cytoplasmic “factories” in a cell infected with reovirus. Micrograph courtesy of B. Fields.

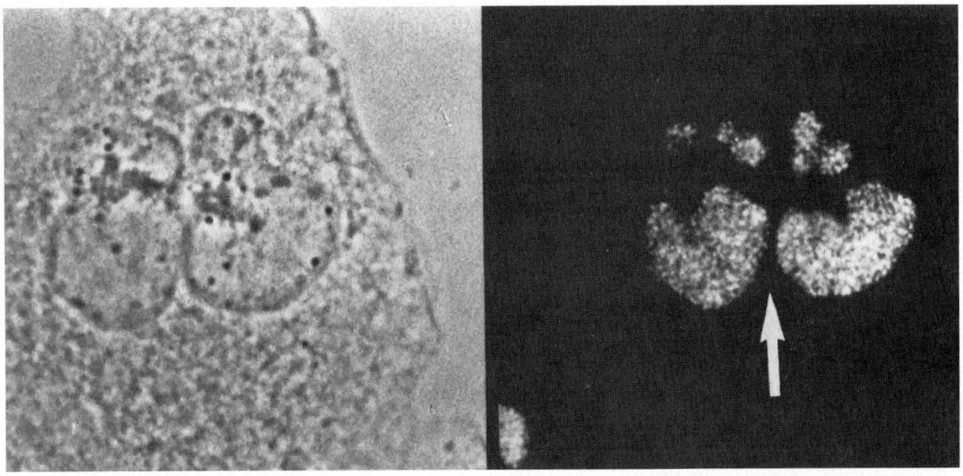

FIG. 11. Immunofluorescence detection of HSV replication compartments in binucleate cells. Micrograph courtesy of A. de Bruyn Kops.

intranuclear compartments in HSV-infected cells are sites of viral DNA replication, late gene transcription, and nucleocapsid assembly.

Studies of the nuclear inclusions in cells infected with HSV have raised several important cell biologic questions related to the assembly of nuclear complexes and structures and compartmentalization of nuclear metabolic processes. First, what signals target viral and cellular proteins to these compartments? Intranuclear localization mechanisms have not been studied extensively. Both viral and host proteins localize to these compartments. The HSV replication proteins, including the ICP8 DNA-binding protein, DNA polymerase, polymerase accessory protein, and helicase-primase complex (39,66,116,199, 202,274) localize to compartments. These proteins undergo multiple interactions with each other; thus, their targeting could involve binding to other proteins in the replication complex, binding to cellular proteins, or other targeting mechanisms. Cellular proteins, including pRb, p53, and DNA pol α (369) and SV40 large T-antigen (378), also localize to replication compartments in HSV-infected cells.

Second, is there a defined assembly pathway for viral protein complexes in these compartments? Experiments examining protein localization in cells infected with mutants defective for each of the HSV DNA replication

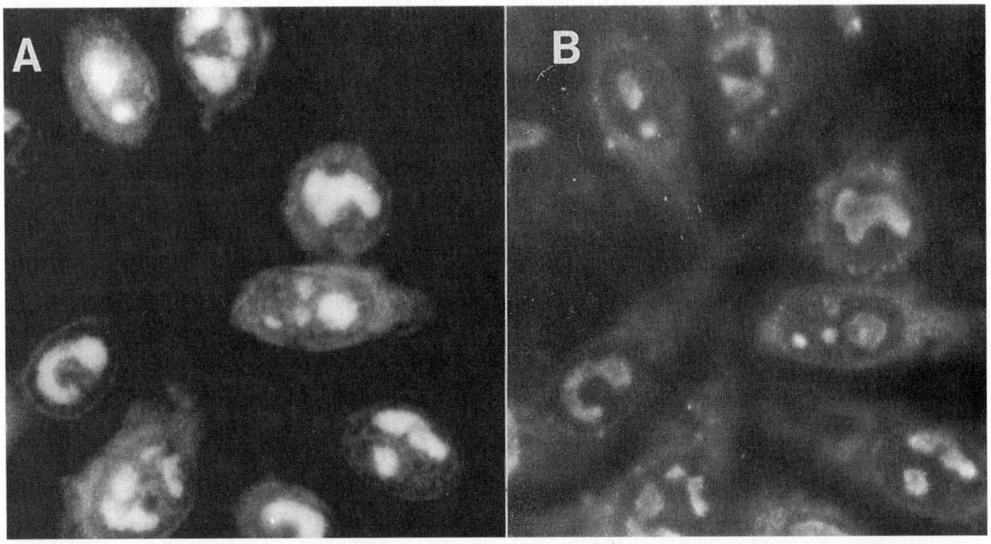

FIG. 12. *In situ* hybridization detection of the location of viral nucleic acids in infected cells. Monkey cells infected with HSV-1 were fixed in formaldehyde, permeabilized in acetone, and incubated with biotin-labeled HSV DNA. The cultures were heated to denature the cellular DNA and the probe, and the culture and solution were allowed to cool. The cells were then reacted with mouse anti-ICP4 monoclonal antibody followed by rhodamine-conjugated goat antimouse immunoglobulin antibody and fluorescein-conjugated avidin. **A:** Rhodamine fluorescence showing the location of the HSV trans-activator protein ICP4. **B:** Fluorescein fluorescence showing the location of HSV DNA in the infected cells. Micrograph courtesy of S. Rice.

proteins have shown that there is a functional order for assembly of HSV DNA replication proteins into nuclear structures (199). The helicase-primase complex of U_L8, U_L42, and U_L52 proteins, the U_L9 origin-binding protein, and the ICP8 ssDNA-binding proteins are the minimal HSV proteins needed to assemble into nuclear structures. The polymerase-U_L42 complex then joins the structure.

Third, is there a receptor on the nuclear framework that anchors viral protein complexes? No cellular molecule has been identified as a receptor for the HSV replication proteins, and nuclear receptors remain an important problem in the targeting of nuclear proteins. One of the few situations where saturable binding of a viral protein to the nuclear matrix has been demonstrated is with the adenovirus preterminal protein (97). The adenoviral preterminal protein interacts with the nuclear matrix, specifically with CAD, a pyrimidine biosynthesis enzyme (5). The identification of a nuclear molecule or receptor that anchors specific proteins in the cell nucleus remains as an important confirmation of the concept of the nuclear matrix, a nuclear structure believed to consist of nuclear lamins under the nuclear envelope and internal fibrous elements.

Fourth, what defines the intranuclear location at which compartments are formed? In binucleate cells infected with HSV, replication compartments often show nearly identical patterns of compartments along a twofold axis of symmetry between many of the sister nuclei (see Fig. 10) (67). Therefore, the location of HSV replication compartments is defined by preexisting nuclear architecture, probably the internal nuclear matrix or receptors thereon. Although the parental HSV genome and DNA replication proteins localize to sites near ND10 sites in the nucleus (216,352), the precise molecular sites of localization remain to be defined.

Nuclear viral inclusions in adenovirus-infected cells (280,331,358) are also sites of viral DNA synthesis and accumulation of progeny DNA (37,212,358) and probably late viral transcription (212,372). Adenoviral inclusions may have an added level of complexity over the HSV nuclear inclusions in that the E1B-55kD/E4-34kD complex of proteins is located in and around the inclusions and is believed to recruit critical components of the host-cell RNA transport process to the sites of late viral RNA synthesis (245).

USE OF THE HOST CELL FOR MATURATION AND BUDDING

As described previously, viruses use the host-cell translational machinery to synthesize the structural proteins for progeny virus production. In addition, viruses may use a cellular polymerase or a virus-encoded polymerase to replicate their genomes. In addition, viruses use cellular proteases, membranes, glycosylation machinery, kinases, and chaperone proteins for their protein maturation (175). Because the sites of viral genome replication—as well as of maturation in general—are different from those where viral protein synthesis takes place, the intracellular trafficking of viral components is crucial for infectious particle formation. Furthermore, it appears that structurally intact cells are essential for efficient virus replication.

The site of assembly and mechanism of progeny virus release from the infected cell depends on the structure of the virus (Fig. 13). Enveloped viruses exit from the infected cell surface either by budding through the

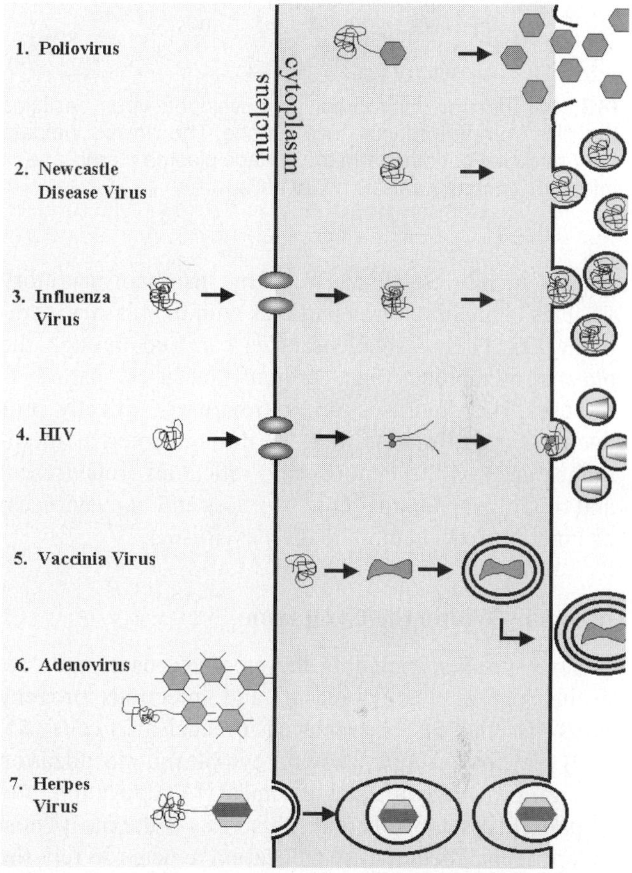

FIG. 13. Pathways of exit from cells for different viruses. Nonenveloped RNA viruses such as poliovirus (*line 1*) and DNA viruses such as adenovirus (*line 6*) leave the cell upon cell lysis. Enveloped viruses that replicate in the cytoplasm such as Newcastle disease virus (*line 2*) exit the cell by budding from the cytoplasmic membrane. Influenza viruses (*line 3*) also leave the cytoplasm in this manner, but the amplified viral ribonucleoprotein (RNP) complexes must first exit the nucleus via the nuclear pore. The amplified genome of HIV (*line 4*) exits the nucleus in a manner similar to influenza virus via the nuclear pore, and the virus buds from the cytoplasmic membrane. Vaccinia virus (*line 5*) replicates in the cytoplasm where it acquires its membrane(s), and in general it remains cell associated. Herpes viruses (*line 7*) acquire envelopes as they bud through the inner membrane of the nuclear envelope. The viral particles are transported within intracellular vesicles to the cytoplasmic membrane, where fusion of the vesicular and cytoplasmic membranes allows release of the virus from the cell. For the sake of clarity, not all viral proteins implicated in exit are shown.

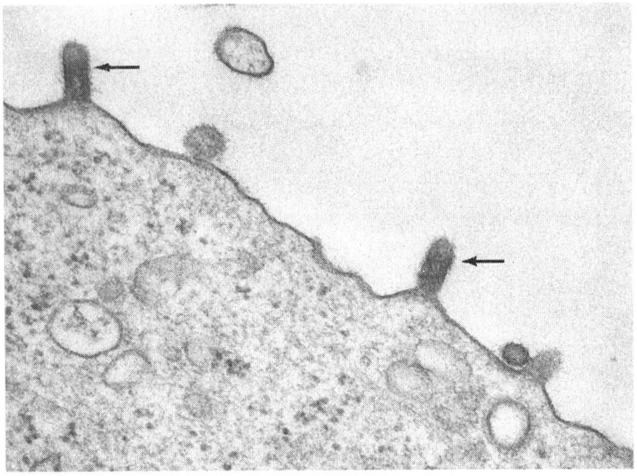

FIG. 14. Electron micrograph of enveloped virus particles budding from the infected cell surface. The *arrows* indicate VSV particles budding from the surface plasma membrane of infected Chinese hamster ovary cells.

plasma membrane (Fig. 14) or by fusion of secretory vesicles containing virus particles with the plasma membrane (326). Thus, nucleocapsids can bud through the plasma membrane (e.g., orthomyxoviruses, paramyxoviruses, rhabdoviruses, and retroviruses), directly producing extracellular virions, or through internal membranes such as the endoplasmic reticulum (rotaviruses) and/or Golgi apparatus (coronaviruses and bunyaviruses) or inner nuclear membrane (herpesviruses).

Assembly Within the Cytoplasm

Some viruses, including the picornaviruses, replicate exclusively in the cytoplasm, and infectious progeny virus particles can be produced in enucleated cells (85, 269). PV, for example, shows a cytoplasmic localization of viral protein synthesis, of viral RNA replication, and of particle assembly. Perhaps this virus is the most "host independent," because its replication appears to rely the least on trafficking within an intact cell. In a landmark paper (226), Wimmer's group showed that an extract of uninfected HeLa cells permitted cell-free translation of naked PV RNA, synthesis of virion RNA, and assembly of infectious PV particles. However, the successful formation of infectious particles required the presence of membranes in the HeLa cell extract (59) and possibly the presence of chaperones such as heat-shock protein 70 (204). Although the efficiency of the cell-free virus replication was low, this experiment revealed that even such a complex process as viral RNA replication and PV encapsidation may be achieved outside a living cell. It has been generally assumed that unenveloped viruses are released by lysis of the cells. However, PV is released almost exclusively from the apical surface of polarized human intestinal epithelial cells (350). Thus, there may be cellular mechanisms used for viruses for active release from the cytoplasm in a polarized fashion (see Fig. 13, line 1).

Assembly Within the Nucleus

The prototypic viruses restricted to assembly within the nucleus are adenovirus and SV40. For adenovirus, synthesis and subsequent transport of the hexon and penton components into the nucleus are essential for virus formation. The transport from cytoplasm to nucleus involves the presence of NLSs on the adenoviral proteins and is accompanied (or followed) by the assembly of the viral components. Although the presence of a viral nonstructural component (the L1 52/55kD protein) appears to be required for encapsidation (129), little is known about which proteins (structures) are involved in the assembly of adenoviruses. Either an empty protein shell is made first, into which the viral DNA is introduced, or the packaging of DNA occurs along with assembly of the viral proteins. Whatever the precise mechanism turns out to be, it is likely that the formation of infectious adenovirus particles requires an intact nucleus (see Fig. 13, line 6).

Even the assembly of the much simpler SV40 virus is quite complex. Despite numerous efforts, the formation of stable SV40 particles through an *in vitro* assembly system has not yet been achieved (300), and, again, efficient packaging seems to require an intact host nucleus. For both adeno- and SV40 viruses, great quantities of virus particles can accumulate in the nucleus, leading eventually to lysis of the cell and release of virus. Like PV, SV40 may also undergo polarized released from epithelial cells (54).

Assembly of Enveloped RNA-Containing Viruses

Many of the RNA viruses that derive their lipid-containing envelopes from the cell's plasma membrane contain single-stranded RNA as their genome. Newcastle disease, vesicular stomatitis, and influenza viruses are prototype viruses of the negative-strand RNA virus group, the study of which has provided us with much of the information presently known about intracellular trafficking of viral glycoproteins and assembly in the plasma membrane. Viral glycoproteins, especially the influenza HA and VSV glycoprotein (G), have been used extensively as prototypes for the study of biogenesis of plasma membrane proteins. These proteins use the signal receptor particle, endoplasmic reticulum enzymes, Golgi apparatus enzymes, and transport mechanisms to realize their proper structure and cell-surface location.

Part of the evidence for the concept that transmembrane proteins are synthesized on membrane-bound polyribosomes and translocated cotranslationally across the endoplasmic reticulum membrane while peripheral membrane proteins are synthesized on free polyribosomes came from the study of virus membrane proteins (176,229). Detailed studies of *in vitro* insertion of viral membrane proteins into the endoplasmic reticulum membrane came from studies of the VSV G protein (292). Detailed genetic study of the VSV G protein has provided evidence for the loop model for signal sequence insertion into the endoplasmic reticulum (311). Transit along the secretory pathway is well described for the glycoproteins of these three viruses, although the ultimate fate of specific viral proteins may depend on specific signals present in the molecule. For example, epithelial cells have apical and basolateral surfaces that can be targeted by specific viral glycoproteins. Influenza virus buds apically and VSV buds basolaterally. This selective localization may be determined by specific transport vesicles that recognize signals in the viral proteins (184,234).

It should also be noted that the neuraminidase cleaves off sialic acid from the host cell and from budding virus particles, thereby preventing binding of the hemagglutinin to cell surfaces and viral surfaces, respectively. Viruses with a temperature-sensitive neuraminidase aggregate on cell surfaces when grown at the nonpermissive temperature or inhibited by neuraminidase inhibitors (190,247–249). Inhibiting this interaction of the viral neuraminidase with the host sialic acid receptor is the basis for drugs recently approved to fight influenza virus infection.

Although the role of the glycoproteins in the efficient assembly of enveloped viruses is well established, it is also thought that the M protein of these viruses may be involved in viral assembly and release. For example, when the matrix (M) protein of VSV is expressed in mammalian cells, it is subsequently released from the cells in the form of lipid vesicles that bud through the plasma membrane (161). Recently it was demonstrated that a highly conserved amino acid motif (PPXY, where P is proline, Y is tyrosine) present within the M protein of VSV and other rhabdoviruses, including rabies virus, may play a functional role in budding. It was found that mutating the PPXY motif in the VSV M protein prevented the release of the protein from cells in this functional budding assay. Interestingly, the PPXY motif within rhabdoviral M proteins was shown to be a ligand for proteins that contain a WW (tryptophan–tryptophan) sequence (136). The hypothesis is that cellular WW proteins interact with the viral M proteins and function as "budding" proteins, facilitating the assembly and release of the viral particles. No such hypothetical budding partners have as yet been identified *in vivo.*

The properties of the PPXY motif in the M proteins of rhabdoviruses are similar to those of the late (L) budding domain identified in the gag-specific protein p2b of Rous sarcoma virus, an avian retrovirus (108,370). In a functional budding assay, the region of the Rous sarcoma virus gag protein (57) containing the proline-rich motif can be replaced by the homologous region of the VSV M protein. However, these PPXY-mediated interactions between viral and cellular proteins are not sufficient to allow virus particles to bud from the cytoplasmic surface. The M and gag proteins appear to possess membrane-association domains (different from the PPXY motifs) that are required for the localization to the cytoplasmic membrane (50,375). The M and gag proteins may also interact with the respective viral glycoproteins, which could lead to an enhanced membrane binding of these viral components. Furthermore, the viral RNAs in the form of ribonucleoprotein complexes must bind to these structures in specific ways to prevent packaging and budding of cellular RNAs rather than viral ones. Many questions remain in this area of study because the precise steps leading to the formation and extracellular release of enveloped RNA viruses remain obscure.

The mouse hepatitis virus, a positive-strand RNA virus, follows an unusual pathway toward infectious particle formation. Rather than budding from the plasma membrane, it appears that murine hepatitis virus replication occurs on late endosomal and/or lysosomal membranes (355). We do not know how the mouse hepatitis virus replication components are targeted to the correct membranes or what the advantage to the virus is of localization in these cytoplasmic compartments. It will be interesting to find answers to these questions in the future.

Assembly of Vaccinia Viruses

Vaccinia virus is known to replicate in the cytoplasm, and it does so within specific regions called factories. What is unusual about the use of the host by vaccinia virus is that the infectious intracellular particle derives two membranes from the Golgi network. This "wrapping" mechanism for forming the intracellular mature virions is not well understood, nor are the cellular components involved in this process well characterized. Some of these virus particles become engulfed by another envelope derived from a post-Golgi or endocytic compartment, which allows fusion with the plasma membrane and eventual release. Thus, there are two forms of infectious particles—one inside the cell and one that is released (see Fig. 13, line 5). In another remarkable process, the intracellular enveloped virions can also become associated with actin tails (60,99). It was found that the viral protein A36R in the viral envelope becomes tyrosine-phosphorylated by cellular Src-family kinases. This phosphorylation results in the recruitment of the cellular adaptor protein Nck and of N-WASP next to the vaccinia particle. The latter two proteins are involved in actin polymerization at the plasma membrane. It thus appears that vaccinia virus mimics the receptor tyrosine kinase signalling observed during actin-based motility of (uninfected) cells. Vaccinia virus particles appear to sit on the tips of actin tails and thereby gain mobility that allows the virus to spread from cell to cell. The actin tails decorated by vaccinia virus (or the virulent smallpox virus) push the virus along and may dip into neighboring cells, thus transferring the virus to a new cell.

Assembly of Herpesviruses

Cellular cytoskeletal structures are exploited by yet another DNA virus for trafficking of viral components. Sodeik et al. (322) showed that the incoming herpesvirus capsids are rapidly transported along microtubules with the help of dynein, a microtubule-dependent motor. Transport of the viral capsids proceeds along microtubules from the cell periphery to the nucleus (see Fig. 5, line 7), involving an interaction of capsid proteins with dynein and microtubules. All herpesvirus capsids acquire a membrane from the inner leaflet of the nuclear membrane when they leave the nucleus. In the reenvelopment model of egress, this enveloped particle loses its envelope after transport into the cytoplasm, and naked capsids travel along (reorganized) microtubules (81,84). What determines directionality of this transport remains undefined. Also, this microtubule-mediated transport may be of great importance for the axonal transport in neurons, where large distances have to be overcome by the virus and its components, and it may be less relevant in other herpesvirus-infected cells (see Fig. 13, line 7a).

A second model describing the interactions of herpesvirus and cellular components during egress is the lumenal model. According to this model, viral capsids acquire their envelopes from the inner leaflet of the nuclear membrane and bud from the cell following the host's secretory pathway without leaving the lumenal spaces of the cell (see Fig. 12, line 7b). Thus, the naked capsids observed by EM, for example, would be "dead end" structures (118) and exocytosis would be independent of the organization of microtubules and/or the organization of the Golgi apparatus (6). The relative importance of these two pathways for herpesvirus egress remains to be defined.

Targeting and Release in Polarized Cells

Finally, release of viruses may be asymmetrical in polarized epithelial cells. Polarized epithelial cells have differentiated apical and basal surface plasma membranes. Thus, viruses budding through the plasma membrane or vesicles containing virus particles can traffic specifically through either membrane. For example, orthomyxoviruses and paramyxoviruses bud at the apical surface, whereas VSV and retroviruses bud at the basal surface. Viral glycoproteins have an intrinsic ability to localize to specific surfaces of polarized cells (159,273, 290,327), and this is thought to be an important factor in deciding the site of virus budding in polarized epithelial cells. Sorting of proteins destined for the different surfaces appears to occur within the Golgi apparatus (326). Studies of the targeting of chimeric glycoproteins expressed from recombinant clones indicate that these targeting signals are complex (349). Some studies indicated that the ectodomain contains the targeting signal (222,291), whereas other studies found that the ectodomain is not sufficient (10,150,273,326). However, targeting of some viruses is not determined by the surface glycoprotein (205).

Once the progeny viruses have been released, they can initiate infection in new cells, and a whole new round of virus replication and interaction with a host cell can begin.

HOST CELL RESPONSES TO VIRAL INFECTION AND HOW VIRUSES COMBAT THESE RESPONSES

As host organisms for virus infection, we have evolved responses that block the replication and spread of viruses. This is apparent at the system level in the immune responses that are made against viruses and other foreign agents. However, host responses are apparent even at the cellular level, and in fact much of the innate immune response to viruses is initiated by host responses at the cellular level.

Interferon

One of the major host responses to viral infection is the production of interferons, components of the innate immune response. Isaacs and Lindenmann (154), during their seminal studies on virus interference, and Nagono and Kojima (231) observed that virus-infected cells produce a secreted factor which mediates the transfer of a virus-resistant state, and furthermore, that the resistance was displayed against both homologous and heterologous viruses. This secreted factor with antiviral activity was called interferon (IFN). It is now known that IFNs comprise a family of cytokines that play a centrally important role in the host response against viral infection.

The IFNs are grouped into two types: type I IFN (viral IFN, IFN-α/β) that includes the large number of α (leukocyte) IFNs and the single β (fibroblast) IFN, all of which act through the IFN-α/β receptor; and, type II IFN (immune IFN, IFN-γ), of which there is a single species that acts through a cognate IFN-γ receptor (297). The IFN response represents an early host defense, one that occurs prior to the onset of the immune response.

Pathogenesis studies utilizing knock-out mice in which the type I IFN-α/β receptor function has been eliminated by targeted gene-disruption illustrate the central importance of the interferon response; IFN-α/β receptor-null mice are unable to establish an antiviral state. These mutant animals are highly susceptible to infection by certain viruses despite the presence of an otherwise intact immune system (106,122,354). IFN-γ possesses unique immunoregulatory activities. Like IFN-α/β, IFN-γ plays an important role in mediating protection against viral infection, especially long-term control of viral infections, as revealed from studies of knock-out mice lacking the type II IFN-γ receptor (42,201). Mice lacking both the type II IFN-γ receptor and the type I IFN-α/β receptor are especially sensitive to viral infection (354).

The discovery that a number of viruses encode gene products that antagonize the antiviral actions of IFNs further illustrates the fundamental importance of the interferon system as a host defense against viral infection. Numerous mechanisms are utilized by viruses to impair the IFN response (Fig. 15). In most cases, the virus-encoded products antagonize one of two stages of IFN action: (a) the IFN signal transduction pathway that leads to transcriptional activation of the 30 or so cellular genes whose products are responsible for the biologic activities of the IFNs, or (b) the biochemical activity of one or a few specific IFN-induced cellular proteins responsible for inhibition of virus replication. A third possible stage of antagonism of the interferon response by viruses is the inhibition of IFN production. However, the viral gene products and biochemical mechanisms responsible for this level of inhibition are generally less well characterized than those responsible for the antagonism of either the signal transduction pathway or the action of IFN-induced proteins.

Several human viruses, including adenovirus, EBV, Sendai virus, and papillomavirus, encode viral proteins that inhibit the IFN-mediated transcriptional activation of cellular genes. The Jak-STAT signaling pathway utilized by IFN is blocked by the adenovirus E1A oncoprotein.

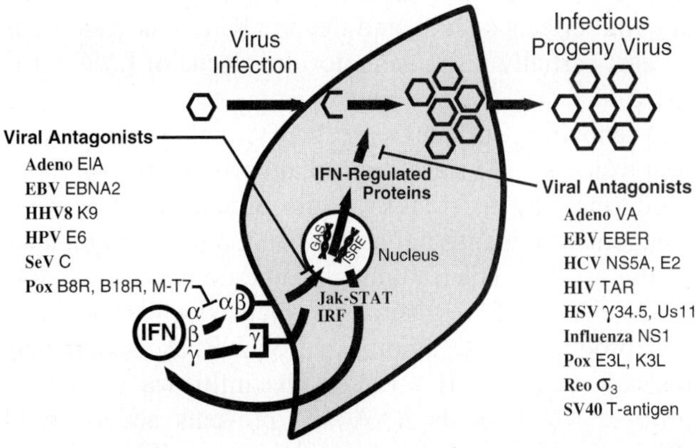

FIG. 15. Antagonism of interferon action by viruses. Virus-coded products that antagonize the IFN signal transduction pathway leading to transcriptional activation of IFN-regulated genes include adenovirus E1A; EBV EBNA2; HHV8 K9; HPV E6; poxvirus B8R, B18R, and M-T7; and Sendai virus C proteins. Virus-coded RNA and protein products that antagonize the biochemical activity of IFN-induced cellular proteins include adenovirus VA, EBV EBER, HCV NS5A and E2, HSV γ34.5 and U_s11, influenza virus NS1, and SV40 T-antigen.

The step affected by E1A appears to reside upstream of the activation of ISGF3, the major transcription factor complex formed of Stat1, Stat2, and IRF-9 (formerly known as p48) in response to IFN-α/β treatment (325), as the DNA-binding ability of ISGF3 is inhibited by the E1A protein (194). Overexpression of the IRF-9 component of ISGF3 restores IFN responses and the transcription of interferon-stimulated response element (ISRE)–driven genes in adenovirus infected cells (194). The Epstein-Barr virus EBNA2 protein also impairs the induction of genes by IFN-α/β but apparently by a mechanism different from that of the adenovirus E1A protein, as formation of the ISGF3 transcriptional activator complex is not significantly affected by EBNA2 (163). Sendai virus, a paramyxovirus that replicates in the cytoplasm of the host, circumvents the IFN-induced antiviral response by interfering with the transcriptional activation of IFN-inducible cellular genes. The C proteins of Sendai virus play a role, because infections with two different C gene mutants eliminate the ability to prevent establishment of an antiviral state against VSV (107). Impairment of the IFN-induced antiviral response appears to be a key determinant of Sendai virus pathogenicity (74,107).

Insight into the biochemical basis of the antagonism of the IFN signal transduction process by impairment of the function of signaling factors other than ISGF3 has been gained from studies of human papillomavirus (HPV) and also adenovirus. IRF-3, a key transcriptional activator affected by viral infection, is constitutively expressed in many cells and tissues. IRF-3 is directly activated by dsRNA or by virus infection, and subsequently plays a role in the activation of the IFN-α and IFN-β promoters and IFN-α/β responsive genes (143). The HPV E6 oncoprotein binds selectively to IRF-3 but only very poorly to other cellular IRFs including IRF-2 and IRF-9. The association of E6 with IRF-3 inhibits the trans-activation function of IRF-3, thereby providing HPV with a mechanism to circumvent the antiviral response (288). Adenovirus E1A protein also inhibits IRF-3–mediated transcriptional activation by a mechanism that depends on the ability of E1A to bind p300. Overexpression of CBP/p300 partially reverses the E1A-mediated inhibition, which is not observed with mutant E1A protein that does not bind p300. CBP/p300 and PCAF histone acetyltransferase (HAT) enzymes are coactivators for several transcription factors including Stat1α, p53, and nuclear hormone receptors; the viral E1A protein represses HAT activity and inhibits p300-dependent transcription and nucleosomal histone modifications by PCAF (45).

There are several known examples in which viruses mimic one or more of the cellular components of the IFN signal transduction pathway. In some instances, this molecular mimicry leads to an antagonism of the IFN signaling process and subsequent impairment of the development of an antiviral state. Virus-coded homologs of IFN signal transduction pathway components include homologs of type I and type II IFN receptors, a viral ISRE-like promoter element that functions as a target of cellular IRF transcription factors, and a viral homolog of the interferon regulatory factor (IRF) family of transcription factors that represses the ISRE element function of IFN-inducible promoters. Soluble viral IFN receptor homologs (vIFN-γRc) encoded by poxviruses are secreted from virus-infected cells and bind IFNs, thereby preventing them from acting through their natural receptors to elicit an antiviral response (320). The first poxvirus receptor homolog identified, the M-T7 protein, was found in myxoma virus–infected cells and acts as a decoy to inhibit the biologic activity of rabbit IFN-γ. The vIFN-γRc gene product is a critical virulence factor for poxvirus pathogenesis. Myxoma virus lacking the M-T7 gene is highly attenuated; infected rabbits survive and do not develop myxomatosis. Other poxviruses also encode soluble IFN-γ receptor homologs, including vaccinia virus in which the B8R gene encodes the IFN-γRc homolog. Vaccinia virus and several other orthopoxviruses also express a soluble vIFN-α/βRc protein that, in the WR strain of vaccinia, is encoded by the B18R gene. The viral type I IFN receptor homolog of vaccinia virus binds several different IFN-α subspecies as well as IFN-β and blocks IFN-α/β signaling activity.

A viral ISRE-like element (vISRE) has been identified in the Q promoter (Qp) of Epstein-Barr virus (384). Qp is used for the transcription of EBV nuclear antigen 1 (EBNA1) during the highly restricted type I latent infection, but it is inactive in type III latency. Constitutive activation of EBV EBNA1 gene transcription is mediated in part by IRF-1 activation of the Qp promoter. Another IRF factor, IRF-7, binds to the vISRE-like sequence in Qp and represses transcriptional activation by both IFN and IRF-1. Expression of IRF-7 is high in type III latency cells but almost undetectable in type I latency, corresponding to the activity of the Qp of EBV in these latency states (384). The Jak-STAT signaling pathway positively regulates Qp activity, and the Zta up-regulation of p53 leads to p53-mediated interference with Jak-STAT activation of Qp (48). Conceivably, the binding of IRFs and Stats at Qp may be mutually exclusive. Interestingly, EBNA2, which is expressed in type III but not type I latency, is reported to have an anti-IFN effect, greatly impairing the induction of IFN-inducible genes (163).

Human herpesvirus 8 (HHV8), a gammaherpesvirus associated with Kaposi's sarcoma, encodes an IFN regulatory factor homolog (vIRF) that functions as a repressor of transcriptional activation induced by α, β, and γ IFNs (105,143). The vIRF product of the K9 ORF of HHV8 forms heterodimers with cellular IRF-1 and competes with binding of IRF-1 to the coactivator p300, thereby down-regulating transcriptional activation by the cellular IRFs. Thus, the HHV8 vIRF protein potentially plays an important role in HHV8 pathogenesis and neoplastic transformation by antagonizing IFN and IRF-mediated transcriptional control. Expression of vIRF antisense RNA in HHV8-infected cells increases IFN-mediated transcriptional activation and down-regulates expression of HHV8 genes. Overexpression of the viral vIRF in NIH3T3 cells induces transformation resulting in morphologic changes, focus formation, and growth in low serum concentrations (105), characteristics similar to the cellular IRF-2 repressor, which likewise mediates transformation of NIH3T3 cells and displays oncogenic potential in the nude mouse model (143).

Several viruses have evolved strategies to block the function of the IFN-inducible, RNA-dependent protein kinase PKR. Antagonism of PKR and the subsequent phosphorylation of eIF-2α have been directly linked to inhibition of the IFN-induced antiviral response of the host (55,102,215,298). Vaccinia virus, for example, can rescue IFN-sensitive viruses such as VSV and encephalomyocarditis virus from the antiviral effects of IFN by antagonizing the biochemical activity of PKR. The vaccinia E3L protein is a potent inhibitor of the PKR kinase and also the 2′,5′-oligoadenylate synthetase (OAS), two IFN-inducible RNA binding proteins (284, 297,314). E3L acts in part by sequestering activator RNA of PKR and 2′5′OAS. Deletion mutants of vaccinia virus lacking the E3L gene are sensitive to the antiviral effects of IFN, but RNA-binding proteins (including the reovirus σ3 protein, RNaseIII, TRBP, rotavirus NSP3, and E3L mutants that retain RNA binding activity) complement the E3L gene deletion and reverse the IFN-sensitive phenotype. Vaccinia mutants that express E3L proteins unable to bind dsRNA are IFN sensitive. Deletion mutants of vaccinia virus lacking the K3L gene, the eIF-2α homolog, are more sensitive to the antiviral effects of IFN than wild-type virus. Complementation studies suggest that the E3L gene product is most likely responsible for the vaccinia virus–mediated rescue of VSV from the antiviral effects of IFN, and that the K3L gene product is at least partially responsible for the rescue of EMC virus (313).

Adenovirus, influenza virus, PV, and SV40 provide four examples of viruses that antagonize the IFN-induced PKR kinase by different strategies. Adenovirus VAI RNA antagonizes the antiviral state of IFN by preventing activation of PKR; deletion mutants that do not express VAI RNA display IFN sensitivity, whereas wild-type virus that produces large amounts of VAI RNA is relatively resistant to type I IFN (214). The influenza virus NS1 protein, which binds RNA and prevents activation of PKR, plays a crucial role in inhibiting IFN-mediated antiviral responses of the host against influenza A virus (102,106,137). PV infection leads to a degradation of PKR (27), although the protease responsible for the down-regulation has not yet been identified. Translation of SV40 early RNA is relatively resistant to the antiviral effects of IFN (297). SV40 large T-antigen antagonizes PKR function but downstream of the kinase activation step (275). The mechanism is not resolved, but one possibility is a T-antigen–mediated enhancement of the phosphatase activity responsible for the dephosphorylation of eIF-2α similar to that observed in HSV-infected cells. In HSV infection, eIF-2α phosphorylation is reduced even though PKR is activated, because of the interaction of the HSV γ34.5 protein with phosphatase 1α (138).

Studies of the genetic evolution of HCV suggest that IFN-α therapy alters virus–host interactions as a result of changes in the nature of circulating HCV quasispecies (253). HCV genotype 1b resistance to IFN-α therapy is associated with changes in the HCV NS5A gene central region quasispecies (254). The HCV second envelope hypervariable region (HVR1), an 81-nucleotide sequence located at the 5′ end of the E2 gene, shows changes in HVR1 quasispecies major variants during and after IFN therapy in patients who failed to clear HCV RNA. Although the underlying mechanisms are unknown, one intriguing possibility is an IFN-mediated selection for resistant viruses mediated by editing of HCV viral RNA catalyzed by the IFN-inducible RNA-editing enzyme ADAR1 (252).

Apoptosis

Apoptosis, or controlled cell death, can serve as a defense mechanism for the host cell to combat viral infection. The apoptotic response involves a cascade of intracellular signals initiated in response to a wide variety of stimuli, including viral infection. Morphologic changes associated with apoptosis of virus-infected cells include condensation of chromatin and vacuolization of the infected cell's cytoplasm, and biochemical changes including activation of cellular proteases and nucleases and degradation of cell DNA to nucleosome-sized fragments. The fundamental importance of apoptosis as a component of the host response to viral infection is illustrated by the fact that a number of viruses encode gene products that either induce or inhibit apoptosis (86,132, 312,339). Untimely early destruction of infected host cells may greatly reduce virus yields. Hence, viruses have evolved strategies to antagonize the apoptotic response by encoding viral gene products that target effector components in the apoptotic cascade. Suppression or delay of apoptosis can extend the period of time available following infection to produce new virions prior to destruction of the host biosynthetic pathways utilized by the virus. The opposite also occurs. Viral gene products have been identified that function as inducers of apoptosis, possibly to facilitate release and spread of progeny virions from the infected host (86,132,312,339).

A wide variety of strategies is used by viruses to affect the balance between growth and death of the infected host cell. The adenovirus E1A gene product stabilizes p53 and induces p53-dependent apoptosis (312,339). This effect of E1A is countered by the adenovirus E1B-19kD, E1B-55kD, and E3 proteins, each of which can antagonize the apoptotic process. The adenovirus E3 gene product promotes the degradation of Fas which prevents apoptosis (345). The E1B-55kD–mediated block of apoptosis involves antagonism of p53 function (340), whereas the E1A-19kD protein is a Bcl-2 homolog that forms heterodimers with proteins such as Bax (365). Bcl-2 is an apoptosis suppressor that prolongs cell survival (25). Among the viral Bcl-2 homologs identified are the LMW5-HL protein of African swine fever virus that functions to antagonize apoptotic cell death, and the BHRF1 protein of EBV that protects human B cells from programmed death (132). The E6 protein of human papilloma virus and SV40 large T-antigen also impair p53-mediated apoptosis (132,312,339).

Cowpox virus blocks apoptosis by encoding CrmA, a serpin family protease inhibitor that blocks the interleukin-1β-converting enzyme (ICE) protease (100). ICE, a cysteine protease, is a key component of the apoptotic response in mammalian cells. The vaccinia virus B13R gene product is homologous to CrmA and inhibits apoptosis induced by Fas or TNFα (75). The baculovirus p35 protein, which prevents apoptosis during infection of insect cells, likewise inhibits the ICE family of proteases (225). Apoptosis via the Fas and TNF death receptors involving death domain (FADD) signaling cascade involves recruitment of several proteins including the procaspase 8 protease FLICE. Lymphotropic γ-herpesviruses (including HHV8, herpesvirus saimiri, equine herpesvirus-2, and bovine herpesvirus-4) encode FLICE-inhibitory proteins known as vFLIPS that are recruited to the activated receptor, but vFLIPS lack proteolytic activity and thus do not activate death signals (348).

Type I IFNs are essential mediators of apoptosis. Primary mouse embryonic fibroblasts undergo apoptosis when infected with EMC virus, VSV, and HSV, but apoptosis induced by these viruses is inhibited by anti-IFN-α/β antibodies and in homozygous null cells lacking either the IFN receptor or the Stat1 signaling factor (335). IFN alone does not induce apoptosis unless the treatment is combined with double-stranded RNA. Two important mediators of the IFN-induced antiviral response, the PKR kinase (334) and the 2′-5′A-dependent RNase L (73,385), play key roles as effectors of apoptosis. Overexpression of wild-type PKR but not catalytically inactive PKR causes apoptosis in the presence of dsRNA (9). Induction of apoptosis by PKR involves eIF-2α and NF-κB, because overexpression of the S51A mutant of eIF-2α or the S32,36A mutant of IκBα led to an inhibition of apoptosis (114). Interestingly, an up-regulation of Fas receptor mRNA accumulation correlates with PKR activation and subsequent apoptosis (77,114). Apoptosis is substantially suppressed following treatment with dsRNA, TNF-α, or lipopolysaccharide of cells from mice with a targeted disruption of either the PKR gene (70) or the RNase L gene (385). Suppression of apoptosis in the PKR null cells was associated with defects in activation of IRF-1 and in Fas mRNA induction (70). Several viral antagonists of PKR function have been described (102,298); presumably, repression of PKR by these viral products would impair the apoptotic response. For example, the antiapoptotic and oncogenic potentials of HCV virus are linked to IFN resistance by viral repression of the PKR protein kinase (103). Resistance to apoptosis is attributed to an HCV NS5A-mediated block in eIF-2α phosphorylation; furthermore, cells expressing NS5A exhibit a transformed phenotype.

SUMMARY

The major points of this chapter can be summarized as follows:

1. The ability of a virus to replicate in a host cell can be determined by the availability of specific macromolecules in that type of cell. These molecules may be external, such as a receptor, or internal, such as a transcription or replication factor.
2. Some of the cytopathic effects of virus infection on a host cell are caused by specific alterations in host-cell metabolism or structure that allow viral replication events. These cytopathic effects are usually not simply toxic effects of virus infection. Instead, viruses have evolved to manipulate the environment of the host cell for their own optimal replication.
3. Interactions of viruses with host cells may involve subtle changes in the host cell, and an understanding of the nature of the interactions between viral gene products and the host-cell molecules often provides insight into the metabolic processes and critical regulatory events of the host cell.
4. The host cell often responds to viral infection, such as by synthesis of IFN and induction of apoptosis. Viruses have evolved to counter these defenses, and this evolutionary chess game continues.

Thus, our challenge continues to be to attempt to relate this information about the interactions of viruses with their host cells to the biology of viruses in their host organisms, and to apply this knowledge to the design of effective antiviral strategies.

REFERENCES

1. Adams A, Lindahl T. Epstein-Barr virus genomes with properties of circular DNA molecules in carrier cells. *Proc Natl Acad Sci U S A* 1975;72:1477–1481.
2. Agris CH, Nemeroff ME, Krug RM. A block in mammalian splicing occurring after formation of large complexes containing U1, U2, U4, U5 and U6 small nuclear ribonucleoproteins. *Mol Cell Biol* 1989;9: 259–267.
3. Aiyar A, Tyree C, Sugden B. The plasmid replicon of EBV consists of multiple cis-acting elements that facilitate DNA synthesis by the cell and a viral maintenance element. *EMBO J* 1998;17:6394–6403.
4. Alam SL, Wills NM, Ingram JA, et al. Structural studies of the RNA pseudoknot required for readthrough of the gag-termination codon of murine leukemia virus. *J Mol Biol* 1999;288:837–852.
5. Angeletti PC, Engler JA. Adenovirus preterminal protein binds to the CAD enzyme at active sites of viral DNA replication on the nuclear matrix. *J Virol* 1998;72:2896–2904.
6. Avitabile E, Di Gaeta S, Torrisi MR, et al. Redistribution of microtubules and Golgi apparatus in Herpes simplex virus-infected cells and their role in viral exocytosis. *J Virol* 1995;69:7472–7482.
7. Babiss LE, Ginsberg HS, Darnell JE. Adenovirus EIB proteins are required for accumulation of late viral mRNA and for effects on cellular mRNA translation and transport. *Mol Cell Biol* 1985;5: 2552–2558.
8. Bagchi S, Raychaudhuri P, Nevins JR. Adenovirus EIA protein can dissociate heteromeric complexes involving the E2F transcription factor: A novel mechanism for EIA trans-activation. *Cell* 1990;62:659–669.
9. Balachandran S, Kim CN, Yeh WC, et al. Activation of the dsRNA-dependent protein kinase, PKR, induces apoptosis through FADD-mediated death signaling. *EMBO J* 1998;17:6888–6902.
10. Ball JM, Mulligan MJ, Compans RW. Basolateral sorting of the HIV type 2 and SIV envelope glycoproteins in polarized epithelial cells: Role of the cytoplasmic domain. *AIDS Res Hum Retroviruses* 1997; 13:665–675.
11. Ballestas ME, Chatis PA, Kaye KM. Efficient persistence of extrachromosonal KSHV DNA mediated by latency-associated nuclear antigen. *Science* 1999;284:641–644.
12. Banerji J, Rusconi L, Schaffner W. Expression of a alpha-globin gene is enhanced by remote SV40 DNA sequences. *Cell* 1981;27:299–308.
13. Barton DJ, Sawicki SG, Sawicki DL. Solubilization and immunoprecipitation of alphavirus replication complexes. *J Virol* 1991;65: 1496–1506.
14. Belsham, GJ, Sonenberg N. RNA-protein interactions in regulation of picornavirus RNA translation. *Microbiol Rev* 1996;60:499–511.
15. Beltz G, Flint SJ. Inhibition of HeLa cell protein synthesis during adenovirus infection: Restriction of cellular messenger jRNA sequences to the nucleus. *J Mol Biol* 1979;131:353–373.
16. Benkirane M, Neuveut C, Chun RF, et al. Oncogenic potential of TAR RNA binding protein TRBP and its regulatory interaction with RNA-dependent protein kinase PKR. *EMBO J* 1997;16:611–624.
17. Benoist C, Chambon P. In vivo sequence requirements of the SV40 early promoter region. *Nature* 1981;290:304–310.
18. Berezney R, Coffey DS. Nuclear protein matrix: Association with newly synthesized DNA. *Science* 1975;189:291–293.
19. Berger EA, Murphy PM, Farber JM. Chemokine receptors as HIV-1 coreceptors: Roles in viral entry, tropism, and disease. *Annu Rev Immunol* 1999;17:657–700.
20. Berger SL, Folk WR. Differential activation of RNA polymerase III-transcribed genes by the polyoma virus enhancer and adenovirus EIA gene products. *Nucleic Acids Res* 1985;13:1413–1428.
21. Berget SM, Moore C, Sharp PA. Spliced segments at the 5′ terminus of adenovirus 2 late mRNA. *Proc Natl Acad Sci U S A* 1977;74: 3171–3175.
22. Berk AJ. Adenovirus promoters and E1a transactivation. *Annu Rev Genet* 1986;20:45–79.
23. Berk AJ, Lee F, Harrison T, et al. Pre-early adenovirus 5 gene product regulates synthesis of early viral messenger RNAs. *Cell* 1979;17: 935–944.
24. Bienz K, Egger D, Pasamontes L. Association of poliovirus proteins of the P2 genomic region with the viral replication complex and virus-induced membrane synthesis as visualized by electron microscopic immunocytochemistry and autoradiography. *Virology* 1987;160: 220–226.
25. Bilbao G, Contreras JL, Zhang HG, et al. Adenovirus-mediated gene expression in vivo is enhanced by the antiapoptotic bcl-2 gene. *J Virol* 1999;73:6992–7000.
26. Black BL, Lyles DS. Vesicular stomatitis virus matrix protein inhibits host cell-directed transcription of target genes in vivo. *J Virol* 1992;66: 4058–4064.
27. Black TL, Barber GN, Katze MG. Degradation of the interferon-induced 68,000-M(r) protein kinase by poliovirus requires RNA. *J Virol* 1993;67:791–800.
28. Blackwell JL, Brinton MA. Translation elongation factor-1 alpha interacts with the 3′ stem-loop region of West Nile virus genomic RNA. *J Virol* 1997;71:6433–6444.
29. Bohmann D, Bos TJ, Admon A, et al. Human proto-oncogene c-*jun*

encodes a DNA binding protein with structural and functional properties of transcription factor AP-1. *Science* 1987;238:1386–1392.
30. Boone RF, Moss B. Sequence complexity and relative abundance of vaccinia virus mRNAs synthesized in vivo and in vitro. *J Virol* 1978;26:554–569.
31. Boshart M, Weber F, Jahn G, et al. A very strong enhancer is located upstream of an immediate-early gene of human cytomegalovirus. *Cell* 1985;41:521–530.
32. Boudin M, Moncany M, D'Halluin J, Boulanger PA. Isolation and characterization of adenovirus type 2 vertex capsomer (penton base). *Virology* 1979;92:125–138.
33. Bouloy M, Plotch SJ, Krug RM. Globin mRNAs are primers for the transcription of influenza viral RNA in vitro. *Proc Natl Acad Sci U S A* 1978;75:4886–4890.
34. Boyle KA, Pietropaolo RL, Compton T. Engagement of the cellular receptor for glycoprotein B of human cytomegalovirus activates the interferon-responsive pathway. *Mol Cell Biol* 1999;19:3607–3613.
35. Brand SR, Kobayashi R, Mathews MB. The Tat protein of human immunodeficiency virus type 1 is a substrate and inhibitor of the interferon-induced, virally activated protein kinase, PKR. *J Biol Chem* 1997;272:8388–8395.
36. Brierley I. Ribosomal frameshifting viral RNAs. *J Gen Virol* 1995;76: 1885–1892.
37. Brigati DJ, Myerson D, Leary JJ, et al. Detection of viral genomes in cultured cells and paraffin-embedded tissue sections using biotin-labeled hybridization probes. *Virology* 1983;126:32–50.
38. Bui M, Whittaker G, Helenius A. Effect of M1 protein and low pH on nuclear transport of influenza virus ribonucleoproteins. *J Virol* 1996; 70:8391–8401.
39. Bush M, Yager DR, Gao M, et al. Correct intranuclear localization of Herpes simplex virus DNA polymerase requires the viral ICP8 DNA-binding protein. *J Virol* 1991;65:1082–1089.
40. Caliguiri LA, Tamm I. Membranous structures associated with translation and transcription of poliovirus RNA. *Science* 1969;166: 885–886.
41. Campbell MEM, Palfreyman JW, Preston CM. Identification of herpes simplex virus DNA sequences which encode a trans-acting polypeptide responsible for stimulation of immediate early transcription. *J Mol Biol* 1984;180:1–19.
42. Cantin E, Tanamachi B, Openshaw H, et al. Gamma interferon (IFN-gamma) receptor null-mutant mice are more susceptible to herpes simplex virus type 1 infection than IFN-gamma ligand null-mutant mice. *J Virol* 1999;73:5196–5200.
43. Cassady KA, Gross M, Roizman B. The herpes simplex virus US11 protein effectively compensates for the gamma1(34.5) gene if present before activation of protein kinase R by precluding its phosphorylation and that of the alpha subunit of eukaryotic translation initiation factor 2. *J Virol* 1998;72:8620–8626.
44. Cattaneo R, Schmid A, Eschle D, et al. Biased hypermutation and other genetic changes in defective measles viruses in human brain infections. *Cell* 1988;55:255–265.
45. Chakravarti D, Ogryzko V, Kao HY, et al. A viral mechanism for inhibition of p300 and PCAF acetyltransferase activity. *Cell* 1999;96:393–403.
46. Challberg MD. A method for identifying the viral genes required for herpesvirus DNA replication. *Proc Natl Acad Sci U S A* 1986;83: 9094–9098.
47. Chardonnet Y, Dales S. Early events in the interaction of adenoviruses with HeLa cells. III. Relationship between an ATPase activity in nuclear envelopes and transfer of core material: A hypothesis. *Virology* 1972;42:342–359.
48. Chen H, Lee JM, Wang Y, et al. The Epstein-Barr virus latency BamHI-Q promoter is positively regulated by STATs and Zta interference with JAK/STAT activation leads to loss of BamHI-Q promoter activity. *Proc Natl Acad Sci U S A* 1999;96:9339–9344.
49. Chen X, Kang H, Shen LX, et al. A characteristic bent conformation of RNA pseudoknots promotes −1 frameshifting during translation of retroviral RNA. *J Mol Biol* 1996;260:479–483.
50. Chong LD, Rose JK. Interactions of normal and mutant vesicular stomatitis virus matrix proteins with the plasma membrane and nucleocapsids. *J Virol* 1994;68:441–447.
51. Chow LT, Gelinas RE, Broker TR, Roberts RJ. An amazing sequence arrangement at the 5′ ends of adenovirus 2 messenger RNA. *Cell* 1977;12:1–8.
52. Cimarelli A, Luban J. Translation elongation factor 1-alpha interacts specifically with the human immunodeficiency virus type 1 Gag polyprotein. *J Virol* 1999;73:5388–5401.
53. Clark ME, Lieberman PM, Berk AJ, Dasgupta A. Direct cleavage of human TATA-binding protein by poliovirus protease 3C in vivo and in vitro. *Mol Cell Biol* 1993;13:1232–1237.
54. Clayson ET, Brando LVJ, Compans RW. Release of simian virus 40 virions from epithelial cells is polarized and occurs without cell lysis. *J Virol* 1989;63:2278–2288.
55. Clemens MJ, Elia A. The double-stranded RNA-dependent protein kinase PKR: structure and function. *J Interferon Cytokine Res* 1997; 17:503–524.
56. Cotter MAN, Robertson ES. The latency-associated nuclear antigen tethers the Kaposi's sarcoma-associated herpesvirus genome to host chromosomes in body cavity-based lymphoma cells. *Virology* 1999; 264:254–264.
57. Craven RC, Harty RN, Paragas J, et al. Late domain function identified in the vesicular stomatitis virus M protein by use of rhabdovirus-retrovirus chimeras. *J Virol* 1999;73:3359–3365.
58. Cripe TP, Haugen TH, Turk JP. Transcriptional regulation of the human papilloma virus-16 E6-E7 promoter by a keratinocyte-depedent enhancer and by viral E2 trans-activator and repressor gene products: Implications for cervical carinogenesis. *EMBO J* 1987;6:3745–3753.
59. Cuconati A, Molla A, Wimmer E. Brefeldin A inhibits cell-free, de novo synthesis of poliovirus. *J Virol* 1998;72:6456–6464.
60. Cudmore S, Cossart P, Griffiths G, Way M. Actin-based motility of vaccinia virus. *Nature* 1995;378:636–638.
61. Cullen BR. Mechanism of action of regulatory proteins encoded by complex retroviruses. *Microbiol Rev* 1992;56:375–394.
62. Dales S, Gomatos PJ, Hsu KC. The uptake and development of reovirus in strain L cells followed with labelled viral ribonucleic acid and ferritin-antibody conjugates. *Virology* 1965;26:193–211.
63. Darlington RW, James C. Biological and morphological aspects of the growth of equine abortion virus. *J Bacteriol* 1966;92:250–257.
64. Das T, Mathur M, Gupta AK, et al. RNA polymerase of vesicular stomatitis virus specifically associates with translation elongation factor-1 alphabetagamma for its activity. *Proc Natl Acad Sci U S A* 1998; 95:1449–1454.
65. Davey J, Dimmock NJ, Colman A. Identification of the sequence responsible for the nuclear accumulation of the influenza virus nucleoprotein in *Xenopus oocytes*. *Cell* 1985;40:667–675.
66. de Bruyn Kops A, Knipe DM. Formation of DNA replication structures in herpes virus-infected cells requires a viral DNA binding protein. *Cell* 1988;55:857–868.
67. de Bruyn Kops A, Knipe DM. Preexisting nuclear architecture defines the intranuclear location of herpesvirus DNA replication structures. *J Virol* 1994;68:3512–3526.
68. DeCaprio JA, Ludlow JW, Figge J, et al. SV40 large tumor antigen forms a specific complex with the product of the retinoblastoma susceptibility gene. *Cell* 1988;54:275–283.
69. Demarchi F, Gutierrez MI, Giacca M. Human immunodeficiency virus type 1 tat protein activates transcription factor NF-kappaB through the cellular interferon-inducible, double-stranded RNA-dependent protein kinase, PKR. *J Virol* 1999;73:7080–7086.
70. Der SD, Yang YL, Weissmann C, Williams BR. A double-stranded RNA-activated protein kinase-dependent pathway mediating stress-induced apoptosis. *Proc Natl Acad Sci U S A* 1997;94:3279–3283.
71. Desai SY, Patel RC, Sen GC, et al. Activation of interferon-inducible 2′-5′ oligoadenylate synthetase by adenoviral VAI RNA. *J Biol Chem* 1995;270:3454–3461.
72. Dever TE, Sripriya R, McLachlin JR, et al. Disruption of cellular translational control by a viral truncated eukaryotic translation initiation factor 2alpha kinase homolog. *Proc Natl Acad Sci U S A* 1998;95: 4164–4169.
73. Diaz-Guerra M, Rivas C, Esteban M. Activation of the IFN-inducible enzyme RNase L causes apoptosis of animal cells. *Virology* 1997;236: 354–363.
74. Didcock L, Young DF, Goodbourn S, Randall RE. Sendai virus and simian virus 5 block activation of interferon-responsive genes: Importance for virus pathogenesis. *J Virol* 1999;73:3125–3133.
75. Dobbelstein M, Shenk T. Protection against apoptosis by the vaccinia virus SPI-2 (B13R) gene product. *J Virol* 1996;70:6479–6485.
76. Dominguez DI, Ryabova LA, Pooggin MM, et al. Ribosome shunting in cauliflower mosaic virus. Identification of an essential and sufficient structural element. *J Biol Chem* 1998;273:3669–3678.

77. Donze O, Dostie J, Sonenberg N. Regulatable expression of the interferon-induced double-stranded RNA dependent protein kinase PKR induces apoptosis and fas receptor expression. *Virology* 1999;256: 322–329.
78. Doohan JP, Samuel CE. Biosynthesis of reovirus-specified polypeptides. Analysis of ribosome pausing during translation of reovirus S1 and S4 mRNAs in virus-infected and vector-transfected cells. *J Biol Chem* 1993;268:18313–18320.
79. Dulbecco R, Harturell LN, Vogt M. Induction of cellular DNA synthesis by polyoma virus. *Proc Natl Acad Sci U S A* 1965;53:403–408.
80. Dunigan DD, Baird S, Lucas-Lenard J. Lack of correlation between the accumulation of plus-strand leader RNA and the inhibition of protein and RNA synthesis in vesicular stomatitis infected mouse L cells. *Virology* 1986;150:231–246.
81. Elliott G, O'Hare P. Herpes simplex virus type 1 tegument protein VP22 induces the stabilization and hyperacetylation of microtubules. *J Virol* 1998;72:6448–6455.
82. Enders JF. Cytopathology of virus infections. *Annu Rev Microbiol* 1954;8:473–502.
83. Enders JF, Weller TH, Robbins FC. Cultivation of the Lansing strain of poliomyelitis virus in cultures of various human embryonic tissues. *Science* 1949;109:85–87.
84. Enquist LW, Husak PJ, Banfield BW, Smith GA. Infection and spread of alphaherpesviruses in the nervous system. *Adv Virus Res* 1998;51: 237–347.
85. Erwin C, Brown DT. Requirement of cell nucleus for Sindbis virus replication in cultured *Aedes albopictus* cells. *J Virol* 1983;45:792–799.
86. Everett H, McFadden G. Apoptosis: An innate immune response to virus infection. *Trends Microbiol* 1999;7:160–165.
87. Everett SF, Ginsberg HS. A toxinlike material separable from type 5 adenovirus particles. *Virology* 1958;6:770–771.
88. Everly DN Jr, Read GS. Mutational analysis of the virion host shutoff gene (U_L41) of herpes simplex virus (HSV): Characterization of HSV type 1 (HSV-1)/HSV-2 chimeras. *J Virol* 1997;71:7157–7166.
89. Farabaugh PJ. Programmed translational frameshifting. *Microbiol Rev* 1996;60:103–134.
90. Feinberg MB, Jarrett RF, Aldovini A, et al. HTLV-II expression and production involve complex regulation at the levels of splicing and translation of viral RNA. *Cell* 1986;46:807–817.
91. Fenwick M, Morse LS, Roizman B. Anatomy of herpes simplex virus DNA. XI. Apparent clustering of functions effecting rapid inhibition of host DNA and protein synthesis. *J Virol* 1979;29:825–827.
92. Fenwick ML, Walker MJ. Suppression of the synthesis of cellular macromolecules by herpes simplex virus. *J Gen Virol* 1978;41:37–51.
93. Ferran MC, Lucas-Lenard JM. The vesicular stomatitis virus matrix protein inhibits transcription from the human beta interferon promoter. *J Virol* 1997;71:371–377.
94. Fornerod M, Ohno M, Yoshida M, Mattaj IW. CRM1 is an export receptor for leucine-rich nuclear export signals [see comments]. *Cell* 1997;90:1051–1060.
95. Fouchier RA, Meyer BE, Simon JH, et al. HIV-1 infection of non-dividing cells: Evidence that the amino-terminal basic region of the viral matrix protein is important for Gag processing but not for post-entry nuclear import. *EMBO J* 1997;16:4531–4539.
96. Fraenkel-Conrat H, Wagner RR. *Viral Cytopathology, Comprehensive Virology.* New York: Plenum Press, 1984.
97. Fredman JN, Engler JA. Adenovirus precursor to terminal protein interacts with the nuclear matrix in vivo and in vitro. *J Virol* 1993;67: 3384–3395.
98. Freed EO, Englund G, Maldarelli F, Martin MA. Phosphorylation of residue 131 of HIV-1 matrix is not required for macrophage infection. *Cell* 1997;88:171–173.
99. Frischknecht F, Moreau V, Rottger S, et al. Actin-based motility of vaccinia virus mimics receptor tyrosine kinase signalling. *Nature* 1999;401:926–929.
100. Gagliardini V, Fernandez PA, Lee RK, et al. Prevention of vertebrate neuronal death by the crmA gene [see comments] [published erratum appears in *Science* 1994;264:1388]. *Science* 1994;263:826–828.
101. Gale M Jr, Blakely CM, Kwieciszewski B, et al. Control of PKR protein kinase by hepatitis C virus nonstructural 5A protein: Molecular mechanisms of kinase regulation. *Mol Cell Biol* 1998;18:5208–5218.
102. Gale M, Katze MG. Molecular mechanisms of interferon resistance mediated by viral-directed inhibition of PKR, the interferon-induced protein kinase. *Pharmacol Ther* 1998;78:29–46.
103. Gale M Jr, Kwieciszewski B, Dossett M, et al. Antiapoptotic and oncogenic potentials of hepatitis C virus are linked to interferon resistance by viral repression of the PKR protein kinase. *J Virol* 1999;73: 6506–6516.
104. Gallay P, Hope T, Chin D, Trono D. HIV-1 infection of nondividing cells through the recognition of integrase by the importin/karyopherin pathway. *Proc Natl Acad Sci U S A* 1997;94:9825–9830.
105. Gao SJ, Boshoff C, Jayachandra S, et al. KSHV ORF K9 (vIRF) is an oncogene which inhibits the interferon signaling pathway. *Oncogene* 1997;15:1979–1985.
106. Garcia-Sastre A, Egorov A, Matassov D, et al. Influenza A virus lacking the NS1 gene replicates in interferon-deficient systems. *Virology* 1998;252:324–330.
107. Garcin D, Latorre P, Kolakofsky D. Sendai virus C proteins counteract the interferon-mediated induction of an antiviral state. *J Virol* 1999;73:6559–6565.
108. Garnier L, Wills JW, Verderame MF, Sudol M. WW domains and retrovirus budding. *Nature* 1996;381:744–745.
109. Gaynor RB, Feldman LT, Berk AJ. Transcription of class III genes activated by viral immediate early proteins. *Science* 1985;230:447–450.
110. Geisberg JV, Chen JL, Ricciardi RP. Subregions of the adenovirus E1A transactivation domain target multiple components of the TFIID complex. *Mol Cell Biol* 1995;15:6283–6290.
111. George CX, Samuel CE. Human RNA-specific adenosine deaminase ADAR1 transcripts possess alternative exon 1 structures that initiate from different promoters, one constitutively active and the other interferon inducible. *Proc Natl Acad Sci U S A* 1999;96:4621–4626.
112. Gerster T, Roeder RG. A herpesvirus trans-activating protein interacts with transcription factor OTF-1 and other cellular proteins. *Proc Natl Acad Sci U S A* 1988;85:6347–6351.
113. Giege R, Frugier M, Rudinger J. tRNA mimics [published erratum appears in *Curr Opin Struct Biol* 1998;8:812]. *Curr Opin Struct Biol* 1998;8:286–293.
114. Gil J, Alcami J, Esteban M. Induction of apoptosis by double-stranded-RNA-dependent protein kinase (PKR) involves the alpha subunit of eukaryotic translation initiation factor 2 and NF-kappaB. *Mol Cell Biol* 1999;19:4653–4663.
115. Gingras AC, Raught B, Sonenberg N. eIF4E initiation factors: Effectors of mRNA recruitment to ribosomes and regulators of translation. *Ann Rev Biochem* 1999;68:913–968.
116. Goodrich LD, Schaffer PA, Dorsky DI, et al. Localization of the herpes simplex virus type 1 65-kilodalton DNA-binding protein and DNA polymerase in the presence and absence of viral DNA synthesis. *J Virol* 1990;64:5738–5749.
117. Gradi A, Svitkin YV, Imataka H, Sonenberg N. Proteolysis of human eukaryotic translation initiation factor eIF4GII, but not eIF4GI, coincides with the shutoff of host protein synthesis after poliovirus infection. *Proc Natl Acad Sci U S A* 1998;95:11089–11094.
118. Granzow H, Weiland F, Jons A, et al. Ultrastructural analysis of the replication cycle of pseudorabies virus in cell culture: A reassessment. *J Virol* 1997;71:2072–2082.
119. Greber UF, Singh I, Helenius A. Mechanisms of virus uncoating. *Trends Microbiol* 1994;53:52–56.
120. Greber UF, Webster P, Weber J, Helenius A. The role of the adenovirus protease in virus entry into cells. *EMBO J* 1996;15:1766–1777.
121. Green MR, Treisman R, Maniatis T. Transcriptional activation of cloned human B-globin genes by viral immediate early genes. *Cell* 1983;35:137–148.
122. Grieder FB, Vogel SN. Role of interferon and interferon regulatory factors in early protection against Venezuelan equine encephalitis virus infection. *Virology* 1999;257:106–118.
123. Griffith GR, Marriot SJ, Rintoul DA, Consilgi RA. Early events in polyomavirus infection: Fusion of monopinocytotic vesicles with mouse kidney cells. *Virus Res* 1988;10:41–51.
124. Grimley PM, Levin JG, Berezesky IK, Friedman RM. Specific membranous structures associated with the replication of group A arboviruses. *J Virol* 1972;10:492–503.
125. Grinnell BW, Wagner RR. Inhibition of DNA-dependent transcription by the leader RNA of vesicular stomatitis virus: Role of specific nucleotide sequences and cell protein binding. *Mol Cell Biol* 1985;5: 2502–2513.
126. Grogan EA, Summers WP, Dowling S, et al. Two Epstein-Barr viral nuclear neoantigens distinguished by gene transfer, serology, and chromosome binding. *Proc Natl Acad Sci U S A* 1983;80:7650–7653.

127. Gruda MC, Zabolotny JM, Xiao JH, et al. Transcriptional activation by simian virus 40 large T antigen: Interactions with multiple components of the transcription complex. *Mol Cell Biol* 1993;13:961–969.
128. Gupta S, De BP, Drazba JA, Banerjee AK. Involvement of action microfilaments in the replication of human parainfluenza virus type 3. *J Virol* 1998;72:2655–2662.
129. Gustin KE, Imperiale MJ. Encapsidation of viral DNA requires the adenovirus L1 52/55 kilodalton protein. *J Virol* 1998;72:7860–7870.
130. Halbert DN, Cutt J, Shenk T. Adenovirus early region 4 encodes functions required for efficient DNA replication, late gene expression, and host cell shut-off. *J Virol* 1985;56:250–257.
131. Hamaguchi M, Nishikawa K, Toyoda T, et al. Transcriptive complex of Newcastle disease virus. *Virology* 1985;147:295–308.
132. Hardwick JM. Viral interference with apoptosis. *Semin Cell Dev Biol* 1998;9:339–349.
133. Hardwicke MA, Sandri-Goldin RM. The herpes simplex virus regulatory protein ICP27 contributes to the decrease in cellular mRNA levels during infection. *J Virol* 1994;68:4797–4810.
134. Hardy WR, Sandri-Goldin RM. Herpes simplex virus inhibits host cell splicing, and regulatory protein ICP27 is required for this effect. *J Virol* 1994;68:7790–7799.
135. Hartley JW, Rowe WP, Huebner RJ. Host range restrictions of murine leukemia viruses in mouse embryo cell cultures. *J Virol* 1970;5: 221–225.
136. Harty RN, Paragas J, Sudol M, Palese P. A proline-rich motif within the matrix protein of vesicular stomatitis virus and rabies virus interacts with WW domains of cellular proteins: Implications for viral budding. *J Virol* 1999;73:2921–2929.
137. Hatada E, Saito S, Fukuda R. Mutant influenza viruses with a defective NS1 protein cannot block the activation of PKR in infected cells. *J Virol* 1999;73:2425–2433.
138. He B, Gross M, Roizman B. The gamma 34.5 protein of herpes simplex virus 1 complexes with protein phosphatase 1 alpha to dephosphorylate the alpha subunit of the eukaryotic translation initiation factor 2 and preclude the shutoff of protein synthesis by double-stranded RNA-activated protein kinase. *Proc Natl Acad Sci U S A* 1997;94: 843–848.
139. Hearing P, Shenk T. The adenovirus type 5 EIA transcriptional control region contains a duplicated enhancer element. *Cell* 1983;33: 695–703.
140. Heinzinger NK, Bukrinsky MI, Haggerty SA, et al. The Vpr protein of human immunodeficiency virus type 1 influences nuclear localization of viral nucleic acids in nondividing host cells. *Proc Natl Acad Sci U S A* 1994;91:7311–7315.
141. Herz C, Stavnezer E, Krug RM, Gurney T. Influenza virus, an RNA virus, synthesizes its messenger RNA in the nucleus of infected cells. *Cell* 1981;26:391–400.
142. Hill VM, Harmon SA, Summers DF. Stimulation of vesicular stomtatis virus in vitro RNA synthesis by microtubule-associated proteins. *Proc Natl Acad Sci U S A* 1986;83:5410–5413.
143. Hiscott J, Pitha P, Genin P, et al. Triggering the interferon response: The role of IRF-3 transcription factor. *J Interferon Cytokine Res* 1999;19:1–13.
144. Hoeffler WK, Roeder RG. Enhancement of RNA polymerase III transcription by the EIA product of adenovirus. *Cell* 1985;41:955–963.
145. Horikoshi N, Maguire K, Kralli N, et al. Direct interaction between adenovirus EIA protein and the TATA box binding transcription factor IID. *Proc Natl Acad Sci U S A* 1991;88:5124–5128.
146. Horikoshi N, Usheva A, Chen J, et al. Two domains of p53 interact with the TATA-binding protein, and the adenovirus 13S E1A protein disrupts the association, relieving p53-mediated transcriptional repression. *Mol Cell Biol* 1995;15:227–234.
147. Horsburgh BC, Kollmus H, Hauser H, Coen DM. Translational recoding induced by G-rich mRNA sequences that form unusual structures. *Cell* 1996;86:949–959.
148. Horwitz M, Brayton C, Baum SG. Synthesis of type 2 adenovirus DNA in the presence of cycloheximide. *J Virol* 1973;11:544–551.
149. Howley PM. The molecular biology of papilloma virus transformation. *Am J Pathol* 1983;113:413–421.
150. Huang QS, Valyi-Nagy T, Kesari S, Fraser NW. beta-Gal enzyme activity driven by the HSV LAT promoter does not correspond to beta-gal RNA levels in mouse trigeminal ganglia. *Gene Ther* 1997;4:797–807.
151. Ilves I, Kivi S, Ustav M. Long-term episomal maintenance of bovine papillomavirus type 1 plasmids is determined by attachment to host chromosomes, which is mediated by the viral E2 protein and its binding sites. *J Virol* 1999;73:4404–4412.
152. Imperiale MJ, Feldman LT, Nevins JR. Activation of gene expression by adenovirus and herpesvirus regulatory genes acting in trans and by a cis-acting adenovirus enhancer element. *Cell* 1983;35:127–136.
153. Inglis SC. Inhibition of host protein synthesis and degradation of cellular mRNAs during infection by influenza and herpes simplex virus. *Mol Cell Biol* 1982;2:1644–1648.
154. Isaacs A, Lindenmann J. Virus interference. I. The interferon. *Proc R Soc Lond B Biol Sci* 1957;147:258–267.
155. Ishov AM, Maul GG. The periphery of nuclear domain 10 (ND10) as site of DNA virus deposition. *J Cell Biol* 1996;134:815–826.
156. Jacks T, Power MD, Masiarz FR, et al. Characterization of ribosomal frameshifting in HIV-1 gag-pol expression. *Nature* 1988;331: 280–283.
157. Jacks T, Varmus HE. Expression of the Rous sarcoma virus pol gene by ribosomal frameshifting. *Science* 1985;230:1237–1242.
158. Jang SK, Krausslich HG, Nicklin MJ, et al. A segment of the 5′ nontranslated region of encephalomyocarditis virus RNA directs internal entry of ribosomes during in vitro translation. *J Virol* 1988;62: 2636–2643.
159. Jones LV, Compans RW, Davis AR, et al. Surface expression of influenza virus neuraminidase, an amino-terminally anchored viral membrane glycoprotein, in polarized epithelical cells. *Cell Biol* 1985; 5:2181–2189.
160. Jones N, Shenk T. An adenovirus type 5 early gene function regulates expression other early viral genes. *Proc Natl Acad Sci U S A* 1979;76: 3665–3669.
161. Justice PA, Sun W, Li Y, et al. Membrane vesiculation function and exocytosis of wild-type and mutant matrix proteins of vesicular stomatitis virus. *J Virol* 1995;69:3156–3160.
162. Kalderon D, Roberts BL, Richardson WD, Smith AE. A short amino acid sequence able to specify nuclear location. *Cell* 1984;39:499.
163. Kanda K, Decker T, Aman P, et al. The EBNA2-related resistance towards alpha interferon (IFN-alpha) in Burkitt's lymphoma cells effects induction of IFN-induced genes but not the activation of transcription factor ISGF-3 [published erratum appears in *Mol Cell Biol* 1993;13:1981]. *Mol Cell Biol* 1992;12:4930–4936.
164. Kaplan AS. A brief review of the biochemistry of herpesvirus-host cell interaction. *Cancer Res* 1973;33:1393–1398.
165. Kartenbeck J, Stukenbrok H, Helenius A. Endocytosis of simian virus 40 into the endoplasmic reticulum. *J Cell Biol* 1989;109:2721–2729.
166. Kates JR, McAuslan B. Messenger RNA synthesis by a "coated" viral genome. *Proc Natl Acad Sci U S A* 1967;57:314–320.
167. Kawagishi-Kobayashi M, Silverman JB, Ung TL, Dever TE. Regulation of the protein kinase PKR by the vaccinia virus pseudosubstrate inhibitor K3L is dependent on residues conserved between the K3L protein and the PKR substrate eIF2alpha. *Mol Cell Biol* 1997;17: 4146–4158.
168. Kawaguchi Y, Bruni R, Roizman B. Interaction of herpes simplex virus 1 alpha regulatory protein ICP0 with elongation factor 1d: ICP0 affects translational machinery. *J Virol* 1997;71:1019–1024.
169. Kawaguchi Y, Matsumura T, Roizman B, Hirai K. Cellular elongation factor 1delta is modified in cells infected with representative alpha-, beta-, or gammaherpesviruses. *J Virol* 1999;73:4456–4460.
170. Kerekatte V, Keiper BD, Badorff C, et al. Cleavage of poly(A)-binding protein by coxsackievirus 2A protease in vitro and in vivo: Another mechanism for host protein synthesis shutoff? *J Virol* 1999;73: 709–717.
171. Kleijn M, Scheper GC, Voorma HO, Thomas AA. Regulation of translation initiation factors by signal transduction. *Eur J Biochem* 1998; 253:531–544.
172. Kleijn M, Vrins CL, Voorma HO, Thomas AA. Phosphorylation state of the cap-binding protein eIF4E during viral infection. *Virology* 1996;217:486–494.
173. Knight DM, Flomerheit FA, Ghrayeb J. Expression of the art/trs protein of HIV and study of its role in viral envelope synthesis. *Science* 1987;236:837–840.
174. Knipe DM. The role of viral and cellular nuclear proteins in herpes simplex virus replication. (Review.) *Adv Virus Res* 1989;37:85–123.
175. Knipe DM. The replication of herpes simplex virus. In: Stanberry LR, ed. *Genital and Neonatal Herpes.* Chichester, UK, John Wiley & Sons, 1996:1–29.
176. Knipe DM, Baltimore D, Lodish HF. Separate pathways of maturation

of the major structural proteins of vesicular stomatitis virus. *J Virol* 1977;21:1128–1139.
177. Knipe DM, Senechek D, Rice SA, Smith JL. Stages in the nuclear association of the herpes simplex virus transcriptional activator protein ICP4. *J Virol* 1987;61:276–284.
178. Kozak M. Initiation of translation in prokaryotes and eukaryotes. *Gene* 1999;234:187–208.
179. Kraus VB, Inostroza JA, Yeung K, et al. Interaction of the Dr1 inhibitory factor with the TATA binding protein is disrupted by adenovirus E1A. *Proc Natl Acad Sci U S A* 1994;91:6279–6282.
180. Kristie TM, Sharp PA. Purification of the cellular C1 factor required for the stable recognition of the Oct-1 homeodomain by the herpes simplex virus alpha-trans-induction factor (VP16). *J Biol Chem* 1993;268:6525–6534.
181. Krug RM. Unique functions of the NS1 protein. In: Nicholson KG, Webster RG, Hay AJ, eds. *Textbook of Influenza.* Oxford, UK: Blackwell Science, 1998:82–92.
182. Krug RM, Alonso-Kaplen FV, Julkunen I, Katze MG. Expression and replication of the influenza virus genome. In: Krug RM, ed. *The Influenza Viruses.* New York: Plenum, 1989:89–152.
183. Kumar M, Carmichael GG. Nuclear antisense RNA induces extensive adenosine modifications and nuclear retention of target transcripts. *Proc Natl Acad Sci U S A* 1997;94:3542–3547.
184. Kundu A, Avalos RT, Sanderson CM, Nayak DP. Transmembrane domain of influenza virus neuraminidase, a type II protein, possesses an apical sorting signal in polarized MDCK cells. *J Virol* 1996;70:6508–6515.
185. Kwong AD, Frenkel N. Herpes simplex virus-infected cells contain a function(s) that destabilizes both host and viral mRNAs. *Proc Natl Acad Sci U S A* 1987;84:1926–1930.
186. Lamb RA, Choppin PW, Chanock RM, Lai CJ. Mapping of the two overlapping genes for polypeptides NS1 and NS2 on RNA segment 8 of influenza virus. *Proc Natl Acad Sci U S A* 1980;77:1857–1861.
187. Lamb RA, Joshi SB, Dutch RE. The paramyxovirus fusion protein forms an extremely stable core trimer: Structural parallels to influenza virus haemagglutinin and HIV-1 gp41. *Mol Membr Biol* 1999;16:11–19.
188. Lamb RA, Lai CJ, Choppin PW. Sequences of mRNAs derived from genomic RNA segment 7 of influenza virus colinear and interrupted mRNAs code for overlapping proteins. *Proc Natl Acad Sci U S A* 1981;78:4170–4174.
189. Lamphear BJ, Rhoads RE. A single amino acid change in protein synthesis initiation factor 4G renders cap-dependent translation resistant to picornaviral 2A proteases. *Biochemistry* 1996;35:15726–15733.
190. Laver WG, Bischofberger N, Webster RE. Disarming flu viruses. *Sci Am* 1999;280:78–87.
191. Lee KAW, Hai TY, Siva Raman L. A cellular protein, activating transcription factor, acivates transcription of multiple E1A-inducible adenovirus early promoters. *Proc Natl Acad Sci U S A* 1987;84:8355–8359.
192. Lee WS, Kao CC, Bryant GO, et al. Adenovirus E1A activation domain binds the basic repeat in the TATA box transcription factor. *Cell* 1991;67:365–376.
193. Lehman CW, Botchan MR. Segregation of viral plasmids depends on tethering to chromosomes and is regulated by phosphorylation. *Proc Natl Acad Sci U S A* 1998;95:4338–4343.
194. Leonard GT, Sen GC. Restoration of interferon responses of adenovirus E1A-expressing HT1080 cell lines by overexpression of p48 protein. *J Virol* 1997;71:5095–5101.
195. Li G, Rice CM. The signal for translational readthrough of a UGA codon in Sindbis virus RNA involves a single cytidine residue immediately downstream of the termination codon. *J Virol* 1993;67:5062–5067.
196. Li JJ, Kelly TJ. Simian virus 40 DNA replication in vitro. *Proc Natl Acad Sci U S A* 1984;81:6973–6977.
197. Lilly F, Pincus T. Genetic control of murine viral leukemogenesis. *Adv Cancer Res* 1973;17:231–277.
198. Lipinski KS, Esche H, Brockmann D. Amino acids 1-29 of the adenovirus serotypes 12 and 2 E1A proteins interact with rap30 (TF(II)F) and TBP in vitro. *Virus Res* 1998;54:99–106.
199. Liptak L, Uprichard SL, Knipe DM. Functional order of assembly of herpes simplex virus DNA replication proteins into prereplicative site structures. *J Virol* 1996;70:1759–1767.
200. Liu Y, Emeson RB, Samuel CE. Serotonin-2C receptor pre-mRNA editing in rat brain and in vitro by splice site variants of the interferon-inducible double-stranded RNA-specific adenosine deaminase ADAR1. *J Biol Chem* 1999;274:18351–18358.
201. Lu B, Ebensperger C, Dembic Z, et al. Targeted disruption of the interferon-gamma receptor 2 gene results in severe immune defects in mice. *Proc Natl Acad Sci U S A* 1998;95:8233–8238.
202. Lukonis CJ, Weller SK. Characterization of nuclear structures in cells infected with herpes simplex virus type 1 in the absence of viral DNA replication. *J Virol* 1996;70:1751–1758.
203. Lusky M, Botchan MR. Characterization of the bovine papilloma virus plasmid maintenance sequences. *Cell* 1984;36:391–401.
204. Macejak DG, Sarnow P. Association of heat shock protein 70 with enterovirus capsid precursor P1 in infected human cells. *J Virol* 1992;66:1520–1527.
205. Maisner A, Klenck HD, Herrler G. Polarized budding of measles virus is not determined by viral surface glycoproteins. *J Virol* 1998;72:5276–5278.
206. Maitra RK, McMillan NA, Desai S, et al. HIV-1 TAR RNA has an intrinsic ability to activate interferon-inducible enzymes. *Virology* 1994;204:823–827.
207. Malim MH, Hauber J, Fenrick R, Cullen BR. Immunodeficiency virus *rev trans*-activator modulates the expression of the viral regulatory genes. *Nature* 1988;335:181–183.
208. Malim MH, Hauber J, Le SY, et al. The HIV *rev trans*–activator acts through a structured target sequence to activate nuclear export of unspliced viral mRNA. *Nature* 1989;338:254–257.
209. Marsden HS, Cross AM, Francis GJ, et al. The herpes simplex virus type 1 UL8 protein influences the intracellular localization of the UL52 but not the ICP8 or POL replication proteins in virus-infected cells. *J Gen Virol* 1996;77:2241–2249.
210. Martin K, Helenius A. Nuclear transport of influenza virus ribonucleoproteins: The viral matrix protein (MI) promotes export and inhibits import. *Cell* 1991;67:117–130.
211. Martin TE, Barghusen SC, Leser GP, Spear PG. Redistribution of nuclear ribonucleoprotein antigens during herpes simplex virus infection. *J Cell Biol* 1987;105:2069–2082.
212. Martinez-Palomo A, Granboulan N. Electron microscopy of adenovirus 12 replication. II. High-resolution autoradiography of infected KB cells labeled with tritiated thymidine. *J Virol* 1967;1:1010–1018.
213. Marvaldi J, Sekellick M, Marcus P, Lucas-Leonard J. Inhibition of mouse L cell protein synthesis by ultraviolet-irradiated vesicular stomatitis virus requires viral transcription. *Virology* 1978;84:127–133.
214. Mathews MB. Adenovirus virus-associated RNA and translational control. *J Virol* 1991;65:5657–5662.
215. Mathews MB. Viral evasion of cellular defense mechanisms: Regulation of the protein kinase DAI by RNA effectors. *Semin Virol* 1993;4:247–257.
216. Maul GG, Ishov AM, Everett RD. Nuclear domain 10 as preexisting potential replication start sites of herpes simplex virus type 1. *Virology* 1996;217:67–75.
217. Maul GG, Tovera G, Vorbrodt A, Abramczuk J. Membrane fusion as a mechanism of simian virus 40 entry into different cellular compartments. *J Virol* 1978;28:936–944.
218. Mazzarelli JM, Mengus G, Davidson I, Ricciardi RP. The transactivation domain of adenovirus E1A interacts with the C terminus of human TAF(II)135. *J Virol* 1997;71:7978–7983.
219. McCormack SJ, Samuel CE. Mechanism of interferon action: RNA-binding activity of full-length and R-domain forms of the RNA-dependent protein kinase PKR—Determination of KD values for VAI and TAR RNAs. *Virology* 1995;206:511–519.
220. McCready SJ, Godwin J, Mason DW, et al. DNA is replicated at the nuclear cage. *J Cell Science* 1980;46:365.
221. Mcknight JLC, Kristie TM, Roizman B. Binding of the virion protein mediating alpha gene induction in herpes simplex virus 1 infected cells to its cis site requires cellular proteins. *Proc Natl Acad Sci U S A* 1987;84:7061–7065.
222. McQueen NL, Nayak DP, Stephens EP, Compans RW. Polarized expression of a chimeric protein in which the transmembrane and cytoplasmic domains of the influenza virus hemagglutinin have been replaced by those of vesicular stomatitits virus G protein. *Proc Natl Acad Sci U S A* 1986;83:9318–9322.
223. Melville MW, Tan SL, Wambach M, et al. The cellular inhibitor of the PKR protein kinase, P58(IPK), is an influenza virus-activated co-chaperone that modulates heat shock protein 70 activity. *J Biol Chem* 1999;274:3797–3803.

224. Merrick WC. Mechanism and regulation of eukaryotic protein synthesis. *Microbiol Rev* 1992;56:291–315.
225. Miller LK. Baculovirus interaction with host apoptotic pathways. *J Cell Physiol* 1997;173:178–182.
226. Molla A, Paul AV, Wimmer E. Cell-free, de novo synthesis of poliovirus. *Science* 1991;254:1647–1651.
227. Morely SM, Curtis PS, Pain VM. eIF-4G: Translation's mystery factor begins to yield its secrets. *RNA* 1997;3:1085–1104.
228. Morgan C, Rosenkranz HS, Mednis B. Structure and development of viruses as observed in the electron microscope. X. Entry and uncoating of adenovirus. *J Virol* 1969;4:777–796.
229. Morrison TG, Lodish HF. Site of synthesis of membrane and non-membrane proteins of vesicular stomatitis virus. *J Biol Chem* 1975; 250:6955–6962.
230. Murakami Y, Wobbe CR, Weissbach L, et al. Role of DNA polymerase alpha and DNA primase in simian virus 40 DNA replication *in vitro. Proc Natl Acad Sci U S A* 1986;83:2869–2873.
231. Nagano Y, Kojima Y. Inhibition de l'infection vaccinale par un facteur liquide dans le tissu intecte par le virus homologue. *C R Soc Biol* 1958;152:1627–1629.
232. Naib ZM, Clepper AS, Elliott SR. Exfoliative cytology as an aid in diagnosis of ophthalmic lesions. *Acta Cytol* 1967;11:295–303.
233. Napthine S, Liphardt J, Bloys A, et al. The role of RNA pseudoknot stem 1 length in the promotion of efficient −1 ribosomal frameshifting. *J Mol Biol* 1999;288:305–320.
234. Nayak DP. A look at assembly and morphogenesis of orthomyxo and paramyxoviruses. *ASM News* 1996;62:411–414.
235. Nemeroff ME, Barabino SM, Li Y, et al. Influenza virus NS1 protein interacts with the cellular 30 kDa subunit of CPSF and inhibits 3′ end formation of cellular pre-mRNAs. *Mol Cell* 1998;1:991–1000.
236. Nemerow GR, Stewart PL. Role of alpha v integrins in adenovirus cell entry and gene delivery. *Microbiol Mol Biol Rev* 1999;63:725–734.
237. Nevins JR. Induction of the synthesis of a 70,000 dalton mammalian heat shock protein by the adenovirus Ela gene product. *Cell* 1982;29: 913–919.
238. Nevins JR. Control of cellular and viral transcription during adenovirus infection. *CRC Crit Rev Biochem* 1986;19:307–322.
239. Nevins JR. E2F: A link between the Rb tumor suppressor protein and viral encoproteins. *Science* 1992;258:424–429.
240. Newton AA. The involvement of nuclear membranes in the synthesis of herpes-type viruses. In: Biggs PM, de The G, Payre LN, eds. *Oncogenesis and Herpesviruses I.* Lyon: International Agency for Research on Cancer Scientific Publications, 1972:489.
241. Nicholson P, Addison C, Cross AM, et al. Localization of the herpes simplex virus type 1 major capsid protein VP5 to the cell nucleus requires the abundant scaffolding protein VP22a. *J Gen Virol* 1994;75: 1091–1099.
242. Nishioka Y, Silverstein S. Requirement of protein synthesis for the degradation of host mRNA in Friend erythroleukemia cells infected with HSV-1. *J Virol* 1978;27:619–627.
243. O'Neill RE, Jaskunas R, Blobel G, et al. Nuclear import of influenza virus RNA can be mediated by viral nucleoprotein and transport factors required for protein import. *J Biol Chem* 1995;270:22701–22704.
244. O'Neill RE, Palese P. NPI-1, the human homolog of SRP-1, interacts with influenza virus nucleoprotein. *Virology* 1995;206:116–125.
245. Ornelles DA, Shenk T. Localization of the adenovirus early region 1B 55-kilodalton protein during lytic infection: Association with nuclear viral inclusions requires the early region 4 34-kilodalton protein. *J Virol* 1991;65:424–429.
246. Oroskar AA, Read GS. A mutant of herpes simplex virus type 1 exhibits increased stability of immediate early (alpha) mRNAs. *J Virol* 1987;61:604–606.
247. Palese P, Compans RW. Inhibition of influenza replication in tissue culture by 2-deoxy2,3-dehydro-N-trifluoroacetylneuraminic acid (FANA) mechanism of action. *J Gen Virol* 1976;33:159–163.
248. Palese P, Schulman L, Bodo G, Meindl P. Inhibition of influenza and parainfluenza virus replication in tissue culture by 2-deoxy2,3-dehydro-N-trifluoroacetylneuraminic acid (FANA). *Virology* 1974;59:490–498.
249. Palese P, Tobita K, Ueda M, Compans RW. Characterization of temperature sensitive influenza virus mutants defective in neuraminidase. *Virology* 1974;61:397–410.
250. Paoletti E, Grady LJ. Transcriptional complexity of vaccinia virus in vivo and in vitro. *J Virol* 1977;23:608–615.
251. Park YW, Wilusz J, Katze MG. Regulation of eukaryotic protein synthesis: Selective influenza viral mRNA translation is mediated by the cellular RNA-binding protein GRSF-1. *Proc Natl Acad Sci U S A* 1999;96:6694–6699.
252. Patterson JB, Samuel CE. Expression and regulation by interferon of a double-stranded RNA-specific adenosine deaminase from human cells: Evidence for two forms of the deaminase. *Mol Cell Biol* 1995; 15:5376–5388.
253. Pawlotsky JM, Germanidis G, Frainais PO, et al. Evolution of the hepatitis C virus second envelope protein hypervariable region in chronically infected patients receiving alpha interferon therapy. *J Virol* 1999;73:6490–6499.
254. Pawlotsky JM, Germanidis G, Neumann AU, et al. Interferon resistance of hepatitis C virus genotype 1b: Relationship to nonstructural 5A gene quasispecies mutations. *J Virol* 1998;72:2795–2805.
255. Pelletier J, Sonenberg N. Internal initiation of translation of eukaryotic mRNA directed by sequence derived from poliovirus RNA. *Nature* 1988;334:320–325.
256. Penman S, Summers D. Effects on host cell metabolism following synchronous infection with poliovirus. *Virology* 1965;27:614–620.
257. Pereira HG. A protein factor responsible for the early cytopathic effect of adenoviruses. *Virology* 1958;6:601–611.
258. Pestova TV, Hellen CUT. Ribosome recruitment and scanning: What's new? *Trends Biochem Sci* 1999;24:85–87.
259. Phelan A, Carmo-Fonseca M, McLaughlan J, et al. A herpes simplex virus type 1 immediate-early gene product, IE63, regulates small nuclear ribonucleoprotein distribution. *Proc Natl Acad Sci U S A* 1993;90:9056–9060.
260. Phelan A, Dunlop J, Patel AH, et al. Nuclear sites of herpes simplex virus type 1 DNA replication and transcription colocalize at early times postinfection and are largely distinct from RNA processing factors. *J Virol* 1997;71:1124–1132.
261. Philipson L, Anderson P, Olshevsky U, et al. Translation of murial leukemia and sarcoma virus RNAs in nuclease-treated reticulocyte extracts enhancement of gag-pol polypeptides with yeast suppressor tRNA. *Cell* 1978;13:189–199.
262. Pilder S, Moore M, Logan J, Shenk T. The adenovirus E1B-55K transforming polypeptide modulates transport or cytoplasmic stabilization of viral and host cell mRNAs. *Mol Cell Biol* 1986;6:470–476.
263. Pinto LH, Holsinger LJ, Lamb RA. Influenza virus M2 protein has ion channel activity. *Cell* 1992;69:517–528.
264. Piron M, Vende P, Cohen J, Poncet D. Rotavirus RNA-binding protein NSP3 interacts with eIF4GI and evicts the poly(A) binding protein from eIF4F. *EMBO J* 1998;17:5811–5821.
265. Planck SR, Mueller GC. DNA chain growth and organization of replicating units in HeLa cells. *Biochemistry* 1977;16:1808.
266. Plotch SJ, Bouloy M, Ulmanen I, Krug RM. A unique cap (m7 GpppXm) dependent influenza virus endoculease cleaves capped RNAs to generate the primers that initiate viral RNA transcription. *Cell* 1981; 23:847–858.
267. Pogo BGT, Dales S. Biogenesis of poxvirus. Inactivation of host DNA polymerase by a component of the invading inoculum partide. *Proc Natl Acad Sci U S A* 1973;70:1726–1729.
268. Pogo BGT, Dales S. Biogenesis of poxvirus. Further evidence for inhibition of host and virus DNA synthesis by component of the invading inoculum particle. *Virology* 1974;58:377.
269. Pollack R, Goldman R. Synthesis of infective poliovirus in BSC-1 monkey cells enucleated with cytochalasin B. *Science* 1973;179: 915–916.
270. Polson AG, Ley HL 3rd, Bass BL, Casey JL. Hepatitis delta virus RNA editing is highly specific for the amber/W site and is suppressed by hepatitis delta antigen. *Mol Cell Biol* 1998;18:1919–1926.
271. Post LE, Mackem S, Roizman B. Regulation of alpha genes of herpes simplex virus: Expression of chimeric genes produced by fusion of thymidine kinase with alpha gene promoters. *Cell* 1981;24:555–565.
272. Preston CM, Frame MC, Campbell MEM. A complex formed between cell components and an HSV structural polypeptide binds to a viral immediate early gene regulatory DNA sequence. *Cell* 1988;52: 425–434.
273. Puddington L, Woodgett C, Rose JK. Placement of the cytoplasmic domain alters sorting of a viral glycoprotein in polarized cells. *Proc Natl Acad Sci U S A* 1987;84:2756–2760.
274. Quinlan MP, Chen LB, Knipe DM. The intranuclear location of a herpes simplex virus DNA-binding protein is determined by the status of viral DNA replication. *Cell* 1984;36:857–868.

275. Rajan P, Swaminathan S, Zhu J, et al. A novel translational regulation function for the simian virus 40 large-T antigen gene. *J Virol* 1995;69: 785–795.
276. Randall RE, Dinwoodie N. Intranuclear localization of herpes simplex virus immediate-early and delayed-early proteins: evidence that ICP 4 is associated with progeny virus DNA. *J Gen Virol* 1986;67: 2163–2177.
277. Rawlins DR, Milman G, Hayward SD, Hayward GS. Sequence specific DNA binding of the Epstein-Barr virus nuclear antigen (EBNA-1) to clustered sites in the plasmid maintenance region. *Cell* 1985;42: 859–868.
278. Read GS, Frenkel N. Herpes simplex virus mutants defective in the virion-associated shutoff of host polypeptide synthesis and exhibiting abnormal synthesis of alpha (immediate early) viral polypeptides. *J Virol* 1983;46:498–512.
279. Rebouillat D, Hovanessian AG. The human 2′,5′–oligoadenylate synthetase family: Interferon-induced proteins with unique enzymatic properties. *J Interferon Cytokine Res* 1999;19:295–308.
280. Reich N, Sarnow P, Duprey E, Levine AJ. Monoclonal antibodies which recognize native and denatured forms of the adenovirus DNA-binding protein. *Virology* 1983;128:480–484.
281. Remm M, Remm A, Ustav M. Human papillomavirus type 18 E1 protein is translated from polycistronic mRNA by a discontinuous scanning mechanism. *J Virol* 1999;73:3062–3070.
282. Rice AP, Roberts BE. Vaccinia virus induces cellular mRNA degradation. *J Virol* 1983;47:529–539.
283. Rice SA, Long MC, Lam V, Spencer CA. RNA polymerase II is aberrantly phosphorylated and localized to viral replication compartments following herpes simplex virus infection. *J Virol* 1994;68:988–1001.
284. Rivas C, Gil J, Melkova Z, et al. Vaccinia virus E3L protein is an inhibitor of the interferon (i.f.n.)-induced 2-5A synthetase enzyme. *Virology* 1998;243:406–414.
285. Rixon FJ, Addison C, McGregor A, et al. Multiple interactions control the intracellular localization of the herpes simplex virus type 1 capsid proteins. *J Gen Virol* 1996;77:2251–2260.
286. Roberts ML, Luxembourg AT, Cooper NR. Epstein-Barr virus binding to CD21, the virus receptor, activates resting B cells via an intracellular pathway that is linked to B cell infection. *J Gen Virol* 1996;77: 3077–3085.
287. Roizman B, Roane PHJ. The multiplication of HSV II. The relation between protein synthesis and the duplication of viral DNA in infected HEp-2 cells. *Virology* 1964;22:262–269.
288. Ronco LV, Karpova AY, Vidal M, Howley PM. Human papillomavirus 16 E6 oncoprotein binds to interferon regulatory factor-3 and inhibits its transcriptional activity. *Genes Dev* 1998;12:2061–2072.
289. Roth J, Dobbelstein M. Export of hepatitis B virus RNA on a Rev-like pathway: Inhibition by the regenerating liver inhibitory factor Ikap paB alpha. *J Virol* 1997;71:8933–8939.
290. Roth MG, Compans RW, Giusti L, et al. Influenza virus hemagglutinin expression is polarized in cells infected with recombinant SV40 viruses carrying cloned hemagglutinin DNA. *Cell* 1983;33:435–443.
291. Roth MG, Gundersen D, Patil N, Rodriguez-Boulan E. The large external domain is sufficient for the correct sorting of secreted or chimeric influenza virus homagglutinins in polarized monkey kidney cells. *J Cell Biol* 1987;104:769–782.
292. Rothman JE, Lodish HF. Synchronized trans-membrane insertion and glycosylation of a nascent membrane protein. *Nature* 1977;269: 755–778.
293. Sachs AB, Sarnow P, Hentze MW. Starting at the beginning, middle and end: Translation initiation in eukaryotes. *Cell* 1997;89:831–838.
294. Sadaie MR, Benter T, Wong-Staal F. Site-directed mutagensis of two trans-regulatory genes (tat-III, tis) of HIV-1. *Science* 1988;239: 910–914.
295. Samuel CE. Mechanism of interferon action: Phosphorylation of protein synthesis initiation factor eIF-2 in interferon-treated human cells by a ribosome-associated kinase possessing site specificity similar to hemin-regulated rabbit reticulocyte kinase. *Proc Natl Acad Sci U S A* 1979;76:600–6044.
296. Samuel CE. Polycistronic animal virus mRNAs. *Prog Nucleic Acid Res Mol Biol* 1989;37:127–153.
297. Samuel CE. Antiviral actions of interferon. Interferon-regulated cellular proteins and their surprisingly selective antiviral activities. *Virology* 1991;183:1–11.
298. Samuel CE. The eIF-2 alpha protein kinases, regulators of translation in eukaryotes from yeasts to humans. *J Biol Chem* 1993;268: 7603–7606.
299. Samuel CE. Reoviruses and the interferon system. *Curr Top Microbiol Immunol* 1998;233:125–145.
300. Sandalon Z, Oppenheim A. Self-assembly and protein-protein interactions between the SV40 capsid proteins produced in insect cells. *Virology* 1997;237:414–421.
301. Sanz-Ezquerro JJ, de la Luna S, Ortin J, Nieto A. Individual expression of influenza virus PA protein induces degradation of coexpressed proteins. *J Virol* 1995;69:2420–2426.
302. Sarnow P, Ho Y-S, Williams J, Levine A. Adenovirus E1b-58kb tumor antigen and SV40 large tumor antingen are physically associated with the same 54kd cellular protein in transformed cells. *Cell* 1982;28: 387–394.
303. Schmechel S, Chute M, Skinner P, et al. Preferential translation of reovirus mRNA by sigma 3-dependent mechanism. *Virology* 1997; 232:62–73.
304. Schneider RJ, Shenk T. Impact of virus infection on host cell protein synthesis. *Annu Rev Biochem* 1987;56:317–332.
305. Schwartz J, Roizman B. Concerning the egress of herpes simplex virus from infected cells: Electron and light microscope observations. *Virology* 1969;38:42–49.
306. Schwartz J, Roizman B. Similarities and differences in the development of laboratory strains and freshly isolated strains of herpes simplex virus in HEp-2 cells: Electron microscopy. *J Virol* 1969;4:879–889.
307. Sedman SA, Mertz JE. Mechanisms of synthesis of virion proteins from the functionally bigenic late mRNAs of simian virus 40. *J Virol* 1988;62:954–961.
308. Sethna PB, Brian DA. Coronavirus genomic and subgenoimic minus-strand RNAs copartition in membrane-protected replication complexes. *J Virol* 1997;71:7744–7749.
309. Sharp TV, Moonan F, Romashko A, et al. The vaccinia virus E3L gene product interacts with both the regulatory and the substrate binding regions of PKR: Implications for PKR autoregulation. *Virology* 1998; 250:302–315.
310. Sharp TV, Raine DA, Gewert DR, et al. Activation of the interferon-inducible (2′-5′) oligoadenylate synthetase by the Epstein-Barr virus RNA, EBER-1. *Virology* 1999;257:303–313.
311. Shaw AS, Rottier PJM, Rose JK. Evidence for the loop model of signal-sequence insertion into the endoplasmic reticulum. *Proc Natl Acad Sci U S A* 1988;85:7592–7596.
312. Shen Y, Shenk TE. Viruses and apoptosis. *Curr Opin Genet Dev* 1995; 5:105–111.
313. Shors ST, Beattie E, Paoletti E, et al. Role of the vaccinia virus E3L and K3L gene products in rescue of VSV and EMCV from the effects of IFN-alpha. *J Interferon Cytokine Res* 1998;18:721–729.
314. Shors T, Kibler KV, Perkins KB, et al. Complementation of vaccinia virus deleted of the E3L gene by mutants of E3L. *Virology* 1997;239: 269–276.
315. Silverman RH. Fascination with 2-5A-dependent RNase: A unique enzyme that functions in interferon action. *J Interferon Res* 1994;14: 101–104.
316. SivaRaman L, Subramanian S, Thimmapaya B. Identification of a factor in HeLa cells specific for an upstream transcriptional control sequence of an E1A-inducible adenovirus promoter and its relative abundance in infected and uninfected cells. *Proc Natl Acad Sci U S A* 1986;83:5914–5918.
317. Skiadopoulos MH, McBride AA. Bovine papillomavirus type 1 genomes and the E2 transactivator protein are closely associated with mitotic chromatin. *J Virol* 1998;72:2079–2088.
318. Smale ST, Tjian R. T-antigen-DNA polymerase alpha complex implicated in simian virus 40 DNA replication. *Mol Cell Biol* 1986;6: 4077–4087.
319. Smith GL, Levin JZ, Palese P, Moss B. Synthesis and cellular location of the ten influenza polypeptides individually expressed by recombinant vaccinia viruses. *Virology* 1987;160:336–345.
320. Smith GL, Symons JA, Alcami A. Poxviruses: Interfering with interferon. *Semin Virol* 1998;8:409–418.
321. Smith RD, Sutherland K. The cytopathology of virus infections. In: Spector S, Lancz GJ, eds. *Clinical Virology Manual.* New York: Elsevier Science, 1986:53–69.
322. Sodeik B, Ebersold M, Helenius A. Dynein mediated transport of incoming herpes simplex virus 1 capsids to the nucleus. *J Cell Biol* 1997;136:1007–1021.

323. Sodroski J, Goh WC, Rosen C, et al. A second post-transcriptional trans-activator gene required for HTLV-III replication. *Nature* 1986; 321:412–417.
324. Stahl H, Droge P, Knippers R. DNA helicase activity of SV40 large tumor antigen. *EMBO J* 1986;5:1939–1944.
325. Stark GR, Kerr IM, Williams BR, et al. How cells respond to interferons. *Annu Rev Biochem* 1998;67:227–264.
326. Stephens EB, Compans RW. Assembly of animal viruses at cellular membranes. In: *Annual Review of Microbiology.* Palo Alto, CA: Annual Reviews, 1988:489–516.
327. Stephens EB, Compans RW, Earl P, Moss B. Surface expression of viral glycoproteins in polarized epithelial cells using vaccinia virus vectors. *EMBO J* 1986;5:237–245.
328. Stewart DL, Cook LN, Rabalais GP. Successful use of extracorporeal membrane oxygenation in a newborn with herpes simplex virus pneumonia. *Pediatr Infect Dis* 1993;12:161–162.
329. Stimac E, Housman D, Huberman JA. Effects of inhibition of protein synthesis on DNA replication in cultured mammalian cells. *J Mol Biol* 1977;115:485.
330. Stoye JP. Fv1, the mouse retrovirus resistance gene. *Rev Sci Tech* 1998;17:269–277.
331. Sugawara K, Gilead Z, Wold WSM, Green M. Immunofluorescence study of the adenovirus type 2 single-stranded DNA binding protein in infected and transformed cells. *J Virol* 1977;22:527–539.
332. Sugrue RJ, Hay AJ. Structural characteristics of the M2 protein of influenza A viruses: Evidence that it forms a tetrameric channel. *Virology* 1991;180:617–624.
333. Svitkin YV, Gradi A, Imataka H, et al. Eukarytoic initiation factor 4GII (eIF4GII), but not eIF4GI, cleavage correlates with inhibition of host cell protein synthesis after human rhinovirus infection. *J Virol* 1999;73:3467–3472.
334. Tan SL, Katze MG. The emerging role of the interferon-induced PKR protein kinase as an apoptotic effector: A new face of death? *J Interferon Cytokine Res* 1999;19:543–554.
335. Tanaka N, Sato M, Lamphier MS, et al. Type I interferons are essential mediators of apoptotic death in virally infected cells. *Genes Cells* 1998;3:29–37.
336. Tang H, Gaietta GM, Fischer WH, et al. A cellular cofactor for the constitutive transport element of type D retrovirus. *Science* 1997;276: 1412–1415.
337. Taube R, Fujinaga K, Wimmer J, et al. Tat transactivation: A model for the regulation of eukaryotic transcriptional elongation. *Virology* 1999; 264:245–253.
338. Taylor DR, Shi ST, Romano PR, et al. Inhibition of the interferon-inducible protein kinase PKR by HCV E2 protein. *Science* 1999;285: 107–110.
339. Teodoro JG, Branton PE. Regulation of apoptosis by viral gene products. *J Virol* 1997;71:1739–1746.
340. Teodoro JG, Branton PE. Regulation of p53-dependent apoptosis, transcriptional repression, and cell transformation by phosphorylation of the 55-kilodalton E1B protein of human adenovirus type 5. *J Virol* 1997;71:3620–3627.
341. Terwilliger E, Burghoff R, Sia R, et al. The art gene product of human immunodficiency virus is required for replication. *J Virol* 1988;62: 655–658.
342. Thomas HC, Torok ME, Foster GR. Hepatitis C virus dynamics in vivo and the antiviral efficacy of interferon alfa therapy. *Hepatology* 1999;29:1333–1334.
343. Thomsen DR, Stenberg RM, Goins WF, Stinski MF. Promoter-regulatory region of the major immediate early gene of human cytomegalovirus. *Proc Natl Acad Sci U S A* 1984;81:659–663.
344. Tjian R. The binding site on SV40 DNA for a T antigen-related protein. *Cell* 1978;13:165–179.
345. Tollefson AE, Hermiston TW, Lichtenstein DL, et al. Forced degradation of Fas inhibits apoptosis in adenovirus-infected cells. *Nature* 1998;392:726–730.
346. Triezenberg SJ, Kingsbury RC, McKnight SL. Functional dissection of VP16, the trans-activator of herpes simplex virus immediate early gene expression. *Genes Dev* 1988;2:718–729.
347. Trono D, Pelletier J, Sonenberg N, Baltimore D. Translation in mammalian cells of a gene linked to the poliovirus 5′ noncoding region. *Science* 1988;241:445–448.
348. Tschopp J, Thome M, Hofmann K, Meinl E. The fight of viruses against apoptosis. *Curr Opin Genet Dev* 1998;8:82–87.
349. Tucker SP, Compans RW. Virus infection of polarized epithelial cells. *Adv Virus Res* 1993;42:187–247.
350. Tucker SP, Thornton CL, Wimmer E, Compans RW. Vectorial release of poliovirus from polarized human intestinal epithelial cells. *J Virol* 1993;67:4274–4284.
351. Tyndall C, LaMantia G, Thacker C, et al. A region of the polyoma virus genome between the replication origin and the protein coding sequence is required in *cis* for both early gene expression and DNA replication. *Nucleic Acids Res* 1981;9:6231–6250.
352. Uprichard SL, Knipe DM. Herpes simplex virus ICP27 mutant viruses exhibit reduced expression of specific DNA replication genes. *J Virol* 1996;70:1969–1980.
353. Valentine RC, Pereira HG. Antigens and structure of the adenoviruses. *J Mol Biol* 1965;13:13–20.
354. van den Broek MF, Muller U, Huang S, et al. Antiviral defense in mice lacking both alpha/beta and gamma interferon receptors. *J Virol* 1995; 69:4792–4796.
355. van der Meer Y, Snijder EJ, Dobbe JC, et al. Localization of mouse hepatitis virus nonstructural proteins and RNA synthesis indicates a role for late endosomes in viral replication. *J Virol* 1999;73: 7641–7657.
356. van der Meer Y, van Tol HG, Krijnse Locker J, Snijder EJ. ORF1a-encoded replicase subunits are involved in membrane association of the arterivirus replication complex. *J Virol* 1998;72:6689–6698.
357. Vodicka MA, Koepp DM, Silver PA, Emerman M. HIV-1 Vpr interacts with the nuclear transport pathway to promote macrophage infection. *Genes Dev* 1998;12:175–185.
358. Voelkerding K, Klessig DF. Identification of two nuclear subclasses of the adenovirus type 5-encoded DNA-binding protein. *J Virol* 1986;60: 353–362.
359. Wagner EK, Roizman B. RNA synthesis in cells infected with herpes simplex virus. II. Evidence that a class of viral mRNA is derived from a high molecular weight precursor synthesized in the nucleus. *Proc Natl Acad Sci U S A* 1969;64:626–633.
360. Wang P, Palese P, O'Neill RE. The NPI-1/NPI-3 (karyopherin alpha) binding site on the influenza a virus nucleoprotein NP is a nonconventional nuclear localization signal. *J Virol* 1997;71:1850–1856.
361. Waskiewicz AJ, Johnson JC, Penn B, et al. Phosphorylation of the cap-binding protein eukaryotic translation initiation factor 4E by protein kinase Mnk1 in vivo. *Mol Cell Biol* 1999;19:1871–1880.
362. Weck P, Wagner R. Transcription of vesicular stomatitis virus is required to shutoff cellular RNA synthesis. *J Virol* 1979;30:410–413.
363. Weissenhorn W, Dessen A, Calder LJ, et al. Structural basis for membrane fusion by enveloped viruses. *Mol Membr Biol* 1999;16:3–9.
364. Westaway EG, Mackenzie JM, Kenney MT, et al. Ultrastructure of Kunjin virus-infected cells: Colocalization of NS1 and NS3 with double-stranded RNA, and NS2B with NS3, in virus-induced membrane structures. *J Virol* 1997;71:6650–6661.
365. White E. Life, death, and the pursuit of apoptosis. *Genes Dev* 1996; 10:1–15.
366. Whittaker GR, Helenius A. Nuclear import and export of viruses and virus genomes. *Virology* 1998;246:1–23.
367. Whyte P, Buchkovich KJ, Horowitz JM, et al. Association between an oncogene and an anti-oncogene: The adenovirus E1A proteins bind to the retinoblastoma gene product. *Nature* 1988;334:124–129.
368. Wickham TJ, Mathias P, Cheresh DA, Nemerow GW. Integrins alpha v beta 3 and alpha v beta 5 promote adenovirus internalization but not virus attachment. *Cell* 1993;73:309–319.
369. Wilcock D, Lane DP. Localization of p53, retinoblastoma and host replication proteins at sites of viral replication in herpes-infected cells. *Nature* 1991;349:429–431.
370. Wills JW, Cameron CE, Wilson CB, et al. An assembly domain of the Rous sarcoma virus gag protein required late in budding. *J Virol* 1994; 68:6605–6618.
371. Wolf R, Wolf D, Ruocco V. Antiviral therapy for recurrent herpes simplex reconsidered. *Dermatology* 1997;194:205–207.
372. Wolgemuth DJ, Hsu M-T. Visualization of nascent RNA transcripts and simultaneous transcription and replication in viral nuceloprotein complexes from adenovirus 2-infected HeLa cells. *J Mol Biol* 1981; 147:247–268.
373. Wu CA, Nelson NJ, McGeoch DJ, Challberg MD. Identification of herpes simplex virus type 1 genes required for origin-dependent DNA synthesis. *J Virol* 1988;62:435–443.
374. Wu L, Rosser DSE, Schmidt MD, Berk A. A TAT box implicated in

E1A transcriptional activation of a simple adenovirus 2 promoter. *Nature* 1987;326:512–515.
375. Xiang Y, Cameron CE, Wills JW, Leis J. Fine mapping and characterization of the Rous sarcoma virus Pr76gag late assembly domain. *J Virol* 1996;70:5695–5697.
376. Xiao H, Neuveut C, Benkirane M, Jeang KT. Interaction of the second coding exon of Tat with human EF-1 delta delineates a mechanism for HIV-1-mediated shut-off of host mRNA translation. *Biochem Biophys Res Commun* 1998;244:384–389.
377. Yates J, Warren N, Reisman D, Sugden B. A cis-acting element from the Epstein-Barr viral genome that permits stable replication of recombinant plasmids in latently infected cells. *Proc Natl Acad Sci U S A* 1984;81:3806.
378. Yeh K-C, Knipe DM. Unpublished results.
379. Yuan H, Yoza BK, Lyles DS. Inhibition of host RNA polymerase II-dependent transcription by vesicular stomatitis virus results from inactivation of TFIID. *Virology* 1998;251:383–392.
380. Yue Z, Shatkin AJ. Double-stranded RNA-dependent protein kinase (PKR) is regulated by reovirus structural proteins. *Virology* 1997;234:364–371.
381. Yueh A, Schneider RJ. Selective translation initiation by ribosome jumping in adenovirus-infected and heat-shocked cells. *Genes Dev* 1996;10:1557–1567.
382. Zelus BD, Stewart RS, Ross J. The virion host shutoff protein of herpes simplex virus type 1: Messenger ribonucleolytic activity in vitro. *J Virol* 1996;70:2411–2419.
383. Zennou V, Petit C, Guetard D, et al. HIV-1 genome nuclear import is mediated by a central DNA flap. *Cell* 2000;101:173–185.
384. Zhang L, Pagano JS. IRF-7, a new interferon regulatory factor associated with Epstein-Barr virus latency. *Mol Cell Biol* 1997;17:5748–5757.
385. Zhou A, Paranjape J, Brown TL, et al. Interferon action and apoptosis are defective in mice devoid of 2′,5′-oligoadenylate-dependent RNase L. *EMBO J* 1997;16:6355–6363.
386. Zhu H, Cong JP, Mamtora G, et al. Cellular gene expression altered by human cytomegalovirus: Global monitoring with oligonucleotide arrays. *Proc Natl Acad Sci U S A* 1998;95:14470–14475.

CHAPTER 8

Virus Assembly

Eric Hunter

Virus assembly, a key step in the replication cycle of any virus, involves a process in which large numbers of chemically distinct macromolecules are transported, often through different transport pathways, to a point within the cell where they are assembled into a nascent viral particle. A diversity of strategies and intracellular assembly sites are employed by members of the various virus families to ensure the efficient production of fully infectious virions. Nevertheless, a virus, irrespective of its molecular structure (membrane enveloped or nonenveloped) or the symmetry with which it assembles (icosahedral, spherical, or helical), must be able to take advantage of the intracellular transport pathways that exist within the cell if it is to achieve this goal. The end product of this selection process is assembly of each virus at a defined point within the cell. This chapter focuses on the cell biology of these intracellular targeting events, the intermolecular interactions that mediate targeting, and the assembly steps themselves.

Most viruses encode a limited number of gene products. They are, therefore, dependent on the cell not only for biosynthesis of the macromolecules that constitute the virus particle but also for the preexisting intracellular sorting mechanisms that the virus uses to achieve delivery of those macromolecules to the sites of virion assembly. Because these are the same sorting mechanisms that the cell uses to delineate its subcellular organelles, the viral macromolecules must possess targeting signals similar to those of the components of those organelles. For a virus such as adenovirus, which assembles its nonenveloped capsids in the nucleus, this means that, after translation in the cytoplasm, each of the structural proteins of the mature virus must have the necessary protein-targeting information to be efficiently routed through the nuclear membrane to the assembly site. The situation is more complicated for a membrane-enveloped virus, such as influenza virus. For this virus, which assembles and releases virions from the apical surface of the epithelial cells that it infects, there is a necessity to ensure that the surface glycoproteins of the virus are correctly sorted by the secretory pathway of the cell to the apical surface. In addition, nucleocapsids, assembled in the nucleus, must be transported into and through the cytoplasm to the same intracellular location. As will be discussed below, the intracellular site at which the final phase of assembly and budding of an enveloped virus takes place is most often defined by the accumulation of the viral glycoproteins at a specific point in the secretory pathway of the cell. This also implies that there is specific molecular recognition of the virally encoded, membrane-spanning envelope components by the cytoplasmic nucleocapsids in order for a productive budding process to occur. Thus, interactions between proteins of viral and cellular origin, between viral proteins and nucleic acids and lipids, as well as between the viral proteins themselves are at the heart of the assembly process.

PARTITIONING OF PROTEINS WITHIN THE CELL

For an actively growing eukaryotic cell, there is a constant need to transport proteins and nucleic acids from their site of synthesis to the specific intracellular domains where they must function (Fig. 1). Proteins synthesized on cytosolic ribosomes, for example, must be transported to specific regions of the cytoplasm, to mitochondria, and into the nucleus, whereas those synthesized on membrane-bound ribosomes enter the secretory pathway and are targeted to specific organelles along the way. At the same time, messenger RNAs (mRNAs) and integral RNA components of the ribosome, ribosomal RNAs (rRNAs), must be transported out of the nucleus. Proteins that participate in these intracellular trafficking processes have evolved to contain specific motifs that ensure the correct localization of the protein within the cell. Viruses have similarly evolved to take advantage of these preexisting pathways to accumulate the necessary components for assembly of a nascent virus in specific locations.

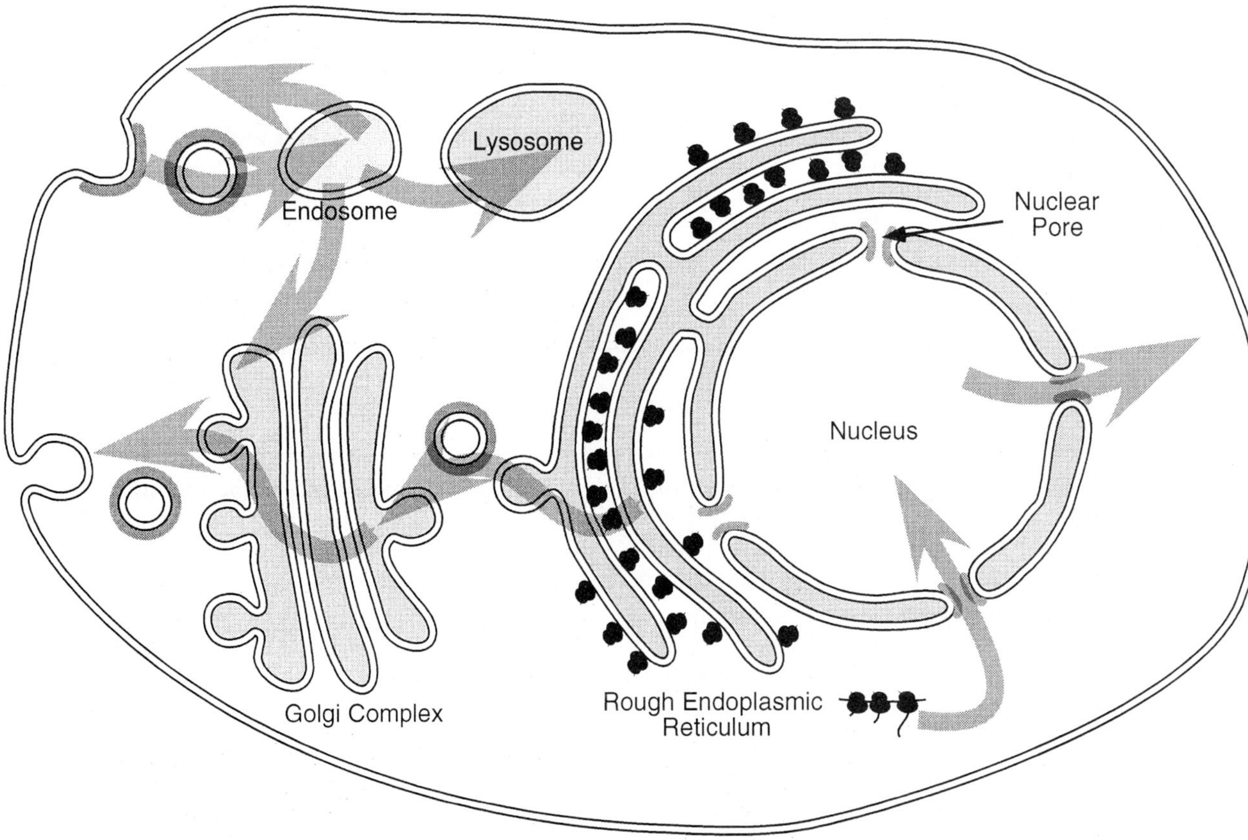

FIG. 1. Protein localization in a mammalian cell. Proteins destined for the plasma membrane traverse the secretory pathway of the cell. They associate with the endoplasmic reticulum (ER) cotranslationally and are translocated across the ER membrane through a proteinaceous pore: the translocon. Proteins are transported from the ER to the Golgi complex and on to the plasma membrane unless they contain specific amino acid motifs that localize or retain them at an intermediate location. Transport from one compartment to the next is by coated vesicles. Some membrane-spanning (integral membrane) proteins contain endocytosis motifs in their cytoplasmic domain that facilitate incorporation into clathrin-coated endocytic vesicles. Such proteins can be sorted back to the plasma membrane, to the *trans*-Golgi compartment of the secretory pathway, or to a lysosome for degradation. Proteins destined for the nucleus contain nuclear localization signals. These are short amino acid sequences that allow interaction with the nuclear pore machinery for transport across the nuclear membrane. Some proteins shuttle between the nucleus and cytoplasm and contain, in addition, a nuclear export signal.

Nuclear Import and Export of Proteins and Nucleic Acids

The Nuclear Pore Complex

Because the nucleus is segregated from the cytoplasm by an inner and outer membrane, access to and egress from this subcellular domain is mediated by specialized structures termed *nuclear pore complexes* (NPCs) (reviewed in 23). There are about 3,000 NPCs on the nuclear envelope of an animal cell, and each provides a proteinaceous channel between the nucleus and cytosol. The NPC itself is a large octagonal structure with a molecular mass exceeding 120×10^6 daltons—about 30 times larger than an 80S ribosome. NPCs can be released from nuclear membranes by detergents and show eightfold symmetry. Negative stain and cryoelectron microscopy reconstructions of these complexes reveal a cagelike structure with upper and lower rings (corresponding to the inner and outer faces of the nuclear membrane) linked by radial spokes that form an inner ring with a diameter of about 48 nm (1,49) (Fig. 2).Inside this is located the transporter, which forms a cylindrical pore of about 10 nm. Attached to both faces of the central framework are peripheral structures, cytoplasmic filaments, and a nuclear basket assembly, which interact with molecules that transit the NPC (54). Small molecules and proteins less than 60 kd in mass may be able to diffuse passively through the eight outer channels formed by the spokes and rings of the NPC (see Fig. 2). Larger proteins and macromolecular assemblages must be actively moved through what is presumably a dynamic, malleable transporter structure that has the capacity to accommodate macromolecular complexes up to about 20 nm in diameter.

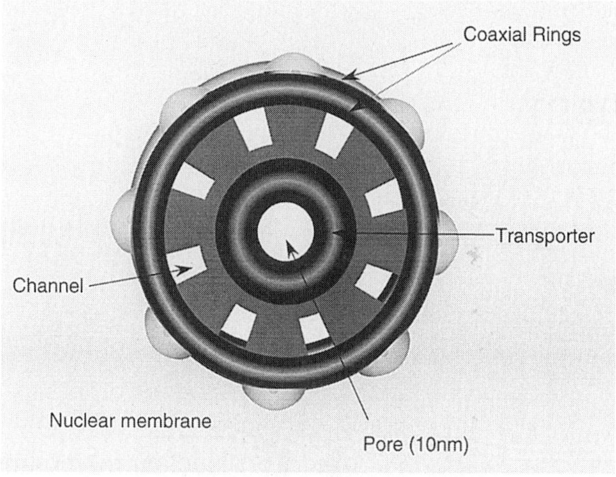

FIG. 2. Schematic representation of a nuclear pore complex. The nuclear pore complex is composed of two ringlike structures that are linked through eight spokes to a central transporter structure. The coaxial rings appear to interact with the outer and inner nuclear membranes. In negative-stain electron microscopy, the pores have a distinct eightfold symmetry. On the cytoplasmic side of the structure, filaments extend outward into the cytoplasm; whereas on the nuclear side, a basket-like structure is formed from the eight filaments that extend from the coaxial ring. Small proteins (5–50 kd) can diffuse into the nucleus, perhaps through the small channels formed by the spokes, whereas larger proteins must be actively transported through the pore.

Nuclear Localization Signals

Proteins that are actively transported into or out of the nucleus are characterized by the presence of amino acid motifs that allow them to interact with the nuclear transport machinery. For import into the nucleus, these motifs are termed *nuclear localization signals* (NLS), and for export, *nuclear export signals* (NES). NLS motifs, such as that first identified in the SV40 T antigen (57), are not only necessary for nuclear localization of the proteins in which they are present but are also sufficient to actively direct large foreign proteins, such as β-galactosidase, into the nucleus. Although there is no conservation of sequence in different NLS motifs, they are generally short (less than 20 amino acids), rich in basic amino acids, and frequently preceded by proline residues (Fig. 3). Some NLS motifs, such as that in the adenovirus DNA-binding protein, are bipartite and require two separate short clusters of basic residues to be functional (137).

To be exported from the nucleus, proteins contain an NES. This nuclear transport signal is also short (about 10 amino acids) and contains a pattern of conserved leucines (83) (see Fig. 3). Some proteins, such as Rev of human immunodeficiency virus type 1 (HIV-1), possess both an NLS and an NES and appear to shuttle back and forth between the cytoplasm and the nucleus (75).

Nuclear Transport Pathways—In and Out

Nuclear import is a two-stage process. In the first stage, the newly synthesized, NLS-containing, protein interacts with cytosolic carrier proteins that then bind to the cytoplasmic side of the NPC; a process referred to as *docking*. This complex is then translocated, in an energy-dependent process, through the nuclear pore into the nucleus, where the complex is disassembled, allowing the transported protein to become functional (39).

The best characterized carrier protein is importin-α or karyopherin-α. After binding its NLS-containing cargo, importin-α interacts with importin-β, which then mediates docking with the NPC through interactions with members of the nucleoporin family of proteins (79). Other import systems use a single molecule, such as transportin or importin-β3, that mediates both binding of the cargo molecule and the docking process (84). Active transport of large molecules in either direction across the nuclear pore involves a family of proteins, known as *nucleoporins,* as well as a small guanosine triphosphate (GTP)-binding protein termed Ran (78) (Fig. 4). The

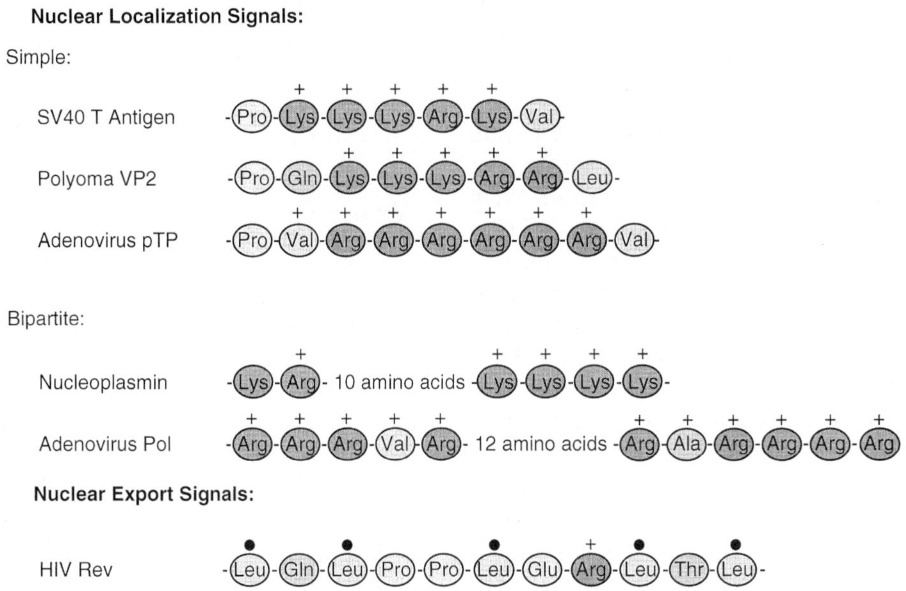

FIG. 3. Nuclear localization and export signals. The amino acid motifs that direct proteins into the nucleus are termed *nuclear localization signals* (NLS). Simple NLS sequences, such as those present in the SV40 virus T antigen or polyomavirus VP2, often contain a proline residue followed by a stretch of basic residues. This short sequence can relocate large proteins, such as β-galactosidase, into the nucleus. Bipartite NLS sequences, such as those present in nucleoplasmin or the adenovirus polymerase, are characterized by two stretches of basic amino acids separated by a variable spacer sequence. These NLS sequences are recognized by import receptor molecules such as importin-α. Proteins that shuttle into and out of the nucleus, such as Rev, possess a second motif, the nuclear export signal (NES). These motifs are characterized by a pattern of conserved leucine residues.

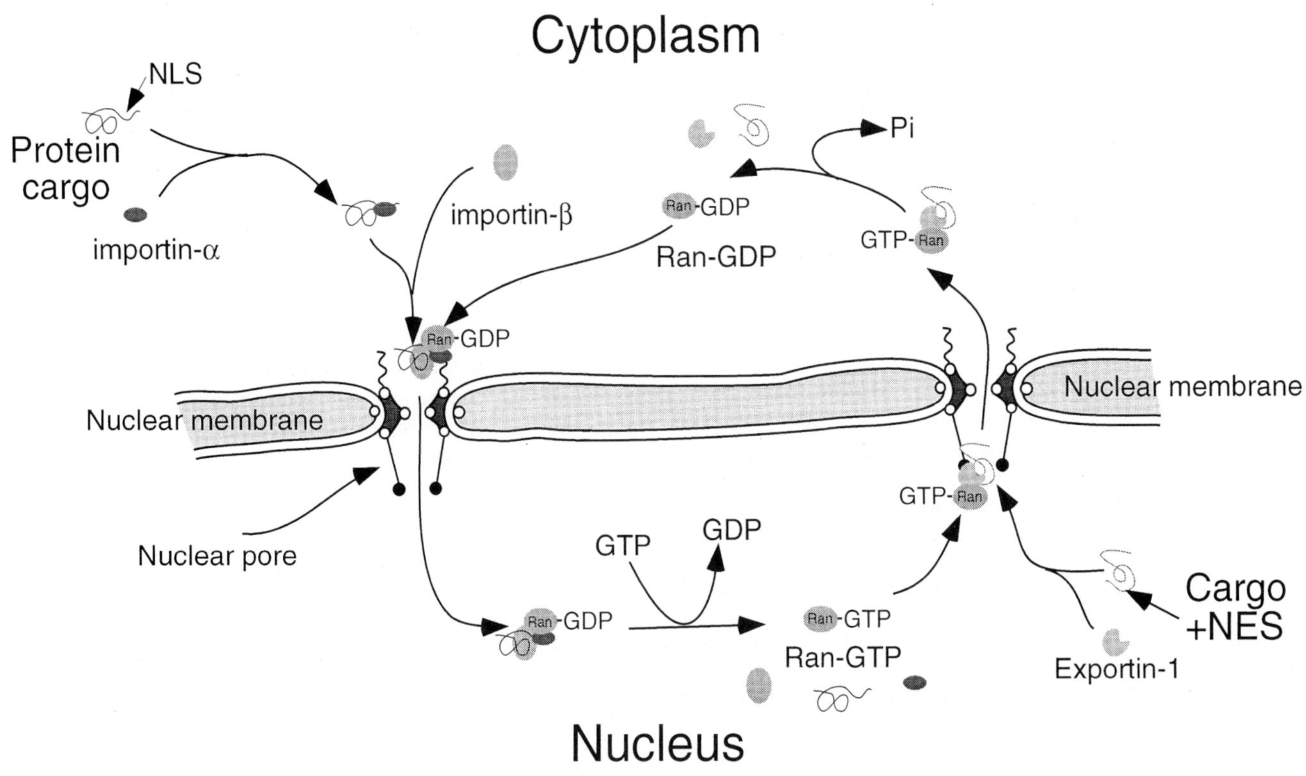

directionality of transport is regulated by whether Ran is complexed with guanosine diphosphate (GDP) or GTP. In the cytosol, Ran-GDP, together with importin-αβ and the cargo, forms a stable transport complex that is subsequently disassembled in the nucleus where GTP replaces GDP. Similarly, stable export complexes that form in the nucleus with Ran-GTP disassociate in the cytosol where a GTPase activity is active. The exact mechanism by which the Ran-GDP and importin–cargo complex is carried through the nuclear pore is not known. It is possible, however, that the process involves a series of docking and release cycles with nucleoporin proteins that make up the transporter machinery.

Export from the nucleus of large proteins and ribonucleoprotein (RNP) complexes involves interactions with an export carrier protein such as exportin-1 (32,118). This molecule binds to the NES sequence of the cargo protein and to Ran-GTP, which in turn mediates interactions with the nucleoporins of the NPC (see Fig. 4).

The Secretory Pathway of the Cell

Proteins of both viral and cellular origin that are destined for the outer membrane of the cell travel along a highly conserved route known as the *secretory pathway.* This complex series of membrane-bound subcellular compartments, through which proteins pass sequentially, includes the endoplasmic reticulum (ER), an intermediate membrane compartment, and the *cis*-, medial-, and *trans*-compartments of the Golgi apparatus (see Fig. 1). Proteins that traverse this pathway, such as the envelope glycoproteins of viruses, enter through the ER. Insertion of proteins into the ER occurs during translation, through a process termed *translocation.* The ER network of tubules and sacs defines a unique environment in which protein modification and folding can occur isolated from the cytoplasm. Regions of the ER membrane where polybosomes are bound tightly and in the process of translating proteins that are translocating into the secretory pathway are known as *rough ER.*

Translocation

Translating ribosomes are directed to the ER membrane by a short sequence in the nascent polypeptide known as the *signal sequence.* In most proteins, this 15- to 30-amino acid sequence, which contains a core of hydrophobic amino acids, is located at the N-terminus of the protein. Shortly after the signal peptide emerges from the ribosome, it is bound by an RNP complex known as the *signal recognition particle* (SRP) (131). Binding of the SRP transiently arrests further translation and directs the ribosome to an SRP receptor on the ER (Fig. 5). Both the SRP and its receptor have GTP-binding components, and the presence of this nucleotide is essential for efficient targeting.

After the initial docking of the translationally arrested complex, the ribosome becomes tightly associated with the ER membrane through the translocon, a gated, aqueous, protein channel that spans the ER membrane (115). Concomitant with this process, the SRP and its receptor are released, the signal peptide is introduced into the channel, and translation resumes. The components of the translocon have been identified through biochemical approaches in mammalian cells and genetic approaches in yeast and are composed of a heterotrimeric complex known as the Sec61p (composed of Sec61 α-, β-, and γ-chains). The complex forms a cylindrical structure, with a diameter of 85 Å and a central pore of 20 Å, which spans the ER membrane and is made up of three or four heterotrimers (44). Additional proteins (e.g., the translocating chain-association membrane [TRAM] protein) are necessary for optimal translocation. It is unlikely that the central pore of the translocon ever allows free diffusion between the cytosol and the lumen of the ER because these compartments are chemically distinct (18). More likely, GRP78/Bip, a member of the Hsp70 family of chaperone proteins, seals the luminal face of the translocon pore until the ribosome forms a tight seal on the cytosolic side. The chaperone is then poised to facilitate the folding of the nascent polypeptide chain as it emerges from the pore, although this binding is not essential for

FIG. 4. Nuclear import and export pathways. A protein bearing an NLS is recognized and bound by importin-α. Importin-β binds to this complex and carries it to the cytoplasmic side of the nuclear pore where it binds initially to nucleoporins in the cytoplasmic filaments. Translocation of the protein complex into the nucleus requires the involvement of the guanine nucleoside–binding protein Ran in the form of Ran–guanosine diphosphate (GDP). Ran binds specifically to certain nucleoporins and is thought to mediate the transfer of the complex from the cytoplasmic face of the nuclear pore to the nuclear face. In the nucleus, a Ran-specific guanine nucleotide exchange protein (Rcc) converts Ran-GDP to Ran–guanosine triphosphate (GTP) and the complex dissociates delivering the protein cargo into the nucleus. Proteins destined for export out of the nucleus bind to exportin-1 through their NES. This complex, together with Ran-GTP, binds to nucleoporins localized to the nuclear basket of the pore complex and initiates translocation into the cytoplasm. Once there, Ran-GTP is converted to Ran-GDP by a Ran-GTPase–activating protein (RanGAP-1), causing the cargo-exportin-1-Ran complex to dissociate, thereby delivering the cargo to the cytoplasm.

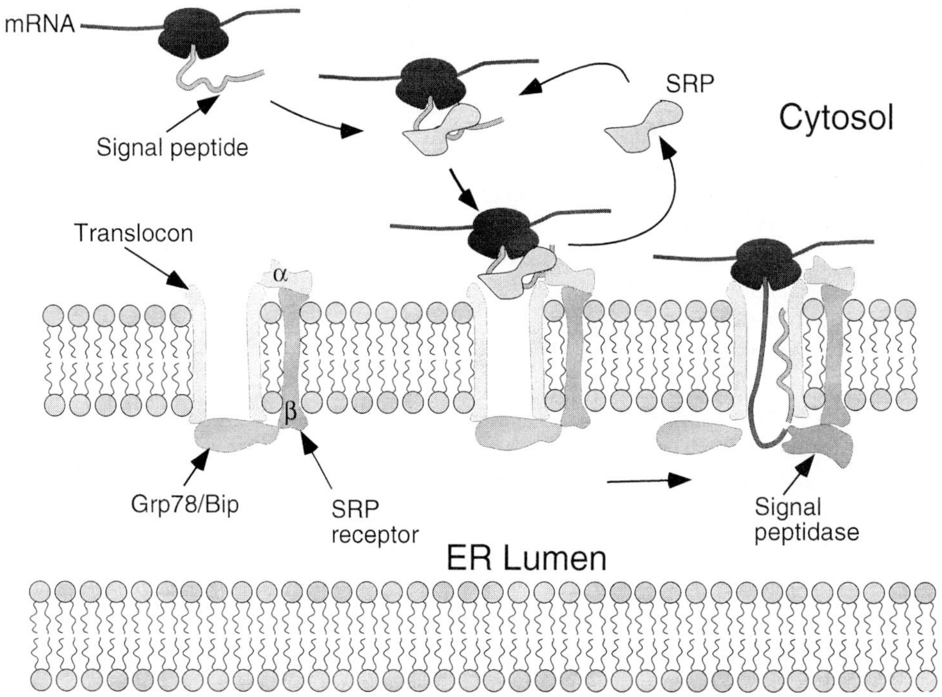

FIG. 5. Protein translocation into the secretory pathway. Translation of a protein destined for the secretory pathway proceeds until the signal peptide exits the ribosome. The signal recognition particle (SRP) binds to the signal peptide and the ribosome and arrests translation. The ribosome–SRP complex moves to the endoplasmic reticulum (ER) membrane where SRP binds to its receptor (*SRP receptor*). This interaction, with concomitant hydrolysis of bound GTP, releases SRP and mediates a tight interaction between the ribosome and a proteinaceous channel, the translocon. The release of SRP and binding of the signal peptide to components of the translocon allows resumption of translation to occur. Grp78/Bip, which appears to block the lumenal side of the translocon before and early in translocation, now allows the extrusion of the nascent polypeptide into the ER as translation continues. The signal peptidase complex removes the signal peptide cotranslationally from those proteins that have a cleavable signal peptide. Secreted proteins continue to traverse the translocon until they are completely located in the lumen of the ER. In contrast, for integral membrane proteins, translocation stops after introduction of the hydrophobic anchor domain into the translocon.

translocation to proceed. The signal peptide, in those proteins with a transient N-terminal sequence, is cleaved from the rest of the polypeptide by a complex of five proteins called the *signal peptidase* shortly after it enters the lumen of the ER (see Fig. 5).

For secreted proteins, translocation of the polypeptide through the translocon continues until the entire protein is present in the lumen of the ER. In contrast, integral membrane proteins, such as the envelope glycoproteins of viruses, contain a stop-transfer, membrane-anchor sequence that is generally located toward the C-terminus of the protein. After the translation of this short (25 amino acids), mostly hydrophobic sequence, the translocon undergoes a conformational change that allows the membrane-spanning domain to be associated directly with the lipid bilayer. The product of this process is a type-I integral membrane protein (Fig. 6), such as the influenza virus hemagglutinin (HA), in which the N-terminal ectodomain is in the lumen of the ER and the C-terminus is in the cytoplasm. In some proteins, such as the influenza virus neuraminidase, a longer N-terminal signal peptide also functions as the membrane anchor. In this case, the signal peptide is not cleaved from the polypeptide chain and the sequences C-terminal to it are translocated into the ER lumen, resulting in a type-II orientation. Multiple membrane-spanning proteins, such as the M protein of the coronaviruses, appear to possess hydrophobic sequences that are alternatively recognized as signal and stop-transfer sequences.

Posttranslational Modifications

Protein Folding and Quality Control

Proteins enter the lumen of the ER in an unfolded state and the process of folding into a transport-competent conformation is facilitated by interactions with molecular chaperones and folding enzymes located there. This collection of proteins includes BiP, calnexin (Cnx), calreticulin (Crt), GRP94, and protein disulfide isomerase (PDI).

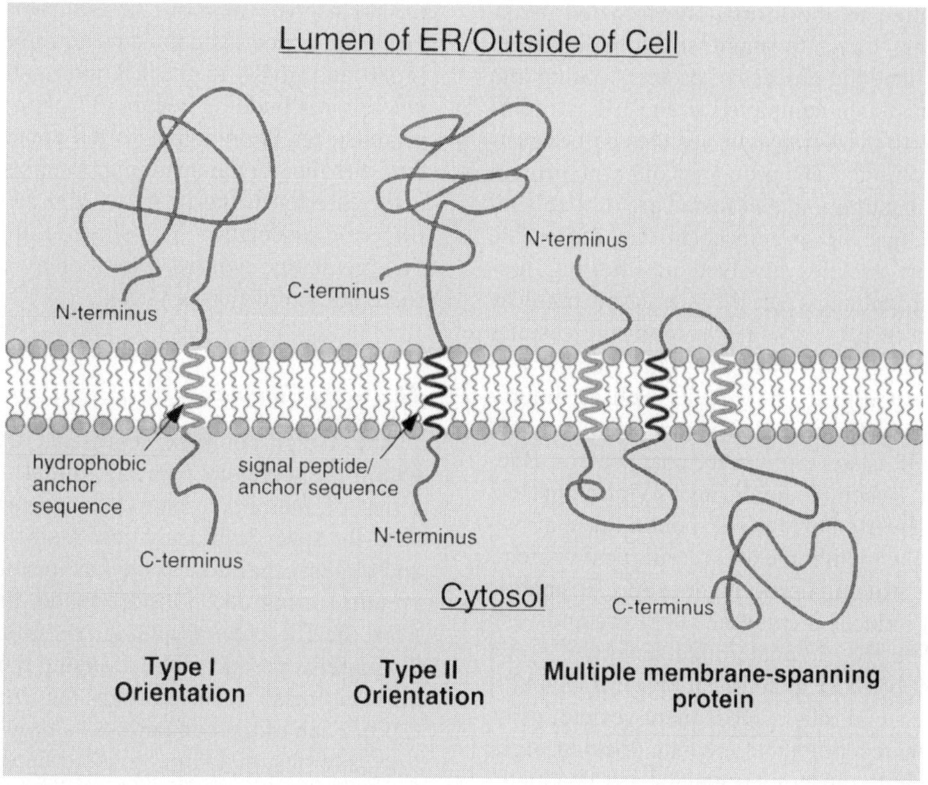

FIG. 6. Protein topology. Proteins with type-I orientation generally have a cleavable N-terminal signal peptide that is removed cotranslationally from the nascent protein. The protein continues to be transferred into the lumen of the endoplasmic reticulum (ER) until a hydrophobic anchor sequence is translated and enters the translocon. Translocation then stops, and the protein transitions from the protein pore into the lipid bilayer. Thus, type-I integral membrane proteins, such as the hemagglutinin of influenza virus, have their C-terminus in the cytoplasm and their N-terminus in the lumen of the ER (topologically equivalent to outside the cell). In type-II proteins, such as the influenza virus neuraminidase, the signal peptide forms the membrane anchor domain, so that at the end of translation, the C-terminal sequences are translocated into the lumen of the ER, leaving the N-terminus in the cytoplasm. For multiple membrane-spanning proteins, such as the M protein of the coronaviruses, translocation is initiated at the first signal peptide sequence and continues until the first anchor domain. It is reinitiated after translation of a subsequent signal sequence and stopped again after translation of a second anchor. The exact mechanism by which this is accomplished without dismantling the translocon at intermediate steps in the process is not understood.

In addition to assisting in folding the nascent molecules, these proteins retain incompletely folded molecules in the lumen and act as a quality control system for the secretory pathway (27). Oligomeric proteins, such as the receptor and fusion proteins of enveloped viruses, also assemble into their quaternary conformation in this compartment. For many of these molecules, oligomerization appears to be a prerequisite for transport out of the ER.

Glycosylation

Most proteins that traverse the secretory pathway are modified by the addition of oligosaccharide side chains either to the amino group of asparagines (*N*-linked glycosylation) or through the hydroxyl group of serines or threonines (*O*-linked glycosylation). *N*-linked moieties are added cotranslationally in the lumen of the ER, where mannose-rich oligosaccharides are transferred from a lipid (dolichol) carrier to asparagine residues present in NXS/T motifs (where X is any amino acid but proline) within the protein. Trimming of terminal glucose and mannose residues from the branched oligosaccharide occurs in the ER and is closely linked with the Cnx- and Crt-mediated quality control process (reviewed in 27). Further trimming of mannose residues followed by addition of other sugars (*N*-acetylglucosamine, galactose, fucose, and sialic acid), to yield complex oligosaccharide structures, occurs in the Golgi complex. *O*-linked oligosaccharides are also added in this organelle.

Transport Through the Secretory Pathway

Transport of soluble and membrane-spanning proteins from one compartment of the secretory pathway to the next is mediated by the formation of coated membrane vesicles that travel to and fuse with the target organelle. Thus, once the process of protein folding and quality control has been completed in the ER, proteins are sequestered into these transport vesicles before transit to the Golgi complex. The processes of cargo protein selection, budding, targeting, and fusion are probably all mediated by the specific protein coats that define the different transport vesicles involved in shuttling proteins between components of the secretory pathway (107). In the case of ER to Golgi transport, the vesicles have COPII coats (3), whereas retrograde transport of vesicles from the Golgi to the ER, as well as anterograde transport through the Golgi, is mediated by COPI coats (69,93). COP is an acronym for coat protein. Budding is initiated when a small myristylated protein (SAR/ARF) is converted to the GTP-bound form, allowing it to bind to the membrane and recruit coat proteins (coatomers) in a stoichiometric manner (3). Formation of the coat itself induces membrane curvature and vesicle budding. The N-ethylmaleimide-sensitive factor (Nsf) and the soluble NSF attachment proteins (SNAPs) appear to play a crucial role in subsequent vesicle fusion events. Membrane receptors that mediate docking of the transport vesicle with the target organelle are also incorporated into the coat and appear to define the specificity with which the cargo protein is delivered. These molecules are termed SNAP receptors or *SNAREs* (117). A target-specific SNARE (t-SNARE) that interacts only with a vesicle specific SNARE (v-SNARE) identifies the target membrane. After docking, Nsf and soluble Nsf attachment proteins SNAPs bind to the SNARE complex. Vesicle membrane fusion is initiated when Nsf hydrolyzes adenosine triphosphate (ATP) and induces a conformational change in the complex (reviewed in 107).

Protein Localization

Subcellular localization of proteins within the secretory pathway appears to be determined by a combination of sorting and targeting signals that mediate interactions with the coat complex for inclusion in a transport vesicle and of retention signals that localize the protein to a specific compartment within the secretory pathway. Localization is enhanced by the interplay of anterograde and retrograde transport that allows retrieval of proteins inadvertently transported beyond their target location. The classic example of this is the KDEL peptide sequence found on soluble proteins that are localized to the lumen of the ER (81). Proteins containing this sequence are efficiently retrieved from the *cis*-Golgi by the KDEL receptor, which is incorporated into COPI vesicles for trafficking back to the ER. Similarly, membrane-spanning proteins localized to the ER have at the C-terminus of the cytoplasmic domain a KKXX amino acid motif that ensures their efficient retrieval from the Golgi complex (53). This type of motif is used by the primate foamy viruses to concentrate the envelope glycoprotein complex (gp80 and gp48) in the ER intermediate compartment, where virus budding occurs (37). For integral membrane proteins, retention signals often appear to be associated with the membrane-spanning domains of the protein, as is the case for the coronavirus M protein, and may reflect preferred association with specific lipid compositions of the membrane within a particular component of the secretory pathway (see later).

The Golgi Complex

The Golgi complex represents a unique organelle within the secretory pathway in that it is composed of a series of membrane-bound compartments that are the sites for specific biochemical modifications to proteins and oligosaccharides, as well as locations where specific protein sorting decisions are made. Proteins transported from the ER enter the Golgi complex through the *cis*-Golgi network, and after traversing the *cis*-, medial-, and *trans*-cisternae, exit through the *trans*-Golgi network (107). Each of the compartments provides a spatially distinct site for maintaining an ordered set of enzymes involved in the process of oligosaccharide maturation. They are also the sites at which proteins undergo *O*-linked glycosylation, through the addition, at certain serines and threonines, of monomeric sugar residues. It is in the *trans*-Golgi and *trans*-Golgi network where viral glycoprotein precursors, such as the Env polyprotein of the retroviruses, are cleaved to their mature forms through the action of members of the furin family of proteinases—enzymes that normally function to process cellular substrates, such as polypeptide hormone precursors. This cleavage event is crucial to the generation of a biologically functional glycoprotein and thus to virus infectivity (60).

INTRACELLULAR TARGETING AND ASSEMBLY OF VIRION COMPONENTS

Viruses can be nominally divided into two groups based on the presence or absence of a lipid bilayer envelope. The nonenveloped viruses can assemble in the cytoplasm or nucleus and generally, for those that propagate in animal cells, exhibit icosahedral symmetry (see Chapter 3). For these viruses, the viral structural proteins and genomic nucleic acid must be targeted to or retained at the subcellular domain at which assembly occurs. Enveloped viruses, by their nature, must acquire a lipid bilayer from one of the cell's membranes during the process of assembly. In a few viruses, such as the herpesviruses and some retroviruses, this envelopment step takes place after the assembly of an intact capsid shell, whereas for others, the processes of envelopment and capsid assembly occur concomitantly. Some viruses undergo transient envelopment and, in certain cases, reenvelopment during the process of assembly.

For nonenveloped viruses, the tightly assembled structure of the icosahedral shell forms a protective coat that prevents degradation of the genome by environmental factors. For enveloped viruses, the integrity of the nucleocapsid structure is less crucial because the membrane provides a barrier to external degradative enzymes.

Assembly of Nonenveloped Viruses in the Nucleus

Adenoviruses are nonenveloped icosahedral viruses, 70 to 100 nm in diameter that have a protein shell surrounding a DNA core. The protein shell (capsid) is composed of 252 capsomeres, of which 240 are hexons and 12 are pentons. Each penton consists of a five-subunit base (polypeptide III) and a trimeric fiber (polypeptide IV) that extends out away from the shell. The hexon capsomeres are composed of trimers of three tightly associated molecules of polypeptide II (Fig. 7).

For a nonenveloped virus such as adenovirus, which replicates exclusively in the nucleus, there is a strong dependence on nuclear targeting and transport pathways to export newly synthesized mRNAs out of the nucleus and to import structural proteins back into the nucleus. Nuclear import of the major capsid protein, polypeptide II, depends on the involvement of a second adenovirus protein, the pVI (precursor) polypeptide (59), which provides the necessary NLS for transporting the trimer into the nucleus. Trimer formation is in turn dependent on yet another virus-encoded, chaperone-like protein, L4 100K, which transiently binds to the newly synthesized hexon monomer and mediates its association with two additional monomers (9,10). Thus, the most abundant structural protein of the adenovirus capsid needs to interact with two additional virus-encoded factors to attain the correct tertiary structure and subcellular location for assembly.

The two other proteins that form the 12 vertices of the capsid, penton, and fiber appear to assemble independently in the cytoplasm. Mutations in the C-terminus of the penton that block assembly into pentamers do not pre-

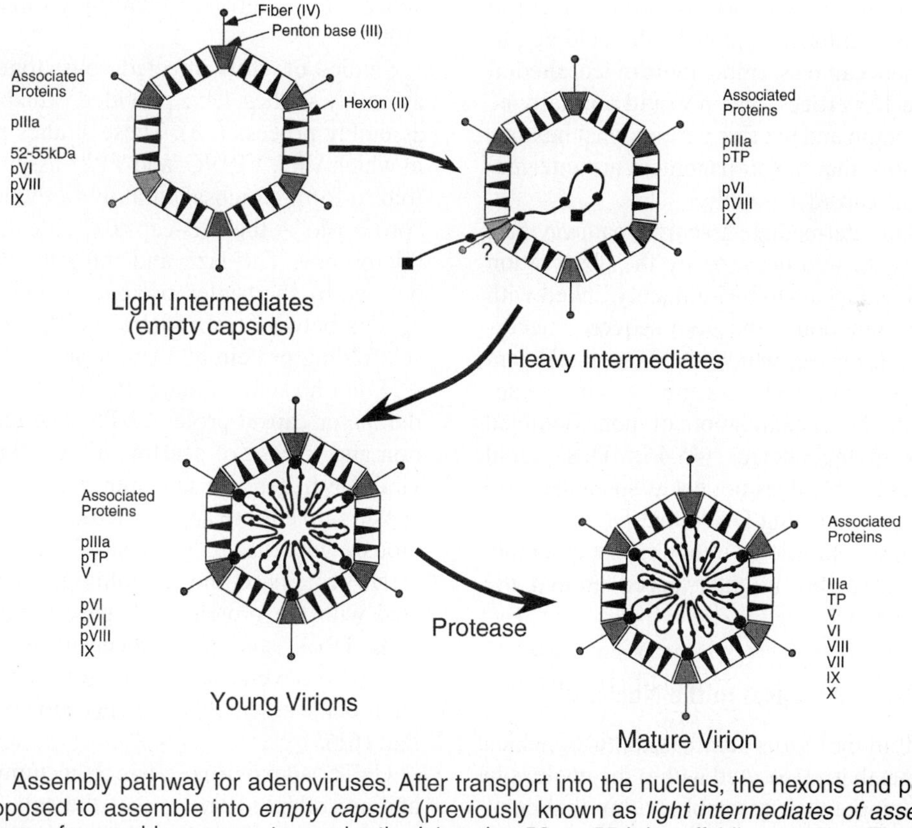

FIG. 7. Assembly pathway for adenoviruses. After transport into the nucleus, the hexons and pentons are proposed to assemble into *empty capsids* (previously known as *light intermediates of assembly*). This stage of assembly appears to require the L1 region 52- to 55-kd scaffolding proteins. These proteins are lost on association with viral DNA, which is inserted into this structure through a packaging sequence at the left end of the genome. The mechanism of insertion is not known. *Heavy intermediate* forms of the capsid probably represent those in which DNA packaging is incomplete and the DNA is fragmented. Precursor core proteins are packaged into the empty capsid along with the genome to form *young virions.* Proteolytic cleavage of the precursor proteins by the viral proteinase yields the mature virion.

vent transport into the nucleus (58), indicating that each monomer has an active NLS. In contrast, the fiber must form trimers to be efficiently transported to the nucleus (91), even though this protein has an active NLS located at its N-terminus (50). It seems likely that the oligomerized penton base and fibers are transported independently into the nucleus and assemble into the intact penton at the site of assembly.

Two distinct pathways for adenovirus capsid assembly have been postulated from a large body of work in this area. Results from experiments that combined kinetic labeling with temperature-sensitive replication mutants yielded an assembly scheme shown in Figure 7, where, in a manner similar to that observed with DNA phages, an empty capsid is first formed. DNA and associated core proteins are then subsequently packaged into these empty shells to yield "young virions" that then undergo proteolytic maturation. Additional viral products appear to act as scaffolding proteins around which shells are assembled and which facilitate the encapsidation process. These proteins are present in the intermediate capsid-like particles but are absent once DNA has been encapsidated (reviewed in 20). Disruption of adenovirus capsids with denaturants results in the release of groups of nine hexons that are associated with the faces of the icosahedron and that lack the peripentonal hexons. Under acid conditions, these nanomers can reassemble to form icosahedral shells that lack the 12 vertices, which would normally be composed of the penton and the five peripentonal hexons, raising the possibility that hexon nanomers are intermediates of adenovirus capsid assembly.

The empty-capsid intermediate assembly pathway has, however, been brought into question by the observation that DNA packaging appears to be intimately linked with capsid assembly. A mutation in the DNA sequence necessary for genomic packaging, which results in inefficient DNA–capsid interactions, blocks assembly of empty capsids and results in the accumulation of nonassembled capsid precursors in the nucleus (45,46). This would argue that capsid assembly does not occur spontaneously in the absence of an interacting DNA, that DNA–protein interactions play a crucial role in initiating the assembly process, and that assembly might proceed around the DNA-containing core.

Assembly of Enveloped Viruses in the Nucleus

Two enveloped animal virus families, both of which use cell components that are located within the nucleus in their replication, initiate their assembly within that compartment. These are the herpesviruses and the orthomyxoviruses. In addition to importing into the nucleus the necessary components for assembly, these viruses must also export large nucleoprotein complexes back out into the cytoplasm.

In some respects, the herpesviruses represent a hybrid between a nonenveloped virus, such as adenovirus, and a more conventional enveloped virus, such as a retrovirus, in that they use the secretory pathway to transport large capsid structures from the nucleus to the outside of the cell. This group of large viruses assemble, within the nucleus, an icosahedral capsid shell that is 160 Å thick and 1,250 Å in diameter. The major component of this protein shell is VP5, which forms both the pentameric and hexameric capsomeres necessary to assemble the icosahedral structure. Associated with the outer surface of the hexamers is the abundant small protein VP26. Two additional proteins, VP19C and VP23, in a 1:2 ratio, form heterotrimeric triplexes, which fit between and link together adjacent capsomeres (87). Scaffolding proteins are essential for herpes simplex virus type 1 (HSV-1) capsid assembly and maturation, and in their absence, incomplete and aberrantly shaped capsids are assembled. As with adenovirus, the major capsid protein lacks a nuclear targeting signal, and its transport into the nucleus requires an interaction with either the scaffolding protein (VP22a) or the triplex protein VP19C, either of which can presumably provide the necessary NLS. VP23 similarly requires VP19C for nuclear localization, whereas VP26 appears to be directed there by its interaction with VP5 (100).

Studies of virus-infected cells, together with *in vitro* assembly studies, have provided valuable insights into the assembly process (88). These studies point to a pathway in which VP5, VP19C, and VP23 assemble around a scaffold to form an icosahedral, but predominantly spherical "procapsid"—the "B-capsids" identified by electron microscopy. The size and integrity of this structure is defined by the triplex proteins, which mediate the interactions between capsomeres (108,127). Cleavage of the scaffolding protein at a site near its C-terminus removes a 25–amino acid sequence that is necessary for binding to the major capsid protein, VP5. The resulting disassociation and release of scaffold allows for packaging of the viral DNA genome and induction of maturation of the capsid into a more angular icosahedral structure, the previously identified "C-capsids." In the absence of an active proteinase, the scaffolding proteins remain associated with the protein shell preventing packaging of the viral DNA, and the procapsid is unable to mature (89,101). Several aspects of this morphogenic pathway parallel the assembly and maturation of the bacteriophage P22 (61).

Unlike adenoviruses, which accumulate in the nucleus and are released on lysis of the cell, herpesviruses exit the nucleus by budding through into the lumen of the nuclear membrane. It is in this way that a herpesvirus initially enters the secretory pathway of the cell; the complexities of this interaction are discussed later in this chapter.

For influenza virus to take advantage of its unusual capacity to "steal" the capped 5′ ends of host cell mRNAs to initiate its own mRNA synthesis, transcription and viral RNA replication must occur in the nucleus (see Chapters 7 and 24). Genomic (minus sense) RNAs are replicated by a different mechanism to yield templates for mRNA synthesis as well as progeny viral genomes. The eight viral RNA segments of this virus are packaged into individual RNPs containing the four proteins of the transcriptase complex (PB1, PB2, PA, and NP, each containing a functional NLS sequence) but are not exported into the cytosol until late in infection when the viral matrix (M1) protein begins to be synthesized (71). Under conditions in which matrix synthesis is inhibited, the viral RNPs (vRNPs) accumulate in the nucleus, tightly associated with the nuclear matrix. The block to export can be relieved by expression of matrix from an independent vector (8). Matrix association with the vRNPs also appears to be important for preventing their reentry into the nucleus because conditions such as acidification or mutations that promote dissociation of M1 allow the RNPs to be reimported (reviewed in 133). Thus, the matrix protein of influenza virus is a key modulator of vRNP transport into and out of the nucleus.

Assembly of Viruses in the Cytoplasm

Although targeting and import of proteins into the nucleus or secretory pathway involves well-characterized motifs on the proteins involved, the processes by which proteins are targeted to destinations within the cytoplasm remains, for the most part, obscure. Most viruses, even those that are nonenveloped, initiate or complete their assembly in association with membranes of the secretory pathway. Nevertheless, the intracellular pathways that function to transport their capsid components and genomes to these sites have not been defined. Reoviruses are the only animal viruses that appear to complete their assembly entirely in the cytoplasm without the involvement of membranes. Both genome replication and virus assembly occur in specialized areas of the cytoplasm known as *virus factories.* Little is known about the establishment and retention of proteins in these sites, but this specialized structure may be a mechanism to avoid the complexities of transporting virion components to a separate cytoplasmic assembly site after translation.

Intracytoplasmic Transport and Assembly of Retroviral Capsids

Retroviruses are enveloped viruses that, for the most part, complete their assembly by budding through the plasma membrane of the infected cell. The immature capsid of the virus is assembled from polyprotein precursors that must be transported through the cytoplasm to the underside of the plasma membrane. The membrane-spanning viral glycoproteins, on the other hand, must be transported through the secretory pathway of the cell to the cell surface, where they co-localize with the nascent, membrane-extruding capsid. All replication competent retroviruses contain four genes that encode the structural and enzymatic components of the virion. These are *gag* (capsid protein), *pro* (aspartyl proteinase), *pol* (reverse transcriptase and integrase enzymes), and *env* (envelope glycoprotein) (see Chapter 27). However, the product of the *gag* gene has been shown to possess all the necessary structural information to mediate intracellular transport, to direct self-assembly into the capsid shell, and to catalyze the process of membrane extrusion known as *budding* (109). In most retroviruses, the nascent Gag polyproteins are transported directly to the plasma membrane, where assembly of the capsid shell and membrane extrusion occur simultaneously (Fig. 8).Viruses that undergo this type C form of morphogenesis include members of the *Alpharetroviruses* and *Gammaretroviruses*. Lentiviruses and *Deltaretroviruses* assemble their capsids in a similar fashion. In the second morphogenic class of viruses, the type B/D class, the Gag precursors appear to be targeted first to an intracytoplasmic site, where capsid assembly occurs. These preassembled immature capsids are then transported to the plasma membrane where they undergo budding and envelopment (see Fig. 8). Viruses that undergo this process of assembly and release include members of the *Betaretroviruse*s. Members of the *spumavirus* genus also assemble immature capsids in the cytoplasm, but they are targeted to the ER for envelopment.

Although the size and protein content of the precursor varies between different retroviral families, at least three *gag*-encoded proteins are found in all retroviruses; these are the matrix protein (MA), the capsid protein (CA), and the nucleocapsid protein (NC). In addition to these functionally conserved domains, the Gag precursor can, depending on the virus encoding it, contain additional peptide sequences (Fig. 9), whose function in virus assembly and future cycles of infection is only now being resolved. Some of these additional domains appear to allow the correct folding of the precursor protein for assembly and subsequent processing into the mature virion proteins.

The detailed mechanisms by which the capsid precursor proteins are directed to the site of assembly remains for the most part unknown, but the process is mediated primarily by the MA domain of the Gag precursor. In most retroviruses, the matrix protein contains two elements involved in plasma membrane targeting. The first of these is an N-terminal myristic acid, which is thought

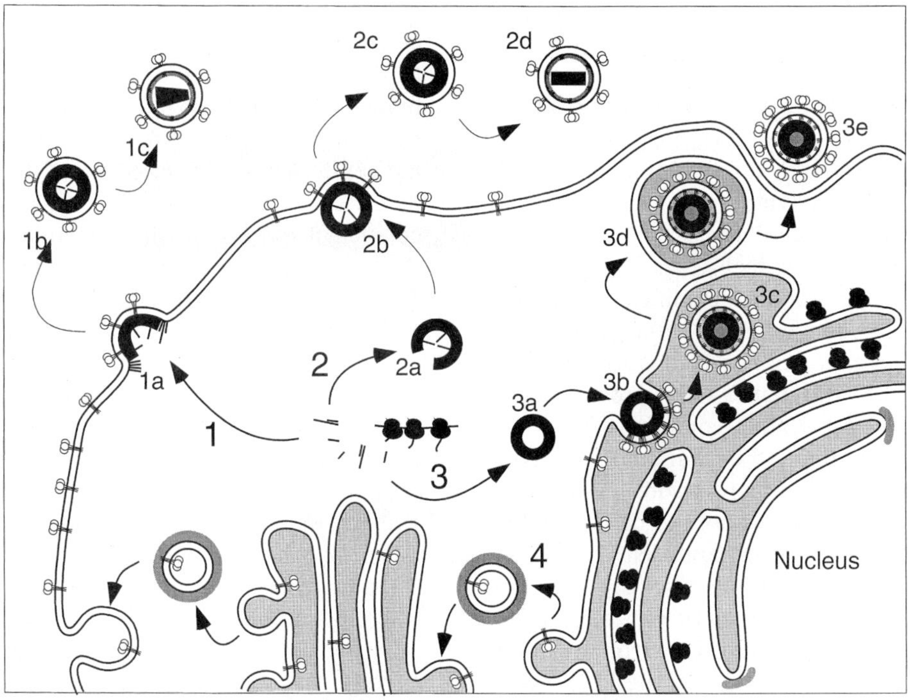

FIG. 8. Assembly of retroviruses. The assembly pathways of retroviruses that exhibit C-type morphogenesis (*Pathway 1*) , B- and D-type morphogenesis (*Pathway 2*) and that of the foamy viruses (*Pathway 3*) are shown. The envelope glycoproteins are translated on membrane-bound polysomes and, for most retroviruses, are transported to the cell surface through the cell's secretory pathway (*Pathway 4*). For all morphogenic classes, the Gag proteins are synthesized on free polysomes. In the case of the C-type morphogenic viruses (i.e., Rous sarcoma virus and human immunodeficiency virus), the Gag and Gag-Pol proteins migrate either individually or in small multimers to the plasma membrane, where immature capsid assembly and envelopment occurs concurrently (*1a*). At some ill-defined point in this pathway, the viral genomic RNAs associate with the Gag and Gag-Pol precursors and are incorporated into the developing capsid. In the case of the B- and D-type viruses, the Gag and Gag-Pol precursors are first transported to an intracytoplasmic assembly site (*2a*), where they assemble into immature capsids. The immature structures are then transported (*2b*) to the plasma membrane, where they associate with the envelope glycoproteins and induce viral budding. For both classes of retroviruses, the capsids of the nascent immature particles appear as doughnut-shaped structures in thin-section electron microscopy and contain unprocessed Gag and Gag-Pol precursors (*1b* and *2c*). The mature virus particles contain electron-dense cores with morphologies characteristic of the virus (*1c* and *2d*). The maturation step is required for infectivity and is the result of the activation of the viral protease, which cleaves the Gag and Gag-Pol precursors into the internal structural and enzymatic proteins of the virus. For the foamy viruses, Gag and Pro-Pol precursors assemble into immature capsids in the cytoplasm (*3a*). Budding primarily occurs at the endoplasmic reticulum membrane where the viral glycoproteins are retained (*3b*). The enveloped virion is presumably transported to the plasma membrane by transport vesicles (*3d*). Maturational cleavage of the immature core is limited to removal of 4 kd from the C-terminus of the precursor; the mature infectious virion maintains an immature morphology (*3e*).

to insert into the hydrophobic lipid bilayer. The second is a surface patch of basic amino acids that are hypothesized to mediate the initial interaction of Gag with the negatively charged, phospholipid head groups of the membrane. The bipartite signal created by these two elements appears to be important for intracellular targeting to the plasma membrane because mutations that interfere with either myristylation or the charged residues can abrogate plasma membrane targeting. In some instances, Gag precursors mutated in these sequences are targeted to internal membranes (reviewed in 33).

In the *Betaretroviruses*, where capsid assembly and virus budding are discrete events, a recent genetic dissection of this process suggests that Gag-containing precursors of these viruses express a dominant sorting signal, identified as a surface loop of the MA domain, that targets the proteins to the initial assembly site. A point mutation within this region of the Mason-Pfizer monkey virus (M-PMV) MA domain abrogates intracytoplasmic targeting and results in the type C–like transport of precursors to the plasma membrane, where efficient capsid assembly occurs. In addition, transfer of the protein motif to the Gag of the C-type virus murine leukemia virus (MuLV) results in its retention and assembly in the cytoplasm (11). These results suggest that the *Betaretroviruses* have evolved to use a transport

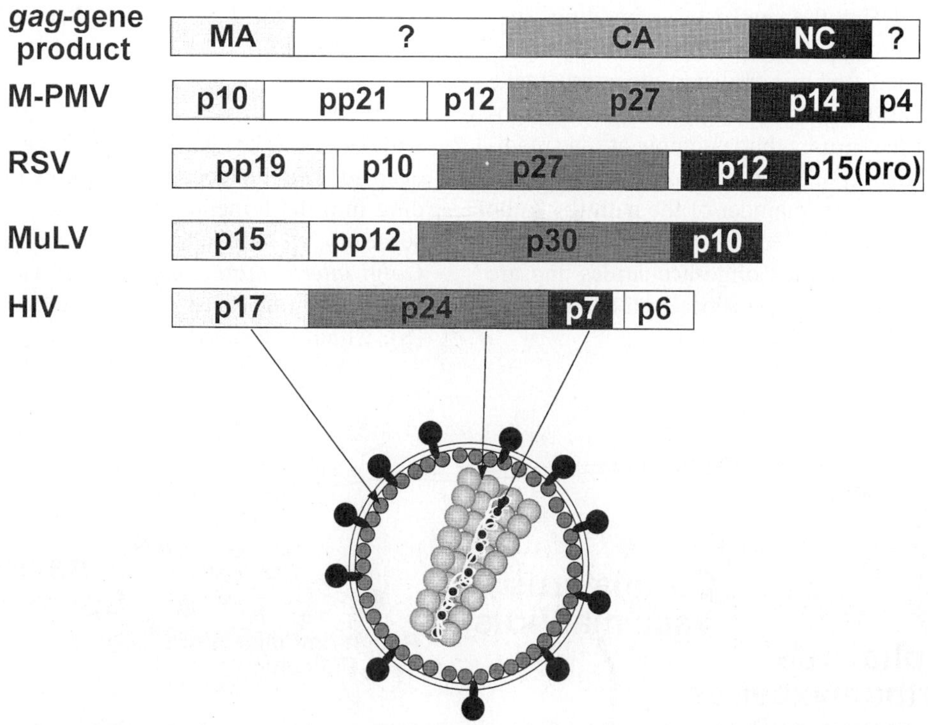

FIG. 9. Organization of the retroviral Gag precursor. The Gag precursor polyproteins of all retroviruses contain, beginning at the N-terminus, matrix (MA), capsid (CA), and nucleocapsid (NC) domains, linked in this order. The *gag* gene products of Mason-Pfizer monkey virus (M-PMV), Rous sarcoma virus (RSV), murine leukemia virus (MuLV), and human immunodeficiency virus (HIV) are shown. The *unshaded boxes* represent regions of the Gag precursor for which no common functions or locations in the mature virion have been established. However, for these three representatives of the alpha-, beta-, and gamma-retroviruses, a "late domain" function required for pinching off of the virus particle from the cell is located between the MA and CA domains. The specific name associated with the Gag cleavage products is derived from their respective apparent molecular weights ($\times 10^{-3}$).

pathway of the cell to target precursors for intracytoplasmic assembly.

By what pathways might preassembled immature capsids of the *Betaretroviruses* or the Gag-containing precursors of the C-type viruses be transported to the plasma membrane? Several studies have suggested that cytoskeletal elements might be involved in this process, but direct evidence for this has not been obtained (reviewed in 62). Recent experiments indicate that the transport process is an active rather than a passive one since it appears to require energy. In cells treated with agents that block ATP synthesis, M-PMV immature capsids are unable to migrate to the plasma membrane from sites deep within the cytoplasm (132).

Irrespective of the assembly site, Gag precursor proteins must associate in a reproducible fashion to assemble into the nascent capsid. Mutational analyses of *gag* genes, as well as *in vitro* assembly studies, have shown that the CA and NC domains of Gag play a crucial role in assembly; MA is dispensable for this process (reviewed in 17 and 33). NC binding to RNA may act to nucleate the capsid assembly process, whereas CA forms a symmetric network of proteins. *In vitro,* the CA protein alone can assemble into tubes that exhibit local sixfold symmetry (hexamers), but cryoelectron microscopy studies of immature capsids has revealed a large heterogeneity in particle size and no evidence of icosahedral symmetry. It is possible, therefore, that the immature capsid has a fullerene-like structure similar to that proposed for the mature core (34,86).

For most retroviruses, capsid assembly drives the process of membrane extrusion known as budding. As discussed later, in order for an infectious virus to be formed, the Gag precursors (or for other viruses, NPs) and surface glycoproteins of the virus must be targeted to the same region of the same membrane. In this way, during virus budding, a proper complement of glycoproteins can be incorporated into the nascent virion.

Assembly of Enveloped Viruses at Cellular Membranes

For most enveloped viruses, the location within the cell at which envelopment takes place is determined by the targeting to or retention of the viral glycoproteins at that site. Indeed, with the exception of the retroviruses, the efficiency of virus budding and particle release is highly dependent on the presence of the envelope glycoprotein, and in its absence, few particles are produced. Because the glycoproteins define the site of virus budding, specific interactions between the viral NP and the glycoproteins, sometimes mediated by a matrix protein, must take place to ensure that the genome of the virus is incorporated. For each of the viruses that assemble at intermediate points within the secretory pathway, fully assembled viruses must traverse the remainder of the pathway to be released from the cell (Fig. 10). Glycoproteins on these released viruses have complex oligosaccharides and are most likely modified by the Golgi-localized enzymes on the way to the cell surface.

Assembly at the Endoplasmic Reticulum Intermediate Compartment

The coronaviruses are positive-stranded RNA viruses with large (30 kb) genomes packaged in a helical nucleocapsid. The nucleocapsid acquires its envelope by budding into the lumen of a pre-Golgi compartment of the secretory pathway termed the *endoplasmic reticulum–Golgi intermediate compartment.* Coronaviruses invariably encode three envelope proteins. The spike protein (S), which determines the host range of the virus, is a

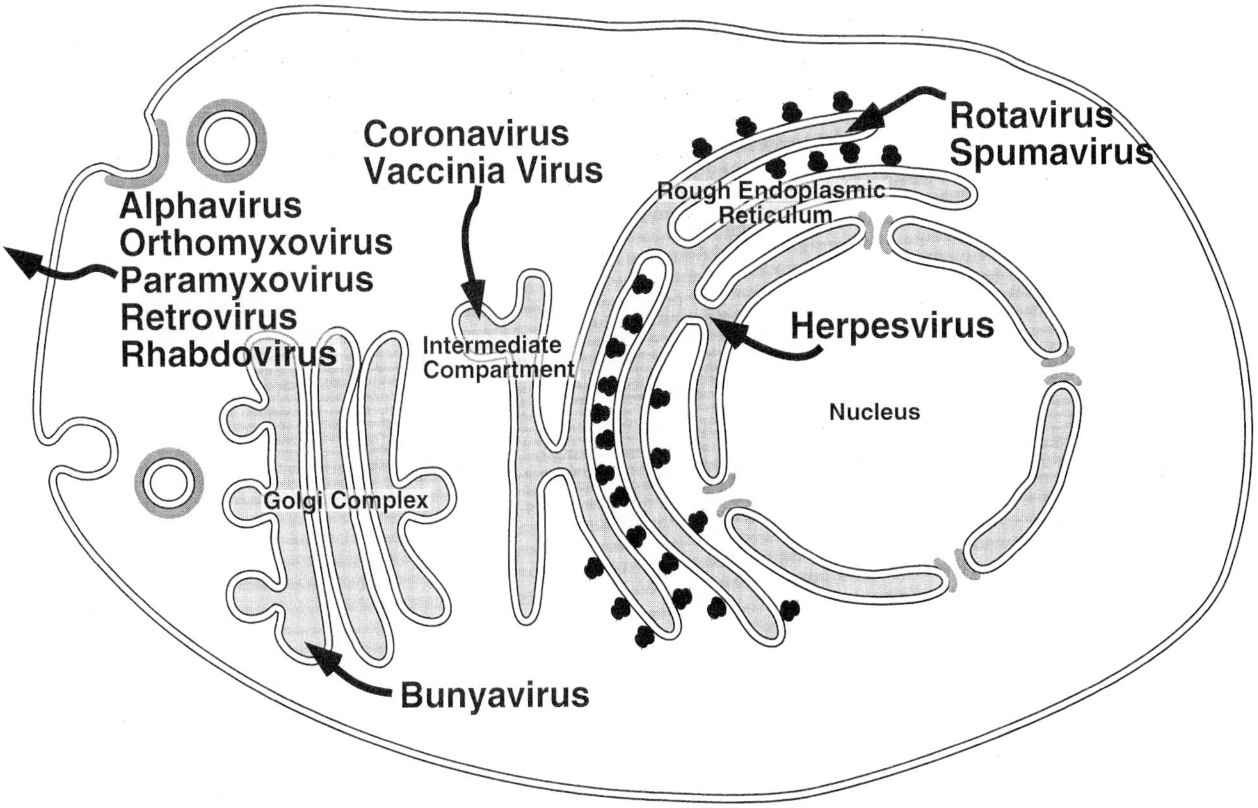

FIG. 10. Viral assembly at cellular membranes. Schematic representation showing the intracellular locations at which enveloped virus assembly takes place. For each virus that is enveloped at organelles within the secretory pathway, the virions must traverse the remainder of the pathway to be released from the cell. For the herpesviruses, two morphogenic pathways have been proposed (see also Fig. 12). In the first, the virus buds into the lumen of the nuclear membrane and is then transported to the cell surface through the secretory pathway. In the second, the virus also buds into the lumen of the nuclear membrane, but then the nascent virus fuses with the outer nuclear membrane to release the capsid, which is then enveloped by membranes derived from the Golgi complex. Rotaviruses appear to use the endoplasmic reticulum (ER) membrane as a scaffold for assembly of virion proteins—the capsids that form during the assembly process are only transiently enveloped, and nonenveloped particles accumulate in the lumen of the ER. Coronaviruses localize the three membrane proteins (E, M, and S) in the ER intermediate compartment, in which virus budding occurs. In contrast, the vaccinia virus nucleocapsid appears to be wrapped by a double membrane derived from this compartment but remains free in the cytoplasm so that it can then be further enveloped by Golgi-derived membranes. The G1 and G2 glycoproteins of bunyaviruses co-localize in the *trans*-Golgi compartment to direct budding of nucleocapsids at this location. For the several families of viruses that assemble at the plasma membrane, the final location of the viral glycoproteins also appears to be important in defining where assembly occurs. Even for the retroviruses, which can assemble and release virus particles in the absence of envelope glycoproteins, these proteins direct virus budding to the basolateral plasma membrane of polarized epithelial cells.

type I glycoprotein that forms the distinct bulbous peplomers of the virus. Expressed independently of the other glycoproteins, S is transported to the plasma membrane and so is unlikely to determine the site of virus assembly. The most abundant virion protein is the membrane (M) glycoprotein. M spans the lipid bilayer three times, exposing a short N-terminal domain outside the virus and a long C-terminus inside the virion. Because of its abundance and because M is transported to the Golgi complex but not to the surface, it was initially thought to define the site at which this family of viruses were enveloped. Recent studies, however, have shown that the small envelope protein (E), which is only a minor component of virions, is the key to defining the site and nature of coronavirus envelopment. E is a hydrophobic type-I membrane protein that localizes to the intermediate compartment of the ER and induces the formation of tubular, convoluted membrane structures characteristic of virus infection (15,98). How E is retained in the intermediate compartment is not known. Coexpression of E, M, and S results in the assembly and release from cells of virus-like particles containing these three viral membrane proteins. The enveloped particles produced by this system form a homogeneous population of spherical particles indistinguishable from authentic virions in size and shape (129). Only M and E are required for efficient particle formation, and expression of E alone can mediate particle release (68). The E protein plays a key role in morphogenesis because mutations in this protein can result in morphologically aberrant viruses (30). The S glycoprotein is thus dispensable for virus particle assembly but is retained in the Golgi by the M protein, which appears to direct its assembly into virions. M protein also directs the incorporation of nucleocapsids containing the genome length RNA into virions, and nucleocapsids associated with newly synthesized M protein have been localized to the budding site in the intermediate compartment (85).

Although most of the retroviruses are enveloped at the plasma membrane of the cell, members of the spumavirus genus bud into the ER intermediate compartment region of the secretory pathway. Expression of the primate foamy virus Env complex, gp80-gp48, in the absence of other structural proteins, results in its localization to the ER. A dilysine ER retrieval motif at the C-terminus of gp48 is responsible for this location, and mutation of either lysine results in efficient transport of the protein to the plasma membrane. Although a greater fraction of capsids bud from the plasma membrane in mutant virus–infected cells, envelopment of capsids at the ER is still observed (37). A second distinguishing feature of foamy viruses is the dependence of capsid envelopment on Env expression. As with the *Betaretroviruses*, immature foamy virus capsids assemble in the cytoplasm. They are then transported to the ER (or plasma membrane) for envelopment. In the absence of foamy virus Env, these preassembled capsids do not associate with membranes or initiate budding (31). Recent experiments have shown that it is the posttranslationally cleaved (148 amino acids long), membrane-spanning, signal peptide domain of the foamy virus Env that mediates capsid membrane association and envelopment and that this protein is incorporated into the virus in the process.

Assembly in the Golgi Complex

Bunyaviruses are negative-stranded, enveloped viruses with a segmented genome that bud into the Golgi complex (see Fig. 10). The glycoprotein spikes of the best-characterized member of this family, Uukuniemi virus, are composed of two type I glycoproteins, G1 and G2, that determine the site of virus budding. G1 and G2 are cotranslationally cleaved from a single precursor protein by signal peptidase, which cleaves after the internal signal sequence that mediates translocation of G2. The two proteins have been shown to fold with distinctly different kinetics, but once properly folded, they form a G1-G2 heterodimer that is transported to the Golgi complex. G2 expressed in the absence of G1 is retained in the ER, whereas G1 expressed alone is targeted to the Golgi (reviewed in 42). The Golgi localization signal of G1 has been mapped, through analysis of mutations and glycoprotein chimeras, to the membrane proximal half of the 98–amino acid long cytoplasmic tail of the protein. Surprisingly, a region of 81 amino acids, between the putative transmembrane domain and the G2 signal peptide at the C-terminus of the G1 cytoplasmic tail, expressed as a soluble protein or as a green fluorescent protein (GFP) fusion, could localize to the cytoplasmic face of the Golgi complex (2). Glycoprotein retention in this case, therefore, appears to depend on interactions between the cytoplasmic tail of G1 in the G1-G2 heterodimer, with components residing on the cytoplasmic side of the Golgi membrane.

During infection by bunyaviruses, the helical nucleoproteins, consisting of the three single-stranded genomic RNA segments and the associated nucleocapsid (N) protein, accumulate in the region of the Golgi and presumably interact with the G1 cytoplasmic domain to initiate the budding of virus particles into the Golgi lumen. The region of the secretory pathway at which G1-G2 heterodimers accumulate clearly defines the budding site because, in the presence of brefeldin, a drug that redistributes Golgi components to the ER, virus budding occurs into the ER (42).

Assembly at the Plasma Membrane

Members of several virus families undergo their envelopment at the plasma membrane. These families include the togaviruses, rhabdoviruses, paramyxoviruses, orthomyxoviruses, and retroviruses. In each of these cases, the viral glycoproteins, either as hetero-oligomeric complexes or homo-oligomers, have traversed the entire secretory pathway to be delivered to the plasma membrane of the cell. Assembly at the plasma membrane obviates the need for the assembled virus to navigate additional compartments of the secretory pathway because virions are released directly into the external milieu of the cell. Alphaviruses are perhaps the best characterized of these different viral systems because a combination of biochemical, genetic, and structural information has been amassed to shed light on the complexity of this assembly process. The major glycoproteins E1 and E2 of the alphaviruses are translated from a subgenomic 26S RNA as a p62, 6K, E1 precursor complex that is transported to the Golgi, where p62 is processed to E2. Stable trimers of E1-E2 heterodimers are then transported to the plasma membrane, where they associate with assembled core structures composed of the capsid (C) protein and genome-length RNA (reviewed in 35). Recent cryoelectron microscopy analyses of mature alphavirus particles have revealed for the first time a detailed structure of this enveloped virion (see Chapters 3 and 19). These studies have shown that both the envelope and the core display icosahedral symmetry. Surprisingly, however, the trimers of E1 and E2 are located at the threefold and quasi-threefold symmetry axes of the pentameric and hexameric order of the nucleocapsid (Fig. 11). Moreover, the heterodimers of each spike splay out above the membrane in a skirtlike fashion, traverse the lipid bilayer individually, and interact with three underlying capsid (C) proteins that belong to three separate capsomeres. This creates a complex network of molecular interactions, where the glycoprotein–capsid protein interactions not only mediate the binding of the nucleocapsid to the spikes but also stabilize the connections between the capsomeres. Above the membrane, the skirts formed by the E1-E2 heterodimers form lateral connections that mimic the pentameric and hexameric arrangement of the capsid. These interactions may facilitate the process of budding by providing a multivalent binding site for the capsid as well as by providing a force for membrane bending (35). Budding, however, requires a cooperative interaction between the glycoproteins and the capsid protein because, in the absence of either, budding does not occur. Moreover, mutations in the cytoplasmic tail of the E2 protein alone can abrogate budding. It has been proposed that alphavirus budding is initiated by NC binding through hydrophobic interactions between the cytoplasmic domain of E2 and the capsid protein to a cluster of E1-E2 trimers at the plasma membrane. The recruitment of additional clusters of glycoprotein heterodimers into the complex by cooperative trimer–trimer and heterodimer–capsid protein interactions would continue until envelopment is completed (35). This model does not, however, take into account a role for the 6K protein, which can clearly influence the budding process and may be present at the cell surface as part of the glycoprotein complex.

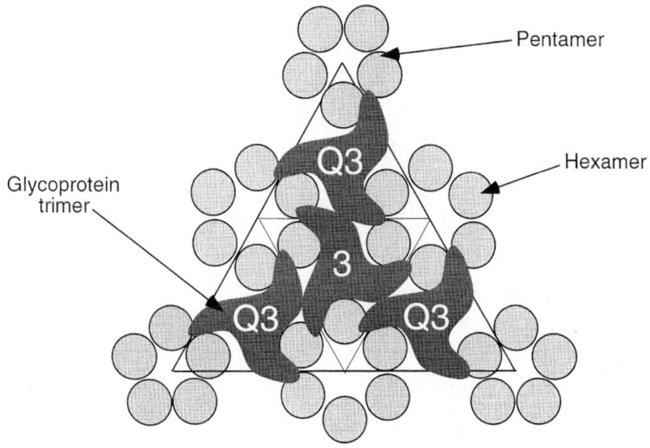

FIG. 11. Alphavirus glycoprotein–capsid interactions. Schematic representation of the interactions between the glycoprotein spikes at the threefold (*3*) and quasi-threefold (*Q3*) axes of the nucleocapsid structure and the capsid proteins of the hexameric and pentameric capsomeres of that structure. The spikes are involved in extensive lateral interactions near the lipid bilayer through their skirts, and through interactions with the capsid protein, they stabilize interactions between capsomeres. (Modified from ref. 35, with permission.)

For the negative-stranded RNA viruses, orthomyxoviruses, paramyxoviruses, and rhabdoviruses, an additional protein, the matrix protein, mediates the interactions between the viral glycoproteins and the RNP and appears to play a key role in envelopment. These proteins are able to bind to membranes through hydrophobic domains or, as with the retroviruses, through a cluster of positively charged residues that initiates electrostatic interactions with the plasma membrane. Cross-linking studies have demonstrated that these M proteins form homo-oligomers in the virus and can self-associate *in vitro* or when expressed at high levels in cells. As discussed earlier, the M1 protein of influenza virus acts to mediate the transport of RNPs from the nucleus to the site of virus assembly on the plasma membrane. Little is known about the intracytoplasmic transport pathways involved in targeting this complex; nevertheless, the RNPs appear to accumulate at regions of the plasma membrane enriched for M1. The importance of the M protein in the paramyxovirus budding process was inferred from the defective measles viruses found in subacute sclerosing panencephalitis (SSPE) that are unable to assemble virus particles and that have mutations in the M protein–coding region (6). However, the recent development of reverse genetics systems for the negative-stranded viruses, in which mutations can be reintroduced into the viral genome, has allowed a more rational approach to examining these questions. Construction of rhabdovirus genomes that lack the M coding region resulted in a dramatic (more than 105-fold) decrease in the release of virus particles, and those that were released lacked the characteristic bullet-shape morphology. The defect could be complemented by expression of M in *trans* (74). Thus, in the rhabdoviruses, the M protein condenses the helical RNP into its characteristic shape and mediates the envelopment process.

Similar approaches have begun to shed light on the role of the G glycoprotein in rhabdovirus assembly. Viruses that lack the G protein–coding domain do assemble and release bullet-shaped particles but at only 3% the efficiency of wild-type viruses (73). Initial studies with G proteins lacking a cytoplasmic tail suggested that this domain might be important in the budding process; however, recent studies have shown that although there is a general requirement for at least a short cytoplasmic tail, it is amino acid sequence independent. Thus, the basis for M protein interactions with G is unresolved. Furthermore, foreign glycoproteins can be efficiently incorporated into rhabdovirus particles, but they do not stimulate budding (102). This is consistent with recent experiments that have identified a domain within the extracellular membrane proximal stem (GS) of vesicular stomatitis virus (VSV) G that is required for efficient VSV budding. Recombinant viruses encoding glycoprotein chimeras with 12 or more membrane proximal residues of the GS, as well as the G protein transmembrane and cytoplasmic tail domains, produced near wild-type levels of particles. In contrast, those with shorter regions produced 10- to 20-fold fewer particles. It is possible, therefore, that this region of the G protein membrane proximal domain modifies the membrane to facilitate the budding process (103).

In influenza virus, the fact that the cytoplasmic domains of both the HA and the neuraminidase (NA) are highly conserved in all subtypes of the virus pointed to a role for this domain in assembly of enveloped virus. Early studies indicated that HA proteins with foreign cytoplasmic tails are not incorporated into virions, although HAs lacking this domain can be incorporated at levels 50% that of wild-type viruses (82). Recent studies using reverse genetics have confirmed these findings and have shown that the short (6 amino acid) cytoplasmic domain of NA also plays an important role in morphogenesis. Viruses encoding the truncated NA protein were released less efficiently and were larger and more filamentous. However, in viruses encoding tail-less versions of both HA and NA, a 10-fold reduction in virus release was observed, and morphogenesis was drastically altered. Virus particles released from these cells were greatly elongated, with an extended irregular shape and a reduced level of viral RNA. Thus, it appears that for influenza virus, the interactions between M1 and the viral glycoproteins are so important for envelopment and morphogenesis that the virus has developed redundant interaction domains in both HA and NA (55,136).

As described earlier, with the exception of the spumaviruses, glycoprotein–capsid interactions are not required for the assembly and release of enveloped retrovirus particles; the Gag precursor alone contains the information necessary to be specifically targeted to the plasma membrane and to drive budding. Moreover, there is contradictory evidence regarding the role of the cytoplasmic domain in directing the envelope glycoprotein into budding virions because Env proteins lacking a cytoplasmic domain can be efficiently incorporated into retrovirus particles and can effectively mediate virus entry into target cells (reviewed in 51). Nevertheless, for members of the lentivirus family, such as HIV and simian immunodeficiency virus (SIV), that encode envelope glycoproteins with a long (150 amino acids or more) cytoplasmic domain, a specific interaction between the tail of TM and the MA domain of the Gag precursor appears to be necessary for Env incorporation. For these viruses, mutations in MA or in the cytoplasmic tail can abrogate Env incorporation (reviewed in 33). Further evidence for this interaction is derived from polarized epithelial cells, in which retroviral glycoproteins define the plasma membrane domain at which virus budding and release occur (see later).

Targeting of Viral Glycoproteins in Polarized Epithelial Cells Defines the Site of Budding

Many viruses initiate their infection of a host by interacting with cells of an epithelial surface. Individual cells within an epithelial layer are tightly connected by junctional complexes that form a barrier to diffusion of molecules throughout the cell membrane and divide the cell surface into two distinct plasma membrane domains: the apical domain, which faces the exterior; and the basolateral domain, which faces the interior. As a result of differential targeting of lipids and protein components to apical and basolateral membranes, epithelial cells in tight monolayers are highly polarized, with each plasma membrane domain having a distinct lipid and protein composition (105). The assembly and release of many viruses from epithelial cells is also highly polarized, occurring selectively at either the apical or basolateral surface. Influenza virus releases newly assembled virions from the apical surface of polarized epithelial cells, whereas VSV and many retroviruses are released from the basolateral membrane. In the absence of other viral proteins, VSV G protein and retroviral Env proteins are transported to the basolateral surface, whereas HA and NA are targeted to the apical membrane. This delivery to specific membranes is consistent with viral glycoproteins directing the site of virus assembly and envelopment (reviewed in 14). Sorting of proteins to one or the other domain occurs in the *trans*-Golgi network, and recent evidence suggests that proteins destined for the basolateral surface contain within their cytoplasmic domain motifs that direct the protein to that membrane. In the VSV G protein, a tyrosine-based motif within the cytoplasmic tail appears to be crucial to basolateral targeting (124). Similarly, tyrosine-based endocytosis motifs in the cytoplasmic domain of both the MuLV and HIV Env proteins are important for their polarized expression and for basolateral budding of their cognate viruses. In the absence of this signal, Env proteins are delivered to and virus buds from both membranes with equal efficiency (65).

Apical transmembrane proteins appear to contain two signals that probably act cooperatively in targeting to the apical surface. Thus, glycosylation in the ectodomain and a signal in the membrane-spanning domain (MSD) function together to ensure association with sphingolipid-cholesterol–enriched membrane domains or rafts. Rafts have been proposed to mediate apical transport in polarized epithelial cells, and the influenza virus HA partitions into these detergent-insoluble glycolipid-rich membrane fractions through sequences in its MSD (111,112). Polarized virus assembly and release may be important in determining the pathogenesis of viral infections because it can influence in a major fashion the pattern of virus spread in the infected host (14).

Complex Interactions with the Secretory Pathway

Although most enveloped viruses undergo assembly and envelopment at a single site within the secretory pathway, some viruses have a more complex interaction that can involve deenvelopment or reenvelopment as part of their assembly pathway.

Rotavirus Assembly Within the Endoplasmic Reticulum

Rotaviruses are nonenveloped viruses that undergo transient envelopment at the ER as an essential step in the formation of the mature double-shelled (triple-layered) virus that is retained within the lumen of the ER until cell lysis. As with the reoviruses, the nucleocapsid, in this case containing 11 double-stranded RNA segments, is assembled in electron-dense areas of the cytoplasm, located close to the ER membrane, known as *viroplasm* (29,90). These double-layered nucleocapsids have an outer icosahedral shell assembled from VP6, the most abundant protein of the virus, surrounding an inner core (see Chapter 54 of *Fields Virology*, 4th ed.). They appear to bud directly into regions of the ER that contain the two outershell proteins VP7 and VP4. A nonstructural protein NSP4, which forms hetero-oligomers with the two outershell proteins, mediates the interaction of the immature particle with the ER membrane (77). A hydrophobic N-terminus anchors this integral membrane protein in the ER, whereas the C-terminal 20 amino acids acts as a receptor for the VP6-containing protein shell. A region of NSP4 near the C-terminus, distinct from the receptor domain, adopts an α-helical coiled-coil structure and mediates the oligomerization of the virus-binding domains into a homotetramer. In this way, presumably, a multivalent receptor for the rotavirus single-shelled particle is connected to an α-helical coiled-coil stalk, which projects from the ER membrane, such that membranes containing NSP4 can bind double-layered particles *in vitro* (92,123).

The exact topology of VP7 in the ER is not known. The mature protein has a cleaved signal peptide but is retained in the ER as if it were an integral membrane protein (56,119). Sequences at the N-terminus of the mature protein, which include the highly conserved LPITGS sequence, are important for its retention (67). VP4 is thought to associate with VP7 and NSP4 just before budding of the nucleocapsid into the ER. Enveloped particles can be observed in the lumen of the ER, which then undergo a process of calcium-dependent deenvelopment, forming in the process an outer icosahedral shell of VP7 and VP4 (97). Thus, this nonenveloped icosahedral virus appears to use the ER membrane transiently as a scaffold on which to assemble an icosahedral shell.

Herpesvirus Transport from the Nucleus

As described earlier, the end product of herpesvirus capsid assembly is a large icosahedral structure that is too large to transit the nuclear pore. To release virus to the exterior of the cell, herpesviruses have evolved to use portions of the secretory pathway. This presumably provides the virus with the ability to propagate progeny virions, whereas the cell and its nucleus remain intact. The precise pathway taken by herpes capsids to the exterior of the cell remains controversial mainly because the bulk of the evidence has come from electron microscopic observations of infected cells (42,99). Nevertheless, there is consensus that the first stage involves budding of the capsid through the inner nuclear membrane into the luminal space. Morphologically, the sites of budding show thickening of the membrane at sites to which viral glycoproteins appear to be targeted (38). Some of these glycoproteins, such as the gB protein of human cytomegalovirus (HCMV), appear to have a novel amino acid motif in their cytoplasmic domain responsible for this intranuclear targeting (76). Little is known, however, about the cellular factors or viral components involved in this envelopment step.

It is equally unclear which of two proposed routes the initially enveloped capsid takes to the exterior (Fig. 12). In the first (Pathway 1: reenvelopment), the membrane of the newly enveloped virus fuses with the outer nuclear

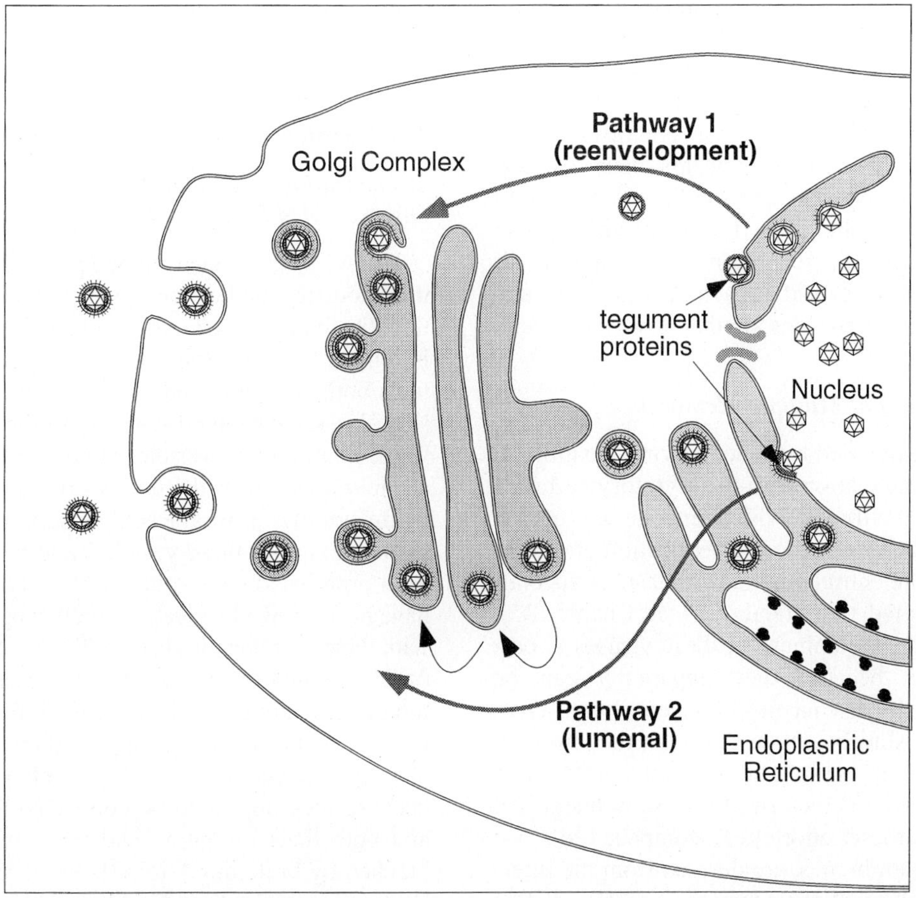

FIG. 12. Herpesvirus assembly. Two pathways are proposed for herpesvirus assembly and release from the cell. In the reenvelopment pathway (*Pathway 1*), nascent assembled capsids bud into the lumen of the nuclear membrane using a subset of virally encoded glycoproteins. These enveloped particles then fuse with and are released from the outer nuclear membrane into the cytoplasm. There, they associate with the tegument proteins and are transported through the cytoplasm to be enveloped by Golgi-derived membranes that contain the full complement of virion glycoproteins. In the lumenal pathway (*Pathway 2*), the nascent capsids associate with tegument proteins in the nucleus before budding through the inner nuclear membrane, which must contain a full complement of virion glycoproteins. The enveloped virus particle now traverses the secretory pathway, and the glycoproteins are modified to their mature form during transit through the Golgi complex.

membrane to release the capsid into the cytoplasm. It is here that *tegument proteins,* a collection of proteins including transcription factors located between the viral capsid and its lipid bilayer in the mature particle, are proposed to associate with the capsid before its reenvelopment by Golgi-derived membrane vesicles. In the second proposed route (Pathway 2: lumenal transport), the virion retains the membrane derived from budding into the lumen of the nuclear membrane and is released into the cytoplasm within a vesicle formed from the outer nuclear membrane or contiguous ER. In this latter pathway, a full complement of viral glycoprotein and tegument proteins must be incorporated into the virus during the nuclear budding step. Maturation of the viral glycoproteins might then be expected to occur after vesicular transport of virions through the Golgi complex.

Although differentiating between the two pathways might seem straightforward, this has not been the case. However, a recent reanalysis of the evidence for each pathway concludes that the balance favors the reenvelopment pathway (28). Some of the clearest evidence comes from the beta-herpesviruses, HCMV, and human herpesvirus type 6 (HHV-6). In these viruses, the tegument is a dense structure that can be observed in electron micrographs. Enveloped virions in the lumen of the nuclear membrane display no evidence of tegument but acquire this layer after loss of the nuclear-derived envelope and release into the cytoplasm (106,125). Studies of the glycoproteins of the gamma-herpesvirus, Epstein-Barr virus, also support this model. Distribution of the viral glycoproteins gp110 and gp350/220 is consistent with the former being incorporated in virions at the nuclear membrane then lost on budding into the cytoplasm, whereas the latter is acquired only during reenvelopment in the Golgi (38). Similarly, studies of the lipid composition of extracellular HSV-1 virions indicate that it is similar to that of the Golgi complex and distinct from that of the nucleus (128). Thus, it appears likely that herpesviruses have evolved to make use of a two-step pathway of release from the cell. It remains to be seen whether different sets of glycoproteins are used to mediate the envelopment of capsid at each of these steps and what the molecular interactions are that drive each event.

Poxvirus Acquisition of Multiple Membranes

Poxviruses, exemplified by vaccinia virus, exhibit an equally complex interaction with the secretory pathway. These large DNA viruses, which encode all of the machinery necessary for genomic replication and transcription, propagate entirely in the cytoplasm in specialized areas designated virus factories (see Chapter 35). The assembly and envelopment of these viruses is particularly complex because they apparently can be enclosed by as many as four lipid bilayers. Initial electron microscopy studies suggested that the crescent membranes that wrap the immature virions are formed *de novo* within the virus factories (21). Subsequently, it was shown that these envelopes, composed of two closely apposed membranes, are derived from the intermediate compartment of the secretory pathway (116). Co-localization of intermediate compartment resident cellular proteins with several vaccinia virus membrane proteins (A17L, A14L, and A13L) known to be crucial to the formation of immature virion membranes supported this model (63,110). The process by which the nucleoprotein and transcription machinery is targeted into these immature envelopes is unclear. Maturation of the immature virion to the infectious intracellular mature virus (IMV) involves a series of proteolytic cleavages of vaccinia structural proteins (80). The mature virus particles are transported out of the assembly areas toward the periphery of the cell, where they become wrapped by additional membranes that are derived from the *trans*-Golgi or early endosomal compartments to form the intracellular enveloped virus (IEV). The membranes of these compartments contain vaccinia proteins that are present in the external enveloped virus (EEV). Wrapping requires the participation of at least one protein present on the IMV and two EEV membrane proteins and thus appears to be driven by interactions between vaccinia-encoded membrane proteins (7,104). The IEV thus contains four concentric membranes, two derived from the intermediate compartment and two from the Golgi and endosome. These particles are then transported through a reorganized actin cytoskeleton (so called actin tails) to the plasma membrane (19), where membrane fusion releases the infectious three-membrane EEV form of the virus.

Modification of the Secretory Pathway

Transcription and Assembly of Poliovirus on a Disassembled Secretory Pathway

Poliovirus is a nonenveloped positive-sense RNA virus that modifies the host cell extensively during its replication. Once introduced into a target cell, the genomic RNA is translated into a long polyprotein precursor that contains both structural and replicative proteins of the virus (Fig. 13; see Chapter 18). Early in the replication of the virus, membranous vesicles appear in the cytoplasm that are found first near the nucleus and then throughout the entire cytoplasm. Viral RNA transcription occurs in close association with these vesicles, and both viral RNA and viral proteins known to be required for RNA replication have been shown by electron microscopy to be associated with their cytoplasmic surface (5,126). Similarly, priming of RNA synthesis by the protein primer, VPg, appears to require membranes (122). Electron microscopy and inhibitor studies initially suggested that the induced vesicles are derived from the host cell secretory pathway because they appear to be connected to ER membranes and both their formation and poliovirus replication are blocked by brefeldin A (5,52). More recent studies have shown that a single poliovirus protein, 3A, which also appears to be responsible for attaching VPg to membranes as a 3AB precursor, induces the formation of these ER-derived vesicles and disassembly of the Golgi complex (26). It is hypothesized that 3A interferes with the assembly of COPII vesicles so that newly synthesized membranes, and those recycled from the Golgi, accumulate in the ER (26).

The formation of vesicular platforms for transcription may also be necessary for efficient capsid assembly. The poliovirus capsid appears to be assembled in a sequential process in which the 5S protomers containing VP1, VP3, and VP0 assemble to form 14S pentamers, which in turn are assembled into virus capsids (see Fig. 13). Pentamers may associate with newly synthesized genomic RNA on intracytoplasmic vesicles, then assemble to form RNA-containing capsids upon completion of the RNA. This assembly pathway is supported by immunoelectron microscopy studies showing that pentamers associated with the replication complex can, if released by detergent, rapidly assemble into empty capsids—arguing that the vesicle prevents assembly of the capsid and keeps the pentamer in an appropriate configuration for association with the RNA (95). In this instance, then, poliovirus appears to have circumvented the problems of intracytoplasmic localization of replicative and structural components by using a membranous organizing center.

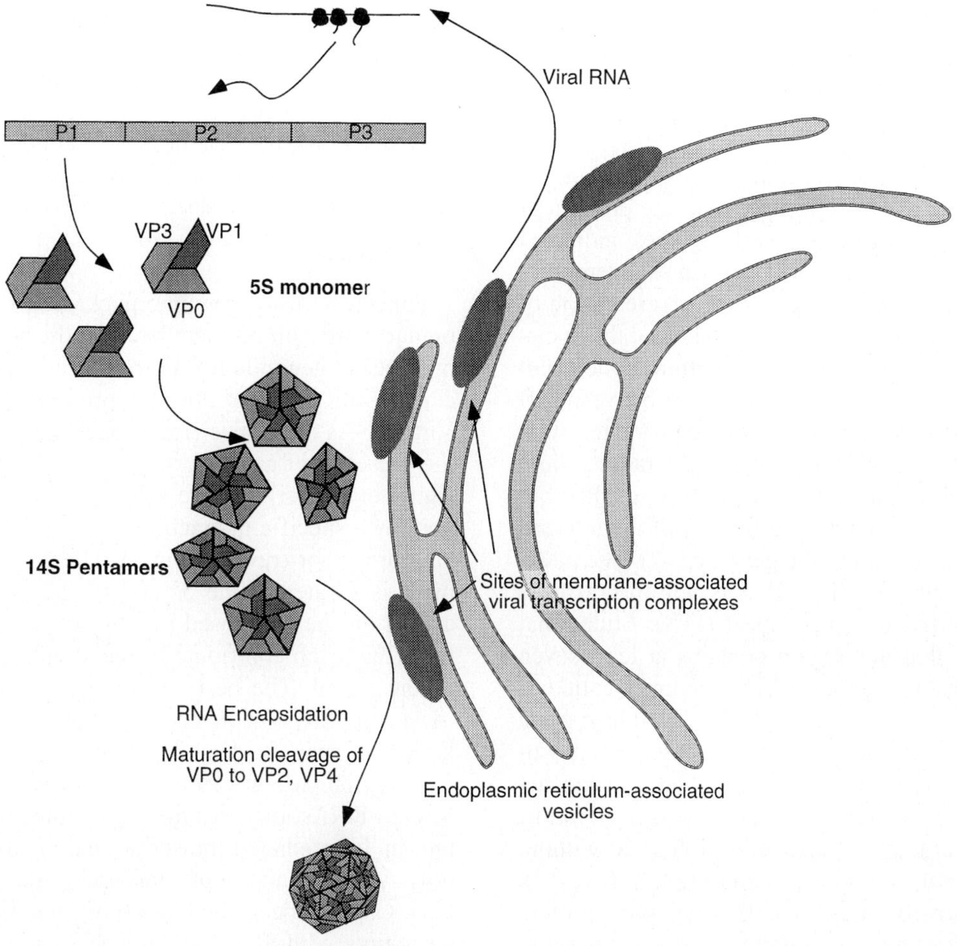

FIG. 13. Poliovirus assembly. The P1 precursor protein is cleaved through an autocatalytic event from the nascent polyprotein and is then cleaved twice by the 3CD-protease to yield VP1, VP3, and VP0. This cleavage is essential for assembly of the 5S monomers into 14S pentamers. It is likely that 12 of these pentamers associate directly with nascent genomic RNA that is being transcribed from membrane-bound transcriptional complexes to assemble an immature 150S provirion. Maturation cleavage of VP0 to yield VP2 and VP4 results in conversion of these immature provirions into the 160S mature virion.

Modification of Post-Golgi Vesicle pH by the Influenza Virus M2 Protein

The influenza HA is synthesized as a precursor protein (HA_0) that, in the case of the avian influenza viruses, is cleaved in the *trans*-Golgi by furin-like proteinases to the biologically functional HA_1-HA_2 heterodimer, three of which in turn form the trimeric HA complex (see Chapters 3 and 24). The influenza virus HA present on an infecting virion is activated to its fusogenic state by the low pH of the endosome. Thus, the similarly low pH of the *trans*-Golgi network and post-Golgi vesicles poses a problem for the virus during the assembly phase of its life cycle, if it is to maintain HA in a functional prefusogenic form. This is apparently solved by the action of the M2 protein, a small tetrameric protein that forms cation-selective ion channels that can increase the pH of the *trans*-Golgi network by pumping out hydrogen ions (96,120).

INCORPORATION OF THE NUCLEIC ACID GENOME DURING THE ASSEMBLY PROCESS

Although the processes involved in the assembly of structural components of a virus are complex and interplay intimately with those of the host cell, they merely provide a mechanism by which the genomic information of the virus can be packaged into a protective environment for transfer to additional host cells. As such, the assembling virus must have evolved to select its genomic nucleic acid efficiently out of the pools of RNA or DNA that are present at the assembly site. Packaging of viral genomes generally involves a cis-acting sequence in the nucleic acid (the so-called packaging sequence) and a structural components of the virus that can recognize and bind this element.

DNA Viruses

As we described earlier, questions remain about the linkage of adenovirus DNA packaging to the process of capsid assembly. Nevertheless, early studies indicated that incomplete virus particles contain subgenomic-length viral DNA that have a large overrepresentation of left-end sequences. Subsequent studies showed that a cis-acting packaging sequence is located within the left 390 base pairs. This region is highly conserved between different adenovirus subtypes and, in Ad 5, overlaps with two distinct enhancer elements for E1A transcription. Deletion of the packaging domain abrogates viability, but infectivity can be restored by substitution of the left-end sequences at the right end of the genome (47). The packaging sequence only functions if it is within 600 base pairs of the inverted terminal repeat (ITS). Mutational analyses showed that this region contains at least seven functional adenosine-thymine (AT)-rich units called *A repeats.* Of the seven, elements I, II, V, and VII have been found to be dominant, and associated 11 base pairs downstream from each of these is a CG motif that also appears crucial to function. Overexpression of an A-repeat multimer results in a dramatic decrease in viral yield without affecting DNA replication or late-transcription (41,114), suggesting the involvement of a limiting viral protein component in packaging. Although this protein has yet to be identified, more recent studies have shown that encapsidation of DNA requires the presence of the nonstructural L1 52/55K protein: empty capsids form in its absence (43). How it might mediate packaging is unclear.

Packaging of the herpesvirus genome is equally complex. As with the large DNA phages, herpesvirus DNA replicates to yield concatamers of genomes in a head-to-tail arrangement, and so packaging must be linked to the generation of genomic length units of DNA. In this virus, two packaging sequences, *pac1* and *pac2,* located within the terminal A repeats, appear to be important for both recognition and cleavage of the DNA (see Chapter 33 and ref. 25). As with the DNA phages, a combination of cleavage recognition sequences and "head-full" packaging appears to ensure the incorporation of unit-length genomes into the procapsid. Studies using a temperature-sensitive protease mutant of HSV-1, which accumulates procapsids (containing an uncleaved scaffolding protein) at the nonpermissive temperature, but which can remove the scaffold and package DNA upon temperature shift to the permissive temperature, have shown that ATP is necessary for DNA packaging to occur but that DNA synthesis is not (12,22). At least seven viral proteins are required for cleavage and packaging of HSV-1 DNA. Sequence analysis reveals that one of these, encoded by the *UL15* gene, shares homology with gp17, the large catalytic subunit of the bacteriophage T4 terminase (134). Thus, the product of this gene may play a direct role in the cleavage of viral DNA replication intermediates into monomers. Moreover, it raises the possibility that herpesviruses assemble a portal and terminase structure, similar to phages such as P22 or λ, for DNA packaging.

RNA Viruses

For retroviruses, genomic packaging represents a particularly difficult problem because the assembling capsid must select genomic RNAs from a large pool of viral and cellular mRNAs that are also present in the cytoplasm. Viral RNAs to be specifically packaged are identified by the presence of an RNA sequence named the packaging signal or ψ (psi) and are selected from the cytoplasmic pool by a specific interaction with the NC domain of the Gag precursor (reviewed in 4). The cis-acting RNA element is located at the 5′ end of the viral genome and appears to be composed of a series of stem-loop structures that each contribute to the strength and specificity of the signal. The best characterized, although perhaps most complex, ψ sequence is that of HIV-1, which is now known to span the first 360 nucleotides of the genome. This region, which can confer packaging specificity on foreign RNAs, includes the TAR sequence that is important in Tat-mediated transcriptional control, the adjacent poly(A) loop, and four stem-loops designated SL1 to SL4. Gag has been shown to bind specifically to the latter region, with SL1, SL3, and SL4 each providing independent high-affinity binding sites. It is likely, although less well documented, that Gag can bind to the 5′ stem-loops also. Disruptive and compensatory mutations within the TAR, poly(A), SL1, and SL3 elements indicate that it is the structure rather than the sequence of the stem-loops that is important for packaging (13,72). Recent nuclear magnetic resonance analyses of SL3 in the presence and absence of the NC protein have begun to provide insights into how Gag might bind this region (24,135).

Given its role in specifying genomic RNA packaging, one might expect the ψ sequence to be located downstream of the splice donor site for subgenomic mRNAs. This is the case for the MuLV and reticuloendotheliosis ψ sequences but is not the case for HIV-1, as shown previously, or for Rous sarcoma virus (RSV). In the case of HIV, the SL3 stem-loop is located in this downstream domain and deletions in this region alone do decrease packaging 5- to 10-fold. In the case of the avian leukosis viruses, however, the entire 5′ ψ sequence is present in both genomic and subgenomic mRNAs; thus, the basis for packaging specificity in this case is unknown (113).

Genomic RNA packaging signals in other RNA viruses are less well defined. In the alphaviruses, this appears to involve direct binding of genomic RNA by the capsid protein. A short (132-nucleotide) segment of RNA in the region of the genome encoding the nonstructural protein NS1 is crucial to this interaction and for packaging of genomic RNA. Like the retroviral ψ sequence, it has also been predicted to form a series of stem-loop structures. The N-terminal third of the capsid protein is basic and is unstructured in the current crystal structure. Nevertheless, a 32–amino acid region (residues 76 to 107) has been shown to be essential for RNA binding in a gel shift assay (113).

For segmented viruses such as the orthomyxoviruses or the reoviruses, genomic packaging requires that a complete set of segments be packaged together in a single virus particle. For influenza virus, reverse genetic approaches have shown that the signals for transcription, replication, and packaging of an RNA segment are located in the 22 5′-terminal and the 26 3′-terminal nucleotides of the RNA (66). These studies do not, however, address how a full complement of RNAs is selected during assembly. Selective packaging of the eight genomic RNAs would presumably require complex recognition systems and molecular interactions. Although there is some evidence to support such a mechanism, the bulk of the evidence appears to be most compatible with a model in which infectious influenza virus particles are formed from random packaging of RNA segments (reviewed in 113).

POSTASSEMBLY MODIFICATIONS AND VIRUS RELEASE

Proteolytic Cleavage and Virus Maturation

Virus-encoded proteolytic enzymes play important roles in the process of assembly for many viruses and in a postassembly maturation steps that are required for the development of an infectious particle for others. These cleavage events can act as molecular switches that introduce flexibility as well as irreversibility into the assembly process.

Proteolytic cleavage in the case of the alphaviruses, for example, is used to allow protein domains, translated from a single mRNA, to enter different transport pathways in the cell. The C protein, which is encoded at the 5′ end of the subgenomic 26S mRNA, folds cotranslationally into an active serine proteinase that cleaves itself from the growing polypeptide chain. This releases the C protein into the cytoplasm for capsid assembly while freeing up the N-terminus of the signal peptide for the p62 glycoprotein precursor, which can then bind SRP and direct the ribosome to the ER.

In the herpesviruses, proteolytic cleavage of the scaffolding protein occurs after assembly of the procapsid is complete and is a prerequisite for DNA packaging. The scaffolding proteins of HSV-1 are encoded by a pair of overlapping genes, *UL26* and *UL26.5*, in which the open reading frame of *UL26* is an in-frame N-terminal extension of that of *UL26.5*. The product of the smaller gene is the abundant scaffolding protein pre-VP22a, whereas the larger gene encodes a protease precursor, which cleaves itself internally to give the proteins VP24 (protease) and VP21. Temperature-sensitive mutants in *UL26* that have an inactive proteinase at the nonpermissive temperature are blocked at the procapsid stage of assembly (reviewed in 99).

A somewhat more complex proteolytic pathway is used by the picornaviruses to regulate the release of both structural and replicative protein components from the single polyprotein precursor that is translated from its positive-stranded RNA genome (see Fig. 13). The initial event in this proteolytic cascade is the primary cleavage in which the P1 structural protein precursor is separated from the P2-P3 precursor. This reaction is catalyzed by the 2A proteinase, which hydrolyzes a Tyr-Gly bond at its own amino-terminus. Although cleavage of the P2-P3 region is carried out by the 3C proteinase at Gln-Gly bonds, the efficient cleavage of the structural protein precursor at the VP0-VP3 and VP3-VP1 boundaries is catalyzed specifically by the 3CD precursor that includes the viral polymerase. Cleavage of the P1 precursor appears to be a prerequisite for entry of the capsid proteins into the assembly pathway. The final processing step is cleavage of VP0 to VP4 and VP2. This autocatalytic, maturational cleavage occurs late in the assembly pathway and appears to be linked to encapsidation of the viral RNA genome. It is likely that the structural alterations that accompany the cleavage event both stabilize the capsid and irreversibly commit the virus to the conformational changes induced on receptor binding that are necessary for productive infection of cells (reviewed in 48).

A similar maturational cleavage is required after assembly and envelopment of retroviral capsids. As described earlier, the retroviral capsid is assembled from polyprotein precursors that are encoded by the *gag* gene. The viral aspartyl proteinase is encoded by the *pro* region of the genome and is translated from unspliced, genome length RNA by a ribosomal frame-shift mechanism as a Gag-Pro or Gag-Pro-Pol precursor protein (see Chapter 27). The presence of the Gag sequences ensures that this key enzyme is targeted to and incorporated into the assembling capsid. The mechanism by which the protease is activated late in the assembly process (most probably after envelopment is complete) is not known. Because the active enzyme is a homodimer of two protease subunits, it has been postulated that dimerization of proteinase precursors in the nascent capsid might allow a functional enzyme to form. However, in the *Betaretroviruses*, the immature capsid contains a full complement of proteinase precursors, which are not activated until late in envelopment at the plasma membrane.

Cleavage of the Gag precursors in the immature capsid is accompanied by a major morphologic rearrangement in which the mature NC protein condenses the genomic

RNA inside a CA shell (see Fig. 8)—the electron-dense core structure of the virus seen in electron micrographs (36). Recent evidence suggests that cleavage at the N-terminus of CA induces a conformational change in the protein, which allows it to assemble the core shell structure (130). Maturational cleavage, as in the case of poliovirus, results in an irreversible commitment to the entry pathway. It prevents a simple reversal of the assembly process and, presumably through the formation of the core, allows the rearrangement of RNA and the reverse transcriptase into a conformation that is optimal for reverse transcription of the genome. In the absence of cleavage, reverse transcription cannot occur, and the virions are noninfectious (reviewed in 121).

Adenoviruses, like retroviruses, undergo a maturational cleavage after assembly that is essential for infectivity. The young virions formed after DNA packaging contain five precursor proteins that must be processed before the mature infectious virion is produced. These include components of the core and the preterminal protein (pTP) used to initiate DNA synthesis. The 23-kd adenovirus proteinase, which is encoded by the L3 region of the genome, is inactive in its purified form. It requires an 11–amino acid peptide present at the carboxyl-terminus of pVI and viral DNA as cofactors for its activity. This unique use of DNA as a cofactor ensures that proteolytic maturation of the virus cannot take place until packaging of DNA is complete (reviewed in 20).

Budding—Role of Viral and Cellular Proteins in Membrane Extrusion

It is clear from the discussions in previous sections that different strategies are used by different enveloped viruses to mediate the process of membrane extrusion that we have termed budding. Envelopment by a lipid bilayer fulfills two functions for a virus: it provides a protective outer layer into which can be embedded the necessary machinery for target cell attachment and entry; and, in most cases, it releases the virus into an environment that is topologically equivalent to the exterior of the cell. The strategies used to drive the budding process can be classified into three general mechanisms (35). In the first, membrane extrusion is driven by envelope glycoproteins alone. This is exemplified by the E protein of the coronaviruses that is capable of inducing the release of virus-like particles in the absence of an RNP. The second strategy is that used by the retroviruses in which the capsid precursors, in the absence of the viral glycoproteins, are able to induce membrane extrusion and particle release efficiently. In this instance, it is hypothesized that the tight interaction between the MA domain of Gag and the lipid bilayer, coupled with the force of Gag-Gag interactions in assembly, drives the budding process. The third mechanism is that of the alphaviruses, which involves interactions between the viral glycoprotein spikes and the assembled capsid. In this case, neither the glycoproteins nor the capsid alone can mediate budding. It appears that lateral interactions between the glycoproteins, coupled with cytoplasmic domain–capsid connections, progressively bend the membrane to form the spherical particle (35,70).

For all of these mechanisms, the final step of budding, the process of pinching off, requires a membrane fusion event. Although for most enveloped viruses, there is no evidence that a viral component is specifically required for pinching off to occur, in the retroviruses, it is clear that this is a separable event that requires the involvement of both viral and host components. Experiments in HIV showed that deletion of the p6 domain at the C-terminus of Gag results in a block to virus release at the pinching-off stage (40). It was later discovered that species within several retrovirus genera encode a similar Gag "late function" domain that is required for efficient release of virions (94). The mechanism by which these "late" domains mediate the pinching-off step is not known, but recent studies of the Yes protein tyrosine kinase have provided a clue. During signal transduction, a PPPY motif on Yes mediates binding through a second amino acid motif called a WW domain—characterized by two widely spaced tryptophan residues—on its partner protein Yap. In the alpha-, beta-, and gamma-retroviruses, the late function of particle release depends on the presence of a PPPY-containing motif that may mediate interactions with WW-containing cellular proteins. The p6 domain in HIV-1 and the late domain of equine infectious anemia virus each appear to bind different cell proteins but can functionally replace the PPPY motif of the *Alpharetroviruses* (reviewed in 121). Interestingly, a similar functional PPPY motif has been found in the matrix protein of VSV, pointing to a similar role for host cell proteins in the release of VSV (16).

Mechanisms to Facilitate the Release of Nascent Particles

If they are to travel efficiently to an uninfected target cell, viruses face one last hurdle after envelopment and release. This is the need to avoid rebinding to receptors on the producing cell. For viruses such as the orthomyxoviruses and paramyxoviruses, which use sialic acid as a receptor on the cell surface, this problem is circumvented by the incorporation of a receptor-destroying enzyme, a sialidase, that can remove these residues during transit through the secretory pathway. For influenza virus, the neuraminidase is crucial to virus release because, in its absence, nascent virus binds to both the cell surface and other virions in large aggregates (64).

Retroviruses have similarly evolved mechanisms to facilitate release and thereby reduce superinfection of a cell. Cells infected with one retrovirus are generally resistant to subsequent infection by a second virus of the same receptor class. The presumed mechanism for this viral interference is the synthesis of viral glycoproteins in large excess over the levels that are incorporated into virions with the effect that cellular receptors that are transported to the cell surface are already occupied by their ligand. This results in removal or down-regulation of the receptor from the cell surface. For HIV-1, down-regulation of the primary receptor CD4 seems to be crucial because the virus has evolved two additional mechanisms to ensure this. Two of the accessory proteins encoded by HIV, Vpu and Nef, act by binding CD4 in the ER and at the cell surface, respectively, and targeting the receptor for degradation (see Chapter 28). In the context of infected tissue, this down-regulation of an abundant receptor could be essential to facilitate spread to adjacent target cells.

REFERENCES

1. Akey CW, Radermacher M. Architecture of the Xenopus nuclear pore complex revealed by three-dimensional cryo-electron microscopy. *J Cell Biol* 1993;122:1–19.
2. Andersson AM, Pettersson RF. Targeting of a short peptide derived from the cytoplasmic tail of the G1 membrane glycoprotein of Uukuniemi virus (Bunyaviridae) to the Golgi complex. *J Virol* 1998;72: 9585–9596.
3. Barlowe C, Orci L, Yeung T, et al. 1994. COPII: A membrane coat formed by Sec proteins that drive vesicle budding from the endoplasmic reticulum. *Cell* 1994;77:895–907.
4. Berkowitz R, Fisher J, Goff SP. RNA packaging. *Curr Top Microbiol Immunol* 1996;214:177–218.
5. Bienz K, Egger D, Pasamontes L. Association of polioviral proteins of the P2 genomic region with the viral replication complex and virus-induced membrane synthesis as visualized by electron microscopic immunocytochemistry and autoradiography. *Virology* 1987;160: 220–226.
6. Billeter MA, Cattaneo R, Spielhofer P, et al. Generation and properties of measles virus mutations typically associated with subacute sclerosing panencephalitis. *Ann N Y Acad Sci* 1994;724:367–377.
7. Blasco R, Moss B. Extracellular vaccinia virus formation and cell-to-cell virus transmission are prevented by deletion of the gene encoding the 37,000-Dalton outer envelope protein. *J Virol* 1991;65:5910–5920.
8. Bui M, Wills EG, Helenius A, et al. Role of the influenza virus M1 protein in nuclear export of viral ribonucleoproteins. *J Virol* 2000;74: 1781–1786.
9. Cepko CL, Sharp PA. Analysis of Ad5 hexon and 100K ts mutants using conformation-specific monoclonal antibodies. *Virology* 1983; 129:137–154.
10. Cepko CL, Sharp PA. Assembly of adenovirus major capsid protein is mediated by a nonvirion protein. *Cell* 1982;31:407–415.
11. Choi G, Park, S, Choi B, et al. Identification of a cytoplasmic targeting/retention signal in a retroviral Gag polyprotein. *J Virol* 1999;73: 5431–5437.
12. Church GA, Dasgupta A, Wilson DW. Herpes simplex virus DNA packaging without measurable DNA synthesis. *J Virol* 1998;72: 2745–2751.
13. Clever JL, Eckstein DA, Parslow TG. Genetic dissociation of the encapsidation and reverse transcription functions in the 5′ R region of human immunodeficiency virus type 1. *J Virol* 1999;73:101–109.
14. Compans RW. Virus entry and release in polarized epithelial cells. *Curr Top Microbiol Immunol* 1995;202:209–219.
15. Corse E, Machamer CE. Infectious bronchitis virus E protein is targeted to the Golgi complex and directs release of virus-like particles. *J Virol* 2000;74:4319–4326.
16. Craven RC, Harty RN, Paragas J, et al. Late domain function identified in the vesicular stomatitis virus M protein by use of rhabdovirus-retrovirus chimeras. *J Virol* 1999;73:3359–3365.
17. Craven RC, Parent LJ. Dynamic interactions of the Gag polyprotein. *Curr Top Microbiol Immunol* 1996;214:65–94.
18. Crowley KS, Liao S, Worrell VE, et al. Secretory proteins move through the endoplasmic reticulum membrane via an aqueous, gated pore. *Cell* 1994;78:461–471.
19. Cudmore S, Reckmann I, Griffiths G, Way M. Vaccinia virus: A model system for actin-membrane interactions. *J Cell Sci* 1996;109: 1739–1747.
20. D'Halluin JC. Virus assembly. *Curr Top Microbiol Immunol* 1995; 199:47–66.
21. Dales S, Mosbach EH. Vaccinia as a model for membrane biogenesis. *Virology* 1968;35:564–583.
22. Dasgupta A, Wilson DW. ATP depletion blocks herpes simplex virus DNA packaging and capsid maturation. *J Virol* 1999;73:2006–2015.
23. Davis LI. The nuclear pore complex. *Annu Rev Biochem* 1995;64: 865–896.
24. De Guzman RN, Wu ZR, Stalling CC, et al. Structure of the HIV-1 nucleocapsid protein bound to the SL3 psi-RNA recognition element. *Science* 1998;279:384–388.
25. Deiss LP, Chou J, Frenkel N. Functional domains within the a sequence involved in the cleavage-packaging of herpes simplex virus DNA. *J Virol* 1986;59:605–618.
26. Doedens JR, Giddings TH Jr, Kirkegaard K. Inhibition of endoplasmic reticulum-to-Golgi traffic by poliovirus protein 3A: Genetic and ultrastructural analysis. *J Virol* 1997;71:9054–9064.
27. Ellgaard L, Molinari M, Helenius A. Setting the standards: Quality control in the secretory pathway. *Science* 1999;286:1882–1888.
28. Enquist LW, Husak PJ, Banfield BW, Smith GA. Infection and spread of alphaherpesviruses in the nervous system. *Adv Virus Res* 1998;51: 237–347.
29. Fabbretti E, Afrikanova I, Vascotto F, Burrone OR. Two non-structural rotavirus proteins, NSP2 and NSP5, form viroplasm-like structures in vivo. *J Gen Virol* 1999;80:333–339.
30. Fischer F, Stegen CF, Masters PS, Samsonoff WA. Analysis of constructed E gene mutants of mouse hepatitis virus confirms a pivotal role for E protein in coronavirus assembly. *J Virol* 1998;72:7885–7894.
31. Fischer N, Heinkelein M, Lindemann D, et al. Foamy virus particle formation. *J Virol* 1998;72:1610–1615.
32. Fornerod M, Ohno M, Yoshida M, Mattaj IW. CRM1 is an export receptor for leucine-rich nuclear export signals [see comments]. *Cell* 1997;90:1051–1060.
33. Freed EO. HIV-1 gag proteins: Diverse functions in the virus life cycle. *Virology* 1998;251:1–15.
34. Ganser BK, Li S, Klishko VY, et al. Assembly and analysis of conical models for the HIV-1 core. *Science* 1999;283:80–33.
35. Garoff H, Hewson R, Opstelten DJE. Virus maturation by budding. *Microbiol Mol Biol Rev* 1998;62:1171–1190.
36. Gelderblom HR, Ozel M, Pauli G. Morphogenesis and morphology of HIV: Structure-function relations. *Arch Virol* 1989;106:1–13.
37. Goepfert PA, Shaw K, Wang G, et al. An endoplasmic reticulum retrieval signal partitions human foamy virus maturation to intracytoplasmic membranes. *J Virol* 1999;73:7210–7217.
38. Gong M, Kieff E. Intracellular trafficking of two major Epstein-Barr virus glycoproteins, gp350/220 and gp110. *J Virol* 1990;64: 1507–1516.
39. Gorlich D, Mattaj IW. Nucleocytoplasmic transport. *Science* 1996; 271:1513–1518.
40. Gottlinger HG, Dorfman T, Sodroski JG, Haseltine WA. Effect of mutations affecting the p6 gag protein on human immunodeficiency virus particle release. *Proc Natl Acad Sci U S A* 1991;88:3195–3199.
41. Grable M, Hearing P. Adenovirus type 5 packaging domain is composed of a repeated element that is functionally redundant. *J Virol* 1990;64:2047–2056.
42. Griffiths G, Rottier P. Cell biology of viruses that assemble along the biosynthetic pathway. *Semin Cell Biol* 1992;3:367–381.
43. Gustin KE, Imperiale MJ. Encapsidation of viral DNA requires the adenovirus L1 52/55-kilodalton protein. *J Virol* 1998;72:7860–7870.
44. Hanein D, Matlack KE, Jungnickel B, et al. Oligomeric rings of the Sec61p complex induced by ligands required for protein translocation [see comments]. *Cell* 1996;87:721–732.
45. Hasson TB, Ornelles DA, Shenk T. Adenovirus L1 52- and 55-kilodalton proteins are present within assembling virions and colocalize with nuclear structures distinct from replication centers. *J Virol* 1992;66:6133–6142.

46. Hearing P, Samulski RJ, Wishart WL, Shenk T. Identification of a repeated sequence element required for efficient encapsidation of the adenovirus type 5 chromosome. *J Virol* 1987;61:2555–2558.
47. Hearing P, Shenk T. The adenovirus type 5 E1A transcriptional control region contains a duplicated enhancer element. *Cell* 1983;33: 695–703.
48. Hellen CUT, Wimmer E. Enterovirus structure and assembly. In: Robart HA, ed. *Human enterovirus infections*. Washington, DC: American Society for Microbiology, 1995:155–174.
49. Hinshaw JE, Carragher BO, Milligan RA. Architecture and design of the nuclear pore complex. *Cell* 1992;69:1133–1141.
50. Hong JS, Engler JA. The amino terminus of the adenovirus fiber protein encodes the nuclear localization signal. *Virology* 1991;185: 758–767.
51. Hunter E. Macromolecular interactions in the assembly of HIV and other retroviruses. *Semin Virol* 1994;5:71–83.
52. Irurzun A, Perez L, Carrasco L. Involvement of membrane traffic in the replication of poliovirus genomes: Effects of brefeldin A. *Virology* 1992;191:166–175.
53. Jackson MR, Nilsson T, Peterson PA. Identification of a consensus motif for retention of transmembrane proteins in the endoplasmic reticulum. *EMBO J* 1990;9:3153–3162.
54. Jarnik M, Aebi U. Toward a more complete 3-D structure of the nuclear pore complex. *J Struct Biol* 1991;107:291–308.
55. Jin H, Leser GP, Zhang J, Lamb RA. Influenza virus hemagglutinin and neuraminidase cytoplasmic tails control particle shape. *EMBO J* 1997;16:1236–1247.
56. Kabcenell AK, Poruchynsky MS, Bellamy AR, et al. Two forms of VP7 are involved in assembly of SA11 rotavirus in endoplasmic reticulum. *J Virol* 1988;62:2929–2941.
57. Kalderon D, Roberts BL, Richardson WD, Smith AE. A short amino acid sequence able to specify nuclear location. *Cell* 1984;39:499–509.
58. Karayan L, Gay B, Gerfaux J, Boulanger PA. Oligomerization of recombinant penton base of adenovirus type 2 and its assembly with fiber in baculovirus-infected cells. *Virology* 1994;202:782–795.
59. Kauffman RS, Ginsberg HS. Characterization of a temperature-sensitive, hexon transport mutant of type 5 adenovirus. *J Virol* 1976;19: 643–658.
60. Kido H, Niwa Y, Beppu Y, Towatari T. Cellular proteases involved in the pathogenicity of enveloped animal viruses, human immunodeficiency virus, influenza virus A and Sendai virus. *Adv Enzyme Regul* 1996;36:325–347.
61. King J, Chiu W. *Procapsid-capsid transition in dsDNA viruses*. New York: Oxford University Press, 1997.
62. Krausslich HG, Welker R. Intracellular transport of retroviral capsid components. *Curr Top Microbiol Immunol* 1996;214:25–63.
63. Krijnse-Locker J, Schleich S, Rodriguez D, et al. The role of a 21-kDa viral membrane protein in the assembly of vaccinia virus from the intermediate compartment. *J Biol Chem* 1996;271:14950–14958.
64. Liu C, Eichelberger MC, Compans RW, Air GM. Influenza type A virus neuraminidase does not play a role in viral entry, replication, assembly, or budding. *J Virol* 1995;69:1099–1106.
65. Lodge R, Delamarre L, Lalonde JP, et al. Two distinct oncornaviruses harbor an intracytoplasmic tyrosine-based basolateral targeting signal in their viral envelope glycoprotein. *J Virol* 1997;71:5696–5702.
66. Luytjes W, Krystal M, Enami M, et al. Amplification, expression, and packaging of foreign gene by influenza virus. *Cell* 1989;59: 1107–1113.
67. Maass DR, Atkinson PH. Retention by the endoplasmic reticulum of rotavirus VP7 is controlled by three adjacent amino-terminal residues. *J Virol* 1994;68:366–378.
68. Maeda J, Maeda A, Makino S. Release of coronavirus E protein in membrane vesicles from virus-infected cells and E protein-expressing cells. *Virology* 1999;263:265–272.
69. Malhotra V, Serafini T, Orci L, et al. Purification of a novel class of coated vesicles mediating biosynthetic protein transport through the Golgi stack. *Cell* 1989;58:329–336.
70. Mancini EJ, Clarke M, Gowen BE, et al. Cryo-electron microscopy reveals the functional organization of an enveloped virus, Semliki Forest virus. *Mol Cell* 2000;5:255–266.
71. Martin K, Helenius A. Nuclear transport of influenza virus ribonucleoproteins: The viral matrix protein (M1) promotes export and inhibits import. *Cell* 1991;67:117–130.
72. McBride MS, Panganiban AT. The human immunodeficiency virus type 1 encapsidation site is a multipartite RNA element composed of functional hairpin structures [published erratum appears in *J Virol* 1997;71(1):858]. *J Virol* 1996;70:2963–2973.
73. Mebatsion T, Konig M, Conzelmann KK. Budding of rabies virus particles in the absence of the spike glycoprotein. *Cell* 1996;84:941–951.
74. Mebatsion T, Weiland F, Conzelmann KK. Matrix protein of rabies virus is responsible for the assembly and budding of bullet-shaped particles and interacts with the transmembrane spike glycoprotein G. *J Virol* 1999;73:242–250.
75. Meyer BE, Malim MH. The HIV-1 Rev trans-activator shuttles between the nucleus and the cytoplasm. *Genes Dev* 1994;8: 1538–1547.
76. Meyer GA, Radsak KD. Identification of a novel signal sequence that targets transmembrane proteins to the nuclear envelope inner membrane. *J Biol Chem* 2000;275:3857–3866.
77. Meyer JC, Bergmann CC, Bellamy AR. Interaction of rotavirus cores with the nonstructural glycoprotein NS28. *Virology* 1989;171:98–107.
78. Moroianu J. Nuclear import and export: Transport factors, mechanisms and regulation. *Crit Rev Eukaryot Gene Expr* 1999;9:89–106.
79. Moroianu J, Blobel G, Radu A. Previously identified protein of uncertain function is karyopherin alpha and together with karyopherin beta docks import substrate at nuclear pore complexes. *Proc Natl Acad Sci U S A* 1995;92:2008–2011.
80. Moss B, Rosenblum EN. Protein cleavage and poxvirus morphogenesis: Tryptic peptide analysis of core precursors accumulated by blocking assembly with rifampicin [letter]. *J Mol Biol* 1973;81:267–269.
81. Munro S, Pelham HR. A C-terminal signal prevents secretion of luminal ER proteins. *Cell* 1987;48:899–907.
82. Naim HY, Roth MG. Basis for selective incorporation of glycoproteins into the influenza virus envelope. *J Virol* 1993;67:4831–4841.
83. Nakielny S, Dreyfuss G. Nuclear export of proteins and RNAs. *Curr Opin Cell Biol* 1997;9:420–429.
84. Nakielny S, Siomi MC, Siomi H, et al. Transportin: Nuclear transport receptor of a novel nuclear protein import pathway. *Exp Cell Res* 1996;229:261–266.
85. Narayanan K, Maeda A, Maeda J, Makino S. Characterization of the coronavirus M protein and nucleocapsid interaction in infected cells. *J Virol* 2000;74:8127–8134.
86. Nermut MV, Hockley DJ, Jowett JB, et al. Fullerene-like organization of HIV gag-protein shell in virus-like particles produced by recombinant baculovirus. *Virology* 1994;198:288–296.
87. Newcomb WW, Brown JC. Structure of the herpes simplex virus capsid: Effects of extraction with guanidine hydrochloride and partial reconstitution of extracted capsids. *J Virol* 1991;65:613–620.
88. Newcomb WW, Homa FL, Thomsen DR, et al. Assembly of the herpes simplex virus capsid: Characterization of intermediates observed during cell-free capsid formation. *J Mol Biol* 1996;263:432–446.
89. Newcomb WW, Trus BL, Cheng N, et al. Isolation of herpes simplex virus procapsids from cells infected with a protease-deficient mutant virus. *J Virol* 2000;74:1663–1673.
90. Nilsson M, von Bonsdorff CH, Weclewicz K, et al. Assembly of viroplasm and virus-like particles of rotavirus by a Semliki Forest virus replicon. *Virology* 1998;242:255–265.
91. Novelli A, Boulanger PA. Deletion analysis of functional domains in baculovirus-expressed adenovirus type 2 fiber. *Virology* 1991;185: 365–376.
92. O'Brien JA, Taylor JA, Bellamy AR. Probing the structure of rotavirus NSP4: A short sequence at the extreme C terminus mediates binding to the inner capsid particle. *J Virol* 2000;74:5388–5394.
93. Orci L, Glick BS, Rothman JE. A new type of coated vesicular carrier that appears not to contain clathrin: Its possible role in protein transport within the Golgi stack. *Cell* 1986;46:171–184.
94. Parent LJ, Bennett RP, Craven RC, et al. Positionally independent and exchangeable late budding functions of the Rous sarcoma virus and human immunodeficiency virus Gag proteins. *J Virol* 1995;69: 5455–5460.
95. Pfister T, Pasamontes L, Troxler M, et al. Immunocytochemical localization of capsid-related particles in subcellular fractions of poliovirus-infected cells. *Virology* 1992;188:676–684.
96. Pinto LH, Holsinger LJ, Lamb RA. Influenza virus M2 protein has ion channel activity. *Cell* 1992;69:517–528.
97. Poruchynsky MS, Maass DR, Atkinson PH. Calcium depletion blocks the maturation of rotavirus by altering the oligomerization of virus-encoded proteins in the ER. *J Cell Biol* 1991;114:651–656.

98. Raamsman MJ, Locker JK, de Hooge A, et al. Characterization of the coronavirus mouse hepatitis virus strain A59 small membrane protein E [in process citation]. *J Virol* 2000;74:2333–2342.
99. Rixon FJ. Structure and assembly of herpesviruses. *Semin Virol* 1993; 4:135–144.
100. Rixon FJ, Addison C, McGregor A, et al. Multiple interactions control the intracellular localization of the herpes simplex virus type 1 capsid proteins. *J Gen Virol* 1996;77:2251–2260.
101. Rixon FJ, McNab D. Packaging-competent capsids of a herpes simplex virus temperature-sensitive mutant have properties similar to those of in vitro-assembled procapsids. *J Virol* 1999;73:5714–5721.
102. Roberts A, Rose JK. Redesign and genetic dissection of the rhabdoviruses. *Adv Virus Res* 1999;53:301–319.
103. Robison CS, Whitt MA. The membrane-proximal stem region of vesicular stomatitis virus G protein confers efficient virus assembly [in process citation]. *J Virol* 2000;74:2239–2246.
104. Rodriguez JF, Smith GL. IPTG-dependent vaccinia virus: Identification of a virus protein enabling virion envelopment by Golgi membrane and egress. *Nucleic Acids Res* 1990;18:5347–5351.
105. Rodriguez-Boulan E, Powell SK. Polarity of epithelial and neuronal cells. *Annu Rev Cell Biol* 1992;8:395–427.
106. Roffman E, Albert JP, Goff JP, Frenkel N. Putative site for the acquisition of human herpesvirus 6 virion tegument. *J Virol* 1990;64: 6308–6313.
107. Rothman JE,. Wieland FT. Protein sorting by transport vesicles. *Science* 1996;272:227–234.
108. Saad A, Zhou ZH, Jakana J, et al. Roles of triplex and scaffolding proteins in herpes simplex virus type 1 capsid formation suggested by structures of recombinant particles. *J Virol* 1999;73:6821–6830.
109. Sakalian M, Hunter E. Molecular events in the assembly of retrovirus particles. *Adv Exp Med Biol* 1998;440:329–339.
110. Salmons T, Kuhn A, Wylie F, et al. Vaccinia virus membrane proteins p8 and p16 are cotranslationally inserted into the rough endoplasmic reticulum and retained in the intermediate compartment. *J Virol* 1997; 71:7404–7420.
111. Scheiffele P, Rietveld A, Wilk T, Simons K. Influenza viruses select ordered lipid domains during budding from the plasma membrane. *J Biol Chem* 1999;274:2038–2044.
112. Scheiffele P, Roth MG, Simons K. Interaction of influenza virus haemagglutinin with sphingolipid-cholesterol membrane domains via its transmembrane domain. *EMBO J* 1997;16:5501–5508.
113. Schlesinger S, Makino S, Linial ML. cis-Acting genomic elements and trans-acting proteins involved in the assembly of RNA viruses. *Semin Virol* 1994;5:39–49.
114. Schmid SI, Hearing P. Bipartite structure and functional independence of adenovirus type 5 packaging elements. *J Virol* 1997;71:3375–3384.
115. Simon SM, Blobel G. A protein-conducting channel in the endoplasmic reticulum. *Cell* 1991;65:371–380.
116. Sodeik B, Doms RW, Ericsson M, et al. Assembly of vaccinia virus: Role of the intermediate compartment between the endoplasmic reticulum and the Golgi stacks. *J Cell Biol* 1993;121:521–541.
117. Sollner T, Whiteheart SW, Brunner M, et al. SNAP receptors implicated in vesicle targeting and fusion [see comments]. *Nature* 1993; 362:318–324.
118. Stade K, Ford CS, Guthrie C, Weis K. Exportin 1 (Crm1p) is an essential nuclear export factor. *Cell* 1997;90:1041–1050.
119. Stirzaker SC, Whitfeld PL, Christie DL, et al. Processing of rotavirus glycoprotein VP7: Implications for the retention of the protein in the endoplasmic reticulum. *J Cell Biol* 1987;105:2897–2903.
120. Sugrue RJ, Hay AJ. Structural characteristics of the M2 protein of influenza A viruses: Evidence that it forms a tetrameric channel. *Virology* 1991;180:617–624.
121. Swanstrom R, Wills JW. 1997. Synthesis, assembly and processing of viral proteins. In: Coffin JM, Hughes SH, Varmus HE, ed. *Retroviruses.* New York: Cold Spring Harbor Laboratory Press, 1997: 263–334.
122. Takegami T, Kuhn RJ, Anderson CW, Wimmer E. Membrane-dependent uridylylation of the genome-linked protein VPg of poliovirus. *Proc Natl Acad Sci U S A* 1983;80:7447–7451.
123. Taylor JA, O'Brien JA, Yeager M. The cytoplasmic tail of NSP4, the endoplasmic reticulum-localized non-structural glycoprotein of rotavirus, contains distinct virus binding and coiled coil domains. *EMBO J* 1996;15:4469–4476.
124. Thomas DC, Roth MG. The basolateral targeting signal in the cytoplasmic domain of glycoprotein G from vesicular stomatitis virus resembles a variety of intracellular targeting motifs related by primary sequence but having diverse targeting activities. *J Biol Chem* 1994; 269:15732–15739.
125. Torrisi MR, Gentile M, Cardinali G, et al. Intracellular transport and maturation pathway of human herpesvirus 6. *Virology* 1999;257: 460–471.
126. Troxler M, Egger D, Pfister T, Bienz K. Intracellular localization of poliovirus RNA by in situ hybridization at the ultrastructural level using single-stranded riboprobes. *Virology* 1992;191:687–697.
127. Trus BL, Booy FP, Newcomb WW, et al. The herpes simplex virus procapsid: Structure, conformational changes upon maturation, and roles of the triplex proteins VP19c and VP23 in assembly. *J Mol Biol* 1996;263:447–462.
128. van Genderen IL, Brandimarti R, Torrisi MR, et al. The phospholipid composition of extracellular herpes simplex virions differs from that of host cell nuclei. *Virology* 1994;200:831–836.
129. Vennema H, Godeke GJ, Rossen JW, et al. Nucleocapsid-independent assembly of coronavirus-like particles by co-expression of viral envelope protein genes. *EMBO J* 1996;15:2020–2028.
130. von Schwedler UK, Stemmler TL, Klishko VY, et al. Proteolytic refolding of the HIV-1 capsid protein amino-terminus facilitates viral core assembly [published erratum appears in *EMBO J* 2000;19(10): 2391]. *EMBO J* 1998;17:1555–1568.
131. Walter P, Lingappa VR. Mechanism of protein translocation across the endoplasmic reticulum membrane. *Annu Rev Cell Biol* 1986;2: 499–516.
132. Weldon RAJ, Parker WB, Sakalian M, Hunter E. Type D retrovirus capsid assembly and release are active events requiring ATP. *J Virol* 1998;72:3098–3106.
133. Whittaker GR, Helenius A. Nuclear import and export of viruses and virus genomes. *Virology* 1998;246:1–23.
134. Yu D, Weller SK. Herpes simplex virus type 1 cleavage and packaging proteins UL15 and UL28 are associated with B but not C capsids during packaging. *J Virol* 1998;72:7428–7439.
135. Zeffman A, Hassard S, Varani G, Lever A. The major HIV-1 packaging signal is an extended bulged stem loop whose structure is altered on interaction with the gag polyprotein [in process citation]. *J Mol Biol* 2000;297:877–893.
136. Zhang J, Leser GP, Pekosz A, Lamb RA. The cytoplasmic tails of the influenza virus spike glycoproteins are required for normal genome packaging. *Virology* 2000;269:325–334.
137. Zhao LJ, Padmanabhan R. Three basic regions in adenovirus DNA polymerase interact differentially depending on the protein context to function as bipartite nuclear localization signals. *New Biol* 1991;3: 1074–1088.

CHAPTER 9

Pathogenesis of Viral Infections

Kenneth L. Tyler and Neal Nathanson

INTRODUCTION

Viral pathogenesis is the process by which viruses produce disease in the host (350,553). Much of our existing knowledge of viral pathogenesis is based on experimental studies using animal models of natural human infections. These are at best imperfect analogs to human infections, but they allow observations and experiments that are not possible in humans and are invaluable in understanding how viruses produce human diseases.

The production of disease, which is the focus of pathogenesis, is in fact a relatively unusual outcome of viral infection of a host (Fig. 1). The virulence of a virus is its capacity, when compared with other closely related viruses, to produce disease in a host. Virulence depends on a variety of viral and host factors, such as the dose of virus, its route of entry, and the host's age, sex, immune status, and species. With many "virulent" viruses, subclinical or inapparent infections often outnumber cases of symptomatic illness. During epidemics of mosquito-borne encephalitis, for example, the ratio of serologically documented infections may exceed cases of acute encephalitis by several hundred fold. However, for certain classic viral infections such as measles, smallpox, rabies, and influenza, almost all infected individuals develop disease.

In addition to acute infection, the interaction between a virus and a host may lead to a variety of other outcomes including the development of persistent or latent infection (see later) and cellular transformation (see Chapter 10). As viral infection proceeds, the virus encounters a constant series of obstacles within the host. Among the most important of these are the various components of the host's specific and nonspecific immunity (see Chapters 11 and 12). Ultimately the interaction between a virus and cell may lead to alterations in host cell function,

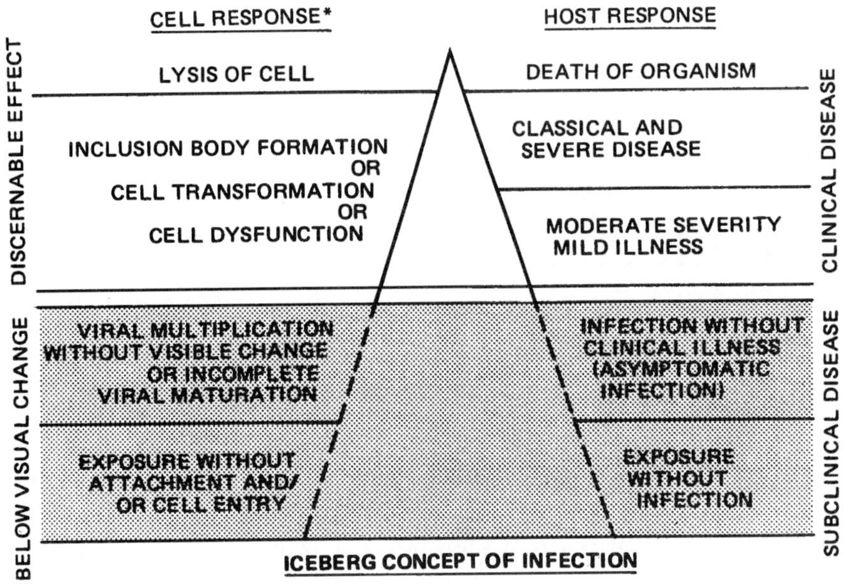

FIG. 1. Varieties of host and cellular responses to virus infection. (From ref. 143, with permission.)

which are discussed in more detail elsewhere (see Chapter 7).

A virus must survive in the environment until it encounters a susceptible host. It must then enter the host, through one of a number of available portals (e.g., the respiratory or the gastrointestinal tract). Once inside the host, the virus undergoes initial replication, typically at a site near its original portal of entry. Viruses that produce localized infections may be released from surface mucosal epithelium or analogous sites and subsequently shed from the host (e.g., in stool or other bodily fluids or through coughing and sneezing). After entering the environment, these viruses may then reinitiate the cycle of virus–host interaction by transmission to a new host.

Viruses that produce systemic rather than localized infections must cross mucosal barriers and spread to distant sites in the host, using defined pathways of spread such as the bloodstream, lymphatics, or nerves. After spreading, or at the site of local infection, viruses are targeted to specific populations of cells within individual organs or tissues (tropism). Each of these stages in viral pathogenesis is discussed in more detail in the following sections.

Each stage of pathogenesis poses a series of biologic obstacles that the virus must overcome to proceed to the subsequent level. The successful completion of all the stages in pathogenesis results in disease, whereas failure to complete these stages results in either abortive, nonproductive, or failed infection. Viral structure has evolved to enable the virus to overcome obstacles successfully at particular stages in pathogenesis. The structure of the virus must enable it to remain infectious after being exposed to conditions such as temperature and humidity that are present in the ambient environment. For many viruses, environmental stability is determined by the envelope or by outer capsid proteins. Once a virus has entered the host, the parts of the virus that ensure environmental stability or promote transmission become nonessential and are often removed as the virus proceeds through subsequent stages in pathogenesis. For example, the proteolytic removal of capsid proteins may, at this stage, actually enhance infectivity rather than attenuate it (381).

ENTRY

The predominant routes by which viruses enter the host include through the skin, or by way of the respiratory, gastrointestinal, or genitourinary systems (377,378) (Fig. 2).

Skin

Breaks in the integrity of the skin or the mucosa of the respiratory, gastrointestinal, or genitourinary tracts facilitate entry of viruses. The outer layer of the epidermis is composed of the dead keratinized cells of the stratum corneum, which do not support viral replication (553). Underneath the stratum corneum are the living cells of the stratum malpighii. Some viruses, such as papillomaviruses—which produce human warts—enter the skin at sites where scrapes or abrasions have resulted in loss of epithelial integrity. Certain animal papillomaviruses are mechanically transmitted by arthropod vectors, and then replicate in epithelial cells at the site of inoculation (see Chapter 66 of *Fields Virology*, 4th ed.). Primary infection begins in the basal cells, and virion replication and maturation occur as these cells differentiate. Mature virions are found in the granular layers and are shed with the dead cells of the stratum corneum.

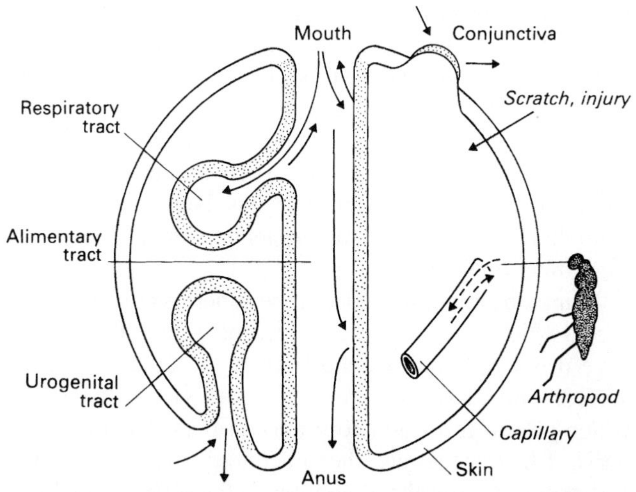

FIG. 2. Portals of entry of viruses into the host, and sites of shedding from the host. (Modified from ref. 350, with permission.)

Sheets of keratinocytes, similar to those used for epithelial cell skin grafts, have been used to study the entry and tropism of viruses that can infect the skin. For example, studies of viral infection of epithelial grafts suggest that cell-free inoculums of human immunodeficiency virus (HIV) do not productively infect keratinocytes, which apparently lack HIV receptors, but cell-associated HIV can initiate productive infection of these cells (415).

Because the epidermal layer is devoid of blood vessels, lymphatics, and nerve fibers, viruses that initiate epidermal infection are typically restricted to the site of entry and only rarely disseminate to produce systemic infections. The system of skin-associated lymphoid tissue (SALT), which includes antigen-presenting Langerhans cells, T cells, and cytokine-producing keratinocytes, may provide a pathway for spread of viruses that can initiate systemic infection after inoculation into the skin. T cells and dendritic cells (Langerhans cells) can circulate between the skin and regional lymph nodes. Both HIV and herpes simplex virus (HSV) can infect Langerhans cells, which can emigrate out of the epidermis to enter regional lymph nodes (342). When macrophage-tropic strains of HIV are inoculated onto abraded epidermis of skin explant grafts, virus can be detected in both epidermal and dermal emigrant cells, which include both T cells and dendritic cells (430). The importance of early dendritic cell infection in the pathogenesis of HIV also can be inferred from the predominance of "macrophage-tropic" viral strains isolated during primary HIV infection (581). Dermal replication in macrophages and fibroblasts also occurs when mouse-, cow-, or rabbit-pox viruses enter the host through traumatic skin lesions in the epidermis (154).

The molecular basis for viral infection of skin remains largely unknown. In the case of varicella-zoster virus (VZV) and HSV, the gC glycoprotein is a critical determinant (354). This suggests that the interaction between viral attachment proteins and specific receptors on skin cells may be critical to initiating epidermal infection.

The bites of arthropod vectors including mosquitoes, mites, ticks, and sand flies allow subcutaneous inoculation of many arthropod-borne viruses (see Chapters 30 and 33 of *Fields Virology*, 4th ed.). Transmission of virus may be purely mechanical, as illustrated by transmission of myxomavirus by the mouthparts of biting insects, or may require replication of the virus within the gut or salivary system of the arthropod vector (205,369,376). Most of the arthropod-borne toga- and flaviviruses, which include the agents of epidemic encephalitis and yellow fever, appear to replicate in the gut of the insect vector, with subsequent spread to salivary tissue. Virus is then inoculated into the host during feeding, and part of the inoculum enters the general circulation, while part remains in the local tissue. Once a virus has reached the dermis, it has access to blood vessels, lymphatics, and dendritic cells, including macrophages present in the skin.

Some viruses are inoculated directly through the epidermis and dermis into deeper tissues. Deep inoculation, into the subcutaneous tissue and muscle, can follow hypodermic needle injections, acupuncture, ear piercing, tattooing, or animal bites. Hepatitis B virus (HBV) may gain access to the host through needle inoculation of various types (313). Infection with both rabies and herpesvirus simiae is characteristically initiated by the bites of infected animals (18,557).

Respiratory Tract

Inhibition of viral entry through the skin depends primarily on the mechanical integrity of the epidermal barrier. By contrast, more complex host defense systems are involved in inhibiting viral entry through mucosal surfaces (1,569). In the respiratory tract, goblet cells secrete mucus that is propelled by the action of ciliated epithelial cells and acts to clear foreign material from the respiratory tract. Clara cells, a type of nonciliated secretory cell, produce trypsin-like proteases that may act to cleave viral proteins such as the hemagglutinin (HA) of influenza virus (269).

Both humoral and cellular immune mechanisms also act to protect the host against mucosal infection (1). Bronchial-associated lymphoid tissue (BALT) includes collections of lymphocytes and macrophages in the tonsils and adenoids as well as in the subepithelial tissue of the nasopharynx and trachea. Specialized epithelial cells known as M cells participate in generating mucosal immunity by delivering antigens to underlying lymphoid tissue (470). Viruses and other microbial pathogens can exploit these cells as transport pathways, enabling them to traverse mucosal surfaces. This has been elegantly demonstrated for reoviruses (360) (reviewed later in the discussion of the analogous pathway in the gastrointestinal tract).

Cytokines also appear to play a critical role in preventing systemic dissemination of some viruses that initiate infection through the respiratory tract. For example, knock-out mice with disruptions in the STAT1, interferon (IFN)α-receptor, or IFNγ genes all show markedly enhanced severity of influenza A infection and systemic dissemination compared with that in their wild-type counterparts (168). Similarly, mice with targeted mutations inactivating the IFNα/β receptor show enhanced spread of measles virus to the lungs and more prominent inflammation than wild-type mice (366).

An additional factor in host defense is the cool temperature of the upper respiratory tract, which acts to inhibit the replication of many viruses (569), but is optimal for the replication of rhinoviruses, a major cause of upper respiratory infections (see Chapter 25 of *Fields Virology*, 4th ed.). The temperature differential between the nose and the body has been exploited in viral vaccine development. Temperature-sensitive (ts) mutants of viruses such as influenza, parainfluenza, and respiratory syncytial virus can replicate in the upper respiratory tract and generate host immune responses, but will not survive higher body temperatures and therefore do not disseminate (569). Despite the nature of host barriers to respiratory infection, a number of viruses including herpesviruses, adenoviruses, myxoviruses, paramyxoviruses, and rhinoviruses can initiate either local or systemic infection via this route.

Viruses that enter the respiratory tract do so primarily in the form of either aerosolized droplets, saliva, or through spread from infected nasal secretions to hands and then subsequently back to the nose (nose–hand–nose transmission). Site of penetration is influenced by droplet size, with only the smallest inhaled droplets reaching the alveoli of the lungs. Initial infection occurs predominantly at the epithelial surface with subsequent spread of virus from cell to cell or by inhalation.

Receptors (see later) for viruses that initiate spread via the respiratory route are predominantly ubiquitous cell-surface molecules such as sialic acid (influenza), and cell adhesion molecules (rhinovirus). In some cases these receptors may be distributed preferentially on certain surfaces of polarized respiratory epithelial cells. For example, the CAR receptor for adenoviruses 2 and 5 and coxsackie B is located predominantly on the basolateral surface of epithelial cells (542), whereas the measles virus receptor CD46 is found preferentially at the apical surface (42). The subsequent propensity of some viruses to produce disease predominantly confined to respiratory mucosal surfaces (e.g., influenza, respiratory syncytial virus), whereas others induce systemic infection after primary replication in respiratory mucosa (e.g., measles, varicella), may be determined in part by the pattern of viral release from infected cells (polarized infection, see later) (98,521). For example, viruses such as influenza and respiratory syncytial virus (436), which are released predominantly from apical surfaces, tend to produce infection confined to the respiratory mucosal surface. Conversely, release of viruses, such as certain murine coronaviruses (447), from the basolateral surface of epithelial cells may facilitate systemic spread (see polarized infection later).

A unique situation occurs in the superior portion of the nares, which contains olfactory receptor cells. These cells have distal rods that extend beyond the outer epithelial surface and proximal axon processes (fila olfactoria), which join to form olfactory nerve fibers. The olfactory nerve fibers penetrate the arachnoid space and form synapses with mitral cell neurons in the olfactory bulb. A variety of experimental studies using polioviruses, herpesviruses, coronaviruses, togaviruses, and rhabdoviruses have shown that these viruses can spread to the central nervous system (CNS) through the olfactory nerve (396,496). This situation, although postulated to explain some cases of human rabies and HSV infection, is probably an extremely unusual route of natural viral infection (251).

Experimental models of natural aerosol infection have been developed, as exemplified by aerosol inoculation of bovine respiratory syncytial virus into calves, and seem to be reasonable facsimilies of natural infection (567). Explant organ cultures, such as those of fetal trachea, and cell cultures of nasal epithelial and adenoidal cells also have been used to study early events in respiratory infection (561,569).

Coughing and sneezing can generate enormous numbers of small aerosolized particles that may travel up to 5 feet at velocities that approach 100 ft/sec. Coughing generates even higher aerosol velocities that can approach 850 ft/sec (569). Particles smaller than 5 μm in diameter can remain airborne for long periods, a property that can be dramatically enhanced by the presence of air currents. The distribution of inhaled aerosol particles within the respiratory tract is largely a function of particle size (277). Large particles rarely escape the filtering action of the nasal turbinates, whereas small particles (<5-μm diameter) are capable of reaching the alveolar spaces.

Environmental factors including air temperature and humidity also influence the stability of aerosolized viral particles (277). The physicochemical properties and structure of virion particles also can influence their stability as aerosols. For example, enveloped viruses are less susceptible to desiccation than are their nonenveloped counterparts. This may provide one explanation for the fact that enveloped viruses (e.g., influenza, parainfluenza, respiratory syncytial virus) are more common causes of lower respiratory tract infections than are their nonenveloped counterparts (e.g., adenovirus, rhinovirus).

The proper functioning of the mucociliary transport system appears to be an important determinant in resistance to viral infection of the respiratory tract. Drugs that inhibit this transport process increase host susceptibility to a number of viral infections (21). Susceptibility to Sendai virus infection in mice has been linked to a genetic polymorphism in mucociliary transport function (58). Patients with HIV infection often have decreased rates of mucociliary clearance, which also facilitates recurrent upper respiratory and sinus infections (347). Acquired ciliary defects, which inhibit host antiviral defense, appear to be a common feature of many other viral upper respiratory infections, even in immunocompetent hosts (75).

Gastrointestinal Tract

Many viruses enter the host via the gastrointestinal (GI) tract, where they may either initiate local infection (e.g., rotaviruses, coronaviruses, adenovirus, and Norwalk agent) or cross the mucosal layer to invade underlying tissues and spread within the host (e.g., enteroviruses, hepatitis A).

The physicochemical environment in the upper GI tract would appear to be extremely inhospitable to invading microorganisms (103). The secretion of acid by gastric parietal cells may reduce the intraluminal pH to 2.0 or lower. In addition, a variety of proteases are secreted by gastric and pancreatic cells, and bile salts enter the duodenum from the biliary tract. Mucus is secreted by both gastric and intestinal cells and may contain both specific [e.g., immunoglobulin A (IgA)] and nonspecific inhibitors of viral infection. To initiate infection via the GI route, a virus would ideally have the properties of acid stability, resistance to loss of infectivity in the presence of bile salts, and resistance to inactivation by proteolytic enzymes. In fact, the majority of viral pathogens that enter via the GI tract generally exhibit all these properties.

Almost all picornaviruses are capable of producing enteric infections in humans. A notable exception to this rule is the rhinoviruses. Unlike other picornaviruses and rotaviruses, rhinoviruses are extremely acid labile and undergo complete inactivation with loss of infectivity at low pH (Chapter 25 of *Fields Virology*, 4th ed.). The pH-induced inactivation appears to result from the loss of the VP4 surface protein and resulting leakage of the viral RNA, which produces noninfectious "empty capsids." Interestingly, many of the enteroviruses undergo an analogous type of degradation under alkaline conditions (263). Similar investigations with reoviruses suggest that under certain circumstances, exposure to alkaline pH can result in the loss of the viral cell-attachment protein from the viral outer capsid (129,130). Changes in the outer capsid structure of rotaviruses also have been observed at both extremely acidic or alkaline pH (Chapter 54 of *Fields Virology*, 4th ed.).

The effect of proteolytic enzymes, such as those present in the GI tract, on the infectivity of enteric viruses also has been investigated. Trypsin, pancreatin, and elastin have all been shown to enhance rotavirus infectivity (92,141) and are routinely incorporated into procedures to isolate and cultivate these viruses. Likewise, inhibition of proteolysis may result in attenuation of rotavirus infection (536), and the importance of proteolytic processing of virions *in vivo* has been demonstrated for reoviruses (24,45). Reovirus particles present in the intestinal lumen are converted into infectious subviral particles (ISVPs) by proteolytic processing of their $\sigma 3$ and $\mu 1C$ outer capsid proteins. ISVPs appear to be the form of the virion responsible for the subsequent initiation of intestinal infection, and inhibition of intraluminal proteolytic digestion dramatically inhibits intestinal infection by reoviruses (7,24,45).

Studies with a number of viruses indicate that host proteases act primarily to alter the viral outer capsid or envelope proteins. For example, proteolytic digestion of rotaviruses with trypsin, pancreatin, or elastase results in cleavage of the outer capsid protein VP4 and the appearance of two cleavage products, VP8 and VP5 (141). Enhancement of coronavirus infectivity also occurs in the presence of proteolytic enzymes (489) and may be due to the cleavage of the E2 peplomer glycoprotein (the viral cell-attachment protein) from an inactive precursor into its active form. Genetic studies with reovirus reassortants derived from parental viruses that differ in their susceptibility to proteolytic digestion indicate that the reovirus major outer capsid protein $\mu 1c$ is the major determinant of protease sensitivity (450).

Detailed studies of the mechanism of action at a molecular level of proteolytic digestion of viral proteins have been made with influenza viruses and Sendai virus (169,174,294,460,559). These studies provide insights into how proteolytic processing of viral proteins can influence viral pathogenicity. Cellular exopeptidases cleave the HA of influenza into two disulfide-bonded subunits (HA_1 and HA_2). After virus enters target cells through the process of receptor-mediated endocytosis, the amino terminus of the HA_2 protein undergoes a pH-dependent conformational change that facilitates the subsequent fusion of the influenza virus envelope with the inner membrane of the endocytic vesicle (473). This in turn results in the escape of the viral nucleocapsid into the target cell's cytoplasm, where replication occurs. If cleavage of the HA does not occur, then influenza virus still binds to cell-surface receptors but is unable to initiate a productive infection. Inhibition of HA cleavage by administration of protease inhibitors results in attenuation of influenza virus infection *in vivo* (502,559).

In the case of measles virus, the fusion glycoprotein gene encodes an inactive precursor protein (F_0) that is cleaved within a region containing a stretch of basic amino acids (108–112) to generate two disulfide-linked active fusion proteins (F_1 and F_2). Cleavage occurs within the trans-Golgi network (TGN) and involves host-cell enzymes belonging to the family of proprotein convertases. Furin has been identified as the likely candidate (46).

Thus many viruses have evolved so that proteolytic processing actually facilitates rather then inhibits viral infection. The mechanisms by which this facilitation occurs are gradually becoming better understood. As a general principle, proteolytic processing of these viruses usually results in partial cleavage of specific viral surface proteins, which in turn facilitates specific events, such as membrane fusion or transcriptional activation, in the viral replicative cycle. Conversely, viruses that are easily inactivated by proteolytic processing are unlikely to initiate infection via sites such as the GI tract where proteolytic enzymes are a prominent part of the internal milieu.

The presence of bile salts in the intestinal lumen also may play an important role in determining the types of viruses that are capable of initiating GI infection. Viral envelopes are derived from host-cell lipoprotein bilayer membranes and are particularly susceptible to dissociation by bile salts. Conversely, the protein capsids of nonenveloped viruses are quite resistant to the action of bile salts. This may explain why, with the exception of coronaviruses, enveloped viruses do not initiate infection via the upper GI tract. Coronaviruses are susceptible to inactivation by bile salts in vitro, and the factors that enable them to survive inactivation *in vivo* remain unknown.

Viruses associated with gastroenteritis can infect a variety of cell types within the GI tract. Some viruses such as adenoviruses, calciviruses, rotaviruses, and coronaviruses infect predominantly the mature nondividing absorptive enterocytes. Other viruses have a predilection for the dividing cells of the crypts (e.g., animal parvoviruses) or infect specialized epithelial cells such as the M (microfold cells) overlying Peyer's patches (e.g., poliovirus, HIV, and reovirus) (103). Factors that determine the capacity of viruses to infect intestinal cells are becoming better understood. In the case of coronaviruses, a critical determinant is the presence of cell-surface receptors such as members of the carcinoembryonic antigen (CEA) family including human biliary glycoprotein and aminopeptidase N (83,227,512,513). Other enteric viruses use more ubiquitously distributed receptors such as sialic acid residues (rotavirus). Some viruses, such as the rotaviruses, produce enteric infections that are typically limited to the intestinal epithelial cells (Chapter 55 of *Fields Virology*, 4th ed.). Local involvement of intestinal epithelial cells also occurs during infection with adenovirus, astrovirus, calcivirus, coronavirus, and parvovirus (110,455).

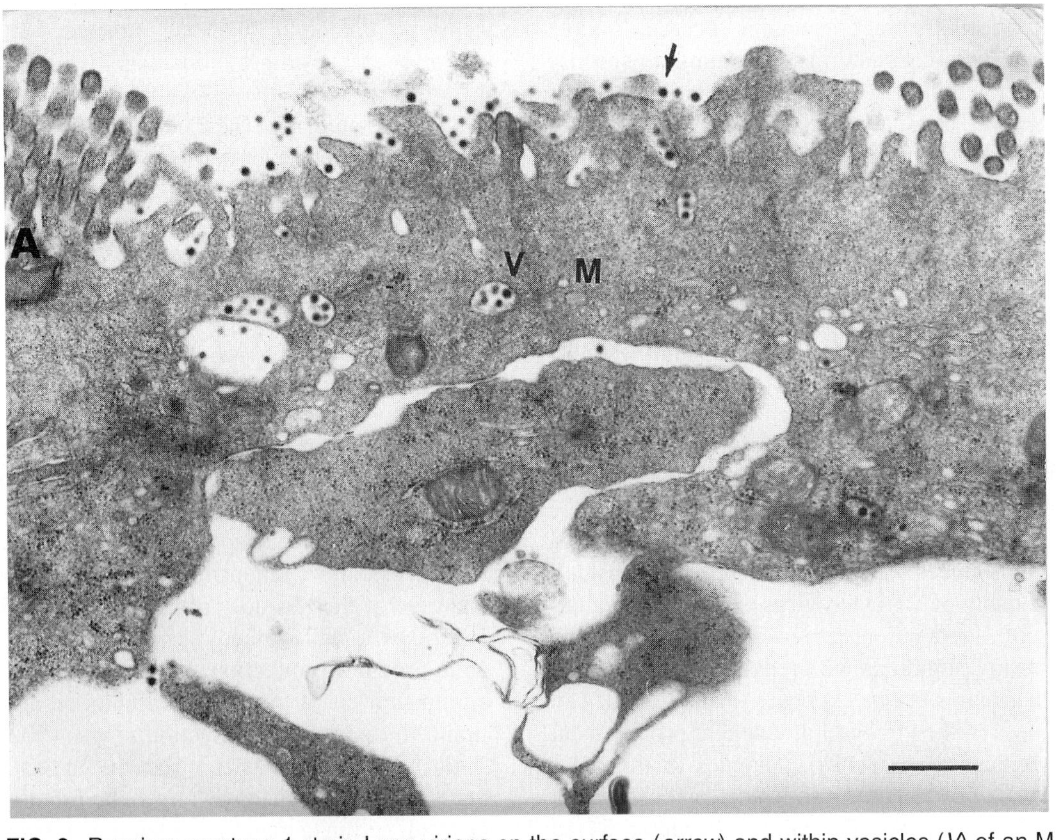

FIG. 3. Reovirus serotype 1 strain Lang virions on the surface (*arrow*) and within vesicles (*V*) of an M cell in the ileal epithelium overlying a Peyer's patch. (From ref. 565, with permission.)

The factors that determine whether viral infection remains limited to the GI tract or spreads to produce systemic illness are largely unknown. Increasing interest has focused on the role of gut-associated lymphoid tissue (GALT) in viral entry. Several enteric viruses, including reoviruses, HIV, and poliovirus, spread from the lumen of the small intestine to collections of submucosal lymphoid tissue known as Peyer's patches (362,470). The early events in the spread of reoviruses after intestinal infection have been investigated extensively using electron microscopy. Virus initially adheres to the surface of specialized intestinal epithelial cells ("M cells") that overlie the surface of Peyer's patches. Reovirions can be sequentially visualized at the surface of M cells, being transported in vesicles through these cells, and subsequently free in the extracellular space of Peyer's patches (26,564,565) (Fig. 3). The M cell pathway also is used by poliovirus and HIV to penetrate the intestinal epithelial barrier (6,282,469), suggesting that this may be a general pathway for the entry of viruses that spread beyond the mucosal surface. Once cells have traversed the epithelial barrier, the macrophages and lymphocytes, present within GALT, may play a role in further dissemination, as has been suggested for reo- and rotaviruses (362).

Additional factors favoring localized infection may be the pattern of release of virus from intestinal epithelial cells with apical release (toward the intestinal lumen) favoring local cell-to-cell spread, as exemplified by rotaviruses (256) and basolateral release facilitating systemic invasion (see later). For example, infection with the porcine coronavirus transmissible gastroenteritis virus (TGEV) occurs at the luminal (apical) surface of epithelial cells, as does release. This facilitates local cell-to-cell spread but reduces the probability of systemic infection. Conversely, the mouse coronavirus mouse hepatitis virus (MHV)-A59 enters cells at the apical surface, but may be preferentially released from the basolateral surface, facilitating systemic spread (447).

The recognition that anal intercourse is a major risk factor for the transmission of HIV infection also has led to the recognition that some viruses that produce systemic disease may gain entry to the host through the lower GI tract. HIV has been detected in bowel epithelium and enterochromaffin cells of patients with HIV, and can infect human colonic cell lines in culture (305,379,397). The mechanisms by which HIV infection is further spread from the lower GI tract remain to be established.

Genitourinary Tract

In addition to the respiratory and GI tracts, other mucosal surfaces may provide sites for viral entry into the host. Sexual activity may produce tears or abrasions in the vaginal epithelium or trauma to the urethra, allowing viral entry via the genitourinary route. Sexually transmitted viruses in humans include HIV, herpes simplex, human papillomaviruses 11, 16, and 18 (the agents responsible for genital warts or condyloma acuminata), and hepatitis B and C (456). In the case of HIV, infection may be facilitated by breaks in the genital epithelial barrier, but the virus also may productively infect cervical epithelial cells and dendritic (Langerhans) cells within the vaginal epithelium (295,296,501). HHV-6 (85) and human papillomavirus (HPV) 16 and 18 also have been shown to infect cervical epithelial cells in culture (566). As might be expected, for sexually transmitted viruses, the degree of sexual promiscuity and the number of sexual partners are risk factors for transmission (456).

The sequence of events that follow vaginally initiated virus infections has not been comprehensively investigated. In a macaque model, after intravaginal inoculation of a simian immunodeficiency virus (SIV)/HIV chimeric virus, virus is first detected in T lymphocytes in the submucosal epithelium, followed by the pelvic and mesenteric lymph nodes within 2 days of inoculation, and virus-infected cells are found in the thymus and spleen within 4 days (248).

Acute hemorrhagic cystitis in young boys has been associated with adenovirus 11 and 21 (Chapter 68 of *Fields Virology*, 4th ed.); however, it is not known whether these viruses reach the bladder directly through the urethra or indirectly via another site of entry. Other viruses, including polyomaviruses, can produce viruria, but this is generally not associated with symptomatic disease. In some of these cases, virus appears to reach the kidney, presumably through the bloodstream, and then enters the urine (Chapter 64 of *Fields Virology*, 4th ed.). Little is known about the nature of host factors that influence viral invasion by these routes. The nature of the cervical mucus, the pH of vaginal secretions, and the chemical composition of the urine all may play a role in host defense against infection.

Conjunctiva

The conjunctiva also may provide a route for the entry of viruses that produce either local disease (conjunctivitis) or more rarely disseminate from this site to produce systemic infection (e.g., paralytic illness with enterovirus 70 and experimental Ebola infection). Direct inoculation of virus onto the conjunctiva during ophthalmologic procedures (e.g., foreign-body removal and tonometry) can produce keratoconjunctivitis, and many cases have been attributed to adenoviruses 8, 19, and 37. Similarly, the conjunctivitis that follows swimming in public areas ("swimming pool conjunctivitis") appears to be frequently due to direct infection most often with adenoviruses (see Chapter 68 of *Fields Virology*, 4th ed.). Conjunctivitis also can occur in association with enteroviral infections (e.g., echo 7, 11; coxsackie A24,

B2) (112). Coxsackie-adenovirus receptor (CAR)-mediated binding of adenoviruses to conjunctival cells via the distal domain of the fiber protein has recently been demonstrated. Mutations at amino acid 240 within the fiber protein can either facilitate or abrogate binding of adenovirus strains to these cells (235).

Systemic spread of virus after conjunctival entry is rare, although as noted, it is an important feature of the acute hemorrhagic conjunctivitis produced by enterovirus 70. This virus can spread from the conjunctiva to the central nervous system, where it can produce poliomyelitis, radiculomyelopathy, or cranial nerve palsies (448). Ebola virus also can be transmitted effectively via the conjunctival route in nonhuman primates, suggesting that this, like the oral route, could be a potential mode of transmission (247).

Conjunctivitis also may occur as part of a systemic viral infection in which virus reaches the conjunctivae after the induction of viremia rather than directly from the external surface. The conjunctivitis associated with acute measles infection is usually considered in this category, but recent experimental studies indicated that systemic measles infection can be produced in rhesus monkeys after conjunctival inoculation with measles, indicating that the conjunctiva also may serve as a portal of entry (335).

SPREAD IN THE HOST

Localized Versus Systemic Infection

Some viruses produce tissue injury predominantly near the site at which they enter the host. This pattern of infection characterizes the upper respiratory infections of influenza, parainfluenza, rhinoviruses, and coronaviruses; the GI infections caused by rotaviruses; and the skin infections of the papillomaviruses. In these cases, spread of virus occurs primarily as a result of contiguous infection of adjacent cells. Virus rarely spreads beyond the epithelial cell layer, although in some cases, involvement of regional lymph nodes and even systemic invasion can occur.

Polarized Infection of Epithelial Cells

Certain viruses preferentially bud from either the apical or basal surfaces of polarized epithelial cells, and this pattern may be an important determinant of whether infection remains localized or becomes systemic (98,99, 521) (Fig. 4). Apical release of virus from epithelial cells lining mucosal surfaces favors the development of localized infection and facilitates cell-to-cell spread along the epithelial layer, whereas basolateral release directs virus toward underlying deeper tissues, facilitating mucosal invasion and the development of systemic infection. This pattern may be further reinforced by differences in the susceptibility of polarized epithelial cells to infection at their apical and basolateral surfaces (427). Finally, in some cases, viruses may preferentially enter cells on one surface and be released from another. This is illustrated by the coronavirus MHV-A59, which enters polarized murine kidney epithelial cells through the apical membrane, whereas progeny virions are released preferentially from the basolateral domain (447). Changes in the patterns of polarized release may dramatically alter viral virulence. For example, wild-type Sendai virus buds from the apical surface of polarized bronchial epithelial cells and produces localized bronchial infection, but mutant viruses with the capacity to bud from basolateral as well as apical surfaces have extended tissue tropism and enhanced virulence in vivo (503).

Examples of viruses with polarized patterns of release from epithelial cells include vaccinia, vesicular stomatitis virus (VSV), and certain retroviruses that are assembled at and bud from the basolateral cell membrane, and influenza, parainfluenza, SV40, poliovirus, rotavirus and Sendai virus which use the apical surface (98). Not all viruses exhibit polarized patterns of infection and release, and some, such as poliovirus, are capable of bidirectional entry into polarized epithelial cells (42,522). Viruses within the same family also may differ in their patterns of release. For example, the Hantavirus Black Creek Canal shows predominantly apical release from polarized epithelial cells, as opposed to the basolateral release characteristic of most other bunyaviruses (427).

In cases of polarized infection by enveloped viruses, envelope glycoproteins are inserted into the appropriate region of the cell membrane before viral budding. This suggests that it is the initial targeting and localization of these proteins to specific regions of the cell membrane that determine the subsequent polarity of viral budding. The information required for appropriate targeting of these proteins to the cell surface is contained in specific regions of the targeted proteins, and even single amino acid substitutions in the appropriate domain can alter polarized delivery (49,236,290,308,506,524).

In the case of retroviruses, including HIV, a tyrosine-based motif located in the intracytoplasmic domain of the envelope glycoprotein is highly conserved and functions as a critical basolateral targeting signal (309). Measles virus may be an exception to the general rule that sorting signals are contained in envelope glycoproteins, as its capacity to bud from apical surfaces of polarized epithelial cells does not appear to depend on prior localization of the H and F surface glycoproteins, which are transported in a nonpolarized fashion (323).

Not all membrane glycoproteins play an equivalent role in determining the site of polarized release. For example, the polarized release of coronaviruses is not determined by the spike (S) glycoprotein, but rather by the membrane (M) and hemagglutinin-esterase (HE) envelope glycoproteins (446).

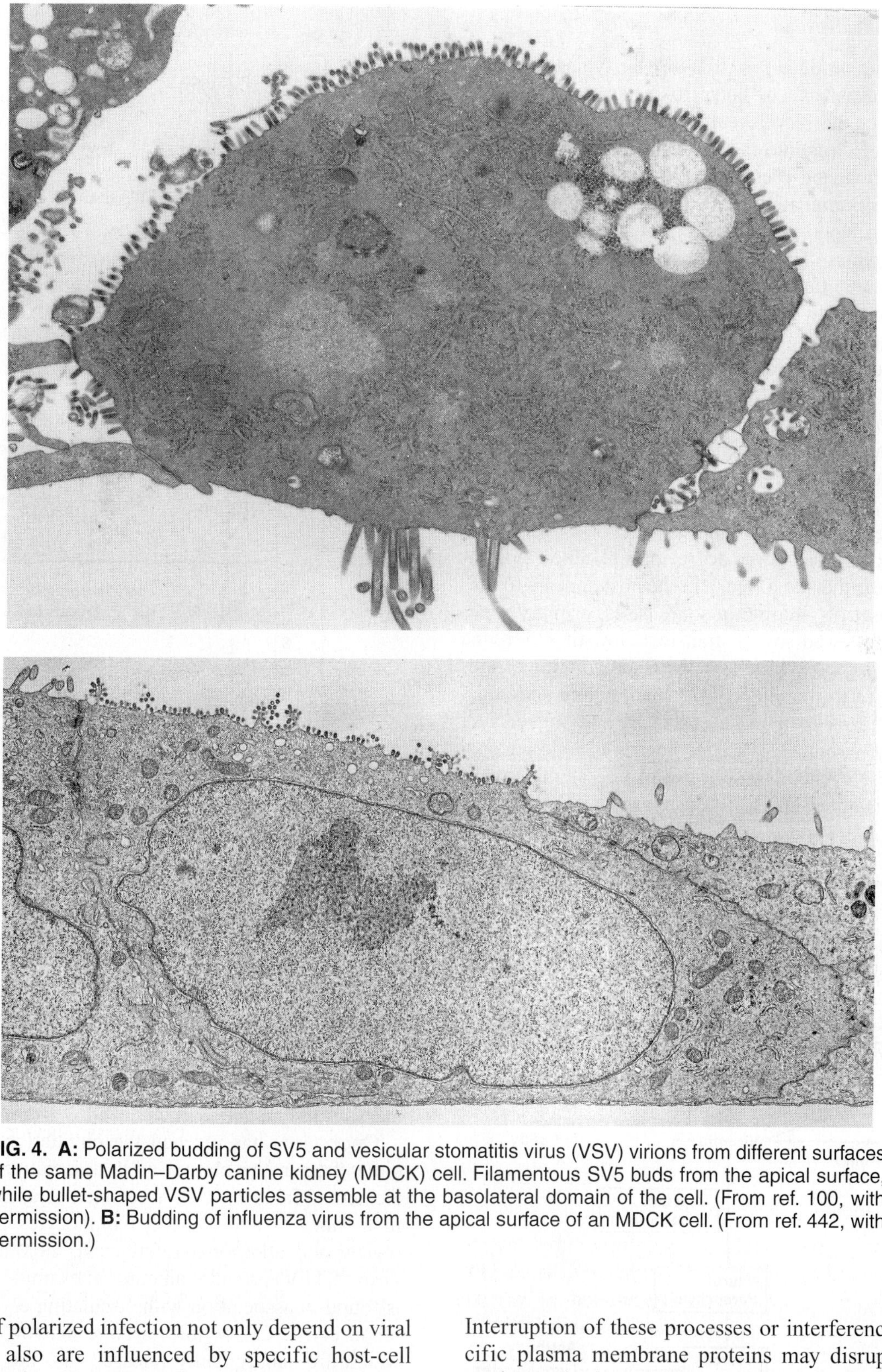

A

B

FIG. 4. A: Polarized budding of SV5 and vesicular stomatitis virus (VSV) virions from different surfaces of the same Madin–Darby canine kidney (MDCK) cell. Filamentous SV5 buds from the apical surface, while bullet-shaped VSV particles assemble at the basolateral domain of the cell. (From ref. 100, with permission). **B:** Budding of influenza virus from the apical surface of an MDCK cell. (From ref. 442, with permission.)

Patterns of polarized infection not only depend on viral factors, but also are influenced by specific host-cell transport proteins. Transport of proteins to the plasma membrane uses specific signal-mediated constitutive pathways through the trans-Golgi network that involve a variety of "cargo" proteins that form transport vesicles. Distinct cytosolic proteins appear to be involved in the assembly of apical and basolateral transport vesicles. Interruption of these processes or interference with specific plasma membrane proteins may disrupt polarized sorting and release of virions. For example, depletion of MAL/VP17 protein, a nonglycosylated cellular membrane protein, from polarized epithelial cells dramatically reduces transport of influenza HA to the apical surface of infected Madin-Darby canine kidney (MDCK) cells (418).

Hematogenous Spread

Viruses that produce systemic disease typically spread from their initial site of entry to distant target tissues through either the bloodstream or inside nerves. Direct inoculation of virus into the bloodstream can occur with the bite of arthropod vectors, through iatrogenic inoculation with a contaminated needle, or by the transfusion of contaminated blood products ("passive viremia"). If the inoculum size is sufficient, a passive viremia may be adequate to initiate infection in target organs without requiring preceding replication. A more common sequence of events, exemplified by viruses such as flaviviruses, measles, and polio, is for virus to undergo primary replication near the site of entry, followed by spread to regional lymph nodes. From the regional lymph nodes, virus can gain access to efferent lymphatics, the thoracic duct, and the systemic circulation. Some viruses can even replicate in lymphatic endothelial cells, further facilitating the development of viremia.

In almost all cases, some degree of replication at a primary site near the site of entry in the host appears to precede the onset of viremia. In some cases, primary replication is followed by a transient low-titer viremia ("primary viremia"), which serves to spread virus to sites such as the reticuloendothelial system, where additional replication leads to a more sustained and higher titer ("secondary viremia"; Fig. 5). Fenner (153) elegantly defined these events in a series of classic studies of the pathogenesis of ectromelia (mousepox; Fig. 6). Although viremia occurs in many human infections (*vide infra*), it is often difficult to demonstrate discrete phases of primary and secondary viremia.

Once virus has reached the circulation, it can travel either free in the plasma or in association with cellular elements (Table 1). Cell-associated viruses can replicate in monocytes and T or B lymphocytes [see (377) for review and additional references]. Colorado tick fever virus (CTFV) provides an unusual example of a virus that is found in association with circulating erythrocytes (red blood cells). CFTV infects bone marrow erythroblasts, which are subsequently released into the circulation as mature erythrocytes. Platelets, their precursor cells (megakaryocyctes), and neutrophils do not typically support virus replication and do not appear to be a significant source of circulating virus *in vivo*. Circulating monocytes can be infected by viruses belonging to a number of viral families (see Table 1) including retro-

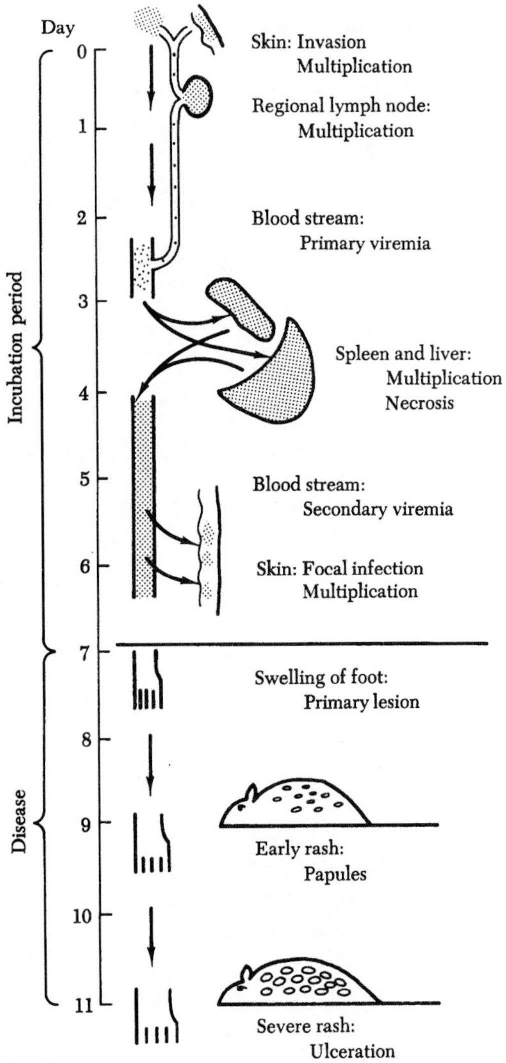

FIG. 6. The pathogenesis of mousepox (ectromelia). (From ref. 153, with permission.)

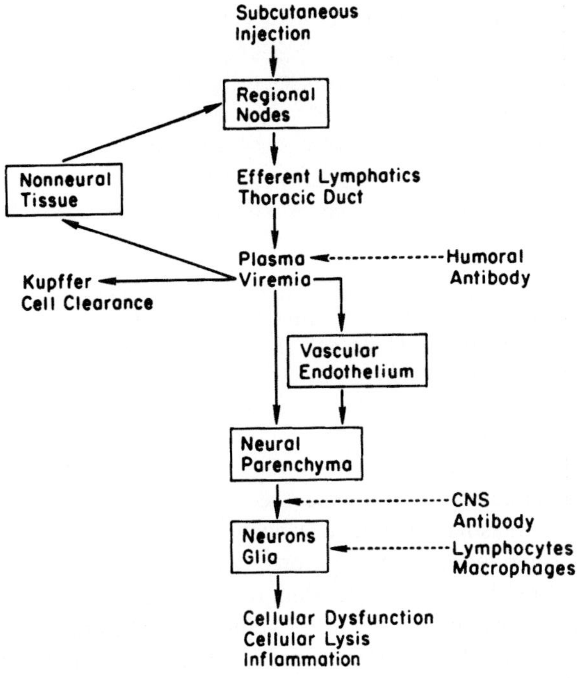

FIG. 5. Stages in the pathogenesis of flavivirus infection. (From ref. 376, with permission.)

TABLE 1. *Selected examples of viruses associated with or replicating in circulating blood cells*

Free in plasma	Togaviruses, picornaviruses
Red cell associated	CTFV
Platelet associated	HSV, LCMV, retroviruses
Lymphocyte associated	CMV, EBV, HBV, HHV 6 & 7, HIV, HTLV-I, JC & BK, LCMV, mumps, measles, rubella
Monocyte/macrophage associated	African swine fever, CMV, dengue, HIV, lentiviruses, LCMV, measles, mousepox (ectromelia), polio, rubella
Neutrophil associated	Influenza

When a virus family is listed, this indicates that one or more members of the family may spread in association with these cellular elements. Association of a virus with a formed element of the blood does not necessarily imply replication or a pathologic effect. See text and ref. 378.

Abbreviations: CMV, cytomegalovirus; CTFV, Colorado tick fever virus; EBV, Epstein-Barr virus; HBV, hepatitis B virus; HHV, human herpesvirus; HIV, human immunodeficiency virus; HSV, herpes simplex virus; HTLV, human T-lymphotropic virus; LCMV, lymphocytic choriomeningitis virus.

viruses (e.g., HIV), herpesviruses [e.g., cytomegalovirus (CMV)], flaviviruses (e.g., dengue), and togaviruses (e.g., measles). Examples of viruses that replicate in lymphocytes include HIV, human T-cell lymphoma virus type I (HTLV-I), and human herpesviruses 6 and 7 (T lymphocytes) and Epstein-Barr virus (EBV; B lymphocytes). Some of the most comprehensive studies of cell-associated viremia have involved HIV. It has been estimated that the percentage of HIV-infected $CD4^+$ T lymphocytes increases from 0.2% to 10% in asymptomatic individuals to as high as 60% in some patients with acquired immunodeficiency syndrome (AIDS). Based on these figures, the blood of asymptomatic HIV^+ individuals contains 5,000 infected cells per milliliter.

The magnitude and duration of viremia reflect the outcome of a series of interactions between the virus and the host. Viral replication at the primary site, and subsequently in a variety of other tissues, provides a continuing source of virus input into the circulation. Important sites of primary replication for viruses that spread through the bloodstream include skeletal muscle for togaviruses, connective tissue, muscle, endothelial cells, and reticuloendothelial organs for flaviviruses, and brown fat for enteroviruses (193,368,376).

At the same time that virus is entering the blood compartment from these sites, a variety of clearance mechanisms are actively removing virus from the circulation. The magnitude of viremia varies as a result of the dynamic interrelationship between the amount of virus entering the blood compartment and the efficiency with which it is removed. The extent to which virus input into the bloodstream exceeds the rate of host clearance determines the magnitude of viremia. Viremia persists for as long as virus input into the bloodstream equals the host's capacity to clear virus from the circulation. The turnover rate for infectious virus in the bloodstream (as opposed to the duration of viremia) varies for different viruses. For example, exogenously infused SIV and HIV particles have been reported to have a plasma half-life that may be as low as 3 (580) to 26 (242) minutes.

Phagocytic cells in the reticuloendothelial system (RES) and serum factors including complement and antibody act in concert to facilitate clearance of virus from the bloodstream. One of the most important determinants of clearance is particle size (351). Rapid clearance (>99.99% of an intravenous inoculum cleared within an hour) is seen after inoculation of a large virus such as vaccinia into the bloodstream of a mouse. A similar pattern of clearance is seen with small viruses opsonized by antibody or complement. The coating of virus with antibody or complement may facilitate clearance by phagocytic cells such as macrophages because of the presence of receptors on these cells for the Fc portion of antibody molecules and for complement (C3 receptor). For example, the plasma half-life of infused cell-free HIV particles is reduced from a range of 13 to 26 minutes in HIV non-immune macaques to 3.9 to 7.2 minutes in animals with high-titer HIV-specific neutralizing antibodies (242).

The nature of the protein(s) on the outer surface of the virus also may be an important determinant of the pattern of clearance. For example, the sialic acid content of the envelope of Sindbis virus appears to influence the degree of viral clearance (217). The net charge on a viral particle also may influence its clearance.

The nature of the interaction between virus and the macrophages of the RES seems to be an important determinant of the development of viremia (351). The capacity of a virus to avoid phagocytosis by macrophages facilitates the maintenance of viremia. Inhibition of the phagocytic capacity of macrophages can serve to amplify viremia and potentiates the severity of experimental viral infections caused by viruses as diverse as yellow fever virus, Semliki Forest virus, and HSV (244). Infection of macrophages with one pathogen may facilitate their infection with another. For example, infection of macrophages with opportunistic pathogens such as *Mycobacterium avium* and *Pneumocystis carinii,* or their exposure to bacterial products such as lipopolysaccharide (LPS), may promote HIV-1 replication through modulation of macrophage cytokine expression and alteration in cell-surface distribution of HIV chemokine coreceptors (361).

Certain viruses may replicate in macrophages, which serves to amplify viremia further rather than terminating it. Viruses known to replicate in macrophages include herpesviruses (e.g., HSV, CMV) (471), togaviruses (e.g., lactate dehydrogenase–elevating virus, Sendai), flaviviruses (e.g., dengue) (87), poxviruses (e.g., ectromelia), lentiviruses (e.g., HIV, visna, equine infectious anemia virus, Aleutian disease virus) (387,398), coronaviruses (e.g., mouse hepatitis virus, human coronavirus OC43)

(97), arenaviruses (e.g., lymphocytic choriomeningitis virus [LCM]), reoviruses, picornaviruses (500), rhabdoviruses (428), and myxo- and paramyxoviruses (e.g., influenza, measles) (299). Because macrophages have receptors for the Fc portion of antibody, these cells may more readily take up viruses coated with antibody. In some cases this facilitated uptake actually leads to an enhanced replication of these viruses in macrophages ("antibody-mediated enhancement"). Antibody-mediated enhancement may play an important role in the pathogenesis of viral infections such as dengue fever and foot-and-mouth disease (27).

Differences in the susceptibility of macrophages to viral infection may account for variation in the age-related susceptibility of animals to certain types of viral infection (216) (see section on host factors). For example, alveolar macrophages derived from young mice will support the replication of HSV. Transfer of adult macrophages to young mice increases their resistance to HSV infection (216,359). More recently it has been suggested that certain HIV strains may differ in their capacity to infect neonatal monocytes as compared with placental macrophages and adult adherent macrophages. This difference may result from maturity-related changes in the levels of HIV coreceptor CCR-5 on macrophages, in combination with differences in HIV gp120 V3 loop sequences (151). Differences in the capacity of Theiler's virus and CMV to infect macrophages after infection also have been correlated with the state of macrophage differentiation (477).

As noted earlier, specific viral proteins may influence the capacity of viral strains to infect macrophages, and this may in turn influence viral pathogenicity and disease expression. Determinants of macrophage infection have been found on envelope proteins, such as the V3 loop of HIV gp120 (151), and on nonenvelope proteins such as the L* protein of Theiler's virus (500) and HIV accessory protein Vpx (218). Examples of macrophage tropism correlating with patterns of pathogenesis have been extensively investigated for HIV (Chapter 28, as well as Chapter 60 of *Fields Virology*, 4th ed.) and lentiviruses such as visna (510) as well as for the Theiler's virus (500).

The interaction between viruses and macrophages also is influenced by both cytokines and chemokines (see Chapter 12 for review and references). Some cytokines, such as γ-IFN, tumor necrosis factor (TNFα), interleukin 2 (IL-2), and IL-16 inhibit replication of viruses such as HIV in macrophages. These cytokines may be secreted by infected macrophages and act via autocrine pathways or be produced by other activated leukocytes including neutrophils, natural killer (NK) cells, or T and B cells. Paradoxically, cytokines also may facilitate the capacity of some viruses to infect macrophages productively. For example, certain opportunistic infections may promote macrophage infection by HIV by modulating chemokine receptor expression. Not surprisingly, viruses have adopted a wide variety of strategies (reviewed in Chapter 11) to circumvent the antiviral defenses of macrophages, including down-regulation of HLA antigens and inhibition of the production of antiviral molecules such as nitric oxide (NO).

Vascular endothelial cells also appear to play an important role in the maintenance of viremia for certain viruses. The capacity of viruses to infect endothelial cells has been studied both *in vitro* and *in vivo* for a large number of viruses (107,157,161,297,334,405,532,541,582). Viruses may differ in their capacity to infect endothelial cells derived from vascular beds in different organs, which may be a factor in their organ-specific tropism and invasion (156). This may be of particular importance in influencing viral invasion of the CNS. For example, mouse hepatitis virus A59 binds to receptors expressed on the endoluminal surface of liver-derived endothelial cells, but fails to bind to endothelial cells derived from brain, which in turn prevents entry of virus into the CNS after intraperitoneal (but not intracerebral) inoculation (179). Conversely, the capacity to infect the CNS and the pattern of disease induced by some strains of adenovirus correlate with their ability to infect cerebral vascular endothelium (81). Viruses that infect circulating cells may enhance their capacity to spread subsequently to endothelial cells by up-regulating integrins such as LFA-1, which facilitate binding of circulating cells to vascular endothelium. This suggests that, in some circumstances, cell-to-cell spread may be an important mechanism of initiating endothelial infection (238).

There is a general correlation between the capacity of blood-borne neurotropic viruses to generate a high-titer viremia and their neuroinvasiveness (376). Similarly, attenuated virulence may reflect incapacity to generate sufficient viremia, even for viruses that are fully virulent after direct CNS inoculation (181). For example, mutants of Semliki Forest virus (SFV) generate high-titer viremia but, unlike their wild-type counterparts, are unable to invade the CNS (13). Thus the capacity to generate a viremia of adequate magnitude and duration may be necessary for neuroinvasiveness, but is not always sufficient. A similar relationship between the degree of virus present in the plasma and clinical outcome has been repeatedly noted in HIV infection, in which plasma viral load at diagnosis correlates with subsequent risk of progression to AIDS and death (341).

Tissue Invasion

The factors that determine the capacity of blood-borne virus to escape the vascular compartment and invade specific organs are poorly understood. The problem has probably been most extensively investigated as it applies to invasion of the CNS by blood-borne viruses (Fig. 7) (251). In most regions of the CNS, tight junctions (zona occludens) join capillary cells of the cerebral microvasculature, and there is an underlying dense basement

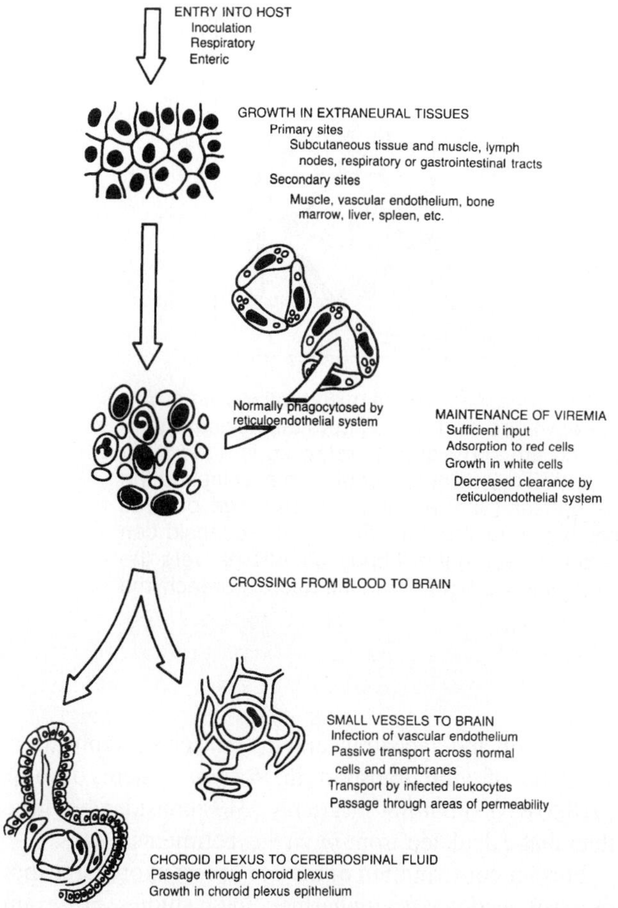

FIG. 7. Pathways of entry of blood-borne viruses into the central nervous system. (From ref. 251, with permission.)

membrane. A notable exception to this pattern occurs in the choroid plexus, where the capillary endothelium is fenestrated and the basement membrane is generally sparse. This was originally postulated as a potential site of invasion for polioviruses, and subsequently established as an important site of infection for lentiviruses such as visna (307). Recent studies suggest that HIV also may infect the choroid plexus (147), and that choroid plexus dendritic cells, which are similar to antigen-presenting dendritic cells elsewhere in the body, may serve as a reservoir and source for CNS disease (203).

Some viruses invade the CNS from the bloodstream by entering the stroma of the choroid plexus through the fenestrated capillary endothelium and then either infecting or being passively transported across the choroid plexus epithelial cells into the cerebrospinal fluid (CSF). Once in the CSF, virus can infect the ependymal cells lining the walls of the ventricles and can then invade the underlying brain tissue. This pattern of infection has been shown for a number of viruses including mumps, arboviruses, and rat virus (251). Visna, a lentivirus, can be shown to infect cultured choroid plexus epithelial cells *in vitro* (372), suggesting that this pathway may be used by this virus *in vivo* as well. In some cases, direct infection of choroid plexus may not be demonstrable, although the sequential appearance of virus in CSF and ependymal cells suggests the possibility that virus has used this route initially to reach the CSF.

A number of viruses that invade the CNS do so by either directly infecting or being passively transported across capillary endothelial cells. Ability to infect endothelial cells has been demonstrated *in vitro* for many viruses (107,161,297,532,541). Infection of endothelial cells has been proposed as a mechanism for CNS invasion of such disparate groups of viruses as picornaviruses (107,582), togaviruses (376), bunyaviruses (252), parvoviruses, and murine retroviruses (336,411). In the case of some murine retroviruses, there is a close association between neuropathogenicity and capacity to bind to brain endothelial capillary cells *in vitro* (334).

Transendothelial transport of viruses including measles, mumps, canine distemper virus, togaviruses, and lentiviruses may provide another route of penetration of the endothelium and may occur via the diapedesis of infected monocytes, leukocytes, and lymphocytes (159, 199). This process may be facilitated by viral modulation of the activity of LFA-1 and other cell-surface adhesion molecules (14,211). Finally, factors that increase vascular permeability, such as vasogenic amines, also may facilitate viral invasion of sites such as the CNS (465).

Neural Spread

Another important route for viral spread is through nerves (251,285) (Fig. 8). Although this was first postulated as a mechanism for the spread of rabies as early as the 18th century (251), it was not clearly demonstrated until the elegant work by Pasteur and his contemporaries (382). During the first half of the 20th century, experiments by Goodpasture, Hurst, Sabin, Bodian, and others established that herpesviruses, polioviruses, and certain arboviruses also were capable of neural spread (183, 234,453). These early observations have been repeatedly confirmed in more modern studies (108,177,291,293, 389,432,495,517,527). The group of neurally spreading viruses has now expanded to include reoviruses (157,363, 525), pseudorabies virus (71,74,573), coronaviruses (23, 407,408), and Borna disease virus (68,358).

Classic experiments on the spread of poliovirus through the sciatic nerve of the monkey by Bodian and Howe (234) established several important principles of neural spread, which have been repeatedly confirmed in other systems (17). They demonstrated that primary replication of virus in extraneural tissues was not an absolute prerequisite for neural spread by showing that poliomyelitis could develop in monkeys after immersion of the cut distal end of the sciatic nerve into a solution containing virus. They also established that the incidence of subsequent neurologic disease, which reflected the efficiency of neural spread, depended on a variety of factors including

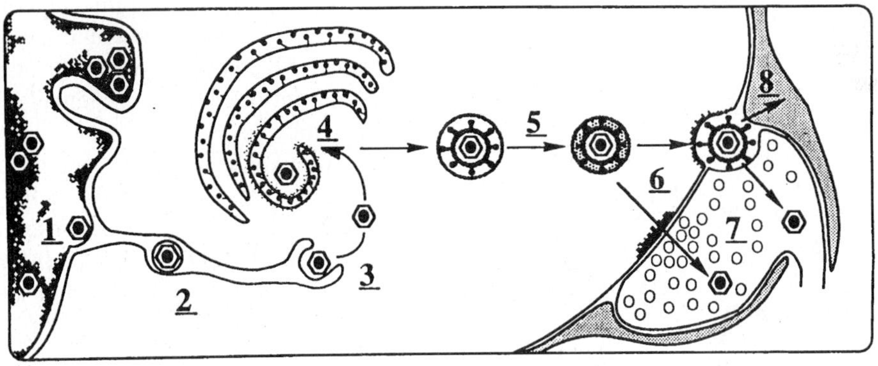

FIG. 8. Significant events that lead to replication and transneuronal passage of pseudorabies virus. Virions replicate in the cell nucleus and acquire a membrane envelope as they bud from the nuclear membrane (*1*), traverse the endoplasmic reticulum (ER) (*2*), and are subsequently released into the cytoplasm after a fusion event between the virion membrane and ER (*3*). Virions acquire an envelope at the Golgi apparatus (*4*), which consolidates and becomes denser (*5*). Transneuronal passage of virus occurs after fusion of the virion envelope with the postsynaptic membrane (*6*); the nucleocapsid can subsequently undergo retrograde axonal transport toward the neuronal cell body (*7*). Alternatively, the virus particle can be released into the extracellular space to infect other cells in the neural parenchyma (*8*). (From ref. 71, with permission.)

the amount of nerve exposed to virus, the duration of this exposure, and the concentration of virus present. Under circumstances of natural infection, direct exposure of a nerve to virus is presumably unusual, and primary replication of virus at peripheral sites, although not essential for subsequent neural spread (108,467), may facilitate this process by amplifying the size of the initial inoculum.

Techniques for localizing viral antigens have been used to document the sequential progression of viral infection along neural pathways (251,291). The direct visualization of herpesvirus and rabies virus particles within axons provided further evidence for intra-axonal transport (214, 245,285,367,420). A natural corollary of these observations was the finding that axonal transport could also be demonstrated in cultured neurons *in vitro* (318,319,518, 519), as well as in isolated nerve preparations (327), and that inhibitors of axonal transport also inhibited the spread of neurally spreading viruses *in vivo* and *in vitro* (39,76,77,283,285,319,516,525).

Both kinetic studies and experiments using pharmacologic inhibitors indicated that most viruses that spread neurally do so via fast axonal transport (285,327,389,525). *In vivo* studies, in which the rate of viral transport is generally measured by dividing the distance traveled by the elapsed time between inoculation and detection at a distant site, have resulted in calculated transport values of 2 to 16 mm/day for viruses as diverse as polio, rabies, herpes simplex, and reovirus T3 Dearing (234,245,285,525). These rates are faster than those associated with slow axonal transport, but far slower than the rate of fast axonal transport (>100 mm/day). The discrepancy may be due to the fact that viral transit times also reflect the time required for a variety of events in addition to transport (e.g., adsorption, penetration and uncoating, and in some cases, replication). The rate of viral transport in *in vitro* systems is often (318,518,519) but not invariably (319) considerably faster than that calculated from *in vivo* experiments.

Further confirmation of the use of fast axonal transport by viruses comes from pharmacologic studies. For example, selective inhibition of fast axonal transport with colchicine, but not the inhibition of slow axonal transport with imidodiproprionitrile (IDPN), inhibits the neural spread of reovirus T3 (525). Colchicine also has been repeatedly shown to inhibit the neural spread of both rabies virus and HSV both to the CNS (39,77) and within the CNS (76). Similarly, taxol, nocodazole, and vinblastine, agents that disrupt the microtubules that serve as the structural guides for fast axonal transport, can inhibit neural spread of viruses *in vivo* and *in vitro* (90,285,319). These results are all consistent with morphologic studies showing a close association between neurally transported viruses and microtubules (258). A selective inhibitor of retrograde axonal transport, erythro-9-3-(2-hydroxynonyl)adenine, also has been shown to inhibit transport of HSV (283), as has an inhibitor of axonal transport in sensory neurons (capsaicin) (482).

The exact mechanism(s) by which axonal transport of viruses occurs has not been established. As described earlier, in the case of several enveloped viruses, such as rabies and herpes simplex, both mature virions and naked nucleocapsids have been visualized within axons. Fast axonal transport typically involves the movement of material contained in vesicles along microtubules. It is easy to see how viruses that initially enter nerve cells via receptor-mediated endocytosis, and thus appear in vesicles, could be transported to the perikaryon in a vesicle-associated fashion. In some cases, virus might be inserted into vesicles via the Golgi apparatus, in a fashion akin to the sorting of certain cellular macromolecules. However, it remains unclear whether virus is transported in this fashion. Some viruses, including reoviruses and adenoviruses, are capable of binding to isolated purified microtubules (16), suggesting that movement of extravesicular virus also could occur.

In vivo studies clearly indicated that viruses can cross the neuromuscular junction and travel transneuronally at both synaptic and nonsynaptic sites (72,284,285,483,490, 527), with the predominant route depending on the virus. In some cases, transneuronal spread may be facilitated by the pattern of viral release from the nerve cell or myocytes. Polarized sorting of viral glycoproteins to the axon and dendrites of cultured neurons, a process analogous to that seen in epithelial cells (*vide supra*), has been described (127), and undoubtedly plays a role in the patterns of viral release and transport in neurons. Rabies virus accumulates in myocytes at the neuromuscular junction (367) and may bind to the nicotinic acetylcholine receptor at the neuromuscular junction (see receptors) (62,202). The synaptic terminals of nerve cells may contain increased numbers of receptors for certain viruses including herpes simplex and rabies (318,319), perhaps explaining how entry at the distal axon terminal is facilitated. Rabies virions also bud from peripheral nerve cells along their axons at the nodes of Ranvier, at the boundary between opposing myelin-producing Schwann cells (367). A related virus, vesicular stomatitis virus (VSV), will preferentially bud from synaptic sites in the presence of antiviral antibody, suggesting that the synaptic region of the axon terminal may have unique structural features that facilitate the exocytosis of some viruses (134).

Viral factors that influence neuron-to-neuron spread are still poorly understood. In the case of herpes simplex virus, it has been suggested that a heterodimer of the envelope glycoproteins gE and gI may be required to facilitate efficient neuron-to-neuron transmission through synaptically linked neural pathways (125).

Different strains of the same virus may show a predilection for retrograde, anterograde, or bidirectional systems of fast axonal transport. This direction-specific predilection has been seen with certain strains of herpes simplex virus and pseudorabies virus (70). The capacity of viruses to spread along discrete neuronal pathways and transneuronally across synapses has made them valuable tools for defining neuroanatomic pathways. Viruses have been used to map synaptically linked interneuronal circuits both within the CNS and between the peripheral and central nervous systems. Injection of virus into a particular target tissue, and sequential study of its central transit, may allow the peripheral and central innervation of these structures to be mapped with exquisite fidelity. HSV and pseudorabies virus have both been used extensively for this purpose (69,71,72, 229,230,291,311,384,483,490).

It is important to recognize that viremia and neural spread are not mutually exclusive processes. Some viruses may use different pathways to reach different organs or different pathways at different stages in pathogenesis. For example, it has been suggested that certain flaviviruses may spread via the bloodstream to reach the neurons of the olfactory bulb and then travel retrogradely via neural spread within these specialized neurons to reach the CNS (355). VZV disseminates to the skin via the bloodstream to produce the classic exanthemal rash of chickenpox but then travels up the axons of sensory neurons to reach sensory ganglia where the virus remains latent. Reactivation of VZV is associated with spread of virus via nerves to reach the skin and the appearance of the dermatomal lesions of shingles (Chapter 79 of *Fields Virology*, 4th ed.).

As discussed earlier, different strains of the same neurotropic virus may differ in their capacity to spread at synaptic versus nonsynaptic sites and to use anterograde or retrograde systems of fast axonal transport. Different strains of the same virus also may differ in the predominant pathway (neural or hematogenous) they use to spread in the host. For example, under experimental conditions, some strains of poliovirus spread to the CNS via nerves (389,432), whereas others do so via the bloodstream (145,234,374,454). Similar differences have been noted for reoviruses, with reovirus serotype 1 strain Lang spreading to the CNS predominantly through the bloodstream, whereas reovirus serotype 3 strain Dearing uses predominantly neural spread (525).

Molecular and Genetic Determinants of Viral Spread

Although the capacity of viruses to spread via different routes in the infected host has been recognized for some time, only recently have the specific viral genes involved in determining this process been identified. Thus several studies with reoviruses indicated that their pattern of spread in the infected host is determined by the nature of the viral S1 gene and the outer capsid protein (σ1) that it encodes. After intramuscular inoculation, reovirus T1 Lang (T1L) spreads to the CNS via the bloodstream, whereas T3 Dearing (T3D) spreads via nerves. The viral S1 gene, which encodes the outer capsid protein σ1, determines the capacity of T1L × T3D reassortants to spread via either the bloodstream or the nerves to reach the CNS (525). T1 and T3 also show different patterns of spread after oral inoculation into mice. T3 does not disseminate to extraintestinal organs, but T1 does. The pattern of spread of T1 suggests that virus initially spreads via local lymphatics and then via the bloodstream. Studies with T1L × T3D reassortants indicate that the capacity of T1 to spread extraintestinally also is determined by the S1 gene (Chapter 53 of *Fields Virology*, 4th ed.).

Genetic factors that influence the capacity of HSV to spread to and invade the CNS also have been investigated. There appear to be numerous factors that influence HSV neuroinvasiveness, neurovirulence, and latency (486). The region of the HSV genome between 0.25 and 0.53 map units (m.u.) appears to contain genes that are critical in allowing HSV-1 to spread to the CNS after footpad inoculation in mice ("neuroinvasiveness") (507). An area contained within this region (0.31–0.44 m.u.) also has been shown to influence the capacity of intertypic HSV-1 × HSV-2 recombinants to spread to the CNS via nerves after corneal inoculation in mice (116). A number of viral proteins including the DNA polymerase, thymidine kinase, the nucleoprotein p40, and the gB envelope glycoprotein are encoded by genes contained in these regions. Mutations in gB may be particularly important in influencing the neuroinvasive capacity of certain HSV strains including KOS and ANG (578). Another genetic mapping study has implicated the DNA polymerase (0.413–0.426 m.u.) (116). The mechanisms by which alterations in the polymerase gene enhance or attenuate neural spread remain speculative. It would appear likely that the effect is an indirect one having to do with replication competence rather than a direct effect on axon transport of virus, because it can be shown that recombinants with differences in this region of the genome vary dramatically in their capacity to replicate in peripheral nervous system tissue.

Mutations within the gD envelope glycoprotein can also influence HSV neuroinvasiveness. For example, the neuroinvasive HSV 1 ANG-path strain differs from its nonneuroinvasive parent by only a single amino acid substitution within gD (246). Finally, as noted earlier, the glycoproteins gE and gI play an important role in determining the capacity of HSV to spread transsynaptically between neurons (125).

These studies suggested that, in the case of HSV, neuroinvasiveness may be affected by mutations involving a number of steps in pathogenesis. Mutations in envelope glycoproteins such as gB and gD may affect viral attachment or penetration. Polymerase mutations and mutations in viral immediate early proteins may hamper viral replication.

Strain-specific patterns in the transport of herpesviruses have been investigated for both HSV and pseudorabies virus (PRV). For example, the PRV-Becker, PRV-Bartha, and PRV-91 strains all differ in their pattern of neuronal uptake and subsequent neural spread (70,74). The PRV-Becker and PRV-91 strains differ only in the deletion of the gene encoding the PRV gI and gp63 glycoproteins, suggesting that the complex formed by these proteins may be critical in determining differences in neuronal uptake and spread (73,272,551).

A number of studies in the bunyavirus system have identified viral genes that are important in the capacity of these viruses to spread from the periphery to the CNS ("neuroinvasiveness"). Comparisons between nonneuroinvasive and neuroinvasive strains indicate that the viral M genome segment, which encodes the two envelope glycoproteins (G1, G2), is the major determinant of the neuroinvasive phenotype (Chapter 49 of *Fields Virology*, 4th ed.). Subsequent studies with monoclonal antibody–resistant bunyavirus variants suggested that the viral G1 glycoprotein may be the important determinant.

Studies with monoclonal antibody–resistant mutants of the flavivirus, Japanese encephalitis virus (JEV) indicated that mutations in the E envelope glycoprotein can reduce the neuroinvasiveness of these variants without altering their virulence after intracranial inoculation (78). Thus studies in a number of viral systems including reoviruses, togaviruses, herpesviruses, and bunyaviruses indicated that viral surface glycoproteins may be critical determinants of the capacity of these viruses to reach the CNS from peripheral sites.

TROPISM

The pattern of systemic illness produced during an acute viral infection depends in large part on the specific host organs infected and in many cases on the capacity of viruses to infect discrete populations of cells within these organs (tropism). The tissue tropism of a virus is influenced by the interaction between a variety of host and viral factors. Although a great deal of attention has focused on the importance of viral cell attachment proteins and specific viral receptors on target cells, it also has become clear that a variety of other virus–host interactions can play an important role in determining the ultimate tropism of a virus (207,385). This fact is clearly indicated by experiments that demonstrate that the mere presence of a functional viral receptor may be insufficient to allow viral infection of target cells, as has been shown with HIV, polio, rotaviruses, measles, and MHV (88,91, 206,383). For example, intracellular factors and the route of viral entry may be important determinants of tropism (see later). Increasing attention also has focused on the importance of "coreceptors" in mediating viral binding and entry. For example, entry of HIV-1 into target cells requires the presence of both CD4 and a second coreceptor protein that belongs to the G-protein–coupled seven-transmembrane receptor family and includes the chemokine receptor proteins CCR5 and CXCR4 (123). As a result, cells expressing CD4 but not the coreceptor are resistant to HIV infection (see earlier).

Binding to Target Cells and Penetration of Cell Membranes

The importance of viral receptors in determining tissue tropism was initially emphasized for polioviruses (224). Since that time, there has been an explosion of knowledge concerning the nature of viral cell-recognition proteins and their target cell receptors. A full discussion of each viral system and its target cell receptor is beyond the scope of this chapter, and readers are directed to the chapters dealing with individual viral families for more detailed information and more com-

TABLE 2. *Cell-surface molecules proposed to play a role in virus binding and entry*

Family	Virus	Putative Virus-Binding Molecule or Co-Receptor (Ref.)
Adenoviridae	Adenovirus type 2	Integrins $\alpha_v\beta_3$ and $\alpha_v\beta_5$ (558)
	Adenoviruses	Coxsackie-adenovirus receptor (CAR) (33,443,457)
Alphaviridae	Sindbis	Laminin receptor (544)
		Heparan sulfate proteoglycan (64)
	Semliki Forest	HLA H2-K, H2-D (208)
Arenaviridae	LCMV, Lassa fever	α-Dystroglycan (66)
Arteriviridae	Lactate dehydrogenase	Ia (243)
Bunyaviridae	Hantaviruses	β_3 Integrins (171)
Coronaviridae	MHV	Carcinoembryonic antigen family (83,138)
	TGEV, HCoV-229E	Aminopeptidase N (513,574)
	HCoV-OC43, BCV	Sialic acid residues (533)
Dependoviridae	Adeno-associated virus 2	Heparan sulfate proteoglycan (494)
		Integrin $\alpha_v\beta_5$ (493)
Flaviviridae	Hepatitis C	Low-density lipoprotein receptor (356)
Herpesviridae	EBV	CD21 (CR2 receptor) (336)
	HSV	Heparan sulfate (468,479)
		HVEM (TNF/NGF receptor family) (357,552)
		Poliovirus receptor–related protein 1 (173)
	CMV	Heparan sulfate (101)
		β_2-Microglobulin/MHC I (572)
	BHV-1, BHV-4	Heparan sulfate (531)
		Poliovirus receptor–related protein 1 (173)
	Pseudorabies	Heparan sulfate (259)
		Poliovirus receptor–related protein 1 (173)
Orthomyxoviridae	Influenza A,B	Sialic acid residues (546)
Papovaviridae	Papillomaviruses	α_6 Group integrins (142)
Paramyxoviridae	Canine distemper virus	CD9 (312)
	Measles	CD46 (59,60,231,371,383)
		Moesin (136)
	Sendai	Gangliosides (329)
		Sialic acid (glycophorin) (571)
		Asialoglycoprotein receptor (41)
Parvoviridae	B19	Erythrocyte P antigen (57)
Picornaviridae	Coxsackievirus A9, Foot-and-mouth-disease, Echovirus 22	Integrin $\alpha_v\beta_3$ (vitronectin receptor) (35,443)
	Coxsackieviruses A21, B1, B3, B5, echo 3, 6, 7, 11–13, 20, 21, 24, 29, 33, Enterovirus 70	Decay-accelerating factor (CD55) (32,144,261,333,466)
	Polio	PVR–IgG superfamily (343,421)
	Coxsackievirus A13, A18, A21, Rhinoviruses (major group)	ICAM-1 (144,190,403,484,509)
	Rhinoviruses (minor group)	Low-density lipoprotein receptor (221,330)
	Echovirus 1, 8	Integrin $\alpha_2\beta_1$ (VLA-2) (271)
	Encephalomyocarditis virus	VCAM-1 (237)
	Coxsackie B viruses	Coxsackievirus–adenovirus receptor (CAR) (33,34)
Poxviridae	Vaccinia	Epidermal growth factor (EGF) receptor (140)
Reoviridae	Reovirus T3 (Dearing)	Sialic acid residues (172,406)
		Epidermal growth factor (EGF) receptor (492)
	Rotavirus SA11, OSU	Gangliosides (445,497)
		Sialic acids (25)
Retroviridae	HIV-1	CD4 (113,274,338,547)
		Galactosylceramide (38,148)
		Chemokine receptors (CXCR5,CCR4) (123,128,345)
	MuLV	y^+ amino acid transporter (270,543)
		PIT-2 Na^+-phosphate co-transporter (441)
	GLV	Phosphate permease (249,548)
	Feline endogenous retrovirus, baboon endogenous retrovirus, avian reticuloendotheliosis virus, simian type D retroviruses	Na-dependent neutral amino acid transporter (426,499)
Rhabdoviridae	Rabies	Acetylcholine receptor (197)
		Neural cell adhesion molecule (497)
		Nerve growth factor receptor (523)
		Gangliosides (497)
		Phospholipids (570)
	VSV	Phosphatidyl serine (461)

Note: The process of virus binding and entry of viral nucleic acids into cells can involve a series of sequential interactions of proteins on the surface of virions with specific molecules on the surface of target cells. Many different types of evidence have been used to identify potential cellular targets of viral attachment proteins. The examples listed here are a partial list of molecules implicated in virus entry. The strength of the evidence supporting the role of each of the listed molecules in virus entry varies considerably, and in some cases, remains controversial or disputed. Additional information about the entry process can be found in the chapters on the various viruses and in the references cited in this table.

plete references. A partial list of virus families and examples of possible associated host cell receptor(s) can be found in Table 2.

As the list of potential receptors for specific viruses becomes more and more complete, it is possible to identify certain common themes. Different viruses may use the same cellular structures as receptors. For example, sialic acid residues have been reported to be components of the receptor for certain coronaviruses (human coronavirus OC43, bovine coronavirus) (533), orthomyxoviruses (influenza A and B) (546), Sendai virus (571), and reoviruses (certain serotype 3 strains and rotaviruses) (172,406). Similarly gangliosides have been implicated as potential receptors for rotaviruses (SA11, OSU) (497), paramyxoviruses (Sendai) (329), and rhabdoviruses (rabies) (498). Sometimes several different viruses belonging to the same family use the same receptor, as appears to be the case with heparan sulfate proteoglycan molecules that are used by HSV-1, human cytomegalovirus, pseudorabies, and bovine herpesvirus-1 for initial attachment. Interestingly, heparan sulfate proteoglycans may also serve as receptors for nonherpesviruses including Sindbis (64) and adeno-associated virus type 2 (AAV-2) (494), demonstrating that the same surface molecule can potentially serve as a receptor for distinct families of viruses. Another example of this shared receptor use is represented by the CAR, which, as its name suggests, serves as a receptor for adenoviruses 2 and 5 as well as Coxsackie B viruses (33). In some cases, even though the receptor molecules are not identical, they may share enough structural similarity to merit inclusion together as part of superfamily. For example, many rhinoviruses, poliovirus, and HIV-1 bind to molecules that are members of the immunoglobulin superfamily (190,343,484,509,556).

Certain types of cell-surface molecules appear to be used as viral receptors far more frequently than would be expected by chance. Among this group are the human membrane cofactor proteins, which include regulators of complement activation such as the measles receptor, CD46 (371), which binds C3b and C4b, the EBV receptor, CD21 (155), which serves as a C3d receptor, the coxsackievirus and enterovirus 70 receptor CD55, another complement regulatory protein also known as decay-accelerating factor (DAF) (261), and the canine distemper virus receptor CD9 (312). HIV-1 and certain other retroviruses bind to CD4 (113).

Major histocompatibility complex (MHC) antigens have been implicated as putative receptors for CMV (196), SFV (208), and lactate dehydrogenase elevating virus (LDEV) (243), although in some cases, the assignment remains controversial (395).

Other cell-surface antigens, including the members of the CEA family (coronaviruses) (138) and the erythrocyte P antigen (parvovirus B19) (57), also serve as viral receptors. Integrins also have been identified as receptors or coreceptors for a large and diverse group of viruses including adenovirus type 2 (558), AAV-2 (493), hantaviruses (171), and papillomaviruses (142).

Receptors for neurotransmitters, growth factors, and extracellular matrix molecules including the acetylcholine receptor (rabies) (197), the epidermal growth factor (EGF) receptor (vaccinia, reovirus T3D) (492), and the laminin receptor (Sindbis) (544) may be involved in virus–cell recognition, although controversy again exists about the validity of certain of these assignments.

Among the new categories of proteins that have been implicated as potential receptors are permeases (Gibbon leukemia virus) (249), aminopeptidases (coronaviruses) (513), amino acid–transporter proteins (Mahoney leukemia virus) (270), α-dystroglycans (66), and lipoprotein receptors (356).

A number of general principles have emerged from studies of virus–receptor interactions (207). Many viruses appear capable of interacting with more than one receptor molecule (see Table 2). HIV-1 binding to different receptors by a single virus may be mediated by either a single cell-attachment protein, or by different proteins. For example, HIV-1 uses the gp120 envelope glycoprotein to bind to both CD4 and to galactosylceramide (see Chapter 28), although different domains of the protein appear to be involved. Adenovirus 2 binds to certain integrin molecules through the penton base, which contains an Arg-Gly-Asp (RGD) sequence of the type recognized by cell-adhesion receptors of the integrin family (19,558). For initial entry into target cells, adenovirus also attaches with high affinity to cell-surface receptors via the fiber protein (186). Similarly, Sindbis virus binds to the high-affinity laminin receptor on many mammalian cells (544), but appears to use a distinct receptor for binding to mouse neuronal cells (526). Single amino acid substitutions in the Sindbis E2 protein can alter binding to neuroblastoma cells but not to BHK cells, suggesting that distinct receptor-binding domains may exist on the E2 spike.

It appears that attachment is often a multiphasic interaction between viral attachment protein(s) and several host-cell receptors. In the case of the alphaherpesviruses, it appears that internalization is better understood in terms of a cascade of events that involve different glycoproteins and different cell-surface molecules at different stages (166,207,385,479). Different cell-surface proteins may be used for initial attachment and entry into target cells and for cell-to-cell spread across closely apposed populations of cells (124). An initial HSV attachment step appears to involve the interaction between gC, and possibly gB, with heparan sulfate molecules (210,287). This is followed by a stable attachment phase that involves gD, and possibly gH, and occurs independent of heparan sulfate binding (166). Other glycoproteins including gE and gI may facilitate cell-to-cell spread across contiguous cell layers (124). An analogous series of events has been postulated to occur with other alphaherpesviruses including pseudorabies (259), human CMV (101), and bovine herpesvirus (BHV-1) (391).

Even for viruses that may use only a single receptor, a progression from weak initial binding to secondary stable attachment ("adhesion strengthening") may occur, as a result of factors such as temperature shifts, or recruitment of receptors to allow multivalent binding (207,385).

For all viruses, initial attachment serves as the first in a series of steps that ultimately delivers the genome to a site in the cell where it can begin replication. For enveloped viruses, penetration of the cytoplasmic membrane takes place after fusion between the viral envelope and the cell membrane. For nonenveloped viruses, penetration of the cytoplasmic membrane is still not completely understood, but involves different strategies (220,331,555). In some cases, as discussed earlier for alphaherpesviruses, initial attachment and subsequent fusion may be mediated, entirely or in part, by different viral proteins. In other cases, the interaction of a virion cell-attachment protein (VAP) with its target cell receptor may initiate conformational changes in other virion proteins that may in turn be essential for subsequent steps in virus–cell interaction including fusion. In some cases, an envelope glycoprotein, such as the vaccinia HA, may have fusion-inhibitory activity, with removal of the protein activating the fusion protein(s) (390). As another example, binding of the alphaviruses Sindbis and SFV to host cells results in structural reorganization of the envelope glycoproteins on the virion surface, which expose previously hidden hydrophobic fusogenic domains (56,158,538). In the case of SFV, dissociation of the E1/E2 heteromer is followed by the appearance of E1 homotrimers that initiate subsequent fusion events (538). In the case of HIV, a conformational change in the gp120 envelope glycoprotein, which serves as the cell-recognition protein, may increase exposure of the N-terminus of the transmembrane (TM) protein, which contains a stretch of nonpolar amino acids that are essential for fusion activity (339). Conformational changes in the envelope glycoproteins required for fusion also may occur after initial receptor binding has resulted in internalization of the virion into acidified vesicles, as occurs with influenza (419,555) and lymphocytic choriomeningitis virus (LCMV) (122). Given these results, it is not surprising that alterations in fusion proteins can dramatically alter viral host range and cell tropism, independent of changes in viral cell-recognition proteins (165,253).

Fusion events may occur under pH-independent or pH-dependent conditions (294,555). The fusions of the envelopes of herpesviruses, coronaviruses, paramyxoviruses, and certain retroviruses with the plasma membrane of target cells are all examples of pH-independent fusion. Conversely, fusion activity may occur only after endocytosis has delivered virions into the acidic environment of endosomal vesicles. This type of pH-dependent fusion is characteristic of orthomyxoviruses, togaviruses, rhabdoviruses, bunyaviruses, and arenaviruses (47,555). It is important to recognize that the type of entry pathway used by a virus may depend on the cell type. For example, EBV entry into lymphoblastoid and epithelial cells seems to occur by direct fusion of the viral envelope with the target cell plasma membrane, whereas entry into normal B cells involves initial internalization into intracellular vesicles (349). In some cases, a single protein serves both as the viral cell-recognition and fusion protein (e.g., the HA of influenza A), whereas in other viruses, these activities are separated (e.g., paramyxoviruses, HIV).

A number of general features of virion fusion proteins have been identified (554,555). For enveloped viruses, typical fusion proteins have external N-termini and internal C-termini, with most of their mass lying outside the viral envelope. Many of these proteins exist as oligomers, typically trimers or less frequently tetramers. This is perhaps best exemplified by the influenza HA, which is a trimer composed of three identical disulfide-linked subunits, each of which is involved in fusion. Many fusion proteins contain a distinctive stretch of apolar amino acids referred to as a fusion sequence, although in some cases, proteins capable of fusion do not have obvious "fusion sequences." Fusion sequences vary from short stretches of three to six amino acids to longer sequences 24 to 36 amino acids in length, and often appear to have a predicted secondary structure either of amphipathic helices with hydrophobic amino acids on one helical face and nonpolar residues on the other, or of stretches of nonpolar amino acids. Because fusion proteins are typically inserted into viral envelopes via apolar transmembrane anchoring segments, the presence of a second apolar region (the fusion peptide sequence) presumably facilitates their simultaneous interaction with the target cell membrane. The fusion sequence may be located at the N-terminal of the fusion protein, as is the case with orthomyxovirus HAs, paramyxovirus F proteins, and many retroviral envelope fusion proteins.

Nonenveloped viruses, like their enveloped counterparts, undergo conformational changes consequent to receptor binding. Intracellular delivery of the viral capsid also may be a complex event involving several viral proteins. For example, in the case of reoviruses, the σ1 outer capsid protein serves as the viral cell-recognition protein (see Chapter 26). Proteolytic removal of other outer capsid proteins, such as occurs during natural infection in the lumen of the intestine, is associated with a change in the σ1 cell-recognition protein from a compact to an extended fibrous form (132). This transition may facilitate subsequent receptor binding. Proteolytic digestion also exposes a fragment on another outer capsid protein, μ1, that is proposed to have a role in membrane penetration (228,511).

During the entry of polioviruses into target cells, conformational transitions also occur that are dependent on binding of the virion to its cell-surface receptor (364).

The VP4 capsid protein and the amino terminus of VP1 are extruded from virion interior (160,364). These proteins appear to play a role in membrane-binding interactions that are important postattachment steps in poliovirus entry.

Viral Gene Expression

For some viruses, the interaction between VAP and host-cell receptors is the principal determinant of tropism (see Table 2). However, as more cellular receptors become identified, it has become apparent that the interaction between a virus and its receptor is not the only determinant. Other important factors, especially for retroviruses and papovaviruses, are the elements in the viral genome that regulate the transcription of viral genes in a cell-, tissue-, or disease-specific fashion, including enhancers and transcriptional activators. A full review of the many examples of viral transcriptional regulatory elements is beyond the scope of this chapter, and readers should refer to the individual chapters dealing with specific viruses for more complete discussion and references.

Both SV40 and polyoma have enhancer elements that show some degree of cell-type specificity (see Chapter 29 for review and references), although they also behave in a "promiscuous" fashion and stimulate viral gene expression to some degree in many varieties of differentiated cells. When the SV40 enhancer and early promoter are linked to a marker gene (CAT, chloramphenicol acetyltransferase), gene expression is about fivefold greater in monkey kidney cells as compared with murine cells. The SV40 enhancer consists of tandemly repeated sequences that contain a number of functionally independent elements, that have distinct patterns of cell-type specificity, which can be mimicked by synthetic oligonucleotides corresponding to the nucleotide sequences of the individual elements.

Wild-type polyomavirus does not replicate in undifferentiated mouse embryonal carcinoma cells (ECs), and there is no early gene expression. Polyoma virus mutants that can infect EC cells have point mutations and duplications within the polyoma enhancer. Polyoma enhancer sequence alterations can alter enhancer-specific viral DNA replication in an organ-specific way and affect acute and persistent infections differently (438). It appears that certain types of EC cells make a negative regulatory factor that represses activity of the wild-type polyomavirus enhancer, but not that of the mutant enhancer. Aging and age-specific transcription factors also affect organ-specific transcription in polyoma virus–infected mice (562).

Another striking example of enhancer-related cell specificity occurs with JC papovavirus, the agent responsible for the neurologic illness progressive multifocal leukoencephalopathy (PML). When the JCV enhancer is coupled to the gene for CAT and this construct is tested for activity in human fetal glial cells and HeLa cells, the enhancer is active only in the glial cells (267). This corresponds well with the fact that, within the CNS, JCV productively infects only oligodendroglia.

Further information on the tissue specificity of papovavirus enhancers has come from studies using transgenic mice (50,474). The offspring of transgenic mice made with early region genes (promoter, enhancer, and T-antigen genes) from JCV develop a neurologic disorder characterized by tremor and seizures. Pathologically, they have abnormalities in CNS myelin due to dysfunction of the myelin-producing oligodendrocytes. Oligodendrocyte dysfunction correlates with the expression of JCV DNA and the presence of high levels of JCV-specified messenger RNA (mRNA) in these cells. It has been suggested that the cell specificity of JCV gene expression is due to the viral enhancer and that cell dysfunction itself is due to expression of virally encoded T antigen.

Transgenic mice made by using the early control region and early genes of SV40 virus often develop choroid plexus epithelial cell tumors. Deletion of the SV40 enhancer region from the microinjected DNA results in a dramatic decrease in the incidence of these tumors, suggesting that the enhancer region may play an important role in the choroid plexus specificity of tumor development, with large-T antigen expression accounting for tumor development (50,399,530). Further studies with polyoma virus indicated that enhancer requirements determine differences in cell-specific control of DNA replication in normal versus transformed pancreas cells (439).

Papillomaviruses also contain enhancers with both inducible and constitutive elements (178). In the case of human papillomavirus 11, the enhancer may play an important role in tissue tropism, as it can be shown that the enhancer is specifically active in keratinocytes (485). Replication and gene expression of papillomaviruses increase as skin cells differentiate from basal cells to mature keratinocytes (29).

The role of enhancer elements in tissue and disease specificity also has been investigated extensively with avian and murine retroviruses and HIV (see Chapters 27 and 28 for review and references). Enhancer elements within the long terminal repeats (LTRs) play a key role in the capacity of avian and murine retroviruses to produce both neoplastic and nonneoplastic diseases. For example, certain strains of avian leukosis virus induce lymphomas, whereas other strains produce osteopetrosis in avian hosts. The capacity of these viruses to produce these different disease patterns is determined by enhancer regions with the LTR region of the viral genome, although non-LTR gene sequences also may play a role. Enhancer regions also determine the disease specificity of murine leukemia viruses. After inoculation into mice, Friend murine leukemia virus (F-MuLV) produces erythroleukemia, and Moloney murine leukemia virus (M-MuLV) produces T-lineage lymphoid cell neoplasms (Chapter 27). When recombinant viruses are made containing the enhancer regions of either F-MuLV or M-MuLV, the pattern of disease production correlates with the enhancer type. Similarly, replacement of the M-MuLV enhancer sequences in the LTR with the enhancer sequences from SV40 results in loss of the capacity of recombinant viruses to produce T-cell lymphomas and the appearance instead of B-lineage lymphomas and acute myeloid leukemia in infected mice. Recombinant polyoma virus that has its B enhancer element replaced with the 72–base pair repeat enhancer from Moloney leukemia virus genome has strong specificity for the pancreas. The LTRs also appear to play a role in the induction of neurodegenerative disease by certain murine retroviruses (404). A variety of cellular factors regulate HIV gene expression and may influence viral load and disease progression (402). These findings indicate that tissue specificity can be achieved by elements within many viral genes.

Enhancer regions also are present in the genomes of herpesviruses (see Chapter 33 for references). EBV virus contains at least two relevant enhancer domains. The A domain is constitutively active in fibroblasts, epithelial cells, and certain myeloid lineage cells but not in B lymphocytes. The B domain is active in B lymphocytes but requires the presence of a viral transactivating factor for activity (Chapter 34).

Viral enhancers also have been found within the hepatitis B virus (HBV) genome (Chapter 35). Some HBV enhancer elements are more active in liver-derived cells (575) compared with nonhepatic cell lines. Transgenic mice injected with the entire HBV genome (15,61) also show a tissue-specific pattern of HBsAg expression, although antigen expression is not exclusively confined to liver tissue.

Site of Entry and Pathway of Spread

The tropism of a virus may depend on both its site of entry and pathway of spread in the infected host. This principle has clearly been illustrated for a number of neurotropic viruses. For example, in a series of classic studies, Howe and Bodian (234) inoculated the Rockefeller MV strain of type 2 poliovirus into rhesus monkeys via various routes and then studied the distribution of lesions within the CNS. Some areas of the brain, including the sensorimotor cortex and certain thalamic nuclei, were always infected regardless of the route of viral inoculation. Other areas, such as the hippocampus and striate cortex, were never involved. Finally, a number of areas were selectively involved only after viral inoculation via specific routes (e.g., the septal nuclei and olfactory bulbs after intranasal inoculation). Similar results have been obtained with a variety of viruses that depend exclusively on neural spread to travel from the site of inoculation to distant target tissues including VSV (453), HSV (8), herpes suis (332), and rabies (18) viruses (see section on neural spread).

The dependence of neural localization on the site of viral inoculation also is illustrated by the appearance of neurally spreading viruses such as herpes simplex, rabies, and reovirus T3D in the region of the spinal cord innervating the skin and muscles at the site of inoculation. The ultimate lesions depend on the neural pathways innervating the site of inoculation.

The effect of portal of entry on the ultimate tropism of viruses has not been extensively investigated for hematogenously spreading viruses. For polyomaviruses, the route of inoculation appears to determine the site of primary replication and the eventual site of persistent replication. The mechanism for this effect has not been clearly established, although the viral VP1 protein type appears to be involved in this effect (133).

For viruses whose ultimate tissue tropism depends on the generation of viremia, it is difficult to understand how route of entry should alter tropism unless inoculation at different sites results in differences in the magnitude or duration of viremia. An interesting and unexplained exception to this rule may be the "provoking effect" described in studies with poliomyelitis. It was shown that if intracardiac injection of poliovirus serotype 1 into a monkey was preceded by an intramuscular injection, paralysis tended to occur more frequently in the injected limb (hence the so-called provoking effect of trauma or intramuscular injection on the subsequent development of paralysis) (234). It was suggested that local trauma could selectively increase the permeability of blood vessels in the region of the spinal cord innervating the traumatized site. This in turn would allow blood-borne virus to localize specifically in that region of the spinal cord and produce preferential paralysis of the traumatized limb. Direct evidence for this sequence of events is lacking, and the mechanism of the provoking effect is still under study (194).

The provoking effect has been suggested as a possible mechanism to explain the high incidence of paralysis in the inoculated limb of individuals injected with incompletely inactivated lots of poliovirus vaccine (375). The provoking effect also has been suggested as a possible mechanism to explain reports of a higher than expected incidence of paralytic poliomyelitis associated with the oral polio vaccine when it was administered within 30 days of intramuscular inoculations (491). The provoking effect may represent an example of the dependence of the tropism of a hematogenously spreading virus on the site of viral inoculation. However, it remains unclear how intramuscularly inoculated poliovirus in humans reaches the CNS. If virus spreads from the site of inoculation to the CNS via nerves, a similar preferential distribution of paralysis also might be expected.

For some viruses, the pathway of spread may vary depending on the site of inoculation, and this difference may in turn influence tropism. This possibility is illustrated by studies in mice with the neurotropic NWS strain of influenza (431). After intraperitoneal inoculation, virus spreads through the bloodstream, and viral antigen is found in the meninges, choroid plexus, ependymal cells, and in perivascular locations in the brain parenchyma. After intranasal inoculation, virus spreads through nerves, and antigen is noted primarily in the olfactory bulbs, trigeminal ganglia, and brainstem. In this instance, the site of inoculation influences the mechanism of viral dissemination, which then determines the ultimate tissue tropism.

PATTERNS OF VIRAL INFECTION

As noted earlier, viral infection of a susceptible host can result in the production of acute infection that may be clinically symptomatic or asymptomatic. Clearance of initial acute infection may be permanent, or conversely, the host may develop periodic reactivations of infection with intervening disease- and symptom-free intervals. Viruses that produce recurrent infection, exemplified by the herpesviridae, have developed strategies for establishing, maintaining, and reactivating from the latent state (117). If the host fails to clear the initial acute infection, it may become chronic or persistent. In persistent active infections, virus is continuously present in infected tissues and may be continuously shed from the infected host. Selected examples of viruses known to cause persistent infections of humans and animals and their major sites of persistence within the host are shown in Tables 3 through 5. Viruses capable of producing persistent infections include both enveloped and

TABLE 3. *Viral strategies for evading the immune system*

Escape Mechanism	Selected Examples
Restricted gene expression (minimal or no expression of viral proteins)	HSV, VZV in latently infected neurons EBV in B cells HIV in resting T cells
Infection of "immunologically privileged sites," or sites not readily accessible to the immune system	HSV, VZV, measles persistence in neurons CMV, JC/BK virus in the kidney Papillomaviruses in the epidermis
Antigenic variation: Mutation of antigenic sites critical for Ab or T-cell recognition	Lentivirus escape variants HIV, EBV, HIV, LCMV T-cell escape variants HIV, HBV T-cell receptor antagonist variants
Interference with antigen processing/presentation	HSV ICP47, HCMV US6, Adeno E3-19K, proteins interfere with TAP HCMV pp65 inhibits processing of IE proteins EBV EBNA-1 inhibits proteosome-mediated processing HIV destruction of helper $CD4^+$ T cells
Altered MHC-I trafficking, expression	Adeno E3-19K, HCMV US3, MCMV m152 Retention of MHC-I in ER HCMV US2, 11 Reverse translocation of MHC-I from ER to cytoplasm HIV Vpu Degradation of MHC-I HIV Nef Accumulation of MHC-I in Golgi
Suppression of cell-surface molecules required for T-cell recognition of MHC class I	Adenovirus E3-19K; CMV US2,3,11; HIV Nef, Vpu; BPV E6, proteins
Viral molecules that inhibit cytokine function	Adenovirus E1A, HCMV block JAK/STAT signal transduction Adenovirus VA, EBV EBER, and HIV TAR RNAs that inhibit IFN function EBV BCRF1 (an IL-10 homolog) that inhibits IL-2, IFN synthesis, and TAP1 expression MCMV inhibits IFN-γ stimulated MHC-II expression
Immunologic tolerance	Clonal deletion/anergy of virus-specific CTLs in HBV carriers, absence of anti-HBsAg
Cell-to-cell spread by syncytia	SSPE (measles), HIV?

Abbreviations: CMV, cytomegalovirus; CNS, central nervous system; CTL, cytotoxic T cell; EBV, Epstein-Barr virus; HbsAg, hepatitis B virus surface antigen; HBV, hepatitis B virus; HIV, human immunodeficiency virus; HSV, herpes simplex virus; IFN, interferon; IL, interleukin; MHC, major histocompatibility complex; TAP, transporter of antigen processing; TNF, tumor necrosis factor; SSPE, subacute sclerosing panencephalitis; VZV, varicella-zoster virus. (Modified from ref. 3 with new information from refs. 54 and 348 and reproduced with permission.)

TABLE 4. *Selected examples representing major categories of persistent viral infections in humans*

Category	Status of Viral Genome	Virus–Cell Interaction	Antiviral Immune Response	Example
Latent	Latent, recurrent activation	Lytic, latent	Present, normal	HSV, VZV
"Tolerant"	Active replication (continuous high level)	Nonlytic	Impaired or absent (to some viral Ags)	HBV
"Breakthrough"	Active replication (continuous but low level)	Lytic, latent	Present (may be reduced or elevated)	SSPE, HIV

Abbreviations: Ags, antigens; HBV, hepatitis B virus; HIV, human immunodeficiency virus; HSV, herpes simplex virus; SSPE, subacute sclerosing panencephalitis; VZV, varicella-zoster virus.

nonenveloped viruses, viruses with DNA and RNA genomes, and members of many viral families.

Persistent Infections

Reduced CPE

For a virus to establish persistent infection [see (84) for review], it must be able to limit its cytolytic effects, maintain its genome within host cells over time, and avoid elimination by the host's immune system (3). It has recently been recognized that numerous viruses are able to induce apoptotic cell death in target cells (429). Conversely, many viruses have developed an extensive variety of strategies to limit or restrict apoptosis in target cells (176) (see also previous references). It has been suggested that inhibition of apoptosis may favor the development of persistent rather than lytic infection (302). Additional factors that may influence the balance between lytic and nonlytic infections include the state of cellular differentiation (301), or the specific type of cell involved. In the case of Sindbis virus, lytic infection occurs in neuroblastoma cells, but differentiation of these cells into mature neurons in the presence of nerve growth factor favors persistent infection. Conversely, CMV causes productive infection in differentiated teratocarcinoma cells, but restricted gene expression in their undifferentiated counterparts. Retinoic acid–induced differentiation of the undifferentiated cells results in a conversion from nonlytic to lytic CMV infection. In a more biologically relevant system, CMV tends to produce nonproductive infection with restricted gene expression in monocytes, but productive infection results when these cells are induced to differentiate into macrophages (504). Like CMV, LDEV also fails to induce permission infection in macrophage precursors, but does so in differentiated cells.

Some viruses, for example, arenaviruses, have evolved to induce predominantly nonlytic infections in their natural hosts (117). For viruses that are normally lytic, persistent infection generally requires restriction of viral gene expression or the generation of attenuated viral variants. For many viruses, the appearance of persistent infection is associated with the generation of defective interfering (DI) particles that are subgenomic deletion mutants lacking one or more components of the wild-type viral genome. These mutant viruses may be unable to generate productive infection, or may act by modulating infection of associated wild-type virus. Viral gene mutations involved in the establishment and maintenance of persistent infection have been studied in reoviruses.

TABLE 5. *Antiviral B-cell and T-cell immune responses*

Recognition System	Target Molecule	Mechanism of Viral Control
Antibody (B-cell product)	Surface glycoproteins Outer capsid proteins Viral glycoproteins expressed on infected cell membranes	Neutralization Opsonization of virus particles ADCC, ACMC Down-regulation of intracellular viral gene expression
$CD4^+$ T cells	Viral peptides presented by MHC class II (10–20 mer peptides derived from exogenous proteins)	Release of antiviral cytokines Activation/recruitment of Mϕ Help for Ab production Help for $CD8^+$ CTL responses Killing of virus-infected cells
$CD8^+$ T cells	Viral peptides presented by MHC class I (8–10 mer proteins derived from endogenous proteins)	Killing of virus-infected cells Release of antiviral cytokines Activation/recruitment of Mϕ

Abbreviations: Ab, antibody; ACMC, antibody-dependent complement-mediated cytotoxicity; ADCC, antibody-dependent cell-mediated cytotoxicity; CTL, cytotoxic T cell; Mϕ, macrophage; MHC, major histocompatibility complex.

(Modified from ref. 3 and reproduced with permission.)

Mutations in the S1 and S4 genes, which encode the virus-attachment protein and a major surface protein, result in alterations in early stages of viral replication and in viral effects on host cell macromolecular synthesis that favor the establishment and maintenance of persistent infection (550). Similarly, coronaviruses, which produce persistent infections in cell culture, frequently contain mutations within the S glycoprotein and show delayed cell penetration (180), and mutations in the Sindbis virus envelope glycoproteins reduce the virus' capacity to induce lytic neuronal infection (301).

In cell culture, persistent infections result from a dynamic interplay between mutations in the infecting virus and alterations in the target cell, as has been reported for reoviruses, coronaviruses, and picornaviruses and parvoviruses (120). This coevolution of cells persistently infected with viruses has been associated with alterations in the expression of cell-surface receptors, or changes in intracellular vesicles.

It has been suggested that a critical factor in the restriction of viral cytolytic effects may be infection of target cells that are only semipermissive. This type of restricted gene expression is characteristic of latent HSV infection of sensory neurons, EBV infection of B cells, and papillomavirus infection of basal skin cells (3). It is important to recognize that noncytolytic persistent infections may be associated with loss of a variety of physiologic cell functions including hormone, cytokine, or neurotransmitter synthesis that may have deleterious effects on the host, even though the infected cells appear anatomically normal (117).

Obviously persistence requires that the viral genome be maintained in infected cells. This is not an issue in nondividing cells, such as mature neurons. Persistent infection of dividing cells requires replication of the viral genome during cell division. Retroviruses, such as HIV (see later), and dependoviruses like AAV (106) integrate their genome directly into the host chromosome, so that each cycle of cell replication also replicates the viral genome. Some viruses, including the herpesviruses HSV and EBV and some papovaviruses, maintain their genome as a circular extrachromosomal "episome" that is readily maintained during latent infection (4).

Evasion of the Immune Response

In addition to developing strategies for avoiding induction of cytolysis, and maintaining their genomes, viruses that persist must also evade host immune responses. The interaction between viruses and the immune system is discussed in detail in Chapter 11, and has been comprehensively reviewed elsewhere (84), but some of the basic strategies used by viruses to avoid host immunity are described later (see Table 4).

Obviously one of the most effective strategies to avoid host immunity is to induce a state of virus-specific immune suppression within the host, by infecting T or B cells and inhibiting their function, by inducing tolerance by deleting virus-specific T cells within the thymus or peripheral lymphoid organs, or by destroying antigen-presenting cells. These mechanisms are discussed in detail in Chapter 11 [see also (84)] and are not considered further. Viruses also have developed specific strategies to evade host cell immunity. Among the more important of these are restricted expression of viral genes and proteins in infected cells, infection of immunoprivileged sites in the host, interference with the effector arm of cellular immunity through down-regulation of MHC molecules or cell-adhesion molecules, interference with antigen processing and presentation, inhibition of cytokine activity, antigenic variation and the development of escape mutants, and spread through syncytial fusion (3).

Latency

Perhaps the best-studied example of limited gene and protein expression is that of HSV (see later). During latent infection, the only viral transcripts that are detected are the latency-associated transcripts (LATs), and no proteins are expressed. Similarly, latent EBV infection is associated only with expression of the EBNA-1 protein. In less dramatic fashion, many viruses appear to show decreased expression of their glycoproteins in persistently infected cells (394).

Privileged Sites

Persistent infection of immunologically privileged sites is perhaps best exemplified by viral infections of the brain, testes, and parts of the eye (488). In the case of the CNS, this may have to do with the specialized nature of the lymphocyte surveillance and trafficking system within the CNS (549). In addition, the absence or markedly reduced expression and induction of MHC molecules on neurons hampers their capacity to serve as effective targets in cytotoxic T lymphocyte (CTL) responses (232,423). In other tissues, including the eye, testes, and possibly CNS, immune privilege also may be maintained in part by the apoptosis of infiltrating activated lymphocytes bearing Fas (CD95) receptor that interact with resident cells bearing Fas ligand on their surface (365,437). In experimental HSV infection, Fas-triggered apoptosis of antiviral lymphocytes may contribute to immune evasion and persistence of HSV (422). The kidney, although not classically considered an immunologically privileged site, is frequently involved in persistent infections (3). This may reflect the fact that although lymphocytes traffic through the kidney, they may have only limited access to epithelial cells because of the presence of a dense basement membrane (9). In some immunologically privileged sites, MHC class I expression may be low or absent, and low levels of transporter proteins may be necessary for antigen processing (see later) (254).

Escape Mutants

Viruses, especially those with RNA genomes, generate mutations resulting in the creation of viral variants with high frequency (225); the potential biologic significance of these viral "quasispecies" is unclear (see 126). Certain quasispecies may replicate better in specific types of cells, as has been shown for LCMV quasispecies in neurons (126). These variants might also facilitate development of persistent infection by avoiding either antibody neutralization (antibody-resistant variants) or by escaping from T-cell recognition (reviewed in 392). The appearance of antibody-resistant variants also is a characteristic of many lentivirus infections including those caused by equine infectious anemia virus, visna virus, caprine arthritis encephalitis virus, and both SIV and HIV. Although the appearance of these variants was once considered a key feature in the pathogenesis of persistent infections, more recent studies suggest they are not in fact essential to the generation of disease (84,317) (see Chapter 61 of *Fields Virology*, 4th ed.).

Just as viruses can escape recognition by the humoral immune system, they can also escape T-cell recognition (392). CTL escape mutants have now been identified in a wide variety of viral systems including arenaviruses (LCMV), herpesviruses (EBV), retroviruses (HIV and SIV), and reoviruses (281). The significance of these viruses in the generation of persistent infections, like that of antibody-escape variants, is difficult to establish. At least in the case of SIV and HIV, these mutants do not appear essential for viral persistence, nor do they typically become the predominant viral species in infected hosts (82).

As noted, one strategy for viruses to evade host antiviral CTLs is to develop mutations within regions of their proteins (epitopes) recognized by virus-specific CTLs (CTL escape mutants) in the context of MHC and the T-cell receptor (TCR). In some cases, viral mutants are still recognized by the TCR, but fail to induce a stimulatory signal, and instead inhibit T-cell responses and induce T-cell anergy (TCR antagonism) (36). HIV variants of this type have been identified with mutations within the gag protein (275).

Decrease in Expression of MHC Molecules

In addition to anergy induced by TCR antagonism, suppression of virus-specific host T-cell responses can result from down-regulation of cell-surface MHC class I (for $CD8^+$ cells) or class II (for $CD4^+$ cells) molecules or other cell-surface molecules essential for efficient induction of T-cell responses including integrins and adhesion molecules (434).

In the MHC class I pathway, viral proteins synthesized within infected target cells are ubiquitinated and then processed within 26S proteosomes into peptide fragments, which are transported to the endoplasmic reticulum (ER) in association with transporter associated with antigen processing (TAP) proteins. These transporter proteins are encoded by two genes (TAP1, TAP2) within the MHC, and have homologies to the adenosine triphosphate (ATP)-binding family of transmembrane transporter proteins. Deficiency of TAP proteins results in a failure to load peptides onto class I MHC molecules and a resultant defect in MHC class I restricted antigen presentation. Once inside the ER, peptide antigens bind to the MHC molecules and the antigen/MHC I complex is then exported through the Golgi and trans-Golgi apparatus to reach the cell surface (162).

In the MHC class II pathway, extracellular soluble viral proteins are taken up by endocytosis and processed within endosomes into peptide fragments. Endosomes containing these peptide antigen fragments fuse with vacuoles containing newly synthesized MHC class II molecules derived via the Golgi and trans-Golgi apparatus from the ER. These antigen/class II complexes are then transported to the cell surface.

Viruses known to down-regulate MHC class I include HSV, CMV (murine and human), EBV, measles, retroviruses including HIV, and adenoviruses (434). A variety of mechanisms, affecting virtually all steps in the MHC class I processing pathway, have been implicated.

Viral proteins, exemplified by EBV EBNA-1, can inhibit ubiquitin-proteosomal protein processing of antigens (303). Similarly, a CMV matrix protein with kinase activity appears to modify other viral proteins in a way that limits their proteolytic processing (175). Viruses also can interfere with the processing and export of the MHC class I molecules. In the case of adenoviruses, the adenovirus E3/19K protein localizes to the ER, where it binds directly with MHC class I molecules and inhibits their terminal glycosylation and processing and blocks their transport out of the ER, so that class I/peptide complexes never reach the surface of infected cells.

Cells infected with human CMV show rapid degradation of the MHC class I molecular complex. Deletion of a viral fragment that encompasses eight genes in the unique short region of the CMV genome abrogates the effects of CMV on MHC expression. These genes appear to encode proteins that act to inhibit the intracellular transport of MHC complex molecules, promoting their retention in the ER and Golgi apparatus and subsequent degradation (162). CMV also encodes a homolog (UL18) of the MHC class I heavy (H) chain protein (146). This protein associates directly with β_2-microglobulin, and was originally postulated to decrease MHC class I expression in CMV-infected cells. More recent studies suggested that this protein may actually result in the appearance of a "decoy" MHC molecule on the cell surface that does not activate CTLs, but does decrease the likelihood that NK cells will recognize the infected cell (119,146,149,162,286,413).

The HSV protein ICP47 binds directly to the TAP molecule within infected cells and prevents the translocation of processed antigen peptides to the ER (213). Down-regulation of TAP also has been seen in cells infected with adenovirus 12 (449). Another strategy is exemplified by HIV, in which the viral tat protein has been shown to decrease MHC class I mRNA transcription. Another HIV protein, Nef, causes down-regulation of MHC class I expression in infected cells by causing the accumulation MHC class I molecules in the Golgi apparatus and then subsequently in clathrin-coated vesicles, where they undergo degradation (298).

Down-regulation of MHC class II has been described after infection with CMV, coronaviruses (JHM), measles, and retroviruses including HIV (434). Down-regulation of MHC class II molecules may involve either the reduction of MHC class II expression or interference with the induction of increased cell-surface expression of class II that usually accompanies virus-induced production of γ-IFN and other cytokines (40). Some viruses encode soluble homologs of cytokine receptors including TNF-R (e.g., poxviruses), or encode cytokine homologs such as IL-10. In both instances, the action of antiviral cytokines such as IL-2 and γ-IFN is inhibited (e.g., EBV) (475). Myxomaviruses encode a secretory protein that binds to γ-IFN and prevents its interaction with its cell-surface receptor. Vaccinia, reovirus, adenovirus, and HIV all encode proteins with double-stranded (ds)-RNA binding activity. These proteins effectively "trap" dsRNA molecules and prevent them from acting to stimulate γ-IFN induction in infected cells (182).

Latency: The HSV Example

An exhaustive discussion of the mechanisms by which viruses establish, maintain, and reactivate from latency is beyond the scope of this chapter. However, the basic principles are well illustrated by HSV latency (537) and HIV latency and persistence (see later).

Primary infection with HSV-1 typically involves epithelial cells of the oropharyngeal mucosa producing gingivostomatitis. Productive infection of epithelial cells at the primary site involves the orderly transcription of α (immediate early), β (early), and γ (late) genes and their cognate proteins. Replication of the viral DNA and structural proteins is then followed by assembly of progeny virions. Progeny virions and/or their nucleocapsids bind to and enter the distal terminals of sensory neurons innervating the oropharynx, and spread through retrograde axonal transport to reach the perikarya of these neurons within the trigeminal ganglion. A similar sequence of events occurs after primary HSV-2 infection of the epithelial cells of the mucosa of the genital tract, with virus spreading to reach sacral dorsal root ganglia.

Once virus reaches the sensory ganglia, it may either produce acute infection with subsequent neuronal cell death or become latent. Acute infection is associated with virus that is easily detectable on direct culture of infected tissue. By contrast, during latent infection, no infectious virus is detectable on direct tissue culture, but virus can be detected when tissues are cocultivated with permissive cells. During the latent state, there is restricted gene expression limited essentially to the production of what are referred to as LATs (43), and minimal or absent expression of any viral proteins. Viral DNA is maintained as a nonreplicating circular episome (340), and probably occurs as between 10 and 1,000 viral genomes per latently infected neuron (212). It has been calculated that 10% or fewer neurons are latently infected (189), although some estimates are substantially higher (424).

The mechanism of reactivation of latent HSV is poorly understood. Reactivation is associated with neuronal injury, stress, fatigue, hormonal changes such as those occurring during menses or lactation, immunosuppression, malnutrition, and exposure to ultraviolet light. Recurrences may be clinical or subclinical, and can occur as frequently as monthly (31). It is presumed that these events trigger the activation of as yet unidentified signal-transduction transcription and kinase pathways within neurons. Reactivation results in initiation of gene transcription and translation, assembly of progeny virions, and their transport through anterograde axonal transport back to mucosal surfaces where active infection results in herpes labialis (cold sores, fever blisters) or herpes genitalis (genital herpes). Under unusual circumstances, reactivated virus may spread to nonmucosal sites including the meninges (herpes meningitis), CNS (herpes encephalitis, myelitis), or eye (herpes keratitis).

The mechanisms responsible for establishment of HSV latency are not yet completely understood. It is possible that special characteristics of neuronal cells, as compared with their epithelial counterparts, may be necessary for HSV to establish latency (280). The key determinant may be the quantity of immediate early and early proteins present within particular neurons. If sufficient quantities of viral α gene products are present, then neurons undergo lytic infection, whereas if only low levels are present, virus becomes latent. This suggests that restriction of HSV α gene transcription within sensory neurons may be a critical determinant in initiating latency (487). This restriction in turn may result from the presence of cellular inhibitors of HSV gene transcription such as the octamer binding proteins Oct-1 and Oct-2 (266), or the absence of cellular transcription factors required for HSV gene transcription (233). In an alternative model, HSV-encoded proteins such as ICP4, 8, or 27 have been suggested to serve as negative regulators of HSV α gene expression in infected neurons (see Chapter 33 for review of HSV replication).

The commitment by virus to latent neuronal infection, as opposed to productive infection (328), appears to occur at an early stage in the virus replication cycle, and does not require an initial cycle of completed viral replication (464). No specific viral product absolutely required for HSV to establish latency has been identified. Viruses lacking functional thymidine kinase, immediate early regulatory genes, and even LATs can all establish latent infection (see Chapter 33), although LAT mutants may be less efficient at establishing latency than are their wild-type counterparts (458).

During latency, no infectious virus can be detected in sensory ganglia by direct culture. Viral DNA is present in a nucleosome-associated circular episomal state (440), and can be detected in infected cells by *in situ* hybridization and polymerase chain reaction (PCR) (264). Neurons are postmitotic cells, and therefore maintenance of latent episomal HSV DNA does not require ongoing DNA replication. Maintenance of the latent state is associated with gene expression limited to the LAT transcripts (43). No protein products of LATs or other HSV genes are detectable in latently infected neurons.

Stimuli that induce reactivation of HSV from latency are well documented, but the mechanism has defied analysis (537). It has been suggested that an early event may be stimulus-induced expression of ICP0, which in turn may lead to a cascade of events starting with the expression of other α gene products including ICP4 and ICP27 (300). ICP0-minus HSV mutants can still reactivate from the latent state, but appear to do so with markedly reduced efficiency compared with their wild-type counterparts (300). LAT-minus mutants also show a similar reduction in efficiency and frequency of reactivation, suggesting a possible role for LATs in this process (515). It appears that frequent reactivation from latency in sensory ganglia can occur without inducing significant neuronal cell loss (105), suggesting that HSV must also have a mechanism for limiting neuronal cell death during reactivation. It is possible that the ICP34.5 protein, which has antiapoptotic activity (89), plays a role in this process.

Persistence: The HIV Example

Another example of persistent infection is provided by HIV (337). In HIV infection, unlike latent HSV infection, high levels of virus are continuously being produced in the infected host. Estimates suggest that patients with advanced AIDS may produce more than 10^7 virions/day (219). The major source of new virus appears to be recently infected cells, rather than chronically infected cells or latently infected cells undergoing reactivation (93). Initial exposure to HIV frequently causes an acute viral syndrome with high levels of HIV cell-free and cell-associated viremia. These levels subsequently decline by 100- to 1,000-fold, but the virus does not disappear, and patients enter a clinically asymptomatic stage of infection (410). During this phase, high levels of virus are detectable in lymphoid organs and extralymphatic follicular dendritic cells, even when plasma viremia is of only modest proportions (139,401).

Although HIV induces a persistent infection associated with continuous production of new virus, latently infected $CD4^+$ lymphocytes also can be detected. After infection of target cells, HIV preintegration complex is transported through nucleopores into the cell nucleus. In nondividing (G_0 phase) T lymphocytes, HIV does not undergo proviral integration, but remains as a nonintegrated extrachromosomal replicative intermediate. In this state of "preintegration" latency, the genome is vulnerable to degradation, and is often rapidly lost from infected cells (337). More commonly, proviral integration occurs, and may then lead to a latent state without production of progeny virions, which has been referred to as "postintegration latency" to distinguish it from preintegration latency (337). After initial inoculation of HIV at skin or mucosal surfaces, the associated local activation of $CD4^+$ T cells, facilitated by their interaction with local skin and mucosal dendritic cells, enhances the likelihood of integration of proviral DNA (416). Stimulation of T cells harboring integrated provirus—by antigen, cytokines, phorbol esters, and other activators of transcription—may then result in active viral production (187). The *nef* gene and its product may play a role in regulating this process, as patients with HIV isolates containing mutations within this gene appear to have markedly reduced levels of productive infection from latently integrated genomes (273).

It has been suggested that there are three distinct broad populations of infected T lymphocytes in lymphoid organs of HIV-infected hosts (337). One population encompasses cells that are actively producing virus, and the other two populations include latently infected cells harboring integrated proviral genomes. Of this latter group, one population includes cells harboring "defective" proviral genomes that appear to be blocked in their capacity to produce virions, and another population carries latent proviral genomes that can produce progeny virions. The body load of HIV presumably reflects a balance between the number of actively infected cells and the rate at which virus spreads to uninfected cells, counterbalanced by the host's ability to destroy productively infected cells. The reservoir of latently infected cells probably plays a minor role except under special circumstances, such as treatment with antiviral drugs. Studies suggested that differences in these various parameters may be one factor accounting for differences in disease progression among infected individuals (67). Based on mRNA expression and RNA-splicing pattern in infected cells, it appears that the proportion of latently infected—as opposed to productively infected—cells declines with advancing disease (346). These shifts from latent to productive infection may reflect factors that trigger proliferation of latently infected cells such as cytokine exposure

(414), or may even result from direct transactivation of the latent HIV genome by co-infection of latently infected cells by opportunistic pathogens (262).

TRANSMISSION OF VIRAL INFECTIONS

After infecting a susceptible host, the virus is shed into the environment, where it encounters a new susceptible host and the infectious cycle begins anew. Many of the basic issues and concepts in the transmission of viral infection are reviewed in Chapter 14 of *Fields Virology*, 4th ed. and are only briefly covered here. Virus transmission typically begins with dissemination from the infected host through respiratory, enteric, or genitourinary secretions. However, there are a number of important exceptions to this general pattern. Arbovirus infections typically involve the ingestion by an arthropod vector of a blood meal from a viremic host, and transmission occurs when the vector feeds on another susceptible host. The transmitting fluid, blood, is never really "shed" from the body. A similar pattern of transmission can occur when contaminated tissues or blood products are removed from an infected individual and transplanted, transfused, or inoculated into a susceptible host. This pattern is exemplified in the transmission of HIV and hepatitis B virus infection by blood, blood products, or between drug addicts sharing blood-contaminated needles. It is important to recognize that both patients and physicians are at risk for viral transmission resulting from needlestick exposure and surgical procedures (314).

A number of factors influence the subsequent likelihood of blood-borne transmission of viral infection. These include the titer of virus in the blood, the duration of the viremic state, the amount of material transmitted, and the route of transmission. Before the advent of adequate tests for screening donated blood, HBV infection was a serious potential complication of transfusion. This reflected the incidence of infection in certain populations (e.g., professional blood donors), the frequency of a chronic carrier state with persisting viremia, and high virus titer (up to 10^7 infectious doses of virus per milliliter) (22). By contrast, posttransfusion infection with hepatitis A virus is an extremely rare event, due to the short duration of viremia and the low virus titer in the blood (226).

Skin

Viral infection of the skin is a hallmark of many types of viral infection including those produced by measles, rubella, certain enteroviruses, herpes simplex, varicella-zoster, various poxviruses, and the HPVs (350). In many of these cases, even though infectious virus can be demonstrated in skin lesions, this does not appear to be a significant source of viral transmission. Exceptions to this rule include the spread of genital herpes simplex and occasionally herpes labialis from infected skin lesions (114), rare cases of chickenpox contacted after exposure to shingles, and the mechanical transmission of HPVs. In the case of certain poxviruses and papillomaviruses of animals, skin lesions provide a source of virus that can infect biting arthropods, which in turn transmit the virus to new hosts (553). Smallpox virus remained infectious in dried skin crusts for extensive periods, and fomites provided an important route of transmission for this disease before its eradication.

Respiratory Tract

Viral transmission from the upper and lower respiratory tracts depends on aerosols generated during coughing or sneezing, or in infected saliva. Some of the factors that influence the stability of viruses in aerosols are reviewed in the section dealing with viral entry. Transmission via infected secretions, which can contain large amounts of infectious virus (400), is important in the genesis of upper respiratory infections, as well as a number of systemic viral infections (e.g., measles, varicella) that enter the host via the respiratory route.

Viruses isolated from saliva include rabies (18,109, 152), EBV (315), CMV (316), HIV, and HTLV (2), human herpesviruses 6, 7, and 8 (316), and hepatitis viruses (86). Rabies is the most widely recognized example of salivary transmission of virus (18). Inoculation of infected saliva through the bite of a rabid animal appears to be the predominant mode of rabies viral entry (109). Infected saliva plays an important role in the transmission of EBV, either through intimate oral contact or possibly by salivary residues left on cups, food, toys, or other objects. Mumps virus is shed in the saliva and can be transmitted after nasal or buccal mucosal inoculation of virus.

Salivary excretion of CMV can frequently be demonstrated, but the importance of oral secretions in disease transmission remains unknown. Hepatitis B, C, and G have all been isolated from saliva, but experimental transmission studies with HBV-infected saliva have demonstrated transmission of hepatitis only after saliva is parenterally inoculated, suggesting that transmission via this route is unusual (321). Saliva has also been shown to contain HIV and HTLV, but salivary secretions have never been shown to play a significant role in viral transmission. Certain murine retroviruses can be isolated from saliva, which may play a role in male-to-male viral transmission when infected saliva is parenterally inoculated during fighting (417).

Enteric Tract

Many viruses are shed in feces. This route of transmission is central to the pathogenesis of enterovirus infection (e.g., polio) (234) and also occurs with rotavirus (433) and hepatitis A virus (577). Enteroviral excretion in feces is prolonged, magnifying the opportunity for person-to-person spread. Transmission to susceptible hosts typically occurs by way of fecal–oral transmission, which is particularly common among young children or institutionalized patients. Colonoscopy also has been implicated as a unusual potential source for transmitting hepatitis C virus between patients (55). Infected stool also can contaminate water supplies when sewage and waste-disposal conditions are substandard. Some viruses, such as HIV (528), that can be detected in feces are not readily transmitted by the enteric route.

Urine

A number of viruses including CMV, hepatitis A, HBV, mumps, polyomaviruses, and HIV have been isolated from urine (11), but are not thought to be transmitted by this fomite. However, urinary excretion is central to zoonotic transmission of many arenaviruses and hantaviruses via human exposure to aerosolized urine-contaminated material.

Sexual Transmission

Sexual transmission plays a critical role in the spread of HIV, HSV, papillomaviruses, and hepatitis B and C viruses (239). Viral infection of semen occurs with HIV (63), herpesviruses including HSV (540), CMV (326), and HHV 8 (44), HPVs (292), and HBV (463). In the case of CMV, virus can be detected in about 5% of cryopreserved semen samples collected for donor insemination (326), although this may not be representative of the prevalence of this virus in the population at large. HSV has been detected in about 3% of semen samples from men with a history of genital herpes, and probably occurs in even higher frequency at the time of clinical reactivation (539).

HIV-infected semen appears to be important in disease transmission. HIV has been found both in cell-free seminal fluid and as cell-associated virus (63) in 85% of HIV^+ men (135). In up to 35% of HIV infections, viral titers in semen are equal to or exceed those found in blood plasma (135). The genotype of HIV found in semen may be genetically distinct from that HIV strains found in blood, suggesting that in some instances, semen and blood compartments are distinct (63,104). HIV-1 can be detected in semen of HIV^+ men who received highly active antiretroviral therapy (HAART), even at times when plasma HIV is undetectable (579), showing that the genital compartment may harbor residual virus. Male-to-female heterosexual transmission of HIV-1 is facilitated by breaks in the cervical, vaginal, or urethral epithelium often associated with sexually transmitted disease, although infection of intact epithelial cells also may occur. Cases of HIV infection related to insemination of women with HIV^+ donor sperm also have been reported (568). Many aspects of HIV transmission parallel events described for the horizontal transmission of murine retroviruses (304).

Several viruses, including HIV and HSV, also have been isolated from the genital secretions and cervix of infected women (415,535,539,563). Infected secretions play a role in female-to-male heterosexual transmission of HIV infection as well as in perinatal vertical transmission from pregnant infected mothers to their neonates (10). Virus shed in vaginal secretions also may play a role in the perinatal transmission of papillomaviruses (505).

Milk

Several viruses, including CMV (201), mumps, rubella, HIV and other retroviruses (478), human herpesviruses (164), hepatitis C (289), certain flaviviruses, and minute virus of mice (MVM), have been isolated from human or animal milk or colostrum. Infected breast milk provides a source of transmission of CMV from mother to child during the perinatal period. In one study (534), it was estimated that up to 85% of CMV-seropositive mothers excrete CMV in breast milk. Nearly 60% of preterm infants born to these mothers will develop CMV infection. Infection of preterm infants born to CMV-seropositive mothers was significantly lower if these infants were not breast fed, indicating that this is an important mode for viral transmission. Hepatitis B and C viruses also can be transmitted from mother to child during the perinatal period. Although this type of transmission is well documented, and virus can be found in the milk of infected mothers, it is unclear what role infected milk plays in disease transmission. In the case of hepatitis C, it appears that the risk of maternal–infant transmission occurs predominantly with symptomatic HCV-infected mothers who breast feed their infants as compared with breast-feeding mothers who were asymptomatic carriers (289). This may reflect the fact that symptomatic mothers had dramatically higher viral loads than did their symptomatic counterparts (289). Maternal milk also has been implicated in the vertical transmission of visna maedi and may play a role in human transmission of HTLV-I.

HIV RNA is detectable by quantitative competitive reverse transcription–PCR (RT-PCR) in the milk of 40% of HIV-1–seropositive women (306). Virus may be either cell-free (306) or present in the T cells and macrophages found in colostrum and milk (478). Recent data showed that 5% to 20% of infants born to HIV-infected mothers may be infected by breast feeding, with transmission occurring up to age 18 months (478). Although mumps virus can be found in human milk, and rare cases of perinatal mumps infection occur (255), infected milk is not important in viral transmission.

Maternal–Child Transmission

Maternal–child transmission can result from intrauterine infection, infection during delivery from virus present in the maternal birth canal, of from neonatal exposure to infected breast milk. Maternal–child transmission of infection has been documented for a number of viral infections (324) as exemplified by HIV, hepatitis B and C, CMV, HSV, human herpesviruses (472), HPVs (505), varicella, measles, mumps, rubella, and human parvoviruses (B19) (279). In the case of HPV, the vertical transmission rate from infected mothers to their infants born vaginally may be as high as 30% (505). Premature rupture of membranes appears to be an important risk factor, with increasing rates of maternal–child transmission being directly correlated with the time elapsing between rupture of membranes and delivery (505). The risk of transmission of parvovirus B19 infection has been estimated to be as high as 50%, but is fortunately only rarely associated with symptomatic disease (279). The risk of transmission for hepatitis C appears significantly lower (2–11%), but may be increased in mothers with associated HIV infection, HCV viremia, and elevated liver-function tests (185).

Perhaps the most extensively studied example of maternal–child viral transmission is that of HIV infection. The risk of transmission of HIV infection from an infected mother to her child appears to be directly proportional to maternal HIV-1 viral load (102,167,353). The risk may be as small as 5% or less in mothers with fewer than 1,000 copies/mL and can reach 40% or higher in those with more than 100,000 copies/mL (102). In another study, the HIV viral load was found to be more than 65,000 copies/mL in mothers who transmitted infection to their children, as compared with 5,139 copies/mL in nontransmitters (412), again indicating a general correlation between the degree of maternal viremia and the risk of transmission. It has been suggested that for each 10-fold increase in maternal HIV RNA level, there is an approximately twofold increased risk of maternal–child transmission (265). Premature delivery, prolonged duration between premature rupture of membranes and delivery, and the presence of genital warts have all been reported to increase the risk of intrapartum transmission of HIV infection (288).

The mechanism by which HIV infection is transmitted transplacentally may involve the presence of maternal chorioamnionitis (529). Infection of placental chorionic villi has been documented in HIV infection (344), although only a subset of the HIV quasispecies found in maternal blood are detectable in chorionic villi (344). This suggests that the capacity of certain HIV strains to infect the placenta may be an important factor in maternal–child transmission. Interestingly, certain HIV-1 p17 matrix protein amino acid sequence motifs appear to be found in nontransmitting HIV isolates as compared with those associated with maternal–child transmission. For example, the p17 matrix protein amino acid sequence K_{103} $IEEQN_{109}$ was found in all HIV B subtype isolates from mothers who had transmitted infection to children, whereas nine of 17 nontransmitting mothers had a $valine_{104}$ in place of the $isoleucine_{104}$ (373).

Organ Transplantation

Organ transplantation has provided an entirely novel method for iatrogenic transmission of viral infections. A full discussion of this subject is beyond the scope of this chapter (192). Transplanted bone marrow, kidneys, livers, and hearts have provided the source for infection with CMV (215), EBV and other herpesviruses (192), and retroviruses including HIV and HTLV-I (409). In one case, HTLV-I–associated myelopathy was attributed to acquisition of infection during cardiac transplantation (184). There also are reports of rabies and hepatitis B transmission resulting from corneal transplantation (222). Increasing use of animal-derived tissues for transplantation (xenotransplantation) has raised fears that these tissues may be the source for transmission of infectious agents (80), although no viral infections have yet been reported.

Little is known about the role played by specific viral genes and the proteins they encode in determining the transmissibility of viral infections (268) (see earlier discussion of maternal–child transmission of HIV). In the case of reoviruses, the capacity of certain strains of virus to spread from an infected mouse to its uninfected littermates is related to both the magnitude of viral growth in intestinal tissues and the amount of virus shed in the stool (268). Studies with reassortant viruses derived from low- and high-transmission reovirus strains indicated that the viral L2 gene, which encodes the core spike protein λ2, is the major determinant of transmission (268). Because this gene also is a major determinant of the capacity of reoviruses to grow in intestinal tissue after peroral inoculation (Chapter 53 of *Fields Virology*, 4th ed.), it may facilitate transmission by increasing viral growth and shedding.

Studies also have been made of the aerosol transmission of influenza virus between mice (462). Although a highly transmissible influenza strain (Jap/305) and a poorly transmissible one (Ao/NWS) grow to equivalent titer in the lungs, the amount of Jap/305 is considerably higher in bronchial secretions and in exhaled air. It was suggested that the neuraminidase protein might account for differences in the amount of virus released from respiratory epithelial cells into bronchial secretions and expelled air, although direct evidence is lacking.

HOST FACTORS

The outcome of viral infection of a particular host depends not only on viral factors but also on a variety of host factors. The role played by host factors in infection has been comprehensively reviewed (553), and interested readers are referred to these sources for more detailed information. The impact of host variation on the epidemiology of viral infection also is discussed in Chapter 14 of *Fields Virology*, 4th ed.

Experience with human infections has repeatedly shown that when a large population is exposed to the same viral pathogen, such as occurs, for example, during epidemics of encephalitis, the result is a range of outcomes varying from asymptomatic infection to significant and even fatal disease. The same pattern has been reproduced in inadvertent natural experiments such as the inoculation of HBV-contaminated lots of yellow fever virus vaccine into 45,000 military personnel (459). Clinical hepatitis occurred in only 2% of those vaccinated (914 cases), and of this group, only a small minority (4%) developed severe disease. The variation in outcomes appears to have been due to differences in host susceptibility, because the amount of HBV inoculated can be presumed to have been fairly uniform among those vaccinated.

In 1955 nearly 120,000 grade-school children were vaccinated with improperly inactivated lots of poliovirus type 1 prepared by Cutter Laboratories (375) ("Cutter incident"). It was subsequently estimated that about 50% of those vaccinated were susceptible to infection (the remainder had preexisting antibody), and of this group, at least 10% to 25% became infected (as estimated by the presence of minor illness or fecal excretion of virus). However, only 60 cases of paralytic poliomyelitis were ultimately documented among those vaccinated. Thus the Cutter incident again emphasizes the fact that when a large population of individuals is inoculated with approximately similar doses of virus, there is a wide range of possible outcomes that presumably depend on a variety of factors specific to the host.

The importance of host factors in determining the outcome of viral infection has been repeatedly demonstrated in animal models (51). Classic studies with VSV infection of mice clearly illustrated the importance of host factors including immune status, genetic background, age, and nutrition in determining the outcome of infection (453). The role of the host immune response and mediators such as cytokines in influencing viral infection are discussed separately (see Chapters 11 and 12).

Genetic Determinants

The genetic constitution of the host is undoubtedly one of the most important factors influencing the outcome of viral infection, and has been extensively investigated using inbred strains of mice (20). It was recognized as early as 1937, by Webster (545), that it was possible to breed selectively strains of mice that differed in their resistance to flaviviruses, including St. Louis encephalitis virus and louping ill. This observation was later extended to a number of other flaviviruses (115) including yellow fever virus and West Nile virus (195). In general, susceptibility correlated with increased levels of viral replication in tissues. In some cases resistant mice appeared to be more susceptible to the antiviral action of IFN (204), although at least one resistance gene (Flv^r) confers flavivirus-specific resistance by an IFN-independent mechanism (52).

Since the early studies with flaviviruses, genetic factors influencing susceptibility to infection have been found for herpesviruses (5), poxviruses (386), papovaviruses (53), rhabdoviruses (310), coronaviruses (48, 278), retroviruses (53), myxoviruses (200), arenaviruses (393), and Borna disease virus (451). In almost all cases, the genes determining resistance to different types of virus appear to segregate independently, suggesting that a variety of mechanisms are involved rather than a single universal type of resistance or susceptibility.

Although it would seem logical that genetic resistance to infection would be linked to host genes controlling the immune response (e.g., H-2 in the mouse), this is surprisingly infrequent. An exception to this rule may be human infection with HTLV type I in which HLA class II alleles are associated with different patterns of disease expression and may influence whether infected individuals develop adult T-cell leukemia (ATL) or HTLV-associated myelopathy (HAM) (325). Transmission of HIV-1 from infected mothers to their offspring also has been linked to the infant's MHC class II allelle (560). Recently it was observed that certain MHC class II haplotypes appear to influence the outcome of SIV infections in rhesus macaques, and that HLA alleles may influence viral load and rate of progression to AIDS after HIV infection in humans (209,452).

Susceptibility to virus infection may be associated with the presence or absence of the appropriate host-cell receptors on target cells. This mechanism may explain the susceptibility of some strains of mice to intestinal infection with MHV (48). However, some strains of mice remain resistant to MHV infection despite the presence of functional virus receptors (576), indicating that other factors also are involved. The recognition of chemokine coreceptors in HIV infection has documented one determinant of susceptibility to HIV infection. Individuals homozygous for a deletion (Δ32) within the chemokine receptor 5 (CCR5) gene have a markedly decreased incidence of HIV infection compared with those with a functional CCR5 gene (209) [see (94) for review]. Polymorphisms within the CCR2 allele also may influence the rate of HIV progression in infected individuals (476). However, factors other than CCR genotype are clearly involved in susceptibility to HIV (370).

Another example of a host gene influencing susceptibility to human viral infection occurs with the TNFα gene encoded within the MHC locus. Polymorphisms within the promoter for this gene have been linked to susceptibility to the development of chronic active hepatitis C infection (223).

The genetic basis for resistance of certain strains of mice to infection with influenza viruses has been extensively investigated. A2G mice are resistant to infection with influenza A. Resistance is inherited as an autosomal dominant trait that is associated with the Mx allele on mouse chromosome 16 (481). Resistance is mediated by the actions of IFN-γ and IFN-β that induce a 72-kd protein (Mx protein) in cells derived from resistant mice. The Mx protein accumulates in the nucleus of cells and inhibits viral replication by inhibiting viral mRNA synthesis (131). Treatment of A2G mice with antibody to interferon renders them susceptible to infection (200). Transfection of cells derived from susceptible mice with cDNA encoding the Mx protein confers protection against influenza A infection *in vitro* (481). Mice that are susceptible to infection appear to have either deletions or nonsense mutations in the Mx gene (480).

Other Physiologic Determinants

Human viral infections provide numerous examples of the correlation between the age of the host and the severity of viral infection. Some viruses tend to produce less severe infection in infants (e.g., varicella, mumps, polio, EBV, hepatitis A), whereas others are more severe (e.g., rotaviruses, RSV, WEE, and measles). Age-related susceptibility to virus infection also occurs in a variety of experimental viral infections in mice (30,188,191,257, 320,562). Conversely, the case/infection ratio is higher in older persons for a few infections such as St. Louis encephalitis (see Chapter 14 of *Fields Virology*, 4th ed.).

The basis for the age dependence of viral infection is poorly understood. Some types of enhanced resistance to viral infection with increasing age may reflect the maturation of both specific and nonspecific components of the host's immune system including phagocytosis, NK activity, cell-mediated cytotoxicity, and antibody production. Organ-specific differences in the immune response may explain why some tissues in adult animals become resistant to viral infection, whereas others do not (562). Finally, age-specific restrictions may reflect changes in the maturity and state of differentiation of target cells, as has been suggested for SFV infection of neurons (396).

For Sindbis (alpha) virus encephalitis, the state of neuronal maturity appears to be an important factor in determining age-related susceptibility (388), whereas immunologic factors play little or no role in this process (191,520). It has recently been shown that changes in the Sindbis E2 glycoprotein can compensate for age-dependent neuronal restriction of replication (520). Dependence of viral infection on the state of cellular differentiation also has been described with coronaviruses (37), herpesviruses (137), polyomaviruses (29,163,322), parvoviruses (198), retroviruses (111), and arenaviruses (118).

Some viruses preferentially infect dividing cells, and differences in the organ distribution of these cells during development and maturation may influence the pattern of disease. For example, prenatal infection of cats with feline parvovirus results in destruction of the germinal cells of the cerebellum and subsequent cerebellar aplasia. Conversely, infection of adult cats involves primarily dividing bone marrow and intestinal epithelial cells and does not result in neurologic illness (250). Induction of cellular damage or injury also may trigger responses that make previously nonpermissive cells able to support viral replication (12).

Hormones also can influence the outcome of viral infection. This may provide one explanation for the frequent observation that male mice are more susceptible to a variety of viral infectious than are their female counterparts (310). A number of infections, including those with polio, hepatitis A and B, and smallpox virus are commonly more severe during pregnancy, although it is not known whether this reflects hormonal alterations or other factors. Reactivation of polyoma virus infection also occurs more commonly during pregnancy, although this typically occurs without associated clinical disease (96). Pregnant mice are more susceptible to intravaginal infection with HSV but not to intraperitoneal or intranasal infection. It has been suggested that this may be due to local hormonal effects. In experimental studies, the administration of both steroid and thyroid hormones can be shown to affect adversely the outcome of certain types of viral infection (reviewed in 350).

The nutritional state of the host also can exert a marked influence on the outcome of viral infection (79). For example, protein malnutrition dramatically exacerbates the severity of measles infection, perhaps by depressing host cellular immunity (79). A similar increase in susceptibility to coxsackievirus and flavivirus infection occurs in experimental infection of malnourished mice. It has been suggested that dietary-induced oxidative stress resulting from deficiency of vitamin E and selenium can increase the severity of certain viral infections, as exemplified by the potentiation of coxsackievirus B3 myocarditis in selenium– and vitamin E–deprived mice (28). Deficiency of vitamin A may result in enhanced severity of respiratory syncytial virus infection in children (380). As a result of these studies, it has been suggested that supplementation with vitamins A, B, C, D, and E may provide an inexpensive form of supplemental therapy for HIV infection, although data directly supporting this approach are still lacking (150). Vitamin A also has been shown to reduce the rate and severity of complications and the duration of hospitalization in children with measles infection (241), and may facilitate healing in HSV keratitis. At the opposite extreme, hyperalimentation and the induction of hypercholesterolemia also may be associated with increased severity of viral infection (65).

Other physiologic factors also may play a role in the severity of viral infection. For example, the severity of influenza is increased in chronic smokers (260), related to the deterioration in mucociliary clearance. Preceding vigorous exercise may worsen the severity of a subsequent bout of poliomyelitis (234), although the mechanism for this has never been clearly established. Experimentally, exercise also can be shown to increase the severity of coxsackievirus infection in mice (170).

The role of host responses such as fever and inflammation in combating viral infection has been examined (435). Classic studies of myxoma infection in rabbits clearly demonstrated that increasing body temperature increased protection against infection and that decreasing temperature increased severity of infection. Similar results have been found with ectromelia and coxsackievirus infections in mice. Blocking the development of fever with drugs (e.g., salicylates) increases the mortality of vaccinia infection in rabbits and increases the shedding of influenza by ferrets (240), providing additional evidence for an antiviral effect of fever. Virus infection exacerbates host stress responses, which in turn may contribute to the pathogenesis of disease. For example, mice infected with Sindbis virus have dramatically increased levels of IFNα/β, TNFα, adrenocorticotropic hormone (ACTH), and corticosteroids. Stress also is associated with high levels of circulating catecholamines including norepinephrine (514). In one recent study, norepinephrine was shown to accelerate HIV replication through its action on protein kinase A–dependent pathways and the subsequent reduction in host levels of several antiviral cytokines including IL-10, IFN-γ, TNFα, IL-1β, and IL-2, -4, and -6 (95).

The importance of host-cell enzymes in influencing the outcome of viral infection was discussed earlier in this chapter. It is well exemplified in the role played by host-cell enzymes in the pathogenesis of myxovirus infection (Chapter 24 as well as Chapter 47 of *Fields Virology*, 4th ed.). Influenza requires cleavage of the viral hemagglutinin from an inactive precursor (HA_0) form into two disulfide-bonded subunits (HA_1 and HA_2) to become infectious. This cleavage is mediated by host-cell trypsin-like proteases, and without this cleavage, virus is avirulent. The HA proteins of mammalian influenza viruses and nonpathogenic avian viruses are susceptible to proteolytic cleavage in a limited number of cell types, whereas the HAs of many pathogenic avian influenza viruses are cleaved by proteases present in many types of host cells (276). Differences in the susceptibilities of these HAs to cleavage is due to the presence of only a single arginine residue at the cleavage site in the mammalian and nonpathogenic avian viruses, whereas the pathogenic avian viruses typically have several basic amino acids present at the cleavage site (276). Mutations in the influenza HA near the cleavage site can dramatically alter both the host range and pathogenicity of influenza viruses (121).

A host-cell protease-mediated cleavage similar to that required for influenza virus is required for activation of the fusion activity of paramyxoviruses such as Sendai virus. Virus containing an uncleaved fusion (F_0) protein does not replicate after inoculation into mice. However, virus will replicate if the F protein has previously been cleaved *in vitro* into the disulfide-bonded F_1 and F_2 subunits by trypsin. Mutant viruses whose F protein can be cleaved by chymotrypsin but not by trypsin also do not produce disease unless the protein is cleaved *in vitro* (352).

Host-cell enzymes also may play an indirect role in susceptibility to Sindbis virus infection. The envelope of the virus contains sialic acid residues derived as the virus buds from host-cell plasma membranes. If the membranes are rich in sialic acid, virus is a more potent activator of complement. Complement activation and subsequent opsonization of virus facilitate viral clearance and thus decreases viral virulence (217). In this example, the biochemical composition of host-cell membranes alters the subsequent virulence of virus.

REFERENCES

1. Abreu-Martin MT, Targan SR. Regulation of immune responses of the intestinal mucosa. *Crit Rev Immunol* 1996;16:277–309.
2. Achiron A, Higuchi I, Takenouchi N, et al. Detection of HTLV type 1 provirus by in situ polymerase chain reaction in mouthwash mononuclear cells of HAM/TSP patients and HTLV type 1 carriers. *AIDS Res Hum Retroviruses* 1997;13:1067–1070.
3. Ahmed R, Morrison LA, Knipe DM, et al., eds. Viral persistence. In: *Viral pathogenesis*. Philadelphia: Lippincott-Raven, 1997:181–205.
4. Akoum A, Lavoie J, Drouin R, et al. Physiological and cytogenetic characterization of immortalized human endometriotic cells containing episomal simian virus 40 DNA. *Am J Pathol* 1999;154:1245–1257.
5. Allan JE, Shellam GR. Genetic control of murine cytomegalovirus infection: viral titres in resistant and susceptible strains of mice. *Arch Virol* 1984;81:139–150.
6. Amerongen HM, Farnet CM, Michetti P, et al. Transepithelial transport of HIV-1 by intestinal M cells: a mechanism for transmission of AIDS. *J Acquir Immune Defic Syndr* 1991;4:760–765.
7. Amerongen HM, Wilson GAR, Fields BN, et al. Proteolytic processing of reovirus is required for adherence to intestinal M cells. *J Virol* 1994;68:8428–8432.
8. Anderson J, Field H. The distribution of herpes simplex virus type 1 antigen in the mouse central nervous system after different routes of inoculation. *J Neurol Sci* 1983;60:181–195.
9. Ando K, Guidotti LG, Cerny A, et al. CTL access to tissue antigen is restricted in vivo. *J Immunol* 1994;153:482–488.
10. Anonymous. Elective caesarean-section versus vaginal delivery in prevention of vertical HIV-1 transmission: a randomised clinical trial. *Lancet* 1999;353:1035–1039.
11. Arthur RR, Shah KV. Occurrence and significance of papovavirus BK and JC in the urine. *Progr Med Virol* 1989;36:42–61.
12. Atencio IA, Shadan FF, Zhou XJ, et al. Adult mouse kidneys become permissive to acute polyomavirus infection and reactivate persistent infections in response to cellular damage and regeneration. *J Virol* 1993;67:1424–1432.
13. Atkins GJ, Sheahan BJ, Dimmock NJ. Semliki Forest virus infection of mice: a model for genetic and molecular analysis of viral pathogenicity. *J Gen Virol* 1985;66:395–408.
14. Attibele N, Wyde PR, Trial J, et al. Measles virus-induced changes in leukocyte function antigen 1 expression and leukocyte aggregation: possible role in measles virus pathogenesis. *J Virol* 1993;67:1075–1079.
15. Babinet CH, Farza H, Morello D, et al. Specific expression of hepatitis B surface antigen (HBsAg) in transgenic mice. *Science* 1985;230:1160–1163.

16. Babiss L, Luftig R, Weatherbee J, et al. Reovirus serotypes 1 and 3 differ in their in vitro association with microtubules. *J Virol* 1979;30: 863–874.
17. Baer GM. Animal models in the pathogenesis and treatment of rabies. *Rev Infect Dis* 1988;10(suppl 4):S739–S750.
18. Baer GM, Bellini WJ, Fishbein DB, et al., eds. Rhabdoviruses. In: *Fields virology.* 2nd ed. New York: Raven Press, 1990:32, 883–930.
19. Bai M, Harfe B, Freimuth P. Mutations that alter an Arg-Gly-Asp (RGD) sequence in the adenovirus type 2 penton base protein abolish its cell-rounding activity and delay virus reproduction in flat cells. *J Virol* 1993;67:5198–5205.
20. Bang F. Genetics of resistance of animal to viruses. I. Introduction and studies in mice. *Adv Virus Res* 1978;23:269–348.
21. Bang F, Bang B, Foard M. Responses of upper respiratory mucosa to drugs and viral infections. *Am Rev Respir Dis* 1966;93(suppl): 5142–5149.
22. Barker LF, Murray R. Relationship of virus dose to incubation time of clinical hepatitis and time of appearance of hepatitis-associated antigen. *Am J Med Sci* 1972;263:27–33.
23. Barnett EM, Perlman S. The olfactory nerve and not the trigeminal nerve is the major site of CNS entry for mouse hepatitis virus, strain JHM. *Virology* 1993;194:185–191.
24. Bass DM, Bodkin D, Dambrauskas R, et al. Intraluminal proteolytic activation plays an important role in replication of type 1 reoviruses in the intestines of neonatal mice. *J Virol* 1990;64:1830–1833.
25. Bass DM, Mackow ER, Greenberg HB. Identification and partial characterization of a rhesus rotavirus binding glycoprotein on murine enterocytes. *Virology* 1991;183:602–610.
26. Bass DM, Trier JS, Dambrauskas R, et al. Reovirus type 1 infection of small intestinal epithelium in suckling mice and its effect on M cells. *Lab Invest* 1988;58:226–235.
27. Baxt B, Mason PW. Foot-and-mouth disease virus undergoes restricted replication in macrophage cell cultures following Fc receptor-mediated adsorption. *Virology* 1995;207:503–509.
28. Beck MA, Levander OA. Dietary oxidative stress and the potentiation of viral infection. *Annu Rev Nutr* 1998;18:93–116.
29. Bedell MA, Hudson JB, Golub TR, et al. Amplification of human papillomavirus genomes in vitro is dependent on epithelial differentiation. *J Virol* 1991;65:2254–2260.
30. Ben-Hur T, Hadar J, Shtram Y, et al. Neurovirulence of herpes simplex virus type 1 depends on age in mice and thymidine kinase expression. *Arch Virol* 1983;78:307–338.
31. Benedetti J, Corey L, Ashley R. Recurrence rates in genital herpes after symptomatic first-episode infection. *Ann Intern Med* 1994;121: 847–854.
32. Bergelson JM, Chan M, Solomon KR, et al. Decay accelerating factor (CD55), a glycosylphosphatidylinositol-anchored complement regulatory protein, is a receptor for several echoviruses. *Proc Natl Acad Sci U S A* 1994;91:6245–6249.
33. Bergelson JM, Cunningham JA, Droguett G, et al. Isolation of a common receptor for coxsackie B viruses and adenoviruses 2 and 5. *Science* 1997;275:1320–1323.
34. Bergelson JM, Krithivas A, Celi L, et al. The murine CAR homolog is a receptor for coxsackie B viruses and adenoviruses. *J Virol* 1998;72: 415–419.
35. Berinstein A, Roivainen M, Hovi T, et al. Antibodies to the vitronectin receptor (integrin $\alpha_v\beta_3$) inhibit binding and infection of foot-and-mouth disease virus to cultured cells. *J Virol* 1995;69:2664–2666.
36. Bertoletti A, Sette A, Chisari FV, et al. Natural variants of cytotoxic epitopes are T cell receptor antagonists for antiviral cytotoxic T cells. *Nature* 1994;369:407–410.
37. Beushausen S, Dales S. In vivo and in vitro models of demyelinating disease. XXI: Relationship between differentiation of rat oligodendrocytes and control of JHMV replication. *Adv Exp Med Biol* 1987; 218:239–254.
38. Bhat S, Spitalnik SL, Gonzalez-Scarano F, et al. Galactosyl ceramide or a derivative is an essential component of the neural receptor for human immunodeficiency virus type 1 envelope glycoprotein gp120. *Proc Natl Acad Sci U S A* 1991;88:7131–7134.
39. Bijlenga G, Heaney T. Post-exposure local treatment of mice infected with rabies with two axonal flow inhibitors, colchicine and vinblastine. *J Gen Virol* 1978;39:381–385.
40. Biron CA. Cytokines in the generation of immune responses and the resolution of virus infection. *Curr Opin Immunol* 1994;6:530–538.
41. Bitzer M, Lauer U, Baumann C, et al. Sendai virus efficiently infects cells via the asialoglycoprotein receptor and requires the presence of cleaved F_0 precursor proteins for this alternative route of cell entry. *J Virol* 1997;71:5481–5486.
42. Blau DM, Compans RW. Entry and release of measles virus are polarized in epithelial cells. *Virology* 1995;210:91–99.
43. Block TM, Hill JM. The latency associates transcript (LAT) of herpes simplex virus: Still no end in sight. *J Neurovirol* 1997;3:313–321.
44. Bobroski L, Bagasra AU, Patel D, et al. Localization of human herpesvirus type 8 (HHV-8) in the Kaposi sarcoma tissues and the semen specimens of HIV-1 infected and uninfected individuals by utilizing in situ polymerase chain reaction. *J Reprod Immunol* 1998;41:149–160.
45. Bodkin D, Nibert ML, Fields BN. Proteolytic digestion of reovirus serotype 1 in the intestinal lumen of neonatal mice. *J Virol* 1989;63: 4676–4681.
46. Bolt G, Pedersen IR. The role of subtilisin-like proprotein convertases for cleavage of the measles virus fusion glycoprotein in different cell types. *Virology* 1998;252:387–398.
47. Borrow P, Oldstone MBA. Mechanism of lymphocytic choriomeningitis virus entry into cells. *Virology* 1994;198:1–9.
48. Boyle JF, Weismiller DG, Holmes KV. Genetic resistance to mouse hepatitis virus correlates with the absence of virus-binding activity on target tissues. *J Virol* 1987;61:185–189.
49. Brewer CB, Roth MG. A single amino acid change in the cytoplasmic domain alters the polarized delivery of influenza virus hemagglutinin. *J Cell Biol* 1991;114:413–421.
50. Brinster R, Chen H, Messing A, et al. Transgenic mice harboring SV40 T-antigen genes develop characteristic brain tumors. *Cell* 1984;37:367–379.
51. Brinton M, Nathanson N, eds. Host susceptibility to viral disease. In: *Viral pathogenesis.* Philadelphia: Lippincott-Raven, 1997:303–328.
52. Brinton M, Blank K, Nathanson N, et al., eds. Host genes that influence susceptibility to viral diseases. In: *Concepts in viral pathogenesis.* New York: Springer-Verlag, 1984:71–78.
53. Brinton M, Nathanson N. Genetic determinants of virus susceptibility: Epidemiologic implications of murine models. *Epidemiol Rev* 1981;3:115–139.
54. Brodsky FM, Lem L, Solache A, et al. Human pathogen subversion of antigen presentation. *Immunol Rev* 1999;168:199–215.
55. Bronowicki JP, Venard V, Botte C, et al. Patient-to-patient transmission of hepatitis C virus during colonoscopy. *N Engl J Med* 1997;337: 237–240.
56. Brown DT, Edwards J. Structural changes in alphaviruses accompanying the process of membrane penetration. *Semin Virol* 1992;3: 519–527.
57. Brown KE, Anderson SM, Young NS. Erythrocyte P antigen: cellular receptor for B19 parvovirus. *Science* 1993;262:114–117.
58. Brownstein D. Resistance/susceptibility to lethal Sendai virus infection genetically linked to a mucociliary transport polymorphism. *J Virol* 1987;61:1670–1671.
59. Bucholz CJ, Koller D, Devaux P, et al. Mapping of the primary binding site of measles virus to its receptor CD46. *J Biol Chem* 1997;272: 22072–22079.
60. Buckland R, Wild TF. Is CD46 the cellular receptor for measles virus? *Virus Res* 1997;48:1–9.
61. Burk RD, DeLoia JA, Elawady MK, et al. Tissue preferential expression of the hepatitis B virus (HBV): surface antigen gene in two lines of HBV transgenic mice. *J Virol* 1988;62:649–654.
62. Burrage TG, Tignor GH, Smith AL. Rabies virus binding at neuromuscular junctions. *Virus Res* 1985;2:273–289.
63. Byrn RA, Kiessling AA. Analysis of human immunodeficiency virus in semen: indications of a genetically distinct virus reservoir. *J Reprod Immunol* 1998;41:161–176.
64. Byrnes AP, Griffin DE. Binding of Sindbis virus to cell surface heparan sulfate. *J Virol* 1998;72:7349–7356.
65. Campbell A, Lorio R, Madge G, et al. Dietary hepatic cholesterol elevation: effects on coxsackie B5 infection and inflammation. *Infect Immun* 1982;37:307–317.
66. Cao W, Henry MD, Borrow P, et al. Identification of α-dystroglycan as a receptor for lymphocytic choriomeningitis virus and Lassa fever virus. *Science* 1998;282:2079–2081.
67. Cao Y, Qin L, Zhang L, Safrit J, et al. Virologic and immunologic characterization of long-term survivors of human immunodeficiency virus type 1 infection. *N Engl J Med* 1995;332:201–208.

68. Carbone KM, Duchala CS, Griffin JW, et al. Pathogenesis of Borna disease virus in rats: evidence that intra-axonal spread is the major route for dissemination and determinant for disease incubation. *J Virol* 1987;61:3431–3440.
69. Card JP. Practical considerations for the use of pseudorabies virus in transneuronal studies of neural circuitry. *Neurosci Biobehav Rev* 1998;22:685–694.
70. Card JP, Levitt P, Enquist LW. Different patterns of neuronal infection after intracerebral injection of two strains of pseudorabies virus. *J Virol* 1998;72:4434–4441.
71. Card JP, Rinaman L, Lynn RB, et al. Pseudorabies virus infection of the rat central nervous system: Ultrastructural characterization of viral replication, transport, and pathogenesis. *J Neurosci* 1993;13: 2515–2539.
72. Card JP, Rinaman L, Schwaber JS, et al. Neurotropic properties of pseudorabies virus: Uptake and transneuronal passage in the rat central nervous system. *J Neurosci* 1990;10:1974–1994.
73. Card JP, Whealy ME, Robbins AK, et al. Pseudorabies virus envelope glycoprotein gI influences both neurotropism and virulence during infection of the rat visual system. *J Virol* 1992;66:3032–3041.
74. Card JP, Whealy ME, Robbins AK, et al. Two alpha-herpesvirus strains are transported differentially in the rodent visual system. *Neuron* 1991;6:957–969.
75. Carson J, Collier AM, Hu SS. Acquired ciliary defects in nasal epithelium of children with viral upper respiratory infections. *N Engl J Med* 1985;312:463–468.
76. Ceccaldi PE, Ermine A, Tsiang H. Continuous delivery of colchicine in the rat brain with osmotic pumps for inhibition of rabies virus transport. *J Virol Methods* 1990;28:79–84.
77. Ceccaldi PE, Gillet JP, Tsiang H. Inhibition of the transport of rabies virus in the central nervous system. *J Neuropathol Exp Neurol* 1989;48:620–630.
78. Cecilia D, Gould EA. Nucleotide changes responsible for loss of neuroinvasiveness in Japanese encephalitis virus neutralization-resistant mutants. *Virology* 1991;181:70–77.
79. Chandra R. Nutrition, immunity, and infection: present knowledge and future directions. *Lancet* 1983;1:688–691.
80. Chapman LE. Guidelines on the risk for transmission of infectious agents during xenotransplants. *Emerg Infect Dis* 1995;1:156.
81. Charles PC, Guida JD, Brosnan C, et al. Mouse adenovirus type-1 replication is restricted to vascular endothelium in the CNS of susceptible strains of mice. *Virology* 1998;245:216–228.
82. Chen AX, Shen L, Miller MD, et al. Cytotoxic T lymphocytes do not appear to select for mutations in an immunodominant epitope of simian immunodeficiency virus gag. *J Immunol* 1992;149: 4060–4066.
83. Chen DS, Asanaka M, Chen FS, et al. Human carcinoembryonic antigen and biliary glycoprotein can serve as mouse hepatitis virus receptors. *J Virol* 1997;71:1688–1691.
84. Chen I, Ahmed R, eds. *Persistent viral infections.* New York: John Wiley & Sons, 1999.
85. Chen M, Popescu N, Woodworth C, et al. Human herpesvirus 6 infects cervical epithelial cells and transactivates human papillomavirus gene expression. *J Virol* 1994;68:1173–1178.
86. Chen M, Sonnerborg A, Johansson B, et al. Detection of hepatitis G virus (GB virus C) in human saliva. *J Clin Microbiol* 1997;35: 973–975.
87. Chen YC, Wang SY, King CC. Bacterial lipopolysaccharide inhibits dengue virus infection of primary human monocytes/macrophages by blockade of virus-entry via a CD14-dependent mechanism. *J Virol* 1999;73:2650–2657.
88. Chesebro B, Buller R, Portis J, et al. Failure of human immunodeficiency virus entry and infection in $CD4^+$ human brain and skin cells. *J Virol* 1990;64:215–221.
89. Chou J, Roizman B. The gamma1.34.5 gene of herpes simplex virus 1 precludes neuroblastoma cells from triggering total shutoff of protein synthesis characteristic of programmed cell death in neuronal cells. *Proc Natl Acad Sci U S A* 1992;89:3266–3270.
90. Cid-Arregui A, Parton RG, Simons K, et al. Nocodazole-dependent transport, and brefeldin A-sensitive processing and sorting, of newly synthesized membrane proteins in cultured neurons. *J Neurosci* 1995; 15:4259–4269.
91. Clapham PR, Blanc D, Weiss RA. Specific cell surface requirements for the infection of $CD4^+$ cells by human immunodeficiency virus types 1 and 2 and by simian immunodeficiency virus. *Virology* 1991; 181:703–715.
92. Clark SM, Roth JR, Clark ML, et al. Tryptic enhancement of rotavirus infectivity: mechanism of enhancement. *J Virol* 1981;39:816–822.
93. Coffin JM. HIV population dynamics in vivo: implications for genetic variation, pathogenesis, and therapy. *Science* 1995;267:483–489.
94. Cohen OJ, Kinter A, Fauci AS. Host factors in the pathogenesis of HIV disease. *Immunol Rev* 1997;159:31–48.
95. Cole SW, Korin YD, Fahey JL, et al. Norepinephrine accelerates HIV replication via protein kinase A-dependent effects on cytokine production. *J Immunol* 1998;161:610–616.
96. Coleman DV, Wolfendale MR, Daniel RA, et al. A prospective study of human polyomavirus infection in pregnancy. *J Infect Dis* 1980;142:1–8.
97. Collins AR. Human macrophages are susceptible to coronavirus OC43. *Adv Exp Med Biol* 1998;440:635–639.
98. Compans RW. Virus entry and release in polarized epithelial cells. *Curr Top Microbiol Immunol* 1995;202:209–219.
99. Compans RW, Srinivas RV. Protein sorting in polarized epithelial cells. *Curr Top Microbiol Immunol* 1991;170:141–181.
100. Compton T, Ivanov IE, Gottlieb T, et al. A sorting signal for the basolateral delivery of vesicular stomatitis virus (VSV) G protein lies in its luminal domain: Analysis of the targeting of VSV G-influenza hemagglutinin chimeras. *Proc Natl Acad Sci U S A* 1989;86:4112–4116.
101. Compton T, Nowlin DM, Cooper NR. Initiation of human cytomegalovirus infection requires initial interaction with cell surface heparan sulfate. *Virology* 1993;193:834–841.
102. Comtopoulos-Ioannidis DG, Ioannidis P. Maternal cell-free viremia in the natural history of perinatal HIV-1 transmission: a meta-analysis. *J Acquir Immune Defic Syndr* 1998;18:126–135.
103. Conner MF, Ramig RF, Nathanson N, eds. Viral enteric diseases. In: *Viral pathogenesis.* Philadelphia: Lippincott-Raven, 1997:713–735.
104. Coombs RW, Speck CE, Hughes JP, et al. Association between culturable human immunodeficiency virus type 1 (HIV-1) in semen and HIV-1 RNA levels in semen and blood: evidence for compartmentalization of HIV-1 between semen and blood. *J Infect Dis* 1998;177: 320–330.
105. Corey L, Wald A, Davis LG. Subclinical shedding of HSV: its potential for reduction by antiviral therapy. *Adv Exp Med Biol* 1996;394: 11–16.
106. Corsini J, Tal J, Winocour E. Directed integration of minute virus of mice DNA into episomes. *J Virol* 1997;71:9008–9015.
107. Couderc T, Barzu T, Horaud F, et al. Poliovirus permissivity and specific receptor expression on human endothelial cells. *Virology* 1990; 174:95–102.
108. Coulon P, Derbin C, Kucera P, et al. Invasion of the peripheral nervous systems of adult mice by the CVS strain of rabies virus and its avirulent derivative Av01. *J Virol* 1989;63:3550–3554.
109. Crepin P, Audry L, Rotivel Y, et al. Intravitam diagnosis of human rabies by PCR using saliva and cerebrospinal fluid. *J Clin Microbiol* 1998;36:1117–1121.
110. Croyle MA, Stone M, Amidon GL, et al. In vitro and in vivo assessment of adenovirus 41 as a vector for gene delivery to the intestine. *Gene Ther* 1998;5:645–654.
111. Czub M, Czub S, McAtee F, et al. Age-dependent resistance to murine retrovirus-induced spongiform neurodegeneration results from central nervous system-specific restriction of viral replication. *J Virol* 1991; 65:2539–2544.
112. Dalapathy S, Lily TK, Roy S, et al. Development and use of nested polymerase chain reaction (PCR) for the detection of adenovirus from conjunctival specimens. *J Clin Virol* 1998;11:77–84.
113. Dalgleish AG, Beverly PCL, Clapham PR, et al. The CD4 (T4) antigen is an essential component of the receptor for the AIDS retrovirus. *Nature* 1985;312:763–767.
114. Daniels CA, LeGoff SG, Notkins AL. Shedding of infectious virus-antibody complexes from vesicular lesions of patients with recurrent herpes labialis. *Lancet* 1975;2:524–528.
115. Darnell M, Koprowski H. Genetically determined resistance to infection with group B arboviruses. II. Increased production of interfering particles in cell cultures from resistant mice. *J Infect Dis* 1974;129: 248–256.
116. Day S, Lausch R, Oakes J. Evidence that the gene for herpes simplex virus type 1 DNA polymerase accounts for the capacity of an intertypic recombinant to spread from eye to central nervous system. *Virology* 1988;163:166–173.

117. De La Torre JC, Oldstone MBA. Anatomy of viral persistence: Mechanisms of persistence and associated disease. *Adv Virus Res* 1996;46: 311–343.
118. De La Torre JC, Rall G, Oldstone C, et al. Replication of lymphocytic choriomeningitis virus is restricted in terminally differentiated neurons. *J Virol* 1993;67:7350–7359.
119. del Val M, Hengel H, Hacker H, et al. Cytomegalovirus prevents antigen presentation by blocking the transport of peptide-loaded major histocompatibility complex class I molecules into the medial-Golgi compartment. *J Exp Med* 1992;176:729–738.
120. Dermody TS, Nibert ML, Wetzel JD, et al. Cells and viruses with mutations affecting viral entry are selected during persistent infection of L cells with mammalian reoviruses. *J Virol* 1993;67:2055–2063.
121. Deshpande K, Fried V, Ando M, et al. Glycosylation affects cleavage of an H5N2 influenza virus hemagglutinin and regulates virulence. *Proc Natl Acad Sci U S A* 1987;84:36–40.
122. Di Simone C, Zandonatti MA, Buchmeier MJ. Acidic pH triggers LCMV membrane fusion activity and conformational change in the glycoprotein spike. *Virology* 1994;189:455–465.
123. Dimitrov RS. How do viruses enter cells? The HIV coreceptors teach us a lesson in complexity. *Cell* 1997;91:721–730.
124. Dingwell KS, Brunetti CR, Hendricks RL, et al. Herpes simplex virus glycoproteins E and I facilitate cell-to-cell spread in vivo and across junctions of cultured cells. *J Virol* 1994;68:834–845.
125. Dingwell KS, Doering LCJ. Glycoproteins E and I facilitate neuron-to-neuron spread of herpes simplex virus. *J Virol* 1995;69:7087–7098.
126. Dockter J, Evans CF, Tishon A, et al. Competitive selection in vivo by a cell for one variant over another: Implications for RNA virus quasispecies in vivo. *J Virol* 1996:70:1799–1803.
127. Dotti CG, Simons K. Polarized sorting of viral glycoproteins to the axon and dendrites of hippocampal neurons in culture. *Cell* 1990;62: 63–72.
128. Dragic T, Litwin V, Allaway GP, et al. HIV-1 entry into $CD4^+$ cells is mediated by the chemokine receptor CC-CKR5. *Nature* 1996;381: 667–673.
129. Drayna D, Fields BN. Biochemical studies on the mechanisms of chemical and physical inactivation of reovirus. *J Gen Virol* 1982;63: 161–170.
130. Drayna D, Fields BN. Genetic studies on the mechanism of chemical and physical inactivation of reovirus. *J Gen Virol* 1982;63:149–159.
131. Dreiding P, Staeheli P, Haller O. Interferon-induced protein Mx accumulates in nuclei of mouse cells expressing resistance to influenza viruses. *Virology* 1985;140:192–196.
132. Dryden KA, Wang G, Yeager M, et al. Early steps in reovirus infection are associated with dramatic changes in supramolecular structure and protein conformation: analysis of virions and subviral particles by cryoelectron microscopy and image reconstruction. *J Cell Biol* 1993; 122:1023–1041.
133. Dubensky TW, Freund R, Dawe CJ, et al. Polyomavirus replication in mice: influences of VP1 type and route of inoculation. *J Virol* 1991; 65:342–349.
134. Dubois-Dalcq M, Hooghe-Peters E, Lazzarini R. Antibody induced modulation of rhabdovirus infection of neurons in vitro. *J Neuropathol Exp Neurol* 1980;39:507–522.
135. Dulioust E, Tachet A, De Almeida M, et al. Detection of HIV-1 in seminal plasma and seminal cells of HIV-1 seropositive men. *J Reprod Immunol* 1998;41:27–40.
136. Dunster LM, Schneider-Schaulies J, Loffler S, et al. Moesin: A cell membrane protein linked with susceptibility to measles virus infection. *Virology* 1994;198:265–274.
137. Dutko F, Oldstone MBA. Cytomegalovirus causes a latent infection in undifferentiated cells and is activated by induction of a cell differentiation. *J Exp Med* 1981;154:1636–1651.
138. Dveskler GS, Dieffenbach CW, Cardellichio CB, et al. Several members of the carcinoembryonic antigen-related glycoprotein family are functional receptors for the coronavirus mouse hepatitis virus A59. *J Virol* 1993;67:1–8.
139. Embretson J, Zupancic M, Ribas JL, et al. Massive covert infection of helper T lymphocytes and macrophages by HIV during the incubation period of AIDS. *Nature* 1993;362:359–362.
140. Eppstein DA, Marsh YV, Schreiber AB, et al. Epidermal growth factor receptor occupancy inhibits vaccinia virus infection. *Nature* 1985; 318:663–665.
141. Estes MK, Graham DY, Mason BB. Proteolytic enhancement of rotavirus infectivity: molecular mechanisms. *J Virol* 1981;39: 879–888.
142. Evander M, Frazer IH, Payne E, et al. Identification of the alpha6 integrin as a candidate receptor for papillomaviruses. *J Virol* 1997;71: 2449–2456.
143. Evans AS, Brachman PS. *Bacterial infections of humans.* New York: Plenum, 1991.
144. Evans DJ, Almond JW. Cell receptors for picornaviruses as determinants of cell tropism and pathogenesis. *Trends Microbiol* 1999;6: 198–202.
145. Faber H. *The pathogenesis of poliomyelitis.* Springfield, IL: Charles C Thomas, 1955.
146. Fahnestock ML, Johnson JL, Feldman RMR, et al. The MHC class I homolog encoded by human cytomegalovirus binds endogenous peptides. *Immunity* 1995;3:583–590.
147. Falangola MF, Hanly A, Galvao-Castro B, et al. HIV infection of human choroid plexus: a possible mechanism of viral entry into the CNS. *J Neuropathol Exp Neurol* 1995;54:497–503.
148. Fantini J, Cook DG, Nathanson N, et al. Infection of colonic epithelial cell lines by type 1 human immunodeficiency virus is associated with cell surface expression of galactosylceramide, a potential alternative gp120 receptor. *Proc Natl Acad Sci U S A* 1993;90:2700–2794.
149. Farrell HE, Vally H, Lynch DM, et al. Inhibition of natural killer cells by a cytomegalovirus MHC class I homologue in vivo. *Nature* 1997; 386:510–514.
150. Fawzi WW, Hunter DJ. Vitamins in HIV disease progression and vertical transmission. *Epidemiology* 1998;9:457–466.
151. Fear WR, Kesson AM, Naif AM, et al. Differential tropism and chemokine receptor expression of human immunodeficiency type 1 in neonatal monocytes, monocyte-derived macrophages and placental macrophages. *J Virol* 1998;72:1334–1344.
152. Fekadu, M, Shaddock JH, Baer GM. Excretion of rabies virus in the saliva of dogs. *J Infect Dis* 1982;145:715–719.
153. Fenner F. Mousepox (infectious ectromelia of mice): A review. *J Immunol* 1949;63:341–373.
154. Fenner F. Poxviruses. In: Fields BN, ed. *Virology.* 2nd ed. New York: Raven Press, 1990:2113–2133.
155. Fingeroth JD, Clabby ML, Strominger JD. Characterization of a T-lymphocyte Epstein-Barr virus/C3d receptor (CD21). *J Virol* 1988;62: 1442–1447.
156. Fish KN, Soderberg-Naucler C, Mills LK, et al. Human cytomegalovirus persistently infects aortic endothelial cells. *J Virol* 1998;72: 5661–5668.
157. Flamand A, Gagner JP, Morrison LA, et al. Penetration of the nervous system of suckling mice by mammalian reoviruses. *J Virol* 1991;65: 123–131.
158. Flynn DC, Meyer WJ, MacKenzie JM, et al. A conformational change in Sindbis virus glycoproteins E1 and E2 is detected at the plasma membrane as a consequence of virus-cell interaction. *J Virol* 1990;64: 3643–3653.
159. Fournier J-G, Tardieu M, Lebon P, et al. Detection of measles virus RNA in lymphocytes from peripheral blood and brain perivascular infiltrates of patients with subacute sclerosing panencephalitis. *N Engl J Med* 1985;313:910–915.
160. Fricks CE, Hogle JM. Cell-induced conformational change in poliovirus: externalization of the amino terminus of VP1 is responsible for liposome binding. *J Virol* 1990;64:1934–1945.
161. Friedman H, Macarek E, MacGregor RA, et al. Virus infection of endothelial cells. *J Infect Dis* 1981;143:266–273.
162. Fruh K, Ahn K, Peterson PA. Inhibition of MHC class I antigen presentation by viral proteins. *J Mol Med* 1997;75:18–27.
163. Fujimura FK, Silbert PE, Eckhart W, et al. Polyoma virus infection of retinoic acid-induced differentiated teratocarcinoma cells. *J Virol* 1981;39:306–312.
164. Fujisaka H, Tanaka-Taya K, Tanabe H, et al. Detection of human herpesvirus 7 (HHV-7) DNA in breast milk by polymerase chain reaction and prevalence of HHV-7 antibody in breast-fed and bottle-fed children. *J Med Virol* 1998;56:275–279.
165. Fujita K, Silver J, Peden K. Changes in both gp120 and gp41 can account for increased growth potential and expanded host range of human immunodeficiency virus type 1. *J Virol* 1992;66:4445–4451.
166. Fuller AO, Lee W-C. Herpes simplex virus type 1 entry through a cascade of virus-cell interactions requires different roles of gD and gH in penetration. *J Virol* 1992;66:5002–5012.

167. Garcia PM, Kalish LA, Pitt J, et al. Maternal levels of plasma human immunodeficiency virus type 1 RNA and the risk of perinatal transmission. *N Engl J Med* 1999;341:441–443.
168. Garcia-Sastre A, Durbin RK, Zheng H, et al. The role of interferon in influenza virus tropism. *J Virol* 1998;72:8550–8558.
169. Garten W, Bosch FX, Linder D, et al. Proteolytic activation of the human influenza virus hemagglutinins: the structure of the cleavage site and the enzyme involved in cleavage. *Virology* 1981;115: 361–374.
170. Gatmaitan B, Chason J, Lerner A. Augmentation of the virulence of murine coxsackie virus B-3 myocardiopathy by exercise. *J Exp Med* 1970;131:1121–1136.
171. Gavrilovskaya IN, Brown EJ, Ginsberg MH, et al. Cellular entry of hantaviruses which can cause hemorrhagic fever with renal syndrome is mediated by beta3 integrins. *J Virol* 1999;73:3951–3959.
172. Gentsch J, Pacitti A. Differential interaction of reovirus type 3 with sialylated components on animal cells. *Virology* 1987;161:245–248.
173. Geraghty RJ, Krummenacher C, Cohen GH, et al. Entry of alphaherpesviruses mediated by poliovirus receptor-related protein 1 and poliovirus receptor. *Science* 1998;280:1618–1620.
174. Gething MJ, White JM, Waterfield MD. Purification of the fusion protein of Sendai virus: Analysis of the NH_2-terminal sequence generated during precursor activation. *Proc Natl Acad Sci U S A* 1978;75: 2737–2740.
175. Gilbert MJ, Riddell SR, Plachter B, et al. Cytomegalovirus selectively blocks antigen processing and presentation of its immediate-early gene product. *Nature* 1996;383:720–722.
176. Gillet G, Brun G. Viral inhibition of apoptosis. *Trends Microbiol* 1996;4:312–316.
177. Gillet JP, Derer P, Tsiang H. Axonal transport of rabies virus in the central nervous system of the rat. *J Neuropathol Exp Neurol* 1986;45: 619–634.
178. Gius D, Grossman S, Bedell M, et al. Inducible and constitutive enhancer domains in the non-coding region of human papillomavirus type 18. *J Virol* 1988;62:665–672.
179. Godfraind C, Havaux N, Holmes KV, et al. Role of virus-receptor bearing endothelial cells of the blood-brain barrier in preventing spread of mouse hepatitis virus A59 into the central nervous system. *J Neurovirol* 1997;3:428–434.
180. Gombold JL, Hingley ST, Weiss SR. Fusion-defective mutants of mouse hepatitis virus A59 contain a mutation in the spike protein cleavage signal. *J Virol* 1993;67:4504–4512.
181. Gonzalez-Scarano F, Jacoby D, Griot C, et al. Genetics, infectivity and virulence of California serogroup viruses. *Virus Res* 1992;24: 123–135.
182. Gooding LR. Virus proteins that counteract host immune defenses. *Cell* 1992;71:5–7.
183. Goodpasture E. The axis-cylinders of peripheral nerves as portals of entry for the virus of herpes simplex in experimentally infected rabbits. *Am J Pathol* 1925;1:11–28.
184. Gout O, Baulac M, Gessain A, et al. Rapid development of myelopathy after HTLV-I infection by transfusion during cardiac transplantation. *N Engl J Med* 1990;322:383–388.
185. Granovsky MO, Minkoff HL, Tess BH, et al. Hepatitis C virus infection in the mothers and infants cohort study. *Pediatrics* 1998;102: 355–359.
186. Greber UF, Willetts M, Webster P, et al. Stepwise dismantling of adenovirus 2 during entry into cells. *Cell* 1993;75:477–486.
187. Greene WC. The molecular biology of human immunodeficiency type 1 virus infection. *N Engl J Med* 1991;324:308–317.
188. Greenlee J. Effect of host age on experimental K virus infection in mice. *Infect Immun* 1981;33:297–303.
189. Gressens P, Martin JR. In situ polymerase chain reaction: localization of HSV-2 DNA sequences in infection of the nervous system. *J Virol Methods* 1994;46:61–83.
190. Greve J, Davis G, Meyer A, et al. The major human rhinovirus receptor is ICAM-1. *Cell* 1989;56:839–847.
191. Griffin DE, Levine B, Tyor WR, et al. Age-dependent susceptibility to fatal encephalitis: Alphavirus infection of neurons. *Arch Virol* 1994;(suppl 9):31–39.
192. Griffiths PD. Viral complications after transplantation. *J Antimicrob Agents Chemother* 1995;36(suppl B):91–106.
193. Grimley P, Friedman R. Arboviral infection of voluntary striated muscles. *J Infect Dis* 1970;122:45–52.
194. Gromeier M, Wimmer E. Mechanism of injury-provoked poliomyelitis. *J Virol* 1998;72:5056–5060.
195. Groschel D, Koprowski H. Development of a virus-resistant inbred mouse strain for the study of innate resistance to arbo B viruses. *Arch Ges Virusforsch* 1965;17:379–391.
196. Grundy JE, McKeating JA, Ward PJ, et al. Beta 2-microglobulin enhances the infectivity of cytomegalovirus and when bound to virus enables class I HLA molecules to be used as a virus receptor. *J Gen Virol* 1987;68:793–803.
197. Gsatka M, Horvath J, Lentz TL. Rabies virus binding to the nicotinic acetylcholine receptor alpha subunit demonstrated by viral overlay protein binding assay. *J Gen Virol* 1996;77:2437–2440.
198. Guetta E, Ron D, Tal J. Developmental-dependent replication of minute virus of mice in differentiated mouse testicular lines. *J Gen Virol* 1986;67:2549–2554.
199. Haase AT. Pathogenesis of lentiviruses infections. *Nature* 1986;322: 130–136.
200. Haller O, Arnheiter H, Lindenmann J, et al. I. Host gene influences sensitivity to interferon action selectively for influenza virus. *Nature* 1980;283:660–662.
201. Hamprecht K, Vochem M, Baumeister A, et al. Detection of cytomegalovirus DNA in human milk cells and cell free milk whey by nested PCR. *J Virol Methods* 1998;70:167–176.
202. Hanham CA, Zhao F, Tignor GH. Evidence from the anti-idiotype network that the acetylcholine receptor is a rabies virus receptor. *J Virol* 1993;67:530–542.
203. Hanly A, Petito CK. HLA-DR positive dendritic cells of the normal human choroid plexus: A potential reservoir of HIV in the central nervous system. *Hum Pathol* 1998;29:88–93.
204. Hanson B, Koprowski H, Baron S, et al. Interferon-mediated natural resistance of mice to arbo B virus infection. *Microbioscience* 1969; 1B:51–68.
205. Hardy JL, Houk EJ, Kramer LD, et al. Intrinsic factors affecting vector competence of mosquitoes for arboviruses. *Annu Rev Entomol* 1983;28:229–262.
206. Harrington RD, Geballe AP. Cofactor requirement for human immunodeficiency virus type 1 entry into a CD4-expressing human cell line. *J Virol* 1993;67:5939–5947.
207. Haywood AM. Virus receptors: Binding, adhesion strengthening, and changes in viral structure. *J Virol* 1994;68:1–5.
208. Helenius A, Morein B, Fries E, et al. Human (HLA-A and HLA-B) and murine (H2K and H2D) histocompatibility antigens are cell surface receptors for Semliki Forest virus. *Proc Natl Acad Sci U S A* 1978;75:3846–3850.
209. Hendel H, Caillat-Zucman S, Lebuanec H, et al. New class I and class II HLA alleles strongly associated with opposite patterns of progression to AIDS. *J Immunol* 1999;162:6942–6946.
210. Herold BC, WuDunn D, Soltys N, et al. Glycoprotein C of herpes simplex virus type 1 plays a principal role in the adsorption of virus to cells and infectivity. *J Virol* 1991;65:1090–1098.
211. Hildreth JEK, Orentas R. Involvement of a leukocyte adhesion receptor (LFA-1) in HIV induced syncytium formation. *Science* 1989;244: 1075–1078.
212. Hill JM, Gebhardt BM, Wen RJ, et al. Quantitation of herpes simplex virus type 1 DNA and latency-associated transcripts in rabbit trigeminal ganglia demonstrates a stable reservoir of viral nucleic acids during latency. *J Virol* 1996;70:3137–3141.
213. Hill JM, Sedarati F, Javier RT, et al. Herpes simplex virus turns off the TAP to evade host immunity. *Nature* 1995;375:411–415.
214. Hill T, Field H, Roome A. Intra-axonal location of herpes simplex virus particles. *J Gen Virol* 1972;15:253–255.
215. Hillyer CD, Snydman DR, Berkman EM. The risk of cytomegalovirus infection in solid organ and bone marrow transplant recipients: Transfusion of blood products. *Transfusion* 1990;30:659–666.
216. Hirsch MS, Zisman B, Allison AC. Macrophages and age-dependent resistance to herpes simplex virus in mice. *J Immunol* 1970;104: 1160–1165.
217. Hirsch RL, Griffin DE, Winkelstein JA. Natural immunity to Sindbis virus is influenced by host tissue sialic acid content. *Proc Natl Acad Sci U S A* 1983;80:548–550.
218. Hirsch VM, Sharkey ME, Brown CR, et al. Vpx is required for dissemination and pathogenesis of SIV(SM) PBJ; evidence of macrophage-dependent viral amplification. *Nat Med* 1998;4:1401–1408.
219. Ho DD, Neumann AU, Perelson AS, et al. Rapid turnover of plasma

virions and CD4 lymphocytes in HIV-1 infection. *Nature* 1995;373: 123–126.
220. Hoekstra D, Kok JW. Entry mechanisms of enveloped viruses: Implications for fusion of intracellular membranes. *Biosci Rep* 1989;9: 273–305.
221. Hofer F, Gruenberger M, Kowalski H, et al. Members of the low density lipoprotein receptor family mediate cell entry of a minor-group common cold virus. *Proc Natl Acad Sci U S A* 1994;91:1839–1842.
222. Hoft RH, Pflugfelder SC, Forster RK, et al. Clinical evidence for hepatitis B transmission resulting from corneal transplantation. *Cornea* 1997;16:132–137.
223. Hohler T, Kruger A, Gerken G, et al. Tumor necrosis factor alpha promoter polymorphism at position -238 is associated with chronic active hepatitis C infection. *J Med Virol* 1998;54:173–177.
224. Holland JJ. Receptor affinities as major determinants of enterovirus tissue tropism in humans. *Virology* 1961;15:312–326.
225. Holland JJ, De La Torre JC, Steinhauer DA. RNA virus populations as quasispecies. *Curr Top Microbiol Immunol* 1992;176:1–20.
226. Hollinger FB, Khan NC, Oefinger PE, et al. Post-transfusion hepatitis A. *JAMA* 1983;250:2313–2317.
227. Holmes KV, Tresnan DB, Zelus BD. Virus-receptor interactions in the enteric tract. *Adv Exp Med Biol* 1997;412:125–133.
228. Hooper JW, Fields BN. Role of the mu 1 protein in reovirus stability and capacity to cause chromium release from host cells. *J Virol* 1996; 70:459–467.
229. Hoover JE, Strick PL. Multiple output channels in the basal ganglia. *Science* 1993;259:819–821.
230. Hoover JE, Strick PL. The organization of cerebellar and basal ganglia outputs to primary motor cortex as revealed by retrograde transneuronal transport of herpes simplex virus type 1. *J Neurosci* 1999;19: 1446–1463.
231. Horvat B, Rivailler P, Varior-Krishnan G, et al. Transgenic mice expressing human measles virus (MV) receptor CD46 provide cells exhibiting different permissivities to MV infection. *J Virol* 1996;70: 6673–6681.
232. Horwitz MS, Evans CF, Klier FG, et al. Detailed in vivo analysis of interferon-gamma induced major histocompatibility complex expression in the central nervous system. *Lab Invest* 1999;79:235–243.
233. Howard MK, Mailhos C, Dent CL, et al. Transactivation by herpes simplex virus virion protein Vmw65 and viral permissivity in a neuronal cell line with reduced levels of the cellular transcription factor Oct-1. *Exp Cell Res* 1993;207:194–196.
234. Howe H, Bodian D. *Neural mechanisms in poliomyelitis.* New York: Commonwealth Fund, 1942.
235. Huang S, Reddy V, Dasgupta N, et al. A single amino acid in the adenovirus type 37 fiber confers binding to human conjunctival cells. *J Virol* 1999;73:2798–2802.
236. Huang XF, Compans RW, Lamb RA, et al. Polarized apical targeting directed by the signal/anchor region of simian virus 5 hemagglutinin-neuraminidase. *J Biol Chem* 1997;272:27598–27604.
237. Huber SA. VCAM-1 is a receptor for encephalomyocarditis virus on murine vascular endothelial cells. *J Virol* 1994;68:3453–3458.
238. Hummel KB, Bellini WJ, Offermann MK. Strain-specific differences in LFA-1 induction on measles-virus infected monocytes and adhesion and viral transmission to endothelial cells. *J Virol* 1998;72: 8403–8407.
239. Huo TI, Wu JC, Huang YH, et al. Evidence for transmission of hepatitis B virus to spouses from sequence analysis of the viral genome. *J Gastroenterol Hepatol* 1998;13:1138–1142.
240. Husseini R, Sweet C, Collie M, et al. Elevation of nasal viral levels by suppression of fever in ferrets infected with influenza viruses of differing virulence. *J Infect Dis* 1982;145:520–524.
241. Hussey GD, Klein M. A randomized controlled trial of vitamin A in children with severe measles. *N Engl J Med* 1990;323:160–164.
242. Igarashi T, Brown C, Azadegan A, et al. Human immunodeficiency virus type 1 neutralizing antibodies accelerate clearance of cell-free virions from blood plasma. *Nat Med* 1999;5:211–216.
243. Inada T, Mims CA. Mouse Ia antigens are receptors for lactate dehydrogenase virus. *Nature* 1984;309:59–61.
244. Irie H, Koyama H, Kubo H, et al. Herpes simplex virus hepatitis in macrophage-depleted mice: the role of massive, apoptotic cell death in pathogenesis. *J Gen Virol* 1998;79:1225–1231.
245. Iwasaki Y, Liu D, Yamamoto T, et al. On the replication and spread of rabies virus in the human central nervous system. *J Neuropathol Exp Neurol* 1985;44:185–195.
246. Izumi KM, Stevens JG. Molecular and biological characterization of a herpes simplex virus type 1 (HSV-1) neuroinvasiveness gene. *J Exp Med* 1990;172:487–496.
247. Jaax NK, Davis KJ, Gesibert TJ, et al. Lethal experimental infection of rhesus monkeys with Ebola-Zaire (Mayinga) virus by the oral and conjunctival route of exposure. *Arch Pathol Lab Med* 1996;120: 140–155.
248. Joag SV, Adany I, Li Z, et al. Animal model of mucosally transmitted human immunodeficiency virus type 1 disease: intravaginal and oral deposition of simian/human immunodeficiency virus in macaques results in systemic infection, elimination of $CD4^+$ T cells, and AIDS. *J Virol* 1997;71:4016–4023.
249. Johann SV, Gibbons JJ, O'Hara B. GLVR1, a receptor for gibbon ape leukemia virus, is homologous to a phosphate permease of *Neurospora crassa* and is expressed at high levels in brain and thymus. *J Virol* 1992;66:1635–1640.
250. Johnson RT. Selective vulnerability of neural cells to viral infection. *Brain* 1980;103:447–472.
251. Johnson RT. *Viral infections of the nervous system.* 2nd ed. Philadelphia: Lippincott-Raven Press, 1998.
252. Johnson RT, Calisher C, Thompson W, eds. Pathogenesis of La Crosse virus in mice. In: *California serogroup viruses.* New York: Alan R. Liss, 1983:139–144.
253. Johnston PB, Dubay JW, Hunter E. Truncations of the simian immunodeficiency virus transmembrane protein confer expanded virus host range by removing a block to virus entry into cells. *J Virol* 1993;67: 3077–3086.
254. Joly E, Mucke L, Oldstone MBA. Viral persistence in neurons explained by lack of major histocompatibility complex class I expression. *Science* 1991;253:1283–1285.
255. Jones JF, Fulginiti VA. Perinatal mumps infection. *J Pediatr* 1980;96: 912–914.
256. Jourdan N, Maurice M, Delautier D, et al. Rotavirus is released from the apical surface of cultured human intestinal cells through nonconventional vesicular transport that bypasses the Golgi apparatus. *J Virol* 1997;71:8268–8278.
257. Jubelt B, Narayan O, Johnson RT. Pathogenesis of human poliovirus infection in mice. II. Age-dependency of paralysis. *J Neuropathol Exp Neurol* 1980;39:149–159.
258. Kalicharran K, Dales S. Involvement of microtubules and the microtubule-associated protein tau in trafficking of JHM virus and components within neurons. *Adv Exp Med Biol* 1995;380:57–61.
259. Karger A, Mettenleiter TC. Glycoproteins gII and gp50 play dominant roles in the biphasic attachment of pseudorabies virus. *Virology* 1993;194:654–663.
260. Kark J, Lubiush M, Rannon L. Cigarette smoking as a risk factor for epidemic A (H1N1) influenza in young men. *N Engl J Med* 1982;307: 1042–1046.
261. Karnauchow TM, Tolson DL, Harrison BA, et al. The HeLa cell receptor for enterovirus 70 is decay-accelerating factor (CD55). *J Virol* 1996;70:5143–5152.
262. Kashanchi F, Thompson J, Sadaie MR, et al. Transcriptional activation of minimal HIV-1 promoter ORF-1 protein expressed from the Sal I-L fragment of human herpesvirus 6. *Virology* 1994;201:95–106.
263. Katagiri S, Aikawa S, Hinuma Y. Stepwise degradation of poliovirus capsid by alkaline treatment. *J Gen Virol* 1971;13:101–109.
264. Katz JP, Bodin ET, Coen DM. Quantitative polymerase chain reaction analysis of herpes simplex virus DNA in ganglia of mice infected with replication-incompetent mutants. *J Virol* 1990;64:4288–4295.
265. Katzenstein DA, Mbizvo M, Zjenah L, et al. Serum level of maternal human immunodeficiency virus (HIV) RNA, infant mortality, and vertcial transmission of HIV in Zimbabwe. *J Infect Dis* 1999;179: 1382–1387.
266. Kemp LM, Dent CL, Latchman DS. Octamer motifs mediate transcriptional repression of HSV immediate-early genes and octamer-containing cellular promoters in neuronal cells. *Neuron* 1990;4: 215–227.
267. Kenney S, Natarajan V, Strike D, et al. JC virus enhancer-promoter active in human brain cells. *Science* 1984;226:1337–1339.
268. Keroack M, Fields B. Viral shedding and transmission between hosts determined by reovirus L2 gene. *Science* 1986;232:1635–1638.

269. Kido H, Yokogoshi Y, Saki K, et al. Isolation and characterization of a novel trypsin-like protease found in rat bronchial epithelial Clara cells. *J Biol Chem* 1992;267:13573–13579.
270. Kim JW, Closs EI, Albritton LM, Cunningham JM. Transport of cationic amino acids by the mouse ecotropic retrovirus receptor. *Nature* 1991;352:725–728.
271. King SL, Cunningham JA, Finberg RW, et al. Echovirus 1 interaction with isolated VLA-2 I domain. *J Virol* 1995;69:3237–3239.
272. Kinman TG, de Wind N, Oei-Lie N, et al. Contribution of single genes within the unique short region of Aujesky's disease virus (suid herpesvirus type 1) to virulence, pathogenesis and immunogenicity. *J Gen Virol* 1992;73:243–251.
273. Kirchoff R, Greenough TC, Brettler DB, et al. Absence of intact *nef* sequences in a long term survivor with nonprogressive HIV infection. *N Engl J Med* 1995;332:2742–2748.
274. Klatzman D, Champagne E, Charmaret S, et al. T-lymphocyte T4 molecule behaves as the receptor for human retrovirus LAV. *Nature* 1984; 312:767–768.
275. Klenerman P, Rowland-Jones S, McAdams S, et al. Cytotoxic T cell activity antagonized by naturally occurring HIV-1 gag variants. *Nature* 1994;369:403–407.
276. Klenk H-D, Rott R. Biology of influenza virus pathogenicity. *Adv Virus Res* 1988;34:247–281.
277. Knight V, Gilbert BE, Wilson SL, et al., eds. Airborne transmission of virus infections. In: *Genetically altered viruses and the environment.* Cold Spring Harbor, NY: Cold Spring Harbor Laboratory, 1985: 73–94.
278. Knobler RL, Taylor BA, Woddell MK, et al. Host genetic control of mouse hepatitis virus type-4 (JHM strain) replication. *Exp Clin Immunogenet* 1984;1:217–222.
279. Koch WC, Harger JH, Barbstein B, et al. Serologic and virologic evidence for frequent intrauterine transmission of human parvovirus B19 with primary maternal infection during pregnancy. *Pediatr Infect Dis J* 1998;17:489–494.
280. Kosz-Vnenchak M, Jacobson J, Coen DM, et al. Evidence for a novel regulatory pathway for herpes simplex virus gene expression in trigeminal ganglion neurons. *J Virol* 1993;67:5383–5393.
281. Koup RA. Viral escape from CTL recognition. *J Exp Med* 1994;180: 779–782.
282. Kraehenbuhl JP. The gut-associated lymphoid tissue: a major site of HIV replication and CD4 cell loss. *Trends Microbiol* 1998;6:419–420.
283. Kristensson K, Lycke E, Ryotta M, et al. Neuritic transport of herpes simplex virus in rat sensory neurons in vitro: Effects of substances interacting with microtubular function and axonal flow (nocodazde, taxol and erythro-9-3(2-hydroxynonyl)adenine). *J Gen Virol* 1986;67: 2023–2028.
284. Kristensson K, Nennesmo I, Persson L, et al. Neuron to neuron transmission of herpes simplex virus. *J Neurol Sci* 1982;54:149–156.
285. Kristensson K, Weiss DG, Gorio A, eds. Implications of axoplasmic transport for the spread of viruses in the nervous system. In: *Axoplasmic transport in physiology and pathology.* New York: Springer-Verlag, 1982:153–158.
286. Kubota A, Kubota S, Farrell HE, et al. Inhibition of NK cells by murine CMV-encoded class I MHC homologue m144. *Cell Immunol* 1999;191:145–151.
287. Kuhn JE, Kramer MD, Willenbacher W, et al. Identification of herpes simplex virus type 1 glycoproteins interacting with the cell surface. *J Virol* 1990;64:2491–2497.
288. Kuhn L, Steketee RW, Weedon J, et al. Distinct risk factors for intrauterine and intrapartum human immunodeficiency virus transmission and consequences for disease progression in infected children. *J Infect Dis* 1999;179:52–58.
289. Kumar RM, Shahul S. Role of breast-feeding in transmission of hepatitis C virus to infants of HCV-infected mothers. *J Hepatol* 1998; 29:191–197.
290. Kundu A, Avalos RT, Sanderson CM, et al. Transmembrane domain of influenza virus neuraminidase, a type II protein, possesses an apical sorting signal. *J Virol* 1996;70:6508–6515.
291. Kuypers HGJM, Ugolini G. Viruses as transneuronal tracers. *Trends Neurosci* 1990;13:72–75.
292. Kyo S, Inoue M, Koyama M, et al. Detection of high-risk human papillomavirus in the cervix and semen of sex partners. *J Infect Dis* 1994;170:682–685.
293. Lafay F, Coulon P, Astic L, et al. Spread of the CVS strain of rabies virus and of the avirulent mutant Av01 along the olfactory pathways of the mouse after intranasal inoculation. *Virology* 1991;183:320–330.
294. Lamb RA. Paramyxovirus fusion: A hypothesis for changes. *Virology* 1993;197:1–11.
295. Langhoff E, Haseltine WA. Infection of accessory dendritic cells by human immunodeficiency virus type 1. *J Invest Dermatol* 1992;99: 89S–94S.
296. Langhoff E, Terwilliger EF, Bos J, et al. Replication of human immunodeficiency virus type 1 in primary dendritic cell cultures. *Proc Natl Acad Sci U S A* 1991;88:7998–8002.
297. Lathey JL, Wiley CA, Verity MA, et al. Cultured human brain capillary endothelial cells are permissive for infection by human cytomegalovirus. *Virology* 1990;176:266–273.
298. Le Gall S, Erdtmann L, Benichou S, et al. Nef interacts with the mu subunit of clathrin adaptor complexes and reveals a cryptic sorting signal in MHC I molecules. *Immunity* 1998;8:483–495.
299. Lehmann C, Sprenger H, Nain M, et al. Infection of macrophages by influenza A virus: Characteristics of tumor necrosis factor alpha (TNF alpha) gene expression. *Res Virol* 1996;147:123–130.
300. Leib DA, Coen DM, Bogard CL, et al. Immediate-early regulatory gene mutants define different stages in the establishment and reactivation of herpes simplex virus latency. *J Virol* 1989;63:759–768.
301. Levine B, Griffin DE. Molecular analysis of neurovirulent strains of Sindbis virus that evolve during persistent infection of SCID mice. *J Virol* 1993;67:6872–6875.
302. Levine B, Huang Q, Isaacs JT, et al. Conversion of lytic to persistent alphavirus infection by the bcl-2 cellular oncogene. *Nature* 1993; 361:739–742.
303. Levitskaya J, Sharipo A, Leonchiks A, et al. Inhibition of the ubiquitin/proteosome-dependent protein degradation pathway by the Gly-Ala repeat domain of the Epstein-Barr virus nuclear antigen 1. *Proc Natl Acad Sci U S A* 1997;94:12616–12621.
304. Levy J, Joyner J, Borenfreund E. Mouse sperm can horizontally transmit type C viruses. *J Gen Virol* 1980;51:439–443.
305. Levy JA, Margaretten W, Nelson J. Detection of HIV in enterochromaffin cells in the rectal mucosa of an AIDS patient. *Am J Gastroenterol* 1989;84:787–789.
306. Lewis P, Nduati R, Kreiss JK, et al. Cell-free human immunodeficiency virus type 1 in breast milk. *J Infect Dis* 1998;177:34–39.
307. List J, Haase AT. Integration of visna virus DNA occurs and may be necessary for productive infection. *Virology* 1997;237:187–197.
308. Lodge R, Delamarre L, Lalonde JP, et al. Two distinct oncornaviruses harbor an intracytoplasmic tyrosine-based basolateral targeting signal in their viral envelope. *J Virol* 1997;71:5696–5702.
309. Lodge R, Lalonde JP, Lemay G, et al. The membrane-proximal intracytoplasmic tyrosine residue of HIV-1 envelope glycoprotein is critical for basolateral targeting of viral budding in MDCK cells. *EMBO J* 1997;16:695–705.
310. Lodmell D. Genetic control of resistance to street rabies virus in mice. *J Exp Med* 1983;157:451–460.
311. Loewy AD. Viruses as transneuronal tracers for defining neural circuits. *Neurosci Biobehav Rev* 1998;22:679–684.
312. Loffler S, Lottspeich F, Lanza F, et al. CD9, a tetraspan transmembrane protein, renders cells susceptible to canine distemper virus. *J Virol* 1997;71:42–49.
313. Long GE, Rickman LS. Infectious complications of tattoos. *Clin Infect Dis* 1994;18:610–619.
314. Lot F, Seguier JC, Fegeux S, et al. Probable transmission of HIV from an orthopedic surgeon to a patient in France. *Ann Intern Med* 1999;130:1–6.
315. Lucht E, Biberfeld P, Linde A. Epstein-Barr virus (EBV) DNA in saliva and EBV serology of HIV-1 infected persons with and without hairy leukoplakia. *J Infect* 1995;31:189–194.
316. Lucht E, Brytting M, Bjerregaard L, et al. Shedding of cytomegalovirus and herpesviruses 6, 7, and 8 in saliva of human immunodeficiency virus type 1 infected patients and healthy controls. *Clin Infect Dis* 1998;27:137–141.
317. Lutley R, Petursson G, Palsson PA, et al. Antigenic drift in visna virus variation during long-term infection of Icelandic sheep. *J Gen Virol* 1983;64:1433–1440.
318. Lycke E, Kristensson K, Svennerhold B, et al. Uptake and transport of herpes simplex virus in neurites of rat dorsal root ganglia cells in culture. *J Gen Virol* 1984;65:55–64.

319. Lycke E, Tsiang H. Rabies virus infection of cultured rat sensory neurons. *J Virol* 1987;61:2733–2741.
320. Maas HJL, DeBoer GF, Groenendal JE. Age-related resistance to avian leukosis virus. 3. Infectious virus, neutralizing antibody, and tumors in chickens inoculated at various ages. *Avian Pathol* 1982;11: 309–327.
321. MacQuarrie MB, Forghani B, Wolochow D, et al. Hepatitis B transmitted by a human bite. *JAMA* 1974;230:723–724.
322. Maione R, Felsani A, Pozzi L, et al. Polyomavirus genome and polyomavirus enhancer-driven gene expression during myogenesis. *J Virol* 1989;63:4890–4897.
323. Maisner A, Klenk H, Herrler G. Polarized budding of measles virus is not determined by viral surface glycoproteins. *J Virol* 1998;72: 5276–5278.
324. Mandelbrot L. Vertical transmission of viral infections. *Curr Opin Obstet Gynecol* 1998;10:123–128.
325. Manns A, Hanchard B, Morgan OS, et al. Human leukocyte antigen class II alleles associated with human T-cell lymphotropic virus type 1 infection and adult T-cell leukemia/lymphoma in a black population. *J Natl Cancer Inst* 1998;90:617–622.
326. Mansat A, Mengelle C, Chalet M, et al. Cytomegalovirus detection in cryopreserved semen samples collected for therapeutic donor insemination. *Hum Reprod* 1997;12:1663–1666.
327. Maratou E, Theophilidis G, Arsenakis M. Axonal transport of herpes simplex virus-1 in an in vitro model based on the isolated nerve of the frog *Rana ridibunda*. *J Neurosci Methods* 1998;79:75–78.
328. Margolis TP, Sedarati F, Dobson AT, et al. Pathways of viral gene expression during acute neuronal infection with HSV-1. *Virology* 1992;189:150–160.
329. Markwell MAK, Svennerholm L, Paulson JC. Specific gangliosides function as host cell receptors for Sendai virus. *Proc Natl Acad Sci U S A* 1981;78:5406–5410.
330. Marlovits TC, Zechmeister T, Gruenberger M, et al. Recombinant soluble low density lipoprotein receptor fragment inhibits minor group rhinovirus infection in vitro. *FASEB J* 1998;12:695–703.
331. Marsh M, Helenius A. Virus entry into animal cells. *Adv Virol Res* 1989;36:107–151.
332. Martin X, Dolivo M. Neuronal and transneuronal tracing in the trigeminal system of the rat using the herpes virus suis. *Brain Res* 1983;273:253–276.
333. Martino TA, Petric M, Brown M, et al. Cardiovirulent coxsackieviruses and the decay accelerating factor (CD55) receptor. *Virology* 1998;244:302–314.
334. Masuda M, Hoffman PM, Ruscetti SK. Viral determinants that control the neuropathogenicity of PVC-211 murine leukemia virus in vivo determine brain capillary endothelial cell tropism in vitro. *J Virol* 1993;67:4580–4587.
335. McChesney MB, Miller CJ, Rota PA, et al. Experimental measles. I. Pathogenesis in the normal and the immunized host. *Virology* 1997; 233:74–84.
336. McClure JE. Cellular receptor for Epstein-Barr virus. *Prog Med Virol* 1992;39:116–138.
337. McCune JM. Viral latency in HIV disease. *Cell* 1995;82:183–188.
338. McDougal JS, Kennedy MS, Sligh JM, et al. Binding of HTLV III/LAV to $T4^+$ T cells by a complex of the 110K viral protein and the T4 molecule. *Science* 1986;231:382–385.
339. McKeating JA, Wiley RL. Structure and function of the HIV envelope. *AIDS* 1989;3(suppl 1):S35–S41.
340. Mellerick DM, Fraser NW. Physical state of the latent herpes simplex virus genome in a mouse model system: evidence suggesting an episomal state. *Virology* 1987;158:265–275.
341. Mellors JW, Rinaldo CR Jr, Gupta P, et al. Prognosis in HIV-1 infection predicted by the quantity of virus in plasma. *Science* 1996;272: 1167–1170.
342. Memar OM, Arany I, Tyring SK. Skin-associated lymphoid tissue in human immunodeficiency-1, human papillomavirus, and herpes simplex virus infections. *J Invest Dermatol* 1995;105(suppl 1):99S–104S.
343. Mendelsohn C, Wimmer E, Racaniello V. Cellular receptor for poliovirus: Molecular cloning, nucleotide sequence, and expression of a new member of the immunoglobulin superfamily. *Cell* 1989;56: 855–865.
344. Menu E, Mbopi-Keou FX, Lagaye S, et al. Selection of maternal human immunodeficiency virus type 1 variants in human placenta. *J Infect Dis* 1999;179:44–51.
345. Michael NL, Louie LG, Rohrbaugh AL, et al. The role of CCR5 and CCR2 polymorphisms in HIV-1 transmission and disease progression. *Nat Med* 1997;3:1160–1162.
346. Michael NL, Mo T, Merzouki A, et al. Human immunodeficiency virus type 1 cellular RNA load and splicing patterns predicts disease progression in a longitudinally studied cohort. *J Virol* 1995;69: 1868–1877.
347. Milgrim LM, Rubin JS, Small CB. Mucociliary clearance abnormalities in the HIV-infected patient: A precursor to acute sinusitis. *Laryngoscope* 1996;105:1202–1208.
348. Miller DM, Sedmark DD. Viral effects on antigen processing. *Curr Opin Immunol* 1999;11:94–99.
349. Miller N, Hutt-Fletcher LM. Epstein-Barr virus enters B cells and epithelial cells by different routes. *J Virol* 1992;66:3409–3414.
350. Mims C, Dimmock NJ, Nash A, et al., eds. *Mims' pathogenesis of infectious disease.* 4th ed. London: Academic Press, 1995.
351. Mims CA, White DO. *Viral pathogenesis and immunology.* Oxford: Blackwell Scientific Publications, 1984.
352. Mochizuki Y, Tashiro M, Homma M. Pneumopathogenicity in mice of a Sendai virus mutant, tsrev-58, is accompanied by in vitro activation with trypsin. *J Virol* 1988;62:3040–3042.
353. Mofenson LM, Lambert JS, Stiehm ER, et al. Risk factors for perinatal transmission of human immunodeficiency virus type 1 in women treated with zidovudine. *N Engl J Med* 1999;341:385–393.
354. Moffat JF, Zerboni L, Kinchington PR, et al. Attenuation of the vaccine Oka strain of varicella-zoster virus and role of glycoprotein C in alphaherpesvirus virulence demonstrated in the SCID-hu mouse. *J Virol* 1998;72:965–974.
355. Monath TP, Cropp C, Harrison A. Mode of entry of a neurotropic arbovirus into the central nervous system. *Lab Invest* 1983;48: 399–410.
356. Monazahian M, Bohme I, Bonk S, et al. Low density lipoprotein receptor as a candidate receptor for hepatitis C virus. *J Med Virol* 1999;57:223–229.
357. Montgomery RI, Warner MS, Lum BJ, et al. Herpes simplex virus-1 entry into cells is mediated by a novel member of the TNF/NGF receptor family. *Cell* 1996;87:427–436.
358. Morales JA, Herzog S, Kompter C, et al. Axonal transport of Borna virus along olfactory pathways in spontaneously and experimentally infected rats. *Med Microbiol Immunol* 1988;177:51–68.
359. Morgensen S. Role of macrophages in natural resistance to virus infection. *Microbiol Rev* 1979;43:1–26.
360. Morin MJ, Warner A, Fields BN. A pathway of entry of reoviruses into the host through M cells of the respiratory tract. *J Exp Med* 1994;180: 1523–1527.
361. Moriuchi M, Moriuchi H, Turner W, et al. Exposure to bacterial products renders macrophages highly susceptible to T-tropic HIV-1. *J Clin Invest* 1998;102:1540–1550.
362. Morrison LA, Fields BN. Parallel mechanisms in neuropathogenesis of enteric virus infections. *J Virol* 1991;65:2767–2772.
363. Morrison LA, Sidman RL, Fields BN. Direct spread of reoviruses from the intestinal lumen to the central nervous system through vagal autonomic fibers. *Proc Natl Acad Sci U S A* 1991;88:3852–3856.
364. Moscufo N, Yafal AG, Rogove A, et al. A mutation in VP4 defines a new step in the late stages of cell entry by poliovirus. *J Virol* 1993;67: 5075–5078.
365. Moulian N, Borrih-Aknin S. FAS/APO-1/CD95 in health and autoimmune disease. *Semin Immunol* 1998;10:449–456.
366. Mrkic B, Pavlovic J, Rulicke T, et al. Measles virus spread and pathogenesis in genetically altered mice. *J Virol* 1998;72:7420–7427.
367. Murphy FA. Rabies pathogenesis: brief review. *Arch Virol* 1977;54: 279–297.
368. Murphy FA, Taylor W, Mims C, et al. Pathogenesis of Ross River virus infection in mice. II. Muscle, heart, and brown fat lesions. *J Infect Dis* 1973;127:129–138.
369. Murphy FA, Whitfield SG, Sudia WD, et al., eds. *Invertebrate immunity.* Orlando: Academic Press, 1979:25.
370. Naif HM, Li S, Alali M, et al. Definition of the stage of host cell genetic restriction of replication of human immunodeficiency virus type 1 in monocytes and monocyte-derived macrophages by using twins. *J Virol* 1999;73:4866–4881.
371. Naniche D, Varior-Krishnan G, Cervoni F, et al. Human membrane cofactor protein (CD46) acts as a cellular receptor for measles virus. *J Virol* 1993;67:6025–6032.

372. Narayan O, Griffin D, Silverstein A. Slow virus infection: replication and mechanisms of persistence of Visna virus in sheep. *J Infect Dis* 1977;135:800–806.
373. Narwa R, Roques P, Courpotin C, et al. Characterization of human immunodeficiency virus type 1 p17 matrix protein motifs associated with mother-to-child transmission. *J Virol* 1996;70:4474–4483.
374. Nathanson N, Bodian D. Experimental poliomyelitis following intramuscular virus injection. I. The effect of neural block on a neurotropic and a pantropic strain. *Bull Johns Hopkins Hosp* 1961;108:308–319.
375. Nathanson N, Langmuir A. The Cutter incident: Poliomyelitis following formaldehyde-inactivated poliovirus vaccination in the United States during the spring of 1955. *Am J Hyg* 1963;78:16–81.
376. Nathanson N, Monath TP, eds. Pathogenesis. In: *St Louis encephalitis*. Washington, DC: American Public Health Association, 1980: 201–236.
377. Nathanson N, Tyler KL, Collier L, eds. Pathogenesis of viral infections. In: *Topley & Wilson's microbiology and microbial infections*. 5th ed. London: Edward Arnold, 1998:149–172.
378. Nathanson N, Tyler KL, Nathanson N, eds. Entry, dissemination, shedding, and transmission of viruses. In: *Viral pathogenesis*. New York: Lippincott-Raven, 1997:13–33.
379. Nelson JA, Wiley CA, Reynolds-Kohler C, et al. Human immunodeficiency virus detected in bowel epithelium from patients with gastrointestinal symptoms. *Lancet* 1988;1:259–262.
380. Neuzil KM, Gruber WC, Chytil F, et al. Serum vitamin A levels in respiratory syncytial virus infection. *J Pediatr* 1994;124:433–436.
381. Nibert ML, Furlong DB, Fields BN. Mechanisms of viral pathogenesis: Distinct forms of reoviruses and their roles during replication in cells and host. *J Clin Invest* 1991;88:727–734.
382. Nicolau S, Mateiesco E. Septinevrites a virus rabique des rues: Preuves de la marche centrifuge du virus dans les nerfs peripheriques des lapins. *CR Acad Sci* 1928;186:1072–1074.
383. Niewiesk S, Schneider-Schaulies J, Ohnimus H, et al. CD46 expression does not overcome the intracellular block of measles virus replication in transgenic rats. *J Virol* 1997;71:7969–7973.
384. Norgren RB, Lehman MN. Herpes simplex virus as a transneuronal tracer. *Neurosci Biobehav Rev* 1998;22:695–708.
385. Norkin LC. Virus receptors: Implications for pathogenesis and the design of antiviral agents. *Clin Microbiol Rev* 1995;8:293–315.
386. O'Neill H, Blanden R. Mechanisms determining innate resistance to ectromelia virus infection in C57BL mice. *Infect Immun* 1983;41: 1391–1394.
387. Oaks JL, McGuire TC, Ulibarri C, et al. Equine infectious anemia virus is found in tissue macrophages during subclinical infection. *J Virol* 1998;72:7263–7269.
388. Ogata A, Nagashima K, Hall WW, et al. Japanese encephalitis virus neurotropism is dependent on the degree of neuronal maturity. *J Virol* 1991;65:880–886.
389. Ohka S, Yang WX, Terada E, et al. Retrograde transport of intact poliovirus through the axon via the fast axonal transport system. *Virology* 1998;250:67–75.
390. Oie M, Shida H, Ichihashi Y. The function of the vaccinia hemagglutinin in the proteolytic activation of infectivity. *Virology* 1990;176: 494–504.
391. Okazaki K, Matsuzaki T, Sugahara Y, et al. BHV-1 adsorption is mediated by the interaction of glycoprotein gIII with heparinlike moiety on the cell surface. *Virology* 1991;181:666–670.
392. Oldstone MBA. How viruses escape from cytotoxic T lymphocytes: Molecular parameters and players. *Virology* 1997;234:179–185.
393. Oldstone MBA, Ahmed R, Buchmeier M, et al. Perturbation of differentiated functions during viral infection in vivo. I. Relationship of lymphocytic choriomeningitis virus and host strains to growth hormone deficiency. *Virology* 1985;142:158–174.
394. Oldstone MBA, Buchmeier MJ. Restricted expression of viral glycoprotein in cells of persistently infected mice. *Nature* 1982;350:360–362.
395. Oldstone MBA, Tishon A, Dutko FJ, et al. Does the major histocompatibility complex serve as a specific receptor for Semliki Forest virus? *J Virol* 1980;34:256–265.
396. Oliver KR, Fazakerley JK. Transneuronal spread of Semliki Forest virus in the developing mouse olfactory system is determined by neuronal maturity. *Neuroscience* 1998;82:867–877.
397. Omary MB, Brenner DA, de Grandpre LA, et al. HIV-1 infection and expression in human colonic cells: Infection and expression in $CD4^+$ and $CD4^-$ cell-lines. *AIDS* 1991;5:275–281.
398. Orenstein J, Fox C, Wahl SM. Macrophages as a source of HIV during opportunistic infections. *Science* 1997;276:1857–1961.
399. Palmiter R, Chen H, Messing A, et al. SV40 enhancer and large-T antigen are instrumental in development of choroid plexus tumors in transgenic mice. *Nature* 1985;316:457–460.
400. Pancic F, Carpentier DC, Came PE. Role of infectious secretions in the transmission of rhinoviruses. *J Clin Microbiol* 1980;12:567–571.
401. Pantaleo G, Graziosi C, Demarest JF, et al. HIV infection is active and progressive in lymphoid tissue during the clinically latent stage of the disease. *Nature* 1993;362:355–358.
402. Pantaleo G, Graziosi C, Fauci AS. The immunopathogenesis of human immunodeficiency virus infection. *N Engl J Med* 1993;328:327–335.
403. Papi A, Johnson SL. Rhinovirus infection induces expression of its own receptor intracellular adhesion molecule 1 (ICAM-1) via increased NF-kappaB-mediated transcription. *J Biol Chem* 1999;274: 9707–9720.
404. Paquette Y, Kay DG, Rassart E, et al. Substitution of the U3 long terminal repeat region of the neurotropic CAS-Br-E retrovirus affects its disease inducing potential. *J Virol* 1990;64:3742–3752.
405. Park BH, Lavi E, Blank KJ, et al. Intracerebral hemorrhages and syncytium formation induced by endothelial infection with a murine leukemia virus. *J Virol* 1993;67:6015–6024.
406. Paul RW, Choi AH, Lee PWK. The alpha-anomeric form of sialic acid is the minimal receptor determinant recognized by reovirus. *Virology* 1989;172:382–385.
407. Perlman S, Evans G, Afifi A. Effect of olfactory bulb ablation on spread of a neurotropic coronavirus into the mouse brain. *J Exp Med* 1990;172:1127–1132.
408. Perlman S, Jacobsen G, Afifi A. Spread of a neurotropic coronavirus into the CNS via the trigeminal and olfactory nerves. *Virology* 1989; 170:556–560.
409. Petersen LR, Simonds RJ, Koistinen J. HIV transmission through blood, tissues, and organs. *AIDS* 1993;7(suppl 1):S99–S107.
410. Piatak M, Saag MS, Yang LC, et al. High levels of HIV-1 in plasma during all stages of infection determined by competitive PCR. *Science* 1993;259:1749–1754.
411. Pitts O, Powers M, Bilello J, et al. Ultrastructural changes associated with retroviral replication in central nervous system capillary endothelial cells. *Lab Invest* 1987;56:401–409.
412. Plaeger S, Bermudez S, Mikyas Y, et al. Decreased CD8 cell-mediated viral suppression and other immunologic characteristics of women who transmit human immunodeficiency virus to their infants. *J Infect Dis* 1999;179:1388–1394.
413. Ploegh HL. Viral strategies of immune evasion. *Science* 1998;280: 248–253.
414. Poli G, Fauci AS. The role of monocytes/macrophages and cytokines in the pathogenesis of human immunodeficiency virus infection. *Pathobiology* 1992;60:246–251.
415. Pomerantz RJ, de la Monte SM, Donnegan SP, et al. Human immunodeficiency virus infection of the human cervix. *Ann Intern Med* 1988;108:321–327.
416. Pope M, Betjes MG, Romani N, et al. Conjugates of dendritic cells and memory T lymphocytes from skin facilitate productive infection with HIV-1. *Cell* 1994;78:389–398.
417. Portis JL, McAtee F, Hayes S. Horizontal transmission of murine retroviruses. *J Virol* 1987;61:1037–1044.
418. Puertollano R, Martin-Belmonte F, Millan J, et al. The MAL proteolipid protein is necessary for normal apical transport and accurate sorting of the influenza virus hemagglutinin in Madin-Darby canine kidney cells. *J Cell Biol* 1999;145:141–151.
419. Puri A, Booy FP, Doms RW, et al. Conformational changes and fusion activity of influenza virus hemagglutinin of the H2 and H3 subtypes: Effects of acid pretreatment. *J Virol* 1990;64:3824–3832.
420. Rabin E, Jenson A, Melnick J. Herpes simplex virus in mice: Electron microscopy of neural spread. *Science* 1968;162:126–129.
421. Racaniello VR. Early events in poliovirus infection: Virus-receptor interactions. *Proc Natl Acad Sci U S A* 1996;93:11378–11381.
422. Raffery MJ, Behrens CK, Muller A, et al. Herpes simplex virus type 1 infection of activated cytotoxic T cells: Induction of fratricide as a mechanism of viral immune evasion. *J Exp Med* 1999;190: 1103–1111.
423. Rall GF, Mucke L, Oldstone MBA. Consequences of cytotoxic T lymphocyte interaction with major histocompatibility complex class I-expressing neurons in vivo. *J Exp Med* 1995;182:1201–1212.

424. Ramakrishnan R, Poliani PL, Levine M, et al. Detection of herpes simplex virus type 1 latency-associated transcript expression in trigeminal ganglia by in situ reverse transcriptase PCR. *J Virol* 1996; 70:6519–6523.
425. Ramarli D, Giri A, Reina S, et al. HIV-1 spreads from lymphocytes to normal human keratinocytes suitable for autologous and allogenic transplantation. *J Invest Dermatol* 1995;105:644–647.
426. Rasko JE, Battini JL, Gottschalk RJ, et al. The RD114/simian type D retrovirus receptor is a neural amino acid transporter. *Proc Natl Acad Sci U S A* 1999;96:2129–2134.
427. Ravkov EV, Nichol ST, Compans RW. Polarized entry and release in epithelial cells of Black Creek Canal virus: A new world hantavirus. *J Virol* 1997;71:1147–1154.
428. Ray NB, Ewalt LC, Lodmell D. Rabies virus replication in primary murine bone marrow macrophages and in human and murine macrophage-like cell lines: Implications for persistence. *J Virol* 1995;69: 764–772.
429. Razvi ES, Welsh RM. Apoptosis in viral infections. *Adv Virus Res* 1995;45:1–60.
430. Reece JC, Handley AJ, Anstee EJ, et al. HIV-1 selection by epidermal dendritic cells during transmission across human skin. *J Exp Med* 1998;187:1623–1631.
431. Reinacher M, Bonin J, Narayan O, et al. Pathogenesis of neurovirulent influenza A virus infection in mice. *Lab Invest* 1983;49:686–692.
432. Ren R, Racaniello VR. Poliovirus spreads from muscle to the central nervous system by neural pathways. *J Infect Dis* 1992;166:747–752.
433. Richardson S, Grimwood K, Gorrell R, et al. Extended excretion of rotavirus and severe diarrhea in young children. *Lancet* 1998;351: 1844–1848.
434. Rinaldo CR JR. Modulation of major histocompatibility antigen expression by viral infection. *Am J Pathol* 1994;144:637–650.
435. Roberts N. Temperature and host defense. *Microbiol Rev* 1979;43: 241–259.
436. Roberts SR, Compans RW, Wertz GW. Respiratory syncytial virus matures at the apical surfaces of polarized epithelial cells. *J Virol* 1995;69:2667–2673.
437. Rocha G, Deschenes J, Rowsey JJ. The immunology of corneal graft rejection. *Crit Rev Immunol* 1998;18:305–325.
438. Rochford R, Moreno JP, Peake ML, et al. Enhancer dependence of polyomavirus persistence in mouse kidneys. *J Virol* 1992;66: 3287–3297.
439. Rochford R, Villarreal LP. Polyomavirus DNA replication in the pancreas and in a transformed pancreas cell line has distinct enhancer requirements. *J Virol* 1991;65:2108–2112.
440. Rock DL, Fraser NW. Detection of HSV-1 genome in the central nervous system of latently infected mice. *Nature* 1983;302:523–525.
441. Rodrigues P, Heard JM. Modulation of phosphate uptake and amphotropic murine leukemia virus entry by posttranslational modifications of PIT-2. *J Virol* 1999;73:3789–3799.
442. Rodriguez-Boulan E, Sabatini DD. Asymmetric building of viruses in epithelial monolayers: a model system for study of epithelial polarity. *Proc Natl Acad Sci U S A* 1978;75:5071–5075.
443. Roelvink PW, Lizonova A, Lee JG, et al. The coxsackievirus-adenovirus receptor protein can function as a cellular attachment protein for adenovirus serotypes from subgroups A, C, D, E, and F. *J Virol* 1998;72:7909–7915.
444. Roivainen M, Pirainen L, Hovi T, et al. Entry of coxsackievirus A9 into host cells: Specific interactions with $\alpha_v v_3$ integrin, the vitronectin receptor. *Virology* 1994;203:357–365.
445. Rolsma MD, Kuhlenschmidt TB, Gelberg HB, et al. Structure and function of a ganglioside receptor for porcine rotavirus. *J Virol* 1998;72:9079–9091.
446. Rossen JW, de Beer R, Godeke GJ, et al. The viral spike protein is not involved in the polarized sorting of coronaviruses in epithelial cells. *J Virol* 1998;72:497–503.
447. Rossen JW, Voorhout WF, Horzinek MC, et al. MHV-A59 enters polarized murine epithelial cells through the apical surface but is released basolaterally. *Virology* 1995;210:54–66.
448. Rotbart HA. Enteroviral infections of the central nervous system. *Clin Infect Dis* 1995;20:971–981.
449. Rotem-Yehudar R, Groettrup M, Soza A, et al. LMP-associated proteolytic activities and TAP-dependent peptide transport for class I MHC molecules are suppressed in cell lines transformed by the highly oncogenic adenovirus 12. *J Exp Med* 1996;183:499–514.
450. Rubin DH, Fields BN. Molecular basis of reovirus virulence: role of the M2 gene. *J Exp Med* 1980;152:853–868.
451. Rubin SA, Waltrip RW, Bautista JR, et al. Borna disease virus in mice: Host-specific differences in disease expression. *J Virol* 1993;67: 548–552.
452. Saah AJ, Hoover DR, Weng S. Association of HLA profiles with early plasma viral load, $CD4^+$ cell count and rate of progression to AIDS following acute HIV-1 infection. *AIDS* 1998;12:2107–2113.
453. Sabin A, Olitsky P. Influence of host factors on neuroinvasiveness of vesicular stomatitis virus. *J Exp Med* 1937;66:15–67, 201–208, 229–249.
454. Sabin AB. Pathogenesis of poliomyelitis: reappraisal in the light of new data. *Science* 1956;123:1151–1157.
455. Saif LJ, Theil KW, eds. Comparative aspects of enteric viral infections. In: *Viral diarrheas of man and animal.* Boca Raton, FL: CRC Press, 1990:9–31.
456. Salleras L, Bruguera M, Vidal J, et al. Importance of sexual transmission of hepatitis C virus in seropositive women: A case- control study. *J Med Virol* 1997;52:164–167.
457. Santis G, Legrand V, Hong SS, et al. Molecular determinants of adenovirus serotype 5 fibre binding to its cellular receptor CAR. *J Gen Virol* 1999;80:1519–1527.
458. Sawtell NM, Thompson RL. Herpes simplex virus type 1 latency-associated transcription unit promotes anatomical site-dependent establishment and reactivation from latency. *J Virol* 1992;66: 2157–2169.
459. Sawyer W, Meyer K, Eaton M, et al. Jaundice in army personnel in the western region of the United States and its relation to vaccination against yellow fever. *Am J Hyg* 1944;39:337–430.
460. Scheid A, Choppin PW, Notkins AL, et al., eds. Proteolytic cleavage and viral pathogenesis. In: *Concepts in viral pathogenesis.* New York: Springer-Verlag, 1984:26–31.
461. Schlegel R, Willingham M, Pastan I. Saturable binding sites for vesicular stomatitis virus on the surface of vero cells. *J Virol* 1982;43: 871–875.
462. Schulman JL. Experimental transmission of influenza virus infection in mice. IV. Relationship of transmissibility of different strains of virus and recovery of airborne virus in the environment of effector mice. *J Exp Med* 1967;125:479–488.
463. Scott RM, Snitbhan R, Bancroft WH, et al. Experimental transmission of hepatitis B virus by semen and saliva. *J Infect Dis* 1980;142:67–71.
464. Sedarati F, Margolis TP, Stevens JG. Latent infection can be established with drastically restricted transcription and replication of the HSV-1 genome. *Virology* 1993;192:687–691.
465. Sellers M. Studies on the entry of viruses into the central nervous system of mice via the circulation: Differential effects of vasoactive amines and CO on virus infectivity. *J Exp Med* 1969;129:719–746.
466. Shafren DR. Viral cell entry mediated by cross-linked decay-accelerating factor. *J Virol* 1998;72:9407–9412.
467. Shankar V, Dietzschold B, Koprowski H. Direct entry of rabies virus into the central nervous system without prior local replication. *J Virol* 1991;65:2736–2738.
468. Shieh MT, WuDunn D, Montgomery RI, et al. Cell surface receptors for herpes simplex virus are heparan sulfate proteoglycans. *J Cell Biol* 1992;116:1273–1281.
469. Sicinski P, Rowinski J, Warchol JB, et al. Poliovirus type 1 enters the human host through intestinal M cells. *Gastroenterology* 1990;98: 56–58.
470. Siebers A, Finlay BB. M cells and the pathogenesis of mucosal and systemic infections. *Trends Microbiol* 1996;4:22–29.
471. Sinzger C, Plachter B, Grefte A, et al. Tissue macrophages are infected by human cytomegalovirus in vivo. *J Infect Dis* 1996;173: 240–245.
472. Sitas F, Newton R, Boshoff C. Increasing probability of mother-to-child transmission of HHV-8 with increasing maternal antibody titer for HHV-8. *N Engl J Med* 1999;340:1923.
473. Skehel JJ, Bayley PM, Brown EB, et al. Changes in the conformation of influenza virus hemagglutinin at the pH optimum of virus mediated membrane fusion. *Proc Natl Acad Sci U S A* 1982;79:968–972.
474. Small J, Scangos G, Cork L, et al. The early region of human papovirus JC induces dysmyelination in transgenic mice. *Cell* 1986; 46:13–18.
475. Smith G, Symons JA, Khanna A, et al. Vaccinia virus immune evasion. *Immunol Rev* 1997;159:137–154.

476. Smith M, Dean M, Carrington M, et al. Contrasting genetic influences of CCR2 and CCR5 variants on HIV-1 infection and disease progression. *Science* 1997;277:959–965.
477. Soderberg-Naucler C, Fish KN, Nelson JA. Interferon-gamma and tumor necrosis factor-alpha specifically induce formation of cytomegalovirus-permissive monocyte-derived macrophages that are refractory to the antiviral activity of these cytokines. *J Clin Invest* 1997;100:3154–3163.
478. Southern SO. Milk-borne transmission of HIV: Characterization of productively infected cells in breast milk and interactions between milk and saliva. *J Hum Virol* 1998;1:328–337.
479. Spear PG. Entry of alphaherpesviruses into cells. *Semin Virol* 1993;4: 167–180.
480. Staeheli P, Grob R, Meier E, et al. Influenza virus-susceptible mice carry MX genes with a large deletion or a non-sense mutation. *Mol Cell Biol* 1988;8:4518–4523.
481. Staeheli P, Pravtcheva D, Lundin LG, et al. Interferon-regulated influenza virus resistance gene Mx is localized on mouse chromosome 16. *J Virol* 1986;58:967–969.
482. Stanberry LR. Capsaicin interferes with the centrifugal spread of virus in primary and recurrent genital herpes simplex virus infections. *J Infect Dis* 1990;162:29–34.
483. Standish A, Enquist LW, Schwaber JS. Innervation of the heart and its central medullary origin defined by viral tracing. *Science* 1994;263: 232–234.
484. Staunton DE, Merluzzi VJ, Rothlein R, et al. A cell adhesion molecule ICAM-1, is the major surface receptor for rhinoviruses. *Cell* 1989;56:849–853.
485. Steinberg BM, Auborn KJ, Bransma JL, et al. Tissue site-specific enhancer function of the upstream regulatory region of human papillomavirus type II in cultured keratinocytes. *J Virol* 1989;63:957–960.
486. Stevens JG. Herpes simplex virus: neuroinvasiveness, neurovirulence, and latency. *Semin Neurosci* 1991;3:141–147.
487. Stevens JG. Overview of herpesvirus latency. *Semin Virol* 1994;5: 191–196.
488. Stevenson PG, Hawke S, Sloan DJ, et al. The immunogenicity of intracerebral virus infection depends on anatomical site. *J Virol* 1997;71:145–151.
489. Storz J, Rott R, Kaluza G. Enhancement of plaque formation and cell fusion of an enteropathogenic coronavirus by trypsin treatment. *Infect Immun* 1981;31:1214–1222.
490. Strack AM, Loewy AD. Pseudorabies virus: A highly specific transneuronal cell body marker in the sympathetic nervous system. *J Neurosci* 1990;10:2139–2147.
491. Strebel PM, Ion-Nedelcu N, Baughman AL, et al. Intramuscular injections within 30 days of immunization with oral poliovirus vaccine: A risk factor for vaccine-associated paralytic poliomyelitis. *N Engl J Med* 1995;332:500–506.
492. Strong JE, Tang D, Lee PWK. Evidence that the epidermal growth factor receptor on host cells confers reovirus infection efficiency. *Virology* 1993;197:405–411.
493. Summerford C, Bartlett JS, Samulski RJ. AlphaVbeta5 integrins: a co-receptor for adeno-associated virus type 2 infection. *Nat Med* 1999;5: 78–82.
494. Summerford C, Samulski RJ. Membrane-associated heparan sulfate proteoglycan is a receptor for adeno-associated virus type 2 virions. *J Virol* 1998;72:1438–1445.
495. Sun N, Cassell MD, Perlman S. Anterograde transneuronal transport of herpes simplex virus type 1 strain H129 in the murine visual system. *J Virol* 1996;70:5405–5413.
496. Sun N, Perlman S. Spread of neurotropic coronavirus to spinal cord white matter via neurons and astrocytes. *J Virol* 1995;69:633–641.
497. Superti F, Donelli G. Gangliosides as binding sites in SA-11 rotavirus infection of LLC-MK2 cells. *J Gen Virol* 1991;72:2467–2474.
498. Superti F, Hauttecoeur B, Morelec MJ, et al. Involvement of gangliosides in rabies virus infection. *J Gen Virol* 1986;67:47–56.
499. Tailor CS, Nouri A, Zhao Y, et al. A sodium-dependent neutral amino acid transporter mediates infection of feline and baboon endogenous retroviruses and simian type D retroviruses. *J Virol* 1999;73: 4470–4474.
500. Takata H, Obuchi M, Yamamoto J, et al. L* protein of the DA strain of Theiler's murine encephalomyelitis virus is important for virus growth in a murine macrophage-like cell line. *J Virol* 1998;72:4950–4955.
501. Tan X, Pearce-Pratt R, Phillips DM. Productive infection of a cervical epithelial cell line with human immunodeficiency virus: Implications for sexual transmission. *J Virol* 1993;67:6447–6452.
502. Tashiro M, Klenk H-D, Rott R. Inhibitory effect of a protease inhibitor, leupeptin, on the development of influenza pneumonia, mediated by a concomitant bacteria. *J Gen Virol* 1987;68:2039–2041.
503. Tashiro MJ, Seto JT, Choosakul S, et al. Budding site of Sendai virus in polarized epithelial cells is one of the determinants for tropism and pathogenicity in mice. *Virology* 1992;187:413–422.
504. Taylor-Wiedeman J, Sissons P, Sinclair J. Induction of endogenous cytomegalovirus gene expression after differentiation of monocytes from healthy carriers. *J Virol* 1994;68:1597–1604.
505. Tenti P, Zappatore R, Migliora P, et al. Perinatal transmission of human papillomaviruses from gravidas with latent infections. *Obstet Gynecol* 1999;93:475–479.
506. Thomas DC, Brewer CB, Roth MG. Vesicular stomatitis virus glycoprotein contains a dominant cytoplasmic sorting signal critically dependent upon a tyrosine. *J Biol Chem* 1993;268:3313–3320.
507. Thompson RL, Cook M, Devi-Rao G, et al. Functional and molecular analysis of the avirulent wild-type herpes simplex virus type 1 strain KOS. *J Virol* 1986;58:203–211.
508. Thoulouze MI, Lafage M, Schachner M, et al. The neural cell adhesion molecule is a receptor for rabies virus. *J Virol* 1998;72: 7181–7190.
509. Tomassini JE, Graham D, Dewitt CM, et al. cDNA cloning reveals that the major group rhinovirus receptor on HeLa cells is intercellular adhesion molecule 1. *Proc Natl Acad Sci U S A* 1989;86:4907–4911.
510. Torsteindottir S, Agnarsdottir G, Matthiasdottir S, et al. In vivo and in vitro infection with two different molecular clones of visna virus. *Virology* 1997;229:370–380.
511. Tosteson MT, Nibert ML, Fields BN. Ion channels induced in lipid bilayers by subvirion particles of the nonenveloped mammalian reoviruses. *Proc Natl Acad Sci U S A* 1993;90:10549–10552.
512. Tresnan DB, Holmes KV. Feline aminopeptidase N is a receptor for all group I coronaviruses. *Adv Exp Med Biol* 1998;440:69–75.
513. Tresnan DB, Levis R, Holmes KV. Feline aminopeptidase N serves as a receptor for feline, canine, porcine, and human coronaviruses in serogroup I. *J Virol* 1996;70:8669–8674.
514. Trgovcich J, Ryman K, Extrom P, et al. Sindbis virus infection of neonatal mice results in a severe stress response. *Virology* 1997;227: 234–238.
515. Trousdale M, Steiner I, Spivack JG, et al. In vivo and in vitro reactivation impairment of a herpes simplex virus type 1 latency-associated transcript variant in a rabbit eye model. *J Virol* 1991;65:6989–6993.
516. Tsiang H. Evidence for intraaxonal transport of fixed and street rabies virus. *J Neuropathol Exp Neurol* 1979;38:286–299.
517. Tsiang H. Pathophysiology of rabies virus infection of the nervous system. *Adv Virus Res* 1993;42:375–412.
518. Tsiang H, Ceccaldi PE, Lycke E. Rabies virus infection and transport in human sensory dorsal root ganglia neurons. *J Gen Virol* 1991;72: 1191–1194.
519. Tsiang H, Lycke E, Ceccaldi PE, et al. The anterograde transport of rabies virus in rat sensory dorsal root ganglia neurons. *J Gen Virol* 1989;70:2075–2085.
520. Tucker PC, Strauss EG, Kuhn RJ, et al. Viral determinants of age-dependent virulence of Sindbis virus for mice. *J Virol* 1993;67: 4605–4610.
521. Tucker SP, Compans RW. Virus infection of polarized epithelial cells. *Adv Virus Res* 1993;42:187–247.
522. Tucker SP, Thornton CL, Wimmer E, et al. Vectorial release of poliovirus from polarized human intestinal epithelial cells. *J Virol* 1993;67:4274–4282.
523. Tuffereau C, Benejean J, Blondel D, et al. Low-affinity nerve-growth factor receptor (P75NTR) can serve as a receptor for rabies virus. *EMBO J* 1998;17:7250–7259.
524. Tugizov S, Maidji E, Xiao J, et al. Human cytomegalovirus glycoprotein B contains autonomous determinants for vectorial targeting to apical membranes of polarized epithelial cells. *J Virol* 1998;72: 7374–7386.
525. Tyler K, McPhee D, Fields B. Distinct pathways of viral spread in the host determined by reovirus S1 gene segment. *Science* 1986;233: 770–774.
526. Ubol S, Griffin DE. Identification of a putative alphavirus receptor on mouse neural cells. *J Virol* 1991;65:6913–6921.
527. Ugolini G, Kuypers HGJM, Strick PL. Transneuronal transfer of her-

pes virus from peripheral nerves to cortex and brainstem. *Science* 1989;243:89–91.
528. van der Hoek L, Goudsmit J, Maas J, et al. Human immunodeficiency virus type 1 in faeces and serum: evidence against independently evolving subpopulations. *J Gen Virol* 1998;79:2455–2459.
529. Van Dyke RB, Korber RT, Popek E, et al. The Ariel project: A prospective cohort study of maternal-child transmission of human immunodeficiency virus type 1 in the era of maternal antiretroviral therapy. *J Infect Dis* 1999;179:319–328.
530. Van Dyke T, Finlay C, Miller D, et al. Relationship between simian virus 40 large tumor antigen expression and tumor formation in transgenic mice. *J Virol* 1987;61:2029–2032.
531. Vanderplasschen A, Bublot M, Dubuisson J, et al. Attachment of the gammaherpesvirus bovine herpesvirus 4 is mediated by the interaction of gp8 glycoprotein with heparinlike moieties on the cell surface. *Virology* 1993;196:232–240.
532. Verdin EM, King GL, Maratos-Flier E. Characterization of a common high-affinity receptor for reovirus serotypes 1 and 3 on endothelial cells. *J Virol* 1989;63:1318–1325.
533. Vlasak R, Luytjes W, Spaan W, et al. Human and bovine coronaviruses recognize sialic acid-containing receptors similar to those of influenza C virus. *Proc Natl Acad Sci U S A* 1988;85:4526–4529.
534. Vochem M, Hamprecht K, Jahn G, et al. Transmission of cytomegalovirus to preterm infants through breast milk. *Pediatr Infect Dis J* 1998;17:53–58.
535. Vogt MW, Will DJ, Craven DE, et al. Isolation of HTLVIII/LAV from cervical secretions of women at risk for AIDS. *Lancet* 1986;1: 525–527.
536. Vonderfecht S, Miskuff R, Wee S, et al. Protease inhibitors suppress the in vitro and in vivo replication of rotaviruses. *J Clin Invest* 1988; 82:2011–2016.
537. Wagner EK, Bloom DC. Experimental investigation of herpes simplex virus latency. *Clin Microbiol Rev* 1997;10:419–443.
538. Wahlberg JM, Bron R, Wilschut J, et al. Membrane fusion of Semliki Forest virus involves homotrimers of the fusion protein. *J Virol* 1992;66:7309–7318.
539. Wald A, Corey L, Cone R, et al. Frequent genital herpes simplex virus 2 shedding in immunocompetent women: effect of acyclovir treatment. *J Clin Invest* 1997;99:1092–1097.
540. Wald A, Matson P, Ryncarz A, et al. Detection of herpes simplex virus DNA in semen of men with genital HSV-2 infection. *Sex Transm Dis* 1999;26:1–3.
541. Waldman WJ, Roberts WH, Davis DH, et al. Preservation of natural cytopathogenicity of cytomegalovirus by propagation in endothelial cells. *Arch Virol* 1991;117:143–164.
542. Walters RW, Grunst T, Bergelson JM, et al. Basolateral localization of fiber receptors limits adenovirus infection from the apical surface of airway epithelia. *J Biol Chem* 1999;274:10219–10226.
543. Wang H, Kavanaugh MP, North RA, et al. Cell-surface receptor for ecotropic murine retroviruses is a basic amino-acid transporter. *Nature* 1991;352:729–731.
544. Wang K-S, Kuhn RJ, Strauss EG, et al. High-affinity laminin receptor is a receptor for Sindbis virus in mammalian cells. *J Virol* 1992;66: 4992–5001.
545. Webster L. Inheritance of resistance of mice to enteric bacterial and neurotropic virus infections. *J Exp Med* 1937;65:261–286.
546. Weis W, Brown J, Cusack S, et al. Structure of the influenza virus hemagglutinin complexed with its receptor, sialic acid. *Nature* 1988; 333:426–431.
547. Weiss RA. Human immunodeficiency virus receptors. *Semin Virol* 1992;3:79–84.
548. Weiss RA, Tailor CS. Retrovirus receptors. *Cell* 1995;82:531–533.
549. Weller RO, Engelhardt B, Phillips MJ. Lymphocyte targeting of the central nervous system: A review of afferent and efferent CNS-immune pathways. *Brain Pathol* 1996;6:275–288.
550. Wetzel JD, Wilson GJ, Baer GS, et al. Reovirus variants selected during persistent infections of L cells contain mutations in the viral s1 and S4 genes and are altered in viral disassembly. *J Virol* 1997;71: 1362–1369.
551. Whealy ME, Card JP, Robbins AK, et al. Specific pseudorabies virus infection of the rat visual system requires both gI and gp63 glycoproteins. *J Virol* 1993;67:3786–3797.
552. Whitbeck JC, Peng C, Lou H, et al. Glycoprotein D of herpes simplex virus (HSV) binds directly to HVEM: a member of the tumor necrosis factor receptor superfamily and a mediator of HSV entry. *J Virol* 1997;71:6083–6093.
553. White DO, Fenner FJ. *Medical virology.* 4th ed. San Diego: Academic Press, 1994.
554. White JM. Viral and cellular membrane fusion proteins. *Annu Rev Physiol* 1990;52:675–697.
555. White JM. Membrane fusion. *Science* 1992;258:917–924.
556. White JM, Littman DR. Viral receptors of the immunoglobulin superfamily. *Cell* 1989;56:725–728.
557. Whitley RJ, Scheld WM, Whitley RJ, eds. B virus. In: *Infections of the central nervous system.* 2nd ed. Philadelphia: Lippincott-Raven, 1997: 139–145.
558. Wickham TJ, Mathias P, Cheresh DA, et al. Integrins alpha$_v$beta$_3$ and alpha$_v$beta$_5$ promote adenovirus internalization but not virus attachment. *Cell* 1993;73:309–319.
559. Wiley DC, Skehel JJ. The structure and function of the hemagglutinin membrane glycoprotein of influenza virus. *Annu Rev Biochem* 1987; 56:365–394.
560. Winchester P, Chen Y, Rose S, et al. Major histocompatibility complex II DR alleles DRB1*1501 and those encoding HLA-DR13 are preferentially associated with a diminution in maternally transmitted human immunodeficiency virus 1 infection in different ethnic groups: Determination by an automated sequence-based typing method. *Proc Natl Acad Sci U S A* 1995;92:12374–12378.
561. Winther B, Gwaltney JM, Hendley JO. Respiratory viral infection of monolayer cultures of human nasal epithelial cells. *Am Rev Respir Dis* 1990;141:839–845.
562. Wirth JJ, Amalfitano A, Gross R, et al. Organ- and age-specific replication of polyomavirus in mice. *J Virol* 1992;66:3278–3286.
563. Wofsy C, Cohen J, Haver L, et al. Isolation of the AIDS-associated retrovirus from vaginal and cervical secretions from women with antibodies to the virus. *Lancet* 1986;1:527–529.
564. Wolf JL, Kauffman RS, Finberg R, et al. Determinants of reovirus interaction with intestinal M cells and absorptive cells of murine intestine. *Gastroenterology* 1983;85:291–300.
565. Wolf JL, Rubin D, Finberg R, et al. Intestinal M cells: a pathway for entry of reovirus into the host. *Science* 1981;212:471–472.
566. Woodworth CD, Bowden PE, Doninger J, et al. Characterization of normal human exocervical epithelial cells immortalized in vitro by papillomavirus types 16 and 18 DNA. *Cancer Res* 1988;48: 4620–4628.
567. Woolums AR, Anderson ML, Gunther RA, et al. Evaluation of severe disease induced by aerosol inoculation of calves with bovine respiratory syncytial virus. *Am J Vet Res* 1999;60:473–480.
568. Wortley PM, Hammett TA, Fleming PL. Donor insemination and human immunodeficiency virus transmission. *Obstet Gynecol* 1998;91:515–518.
569. Wright PF, Nathanson N, eds. Respiratory diseases. In: *Viral pathogenesis.* Philadelphia: Lippincott-Raven, 1997:703–711.
570. Wunner WH, Reagan KJ, Koprowski H. Characterization of saturable binding sites for rabies virus. *J Virol* 1984;50:691–697.
571. Wybenga LE, Epand RF, Nir S, et al. Glycophorin as a receptor for Sendai virus. *Biochemistry* 1996;35:9513–9518.
572. Wykes MN, Shellam GR, McCluskey J, et al. Murine cytomegalovirus interacts with major histocompatibility complex class I molecules to establish cellular infection. *J Virol* 1993;67:4182–4189.
573. Yang M, Card JP, Tirabassi RS, et al. Retrograde transneuronal spread of pseudorabies virus in defined neuronal circuitry of the rat brain is facilitated by gE mutations that reduce virulence. *J Virol* 1999;73: 4350–4359.
574. Yeager CL, Ashmun RA, Williams RK, et al. Human aminopeptidase N is a receptor for human coronavirus 229E. *Nature* 1992;357: 420–422.
575. Yee JK. A liver-specific enhancer in the core promoter region of the human hepatitis B virus. *Science* 1989;246:658–661.
576. Yokomori K, Lai MC. The receptor for mouse hepatitis virus in the resistant mouse strain SJL is functional: Implications for the requirement of a second factor for viral infection. *J Virol* 1992;66: 6931–6938.
577. Yotsuyanagi H, Koike K, Yasuda K, et al. Prolonged fecal excretion of hepatitis A virus in adult patients with hepatitis A as determined by polymerase chain reaction. *Hepatology* 1996;24:10–13.

578. Yuhasz SA, Stevens JG. Glycoprotein B is a specific determinant of herpes simplex virus type 1 neuroinvasiveness. *J Virol* 1993;67: 5948–5954.
579. Zhang H, Dornadula G, Beumont M, et al. Human immunodeficiency virus type 1 in the semen of men receiving highly active antiretroviral therapy. *N Engl J Med* 1998;339:1803–1809.
580. Zhang L, Dailey PJ, He T, et al. Rapid clearance of simian immunodeficiency virus particles from plasma of rhesus macaques. *J Virol* 1999;73:855–860.
581. Zhu T, Mo T, Wang N, et al. Genotypic and phenotypic characterization of HIV-1 in patients with primary infection. *Science* 1993;261: 1179–1181.
582. Zurbriggen A, Fujinami R. Theiler's virus infection in nude mice: Viral RNA in vascular endothelial cells. *J Virol* 1988;62:3589–3596.

CHAPTER 10

Cell Transformation by Viruses

Joseph R. Nevins

GENERAL FEATURES OF VIRUS-INDUCED CELL TRANSFORMATION AND ONCOGENESIS

The science of virology includes studies directed at understanding the mechanisms by which pathogenic viruses cause disease. In addition, viruses serve as simple model systems to explore complex cellular events. Also, the ability of the oncogenic viruses to deregulate or disrupt cellular biochemical pathways has led to a better understanding of the role of these pathways in cell growth and differentiation.

Viruses that induce cell transformation and tumor formation can be found in several taxonomic groups. All RNA tumor viruses belong to the retrovirus family and in general represent the generation of viruses that have developed an oncogenic capacity by acquiring and modifying cellular genetic material. There are exceptions, such as the viruses that induce tumors by inserting next to key cellular genes and human T lymphotropic virus-I (HTLV-I), in which the oncogenic activity is due to the action of an essential viral gene. But in the majority of cases, the RNA tumor viruses can be seen as cloning events that select for cellular genes with the capacity to transform when deregulated. The replication of oncogenic retroviruses is not cytocidal, and therefore oncogenic transformation is compatible at the cellular level with the production of infectious progeny virus. However, virus production is not a prerequisite of oncogenesis (115,241).

The DNA tumor viruses come from seven different groups encompassing both nonenveloped and enveloped

TABLE 1. *Oncogenic viruses*

Taxonomic Grouping	Examples	Tumor Types
1. RNA viruses		
Retroviridae		
Mammalian B type	Mouse mammary tumor virus	Mammary carcinoma T-cell lymphoma
Mammalian C type	Murine leukemia viruses Gross leukemia virus Moloney leukemia virus Graffi leukemia virus Friend leukemia virus Moloney sarcoma virus Kirsten sarcoma virus Harvey sarcoma virus Feline leukemia viruses Gardner-Amstein feline sarcoma virus McDonough feline sarcoma virus Simian sarcoma virus	Leukemia, lymphoma, sarcoma, various other malignancies and pathologic conditions
Avian C type	Avian leukosis and sarcoma viruses Rous sarcoma virus Rous-associated viruses (RAV) Avian leukosis viruses Avian myeloblastosis virus Avian erythroblastosis virus Mill-Hill 2 virus Myelocytoma virus MC29	Sarcoma, B-cell lymphoma, myeloid and erythroid leukemia, various carcinomas and other tumors
HTLV-BLV	Human T-lymphotropic virus Bovine leukemia virus	T-cell leukemia[a] B-cell lymphoma
II. DNA viruses		
Adenoviridae	All types	Various solid tumors
Hepadnaviridae	Hepatitis B	Hepatocellular carcinoma[a]
Herpesviridae	EBV	Burkitt's lymphoma (African),[a] nasopharyngeal carcinomas[a]
Papovaviridae		
Polyomaviruses	SV40, polyoma	Various solid tumors
Papillomaviruses	HPV, Shope papillomavirus	Papillomas, carcinomas[a]
Poxviridae	Shope fibroma	Myxomas, fibromas

[a]Human tumors

viruses (Table 1). Regardless of taxonomic provenance, the oncogenic potential of the DNA tumor virus is tightly linked to the genetic strategy of virus replication. In general, the synthesis of infectious progeny is linked to cell death; hence oncogenic transformation can occur only if the viral life cycle is aborted (354).

Some viruses can act as carcinogens in the natural setting, whereas others reveal their oncogenic potential only in experimental systems. The potency of viruses as inducers of tumors varies widely. The most effective retroviruses can initiate tumorous growth in virtually all infected animals within a matter of days. Most other viruses, however, require a much longer latent period, and only a small fraction of the infected hosts eventually develop the virus-induced malignancy. All human tumors associated with virus infections belong in this category. The fact that tumor formation is not an inevitable consequence of virus infection reflects the multistep nature of oncogenesis, in which each step constitutes an independent and irreversible genetic change that incrementally contributes to the deregulation of cell growth. Viral infection represents one of these steps; only if the others occur in the same cell does a cancer develop. In cell culture, viruses can transform cells to a fully oncogenic phenotype. Such cells display all the altered properties of the tumor cell and are capable of initiating a cancer in a susceptible host animal. In some instances, however, the transformation is only partial, discernible in culture by changes in morphology and growth properties but not capable of inducing a tumor *in vivo.*

Virus-induced transformation in cell culture has played a major role in the conversion of modern cancer research into a genetic science. Much of what we know today about molecular mechanisms of oncogenesis has its origin in the study of tumor viruses. These studies have led to an almost universal consensus among cancer researchers that the oncogenic phenotype results from discrete changes in key cellular control genes. Detailed mechanisms of virus-induced oncogenic transformation diverge widely, but all have important characteristics in common. These include a single infectious virus particle is sufficient for transformation: virus-induced transformation is a "single hit" process; all or part of the viral genome persists in the transformed cell, although there is often no production of infectious progeny virus; in virtually all cases of virus-induced transformation, at least part of the viral genome is expressed in the transformed cell; transformation results from corruption of normal cellular growth signals; and reversion of the transformed cellular phenotype can be achieved by specific interference with the function of viral effector molecules (e.g., by transdominant negative mutants of oncogenes).

Viral mutants that are temperature sensitive in their transforming potential can be used to compare cellular properties at the permissive temperature, when the cell is transformed, with the nonpermissive temperature, when the cell is not transformed, but all viral functions not required for the maintenance of transformation are still active. Expression vectors carrying single viral oncogenes have likewise been instrumental in determining the effects of these genes on cellular properties. The alteration of cellular parameters accompanying transformation can be divided into changes in cell growth and changes in cell morphology; the latter affect the cytoskeleton, the cell surface, and extracellular matrix (Table 2). Both kinds of change are interrelated, but not all of the changes are seen in every type of transformed cell.

Alterations in cell growth affect three parameters: saturation density, growth-factor requirements, and anchorage dependence. When normal cells replicate to form a confluent layer, covering the available solid substrate surface, they stop dividing, even if ample nutrients are supplied. This saturation density of a culture is significantly higher when the same cells are transformed, reflecting an enhanced ability of the transformed cells to pile up and to grow in multiple layers (20). If a monolayer of normal cells is infected and transformed by a few individual virus particles, these changes in cellular growth behavior lead to the outgrowth of microtumors, referred to as transformed cell foci (349). Normal cells also are highly dependent for their growth on the presence of growth factors in the culture medium. Viral transformation often abrogates or reduces these growth-factor requirements.

TABLE 2. *The transformed cellular phenotype*

Cellular Property	Oncogenic Change or Component
Growth	Increase in saturation density Reduced growth factor requirement Increased nutrient transport Anchorage independence of growth
Cytoskeleton	Loss of "stress fibers" Redistribution of microfilaments
Cell surface	Increased agglutinability by lectins Increased lateral mobility of transmembrane protein Increased production of surface proteases Decreased adhesion to solid substrates
Extracellular matrix	Decreased levels of fibronectins

Normal fibroblasts and epithelial cells must have a solid glass or plastic surface on which to spread before they can grow and divide. Transformation leads to a loss of this anchorage dependence. Transformed cells are able to form colonies if suspended in a semisolid gel nutrient medium. This anchorage independence allows the selection of a few transformed cells occurring within a population of mostly normal cells (219). The latter will survive in the nutrient gel for a few days, but will not grow and form colonies. In contrast to fibroblasts and epithelial cells, normal hematopoietic cells can often form colonies in semisolid medium, provided the appropriate growth factors are supplied.

As the name implies, transformation also leads to changes in cell morphology. These changes affect the cytoskeleton, the cell surface, and the extracellular matrix (354,374). Cytoskeletal changes are detectable by light-microscopic inspection and show up as a loss of "stress fibers." At the electron-microscopic level, they are seen as a rearrangement and redistribution of microfilaments. Several proteins are involved in this reorganization. The major structural components are actin, myosin, and tropomyosin, and near the plasma membranes, α-actinin, vinculin, and talin (50,341). For instance, actin cables prominent in normal fibroblasts disappear on transformation; the actin becomes diffusely distributed in the cytoplasm. Particularly important in the process of maintenance of cell morphology through the interaction with the extracellular matrix is the action of the focal adhesion kinase, a nonreceptor tyrosine kinase that is intimately involved in the processing of signals from the cell–matrix interaction involving recruitment of the Src kinase (66,153).

Changes in cell-surface glycoproteins make transformed cells agglutinable by lectins such as wheat germ agglutinin or concanavalin A (276). Viral transformation also stimulates the production of surface bound and secreted proteases (59,62,251). These have a mitogenic effect on the cell and facilitate tumor invasion and metastasis in the animal. Finally, cells synthesize macromolecules that form an extracellular matrix important in the attachment, spreading, and movement of the cell. Major components of this matrix are fibronectin, laminin, and collagen. Matrix molecules bind to specific cell-surface receptors called integrins, heterodimeric transmembrane proteins that form a connection between the extracellular matrix and the cytoskeleton (162). Transformed cells show decreased levels of fibronectin because of the action of extracellular proteases, reduced fibronectin synthesis, and reduced expression of fibronectin receptors (61,161,162,249).

VIRUS-INDUCED TRANSFORMATION: MODELS FOR CELL-CYCLE CONTROL AND SIGNAL-TRANSDUCTION PATHWAYS

Much of our present understanding of the cell cycle and cell growth control events derives from an elegant combination of genetics and biochemistry that the budding and fission yeast have provided (143). The ability to identify critical regulatory activities through mutation, to identify the genes that specify these activities, and then to understand the biochemical mechanisms of action of these gene products has been enormously productive. Although the study of the cell cycle in mammalian cells clearly suffers from the limited genetic analysis possible in mammalian systems, studies of the oncogenic action of the proteins encoded by the tumor viruses, particularly the DNA tumor viruses, have provided important insights into the mechanisms controlling mammalian cell growth. Such studies have helped to elucidate roles for the retinoblastoma and p53 tumor-suppressor proteins as regulators of mammalian cell growth (Fig. 1). Each of these proteins controls the progression of cells through the G_1 phase of the cell cycle. The p53 gene plays an additional role in triggering programmed cell death (apoptosis) in response to various signals. In each case, DNA tumor virus oncoproteins act to inhibit the action of these two key tumor-suppressor proteins, thereby driving an otherwise quiescent cell to enter S phase. Indeed, this is the key to understanding the link between the replication strategy of the DNA tumor viruses and their oncogenic potential. The natural host cell for the viruses is a quiescent, differentiated cell that presents an environment that is not conducive to viral DNA replication. Thus the strategy of these viruses is to alter this environment, by deregulating the normal cell-cycle control of entry to S phase to induce the genes encoding activities necessary for DNA replication. In the normal replicative infection by these viruses, this cell-cycle deregulation is of no consequence because the infected cell eventually dies. However, when the infection is in some way impaired, then the events causing deregulation of the cell cycle contribute to oncogenic transformation.

In many respects, the virus-mediated disruption of a cell growth control pathway is analogous to the genetic analysis afforded by yeast. For instance, the inactivation of p53 function through the action of the adenovirus E1B protein is, in principle, equivalent to the isolation of a p53 mutant cell; in essence, the viral protein is a mutagen. Moreover, the ability to understand this "mutation" in the context of a viral infectious cycle provides an additional physiologic context, the evolution of a viral replication strategy, in which to view the mutation.

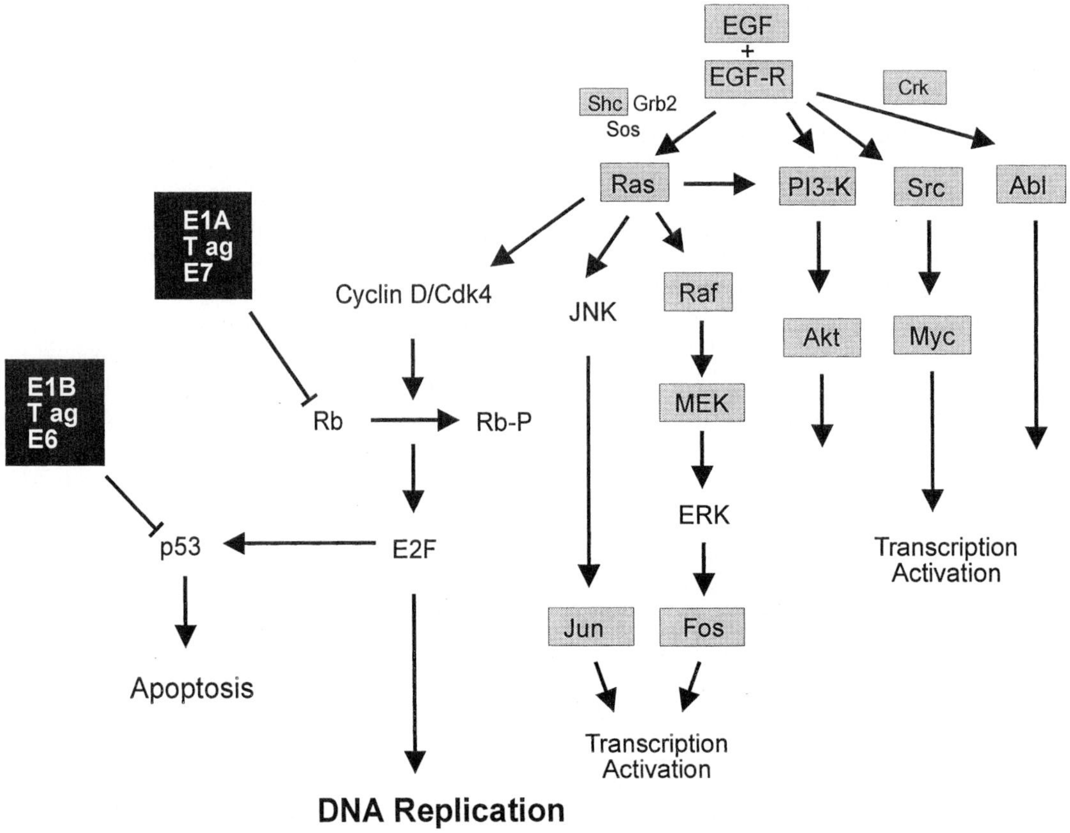

FIG. 1. Cell growth-regulatory pathways, activated by growth factor–receptor activation, which are targets of viral oncoproteins. The DNA tumor virus oncoproteins (*black boxes*) target the Rb and p53 tumor suppressors, leading to an inactivation of their function and deregulation of the G_1 cell-cycle pathway and the apoptotic response pathway. In contrast, the transforming genes found in the RNA tumor viruses (*gray boxes*) represent activated oncogenes, encoding various proteins that function in growth factor–signaling pathways.

Likewise, the analysis of the oncogenes recovered in the RNA tumor viruses has been particularly important for the elucidation of signal-transduction pathways linking the cell surface with the regulation of the genetic apparatus in the nucleus. Unlike the DNA tumor viruses that have adopted a strategy of inactivation of key tumor-suppressor proteins, the RNA tumor viruses have identified oncogenes, the products of which function to drive cell proliferation when deregulated. Perhaps most striking is the fact that the oncogenes recovered in the RNA tumor viruses encode proteins involved in virtually every step in the pathway of signal transduction (see Fig. 1). Indeed, the study of these viral oncogenes has identified many of the participants in these complex pathways. Unlike the oncogenes of the DNA tumor viruses, the RNA tumor virus oncogenes are not essential viral genes but rather, in most cases, are cellular genes that have been acquired during viral replication and selected based on transforming function. As such, the study of these genes cannot be placed in the context of a strategy of viral replication. The presence of these genes usually renders the virus defective for replication. Nevertheless, the real utility of the RNA tumor viruses is the facility with which cellular genes encoding proteins that participate in cell growth control are trapped within the viral genome, altered in the process, and converted to a form that can radically change cell growth properties. The power of this approach is enormous, as evidenced by the sheer number of cellular genes so identified.

Without question, the study of these tumor viruses has been of immense value in elucidating events of cell growth control, providing reagents for further dissection of pathways, and in providing a perspective in which to view the action of various regulatory events. The contributions of the DNA tumor viruses and the RNA tumor viruses are distinct, each group providing unique advantages and approaches to the elucidation of mechanisms of oncogenesis. Indeed, the nature of the oncogenic activities of the two groups of viruses defines the two distinct events of oncogenesis seen in cancer cells: the RNA tumor viruses create oncogenes, whereas the DNA tumor viruses encode proteins that inactivate tumor suppressors. Like the combination of yeast genetics and biochemical analysis that has propelled the analysis of the cell cycle, the combination of these two viral oncogenic systems has provided a wealth of information and afforded an enormously valuable approach to the study of cell growth control and differentiation and the disruption of this control that is evident during oncogenic transformation.

MECHANISMS OF CELL TRANSFORMATION BY THE RNA TUMOR VIRUSES

Since early in the 20th century, retroviruses have been known to cause cancer in animals. Lymphoid tumors in chickens were among the first diseases to be recognized as having a viral etiology; shortly thereafter, virus-induced sarcoma in fowl was discovered (106,295). But these tumors were regarded as somewhat of an oddity, having uncertain relevance for our understanding of cancer in higher animals, let alone cancer in humans. Only when mammary tumors, leukemias, and sarcomas in mice were traced to virus infections did the idea of virus-induced tumors gain some measure of acceptance and respectability as a worthwhile and relevant subject matter for cancer research (34,118,134,137,142,183,233).

The single most important development to open the field of tumor virology as a quantitative science was the advent of cell culture, making it possible to induce oncogenic transformation of individual cells inoculated with cell-free virus. These *in vitro* transformation assays, first established for Rous sarcoma virus (220, 349), provided the basis for cellular and molecular studies that distinguished RNA from DNA tumor viruses and set RNA tumor viruses apart as a unique group of microbes (206,357,375). The salient features of the RNA tumor virus life cycle include reverse transcription of the single-strand RNA viral genome into double-strand DNA; integration of this DNA into the host chromosome; and expression of the integrated provirus under the control of viral transcriptional regulatory sequences. It is the process of reverse transcription that has given this viral group the name retroviruses. Integration into the host genome, together with an absence of cytocidal action, is the basis for the genetic permanence of retroviral infection. Retroviral genomes that become established in the germline are then transmitted as a set of mendelian genetic elements. Of particular importance for oncogenesis are two additional features of the retroviral growth cycle that are direct consequences of integration into the host genome: the ability to acquire and transduce cellular genetic material and the insertional activation (and occasional inactivation) of cellular genes by the integrated provirus. The analysis of retrovirus-induced transformation in cell culture and in animals led to the discovery of a set of cellular genes, called oncogenes, that function as effectors of viral carcinogenesis and play key roles in the control of cell growth and differentiation (for reviews, see refs. 31, 46,282,358,370,371). Retroviruses, through their interaction with oncogenes, have provided independent and often exclusive access to these important regulatory elements of the cell. Today, retroviruses are recognized as significant natural carcinogens in several animal species: fowl, mice, cats, cattle, and monkeys. A rare but aggressive form of human leukemia has been linked to infection with a retrovirus, HTLV-I (122,232,263).

Retroviruses transform cells and induce tumors by three distinct mechanisms (Table 3). Most retroviruses effect oncogenesis through the action of cellular oncogenes. This majority comprises two well-defined

TABLE 3. *Retroviruses: Mechanisms of Oncogenicity*

Virus Category	Tumor Latency Period	Efficiency of Tumor Formation	Oncogenic Effector	State of Viral Genome	Ability to Transform Cultured Cells
Transducing retroviruses	Short (days)	High (can reach 100% of animals)	Cell-derived oncogene carried in viral genome	Viral–cellular chimera, replication defective	Yes
Cis-activating	Intermediate (wk, mo)	High to intermediate	Cellular oncogene activated *in situ* by provirus insertion	Intact, replication competent	No
Trans-activating	Long (mo, yr)	Very low (<5%)	Virus-coded transcriptional regulatory protein	Intact, replication competent	No

groups: retroviruses that carry a cellular oncogene within their genomes, called *transducing retroviruses,* and retroviruses that lack cellular information but transform by integrating in the vicinity of a cellular oncogene, the *cis-activating retroviruses.* Almost all of the transducing retroviruses have lost some viral coding information in exchange for cellular sequences. Consequently they are defective with respect to the production of progeny virus and depend on the co-infection by a closely related helper virus for reproduction. They also are highly efficient carcinogens that transform cells in culture and cause tumors with short latent periods, often within days after infection. All of the cis-activating retroviruses retain the full complement of viral genes and multiply efficiently in solitary infection. Characteristically, they induce tumors more slowly, within weeks or months. In cell culture, these cis-activating retroviruses fail to cause oncogenic transformation. Although the establishment of infection by transducing and by cis-activating retroviruses is dependent on viral coding sequences, such viral coding information does not play an essential and direct role in the processes of oncogenesis induced by these viruses. Transducing retroviruses often have none of their basic coding domains intact, and in cis-activating retroviruses, these also become expendable once the provirus integrates near a cellular oncogene.

Although only poorly understood, a third mechanism of retroviral oncogenesis involves the action of nonstructural viral regulatory proteins that function primarily to enhance transcription from the viral long terminal repeat (LTR). An example is seen in the HTLV-I virus, associated with the development of adult T-cell leukemia, where the viral *Tax* gene, responsible for activation of viral LTR-dependent transcription, has been implicated in oncogenesis. Such a mechanism, involving the action of a viral protein that is essential for viral replicative growth, is analogous to transformation by the DNA tumor viruses. However, in contrast to the DNA viruses in which expression of the viral gene can be observed in the tumor, HTLV-I *Tax* expression is not found in tumors. Moreover, the precise mechanism of action of *Tax,* particularly with respect to how it might contribute to cell transformation, is not understood.

Retrovirus-Mediated Oncogenesis Defines Components of Cellular Regulatory Systems That Control Growth and Differentiation

The vast majority of the oncogenes found in the genomes of retroviruses are derived from the cell. Most cellular proto-oncogenes or c-oncogenes are conserved over long evolutionary distances. For instance, the *ras* oncogene and parts of the *jun* oncogene are found in eukaryotes ranging from yeast to humans. This evolutionary conservation of proto-oncogene sequences suggests that they are indispensable for a broad spectrum of life forms, fulfilling some fundamental function that permits little change. All known oncogenes encode protein products, referred to as *oncoproteins.* There are no cell-derived oncogenes that consist only of noncoding, regulatory sequences. Oncoproteins must, by definition, harbor the potential for inducing oncogenic cellular transformation.

The carcinogenic action of oncogenes is usually a corruption, or deregulation, of their normal physiologic function. To understand oncogene-mediated viral carcinogenesis, it is therefore important to uncover the normal functions of cellular oncogenes. In many instances, the function of the normal cellular gene counterpart has been determined, whereas for a significant fraction of oncogenes, information on physiologic roles remains general and tentative. In general, these genes are involved in the regulation of cell growth, representing components of signaling networks that receive input from outside the cell and propagate the signal to the nucleus, where the information is converted into patterns of gene activity.

A typical growth signal may arrive at the cell surface in the form of a polypeptide growth factor and bind to its specific receptor (see Fig. 1). The receptor, often an integral membrane protein with tyrosine-specific kinase activity, becomes activated by binding to the ligand. It may dimerize, leading to activation of kinase activity and autophosphorylation of specific cytoplasmic residues of the receptor molecule. The signal is further propagated by sequential and specific protein–protein interactions involving numerous participants and ending in the nucleus. The ultimate recipients of incoming signals are transcription factors that control the expression of specific sets of genes.

Of special importance in the transduction of cellular signals are two protein domains that were first recognized in the Src oncoprotein: SH2 (Src homology region 2) and SH3 (Src homology region 3). These domains occur on several protein components of signal-transduction chains; they mediate specific binding of interacting proteins. The SH2 domains bind to phosphotyrosine-containing sequences. The binding specificity is determined by the SH2 sequences in one molecule and the amino acid context of the phosphotyrosine in the other. SH3 domains have an affinity for proline-rich sequences. Proteins carrying SH2 or SH3 domains often also have an enzymatic activity, such as the Src protein tyrosine kinase, but some of these proteins are devoid of any catalytic activity; they function as linker–adaptor molecules and as regulators in binding to and controlling the activity of key enzymes (37,229,236,307).

Table 4 lists the principal retroviral oncogenes, arranged according to function. The *sis* oncogene is

TABLE 4. *Oncogenes recovered in transducing retroviral genomes*

Oncogene	Retrovirus	Oncoprotein[a]	Notes
Growth factors			
sis	Simian sarcoma virus (SSV)	p28$^{env\text{-}sis}$	PDGF
Tyrosine kinase growth-factor receptors			
*erb*B	Avian erythroblastosis virus (AEV)-ES4,[b] AEV-R,[b] AEV-H	gp65^{erbB}	EGF receptor
fms	McDonough feline sarcoma virus (FeSV)	gp180$^{gag\text{-}fms}$	CSF-1 receptor
sea	S13 avian erythroblastosis virus	gp160$^{env\text{-}sea}$	Receptor; ligand unknown
kit	Hardy–Zuckerman-4 FeSV	gp80$^{gag\text{-}kit}$	Hematopoietic receptor; product of the mouse W locus
ros	UR2 avian sarcoma virus (ASV)	p68$^{gag\text{-}ros}$	Receptor, ligand unknown
mpl	Mouse myeloproliferative leukemia virus	p31$^{env\text{-}mpl}$	Member of the hematopoietin receptor family
eyk	Avian retrovirus RPL30	gp37^{eyk}	Receptor, ligand unknown
Hormone receptors			
erbA	AEV-ES4,[b] AEV-R[b]	p75$^{gag\text{-}erbA}$	Thyroid hormone receptor
G proteins			
H-*ras*	Harvey murine sarcoma virus (MSV)	p21^{ras}	
K-*ras*	Kirsten MSV	p21^{ras}	
Adaptor protein			
crk	CT10, ASV-1	p47$^{gag\text{-}crk}$	
Nonreceptor tyrosine kinases			
src	Rous sarcoma virus (RSV)	pp60^{src}	
abl	Abelson murine leukemia virus (MuLV)	p160$^{gag\text{-}abl}$	
fps[c]	Fujinami ASV	p130$^{gag\text{-}fps}$	
	PRC 11 ASV	p105$^{gag\text{-}fps}$	
Fes[c]	Snyder–Theilen FeSV	p85$^{gag\text{-}fes}$	
	Gardner–Amstein FeSV	p110$^{gag\text{-}fes}$	
fgr	Gardner–Rasheed FeSV	p70$^{gag\text{-}actin\text{-}fgr}$	
yes	Y73 ASV	p90$^{gag\text{-}yes}$	
	Esh ASV	p80$^{gag\text{-}yes}$	
Serine–threonine kinases			
mos	Moloney MSV	p37$^{env\text{-}mos}$	
raf[d]	3611-MSV	p75$^{gag\text{-}raf}$	
mil[d]	MH2 avian myelocytoma virus[b]	p100$^{gag\text{-}mil}$	
Transcription factors			
jun	ASV17	p65$^{gag\text{-}jun}$	
fos	Finkel–Biskis–Jenkins MSV	p55^{fos}	
myc	MC29 avian myelocytoma virus	p100$^{gag\text{-}myc}$	
	CMII avian myelocytoma virus	p90$^{gag\text{-}myc}$	
	OK10 avian leukemia virus	p200$^{gag\text{-}pol\text{-}myc}$	
	MH2 avian myelocytoma virus[b]	p59$^{gag\text{-}myc}$	
myb	Avian myeloblastosis virus (AMV) BAI/A, AMV-E26[b]	p45^{myb} p135$^{gag\text{-}myb\text{-}ets}$	
ets	AMV-E26[b]	p135$^{gag\text{-}myb\text{-}ets}$	
rel	Avian reticuloendotheliosis virus T	p64^{rel}	
maf	Avian retrovirus AS42	p100$^{gag\text{-}maf}$	
ski	SKV ASV	p110$^{gag\text{-}ski\text{-}pol}$	
qin	Avian retrovirus ASV31	p90$^{gag\text{-}qin}$	

[a]The nomenclature of viral oncoproteins refers to basic structural data: p, protein; gp, glycoprotein; and pp, phosphoprotein; the numbers designate the molecular weight in kilodaltons; the superscript indicates the genes from which the coding information is derived in a 5′ to 3′ direction.

[b]Transducing retrovirus containing two oncogenes.

[c]*fps* and *fes* are the same oncogene derived from the avian and feline genomes, respectively.

[d]*raf* and *mil* are the same oncogene derived from the murine and avian genomes, respectively.

derived from the gene encoding the platelet-derived growth factor (PDGF) (95,369). The *int-2* oncogene, which has not been found in a retrovirus genome but which can be cis-activated by mouse mammary tumor virus (MMTV), codes for a protein related to fibroblast growth factor (FGF) (91). *ErbB, fms, kit,* and *mpl* code for altered growth-factor receptors with known ligands (97,124,245,328,337); several other oncogenes produce proteins that have the general structure of a polypeptide growth-factor receptor, but specific ligands remain to be identified. The products of the *ras* genes belong to a family of small guanosine triphosphatases (GTPases) that occupy central positions in signal transduction (38,42, 128,228,330). The precise functions of *src, abl,* and other genes coding for nonreceptor tyrosine kinases are not clear; they may be active in the amplification stage of growth signals (49,70,72,262,316).

Another class of signaling molecules are those involved in phosphoinositol signaling, initiated by the activation of phosphatidylinositol 3-kinase (PI-3K) after growth factor–receptor activation. PI-3K activity is stimulated in many cell types in response to extracellular signals, generating a variety of phosphoinositides. One downstream target for PI-3K signaling is the Akt protein kinase, a serine/threonine kinase that is activated by phosphoinositides. A number of lines of study have implicated Akt in signaling pathways that control cell fate, in part through control of GSK-3 activity, but likely other targets as well. Although not initially identified by retroviral transduction, both PI-3K and Akt have been recovered in transforming retroviruses (7,55).

A number of oncogenes code for cytoplasmic kinases that are either tyrosine (*fps*) or serine/threonine specific (*raf, mos*). The oncogene, *crk,* is of interest because it lacks enzymatic activity but contains both SH2 and SH3 domains. Similar to the Grb-2 protein, it belongs to a class of linker–adaptor molecules that connect various catalytic steps of signal transduction (227). Finally, a large number of oncogenes encode proteins that control transcription. Notable are the Jun and Fos proteins that make up the AP-1 transcription factor, Rel, a member of the NF-κB family, and Myc, of interest because of its frequent involvement in human tumors (5,29,39,75,125, 319). Other oncogenes are related to the control of development, such as *wnt*-1 and *qin. Wnt*-1 is frequently activated in MMTV-induced tumors. It shows a striking tissue-specific distribution during mammalian embryogenesis and is homologous to the *Drosophila* gene *wingless,* which participates in the control of segmentation polarity in *Drosophila* embryos (286). Qin is a transcription factor with homology to the *Drosophila* forkhead gene product, which controls fore- and hindgut development in the early embryo (208). It is self-evident that qualitative or quantitative alterations of these growth regulatory genes carry the risk of uncontrolled growth.

Cellular Transformation by Retroviral Transduction of an Oncogene

With a combination of genetic and biochemical studies, mutants of Rous sarcoma virus (RSV) were isolated that are temperature sensitive for transformation; additional mutants were isolated that nonconditionally lost transforming capacity (222,224,355,363). The temperature-sensitive transformation mutants fail to induce or maintain oncogenic transformation at the nonpermissive temperature, while remaining fully oncogenic at the permissive temperature. Their replication is not temperature sensitive. These temperature-sensitive mutants provide unequivocal evidence for the dependence of oncogenesis on viral genetic information. The properties of these mutants also show that viral information must be expressed continuously to maintain the transformed phenotype. The nonconditionally transformation-defective RSV represents a deletion mutant that has lost about 20% of the genome. This loss does not affect the replicative properties of the virus; the deleted sequences, although essential for transformation, are therefore dispensable for virus production. This nonessential characteristic of transforming information for the viral growth cycle presaged the cellular origin of retroviral oncogenes. In temperature-sensitive and transformation-defective mutants, the same gene is affected: the two types of mutants cannot complement each other or form wild-type virus by recombination (25). The gene of RSV initially defined by these mutants is now known as the *src* gene. The deletion of *src* sequences in transformation-defective RSV also allowed the production of the first nucleic acid probe specific for *src.* A cDNA transcript of wild-type virus was generated and then was hybridized to the genome of the transformation-defective deletion mutant lacking the *src* gene. The nonhybridizing single-strand cDNA sequences of this reaction were separated from the double-strand hybrids. These single-strand sequences represented the viral oncogenic information. The cDNA *src* probe was found to hybridize to cellular DNA, providing conclusive evidence that *src* is not a viral but a cellular gene (340).

The basic characteristics discovered with the *src* gene apply to transduced retroviral oncogenes in general (32,282,358,370). All are derived from the cellular genome, and all are nonessential for virus replication. The virus serves as a vehicle of transduction, but it also exercises transcriptional control over the transduced oncogene. The cellular origin of retroviral oncogenes is of far-reaching significance because the transforming potential of a cellular oncogene can become activated independent of any viral intervention. Point mutations, gene amplification, and chromosomal rearrangements that can affect transcriptional regulation, as well as altering protein structure and function, can uncover the oncogenic potential of an otherwise normal gene. Activated oncogenes play important roles in nonviral, as well as viral, carcinogenesis; they may be the common denominator of all kinds of cancer.

In several cases, isolated temperature-sensitive as well as nonconditional mutants convincingly show that the gene is required for the initiation and maintenance of the transformed cellular phenotype (27,28,180,222,258,331, 355,388). Transduced oncogenes also can be excised from their native viral genomes and inserted into an expression vector (156,157). They then confer oncogenicity on this new vector. In the transducing retrovirus, the cell-derived oncogene is the only coding information that is needed for oncogenicity. Most or all retroviral coding information may be either nonfunctional or deleted without affecting the oncogenicity.

Transduced retroviral oncogenes cause transformation within a very short time; moreover, in appropriate target cells, transformation is an inevitable consequence of infection and of expression of the oncogene. With some retroviruses (e.g., RSV), it is possible to transform all cells of a culture synchronously with one inoculum in the first round of infection. Because transformation occurs with high frequency, tumors induced by transducing retroviruses are usually polyclonal in origin. Unlike most cancers that result from a multistep transformation process, the tumors caused by transducing retroviruses probably result from single-step carcinogenesis. Some retroviruses are vectors for two oncogenes; for instance, avian erythroblastosis virus strain R carries the *erbA* and *erbB* genes, and MH2 avian carcinoma virus transduces *raf* and *myc* (33). In these cases, one of the two oncogenes is sufficient to induce transformation (*erbB* or *myc* in the earlier examples). The second enhances oncogenicity of the virus and conveys greater nutritional and growth-factor independence on the tumor cells. This is interesting in the case of MH2, which carries the *mil* gene together with *myc,* in that biochemical experiments have shown that the stability of the Myc protein is significantly extended by the action of Raf (the murine equivalent of avian Mil), leading to an enhanced accumulation of active Myc (314).

Mechanism of Acquisition of Cellular Sequences by Retroviruses

Because incorporation of an oncogene into a retroviral genome is a rare event, it can be studied only after the fact. A plausible model involves the integration of a retrovirus upstream of a potential cellular oncogene. The provirus has a deletion that includes its 3′ LTR and is integrated in the same transcriptional orientation as the adjacent oncogene (67,131,343). Transcription from the 5′ LTR will extend through the oncogene, creating a chimeric RNA that contains the packaging signal located near the 5′ terminus of the viral genome. Complete introns are removed from this transcript, and the processed RNA can be exported in virus particles. The model also envisages infection of the same cell by a second virus that has not had a deletion and replicates complete progeny RNA as well as all structural proteins. Because retroviruses are diploid, such a cell will produce heterozygous progeny virus containing a complete viral genome and the defective chimeric RNA. In the next round of infection during reverse transcription of such a heterozygous particle, nonhomologous recombination between the two virion RNAs may take place, possibly as a result of template switching by the polymerase.

This model proposes two formal steps of recombination. The first step involves the integration of the defective provirus near the cellular oncogene, the formation of the 5′ junction of cellular with viral sequences, and the generation of the packageable chimeric RNA. This recombination event occurs at the DNA level. The second recombination event takes place during reverse transcription and involves the formation of the 3′ junction of cellular sequence with viral information. The resulting recombinant is a provirus with two LTRs and 5′ coding information derived from the chimeric RNA; 3′ sequences come from the nondefective retrovirus. Recent evidence supports this model (109,110). If chicken neuroretina cells are infected with the avian leukemia virus RAV-1, their growth is stimulated, and the culture releases a virus that transduces the *raf* oncogene. The identifiable steps in this acquisition of a cellular gene are in accord with this model. However, other possible models, suggested by exceptional provirus structures, have not been ruled out. RNA splicing of viral and cellular sequences would be an alternative mechanism for recombination (164,225). A third possibility is that viral–cellular recombinants derive from packaged read-through transcripts of a nondefective retroviral genome and an oncogene located downstream (150). It also is possible that transducing retroviruses can be generated by more than one mechanism.

The defectiveness of transducing retroviruses is caused by the replacement of viral coding sequences with cellular oncogene sequences. There are only rare exceptions including some strains of RSV, in which the *src* oncogene is added to a complete viral genome (Fig. 2). In contrast, the MC29 virus has acquired the *c-myc* gene at the expense of viral *pol* and part of *gag*. The defective viruses go through a partial life cycle that includes reverse transcription, integration, RNA synthesis, and translation. The expression of the defective provirus leads to oncogenic transformation; however, because one or several of the essential virion proteins cannot be synthesized, no infectious progeny are made. Only if the same cell is infected by a replication-competent retrovirus that supplies the missing protein(s) in *trans* is infectious transforming virus released. This transforming progeny virus remains, however, genetically defective and helper dependent.

It is interesting that cellular oncogenes have been found only in one subfamily of retroviruses, appropri-

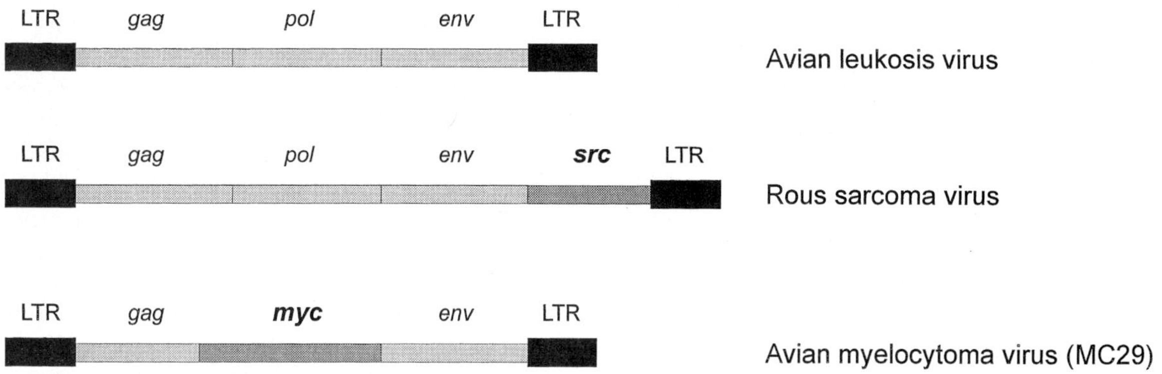

FIG. 2. Genomic structure of avian leukosis virus (ALV) and two transducing retroviruses. In addition to the long terminal repeat (LTR) sequences that provide transcriptional regulatory elements, the normal genome of ALV contains three major coding regions including *gag, pol,* and *env. Gag* encodes structural proteins of the virus, *pol* encodes enzymes involved in reverse transcription and integration, and *env* encodes the virion surface glycoproteins. In Rous sarcoma virus, the cellular *src* sequences are added to an otherwise intact retroviral genome. In contrast, in the MC29 virus, the addition of *myc* sequence is at the expense of the entire *pol* gene and parts of both *gag* and *env.*

ately called the oncornaviruses. They have not been seen in the genomes of the lenti- and spumaviruses, although the steps of replication that are thought to favor acquisition of cellular sequences are the same for all retroviruses. A possible explanation is the greater complexity of the lenti- and spumaviral genomes. Oncoviruses efficiently replicate without virus-coded regulatory proteins, whereas lenti- and spumavirus replication depends on nonvirion proteins that are generated from the provirus by way of multiply spliced messages. Generation of these messages and their cis-acting targets would be destroyed by a cellular genetic insert, essentially inactivating the virus. Oncornavirus genomes, conversely, can accept cellular inserts without such debilitating effects (31,33,40, 282,361,370).

Activation of the Transforming Potential of Oncogenes by Retroviral Transduction

Part of the process of turning an otherwise normal cellular gene into an oncogene is simply the process of viral transduction, resulting in misexpression of the gene due to control by the viral LTR in a cell when it would normally not be expressed. There are proto-oncogenes that, if sufficiently overexpressed, can transform cells. The *mos* gene is an example of this category (385). For such oncogenes, structural changes of the transduced or insertionally activated oncogene are not essential to bring forth the oncogenic potential, although they may contribute to it. Increased dosage is then the main factor in oncogenesis.

In many cases, the mere insertion of a proto-oncogene into a retroviral vector, resulting in expression at levels comparable to the viral gene, is not, in and of itself, suf-

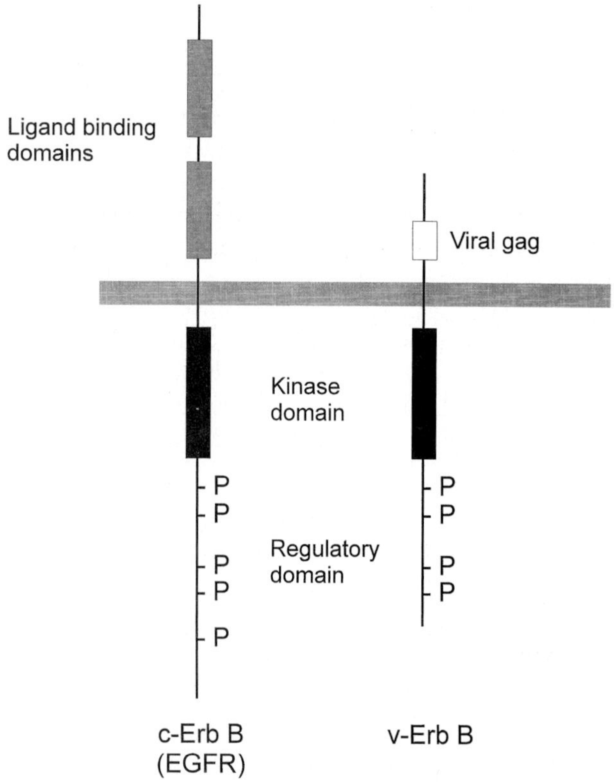

FIG. 3. Structural comparison of the cellular Erb B protein (the epidermal growth factor receptor, EGFR) with the transduced retroviral version, the v-Erb B protein of avian erythroblastosis virus H (AEV-H). The oncogenic v-Erb B lacks a regulatory phosphorylation site in the carboxyl terminal of the protein and has lost the extracellular ligand-binding domain. It functions as a constitutively activated EGFR.

ficient to transform cells. Thus specific structural changes in the viral version must be responsible for eliciting the transforming potential. For example, the cellular *src* gene, overexpressed in a retrovirus vector, does not induce oncogenic transformation (163,255,320). As outlined later, specific changes in *c-src* are necessary to reveal its oncogenic trait. Another example is the ErbB oncoprotein, derived from the avian erythroblastosis virus, in which the ligand-binding domain of the EGF receptor has been deleted and replaced with a fused viral *gag* sequence (Fig. 3).

Various approaches have defined oncogenically relevant structural changes for a number of oncogenes (e.g., *src, ras,* and *fms*) (282,370). These changes are always found in the oncogene proper; the viral sequences that are sometimes fused to it may facilitate oncogenicity by increasing the stability of the oncoprotein, determining the cellular localization, or enhancing efficiency of translation, but they do not participate directly in the transformation process.

It also is true that a comparison of activated oncogenes and their cellular counterparts often reveals structural and functional changes. Transduced oncogenes are usually truncated at one or both ends (for reviews, see refs. 282,370). The remaining coding sequences carry point mutations and sometimes deletions. They are often fused with viral sequences that are themselves truncated. Commonly, the viral sequences constitute the 5′ end of the chimeric transcription unit, providing splice acceptor site and initiation codon. Occasionally, the oncogene sequences also may be fused to other, unrelated cellular sequences as, for instance, in viral *src* (345).

Examples of Oncogenes Identified by Retrovirus-Mediated Transduction

It is now clear that deregulation of virtually any step in the process of growth factor–mediated signal transduction can represent an oncogenic event. This can be seen from the identification of mutations in tumors but also from the recovery of oncogenic retroviruses. The isolation and analysis of transforming retroviruses has illuminated many of the details of signaling pathways critical for cell growth. Starting from the extracellular environment and working through the cell to the nucleus, examples will illustrate the process.

Sis: *Growth Factor and Autocrine-Mediated Transformation*

Sis is the oncogene of simian sarcoma virus (SSV) (for reviews, see refs. 289,377,383); it is an insert that was acquired from the genome of the woolly monkey, a New World monkey. A homologous oncogenic determinant derived from the genome of a cat was discovered in the Parodi Irgens feline sarcoma virus (FeSV). The amino acid sequence of the SSV Sis protein shows about 88% identity with the sequence of the B-chain of the human PDGF. The discovery of this homology provided the first direct and exciting link between oncogenes and cellular growth signals. The immediate cellular precursor of the *sis* gene is most likely the PDGF-B gene of the woolly monkey genome, with the deviation from the human sequence being a species difference.

Sequence analysis of the SSV genome shows that *v-sis* is expressed as a fusion product containing, at its N-terminus, sequences derived from the retroviral envelope (Env) protein, including the Env signal sequence that effects the translocation of the Env-Sis protein into the vesicles of the endoplasmic reticulum. The initial *v-sis* product is a 28-kd glycoprotein that is rapidly dimerized to a gp56 dimer and then proteolytically processed to become a p24 homodimer, similar in structure to the homodimer of the PDGF-B chain. This Sis protein is firmly associated with cellular membrane fractions, but only about 1% is secreted by the SSV-transformed cell. Primary and processed *v-sis* products show PDGF-like activity: they react with anti-PDGF antibodies, bind to PDGF receptors, induce internalization of the receptor–ligand complex, induce phosphorylation of the receptor on a tyrosine residue, and stimulate the mitogenic response of the cell. This biologic activity of the *v-sis* product suggests an autocrine transforming mechanism for SSV-infected cells. Additional support for this suggestion comes from the following observations: SSV transforms only those cells that express a PDGF receptor. Transformation appears to be dependent on the interaction of the *v-sis* product with the PDGF receptor. In addition, the nascent *v-sis* product must be translocated into the endoplasmic reticulum to be transforming. Deletion of the Env signal sequence from the Env-Sis fusion protein abolishes transforming activity. Because the v-Sis protein is functionally equivalent to PDGF, the cellular PDGF gene also can function as an oncogene by autocrine mechanisms similar to those of v-Sis: The PDGF B-chain expressed under the control of a strong retroviral promoter induces oncogenic transformation in cells expressing the PDGF receptor.

The transforming signal of Sis could be generated by binding to receptors at the cell surface, but intracytoplasmic receptor binding also may play a role in transformation. The PDGF receptor is processed along the same cellular compartments as is the v-Sis protein, and it is conceivable that the two interact before reaching the cell surface. SSV-transformed cells, exposed to antibody against Sis, sometimes assume a near-normal phenotype. This observation was interpreted to suggest that the relevant interaction between growth factor and receptor, leading to transformation, is a cell-surface event. However, if a signal sequence (KDEL) that effects retention in the endoplasmic reticulum is added to the PDGF-B chain, the transforming potential for PDGF receptor–expressing cells is not abolished. Therefore PDGF may interact with the receptor intracellularly and then become translocated to the cell surface as a complex.

ErbB *and* Fms: *Growth Factor Receptors and Constitutive Mitotic Signals*

The oncogene *erbB* has been studied in two avian retroviruses that cause erythroblastosis and fibrosarcoma in chickens: avian erythroblastosis virus strain H (AEV-H) and strain ES4 (for reviews, see refs. 146,223,359). AEV-H contains *erbB* as its only oncogene. AEV strain ES4 carries, in addition to *erbB,* the *erbA* oncogene derived from a thyroid hormone–receptor gene (373). However, *erbB* alone is both necessary and sufficient to induce the pathogenic effects associated with AEV infections, erythroblastosis, and fibrosarcoma.

The nucleotide sequence of *erbB* shows close homology to that of the epidermal growth-factor receptor (EGFR) gene (95). The *erbB* of AEV strains H and ES4 is derived from the chicken *EGFR* gene. The EGFR contains four major structural and functional domains: an amino-terminal extracellular ligand-binding domain, a transmembrane segment, a kinase domain, and a carboxyl-terminal regulatory segment with at least five tyrosine phosphorylation sites: P1 through P5 (see Fig. 3). In *erbB,* most of the growth-factor–binding domain is deleted. Furthermore, carboxyl-terminal deletions have removed P1 from the *erbB* of AEV-H and have removed P1 as well as P2 from *erbB* of AEV ES4.

The mechanism of *erbB*-induced oncogenesis probably includes elements of the same mitotic signal that is initiated by the binding of epidermal growth factor (EGF) to its receptor (see Fig. 1). Ligand binding appears to induce an allosteric change and oligomerization of the receptor (305–307). The kinase activity of EGFR is elevated, and the protein becomes autophosphorylated on tyrosine residues at its carboxyl-terminal regulatory sites. EGFR substrates of potential importance in mitotic signaling include the SHC proteins (containing an SH2 domain but no recognizable catalytic domain), GAP (GTPase activating protein), PI-3K, and phospholipase C. At least one of the phosphotyrosines in the cytoplasmic tail of EGFR is recognized and bound by the SH2 domain of a small adaptor protein called Grb2 that also binds with its SH3 domains to the nucleotide releasing factor Sos. Sos, in turn, interacts with the product of the proto-oncogene *ras,* leading to an exchange of the Ras-bound guanosine diphosphate (GDP) for GTP, thereby activating the Ras protein. From Ras the signal is propagated through a kinase cascade involving the product of the proto-oncogene *raf* and the MAP kinase (mitogen-activated protein kinase) among other kinases. Translocation of the signal into the nucleus and activation of the ultimate recipient of the signal pathway, presumably a transcription factor, are still poorly understood. The tyrosine-specific kinase activity of EGFR is essential for the mitogenic effect of EGF. Binding of EGF to the receptor is followed by internalization of the receptor–ligand complex. This process removes available EGFR from the cell surface and results in a down-regulation of EGF responsiveness. Reduced EGF responsiveness also can be caused by an activated protein kinase C, probably through phosphorylation of a threonine residue near the EGFR kinase domain.

The transforming activity of *erbB* has been analyzed with the help of several conditional and nonconditional mutants of AEV (133,244). Transforming activity of ErbB requires localization of the protein at the plasma membrane as well as truncation of the carboxyl-terminal regulatory domain. The ErbB protein is glycosylated. Intracellular forms are gp65 and gp68 proteins; the mature cell-surface molecule is a gp74. The *erbB* coding information lacks a conventional signal sequence, so targeting to the plasma membrane appears to be a function of the transmembrane domain. Temperature-sensitive mutants of AEV ES4 that prevent membrane localization at the nonpermissive temperature also are temperature sensitive for the transformed cellular phenotype. Deletions from the carboxyl-terminal end of the c-ErbB protein have shown that loss of the P1 phosphorylation site is important for both erythroblast and fibroblast transformation. As the size of the carboxyl-terminal deletion increases, there is a loss of erythroblast transformation, while still retaining fibroblast transformation.

A somewhat different picture emerges from the study of AEVs that have recently acquired *erbB* (230,273,274) (see section entitled cis-activation of oncogenes). These newer *erbB*-transducing agents carry a version of c-*erbB* that lacks the ligand-binding domain of EGFR, but some have an intact carboxyl terminus and yet can induce erythroblastosis in a highly susceptible chicken line. They do, however, fail to transform fibroblasts. A separate analysis of fibroblast transformation using mutants of AEV ES4 has shown that an intact kinase domain is essential for this biologic effect. These observations are compatible with the proposal that ErbB transforms cells as a constitutively activated EGFR. Membrane localization and kinase activity are essential.

Ligand-independent activation of receptor tyrosine kinase also plays an important role in the oncogenicity of v-*fms* (for reviews, see refs. 283,292,293,326,327). *Fms* is the oncogene of the McDonough strain of feline sarcoma virus (SM FeSV). It also has been found as the oncogenic insert in the Hardy Zuckerman 5 (HZ5) FeSV. *Fms* is derived from the gene of the receptor for the macrophage colony-stimulating factor CSF-1 (328). In SM FeSV, it replaces most of the viral *gag* and practically all of the *pol* gene, whereas the *env* gene of the virus has remained intact. *Fms* is fused in frame to the partial *gag* sequences. The crossover point in the *fms* gene is located in the 5′ untranslated region of c-*fms* messenger RNA and preserves the signal sequence of c-*fms*. The 3′ recombination point in *fms* is located 120 nucleotides upstream of the c-*fms* termination codon. SM-FeSV and HZ5-FeSV induce fibrosarcomas in cats but no hematopoietic malignancies, notwithstanding the normal function of CSF-1 as a hematopoietic growth factor.

The CFS-1 receptor has a structure similar to that of growth-factor receptors such as the PDGF receptor, the Kit protein and Flt (26,151,329,390). The extracellular domain consists of five immunoglobulin-like repeats; the three amino-terminally located of these repeats form the ligand-binding region. The fourth immunoglobulin-like domain functions in receptor dimerization; the point mutations contributing to the oncogenicity of v-*fms* are in or near this domain. Important cytoplasmic regions of Fms are the tyrosine kinase domain and the C-terminal tail, which contains targets for negative regulation. Activation of Fms by ligand or by mutation results in autophosphorylation of several tyrosines in the cytoplasmic domain of the receptor. These phosphotyrosines are then bound by the SH2 regions of effector molecules including PI-3 kinase, members of the Src family of proteins, and Grb2. From Grb2, propagation of the signal continues via SOS-1, Ras and Raf, and the MAPK cascade. An alternative pathway to the nucleus may involve the interferon-stimulated gene factor 3, but molecular details of this signal chain are still sketchy.

The v-*fms* genes of SM-FeSV and of HZ5-FeSV differ from c-*fms* by several point mutations leading to amino acid substitutions and by a deletion that removes the 50 carboxyl-terminal amino acids from the protein. The deleted residues are replaced in SM- and HZ5-FeSV by 14 and 11 unrelated amino acids, respectively. The oncogenicity of the v-*fms* genes can be attributed to two point mutations in the extracellular domain and to the carboxyl-terminal deletion. The deletion removes phosphorylation sites that negatively regulate the kinase activity of the receptor, and the point mutations in the extracellular domain lead to a ligand-independent activation of the receptor.

Src *and* Abl: *Membrane-Bound Nonreceptor Tyrosine Kinases*

Src was the first retroviral oncogene discovered and defined (for reviews, see refs. 130,316). It was also the first whose origin from the cellular genome was recognized and the first for which a protein product was identified (49,340). The discovery of the *src* gene product was soon followed by observations that showed that this protein is a tyrosine-specific protein kinase, providing suggestive evidence for a regulatory function of Src and raising hopes for an immediate understanding of its oncogenic action (68,160,205). Throughout this period of rapidly expanding work on oncogenes, *src* has served as an important and pace-setting model. Yet despite this paradigmatic role and despite much additional data on structural and functional properties of cellular and viral *src,* the mechanism by which Src transforms cells is only now emerging. *Src* codes for a 60-kd phosphoprotein that is bound to cytoplasmic membranes. (This protein has been termed $pp60^{src}$; we will refer to it as Src protein, to remain consistent with the terminology applied to other oncoproteins.) The cellular Src protein contains several well-defined functional domains: an amino-terminal myristilation domain, followed by a region that diverges among related nonreceptor tyrosine kinases, an SH3 and an SH2 domain, a catalytic domain, and a C-terminal regulatory region. The viral Src protein shows the same general structure but has had a deletion in the carboxyl-terminal regulatory domain. Because c-Src expressed at levels comparable to transduced v-Src does not transform cells (163,255,320), structural differences between the cellular and viral version of the Src protein must activate oncogenic potential. The oncogenicity of Src requires binding to the plasma membrane and is correlated with increased kinase activity. The kinase activity of Src is controlled positively by phosphorylation of tyrosine 416 in the catalytic region and negatively by phosphorylation of tyrosine 527 in the C-terminal regulatory region. Tyrosine 527 is the target of Csk (C-terminal Src kinase), which appears to be a specific regulator of Src family kinases. The phosphotyrosine 527 is most likely bound intramolecularly by the SH2 domain of the Src protein. This folding of the Src protein is believed to affect the catalytic domain and to turn off kinase activity. Significantly, the viral Src lacks tyrosine 527 and is constitutively active as a kinase. Activation of Src in the presence of tyrosine 527 may involve dephosphorylation of this residue by a specific phosphatase. However, access to tyrosine 527 may depend on an allosteric change of the molecule that includes dissociation of phosphotyrosine 527 from the SH2 domain. Consequently, such allosteric interactions could target the SH2 and SH3 domains of Src that connect to other members of the signal transmission chains. Accordingly, oncogenic activation of Src can result from mutations in SH3, SH2, the kinase domain, and the C-terminal tail (69,256,348), suggesting that all of these may be important in the allosteric transitions that affect Src kinase activity.

Over the years, numerous proteins have been identified that can serve as downstream targets and substrates of Src. Most of these are probably not relevant in oncogenic transformation. Exceptions appear to be an SH2-containing protein (SHC) and focal adhesion kinase (FAK) (66,154,229,278,294). SHC is an adaptor protein that is phosphorylated by Src and related kinases and then binds to Grb-2; the SHC–Grb-2 complex then interacts with the SOS, making a nucleotide exchange factor that activates Ras. FAK is bound by the SH2 domain of Src, and this interaction appears to keep FAK in the activated state. The resulting overphosphorylation of cytoskeletal proteins may be responsible for the poor adhesion and altered shape of Src-transformed cells.

Src is highly expressed in some cell types such as blood platelets, neurons, and osteoclasts. Src-deficient mice develop osteopetrosis, the result of dysfunctional osteoclasts, but show no other major abnormalities in development and growth, possibly because the Src defect can be compensated by related kinases (336).

The product of the oncogene *abl* shares with the Src protein two important properties: attachment to the cytoplasmic face of the plasma membrane by a myristic acid residue and tyrosine-specific protein kinase activity (for reviews, see refs. 281,287,384). *Abl* was first identified as the oncogene of the Abelson murine leukemia virus (A-MuLV). More recently, it also has been found as a cell-derived oncogenic insert in the Hardy–Zuckerman HZ2 FeSV. In A-MuLV (with which most of the work on *abl* has been carried out), the *abl* gene is merged to partial *gag* sequences and is expressed as a Gag–Abl fusion protein. The *abl* insert in A-MuLV is truncated at its 5′ terminus as compared with the cellular gene, but the *abl* coding sequences in p160v-abl begin downstream of the SH3 domain. Point mutations also are found in the *abl* sequences in v-abl. The v-Abl protein contains three domains: the amino-terminal Gag domain, an SH2 and SH3 domain mediating interactions with other signal-transduction proteins, and a catalytic domain that is homologous to the corresponding domain of other tyrosine kinases. Mutational analysis of the *abl* gene shows that for oncogenic transformation to occur, two properties are essential: membrane association through myristilation and elevated tyrosine kinase activity. In the v-Abl protein, the Gag domain provides the myristilation signal and therefore becomes indispensable for transformation—in contrast to the Gag domain of most other oncoproteins, which can be deleted without affecting oncogenicity. The Gag sequences of v-Abl also increase the half-life of the protein in hematopoietic cells. The c-Abl protein localizes to both the cytosol and the nucleus, and it is phosphorylated in a cell cycle–dependent manner (181,182). In some cell types (for example, primary neuronal and epithelial cells), c-Abl is primarily cytoplasmic, whereas in other cell types (for example, hematopoietic cells), the protein is largely nuclear. Recent observations suggest that it may function as a negative regulator of cell growth; transdominant negative mutants of c-*abl* disrupt the control of the cell cycle and enhance cellular susceptibility to oncogenic transformation (302). The SH2 and SH3 domains of Abl have complex regulatory functions. The SH3 domain appears to be the target of a negative control mechanism; deletion of this domain activates the oncogenic potential of Abl. The SH2 domain of Abl may have multiple functions—controlling the kinase activity of Abl by intramolecular binding to phosphotyrosine residues and interacting with signal-transduction proteins apparently in a phosphotyrosine-independent manner. Replacement of the Abl SH2 domain with a heterologous SH2 domain also may activate the oncogenic potential of this nonreceptor kinase (65,236,237). A-MuLV is an effective transforming agent for early B cells. Other hematopoietic cells can be transformed, but special conditions and additional selective pressure are required to reveal these less frequent transforming events. A-MuLV also can transform fibroblasts. The HZ2 FeSV induces only sarcomas and does not transform hematopoietic cells either *in vitro* or *in vivo*. An activated *abl* oncogene also is found in human chronic myelogenous leukemia. The leukemic cells carry a chromosomal translocation that gives rise to the marker Philadelphia chromosome and joins *abl* sequences of chromosome 9 to *bcr* (breakpoint cluster region) sequences of chromosome 22 (149,333). *Bcr* and *abl* sequences are found in a single, fused transcript in leukemic cells. Although the junction point between *bcr* and *abl* varies in different patients, the regularity with which this translocation occurs in chronic myelogenous leukemia strongly suggests that the Bcr-Abl protein conveys a growth advantage to the leukemic cells.

Ras: *Growth-Regulatory GTPase*

Mammalian cells contain three *ras* genes: H-*ras*, K-*ras*, and N-*ras* (for reviews, see refs. 38,44,45,204). All three are composed of four coding exons that contain information for a protein of about 190 amino acids, or 21 kd, plus an upstream noncoding exon. The amino-terminal halves of these cellular p21 proteins are virtually identical. About two thirds of the carboxyl-terminal halves are also closely related, and only the most 25-carboxyl-terminal amino acids show divergence. Two of the mammalian *ras* genes—H-*ras* and K-*ras*—have been found transduced by retroviruses; N-*ras* has not been detected in a naturally occurring virus. More than half a dozen independently isolated retroviruses that transduce a *ras* gene; the best studied are Harvey and Kirsten murine sarcoma viruses (H-MuSV and K-MuSV). Their *ras* inserts are derived from the rat genome and carry sequences of an endogenous rat retrovirus VL30.

Ras proteins are GTPases that act as nodal points in cellular growth control, receiving inputs from several signal-transmission chains and propagating the signal through kinase cascades toward the nucleus. Ras proteins belong to a superfamily of low-molecular-weight GTPases that also encompasses the Rho proteins, important in the control of the cytoskeleton, and the Rab proteins, which function in membrane protein trafficking. Other related proteins with GTPase activity and homology to Ras are the heterotrimeric G proteins involved in signal transduction and the elongation and initiation factors of the protein-synthesizing machinery.

Ras proteins must be anchored in cellular membranes for proper functioning. They are posttranslationally modified by covalent attachment of prenyl groups to cysteines near their C-terminus, providing a lipophilic tail. Ras proteins can be considered as binary switches that are either on (bound to GTP) or off (bound to GDP). They are regulated by at least three types of proteins; the guanine nucleotide exchange factors (GEFs), the GTPase-activating proteins (GAPs), and guanine nucleotide dissociation inhibitors (GDIs) (38). GEF proteins activate Ras through exchange of Ras-bound GDP for GTP. An example of a GEF is the SOS protein, which is instrumental in transmitting growth signals from tyrosine kinases to Ras. Gap proteins have an attenuating effect on Ras. They stimulate the conversion of active GTP Ras to the inactive GDP Ras. They are represented by p120 GAP and by NF1 (neurofibromin). The GDI proteins are the least understood regulators of Ras. They bind to GDP Ras, thereby interfering with the action of GEF activators and possibly also with GAP-like attenuators.

Oncogenicity of Ras is greatly elevated by specific point mutations, notably in codons 12, 13, and 61. These mutations inhibit the binding of GAP proteins to activated Ras and thus prevent the stimulation of Ras GTPase activity. The mutant Ras proteins remain bound to GTP and are constitutively active, contributing to oncogenic transformation. Retroviral Ras proteins carry these activating mutations. Additionally, the transforming potential of Ras can be elicited by changes in upstream nontranslated regions; the endogenous VL30 sequences also can have an enhancing effect on transformation.

Activated Ras with a mutation in one of the critical codons also is found in human cancers, notably in carcinomas of the bladder, colon, and lung. A significant minority of the primary tumors in these sites contain the mutated oncogene. Normal tissue surrounding the tumor is free of the mutation. The possibility that activated Ras plays an important role in human tumor development also is supported by animal studies. Virtually all tumors induced by certain chemical carcinogens contain an activated *ras* gene (19,342). Examples are mammary carcinomas in the rat induced by nitrosomethylurea and skin carcinomas in the mouse caused by dimethylbenzanthrazene.

Mos *and* Raf: *Cytoplasmic Serine/Threonine Kinases*

The *mos* oncogene was originally found in Moloney sarcoma virus as a cell-derived insert into the retroviral *env* gene (for reviews, see refs. 40,318,394). Moloney sarcoma virus induces rhabdomyosarcomas in mice and transforms cultured murine fibroblasts. The viral Mos protein is an Env–Mos fusion product; it has a molecular mass of 37 kd, and its first five codons are derived from the 5′ end of the retroviral *env* gene. The v-Mos protein is localized in the soluble portion of the cytoplasm. Several strains of the Moloney murine sarcoma virus differ by point mutations and deletions. The HT1 strain, which is probably closest to the original isolate, carries a *mos* insert that is identical to c-*mos* if amino acid sequences are compared. Another *mos*-containing retrovirus, myeloproliferative sarcoma virus, has a frameshift mutation and appears to initiate *mos* translation from an internal site downstream of this mutation.

The cellular *mos* gene can transform cells in culture with virtually the same efficiency as the viral gene, suggesting that the transforming potential of this gene can be activated by deregulated expression of the cellular product (385). *Mos* shows homology to cyclic adenosine monophosphate (AMP)-dependent protein kinase and to the Src family of tyrosine kinases. The Mos protein is a serine–threonine kinase; the cellular *mos* is an intronless gene that is expressed at very low levels (less than one copy of *mos* RNA per cell) in most tissues. Notable exceptions are germ cells, where *mos* is highly expressed (132,269,299). Recent investigations show that the cellular Mos protein is a regulator of meiotic maturation. It is required for meiosis, and as a component of the cytostatic factor (CSF), it is essential for the normal arrest of meiosis at metaphase II. Mos also stabilizes maturation-promoting factor (MPF $p34^{cdc2}$) in meiosis. It further associates with and phosphorylates tubulin and can activate MAP kinase. One hypothesis of *mos*-induced oncogenic transformation suggests that Mos imposes a mitotic program onto the interphase cell and thus contributes to reduced adhesiveness, cell rounding, and cytoskeletal reorganization, all part of the transformed phenotype (394).

The *raf* oncogene has been found to be the sole oncogenic determinant in murine sarcoma virus 3611 but has also been isolated as a second oncogene, together with *myc,* from the genome of the MH2 avian carcinoma virus (for reviews, see refs. 147,277). This avian homolog is still sometimes referred to as *mil.* In the mammalian genome, other *raf*-related genes have been identified, among them A-*raf* and B-*raf.* Cellular *raf* sequences inserted into a retroviral vector induce oncogenic transformation. These sequences are truncated at the 5′ end, a modification that is probably instrumental in activating the oncogenic potential. In cells infected with the 3611 murine sarcoma virus, Raf is expressed as a 79-kd Gag–Raf fusion protein. This protein is myristilated in its Gag domain and is phosphorylated on serines and threonines. Because the murine Gag protein also occurs in a glycosylated form, there is a corresponding Gag–Raf glycoprotein in cells transformed by virus 3611. In contrast to the mammalian *raf* genes, the avian homolog *mil* does not induce transformation on its own. The *mil* insert of the MH2 avian carcinoma virus also is expressed as a fusion product with Gag. The 100-kd Gag–Mil and the 70-kd Gag–Raf proteins are both cytoplasmic serine–threonine kinases, and they show some homology to the Src family of tyrosine kinases. Raf is emerging as a second important nodal point besides Ras for the propagation of growth signals. Raf is distal to Ras but upstream of the MAP kinase cascade. Activated Ras binds to the amino terminal regulatory domain of Raf, and there is a suggested association of Raf with MAP kinase kinase.

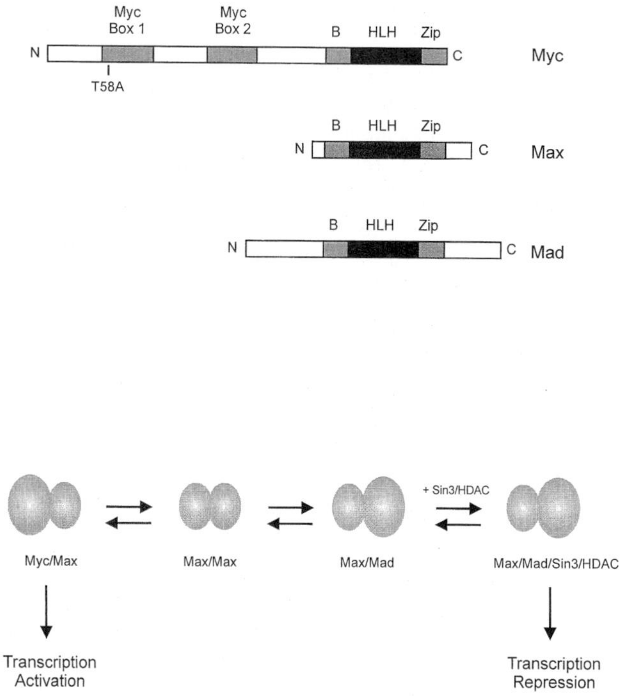

FIG. 4. Comparison of the Myc protein, the dimerization partner Max, and the alternate Max partner Mad. Myc and Max, as well as Max and Mad, associate through the leucine zipper helix–loop–helix domains. The heterodimers bind to the sequence CACGTG. Association with Max is necessary for transcriptional regulation and for transformation by Myc. Myc box-1 and -2, and the acidic region represent sequences conserved in various *myc* genes. The threonine 58 residue (corresponding to threonine 61 in avian Myc), which is a site for phosphorylation, is the most frequent site of mutation in oncogenic forms of *myc* recovered in viruses and is often found in Burkitt's lymphomas (1). Shown is a schematic depiction of the relationship between the various interacting proteins, changing the function from one of transcription activation (Myc–Max) to one of transcription repression (Mad–Max).

Fos, Jun, *and* Myc*: Transcriptional Regulatory Proteins*

Finally, a large number of oncogenic retroviruses have been recovered that encode nuclear proteins that act as transcription factors. In this category belong *myc, myb, fos, rel, ski, jun, erbA, maf,* and *qin* (6,76,77,80,102,108, 152,253,267,280,339,359,365).

Myc is the oncogenic determinant in avian retroviruses MC29, CMII, MH2, and OK10 (108). Besides c-*myc*, the human genome contains several other *myc*-related genes including N-*myc* and L-*myc*: the latter two have not been found as oncogenes in retroviruses. *Myc* plays an important role in a number of human cancers. In all Burkitt lymphomas, *myc* is translocated into the vicinity of an immunoglobulin gene and, unlike the nontranslocated allele, is actively expressed in B cells (139). An understanding of the Myc protein has been advanced with the discovery of a small Myc dimerization partner, the Max protein (36,216,266) and a variety of other interacting proteins that determine the function of Myc and related complexes (Fig. 4). Max associates with Myc by a helix–loop–helix and a leucine zipper motif. Genetic experiments show that dimerization with Max is required, not only for Myc DNA binding (consensus sequence CACGTG) but also for oncogenic transformation and for Myc-induced apoptosis (3,4). Through the use of protein-interaction assays, an additional Max-interacting partner was termed the Mad protein (11). Further studies have shown that, depending on the growth and differentiation state of a cell, there exists an equilibrium between homodimers of Max and heterodimers of Myc–Max or Mad–Max (10). Whereas the Myc–Max heterodimer is associated with transcription activation, no unique activity has been attributed to the Max–Max homodimer. In contrast, various experiments have now shown that the Mad–Max heterodimer functions as a transcription repressor through the recruitment of the Sin 3 protein and a histone deacetylase (12,195).

Myb is the oncogene of avian myeloblastosis virus AMV BAI-1 and of the avian leukemia virus E26; it binds to a specific DNA sequence, and the viral oncogenic version of the gene may transform by interference with normal transcriptional control (29,93,217,324). The cellular *myb* gene is preferentially expressed in hematopoietic tissues, controls the expression of myeloid-specific genes, and is required for normal fetal hematopoiesis (235,272,280,312).

The *rel* oncogene of avian reticular endotheliosis virus belongs to the NF-κB transcription factor family. The viral version of this gene corrupts normal transcriptional regulation by NF-κB (210,285). The *ets* oncogene is the second oncogene of E26 AMV. It is a member of an important transcription factor family (167,253,368) and can be activated by insertional mutagenesis as well as by transduction (21). *Fos* is the oncogene of the FBJ and FBR murine osteosarcoma viruses. It is a component of the cellular AP-1 transcription factor complex, and like other transcription factor oncoproteins, it transforms by altering normal transcriptional controls (77,113). The product of the *maf* oncogene is structurally and functionally related to the AP-1 family of transcription factors. *Maf* was originally found in avian retrovirus AS42; it can interact with AP-1 proteins (178). *Qin,* the oncogene of avian sarcoma virus 31, codes for a transcription factor of the fork head/HNF-3 family. Fork-head proteins are important regulators of embryonal development (208).

Jun is the cell-derived insert in the genome of avian sarcoma virus 17 (6,77,365). In cells transformed by this virus, *jun* is expressed as a 65-kd Gag–Jun fusion protein concentrated in the nucleus. Together with Fos, the cellular Jun protein is a component of the AP-1 transcription factor complex (5,39). It belongs to a multigene family together with the related genes *junB* and *junD* (154,296). Areas of homology among these genes roughly correspond to functional domains: a carboxyl-terminal leucine zipper dimerization domain, an adjacent basic region that makes contact with DNA, and an amino-terminal domain required for transcriptional activation (77,196,248). Jun proteins can form homodimers, but under physiologic conditions are usually found in heterodimers with Fos family proteins, with proteins of the ATF transcription factor family, and with other leucine zipper proteins. In the heterodimers, the leucine zipper of Jun joins with that of the partner protein in a coiled structure (64,126,138, 187,310,356). The DNA contact domain extends from the leucine zipper, forming a fork that interacts with the major groove for the DNA double helix. The principal functions of Jun show a hierarchic dependence: dimerization is a prerequisite for DNA binding and transactivation, and DNA binding is required for transactivation. All three domains, for dimerization, DNA binding, and transactivation, are needed in oncogenic transformation.

Transformation by Jun reflects a disturbance of normal transcriptional controls (364), but the molecular details of this process are still unknown. Viral Jun differs from cellular Jun by a 27-amino-acid deletion in the transactivation domain, by two amino acid substitutions affecting important regulatory sites of the molecule, and by the loss of the 3′ untranslated region, which appears to be responsible for the short half-life of *jun* messenger RNA (Fig. 5). All these mutations contribute to the oncogenic potential of *jun*. *Jun* acts as a single oncogene in transforming avian cells, and there appears to be no requirement for auxiliary genetic changes. In mammalian cells, *jun* transforms only in cooperation with a second oncogene such as activated *ras* or another growth-stimulatory gene. Transactivation by the Jun protein is regulated through phosphorylation. Phosphorylation of amino-terminal serines and threonines increases transactivation potential, and phosphorylation of a serine and a DNA-binding domain inhibits transactivation. Transformation depends on the presence of the transactivation domain, but it is not correlated with a general increase in AP-1–dependent transcription that is controlled by AP-1 consensus sequences. The transforming potential of Jun reflects more subtle changes that may involve altered preference for heterodimer partners, for DNA consensus sequences, and hence for target genes. Although numerous target genes responsive to AP-1 are known, the target genes important in the oncogenic action of Jun have not been identified. The possibility that the oncogenic change in Jun reflects a loss of function rather than a gain of function also has not been ruled out.

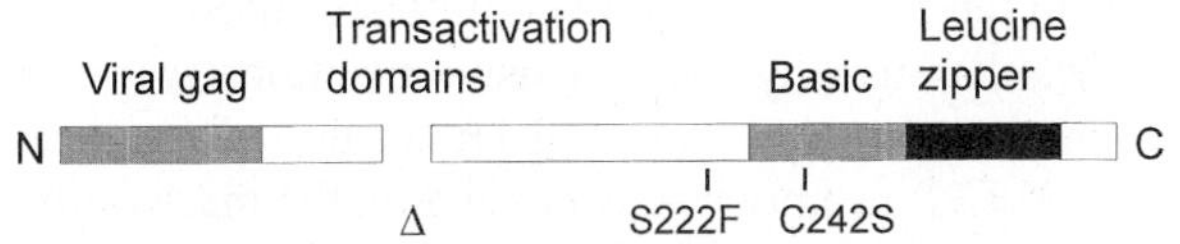

FIG. 5. Alterations in the *jun* sequences recovered in avian sarcoma virus 17. The viral *jun* differs from the cellular progenitor found in chicken cells in the following ways: v-*jun* has fused at its amino terminal partial Gag sequences derived from an avian retrovirus. It has a 27-amino-acid deletion affecting the transactivation domains. Two amino acid substitutions interfere with normal posttranslational regulation, and an absence of 3′ untranslated sequences in the message contributes to the greater stability of the v-Jun mRNA. With the exception of the Gag sequences, all changes seen in viral Jun contribute to its enhanced transforming activity as compared with cellular Jun.

An entirely different regulator of transcription is the product of the oncogene *erbA* (for reviews, see refs. 80,133). *ErbA* occurs as the second oncogene in AEV strains ES4 and R, which also carry the *erbB* oncogene. *ErbB* alone is sufficient for the induction of erythroblastosis and sarcoma. In cultured erythroblasts, expression of the v-*erbB* oncogene induces a high rate of self-renewal without completely blocking a low incidence of spontaneous differentiation to erythrocytes. V-*erbA* does not induce proliferation in erythroblasts, but it blocks spontaneous differentiation and allows cell growth in a wide range of Na^+ concentrations and pH. Erythroblasts transformed by *erbB* and *erbA* together are nutritionally less fastidious than are erythroblasts transformed by *erbB* alone. Through its inhibitory effect on differentiation and by inducing nutritional vigor, *erbA* augments the oncogenicity of *erbB*. *ErbA* is the homolog of the thyroid hormone receptor (300,372,373,397). It belongs to a protein family that also includes receptors for glucocorticoid hormones, retinoic acid, and estrogen. These receptor proteins are related in structure and mechanism of action. They contain a ligand-binding domain, a transactivation domain, and a DNA-binding domain with two zinc fingers. They bind to similar, but not identical palindromic DNA consensus sequences. Initially the homology of v-*erbA* to the gene encoding thyroid hormone receptor led to the suggestion that the oncogenic effect of the *erbA* is due to its interference with the thyroid receptor function. Indeed, the v-ErbA protein can act as a repressor of thyroid hormone–dependent transcription, functioning as a transdominant negative mutant. However, recent investigations have shown that the oncogenic potential of v-*erbA* is primarily due to its inhibitory effect of the retinoic acid receptor rather than the thyroid hormone receptor (309,322). The transformation-related target genes that are retinoic acid (and possibly thyroid hormone) dependent and affected by the v-*erbA* still remains to be determined.

Oncogene Activation by Retrovirus Insertion

Many retroviruses that do not carry an oncogene are nevertheless capable of inducing tumors in animals (for reviews, see refs. 192,193,247). The kinds of tumor seen with these viruses are similar to the ones caused by transducing retroviruses. They include sarcomas, various forms of leukemia, and carcinomas. However, a uniform difference with respect to the tumors induced by transduction is the latent period of tumor formation. Nondefective retroviruses lacking a transduced oncogene induce tumors only after a long latent period of several weeks to several months. None of these viruses induces oncogenic transformation in cell culture. These differences largely reflect the mechanism by which viruses induce transformation. As discussed in detail later, transformation results from the cis-activation of a proto-oncogene by the insertion of the retrovirus. Thus the long latency *in vivo,* as well as the absence of transformation *in vitro,* is due to the infrequency with which an insertion occurs adjacent to a potential oncogene.

The tumors caused by these nontransducing retroviruses have several common properties that are important in understanding their origin. They all contain an integrated provirus. The proviral sequences are found in the same chromosomal site in all cells of a given tumor; hence each tumor is monoclonal, having originated from a single transformed cell. Although infection is initiated with a nondefective virus that undergoes multiple rounds of replication, the proviruses seen in tumors are usually defective, containing only part of the viral genome. The part that is always present and conserved is at least one LTR, whereas a portion or all of the viral coding sequences may be missing. This observation suggests that viral coding sequences are not required for the maintenance of the transformed state. Most important in the genesis of these tumors is the fact that viral sequences are integrated at preferred sites of the cellular genomes. In several tumor systems, these sites are located in the immediate vicinity of a cellular oncogene that has also been found in transducing retroviruses. As a result of retroviral integration nearby, the transcription of the cellular oncogene is elevated in the tumor cells. This is referred to as insertional activation, or cis-activation, of an oncogene.

The active replication of a nontransducing competent retrovirus in a susceptible host and the presumably accidental insertional mutation or cis-activation of a cellular oncogene are not the only factors important in tumorigenesis by nontransducing retroviruses.

A systematic genetic analysis of the nontransducing retrovirus genomes for oncogenic potential has revealed a surprising multiplicity of important sequences and has demonstrated the complexity of their interactions. Among both avian and murine retroviruses, there are strains of high and low leukemogenicity. Recombinants between these strains, as well as mutants of these strains, show that the LTR is a major determinant (but not the sole one) of oncogenicity (48,89,290,291). The coding information for *gag, pol,* and *env* can be involved to varying degrees as well. In some murine leukemia viruses (e.g., Moloney leukemia virus), viral replication during the latent period of the disease gives rise to recombinants with endogenous retroviral information in the *env* gene (67,142). These recombinant "MCF" viruses multiply more actively in hematopoietic target tissue than does parental virus, and this increased replication is an important factor in leukemogenicity. The multiplicity of contributing factors suggests that every step of virus replication—from efficient entry into specific target cells to active transcription of the provirus and maturation of highly infectious progeny—is important in increasing the probability of cis-activation.

A number of questions on the mechanism of cis-activation remain to be answered. For instance, although the insertional activation of the cellular oncogene is a rare event, it does not account for the fixed minimal duration of the latent period, suggesting that some sort of threshold condition has to be met. The monoclonality of the tumors indicates that the transformation to the oncogenic phenotype is rare. It is compatible with the idea that two or more independent events are necessary to convey tumorigenicity to the infected cell. The possibility of more than one necessary event also is suggested by the fact that retroviruses that cause cancer through cis-activation of a cellular oncogene have not been found to induce transformation in cell culture. If a single cis-activating event were sufficient, it should be detectable *in vitro.* Another puzzling aspect in cis-activation is the tissue tropism of oncogenesis. It is not clear why RAV activates the *myc* gene in some chicken lines and the *erbB* gene in others or why some mouse strains develop B-cell and others T-cell or myeloid lymphomas in response to infection with the same murine leukemia virus.

Two principal mechanisms of cis-activation have been identified: promoter insertion and enhancer insertion. In promoter insertion, a chimeric mRNA is generated that combines R and U5 sequences of the viral LTR with sequences of the cellular oncogene. If the transcripts originate in the 5′ LTR of the provirus, they also may contain partial viral coding sequences. However, transcription starts in the 3′ LTR are more common; in these cases, the provirus has usually had extensive deletions that extend into, and may include, the 5′ LTR. In fact, the activation of the 3′ LTR promoter may depend on the inactivation of the 5′ promoter. The preferred integration sites of promoter insertions may lie within the cellular oncogene and either truncate the coding sequences or effectively remove noncoding domains that contain negative regulatory elements. For enhancer insertion, the provirus need not be integrated in the transcriptional orientation of the cellular oncogene, and its position may also be downstream of the cellular gene. In enhancer insertion, the oncogene transcripts do not contain viral sequences. To illustrate the essential aspects of insertional oncogenesis, selected representative examples will be discussed.

Myc *and* **ErbB** *Are Activated by Insertion of Avian Leukosis Virus*

The Rous-associated viruses types 1 and 2 (RAV-1 and RAV-2) are replication-competent avian retroviruses that do not carry a cell-derived oncogene. In young chickens, these avian leukosis viruses induce B-cell tumors originating in the bursa of Fabricius. The tumors arise after a prolonged latent period, they are monoclonal with respect to proviral integration site, and they overexpress c-*myc*. Most contain a defective provirus that has suffered a 5′ deletion. The provirus is integrated in the vicinity of the cellular *myc* gene (147,258). The exact integration site varies from tumor to tumor. Most commonly, the integrations are located between exon 1 (which is noncoding) and exon 2 of c-*myc* or within exon 1 (Fig. 6). The cis-activation of c-*myc* then occurs by promoter insertion, generating a chimeric viral–cellular fusion transcript that starts in the 3′ viral LTR. In some tumors, the provirus is found downstream of *myc,* and it may also be integrated in the opposite transcriptional orientation. These situations suggest that viral enhancer activity elevates *myc* transcription; the *myc* transcripts do not contain viral sequences. Although provirus insertion often leads to a truncation of the *myc* gene, the deleted sequences are noncoding. Their removal or inactivation seems to contribute to the elevated expression of c-*myc*. The Myc protein in avian B-cell lymphomas has been found to contain point mutations, but there is no evidence that these are necessary for transforming activity. The part played by *myc* in avian lymphomagenesis requires only overexpression of the normal cellular gene. Insertional activation of c-*myc* also is seen in murine and in feline leukemias induced by nontransducing, replication-competent retroviruses.

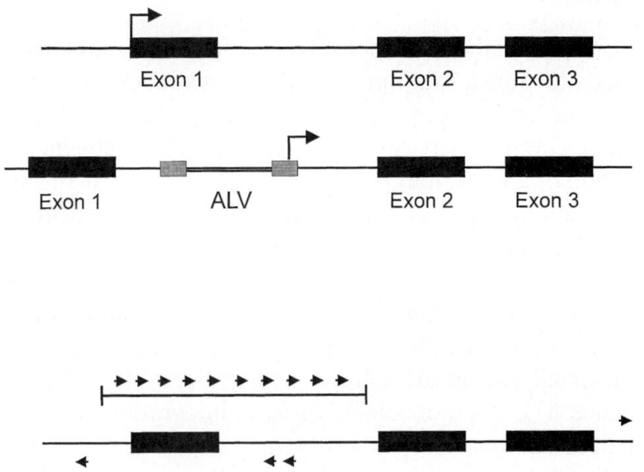

FIG. 6. Integration sites (*black triangles*) in avian B-cell lymphoma. The majority of integrations (*bracketed region*) are clustered in the noncoding exon 1 of the cellular *myc* gene and in intron 1. Most of the proviruses are integrated in the orientation of myc transcription (*triangles pointing to the right*), but some are found in opposite orientation.

In certain lines of chicken, notably those with the B5 MHC haplotype, RAV-1 induces erythroblastosis instead of lymphoma (119,230,273). These tumors also appear after a long latent period of almost 3 months, and they are monoclonal. Unlike the lymphomas, however, they contain an intact, nondefective provirus, integrated near the cellular *erbB* gene, and *erbB* expression is elevated in the tumor cells. The provirus integration sites in *erbB* are tightly clustered in a region that corresponds to the carboxyl terminus of the ligand-binding domain of the EGF receptor. Primary read-through transcripts are synthesized containing the entire proviral sequences and the truncated c-*erbB* sequences. RNA processing then creates an mRNA of uniform size with R, U5, partial *gag, env,* and *erbB* sequences. This overexpressed *erbB* mRNA codes for an EGF receptor that has deleted the ligand-binding domain at the same site as transduced viral *erbB.* The mechanism of transformation is probably similar to that of v-*erbB*: a constitutive mitogenic signal originating from the truncated EGF receptor. However, unlike v-*erbB*, the cis-activated gene contains the complete 3′ terminus, and the resulting protein retains the regulatory tyrosine phosphorylation sites of the EGF receptor. The absence of some of these sites in the *erbB* insert of AEV is therefore not the only factor determining increased tyrosine kinase and oncogenic activity. In RAV-1–induced erythroblastosis, the activated *erbB* gene also is incorporated into the viral genome with comparatively high frequency. This results in the generation of new *erbB*-transducing viruses that now induce polyclonal erythroblastosis within a short latent period.

Activation of **Wnt-*1*** *by Mouse Mammary Tumor Virus Integration*

Another retrovirus that does not carry an oncogene in its genome and induces tumors by insertional activation of a cellular oncogene is the MMTV. MMTV has several preferred integration sites in tumor target cells. Those most frequently used are close to three cellular genes *int*-1, *int*-2, and *int*-3 (for reviews, see refs. 193,246,247, 259). These genes are located on different chromosomes; furthermore, despite the identical names, there is no sequence relationship between the three. The integrated MMTV provirus enhances transcription of the adjacent cellular *int* locus in the mammary tumors, and this increased expression probably plays a key role in tumor development. Although none of the *int* sequences has been found as transduced oncogenes in naturally occurring retroviruses, there are good reasons to believe that these cellular loci represent oncogenes.

Int-1, now referred to as *wnt*-1 (an abbreviation derived from the name of the homologous *Drosophila* segment polarity gene *wingless* and *int*), belongs to a gene family that fulfills important functions in pattern formation during embryonal development from *Drosophila* to mammals (193,286). *Wnt*-1 codes for a glycoprotein that is secreted but remains closely associated with the cell of origin. It is probably a component of a short-range developmental signal. Ectopic expression of *wnt*-1 in mammary cell lines induces at least partial oncogenic transformation (47).

Int-2 codes for a protein that belongs to the FGF family (91). It also appears to be a secreted protein and may act as a growth factor. Another member of this family, *hst,* is occasionally activated in mammary tumors. *Hst* also has been isolated from human tumors (Kaposi's sarcoma and stomach cancer) as a transforming oncogene (87,344). The *int*-3 oncogene also codes for a protein with presumed developmental function and belongs to the notch family of developmental regulators (288).

Transformation by Molecular Mimicry and Insertional Mutagenesis: Friend Leukemia Virus

The Friend leukemia virus occupies a unique position among retroviruses with respect to mechanism of oncogenic transformation. Key factors in this process are an altered viral envelope protein and preferred sites of provirus integration that lead to cis-activation. However, Friend virus also inactivates the cellular p53 tumor-suppressor gene, and some of this inactivation occurs by insertional mutagenesis. Friend leukemia virus causes erythroid malignancies that result from a two-step transformation (for reviews, see refs. 21,173). Virus stocks contain two agents: a replication-competent retrovirus and a replication-defective virus called spleen focus-forming virus (SFFV), with the former acting as a helper virus for the latter. Infection of mice with SFFV and its helper leads first to a polyclonal proliferation of infected erythroblasts, causing pronounced splenomegaly. The replicating erythroblasts are neither immortal nor transplantable in syngeneic animals. The pool of dividing cells is maintained and increased through recruitment of new target erythroblasts by replicating virus. The second step of transformation in Friend disease occurs in only one or a few cells in an infected animal. It results in immortality and tumorigenicity and is due to a discrete genetic change.

A molecular analysis of this two-step leukemogenesis has revealed complex interactions between SFFV, helper virus, and target cells and tissues. Helper-free stocks of SFFV have been produced in packaging cell lines. These cell lines contain helper virus information necessary to produce infectious SFFV, but cannot synthesize infectious helper virus. Helper-free SFFV infects cells but does not produce infectious progeny. Its pathogenicity appears to be restricted to the first stage of Friend disease. Mutant analysis of the SFFV genome indicates that this initial, polyclonal proliferation of erythroblasts is caused by the expression of the altered Env protein of SFFV, gp55. Gp55 is the only gene product of SFFV, and it acts as a mitogen for erythroblasts, by binding to and activating the erythropoietin receptor (78,207). As we shall see later in the discussion of the DNA tumor viruses, this is not a unique situation—in many respects, the suspected action of the SFFV gp55 protein is analogous to the action of the E5 product of bovine papillomaviruses (see Fig. 11). The E5 protein, a transmembrane protein that interacts with the PDGF receptor, has been to shown to activate the PDGF receptor–mediated signaling by causing a ligand-independent dimerization of the receptor.

The second step in Friend virus–induced leukemia is due to a rare event that leads to the development of a monoclonal tumor consisting of transplantable, immortal, transformed erythroblasts. Second-stage Friend virus–induced malignancies have two important properties in common: the provirus is integrated in either one of two preferred loci, referred to as *fli*-1 and *spi*-1, and a high percentage of Friend virus–induced leukemias also show inactivation of p53. The cellular *fli*-1 and *spi*-1 genes code for members of the Ets family of transcription factors; the Fli-1 and Spi-1 proteins are functionally distinct; their activation is associated with different variants of Friend virus disease. Some of the p53 inactivation events are the result of proviral integration in one of the p53 alleles with consequent loss of wild-type function and reduction to inactivated homozygous state (21,169). The activation of Ets-related transcription factors and inactivation of p53 represent rare genetic changes probably contingent on continuous helper virus–dependent replication that increases the probability for critical integration events.

Oncogenesis Mediated by Essential Retroviral Proteins

Although the vast majority of oncogenic retroviruses mediate transformation by either transducing an oncogene or activating a gene after insertion, there is at least one example whereby oncogenesis is the consequence of action of an essential viral gene product. Specifically, the *tax* gene product of HTLV-I has been implicated in the development of adult T-cell leukemia (ATL) (for review, see refs. 122,240,311). The fundamental features of HTLV-I in ATL are as follows: all cases of ATL harbor the HTLV-I provirus; the provirus is found in the same chromosomal site in all cells of a given case of ATL, and hence ATL is a monoclonal disease; integration of HTLV-I does not occur in preferred sites of the host genome; HTLV-I does not carry a cell-derived oncogene within its genome; the HTLV-I provirus is not expressed in ATL cells; and if ATL cells are placed in culture, viral gene expression is turned on.

The presence of HTLV-I provirus in all cases of ATL indicates an etiologic association between HTLV-I and

ATL. The monoclonality of the tumors indicates that oncogenic transformation is a rare, and by no means inevitable, consequence of infection. It also suggests the necessity for second and possibly third contributing event. Fewer than 0.1% of all individuals infected with HTLV-I later develop ATL; the latent period can be in excess of 20 years. The absence of a preferred integration site for HTLV-I in ATL shows that there is no cis-activation of a cellular oncogene; because there is no transduced oncogene in the HTLV-I genome, ATL must be caused by a unique mechanism of viral transformation. The lack of viral expression distinguishes ATL from most other retroviral tumors and implies that although a viral gene product may be required for the initiation of transformation, it is not required for the maintenance of the transformed phenotype. The absence of viral gene expression in the fully developed leukemia also supports the probable necessity for additional events that make the growth of the leukemic cell independent of continuous viral intervention.

The HTLV-I genome contains coding information for several nonstructural proteins (Fig. 7). The best studied of these is the p40 product of the *tax* gene (58). This protein functions as a transcriptional activator for the HTLV-I genome, probably in conjunction with cellular transcription factors. The target sequences are located in the LTR of the virus. The possibility that Tax could affect the transcription of cellular genes has received support by work with transgenic mice carrying *tax* as a transgene under the control of the HTLV-I LTR. A group of these animals expressed p40 in muscle tissue. These mice developed multiple soft-tissue sarcomas of independent origin (239). The Tax protein also has been shown to transform fibroblasts in culture together with Ras (265). Similar results have also been obtained with transgenic mice that carry the *tat* gene of human immunodeficiency virus (HIV). These animals develop Kaposi's sarcoma (362).

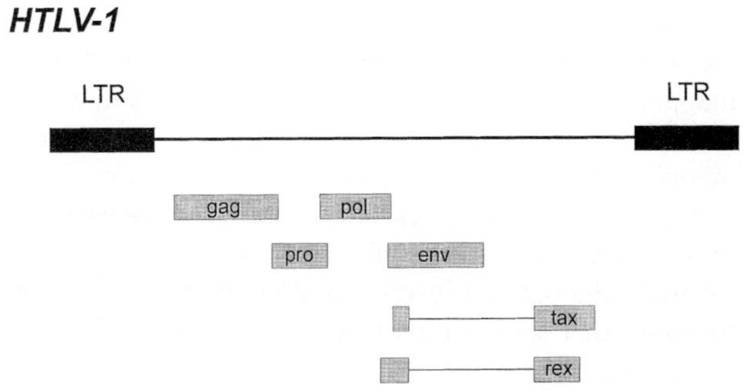

FIG. 7. Coding organization of human T-lymphotrophic virus I (HTLV-I). Gag and Env code for the major structural virion proteins; Pro for a protease, and Pol for the reverse transcriptase. Two nonstructural proteins are Tax and Rex. Tax is suspected of playing a role in HTLV-induced leukemogenesis.

Could *tax, tat,* and other regulatory genes of retroviruses function as oncogenes? Because *tax* is a viral gene without a cellular homolog and is required for efficient replication of HTLV, the situation is formally similar to that of DNA-virus–induced transformation, where the oncogenic effectors also are essential viral genes. The data on ATL and on transgenic mice are compatible with the proposal that the Tax protein affects the expression of some key cellular regulatory genes. In the case of ATL, important targets appear to be the transcription factors CREB/ATF and NF-κB, which become stably up-regulated. Inhibition of NF-κB in leukemic cells with antisense constructs leads to tumor regression in the nude mouse model (184,334).

MECHANISMS OF CELL TRANSFORMATION BY DNA TUMOR VIRUSES

Each major DNA virus family, except the parvoviruses, includes viruses that have the capacity to elicit cellular transformation (see Table 1). This represents an extremely diverse group of viruses with very different structures, genome organizations, and strategies of replication. In some cases, the DNA viruses have been shown to be responsible for inducing tumors in their natural hosts, including the induction of human cancers, whereas in other cases, they are known only to induce transformation of cells in culture and form tumors in experimental animal systems. For instance, a variety of data strongly implicate various types of the human papillomaviruses (HPVs) with the development of almost all cervical carcinomas (400). Epstein-Barr virus (EBV) has long been associated with the development of Burkitt's lymphoma as well as nasopharyngeal carcinoma, and epidemiologic data provide compelling evidence for a role of hepatitis B virus in the development of hepatocellular carcinoma (401). In contrast, although adenoviruses can form tumors in rodents and the viral genes E1A and E1B can transform human cells in culture, there is no evidence that adenoviruses are responsible for any human cancers (218). Likewise, SV40 and polyomavirus, which are clearly capable of forming tumors in experimental settings, have not been shown to be oncogenic in a natural setting. Nevertheless, it is these small DNA tumor viruses, which includes the adenoviruses, polyomaviruses, and papillomaviruses, that have been studied in greatest depth and that have provided much of our current understanding of virus-mediated oncogenic transformation. This is principally due to the small genome size and utility of these viruses as model systems for the study of gene expression and DNA replication, to name but two examples. The understanding of the oncogenic process has been aided by the concurrent elucidation of molecular mechanisms of action of the tumor virus oncoproteins. Because of the role these viruses have played in uncovering many of the details of cell-growth control, and the elucidation of the mechanisms that couple cell proliferation with cell-fate determination, the discussion focuses on the properties of cell transformation by the small DNA tumor viruses. For further discussion of the particulars of oncogenesis by either EBV or hepatitis B virus, please refer to Chapter 34 as well as Chapters 75 and 87 of *Fields Virology*, 4th ed.

Transformation by the DNA Tumor Viruses: The Relationship to the Viral Replication Cycle

With the exception of HTLV-I, the oncogenic properties of the retroviruses (RNA tumor viruses) are unrelated to the requirements for productive viral growth. In the vast majority of cases, the oncogenic retroviruses are defective for replication because of the loss of essential viral sequences during the formation of the oncogenic virus. In sharp contrast, the oncogenic properties of the DNA tumor viruses are intimately associated with the ability of these viruses to carry out a productive infection. Whereas the oncogenes of the retroviruses are cellular genes that have been acquired as a consequence of the integration of the viral genome into the host cell chromosome, and then selected by virtue of their oncogenic activity, the DNA tumor virus oncogenes are essential viral genes that bear little or no relationship to cellular counterparts. Thus infection of a cell that is permissive for viral replication will generally result in a productive infection, liberating increased numbers of viral particles, and eventual cell death. A transformation event that may have been initiated would never be scored. It is only when the viral infection takes place under nonpermissive circumstances, in which the viral replication process is aborted, that a transformation event can be observed.

The frequency of cellular transformation after infection of a nonpermissive cell by adenovirus, SV40, or polyomavirus is very low, usually less than 10^{-5}. In large part, this inefficiency reflects the lack of a specific mechanism for integration of the DNA tumor virus genome into the host cell chromosome. Thus the transformation process is extremely inefficient because of the low probability that the viral genes that are essential for transformation will integrate intact and in a state that will allow transcription at appropriate levels. The lack of a system for analyzing a productive papillomavirus infection precludes such determinations for this virus group.

The oncogenic events mediated by the DNA tumor virus oncoproteins reflect the ability of these viruses to stimulate a quiescent, nongrowing cell to enter the cell cycle. For instance, a normal target for infection by adenovirus is a terminally differentiated epithelial cell that lines the upper respiratory tract. Because this cell is not in the cell cycle, the essential substrates for the replication of both viral and cellular DNA are in short supply and thus limiting. In particular, the levels of deoxyribonucleotides are tightly regulated during the cell cycle, and increase to non–rate-limiting levels only during S phase (351). The ability of the virus to stimulate such a cell to enter S phase, creating an environment for DNA replication, is thus critical for the efficient replication of the virus. This virus-mediated S-phase induction is dependent on the viral genes that also elicit transformation in other contexts. Thus if the infection does not proceed to completion, either because of a nonpermissive cell type or as a consequence of a viral mutation that blocks viral growth, the disruption of cell-growth control that was intended to prepare the cell for viral DNA replication may instead lead to the development of a transformed cell. It is the elucidation of the mechanisms of action of these viral proteins, and in particular the cellular pathways that are targeted by the action of these viral proteins, that has propelled much of the knowledge of mammalian cell-growth control.

The DNA Tumor Virus Oncogenes

A viral infection can be divided into an early and late phase, as defined by the timing of viral gene expression relative to viral DNA replication. In general, the early genes encode proteins that prepare the infected cell to replicate viral DNA, whereas the late gene products include the structural components of the virion. For the DNA tumor viruses, these early gene products, or at least a subset of the early products, are responsible for oncogenic transformation. What follows is a general description of the adenovirus, polyomavirus, and papillomavirus genes that encode the transforming activities. For a more detailed description of these viral genes and gene products, refer to the appropriate sections in the chapters on the specific viruses.

Adenovirus

The identification of the adenovirus genes responsible for oncogenic transformation was accomplished by the mapping of viral sequences that were retained in an integrated state in transformed cells (94,121), as well as by mapping the viral transcripts present in the transformed cell (323). Such analyses indicated that a full range of viral DNA sequences could be recovered from transformed cells but that it was the left end of the viral chromosome that was common in every case. Transfection assays provided a direct demonstration that these viral sequences could indeed mediate transformation (135, 136). Subsequent studies identified two distinct transcription units within this region that encode stable mRNAs found in the cytoplasm of transformed cells, as well as during the early phase of a productive infection

(24). The two transcription units, termed E1A and E1B, each encode two major messenger RNAs through alternative splicing of the two primary transcripts (Fig. 8).

The major products of the E1A gene include proteins of 289 and 243 amino acids, encoded by the so-called $E1A_{13S}$ and $E1A_{12S}$ mRNAs, respectively, that are identical in sequence except for the additional 43 amino acids found in the middle of the $E1A_{13S}$ product. The $E1A_{13S}$ product is critical for the activation of viral transcription during a lytic infection (23,171), dependent on the CR3 sequences unique to this protein (284). This activity is not important, however, for transformation. Rather, the ability of distinct domains of the protein to interact with a series of cellular proteins, including the retinoblastoma gene product (Rb), does coincide with the transforming activity. The two major E1B gene products, a 55-kd protein of 495 amino acids and a 19-kd protein of 175 amino acids, are encoded by alternatively spliced mRNAs. The two E1B proteins do not share sequence, and they appear to perform distinct although related functions. The 55-kd E1B protein, in concert with a 34-kd product of the early region 4 gene, functions to facilitate transport of viral mRNA from the nucleus to the cytoplasm (13,201,261). In addition, the 55-kd protein interacts with at least one cellular protein, the p53 tumor suppressor (301), and it is this latter activity that correlates with transforming function (395).

Polyomaviruses

Although this group includes a large number of viruses that infect a variety of cell types and host species, the two best studied viruses include the mouse polyomavirus and the monkey SV40 virus. These two viruses are very closely related in genome structure and DNA sequence, but they differ with respect to the organization and function of the early genes that carry the

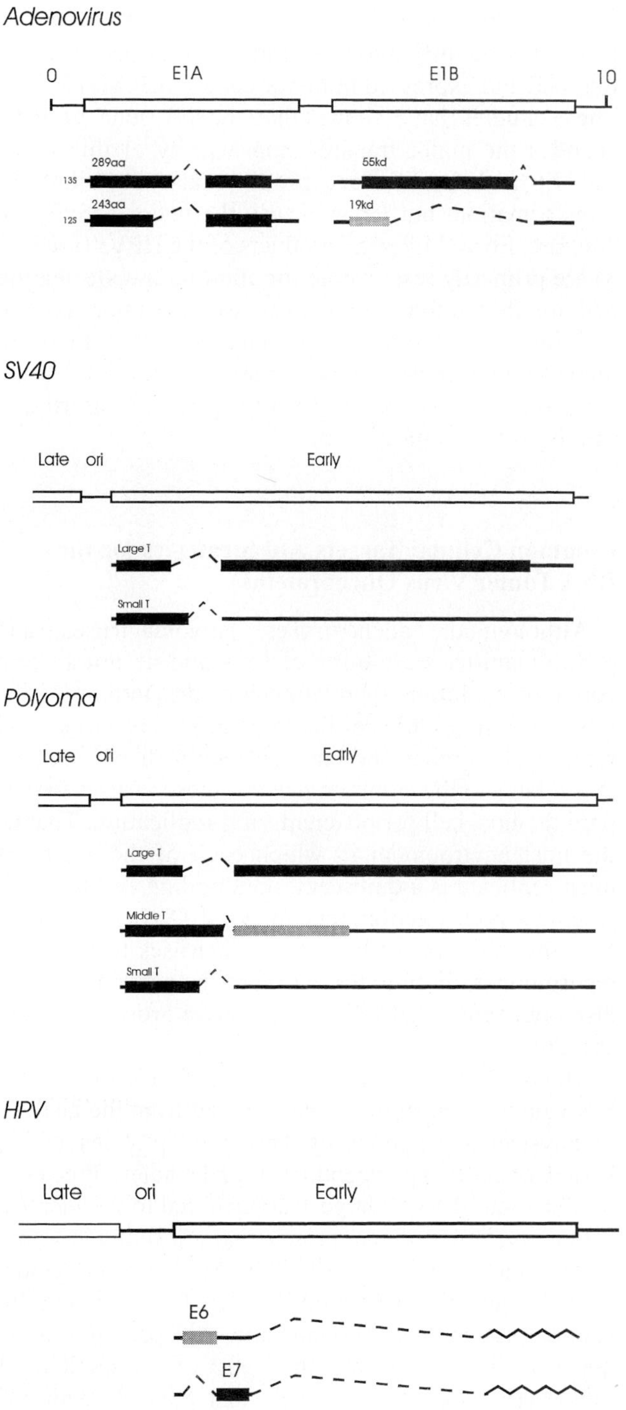

FIG. 8. The DNA tumor virus transforming genes. The left end of the adenovirus chromosome (0 to 10 map units) includes the E1A and E1B transcription units. The major mRNA products of each region are depicted, as well as the coding sequences contained within each (*black boxes*). The E1A mRNAs are commonly referred to by their sedimentation coefficients (13S and 12S), and the protein products by the amino acid residues. The E1B products are generally identified by their molecular weights. The early regions of SV40 and polyomavirus are depicted, together with the major mRNA products. The region between the early and late coding sequences referred to as "ori" contains the origin of DNA replication as well as transcriptional regulatory sequences. Coding sequences for large, middle, and small T antigen are shown by the *boxes*. The splice acceptor for polyoma large T and middle T are distinct, resulting in a change in the reading frame. The early region of the human papillomavirus genome is depicted, together with the structures of the major mRNAs that encode the E6 and E7 products. Both RNAs derive from a common promoter that starts transcription at nucleotide 97. The *wavy lines* representing 3′ sequence in the mRNAs reflect the use of splice acceptors found in cellular sequences at the site of integration of the viral DNA.

transforming activity of the virus (see Fig. 8). Both viruses encode a multifunctional protein, termed large T antigen, directly involved in the initiation of viral DNA replication through specific binding to the origin of replication (88,170). Although the origin binding capacity, as well as associated ATPase (127,353) and helicase (82,338) activities, are essential for DNA replication and a productive infection, these activities are not important for transformation (9,129,174,221,268). Rather, the ability of the viral protein to bind to a variety of cellular proteins is critical for transformation. In this regard, the function of large T antigen of SV40 and polyomavirus overlap but also are distinct. Specifically, although both bind to Rb, only SV40 large T antigen binds to p53.

In addition, both viruses encode a low-molecular-weight protein termed small t antigen that contains sequence in common with the amino terminus of large T antigen, in addition to a unique sequence. Two activities have been associated with the small t antigen: the ability to bind to the PP2A cellular protein phosphatase (252, 367), inhibiting activity for some substrates (392), and the capacity to activate polymerase II– and polymerase III–dependent transcription (212). At least one target for this transcription activation is the E2F transcription factor (213), which also is a target for activation by adenovirus E1A, SV40 large T antigen, and the HPV E7 protein (242). Although small t antigen does not appear to be essential in a lytic infection of tissue culture cells, it does contribute to transformation efficiency in conjunction with large T antigen (30,43).

Unlike SV40, polyomavirus encodes a distinct third early protein, termed middle T antigen, that is the principal transforming activity of the virus. Middle T antigen also shares sequence with the N terminus of large T antigen and small T antigen, but then as a result of the use of an alternative splice acceptor, the reading frame is changed from that used to encode the large T antigen (see Fig. 8). Unlike the other polyomavirus and adenovirus transforming proteins, which are localized in the nucleus, the polyoma middle T antigen is an integral membrane protein primarily associated with the plasma membrane (166,317). As we shall see later, middle T antigen binds to and activates *src* family tyrosine kinases as well as the phosphatidylinositol-3 kinase, PI-3 kinase (74,185,186, 240,347).

Papillomavirus

Although the papillomaviruses are grouped within the general category of the papovaviruses, they are quite distinct from the polyomaviruses with respect to structure, gene organization, and nucleotide sequence. The majority of initial work directed at papillomavirus-mediated transformation focused on the bovine papillomaviruses, particularly BPV-1. Attention has now tended to shift to the study of the HPVs, particularly given their association with human cervical carcinoma, as well as the realization of the mechanistic similarities with the adenovirus and SV40 oncogene products.

The papillomavirus genetic information is read from only one strand, with distinct transcripts being produced by alternative transcription start sites, alternative splicing, and alternative polyadenylation (refer to Chapter 30). The genes responsible for oncogenic transformation have been identified through transfection assays using *in vitro* cell-culture systems (99,215), as well as from the identification of viral sequences that are retained and expressed in tumor cells (16,308,313,335). These studies have shown that the E5 gene of BPV encodes the major transforming activity of this virus. The E6 and the E7 gene products also contribute to transformation, but E5 is clearly the major activity. In contrast, E6 and E7 gene products of the HPVs (see Fig. 8) are primarily responsible for eliciting transformation and are always found to be expressed in tumor cells. In addition, the integrated papillomavirus DNA found in human tumor cells usually is disrupted in the E2 gene, the product of which negatively regulates transcription of the E6,E7 promoter (16).

Common Cellular Targets and Strategies for the DNA Tumor Virus Oncoproteins

Although the adenoviruses, polyomaviruses, and papillomaviruses are quite distinct and do not share a common evolutionary relationship, the actions of the transforming proteins of the three groups of viruses are remarkably similar and have defined a shared strategy that relates to the common need of these viruses to prepare the host cell for efficient viral replication. That is, the host environment in which each of these viruses must replicate is a quiescent, nondividing cell that represents a poor environment for viral DNA replication. It is the common ability of these viruses to alter this environment, through the action of the proteins that are also oncogenic, that relates replicative growth to oncogenicity.

Much of the current understanding of the actions of the DNA tumor virus proteins has derived from the analysis of physical associations of these viral proteins with a variety of cellular polypeptides. Initial studies, directed at the function of SV40 large T antigen, led to the identification of a 53-kd cellular protein that was found in T antigen immunoprecipitates (197,209). Further work demonstrated a specific interaction between T antigen and this cellular protein, which became known as p53, and subsequent studies have shown that most of the small DNA tumor viruses encode a protein that interacts with p53

(Table 5). The one clear exception among the small DNA tumor viruses is polyomavirus, which shows no evidence of encoding a protein that binds to p53. Most important, the ability of the adenovirus 55-kd E1B protein, the HPV E6 product, and SV40 T antigen to associate with p53 coincides with the transforming activity of the viral proteins (197,209,376,395).

Similar studies identified a large number of cellular polypeptides associated with the adenovirus E1A product (140,393). Analysis of E1A sequences essential for binding to these cellular proteins revealed two domains of interaction. One, involving N-terminal sequence and a portion of the CR1 domain, bound to a 300-kd protein, whereas the other, including the CR1 and CR2 domains, bound to a series of proteins ranging in molecular mass from 130 kd to 33 kd. Two subsequent findings with respect to these E1A interactions were of enormous significance, with respect to developing an understanding of the action of both the DNA tumor virus oncoproteins and normal mechanisms of cell-growth control. First, one of the E1A-associated proteins, a polypeptide of 105 kd, was identified as the product of the retinoblastoma susceptibility gene (382). This simple finding had immediate and far-reaching implications, because this was the first suggestion that the action of a DNA tumor virus transforming protein could be viewed as inactivating the function of a cellular growth-suppressing protein.

Second, it soon became evident that the binding of the adenovirus E1A protein to the Rb tumor-suppressor protein was an activity shared with the other DNA tumor viruses (see Table 2). SV40 and polyomavirus large T antigen, as well as the E7 product of the HPVs, were all found to bind to Rb (84,101). Moreover, the ability of each viral protein to bind to Rb was found to be dependent on viral sequences that were also important for oncogenic activity. Comparison of sequences of the viral proteins revealed a short region of homology that included the sequence important for binding to Rb (111) (Fig. 9). Although the homology between the viral proteins is limited to these sequences and is not consistent

TABLE 5. *Cellular targets of the DNA tumor virus oncoproteins*

Virus	Gene Product	Cellular Target
Adenovirus	E1A	Rb
	E1B	p53
SV40	Large T antigen	Rb, p53
Polyomavirus	Large T antigen	Rb
	Middle T antigen	Src, PI 3-K
Papillomavirus	E7	Rb
	E6	p53
	E5	PDGF receptor

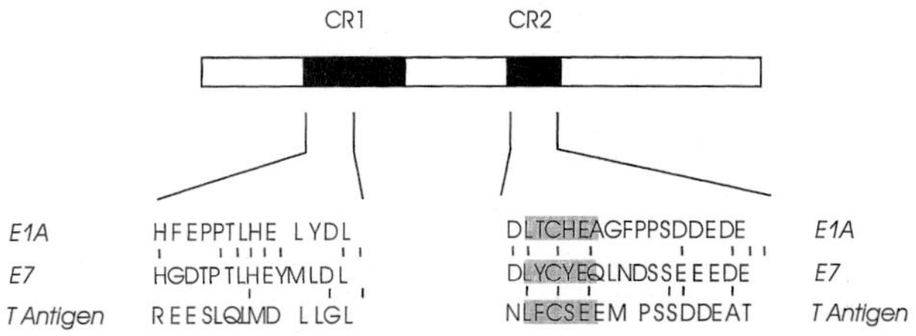

FIG. 9. Homology in the viral sequences involved in binding to the Rb family of proteins. The regions in E1A that exhibit homology with sequences in SV40 T antigen and HPV E7 are depicted (111). The L-X-C-X-E motif found in the CR2 region of E1A, that is also shared with various cellular proteins (85) including the D-type cyclins (227,390), is indicated by the *hatched box.*

with an evolutionary relationship among the viruses, it does suggest that the viruses have each acquired a common activity.

Given that the ability of the various DNA tumor virus proteins to interact with Rb and p53 coincides with the transforming activity of the viral proteins, together with the fact that it is the loss of Rb and p53 gene function that is associated with the development of tumors, implies that the viral proteins achieve the same result by binding to the cellular regulatory proteins. This point is further emphasized by the relationship between HPV gene expression and the state of the Rb and p53 genes in cervical carcinoma cell lines. The vast majority of cervical carcinomas are associated with the so-called high-risk types of HPV, primarily HPV 16 and HPV 18 (400). An analysis of cell lines derived from cervical carcinomas revealed the presence of normal, wild-type Rb and p53 genes in those cells that were HPV positive and that expressed the E6 and E7 viral gene products, whereas mutations were found in the Rb and p53 genes in cell lines that were HPV negative (303). It is apparent from these results that loss of Rb and p53 function is a common event in the development of these human tumors, either as a result of mutation or through the action of the viral proteins.

Common Mechanisms of Action of the DNA Tumor Virus Oncoproteins

The physical association of the DNA tumor virus proteins with the same two cellular growth-regulatory proteins implies that these otherwise diverse viruses share a common need. Although the inactivation of Rb and p53 is most often viewed in the context of oncogenesis, the targeting of these proteins by DNA virus regulatory proteins implies a role in facilitating a productive infection. Given the common properties of the DNA tumor virus oncoproteins in the binding to key cellular growth-regulatory proteins, we discuss the common aspects of their function rather than discussing each individual viral protein in isolation.

Inactivation of Retinoblastoma Protein Function

As described earlier, adenovirus E1A, SV40 large T antigen, and HPV E7 physically interact with the retinoblastoma protein. A variety of studies have now shown that these interactions involve viral protein sequences that also are critical for transforming activity, and thus it is clear that this association is part of the transforming function. A very large body of work has now elucidated the role of the Rb protein in normal cell-growth control and provided a rationale for the strategy of the DNA tumor virus oncoproteins in disrupting this function (see Fig. 1).

Studies directed at the action of the E1A proteins in viral transcription activation during a lytic infection led to the identification of a cellular transcription factor, termed E2F, that was important for transcription of the adenovirus E2 gene (188). Subsequent studies revealed that this cellular transcription factor was normally complexed to other cellular proteins in most cell types, that these interactions prevented the activation of E2 transcription, and that the E1A protein possessed the capacity to disrupt these complexes, releasing E2F that could be used for E2 transcription (14). The ability of E1A to carry out this dissociation was found to be dependent on viral sequences that were known to be important for oncogenic activity, including binding to the Rb protein (279). This finding suggested the relationship depicted in Fig. 10A, in which the interaction of E1A with a cellular protein such as Rb, as previously described by immunoprecipitation assays, results in disruption of the E2F complex. A variety of experiments have now shown that the Rb protein, along with the majority of the other proteins previously identified as E1A-binding proteins, is a component of the E2F complexes (15,17,18,53,57,90,332). Moreover, not only does E1A have the capacity to release E2F from interactions with Rb and Rb-family proteins, but so also do the other DNA tumor virus oncoproteins including T antigen and E7 (56).

The realization that E2F was a target for control by Rb, together with the observation that Rb function was controlled by the action of G_1 cyclin-dependent kinases, led to the eventual delineation of a G_1 regulatory pathway that ultimately controls the accumulation of E2F activity. The G_1 cyclin-dependent kinase–mediated phosphorylation abolishes the ability of Rb to interact with E2F proteins; thus the physiologic control of Rb function is mediated by G_1 CDK phosphorylation. The viral oncoproteins E1A, Tag, and E7 effect an inactivation of Rb through a direct physical interaction, independent of phosphorylation. Interestingly, the mechanism for recognition of Rb by either the viral oncoproteins or the G_1 cyclin may be similar. As

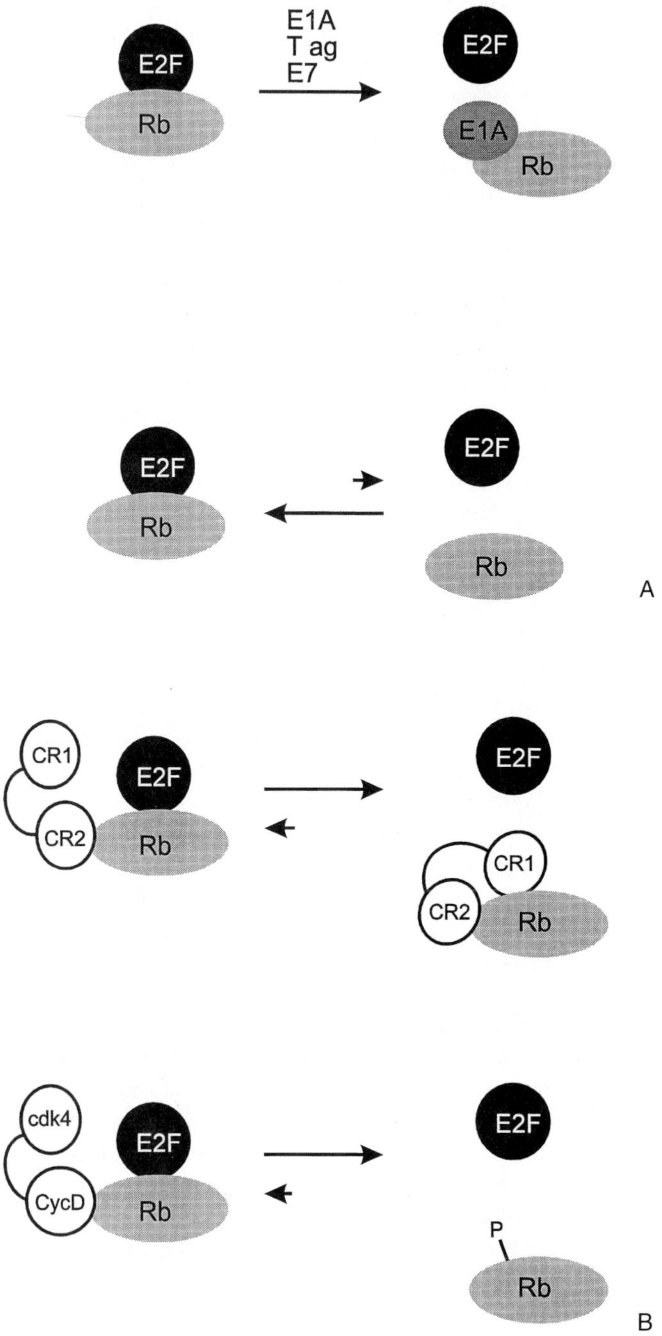

FIG. 10. Inactivation of Rb-mediated control of E2F activity. **A:** Depicted is the process of E1A (and T antigen and E7) mediated release of E2F from the complex with Rb. This action leaves the viral protein firmly associated with Rb, releasing a transcriptionally active E2F. **B:** A mechanism for E1A or D/cdk4-mediated disruption of E2F–Rb interaction.

depicted in Fig. 10B, the E1A-mediated disruption of the E2F–Rb complex would appear to involve first the recognition of Rb by the CR2 domain of E1A, followed by interaction of the CR1 domain with a site on Rb involved in E2F interaction (165). The conserved LXCXE sequence element found in CR2, which is shared in the other DNA tumor virus oncoproteins (see Fig. 8), also is found in the cyclin D1 protein and has been shown to be important for the interaction of cyclin D1 with Rb (96). Thus the LXCXE motif may be responsible for targeting either a viral protein or a kinase to Rb to achieve an inactivation of function.

The consequence of inactivation of Rb, either by phosphorylation or by binding of a viral oncoprotein, is to allow the accumulation of E2F activity. A large body of work has now shown that the genes subject to E2F control include the majority, if not all, of the genes encoding proteins essential for DNA replication (100,243). These include components of the enzymatic machinery such as DNA polymerase α and PCNA as well as the enzymes generating the necessary deoxyribonucleotide substrates such as ribonucleotide reductase, thymidine kinase, and dihydrofolate reductase. Moreover, it also is now clear that the majority of genes encoding proteins that function at the origins of replication, including the proteins of the origin recognition complex (ORC), the Mcm proteins, and Cdc6 are all E2F targets (200). Thus the Rb/E2F pathway, which is normally controlled by the action of G_1 cyclin-dependent kinases in response to a growth stimulus, or deregulated by the action of the DNA tumor virus oncoproteins, is responsible for the synthesis of the apparatus of DNA replication.

Numerous previous experiments have shown that the infection of quiescent cells by adenovirus, SV40, and polyoma results in the activation of S phase in these infected cells and that this coincides with the induction of the activities normally associated with entry into S phase and that are now known to be E2F targets (98,116,177, 198,391). Very likely, this activation reflects the need of the virus to create an environment appropriate for viral DNA synthesis. Thus when a DNA tumor virus infects a quiescent, nongrowing cell, which is the normal target for infection by these viruses, the environment for DNA replication, whether it be viral or cellular, is not suitable. For instance, the levels of deoxynucleotides are very low in quiescent cells and they only increase as a consequence of the induction of ribonucleotide reductase activity when such cells are stimulated to grow and enter S phase (35,107). Thus through the ability to activate genes encoding the enzymes that create the appropriate environment, the virus is then able to achieve efficient replication of viral DNA.

Inactivation of p53 Function

After the discovery of p53 as a protein in association with SV40 T antigen (197,209), various analyses suggested that p53 functioned as an oncoprotein (105,168, 254). Thus early speculation centered on a role for the association of the viral protein with p53 in stimulating or somehow augmenting the action of this oncoprotein. A radical change in thinking occurred when it was realized that the p53 gene used for the initial studies of transformation was in fact a mutated version and that the transforming activity of the previously assayed p53 gene was dependent on this mutation (104,113). Moreover, assays of the normal wild-type version of p53 revealed that it possessed characteristics of a tumor-suppressor molecule (112). It is now clear that the loss of p53 function, as a result of mutation or deletion of the gene, occurs during the development of a large number of human cancers (202). These studies suggest that loss of p53 function may be an event involved in the majority of human tumors.

Once again, each of the DNA tumor viruses encodes a protein that has the ability to interact with p53 and, as a consequence of this interaction, inactivate p53 function. In contrast to the targeting of Rb, however, the viral protein sequences involved in these interactions, as well as the result of the interaction, appear to be distinct among the different viruses. That is, an examination of amino acid sequences known to be involved in the targeting of p53 in adenovirus E1B, SV40 T-antigen, and HPV E6 show no evidence for sequence similarity. Moreover, it would appear that distinct domains of the p53 protein are recognized by the viral proteins. Finally, it also is apparent that the targeting of p53 represents a point of divergence in the polyomavirus group, in that the primate polyomavirus SV40 has evolved a protein to target the p53 molecule, whereas the mouse polyomavirus lacks this function and shows no evidence of perturbing the function of p53.

Although the actual mechanism by which E1B, T antigen, and E6 target p53 does not appear to be conserved, the ultimate consequence of the interaction of these viral proteins with p53 is the same: a loss of p53 function. For instance, whereas T-antigen interaction with p53 appears to stabilize the p53 protein, presumably in an inactive state, the interaction of the HPV E6 protein with p53 triggers a ubiquitin-mediated degradation of the p53 protein (304). The process of E6-mediated degradation of p53 has been studied in some detail because these events can be assayed in cell-free extracts. These studies have led to the identification of an additional cellular protein, termed E6-AP (E6-associated protein), that functions in concert with E6 to target p53 for destruction (158,159). E6-AP functions as an E3 ubiquitin protein ligase and may be targeted to p53 through the interaction with E6, because E6-AP does not appear to be involved in p53 degradation in the absence of E6 (346).

What normal function of p53 is disrupted by these viral oncoproteins? Most likely, it is the ability of p53 to function as a transcription factor that is targeted by the viral proteins. The p53 protein has been shown to bind to DNA in a sequence-specific manner (180) and, as a consequence of this binding, activates transcription if the binding site is part of a promoter element (120,396). The *WAF1* gene, which encodes the p21 cyclin kinase inhibitor (141), was originally identified as a target for p53 transcriptional activation (103). Thus the p53-mediated suppression of cell growth may be due in part to the inhibition of G_1 cyclin-dependent kinases, the activity of which is critical for G_1 progression and cell growth.

p53 Has been extensively characterized as a transcription factor that can contribute to the activation of many genes as well as the repression of others. The transcriptional activity of p53 appears to underlie its ability to induce growth arrest, and at least in some contexts, its ability to induce apoptosis. p53 Binds DNA as a tetramer, recognizing a DNA consensus consisting of two inverted repeats of 5′-PuPuPuC(A/T)-3′. p53 Directly regulates, through p53 binding sites in the promoters, the expression of several genes involved in cell-cycle control, apoptosis, and the response to cellular stress, including p21, Bax, GADD45, IGF-BP3, and 14-3-3γ (185,203). p53 Also can repress the expression of other genes lacking p53 binding sites in their promoters, including the antiapoptotic *Bcl2* gene, apparently by interacting with the TATA-containing basal promoter (185,203). Transcriptional repression by p53 may be important for its proapoptotic function, as the expression of *Bcl2* or E1B 19K blocks p53-dependent apoptosis and transcriptional repression without affecting transcriptional activation (297,325). As a further indication that p53-dependent growth arrest and apoptosis are genetically separable, p53 that is deleted of its proline-rich domain (amino acids 62–91) retains the ability to induce growth arrest, but is deficient in the induction of apoptosis (360). Interestingly, this p53 mutant can still transactivate some genes such as *mdm2*, *p21*, and *bax*, but fails to activate the PIG3 redox enzyme gene or to repress the transcription of genes normally repressed by p53.

The importance of transcriptional control by p53 is highlighted by the fact that most mutational hotspots found in human cancers map to the DNA-binding domain of p53 (185). Nonetheless, DNA damage-induced p53-dependent apoptosis can occur in the presence of inhibitors of RNA and protein synthesis (51,366), and overexpression of transactivation-defective p53 can induce apoptosis in HeLa cells (145). In other contexts, however, such as apoptosis induced by the adenoviral E1A oncoprotein, apoptosis is abrogated when the expressed p53 possesses mutations that reduce DNA binding or transactivation (8,298). Thus p53 appears to mediate both transcription-dependent and transcription-independent apoptosis.

The Actions of the DNA Tumor Virus Proteins Suggest a Functional Link Between the Rb and p53 Pathways

Although the combined action of adenovirus E1A and E1B leads to the oncogenic transformation of susceptible cells in culture, E1A expression alone most often leads to cell death as a result of apoptosis (275,380). Expression of the adenovirus E1B gene suppresses this E1A-induced apoptosis response, allowing the cells to become stably transformed. This phenomenon was first observed in cells infected by adenovirus E1B mutants, in which the infection led to the degradation of both viral and cellular DNA (260,379), a hallmark of the apoptosis response.

Further studies have shown that the induction of apoptosis in an adenovirus infection not only is dependent on E1A expression but also involves an induction of the p53 tumor-suppressor protein. In particular, there is no such apoptotic response in cells that are lacking a functional p53 gene, but the response can be restored on transfection of the wild-type p53 gene (83). It is now evident that the action of E1A to induce apoptosis is tightly linked to its ability to deregulate the Rb pathway. Direct evidence for this has come from studies of E1A mutants, in which it is clear that the ability of E1A to promote apoptosis and induce p53 accumulation is dependent on the domains involved in Rb binding (214). As discussed previously, the inactivation of Rb leads to deregulation of E2F. Indeed, overexpression of the E2F1 protein, a key target for Rb control, leads not only to an induction of S phase but also to an induction of apoptosis, which is largely p53 dependent (190,270,321,387). Further work has shown that the ability of E2F to induce apoptosis when expressed in quiescent cells is an activity unique to E2F1 (86). Moreover, E2F1, but not E2F2, also induces an accumulation of p53 protein (189). Thus one can now envision the apoptotic response and the induction of p53 accumulation as a response to the deregulation of the Rb pathway, with the E2F1 protein providing a signal to trigger p53 accumulation.

The inactivation of p53 function by the viral oncoproteins may mimic the normal activity of the product of the cellular *mdm2* gene. *Mdm2* was originally identified as a gene amplified in various tumors, primarily sarcomas (52). Subsequent studies revealed that the Mdm2 protein could physically interact with p53 and inhibit the transactivation function of p53 (60,250). In addition, it is now evident that Mdm2 functions to target p53 for ubiquitin-mediated degradation (144,191). Thus like the HPV E6 protein, Mdm2 can control the accumulation of p53 by controlling the stability of the protein.

A variety of studies have now elucidated a pathway that links the deregulation of the Rb pathway with the induction of p53 accumulation. A key component in this pathway is the $p19^{ARF}$ gene product. ARF (alternate reading frame) was identified as an alternate reading frame contained within the locus encoding the p16 cyclin kinase inhibitor (271). ARF has now been shown to interact with and control the activity of Mdm2; specifically, ARF prevents Mdm2 from targeting p53 for degradation (81,175,264,400,401). Moreover, other work has demonstrated that the $p19^{ARF}$ gene is activated by E2F1 (86), thus linking the deregulation of the Rb pathway with the activation of ARF, inactivation of Mdm2, and thus the accumulation of p53 protein (see Fig. 11).

Mdm2 may play a normal role in regulating the action of p53, possibly during normal growth stimulation (386). Although it is straightforward to envision the E2F1–ARF–Mdm2 pathway as a mechanism to monitor the integrity of the Rb pathway, triggering cell death when mutations or viral oncoproteins disrupt the normal control of the pathway, it also is possible that the balance of these two regulatory pathways (Rb and p53) plays an important role in normal cell growth and tissue homeostasis. Perhaps the most striking observation relating Mdm2 to p53 in the context of normal physiology is the analysis of mice bearing deletions of the p53 or Mdm2 locus. Targeted deletion of the Mdm2 gene leads to an early embryonic lethality, with mice not surviving beyond embryonic day 6. Although loss of p53 is without discernible effect during embryonic development, combining the p53 deletion with the Mdm2 null leads to a complete suppression of the Mdm2 lethality (172,234). Thus under circumstances in which there is likely to be no DNA damaged–induced p53 response, or oncogene activation, p53 and Mdm2 are seen to function in relation to one another. Given the fact that normal proliferation leads to the accumulation of E2F1 as a consequence of Rb phosphorylation, it may be necessary to block the ARF–Mdm2–p53 pathway each time cells are stimulated to grow.

The paradigm established by the analysis of the DNA tumor virus oncoproteins, whereby the dual inactivation of Rb and p53 can be seen as a mechanism to deregulate cell proliferation (inactivation of Rb) and block the response to this deregulation (inactivation of p53), may

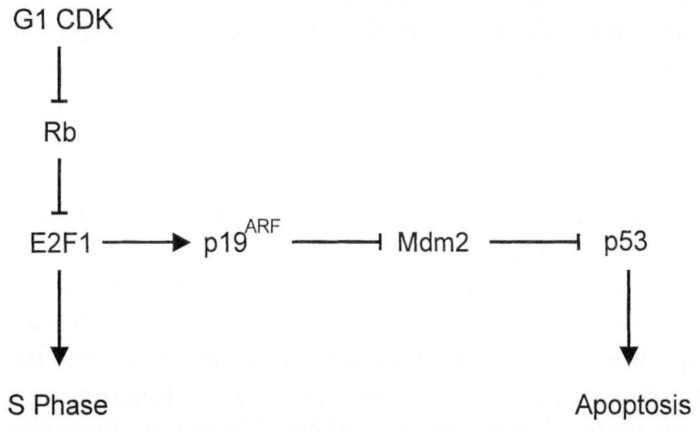

FIG. 11. The E2F1/ARF/Mdm2/p53 pathway. The accumulation of E2F1 protein, after inactivation of Rb by G_1 cyclin–dependent kinase action, leads to the activation of transcription of the $p19^{ARF}$ gene. The ARF protein has been shown to interfere with the ability of Mdm2 to target p53 for ubiquitin-mediated degradation. Thus as a result of activation of the ARF pathway, p53 levels increase due to reduced turnover.

reflect events occurring during the development of human tumors. With the exception of colon cancer, virtually all human cancers exhibit a deregulation of the Rb pathway. This might take the form of amplification of a D-type cyclin gene, amplification of the cyclin-dependent kinase gene, loss of a cyclin kinase inhibitor, or loss of Rb. Even in colon cancer, the pathway may be deregulated, because recent data have shown that loss of the APC tumor suppressor, which controls the β-catenin/TCF transcription factor, leads to an activation of Myc (148) as well as D cyclin transcription (350). Certainly, a role for TCF in the activation of D cyclin transcription provides one direct connection to the Rb/E2F pathway, but, in addition, other experiments provide evidence for a direct role for Myc in the activation of E2F genes (199,315).

In addition to the fact that virtually all tumors exhibit a loss of Rb pathway control, roughly half of all human tumors exhibit an inactivation of p53, resulting from either inactivating mutations or generation of dominant negative mutant forms of p53. Amplification of the Mdm2 gene is seen in a fraction of those tumors that appear to be p53 wild-type, and recent data indicated that loss of ARF is frequently seen in p53 wild-type tumors. Thus as is the case for the Rb pathway, one way or another there is a loss of p53 function. One might speculate that the deregulation of the Rb pathway, leading to loss of proliferative restraint, coupled with loss of the p53 pathway that abolishes the response to loss of Rb, are events that will always be found in the course of tumorigenesis.

Other DNA Tumor Virus–Transforming Activities

Although the inactivation of Rb and p53 function is an activity that is common to the small DNA tumor viruses, at least two other virus-specific activities have evolved that do not appear to be shared in common among the DNA tumor viruses, but that do clearly contribute to the transforming capacity of the viruses. In one instance, the activity may represent an alternate path to p53 inactivation.

Although the bovine papillomaviruses (BPVs) show considerable homology and related function to the human viruses, the major transforming activity of BPV is the product of the E5 gene, a 44-amino-acid transmembrane protein. Studies of the mechanism of action of the E5 protein has revealed a role in activating tyrosine kinase signaling. In particular, the E5 homodimer interacts with, and promotes dimerization of, the PDGF receptor, leading to the activation of kinase activity of the receptor and thus the signaling cascade normally activated by binding of PDGF (see Fig. 12) (for review, see ref. 92). As such, the E5 protein can be seen to act as a molecular mimic of a growth factor, providing a growth stimulus in the absence of the normal proliferative signal. This action of E5 is quite analogous to the action of the SFFV gp55 pro-

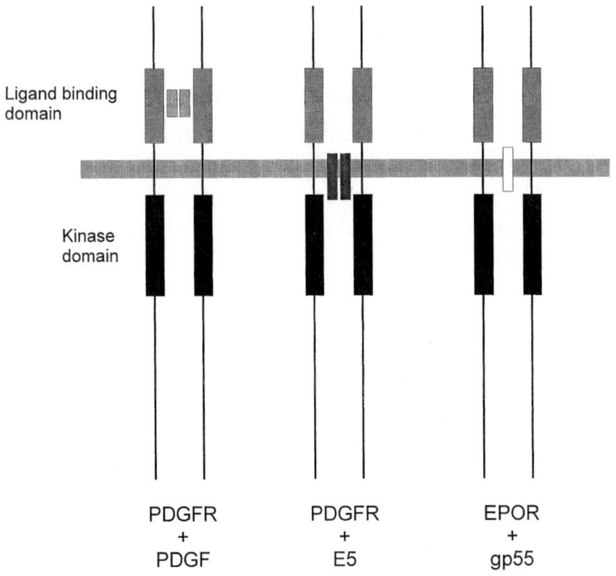

FIG. 12. Oncogenesis by molecular mimicry. The platelet-derived growth factor (PDGF) receptor is normally activated by PDGF-mediated receptor dimerization, which then activates the tyrosine kinase activity of the receptor and initiates a signal-transduction cascade. The E5 transmembrane protein of bovine papillomavirus provides a mimic of the PDGF signal by inducing a ligand-independent dimerization of the receptor through a direct interaction. Although not proven in detail, the gp55 protein of SFFV may act similarly to activate the EPO receptor independent of erythropoietin.

tein, also a transmembrane protein that leads to a ligand-independent activation of the Epo receptor.

A second example of virus-mediated activation of a kinase signaling pathway, independent of normal proliferative signals, can be seen in the analysis of the polyomavirus transformation. The polyomavirus middle T antigen, a product unique to polyoma, revealed the association of this viral protein with the c-*src* proto-oncogene (73,74). The interaction of middle T with the c-*src* product results in an activation of the tyrosine kinase activity of the Src protein (41,71), as a consequence of the prevention of a phosphorylation-mediated inhibition of the Src kinase (54,71). Subsequent experiments have revealed that middle T can complex with other members of the Src kinase family including the Yes and Fyn kinases (63,155,186,194). In addition, formation of the middle T antigen/Src kinase complex leads to a recruitment of the PI-3 kinase (176,381), resulting in the formation of a ternary complex involving middle T, Src, and the PI-3 kinase. The formation of this complex is dependent on the phosphorylation of middle T at tyrosine 315 by the Src kinase (347). One role for the middle T–mediated activation of Src kinase activity for a lytic viral infection would appear to be the promotion of phosphorylation of the late viral capsid protein VP1, an essential modification for viral morphogenesis (123).

The interaction of middle T with Src family kinases and the PI-3 kinase appears to be a unique feature of polyomavirus, because an equivalent interaction is not found with proteins encoded by SV40, adenovirus, or papillomavirus. Moreover, this association and concomitant activation of Src kinase activity appear to be sufficient for transformation by polyomavirus. Given that this activity does mediate transformation, together with the observations that the common aspect of the other small DNA tumor viruses appears to involve an ability to drive quiescent cells into a cell cycle, one suspects that the action of middle T in activating the Src kinase pathway achieves a similar result: the creation of a proliferating cell environment that is conducive to viral replication. Indeed, analysis of a polyomavirus mutant that is defective in binding and activating PI-3 kinase suggests that this activity of middle T is important for the ability of polyomavirus to prevent apoptosis (79).

A number of previous experiments have identified polyomavirus mutants that exhibit a host range and transformation defective phenotype (hr-t) (22) that have mutations in the small and middle T specific sequences. These mutants are unable to induce a permissive state for virus replication in certain cell types, presumably a reflection of the requirement for middle T function in altering the growth properties of the target cell. Although in most instances there is a tight link between the two phenotypes, isolate middle T mutants continue to grow but fail to transform (123).

The analysis of middle T antigen–mediated transformation and tumor induction *in vivo* has shown that the presence of the src kinase is not essential for this activity because infection of src-negative mice with a middle T–expressing retrovirus led to the formation of tumors with a frequency nearly the same as that for Src-positive mice (352). Nevertheless, although the association of middle T with Src may not be absolutely critical, it is certainly possible that other Src family kinases compensate for the loss of Src because middle T is found in association with *yes* and *fyn*. These results do raise the question, however, of the nature of the underlying specificity in the interaction of middle T with one of the kinases.

Finally, although the action of middle T antigen is clearly sufficient to transform cells, one suspects that the ability of polyoma large T antigen to bind to and inactivate the Rb protein may well contribute in some circumstances. For instance, although polyomavirus mutants that are defective in large T function with respect to Rb binding are still capable of transformation and induction of tumor formation, they are defective in immortalization assays (117). Thus it may well be true that it is the combination of large T function in inactivating Rb together with the action of middle T in activating the Src kinase pathway that is necessary to facilitate fully the creation of a suitable environment for polyomavirus replication.

EVOLUTION OF COMMON STRATEGIES OF THE DNA TUMOR VIRUSES

Given that the small DNA tumor viruses represent a diverse group of viruses with little or no evolutionary relationship, it is striking that they share common targets and strategies for replication and transformation. Although the inactivation of Rb and p53 by the DNA tumor virus oncoproteins is generally considered in the context of oncogenic transformation, these events must be important for the normal process of a productive infection by these viruses, because it is the ability to replicate that provides the driving force for the evolution of these viral genes. Clearly, these evolutionarily distinct viruses share a common need and have developed a common strategy, not to transform cells, but to replicate.

As discussed previously, these otherwise diverse viruses do have a common need to induce a quiescent, nondividing cell to enter S phase so as to create an environment that is favorable for viral DNA replication. The inactivation of Rb function through the action of E1A, T antigen, or E7 would appear to facilitate this process by activating the E2F transcription factor and possibly the D type G_1 cyclins. At least for E2F activation, this would lead to an induction of various genes that create the environment for DNA replication.

The virus-mediated inactivation of p53 function also appears to facilitate entry to S phase, because expression of p53 can result in a G_1 arrest, particularly in response to DNA-damaging events (211), or to initiate a pathway of programmed cell death in response to various proliferative signals (378). As discussed in previous sections, the ability of E1A to stimulate S phase also coincides with the induction of apoptosis. The mechanism for this response remains to be determined, but it does involve the p53 tumor-suppressor protein. Indeed, there is an induction of p53 expression in cells expressing E1A. The E1B 55-kd protein, SV40 T antigen, and HPV E6 all block the action of p53 and thus block the apoptosis pathway. Thus one might view these actions as "allowing" the E1A-mediated process of S-phase induction to continue.

Given the common activities exhibited by adenovirus, SV40, and HPV, it is perhaps equally striking to find a distinct activity that is unique to polyomavirus, the middle T antigen–mediated induction of tyrosine kinase activity. Presumably polyomavirus has evolved a mechanism to accomplish the same result, the creation of a favorable environment for viral replication, without the need of eliminating the Rb and p53 suppression events. Nevertheless, it also is true that polyoma large T antigen does target Rb, and given the pairwise relationship between Rb inactivation and p53 inactivation seen with the other viral oncoproteins, one wonders if the ultimate action of middle T might lead to the same result.

Finally, if the small DNA tumor viruses have evolved a common mechanism to drive a quiescent cell into S phase to allow efficient viral DNA replication, one might also anticipate that other DNA viruses that must replicate DNA at a high level, such as the herpesviruses or the poxviruses, would also find this to be a beneficial event, yet there is no compelling evidence that any of the herpesviruses or poxviruses encode proteins that inactivate Rb or p53. It is striking, however, that many of the genes whose products create the S-phase environment, and that are suspected to be activated as a consequence of the release of E2F from inhibition by Rb, are also found within the genomes of the large viruses of the herpesvirus and poxvirus family (2). Although it is clear that the entire complement of genes is not found within every virus of these groups, it is nevertheless true that each virus contains a ribonucleotide reductase, the rate-limiting enzyme in deoxynucleotide biosynthesis (351). Thus a common strategy of the DNA viruses, whether oncogenic or not, may be to induce activities that create the appropriate environment for viral DNA replication to take place in an efficient manner. If this involves the disruption of normal cell-growth control events to force a quiescent cell into S phase, then transformation can result if the infection does not go to completion.

CONCLUSIONS

The study of virus-induced oncogenic transformation has defined paradigmatic changes that differentiate cancer cells from their normal progenitors. These changes affect the components of signal-transduction pathways and circuits that control the cell cycle. RNA tumor viruses mutate the sequence information of growth-regulatory genes. These mutations are causative events in oncogenesis. DNA tumor viruses, conversely, disrupt various growth regulatory events as a consequence of the interaction of viral proteins with cellular regulatory proteins, temporarily inactivating the function of the cellular protein. The genes encoding these cellular proteins remain unaltered.

We have seen from the study of the RNA and DNA tumor viruses that the induction of oncogenic transformation results from the targeting of two distinct classes of cellular genes and their products: oncogenes and tumor-suppressor genes. Oncogenes encode components of cellular signal transduction, and their activation leads to a constitutive growth signal. Most often, it is this process that is seen in the retroviruses. By contrast, tumor-suppressor genes encode negative regulators of cell growth, particularly the cell cycle, and their inactivation removes such attenuating controls. The oncogenic activities of the DNA tumor viruses most often target the tumor suppressors.

The activation of cellular oncogenes can occur by all manner of mutagenic events, which include, besides viral intervention, point mutation, and chromosomal translocation and amplification. DNA-transfection techniques have identified numerous genes that can confer oncogenic properties of recipient cells. Some of these genes are closely related to the oncogenes that have also been identified in retroviruses. Many others, however, have no known association with viruses. However, the normal functions of all these genes are related to the control of cell growth, providing strong evidence for their oncogenic potential as altered control elements.

The genetic inactivation of tumor-suppressor genes clearly plays an important role in the heritable forms of human cancer. Although the action of the tumor virus proteins in achieving a phenotypic inactivation of these gene products is clearly not relevant to the understanding of the genetic basis of human cancer, it is true that somatic mutations of tumor-suppressor genes are also increasingly recognized as critical factors in sporadic cancers. Virus-induced and genetic inactivation of tumor suppressors have the same net effect as most dramatically seen in the case of cervical carcinomas: the loss of tumor-suppressor activity and thus the study of the events after inactivation by viral proteins has been and will continue to be an important approach for the study of human cancer.

Finally, despite strong evidence for the genetic etiology of cancer, it is likely that epigenetic factors also play important, but much less well defined and understood roles. In certain circumstances, such factors can exert a dominant effect, thereby converting tumor cells into normal cells. A dramatic demonstration of such epigenetic reversion is seen with murine embryonal carcinoma cells that, when injected into a normal mouse blastocyst, become subject to developmental control and contribute to the development of normal mouse tissues (231). Because molecular biology is biased in favor of genetic analysis and interpretation, it is especially important to keep a watchful eye for such epigenetic phenomena. Although the influence of these events on the development of a tumor is often difficult to measure, it is nevertheless true that these epigenetic factors also will influence the development of virally induced tumors, and thus one might expect that use of tumor viruses will play a role in the understanding of these more subtle events.

REFERENCES

1. Albert T, Urlbauer B, Kohlhuber F, et al. Ongoing mutations in the N-terminal domain of c-Myc affect transactivation in Burkitt's lymphoma cell lines. *Oncogene* 1994;9:759–763.
2. Albrecht JC, Nicholas J, Biller D, et al. Primary structure of the herpesvirus saimiri genome. *J Virol* 1992;66:5047–5058.
3. Amati B, Brooks MW, Levy N, et al. Oncogenic activity of the c-Myc protein requires dimerization with Max. *Cell* 1993;72:233–245.
4. Amati B, Littlewood TD, Evan GI, et al. The c-Myc protein induces cell cycle progression and apoptosis through dimerization with Max. *EMBO J* 1993;12:5083–5087.
5. Angel P, Allegretto EA, Okino ST. Oncogene jun encodes a sequence-specific trans-activator similar to AP-1. *Nature* 1988;332:166–171.
6. Angel P, Karin M. The role of jun, fos and the AP-1 complex in cell proliferation and transformation. *Biochim Biophys Acta* 1991;1072:129–157.
7. Aoki M, Batista O, Bellacosa A, et al. The akt kinase: molecular determinants of oncogenicity. *Proc Natl Acad Sci U S A* 1998;95:14950–14955.
8. Attardi LD, Lowe SW, Brugarolas J, et al. Transcriptional activation by p53, but not induction of the p21 gene, is essential for oncogene-mediated apoptosis. *EMBO J* 1996;15:3693–3701.
9. Auborn K, Guo M, Prives C. Helicase, DNA binding, and immunological properties of replication defective simian virus 40 mutant T antigens. *J Virol* 1989;63:912–918.
10. Ayer DE, Eisenman RN. A switch from Myc:Max to Mad:Max heterocomplexes accompanies monocyte/macrophage differentiation. *Genes Dev* 1993;7:2110–2119.
11. Ayer DE, Kretzner L, Eisenman RN. Mad: a heterodimeric partner for Max that antagonizes Myc transcriptional activity. *Cell* 1993;72:211–222.
12. Ayer DE, Lawrence QA, Eisenman RN. Mad-Max transcriptional repression is mediated by ternary complex formation with mammalian homologs of yeast repressor sin3. *Cell* 1995;80:767–776.
13. Babiss LE, Ginsberg HS, Darnell JE Jr. Adenovirus E1B proteins are required for accumulation of late viral mRNA and for effects on cellular mRNA translation and transport. *Mol Cell Biol* 1985;5:2522–2558.
14. Bagchi S, Raychaudhuri P, Nevins JR. Adenovirus E1A proteins can dissociate heteromeric complexes involving the E2F transcription factor: a novel mechanism for E1A trans-activation. *Cell* 1990;62:659–669.
15. Bagchi S, Weinmann R, Raychaudhuri P. The retinoblastoma protein copurifies with E2F-I: an E1A-regulated inhibitor of the transcription factor E2F. *Cell* 1991;65:1063–1072.
16. Baker CC, Phelps WC, Lindgren V, et al. Structural and transcriptional analysis of human papillomavirus type 16 sequences in cervical carcinoma cell lines. *J Virol* 1987;61:962–971.
17. Bandara LR, Adamczewski JP, Hunt T, et al. Cyclin A and the retinoblastoma gene product complex with a common transcription factor. *Nature* 1991;352:249–251.
18. Bandara LR, La Thangue NB. Adenovirus E1a prevents the retinoblastoma gene product from complexing with a cellular transcription factor. *Nature* 1991;351:494–497.
19. Barbacid M. Involvement of ras oncogenes in the initiation of carcinogen-induced tumors. In: Aronson SA, Bishop M, Sugimura T, et al., eds. *Oncogenes and cancer.* Tokyo: Japan Scientific Society, 1987:43–53.
20. Baserga R. The biology of cell reproduction. In: *The biology of cell reproduction.* Boston: Harvard University Press, 1985.
21. Ben-David Y, Bernstein A. Friend virus-induced erythroleukemia and the multistage nature of cancer. *Cell* 1991;66:831–834.
22. Benjamin TL. Host range mutants of polyoma virus. *Proc Natl Acad Sci U S A* 1970;67:394–399.
23. Berk AJ, Lee F, Harrison T, et al. Pre-early adenovirus 5 gene product regulates synthesis of early viral messenger RNAs. *Cell* 1979;17:935–944.
24. Berk AJ, Sharp PA. Sizing and mapping of early adenovirus mRNAs by gel electrophoresis of S1 endonuclease digested hybrids. *Cell* 1977;12:721–732.
25. Bernstein A, MacCormick R, Martin GS. Transformation-defective mutants of avian sarcoma viruses: the genetic relationship between conditional and nonconditional mutants. *Virology* 1976;170:206–209.
26. Besmer P. The kit ligand encoded at the murine Steel locus: a pleiotropic growth and differentiation factor. *Curr Opin Cell Biol* 1991;3:939–946.
27. Beug H, Graf T. Transformation parameters of chicken embryo fibroblasts infected with the ts34 mutant of avian erythroblastosis virus. *Virology* 1980;100:348–356.
28. Beug H, Leutz A, Kahn P, et al. Ts mutants of E26 leukemia virus allow transformed myeloblasts, but not erythroblasts or fibroblasts, to differentiate at the nonpermissive temperature. *Cell* 1984;39:579–588.
29. Biedenkapp H, Borgmeyer U, Sippel AE, et al. Viral myb oncogene encodes a sequence-specific DNA-binding activity. *Nature* 1988;335:835–837.
30. Bikel I, Montano X, Agha ME, et al. SV40 small t antigen enhances the transformation activity of limiting concentrations of SV40 large T antigen. *Cell* 1987;48:321–330.

31. Bishop JM. Cellular oncogenes and retroviruses. *Annu Rev Biochem* 1983;52:301–354.
32. Bishop JM. Viral oncogenes. *Cell* 1985;42:23–38.
33. Bister K. Multiple cell-derived sequences in single retroviral genomes. *Adv Viral Oncol* 1986;6:45–70.
34. Bittner JJ. Some possible effects of nursing on the mammary gland tumor incidence in mice. *Science* 1936;84:162.
35. Bjorklund S, Skog S, Tribukait B, et al. S-phase-specific expression of mammalian ribonucleotide reductase R1 and R2 subunit mRNAs. *Biochemistry* 1990;29:5452–5458.
36. Blackwood EM, Kretzner L, Eisenman RN. Myc and Max function as a nucleoprotein complex. *Curr Opin Genet Dev* 1992;2:227–235.
37. Blenis J. Signal transduction via the MAP kinases: proceed at your own RSK. *Proc Natl Acad Sci U S A* 1993;90:5889–5892.
38. Boguski MS, McCormick F. Proteins regulating Ras and its relatives. *Nature* 1993;336:643–654.
39. Bohmann D, Bos TJ, Admon A, et al. Human proto-oncogene c-jun encodes a DNA binding protein with structural and functional properties of transcription factor AP-1. *Science* 1987;238:1386–1392.
40. Bold RJ, Hannink M, Donoghue DJ. Functions of the *mos* oncogene. *Cancer Surv* 1986;5:243–256.
41. Bolen SB, Thiele CJ, Israel MA, et al. Enhancement of cellular src gene product associated tyrosine kinase activity following polyoma virus infection and transformation. *Cell* 1984;38:767–777.
42. Bollag G, McCormick F. Regulators and effectors of *ras* proteins. *Annu Rev Cell Biol* 1991;7:601–632.
43. Bouck N, Bealer N, Shenk T, et al. New region of simian virus 40 genome required for efficient viral transformation. *Proc Natl Acad Sci U S A* 1978;75:2473–2477.
44. Bourne HR, Sanders DA, McCormick F. The GTPase superfamily: a conserved switch for diverse cell functions. *Nature* 1990;348: 125–132.
45. Bourne HR, Sanders DA, McCormick F. The GTPase superfamily: conserved structure and molecular mechanism. *Nature* 1991;349: 117–127.
46. Bradshaw RA, Prentis S. Oncogenes and growth factors. In: *Oncogenes and growth factors*. Amsterdam: Elsevier, 1987.
47. Brown AMC, Wildin RS, Prendergast TJ, et al. A retrovirus vector expressing the putative mammary oncogene *int*-1 causes partial transformation of a mammary epithelial cell line. *Cell* 1986;46:1001–1009.
48. Brown DW, Blais BP, Robinson HL. Long terminal repeat (LTR) sequences, *env,* and a region near the 5′ LTR influence the pathogenic potential of recombinants between Rous-associated virus type 0 and 1. *J Virol* 1988;62:3431–3437.
49. Brugge JS, Erikson RL. Identification of a transformation-specific antigen induced by an avian sarcoma virus. *Nature* 1977;269: 346–348.
50. Burridge K. Substrate adhesions in normal and transformed fibroblasts: organization and regulation of cytoskeletal, membrane and extracellular matrix components at focal contacts. *Cancer Rev* 1986; 4:18–78.
51. Caelles C, Heimberg A, Karin M. p53-dependent apoptosis in the absence of p53-target genes. *Nature* 1994;370:220–223.
52. Cahilly-Snyder L, Yang-Feng T, Francke U, et al. Molecular analysis and chromosomal mapping of amplified genes isolated from a transformed mouse 3T3 cell line. *Somat Cell Mol Genet* 1987;13:235–244.
53. Cao L, Faha B, Dembski M, et al. Independent binding of the retinoblastoma protein and p107 to the transcription factor E2F. *Nature* 1992;355:176–179.
54. Cartwright CA, Kaplan PlL, Cooper JA, et al. Altered sites of tyrosine phosphorylation in pp60c-src associated with polyoma virus middle tumor antigen. *Mol Cell Biol* 1986;6:1562–1570.
55. Chang HW, Aoki M, Fruman D, et al. Transformation of chicken cells by the gene encoding the catalytic subunit of PI 3-kinase. *Science* 1997;276:1848–1850.
56. Chellappan S, Kraus VB, Kroger B, et al. Adenovirus E1A, simian virus 40 tumor antigen, and human papillomavirus E7 protein share the capacity to disrupt the interaction between transcription factor E2F and the retinoblastoma gene product. *Proc Natl Acad Sci U S A* 1992;89:4549–4553.
57. Chellappan SP, Hiebert S, Mudryj M, et al. The E2F transcription factor is a cellular target for the RB protein. *Cell* 1991;65:1053–1061.
58. Chen ISY, Wachsman W, Rosenblatt JD, et al. The role of the *x* gene in HTLV associated malignancy. *Cancer Surv* 1986;5:329–341.
59. Chen J-M, Chen W-T. Fibronectin-degrading proteases from the membranes of transformed cells. *Cell* 1987;48:193–203.
60. Chen JD, Lin JY, Levine AJ. Regulation of transcription functions of the p53 tumour suppressor by the *mdm-2* oncogene. *Mol Med* 1995;1:141–152.
61. Chen LB, Gallimore PH, McDougall JK. Correlation between tumor induction and the large external transformation sensitive protein on the cell surface. *Proc Natl Acad Sci U S A* 1976;73:3570–3574.
62. Chen W-T, Olden K, Bernard BA, et al. Expression of transformation-associated protease(s) that degrade fibronectin at cell contact sites. *J Cell Biol* 1984;98:1546–1555.
63. Cheng SH, Harvey R, Espino PC, et al. Peptide antibodies to the human c-fyn gene product demonstrate pp59c-fyn is capable of complex formation with the middle-T antigen of polyomavirus. *EMBO J* 1988;7:3845–3855.
64. Chiu R, Boyle WJ, Meek J, et al. The c-Fos protein interacts with c-Jun/AP-1 to stimulate transcription of AP-1 responsive genes. *Cell* 1988;54:541–552.
65. Cicchetti P, Mayer BJ, Thiel G, et al. Identification of a protein that binds to the SH3 region of Abil and is similar to Bcr and GAP-rho. *Science* 1992;257:803–806.
66. Cobb BS, Schaller MD, Leu T-H, et al. Stable association of pp60*src* and pp59*fyn* with the focal adhesion-associated protein tyrosine kinase, p125*FAK*. *Mol Cell Biol* 1994;14:147–155.
67. Coffin JM. Genetic diversity and evolution of retroviruses. *Curr Topics Microbiol Immunol* 1992;176:143–164.
68. Collett MS, Erikson RL. Protein kinase activity associated with the avian sarcoma virus *src* gene product. *Proc Natl Acad Sci U S A* 1978; 75:2021–2024.
69. Cooper JA, Howell B. The when and how of Src regulation. *Cell* 1993; 73:1051–1054.
70. Courtneidge SA. Activation of the pp60 c-src kinase by middle T antigen binding or by dephosphorylation. *EMBO J* 1985;4:1471–1477.
71. Courtneidge SA. Further characterisation of the complex containing middle T antigen and pp60. *Curr Topics Microbiol Immunol* 1989;144:121–128.
72. Courtneidge SA, Heber A. An 81 kd protein complexed with middle T antigen and pp60$^{c\text{-}src}$: a possible phosphatidylinositol kinase. *Cell* 1987;50:1031–1037.
73. Courtneidge SA, Kypta RM, Ulug ET. Interactions between the middle T antigen of polyomavirus and host cell proteins. *Cold Spring Harbor Symp Quant Biol* 1988;53:153–160.
74. Courtneidge SA, Smith AE. Polyoma virus transforming protein associates with the product of the c-src cellular gene. *Nature* 1983;303: 435–439.
75. Croce CM. Molecular biology of lymphomas. *Semin Oncol* 1993;20: 31–46.
76. Curran T. The *fos* oncogene. In: Reddy EP, Skalka AM, Curran T, eds. *The oncogene handbook.* Amsterdam: Elsevier, 1988:307–325.
77. Curran T, Vogt PK. Dangerous liaisons: Fos and Jun: oncogenic transcription factors. In: McKnight SL, Yamamota KR, eds. *Transcriptional regulation.* Cold Spring Harbor, NY: CSH Laboratory Press, 1991:797–831.
78. D'Andrea AD. The interaction of the erythropoietin receptor and gp55. *Cancer Surv* 1992;15:19–36.
79. Dahl J, Jurczak A, Cheng LA, et al. Evidence of a role for phosphatidylinositol 3-kinase activation in the blocking of apoptosis by polyomavirus middle T antigen. *J Virol* 1998;72:3221–3226.
80. Damm K. c-erbA: protooncogene or growth suppressor gene? *Adv Cancer Res* 1992;59:89–113.
81. de Stanchina E, McCurrach ME, Zindy F et al. E1A signaling to p53 involves the p19^{ARF} tumor suppressor. *Genes Dev* 1998;12: 2434–2442.
82. Dean FB, Bullock P, Murakami Y, et al. Simian virus 40 (SV40) DNA replication: SV40 large T antigen unwinds DNA containing the SV40 origin of replication. *Proc Natl Acad Sci U S A* 1987;84:16–20.
83. Debbas M, White E. Wild-type p53 mediates apoptosis by E1A, which is inhibited by E1B. *Genes Dev* 1993;7:546–554.
84. DeCaprio JA, Ludlow JW, Figge J, et al. SV40 large tumor antigen forms a specific complex with the product of the retinoblastoma susceptibility gene. *Cell* 1988;54:275–283.
85. Defeo-Jones D, Huang PS, Jones RE, et al. Cloning of cDNAs for cellular proteins that bind to the retinoblastoma gene product. *Nature* 1991;352:251–254.

86. DeGregori J, Leone G, Miron A, et al. Distinct roles for E2F proteins in cell growth control and apoptosis. *Proc Natl Acad Sci U S A* 1997;94:7245–7250.
87. Delli-Bovi P, Curatola AM, Kern FG, et al. An oncogene isolated by transfection of Kaposi's sarcoma DNA encodes a growth factor that is a member of the FGF family. *Cell* 1987;50:729–737.
88. DeLucia AL, Lewton BA, Tjian R, et al. Topography of simian virus 40A protein-DNA complexes: arrangement of pentanucleotide interaction sites at the origin of replication. *J Virol* 1983;46:143–150.
89. DesGroseillers L, Jolicoeur P. The tandem direct repeats within the long terminal repeat of murine leukemia viruses are the primary determinant of their leukemogenic potential. *J Virol* 1984;52:945–952.
90. Devoto SH, Mudryj M, Pines J, et al. A cyclin A-protein kinase complex possesses sequence-specific DNA binding activity: p33cdk2 is a component of the E2F-cyclin A complex. *Cell* 1992;68:167–176.
91. Dickson C, Peters G. Potential oncogene product related to growth factors. *Nature* 1987;326:833.
92. DiMaio D, Lai CC, Klein O. Virocrine transformation: the intersection between viral transforming proteins and cellular signal transduction pathways. *Annu Rev Microbiol* 1998;52:397–421.
93. Dini PW, Lipsick JS. Oncogenic truncation of the first repeat of c-Myb decreases DNA binding in vitro and in vivo. *Mol Cell Biol* 1993; 13:7334–7348.
94. Doerfler W. The fate of the DNA of adenovirus type 12 in baby hamster kidney cells. *Proc Natl Acad Sci U S A* 1968;60:636.
95. Doolittle RF, Hunkapiller MW, Hood LE, et al. Simian sarcoma virus *onc* gene, v-*sis*, is derived from the gene (or genes) encoding a platelet-derived growth factor. *Science* 1983;221:275–277.
96. Dowdy SF, Hinds PW, Louie K, et al. Physical interaction of the retinoblastoma protein with human D cyclins. *Cell* 1993;73:499–511.
97. Downward J, Yarden Y, Mayes E. Close similarity of epidermal growth factor receptor and v-*erbB* oncogene protein sequences. *Nature* 1984; 307:521–527.
98. Dulbecco R, Hartwell LH, Vogt M. Induction of cellular DNA synthesis by polyoma virus. *Proc Natl Acad Sci U S A* 1965;53:403.
99. Dvoretzky I, Shober R, Chattopadhyay SK, et al. A quantitative in vitro focus assay for bovine papillomavirus. *Virology* 1980;103:369–375.
100. Dyson N. The regulation of E2f by pRB-family proteins. *Genes Dev* 1998;12:2245–2262.
101. Dyson N, Howley PM, Munger K, et al. The human papilloma virus-16 E7 oncoprotein is able to bind to the retinoblastoma gene product. *Science* 1989;243:934–937.
102. Eisenman RN. Nuclear oncogenes. In: Weinberg RA, ed. *The oncogenes.* Cold Spring Harbor, NY: CSH Laboratory Press, 1989:175–221.
103. El-Deiry WS, Tokino T, Velculescu VE, et al. WAF1, a potential mediator of p53 tumor suppression. *Cell* 1993;75:817–825.
104. Eliyahu D, Goldfinger N, Pinhasi-Kimhi O, et al. Meth A fibrosarcoma cells express two transforming mutant p53 species. *Oncogene* 1988;3:313–321.
105. Eliyahu D, Raz A, Gruss P, et al. Participation of p53 cellular tumour antigen in transformation of normal embryonic cells. *Nature* 1984; 312:646–649.
106. Ellermann V, Bang O. Experimentelle Leukamie bei Huhnern. *Zentralb Bakteriol* 1908;46:595–609.
107. Engstrom Y, Eriksson S, Jildevik I, et al. Cell cycle-dependent expression of mammalian ribonucleotide reductase: differential regulation of the two subunits. *J Biol Chem* 1985;260:9114–9116.
108. Ersman MD, Astrin SM. The *myc* oncogene. In: Reddy EP, Skalka AM, Curran T, eds. *The oncogene handbook.* Amsterdam: Elsevier, 1988:341–379.
109. Felder M-P, Eychene A, Barnier JV, et al. Common mechanism of retrovirus activation and transduction of c-*mil* and c-R*mil* in chicken neuroretina cells infected with Rous-associated virus type 1. *J Virol* 1991;65:3633–3640.
110. Felder M-P, Laugier D, Eychene A, et al. Occurrence of alternatively spliced leader-delta*onc*Poly(a) transcripts in chicken neuroretina cells infected with Rous-associated virus type 1: implication in transduction of the c-*mil*/c-*raf* and c-R*mil*/B-*raf* oncogenes. *J Virol* 1993;67: 6853–6856.
111. Figge J, Webster T, Smith TF, et al. Prediction of similar transforming regions in simian virus 40 large T, adenovirus E1A, and myc oncoproteins. *J Virol* 1988;62:1814–1818.
112. Finlay CA, Hinds PW, Levine AJ. The p53 proto-oncogene can act as a suppressor of transformation. *Cell* 1989;57:1083–1093.
113. Finlay CA, Hinds PW, Tan TH, et al. Activating mutations for transformation by p53 produce a gene product that forms an hsc70-p53 complex with an altered half-life. *Mol Cell Biol* 1988;8:531–539.
114. Forrest D, Curran T. Crossed signals: oncogenic transcription factors. *Curr Opin Genet Dev* 1992;2:19–27.
115. Fraser NW, Nevins JR, Ziff E, et al. The major late adenovirus type-2 transcription unit: termination is downstream from the last poly(A) site. *J Mol Biol* 1979;129:643–656.
116. Frearson PM, Kit S, Dubbs DR. Induction of dehydrofolate reductase activity by SV40 and polyoma virus. *Cancer Res* 1966;26:1653.
117. Freund R, Bronson RT, Benjamin TL. Separation of immortalization from tumor induction with polyoma large T mutants that fail to bind to retinoblastoma gene product. *Oncogene* 1992;7:1979–1987.
118. Friend C. Cell-free transmission in adult Swiss mice of a disease having the character of a leukemia. *J Exp Med* 1957;105:307–319.
119. Fung Y-KT, Lewis WG, Crittenden LB, et al. Activation of the cellular oncogene c-*erbB* by LTR insertion: molecular basis for induction of erythroblastosis by avian erythroblastosis virus. *Cell* 1983;33: 357–368.
120. Funk WD, Pak DT, Karas RH, et al. A transcriptionally active DNA-binding site for human p53 protein complexes. *Mol Cell Biol* 1992;12: 2866–2871.
121. Gallimore PH, Sharp PA, Sambrook J. Viral DNA in transformed cells. II. A study of the sequences of adenovirus 2 DNA in 9 lines of transformed rat cells using specific fragments of the viral genome. *J Mol Biol* 1974;89:49.
122. Gallo RC. The first human retrovirus. *Sci Am* 1986;255:88–98.
123. Garcea RL, Talmage DA, Harmatz A, et al. Separation of host range from transformation functions of the hr-t gene of polyomavirus. *Virology* 1989;168:312–319.
124. Geissler EN, Ryan MA, Housman DE. The dominant-white spotting (W) locus of the mouse encodes the c-*kit* proto-oncogene. *Cell* 1988; 55:185–192.
125. Gelinas C, Temin HM. The v-*rel* oncogene encodes a cell-specific transcriptional activator of certain promoters. *Oncogene* 1988;3: 349–355.
126. Gentz R, Rauscher FJI, Abate C, et al. Parallel association of *Fos* and *Jun* leucine zippers juxtaposes DNA binding domains. *Science* 1989; 243:1695–1699.
127. Giacherio D, Hager LP. A poly(dT)-stimulated ATPase activity associated with simian virus 40 large T antigen. *J Biol Chem* 1979;254: 8113–8116.
128. Gilman AG. G proteins: transducers of receptor-generated signals. *Annu Rev Biochem* 1987;56:615–649.
129. Gluzman Y, Davison T, Oren M, et al. Properties of permissive monkey cells transformed by UV-irradiated simian virus 40. *J Virol* 1977; 22:256–266.
130. Golden A, Brugge JS. The *src* oncogene. In: Reddy EP, Skalka AM, Curran T, eds. *The oncogene handbook.* Amsterdam: Elsevier, 1988: 149–173.
131. Goldfarb MP, Weinberg RA. Generation of novel biologically active Harvey sarcoma viruses via apparent illegitimate recombination. *J Virol* 1981;38:136–150.
132. Goldman DS, Kiessling AA, Millette CF, et al. Expression of c-*mos* RNA in germ cells of male and female mice. *Proc Natl Acad Sci U S A* 1987;84:4509–4513.
133. Graf T, Beug H. Role of the v-*erbA* and v-*erbB* oncogenes of avian erythroblastosis virus in erythroid cell transformation. *Cell* 1983;34: 7–9.
134. Graffi A, Bielka H, Fey F, et al. Gehyauauftes Auftreten von Leukyauamien nach Injektion von Sarkom-Filtraten. *Wien Klin Wochenschr* 1955;105:61–64.
135. Graham FL, Abrahams PJ, Mulder C. Studies on in vitro transformation by DNA and DNA fragments of human adenoviruses and SV40. *Cold Spring Harbor Symp Quant Biol* 1974;39:637–650.
136. Graham FL, Abrahams PS, Mulder C, et al. Studies on in vitro transformation by DNA and DNA fragments of human adenoviruses and simian virus 40. *Cold Spring Harbor Symp Quant Biol* 1975;39:637.
137. Gross L. Development and serial cell-free passage of a highly potent strain of mouse leukemia virus. *Proc Soc Exp Biol Med* 1957;94:767–771.
138. Hai T, Curran T. Cross-family dimerization of transcription factors Fos/Jun and ATF/CREB alters DNA binding specificity. *Proc Natl Acad Sci U S A* 1991;88:3720–3724.

139. Haluska FG, Tsujimoto Y, Croce CM. Mechanisms of chromosome translocation in B- and T-cell neoplasia. *Trends Genet* 1987;3:11–15.
140. Harlow E, Whyte P, Franza BR Jr, et al. Association of adenovirus early-region 1A proteins with cellular polypeptides. *Mol Cell Biol* 1986;6:1579–1589.
141. Harper JW, Adami GR, Wei N, et al. The p21 cdk-interacting protein Cip1 is a potent inhibitor of G1 cyclin-dependent kinases. *Cell* 1993; 75:805–816.
142. Hartley JW, Wolford NK, Old LJ, et al. A new class of murine leukemia virus associated with development of spontaneous lymphomas. *Proc Natl Acad Sci U S A* 1977;74:789–792.
143. Hartwell LH, Weinert TA. Checkpoints: controls that ensure the order of cell cycle events. *Science* 1989;246:629–633.
144. Haupt Y, Maya R, Kazaz A, et al. Mdm2 promotes the rapid degradation of p53. *Nature* 1997;387:296–299.
145. Haupt Y, Rowan S, Shaulian E, et al. Induction of apoptosis in HeLa cells by transactivation-deficient p53. *Genes Dev* 1995;9:2170–2183.
146. Hayman MJ. *erb*-B: growth factor receptor turned oncogene. In: Bradshaw RA, Prentis S, eds. *Oncogenes and growth fac*tors. Amsterdam: Elsevier, 1989:81–89.
147. Hayward WS, Neel BG, Astrin SM. Activation of a cellular *onc* gene by promoter insertion in ALV-induced lymphoid leukosis. *Nature* 1981;290:475–480.
148. He T-C, Sparks AB, Rago C, et al. Identification of c-*Myc* as a target of the APC pathway. *Science* 1998;281:1509–1512.
149. Heisterkamp N, Stam K, Groffen J, et al. Structural organization of the *bcr* gene and its role in the Ph1 translocation. *Nature* 1985;315:758–761.
150. Herman SA, Coffin JM. Efficient packaging of read-through RNa in ALV: implications for oncogene transduction. *Science* 1987;236: 845–848.
151. Herren B, Rooney B, Weyer KA, et al. Dimerization of extracellular domains of platelet-derived growth factor receptors: a revised model of receptor-ligand interaction. *J Biol Chem* 1993;268:15088–15095.
152. Herrlich P, Ponta H. "Nuclear" oncogenes convert extracellular stimuli into changes in the genetic program. *Trends Genet* 1989;5: 112–115.
153. Hildebrand JD, Schaller MD, Parsons JT. Identification of sequences required for the efficient localization of the focal adhesion kinase. *J Cell Biol* 1993;123:993–1005.
154. Hiral SI, Ryseck R-P, Mechta F, et al. Characterization of *jun D*: a new member of the *jun* protooncogene family. *EMBO J* 1989;8:1433–1439.
155. Horak ID, Kawakami T, Gregory F, et al. Association of p60fyn with middle tumor antigen in murine polyomavirus-transformed rat cells. *J Virol* 1989;63:2343–2347.
156. Hughes S, Greenhouse JJ, Petropoulos CJ, et al. Adapter plasmids simplify the insertion of foreigh DNA into helper-independent retroviral vectors. *J Virol* 1987;61:3004–3012.
157. Hughes S, Kosik E. Mutagenesis of the region between env and src of the SR-A strain of Rous sarcoma virus for the purpose of constructing helper-independent vectors. *Virology* 1984;136:89–99.
158. Huibregtse JM, Scheffner M, Howley PM. A cellular protein mediates association of p53 with the E6 oncoprotein of human papillomavirus types 16 or 18. *EMBO J* 1991;10:4129–4135.
159. Huibregtse JM, Scheffner M, Howley PM. Localization of the E6-AP regions that direct human papillomavirus E6 binding, association with p53, and ubiquitination of associated proteins. *Mol Cell Biol* 1993;13: 4918–4927.
160. Hunter T, Sefton BM. Transforming gene product of Rous sarcoma virus phosphorylates tyrosine. *Proc Natl Acad Sci U S A* 1980;77: 1311–1315.
161. Hynes RO. Role of surface alterations in cell transformation: the importance of proteases and surface proteins. *Cell* 1974;1:147–156.
162. Hynes RO. Integrins: versatility, modulation, and signalling in cell adhesion. *Cell* 1992;69:11–25.
163. Iba H, Takeya T, Cross F, et al. Rous sarcoma virus variants which carry the cellular *src* gene instead of the viral *src* gene cannot transform chicken embryo fibroblasts. *Proc Natl Acad Sci U S A* 1984;81: 4424–4428.
164. Ikawa S, Hagino-Yamagishi K, Kawai S, et al. Activation of the cellular *src* gene by transducing retrovirus. *Mol Cell Biol* 1986;6: 2420–2428.
165. Ikeda M-A, Nevins JR. Identification of distinct roles for separate E1A domains in the disruption of E2F complexes. *Mol Cell Biol* 1993;13:7029–7035.
166. Ito Y, Brocklehurst JR, Dulbecco R. Virus-specific proteins in the plasma membrane of cells lytically infected or transformed by polyoma virus. *Proc Natl Acad Sci U S A* 1977;74:4666–4670.
167. Janknecht R, Nordheim A. Gene regulation by Ets proteins. *Biochim Biophys Acta* 1993;1155:346–356.
168. Jenkins JR, Rudge K, Currie GA. Cellular immortalization by a cDNA clone encoding the transformation associated phosphoprotein p53. *Nature* 1984;312:651–654.
169. Johnson P, Benchimol S. Friend virus induced murine erythroleukaemia: the p53 locus. *Cancer Surv* 1992;12:137–151.
170. Jones KA, Tjian R. Essential contact residues within SV40 large T antigen binding sites I and II identified by alkylation-interference. *Cell* 1984;36:155–162.
171. Jones N, Shenk T. An adenovirus type 5 early gene function regulates expression of other early viral genes. *Proc Natl Acad Sci U S A* 1979; 76:3665–3669.
172. Jones SN, Roe AE, Donehower LA, et al. Rescue of embryonic lethality in Mdm2-deficient mice by absence of p53. *Nature* 1995;378: 206–208.
173. Kabat D. Molecular biology of Friend viral erythroleukemia. *Curr Top Microbiol Immunol* 1989;148:1–42.
174. Kalderon D, Smith AE. In vitro mutagenesis of a putative DNA binding domain of SV40 large-T. *Virology* 1984;139:109–137.
175. Kamijo T, Weber JD, Zambetti G, et al. Functional and physical interactions of the ARF tumor suppressor with p53 and Mdm2. *Proc Natl Acad Sci U S A* 1998;95:8292–8297.
176. Kaplan DR, Whitman M, Schaffhausen B. Phosphatidylinositol metabolism and polyoma-mediated transformation. *Proc Natl Acad Sci U S A* 1986;83:3624–3628.
177. Kara J, Weil R. Specific activation of the DNA synthesizing apparatus in contact inhibited cells by polyoma virus. *Proc Natl Acad Sci U S A* 1967;57:63.
178. Kataoka K, Nishizawa M, Kawai S. Structure-function analysis of the maf oncogene product, a member of the b-Zip protein family. *J Virol* 1993;67:2133–2141.
179. Kawai S, Hanafusa H. The effects of reciprocal changes in the temperature on the transformed state of cells infected with a Rous sarcoma virus mutant. *Virology* 1971;46:470–479.
180. Kern SE, Kinzler KW, Bruskin A, et al. Identification of p53 as a sequence specific DNA binding protein. *Science* 1991;252:1707–1711.
181. Kipreos ET, Wang JYJ. Differential phosphorylation of c-*Abl* in cell cycle determined by cdc2 kinase and phosphatase activity. *Science* 1990;248:217–220.
182. Kipreos ET, Wang JYJ. Cell cycle-regulated binding of c-Abl tyrosine kinase to DNA. *Science* 1992;256:382–385.
183. Kirsten WH, Mayer LA. Morphologic responses to a murine erythroblastosis virus. *J Natl Cancer Inst* 1967;39:311–355.
184. Kitajima I, Shinohara T, Bilakovics J, et al. Ablation of transplanted HTLV-I tax-transformed tumors in mice by antisense inhibition of MF-kappa B. *Science* 1992;258:1792–1795.
185. Ko LJ, Prives C. p53: puzzle and paradigm. *Genes Dev* 1996;10: 1054–1072.
186. Kornbluth S, Sudol M, Hanafusa H. Association of the polyomavirus middle-T antigen with c-yes protein. *Nature* 1987;325:171–173.
187. Kouzarides T, Ziff E. The role of the leucine zipper in the *fos-jun* interaction. *Nature* 1988;336:646–651.
188. Kovesdi I, Reichel R, Nevins JR. Identification of a cellular transcription factor involved in E1A trans-activation. *Cell* 1986;45:219–228.
189. Kowalik TF, DeGregori J, Leone G, et al. E2F1-specific induction of apoptosis and p53 accumulation is modulated by mdm2. *Cell Growth Differ* 1998;9:113–118.
190. Kowalik TF, DeGregori J, Schwarz JK, et al. E2F1 overexpression in quiescent fibroblasts leads to induction of cellular DNA synthesis and apoptosis. *J Virol* 1995;69:2491–2500.
191. Kubbutat MHG, Jones SN, Vousden KH. Regulation of p53 stability by Mdm2. *Nature* 1997;387:299–302.
192. Kung H-J, Maihle NJ. Molecular basis of oncogenesis by nonacute avian retroviruses. In: de Boer GF, ed. *Avian leukosis*. Boston: Martinus Nijhoff, 1987:77–99.
193. Kung HJ, Vogt P. Retroviral insertion and oncogene activation. *Curr Top Microbiol Immunol* 1991.
194. Kypta RM, Hemming A, Courtneidge SA. Identification and characterization of p59fyn (a src-like protein tyrosine kinase) in normal and polyoma virus transformed cells. *EMBO J* 1988;7:3837–3844.

195. Laherty CD, Yang W-M, Sun J-M, et al. Histone deacetylases associated with the mSin3 corepressor mediate mad transcriptional repression. *Cell* 1997;89:349–356.
196. Landschulz WH, Johnson PF, McKnight SL. The leucine zipper: a hypothetical structure common to a new class of DNA binding proteins. *Science* 1988;240:1759–1764.
197. Lane DP, Crawford LV. T antigen is bound to a host protein in SV40-transformed cells. *Nature* 1979;278:261–263.
198. Ledinko N. Enhanced deoxyribonucleic acid polymerase activity in human embryonic kidney cultures infected with adenovirus 2 and 12. *J Virol* 1968;2:89–98.
199. Leone G, DeGregori J, Sears R, et al. Myc and Ras collaborate in inducing accumulation of active cyclin E/Cdk2 and E2F. *Nature* 1997;387:422–426.
200. Leone G, DeGregori J, Yan Z, et al. E2F3 activity is regulated during the cell cycle and is required for the induction of S phase. *Genes Dev* 1998;12:2120–2130.
201. Leppard KN, Shenk T. The adenovirus E1B 55 kd protein influences mRNA transport via an intranuclear effect on RNA metabolism. *EMBO J* 1989;8:2329–2336.
202. Levine AJ. The tumor suppressor genes. *Annu Rev Biochem* 1993;62: 623–651.
203. Levine AJ. p53, the cellular gatekeeper for growth and division. *Cell* 1997;88:323–331.
204. Levinson AD. Normal and activated *ras* oncogenes and their encoded products. In: Bradshaw RA, Prentis S, eds. *Oncogenes and growth factors*. Amsterdam: Elsevier, 1987:74–83.
205. Levinson AD, Oppermann H, Levintow L, et al. Evidence that the transforming gene of avian sarcoma virus encodes a protein kinase associated with a phosphoprotein. *Cell* 1978;15:561–572.
206. Levy JA. The retroviridae. In: *The retroviridae*. New York: Plenum Press, 1992:1.
207. Li J-P, D'Andrea A, Lodish HF, et al. Activation of cell growth by binding of Friend spleen focus-forming virus gp55 glycoprotein to the erythropoietin receptor. *Nature* 1990;343:762–764.
208. Li J, Vogt P. The retroviral oncogene *qin* belongs to the transcription factor family that includes the homeotic gene fork head. *Proc Natl Acad Sci U S A* 1993;90:4490–4494.
209. Linzer DI, Levine AJ. Characterization of a 54K dalton cellular SV40 tumor antigen present in SV40-transformed cells and uninfected embryonal carcinoma cells. *Cell* 1979;17:43–52.
210. Liou HC, Baltimore D. Regulation of the NF-Kappa B/rel transcription factor and I kappa B inhibitor system. *Curr Opin Cell Biol* 1993;5:477–487.
211. Livingstone LR, White A, Sprouse J, et al. Altered cell cycle arrest and gene amplification potential accompany loss of wild-type p53. *Cell* 1992;70:923–935.
212. Loeken M, Bikel I, Livingston DM, et al. Trans-activation of RNA polymerase II and III promoters by SV40 small t antigen. *Cell* 1988; 55:1171–1177.
213. Loeken MR. Simian virus 40 small t antigen trans activates the adenovirus E2A promoter by using mechanisms distinct from those used by adenovirus E1A. *J Virol* 1992;66:2551–2555.
214. Lowe SW, Ruley HE. Stabilization of the p53 tumor suppressor is induced by adenovirus 5 E1A and accompanies apoptosis. *Genes Dev* 1993;7:535–545.
215. Lowy DR, Dvoretzky I, Shober R, et al. In vitro tumorigenic transformation by a defined sub-genomic fragment of bovine papilloma virus DNA. *Nature* 1980;287:72–74.
216. Luscher B, Eisenman RN. New light on Myc and Myb. Part I. Myc. *Genes Dev* 1990;4:2025–2035.
217. Luscher B, Eisenman RN. New light on Myc and Myb. Part II. Myb. *Genes Dev* 1990;4:2235—2241.
218. Mackey JK, Rigden PM, Green M. Do highly oncogenic group A human adenoviruses cause human cancer? Analysis of human tumors for adenovirus 12 transforming DNA sequences. *Proc Natl Acad Sci U S A* 1976;73:4657–4661.
219. Macpherson I, Montagnier L. Agar suspension culture for the selective assay of cells transformed by polyoma virus. *Virology* 1964;23: 291–294.
220. Manaker RA, Groupe V. Discrete foci of altered chicken embryo cells associated with Rous sarcoma virus in tissue culture. *Virology* 1956; 2:838–840.
221. Manos MM, Gluzman Y. Genetic and biochemical analysis of transformation-competent, replication-defective simian virus 40 large T antigen mutants. *J Virol* 1985;53:120–127.
222. Martin GS. Rous sarcoma virus: a function required for the maintenance of the transformed state. *Nature* 1970;227:1021–1023.
223. Martin GS. The *erbB* gene and the EGF receptor. *Nature* 1970;227: 1021–1023.
224. Martin GS, Duesberg PH. The *a* subunit in the RNA of transforming avian tumor viruses. I. Occurrence in different virus strains. II. Spontaneous loss resulting in nontransforming variants. *Virology* 1972;47: 494–497.
225. Martin P, Henry C, Ferre F. Characterization of a *myc*-containing retrovirus generated by propagation of an MH2 viral subgenomic RNA. *J Virol* 1986;57:1191–1194.
226. Matsushime H, Roussel MF, Ashmun RA, et al. Colony-stimulating factor 1 regulates novel cyclins during the G1 phase of the cell cycle. *Cell* 1991;65:701–713.
227. Mayer BJ, Hamaguchi M, Hanafusa H. A novel viral oncogene with structural similarity to phospholipase C. *Nature* 1988;332:272–278.
228. McCormick F. *ras* GTPase activating protein: signal transmitter and signal terminator. *Cell* 1989;56:5–8.
229. McGlade J, Cheng A, Pelicci G, et al. Shc proteins are phosphorylated and regulated by the v-Src and v-Fps protein-tyrosine kinases. *Proc Natl Acad Sci U S A* 1992;89:8869–8873.
230. Miles DB, Robinson HL. High frequency of transduction of c-*erbB* in avian leukosis virus-induced erythroblastosis. *J Virol* 1985;54: 295–303.
231. Mintz B, Illmensee K. Normal genetically mosaic mice produced from malignant teratocarcinoma cells. *Proc Natl Acad Sci U S A* 1975; 72:3585–3589.
232. Miyoshi I, Kubonishi I, Yoshimoto S. Type C virus particles in a cord blood T-cell line derived from cocultivating normal human cord leukocytes and human leukaemic T cells. *Nature* 1981;294:770–771.
233. Moloney JB. A virus-induced rhabdomyosarcoma of mice. *Natl Cancer Inst Monogr* 1966;22:139–142.
234. Montes de Oca Luna R, Wagner DS, Lozano G. Rescue of early embryonic lethality in *mdm2*-deficient mice by deletion of p53. *Nature* 1995;378:203–206.
235. Mucenski M, McLain K, Kier AB, et al. A functional c-*myb* gene is required for normal murine fetal hepatic hematopoiesis. *Cell* 1991;65: 677–689.
236. Muller AJ, Pendergast AM, Havlik MH, et al. A limited set of SH2 domains binds BCR through a high-affinity phosphotyrosine-independent interaction. *Mol Cell Biol* 1992;12:5087–5093.
237. Muller AJ, Pendergast AM, Parmar K, et al. En bloc substitution for the Src homology region 2 domain activates the transforming potential of the c-Abl protein tyrosine kinase. *Proc Natl Acad Sci U S A* 1993;90:3457–3461.
238. Neill SD, Hemstrom C, Virtanen A, et al. An adenovirus E4 gene product trans-activates E2 transcription and stimulates stable E2F binding through a direct association with E2F. *Proc Natl Acad Sci U S A* 1990;87:2008–2012.
239. Nerenberg M, Hinrichs SH, Reynolds RK, et al. The *tat* gene of human T-lymphotropic virus type 1 induces mesenchymal tumors in transgenic mice. *Science* 1987;237:1324–1329.
240. Nerenberg MI. Biological and molecular aspects of HTLV-1-associated diseases. *Mol Neurovirol* 1992;225–247.
241. Nevins JR. Processing of late adenovirus nuclear RNA to mRNA: kinetics of formation of intermediates and demonstration that all events are nuclear. *J Mol Biol* 1979;130:493–506.
242. Nevins JR. E2F: A link between the Rb tumor suppressor protein and viral oncoproteins. *Science* 1992;258:424–429.
243. Nevins JR. Toward an understanding of the functional complexity of the E2F and Retinoblastoma families. *Cell Growth Differ* 1998;9:585–593.
244. Ng M, Privalsky ML. Structural domains of the avian erythroblastosis virus *erbB* protein required for fibroblast transformation: dissection by in-frame insertional mutagenesis. *J Virol* 1986;58:542–553.
245. Nocka K, Majumder S, Chabot B, et al. Expression of c-*kit* gene products in known cellular targets of W mutations in normal and W mutant mice—evidence for an impaired c-*kit* kinase in mutant mice. *Genes Dev* 1989;3:816–826.
246. Nusse R. The *int* genes in mammary tumorigenesis and in normal development. *Trends Genet* 1988;4:291–295.
247. Nusse R. The Wnt gene family in tumorigenesis and in normal development. *J Steroid Biochem Mol Biol* 1992;43:9–12.

248. O'Shea EK, Rutkowski R, Kim PS. Evidence that the leucine zipper is a coiled coil. *Science* 1989;243:538–542.
249. Olden K, Yamada KM. Mechanism of the decrease in the major cell surface protein of chick embryo fibroblasts after transformation. *Cell* 1977;11:957–969.
250. Oliner JD, Kinzler KW, Meltzer PS, et al. Amplification of a gene encoding a p53-associated protein in human sarcomas. *Nature* 1992; 358:80–83.
251. Ossowski L, Quigley JP, Kellerman GM, et al. Fibrinolysis associated with oncogenic transformation. *J Exp Med* 1973;138:1056–1064.
252. Pallas DC, Shahrik LK, Martin BL, et al. Polyoma small and middle T antigens and SV40 small t antigen form stable complexes with protein phosphatase 2A. *Cell* 1990;60:167–176.
253. Papas TS, Blair DG, Fisher RJ. The *ets* oncogene. In: Reddy EP, Skalka AM, Curran T, eds. *The oncogene handbook*. Amsterdam: Elsevier, 1988:467–485.
254. Parada LF, Land H, Weinberg RA, et al. Cooperation between gene encoding p53 tumour antigen and ras in cellular transformation. *Nature* 1984;312:649–651.
255. Parker R, Varmus HE, Bishop JM. Expression of v-*src* and chicken c-*src* in rat cells demonstrates qualitative differences between pp60$^{v\text{-}src}$ and pp60$^{v\text{-}src}$. *Cell* 1984;37:131–139.
256. Parsons JT, Weber MJ. Genetics of *src: structure and functional organization of a protein tyrosine kinase.* Curr Top Microbiol Immunol 1989;147:79–127.
257. Pawson T, Guyden J, King T-H, et al. A strain of Fujinami sarcoma virus which is temperature-sensitive in protein phosphorylation and cellular transformation. *Cell* 1980;22:767–775.
258. Payne GS, Bishop JM, Varmus HE. Multiple arrangements of viral DNA and an activated host oncogene in bursal lymphomas. *Nature* 1982;259:209–214.
259. Peters G. The *int* oncogenes. In: Reddy EP, Skalka AM, Curran T, eds. *The oncogene handbook.* Amsterdam: Elsevier, 1988:487–494.
260. Pilder S, Logan J, Shenk T. Deletion of the gene encoding the adenovirus 5 early region 1b 21,000-molecular-weight polypeptide leads to degradation of viral and host cell DNA. *J Virol* 1984;52: 664–671.
261. Pilder S, Moore M, Logan J, et al. The adenovirus E1B-55K transforming polypeptide modulates transport or cytoplasmic stabilization of viral and host cell mRNAs. *Mol Cell Biol* 1986;6:470–476.
262. Plattner R, Kadlec L, DeMali KA, et al. c-Abl is activated by growth factors and Src family kinases and has a role in the cellular response to PDGF. *Genes Dev* 1999; in press.
263. Poiesz BJ, Ruscetti FW, Gazdar AF, et al. Detection and isolation of type C retrovirus particles from fresh and cultured lymphocytes of a patient with cutaneous T-cell lymphoma. *Proc Natl Acad Sci U S A* 1980;77:7415–7419.
264. Pomerantz J, Schreiber-Agus N, Liegeois NJ, et al. The *Ink4a* tumor suppressor gene product, p19^{Arf}, interacts with MDM2 and neutralizes MDM2's inhibition of p53. *Cell* 1998;92:713–723.
265. Pozzatti R, Vogel J, Jay G. The human T-lymphotropic virus type I tax gene can cooperate with the ras oncogene to induce neoplastic transformation of cells. *Mol Cell Biol* 1990;10:413–417.
266. Prendergast GC, Ziff EB. A new bind for Myc. *Trends Genet* 1992;8: 91–96.
267. Privalsky ML. v-erb A, nuclear hormone receptors, and oncogenesis. *Biochim Biophys Acta* 1992;1114:51–62.
268. Prives C, Covey L, Scheller A, et al. DNA-binding properties of simian virus 40 T-antigen mutants defective in viral DNA replication. *Mol Cell Biol* 1983;3:1958–1966.
269. Propst F, Van de Woude GF. Expression of c-*mos* proto-oncogene transcripts in mouse tissues. *Nature* 1985;315:516–518.
270. Qin X-Q, Livingston DM, Kaelin WG, et al. Deregulated transcription factor E2F-1 expression leads to S-phase entry and p53-mediated apoptosis. *Proc Natl Acad Sci U S A* 1994;91:10918–10922.
271. Quelle DE, Zindy F, Ashmun RA, et al. Alternative reading frames of the *INK4a* tumor suppressor gene encode two unrelated proteins capable of inducing cell cycle arrest. *Cell* 1995;83:993–1000.
272. Queva C, Ness SA, Grasser FA, et al. Expression patterns of c-myb and of v-myb induced myeloid-1 (min-1) gene during the development of the chick embryo. *Development* 1992;114:125–133.
273. Raines MA, Haihle NJ, Moscovici C, et al. Molecular characterization of three *erbB* transducing viruses generated during avian leukosis virus-induced erythroleukemia: extensive internal deletion near the kinase domain activates the fibrosarcoma- and hemangioma-inducing potentials of *erbB. J Virol* 1988;62:2444–2452.
274. Raines MA, Maihle NJ, Moscovici C, et al. Mechanism of c-*erbB* transduction: newly released transducing viruses retain Poly(A) tracts of *erbB* transcripts and encode C-terminally intact *erbB* proteins. *J Virol* 1988;62:2437–2443.
275. Rao L, Debbas M, Sabbatini P, et al. The adenovirus E1A proteins induce apoptosis, which is inhibited by the E1B 19-kDa and Bcl-2 proteins [published erratum appears in *Proc Natl Acad Sci U S A* 1992;89:9974]. *Proc Natl Acad Sci U S A* 1992;89:7742–7746.
276. Rapin AMC, Burger MM. Tumor cell surfaces: general alterations detected by agglutinins. *Adv Cancer Res* 1974;20:1–91.
277. Rapp UR, Cleveland JL, Bonner TI, et al. The *raf* oncogene. In: *The oncogene handbook.* Amsterdam: Elsevier, 1988:213–253.
278. Ravichandran KS, Lee KK, Songyang Z, et al. Interaction of Shc with the zeta chain of the T cell receptor upon T cell activation. *Science* 1993;262:902–905.
279. Raychaudhuri P, Bagchi S, Devoto SH, et al. Domains of the adenovirus E1A protein required for oncogenic activity are also required for dissociation of E2F transcription factor complexes. *Genes Dev* 1991;5:1200–1211.
280. Reddy EP. The *myb* oncogene. In: Reddy EP, Skalka AM, Curran T, eds. *The oncogene handbook.* Amsterdam: Elsevier, 1988:327–340.
281. Reddy EP. The Abelson leukemia viral oncogene. In: Deisseroth AB, Arlinghaus RB, eds. *Chronic myelogenous leukemia.* New York: Marcel Dekker, 1991:153–165.
282. Reddy EP, Skalka AM, Curran T, eds. *The oncogene handbook.* Amsterdam: Elsevier, 1988.
283. Rettenmier CW, Sherr CJ. The *fms* oncogene. In: Reddy EP, Skalka AM, Curran T, eds. *The oncogene handbook.* Amsterdam: Elsevier, 1988:73–99.
284. Ricciardi RP, Jones RL, Cepko CL, et al. Expression of early adenovirus genes requires a viral encoded acidic polypeptide. *Proc Natl Acad Sci U S A* 1981;78:6121–6125.
285. Rice NR, Gilden RV. The *rel* oncogene. In: Reddy EP, Skalka AM, Curran T, eds. *The oncogene handbook.* Amsterdam: Elsevier, 1988: 495–508.
286. Rijsewijk F, Schuermann M, Wagenaar E, et al. The *Drosophila* homolog of the mouse mammary oncogene *int*-1 is identical to the segment polarity gene *wingless. Cell* 1987;50:649–657.
287. Risser R, Holland GD. Structures and activities of activated *abl* oncogenes. *Curr Top Microbiol Immunol* 1989;147:129–153.
288. Robbins J, Blondel BJ, Gallahan D, et al. Mouse mammary tumor gene *int*-3: a member of the notch gene family transforms mammary epithelial cells. *J Virol* 1992;66:2594–2599.
289. Robbins KC, Aaronson SA. The *sis* oncogene. In: Reddy EP, Skalka AM, Curran T, eds. *The oncogene handbook.* Amsterdam: Elsevier, 1988:427–452.
290. Robinson HL, Blais BM, Tsichlis PN, et al. At least two regions of the viral genome determine the oncogenic potential of avian leukosis viruses. *Proc Natl Acad Sci U S A* 1982;79:1225–1229.
291. Robinson HL, Jensen L, Coffin JM. Sequences outside of the long terminal repeat determine the lymphomagenic potential of Rous-associated virus type 1. *J Virol* 1985;55:752–759.
292. Rohrschneider LR. The macrophage-colony stimulating factor (M-CSF) receptor. In: Nicola NA, ed. *Guidebook to cytokines and their receptors*. New York: Oxford University Press, 1994.
293. Rohrschneider LR, Woolford J. Structural and functional comparison of viral and cellular *fms. Semin Virol* 1991;2:385–395.
294. Rosakis-Adcock M, McGlade J, Mbamalu G, et al. Association of the Shc and Grb2/Sem5 SH2-containing proteins is implicated in activation of the Ras pathway by tyrosine kinases. *Nature* 1992;360: 689–692.
295. Rous P. A transmissible avian neoplasm: sarcoma of the common fowl. *J Exp Med* 1910;12:696–705.
296. Ryder K, Lau LF, Nathans DA. A gene activated by growth factors is related to the oncogene v-*jun. Proc Natl Acad Sci U S A* 1988;85: 1487–1491.
297. Sabbatini P, Chiou S-K, Rao L, et al. Modulation of p53-mediated transcriptional repression and apoptosis by the adenovirus E1B 19K protein. *Mol Cell Biol* 1995;15:1060–1070.
298. Sabbatini P, Lin J, Levine AJ, et al. Essential role for p53-mediated transcription in E1A-induced apoptosis. *Genes Dev* 1995;9: 2184–2192.

299. Sagata N, Oskarsson M, Copeland T, et al. Function of c-*mos* proto-oncogene product in meiotic maturation in *Xenopus* oocytes. *Nature* 1988;335:519–525.
300. Sap J, Munoz A, Damm K. The c-*erb*-A protein is a high-affinity receptor for thyroid hormone. *Nature* 1986;324:635–640.
301. Sarnow P, Ho YS, Williams J, et al. Adenovirus E1b-58kd tumor antigen and SV40 large tumor antigen are physically associated with the same 54kd cellular protein in transformed cells. *Cell* 1982;28:387–394.
302. Sawyers CL, McLaughlin J, Goga A, et al. The nuclear tyrosine kinase C-ABL negatively regulates cell growth. *Cell* 1994;77:121–131.
303. Scheffner M, Munger K, Byrne JC, et al. The state of the p53 and retinoblastoma genes in human cervical carcinoma cell lines. *Proc Natl Acad Sci U S A* 1991;88:5523–5527.
304. Scheffner M, Werness BA, Huibregtse JM, et al. The E6 oncoprotein encoded by human papillomavirus types 16 and 18 promotes the degradation of p53. *Cell* 1990;63:1129–1136.
305. Schlessinger J. Allosteric regulation of the epidermal growth factor receptor kinase. *J Cell Biol* 1986;103:2067–2072.
306. Schlessinger J. Signal transduction by allosteric receptor oligomerization. *Trends Biochem Sci* 1988;13:443–447.
307. Schlessinger J. How receptor tyrosine kinases activate Ras. *Trends Biochem Sci* 1993;18:273–275.
308. Schnieder-Gadicke A, Schwarz E. Different human cervical carcinoma cell lines show similar transcription patterns of human papillomavirus type 18 early genes. *EMBO J* 1986;5:2285–2292.
309. Schroeder C, Gibson L, Beug H. The v-erbA oncogene requires cooperation with tyrosine kinase to arrest erythroid differentiation induced by ligand-activated endogenous c-erbA and retinoic acid receptor. *Oncogene* 1992;7:203–216.
310. Schuermann M, Neuberg M, Hunter JB. The leucine repeat motif in *Fos* protein mediates complex formation with *Jun*/AP-1 and is required for transformation. *Cell* 1988;56:507–516.
311. Schupbach J. *Human retrovirology facts and concepts.* Heidelberg: Springer Verlag, 1989.
312. Schwab M. The *myc*-box oncogenes. In: Reddy EP, Skalka AM, Curran T, eds. *The oncogene handbook.* Amsterdam: Elsevier, 1988:381–388.
313. Schwarz E, Freese UK, Gissman L. Structure and transcription of human papillomavirus sequences in cervical carcinoma cells. *Nature* 1985;314:111–114.
314. Sears R, Leone G, DeGregori J, et al. Ras enhances Myc protein stability. *Mol Cell Biol* 1999;3:169–179.
315. Sears R, Ohtani K, Nevins JR. Identification of positively and negatively acting elements regulating expression of the E2F2 gene in response to cell growth signals. *Mol Cell Biol* 1997;17:5227–5235.
316. Sefton BM, Hunter T. From c-*src* to v-*src*, or the case of the missing C terminus. *Cancer Surv* 1986;5:159–171.
317. Segawa K, Ito Y. Differential subcellular localization of in vivo-phosphorylated and non-phosphorylated middle-sized tumor antigen of polyoma virus and its relationship to middle-sized tumor antigen phosphorylating activity in vitro. *Proc Natl Acad Sci U S A* 1982;79:6812–6816.
318. Seth A, Vande Woude GF. The *mos* oncogene. In: Reddy EP, Skalka AM, Curran T, eds. *The oncogene handbook.* Amsterdam: Elsevier, 1988:195–211.
319. Setoyama C, Frunzio R, Liau G, et al. Transcriptional activation encoded by the v-fos gene. *Proc Natl Acad Sci U S A* 1986;83:3213–3217.
320. Shalloway D, Coussens PM, Yaciuk P. Overexpression of the c-*src* protein dies not induce transformation of NIH 3T3 cells. *Proc Natl Acad Sci U S A* 1984;81:7071–7075.
321. Shan B, Lee W-H. Deregulated expression of E2F-1 induces S-phase entry and leads to apoptosis. *Mol Cell Biol* 1994;14:8166–8173.
322. Sharif M, Privalsky ML. v-ErbA oncogene function in neoplasia correlates with its ability to repress retinoic acid receptor action. *Cell* 1991;166:885–893.
323. Sharp PA, Pettersson U, Sambrook J. Viral DNA in transformed cells. I. A study of the sequences of adenovirus 2 DNA in a line of transformed rat cells using specific fragments of the viral genome. *J Mol Biol* 1974;86:709.
324. Shen-Ong GL. The myb oncogene. *Biochem Biophys Acta* 1990;1032:39–52.
325. Shen Y, Shenk T. Relief of p53-mediated transcriptional repression by the adenovirus E1B 19-kDa protein or the cellular Bcl-2 protein. *Proc Natl Acad Sci U S A* 1994;91:8940–8944.
326. Sherr CJ. The *fms* oncogene. *Biochim Biophys Acta* 1988;948:225–243.
327. Sherr CJ, Rettenmier CW. The *fms* gene and the CSF-1 receptor. *Cancer Surv* 1986;5:225–231.
328. Sherr CJ, Rettenmier CW, Sacca R, et al. The c-*fms* proto-oncogene product is related to the receptor for the mononuclear phagocyte growth factor, CSF-1. *Cell* 1985;41:665–676.
329. Shibuya M, Yamaguchi S, Yamane A, et al. Nucleotide sequence and expression of a novel human receptor-type tyrosine kinase gene (flt) closely related to the fms family. *Oncogene* 1990;5:519–524.
330. Shih TY, Papageorge AG, Stokes PE, et al. Guanine nucleotide-binding and autophosphorylating activities associated with the p21 *src* protein of Harvey murine sarcoma virus. *Nature* 1980;287:686–691.
331. Shih TY, Weeks MO, Young HA, et al. p21 of Kirsten murine sarcoma virus is thermolabile in a viral mutant temperature sensitive for the maintenance of transformation. *J Virol* 1979;31:546–556.
332. Shirodkar S, Ewen M, DeCaprio JA, et al. The transcription factor E2F interacts with the retinoblastoma product and a p107-cyclin A complex in a cell cycle-regulated manner. *Cell* 1992;68:157–166.
333. Shtivelman E, Lifshitz B, Gale RP, et al. Fused transcript of *abl* and *bcr* genes in chronic myeloid leukaemia. *Nature* 1985;315:550–554.
334. Smith MR, Green WC. Type I human T cell leukemia virus tax protein transforms rat fibroblasts through the cyclic adenosine monophosphate response element binding protein/activating transcription factor pathway. *J Clin Invest* 1991;88:1038–1042.
335. Smotkin D, Wettstein FO. Transcription of human papillomavirus type 16 early genes in a cervical cancer and a cancer-derived cell line and identification of the E7 protein. *Proc Natl Acad Sci U S A* 1986;83:4680–4684.
336. Soriano P, Montgomery C, Geske R, et al. Targeted disruption of the c-*src* proto-oncogene leads to osteopetrosis in mice. *Cell* 1991;64:693–702.
337. Souyri M, Vigon I, Penciolelli JF, et al. A putative truncated cytokine receptor gene transduced by the myeloproliferative leukemia virus immortalizes hematopoietic progenitors. *Cell* 1990;63:1137–1147.
338. Stahl H, Droge P, Knippers R. DNA helicase activity of SV40 large tumor antigen. *EMBO J* 1986;5:1939–1944.
339. Stavnezer E. The *ski* oncogenes. In: Reddy EP, Skalka AM, Curran T, eds. *The oncogene handbook.* Amsterdam: Elsevier, 1988:393–401.
340. Stehelin D, Varmus HE, Bishop JM, et al. DNA related to the transforming gene(s) of avian sarcoma viruses is present in normal avian DNA. *Nature* 1976;260:170–173.
341. Stossel TP, Chaponnier C, Ezzell RM. Nonmuscle actin-binding proteins. *Annu Rev Cell Biol* 1985;1:353–402.
342. Sukumar S. *Ras* oncogenes in chemical carcinogenesis. *Curr Top Microbiol Immunol* 1989;148:93–114.
343. Swanstrom R, Parker RC, Varmus HE, et al. Transduction of a cellular oncogene: the genesis of Rous sarcoma virus. *Proc Natl Acad Sci U S A* 1983;80:2519–2523.
344. Taira M, Yoshida T, Miyagawa K, et al. cDNA sequence of human transforming gene hst and identification of the coding sequence required for transforming activity. *Proc Natl Acad Sci U S A* 1987;84:2980–2984.
345. Takeya T, Hanafusa H. Nucleotide sequence of c-*src*. *Cell* 1983;32:881–890.
346. Talis AL, Huibregtse JM, Howley PM. The role of E6AP in the regulation of p53 protein levels in human papillomavirus (HPV)-positive and HPV-negative cells. *J Biol Chem* 1998;273:6439–6445.
347. Talmage DA, Freund R, Young AT, et al. Phosphorylation of middle T by pp60 c-src: a switch for binding of phosphatidylinositol 3-kinase and optimal tumorigenesis. *Cell* 1989;59:55–65.
348. Taylor SJ, Shalloway D. The cell cycle and c-Srf. *Curr Opin Gen Dev* 1993;3:26–34.
349. Temin HM, Rubin H. Characteristics of an assay for Rous sarcoma virus and Rous sarcoma cells in tissue culture. *Virology* 1958;6:669–688.
350. Tetsu O, McCormick F. Beta-catenin regulates expression of cyclin D1 in colon carcinoma cells. *Nature* 1999;398:422–426.
351. Thelander L, Reichard P. Reduction of ribonucleotides. *Annu Rev Biochem* 1979;48:133–158.
352. Thomas JE, Aguzzi A, Soriano P, et al. Induction of tumor formation and cell transformation by polyoma middle T antigen in the absence of Src. *Oncogene* 1993;8:2521–2529.

353. Tjian R, Robbins A. Enzymatic activities associated with a purified simian virus 40 T antigen-related protein. *Proc Natl Acad Sci U S A* 1979;76:610–614.
354. Tooze J. *DNA tumor viruses: molecular biology of tumor viruses*. 2nd ed. New York: Cold Spring Harbor, 1981.
355. Toyoshima K, Vogt PK. Temperature sensitive mutants of an avian sarcoma virus. *Virology* 1969;39:930–931.
356. Turner R, Tjian R. Leucine repeats and an adjacent DNA binding domain mediate the formation of functional c*Fos*-c*Jun* heterodimers. *Science* 1989;243:1689–1694.
357. Varmus H. Retroviruses. *Science* 1988;240:1427–1435.
358. Varmus HE. The molecular genetics of cellular oncogenes. *Annu Rev Genet* 1984;d18:553–612.
359. Vennstrom B, Damm K. The *erbA* and *erbB* oncogenes. In: Reddy EP, Skalka AM, Curran T, eds. *The oncogene handbook.* Amsterdam: Elsevier, 1988:25–37.
360. Venot C, Maratrat M, Dureuil C, et al. The requirement for the p53 proline-rich functional domain for mediation of apoptosis is correlated with specific PIG3 gene transactivation and with transcriptional repression. *EMBO J* 1998;17:4668–4679.
361. Verma IM. Proto-oncogene *fos:* a multifaceted gene. In: Bradshaw RA, Prentis S, eds. *Oncogenes and growth factors*. Amsterdam: Elsevier, 1987:67–73.
362. Vogel J, Hinrichs SH, Reynolds RK, et al. The HIV *tat* gene induces dermal lesions resembling Kaposi's sarcoma in transgenic mice. *Nature* 1988;335:606–611.
363. Vogt PK. Spontaneous segregation of nontransforming viruses from cloned sarcoma viruses. *Virology* 1971;46:939–946.
364. Vogt PK. Oncogenic transformation by *jun.* In: Angel P, Herrlich P, eds. *The Fos and Jun families of transcription factors.* Boca Raton, FL: CRC Press, 1994:203–220.
365. Vogt PK, Bos TJ. *Jun:* oncogene and transcription factor. *Adv Cancer Res* 1990;55:1–35.
366. Wagner AJ, Kokontis JM, Hay N. Myc-mediated apoptosis requires wild-type p53 in a manner independent of cell cycle arrest and the ability of p53 to induce *p21waf1/cip1*. *Genes Dev* 1994;8:2817–2830.
367. Walter G, Ruediger R, Slaughter C, et al. Association of protein phosphatase 2A with polyoma virus medium T antigen. *Proc Natl Acad Sci U S A* 1990;87:2521–2525.
368. Wasylyk B, Hahn SL, Giovane A. The Ets family of transcription factors. *Eur J Biochem* 1993;211:7–18.
369. Waterfield MD, Scrace GT, Whittle N. Platelet-derived growth factor is structurally related to the putative transforming protein $p28^{sis}$ of simian sarcoma virus. *Nature* 1983;304:35–39.
370. Weinberg R, Wigler M. *Oncogenes and the molecular origins of cancer.* Cold Spring, NY: Cold Spring Harbor Press, 1989.
371. Weinberg RA. The action of oncogenes in the cytoplasm and nucleus. *Science* 1985;230:770–776.
372. Weinberger C, Hollenberg SM, Rosenfeld MG, et al. Domain structure of human glucocorticoid receptor and its relationship to the v-*erbA* oncogene product. *Nature* 1985;318:670–672.
373. Weinberger C, Thompson CC, Ong ES, et al. The c-*erb-A* gene encodes a thyroid hormone receptor. *Nature* 1986;324:641–646.
374. Weiss R. Human T-cell retroviruses. In: *RNA tumor viruses:* molecular biology of tumor viruses. Cold Spring Harbor, NY: Cold Spring Harbor Press, 1985:405–485.
375. Weiss R, Teich N, Varmus HE, et al. *RNA tumor viruses: molecular biology of tumor viruses.* Cold Spring, NY: Cold Spring Harbor Press, 1985.
376. Werness BA, Levine AJ, Howley PM. Association of human papillomavirus types 16 and 18 E6 proteins with p53. *Science* 1990;248:76–79.
377. Westermark B, Heldin C-H. Platelet-derived growth factor in autocrine transformation. *Cancer Res* 1991;51:5087–5092.
378. White E. Death-defying acts: a meeting review on apoptosis. *Genes Dev* 1993;7:2277–2284.
379. White E, Grodzicker T, Stillman BW. Mutations in the gene encoding the adenovirus early region 1B 19,000-molecular-weight tumor antigen cause the degradation of chromosomal DNA. *J Virol* 1984;52:410.
380. White E, Sabbatini P, Debbas M, et al. The 19-kilodalton adenovirus E1B transforming protein inhibits programmed cell death and prevents cytolysis by tumor necrosis factor alpha. *Mol Cell Biol* 1992;12:2570–2580.
381. Whitman M, Kaplan DR, Schaffhausen B, et al. Association of phosphatidylinositol kinase activity and polyoma middle T competent for transformation. *Nature* 1985;315:239–242.
382. Whyte P, Buchkovich KJ, Horowitz JM, et al. Association between an oncogene and an anti-oncogene: the adenovirus E1A proteins bind to the retinoblastoma gene product. *Nature* 1988;334:124–129.
383. Williams LT. The *sis* gene and PDGF. *Cancer Surv* 1986;5:231–241.
384. Witte ON. Functions of the *abl* oncogene. *Cancer Surv* 1986;5:183–197.
385. Wood TG, McGeady ML, Baroudy BM, et al. Mouse c-*mos* oncogene activation is prevented by upstream sequences. *Proc Natl Acad Sci U S A* 1984;81:7817–7821.
386. Wu X, Bayle JH, Olson D, et al. The p53-mdm-2 autoregulatory feedback loop. *Genes Dev* 1993;7:1126–1132.
387. Wu X, Levine AJ. p53 and E2F-1 cooperate to mediate apoptosis. *Proc Natl Acad Sci U S A* 1994;91:3602–3606.
388. Wyke JA. The selective isolation of temperature-sensitive mutants of Rous sarcoma virus. *Virology* 1973;52:587–590.
389. Xiong Y, Connolly T, Futcher B, et al. Human D type cyclin. *Cell* 1991;65:691–699.
390. Yamaguchi TP, Dumont DJ, Conlon RA, et al. Elk-1, an flt-related receptor tyrosine kinase is an early marker for endothelial cell precursors. *Development* 1993;118:489–498.
391. Yamashita T, Shimojo H. Induction of cellular DNA synthesis by adenovirus 12 in human embryo kidney cells. *Virology* 1969;38:351–355.
392. Yang S-I, Lickteig RL, Estes R, et al. Control of protein phosphatase 2A by simian virus 40 small-t antigen. *Mol Cell Biol* 1991;11:1988–1995.
393. Yee S, Branton PE. Detection of cellular proteins associated with human adenovirus type 5 early 1A polypeptides. *Virology* 1985;147:142–153.
394. Yew N, Strobel M, Vande Woude GF. Mos and the cell cycle: the molecular basis of the transformed phenotype. *Curr Opin Genet Dev* 1993;3:19–25.
395. Yew PR, Berk AJ. Inhibition of p53 transactivation required for transformation by adenovirus early 1B protein. *Nature* 1992;357:82–85.
396. Zambetti GP, Bargonetti J, Walker K, et al. Wild-type p53 mediates positive regulation of gene expression through a specific DNA sequence element. *Genes Dev* 1992;6:1143–1152.
397. Zenke M, Kahn P, Disela C. v-*erb A* specifically suppresses transcription of the avian erythrocyte anion transporter (band 3) gene. *Cell* 1988;52:107–119.
398. Zhang Y, Xiong Y, Yarbrough WG. ARF promotes MDm2 degradation and stabilizes p53: *ARF-INK4a* locus deletion impairs both the Rb and p53 tumor suppressor pathways. *Cell* 1998;92:725–734.
399. Zindy F, Eischen CM, Randle DH, et al. Myc signaling via the ARF tumor suppressor regulates p53-dependent apoptosis and immortalization. *Genes Dev* 1998;12:2424–2433.
400. zur Hausen H. Human papillomaviruses in the pathogenesis of anogenital cancer. *Virology* 1991;184:9–13.
401. zur Hausen H. Viruses in human cancers. *Science* 1991;254:1167–1173.

CHAPTER 11

The Immune Response to Viruses

J. Lindsay Whitton and Michael B.A. Oldstone

Virus infections have long been a major cause of human morbidity and mortality, at times substantially affecting the course of human history (167). However, due mainly to the astonishing benefits of antiviral vaccination in the past 50 years, smallpox has been eliminated, worldwide polio eradication is on the horizon, and at least in the "developed" countries, many of the childhood illnesses (measles, mumps, rubella, chickenpox, etc.) appear under control. Therefore as we reach the millenium, it is tempting to become sanguine, to conclude that we are close to completing the catalog of viruses and their associated diseases, and perhaps even to suggest that virus infections no longer pose a significant threat to human health. Nothing could be further from the truth. First, viruses still exact a heavy toll in human suffering, increasingly so with the spread of human immunodeficiency virus (HIV), which in 1998 became the fourth leading cause of death worldwide (behind ischemic heart disease, cerebrovascular disease, and acute lower respiratory tract infections). Second, new (or at least newly recognized) diseases continue to appear, most tragically demonstrated by the mushrooming acquired immunodeficiency syndrome (AIDS) epidemic, first recognized 18 years ago, and for which the causative virus was identified in 1983 (11). More recently, an outbreak of a "mysterious virus" occurred in Malaysia, killing more than 100 people (1).

This virus is related to, but distinct from, Hendra virus, an equine morbillivirus first isolated in stables in Hendra, Australia, which had high pathogenicity in humans (214). Whereas Hendra virus is associated with horses, and may be spread by cats and bats (276), the Malaysian paramyxovirus is associated with pigs. Third, diseases that in the past have been geographically constrained may plausibly be spread worldwide by rapid intercontinental travel (e.g., Ebola, Lassa). Fourth, we must be continually wary of the reappearance of old foes; there were 90 deaths from measles in the United States in 1990 (200) and over 150,000 cases in 1998, 1999, and 200 in Japan, as a result of reduced vaccine compliance; and the 1997 outbreak (fortunately limited) of influenza in Hong Kong had a 30% fatality rate (219). Fifth, it is becoming increasingly clear that virus infections are associated with various cancers; for example, human papillomavirus with cervical carcinoma; human herpesvirus 8 with Kaposi's sarcoma; and hepatocellular carcinoma may be causally associated with hepatitis B virus (149), which infects hundreds of millions. Finally, there remain many diseases whose causes are undefined, and for which undiscovered viruses remain prime etiologic candidates.

To counter the continuing threat, it is vital that we understand the antiviral immune response. Studies of antiviral immunity can help us evaluate clinical problems (at the most basic level, our knowledge of the kinetics of the antibody response has been the basis of many viral diagnostic procedures, at least until recently). Furthermore, in the last decade we have begun to uncover the mechanisms that underlie the success of antiviral vaccines, and with this knowledge in hand, we may now be able to design better vaccines. In addition, viruses are powerful tools with which to probe the workings of the host immune system, and the knowledge that accrues may yield benefits in diverse fields. For example, the relationship between virus infection and subsequent immunity was noted more than 200 years ago by Jenner (85), whereas virus-induced immunosuppression was first suspected more than 90 years ago by von Pirquet (260). Major histocompatibility complex (MHC) restriction—described later in this chapter—was discovered with a viral model system (286); so pivotal was this finding to almost all aspects of antigen-specific immunity (not only in virology, but also in tumor immunology and autoimmunity) that its discoverers were awarded the 1996 Nobel Prize in Medicine.

OVERVIEW OF THE IMMUNE RESPONSE TO VIRUS INFECTION

Virus infections are countered by host immune responses. Acute virus infections represent a race between viral replication and host immunity; the usual outcome is either death of the host or termination of infection followed by recovery. In chronic virus infections, the time scale is lengthened, and both ongoing virus replication and a continuous host immune response may be present. In both acute and chronic infections, the antiviral immune response can itself be harmful to the host; this is termed immunopathology. For example, host responses may kill virus-infected cells, perhaps eradicating the agent, but at the cost of local tissue destruction. In addition many of the systemic clinical signs and symptoms manifested during viral infection are a consequence not of virus replication *per se,* but rather of the host immune reaction; cytokines released in response to infection may cause systemic symptoms (fever, headache, myalgia, anorexia, weight loss, etc.) (248,255). Furthermore, particularly during chronic infection, viral antigen–antibody complexes may form with subsequent manifestations of immune complex disease. Finally, the immune response triggered by the virus may be aberrant, focusing not on the virus but instead on self proteins, and possibly causing autoimmune disease (166,273).

The immune response can be subdivided in several ways, the two most useful of which are shown in Fig. 1. Immune responses may be categorized either by the *nature of the effector function* or by the *antigen specificity of the response.*

By effector function. Effector functions carried out directly by cells [e.g., natural killer (NK) cells, T cells] are classified as "cellular" immunity. When the effector functions are fluid-borne, they are termed "humoral" immunity; this term is often wrongly thought to be synonymous with antibodies, but in fact it encompasses all fluid-borne effector molecules (antibodies, cytokines, chemokines, complement, etc.). These divisions are obviously overlapping; cellular immunity can involve cytokine secretion, which is itself humoral. Finally, physicochemical defenses are termed "barrier" immunity.

By antigen specificity. Immune responses may be termed antigen specific (adaptive) or non–antigen specific (innate); as the names indicate, the former (mediated by lymphocytes) recognize specific antigenic motifs, as described later, whereas the latter (e.g., interferons, natural killer cells, mucociliary responses) are incapable of doing so. However, the key distinction between antigen-specific and nonspecific immunity is that only the former has "memory." On first exposure to a virus, both nonspecific and antigen-specific responses are activated, and the infection is (we hope) cleared. However, on second exposure to the same agent, the antigen-specific response occurs much more rapidly, and is much stronger, because of amplification of memory cells, whereas the nonspecific response occurs almost precisely as before. The beneficial effects of vaccination rely on the induction of memory cells.

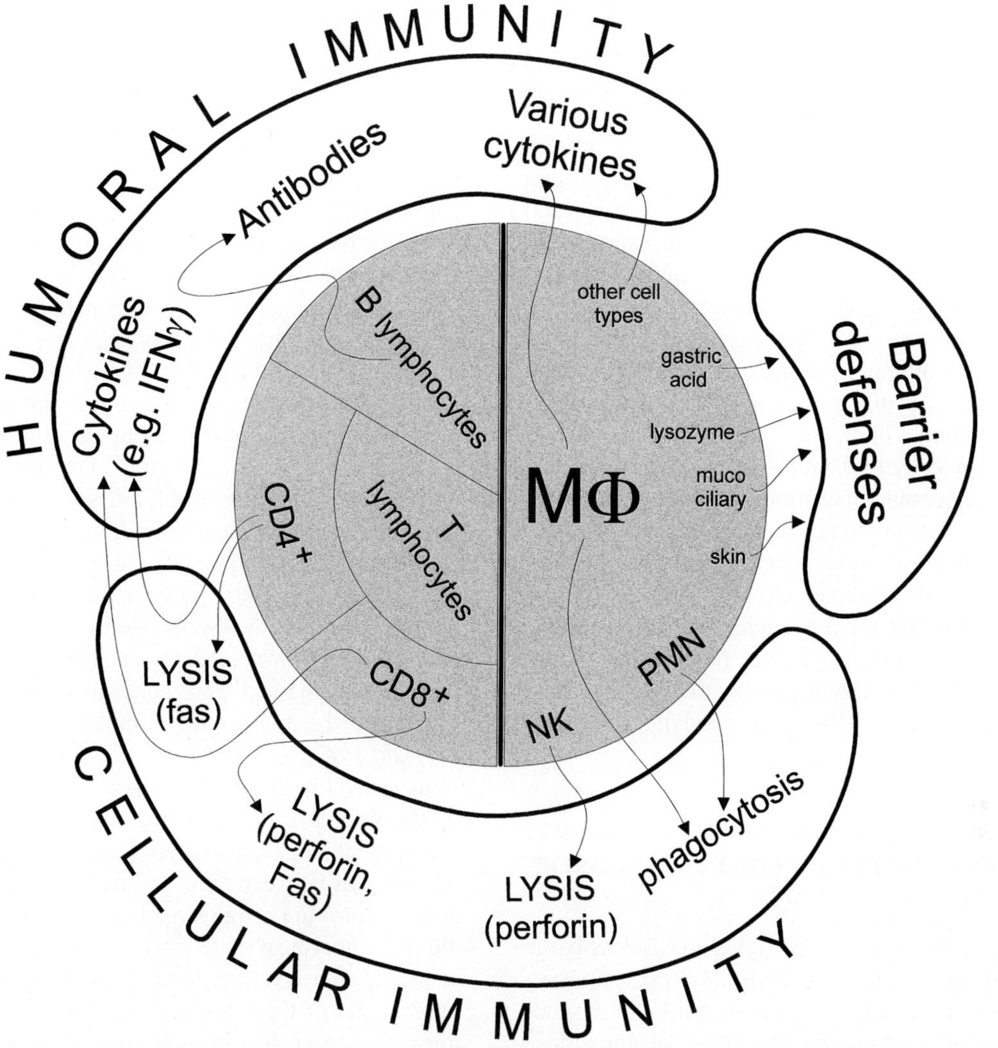

FIG. 1. Cutting the immunological cake. The central gray circle represents the immune response, which can be subdivided into antigen-specific responses (*left half*) and innate or non-specific immunity (*right half*). The correlations of these responses with an alternative means of classifying immunity (cellular, humoral, and barrier) are shown, as are some of the effector functions involved (lysis, cytokine release, etc.). *MΦ*, macrophages; *NK*, natural killer cells; *PMN*, polymorphonuclear leukocytes; *IFN*, interferon.

Both innate and adaptive immunity are important in clearing virus infection. Innate responses, and their effector functions, are described later in the chapter; we focus first on adaptive (antigen-specific) immunity. As shown in Fig. 1, this relies on lymphocytes, of which there are two classes, T (thymus-derived) lymphocytes and B lymphocytes (which give rise to antibody-producing plasma cells). Antibodies act mainly to diminish the infectivity of free virus, whereas T cells recognize (and often kill) infected cells. Thus antibodies and T lymphocytes act in a complementary manner: antibodies reduce the infectivity of free virus in fluid phase, thereby decreasing the number of infected cells that T lymphocytes must deal with, and T lymphocytes kill infected cells before virus maturation has occurred, minimizing the release of infectious virus and thus easing the load on antibodies. Primary virus infection (when the host is first exposed to the wild virus or to a vaccine containing viral antigens) in many cases induces readily detectable antiviral antibody and T-cell responses. At the peak of the T-cell response (usually 7–10 days), some 50% to 60% of $CD8^+$ cells are virus specific (26,147); this number decreases (often in parallel with the resolving virus infection), and by 3 to 4 weeks after infection, the cell numbers have decreased, although a significant proportion (1–10%) of splenic $CD8^+$ cells are virus-specific (memory) cells. Antibody responses usually peak later than T-cell responses; antibodies are often barely detectable in the acute (symptomatic) stage of infection, but increase in number over a period of 2 to 4 weeks to a readily measurable level that often lingers for weeks or months, depending on the host and virus. Antibodies to some viruses (e.g., yellow fever and measles) can linger for a lifetime. Because antibody molecules have half-lives measured in weeks, the lifelong presence of antibody implies ongoing production, which may be stimulated by reexposure to related viruses circulating in the population. Long-term antibody production can be effected by long-lived plasma cells (224). After a second exposure to the same antigen(s) (i.e., reexposure to the wild virus, or initial exposure to wild virus after appropriate vaccination), both classes of lymphocytes display antigen-specific memory. The classic "anamnestic" or memory antibody response is seen, with antibody levels climbing more rapidly and higher than before, and usually being maintained for a longer time. Secondary cytotoxic T-cell responses, too, are brisk, because of the presence of the memory T cells, which proliferate on antigen contact. The molecular requirements for T-cell memory remain somewhat controversial. Some workers argue that specific antigen must persist to restimulate memory T cells continuously (157), but persuasive evidence indicates that memory cells can persist in the absence of specific antigen (81,114), perhaps being sporadically stimulated in a nonspecific manner by local cytokine release during other, antigenically unrelated, immune reactions.

THE IMMUNE SYSTEM HAS BEEN SHAPED BY THE TYPES OF MICROBES THAT CHALLENGE IT

The vertebrate immune system fights a ceaseless battle against infectious agents, and both of these opposing forces have been shaped by the constant conflict. Immunological pressures bear on mutable microbes, selecting those best able to escape the unwelcome attentions of the immune system. Microbial evolution is thus driven, at least in part, by the efforts of the immune response to eradicate infection. These enforced microbial changes are mirrored in the vertebrate hosts: the immune system is molded by the nature of the microbes that it faces. For example, hosts whose immune systems are less able to counter a specific infectious agent may die; those that live (and their progeny) are better able to resist similar organisms. Hence, the vertebrate gene pool is altered by exposure to specific microbes. This battle for evolutionary supremacy places the virus in a difficult situation. If the virus is too readily eliminated by host immunity, and is in consequence unable to maintain itself in the host population, it becomes extinct. Conversely, if a virus is too virulent and cannot be controlled by host immunity, it may result in eradication of the host and thus, theoretically, viral extinction. Thus from the virus' viewpoint, it is best to be sufficiently virulent to allow transfer from an infected to an uninfected host, but to temper its pathogenicity to ensure that the host will survive long enough to permit the transfer. At either extreme, the virus may be eliminated. Frequently the initial virulence of a virus is diminished by mutation to a less virulent form, and this, in concert with the selection of more resistant hosts, results in a fluctuating equilibrium, in which both host and microbe coexist. Many examples of microbial and host changes have been documented. For example, influenza virus is the quintessence of antigenic variation in the face of host immunity, and those influenza viruses best able to evade host responses have fueled outbreaks of epidemic or pandemic proportions. The complementary outcome, in which the microbes select for survival those hosts best able to counter their pathogenic effects, is best demonstrated when the offspring have enhanced survival prospects. Such improved resistance in the progeny may, of course, be in part conferred by passive (maternally derived) immunity rather than by genetic fitness, but there are clear examples of the latter. For instance, wild Australian rabbits that survived the first onslaught by myxoma virus (a poxvirus deliberately administered in an attempt to control the exponential increase in the rabbit population) bred hardy offspring more resistant to the agent (46). Natives of the New World were devastated by smallpox and measles, introduced by the European invaders, and those who remained were better able to survive infection (135); and the appearance in dolphins (12,251) and seals (177,258) of a morbillivirus related to canine distemper virus caused high initial morbidity, which now appears to be decreasing. It has been suggested that a contemporary example of such an evolving host–parasite relationship may be that between HIV and its human host. Many host gene systems are responsible for determining the ability of the individual host to respond to an infectious agent, and several have been characterized in experimental model systems; some of them are discussed later. In summary, the immune system has been shaped at least in part by the nature of the challenges it has faced. We cited some specific examples of such evolutionary sculpture, but can we discern a more global effect whereby different classes of organisms (e.g., viruses compared with bacteria) have caused the immune system to evolve in a particular way? We shall argue later that this is indeed the case; that the two different facets of the antigen-specific immune response (antibodies and T cells) have evolved to control infection, depending on the replication site of the infecting organism (i.e., whether it is intracellular or extracellular); and that the deciding factor in determining which component of the immune response will predominate (i.e., antibody or T cell) is which of the two antigen-presentation pathways the microbial antigens best can enter.

THE ROLES OF ANTIBODIES AND T CELLS IN THE CONTROL OF MICROBIAL INFECTIONS: POINTERS FROM EXPERIMENTS OF NATURE

Antibody responses have long been recognized as important indicators of recent virus infection. Historically, a patient with an acute illness had blood drawn (acute-phase serum sample), and at a later date, often 2 to 4 weeks later, after clinical recovery, a second sample was gathered (convalescent-phase serum sample). For various candidate viruses, the levels of specific antibodies in the two samples were compared, and an increase of more than fourfold was usually considered diagnostic of recent infection. Diagnosis of a current infection requires virus isolation and growth or, nowadays, polymerase chain reaction (PCR)-based identification. The ready detection of antiviral antibodies, and the demonstration that some of them were capable on inactivating the virus, led to the reasonable assumption that antibodies were important in combating primary virus infections. This position was proven by many studies that showed that several acute virus infections could be modified or prevented by transfer of serum from an immune source. Passive antibody therapy can protect against or modify the course of several human virus infections. For example, infusion of antibodies specific for the Junin arenavirus is beneficial in Argentinian hemorrhagic fever (42,130), whereas post-exposure rabies prophylaxis relies on vaccination and concurrent administration of virus-specific immunoglobulins (Igs) (122). Furthermore, in experimental models, antibodies can reduce viral titers and modulate disease. For instance, recovery from ocular herpesvirus infection is hastened by administration of anti-HSV antibody (115). Similarly, the role of antiviral antibodies in vaccination has long been unquestioned. It is important to note that the studies cited earlier showed convincingly that antibodies are sufficient for protective immunity against some viruses; they did not show that antibodies are required. Nevertheless these findings, along with the excellent correlation between vaccine immunogenicity (as judged by induction of high levels of specific antibody) and vaccine efficacy (as judged by the vaccine's protective effect) has led some workers to the misguided conclusion that antibodies alone contribute to vaccine-induced protection. "Experiments of nature" in humans strongly suggest that, for some viral infections, antiviral antibody responses can be dispensed with at little cost to the host. For example, children born with genetically determined deficiencies in antibody production, with no detectable Igs, do not show an increased susceptibility to most viral diseases, with the exception of rare enteroviral meningitides, caused most often by picornaviruses such as coxsackievirus (58,76) and echovirus type 9 or 11 (134,142). Indeed the picornavirus family is the exception that proves the rule. Before the disorder was diagnosed, a patient with common variable immunodeficiency syndrome (a defect in antibody formation) was given oral (live) polio vaccine; the patient developed paralytic disease, and continues to shed infectious poliovirus many years later (102). In addition, coxsackievirus infection of mice lacking B cells leads to a lifelong chronic infection, confirming that antibodies are required to control picornaviruses (136). However, for most viruses, the incidence of viral disease, and disease severity, are similar in antibody-deficient individuals and normal children. These data suggest that—even though they are capable of conferring antiviral protection—antibodies are expendable in resolving some virus infections. In contrast to their ability to clear virus infections, agammaglobulinemic children show a marked increase in susceptibility to bacterial infection (60,61). Similarly, children with genetic defects in components of the complement cascade (a final effector mechanism in some antibody-mediated responses) are less able to cope with bacterial, particularly meningococcal, challenge, but their resistance to virus infection and disease appears normal (133,176). Thus antibodies are required primarily to control bacterial, not viral, infection. In the absence of antibodies, the host has an alternative means of controlling viruses: T cells. That T cells can play a critical part in eradicating human viral infections is suggested by several observations. The frequency and severity of virus infections are markedly increased in humans with impaired T-cell responses [for example, in patients with Di George's syndrome (congenital thymic aplasia), AIDS, leukemia, or recipients of immunosuppressive therapy] (60). In many of these cases, however, there also is some impairment of antibody response, and so it is difficult to draw firm conclusions. In animals, models have been developed with clean mutations in various aspects of antibody or T-cell function; these are discussed later in this chapter. However, measles infection provides an excellent example of the importance of T cells in controlling virus infections in humans. In normal children, the disease is typified by the characteristic rash, and complete recovery is usual. In contrast, in T cell–deficient children, the disease is often fatal (64,148,221). The rash itself is T-cell mediated and does not develop in severely immunosuppressed children; indeed, the presence of a rash in an immunosuppressed child (e.g., in a child with leukemia who contracts measles) is considered a positive prognostic indicator (101). In agammaglobulinemic children, the rash develops normally, and the course of the disease is unaltered by the absence of antibody responses. Furthermore, agammaglobulinemic children are subsequently immune to measles; thus antibodies in this instance are required neither for control of the primary infection nor for resistance to secondary disease (61). In summary, as outlined at the beginning of this section, overwhelming evidence shows that antibodies can control many virus infections; nevertheless, they are sometimes expendable.

Thus although both antibodies and T cells play important roles in the control of virus infection, disruption of the former has less effect on the host's ability to control virus infections but dramatically reduces the host's capacity to counter bacterial challenges. What is the molecular explanation for this phenomenon? To understand this question, it is necessary to review how antibodies and T cells see virus antigens on the virus particle or at the surface of an infected cell and to describe in some detail how these virus antigens get there. We approach this issue in the form of an overview, and then describe in greater detail the individual genes and gene families involved.

THE ROLES OF ANTIBODIES AND T CELLS IN THE CONTROL OF MICROBIAL INFECTIONS: THE IMPORTANCE OF HOW ANTIGENS ARE RECOGNIZED

Antigen Recognition by Antibodies

Antibodies recognize antigen by using regions of hypervariable sequence. The antibody–antigen union has been subjected to crystallographic analyses (7,199), which indicated that the union is more "hand-in-glove" (in which components can, to some extent, alter their conformation to accommodate one another) than "lock and key" (in which both elements are fixed, each unable to modulate to the other). Antibodies recognize intact proteins. Thus antibodies can recognize free bacteria and viruses, as well as viral proteins (most often glycoproteins), expressed on the surface of infected cells. It is therefore easy to imagine how antibodies can play a major role in the control of viruses and bacteria, by inactivating them as free extracellular entities.

However, what happens when a microbe can evade antibody recognition by locating itself within a host cell? Few bacteria can accomplish this, but viruses are obligate intracellular parasites; their replication is intracellular, often relying on subversion of host machinery. How can antibodies exert an antiviral effect at this stage? One obvious mechanism is the recognition of viral proteins on the surface of infected cells. However, many viruses delay the display of cell-surface proteins until late in the infective cycle, by which time viral maturation may have occurred, and antibody-mediated cell lysis would simply release the infectious progeny.

How can a host detect an infected cell early in the infectious process, thus maximizing its immunological advantage? Here antibodies are less effective, being limited by their recognition requirements, whereas T cells play a critical role. T cells, as will be detailed later, can recognize almost any viral protein, including those made immediately on infection; when this early-recognition capacity is allied to the ability to destroy such infected cells, T cells become a formidable component of the antiviral armamentarium.

Antigen Recognition by T Cells

T cells can be subdivided by the surface marker proteins (CD4/CD8) they express. The majority of $CD8^+$ cells are cytotoxic T lymphocytes (CTLs), although some $CD8^+$ cells exert their antiviral effects mainly by cytokine release (204), whereas most $CD4^+$ cells are helper cells that secrete cytokines to assist B-cell maturation.

T cells recognize antigens via a cell-surface heterodimer, the T-cell receptor (TcR). This molecule is structurally reminiscent of the Fab portion of an antibody molecule, but the nature of T-cell recognition differs from that of antibody recognition in one critical aspect: whereas antibodies recognize antigen in isolation, T cells react to antigen in the form of a short peptide presented by a host glycoprotein encoded in the MHC. This phenomenon, named MHC restriction, was discovered by analyses of host responses to virus infection (285,286). There are two major classes of MHC molecule (class I and class II), and there is a tight relationship between the class of MHC/peptide complex recognized by a T cell and the surface marker (CD4 or CD8) borne by the T cell. MHC class I molecules are the "classic" molecules associated with graft rejection (the phenomenon that gave the MHC its name); they are expressed on most somatic cells [neurons being a rare exception (88)], and they interact with T cells bearing the CD8 surface marker. In contrast, MHC class II molecules, previously termed Ia or Ir (immune response gene) molecules, have a much more restricted expression, being found only on specialized antigen-presenting cells (APCs; e.g., macrophages, B lymphocytes, dendritic cells), and they interact with T cells carrying the CD4 surface marker. The relationships between surface marker, MHC class, and cell function are summarized in Table 1. The CD4/II and CD8/I relationships are determined by direct interactions between the respective molecules: CD4 binds to a specific conserved region of MHC class II (109,256), and a similar interaction occurs between CD8 and class I (57,212).

So evolution has produced two classes of T cells, and the major feature distinguishing them is which of the two MHC/peptide complexes each can recognize. It is clear how T cells distinguish between class I and class II (using the CD4/8 proteins); but what is the importance of their being able to make this distinction? Presumably there is some vital and fundamental difference between the class I and class II complexes, and the ability of the immune response to detect and respond to this class I/class II difference is of prime importance.

At the target cell surface, class I and class II molecules are similar in overall structure. The molecules are heterodimers, with four domains: two Ig-like domains at the cell membrane and two distal domains. The class I heterodimer comprises the class I heavy (H) chain (three domains) closely complexed with a non–MHC-encoded protein, β_2-microglobulin (β_2M). Stable expression of the class I H chain on the cell surface usually requires β2M. The class II heterodimer consists of two similar chains, α and β, each with two domains and encoded in the MHC. For both class I and class II, the two membrane-distal domains together form a structure graphically described

TABLE 1. *Recognition requirements and functions of CD4+ AND CD8+ T Cells*

	$CD8^+$ T cells	$CD4^+$ T cells
MHC class that presents the antigen to T cells	MHC class I	MHC class II
Cell types that bear the MHC molecule and thus can present antigen to the T cells	Almost all nucleated cells, with the exception of neurons	Specialized antigen-presenting cells (e.g., macrophages, dendritic cells, B lymphocytes)
Source of antigen recognized	Usually endogenous antigen, made within the presenting cell	Usually exogenous antigen, taken into the presenting cell by endocytosis
Such an antigen will be made during infection by	Intracellular organisms (e.g., viruses), a few bacteria (e.g., *Listeria, Mycobacteria*), and some parasites	Viruses, bacteria, and other parasites; infection results in microbial proteins being shed into the fluid phase
T-cell functions	Usually cytotoxic, killing target cells. Other mechanisms of antiviral activity (e.g., cytokine release)	Usually provide "help" in the form of cytokines to B cells, thereby helping in antibody production

as a "Venus fly trap," the "groove" of which binds the antigenic peptide in a sequence-specific manner and displays it on the cell surface for the perusal of T cells (18,19). The MHC molecule is hence said to "present" the antigenic peptide. MHC molecules (both I and II) are polymorphic, and many alleles exist in the population. Much of the polymorphism lies at or near the peptide-binding groove; as a result, different MHC molecules bind different peptides. Because MHC differs among different individuals, different people will present different parts (epitopes) of a given antigen (e.g., a virus) and therefore will mount T-cell responses of different epitope specificities. Thus there are many common features between class I and class II complexes: both have four domains, both have a groove that presents antigenic peptide, and both are polymorphic around this groove.

What is the evolutionary benefit of producing two such apparently similar molecular complexes? Presumably it relates to their interactions with the specific T-cell subsets. What, then, is the essential difference between the class I/peptide complex and the class II/peptide complex, and why is it important that T cells can distinguish between them? The critical difference between the two complexes lies not in the complex itself but instead in how the MHC/peptide complex reaches the cell surface. The two classes of MHC reflect two different antigen-processing pathways (described later), one of which (class I) is optimized to present intracellular antigen and the other (class II) to present extracellular antigen. Thus when T cells distinguish between a peptide/class I complex and a peptide/class II complex, they are really discriminating based on the source of the peptide: from protein made within the APC, or from protein taken up from the extracellular milieu.

ANTIGEN PROCESSING: CLASSICAL AND NON-CLASSICAL PATHWAYS

There are two "classical" pathways of antigen presentation: (a) the class I pathway, in which endogenous antigen (usually made within the target cell) is processed, eventually to appear as a peptide fragment in the class I groove on the cell surface, and (b) the class II pathway, in which exogenous antigen, usually soluble protein applied to the outside of the presenting cell, is internalized and eventually also finds itself presented on the cell surface in an MHC/peptide complex. The key here is the location of the antigen; endogenous antigens are presented by class I MHC, and exogenous antigens, by class II MHC. As with most generalizations, this division is not absolute; there are examples of *de novo* synthesized antigen that enters the class II pathway, and of protocols to introduce exogenous antigens into the class I pathway. By and large, however, this generalization holds. Figure 2 summarizes the two pathways. A cell is shown, bisected by a dotted line; this hypothetical cell expresses both classes of MHC (it could therefore be, for example, an activated macrophage or dendritic cell). Below and to the right of the dotted line, the class I antigen processing/presentation pathway

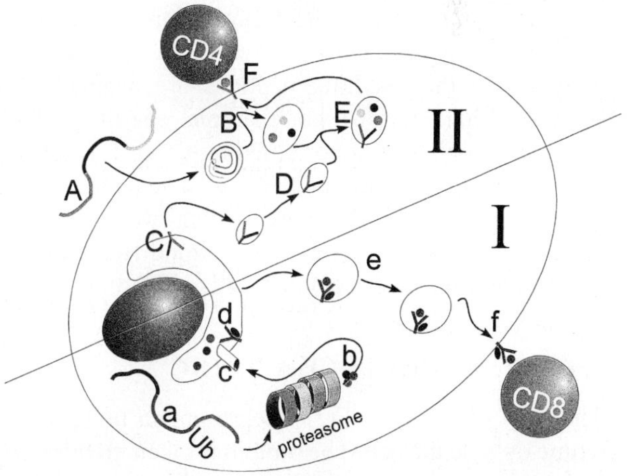

FIG. 2. Antigen-processing pathways. A cell capable of presenting antigen via both class I and class II pathways is shown, bisected by a line which separates the pathways. The letters identify various stages in the pathways, described in the text. A–F, class II; a–f, class I; Ub, ubiquitin (see text).

is outlined, and above and to the left of the line, the class II pathway is shown.

Antigen Presentation by Class I MHC

The thick line (a) in Fig. 2 represents a virus protein, newly synthesized in the cell cytoplasm. A certain proportion of all intracellular proteins are "tagged" for destruction by the covalent attachment of the 76-amino-acid cellular protein ubiquitin (Ub in Fig. 2). Ubiquitin covalently attaches, via its C-terminal glycine residue G76, to a lysine on the target protein; a second ubiquitin then attaches to a lysine residue on the first, and then a third ubiquitin attaches to the second, and so on. The doomed protein is therefore marked with a poly-ubiquitin chain, and this complex is taken to the proteasome (b), where it is degraded to generate shorter peptides (150). The ubiquitin system can be manipulated to increase protein degradation, resulting in enhanced induction of MHC class I–restricted T-cell responses (203,205,245, 278). The peptides are next passed into the endoplasmic reticulum (ER) by a transporter mechanism, the TAP (transporter associated with antigen presentation) proteins (c), which belong to the ABC transporter family and are encoded within the MHC (100,186,249). Three peptides are shown in the ER, where they encounter the heterodimeric MHC class I complex (d) [comprising the class I protein and an accessory protein β_2-microglobulin (β_2m)]; one peptide is selected by the class I MHC heterodimer (on the basis of binding affinity in the MHC groove), and assembly of the class I/peptide complex occurs. These events have been recently reviewed in some detail (48,202). The complex passes into the Golgi apparatus (e), finally reaching the cell surface (f), where the peptide/MHC complex is recognized by a CD8$^+$ T cell–bearing TcR of the appropriate specificity. Note that peptides can reach class I molecules by a TAP-independent route, not shown in the figure; signal sequences, when clipped by signal peptidases in the ER, can be degraded, and the resulting peptides are available for MHC class I loading (73). For example, one of the CTL epitopes of lymphocytic choriomeningitis virus (LCMV) (272) is located within a putative signal sequence in the viral glycoprotein. Furthermore, recent work suggests that some class I proteins can present modified peptides (for example, glycopeptides) to T cells (230).

Antigen Presentation by Class II MHC

The thick line (A) in Fig. 1 represents a protein, but this time outside the cell. The protein is taken up by endocytosis and eventually reaches an acidic compartment, where it is degraded by proteases, generating peptides (B). Meanwhile, the class II molecule is synthesized within the ER (C) and is transported out through the Golgi/trans-Golgi (D). The class II vacuole fuses with the endosome containing the fragmented internalized protein (E), and a peptide is bound in the MHC class II groove, again selected on the basis of affinity. The mature complex is passed onto the cell membrane (F), where it is recognized by the TcR of a CD4$^+$ T cell. Note that the class II molecule in the ER (class II, C) does not bind peptides introduced by the transporters (class I, d) because the class II molecule in the ER is attached to another protein, the invariant chain (not shown), which prevents peptide binding. The invariant chain is lost as the class II molecule undergoes transport, so when fusion occurs with the endosome (class II, E), the class II molecule can bind to the peptide fragments therein (240). A recent review of presentation of exogenous antigen is available (156).

Biological Importance of the Difference Between the Two Classical Antigen-Presentation Pathways

From this it can be seen that T-cell recognition distinguishes between intracellular and extracellular sources of antigen; CD8$^+$ T cells, usually CTLs, recognize peptides from endogenously synthesized proteins, and CD4$^+$ T cells, usually helpers, detect peptides derived from exogenously applied proteins. Why is it important for the different T-cell subsets to respond differently, depending on the source of antigen? Organisms that replicate intracellularly (viruses, as well as some bacteria and other parasites) will feed antigens into the class I pathway, as well as into the class II pathway (when antigens are shed, e.g., during cell death). Conversely, obligate extracellular organisms (most bacteria) will be limited to introducing antigen mainly into the class II pathway. Therefore bacteria (extracellular) will induce mainly CD4$^+$ T-cell and antibody responses, but few CD8$^+$ T cells; whereas the response to viruses will include CD8$^+$ T cells in addition to CD4$^+$ T cells and antibodies. These considerations allow the experiments of nature to be viewed in a more molecular light. The absence of antibodies in patients with agammaglobulinemia will markedly reduce the host's ability to control bacterial infection, because this ability relies primarily on antibodies, and there is no "backup" available if antibodies are absent. In contrast, agammaglobulinemia will have much less effect on most antiviral responses because the CD8$^+$ T-cell response, effective against intracellular organisms, remains intact. Furthermore, if CD8$^+$ T cells have evolved in part to control infections by intracellular organisms, then the removal of the T-cell arm might be expected to most severely disable the host's capacity to combat such infections; this is the case. However, there are no clinical syndromes in which the class I presentation pathway alone is defective, and so it is difficult to infer how well antibody and CD4$^+$ T-cell responses could cope with virus infection in the absence of CD8$^+$ T cells. This question has been addressed experimentally in several transgenic mouse knock-out models. For example, mice lacking

β_2M express little or no MHC class I on their cell surfaces and, because CD8$^+$ T-cell maturation requires thymic expression of MHC class I, these mice develop very few CD8$^+$ T cells. Such mice mount extremely limited CD8$^+$ CTL responses, but develop readily detectable CD4$^+$ CTLs (80,146). The outcome of virus infection in these CD8$^-$CD4$^+$ mice varies with the virus used, but in general, there is delayed clearance of several viruses (50). These studies support the contention that CD8$^+$ CTLs play an important role in controlling virus infection, because their ablation reduces the host's ability to clear virus; however, the second pathway (CD4$^+$ T cells and antibodies) provides a certain degree of antiviral protection.

Thus there is an evolutionary relationship between the type of invading microbe, the MHC pathways that present its antigens, and the T cells that respond. Evolution appears to have honed the interactions to ensure that, upon infection, the immune response which predominates is that best suited to deal with the specific type of organism being faced. The fulcrum upon which this decision balances is the MHC antigen-presentation pathway. Most bacterial (extracellular) infections will present antigen through the class II pathway and in consequence will induce a predominantly CD4$^+$ T-cell and antibody response; antibodies can recognize intact antigen, and use various effector mechanisms (e.g., opsonization, agglutination, and complement fixation) to destroy the bacteria. In contrast, during bacterial infection, CD8$^+$ T cells, which recognize antigen only if associated with MHC class I, are infrequently induced and of limited value. Conversely, viral (intracellular) infections are susceptible to both antibodies and CD8$^+$ T cells, both of which are induced, and play important roles in recovery from infection. The explanation advanced earlier focuses on the induction phase of the immune response. However, the situation is not quite as straightforward as it at first appears. T-cell responses can be efficiently induced only by APCs, and the induction of virus-specific responses therefore requires that virus proteins be presented by the MHC class I pathway in this cell population. It has been argued that most viruses cannot infect specialized APCs, although in fact many types of virus can do so; for example, dendritic cells can be infected by retroviruses including HIV (179); RNA viruses such as measles virus (96), LCMV (20), and influenza virus (13); and DNA viruses such as pox viruses [e.g., ectromelia (232)] and African swine fever virus (65). However, many viruses do have quite tightly restricted tissue tropisms, and it appears unlikely that all viruses can infect APCs; how, then, can CD8$^+$ T cells be induced? Here we encounter the phenomenon of "cross priming," in which exogenous proteins can be taken up by APCs and introduced into the MHC class I pathway. Several studies have clearly demonstrated that cross-priming can occur in specialized cells (201), and it has been suggested that cross-priming, far from being unusual, may be the major mode of induction of virus-specific CD8$^+$ T cells (29). Extending this cross-priming idea, it has been suggested that endogenous synthesis is important only in the recognition phase of the immune response, rather than in the induction phase (216). By this argument, antiviral CD8$^+$ T cells can be induced by exogenous protein taken up by specialized APCs (i.e., by cross priming). However, the vast majority of infected cells are not specialized APCs, and therefore cannot be "cross primed"; therefore, if the CD8$^+$ cells are to exert their effector functions, these cells must be able to present the internal antigens, and they do so via the pathway of endogenous synthesis. A recent study using transgenic mice provides strong support for the hypothesis (222), although it remains open to interpretation. Many questions remain about the true biological relevance of cross priming. For example, bacteria shed abundant protein into the extracellular milieu and are phagocytosed by APCs; if cross priming is so efficient, why do we not see brisk CD8$^+$ T-cell induction during bacterial infections?

Certain aspects of the CD8$^+$ CTL response appear particularly well suited to combat viral infections. First, the MHC allows the cell to present a fragment from a viral protein made at a very early stage of infection. Thus a cell can signal its infected status before the virus has had a chance to replicate, and lysis of the cell by CTLs is beneficial to the host, as potential virus factories are eliminated. In contrast to the ability of CTLs to recognize early transcribed (usually nonstructural) antigens, antibodies usually recognize viral cell-surface proteins, often made late in the viral life cycle during virus maturation. Second, CD8$^+$ T cells are more likely to be of direct antiviral benefit than are their CD4$^+$ counterparts because almost all cells [excepting neurons (88)] express class I molecules. Conversely, most cells are class II negative, and virus in these cells would be "invisible" to CD4$^+$ T cells. These evolutionary lessons have implications for the design of antiviral vaccines.

Non-classical Antigen-Presentation Pathways

The two classical pathways described earlier allow the host to present short peptides for the perusal of the cellular immune system. However, evolution often provides variety, and growing evidence points to the existence of alternative antigen-presentation pathways which expand the epitope universe against which the host can respond. For example, as described later, the MHC class I genes can be subdivided into two groups, class Ia genes (encoding the classical class I proteins discussed earlier) and class Ib genes which encode proteins similar to, but structurally distinct from, class Ia. Somewhat surprisingly, deletion of the class Ia genes does not completely eradicate the ability of the host to mount CD8$^+$ T-cell responses (261), and class Ia knock-out mice cope well with certain microbial challenges (213), in part because some of the class Ib proteins appear able to present modified peptide antigens to $CD8^+$ T cells (178). In mice, the class Ib MHC molecule H-2M3 is able to bind and present a peptide from the bacterium *Listeria monocytogenes* (178). It has been suggested that this molecule may present *N*-formylated peptides, characteristic of prokaryotes (110), but viral proteins too may be presented by class Ib MHC molecules (141). No equivalent of H-2M3 has yet been identified in humans. The class Ia and Ib genes are described in more detail later.

For many years, antigen presentation at the cell surface has been seen as the sole purview of the MHC locus. However, a fascinating new family of antigen-presentation molecules, not encoded in the MHC locus, has been identified. This CD1 family comprises proteins which are structurally related to classes I and II but, rather remarkably, present non-peptide antigens to T cells. CD1 glycoproteins are—like MHC class I—expressed on the cell membrane in association with β_2M but, like MHC class II, they find their way into acidic endosomal compartments where they encounter their non-peptide antigens (190). The antigens include lipids and glycolipids, which bind in the CD1 groove and are specifically recognized by $CD8^+$ T cells. CD1 proteins can present microbial antigens or self antigens. In the former case, glycolipids (from, for example, mycobacteria) are presented by CD1 to $CD8^+$ T cells bearing an apparently "normal" TcR, which confers dual specificity for the lipid antigen and the CD1 gene product (63). Certain CD1 proteins present a self molecule, glycosylceramide, which is recognized by the TcR of NK T (NKT) cells, an unusual class of mononuclear cell which expresses the NK1.1 surface marker (characteristic of NK cells) along with a TcR of very limited polymorphism (99,137). Mouse model studies show that NKT cells may be important in tumor rejection (35), and similar cells have been identified in humans (155).

SOME HOST GENES INVOLVED IN THE IMMUNE RESPONSE

Current immunological mechanisms have evolved in response to the variety of pathogenic challenges imposed on their predecessors; implicit in this assumption is the existence of primordial genes from which present-day genes have evolved. Molecular analyses of the host genes described in the following section show that many of these genes are evolutionarily related, containing domains of similar protein folding. This has led to the inclusion of many of the genes in an Ig superfamily. The primitive gene(s) from which this superfamily has descended remains unidentified but presumably resided in a less complex organism, perhaps subserving an intercellular recognition function.

This Ig superfamily contains several families of proteins involved in the generation of an effective immune response. These include the class I and class II glycoproteins of the MHC; the CD1 glycoproteins, which present lipid antigens; the TcR proteins, present in the membranes of T cells and responsible for the antigen-specific recognition of peptide in the context of the earlier mentioned MHC and CD1 glycoproteins; proteins present in the TcR complex and necessary for T-cell function but which are not antigen specific; and of course, the Ig molecules themselves, the mediators of specific humoral immunity. Other genes, not members of the Ig superfamily but important to the immune response, also are discussed later. These genes encode the TAP transporter proteins, which lie in the MHC and are responsible for shuttling peptides from the cytoplasm into the ER, and proteins involved in antigen processing and cleavage.

The MHC Locus

The MHC loci of mice and humans, although not identical, bear strong similarities both in the overall organization of genes within the complexes and in the structure and sequences of individual genes. The murine MHC locus (on chromosome 17) comprises two regions (H-2 and Tla), whereas the human MHC locus (four megabases on chromosome 6, encoding >200 genes) is termed human leukocyte antigen (HLA). The loci have not been fully sequenced, and the cloning of the complete mouse MHC on a yeast artificial chromosome (4) doubtless will allow many interesting secrets to be unveiled. The genes within the MHC locus are divided into three classes on the basis of structure and function. The first two MHC classes, I and II, were introduced earlier and are described in more detail later. Although structurally unrelated to the class I and class II MHC genes, some of the additional genes within the MHC complex encode immunological functions (e.g., complement proteins, tumor necrosis factor, transporter proteins) and are loosely termed "class III" genes. The linkage of the class III genes to the class I/II families may be incidental or may reflect evolutionarily selected cosegregation.

MHC Class I Genes

Many texts refer to the MHC class I genes as a homogeneous group, but in fact, the group supports at least one further subdivision, into classes a and b. Class Ia proteins, by far the most studied class I molecules (and those referred to whenever the generic term class I is used) are the transplantation antigens, which led to the discovery of the MHC. These are the proteins that control MHC restriction, a phenomenon central to the specificity of cellular immune responses not only to transplanted tissues but also to virus-infected cells and tumor cells. Class Ib proteins are structurally similar to the class Ia molecules, and their functions are now being revealed. The numbers of both class Ia and class Ib genes vary between different individuals.

Three class Ia loci have been defined; K, D, and L in mice and A, B, and C in humans. The precise number of genes at each locus varies (e.g., some mouse strains lack an L gene locus; some strains have four D genes, whereas others have a single D gene), which is consistent with the occurrence of gene duplication/deletion events. Sequence homology occurs among these genes both within and between species, suggesting evolution from a common ancestor. The interspecies sequence similarities extend to the functional level because a human HLA gene expressed in a transgenic mouse appears to function similarly to the endogenous murine proteins. All share a genomic layout of eight exons that undergo splicing to generate a mature messenger RNA encoding the class I molecule, a glycoprotein of 350 amino acids. This molecule has five domains: three extracellular (α1, α2, and α3), one transmembrane, and one cytoplasmic. The class I molecules are expressed on the cell membrane in association with β_2M, a 12-kd protein encoded outside the MHC. The crystallographic structure of the MHC class I molecule has been solved. The α3 domain and the β_2M molecule, both of which are evolutionarily related to the constant region of Ig, are in intimate contact with the cell membrane, whereas the α1 and α2 domains interact at the top of the molecule to form the groove that presents the short peptides, most often nonameric, to $CD8^+$ T cells. Class I molecules are found in the membrane of almost all nucleated cells, which are therefore presumably able to present antigen. Neurons, an exception to this rule, transcribe β_2m but fail to transcribe the MHC heavy chain (88).

The peptides presented by class I MHC can originate from almost any protein synthesized within the cell, including self, tumor, and microbial proteins. It has been estimated that a single cell can display from 1,000 to 10,000 different peptides at any one time (84) and that $CD8^+$ T cell induction most often requires a threshold presentation of at least 100 MHC/peptide complexes per cell (31), although one report suggests that T cells can be activated by a single MHC/peptide complex (238). Essentially all viral proteins (including nucleoproteins, polymerases, and glycoproteins) can provide sequences to be presented to the cellular immune system. This provides a marked advantage to the host by allowing the entire coding region of the virus genome to be exposed to immune surveillance. Furthermore, the system allows presentation of virus antigens expressed early in infection. These often are non-membrane proteins, "invisible" to antibodies, and the MHC system thus provides a selective advantage to the host by permitting detection and removal of infected cells before virion particles have been produced. Analyses of MHC structure/function relationships provide a molecular explanation for the variability of T-cell responses in different mouse strains and in different individuals in a random-bred (e.g., human) population. The MHC class I proteins are highly polymorphic (i.e., there are many functionally distinct alleles at each locus). Sequencing studies of many different alleles show that the variable residues cluster around sites close to the antigen-presenting groove. Thus the functional polymorphism is caused by alterations affecting the nature of antigen binding and presentation by individual MHC molecules; different MHC molecules will bind and present peptides of different sequence. Hence, one variable in the immune response is the ability of the host class I molecule to bind microbial sequences and present them to the T-cell repertoire. If a host, when challenged with a particular virus, lacks the class I sequences necessary to bind and present viral peptides, then that host will be unable to mount class I–restricted CTL responses, and therefore will probably be more susceptible to disease caused by the agent in question. In contrast, a host whose genotype encodes MHC molecules capable of binding and presenting a peptide from this particular virus is more likely to be able to mount a CTL response that will limit viral replication, dissemination, and virus-induced disease. Given the risk of failure to present, one might ask why we have not retained more than the six or so MHC class I alleles in each diploid host cell; if an individual could instead express, for example, 20 class I alleles, the risk of being unable to present epitopes from any microbe would be greatly reduced. The reason is straightforward. Some 98% of lymphocytes entering the thymus fail to develop into mature T cells, and a major cause of this attrition is negative selection, in which T cells with excessive affinity for self molecules (i.e., for MHC molecules associated with self peptides) are deleted. Thus the more MHC alleles we carry, the more self peptides we can present; and as more self peptides are presented, so we clonally delete more T cells in the thymus. With our present complement of MHC alleles (about six per person), we already delete some 98% of all of our T-cell specificities; increasing our MHC representation would most probably reduce our T-cell repertoire below effective levels. We are, therefore, in a state of equilibrium: our T-cell repertoire is balanced against our ability to present antigen for the perusal of T cells. We must present just the correct number of antigens; too many (too many MHC alleles) would decimate our population of mature T cells, whereas too few (too few MHC alleles) would increase the risk that we would be unable to present antigen to our T cells.

Early attempts to predict viral (or other) sequences that might bind class I MHC molecules were not consistent and thus were unsuccessful, probably because they attempted to predict the viral epitopes without taking into consideration the specific polymorphism (i.e., allelism) of the MHC molecules. However, two factors allowed more consistently correct predictive motifs to emerge for specific MHC alleles. First, the increasing database of

CTL epitopes for the individual MHC alleles allowed comparison of the peptide sequences they presented, and allele-specific consensus sequences could be deduced. Second, work by the Rammensee and Nathenson groups showed that peptides can be eluted from MHC molecules and their sequences inferred or directly determined (84, 207,208,251). By a combination of these two approaches, specific motifs have been identified for several murine and human MHC class I alleles. Most, but not all, peptide epitopes are nonameric, with two highly conserved anchor residues critical for binding of the peptide to the MHC molecule. The MHC class I/peptide complex has been studied at high resolution, allowing the detailed analysis of the interaction between MHC class I molecular grooves and the peptides found therein (18,19,51,132, 277). The MHC groove contains several binding pockets, the most critical of which is that which binds the C-terminal residue of the peptide. The MHC residues that form this binding pocket have been identified, and their nature allows fairly confident prediction of which C-terminal residues will be favorable for a particular MHC pocket. Because the polymorphism of the amino acids forming this MHC pocket is fairly restricted, so too are the C-terminal amino acids of the binding peptides. Thus the great majority of peptides have as their C-terminal residue one of seven amino acids (I, L, V, R, K, Y, or F). Another pocket, located in the middle of the groove, appears important in determining allele-specific binding (i.e., in conferring fine specificity for specific peptide sequences) (132).

The "non-classical" class Ib MHC molecules are less well studied, but their functions are being slowly uncovered. In humans, four genes were identified and named HLA-E, -F, -G, and -H. In mice, three class Ib gene clusters, named Q, T, and M, have been found, but remain incompletely characterized. HLA-H is now known to be the gene related to 90% of cases of hereditary hemochromatosis (HH), and the HLA-H designation has therefore been replaced by HLE, the original name given to the gene conferring HH susceptibility; the protein is topologically similar to class I MHC, but its groove is too narrow to bind peptide. Thus it appears that this class Ib gene subserves no immunological function. The tissue distribution of HLA-E is similar to that of the class Ia proteins—that is, almost ubiquitous. Intriguingly, expression of this protein on the cell surface is greatly enhanced when its groove is loaded with a nonameric peptide derived from the leader sequence of class Ia molecules, ensuring that its surface expression is coordinately regulated with that of the classical molecules. In contrast to the groove of class Ia proteins, the HLA-E groove is relatively non-polymorphic, consistent with its role in binding a nonameric sequence which varies only slightly among the different class I leader sequences. HLA-E has been implicated in regulation of NK-cell activity (23), and it is possible that the very limited polymorphism allows it to interact with subtly different receptors on the NK cells (NK receptors are discussed later in this chapter). HLA-G has been implicated in antigen presentation, but it differs from other class I molecules in its distribution, being found mainly at the maternal/fetal interface; it has been implicated in protecting the fetus from rejection (113,116). The function of HLA-F remains obscure.

MHC Class II Genes

The existence in the mouse MHC of genes that regulate the humoral responses to antigen was clearly demonstrated more than 30 years ago. They were initially termed immune response (Ir) genes, subsequently termed Ia genes (easily confused with class Ia), and both terms have now been replaced by the term class II MHC glycoproteins. The class II locus of humans is termed HLA-D; and in mice, H-2I. Like their class I counterparts, the overall structure and function of class II genes appear similar in both humans and mice. Mature class II molecules are membrane-bound heterodimers resulting from the association of two MHC-encoded class II proteins, an α chain and a β chain (Fig. 3). Six α and seven β genes have been identified in the HLA-D region, divided into

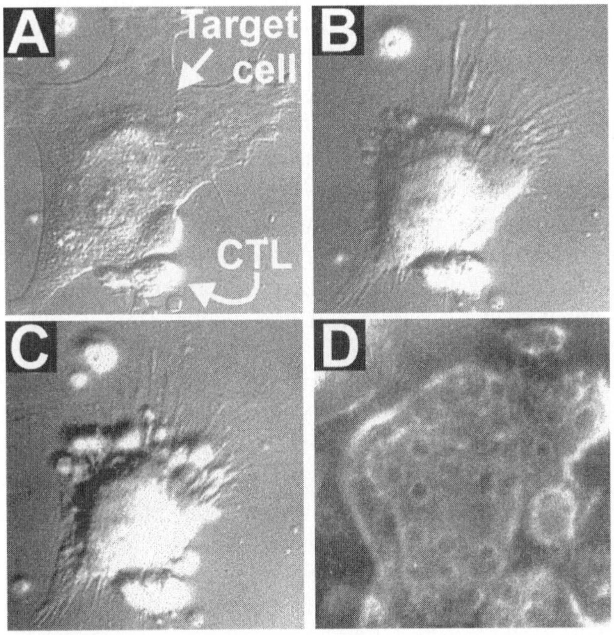

FIG. 3. Cytotoxic T lymphocytes (CTLs) kill target cells and insert perforin pores into the target cell membrane. Video-capture photographs (**A–C**) and an electron micrograph (**D**) are shown. **A:** A CTL encounters a target cell expressing an appropriate peptide/class I major histocompatibility complex (MHC), and within minutes the target cell begins to contract (**B**), and to show extensive blebbing of the cytoplasmic membrane (**C**). The CTL releases perforin, which self-assembles within the target cell cytoplasmic membrane, generating pores (visible in **D**), which permit entry of effector molecules, and also cause the cell to become hypoosmolar.

three clusters termed DR, DQ, and DP. Murine equivalents are present in the H-2 I region: two α and five β genes divided into two clusters termed A and E. The genes encoding the α and β chains are similar, although some variation between exon numbers is seen, even within a chain type. The resultant α or β proteins have two extracellular domains, a transmembrane region and a cytoplasmic domain. The top (membrane-distal) domain is named α1 (β1), whereas the lower one, adjacent to the membrane, is termed α2 (β2). The membrane-proximal paired α2 and β2 domains share significant homology with the class I α3/β_2M pairing, indicating once again common ancestry and possible functional relatedness. Indeed, there are many similarities in the overall topology of the two cell-surface MHC classes. Both classes have four extracellular domains; both the membrane-proximal domains are similar to Ig constant region, and the two distal domains interact to provide a groove for antigen presentation. The location of disulfide bridges is similar. The crystallographic structure of the class II molecule has been solved and appears similar to that of the class I heterodimer (25). Peptides bound by class II molecules are derived from a different processing pathway (see earlier) and are longer, usually between 15 and 20 amino acids. Unlike the class I peptides, in which the C-terminal residue is firmly anchored, class II–bound peptides protrude at both ends of the groove. Some motifs have begun to emerge for peptide binding to specific class II dimers, but this work lags behind the class I studies (210).

The polymorphism of class II molecules varies from gene to gene; for example, DQ α1 is highly polymorphic, DQ α2 much less so. However, the low polymorphism at certain loci is offset by the ability of class II genes to reassort. Thus in theory, the haploid genome encoding six α and seven β genes might make 42 different class II molecules, although in practice, reassortment is not entirely unrestricted. Reassortment cannot, of course, operate for the class I molecules because the heterodimer includes one monomorphic molecule (β_2M). The tissue distribution of class II molecules is markedly more restricted than that of class I. They are most abundant on B and T lymphocytes and cells of the macrophage/monocyte lineage. The class II/peptide complex is recognized by T cells bearing the CD4 surface marker; these cells are most frequently helper T cells rather than cytotoxic T cells.

CD1 Genes

The CD1 family encodes five proteins in humans (CD1a–CD1e), and the human CD1d gene has two homologs in mice (mCD1d1 and mCD1d2) (184). The intron/exon organization of these genes is similar to the MHC class I genes, and crystallographic analyses of the mouse CD1d1 protein revealed a strong similarity to the classical MHC structures, although the binding groove is deeper, presumably to accommodate the non-peptide (usually lipid/glycolipid) antigen described earlier (282). The tissue distribution of the CD1 proteins is severely restricted; like MHC class II genes, most CD1 proteins are expressed in professional APCs including B lymphocytes, macrophages, and dendritic cells.

TcR Genes

TcR genes belong to the Ig superfamily. Antigen specificity of T lymphocytes is bestowed by a heterodimeric surface-bound glycoprotein, the TcR. Four distinct genomic regions encode different TcR chains, which have been named α, β, γ, and δ. The great majority of circulating T cells, regardless of their helper/cytotoxic phenotype or MHC restrictions, bear αβ receptors; γδ receptor–bearing T cells have been identified quite recently, are far less well characterized, and are not discussed further in this chapter. The TcR genes are, like the Ig genes, products of somatic rearrangements that appose noncontiguous germline gene segments. The mature gene usually results from joining of V, D, J, and C regions; each chain type draws from its own pool of germline segments. The germline copy number of each of these regions varies among the chains but appears sufficient, when both combinatorial rearrangement and other V-region diversification mechanisms are invoked, to provide a TcR repertoire at least as large as that of antibodies. The mature TcR chains are glycoproteins of 260 to 300 residues in length, comprising a short cytoplasmic tail, a transmembrane region, and two extracellular domains, one constant and one variable. The antigen-recognition site, which recognizes the complex of antigenic peptide and MHC, thus consists of the Vα and Vβ regions. The crystallographic structures of several TcR/MHC class I/peptide complexes have been solved, and show that the TcR lies diagonally across the MHC/peptide complex; there is a degree of plasticity in the interaction, in which the TcR can to some extent conform to the peptide/MHC with which it interacts (55,56). In overall structure, the TcR molecule is similar to the distal (Fab) portion of an antibody molecule. However, the TcR differs from antibodies in several aspects. First, the effector function of an antibody is imposed on it by the constant region used in its generation, and there are multiple nonallelic constant-region genes to which the antibody-variable regions can be linked. In contrast, the copy number of TcR constant-region genes is very low, and the same C regions are represented in both CTLs and T helper (Th) cells. Thus the TcR C region does not dictate the T cell's effector function. The same Vα and Vβ gene pools are used in both class I and class II restricted T cells, indicating that the TcR does not fundamentally distinguish between the two classes of MHC molecule. Rather, the TcR recognizes the antigen/MHC complex, and other T-cell components determine the MHC class specificity (CD4/class II and CD8/class I) and the effector function (helper/cytotoxic) of the cell.

How restricted at the molecular level are T-cell responses to virus infection? This has been studied at the level of *in vitro* specificity of T-cell lines and clones, but much more rigorous analysis can be achieved by studying the TcR sequences of individual clones. This allows us to ask if responses to immunological stimuli are monoclonal or polyclonal, which is interesting not only at an academic level, but also at a practical one. If responses are monoclonal (i.e., if all TcRs are identical), then it may be possible to ablate specifically cells bearing that TcR, thus potentially diminishing immunopathological effects related to the antiviral immune response. In contrast, if such responses are polyclonal, such intervention is likely to be difficult and unrewarding. The VDJ gene use in TcRs of cells responding to a variety of stimuli have been determined. In general, response to certain model antigens, such as cytochrome c, have shown quite restricted VDJ uses, but responses to virus infection have shown much broader use (79,279). Thus it appears unlikely that TcR-specific ablation will be a valuable therapeutic approach in control of virus-induced pathology. The catholic use of Vα and Vβ chains during acute infection extends also to the memory response. Certain T cells in an acute response will act as progenitors of the memory T-cell pool (175), and the selection process appears to be stochastic (228).

T-Cell Accessory Molecules

At the T-cell surface, both αβ and γδ receptors are intimately associated with several other proteins, collectively referred to as the CD3 complex. The CD3 complex comprises at least four transmembrane proteins that relay a signal across the T-cell membrane when the TcR is appropriately stimulated. Also on the T-cell surface, although not stably linked to the CD3/TcR complex, are the CD4 and CD8 molecules, which play critical roles in T-cell function. These nonpolymorphic glycoproteins, again members of the Ig superfamily, are differentially expressed during ontogeny, but mature circulating T cells generally express only one of the two molecules. There is a very strong correlation between the CD4/CD8 characteristic of a T cell and the MHC class that presents the antigen to that T cell. Thus almost all $CD4^+$ T cells are class II MHC restricted, whereas $CD8^+$ cells are class I restricted. There also is a correlation, although less absolute than the earlier one, between the T cell's CD4/CD8 characteristic and its effector function; most $CD4^+$ (class II–restricted) T cells are of the helper phenotype, whereas most $CD8^+$ (class I–restricted) T cells are of the cytotoxic phenotype. The CD4/CD8 molecules recognize specific regions of the MHC glycoproteins and may play a role in activating the transmembrane signal relayed by the CD3 complex (57). However, the outcome of signal transduction (help or cytotoxicity) is independent of the nature of the CD4/CD8 molecule or TcR; thus there are examples of $CD4^+$, MHC class II–restricted cytotoxic T cells. Interestingly, in animal model systems, these cells appear to modulate the outcome of virus infection, despite their presumed inability to recognize the great majority of infected cells (which will be class II negative) (39,80,146).

Immunoglobulin Genes

The humoral response to virus infection plays an important role not only in promoting clearance of primary infection but also in preventing the establishment of widespread infection on secondary exposure to the agent. All antibodies have a similar overall monomeric structure, comprising two disulfide-linked identical heavy (H) chains, each of which is flanked by a light (L) chain. The centrally located H chains usually have four domains: three constant and one N-terminal variable. The L chains contain one constant domain and one variable domain. The variable regions of each L+H pair combine to form a single antigen-binding site: an antibody monomer is thus divalent in terms of antigen recognition. The L proteins are segmentally encoded in the germline, as variable (V), joining (J), and constant (C) regions, and are linked by somatic recombination. The H proteins are similarly arrayed, although they also have diversity (D) regions. Variability at the antigen-binding site is brought about by a variety of mechanisms during somatic recombination (as for TcR). The rearranged VDJ region is then apposed to one of the constant regions; the nature of the constant region determines the class (and therefore the function) of antibody that results. There are five general classes of antibody, differing in function, time of appearance, and distribution in the body. Structurally, the classes differ in the constant region of their H chains. The classes are IgM (H chain is Cμ), IgG (Cγ), IgD (Cδ), IgE (Cε), and IgA (Cα). First exposure to a virus induces a rapid IgM response, which is usually independent of Th cells, and a slightly delayed IgG response, usually Th dependent and thus requiring antigen to be presented via MHC class II molecules.

In contrast, secondary exposure results in a similar IgM response but a much more rapid and massive IgG response. In many instances, the precise specificity of the secondary IgG antibodies is identical to that of the initial IgM molecules: that is, the antigen-binding sites have been retained, but the remainder of the molecule (which determines its effector functions) has been altered. This "class switching" occurs when, for example, an H chain VDJ region is moved from the Cμ gene to the Cγ region; the new H chain has the same V region but a different C region. Two of these chains, in association with two unchanged L chains, generate an antibody identical to the original in specificity but different in effector function; it is now an IgG rather than an IgM. Initially, all B cells express membrane-bound IgM, but on exposure to specific antigen, they develop into plasma cells, usually undergoing class switching. The five classes of antibody subserve distinct effector functions, but only three are thought to play a role in opposing virus infection. IgM molecules form pentameric masses, each with 10 antigen-binding sites. These molecules are effective mediators of virus aggregation; they also activate both macrophages and the complement system. IgG, the main serum antibody, is monomeric, activates macrophages and complement, and can cross the placental barrier. IgA can exist as monomer, dimer, or trimer; it is transmitted to luminal surfaces (in saliva, tears, and intestinal and other secretions) to provide an initial defense against infection. IgE may play a role in immunity to parasite infection, but its major recognized task is the initiation of many allergic reactions, acting through histamine release from mast cells. The IgE-mediated release of histamine and other factors probably contributes to some of the respiratory manifestations of virus infection. The function of IgD remains obscure.

Genes Involved in Antigen Degradation in the MHC Class I and Class II Pathways

Many (but not all) of the peptides that eventually encounter MHC class I are generated by the proteasome, a multiprotein cytoplasmic organelle, the constitution of which is regulated by interferon γ (IFN-γ); this cytokine induces expression of three proteins, LMP (low-molecular-weight polypeptide)-2, LMP-7, and MECL-1 (multicatalytic endopeptidase complex-like), which replace three constitutive catalytic components of the "normal" proteasome, generating the "immunoproteasome" (52). Whereas MECL-1 is encoded outwith the MHC, both LMP-2 and LMP-7 are encoded next to the TAP genes, and should be considered MHC class III genes. Although several genes related to class I antigen presentation are MHC encoded, this is not true for some important genes related to the class II pathway; in both man and mouse, several genes encoding cathepsins [proteases vital to antigen degradation in the class II pathway (252)] are scattered throughout the genome (38,217).

Genes Involved in Peptide Transport and in Assembly of the Peptide/MHC Complex

Two TAP transporter genes are encoded in the MHC, called TAP-1 and -2; one copy of each combines to form a functional heterodimeric transporter. The role of these proteins in antigen presentation has been clearly demonstrated (247). Cell lines defective in transport are unable to present endogenously synthesized antigen in a normal fashion, but when the defective TAP is restored, antigen presentation proceeds (8,189). *In vivo* studies confirm these observations: TAP knock-out mice exhibit the expected phenotypes, having little or no cell-surface MHC and no mature $CD8^+$ T cells (253). There is some selectivity in the peptides transported by these molecules, as demonstrated in the rat; the class I modifier (cim) locus contains (at least) two genes (named mtp-1 and mtp-2), the latter of which has (at least) two alleles that result in presentation of different peptides by identical MHC molecules. The cim locus encodes a transporter, and the two alleles permit the passage of different peptides, thus providing the MHC class I molecules in the ER with different peptide populations from which to select (124,125,187,188). Direct evidence has been obtained showing that different transporter proteins display preferences for specific peptide sequences (153); one cim allelic product could transport peptides terminating in H, K, or R, whereas the other could not (70). Allelism has been identified in humans by sequencing the human TAP equivalents (186). Thus although the major contributor to epitope selection probably remains the class I molecule, the transporter proteins may play some role in limiting the range of peptides to which the class I molecules are exposed. However, this role is likely to be minor, for several reasons. First, many cell lines have been transfected with non-homologous MHC alleles, but these MHC molecules continue to present the same CTL epitopes as they did in their own background, suggesting that there is no major difference in the peptide pools generated in the differing backgrounds. Second, transporter heterodimers in which one component is murine and the other human appear to function the same as either of the natural heterodimers (280). Within the ER, several proteins are important to assembly of the class I/peptide complex (48). Four are quite well characterized: tapasin, which ensures association between the TAP transporter complex and the empty MHC-β_2M heterodimer, is encoded close to the MHC locus (75), whereas the genes encoding three chaperones (BiP, calnexin, and calreticulin) are not MHC linked.

CELL-MEDIATED EFFECTOR MECHANISMS

We have outlined our current understanding of immune responsiveness at the molecular level. In the following section, we discuss immune responsiveness at the organismal level, describing the biological roles of several different cell types and the effector mechanisms through which they act.

Virus-Specific $CD8^+$ T Cells

These cells have been extensively characterized in the mouse, and the results equate well with those obtained with human cells. First, the vast majority of these cells are restricted by class I MHC proteins, although a few have been identified that are restricted by class II or by CD1. The importance of these cells in the control and eradication of virus has been documented for several experimental infections. In the mouse, they are critical in combating infection with LCMV (272). In this case (105, 106) and in murine cytomegalovirus (MCMV) infection (92), it is possible to fully protect a naive animal from virus challenge by immunization with a recombinant vaccinia virus (VV) expressing a single viral internal (i.e., nonmembrane) protein; the protection is mediated solely by CD8$^+$ T cells. Recombinant vaccines containing minigenes encoding isolated CTL epitopes as short as 11 residues can confer protection against normally lethal doses of challenge virus, and different epitopes can be linked on a "string of beads" to protect on several MHC backgrounds (5,6). No LCMV-specific antibody responses are induced by these vaccines, proving that protective effects can be mediated by cellular immune responses. In humans, it is clear that CTL responses can be generated against similar proteins. For example, the major CTL response to human cytomegalovirus (HCMV) is to a protein expressed immediately upon infection; a similar situation exists for varicella-zoster virus (VZV) and herpes simplex virus (HSV). Epstein–Barr virus (EBV) infects and transforms human B lymphocytes, and the control of this cell population appears to be managed in large part by class I MHC–restricted CTLs. Indeed some immunosuppressed individuals may develop EBV$^+$ lymphomata (198). Influenza virus infection induces CTLs directed against most viral components, but the major group is specific for the virus nucleoprotein. These CTLs, unlike anti-influenza antibodies, are cross-reactive; that is, they lyse HLA-matched target cells infected with a serologically distinct strain of influenza virus. However, their presence fails to confer absolute immunity to infection and disease caused by a serotypically distinct influenza virus. These results are sometimes used to challenge the hypothesis that the presence of virus-specific CD8$^+$ cells confers protection against virus-induced disease. It is important to understand that CD8$^+$ T cells cannot prevent infection; on the contrary, recognition by these cells requires that the target cell be infected. Only antibodies can prevent infection, whereas CD8$^+$ T cells limit virus production and dissemination; together they protect against disease. Thus the preexisting antiinfluenza CTLs, although failing to prevent infection, may diminish the ensuing morbidity (disease) and mortality (death). CTLs also have been found against measles virus, mumps, respiratory syncytial virus (RSV), and other agents. In patients with AIDS-related complex and AIDS, CTLs are detectable against gag, pol, and env proteins. CTLs to env correlate with clearance of initial viral load, and their absence heralds a return to high viral titers and AIDS. Antigen-specific recognition mediated by the TcR initiates a series of events including signal transduction across the cell membrane, which activates the CD8$^+$ T cell's effector functions. Several mechanisms have been proposed to explain the *in vivo* antiviral effects of virus-specific CD8$^+$ T cells.

CTLs Usually Release Perforin, a Pore-Forming Protein

CTLs contain granules, which align with the target cell upon recognition, and whose contents are released in a calcium-dependent manner onto the target cell membrane. These granules include a protein called perforin (183), which undergoes assembly into trans-membrane pores and thus punches holes in the cytoplasmic membrane of the target cell. Perforin shares immunological cross-reactivity with the C9 component of complement, and cloning of the murine perforin gene has allowed identification of a short stretch of amino acid homology between the two proteins. The membrane lesions caused by perforin are similar to those induced by the complement C9 complex. Thus CTLs and complement-mediated lysis seem to share one common mechanism of action. The importance of perforin in CTL activity *in vivo* has been demonstrated. Transgenic mice with a dysfunctional perforin gene are much less effective in controlling infection by some (though not all) viruses (94,95,262).

CD8$^+$ T Cells Can Induce Apoptosis in Target Cells

Apoptosis, or programmed cell death, is a well-recognized phenomenon responsible for several developmental processes, including the clonal deletion of T cells in the thymus. Its most characteristic features are nuclear blebbing and disintegration, resulting in a nucleosome stepladder of fragmented DNA. CD8$^+$ (and sometimes CD4$^+$) T cells can induce apoptosis when the fasL protein, expressed on the T-cell membrane (237), interacts with Fas protein on the target cell, initiating a signaling cascade which ends in target cell apoptosis. Virus-specific T cells may induce this process in infected target cells (220,269,287). A graphic representation of CTL–target cell interactions is provided in Fig. 3. In panel A, the CTL (small cell, bottom of panel) has just encountered a larger target cell expressing the appropriate peptide/MHC class I complex. Within minutes, the target cell contracts (B), and extensive membrane blebbing occurs (C). An electron micrograph shows the target cell membrane studded with pores, after CTL contact and perforin release (Fig. 3D).

CD8$^+$ T Cells Release Antiviral Cytokines

Many CD8$^+$ T cells are capable of releasing high levels of cytokines, for example, interferon-γ (IFN-γ) and tumor necrosis factor-α (TNF-α). Mice lacking the IFN-γ receptor have increased susceptibility to several infections, despite apparently normal CTL and Th responses

(83). It has been cogently argued that a major role of the TcR/MHC/peptide interaction is simply to hold CD8$^+$ T cells in the immediate proximity of virus-infected cells, thus focusing cytokines on the infected cell (193,209), and convincing data from mice persistently infected with LCMV (168,242), from hepatitis B virus (HBV) transgenic mice (66,67), and from HBV-infected primates (68) has shown that viral materials can be eradicated *in vivo* from neurons (168,242) and hepatocytes (66,67) in the absence of cytolysis. We have recently shown that, even at the peak of the immune response, the great majority of virus-specific CD8$^+$ T cells are not producing cytokines; however, these virus-specific cells are exquisitely sensitive to antigen contact, initiating cytokine synthesis immediately upon encountering an infected cell, and terminating production the instant the contact is broken (225). This tight regulation is important because cytokines can be toxic to the host, and indeed, systemic cytokine release is responsible for many of the symptoms of microbial infection, and for the extensive weight loss seen in certain cancers.

Natural Killer Cells

Although our understanding of NK cells is in its infancy compared with that of T cells, significant advances have been made in the last 2 years (195). NK cells play an important role in the control of certain virus infections, as established by clinical studies in humans and experimental manipulations of mice. NK cell development normally occurs extrathymically; these cells are not antigen specific and therefore do not exhibit immunological memory. NK cells carry several non–antigen-specific receptors, through which they can be activated by a variety of mechanisms (112), and they kill susceptible target cells by perforin-mediated lysis. In addition to receptors through which they are activated, NK cells carry inhibitory receptors whose engagement with a specific molecule on a non-susceptible target cell *prevents* the NK cell's effector function. What might this inhibitory ligand be? Early work showed that NK cells had somewhat varied specificities (270) and could very effectively lyse target cells lacking MHC class I (265). Incubation of target cells with IFN-γ increased their sensitivity to CTL, but diminished their sensitivity to NK cells (268). In 1990, the "missing self" hypothesis was proposed, which argued that NK cells are inhibited by the presence of self MHC class I, and that the absence of such molecules permits target cell lysis by NK cells (126). This is an intrinsically attractive idea, for the following reason. As stated earlier, MHC class I is vital to the control of most virus infections (and also for eradication of many tumors), and one might imagine that viruses (or tumors) that could down-regulate MHC expression would be at a selective advantage. However, such down-regulation, while protecting the cells from CD8$^+$ T cells, would make the cells more sensitive to NK-mediated lysis. Thus NK cells and antigen-specific CD8$^+$ cells together span the MHC expression spectrum.

Early studies of NK receptors and ligands were somewhat confusing, showing that only certain class I MHC molecules could inhibit recognition by certain NK cells (i.e., there was some form of MHC restriction, albeit different from that involved in T-cell recognition). These studies have been borne out, and greatly extended, by the identification of three families of inhibitory receptor proteins on NK cells, and of the target molecules with which they interact. The three NK inhibitory receptor families are (a) the CD94-NKG2 family (common to humans and rodents), (b) the Ly49 family (only in rodents), and (c) the KIR family (killer inhibitory receptor, only in humans) (112).

The first two families are members of the C-lectin superfamily and lie in an "NK complex" on mouse chromosome 6 or human chromosome 12. Despite being in the same superfamily, these two families are quite distinct. The CD94-NKG2 proteins are expressed on the NK cell surface as heterodimers of the monomorphic CD94 molecule (encoded by a single gene in the NK complex) along with one of the products of the four NKG2 genes.

In contrast, the mouse Ly49 locus contains at least nine genes, and the protein products are expressed on the cell surface as homodimers. As yet there is no evidence to suggest that different Ly49 alleles can interact to form a heterodimer, but the polymorphism of the Ly49 homodimers is increased by alternative splicing.

The KIR family is a member of the Ig superfamily, and probably includes about 12 genes; mouse equivalents have not been found. The target cell ligands with which these receptors interact are varied.

1. CD94-NKG2 receptors in humans interact mainly with the MHC class Ib molecule HLA-E (23) which, as described earlier, carries in its groove a peptide from the leader sequence of classical class I MHC proteins. Because the leader peptides vary slightly, it is possible that each different peptide/HLA-E combination is recognized by only one of the four NKG2 gene products (in association with CD94). In the majority of cases, these interactions inhibit NK cell activity (although, to complicate matters, there are reports that certain interactions can stimulate NK effector functions).
2. At least some of the Ly49 proteins interact with sites on the $\alpha 1$ or $\alpha 2$ domains of classical MHC class I molecules in mice. For example, Ly49A recognizes H-$2D^d$ and H-$2D^k$, whereas Ly49C may recognize several ligands on the H-2b and H-2d backgrounds (24). The importance of MHC-bound peptide in these interactions is somewhat unclear.
3. Most of the KIR proteins interact with the $\alpha 1$ domain of the classical HLA class I molecules HLA-A, -B or -C, and some reports suggest that the MHC-bound peptide may alter NK recognition. Recent data (191) sug-

gest that one of the KIR proteins is the NK receptor that interacts with HLA-G, which, as stated earlier, is expressed extensively at the fetal/maternal interface.

Thus the target cell ligands for all three NK receptors families appear to be MHC class I molecules of one sort or another, consistent with the missing self hypothesis. However, individual NK cells express on average five of the possible receptors (250), and different NK cells in an individual can express different receptor subsets. The regulation of NK receptor expression is poorly understood, and several conflicting hypotheses exist, comparison of which is beyond the scope of this chapter. Perhaps the most popular idea is the "at least one" hypothesis, which dictates that NK cells will (perhaps randomly) express one receptor, then a second, and so on, until at least one receptor has been expressed which can interact with a self MHC molecule, thus ensuring that the NK cell will not attack the host. In this model, the expression of an NK receptor able to interact with self MHC will then prevent the subsequent expression of still more NK receptor types. Consistent with this, NK cells in MHC-deficient mice expressed a wider variety of NK receptors.

Definitive studies on the role of NK cells in viral infections have been performed in the mouse model. Depletion of NK cells *in vivo* by administration of anti-NK cell antibodies leads to enhanced synthesis of some viruses, such as MCMV and VV, but not of other viruses, such as LCMV (266). NK cell–mediated resistance to MCMV is particularly profound. An age-dependent resistance to MCMV occurs in mice at about the third week of age, and coincides with the maturing NK cell response. Furthermore, adoptive transfers of NK cells into suckling mice protect them from severe MCMV infection. Lymphokine-activated killer (LAK) cells, which are NK cells highly activated by growth in culture in the presence of interleukin-2 (IL-2) and which have been used in a variety of clinical and animal model tumor therapy protocols, protect suckling mice against MCMV. The presence of prolonged NK cell activity during persistent infections may select for NK cell–resistant viruses; establishment of a persistent infection in severe combined immunodeficient (SCID) mice with an NK cell–sensitive variant of Pichinde virus resulted in the conversion of the virus into an NK cell–resistant genotype(s). The related arenavirus, LCMV, normally causes a persistent infection in mice in nature and is also NK cell resistant.

In general, NK cell activity peaks earlier than that of T cells (2–3 days) and diminishes rapidly thereafter. Clinical correlations have been observed between decreased NK cell activity as a consequence of disease or drug therapy and susceptibility to infections with HCMV and HSV-1. Examples of individuals with complete NK cell defects are rare, perhaps attesting to the importance of NK cells, but one adolescent with a complete and selective deficiency in NK cells presented with unusually severe infections with VZV, HCMV, and HSV-1 (17). Although the VZV and HCMV infections were life threatening, each infection resolved completely, probably because T-cell and B-cell immunity was normal in this individual.

We have now reviewed the most relevant aspects of cellular immunity, including T cells and NK cells. At this point, it is appropriate to present a tabular summary of the antigen-presenting molecules, the elements presented, the responding cells, and the nature of the responding cells' receptor (Table 2).

Antibody-Dependent Cell-Mediated Cytotoxicity

Antibody-dependent cell-mediated cytotoxicity (ADCC) may be mediated either by T lymphocytes or by NK cells. In the latter case, the antibody, usually IgG, is specific for a structure on the target-cell membrane. The antibody "coats" the target cell, and the NK cell then attaches by its Fc receptors, triggering release of perforin, and target cell death. ADCC can be brought about in a different way if the target cell bears Fc receptor. Incubation of uninfected cells with antibody to either the CD3 complex or the TcR idiotype itself causes a cytotoxic

TABLE 2. *Summary of antigen-presenting molecules, the materials presented, the cells that recognize them, and the cells' receptors*

Presenting Molecule	Antigen Presented	To (Cell Type)	Responding Cell's Receptor
MHC class Ia	Peptide	$CD8^+$ T cells	Normal TcR
	Glycopeptide	$CD8^+$ T cells	Normal TcR
	Peptide (?)	NK cells	Ly49 and KIR families
MHC class Ib			
H2M3	Formylated peptide	$CD8^+$ T cells	Normal TcR
HLA-E	Peptide from class Ia leader	NK cells	CD94/NKG2
HLA-F	Unknown		
HLA-G	? Fetal/maternal peptides	? NK cells	? Specific KIR
HLA-H	No immune function		
MHC class II	Peptides	$CD4^+$ T cells	Normal TcR
CD1	Microbial lipid & glycolipid	$CD8^+$ T cells	Normal TcR
	Glycosylceramide (self)	NK T cells	TcR of limited polymorphism

lymphocyte to attach to the target cell and lyse it. Note that in both cases, the specificity is conferred on the reaction by antibody; in one instance, the antibody is target cell specific, whereas in the other, it is effector cell specific. Although ADCC can commonly be identified *in vitro,* its contribution *in vivo* is still not known.

Macrophages

Mononuclear phagocytes (blood monocytes, tissue macrophages) are principal cellular players in the clearance and inactivation of most microbial pathogens. Interestingly, these same cells also represent a major target cell and infectious reservoir for many viruses that persist [e.g., measles, lentiviruses, and cytomegaloviruses (45, 93,227), and see relevant chapters in these volumes]. There are at least four complications of infection of these cells. First, infectious virus can be transported by these cells to distant parts of the body where infection can continue.

Second, activated monocytes/macrophages are APCs, taking up, processing, and delivering viral antigens to T cells in regional lymph nodes (62,211). *In vitro* studies indicate that activated macrophages are 10- to 100-fold less efficient in antigen presentation compared with the major professional APC, the dendritic cell (see later), but are 10 to 100 times more efficient than antigen-presenting B cells. During certain virus infections, their ability to present antigens, or to initiate immune responses, can be compromised.

Third, viruses can interfere with the macrophage's capacity to degrade other microbial agents. For example, the microbe *Histoplasma capsulatum* normally replicates in quiescent macrophages, and is degraded upon macrophage activation. Activation depends, in part, on IFN-γ. In a model system, persistent infection of macrophages by lymphocytic choriomeningitis virus clone 13 prevented IFN-γ activation of macrophages; as a result, the mice succumbed to a normally sublethal dose of *Histoplasma* (257). This may be one reason that a number of virus infections are associated with secondary infections by microbes that are usually phagocytosed and inactivated by macrophages.

Fourth, the infection of macrophages or microglia (brain cells of macrophage lineage) can lead to pathology. For example, HIV primarily infects microglia in the central nervous system (CNS) (275) and indirectly, presumably by release of cytokines and perhaps other toxic molecules, leads to neuronal dysfunction mirrored clinically as AIDS dementia (123). Macrophages also can restrict virus infection or replication by acting as nonspecific effector cells for ADCC. The outcome of a macrophage–virus interaction is determined by a complex series of reactions that may dramatically affect the ability of macrophages to act as scavenger cell, immune effector cell, or susceptible target cell for virus replication. Mononuclear phagocytes have a vigorous phagocytic ability enabling them to eliminate virus from the circulation after a blood-borne infection. Their scavenger function constitutes an early line of defense for reducing the virus load either initially or in concert with the specific immune response. Monocytes and macrophages also can initiate a series of immune reactions through the cytokine network (see later) that assists or injures the host. Macrophages may be activated for enhanced antiviral activity by cytokines produced by virus-specific T cells.

Dendritic Cells

Recent attention in virology and immunology has focused on the dendritic cell. These are bone marrow–derived cells that are located in blood and lymph as well as in most tissues. They include Langerhans cells in the skin and mucous membranes, dermal dendritic cells, tissue-resident dendritic cells, and interdigitating dendritic cells in the thymic medulla, splenic white pulp, and lymph nodes (9,62,107). Activated dendritic cells express high levels of MHC molecules (classes I and II) together with accessory (co-stimulatory) molecules (e.g., CD80, CD86, CDIA, CD83) and, by producing a variety of chemokines, attract naive T cells. Infection or inflammation leads to the maturation of immature dendritic cells. For example, after a respiratory virus infection, immature dendritic cells lining the respiratory mucosa are infected, become activated, and carry viral antigens to T cell–dependent areas. These cells now appear as interdigitating dendritic cells and efficiently stimulate naive T cells, producing antigen-specific responses. *In vitro* studies show that only a few dendritic cells are required to provoke strong T-cell responses; for example, one dendritic cell can stimulate 10^2 to 3×10^3 T cells in a mixed lymphocyte reaction. Recent *in vivo* evidence revealed that adoptive transfer of only 10^2 to 10^3 activated dendritic cells to an immunologically naive animal could generate $CD8^+$ CTL-mediated protective immunity. In this study, transferred dendritic cells expressing an LCMV CTL epitope transgene were able to induce $CD8^+$ CTLs that were protective as early as 2 days after immunization, and lasted for at least 60 days (128).

Because dendritic cells play a primary role in the initiation of antigen presentation leading to immunity, a number of viruses can be expected to have evolved mechanisms to exploit these cells. The two best examples are HIV and LCMV. In the case of HIV, two conflicting events occur. First, it is likely that dendritic cells in the mucosal membrane are infected initially by HIV and migrate to lymphoid organs where effective presentation of HIV antigens triggers both $CD8^+$ and $CD4^+$ T-cell responses for the host's benefit. However, concurrently the dendritic cell has transported live HIV into lymph nodes, where it is believed to contribute to the spread of virus to $CD4^+$ T cells (107). LCMV has a different strategy. LCMV Armstrong clone 13 causes immunosuppression in adult mice (20) by preferentially replicating in the interdigitating dendritic cells in the T cell–dependent (white pulp) area. This leads to an early host antiviral $CD8^+$ T-cell response, which then destroys these infected professional APCs (an example of immunopathology). The result is generalized host immunosuppression. Evidence is accumulating that other viruses also can infect dendritic cells and alter their function, with resulting immunosuppression. Currently these reports are restricted primarily to *in vitro* studies, and *in vivo* confirmation is needed (for example, in measles virus/dendritic cell interactions) (104). However, owing to the olympian properties and role played by dendritic cells in acquired immunity, it is reasonable to predict that more examples of virus manipulation of dendritic cells will emerge. Furthermore, it seems likely that dendritic cells (or viruses that home to them) will prove useful for immunization.

CYTOKINES

Cytokines (for the purpose of this chapter, lymphokines and monokines) are proteins made by cells of the immune system, usually during cell activation. As soluble factors, they assist in regulation of the immune response and in elimination of viruses and other pathogens. Their activities and structure are reviewed elsewhere in this volume. Immune responses to particular antigens or microbes are often distinguished by a relatively distinct pattern of cytokines production by $CD4^+$ Th cell subsets. This in turn drives the immune system toward a predominant cell-mediated or humoral immune response (144). The subsets have been described in humans and mice. Th1 cells secrete IL-2, IFN-γ, and lymphotoxin. They promote CTL-type and other delayed-type hypersensitivity reactions frequently required for clearance of intracellular organisms. Th2 cells produce IL-4, IL-5, IL-6, IL-10, and IL-13. They promote allergic-type responses and stimulate the differentiation of B lymphocytes, mast cells, and eosinophils. The role and balance of Th1 and Th2 cells and their cytokines in viral infections is believed to be important in pathogenesis and immunity. Viruses themselves can use cytokines, or cytokine homologs, to their own advantage. Certain viruses contain genes encoding cytokine homologs, the expression of which potentially enables the viruses to modify immune responses to their own advantage. Some examples are provided later in this chapter. In addition, cytokines released from T cells, especially IFN-γ, have been implicated in clearance of virus from infected cells in the absence of $CD8^+$ T cell–mediated lysis (30,67,168,242).

HUMORAL EFFECTOR MECHANISMS

Generation of B-Cell Responses and Antibody

The B-cell receptor for antigen is Ig, which is initially expressed as a membrane protein. The structure and genetics of Ig are well defined and were described earlier. During their development, B cells initially express IgM on their surface, followed by expression of different H chain classes IgG(γ), IgA(α), or IgD(δ). IgM and IgD may be expressed in all B cells, but once a cell has expressed an H chain class other than IgM, it remains committed to secrete that class of Ig. When a B cell encounters antigen, it usually differentiates into a mature plasma cell, secreting specific antibody as a single Ig class; memory B cells also are generated. This differentiation of B cells is controlled by specific B-cell growth and differentiation factors produced by T cells, analogous to the factors involved in the differentiation of T cells themselves. It has been suggested that B-cell responses to some viral antigens are more brisk than are those to isolated antigens because of the densely packed, paracrystalline nature of certain viral structures (284). Antibodies of all classes are usually generated in response to virus infection.

How Do the Various Antibody Classes Exert Their Antiviral Effects?

Antibodies neutralize viruses in a number of ways.

1. They may bind to the part of the virus that interacts with its cell-surface receptor, preventing virus attachment to the cell.
2. They may agglutinate many infectious particles into a single "clump," thus reducing the number of cells that will become infected.
3. They may bind to virus glycoproteins on the cell surface, lysing the infected cell in association with complement, or modulating the intracellular viral replication.
4. Viruses may activate complement, releasing chemotactic factors such as C5a or C3q.

Recent animal experiments studying the effects of antiviral monoclonal antibodies on a wide variety of DNA and RNA infections have led to a new and important conceptual distinction between *in vitro* neutralization and *in vivo* protection. First, monoclonal antibodies that do not neutralize *in vitro* may nevertheless afford protection on *in vivo* transfer. Second and conversely, antibodies that have high neutralizing activity *in vitro* may not provide protection when adoptively transferred *in vivo.* Nevertheless, *in vitro* studies have provided much information regarding the probable mechanisms underlying the antiviral efficacy of each antibody class, and there often is a correlation between *in vitro* and *in vivo* efficacy. Note that intact antibodies are not a prerequisite for antiviral effectiveness; Fab fragments specific for RSV F glycoprotein, when instilled into the lungs of infected mice, were therapeutically effective (34). Such approaches hold promise, particularly in light of recent advances in technologies that allow the rapid production of antibodies of any desired specificity (10,97).

Immunoglobulin A

During natural infection, most viruses gain entry via mucosal surfaces, so it is not surprising that mucosal immunity plays an important role in control of viral infections (158). Development of mucosal immunity and secretory IgA are important in preventing mucosally restricted viral respiratory and enteric infections, and virus-specific circulating antibody plays an important role in limiting viremia and thereby aborting spread of virus to systemic sites. For successful induction of a secretory IgA response in the gut, virus must come into contact with a Peyer's patch, the gut-associated lymphoid tissue. Once a local response has been generated, IgA-producing memory B cells recirculate to other areas in the gut. This has been demonstrated in humans by using oral polio vaccine. The protective effects of IgA are usually attributable to antibody directly preventing virus binding to the mucosa. The approaches and concepts are discussed in detail elsewhere in this volume.

Immunoglobulin G

There are several IgG subclasses in humans and mice. For example, human IgG falls into four subclasses (IgG1, IgG2, IgG3, and IgG4), which normally constitute 70%, 20%, 8%, and 2% of the total IgG, respectively. However, IgG subclass–specific antiviral antibodies are generated in different amounts in acute or persistent infections. For example, IgG1 is the dominant IgG isotype found in HIV-infected individuals during the quiescent stage of disease, but it declines in those with progressive illness, perhaps because of a decrease in $CD4^+$ T-helper cells. IgG1 is the major complement-binding and opsonizing antibody in humans (231), and in patients recovering from acute hepatitis B virus infection, IgG1 and IgG3 dominate, with a switch from IgG3 to IgG4 (a non–complement-binding antibody) during chronic infection. IgG1 in humans corresponds to mouse IgG2a (major complement-binding and opsonizing antibody). In experimental mouse infection with LCMV, IgG2a antibody is the predominant isotype raised in acute infection with subsequent viral clearance (>90% of IgG isotype). However, during persistent LCMV infection, there is a switch to more than 90% of IgG1, a non–complement-binding antibody (243). This switch may be related to activation of different Th subsets and the cytokines they produce: in the mouse, IgG2a is associated with the Th1 subset (IFN-γ, IL-2, and lymphotoxin production), whereas IgG1 is associated with the Th2 subset and low levels of IFN-γ. Complexing of viruses with IgG antibody also will facilitate their phagocytosis by mononuclear cells and polymorphonuclear leukocytes via Fc receptors on these phagocytic cells. However, this latter process may actually enhance the infectivity of some viruses (185). Sindbis virus infection of mice provides an interesting animal model demonstrating the antiviral effect of IgG. Sindbis virus, an alphavirus, can establish persistent infection of mouse neurons. Because neurons express little or no class I MHC (88,89), the virus is effectively hidden from $CD8^+$ T cells, but infusion of antiviral antibodies, or even of antiviral Fab'_2 fragments, clears virus infection almost entirely (118). The mechanism is unclear, but may involve modulation of viral replication, as demonstrated for measles virus in tissue culture (171).

Immunoglobulin M

This pentameric, decavalent molecule is produced early after virus infection, is usually independent of T-cell help, and acts as the initial antibody-mediated antiviral response. Later in infection, and on secondary exposure, most IgM-producing cells switch classes to IgG but retain antigen specificity. There is good *in vitro* evidence that IgM is effective in neutralizing the infectivity of virus in the fluid phase. This may result from the antibody preventing virus attachment to specific cellular receptors and from the aggregation of virus particles, thereby reducing the number of infectious particles.

Immunoglobulin E

IgE antibody is present at low concentration in serum; its principal biological activity appears to be mediated by binding to mast cells via specific receptors. When antigen reacts with the cell-bound IgE, inflammatory mediators are released from the mast cell. This IgE-dependent mechanism accounts for several of the clinical features of allergy, including wheezing with respiratory infections and pharmacologic relief with antihistamines. There has been little study of the antiviral IgE response or of the molecular mechanism(s) underlying its role in clinical disease.

Role of Complement

The human complement system comprises more than 20 plasma proteins, and most aspects of their interaction are now well understood (27,145). The classical pathway of complement is activated by the C1 macromolecule binding to IgG or IgM complexed to antigen. Attachment occurs via the Fc portion of Ig interacting with the C1q subunit of C1. C1r and C1s, two highly specific serine proteases, become activated in this process. C1s sequentially cleaves C4 and C2 with resultant assembly of C4b2a, the C3-cleaving enzyme or convertase of the classical pathway. C4b binds covalently to the target, whereas C2a carries the catalytic domain. The activity of C4b2a is restrained by the lability of C2b and to a lesser extent by specific regulatory proteins that inactivate C4b (these are the C4-binding protein and factor I). The more recently discovered mannan binding or lectin pathway of complement activation is similar to the classical pathway, except that it is triggered by the interaction of mannan- or lectin-binding proteins with sugars on microorganisms. A distinct plasma protease, analogous to C1s, is used to cleave C4 and C2.

The major difference involved in the initiation of the alternative, or amplification, pathway of complement activation is that it does not depend on antibody. The internal thioester linkage of C3 undergoes slow spontaneous hydrolysis in plasma, producing a C3b-like molecule. Although most of these C3b-like molecules are rapidly inactivated by factor H and factor I, some may bind directly to a target, and a proportion interact with factors B and D to form a C3-cleaving enzyme. The C3b generated by this transient fluid phase C3 convertase can then bind to surfaces. Most so-called "activators" of the alternative pathway, such as microbes and foreign surfaces, lack the membrane regulatory proteins expressed by host tissue. Therefore deposition of C3b on their membranes can trigger the alternative pathway. One property shared by activators of the alternative pathway, which are mostly particulate, is that when C3b is deposited on their surface from the fluid phase, it is relatively protected from inactivation by factors H and I. This protected C3b covalently attached to a target can then bind factor B, which is cleaved by factor D (a 25-kd serine protease in plasma) to give C3bBb, the C3-cleaving enzyme of the alternative pathway. This convertase has its catalytic site on the Bb fragment and decays rapidly, but the half-life of the enzyme is prolonged by properdin, which binds to the enzyme complex and retards this decay. An important point about the alternative pathway is that C3b, however generated (whether by the classical pathway, spontaneous hydrolysis, or cleavage of C3 by other proteolytic enzymes), serves to initiate the amplification of C3 cleavage. Thus the presence of an activator surface, lacking membrane regulators, unleashes a powerful biological positive-feedback loop. This emphasizes the importance of the regulatory proteins in the fluid phase and on cell surfaces, without which trivial amounts of C3b would result in unrestrained activation of the pathway, even in the absence of an activator surface. After cleavage of C3, additional C3b molecules may be incorporated into either C3bBb or C4b2a, giving C3bnBb or C4b2a3b; these complexes have C5-cleaving activity and are called C5 convertases. After C5 cleavage, sequential nonenzymatic binding of C5b to C6, C7, C8, and five to 10 C9 molecules results in assembly of the C5b-9 terminal complex. This membrane attack unit inserts into the lipid bilayer of cell membranes, where it can lead to osmotic lysis. By electron microscopy, the familiar lesion is visualized as a doughnut-shaped pore, and is similar to the lesion caused by CTL and NK cells when they release perforin, a protein with homology to C9.

In addition to the proteins of the classical and alternative pathways and the C5b-9 membrane attack complex, the complement system also includes cell-surface molecules that specifically bind activated or cleaved complement molecules in a receptor-mediated manner. These include receptors for C3b (CR1, CD35), iC3b (CR3, Mac-1, CD11b/CD18), and C3dg (CR2, CD21). The complement system is regulated by a number of plasma proteins (factors H and I, C1 inhibitor, C4-binding protein, S protein) and cell-membrane proteins [CD46 or membrane cofactor protein (MCP), CD55 or decay accelerating factor (DAF), and CD59, the membrane inhibitor of the membrane attack complex]. These regulatory molecules restrict inappropriate complement activation by sequestering activation fragments and/or facilitating their inactivation. The regulatory molecules do not block appropriate complement activation. They do, however, prevent chronic activation and restrict inappropriate activation (e.g., in plasma or on autologous tissue).

The major function of the complement system is to modify foreign membranes by opsonization or, less commonly, by lysis. Its second function is to promote the inflammatory response. Low-molecular-weight cleavage fragments (e.g., the C3a and C5a anaphylatoxins) induce chemokinesis and chemotaxis, mast cell degranulation, and other types of cell activation.

Complement is involved in innate as well as adaptive immunity. Complement enhances the neutralization of viruses by antibody. This is achieved by at least four different mechanisms. First, complement can blanket the sensitized (antibody-coated) virion, thus rendering it incapable of binding to its receptor. Second, complement can aggregate or clump sensitized virions, thereby reducing the number of infectious units. Third, by incorporating C3b into virus/antibody complexes, such sensitized virions can bind to C3b receptors on phagocytic cells, leading to their ingestion and degradation by these cells. Fourth, antibody and complement can directly lyse viruses possessing a lipid envelope. Complement likely plays an important role early during infection when small amounts of low-avidity antibody are made. [For a comprehensive review of the area, the reader should consult reference (78)]. Complement alone can inactivate certain viruses directly in the absence of antibody. Retroviruses from several species are lysed by human complement, in association with an anti-α-galactosyl natural antibody (206,267). This occurs because a viral protein alone (rather than an Ab/Ag complex) can act as a receptor for C1q. The alternative pathway of complement can be activated on the surface of a variety of microorganisms, including bacteria and yeasts. Thus an additional principal function of the complement pathway is as a nonspecific mechanism of host defense, capable of opsonizing or lysing a variety of microorganisms before the generation of specific immune responses. Hence it is not surprising that some viruses, notably the pox and herpes families, contain genes that interfere with selected complement molecules (36,127,226). Finally, at least three of the complement proteins are used as receptors by viruses. These include the C3d receptor (CR2 or CD21) used by EBV (47,90,154), the CD46 protein or MCP used by measles virus (41,131,151), and DAF, which appears to be used (probably as a co-receptor) by coxsackieviruses (15,215) and echoviruses (14). It is not known whether using complement proteins as a receptor confers any selective advantage to the virus. Possibilities include cell signaling via the complement protein, or protecting itself from complement attack.

Lysis of Virus-Infected Cells by Antibody and Complement

Antibody and complement can kill virus-infected cells *in vitro.* A variety of human cell lines (epithelioid, neural, and lymphoid) infected with a wide variety of human DNA and RNA viruses and expressing viral antigens on their surfaces are lysed by human serum when it contains both specific antibody to the virus and functional complement. Here, lysis appears primarily dependent on an intact alternative pathway of complement (33,223). A detailed analysis of this system using measles virus–infected cells as a model showed that the infected cell activates the alternative pathway in the absence of antibody, but that antibody is needed for lysis to occur. Despite the activation of the alternative pathway being independent of antibody, IgG enhances C3 deposition and thus facilitates lysis. The involvement of multiple cell types and viruses in similar events indicates the generality of the phenomenon. Although it is difficult to quantitate this mechanism *in vivo,* it is likely that cellular injury can be produced by antibody and complement *in vivo.*

Idiotypes and the Network Theory

The antigen-combining site of each Ig molecule itself represents a novel antigenic determinant known as an idiotype. Idiotypes can be recognized by other antibodies, and these latter "anti-idiotypic" antibodies often represent an "internal image" of the antigen to which the original antibody (bearing the idiotype) was directed. The "network theory," formulated by Jerne (86), and for which he received the Nobel prize, stated this concept and extended it to view the whole immune system as a network of interacting idiotypes and anti-idiotypes. Simply put, all antibodies are anti-idiotypes, which also react with specific external antigens. When external antigen enters the system and produces expansion of specific clones of cells being particular idiotypes, the system is perturbed, and expansion of anti-idiotypic, anti–anti-idiotypic antibodies, and so on ensues. These were postulated to play a regulatory role in modulating the immune response. The same principles would apply to TcRs, which also bear idiotypes. These ideas have stimulated much current research. Anti-idiotypic antibodies have been demonstrated in some human autoimmune diseases and infections.

Does the network theory have any specific relevance for virus infections? Apart from their regulatory role in the immune response, anti-idiotypic antibodies that have the "image" of antigen may compete with that antigen for specific cellular receptors. For example, anti-idiotypic antibodies raised against antibody to reovirus glycoprotein can prevent the adsorption of the reovirus to its specific receptor on the cell surface, presumably because the anti-idiotype can itself bind to the receptor. In addition, anti-idiotype antibodies (which look like the original antigen) have been used as vaccines, because they induce anti–anti-idiotype antibodies, which can cross-react with the microbe, thus avoiding inoculation with the microorganism.

VIRUS STRATEGIES TO EVADE THE HOST IMMUNE RESPONSE

Viruses are relatively unstable outside a competent host, and for a virus to remain in circulation, it must be able to move efficiently among different hosts and/or to persist in an individual host. The virus' ability to evade host immunity is critical to the virus' survival both in the population and in the individual. For example, if there is widespread immunity in a population, a virus able to evade that pre-existing immunity will have an increased pool of susceptible targets. In the individual host, evasion of immunity is necessary to permit virus persistence, and immune evasion also may allow the virus to replicate to higher titers in the host, perhaps increasing its chance of transmission to a susceptible recipient.

Virus-induced immunosuppression is often directed against that component of the immune response which is most important in limiting the virus infection. For example, influenza viruses are highly sensitive to neutralizing antibodies, and this virus provides one of the best examples of antibody evasion; HSVs are controlled in large part by T cells, and HSV can inhibit antigen presentation by MHC class I; and NK cells combat primary cytomegalovirus infections, and this virus encodes an MHC homolog which may inhibit NK activity. These observations underline our contention that the intimate relationships between viruses and host immunity has been central to the evolution of both protagonists.

As with our overview of the immune response (Fig. 1), the array of viral evasion mechanisms could be categorized in a number of ways. We have chosen to classify the viral strategies as either "avoidance" (in which the virus "hides" from host immunity but does not actively interrupt it) or "inhibition" (in which the virus actively disrupts host immunity). This classification (the various underlying mechanisms of which are summarized in Table 3 and are discussed later) may have some clinical

TABLE 3. *Overview of how viruses can evade the host immune response*

Evasion Technique	Mechanism
Avoidance: Virus hides from the immune system but does not actively disturb host immune responses	Infection of immune privileged sites Down-regulation of viral gene expression Virus protein structure limits its immunogenicity Mutation or reassortment of genetic material
Inhibition: Virus inhibits either the induction or the effector phase of the immune response	Infection of thymus, leading to deletion of high-affinity T cells (negative selection), inducing partial tolerance Destruction of specialized APCs Inhibition of antigen presentation Expression of proteins that inhibit effector-cell function Expression of proteins that delay target-cell death Infection of T or B lymphocytes

significance, because the active inhibition of immunity may have serious consequences for the host.

Evasion by Avoiding the Immune Response

Infection of Immune-Privileged Sites

Certain regions of the body appear to be immune privileged, that is, not subject to the same rigorous immune surveillance as most somatic sites. Examples include the anterior chamber of the eye, perhaps because immune infiltration would be catastrophic to vision. Of all somatic cell types, perhaps we can least afford the wholesale destruction of neurons, which not only subserve critical functions, but also have very limited regenerative capacity. The CNS is protected by the blood–brain barrier, and has long been considered relatively immune privileged, but it is clear that it is accessible to activated T cells and cellular immunity and, if injured, to the passage of antibodies. Perhaps in part to ensure that neurons are less susceptible to immune-mediated destruction, they are one of the few somatic cell types that do not express class I MHC (88,89). Viruses have been quick to take advantage of this, and many viruses can infect neuronal cells (for example, polioviruses, coxsackieviruses, mengoviruses, LCMV, measles, alphaviruses). Several virus families have further exploited the loophole by using neurons as their site of persistent infection or latency. The best-characterized example, albeit still incompletely understood, is the herpesvirus family, several members of which (HSV, VZV) establish latent infection in sensory nerve ganglia. The costs and benefits of low neuronal class I expression have been recently reviewed (192).

Down-Regulation of Viral Gene Expression

How might viruses hide within cells that express class I MHC? Viruses may selectively reduce the level of expression of cell-surface glycoproteins, sometimes down-regulating them manifold in comparison with other, non-surface, viral products (169). This may help evade antibody-mediated detection, but, as has been stressed throughout this chapter, the detection of intracellular viral proteins is the major remit of T cells, in concert with the MHC. Thus the major problem facing intracellular virus is the evasion of this aspect of the host's detection systems. T-cell recognition requires as few as 1 to 100 MHC/peptide complexes to be displayed on the target cell, and this can be achieved with low levels of protein expression; it may therefore be difficult for viruses to down-regulate expression to a level preventing MHC presentation. Some viruses, such as herpesviruses, may be able to shut down protein synthesis during latency in neurons, but this luxury is available to only a few virus families. The inability to terminate protein synthesis completely is, presumably, one of the selective pressures which has driven many viruses (including even HSV) to inhibit actively MHC class I antigen presentation, as discussed later.

Virus proteins may be refractory to immune recognition. Virus proteins have been honed by constant interactions with the immune system, and over the millennia, many immunogenic sequences doubtless have been hidden or lost; those sites still recognized may reasonably be considered the residue. The intrinsic structure of a virus protein can render the protein less digestible to some part of the MHC class I processing pathway; the Gly-Ala repeats of the EBV antigen EBNA-1 act in cis to render the protein relatively resistant to proteasomal degradation (119). Furthermore, post-translational modifications can play a role. Many potential antibody epitopes on viral glycoproteins are masked by the glycosylation event (although the virus pays the price of inducing carbohydrate-specific antibodies). Although some modified peptides [e.g., glycopeptides (230)] can be presented by class I MHC molecules, it is plausible to suggest that certain modifications might prevent the protein's presentation, even if they do not actively inhibit the cells' ability to process other antigens. Consistent with this, an HCMV matrix protein appears to selectively inhibit processing of

HCMV IE proteins, perhaps by phosphorylation of the IE products (59).

Mutation of Viral Gene Sequences

RNA viruses may be at a particular advantage, because the high mutation rate of RNA polymerases provides a rich diversity of virus mutants from which variants can be selected.

Evasion of Antibody Responses by Gene Mutation

This strategy is best exemplified by influenza virus, which contains a segmented RNA genome encased in a viral envelope studded with influenza proteins [hemagglutinin (HA) and neuraminidase (N)]. These proteins are critical for binding to, and entry into, target cells, and are obvious targets for the host antibody response; the host takes full advantage of the opportunity by producing neutralizing antibodies targeted to both proteins. The virus responds by generating mutant HA and N sequences, thus providing itself with the opportunity to evolve. This evolution is driven by two requirements: the mutant proteins must retain their function (i.e., the virus must be viable), but they should be able to escape detection by the preexisting antibodies. The resultant virus often has fairly subtle immunological changes, but these are sufficient to give it a temporary edge in the battle; it may have an expanded pool of susceptible hosts, because it should be able to infect individuals carrying the original set of antibodies. This phenomenon has been termed antigenic drift and plays a role in influenza epidemics, which occur sporadically. The process of antibody escape through mutation of viral target proteins is not restricted to influenza virus. Examples have been found in almost all viruses in which they have been sought, and indeed the need to escape antibodies doubtless has driven the diversification of many viruses into the different strains or serotypes that we recognize today. When we categorize viruses by the antibodies that do or do not recognize them, we are simply using the results of this ongoing evolutionary interplay.

Evasion of T-Cell Responses by Gene Mutation

In a manner analogous to evasion of antibody responses, viruses can mutate those sequences presented to the immune system as T-cell epitopes. The process of viral mutation toward CTL escape has been less widely studied than the antibody equivalent. Mice immunized with a minigene vaccine encoding a single LCMV CTL epitope, and later infected with LCMV, rapidly generate LCMV variants in which the vaccine epitope has been mutated (263), and CTL escape variants of LCMV replicate to higher levels in the host, although the viruses are eventually cleared (120). Studies using HIV have shown that viruses can mutate *in vivo,* in a natural infection, into CTL escape variants (181), and that this escape has important biological consequences (21). Finally, evidence of CTL escape variants comes from studies of a specific CTL epitope in EBV, presented by the HLA-A11 allele. This epitope is present in EBV strains circulating in a population in which the HLA-A11 allele is infrequent, but is mutated in virus circulating in an A11-rich population, and cannot bind to the A11 molecule (37).

Wholesale Replacement of Viral Proteins

In addition to gene mutation, which many viruses exploit, influenza virus escapes host immunity by using a second method, which is available only to virus families with a segmental genome structure. The influenza virus genome has eight RNA segments, and during co-infection of a single cell by two viruses (1 and 2), the segments from both infecting viruses can mix (reassort). The majority of RNA segments in the resulting virus may come from virus 1, but (for example) its HA-encoding segment may come from virus 2. In nature, such molecular reassortment appears to take place in non-human hosts, most probably porcine or avian, when there is co-infection of a human virus (which will infect pigs or birds only rarely) and an avian virus. The biological consequences of this event are difficult to predict, but if one of the resulting reassortants carries the avian HA but is able to infect humans, this virus may be immunologically unknown to, and highly pathogenic in, humans. It appears likely that such antigenic shift is the cause of severe influenza epidemics and pandemics.

Evasion by Active Inhibition of Immunity

Viruses have a developed a plethora of approaches to actively inhibit the development of host immunity, as outlined in Table 3.

Thymic Infection May Induce Tolerance

If viruses infect the thymus, the viral antigen presented by MHC in the thymic stroma may cause clonal deletion of virus-specific T cells (i.e., the virus is viewed as self). Thus no virus-specific cells will exit the thymus, and neither antibody nor T-cell responses will be induced by viral challenge; there is no generalized immune suppression, and the inhibition of immunity will be specific to the infecting virus. Congenital infection of mice with LCMV results in thymic infection, which begins in the fetus and is maintained for the life of the mouse. The mouse is persistently infected and cannot mount an LCMV-specific $CD8^+$ T-cell response. If the virus is eradicated (e.g., by adoptive transfer of LCMV-specific $CD8^+$ T cells), then the ability of the host to mount LCMV-specific responses is restored (103), because the transferred CTLs remove thymic cells expressing viral peptide/MHC complexes, and naive host T-cell precursors bearing TcR with specificity for the virus/MHC complex will no longer be deleted, and instead mature and exit the thymus. Recent studies indicate that, despite viral replication in the thymus, negative selection may be incomplete, with virus-specific T cells escaping to the peripheral lymphoid organs, and antiviral antibodies being generated. This occurs experimentally in LCMV infection and may similarly occur in HBV carriers. In both instances, antiviral antibodies are generated, and CTL can be induced by vaccination (162,170,180).

Destruction of Specialized Antigen-Presenting Cells

Many viruses can infect specialized APCs (dendritic cells, macrophages), the destruction of which may lead to generalized immunosuppression. Infection of, or absorption to, follicular dendritic cells by HIV-1 has been demonstrated and was proposed as the underlying cause of the late immune failure that characterizes AIDS (179,264). Certain variants of LCMV rapidly infect interdigitating dendritic cells, the major APCs, and the resulting antiviral CTL response destroys APCs and causes a transient global immunosuppression (20,283) affecting both antibodies (143) and T cells.

Inhibition of Antigen Presentation

Rather than destroying the infected professional APCs, viruses may instead inhibit antigen processing, thus providing themselves with a safe haven in which to produce progeny. This would apply not only to virus-infected specialized APCs (which express MHC classes I and II) but also to somatic cells, which can present antigen only via the class I pathway. Given that the vast majority of virus-infected cells are somatic cells, not specialized APCs, one might predict that viruses would have developed more tricks to inhibit MHC class I presentation than to disrupt the MHC class II pathway; this is the case, as recently reviewed (139). Herpesviruses are particularly skillful, blocking the class I pathway at almost every stage (87). The HSV IE protein ICP47 binds to the cytosolic surface of TAP and inhibits transport of peptides into the ER (77), whereas the HCMV US6 protein binds to the luminal aspect of TAP, to similar effect (3). The HCMV US3 gene product retains peptide/MHC complexes in the ER (91), and the US2 and US11 proteins cause rapid degradation of class I heavy chains by the proteasome (274). Finally, IFN-γ–mediated stimulation of MHC expression is inhibited by MCMV (71) and HCMV (138). Similar strategies are found in other viruses. Adenoviruses encode a 19-kd protein that binds to class I MHC and prevents its transport to the cell surface (111,229), rendering the adenovirus-infected cell relatively refractory to T-cell recognition. Although most examples of antigen presentation blockade involve class I MHC, some viruses do appear to inhibit MHC class II; for example, the EBV BZLF2 gene product binds to the HLA-DR molecule, inhibiting MHC class II antigen presentation (234) [and aiding entry of the virus into B cells (121)], as does the CMV-induced defect in IFN-γ signaling mentioned earlier.

Expression of Proteins That Inhibit Effector Cell Function

Many years ago, it was shown that the pathogenicity of vaccinia virus could be modulated by addition of a host cytokine gene such as IL-2 (194). It now transpires that several poxviruses needed no help from us; they encode their own cytokine homologs, which can modulate the immune response (32,233,235). In addition, EBV encodes a potent equivalent to IL-10 (82). Finally, the HCMV UL18 protein is an MHC class I homolog expressed on the cell surface in association with β_2M; some studies have suggested that this molecule can engage inhibitory NK receptors, protecting the cell from NK lysis (197), although this is controversial (117).

Expression of Proteins Which Delay Target Cell Death

Antiviral $CD8^+$ T cells [and sometimes antiviral $CD4^+$ T cells (281)] can eradicate infected cells by induction of apoptosis. It would benefit the virus to retain cellular integrity for as long as possible, and many viruses have developed means to delay the apoptotic process. The EBV BHRF1 gene product encodes a bcl-2 homolog which prevents cell death (74), as does the adenovirus E1B/19k protein (271). The p53 and Rb proteins, important cell-cycle regulators that can drive cells into apoptosis, can be bound by SV40 T antigen (129,239), with resulting survival and proliferation of the infected cell, and the product of the poxvirus molluscum contagiosum gene MC159 protects cells from Fas-mediated apoptosis (16). Finally, reactive oxygen metabolites (free radicals) can be harmful to both viruses and cells; molluscum contagiosum virus gene MC066L encodes a selenoprotein with antioxidant functions (218).

Infection of T or B Lymphocytes

The simplest and most direct means by which viruses can disrupt immune effector mechanisms is by infecting the immune cells. As shown in Table 4, many acute virus infections, and the vast majority of persistent virus infections, involve cells of the immune system. HIV-1 infects $CD4^+$ T cells, causing their destruction directly, or through immunopathological attack. EBV infects B lymphocytes, as does coxsackievirus B3, perhaps another example of a virus “attempting” to counter that aspect of host immunity which most threatens it (136). An interest-

TABLE 4. *Viruses that infect lymphocytes and monocytes*

Virus	Host	Infected Cells
Double-stranded DNA viruses		
Hepatitis B virus	Human, monkey	PBMCs, T and B lymphocytes
Woodchuck hepatitis virus	Woodchuck	PBMCs, bone marrow
Papovavirus	Human, monkey	PBMCs
Group C adenoviruses	Human	T, B, and null lymphocytes
Herpes simplex virus	Human	T lymphocytes
Epstein-Barr virus	Human	B lymphocytes
Cytomegalovirus	Human	Lymphocytes, monocytes
Pox virus	Rabbit	Spleen cells
Single-stranded DNA viruses		
Porcine parvovirus	Pig	Spleen cells
Minute virus of mice	Mouse	Lymphocytes
Postive-strand RNA viruses		
Poliovirus	Human	Lymphocytes, monocytes
Rubella	Human	T and B lymphocytes
Negative-strand RNA viruses		
Measles	Human, monkey	T and B lymphocytes, monocytes
Mumps	Human	T and B lymphocytes
Respiratory syncytial virus	Human	Lymphocytes, monocytes
Vesicular stomatitis virus	Human, mouse	T lymphocytes
Influenza A	Human	Lymphocytes, monocytes
Parainfluenza	Human	Lymphocytes, monocytes
Ambisense RNA viruses		
Lymphocytic choriomeningitis virus	Mouse	T and B lymphocytes, monocytes
Junin virus	Human	Peripheral blood mononuclear cells
Retroviruses		
Murine leukemia virus	Mouse	B lymphocytes
Feline leukemia virus	Cat	T and B lymphocytes, monocytes
HTLV-I, -II	Human	T, B, and null lymphocytes
HIV-I	Human	T and B lymphocytes, monocytes
SIV	Monkey	PBMCs, macrophages
Endogenous C-type virus	Mouse	Spleen cells
Bovine leukemia virus	Cow	PBMCs

ing mode of B-cell disruption is practiced by LCMV. The virus infects B cells which express surface IgM capable of binding to neutralizing epitopes on the viral glycoprotein, and these B cells present the viral epitopes on their class I MHC and are promptly killed by virus-specific CTLs; as a result, infected animals make very little neutralizing antibody (182). The specificity of this interaction is nicely shown by the fact that anti-NP antibody is produced in abundance, because B cells bearing NP-specific IgM are not selectively infected by the virus (because NP is not present on the surface of the infectious particle). LCMV also infects $CD4^+$ and $CD8^+$ T cells. During persistent infection, viral sequences and infectious virus (detected by infectious center assay) are found mainly in the $CD4^+$ population (2,22,244). Measles virus infects T cells, B lymphocytes, and APCs. Acute measles virus infection is a well-recognized cause of immunosuppression (indeed in the earlier part of this century, measles infection was used to treat certain immune-mediated diseases), and although the precise cause of the suppression remains unclear, the virus ability to infect T and B cells (and APCs) may be in some way involved.

IMMUNOPATHOLOGY OF VIRAL INFECTIONS: VIRUS-INDUCED IMMUNE COMPLEX DISEASE

One of the most common immunopathologic manifestations associated with viral infection (acute or persistent) is virus-induced immune complex formation. In many virus infections, antiviral antibody interacts with virus in the fluid phase, or with viral antigens on cells forming complexes that are shed into the fluid phase, resulting in the formation of virus/antibody (V-Ab) immune complexes. Such V-Ab complexes occur in most infections. Circulating complexes carry infectious virus, which can enter cells that express Fc or complement receptors (e.g., macrophages, activated lymphocytes). However, the production of circulating complexes does not inevitably lead to disease, as long as mesangial cells and macrophages can remove them sufficiently rapidly to prevent their deposition. When the infection is chronic, the continuous trapping of the complexes in renal glomeruli, arteries, and choroid plexus leads to arteritis, glomerulonephritis, and choroiditis. V-Ab immune complex disease is the common pathogenic mechanism of animal nephritides, vasculitis associated with HBV infection, and glomerulonephritis seen in several chronic human infections, all presenting an immunopathologic picture similar to that seen in chronic human nephritis of unknown cause.

However, even in the face of persistent immune complex formation, some individuals escape disease. Why is that? It is a matter of genetics. Genetic studies of different mouse strains that displayed high or low levels of immune complexes revealed that high levels of complexes was a dominant trait. Backcrossing of F_1 mice to their parents mapped the effect to a single gene in the MHC locus (174). Additional studies using recombinant inbred mice mapped the effect to the MHC class II locus (IA in mouse, equivalent HLA-DR in humans). Thus the immune-response gene(s) control the antiviral antibody response and, at a certain antibody–antigen ratio, immune complexes can result.

The presence of immune complex disease is best documented by identification of viral antigen, host Ig, and complement in a granular pattern along the basement membrane of glomeruli or capillaries, or in the intima or media of arteries. Identification and quantitation of specific antiviral antibodies are accomplished by elution of Ig by low-ionic, high-ionic, or low-pH buffers to disassociate the V-Ab complex, recovery, and quantitation of the eluted Ig and determining the specific antiviral activity of the total Ig eluted (usually >75% compared with <1% specific viral Ig in circulation). Such immune complex depositions are constant companions of persistent viral infection of humans and animals (160,161).

VIRUS-INDUCED AUTOIMMUNE DISEASE

Viruses have been implicated in autoimmunity by three findings. First, human autoimmune responses are made *de novo* in, or are enhanced during, infection by a wide variety of DNA and RNA viruses (164,165). Second, in experimental animal models, both acute and persistent virus infections can induce, accelerate, or enhance autoimmune disease in high-responder mice (246). Third, investigation of molecular mimicry (one potential mechanism whereby microbes may cause autoimmunity) indicates that a number of etiologic agents may cause autoimmune disease (163,166).

How can viruses induce autoimmune responses? Certain viruses [or their protein(s)] have a mitogenic effect on unique lymphocyte subsets and hence act as polyclonal activators. However, because agents such as mycoplasma also can activate lymphocytes and may contaminate viral stocks, stringent evidence must be presented that the activation is due to the virus, and not to mycoplasma contamination. Viruses also can infect lymphocytes and macrophages, causing release of cytokines and chemokines. These molecules can modulate immune responses in a variety of ways (e.g., as growth or differentiation factors, or by regulating MHC class I and/or class II expression on cells). Finally, microbial agents share determinants with host (self) proteins (molecular mimicry). In this instance, an immune response mounted by the host against a specific determinant of the infecting agent may cross-react with the shared host sequence, leading to autoimmunity and, in some cases, tissue injury and disease. Many viral proteins share epitopes with host proteins, as determined by computer sequence analysis, or by analysis of monoclonal antibodies raised against a large panel of DNA and RNA viruses in which nearly 4% of more than 800 tested showed cross-reaction with host determinants expressed on uninfected tissues (236). The evidence that mimicry could cause disease came from experiments in which inoculation of a viral peptide homologous to the encephalitogenic site of myelin basic protein was able to cause the autoimmune disease, allergic encephalomyelitis (53). These observations suggest that the human viral encephalopathies which occur after measles, mumps, vaccinia, or herpes zoster viral infection, in which recovery of a virus is unusual, may have a similar pathogenic mechanism. In these instances, autoimmunity would occur only when the microbial and host determinants are similar enough to cross-react, yet different enough to break immunological tolerance. The induction and breaking of tolerance at both the B- and T-cell levels have been established in heterologous serum protein models, and the same kinetics would likely govern the establishment and the break of tolerance to microbial agents cross-reacting with host proteins. Such cross-reactions could occur either through antibody- or cell-mediated immune responses. Another process implicated in the pathogenesis of autoimmune disease is "epitope spreading," initiated by an appropriate immune response to an infectious agent, but spreading to epitopes encoded on host proteins (140,254). For example, during the demyelination seen in Theiler's murine encephalomyelitis virus infection, the original virus-specific T-cell response extends to include T cells specific for self epitopes on myelin basic protein and proteolipid protein, and these autoreactive cells contribute to disease. It will be interesting to see if this process applies also to human autoimmune disease associated with virus infections.

VACCINE CONSIDERATIONS

At a time when new vaccines are being sought to counter new challenges (HIV, and even tumor vaccines) and because new methods of subunit vaccination are being suggested as replacements for older vaccines that have performed extremely well (e.g., live attenuated viruses), it is critical that we carefully determine the role of each aspect of the immune response in combating primary virus infection, and in preventing and/or limiting subsequent infection in an immune host. This can now be viewed in light of the foregoing discussion. Historically, two approaches have been taken to developing antiviral vaccines. First, live vaccines have been developed, usually by attenuating the pathogenic virus by tissue-culture passage in a variety of cell lines. Attenuation was then tested in animal models. When pathogenicity was sufficiently reduced, the attenuated virus was considered a candidate. Second, the pathogenic virus could be inactivated (e.g., by formalin treatment), and the killed vaccine tested for immunogenicity. A major difference is evident between these two groups: the antigens of live vaccines will be presented by both class I and class II MHCs, whereas those in killed vaccines will be presented mainly by the class II pathway. In Table 5 are listed the major vaccines in current use and their nature [live or dead (we have avoided the adjective "killed" because the hepatitis B vaccine is a recombinant protein, and thus killing of the hepatitis virus itself was not required for this vaccine)]. Included also are some of the immunological findings associated with each type of vaccine. Each vaccine has costs and benefits. Live vaccines give longer-lasting immune responses against most or all viral antigens (partly because the vaccine replicates to give a large antigenic dose), and they induce a balanced response that includes $CD8^+$ T-cell responses as well as $CD4^+$ T-cell and antibody responses. The induction of $CD8^+$ T cells may be in part responsible for the astonishing efficacy of the live vaccines listed earlier. Live vaccines carry the risk of vaccine-associated viral disease, caused by reversion to pathogenicity of the vaccine strain during its replication in the vaccinee. For example, several cases of adult polio occur annually in developed countries and are almost invariably vaccine associated; that is, the victims have been in recent close contact with vaccinees. Molecular analyses of the viruses shed in the feces of recently vaccinated infants demonstrated that the vaccine virus had rapidly reverted toward neurovirulence (28,44). In contrast, killed vaccines should carry no real risk of revertant-associated disease, although if inactivation is inadequate, as in an early batch of the Salk polio vaccine (152), then vaccinees may receive virulent virus. However, dead vaccines do not induce good $CD8^+$ T-cell responses; the immunity is short-lasting and often not detectable against all of the viral antigens (in part because inactivation may selectively modify or destroy the immunogenicity of the various virus proteins). Furthermore, there is a risk of disease potentiation. Vaccinees who are subsequently exposed to the wild virus may get much more severe disease than do unvaccinated individuals. This has been well documented for killed measles (54) and RSV vaccines (98), which were withdrawn in large part for this reason. Such disease potentiation has rarely been shown for live vaccines, although recent experience with high-dose measles vaccine in Africa has indicated that occasional unpredictable problems might arise, thus counseling caution in use of new vaccines and mandating the continual monitoring of vaccinee status. The "ideal" vaccine therefore would combine the best features of both, while omitting the problems. It should deliver antigen into both class I and class II pathways to induce a balanced, long-lasting, and cross-reactive immunity without significant vaccine-associated risks. Since the last version of this chapter was written, many articles have been published on DNA immunization, which combines some of the advantages of both live and dead vaccines; several reviews are available (40,69,241). To date the approach has shown itself to be wonderfully adaptable and moderately successful. However, enhancements are needed, as the immunity induced by a DNA vaccine alone is usually less than that induced by a conventional vaccine.

TABLE 5. *Summary of currently available antiviral vaccines*

	Live	Dead
	Polio (Sabin) Measles Mumps Rubella Yellow fever Vaccinia Varicella	Influenza Rabies Hepatitis B Polio (Salk)
Antibody induction	+++	+++
CD4 T cell	+++	+++
CD8 T cell	+++	–
All viral antigens?	Usually	Often not
Longevity of immunity	Mo/yr	Mo
Cross-reactivity among viral strains	+++	+
Disease potentiation	? High-dose measles	RSV, measles
Risk of viral disease	+	–

RSV, respiratory syncytial virus.

TRANSGENIC MODELS OF VIRUS–IMMUNE SYSTEM INTERACTIONS

The ability to generate transgenic mice and mice with targeted gene deletions introduced by homologous recombination (known as knock-out mice) has already provided, and will continue to provide, unique opportunities to understand both the biology of virus infections and the molecular basis of virus-immune interactions. For several important human viruses (e.g., poliovirus, measles virus, and hepatitis B virus), small animal models of disease did not exist because of restricted host tropism of the virus. Transgenic mouse lines were created that express the human cellular receptor for either poliovirus [poliovirus receptor molecule (PVR) (108, 196)] or measles virus [CD46 molecule (172)]. Transgenic mice expressing PVR are susceptible to poliovirus infection, and replication of virus in neurons gives rise to poliomyelitis. Measles virus infects transgenic mice expressing the measles virus receptor and gives rise to suppression of both cellular and humoral immune responses. Both models now allow probing of the generation and effect of the antiviral immune response in a well-defined genetic host (the mouse) in which various T and B lymphocytes, MHC class I and II molecules, activation and co-stimulatory molecules, and cytokine genes can be knocked out. However, neither the poliomyelitis nor the measles virus model totally recapitulates the natural human infection because, when the respective virus is provided by the natural route, little or no infection occurs. A third valuable transgenic model is that for HBV. Unlike the polio or measles virus approach, transgenic mice that express HBV sequences have been established by use of liver-associated promoters (metallothionein and/or albumin promoters) (30). Using these models, Chisari et al. (49,67) have shown the role played by both $CD8^+$ and $CD4^+$ T cells in control of HBV, and have demonstrated that IFN-γ and TNF-α secreted by CTLs play a prominent role in clearing HBV sequences from the vast majority of hepatic cells. IFN-γ and TNF-α triggered the down-regulation of HBV gene expression by a post-transcriptional mechanism, in which HBV RNA levels in hepatocytes are controlled by stabilizing (or destabilizing) influences of several HBV RNA-binding host proteins, whose activity is regulated through cytokine-induced signal pathways (72).

By a different approach, focal expression of a viral gene in a selected cell with a cell-specific promoter can be used as a means to evaluate virus-induced autoimmune disease (43,173,259). The viral transgene is integrated into the host's genome and passed on to progeny, essentially becoming a "self" antigen. This approach has been used to express a viral gene in the beta cells of the islets of Langerhans [a model for diabetes (159,173,259)] or in oligodendrocytes [a demyelination model for multiple sclerosis (43)]. Subsequent infection of the transgenic mouse with the appropriate virus allows one to determine whether related or unrelated viruses induce responses to the transgene, and how cytokines, or co-stimulatory molecules, might initiate or enhance autoimmune disease of the pancreas or CNS.

Gene dysfunction (knock-out) studies allow the generation of mice lacking specific immune cell populations (e.g., B cells, $CD4^+$ or $CD8^+$ T lymphocytes), T-cell effector molecules (e.g., perforin, IFN-γ, TNF-α), and a litany of other molecules including specific MHC class I or class II molecules, cytokines, chemokines, activation and co-stimulatory, and adhesion molecules. Using such mice, the role of specific genes and their products can be defined during a virus infection; however, the redundancy of the genome, and the resultant capacity for compensatory changes, indicate that the results obtained with knock-out mice should be interpreted with some caution. For instance, there are several examples in which deletion of the gene has given results very different from prior studies that used monoclonal antibodies to inactivate the gene product in a developmentally normal mouse. It is not clear which of the two approaches has given us the "correct" result. With this caveat, the various knock-out and expresser models presently available should help us to identify the roles played by various components in immunization and immunopathology, which in turn may lead to therapeutic strategies to optimize vaccination and to limit immunopathologic injury and disease.

REFERENCES

1. Outbreak of Hendra-like virus—Malaysia and Singapore, 1998-1999. *MMWR* 1999;48:265–269.
2. Ahmed R, King CC, Oldstone MBA. Virus-lymphocyte interactions. T cells of the helper subset are infected with lymphocytic choriomeningitis virus during persistent infection in vivo. *J Virol* 1987;61: 1571–1576.
3. Ahn K, Gruhler A, Galocha B, et al. The ER-luminal domain of the HCMV glycoprotein US6 inhibits peptide translocation by TAP. *Immunity* 1997;6:613–621.
4. Amadou C, Kumanovics A, Jones EP, et al. The mouse major histocompatibility complex: Some assembly required. *Immunol Rev* 1999; 167:211–221.
5. An LL, Whitton JL. A multivalent minigene vaccine, containing B cell, CTL, and Th epitopes from several microbes, induces appropriate responses in vivo, and confers protection against more than one pathogen. *J Virol* 1997;71:2292–2302.
6. An LL, Whitton JL. Multivalent minigene vaccines against infectious disease. *Curr Opin Mol Ther* 1999;1:16–21.
7. Arevalo JH, Taussig MJ, Wilson IA. Molecular basis of crossreactivity and the limits of antibody-antigen complementarity. *Nature* 1993; 365:859–863.
8. Attaya M, Jameson S, Martinez CK, et al. Ham-2 corrects the class I antigen-processing defect in RMA-S cells. *Nature* 1992;355:647–649.
9. Banchereau J, Steinman RM. Dendritic cells and the control of immunity. *Nature* 1998;392:245–252.
10. Barbas CF, Kang as, Lerner RA, et al. Assembly of combinatorial antibody libraries on phage surfaces: The gene III site. *Proc Natl Acad Sci U S A* 1991;88:7978–7982.
11. Barre-Sinoussi F, Chermann JC, Rey F, et al. Isolation of a T-lymphotropic retrovirus from a patient at risk for acquired immune deficiency syndrome (AIDS). *Science* 1983;220:868–871.
12. Barrett T, Visser IK, Mamaev L, et al. Dolphin and porpoise morbilliviruses are genetically distinct from phocine distemper virus. *Virology* 1993;193:1010–1012.
13. Bender A, Albert M, Reddy A, et al. The distinctive features of influenza virus infection of dendritic cells. *Immunobiology* 1998;198: 552–567.
14. Bergelson JM, Chan M, Solomon KR, et al. Decay-accelerating factor (CD55), a glycosylphosphatidylinositol-anchored complement regulatory protein, is a receptor for several echoviruses. *Proc Natl Acad Sci U S A* 1994;91:6245–6249.
15. Bergelson JM, Mohanty JG, Crowell RL, et al. Coxsackievirus B3 adapted to growth in RD cells binds to decay-accelerating factor (CD55). *J Virol* 1995;69:1903–1906.
16. Bertin J, Armstrong RC, Ottilie S, et al. Death effector domain-containing herpesvirus and poxvirus proteins inhibit both Fas- and TNFR1-induced apoptosis. *Proc Natl Acad Sci U S A* 1997;94: 1172–1176.
17. Biron CA, Byron KS, Sullivan JL. Severe herpesvirus infections in an adolescent without natural killer cells. *N Engl J Med* 1989;320: 1731–1735.
18. Bjorkman PJ, Saper MA, Samraoui B, et al. Structure of the human class I histocompatibility antigen HLA-A2. *Nature* 1987;329: 506–512.
19. Bjorkman PJ, Saper MA, Samraoui B, et al. The foreign antigen binding site and T cell recognition regions of class I histocompatibility antigens. *Nature* 1987;329:512–518.
20. Borrow P, Evans CF, Oldstone MBA. Virus-induced immunosuppression: Immune system-mediated destruction of virus-infected dendritic cells results in generalized immune suppression. *J Virol* 1995;69: 1059–1070.

21. Borrow P, Lewicki H, Wei X, et al. Antiviral pressure exerted by HIV-1-specific cytotoxic T lymphocytes (CTLs) during primary infection demonstrated by rapid selection of CTL escape virus. *Nat Med* 1997; 3:205–211.
22. Borrow P, Tishon A, Oldstone MBA. Infection of lymphocytes by a virus that aborts cytotoxic T lymphocyte activity and establishes persistent infection. *J Exp Med* 1991;174:203–212.
23. Braud VM, Allan DS, O'Callaghan CA, et al. HLA-E binds to natural killer cell receptors CD94/NKG2A, B and C. *Nature* 1998;39: 795–799.
24. Brennan J, Mahon G, Mager DL, et al. Recognition of class I major histocompatibility complex molecules by Ly- 49: Specificities and domain interactions. *J Exp Med* 1996;183:1553–1559.
25. Brown JH, Jardetzky TS, Gorga JC, et al. Three-dimensional structure of the human class II histocompatibility antigen HLA-DR1. *Nature* 364:33–39.
26. Butz EA, Bevan MJ. Massive expansion of antigen-specific CD8+ T cells during an acute virus infection. *Immunity* 1998;8:167–175.
27. Campbell RD, Law SK, Reid KB, et al. Structure, organization, and regulation of the complement genes. *Annu Rev Immunol* 1988;6: 161–195.
28. Cann AJ, Stanway G, Hughes PJ, et al. Reversion to neurovirulence of the live-attenuated Sabin type 3 oral poliovirus vaccine. *Nucleic Acids Res* 1984;12:7787–7792.
29. Carbone FR, Kurts C, Bennett SR, et al. Cross-presentation: A general mechanism for CTL immunity and tolerance. *Immunol Today* 1998; 19:368–373.
30. Chisari FV. Hepatitis B virus transgenic mice: Models of viral immunobiology and pathogenesis. *Curr Top Microbiol Immunol* 1996;206:149–173.
31. Christinck ER, Luscher MA, Barber BH, et al. Peptide binding to class I MHC on living cells and quantitation of complexes required for CTL lysis. *Nature* 1991;352:67–70.
32. Comeau MR, Johnson R, DuBose RF, et al. A poxvirus-encoded semaphorin induces cytokine production from monocytes and binds to a novel cellular semaphorin receptor, VESPR. *Immunity* 1998;8: 473–482.
33. Cooper NR, Oldstone MBA. Virus infected cells, IgG and the alternative complement pathway. *Immunol Today* 1983;4:107–108.
34. Crowe JE, Murphy BR, Chanock RM, et al. Recombinant human RSV monoclonal antibody Fab is effective therapeutically when introduced directly into the lungs of respiratory syncytial virus-infected mice. *Proc Natl Acad Sci U S A* 1994;91:1386–1390.
35. Cui J, Shin T, Kawano T, et al. Requirement for Valpha14 NKT cells in IL-12-mediated rejection of tumors. *Science* 1997;278:1623–1626.
36. Davis-Poynter NJ, Farrell HE. Masters of deception: A review of herpesvirus immune evasion strategies. *Immunol Cell Biol* 1996;74: 513–522.
37. de Campos-Lima PO, Gavioli R, Zhang Q-J, et al. HLA-A11 epitope loss isolates of Epstein-Barr virus from a highly A11+ population. *Science* 1993;260:98–100.
38. Deussing J, Roth W, Rommerskirch W, et al. The genes of the lysosomal cysteine proteinases cathepsin B, H, L, and S map to different mouse chromosomes. *Mamm Genome* 1997;8:241–245.
39. Doherty PC, Hou S, Southern PJ. Lymphocytic choriomeningitis virus induces a chronic wasting disease in mice lacking class I MHC glycoproteins. *J Neuroimmunol* 1993;46:11–17.
40. Donnelly JJ, Ulmer JB, Liu MA. DNA vaccines. *Life Sci* 1997;60: 163–172.
41. Dorig RE, Marcil A, Chopra A, et al. The human CD46 molecule is a receptor for measles virus (Edmonston strain). *Cell* 1993;75:295–305.
42. Enria DA, Fernandez NJ, Briggiler AM, et al. Importance of dose of neutralizing antibodies in treatment of Argentine hemorrhagic fever with immune plasma. *Lancet* 1984;2:255–256.
43. Evans CF, Horwitz MS, Hobbs MV, et al. Viral infection of transgenic mice expressing a viral protein in oligodendrocytes leads to chronic central nervous system autoimmune disease. *J Exp Med* 1996;184: 2371–2384.
44. Evans DM, Dunn G, Minor PD, et al. Increased neurovirulence associated with a single nucleotide change in a noncoding region of the Sabin type 3 poliovaccine genome. *Nature* 1985;314:548–550.
45. Fauci AS. Host factors and the pathogenesis of HIV-induced disease. *Nature* 1996;384:529–534.
46. Fenner F. Myxomatosis in Australian wild rabbits: Evolutionary changes in an infectious disease. *Harvey Lectures* 1959;53:25–55.
47. Fingeroth J, Weis JJ, Tedder TF, et al. Epstein-Barr virus receptor of human B lymphocytes is the C3d receptor CR2. *Proc Natl Acad Sci U S A* 1984;81:4510–4514.
48. Fourie AM, Yang Y. Molecular requirements for assembly and intracellular transport of class I major histocompatibility complex molecules. *Curr Top Microbiol Immunol* 1998;232:49–74.
49. Franco A, Guidotti LG, Hobbs MV, et al. Pathogenetic effector function of CD4-positive T helper 1 cells in hepatitis B virus transgenic mice. *J Immunol* 1997;159:2001–2008.
50. Frelinger JA, Serody J. Immune response of beta 2-microglobulin-deficient mice to pathogens. *Curr Top Microbiol Immunol* 1998;232: 99–114.
51. Fremont DH, Matsumura M, Stura EA, et al. Crystal structures of two viral peptides in complex with murine MHC class I H-2K^{b}. *Science* 1992;257:919–927.
52. Fruh K, Yang Y. Antigen presentation by MHC class I and its regulation by interferon γ. *Curr Opin Immunol* 1999;11:76–81.
53. Fujinami RS, Oldstone MBA. Amino acid homology between the encephalitogenic site of myelin basic protein and virus: Mechanism for autoimmunity. *Science* 1985;230:1043–1045.
54. Fulginiti VA, Eller JJ, Downie A, et al. Atypical measles in children previously immunized with inactivated measles virus vaccine. *JAMA* 1967;202:1075–1080.
55. Garboczi DN, Ghosh P, Utz U, et al. Structure of the complex between human T-cell receptor, viral peptide and HLA-A2. *Nature* 1996;384: 134–141.
56. Garcia KC, Degano M, Pease RL, et al. Structural basis of plasticity in T cell receptor recognition of a self peptide-MHC antigen. *Science* 1998;279:1166–1172.
57. Garcia KC, Scott CA, Brunmark A, et al. CD8 enhances formation of stable T-cell receptor/MHC class I molecule complexes. *Nature* 1996; 384:577–581.
58. Geller TJ, Condie D. A case of protracted coxsackievirus meningoencephalitis in a marginally immunodeficient child treated successfully with intravenous immunoglobulin. *J Neurol Sci* 1995;129:131–133.
59. Gilbert MJ, Riddell SR, Plachter B, et al. Cytomegalovirus selectively blocks antigen processing and presentation of its immediate-early gene product. *Nature* 1996;383:720–722.
60. Good RA. Experiments of nature in the development of modern immunology. *Immunol Today* 1991;12:283–286.
61. Good RA, Zak SZ. Disturbance in gamma-globulin synthesis as "experiments of nature." *Pediatrics* 1956;18:109–149.
62. Gordon S. The role of the macrophage in immune regulation. *Res Immunol* 1998;149:685–688.
63. Grant EP, Degano M, Rosat JP, et al. Molecular recognition of lipid antigens by T cell receptors. *J Exp Med* 1999;189:195–205.
64. Gray MM, Hann IM, Glass S, et al. Mortality and morbidity caused by measles in children with malignant disease attending four major treatment centres: A retrospective review. *Br Med J [Clin Res]* 1987; 295:19–22.
65. Gregg DA, Schlafer DH, Mebus CA. African swine fever virus infection of skin-derived dendritic cells in vitro causes interference with subsequent foot-and-mouth disease virus infection. *J Vet Diagn Invest* 1995;7:44–51.
66. Guidotti LG, Chisari FV. To kill or to cure: Options in host defense against viral infection. *Curr Opin Immunol* 1996;8:478–483.
67. Guidotti LG, Ishikawa T, Hobbs MV, et al. Intracellular inactivation of the hepatitis B virus by cytotoxic T lymphocytes. *Immunity* 1996;4: 25–36.
68. Guidotti LG, Rochford R, Chung J, et al. Viral clearance without destruction of infected cells during acute HBV infection. *Science* 1999;284:825–829.
69. Hassett DE, Whitton JL. DNA immunization. *Trends Microbiol* 1996; 4:307–312.
70. Heemels M-T, Schumacher TNM, Wonigeit K, et al. Peptide translocation by variants of the transporter associated with antigen processing. *Science* 1993;262:2059–2063.
71. Heise MT, Connick M, Virgin HW. Murine cytomegalovirus inhibits interferon gamma-induced antigen presentation to CD4 T cells by macrophages via regulation of expression of major histocompatibility complex class II-associated genes. *J Exp Med* 1998;187:1037–1046.
72. Heise T, Guidotti LG, Cavanaugh VJ, et al. Hepatitis B virus RNA-binding proteins associated with cytokine-induced clearance of viral RNA from the liver of transgenic mice. *J Virol* 1999;73:474–481.
73. Henderson RA, Michel H, Sakaguchi K, et al. HLA2.1-associated

peptides from a mutant cell line: A second pathway of antigen presentation. *Science* 1992;255:1264–1266.
74. Henderson S, Huen D, Rowe M, et al. Epstein-Barr virus-coded BHRF1 protein, a viral homologue of Bcl-2, protects human B cells from programmed cell death. *Proc Natl Acad Sci U S A* 1993;90: 8479–8483.
75. Herberg JA, Sgouros J, Jones T, et al. Genomic analysis of the Tapasin gene, located close to the TAP loci in the MHC. *Eur J Immunol* 1998; 28:459–467.
76. Hertel NT, Pedersen FK, Heilmann C. Coxsackie B3 virus encephalitis in a patient with agammaglobulinaemia. *Eur J Pediatr* 1989;148: 642–643.
77. Hill A, Jugovic P, York I, et al. Herpes simplex virus turns off the TAP to evade host immunity. *Nature* 1995;375:411–415.
78. Hirsch RL. The complement system: its importance in the host response to viral infection. *Microbiol Rev* 1982;46:71–85.
79. Horwitz MS, Yanagi Y, Oldstone MBA. T-cell receptors from virus-specific cytotoxic T lymphocytes recognizing a single immunodominant nine-amino-acid viral epitope show marked diversity. *J Virol* 1994;68:352–357.
80. Hou S, Doherty PC, Zijlstra M, et al. Delayed clearance of Sendai virus in mice lacking class I MHC-restricted CD8$^+$ T cells. *J Immunol* 1992;149:1319–1325.
81. Hou S, Hyland L, Ryan KW, et al. Virus-specific CD8$^+$ T-cell memory determined by clonal burst size. *Nature* 1994;369:652–654.
82. Hsu DH, de Waal MR, Fiorentino DF, et al. Expression of interleukin-10 activity by Epstein-Barr virus protein BCRF1. *Science* 1990;250: 830–832.
83. Huang S, Hendriks W, Althage A, et al. Immune response in mice that lack the interferon-γ receptor. *Science* 1993;259:1742–1745.
84. Hunt DF, Henderson RA, Shabanowitz J, et al. Characterization of peptides bound to the class I MHC molecule HLA2.1 by mass spectrometry. *Science* 1992;255:1261–1263.
85. Jenner E. *An inquiry into the causes and effects of the variolae vaccine, a disease discovered in some western counties of England, particularly Gloucestershire, and known by the name of cowpox.* London: Cassell, 1896.
86. Jerne NK. The generative grammar of the immune system. *Science* 1985;229:1057–1059.
87. Johnson DC, Hill AB. Herpesvirus evasion of the immune system. *Curr Top Microbiol Immunol* 1998;232:149–177.
88. Joly E, Mucke L, Oldstone MBA. Viral persistence in neurons explained by lack of major histocompatibility class I expression. *Science* 1991;253:1283–1285.
89. Joly E, Oldstone MBA. Neuronal cells are deficient in loading peptides onto MHC class I molecules. *Neuron* 1992;8:1185–1190.
90. Jondal M, Klein G, Oldstone MBA, et al. Surface markers on human B and T lymphocytes. VIII. Association between complement and Epstein-Barr virus receptors on human lymphoid cells. *Scand J Immunol* 1976;5:401–410.
91. Jones TR, Wiertz EJ, Sun L, et al. Human cytomegalovirus US3 impairs transport and maturation of major histocompatibility complex class I heavy chains. *Proc Natl Acad Sci U S A* 1996;93:11327–11333.
92. Jonjic S, del Val M, Keil GM, et al. A nonstructural viral protein expressed by a recombinant vaccinia virus protects against lethal cytomegalovirus infection. *J Virol* 1988;62:1653–1658.
93. Joseph BS, Lampert PW, Oldstone MBA. Replication and persistence of measles virus in defined subpopulations of human leukocytes. *J Virol* 1975;16:1638–1649.
94. Kagi D, Ledermann B, Burki K, et al. Cytotoxicity mediated by T cells and natural killer cells is greatly impaired in perforin-deficient mice. *Nature* 1994;369:31–37.
95. Kagi D, Vignaux F, Ledermann B, et al. Fas and perforin pathways as major mechanisms of T cell-mediated cytotoxicity. *Science* 1994;265: 528–530.
96. Kaiserlian D, Grosjean I, Caux C. Infection of human dendritic cells by measles virus induces immune suppression. *Adv Exp Med Biol* 1997;417:421–423.
97. Kang AS, Barbas CF, Janda KD, et al. Linkage of recognition and replication functions by assembling combinatorial antibody Fab libraries along phage surfaces. *Proc Natl Acad Sci U S A* 1991;88: 4363–4366.
98. Kapikian AZ, Mitchell RH, Chanock RM, et al. An epidemiologic study of altered clinical reactivity to respiratory syncytial (RS) virus infection in children previously vaccinated with an inactivated RS vaccine. *Am J Epidemiol* 1969;89:404–421.
99. Kawano T, Cui J, Koezuka Y, et al. CD1d-restricted and TCR-mediated activation of valpha14 NKT cells by glycosylceramides. *Science* 1997;278:1626–1629.
100. Kelly A, Powis SH, Kerr LA, et al. Assembly and function of the two ABC transporter proteins encoded in the human major histocompatibility complex. *Nature* 1992;355:641–644.
101. Kernahan J, McQuillin J, Craft AW. Measles in children who have malignant disease. *Br Med J [Clin Res]* 1987;295:15–18.
102. Kew OM, Sutter RW, Nottay BK, et al. Prolonged replication of a type 1 vaccine-derived poliovirus in an immunodeficient patient. *J Clin Microbiol* 1998;36:2893–2899.
103. King CC, Jamieson BD, Reddy K, et al. Viral infection of the thymus. *J Virol* 1992;66:3155–3160.
104. Klagge IM, Schneider-Schaulies S. Virus interactions with dendritic cells. *J Gen Virol* 1999;80(Pt 4):823–833.
105. Klavinskis LS, Oldstone MBA, Whitton JL. Designing vaccines to induce cytotoxic T lymphocytes: Protection from lethal viral infection. In: Brown F, Chanock R, Ginsberg H, Lerner R, eds. *Vaccines 89: Modern approaches to new vaccines including prevention of AIDS.* New York: Cold Spring Harbor Laboratory, 1989:485–489.
106. Klavinskis LS, Whitton JL, Oldstone MBA. Molecularly engineered vaccine which expresses an immunodominant T-cell epitope induces cytotoxic T lymphocytes that confer protection from lethal virus infection. *J Virol* 1989;63:4311–4316.
107. Knight SC, Patterson S. Bone marrow-derived dendritic cells, infection with human immunodeficiency virus, and immunopathology. *Annu Rev Immunol* 1997;15:593–615.
108. Koike S, Taya C, Kurata T, et al. Transgenic mice susceptible to poliovirus. *Proc Natl Acad Sci U S A* 1991;88:951–955.
109. Konig R, Huang LY, Germain RN. MHC class II interaction with CD4 mediated by a region analogous to the MHC class I binding site for CD8. *Nature* 1992;356:796–798.
110. Kurlander RJ, Shawar SM, Brown ML, et al. Specialized role for a murine class I-b MHC molecule in prokaryotic host defenses. *Science* 1992;257:678–679.
111. Kvist S, Ostberg L, Curman B, et al. Molecular association of a virus protein and transplantation antigens on tumor cell lines. *Scand J Immunol* 1978;8:162–162.
112. Lanier LL. NK cell receptors. *Annu Rev Immunol* 1988;16:359–393.
113. Lanier LL. Natural killer cells fertile with receptors for HLA-G? *Proc Natl Acad Sci U S A* 1999;96:5343–5345.
114. Lau LL, Jamieson BD, Somasundaram T, et al. Cytotoxic T-cell memory without antigen. *Nature* 1994;369:648–652.
115. Lausch RN, Staats H, Metcalf JF, et al. Effective antibody therapy in herpes simplex virus ocular infection: Characterization of recipient immune response. *Intervirology* 1990;31:159–165.
116. Le Bouteiller P, Blaschitz A. The functionality of HLA-G is emerging. *Immunol Rev* 1999;167:233–244.
117. Leong CC, Chapman TL, Bjorkman PJ, et al. Modulation of natural killer cell cytotoxicity in human cytomegalovirus infection: The role of endogenous class I major histocompatibility complex and a viral class I homolog. *J Exp Med* 1998;187:1681–1687.
118. Levine B, Hardwick JM, Trapp BD, et al. Antibody-mediated clearance of alphavirus infection from neurons. *Science* 1991;254: 856–860.
119. Levitskaya J, Coram M, Levitsky V, et al. Inhibition of antigen processing by the internal repeat region of the Epstein-Barr virus nuclear antigen-1. *Nature* 1995;375:685–688.
120. Lewicki HA, von Herrath MG, Evans CF, et al. CTL escape viral variants II. Biologic activity in vivo. *Virology* 1995;211:443–450.
121. Li Q, Spriggs MK, Kovats S, et al. Epstein-Barr virus uses HLA class II as a cofactor for infection of B lymphocytes. *J Virol* 1997;71: 4657–4662.
122. Lin FT, Chen SB, Wang YZ, et al. Use of serum and vaccine in combination for prophylaxis following exposure to rabies. *Rev Infect Dis* 1988;10(suppl 4):S766–S770.
123. Lipton SA. Neuronal injury associated with HIV-1: Approaches to treatment. *Annu Rev Pharmacol Toxicol* 1998;38:159–177.
124. Livingstone AM, Powis SJ, Diamond AG, et al. A trans-acting major histocompatibility complex-linked gene whose alleles determine gain and loss changes in the antigenic structure of a classical class I molecule. *J Exp Med* 1989;170:777–795.

125. Livingstone AM, Powis SJ, Gunther E, et al. Cim: An MHC class II-linked allelism affecting the antigenicity of a classical class I molecule for T lymphocytes. *Immunogenetics* 1991;34:157–163.
126. Ljunggren HG, Karre K. In search of the "missing self": MHC molecules and NK cell recognition. *Immunol Today* 1990;11:237–244.
127. Lubinski J, Nagashunmugam T, Friedman HM. Viral interference with antibody and complement. *Semin Cell Dev Biol* 1998;9:329–337.
128. Ludewig B, Ehl S, Karrer U, et al. Dendritic cells efficiently induce protective antiviral immunity. *J Virol* 1998;72:3812–3818.
129. Ludlow JW. Interactions between SV40 large-tumor antigen and the growth suppressor proteins pRB and p53. *FASEB J* 1993;7:866–871.
130. Maiztegui JI, Fernandez NC, de Damilano AJ. Efficacy of immune plasma in treatment of Argentine haemorrhagic fever and association between treatment and a late neurological syndrome. *Lancet* 1979;2: 1216–1217.
131. Manchester M, Liszewski MK, Atkinson JP, et al. Multiple forms of CD46 (membrane cofactor protein) serve as receptors for measles virus. *Proc Natl Acad Sci U S A* 1994;91:2161–2165.
132. Matsumura M, Fremont DH, Peterson PA, et al. Emerging principles for the recognition of peptide antigens by MHC class I molecules. *Science* 1992;257:927–934.
133. McBride SJ, McCluskey DR, Jackson PT. Selective C7 complement deficiency causing recurrent meningococcal infection. *J Infect* 1991; 22:273–276.
134. McKinney REJ, Katz SL, Wilfert CM. Chronic enteroviral meningoencephalitis in agammaglobulinemic patients. *Rev Infect Dis* 1987; 9:334–356.
135. McNeill WH. *Plagues and peoples:* A natural history of infectious diseases. Garden City, NY: Anchor Press, Doubleday, 1976.
136. Mena I, Perry CM, Harkins S, et al. The role of B lymphocytes in coxsackievirus B3 infection. *Am J Pathol* 1999;155:1205–1215.
137. Mendiratta SK, Martin WD, Hong S, et al. CD1d1 mutant mice are deficient in natural T cells that promptly produce IL-4. *Immunity* 1997;6:469–477.
138. Miller DM, Rahill BM, Boss JM, et al. Human cytomegalovirus inhibits major histocompatibility complex class II expression by disruption of the Jak/Stat pathway. *J Exp Med* 1998;187:675–683.
139. Miller DM, Sedmak DD. Viral effects on antigen processing. *Curr Opin Immunol* 1999;11:94–99.
140. Miller SD, Vanderlugt CL, Begolka WS, et al. Persistent infection with Theiler's virus leads to CNS autoimmunity via epitope spreading. *Nat Med* 1997;3:1133–1136.
141. Milligan GN, Flaherty L, Braciale VL, et al. Nonconventional (TL-encoded) major histocompatibility complex molecules present processed viral antigen to cytotoxic T lymphocytes. *J Exp Med* 1991; 174:133–138.
142. Misbah SA, Spickett GP, Ryba PC, et al. Chronic enteroviral meningoencephalitis in agammaglobulinemia: Case report and literature review. *J Clin Immunol* 1992;12:266–270.
143. Moskophidis D, Pircher, Ciernik I, et al. Suppression of virus-specific antibody production by $CD8^+$ class I-restricted antiviral cytotoxic T cells in vivo. *J Virol* 1992;66:3661–3668.
144. Mosmann TR, Coffman RL. Heterogeneity of cytokine secretion patterns and functions of helper T cells. *Adv Immunol* 1989;46:111–147.
145. Muller-Eberhard HJ. The membrane attack complex of complement. *Annu Rev Immunol* 1986;4:503–528.
146. Muller D, Koller BH, Whitton JL, et al. LCMV-specific, class II-restricted cytotoxic T cells in β2-microglobulin-deficient mice. *Science* 1992;255:1576–1578.
147. Murali-Krishna K, Altman JD, Suresh M, et al. Counting antigen-specific CD8 T cells: A reevaluation of bystander activation during viral infection. *Immunity* 1998;8:177–187.
148. Nahmias AJ, Griffith D, Salsbury C, et al. Thymic aplasia with lymphopenia, plasma cells, and normal immunoglobulins: Relation to measles virus infection. *JAMA* 1967;201:729–734.
149. Nakamoto Y, Guidotti LG, Kuhlen CV, et al. Immune pathogenesis of hepatocellular carcinoma. *J Exp Med* 1998;188:341–350.
150. Nandi D, Marusina K, Monaco JJ. How do endogenous proteins become peptides and reach the endoplasmic reticulum? *Curr Top Microbiol Immunol* 1998;232:15–47.
151. Naniche D, Varior-Krishnan G, Cervoni F, et al. Human membrane cofactor protein (CD46) acts as a cellular receptor for measles virus. *J Virol* 1993;67:6025–6032.
152. Nathanson N, Langmuir AD. The Cutter incident: Poliomyelitis following formaldehyde-inactivated poliovirus vaccination in the United States during the spring of 1955. II. Relationship of poliomyelitis to Cutter vaccine [classic article]. *Am J Epidemiol* 1963;142:109–140.
153. Neefjes JJ, Momburg F, Hammerling GJ. Selective and ATP-dependent translocation of peptides by the MHC-encoded transporter. *Science* 1993;261:769–771.
154. Nemerow GR, Wolfert R, McNaughton ME, et al. Identification and characterization of the Epstein-Barr virus receptor on human B lymphocytes and its relationship to the C3d complement receptor (CR2). *J Virol* 1985;55:347–351.
155. Nieda M, Nicol A, Koezuka Y, et al. Activation of human Valpha24NKT cells by alpha-glycosylceramide in a CD1d-restricted and Valpha24TCR-mediated manner. *Hum Immunol* 1999;60:10–19.
156. Nordeng TW, Gorvel JP, Bakke O. Intracellular transport of molecules engaged in the presentation of exogenous antigens. *Curr Top Microbiol Immunol* 1998;232:179–215.
157. Oehen S, Waldner H, Kundig TM, et al. Antivirally protective cytotoxic T cell memory to lymphocytic choriomeningitis virus is governed by persisting antigen. *J Exp Med* 1992;176:1273–1281.
158. Ogra PL, Garofalo R. Secretory antibody response to viral vaccines. *Prog Med Virol* 1990;37:156–189.
159. Ohashi PS, Oehen S, Buerki K, et al. Ablation of tolerance and induction of diabetes by virus infection in viral antigen transgenic mice. *Cell* 1991;65:305–318.
160. Oldstone MBA. Virus neutralization and virus-induced immune complex disease: Virus-antibody union resulting in immunoprotection or immunologic injury: Two sides of the same coin. *Prog Med Virol* 1975;19:84–119.
161. Oldstone MBA. Virus induced immune complex formation and disease: Definition, regulation and importance. In: Notkins AL, Oldstone MBA, eds. *Concepts in viral pathogenesis.* New York: Springer Verlag, 1984:201–209.
162. Oldstone MBA, ed. Current topics in microbiology and immunology. In: *Arenaviruses:* biology and immunotherapy. New York: Springer Verlag, 1987:134.
163. Oldstone MBA. Molecular mimicry and autoimmune disease. *Cell* 1987;50:819–820.
164. Oldstone MBA. Viral alteration of cell function. *Sci Am* 1989;261: 42–48.
165. Oldstone MBA. Viruses can cause disease in the absence of morphological evidence of cell injury implication for uncovering new diseases in the future. *J Infect Dis* 1989;159:384–389.
166. Oldstone MBA. Molecular mimicry and immune-mediated diseases. *FASEB J* 1998;12:1255–1265.
167. Oldstone MBA. *Viruses, plagues and history.* Oxford: Oxford University Press, 1998.
168. Oldstone MBA, Blount P, Southern PJ, et al. Cytoimmunotherapy for persistent virus infection reveals a unique clearance pattern from the central nervous system. *Nature* 1986;321:239–243.
169. Oldstone MBA, Buchmeier MJ. Restricted expression of viral glycoprotein in cells of persistently infected mice. *Nature* 1982;350: 360–362.
170. Oldstone MBA, Dixon FJ. Lymphocytic choriomeningitis: production of antibody by "tolerant" infected mice. *Science* 1967;158: 1193–1195.
171. Oldstone MBA, Fujinami RS, Lampert PW. Membrane and cytoplasmic changes in virus infected cells induced by interactions of anti viral antibody with surface viral antigen. *Prog Med Virol* 1980; 26:45–93.
172. Oldstone MBA, Lewicki HA, Thomas D, et al. Measles virus infection in a transgenic model: Virus-induced immunosuppression and CNS disease. *Cell* 1999;98:629–640.
173. Oldstone MBA, Nerenberg N, Southern PJ, et al. Virus infection triggers insulin-dependent diabetes mellitus in a transgenic model: Role of anti-self (virus) immune response. *Cell* 1991;65:319–331.
174. Oldstone MBA, Tishon A, Buchmeier MJ. Virus induced immune complex disease: Genetic control of complement C1q binding complexes in the circulation of mice persistently infected with lymphocytic choriomeningitis virus. *J Immunol* 1983;130:912–918.
175. Opferman JT, Ober BT, Ashton-Rickardt PG. Linear differentiation of cytotoxic effectors into memory T lymphocytes. *Science* 1999;283: 1745–1748.
176. Orren A, Potter PC, Cooper RC, et al. Deficiency of the sixth component of complement and susceptibility to *Neisseria meningitidis* infec-

tions: Studies in 10 families and five isolated cases. *Immunology* 1987;62:249–253.
177. Osterhaus AD, Vedder EJ. Identification of virus causing recent seal deaths. *Nature* 1988;335:20.
178. Pamer EG, Wang CR, Flaherty L, et al. H-2M3 presents a *Listeria monocytogenes* peptide to cytotoxic T lymphocytes. *Cell* 1992;70: 215–223.
179. Patterson S, Knight SC. Susceptibility of human peripheral blood dendritic cells to infection by human immunodeficiency virus. *J Gen Virol* 1987;68(Pt 4):1177–1181.
180. Penna A, Chisari FV, Bertoletti A, et al. Cytotoxic T lymphocytes recognize an HLA-A2-restricted epitope within the hepatitis B virus nucleocapsid antigen. *J Exp Med* 1991;174:1565–1570.
181. Phillips RE, Rowland-Jones S, Nixon DF, et al. Human immunodeficiency virus genetic variation that can escape cytotoxic T cell recognition. *Nature* 1991;354:453–459.
182. Planz O, Seiler P, Hengartner H, et al. Specific cytotoxic T cells eliminate cells producing neutralizing antibodies. *Nature* 1996;382: 726–729.
183. Podack ER, Lowrey DM, Lichtenheld M, et al. Function of granule perforin and esterases in T cell-mediated reactions: Components required for delivery of molecules to target cells. *Ann N Y Acad Sci* 1998;532:292–302.
184. Porcelli SA, Segelke BW, Sugita M, et al. The CD1 family of lipid antigen-presenting molecules. *Immunol Today* 1998;19:362–368.
185. Porterfield J, Cardosa MJ. Host range and tissue tropism: Antibody-dependent mechanism. In: Notkins AL, Oldstone MBA, eds. *Concepts in viral pathogenesis.* New York: Springer Verlag, 1984:117–122.
186. Powis SH, Mockridge I, Kelly A, et al. Polymorphism in a second ABC transporter gene located within the class II region of the human major histocompatibility complex. *Proc Natl Acad Sci U S A* 1992;89:1463–1467.
187. Powis SJ, Deverson EV, Coadwell WJ, et al. Effect of polymorphism of an MHC-linked transporter on the peptides assembled in a class I molecule. *Nature* 1992;357:211–215.
188. Powis SJ, Howard JC, Butcher GW. The major histocompatibility complex class II-linked cim locus controls the kinetics of intracellular transport of a classical class I molecule. *J Exp Med* 1991;173:913–921.
189. Powis SJ, Townsend ARM, Deverson EV, et al. Restoration of antigen presentation to the mutant cell line RMA-S by an MHC-linked transporter. *Nature* 1991;354:528–531.
190. Prigozy TI, Sieling PA, Clemens D, et al. The mannose receptor delivers lipoglycan antigens to endosomes for presentation to T cells by CD1b molecules. *Immunity* 1997;6:187–197.
191. Rajagopalan S, Long EO. A human histocompatibility leukocyte antigen (HLA)-G-specific receptor expressed on all natural killer cells. *J Exp Med* 1999;189:1093–1100.
192. Rall GF. CNS neurons: The basis and benefits of low class I major histocompatibility complex expression. *Curr Top Microbiol Immunol* 1998;232:115–134.
193. Ramsay AJ, Ruby J, Ramshaw IA. A case for cytokines as effector molecules in the resolution of virus infection. *Immunol Today* 1993; 14:155–157.
194. Ramshaw IA, Andrew ME, Phillips SM, et al. Recovery of immunodeficient mice from a vaccinia virus/IL-2 recombinant infection. *Nature* 1987;329:545–546.
195. Raulet DH. Development and tolerance of natural killer cells. *Curr Opin Immunol* 1999;11:129–134.
196. Ren RB, Costantini F, Gorgacz EJ, et al. Transgenic mice expressing a human poliovirus receptor: A new model for poliomyelitis. *Cell* 1990; 63:353–362.
197. Reyburn HT, Mandelboim O, Vales-Gomez M, et al. The class I MHC homologue of human cytomegalovirus inhibits attack by natural killer cells. *Nature* 1997;386:514–517.
198. Rickinson AB, Murray RJ, Brooks J, et al. T cell recognition of Epstein-Barr virus associated lymphomas. *Cancer Surv* 1992;13: 53–80.
199. Rini JM, Schulze-Gahmen U, Wilson IA. Structural evidence for induced fit as a mechanism for antibody-antigen recognition. *Science* 1992;255:959–965.
200. Robbins AS. Controversies in measles immunization recommendations. *West J Med* 1993;158:36–39.
201. Rock KL. A new foreign policy: MHC class I molecules monitor the outside world. *Immunol Today* 1996;17:131–137.
202. Rock KL, Goldberg AL. Degradation of cell proteins and the generation of MHC class I-presented peptides. *Annu Rev Immunol* 1999;17: 739–779.
203. Rodriguez F, An LL, Harkins S, et al. DNA immunization with minigenes: Low frequency of memory CTL and inefficient antiviral protection are rectified by ubiquitination. *J Virol* 1998;72: 5174–5181.
204. Rodriguez F, Slifka MK, Harkins S, Whitton JL, et al. Two overlapping subdominant epitopes identified by DNA immunization induce protective CD^{8+} T cell populations with differing cytolytic activities. *J Immunol* (in press).
205. Rodriguez F, Zhang J, Whitton JL. DNA immunization: Ubiquitination of a viral protein enhances CTL induction, and antiviral protection, but abrogates antibody induction. *J Virol* 1997;71:8497–8503.
206. Rother RP, Fodor WL, Springhorn JP, et al. A novel mechanism of retrovirus inactivation in human serum mediated by anti-alpha-galactosyl natural antibody. *J Exp Med* 1995;182:1345–1355.
207. Rotzschke O, Falk K. Naturally occurring peptide antigens derived from the MHC class-I-restricted processing pathway. *Immunol Today* 1991;12:447–455.
208. Rotzschke O, Falk K, Deres K, et al. Isolation and analysis of naturally processed viral peptides as recognized by cytotoxic T cells. *Nature* 1990;348:252–254.
209. Ruby J, Ramshaw IA. The antiviral activity of immune $CD8^+$ T cells is dependent on interferon-gamma. *Lymphokine Cytokine Res* 1991; 10:353–358.
210. Rudensky AY, Preston-Hurlburt P, Al-Ramadi BK, et al. Truncation variants of peptides isolated from MHC class II molecules suggest sequence motifs. *Nature* 1992;359:429–431.
211. Russell SW, Gordon S, eds. Macrophage biology and activation. *Curr Top Microbiol Immunol* 1992;181.
212. Salter RD, Benjamin RJ, Wesley PK, et al. A binding site for the T cell co-receptor CD8 on the $\alpha 3$ domain of HLA-A2. *Nature* 1990;345: 41–46.
213. Seaman MS, Perarnau B, Lindahl KF, et al. Response to *Listeria monocytogenes* in mice lacking MHC class Ia molecules. *J Immunol* 1999;162:5429–5436.
214. Selvey LA, Wells RM, McCormack LG, et al. Infection of humans and horses by a newly described morbillivirus. *Med J Aust* 1995;162: 642–645.
215. Shafren DR, Bates RC, Agrez MV, et al. Coxsackieviruses B1, B3, and B5 use decay accelerating factor as a receptor for cell attachment. *J Virol* 1995;69:3873–3877.
216. Shen H, Miller JF, Fan X, et al. Compartmentalization of bacterial antigens: Differential effects on priming of CD8 T cells and protective immunity. *Cell* 1998;92:535–545.
217. Shi GP, Webb AC, Foster KE, et al. Human cathepsin S: Chromosomal localization, gene structure, and tissue distribution. *J Biol Chem* 1994;269:11530–11536.
218. Shisler JL, Senkevich TG, Berry MJ, et al. Ultraviolet-induced cell death blocked by a selenoprotein from a human dermatotropic poxvirus. *Science* 1998;279:102–105.
219. Shortridge KF, Zhou NN, Guan Y, et al. Characterization of avian H5N1 influenza viruses from poultry in Hong Kong. *Virology* 1998; 252:331–342.
220. Shresta S, Pham CT, Thomas DA, et al. How do cytotoxic lymphocytes kill their targets? *Curr Opin Immunol* 1998;10:581–587.
221. Siegel MM, Walter TK, Ablin RA. Measles pneumonia in childhood leukemia. *Pediatrics* 1977;60:38–40.
222. Sigal LJ, Crotty S, Andino R, et al. Cytotoxic T-cell immunity to virus-infected non-haematopoietic cells requires presentation of exogenous antigen. *Nature* 1999;398:77–80.
223. Sissons JGP, Oldstone MBA. Antibody-mediated destruction of virus-infected cells. *Adv Immunol* 19980;929:209–260.
224. Slifka MK, Antia R, Whitmire JK, et al. Humoral immunity due to long-lived plasma cells. *Immunity* 1998;8:363–372.
225. Slifka MK, Rodriguez F, Whitton JL. Rapid on/off cycling of cytokine production by virus-specific $CD8^+$ T cells. *Nature* 1999;40:76–79.
226. Smith GL, Symons JA, Khanna A, et al. Vaccinia virus immune evasion. *Immunol Rev* 1997;159:137–154.
227. Soderberg-Naucler C, Fish KN, Nelson JA. Reactivation of latent human cytomegalovirus by allogeneic stimulation of blood cells from healthy donors. *Cell* 1997;91:119–126.
228. Sourdive DJ, Murali-Krishna K, Altman KD, et al. Conserved T cell

receptor repertoire in primary and memory CD8 T cell responses to an acute viral infection. *J Exp Med* 1998;188:71–82.
229. Sparer TE, Gooding RL. Suppression of MHC class I antigen presentation by human adenoviruses. *Curr Top Microbiol Immunol* 1998; 232:135–147.
230. Speir JA, Abdel-Motal UM, Jondal M, et al. Crystal structure of an MHC class I presented glycopeptide that generates carbohydrate-specific CTL. *Immunity* 1999;10:51–61.
231. Spiegelberg HL. The role of interleukin-4 in IgE and IgG subclass formation. *Springer Semin Immunopathol* 1990;12:365–383.
232. Spohr dF, Gierynska IM, Niemialtowski MG, et al. Ectromelia virus establishes a persistent infection in spleen dendritic cells and macrophages of BALB/c mice following the acute disease. *Adv Exp Med Biol* 1995;378:257–261.
233. Spriggs MK. One step ahead of the game: Viral immunomodulatory molecules. *Annu Rev Immunol* 1996;14:101–130.
234. Spriggs MK, Armitage RJ, Comeau MR, et al. The extracellular domain of the Epstein-Barr virus BZLF2 protein binds the HLA-DR beta chain and inhibits antigen presentation. *J Virol* 1996;70: 5557–5563.
235. Spriggs MK, Hruby DE, Maliszewski CR, et al. Vaccinia and cowpox viruses encode a novel secreted interleukin-1-binding protein. *Cell* 1992;71:145–152.
236. Srinivasappa J, Saegusa J, Prabhakar BS, et al. Molecular mimicry: Frequency of reactivity of monoclonal antiviral antibodies with normal tissues. *J Virol* 1986;57:397–401.
237. Suda T, Nagata S. Purification and characterization of the Fas-ligand that induces apoptosis. *J Exp Med* 1994;179:873–879.
238. Sykulev Y, Joo M, Vturina I, et al. Evidence that a single peptide-MHC complex on a target cell can elicit a cytolytic T cell response. *Immunity* 1996;4:565–571.
239. Tevethia MJ, Lacko HA, Kierstead TD, et al. Adding an Rb-binding site to an N-terminally truncated simian virus 40 T antigen restores growth to high cell density, and the T common region in trans provides anchorage-independent growth and rapid growth in low serum concentrations. *J Virol* 1997;71:1888–1896.
240. Teyton L, O'Sullivan D, Dickson PW, et al. Invariant chain distinguishes between the exogenous and endogenous antigen presentation pathways. *Nature* 1990;348:39–44.
241. Tighe H, Corr M, Roman M, et al. Gene vaccination: Plasmid DNA is more than just a blueprint. *Immunol Today* 1998;19:89–97.
242. Tishon A, Lewicki H, Rall G, et al. An essential role for type 1 interferon-gamma in terminating persistent viral infection. *Virology* 1995; 212:244–250.
243. Tishon A, Salmi Ahmed R, et al. Role of viral strains and host genes in determining levels of immune complexes in a model system: Implications for HIV infection. *AIDS Res Hum Retroviruses* 1991;7:963–969.
244. Tishon A, Southern PJ, Oldstone MBA. Virus-lymphocyte interactions II. Expression of viral sequences during the course of persistent lymphocytic choriomeningitis virus infection and their localization to the L3T4 (CD4$^+$) lymphocyte subset. *J Immunol* 1988;140:1280–1284.
245. Tobery TW, Siliciano RF. Targeting of HIV-1 antigens for rapid intracellular degradation enhances cytotoxic T lymphocyte (CTL) recognition and the induction of de novo CTL responses in vivo after immunization. *J Exp Med* 1997;185:909–920.
246. Tonietti G, Oldstone MBA, Dixon FJ. The effect of induced chronic viral infections on the immunologic diseases of New Zealand mice. *J Exp Med* 1970;132:89–109.
247. Townsend ARM, Trowsdale J. The transporters associated with antigen presentation. *Semin Cell Biol* 1993;4:53–61.
248. Tracey KJ, Beutler B, Lowry SF, et al. Shock and tissue injury induced by recombinant human cachectin. *Science* 1986;234:470–474.
249. Trowsdale J, Hanson I, Mockridge I, et al. Sequences encoded in the class II region of the MHC related to the abc superfamily of transporters. *Nature* 1990;348:741–744.
250. Valiante NM, Uhrberg M, Shilling HG, et al. Functionally and structurally distinct NK cell receptor repertoires in the peripheral blood of two human donors. *Immunity* 1997;7:739–751.
251. Van Bleek GM, Nathenson SG. Isolation of an endogenously processed immunodominant viral peptide from the class I H-2 Kb molecule. *Nature* 1990;348:213–216.
252. van der Drift AC, van Noort JM, Kruse J. Catheptic processing of protein antigens: Enzymic and molecular aspects. *Semin Immunol* 1990; 2:255–271.
253. Van Kaer L, Ashton-Rickardt PG, Ploegh HL, et al. TAP1 mutant mice are deficient in antigen presentation, surface class I molecules, and CD4-8$^+$ T cells. *Cell* 1992;71:1205–1214.
254. Vanderlugt CL, Begolka WS, Neville WL, et al. The functional significance of epitope spreading and its regulation by co-stimulatory molecules. *Immunol Rev* 1998;164:63–72.
255. Vassalli P. The pathophysiology of tumor necrosis factors. *Annu Rev Immunol* 19923;10:411–452.
256. Vignali DA, Moreno J, Schiller D, et al. Species-specific binding of CD4 to the beta 2 domain of major histocompatibility complex class II molecules. *J Exp Med* 1992;175:925–932.
257. Villarete L, de Fries R, Kolhekar S, et al. Impaired responsiveness to gamma interferon of macrophages infected with lymphocytic choriomeningitis virus clone 13: Susceptibility to histoplasmosis [published erratum appears in *Infect Immun* 1995;63:3748]. *Infect Immun* 1995;63:1468–1472.
258. Visser IK, van Bressem MF, van de Bildt MW, et al. Prevalence of morbilliviruses among pinniped and cetacean species. *Rev Sci Tech* 1993;12:197–202.
259. von Herrath MG, Dockter J, Oldstone MBA. How virus induces a rapid or slow onset insulin-dependent diabetes mellitus in a transgenic model. *Immunity* 1994;1:231–242.
260. von Pirquet C. Das ver halten der kutanen tuberkulin-reaktion wahren der masern. *Dtsch Med Wochenschr* 1908;37:1297.
261. Vugmeyster Y, Glas R, Perarnau B, et al. Major histocompatibility complex (MHC) class I KbDb –/– deficient mice possess functional CD8$^+$ T cells and natural killer cells. *Proc Natl Acad Sci U S A* 1998; 95:12492–12497.
262. Walsh CM, Matloubian M, Liu CC, et al. Immune function in mice lacking the perforin gene. *Proc Natl Acad Sci U S A* 1994;91: 10854–10858.
263. Weidt G, Deppert W, Utermohlen O, et al. Emergence of virus escape mutants after immunization with epitope vaccine. *J Virol* 1995;69: 7147–7151.
264. Weissman D. Fauci AS. Role of dendritic cells in immunopathogenesis of human immunodeficiency virus infection. *Clin Microbiol Rev* 1997;10:358–367.
265. Welsh RM. Cytotoxic cells induced during lymphocytic choriomeningitis virus infection of mice. 1. Characterization of natural killer cell induction. *J Exp Med* 1978;148:163–181.
266. Welsh RM. Regulation of virus infections by natural killer cells a review. *Nat Immun Cell Growth Regul* 1986;5:169–199.
267. Welsh RM, Cooper NR, Jensen FC, et al. Human serum lyses RNA tumour viruses. *Nature* 1975;257:612–614.
268. Welsh RM, Karre K, Hansson M, et al. Interferon-mediated protection of normal and tumor target cells against lysis by mouse natural killer cells. *J Immunol* 1981;126:219–225.
269. Welsh RM, Nishioka WK, Antia R, et al. Mechanism of killing by virus-induced cytotoxic T lymphocytes elicited in vivo. *J Virol* 1990; 64:3726–3733.
270. Welsh RM, Zinkernagel RM. Heterospecific cytotoxic cell activity induced during the first three days of acute lymphocytic choriomeningitis virus infection in mice. *Nature* 1977;268:646–648.
271. White E, Sabbatini P, Debbas M, et al. The 19-kilodalton adenovirus E1B transforming protein inhibits programmed cell death and prevents cytolysis by tumor necrosis factor alpha. *Mol Cell Biol* 1992;12: 2570–2580.
272. Whitton JL. Lymphocytic choriomeningitis virus CTL. *Semin Virol* 1990;1:257–262.
273. Whitton JL, Fujinami RS. Viruses as triggers of autoimmunity: Facts and fantasies. *Curr Opin Microbiol* 1999;2:392–397.
274. Wiertz EJHJ, Tortorella D, Bogyo M, et al. Sec61-mediated transfer of a membrane protein from the endoplasmic reticulum to the proteasome for destruction. *Nature* 1996;384:432–438.
275. Wiley CA, Schrier RD, Nelson JA, et al. Cellular localization of human immunodeficiency virus infection within the brains of acquired immune deficiency syndrome patients. *Proc Natl Acad Sci U S A* 1986;83:7089–7093.
276. Williamson MM, Hooper PT, Selleck PW, et al. Transmission studies of Hendra virus (equine morbillivirus) in fruit bats, horses and cats. *Aust Vet J* 1998;76:813–818.
277. Wilson IA, Fremont DH. Structural analysis of MHC class I molecules with bound peptide antigens. *Semin Immunol* 1993;5:75–80.
278. Wu Y, Kipps TJ. Deoxyribonucleic acid vaccines encoding antigens

with rapid proteasome-dependent degradation are highly efficient inducers of cytolytic T lymphocytes. *J Immunol* 1997;159:6037–6043.
279. Yanagi Y, Tishon A, Lewicki H, et al. Diversity of T-cell receptors in virus-specific cytotoxic T lymphocytes recognizing three distinct viral epitopes restricted by a single major histocompatibility complex molecule. *J Virol* 1992;66:2527–2531.
280. Yewdell JW, Esquivel F, Arnold D, et al. Presentation of numerous viral peptides to mouse major histocompatibility complex (MHC) class I-restricted T lymphocytes is mediated by the human MHC-encoded transporter or by a hybrid mouse-human transporter. *J Exp Med* 1993;177:1785–1790.
281. Zajac AJ, Quinn DG, Cohen PL, et al. Fas-dependent $CD4^+$ cytotoxic T-cell-mediated pathogenesis during virus infection. *Proc Natl Acad Sci U S A* 1995;93:14730–14735.
282. Zeng Z, Castano AR, Segelke BW, et al. Crystal structure of mouse CD1: An MHC-like fold with a large hydrophobic binding groove. *Science* 1997;277:339–345.
283. Zinkernagel RM. Virus-induced acquired immune suppression by cytotoxic T cell-mediated immunopathology. *Vet Microbiol* 1992;33:13–18.
284. Zinkernagel RM. Protective antibody responses against viruses. *Biol Chem* 1997;378:725–729.
285. Zinkernagel RM, Doherty PC. Immunological surveillance against altered self components by sensitised T lymphocytes in lymphocytic choriomeningitis. *Nature* 1974;251:547–548.
286. Zinkernagel RM, Doherty PC. Restriction of in vitro T cell-mediated cytotoxicity in lymphocytic choriomeningitis within a syngeneic or semiallogeneic system. *Nature* 1974;248:701–702.
287. Zychlinsky A, Zheng LM, Liu CC, et al. Cytolytic lymphocytes induce both apoptosis and necrosis in target cells. *J Immunol* 1991; 146:393–400.

CHAPTER 12

Interferons and Other Cytokines

Christine A. Biron and Ganes C. Sen

GENERAL FEATURES OF CYTOKINES

Cytokines are protein factors made by cells to act on cells. The family of these includes a large and growing number of molecules acting on nonimmune and immune cells to mediate a variety of functions. Although their properties cannot be described briefly, certain characteristics are shared by most cytokines (Table 1). In general, cytokines are soluble, but there are examples of membrane-bound forms. They are structurally and biochemically similar to polypeptide hormones and growth factors (1,297). In particular, specific receptors for cytokines are expressed at cell surfaces, and cytokine binding to these activates intracellular signaling pathways. In addition, cytokines typically mediate autocrine and paracrine effects in a short radius, but they can also have endocrine effects under extreme conditions. Finally, some cytokines can themselves act as growth factors. One major difference between cytokines and their hormone and growth factor relatives, however, is that cytokines are tightly regulated for limited expression under basal conditions and are induced in response to host challenges, particularly microbial infections.

In terms of functions, cytokines are generally pleiotropic, activating multiple distinct consequences, but different cytokines can mediate overlapping functions. They are frequently observed in cascade responses with simultaneous or sequential expression of several kinds. This is because clusters of cytokines are sometimes induced by the same signals and because certain cytokines induce downstream activation of other cytokines. Because they can have synergistic or antagonistic interactions, the interactive biologic effects of the multiple cytokines elicited during infections may be more important than effects mediated by any single factor. After challenges with particular classes of infectious agents, such as viruses, bacteria, or parasites, unique or dominant cytokine responses can be induced and linked to help drive a cascade of initial to innate to adaptive subset cytokine and immune responses that are most effective in defense against the particular agent (Fig. 1). The earliest events appear to be controlled by stimulation of host receptors recognizing unique structures expressed by

TABLE 1. *General characteristics of cytokines*

Most cytokines are simple polypeptides or glycoproteins ≤ 30 kd in size. Some cytokines form homodimers or homotrimers. One cytokine is a known heterodimer.
Cytokines are tightly regulated for limited expression under basal conditions. Various stimuli induce cytokine expression at the level of transcription, translation, or posttranslational protein processing.
Cytokine production is transient. The action radius is usually short, resulting in autocrine or paracrine functions. After profound conditions of stimulation or during systemic infections, however, some cytokines are found at circulating levels with endocrine functions.
Cytokines mediate their actions by binding to specific cell surface receptors (Kd in the range of 10^{-9}–10^{-12} M). Target cell responsiveness to a particular cytokine is dependent upon expression of receptors for the factor.
Most cytokine actions can be attributed to altered patterns of gene expression in target cells. Phenotypically, cytokine stimulation leads to an increase (or decrease) in the rate of cell proliferation, change in cell differentiation state, or change in the expression of some differentiated function.
Cytokines often act by regulating expression of other cytokines through the mechanism of inducing other cytokines in cascade responses or of decreasing certain other cytokines. Alternatively or additionally, cytokines can regulate the functions of other cytokines by positively or negatively modulating their receptors.
Structurally dissimilar cytokines sometimes mediate overlapping actions (*redundant*), but structurally similar cytokines sometimes mediate different actions.
A single cytokine often has multiple target cells and multiple actions (*pleiotropic*).
Cytokines can have synergistic or antagonistic interactions. Because cells and tissues in the body are rarely, if ever, exposed to a single cytokine at a time, important biologic functions are likely to be the result of such interactions.

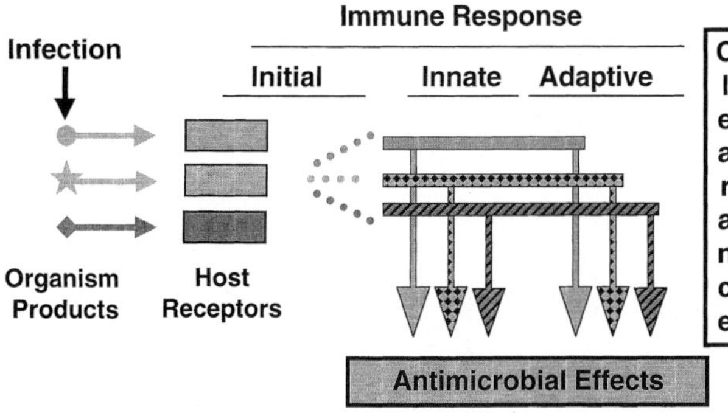

FIG. 1. General pathways of initial to innate to adaptive immune responses during infections. The picture emerging is that initial host responses to infectious agents are induced as a result of recognition, by specific receptors for unique microbial structures that are expressed in or on host cells. As a result of sensing structures expressed by classes of agents, these receptors activate a cascade of events, inducing subsets of innate and adaptive immune responses most effective in defense against the organism being encountered. Particular initial/innate cytokine responses (represented as broken lines) are major mediators in shaping the downstream immune responses.

classes of infectious organisms but distinct from host determinants (23,24,181). Thus, there are many different kinds of cytokines, but expression of particular subsets appears to be regulated by host responses to unique conditions of challenge.

Cytokine nomenclature reflects the evolution of knowledge from varied areas of investigations. Many of the factors have derived names from the biologic functions originally assigned to them. Examples are the interferons (IFNs), first identified by their ability to interfere with virus replication (222,297), and the tumor necrosis factors (TNF), which were demonstrated to induce necrosis of tumors (134,304). The first demonstrated function, however, is not always the most or only important one. The name interleukin (IL) was adapted for a number of cytokines originally thought to be leukocyte produced to act on other leukocytes. This has led to a long list of numbered factors (currently IL-1 through IL-18). Many of these, however, are now known to be made by, and act on, cells other than leukocytes.

Cytokines can be divided into four major groups based on general induction and function characteristics: (a) initial and innate cytokines, (b) adaptive cytokines, (c) chemokines, and (d) hematopoietic growth factors (1). The first three groups have well-characterized functions associated with abilities to mediate defense against infections by activating biochemical antimicrobial mechanisms or by regulating endogenous immune responses. These are reviewed in Table 2. Generally, initial and innate cytokines are associated during primary infections with early events; depend on nonimmune cells or cells of the innate immune system, such as polymorphonuclear leukocytes (PMNs), monocyte-macrophages (monocytic cells), natural killer (NK) cells, or dendritic cells (DCs), for expression; and contribute to innate immunity. In contrast, adaptive cytokines are associated with later events, depend on T and B cells of the adaptive immune system for expression, and contribute to adaptive immunity. Chemokines are associated with inflammation occurring during either innate or adaptive immune responses. These cytokines and their functions are discussed in more detail below. The fourth group is composed of mediators of leukocyte growth and differentiation. Although some of these factors may be induced during infections, they have been characterized primarily for function in normal leukocyte development, and such information is beyond the scope of this chapter.

The focus of the material presented is current understanding of cytokine expression and function in the context of viral challenge. First, an overview is presented of important biologic functions mediated by, and kinetics of induction for, cytokine responses. This is a "low-power"

TABLE 2. *List of important cytokines and chemokines*

Group (Class)	Cytokine (chemokine)	Abbreviation subtypes	Size	Cell source(s)	Target cells	Primary effects activated
Initial and innate	Type 1 interferons	IFN-α/β	18 kd	All	All	Antiviral, NK cell cytotoxicity, induction of class I MHC
	Interleukin-15	IL-15	14–15 kd	Monocytic cells, others	NK and T cells	Proliferation, differentiation
	Tumor necrosis factor	TNF-α	17 kd	Monocytic cells, NK cells, others	PMNs, endothelial cells, hypothalamus, others	Activation of adhesion, inflammation, fever, cell death, antiviral, induction of class I MHC
	Interleukin-1	IL-1 α and β	17 kd	Monocytic cells, others	Endothelial cells, hypothalamus, others	Inflammation, fever
	Interleukin-6	IL-6	26 kd	Monocytic cells, others	B cells, liver	Growth, acute-phase reactants
	Interleukin-12	IL-12	35 kd + 40 kd	Moncytic cells, granulocytes, dendritic cells	NK and T cells	IFN-γ production, CD4 T-cell differentiation
	Interferon-γ	IFN-γ	21 kd	NK cells, NKT cells (?)	Monocytic cells, most others	Activation, induction of class II MHC, CD4 T-cell differentiation
	Interleukin-18	IL-18	18 kd	Monocytic cells, few others	NK and T cells	Enhances IFN-γ production
Initial and innate or adaptive (?)	Interleukin-10	IL-10	20 kd	Monocytic cells, T cells	Monocytic cells, many others	Inhibits IL-12, Inhibits IFN-γ
	Transforming growth factor-β	TGF-β	14 kd	Monocytic cells, T cells, others	NK and T cells, many others	Inhibits IFN-γ expression, proliferation
Adaptive	Interleukin-2	IL-2	14 kd	Primarily CD4 T cells	T cells (less NK cells)	Proliferation, IFN-γ production
	Interferon-γ	IFN-γ	21 kd	CD4 and CD8 T cells, NKT cells (?)	Monocytic cells, most others	Activation, induction of class II MHC, isotypes switching to particular IgGs
	Interleukin-4	IL-4	20 kd	CD4 T cells (NKT cells, mast cells)	B cells, T cells	Isotype switching to IgE, growth and differentiation
	Interleukin-13	IL-13	15 kd	T cells, NK cells (?)	Monocytes, T cells	Differentiation, anti-inflammatory
	Interleukin-5	IL-5	20 kd	T cells	Eosinophils	Activation, differentiation
	Lymphotoxin	LT	24 kd	T cells, others	Endothelial cells, others	Activation, cell death, lymphomorphogenesis
C type chemokine	Lymphotactin	Ltn	12–18 kd	Lymphocytes	NK cells, T cells	Chemoattractant
CC type chemokine	Monocyte chemotactic protein 1	MCP-1 (CCL2)	8–9 kd	Monocytic cells	Monocytes, T cells, NK cells, others	Chemoattractant
	Monocyte chemotactic protein 2	MCP-2 (CCL8)	9 kd	Monocytic cells	Monocytes, T cells, eosinophils, basophils, NK cells	Chemoattractant
	Monocyte chemotactic protein 3	MCP-3 (CCL7)	9 kd	Monocytic cells	Monocytes, T cells, eosinophils, basophils, NK cells, dendritic cells	Chemoattractant
	RANTES	RANTES (CCL5)	7–8 kd	T cells, NK cells	T cells, others	Chemoattractant, antiviral for HIV
	Macrophage inflammatory protein-1α	MIP-1α (CCL3)	7–8 kd	Monocytic cells, T cells, NK cells, others	Monocytes, T cells, NK cells, others	Chemoattractant, promotes antiviral states, antiviral for HIV
	Macrophage inflammatory protein-1β	MIP-1β (CCL4)	7–8 kd	Monocytic cells, others	Monocytes, T cells, others	Chemoattractant
	Eotaxin		8–8 kd	Epithelial cells, phagocytic cells	Eosinophils	Chemoattractant
	Others					
CXC type chemokine	Interleukin 8	IL-8 (CXCL8)	8 kd	Moncytic cells, many	Neutrophils	Chemoattractant
	Gro (α, β, γ)	Gro	8 kd	Fibroblasts, monocytic cells, others	Neutrophils, others	Chemoattractant
	Interferon-γ–induced protein-10	IP-10 (CXCL10)	8–9 kd	Endothelial cells, many	(?) Lymphocytes	Chemoattractant, angiogenesis
	Monokine-induced by interferon-γ	Mig (CXCL9)	11–12 kd	Monocytic cells	Activated T cells, others (?)	Chemoattractant, promotes antiviral states, angiogenesis
	Others					
CX_3C chemokine	Fractalkine	(CX3CL1)	8–9 kd	Endothelial cells	Monocytes, T cells, NK cells	Leukocyte adhesion and extravasation (?)

NK, natural killer; PMN, polymorphonuclear leukocyte; MHC, major histocompatibility complex; IgG, immunoglobulin G; IgE, immunoglobulin E; RANTES, a factor *r*egulated upon *a*ctivation, *n*ormal *T* *e*xpressed and *s*ecreted.

Source: Adapted and modified from ref. 1.

view because events are considered in the context of the intact host and because the existing understanding at this level is still primarily extracellular. Known induction mechanisms and pathways accessed for mediating direct antiviral or direct and indirect immunoregulatory effects are discussed. Because the IFN cytokines induced by viral infections, such as the type I IFN family, appear to be expressed at particular high levels as well as to have unique or uniquely dominant roles in mediating direct antiviral functions and regulating immune responses, these factors are described in extensive detail. Review of type I IFN is at a "higher power" because the intracellular biochemical pathways inducing expression of these factors and delivering their antiviral functions are being precisely defined at the molecular level. The chapter concludes with general discussions of strategies evolved by viruses to avoid or utilize cytokine functions and of cytokine contributions to virus-induced disease.

SPECIFIC CYTOKINE CHARACTERISTICS, IMMUNOREGULATORY FUNCTIONS, AND FACTOR INDUCTION DURING VIRAL INFECTIONS

The immune system traditionally has been divided into innate and adaptive components based on kinetics of responses following primary challenges with infectious agents and on specificity for antigenic determinants associated with protection against secondary challenges. Innate cells, including monocytic cells, NK cells, PMNs, and DCs, express receptors with limited diversity, and tend to respond rapidly as large populations of cells. In contrast, adaptive T- and B-lymphocyte populations express an extensive range of antigen-specific receptors. Primary responses of T and B lymphocytes are delayed because specific subsets of low-frequency cells must be expanded. Innate immunity mediates defense, at times preceding activation of adaptive defense mechanisms. Innate events also make important contributions to shaping downstream immune responses. Such immunoregulatory functions are significant because only subsets of the various component immune responses activate mechanisms most effective in defense against particular challenges. Adaptive immunity is required to clear infections and mediate long-term memory defense. Thus, innate to adaptive responses are cascades in place both to mediate defense during each of the phases and to activate protective downstream immune responses (see Fig. 1). Cytokine constituent responses are known to be of major importance in delivery of both functions. Cell targets for cytokine actions express specific receptors for the factors.

To induce the chain of events activating immune responses most beneficial in defense against a particular infectious organism, the host links information available during the earliest times of infection to subset cascades. Unique microbial structures, distinct from host determinants, provide the early information. The known structures of this type are shared, and tightly conserved, by groups of pathogens sensitive to the same or similar defense mechanisms (181,319). Examples of unique microbial structures of this class are the lipopolysaccharide (LPS) structures on gram-negative bacteria, unmethylated CpG DNA motifs synthesized by invertebrate organisms, and other unique nucleic acid structures, such as double-stranded RNA (dsRNA), not detectable in normal cells but expressed in virus-infected host cells. These structures are sensed through receptors expressed by nonimmune or immune cells and result in activation of particular initial and innate cytokine cascade responses with shaping of downstream innate and adaptive immune responses.

It is difficult to assign responses to either initial or innate response phases. Initial events can be defined as those directly elicited by products of infectious agents, and innate components as those activated by initial response products. The adaptive phase depends on T or B cells. By these definitions, a particular cytokine may be part of all three phases if its expression can be stimulated directly by microbial products, and it can be produced by downstream innate and adaptive responses. Certain cytokines classified as initial or innate (e.g., IFN-α/β, TNF-α, IL-1, and IL-6) are induced in response to microbial products in both nonimmune cells and cells of the innate immune system. Other cytokines can be products of both innate and adaptive immune cells, such as IFN-γ produced by NK cells as well as T cells. A few cytokines, such as IL-2, are exclusively assigned to one phase. These tend to be factors made only or predominantly by cells of the adaptive immune system. Cytokines can be related in terms of genetic homology, structural similarities, and overlapping use of receptor components.

Although much remains to be learned, initial and innate induction of high levels of the type I IFN family of cytokines (e.g., IFN-α/β) appears to be a unique or uniquely dominant characteristic of many viral infections (23,24). Other cytokine cascades often associated with responses to nonviral challenges, however, can sometimes be detected in the context of viral infections (Fig. 2). The cytokines known to be induced and functioning in the different phases of responses to primary viral infections are reviewed here (Table 3). The reader should keep in mind that the material is presented in idealized patterns based on results from infections studied in depth. Not all responses fit into these patterns because the host adapts to different conditions of viral infections, subtle or extreme, to access more appropriate defense mechanisms. Thus, many variations can arise.

Initial and Innate Cytokines

At least two clear pathways induce initial to innate cytokine responses. The first leads to IFN-α/β production

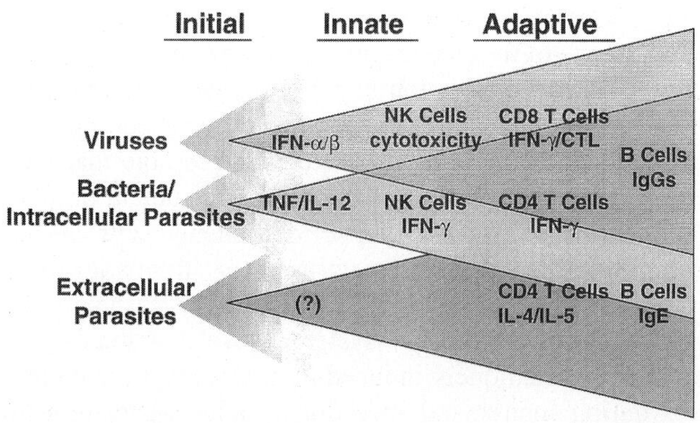

FIG. 2. Key known and proposed cytokine-regulated pathways shaping endogenous immune responses during infection with viruses, bacteria, and intracellular and extracellular parasites. Immune responses to bacteria or intracellular protozoan parasitic infections have dominant innate responses composed of interleukin-12 (IL-12) and natural killer (NK) cell interferon-γ (IFN-γ) production for shaping of downstream T_H1 type responses with CD4 T-cell IFN-γ production. Challenges with certain organisms of these classes also are know to induce an innate cascade of proinflammatory cytokines, including tumor necrosis factor (TNF), IL-1, and IL-6. Responses to extracellular parasites of the helminth group fail to elicit an early IL-12 production and are linked to T_H2 responses with CD4 T-cell IL-4 and IL-5 production. Although responses to viruses have certain characteristics in common with T_H1 responses, they can also have dominant initial IFN-α/β production induced by unique viral products. This response is associated with NK cell cytotoxicity but not IFN-γ production and is frequently accompanied by prominent downstream CD8 T-cell responses, including IFN-γ production and cytotoxic T-lymphocyte (CTL) function. The patterns are idealized, and there can be overlap (represented by triangle overlap). This is clearly demonstrated during certain viral infections by induction of proinflammatory innate cytokine responses with IL-12 and NK cell IFN-γ production and with mixed T-cell cytokine responses.

and is elicited during many viral infections. The second leads to TNF, IL-6, IL-12, and downstream innate IFN-γ and is elicited during many nonviral and certain viral infections. Numbers of other cytokines have been reported to be produced at the same time as, or to facilitate, these pathways. They include IL-1, IL-15, and IL-18. Still others, including IL-10 and transforming growth factor-β (TGF-β), have the potential to regulate particular innate cytokine responses negatively.

Interferon-α/β Cascade and a Potential Interleukin-15 Branch

Interferon-α/β

The type I IFNs are a superfamily with four subfamilies: IFN-α, IFN-β, IFN-ω, and IFN-τ. The IFN-α/β members are the best characterized and are known to be induced in response to viral infections. The factors are products of a single IFN-β and multiple IFN-α genes (222,297). They can be made by virtually any cell type in response to appropriate stimulation, and intracellular infections with viruses can be potent stimulators of IFN-α/β. These cytokines were first identified by their antiviral functions.

The transcriptional activation of the IFN-α and IFN-β genes is being extensively defined in regard to various mechanisms underlying stimulation during infections. Regulation of IFN-α/β genes is complex with potential for many pathways to expression. A well-characterized pathway is from one microbial product, that is, dsRNA, expressed in certain virus-infected, but not in uninfected, cells. Others, however, including interactions between certain viruses and their receptors and intracellular expression of particular viral proteins, exists (100,306). Several positive and negative regulatory gene elements

TABLE 3. *Cytokines induced during viral infections*

	Cytokine expression	
Virus	Initial and innate	Adaptive
Lymphocytic choriomeningitis virus	IFN-α/β	IFN-γ, IL-2 IL-4, TGF-β
Murine cytomegalovirus	IFN-α/β TNF, IL-1α, IL-6 IL-12, IFN-γ	IFN-γ, IL-2
Herpes simplex virus type 1	IFN-α/β TNF, IL-1α, IL-6 IL-12, IFN-γ	IFN-γ, IL-2 IL-4, IL-5
Influenza	IFN-α/β TNF, IL-18 IL-12, IFN-γ	IFN-γ, IL-2 IL-4, IL-5, IL-10
Human immunodeficiency virus	?	IFN-γ, IL-2 IL-4, IL-5, IL-10
Respiratory syncytial virus	IFN-γ IL-1, IL-6	IFN-γ, IL-2 IL-4, IL-5, IL-10

IFN, interferon; IL, interleukin; TGF, transforming growth factor; TNF, tumor necrosis factor.

participate in the transcriptional regulation process by binding specific transcription factors activated upon virus infections. The transcription factors are present in inactive forms in the cytoplasm of all cells. Their activation often requires phosphorylation of specific serine and threonine residues. The protein kinases involved in this process remain elusive, although participation of the IκB kinase complex and protein kinase R (PKR) in activating the NFκB transcription factor has been demonstrated (172). NFκB is one of the factors required for inducing transcription of the IFN-β gene and certain IFN-α genes. The other activated factors needed for induction of all IFN genes constitute the family of interferon regulatory factors (IRFs). There are at least 10 members of the IRF family (198). These molecules contain DNA-binding domains recognizing specific DNA elements (the interferon response element) in the IFN genes and in many IFN-inducible genes. The IRFs also contain transcriptional regulatory domains to activate or repress transcription, depending on the cell and gene context. Some IRFs are constitutively present in cells, whereas others are induced by IFNs. A few IRFs have cell type–dependent expression. The two IRFs most relevant for induction of the IFN genes are IRF-3 and IRF-7. A virus-activated factor that also mediates this process contains IRF-3, IRF-7, and the transcriptional coactivators p300 and the creb-binding protein (CBP) (306). This complex, in conjunction with NFκB and Atf-2/c-Jun, is recruited to the promoter region of the IFN-β gene to activate its transcription.

An interesting cascade operating in the IFN gene induction process has been recently discovered (173). The first members of this cascade are the IFN-β and specific IFN-α genes. They are activated by virus infection through the use of ubiquitously present IRF-3. These IFNs are then secreted and act through the IFN-α/β receptor to induce synthesis of IRF-7, not usually present in untreated cells. IRF-7, in turn, is used for the induction of other IFN-α members whose genes cannot be induced by IRF-3. This observation provides a molecular explanation for the phenomenon of priming for viral infection–induced IFN production by pretreating cells with a low IFN dose. It also couples, in a physiologic sense, the signal transduction pathways and the transcriptional induction mechanisms used by IFN and IFN-inducible genes. Thus, the direct intracellular signaling pathways for initial IFN-α/β induction, in response to infections, are being delineated clearly, and secondary type I IFN responses are induced in innate response to expression of the initial IFN-α/β gene products.

There are likely to be many additional mechanisms for IFN induction. The existence of the complex gene family may in fact be in place to respond to different stimulatory pathways. Several other biochemical pathways to IFN-α/β expression being identified include pathways induced during nonviral infections (66) or in response to the CpG DNA motifs synthesized by bacteria (15,277, 288). Some of these mechanisms may preferentially stimulate IFN-α/β expression in particular cell types because they are preferred targets or are uniquely equipped to respond. In this regard, it is interesting to note that low-frequency populations of human DCs are potent producers of type I IFN in response to challenge with herpes simplex virus or influenza virus or to stimulation with CD40L (40,73,264). Much remains to be learned about IFN-α/β expression, but systemic levels of the factors appear to be uniquely induced to high and sustained levels during many viral infections, including those with lymphocytic choriomeningitis virus (LCMV) and murine cytomegalovirus (MCMV) (22,24). Production at this level is likely to be in part the result of recruiting large numbers of cells, including nonimmune cell types such as fibroblasts and vascular endothelial cells, into IFN-α/β production. Major functions for such systemic and sustained IFN-α/β responses are to protect the many different host compartments and distal sites at risk for spreading or for secondary waves of infections. The conditions, however, are also likely to exert unique immunoregulatory effects on ongoing and developing immune responses (see later). A few viruses are reported to be poor inducers of IFN-α/β—most notably, respiratory syncytial virus (RSV) (45,232).

All nucleated cells express IFN-α/βRs. These are heterodimers comprised of IFNAR1 and IFNAR2c chains. A variety of generalized antiviral and cell-type specific immunoregulatory functions are activated as a result of binding the IFN-α/β forms to these receptors. The information available on the intracellular biochemical pathways activated through the IFN-α/βRs and on the complex potential and known immunoregulatory functions of IFN-α/β is reviewed later. Many IFN-α/β actions have been identified in vivo. Although some of these are direct, others are likely to be secondary effects. IFN-α/β cytokines can regulate expression of a number of other cytokines and cytokine receptors and, as a result, modify downstream consequences mediated by other factors.

Interleukin-15

In the context of cytokine cascades, IFN-α/β expression has a possible link to the induction of another innate cytokine, IL-15 (299). This factor was first identified as a stimulator of T-cell responses but is now known to activate both NK and T cells to proliferate, to be important for NK cell development, and to have a variety of other immunoregulatory functions. It is thought to be made by a number of different cell types and is known to be produced by monocytic cells in response to appropriate stimulation. The high-affinity receptor for IL-15 is a trimer (IL-15R) with α, β, and γ chains (299). The IL-15Rα chain is specific for IL-15, but the β and γ chains also bind the adaptive cytokine, IL-2, with a lower affinity and associate with an IL-2Rα chain to form the high-affinity IL-2R receptor. IL-15 can be made by a variety of cells, including monocytic cells. This cytokine may be induced with other proinflammatory cytokines (37). Its induction at the mRNA level, however, has also been observed after stimulation with type I IFNs, chemical inducers of type I IFNs, or viral infections (12,75,322). Expression of IL-15 is dependent on IRF-1, and this transcription factor can be activated by stimulation with IFN-α/β. Thus, there is a potential for IL-15 to be induced during viral infections either through direct stimulation or indirectly as a result of IFN-α/β–mediated effects.

Other Immunoregulatory Functions of Interferon-α/β

IFN-α/β can positively or negatively regulate other cytokine functions by modulating expression of these factors or their receptors. Of particular relevance during innate responses, type I IFNs can inhibit expression of IL-12 (52,124,180). Other early changes induced by or associated with IFN-α/β expression are modifications in immune cell distribution *in vivo* (22,24,99,115), activation of NK cell cytotoxic activity (22), inhibition of NK cell responsiveness to IL-12 (200), *in vivo* induction of modest NK cell and memory CD8 T-cell proliferation (22,289), enhancement of pathways for presenting antigen on class I molecules of the major histocompatibility complex (MHC) (see later), and facilitation of T-cell IFN-γ responses (31,53,234,235,251). Thus, the products of the initial and innate induction of the IFN-α/β cascade have the potential to regulate a variety of downstream innate and adaptive immune responses. Moreover, at extremely high concentrations, IFN-α/β inhibits the proliferation of a variety of cell types.

The Tumor Necrosis Factor-α, Interleukin-1, Interleukin-6 Cascade and an Interleukin-12, Interferon-γ Branch

Other initial and innate cytokine responses may include a cascade of TNF-α, IL-1, and IL-6. This clustered response has been best characterized after stimulation with LPS components from gram-negative bacteria (1). TNF-α expression appears to be a major regulator of the cascade because treatment with factor alone induces the other two cytokines, but LPS can induce IL-1 in the absence of TNF-α. Often called the proinflammatory cytokine cascade, this response is generally detectable during inflammation. IFN-α can sometimes be seen under these conditions (86), but it is not clear that the factor is induced to the levels elicited by viral infections. Additional cytokines, such as IL-12, IL-15, IL-18, and NK cell–produced IFN-γ, have also been reported to be associated with the innate TNF-α, IL-1, and IL-6 cascade under particular conditions, most notably stimulation with bacteria and bacterial products. An understanding of pathways to induction of this cytokine cluster is advancing. For example, CD14 and Toll-related receptors act in concert to bind LPS to induce signal transduction cascades, ultimately activating expression of the TNF-α, IL-1, and IL-6 genes (135,319).

Although the list of conditions under which certain of these proinflammatory cytokines are produced during viral infections is growing, less is known about how viruses elicit them. Expression of messenger RNA (mRNA) or protein is elevated for TNF-α, two major forms of IL-1, IL-6, and the two chains of heterodimeric IL-12 during infections with a variety of viruses, particularly the herpesviruses, including cytomegalovirus (CMV) (see Table 3) (2,121,122,192,207,208,226,243,244). TNF-α, IL-6, and IL-12 proteins are all expressed in the circulation during some viral infections and IL-18 has been detected during MCMV infection (223). The IL-1 cytokines are not readily detectable at the protein level. Induction of biologically active IL-12 during initial and innate immune responses elicits downstream induction of IFN-γ production by NK cells, and NK cell–produced IFN-γ can also be detected in the circulation during MCMV infections (208,209,243). The systemic TNF-α, IL-1, and IL-6, as well as the IL-12–to–IFN-γ branch, cascade responses are likely to be in place to induce antimicrobial functions, promote inflammation at distal sites, and communicate with other organs, such as the brain and liver, to elicit secondary responses. As is the case with most cytokines, these responses must be tightly controlled. Under conditions of profound stimulation, including bacterial sepsis and certain viral infections, constituents of the proinflammatory cascade can be produced systemically, reach high levels in serum, and induce toxic shock conditions with coagulation, vascular collapse, and death.

TNF-α

Many of the important biologic functions mediated by TNF-α are related to its inflammation-promoting activity, that is, induction of enhanced adhesive properties of vascular endothelial cells and PMNs as well as vascular permeability (1,134,300). TNF-α mediates a variety of additional immunoregulatory and antiviral functions. Cell death (320), activation of monocytic cell functions (1), DC migration (231,302), enhancement of IFN-γ responses (1), up-regulation of class I MHC expression (1,296), and activation of certain antiviral pathways (91,159,197,314) are among the responses known to be induced by or associated with TNF-α expression. Under toxic shock conditions, TNF-α is required for disease induction and the detrimental conditions resulting in death (105,134). During systemic responses, the cytokine can also function as an "endogenous pyrogen" to communicate with hypothalamic regions of the brain and induce fever (1). TNF-α is made by a number of cell types, but activated monocytic cells are often the major producers. It is a member of a cytokine family including a related form, called lymphotoxin (LT), made primarily as an adaptive cytokine (41). TNF-α is synthesized as a type II membrane protein. The released form of the molecule is produced by proteolytic cleavage at an extracellular, membrane-proximal site. Both membrane-bound and released forms can mediate biologic functions. A number of different receptors for TNF-α, including TNF receptors type 1 (TNFR1) and 2 (TNFR2), are expressed on diverse cell types (283).

Interleukin-1 and Interleukin-6

The other members of this cascade, IL-1 and IL-6, are also made by both nonimmune cells and cells of the immune system. In comparison to TNF-α, however, they appear to be induced more readily in particular nonimmune cells (1). There are three gene products in the IL-1 family: IL-1α and IL-1β, functioning as stimulatory factors, and an IL-1 receptor antagonist, IL-1ra. Both IL-1α and IL-1β are synthesized as precursor molecules requiring proteolytic cleavage to generate mature forms. The IL-1α precursor may have some biologic activity, but the IL-1β form has to be cleaved to acquire function. An IL-1 protease, called the IL-1β-converting enzyme (ICE), or caspase 1, is responsible for most of the IL-1β processing (71,150). All three products of the IL-1 gene family can bind to two different characterized receptors. A type 1 receptor, however, may have higher affinity for IL-1β and is primarily responsible for IL-1–mediated responses. The type 1 receptor is expressed on virtually all cell types. A type 2 receptor can competitively inhibit IL-1 binding to the functional type 1 receptor and may be expressed on a more limited range of cell types. The functions mediated by IL-1 overlap with those mediated by TNF, in that the factor has been reported to enhance inflammatory and IFN-γ responses and to be an endogenous pyrogen. In contrast to TNF-α, however, it does not appear to be required for many of the detrimental effects induced during cascade responses but can be a major contributor to eliciting IL-6. The two best-characterized functions of IL-6 are to promote B-cell growth and activate hepatocytes (1). Thus, prominent features of the proinflammatory cascade in total are (a) toxic potential of TNF-α, (b) overlapping functions for TNF-α and IL-1 in promoting inflammation and communication with the brain, (c) IL-1 induction of IL-6, and (d) unique IL-6–dependent links to other immune and hepatic responses.

Interleukin-12

Expression of IL-12, IFN-γ, IL-15, and IL-18 can also be induced under conditions of LPS stimulation (37,279,317). In contrast to the expression of TNF-α, IL-1, and IL-6 by a variety of cell types, IL-12 appears to be primarily produced by monocytic cells, certain DCs, and PMNs (290). IL-12 is unusual among cytokines because it is a heterodimeric molecule composed of 35-kd (p35) and 40-kd (p40) subunits. Generally, the p35 subunit is constitutively expressed, and the p40 subunit is induced in response to challenge. Biologic activity is dependent on the presence of both chains. The receptor for IL-12 is composed of two subunits, the β1 and β2 chains, and is primarily expressed by NK and T cells (290). IL-12 was originally identified as a potent inducer of cytotoxicity and IFN-γ production by NK cells and activated T cells. It is now clear that a major function for the factor is induction of NK cell IFN-γ production under conditions of challenge with a variety of agents (21). It also appears to promote a particular subset of CD4 T-cell responses associated with IL-2 and IFN-γ production (21,170,290).

Interferon-γ

IFN-γ was originally called type II because it can induce antiviral states. It was called immune IFN because, in contrast to the type I IFNs, it is made exclusively by cells of the immune system (29). IFN-γ is primarily an NK cell product during innate responses, but it can be made by T cells during adaptive responses. A heterodimeric IFN-γ receptor, distinct from the IFN-α/β receptor with IFNGR1 and IFNGR2 molecules, is expressed on virtually all nucleated cells. Despite the use of different receptors, certain IFN-α/β and IFN-γ functions are shared because the signal transduction pathways activated through these receptors partly overlap (see later). However, IFN-γ can mediate a number of unique immunoregulatory functions. Activation of monocytic cells to deliver antimicrobial defense mechanisms is an extremely important IFN-γ function. After exposure to this cytokine, mononuclear phagocytes are induced to synthesize enzymes required for reactive oxygen intermediates contributing to the killing of phagocytosed organisms, particularly bacteria. IFN-γ can act alone to induce nitric oxide synthase 2 (NOS2 or iNOS) (165). This enzyme contributes to the production of NO radicals for antimicrobial defense against a variety of agents, including viruses. TNF can enhance iNOS induction by either IFN-γ or IFN-α/β, but the IFN-γ effects are more potent. Thus, IFN-γ is an important intermediary in induction of known effector mechanisms contributing to resistance against infections. Because there is a growing list of other enzyme responses to IFN-γ, including the induction of a series of molecules having homologies to enzymes dephosphorylating guanosine triphosphate (GTP), that is, GTPases (28,36,286, 287), there are likely to be additional or alternative mechanisms for IFN-γ–induced antimicrobial defense. IFN-γ can promote and amplify inflammatory responses by upregulating expression of TNF receptors to potentiate the effects of this cytokine and by activating vascular endothelial cells. Finally, IFN-γ enhances expression of a particular subset of chemokines. All of the effector mechanisms and inflammatory pathways are important consequences of IFN-γ induction during either innate or adaptive responses.

A number of other immunoregulatory functions can be mediated or induced by IFN-γ. IFN-γ can activate NK cell cytotoxicity, but this may be of less importance than IFN-α/β activation during viral infections (22,92,208,211). Many other immunoregulatory functions appear to be in place to shape the development of adaptive immune responses. In particular, IFN-γ induces increased class I and class II MHC expression on a wide variety of cell types (164), enhances CD4 T-cell differentiation to responses associated with IL-2 and IFN-γ production by promoting expression of the IL-12 receptor (92,235,278), and acts on B cells to facilitate immunoglobulin class switching to particular subclasses, most notably immunoglobulin G2a (IgG2a) in the mouse (21). Taken together with the enhancement of mononuclear phagocytic cell functions, these immunoregulatory effects of IFN-γ are likely to be most important in promoting antigen processing and presentation to CD4 T cells and in helping particular antibody responses against extracellular pathogens.

Interleukin-18

Less is known about the induction and function of IL-15 and IL-18. The IL-15 characteristics and proposed IFN-α/β induction were reviewed earlier. IL-18 was identified by its ability to promote IFN-γ expression, and as a result, it was first named IFN-γ–inducing factor (IGIF) (204). It is also sometimes called IL-1γ because it has structural and biochemical similarities to the other IL-1 molecules. In particular, it is synthesized as an inactive precursor molecule and requires proteolytic cleavage by ICE (or other caspases) for release of the active form (71,87,101). Although only limited information is available concerning the IL-18 receptor, it is known to be different from those binding IL-1. It appears to be expressed on NK, T, and B cells. IFN-γ expression can be induced by IL-18 alone or in synergy with IL-12. Most of the work characterizing induction of IL-18 expression has been done following stimulation with Propionibacterium acnes and LPS challenges. The cytokine appears to be readily elicited in response to this stimulation protocol and is found at high levels in liver (176,279). A natural soluble binding factor exists, IL-18–binding protein (203). IL-18 may not be required for driving T-cell IL-2 and IFN-γ responses, but it can enhance them by facilitating IFN-γ production and T-cell IL-12 receptor expression (233). In addition, there are intriguing data that indicate that IL-18 can act with IFN-α/β in promoting T-cell IFN-γ responses (251).

Other Innate Cytokines

A number of other cytokines made by nonimmune or innate immune cells have the potential to mediate immunoregulatory functions during infections, including IL-10 and TGF-β, factors known to be potent inhibitors of IFN-γ expression (163,239). These cytokines are induced under particular conditions of viral infections (250,276). Nonadaptive immune cell populations can be sources of the factors, but IL-10 and TGF-β have been more frequently observed at times of adaptive immune responses to viral infections.

Two other cytokines, IL-4 and IL-13, have structural similarities, share receptor components for intracellular signaling, induce overlapping biologic responses, and have potential to inhibit IFN-γ expression and promote a subset of CD4 T-cell responses associated with IL-4, IL-13, and IL-5 production (44). These cytokines can be produced during adaptive immune responses and are induced at times of T-cell responses to certain viral infections. Little is known, however, about their expression during innate responses. Populations of mast cells and NK T cells, with similarities to classic NK cells but also expressing T-cell receptors for antigens, can be induced to make IL-4 under particular conditions of stimulation (18). It is not yet clear, however, whether these responses are activated during innate immune responses to challenge, and there is no definitive evidence for IL-4 stimulation during innate responses to viral infections. Likewise, although NK cell subsets making IL-5 or IL-13, but not IFN-γ (22,110,220), have been identified, infection conditions under which such populations would be induced have not yet been defined.

Adaptive Cytokines

In comparison with initial and innate cytokine responses, adaptive cytokine responses are delayed and are associated with T-cell activation. A number of cytokines are produced during adaptive immune responses. Some of these are made exclusively by T cells. Some, however, are also made by other cell types but are produced at moderate or high levels by activated T cells. T-cell subsets can develop to produce preferentially particular adaptive cytokines, and the subset responses have been shown to be associated with defense against particular types of agents (see Fig. 2) or types of cytokine-mediated disease. For example, helper T-cell subtype 1 (T_H1) responses result in high production of IL-2 and IFN-γ, are major contributors to delayed type hypersensitivity, and contribute to defense against bacterial or intracellular protozoan parasite infections (21,130,218). In contrast, helper T-cell subtype 2 (T_H2) responses result in IL-4, IL-13, and IL-5 production; are associated with antigen-induced airway hyperresponsiveness (asthma); and contribute to defense against certain parasitic infections (218,313). In general, polarization toward T_H1 responses is beneficial in defense against nonviral intracellular pathogens because IFN-γ activates macrophage-dependent antimicrobial functions against such organisms. Development of T_H2 responses is beneficial in defense against extracellular parasitic pathogens, such as helminths, in part because IL-5 elicits production and recruitment of eosinophils and defense mechanisms delivered by these cells. Both cytokine profiles can promote B-cell production of antibody but are associated with different classes of antibody isotype production. High-level production of IgE is a characteristic of T_H2 responses.

The picture emerging from *in vitro* experiments and studies of nonviral infections is that development of a particular adaptive cytokine response is dependent on activation of T cells through their receptors for antigen (TCRs), the magnitude of stimulation, and the cytokine milieu in which the T cells are stimulated (2,25,92,235, 260,278). For the most part, "polarized" subset responses have been characterized with CD4 T cells. Antigens for their activation are processed from extracellular forms and presented by class II MHC molecules. They are called helper responses because they promote T- or B-cell responses. As stated earlier, induction of IL-12 and IFN-γ during innate immune responses preferentially promotes T_H1 CD4 T cells. In contrast, T_H2 CD4 T cells are promoted by the absence of IL-12 and IFN-γ and the presence of IL-4 and IL-10 (218). A variety of infections with nonviral agents have been shown to result in polarized T_H1 or T_H2 profiles, but the T-cell cytokine responses characterized during a number of viral infections appear to be of a more mixed phenotype (see Fig. 2 and Table 3). In addition, some infections, particularly viral, induce CD8 T-cell responses. Antigens for activation of these cells are usually processed from intracellular forms and presented by class I MHC molecules. CD8 T-cell responses are generally associated with IFN-γ expression and MHC class I–restricted, cytotoxic T-lymphocyte (CTL) function. Our understanding of the innate response conditions promoting particular CD8 T-cell functions is still limited.

Type 1 T-Cell Cytokine Responses

Interleukin-2

T cells produce IL-2, and a major function for this factor is promoting T-cell proliferation. Activated T cells express the high-affinity trimeric form of IL-2R, comprised of the γ and β chains shared with IL-15R and a specific IL-2Rα chain (299). NK cells generally express the γ and β chains but are infrequently found with the high-affinity form of IL-2R. As a result, NK cells can be activated in response to IL-2 but are much less efficient than activated T cells in binding and utilizing the factor at the major times of production. In addition to acting as an autocrine growth factor for T cells, IL-2 is a potent inducer or facilitator of T-cell IFN-γ production (51,271). B cells can respond to IL-2, and the factor promotes antibody synthesis. Viral infections have been shown to induce IL-2 expression (see Table 3). CD4 T cells are major producers, but CD8 T cells can express IL-2 under conditions of profound activation and during certain viral infections (2,51,128,129,275).

Interferon-γ

Given its roles in supporting T-cell expansion and enhancing IFN-γ expression, it is not a coincidence that IL-2 production is associated with T-cell IFN-γ responses. T-cell IFN-γ production is an important contributor to antiviral defense, and the pathways accessed for this are similar to those used by NK cell–produced IFN-γ. The same cytokine is simply being made by two different cell types. The immunoregulatory functions, including facilitating switching of immunoglobulin classes and enhancement of antigen processing and presentation on MHC molecules, also predictably overlap. A major difference between NK cell and T-cell responses, however, is that T-cell responses are sustained for longer periods of time. As a result, there is potential for continued access to T-cell IFN-γ production. Another apparent difference is that in contrast to the systemic NK cell IFN-γ responses sometimes observed early during infections, T-cell IFN-γ responses appear to be more often restricted to particular compartments. A likely contributing factor is the profound stimulatory effect for IFN-γ expression mediated through TCR engagement (2,38). This signaling pathway needs T-cell exposure to antigen presented on MHC molecules. As a result, it provides an intrinsic regulation for need; that is, if viral antigen is cleared in vivo, T cells will not be stimulated through their TCRs.

A chain of events with innate IL-12 and NK cell IFN-γ responses facilitating adaptive CD4 T-cell IFN-γ responses is required to achieve optimal protection against nonviral, intracellular bacterial infections such as those with Listeria monocytogenes (130). Through this pathway, an NK cell IFN-γ response can "pass off" a major function to a longer lasting-lymphocyte subset with different conditions for responding. It is not clear that such a pathway is needed during viral infections. CD4 T cells are induced to produce IFN-γ, but T-cell IFN-γ responses have been observed in the absence of endogenous biologically active IL-12, during a number of viral infection (53,188,207,213,258). This may be in part because many viruses elicit specific CD8 T-cell responses primed to produce high levels of IFN-γ upon engagement of their TCRs. Most notable among these are infections of humans with Epstein-Barr virus (EBV) (141), influenza virus (55), and human immunodeficiency virus (HIV) (55,116) and infections of mice with LCMV (34,53,194), influenza virus (78), polyomavirus (160), and murine gamma-herpesvirus 68 (MHV-68) (274). Studies in culture suggest that the requirements for IFN-γ expression in response to TCR stimulation are different for CD8 than for CD4 T cells, or that CD8 T cells may be more readily induced to produce IFN-γ (38). Another pathway with IFN-α/β promoting CD8 T-cell IFN-γ responses is being defined in the context of viral infections (see later).

Type 2 T-Cell Cytokine Responses

Interleukin-4 and Interleukin-13

As stated earlier, IL-4 and IL-13 have structural and functional similarities. T cells are major producers of both cytokines. IL-4 was first identified by its function in promoting B-cell responses. It is now know to be important in regulating IgE production and mast cell and eosinophil functions (1). IL-13 mediates overlapping functions, and both cytokines appear to contribute to recruitment of cells into tissues during allergic reactions (1,313). The cytokines use a common dimeric receptor expressed largely on nonlymphoid cells, including macrophages and vascular endothelial cells. One of these chains, however, can pair with the γ chain common to the IL-15 and IL-2 receptors to form a specific IL-4 receptor on lymphocytes. Although polarized T_H1 and T_H2 responses are induced during certain nonviral infections, a number of different viral infections have been reported to express some level of IL-4 along with IL-2 and IFN-γ (see Table 3). For the most part, IL-4 appears to be expressed at very low levels. Little information is available concerning the induction and function of IL-13 during viral challenges.

Interleukin-5

The major known function of IL-5 is induction and activation of eosinophils. These populations have not been observed frequently, or reported to mediate defense, during viral infections. They have been detected during respiratory viral infections, in particular those with RSV, and a predisposition for IL-5 expression after infectious challenge is induced by vaccination with the heavily glycosylated RSV G protein (see Table 3) (107,112, 206,269).

Other Cytokines Made by T Cells

Lymphotoxin

T cells make a variety of other cytokines, including TGF-β and IL-10. They can make TNF-α but do not appear to be a major source of the factor under most conditions of in vivo challenge. They are important producers of a related cytokine, LT. LT has been called TNF-β because of its homology to TNF-α. It can compete for binding to TNF receptors. As a result of binding to these, it can induce functions overlapping with TNF. However, LT can also form a unique complex recognized by a different receptor identified as the LT β-receptor. This cytokine is often produced along with IFN-γ by activated T cells and is generally considered part of T_H1 responses. A major unique function of LT is promotion of lymphomorphogenesis (41). Induction of LT expression at the mRNA level has been reported during a number of infections, but protective functions specifically mediated by LT under these conditions have not been defined.

UNFOLDING OF ENDOGENOUS IMMUNE RESPONSES DURING VIRAL INFECTIONS

The kinetics of virus-induced immune responses, as revealed during primary purposeful infections of mice and natural human infections, is schematically presented in Figure 3. Certain viruses activate component responses overlapping with those characterized as T_H1, but they also appear to elicit unique components. In particular, during initial and innate immune responses, uniquely dominant characteristics include prominent initial and innate IFN-α/β release and NK cell cytotoxicity (22,208). In LCMV infections of immunocompetent mice, IFN-α/β responses are observed without induction of detectable IL-12 (52,207). Moreover, although there are examples of both IFN-α/β and IL-12 initial and innate responses after infections with MCMV or influenza virus (188,207), they have dichotomous functions. During MCMV infections, IFN-α/β is necessary for induction of NK cell–mediated cytotoxicity but not IFN-γ production. Conversely, and in contrast to the IL-12 role in activation of both NK cell responses during certain nonviral infections (23,256), IL-12 is required for MCMV infection–induced NK cell IFN-γ production but not cytotoxic activity (207,208). Many of the NK cell–mediated antiviral effects depend on their being induced to make IFN-γ (22,207,210), but the contribution of NK cell–mediated cytotoxicity to defense is less well documented (22,284). Thus, there are examples of initial and innate cytokine responses to viral infections sharing characteristics with those setting up for T_H1 responses during nonviral infections. These are associated with induction of NK cell–mediated antiviral effects, but there is also induction of IFN-α/β under these conditions. Moreover, certain viral infections induce IFN-α/β but fail to induce detectable IL-12.

In addition to the differences observed during initial and innate events, adaptive immune responses to viral infections can be contrasted with those to nonviral infections in terms of CD4 T_H1 and T_H2 and magnitudes of CD8 T-cell responses. Studies examining expression of the T_H1 cytokines, IL-2 and IFN-γ, and the T_H2 cytokines, IL-4 and IL-5, indicate that T-cell responses to viral infections can be of mixed phenotypes with high IFN-γ, moderate IL-2, and low IL-4 levels (35,97,112,166,167,187, 201,237,250,275,310) (see Table 3). Moreover, CD8 T-cell responses can be induced to uniquely high levels with profound expansion, along with priming and activation of

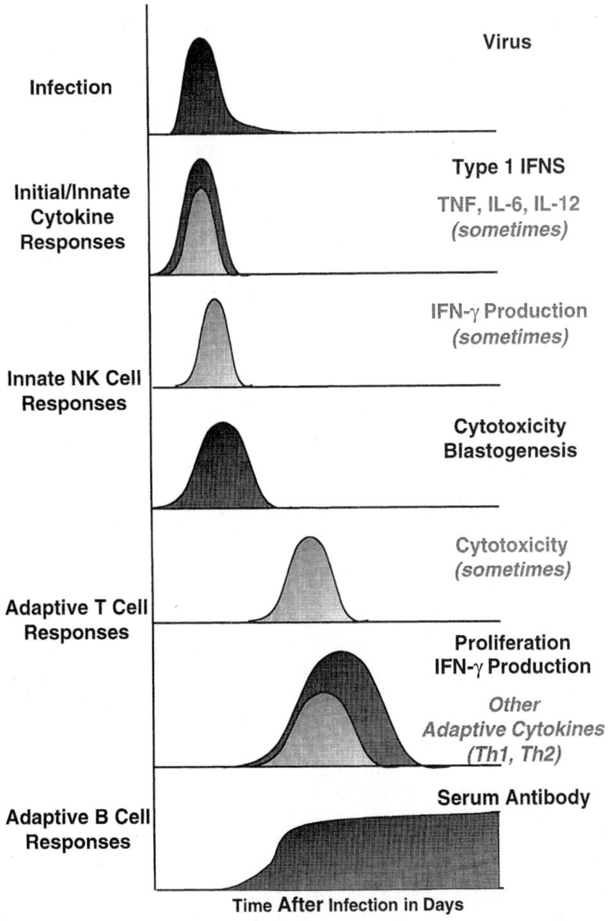

FIG. 3. Kinetics of known endogenous cytokine and cellular immune responses to viral infections during primary challenges. Initial events can include induction of prominent interferon (IFN)-α/β responses. Some viral infections also induce detectable tumor necrosis factor (TNF), interleukin-6 (IL-6), and IL-12 responses with an associated natural killer (NK) cell IFN-γ production. NK cell cytotoxicity and blastogenesis are elicited as a result IFN-α/β responses. Adaptive responses include CD4 and CD8 T-cell responses with high-level expression of IFN-γ, moderate expression of the T_H1 cytokine IL-2, and low-level production of the T_H2 cytokine IL-4. Dramatic CD8 T-cell proliferation with IFN-γ production can be induced in a wide range of infections. Class I–restricted and virus-specific cytotoxicity mediated by CD8 T cells can be detected during some viral infections. B-cell antibody responses are extended for long periods of time.

IFN-γ production and cytotoxicity (2,6,34,53,78,194, 274). Because these CD8 T-cell responses contribute to antiviral defense, their induction is important to the host. Remarkably, IL-12–independent T-cell IFN-γ responses have been demonstrated during LCMV (53,207,213), influenza virus (188), and MHV (258) infections. Moreover, patients with deficiencies in IL-12 responsiveness have notably increased susceptibility to bacterial, but not viral, infections (5,62). Thus, the paradigm emerging from the studies of nonviral agents—that IL-12 is a required innate cytokine for promoting critical T-cell IFN-γ responses—cannot be applied to the viral infections studied to date.

Given the direct pathways to IFN-α/β induction and the many immunoregulatory functions of cytokines, these factors are good-candidate molecules for dominant regulators of endogenous adaptive immune responses to viral infections; that is, they provide the key link between information available at early times during the infection and downstream immune responses. As stated previously, their expression results in profound early changes in cell distributions and modifies expression and function of other cytokines. By recruiting T- and B-cell repertoires into specialized areas for antigen presentation, the IFN-α/β–induced trafficking changes may increase the likelihood of activation of low-frequency antigen specific cells. Alternatively or additionally, they may localize adaptive cell populations into specific cytokine milieus elicited during innate responses to viral infections, and these could in turn mediate immunoregulatory functions directing downstream immune responses.

They may also uniquely regulate the endogenous cytokine milieu to promote the particular T-cell subset responses needed during viral infections. IFN-α/β set up conditions actively inhibiting IL-12–regulated pathways because they block IL-12 induction (52,53,124,180). This may be important to protect against viral infection–enhanced sensitivity to IL-12–induced toxicities (210, 212) but would also limit access to a pathway promoting CD4 T-cell IFN-γ responses. On the other hand, IFN-α/β may drive preferential stimulation of CD8 T-cell responses by enhancing class I MHC presentation, or IFN-α/β–induced NK cell-mediated cytotoxicity may negatively regulate T-cell responses (22,273). Finally, recent studies of a limited number of viral infections—influenza virus (83), herpes simplex virus (HSV) (144), and Sindbis virus (245)—in mice deficient in IFN-α/β functions show that these cytokines modulate viral cell tropism. If so, the characteristics of the primary host immune responses might be altered because of differences in antigen presentation or cytokine production resulting from infection of different target cells. Thus, many of the effects mediated by IFN-α/β have the potential to promote particular T-cell subset responses during viral infections.

Nevertheless, understanding of exactly how CD8 T cells are regulated *in vivo* is still limited. IFN-α/β can enhance human T-cell IFN-γ production under certain specific conditions in culture. However, experiments to date have examined only IFN-γ roles for modest effects in association with IL-12 (169), for CD4 T-cell subset IFN-γ responses (31,234,235), and for dramatic effects in association with IL-18 (251). Studies of the effects of blocking endogenous IFN-α/β functions during infections of mice with LCMV indicate that two divergent supporting pathways can act to promote CD8 T-cell

IFN-γ responses (53). Under normal conditions of infections, the CD8 T-cell IFN-γ response is dependent on endogenous IFN-α/β effects but is IL-12 independent. In contrast, in the absence of IFN-α/β functions, an IL-12 response is revealed to substitute an alternative pathway to IFN-γ. Thus, there appear to be important IFN-α/β–controlled pathways uniquely shaping T-cell IFN-γ responses during viral infections, but the immune system has plasticity for accessing divergent innate mechanisms to achieve the same goal.

Although there are mechanisms by which IFN-α/β may promote activation of CD8 T cells and CD8 T-cell IFN-γ responses, the cytokines are not essential for induction of CD8 T-cell cytotoxic function. Deficiencies in IFN-α/β functions are associated with poor detectable CTL responses during LCMV, but not vaccinia virus (VV), infections (193,294). CD8 T-cell cytotoxicity is essential for antiviral defense during certain viral infections (118), but the requirements for eliciting CTLs *in vivo* are poorly understood. IL-2 promotes CD8 T-cell expansion *in vivo* and enhances IFN-γ production by these cells (51,275). As a result of supporting cell expansion, the factor also enhances the magnitude of CTL responses (51). It is not, however, absolutely required for *in vivo* induction of CD8 T-cell–mediated cytotoxicity (51,137). This may be in part because mixed cytokine responses can be observed during viral infections and because IL-4 can support certain CD8 T-cell responses (14). Alternatively or additionally, IL-15 made by non–T-cell populations may help promote CD8 T-cell responses (299). CD4 T-cell help for induction of acute CD8 T-cell responses is observed in some but not all viral infections (68,191,227), but CD4 T cells or IFN-γ responses may be important for the general maintenance of CD8 T-cell memory (2,298). IFN-γ does not appear to be required for CTL induction (96).

Acute and vaccine-induced changes in the conditions of RSV infections merit special consideration. Responses to respiratory infections with this virus appear to stand out from those characterized during many other viruses because RSV is a poor IFN-α/β inducer (45,232), eosinophils can sometimes be observed during infections with this agent (85), and vaccination with the highly glycosylated RSV G protein can predispose host responses upon challenge with the infectious agent to include IL-5 production and an accompanying lung pathology (7,94,206,269,304). Surprisingly, vaccination with one RSV antigen epitope presented to CD8 T cells as well as the G protein can enhance IFN-γ production and protect against priming for the detrimental IL-5 response and disease (268). These observations suggest that there may be a particular requirement for inducing CD8 T-cell IFN-γ responses at times of secondary CD4 T-cell responses to drive T_H1 over T_H2 responses preferentially to RSV. Although highly speculative, it is possible that the requirement is a result of the fact that alternative IFN-α/β–facilitated CD8 T-cell IFN-γ responses are missing during infections with this virus.

CHEMOKINES

A group of low-molecular-weight cytokines, about 8 to 12 kd in size, with chemotactic functions are being described (see Table 2) (236,240,255). Because they are chemotactic cytokines, the mediators are called chemokines. This area of research is in a dramatic expansion period, and many newly identified factors are likely to be added to this group. The factors have important proinflammatory functions and can be induced in response to challenge with a number of infectious agents and their products and in response to particular cytokines. Although characterization of production has largely focused on immune cells, particular chemokines can be made by a variety of immune and nonimmune cells. The factors are broadly distributed into four families, C, C-C, C-X-C, and C-X3-C, based on their amino acid sequences. The C family has only one known member, lymphotactin. This factor targets lymphocytes for chemotactic responses. Many of the members of the C-C chemokine family are known to be produced by activated T cells and monocytes, but at least two members—the macrophage inflammatory protein-1α (MIP-1α) and a factor *r*egulated upon *a*ctivation, *n*ormal *T* *e*xpressed and *s*ecreted (RANTES)—can also be made by NK cells (26,72,205). C-C chemokine cell targets include monocytes, lymphocytes, and NK cells. The C-X-C chemokines are largely produced by activated monocytes, but certain family members can be produced by other cell types. A C-X-C chemokine, with a particular requirement for IFN-γ in induction, is the monokine induced by IFN-γ (Mig) (8,32,315,316). This factor may be uniquely restricted for, and especially potent at, induction of activated T-cell migration. Major target cells of the C-X-C chemokines include neutrophils, monocytes, and lymphocytes. The C-X3-C family has one known member, fractalkine. Monocytes and lymphocytes are major target cells of this factor.

Identification of specific roles for particular chemokines is complicated by the fact that they bind to and utilize different, but overlapping, receptors, and that the expression of multiple cytokines is generally induced simultaneously. As an example, the ligands MIP-1α, RANTES, and the monocyte chemotactic protein-1 (MCP-1) can all bind to the CC chemokine receptor CCR5 in culture systems (236). Moreover, conditions associated with MIP-1α induction are reported to induce other CC chemokines, including RANTES, during infections with VV (8), LCMV (11), mouse hepatitis virus (MHV) (142), HSV, and HIV (26,72). Nevertheless, there is good evidence supporting a specific requirement for a single chemokine (MIP-1α) during inflammatory responses *in vivo*. MIP-1α is crucial to migration of protective NK cells into infected livers during innate responses to MCMV infection (249). This results in local IFN-γ driven Mig production (248). In addition, the chemokine is required for tissue inflammation at times associated with adaptive immune responses to influenza virus, coxsackievirus (50), and HSV infections (291).

Under the specific conditions of HIV infection, particular chemokines can also mediate direct antiviral functions (48). This is because HIV strains use the chemokine receptors CXCR4 and CCR5 as coreceptors with CD4 molecules for virus infection and because the natural chemokine ligands for these specific receptors can block HIV infection (4,19). The ligands include RANTES and MIP-1α. Both T and NK cells are capable of delivering this chemokine-mediated mechanism of protection.

CYTOKINE RECEPTORS AND SIGNALING PATHWAYS

Most cytokines use similar mechanisms to signal from the extracellular milieu to specific genes in the nucleus (113,281). The cellular receptors to which cytokines bind are generally type I ectoproteins with a single transmembrane domain (Fig. 4). Functional receptors may be composed of one, two, or three distinct protein subunits, each of which is a transmembrane protein. Particular subunits may be common to receptors of several cytokines. In some cases, one subunit binds the cytokine with high affinity, whereas in other cases, only composite multisubunit receptors do so. Structurally, the extracellular regions of these receptors contain fibronectin type III–like domains, cysteine-rich immunoglobulin-like domains, or combinations thereof. The carboxyl-terminal region of at least one of the receptor proteins forms a cytoplasmic tail used to recruit particular and crucial signaling proteins to provide specificity of intracellular signaling. Unlike many growth factor and hormone receptors, the cytoplasmic domains of cytokine receptors do not have intrinsic enzyme activity. Instead, they recruit specific tyrosine kinases, which are activated through events at the extracellular domains, resulting in ligand binding and receptor dimerization. A common family of such tyrosine kinases is the Janus kinase (Jak) group. One or more members of the Jaks are bound to specific sites on the cytoplasmic domain of different cytokine receptors. Ligand-bound receptors activate the Jaks, causing phosphorylation of specific tyrosine residues on the receptor subunits and on the Jaks themselves. Other tyrosine kinases, such as members of the sarcoma (Src) family, are also associated with particular cytokine receptors. Tyrosine phosphorylation of receptors and receptor-associated tyrosine kinases triggers a chain of events with cytoplasmic proteins containing Src-homology 2 (SH2) domains, to recognize phosphorylated tyrosines, recruited to the receptor and subsequently tyrosine phosphorylated. The most important signal transducing proteins for gene induction by cytokines are the signal transducers and activators of transcription (STATs). (Particular cytokine–cytokine receptor interactions associated with major specific STAT molecules are listed in Table 4.) Tyrosine phosphorylated STATs form homodimers or heterodimers and translocate to the nucleus, where they, by themselves or in association with other

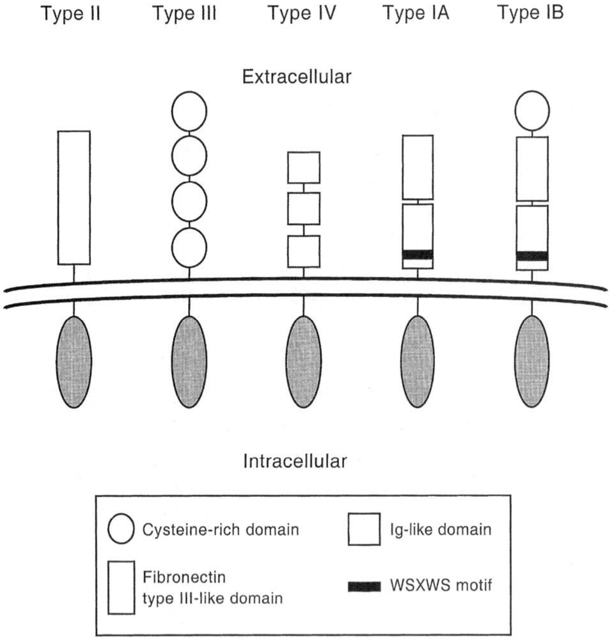

FIG. 4. Shared structural features among various cytokine receptors. The receptors are divided in groups by the nature of structural motifs present in their ligand-binding extracellular domains. Four such motifs are shown here. Type II receptors include those for type I and type II interferons (IFNs); these receptors are discussed in more detail in Figure 5. IL-10R is also a type II receptor. Type III receptors include TNF-RI and TNF-RII. Type IV receptors include IL-1RI and IL-1RII. Type IA receptors include IL-2Rβc, IL-2Rβc, IL-3Rα, IL-3Rβc, IL-4Rα, IL-5Rα, IL-7Rα, IL-9Rα. Type IB receptors include IL-6Rα, IL-6Rβ, and IL-12Rβ.

TABLE 4. *Activation of JAK and STAT by various cytokines*

Cytokine	Jak	STAT
IFN-α/β	Tyk2, Jak1	1, 2, 3, (4)
IFN-γ	Jak1, Jak2	1
IL-2	Jak1, Jak3	(1), 3, 5
IL-3	Jak1, Jak2	5, 6
IL-4	Jak1, Jak3	6
IL-5	Jak2	
IL-6	Tyk2, Jak1, Jak2	1, 3
IL-7	Jak1, Jak3	
IL-9	Jak1, Jak3	3
IL-10	Tyk2, Jak1	1, 3
IL-11	Jak1	3
IL-12	Tyk2, Jak2	3, 4
IL-13	Jak1	6
IL-15	Jak1, Jak3	(1), 3, 5

IFN, interferon; IL, interleukin.
Parentheses denote cell-type specific activation.

specific proteins, bind to specific DNA elements in cytokine-inducible genes to activate transcription. Thus, STATs are the true messengers carrying activation signals from specific receptors on the cell surface to specific genes in the nucleus.

Because the Jak–STAT pathways were discovered through analysis of the mechanisms used by IFNs (271), signaling by these cytokines is described in detail. The pathways used by TNF also are discussed in brief because of their distinct nature. Little is known about the pathways used by cytokines for activating many of the immunoregulatory functions described earlier. Moreover, as most of the work characterizing these pathways has been done in culture, much remains to be learned about how they function in the context of the mixed cytokine responses elicited during viral infections in the host.

Interferon Receptors and Cell Signaling

IFN-specific intracellular signaling processes culminate in transcriptional activation of a set of IFN-inducible genes. Many of these genes are also induced in virus-infected cells by dsRNA or other viral products. The genes encoding the Jaks and the STATs themselves are often transcriptionally regulated by cytokines, thus providing positive feedback loops to the signaling systems. The intricate and partially overlapping signaling pathways used by IFNs and other cytokines provide opportunities for "cross-talking" among them, causing either synergistic or antagonistic outcomes. The cross-talking is physiologically relevant because a single cytokine is never induced in isolation in a virus-infected organism. Instead, cells are exposed *in vivo* to mixtures of cytokines simultaneously, and resultant changes in their gene expression reflect equilibrium between the multiple activated signaling pathways.

Interferon Receptors

Cells of all lineages, except possibly mature erythrocytes, express cell surface receptors for both type I IFNs (IFN-α, IFN-β, IFN-ω) and type II IFN (IFN-γ). Receptor numbers vary from 100 to 2000 per cell, and ligand-binding constants vary between 10^{-11} and 10^{-9} M. The receptors are multimeric transmembrane glycoproteins whose extracellular domains bind IFNs and whose cytoplasmic domains bind Jaks, STATs, and other signaling proteins. The type I IFNs bind to a receptor that has two major subunits, IFNAR1, a protein with 530 residues, and IFNAR2c, a protein with 315 residues (162). Neither subunit alone can bind IFN-α/β with high affinity, but the receptor complex can (49). The two IFNAR subunits associate with the tyrosine kinases Tyk2 and Jak1, respectively. Fully functional type I IFN receptors may contain additional transmembrane protein components because several other proteins coprecipitate with the ligand–receptor complex and because certain biochemical events cannot be reconstituted with the IFNAR1 and IFNAR2 molecules alone. The IFN-γ receptor has two different subunits, IFNGR1 and IFNGR2, whose intracellular domains respectively bind the Jak1 and Jak2 kinases. IFNGR1 has 472 residues, whereas IFNGR2 has 315 residues (58). Functional IFN-γ is a dimer binding to two IFNGR1 subunits to generate binding sites for two IFNGR2 subunits. Thus, the occupied, active receptor complex consists of two molecules each of IFN-γ, IFNGR1, and IFNGR2. The crucial events in both type I IFN and IFN-γ signaling are IFN-driven dimerizations of receptors. This leads to a cascade of tyrosine phosphorylation of proteins bound to the cytoplasmic domains of the receptor subunits.

Intracellular Signaling by Interferons

Both type I and II IFNs use similar principles in cellular signaling (Fig. 5). Specific protein tyrosine kinases of the Jak family are associated with cytoplasmic domains of the receptors, and ligand binding to receptor extracellular domains causes their activation to initiate a cascade of protein tyrosine phosphorylation events, with the STATs among the phosphorylated proteins (271). Once phosphorylated, STATs can form specific multimeric complexes that translocate to the nucleus and bind to specific cis-acting DNA elements present in the 5′ regulatory regions of IFN-inducible genes. Thus, strong and specific transcriptional signals are transmitted from the outside of cells to specific genes in the nucleus. These signals are generated within minutes of ligand binding to the receptors. The effects are transient, decaying within hours of initiation. As a result, target gene transcription is activated in responding cells for only short periods of time.

At least seven proteins are essential for IFN-α/β signaling, including the two subunits of the receptor, two members of the Jak family of protein tyrosine kinases (Jak1 and Tyk2), two members of the STAT family (most notably STAT1 and STAT2), and a specific member of the IRF family, P48 (117,136,151,247,271). The interferon-stimulated response element (ISRE), cis-acting DNA sequences present in the regulatory regions of the IFN-α/β inducible genes to receive the stimulatory signal, has been defined (58). The relevant transcription factor binding to ISRE is ISGF3, a complex composed of three proteins, STAT1, STAT2, and P48. All of these proteins preexist in untreated cells, but the ISGF3 complex is formed only in IFN-treated cells after tyrosine phosphorylation of STAT1 and STAT2. P48 is a member of the IRF family of proteins, all capable of specifically binding to ISRE (198). Some IRF members stimulate transcription, whereas others repress it. Although the initial phase of positive signaling is transmitted to the ISRE by ISGF3, transcription of the IFN-stimulated genes (ISGs) may be sustained by specific IRF members, such

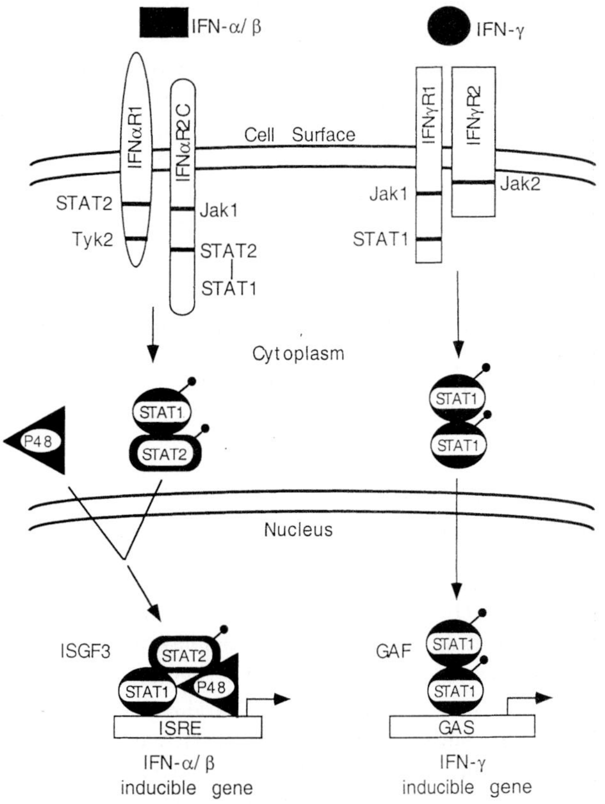

FIG. 5. Interferon (IFN)-signaling pathways. Binding of the IFN-α/β ligands to the extracellular domain of their receptor causes activation of Jak1 and Tyk2 and resultant Tyr-phosphorylation of STAT1 and STAT2. The phosphorylated STATs form a heterodimer and translocate to the nucleus, where they form a trimeric complex (ISGF3) with P48. ISGF3 binds to the ISRE elements of the promoters in IFN-α– and -β–inducible genes to activate their transcription. IFN-γ binds to a different heterodimeric receptor, the intracellular domains of which bind to Jak1, Jak2, and STAT1. Ligand-induced activation of the tyrosine kinase causes STAT1 Tyr-phosphorylation, its dimerization, and nuclear translocation. The STAT1 homodimer (GAF) binds to the GAS elements of IFN-γ–inducible genes and activates their transcription.

as IRF-1. In addition to these proteins, the protein tyrosine phosphatase SHP-2 may also be involved in IFN-α/β signaling (69,117).

The previously described Jak–STAT pathway is thought to be the major signaling cascade used by IFN-α/β, but there is experimental evidence to implicate other STAT molecules, such as STAT4 (43,58). Moreover, cytosolic phospholipase A2 may be activated under particular conditions of IFN-α/β stimulation (76). An additional subtype-specific signaling pathway may be in place because a mutant cell line lacking Tyk2 cannot respond to IFN-α1 or α2 but retains a partial response to IFN-β and IFN-α8 (80). The possible existence of an IFN-β–specific pathway is supported by identification of a gene preferentially induced by IFN-β, that is, βR1 (228). IFN-α/β also activate the mitogen-activated protein (MAP) kinase pathway. This could be initiated by tyrosine phosphorylation and activation of an IFNAR1-associated MAP kinase identified as ERK2 (59).

The major IFN-γ signaling pathway requires at least five cellular proteins: the two subunits of the receptor, the protein tyrosine kinases Jak1 and Jak2, and STAT1 (13,301). These receptor-bound STATs are also phosphorylated by the Jaks to cause their dissociation from the receptor complex (259,262,263). The dissociated Tyr-phosphorylated STAT1 proteins form a reciprocal homodimer, called the γ-activated factor (GAF), and GAF translocates to the nucleus. The most commonly used cis element in IFN-γ–responsive genes is called γ-activated sequence (GAS) (61). GAF binds to GAS to promote gene transcription (see Fig. 5). Optimal transcriptional activation, however, requires further phosphorylation of STAT1 homodimers at Ser727 (59,309,316). The Pyk2 kinase with a MAP kinase–like specificity has been implicated in this process. IFN-γ can also signal to ISRE and other elements. The compositions of the corresponding trans-acting factors remain to be determined. The IFN-γ signal to ISRE may not be as strong as that mediated by IFN-α/β. Conversely, although ISGF3 is the major effector of IFN-α/β signaling, STAT1 homodimers are also formed under these conditions and can bind to GAS elements to drive transcription of some ISGs, such as the IRF-1 gene. Because only a subset of ISGs are induced, this pathway appears to be less prominent that the one induced by IFN-γ. The STATs present in ISGF3 or GAF can interact with the basic transcriptional machinery by binding to the universal coactivator with its CBP/p300 components (323). Because induction of many genes by IFN-γ, such as 9-27, P48, and class II MHC (see later), is not mediated by GAS elements, additional signaling pathways must exist. Although some features of these alternative pathways have been reported, their full descriptions await further investigation (27,157,230).

The mechanisms used by cells to down-regulate and terminate IFN signaling are not well understood. It is clear, however, that many components of the signaling pathway are inactivated in the process. Receptors are dephosphorylated (98) and down-regulated from the cell surface (221), and activated Jaks are inhibited by the suppressors of cytokine signaling (SOCS) family of proteins whose expression is induced by IFN (69,195,272). In addition, activated STAT1 is dephosphorylated by SHP-1 or similar tyrosine phosphatases (60) and possibly degraded by a proteasome-mediated process (131).

Interferon-Independent Signaling for Gene Expression in Virus-Infected Cells

Many IFN-α/β–stimulated genes are activated in virus-infected cells through signaling pathways independent of IFN. The IFN-independent pathways can be activated by dsRNA produced in cells infected with many viruses. These pathways are most convincingly demonstrated in cells devoid of type I IFN genes or incapable of responding to IFNs (16). The dsRNA-elicited signal is also received by the ISRE element. However, dsRNA-signaling does not require STAT1, STAT2, Jak1, Tyk2, or P48 used by IFN-α/β. Instead, dsRNA or virus-signaling is mediated by the dsRNA-activated factor (DRAF) (57) or virus-activated factor (VAF) (56) complexes binding to ISRE. The protein constituents of these factors are not as well defined as those of ISGF3 but contain IRF-3 and CBP/p300 (152,175,307,321). Regulation of these factors is poorly understood. IRF-3 phosphorylation is required, but the cognate protein kinase has not yet been identified. The dsRNA-dependent protein kinase PKR is likely to be involved in a cascade leading to activation. The pathway used by dsRNA to signal to ISRE is not well defined, but it and the ISGF3 pathway used by IFNs are distinct (143). Viruses may use yet another pathway to activate transcription from the same cis element because binding of virions or the relevant viral glycoproteins to the cell surface receptors can be sufficient to trigger transcription of specific ISGs (30,196,326).

Signaling by Tumor Necrosis Factor

There are two distinct TNF receptors to which both TNF-α and LT (also called TNF-β or LT-α) bind: TNFR1 or P55 and TNFR2 or P75. Their extracellular domains have homologies to many other cell surface receptors, such as Fas, nerve growth factor (NGF) receptors, and two poxvirus decoy TNF receptors, T2 and A53R. The cytoplasmic domains of the two TNF receptors are quite distinct, indicating that they elicit different intracellular signals. In general, TNFR1-generated signals cause cytotoxicity, increased cell proliferation, and antiviral activity, whereas TNFR2-generated signals are important in hematopoietic cells for specific functions (282,283). TNF binding to cell surface receptors causes pleiotropic intracellular responses, including activation and induced synthesis of transcription factors such as NF-κB and AP-1. As a result, transcription of many cellular genes is induced or repressed (296). The specific pathways used by TNF for signaling are not well characterized. MAP kinase is activated (295). Under most of the conditions studied to date, the Jak–STAT pathway does not appear to be activated by TNF. There are reports that TNF causes sphingomyelin hydrolysis generating lipid ceramide that activates a specific protein kinase to transmit the signal (133). The supporting evidence is, however, incomplete.

Because signaling by TNFR1 can cause apoptosis, it has been classified as a death receptor and has a characterized death domain in its cytoplasmic tail. Binding of TNF to the receptor causes its aggregation and the recruitment of intracellular signal transducers. One class of such proteins contains death domains as well (111). The TNFR1-associated death domain (TRADD) molecule is an example of a protein binding to the death domain of TNFR1. The second class of proteins, including those identified as TNF-receptor associated factors (TRAFs), do not contain death domains (114,242). They interact with each other and the receptor via a conserved C-terminal domain. A general picture of the signaling processes suggest that they lead to either apoptosis primarily through TRADD or activation of NFκB and cell survival through TRAFs (241,320). The balance between the two opposite outcomes depends on cell type. Thus, most normal cells are not killed by TNF, probably because strong NF-κB activation protects the cells from apoptotic effects. TRAF2 mediates both NF-κB activation and C-Jun N-terminus kinase (JNK) activation by TNF.

ACTIONS OF CYTOKINES ON VIRAL REPLICATION AND IMMUNE RESPONSES

Many cellular actions of cytokines are mediated by differentially induced proteins. These molecules are not expressed, or are expressed at a low level, in untreated cells. Most are products of genes whose transcription is directly induced, but some are products of genes requiring ongoing protein synthesis for expression. The latter proteins are likely to represent a second stage of a gene induction cascade. A variety of approaches, including gene array technology (63), have revealed that IFNs induce synthesis of a surprisingly large number of cellular proteins, counting in the hundreds. Type I and II IFNs induce two partially overlapping sets of proteins. Many of the type I IFN-inducible proteins can also be induced by host cell responses to dsRNA or virus infection (326). Although IFN-α and IFN-β primarily induce the same proteins, some proteins may be induced by one better than the other.

The characteristics of a few extensively studied IFN-induced proteins are described later. Their biochemical and cellular regulatory functions are well understood, and many of them play major roles in the antiviral functions of IFNs (Fig. 6). Particularly active in antiviral defense are certain enzymes with binding activity for dsRNA and molecules called Mx proteins. Progress is also being made toward understanding the induction and function of MHC molecules in response to IFNs. By promoting antigen processing and presentation, these effects can facilitate the development of adaptive T-cell responses. (TNF-α is also known to induce certain of these, but the pathways for induction are not as thoroughly characterized.) Exciting new information is becoming available about the biochemical pathways of IFN-mediated regulation of cell proliferation. These effects are likely to be important in shaping endogenous immune responses and in therapeutic effects resulting from IFN-α/β treatments of cancers. Finally, although less well characterized, IFN or TNF-α activates pathways inducing a nitric oxide synthase important in antiviral defense.

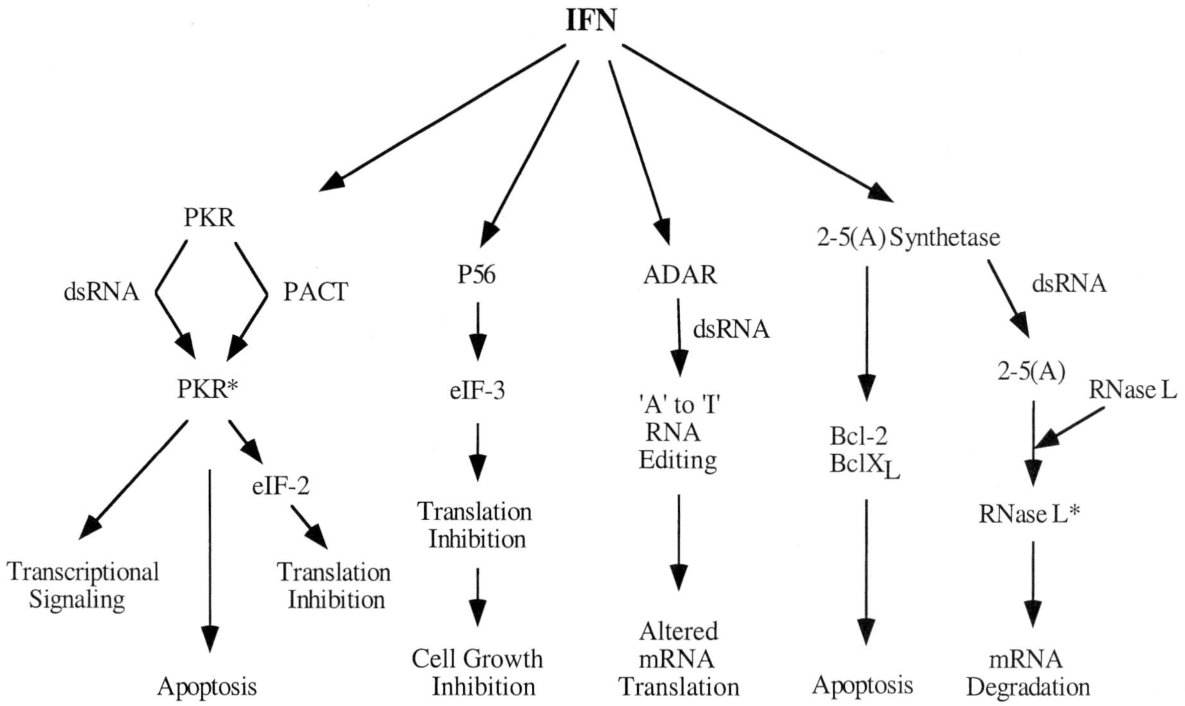

FIG. 6. Interferon (IFN)-induced biochemical pathways affecting cell growth and metabolism. Among the many proteins induced by IFNs are PKR, P56, ADAR, and 2-5(A) synthetase. IFN-induced PKR is inactive as such and requires either dsRNA or another cellular protein, PACT, for its activation by autophosphorylation. Activated PKR (PKR*) is a protein kinase with stringent substrate specificity. It can phosphorylate eIF-2α to inhibit protein synthesis. It can also cause cellular apoptosis and participate in specific transcriptional signaling pathways. The IFN-induced protein, P56, binds to the P48 subunit of eIF-3 and inhibits its function, causing translation inhibition and cell growth inhibition. The IFN-induced ADAR adenosine diaminase edits (A to I) dsRNA structures in viral and cellular RNAs, thereby changing their coding properties. The IFN-induced 2-5(A) synthetases are a family of enzymes, all of which are activated by dsRNA to synthesize 2′-5′–linked oligoadenylates [2-5(A)]. 2-5(A) binds and dimerizes inactive RNase L, causing its activation (RNase L*), and activated RNase L degrades mRNA. A specific isozyme, 9-2, of 2-5(A) synthetase has an additional cellular activity. It binds to the Bcl-2 family of proteins and causes cellular apoptosis.

Enzymes Dependent on Double-Stranded RNA

Studies of the IFN-induced proteins have led to the discovery of three interesting classes of enzymes, all of which bind to and require dsRNA for their functions: (a) the family of 2-5(A) synthetases (229) whose products, the 2′-5′-oligoadenylates, activate a latent ribonuclease, RNase L, to cleave cellular and viral RNAs (265); (b) the PKR, affecting many cellular processes and resulting in inhibition of viral replication (312); and (c) an isoform of dsRNA-specific adenosine deaminase, which converts adenosines to inosines (217). The functions of these enzymes are known to be important for induction of an antiviral state by IFNs, and the mechanisms for induction of the antiviral effects have been extensively studied.

As a result of binding dsRNA, the 2′-5′-oligoadenylate [2-5(A)] synthetases are activated to polymerize adenosine triphosphate (ATP) into 2′-5′–linked oligoadenylates. All 2-5(A) synthetase proteins are IFN induced, although basal levels are present in many cell lines. There are three size classes of these enzymes: small, in the 40-kd range; medium, in the 70-kd range; and large, in the 100-kd range (229,254). Each class is encoded by separate genes, which are all clustered in one genetic locus. Within each class, multiple isozymes are produced by alternative splicing of primary transcripts. Different isozymes have different posttranslational modifications and different subcellular locations. Studies with natural and recombinant proteins have shown that the three classes have different dsRNA optima and synthesize 2-5(A) of different lengths (90,252). Many small viral RNAs, such as adenoviral VAI RNA, EBV EBER RNA, and HIVI TAR RNA, can also activate these enzymes (64,168,261). Oligomerization of the small and medium proteins is essential for their enzyme activity (90,253). Recent studies with a medium isozyme, P69, have revealed that the catalytic domains of these proteins have an $\alpha\beta\beta\alpha\beta\beta\beta$ structure similar to the catalytic domain of

DNA polymerase β. Three Asp residues in this domain form the catalytic triad, and their mutation inactivates the enzyme without affecting ATP and dsRNA binding (253). The residues responsible for dimerization of P69 have also been identified.

The 2-5(A) product molecules activate RNase L by causing dimerization of inactive monomeric RNase L (265). The N-terminal half of the protein containing P-loop motifs and ankyrin repeats binds 2-5(A) and serves as a repressor of enzyme function. The C-terminal half contains a region of protein kinase homology, a cysteine-rich domain, and the ribonuclease domain. Trimeric 2-5(A) is required for the activation of RNase L, dimers are inactive, and much longer oligomers of 2-5(A) may have inhibitory activity. The 2-5(A) synthetase–RNase L system has been shown to inhibit replication of specific families of viruses, especially picornaviruses. Constitutive expression of either the small or the medium isozyme causes inhibition of replication of encephalomyocarditis virus (EMCV) but not vesicular stomatitis virus (VSV) (42,89). Cells expressing a dominant negative mutant of RNase L and RNase L–null mice are deficient in the anti-EMCV effect of IFN-α/β (324). The constituents of the 2-5(A) synthetase–RNase L system can also affect cell growth. RNase L has been implicated in apoptotic pathways (324); and a small isozyme of 2-5(A) synthetase, 9-2, causes cellular apoptosis (88). The 9-2 activity is unique to this form of the 2-5(A) synthetase family and unrelated to 2-5(A) synthesis and RNase L binding. The function has been traced to a unique C terminus of 9-2 acquired by alternative splicing. This region contains a Bcl-2 homology 3 (BH3) domain, which enables it to interact with the antiapoptotic proteins Bcl2 and BclxL. Much remains to be learned about the effects on cell growth and death, however, because constitutive overexpression of P69 can cause a contrasting dose-dependent increase in cell doubling time and the formation of multinucleated cells (89).

Another dsRNA-activated enzyme is PKR (312). This enzyme is expressed in all cells at a low level but is induced to a higher level upon IFN treatment. The protein is inactive, but dsRNA binding activates it to cause its autophosphorylation in serine-threonine residues. Phosphorylated PKR can phosphorylate other proteins. The PKR dsRNA-binding domain is at the N-terminal half and the catalytic domain is in the C-terminal half of the molecule. The dsRNA-binding domain contains two dsRNA-binding motifs of about 70 residues. These motifs are present in other members of this family of dsRNA-binding proteins but not in 2-5(A) synthetases. The domain also mediates direct protein–protein interaction, causing PKR homodimerization (215) or allowing heterodimerization among different members of this family of proteins. The kinase domain contains the usual kinase subdomains and an insert domain shared with other eIF-2α kinases. PKR can be activated by other cellular and viral RNAs with partial double-stranded structures and heparin or other polyanionic compounds as well as by authentic dsRNA. Recently, a protein activator of PKR, PACT, has been identified (214). PACT also has the dsRNA-binding motifs and dimerizes with PKR. Activation of PKR by PACT is independent of dsRNA. Low concentration of dsRNA can activate PKR, whereas higher concentrations inhibit it. Many viruses, such as adenovirus, exploit this property by producing a large quantity of VAI RNA that inhibits PKR (280). Binding of dsRNA causes a conformational change in PKR, exposing the ATP-binding site and autophosphorylation. The most well-characterized PKR substrate is the translation initiation factor eIF-2α. Its phosphorylation inhibits the function of eIF-2 and causes an inhibition of translation. Thus, activation or overexpression of PKR causes an inhibition of cellular protein synthesis, and this is one mechanism for IFN-induced inhibition of viral replication. PKR can also phosphorylate histones, HIV Tat protein and IκB *in vitro* (312). It interacts with STAT1, STAT3, and P53 as well but does not phosphorylate them. A new nuclear dsRNA-binding protein substrate of PKR, DRBP76, has recently been identified (216).

Overexpression of PKR leads to inhibition of EMCV replication, and a dominant-negative PKR mutant or an antisense PKR cDNA suppresses the anti-EMCV action of IFN-α and IFN-β. To circumvent the actions of PKR, many viruses have evolved different mechanisms to inhibit its function. These viral evasion strategies are discussed in a separate section later. There are other cellular functions of PKR in addition to its antiviral effects. PKR has been shown to be required in transcriptional signaling by dsRNA (312). Through an as yet undefined pathway, dsRNA-activated PKR activates the IκK complex and causes degradation of IκB. PKR is also involved in cellular signaling by TNF-α, LPS, and IFN-γ. There are suggestions that PKR may act upstream of the MAP kinase P38. Because PKR is a cell growth inhibitor, its trans-dominant inhibitors can promote unregulated cell growth and transformation of NIH/3T3 cells. In virus-infected cells, PKR promotes cellular apoptosis. Viruses encode or induce many antiapoptotic proteins to keep the cells alive during replication. One such inhibitor, P58IPK, is a cellular protein induced by influenza virus (280).

The IFN-inducible dsRNA-specific adenosine deaminase, ADAR, differs from 2-5(A) synthetases and PKR in the role dsRNA plays. The dsRNA structures are substrates of ADAR, whereas they are regulatory factors activating or antagonizing enzymatic functions of the other molecules. ADAR catalyzes C6 deamination of adenosine to inosine in viral and cellular RNAs (156,217). Consequences of this IFN-induced RNA editing are changes in target RNA coding capacities. Such site-specific editing can cause amino acid substitution and, as a result, synthesis of proteins with altered functions (155,156).

Mx and Guanylate-Binding Proteins

The Mx proteins and other guanylate-binding proteins are abundantly induced by IFNs in a number of species (270). The human MxA and MxB proteins are induced primarily by type I IFNs. These proteins belong to the dynamin superfamily of GTPase involved in endocytosis and vesicle transport (109). The Mx proteins were originally discovered as IFN-induced proteins with the ability to block replication of influenza viruses. Later, they were shown to be capable of inhibiting many other RNA viruses, including members of the Orthomyxoviridae, Paramyxoviridae, Rhabdoviridae, Bunyaviridae, and Togaviridae families (106). The Mx proteins are thought to interfere with virus replication through a dynamin-like force–generating mechanism by wrapping around viral nucleocapsids. The MxA protein associates, in the GTP-bound form, with the nucleoprotein component of Thogoto virus to cause an inhibition in nuclear transport of the viral nucleocapsids and viral genome transcription (132). The existence of considerable residual effects of IFN-α/β against EMCV in mice lacking functional RNase L, PKR, and Mx suggest the presence of additional pathways (325). Another family of IFN-induced proteins includes the guanylate-binding proteins, GBP-1 and GBP-2. They bind and hydrolyze GTP; that is, they have GTPase functions and may have mild antiviral activities (9).

Major Histocompatibility Complex Expression

Among the IFN-induced proteins playing major roles in recognition of virus antigens by cells of the immune system are the MHC proteins (29,153). The class I MHC proteins are induced by both types of IFNs, but the class II proteins are induced by IFN-γ only. Enhanced surface expression of class I MHC proteins facilitates activation of CD8 T cells. Along with the class I proteins, IFNs promote the expression of other proteins that help constitute the class I MHC, including β_2-microglobulin, three subunits of the proteasome LMP-2, LMP-8 and LMP-10, PA28, TAP, tapsin, and gp96 (185). The IFN-γ–induced class II MHC response promotes CD4 T-cell activation. IFN-γ up-regulates the class II MHC heterodimer, the invariant chain protein, two DM proteins that assist in assembly of the class II complex, and the transcription factor CIITA that is required for transcription of these genes (164). IFN-γ regulates the expression of three cathepsins believed to be responsible for cleavage-processing of exogenous proteins into peptides for loading onto the class II MHC complex. IFN-γ also induces the high-affinity Fcγ receptor and the components of the complement system (54). PML and SP11, two human proteins localized in nuclear bodies within the nucleus, are IFN inducible (303).

P200 Gene Family

In mice, type I IFNs strongly induce synthesis of various members of the *P200* gene family (145). The cluster contains at least six IFN-regulated linked genes. The protein products of these genes are related in that they all contain at least one unit of a conserved domain of about 200 amino acids. The p202 protein inhibits cell proliferation by binding to and inhibiting the functions of a number of transcription factors, including NFκB, E2F, P53, c-fos, c-jun, and the retinoblastoma protein Rb (47). The p204 protein, on the other hand, inhibits rRNA transcription by binding to the UBF1 transcription factor that is required for ribosomal RNA synthesis (154). Genes from the homologous human locus are also induced by IFNs. Their products, IFI16 and MNDA, are DNA-binding nuclear proteins.

ISG56 Gene Family

In humans, a genetic locus encodes several proteins that are strongly induced by type I IFNs. They include P56, P54, P60, and P58 of the *ISG56* gene family (305). The corresponding mouse proteins also are known. These proteins are structurally related. They contain multiple tetratricopeptide domains thought to mediate protein–protein interactions. P56 is the product of gene *561* or *ISG56* (139). This gene is not expressed in untreated cells but induced very rapidly upon IFNα/β treatment. It is also induced by dsRNA or by infection with viruses. Both the mRNA and the protein are relatively short lived, and the protein, P56, is primarily cytoplasmic (103). The P56 cellular function is still poorly understood, but the molecule interacts with Int-6. The Int-6 protein has cytoplasmic and nuclear isoforms, arising from alternative translation initiation sites. The full-length cytoplasmic protein has a nuclear export signal at the N terminus and a nuclear localization signal near the C terminus (102). An internally initiated protein lacks the nuclear export signal and hence stays in the nucleus. P56 interacts with both proteins and keeps the nuclear isoform sequestered in the cytoplasm. Int-6 is identical to P48, a subunit of the translation initiation factor eIF-3 (10). As expected, P56 binds eIF-3, and purified recombinant P56 inhibits *in vitro* translation by blocking eIF-3 function (104). *In vivo* P56 and P48 are colocalized in the cytoplasm. When P56 is overexpressed in cells, the rate of protein synthesis is decreased, and the rate of cell growth is affected as a consequence.

Inducible Nitric Oxide Synthase

The inducible nitric oxide synthase (iNOS), alternatively identified as nitric oxide synthase 2 (NOS2), can be expressed in activated macrophages to mediate a variety of antimicrobial functions. Much of the work characterizing iNOS induction has been done in mice and in response to IFN-γ or LPS stimulation. Inflammatory macrophages from humans, however, also express iNOS (165). Signaling for iNOS induction is incompletely characterized. The promoter regions of both mouse and human genes are complex, and there are likely to be multiple pathways to iNOS induction. The transcription factor, NFκB, can play a role in induction elicited by LPS. Moreover, the absence of IRF-1 results in significant iNOS deficiencies, and the absence of IFN-γ induction of IRF-1 is likely to be a pathway to this effect (120). Although IFN-γ is a potent inducer, TNF-α and TNF-α in synergy with IFN-α/β can also act as inducers of the enzyme (165). Through biochemical pathways with NADPH to oxidize and consume L-arginine, NOS enzymes catalyze production of NO, with L-citruline as a second product (165). NO is a lipid- and water-soluble gas that reacts with oxygen and its intermediates to yield other reactive molecules. The iNOS-dependent pathways have been shown to contribute to defense during a range of infections, including those with the RNA virus, VSV, and the DNA viruses, VV, EBV, HSV, and MCMV (2,126,127,165,182,284). Because of the variety of reactive intermediates and products, NO has the potential to mediate antiviral activity by modifying downstream target molecules. It has been shown to promote maintenance of EBV latency by down-regulating an intermediate-early transactivator protein (171) and to interrupt VV replication and protein synthesis by blocking required enzymes and intermediates (126,182).

VIRAL STRATEGIES FOR COUNTERACTING OR TAKING ADVANTAGE OF CYTOKINE AND CHEMOKINE ACTION

Viruses have evolved many strategies either to inhibit cytokine- or chemokine-mediated effects detrimental to their replication or to take advantage of cytokine and chemokine functions to promote viral propagation and spread in the host. In particular, viruses constantly try to evade antiviral IFN action. A virus that is a potent inducer of IFN and also highly sensitive to its antiviral effects will reproduce poorly and hence be at an evolutionary disadvantage. Thus, in nature, equilibrium is maintained between viruses and the IFN system. In the laboratory, this equilibrium can be shifted either way by increasing IFN concentration or viral multiplicity of infection: at high virus load, IFN is ineffective, and at high IFN dose, virus replication is totally shut off. A global strategy used by many virulent viruses is to inhibit cellular RNA and protein synthesis. As a result, both IFN synthesis and synthesis of IFN-induced proteins are impaired. Other viruses have developed more targeted and sophisticated strategies to interfere with different steps of the IFN and other cytokine systems (Table 5). These strategies are discussed subsequently.

Inhibition of Interferon Synthesis

IFN synthesis is inhibited by some viral gene products. Hepatitis B virus ORF-C product inhibits IFN-β gene induction, as does the viral terminal protein (307). For IFN induction by VSV, mutations in the M protein may dictate this capacity of the virus (74). African swine fever virus that infects macrophages inhibits phorbol myristil acetate (PMA)-induced synthesis of IFN-α and TNF-α. Here, the product of the viral A238L gene encodes a homolog of IκB to inhibit NFκB actions in cytokine induction (224). Other viruses produce cytokine homologs. The myxoma virus MT-7 protein can bind IFN-γ and serve as its decoy receptor. This protein can also bind several chemokines (252). VV encodes a homolog of IFN-α/β receptor that, unlike the cellular receptor, can bind type I IFN of many species (3,179). Tanapox virus–infected cells secrete a protein that can bind to and inactivate IFN-γ, IL-2, and IL-5 (70).

Inhibition of Interferon Signaling

Another common step of interference by different viruses is at the level of signal transduction by IFNs. The Jak–STAT pathway loses its regulation and is constitutively activated by human T-lymphotrophic virus (HTLV) tax proteins (183) and by spleen focus-forming viral envelope protein gp55 that binds to the erythropoietin receptor (318). Herpesvirus saimiri activates the Jak–STAT pathway using lck, a src-related tyrosine kinase (161). In the opposite scenario, many viral proteins inhibit the Jak–STAT pathway. Infection with HCMV appears to decrease Jak1 levels in infected cells by enhancing degradation of the protein, and a consequence of this effect is disruption of induction of class II MHC expression on the surface of infected cells (184). Murine polyomavirus large T antigen binds to Jak1 and inhibits IFN signaling. This activity requires the pRB binding sites of the large T molecule. As a result, ISGF3 is not activated in response to IFN-α/β, and consequently, other viruses such as VSV are also not inhibited by IFN in cells expressing large T (308).

The most thoroughly studied example of interference with IFN signaling is that mediated by the adenoviral E1A proteins. Adenoviruses are insensitive to IFNs because several adenoproteins counteract the IFN system at multiple steps, with the earliest step at an IFN-signaling block by E1A. As a result of the E1A-mediated effect, IFN also cannot inhibit the replication of other viruses. E1A expression does not allow ISGF3 formation. The defect can be ascribed to a lowered cellular level of one or more of the signaling proteins, including STAT1 and P48 (146,147). E1A also disrupts the interactions between the STAT proteins and CBP/P300 required for ISG transcription by interacting with both STAT1 and STAT2 (20). Other DNA viruses can interfere with IFN-signaling. The hepatitis B

TABLE 5. *Viral interference with cytokines*

Nature of action	Viral protein	Affected cellular protein
Homologs of cytokine receptors	Poxvirus	
	MT7	IFNγR
	MT2	TNFR
	B18R	IFN α/βR
	B28R	IL-1R
	SPV-K2R	IL-8R
	EB virus	
	LMP	CSF-IR
Inhibition of synthesis	HBV ORF-C	IFN-β
	African swine fever virus	IFN-α, TNF-α
	A238L	IL-8
	HPV-16 E6	IFN-β
	Herpesvirus 8	IFN-β
Inhibition of gene induction by IFN	Adenovirus E1A	STAT1, P48
	HBV TP	
	EBNA1	
	HPV E7	P48
	Ebola virus	
	Sendai virus C protein	
	SV5 V protein	
	Polyomavirus large T	Jak1
	HCMV	Jak1
Inhibition of IFN-induced protein actions	Adenovirus VAI RNA	PKR, ADAR
	EBV EBER RNA	PKR
	HIV TAR RNA	PKR
	Vaccinia virus E3L	PKR, 2-5(A) synthetase
	Vaccinia virus K3L	PKR
	Influenza virus NSI	PKR
	Reovirus sigma 3	PKR
	HSV-1, γ 34•5	PKR
	HCV NS5A, E2	PKR
	Poliovirus	PKR
	HSV-1	RNase L

CSF, colony-stimulating factor; HBV, hepatitis B virus; HPV, human papillomavirus; HCMV, human cytomegalovirus; EBV, Epstein-Barr virus; HIV, human immunodeficiency virus; HSV, herpes simplex virus; HCV, hepatitis C virus.

virus (HBV) polymerase protein or its subdomain TP blocks ISGF3 activation (79). The EBV EBNA1 oncogene blocks gene induction and cell growth inhibition by IFN without interfering with the activation of ISGF3, indicating that the block may be at the level of ISGF3–coactivator interactions (123). The human papillomavirus E7 protein abrogates IFN-α signaling and blocks ISGF3 activation. In this case, E7 directly binds to P48 and inhibits its translocation to the nucleus (17). Numerous RNA viruses have also been shown to interfere with IFN signaling. Ebola virus inhibits both IFN-α and IFN-γ signaling in endothelial cells (108). Sendai virus C proteins prevent the antiviral action of IFN, possibly by interfering with signaling (84). One specific C protein appears to be responsible. A similar virus, SV5, has a viral V protein blocking the activation of ISGF3 in response to IFN-α/β and GAF in response to IFN-γ (65). This dual block is achieved by targeting STAT1 for proteasome-mediated degradation. Several viruses have strategies to block other steps. The HPV16 E6 oncoprotein binds to IRF-3 and blocks its transactivation functions (238). IRF-3 is activated in response to dsRNA and virus infection and promotes transcription of IFN genes and many ISGs. In the presence of E6, IFN-β is not induced by Sendai virus infection. Human herpesvirus type 8 (HHV-8) encodes a transcription factor similar to the IRF proteins (189). The viral IRF interferes with the actions of cellular IRF proteins and thereby blocks IFN and ISG expression. Thus, a variety of viruses have evolved to overcome potent antiviral effects induced by IFNs by blocking IFN-signaling pathways.

Interference with Functions of Interferon-Induced Proteins

Many viruses have developed mechanisms to counteract specific functions of various IFN-induced proteins. There are known viral inhibitors of the two well-studied IFN-induced antiviral pathways requiring dsRNA for activation. EMCV infection causes an inhibition of binding of 2-5(A) to RNase L, although IFN pretreatment overcomes this inhibition. Analogs of 2-5(A), which block activation of RNase L, are synthesized in herpesvirus- or SV40-infected cells (39). The most frequent IFN-induced antiviral mechanisms targeted, however, are those mediated through activation and function of PKR (119). Adenovirus produces abundant amounts of spoiler VAI RNA that bind to the dsRNA-binding domain of PKR but do not activate it. Similarly, EBV produces EBER RNA, and HIV-1 produces TAR RNA; at high concentrations, these viral products block PKR activation. The VV E3L protein, influenza virus NS1 protein, and reovirus sigma 3 protein, on the other hand, prevent PKR activation by binding dsRNA. VV also encodes K3L, which functions as a decoy of eIF-2 and an alternative substrate of PKR. A phosphoprotein of HSV-1 neutralizes PKR action by inhibiting phosphorylation of eIF-2 (46). The HSV-1 $\gamma 34 \cdot 5$ protein complexes with protein phosphatase 1α (PP1α) to promote dephosphorylation of eIF-2α. PP1α may also be responsible for inactivating the enzyme itself by causing PKR dephosphorylation. Influenza virus activates a novel cellular chaperone protein, P58IPK, which inhibits PKR, possibly by interfering with its dimerization. Poliovirus and HIV promote degradation of PKR through unknown mechanisms. Hepatitis C virus encodes two proteins interfering with PKR action. The NS5A protein binds to the dimerization domain of PKR to block its activation (81), and differences in natural resistance to IFNs between different strains of HCV can be attributed to mutations in the NS5A protein. Another protein of HCV, the E2 glycoprotein, has also been shown to inhibit PKR (285). E2 contains a sequence identical to the phosphorylation sites of PKR and eIF-2 and binds to PKR to inhibit its action. The previous examples of many viruses evolving a variety of mechanisms to inhibit PKR support the notion that PKR functions as a major antiviral enzyme in the IFN system.

Other Mechanisms

In addition to those directed at IFN functions, viruses have evolved a number of other far-reaching mechanisms to counteract or take advantage of host cytokines or their actions (93,266,267). Although it is not possible to review all of these in detail, a few examples are given here. The large poxviruses are packed with genes having potential to inhibit or modify host immune responses. One of these is the T2 protein, which can protect virus-infected cells from the antiviral effects of TNF actions (93,158). The myxoma virus MT-2 molecule is a homolog of the cellular receptor for TNF and is released from infected cells to serve as a binding decoy and block signaling through functional host TNF receptors. Myxoma virus also produces a homolog of EGF/TGF-α (3). HHV-8 encodes a cytokine similar to IL-6, which promotes the growth of transformed B cells (33). The EBV BCRF-1 protein is highly homologous to mammalian IL-10 (186). The viral protein is biologically active and is thought to aid viral pathogenicity by suppressing production of immunostimulatory cytokines and by promoting B-cell growth and transformation. This gene function is essential for the transforming capacity of EBV. A VV gene for an enzyme promoting steroid production may act to inhibit endogenous immune responses by accessing the immunoregulatory pathways induced by these hormones (190). A different mechanism is used by the cow poxvirus to block IL-1β. It encodes an inhibitor of IL-1β converting enzyme that is required for the production of IL-1β by proteolytic cleavage from a larger precursor. Finally, there is an example of one virus, measles, using as its receptor a cell surface molecule delivering a signal to regulate IL-12 expression negatively (125).

Certain viruses also have genes with homology to host chemokines or chemokine receptors and other gene products with chemokine-binding activities (82,95,140,177, 219,266,293). It is not yet clear whether all of these function to help virus escape from immune defense or whether they might also act to promote viral replication. In soluble forms, the chemokine receptor homologs could act as natural chemokine receptor antagonists or blockers. This appears to be the case during myxoma virus infections, in which certain viral products with chemokine-binding activity are virulence factor for infections and interfere with recruitment of leukocytes into virus-infected tissues. In contrast, chemokine homologs might promote virus spread by calling in cell for infection, and this appears to be the case with a chemokine homolog expressed by MCMV (77,246).

CYTOKINE-MEDIATED PATHOLOGY

Although characterization of immunopathology during viral infections has traditionally focused on adaptive immune responses resulting in particular antibody-dependent immune complex– or CTL-mediated diseases, cytokines can also contribute to immunopathology. This has been long appreciated in the case of bacterial infections. Cytokine-dependent consequences detrimental to the host have been clearly delineated during gram-negative bacterial sepsis and after exposure to LPS (105) as well as in response to gram-positive bacterial toxins such as the staphylococcal enterotoxins (174). High-level exposure to the first class of agents induces proinflammatory cytokines by innate immune response mechanisms. These conditions are associated with high systemic levels of TNF-α, IL-1, IL-6, IL-12, and IFN-γ and with TNF-α essential for the detrimental effects and most of the other factors acting to increase sensitivity to TNF-α. Exposure to the bacterial endotoxins activates large proportions of T-cell subsets to produce cytokines amplifying the proinflammatory innate cytokine cascades. If uncontrolled, the conditions can result in coagulation, vascular collapse, and multiple-organ failure. Remarkably, the functions of certain of the proinflammatory cytokines, such as TNF-α, IL-1, and IL-6, include alerting the neuroendocrine system to the problem and activating the hypothalamic–pituitary–adrenal axis to induce the release of glucocorticoid (GC) hormones from the adrenal glands (178). The GC hormones can mediate a number of immunoregulatory effects to limit detrimental consequences of the endogenous cytokine responses. In particular, they can inhibit the expression of certain of the cytokines (2,178,202,257).

Little attention has been paid to potential cytokine-mediated diseases during viral infections. Recently, MCMV infections have been shown to induce systemic proinflammatory cytokines overlapping with, but not exactly identical to, those known to be induced under conditions of LPS exposure, that is, significant serum levels of TNF-α, IL-6, IL-12, and IFN-γ but low or undetectable IL-1 responses (243,244). Under these conditions, an adaptive immune response–independent, but TNF-dependent, liver necrosis is induced and results in significant organ damage (209). Such a pathway may contribute to liver disease during other viral infections. In particular, infections with mouse hepatitis virus type 3 (MHV-3) also induce liver necrosis and disease associated with macrophage activation and coagulation (67,148,149). The conditions of systemic cytokine induction during MCMV infection result in an IL-6–dependent induction of endogenous GC production (243), and the GC response acts to protect the host from a TNF-dependent lethality during the infection (244).

Results of treatments with IL-12 (210,212) or challenge with LPS (199) suggest that there may be conditions under which T-cell responses to viral infections promote cytokine-mediated or cytokine-dependent disease during viral infections. Such pathways are likely to contribute to pathology during infections with Dengue virus (138) and perhaps Hantaan viruses, but this remains to be thoroughly investigated. Recent evidence suggests that effects mediated through the LT β-receptor also may contribute to viral pathogenesis (225).

SUMMARY

This chapter has reviewed current understanding of cytokine responses and functions during viral infections.

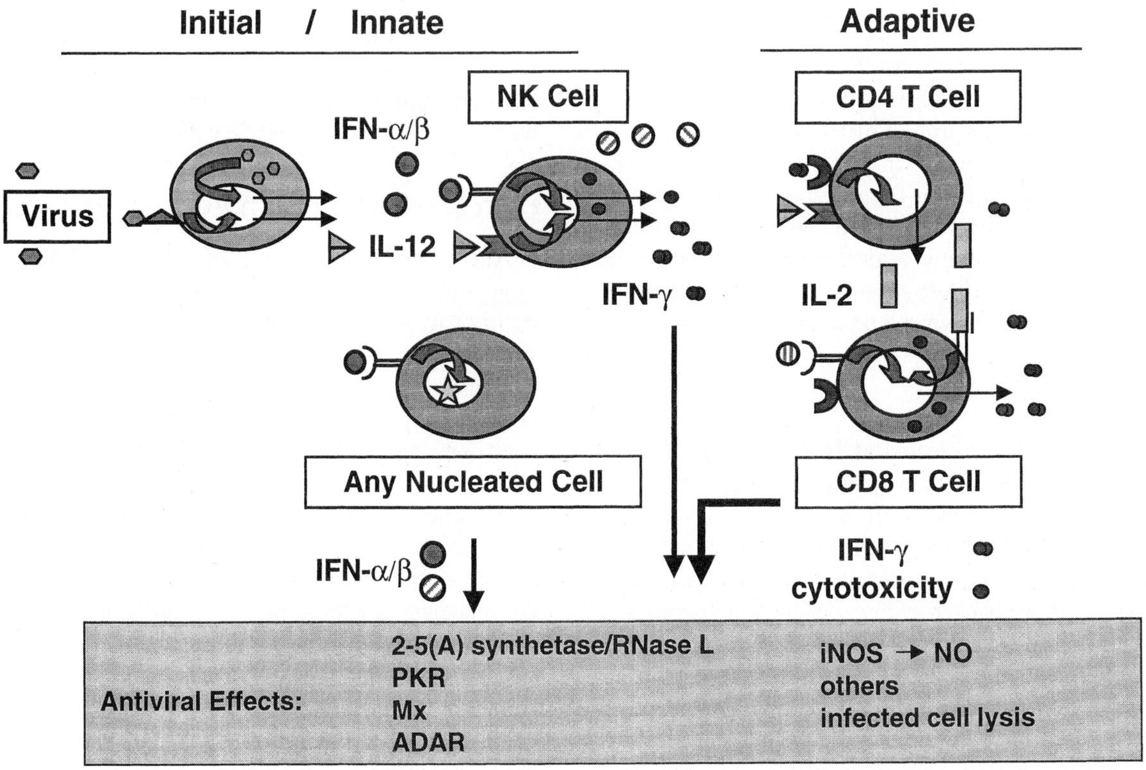

FIG. 7. Summary of known specific responses and their effects during viral infections. Initial events during infections include induction of interferon (IFN)-α/β (●⊘) in response to viral products. These cytokines then activate a variety of biochemical events through receptor stimulation of a Jak/STAT signaling pathway with activation of the ISGF transcriptional complex (★) and lead to expression of proteins contributing to antiviral defense mechansims, including, but not limited to, 2-5 (A) synthetase/RNase L, PKR, and Mx. The IFN-a/b cytokines also promote the induction of innate natural killer (NK) cell cytotoxicity (⬬) and can enhance adaptive T-cell IFN-γ (⬬⬬) responses. Certain viral infections also induce an initial or innate interleukin-12 (IL-12) response (▶) response. This factor is associated with NK cell IFN-g production. Many viral infections induce profound CD8 T-cell expansion with activation of CD8 T-cell IFN-g production and cytotoxic T-lymphocyte (CTL) functions. T-cell IFN-g responses can be IL-12 independent during viral infections. IL-2 (▮) can promote CD8 T-cell expansion and facilitate optimal responses mediated by these populations.

We have attempted to present the broad picture, but emphasis has been on unique pathways activated by and during viral infections. A focus has been on IFN-α/β. Key aspects of the integrated responses are schematically represented in Figure 7. Many viruses have evolved specific mechanisms to exert control over the responses and their functions. The overall balance is crucial to the host. As the material reviewed shows, our understanding is becoming sophisticated, but much remains to be learned. This is an active period of investigation. The authors look forward to the next few years of study and the knowledge to be derived from the results of this work, particularly in the areas of understanding how the systems work at the biochemical level to regulate immune responses *in vivo.*

REFERENCES

1. Abbas AK, Lichtman AH, Pober JS. *Cellular and molecular immunology.* Philadelphia: WB Saunders, 1997.
2. Ahmed R, Biron CA. Immunity to viruses. In: Paul WE, ed. *Fundamental immunology,* 4th ed. Philadelphia: Lippincott-Raven, 1998: 1295–1334.
3. Alcami A, Smith GL. Cytokine receptors encoded by poxviruses: A lesson in cytokine biology. Immunol Today 1995;16:474-478.
4. Alkhatib G, Combadiere C, Broder CC, et al. CC CKR5: A RANTES, MIP-1alpha, MIP-1beta receptor as a fusion cofactor for macrophage-tropic HIV-1. *Science* 1996;272:1955–1958.
5. Altare F, Durandy A, Lammas D, et al. Impairment of mycobacterial immunity in human interleukin-12 receptor deficiency. *Science* 1998;280:1432–1435.
6. Altman JD, Moss PAH, Goulder PJR, et al. Phenotypic analysis of antigen-specific T lymphocytes. *Science* 1996;274:94–96.
7. Alwan WH, Kozlowska WJ, Openshaw PJ. Distinct types of lung disease caused by functional subsets of antiviral T cells. *J Exp Med* 1994;179:81–89.
8. Amichay D, Gazzinelli RT, Karupiah G, et al. Genes for chemokines MuMig and Crg-2 are induced in protozoan and viral infections in response to IFN-gamma with patterns of tissue expression that suggest nonredundant roles in vivo. *J Immunol* 1996;157:4511–4520.
9. Anderson SL, Carton JM, Lou J, et al. Interferon-induced guanylate binding protein-1 (GBP-1) mediates an antiviral effect against vesicular stomatitis virus and encephalomyocarditis virus. *Virology* 1999;256:8–14.
10. Asano K, Merrick WC, Hershey JW. The translation initiation factor eIF3-p48 subunit is encoded by int-6, a site of frequent integration by the mouse mammary tumor virus genome. *J Biol Chem* 1997;272: 23477–23480.
11. Asensio VC, Campbell IL. Chemokine gene expression in the brains of mice with lymphocytic choriomeningitis. *J Virol* 1997;71:7832–7840.
12. Atedzoe BN, Ahmad A, Menezes J. Enhancement of natural killer cell cytotoxicity by the human herpesvirus-7 via IL-15 induction. *J Immunol* 1997;159:4966–4972.
13. Bach EA, Aguet M, Schreiber RD. The IFN gamma receptor: A paradigm for cytokine receptor signaling. *Annu Rev Immunol* 1997;15: 563–591.
14. Bachmann MF, Schorle H, Kuhn R, et al. Antiviral immune responses in mice deficient for both interleukin-2 and interleukin-4. *J Virol* 1995;69:4842–4846.
15. Ballas ZK, Rasmussen WL, Krieg AM. Induction of NK activity in murine and human cells by CpG motifs in oligodeoxynucleotides and bacterial DNA. *J Immunol* 1996;157:1840–1845.
16. Bandyopadhyay S, Leonard GT Jr, Bandyopadhyay T, et al. Transcriptional induction by double-stranded RNA is mediated by interferon-stimulated response elements without activation of interferon-stimulated gene factor 3. *J Biol Chem* 1995;270:19624–19629.
17. Barnard P, McMillan NA. The human papillomavirus E7 oncoprotein abrogates signaling mediated by interferon-α. *Virology* 1999;259: 305–313.
18. Bendelac A, Rivera MN, Park SH, Roark JH. Mouse CD1-specific NK1 T cells: Development, specificity, and function. *Annu Rev Immunol* 1997;15:535–562.
19. Berger EA. HIV entry and tropism: The chemokine receptor connection. *AIDS* 1997;11:S3–S16.
20. Bhattacharya S, Eckner R, Grossman S, et al. Cooperation of Stat2 and p300/CBP in signaling induced by interferon-alpha. *Nature* 1996; 383:344–347.
21. Biron CA, Gazzinelli RT. Effects of IL-12 on immune responses to microbial infections: A key mediator in regulating disease outcome. *Curr Opin Immunol* 1995;7:485–496.
22. Biron CA, Nguyen KB, Pien GC, et al. Natural killer cells in antiviral defense: Function and regulation by innate cytokines. *Annu Rev Immunol* 1999;17:189–220.
23. Biron CA. Initial and innate responses to viral infections: Pattern setting in immunity or disease. *Curr Opin Microbiol* 1999;2:374–381.
24. Biron CA. Role of early cytokines, including alpha and beta interferons (IFN-α/β), in innate and adaptive immune responses to viral infections. *Semin Immunol* 1998;10:383–390.
25. Bix M, Locksley RM. Independent and epigenetic regulation of the interleukin-4 alleles in CD4+ T cells. *Science* 1998;281:1352–1354.
26. Bluman EM, Bartynski KJ, Avalos BR, Caligiuri MA. Human natural killer cells produce abundant macrophage inflammatory protein-1α in response to monocyte-derived cytokines. *J Clin Invest* 1996;97: 2722–2727.
27. Bluyssen HA, Muzaffar R, Vlieststra RJ, et al. Combinatorial association and abundance of components of interferon-stimulated gene factor 3 dictate the selectivity of interferon responses. *Proc Natl Acad Sci U S A* 1995;92:5645–5649.
28. Boehm U, Guethlein L, Klamp T, et al. Two families of GTPases dominate the complex cellular response to IFN-gamma. *J Immunol* 1998;161:6715–6723.
29. Boehm U, Klamp T, Groot M, Howard JC. Cellular responses to interferon-gamma. *Annu Rev Immunol* 1997;15:749–795.
30. Boyle KA, Pietropaolo RL, Compton T. Engagement of the cellular receptor for glycoprotein B of human cytomegalovirus activates the interferon-responsive pathway. *Mol Cell Biol* 1999;19:3607–3613.
31. Brinkmann V, Geiger T, Alkan S, Heusser CH. Interferon alpha increases the frequency of interferon gamma-producing human CD4+ T cells. *J Exp Med* 1993;178:1655–1663.
32. Bukowski RM, Rayman P, Molto L, et al. Interferon-gamma and CXC chemokine induction by interleukin 12 in renal cell carcinoma. *Clin Cancer Res* 1999;5:2780–2789.
33. Burger R, Neipel F, Fleckenstein B, et al. Human herpesvirus type 8 interleukin-6 homologue is functionally active on human myeloma cells. *Blood* 1998;91:1858–1863.
34. Butz EA, Bevan MJ. Massive expansion of antigen-specific CD8+ T cells during an acute virus infection. *Immunity* 1998;8:167–175.
35. Carding SR, Allan W, McMickle A, Doherty PC. Activation of cytokine genes in T cells during primary and secondary murine influenza pneumonia. *J Exp Med* 1993;177:475–482.
36. Carlow DA, Teh SJ, Teh HS. Specific antiviral activity demonstrated by TGTP, a member of a new family of interferon induced GTPases. *J Immunol* 1998;161:2348–2355.
37. Carson WE, Ross ME, Baiocchi RA, et al. Endogenous production of interleukin 15 by activated human monocytes is critical for optimal production of interferon-gamma by natural killer cells in vitro. *J Clin Invest* 1995;96:2578–2582.
38. Carter LL, Murphy KM. Lineage-specific requirement for signal transducer and activator of transcription (Stat)4 in interferon gamma production from CD4(+) versus CD8(+) T cells. *J Exp Med* 1999; 189:1355–1360.
39. Cayley PJ, Davies JA, McCullagh KG, Kerr IM. Activation of the ppp(A2′p)nA system in interferon-treated, herpes simplex virus-infected cells and evidence for novel inhibitors of the ppp(A2′p)nA-dependent RNase. *Eur J Biochem* 1984;143:165–174.
40. Cella M, Jarrossay D, Facchetti F, et al. Plasmacytoid monocytes migrate to inflamed lymph nodes and produce large amounts of type 1 interferon. *Nat Med* 1999;5:919–923.
41. Chaplin DD, Fu Y. Cytokine regulation of secondary lymphoid organ development. *Curr Opin Immunol* 1998;10:289–297.
42. Chebath J, Benech P, Revel M, Vigneron M. Constitutive expression of (2′-5′) oligo A synthetase confers resistance to picornavirus infection. *Nature* 1987;330:587–588.
43. Cho SS, Bacon CM, Sudarshan C, et al. Activation of STAT4 by IL-12 and IFN-α: Evidence for the involvement of ligand-induced tyrosine and serine phosphorylation. *J Immunol* 1996;157:4781–4789.

44. Chomarat P, Banchereau J. Interleukin-4 and interleukin-13: Their similarities and discrepancies. *Int Rev Immunol* 1998;17:1–52.
45. Chonmaitree T, Roberts NJ Jr, Douglas RG Jr, et al. Interferon production by human mononuclear leukocytes: Differences between respiratory syncytial virus and influenza viruses. *Infect Immunol* 1981; 32:300–303.
46. Chou J, Chen JJ, Gross M, Roizman B. Association of a M(r) 90,000 phosphoprotein with protein kinase PKR in cells exhibiting enhanced phosphorylation of translation initiation factor eIF-2 alpha and premature shutoff of protein synthesis after infection with gamma 134.5– mutants of herpes simplex virus 1. *Proc Natl Acad Sci U S A* 1995;92:10516–10520.
47. Choubey D, Li SJ, Datta B, et al: Inhibition of E2F-mediated transcription by p202. *EMBO J* 1996;15:5668–5678.
48. Cocchi F, DeVico AL, Garzino-Demo A, et al. Identification of RANTES, MIP-1 alpha, and MIP-1 beta as the major HIV-suppressive factors produced by CD8+ T cells. *Science* 1995;270:1811–1815.
49. Cohen B, Novick D, Barak S, Rubinstein M. Ligand-induced association of the type I interferon receptor components. *Mol Cell Biol* 1995;15:4108–4214.
50. Cook DN, Beck MA, Coffman TM, et al. Requirement of MIP-1α for an inflammatory response to viral infection. *Science* 1995;269: 1583–1585.
51. Cousens LP, Orange JS, Biron CA. Endogenous IL-2 contributes to T cell expansion and IFN-γ production during lymphocytic choriomeningitis virus infection. *J Immunol* 1995;155:5690–5699.
52. Cousens LP, Orange JS, Su HC, Biron CA. Interferon-α/β inhibition of interleukin 12 and interferon-γ production in vitro and endogenously during viral infection. *Proc Natl Acad Sci U S A* 1997;94: 634–639.
53. Cousens LP, Peterson R, Hsu S, et al. Two roads diverged: Interferon α/β- and interleukin-12- mediated pathways in promoting T cell interferon γ responses during viral infection. *J Exp Med* 1999;189: 1315–1328.
54. Daeron M. Fc receptor biology. *Annu Rev Immunol* 1997;15:203–234.
55. Dalod M, Sinet M, Deschemin JC, et al. Altered ex vivo balance between CD28+ and CD28– cells within HIV-specific CD8+ T cells of HIV-seropositive patients. *Eur J Immunol* 1999;29:38–44.
56. Daly C, Reich NC. Characterization of specific DNA-binding factors activated by double-stranded RNA as positive regulators of interferon α/β-stimulated genes. *J Biol Chem* 1995;270:23739–23746.
57. Daly C, Reich NC. Double-stranded RNA activates novel factors that bind to the interferon-stimulated response element. *Mol Cell Biol* 1993;13:3756–3764.
58. Darnell JE Jr, Kerr IM, Stark GR. Jak-STAT pathways and transcriptional activation in response to IFNs and other extracellular signaling proteins. *Science* 1994;264:1415–1421.
59. David M, Petricoin E 3rd, Benjamin C, et al. Requirement for MAP kinase (ERK2) activity in interferon alpha- and interferon beta-stimulated gene expression through STAT proteins. *Science* 1995;269: 1721–1723.
60. David M, Zhou G, Pine R, et al. The SH2 domain-containing tyrosine phosphatase PTP1D is required for interferon alpha/beta-induced gene expression. *J Biol Chem* 1996;271:15862–15865.
61. Decker T, Kovarik P, Meinke A. GAS elements: A few nucleotides with a major impact on cytokine-induced gene expression. *J Interferon Cytokine Res* 1997;17:121–134.
62. de Jong R, Altare F, Haagen IA, et al. Severe mycobacterial and Salmonella infections in interleukin-12 receptor-deficient patients. *Science* 1998;280:1435–1438.
63. Der SD, Zhou A, Williams BR, Silverman RH. Identification of genes differentially regulated by interferon α, β, or γ using oligonucleotide arrays. *Proc Natl Acad Sci U S A* 1998;95:15623–15628.
64. Desai SY, Patel RC, Sen GC, et al. Activation of interferon-inducible 2′-5′ oligoadenylate synthetase by adenoviral VAI RNA. *J Biol Chem* 1995;270:3454–3461.
65. Didcock L, Young DF, Goodburn S, Randall RE. The V protein of simian virus 5 inhibits interferon signaling by targeting STAT1 for proteasome-mediated degradation. *J Virol* 1999;73:9928–9933.
66. Diefenbach A, Schindler H, Donhauser N, et al. Type 1 interferon (IFN-α/β) and type 2 nitric oxide synthase regulate the innate immune response to a protozoan parasite. *Immunity* 1998;8:77–87.
67. Ding JW, Ning Q, Liu MF, et al. Fulminant hepatic failure in murine hepatitis virus strain 3 infection: Tissue-specific expression of a novel fgl2 prothrombinase. *J Virol* 1997;71:9223–9230.
68. Doherty PC, Topham DJ, Tripp RA, et al. Effector CD4+ and CD8+ T-cell mechanisms in the control of respiratory virus infections. *Immunol Rev* 1997;159:105–117.
69. Endo TA, Masuhara M, Yokouchi M, et al. A new protein containing an SH2 domain that inhibits JAK kinases. *Nature* 1997;387:921–924.
70. Essani K, Chalasani S, Eversole R, et al. Multiple anti-cytokine activities secreted from tanapox virus-infected cells. *Microb Pathol* 1994;17:347–353.
71. Fantuzzi G, Dinarello CA. Interleukin-18 and interleukin-1 beta: Two cytokine substrates for ICE (caspase-1). *J Clin Immunol* 1999;19: 1–11.
72. Fehniger TA, Herbein G, Yu H, et al. Natural killer cells from HIV-1+ patients produce C-C chemokines and inhibit HIV-1 infection. *J Immunol* 1998;161:6433–6438.
73. Feldman SB, Ferraro M, Zheng HM, et al. Viral induction of low frequency interferon-α producing cells. *Virology* 1994;204:1–7.
74. Ferran MC, Lucas-Lenard JM. The vesicular stomatitis virus matrix protein inhibits transcription from the human beta interferon promoter. *J Virol* 1997;71:371–377.
75. Flamand L, Stefanescu I, Menezes J. Human herpesvirus-6 enhances natural killer cell cytotoxicity via IL-15. *J Clin Invest* 1996;97: 1373–1381.
76. Flati V, Haque SJ, Williams BR. Interferon-alpha-induced phosphorylation and activation of cytosolic phospholipase A2 is required for the formation of interferon-stimulated gene factor three. *EMBO J* 1996; 15:1566–1571.
77. Fleming P, Davis-Poynter N, Degli-Esposti M, et al. The murine cytomegalovirus chemokine homolog, m131/129, is a determinant of viral pathogenicity. *J Virol* 1999;73:6800–6809.
78. Flynn KJ, Belz GT, Altman JD, et al. Virus-specific CD8+ T cells in primary and secondary influenza pneumonia. *Immunity* 1998;8: 683–691.
79. Foster GR, Ackrill AM, Goldin RD, et al. Expression of the terminal protein region of hepatitis B virus inhibits cellular responses to interferons α and γ and double-stranded RNA. *Proc Natl Acad Sci U S A* 1991;88:2888–2892.
80. Foster GR, Rodrigues O, Ghouze F, et al. Different relative activities of human cell-derived interferon-alpha subtypes: IFN-alpha 8 has very high antiviral potency. *J Interferon Cytokine Res* 1996;16: 1027–1033.
81. Gale MJ Jr, Korth MJ, Tang NM, et al. Evidence that hepatitis C virus resistance to interferon is mediated through repression of the PKR protein kinase by the nonstructural 5A protein. *Virology* 1997;230: 217–227.
82. Gao JL, Murphy PM. Human cytomegalovirus open reading frame US28 encodes a functional beta chemokine receptor. *J Biol Chem* 1994;269:28539–28542.
83. Garcia-Sastre A, Durbin RK, Zheng H, et al. The role of interferon in influenza virus tissue tropism. *J Virol* 1998;72:8550–8558.
84. Garcin D, Latorre P, Kolakofsky D. Sendai virus C proteins counteract the interferon-mediated induction of an antiviral state. *J Virol* 1999;73:6559–6565.
85. Garofalo R, Kimpen JL, Welliver RC, Ogra PL. Eosinophil degranulation in the respiratory tract during naturally acquired respiratory syncytial virus infection. *J Pediatr* 1992;120:28–32.
86. Gessani S, Belardelli F, Borghi P, et al. Correlation between the lipopolysaccharide response of mice and the capacity of mouse peritoneal cells to transfer an antiviral state: Role of endogenous interferon. *J Immunol* 1987;139:1991–1998.
87. Ghayur T, Banerjee S, Hugunin M, et al. Caspare-1 processes IFN-gamma-inducing factor and regulates LPS-induced IFN-gamma production. *Nature* 1997 386:619–623.
88. Ghosh A, Sarkar S, Sen G. A new isozyme-specific cellular effect of 2-5 (A) sythetase. *J Interferon Cytokine Res* 1999;19:S68.
89. Ghosh A, Sarkar S, Sen G. Cell growth regulatory and anti-viral effects of the P69 isozyme of 2-5 (A) synthetase. *Virology* 2000;266:319–328.
90. Ghosh A, Sarkar SN, Guo W, et al. Enzymatic activity of 2′-5′-oligoadenylate synthetase is impaired by specific mutations that affect oligomerization of the protein. *J Biol Chem* 1997;272: 33220–33226.
91. Gilles PN, Fey G, Chisari FV. Tumor necrosis factor alpha negatively regulates hepatitis B virus gene expression in transgenic mice. *J Virol* 1992;66:3955–3960.
92. Gollob JA, Kawasaki H, Ritz J. Interferon-gamma and interleukin-4 regulate T cell interleukin-12 responsiveness through the differential

modulation of high-affinity interleukin-12 receptor expression. *Eur J Immunol* 1997;27:647–652.

93. Goodling LR. Virus proteins that counteract host immune defenses. *Cell* 1992;71:5–7.
94. Graham BS. Pathogenesis of respiratory syncytial virus vaccine-augmented pathology. *Am J Respir Crit Care Med* 1995;152:S63–66.
95. Graham KA, Lalani AS, Macen JL, et al. The T1/35 kDa family of poxvirus-secreted proteins bind chemokines and modulate leukocyte influx into virus-infected tissues. *Virology* 1997;229:12–24.
96. Graham MB, Dalton DK, Giltinan D, et al. Response to influenza infection in mice with a targeted disruption in the interferon gamma gene. *J Exp Med* 1993;178:1725–1732.
97. Graziosi C, Pantaleo G, Gantt KR, et al. Lack of evidence for the dichotomy of TH1 and TH2 predominance in HIV-infected individuals. *Science* 1994;265:248–252.
98. Greenlund AC, Farrar MA, Viviano BL, Schreiber RD. Ligand-induced IFN gamma receptor tyrosine phosphorylation couples the receptor to its signal transduction system (p91). *EMBO J* 1994;13:1591–1600.
99. Gresser I, Guy-Grand D, Maury C, Maunoury MT. Interferon induces peripheral lymphademopathy in mice. *J Immunol* 1981;127: 1569–1575.
100. Gronowski AM, Hilbert DM, Sheehan KC, et al. Baculovirus stimulated antiviral effects in mammalian cells. *J Virol* 1999;73:9944–9951.
101. Gu Y, Kuida K, Tsutsui H, et al. Activation of interferon-gamma inducing factor mediated by interleukin-1beta converting enzyme. *Science* 1997;275:206–209.
102. Guo J, Sen GC. Characterization of the interaction between the interferon-induced protein P56 and the Int-6 protein encoded by a locus of insertion of the mouse mammary tumor virus. *J Virol* 74:1892–1899.
103. Guo J, Peters K, Sen GC. Induction of the human protein P56 by interferon, double-stranded RNA or virus infection. *Virology* 267: 209–219.
104. Guo J, Hui D, Merrick WC, Sen GC. A new pathway of translational regulation mediated by enkaryotic initiation factor 3. *EMBO J* 2000; 19:6891–6899.
105. Gutierrez-Ramos JC, Bluethmann H. Molecules and mechanisms operating in septic shock: Lessons from knockout mice. *Immunol Today* 1997;18:329–334.
106. Haller O, Frese M, Kochs G. Mx proteins: Mediators of innate resistance to RNA viruses. *Rev Sci Tech* 1998;17:220–230.
107. Hancock GE, Speelman DJ, Heers K, et al. Generation of atypical pulmonary inflammatory responses in BALB/c mice after immunization with the native attachment (G) glycoprotein of respiratory syncytial virus. *J Virol* 1996;70:7783–7791.
108. Harcourt BH, Sanchez A, Offermann MK. Ebola virus selectively inhibits responses to interferons, but not to interleukin-1β, in endothelial cells. *J Virol* 1999;73:3491–3496.
109. Horisberger MA. Interferon-induced human protein MxA is a GTPase which binds transiently to cellular proteins. *J Virol* 1992;66: 4705–4709.
110. Hoshino T, Winkler-Pickett RT, Mason AT, et al. IL-13 production by NK cells: IL-13-producing NK and T cells are present in vivo in the absence of IFN-γ. *J Immunol* 1999;162:51–59.
111. Hsu H, Xiong J, Goeddel DV. The TNF receptor 1-associated protein TRADD signals cell death and NF-κ B activation. *Cell* 1995;81: 495–504.
112. Hussell T, Spender LC, Georgiou A, et al. Th1 and Th2 cytokine induction in pulmonary T cells during infection with respiratory syncytial virus. *J Gen Virol* 1996;77:2447–2455.
113. Ihle J. Cytokine receptor signaling. *Nature* 1995;377:591–594.
114. Ishida TK, Tojo T, Aoki T, et al. TRAF5, a novel tumor necrosis factor receptor-associated factor family protein, mediates CD40 signaling. *Proc Natl Acad Sci U S A* 1996;93:9437–9442.
115. Ishikawa R, Biron CA. IFN induction and associated changes in splenic leukocyte distribution. *J Immunol* 1993;150:3713–3727.
116. Jassoy C, Harrer T, Rosenthal T, et al. Human immunodeficiency virus type 1-specific cytotoxic T lymphocytes release gamma interferon, tumor necrosis factor alpha (TNF-alpha), and TNF-beta when they encounter their target antigens. *J Virol* 1993;67:2844–2852.
117. John J, McKendry R, Pellegrini S, et al. Isolation and characterization of a new mutant human cell line unresponsive to alpha and beta interferons. *Mol Cell Biol* 1991;11:4189–4195.
118. Kägi D, Ledermann B, Burki K, et al. Cytotoxicity mediated by T cells and natural killer cells is greatly impaired in perforin-deficient mice. *Nature* 1994;369:31–37.
119. Kalvakolanu DV. Virus interception of cytokine-regulated pathways. *Trends Microbiol* 1999;7:166–171.
120. Kamijo R, Harada H, Matsuyama T, et al. Requirement for transcription factor IRF-1 in NO synthase induction in macrophages. *Science* 1994;263:1612–1615.
121. Kanangat S, Babu JS, Knipe DM, Rouse BT. HSV-1-mediated modulation of cytokine gene expression in a permissive cell line: Selective upregulation of IL-6 gene expression. *Virology* 1996;219:295–300.
122. Kanangat S, Thomas J, Gangappa S, et al. Herpes simplex virus type 1-mediated up-regulation of IL-12 (p40) mRNA expression: Implications in immunopathogenesis and protection. *J Immunol* 1996;156: 1110–1116.
123. Kanda K, Decker T, Aman P, et al. The EBNA2-related resistance towards a interferon (IFN-α) in Burkitt's lymphoma cells effects induction of IFN-induced genes but not the activation of transcription factor ISGF-3. *Mol Cell Biol* 1992;12:4930–4936.
124. Karp CL, Biron CA, Irani DN. Interferon-β in multiple sclerosis: Is IL-12 suppression the key? *Immunol Today* 2000;21:24–28.
125. Karp CL, Wysocka M, Wahl LM, et al. Mechanism of suppression of cell-mediated immunity by measles virus. *Science* 1996;273:228–231.
126. Karupiah G, Harris N. Inhibition of viral replication by nitric oxide and its reversal by ferrous sulfate and tricarboxylic acid cycle metabolites. *J Exp Med* 1995;181:2171–2179.
127. Karupiah G, Xie QW, Buller RM, et al. Inhibition of viral replication by interferon-gamma-induced nitric oxide synthase. *Science* 1993; 261:1445–1448.
128. Kasaian MT, Biron CA. Effects of cyclosporin A on IL-2 production and lymphocyte proliferation during infection of mice with lymphocytic choriomeningitis virus. *J Immunol* 1990;144:299–306.
129. Kasaian MT, Biron CA. The activation of IL-2 transcription in L3T4+ and Lyt-2+ lymphocytes during virus infection in vivo. *J Immunol* 1989;142:1287–1292.
130. Kaufmann SHE. Immunity to intracellular bacteria. In: Paul WE, ed. *Fundamental immunology,* 4th ed. Philadelphia: Lippincott-Raven, 1998:1335–1371.
131. Kim TK, Maniatis T. Regulation of interferon-gamma-activated STAT1 by the ubiquitin-proteasome pathway. *Science* 1996;273:1717–1719.
132. Kochs G, Haller O. Interferon-induced human MxA GTPase blocks nuclear import of Thogoto virus nucleocapsids. *Proc Natl Acad Sci U S A* 1999;96:2082–2086.
133. Kolesnick R, Golde DW. The sphingomyelin pathway in tumor necrosis factor and interleukin-1 signaling. *Cell* 1994;77:325–328.
134. Kollias G, Douni E, Kassiotis G, Kontoyiannis D. On the role of tumor necrosis factor and receptors in models of multiorgan failure, rheumatoid arthritis, multiple sclerosis and inflammatory bowel disease. *Immunol Rev* 1999;169:175–194.
135. Kopp EB, Medzhitov R. The Toll-receptor family and control of innate immunity. *Curr Opin Immunol* 1999;11:13–18.
136. Krishnan K, Yan H, Lim JT, Krolewski JJ. Dimerization of a chimeric CD4-interferon-alpha receptor reconstitutes the signaling events preceding STAT phosphorylation. *Oncogene* 1996;13:125–133.
137. Kündig TM, Schorle H, Bachmann MF, et al. Immune responses in interleukin-2-deficient mice. *Science* 1993;262:1059–1061.
138. Kurane I, Innis BL, Nimmannitya S, et al. Activation of T lymphocytes in dengue virus infections: High levels of soluble interleukin 2 receptor, soluble CD4, soluble CD8, interleukin 2, and interferon-γ in sera of children with dengue. *J Clin Invest* 1991;88:1473–1480.
139. Kusari J, Sen GC. Regulation of synthesis and turnover of an interferon-inducible mRNA. *Mol Cell Biol* 1986;6:2062–2067.
140. Lalani AS, Graham K, Mossman K, et al. The purified myxoma virus gamma interferon receptor homolog M-T7 interacts with the heparin-binding domains of chemokines. *J Virol* 1997;71:4356–4363.
141. Lalvani A, Brookes R, Hambleton S, et al. Rapid effector function in CD8+ memory T cells. *J Exp Med* 1997;186:859–865.
142. Lane TE, Asensio VC, Yu N, et al. Dynamic regulation of alpha- and beta-chemokine expression in the central nervous system during mouse hepatitis virus-induced demyelinating disease. *J Immunol* 1998;160:970–978.
143. Leaman DW, Salvekar A, Patel R, et al. A mutant cell line defective in response to double-stranded RNA and in regulating basal expression of interferon-stimulated genes. *Proc Natl Acad Sci U S A* 1998;95: 9442–9447.
144. Leib DA, Harrison TE, Laslo KM, et al. Interferons regulate the phenotype of wild-type and mutant herpes simplex viruses in vivo. *J Exp Med* 1999;189:663–672.

145. Lengyel P, Choubey D, Li S, Datta B. The interferon-activatable gene 200 cluster: From structure toward function. *Semin Virol* 1995;6: 202–213.
146. Leonard GT, Sen GC. Effects of adenovirus E1A protein on interferon-signaling. *Virology* 1996;224:25–33.
147. Leonard GT, Sen GC. Restoration of interferon responses of adenoviruses E1a-expressing HT 1080 cell lines by overexpression of p48 protein. *J Virol* 1997;71:5095–5101.
148. Levy GA, Leibowitz JL, Edgington TS. Induction of monocyte procoagulant activity by murine hepatitis virus type 3 parallels disease susceptibility in mice. *J Exp Med* 1981;154:1150–1163.
149. Li C, Fung LS, Chung S, et al. Monoclonal antiprothrombinase (3D4.3) prevents mortality from murine hepatitis virus (MHV-3) infection. *J Exp Med* 1992;176:689–697.
150. Li P, Allen H, Banerjee S, et al. Mice deficient in IL-1 beta-converting enzyme are defective in production of mature IL-1 beta and resistant to endotoxic shock. *Cell* 1995;80:401–411.
151. Li X, Leung S, Kerr IM, Stark GR. Functional subdomains of STAT2 required for preassociation with the alpha interferon receptor and for signaling. *Mol Cell Biol* 1997;17:2048–2056.
152. Lin R, Heylbroeck C, Pitha P, Hiscott J. Virus-dependent phosphorylation of the IRF-3 transcription factor regulates nuclear translocation, transactivation potential, and proteasome-mediated degradation. *Mol Cell Biol* 1998;18:2986–2996.
153. Lindahl P, Gresser I, Leary P, Tovey M. Interferon treatment of mice: Enhanced expression of histocompatibility antigens on lymphoid cells. *Proc Natl Acad Sci U S A* 1976;73:1284–1287.
154. Liu CJ, Wang H, Lengyel P. The interferon-inducible nucleolar p204 protein binds the ribosomal RNA-specific UBF1 transcription factor and inhibits ribosomal RNA transcription. *EMBO J* 1999;18: 2845–2854.
155. Liu Y, Emerson RB, Samuel CE. Serotonin-2C receptor pre-mRNA editing in rat brain and in vitro by splice site varients of the interferon-inducible double-stranded RNA-specific adenosinase ADAR1. *J Biol Chem* 1999;274:18351–18358.
156. Liu Y, Samuel CE. Mechanism of interferon action: Functionally distinct RNA-binding and catalytic domains in the interferon-inducible, double-stranded RNA-specific adenosine deaminase. *J Virol* 1996;70: 1961–1968.
157. Look DC, Pelletier MR, Tidwell RM, et al. Stat1 depends on transcriptional synergy with Sp1. *J Biol Chem* 1995;270:30264–30267.
158. Loparev VN, Parsons JM, Knight JC, et al. A third distinct tumor necrosis factor receptor of orthopoxviruses. *Proc Natl Acad Sci U S A* 1998;95:3786–3791.
159. Lucin P, Jonjic S, Messerle M, et al. Late phase inhibition of murine cytomegalovirus replication by synergistic action of interferon-gamma and tumour necrosis factor. *J Gen Virol* 1994;75:101–110.
160. Lukacher AE, Moser JM, Hadley A, Altman JD. Visualization of polyoma virus-specific CD8+ T cells in vivo during infection and tumor rejection. *J Immunol* 1999;163:3369–3378.
161. Lund TC, Garcia R, Medveczky MM, et al. Activation of STAT transcription factors by herpesvirus Saimiri Tip-484 requires p56lck. *J Virol* 1997;71:6677–6682.
162. Lutfalla G, Holland SJ, Cinato E, et al. Mutant U5A cells are complemented by an interferon-alpha beta receptor subunit generated by alternative processing of a new member of a cytokine receptor gene cluster. *EMBO J* 1995;14:5100–5108.
163. Macatonia SE, Doherty TM, Knight SC, O'Garra A. Differential effect of IL-10 on dendritic cell induced T cell proliferation and IFN-gamma production. *J Immunol* 1993;150:3755–3765.
164. Mach B, Steimle V, Martinez-Soria E, Reith W. Regulation of MHC class II genes: Lessons from a disease. *Annu Rev Immunol* 1996;14: 301–331.
165. MacMicking J, Xie QW, Nathan C. Nitric oxide and macrophage function. *Annu Rev Immunol* 1997;15:323–350.
166. Maggi E, Manetti R, Annunziato F, et al. Functional characterization and modulation of cytokine production by CD8+ T cells from human immunodeficiency virus-infected individuals. *Blood* 1997;89: 3672–3681.
167. Maggi E, Mazzetti M, Ravina A, et al. Ability of HIV to promote a Th1 to Th0 shift and to replicate preferentially in Th2 and Th0 cells. *Science* 1994;265:244–248.
168. Maitra RK, McMillan NA, Desai S, et al. HIV-1 TAR RNA has an intrinsic ability to activate interferon-inducible enzymes. *Virology* 1994;204:823–827.
169. Manetti R, Annuziato F, Tomasevic L, et al. Polyinosinic acid: Polycytidylic acid promotes T helper type 1-specific immune responses by stimulating macrophage production of interferon-alpha and interleukin-12. *Eur J Immunol* 1995;25:2656–2660.
170. Manetti R, Parronchi P, Giudizi MG, et al. Natural killer cell stimulatory factor (interleukin 12 (IL-12)) induces T helper type 1 (Th1)-specific immune responses and inhibits the development of IL-4-producing Th cells. *J Exp Med* 1993;177:1199–1204.
171. Mannick JB, Asano K, Izumi K, et al. Nitric oxide produced by human B lymphocytes inhibits apoptosis and Epstein-Barr virus reactivation. *Cell* 1994;79:1137–1146.
172. Maran A, Maitra RK, Kumar A, et al. Blockage of NF-kappa B signaling by selective ablation of an mRNA target by 2-5A antisense chimeras. *Science* 1994;265:789–792.
173. Marie I, Durbin JE, Levy DE. Differential viral induction of distinct interferon-α genes by positive feedback through interferon regulatory factor-7. *EMBO J* 1998;17:6660–6669.
174. Marrack P, Kappler J. The staphylococcal enterotoxins and their relatives. *Science* 1990;705–711.
175. Masumi A, Wang IM, Lefebure B, et al. The histone acetylase PCAF is a phorbol-ester-inducible coactivator of the IRF family that confers enhanced interferon responsiveness. *Mol Cell Biol* 1999;19: 1810–1820.
176. Matsui K, Yoshimoto T, Tsutsui H, et al. Propionibacterium acnes treatment diminishes CD4+ Nk1.1+ T cells but induces type 1 T cells in the liver by induction of IL-12 and IL-18 production from Kupffer cells. *J Immunol* 1997;159:97–106.
177. McDonald MR, Li XY, Virgin HW. Late expression of a beta chemokine homolog by murine cytomegalovirus. *J Virol* 1997;71: 1671–1678.
178. McEwen BS, Biron CA, Brunson KW, et al. The role of adrenocorticoids as modulators of immune function in health and disease: neural, endocrine and immune interactions. *Brain Res Rev* 1997;23:79–133.
179. McFadden G, Graham K, Ellison K, et al. Interruption of cytokine networks by poxviruses: Lessons from myxoma virus. *J Leukoc Biol* 1995;57:731–738.
180. McRae BL, Semnani RT, Hayes MP, Seventer GA. Type 1 IFNs inhibit human dendritic cell IL-12 production and Th1 cell development. *J Immunol* 1998;160:4298–4304.
181. Medzhitov R, Janeway CA Jr. Innate immune recognition and control of adaptive immune responses. *Semin Immunol* 1998;10:351–353.
182. Melkova Z, Esteban M. Inhibition of vaccinia virus DNA replication by inducible expression of nitric oxide synthase. *J Immunol* 1995;155: 5711–5718.
183. Migone T-S, Lin JX, Cereseto A, et al. Constitutively activated Jak-STAT pathway in T cells transformed with HTLV-I. *Science* 1995;269:79–81.
184. Miller DM, Rahill BM, Boss JM, et al. Human cytomegalovirus inhibits major histocompatibility complex class II expression by disruption of the JAK/Stat pathway. *J Exp Med* 1998;187:675–683.
185. Min W, Pober JS, Johnson DR. Kinetically coordinated induction of TAP1 and HLA class I by IFN-γ: The rapid induction of TAP1 by IFN-gamma is mediated by Stat1 alpha. *J Immunol* 1996;156:3174–3183.
186. Miyazaki I, Cheung RK, Dosch HM. Viral interleukin 10 is critical for the induction of B cell growth transformation by Epstein-Barr virus. *J Exp Med* 1993;178:439–447.
187. Mo XY, Sarawar SR, Doherty PC. Induction of cytokines in mice with parainfluenza pneumonia. *J Virol* 1995;69:1288–1291.
188. Monteiro JM, Harvey C, Trinchieri G. Role of interleukin-12 in primary influenza virus infection. *J Virol* 1998;72:4825–4831.
189. Moore PS, Boshoff C, Weiss RA, Chang Y. Molecular mimicry of human cytokine and cytokine response pathway genes by KSHV. *Science* 1996;274:1739–1744.
190. Moore JB, Smith GL. Steroid hormone synthesis by a vaccinia enzyme: A new type of virus virulence factor. *EMBO J* 1992;11: 3490–3494.
191. Moskophidis D, Cobbold SP, Waldmann H, Lehmann-Grube F. Mechanism of recovery from acute virus infection: Treatment of lymphocytic choriomeningitis virus-infected mice with monoclonal antibodies reveals that Lyt-2+ T lymphocytes mediate clearance of virus and regulate the antiviral antibody response. *J Virol* 1987;61:1867–1874.
192. Moskophidis D, Frei K, Lohler J, et al. Production of random classes of immunoglobulins in brain tissue during persistent viral infection paralleled by secretion of interleukin-6 (IL-6) but not IL-4, IL-5, and gamma interferon. *J Virol* 1991;65:1364–1369.
193. Müller U, Steinhoff U, Reis LFL, et al. Functional role of type I and

type II interferons in antiviral defense. *Science* 1994;264:1918–1921.
194. Murali-Krishna K, Altman JD, Suresh M, et al. Counting antigen-specific CD8 T cells: A reevaluation of bystander activation during viral infection. *Immunity* 1998;8:177–187.
195. Naka T, Narazaki M, Hirata M, et al. Structure and function of a new STAT-induced STAT inhibitor. *Nature* 1997;387:924–929.
196. Navarro L, Mowen K, Rodems S, et al. Cytomegalovirus activates interferon immediate-early response gene expression and an interferon regulatory factor 3-containing interferon-stimulated response element-binding complex. *Mol Cell Biol* 1998;18:3796–3802.
197. Neuzil KM, Tang YW, Graham BS. Protective role of TNF-alpha in respiratory syncytial virus infection in vitro and in vivo. *Am J Med Sci* 1996;311:201–204.
198. Nguyen H, Hiscott J, Pitha PM. The growing family of interferon regulatory factor. *Cytokine Growth Factor Rev* 1997;8:293–312.
199. Nguyen KB, Biron CA. Synergism for cytokine-mediated disease during concurrent endotoxin and viral challenges: Roles for NK and T cell IFN-γ production. *J Immunol* 1999;162:5238–5246.
200. Nguyen KB, Cousens LP, Doughty LA, et al. Interferon α/β-mediated inhibition and promotion of IFN-γ: STAT1 resolves a paradox. *Nat Immunol* 2000;1:70–76.
201. Niemialtowski MG, Rouse BT. Predominance of Th1 cells in ocular tissues during herpetic stromal keratitis. *J Immunol* 1992;149: 3035–3039.
202. Northrop JP, Crabtree GR, Mattila PS. Negative regulation of interleukin 2 transcription by the glucocorticoid receptor. *J Exp Med* 1992;175:1235–1245.
203. Novick D, Kim SH, Fantuzzi G, et al. Interleukin-18 binding protein: A novel modulator of the Th1 cytokine response. *Immunity* 1999;10: 127–136.
204. Okamura H, Tsutsui H, Kashiwamura S, et al. Interleukin-18: A novel cytokine that augments both innate and acquired immunity. *Adv Immunol* 1998;70:281–312.
205. Oliva A, Kinter AL, Vaccarezza M, et al. Natural killer cells from human immunodeficiency virus (HIV)-infected individuals are an important source of CC-chemokines and suppress HIV-1 entry and replication in vitro. *J Clin Invest* 1998;102:223–231.
206. Openshaw PJ, Clarke SL, Record FM. Pulmonary eosinophilic response to respiratory syncytial virus infection in mice sensitized to the major surface glycoprotein G. *Int Immunol* 1992;4:493–500.
207. Orange JS, Biron CA. An absolute and restricted requirement for IL-12 in natural killer cell IFN-γ production and antiviral defense: Studies of natural killer and T cell responses in contrasting viral infections. *J Immunol* 1996;156:1138–1142.
208. Orange JS, Biron CA. Characterization of early IL-12, IFN-α/β, and TNF effects on antiviral state and NK cell responses during murine cytomegalovirus infection. *J Immunol* 1996;156:4746–4756.
209. Orange JS, Salazar-Mather TP, Opal SM, Biron CA. Mechanisms for virus-induced liver disease: Tumor necrosis factor-mediated pathology independent of natural killer and T cells during murine cytomegalovirus infection. *J Virol* 1997;71:9248–9258.
210. Orange JS, Salazar-Mather TP, Opal SM, et al. Mechanism of interleukin 12-mediated toxicities during experimental viral infections: Role of tumor necrosis factor and glucocorticoids. *J Exp Med* 1995; 181:901–914.
211. Orange JS, Wang B, Terhorst C, Biron CA. Requirement for natural killer (NK) cell-produced interferon γ in defense against murine cytomegalovirus infection and enhancement of this defense pathway by interleukin 12 administration. *J Exp Med* 1995;182:1045–1056.
212. Orange JS, Wolf SF, Biron CA. Effects of IL-12 on the response and susceptibility to experimental viral infections. *J Immunol* 1994;152: 1253–1264.
213. Oxenius A, Karrer U, Zinkernagel RM, Hengartner H. IL-12 is not required for induction of type 1 cytokine responses in viral infections. *J Immunol* 1999;162:965–973.
214. Patel RC, Sen GC. PACT, a protein activator of the interferon-induced protein kinase, PKR. *EMBO J* 1998;17:4379–4390.
215. Patel RC, Stanton P, McMillan NM, et al. The interferon-inducible double-stranded RNA-activated protein kinase self associates in vitro and in vivo. *Proc Natl Acad Sci U S A* 1995;92:8283–8287.
216. Patel RC, Vestal DJ, Xu Z, et al. DRBP76, a double-stranded RNA-binding nuclear protein, is phosphorylated by the interferon-induced protein kinase, PKR. *J Biol Chem* 1999;274:20432–20437.
217. Patterson JB, Samuel CE. Expression and regulation by interferon of a double-stranded-RNA-specific adenosine deaminase from human cells: Evidence for two forms of the deaminase. *Mol Cell Biol* 1995; 15:5376–5388.
218. Pearce EJ, Scott PA, Sher A. Immune regulation in parasitic infection and disease. In: Paul WE, ed. *Fundamental immunology,* 4th ed. Philadelphia: Lippincott-Raven, 1998:1271–1294.
219. Penfold ME, Dairaghi DJ, Duke GM, et al. Cytomegalovirus encodes a potent alpha chemokine. *Proc Natl Acad Sci U S A* 1999;96: 9839–9844.
220. Peritt D, Robertson S, Gri G, et al. Differentiation of human NK cells into NK1 and NK2 subsets. *J Immunol* 1998;161:5821–5824.
221. Pernis A, Gupta S, Gollob KJ, et al. Lack of interferon gamma receptor beta chain and the prevention of interferon gamma signaling in TH1 cells. *Science* 1995;269:245–247.
222. Pfeffer LM, Dinarello CA, Herberman RB, et al. Biological properties of recombinant alpha-interferons: 40th Anniversary of the discovery of interferons. *Cancer Res* 1998;58:2489–2499.
223. Pien GC, Satoskar AR, Takeda K, et al. Selective IL-18 requirements for induction of compartmental IFN-γ responses during viral infection. *J Immunol* 2000;165:4787–4791.
224. Powell PP, Dixon LK, Parkhouse RM. An IκB homolog encoded by African swine fever virus provides a novel mechanism for downregulation of proinflammatory cytokine responses in host macrophages. *J Virol* 1996;70:8527–8533.
225. Puglielli MT, Browning JL, Brewer AW, et al. Reversal of virus-induced systemic shock and respiratory failure by blockade of the lymphotoxin pathway. *Nat Med* 1999;5:1370–1374.
226. Pulliam L, Moore D, West DC. Human cytomegalovirus induces IL-6 and TNF alpha from macrophages and microglial cells: Possible role in neurotoxicity. *J Neurovirol* 1995;1:219–227.
227. Rahemtulla A, Fung-Leung WP, Schilham MW, et al. Normal development and function of CD8+ cells but markedly decreased helper cell activity in mice lacking CD4. *Nature* 1991;353:180–184.
228. Rani MRS, Foster GR, Leung S, et al. Characterization of beta-R1, a gene that is selectively induced by interferon beta (IFN-beta) compared with IFN-alpha. *J Biol Chem* 1996;271:22878–22884.
229. Rebouillat D, Howvanessian AG. The human 2′,5′-oligoadenylate synthetase family: Interferon-induced proteins with unique enzymatic properties. *J Interferon Cytokine Res* 1999;19:295–308.
230. Reid LE, Brasnett AH, Gilbert CS, et al. A single DNA response element can confer inducibility by both alpha- and gamma-interferons. *Proc Natl Acad Sci U S A* 1989;86:840–844.
231. Roake JA, Rao AS, Morris PJ, et al. Dendritic cell loss from nonlymphoid tissues after systemic administration of lipopolysaccharide, tumor necrosis factor, and interleukin 1. *J Exp Med* 1995;181: 2237–2247.
232. Roberts NJ Jr, Hiscott J, Signs DJ. The limited role of the human interferon system response to respiratory syncytial virus challenge: Analysis and comparison to influenza virus challenge. *Microb Pathog* 1992; 12:409–414.
233. Robinson D, Shibuya K, Mui A, et al. IGIF does not drive Th1 development but synergizes with IL-12 for interferon-gamma production and activates IRAK and NFkappaB. *Immunity* 1997;7:571–581.
234. Rogge L, Barberis-Maino, Biffi M, et al. Selective expression of an interleukin-12 receptor component by human T helper 1 cells. *J Exp Med* 1997;185:825–831.
235. Rogge L, D'Ambrosio D, Biffi M, et al. The role of STAT4 in species-specific regulation of Th cell development by type 1 IFNs. *J Immunol* 1998;161:6567–6574.
236. Rollins BJ. Chemokines. *Blood* 1997;90:909–928.
237. Romagnani S, Del-Prete G, Manetti R, et al. Role of TH1/TH2 cytokines in HIV infection. *Immunol Rev* 1994;140:73–92.
238. Ronco LV, Karpova AY, Vidal M, Howley PM. Human papillomavirus 16 E6 oncoprotein binds to interferon regulatory factor-3 and inhibits its transcriptional activity. *Genes Dev* 1998;12:2061–2072.
239. Rook AH, Kehrl JH, Wakefield LM, et al. Effects of transforming growth factor beta on the functions of natural killer cells: Depressed cytolytic activity and blunting of interferon responsiveness. *J Immunol* 1986;136:3916–3920.
240. Rossi D, Zlotnik A. The biology of chemokines and their receptors. *Ann Rev Immunol* 2000;18:217–242.
241. Rothe M, Sarma V, Dixit VM, Goeddel DV. TRAF2-mediated activation of NF-κ B by TNF receptor 2 and CD40. *Science* 1995;269:1424–1427.
242. Rothe M, Wong SC, Henzel WJ, Goeddel DV. A novel family of putative signal transducers associated with the cytoplasmic domain of the 75 kDa tumor necrosis factor receptor. *Cell* 1994;78:681–692.

243. Ruzek MC, Miller AH, Opal SM, et al. Characterization of early cytokine responses and an interleukin (IL)-6-dependent pathway of endogenous glucocorticoid induction during murine cytomegalovirus infection. *J Exp Med* 1997;185:1185–1192.
244. Ruzek MC, Pearce BD, Miller AH, Biron CA. Endogenous glucocorticoids protect against cytokine-mediated lethality during viral infection. *J Immunol* 1999;162:3527–3533.
245. Ryman KD, Klimstra WB, Nguyen KB, et al. Type 1 interferon protects adult mice from fatal Sindbis virus infection and is an important determinant of cell and tissue tropism. *J Virol* 2000;74:3366–3378.
246. Saederup N, Lin YC, Dairaghi DJ, et al. Cytomegalovirus-encoded beta chemokine promotes monocyte-associated viremia in the host. *Proc Natl Acad Sci U S A* 1999;96:10881–10886.
247. Sakatsume M, Igarashi K, Winestock KD, et al. The Jak kinases differentially associate with the alpha and beta (accessory factor) chains of the interferon gamma receptor to form a functional receptor unit capable of activating STAT transcription factors. *J Biol Chem* 1995; 270:17528–17534.
248. Salazar-Mather TP, Hamiltn TA, Biron CA. A chemokine-to-cytokine-to-chemokine cascade critical in antiviral defense. *J Clin Invest* 2000;105:985–993.
249. Salazar-Mather TP, Orange JS, Biron CA. Early murine cytomegalovirus (MCMV) infection induces liver natural killer (NK) cell inflammation and protection through macrophage inflammatory protein 1α (MIP-1α)-dependent pathways. *J Exp Med* 1998;187:1–14.
250. Sarawar SR, Doherty PC. Concurrent production of interleukin-2, interleukin-10, and gamma interferon in the regional lymph nodes of mice with influenza pneumonia. *J Virol* 1994;68:3112–3119.
251. Sareneva T, Matikainen S, Kurimoto M, Julkunen I. Influenza A virus-induced IFN-α/β and IL-18 synergistically enhance IFN-γ gene expression in human T cells. *J Immunol* 1998;160:6032–6038.
252. Sarkar SN, Bandyopadhyay S, Ghosh A, Sen GC. Enzymatic characteristics of recombinant medium isozyme of 2′-5′ oligoadenylate synthetase. *J Biol* Chem 1999;274:1848–1855.
253. Sarkar SN, Ghosh A, Wang HW, et al. The nature of the catalytic domain of 2′-5′-oligoadenylate synthetases. *J Biol Chem* 1999;274: 25535–25542.
254. Sarkar SN, Sen GC. Production, purification, and characterization of recombinant 2′,5′-oligoadenylate synthetases. *Methods* 1998;15:233–242.
255. Schall TJ, Bacon KB. Chemokines, leukocyte trafficking, and inflammation. *Curr Opin Immunol* 1994:6:865–873.
256. Scharton-Kersten T, Afonso LC, Wysocka M, et al. IL-12 is required for natural killer cell activation and subsequent T helper 1 cell development in experimental leishmaniasis. *J Immunol* 1995;154:5320–5330.
257. Scheinman RI, Cogswell PC, Lofquist AK, Baldwin AS Jr. Role of transcriptional activation of I kappa B alpha in mediation of immunosuppression by glucocorticoids. *Science* 1995;270:283–286.
258. Schijns VECJ, Haagmans BL, Wierda CMH, et al. Mice lacking IL-12 develop polarized Th1 cells during viral infection. *J Immunol* 1998; 160:3958–3964.
259. Schindler C, Shuai K, Prezioso VR, Darnell JE Jr. Interferon-dependent tyrosine phosphorylation of a latent cytoplasmic transcription factor. *Science* 1992;257:809–813.
260. Seder RA, Gazzinelli R, Sher A, Paul WE. IL-12 acts directly on CD4+ T cells to enhance priming for IFN-g production and diminishes IL-4 inhibition of such priming. Proc Natl Acad Sci U S A 1993; 90:10188–10192.
261. Sharp T, Raine DA, Gewert DR, et al. Activation of the interferon-inducible (2′-5′) oligoadenylate synthetase by the Epstein-Barr Virus RNA, EBER-1. *Virology* 1999;257:303–313.
262. Shuai K, Schindler C, Prezioso VR, Darnell JE Jr. Activation of transcription by IFN-gamma: Tyrosine phosphorylation of a 91-kD DNA binding protein. *Science* 1992;258:1808–1812.
263. Shuai K, Stark GR, Kerr IM, Darnell JE Jr. A single phosphotyrosine residue of Stat91 required for gene activation by interferon-gamma. *Science* 1993;261:1744–1746.
264. Siegal FP, Kadowaki N, Shodell M, et al. The nature of the principal type 1 interferon-producing cells in human blood. *Science* 1999;284: 1835–1837.
265. Silverman RH, Cirino NM. mRNA metabolism and post-transcriptional gene regulation. In: Morris DR, Harford JB, eds. *Gene regulation.* New York: John Wiley & Sons, 1997:295–309.
266. Smith GL. Virus proteins that bind cytokines, chemokines or interferons. *Curr Opin Immunol* 1996;8:467–471.
267. Spriggs MK. Cytokine and cytokine receptor genes "captured" by viruses. *Curr Opin Immunol* 1994;6:526–529.
268. Srikiatkhachorn A, Braciale TJ. Virus-specific CD8+ T lymphocytes downregulate T helper cell type 2 cytokine secretion and pulmonary eosinophilia during experimental murine respiratory syncytial virus infection. *J Exp Med* 1997;186:421–432.
269. Srikiatkhachorn A, Braciale TJ. Virus-specific memory and effector T lymphocytes exhibit different cytokine responses to antigens during experimental murine respiratory syncytial virus infection. *J Virol* 1997;71:678–685.
270. Staeheli P. Interferon-induced proteins and the antiviral state. *Adv Virus Res* 1990;38:147–200.
271. Stark GR, Kerr IM, Williams BR, et al. How cells respond to interferons. *Annu Rev Biochem* 1998;67:227–264.
272. Starr R, Willson TA, Viney EM, et al. A family of cytokine-inducible inhibitors of signalling. *Nature* 1997;387:917–921.
273. Stepp S, Dufourcq-Lagelaouse R, Le Deist F, et al. Perforin gene defects in familial hemophagocytic lymphohistiocytosis. *Science* 1999;286:1957–1959.
274. Stevenson PG, Doherty PC. Kinetic analysis of the specific host response to a murine gammaherpesvirus. *J Virol* 1998;72:943–949.
275. Su HC, Cousens LP, Fast LD, et al. CD4+ and CD8+ T cell interactions in IFN-γ and IL-4 responses to viral infections: Requirements for IL-2. *J Immunol* 1998;160:5007–5017.
276. Su HC, Leite-Morris KA, Braun L, Biron CA. A role for transforming growth factor-β1 in regulating natural killer cell and T lymphocyte proliferative responses during acute infection with lymphocytic choriomeningitis virus. *J Immunol* 1991;147:2717–2727.
277. Sun S, Zhang X, Tough DF, Sprent J. Type 1 interferon-mediated stimulation of T cells by CpG DNA. *J Exp Med* 1998;188:2335–2342.
278. Szabo SJ, Dighe AS, Gubler U, Murphy KM. Regulation of the interleukin (IL)-12R beta 2 subunit expression in developing T helper 1 (Th1) and Th2 cells. *J Exp Med* 1997;185:817–824.
279. Takeda K, Tsutsui H, Yoshimoto T, et al. Defective NK cell activity and Th1 response in IL-18-deficient mice. *Immunity* 1998;8: 383–390.
280. Tan SL, Katze MG. The emerging role of the interferon-induced PKR protein kinase as an apoptotic effector: A new face of death? *J Interferon Cytokine Res* 1999;19:543–554.
281. Taniguchi T. Cytokine signaling through nonreceptor protein tyrosine kinases. *Science* 1995;268:251–255.
282. Tartaglia LA, Ayres TM, Wong GH, Goeddel DV. A novel domain within the 55kd TNF receptor signals cell death. *Cell* 1993;74:845–853.
283. Tartaglia LA, Goeddel DV. Two TNF receptors. *Immunol Today* 1992; 13:151–153.
284. Tay CH, Welsh RM. Distinct organ-dependent mechanisms for the control of murine cytomegalovirus infection by natural killer cells. *J Virol* 1997;71:267–275.
285. Taylor DR, Shi ST, Romano PR, et al. Inhibition of the interferon-inducible protein kinase PKR by HCV E2 protein. *Science* 1999; 285:107–110.
286. Taylor GA, Collazo-Custodio CM, Yap GS, et al. Pathogen specific loss of host resistance in mice lacking the interferon-γ-inducible gene IGTP. *Proc Natl Acad Sci U S A* 2000;97:751–755.
287. Taylor GA, Jeffers M, Largaespada DA, et al. Identification of a novel GTPase, the inducibly expressed GTPase, that accumulates in response to interferon gamma. *J Biol Chem* 1996;271:20399–20405.
288. Tokunaga T, Yano O, Kuramoto E, et al. Synthetic oligonucleotides with particular base sequences from the cDNA encoding proteins of *Mycobacterium bovis* BCG induce interferons and activate natural killer cells. *Microbiol Immunol* 1992;36:55–66.
289. Tough DF, Borrow P, Sprent J. Induction of bystander T cell proliferation by viruses and type I interferon in vivo. *Science* 1996;272:1947–1950.
290. Trinchieri G. Interleukin-12: A cytokine at the interface of inflammation and immunity. *Adv Immunol* 1998;70:83–243.
291. Tumpey TM, Cheng H, Cook DN, et al. Absence of macrophage inflammatory protein-1α prevents the development of blinding herpes stromal keratitis. *J Virol* 1998;72:3705–3710.
292. Ulevitch RJ, Tobias PS. Receptor-dependent mechanisms of cell stimulation by bacterial endotoxin. *Annu Rev Immunol* 1995;13:437–457.
293. Upton C, Mossman K, McFadden G. Encoding of a homolog of the IFN-gamma receptor by myxoma virus. *Science* 1992;258: 1369–1372.
294. van den Broek MF, Müller U, Huang S, et al. Antiviral defense in mice

lacking both alpha/beta, and gamma interferon receptors. *J Virol* 1995; 69:4792–4796.
295. Vietor I, Schwenger P, Li W, et al. Tumor necrosis factor-induced activation and increased tyrosine phosphorylation of mitogen-activated protein (MAP) kinase in human fibroblasts. *J Biol Chem* 1993;268: 18994–18999.
296. Vilcek J, Lee TH. Tumor necrosis factor: New insights into the molecular mechanisms of its multiple actions. *J Biol Chem* 1991;266: 7313–7316.
297. Vilcek J, Sen GC. Interferons and other cytokines. In: Fields BN, Knipe DM, Howley PM, eds. *Fundamental virology,* 3rd ed. Philadelphia: Lippincott-Raven, 1996:341–365.
298. von Herrath MG, Yokoyama M, Dockter J, et al. CD4-deficient mice have reduced levels of memory cytotoxic T lymphocytes after immunization and show diminished resistance to subsequent virus challenge. *J Virol* 1996;70:1072–1079.
299. Waldmann TA, Tagaya Y. The multifaceted regulation of interleukin-15 expression and the role of this cytokine in NK cell differentiation and host response to intracellular pathogens. *Annu Rev Immunol* 1999; 17:19–49.
300. Wallach D, Varfolomeev EE, Malinin NL, et al. Tumor necrosis factor receptor and Fas signaling mechanisms. *Annu Rev Immunol* 1999;17: 331–367.
301. Walter MR, Windsor WT, Nagabhushan TL, et al. Crystal structure of a complex between interferon-gamma and its soluble high-affinity receptor. *Nature* 1995;376:230–235.
302. Wang B, Fujisawa H, Zhuang L, et al. Depressed Langerhans cell migration and reduced contact hypersensitivity response in mice lacking TNF receptor p75. *J Immunol* 1997;159:6148–6155.
303. Wang ZG, Ruggero D, Ronchetti S. PML is essential for multiple apoptotic pathways. *Nat Genet* 1998;20:266–272.
304. Waris ME, Tsou C, Erdman DD, et al. Respiratory syncytial virus infection in BALB/c mice previously immunized with formalin-inactivated virus induces enhanced pulmonary inflammatory response with a predominant Th2-like cytokine pattern. *J Virol* 1996;70:2852–2860.
305. Wathelet MG, Clauss IM, Content J, Huez GA. The IFI-56K and IFI-54K interferon-inducible human genes belong to the same gene family. *FEBS Lett* 1988;231:164–171.
306. Wathelet MG, Lin CH, Parekh BS, et al. Virus infection induces the assembly of coordinately activated transcription factors on the IFN-beta enhancer in vivo. *Mol Cells* 1998;1:507–518.
307. Weaver BK, Kumar KP, Reich NC. Interferon regulatory factor 3 and CREB-binding protein/p300 are subunits of double-stranded RNA-activated transcription factor DRAF1. *Mol Cell Biol* 1998;18:1359–1368.
308. Weihua X, Ramanujam S, Lindner DJ, et al. The polyoma virus T antigen interferes with interferon-inducible gene expression. *Proc Natl Acad Sci U S A* 1998;95:1085–1090.
309. Wen Z, Zhong Z, Darnell JE Jr. Maximal activation of transcription by Stat1 and Stat3 requires both tyrosine and serine phosphorylation. *Cell* 1995;82:241–250.
310. Wesselingh SL, Levine B, Fox RJ, et al. Intracerebral cytokine mRNA expression during fatal and nonfatal alphavirus encephalitis suggests a predominant type 2 T cell response. *J Immunol* 1994;152:1289–1297.
311. Whitten TM, Quets AT, Schloemer RH. Identification of the hepatitis B virus factor that inhibits expression of the beta interferon gene. *J Virol* 1991;65:4699–4704.
312. Williams BR. PKR, a sentinel kinase for cellular stress. *Oncogene* 1999;18:6112–6120.
313. Wills-Karp M. Immunologic basis of antigen-induced airway hyperresponsiveness. *Annu Rev Immunol* 1999;17:255–281.
314. Wong GHW, Goeddel DV. Tumor necrosis factors alpha and beta inhibit virus replication and synergize with interferons. *Nature* 1986; 323:819–822.
315. Wong P, Severns CW, Guyer NB, Wright TM. A unique palindromic element mediates gamma interferon induction of mig gene expression. *Mol Cell Biol* 1994;14:914–922.
316. Wright TM, Farber JM. 5′ Regulatory region of a novel cytokine gene mediates selective activation by interferon γ. *J Exp Med* 1991;173: 417–422.
317. Wysocka M, Kubin M, Vieira LQ, et al. Interleukin-12 is required for interferon-γ production and lethality in lipopolysaccharide-induced shock in mice. *Eur J Immunol* 1995;25:672–676.
318. Yamamura Y, Sendra H, Noda M, Ikawa Y. Activation of the JAK1-STAT5 pathway by binding of the Friend Virus gp55 glycoprotein to the erythropoietin receptor. *Leukemia* 1997;11:432–434.
319. Yang RB, Mark MR, Gray A, et al. Toll-like receptor 2 mediates lipopolysaccharide-induced cellular signalling. *Nature* 1998;395:284–288.
320. Yeh W, Hakem R, Woo M, Mak TW. Gene targeting in the analysis of mammalian apoptosis and TNF receptor superfamily signaling. *Immunol Rev* 1999;169:283–302.
321. Yoneyama M, Suhara W, Fukuhara Y, et al. Direct triggering of the type I interferon system by virus infection: Activation of a transcription factor complex containing IRF-3 and CBP/p300. *EMBO J* 1998;17:1087–1095.
322. Zhang X, Sun S, Hwang I, et al. Potent and selective stimulation of memory-phenotype CD8+ T cells in vivo by IL-15. *Immunity* 1998; 8:591–599.
323. Zhang JJ, Vinkemeier U, Gu W, et al. Two contact regions between Stat1 and CBP/p300 in interferon gamma signaling. *Proc Natl Acad Sci U S A* 1996;93:15092–15096.
324. Zhou A, Paranjape J, Brown TL, et al. Interferon action and apoptosis are defective in mice devoid of 2′,5′-oligoadenylate-dependent RNase L. *EMBO J* 1997;16:6355–6363.
325. Zhou A, Paranjape JM, Der SD, et al. Interferon action in triply deficient mice reveals the existence of alternate antiviral pathways. *Virology* 1999;258:435–440.
326. Zhu H, Cong J, Shenk T. Use of differential display analysis to assess the effect of human cytomegalovirus infection on the accumulation of cellular RNAs: Induction of interferon-responsive RNAs. *Proc Natl Acad Sci U S A* 1997;94:13985–13990.

CHAPTER 13

Virus Vectors and Their Applications

Alexander Pfeifer and Inder M. Verma

Gene therapy is a novel form of molecular medicine that is likely to have a major impact on human health in the coming century. Rarely has a medical technology elicited so much excitement, although that excitement is tempered by unfulfilled expectations. Excitement originates from the simplicity of the concept—introduce the gene and its product should have the ability to correct a genetic disorder and slow the progression of a disease. Disappointment stems from the inability to execute this task. How does one deliver genes into a wide variety of cells, organs, and whole animals? How long is the foreign gene expressed in its new milieu? Are there adverse immunologic consequences of both the delivery vehicle and its cargo? The quest for the perfect delivery vehicle is still incomplete!

The currently available delivery vehicles fall into two categories: The first consists of viral vectors, which take advantage of a variety of naturally occurring viruses to shuttle the foreign cargo either to be integrated permanently into the host's chromosome or to masquerade as an autonomous unit. The second category of delivery vehicles is made up of the nonviral vectors, which rely on direct delivery of either naked DNA or a mixture of genes with cationic lipids (liposomes). In this chapter, the currently available and widely used viral vectors, and their advantages and limitations, will be discussed.

RETROVIRAL VECTORS

Retroviruses can be classified into two categories (160): Simple retroviruses, encompassing the murine leukemia–related viral group [e.g., murine leukemia virus (MuLV)], and a group of complex retroviruses such as lentiviruses [e.g., human immunodeficiency virus (HIV)]. Gene therapy vectors have been developed from both groups of retroviruses and will be covered in separate sections.

Retroviral vectors based on MuLV were the first viral vectors to be used in a gene therapy trial that started a decade ago, with the aim to treat two children suffering from severe combined immunodeficiency (SCID) (16). Although the efficacy of this treatment and whether the disease was indeed cured by gene therapy could not be clearly ascertained because the patients received supportive conventional therapy during the trial, the retroviral gene transfer into the target cells (T cells) was partially successful.

Further underlining the potential of this class of gene delivery vehicles is the success of a clinical trial that resulted in the full correction of a disease phenotype (24). In this trial, CD34+ bone marrow cells were isolated from SCID patients and infected *ex vivo* with a MuLV-based retroviral vector carrying the cytokine receptor gene, which is mutated in these SCID patients. Cavazzano-Calvo et al. (24) were able to demonstrate expression and function of the transgene over a 10-month period, and most important, they showed the development and sustained function of the immune system, resulting in clinical improvement of the patients receiving gene therapy.

In principal, gene therapy vectors are either replication competent or they are rendered replication defective by deletion of essential viral genes from the vector. Replication-defective vectors are able to perform only one initial infectious cycle within the target cell. Although replication-competent retroviral vectors have been designed—especially in the early days of vector development—that are able to productively infect the target cell (106), replication of the viral vectors is unwanted in most gene therapy approaches, to avoid spreading of the recombinant virus.

Replication-Defective Retroviral Vectors

Most of the retroviral vectors (106,176) presently used in gene therapy approaches are derived from MuLV. To generate replication-defective MuLV, all of the protein-encoding sequences are removed from the virus and replaced by the transgene of interest (Fig. 1A,B).

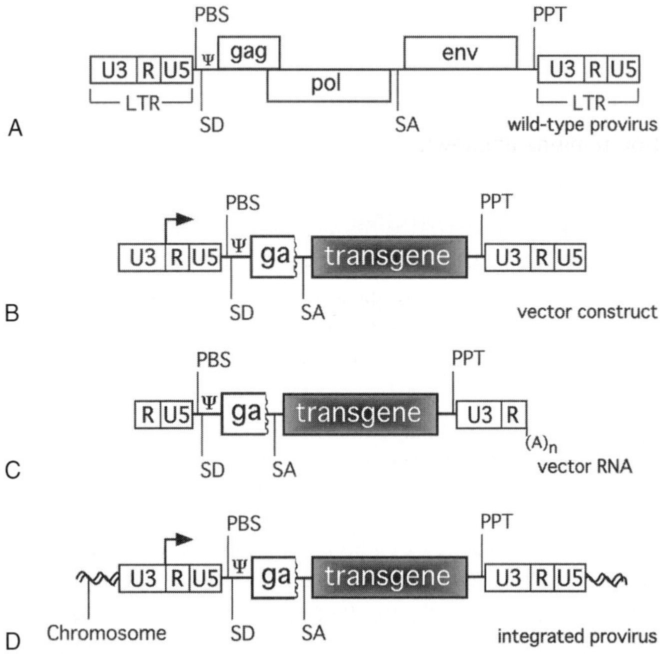

FIG. 1. Retroviral vectors. **A:** Schematic representation of the retroviral provirus. PBS, primer binding site; SD, splice donor; Ψ, packaging signal; SA, splice acceptor; PPT, poly purine tract; LTR, long terminal repeat. **B:** Retroviral vector. The transgene replaces the viral genes and is flanked by the retroviral LTRs. Apart from the minimal packaging signal (Ψ), portions of 5′ *gag* sequences are included to increase packaging efficacy. **C:** Vector RNA packaged into virions in the producer/packaging cells. **D:** Integrated provirus. The transgene of interest is transcribed from the promoter/enhancer region within the U3 of the 5′ LTR (*arrow*).

However, the sequences required for encapsidation of the vector RNA [i.e., a packaging signal (Ψ)] have to be included in the vector construct. The absolute minimal MuLV packaging signal has been narrowed down to a region encompassing bases 215 to 355 (96,97). In addition, the 5′ end of the *gag* gene has been shown to carry sequences that are required for efficient encapsidation of the vector RNA. Inclusion of this region [nucleotides 215 to 1,039 (10)] resulted in so-called Ψ^+ or gag^+ vectors with a 50- to 200-fold increase of vector titers (7,10) compared to vectors containing only the minimal Ψ signal. To ensure reverse transcription and integration of the vector DNA into the host genome, the long terminal repeats (LTRs), the primer transfer RNA (tRNA) binding site (PBS), and the polypurine tract (PPT) have to be incorporated into the vector construct (see Fig. 1B). The proteins needed for production of infectious viral particles can be supplied in trans in packaging/producer cells (see next section, Packaging of Retroviral Vectors).

Although the retroviruses and their genomic organization are described in detail in Chapters 27, 28 and Chapters 60 to 62 in *Fields Virology*, 4th ed., the life cycle of a retroviral vector is briefly summarized here (see Fig. 1B–D). The vector DNA is transcribed into RNA in the producer cells and packaged into viral particles. The promoter/enhancer regions of the 5′ U3 region are not transcribed, and the U5 sequences of the 3′ LTR are replaced by a polyadenylation [poly(A)] tail as a result of the presence of a poly(A) signal in the R region (see Fig. 1C). In the infected cell, the vector RNA genome is reverse transcribed and the provirus DNA integrates into the host genome. The U3 regions of the 5′ and the 3′ LTR of the provirus are derived from the U3 regions of the 3′ LTR originally present in the vector RNA, and both U5 regions are derived from the 5′ LTR originally present at 5′ end of the vector RNA (see Fig. 1C,D). This has important practical implications for the vector design. The transgene should not contain a poly(A) signal sequence, as this would lead to the replacement of the 3′ U3/R region with a poly(A) tail during transcription of the vector RNA (106). Furthermore, the duplication of the 3′ U3 region during reverse transcription is also the basis for the development of self-inactivating vectors (see later).

Several changes of the 5′ as well as the 3′ LTR region have been introduced into the retroviral vectors to increase vector yield and to improve the biosafety of the vectors, respectively. Among the most important changes concerning the efficacy of virus production is the replacement of the U3 region of the 5′ LTR with the immediate-early region of the human cytomegalovirus (CMV) enhancer-promoter (Fig. 2A), which results in a CMV/LTR hybrid that has a high transcriptional activity when introduced into the appropriate cell line (47), such as human embryonic kidney (HEK) 293 cells. This cell line expresses the adenoviral E1 gene products (59),

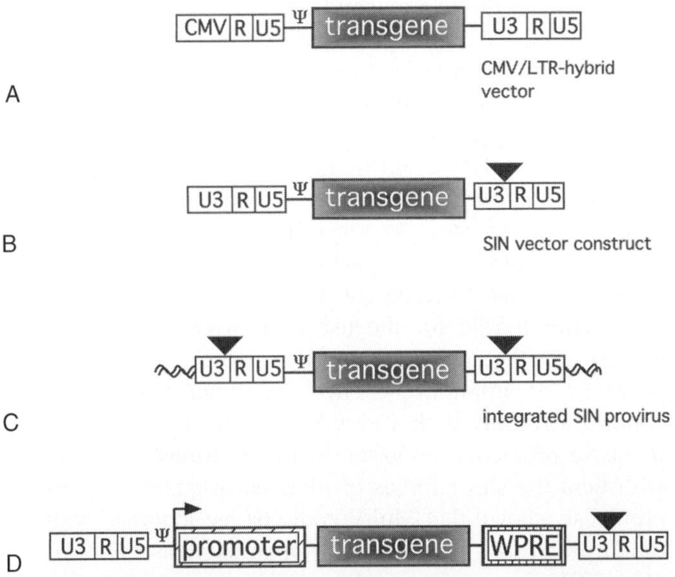

FIG. 2. Retroviral vector development. **A:** The CMV/LTR-hybrid vector system [e.g., r*kat* or pCL vectors (47,120)] allows a high-titer vector production in 293 cells. **B,C:** Retroviral SIN (self-inactivating) vectors with deletions (*black triangle*) of the promoter/enhancer regions of the 3′ LTR of the vector construct, which replaces the 5′ U3 region in the final integrated SIN provirus. **D:** An internal, heterologous promoter can be included in the vector construct to increase transgene expression in the target cell and/or to restrict transgene expression to certain cell types and tissues. To avoid interference with the promoter/enhancer of the viral LTRs, a SIN vector can be used. Incorporation of the WPRE into the vector enhances transgene expression.

which have been shown to superactivate the CMV promoter (55). After transient transfection of CMV/LTR vectors (47,120) together with CMV-driven packaging constructs (47,120) in 293 cells, this vector system yielded titers that were 100-fold higher than those obtained with retroviral vectors carrying the parental MuLV 5′ LTR.

To improve the biosafety of the retroviral vectors, deletion mutations were introduced into essential regions of the 3′ LTR. Because the U3 promoter/enhancer region of the 5′ LTR of the integrated provirus is derived from the 3′ LTR of the vector construct, deletion of promoter activity from the 3′ LTR should be carried over to the 5′ LTR during reverse transcription in the target cell (see Fig. 2B,C). This concept of transcriptional inactivation of the provirus is also termed self-inactivation, and these vectors are known as SIN (self-inactivating) vectors (178,182). Because the transcriptional activity of wild-type LTRs can affect the expression of host proto-oncogenes, the SIN strategy is a major improvement in the biosafety of the vectors. The drawback of the inactivation of the transcriptional regulatory elements of the proviral LTRs is a substantial loss in viral titer, which was at least 10- to 100-fold lower than the parental retroviral vector (178,182). On the other hand, partially disabled vectors (178) with an intact TATA box still exhibit a low level of LTR-driven transcription (0.1% to 1%).

The use of SIN vectors may be necessary to avoid interference of the viral promoter and enhancer regions with internal promoters of the vector in the target cells. In the most simple vector design, the 5′ LTR of the integrated provirus drives the expression of the transgene (see Fig. 1D). To achieve a higher level of transgene expression and/or specific expression in certain cell types and tissues, heterologous promoters can be placed internally in the retroviral transcription unit to drive transgene transcription (see Fig. 2D). However, the transcriptional activity of the proviral 5′ LTR can interfere with the activity of internal promoters (42). Thus, elimination of the promoter and enhancer functions of the proviral 5′ LTR may be necessary, and this can be achieved by using SIN vectors (see Fig. 2D).

Another improvement of transgene expression can be achieved by inclusion of cis-acting posttranscriptional regulatory elements (PRE) (186). PREs are present in herpes simplex and hepatitis B virus, and the latter has been shown to enhance expression of a heterologous cDNA (e.g., β-globin cDNA). Incorporation of the PRE of the woodchuck hepatitis virus (WPRE) 3′ of the transgene (see Fig. 2D) increased gene expression at least fivefold in MuLV-derived vectors (186). Interestingly, the enhancement of transgene expression by the WPRE was independent of the cell type or the cell cycle status of the target cells (186). The precise mechanism of WPRE function remains unknown.

Packaging of Retroviral Vectors

To package the replication-defective vector into virions, the viral proteins required are provided in trans in the packaging cell (Figs. 3 and 4). Retroviral packaging constructs are either transfected transiently into the packaging cells, or a cell line is established that stably expresses the viral proteins. The first-generation packaging cell lines (such as Ψ-2) carried a mutant MuLV virus with deletion mutations of the essential Ψ sequence (97) (see Fig. 3B). Deletion of Ψ results in a dramatic reduction of encapsidation of MuLV. In addition, the host range of vector particles produced by this packaging cell line was rather small. The tropism of MuLV is defined by Env and the species distribution of its receptor (see Chapter 27). Ecotropic viruses—such as MuLV—can infect only murine cells that express the receptor for Env [a sodium-independent cationic amino acid transporter (2)]. Since Ψ-2 cells carry the ecotropic *env* of MuLV, only murine cells could be infected with viral vectors produced by these cells. The host range of the vectors can be expanded by replacing the MuLV *env* gene with envelope sequences from amphotropic viruses (see Chapter 27; and refs. 32,108). These chimeric retroviruses contain *gag* and *pol*

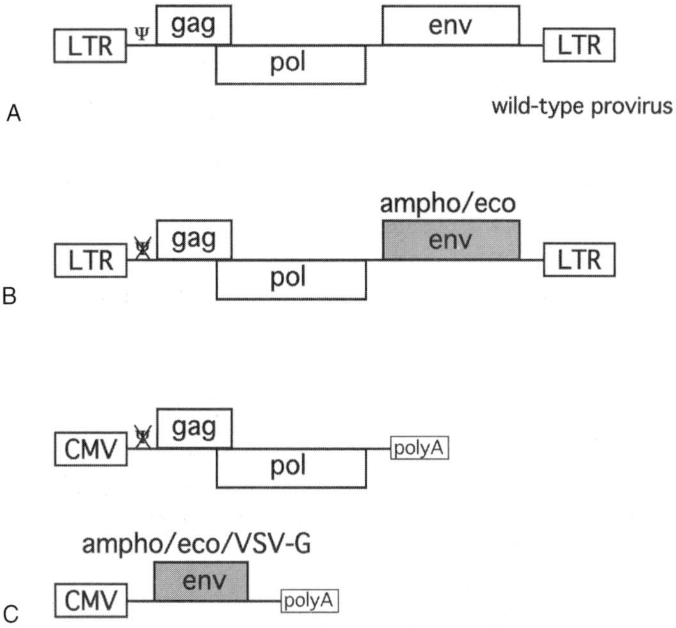

FIG. 3. Retroviral packaging system. **A:** Schematic representation of the wild-type retroviral provirus. **B:** First-generation packaging strategy with deletion mutations of the packaging signal (Ψ). Replacement of the wild-type *env* gene (*eco*) with, for example, amphotropic *env* (*amph*) results in a broadened host range. **C:** Split-genome packaging strategy: *gag*/*pol* and *env* are encoded on separate plasmids.

sequences from MuLV and the *env* gene from the amphotropic viruses (e.g., 4070A) (see Fig. 3B). Transfection of NIH3T3 with these chimeric packaging constructs, which lack the encapsidation signal, together with a retroviral vector, resulted in the production of high-titer [$>10^5$ transducing units (T.U.)/mL] stocks of helper-free recombinant retrovirus with amphotropic host range, able to infect murine and human cells (32).

An important biosafety issue of these early generations of packaging systems was contamination with replication-competent recombinants (RCRs), also called helper viruses. This problem was addressed by introducing further deletions into the packaging construct: the 3′ LTR and the PPT site (see Fig. 1A) were replaced with the simian virus 40 (SV40) poly(A) signal (107). Thus, in the rare case of encapsidation of the packaging construct into infectious virions, the packaging RNA will not be completely reverse-transcribed because it lacks the site for initiation of second-strand DNA synthesis. In addition, the 5′ end of the 5′ LTR that contains the cis-acting signal sequence required for integration (also called *att* element; see Chapter 27 for details) was removed. This deletion mutation should prevent integration of recombinant viruses that contain the 5′ part of the packaging construct. However, there was still a considerable amount of homology between the packaging construct and the retroviral vector, which could lead to the production of helper virus after a single recombination event between the two plasmids. Therefore, a packaging strategy based on split packaging constructs, one containing the *gag* and *pol* genes and the other carrying the *env* gene, was introduced (see Fig. 3C) (36,98). Splitting the packaging genome into multiple units not only increases the safety of retroviral vectors, but also facilitates pseudotyping of retroviral vectors with the envelope of other viruses, because different envelope genes can be included in the packaging cells by a simple exchange of the envelope construct.

A major hurdle for the use of retroviral vectors in human gene therapy was that virions, which incorporated ecotropic or amphotropic envelope proteins, could be concentrated only with a very low efficiency and labor-intensive protocols. Importantly, these virions could not withstand the shear forces of ultracentrifugation. It was previously shown that MuLV could be pseudotyped with the G protein of the vesicular stomatitis virus (VSV-G) (43). VSV-G mediates viral entry by membrane fusion via the interaction with phospholipid components of the cell membrane, and therefore it has a broad host range. Additionally, VSV-G-pseudotyped vectors can be concentrated 100- to 300-fold by ultracentrifugation to titers above 10^9 infectious units (IU)/mL (21). The major disadvantage of using VSV-G as an envelope is its toxic effects in the packaging cells, especially as high levels of VSV-G expression are required for high-titer virus production (21). The packaging cells express the VSV-G protein also on their cell surface, which leads to the formation of syncytia and cell death after several days of transfection with the VSV-G plasmid (21). Because of the toxicity of VSV-G, attempts to produce retroviral vectors from cell lines stably expressing VSV-G failed until inducible expression strategies (26,124) were developed using the tetracycline-repressed regulatable system (TrRS) (57).

The TrRS is based on the tetracycline resistance operon of *Escherichia coli* and combines the specificity of the tet repressor (tetR) for the tet operator sequence (*tet*O) with the activity of the herpes simplex virus transactivator (VP16) in eukaryotic cells. A conditionally active tetracycline transactivator (tTA) was created by fusion of the C-terminus of VP16 to the C-terminus of the tetR protein. Alternatively, tetR can also be fused to the ligand-binding domain of the estrogen receptor, leading to hormone-dependent function of the fusion protein (26). In the absence of tetracycline, the tetR domain of tTA binds to a tetracycline-regulated promoter (tRP), consisting of seven *tet*O repeats placed upstream of a minimal CMV promoter, and activates transcription of the transgene. Binding of tetracycline to tTA leads to a conformational change and highly reduced affinity of tTA for tRP, and the transgene expression is switched off. This strategy is also known as tet-off system (see Fig. 5D). The tetracycline system exhibits an impressive degree of regulation and can be turned off and on within

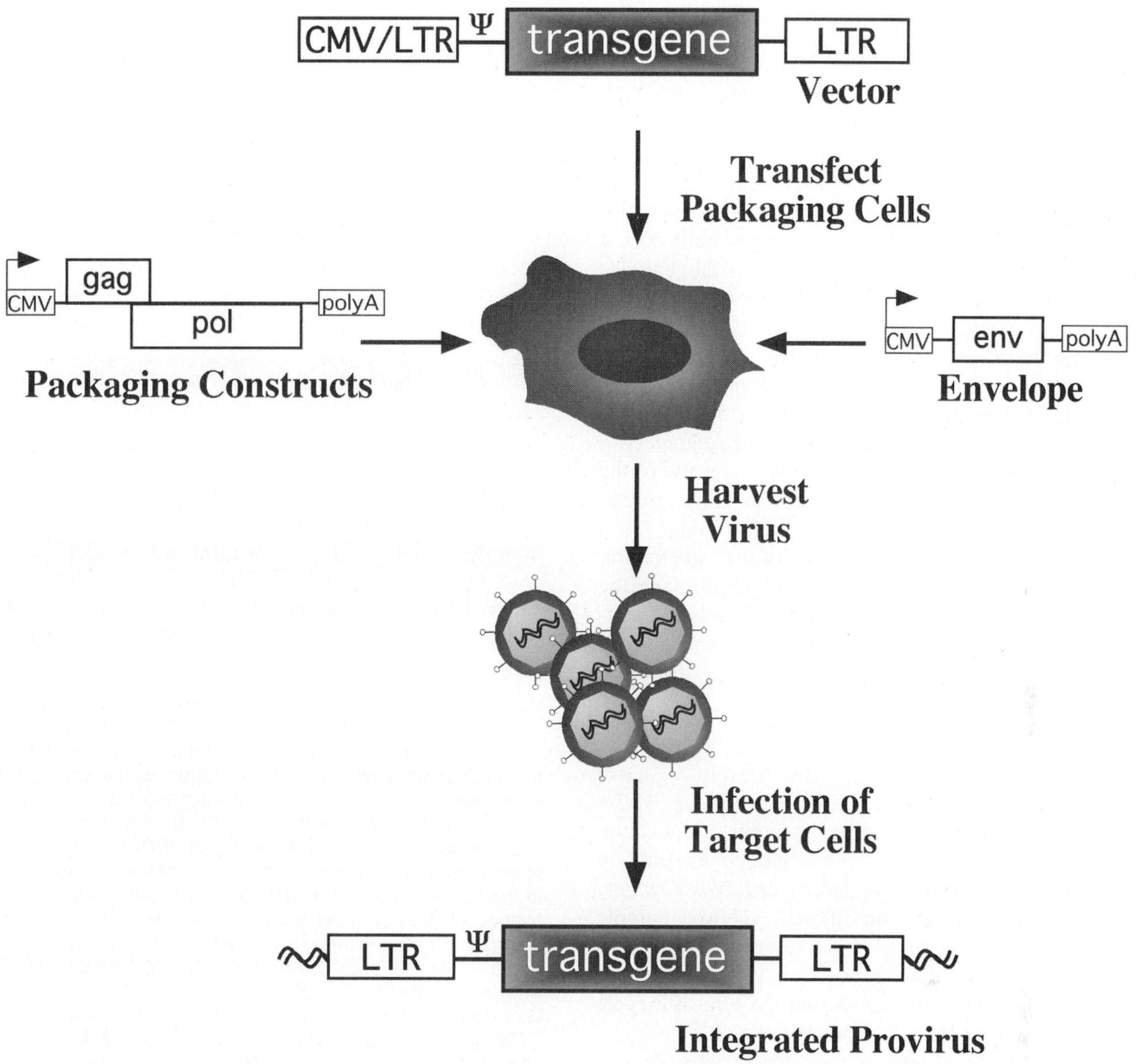

FIG. 4. Production of retroviral vector particles. Retroviral vectors can be produced by transient co-transfection of the vector plasmid (containing a hybrid CMV-LTR promoter/enhancer at the 5′ LTR position) with packaging constructs (coding for *gag* and *pol*) together with the envelope plasmid (a total of three plasmids are transfected) into packaging cells (e.g., 293 cells). The CMV promoter drives the expression of the different expression cassettes in the packaging cells. After infection of the target cells, the integrated provirus containing the foreign gene is transcribed from the 5′ LTR.

24 hours (77). The two components of this regulatory system, the transactivator tTA and the regulated promoter tRP, together with the VSV-G expression cassette were transfected into 293 (HEK) cells that stably express *gag* and *pol* [293GP cells (21)], and stable clones were selected (26,124). Finally, the retroviral vector is introduced into the stable packaging cell clones, either by infection with a recombinant virus (SIN vectors cannot be used for this purpose) or by transfection of the vector construct. Withdrawal of tetracycline induces a VSV-G expression in the packaging cells (26,124), with maximal virus production between 48 and 96 hours after removal of tetracycline (124).

Taken together, the recent improvements of the retroviral vector and packaging system are important steps toward using retroviral vectors for gene therapy trials in humans. The stable packaging cell lines allow the standardized production of retroviral vectors that can be screened for the presence of helper virus contamination. The split-genome approach to packaging (see Fig. 4) is an important safety feature that reduces the risk of such contamination. Pseudotyping of the virions with VSV-G broadens the host range and allows concentration of the virus with easy ultracentrifugation protocols. The toxic effects of the VSV-G protein in the packaging cells can be controlled by inducible expression strategies (e.g., the tetracycline-regulated system). The development of human-derived packaging cell lines (based on 293 cells) allows the production of clinical-grade virus preparations and offers several advantages over the—so far—frequently used NIH3T3 cells: Human-derived cells do not harbor a large number of endogenous retroviral genomes that could participate in recombination events to generate replication-competent viral mutants (147). Retroviral vectors produced from murine cells have been shown to be inactivated by human serum (natural antibodies and complement). The use of vectors that carry a CMV–LTR hybrid (see Fig. 2A) and CMV-driven packaging constructs (see Figs. 3C and 4) in 293 cells makes use of the fact that 293 cells express the adenoviral E1A protein, which stimulates of CMV-dependent transcription.

Furthermore, transient transfection of the viral vector, the packaging construct (carrying *gag* and *pol*), and the envelope construct (e.g., VSV-G) into 293 cells is a suitable way to generate high-titer (>10^9 IU/mL) preparations of many different viral vectors for laboratories that work on animal models for gene therapy (177).

LENTIVIRAL VECTORS

Lentiviruses belong to the family *Retroviridae*, whose characteristics—virion structure, genome, replication strategy, and host spectrum—are described in detail in Chapters 28 and Chapters 60 and 61 in *Fields Virology*, 4th ed. An important genetic difference between simple retroviruses and lentiviruses is the presence of regulatory (*tat* and *rev*) and auxiliary genes (*vpr*, *vif*, *vpu*, and *nef*) that have important functions during the viral life cycle and are relevant for lentiviral pathogenesis.

In contrast to simple retroviruses, lentiviruses are able to infect nondividing, terminally differentiated mammalian cells. This feature of lentiviruses makes them a very attractive tool for gene delivery (119,159).

The development of lentiviral vectors is based on the techniques and strategies developed for vectors studied in simple retroviruses. Previous experiences with retroviral vectors proved to be very helpful in the development of lentiviral vectors.

Replication-Defective Lentiviral Vectors

Like murine retroviral vectors, replication-deficient lentiviral vectors were designed by splitting the viral genome into cis- and trans-acting components necessary for gene transfer into the target cells (Figs. 5 and 6). The viral proteins required for the infection of the target cells are provided in trans by producer/packaging cells, which package the transfer vector that contains the transgene into infectious viral particles. In the vector constructs, the transgene is flanked by viral LTRs that contain cis-acting sequences necessary for packaging, integration, transcription, and polyadenylation (see Fig. 5).

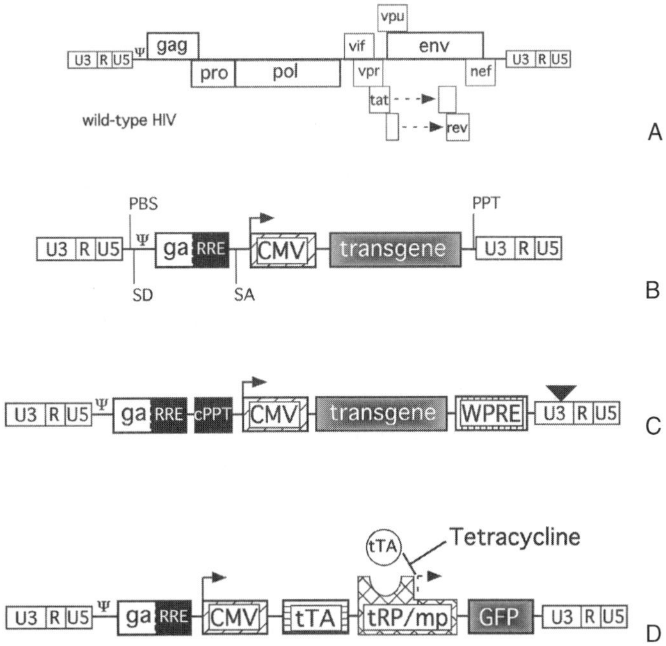

FIG. 5. Lentiviral vectors. **A:** Schematic representation of the wild-type HIV provirus. **B:** Lentiviral vector containing the lentiviral LTRs, a packaging signal (Ψ), the primer tRNA binding site (*PBS*), and a polypurine tract. 5′ *gag* sequences and the Rev-responsive element (*RRE*) are included to increase packaging efficacy and to allow efficient transcription and cytoplasmic export of full-length vector transcripts. **C:** The most advanced lentiviral vector construct with improved performance is a result of the incorporation of a central polypurine tract (*cPPT*) to enhance nuclear translocation of the vector in the target cell. In addition, the WPRE is included to improve transgene expression in the target cell and deletions in the U3 region of the 3′ LTR (*triangle*) to achieve self-inactivation of the vector in the target cell. **D:** Lentiviral vector incorporating the tetracycline-regulated system. The vector contains the tetracycline transactivator (*tTA*) (a fusion of tetR and VP16) and the tetracycline-regulated promoter (*tRP*), consisting of *tet*O repeats placed upstream of a minimal CMV promoter (*mp*). Expression of the tetracycline responsive elements is driven by a CMV promoter. Binding of tetracycline to tTA inhibits tRP-dependent gene expression; the transgene (e.g., GFP) expression is switched off.

As in the MuLV-based vectors, inclusion of sequences extending further into the *gag* gene (up to 722 nucleotides) significantly increased vector propagation and gene transfer efficiency (19,128). In addition, incorporation of the Rev-responsive element (RRE) of *env* (see Fig. 5B) increases encapsidation and transfer efficacy (128,137). Analysis of the ratio of unspliced to spliced cytoplasmic vector RNAs in packaging cells showed a significant reduction of unspliced RNA in the HIV-based vectors lacking the RRE compared to vectors containing the RRE (128).

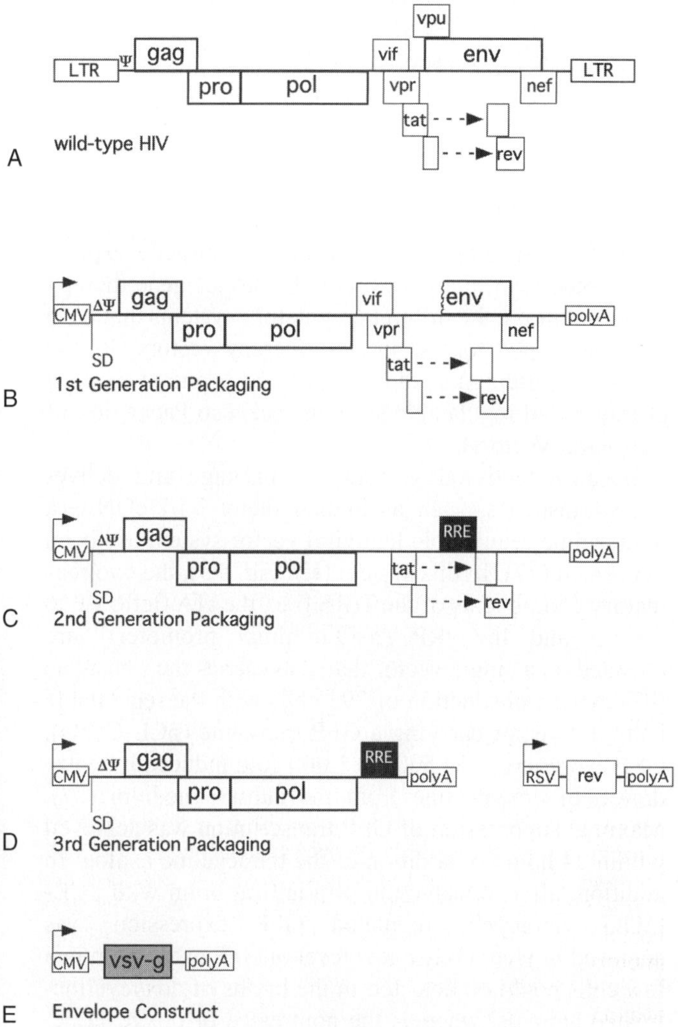

FIG. 6. HIV-derived packaging constructs. **A:** HIV-1 provirus. **B:** First-generation packaging plasmid. The reading frames of *env* and *vpu* are blocked, and the 5′ and 3′ LTRs are replaced with the CMV promoter and a polyadenylation [poly(A)] site, respectively [e.g., pCMVΔR9 (118)]. **C:** Deletion of *env, vif, vpr, vpu,* and *nef* resulted in the second generation of packaging construct [e.g., pCMVΔR8.91 (188)]. **D:** Tat-free, nonoverlapping split genome packaging system. In this third generation of an HIV-based packaging system, *gag* and *pol* are encoded on one plasmid [e.g., pMDLg/pRRE (40)], and *rev* is expressed in trans from another plasmid [e.g., RSV-REV (40)]. **E:** The envelope of the lentiviral vector is provided by a plasmid containing the VSV-G coding region flanked by the CMV promoter and a poly(A) signal [e.g., pMD.G (118)]. Ψ, packaging signal; RRE, Rev-responsive element; SD, splice donor.

The ability of lentiviruses to infect nondividing and terminally differentiated cells has been extensively studied, but the precise mechanism by which lentiviruses transduce nondividing cells remains elusive. The preintegration nucleoprotein complex (PIC) is recognized by the nuclear import machinery of the target cell and actively transported through the nucleopore (see Chapter 28 and Chapters 60 and 61 in *Fields Virology*, 4th ed.). HIV-1 contains multiple nucleophilic determinants that allow the nuclear entry of the lentiviral PIC. Three karyophilic proteins have been identified in HIV-1: the *gag*-encoded matrix protein (MA) (20), integrase (IN) (52), and Vpr (69). The MA contains two nuclear localization signal (NLS) motifs (65), and inactivation of both of them renders the mutant virus defective in nuclear transport, even in the presence of Vpr and IN. IN also harbors sequence homologies to NLS (51,130), and mutation of these regions has caused nuclear exclusion of IN but not of the HIV PIC (130). Both MA and IN are included in the HIV-based lentiviral vectors, but the multiply attenuated lentiviral vectors produced with the second- (see Fig. 6C) (188) or third-generation packaging systems (40) (see Fig. 6D) lack Vpr (see later section, Development of Lentiviral Packaging Systems). At least for the gene transfer into the central nervous system, Vpr is completely dispensable, as Vpr-deficient (Vpr^-) vectors transduce a similar number of adult rat neurons as Vpr-positive vectors (75,188). In addition, quiescent human and murine hematopoietic stem cells are transduced by Vpr^- vectors (23,99). However, the requirement of lentiviral accessory genes for the transduction of other cells such as macrophages may differ, as Vpr can rescue the ability of MA NLS-mutant viruses to infect nondividing macrophages (69).

Apart from these karyophilic viral proteins, HIV-1 genomic cis-acting sequences have recently been found to enhance the nuclear DNA import (50,183). In addition to the 3′ PPT, located just 5′ of the U3 region of the LTR (see Fig. 5B), all lentiviruses contain a central copy of the PPT (cPPT), at which synthesis of the downstream plus strand is initiated (183). Inclusion of the upstream cPPT element (see Fig. 5C) enhances nuclear import of the HIV-1-derived vector genome (50,183). Because the cPPT element is situated in the *pol* gene, the HIV-based gene transfer vectors devoid of *pol* lack this sequence, and the nuclear import of these vectors should be retarded as compared to wild-type HIV-1. Interestingly, *pol*-deficient lentiviral vectors are able to transduce terminally differentiated, nondividing cells such as neurons (118), muscle (75), hepatocytes (75), retinal photoreceptors (112,156), and hematopoietic stem cells (23,111), showing that at least in these cell types the cPPT is not necessary for nuclear import. An important difference between the $cPPT^-$ and $cPPT^+$ vectors is the time course of the transgene expression *in vitro* and *in vivo* and the total amount of protein expression achieved (50): After intravenous injection of $cPPT^+$ vectors carrying a CMV-driven expression cassette encoding human factor IX into SCID mice, the plasma level was twice as high as that achieved after injection of the $cPPT^-$ vector. Interestingly, inclusion of a cPPT has also been shown to enhance two- to threefold the transduction efficacy of simian immunodeficiency (SIV)-based vectors (95). Thus, the inclusion of a cPPT-element into lentiviral vectors improves their performance *in vivo* (50,183).

Enhancement of Lentiviral Transgene Expression

Vector performance can also be improved by increasing transgene expression after integration of the recombinant lentivirus into the host genome using cis-acting transcriptional regulatory elements. Inclusion of the post-transcriptional regulatory element of WPRE in HIV-derived vectors increased the reporter gene (green fluorescent protein [GFP] and luciferase) expression five- to eightfold after transduction of both dividing and arrested 293T cells (186). The WPRE has to be present within the transgene transcript in sense orientation, and it is placed 3′ of the transgene cDNA upstream of the 3′ LTR (see Fig. 5C).

SIN Lentivectors

As in all retroviruses, the U3 and U5 LTR regions of the lentiviral provirus are derived by duplication of the 5′ U5 and the 3′ U3 regions of the viral RNA during reverse transcription. Therefore, the same principal used to generate retroviral SIN vectors (see earlier and Figs. 1 and 2) can be employed for the production of lentiviral SIN vectors. SIN lentivectors (see Fig. 5C) were designed by incorporating extensive deletions (133 to 400 bp) in the 3′ U3 region of HIV-1 LTR, leaving intact the *att* element at the 5′ end of the U3 that is required for integration into the host genome (110,187). The deleted U3 regions include the TATA box, the three SP1 binding sites, the NFκb sites (110) up to the NF-ATc sites located further upstream, and the so-called negative response element (187). Co-transfection of the SIN vectors with packaging constructs resulted in titers that were similar to those obtained with the original vector plasmid without U3 deletions (110,187). Analysis of the effect of the U3 deletions on SIN lentivirus–derived RNA production in the target cells revealed an almost complete loss of the LTR promoter activity (187). Importantly, using a sensitive virus rescue assay, it was shown that the amount of virus rescued from SIN vector–infected cells was 10,000-fold lower than from cells infected with the parental vector without SIN mutations (110). Thus, the use of SIN vectors reduces the risk of mobilization of integrated provirus by replication-competent virus, minimizing the risk of vector virus spread.

Furthermore, after one round of viral replication, the U3 regions in both LTRs are derived from the U3 region of the 3′ LTR (see Fig. 1), thus allowing the replacement of the U3 region of the 5′ LTR with the CMV promoter in the vector plasmid (110,187). This modification of the 5′ LTR is important because SIN vectors combined with hybrid CMV-LTR contain only one U3 region (with deletions). Thus, recombination to generate a wild-type U3 region is not likely. In addition, replacement of the U3 region of the 5′ LTR with the CMV promoter resulted in Tat-independent transcription (110,187). This allows the production of HIV-derived vectors in the absence of Tat (see later).

Regulated Gene Expression

Spatial and temporal regulation of transgene expression would be a highly desirable feature of gene therapy vectors. Among the different regulatory systems that have been developed for use in gene therapy vectors (1), the TrRS (57) offers many advantages and is one of the best characterized regulatable systems (see also Packaging of Retroviral Vectors).

Because lentiviral vectors can package and deliver large transgenes, such as human factor VIII cDNA, a tetracycline-regulatable lentiviral vector system has been developed (77). In this system (see Fig. 5D), the two regulatory components of the TrRS [i.e., the tTA (tetR/VP16 fusion) and the tRP (*tet*O/minimal promoter)] are encoded on a single vector that also carries the transgene (77). After transduction of 293 cells with the regulatable lentiviral vector carrying a GFP transgene (pCL-CTIG), GFP expression was 500- to 1,000-fold induced by withdrawal of doxycycline from the culture medium (77). Maximal suppression of GFP transcription was achieved within 24 hours of addition of the tetracycline analog. In addition, after transduction of adult rat brain with pCL-CTIG, tetracycline-regulated GFP expression was achieved *in vivo*: Only a low level of GFP expression in a few cells could be detected in the brains of doxycycline-treated animals, whereas the nontreated or doxycycline-removal group demonstrated a very high level of GFP, as far as 2 to 3 mm from the site of virus injection.

So far, only the tetracycline-regulated system has been used in combination with lentiviral vectors, but studies are underway that employ the insect hormone ecdysone (121) or other nuclear hormone receptors as regulatory elements in the context of lentiviral vectors. Also, the rapamycin (FK506) system (138), which has been shown to function in an adeno-associated viruses (AAV)-inducible system (139,175), holds great promise, because it exhibits low baseline expression and a high induction ratio, as well as control by an orally bioavailable small-molecule drug.

Development of the Lentiviral Packaging System

Like retroviral packaging cells, all lentivirus proteins necessary for virus production are provided in trans by packaging plasmids, and virus particles are assembled by expressing viral proteins in producer/packaging cells (see Fig. 4). As a result of biosafety concerns, the packaging constructs lack cis-acting sequences required for the transfer of the viral genome to target cells (see Fig. 6).

The aim is to identify the minimal number of viral genes required for efficient virus production and to minimize the number of lentiviral genes present in the packaging plasmids.

The first genuine lentiviral packaging constructs (19,128,133,149) carried a deletion mutation of Ψ, and/or lacked the 5′ and 3′ LTRs (which were replaced by the CMV promoter and a polyadenylation signal, respectively). Although deletion of LTR and Ψ eliminated the sequences crucial for packaging—reverse transcription and integration of transcripts derived from the packaging plasmids—these packaging constructs still contained more than 90% of the HIV genome. Because these initial packaging systems incorporated the endogenous HIV envelope, the host range of these vectors was restricted to CD4-positive cells, and there was a risk of generating wild-type HIV. In addition, only low infectious titers [in the range of 10^1 to 10^2 IU/mL (19,128)] were obtained, and the vector particles could not be efficiently concentrated.

A crucial step for the advancement of lentiviral gene transfer was the incorporation of envelope proteins of other viruses. Dual infection of cells with HIV and a murine amphotropic retrovirus led to the production of HIV virus that carried the amphotropic envelope, demonstrating that HIV-1 can be pseudotyped with heterologous envelopes (151). By using replication-defective HIV-1 mutants that carry deletions of gp160, it was shown that the HIV enevelope can be provided in trans (125). Expression of the envelope gene of an amphotropic virus or of the human T-cell leukemia virus in cells transfected with the gp160-deficient HIV mutant resulted in the production of infectious viral particles (88,125).

Replacement of the HIV envelope glycoprotein with VSV-G (see Fig. 6B,E) expanded the host range of the HIV vectors (117,136). After transient co-transfection of packaging and vector plasmids, the virus can be harvested by collection of the culture medium of the 293T producer cells and concentrated to titers of up to 10^8 IU/mL by using a facile ultracentrifugation procedure (117,136). First-generation, VSV-G pseudotyped lentiviral vectors (see Fig. 6B,E) were able to transduce nondividing, G1/S- and G2-arrested HeLa cells (118). Furthermore, comparison of the transduction efficiency of MuLV-based with HIV-based VSV-G pseudotyped vector in unstimulated human peripheral blood CD34+ cells, which are highly enriched for G0/G1 cells, revealed an eightfold higher number of transduced cells after infection with the lentiviral vector (136). More importantly, lentiviral vectors (10^8 IU/mL) were able to transduce terminally differentiated, nondividing neurons *in vivo* (118).

With an approach similar to that used for HIV-1-based vectors, packaging systems for vectors based on feline immunodeficiency (FIV) (132), SIV (95), HIV-2 (131), and equine infectious anemia virus (123) have been developed, achieving titers (after concentration by ultracentrifugation) in the range of 10^7, 10^7, 10^8, and 10^6 IU/mL, respectively. Because HIV-1-based vectors have been exploited more extensively, we have used them as a model system for discussion of lentiviral vectors.

The initial packaging plasmids contain most of the lentivirus genes except for *env* (see Fig. 6B). In an effort to improve safety, a second version of the packaging system was introduced with extensive deletions of the viral genome (see Fig. 6C). Because it was shown that accessory genes of HIV-1 (*vpr*, *vpu*, *vif*, and *nef*) are not required for efficient production of viral particles (188), a packaging system containing only the *gag*, *pol*, *tat*, and *rev* genes of HIV-1 was developed (75,188). Thus, these packaging constructs are devoid of all the accessory genes required for efficient replication in human cells. HIV-based vectors packaged with this system are able to deliver genes into dividing and nondividing cells *in vitro*, and to transduce adult neurons and muscle *in vivo* (75,188).

In the latest, third generation of packaging strategies, the *tat* gene is deleted (40) (see Fig. 6D). Tat is a strong transcriptional activator of the HIV-1 LTR promoter element and is essential for viral replication (34,41). Tat expression in the packaging cells is necessary for the production of high-titer HIV-vectors (40), because interaction of Tat with the LTR promoter region is essential for the transcription of the vector plasmids in the packaging cells. Transcription from the HIV LTR in the absence of Tat was 10- to 20-fold reduced compared to the levels obtained in the presence of Tat in the first and second generation of packaging systems. This limitation of the Tat-free system was overcome by the inclusion of strong constitutive promoters, such as CMV (40,110) or respiratory syncytial virus (RSV) promoters (40), in the U3 region of the 5′ LTR of the vector constructs, resulting in CMV/RSV–HIV hybrid LTRs.

Another prominent feature of the third-generation packaging system is a split genome strategy (40). Initially, only the *gag* and *pol* genes (without the sequences upstream of the *gag* initiation codon) were cloned into one plasmid. However, transfection of this construct resulted in almost no detectable expression (40). Efficient expression was achieved after Dull et al. (40) inserted the HIV RRE 3′ of *pol* (see Fig. 6D) and included the *rev* gene—on a separate plasmid—in the packaging system. This minimized HIV-genome, split-genome packaging strategy is a significant improvement of the biosafety of the viral vectors.

Stable Packaging Cell Lines

Most of the studies using lentiviral vectors published so far rely on transient transfection of packaging and vector plasmids for vector production. Using the highly transfectable 293T cells, one routinely obtains titers of 10^9 to 10^{10} IU/mL after transient transfection with the latest generations of packaging (containing VSV-G) and vector constructs followed by concentration of the virus particles by ultracentrifugation. However, standardization of the virus production is not easily achieved with transient transfections. Given the problem of possible contaminations of the lentivirus preparations with RCRs and cellular debris (e.g., proteins and lipids shed by apoptotic producer cells), stable producer cell lines may be necessary to address biosafety concerns before HIV-derived vectors are used in clinical trials.

The development of a packaging cell line for lentiviral vectors was curtailed by the fact that VSV-G and some lentiviral proteins inhibit cell proliferation (e.g., Vpr) and/or exhibit cytotoxic effects (Vpr, Gag, and Tat). Because a long-term, stable expression of these proteins is not feasible, cell lines that carry deletion mutations of most of the accessory genes and that do not contain the VSV-G envelope gene were developed (22,33,181). However, these cell lines produced only low-titer virus with a limited host range. A very promising approach to address this problem is the development of cell lines that express the toxic components from inducible plasmids (78,181). The first inducible packaging cell line for the production of HIV-based vectors was described by Yu et al. (181). In this cell line, the expression of HIV genes is regulated by a dual system: HIV *rev* and *env* are encoded on a plasmid that carries the tetracycline-regulated system (see preceding section, Packaging of Retroviral Vectors), whereas the HIV late transcripts Gag, Pol, Tat, and Vif are expressed from a second plasmid that lacks the 3′ LTR, Ψ, and the other HIV proteins. Only in the absence of tetracycline, is Rev expressed, which in turn up-regulates the expression of the other HIV proteins (i.e., Gag, Pol, Tat, and Vif). In the presence of tetracycline, no infectious particles were detected (by measuring reverse transcriptase activity after stable transfection with the vector plasmid) (181), because of the regulatory function of Rev for the expression of late HIV transcripts.

In the packaging cell line developed by Kafri et al. (78), all HIV-1 genes (except the HIV envelope) are transcribed from a single expression cassette that is regulated by the tetracycline-regulated promoter. In addition, the VSV-G gene too is under the control of the tetracycline-responsive system. Withdrawal of tetracycline after transduction with the vector constructs results in the production of vector particles at titers greater than 10^6 IU/mL for 3 to 4 days, after which cell viability declines dramatically (78). Recently, a third-generation lentiviral packaging cell line has been generated (82) (T. Kafri, personal communication, 2000).

Transduction of Nondividing Cells

VSV-G pseudotyped lentiviral vectors derived from HIV-1 have been shown to transduce a broad spectrum of terminally differentiated, nondividing cells *in vivo*, such as neurons (118) and retinal (110,156), hepatic (75), and muscle cells (75). The absence of a cellular immune response at the site of injection, as measured by staining for CD4+ T lymphocytes or macrophages, after injection of lentiviral vectors (1 to 3×10^7 IU/mL) into the liver and muscle of the rat, indicates that lentiviral vectors might constitute immune-tolerated vectors. However, higher vector concentrations (>10^9 vector genomes) and different tissues have to be tested, especially in higher mammals, and also the humoral immune response has to be assessed.

The fact that lentiviral vectors transduce human CD34+ hematopoietic stem cells *in vitro* without cytokine prestimulation is of high clinical relevance and a clear advantage in comparison to MuLV-based retroviral vectors (23,50,111). The transduced CD34+ cells provided long-term repopulation and were capable of engrafting and differentiation into multiple hematopoietic lineages after transplantation into nonobese diabetic (NOD)/SCID mice (111).

The correction of several human genetic diseases by gene therapy will require the delivery of large DNA fragments. For instance, sickle cell anemia and β-thalassemia, two genetic disorders of the β-globin gene, will require high-level expression of the β-globin gene in hematopoietic and erythroid (31) cells. To achieve this, introns of the β-globin gene and parts of the locus control region (LCR) of the human β-globin gene (122) will have to be included in the vector. Viral vectors based on simple retroviruses exhibit genetic instability if genomic fragments, such as introns, are included in the vector DNA. Therefore, retroviral vectors containing β-globin transcription units and LCR fragments are very unstable, with multiple rearrangements on transmission of the provirus (91,122). Genetic instability of retroviruses occurs by (a) inappropriate splicing or polyadenylation of the viral genome, and/or by (b) rearrangements during reverse transcription (91). In contrast, lentiviruses such as HIV-1 have the ability to package unspliced viral genomes, and Rev has been shown to permit the nuclear export of unspliced or incompletely spliced HIV-1 RNAs (94). Because RRE is included in HIV-based lentiviral vectors (118), it was speculated that lentiviral vectors might overcome the problem of retroviral instability.

It has recently been shown that the use of HIV-based viral vectors enables the efficient transfer and faithful integration of the human β-globin gene together with large parts of its LCR into hematopoietic stem cells (99). The high efficiency of the lentiviral gene transfer, together with an optimized β-globin-LCR configuration and the absence of vector rearrangements, yielded human β-globin expression in the therapeutic range in a mouse model of β-thalassemia after bone marrow transplantation of transduced stem cells. In summary, lentiviral vectors clearly fulfill many of the promises of a suitable gene delivery vehicle.

ADENO-ASSOCIATED VIRUS

Adeno-associated viruses are nonpathogenic, nonenveloped DNA viruses that belong to the parvovirus family. AAV virions contain a single-stranded DNA genome of only 4,680 bases, which is flanked by two inverted terminal repeats (ITRs). Because productive (lytic) infection with AAV normally requires co-infection with an unrelated helper virus, either adenovirus or herpesvirus, these viruses were also termed dependoviruses (for a detailed description, see Chapter 32 and Chapter 70 in *Fields Virology*, 4th ed.). In the absence of helper virus, AAV establishes a latent infection and integrates into a host chromosome via its ITRs. The ITR consists of 145 nucleotides, with the first 125 bases forming a palindromic sequence that forms a Y- or T-shaped structure. The ITR plays a crucial role in the AAV life cycle: It is involved in integration of the AAV genome and its rescue from the integration site. Latent infection in human cells with wild-type AAV results in site-specific integration into the AAV-S1 region of chromosome 19 (86,146). The integration sites are clustered, and they show microhomologies between the host DNA and the ITR (173). Because the integrated AAV provirus can be mobilized by subsequent superinfection of the host with a helper virus, latent infection seems to be a mechanism for ensuring the survival of AAV in the absence of helper virus. On the other hand, the helper-free life cycle of AAV is the basis for the development of AAV-based gene therapy vectors (12,61,113,114,145,152).

Adeno-Associated Viral Vectors

So far, six serotypes of AAV have been found in primates (AAV-1 to AAV-6). Type 2 is the best-characterized primate serotype, and it was the first AAV used for the development of vectors for gene transfer (103,144). Most of the vectors currently in use are derived from AAV-2, but vectors based on AAV-1 have been recently described (169).

In contrast to retro- and lentiviral vectors, in which vector development not only resulted in different versions but also achieved significant improvements of transduction efficacy and biosafety, the original design of AAV vectors has not changed over the last decade. The AAV-2-based vectors contain only the left and right ITRs, and 139 (103) or 45 (144) nucleotides of nonrepeated AAV sequences adjacent to the right terminal repeat, respectively. Samulski et al. (143) were able to show that all the cis-acting AAV functions required for replication and virion production are located within the ITR and the immediately adjacent 45 nucleotides. In the AAV-based vectors, the two viral open reading frames (ORFs), which code for the capsid proteins (VP1, 2, and 3) and the four nonstructural Rep proteins (Rep78/68 and Rep52/40) are replaced with the transgene of interest and its promoter (Fig. 7B,C) and then transfected into the producer cells, where the viral genes necessary for virus production and packaging of the vector genome are provided in trans by packaging plasmids and helper viruses/plasmids (see next section, AAV-Vector Packaging Strategies).

One disadvantage of AAV-based vectors is their size limitation: The optimal size for AAV vectors lies between 4.1 and 4.9 kb (37). Although larger genomes can be packaged, the packaging efficacy is sharply reduced and the maximal size of the vector genome (including the two ITRs) is 5.2 kb (37). Because of this size limitation, a dual vector, trans-splicing AAV vector system was developed (39,116,155,172), which allows the transduction of target cells and tissues with two AAV vectors that contain a split expression cassette. This promising approach to AAV-based gene transfer is based on the finding that episomal recombinant AAV (rAAV) genomes form circular multimers that concatamerize in a head-to-tail orientation (38). The dual-vector strategy functions as follows: After

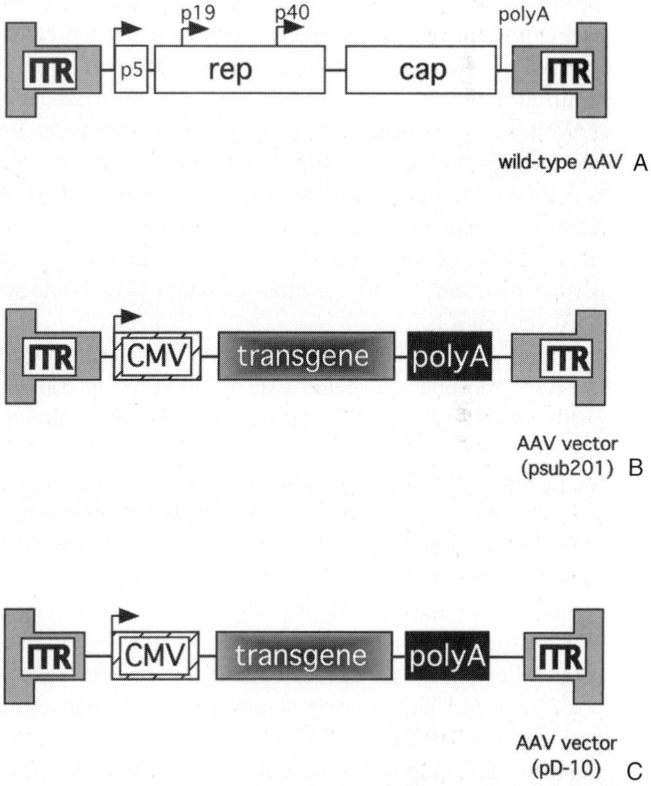

FIG. 7. Adeno-associated viral vectors. **A:** Scheme depicting wild-type AAV. The inverted terminal repeats (*ITRs*) and the promoters (*p5*, *p19*, and *p40*) of the *rep* gene are indicated. **B:** Recombinant AAV vector [e.g., p*sub*201 (143)]. The viral *rep* and *cap* genes are replaced with the transgene of interest, its promoter (e.g., CMV) and a polyadenylation signal sequence [*poly(A)*]. **C:** AAV vector carrying deletion mutations of the ITRs [e.g., pD-10 (164)] to minimize recombination between the vector and packaging/helper plasmids carrying adenoviral terminal repeats.

co-infection of the target cells, the two AAV vectors that carry the split genome form head-to-tail heterodimers through sequence homology of the ITRs, thereby rejoining the split gene into one continuous DNA molecule. Although such rejoining leads to the disruption of the gene-coding sequence by the AAV ITR, this problem can be overcome by inclusion of eukaryotic splicing signals to remove the ITR sequences during RNA maturation. With this novel dual-vector approach, the *E. coli lacZ* transgene (116,155), a luciferase reporter gene (39), and the human erythropoietin (172) gene were successfully delivered *in vitro* and *in vivo* (to muscle and liver of the mouse). Although the efficacy of gene delivery in the dual-vector system was consistently reported to be lower than in the unsplit, conventional AAV vector system, the individual efficacies vary between 16% (155) and 70% (116) as compared to unsplit vectors.

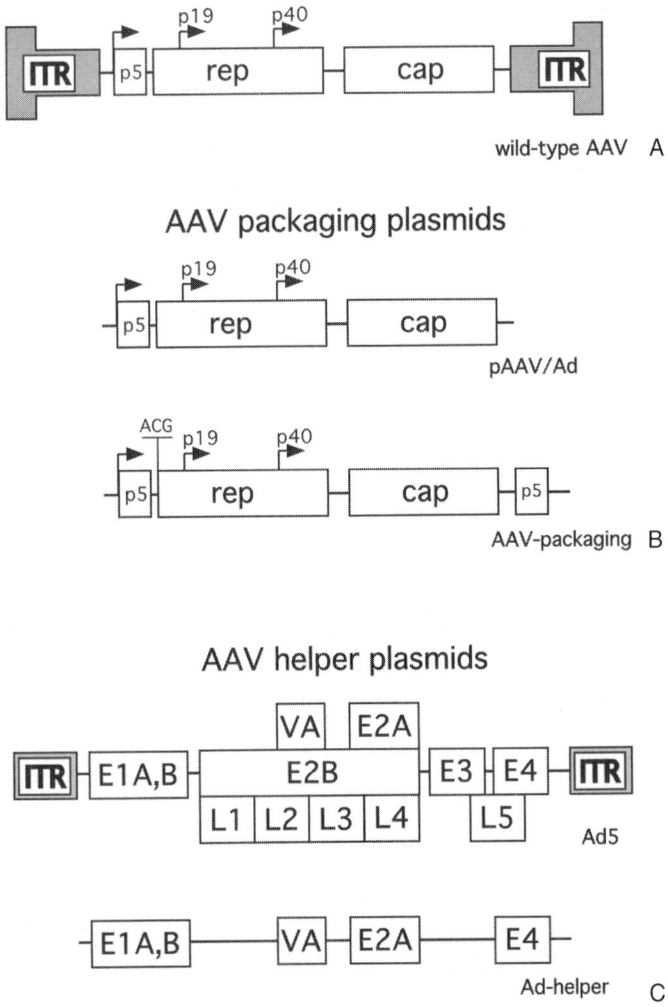

FIG. 8. AAV packaging/helper constructs. **A:** Wild-type AAV. **B:** AAV packaging constructs of the first [e.g., pAAV/Ad (144)] (*top*) and of the second generation [e.g., pXX2 (171)] (*bottom*); the latter contains a mutation of the start ATG to ACG, and two p5 promoter/enhancer elements to optimize *rep* and *cap* expression. **C:** Ad5 (*top*) can be used as an AAV helper virus. The use of adenovirus-derived helper plasmids [e.g., pXX6 (171)] that contain the required viral genes minimizes the risk of helper-virus contamination.

AAV-Vector Packaging Strategies

The basic principal of the AAV packaging system is the same as in other vectors: The vector plasmid contains the required cis-acting viral sequences necessary for packaging and integration and the transgene, while the packaging plasmids provide the viral components required for virus production in *trans*. However, because AAV is a dependovirus, its propagation depends on the functions provided by a helper virus (adenovirus or herpesvirus). Although replication has been described to occur in a helper-independent fashion if the host cells are stressed with genotoxic agents such as irradiation, adenovirus infection is still the most efficient way to induce AAV replication.

The initial studies with AAV vectors revealed that both the AAV *rep* and *cap* genes can be provided in trans in producer cells (103,144), and this resulted in the first generation of packaging systems (103,144). In this system, the packaging plasmid [pAAV/Ad (144)] encodes the *rep* and *cap* genes, and the essential helper functions are provided by the adenovirus (Fig. 8). Transfection of the AAV packaging construct together with the vector plasmid into adenovirus-infected packaging/helper cells results in excision of the ITR-flanked transgene from the vector plasmid, followed by its amplification and packaging into AAV capsids. This first generation of AAV packaging yielded up to 102 rAAV particles per cell, but there is a major disadvantage: the coproduction of wild-type adenovirus along with the AAV vector particles. Although these AAV preparations can be purified [e.g., by centrifugation in multiple cesium chloride (CsCl) gradients] and/or the adenovirus contamination can be inactivated (e.g., by heating the preparations for 30 minutes at 56°C), a complete removal of adenoviral capsid components is not always possible. In addition, this may lead to a loss in the activity of the AAV particles. Given the fact that viral proteins derived from inactivated adenovirus preparations elicit a cytotoxic T lymphocyte (CTL) immune response at the site of injection (76), it is clear that this packaging system is suboptimal, at least for clinical use.

To overcome this problem, a packaging system was developed (171) that is free of adenovirus. The adenoviral genes that provide essential helper functions during the productive life cycle of AAV are the E1A, E1B, E2A, E4, and VA RNA genes (reviewed in Chapter 32 and ref. 114). E1A functions as a transactivator of AAV *rep* and *cap* transcription. Interaction of E1B with E4 stabilizes AAV mRNAs and/or facilitates the mRNA transport to the cytoplasm. A similar role has been described for E2A and VA RNA. By cloning of the E2A, E4, and VA RNA genes into a high-copy plasmid, Xiao et al. (171) generated a helper plasmid (pXX6) that contains all the essential helper genes but lacks the adenovirus structural and replication genes and the adenoviral terminal repeats (see Fig. 8C). The missing E1 gene products are provided by using 293 producer cells (59). Surprisingly, supplying the adenoviral helper functions from a plasmid that resulted from deleting most of the adenoviral genome significantly increased AAV vector production (171). This is presumably the result of the lack of competition between the AAV and adenovirus for adenoviral gene products in the packaging cells, in addition to the removal of the lytic action of the helper virus (145).

A further, major improvement of AAV vector production was the development of a second generation of packaging constructs (171): Because *rep* expression has been shown to cause a paradoxical inhibition of rAAV production if the Rep68/78 proteins are overexpressed in the producer cells (92), the ATG translation start codon of the *rep* gene was mutated into an inefficient ACG codon to achieve attenuation of Rep68/78 synthesis (see Fig. 8B). Because the p5 promoter exerts positive effects on p19 and p40 but negatively regulates its own transcription (100,129), Xiao et al. (171) reasoned that inclusion of a second copy of the p5 promoter/enhancer element 3′ of the *cap* gene might have positive effects on AAV vector production (see Fig. 8B). Indeed, these changes increase vector yields approximately 15-fold over the conventional packaging plasmid pAAV/Ad. Thus, co-transfection of 293 cells with this second-generation packaging system, containing three plasmids (the vector, the pXX2 packaging plasmid, and the pXX6 helper construct) results in viral titers of up to 10^{10}/10-cm plate (171).

A problem with this packaging system is that the adenoviral terminal repeats present in pAAV/Ad and pXX2 have been shown to be involved in illegitimate recombination with the AAV ITRs. This recombination between the AAV vector and the packaging plasmids can lead to the production of wild-type AAV-2 particles in the range of 4% of the total physical titer (164). However, removal of the distal 10 nucleotides (in the D sequence of the ITR; see also Chapter 32) of the AAV vector ITRs [pD-10 vector construct (164)] reduced the amount of wild-type AAV contaminants to below the detection level, when a packaging plasmid was used that lacked adenoviral ITRs (164). The elimination of replication-competent wild-type AAV and helper virus (e.g., adenovirus) contaminations from the rAAV preparations is an important step toward the generation of clinical-grade vectors.

Packaging Cell Lines for AAV

Adeno-associated-virus vector production in stable cell lines has to overcome several problems associated with the toxicity of viral proteins and the viral life cycle. The Rep proteins exert an antiproliferative effect on mammalian cells (174), and they have a negative effect on heterologous gene expression (92). Therefore, it was not surprising that initial attempts to establish a stable cell line containing AAV-2 *rep* and *cap* (30,157) were not very successful. The initial AAV cell lines gave titers of 30 IU/cell (30), whereas transient transfection of the second generation of packaging/helper system yields up to 1,000 IU/cell (171). Recently, a number of promising inducible cell lines have been developed, in which the expression of Rep and Cap proteins is regulated by the tetracycline-inducible system (73) (see earlier section, Packaging of Retroviral Vectors). Infection of the cell line with adenovirus after the addition of tetracycline or doxycycline to the medium resulted in AAV vector production with titers 10 times higher (i.e., 10,000 IU/cell) than those obtained by transient transfection. However, after 3 to 4 days in doxycycline, the number of particles per cell dropped dramatically (73).

A major drawback of the presently available packaging cell lines is the requirement for the infection with a helper virus, and an extensive purification procedure has to be applied to minimize the amount of helper virus contamination. In addition, an important problem with stable cell lines for AAV vector production is that expression of the helper viral genes leads to the excision of the vector genome from the integration site, and thus prolonged expression of helper virus genes might disturb the genomic stability of the packaging/producer cells.

Purification of Recombinant AAV and Titering

In contrast to retroviral vector particles that are secreted into the culture medium of the packaging/producer cells, rAAV accumulates intracellularly and has to be purified from the producer cells. Lysis of the producer cells (e.g., by freeze/thaw cycles) is necessary if a packaging/helper system is used that is devoid of lytic helperviruses. The conventional purification protocol involves a step-wise precipitation of AAV particles with ammonium sulfate, followed by up to three rounds of CsCl density gradient centrifugation (170). After each round of CsCl centrifugation, the gradient is fractionated and the active fractions are identified by dot-blot hybridization or polymerase chain reaction analysis. Because this purification method is labor intensive and often results in substantial loss of viral particles, new methods have been developed to purify rAAV using gradient media other than CsCl or column chromatography (29,157,185). A major improvement of AAV purification is the iodixanol method developed by Zolotukhin et al. (185), which decreases toxicity from rAAV aggregates and avoids the toxicity of residual hyperosmotic CsCl. Iodixanol is an iso-osmotic, inert x-ray contrast reagent that has been extensively tested. Crude producer cell lysates can be purified at least 100-fold, and 70% to 80% of the starting infectious particles are recovered. With this method, lysates obtained from 2.5×10^9 cells can generate 10^{14} virus particles or 10^{12} IU/mL (185).

An important further step toward clinical-grade virus preparations was the development of ligand affinity chromatography purification techniques. Two laboratories have developed heparin affinity chromatography procedures using commercially available heparin columns (29,185). This approach exploits the fact that heparan sulfate proteoglycan acts as a cellular receptor for AAV-2 (154). Furthermore, it appears to be superior to earlier attempts to purify AAV using ion exchange or size-exclusion columns (29,157). The combined iodixanol/heparin chromatography procedure results in 50% to 70% recovery of virus that is better than 99% pure and is more infectious than the CsCl method (particle-to-infectivity ratios are less than 100:1 for iodixanol/heparin, versus 1,000:1 for the traditional purification strategies) (185). Recently, an immunoaffinity column chromatography approach to AAV purification has also been explored (60).

Host Range and Infection of Nondividing Cells

AAV-2-derived viral vectors exhibit a broad host range and infect a wide variety of tissues and cells. Furthermore, AAV is a nonpathogenic virus and is able to transduce nondividing cells such as muscle cells (170), hepatocytes (150), and neurons (101). These cells are terminally differentiated, and progression through the cell cycle seems not to be a prerequisite for transduction, as indicated by analysis of 5′-bromo-2′-deoxyuridine (BrdU) labeling of livers infected with rAAV (104). However, it has been reported that transduction efficacy is influenced by the cell cycle phase of the target cells and that the transduction frequency is significantly higher in cells in S phase (142). In addition, there appears to be a preference of rAAV for certain cell types: For example, rAAV infects neurons, but no transgene expression was found in astrocytes or microglia after infusion of AAV vectors into the adult rat brain (9). Furthermore, neuronal AAV infection was reported to be restricted to certain areas of the brain (e.g., the hippocampus), whereas neurons in the cerebral cortex were not transduced (101). Possible explanations are that rAAV might require a certain metabolic state, or that the receptors needed for AAV attachment and entry are not expressed on cells refractory to AAV transduction. The latter notion received further attention when the cellular receptor and coreceptors for AAV were identified. Heparan sulfate proteoglycan has been identified as the primary receptor for AAV (154) that mediates attachment of AAV-2 to the cell membrane of the target cell. In addition, integrin $\alpha_v\beta_5$ and the fibroblast growth factor receptor 1 (FGFR1) have been identified as coreceptors for AAV infection (134,153). Interestingly, coreceptors have been identified for both adenoviruses (Chapter 31 and Chapter 68 in *Fields Virology*, 4th ed.) and herpes simplex viruses (Chapter 33 and Chapter 73 in *Fields Virology*, 4th ed.). Thus, AAV may have acquired coreceptor dependency as a mechanism for co-infection with its helper viruses that allows the optimal production of progeny virions (153).

Apart from the cell cycle phase and the requirement for AAV receptor, expression of helper virus genes (46) and exposure to agents that induce genotoxic stress (e.g., irradiation) and DNA repair (46,140) can significantly increase transduction efficiency. Not only does adenovirus help wild-type AAV to initiate productive infection, it also enhances rAAV transduction (reviewed in ref. 145). It has been shown that the E4 protein is directly involved in this process, and that the E4- and genotoxic stress-induced increase in rAAV transduction is caused by enhanced second-strand synthesis (46). The latter is of importance for AAV-based gene delivery, because the conversion of the single-stranded AAV genome to duplex is the rate-limiting step for rAAV transduction in many cell types (145).

Integration Versus Episomal Persistence of rAAV

Site-specific integration would be a highly desirable feature of a gene therapy vector, as it would ensure long-term (theoretically even life-long) expression of the transgene and minimize the mutagenic and carcinogenic potential—major drawbacks of random integrating vectors based on retroviruses. Although the ITRs are the only genomic elements necessary for integration, efficient integration and site specificity require the presence of the viral Rep protein (165). Because AAV vectors lack the Rep expression cassette, it comes as no surprise that AAV vectors integrate with low efficacy and low specificity into the host genome. Integration of rAAV has been observed in dividing cells (e.g., HeLa cells) (173), as well as in nondividing cells *in vitro* (human neuronal cell lines) (168). Nakai et al. (115) provide direct evidence for integration of rAAV into the mouse genome. Further analysis by pulse-field electrophoresis and fluorescence in-situ hybridization (FISH) showed integration of the rAAV in approximately 5% of liver cells (105).

Apart from integration into the host genome, the presence of episomal forms of rAAV has been demonstrated *in vivo* (38,49,115). Several studies demonstrated the presence of AAV vector DNA in an episomal circular form in muscle and brain tissue transduced with AAV vectors (38,115). Because this form of episomal AAV DNA persists for up to 9 months (38,115), the episomal AAV DNA might be a major contributor to the long-term expression of transgenes delivered with AAV vectors. The characteristic feature of these circular genomes is that they contain two viral ITRs in a head-to-tail orientation, which appears to confer an increased persistence of episomal DNA at least in certain cell types (e.g., HeLa cells) (38). Presently, not much is known about the exact mechanisms that lead to the formation of these concatamers, but it appears to involve recombination events between separate viral genomes. This inherent ability of AAV to form concatamers fusing the 5′ and 3′ ends of two genomes of two viruses is the basis for the development of trans-splicing, dual-vector systems (39,116,155,172).

In summary, completion of second-strand synthesis appears to be the rate-limiting step of rAAV infection (recently reviewed in refs. 113,141), and it is associated with an increase in transgene expression, which can take several weeks after administration *in vivo*. Long-term (i.e., several months) transgene expression could be achieved by integrated concatamers, or by stable concatameric episomes, or both.

Immune Response Against AAV in Humans

Single administration of rAAV into the muscle of immune-competent mice does not result in a detectable cellular immune response as determined by staining for CTLs (170). However, a detailed analysis of the immune response in mice that received rAAV via intramuscular (i.m.), intraperitoneal (i.p.), intravenous (i.v.), and subcutaneous (s.c.) injection revealed that all these different routes of administration elicited a humoral response (17). Interestingly, a potent transgene-specific CTL response was detected after i.p., i.v., and s.c. injection, whereas only a minimal CTL activity was observed after i.m. administration (17).

The preexisting humoral immunity against AAV in humans is likely to be a hurdle for many gene therapy approaches in humans. A recent study by Chirmule et al. (27) showed that virtually all patients had antibodies to AAV-2, and in 32% of the cases neutralizing antibodies were found. In addition, 5% of the subjects had peripheral blood lymphocytes that proliferated in response to AAV-2 antigens. All patients enrolled in the first clinical trial of intramuscular injection of an AAV vector carrying human factor IX in patients with hemophilia B (79) had detectable titers of neutralizing antibodies against AAV before treatment. However, factor IX expression was demonstrated in muscle biopsies even in the patient with the highest pretreatment antibody titer. Administration of the AAV vector elicited a 10- to 1,000-fold increase in the neutralizing antibody titer.

Therefore, especially if vectors are readministered, efforts to overcome the humoral immunity against AAV have to be considered. Temporary block of CD4 T cell function to inhibit memory B cells (28), and the selective modification of the AAV capsid (54) are additional approaches. The latter is also a way to alter AAV-2 tropism and may be employed for targeting of AAV vectors *in vivo*.

ADENOVIRAL VECTORS

Adenoviruses are medium-sized DNA viruses that have been isolated from avian and mammalian species. Their genomic organization and virion structure are described in detail in Chapter 31 and Chapter 68 in *Fields Virology*, 4th ed.. The double-stranded linear DNA genome is 36 kb long and is flanked by two ITRs that contain the origin of replication (Fig. 9A). The Ad genome is packaged in a nonenveloped icosahedral protein capsid. On infection of permissive cells, the viral genome is replicated and transcribed in two major stages: an early and a late phase. The boundaries of the two phases are delineated by viral replication. The early genes lie in five noncontiguous regions designated as early region 1A (E1A), E1B, E2, E3, and E4. Most late transcripts are initiated from the major late promoter and are subsequently processed to generate five families of transcripts (L1 to L5) that share the same carboxyl terminus.

Development of Adenoviral Vectors

Of the approximately 50 known serotypes of human adenovirus, which are categorized into six subgroups, most adenoviral vectors (63,71,166) have been derived from serotype 5 (Ad5) of subgroup C. An important finding for the development of adenoviral vectors was that Ad5 carries a cis-acting DNA encapsidation signal at the end of the viral chromosome, and that recombinant viral genomes lacking these signal sequence cannot be packaged into viral particles, although normal levels of viral proteins were synthesized from these mutants (68). Two other important findings are (a) that Ad DNA can circularize in infected cells and that circular Ad genomes can be propagated as bacterial plasmids (reviewed in ref. 13), and (b) that co-transfection of two plasmids with overlapping sequences can generate infectious viral particles via homologous recombination *in vivo*.

Based on these findings, the first generation of Ad-derived vectors were designed by replacing adenoviral coding regions E1 and/or E3 with foreign genes. Because the E1A proteins are essential for transcription of other early viral genes and promote the expression of host cell proteins needed for DNA replication, deletion of the E1 region should render the vector replication-defective. The E1-deleted vectors can be propagated in 293 cells, which express 11% of the Ad5 genome and complement for E1 function (59). Thus, nearly all the E1 coding sequences (up to 3,181 nucleotides) can be removed (13), as long as the packaging signal and the coding sequence of protein IX, which is colinear with E1B but uses a different promoter (see Chapter 31), is not affected. Because the packaging capacity of Ad5 virions is 105% of the wild-type genome (14), transgenes of up to 4.7 to 4.9 kb can be accommodated in E1-deleted adenoviral vectors. The capacity of the viral vectors can be further increased by

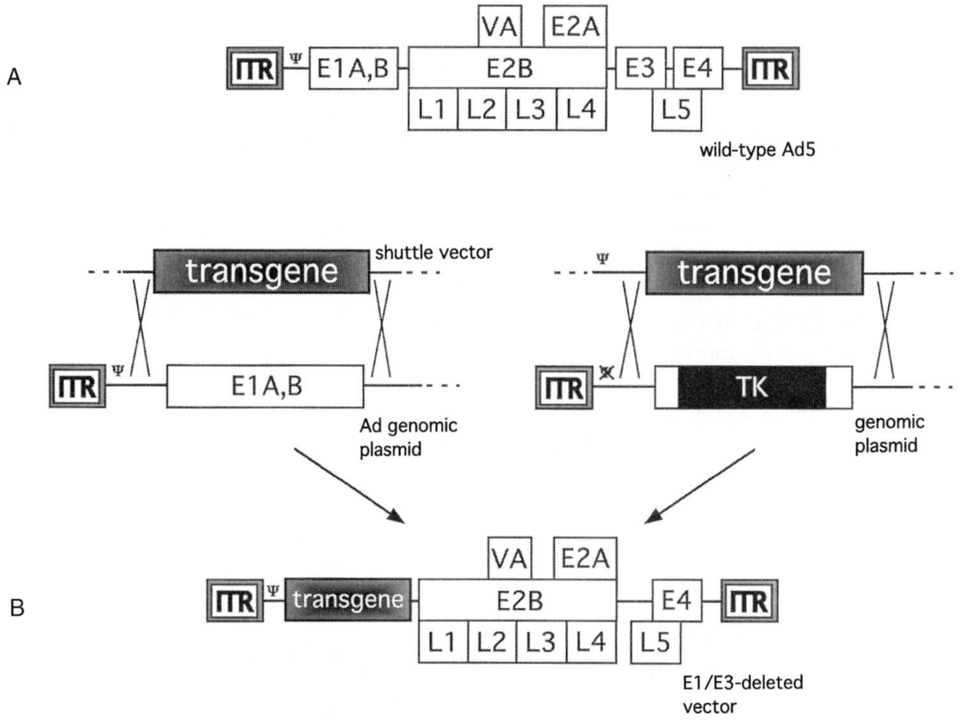

FIG. 9. Adenoviral vectors. **A:** Wild-type adenovirus (Ad5). **B:** First generation of adenoviral vectors. *Left:* Homologous recombination of the shuttle vector that carries the transgene flanked by adenoviral genomic sequences with the genomic plasmid results in the replacement of the E1 region with the transgene in the recombinant Ad vector (*bottom*). *Right:* Deletion of the packaging signal and/or insertion of a selection marker such as thymidine kinase (TK) reduces the amount of contamination with unrecombined parental virus.

deletion of the E3 region (11,66), which is not essential for viral replication and growth in cell culture. However, for gene therapy vectors, the E3 protein is of relevance, as it has immunosuppressive functions (71): From the seven proteins encoded by the E3 region, the gp 19-kd protein binds to MHC class molecules and the 14.7/10.4-kd proteins inhibit apoptosis. The largest viable E3 deletion described so far is 3.1 kb (13). A combination of both E1 and E3 deletions in one mutant virus results in a cloning capacity of 8.3 kb.

Several strategies have been developed to insert the transgenes of interest into the Ad vectors. The most commonly used strategy relies on homologous recombination in the 293 producer cells (see Fig. 9). The transgene is inserted into a shuttle vector that contains adenoviral genomic sequences that flank the recombination target site (i.e., the E1 coding region) in the recipient Ad genomic plasmid. Through homologous recombination in the 293 cells, the transgene sequence is integrated into the Ad vector DNA, replacing the E1 gene. This E1-deleted Ad vector is able to replicate in the 293 cells because of their E1 helper function, and it is possible to produce up to 10^{11} viral particles per 10-cm cell culture dish.

A drawback of this first generation of Ad vectors is the contamination with wild-type virus. Two major changes have been incorporated into the Ad genomic plasmids to solve this problem (see Fig. 9): (a) removing the packaging signal (13), or increasing its size beyond the maximum that can be packaged (102), thereby inhibiting packaging of the parental genome, and (b) incorporating a selection marker (e.g., by replacing the E1 region with the thymidine kinase gene) that allows for the selection against wild-type virus (72). In addition, strategies have been designed for the production of recombinant viral DNA that do not rely on recombination with parental infectious viral genomes in 293 cells. Instead, Ad genomic DNA can be manipulated in yeast (80) and bacteria (25). The recombinant Ad genome can then be purified from these hosts and used to produce virus in 293 cells.

A recurrent problem with the first generation of Ad vectors is the generation of replication-competent adenovirus (RCA). To address this problem, further deletions of viral genes were introduced into the vector backbone, resulting in the second generation of Ad vectors. Reduction of the number of viral genes present in the Ad vector should also reduce the immune response against the vector and vector-infected cells. These second-generation vectors (71,161) are based on deletion of the E2 and/or E4 regions within the E1-deleted vectors. The E2 region encodes proteins required for the replication of the viral chromosome: the precursor terminal protein, DNA polymerase, and DNA-binding protein (DBP). The first attempts to delete the E2 region were hampered by the fact that the production of the E2-deleted vectors require expression of E2 in trans, which is not easily achieved because of the toxicity of the E2 protein (83). Therefore, Engelhardt et al. (44) constructed an E1-deleted adenoviral vector that harbors a temperature-sensitive mutation of DBP. This mutation reduces the ability of the virus to replicate at 39°C. Because of the "leakiness" of this system and the conflicting results regarding persistence of transgene expression [especially at a later time (beyond 7 days) (44,45)], vectors with deletions of DBP (56), of adenoviral DNA polymerase (5), and of the precursor terminal protein (148) were designed that can be produced in packaging cell lines that complement for the deleted protein (4,56,89,184).

E4 is the other genomic region that has been targeted for the development of second-generation vectors. Located at the right end of the Ad genome (see Fig. 9A), E4 encodes proteins that are required for viral DNA replication, mRNA splicing and accumulation, late protein synthesis, and inhibition of host cell protein synthesis. Deletion of the entire E4 region is theoretically possible; however, in practice such vectors have been shown to result in a significant drop in vector yield (18). The mechanism for this decrease in viral titer of E4-deleted vectors is not completely understood, but it was shown that total deletion of E4 causes a reduction in the expression of late region 5 (L5) mRNA. It was postulated that the spatial organization of E4, L5, and the right ITR itself might be of importance for the regulation of L5. The defect of E4-deleted vectors was overcome either by insertion of spacer sequences into the E4 locus (18) or by only partially deleting the E4 region (53,162,179). To propagate the E1/E4-deleted vectors, E4-complementing cell lines have been developed. An important aspect of E4 function is the discovery that the product of ORF6 can substitute for the entire E4 region. Because expression of E4 ORF6 together with E1B is detrimental to the packaging cells, inducible E4 expression systems have been developed (87,163). Although deletion of the majority of E4 should decrease the host immune response and increase the cloning capacity of the Ad vector, the E4 region may be required for long-term expression, especially if the CMV promoter is used as internal promoter in the vector construct (6,8).

High-Capacity, Helper-Dependent Vectors

The third-generation Ad vectors (63,71,84) have been termed, according to their characteristics, high-capacity, helper-dependent, mini, and "gutless" adenoviral vectors. They were designed to minimize the amount of Ad viral genes present in the vector. This would increase the cloning capacity of the vector and should reduce the host immune responses against the Ad vector-transduced cells.

Earlier attempts (48,64,109) to divide the adenovirus genome into separate cis- and trans-acting functions to establish clearly separated vector and packaging/helper constructs were successful. However, two major problems were encountered (71): The vector preparations were highly contaminated with up to a 1,000-fold excess of helper virus (48). Vectors that are significantly below the size of the wild-type Ad genome proved to be unstable and undergo DNA rearrangements (48,64). Parks and Graham (127) analyzed the size constraints of Ad vectors: The optimal DNA packaging length ranges from 75% to 105% of the wild-type (36-kb) genome. Vectors smaller than 75% were packaged with a much lower efficacy, and were unstable (127).

An important step in the production of helper-dependent vectors was the introduction of the Cre/*loxP*-strategy in the Ad system to remove viral DNA sequences (67,93,126). The Cre-recombinase of bacteriophage P1 excises DNA sequences that are flanked by *loxP* recognition sites and has been successfully used for gene targeting experiments in mice (62). The Cre/*loxP* systems allows even the manipulation of mammalian chromosomal regions (up to 3 to 4 cM) (135). Insertion of *loxP* sites so that they flank the genomic region to be deleted is a promising way to restrict the Ad genome (Fig. 10). Lieber et al. (93) deleted 25 kb of adenoviral genome encompassing the pIX, the E2, and the L1 to L4 regions by infection of 293 cells stably expressing the Cre recombinase (293-cre) with an Ad vector that contained *loxP* sites flanking the region to be deleted. These authors (93) introduced the *loxP* sites into an E1-deleted vector backbone that carried a transgene in the place of the E1 region, and the final result after Cre-mediated excision was a 9-kb vector that contained only the transgene, a *loxP* site, the packaging signal, and the E4 region flanked by ITRs (see Fig. 10). Unfortunately, this vector was unstable, presumably because of its size, and it provided only limited transgene expression *in vivo*.

An alternative Cre/*loxP* system was designed that targeted the sequences essential for packaging of the helper virus to prevent its packaging (67,126). Previous studies (85) had shown that using a helper virus that carried a deletion of 91 bp of the Ad packaging signal, together with a helper-dependent Ad vector, resulted in a considerable improvement of the helper virus contamination, reducing it to less than 1% after CsCl purification. The helper virus with the *loxP*-flanked packaging signal can be easily propagated in conventional 293 cells. After infection of 293-cre cells with this helper virus, the packaging signal is excised, and the helper virus retains its capability to provide the Ad functions required for replication and packaging of the helper-dependent virus. With this system, Parks et al. (126) obtained about 10^{10} IU, with less than 0.01% of total virus being helper virus.

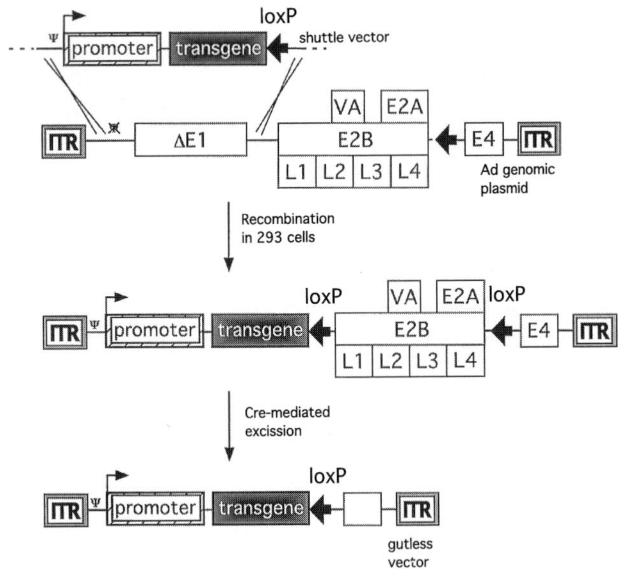

FIG. 10. High-capacity adenoviral vectors. High-capacity, adenovirus vectors can be obtained by introduction of two *loxP* sites (*black arrows*) into an Ad genomic plasmid that carries deletions in the packaging signal, in the E1 region, and in the E3 region (93) (*top*). Infection of 293-cre cells that express the Cre recombinase leads to the excision of the sequences flanked by the *loxP* sites (*middle*), thereby deleting almost all viral sequences. The resulting "gutless" vector contains only the ITRs, the packaging signal, the viral E4 region, and the transgene and the internal promoter.

The principal advantage of helper-dependent vectors over first- and second-generation Ad vectors and other gene therapy vectors is their enlarged cloning capacity: If all viral genes are deleted, up to about 35 kb of DNA could be packaged in the Ad5 virion. The cis-acting elements required for replication and packaging (i.e., the packaging signal and the ITRs) of the vector are contained within 500 bp at the end of the Ad genome (58). In addition, the removal of viral genes from the vector is a promising way to avoid the host immune response.

Replication-Competent Adenoviral Vectors

Although replication of Ad vectors is unwanted in most gene therapy approaches, viral replication, virus assembly, and release of the progeny virus by lysis of the infected cell can be exploited for cancer gene therapy. To use adenoviruses for oncolytic gene therapy, conditionally replicative adenoviruses have been developed that replicate exclusively in tumor cells (3). An example of such a virus is an Ad mutant that replicates selectively in p53-deficient cells (called dl1520 or ONYX-015) (15,70). The dl1520 is a human subgroup C Ad that carries an 827-bp deletion and a point mutation in the E1B region that prevents expression of the E1B-encoded 55-kd (E1B-55K) protein. E1B-55K normally binds and inactivates the tumor suppressor p53 (180) and contributes to oncogenic transformation by Ad. Because p53 function must be blocked to allow efficient virus replication, it was hypothesized that replication of the E1B-55K-deficient Ad virus would be suppressed in normal cells, whereas cancer cells that lack p53 would support viral replication. Indeed, the E1B-55K-deficient virus was subsequently shown to productively infect a broad spectrum of human tumors with p53 abnormalities (e.g., p53 mutations and/or deletions) and to exert a replication-dependent cytopathic effect in these tumors *in vitro* and *in vivo* (70). On the other hand, human cells with functional p53 were highly resistant to the E1B-55K-deficient virus (70). Given this promising result, a phase II clinical trial was started with intratumoral administration of E1B-55K-deficient Ad mutant in combination with standard i.v. chemotherapy in patients with recurrent squamous cell carcinoma of the head and neck (81). The combined therapy caused a more than 50% decrease in tumor volume in 63% of the patients, and none of the responding tumors progressed for 6 months, whereas all tumors treated with chemotherapy alone did progress. Thus, the approach of using specially engineered replication-competent Ad vectors in the treatment of cancer is a promising direction for gene therapy.

Immunologic Impediments

The ability to generate high-titer (10^{14} particles/mL) recombinant Ad vectors (RAd) and their efficient transduction of both dividing and nondividing cells boded well for a very successful vector. Unfortunately, length of expression of the transgene was transient (7 to 10 days) (35). It soon emerged that transient expression was caused by an immune response, because in immunocompromised animals, expression in slow-turnover cells such as muscle and neurons is observed for long periods of time. It is now generally accepted that cells transduced by RAd vectors are eliminated by CTLs generated against viral proteins or the transgene (76,158). It was for this reason that a number of investigators generated second- and third-generation vectors in which chances of synthesis of viral proteins are minimized. Unfortunately, RAd vectors present a unique problem because even the inactivated RAd vector can elicit potent CTLs against viral proteins (76). Furthermore, the RAd vectors elicit a potent humoral response that will effectively eliminate all subsequent transduction. This is even more pertinent to adenoviral vectors because they do not integrate, and hence they suffer loss by cell division and by DNA degradation, necessitating a repeat infection with the vector. Because there are scores of adenoviral serotypes, one strategy to overcome this problem might be to use different serotypes.

The high-titer recombinant adenoviruses are potentially toxic, even though the precise mechanism associated with this toxicity remains uncertain. The death of a patient directly associated with recombinant adenoviruses is a tragic warning sign that signals the need for further improvement of viral gene therapy. The RAd vectors will, however, continue to be utilized in situations where a high-level but transient expression of the foreign gene is required—for example, restenosis and cancer.

OTHER VECTORS

Our emphasis in this chapter was on most commonly used viral vectors, but there are other viral vectors based on SV40, Sindbis virus, herpes viruses, and others. Among these, the herpes virus–based vectors have the best potential for clinical applications. The presently available herpes viral vectors, where viral immediate-early genes have been deleted, appear to be nontoxic and therefore likely to be useful for clinical applications. We refer the reader to excellent reviews on the subject of emerging vectors (74) and herpes viral vectors (90,167).

The last two decades have witnessed the birth of the field of gene therapy, which has generated great hopes and great hypes. The promise of influencing the outcome of a vast array of diseases, ranging from birth defects to neurological disorders and from cancer to infectious disease, although far-reaching, is not beyond reach. With the completion of the sequence of the human genome, over 50,000 genes will be available to the practitioners of gene therapy. The potential benefits for human health are vast. Gene therapy has many challenges and hurdles ahead, but they are surmountable. It will continue to remain an exciting field of research.

REFERENCES

1. Agha-Mohammadi S, Lotze MT. Regulatable systems: Applications in gene therapy and replicating viruses. *J Clin Invest* 2000;105:1177–1183.
2. Albritton LM, Tseng L, Scadden D, Cunningham JM. A putative murine ecotropic retrovirus receptor gene encodes a multiple membrane-spanning protein and confers susceptibility to virus infection. *Cell* 1989;57:659–666.
3. Alemany R, Balague C, Curiel DT. Replicative adenoviruses for cancer therapy. *Nat Biotechnol* 2000;18:723–727.
4. Amalfitano A, Begy CR, Chamberlain JS. Improved adenovirus packaging cell lines to support the growth of replication-defective gene-delivery vectors. *Proc Natl Acad Sci U S A* 1996;93:3352–3356.
5. Amalfitano A, Hauser MA, Hu H, et al. Production and characterization of improved adenovirus vectors with the E1, E2b, and E3 genes deleted. *J Virol* 1998;72:926–933.
6. Armentano D, Smith MP, Sookdeo CC, et al. E4ORF3 requirement for achieving long-term transgene expression from the cytomegalovirus promoter in adenovirus vectors. *J Virol* 1999;73:7031–7034.
7. Armentano D, Yu SF, Kantoff PW, et al. Effect of internal viral sequences on the utility of retroviral vectors. *J Virol* 1987;61:1647–1650.
8. Armentano D, Zabner J, Sacks C, et al. Effect of the E4 region on the persistence of transgene expression from adenovirus vectors. *J Virol* 1997;71:2408–2416.
9. Bartlett JS, Samulski RJ, McCown TJ. Selective and rapid uptake of adeno-associated virus type 2 in brain. *Hum Gene Ther* 1998;9:1181–1186.
10. Bender MA, Palmer TD, Gelinas RE, Miller AD. Evidence that the packaging signal of Moloney murine leukemia virus extends into the gag region. *J Virol* 1987;61:1639–1646.
11. Berkner KL, Sharp PA. Generation of adenovirus by transfection of plasmids. *Nucleic Acids Res* 1983;11:6003–6020.
12. Berns KI, Linden RM. The cryptic life style of adeno-associated virus. *Bioessays* 1995;17:237–245.
13. Bett AJ, Haddara W, Prevec L, Graham FL. An efficient and flexible system for construction of adenovirus vectors with insertions or deletions in early regions 1 and 3. *Proc Natl Acad Sci U S A* 1994;91:8802–8806.
14. Bett AJ, Prevec L, Graham FL. Packaging capacity and stability of human adenovirus type 5 vectors. *J Virol* 1993;67:5911–5921.
15. Bischoff JR, Kirn DH, Williams A, et al. An adenovirus mutant that replicates selectively in p53-deficient human tumor cells. *Science* 1996;274:373–376.
16. Blaese RM, Culver KW, Miller AD, et al. T lymphocyte-directed gene therapy for ADA-SCID: Initial trial results after 4 years. *Science* 1995;270:475–480.
17. Brockstedt DG, Podsakoff GM, Fong L, et al. Induction of immunity to antigens expressed by recombinant adeno-associated virus depends on the route of administration. *Clin Immunol* 1999;92:67–75.
18. Brough DE, Lizonova A, Hsu C, et al. A gene transfer vector-cell line system for complete functional complementation of adenovirus early regions E1 and E4. *J Virol* 1996;70:6497–6501.
19. Buchschacher GL Jr, Panganiban AT. Human immunodeficiency virus vectors for inducible expression of foreign genes. *J Virol* 1992;66:2731–2739.
20. Bukrinsky MI, Haggerty S, Dempsey MP, et al. A nuclear localization signal within HIV-1 matrix protein that governs infection of non-dividing cells. *Nature* 1993;365:666–669.
21. Burns JC, Friedmann T, Driever W, et al. Vesicular stomatitis virus G glycoprotein pseudotyped retroviral vectors: Concentration to very high titer and efficient gene transfer into mammalian and nonmammalian cells. *Proc Natl Acad Sci U S A* 1993;90:8033–8037.
22. Carroll R, Lin JT, Dacquel EJ, et al. A human immunodeficiency virus type 1 (HIV-1)-based retroviral vector system utilizing stable HIV-1 packaging cell lines. *J Virol* 1994;68:6047–6051.
23. Case SS, Price MA, Jordan CT, et al. Stable transduction of quiescent CD34(+)CD38(−) human hematopoietic cells by HIV-1-based lentiviral vectors. *Proc Natl Acad Sci U S A* 1999;96:2988–2993.
24. Cavazzana-Calvo M, Hacein-Bey S, de Saint Basile G, et al. Gene therapy of human severe combined immunodeficiency (SCID)-X1 disease. *Science* 2000;288:669–672.
25. Chartier C, Degryse E, Gantzer M, et al. Efficient generation of recombinant adenovirus vectors by homologous recombination in *Escherichia coli*. *J Virol* 1996;70:4805–4810.
26. Chen ST, Iida A, Guo L, et al. Generation of packaging cell lines for pseudotyped retroviral vectors of the G protein of vesicular stomatitis virus by using a modified tetracycline inducible system. *Proc Natl Acad Sci U S A* 1996;93:10057–10062.
27. Chirmule N, Propert K, Magosin S, et al. Immune responses to adenovirus and adeno-associated virus in humans. *Gene Ther* 1999;6:1574–1583.
28. Chirmule N, Xiao W, Truneh A, et al. Humoral immunity to adeno-associated virus type 2 vectors following administration to murine and nonhuman primate muscle. *J Virol* 2000;74:2420–2425.
29. Clark KR, Liu X, McGrath JP, Johnson PR. Highly purified recombinant adeno-associated virus vectors are biologically active and free of detectable helper and wild-type viruses. *Hum Gene Ther* 1999;10:1031–1039.
30. Clark KR, Voulgaropoulou F, Fraley DM, Johnson PR. Cell lines for the production of recombinant adeno-associated virus. *Hum Gene Ther* 1995;6:1329–1341.
31. Collis P, Antoniou M, Grosveld F. Definition of the minimal requirements within the human beta-globin gene and the dominant control region for high level expression. *EMBO J* 1990;9:233–240.
32. Cone RD, Mulligan RC. High-efficiency gene transfer into mammalian cells: Generation of helper-free recombinant retrovirus with broad mammalian host range. *Proc Natl Acad Sci U S A* 1984;81:6349–6353.
33. Corbeau P, Kraus G, Wong-Staal F. Efficient gene transfer by a human immunodeficiency virus type 1 (HIV-1)-derived vector utilizing a stable HIV packaging cell line. *Proc Natl Acad Sci U S A* 1996;93:14070–14075.
34. Cullen BR. HIV-1 auxiliary proteins: Making connections in a dying cell. *Cell* 1998;93:685–692.
35. Dai Y, Schwarz EM, Gu D, et al. Cellular and humoral immune

responses to adenoviral vectors containing factor IX gene: Tolerization of factor IX and vector antigens allows for long-term expression. *Proc Natl Acad Sci U S A* 1995;92:1401–1405.

36. Danos O, Mulligan RC. Safe and efficient generation of recombinant retroviruses with amphotropic and ecotropic host ranges. *Proc Natl Acad Sci U S A* 1988;85:6460–6464.
37. Dong JY, Fan PD, Frizzell RA. Quantitative analysis of the packaging capacity of recombinant adeno-associated virus. *Hum Gene Ther* 1996;7:2101–2112.
38. Duan D, Sharma P, Yang J, et al. Circular intermediates of recombinant adeno-associated virus have defined structural characteristics responsible for long-term episomal persistence in muscle tissue. *J Virol* 1998;72:8568–8577.
39. Duan D, Yue Y, Yan Z, Engelhardt JF. A new dual-vector approach to enhance recombinant adeno-associated virus-mediated gene expression through intermolecular cis activation. *Nat Med* 2000;6:595–598.
40. Dull T, Zufferey R, Kelly M, et al. A third-generation lentivirus vector with a conditional packaging system. *J Virol* 1998;72:8463–8471.
41. Emerman M, Malim MH. HIV-1 regulatory/accessory genes: Keys to unraveling viral and host cell biology. *Science* 1998;280:1880–1884.
42. Emerman M, Temin HM. Genes with promoters in retrovirus vectors can be independently suppressed by an epigenetic mechanism. *Cell* 1984;39:449–467.
43. Emi N, Friedmann T, Yee JK. Pseudotype formation of murine leukemia virus with the G protein of vesicular stomatitis virus. *J Virol* 1991;65:1202–1207.
44. Engelhardt JF, Ye X, Doranz B, Wilson JM. Ablation of E2A in recombinant adenoviruses improves transgene persistence and decreases inflammatory response in mouse liver. *Proc Natl Acad Sci U S A* 1994; 91:6196–6200.
45. Fang B, Wang H, Gordon G, et al. Lack of persistence of E1-recombinant adenoviral vectors containing a temperature-sensitive E2A mutation in immunocompetent mice and hemophilia B dogs. *Gene Ther* 1996;3:217–222.
46. Ferrari FK, Samulski T, Shenk T, Samulski RJ. Second-strand synthesis is a rate-limiting step for efficient transduction by recombinant adeno-associated virus vectors. *J Virol* 1996;70:3227–3234.
47. Finer MH, Dull TJ, Qin L, et al. *kat*: A high-efficiency retroviral transduction system for primary human T lymphocytes. *Blood* 1994;83: 43–50.
48. Fisher KJ, Choi H, Burda J, et al. Recombinant adenovirus deleted of all viral genes for gene therapy of cystic fibrosis. *Virology* 1996;217: 11–22.
49. Fisher KJ, Jooss K, Alston J, et al. Recombinant adeno-associated virus for muscle directed gene therapy. *Nat Med* 1997;3:306–312.
50. Follenzi A, Ailles LE, Bakovic S, et al. Gene transfer by lentiviral vectors is limited by nuclear translocation and rescued by HIV-1 pol sequences. *Nat Genet* 2000;25:217–222.
51. Gallay P, Hope T, Chin D, Trono D. HIV-1 infection of nondividing cells through the recognition of integrase by the importin/karyopherin pathway. *Proc Natl Acad Sci U S A* 1997;94:9825–9830.
52. Gallay P, Swingler S, Song J, et al. HIV nuclear import is governed by the phosphotyrosine-mediated binding of matrix to the core domain of integrase. *Cell* 1995;83:569–576.
53. Gao GP, Yang Y, Wilson JM. Biology of adenovirus vectors with E1 and E4 deletions for liver-directed gene therapy. *J Virol* 1996;70: 8934–8943.
54. Girod A, Ried M, Wobus C, et al. Genetic capsid modifications allow efficient re-targeting of adeno-associated virus type 2. *Nat Med* 1999; 5:1438.
55. Gorman CM, Gies D, McCray G, Huang M. The human cytomegalovirus major immediate early promoter can be trans-activated by adenovirus early proteins. *Virology* 1989;171:377–385.
56. Gorziglia MI, Kadan MJ, Yei S, et al. Elimination of both E1 and E2 from adenovirus vectors further improves prospects for *in vivo* human gene therapy. *J Virol* 1996;70:4173–4178.
57. Gossen M, Bujard H. Tight control of gene expression in mammalian cells by tetracycline-responsive promoters. *Proc Natl Acad Sci U S A* 1992;89:5547–5551.
58. Grable M, Hearing P. Cis and trans requirements for the selective packaging of adenovirus type 5 DNA. *J Virol* 1992;66:723–731.
59. Graham FL, Smiley J, Russell WC, Nairn R. Characteristics of a human cell line transformed by DNA from human adenovirus type 5. *J Gen Virol* 1977;36:59–74.
60. Grimm D, Kern A, Rittner K, Kleinschmidt JA. Novel tools for production and purification of recombinant adenoassociated virus vectors. *Hum Gene Ther* 1998;9:2745–2760.
61. Grimm D, Kleinschmidt JA. Progress in adeno-associated virus type 2 vector production: Promises and prospects for clinical use. *Hum Gene Ther* 1999;10:2445–2450.
62. Gu H, Zou YR, Rajewsky K. Independent control of immunoglobulin switch recombination at individual switch regions evidenced through Cre-*loxP*-mediated gene targeting. *Cell* 1993;73:1155–1164.
63. Hackett NR, Crystal RG. Adenovirus vectors for gene therapy. In: Templeton NS, Lasic DD, eds. *Gene Therapy.* New York: Marcel Dekker, 2000:17–39.
64. Haecker SE, Stedman HH, Balice-Gordon RJ, et al. *In vivo* expression of full-length human dystrophin from adenoviral vectors deleted of all viral genes. *Hum Gene Ther* 1996;7:1907–1914.
65. Haffar OK, Popov S, Dubrovsky L, et al. Two nuclear localization signals in the HIV-1 matrix protein regulate nuclear import of the HIV-1 pre-integration complex. *J Mol Biol* 2000;299:359–368.
66. Haj-Ahmad Y, Graham FL. Development of a helper-independent human adenovirus vector and its use in the transfer of the herpes simplex virus thymidine kinase gene. *J Virol* 1986;57:267–274.
67. Hardy S, Kitamura M, Harris-Stansil T, et al. Construction of adenovirus vectors through Cre-lox recombination. *J Virol* 1997;71: 1842–1849.
68. Hearing P, Samulski RJ, Wishart WL, Shenk T. Identification of a repeated sequence element required for efficient encapsidation of the adenovirus type 5 chromosome. *J Virol* 1987;61:2555–2558.
69. Heinzinger NK, Bukinsky MI, Haggerty SA, et al. The Vpr protein of human immunodeficiency virus type 1 influences nuclear localization of viral nucleic acids in nondividing host cells. *Proc Natl Acad Sci U S A* 1994;91:7311–7315.
70. Heise C, Sampson-Johannes A, Williams A, et al. ONYX-015, an E1B gene-attenuated adenovirus, causes tumor-specific cytolysis and antitumoral efficacy that can be augmented by standard chemotherapeutic agents. *Nat Med* 1997;3:639–645.
71. Hitt MM, Parks RJ, Graham FL. Structure and genetic organization of adenovirus vectors. In: Friedmann T, ed. *The Development of Human Gene Therapy.* New York: Cold Spring Harbor Laboratory Press, 1999:61–86.
72. Imler JL, Chartier C, Dieterle A, et al. An efficient procedure to select and recover recombinant adenovirus vectors. *Gene Ther* 1995;2: 263–268.
73. Inoue N, Russell DW. Packaging cells based on inducible gene amplification for the production of adeno-associated virus vectors. *J Virol* 1998;72:7024–7031.
74. Jolly DJ. Emerging viral vectors. In: Friedmann T, ed. *The Development of Human Gene Therapy.* New York: Cold Spring Harbor Laboratory Press, 1999:209–240.
75. Kafri T, Blomer U, Peterson DA, et al. Sustained expression of genes delivered directly into liver and muscle by lentiviral vectors. *Nat Genet* 1997;17:314–317.
76. Kafri T, Morgan D, Krahl T, et al. Cellular immune response to adenoviral vector infected cells does not require de novo viral gene expression: Implications for gene therapy. *Proc Natl Acad Sci U S A* 1998; 95:11377–11382.
77. Kafri T, van Praag H, Gage FH, Verma IM. Lentiviral vectors—Regulated gene expression. *Mol Ther* 2000;1:516–521.
78. Kafri T, van Praag H, Ouyang L, et al. A packaging cell line for lentivirus vectors. *J Virol* 1999;73:576–584.
79. Kay MA, Manno CS, Ragni MV, et al. Evidence for gene transfer and expression of factor IX in haemophilia B patients treated with an AAV vector [see comments]. *Nat Genet* 2000;24:257–261.
80. Ketner G, Spencer F, Tugendreich S, et al. Efficient manipulation of the human adenovirus genome as an infectious yeast artificial chromosome clone. *Proc Natl Acad Sci U S A* 1994;91:6186–6190.
81. Khuri FR, Nemunaitis J, Ganly I, et al. A controlled trial of intratumoral ONYX-015, a selectively-replicating adenovirus, in combination with cisplatin and 5-fluorouracil in patients with recurrent head and neck cancer. *Nat Med* 2000;6:879–885.
82. Klages N, Zufferey R, Trono D. A stable system for the high-titer production of multiply attenuated lentiviral vectors. *Mol Ther* 2000;2: 170–176.
83. Klessig DF, Brough DE, Cleghon V. Introduction, stable integration, and controlled expression of a chimeric adenovirus gene whose prod-

uct is toxic to the recipient human cell. *Mol Cell Biol* 1984;4: 1354–1362.
84. Kochanek S. High-capacity adenoviral vectors for gene transfer and somatic gene therapy. *Hum Gene Ther* 1999;10:2451–2459.
85. Kochanek S, Clemens PR, Mitani K, et al. A new adenoviral vector: Replacement of all viral coding sequences with 28 kb of DNA independently expressing both full-length dystrophin and beta-galactosidase. *Proc Natl Acad Sci U S A* 1996;93:5731–5736.
86. Kotin RM, Siniscalco M, Samulski RJ, et al. Site-specific integration by adeno-associated virus. *Proc Natl Acad Sci U S A* 1990;87:2211–2215.
87. Krougliak V, Graham FL. Development of cell lines capable of complementing E1, E4, and protein IX defective adenovirus type 5 mutants. *Hum Gene Ther* 1995;6:1575–1586.
88. Landau NR, Page KA, Littman DR. Pseudotyping with human T-cell leukemia virus type I broadens the human immunodeficiency virus host range. *J Virol* 1991;65:162–169.
89. Langer SJ, Schaack J. 293 cell lines that inducibly express high levels of adenovirus type 5 precursor terminal protein. *Virology* 1996;221: 172–179.
90. Laquerre S, Goins WF, Moriuchi S, et al. Gene-transfer tool: Herpes simplex virus vectors. In: Friedmann T, ed. *The Development of Human Gene Therapy.* New York: Cold Spring Harbor Laboratory Press, 1999:173–208.
91. Leboulch P, Huang GM, Humphries RK, et al. Mutagenesis of retroviral vectors transducing human beta-globin gene and beta-globin locus control region derivatives results in stable transmission of an active transcriptional structure. *EMBO J* 1994;13:3065–3076.
92. Li J, Samulski RJ, Xiao X. Role for highly regulated *rep* gene expression in adeno-associated virus vector production. *J Virol* 1997;71: 5236–5243.
93. Lieber A, He CY, Kirillova I, Kay MA. Recombinant adenoviruses with large deletions generated by Cre-mediated excision exhibit different biological properties compared with first-generation vectors *in vitro* and *in vivo*. *J Virol* 1996;70:8944–8960.
94. Malim MH, Hauber J, Le SY, et al. The HIV-1 rev trans-activator acts through a structured target sequence to activate nuclear export of unspliced viral mRNA. *Nature* 1989;338:254–257.
95. Mangeot PE, Negre D, Dubois B, et al. Development of minimal lentivirus vectors derived from simian immunodeficiency virus (SIVmac251) and their use for gene transfer into human dendritic cells. *J Virol* 2000;74:8307–8315.
96. Mann R, Baltimore D. Varying the position of a retrovirus packaging sequence results in the encapsidation of both unspliced and spliced RNAs. *J Virol* 1985;54:401–407.
97. Mann R, Mulligan RC, Baltimore D. Construction of a retrovirus packaging mutant and its use to produce helper-free defective retrovirus. *Cell* 1983;33:153–159.
98. Markowitz D, Goff S, Bank A. A safe packaging line for gene transfer: Separating viral genes on two different plasmids. *J Virol* 1988;62: 1120–1124.
99. May C, Rivella S, Callegari J, et al. Therapeutic haemoglobin synthesis in beta-thalassaemic mice expressing lentivirus-encoded human beta-globin. *Nature* 2000;406:82–86.
100. McCarty DM, Christensen M, Muzyczka N. Sequences required for coordinate induction of adeno-associated virus p19 and p40 promoters by Rep protein. *J Virol* 1991;65:2936–2945.
101. McCown TJ, Xiao X, Li J, et al. Differential and persistent expression patterns of CNS gene transfer by an adeno-associated virus (AAV) vector. *Brain Res* 1996;713:99–107.
102. McGrory WJ, Bautista DS, Graham FL. A simple technique for the rescue of early region I mutations into infectious human adenovirus type 5. *Virology* 1988;163:614–617.
103. McLaughlin SK, Collis P, Hermonat PL, Muzyczka N. Adeno-associated virus general transduction vectors: Analysis of proviral structures. *J Virol* 1988;62:1963–1973.
104. Miao CH, Nakai H, Thompson AR, et al. Nonrandom transduction of recombinant adeno-associated virus vectors in mouse hepatocytes *in vivo*: Cell cycling does not influence hepatocyte transduction. *J Virol* 2000;74:3793–3803.
105. Miao CH, Snyder RO, Schowalter DB, et al. The kinetics of rAAV integration in the liver. *Nat Genet* 1998;19:13–15.
106. Miller AD. Development and application fo retroviral vectors. In: Coffin JM, Hughes SH, Varmus HE, eds. *Retroviruses.* New York: Cold Spring Harbor Laboratory Press, 1997:437–473.
107. Miller AD, Buttimore C. Redesign of retrovirus packaging cell lines to avoid recombination leading to helper virus production. *Mol Cell Biol* 1986;6:2895–2902.
108. Miller AD, Law MF, Verma IM. Generation of helper-free amphotropic retroviruses that transduce a dominant-acting, methotrexate-resistant dihydrofolate reductase gene. *Mol Cell Biol* 1985;5:431–437.
109. Mitani K, Graham FL, Caskey CT, Kochanek S. Rescue, propagation, and partial purification of a helper virus-dependent adenovirus vector. *Proc Natl Acad Sci U S A* 1995;92:3854–3858.
110. Miyoshi H, Blomer U, Takahashi M, et al. Development of a self-inactivating lentivirus vector. *J Virol* 1998;72:8150–8157.
111. Miyoshi H, Smith KA, Mosier DE, et al. Transduction of human CD34+ cells that mediate long-term engraftment of NOD/SCID mice by HIV vectors. *Science* 1999;283:682–686.
112. Miyoshi H, Takahashi M, Gage FH, Verma IM. Stable and efficient gene transfer into the retina using an HIV-based lentiviral vector. *Proc Natl Acad Sci U S A* 1997;94:10319–10323.
113. Monahan PE, Samulski RJ. AAV vectors: Is clinical success on the horizon? *Gene Ther* 2000;7:24–30.
114. Muzyczka N. Use of adeno-associated virus as a general transduction vector for mammalian cells. *Curr Top Microbiol Immunol* 1992;158: 97–129.
115. Nakai H, Iwaki Y, Kay MA, Couto LB. Isolation of recombinant adeno-associated virus vector-cellular DNA junctions from mouse liver. *J Virol* 1999;73:5438–5447.
116. Nakai H, Storm TA, Kay MA. Increasing the size of rAAV-mediated expression cassettes *in vivo* by intermolecular joining of two complementary vectors. *Nat Biotechnol* 2000;18:527–532.
117. Naldini L, Blomer U, Gage FH, et al. Efficient transfer, integration, and sustained long-term expression of the transgene in adult rat brains injected with a lentiviral vector. *Proc Natl Acad Sci U S A* 1996;93: 11382–11388.
118. Naldini L, Blomer U, Gallay P, et al. *In vivo* gene delivery and stable transduction of nondividing cells by a lentiviral vector. *Science* 1996; 272:263–267.
119. Naldini L, Verma IM. Lentiviral vectors. In: Friedmann T, ed. *The Development of Human Gene Therapy.* New York: Cold Spring Harbor Laboratory Press, 1999:47–60.
120. Naviaux RK, Costanzi E, Haas M, Verma IM. The pCL vector system: Rapid production of helper-free, high-titer, recombinant retroviruses. *J Virol* 1996;70:5701–5705.
121. No D, Yao TP, Evans RM. Ecdysone-inducible gene expression in mammalian cells and transgenic mice. *Proc Natl Acad Sci U S A* 1996;93:3346–3351.
122. Novak U, Harris EA, Forrester W, et al. High-level beta-globin expression after retroviral transfer of locus activation region-containing human beta-globin gene derivatives into murine erythroleukemia cells. *Proc Natl Acad Sci U S A* 1990;87:3386–3390.
123. Olsen JC. Gene transfer vectors derived from equine infectious anemia virus. *Gene Ther* 1998;5:1481–1487.
124. Ory DS, Neugeboren BA, Mulligan RC. A stable human-derived packaging cell line for production of high titer retrovirus/vesicular stomatitis virus G pseudotypes. *Proc Natl Acad Sci U S A* 1996;93: 11400–11406.
125. Page KA, Landau NR, Littman DR. Construction and use of a human immunodeficiency virus vector for analysis of virus infectivity. *J Virol* 1990;64:5270–5276.
126. Parks RJ, Chen L, Anton M, et al. A helper-dependent adenovirus vector system: Removal of helper virus by Cre-mediated excision of the viral packaging signal. *Proc Natl Acad Sci U S A* 1996;93: 13565–13570.
127. Parks RJ, Graham FL. A helper-dependent system for adenovirus vector production helps define a lower limit for efficient DNA packaging. *J Virol* 1997;71:3293–3298.
128. Parolin C, Dorfman T, Palu G, et al. Analysis in human immunodeficiency virus type 1 vectors of cis-acting sequences that affect gene transfer into human lymphocytes. *J Virol* 1994;68:3888–3895.
129. Pereira DJ, McCarty DM, Muzyczka N. The adeno-associated virus (AAV) Rep protein acts as both a repressor and an activator to regulate AAV transcription during a productive infection. *J Virol* 1997;71: 1079–1088.
130. Petit C, Schwartz O, Mammano F. The karyophilic properties of human immunodeficiency virus type 1 integrase are not required for nuclear import of proviral DNA. *J Virol* 2000;74:7119–7126.

131. Poeschla E, Gilbert J, Li X, et al. Identification of a human immunodeficiency virus type 2 (HIV-2) encapsidation determinant and transduction of nondividing human cells by HIV-2-based lentivirus vectors. *J Virol* 1998;72:6527–6536.
132. Poeschla EM, Wong-Staal F, Looney DJ. Efficient transduction of nondividing human cells by feline immunodeficiency virus lentiviral vectors. *Nat Med* 1998;4:354–357.
133. Poznansky M, Lever A, Bergeron L, et al. Gene transfer into human lymphocytes by a defective human immunodeficiency virus type 1 vector. *J Virol* 1991;65:532–536.
134. Qing K, Mah C, Hansen J, et al. Human fibroblast growth factor receptor 1 is a co-receptor for infection by adeno-associated virus 2. *Nat Med* 1999;5:71–77.
135. Ramirez-Solis R, Liu P, Bradley A. Chromosome engineering in mice. *Nature* 1995;378:720–724.
136. Reiser J, Harmison G, Kluepfel-Stahl S, et al. Transduction of nondividing cells using pseudotyped defective high-titer HIV type 1 particles. *Proc Natl Acad Sci U S A* 1996;93:15266–15271.
137. Richardson JH, Child LA, Lever AM. Packaging of human immunodeficiency virus type 1 RNA requires cis-acting sequences outside the 5′ leader region. *J Virol* 1993;67:3997–4005.
138. Rivera VM, Clackson T, Natesan S, et al. A humanized system for pharmacologic control of gene expression. *Nat Med* 1996;2:1028–1032.
139. Rivera VM, Ye X, Courage NL, et al. Long-term regulated expression of growth hormone in mice after intramuscular gene transfer. *Proc Natl Acad Sci U S A* 1999;96:8657–8662.
140. Russell DW, Alexander IE, Miller AD. DNA synthesis and topoisomerase inhibitors increase transduction by adeno-associated virus vectors. *Proc Natl Acad Sci U S A* 1995;92:5719–5723.
141. Russell DW, Kay MA. Adeno-associated virus vectors and hematology. *Blood* 1999;94:864–874.
142. Russell DW, Miller AD, Alexander IE. Adeno-associated virus vectors preferentially transduce cells in S phase. *Proc Natl Acad Sci U S A* 1994;91:8915–8919.
143. Samulski RJ, Chang LS, Shenk T. A recombinant plasmid from which an infectious adeno-associated virus genome can be excised *in vitro* and its use to study viral replication. *J Virol* 1987;61: 3096–3101.
144. Samulski RJ, Chang LS, Shenk T. Helper-free stocks of recombinant adeno-associated viruses: Normal integration does not require viral gene expression. *J Virol* 1989;63:3822–3828.
145. Samulski RJ, Sally M, Muzyczka N. Adeno-associated viral vectors. In: Friedmann T, ed. *The Development of Human Gene Therapy.* New York: Cold Spring Harbor Laboratory Press, 1999:131–172.
146. Samulski RJ, Zhu X, Xiao X, et al. Targeted integration of adeno-associated virus (AAV) into human chromosome 19. *EMBO J* 1991;10: 3941–3950.
147. Scadden DT, Fuller B, Cunningham JM. Human cells infected with retrovirus vectors acquire an endogenous murine provirus. *J Virol* 1990;64:424–427.
148. Schaack J, Guo X, Langer SJ. Characterization of a replication-incompetent adenovirus type 5 mutant deleted for the preterminal protein gene. *Proc Natl Acad Sci U S A* 1996;93:14686–14691.
149. Shimada T, Fujii H, Mitsuya H, Nienhuis AW. Targeted and highly efficient gene transfer into CD4+ cells by a recombinant human immunodeficiency virus retroviral vector. *J Clin Invest* 1991;88: 1043–1047.
150. Snyder RO, Miao CH, Patijn GA, et al. Persistent and therapeutic concentrations of human factor IX in mice after hepatic gene transfer of recombinant AAV vectors. *Nat Genet* 1997;16:270–276.
151. Spector DH, Wade E, Wright DA, et al. Human immunodeficiency virus pseudotypes with expanded cellular and species tropism. *J Virol* 1990;64:2298–2308.
152. Srivastava A. Parvovirus-based vectors for human gene therapy. *Blood Cells* 1994;20:531–536.
153. Summerford C, Bartlett JS, Samulski RJ. AlphaVbeta5 integrin: A coreceptor for adeno-associated virus type 2 infection. *Nat Med* 1999;5: 78–82.
154. Summerford C, Samulski RJ. Membrane-associated heparan sulfate proteoglycan is a receptor for adeno-associated virus type 2 virions. *J Virol* 1998;72:1438–1445.
155. Sun L, Li J, Xiao X. Overcoming adeno-associated virus vector size limitation through viral DNA heterodimerization. *Nat Med* 2000;6: 599–602.
156. Takahashi M, Miyoshi H, Verma IM, Gage FH. Rescue from photoreceptor degeneration in the rd mouse by human immunodeficiency virus vector-mediated gene transfer. *J Virol* 1999;73:7812–7816.
157. Tamayose K, Hirai Y, Shimada T. A new strategy for large-scale preparation of high-titer recombinant adeno-associated virus vectors by using packaging cell lines and sulfonated cellulose column chromatography. *Hum Gene Ther* 1996;7:507–513.
158. Tripathy SK, Black HB, Goldwasser E, Leiden JM. Immune responses to transgene-encoded proteins limit the stability of gene expression after injection of replication-defective adenovirus vectors. *Nat Med* 1996;2:545–550.
159. Trono D. Lentiviral vectors: Turning a deadly foe into a therapeutic agent. *Gene Ther* 2000;7:20–23.
160. Vogt PK. Historical introduction to the general properties of retroviruses. In: Coffin JM, Hughes SH, Varmus HE, eds. *Retroviruses.* New York: Cold Spring Harbor Laboratory Press, 1997:1–25.
161. Wang Q, Finer MH. Second-generation adenovirus vectors. *Nat Med* 1996;2:714–716.
162. Wang Q, Greenburg G, Bunch D, et al. Persistent transgene expression in mouse liver following *in vivo* gene transfer with a delta E1/delta E4 adenovirus vector. *Gene Ther* 1997;4:393–400.
163. Wang Q, Jia XC, Finer MH. A packaging cell line for propagation of recombinant adenovirus vectors containing two lethal gene-region deletions. *Gene Ther* 1995;2:775–783.
164. Wang XS, Khuntirat B, Qing K, et al. Characterization of wild-type adeno-associated virus type 2-like particles generated during recombinant viral vector production and strategies for their elimination. *J Virol* 1998;72:5472–5480.
165. Weitzman MD, Kyostio SR, Kotin RM, Owens RA. Adeno-associated virus (AAV) Rep proteins mediate complex formation between AAV DNA and its integration site in human DNA. *Proc Natl Acad Sci U S A* 1994;91:5808–5812.
166. Wivel NA, Gao G-P, Wilson JM. Adenovirus vectors. In: Friedmann T, ed. *The Development of Human Gene Therapy.* New York: Cold Spring Harbor Laboratory Press, 1999:87–111.
167. Wolfe D, Goins WF, Fink DJ, Glorioso JC. Desing and use of herpes simplex viral vectors for gene therapy. In: Templeton NS, Lasic DD, ed. *Gene Therapy.* New York: Marcel Dekker, 2000:81–108.
168. Wu P, Phillips MI, Bui J, Terwilliger EF. Adeno-associated virus vector-mediated transgene integration into neurons and other nondividing cell targets. *J Virol* 1998;72:5919–5926.
169. Xiao W, Chirmule N, Berta SC, et al. Gene therapy vectors based on adeno-associated virus type 1. *J Virol* 1999;73:3994–4003.
170. Xiao X, Li J, Samulski RJ. Efficient long-term gene transfer into muscle tissue of immunocompetent mice by adeno-associated virus vector. *J Virol* 1996;70:8098–8108.
171. Xiao X, Li J, Samulski RJ. Production of high-titer recombinant adeno-associated virus vectors in the absence of helper adenovirus. *J Virol* 1998;72:2224–2232.
172. Yan Z, Zhang Y, Duan D, Engelhardt JF. From the cover: Trans-splicing vectors expand the utility of adeno-associated virus for gene therapy. *Proc Natl Acad Sci U S A* 2000;97:6716–6721.
173. Yang CC, Xiao X, Zhu X, et al. Cellular recombination pathways and viral terminal repeat hairpin structures are sufficient for adeno-associated virus integration *in vivo* and *in vitro*. *J Virol* 1997;71: 9231–9247.
174. Yang Q, Chen F, Trempe JP. Characterization of cell lines that inducibly express the adeno-associated virus Rep proteins. *J Virol* 1994;68:4847–4856.
175. Ye X, Rivera VM, Zoltick P, et al. Regulated delivery of therapeutic proteins after *in vivo* somatic cell gene transfer. *Science* 1999;283:88–91.
176. Yee J-K. Retroviral vectors. In: Friedmann T, ed. *The Development of Human Gene Therapy.* New York: Cold Spring Harbor Laboratory Press, 1999:21–46.
177. Yee JK, Miyanohara A, LaPorte P, et al. A general method for the generation of high-titer, pantropic retroviral vectors: Highly efficient infection of primary hepatocytes. *Proc Natl Acad Sci U S A* 1994;91: 9564–9568.
178. Yee JK, Moores JC, Jolly DJ, et al. Gene expression from transcriptionally disabled retroviral vectors. *Proc Natl Acad Sci U S A* 1987;84: 5197–5201.
179. Yeh P, Dedieu JF, Orsini C, et al. Efficient dual transcomplementation of adenovirus E1 and E4 regions from a 293-derived cell line expressing a minimal E4 functional unit. *J Virol* 1996;70:559–565.

180. Yew PR, Berk AJ. Inhibition of p53 transactivation required for transformation by adenovirus early 1B protein. *Nature* 1992;357:82–85.
181. Yu H, Rabson AB, Kaul M, et al. Inducible human immunodeficiency virus type 1 packaging cell lines. *J Virol* 1996;70:4530–4537.
182. Yu SF, von Ruden T, Kantoff PW, et al. Self-inactivating retroviral vectors designed for transfer of whole genes into mammalian cells. *Proc Natl Acad Sci U S A* 1986;83:3194–3198.
183. Zennou V, Petit C, Guetard D, et al. HIV-1 genome nuclear import is mediated by a central DNA flap. *Cell* 2000;101:173–185.
184. Zhou H, O'Neal W, Morral N, Beaudet AL. Development of a complementing cell line and a system for construction of adenovirus vectors with E1 and E2a deleted. *J Virol* 1996;70:7030–7038.
185. Zolotukhin S, Byrne BJ, Mason E, et al. Recombinant adeno-associated virus purification using novel methods improves infectious titer and yield. *Gene Ther* 1999;6:973–985.
186. Zufferey R, Donello JE, Trono D, Hope TJ. Woodchuck hepatitis virus posttranscriptional regulatory element enhances expression of transgenes delivered by retroviral vectors. *J Virol* 1999;73:2886–2892.
187. Zufferey R, Dull T, Mandel RJ, et al. Self-inactivating lentivirus vector for safe and efficient *in vivo* gene delivery. *J Virol* 1998;72:9873–9880.
188. Zufferey R, Nagy D, Mandel RJ, et al. Multiply attenuated lentiviral vector achieves efficient gene delivery *in vivo*. *Nat Biotechnol* 1997;15:871–875.

CHAPTER 14

Plant Viruses

Sondra G. Lazarowitz

HISTORY

The oft cited color variegation in tulip flowers, caused by tulip breaking virus, is probably the most splendid example of disease symptoms produced by a viral infection of plants. Tulips, with their naturally solid colored flowers, acquired this infection when introduced from Constantinople to the Netherlands in 1551. The spectacular floral patterns that resulted were so highly coveted that a tulip bulb could command an astonishingly high price: 5,200 guilders were reportedly paid for a tulip bulb in 1637, whereas Rembrandt's fee for his masterpiece "The Night Watch" in 1642 was a mere 1,600 guilders (59). Given the tulip mania that seized the Netherlands, the affected tulips were reproduced in great numbers by noted 17th-century Dutch painters and growers alike (Fig. 1). Although considered an example of the beneficial consequences of some virus infections, most plants do no fare as well in the face of virus infection. Indeed, viruses are currently responsible for severe losses in crop plants of every type worldwide (Table 1). It is difficult to place a precise dollar figure on the total losses annually, but a single virus, such as tomato spotted wilt virus (TSVW), is estimated to cause annual crop losses in excess of $1 billion.

The origins of the science of virology in general are rooted in research at the end of the 19th century on tobacco mosaic disease, caused by what came to be called tobacco mosaic virus (TMV). The interest in TMV at the time was economic: the diseased tobacco leaves were not suitable for making cigars. Adolf Mayer, Director of the Agricultural Research Station at Wageningen, was investigating this tobacco mosaic syndrome and in 1886 showed that he could transfer the disease by injecting healthy tobacco plants with leaf extracts from diseased plants (222). Thus, he had established the infectious nature of this disease, but he failed to identify the pathogenic agent. In 1892, Dmitrii Ivanowski, working in the Crimea, reported that such extracts from mosaic-diseased tobacco, when passaged through candle filters that would exclude bacteria, were still infectious (157), thereby establishing the cause of this disease as a "filterable agent." However, despite this and additional evidence from his own work, he wrongly concluded that the causal agent was a toxin or bacterial agent that could still pass through the filters. It was Martinus Beijerinck at the Technical School of Delft, repeating and extending these filtration studies, who made the conceptual leap to report in 1898 (22) that this mosaic disease of tobacco was caused by a "contagium vivum fluidum"—a contagious living fluid. Thus, TMV was the first of the new class of "filterable agents" of disease, which eventually would simply be called *viruses,* to be identified, in the same year that Loeffler and Frosch reached similar conclusions for the cause of foot-and-mouth disease in livestock.

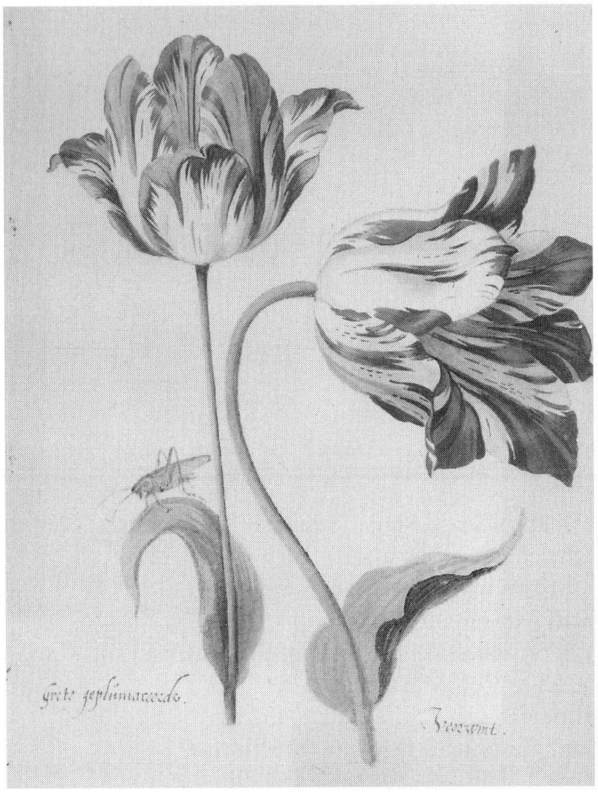

FIG. 1. "Study of Tulips" by the Dutch botanical artist Jacob Marrel (1614–1681). Reprinted with permission of the Metropolitan Museum of Art, New York, Rogers Fund, 1968 (66,68).

During the first half of the 20th century, TMV remained a central player in the development of modern virology, in general, and plant virology in particular. This was due in part to the ease of infecting and propagating a virus in plants (as opposed to obtaining human volunteers as did Reed and Carroll in their studies of yellow fever) and largely to the stability of TMV and the large amounts of virus that could readily be purified from infected tobacco plants. TMV was the first virus to be purified in a crystalline state and shown to consist of ribonucleoprotein (RNP) particles (19,325), and the first for which the architecture of the particles was revealed by electron microscopy and x-ray diffraction (25,44,107,168). It was the first virus shown to reassemble into infectious particles *in vitro* from viral RNA and coat protein (105) and the first for which the intrinsic infectivity of the virion RNA was demonstrated (118). As studies became more molecular, TMV has continued to be in the forefront of the development of techniques and concepts in modern plant virology. Techniques to prepare plant protoplasts and infect these with TMV were a major technical breakthrough in plant virology (15,338). The concept that plant virus movement between cells was an active process facilitated by a viral-encoded "movement protein" was established based on studies of temperature-sensitive mutants of TMV (244). The first successful example of pathogen-derived resistance was the engineering of transgenic plants resistant to TMV infection based on the expression of the viral coat protein gene (270), and much of our current thinking about the function of virus movement proteins derives from the initial demonstration that the TMV movement protein could alter the gating properties of plasmodesmata (376). Just as for animal viruses, research on plant viruses has been both applied and basic, with very similar goals: to understand how plant viruses cause diseases so as to prevent these and their impact economically and in terms of human and animal nutrition, and to use them as models to investigate plant cell biology and gene expression. In contrast to animal viruses, this latter goal has taken longer to realize because of technical limitations in investigating plant viruses.

REVERSE GENETICS AND THE MODERN ERA OF PLANT VIROLOGY

From the mid-1950s on, the availability of animal cell tissue culture systems meant that clonal isolates of animal viruses, essential for genetic studies, could be readily obtained and that synchronous infections could be done to dissect viral multiplication cycles. Thus, investigations of animal viruses became more molecular, and our knowledge of animal virus–host interactions advanced. Lacking appropriate tissue culture systems, plant virus studies relied on the ability to infect plants by mechanical

TABLE 1. *Viruses that cause severe crop losses worldwide*

Virus disease	Geographic distribution	Host crop
Sugarcane mosaic	Worldwide	Sugarcane, corn
Cassava mosaic	Africa	Cassava
Citrus quick decline (tristeza)	Africa, Americas	Trees[a]
Swollen shoot of cacao	Africa	Cacao (heavy losses)
Plumpox (sharka)[b]	Europe	Plums, peaches, apricots
Barley yellow dwarf	Worldwide	Grains
Tomato yellow dwarf	Mediterranean, Caribbean	Tomatoes, beans
Tomato spotted wilt	Worldwide	Tomatoes, tobacco, peanuts, ornamentals, others[c]

[a]Tens of millions of trees infected as of 1997.
[b]Severe, spreading epidemic.
[c]Extremely broad host range.

means—rubbing a suspension of virus particles onto a leaf with a finger or spatula, often in the presence of an abrasive agent such as fine-grade carborundum—or using appropriate vectors, usually insects. For a number of plant viruses, protoplasts (isolated plants cells from which the walls had been enzymatically removed) could be transfected with the viral genome or, in some cases, virions. However, this advance did not occur until 1968, at which point plant virus studies began to focus more on virus replication and on the synthesis and translation of viral messenger RNAs (mRNAs). In particular, advances were reported for positive-sense RNA plant viruses (including TMV) that could be readily propagated because the purified viral genome was infectious, often multipartite (i.e., segmented), and could be translated *in vitro* using available rabbit reticulocyte and wheat germ extracts, or when injected into oocytes from frogs or toads. Thus, from the 1970s to the early 1980s, knowledge about virus replication was advanced for those positive-sense RNA viruses that accumulated to high levels in infected plants and could be easily purified. The coat proteins of brome mosaic virus (BMV) and TMV were shown to be translated from a subgenomic mRNA (152,317). Protoplast studies began to identify nonstructural proteins encoded by these viruses and other viruses, and genetic studies began to identify specific viral genes through the study of temperature-sensitive mutants and genetic reassortment studies for viruses having segmented genomes.

Against this background of technical limitations, the impact of reverse genetics on the investigation of plant viruses in the early 1980s was immense, ushering in the current era of research on plant virus–host interactions at the cellular level. Ahlquist and colleagues (8) were the first to report the generation of infectious plant virus transcripts from cloned complementary DNA (cDNA) of the genome of BMV. Their success was facilitated by the fact that the BMV genome consists of three segments of positive-sense RNA, the largest being 3.2 kb. Their approach was to clone each of the three BMV cDNAs behind a modified bacteriophage lambda P_R promoter such that transcription would correctly initiate at the first nucleotide of the inserted sequence. Transcripts of each segment with correct 5′ and 3′ ends were generated *in vitro* using *Escherichia coli* RNA polymerase, and these proved to be infectious when mechanically inoculated onto susceptible host plants or transfected into plant protoplasts. Generating full-length cDNAs that could be transcribed into an infectious transcript for the larger (at least in terms of contiguous nucleotides) genomes of RNA plant viruses like TMV (6.4 kb) and the potyviruses tobacco vein mottling virus and plum pox virus (~10 kb) proved to be more difficult, but followed within a few years (83,288).

It was more straightforward to clone infectious DNA copies for plant viruses with DNA genomes like the geminiviruses with their single-stranded DNA (ssDNA) genomes, or the pararetrovirus cauliflower mosaic virus (CaMV) with its double-stranded DNA (dsDNA) genome. However, here the problem was how to efficiently infect plants with these cloned DNAs. The same issue in principle existed for positive-sense RNA viruses like the luteoviruses that could not be mechanically transmitted to plants, and for the negative-sense plant rhabdoviruses and tospoviruses (in the *Bunyaviridae*), in which the genome alone would not be infectious. The earliest solution was developed in studies of CaMV and the geminivirus tomato golden mosaic virus (TGMV) and took advantage of the ability of *Agrobacterium tumefaciens,* the bacteria that causes crown gall tumors on plants, to transfer its tumor-inducing (Ti) plasmid into plant cells by a mechanism that resembles bacterial conjugal DNA transfer (126). In crown gall tumor, bacterial Ti plasmid sequences are integrated into the plant chromosome, and studies to define the mechanism by which this occurs led to the development of vectors that are commonly used to generate transgenic plants. In the agroinfection procedure that was developed, the CaMV or TGMV genomes were each cloned into vectors that would autonomously replicate in *A. tumefaciens.* These would be transferred into plant cells by the same mechanism as Ti plasmid transfer when the bacteria were either injected into the plants or introduced at wounded sites (Fig. 2). Once inside the plant cells, infection was initiated when inserted viral sequences would replicate or recombine out of the bacterial vector to reform the virus

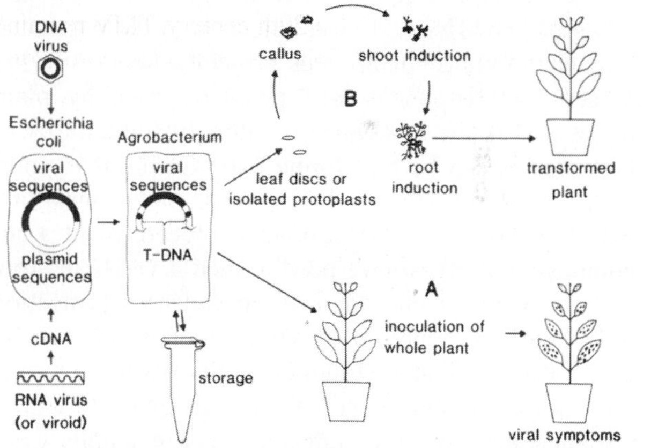

FIG. 2. Agroinfection: transfer of a viral genome or viroid RNA to plants. The gene or genome of interest is cloned into a plasmid that can replicate in *Agrobacterium tumefaciens.* It contains at least the Ti plasmid right border sequence; thus, it can be transferred into plant cells by the action of the bacterial *Vir* genes. The outcome of infection, or integration to create a transgenic plant, is determined by the Ti plasmid having a left as well as a right border sequence (integration) and on whether the introduced plasmid contains a viral sequence that can autonomously replicate when released from the plasmid in the plant. (From Grimsley N, Bisaro DM. Agroinfection. In: Hohn TH, Schell J, eds. *Plant DNA infectious agents.* New York: Springer-Verlag, 1987:87—107, with permission.)

genome. This same general approach can be used to infect plants with the cloned cDNA copies of RNA virus genomes and viroids, as well as to generate transgenic plants that contain specific viral sequences (126). The introduction of biolistic bombardment in the early 1990s to "shoot" cloned DNAs into plant cells provided an alternative approach to using *A. tumefaciens* to transform plants, as well as to infect them with cloned plant virus genomes or introduce reporter gene constructs for transient expression assays.

The impact of reverse genetics on plant virology cannot be overstated. Having clonal isolates of plant virus genomes and the techniques in place to introduce these back into plants in the absence of a vector meant that defined mutations could be introduced and studied for their effects on the virus replication, transcription, and host interactions. Thus, individual viral genes could be readily identified and functions assigned to these. Viral genomes and genes were used for *in situ* hybridization to track virus multiplication and infection in the plant and were expressed in *E. coli* to generate antisera for identifying and localizing individual virus-encoded proteins in infected plants. Sequence analysis and hybridization studies established the relationships among viruses and, extended through the use of the polymerase chain reaction (PCR), have produced a veritable growth industry in the identification and cloning of new plant viruses, which has profoundly affected studies on plant virus epidemiology. β-Glucuronidase (GUS) and the jellyfish green fluorescent protein (GFP) expressed from plant virus genomes have provided visual reporters to trace the path and tissue specificity of virus infection in the plant and, fused to individual plant virus proteins, are identifying the cellular components and pathways used by plant viruses. Given the relative ease with which a number of plant species can be transformed, the functions of individual plant virus genes and their role in pathogenesis are being studied in transgenic plants. Indeed, plant virus genomes themselves have been termed a veritable "tool box" for plant genetic engineering and crop protection (374), being the source of strong promoters and translational enhancers that are routinely used to express foreign genes in plants, and of individual virus genes to confer resistance against virus infection. For example, it is almost impossible to read about transgenic plants without coming across reference to the strong CaMV 35S promoter (24). What we have learned is that plant viruses are not fundamentally different from animal viruses in their basic replication and gene expression strategies, which is logical because they are after all eukaryotic viruses. However, because of fundamental differences in the structure of plant and animal cells and in the physiology of plants and animals, plant viruses are fundamentally different in how they enter and exit from cells and systemically invade their hosts, and they have evolved some clever strategies to deal with these problems.

In the previous edition of this textbook, it was noted that interactions between plant viruses and their vectors or the earliest events in the infection process were poorly understood, that detailed information about plant virus replication and cell-to-cell movement was just beginning to accumulate, and that the mechanisms by which plant viruses induce disease responses had not been determined (313). Yet, John Shaw in writing this was optimistic that it seemed "certain that the increasingly powerful techniques of molecular and cellular biology should provide us with explanations of these phenomena within a relatively short period of time." His optimism was not misplaced. Since 1996, when the last edition of this text was published, we have made major advances in all of these areas. This chapter focuses on the molecular and cellular details of plant virus replication and pathogenesis, highlighting the studies of a number of representative model plant viruses that have advanced our understanding of how plant viruses interact with their insect vectors, how different plant viruses replicate and regulate their gene expression, how these viruses move from cell to cell to systemically infect the host, and the interplay between virus and plant that results in disease or resistance of the host. An excellent overview of the families and genera of plant viruses, with descriptions of representative viruses within each group, can be found in the third edition of this book (313). The *Seventh Report of the International Committee on Taxonomy of Viruses* (ICTV) (347) and the *Encyclopedia of Virology* (123) present more detailed descriptions of all known viruses and viroids and their current classification. Additional excellent texts and reviews that describe the diseases caused by and the epidemiology of different plant viruses, as well as subviral agents (viroids and satellites) that infect plants, are also available (5,73,294).

THE PLANT VIRUS FAMILIES

According to the latest ICTV report (347), the number of recognized viruses is 3,618, of which ~25% (957) are plant viruses. In addition, there are subviral agents (formerly called *unconventional agents*) that can infect plants, namely viroids and satellites. Satellites are analogous to the δ-agent of hepatitis B virus, being encapsidated RNAs that are not essential for the infectivity of a particular plant virus "partner" but can modulate the pathogenicity of that virus (294). Viroids, now classified in seven different genera, are small (~250 to 370 nt), highly structured RNAs that are responsible for a number of important diseases in plants, including potato spindle tuber disease, coconut cadang-cadang, and avocado sunblotch.

As for animal viruses, a system based on the use of Latin names has been adopted to classify plant viruses into families and subfamilies. Genera within these are based on running together the first few letters of the name of the virus that is considered to be the "type member" for that group. For example, *Tobamovirus* comes from *toba*cco *mo*saic virus, *Potexvirus* from *pot*ato virus *X*, and *Tospovirus* from *to*mato *spo*tted wilt virus (Fig. 3). This approach to classification has at times led to vigorous debate because the genera designations are not necessarily intuitive for the nonexpert, and even those in the field can find them difficult to remember. As is the case for animal viruses, researchers generally use common names to refer to individual viruses.

Figure 3 illustrates several important points about plant viruses in relation to animal viruses. The vast majority of plant viruses are nonenveloped positive-sense ssRNA viruses. There are few enveloped plant viruses, and these are negative-sense (the rhabdoviruses) or ambisense (the tospoviruses and tenuiviruses) ssRNA viruses. There are few DNA plant viruses, and none of these are true dsDNA viruses. Thus, there are no simple dsDNA viruses corresponding to the papovaviruses, and there are no dsDNA viruses of the complexity of the adenoviruses, herpesviruses, or vaccinia viruses. The caulimoviruses and badnaviruses have dsDNA genomes of ~7.2 to 8.2 kb in size but employ a reverse-transcribing replication strategy through a positive-sense ssRNA intermediate, as do the hepadnaviruses (see Chapter 36). The geminiviruses and

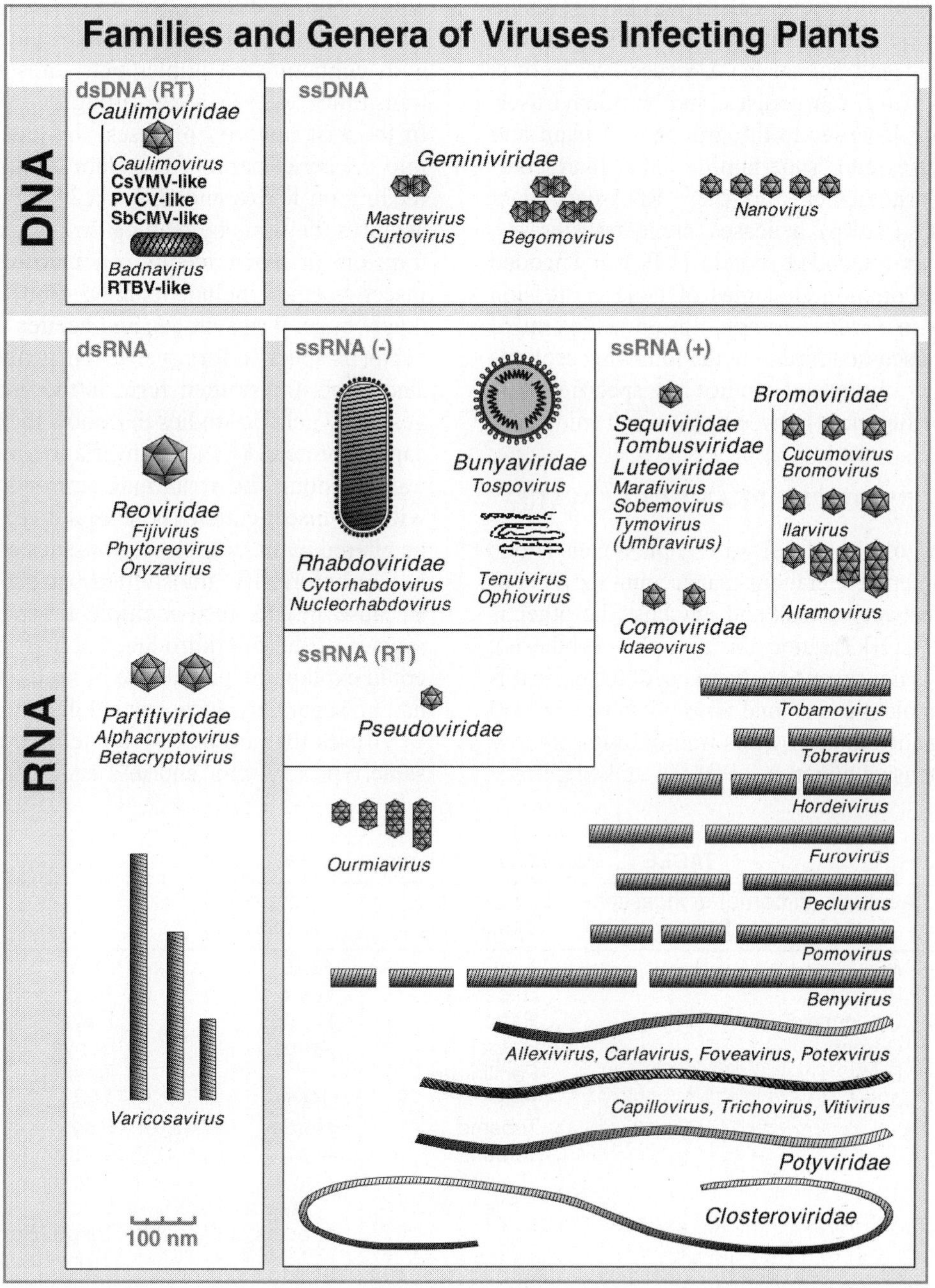

FIG. 3. Classification of plant viruses. (From ref. 347, with permission.)

the nanoviruses have small multicomponent circular ssDNA genomes (one or two genome segments of ~2.6 to 2.9 kb for geminiviruses, and at least six genome segments of ~1.0 to 1.2 kb for nanoviruses) and, like the parvoviruses, replicate through dsDNA intermediates. In contrast to animal viruses, in which segmented genomes are encapsidated in a single particle, the majority of plant viruses (positive-sense ssRNA, and ssDNA) have segmented genomes (referred to as *multicomponent*), with each genome segment encapsidated in a distinct particle. Only a few plant viruses belong to recognized families of animal viruses: *Reoviridae, Rhabdoviridae,* and *Bunyaviridae.* The diversity of plant virus families and genera classified according to the scheme in Figure 3 is striking. Yet despite this diversity, sequence analyses have revealed striking similarities, both among the RNA plant viruses and between plant and animal RNA viruses, as well as among caulimoviruses, retroviruses, and hepadnaviruses. Such comparisons have led to the grouping of plant and animal RNA viruses into "superfamilies" that share common sequence arrangements in their RNA-dependent RNA polymerases (RdRp), helicases, methyltransferases, genome-linked viral-encoded protein (VPg) or encoded proteinases, and common strategies of gene expression (see Chapter 13 in *Fields Virology*, 4th ed.). Several of these points are discussed further in the following sections in the context of functional studies on specific plant viruses and the differences between plants and animals.

CONSEQUENCES OF THE PLANT CELL WALL

The production of a rigid cell wall by plant cells is one of the two fundamental alterations that account for most of the differences between plants and animals (the other is carbon dioxide [CO_2] fixation through photosynthesis). Thus, perhaps it is not surprising that most of the basic differences between plant and animal viruses can be traced to plant cells being surrounded by this wall of long cellulose microfibrils (extensive polymers of β1→4–linked glucose residues) embedded in a matrix of branched polysaccharides (hemicellulose) and pectins, and the resultant rather sedentary lifestyle this imposes on plants. The plant cell wall is an effective barrier to virus entry and spread within the plant. External surface layers composed of cutin and waxes provide an additional protective barrier for the plant as a whole. Thus, to enter the plant initially and establish infection in a cell, a virus must mechanically breach these barriers. In addition, the virus will have to be delivered to the plant.

Plant-to-Plant Transmission

Although in nature a few plant viruses have been reported to be transmitted by direct plant-to-plant contact, and some can be introduced by mechanical abrasion with contaminated implements, most plant viruses are transmitted to their hosts through the action of a vector. In the vast majority of cases, this involves introduction into the aerial parts of the plant by the action of insects feeding on leaves and stems (124) (Table 2). The insect acquires the virus by feeding on infected plants and then transmits it when feeding on uninfected plants. These insect vectors include aphids, whiteflies, leafhoppers, mealy bugs, thrips, mites, and beetles. The type of insect vector is specific for a particular genus of plant viruses. The insect-transmitted form is the virion itself, as suggested by genetic studies that show the plant virus coat or capsid protein (CP) is invariably required for insect transmission. The virus may simply become associated with the insect cuticle (noncirculative), or it may have to be altered by passing through tissues of the insect (circulative) before it is transmitted back to plants (Table 3). Because insects feed multiple times on a given plant, viruses are usually introduced at high multiplicities. This could explain the prevalence of multipartite plant viruses having separately encapsidated genome components.

Viruses that are closely related are transmitted by the same type of vector and in a similar manner. For exam-

TABLE 2. *Transmission of viruses between hosts*[a]

	Aerosols (airborne) or ingestion (waterborne or foodborne)	Fluids (direct contact)	Parent to offspring	Vectors
Animal viruses	*Most*	*Few*	*Few*	*Many*
	Picorna	Hepadna	Retro	Toga
	Orthomyxo	Retro	Herpes	Flavi
	Corona	Herpes	Arena	Bunya
	Reo	Papilloma		Rhabdo
Plant viruses	*None*	*Few*	*Many*	*Most*
		Tobamo	Hordei	Poty
		Tombus	Ilar	Potex
		(water,	Poty	Gemini
		mechanical)	(seeds, pollen,	Luteo
			bulbs, cuttings)	Tospo (Bunya)
				(insects, nematodes, fungi)

[a]Examples indicate that some, not necessarily all, viruses within the family are transmitted by the given mode. (Based on ref. 124.)

TABLE 3. *Modes of plant virus insect transmission*

	Noncirculative (cuticle associated)		Circulative (tissue associated)	
	Stylet-borne (nonpersistent)	Foregut-borne (semipersistent)	Nonpropagative (persistent)	Propagative (persistent)
Example	Potyviruses	Caulimoviruses	Luteoviruses	Tospoviruses
Acquire[a]	Seconds	Minutes	Hours	
Inoculate[b]	Seconds	Minutes	Hours	
Retain[c]	Hours	Days	Days	
Latent period[d]	No	No	Yes	

Minimum feeding time required for an insect to acquire[a] or transmit[b] a virus.
[c]Period of time for which an insect retains the ability to transmit a virus.
[d]Lag between the time an insect acquires a virus and the time it becomes competent to transmit that virus.
Based on ref. 124.

ple, luteoviruses and potyviruses are both transmitted by aphids, but their relationships to the aphid differ. For potyviruses, the aphid is similar in principle to a flying syringe, although the interaction is more specific. The virus binds to a receptor(s) in the aphid stylet (the feeding probe), but the aphid is not a host for the virus: it simply serves to inject the virus into a plant during feeding, probably by a process of ingestion and salivation (124). This type of transmission mode has been termed *nonpersistent* and is now referred to as *stylet borne.* It is characterized by rapid insect acquisition and inoculation times (on the order of seconds), and the insect retains the ability to transmit the virus for only a few hours (see Table 3). In contrast, luteoviruses have to circulate through the aphid, passing from the insect midgut to the hindgut and crossing the hindgut wall to enter the hemocoel. From the hemocoel, the virus moves to the salivary glands and then enters the salivary canal, from which it will be inoculated into plants during aphid feeding. Thus, there is an obligatory biological relationship between the luteovirus and the aphid, one in which the acquired virus is altered in preparation for transmission. There is evidence to suggest that this alteration may involve proteolytic cleavage of a proline-rich extension in a subset of the viral CP subunits that make up the viral capsid. Although luteoviruses do not in fact multiply in the aphid, the insect is referred to as a "host," but a nonpropagative one (see Table 3), and it is considered "infected" with the virus. This circulative mode of transmission is characterized by long acquisition and plant inoculation times, on the order of hours. It was formerly referred to as "persistent" because the insect can transmit the virus for many days, and potentially throughout its life, once it has acquired the virus.

A number of plant viruses that are transmitted by the circulative mode have been shown to multiply in their insect vector, thus infecting the insect in the more conventional sense. The insect in these cases is termed a *propagative host* (see Table 3). Perhaps not surprisingly, most of these plant viruses, which when viewed from their ability to multiply in the insect could be considered to be "animal viruses," belong to well-recognized animal virus families—*Reoviridae, Rhabdoviridae,* and *Bunyaviridae*—although some apparently do not (marafiviruses) (see Table 3). The tospoviruses, named for the type member TSWV, are a genera within the *Bunyaviridae,* and TSWV illustrates at least some of the adaptations a plant virus may evolve to achieve this dual lifestyle.

TSWV, like the animal-infecting *Bunyaviridae,* has a tripartite ssRNA genome encapsidated in three nucleocapsids, which are surrounded by an envelope. The envelope contains heterodimeric spikes composed of the viral-encoded G1 and G2 glycoproteins. TSWV is transmitted by thrips in a circulative and propagative manner. The virus, once ingested, passes to the thrip midgut, where it may bind to a receptor(s) (17), and crosses the midgut wall, apparently by endocytosis. TSWV multiplies in the infected thrip, eventually reaching the salivary glands and salivary canal, from which it is transmitted to other plants. Comparison of the TSWV genome organization with that of the animal-infecting *Bunyaviridae* shows that its M segment, which encodes G1 and G2 in all *Bunyaviridae,* is uniquely ambisense, being transcribed into a subgenomic RNA that is translated into a plant virus-specific NSm protein (see Chapter 25). Both the glycoproteins and NSm are needed for TSWV to exit from an infected cell, but in very different ways. G1 and G2, indeed the entire enveloped structure, are required for multiplication in and transmission by thrips, but are completely dispensable for infecting plants. This was graphically shown by the studies in which TSWV was serially passaged in tobacco plants by mechanical abrasion in the complete absence of the insect vector (285). After a number of passages, virus was obtained that was highly infectious when mechanically inoculated on plants but could not be transmitted by thrips. This mutated TSWV would still react with antinucleocapsid antisera but was no longer recognized by either anti-G1 or anti-G2 antisera, suggesting that the glycoproteins were absent. This was confirmed and extended in electron microscopic studies that showed these mutant TSWV preparations consisted of the typical viral RNPs, with no enveloped particles being present. Molecular studies in insect cells and gel overlay assays with tissue extracts from thrips suggest that the glycoprotein spikes are required for attachment and penetration in the thrips vector (17,171). NSm is not required for insect transmission or replication of the viral genome (272). Rather, it is a unique plant virus protein—a movement protein—that is needed for the virus to cross the cell wall and systemically infect the plant.

The specificity of the virus–insect interaction requires virus-encoded protein and presumably a receptor protein(s) in the insect, although few such candidate receptors have been identified. As shown for the geminiviruses, in nonenveloped viruses, the CP can be the only virus-encoded protein required for the specificity of interaction with the insect vector. There are different genera of geminiviruses, and the begomoviruses, such as African cassava mosaic virus (ACMV), are transmitted by whiteflies, whereas the curtoviruses, such as beet curly top virus (BCTV), and the mastreviruses, such as maize streak virus, are transmitted by different leafhopper species (see Fig. 3). When ACMV was engineered to express the BCTV CP in place of its own, the recombinant ACMV genome encapsidated in the BCTV CP was now transmitted by leafhoppers, and not by whiteflies, which demonstrated a direct role of the geminivirus CP in insect recognition (31). However, for some nonenveloped plant viruses, a virus-encoded transmission accessory or "helper" factor is required, in addition to the CP, for the specific interaction with receptors in the insect. This is the case for the potyviruses and their aphid vectors, where it has been suggested that a dimeric form of the viral-encoded helper factor (helper component, the HC domain of HC-Pro) acts as a bridging molecule between the virion capsid and receptor(s) in the cuticle lining the aphid stylet (264). The viral spikes in TSWV appear to bind directly to candidate receptor proteins in thrips (17,171), and it is reasonable to think that this may be generally true for all enveloped plant viruses that are transmitted by insects. Our understanding of plant virus attachment to and passage through, or replication in, the insect vector is currently rudimentary owing to the general lack of stable virus mutants that are defective in insect transmission, and of cultured insect cells in which to study plant virus attachment and replication. The functions in virus penetration or circulation of the few candidate receptor molecules that have been identified remains to be defined. Recent technical advances, such as the establishment of cultured thrips and leafhopper cell lines for replication studies, and genetic approaches to generate stable virus mutants (172,241,279) should aid in addressing these questions and increase our knowledge of how virions are altered as they pass through their insect vectors.

Elementary as our knowledge is about insect transmission of plant viruses, we understand even less about the transmission of plant viruses by fungi or nematodes, or their horizontal transmission through seed or pollen (see Table 2). In those instances in which it has been is studied, both virus-encoded and host-encoded components appear to be important in these modes of transmission. As for insect transmission, the evidence suggests that virus particles are transmitted by nematodes and fungi because, in the few cases in which it has been investigated, at least the viral CP is required for transmission by these vectors (125,212). About 18% of plant viruses can be transmitted through seeds in at least one host, a process that is more significant in terms of economic and epidemiologic impact than this number might imply once one considers the number of infected seeds that can be produced by a field of plants. In all cases, except for TMV, seed transmission requires that the embryo be infected either directly or indirectly through infection of the gametes prior to fertilization (221). Molecular studies of barley stripe mosaic virus (a hordeivirus), the potyvirus pea seed-borne mosaic virus, and the tobravirus pea early browning virus indicate that the process is complex. Nevertheless, in two of these cases, a viral-encoded protein that is a "pathogenicity determinant" has been identified as a determinant of seed transmission (96,162,362). This suggests that perhaps efficient systemic invasion of the host is a factor in the ability of some plant viruses to overcome tissue barriers and invade the developing embryo.

Adaptation to the Cell Wall: The Fundamental Difference Between Plant and Animal Viruses

Once mechanically introduced into a plant, by insect feeding or other means, plant viruses will initiate infection of the inoculated cells, most commonly within a leaf. However, the problem of the plant cell wall does not end here because it is an effective barrier to plant viruses exiting from as well as entering a cell. The virus must do this to spread from cell to cell within the inoculated leaf and then invade the growing plant, a process termed *systemic infection.* A fundamental distinction from bacteriophage, which also have to negotiate their way across cell walls, is that plant viruses infect and invade an integrated multicellular host, not a population of autonomously functioning walled cells. Plant cells, although surrounded by walls, are connected by transwall channels termed *plasmodesmata,* the formation and function of which can be developmentally regulated. Through these channels, all plant cells are potentially in communication with each other through the passage of solutes and small molecules, and recent studies suggest that even rather large proteins may pass through plasmodesmata at certain developmental stages (252,291). The term *symplasm* was coined to reflect this potential cytoplasmic continuity among plant cells. The spaces between plant cells constitute the *apoplasm.* If plant viruses were to adapt the solution of most phage (except f1/M13) of encoding the equivalent of a lysozyme function (a "cellulase") to dissolve the wall of the infected cell, they would find themselves in the apoplasm facing the next cell wall. Worse yet, the "cellulase" could digest the walls of the surrounding cells, which, given their high internal hydrostatic pressure, would burst—not a useful outcome for the virus.

Although the cell wall presents a barrier, the plasmodesmata present an opportunity for the plant virus to move directly from cell to cell without having to go through an extracellular phase. This is similar in principle to cell-to-cell spread of vaccinia virus or human immunodeficiency virus (HIV), but in a manner that is potentially less destructive to the plant cells. All plant viruses encode a unique class of proteins termed movement proteins (MPs), which modify or alter plasmodesmata so that the virus genome can spread directly from cell to cell, effectively "tunneling" through the cell wall in a nondestructive way. The MP is essential for this process, as indicated by the name, which originates from the genetic studies that first identified the genes encoding such proteins. A plant virus that is mutated in the gene encoding this MP will still replicate in individual plant cell protoplasts and assemble virus particles, but this virus will be defective in spreading within the inoculated leaf and systemically infecting the host. The classic studies on the TMV temperature-sensitive *Ls1* mutant (245) were among the first to show that such MPs exist. TMV *Ls1* can systemically infect tomato plants at 22°C but will not do so when the plants are grown at 32°C, although it replicates well at both temperatures. When tomato plant leaflets mechanically inoculated with this *Ls1* mutant were grown for 24 hours at 22°C or 32°C and stained with fluorescently tagged antivirus antibody that would detect TMV CP, fields of large numbers of adjoining infected cells that accumulated viral CP could be seen at the permissive temperature of 22°C. This was also true for leaflets at both temperatures inoculated with wild-type TMV. In contrast, only individual single cells were found to accumulate CP in the *Ls1*-inoculated leaflets grown at 32°C. This demonstrated that the *Ls1* mutant could replicate at the nonpermissive temperature because it was synthesizing viral CP. However, the fact that only individual single cells were seen to be infected, rather than fields of contiguous cells, showed that this *Ls1* mutant was defective at the high temperature in moving from the inoculated cell into neighboring cells within the leaf. As described in more detail later, we now know that this *Ls1* mutant has a missense mutation in the 30-kd MP of TMV (71).

Although the MP is essential for this cell-to-cell movement, the viral CP may or may not be required. TMV and several other positive-sense RNA viruses do not require CP to move locally from cell to cell within the infected leaf. Neither do the ssDNA bipartite geminiviruses (begomoviruses). As discussed later, although the mechanisms differ, the genomes of these viruses can move from cell to cell in a complex with a movement protein. Other plant viruses, such as TSWV, CaMV, and potato virus X (PVX), require CP in addition to movement proteins to move locally from cell to cell, moving as virions or subviral particles. Thus, although plant viruses are transmitted from plant to plant in the form of virus particles, virions are not necessarily the form in which the plant virus genome is transmitted directly from cell to cell, at least within an infected leaf (194). This is in stark contrast to animal viruses and phage. This does not mean that virus particles do not play a role in systemic infection of the plant. For most plant viruses, movement out of the inoculated leaf to distant parts of the plant to establish systemic infection occurs through the nutrient transport system of the plant, the phloem, by way of companion cells connected to the sieve elements or "tubes" that form the conduits for long distance transport of nutrients. Evidence suggests that most plant viruses require CP for this long-distance movement, although whether this occurs in the form of stable assembled virions in all cases remains to be shown.

As suggested from the preceding considerations, an additional distinct feature of plant viruses when compared to animal viruses and phage is that there is no evidence for the attachment of virus particles to specific receptors on the surface of plant cells to initiate infection. Such virus–receptor interactions do appear to be important for recognition of plant viruses by their insect vectors, and perhaps other agents, for transmission. It also seems likely that within the vector, receptor-mediated endocytosis or receptor binding, followed by cell surface fusion, will be used by plant viruses that infect their insect vectors such as the topsoviruses and plant rhabdoviruses. Whether this represents another plant virus adaptation to the presence of the plant cell wall or the physiology of the plant, such an interaction has not been demonstrated to play a role in virus infection of a plant host. Few studies have focused on the mechanism by which plant virus particles or the genome in some other packaged form moves out of phloem sieve elements to penetrate plant cells when invading a new leaf, or on the uncoating of the plant virus genome, and we understand little about these processes.

PLANT VIRUS GENE EXPRESSION AND REPLICATION STRATEGIES

Given the relatively compact nature of their genomes, plant viruses, like animal viruses, have devised a variety of strategies to expand their coding capacity and regulate their gene expression while adhering to the rules for the translation of mRNAs in their eukaryotic hosts. These strategies, and the viral replication schemes, are all found among the animal viruses. Plant viruses with ssRNA genomes each replicate through an antigenomic or complementary strand, which serves as template for the synthesis of progeny strand genome ssRNA: the antigenomic replication template is negative-sense for a positive-sense RNA virus and the same polarity as mRNA (positive) for a negative-sense ssRNA virus, but it is not translated. Thus, exactly like ssRNA animal viruses, plant ssRNA viruses have to reconcile their genome structure with the requirement for monocistronic mRNAs in eukaryotic cells. In doing so, positive-sense ssRNA plant viruses regulate their gene expression at the level of transcription, through the production of subgenomic RNA (sgRNA); and at the level of translation, through polyprotein synthesis, leaky ribosome scanning, suppression of termination (called *readthrough translation*), ribosomal frameshifting, or internal ribosome entry (see Chapter 5). The production of sgRNA is the most common strategy employed; however, most positive-sense ssRNA plant viruses use more than a single strategy to regulate and optimize their gene expression. The ambisense tospoviruses, in the *Bunyaviridae* (see Chapter 25), regulate their expression at the transcriptional level through cap snatching and the production of sgRNA, and by a polyprotein strategy at the translational level. The negative-sense plant rhabdoviruses probably employ a strictly monocistronic transcriptional strategy, as do the animal rhabdoviruses (see Chapter 22). Reinitiation of translation and RNA editing, strategies employed along with these others by different animal ssRNA viruses, have not been reported for ssRNA plant viruses.

In terms of plant DNA viruses, geminivirus circular ssDNA genomes are replicated through dsDNA intermediates by a rolling circle mechanism, as has been shown for the replication of the ssDNA genome of bacteriophage ϕX174 and proposed for the replication of herpesvirus dsDNA (see Chapters 17 and 33). The geminivirus dsDNA forms are also templates for the transcription of viral mRNAs, and gene expression is temporally regulated through transcriptional cascades, as it is in animal DNA viruses, such as the papovaviruses, adenoviruses, and herpesviruses, and in DNA bacteriophage. Alternative splicing of transcripts, as is found in many DNA animal viruses and the retroviruses, also regulates gene expression in some geminiviruses and in the caulimoviruses, such as CaMV and figwort mosaic virus (FMV). For these latter viruses, and the badnaviruses, the dsDNA genome is replicated by a reverse-transcribing mechanism through a positive-sense ssRNA in a manner similar to the hepadnaviruses (see Chapter 36). CaMV also regulates its gene expression through ribosome shunting (also used by adenovirus type 2) and the use of two promoters, and a virus-encoded transactivator acts to couple the translation of genes so that the viral 35S transcript is translated as a polycistronic mRNA even though it uses the eukaryotic translation machinery.

These strategies and principles are illustrated in the following sections by examining in detail the multiplication of plant viruses within several genera in an attempt to present the current state of our knowledge and highlight the experimental approaches being used. The particular viruses are not necessarily the most important in terms of disease potential and economic impact, but rather were chosen because they have been extensively characterized at the molecular, biochemical, and/or cellular levels and each illustrates particular points about the regulation of gene expression and virus interactions with plant cells. All plant viruses that have been sequenced and characterized to date employ some combination of the strategies that are discussed in these sections. Unsegmented (monopartite) positive-sense ssRNA viruses are presented first, chosen to illustrate the spectrum of positive-sense RNA virus strategies in a variety of combinations. These are followed by an example of a positive-sense ssRNA plant virus with a segmented genome, enveloped plant viruses, and plant DNA viruses. All of the RNA viruses in the following sections, except for some of the rhabdoviruses, are cytoplasmic viruses. In addition, all of the viruses that are presented, save for the *Luteoviridae* and *Geminiviridae*, infect and replicate in mesophyll cells (the cells between the veins that make up the bulk of a leaf). Viruses in the family *Luteoviridae* are limited to infecting the phloem tissue within the veins, and this is also true for a number of the *Geminiviridae*.

Positive-Sense Single-Stranded RNA Viruses

Potyviruses: Polyprotein Strategy

The largest of the plant virus families, the *Potyviridae,* encompasses the potyviruses, rymoviruses, and bymoviruses, along with several other genera (347). The potyviruses themselves constitute the largest genus of known plant viruses (~30%) and as a group are responsible for the highest losses of crop plants worldwide (5). Although *pot*ato virus *Y* is the type member for this genus (hence "poty"), other potyviruses, such as tobacco etch virus (TEV), tobacco vein mottling virus (TVMV), and plum pox virus (PPV), have been better characterized at the molecular level. The virions are flexuous filamentous rods 11 to 15 nm in diameter and 680 to 900 nm in length (see Fig. 3) and are transmitted by aphids. The capsid is assembled from subunits of a single protein, the viral-encoded coat protein (CP). The potyviral genome is an unsegmented (monopartite) positive-sense ssRNA of ~10 kb that has a viral-encoded protein (VPg) covalently linked to its 5′ end and is polyadenylated at its 3′ end (reviewed in 290). With the initial complete sequencing of the genomes of TEV, TVMV, and PPV, it became clear that the potyvirus genomic RNA encodes a single open reading frame (ORF), which could be translated into one large polyprotein of 340 to 370 kd, similar to the animal picornaviruses. This, and similarities with picornaviruses and flaviviruses, as well as plant nepoviruses and comoviruses, in predicted amino acid sequence motifs, and the organization of proteins potentially involved in RNA replication, eventually led to the proposed superfamily of picorna-like plant and animal viruses (120) (see Chapter 13 in *Fields Virology*, 4th ed.).

Prior to the availability of complete genome sequences and infectious clones, several of the potyvirus-encoded proteins were identified by a combination of biochemical and immunological studies of virions, insect (aphid) transmission, and infected plant tissue, and their names reflect these original associations. Thus, the viral CP was originally "Cap" for capsid protein, VPg is the genome-linked viral protein, and HC is the "helper component" N-terminal domain of HC-Pro (found in amorphous cytoplasmic inclusions) that is required as an accessory factor for insect transmission of virions (this has been extensively characterized, as reviewed in 264). Three additional viral proteins were associated with characteristic inclusions in infected cells: CI with cytoplasmic *cylindrical inclusions,* and NIa and NIb with *nuclear inclusions*.

The single polyprotein encoded by the potyvirus genomic RNA is cotranslationally and posttranslationally cleaved to produce all of the mature viral proteins by the action of three viral-encoded proteinases: P1, HC-Pro, and NIa (39,40,116,135,353) (Fig. 4). P1 and HC-Pro are responsible for two distinct autoproteolytic (*cis*) cleavages within the N-terminal region of the polyprotein. NIa, which resembles the picornavirus 3C proteinase, carries out the remaining cleavages (both in *cis* and in *trans*) within the C-terminal two-thirds of the polyprotein. NIa is composed of an N-terminal VPg domain and a C-terminal proteinase domain. This proteinase domain, and the C-terminal proteinase domain of P1, are both structurally related to the chymotrypsin class of serine proteinases. HC-Pro, also having a C-terminal proteinase domain, is a papain-like cysteine proteinase. P1, HC-Pro, and NIa are not only required for the correct proteolytic processing of the viral-encoded polyprotein: each proteinase is a multifunctional protein with additional roles in the virus life cycle. This multifunctionality appears to be true for most of the potyvirus proteins.

P1 autoproteolytically separates itself from HC-Pro (see Fig. 4). This proteolytic cleavage is essential for virus infectivity, but P1 proteolytic activity *per se* is not. This was shown in studies with TEV using mutants that were nonviable because each encoded a processing-defective P1 proteinase. Each mutant could be restored to infectivity by the insertion of an NIa cleavage site between P1 and HC-Pro (350). P1 can bind ssRNA *in vitro* (30,352), and based on this and sequence comparisons, it was long speculated that P1 might be an MP. To address this point, a modified strain of TEV was engineered to express the bacterial *GUS* gene (TEV-GUS) as a reporter. When protoplasts prepared from tobacco plants are transfected with TEV-GUS RNA, the level of virus replication can be determined based on a fluorometric assay to detect GUS activity, produced from the

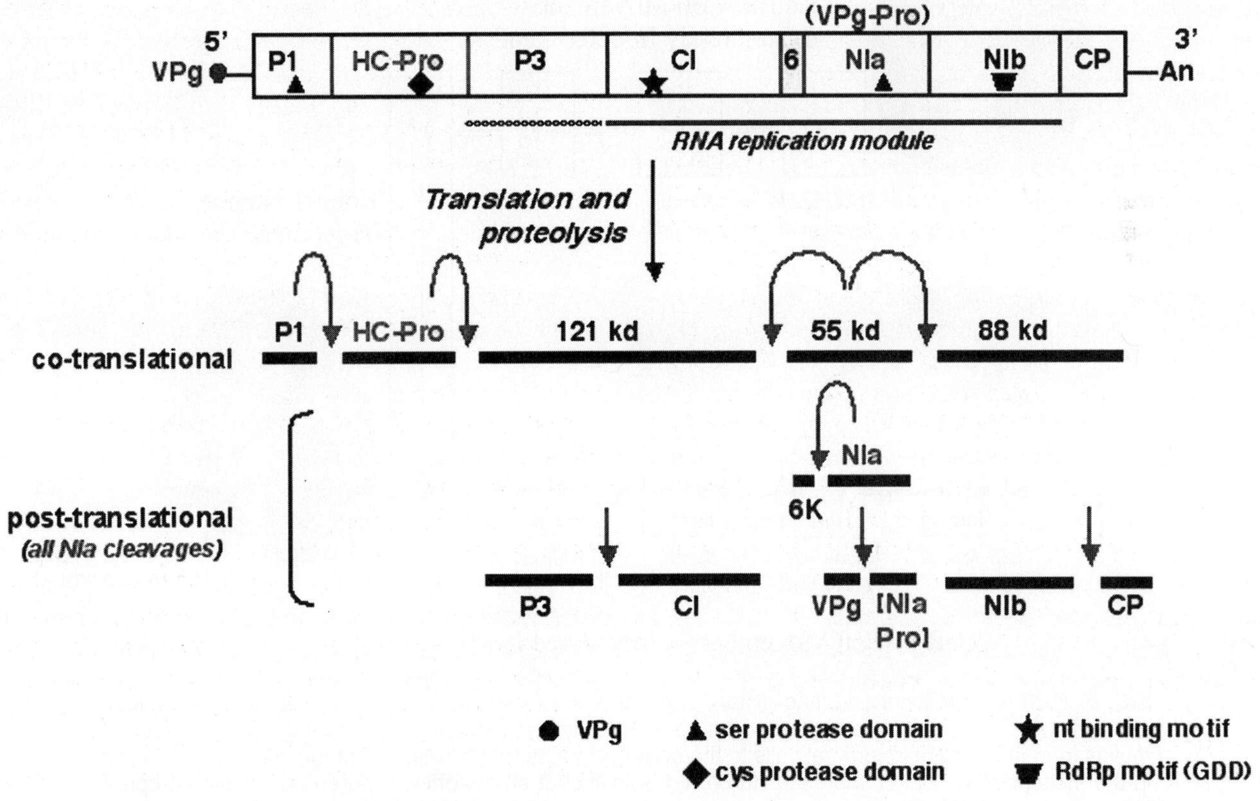

FIG. 4. Genome organization and polyprotein processing of tobacco etch virus (TEV). (Adapted from refs. 287 and 290, with permission.)

viral genome, in cell extracts. When plants are inoculated with TEV-GUS, in addition to quantitating GUS activity in leaf extracts using this assay, intact leaves can be fixed and stained for GUS activity using a histochemical substrate (X-gluc) that will stain GUS-expressing cells blue (Fig. 5). Thus, using this GUS-expressing virus, mutations in P1, or in any other viral protein, can be directly assayed in plants for their effects on virus movement as well as virus replication. A mutant in which the P1 coding sequence was deleted from TEV-GUS replicated to low levels in protoplasts (~3% wild-type levels), suggesting that while P1 was not essential for replication, it did play an accessory role. Despite this poor replication, this mutant was capable of cell-to-cell and leaf-to-leaf (systemic) movement in inoculated plants (351). The level of replication in protoplasts could be increased if the protoplasts were prepared from transgenic plants engineered to express P1. Thus, P1 is not an MP but may be a *trans*-acting accessory factor that stimulates viral genome amplification. P1 could exert this effect directly by interacting with viral RNA or proteins in the replication complex, or more analogous to the 2A proteinase of picornaviruses, could indirectly affect genome amplification by stimulating viral RNA translation (351) (see Chapter 18).

The CI-6K-NIa-NIb region of the potyviral polyprotein is similar in sequence and organization to the 2C-3A-3B-3C-3D region of the picornavirus polyprotein, which led to its original designation as the RNA replication module (290) (see Fig. 4). Molecular genetic and biochemical studies have established that this similarity extends to function as well, with NIa (VPg-proteinase) playing an essential regulatory role similar to that of the picornavirus 3C proteinase (see Chapter 18). Potyvirus replication occurs in the cytoplasm, apparently in association with endoplasmic reticulum (ER)-derived membranes (Fig. 6). Several lines of evidence suggest that the 6K protein, probably in the form of the 6K-NIa polyprotein (see Fig. 4), may act to target and anchor replication complexes to these membrane sites. TEV infection causes a collapse of the ER network into aggregated structures, and 6K appears to be associated with these ER-derived membranes. This was shown by expressing a fusion of 6K and the jellyfish green fluorescent protein (GFP:6K) in living cells from plasmids or the TEV genome, which could be

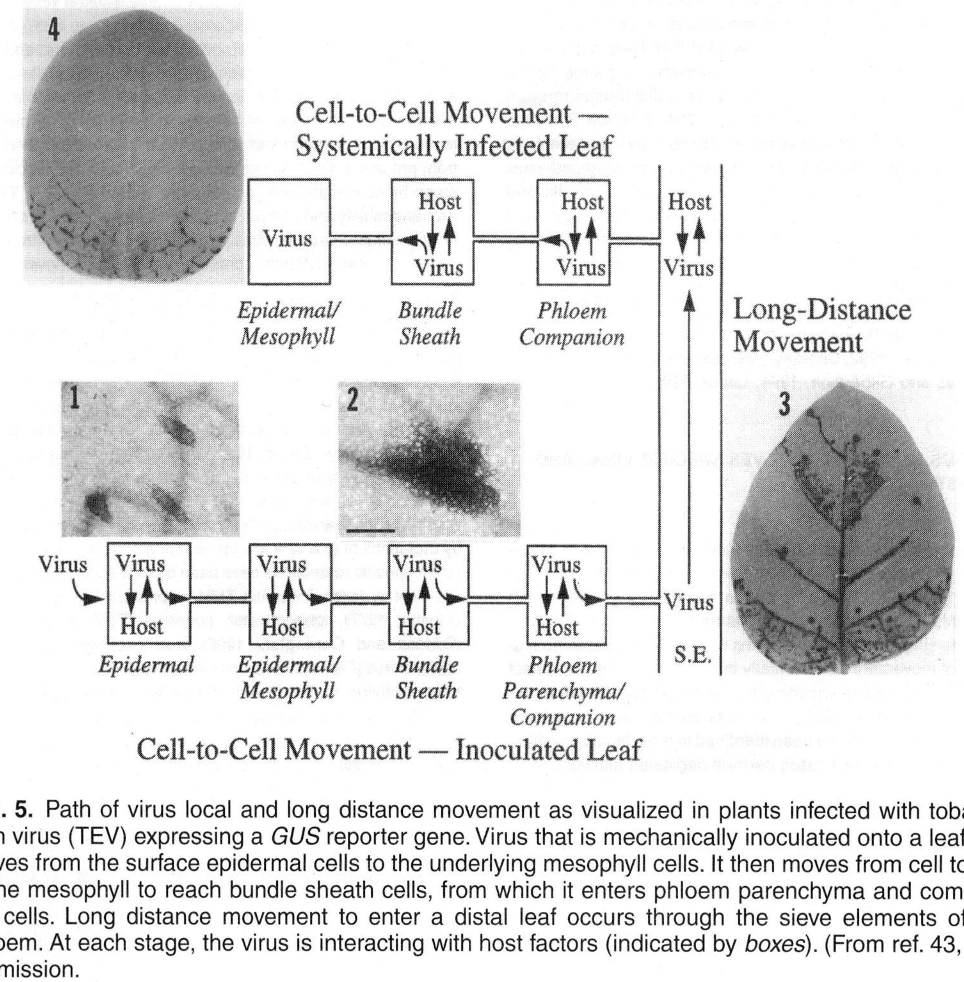

FIG. 5. Path of virus local and long distance movement as visualized in plants infected with tobacco etch virus (TEV) expressing a *GUS* reporter gene. Virus that is mechanically inoculated onto a leaf first moves from the surface epidermal cells to the underlying mesophyll cells. It then moves from cell to cell in the mesophyll to reach bundle sheath cells, from which it enters phloem parenchyma and companion cells. Long distance movement to enter a distal leaf occurs through the sieve elements of the phloem. At each stage, the virus is interacting with host factors (indicated by *boxes*). (From ref. 43, with permission.

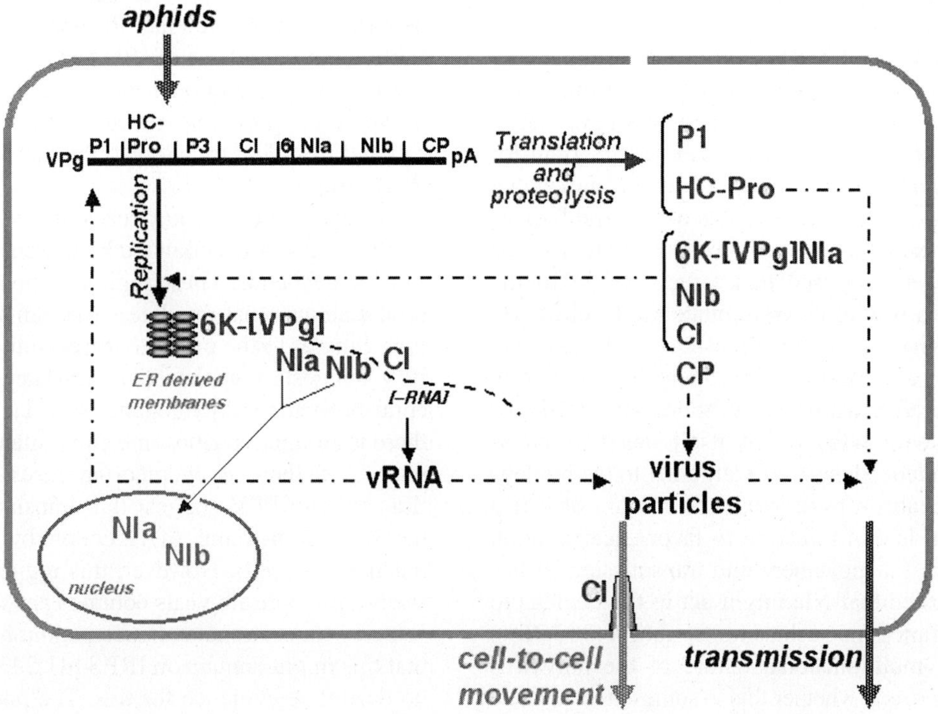

FIG. 6. Multiplication of tobacco etch virus (TEV). See Fig. 4 for the proteolytic events catalyzed by P1, HC-Pro, and NIa to process the TEV polyprotein into the individual encoded proteins.

introduced into leaf cells by biolistic bombardment, transfected into protoplasts, or inoculated onto plants. Using confocal microscopy and immune staining for marker proteins known to be located in the ER or Golgi, the GFP:6K was shown to localize to ER-derived membrane vesicles, and subcellular fractionation studies showed that both replication complexes and the 6K protein were associated with ER-like membranes (304).

Proteolytic processing by NIa, as well as NIa interacting with NIb, the viral RdRp (100,207), appear to be critical in orchestrating these events, with NIa acting in *cis* and NIb in *trans* (see Fig. 6). The latter conclusion is based on the finding that NIa mutants cannot be rescued for replication when transfected into protoplasts prepared from transgenic plants that express NIa, but NIb mutants can be rescued in transgenic protoplasts that express NIb (206,303). NIa can bind RNA *in vitro* (58), and TEV and TVMV NIa have also been shown to interact with NIb in yeast two-hybrid and *in vitro* binding assays (100,146, 207). Genetic studies indicate that NIa–NIb interaction is essential for virus replication (57). TEV NIa cleaves sites that contain the consensus heptapeptide motif Glu-X-X-Tyr-X-Gln↓Gly/Ser at differing rates, and it shows *cis*-preferential cleavage at a number of sites in the polyprotein, including those at CI/6K, 6K/NIa, and NIa/NIb. Whether NIa is retained in the cytoplasm or transported to the nucleus appears to be regulated by its association with 6K: the 6K-NIa polyprotein is retained in the cytoplasm, apparently because 6K masks the nuclear localization signal (NLS) which is present in NIa. However, after cleavage to produce the two separate proteins, NIa itself is efficiently transported to the nucleus mediated by its NLS, which is located in the VPg domain of the NIa (287). A suboptimal site that is slowly processed separates the VPg and proteinase domains of NIa itself. Mutants altered at this site to accelerate autocleavage by NIa are defective in amplifying the viral genome, as are mutants in the VPg linkage site (Tyr-62), the NIa (VPg) NLS, or the proteinase active site (303). Thus, nuclear targeting of NIa and slow internal processing between the VPg and proteinase domains, as well as VPg (or NIa) linkage to the viral genome and NIa proteinase activity, are required for viral RNA replication. The model that is consistent with these findings is that the 6K-NIa polyprotein bound to viral RNA by its NIa (VPg-proteinase) domain is anchored to ER-derived membranes through the 6K domain. NIb (RdRp) would be recruited to these replication complexes through a protein–protein interaction with NIa, which would position it next to the VPg domain to stimulate polymerase activity and protein priming of RNA synthesis (57), analogous to what has been proposed for picornavirus RNA replication. Whether VPg acts as a protein primer in potyvirus replication remains to be demonstrated. CI, which *in vitro* has been shown to have the properties of a helicase (95,188), is also required for genome replication (42,177). Such helicase activity is generally needed by large RNA viruses for their replication.

Given the functions of NIa and NIb in replication, why are both found to accumulate in the nucleus? It may be a consequence of the viral polyprotein strategy. CP is needed in large amounts to encapsidate the genome for insect transmission as well as for cell-to-cell movement (see below). Thus, very large amounts of NIa and NIb, as well as the other viral-encoded proteins, will also be made. It has been proposed that targeting NIa to the nucleus may be a way to down-regulate the level of NIa proteinase activity in the cytoplasm by, in essence, removing NIa to a separate compartment. This could be mediated by the NLS within the VPg domain of NIa, or an association with NIb, which itself has two NLSs (57,207,303). Independently, NIb targeting to the nucleus would be a mechanism to decrease the amount of RdRp in the cytoplasm late in infection to favor encapsidation of viral genomes for movement and transmission. It has also been suggested that NIa might act in the nucleus to affect host cell functions such as transcription (303,363).

The reported multifunctional nature of the potyvirus proteins is striking, and whether this to some extent reflects the polyprotein strategy of these viruses is an interesting point to ponder. At least CI and CP are not so different in this regard from other plant virus–encoded proteins as their multifunctional nature may reflect the particular requirements for virus movement. As discussed in the section on movement proteins, studies during the past several years have broadened our view beyond these simply being proteins that move the virus genome across the cell wall: movement proteins coordinate replication of the viral genome with its directed movement within and between plant cells (194). Genetic and ultrastructural studies suggest that CI, the virus-encoded helicase, is the potyvirus MP, associated with cone-shaped structures that align with plasmodesmata in infected cells (42,293). CP is also required for movement apparently because the viral genome is transported either as virus particles or in an RNP-complex with CP (81). Its role in aphid transmission is similarly explained by the fact that virus particles are the form transmitted, in a process that requires the helper component N-terminal domain of HC-Pro (reviewed in 264). Genetic studies suggest that the VPg domain of NIa, as well as HC-Pro, are "factors" involved in virus long distance (systemic) movement as well as genome amplification (55,166,177,282,305), but such studies do not distinguish between these proteins directly or indirectly affecting these processes. For HC-Pro, the effects seem to be the consequence of its role as a "pathogenicity factor," and indeed HC-Pro may be the most impressive example of a truly multifunctional protein (277,316). It is undoubtedly the helper component for aphid transmission and a proteinase for viral polyprotein processing. However, its effects on virus replication and systemic movement are now known to reflect an additional role of HC-Pro as a viral counterstrategy against a host RNA–mediated defense response (see Plant Responses to Virus Infection). Sorting out the effects of VPg mutations on long distance movement will require a better understanding of the forms in which the potyvirus genome moves, both from cell to cell and from leaf to leaf, and the mechanism of systemic movement.

Similar to the picornaviruses, the coding region of the potyvirus genome is flanked by untranslated sequences at its 5′ and 3′ ends. These regions appear to contain structural elements that regulate virus translation and replication. Similar to the picornaviruses, mutational analysis of PPV suggests that the 5′-untranslated region (5′-UTR) contributes to viral pathogenesis (211). However, whether there is an internal ribosome entry site (IRES) within this region, as there is in picornaviruses, remains unclear. Studies with PPV suggest that translation is initiated at the second in-frame AUG codon by a leaky-scanning mechanism (289). However, this region in TEV and pea seed–borne mosaic virus contains an AU-rich region that acts as a translational enhancer, and it has been suggested that this might contain an IRES (41,243). To date, there is no definitive evidence for this. The potyvirus 5′-UTR is less than 200 nt in length, much shorter that that found in picornaviruses, and it is predicted to be less structured (214). The 3′-UTR of the genome is predicted to contain secondary structures, and mutational studies with TVMV suggest that these may contribute to viral pathogenesis. Studies that compared the effects on virus replication of frameshift-stop codon mutations and deletions within the CP coding sequence of TEV suggest that translation through at least the first half of the CP coding sequence was required for efficient replication to occur (213), perhaps because passage of the translational apparatus alters secondary structure, which facilitates initiation of replication at the 3′ end of the genome. These studies also identified a structural element within the 3′ end of the CP coding sequence that was essential for replication, although whether this element interacts with *cis* or *trans* factors involved in genome replication or promotes stability of the viral genome remains to be determined (213).

Potexviruses: Subgenomic RNA and Leaky Ribosome Scanning

There are about ~30 viruses in the genus *Potexvirus,* of which PVX is the type member and one of the best characterized at the molecular level. In addition to its role in defining the potexvirus multiplication cycle, PVX has been important both historically and recently in studies on the synergistic enhancement of virulence that occurs when certain unrelated viruses co-infect a plant, and as a vector for gene expression studies in plants (47). Although individual potexviruses have a limited host range, as a group the potexviruses infect a range of monocotyledonous and dicotyledonous plants from bamboo and lilies to papaya, strawberry, cassava, and potato (1). The virions are flexuous filamentous rods ~14 nm in diameter and 470 to 580 nm in length (see Fig. 3) and appear to be one of the few groups of plant viruses directly transmitted by the mechanical mode. The capsid is assembled from subunits of a single protein, the viral-encoded CP. The potexvirus genome is an unsegmented positive-sense ssRNA of ~5.8 to 7 kb with a 5′-terminal cap (m^7GpppG) and is polyadenylated at its 3′ terminus.

The PVX genomic RNA contains five ORFs (151), which encode (in 5′-to-3′ order) the viral RdRp (166K), a so-called triple gene block (TGB) cluster of three proteins required for virus movement (25K, 12K, and 8K), and the viral CP (25 kd) (Fig. 7). Following uncoating in a plant cell, the viral genomic RNA is translated as a monocistronic mRNA to produce the RdRp (encoded by the 5′-proximal ORF), which then copies the viral genomic positive-sense RNA to produce full-length complementary negative-stranded RNA. This is then transcribed by the RdRp to produce additional copies of full-length genomic positive-sense RNA, or if the RdRp uses internal subgenomic promoters, a set of 3′-collinear sgRNAs. Each of the sgRNAs contains sequences identical to the 3′ end of the viral genome, and these function as the mRNAs for the viral movement proteins (TGB) and CP (see Fig. 7). A variety of *in vivo* and *in vitro* experimental studies support this mechanism for sgRNA synthesis and this view of potexvirus replication and expression (reviewed in 1 and 214). This strategy in general generates a family of 3′-co-terminal sgRNAs such that each gene to be expressed is located at the 5′ end of one of the sgRNAs (i.e., they are each functionally a monocistronic mRNA). In the case of PVX, the largest (2.1 kb) and the smallest (0.9 kb, encoding CP) sgRNAs are monocistronic and the major sgRNAs, and these encode the 25-kd movement protein and CP, respectively. However, the third sgRNA (1.4 kb), which is less abundant, functions as a bicistronic mRNA. It is translated by leaky ribosome scanning to produce the 12K and 8K proteins (349).

For PVX and other potexviruses, the first and largest ORF was originally predicted to encode the viral replicase (RdRp = 166K protein) based on sequence comparisons that showed it contained the conserved motifs characteristic of the methyltransferase/helicase/polymerase arrangement of the alphavirus supergroup (see Chapter 13 in *Fields Virology*, 4th ed.). Mutational studies show that the 166K protein is the only viral protein that is absolutely required for PVX RNA synthesis. In particular, mutation of the GKS nucleotide binding motif characteristic of helicases or the conserved GDD motif found in viral RdRps eliminates virus replication and infectivity in plants (61,210). Viral genome length positive- and negative-sense ssRNAs and the three sgRNAs, as well as the corresponding dsRNA forms, have been identified in PVX-infected protoplasts or plants (80,236,271,349). Consistent with its function as an mRNA, the viral genomic RNA from PVX and other potexviruses is infectious and is translated *in vitro* into the RdRp encoded by the first ORF (23,136). The largest (2.1 kb) and smallest

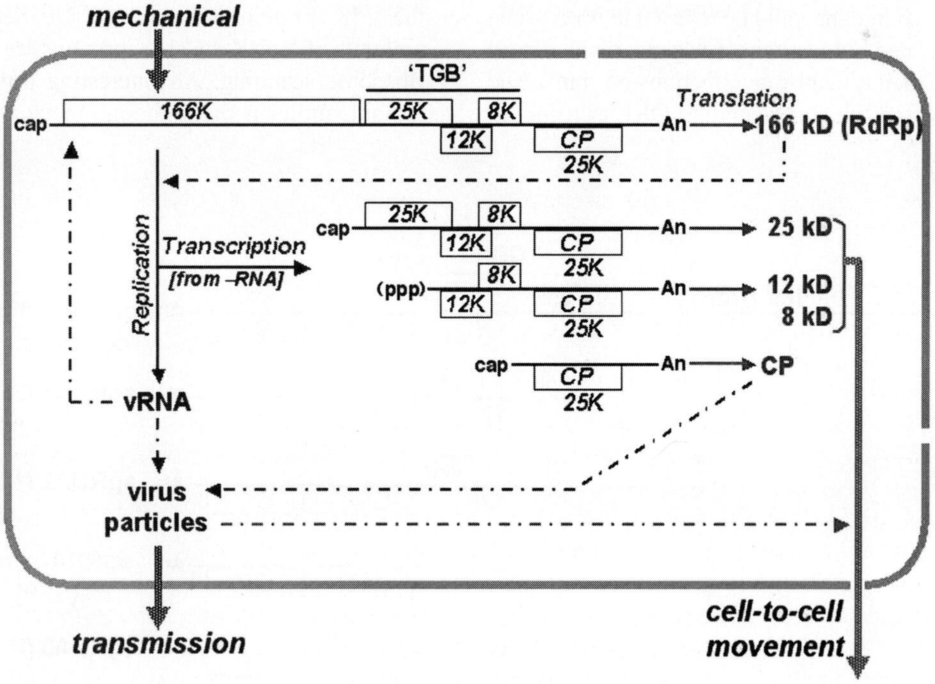

FIG. 7. Multiplication of potato virus X (PVX).

(0.9 kb) sgRNAs, as well as the viral genomic RNA, are capped and polyadenylated, and infectivity studies, as well as *in vitro* translation studies, show that the 5′-cap structure is necessary for efficient infection (1,136,236). Whether the low abundance PVX 1.4-kb sgRNA that encodes the 12K and 8K proteins is capped has not been directly determined. In general, sgRNAs commonly have the same 5′ and 3′ modifications as do the genomic RNA, but this is not always the case.

The PVX 1.4-kb sgRNA functions as a bicistronic mRNA, with the 12K and 8K proteins being translated by a leaky ribosome scanning mechanism. This was shown in *in vivo* studies using PVX engineered to express either GUS or GFP as a visual marker for virus movement, and transgenic plants that expressed different combinations of the TGB-encoded proteins (349). Because of the PVX expression strategy, the gene encoding GUS or GFP could be cloned just upstream of the *CP* gene so that it would be expressed from a duplicated copy of the CP subgenomic promoter. Thus, during infection the marker protein would be translated from an sgRNA separate from the other virus proteins (Fig. 8). Because PVX has a helical capsid, such engineered genomes can also be encapsidated into infectious virus particles.

Mutant PVX-GUS virus or transcripts that could not express either the 25K (Δ25K), the 12K (Δ12K) or the 8K protein (Δ8K, engineered by inserting a premature stop codon so that the overlapping *12K* ORF would not be affected) were not infectious when inoculated onto wild-type plants. Histochemical staining of inoculated leaves for GUS activity showed that each of these mutants is defective in cell-to-cell movement: GUS activity is restricted to the single initially infected cells. The cell-to-cell movement defect of each mutant could be rescued in *trans* when these were inoculated onto certain transgenic plants. In all cases, save one, each mutant was infectious on transgenic plants that expressed the corresponding ORF as a monocistronic mRNA or from a bicistronic or tricistronic mRNA in which this ORF was the 5′-most ORF in the transgene. Thus, for example, the Δ12K mutant was infectious on transgenic plants expressing either the *12K* ORF alone or the bicistronic *12K-8K* transgene but was not rescued on transgenic plants that expressed the tricistronic *25K-12K-8K* transgene in which the *12K* ORF was internal. The one exception was the Δ8K mutant: this was rescued on transgenic plants that expressed either the *8K* ORF alone or the bicistronic *12K-8K* transgene, thus showing that it is translated from a bicistronic mRNA (see Fig. 7). Inspection of the sequences surrounding the *12K* ORF initiation codon showed that it was in a suboptimal context for translation initiation, consistent with its being translated by leaky ribosome scanning. This was shown by constructing a set of PVX-GFP mutants in which the *12K* ORF was internally deleted (to remove any IRES), or its initiation codon was eliminated, or mutated to a stop codon or optimized initiation sequence. Because most of these mutations would eliminate translation of the 12K protein, each mutant was tested for infectivity on transgenic tobacco plants that expressed the *12K* ORF. The only mutant that could not be rescued on these transgenic plants was that in which the 12K initiation codon had been mutated to an optimized context. This mutant could be rescued only on transgenic plants that expressed the bicistronic *12K-8K* transgene, showing that the 8K protein is translated by leaky ribosome scanning (349). Thus, it appears that the amounts of the 12K and 8K proteins are regulated, relative to the 25K protein and other viral proteins, in at least two different ways. First, the bicistronic sgRNA encoding the 12K and 8K proteins is present at much lower levels in infected cells than are the mRNAs for the 25K protein, CP, and RdRp. Second, the relative amounts of the 8K and 12K proteins are regulated by leaky ribosome scanning. An interesting aspect of these PVX mutant studies is that although the appropriate transgenic

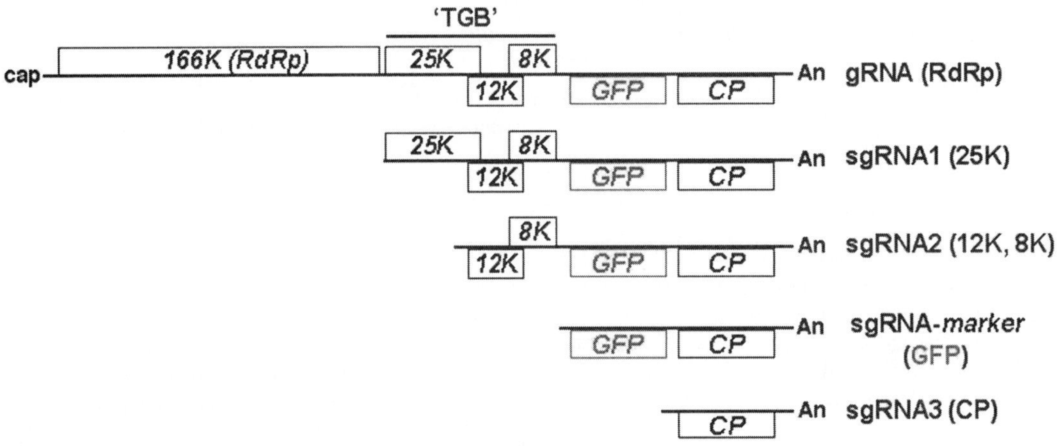

FIG. 8. Strategy to express a foreign gene using potato virus X (PVX).

lines could rescue PVX mutants for local cell-to-cell movement, in no case was there complementation for long distance systemic infection.

PVX sgRNAs, genomic RNA, and full-length complementary negative-sense RNA can be synthesized *in vitro* using membrane-containing extracts from infected plants (86). This suggests that PVX replicates in association with cytoplasmic membranes, like most if not all positive-sense plant and animal RNA viruses, including TEV and TMV (35). Consistent with this, virus replication appears to occur associated with virus-induced cytoplasmic laminate inclusions ("viroplasms") in plant cells (1,62). PVX genomic RNA contains an 84-nt 5′-UTR and a 72-nt 3′-UTR. The 3′-UTR contains cis-acting sequence elements important for initiation of RNA negative-strand synthesis. These include a hexanucleotide sequence (5′-ACUUAA-3′) that is conserved among potexviruses and a downstream U-rich motif (5′-UAUUUUCU-3′) that has been identified in PVX and reported to bind host proteins from tobacco (322,372). The PVX 5′-UTR includes an AC-rich region (nucleotides 1 to 41) and contains cis-acting elements required for efficient translation (268,387) and presumably virus assembly, this last inferred from studies of papaya mosaic virus assembly (319). By analyzing positive- and negative-strand RNA accumulation in tobacco protoplasts that had been transfected with PVX transcripts, mutational studies have shown that multiple sequence and structural elements in the 5′-UTR affect the accumulation of both genomic RNA and sgRNA, without significantly affecting levels of negative-strand RNA (173,227). In particular, thermodynamic predictions and the analysis of solution structure by chemical modification and RNase digestion suggest that nucleotides 1 to 203 contains two well-defined stem-loop structures (SL1 and SL2), both of which terminate in stable GAAA tetraloops, a motif shown in other studies to enhance RNA stability (Fig. 9). Site-directed mutations introduced into SL1 show that both its sequence and structure are required for positive-strand RNA accumulation, with the internal loop C (closest to the terminal tetraloop) and its two flanking stems being particularly critical. Both the formation of and specific nucleotides within loop C were essential for positive-strand RNA accumulation, as was base-pairing within and the length of the flanking stems. Increasing the length or stability of these two stems drastically reduced positive-strand RNA accumulation (both genomic and sgRNA), suggesting that they may function to position other elements to interact with viral and/or host proteins. The sequence of the tetraloop was also important beyond just stabilizing structure (227).

The relevance of these findings to virus genomic and sgRNA replication was shown by inoculating PVX mutants with specific alterations within SL1 in the 5′-UTR onto plants and analyzing revertants that accumulated following serial passages (226). Mutational studies using the protoplast replication assay also showed that conserved octanucleotide sequence elements located upstream of the two major PVX sgRNAs (2.1 kb and 0.9 kb) and the location of each element relative to the sgRNA start site were essential for sgRNA accumulation (174). Notably, these octanucleotide elements contain the

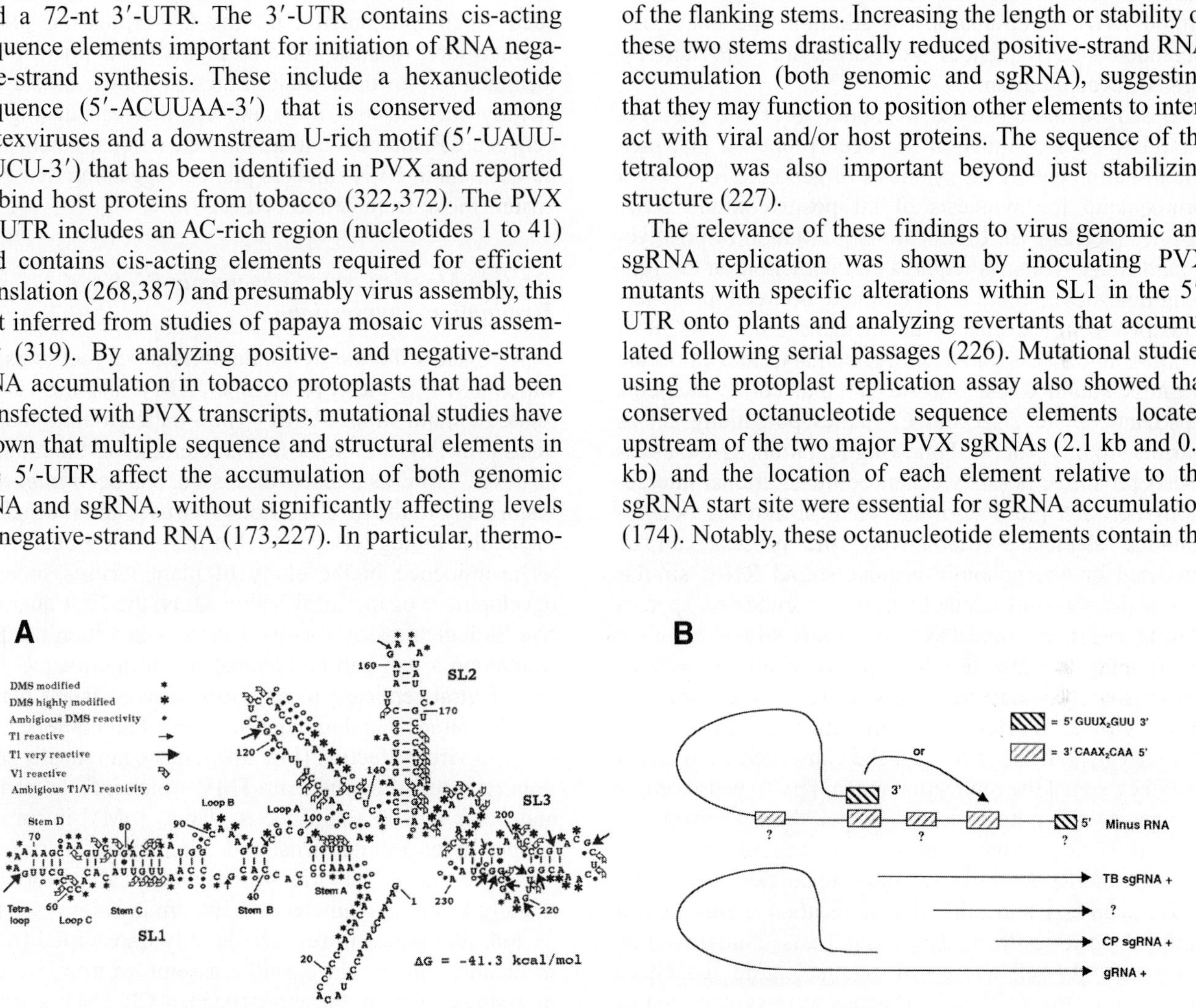

FIG. 9. A: Structure of the 5′ end of potato virus X (PVX) genomic RNA. Shown are three predicted stem-loop structures (SL1, SL2, SL3) as determined by a variety of *in vitro* chemical methods (indicated by *symbols*). Labeled in SL1 are the tetraloop and specific stems and loops discussed in the text. **B:** Model for PVX positive-strand (+) RNA synthesis from the viral negative-strand (–) RNA. Shown are the PVX -RNA and the +RNA products (full-length and subgenomic RNAs (sgRNAs). The *black hatched box* corresponds to the element located 4 nucleotides from the 3′ end of the –RNA (5′-GUUUAGUU-3′). The *gray hatched boxes* mark the locations of the octanucleotide elements (3′-CAAUUCAA-5′) upstream of the triple gene block (TGB) and coat protein (CP) open reading frames (ORFs). The putative octanucleotide element near the 12K ORF and corresponding sgRNA for the 12K and 8K proteins are also shown (indicated by ?). An additional putative octanucleotide element within the 166K ORF is also marked with a "?" below it. (A from ref. 226, with permission; B from ref. 175, with permission.)

conserved hexanucleotide element that is in the 3′-UTR of potexvirus genomic RNA, and they also exhibit complementarity to sequences in an apparently unstructured region of the 5′-UTR. The importance of this complementarity and of the sequence of the conserved octanucleotide elements was shown by inoculating protoplasts or plants with PVX transcripts that contained mutations within these elements, as well as compensatory mutations. Complementarity between the 5′ terminus (which would be the 3′ terminus of the negative-strand RNA) and the conserved octanucleotide elements is important for accumulation of both genomic RNA and sgRNA, and long distance interaction is required for all positive-strand RNA accumulation. In addition, the conserved octanucleotide sequences themselves are important for sgRNA accumulation.

Based on these studies, a model for PVX positive-strand RNA accumulation has been proposed in which the initiation events for synthesis of genomic RNA are a prerequisite for synthesis of all positive-strand RNA species (see Fig. 9). In this model, initiation of positive-strand RNA synthesis requires an interaction on the full-length negative-strand RNA template between the 3′-terminal element (defined by the element in the 5′-UTR of the genomic RNA) and a complementary element on the negative-strand RNA. The two octanucleotide elements upstream of the *TGB* and *CP* genes potentially act as partners in this process. Following initiation, sgRNA synthesis proceeds, possibly enhanced by additional interactions between the 3′-terminal element and the octanucleotide elements. Alternatively, the process can be modeled on the genomic positive-strand RNA: similar interactions would occur to generate truncated species during negative-strand RNA synthesis, with these then functioning as templates for sgRNA synthesis, as proposed for coronaviruses (see Chapter 21) and for the plant virus red clover necrotic mosaic virus (175). Another hypothesized role for the conserved elements is that they signal the replication machinery to pause or terminate RNA synthesis. In this model, the conserved element (GU-rich) at the 3′ terminus of the replicating negative-strand RNA would act to terminate negative-strand RNA synthesis and allow the replication complexes to initiate positive-strand RNA synthesis. Subsequently, once the GU-rich conserved octanucleotide sequences upstream of the *TGB* and *CP* genes were synthesized as the positive-strand RNA was made, these would cause pausing or termination and thus reinitiation to synthesize the sgRNAs.

Viral CP is required for cell-to-cell movement of PVX, and several lines of evidence suggest that PVX moves from cell to cell in the form of encapsidated virus particles. When plants are inoculated with a PVX mutant in which the *CP* gene is replaced with the gene encoding GFP (PVX-GFPΔCP) so that infected cells can be visualized by confocal microscopy, the virus is not infectious and is found to be limited to single inoculated cells (253). Mutational studies also show a correlation between the ability of altered CP to assemble virus particles and the ability of such mutants to spread on inoculated leaves (46). CP is detected in the central cavity of plasmodesmata when thin sections of leaves from PVX-infected tobacco plants are immunogold labeled to detect viral CP and examined by electron microscopy. In contrast, in transgenic tobacco plants that express the PVX CP, immunogold staining shows that CP is found throughout the cytoplasm and not localized to plasmodesmata. These transgenic plants make functional CP since the defective PVX-GFPΔCP mutant that is missing the *CP* gene is rescued when inoculated onto the CP-expressing plants. Furthermore, in these infected plants CP is again found localized to plasmodesmata. Extending these studies, an affinity-purified antivirion antisera that can distinguish between CP subunits and assembled virions, labels plasmodesmata in PVX-infected plants, suggesting that PVX virions move from cell to cell (300).

Tobacco Mosaic Virus: Subgenomic RNA and Termination Suppression

The genus *Tobamovirus* comprises 15 members, of which TMV is the type member. TMV and the closely related tomato strain of TMV (now called tomato mosaic virus [ToMV]) are the best characterized on the molecular level. TMV, as already discussed, has been important historically in the investigation of viruses and the field of molecular biology. Beyond what has already been cited, its prominence in the study of plant viruses includes development of the local lesion assay, the first quantitative biological assay for plant viruses in which necrotic lesions on a leaf can be counted much like plaques; the use of viral replicase to engineer virus-resistant plants; and the nature of a dominant host gene that confers resistance to virus infection (Fig. 10). The economically most important tobamoviruses are TMV, which infects tobacco and other mostly solanaceous plants, ToMV in tomato, pepper green mottle virus, and odontoglossum ringspot virus in orchids. The virions are rigid helical rods approximately 18 nm in diameter and 300 nm in length (see Fig. 3) and, like potexviruses, are directly transmitted by the mechanical mode. The capsid is assembled from subunits of a single protein, the viral-encoded CP. TMV is extraordinarily stable: it not only persists in dead plant matter in the soil and on contaminated seeds, but has also been reported to exist for years in cigars and cigarettes made from infected tobacco leaves (5). The tobamovirus genome is an unsegmented positive-sense ssRNA of ~6.4 to 6.6 kb with a 5′-terminal cap (m^7GpppG) followed by an AU-rich 5′-UTR of about 70 nt. The 3′-UTR consists of sequences that can fold into a number of pseudoknots followed by a transfer RNA (tRNA)-like structure at the terminus, which in TMV and most tobamoviruses, can

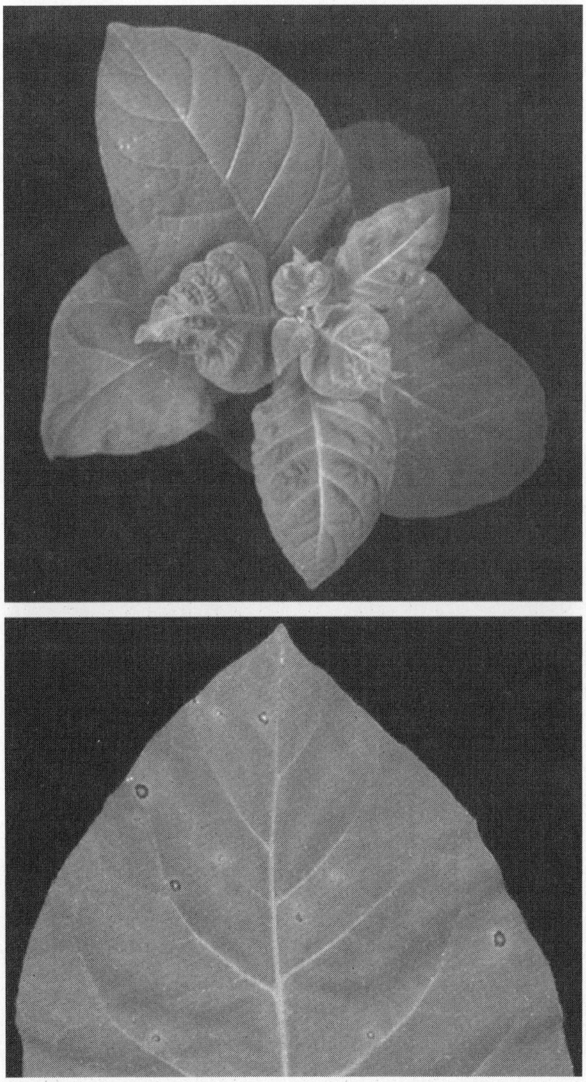

FIG. 10. Tobacco mosaic virus (TMV) infection of plants with or without the dominant *N* gene. **Top:** Systemic mosaic symptoms of TMV infection on *nn* tobacco plants. **Bottom:** Localized necrotic lesions typical of the hypersensitive response (HR) on a leaf from a TMV-infected tobacco plant carrying the *N* gene. (Photographs courtesy of Dr. Milton Zaitlin, Cornell University.)

accept histidine *in vitro*. In TMV, the 3′-UTR contains five pseudoknots, two of which are in the tRNA-like terminus (204,313). Positive-sense RNA plant viruses in a number of genera have a 3′ terminus that, like that of the TMV genome, can fold into a tRNA-like structure that encompasses pseudoknots: Watson-Crick base pairing between a loop and a single strand region in the same RNA molecule. This distinguishes them from tRNAs, which do not contain pseudoknots. The significance of pseudoknots is that they introduce structure into RNA molecules, which can potentially provide specificity in terms of interactions with proteins or catalytic reactions. The 3′ tRNA-like structures in those positive-sense RNA plant viruses in which they are found have been shown to be important for negative-strand RNA synthesis. They can be aminoacylated *in vitro* and *in vivo*, but only three specificities have been reported for different plant viral RNAs: histidine, valine, or tyrosine.

The TMV genomic RNA contains four ORFs (119), which encode (5′ to 3′): a methyltransferase/helicase and RdRp (126K and 183K, respectively), the MP (30K, referred to as the 30-kd protein), and the viral CP (17.5K) (Fig. 11). The viral genomic RNA is infectious (63,118), consistent with its initial role as an mRNA for translation of the viral RdRp (183K + 126K proteins). Following entry into the cell, the removal of a few CP subunits from the virion end that contains the 5′ terminus of the genome appears to initiate uncoating. *In vitro*, this can be accomplished by incubating virions at pH 8.0 or for brief periods in low levels of sodium dodecylsulfate (SDS) (238,375). Because some cations can slow or prevent this process, it has been suggested that removal of Ca^{2+} when virions encounter the low Ca^{2+} concentrations inside the cell may induce a conformational change and removal of these few CP subunits. After this, disassembly of about three-fourths of the genome rapidly proceeds cotranslationally as ribosomes translate the 126K and 183K proteins. This was first shown to occur *in vitro* by incubating pH 8.0 treated TMV virions in rabbit reticulocyte cell-free protein synthesizing extracts. It was subsequently shown *in vivo*, both by examining extracts from tobacco epidermal cells that had been inoculated with radioactively labeled virions, and in time course studies in which reverse transcription and PCR were used to analyze the parts of the viral genome that remained encapsidated at different times following inoculation of tobacco protoplasts (314,375,380). Following this 5′-to-3′ disassembly, the remainder of the genome is coreplicationally disassembled in the 3′-to-5′ direction as replication of complementary negative-sense RNA is initiated. This was concluded from protoplast studies again, in which it was shown that particles from which large regions of the *126K* and *183K* ORFs have been deleted cannot undergo 3′-to-5′ disassembly. However, these will fully disassemble if the protoplasts are co-inoculated with TMV genomic RNA that can provide the 126K and 183K proteins in trans. Furthermore, virions in which the genomic RNA is mutated in sequences in or near the conserved methyltransferase and helicase motifs within the 126K protein are also defective in final 3′-to-5′ disassembly (379).

As described previously, following initial 5′-to-3′ disassembly, the 126K and 183K proteins are translated from the genomic RNA. The 183K protein is produced by readthrough translation approximately 5% to 10% of the time of the UAG codon that terminates the 126K protein. This was first shown *in vitro* using rabbit reticulocyte extracts primed with TMV genomic RNA (260), and it was subsequently reported that tobacco plants contain two suppressor $tRNA^{tyr}$ having a 5′-GΨA-3′ anticodon

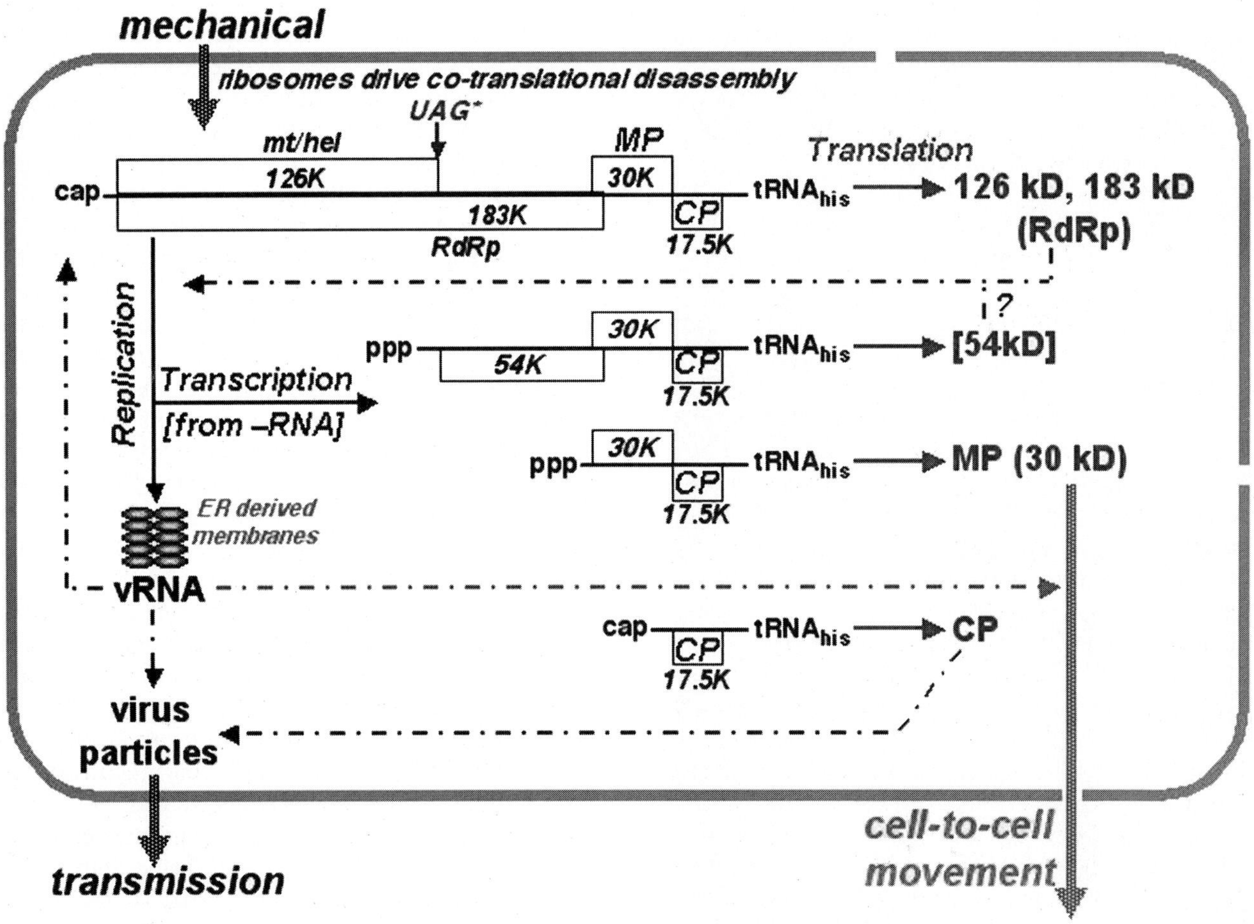

FIG. 11. Multiplication of tobacco mosaic virus (TMV).

that can accomplish this (21). Readthrough (more properly termination suppression) is context dependent: in TMV the two codons just downstream of the suppressed UAG are critical for efficient readthrough *in vitro* and *in vivo* (320,344). As a result of this readthrough translation, the two proteins are read in the same frame and the amino acid sequence of the 126K protein is contained within the N-terminus of the 183K protein. The efficiency of readthrough regulates the relative amounts of the 183K and 126K proteins made. The sequence of the TMV genomic RNA first showed that the 126K (and thus the N-terminal region of the 183K) protein contains conserved motifs typical of methyltransferases and helicases, and the 183K readthrough domain contains in addition the GDD motif typical of a viral RdRp, with the arrangement of these motifs being characteristic of that found in the alphavirus superfamily (see Chapter 13 in *Fields Virology*, 4th ed.). The 126K protein has also been shown to covalently bind [α-^{32}P]GTP (93). This, combined with the studies described previously and additional mutational studies in which deletion of the *MP* and *CP* ORFs was shown not to inhibit replication (225), led to the suggestion that the 183K protein, perhaps together with the 126K protein, is required for viral replication and that these two proteins make up the subunits of the replicase. Consistent with this, the 126K and 183K proteins are found in membrane-associated preparations of viral replicase and copurify with viral RdRp activity. Antibodies against different regions of the 126K protein also inhibit RdRp activity *in vitro* (256,257). Using a complementing system in which the 183K and 126K proteins could be expressed from separate RNAs, it has recently been shown that the 183K protein is apparently the RdRp and can act in *trans* because mutants that express only this readthrough form can replicate all forms of viral positive- and negative-sense RNA, and can synthesize the viral proteins, move from cell to cell, and replicate defective deleted forms of the genomic RNA that themselves do not encode the 126K or 183K proteins (205). The 126K protein seems to increase the efficiency of replication approximately 10-fold, apparently acting in cis. Whereas expression of the 126K protein from a defective RNA does not increase replication of the helper virus expressing the 183K protein, the 126K-expressing defective

RNA itself is efficiently replicated in the presence of this helper virus. This 126K-expressing defective RNA, however, is not efficiently replicated by wild-type TMV that expresses both the 126K and 183K proteins. This suggests that efficient TMV replication requires the 183K protein to form a heterodimer with the 126K protein that itself is already bound to the template RNA (205).

Following initial translation of the 126K and 183K proteins, these act to replicate full-length complementary negative-strand RNA. This then serves as the template for the synthesis of additional copies of the full-length genomic RNA or, if the RdRp (183K + 126K) recognizes internal subgenomic promoters, three subgenomic RNAs, each of which is functionally monocistronic (204,313) (see Fig. 11). Unlike the potexviruses, there are not any conserved sequences that aid in identifying the viral subgenomic promoters. The smallest sgRNA is the most abundant and is translated into the viral CP. The middle-sized sgRNA, which accumulates to much lower levels than the CP sgRNA, is translated into the viral MP. Mutational studies, and complementation studies using mutant viruses and transgenic plants that express the MP, show that MP is the only viral protein essential for cell-to-cell movement (71,225). The CP, although not required for cell-to-cell movement, is required for systemic infection of the plant through the phloem (64). As is the case for the potexviruses, the sgRNAs serve to regulate expression of the MP and CP both temporally and quantitatively. Whereas CP is produced late during infection and in extremely large amounts, MP is produced early, accumulates to low levels, and decreases at late times following infection (16,65). In addition to differences in the accumulated levels of the two sgRNAs, the sgRNA for the MP is not capped and has a long 5′-UTR. In contrast, the sgRNA for the CP is capped and has a short AU-rich 5′-UTR, which together appear to make it an efficient mRNA (204). The longest sgRNA found in TMV-infected cells accumulates to low levels and is predicted to encode a 54-kd protein with the same sequence as the readthrough domain of the 183K protein. Although such a protein is translated from this sgRNA *in vitro*, this 54-kd protein has never been detected in infected plants or in protoplasts (37,329). The predicted protein is also not detected in transgenic plants that are engineered to express this sgRNA, despite the fact that these plants are resistant to TMV infection (121). The studies that have been done suggest that this sgRNA for the 54-kd protein is translated: it is associated with polyribosomes in infected cells, and analysis of mutant forms in infected protoplasts indicates that its translation, not simply the presence of the sgRNA, is required to inhibit virus replication (37,329). Thus, although it stands as the first example of replicase-mediated resistance as an approach to engineer virus-resistant plants, the 54-kd protein remains enigmatic. Comparing TMV to another alphavirus, namely Sindbis (see Chapter 30 in *Fields Virology*, 4th ed.), in which the replicase subunits are generated by a combination of readthrough and proteolytic processing by the viral-encoded proteinase nsp2, and considering that the predicted 54-kd protein would be the equivalent of nsp4 in Sindbis, it is tempting to speculate that the 54-kd protein is highly labile and may play a regulatory role in suppressing the synthesis of full-length negative-strand RNA during TMV infection while allowing the synthesis of all forms of positive-sense RNA (sgRNA and genomic RNA) to continue, analogous to what occurs during Sindbis replication. Just like Sindbis, TMV negative-strand RNA replication ceases early in infection, as the replication of genomic RNA and sgRNAs continues, so that late in TMV infection there is an asymmetric production of the viral positive-strand RNAs. Studies of TMV replication using recently described *in vitro* template-dependent membrane-associated RNA polymerase preparations from infected tomato plants (256) should help to solve this mystery of the 54K protein and better define the functions of the 183K protein alone, or as a heterodimer with the 126K protein, in regulating the synthesis of the different form of viral RNA.

Like other cytoplasmic positive-sense RNA viruses, TMV replication occurs in association with cytoplasmic membranes. This was first suggested by ultrastructural studies of so-called X bodies or viroplasms as sites of virus replication and protein synthesis (99), which were described as being composed of ER, ribosomes, virus rods, and bundles of tubules. Purified preparations capable of directing TMV replication in a template-dependent manner have now been shown to be membrane-bound complexes (256). The effects of TMV infection on the organization of the ER have been examined by infecting transgenic tobacco plants that expressed an ER targeted GFP fused to the retention signal HDEL so that GFP accumulated in the ER and ER structure could be examined by confocal microscopy (284). Early in infection, the ER tubular network is converted into large cytoplasmic aggregates. Remarkably, late in infection these aggregates disappear and the normal ER network is reformed (284). That these ER-derived membranes are sites of virus replication has been shown by indirect immune fluorescence staining with antibodies against the TMV RdRp and *in situ* hybridization for viral RNA. These approaches show that the replicase and viral RNA are found associated with ER membrane and the ER-derived aggregates (219,284). Based on localization of a TMV GFP:MP fusion protein in infected plant cells and infected protoplasts, it appears that the MP plays a central role in establishing these ER-associated replication sites and in the transient reorganization of the ER membrane network (see Virus Movement) (134,284). Two different approaches have also implicated host proteins in TMV replication. The analysis of TMV recombinant viruses and mutants that could induce or overcome the so-called gene-for-gene resistance response (see Plant Responses to Virus Infection) in tobacco plants that contain the dominant *N* gene have identified the helicase domain in the 126K/183K RdRp as being responsible for induction of the hypersensitive response that characterizes this type of host defense response (98,259). This suggests that the TMV RdRp interacts with the *N* gene product or other host factor in the *N* gene–mediated signal transduction pathway. The analysis of proteins that copurify with TMV RdRp activity from infected tomato plants has implicated a protein related to yeast GCD10, the RNA-binding subunit of yeast eIF-3, in virus replication. An antibody-linked polymerase assay was used to show that active TMV RdRp complexes bind to antibodies against the yeast GCD10 protein. Furthermore, these anti-GCD10 antibodies inhibited *in vitro* synthesis of viral ssRNA and dsRNA by the purified RdRp, and this could be reversed by prior addition of GCD10 itself (257).

Cis-acting sequences in the 5′-UTR and 3′-UTR of the TMV genome have been implicated in efficient viral translation and replication. The study of virus mutants and recombinant viruses has shown that within the 205 nt 3′-UTR, the $tRNA_{his}$ structure and the 3′-most pseudoknot just upstream of this structure are both involved in negative-strand RNA replication (63,337). Sequence elements in both the 68 nt 5′-UTR and the 3′-UTR, together with the 5′ cap, are required for efficient translation of the viral genome. In this regard, the 3′-UTR appears to substitute for the lack of a poly(A) tail in synergistically interacting with the cap to facilitate translation. The 5′-UTR (also called the *leader sequence*) appears to lack any stable secondary structure and acts as an efficient translational enhancer *in vitro* and *in vivo* when fused to a reporter gene (87,114). The 5′-UTR of many TMV strains contains two conserved regions—three copies of an 8 nt direct repeat element and a (CAA)n repeat region—and mutational studies suggest that these are functionally redundant in their effects on translation. By fusing different combinations of these two elements as a leader to a GUS reporter gene and expressing these mRNA constructs in carrot protoplasts, it has been shown that the core regulatory element consists of one copy of the 8 nt direct repeat and a 25 nt (CAA)n region, with the (CAA)n region being the more critical one. Furthermore, by combining such constructs with sequences from the TMV 3′-UTR, a 72 nt region that contains the three pseudoknots located just upstream of the $tRNA_{his}$ was also shown to be required for efficient translation (115,198). This synergism in translation involves interactions with both the 5′ cap and the translational enhancer region within the 5′-UTR, with sequences within as well as the structure of the pseudoknots being important (198). These studies suggest that the 5′ and 3′ ends of the viral genome interact with each other to regulate translation, and perhaps replication. Consistent with this, a 102-kd protein that binds to both the (CAA)n region and the 72 nt 3′-UTR pseudoknot region has been identified in wheat germ extracts (339). The precise nature of these interactions, and whether the 3′-terminal $tRNA_{his}$ may also interact with sequences in or complexes formed at the 5′ end of the genome to potentially regulate replication and translation, has not been determined. Further biochemical studies are needed to address these questions.

With the report in 1955 that TMV virus particles could be assembled *in vitro* from the component viral RNA and CP (105), this assembly process has been extensively studied *in vitro*. The *in vivo* studies that have been done (378) are compatible with the model that has been developed based on *in vitro* analyses (36,199). Encapsidation initiates at a sequence-specific stem-loop structure within an origin of assembly that is located within the *MP* ORF for most tobamoviruses (Fig. 12). Fusion of this assembly origin to nonviral RNAs will direct their assembly into virus-like particles. Loop 1 of the assembly origin interacts with and is threaded through the center of a two-layered disk composed of CP, with both the 3′-to-5′ends of the viral RNA trailing from one side of the disk. The association of the RNA with a central groove between the two layers of the disk causes a conformational change in the disk to a so-called lockwasher configuration (see Fig. 12). Elongation rapidly proceeds in the 3′-to-5′ direction as additional disks are added and lengths of the genome bearing the 5′ end are looped through the central cavity of the new disk and inserted into the central groove, inducing a change to the lockwasher configuration with each new addition as the helix is assembled. Encapsidation of the exposed 3′ end of the genome appears to occur more slowly by the addition of smaller aggregates (the so-called A form) of CP subunits, although there is some disagreement as to how this occurs. A consequence of the assembly origin being located within the *MP* ORF (or the *CP* ORF for two tobamoviruses) is that the corresponding sgRNA is also encapsidated, the amount found in virus preparations being determined by the relative level of expression of the sgRNA.

Turnip Yellow Mosaic Virus (TYMV): Subgenomic RNA, Polyprotein, and Independent Initiation

There are ~20 viruses in the genus *Tymovirus,* of which *t*urnip *y*ellow *mo*saic virus (TYMV) is the type member and best characterized on the molecular level. Tymoviruses are naturally found in uncultivated dicotyledonous plants and are transmitted by beetles. Each virus has a narrow host range, and none has been reported to cause economically important diseases of crop plants (117). TYMV has been important historically as one of the earliest examples of the infectious nature of viral RNA and as a model for investigating the structure of isometric virus particles (215,313). TYMV virions are T=3 icosahedral particles that are 29 nm in diameter and composed of 180 copies of a single protein, the 20-kd CP. Each CP subunit is folded into an eight-stranded antiparallel (jellyroll) β-bar-

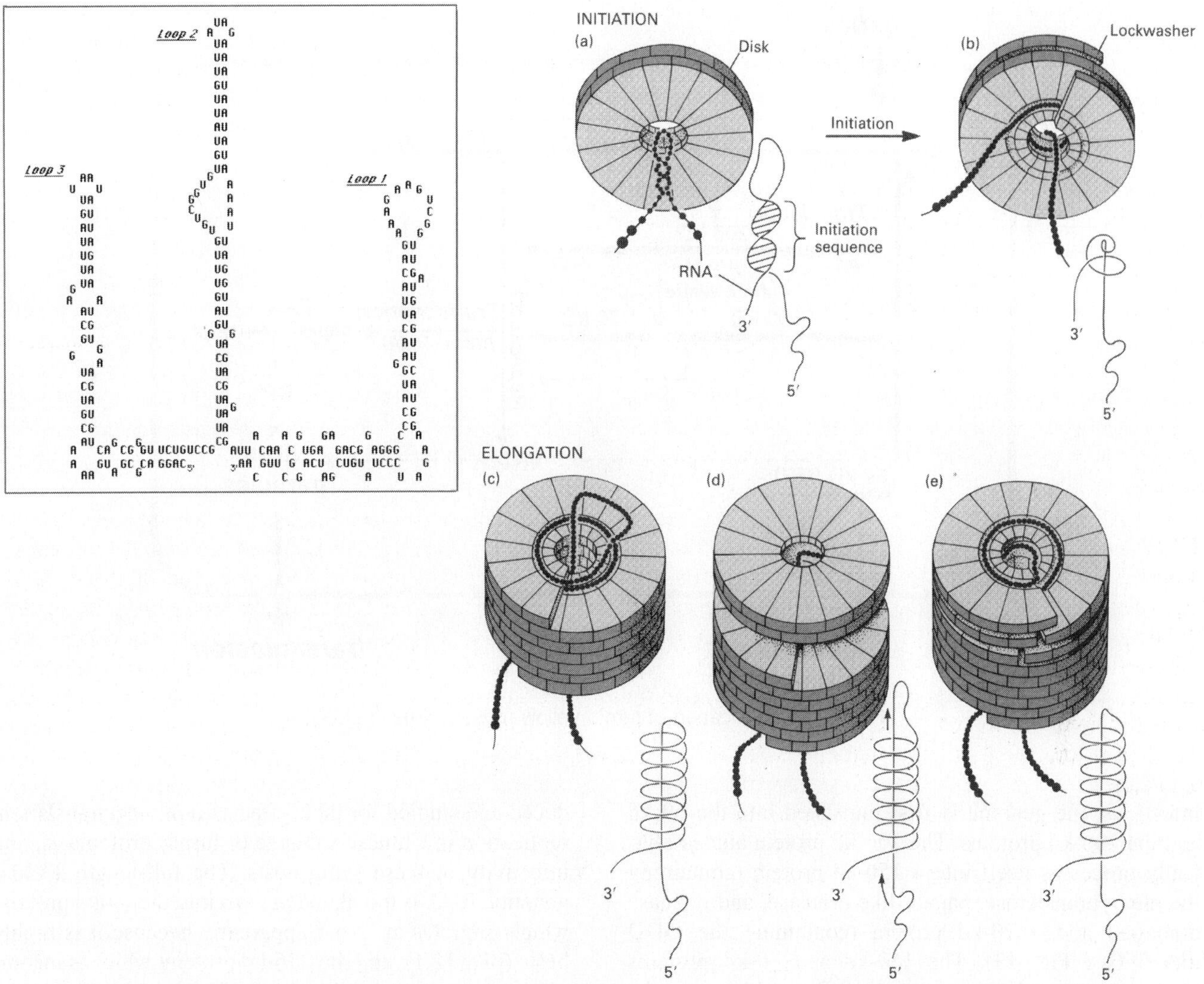

FIG. 12. Assembly of tobacco mosaic virus (TMV). **Inset:** Origin of assembly of TMV. (From Darnell JE, Lodish H, and Baltimore D. *Molecular cell biology,* 1st ed. New York: Scientific American, 1986, with permission; **inset** adapted from ref. 220, with permission.)

rel, and these are arranged in pentameric clusters at the vertices of the virus particles. The genome is an unsegmented positive-sense ssRNA of ~6.3 kb with a 5′-terminal cap (m^{7}GpppGp) and a 3′ terminus that can form a tRNA-like structure (Fig. 13). TYMV was the first virus for which it was shown that this type of tRNA-like 3′-terminal end could accept an amino acid, in this case valine (263), and it has recently served as a model for unraveling the role of such structures in directing the viral RdRp to recognize the viral 3′ end and initiate RNA negative-strand synthesis.

The TYMV genome contains three ORFs, which encode (5′ to 3′) the MP (*69K*), the RdRp (*206K*), and the viral CP (*20K*) (88) (see Fig. 13). It is a very compact coding arrangement. The 5′-UTR is 87 nt, with the *69K* ORF initiating at nucleotide 88. This ORF extensively overlaps the *206K* ORF, which initiates only 7 nt downstream in a different reading frame at nucleotide 95. There is only a short intergenic region (~15 nt, depending on the isolate) between the end of the *206K* ORF and the start of the CP (*20K*) ORF, which is followed by a 107 nt 3′-UTR. The 206-kd protein contains (starting from its N terminus) a methyltransferase motif, a helicase nucleotide binding site motif (GXGKT), a papain-like protease domain, and the GDD motif characteristic of a viral RdRp. Sequence similarities and the arrangement of the methyltransferase, helicase, and GDD motifs place TYMV in the alphavirus family. It has been suggested that upon entering a cell, deprotonation of histidine residues in the CP may aid in virion disassembly (117).

The TYMV multiplication cycle has been deduced based on *in vitro* translation of both virion RNA and infectious transcripts of cloned full-length genomic cDNA, as well as identification of viral RNA in infected plants. Consistent with the virion genomic RNA being

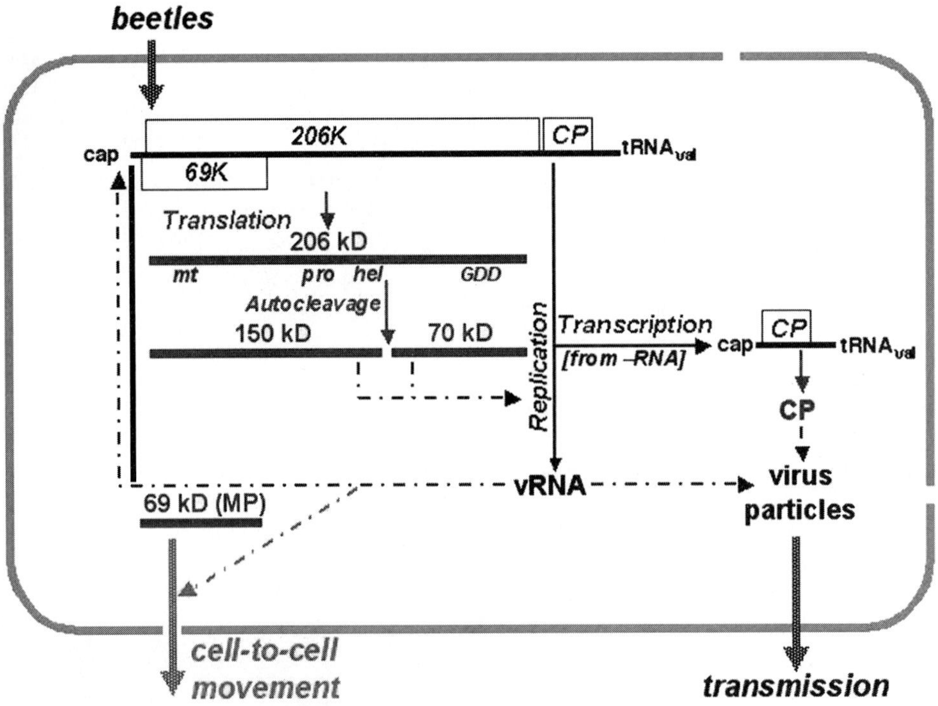

FIG. 13. Multiplication of turnip yellow mosaic virus (TYMV).

infectious, the genome is first translated into the 69-kd and the 206-kd proteins. The 206-kd protein autocatalytically processes itself into a 150-kd protein (containing the methyltransferase, papain-like protease, and helicase domains) and a 70-kd protein (containing the GDD motif) (see Fig. 13). The 150-kd and 70-kd proteins together apparently constitute the RdRp, which uses the genomic positive-strand RNA as the template to replicate full-length complementary negative-strand RNA. This then functions as the template for the replication of viral positive-strand RNAs, both full-length genomic RNA or, if the internal subgenomic promoter is recognized, an sgRNA that is translated into CP. The CP sgRNA is encapsidated into virus particles; hence, its translation into CP was demonstrated *in vitro* using virion RNA in cell-free protein synthesizing lysates from rabbit reticulocytes or wheat germ. The CP sgRNA has also been detected associated with polyribosomes in infected plants (220). Viral RNA replication takes place in the cytoplasm, associated with membranes. However, unlike TEV, PVX, or TMV replication, these membranes appear to be derived from the chloroplast outer membrane. TYMV infection causes clumping of chloroplasts and invagination of the chloroplast outer membrane. Both viral RNA and RdRp localize to these chloroplast-associated peripheral vesicles in infected cells (220).

Most of the details of TYMV multiplication have been deduced using infectious transcripts of the cloned TYMV genomic cDNA, into which mutations could be introduced and studied for their effects on *in vitro* translation, replication in Chinese cabbage or turnip protoplasts, and infectivity in these same hosts. The full-length TYMV genomic RNA is translated *in vitro* into the 69-kd protein, which migrates at 75 kd apparently because it is highly basic (pI = 12.1), and the 206-kd protein, which is incompletely processed *in vitro* to the 150-kd and 70-kd proteins. In contrast to what one would expect for leaky ribosome scanning, mutations of the initiation codon for the 69-kd protein (nucleotides 88 to 90) have no effect on expression of the 206-kd protein, but mutations of the initiation codon for the latter (nucleotides 95 to 97) significantly increase expression of the 69-kd protein (88). It has been suggested that similar to influenza virus B segment 6, in which the initiation codons for the overlapping *NB* and *NA* ORFs are only 4 nt apart (see Chapter 24), translation of the 69-kd and the 206-kd proteins is initiated by random ribosome movement in which the 40S subunit moves both 5′→3′ and 3′→5′ until the AUG initiation codon is encountered. The identification of the *69K* ORF as encoding the viral MP is based on mutations that eliminated the initiation codon at nucleotide 88 or caused premature termination of its translation: such mutants replicate normally in protoplasts but fail to form local lesions on inoculated leaves or systemically infect plants, thus suggesting that they are defective in cell-to-cell movement. Consistent with its proposed role as an MP, antisera specific for the 69-kd protein has detected the protein associated with an insoluble cell wall fraction from TYMV systemically infected leaves, and it appears to be maximally expressed in young, expanding systemically infected leaves (29). The CP is not needed for local cell-to-cell movement. A TYMV mutant in which two-thirds of the *CP* ORF is deleted can replicate normally in protoplasts and produce chlorotic local lesions on inoculated leaves (88). However, this mutant does not systemically infect the host, showing that in addition to beetle transmisson, the CP is needed for systemic infection via the phloem.

Using antisera specific for the N- and C-terminal regions of the 206-kd protein, it was shown *in vitro* that the 206-kd protein is processed into a 150-kd protein (recognized by the N-terminal–specific antisera) and an apparently unstable 70-kd protein (recognized by the C-terminal–specific antisera) (88). This resembles the processing of Sindbis virus RdRp by autocatalytic proteolysis to nsp123 and nsp4, with the TYMV 70-kd protein corresponding to Sindbis nsp4 (see Chapter 30 in *Fields Virology*, 4th ed.). Whether there is additional processing *in vivo* of the 150-kd protein, analogous to the processing of nsp123 during Sindbis infection, is not clear as there is disagreement about a viral 115-kd protein being a subunit of the RdRp. Further studies are needed to determine whether the 150-kd protein is further processed and what role, if any, processing of the 206-kd protein and its products plays in regulating the levels of newly synthesized viral positive- and negative-sense RNA. Mutational studies have mapped the protease domain (amino acids 670 to 885) and the cleavage site within the 206-kd protein. Consistent with its proposed function as a papain-like proteinase, mutation of Cys^{783} and His^{869} within the protease domain of the 206-kd protein prevent its autocatalytic cleavage to the 150-kd and 70-kd proteins (88). Furthermore, TYMV missense mutants in which the initiation codon for the *206K* ORF is eliminated, or the helicase or GDD motifs are mutated, are noninfectious and do not replicate in protoplasts. This is consistent with both proteins being required for replication, with the 150-kd protein having helicase activity and the 70-kd protein being an RdRp. Complementation studies using the TYMV helicase and GDD mutants together, or each mutant complemented with a helper TYMV in which the CP was deleted, further suggest that the 150-kd and 70-kd proteins may function as a heterodimeric complex and act in a *cis*-preferential manner (371). The complementing helicase and GDD mutants can support the replication of each other in *trans*, but they do so poorly. When each mutant is complemented with the helper virus, they replicate to 20% or less of the level of the helper RNA. However, if a TYMV deletion mutant that cannot make the 70-kd protein is substituted for the GDD missense mutant that produces a defective 70-kd protein, the deletion mutant does accumulate to high levels, comparable to the helper virus. This deletion mutant could also complement the defective helicase missense (150-kd) mutant; however, again the 70-kd protein deletion mutant replicated to approximately 10-fold higher levels than did the helicase mutant. This suggests that the 70-kd protein can act in *trans* but that the 150-kd protein acts in a *cis*-preferential manner, leading to a model similar to that proposed for the TMV 183-kd and 126-kd proteins: the 150-kd protein binds to the negative strand promoter in *cis*, and the 70-kd protein, also showing some *cis* preference, forms a stable heterodimeric complex with the 150-kd protein, thus favoring replication of the RNA encoding the active complex.

It appears that TYMV virion RNA is rapidly packaged following replication so that it is not accessible to the host cell CCA-tRNA nucleotidyltransferase. Thus, the tRNA-like structure at the 3′ end of the virion RNA terminates in 5′-CC-3′ but is efficiently adenylated to 5′-CCA-3′ *in vitro* by CCA-tRNA nucleotidyltransferase. In this form, it is an active *in vitro* substrate for aminoacylation with valine by valyl-tRNA synthetase from yeast or wheat germ (88). Valylated TYMV RNA has also been detected in infected plant cells. Although this tRNA-like structure has only limited sequence similarity to higher plant $tRNA^{val}$, it does have a valine -CAC- anticodon and an -ACAC- present in the anticodon loop of all eukaryotic $tRNA^{val}$, and it structurally resembles tRNAs on the secondary and tertiary levels. As discussed for TMV, the TYMV tRNA-like structure is distinct from cellular tRNAs in having a pseudoknot, which is involved in building the amino acid acceptor stem. The role of the TYMV $tRNA_{val}$-like structure in virus replication has been extensively investigated, using either the viral genomic RNA or an *in vitro* transcript comprising a 3′-terminal fragment of the genomic RNA. *In vitro*, the valylated TYMV tRNA-like structure tightly binds elongation factor eEF1α from wheat germ or EF-Tu from *E. coli.* Initial mutational studies showed a direct correlation between valylation and TYMV RNA replication in protoplasts or viral infectivity in plants. In addition, mutation of the TYMV aminoacylation specificity from valine to methionine, a novel specificity for viral tRNA-like structures, produced infectious virus, and there was now a direct correlation between the ability of mutated forms of this altered TYMV genome to accept methionine and replicate (88,90). Thus, the valine specificity does not appear to be crucial here, and the results suggested that aminoacylation might be required for efficient replication of TYMV RNA.

However, tymovirus genomic RNAs exhibit a wide range of tRNA mimicry, from highly developed, as in the case of TYMV, to minimal, and it was possible to construct infectious variants of TYMV that were not aminoacylated (89,122). The starting point for these variants was a chimeric TYMV genomic RNA in which the 3′-$tRNA_{val}$–like structure had been replaced with 3′-sequences from TMV. Although it could accept histidine *in vitro*, this chimeric TYMV-TMV genome was not infectious, but it did replicate to ~3% the level of wild-type TYMV in protoplasts. Adding back TYMV sequences from the anticodon loop and amino acid acceptor stem to the 3′ region of this chimeric genome increased its replication a few fold. Two of these chimeric genomes could be serially passaged in plants, eventually giving rise to two highly infectious TYMV-TMV variant viruses which had accumulated some minor additional changes in their 3′-end sequences. Unexpectedly, these two infectious TYMV-TMV variants, both of which now contained the valine-specific anticodon loop, could be adenylated to produce -CCA-3′ ends *in vitro*, but they could not be aminoacylated. Thus, aminoacylation is not obligatory for virus replication. This suggests that a number of structural features of the viral 3′ end can contribute to genome amplification and infectivity, and that these have the ability to compensate for lack of aminoacylation (122). Of course, some of the TYMV 3′-terminal sequences added back to these chimeras could have included critical promoter elements needed for negative strand synthesis that would be recognized by replicator complexes and overlap the determinants for valylation. However, the ability of the TYMV RdRp to efficiently transcribe a range of unmodified tRNAs and tRNA-like structures, some quite short, in addition to the heterogeneity in the 3′-terminal sequences of the TYMV-TMV chimeras themselves, brought into question the very existence of such specific promoter elements, either in terms of sequence or structure, to direct negative strand synthesis. Using a TYMV RdRp preparation from infected plants to transcribe different RNA templates *in vitro*, it was determined that a 27 nt fragment encompassing the 3′ terminus and pseudoknotted acceptor stem, or a 21 nt fragment encompassing this 3′ end and adjacent hairpin, were efficiently transcribed, each correctly initiating at the penultimate C in the unpaired terminal 5′-CCA-3′ sequence (68,318). By testing additional truncated, mutated, and duplicated templates, as well as unstructured C-rich templates or a 12 nt (CCA)n template, the minimal template requirement for initiation of negative-sense RNA synthesis by the TYMV RdRp has been defined. The surprising answer is that the TYMV RdRp can recognize any sterically accessible 5′-CC(A/G)-3′ triplet; indeed, it will accurately initiate at multiple internal sites on unstructured C-rich or (CCA)n templates. However, the introduction of nonspecific secondary structure into such templates can confer specificity in terms of the 5′-CC(A/G)-3′ triplets at which the RdRp will initiate transcription (68,318). Thus, there are no specific promoter elements within the acceptor stem and upstream regions of the TYMV tRNA-like structure: the specific target for initiation by the TYMV RdRp appears to be 5′-CC(A/G)-3′. The function of the tRNA-like structure would appear to be to prevent internal initiation of negative-strand RNA synthesis and place the 3′-terminal correct initiation site (-ACCA-) in a very accessible location. In addition, tRNA mimicry becomes important here for viral negative-strand RNA synthesis. The TYMV genome terminates in 5′-CC-3′. However, the 3′-terminal A is essential for initiation of negative-strand RNA synthesis, and this is added by the host CCA-tRNA nucleotidyltransferase, which recognizes the viral 3′ tRNA-like structure and adenylates it. Thus, tRNA mimicry creates the proper 5′-CCA-3′ terminus for the viral RdRp to initiate negative strand synthesis. Recent studies show that the RdRp of turnip crinkle virus (a carmovirus in the family *Tombusviridae*) and phage Qβ replicase can also, to varying degrees, initiate transcription *in vitro* at CCA sequences without unique promoter elements. Thus, initiation at CCA sites with specificity being conferred by preference for 3′initiation sites and RNA structure may be common among the RdRps encoded by positive-sense RNA viruses (384).

Luteoviruses: Subgenomic RNA, Frameshift, Leaky Ribosome Scanning, Termination Suppression, and Polyprotein

The viruses that were formerly grouped as luteoviruses ("luteo" is Latin for "yellow", referring to a characteristic symptom produced by these viruses) have recently been reclassified within two genera in the new family of *Luteoviridae: Luteovirus* (formerly subgroup I) and *Polerovirus* (formerly subgroup II) (347). *Enamovirus* is a third genus in this family and consists solely of pea enation mosaic virus type 1 (PEMV1). PEMV1 exists in an interdependent relationship with a second virus, PEMV2. The genome organization of PEMV1 resembles that of the poleroviruses; however, PEMV2 is classified as an umbravirus. Only the luteoviruses and poleroviruses will be discussed here. Viruses within these two genera are grouped as *Luteoviridae* because of their biological properties, and they are clearly similar in the genes encoded in the 3′ halves of the viral genomes. However, the genetic organization of the 5′ halves of the luteovirus and polerovirus genomes is quite distinct. The luteovirus-encoded RdRp is similar to the RdRp encoded by tombusviruses and umbraviruses, among others; but the polerovirus-encoded RdRp resembles that of the sobemoviruses. The divergent nature of the 5′ halves of the luteovirus and polerovirus genomes has led to the suggestion that these two genera were generated by horizontal gene transfer (229).

Of the ~20 viruses in these two genera, barley yellow dwarf virus (BYDV) (luteovirus, although some isolates may be poleroviruses), and the poleroviruses potato leaf roll virus (PLRV), beet western yellows virus (BWYV), and cereal yellow dwarf virus (CYDV) occur worldwide and cause significant losses in crops of economic importance. Although PLRV infects only potatoes, it can cause devastating disease and high losses. BYDV and CYDV affect a wide range of grains, including barley, oats, wheat, and rye, causing significant losses in these crops annually. The viruses are transmitted in nature by aphids. With the exception of BWYV, most luteoviruses and poleroviruses have very narrow host ranges. This, combined with their phloem restriction, have made them difficult to study. Although complete cDNA clones have been generated for a few of the viral genomes (202,275,385), the phloem limitation of virus infection means that, in contrast to viruses that infect mesophyll cells, neither the cDNAs nor the virions can be mechanically transmitted to plants for experimental studies. Agroinfection has been successfully used to infect plants with the cDNA clone for BWYV (202), but this approach does not efficiently work for many monocotyledonous plants, such as those infected by BYDV. PLRV gene functions have been, in part, studied by expressing the viral genome or individual ORFs in transgenic plants (275). The virions are T=3 icosahedral particles that are 24 to 30 nm in diameter and composed of 180 copies of the 22-kd CP, some fraction of which has a C-terminal extension of ~50 kd (CP-AT) (229). BYDV-PAV (luteoviruses), and PLRV and BWYV (poleroviruses), are the best characterized *Luteoviridae* at the molecular level. Each virus has a genome of unsegmented positive-sense ssRNA of ~6 kb. The PLRV genomic RNA has a genome-linked viral-encoded protein (VPg) of 7 kd covalently attached to its 5′ terminus. In contrast, the BYDV-PAV genome does not have this or any other known modification at its 5′ terminus (12). The luteovirus and polerovirus genomes do not contain either a poly(A) tail or a tRNA-like structure at their 3′ end. A combination of approaches has been used to investigate the multiplication of these viruses. These include transfection of protoplasts with virion genomic RNA and transcripts of cloned cDNA, expression of cloned ORFs in *E. coli* (which also provides viral proteins for generating specific antisera), hybridization studies with sequence-specific probes and immunoblot studies with specific antisera to detect viral RNAs and proteins in infected plants and protoplasts, and *in vitro* translation of genomic and sgRNAs. Given that infected protoplasts can produce virions, aphids can be fed on protoplast extracts through a membrane to acquire virions with mutated genomes and transmit these to plants. This has allowed for mutational and complementation studies to study the functions of some of the viral proteins in aphid transmission and in systemic infection of plant hosts.

BYDV-PAV genomic RNA encodes six ORFs, numbered 1 through 6 (5′ to 3′) (Fig. 14). ORF 2 (*60K*) is pre-

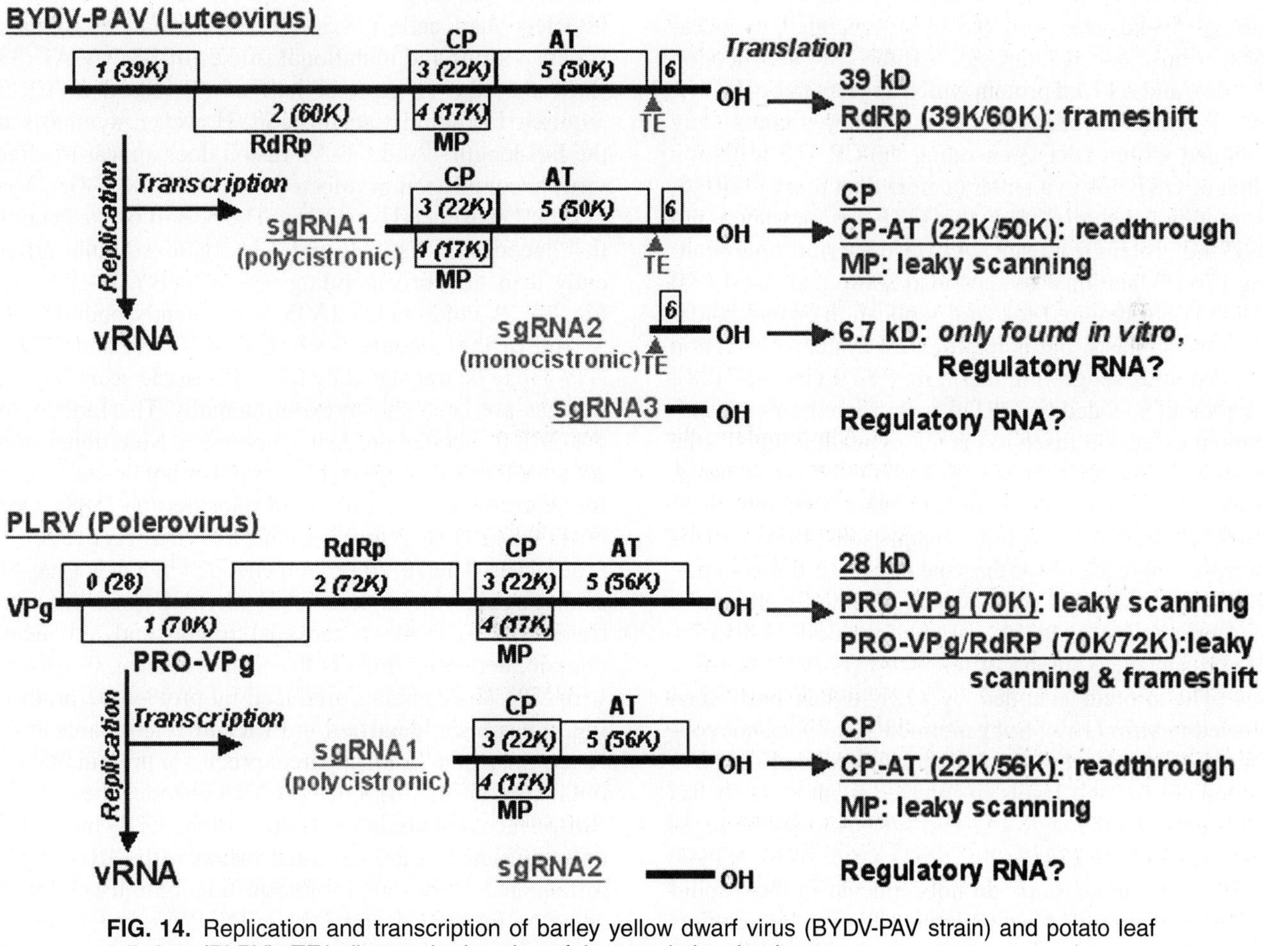

FIG. 14. Replication and transcription of barley yellow dwarf virus (BYDV-PAV strain) and potato leaf roll virus (PLRV). *TE* indicates the location of the translational enhancer.

dicted to encode a protein containing the GDD motif characteristic of a viral RdRp. It is translated from the genomic RNA both *in vivo* and *in vitro* only as a C-terminal fusion to the protein (39 kd) encoded by ORF 1 by a −1 ribosomal frameshift (72,233). These are the only proteins translated directly from the genome. Consistent with the presence of the GDD motif within the C-terminus of this fused protein, deletion studies show that both ORFs 1 and 2 are essential for viral replication in plant protoplasts (233). Because the ribosomal frameshift appears to occur ≤8% of the time in BYDV-PAV, the majority of the time, ORF 1 is translated into a 39-kd protein, the function of which alone is unknown. Although the 39-kd protein has been proposed to be a helicase, it does not appear to have homology to any known helicases (233). By analogy to other positive-sense viruses, it is assumed that following translation of the genomic RNA, the RdRp (99 kd), perhaps together with the 39-kd protein, uses the genomic positive-strand RNA as a template to synthesize full-length complementary negative-strand RNA, which then serves as template for the replication of additional genomic positive-sense RNA and three 3′ coterminal sgRNAs (see Fig. 14), all of which have been detected in infected plants (169). The largest of these (sgRNA1) functions as a tricistronic mRNA. It is translated into the CP (22 kd), a small amount of CP with a C-terminal 50-kd extension (CP-AT) generated by occasional ribosomal readthrough of the CP stop codon (50,102), and a 17-kd protein which appears to be the MP. ORF 4, which encodes the 17-kd protein, is completely contained within ORF 3 encoding the CP. The initiation codon of ORF 4 is in a better context than that of ORF 3, and mutational studies show that ORF 4 is translated into the 17-kd protein from sgRNA1 by leaky ribosome scanning (76). Mutational studies also show that the 17-kd protein is not required for viral replication or encapsidation in protoplasts, but is required for systemic infection of plants, thus suggesting that it may be a viral MP (48). The protein encoded by ORF 5 is translated only as a C-terminal extension fused to the CP by readthrough of the CP stop codon; thus, it is called *RTD,* for *readthrough domain.* Mutational and complementation studies show that it is required for aphid transmission (48), and it is referred to here as *AT* for the sake of clarity. Subgenomic RNA2 contains only ORF 6, which potentially encodes a small protein that is highly variable in length (4.3 to 7.1 kd) and sequence among different BYDV-PAV–like isolates. The protein encoded by ORF 6 has only been detected *in vitro* (169). Subgenomic RNA3 does not contain any ORFs. Nevertheless, both sgRNA2 and sgRNA3 accumulate to high levels in infected plant cells. It has been suggested that sgRNA2 and sgRNA3 may be regulatory RNAs (229,230).

Although *Luteoviridae* do not replicate in their aphid vectors, they do follow a circulative pathway that requires virions to be transported across three barriers following acquisition: the hindgut epithelium, across which virions enter the hemocoel, and the basal lamina and plasma membrane of the accessory salivary glands, to which they are actively transported from the hemolymph. Virions are then introduced into the phloem of a plant through the salivary duct as the aphids feed. Electron microscopic studies suggest that virion transport across the hindgut epithelium and accessory salivary gland plasma membrane may occur by receptor-mediated endocytosis (229). Mutational studies with BYDV-PAV suggest that the AT extension in the CP-AT subunits is required for transport of virions from the hemolymph into the salivary glands (48). This transport is an interesting example of the virus taking advantage of a symbiotic relationship. The aphid hemocoel contains a high level of proteins called *symbionins* that are produced by intracellular endosymbiotic bacteria (*Buchnera* species) and are homologs of the *E. coli* chaperonin groEL. Symbionins have been shown to bind the AT readthrough domain in BYDV-PAV, PLRV, and BWYV *in vitro*, and aphid transmission studies with viral mutants suggest that binding of symbionins to the virus particle may protect it from degradation in the aphid (101,143,345). The few CP-AT subunits incorporated into virions are found as a ~58-kd cleavage product that contains CP fused to the N-terminal half of AT, although full-length 72-kd CP-AT can be found in infected plant cells (48,50,233,365). Analysis of these BYDV virions and mutational studies of BWYV AT (33) show that the N-terminal half of AT, fused to CP, is required for aphid transmission. However, synthesis of the full-length 72-kd CP-AT fusion does appear to affect virus accumulation in infected plants (33,48,388).

PLRV also encodes 6 ORFs. The 5′ half of the genome that encodes ORFs 0, 1, and 2 is organized quite differently than the corresponding region of BYDV-PAV (see Fig. 14). A viral-encoded VPg is covalently bound to the 5′ end of the genome RNA. ORF 0 (*28K*) and ORF 1 (*70K*) may be translated by leaky ribosome scanning, but this has not been shown experimentally. The function of the ORF 0 encoded product is unknown. Mutational studies with BWYV suggest that ORF 0 is not needed, either for systemic infection or aphid transmission (388). Only ORF 1 and ORF 2 are essential for virus replication in protoplasts. The 70-kd protein encoded by ORF 1 has the catalytic triad characteristic of chymotrypsin-like proteases (PRO) in its N-terminal region and a helicase domain, between which is the VPg sequence. Consistent with VPg (7 kd) being produced by proteolytic processing, it has been identified in PLRV-infected plants at the N-terminus of a 25-kd apparent precursor protein that can bind RNA (274,276). ORF 3 (*72K*) encodes the putative RdRp since it is predicted to contain the GDD motif. It is only translated as a C-terminal fusion with PRO-VPg by infrequent −1 ribosomal frameshifting, reminiscent of the situation for ORF 1 and 2 in BYDV-PAV (187). Thus, in contrast to viruses like TEV and poliovirus, it would appear that PLRV VPg is produced in great excess over the RdRp.

In contrast to this divergence in the 5′ end of the genome, ORF 3 (*22K*), ORF 4 (*17K*), and ORF 5 (*56K*) correspond to the same ORFs in BYDV-PAV and are also expressed from a subgenomic RNA (sgRNA1) to encode CP, a proposed MP, and AT, respectively (see Fig. 14), with AT only translated as the fused CP-AT as the result of occasional readthrough of the CP stop codon (143,223, 228,334,336). There is also a second subgenomic RNA (sgRNA2), which in this case is not predicted to encode any ORFs. The PLRV 17K protein (ORF 4) is proposed to be an MP based on its having properties similar to those of other well-characterized MPs such as the TMV 30-kd protein. In particular, the PLRV 17-kd protein can nonspecifically bind single-stranded nucleic acid *in vitro*, is phosphorylated, and has been reported to localize to plasmodesmata in infected plants or when expressed in transgenic plants (309,335,336). This corresponds to the suggestion that BYDV-PAV ORF 4 encodes an MP. However, mutational studies of BWYV using agroinfection to introduce the mutated cDNAs into tobacco led to a very different conclusion: that ORF 4 was dispensable for virus systemic infection and aphid transmission, but that the C-terminal half of AT was required for systemic infection and a potential MP (33,388). Thus, the picture is confusing in terms of movement. Given the technical limitations involved in investigating luteovirus infection in plants, studies of BYDV-PAV, PLRV, and BWYV have not directly studied virus movement, nor do they distinguish between local cell-to-cell movement and systemic infection. In addition, the potential functions of the CP in local or long-distance systemic movement have not been addressed, although for BWYV it was concluded that the CP is needed for systemic infection (388). A better understanding of the phloem cell types between which these viruses move and the functions of CP in local and long-distance movement, coupled with direct investigation of luteovirus and polerovirus movement, should clarify this situation.

Luteoviruses and poleroviruses are notable for the sheer number of strategies they employ to regulate and maximize their gene expression: (a) sgRNAs, some of which appear to be regulatory molecules rather than mRNAs; (b) leaky scanning to produce CP and MP (ORF 4), and likely translate ORFs 0 and 1; (c) polyprotein synthesis and autocatalytic processing (poleroviruses) of PRO-VPg, and likely PRO-VPg-RdRp, to produce VPg, probably in different functional forms analogous to TEV and poliovirus; (d) −1 ribosomal frameshifting to produce RdRp; and (e) readthrough to produce CP-AT, the capsid subunit essential for aphid transmission. Beyond the number of strategies, there are some novel luteovirus twists here that have been reported in studies of BYDV-PAV. Frameshifting to produce RdRp occurs at a shifty heptanucleotide sequence (5′-GGGUUUU-3′ in BYDV-PAV, 5′-GGGAAAC-3′ in PLRV) and involves a downstream pseudoknot or hairpin structure (230), as reported for other viruses. However, a higher rate of frameshift was found when the intact BYDV genome was translated *in vitro* in wheat germ extracts than when a reporter gene, in which the BYDV frameshift site was inserted so that the coding sequence was mostly in the −1 frame, was used (72). Mutational studies identified sequences 4 kb downstream in the 3′-UTR of the BYDV-PAV genome that appear to be required for efficient frameshifting (367). Readthrough to produce CP-AT in BYDV-PAV requires at least five copies of a series of tandem repeats of the sequence 5′-CCN NNN-3′, beginning 12 to 21 nt downstream of the CP stop codon, with no apparent secondary structure in this region. Deletion studies further identify an additional element ~700 nt downstream within ORF 5 that is also needed for readthrough (32). Even given all of this, perhaps one of the most puzzling aspects of BYDV translation is its cap-independent nature, and the solution here may be the most novel of all.

A 109 nt sequence element located in the 3′-UTR of BYDV-PAV between ORFs 5 and 6 has been identified as a translational enhancer, and thus named 3′TE (see Fig. 14). It appears to mimic a 5′ cap in interacting with eIF4F, either directly or indirectly, to facilitate efficient translation of uncapped mRNAs (366). This conclusion is based on *in vitro* and *in vivo* studies using a GUS reporter gene that contained different 5′-UTR sequences (BYDV, TMV, or plasmid) that were or were not capped, in combination with different 3′-UTR sequences [BYDV or plasmid with poly(A) tail]. Without a 5′ cap, the GUS reporter gene is very inefficiently translated *in vitro*, whether or not a poly(A) tail is present. However, if the GUS reporter is flanked by the 5′-UTR from BYDV upstream and the 3′TE inserted in its 3′-UTR, it is efficiently translated *in vitro* without a cap, with the level of translation being comparable to that of GUS with a 5′-cap but lacking the 3′TE. The relative enhancing effect of the 3′TE is the same *in vitro* and *in vivo* in oat protoplasts, although additional BYDV 3′-UTR sequences are needed *in vivo* to substitute for a poly(A) tail, whether the 3′TE or a 5′ cap is present. The 3′TE within the 3′-UTR enhances translation of uncapped mRNA when the BYDV 5′-UTR is present upstream of the GUS reporter, but has the same effect without the BYDV 5′-UTR sequences if the 3′TE itself is placed in the 5′-UTR region upstream of the GUS coding sequence. Thus, the 3′TE can functionally substitute for a 5′ cap in this position and, in either position, it was found to decrease the amount of eIF4F needed for maximum translation *in vitro*. Furthermore, in competition studies, excess 3′-TE RNA inhibits *in vitro* translation of capped GUS mRNA in *trans*, and this effect is reversed by addition of excess eIF4F. Thus, the 3′TE appears to act to recruit translation factors and ribosomes by interacting with eIF4F, either directly or indirectly. The BYDV 5′-UTR is proposed to function for long distance

3′–5′ interactions, probably by also interacting with eIF4F or other host factors rather than through direct base pairing, to position the recruited translation machinery at the 5′ end of the viral genome (366). The significance of this translational enhancer being located between ORFs 5 and 6 (see Fig. 14) is that it would act to enhance translation of the genome and sgRNA1 to produce BYDV proteins. At the same time, its presence at the 5′-end of sgRNA2, which accumulates to high levels later in infection, could inhibit translation of genomic RNA by effectively competing for eIF4F and translation factors to favor replication and encapsidation. Of course, it could eventually act to inhibit translation of sgRNA1 as well.

Brome Mosaic Virus: Multipartite, Subgenomic RNA

The *Bromoviridae* comprise five genera: *Bromovirus, Cucumovirus, Alfamovirus, Ilarvirus,* and *Oleavirus* (347). All of these viruses have positive-sense tripartite genomes that consist of three separate segments of positive-sense ssRNA. The three genomic segments are separately encapsidated in distinct particles. This separation of gene function on physically distinct RNAs was historically a major advantage before the development of recombinant DNA approaches. Genetic reassortment of the genomic segments between different strains or mutants of the same virus, or different related viruses within these genera, made mapping gene functions relatively straightforward. In addition, studies of viral replication were facilitated by the components of the RdRp being encoded on two different segments distinct from the third genomic RNA that encodes the MP and CP. Thus, the RdRp activities could be mutated separately from promoters for positive-strand RNA and negative-strand RNA synthesis on the third genomic RNA, in effect using this third RNA as a reporter to identify essential replication functions in the RdRp and to investigate the mechanisms of genomic RNA, complementary RNA, and sgRNA synthesis. BMV, the type member of the bromoviruses, together with cowpea chlorotic mottle virus (CCMV) (bromovirus), cucumber mosaic virus (CMV) (cucumovirus), and alfalfa mosaic virus (alfamovirus) are among the best characterized viruses in the *Bromoviridae*. BMV illustrates many of the principles governing gene expression of multipartite plant viral genomes, and is the focus here. Although BMV combines expression of a sgRNA with the multipartite strategy, different multipartite positive-sense ssRNA plant viruses combine a number of the strategies that have been discussed, with their segmented genome approach, such as polyprotein synthesis and processing by a viral-encoded proteinase (comoviruses); readthrough and sgRNA (tobraviruses); or sgRNA, readthrough, and leaky scanning (hordeiviruses) (123). Multipartite viruses that use the polyprotein approach can have a viral VPg linked to the 5′ ends of the genomic RNAs and 3′ poly(A) tails, as do the comoviruses. The others, in general, have 5′ caps combined with a poly(A) tail, a tRNA-like structure, or no known modification at the 3′ ends of their genome segments.

BMV, although not of major economic importance, is historically important as the first RNA virus for which infectious genomic transcripts were generated *in vitro* from cDNA clones (8) and a model for investigating how positive-sense RNA plant viruses replicate their genomes and transcribe sgRNA (6,231). More recently, the demonstration that BMV can replicate in yeast has led to a novel approach to study virus replication *in vivo* and use yeast genetics to identify host factors involved in BMV replication (159). There appear to be no efficient invertebrate vectors for bromoviruses, although beetles and nematodes have been experimentally shown to transmit them. The viruses can be mechanically transmitted, in both the laboratory and field. The virions have T=3 quasi-icosahedral symmetry and are about ~28 nm in diameter. These are composed of 180 copies of the viral 20-kd CP, with each subunit having a β-barrel structure that is uncharacteristically perpendicular to the capsid surface so that the pentameric and hexameric subunit clusters have a bulging knoblike appearance (7,186). The N-termini of the CP subunits are internal and appear to interact with the encapsidated viral genomic RNA. The BMV genome consists of three distinct segments of positive-sense ssRNA that are 3.2 kb (RNA1), 2.9 kb (RNA2), and 2.1 kb (RNA3) in size, each with a 5′ cap (m^7GpppGp) and a 3′ tRNA-like structure that contains a pseudoknot and can accept tyrosine *in vitro* (Fig. 15). Density gradient centrifugation shows that these, together with the subgenomic RNA encoding the viral CP (RNA 4), are separately encapsidated into three different particles: (a) 3.2-kb genomic RNA (gRNA) in the highest density particles; (b) 2.9-kb gRNA in the intermediate density particles; and (c) 2.1-kb gRNA and 0.9-kb sgRNA in the lowest density particles (7). The CP sgRNA, like the genomic RNAs, has a 5′ cap and a 3′ $tRNA_{tyr}$-like structure (see Fig. 15).

How the virions are uncoated is not well understood. What is clear is that the three genomic RNAs and subgenomic RNA4 (hereafter [sg]RNA4) are each monocistronic and translated into the protein encoded by the single or the 5′-proximal gene. RNA1 and RNA2 are the only genome segments required for virus replication, as shown by direct transfection of plant protoplasts. These are translated, respectively, into proteins 1a (109 kd) and 2a (94 kd) (see Fig. 15), which coordinately act to replicate all three genomic RNAs by way of negative strand intermediates, as well as recognize an internal promoter on RNA3 to transcribe it into the 0.9-kb [sg]RNA4 that encodes the CP. RNA3 itself is translated into the viral MP (32 kd). Consistent with BMV having a positive-sense ssRNA genome and the previously described picture, the three genomic RNAs together are infectious, and each of these, as well as [sg]RNA4, is translated into the corresponding protein *in vitro* (6). This view of BMV

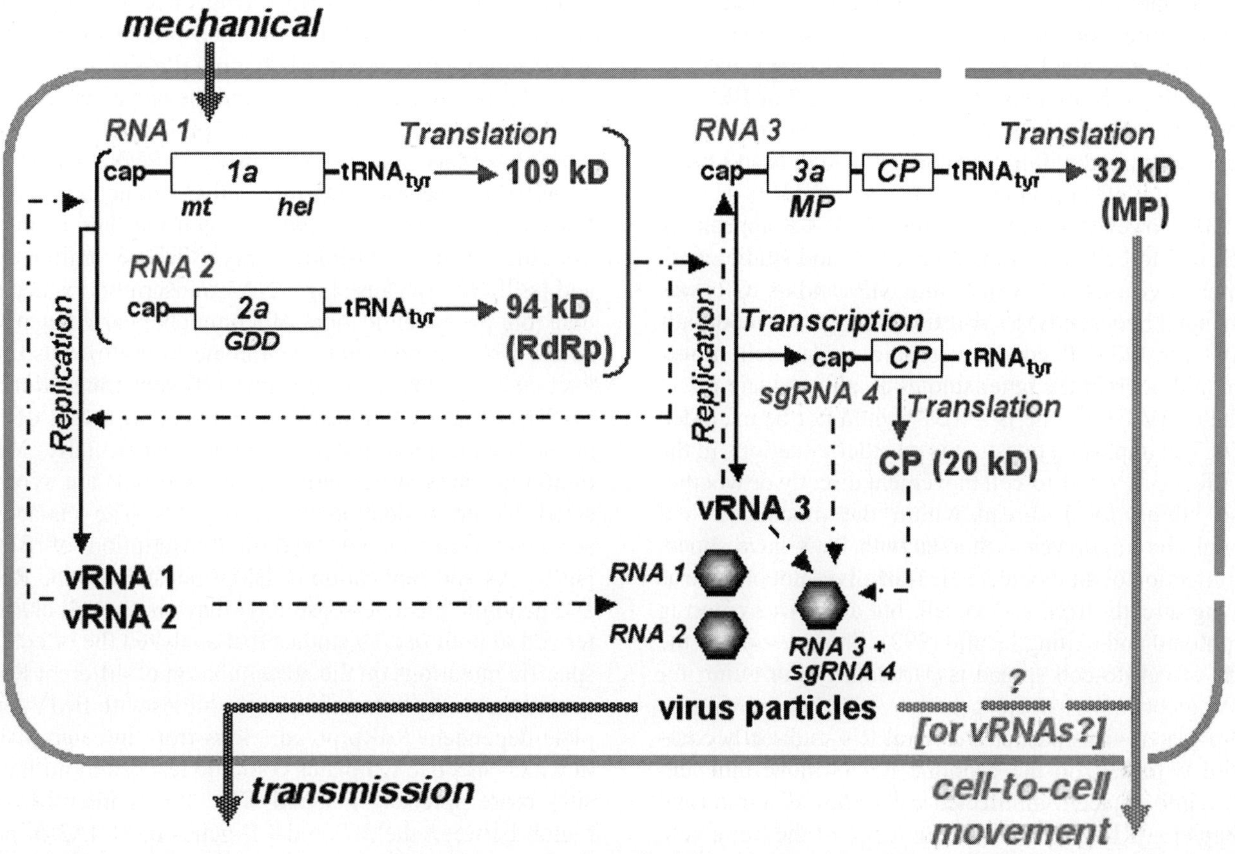

FIG. 15. Multiplication of brome mosaic virus (BMV).

multiplication and gene expression is supported by a variety of experimental studies that were facilitated by the generally high efficiency with which RNA can be transfected into protoplasts and the ability to prepare highly active template-dependent replicase-containing extracts from BMV-infected plants (232), in addition to the segmented nature of the BMV genome. Protein 1a contains conserved motifs characteristic of RNA methyltransferases (N-terminal domain) and helicases (C-terminal domain), and the central region of protein 2a contains the GDD motif characteristic of a viral RdRp. The arrangement and sequences of these resemble those in Sindbis and other alphaviruses, placing BMV in the alphavirus superfamily. Mutations in any of these conserved domains of 1a or 2a block or alter virus RNA replication and sgRNA transcription (6). Consistent with the N-terminus of 1a (methyltransferase) having a role in capping viral genomic and subgenomic RNA, 1a expressed in *E. coli* or yeast has been shown to methylate GTP at the 7 position of guanine in a reaction requiring *S*-adenosylmethionine and to form an adduct with m(7)GMP (10,178). Evidence further suggests that proteins 1a and 2a interact. Pseudorecombinant studies in which RNA1 and RNA2 from BMV and the bromovirus CCMV were exchanged first suggested that 1a and 2a had to be "compatible": such pseudorecombinants do not replicate in protoplasts, not even supporting the replication of BMV RNA3, which can be replicated by either homologous *1a/2a* gene combination (75). In addition, antisera against BMV 1a coprecipitates 1a and 2a from BMV RdRp-containing extracts (280). The C-terminal helicase region of 1a has been shown to interact with the N-terminal region of 2a by Far Western blotting and yeast two-hybrid assays (9,248), and recombinant studies suggest that the core RdRp region of 2a interacts with 1a as well (321). That the 32-kd protein encoded by the *3a* gene is the MP is suggested by several lines of evidence. RNA3 is not needed for viral replication in protoplasts but is essential for virus infectivity in plants. In addition, genetic studies show that deletions in the *3a* gene confine virus infection to individual cells; such mutations prevent the appearance of local necrotic lesions on the inoculated leaves of an appropriate plant host (234). The 32-kd protein also has properties reported for other viral MPs, such as the TMV 30-kd protein: it cooperatively binds single-stranded nucleic acids *in vitro* in a sequence-nonspecific manner, and it has been immunolocalized to plasmodesmata in BMV-infected plants (109,161).

Mutational studies also show that the CP is needed for systemic infection via the phloem, but whether it is required as well for local cell-to-cell movement has not been resolved. Mutations that disrupt the CP of BMV or CCMV have been reported to slow down, but not eliminate, virus spread within the inoculated leaf, based again on the rate of appearance and size of local lesions (7,103). However, mutation of the BMV CP appears to block cell-to-cell spread in some hosts, and studies with chimeric viruses in which the MP and/or CP was exchanged between BMV and CMV suggest a "compatibility" for MP–CP combinations in cell-to-cell movement, although in the latter studies an antagonistic effect of the CMV CP on the BMV MP could not be excluded (239). The important question is whether mutations in the CP affect BMV cell-to-cell movement directly or whether these inhibit local spread within the inoculated leaf through the minor veins. Studies with PVX have shown that infection of an inoculated leaf involves not only virus moving directly from cell to cell, but also virus entering the phloem and exiting locally (292). The question of the mode of cell-to-cell spread is particularly intriguing for BMV given its tripartite genome. Whether moving as encapsidated virus particles or viral RNAs directly complexed with MP, do the genomic RNAs move independently into adjacent uninfected cells until all three (and perhaps [sg]RNA4 as well) accumulate in the same cell, or is there a mechanism to coordinate movement of the three genomic RNAs as they move from cell to cell?

BMV replication occurs in the cytoplasm in association with ER-derived membranes, as reported for other positive-sense RNA viruses. Viral RdRp activity isolated from BMV-infected plants is membrane associated. In addition, immune staining with specific antisera against 1a, 2a, or ER marker proteins, or to detect 5-bromouridine incorporation into replicating viral RNA, show that 1a, 2a, and nascent viral RNA colocalize to cytoplasmic vesicles that also contain ER marker proteins (286). The BMV multiplication cycle is temporally regulated at the level of positive-sense RNA and negative-sense RNA synthesis, and the transcription of [sg]RNA4 to produce the CP, as has also been shown for PVX, TMV, and TYMV. The accumulation of positive-and negative-sense RNA is independently regulated such that late in infection, there is an ~100-fold excess of the genomic RNAs and [sg]RNA. Because [sg]RNA4 transcription is dependent on prior replication of complementary negative-strand RNA, it does not accumulate to high levels until later in infection, at which time efficient translation of [sg]RNA4 into CP appears to compete with that of the nonstructural proteins (1a, 2a, and particularly MP), inhibiting these while large amounts of CP are synthesized for encapsidation of virions (7). The cis-acting sequence elements involved in transcription of BMV [sg]RNA4 and replication of BMV negative-strand RNA and genomic positive-sense RNA have been well characterized in both *in vivo* studies that analyzed the effects of specific mutations on the accumulation of different RNA species in protoplasts and *in vitro* studies with BMV template-dependent RdRp preparations from infected plants in which specific templates could be tested and initiation sites more precisely mapped. The 250 nt intercistronic region between the *MP* and *CP* genes on RNA3 in particular contains important sequence elements for the regulation of replication as well as transcription. Transcription of [sg]RNA4 initiates internally on negative strand copies of RNA3 within a 100 nt sequence in this intercistronic region located upstream of the *CP* gene (231) (Fig. 16). This subgenomic promoter consists of a core promoter of 20 nt located immediately upstream of the *CP* gene that directs specific basal transcription of [sg]RNA4, and additional upstream activating sequences

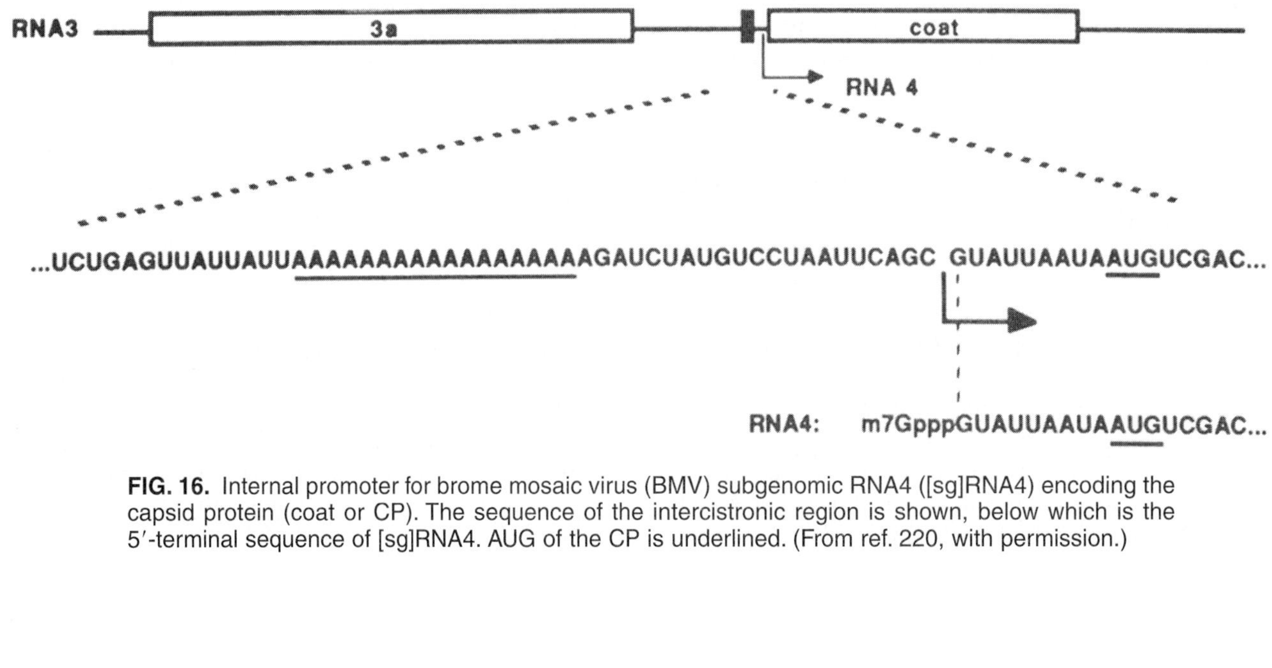

FIG. 16. Internal promoter for brome mosaic virus (BMV) subgenomic RNA4 ([sg]RNA4) encoding the capsid protein (coat or CP). The sequence of the intercistronic region is shown, below which is the 5′-terminal sequence of [sg]RNA4. AUG of the CP is underlined. (From ref. 220, with permission.)

that consist of an oligo(A) tract and partial repeats of core promoter sequences that act to increase levels of [sg]RNA4 transcription (108,216).

Replication of BMV RNAs involves cis-acting sequences within the 5′-UTR and 3′-UTR of RNA1, RNA2, and RNA3, as well as internal sequences within the *2a* gene of RNA2 and a 150 nt sequence within the intercistronic region of RNA3. This 150 nt sequence is located upstream of the oligo(A) tract and most of the subgenomic promoter, overlapping sequences at the 5′ end of the activating region. The promoter sequences for negative strand RNA synthesis have been mapped to the 3′-terminal 200 nt of the genomic RNAs that include the $tRNA_{tyr}$-like structure (6). Unlike TYMV, encapsidated BMV genomic RNAs terminate in 5′-CCA-3′, but *in vitro* transcribed genomic RNAs that lack the 3′-terminal A residue can be adenylated by cellular CCA-tRNA nucleotidyltransferase *in vitro*. Like TYMV, BMV negative-strand RNA synthesis starts at the penultimate C within this terminal 5′-CCA-3′ sequence, and thus it is assumed that adenylation of the 3′ end of BMV positive strand RNAs by host CCA-tRNA nucleotidyltransferase must normally occur *in vivo*. The role of tRNA mimicry in BMV replication has not been as extensively studied biochemically as it has for TYMV. Interestingly, a recent study of the template requirements for initiation by the RdRp of TYMV and BMV reported that BMV RdRp can initiate synthesis internally at 5′-ACCA-3′ sequences, but does so inefficiently. However, it could efficiently initiate at internal 5′-AUGC-3′ sequences (69). The *cis*-acting sequences within the 5′-UTR regions of the BMV genomic RNAs are presumed to be involved in initiation of positive-strand RNA synthesis. These, and the 150 nt internal intercistronic sequence required for efficient accumulation of BMV RNA3, all contain a sequence similar to the motif 5′-GGUUCAAyyCC-3′ (y = U or C), which is one of two consensus elements (Box B) found in cell RNA pol III promoters and also corresponds to the invariant residues of tRNA TΨC loops (7). Mutations in this sequence within the 5′-UTR of RNA2 or the intercistronic region of RNA3 each reduce the accumulation of the corresponding RNA *in vivo*, and several proteins from barley extracts have been reported to bind to the Box B–like element within the 5′-UTR of RNA2 or the complement of this element within the 3′-UTR of the negative strand of RNA2 (92,265).

The involvement of Box B–like elements in the replication and/or accumulation of BMV RNA, the binding of host proteins to these elements, and the presence of cellular proteins in partially purified preparations of BMV RdRp (280,281) have been cited as circumstantial evidence for the involvement of host proteins in BMV replication. More direct evidence for this, as well as more detailed analysis of viral replication, has been obtained through studies of BMV replication in yeast (154,155,159). In this system, BMV proteins 1a and 2a are each expressed from separate yeast 2-μ plasmids having an *HIS3* (for 1a) or *LEU2* (for 2a) selectable marker so that the transformed yeast strain (*his3⁻ leu2⁻ trp1⁻ ura3⁻*) can be selected for growth in the absence of histidine and leucine. These are constructed such that the mRNAs encoding 1a or 2a are transcribed from the yeast *ADH* promoter; however, most of the 5′-UTR and 3′-UTR from RNA1 and RNA2 are missing, so these RNAs cannot be replicated. Replication is assayed by introducing RNA3, either by transfecting yeast coexpressing 1a and 2a with *in vitro* transcripts of RNA3, or by *in vivo* transcription of a RNA3 cDNA from a yeast *CEN4* plasmid (*TRP1* selectable marker) or chromosomal insertion (Fig. 17). In these latter two cases, RNA3 cDNA is flanked by the *GAL1* promoter and the self-cleaving ribozyme from hepatitis δ virus. Growth in galactose induces transcription of RNA3, and the ribozyme cleaves the transcript at its natural 3′ end. In the presence of BMV 1a and 2a, this RNA3 transcript, which is complete with its natural 5′-UTR and 3′-UTR, is correctly replicated in yeast via its complementary strand, and [sg]RNA4 is transcribed. For purposes of selection or screening, the *CP* gene on RNA3 can be replaced with the yeast *URA3* gene or the bacterial GUS or choramphenicol acetyltransferase (CAT) coding sequence. These will be translated from [sg]RNA4, thus allowing for selection of yeast replicating RNA3 (in the case of transfection of *in vitro* transcripts) based on uracil-independent growth of

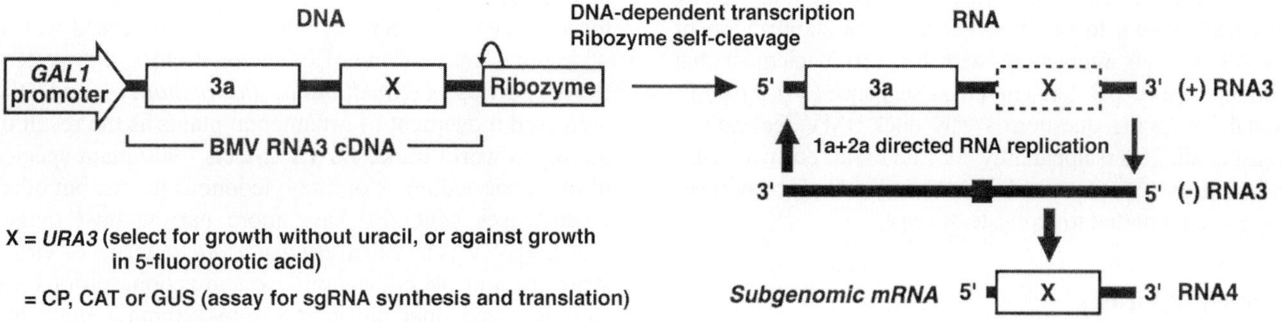

FIG. 17. A yeast system to study brome mosaic virus (BMV) RNA replication. (From ref. 154, with permission.)

the appropriate yeast strain, or screening of RNA3 replication based on GUS or CAT assays. Selection against expression of the *URA3* gene (growth in 5-fluoroorotic acid) can also be used to isolate mutants defective in BMV 1a- and 2a-dependent replication of RNA3 (154). The *MP* coding sequence has also been replaced by *CAT* to assay for translation of RNA3 relative to its replication, the latter determined by Southern blotting with appropriate probes (160).

The intriguing finding is that RNA3 is faithfully replicated and transcribed in the presence of 1a and 2a in yeast. This suggests that whatever host factors may be involved in BMV replication, yeast must contain equivalent factors that can substitute for those present in plants (159). Beyond this finding, the power of the yeast system is the ability to investigate the independent as well as the coordinate effects of 1a or 2a on replication and transcription of RNA3 and to select for host mutants that block different stages of RNA3 replication and transcription. Using this system, it was found that BMV 1a alone acts to stabilize RNA3 positive-sense transcripts expressed from the *GAL1* promoter, increasing their half-life from 5-to-10 minutes to greater than 3 hours. Using a *CAT* reporter gene in place of the *MP* coding sequence, this 1a stabilization appeared to block translation of RNA3, which led to the suggestion that 1a interacts with RNA3 to recruit it (and by inference RNA2 and RNA1) away from translation and into RNA replication (160). What sequences does 1a interact with in RNA3?: The intercistronic 150-nt "replication signal" that includes the consensus Box B–like element. Mutational analysis of RNA3 in this 1a-dependent yeast system shows that this 150-nt "enhancer of RNA3 replication" is required for this 1a stabilization of RNA3, and beyond this is sufficient to confer 1a-dependent stabilization when fused to the 5′ end of β-globin RNA (328). Using 5-fluoroorotic acid to select against replication of a chromosomal insertion of RNA3 that expresses the *URA3* gene in place of the *CP* gene, recessive mutations in a number of yeast genes have now been identified that inhibit this BMV 1a- and 2a-dependent replication and transcription of RNA3. Characterization of these and other yeast genes that affect BMV replication and transcription in yeast is a powerful approach for deciphering the involvement of host proteins in RNA virus replication. One yeast protein, Lsm1p, a cytoplasmic protein related to core RNA splicing factors, has been shown to be involved in the 1a stabilization of RNA3 through interactions with the 150-nt element that contains the Box B–like consensus sequence (74). An additional interesting question is why does BMV replicate in yeast at all. This is apparently not true for all positive-sense RNA viruses: to date, only BMV and a few nodaviruses have been reported to replicate in yeast.

Enveloped Viruses

Given the plant cell wall and the movement of plant viruses from cell to cell without going through an extracellular phase, the existence of enveloped plant viruses raises a number of interesting questions in terms of viral adaptation. At what site(s)within the plant cell will these viruses bud to acquire their envelope? Surely the plant cell wall poses problems for budding at the plasma membrane, the site of maturation for most, although not all, enveloped animal viruses. Why would a plant virus have an envelope? Does the envelope and its associated glycoproteins have a role in infecting the plant host, or do they serve a separate function? What is the relationship between the form of the virus that moves from cell to cell to infect the plant and the virion? As already alluded to for tospoviruses such as TSWV (see Plant-to-Plant Transmission), and described in more detail later, the enveloped virion with its glycoproteins may represent an adaptation to a dual lifestyle: that of an "animal-infecting virus" as well as a plant virus. The genomic organization of the tospoviruses, and plant-infecting rhabdoviruses that have been characterized, suggests that they are "animal viruses" that encode one extra, unique protein—a movement protein needed for the virus to invade and infect plants. An important issue then becomes how virus maturation may be regulated in infected plant cells. Being negative-sense (nucleorhabdoviruses and cytorhabdoviruses) or ambisense (tospoviruses), transcripts of cDNA clones are not infectious. Thus, the interactions of these viruses with their hosts have been difficult to study, and a number of the details of their replication are sketchy or inferred by analogy to other, better characterized animal viruses within the same family. These particular plant viruses are included here, not to focus on the details of their replication, but to illustrate possible adaptations of enveloped viruses when infecting a plant.

Tomato Spotted Wilt Virus

Topsoviruses, a genus in the *Bunyaviridae*, have emerged as serious pathogens of crops in the past 20 years. In nature, the viruses are transmitted by thrips, but they can be mechanically transmitted in the laboratory. TSWV, the type member and best characterized of the tospoviruses, is in the current "top ten" of plant viruses in terms of economic losses worldwide (272). The recent emergence of TSWV, as well as a number of other tospoviruses, has been attributed to the increased worldwide prevalence of one of its major vectors, the western flower thrips (*Frankliniella occidentalis*), and the increased movement of ornamental plants as the result of increased world trade. TSWV infects >900 plant species of monocotyledonous or dicotyledonous plants, but other topsoviruses generally have more narrow host ranges (237). TSWV is a typical *Bunyaviridae* in terms of virion structure and overall genomic organization. Virions are spherical enveloped particles ~80-to-120 nm in diameter, with surface projections (spikes) composed of two viral-encoded glycoproteins, G1 and G2. The three genomic segments of the viral tripartite genome are associated with the nucleoprotein N and a few copies of the viral RdRp (L protein) to form three separate nucleocapsids within the enveloped particles (see Chapter 25). There is no matrix protein.

TSWV has three genomic ssRNA segments designated *L* (large), *M* (middle), and *S* (small) (Fig. 18) that are organized and expressed overall as are the genomic segments of the animal-infecting *Bunyaviridae* (see Chapter 25). The L segment encodes a single protein, L (330 kd), shown to be the viral RdRp in several animal-infecting *Bunyaviridae.* The TSWV M segment encodes the viral glycoproteins, G1 and G2, on the complementary strand, and a nonstructural protein NSm (33.6 kd), which is translated from an sgRNA that is 5′ coterminal with the viral genomic M segment. The S segment encodes the nucleoprotein N (30 kd) on the complementary strand, and a nonstructural protein NSs (54 kd), which like NSm, is translated from an sgRNA that corresponds to the 5′ end of the viral genomic S segment. Thus, both the M and S segments of TSWV are expressed by an ambisense strategy (67,180,181) (see Fig. 18). All of the *Bunyaviridae* are principally negative sense viruses in terms of their replication strategy. Thus, TSWV, like other *Bunyviridae* and negative sense RNA viruses, contains the viral-encoded RdRp (L protein) associated with the nucleocapsids in the enveloped virus particles and in infected plant cells (346). L is the putative RdRp of TSWV based on sequence similarity to the RdRp of other *Bunyaviridae* and negative sense RNA viruses (66). Consistent with this, detergent-disrupted TSWV virions have been shown to contain an RdRp activity *in vitro* (4). The L protein is an endonuclease as well as an RdRp. The endonucleolytic activity is required because *Bunyviridae,* like the segmented negative strand influenza viruses and "ambisense" arenaviruses, require capped primers to initiate transcription of mRNAs. These are acquired from host mRNAs in the cytoplasm, not the nucleus, by a "cap snatching" mechanism (see Chapter 25). For TSWV, primer extension analysis has shown that the two mRNAs transcribed from the S segment contain nonviral sequences 12 to 20 nt in length at their 5′ ends (184) (see Fig. 18). In addition, when plants are co-infected with TSWV and alfalfa mosaic virus (AMV) (a *Bromoviridae* with a genome organization like BMV), the heterogeneous 5′ ends of the TSWV mRNAs can be acquired from the co-infecting AMV RNAs, thus clearly showing that this cap-snatching does occur in the cytoplasm. By analogy to other well-characterized negative strand RNA viruses such as vesicular stomatis virus (VSV), it is generally assumed that the TSWV N protein regulates the switch from mRNA transcription to viral genome replication (see Fig. 18). Consistent with this, both TSWV genomic and full-length complementary RNAs are found associated with N protein in RNP particles in infected plants (181). Using antisera generated against NSs expressed from a baculovirus vector in insect cells, NSs has been found associated with what has been described as fibrous structures or paracrystalline arrays in the cytoplasm of infected TSWV plant cells (182,237). Its function remains unknown. It is also not known how the viral nucleocapsids are released from virions following their introduction into plant cells by thrips. It is generally assumed by analogy with other enveloped viruses that they are taken up in cytoplasmic

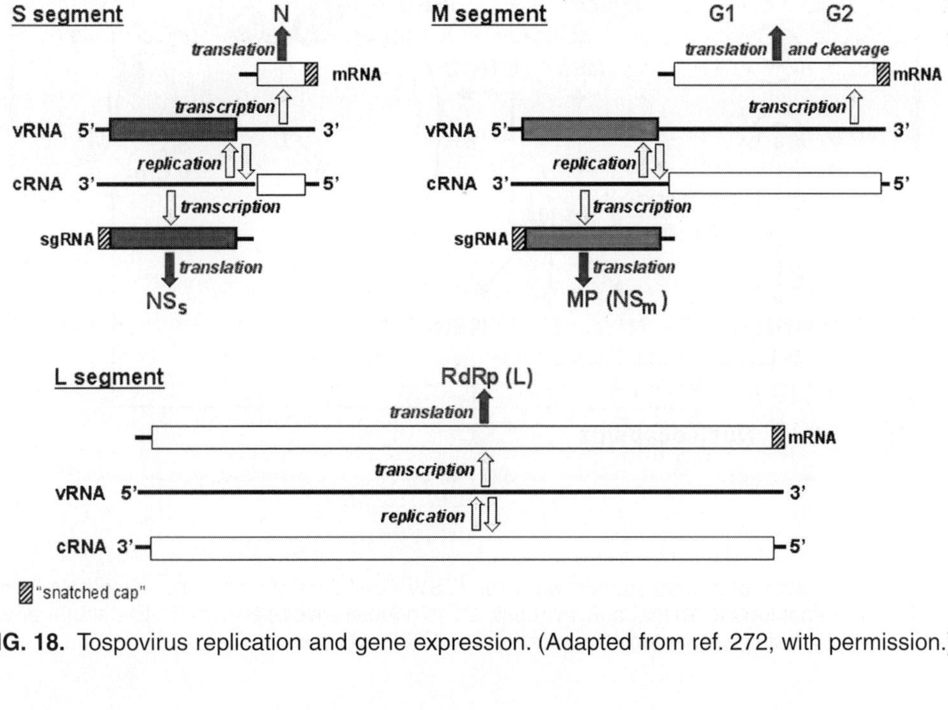

FIG. 18. Tospovirus replication and gene expression. (Adapted from ref. 272, with permission.)

vesicles, with release occurring by fusion of the viral envelope with the vesicle membrane (Fig. 19).

The distinctive feature of the genomic organization of TSWV when compared with that of the animal-infecting *Bunyaviridae* is the presence of an additional virus-sense gene in the M segment, which is expressed from an sgRNA (see Fig. 18). Evidence suggests that this encodes the viral MP. In infected plant cells, viral RNPs are seen associated with unique large tubular structures that extend into adjacent cells from what appear to be highly modified plasmodesmata. NSm immunolocalizes to these unique tubules, and has been shown to be necessary and sufficient to induce such tubules when transiently expressed in plant protoplasts or insect cells. In addition, NSm immunolocalizes to plasmodesmata in transgenic plants that express this protein (183,273,327). Although viral RNPs are associated with or within these tubules, transient expression studies in plant protoplasts show that N protein is not required for the formation of the tubules. Thus, it has been suggested that viral RNPs move from cell to cell in the plant through these MP-containing tubules (see Fig. 19). This picture of TSWV movement in infected plants envisions a pathway quite distinct from and clearly not involving enveloped virions with their associated G1 and G2 glycoproteins. As already discussed, the enveloped virion structure and G1 and G2 glycoproteins are required for thrips recognition and acquisition of TSWV but not for plant infection, as clearly demonstrated by the fact that plant-infectious TSWV lacking the envelope structure and glycoproteins can be generated by repeated mechanical passage in plants (285) (see Plant-to-Plant Transmission). Only thrips in the larval stage can acquire the virus, which they ingest during feeding on plants. Ultrastructural studies show that virions are transported along the lumen of the thrips digestive tract to the midgut, where they appear to cross the midgut wall by endocytosis to enter the hemocoel. From the hemocoel, they invade the salivary glands. However, unlike the *Luteoviridae,* topsoviruses replicate in their thrips hosts, persistently infecting the insects without being pathogenic. Evidence for this includes the detection of the nonstructural protein NSs in infected thrips and the identification of viral inclusions in endothelial cells, muscle cells, and the salivary glands (237). Using gel overlay and immune labeling assays, two candidate thrips receptor proteins that recognize TSWV glycoproteins have been identified: a midgut protein that can bind both G1 and G2, and a protein found in all tissues except the midgut that recognizes G2 (17,171). The functions of these thrips proteins in virus acquisition and circulation has not been determined.

Where does TSWV virion assembly occur in infected plant cells? For those animal-infecting *Bunyaviridae* where it has been investigated, the viral G1/G2 polyprotein precursor has a signal sequence so that it is cotranslationally transported into the ER lumen, being processed to G1 and G2 by host cell peptidases and glycosylated as it transits from the ER to the Golgi stacks. The het-

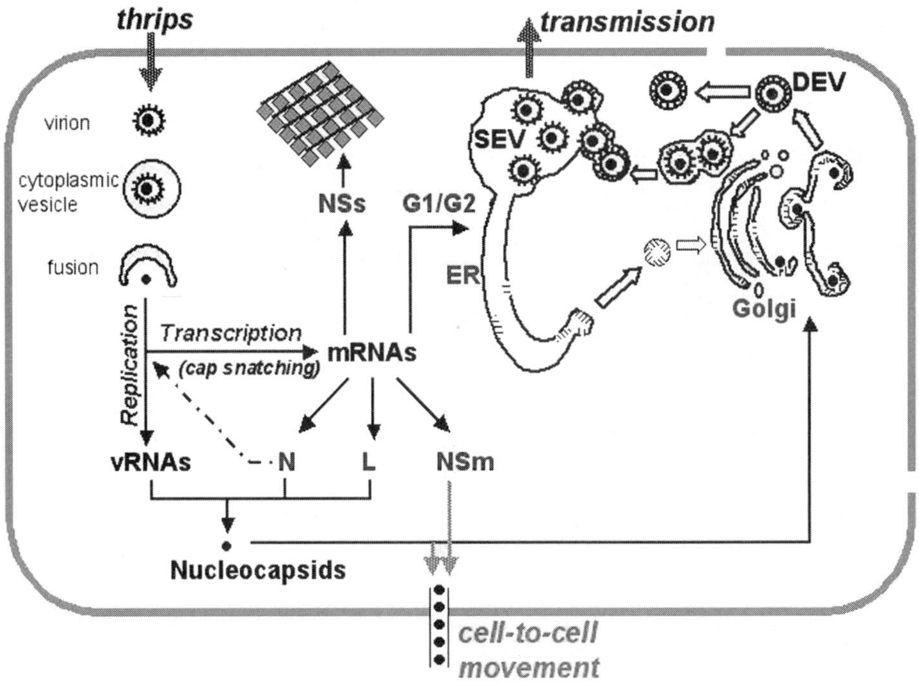

FIG. 19. Multiplication of tomato spotted wilt virus (TSWV). Stages of virion uncoating have been proposed based on analogy to animal bunyaviruses. DEV, double-enveloped virus; SEV, single-enveloped virus. See text for details. (Adapted from refs. 170 and 272, with permission.)

erodimeric G1:G2 complex contains a Golgi-retention signal, so that virion assembly occurs by viral RNPs associating with G1:G2-containing areas of Golgi membranes and budding into the Golgi. These assembled virions are then transported to the cell surface in vesicles, where they are released from the cell as the vesicles fuse with the plasma membrane (see Chapter 25). Until recently, the pathway for TSWV virion morphogenesis in plant cells has not been clear. The TSWV G1/G2 precursor is predicted to contain a signal peptide and has been shown to be processed when expressed in insect cells, where it was also reported to be associated with cellular membranes, including the plasma membrane (3). However, this study done in insect cells does not answer the question concerning where virions mature in infected plant cells. Ultrastructural and immune labeling studies have reported virus particles or virion proteins associated with what morphologically appeared to be ER membrane in infected plants cells or Golgi-like structures in infected thrips cells, leading different authors to state that TSWV acquires its envelope by budding into the ER or the Golgi. However, the identity of these membrane structures was never determined by immune labeling for appropriate ER and Golgi marker proteins. A major advance in this area is the recent development of a plant protoplast system for investigating TSWV infection in which more than >50% of the cells (*Nicotiana rustica* tobacco cells) can be infected with TSWV particles and maintained for several days (172). Using this synchronous infection system for ultrastructural studies and immune staining for compartment-specific marker proteins, the TSWV glycoproteins G1 and G2 were found to accumulate in Golgi membranes. These areas of the Golgi then appear to wrap around viral RNPs in the cytoplasm to form double-enveloped particles (DEV) (see Fig. 19). At later stages of infection, both in the infected protoplasts and in cells in TSWV-infected plants, these cytoplasmic DEV double-enveloped particles can be found fused to each other and fusing to ER membrane to form single-enveloped particles (SEV, the virions) clustered in membrane-bound bodies in the cytoplasm or in the ER (170) (see Fig. 19). Thus, rather than be transported in Golgi-derived vesicles to the plant plasma membrane with its cell wall, TSWV appears to have adapted a strategy that allows mature virions to move back from the Golgi to the ER and accumulate there, as well as in the cytoplasm. It is suggested that when thrips feed, they acquire TSWV virions from these sites of accumulation in the ER (170).

Rhabdoviruses: Sonchus Yellow Net Virus and Lettuce Necrotic Yellows Virus

Plant viruses have historically been categorized as rhabdoviruses based on ultrastructural examination of infected plant cells or virus preparations, which identify enveloped virus particles that are bullet shaped in unfixed preparations or bacilliform when fixed (Fig. 20). Virions are 45 to 100 nm wide and 130 to 250 nm long, and in nature are transmitted by aphids, leafhoppers, or planthoppers, depending on the virus. Like the tospoviruses, these viruses infect and multiply in their insect vectors, thus leading a dual lifestyle as an animal-infecting and

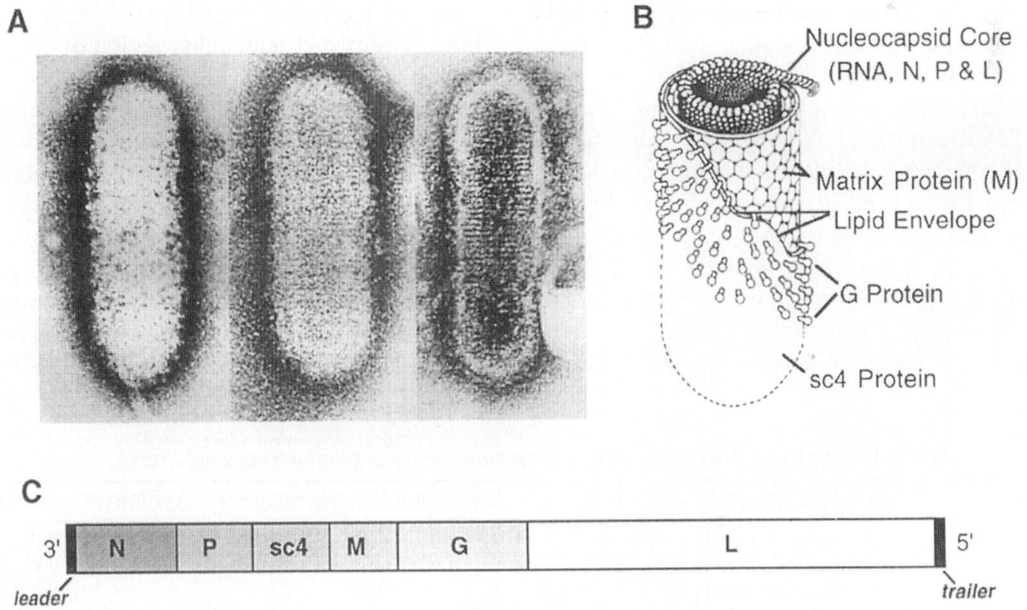

FIG. 20. Structure and genome organization of sonchus yellow net virus (SYNV), a nucleorhabdovirus. (From ref. 158, with permission.)

plant-infecting virus. Approximately 75 plant viruses are currently listed as possible rhabdoviruses, although it is not clear that all of these represent distinct viruses or are in fact rhabdoviruses. About 15 of these viruses have been sufficiently characterized in terms of virion structure and composition, host range, vector transmission, serology, nucleic acid hybridization, and ultrastructural alterations in infected plant cells to be placed in the genus *Cytorhabdovirus* or *Nucleorhabdovirus* (158). As these names imply, the plant rhabdoviruses are grouped based on the site of virus multiplication, as determined by electron microscropic examination of infected plant cells. Nucleorhabdoviruses form nuclear inclusions and appear to bud from the inner nuclear envelope to accumulate in perinuclear spaces. Cytorhabdoviruses are seen to form at cytoplasmic membranes and accumulate in the cytoplasm. Of these, sonchus yellow net virus (SYNV; a nucleorhabdovirus) and lettuce necrotic yellow virus (LNYV; a cytorhabdovirus) are the best characterized in terms of sequence analysis.

Electron microscopy of purified virions, combined with detergent disruption, gel analysis of viral proteins, and RNA analyses, show that plant rhabdoviruses, as typified by SYNV and LNYV, resemble VSV in structure and composition (158) (see Fig. 20). Virions are composed of a lipid envelope from which project spikes made of the viral-encoded G glycoprotein, which is presumed to exist in a trimeric form as in VSV. Within the envelope, the virion core is composed of a helical RNP that consists of the viral genomic unsegmented negative-sense ssRNA (~11 to 14 kb) surrounded by N protein to form the nucleocapsid, in association with a few copies of the viral P and L proteins that make up the RdRp (see Fig. 20). The location of the matrix protein M has not been unambiguously determined, but like VSV, it is assumed to be involved in coiling the nucleocapsid and interacting with the internal domains of G (see Chapter 22). The available evidence suggests that replication of the plant rhabdoviruses resembles that of VSV. Treatment of LYNV virions with nonionic detergent activates a viral RdRp that transcribes RNAs complementary to the viral genome *in vitro* (158). The RdRp activity is associated with loosely coiled nucleocapsids that contain N, L, and P, in addition to the virion ssRNA. Interestingly, similar treatment of SYNV virions does *not* activate RdRp activity, but such an activity can be extracted from the nuclei of plant cells infected with SYNV (358). This SYNV RdRp activity co-sediments with viral nucleocapsid cores and contains the viral N, L and P proteins, based on copurification and immune precipitation studies (359). Antibody inhibition studies show that L is a functional component of the RdRp activity. Kinetic analysis of the products transcribed *in vitro* shows that like VSV, SYNV transcription occurs by a stop-start mechanism in which the individual mRNAs for each gene are sequentially transcribed starting at the 3′ end of the viral genome and continuing through to the 5′ end, with the RdRp pausing at intergenic regions between each gene to polyadenylate and terminate the upstream gene, and then transcribe the next gene in order (see Chapter 17). Also like VSV, the relative abundance of each mRNA is determined by the gene order in the viral genome, with the 3′-proximal N mRNA being most abundant and the 5′-proximal L mRNA being transcribed in the lowest amount (359). All of the mRNAs are polyadenylated by the viral RdRp activity. Like VSV, a positive-sense short leader RNA is transcribed from the 3′ end of the genomic RNA; but unlike VSV, the SYNV leader RNA is also polyadenylated (359). Thus, while the picture is one of virions containing RNP cores that can initiate transcription upon uncoating, as one would expect for a negative-sense RNA virus, the SYNV core-associated RdRp appears to require activation within the host cell. This, along with the polyadenylation of the SYNV leader RNA, appears to reflect adaptations necessary for the nuclear multiplication of this virus.

The complete sequence of the SYNV genome shows an organization that is the same as VSV, with one additional gene *sc4* not found in VSV (reviewed in 358) (see Fig. 20). The 3′ leader sequence is followed by the genes encoding N, P, M, G, and L in the same order as they occur in VSV (see Chapter 17). The *sc4* gene is located between the P and M genes (see Fig. 20). The 3′ leader and 5′-proximal noncoding region of SYNV are distinct from those in VSV and other animal-infecting rhabdoviruses, but the intergenic gene junctions are highly conserved (158) (Table 4). The sc4 protein is found in virions (see Fig. 20) and appears to be phosphorylated *in vivo*. Although its precise location is unknown, it is solubilized from virions by treatment with nonionic detergents. It has been suggested that sc4 might be the viral MP, although it could also play a role in aphid transmission (158). SYNV induces the formation of viroplasms in the nuclei of infected plant cells. The viral N, L, and P

TABLE 4. *Sequence elements in the intergenic regions of plant and animal rhabdoviruses*

Virus	Element I [upstream poly (U) tract]	Element II (nontranscribed)	Element III (mRNA start site)
VSV	ACUUUUUUU	$^{G}_{C}$U	UUGUC
Rabies virus	ACUUUUUUU	C(N)x	UUGU$^{A}_{G}$
SYNV	AUUCUUUUU	GG	UUG$^{AA}_{UC}$
LNYV	AUUCUUUU	G(N)x	CU$^{AAG}_{UUU}$

VSV, vesicular stomatis virus; SYNV, sonchus yellow net virus; LNYV, lettuce necrotic yellow virus.
Adapted from ref. 158, with permission.

proteins have been immunolocalized to these nuclear viroplasms, which appear to be the sites of viral replication and the source of the RdRp activity that can be extracted from nuclei of infected cells (217,359). N and P also appear to contain NLSs: when N or P are individually expressed from a PVX vector (see Fig. 8), each accumulates in the nucleus, and if expressed as fusions to GUS, the GUS:N and the GUS:P fusion proteins are also targeted to nuclei (217). Ultrastructural studies show SYNV virions budding at the inner nuclear membrane to accumulate in swollen perinuclear spaces between the inner and outer nuclear envelopes. Thus, the rather striking adaptation to replicate in nuclei, as opposed to VSV, which replicates in the cytoplasm, appears to be a strategy to acquire the viral envelope from the inner nuclear envelope rather than the plant cell plasma membrane. The current model for SYNV multiplication (Fig. 21A) proposes that upon entering a cell, the viral nucleocapsid cores are released into the cytoplasm, possibly in association with the ER, and these are transported into the nucleus, where the SYNV RdRp is activated and primary transcription occurs. Viral mRNAs are transported to the cytoplasm, where they are translated, and newly synthesized N, L, and P are transported into the nucleus to continue transcription of viral mRNAs and replicate the viral genome. Presumably, newly synthesized viral M and sc4 proteins also have to be transported to the nucleus: M for virion assembly and sc4 since it is present in virions. Because tunicamycin interrupts SYNV budding at the nuclear envelope and causes nucleocapsids to accumulate at the nuclear periphery, it is proposed that newly synthesized G is transported to the inner nuclear envelope, and virus buds at these sites into the perinuclear space between the inner and outer nuclear membranes (158). This model envisions that viral cores lacking an envelope are exported from the nucleus and move cell to cell, presumably through plasmodesmata, as an alternative to virion assembly (see Fig. 21), as is the case for TSWV.

In the context of the nuclear replication of SYNV, the presence of an inactive form of the RdRp within virions and the polyadenylation of the leader RNA make sense. Packaging of an inactive RdRp provides a mechanism to prevent premature transcription from occurring in the cytoplasm before nucleocapsid cores are transported to the nucleus. Host activation of the RdRp could involve a posttranslational modification, such as phosphorylation

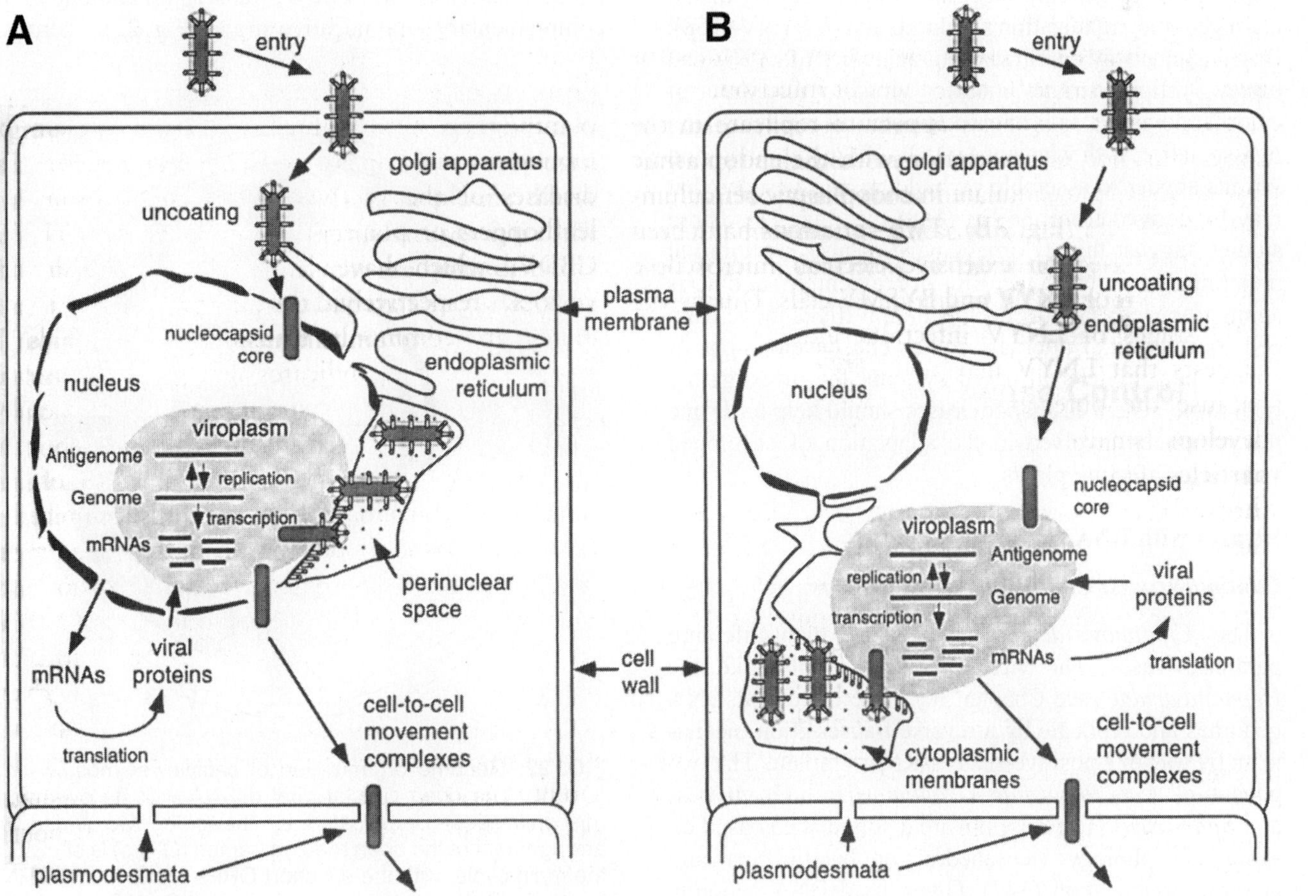

FIG. 21. Multiplication of **(A)** nucleorhabdoviruses and **(B)** cytorhaboviruses. (From ref. 158, with permission.)

of L or P within the RdRp complex, or of the core structure such that it can be transported into the nucleus. Polyadenylation of the leader sequence may prevent this RNA from being degraded within the nucleus. Although there are some biochemical and immune localization studies to support aspects of this model, the proposed pathways for viral assembly and movement are primarily based on ultrastructural studies. Cell biological and additional biochemical studies are needed to investigate the interesting questions raised by this model. Essentially nothing is known about the form in which the virus moves from cell to cell to invade the plant, or the process of movement. Perhaps M is required only for virion assembly at the inner nuclear envelope, and flexible nucleocapsids, in association with sc4 as well as P and L, are the form that exits from the nucleus and moves from cell to cell. What regulates whether genomic RNPs are packaged into virions or transported from cell to cell? Could it be posttranslational modifications of sc4, such as phosphorylation or dephosphorylation? If sc4 is not the viral MP, what is the MP? As is clear from studies of TSWV, appropriate mutational studies and cell-based systems are needed to investigate viral morphogenesis and movement, for both the nucleorhabdoviruses and the cytorhabdoviruses. LYNV has not been completely sequenced, but genome mapping studies suggest that it has a genome organization similar to that of SYNV (158). Based exclusively on ultrastructural studies of LYNV and barley yellow striate mosaic virus, replication of cytorhabdoviruses is proposed to occur in the cytoplasm in association with what appear to be ER membranes, and virions appear to assemble by budding into vesicles that may be derived from the ER (158) (see Fig. 21). These studies suggest that cytorhabdoviruses also use internal membranes—perhaps the ER—for assembly, and it is again proposed that nonenveloped viral RNPs move from cell to cell by an alternate route. The development of appropriate model cell-based systems for investigating both these genera of rhabdoviruses should help to define the principles involved in the adaptation of enveloped viruses to infecting plants.

Viruses with DNA Genomes

Caulimoviruses: Cauliflower Mosaic Virus

The *Caulimoviridae* comprises the plant-infecting pararetroviruses. The viruses in this family, like the *Hepadnaviridae* (see Chapter 36), have circular dsDNA genomes and replicate by a reverse transcription mechanism by way of a positive-sense ssRNA template. The two genera of *Caulimoviridae*—*Caulimovirus* (12 viruses) and *Badnavirus* (13 viruses)—are distinguished based on virion morphology (icosahedral or bacilliform) and genome organization (347). Given its dsDNA genome, CaMV, the type member of the caulimoviruses, was the first plant virus to be cloned and sequenced. Thus, it has been extensively characterized in terms of its molecular biology and host interactions. CaMV, in addition to providing what is still generally the promoter of choice for generating transgenic plants (the 35S promoter), has been a model for investigating the replication and gene expression strategies of the caulimoviruses in particular, and mechanisms of translational control in general. Caulimovirus particles are icosahedral (T=7), 45 to 50 nm in diameter, with the capsid being composed of subunits of a single protein, CP, which in CaMV exists in two processed forms of 37 kd and 44 kd. CaMV particles also contain minor amounts of three additional viral-encoded proteins: a 15-kd nucleic acid–binding protein, and a protease (PR) and reverse transcriptase (RT) that are synthesized as the PRO-RT polyprotein product of a single ORF. Most caulimoviruses are transmitted in nature by aphids in a noncirculative manner, neither circulating in nor infecting the vector. Although each virus has a fairly narrow host range, individual caulimoviruses cause serious yield losses in economically important crops, such as cauliflower, turnips, and blueberries (144,310). CaMV infects crucifers, including *Brassica* species, such as turnip and cauliflower.

The CaMV circular dsDNA genome is 8 kb and contains three discontinuities: two in the viral positive strand (same polarity as viral mRNA transcripts) and one in the complementary viral negative strand (Fig. 22). There is a

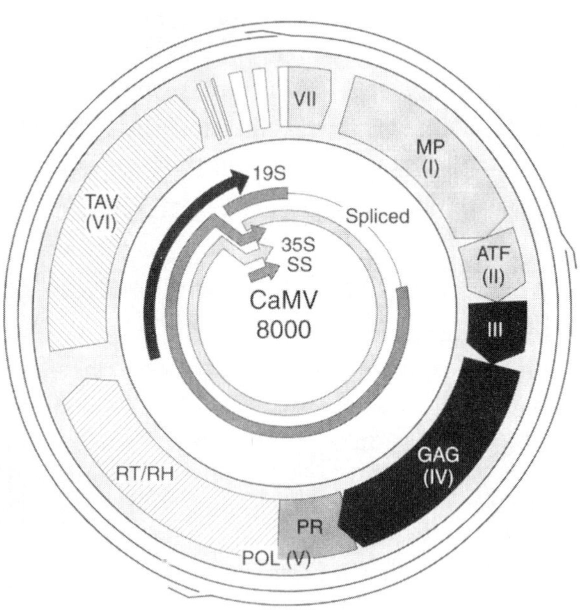

FIG. 22. Genome organization of cauliflower mosaic virus (CaMV). The open circular viral dsDNA with its overhangs (discontinuities) is indicated by the *outer two lines.* The arrangement of the open reading frames (ORFs) is shown on the main circle, with the six short ORFs within the 35S RNA leader indicated by *white boxes.* The 35S, 19S, short stop (SS) and essential spliced transcripts are each indicated by the *inner circular arrows.* (From ref. 144, with permission.)

short 5′ overlap at each discontinuity, with ribonucleotides often attached to the 5′ ends. These discontinuities are formed by strand displacement synthesis during reverse transcription of the 35S pregenomic positive strand RNA. CaMV encodes seven major ORFs (I to VII). Mutational studies show that ORFs I through VI are essential for viability and infectivity. These encode: the viral MP (I, 45 kd), an aphid transmission factor (ATF, II, 18 kd), a minor capsid component (pIII, 15 kd), a precursor of the capsid protein (pre-CP = GAG, IV, 56 kd), a polyprotein (V, POL, 80 kd) that is processed to an aspartic proteinase (PR) and reverse transcriptase (RT) with an RNase H domain (RH), and a multifunctional translational transactivator (TAV, VI, 62 kd) (144) (see Fig. 22). These functional assignments are supported by a large number of experimental studies. ORF I is essential for cell-to-cell movement and systemic infection of the plant. The encoded MP has been localized to unique large tubules that contain virus-like particles and extend from plasmodesmata in infected cells, and it can induce these tubules when expressed in cultured cells (208,261,340). ATF forms inclusion bodies in infected cells and has been shown to bind to virus particles. CaMV ATF mutants are infectious when mechanically inoculated onto plants, but they cannot be transmitted by aphids. It is not precisely known how ATF acts. However, aphids which are fed ATF can acquire and transmit ATF-defective CaMV, suggesting that ATF may interact with the cuticular lining of the aphid stylet (307,310). pIII, found associated with virus particles, can bind DNA in a sequence-nonspecific manner and appears to function as a tetramer. It has been suggested that it compacts the viral genomic DNA during virion assembly (60,200). GAG, or pre-CP, as synthesized, contains highly acidic N- and C-terminal regions, which are removed by the viral aspartic proteinase (PR) to form the mature capsid proteins of 44 kd and 37 kd: the 37-kd protein is contained within the 44-kd protein sequence. It is not known whether one or both of these CP forms is the functional capsid protein (144). The polyprotein product of ORF V (POL = PR-RT) if expressed in *E. coli* or translated *in vitro* in reticulocyte extracts, self-cleaves into the N-terminal PR (20 to 22 kd) and C-terminal RT (56 kd). PR contains the consensus motif found in aspartic proteinases, and mutation of this motif destroys proteolytic activity and is lethal for the virus. PR processes both the POL polyprotein to PR and RT and the pre-CP (GAG) (341). The expected RNA:DNA replication intermediates and RT, activity have been identified in the cytoplasm of infected cells, and the RT activity has been characterized (27,262). TAV is a translational activator required for the 35S pregenomic RNA to be translated as a polycistronic mRNA (112,311). It also forms inclusion bodies, distinct from the ATF inclusions, that appear to be the site of virus assembly and reverse transcription. Virus particles, pregenomic RNA, and reverse transcriptase all copurify with these inclusions (262,315).

Although the early events of caulimovirus uncoating are not well understood, it appears that upon infection, virus particles deliver the viral dsDNA to the nuclear pore, where it is released into the nucleus and the discontinuities are sealed by host enzymes to form a supercoiled minichromosome. Host RNA pol II complexes transcribe these minichromosomes. Transcription is unidirectional, using two viral promoters to produce two major capped and polyadenylated transcripts that are named for their sedimentation characteristics: the 35S RNA (also termed the *35S pregenomic RNA*), which is transcribed from the 35S promoter, and the 19S RNA, transcribed from the 19S promoter (Figs. 22 and 23). The relative amounts of these transcripts are determined by the promoter strength. The 35S promoter is very strong owing to the presence of several enhancer elements, which in combination make it a constitutive promoter in most plant cell types. The 19S promoter is relatively weak *in vitro*, but *in vivo* could be influenced by the enhancer elements within the 35S promoter region (54,91,129,249,250). The 19S RNA is monocistronic and is translated into TAV. The 35S RNA is translated into the remaining five essential proteins (MP, ATV, pIII, pre-CP [GAG], POL [PR-RT]) by two unusual mechanisms in eukaryotic cells: ribosome shunting (84,113) and reinitiation, the latter of which makes it functionally a polycistronic mRNA (112,311) (see Fig. 23). The 35S RNA has 180-nt terminal repeats and, similar to hepadnaviruses and retroviruses, functions both as the major viral mRNA and the template for reverse transcription to synthesize the viral dsDNA. The polyadenylation signal for both the 19S RNA and the 35S RNA is located 180 base pairs downstream of the transcription start site for the 35S RNA. The 180-nt terminal repeats at the ends of the 35S RNA are created by RNA pol II ignoring this polyadenylation signal on its first passage to transcribe around the circular genome and terminate on the second encounter with this signal. The polymerase will occasionally recognize the polyadenylation signal on its first encounter, thus producing a 180 nt "short stop" RNA, the function of which is not known (144) (see Fig. 22). Alternatively spliced transcripts of the 35S RNA have also been detected using reporter gene constructs in transiently transfected protoplasts and in CaMV-infected cells. All of these use an acceptor site within ORF II, but differ in using a donor site near the end of the RNA leader region or at sites within ORF I (Fig. 22). The function of these spliced transcripts is not known, but mutation of the common splice acceptor site suggests that splicing is essential for viral infectivity (176).

Whereas the 19S RNA can be translated *in vitro*, the 35S RNA, and most of its spliced variants, cannot because of its polycistronic nature and a long highly structured 600-nt leader. This leader prevented *in vitro* translation of the 35S RNA until the recent development of a cell-free wheat germ system in which ribosome shunting could occur (138,308). Thus, most of the studies

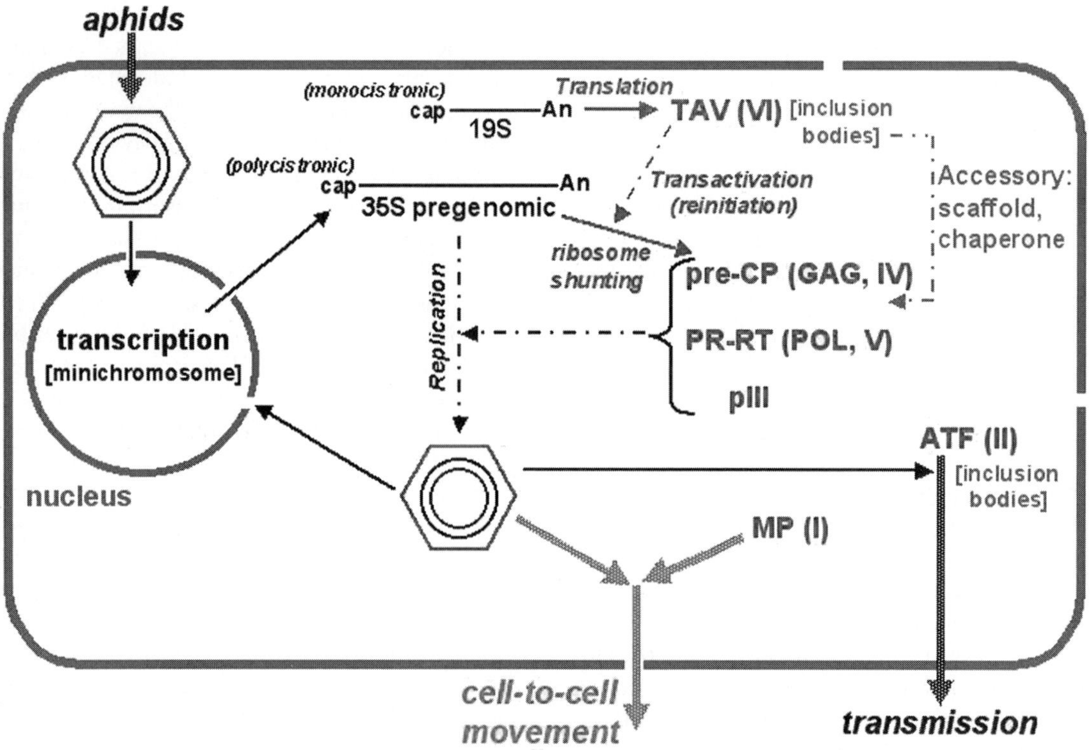

FIG. 23. Multiplication of cauliflower mosaic virus (CaMV).

on the translation of the 35S RNA have been done by expressing appropriate dicistronic and polycistronic reporter gene constructs transiently in plant protoplasts or in transgenic plants. The earliest indication that the 35S RNA was polycistronic was the polar effects that certain mutations in ORF VII or *ATF* had on the expression of viral proteins encoded by the downstream ORFs (145 and citations therein). Most of the ORFs downstream of ORF VII are poorly expressed in protoplasts or transgenic plants unless TAV is present. In particular, transient expression studies with CAT or GUS reporter genes inserted in dicistronic constructs derived from the CaMV 35S RNA or at different sites along the 35S RNA transcript from figwort mosaic virus (also a caulimovirus) showed that these could be expressed, but only if TAV was provided in *cis* or in *trans* (112,311). Activation by TAV is specific for downstream ORFs and does not require virus-specific sequence elements, nor does TAV induce internal ribosome binding or ribosome shunting. Rather, TAV acts on ribosomes migrating through and apparently translating regions upstream of the reporter gene, thus suggesting that it acts by allowing ribosomes to reinitiate translation at a downstream ORF.

The 600-nt leader of the CaMV 35S RNA contains seven to nine short ORFs (sORFs) depending on the strain, and both chemical and enzymatic probing show this region to be highly structured (138) (Figs. 22 and 24). Normally in eukaryotic translation, the presence of such features will inhibit ribosome scanning unless there is an IRES (see Chapter 18) or the ribosomes can bypass or "shunt" around the sORFs and structured region. Expression studies with appropriate reporter gene constructs in protoplasts and transgenic plants first suggested that ribosome shunting is the mechanism by which translation is initiated on the first ORF (VII) in the CaMV 35S RNA (see Fig. 24). Of the six sORFs shown within the 35S RNA leader in Figure 24, A to D are only 2 to 8 codons each, but E and F are 26 and 33 codons, respectively. Transient expression studies first showed that some regions of the 35S leader are more inhibitory to translation than other regions or the intact 600-nt leader. In particular, the very short sORFs A to D do not inhibit translation of a downstream reporter gene, but E and F are strongly inhibitory to translation of ORF VII or a downstream reporter gene. Insertion of a stable stem-loop structure near the cap or within a duplication of the first 60 nt of the leader inhibits translation, but insertion of the stem-loop or the GUS coding sequence in the middle of the leader does not. That this is not a linear process was shown by expressing the capped 5′ half of the leader and the 3′ half fused to a CAT reporter gene as two distinct molecules in protoplasts: CAT was expressed only when both transcripts were expressed in the same cell. These studies suggested that ribosomes initiate translation on the 35S RNA by cap-dependent scanning, but can bypass or shunt around the central region of the leader. By inserting AUGs at different positions within the leader, the shunt donor site was located in the first 100 nt of the

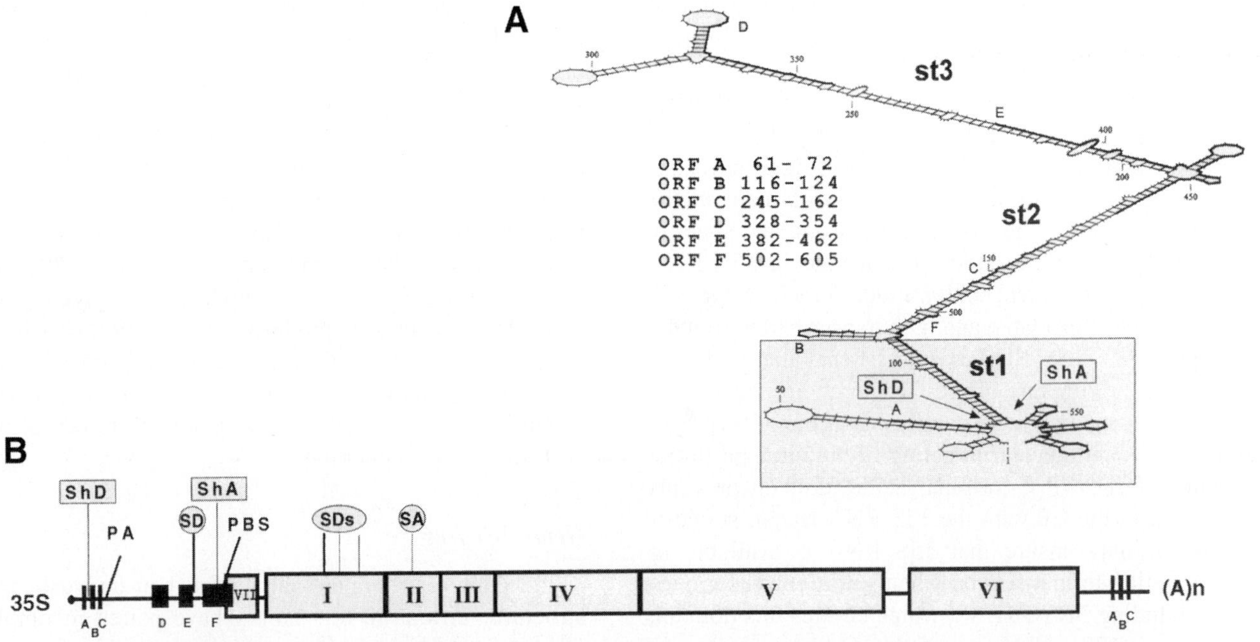

FIG. 24. A: Extensive secondary structure of the CaMV 35S RNA leader. Shunt donor (*ShD*) and Shunt acceptor (*ShA*) sites and stems (*st*) are indicated. **B:** CaMV 35S RNA. *Black boxes* represent small open reading frames. (From ref. 84, with permission.)

leader, past the termination codon of sORF A, and the shunt acceptor site was mapped to within sORF F (111,113). The development of an *in vitro* wheat germ translation system in which ribosome shunting can occur has led to a more detailed examination of the shunting mechanism (308). In particular, insertion of the leader between the coding sequences for GUS upstream and CAT downstream prevents expression of CAT activity, clearly showing that an IRES is not present within the leader sequence. By constructing an in-frame fusion of sORF F with the CAT coding sequence, the relative rates of scanning through the leader (translation of the longer F:CAT fusion protein) and shunting (translation of the shorter CAT protein) could be determined, and mutational studies showed that the structure of stem 1 (see *st1,* Fig. 24) is important for shunting to occur. Mutations that abolish stem 1 drastically reduce CAT expression, and compensatory mutations that restore stem 1 structure restore CAT expression. In fact, stem 1 and flanking sequences alone will allow shunting, and sORF A preceding stem 1 enhances shunting (84).

The importance of sORF A was further shown by constructing viruses with mutations that eliminated the various sORFs or structures within the leader. Viable mutants were obtained that were very delayed in the time of appearance of symptoms. Serial mechanical passage of these in turnip plants produced phenotypic revertants that resembled wild-type CaMV in their disease production. Analysis of these showed that sORF A and secondary structure within the central region of the leader are important for viral infectivity and thus presumably ribosome shunting (266). Further investigation of ribosome shunting by *in vitro* translation in reticulocyte as well as wheat germ extracts and expression of reporter constructs in plant protoplasts showed that proper translation and termination of a short upstream ORF is required for shunting to occur and that TAV increases shunting efficiency (137,267,295). Thus, the shunt-mediated translation appears to require reinitiation, which can be facilitated in the presence of TAV. As to the mechanism of ribosome shunting, a model has been proposed in which scanning 40S subunits and 80S ribosomes translating through sORF A stall when they encounter the stable hairpin structure. Proper termination of translation of sORF A by the 80S ribosomes promotes reinitiation, such that on release of the encoded peptide and dissociation of the 60S subunit, the reinitiation-competent 40S subunit skips over the stem and resumes scanning downstream (137). Why have this elongated 480-nt hairpin in the middle of the leader in the first place, necessitating ribosome shunting at all? Yeast three-hybrid studies show that CP specifically interacts with a purine-rich sequence at the top of this elongated hairpin (128). Thus, ribosome shunting ensures, in the context of this structure, that translation of the 35S RNA and its encapsidation as a template for reverse transcription of the viral dsDNA can both occur.

CaMV replicates by reverse transcription of the 35S RNA. Unlike retroviruses, and more similar to hepadnaviruses, the CaMV dsDNA is packaged into virions, and it does not integrate into host chromosome during normal multiplication. Rather, it exists as autonomously replicating circular minichromosomes in the nuclei of infected cells. However, the mechanism of reverse transcription is more similar in several respects to that of the retroviruses (see Chapter 27) than the hepadnaviruses. Reverse transcription occurs in the cytoplasm. Yeast three-hybrid studies show that the zinc finger motif (C-X_2-C-X_4-H-X_4-C) and an adjacent basic domain in the central region of CP are essential for strong and specific interaction with the purine-rich sequence in 35S RNA leader. This is consistent with a model in which the 35S RNA is first encapsidated and then transcribed within the virus particle (128). Studies suggest that the acidic C- and N-terminal regions of pre-CP, which are cleaved by the viral PR, may regulate packaging of the 35S (pregenomic) RNA and nuclear targeting of the virus particles. Presence of the CP C-terminal acidic domain prevents interaction of the CP with the 35S RNA leader, suggesting that it may ensure that 35S RNA is available as mRNA until late in infection when sufficient virion proteins, including PR (ORF V), which cleaves this domain, are present (128). Cleavage of this C-terminal domain would allow CP binding to and encapsidation of 35S RNA, presumably together with bound RT. Like retroviruses, reverse transcription is initiated from a tRNA primer ($tRNA_{met}$), which binds to a primer binding site on the 35S RNA at a position ~600 nt downstream of the 35S promoter, which is ~400 nt downstream of the end of the first terminal repeat at the 5′ end of the 35S RNA. Synthesis of the complementary DNA negative strand proceeds to the end of the 35S RNA, where the template switch occurs as the 3′ end of this newly synthesized negative strand DNA melts from the 5′ end of the 35S RNA template and anneals to the terminal repeat at the 3′ end of the same or another 35S RNA. Synthesis of the DNA negative strand continues along the 35S RNA, passing the primer binding site and the 5′ end of the of the molecule (overshooting) to create the 8-nt discontinuity or terminal repeat at the ends of the negative strand DNA. As this proceeds, regions of the RNA template that have been reverse transcribed are digested by RNase H, except for oligo(G) stretches—two for the genome shown in Figure 22—which are resistant and serve as primers for DNA positive strand synthesis. Again, the polymerase will overshoot, creating the two discontinuities or short terminal redundancies in the viral positive strand DNA (27, 262) (see Fig. 22). Encapsidation of the 35S RNA and reverse transcription within the virus particles appear to occur within the TAV inclusion bodies, and it has been suggested that the TAV matrix may provide accessory scaffolding or chaperone functions important in virus assembly. At this point, the virus particles with their dsDNA can either target back to the nucleus, contributing to the transcription pool, or move from cell to cell, apparently through the plasmodesmal-associated tubules that contain the viral MP (see Fig. 23). The fully processed virus CP contains an N-terminal NLS, which is exposed on the surface of virus particles but is masked if the N-terminal acidic domain of pre-CP is present. Thus, the presence of the N-terminal acidic domain keeps pre-CP in the cytoplasm, where it can be targeted to inclusion bodies for virus assembly. Once particles are assembled, cleavage of this domain by the viral PR exposes the CP NLS, and the virus particle can be transported to the nucleus (201). The CP is also phosphorylated by a host casein kinase II, which apparently stabilizes it (201), and it has been reported to be methylated and glycosylated. Not addressed by this model is the question of whether the presence of the N-terminal acidic domain of pre-CP or other CP modifications may play a role in the virus particles being directed to move from cell to cell or bind ATF for aphid acquisition.

Geminiviruses

The *Geminiviridae* are named for their unusual capsid structure. Virions in this family have paired incomplete (T=1) icosahedral capsids (gemini = twin moons), ~18 × 30 nm, composed of subunits of a single CP (29 kd) (Fig. 25). The viral genomes are covalently closed circular ssDNA (~2.5 to 3.0 kb), with a single ssDNA molecule encapsidated in each geminate particle (193). *Geminiviridae* comprise three genera based on genome organization, vector specificity, and host range properties (Fig. 26). Mastreviruses (type member, maize streak virus [MSV]) have a single genomic component of ssDNA, are transmitted by different leafhopper species and, with two exceptions (bean yellow dwarf virus [BYDV] and tomato yellow dwarf virus [TYDV]), infect monocotyledonous plants. Begomoviruses (type member, bean golden mosaic virus) are transmitted by whiteflies (*Bemicia tabaci,* A and B biotypes), infect dicotyledonous plants and, with a few exceptions (e.g., some isolates of tomato yellow leaf curl virus [TYLCV]), have two distinct genomic components (A and B) that are both required for

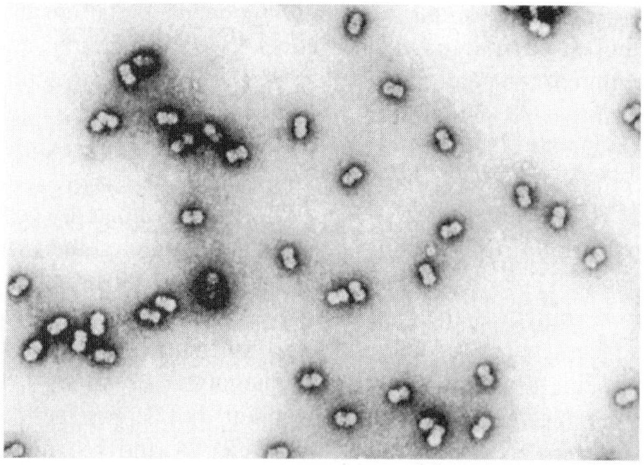

FIG. 25. Electron micrograph of virions of bean golden mosaic virus, a begomovirus. (From ref. 5, with permission.)

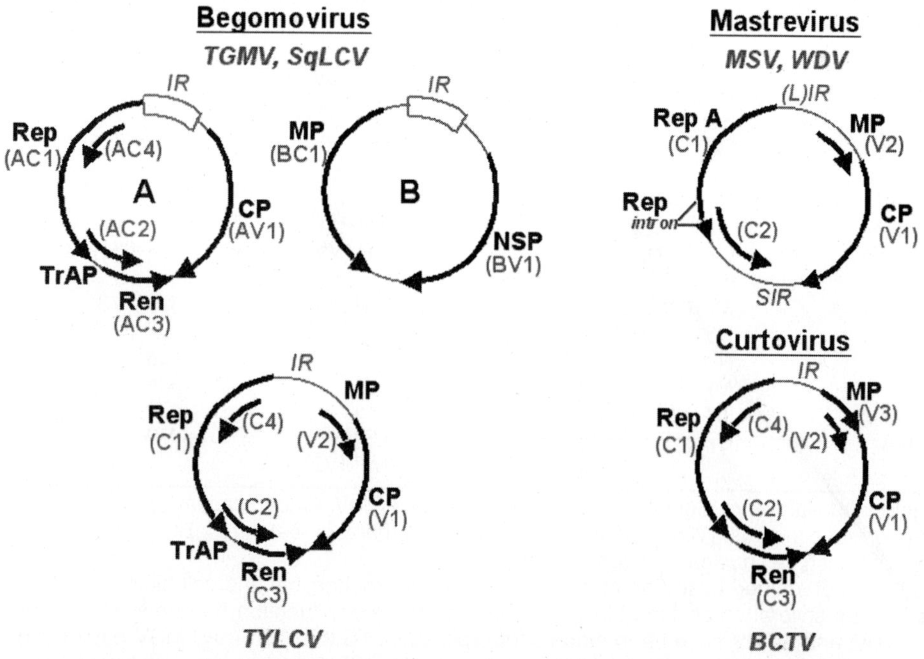

FIG. 26. Genome organization of different genera in the *Geminiviridae.*

infectivity and separately encapsidated. TYLCV has a single genomic component that is similar in its overall organization and sequence of the CP to the A component of the begomoviruses. Curtoviruses (type member, beet *curly top* virus [BCTV]), like mastreviruses, are transmitted by leafhopper species (except for tomato pseudo-curly top virus, which is transmitted by planthoppers) and have a single genomic component, the organization of which looks like a hybrid of the mastrevirus virion-sense (V) ORFs and the begomovirus complementary-sense (C) ORFs (see Fig. 26). Like the begomoviruses, curtoviruses infect dicotyledonous plants (34). With the notable exception of BCTV, individual *Geminiviridae* have narrow host ranges. Nevertheless, they have emerged in recent years as one of the most serious groups of plant viral pathogens worldwide because of the widespread expansion of the B biotype of *B. tabaci* and the ability of viruses in mixed infection to give rise to new strains and isolates through recombination (141,150).

Viral genes are transcribed bidirectionally from an intergenic region (IR), named the *long intergenic region* (LIR) in mastreviruses (see Fig. 26). Genome sequences for several begomoviruses first showed that this 200-nt IR was identical in the A and B components, and thus it has been called the *common region* in these bipartite viruses (193). The encapsidated ssDNA is the virion-sense positive strand. Viral ORFs were traditionally named based on their being encoded on the virion-sense (V) strand or the complementary-sense (C) strand, which for some viruses were referred to as the *rightward* (R) or *leftward* (L) transcribed ORFs (see *arrows* in Fig. 26). For example, AC1 and AL1 referred to the same ORF. Adding to this confusion, ORFs with the same name did not always encode the same function. Thus, CP was encoded by the AV1 or AR1 ORF in begomoviruses, but by ORF V2 in MSV. The nomenclature in Figure 26 represents an emerging consensus for naming the viral ORFs. For clarity, individual gene functions, when known, will be referred to. These are summarized in Table 5 for the different virus groups, based on mutational and infectivity studies, transient expression assays in protoplasts, and cell-based assays in infected and transgenic plants.

The bipartite begomoviruses, such as TGMV, ACMV, and squash leaf curl virus (SqLCV), encode proteins needed for replication (Rep, Ren), transcriptional regulation (TrAP), and encapsidation (CP) on their A component, and two essential movement proteins (MP and NSP) on the B component (see Fig. 26 and Table 5). In some begomoviruses, there is an additional ORF, *AC4,* which for TGMV has been reported to repress transcription of *AL1* weakly in transient expression assays in plant protoplasts. However, mutational studies of TGMV show that *AC4* is dispensable for virus infection (94,127,269). Mutational and transient expression studies show that Rep (replication initiation) is essential for virus replication. Ren (replication enhancer) is not essential for replication, but it interacts with Rep to increase the efficiency of viral replication (97,312,333). Using appropriate GUS reporter gene constructs in transiently expressing plant protoplasts, TGMV TrAP (transcriptional activator protein) has been shown to activate transcription of the V genes encoding CP and NSP on the A and B component, respectively. TrAP binds ssDNA in a sequence-nonspecific manner,

TABLE 5. *Geminivirus gene function*

Function	Begomovirus[a] TGMV, SqLCV, ACMV	Begomovirus[a] TYLCV	Curtovirus[a]	Mastrevirus[a]
Replication	Rep (AL1, AC1) Ren (AL3, AC3)	Rep (C1) Ren (C3)	Rep (C1) Ren (C3)	Rep (C1:2) Rep A (C1)
Transcription				
Repress Rep	Rep (AL1, AC1), (AL4, AC4)			
Activate late (V) genes	TrAP (AL2, AC2)	TrAP (C2)		Rep A (C1)
Encapsidation and Insect Transmission	CP (AR1, AV1)	CP (V1)	CP (V1)	CP (V1)
Movement	MP (BL1, BC1) NSP (BR1,BV1)	MP (V2) CP (V1)	MP (V3) CP (V1)	MP (V2) CP (V1)
Host activation[b]	Rep (AL1, AC1)		C4	Rep A
Symptoms	MP (BL1, BC1)	C4	C4	MP (V2)
Suppress host defenses	TrAP (AL2, AC2)		C2	
Regulate viral ssDNA accumulation	CP (AR1, AV1)	CP (V1) MP (V2)	V2	CP (V1)

TGMV, tomato golden mosaic virus; SqLCV, squash leaf curl virus; ACMV, African cassava mosaic virus; TYLCV, tomato yellow leaf curl virus; WDV, wheat dwarf virus; MSV, maize streak virus; BCTV, beet curly top virus; PCNA, proliferating cell nuclear antigen

[a]Functions have been determined based on mutational, infectivity, biochemical and cell biological studies with these, as well as several other, bipartite geminiviruses. Not every function has been shown for each virus. TGMV, WDV, and ACMV have been models for replication. TGMV, WDV, and MSV have been models for transcription. SqLCV has been a model for virus movement. BCTV has been a model curtovirus. See recent reviews for additional details and references 34, 130, 132, and 194.

[b]Activation of PCNA transcription, initiation of cell division, and/or bind Rb based on studies with TGMV, BCTV, WDV.

and only weakly binds dsDNA (133,246, 330). The biochemical properties of TGMV TrAP expressed from a baculovirus vector in insect cells have been studied. TrAP is a phosphoprotein that binds and requires zinc for optimal interactions with ssDNA. The highly acidic C-terminal domain of TrAP acts as a transcriptional activator. When fused to the DNA binding domain of the yeast transcriptional activator GAL4, it specifically activates expression of a *CAT* reporter gene driven by a minimal adenovirus E1B promoter with GAL4 binding sites in mouse cells, or of an *E. coli lacZ* gene expressed from the GAL1 promoter in yeast (133). Thus, it has been suggested that TrAP, like adenovirus E1A (289R) or herpes simplex virus VP16, may act as a transcriptional coactivator, interacting with cellular transcription factors bound to sequence-specific promoter elements to cooperatively recruit the basal transcription machinery. Transcriptional regulation by TrAP is complicated. Analysis of the expression of GUS reporter gene constructs in transgenic plants shows that TrAP activates transcription of the CP promoter in mesophyll cells but derepresses the expression of this promoter in phloem cells (331). CP is required for encapsidation, and studies in which the CP of the curtovirus BCTV was substituted for that of the begomovirus ACMV showed that CP is required for insect acquisition and transmission (31) (see Plant-to-Plant Transmission). The B component encodes two movement proteins because, like most animal DNA viruses, geminiviruses replicate in the nucleus. Thus, NSP and MP are required to cooperate in moving the viral genome across the nuclear envelope, through the cytoplasm, and across the cell wall. Studies with SqLCV show that NSP is a *n*uclear *s*huttle *p*rotein that binds viral ssDNA and transports it between the nucleus and cytoplasm. Like many other rapidly shuttling nuclear proteins, including HIV Rev and adenovirus E1B-55 kd and E4-34 kd, SqLCV NSP contains nuclear localization signals and a leucine-rich nuclear export signal (NES). MP traps NSP-genome complexes in the cytoplasm and, analogous to the MPs encoded by the RNA viruses discussed in this chapter, acts to move these across the cell wall through what appear to be modified plasmodesmata (194). The bipartite begomovirus CP is not required for systemic infection of natural hosts. Mutational and functional studies for TYLCV, including the finding that TYLCV can complement a TGMV TrAP mutant in tobacco protoplasts, suggest that each of the ORFs on its single genomic component encodes functions analogous to the bipartite virus A component (133,164,246,247,370), except for the extra *V2* (MP) ORF and perhaps *C4* (see Fig. 26). Mutational studies suggest that *V2* may encode the MP, and in contrast to the bipartite begomoviruses, CP is also needed for viral movement. *C4* affects TYLCV infection, depending on the host, showing that it is does not encode an essential movement protein. It appears to play a role in the development of symptoms (163,370).

Mastreviruses, such as MSV and wheat dwarf virus (WDV), while having a distinct genome organization from the begomoviruses, encode proteins that carry out analogous functions in viral replication (Rep), transcriptional activation (Rep A and/or Rep), movement (MP), and encapsidation and insect transmission (CP) (see Fig. 26 and Table 5). One major distinction from the begomoviruses is the processing of viral transcripts. All geminiviral genomes are bidirectionally transcribed to produce mRNAs that are polyadenylated and are likely to be capped; and all of the viral promoters are in the IR (LIR), except those for *TrAP* and *Ren,* and perhaps *AC4,* in begomoviruses. For the TGMV A and B components, a single unspliced V-sense transcript is translated into CP or NSP. The pattern of C-sense transcripts is complicated, but only TrAP and Ren appear to be translated from a bicistronic mRNA, and none of the transcripts is spliced (34,132). In contrast, splicing is essential in MSV and WDV. Rep, which is essential for viral replication, is translated from a spliced transcript that fuses ORFs C1 and C2 (306,377) (see Fig. 26). The corresponding unspliced transcript is translated into Rep A (C1), which shares ~200 N-terminal residues with Rep and alone, or together with Rep, activates expression of the V-encoded genes (45,53,142). This is analogous to the role of TrAP in activating *CP* and *NSP* transcription, although the mechanisms may not be identical. For WDV, only a single V-sense transcript has been detected that would be translated into MP and CP, but how CP is translated is not known. In MSV, there are two V-sense transcripts that initiate either 1 or 142 nt upstream of the MP coding sequence. Both of these are spliced within the MP coding sequence. It appears that MSV CP is translated from an abundant spliced form of the former (shorter) transcript, and MP is translated from a low abundance unspliced form of the latter with a 142 nt leader sequence (377). Mutational studies show that both MSV MP and CP are needed for systemic infection (28,195), and transient expression studies in plant protoplasts or plants biolistically bombarded with a GFP:MP fusion suggest that MSV MP has an analogous function to MP in the bipartite begomoviruses, but CP carries out the nuclear shuttling role of NSP (185,209). MSV MP is predicted to have a transmembrane domain, making it quite distinct from the bipartite virus MP. The curtovirus BCTV, like the mastreviruses, produces several V-sense transcripts, consistent with its complex genome organization (see Fig. 26). Based on mutational and transient expression studies, BCTV Rep (C1), Ren (C3), and CP (V1) are analogous to these same proteins in begomoviruses or mastreviruses (148,149,324). Like the mastreviruses, BCTV MP (V3) and CP (V1) are both required for systemic infection and thus may perform analogous roles to the SqLCV MP and NSP, or the MSV MP and CP, respectively. BCTV C2 is not analogous to TrAP in that it is not a transcriptional activator. However, both BCTV C2 and TrAP may play a similar role in counteracting host defenses against infection (149,356) (see Plant Responses to Virus Infection). C4 appears to induce cell division in BCTV-infected vascular cells and could function in inducing cells into S phase, as does Rep (189). V2 is unique to the curtoviruses and has been reported to be involved in regulating viral ssDNA accumulation (324).

Following introduction by the vector, how the viral genome is uncoated and delivered to the nucleus is not known. The identification of viral circular dsDNA as well as genomic ssDNA in infected plants was the first indication that the viral genome replicates through a dsDNA intermediate, as one might expect (Fig. 27). Since virion ssDNA is infectious, it appears that the dsDNA replicative form is synthesized from the incoming viral ssDNA genome (the positive strand) by host DNA replication enzymes, with cellular DNA polymerase α-primase complex also synthesizing the primer for synthesis of the complementary DNA strand. In the mastreviruses, such a primer—a ~75-to-80 nt oligodeoxyribonucleotide that contains several ribonucleotides at its 5′ end—is found bound to the viral genome within the *small intergenic region* (SIR) in virions (see Fig. 26). This serves as a primer for synthesis of the viral complementary DNA strand *in vitro* (34,193). Such a primer is not present in virion ssDNA of begomoviruses or curtoviruses, suggesting that it would have to be synthesized by host enzymes upon infection. Studies of ACMV replication intermediates suggest that such an RNA primer may be synthesized within the IR (302). As shown in Figure 27 for the begomoviruses, geminivirus multiplication involves the same nucleocytoplasmic trafficking of viral mRNAs and proteins, and the same temporal regulation of viral gene expression, as the multiplication of nuclear-replicating animal DNA viruses. It is assumed that host RNA pol II complexes transcribe the viral dsDNA template into viral mRNAs. These are then transported to the cytoplasm, where they are translated. The C-sense genes (*Rep, TrAP, Ren, MP,* and *C4,* if present) are transcribed first. With the exception of the plant virus–specific MP, these correspond to the early genes found in DNA animal viruses and phage, encoding nonstructural proteins for regulating viral gene expression and initiating viral DNA replication. Trap, Rep and Ren are transported to the nucleus, where Rep and Ren initiate synthesis of viral genomic ssDNA by rolling circle replication, apparently in much the same way as the ssDNA phage ϕX174 (see Chapter 17) (301,326). Probably early in infection, the newly synthesized viral ssDNA positive strands are copied to make additional dsDNA templates for transcription. TrAP (Rep A, Rep, or both, in mastreviruses) will activate transcription of the *CP* and *NSP* (late) genes, and as Rep accumulates, it will repress its own transcription (147,332). CP and NSP are synthesized in the cytoplasm and transported to the nucleus. Studies with SqLCV suggest that initially, CP sequesters genomic ssDNA away from the viral dsDNA replication pool without encapsidating it, to make it available for NSP binding (278). NSP–genome complexes are exported to the cytoplasm, where MP will trap them and move them across the cell wall. As CP accumu-

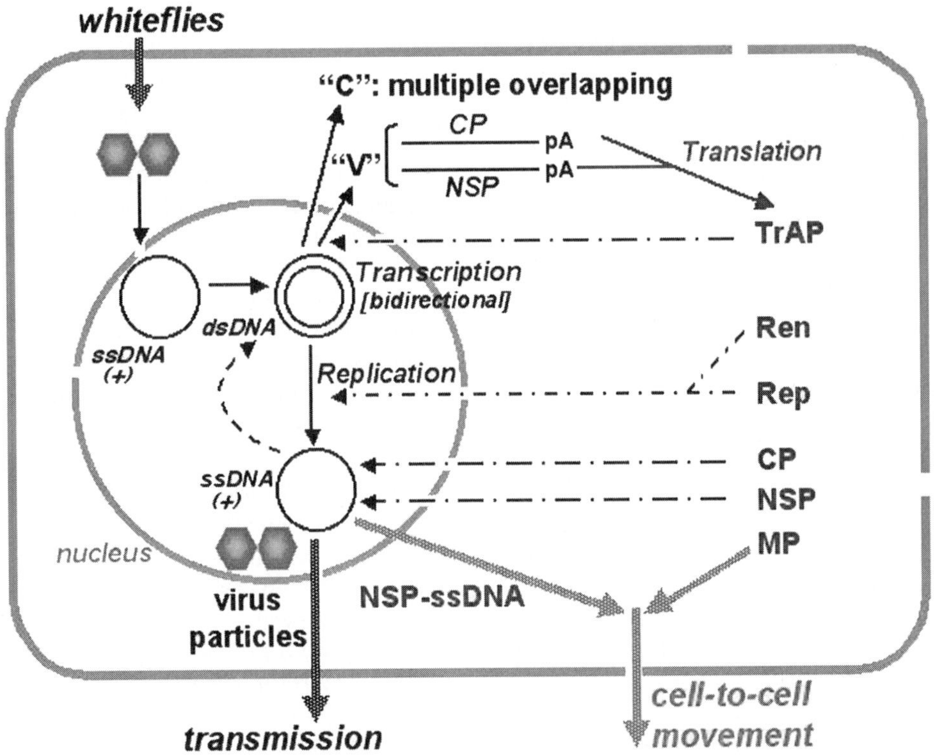

FIG. 27. Multiplication of begomoviruses.

lates, virus particles will be assembled in the nucleus (34,193). In mastreviruses, and perhaps curtoviruses, CP appears to serve a dual role of exporting newly replicated viral ssDNA genomes to the cytoplasm for movement by MP and encapsidating these into virions within the nucleus for insect transmission (185,209).

The sequence identity of the IRs (common regions) in the A and B components of the bipartite begomoviruses such as TGMV and ACMV first suggested that the viral replication origin was located within this region. This was further reinforced by the fact that the IR (or LIR) in all geminiviruses contains a potential stem-loop structure with a conserved nonanucleotide sequence in the loop, 5′-TAATATTAC-3′, which resembles the origin for positive strand synthesis in ϕX174 and bacterial plasmids that replicate by a rolling circle mechanism. Two approaches first showed that geminiviruses replicate by this mode. Two-dimensional gel electrophoresis of extracts from ACMV-infected plants identified the expected DNA intermediates for rolling circle replication (301). In separate studies, plants were inoculated with plasmids that contained heterodimers of WDV or ACMV, or the genomes of two strains of BCTV cloned as tandem direct repeats in the two possible combinations. In the BCTV studies, two predominant types of progeny genomes were recovered, depending on the order in which the two BCTV strains were cloned, and the sequences of these progeny were consistent with rolling circle replication initiating within the conserved stem-loop structure in the IR (326). The same conclusion was drawn in the WDV and ACMV studies (139,323), and the latter mapped the initiation site for viral positive strand ssDNA synthesis to the conserved nonanucleotide sequence TAATATT↓AC. *In vitro* biochemical studies show that Rep from WDV, TYLCV, and TGMV is an endonuclease that nicks virion sense ssDNA at this same position (140, 191,255). Further biochemical characterization of WDV and TYLCV Rep using appropriately end-labeled ssDNA substrates show that Rep is also a ligase, capable of catalyzing a strand transfer reaction following cleavage at the viral replication origin *in vitro*. The reaction intermediate is Rep covalently linked to the 5′-end of the cleaved DNA through a phosphodiester bond to tyrosine-103, which identifies this residue as the one mediating DNA cleavage (140, 190,191). Thus, analogous to ϕX174 rolling circle replication, these studies suggest that Rep nicks the viral origin in the positive strand of the dsDNA to initiate replication and remains bound to the 5′ end of the nicked strand as a new virion-sense ssDNA is copied from the complementary strand, presumably by host DNA replication complexes. Rep is also the terminase, with its endonuclease and ligase activities resolving the nascent virion ssDNA into genome-length units and reinitiating synthesis of a new ssDNA positive strand after each round of rolling circle replication. Although TYLCV and TGMV Rep have ATPase activity *in vitro*, this activity is not DNA dependent, and Rep has only weak homology to consensus helicase motifs.

The conserved potential stem-loop structure containing the invariant nonanucleotide sequence is essential for replication (197,255) and the only element common to the positive strand origins of geminiviruses. However, geminivirus replication origins are, in general, virus specific, a consequence at least in part of Rep being a sequence-specific dsDNA binding protein. The TGMV Rep binding site is a 13-bp element that contains two pentanucleotide repeats (*underlined*): 5′-GGTAGTAATAG-GTAG-3′. It is located upstream of the conserved potential stem-loop, between the TATA box and transcriptional start site for Rep mRNA, and Rep binding to this motif also represses Rep transcription (reviewed in 132). Related but not identical elements located in a similar position are also found in the IR of curtoviruses and other begomoviruses, and the Rep binding site is necessary, but not sufficient, for virus-specific origin recognition in these viruses (51,104). The Rep binding site and a palindromic AG motif, located between the binding site and conserved potential stem-loop, are also essential for origin function in TGMV, (132). Mutations in the TATA box of the Rep promoter, a G box motif, and a CA motif decrease the efficiency of TGMV replication, but whether the contribution of these sequences involves binding of transcription factors or other host factors has not been determined (254). TGMV appears to bind DNA as a dimer but exists in solution as an octamer.

The modular structure of the geminivirus positive strand replication origin is also evident in studies of WDV, although there are multiple rather than a single Rep-binding site (consensus: GTGTGA$N_{22\text{-}23}$GTG(G)TC) (130). A detailed study of WDV Rep binding to its own LIR using gel-shift assays, electron microscopy, and DNase footprinting identifies three distinct Rep-DNA complexes: two high-affinity complexes located in the regions of the two divergent TATA boxes for C-sense and V-sense transcription (see Fig. 26), and a low-affinity complex that assembles in the region containing the conserved stem-loop under conditions supporting site-specific cleavage of the invariant sequence TAATATT↓AC (45). The WDV stem-loop would form a dsDNA region containing the sequence GTGG(T)GG, and it is proposed that this half binding site directs formation of the low-affinity complex, which would be capable of producing the sequence-specific cleavage within the loop. It is also proposed that the high-affinity complexes in the regions of the V-sense and C-sense TATA boxes may function, respectively, in up-regulation of V-sense transcription and repression of C-sense transcription, although the latter has not been shown to be a property of mastrevirus Rep. The latter high-affinity complex is essential for origin activity, suggesting that a Rep oligomeric complex formed at this site could also contact the low-affinity site, thus bending the DNA and positioning the Rep complex to initiate replication by site-specific nicking of the positive strand (45). A similar bent structure has been proposed for TGMV Rep, mediated by Rep–Ren interactions (132). The DNA binding domain is present in both WDV Rep and Rep A. Thus, an interesting possibility is that Rep A–Rep hetero-oligomers, as well as homo-oligomers of each protein, have the potential to finely regulate different aspects of viral replication and transcription. The involvement of cellular proteins in any or all of these interactions is one area yet to be explored. The situation described for WDV Rep interacting with the LIR resembles in a number of respects that of SV40 large T interacting with the viral origin region (see Chapter 29).

A problem that geminiviruses have in common with the majority of animal DNA viruses is that fully differentiated plant cells lack detectable levels of the DNA replication enzymes that the virus will need for its own replication. DNA replication and cell division in mature plants is restricted to meristems at the growing points of the plant, developing leaves and roots, and the cambium that gives rise to the vascular system. Infection by a number of geminiviruses, such as SqLCV, BCTV, and Abutilon mosaic virus (AbMV), is restricted to the phloem. Studies with SqLCV suggest that, in this situation, the virus replicates in actively dividing procambial cells (developing phloem cells) that will differentiate into phloem (369). Other geminiviruses, such as TGMV and MSV, can infect a variety of differentiated plant cells, and studies suggest that these viruses, similar to DNA animal viruses, may induce cells to synthesize S-phase replication enzymes by a number of possible mechanisms, but without necessarily inducing cell proliferation. Studies of TGMV-infected tobacco plants and of transgenic plants that express TGMV Rep showed that Rep induces synthesis of proliferating cell nuclear antigen (PCNA), the processivity factor for DNA polymerase δ (240), although the cells are not induced to divide. Whether this is a direct or indirect effect of Rep on PCNA transcription is not known. A common strategy of DNA animal viruses such as SV40, adenoviruses, and some human papillomaviruses, is to induce cells into S phase by encoding an immediate early or early protein with the consensus LXCXE motif that will bind to the pocket of the tumor suppressor Rb (and the related p107 and p130) to sequester Rb or target it for degradation (see Chapters 29 and 31). Plant proteins related to RB have been identified (termed *RBR*, for Rb-related protein). The Rep and Rep A of mastreviruses contain an LXCXE motif, and WDV Rep A (but not Rep) interacts with a plant RBR by means of this motif in yeast two-hybrid assays. The functional significance of this interaction is suggested by studies in wheat protoplasts. Mutation of the LXCXE motif in RepA/Rep complexes reduces the ability of WDV to replicate in these cells. Furthermore, wild-type WDV replication is reduced when these protoplasts are cotransfected with a plasmid that will produce high levels of either the maize RBR ZmRb1 or the human pocket protein p130 (381,382). TGMV Rep has also been reported to interact with a maize RBR in yeast two-hybrid studies, or using a GST pull-down assay to identify complexes when Rep is coexpressed with a GST:RBR fusion protein in insect cells (2). However, this TGMV Rep–RBR interaction appears to be about 10-fold weaker than that of SV40 large T with RBR (179). Begomovirus Rep proteins do not contain the pocket binding motif LXCXE. Deletion studies map the interaction domain in TGMV Rep to 80 residues that overlap the DNA cleavage/ligation, DNA binding, and oligomerization domains of Rep. These 80 residues have no homology to any known plant RBR binding proteins or any other proteins, except for begomovirus Rep proteins, suggesting that whatever the sequences involved in this RBR interaction, it is a novel or previously unrecognized motif (179). Additional studies should establish whether these Rep proteins directly interact with RBRs *in vitro*. To date, there is no evidence for direct interaction of WDV Rep or TGMV Rep with RBRs in plant cells, nor have the plant RBRs been shown to function in cell cycle control in plants as do Rb and other pocket domain proteins in mammalian cells. The geminiviruses are good models for investigating these aspects of cell cycle control, as well as regulation of DNA replication in plant cells.

VIRUS MOVEMENT

For virus infection to disseminate throughout the plant, the virus first moves from cell to cell within the inoculated leaf and enters the vascular system. For the majority of plant viruses, with the exception of phloem-restricted viruses like the luteoviruses and certain geminiviruses, this involves moving from infected mesophyll cells to bundle sheath cells, and from these into phloem parenchyma and/or companion cells, from which the virus will enter the sieve elements. From the sieve elements, the virus can infect additional sites within the inoculated leaf, as well as follow photoassimilate flow to move to distant leaves and systemically infect the plant (242) (see Fig. 5). Phloem-restricted viruses appear to move locally between companion cells, phloem parenchyma, and bundle sheath cells, and from leaf to leaf through the sieve elements. Some viruses also move from leaf to leaf through xylem. The study of plant virus-encoded MPs has revealed how viruses can alter plasmodesmata to move from cell to cell and enter phloem tissue. We understand less about how viruses enter into and exit from sieve elements or the xylem to systemically invade the plant.

Movement proteins do more than simply move the viral genome across the barrier of the plant cell wall. They coordinate replication of the viral genome with its directed movement within, as well as between, plant cells. In doing this, MPs use the cellular machinery for trafficking macromolecules. The final act of crossing the cell wall is preceded by a series of regulated events in which MPs interact not only with replicating viral genomes but also with the endomembrane system, the cytoskeletal network, and in the case of geminiviruses, the nuclear import and export machinery. Thus, the study of MP function in the past decade has been to a large extent an investigation of intracellular and intercellular transport in plants. Genetic studies have established that MPs are critical determinants of plant virus host range and pathogenic properties. Thus, as knowledge has been gained about MP function, this has also suggested new approaches for engineering virus-resistant plants.

Approaches to Investigating Virus Movement

A variety of approaches, each designed to address different questions, have been used to investigate MP function (reviewed in 43 and 194). Genetic studies identified the viral gene(s) encoding the MP(s) and defined the role of the MP(s) in infectivity, host range, and pathogenesis. MP null mutants were noninfectious in all host plants, but could replicate and assemble virions in protoplasts. Partially defective MP missense mutants, such as alanine-scanning mutants, could be altered in their host range phenotype, still infecting some host plants but not others, and produce attenuated symptoms. This role in pathogenesis was underscored by the finding that transgenic plants that expressed one of a number of viral MPs phenotypically resembled virus-infected plants. By inserting a *GUS* or *GFP* reporter gene into the viral genome, the precise stage at which virus infection was blocked could be determined. This approach identified the path followed by the virus in infecting a leaf and moving long distance from leaf to leaf, and the role of other proteins, such as CP, in affecting virus movement locally or systemically could also be examined (see Fig. 5). Immunogold labeling of systemically infected leaves or protoplasts, usually using antisera raised against MPs overexpressed from plasmids in *E. coli,* and subcellular fractionation of infected plant tissue provided information about MP function based on where the MP was found. In virus-infected or transgenic plants that expressed the MP, some MPs encoded by viruses like TMV or red clover necrotic mosaic virus (RCNMV; a dianthovirus) were localized to plasmodesmata that were not morphologically altered, and there was no evidence of virus particles being present. The MPs encoded by other viruses like CaMV and TSWV were localized to tubules that extended from what appeared to be altered plasmodesmata, and virus-like particles were associated with or within these tubules, consistent with a requirement for CP in cell-to-cell movement. For PVX, virus particles were associated with "swollen" plasmodesmata, but no tubules were present. Consistent with this association with plasmodesmata, most viral MPs (with the exception of SqLCV NSP) cofractionated with cell wall and plasma membrane fractions from infected or transgenic plants. The TMV 30-kd MP and SqLCV MP also cofractionated with ER membrane. Indirect immune fluorescence staining of plant protoplasts infected with the virus or expressing the viral MP and confocal microscopy further showed association of the TMV MP with microtubules, actin filaments, and ER membrane, and the SqLCV MP and NSP with ER membrane and nuclei, respectively. *In vitro* binding assays showed that a common property of most viral MPs was the ability to bind nucleic acids cooperatively and in a sequence-nonspecific manner, consistent with their role in moving the viral genome. Thus, as first shown for the TMV and RCNMV MPs, the MPs encoded by many positive-sense RNA viruses bound ssRNA and ssDNA *in vitro*. The begomovirus SqLCV NSP was shown to be an ssDNA binding protein. For viruses, such as TSWV, in which CP is also required for local cell-to-cell movement, the MP (NSm) has been shown to interact with the nucleocapsid protein (N).

The dynamics of MP function and the effects of MPs on plasmodesmata have been investigated using two basic approaches in plants and model studies in plant protoplasts. Dye-coupling studies in which fluorescently tagged dextrans of different sizes were microinjected into tobacco mesophyll cells of transgenic plants that expressed an MP, or co-injected with an *E. coli*–expressed MP into mesophyll cells in leaves of wild-type plants, were designed to test a particular property of MPs, namely their ability to affect the gating properties of plasmodesmata in the absence of virus infection (Fig. 28). By microinjecting fluorescently labeled MP, or unlabeled MP together with RNA or DNA fluorescently labeled with TOTO-1 iodide, the movement of the MP itself or its ability to move nucleic acids in *trans* could also be tested. As first shown for TMV and RCNMV, the ability to increase the size exclusion limits of plasmodesmata was a common feature of MPs encoded by a number of plant viruses, and the MPs could themselves move from cell to cell and facilitate movement of nucleic acids as well (110,361,376). Concerns about possible artifacts as the result of the high pressure microinjection techniques used in these studies, as well as the effects of posttranslational modifications (most, if not all, MPs are phosphorylated), led to the examination of GFP:MP fusion proteins expressed within mesophyll cells from plasmids that were introduced by biolistic bombardment, or expressed from a PVX vector (Fig. 29**A**), with generally the same results (156). A complication in all of these studies was the growing recognition that the gating properties of plasmodesmata were developmentally regulated and that large proteins could move between mesophyll cells at certain developmental stages (156,252). This, and mutational and subcellular fractionation studies that showed that MP expression and function were regulated during infection, led to investigations of mesophyll cells in plants, and plant protoplasts, infected with a virus that expressed either free GFP or a GFP:MP fusion protein (reviewed in 194). Using confocal microscopy, in combination with immunostaining for appropriate marker proteins, the TMV MP was shown to form specific associations with microtubules and microfilaments, as well as the ER, both in infected protoplasts and plants (134,218,224,284). Time course studies could be done in single protoplasts embedded in agarose, or in expanding local lesions on leaves inoculated with the GFP-expressing TMV, because the visibly expanding necrotic lesion and GFP allowed the precise identification of the infected

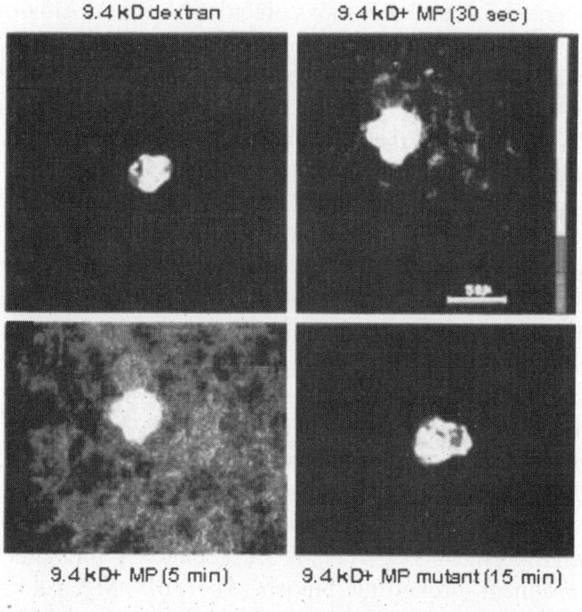

FIG. 28. Dye-coupling studies of red clover necrotic mosaic virus (RCNMV) movement protein (MP) co-injected with 9.4-kd fluorescently tagged dextran into tobacco mesophyll cells. The dextran, when injected alone or with a nonfunctional MP mutant protein, remains in the microinjected cell. When co-injected with wild-type MP, it rapidly moves to surrounding mesophyll cells, indicating that the plasmodesmal gating properties have be altered to allow the passage of larger molecules. (From ref. 110, with permission.)

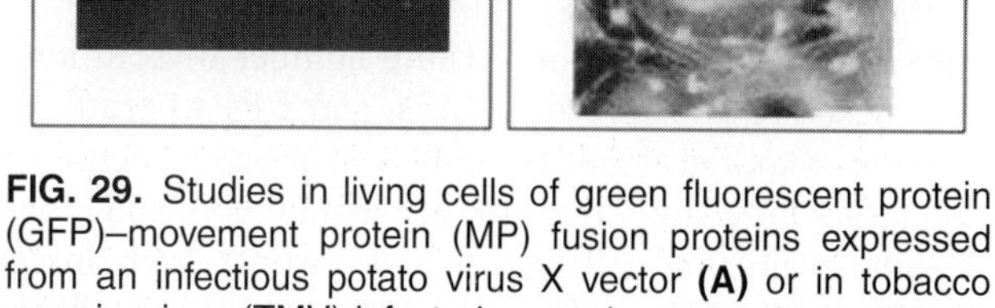

FIG. 29. Studies in living cells of green fluorescent protein (GFP)–movement protein (MP) fusion proteins expressed from an infectious potato virus X vector **(A)** or in tobacco mosaic virus (TMV)-infected protoplasts or plants **(B)**. (**A** courtesy of Dr. Karl Oparka, Scottish Crop Research Institute, Dundee; **B** from ref. 134, with permission.)

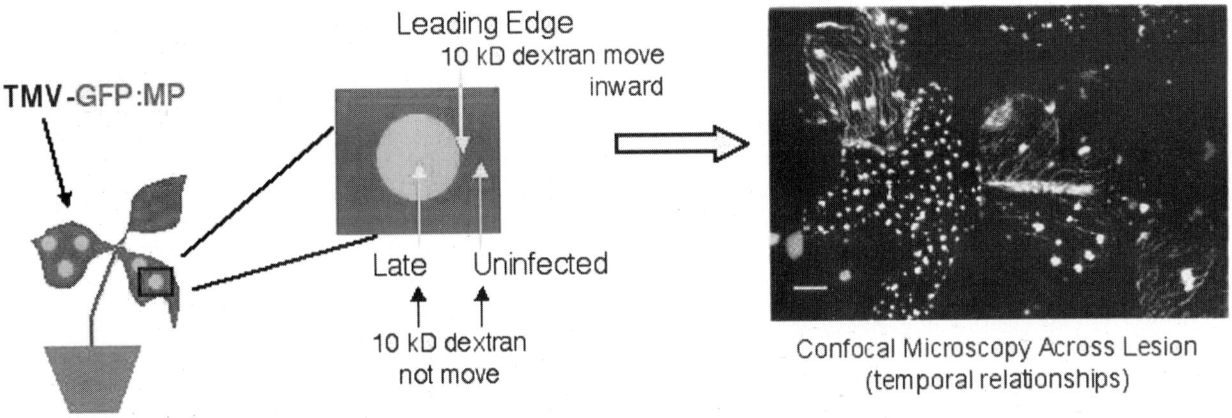

FIG. 30. Time course of tobacco mosaic virus (TMV) green fluorescent protein (GFP)–movement protein (MP) effects on plasmodesmal gating and associations with the cytoskeleton (microtubules and actin filaments) and endoplasmic reticulum (aggregates) in different cells within an expanding lesion. Because virus is moving outward from the center, cells at the leading edge are at early stages in infection, whereas those at the center are at late stages in infection. (Cartoon based on ref. 134, with permission; figure from Oparka KJ, Boevink P, Santa Cruz S. *Tr Plant Sci* 1996;1:412–418, with permission.)

cells visually and by confocal microscopy (134,218) (Fig. 30). These studies showed that MP function was regulated. MP did not move beyond the leading edge of the infection front, nor were the gating properties of plasmodesmata altered in cells beyond the expanding lesion, in contrast to the results of microinjection and bombardment studies. In addition, the size exclusion limits of plasmodesmata early in infection (leading edge of the lesion) were increased so that 10-kd dextrans would move from cell to cell, but these had returned to normal late in infection (center of lesion). The associations of the MP with the cytoskeleton and endomembrane system were also found to be temporally regulated, as the MP associated with replicated viral RNA at ER-membrane derived sites and moved the genomes along microtubules and actin filaments to plasmodesmata (134,251,284). Other aspects of the dynamics of movement and subcellular associations could also be studied in protoplasts expressing viral MPs. The MP encoded by TSWV, CaMV, and other viruses was shown to induce the formation of tubules in transfected protoplasts (reviewed in 194), and the nuclear shuttling of SqLCV NSP and its interactions with MP to redirect NSP to the periphery of the cell were also shown (298,368).

These studies demonstrate that whereas different viruses may solve the problem of moving the viral genome across the cell wall in a number of different ways, there appears to be a finite number of solutions, and these are not unrelated. MPs, and CPs where these are also required, identify replicated progeny genomes and target these away from the replication pool and along a path toward the cell wall that is distinct from insect transmission. MPs alter plasmodesmata to facilitate movement of the viral genome from cell to cell, sometimes morphologically altering them or affecting their formation as well as function. For a few MPs where it has been investigated, specific associations with ER have been reported. This may not be coincidental since the desmotubule at the center of a plasmodesmata is originally derived from the ER. Similarly, given that actin filaments have been shown to be involved in regulating plasmodesmal function, specific associations of MPs with the cytoskeletal network where these have been documented are probably not coincidental either. Although the same studies have not been done for all plants viruses, there are four well-developed models for the function of MPs encoded by different virus groups. As additional studies are done, these models will be refined, and a few more may be added.

Cell-to-Cell Movement

Studies of the TMV 30-kd protein established the paradigm for MP function, first showing that contrary to a then commonly held view, plasmodesmata were not just boring holes in the plant cell wall, but rather could be modified by a viral MP. This presented a more dynamic view of plasmodesmata than had been previously held (78). TMV represents the simplest case of a virus that needs only one MP and does not require CP for cell-to-cell movement (Fig. 31A). It does require CP for systemic movement through the phloem. The TMV MP has been more extensively characterized than other viral MPs in terms of its effects on the size exclusion limits of plasmodesmata and the details of its regulation and cellular interactions during virus infection (194). In addition to binding viral RNA, the MP interacts with the ER, microtubules, and actin filaments at different stages during the progression of TMV infection. Immune colocalization studies have also localized the TMV MP to sites of viral

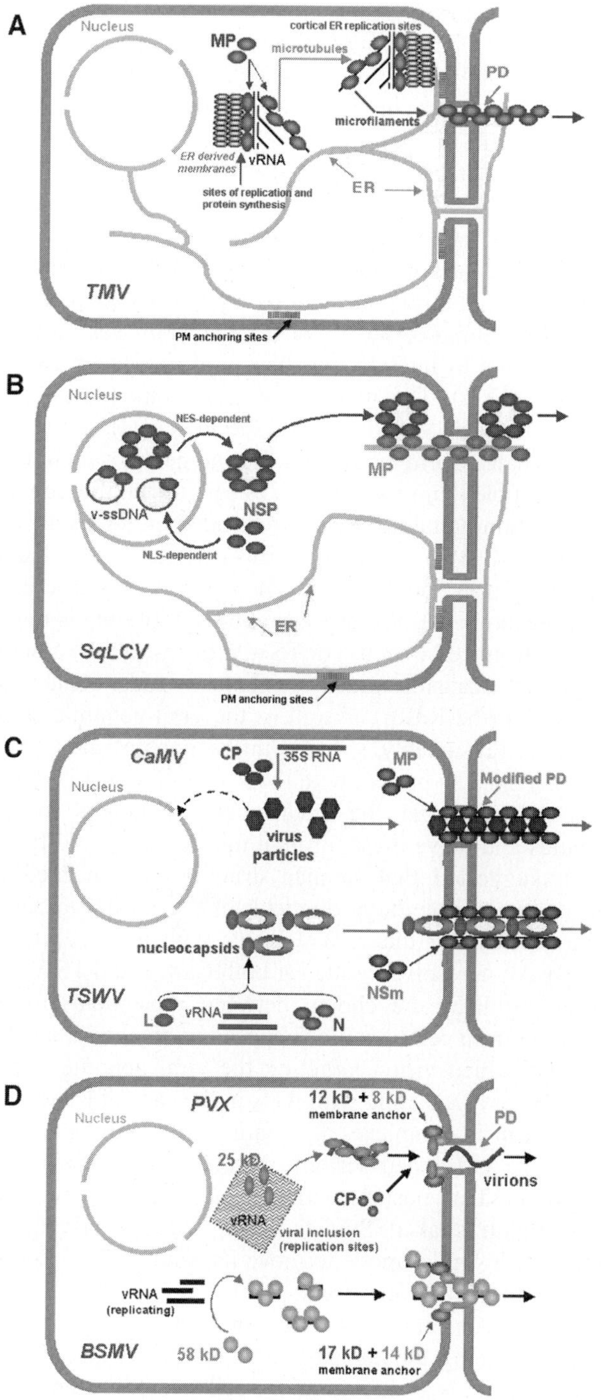

FIG. 31. Models for virus cell-to-cell movement. (**A**) TMV, (**B**) SqLCV, (**C**) CaMV and TSWV, where the MP forms tubules for the movement of encapsidated genomes, and (**D**) examples of triple gene block proteins for a virus that requires (PVX) or does not require (BSMV) CP for local movement. (Modified from ref. 194, with permission.)

replication (134,218). The model that has been proposed is that the TMV 30-kd MP binds to replicating viral genomic RNA at ER-anchored replication sites (so-called X bodies) and, at early stages, tracks these along microtubules to establish additional replication sites within the cell. It is suggested that this is the period during which the ER network is disrupted and forms aggregates. From replication sites established in the cortical region of the cell (the periphery), the MP bound to the viral genome is proposed to target it along actin microfilaments to plasmodesmata, where the MP acts to increase the size exclusion limits and move the viral genome into adjacent uninfected cells. The plasmodesmata do not appear to be altered morphologically, and studies suggest that the MP may act like a chaperone to extend the viral genome into a configuration that is compatible with passing through plasmodesmata. Mutational and expression studies show that TMV MP function is regulated in terms of both its synthesis and posttranslational modification. The TMV MP accumulates to high levels early in infection, after which it declines. This appears to be a common property of viral MPs: it has also been documented for other plant viral MPs, including SqLCV NSP and TSWV NSm (183,235,369). Mutational studies suggest that TMV MP function may be regulated by changes in its phosphorylation state (52,360). Temporal regulation of its activity is also evident from studies in expanding TMV lesions. Although the MP localizes to plasmodesmata at both early (leading edge) and late (lesion center) stages of infection, it acts to increase the size exclusion limits of infected cells in the early stage cells at the leading edge, and not at the center (251) (see Fig. 30). Recent studies suggest that the TMV MP interacts with a cell wall–associated pectin methylesterase, and mutational studies indicate that this interaction is important for TMV MP function (49).

The bipartite begomoviruses, such as SqLCV, encode two nonstructural movement proteins (NSP and MP) that are required for cell-to-cell movement and, like TMV, do not require CP for local movement. In contrast to TMV and many other plant viruses, these viruses also do not require CP to systemically infect their natural hosts, and it has been suggested that NSP–ssDNA genome complexes may be the form that moves long distance through the phloem, as well as from cell to cell (153,298). As already discussed, NSP and MP are both required to cooperate in moving the viral ssDNA genome from its site of replication in the nucleus, to and through the cytoplasm, and across the cell wall (see Fig. 31B). SqLCV is phloem limited, which is clearly shown by infecting plants with SqLCV engineered to express free GFP (196). Consistent with this, SqLCV NSP and MP are found only in phloem cells in systemically infected leaves, and it appears that SqLCV infects and replicates in procambial cells. In these immature phloem cells, immunogold labeling shows that MP is associated with unique tubules that extend from and cross the cell walls

(369). There are no virus-like particles associated with these tubules, consistent with CP not being needed for movement. These tubules, which are not found in normal uninfected cells, are also labeled with antisera against the ER lumenal binding protein BiP, suggesting that they are derived from the ER. Consistent with this, SqLCV MP cofractionates with ER membrane from infected plants. The cooperative interaction of NSP and MP has been studied using transient expression assays in tobacco protoplasts, where it was also shown that this interaction is regulated (297,298). When each protein is expressed alone, NSP localizes to the nucleus, and MP is found in the cortical cytoplasm at the cell periphery, apparently the consequence of its targeting to the cortical ER (194). However, when NSP is coexpressed with MP in the same cells, NSP is relocalized from the nucleus to the cortical cytoplasm, where it now colocalizes with MP. This interaction is regulated. At late times after cotransfection of these cells, NSP no longer interacts with MP, but rather is found in the perinuclear region of these cells, although MP remains in the cortical cytoplasm (296,298). The model that has been proposed is that NSP, as a nuclear shuttle protein, binds newly replicated viral ssDNA genomes in the nucleus and moves these between the nucleus and cytoplasm. MP, associated with ER-derived tubules, traps these complexes in the cytoplasm and directs them to and across the cell wall. In adjacent uninfected cells, the NSP–genome complex is released, which then targets the viral ssDNA genome to the perinuclear region and delivers it across nuclear pores to initiate a new round of replication (194). The apparent ER origin of the MP-associated tubules and the fact that SqLCV is replicating in actively dividing procambial cells have led to the suggestion that the tubules may be the analog of the desmotubule core of plasmodesmata. Thus, MP is proposed to associate with regions of ER that are destined to form desmotubule, perhaps altering plasmodesmata as they are being formed in the walls of these cells (369). The regulated interaction of NSP with MP, as observed in protoplasts, further suggests that NSP is posttranslationally modified as a consequence of interacting with MP, and it has been proposed that this may involve alterations in the phosphorylation of NSP.

Unlike TMV and SqLCV, TSWV, CaMV, as well as comoviruses and nepoviruses, require CP in addition to a dedicated MP for cell-to-cell movement. All of these viruses, like TMV, infect fully differentiated mesophyll cells. The MP encoded by each of these viruses has been immunolocalized in infected plants to large tubular structures that extend from what appear to be modified plasmodesmata that lack a central desmotubule (see Fig. 31C). These tubules characteristically extend from the walls of infected cells into neighboring cells and have virus-like particles associated with or within them (reviewed in 43 and 194). The role, if any, of cellular components in the formation of these tubular structures remains unknown. Studies that have been done do not show an association with ER, microtubules, or microfilaments. The tubular structures have been reported to form in plant protoplasts or insect cells that transiently express the MP of TSWV (NSm), CaMV (I), or cowpea mosaic virus. These studies show that the MP in each case is necessary and sufficient to induce the formation of these tubules, and neither CP, plasmodesmata, nor any unique plant cell factors are apparently required for this process. CP is required for the formation of the virus-like particles within the tubules (167). The TSWV NSm has recently been shown to interact with the viral nucleocapsid (N) protein (321a). The model that has been proposed, as shown for CaMV and TSWV (see Fig. 31C), is that an encapsidated form of the viral genome—a subviral or viral particle—moves from cell to cell guided through the MP-containing tubular structures and altered plasmodesmata. For CaMV, icosahedral virus particles assembled in the cytoplasm and containing newly reverse transcribed viral genomic dsDNA appear to be the form that is transported from cell to cell. For TSWV, this would be assembled nucleocapsids, which are flexuous rods, containing L protein (the RdRp) as well as the viral genomic components. Presumably, specific interactions of the CaMV CP or TSWV N protein with the MP within the tubules is required to target the encapsidated genomes to the tubules and move these through into the next cell. It has been suggested that tubular structures are needed to accommodate the large diameter of the CaMV icosahedral particles or the TSWV RNPs with their L protein (300). An unresolved issue for both CaMV and TSWV is what regulates the choice between movement of the genome from cell to cell as opposed to an alternate path: the assembled virion targeting the viral genome to the nucleus or associating with ATF, in the case of CaMV; or nucleocapsid complexes associating with Golgi stacks to assemble enveloped virions, in the case of TSWV. It might be that posttranslational modifications regulate which path is taken. Studies of TEV suggest that it, too, may use a similar mode to move its genome from cell to cell, with the CI cone structures that align with plasmodesmata performing a function similar to that of the large MP-containing tubular structures in CaMV and TSWV (42,293). CP is also required for cell-to-cell movement of TEV. Although it has not been determined whether the TEV genome is transported from cell to cell as virus particles or as a distinct RNA-CP complex, the finding that cell-to-cell movement requires an assembly-competent CP is consistent with virus particles being transported between cells (81,82).

Requiring CP for cell-to-cell movement does not necessarily require the formation of tubular structures. PVX requires CP, as well as the TGB-encoded proteins, for cell-to-cell movement but moves in the absence of any tubular structures. A number of distinct plant viruses encode an analogous set of essential TGB movement proteins, and it is intriguing that some of these, such as barley stripe mosaic virus (BSMV; a hordeivirus) do not require CP for cell-to-cell movement (192). In fact, like SqLCV, BSMV does not require CP for systemic infection of natural hosts. In the case of PVX, a viral mutant in which *GFP* replaced the *CP* gene was found to be confined to single inoculated cells, thus establishing the requirement for CP in cell-to-cell movement. Immune localization studies of infected plant cells and confocal imaging of plants inoculated with PVX that expressed a GFP:CP fusion show that CP localizes to plasmodesmata. Using a virion-specific antiserum, immune electron microscopy further identifies virions within the plasmodesmata of all PVX-infected cell types, leading to the conclusion that PVX virus particles move from cell to cell. However, dye-coupling studies using transgenic plants that express PVX CP show that CP does not affect the gating properties of plasmodesmata (253, 299,300). The PVX TGB-encoded 25-kd protein (25K) does affect plasmodesmal gating properties. This was first shown in dye-coupling studies in which PVX viruses that expressed a GUS reporter gene were microinjected into tobacco trichome cells these viruses remained confined to single cells when the 25K protein was not expressed, and only the smallest sized dextrans (4.4 kd as opposed to 10 kd) could now move out of the infected cells (14). However, in infected plant cells, the 25K protein localizes to viral inclusion bodies in the cytoplasm, whereas the TGB-encoded 8-kd (8K) protein localizes to the cell wall. It has been suggested that both the TGB 8-kd and 12-kd proteins may function as membrane anchors since they contain potential transmembrane domains and associate with membranes. In recent studies, plasmids that expressed the PVX 25K protein fused to GFP (GFP:25K) were introduced by biolistic bombardment into transgenic plants that expressed CP, or the TGB 8-kd or 12-kd proteins. The GFP:25K fusion moved from cell to cell in wild-type tobacco plants and tobacco plants that expressed either the 8K or 12K proteins, but it did not move in transgenic plants that expressed either CP or both the 8K and 12K proteins (383).

One model that is consistent with the data is shown in Figure 31D, although other models are possible. This model is based, in part, on the 25K protein binding RNA *in vitro* and having properties similar to the largest TGB protein encoded by BSMV (58 kd) and other viruses. In this model, the 8K and 12K proteins act as membrane anchors. Replicated viral genomic RNA associated with the 25K protein is targeted to the plasma membrane and plasmodesmata through interactions of the 25K protein with the 8K/12K anchors. This interaction somehow facilitates exchange of the CP for the 25K protein bound to the viral genome, while the 25K protein acts to increase the size exclusion limits of the plasmodesmata and the assembled virions move into neighboring cells. The 25K protein is retained in the infected cell through binding to the 8K/12K membrane-anchored complexes and/or because viral CP occludes plasmodesmal sites to prevent its moving through. It has been suggested that early in infection, before CP and the 8K and 12K proteins accumulate, the 25K protein could itself move from cell to cell, creating a "preconditioned" state conducive to virus movement (383). It is also formally possible that the 35K protein and CP both associate with replicated viral genomic RNA as RNPs and, together with the 8K and 12K proteins, participate in assembly of virion complexes once the RNPs are targeted to the membrane sites, or that at sites of replication, CP and viral RNA assembled into virions associate with 25K, and these complexes are then targeted to the cell membrane and wall through interactions of 25K with the 8K/12K complexes. The BSMV TGB-encoded proteins that are analogous to those in PVX are 58 kd (βb), 17 kd (βc) and 14 kd (βd). In BSMV, the 58-kd protein is essential for cell-to-cell movement, and its ability to bind RNA appears to be required for this function (85). RNPs containing BSMV genomic RNA complexed with the 58-kd protein can be isolated from infected plant cells. The 17-kd and 14-kd proteins have potential transmembrane domains and appear to be similar to the PVX 12-kd and 8-kd proteins. A model consistent with the studies of BSMV (85,192) that also draws on parallels to PVX (see Fig. 31D) is that the 17-kd and 14-kd proteins act as membrane anchors. The 58-kd protein forms RNP complexes with replicated viral genomic RNA, which are targeted to the plasma membrane and plasmodesmata through interactions with the 17-kd/14-kd anchors. The 58-kd protein, like the TMV MP, then acts to increase the size exclusion limits of the plasmodesmata, and the 58-kd protein genome complexes move into adjacent cells. Other models are also possible, and as for PVX and other viruses encoding TGB proteins, biochemical and cellular studies of the TGB proteins are required to fully understand how these proteins function and interact to facilitate movement.

Long-Distance Movement

Little is understood about how viruses enter, move through, and exit from the phloem, owing largely to technical difficulties associated with investigating phloem cells without damaging them. Most of what is known is based on immunocytochemical and ultrastructural studies, and the analysis of virus mutants or host range variants (242). A complicating factor in determining the role of MPs in viruses entering the phloem and moving systemically is their requirement in cell-to-cell movement, which is a prerequisite for systemic infection. This is also an issue for those viruses in which CP is also needed for cell-to-cell movement. In addition, in analyzing viral mutants it is difficult to discern whether effects on phloem entry or systemic infection directly involve a stage in vascular transport or are the general consequence of a decrease in virus accumulation and efficiency of infection. This becomes an issue if a threshold level of virus accumulation must be reached for systemic spread to successfully occur, or if a lower efficiency in spread allows time for the host to mount a defense response. Some plant viruses are transported through the xylem. We know even less about this process than about phloem transport of viruses, and it will not be discussed here. Whether phloem-restricted viruses follow the same routes that evidence suggests are used by viruses not so restricted has also not been studied in detail.

It has generally been accepted that viruses that infect mesophyll cells and move through the phloem do so along with the flow of nutrients (photoassimilates), exiting from mature leaves by the same path and at the same sites that photoassimilates are exported (the minor veins), and entering developing leaves by the same path and at the same sites (major or "lower order" veins) as photoassimilates are imported. This was suggested by classic studies that showed that plant viruses rapidly move toward the growing regions or young leaves in infected plants, and by more recent studies of CaMV infection in which virus accumulation in systemically infected leaves was found to be similar to that of photoassimilate import (203). This has now been directly shown for PVX infection in tobacco, by comparing spread of PVX expressing GFP with that of carboxyfluorescein (CF), a membrane-impermeant fluorescent solute that is transported through phloem in a manner similar to photoassimilate (292). Although virus transport was slower than that of CF, PVX exited from the same lower order veins (class III) into importing regions of developing leaves as did CF, and following infection of mesophyll cells, moved into the minor veins when these matured. The virus, as well as CF, was unable to enter regions of a leaf that were already actively exporting photoassimlate at the time of virus entry into the leaf.

Studies of the progression of infection for a number of plant virus variants and mutants have identified barriers or "control points" for virus movement from bundle sheath cells into phloem parenchyma cells, or from these into companion cells and then into the sieve elements. Plasmodesmal function between these cell types is also regulated (77); thus, not surprisingly, it appears that both viral and host cell factors control virus entry into the phloem. The majority of plant viruses require CP for long distance movement, whether they require CP for cell-to-cell movement or not. Analysis of CP mutants for a number of these viruses, including TMV, TEV, and RCNMV, suggests that CP is essential for entry into and/or spread through the sieve elements of the phloem, probably in the form of virions (242). In the case of TMV and RCNMV, the ability to assemble virions correlated with efficient systemic infection. Immunocytochemical analysis of infection by TMV CP mutants suggested that CP and encapsidation were not required for movement into minor veins but did appear to increase the efficiency of movement from companion cells into sieve elements (79,343). For PVX, a mutant that lacked CP but expressed GFP was inoculated onto transgenic plants that expressed viral CP, and its movement into grafted leaves that did not express CP was examined (300). The PVX mutant systemically infected the CP transgenic rootstock and moved into the grafted nontransgenic leaves, where it remained confined to cells close to major veins because of the lack of CP in the nontransgenic tissue. These studies showed that PVX CP, presumably assembled into virions, is transported through the phloem.

A detailed study using quantitative immune electron microscopy and an MP:GFP fusion to examine cucumber mosaic virus (CMV, a cucumovirus) progression into the minor veins of tobacco raised the interesting possibility that virions may be assembled in sieve elements (26). CMV needs MP (the 3a protein) and CP for cell-to-cell movement. The CMV MP was found associated with plasmodesmata whether it was expressed from infectious CMV or from PVX as an MP:GFP fusion. In minor veins, the MP was clearly present in plasmodesmata connecting companion cells and sieve elements, and in fibrillar formations within the sieve elements. However, in CMV-infected plants, virions were not detected in plasmodesmata, including those between the companion cells and sieve elements, but were found as large aggregates associated with the MP in the sieve elements. It was suggested that the viral genomic RNA, CP, and MP move into the sieve elements as an RNP complex and that virions are subsequently assembled within the sieve elements. Despite the evidence supporting the idea that where CP is required for systemic infection, virions may move through sieve elements, it remains an open point as to whether virions, as such, could pass through the plasmodesmata between sieve elements and companion cells to exit from the phloem.

It has been difficult to distinguish potential functions of MP in phloem entry and systemic movement from its role in cell-to-cell movement. A recent study with RCNMV took advantage of the ability to create partially defective MP mutants using alanine-scanning mutagenesis to identify functions of the viral MP in long distance movement that were distinct from its requirement for cell-to-cell movement (364). Immunocytochemical studies of three different host plants infected with different RCNMV MP mutants showed that MP was required for viral entry into the phloem for systemic infection, acting to facilitate viral movement from phloem parenchyma into companion cells independent of its function in cell-to-cell movement within mesophyll, bundle sheath, and phloem parenchyma.

PLANT RESPONSES TO VIRUS INFECTION

Although plants do not have an immune system, they are not completely defenseless in the face of virus infection. Plants can be nonhosts for or tolerant of infection by particular viruses. In the former instance, there is no evidence of virus replication in the plant, whereas in the latter, virus replicates and can move, but the host shows no or mild disease symptoms and continues to grow. Historically, it has been presumed that in these situations the infecting virus cannot interact with host factors that are involved in its replication or movement. While this may be true in a number of virus–host interactions, the recent demonstration of an innate plant defense response to virus infection suggests other possibilities as well. Potentially susceptible species of plants can also be resistant to infection by viral, bacterial, and fungal pathogens if they contain a dominant or recessive resistance gene, and these have been successfully used in breeding. Little is known about the action of recessive resistance genes; however, dominant resistance (*R*) genes have been shown to respond to a corresponding avirulence (*Avr*) gene in the attacking pathogen. This so-called gene-for-gene interaction induces a hypersensitive response that is usually evident by the local production of necrotic lesions (see Fig. 10) and involves a series of responses in the plant that include the local production of reactive oxygen species and induction of an apoptotic response, and systemic signaling to induce pathogenesis-related proteins. This hypersensitive response eliminates local infection and protects the plant against further attack. A number of *R* genes have been cloned in the past few years, and they appear to be involved in signal transduction pathways (reviewed in 56). One of the best characterized *R* gene responses to virus infection is that of the *N* gene in tobacco in conferring resistance to TMV, in which the corresponding *Avr* gene product has been shown to be the viral 126-kd component of the RdRp (258,259). The *N* gene has been cloned by transposon tagging and, in common with a number of other cloned *R* genes, it appears to encode a cytoplasmic protein that contains a nucleotide binding site and a region of leucine-rich repeats. Such repeats are known to be important in protein–protein interactions. Strikingly, the amino-terminal domain of the *N* gene–encoded protein is similar to the cytoplasmic domain of the *Drosophila* Toll protein and the mammalian interleukin-1 receptor, suggesting that it mediates resistance through a Toll–interleukin-1–type pathway (373).

Mixed virus infections in plants are common. If the two infecting viruses are related (e.g., different strains of a particular virus), one outcome can be the phenomenon of cross protection. As typified in studies of TMV, inoculating plants first with a mild tomato strain of TMV will protect plants against subsequent infection by more virulent strains of TMV. This cross protection response involves the CP of TMV, and it provided the first example of so-called pathogen-derived resistance in which transgenic plants that expressed a viral gene or protein, in this case the TMV CP, were shown to be resistant to virus infection (reviewed in 20 and 70). Subsequently, other viral genes encoding CP, as well as different viral RdRps and MPs, have been used to engineer virus-resistance plants, as have genes encoding known plant antiviral proteins, such as pokeweed antiviral proteins, a class of ribosome-inactivating proteins found in a wide variety of plants (342). The studies of the mechanism of pathogen-derived resistance quickly made it apparent that although, at times, such as with transgenic plants expressing the TMV CP, the resistance is mediated by expression of a viral protein, in most cases it is conferred by RNA (RNA-mediated resistance). The expressed viral transgene induces a homology-dependent degradation of the infecting virus genome that is mechanistically related to posttranscriptional cosuppression of a nonviral transgene and corresponding cellular gene in transgenic plants, and homology-dependent posttranscriptional gene silencing in plants (PTGS) (18). These, and other studies (11,283), suggested that plant viruses could be initiators as well as targets of PTGS, also called *RNA interference* (RNAi), a phenomenon that occurs in plants, animals (e.g., *Caenorhabditis elegans* and *Drosophila*) and fungi. As can happen in science, these studies on RNA-mediated resistance and investigation of the phenomenon of plant virus synergy converged to show that PTGS is a plant defense against virus infection and that, not unexpectedly, plant viruses can encode suppressors of PTGS as a counterstrategy.

In contrast to the antagonistic interaction in cross protection, mixed infection of plants by two usually unrelated viruses can be synergistic, producing more severe disease symptoms than would be caused by either virus alone and enhancing the replication and/or spread of one or both viruses. This synergistic interaction occurs in a number of mixed plant virus infections. Many of these involve a potyvirus and any of a number of unrelated viruses, which suggested that rather than the potyvirus affecting replication of the co-infecting virus directly, it was more likely to do so indirectly by modulating host functions. Recent studies of the interactions of potyviruses PVY, TEV, and TVMV with PVX, using viral mutants and transgenic plants, showed that the P1/HC-Pro region of the potyvirus genome is responsible for this synergism (277,348). This was directly shown in two ways. Infectious PVX engineered to express the P1/HC-Pro or HC-Pro of TEV was found to have enhanced pathogenicity in tobacco plants (Fig. 32). Similarly, transgenic plants that express the P1/HC-Pro region of TEV or TVMV showed enhanced symptoms when infected with wild-type PVX, which normally produces only mild symptoms on wild-type tobacco. Mutational studies showed that the region of HC-Pro that had been implicated in affecting replication, long distance movement, and pathogenicity of TEV was necessary and sufficient to produce the synergistic increase in disease symptoms, and that both P1 and HC-Pro were required for the increased replication of PVX (277). At the same time, in an attempt to develop a transient assay for investigating PTGS, it was discovered that local injection of *A. tumefaciens* expressing a 35S-GFP construct not only would

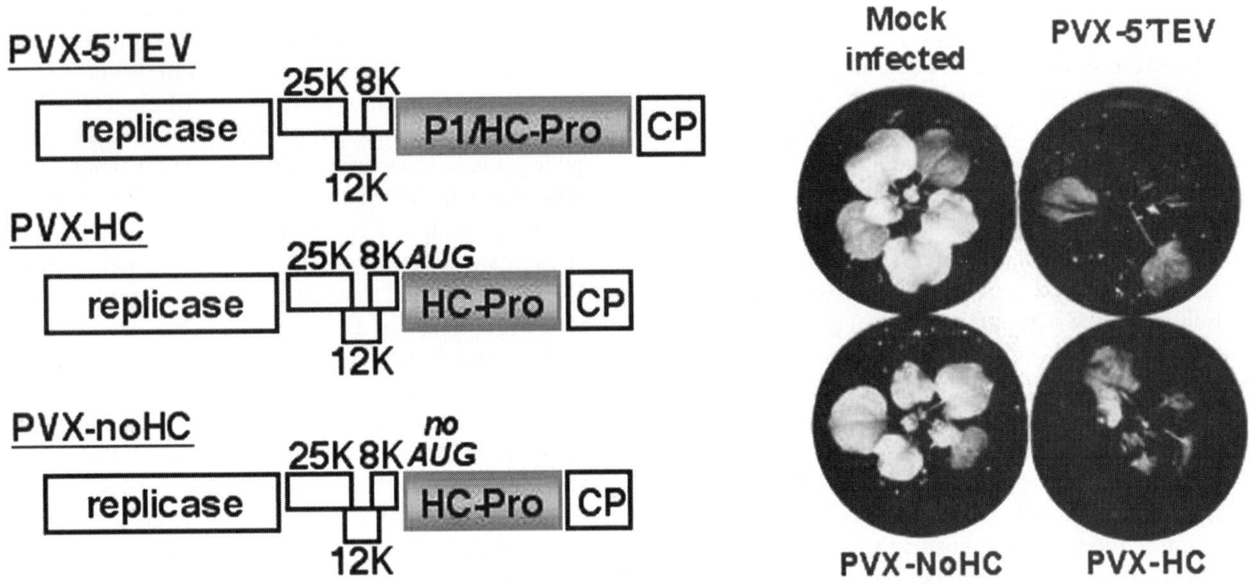

FIG. 32. PVX viruses that express TEV P1/HC-Pro or HC-Pro show enhanced pathogenicity (PVX-5′TEV, PVX-HC). Expression of P1/HC-Pro or HC-Pro protein is required, since PVX expressing HC-Pro without a start codon (PVX-NoHC) does not show enhanced pathogenicity. (From ref. 277, with permission.)

silence GFP expression in a transgenic plant locally in the inoculated leaf, as hoped, but also would induce PTGS of the GFP expression systemically throughout the entire plant. This was evident by the fact that these plants were no longer fluorescent under ultraviolet light (354). These and subsequent studies showed that PTGS in plants can be triggered by a systemically transmitted signal that is presumed to be nucleic acid (354,357). By infecting these GFP-silenced transgenic plants with PVX vectors expressing different forms of HC-Pro, or using transgenic tobacco plants that contain a preexisting silenced *GUS* transgene, it was shown that HC-Pro could suppress the PTGS of GFP or GUS (13,165,357). Small RNAs approximately 23 nt in length that correspond to both sense and antisense strands are associated with PTGS, and it has been proposed that these provide the specificity for targeted RNA degradation through association with an RNAse III–like enzyme (131,386). Additional studies have shown that encoding such a suppressor of PTGS is a strategy employed by a number of diverse plant viruses, including TMV, CMV (2b), TGMV (TrAP), cowpea mosaic virus (comovirus), a number of potexviruses (although not PVX), tobacco rattle virus (tobravirus), and tomato bushy stunt virus (tombusvirus, 19K) (356,357). In some cases, the viral-encoded suppressor has been identified (shown in parentheses). Thus, not every plant virus encodes such an RNAi suppressor, or counteracts this defense response in the same way. For viruses that do not, like PVX, it has been suggested that the virus can partially evade this host defense, although it clearly does not replicate at its maximal potential in those host plants in which this has been studied. The viral proteins identified as suppressing PTGS had each been identified in mutational studies as a "pathogenicity" factor that affected virus replication, movement, and/or pathogenesis, driving home the point that the roles of a number of these proteins, such as HC-Pro and CMV 2b, in systemic infection and phloem-dependent transport could be explained by suppression of the host PTGS defense response, rather than the protein directly facilitating active virus movement through plasmodesmata. This raises the possibility that some viral MPs could facilitate cell-to-cell movement by hindering intercellular communication required for spread of a PTGS defense (38). Recent studies with PVX suggest that the 25-kd protein, one of the TGB-encoded movement proteins, can block systemic spread of the PTGS signal (355), thus being responsible for the proposed PVX evasion of the PTGS response. Current studies are identifying host genes involved in PTGS. As the functions of these host genes are determined, we will begin to understand the signaling pathways by which PTGS is induced and how it can be suppressed or evaded.

REFERENCES

1. AbouHaidar MG, Gellatly D. Potexviruses. In: Granoff A, Webster RG, eds. *Encyclopedia of virology,* vol. 3. San Diego: Academic Press, 1999;1364–1368.
2. Ach RA, Durfee T, Miller AB, et al. RRB1 and RRB2 encode maize retinoblastoma-related proteins that interact with a plant D-type cyclin and geminivirus replication protein. *Mol Cell Biol* 1997;17: 5077–5086.
3. Adkins S, Choi TJ, Israel BA, et al. Baculovirus expression and processing of tomato spotted wilt tospovirus glycoproteins. *Phytopathology* 1996;86:849–855.
4. Adkins S, Quadt R, Choi TJ, et al. An RNA-dependent RNA poly-

merase activity associated with virions of tomato spotted wilt virus, a plant- and insect-infecting bunyavirus. *Virology* 1995;207:308–311.
5. Agrios GN. *Plant pathology*. San Diego, Academic Press, 1997.
6. Ahlquist P. Bromovirus RNA replication and transcription. *Curr Opin Genet Dev* 1992;2:71–76.
7. Ahlquist P. Bromoviruses (*Bromoviridae*). In: Granoff A, Webster R, eds. *Encyclopedia of virology*, vol. 1. San Diego: Academic Press, 1999:198–204.
8. Ahlquist P, French R, Janda M, Loesch-Fries LS. Multicomponent RNA plant virus infection derived from cloned viral cDNA. *Proc Natl Acad Sci U S A* 1984;81:7066–7070.
9. Ahlquist P, Wu SX, Kaesberg P, et al. Protein-protein interactions and glycerophospholipids in bromovirus and nodavirus RNA replication. *Arch Virol Suppl* 1994;9:135–145.
10. Ahola T, Ahlquist P. Putative RNA capping activities encoded by brome mosaic virus: Methylation and covalent binding of guanylate by replicase protein 1a. *J Virol* 1999;73:10061–10069.
11. Al-Kaff NS, Covery SN, Kreike MM, et al. Transcriptional and post-transcriptional plant gene silencing in response to a pathogen. *Science* 1998;279:2113–2115.
12. Allen E, Wang S, Miller WA. Barley yellow dwarf virus RNA requires a cap-independent translation sequence because it lacks a 5′ cap. *Virology* 1999;253:139–144.
13. Anandalakshmi R, Pruss GJ, Ge X, et al. A viral suppressor of gene silencing in plants. *Proc Natl Acad Sci U S A* 1998;95:13079–13084.
14. Angell SM, Davies C, Baulcombe DC. Cell-to-cell movement of potato virus X is associated with a change in the size-exclusion limit of plasmodesmata in trichome cells of *Nicotiana clevelandii*. *Virology* 1996;216:197–201.
15. Aoki S, Takebe I. Infection of tobacco mesophyll protoplasts by tobacco mosaic virus. *Virology* 1969;39:439–448.
16. Atkins D, Hull R, Wells B, et al. The tobacco mosaic virus 30K movement protein in transgenic tobacco plants is localized to plasmodesmata. *J Gen Virol* 1991;72:209–211.
17. Bandla MD, Campbell LR, Ullman DE, Sherwood JL. Interaction of tomato spotted wilt tospovirus (TSWV) glycoproteins with a thrips midgut protein, a potential cellular receptor for TSWV. *Phytopathology* 1998;88:98–104.
18. Baulcombe DC. Mechanisms of pathogen-derived resistance to viruses in transgenic plants. *Plant Cell* 1996;8:1833–1844.
19. Bawden FC, Pirie NW, Bernal JD, Fankuchen I. Liquid crystalline substances from virus-infected plants. *Nature* 1936;138:1051–1052.
20. Beachy RN. Mechanisms and applications of pathogen-derived resistance in transgenic plants. *Curr Opin Biotechnol* 1997;8:215–220.
21. Beier H, Barciszewska M, Krupp G, et al. UAG readthrough during TMV RNA translation: Isolation and sequence of two $tRNA^{Tyr}$ with suppressor activity from tobacco plants. *EMBO J* 1984;3:351–356.
22. Beijerinck MW. Uber ein contagium vivum fluidum als ursache der flechenkrankheit der tabaksblatter. 1898. *Verh K Acad Wettensch Amst* 1989;65:3–21.
23. Bendena WG, Mackie GA. In vitro translation of potexvirus gRNA. *Virology* 1986;153:220–229.
24. Benfey PN, Chua NH. The cauliflower mosaic virus 35S promoter: combinatorial regulation of transcription in plants. *Science* 1990;250: 959–966.
25. Bernal JD, Fankuchen I. X-ray and crystallographic studies of plant virus preparations. III. *J Gen Physiol* 1941;25:147–165.
26. Blackman LM, Boevink P, Cruz SS, et al. The movement protein of cucumber mosaic virus traffics into sieve elements in minor veins of *Nicotiana clevelandii*. *Plant Cell* 1998;10:525–537.
27. Bonneville J, Hohn T. A reverse transcriptase for cauliflower mosaic virus. The state of the art, 1991. In: Skalka N, Goff S, eds. *Reverse transcriptase*. Cold Spring Harbor, NY: Cold Spring Harbor Laboratory Press, 1993:357–390.
28. Boulton MI, Steinkellner H, Donson J, et al. Mutational analysis of the virion-sense genes of maize streak virus. *J Gen Virol* 1989;70: 2309–2323.
29. Bozarth CS, Weiland JJ, Dreher TW. Expression of ORF-69 of turnip yellow mosaic virus is necessary for viral spread in plants. *Virology* 1992;187:124–130.
30. Brantley JD, Hunt AG. The N-terminal protein of the polyprotein encoded by the potyvirus tobacco vein mottling virus is an RNA binding protein. *J Gen Virol* 1993;74:1157–1162.
31. Briddon RW, Pinner MS, Stanley J, Markham PG. Geminivirus coat protein gene replacement alters insect specificity. *Virology* 1990;177: 85–94.
32. Brown CM, Dinesh-Kumar SP, Miller WA. Local and distant sequences are required for efficient readthrough of the barley yellow dwarf virus PAV coat protein gene stop codon. *J Virol* 1996;70: 5884–5892.
33. Bruyere A, Brault V, Ziegler-Graff V, et al. Effects of mutations in the beet western yellows virus readthrough protein on its expression and packaging and on virus accumulation, symptoms, and aphid transmission. *Virology* 1997;230:323–334.
34. Buck K. Geminiviruses (*Geminiviridae*). In: Granoff A, Webster RG, eds. *Encyclopedia of virology*, vol. 1. San Diego: Academic Press, 1999:597–606.
35. Buck KW. Comparison of the replication of positive-stranded RNA viruses of plants and animals. *Adv Virus Res* 1996;47:159–251.
36. Butler PJG, Finch JT, Zimmern D. Configuration of tobacco mosaic virus RNA during virus assembly. *Nature* 1977;265:217–219.
37. Carr JP, Marsh LE, Lomonossoff GP, et al. Resistance to tobacco mosaic virus induced by the 54-kDa gene sequence requires expression of the 54-kDa protein. *Mol Plant Microbe Interact* 1992;5: 397–404.
38. Carrington JC. Reinventing plant virus movement. *Trends Microbiol* 1999;7:312–313.
39. Carrington JC, Cary SM, Dougherty WG. Mutational analysis of tobacco etch virus polyprotein processing: cis and trans proteolytic activities of polyproteins containing the 49-kilodalton proteinase. *J Virol* 1988;62:2313–2320.
40. Carrington JC, Cary SM, Parks TD, Dougherty WG. A second proteinase encoded by a plant potyvirus genome. *EMBO J* 1989;8: 365–370.
41. Carrington JC, Freed DD. Cap-independent enhancement of translation by a plant potyvirus 5′ nontranslated region. *J Virol* 1990;64: 1590–1597.
42. Carrington JC, Jensen PE, Schaad MC. Genetic evidence for an essential role for potyvirus CI protein in cell-to-cell movement. *Plant J* 1998;14:393–400.
43. Carrington JC, Kasschau KD, Mahajan SK, Schaad MC. Cell-to-cell and long-distance transport of viruses in plants. *Plant Cell* 1996; 8:1669–1681.
44. Caspar DLD. Radial density distribution in the tobacco mosaic virus particle. *Nature* 1956;177:928.
45. Castellano MM, Sanz-Burgos AP, Gutierrez C. Initiation of DNA replication in a eukaryotic rolling-circle replicon: Identification of multiple DNA-protein complexes at the geminivirus origin. *J Mol Biol* 1999;290:639–652.
46. Chapman S, Hills G, Watts J, Baulcombe D. Mutational analysis of the coat protein gene of potato virus X: Effects on virion morphology and viral pathogenicity. *Virology* 1992;191:223–230.
47. Chapman SN, Kavanagh TA, Baulcombe DC. Potato virus X as a vector for gene expression in plants. *Plant J* 1992;2:549–557.
48. Chay CA, Gunasinge UB, Dinesh-Kumar SP, et al. Aphid transmission and systemic plant infection determinants of barley yellow dwarf luteovirus-PAV are contained in the coat protein readthrough domain and 17-kDa protein, respectively. *Virology* 1996;219:57–65.
49. Chen MH, Sheng J, Hind G, et al. Interaction between the tobacco mosaic virus movement protein and host cell pectin methylesterases is required for viral cell-to-cell movement. *EMBO J* 2000;19:913–920.
50. Cheng SL, Domier LL, D'Arcy CJ. Detection of the readthrough protein of barley yellow dwarf virus. *Virology* 1994;202:1003–1006.
51. Choi IR, Stenger DC. The strain-specific cis-acting element of beet curly top geminivirus DNA replication maps to the directly repeated motif of the ori. *Virology* 1996;226:122–126.
52. Citovsky V, McLean BG, Zupan JR, Zambryski P. Phosphorylation of tobacco mosaic virus cell-to-cell movement protein by a developmentally regulated plant cell wall-associated protein kinase. *Genes Dev* 1993;7:904–910.
53. Collin S, Fernandez-Lobato M, Gooding PS, et al. The two nonstructural proteins from wheat dwarf virus involved in viral gene expression and replication are retinoblastoma-binding proteins. *Virology* 1996;219:324–329.
54. Covey SN, Lomonossoff GP, Hull R. Characterization of cauliflower mosaic virus DNA sequences which encode major polyadenylated transcripts. *Nucleic Acids Res* 1981;24:6735–6747.
55. Cronin S, Verchot J, Haldeman-Cahill R, et al. Long-distance move-

ment factor: A transport function of the potyvirus helper component proteinase. *Plant Cell* 1995;7:549–559.
56. Dangl JL. Piéce de résistance: Novel classes of plant disease resistance genes. *Cell* 1995;80:363–366.
57. Daros JA, Schaad MC, Carrington JC. Functional analysis of the interaction between VPg-proteinase (NIa) and RNA polymerase (NIb) of tobacco etch potyvirus, using conditional and suppressor mutations. *J Virol* 1999;73:8732–8740.
58. Daros JA, Carrington JC. RNA binding activity of NIa proteinase of tobacco etch potyvirus. *Virology* 1997;237:327–336.
59. Dash M. *Tulipomania: The story of the world's most coveted flower and the extraordinary passions it aroused.* New York: Crown Publishers, 1999.
60. Dautel S, Guidasci T, Pique M, et al. The full-length product of cauliflower mosaic virus open reading frame III is associated with the viral particle. *Virology* 1994;202:1043–1045.
61. Davenport GF, Baulcombe DC. Mutation of the GKS motif of the RNA-dependent RNA polymerase from potato virus X disables or eliminates virus replication. *J Gen Virol* 1997;78:1247–1251.
62. Davies C, Hills G, Baulcombe DC. Sub-cellular localization of the 25-kDa protein encoded in the triple gene block of potato virus X. *Virology* 1993;197:166–175.
63. Dawson WO, Beck DL, Knorr DA, Grantham GL. cDNA cloning of the complete genome of tobacco mosaic virus and production of infectious transcripts. *Proc Natl Acad Sci U S A* 1986;83:1832–1836.
64. Dawson WO, Bubrick P, Grantham GL. Modifications of the tobacco mosaic virus coat protein gene affecting replication, movement and symptomatology. *Phytopathology* 1988;78:783–789.
65. Dawson WO, Lehto KM. Regulation of tobamovirus gene expression. *Adv Virus Res* 1990;38:307–342.
66. de Haan P, Kormelink R, de Oliveira Resende R, et al. Tomato spotted wilt virus L RNA encodes a putative RNA polymerase. *J Gen Virol* 1991;72:2207–2216.
67. de Haan P, Wagemakers L, Peters D, Goldbach R. The S RNA segment of tomato spotted wilt virus has an ambisense character. *J Gen Virol* 1990;71:1001–1007.
68. Deiman BA, Koenen AK, Verlaan PW, Pleij CW. Minimal template requirements for initiation of minus-strand synthesis *in vitro* by the RNA-dependent RNA polymerase of turnip yellow mosaic virus. *J Virol* 1998;72:3965–3972.
69. Deiman BA, Verlaan PW, Pleij CW. *In vitro* transcription by the turnip yellow mosaic virus RNA polymerase: A comparison with the alfalfa mosaic virus and brome mosaic virus replicases. *J Virol* 2000;74:264–271.
70. Deom CM. Engineered resistance. In: Granoff A, Webster RG, eds. *Encyclopedia of virology,* vol 2. San Diego: Academic Press, 1999:1307–1314.
71. Deom CM, Oliver MJ, Beachy RN. The 30-kilodalton gene product of tobacco mosaic virus potentiates virus movement. *Science* 1987;237:389–394.
72. Di R, Dinesh-Kumar SP, Miller WA. Translational frameshifting by barley yellow dwarf virus RNA (PAV serotype) in *Escherichia coli* and in eukaryotic cell-free extracts. *Mol Plant Microbe Interact* 1993;6:444–452.
73. Diener TO, Owens RA, Hammond RW. Viroids: The smallest and simplest agents of infectious disease. How do they make plants sick? *Intervirology* 1993;35:186–195.
74. Diez J, Ishikawa M, Kaido M, Ahlquist P. Identification and characterization of a host protein required for efficient template selection in viral RNA replication. *Proc Natl Acad Sci U S A* 2000;97:3913–3918.
75. Dinant S, Janda M, Kroner PA, Ahlquist P. Bromovirus RNA replication and transcription require compatibility between the polymerase- and helicase-like viral RNA synthesis proteins. *J Virol* 1993;67:7181–7189.
76. Dinesh-Kumar SP, Miller WA. Control of start codon choice on a plant viral RNA encoding overlapping genes. *Plant Cell* 1993;5:670–692.
77. Ding B. Intercellular protein trafficking through plasmodesmata. *Plant Molec Biol* 1998;38:279–310.
78. Ding B, Turgeon R, Parthasarathy MV. Substructure of freeze-substituted plasmodesmata. *Protoplasma* 1992;169:28–41.
79. Ding X, Shintaku MH, Carter SA, Nelson RS. Invasion of minor veins of tobacco leaves inoculated with tobacco mosaic virus mutants defective in phloem-dependent movement. *Proc Natl Acad Sci U S A* 1996;93:11155–11160.
80. Dolja VV, Grama DP, Morozov SY, Atabekov JG. Potato virus X-related single-stranded and double-stranded RNAS. *FEBS Lett* 1987;214:308–312.
81. Dolja VV, Haldeman R, Robertson NL, et al. Distinct functions of capsid protein in assembly and movement of tobacco etch potyvirus in plants. *EMBO J* 1994;13:1482–1491.
82. Dolja VV, Haldeman-Cahill R, Montgomery AE, et al. Capsid protein determinants involved in cell-to-cell and long distance movement of tobacco etch virus. *Virology* 1995;207:1007–1016.
83. Domier LL, Franklin KM, Hunt AG, et al. Infectious *in vitro* transcripts from cloned cDNA of a potyvirus, tobacco vein mottling virus. *Proc Natl Acad Sci U S A* 1989;86:3509–3513.
84. Dominguez DI, Ryabova LA, Pooggin MM, et al. Ribosome shunting in cauliflower mosaic virus: Identification of an essential and sufficient structural element. *J Biol Chem* 1998;273:3669–3678.
85. Donald RG, Lawrence DM, Jackson AO. The barley stripe mosaic virus 58-kilodalton bb protein is a multifunctional RNA binding protein. *J Virol* 1997;71:1538–1546.
86. Doronin SV, Hemenway C. Synthesis of potato virus X RNAs by membrane-containing extracts. *J Virol* 1996;70:4795–4799.
87. Dowson Day MJ, Ashurst JL, Mathias SF, et al. Plant viral leaders influence expression of a reporter gene in tobacco. *Plant Mol Biol* 1993;23:97–109.
88. Dreher TW, Bozarth CS, Bransom KL, et al. The replication and gene expression of turnip yellow mosaic virus. In: Bills DD, Kung SD, eds. *Biotechnology and plant protection.* Singapore: World Scientific Press, 1995:47–67.
89. Dreher TW, Goodwin JB. Transfer RNA mimicry among tymoviral genomic RNAs ranges from highly efficient to vestigial. *Nucleic Acids Res* 1998;26:4356–4364.
90. Dreher TW, Tsai CH, Skuzeski JM. Aminoacylation identity switch of turnip yellow mosaic virus RNA from valine to methionine results in an infectious virus [see Comments]. *Proc Natl Acad Sci U S A* 1996;93:12212–12216.
91. Driesen M, Benito-Moreno R, Hohn T, Fütterer, J. Transcription from the CaMV 19S promoter and autocatalysis of translation from CaMV RNA. *Virology* 1993;195:203–210.
92. Duggal R, Hall TC. Interaction of host proteins with the plus-strand promoter of brome mosaic virus RNA-2. *Virology* 1995;214:638–641.
93. Dunigan DD, Zaitlin M. Capping of tobacco mosaic virus RNA: Analysis of a viral-coded guanylyltransferase-like activity. *J Biol Chem* 1990;265:7779–7786.
94. Eagle PA, Hanley-Bowdoin L. Cis elements that contribute to geminivirus transcriptional regulation and the efficiency of DNA replication. *J Virol* 1997;71:6947–6955.
95. Eagles RM, Balmori-Melián E, Beck DL, et al. Characterization of NTPase, RNA-binding and RNA helicase activities of the cytoplasmic inclusion protein of tamarillo mosaic potyvirus. *Eur J Biochem* 1994;224:677–684.
96. Edwards MC. Mapping of the seed transmission determinants of barley stripe mosaic virus. *Mol Plant Microbe Interact* 1995;8:906–915.
97. Elmer JS, Brand L, Sunter G, et al. Genetic analysis of the tomato golden mosaic virus II: The product of the AL1 coding sequence is required for replication. *Nucleic Acids Res* 1988;16:7043–7060.
98. Erickson FL, Holzberg S, Calderon-Urrea A, et al. The helicase domain of the TMV replicase proteins induces the N-mediated defence response in tobacco. *Plant J* 1999;18:67–75.
99. Esau K, Cronshaw J. Relation of tobacco mosaic virus to the host cells. *J Cell Biol* 1967;33:665–678.
100. Fellers J, Wan J, Hong Y, et al. *In vitro* interactions between a potyvirus-encoded, genome-linked protein and RNA-dependent RNA polymerase. *J Gen Virol* 1998;79:2043–2049.
101. Filichkin SA, Brumfield S, Filichkin TP, Young MJ. *In vitro* interactions of the aphid endosymbiotic SymL chaperonin with barley yellow dwarf virus. *J Virol* 1997;71:569–577.
102. Filichkin SA, Lister RM, McGrath PF, Young MJ. *In vivo* expression and mutational analysis of the barley yellow dwarf virus readthrough gene. *Virology* 1994;205:290–299.
103. Flasinski S, Dzianott A, Pratt S, Bujarski JJ. Mutational analysis of the coat protein gene of brome mosaic virus: Effects on replication and movement in barley and in *Chenopodium hybridum*. *Mol Plant Microbe Interact* 1995;8:23–31.
104. Fontes EP, Gladfelter HJ, Schaffer RL, et al. Geminivirus replication origins have a modular organization. *Plant Cell* 1994;6:405–416.

105. Fraenkel-Conrat H, Williams RC. Reconstitution of active tobacco mosaic virus from its inactive protein and nucleic acid components. *Proc Natl Acad Sci U S A* 1955;41:690–698.
106. Deleted in page proofs.
107. Franklin RE. Location of the ribonucleic acid in the tobacco mosaic virus particle. *Nature* 1956;177:928–920.
108. French R, Ahlquist P. Characterization and engineering of sequences controlling *in vivo* synthesis of brome mosaic virus subgenomic RNA. *J Virol* 1988;62:2411–2420.
109. Fujita M, Mise K, Kajiura Y, et al. Nucleic acid-binding properties and subcellular localization of the 3a protein of brome mosaic bromovirus. *J Gen Virol* 1998;79:1273–1280.
110. Fujiwara T, Giesman-Cookmeyer D, Ding B, et al. Cell-to-cell trafficking of macromolecules through plasmodesmata potentiated by the red clover necrotic virus movement protein. *Plant Cell* 1993;5: 1783–1794.
111. Fütterer J, Gordon K, Sanfaçon H, et al. Positive and negative control of translation by the leader of cauliflower mosaic virus pregenomic 35S RNA. *EMBO J* 1990;9:1697–1707.
112. Fütterer J, Hohn T. Translation of a polycistronic mRNA in the presence of cauliflower mosaic virus transactivator protein. *EMBO J* 1991;10:3887–3896.
113. Fütterer J, Kiss-László A, Hohn T. Nonlinear ribosome migration on cauliflower mosaic virus 35S RNA. *Cell* 1993;73:789–802.
114. Gallie DR, Sleat DE, Watts JW, et al. The 5′-leader sequence of tobaccomosaic virus RNA enhances the expression of foreign gene transcripts *in vitro* and *in vivo*. *Nucleic Acids Res* 1997;15:3257–3273.
115. Gallie DR, Walbot V. Identification of the motifs within the tobacco mosaic virus 5′-leader responsible for enhancing translation. *Nucleic Acids Res* 1992;20:4631–4638.
116. García JA, Riechmann JL, Laín S. Proteolytic activity of the plum pox virus NIa-like protein in *Escherichia coli*. *Virology* 1989;170: 362–369.
117. Gibbs A. Tymoviruses. In: Granoff A, Webster RG, eds. *Encyclopedia of virology*, vol. 3. San Diego: Academic Press, 1999:1850–1853.
118. Gierer A, Schramm G. Infectivity of ribonucleic acid from tobacco mosaic virus. *Nature* 1956;177:702–703.
119. Goelet P, Lomonossoff GP, Butler PJG, et al. Nucleotide sequence of tobacco mosaic virus RNA. *Proc Natl Acad Sci U S A* 1982;79: 5818–5822.
120. Goldbach R, Eggen R, de Jager C, van Kammen A. Genetic organization, evolution and expression of plant viral RNA genomes. In: Fraser RSS, ed. *Recognition and response in plant-virus interactions*. Heidelberg: Springer-Verlag, 1990:147–162.
121. Golemboski DB, Lomonossoff GP, Zaitlin M. Plants transformed with a tobacco mosaic virus nonstructural gene sequence are resistant to the virus. *Proc Natl Acad Sci U S A* 1990;87:6311–6615.
122. Goodwin JB, Skuzeski JM, Dreher TW. Characterization of chimeric turnip yellow mosaic virus genomes that are infectious in the absence of aminoacylation. *Virology* 1997;230:113–124.
123. Granoff A, Webster RG. *Encyclopedia of virology*. San Diego: Academic Press, 1999:1997.
124. Gray SM, Banerjee N. Mechanisms of arthropod transmission of plant and animal viruses. *Microbiol Mol Biol Rev* 1999;63:128–148.
125. Gray SM, Rochon D. Vector transmission of plant viruses. In: Granoff A, Webster RG, eds. *Encyclopedia of virology*, vol. 3. San Diego: Academic Press, 1999:1899–1910.
126. Grimsley N, Hohn B, Hohn T, Walden R. "Agroinfection," an alternative route for viral infection of plants by using the Ti plasmid. *Proc Natl Acad Sci U S A* 1986;83:3282–3286.
127. Groning BR, Hayes RJ, Buck KW. Simultaneous regulation of tomato golden mosaic virus coat protein and AL1 gene expression: Expression of the AL4 gene may contribute to suppression of the AL1 gene. *J Gen Virol* 1994;75:721–726.
128. Guerra-Peraza O, de Tapia M, Hohn T, Hemmings-Mieszczak M. Interaction of the cauliflower mosaic virus coat protein with the pregenomic RNA leader. *J Virol* 2000;74:2067–2072.
129. Guilley H, Dudley RK, Jonard G, et al. Transcription of cauliflower mosaic virus DNA: Detection of promoter sequences, and characterization of transcripts. *Cell* 1982;30:763–773.
130. Gutierrez C. DNA replication and cell cycle in plants: Learning from geminiviruses. *EMBO J* 2000;19:792–799.
131. Hamilton AJ, Baulcombe DC. A species of small antisense RNA in posttranscriptional gene silencing in plants. *Science* 1999;286:950–952.
132. Hanley-Bowdoin L, Settlage SB, Orozco BM, et al. Geminiviruses: Models for plant DNA replication, transcription, and cell cycle regulation. *Crit Rev Plant Sci* 1999;18:71–106.
133. Hartitz MD, Sunter G, Bisaro DM. The tomato golden mosaic virus transactivator (TrAP) is a single-stranded DNA and zinc-binding phosphoprotein with an acidic activation domain. *Virology* 1999;263: 1–14.
134. Heinlein M, Padgett HS, Gens JS, et al. Changing patterns of localization of the tobacco mosaic virus movement protein and replicase to the endoplasmic reticulum and microtubules during infection. *Plant Cell* 1998;10:1107–1120.
135. Hellmann GM, Shaw JG, Rhoads RE. *In vitro* analysis of tobacco vein mottling virus NIa cistron: Evidence for virus-encoded protease. *Virology* 1988;163:554–562.
136. Hemenway C, Weiss J, O'Connel K, Tumer NE. Characterization of infectious transcripts from a potato virus X cDNA clone. *Virology* 1990;175:365–371.
137. Hemmings-Mieszczak M, Hohn T, Preiss T. Termination and peptide release at the upstream open reading frame are required for downstream translation on synthetic shunt-competent mRNA leaders. *Mol Cell Biol* 2000;20:6212–6223.
138. Hemmings-Mieszczak M, Steger G, Hohn T. Alternative structures of the cauliflower mosaic virus 35 S RNA leader: Implications for viral expression and replication. *J Mol Biol* 1997;267:1075–1088.
139. Heyraud F, Matzeit V, Schaefer S, et al. The conserved nonanucleotide motif of the geminivirus stem-loop sequence promotes replicational release of virus molecules from redundant copies. *Biochimie* 1993;75: 605–615.
140. Heyraud-Nitschke F, Schumacher S, Laufs J, et al. Determination of the origin cleavage and joining domain of geminivirus Rep proteins. *Nucleic Acids Res* 1995;23:910–916.
141. Hill JE, Strandberg JO, Hiebert E, Lazarowitz SG. Asymmetric infectivity of pseudorecombinants of cabbage leaf curl virus and squash leaf curl virus: Implications for bipartite geminivirus evolution and movement. *Virology* 1998;250:283–292.
142. Hofer JM, Dekker EL, Reynolds HV, et al. Coordinate regulation of replication and virion sense gene expression in wheat dwarf virus. *Plant Cell* 1992;4:213–223.
143. Hogenhout SA, van der Wilk F, Verbeek M, et al. Potato leafroll virus binds to the equatorial domain of the aphid endosymbiotic GroEL homolog. *J Virol* 1998;72:358–365.
144. Hohn T. Caulimoviruses: Molecular biology. In: Granoff A, Webster RG, eds. *Encyclopedia of virology*, vol. 2. San Diego: Academic Press, 1999:1281–1285.
145. Hohn T, Dominguez DI, Schärer-Hernández N, et al. Ribosome shunting in eukaryotes: What the viruses tell me. In: Gallie JBS, ed. *A look beyond transcription:* Mechanisms determining mRNA stability and translation in plants. Bethesda, Md: American Society of Plant Physiology, 1998:84–95.
146. Hong Y, Levay K, Murphy JF, et al. The potyvirus polymerase interacts with the viral coat protein and VPg in yeast cells. *Virology* 1995; 214:159–166.
147. Hong Y, Stanley J. Regulation of African cassava mosaic virus complementary-sense gene expression by N-terminal sequences of the replication-associated protein AC1. *J Gen Virol* 1995;76:2415–2422.
148. Hormuzdi SG, Bisaro DM. Genetic analysis of beet curly top virus: Evidence for 3 virion sense genes involved in movement and regulation of single-stranded and double-stranded DNA levels. *Virology* 1993;193:900–909.
149. Hormuzdi SG, Bisaro DM. Genetic analysis of beet curly top virus: Examination of the roles of L2 and L3 genes in viral pathogenesis. *Virology* 1995;206:1044–1054.
150. Hou YM, Gilbertson RL. Increased pathogenicity in a pseudorecombinant bipartite geminivirus correlates with intermolecular recombination. *J Virol* 1996;70:5430–5436.
151. Huisman MJ, Linthorst HJM, Bol JF, Cornelissen BJC. The complete nucleotide sequence of potato virus X and it homologies at the amino acid level with various plus-stranded RNA viruses. *J Gen Virol* 1988; 69:1789–1798.
152. Hunter TR, Hunt T, Knowland J, Zimmern D. Messenger RNA for the coat protein of tobacco mosaic virus. *Nature* 1976;260:759–764.
153. Ingham DJ, Pascal E, Lazarowitz SG. Both geminivirus movement proteins define viral host range, but only BL1 determines viral pathogenicity. *Virology* 1995;207:191–204.

154. Ishikawa M, Diez J, Restrepo-Hartwig M, Ahlquist P. Yeast mutations in multiple complementation groups inhibit brome mosaic virus RNA replication and transcription and perturb regulated expression of the viral polymerase-like gene. *Proc Natl Acad Sci U S A* 1997;94: 13810–13815.
155. Ishikawa M, Janda M, Krol MA, Ahlquist P. *In vivo* DNA expression of functional brome mosaic virus RNA replicons in *Saccharomyces cerevisiae*. *J Virol* 1997;71:7781–7790.
156. Itaya A, Woo YM, Masuta C, et al. Developmental regulation of intercellular protein trafficking through plasmodesmata in tobacco leaf epidermis. *Plant Physiol* 1998;118:373–385.
157. Ivanowski D. Uber die mosaickkranheit der tabakspflanze St. Petersb. *Acad Imp Sci Bull* 1892;35:67–70.
158. Jackson AO, Goodin M, Moreno I, et al. Plant rhabdoviruses. In: Granoff A, Webster RG, eds. *Encyclopedia of virology*, vol. 3. San Diego: Academic Press, 1999:1531–1541.
159. Janda M, Ahlquist P. RNA-dependent replication, transcription, and persistence of brome mosaic virus RNA replicons in *S. cerevisiae*. *Cell* 1993;72:961–970.
160. Janda M, Ahlquist P. Brome mosaic virus RNA replication protein 1a dramatically increases *in vivo* stability but not translation of viral genomic RNA3. *Proc Natl Acad Sci U S A* 1998;95:2227–2232.
161. Jansen KA, Wolfs CJ, Lohuis H, et al. Characterization of the brome mosaic virus movement protein expressed in *E. coli*. *Virology* 1998; 242:387–394.
162. Johansen IE, Dougherty WG, Keller KE, et al. Multiple determinants affect seed transmission of pea seedborne mosaic virus in *Pisum sativum*. *J Gen Virol* 1996;77:3149–3154.
163. Jupin I, De Kouchkovsky F, Jouanneau F, Gronenborn B. Movement of tomato yellow leaf curl geminivirus (TYLCV): Involvement of the protein encoded by ORF C4. *Virology* 1994;204:82–90.
164. Jupin I, Hericourt F, Benz B, Gronenborn B. DNA replication specificity of TYLCV geminivirus is mediated by the amino-terminal 116 amino acids of the Rep protein. *FEBS Lett* 1995;362:116–120.
165. Kasschau KD, Carrington JC. A counterdefensive strategy of plant viruses: suppression of posttranscriptional gene silencing. *Cell* 1998; 95:461–470.
166. Kasschau KD, Cronin S, Carrington JC. Genome amplification and long-distance movement functions associated with the central domain of tobacco etch potyvirus helper component-proteinase. *Virology* 1997;228:251–262.
167. Kasteel DTJ, Wellink J, Goldbach RW, vanLent JWM. Isolation and characterization of tubular structures of cowpea mosaic virus. *J Gen Virol* 1997;78:3167–3170.
168. Kausche GA, Pfankych E, Ruska H. Die sichtbarmachung von pflanzlichem virus im übermikroskop. *Naturwissenschaften* 1939;27: 292–299.
169. Kelly L, Gerlach WL, Waterhouse PM. Characterisation of the subgenomic RNAs of an Australian isolate of barley yellow dwarf luteovirus. *Virology* 1994;202:565–573.
170. Kikkert J, van Lent J, Storms M, et al. Tomato spotted wilt virus particle morphogenesis in plant cells. *J Virol* 1999;73:2288–2297.
171. Kikkert M, Meurs C, van de Wetering F, et al. Binding of tomato spotted wilt virus to a 94-kDa thrips protein. *Phytopathology* 1998;88: 63–69.
172. Kikkert M, van Poelwijk F, Storms M, et al. A protoplast system for studying tomato spotted wilt virus infection. *J Gen Virol* 1997;78: 1755–1763.
173. Kim KH, Hemenway C. The 5′ nontranslated region of potato virus X RNA affects both genomic and subgenomic RNA synthesis. *J Virol* 1996;70:5533–5540.
174. Kim KH, Hemenway C. Mutations that alter a conserved element upstream of the potato virus X triple block and coat protein genes affect subgenomic RNA accumulation. *Virology* 1997;232:187–197.
175. Kim KH, Hemenway CL. Long-distance RNA-RNA interactions and conserved sequence elements affect potato virus X plus-strand RNA accumulation. *RNA* 1999;5:636–645.
176. Kiss-Laszlo Z, Blanc S, Hohn T. Splicing of cauliflower mosaic virus 35S RNA is essential for viral infectivity. *EMBO J* 1995;14: 3552–3562.
177. Klein PG, Klein RR, Rodríguez-Cerezo E, et al. Mutational analysis of the tobacco vein mottling virus genome. *Virology* 1994;204: 759–769.
178. Kong F, Sivakumaran K, Kao C. The N-terminal half of the brome mosaic virus 1a protein has RNA capping-associated activities: Specificity for GTP and S-adenosylmethionine. *Virology* 1999;259: 200–210.
179. Kong LJ, Orozco BM, Roe JL, et al. A geminivirus replication protein interacts with the retinoblastoma protein through a novel domain to determine symptoms and tissue specificity of infection in plants. *EMBO J* 2000;19:3485–3495.
180. Kormelink R, de Haan P, Meurs C, et al. The nucleotide sequence of the M RNA segment of tomato spotted wilt virus, a bunyavirus with two ambisense RNA segments [published erratum appears in *J Gen Virol* 1993;74:790]. *J Gen Virol* 1992;73:2795–2804.
181. Kormelink R, de Haan P, Peters D, Goldbach R. Viral RNA synthesis in tomato spotted wilt virus-infected Nicotiana rustica plants. *J Gen Virol* 1992;73:687–693.
182. Kormelink R, Kitajima EW, De Haan P, et al. The nonstructural protein (NSs) encoded by the ambisense S RNA segment of tomato spotted wilt virus is associated with fibrous structures in infected plant cells. *Virology* 1991;181:459–468.
183. Kormelink R, Storms M, van Lent J, et al. Expression and subcellular localization of the NSM protein of tomato spotted wilt virus (TSWV), a putative viral movement protein. *Virology* 1994;200:56–65.
184. Kormelink R, van Poelwijk F, Peters D, Goldbach R. Non-viral heterogeneous sequences at the 5′ ends of tomato spotted wilt virus mRNAs. *J Gen Virol* 1992;73:2125–2128.
185. Kotlizky G, Boulton MI, Pitaksutheepong C, et al. Intracellular and intercellular movement of maize streak geminivirus V1 and V2 proteins transiently expressed as green fluorescent protein fusions. *Virology* 2000;274:32–38.
186. Krol MA, Olson NH, Tate J, et al. RNA-controlled polymorphism in the *in vivo* assembly of 180-subunit and 120-subunit virions from a single capsid protein. *Proc Natl Acad Sci U S A* 1999;96: 13650–13655.
187. Kujawa AB, Drugeon G, Hulanicka D, Haenni AL. Structural requirements for efficient translational frameshifting in the synthesis of the putative viral RNA-dependent RNA polymerase of potato leafroll virus. *Nucleic Acids Res* 1993;21:2165–2171.
188. Laín S, Riechmann JL, García JA. RNA helicase: A novel activity associated with a protein encoded by a positive-strand RNA virus. *Nucleic Acids Res* 1990;18:7003–7006.
189. Latham JR, Saunders K, Pinner MS, Stanley J. Induction of plant cell division by beet curly top virus gene C4. *Plant J* 1997;11:1273–1283.
190. Laufs J, Schumacher S, Geisler N, et al. Identification of the nicking tyrosine of geminivirus Rep protein. *FEBS Lett* 1995;377:258–262.
191. Laufs J, Traut W, Heyraud F, et al. *In vitro* cleavage and joining at the viral origin of replication by the replication initiator protein of tomato yellow leaf curl virus. *Proc Natl Acad Sci U S A* 1995;92:3879–3883.
192. Lawrence DM, Jackson AO. Hordeiviruses. In: Granoff A, Webster RG, eds. *Encyclopedia of virology*, vol. 2. San Diego: Academic Press, 1999:749–753.
193. Lazarowitz SG. Geminiviruses: Genome structure and gene function. *Crit Rev Plant Sci* 1992;11:327–349.
194. Lazarowitz SG, Beachy RN. Viral movement proteins as probes for investigating intracellular and intercellular trafficking in plants. *Plant Cell* 1999;11:535–548.
195. Lazarowitz SG, Pinder AJ, Damsteegt VD, Rogers SG. Maize streak virus genes essential for systemic spread and symptom development. *EMBO J* 1989;8:1023–1032.
196. Lazarowitz SG, Ward BM, Sanderfoot AA, Laukaitis CM. Intercellular and intracellular trafficking: What we can learn from geminivirus movement. In: Lo Schiavo F, Last RL, Morelli G, Raikhel NV, eds. *Cellular integration of signalling pathways in plant development*, vol. H104. Berlin: Springer-Verlag, 1998.
197. Lazarowitz SG, Wu LC, Rogers SG, et al. Sequence specific interaction with the viral AL1 protein identifies a geminivirus DNA replication origin. *Plant Cell* 1992;4:799–809.
198. Leathers V, Tanguay R, Kobayashi M, Gallie DR. A phylogenetically conserved sequence within viral 3′ untranslated RNA pseudoknots regulates translation. *Mol Cell Biol* 1993;13:5331–5347.
199. Lebeureir G, Nicolaieff A, Richards KE. Inside-out model for self-assembly of tobacco mosaic virus. *Proc Natl Acad Sci U S A* 1977;74: 149–153.
200. Leclerc D, Burri L, Kajava AV, et al. The open reading frame III product of cauliflower mosaic virus forms a tetramer through a N-terminal coiled-coil. *J Biol Chem* 1998;273:29015–29021.

201. Leclerc D, Chapdelaine Y, Hohn T. Nuclear targeting of the cauliflower mosaic virus coat protein. *J Virol* 1999;73:553–560.
202. Leiser RM, Ziegler-Graff V, Reutenauer A, et al. Agroinfection as an alternative to insects for infecting plants with beet western yellows luteovirus. *Proc Natl Acad Sci U S A* 1992;89:9136–9140.
203. Leisner SM, Turgeon R, Howell SH. Long distance movement of cauliflower mosaic virus in infected turnip plants. *Mol Plant Microbe Interact* 1992;5:41–47.
204. Lewandowski DJ, Dawson WO. Tobamoviruses. In: Granoff A, Webster RG, eds. *Encyclopedia of virology,* vol. 3. San Diego: Academic Press, 1999:1780–1783.
205. Lewandowski DJ, Dawson WO. Functions of the 126- and 183-kDa proteins of tobacco mosaic virus. *Virology* 2000;271:90–98.
206. Li XH, Carrington JC. Complementation of tobacco etch potyvirus mutants by active RNA polymerase expressed in transgenic cells. *Proc Natl Acad Sci U S A* 1995;92:457–461.
207. Li XH, Valdez P, Olvera RE, Carrington JC. Functions of the tobacco etch virus RNA polymerase (NIb): Subcellular transport and protein-protein interaction with VPg/proteinase (NIa). *J Virol* 1997;71: 1598–1607.
208. Linstead PJ, Hills GJ, Plaskitt KA, et al. The subcellular localization of the gene 1 product of cauliflower mosaic virus is consistent with a function associated with virus spread. *J Gen Virol* 1988;69: 1809–1818.
209. Liu H, Boulton MI, Thomas CL, et al. Maize streak virus coat protein is karyophyllic and facilitates nuclear transport of viral DNA. *Mol Plant Microbe Interact* 1999;12:894–900.
210. Longstaff M, Brigneti G, Boccard F, et al. Extreme resistance to potato virus X infection in plants expressing a modified component of the putative viral replicase. *EMBO J* 1993;12:379–386.
211. López-Moya JJ, García JA. Potyviruses (*Potyviridae*). In: Granoff A, Webster RG, eds. *Encyclopedia of virology,* vol. 3. San Diego: Academic Press, 1999:1369–1375.
212. MacFarlane SA, Wallis CV, Brown DJF. Multiple virus genes involved in the nematode transmission of pea early browning virus. *Virology* 1996;219:417–422.
213. Mahajan S, Dolja VV, Carrington JC. Roles of the sequence encoding tobacco etch virus capsid protein in genome amplification: Requirements for the translation process and a cis-active element. *J Virol* 1996;70:4370–4379.
214. Maia IG, Seron K, Haenni AL, Bernardi F. Gene expression from viral RNA genomes. *Plant Mol Biol* 1996;32:367–391.
215. Markham R, Smith KM. Studies on the virus of turnip yellow mosaic. *Parasitology* 1949;39:330–342.
216. Marsh LE, Dreher TW, Hall TC. Mutational analysis of the core and modulator sequences of the BMV RNA3 subgenomic promoter. *Nucleic Acids Res* 1988;16:981–995.
217. Martins CR, Johnson JA, Lawrence DM, et al. Sonchus yellow net rhabdovirus nuclear viroplasms contain polymerase-associated proteins. *J Virol* 1998;72:5669–5679.
218. Mas P, Beachy RN. Distribution of TMV movement protein in single living protoplasts immobilized in agarose. *Plant J* 1998;15:835–842.
219. Mas P, Beachy RN. Replication of tobacco mosaic virus on endoplasmic reticulum and role of the cytoskeleton and virus movement protein in intracellular distribution of viral RNA. *J Cell Biol* 1999;147:945–958.
220. Matthews REF. *Plant virology*. San Diego: Academic Press, 1991.
221. Maule AJ, Wang D. Seed transmission of plant viruses: A lesson in biological complexity. *Trends Microbiol* 1996;4:153–158.
222. Mayer A. Uber die mosaikkrankheit des tabaks. *Die Landwirtschaftlichen Versuchs-Stationen* 1886;32:451–467.
223. Mayo MA, Robinson DJ, Jolly CA, Hyman L. Nucleotide sequence of potato leafroll luteovirus RNA. *J Gen Virol* 1989;70:1037–1051.
224. McLean BG, Zupan J, Zambryski PC. Tobacco mosaic virus movement protein associates with the cytoskeleton in tobacco cells. *Plant Cell* 1995;7:2101–2114.
225. Meshi T, Watanabe Y, Saito T, et al. Function of the 30 kd protein of tobacco mosaic virus: Involvement in cell to cell movement and dispensibility for replication. *EMBO J* 1987;6:2557–2563.
226. Miller ED, Kim KH, Hemenway C. Restoration of a stem-loop structure required for potato virus X RNA accumulation indicates selection for a mismatch and a GNRA tetraloop. *Virology* 1999;260:342–353.
227. Miller ED, Plante CA, Kim KH, et al. Stem-loop structure in the 5′ region of potato virus X genome required for plus-strand RNA accumulation. *J Mol Biol* 1998;284:591–608.
228. Miller JS, Mayo MA. The location of the 5′ end of the potato leafroll luteovirus subgenomic coat protein mRNA. *J Gen Virol* 1991;72: 2633–2638.
229. Miller WA. Luteovirus (*Luteoviridae*). In: Granoff A, Webster RG, eds. *Encyclopedia of virology,* vol. 2. San Diego: Academic Press, 1999:901–908.
230. Miller WA, Brown CM, Wang S. New punctuation for the genetic code: Luteovirus gene expression. *Semin Virol* 1997;8:3–13.
231. Miller WA, Dreher TW, Hall TC. Synthesis of brome mosaic virus subgenomic RNA *in vitro* by internal initiation on (−)-sense genomic RNA. *Nature* 1985;313:68–70.
232. Miller WA, Hall TC. Use of micrococcal nuclease in the purification of highly template-dependent RNA-dependent RNA polymerase from brome mosaic virus-infected barley. *Virology* 1983;125:236–241.
233. Miller WA, Raschova L. Barley yellow dwarf viruses. *Annu Rev Phytopathol* 1997;35:167–190.
234. Mise K, Allison RF, Janda M, Ahlquist P. Bromovirus movement protein genes play a crucial role in host specificity. *J Virol* 1993;67: 2815–2823.
235. Moore PJ, Fenczik CA, Deom CM, Beachy RN. Developmental changes in plasmodesmata in transgenic tobacco expressing the movement protein of tobacco mosaic virus. *Protoplasma* 1992;170: 115–127.
236. Morozov SY, Miroshnichenko NA, Solovyev AG, et al. Expression strategy of the potato virus X triple gene block. *J Gen Virol* 1991;72: 2039–2042.
237. Moyer JW. Tospoviruses (*Bunyaviridae*). In: Granoff A, Webster RG, eds. *Encyclopedia of virology,* vol. 3. San Diego: Academic Press, 1999:1803–1807.
238. Mundry KW, Watkins PAC, Ashfield T, et al. Complete uncoating of the 5′ leader sequence of tobacco mosaic virus RNA occurs rapidly and is required to initiate cotranslational disassembly *in vitro*. *J Gen Virol* 1991;72:769–777.
239. Nagano H, Mise K, Okuno T, Furusawa I. The cognate coat protein is required for cell-to-cell movement of a chimeric brome mosaic virus mediated by the cucumber mosaic virus movement protein. *Virology* 1999;265:226–234.
240. Nagar S, Pedersen TJ, Carrick KM, et al. A geminivirus induces expression of a host DNA synthesis protein in terminally differentiated plant cells. *Plant Cell* 1995;7:705–719.
241. Nagata T, Storms MMH, Goldbach R, Peters D. Multiplication of tomato spotted wilt virus in primary cell cultures derived from two thrips species. *Virus Res* 1997;49:59–66.
242. Nelson RE, van Bel AJE. The mystery of virus trafficking into, through and out of vascular tissue. *Prog Botany* 1998;59:476–533.
243. Nicolaisen M, Johansen E, Poulsen GB, Borkhardt B. The 5′ untranslated region from pea seedborne mosaic potyvirus RNA as a translational enhancer in pea and tobacco protoplasts. *FEBS Lett* 1992;303: 169–172.
244. Nishiguchi M, Motoyoshi F, Oshima N. Behaviour of a temperature sensitive strain of tobacco mosaic virus in tomato leaves and protoplasts. *J Gen Virol* 1978;39:53–61.
245. Nishiguchi M, Motoyoshi F, Oshima N. Further investigation of a temperature-sensitive strain of tobacco mosaic virus: Its behavior in tomato leaf epidemis. *J Gen Virol* 1980;46:487–500.
246. Noris E, Jupin I, Accotto GP, Gronenborn B. DNA-binding activity of the C2 protein of tomato yellow leaf curl virus. *Virology* 1996;217: 607–612.
247. Noris E, Vaira AM, Caciagli P, et al. Amino acids in the capsid protein of tomato yellow leaf curl virus that are crucial for systemic infection, particle formation, and insect transmission. *J Virol* 1998;72: 10050–10057.
248. O'Reilly EK, Paul JD, Kao CC. Analysis of the interaction of viral RNA replication proteins by using the yeast two-hybrid assay. *J Virol* 1997;71:7526–7532.
249. Odell JT, Dudley RK, Howell SH. Structure of the 19 S RNA transcript encoded by the cauliflower mosaic virus genome. *Virology* 1981;111:377–385.
250. Odell JT, Nagy F, Chua NH. Identification of DNA sequences required for activity of the cauliflower mosaic virus 35S promoter. *Nature* 1985;313:810–812.
251. Oparka KJ, Prior DA, Santa Cruz S, et al. Gating of epidermal plasmodesmata is restricted to the leading edge of expanding infection sites of tobacco mosaic virus (TMV). *Plant J* 1997;12:781–789.

252. Oparka KJ, Roberts AG, Boevink P, et al. Simple, but not branched, plasmodesmata allow the nonspecific trafficking of proteins in developing tobacco leaves. *Cell* 1999;97:743–754.
253. Oparka KJ, Roberts AG, Roberts IM, et al. Viral coat protein is targeted to, but does not gate, plasmodesmata during cell-to-cell movement of potato virus X. *Plant J* 1996;10:805–813.
254. Orozco BM, Gladfelter HJ, Settlage SB, et al. Multiple cis elements contribute to geminivirus origin function. *Virology* 1998;242: 346–356.
255. Orozco BM, Hanley-Bowdoin L. A DNA structure is required for geminivirus replication origin function. *J Virol* 1996;70:148–158.
256. Osman TA, Buck KW. Complete replication *in vitro* of tobacco mosaic virus RNA by a template-dependent, membrane-bound RNA polymerase. *J Virol* 1996;70:6227–6234.
257. Osman TA, Buck KW. The tobacco mosaic virus RNA polymerase complex contains a plant protein related to the RNA-binding subunit of yeast eIF-3. *J Virol* 1997;71:6075–6082.
258. Padgett HS, Beachy RN. Analysis of a tobacco mosaic virus strain capable of overcoming N gene- mediated resistance. *Plant Cell* 1993; 5:577–586.
259. Padgett HS, Watanabe Y, Beachy RN. Identification of the TMV replicase sequence that activates the N gene-mediated hypersensitive response. *Mol Plant Microbe Interact* 1997;10:709–715.
260. Pelham H. Leaky UAG termination codon in tobacco mosaic virus RNA. *Nature* 1978;272:469–471.
261. Perbal MC, Thomas CL, Maule AJ. Cauliflower mosaic virus gene I product (P1) forms tubular structures which extend from the surface of infected protoplasts. *Virology* 1993;195:281–285.
262. Pfeiffer P, Hohn T. Involvement of reverse transcription in the replication of cauliflower mosaic virus: A detailed model and test of some aspects. *Cell* 1983;33:781–789.
263. Pinck M, Yot P, Chapeville F, Duranton H. Enzymatic binding of valine to the 3′-end of TYMV RNA. *Nature* 1970;226:954–956.
264. Pirone TP, Blanc S. Helper-dependent vector transmission of plant viruses. *Annu Rev Phytopathol* 1996;34:227–247.
265. Pogue GP, Marsh LE, Hall TC. Point mutations in the ICR2 motif of brome mosaic virus RNAs debilitate (+)-strand replication. *Virology* 1990;178:152–160.
266. Pooggin MM, Hohn T, Futterer J. Forced evolution reveals the importance of short open reading frame A and secondary structure in the cauliflower mosaic virus 35S RNA leader. *J Virol* 1998;72: 4157–4169.
267. Pooggin MM, Hohn T, Futterer J. Role of a short open reading frame in ribosome shunt on the cauliflower mosaic virus RNA leader. *J Biol Chem* 2000;275:17288–17296.
268. Pooggin MM, Skryabin KG. The 5′-untranslated sequence of potato virus X RNA enhances the expression of a heme gene *in vivo*. *Mol Gen Genet* 1992;234:329–331.
269. Pooma W, Petty ITD. Tomato golden mosaic virus open reading frame AL4 is genetically distinct from its C4 analogue in monopartite geminiviruses. *J Gen Virol* 1996;77:1947–1951.
270. Powell-Abel P, Nelson RS, De B, et al. Delay of disease development in transgenic plants that express the tobacco mosaic virus coat protein gene. *Science* 1986;232:738–743.
271. Price M. Examination of potato virus X proteins synthesized in infected tobacco plants. *J Virol* 1992;66:5658–5661.
272. Prins M, Goldbach R. The emerging problem of tospovirus infection and nonconventional methods of control. *Trends Microbiol* 1998; 6:31–35.
273. Prins M, Storms MMH, Kormelink R, et al. Transgenic tobacco plants expressing the putative movement protein of tomato spotted wilt tospovirus exhibit aberrations in growth and appearance. *Transgenic Res* 1997;6:245–251.
274. Prufer D, Kawchuk L, Monecke M, et al. Immunological analysis of potato leafroll luteovirus (PLRV) P1 expression identifies a 25 kDa RNA-binding protein derived via P1 processing. *Nucleic Acids Res* 1999;27:421–425.
275. Prufer D, Schmitz J, Tacke E, et al. *In vivo* expression of a full-length cDNA copy of potato leafroll virus (PLRV) in protoplasts and transgenic plants. *Mol Gen Genet* 1997;253:609–614.
276. Prufer D, Tacke E, Schmitz J, et al. Ribosomal frameshifting in plants: A novel signal directs the –1 frameshift in the synthesis of the putative viral replicase of potato leafroll luteovirus. *EMBO J* 1992;11: 1111–1117.
277. Pruss G, Ge X, Shi XM, et al. Plant viral synergism: The potyviral genome encodes a broad-range pathogenicity enhancer that transactivates replication of heterologous viruses. *Plant Cell* 1997;9:859–868.
278. Qin S, Ward BM, Lazarowitz SG. The bipartite geminivirus coat protein aids BR1 function in viral movement by affecting the accumulation of viral single-stranded DNA. *J Virol* 1998;72:9247–9256.
279. Qiu WP, Geske SM, Hickey CM, Moyer JW. Tomato spotted wilt Tospovirus genome reassortment and genome segment-specific adaptation. *Virology* 1998;244:186–194.
280. Quadt R, Jaspars EMJ. Purification and characterization of brome mosaic virus RNA-dependent RNA polymerase. *Virology* 1990;178: 189–194.
281. Quadt R, Kao CC, Browning KS, et al. Characterization of a host protein associated with brome mosaic virus RNA-dependent RNA polymerase. *Proc Natl Acad Sci U S A* 1993;90:1498–1502.
282. Rajamaki ML, Valkonen JP. The 6K2 protein and the VPg of potato virus A are determinants of systemic infection in *Nicandra physaloides*. *Mol Plant Microbe Interact* 1999;12:1074–1081.
283. Ratcliffe R, Harrison BD, Baulcombe DC. A similarity between viral defence and gene silencing in plants. *Science* 1997;276:1558–1560.
284. Reichel C, Beachy RN. Tobacco mosaic virus infection induces severe morphological changes of the endoplasmic reticulum. *Proc Natl Acad Sci U S A* 1998;95:11169–11174.
285. Resende RDO, de Haan P, de Avila AC, et al. Generation of envelope and defective interfering RNA mutants of tomato spotted wilt virus by mechanical passage. *J Gen Virol* 1991;72:2375–2383.
286. Restrepo-Hartwig MA, Ahlquist P. Brome mosaic virus helicase- and polymerase-like proteins colocalize on the endoplasmic reticulum at sites of viral RNA synthesis. *J Virol* 1996;70:8908–8916.
287. Restrepo-Hartwig MA, Carrington JC. Regulation of nuclear transport of a plant potyvirus protein by autoproteolysis. *J Virol* 1992;66:5662–5666.
288. Riechmann JL, Laín S, García JA. Infectious *in vitro* transcripts from a plum pox potyvirus cDNA clone. *Virology* 1990;177:710–716.
289. Riechmann JL, Laín S, García JA. Identification of the initiation codon of plum pox potyvirus genomic RNA. *Virology* 1991;185: 544–552.
290. Riechmann JL, Laín S, García JA. Highlights and prospects of potyvirus molecular biology. *J Gen Virol* 1992;73:1–16.
291. Robards AW, Lucas WJ. Plasmodesmata. *Annu Rev Plant Phys* 1990; 41:369–419.
292. Roberts AG, Santa Cruz S, Roberts IM, et al. Phloem unloading in sink leaves of *Nicotiana benthamiana:* Comparison of a fluorescent solute with a fluorescent virus. *Plant Cell* 1997;9:1381–1396.
293. Rodriguez-Cerezo E, Findlay K, Shaw JG, et al. The coat and cylindrical inclusion proteins of a potyvirus are associated with connections between plant cells. *Virology* 1997;236:296–306.
294. Roossinck MJ, Sleat D, Palukaitis P. Satellite RNAs of plant viruses: Structures and biological effects. *Microbiol Rev* 1992;56:265–279.
295. Ryabova LA, Hohn T. Ribosome shunting in the cauliflower mosaic virus 35S RNA leader is a special case of reinitiation of translation functioning in plant and animal systems. *Genes Dev* 2000;14: 817–829.
296. Sanderfoot AA, Ingham DJ, Lazarowitz SG. A viral movement protein as a nuclear shuttle: The geminivirus BR1 movement protein contains domains essential for interaction with BL1 and nuclear localization. *Plant Physiol* 1996;110:23–33.
297. Sanderfoot AA, Lazarowitz SG. Cooperation in viral movement: The geminivirus BL1 movement protein interacts with BR1 and redirects it from the nucleus to the cell periphery. *Plant Cell* 1995;7: 1185–1194.
298. Sanderfoot AA, Lazarowitz SG. Getting it together in plant virus movement: Cooperative interactions between bipartite geminivirus movement proteins. *Trends Cell Biol* 1996;6:353–358.
299. Santa Cruz S, Chapman S, Roberts AG, et al. Assembly and movement of a plant virus carrying a green fluorescent protein overcoat. *Proc Natl Acad Sci* 1996;93:6286–6290.
300. Santa Cruz S, Roberts AG, Prior DAM, et al. Cell-to-cell and phloem-mediated movement of potato virus X: The role of virions. *Plant Cell* 1998;10:495–510.
301. Saunders K, Lucy A, Stanley J. DNA forms of the geminivirus African cassava mosaic virus consistent with a rolling circle mechanism of replication. *Nucleic Acids Res* 1991;19:2325–2330.
302. Saunders K, Lucy A, Stanley J. RNA-primed complementary-sense

DNA synthesis of the geminivirus African cassava mosaic virus. *Nucleic Acids Res* 1992;20:6311–6315.
303. Schaad MC, Haldeman-Cahill R, Cronin S, Carrington JC. Analysis of the VPg-proteinase (NIa) encoded by tobacco etch potyvirus: Effects of mutations on subcellular transport, proteolytic processing, and genome amplification. *J Virol* 1996;70:7039–7048.
304. Schaad MC, Jensen PE, Carrington JC. Formation of plant RNA virus replication complexes on membranes: Role of an endoplasmic reticulum-targeted viral protein. *EMBO J* 1997;16:4049–4059.
305. Schaad MC, Lellis AD, Carrington JC. VPg of tobacco etch potyvirus is a host genotype-specific determinant for long distance movement. *J Virol* 1997;71:8624–8631.
306. Schalk HJ, Matzeit V, Schiller B, et al. Wheat dwarf virus, a geminivirus of graminaceous plants needs splicing for replication. *EMBO J* 1989;8:359–364.
307. Schmidt I, Blanc S, Esperandiwu P, et al. Interaction between the aphid transmission factor and virus particles is a part of the molecular mechanism of cauliflower mosaic virus aphid transmission. *Proc Natl Acad Sci U S A* 1994;91:8885–8889.
308. Schmidt-Puchta W, Dominguez D, Lewetag D, Hohn T. Plant ribosome shunting *in vitro*. *Nucleic Acids Res* 1997;25:2854–2860.
309. Schmitz J, Stussi-Garaud C, Tacke E, et al. *In situ* localization of the putative movement protein (pr17) from potato leafroll luteovirus (PLRV) in infected and transgenic potato plants. *Virology* 1997;235: 311–322.
310. Schoelz JE, Bourque JE. *Caulimoviruses:* General features. In: Granoff A, Webster RG, eds. *Encyclopedia of virology,* vol. 2. San Diego: Academic Press, 1999:1275–1281.
311. Scholthof HB, Gowda S, Wu FC, Shepherd RJ. The full-length transcript of a caulimovirus is a polycistronic mRNA whose genes are transactivated by the product of gene VI. *J Virol* 1992;66:3131–3139.
312. Settlage SB, Miller AB, Hanley-Bowdoin L. Interactions between geminivirus replication proteins. *J Virol* 1996;70:6790–6795.
313. Shaw JG. *Plant viruses*. In: Fields BN, Knipe DM, Howley PM, et al, eds. *Fundamental virology*. Philadelphia: Lippincott-Raven, 1996: 367–400.
314. Shaw JG, Plaskitt KA, Wilson TMA. Evidence that tobacco mosaic virus particles disassemble cotranslationally *in vivo*. *Virology* 1986; 148:326–336.
315. Shepherd RJ, Richins RD, Shalla TA. Isolation and properties of the inclusion bodies of cauliflower mosaic virus. *Virology* 1979;102: 389–400.
316. Shi XM, Miller H, Verchot J, et al. Mutations in the region encoding the central domain of helper component-proteinase (HC-Pro) eliminate potato virus X/potyviral synergism *Virology* 1997;231:35–42.
317. Shih DS, Lane LC, Kaesberg P. Origin of the small component of brome mosaic virus RNA. *J Mol Biol* 1972;64:353–362.
318. Singh RN, Dreher TW. Specific site selection in RNA resulting from a combination of nonspecific secondary structure and -CCR- boxes: Initiation of minus strand synthesis by turnip yellow mosaic virus RNA-dependent RNA polymerase. *RNA* 1998;4:1083–1095.
319. Sit TL, Leclerc D, AbouHaidar MG. The minimal 5′ sequence for *in vitro* initiation of papaya mosaic potexvirus assembly. *Virology* 1994; 199:238–242.
320. Skuzeski JM, Nichols LM, Gesteland RF, Atkins JF. The signal for a leaky UAG stop codon in several plant viruses includes the two downstream codons. *J Mol Biol* 1991;218:365–373.
321. Smirnyagina E, Lin NS, Ahlquist P. The polymerase-like core of brome mosaic virus 2a protein, lacking a region interacting with viral 1a protein *in vitro*, maintains activity and 1a selectivity in RNA replication. *J Virol* 1996;70:4729–4736.
321a. Soellick T, Uhrig JF, Bucher GL, et al. The movement protein NSm of tomato spotted *wilt topsovirus* (TSWV): RNA binding, interaction with the TSWV N protein, and identification of interacting plant proteins. *Proc Natl Acad Sci USA* 2000;97:2373–2378.
322. Sriskanda VS, Pruss G, Ge X, Vance VB. An eight-nucleoide sequence in the potato virus X 3′ untranslated region is required for both host protein binding and viral multiplication. *J Virol* 1996;70:5266–5271.
323. Stanley J. Analysis of African cassava mosaic virus recombinants suggests strand nicking occurs within the conserved nonanucleotide motif during the initiation of rolling circle DNA replication. *Virology* 1995; 206:707–712.
324. Stanley J, Latham JR, Pinner MS, et al. Mutational analysis of the monopartite geminivirus beet curly top virus. *Virology* 1992;191:396–405.
325. Stanley WM. Isolation of a crystalline protein possessing the properties of tobacco-mosaic virus. *Science* 1935;81:644–645.
326. Stenger DC, Revington G, Stevenson MC, Bisaro DM. Replicational release of geminivirus genomes from tandemly repeated copies: Evidence for rolling circle replication of a plant viral DNA. *Proc Natl Acad Sci U S A* 1991;88:8029–8033.
327. Storms MMH, Kormelink R, Peters D, et al. The nonstructural NSm protein of tomato spotted wilt virus induces tubular structures in plant and insect cells. *Virology* 1995;214:485–493.
328. Sullivan ML, Ahlquist P. A brome mosaic virus intergenic RNA3 replication signal functions with viral replication protein 1a to dramatically stabilize RNA *in vivo*. *J Virol* 1999;73:2622–2632.
329. Sulzinski MA, Gabard KS, Palukaitis P, Zaitlin M. Replication of tobacco mosaic virus VIII: Characterization of a third subgenomic TMV RNA. *Virology* 1985;145:132–140.
330. Sunter G, Bisaro DM. Transactivation of geminivirus AR1 and BR1 gene expression by the viral AL2 gene product occurs at the level of transcription. *Plant Cell* 1992;4:1321–1331.
331. Sunter G, Bisaro DM. Regulation of a geminivirus coat protein promoter by AL2 protein (TrAP): Evidence for activation and derepression mechanisms. *Virology* 1997;232:269–280.
332. Sunter G, Hartitz MD, Bisaro DM. Tomato golden mosaic virus leftward gene expression: Autoregulation of geminivirus replication protein. *Virology* 1993;195:275–280.
333. Sunter G, Hartitz MD, Hormuzdi SG, et al. Genetic analysis of tomato golden mosaic virus: ORF AL2 is required for coat protein accumulation while ORF AL3 is necessary for efficient DNA replication. *Virology* 1990;179:69–77.
334. Tacke E, Prufer D, Salamini F, Rohde W. Characterization of a potato leafroll luteovirus subgenomic RNA: Differential expression by internal translation initiation and UAG suppression. *J Gen Virol* 1990; 71:2265–2272.
335. Tacke E, Prufer D, Schmitz J, Rohde W. The potato leafroll luteovirus 17K protein is a single-stranded nucleic acid-binding protein. *J Gen Virol* 1991;72:2035–2038.
336. Tacke E, Schmitz J, Prufer D, Rohde W. Mutational analysis of the nucleic acid-binding 17 kDa phosphoprotein of potato leafroll luteovirus identifies an amphipathic alpha-helix as the domain for protein/protein interactions. *Virology* 1993;197:274–282.
337. Takamatsu N, Watanabe Y, Meshi T, Okada Y. Mutational analysis of the pseudoknot region in the 3′-noncoding region of tobacco mosaic virus RNA. *J Virol* 1990;64:3686–3693.
338. Takebe I, Otsuki Y, Aoki S. Isolation of tobacco mesophyll cells in intact and active state. *Plant Cell Physiol* 1968;9:115–124.
339. Tanguay RL, Gallie DR. Isolation and characterization of the 102-kilodalton RNA-binding protein that binds to the 5′ and 3′ translational enhancers of tobacco mosaic virus RNA. *J Biol Chem* 1996; 271:14316–14322.
340. Thomas CL, Maule AJ. Identification of structural domains within the cauliflower mosaic virus movement protein by scanning deletion mutagenesis and epitope tagging. *Plant Cell* 1995;7:561–572.
341. Torruella M, Gordon K, Hohn T. Cauliflower mosaic virus produces an aspartic proteinase to cleave its polyproteins. *EMBO J* 1989;8: 2819–2825.
342. Tumer NE, Hudak K, Di R, et al. Pokeweed antiviral protein and its applications. *Curr Top Microbiol Immunol* 1999;240:139–158.
343. Vaewhongs AA, Lommel SA. Virion formation is required for the long-distance movement of red clover necrotic mosaic virus in movement protein transgenic plants. *Virology* 1995;212:607–613.
344. Valle RP, Drugeon G, Devignes-Morch MD, et al. Codon context effect in virus translational readthrough: A study *in vitro* of the determinants of TMV and Mo-MuLV amber suppression. *FEBS Lett* 1992;306:133–139.
345. van den Heuvel JF, Bruyere A, Hogenhout SA, et al. The N-terminal region of the luteovirus readthrough domain determines virus binding to Buchnera GroEL and is essential for virus persistence in the aphid 1997. *J Virol* 1997;71:7258–7265.
346. van Poelwijk F, Boye K, Oosterling R, et al. Detection of the L protein of tomato spotted wilt virus. *Virology* 1993;197:468–470.
347. Van Regenmortel MHV, Fauquet CM, Bishop D, et al. Virus taxonomy. *Seventh Report of the International Committee on Taxonomy of Viruses.* San Diego: Academic Press, 1999.
348. Vance VB, Berger PH, Carrington JC, et al. 5′ Proximal potyviral sequences mediate potato virus X/potyviral synergistic disease in transgenic tobacco. *Virology* 1995;206:583–590.

349. Verchot J, Angell SM, Baulcombe DC. *In vivo* translation of the triple gene block of potato virus X requires two subgenomic mRNAs. *J Virol* 1998;72:8316–8320.
350. Verchot J, Carrington JC. Debilitation of plant potyvirus infectivity by P1 proteinase-inactivating mutations and restoration by second-site modifications. *J Virol* 1995;69:1582–1590.
351. Verchot J, Carrington JC. Evidence that the potyvirus P1 proteinase functions in trans as an accessory factor for genome amplification. *J Virol* 1995;69:3668–3674.
352. Verchot J, Herndon KL, Carrington JC. Mutational analysis of the tobacco etch potyviral 35-kDa proteinase: Identification of essential residues and requirements for autoproteolysis. *Virology* 1992;190: 298–306.
353. Verchot J, Koonin EV, Carrington JC. The 35-kDa protein from the N-terminus of a potyviral polyprotein functions as a third virus-encoded proteinase. *Virology* 1991;185:527–535.
354. Voinnet O, Baulcombe DC. Systemic signalling in gene silencing. *Nature* 1997;389:553.
355. Voinnet O, Lederer C, Baulcombe DC. A viral movement protein prevents spread of the gene silencing signal in *Nicotiana benthamiana*. *Cell* 2000;103:157–167.
356. Voinnet O, Pinto YM, Baulcombe DC. Suppression of gene silencing: A general strategy used by diverse DNA and RNA viruses of plants. *Proc Natl Acad Sci U S A* 1999;96:14147–14152.
357. Voinnet O, Vain P, Angell S, Baulcombe DC. Systemic spread of sequence-specific transgene RNA degradation in plants is initiated by localized introduction of ectopic promoterless DNA. *Cell* 1998;95: 177–187.
358. Wagner JDO, Choi TJ, Jackson AO. Extraction of nuclei from sonchus yellow net rhabdovirus-infected plants yields a polymerase that synthesizes viral mRNAs and polyadenylated plus-strand leader RNA. *J Virol* 1996;70:468–477.
359. Wagner JDO, Jackson AO. Characterization of the components and activity of sonchus yellow net rhabdovirus polymerase. *J Virol* 1997; 71:2371–2382.
360. Waigmann E, Chen MH, Bachmaier R, et al. Regulation of plasmodesmal transport by phosphorylation of tobacco mosaic virus cell-to-cell movement protein. *EMBO J* 2000;19:4875–4884.
361. Waigmann E, Lucas WJ, Citovsky V, Zambryski P. Direct functional assay for tobacco mosaic virus cell-to-cell movement protein and identification of a domain involved in increasing plasmodesmal permeability. *Proc Natl Acad Sci U S A* 1994;91:1433–1437.
362. Wang D, MacFarlane SA, Maule AJ. Viral determinants of pea early browning virus seed transmission in pea. *Virology* 1997;234:112–117.
363. Wang D, Maule AJ. Inhibition of host gene expression associated with plant virus replication. *Science* 1995;267:229–231.
364. Wang HL, Wang Y, Giesman-Cookmeyer D, et al. Mutations in viral movement protein alter systemic infection and identify an intercellular barrier to entry into the phloem long-distance transport system. *Virology* 1998;245:75–89.
365. Wang JY, Chay C, Gildow FE, Gray SM. Readthrough protein associated with virions of barley yellow dwarf luteovirus and its potential role in regulating the efficiency of aphid transmission. *Virology* 1995; 206:954–962.
366. Wang S, Browning KS, Miller WA. A viral sequence in the 3′-untranslated region mimics a 5′ cap in facilitating translation of uncapped mRNA. *EMBO J* 1997;16:4107–4116.
367. Wang S, Miller WA. A sequence located 4.5 to 5 kilobases from the 5′ end of the barley yellow dwarf virus (PAV) genome strongly stimulates translation of uncapped mRNA. *J Biol Chem* 1995;270: 13446–13452.
368. Ward BM, Lazarowitz SG. Nuclear export in plants: Use of geminivirus movement proteins for an *in vivo* cell based export assay. *Plant Cell* 1999;11:1267–1276.
369. Ward BM, Medville R, Lazarowitz SG, Turgeon R. The geminivirus BL1 movement protein is associated with endoplasmic reticulum-derived tubules in developing phloem cells. *J Virol* 1997;71: 3726–3733.
370. Wartig L, Kheyr-Pour A, Noris E, et al. Genetic analysis of the monopartite tomato yellow leaf curl geminivirus: Roles of V1, V2, and C2 ORFs in viral pathogenesis. *Virology* 1997;228:132–140.
371. Weiland JJ, Dreher TW. cis-Preferential replication of the turnip yellow mosaic virus RNA genome. *Proc Natl Acad Sci U S A* 1993; 90:6095–6099.
372. White KA, Bancroft JB, Mackie GA. Mutagenesis of a hexanucleotide sequence conserved in potexvirus RNAs. *Virology* 1992; 189:817–820.
373. Whitham S, Dinesh-Kumar SP, Choi D, et al. The product of the tobacco mosaic virus resistance gene N: Similarity to toll and the interleukin-1 receptor. *Cell* 1994;78:1101–1115.
374. Wilson TM. Strategies to protect crop plants against viruses: Pathogen-derived resistance blossoms. *Proc Natl Acad Sci U S A* 1993;90:3134–3141.
375. Wilson TMA. Cotranslational disassembly of tobacco mosaic virus *in vitro*. *Virology* 1984;137:255–265.
376. Wolf S, Deom CM, Beachy RN, Lucas WJ. Movement protein of tobacco mosaic virus modifies plasmodesmatal size exclusion limit. *Science* 1989;246:377–379.
377. Wright EA, Heckel T, Groenendijk J, et al. Splicing features in maize streak virus virion- and complementary-sense gene expression. *Plant J* 1997;12:1285–1297.
378. Wu X, Shaw JG. Bidirectional uncoating of the genomic RNA of a helical virus. *Proc Natl Acad Sci U S A* 1996;93:2981–2984.
379. Wu X, Shaw JG. Evidence that a viral replicase protein is involved in the disassembly of tobacco mosaic virus particles *in vivo*. *Virology* 1997;239:426–434.
380. Wu X, Xu Z, Shaw JG. Uncoating of tobacco mosaic virus RNA in protoplasts. *Virology* 1994;200:256–262.
381. Xie Q, Sanz-Burgos AP, Hannon GJ, Gutierrez C. Plant cells contain a novel member of the retinoblastoma family of growth regulatory proteins. *EMBO J* 1996;15:4900–4908.
382. Xie Q, Suarez-Lopez P, Gutierrez C. Identification and analysis of a retinoblastoma binding motif in the replication protein of a plant DNA virus: Requirement for efficient viral DNA replication. *EMBO J* 1995;14:4073–4082.
383. Yang Y, Ding B, Baulcombe DC, Verchot J. Cell-to-cell movement of the 25K protein of potato virus X is regulated by three other viral proteins. *MPMI* 2000;13:599–605.
384. Yoshinari S, Nagy PD, Simon AE, Dreher TW. CCA initiation boxes without unique promoter elements support *in vitro* transcription by three viral RNA-dependent RNA polymerases. *RNA* 2000;6:698–707.
385. Young JL, Kelly L, Larkin PJ, Waterhouse PM. Infectious *in vitro* transcripts from a cloned cDNA of barley yellow dwarf virus. *Virology* 1991;180:372–379.
386. Zamore PD, Tuschi T, Sharp PA, Bartel DP. RNAi: Double-stranded RNA directs the ATP-dependent cleavage of mRNA at 21 to 23 nucleotide intervals. *Cell* 2000;101:25–33.
387. Zelenina DA, Kulaeva OI, Smirnyagina EV, et al. Translation enhancing properties of the 5′-leader of potato virus X genomic RNA. *FEBS Lett* 1992;296:267–270.
388. Ziegler-Graff V, Brault VDM, Simonis MT, et al. The coat protein of beet western yellows luteovirus is essential for systemic infection but the viral gene products p29 and p19 are dispensable for systemic infection and aphid transmission. *Mol Plant Microbe Interact* 1996;9:510.

CHAPTER 15

Insect Viruses

Paul D. Friesen and Lois K. Miller

HISTORY OF INSECT VIRUSES

It is likely that insect viruses have existed as long as the insects themselves and have therefore evolved for 350 million years. Insect viruses have long been of interest and concern to humans, as first indicated by scientific reports and literature of the 16th and 17th centuries, which describe insect diseases. In the early 19th century, crystalline polyhedral-shaped bodies called polyhedra were first discovered in association with the "wilting" disease of silkworms. It was subsequently established that the polyhedra were the causal agents of the disease, and by 1920, the silkworm disease was attributed to a filterable virus (reviewed in 14). Finally in 1947, Gernot Bergold (15) made the landmark discovery that the protein matrix of the polyhedra contained rod-shaped virions that are characteristic of the baculoviruses.

Studies in the 1940s and 1950s set the stage for development of insect pathogens as biologic pesticides. Important candidates were the insect viruses, especially the baculoviruses (246). The list of viral candidates was expanded in the 1960s through the discovery of new families of insect viruses, including the iridoviruses, nodaviruses, polydnaviruses, and entomopoxviruses. In the 1960s, significant progress also was made in establishing insect cell lines, and by 1973, a plaque assay for baculoviruses was available (100,131,132). Thus studies of the molecular biology and genetics of virus replication under controlled conditions were possible. Ultimately, the first insect virus (a baculovirus) was registered as a pesticide for use against the cotton bollworm by the United States Environmental Protection Agency in 1975 (reviewed in 192).

The mid-1970s marked the beginning of modern research on the molecular biology of insect viruses. Pioneering studies during this period triggered great interest in diverse applications of invertebrate viruses, including their use as vectors for foreign gene expression and as genetically improved biopesticides. To date, molecular studies on the replication, assembly, and host interactions of insect viruses have contributed enormously to molecular, cellular, and organismal biology.

CURRENT IMPACT OF INSECT VIRUSES

Insect Control

Insects comprise more than 80% of the existing animal species, outnumbering *Homo sapiens* 200 million to 1. Often considered the most successful animals on earth, many insect species are of serious biomedical concern to humans and represent significant pests in agricultural and forestry settings. It is not surprising that throughout history, humans have sought to control the insects. In nature, insect populations are held in balance by diverse factors, including predation, parasitism, and microbial (viral and fungal) infections. Of these regulatory forces, viral diseases can have profound effects.

Viruses can cause widespread epizootics and morbidity in insects, especially within dense populations. In contrast, some viruses have little or no overt effects, but can influence the "health" of a species by stressing the general population. Viral diseases occur in pest insects (gypsy moths, corn earworms, and mosquitoes, among others) as well as beneficial species (honey bees, silkworms, and parasitoids). Diseases of beneficial insects can cause economic and ecologic problems, whereas diseases of pest species can alleviate economic hardship and reduce medical concerns. Natural epizootics by viruses have been frequently observed in agricultural and forest settings, especially when insect populations are high. One of the most dramatic episodes of virus-mediated insect control occurred in North America during infestations of the European spruce sawfly. On accidental introduction of the sawfly baculovirus in the 1930s, sawfly populations declined sharply and remained low because of the continued presence of the virus (4). Such dependence on natural epizootics for insect pest control in agriculture, however, is generally impractical, because crop damage exceeds economically acceptable levels before virus-mediated reduction occurs.

Much effort has been invested at the academic and industrial levels in the development of virus-based biopesticides for the purpose of reducing agricultural dependence on broad-range, environmentally toxic chemical insecticides. Currently in Brazil, more than a million hectares of land are treated annually with a baculovirus to control the soybean looper. In Europe, a different baculovirus is used to control the codling moth, a common pest of fruit crops (192). In the South Pacific, a nudivirus is used for effective control of the rhinoceros beetle on coconut plantations (297). Several baculoviruses are currently registered as pesticides in the U.S., but their implementation has been pursued primarily by government agencies such as the U.S.D.A. Forest Service. Industrial interest in commercial development of virus insecticides has been sporadic, in part because of restricted markets and limitations in efficacy of these biopesticides. However, as environmental concerns increase and insects acquire resistance to chemical pesticides, it is expected that viral insecticides will have an expanded role in integrated pest-management programs. In particular, the capacity to improve insecticidal efficacy by genetic manipulation of baculoviruses through the insertion of insect-specific toxin or hormone genes holds much promise (118,183,247,266). Field tests of genetically improved baculovirus pesticides have already been conducted in the U.S. and the United Kingdom and have involved participation by multiple companies (reviewed in 20,192).

Foreign Gene Expression Vectors

Baculoviruses are popularly known for their use as highly efficient vectors for foreign gene expression in eukaryotic (insect) cells (reviewed in 144,155,199). This important and widely used application is the direct result of molecular studies on these large DNA viruses and is a striking example of the utility of insect viruses for biotechnology and basic research. Baculovirus expression vectors are distinguished by their capacity to produce unusually high levels of biologically active foreign proteins. Posttranslational modifications and protein folding in infected insect cells parallel those in mammalian cells and thereby provide abundant proteins for applications in vaccine development, therapeutic and diagnostic purposes, and structure/function studies. To date, several thousand genes have been expressed by using baculovirus vectors, which themselves have been recently improved for ease of use and increased protein yields. The biologic activity of these foreign proteins often can be tested directly in the vector-infected insect cells, providing a reliable and efficient system for functional analysis. The unique properties of other insect viruses, including the entomopoxviruses, nodaviruses, densoviruses, and alphaviruses, also are being exploited for use as expression vectors.

Recently the nucleopolyhedroviruses (NPVs) have been evaluated as gene-transfer vectors in mammals and insects (reviewed in 155). Reporter genes placed under control of mammalian promoters and inserted into the virus genome are readily expressed after inoculation of certain mammalian cell lines (26,52,134). Moreover, it has been demonstrated that a recombinant NPV can be used to stably deliver functional genes to the germline of the silkworm *Bombyx mori* (291), suggesting that baculoviruses will provide a useful vector for targeted gene insertion and gene disruption in transgenic insects.

Cell Biology, Host–Virus Interactions, and Evolution

The study of insect viruses has provided unique insights into fundamental biologic processes. Examples include the discovery of the 7-methyl guanosine cap structure of eukaryotic mRNAs by using the insect cypoviruses of *Reoviridae* (89). Studies on translation of cricket paralysis–like viruses have revealed a new mechanism for initiation of protein synthesis (235, 282). The polydnaviruses have revealed a novel symbiotic relationship between virus and host that involves virus-mediated immune suppression. Insect viruses also are providing unique opportunities to investigate antivirus defense strategies. Because of their capacity to induce and suppress apoptosis, baculoviruses have provided insight into the role played by programmed cell death as an antivirus defense mechanism and as a contributor to viral pathogenesis. Recombinant baculoviruses also have been used to trap host cell apoptotic regulators (243), providing information on regulation of programmed cell death. Last, apoptotic suppressors of these insect viruses are being used in antiapoptosis therapies involving transgenic organisms (58,133, 270).

Insect viruses also have provided unique insight into virus evolution. The close association of insects with plants and higher animals has allowed the natural exchange of viruses, thus contributing to virus evolution. Many insect viruses within the families *Poxviridae, Rhabdoviridae, Reoviridae, Picornaviridae*, and *Parvoviridae* have vertebrate counterparts, spurring speculation that viruses of higher animals evolved from ancient insect viruses. It is therefore likely that understanding the evolution of vertebrate viruses will depend on knowledge of their invertebrate relatives. In addition, some insect viruses have coevolved with viruses of unrelated families. For example, the unusual conservation of specific genes found in baculoviruses, entomopoxviruses, and orthomyxoviruses suggests an evolutionary link between these diverse virus families. Last, certain insect viruses (baculoviruses) readily accommodate host transposons, which are especially abundant and diverse in arthropods. Stable insertion of such host-derived genetic elements accelerates virus evolution and may contribute to the horizontal exchange of genes between invertebrate species.

CLASSIFICATION OF INSECT VIRUSES

Insects are susceptible to highly diverse families of RNA and DNA viruses (Table 1). Many members of these insect virus families have counterparts in vertebrates. Others are unique to arthropods. Nonetheless, insect-specific members of these virus families have novel properties that are conserved between families. A striking example is the use of an occluded form of infectious virus that is required for virus transmission between insect hosts and is conserved among diverse virus families, including the baculoviruses, entomopoxviruses, and cypoviruses.

This chapter focuses on those virus families that are found primarily or exclusively in insects: *Baculoviridae, Nudiviridae, Polydnaviridae, Ascoviridae, Nodaviridae, Tetraviridae,* and the cricket paralysis–like viruses. Viruses in which insects are used as temporary hosts during transmission (e.g., arboviruses) are not included, nor are virus families that have well-

TABLE 1. *Families of viruses infecting invertebrates*

Characteristics	Virus family	Genus	Representative member
dsDNA, enveloped	*Baculoviridae*	Nucleopolyhedrovirus (NPV)	*Autographa californica* MNPV (AcNMPV)
		Granulovirus (GV)	*Cydia pomonella* GV (TnGV)
	Nudiviruses[a]	Nonoccluded virus	Hz-1, *Oryctes rhinoceros* virus
	Polydnaviridae	Ichnovirus	*Campoletis sonorensis* virus (CsV)
		Bracovirus	*Cotesia melanoscela* virus (CmV)
	Poxviridae	Entomopoxvirus A	*Melontha melontha* entomopoxvirus
		Entomopoxvirus B	*Amsacta moorei* entomopoxvirus
		Entomopoxvirus C	*Chironomus luridus* entomopoxvirus
	Ascoviridae	Ascovirus	*Spodoptera frugiperda* ascovirus (SAV)
dsDNa, nonenveloped	*Iridoviridae*	Iridovirus	*Chilo* iridescent virus
		Chloriridovirus	Mosquito iridescent virus
ssDNA, nonenveloped	*Parvoviridae*	Densovirus	*Galleria* densovirus
dsRNA, nonenveloped	*Reoviridae*	Orbivirus	Bluetongue virus
		Cypovirus	Cytoplasmic polyhedrosis viruses (CPVs)
		Coltivirus	Colorado tick fever virus
	Birnaviridae	Birna virus	Drosphila X virus
ssRNA, enveloped	*Togaviridae*	Alphavirus	Sindbis virus
	Flaviviridae	Flavivirus	Yellow fever virus
	Rhabdoviridae	Vesiculovirus	Carajas virus
		Lyssavirus	Humpty Doo, Sigma virus
	Bunyaviridae	Bunyavirus	Anopheles A group
		Phlebovirus	Sandfly fever virus
		Nairovirus	Crimean-Congo hemorrhagic fever virus
ssRNA, nonenveloped	*Nodaviridae*	Alphanodavirus	Nodamura virus, Flock House Virus
	Tetraviridae	Betatetravirus	Nudaurelia capensis β virus
		Omegatetravirus	Nudaruelia capensis ω virus
	Cricket paralysis-like[a]	Cricket paralysis-like	Cricket paralysis virus
			Drosophila C virus

[a]These viruses are currently listed as unclassified by the ICTV.

characterized vertebrate members described in other chapters. These insect viruses and others (entomopoxviruses, iridescent viruses, densoviruses, and cypoviruses) are described by recent reviews (189).

DESCRIPTION OF INSECT VIRUS FAMILIES

Baculoviridae

Classification of Baculoviruses

Members of the family *Baculoviridae* are taxonomically characterized by their large, circular genome of double-stranded DNA, which is packaged into an enveloped, rod-shaped virion. The family name is derived from the Latin term *baculum,* meaning rod or stick, to describe the virion. Baculoviruses also are distinguished by their two morphologically distinct forms of infectious particles: occluded virus (OV), comprising enveloped virions embedded within a crystalline matrix of protein, and budded virus (BV), comprising a single virion enveloped by a plasma membrane. Baculoviruses are divided into two genera: the nucleopolyhedroviruses (NPVs) and granuloviruses (GVs), previously known as nuclear polyhedrosis viruses and granulosis viruses, respectively. For GVs, a single virion is embedded within each ovicylindrical OV particle, which collectively have a "granular" appearance in the light microscope. In contrast, NPVs have numerous (>20) virions per polyhedral OV particle (polyhedra) which are several microns in diameter and thus easily visualized by light microscopy. OV is produced in the nucleus of NPV-infected cells, whereas OV generally forms after loss of the nuclear membrane in GV-infected cells.

Baculovirus diseases have been reported in more than 500 different insect species. Individual viruses are most often named according to the species of host insect from which they were isolated. For example, *Autographa californica* nucleopolyhedrovirus (Ac*M*NPV) was isolated from the alfalfa looper *Autographa californica,* and *Cydia pomonella* granulovirus (CpGV) was isolated from the codling moth *Cydia pomonella.* In general, baculoviruses have distinct and relatively narrow host ranges that are limited to invertebrate species within a single genus or family. However, certain baculoviruses, including Ac*M*NPV, have broader host ranges, infecting more than 30 different lepidopteran (moth and butterfly) species.

Baculovirus Structure: OV and BV

Baculoviruses sequentially produce BV and OV in their unique, biphasic multiplication cycle. These infectious forms (Fig. 1) contain one or more virions comprising a rod-shaped nucleocapsid that is 250 to 300 nm long and 30 to 60 nm in diameter (recently reviewed in 88). The nucleocapsid is composed of a nucleoprotein core surrounded by a bacilliform proteinaceous sheath, referred to as the capsid. The capsid contains ring-like subunits stacked every 4.5 mm in the longitudinal axis (12). A distinctive morphology at the apical end of the capsid suggests a specialized function, for either DNA packaging, virion budding, nuclear entry, or uncoating (77,269). An essential 78-kd phosphoprotein is associated with this end structure (269). The capsid contains one major 35- to 40-kd capsid protein and additional minor proteins (213,258,264,269). The nucleoprotein core consists of a single molecule of circular, double-stranded DNA associated with protein. The major core protein is a 6.9-kd protamine-like protein, rich in arginine (150,268,285).

A distinctive feature of the baculoviruses is the large size (0.15 to 15 μm) and polyhedral or oval shape of the OV particles (see Fig. 1). The OV mediates virus transmission between insect larvae, the developmental stage most susceptible to viral infection. On ingestion by a larva, the OV protein matrix is dissolved by the alkaline pH of the midgut, releasing the occlusion-derived virions (ODVs), which initiate infection of the midgut epithelium. Within the OV particle, these virions are embedded in a crystalline matrix consisting of a single 29-kd protein, designated polyhedrin or granulin for the NPVs and GVs, respectively. Both matrix proteins are closely related. Within the matrix of NPVs (see Fig. 1A and B), either a single nucleocapsid (*S*NPVs) or multiple nucleocapsids (*M*NPVs) are bundled together and surrounded by a membrane envelope with virus-encoded proteins (88). The intranuclear membranes used for envelopment may be synthesized *de novo* or represent a modified form of the nuclear membrane (29,250). On their surface, mature OVs have an additional covering of protein and carbohydrate, known as the polyhedron envelope or calyx.

The BV form of baculoviruses consists of a nucleocapsid surrounded by a loose-fitting membrane envelope acquired by budding at the plasma membrane surface of the host cell (see Fig. 1C). The membrane envelope of BVs is thus distinct from that which envelops nucleocapsids embedded within OV. BV is the infectious unit responsible for cell-to-cell transmission within the insect and in cell culture. The envelope fusion protein (EFP) gp64 is the major virus-specific protein associated with the BV envelope of some NPVs (272). Antiserum to EFP gp64 neutralizes BV infectivity (275), suggesting that this protein participates in host cell–receptor interaction. Indeed, EFP gp64 is required for cell-to-cell infectivity (190). Envelope proteins unrelated to gp64 appear to mediate infectivity of other NPVs (211).

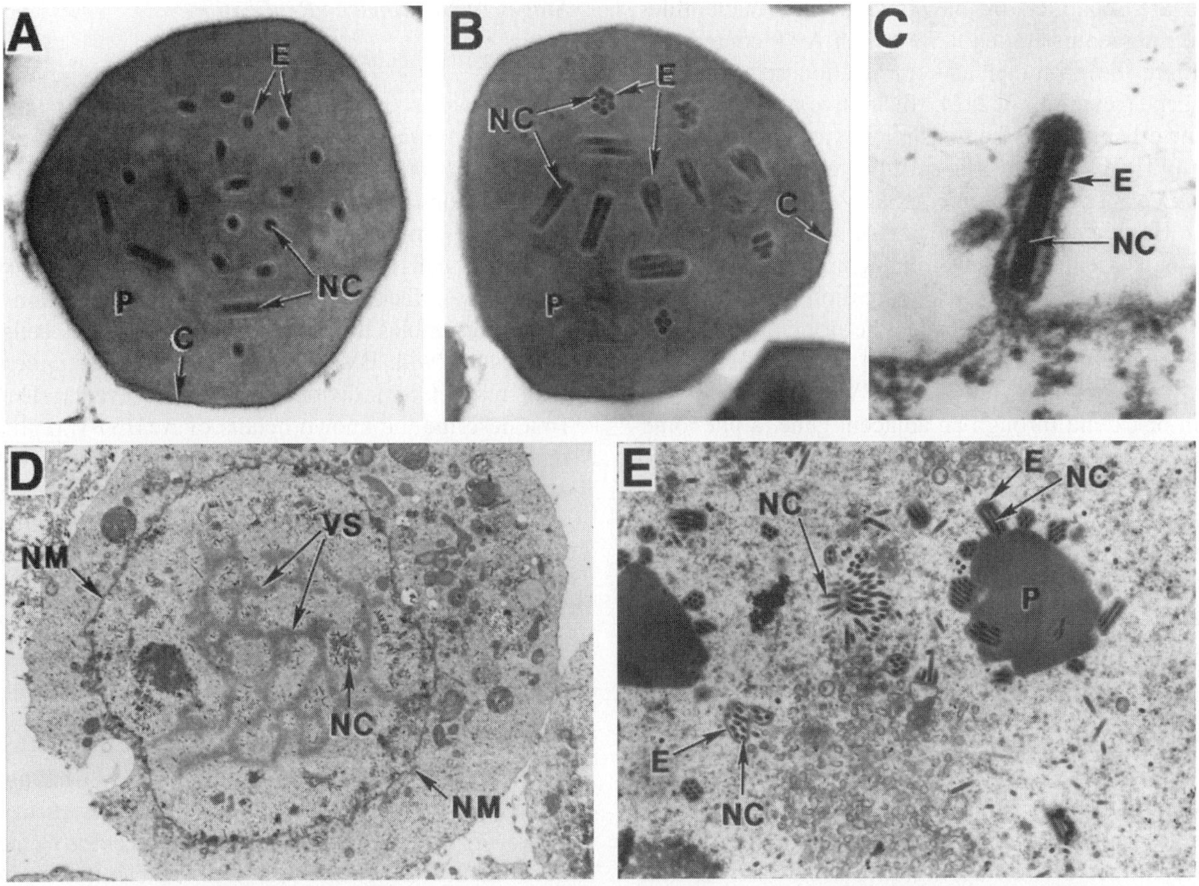

FIG. 1. OV and BV structure of the nucleopolyhedroviruses. **A:** Cross section of the OV particle (2-mm diameter) of a single capsid NPV (*S*NPV). Individual nucleocapsids (*NC*) within a unit membrane envelope (*E*) are embedded within a matrix of polyhedrin protein (*P*). The OV external surface is covered by the thin carbohydrate-rich calyx (*C*). **B:** Cross section of the OV particle (3-mm diameter) of a multicapsid NPV (*M*NPV). Envelopes (*E*) containing two or more nucleocapsids (*NC*) are embedded within the polyhedrin matrix (*P*). **C:** A nucleocapsid budding from the plasma membrane of an NPV-infected cell. The budded virus form (*BV*) of *M*NPVs and *S*NPVs contain a single nucleocapsid (*NC*) of the same dimensions (30 × 250 nm) as OV-derived nucleocapsids (**A, B**). **D:** Thin section of an *M*NPV-infected cell during the late phase of replication. The nucleus, surrounded by the nuclear membrane (*NM*), contains the virogenic stroma (*VS*) with associated nucleocapsids (*NC*). **E:** Nucleus of an *M*NPV-infected cell at the beginning of the very late, occlusion phase. Newly assembled nucleocapsids (*NC*) associate with intranuclear membrane envelopes (*E*), then become enveloped, and are embedded within a polyhedrin matrix (*P*). Electron micrographs were kindly provided by Dr. Malcolm J. Fraser, Jr., University of Notre Dame.

Baculovirus Genome Structure

The baculovirus genome is a large (90 to 160 bp) covalently closed, supercoiled circle of double-stranded DNA. To date, the complete nucleotide sequence of six baculoviruses has been reported, including that of *Autographa californica M*NPV (Ac*M*NPV), *Bombyx mori S*NPV (BmNPV), *Orgyia pseudotsugata M*NPV (Op*M*NPV), *Lymantria dispar M*NPV (Ld*M*NPV), *Xestia c-nigrum* granulovirus (XcGV), and *Cydia pomonella* granulovirus (CpGV) (2,3,95,126,163,200). Extensive transcriptional mapping of several baculoviruses has provided a broad picture of gene organization and regulation of expression. Ac*M*NPV is the best studied and represents the prototype NPV.

The AcMNPV genome (133,894 bp) consists almost entirely of unique DNA sequences, encoding 337 open reading frames (ORFs) of 150 nucleotides or more (3). The ORFs are closely spaced on both DNA strands with no apparent organization with respect to temporal expression during infection. Early, late, and very late genes are interspersed throughout the genome. Most

ORFs are separated by only two to 200 nucleotides. These intergenic regions have a high A+T content and constitute the promoter and termination sequences for each gene (reviewed in 216). Illustrative of the economy of gene organization, the translational termination codon (usually **UAA**) often overlaps the polyadenylation signal, AA**UAA**A. There also are examples of overlapping ORFs. However, because splicing of baculovirus RNA is rare, there are few if any introns in the genome. An example of splicing involves expression of the *ie-0*/*ie-1* gene (see later), which encodes the principal transcriptional regulator of baculoviruses (45,157,212). Frequently transcripts of one AcMNPV gene initiate from within or extend through an adjacent gene, a phenomenon especially prevalent among viral RNAs late in infection (81,179). Thus numerous genes are transcribed into bi- or multicistronic RNAs in which the upstream ORF is translated. In addition, there are multiple examples of the transcription of overlapping, antisense RNAs. The potential regulatory role of such antisense RNAs is unclear. Evidence exists that the interspersion of different temporal classes of transcripts may have functional significance. For example, activation of the very late promoter of *polh*, the gene encoding the major OV protein polyhedrin, down-regulates overlapping, antisense RNAs initiated downstream of *polh* (204). However, no evidence of this type of promoter interference occurs for a different set of overlapping RNAs that are all transcribed in the same direction (104).

A distinguishing feature of the baculovirus genome is the presence of multiple copies of interspersed repetitive sequences, known as homologous regions (*hrs*) (51,108). The *hrs* function as transcriptional enhancers (108,112) and are likely origins of viral DNA replication (154,210). Ac*M*NPV contains eight *hrs*, ranging in size from 30 to 800 bp and accounting for 3% to 4% of the genome. The *hrs* have a complex modular organization consisting of 60-bp repeats, each with a highly conserved 28-bp imperfect palindrome (28-*mer*). The 28-*mer* is the minimal sequence required for orientation- and position-independent enhancement of promoter activity and DNA replication (169,231). The *hrs* bind host- and virus-specific proteins. In particular, the transcriptional activator IE1 binds as a dimer to the palindromic 28-*mer*, which is required for IE1-mediated stimulation of enhancer activity (156,169,232). Deletion of a single *hr* (*hr5*) from the Ac*M*NPV genome reduces transcription of proximal genes, but has no obvious effect on virus replication, suggesting that these elements are functionally redundant (231). Nonetheless, the novel distribution and repetition of the *hrs* or *hr*-like elements within multiple baculovirus genomes suggest that these sequences play a critical role in the virus life cycle.

Stages of Baculovirus Replication

Primary and Secondary Infection

Baculovirus multiplication in the insect larva is divided into primary and secondary stages to describe the initial infection of midgut cells and the subsequent infection of secondary tissues, respectively (Fig. 2A and B). In both stages, infection is initiated by the binding of virus to the host cell. However, multiple aspects of primary and secondary infections differ. Secondary infection most closely resembles that which occurs in cultured cells after inoculation with BV, a process that is better understood with respect to individual replication events. Thus we first describe the known details of Ac*M*NPV replication in a high-multiplicity infection of cultured SF21 (or SF9) cells, a well-studied and fully permissive cell line derived from the nocturnal moth, *Spodoptera frugiperda* (Lepidoptera; Noctuidae). Subsequently, aspects unique to primary infection in the midgut of permissive caterpillars are described. It should be noted that the timing of replication events varies with the virus and insect host.

Attachment, Endocytosis, and Uncoating

BV enters the host cell (see Fig. 2A) by what appears to be receptor-mediated endocytosis (reviewed in 280). However, the participating host-cell receptor(s) has not been identified. A second, less efficient, membrane-fusion mechanism also may allow virus entry (273). The major glycoprotein of BV, gp64 EFP, is required for receptor interaction and fusion with the endosomal membrane (25,127,274). After release within the cytoplasm, nucleocapsids migrate to the nucleus in conjunction with virus-induced actin polymerization (41). Ac*M*NPV nucleocapsids interact end-on with the nuclear pore, enter the nucleus, and uncoat. In this process, the capsid sheath of the nucleocapsid is released from the nucleoprotein core (268). It is unknown whether the 6.9K protamine-like core protein remains associated with the viral chromosome, but phosphorylation by a virus-encapsidated protein kinase may induce its release (284). Uncoating occurs rapidly because new synthesis of viral RNAs can be detected within the first 15 minutes after inoculation (45,113,140,160,195,260).

Early Phase

By definition, the early replication phase (from 0 through 6–9 hours) precedes virus DNA replication. During this period, baculoviruses express genes encoding transcriptional activators, a virus-specific RNA polymerase activity, DNA replication factors, apoptotic suppressors, and others. These early gene products prepare the cell for the enormous burden imposed by the synthe-

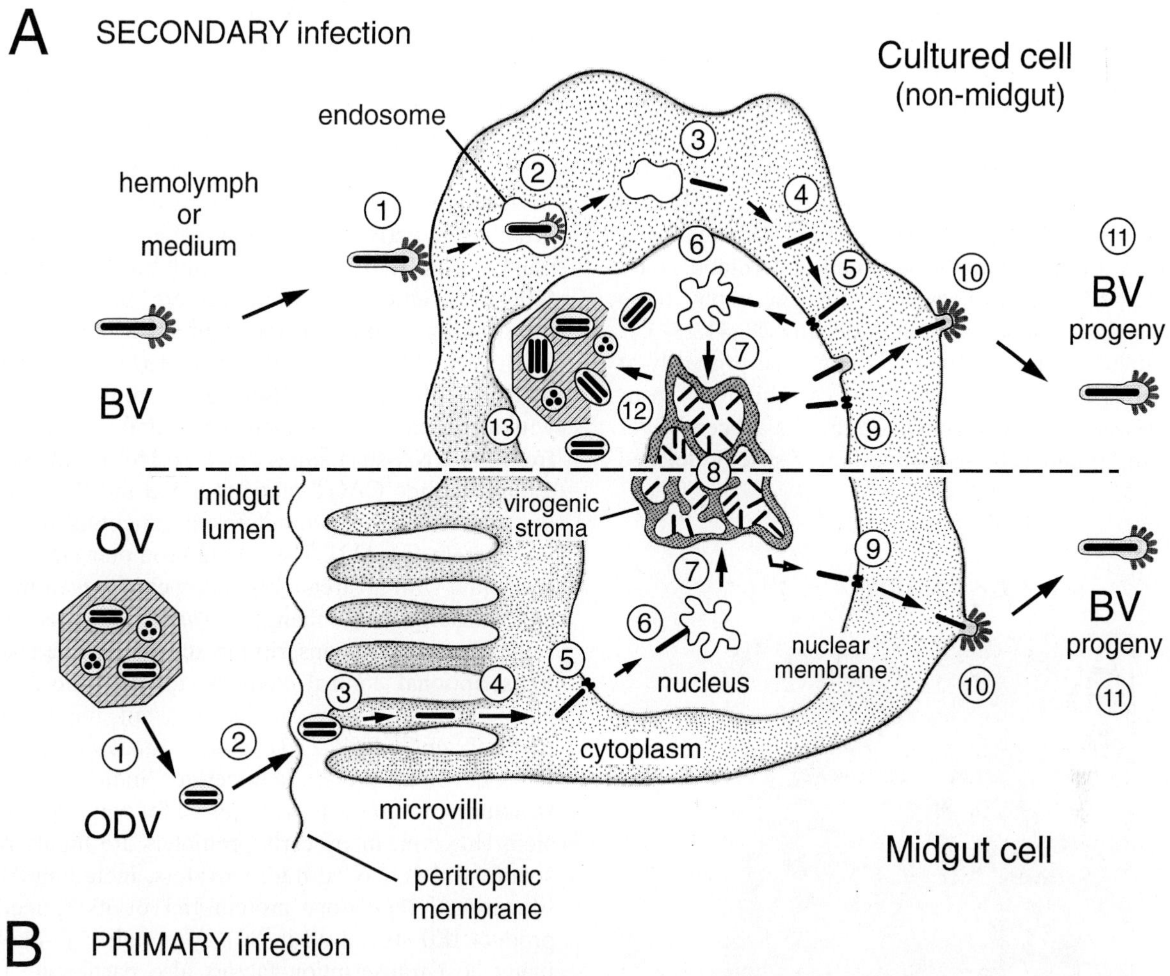

FIG. 2. Multiplication cycle of a baculovirus (*M*NPV). **A:** Infection of a cultured or nonmidgut cell by BV (secondary phase of infection). Enveloped BV attaches to receptors on the cell surface *(step 1)* and enters by endocytosis (*step 2*). As the endosome acidifies, virus and endosomal envelopes fuse (*step 3*), releasing nucleocapsids into the cytoplasm. Nucleocapsids proceed to the nucleus (*step 4*), where they interact end-on with the nuclear pore (*step 5*). On entering the nucleus, the DNA is released from the virion (*step 6*), and transcription begins (*step 7*). In association with the newly formed virogenic stroma, viral DNA is replicated and packaged into nucleocapsids (*step 8*). During the late phase, nucleocapsids exit the nucleus (*step 9*), migrate to the plasma membrane, and bud (*step 10*), thereby acquiring virus envelope proteins and producing infectious BV (*step 11*). During the very late phase, nucleocapsids are retained in the nucleus, acquire an envelope (*step 12*), and are embedded within a crystalline matrix of polyhedrin (*step 13*) to form OV particles. Mature OV are released by cell lysis. **B:** Infection of a midgut epithelial cell by OV (primary phase of infection). The polyhedrin matrix of an ingested OV particle dissolves in the midgut lumen *(step 1)*, releasing occlusion-derived virions (*ODV*), which crosses the peritrophic membrane (*step 2*) to gain access to the columnar epithelial cells. The enveloped ODV fuses with the microvilli membranes (*step 3*), releasing nucleocapsids into the cytoplasm, whereupon they migrate to the nucleus (*step 4*). The remaining replication events (*steps 5 to 11*) are similar to those in cultured cells (**A**).

sis of viral nucleic acid and structural components that can constitute more than a third of the infected cell's mass (Fig. 3A). The level and timing of both early and late gene expression is orchestrated to ensure proper temporal assembly of infectious BV and OV. Early viral gene products also block cell-cycle progression, causing infected cells to accumulate in S and G_2/M phases (28,142). In addition, the cell's cytoskeletal structure is dramatically rearranged. Both filamentous actin and microtubules are redistributed, leading to a characteristic hypertrophy of the nucleus and cell rounding during infection (40,41,234).

Baculovirus gene expression is regulated primarily at the level of transcription and involves a highly coordinated cascade of gene-activation events (recently reviewed in 80 and 178). Transcription of strictly defined early genes usually peaks between 6 and 12 hours after infection and declines thereafter, as late viral transcription accelerates. During this early time, the viral DNA genome adopts a nucleosome-like structure (286). The level of viral early RNAs is usually lower than that of late RNAs, which are transcribed by a novel virus-encoded RNA polymerase (RNA pol) specific for late genes. Suggesting that early transcription is mediated by host RNA pol II, early RNA synthesis is inhibited by α-amanitin (106,141), and early promoters are active in cell-free transcription extracts from uninfected cells (21,93,135, 223). Moreover, the structure of early viral promoters resembles that of host RNA pol II promoters, complete with a consensus TATA element located ~30 bp upstream from the RNA start site (22,61,110,159,175,223,260). A tetranucleotide CAGT motif found at the RNA start site is common to early promoters and functions as an initiator element (21,222). These core promoter elements also cooperate with upstream activating elements or more distal transcription enhancers (*hr*s) to interact with sequence-specific transcription activators. The cis-acting transcriptional control elements for multiple Ac*M*NPV early genes have been studied in detail, including those for *ie-1, gp64* EFP, *pp31* (39K), *he65*, and *p35*. Viral DNA devoid of protein is infectious, indicating that viral structural proteins are not required for early gene expression. However, many early promoters are highly responsive to virus-encoded transactivators, including the multifunctional regulatory protein IE1 or its spliced gene product IE0 (reviewed in 80). Although it is likely that many host transcription factors also participate in promoting viral transcription, few cellular factors have been identified (92,151,159,228).

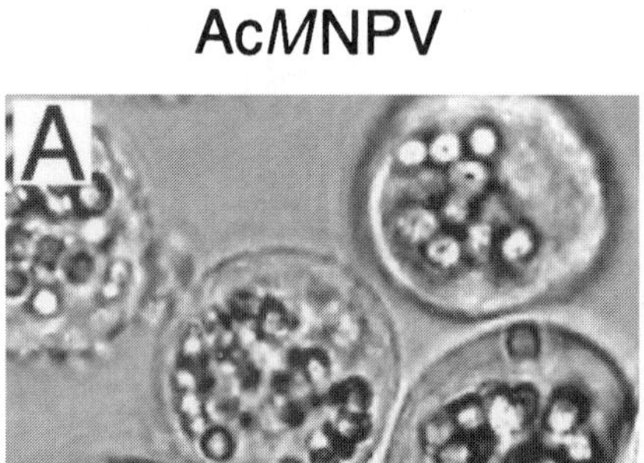

FIG. 3. Ac*M*NPV-infected SF21cells and apoptosis. **A:** Infection with wild-type Ac*M*NPV. Very late in infection the highly refractile OV particles *(arrow)* accumulate in the hypertrophied nucleus of each cell. **B:** Late stages of apoptotic blebbing. A single cell has undergone apoptosis forming a cell mass surrounded by membrane-enveloped apoptotic bodies *(arrow)*. Magnification, 200x. Micrographs provided by Gulam Manji, University of Wisconsin-Madison.

IE1 is the principal transcriptional regulator of early baculovirus genes. When assayed by plasmid transfections, IE1 stimulates early, but not late baculovirus promoters (22,110,111,158,162,175,195,209,229,260). This highly conserved, 67-kd transregulator has a modular structure consisting of an acidic transactivation domain(s) within its N-terminal half and DNA binding and oligomerization domain(s) at its C terminus (156, 233,244). IE1 also augments expression of genes that are cis-linked to the *hr* elements by interacting with the 28-bp palindromes within these enhancers (108,112,156, 169,195,232). By virtue of its interaction with the *hr*s, the co-localization of IE1 and DNA replication factors (202), and the requirement for IE1 in plasmid replication assays (see later), it is postulated that IE1 also contributes to viral DNA replication. However, the exact functions of IE1 during infection are still unclear (229).

Baculoviruses encode additional transcription activators, including IE0, IE2, and PE38. Although these proteins are conserved among baculoviruses, their role during infection is poorly understood. Derived by RNA splicing, IE0 is identical to IE1, except for 54 additional residues at its N terminus. It therefore has regulatory activities similar to those of IE1 (45,158,212,232). IE2 is a 47-kd leucine zipper, RING finger-containing transactivator that is also conserved among baculoviruses (35,261,293). Ac*M*NPV mutants containing loss-of-function *ie-2* alleles are viable, but exhibit delays in virus replication (218). On overexpression in transfected cells, *ie-2* causes cell-cycle arrest (220), but the significance of this activity is unknown. IE2 and the transregulator PE38 co-localize to punctate nuclear structures in transfected cells (161). PE38, which also contains a leucine zipper and RING finger, is capable of promoter-specific transactivation in plasmid transfection assays (160,175,209).

In general, the promoters for the immediate early baculovirus genes are highly active in the absence of virus proteins (158,161,223,261). As a consequence, several of these promoters including those for IE1 and IE2 have been used extensively for high-level gene expression in diverse lepidopteran and dipteran insects by stable or transient transfection protocols.

Late Phase

The late phase of the baculovirus life cycle is initiated by viral DNA replication, which begins between 6 and 12 hours after infection. The synthesis of new genomic DNA and the expression of late structural genes are necessary for the production of BV, the predominant infectious form generated during this period. Viral late gene expression is dependent on proper viral DNA replication. For example, inhibition of viral DNA synthesis by using a temperature-sensitive (*ts*) mutant in the helicase *p143* gene (see later) blocks DNA replication at the nonpermissive temperature and abrogates late gene expression and BV production (96). Likewise, treatment of infected cells with aphidicolin, which inhibits viral and host DNA polymerases, prevents viral DNA synthesis and blocks late viral transcription (230). The molecular basis for the coupling of late gene expression to DNA replication is unknown, but is common among large DNA viruses. At least five baculovirus genes (*ie-1, p143, lef-1, lef-2,* and *lef-3*) are required for DNA replication (Table 2). These genes were identified by using transient DNA replication assays conducted with plasmids containing an *hr* element/origin (152,177). The essential function of several replication genes during infection has been confirmed through the use of conditionally lethal mutants (see Table 2). Replication factors include a DNA-binding helicase (p143), a putative primase (LEF-1), a primase-associated protein (LEF-2), and a single-stranded DNA binding protein (LEF-3). The transactivator IE1 may stimulate transcription of the early replication genes and act as a DNA origin (*hr*)-binding protein (176). Five other genes (*dnápol, ie-2, lef-7, pe38,* and *p35*) directly or indirectly stimulate replication in this transient replication assay (reviewed in 176). A virus-specific DNA polymerase activity has been characterized (120,267), but the exact role of virus-encoded *dnapol* during infection is unclear. Viral factors localize to cen-

TABLE 2. *Baculovirus DNA replication and late expression factors*

Gene	DNA replication	LATE expression	Function/Homology	Virus mutants
ie-1	+	+	Transcription transactivator, DNA origin binding protein	*ts*B821
ie-2	+	+	Transcription transactivator, cell line–specific cell cycle regulator	
p47	–	+	Late RNA pol component	*ts*317
p143	+	+	Helicase, DNA binding, ATP-binding motif	*ts*8
dnapol	?	+	DNA polymerase, 5′→3′ exonuclease	
pp31	–	+	Virogenic stroma association	
p35	+	+	Apoptosis suppressor	
lef-1	+	+	Primase homology (WVVDAD motif), LEF2 association	
lef-2	+	+	Primase-associated protein? Late, VL expression	VLD1
lef-3	+	+	ssDNA binding, p143 association	
lef-4	–	+	Late RNA pol component, guanyl transferase, 5′ triphosphatase	*ts*538
lef-5	+	+	Unknown	
lef-6	+	+	Vaccinia virus RNA pol homology	
lef-7	+	+	Cell line–specific DNA replication	vlef-7-AG
lef-8	–	+	Late RNA pol component	*ts*S1
lef-9	–	+	Late RNA pol component	
lef-10	–	+	Unknown	
lef-11	–	+	Unknown	
lef-12	–	+	Unknown	
pe38	+	+	Transactivator of p143	
hcf-1	+	+	Cell line-specific, late, and VL expression	
vlf-1	–	–	VL expression, integrase/resolvase homology	*ts*B837

ters of viral DNA replication within the virogenic stroma appearing with the nucleus (see later) (202).

The mechanisms of baculovirus DNA replication are less well understood. Although the *hr* sequences are likely origins of viral DNA replication (154,169,210), it remains to be demonstrated that they act as origins during infection. The *hr*s are functionally redundant and do not affect late gene expression (210,229,231). Other non-*hr* sequences within the genome also have been implicated as replication origins (153,167,288). As suggested by the presence of multiple unit-length genome fragments and concatamers of defective genomes in cells (167,207), the large DNA genome may be replicated by a rolling-circle mechanism. Newly replicated, unit-length circles of DNA are packaged within nucleocapsids. During the late phase, the viral DNA adopts a nucleoprotein organization distinct from the host DNA that remains in a typical nucleosomal structure (286). The replicative or transcriptional function of this viral nucleoprotein structure is unknown.

Nineteen baculovirus genes are required for late gene expression (see Table 2), as first determined for Ac*M*NPV (173,177,227). These genes, designated late expression factors (*lefs*), were identified by their ability to support high-level expression of a reporter gene placed under control of a virus late promoter and cis-linked to an *hr* origin/enhancer element (209). The function and role of the *lefs* in baculovirus replication is the subject of ongoing research in this field (reviewed in 178). Because of the link between DNA replication and late gene expression, several genes required for late gene expression (*ie-1, p143, lef-1, lef-2,* and *lef-3*) are required DNA replication factors (see Table 2). Multiple *lef*s (*ie-2, lef-7,* and *hcf-1*) confer tissue or species specificity, because they are dispensable for late gene expression in certain cell lines. In addition, a variety of viral genes contribute to host range, including helicase *p143* and host range factor-1 (*hrf-1*) (42,53,148). Several *lefs* function directly or indirectly at the level of transcription or mRNA stabilization (see Table 2). Of these genes, four (*p47, lef-4, lef-8,* and *lef-9*) have been shown to encode components or subunits of the viral RNA polymerase (114) specific for late and very late gene expression (see later). The role of transcription-specific *lef*s during infection also has been characterized by using conditionally lethal mutations (see Table 2).

Unique among the nuclear-replicating DNA viruses, the baculoviruses switch from host RNA pol II for early transcription to a novel RNA polymerase for selective transcription of late and very late genes. The virus-encoded RNA polymerase retains its specificity for late virus promoters when assayed by using *in vitro* transcription extracts and is distinguished from other host RNA polymerases by its resistance to α-amanitin and tagetitoxin, inhibitors of RNA pol II and III, respectively (87,93,140,289). Chromatographic analyses of the late RNA polymerase activity indicated that the core of the complex comprises p47, LEF-4, LEF-8, and LEF-9, and is associated with additional proteins (13,114).

Late RNA transcripts initiate from a nucleotide motif containing the sequence (A/G/T)TAAG, which is the primary element for late and very late promoter activity (reviewed in 178). All genes encoding proteins synthesized in abundance during the late phase, including the major capsid protein vp39, the 6.9K basic core protein, and gp64 EFP, possess this late promoter motif. Nucleotide substitutions within the TAAG motif cause a dramatic loss of late promoter activity (191). Moreover, fewer than 18 nucleotides surrounding this initiation site are sufficient to direct high-level late gene expression. This simple promoter organization is reminiscent of yeast mitochondrial promoters and the T-odd bacteriophage promoters. Interestingly, certain late genes have multiple TAAG motifs, each serving as an independent RNA initiation site. For example, the *vp39* capsid gene is transcribed from three autonomous TAAG motifs at −57, −105, and −321 relative to the ORF (264). Such an arrangement may boost transcription levels needed for highly expressed genes. It is noteworthy that some early genes (*p35, gp64, pp31,* and *ie-1*) are also transcribed late in infection. This late transcription is most often accomplished by the use of late TAAG-containing elements that overlap the early promoter elements (22,110,195,222).

Very Late Phase

The final, very late stage of infection is characterized by the hyperexpression of occlusion-specific genes and the production of mature OV from 18 through 76 hours after infection or until cell lysis (Figs. 3A and 4). The very late phase is marked by a dramatic increase in transcription of *polh*, which encodes the major matrix protein of the OV. The temporally regulated hyperexpression of *polh* and its nonessential nature for BV production were the basis for development of the baculoviruses as highly efficient and productive vectors for foreign gene expression (reviewed in 144, 155, 186, and 199). In early vectors, foreign genes were placed under control of the *polh* promoter replacing the *polh* ORF to obtain high levels of expression very late in infection of cultured cells or whole larvae (180,215,245). More recently, the expression system has been extended to include other promoters, including that of the *p10* gene (see later).

Very late genes also are transcribed by the baculovirus α-amanitin-insensitive RNA polymerase. The promoters of these hypertranscribed genes, which include *polh* and *p10*, contain the late TAAG motif, which is the critical transcriptional element as shown by mutational analyses. However, these very late promoters also are positively regulated by the 50 nucleotides constituting the noncoding leader of their gene (191,205,279). This region between the TAAG and the ORF is responsible for the very late burst of transcriptional activity that distinguishes very late genes from late genes. Interestingly, insertion of the "burst" sequences immediately downstream from a late promoter was not sufficient to convert it to a very late promoter (191). These sequences may interact with activation factors responsible for the stimulation of transcription at this late time. Genetic evidence (184) suggests that virus-encoded very late factor-1 (VLF-1) is a likely candidate for the positive activator (see Table 2). VLF-1 forms a complex with the burst sequences, but the mechanism of transcriptional enhancement is not known (292). Host factors also may participate in transcription of very late genes (92).

The p10 gene is also the other hyperexpressed during the very late phase (reviewed in 196). It encodes a small coiled coil-domain protein (P10) that associates with expansive fibrillar structures that assemble in the nucleus and cytoplasm late in infection (see Fig. 4). P10 is nonessential for NPV replication, including OV formation (271,281). However, it may contribute to disruption of the nuclear membrane and may function at the tissue or organismal levels.

Virus Assembly, Budding, and Occlusion

Nucleocapsids assemble during the late and very late phases of infection. New capsids appear at the edge of the stromal matte located in the virogenic stroma (see Fig. 1D), a virus-specific nucleoprotein structure centered within the nucleus (123,294). Partially filled nucleocapsids with DNA strands connecting the core with the virogenic stroma have been observed, suggesting that the virogenic stroma may be the site of viral DNA replication, condensation, and encapsulation (77,294). A major viral protein associated with the virogenic stroma is phosphoprotein pp31, which is capable of DNA binding by a phosphorylation-regulated mechanism (30,31). RNA also may serve as a structural component of the virogenic stroma (294). Little else is known about this critically important virus-replication center. Newly assembled nucleocapsids exit the nucleus by budding or by transport through nuclear pores (see Fig. 2) (reviewed in 280). Nucleocapsid maturation is sensitive to the actin-depolymerizing drug cytochalasin D, suggesting a critical role for actin in this morphogenic process (40,201). Although enveloped nucleocapsids have been observed in the cytoplasm, the nuclear envelope is removed when the plasma membrane is reached. By interacting end-on with the plasma membrane that is associated with the envelope fusion protein EFP gp64, single nucleocapsids bud from the cell surface to produce extracellular BV (see Fig. 1C). EFP gp64 is required for budding of Ac*M*NPV (206). The rate of BV release from Ac*M*NPV-infected cells increases exponentially from 10 to 20 hours and then declines through 36 hours (166). The kinetics of BV production varies between baculoviruses.

OV particles accumulate in the nucleus of Ac*M*NPV-infected cells (see Figs. 3A and 4) starting ~18 hours after infection. OV production accelerates as BV production shuts down. Virion occlusion involves a number of processes, including virus-induced modification of the nuclear membrane and nuclear transport of polyhedrin, the OV matrix protein (145,280). Nucleocapsids align along nuclear membrane segments and acquire an envelope before condensation of polyhedrin, which encases the enveloped virions (see Fig. 1E). OV formation begins on the inside edge of the infected nucleus (see Fig. 4). Time-lapse video microscopy has indicated that the number of OV particles per cell is established early, and with time, each particle increases in size (181). Maturation of the OV includes deposition of the polyhedron envelope (calyx) over the particle's surface. OV is released from the nucleus on cytolysis very late in infection. Multiple virus genes are likely involved in OV production. For example, loss of function of the 25K protein gene of Ac*M*NPV causes the easily recognized "few polyhedra" (FP) phenotype, which is characterized by reduced OV accumulation, limited intranuclear envelopment of nucleocapsids, and increased production of BV (10,27,124). The exact function of the cytoplasmic 25K protein remains unknown. A gene involved in calyx formation also has been identified (94).

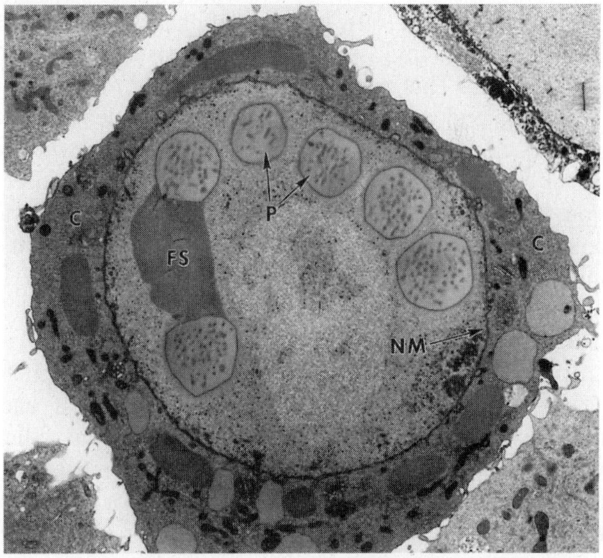

FIG. 4. The very late, occlusion stage of Ac*M*NPV infection. During the very late, occlusion phase, multiple OV particles of polyhedrin (*P*) form on the inside edge of the enlarged nucleus, defined by an intact nuclear membrane (*NM*). Dense fibrillar structures (*FS*) often form in the nucleus and the cytoplasm (*C*). Electron micrograph was provided by Dr. Peter Faulkner and Dr. Gregory Williams, Queens University.

Disease Progression in the Insect

Horizontal transmission of baculoviruses occurs through the OV, the form of the virus that is most stable and resistant to environmental degradation. Primary infection occurs in the midgut epithelium of the insect larva (reviewed in 69). Infection is initiated by larval ingestion of virus-contaminated food. On entry into the midgut lumen (see Fig. 2B), the OV particles dissolve in response to the alkaline environment, thereby releasing the ODV. These virions pass through the peritrophic membrane, facilitated by the activity of virus-encoded proteases (enhancins), first discovered in the GVs (170). ODVs subsequently bind to the brush-border membrane of columnar epithelial cells and enter, apparently by direct fusion with the plasma membranes (see Fig. 2B). Infection proceeds in a manner similar to that of BV-infected cell cultures, with the interesting exception that formation of OV in midgut cells of most lepidopteran hosts is rare (76). In addition, there is a distinct polarity in the intracellular transport of EFP gp64, which is directed primarily to the basal membrane side of the midgut cell (149). This directionality likely dictates nucleocapsid budding to the basal lamina, allowing access of BV to the hemocoel and tracheal epithelium for rapid systemic spread. Certain baculoviruses, such as the mosquito (Diptera) NPVs, are restricted to the midgut.

Secondary infection is achieved by BV produced in midgut cells (see Fig. 2A). Virus is spread by hemocytes (blood cells), the epithelial cells lining the tracheal network, or both (65,101). With highly susceptible hosts, secondary infection can affect virtually all the internal tissues of the larva (69). In the final phases, the larva is converted into a milky white liquid, consisting mostly of OV particles. This process, referred to as "melting" or "liquification," is facilitated by a virus-encoded cathepsin and chitinase, which cooperate to break down the larval cuticle (skin) (125). In a typical Ac*M*NPV infection, more than 10^8 OV particles are produced per larva, constituting more than 10% of the dry weight of the insect. On rupture of the cuticular exoskeleton, OV is released into the environment for transmission to other insects.

It is noteworthy that not all baculoviruses are lethal. There are several reports of persistent or latent baculovirus infections in seeming healthy insects. Such viruses may be transmitted vertically. The most thoroughly described virus/host system is that of a *Mamestra brassicae* NPV that persists in a laboratory insect colony without causing significant mortality (139).

Baculovirus-Mediated Alterations of the Host

Baculoviruses have dramatic effects on the host cell, altering both cytoskeletal and nuclear structure (see earlier) and causing shutdown of host protein and RNA synthesis (36,203). However, these viruses also can control their insect hosts at the physiologic and behavioral levels (reviewed in 196). For example, infected larvae often display the abnormal behavior of wandering away from their food supply or climbing to the top of the vegetation, where they succumb hanging from a leaf or branch. This strategy may facilitate virus dispersal. In another example, baculoviruses arrest development of their larval hosts by controlling the activity of ecdysone, the steroid hormone that triggers molting (197). The baculovirus *egt* gene encodes an ecdysteroid uridine diphosphate (UDP)-glucose/galactose transferase, which is secreted from infected cells and transfers glucose or galactose to the hydroxyl group at position C22 of these ecdysteroids. Evidence exists that viral *egt* blocks larval molting (reviewed in 196). Larval developmental arrest is correlated with increased virus production, because on deletion of *egt*, infected larvae attempt to molt, but die sooner and produce less virus (198). The overall effect of *egt* depends on virus dose and the developmental stage at the time of inoculation.

Apoptosis and Apoptotic Suppressors

The replicative success of baculoviruses depends on active suppression of host-cell apoptosis, a process that may represent an antivirus defense strategy by the host. Apoptosis or programmed cell death (PCD) is a highly conserved mechanism for cellular self-destruction that is critically important in normal development, tissue homeostasis, and virus pathogenesis. To counteract the apoptotic suicide response and prolong cell viability, the baculoviruses encode novel apoptotic suppressors, which block virus-induced apoptosis (reviewed in 47 and 187). Because these same proteins function in phylogenetically diverse organisms, baculoviruses have provided important insight into the biochemical components of PCD and its regulation.

Ac*M*NPV mutants that lack PCD suppressors cause widespread apoptosis (48,49,129). Apoptosis of cultured *Spodoptera frugiperda* SF21 cells, a model system for studies of invertebrate PCD, is characterized by fragmentation of cellular and viral DNA and dismemberment of the infected cell into extracellular vesicles called apoptotic bodies (see Fig. 3B) (48,164,181). SF21 cells are highly sensitive to a variety of apoptotic stimuli, including UV radiation, actinomycin D, calcium ionophores, okadaic acid, and hydrogen peroxide (Fig. 5A). In cultured cells, apoptosis reduces the yield of infectious virus by as much as 10,000-fold (49,129). Moreover, the infectivity of apoptosis-causing Ac*M*NPV mutants in larvae is 25- to 1,000-fold lower than that of wild-type virus (49), suggesting that apoptosis impedes baculovirus multiplication in larvae. Interestingly, baculovirus-induced apoptosis is tissue or species specific. For example, cultured *Trichoplusia ni* TN368 cells fail to undergo apoptosis when infected by Ac*M*NPV mutants that cause apoptosis of SF21 cells (49,129). In *T. ni* larvae, the infectivity of these mutants is comparable to that of wild-type virus. The molecular basis of this cellular resistance to virus-induced apoptosis is not understood.

It is likely that multiple mechanisms are responsible for triggering apoptosis during baculovirus infection. Virus binding to cellular receptors is not sufficient. Rather, viral gene expression is required (50,164). After Ac*M*NPV infection, the earliest of detected apoptotic events (see Fig. 5A) is the activation of host-cell caspases (16,165). The caspases are a highly conserved family of **c**ysteinyl **asp**artate–specific prote**ases** that are critical and necessary effectors of apoptosis (reviewed in 265). Proteolytic activation of the proenzyme form of *Sf*-caspase-1, the principal executioner caspase in SF21 cells, coincides with the initiation of virus DNA replication (164,165,182,242). Thus apoptotic signaling must occur at or before this time, suggesting that viral DNA replication, late gene products, or shutdown of host RNA or protein synthesis may trigger apoptosis (50,164). Early gene expression also can contribute to apoptotic signaling (164). In particular, transactivator IE1 is sufficient to induce limited apoptosis in SF21 cells on overexpression by plasmid transfection (219). However, the mechanism by which IE1 induces apoptosis and its role in baculovirus-induced apoptosis are unclear (229).

The baculoviruses encode two mechanistically distinct types of apoptotic suppressors (see Fig. 5B), the inhibitors of apoptosis (IAPs) and the caspase inhibitors (P35 and P49). These proteins prevent premature host-cell death and thereby promote virus multiplication (reviewed in 47 and 187). Identification of functional *iap genes* in lepidopteran insects (see Fig. 5B) suggests that baculoviruses originally acquired these apoptotic regulators from the host cell (138,243). This possibility is consistent with the strong selective advantage conferred to the virus by the capacity to prevent virus-induced apoptosis (172). Although baculoviruses encode multiple apoptotic suppressors, usually one is sufficient per genome. For example, Ac*M*NPV encodes one functional copy of *p35* and two copies of *iap* (*iap1* and *iap2*), which are nonfunctional for blocking virus-induced apoptosis (50,103). Lacking *p35,* Op*M*NPV encodes one functional (*iap3*) and three nonfunctional *iaps* (19).

Baculovirus IAPs were the first discovered members of the IAP family, which now includes related proteins from invertebrates and vertebrates (reviewed in 47, 59, and 187). IAPs are distinguished by their highly conserved Cys/His-containing motif called the BIR (**b**aculovirus **i**ap **r**epeat) (see Fig. 5B). This defining ~65-

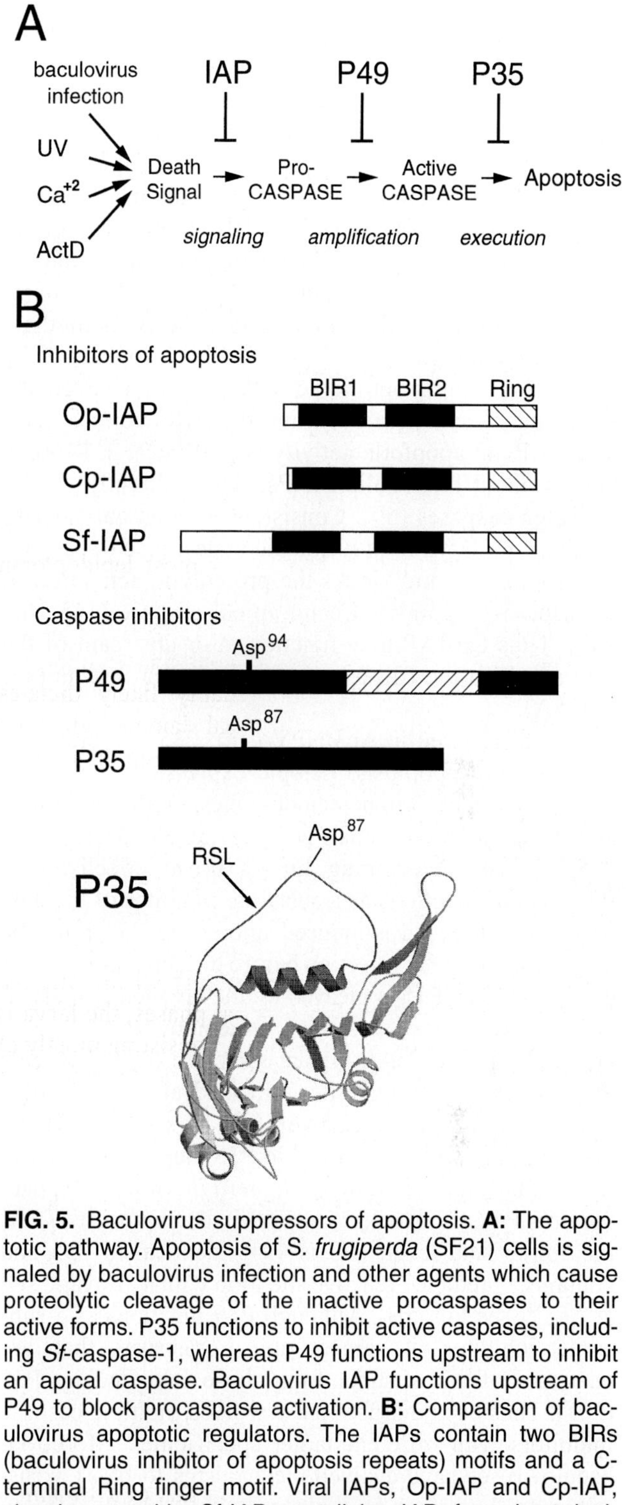

FIG. 5. Baculovirus suppressors of apoptosis. **A:** The apoptotic pathway. Apoptosis of *S. frugiperda* (SF21) cells is signaled by baculovirus infection and other agents which cause proteolytic cleavage of the inactive procaspases to their active forms. P35 functions to inhibit active caspases, including *Sf*-caspase-1, whereas P49 functions upstream to inhibit an apical caspase. Baculovirus IAP functions upstream of P49 to block procaspase activation. **B:** Comparison of baculovirus apoptotic regulators. The IAPs contain two BIRs (baculovirus inhibitor of apoptosis repeats) motifs and a C-terminal Ring finger motif. Viral IAPs, Op-IAP and Cp-IAP, closely resemble Sf-IAP, a cellular IAP from host lepidopteran *S. frugiperda.* Caspase inhibitors P49 and P35 are 49% identical and contain aspartate residues (Asp^{94} and Asp^{87}) required for caspase cleavage. P49 contains a 120 residue insertion (crosshatched) unrelated to P35. The P35 crystal structure (bottom) illustrates its reactive site loop (RSL) in which Asp^{87} is located at the apex for caspase cleavage and interaction.

residue motif coordinates a Zn atom and is required for IAP antiapoptotic function. Baculovirus Op-IAP (31 kd) and Cp-IAP (31 kd) from Op*M*NPV and CpGV, respectively, contain two BIRs and a C-terminal RING finger motif (19,54). Suggesting that they function at a conserved step in the apoptotic pathway, the viral IAPs prevent apoptosis induced by diverse signals in insect and mammalian cells (47,187). The BIR motif is required for interaction with cellular proapoptotic factors, including Reaper, Hid, and Grim from *Drosophila melanogaster* (276,277). In addition, the BIRs mediate homo-oligomerization of Op-IAP, which appears to be required for antiapoptotic activity (137). However, the molecular mechanism by which the BIRs contribute to viral IAP antiapoptotic activity is still unclear. More is known about mammalian IAPs, which directly inhibit activated caspases (59). Consistent with an anticaspase mechanism, Op-IAP prevents the appearance of caspase activity *in vivo* and blocks the proteolytic activation of *Sf*-caspase-1 by an upstream, apical caspase (165,182, 242). Thus Op-IAP may function at or upstream of the step at which the caspases are activated in insects (see Fig. 5A).

First discovered in Ac*M*NPV (48), P35 is a universal suppressor of apoptosis. Ectopic expression of the *p35* gene prevents PCD in nematodes, flies, moths, and mice, as well as cultured human cells (37,50,58,133,143,224, 225,257,270). Accounting for its broad effectiveness, P35 (35 kd) functions as a substrate inhibitor of the caspases. To block virus-induced apoptosis, P35 must be synthesized early in infection before the activation of host caspases (130). P35 is cleaved by the targeted caspase at Asp^{87} and forms a stable, stoichiometric complex (16,32,298). The 2.2-Å crystal structure of P35 reveals that the Asp^{87} cleavage site is located at the apex of a novel solvent-exposed reactive site loop (see Fig. 5B), the orientation of which is critical to P35's anticaspase activity (72,300). Identified in *Spodoptera littoralis* NPV, baculovirus P49 also blocks virus-induced apoptosis (63). At the amino acid level, P49 is 49% identical to P35 and contains a predicted reactive site loop with a cleavage site at Asp^{94} (see Fig. 5B). Although P49 functions as a substrate inhibitor, it targets apical caspases that are upstream of and distinct from those inhibited by P35 (301). Thus baculoviruses have evolved multiple caspase inhibitors with different target specificities. Moreover, baculoviruses have evolved mechanisms to block virus-induced apoptosis at multiple steps in the death pathway (see Fig. 5A). No cellular homologs of *p35* or *p49* have been identified.

Host Transposons

The baculoviruses are one of the few families of animal viruses that accommodate the frequent and spontaneous insertion of host-derived transposable elements (reviewed in 79). By virtue of their nuclear replication and flexibility with respect to size of their DNA genome, baculoviruses are vulnerable to the insertion of resident transposons. Because of their relative abundance and mobility, arthropod transposons represent important insertional mutagens and can have a significant influence on virus and host evolution. Transposon insertion provides genetic diversity and potentially novel genes to the recipient virus. The baculovirus' capacity to act as a landing platform for these elements has led to the identification of new families of lepidopteran transposons.

Baculovirus mutants with transposon insertions are often distinguished by their altered plaque morphology, especially the "few polyhedra" (FP) phenotype, which exhibits reduced OV accumulation (see earlier). Several FP-causing lepidopteran transposons, including IFP2, IFP2.2, IFP1.6, TFP3, and hitchhiker, have been identified by their insertion at or near the FP locus that encodes the 25K protein gene (9–11,38,78). These middle to highly repetitive elements are characterized by their small size and terminal inverted repeats that sometimes flank a transposase-like ORF. Significantly, IFP2 (also called PiggyBac) is a 2.5-kb autonomous transposon from the moth *T. ni,* which is capable of stable germline transformation of the Mediterranean fruit fly from the order Diptera (119). Thus PiggyBac and other lepidopteran elements have the potential for gene transfer in non-drosophilid insects.

Also discovered as a baculovirus insertion, TED (transposable element D) is a 7.5-kb, middle-repetitive retrotransposon of *T. ni* (82,185). TED has a retrovirus-like organization with *gag, pol,* and *env* genes that are flanked by long terminal repeats, and thus is a member of the gypsy family of retroelements (79). Unlike the smaller lepidopteran transposons, TED assembles virus-like *gag*-containing particles, complete with protease and reverse transcriptase activities (115,171). Moreover, the TED *env* gene encodes a membrane-associated glycoprotein that could function as a viral envelope protein (208). Thus TED and other *env*-carrying gypsy elements are likely insect retroviruses. As such, integration within the baculovirus genome could facilitate interspecies shuttling of these passenger viruses (79,185).

Nudiviruses

Classification and Structure of Nudiviruses

The nudiviruses were previously categorized as "nonoccluded" baculoviruses, but are currently unclassified. Like the baculoviruses, they have rod-shaped, enveloped nucleocapsids that contain a large circular, double-stranded DNA genome (recently reviewed in 33).

The envelope is acquired in the nucleus, and in some cases, a second unit membrane is obtained by budding from the plasma membrane of the infected cell. In contrast to the baculoviruses, the nudiviruses lack an occluded form. This difference limits their survival outside the host and may contribute to their persistence or latency in infected insects. Because of the paucity of nucleotide sequence information, the relatedness between individual nudiviruses or baculoviruses is unknown. The nudiviruses could be an aggregate of genetically diverse viruses.

Nudivirus Transmission and Persistence

Nudiviruses can exert dramatic effects on insect populations. Oryctes virus, a nudivirus infecting the rhinoceros beetle *Oryctes rhinoceros,* causes a potentially fatal infection that initiates in the midgut of adult beetles and their larvae (295,296). This virus has been enormously successful as a control agent of the rhinoceros beetle in coconut plantations in the South Pacific (297). Virus transmission occurs primarily through contaminated food sources, but also can occur through mating. Another nudivirus, Gonad Specific Virus (GSV), infects gonadal tissue (ovarian and testicular organs) of adult moths and causes sterility (116,226). GSV appears to be transmitted by asymptomatic carriers within the insect population and can be vertically transmitted from eggs, probably in a persistent or latent state. Virus replication is hormonally activated in adult gonadal tissue. Hormonal or developmental activation also occurs with other viruses, including the polydnaviruses (see later). GSV can be propagated in cell culture, and persistently infected cell lines have been established (34).

Hz-1 is the most extensively studied nudivirus at the molecular level. This complex, nonoccluded virus has provided a useful model for insect virus persistence and latency (reviewed in 33). Hz-1 was originally isolated from a persistently infected cell line established from adult ovarian tissue of the corn earworm *Heliothis zea* (102). It has an unusually large (230 kbp) circular, double-stranded DNA genome. Hz-1 establishes persistent infections of cultured cells where replication occurs at low levels and produces defective interfering particles. Virus from persistent infections can cause lytic infection of naive cells not previously exposed to virus. The genome of persistently infected cells can harbor stably integrated Hz-1 DNA (174). The establishment or maintenance of viral persistence is associated with the synthesis of a single 2.9-kb RNA transcript from Hz-1, referred to as the persistency-associated transcript (PAT1) (39). The function of PAT1 and whether it encodes a protein(s) is unknown. Hz-1–infected cells also are resistant to superinfection. This immunity is not due to an acquired resistance to virus-induced apoptosis (168).

Polydnaviridae

Classification and Structure of Polydnaviruses

The polydnaviruses are distinguished by their obligate and mutualistic association with their host, the endoparasitic wasps (Order Hymenoptera). The family *Polydnaviridae* derives its name from the taxonomically characteristic "polydisperse" DNAs composing its multi-segmented genome. Virions contain numerous double-stranded, supercoiled DNA molecules with sizes ranging from 2 to 28 kbp (reviewed in 248 and 278). Depending on the virus, there are 15 to 30 different DNA molecules with an estimated genomic complexity of 75 to 200 kbp. Virion DNA is derived from proviral DNA integrated within the host wasp, where the virus is transmitted vertically. Current evidence indicates that the proviral DNA is also polydisperse within the host genome where certain DNAs are the linear equivalent of circular segments packaged within virions (55,74, 105,290). Because polydnaviruses are not known to replicate outside the host wasp, it is not yet clear that virion DNA represents the entire virus genome.

The only characterized polydnaviruses are from endoparasitic wasps. These predatory insects lay their eggs inside the bodies of other living insects, often in the larval stage, where the eggs hatch and the young parasites develop. Polydnaviruses have been isolated from the Ichneumonidae and Braconidae families of wasps and are correspondingly divided into two genera, the ichnoviruses and bracoviruses (278). Although polydnavirus-like particles have been observed in other parasitoids, they remain unclassified.

The ichnoviruses and bracoviruses are morphologically distinct. The only feature shared by the two genera may be their polydisperse virion DNA and their novel life cycle. The ichnovirus virion is complex, resembling that of the ascoviruses (see later). The virions are ellipsoid or quasi-cylindrical, with a uniform size of 90 × 300 nm (Fig. 6A and B). The nucleocapsid is enveloped by two unit membranes, one derived from the nucleus during virion morphogenesis and the other by budding from the plasma membrane of the host cell. Resembling the baculoviruses, bracovirus nucleocapsids are rod-shaped with a uniform diameter (35–40 nm) and variable length (30–200 nm). They have a single membrane envelope, which is derived from the nucleus and surrounds one or more nucleocapsids (see Fig. 6C). Polydnavirus particles contain 20 different polypeptides. The minimal genetic information needed to encode these structural proteins is about 30 kb. However, evidence exists that some structural proteins may be produced by

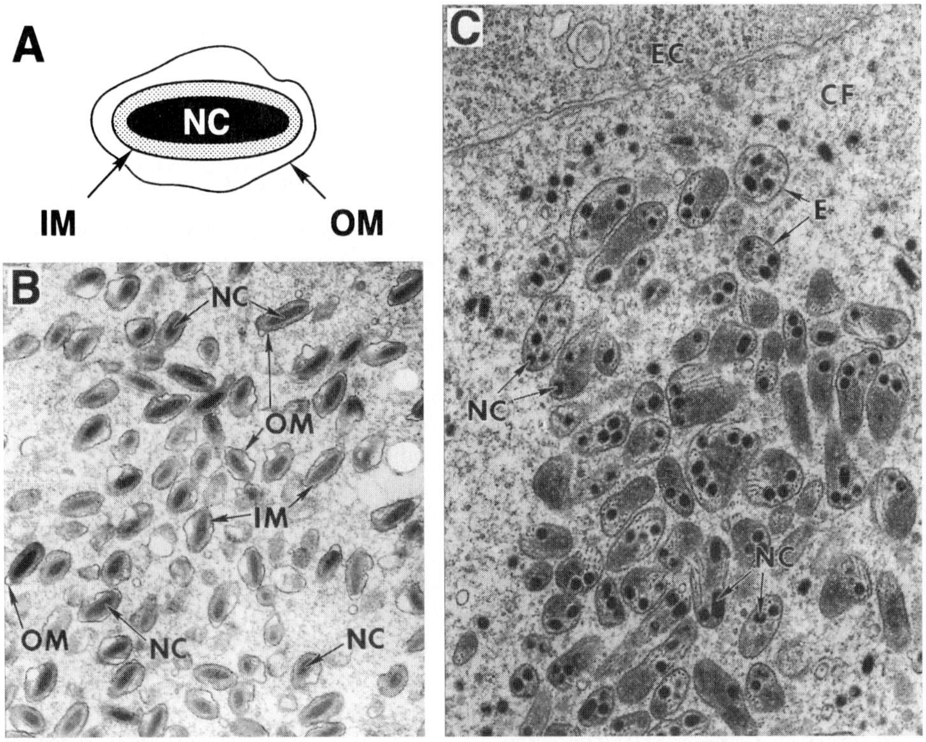

FIG. 6. Morphological features of polydnaviruses. **A:** Schematic view of the ichnovirus structure. The nucleocapsid (*NC*) is surrounded by an inner (*IM*) and outer (*OM*) membrane. **B:** Ichnovirus preparation. Lenticular nucleocapsids (*NC*) of uniform size are enveloped by inner and outer membranes (*IM* and *OM*). **C:** Bracoviruses in the calyx fluid (*CF*) of an adult female parasitoid wasp. Nucleocapsids (*NC*) are observed end-on and in lateral view. Multiple nucleocapsids are surrounded by a unit membrane envelope (*E*). An epithelial cell (*EC*) of the calyx is also observed. Electron micrographs provided by Dr. Donald B. Stoltz, Dalhousie University. Modified with permission from (251).

the expression of integrated, proviral DNA, rather than virion DNA (278).

Obligate Mutualism of Virus and Host

The polydnaviruses play a critical role in the life cycle of their host wasp. This mutualistic participation is central to the multiplication strategy and genetic organization of these novel viruses. The polydnaviruses replicate asymptomatically in the oviducts of female wasps, as a normal step in the development of the reproductive tract (Fig. 7). Proviral DNA is present as dispersed, integrated segments and is inherited in a mendelian fashion (249). On replication, polydnavirus particles accumulate to high density in the calyx fluid of the oviduct. On parasitization, virus and the wasp's egg is delivered to the recipient caterpillar (see Fig. 7). Normally, the caterpillar mounts an immune response that is mediated in part by hemocytes of the open circulatory system, which encapsulate the intruding egg, thereby destroying it. However, in the case of polydnavirus-carrying ichneumonid and braconid wasps, encapsulation is counteracted or repressed by the accompanying virus. As a result, development of the parasitic egg is ensured. Demonstrating a definitive role for virus-mediated abrogation of the host immune response, the wasp egg is destroyed within the larva when introduced in the absence of virus (64). Thus the relationship between polydnavirus and wasp is mutualistic. The wasp requires the virus to provide protection against the immune response of the parasitized insect, and the virus requires the wasp for replication and survival of its genome.

Polydnavirus Genome Organization

The polydnavirus genome is highly complex. Virion DNAs (designated by letters) are nonequimolar, polymorphic in length, and present in multiple topologic forms (superhelical, relaxed circular, etc.) (reviewed in 278). For example, the genome of *Campoletis sonorensis* polydnavirus (CsPDV), the ichnovirus prototype, consists of 28 to 30 different DNAs, ranging in size from 5.5 to 21 kbp, with a collective size of 200 to 250 kbp. It is not known how many viral DNAs are packaged within each virion or whether each virion contains

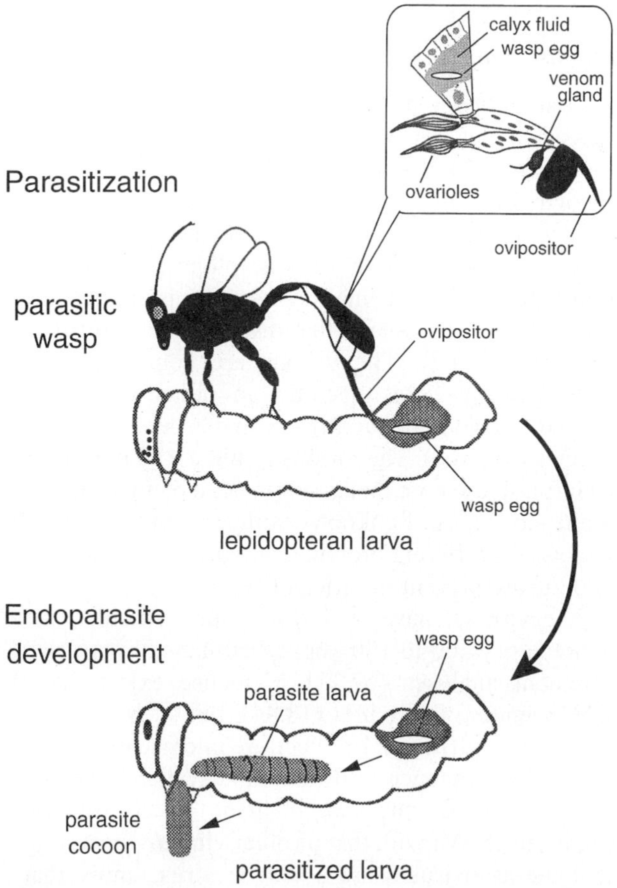

FIG. 7. Polydnavirus life cycle. Polydnavirus particles form in the epithelial cells of adult female ovaries and are released into the calyx fluid where they accumulate to high densities (*top inset*). As the first step in parasitization (*top*), the wasp egg along with virus and venom are injected into a lepidopteran larva during oviposition. During endoparasite development (*bottom*), polydnavirus activity suppresses the larval immune response allowing the wasp egg to develop within the parasitized larva. After development, the wasp larva emerges, spins a cocoon, pupates, and emerges as an adult to repeat the process in a new host. From Dr. Bruce A. Webb, University of Kentucky; modified with permission.

all or a subset of DNA segments. Particles of CsPDV (see Fig. 6) have a uniform size and density and thus may have similar DNA contents. In contrast, bracovirus virions vary in length and may contain different quantities of DNA. In addition, certain ichnovirus DNA segments are likely derived from recombination events within larger segments, which are referred to as "nested" segments (55,290). The presence of nested segments may reduce the effective complexity of virion DNA. However, complete determination of genetic complexity will require characterization of all genomic DNA segments.

From the few cases in which the relationship between virion and proviral DNA is known, the largest or "master" DNA segments within the wasp genome are flanked by direct repeats. The 16-kbp integrated W segment of CsPDV has long terminal repeats of 1.2 kb (55). Additional 350-bp repeats within this segment are apparently responsible for generating nested R and M segments through homologous recombination during amplification of circular DNA segments in the female wasp. Within the wasp genome, the termini of CsPDV segment B are flanked by 59-bp direct repeats and are removed during excision and circularization of this DNA (74). This finding and others suggest that proviral segments are excised from the wasp genome by recombination before amplification (105). Other sequences are repeated between CsPDV DNA segments, but may not be involved in recombination (262).

Virion DNA from the polydnaviruses carry genes that participate in suppression of the immune response of parasitized caterpillar. Several gene families have been identified (23,60,256,290). One family within CsPDV encodes proteins with sequence similarity to omega-conotoxins of marine snail venoms (60). One of the conotoxin-like proteins has been implicated in the suppression of the encapsulation response (reviewed in 278). Moreover, a functional relationship between the viral toxins and wasp venom peptides may explain the independence of the ichnoviruses from venom gland secretions of the wasp for immune suppression. Another gene family with sequence similarity to epidermal growth factors has been identified in *Microplitis demolitor* polydnavirus (MdPDV) (256). The nature and function of these gene products are unclear. It also is unknown whether virions contain all the genes required for virion assembly, because only a few polydnavirus structural genes have been characterized.

Polydnavirus Life Cycle and Host Effects

The formation of polydnavirus virions occurs primarily, if not exclusively, in the nuclei of epithelial calyx cells composing the oviducts of female wasps (see Fig. 7). Virus replication is under hormonal control and is first detected at a specific stage in wasp pupal development (reviewed in 278). Proviral DNA segments may be amplified in an "onion skin" fashion from within the wasp chromosome and then circularized. Alternatively, proviral DNA may be excised first, circularized, and then amplified. The presence of chromosomal sites lacking proviral DNA in tissues supporting viral replication is consistent with the latter mechanism (105). In mature females, the virions are released from the calyx cells into the oviduct lumen, either by budding (ichnoviruses) or by cell lysis (bracoviruses). The calyx fluid contains massive numbers of polydnavirus particles (see Fig. 6C), which are deposited along with the egg and wasp secretions such as venom from accessory glands during oviposition.

Despite the presence of high concentrations of virions, polydnaviruses cause no obvious pathology in wasps. RNA transcripts from some genomic segments have been detected in wasp ovaries, and there is evidence that some of the viral RNAs produced in wasps differ from those produced in parasitized hosts (23,262). Although virus particles are confined to the female reproductive tract, viral DNA also is present in many tissues of adult females and males (75). The predominant form of the viral DNA in males is the integrated proviral form, but a minor component of extrachromosomal DNA also has been detected.

The most obvious physiologic effect of the polydnaviruses is in the parasitized insect host, where larval immunity and development are altered (reviewed in 254 and 278). The mechanisms of virus-mediated immune suppression are not yet understood. Polydnavirus suppression of encapsulation involves physiologic changes in hemocytes that participate in capsule formation, including granulocytes and plasmatocytes (252). On virus entry, viral gene expression occurs in hemocytes and possibly other tissues. Many hemocytes survive throughout parasitization and continue to support virus gene expression. Some viral gene products are secreted and are thought to affect other hemocytes and tissues. In MdPDV, virus gene products induce apoptosis in a specific subclass of hemocytes, which are involved in the encapsidation response (255). Other aspects of larval physiology also are affected, either directly by polydnavirus-specific proteins or indirectly as result of infection of normal cells.

There is no evidence for polydnavirus replication in the parasitized larva. Neither synthesis of virion DNA nor assembly of virions has been detected. Nonetheless, virion DNA is long-lived, and viral RNA transcription occurs throughout parasitization. In the ichnovirus CsPDV, 12 different polyadenylated RNAs have been identified in parasitized or virion-injected larvae (23,24). Some of these viral RNAs are spliced. CsPDV transcripts are detected within 2 hours and persist throughout development and emergence of the parasite wasp 9 days after oviposition. Several virion gene products have been detected (reviewed in 278). A similar strategy of gene expression and persistence of the bracovirus MdPDV occurs in parasitized and virus-injected *Pseudoplusia includens* larvae (253,256). Viral DNA persists for 6 days, but is not amplified. At least six different classes of MdPDV RNA are synthesized primarily in hemocytes, which may be the principal target for immune suppression. The identification and functional characterization of polydnavirus gene products that modulate the lepidopteran immune system remain the areas of intense interest.

Ascoviridae

Classification and Structure

First discovered in the 1970s, the ascoviruses are classified as a single genus, ascovirus, within the family *Ascoviridae* (reviewed in 70 and 188). The name ascovirus is derived from the Greek word *askós*, meaning sac, to describe the large membrane-bound vesicles that are associated with virus development. The formation of these virion-containing vesicles is unique among viruses and represents the distinguishing feature of *Ascoviridae* (67). The virions are complex, double-enveloped particles having an allantoid (kidney-shaped), ovoidal, or bacilliform shape, depending on the species (Fig. 8A). The virions (~400 × 130 nm) have an electron-dense core that is surrounded by two unit membrane envelopes of unknown composition (see Fig. 8B). At least 12 different proteins, ranging in size from 11 to 200 kd, are present in virions (71).

Ascoviruses have a large, double-stranded DNA genome of ~100 to 180 kbp, as estimated by restriction fragment analyses (67,71). Evidence exists that the DNA genome is circular (18,44), but such forms have not been confirmed by electron microscopy. Limited nucleotide sequence information is available. Sequence comparisons of the *dnapol* gene of *S. frugiperda* ascovirus (SAV) with that of other viral *dnapol*s suggest that the ascoviruses are a unique virus family that is most closely related to the iridoviruses (214). Short imperfect repeats also have been identified within the ascovirus genome (18).

Replication Stages

Studies on ascovirus replication have been limited to cytologic observations in tissues of infected moth larvae (188). The first sign of infection is nuclear and cellular hypertrophy, in which the diameter of the infected cell increases from fivefold to 10-fold (67). As replication proceeds, the nucleus fragments, and the cell separates into 20 to 30 membrane-bound vesicles that contain assembling virions (see Fig. 8C). This unusual process involves extensive invagination of the plasma membrane, similar to that of a cell undergoing apoptosis. Once formed, the vesicles dissociate from the cell and are released into the hemolymph. As the vesicles accumulate, basement membranes surrounding the tissue are disrupted, and the hemocoel becomes filled with $\sim 10^8$ vesicles/mL, a process that turns the hemolymph a milky white color.

Ascovirus Transmission and Disease Progression

In the laboratory, ascovirus transmission is accomplished by pricking the host with a fine pin contami-

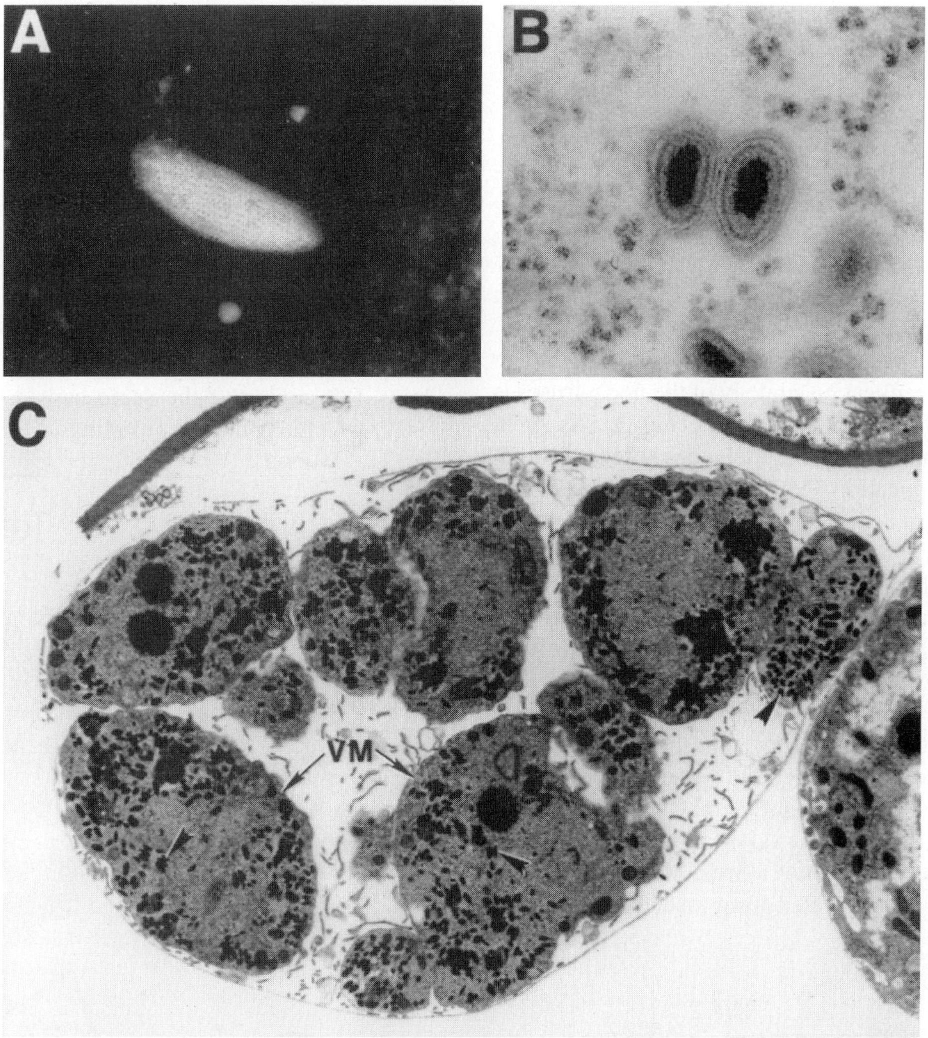

FIG. 8. Ascoviruses. **A:** An individual kidney-shaped nucleocapsid of the ascovirus from the moth *Trichoplusia ni.* The surface is reticular in appearance. **B:** Cross-section of two adjacent virions of the *Scotogramma* ascovirus. A multi-layered membrane envelope surrounds the nucleocapsid. **C:** Remnants of an ascovirus-infected cell. Dark-staining bodies are membrane-bound vesicles (*VM*) that contain *Autographa precationis* ascovirus particles (arrowheads). Different-sized vesicles are collectively bordered by a basement membrane. Provided by Dr. Brian A. Federici, University of California-Riverside, and Dr. J. J. Hamm, USDA-ARS, Tifton, GA; modified with permission from (68,70)

nated with virus-containing vesicles. A dose of 10 vesicles is sufficient to infect more than 90% of inoculated insects. In nature, ascoviruses are probably transmitted by female endoparasitic wasps through virus contamination of their ovipositor during egg laying. For example, *Diadromus pulchellus* ascovirus (DpAV) is vectored by the ichneumonid wasp *Diadromus pulchellus* during oviposition of leek moth pupae, where the virus multiplies during parasitization (18). DpAV can be found in the wasp reproductive tract, but appears to replicate poorly there. DpAV DNA is found in both male and female wasps. A mutualistic relationship between the ascovirus and its wasp vector is suspected, because survival of *D. pulchellus* wasps in the laboratory is positively correlated with the presence of DpAV (17). The host range of ascoviruses may include only a few closely related species or may extend to species in different families (117).

Ascoviruses cause a slow, chronic infection in lepidopteran (moth) larvae or pupae. The disease causes reduced feeding, aberrant development, and death within 2 to 6 weeks (reviewed in 188). During the early stages, there is little obvious pathology. In the later stages, the most notable disease symptom is developmental arrest. Some larvae exhibit a milky discoloration. Different ascoviruses exhibit different tissue tropisms. For example, SAV selectively multiplies in fat body, whereas other viruses multiply in diverse tissues.

Nodaviridae

Classification of Nodaviruses

The *Nodaviridae* are small riboviruses with a single-stranded, positive-sense genome of two RNAs. The bipartite genome is packaged within a single, nonenveloped virion (~30 nm diameter) with T=3 icosahedral symmetry (recently reviewed in 8, 146, and 238). The genome organization and replication strategy of the nodaviruses is among the simplest of known viruses (Fig. 9). As such, the nodaviruses are powerful models for exploring strategies of virus replication, host interactions, and virion assembly.

The nodaviruses are divided into two genera (alpha and beta), which infect insects and fish, respectively. The family name originated from Nodamura virus, the first discovered family member isolated from mosquitoes near the Japanese village of Nodamura (236). The best-studied insect nodaviruses include Nodamura virus (NoV), black beetle virus (BBV), and flock house virus (FHV), each of which has been fully characterized at the molecular level. Other alpha members include New Zealand virus, Boolarra virus, Manawatu virus, and gypsy moth (*Lymantria ninayi*) virus. Most members of the alpha genus were isolated from insects of Australasia. NoV is the only nodavirus with the capacity to multiply in vertebrates (8). Nonetheless, on transfection of genomic RNA, nodaviruses can replicate in mammalian, yeast (*Saccharomyces cerevisae*), and plant cells (5,217,240).

Virion Structure of the Nodaviruses

The nodaviruses have provided enormous insight into icosahedral virus assembly and maturation. The structures of BBV, FHV, and NoV have been determined at atomic resolution (73,136,299). Each virion contains 180 copies of the same capsid protein (Fig. 10). Sixty triangular units, consisting of three similarly fold-

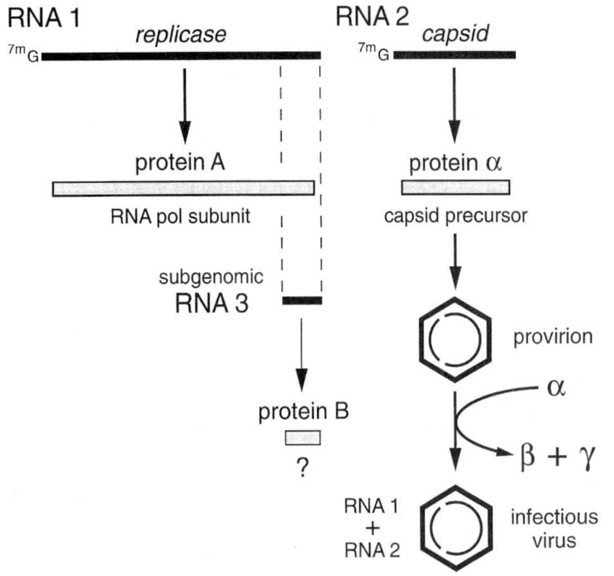

FIG. 9. Nodavirus replication strategy. The two genomic RNA segments (RNAs 1 and 2) encode the replicase (protein A) and capsid precursor protein (protein α), respectively. RNA 1 also specifies subgenomic RNA 3 which encodes protein B of unknown function. Assembled from capsid precursor α, provirions undergo a maturation cleavage producing capsid proteins β and κ. Infectious virions contain both genomic RNAs.

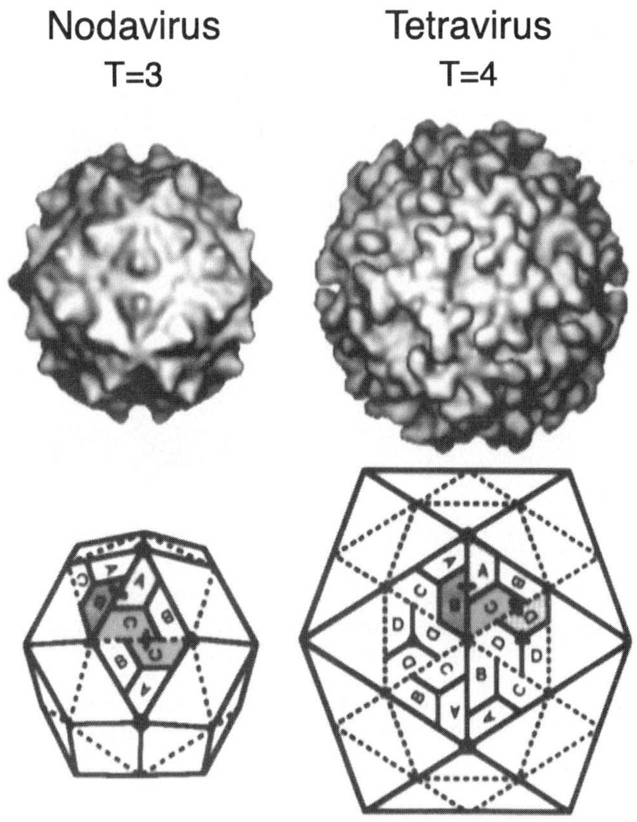

FIG. 10. Comparison of nodavirus and tetravirus structures. *Top:* Image reconstructions of the virion of a nodavirus (Flock House virus, *left*) and a tetravirus (Nudaurelia omega virus, *right*). The average particle diameter for the nodaviruses and tetraviruses is 320 Å and 415 Å, respectively. *Bottom*: Diagrammatic illustration of the subunit assembly of the T=3 nodavirus (*left*) and the T=4 tetravirus (*right*) virions. Each subunit (A, B, C, and D) is indicated by a trapezoid. Nodaviruses contain 60 subunits of three similarly folded capsid proteins that form a prominent peak at the quasi-three-fold axis (*top*). In contrast, tetraviruses contain 240 capsid protein subunits, twelve of which comprise each triangular face of the virion. Structural images are available at http://www.bocklabs.wisc.edu/virusviz1.html at the Institute for Molecular Virology, University of Wisconsin-Madison. Adapted with permission from Dr. John E. Johnson, Scripps Research Institute, La Jolla, CA.

ed capsid proteins, form an icosahedral lattice with T=3 symmetry and a radius of 156 Å (recently reviewed in 146 and 238). The three capsid proteins form a prominent peak at the quasi-threefold axis (see images at www.bocklabs.wisc.edu/virusviz1.html). At the twofold axes, conserved C-terminal residues of the capsid protein make contact with duplexed genomic RNA that is highly ordered and stabilize the capsid protein interface (73). C-terminal residues of the capsid protein also are required for RNA encapsulation (237). At the fivefold axes, the capsid proteins form a pentameric helical bundle that has been proposed to participate in release of the genomic RNA on virus penetration into the host cell's cytosol (43).

The nodavirus provirion is assembled from 180 copies of the ~43-kd capsid precursor α. During virus morphogenesis (see Fig. 9), α is cleaved very near its C terminus to generate capsid proteins β and γ (84,91, 136). For FHV, this postassembly cleavage occurs autocatalytically between Asn^{363} and Ala^{364}, located on the inside surface of the virion. This cleavage is required for infectivity and virion stability (91,239). In addition, the maturation cleavage may be necessary for an undefined event occurring between cell attachment and cytosolic release of the RNAs.

Nodavirus genome organization

The nodavirus genome consists of two single-stranded, messenger-active RNAs (RNA 1 and 2) that are ^{7m}G-capped, but not polyadenylated (see Fig. 9). An unknown structure or factor blocks the 3′ ends. RNA 1 (~3.1 kb) encodes the functions required for RNA transcription and replication, whereas RNA 2 (~1.4 kb) encodes capsid precursor α. Both RNAs are required for infectivity and are packaged within the same virion (241). Infectious RNA transcripts from full-length cDNAs of the nodavirus genomic RNAs have been generated (57), and genetic functions have been determined by *in vitro* translation of the messenger-active RNAs and expression of cDNAs in heterologous systems, including baculovirus and vaccinia virus vectors and yeast cultures (5,62,84,217).

RNA 1 carries the information for at least two polypeptides, proteins A and B (see Fig. 9). Protein A (~112 kd) contains known RNA polymerase motifs and is required for nodavirus RNA replication. Most likely, protein A is an RNA-dependent RNA polymerase (RdRp) or a subunit thereof (7,90,109,217,287). Encoded by the 3′ end of RNA 1 (see Fig. 9), protein B (~12 kd) is translated from subgenomic RNA 3 that is abundant in infected cells, but not packaged into virions (83,107). Although its exact function is unknown, protein B may play a role in RNA replication (8). RNA 1 encodes all the information necessary for autonomous replication (90). In contrast, RNA 2 encodes only capsid protein α. Thus the functions necessary for genome replication and virus transmission are segregated onto different genetic elements.

Stages of Replication

FHV and closely related BBV multiply prolifically in *Drosophila melanogaster* cell lines (86,91,241), thereby providing a highly tractable system by which to dissect virus replication. The mechanisms of nodavirus attachment and entry are unknown. Virus replication is cytoplasmic. Uncoated genomic RNA 1 is translated to produce the protein A–containing RdRp, which is insensitive to actinomycin D. Newly synthesized viral RNAs are detected by 2 hours after inoculation and continue to accumulate through 20 hours, eventually composing up to 50% of the total cellular RNA (84,85,91). Despite the presence of an equimolar ratio of RNA 1 and 2 throughout infection, synthesis of capsid protein α predominates because of the ability of RNA 2 to outcompete RNA 1 for rate-limiting translation factors (85). Nodavirus RNA synthesis also is regulated. RNA 1 and 2 replication is coupled, ensuring the production of an equal ratio of both genomic RNAs. During infection, RNA 1 must be generated before RNA 2 (6), which subsequently represses synthesis of subgenomic RNA 3 (90). Cis-acting sequences required for (+) and (–) strand RNA transcription and RNA 3 suppression have been identified (reviewed in 8). Virion assembly copackages an equimolar ratio of RNA 1 and 2 by an unknown mechanism. Owing to the segmented genome, reassortment of genomic RNAs has been detected on mixed infections of cultured cells. Moreover, the nodaviruses can generate defective interfering particles at high multiplicities of infection and can establish persistent infections in cell cultures that are resistant to superinfection (56).

Tetraviridae

Classification of Tetraviruses

The tetraviruses, formerly known as the Nudaurelia β virus (NβV) group, contain a single-stranded, positive-sense RNA genome that is packaged into an nonenveloped, icosahedral virion. The virions (~40 nm diameter) have T=4 symmetry, which forms the basis of the family name ("tetra" from Greek *tettares,* meaning "four"). The tetraviruses are the only known nonenveloped viruses with T=4 symmetry (reviewed in 97, 128, and 146). All tetraviruses have been isolated from insects of the order Lepidoptera (moths and butterflies). Nine viruses have been assigned to the family on the basis of serologic relatedness or the presence of a similar-sized capsid protein of more than 62 kd (97). Ten other viruses are likely members. The family is divided into betatetravirus and omegatetravirus genera. The genome of the betatetraviruses consists of a single (monopartite) RNA of ~5.5-kb, whereas the genome of the omegatetraviruses consists of two (bipartite) RNAs of ~2.5 and 5.5 kb. For example, the betatetravirus NβV has a single RNA, whereas the omegatetraviruses Nudaurelia omega virus (NωV) and *Helicoverpa armigera* stunt virus (HaSV) have two RNAs.

Virion Structure

Cryo-EM reconstructions have distinguished the basic structural features of the T=4 symmetry of the tetraviruses (see Fig. 10) (recently reviewed in 146). In addition, the structure of NωV has been resolved in atomic detail (193,194), providing the first structure of a T=4 virus. Tetravirus particles are composed of 240 capsid protein subunits. Twelve chemically identical capsid proteins compose each triangular face of the virion (see Fig. 10). The NωV capsid precursor is cleaved after Asn^{570} near the C terminus in a postassembly mechanism that is analogous to the cleavage of nodavirus capsid precursors required for virus infectivity (see earlier). The T=4 capsid protein arrangement of tetraviruses (~40 nm diameter) is readily distinguished from the T=3 arrangement of the nodaviruses (30 nm diameter), which have 60 fewer capsid proteins per particle (see Fig. 10). Nonetheless, the tertiary structure of capsid proteins of both virus families is strikingly similar. This conservation and the requirement for a postassembly cleavage of capsid proteins suggests that the tetraviruses and nodaviruses evolved from a common ancestor (146).

Tetravirus Genome Structure and Replication

The tetravirus RNA genome is either mono- or bipartite. The genomic RNAs are capped at their 5′ end and have a unique tRNA-like structure at their 3′ end (1,122). The genomes of several members of the beta and omega genera have been sequenced.

The 6,625-nucleotide NβV genome RNA contains two large ORFs (99). The 5′ proximal ORF has the potential to encode a 214-kd protein containing domains characteristic of an RNA-dependent RNA polymerase with methyltransferase, nucleotide binding/helicase, and RNA polymerase motifs. The proteolytic processing steps of this predicted polyprotein are unknown. The 66-kd NβV capsid protein is encoded by the 3′ proximal ORF, which is almost entirely overlapped by the replicase ORF, but in a different (+1) reading frame. It is therefore likely that the capsid protein is translated from a 2.5-kb subgenomic RNA that has been detected in preparations of virion RNA (99). *Thosea asigna* virus (TaV), a related betatetravirus, synthesizes a 2.5-kb subgenomic RNA, which also encodes the capsid protein (221).

The omegatetravirus HaSV contains two genomic RNAs of 5,300 and 2,478 nucleotides (98,122). RNA1 possesses a single ORF (1,704 codons) covering 96% of the RNA and likely encodes the RNA replicase. RNA2 encodes the 71-kd HaSV capsid protein, which is closely related (66% identical) to the capsid protein of NωV (1). During assembly, the capsid precursor is cleaved near its C terminus to generate a 62-kd capsid protein and a smaller 7-kd sister polypeptide. RNA2 of HaSV also contains a 5′ proximal ORF, which encodes a 17-kd protein of unknown function (122). It is not known whether both RNAs 1 and 2 of the omegatetraviruses are packaged within the same particle.

Stages of Replication

Tetravirus replication occurs in the cytoplasm of infected cells, and crystalline arrays of virus particles accumulate within cytoplasmic vesicles (128). However, because of the lack of permissive cell cultures, the stages of virus replication are unknown (97). Nonetheless, it is likely that tetravirus replication strategies resemble those of the nodaviruses and alphaviruses.

Tetravirus Transmission, Pathology, and Ecology

The tetraviruses are the only known RNA viruses restricted to insects, specifically those within the order Lepidoptera. Infection of larvae can be initiated by the ingestion of virus-contaminated foods (121). Virus multiplication is most often restricted to the foregut and midgut cells, even on injection of infectious virus into the hemolymph of larvae. Virus-mediated killing of midgut cells may account for the stunting pathology associated with HaSV. In general, susceptible insect larvae exhibit a wide range of pathogenic effects that include rapid death, an extended wasting disease, or a delay in pupation (97). NβV also has been isolated from pupae and adult moths. Larval death occurs within 4 to 7 days and is usually accompanied by discoloration, flaccidity, and sometimes liquefaction that resembles baculovirus-mediated melting. Tetravirus pathogenesis can be influenced by the presence of other viruses, latent or otherwise.

Tetravirus infections occur sporadically in natural populations. Thus ecologic aspects of virus spread and the existence of virus reservoirs are poorly understood. Nonetheless, these insect viruses function as natural biopesticides and have participated in natural control of certain insect pests. *Darna trima* virus and *Thosea asigna* (or *Setothosea asigna*) virus have been successfully used as pest-control agents in oil palm plantations. Although tetraviruses have been only isolated from insects, antibodies cross-reacting with some tetraviruses have been detected in wild and domestic animals and humans. Thus far, development of these viruses as biopesticides has been limited (97).

Cricket Paralysis–Like Viruses

Classification

The cricket paralysis–like viruses are small, nonenveloped riboviruses with icosahedral symmetry. Because their biophysical properties resemble those of the vertebrate picornaviruses, they were originally classified as members of *Picornaviridae* (recently reviewed by 46). However, more recent nucleotide sequence determinations (147,259,283) indicated that these invertebrate viruses are members of a taxonomically distinct family that remains unclassified (see Table 1). The best characterized members include Cricket paralysis virus (CrPV) and serologically related *Drosophila* C virus. Because of its ability to cause paralysis of the hindlimbs of early-instar cricket nymphs, CrPV is appropriately named. Other members of the CrPV-like virus family include *Plantia stili* intestine virus, himetobi P virus, and *Rhopulosiphum* virus (46).

Virion Structure

The physicochemical properties of the virions of the cricket paralysis–like viruses are strikingly similar to those of the vertebrate picornaviruses. These icosahedral riboviruses (<40 nm diameter, ρ =1.35 to 1.37 g/mL) contain four capsid proteins (VP1, VP2, VP3, and VP4) that are arranged in a pseudo T=3 lattice (259). The 2.4-Å resolution crystal structure of CrPV reveals a capsid conformation and virion morphology that is nearly identical to that of the vertebrate picornaviruses (259). However, unlike the human enteroviruses, CrPV lacks the distinguishing deep depression (canyon) at the fivefold axis or a VP1 pocket. These differences suggest that the mechanism of receptor binding is distinct from that of the picornaviruses. Interestingly, the proteolytic processing of VP0 $\rightarrow$ VP3 + VP4 appears to be autocatalytic, which suggests that CrPV capsid assembly and processing more closely resemble those of the insect nodaviruses and tetraviruses than of the vertebrate picornaviruses (259).

Genome Organization and Novel Translation Initiation

CrPV and DCV possess single-stranded, messenger-sense RNA genomes of 9,185 and 9,264 nucleotides, respectively (147,283). The genomes are divided into two major ORFs (Fig. 11), which when translated generate two separate polyproteins that undergo proteolytic processing. Preceded by a 5′ UTR, ORF1 encodes proteins with predicted RNA helicase, picornavirus 3C–like protease, and RNA-dependent RNA polymerase activities. ORF2 is preceded by an intergenic UTR (~200 nucleotides) and encodes the virion capsid proteins. Thus unlike the vertebrate picornaviruses, the capsid proteins are encoded within the 3′ half of the genome, whereas nonstructural replication proteins are encoded within the 5′ half (see Fig. 11).

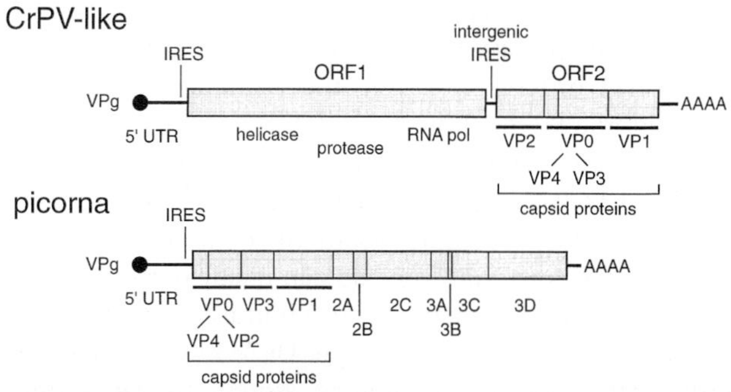

FIG. 11. Genome organization of the Cricket paralysis-like riboviruses. The single-stranded RNA genome of CrPV and DCV possess two open reading frames (ORF1 and ORF2) separated by a ~200 nucleotide spacer. Each ORF is preceded by an internal ribosome entry site (IRES). ORF1 encodes replicative functions (helicase, protease, and RNA-dependent RNA polymerase), whereas ORF2 encodes capsid proteins VP0, VP1, and VP2. VP3 and VP4 are generated by processing of precursor VP0 (259). VPg and an untranslated region (5' UTR) are located at the 5' end of the genomic RNA. The genome organization of the vertebrate picornaviruses differs from the CrPV-like viruses by possessing a single ORF which encodes capsid proteins and replicative functions at the 5' and 3' ends, respectively.

During infection, CrPV and DCV capsid proteins are produced in significant excess compared with the nonstructural proteins (46), a phenomenon that differs from that of the picornaviruses, which produce equimolar amounts of both structural and nonstructural proteins from their single ORF. Accounting for the differential levels of expression, CrPV possesses two internal ribosome entry sites, each located upstream from the nonoverlapping ORFs (283). Thus the CrPV genome represents a rare but naturally occurring bicistronic messenger RNA in eukaryotes. Most interestingly, ORF2 begins with a noncognate CCU triplet rather than AUG, suggesting a novel mechanism for translation initiation (283). Recent evidence indicates that the IRES within the intergenic UTR (see Fig. 11) can assemble an 80S ribosome in the absence of initiator Met-tRNA$_i$ and canonic initiation factors to initiate protein synthesis from the second triplet (GCU), which is positioned within the A site of the ribosome (235,282). This novel mechanism for translation initiation appears to involve the participation of a pseudoknot-like structure within the IRES that can substitute for the usual interactions between Met-tRNA$_i$ and the P-site initiator codon.

CrPV-like Virus Ecology and Transmission

CrPV was originally isolated in 1970 from Australian crickets *Teleogryllus oceanicus* and *T. commodus.* It has one of the widest experimental host ranges of the insect viruses and is capable of infecting invertebrate species of diverse orders, including the Diptera, Lepidoptera, Orthoptera, Hymenoptera, and Hemiptera (46). However, little is known of the distribution of CrPV in nature. Experimental inoculation by injection leads to virus multiplication and death of a number of insect hosts. CrPV transmission also can occur *per os* through contaminated food sources. In contrast to CrPV, DCV has a more restricted host range. DCV has been isolated only from wild or laboratory strains of *Drosophila melanogaster* (46). DCV can be transmitted *per* os to adult flies or larvae, causing death. In addition, DCV is transmitted horizontally between infected and uninfected adults.

This chapter is dedicated to the memory of Lois K. Miller, a friend and mentor, pioneer in baculovirology, and champion for studies of insect viruses and their application.

REFERENCES

1. Agrawal DK, Johnson JE. Sequence and analysis of the capsid protein of *Nudaurelia capensis* omega virus, an insect virus with T=4 icosahedral symmetry. *Virology* 1992;190:806–814.
2. Ahrens CH, Russell RL, Funk CJ, et al. The sequence of the *Orgyia pseudotsugata* multinucleocapsid nuclear polyhedrosis virus genome. *Virology* 1997;229:381–399.
3. Ayres MD, Howard SC, Kuzio J, et al. The complete DNA sequence of *Autographa californica* nuclear polyhedrosis virus. *Virology* 1994; 202:586–605.
4. Balch RE, Bird FT. A disease of the European spruce sawfly, *Gilpinia hercyniae* (Htg.) and its place in natural control. *Sci Agric* 1944;25: 65–73.
5. Ball LA. Cellular expression of a functional nodavirus RNA replicon from vaccinia virus vectors. *J Virol* 1992;66:2335–2345.
6. Ball LA. Replication of the genomic RNA of a positive-strand RNA animal virus from negative-sense transcripts. *Proc Natl Acad Sci U S A* 1994;91:12443–12447.
7. Ball LA. Requirements for the self-directed replication of flock house virus RNA 1. *J Virol* 1995;69:720–727 [published erratum appears in *J Virol* 1995;69:2722].
8. Ball LA, Johnson KL. Nodaviruses of insects. In: Miller LK, Ball LA, eds. *The insect viruses.* New York: Plenum, 1998:225–267.
9. Bauser CA, Elick TA, Fraser MJ. Characterization of hitchhiker, a transposon insertion frequently associated with baculovirus FP mutants derived upon passage in the TN-368 cell line. *Virology* 1996; 216:235–237.
10. Beames B, Summers MD. Location and nucleotide sequence of the 25K protein missing from baculovirus few polyhedra (FP) mutants. *Virology* 1989;168:344–353.
11. Beames B, Summers MD. Sequence comparison of cellular and viral copies of host cell DNA insertions found in *Autographa californica* nuclear polyhedrosis virus. *Virology* 1990;174:354–363.
12. Beaton CD, Fishie BK. Comparative ultrastructural studies of insect granulosis and nuclear polyhedrosis viruses. *J Gen Virol* 1976;31: 151–164.
13. Beniya H, Funk CJ, Rohrmann GF, et al. Purification of a virus-induced RNA polymerase from *Autographa californica* nuclear polyhedrosis virus-infected *Spodoptera frugiperda* cells that accurately initiates late and very late transcription in vitro. *Virology* 1996;216: 12–19.
14. Benz GA. Introduction: Historical perspectives. In: Granados RR, Federici BA, eds. *The biology of baculoviruses.* Boca Raton, FL: CRC Press, 1986:1–35.
15. Bergold GH. Die Isolierung des polyeder-virus und die natur der polyeder. *Z Naturforsch Teil B* 1947;2b:122–143.
16. Bertin J, Mendrysa SM, LaCount DJ, et al. Apoptotic suppression by baculovirus P35 involves cleavage by and inhibition of a virus-induced CED-3/ICE-like protease. *J Virol* 1996;70:6251–6259.
17. Bigot Y, Rabouille A, Doury G, et al. Biological and molecular features of the relationships between *Diadromus pulchellus* ascovirus, a parasitoid hymenopteran wasp (*Diadromus pulchellus*) and its lepidopteran host, *Acrolepiopsis assectella. J Gen Virol* 1997;78: 1149–1163.
18. Bigot Y, Rabouille A, Sizaret PY, et al. Particle and genomic characteristics of a new member of the Ascoviridae: *Diadromus pulchellus* ascovirus. *J Gen Virol* 1997;78:1139–1147.
19. Birnbaum MJ, Clem RJ, Miller LK. An apoptosis-inhibiting gene from a nuclear polyhedrosis virus encoding a polypeptide with Cys/His sequence motifs. *J Virol* 1994;68:2521–2528.
20. Black BC, Brennan LA, Dierks PM, et al. Commercialization of baculovirus insecticides. In: Miller LK, ed. *The baculoviruses.* New York: Plenum, 1997:341–381.
21. Blissard GW, Kogan PH, Wei R, et al. A synthetic early promoter from a baculovirus: Roles of the TATA box and conserved start site CAGT sequence in basal levels of transcription. *Virology* 1992;190:783–793.
22. Blissard GW, Rohrmann GF. Baculovirus gp64 gene expression: Analysis of sequences modulating early transcription and transactivation by IE1. *J Virol* 1991;65:5820–5827.
23. Blissard GW, Smith OP, Summers MD. Two related viral genes are located on a single superhelical DNA segment of the multipartite *Campoletis sonorensis* virus genome. *Virology* 1987;160:120–134.
24. Blissard GW, Vinson SB, Summers MD. Identification, mapping, and in vitro translation of *Campoletis sonorensis* virus mRNAs from parasitized *Heliothis virescens* larvae. *J Virol* 1986;57:318–327.
25. Blissard GW, Wenz JR. Baculovirus gp64 envelope glycoprotein is sufficient to mediate pH-dependent membrane fusion. *J Virol* 1992; 66:6829–6835.
26. Boyce FM, Bucher NL. Baculovirus-mediated gene transfer into mammalian cells. *Proc Natl Acad Sci U S A* 1996;93:2348–2352.
27. Braunagel SC, Burks JK, Rosas-Acosta G, et al. Mutations within the *Autographa californica* nucleopolyhedrovirus FP25K gene decrease the accumulation of ODV-E66 and alter its intranuclear transport. *J Virol* 1999;73:8559–8570.
28. Braunagel SC, Parr R, Belyavskyi M, et al. *Autographa californica* nucleopolyhedrovirus infection results in Sf9 cell cycle arrest at G_2/M phase. *Virology* 1998;244:195–211.
29. Braunagel SC, Summers MD. *Autographa californica* nuclear polyhedrosis virus, PDV, and ECV viral envelopes and nucleocapsids: Structural proteins, antigens, lipid and fatty acid profiles. *Virology* 1994; 202:315–328.
30. Broussard DR, Guarino LA, Jarvis DL. Dynamic phosphorylation of *Autographa californica* nuclear polyhedrosis virus pp31. *J Virol* 1996;70:6767–6774.
31. Broussard DR, Guarino LA, Jarvis DL. Mapping functional domains in AcMNPV pp31. *Virology* 1996;222:318–331.
32. Bump NJ, Hackett M, Hugunin M, et al. Inhibition of ICE family proteases by baculovirus antiapoptotic protein p35. *Science* 1995;269: 1885–1888.
33. Burand JP. Nudiviruses. In: Miller LK, Ball LA, eds. *The insect viruses.* New York: Plenum, 1998:69–90.
34. Burand JP, Lu H. Replication of a gonad-specific insect virus in TN-368 cells in culture. *J Invert Pathol* 1997;70:88–95.
35. Carson DD, Guarino LA, Summers MD. Functional mapping of an AcNPV immediately early gene which augments expression of the IE-1 trans-activated 39K gene. *Virology* 1988;162:444–451.
36. Carstens EB, Tjia ST, Doerfler W. Infection of *Spodoptera frugiperda* cells with *Autographa californica* nuclear polyhedrosis virus. I. Synthesis of intracellular proteins after virus infection. *Virology* 1979;99: 386–398.
37. Cartier JL, Hershberger PA, Friesen PD. Suppression of apoptosis in insect cells stably transfected with baculovirus *p35: Dominant interference by N-terminal sequences* p35(1-76). *J Virol* 1994;68: 7728–7737.
38. Cary LC, Goebel M, Corsaro BG, et al. Transposon mutagenesis of baculoviruses: Analysis of *Trichoplusia ni* transposon IFP2 insertions within the FP-locus of nuclear polyhedrosis viruses. *Virology* 1989; 172:156–169.
39. Chao YC, Lee ST, Chang MC, et al. A 2.9-kilobase noncoding nuclear RNA functions in the establishment of persistent Hz-1 viral infection. *J Virol* 1998;72:2233–2245.
40. Charlton CA, Volkman LE. Sequential rearrangement and nuclear

polymerization of actin in baculovirus-infected *Spodoptera frugiperda* cells. *J Virol* 1991;65:1219–1227.
41. Charlton CA, Volkman LE. Penetration of *Autographa californica* nuclear polyhedrosis virus nucleocapsids into IPLB Sf21 cells induces actin cable formation. *Virology* 1993;197:245–254.
42. Chen CJ, Quentin ME, Brennan LA, et al. *Lymantria dispar* nucleopolyhedrovirus *hrf-1* expands the larval host range of *Autographa californica* nucleopolyhedrovirus. *J Virol* 1998;72:2526–2531.
43. Cheng RH, Reddy VS, Olson NH, et al. Functional implications of quasi-equivalence in a T = 3 icosahedral animal virus established by cryo-electron microscopy and X-ray crystallography. *Structure* 1994; 2:271–282.
44. Cheng XW, Carner GR, Brown TM. Circular configuration of the genome of ascoviruses. *J Gen Virol* 1999;80:1537–1540.
45. Chisholm GE, Henner DJ. Multiple early transcripts and splicing of the *Autographa californica* nuclear polyhedrosis virus IE-1 gene. *J Virol* 1988;62:3193–3200.
46. Christian PD, Scotti PD. Picornalike viruses of insects. In: Miller LK, Ball LA, eds. *The insect viruses.* New York: Plenum, 1998: 301–336.
47. Clem RJ. Regulation of programmed cell death by baculoviruses. In: Miller LK, ed. *The baculoviruses.* New York: Plenum, 1997:237–261.
48. Clem RJ, Fechheimer M, Miller LK. Prevention of apoptosis by a baculovirus gene during infection of insect cells. *Science* 1991;254: 1388–1390.
49. Clem RJ, Miller LK. Apoptosis reduces both the in vitro replication and the in vivo infectivity of a baculovirus. *J Virol* 1993;67: 3730–3738.
50. Clem RJ, Miller LK. Control of programmed cell death by the baculovirus genes *p35* and *iap*. *Mol Cell Biol* 1994;14:5212–5222.
51. Cochran MA, Faulkner P. Location of homologous DNA sequences interspersed at five regions in the baculovirus *Autographa californica* nuclear polyhedrosis virus genome. *J Virol* 1983;45:961–970.
52. Condreay JP, Witherspoon SM, Clay WC, et al. Transient and stable gene expression in mammalian cells transduced with a recombinant baculovirus vector. *Proc Natl Acad Sci U S A* 1999;96:127–132.
53. Croizier G, Croizier L, Argaud O, et al. Extension of *Autographa californica* nuclear polyhedrosis virus host range by interspecific replacement of a short DNA sequence in the p143 helicase gene. *Proc Natl Acad Sci U S A* 1994;91:48–52.
54. Crook NE, Clem RJ, Miller LK. An apoptosis-inhibiting baculovirus gene with a zinc finger-like motif. *J Virol* 1993;67:2168–2174.
55. Cui L, Webb BA. Homologous sequences in the *Campoletis sonorensis* polydnavirus genome are implicated in replication and nesting of the W segment family. *J Virol* 1997;71:8504–8513.
56. Dasgupta R, Selling B, Rueckert R. Flock house virus: A simple model for studying persistent infection in cultured *Drosophila* cells. *Arch Virol* 1994;9(suppl):121–132.
57. Dasmahapatra B, Dasgupta R, Saunders K, et al. Infectious RNA derived by transcription from cloned cDNA copies of the genomic RNA of an insect virus. *Proc Natl Acad Sci U S A* 1986;83:63–66.
58. Davidson FF, Steller H. Blocking apoptosis prevents blindness in *Drosophila* retinal degeneration mutants. *Nature* 1998;391:587–591.
59. Deveraux QL, Reed JC. IAP family proteins: Suppressors of apoptosis. *Genes Dev* 1999;13:239–252.
60. Dib-Hajj SD, Webb BA, Summers MD. Structure and evolutionary implications of a "cysteine rich" *Campoletis sonorensis* polydnavirus gene family. *Proc Natl Acad Sci U S A* 1993;90:3765–3769.
61. Dickson JA, Friesen PD. Identification of upstream promoter elements mediating early transcription from the 35,000-molecular-weight protein gene of *Autographa californica* nuclear polyhedrosis virus. *J Virol* 1991;65:4006–4016.
62. Dong XF, Natarajan P, Tihova M, et al. Particle polymorphism caused by deletion of a peptide molecular switch in a quasiequivalent icosahedral virus. *J Virol* 1998;72:6024–6033.
63. Du Q, Lehavi D, Faktor O, et al. Isolation of an apoptosis suppressor gene of the *Spodoptera littoralis* nucleopolyhedrovirus. *J Virol* 1999; 73:1278–1285.
64. Edson KM, Vinson SB, Stoltz DB, et al. Virus in a parasitoid wasp: Suppression of the cellular immune response in the parasitoid's host. *Science* 1981;211:582–583.
65. Engelhard EK, Kam-Morgan LNW, Washburn JO, et al. The insect tracheal system: A conduit for the systemic spread of *Autographa californica* M nuclear polyhedrosis virus. *Proc Natl Acad Sci U S A* 1994; 91:3224–3227.
66. Federici BA. A new type of insect pathogen in larvae of the clover cutworm *Scotogramma trifolii*. *J Invert Pathol* 1982;40:41–54.
67. Federici BA. Enveloped double-stranded DNA insect virus with novel structure and cytopathology. *Proc Natl Acad Sci U S A* 1983;80: 7664–7668.
68. Federici BA. Viral pathobiology in relation to insect control. In: Beckage NE, Thompson SN, Federici BA, eds. *Parasites and pathogens of insects.* San Diego, CA: Academic Press, 1993:81–101.
69. Federici BA. Baculovirus pathogenesis. In: Miller LK, ed. *The baculoviruses.* New York: Plenum, 1997:33–59.
70. Federici BA, Hamm JJ, Styer EL. Ascoviridae. In: Adams JR, Bonami JR, eds. *Atlas of invertebrate viruses.* Boca Raton, FL: CRC Press, 1991:339–349.
71. Federici BA, Vlak JM, Hamm JJ. Comparative study of virion structure, protein composition and genomic DNA of three ascovirus isolates. *J Gen Virol* 1990;71:1661–1668.
72. Fisher AJ, Cruz W, Zoog SJ, et al. Crystal structure of baculovirus P35: Role of a novel reactive site loop in apoptotic caspase inhibition. *EMBO J* 1999;18:2031–2039.
73. Fisher AJ, Johnson JE. Ordered duplex RNA controls capsid architecture in an icosahedral animal virus. *Nature* 1993;361:176–179.
74. Fleming JG, Summers MD. Polydnavirus DNA is integrated in the DNA of its parasitoid wasp host. *Proc Natl Acad Sci U S A* 1991; 88:9770–9774.
75. Fleming JGW, Summers MD. *Campoletis sonorensis* endoparasitic wasps contain forms of *C. sonorensis* virus DNA suggestive of integrated and extrachromosomal polydnavirus DNAs. *J Virol* 1986;57: 552–562.
76. Flipsen JTM, Vanlent JWM, Goldbach RW, et al. Expression of polyhedrin and p10 in the midgut of AcMNPV-infected *Spodoptera exigua* larvae: An immunoelectron microscope investigation. *J Invert Pathol* 1993;61:17–23.
77. Fraser MJ. Ultrastructural observations of virion maturation in *Autographa californica* nuclear polyhedrosis virus infected *Spodoptera frugiperda* cell cultures. *J Ultrastruct Mol Struct Res* 1986;95: 189–195.
78. Fraser MJ, Smith GE, Summers MD. Acquisition of host cell DNA sequences by baculoviruses: Relationship between host DNA insertions and FP mutants of *Autographa californica* nuclear polyhedrosis virus and *Galleria mellonella* nuclear polyhedrosis viruses. *J Virol* 1983;47:287–300.
79. Friesen PD. Invertebrate transposable elements in the baculovirus genome: Characterization and significance. In: Beckage NE, Thompson SN, Federici BA, eds. *Parasites and pathogens of insects.* San Diego, CA: Academic Press, 1993:147–178.
80. Friesen PD. Regulation of baculovirus early gene expression. In: Miller LK, ed. *The baculoviruses.* New York: Plenum, 1997:141–166.
81. Friesen PD, Miller LK. Temporal regulation of baculovirus RNA: Overlapping early and late transcripts. *J Virol* 1985;54:392–400.
82. Friesen PD, Nissen MS. Gene organization and transcription of TED, a lepidopteran retrotransposon integrated within the baculovirus genome. *Mol Cell Biol* 1990;10:3067–3077.
83. Friesen PD, Rueckert RR. Black beetle virus: Messenger for protein B is a subgenomic viral RNA. *J Virol* 1982;42:986–995.
84. Friesen PD, Rueckert RR. Synthesis of black beetle virus proteins in cultured *Drosophila* cells: Differential expression of RNAs 1 and 2. *J Virol* 1981;37:876–886.
85. Friesen PD, Rueckert RR. Early and late functions in a bipartite RNA virus: Evidence for translational control by competition between viral mRNAs. *J Virol* 1984;49:116–124.
86. Friesen PD, Scotti P, Longworth J, et al. Propagation in *Drosophila* line 1 cells and an infection-resistant subline carrying endogenous black beetle virus-related particles. *J Virol* 1980;741:741–747.
87. Fuchs LY, Woods MS, Weaver RF. Viral transcription during *Autographa californica* nuclear polyhedrosis virus infection: A novel RNA polymerase induced in infected *Spodoptera frugiperda* cells. *J Virol* 1983;43:641–646.
88. Funk CJ, Braunagel SC, Rohrmann GF. Baculovirus structure. In: Miller LK, ed. *The baculoviruses.* New York: Plenum, 1997:7–27.
89. Furuichi Y, Miura K. A blocked structure at the 5′ terminus of mRNA from cytoplasmic polyhedrosis virus. *Nature* 1975;253:374–375.
90. Gallagher TM, Friesen PD, Rueckert RR. Autonomous replication and expression of RNA 1 from black beetle virus. *J Virol* 1983;46: 481–489.
91. Gallagher TM, Rueckert RR. Assembly-dependent maturation cleav-

age in provirions of a small icosahedral insect ribovirus. *J Virol* 1988; 62:3399–3406.
92. Ghosh S, Jain A, Mukherjee B, et al. The host factor polyhedrin promoter binding protein (PPBP) is involved in transcription from the baculovirus polyhedrin gene promoter. *J Virol* 1998;72:7484–7493.
93. Glocker B, Hoopes RR Jr, Hodges L, et al. In vitro transcription from baculovirus late gene promoters: Accurate mRNA initiation by nuclear extracts prepared from infected *Spodoptera frugiperda* cells. *J Virol* 1993;67:3771–3776.
94. Gombart AF, Pearson MN, Rohrmann GF, et al. A baculovirus polyhedral envelope-associated protein: Genetic location, nucleotide sequence, and immunocytochemical characterization. *Virology* 1989; 169:182–193.
95. Gomi S, Majima K, Maeda S. Sequence analysis of the genome of *Bombyx mori* nucleopolyhedrovirus. *J Gen Virol* 1999;80: 1323–1337.
96. Gordon JD, Carstens EB. Phenotypic characterization and physical mapping of a temperature-sensitive mutant of *Autographa californica* nuclear polyhedrosis virus defective in DNA synthesis. *Virology* 1984;138:69–81.
97. Gordon KHJ, Hanzlik TN. Tetraviruses. In: Miller LK, Ball LA, eds. *The insect viruses.* New York: Plenum, 1998:269–295.
98. Gordon KHJ, Johnson KN, Hanzlik TN. The larger genomic RNA of *Helicoverpa armigera* stunt tetravirus encodes the viral RNA polymerase and has a novel 3′-terminal tRNA-like structure. *Virology* 1995;208:84–98.
99. Gordon KHJ, Williams MR, Hendry DA, et al. Sequence of the genomic RNA of *Nudaurelia* beta virus (Tetraviridae) defines a novel virus genome organization. *Virology* 1999;258:42–53.
100. Grace TDC. Establishment of four strains of cells from insect tissues grown in vitro. *Nature* 1962;195:788–789.
101. Granados RR, Lawler KA. In vivo pathway of *Autographa californica* baculovirus invasion and infection. *Virology* 1981;108:297–308.
102. Granados RR, Nguyen T, Cato B. An insect cell line persistently infected with a baculovirus-like particle. *Intervirology* 1978;10: 309–317.
103. Griffiths CM, Barnett AL, Ayres MD, et al. In vitro host range of *Autographa californica* nucleopolyhedrovirus recombinants lacking functional *p35, iap1* or *iap2. J Gen Virol* 1999;80:1055–1066.
104. Gross CH, Rohrmann GF. Analysis of the role of 5′ promoter elements and 3′ flanking sequences on the expression of a baculovirus polyhedron envelope protein gene. *Virology* 1993;192:273–281.
105. Gruber A, Stettler P, Heiniger P, et al. Polydnavirus DNA of the braconid wasp *Chelonus inanitus* is integrated in the wasp's genome and excised only in later pupal and adult stages of the female. *J Gen Virol* 1996;77:2873–2879.
106. Grula MA, Buller PL, Weaver RF. α-Amanitin-resistant viral RNA synthesis in nuclei isolated from nuclear polyhedrosis virus-infected *Heliothis zea* larvae and *Spodoptera frugiperda* cells. *J Virol* 1981; 38:916–921.
107. Guarino LA, Ghosh A, Dasmahapatra B, et al. Sequence of the black beetle virus subgenomic RNA and its location in the viral genome. *Virology* 1984;139:199–203.
108. Guarino LA, Gonzalez MA, Summers MD. Complete sequence and enhancer function of the homologous DNA regions of *Autographa californica* nuclear polyhedrosis virus. *J Virol* 1986;60:224–229.
109. Guarino LA, Kaesberg P. Isolation and characterization of an RNA-dependent RNA polymerase from black beetle virus-infected *Drosophila melanogaster* cells. *J Virol* 1981;40:379–386.
110. Guarino LA, Smith M. Regulation of delayed-early gene transcription by dual TATA boxes. *J Virol* 1992;66:3733–3739.
111. Guarino LA, Summers MD. Functional mapping of a trans-activating gene required for expression of a baculovirus delayed-early gene. *J Virol* 1986;57:563–571.
112. Guarino LA, Summers MD. Interspersed homologous DNA of *Autographa californica* nuclear polyhedrosis virus enhances delayed-early gene expression. *J Virol* 1986;60:215–223.
113. Guarino LA, Summers MD. Nucleotide sequence and temporal expression of a baculovirus regulatory gene. *J Virol* 1987;61:2091–2099.
114. Guarino LA, Xu B, Jin J, et al. A virus-encoded RNA polymerase purified from baculovirus-infected cells. *J Virol* 1998;72:7985–7991.
115. Hajek KL, Friesen PD. Proteolytic processing and assembly of gag and gag-pol proteins of TED, a baculovirus-associated retrotransposon of the gypsy family. *J Virol* 1998;72:8718–8724.
116. Hamm JJ, Carpenter JE, Styer EL. Oviposition day effect on incidence of gonadal progeny of *Helicoverpa zea* [Lepidoptera: Noctuidae] infected with a virus. *Ann Entomol Soc Am* 1996;89:266–278.
117. Hamm JJ, Styer EL, Federici BA. Comparison of field-collected ascovirus isolates by DNA hybridization, host range, and histopathology. *J Invert Pathol* 1998;72:138–146.
118. Hammock BD, Bonning BC, Possee RD, et al. Expression and effects of the juvenile hormone esterase in a baculovirus vector. *Nature* 1990;344:458–461.
119. Handler AM, McCombs SD, Fraser MJ, et al. The lepidopteran transposon vector, piggyBac, mediates germ-line transformation in the Mediterranean fruit fly. *Proc Natl Acad Sci U S A* 1998;95:7520–7525.
120. Hang X, Guarino LA. Purification of *Autographa californica* nucleopolyhedrovirus DNA polymerase from infected insect cells. *J Gen Virol* 1999;80:2519–2526.
121. Hanzlik TN, Dorrian SJ, Gordon KHJ, et al. A novel small RNA virus isolated from the cotton bollworm, *Helicoverpa armigera. J Gen Virol* 1993;74:1805–1810.
122. Hanzlik TN, Dorrian SJ, Johnson KN, et al. Sequence of RNA2 of the *Helicoverpa armigera* stunt virus (Tetraviridae) and bacterial expression of its genes. *J Gen Virol* 1995;76:799–811.
123. Harrap KA. The structure of nuclear polyhedrosis viruses. III. Virus assembly. *Virology* 1972;50:133–139.
124. Harrison RL, Jarvis DL, Summers MD. The role of the AcMNPV 25K gene, "FP25," in baculovirus *polh* and *p10* expression. *Virology* 1996;226:34–46.
125. Hawtin RE, Zarkowska T, Arnold K, et al. Liquefaction of *Autographa californica* nucleopolyhedrovirus-infected insects is dependent on the integrity of virus-encoded chitinase and cathepsin genes. *Virology* 1997;238:243–253.
126. Hayakawa T, Ko R, Okano K, et al. Sequence analysis of the *Xestia c-nigrum* granulovirus genome. *Virology* 1999;262:277–297.
127. Hefferon KL, Oomens AG, Monsma SA, et al. Host cell receptor binding by baculovirus GP64 and kinetics of virion entry. *Virology* 1999;258:455–468.
128. Hendry D, Agrawal D. Small RNA viruses of insects: Tetraviridae. In: Webster RG, Granoff A, eds. *Encyclopedia of virology.* London: Academic Press, 1994:1416–1422.
129. Hershberger PA, Dickson JA, Friesen PD. Site-specific mutagenesis of the 35-kilodalton protein gene encoded by *Autographa californica* nuclear polyhedrosis virus: Cell line-specific effects on virus replication. *J Virol* 1992;66:5525–5533.
130. Hershberger PA, LaCount DL, Friesen PD. The apoptotic suppressor P35 is required early during baculovirus replication and is targeted to the cytosol of infected cells. *J Virol* 1994;68:3467–3477.
131. Hink WF. Established insect cell line from the cabbage looper, *Trichoplusia ni. Nature* 1970;226:466–467.
132. Hink WF, Vail PV. A plaque assay for titration of alfalfa looper nuclear polyhedrosis virus in a cabbage looper TN-368 cell line. *J Invert Pathol* 1973;22:168–174.
133. Hisahara S, Araki T, Sugiyama F, et al. Targeted expression of baculovirus p35 caspase inhibitor in oligodendrocytes protects mice against autoimmune-mediated demyelination. *EMBO J* 2000;19: 341–348.
134. Hofmann C, Sandig V, Jennins G, et al. Efficient gene transfer into human hepatocytes by baculovirus vectors. *Proc Natl Acad Sci U S A* 1995;92:10099–10103.
135. Hoopes RR, Rohrmann GF. In vitro transcription of baculovirus immediate early genes: Accurate messenger RNA initiation by nuclear extracts from both insect and human cells. *Proc Natl Acad Sci U S A* 1991;88:4513–4517.
136. Hosur MV, Schmidt T, Tucker RC, et al. Structure of an insect virus at 3.0 Å resolution. *Proteins* 1987;2:167–176.
137. Hozak RR, Manji GA, Friesen PD. The BIR motifs mediate dominant interference and oligomerization of inhibitor of apoptosis Op-IAP. *Mol Cell Biol* 2000;20:1877–1885.
138. Huang Q, Deveraux QL, Maeda S, et al. Evolutionary conservation of apoptosis mechanisms: Lepidopteran and baculoviral inhibitor of apoptosis proteins are inhibitors of mammalian caspase-9. *Proc Natl Acad Sci U S A* 2000;97:1427–1432.
139. Hughes DS, Possee RD, King LA. Activation and detection of a latent baculovirus resembling *Mamestra brassicae* nuclear polyhedrosis virus in *M. brassicae* insects. *Virology* 1993;194:608–615.
140. Huh NE, Weaver RF. Categorizing some early and late transcripts directed by the *Autographa californica* nuclear polyhedrosis virus. *J Gen Virol* 1990;71:2195–2200.

141. Huh NE, Weaver RF. Identifying the RNA polymerases that synthesize specific transcripts of the *Autographa californica* nuclear polyhedrosis virus. *J Gen Virol* 1990;71:195–202.
142. Ikeda M, Kobayashi M. Cell-cycle perturbation in Sf9 cells infected with *Autographa californica* nucleopolyhedrovirus. *Virology* 1999; 258:176–188.
143. Izquierdo M, Grandien A, Criado LM, et al. Blocked negative selection of developing T cells in mice expressing the baculovirus p35 caspase inhibitor. *EMBO J* 1999;18:156–166.
144. Jarvis DL. Baculovirus expression vectors. In: Miller LK, ed. *The baculoviruses.* New York: Plenum, 1997:389–431.
145. Jarvis DL, Bohlmeyer DA, Garcia AJ. Requirements for nuclear localization and supramolecular assembly of a baculovirus polyhedrin protein. *Virology* 1991;185:795–810.
146. Johnson JE, Reddy V. Structural studies of nodaviruses and tetraviruses. In: Miller LK, Ball LA, eds. *The insect viruses.* New York: Plenum, 1998:171–221.
147. Johnson KN, Christian PD. The novel genome organization of the insect picorna-like virus *Drosophila* C virus suggests this virus belongs to a previously undescribed virus family. *J Gen Virol* 1998; 79:191–203.
148. Kamita SG, Maeda S. Sequencing of the putative DNA helicase-encoding gene of the *Bombyx mori* nuclear polyhedrosis virus and fine-mapping of a region involved in host range expansion. *Gene* 1997;190:173–179.
149. Keddie BA, Aponte GW, Volkman LE. The pathway of infection of *Autographa californica* nuclear polyhedrosis virus in an insect host. *Science* 1989;243:1728–1730.
150. Kelly DC, Brown DA, Ayres MD, et al. Properties of the major nucleocapsid protein of *Heliothis zea* singly enveloped nuclear polyhedrosis virus. *J Gen Virol* 1983;64:399–408.
151. Kogan PH, Blissard GW. A baculovirus gp64 early promoter is activated by host transcription factor binding to CACGTG and GATA elements. *J Virol* 1994;68:813–822.
152. Kool M, Ahrens CH, Goldbach RW, et al. Identification of genes involved in DNA replication of the *Autographa californica* baculovirus. *Proc Natl Acad Sci U S A* 1994;91:11212–11216.
153. Kool M, Goldbach RW, Vlak JM. A putative non-hr origin of DNA replication in the *Hin*dIII-K fragment of *Autographa californica* multiple nucleocapsid nuclear polyhedrosis virus. *J Gen Virol* 1994;75: 3345–3352.
154. Kool M, Voeten JT, Goldbach RW, et al. Identification of seven putative origins of *Autographa californica* multiple nucleocapsid nuclear polyhedrosis virus DNA replication. *J Gen Virol* 1993;74:2661–2668.
155. Kost TA, Condreay JP. Recombinant baculoviruses as expression vectors for insect and mammalian cells. *Curr Opin Biotechnol* 1999; 10:428–433.
156. Kovacs GR, Choi J, Guarino LA, et al. Functional dissection of the *Autographa californica* nuclear polyhedrosis virus immediate-early 1 transcriptional regulatory protein. *J Virol* 1992;66:7429–7437.
157. Kovacs GR, Guarino LA, Graham BL, et al. Identification of spliced baculovirus RNAs expressed late in infection. *Virology* 1991;185: 633–643.
158. Kovacs GR, Guarino LA, Summers MD. Novel regulatory properties of the IE1 and IE0 transactivators encoded by the baculovirus *Autographa californica* multicapsid nuclear polyhedrosis virus. *J Virol* 1991;65:5281–5288.
159. Krappa R, Behn-Krappa A, Jahnel F, et al. Differential factor binding at the promoter of early baculovirus gene PE38 during viral infection: GATA motif is recognized by an insect protein. *J Virol* 1992;66: 3494–3503.
160. Krappa R, Knebel-Mörsdorf D. Identification of the very early transcribed baculovirus gene PE-38. *J Virol* 1991;65:805–812.
161. Krappa R, Roncarati R, Knebel-Mörsdorf D. Expression of PE38 and IE2, viral members of the C3HC4 finger family, during baculovirus infection: PE38 and IE2 localize to distinct nuclear regions. *J Virol* 1995;69:5287–5293.
162. Kremer A, Knebel-Mörsdorf D. The early baculovirus he65 promoter: On the mechanism of transcriptional activation by IE1. *Virology* 1998;249:336–351.
163. Kuzio J, Pearson MN, Harwood SH, et al. Sequence and analysis of the genome of a baculovirus pathogenic for *Lymantria dispar. Virology* 1999;253:17–34.
164. LaCount DJ, Friesen PD. Role of early and late replication events in induction of apoptosis by baculoviruses. *J Virol* 1997;71:1530–1537.
165. LaCount DJ, Hanson SF, Schneider CL, et al. Caspase inhibitor P35 and inhibitor of apoptosis Op-IAP block in vivo proteolytic activation of an effector caspase at different steps. *J Biol Chem* 2000;275: 15657–15664.
166. Lee HH, Miller LK. Isolation, complementation, and initial characterization of temperature sensitive mutants of the baculovirus *Autographa californica* nuclear polyhedrosis virus. *J Virol* 1979;31:240–252.
167. Lee HY, Krell PJ. Generation and analysis of defective genomes of *Autographa californica* nuclear polyhedrosis virus. *J Virol* 1992;66: 4339–4347.
168. Lee JC, Chao YC. Apoptosis resulting from superinfection of *Heliothis zea* virus 1 is inhibited by *p35* and is not required for virus interference. *J Gen Virol* 1998;79:2293–2300.
169. Leisy DJ, Rasmussen C, Kim HT, et al. The *Autographa californica* nuclear polyhedrosis virus homologous region 1a: Identical sequences are essential for DNA replication activity and transcriptional enhancer function. *Virology* 1995;208:742–752.
170. Lepore LS, Roelvink PR, Granados RR. Enhancin, the granulosis virus protein that facilitates nucleopolyhedrovirus (NPV) infections, is a metalloprotease. *J Invert Pathol* 1996;68:131–140.
171. Lerch RA, Friesen PD. The baculovirus-integrated retrotransposon TED encodes gag and pol proteins that assemble into viruslike particles with reverse transcriptase. *J Virol* 1992;66:1590–1601.
172. Lerch RA, Friesen PD. The 35-kilodalton protein gene (p35) of *Autographa californica* nuclear polyhedrosis virus and the neomycin resistance gene provide dominant selection of recombinant baculoviruses. *Nucleic Acids Res* 1993;21:1753–1760 [published erratum in *Nucleic Acids Res* 1993;21:2962].
173. Li L, Harwood SH, Rohrmann GF. Identification of additional genes that influence baculovirus late gene expression. *Virology* 1999;255: 9–19.
174. Lin CL, Lee JC, Chen SS, et al. Persistent Hz-1 virus infection in insect cells: Evidence for insertion of viral DNA into host chromosomes and viral infection in a latent status. *J Virol* 1999;73:128–139.
175. Lu A, Carstens EB. Immediate-early baculovirus genes transactivate the p143 gene promoter of *Autographa californica* nuclear polyhedrosis virus. *Virology* 1993;195:710–718.
176. Lu A, Krell PJ, Vlak JM, et al. Baculovirus DNA replication. In: Miller LK, ed. *The baculoviruses.* New York: Plenum, 1997:171–191.
177. Lu A, Miller LK. The roles of eighteen baculovirus late expression factor genes in transcription and DNA replication. *J Virol* 1995;69: 975–982.
178. Lu A, Miller LK. Regulation of baculovirus late and very late gene expression. In: Miller LK, ed. *The baculoviruses.* New York, Plenum, 1997:193–211.
179. Lübbert H, Doerfler W. Mapping of early and late transcripts encoded by the *Autographa californica* nuclear polyhedrosis virus genome: Is viral RNA spliced? *J Virol* 1984;50:497–506.
180. Maeda S, Kawai T, Obinata M, et al. Production of human *alpha*-interferon in silkworm using a baculovirus vector. *Nature* 1985;315: 592–594.
181. Manji GA, Friesen PD. (submitted).
182. Manji GA, Hozak RR, LaCount DJ, et al. Baculovirus inhibitor of apoptosis functions at or upstream of the apoptotic suppressor P35 to prevent programmed cell death. *J Virol* 1997;71:4509–4516.
183. McCutchen BF, Choudary PV, Crenshaw R, et al. Development of a recombinant baculovirus expressing an insect-selective neurotoxin: potential for pest control. *Biotechnology* 1991;9:848–852.
184. McLachlin JR, Miller LK. Identification and characterization of *vlf-1,* a baculovirus gene involved in very late gene expression. *J Virol* 1994;68:7746–7756.
185. Miller DW, Miller LK. A virus mutant with an insertion of a copia-like transposable element. *Nature* 1982;299:562–564.
186. Miller LK. Baculoviruses: High level expression in insect cells. *Curr Opin Genet Dev* 1993;3:97–101.
187. Miller LK. Baculovirus regulation of apoptosis. *Semin Virol* 1998;8: 445–452.
188. Miller LK. Ascoviruses. In: Miller LK, Ball LA, eds. *The insect viruses.* New York: Plenum, 1998:91–102.
189. Miller LK, Ball LA, eds. *The insect viruses.* New York: Plenum, 1998.
190. Monsma SA, Oomens AG, Blissard GW. The GP64 envelope fusion protein is an essential baculovirus protein required for cell-to-cell transmission of infection. *J Virol* 1996;70:4607–4616.
191. Morris TD, Miller LK. Mutational analysis of a baculovirus major late promoter. *Gene* 1994;140:147–153.

192. Moscardi F. Assessment of the application of baculoviruses for control of lepidoptera. *Annu Rev Entomol* 1999;44:257–289.
193. Munshi S, Liljas L, Cavarelli J, et al. The 2.8 Å structure of a T = 4 animal virus and its implications for membrane translocation of RNA. *J Mol Biol* 1996;261:1–10.
194. Munshi S, Liljas L, Johnson JE. Structure determination of *Nudaurelia capensis* omega virus. *Acta Crystallogr D Biol Crystallogr* 1998; 54:1295–1305.
195. Nissen MS, Friesen PD. Molecular analysis of the transcriptional regulatory region of an early baculovirus gene. *J Virol* 1989;63:493–503.
196. O'Reilly DR. Auxiliary genes of baculoviruses. In: Miller LK, ed. *The baculoviruses.* New York: Plenum, 1997:267–300.
197. O'Reilly DR, Miller LK. A baculovirus blocks insect molting by producing ecdysteroid UDP-glucosyl transferase. *Science* 1989;245: 1110–1112.
198. O'Reilly DR, Miller LK. Improvement of a baculovirus pesticide by deletion of the egt gene. *Biotechnology* 1991;9:1086–1089.
199. O'Reilly DR, Miller LK, Luckow VA. *Baculovirus expression vectors:* A laboratory manual. New York: WH Freeman, 1992.
200. O'Reilly DR, Winstanley D. Personal communication.
201. Ohkawa T, Volkman LE. Nuclear F-actin is required for AcMNPV nucleocapsid morphogenesis. *Virology* 1999;264:1–4.
202. Okano K, Mikhailov VS, Maeda S. Colocalization of baculovirus IE-1 and two DNA-binding proteins, DBP and LEF-3, to viral replication factories. *J Virol* 1999;73:110–119.
203. Ooi BG, Miller LK. Regulation of host RNA levels during baculovirus infection. *Virology* 1988;166:515–523.
204. Ooi BG, Miller LK. Transcription of the baculovirus polyhedrin gene reduces the levels of an antisense transcript initiated downstream. *J Virol* 1990;64:3126–3129.
205. Ooi BG, Rankin C, Miller LK. Downstream sequences augment transcription from the essential initiation site of a baculovirus polyhedrin gene. *J Mol Biol* 1989;210:721–736.
206. Oomens AG, Blissard GW. Requirement for GP64 to drive efficient budding of *Autographa californica* multicapsid nucleopolyhedrovirus. *Virology* 1999;254:297–314.
207. Oppenheimer DI, Volkman LE. Evidence for rolling circle replication of *Autographa californica* M nucleopolyhedrovirus genomic DNA. *Arch Virol* 1997;142:2107–2113.
208. Ozers MS, Friesen PD. The Env-like open reading frame of the baculovirus-integrated retrotransposon TED encodes a retrovirus-like envelope protein. *Virology* 1996;226:252–259.
209. Passarelli AL, Miller LK. Three baculovirus genes involved in late and very late gene expression: *ie-1, ie-n,* and *lef-2. J Virol* 1993;67: 2149–2158.
210. Pearson MN, Bjornson RM, Pearson GD, et al. The *Autographa californica* baculovirus genome: evidence for multiple replication origins. *Science* 1992;257:1382–1384.
211. Pearson MN, Groten C, Rohrmann GF. Identification of the *Lymantria dispar* nucleopolyhedrovirus envelope fusion protein provides evidence for a phylogenetic division of the Baculoviridae. *J Virol* 2000; 74:6126–6131.
212. Pearson MN, Rohrmann GF. Splicing is required for transactivation by the immediate early gene 1 of the *Lymantria dispar* multinucleocapsid nuclear polyhedrosis virus. *Virology* 1997;235:153–165.
213. Pearson MN, Russell RLQ, Rohrmann GF, et al. P39, a major baculovirus structural protein: Immunocytochemical characterization and genetic location. *Virology* 1988;167:407–413.
214. Pellock BJ, Lu A, Meagher RB, et al. Sequence, function, and phylogenetic analysis of an ascovirus DNA polymerase gene. *Virology* 1996;216:146–157.
215. Pennock GD, Shoemaker C, Miller LK. Strong and regulated expression of *Escherichia coli* β-galactosidase in insect cells with a baculovirus vector. *Mol Cell Biol* 1984;4:399–406.
216. Possee RD, Rohrmann GF. Baculovirus genome organization and evolution. In: Miller LK, ed. *The baculoviruses.* New York: Plenum, 1997:109–140.
217. Price BD, Rueckert RR, Ahlquist P. Complete replication of an animal virus and maintenance of expression vectors derived from it in *Saccharomyces cerevisiae. Proc Natl Acad Sci U S A* 1996;93: 9465–9470.
218. Prikhod'ko EA, Lu A, Wilson JA, et al. In vivo and in vitro analysis of baculovirus *ie-2* mutants. *J Virol* 1999;73:2460–2468.
219. Prikhod'ko EA, Miller LK. Induction of apoptosis by baculovirus transactivator IE1. *J Virol* 1996;70:7116–7124.
220. Prikhod'ko EA, Miller LK. Role of baculovirus IE2 and its RING finger in cell cycle arrest. *J Virol* 1998;72:684–692.
221. Pringle FM, Gordon KH, Hanzlik TN, et al. A novel capsid expression strategy for *Thosea asigna* virus (Tetraviridae). *J Gen Virol* 1999;80: 1855–1863.
222. Pullen SS, Friesen PD. The CAGT motif functions as an initiator element during early transcription of the baculovirus transregulator *ie-1. J Virol* 1995;69:3575–3583.
223. Pullen SS, Friesen PD. Early transcription of the *ie-1* transregulator gene of *Autographa californica* nuclear polyhedrosis virus is regulated by DNA sequences within its 5′ noncoding leader region. *J Virol* 1995;69:156–165.
224. Qi XM, He HL, Zhong HY, et al. Baculovirus *p35* and Z-VAD-fmk inhibit thapsigargin-induced apoptosis of breast cancer cells. *Oncogene* 1997;15:1207–1212.
225. Rabizadeh S, LaCount DJ, Friesen PD, et al. Expression of the baculovirus *p35* gene inhibits mammalian neural cell death. *J Neurochem* 1993;61:2318–2321.
226. Raina AK, Adams JR. Gonad-specific virus of corn earworm. *Nature* 1995;374:770.
227. Rapp JC, Wilson JA, Miller LK. Nineteen baculovirus open reading frames, including LEF-12, support late gene expression. *J Virol* 1998;72:10197–10206.
228. Rasmussen C, Rohrmann GF. Characterization of the *Spodoptera frugiperda* TATA-binding protein: Nucleotide sequence and response to baculovirus infection. *Insect Biochem Mol Biol* 1994;24:699–708.
229. Ribeiro BM, Hutchinson K, Miller LK. A mutant baculovirus with a temperature-sensitive IE-1 transregulatory protein. *J Virol* 1994;68: 1075–1084.
230. Rice WC, Miller LK. Baculovirus transcription in the presence of inhibitors and in nonpermissive *Drosophila* cells. *Virus Res* 1986;6: 155–172.
231. Rodems SM, Friesen PD. The *hr*5 transcriptional enhancer stimulates early expression from the *Autographa californica* nuclear polyhedrosis virus genome but is not required for virus replication. *J Virol* 1993;67:5776–5785.
232. Rodems SM, Friesen PD. Transcriptional enhancer activity of *hr*5 requires dual-palindrome half sites that mediate binding of a dimeric form of the baculovirus transregulator IE1. *J Virol* 1995;69:5368–5375.
233. Rodems SM, Pullen SS, Friesen PD. DNA-dependent transregulation by IE1 of *Autographa californica* nuclear polyhedrosis virus: IE1 domains required for transactivation and DNA binding. *J Virol* 1997; 71:9270–9277.
234. Roncarati R, Knebel-Mörsdorf D. Identification of the early actin-rearrangement-inducing factor gene, *arif-1,* from *Autographa californica* multicapsid nuclear polyhedrosis virus. *J Virol* 1997;71: 7933–7941 [published erratum *J Virol* 1998;72:7888–7889].
235. Sasaki J, Nakashima N. Methionine-independent initiation of translation in the capsid protein of an insect RNA virus. *Proc Natl Acad Sci U S A* 2000;97:1512–1515.
236. Scherer WF, Hurlbut HS. Nodamura virus from Japan: A new and unusual arbovirus resistant to diethyl ether and chloroform. *Am J Epidemiol* 1967;86:271–285.
237. Schneemann A, Marshall D. Specific encapsidation of nodavirus RNAs is mediated through the C terminus of capsid precursor protein alpha. *J Virol* 1998;72:8738–8746.
238. Schneemann A, Reddy V, Johnson JE. The structure and function of nodavirus particles: A paradigm for understanding chemical biology. *Adv Virus Res* 1998;50:381–446.
239. Schneemann A, Zhong WD, Gallagher TM, et al. Maturation cleavage required for infectivity of a nodavirus. *J Virol* 1992;66:6728–6734.
240. Selling BH, Allison RF, Kaesberg P. Genomic RNA of an insect virus directs synthesis of infectious virions in plants. *Proc Natl Acad Sci U S A* 1990;87:434–438.
241. Selling BH, Rueckert RR. Plaque assay for black beetle virus. *J Virol* 1984;51:251–253.
242. Seshagiri S, Miller LK. Baculovirus inhibitors of apoptosis (IAPs) block activation of Sf-caspase-1. *Proc Natl Acad Sci U S A* 1997;94: 13606–13611.
243. Seshagiri S, Vucic D, Lee J, et al. Baculovirus-based genetic screen for antiapoptotic genes identifies a novel IAP. *J Biol Chem* 1999;274: 36769–36773.
244. Slack JM, Blissard GW. Identification of two independent transcriptional activation domains in the *Autographa californica* multicapsid nuclear polyhedrosis virus IE1 protein. *J Virol* 1997;71:9579–9587.

245. Smith GE, Summers MD, Fraser MJ. Production of human β-interferon in insect cells infected with a baculovirus expression vector. *Mol Cell Biol* 1983;3:2156–2165.
246. Steinhaus EA. *Principles of insect pathology.* New York: McGraw-Hill, 1947.
247. Stewart LMD, Hirst M, Ferber ML, et al. Construction of an improved baculovirus insecticide containing an insect-specific toxin gene. *Nature* 1991;352:85–88.
248. Stoltz DB. The polydnavirus life cycle. In: Beckage NE, Thompson SN, Federici BA, eds. *Parasites and pathogens of insects.* San Diego, CA: Academic Press, 1993:167–187.
249. Stoltz DB, Guzo D, Cook D. Studies on polydnavirus transmission. *Virology* 1986;155:120–131.
250. Stoltz DB, Pavan C, Da Cunha AB. Nuclear polyhedrosis virus: A possible example of *de novo* intranuclear membrane morphogenesis. *J Gen Virol* 1973;19:145–150.
251. Stoltz DB, Vinson SB. Viruses and parasitism in insects. *Adv Virus Res* 1979;24:125–171.
252. Strand MR. *Microplitis demolitor* polydnavirus infects and expresses in specific morphotypes of *Pseudoplusia includens* haemocytes. *J Gen Virol* 1994;75:3007–3020.
253. Strand MR, McKenzie DI, Grassl V, et al. Persistence and expression of *Microplitis demolitor* polydnavirus in *Pseudoplusia includens. J Gen Virol* 1992;73:1627–1635.
254. Strand MR, Pech LL. Immunological basis for compatibility in parasitoid-host relationships. *Annu Rev Entomol* 1995;40:31–56.
255. Strand MR, Pech LL. *Microplitis demolitor* polydnavirus induces apoptosis of a specific haemocyte morphotype in *Pseudoplusia includens. J Gen Virol* 1995;76:283–291.
256. Strand MR, Witherell RA, Trudeau D. Two *Microplitis demolitor* polydnavirus mRNAs expressed in hemocytes of *Pseudoplusia includens* contain a common cysteine-rich domain. *J Virol* 1997;71:2146–2156.
257. Sugimoto A, Friesen PD, Rothman JH. Baculovirus *p35* prevents developmentally programmed cell death and rescues a *ced-9* mutant in the nematode *Caenorhabditis elegans. EMBO J* 1994;13:2023–2028.
258. Summers MD, Smith GE. Baculovirus structural polypeptides. *Virology* 1978;84:390–402.
259. Tate J, Liljas L, Scotti P, et al. The crystal structure of cricket paralysis virus: The first view of a new virus family. *Nat Struct Biol* 1999; 6:765–774.
260. Theilmann DA, Stewart S. Identification and characterization of the IE-1 gene of *Orgyia pseudotsugata* multicapsid nuclear polyhedrosis virus. *Virology* 1991;180:492–508.
261. Theilmann DA, Stewart S. Molecular analysis of the trans-activating IE-2 gene of *Orgyia pseudotsugata* multicapsid nuclear polyhedrosis virus. *Virology* 1992;187:84–96.
262. Theilmann DA, Summers MD. Identification and comparison of *Campoletis sonorensis* virus transcripts expressed from four genomic segments in the insect hosts *Campoletis sonorensis* and *Heliothis virescens. Virology* 1988;167:329–341.
263. Theilmann DA, Summers MD. Physical analysis of the *Campoletis sonorensis* virus multipartite genome and identification of a family of tandemly repeated elements. *J Virol* 1987;61:2589–2598.
264. Thiem SM, Miller LK. Identification, sequence, and transcriptional mapping of the major capsid protein gene of the baculovirus *Autographa californica* nuclear polyhedrosis virus. *J Virol* 1989;63: 2008–2018.
265. Thornberry NA, Lazebnik Y. Caspases: Enemies within. *Science* 1998;281:1312–1316.
266. Tomalski MD, Miller LK. Insect paralysis by baculovirus-mediated expression of a mite neurotoxin gene. *Nature* 1991;352:82–85.
267. Tomalski MD, Wu JG, Miller LK. The location, sequence, transcription and regulation of a baculovirus DNA polymerase gene. *Virology* 1988;167:591–600.
268. Tweeten KA, Bulla LAJ, Consigli RA. Characterization of an extremely basic protein derived from granulosis virus nucleocapsids. *J Virol* 1980;33:866–876.
269. Vialard JE, Richardson CD. The 1,629-nucleotide open reading frame located downstream of the *Autographa californica* nuclear polyhedrosis virus polyhedrin gene encodes a nucleocapsid-associated phosphoprotein. *J Virol* 1993;67:5859–5866.
270. Viswanath V, Wu Z, Fonck C, et al. Transgenic mice neuronally expressing baculoviral *p35* are resistant to diverse types of induced apoptosis, including seizure-associated neurodegeneration. *Proc Natl Acad Sci U S A* 2000;97:2270–2275.
271. Vlak JM, Klinkenberg FA, Zaal KJM, et al. Functional studies on the *p10* gene of *Autographa californica* nuclear polyhedrosis virus using a recombinant expressing a *p10*-β-galactosidase fusion gene. *J Gen Virol* 1988;69:765–776.
272. Volkman LE. The 64K envelope protein of budded *Autographa californica* nuclear polyhedrosis virus. In: Doerfler W, Bohm P, eds. *Current topics in microbiology and immunology:* The molecular biology of baculoviruses. New York: Springer-Verlag, 1986:103–118.
273. Volkman LE, Goldsmith PA. Mechanism of neutralization of budded *Autographa californica* nuclear polyhedrosis virus by a monoclonal antibody inhibition of entry by adsorptive endocytosis. *Virology* 1985; 143:185–195.
274. Volkman LE, Goldsmith PA, Hess RT, et al. Neutralization of budded *Autographa californica* NPV by a monoclonal antibody: Identification of the target antigen. *Virology* 1984;133:354–362.
275. Volkman LE, Goldsmith PA, Hess RT. Alternate pathway of entry of budded *Autographa californica* nuclear polyhedrosis virus fusion at the plasma membrane. *Virology* 1986;148:288–297.
276. Vucic D, Kaiser WJ, Harvey AJ, et al. Inhibition of reaper-induced apoptosis by interaction with inhibitor of apoptosis proteins (IAPs). *Proc Natl Acad Sci U S A* 1997;94:10183–10188.
277. Vucic D, Kaiser WJ, Miller LK. Inhibitor of apoptosis proteins physically interact with and block apoptosis induced by *Drosophila* proteins HID and GRIM. *Mol Cell Biol* 1998;18:3300–3309.
278. Webb BA. Polydnavirus biology, genome structure, and evolution. In: Miller LK, Ball LA, eds. *The insect viruses.* New York: Plenum, 1998: 105–139.
279. Weyer U, Possee RD. Functional analysis of the *p10* gene 5′ leader sequence of the *Autographa californica* nuclear polyhedrosis virus. *Nucleic Acids Res* 1988;16:3635–3654.
280. Williams GV, Faulkner P. Cytological changes and viral morphogenesis during baculovirus infection. In: Miller LK, ed. *The baculoviruses.* New York: Plenum, 1997:61–107.
281. Williams GV, Rohel DZ, Kuzio J, et al. A cytopathological investigation of *Autographa californica* nuclear polyhedrosis virus *p10* gene function using insertion-deletion mutants. *J Gen Virol* 1989;70:187–202.
282. Wilson JE, Pestova TV, Hellen CUT, et al. Initiation of protein synthesis from the A site of the ribosome. *Cell* 2000;102:511–520.
283. Wilson JE, Powell MJ, Hoover SE, et al. Naturally occurring dicistronic cricket paralysis virus RNA is regulated by two internal ribosome entry sites. *Mol Cell Biol* 2000;20:4990–4999.
284. Wilson ME, Consigli RA. Functions of a protein kinase activity associated with purified capsids of the granulosis virus infecting *Plodia interpunctella. Virology* 1985;143:526–535.
285. Wilson ME, Mainprize TH, Friesen PD, et al. Location, transcription, and sequence of a baculovirus gene encoding a small arginine-rich polypeptide. *J Virol* 1987;61:661–666.
286. Wilson ME, Miller LK. Changes in the nucleoprotein complexes of a baculovirus DNA during infection. *Virology* 1986;151:315–328.
287. Wu SX, Ahlquist P, Kaesberg P. Active complete in vitro replication of nodavirus RNA requires glycerophospholipid. *Proc Natl Acad Sci U S A* 1992;89:11136–11140.
288. Wu Y, Carstens EB. Initiation of baculovirus DNA replication: Early promoter regions can function as infection-dependent replicating sequences in a plasmid-based replication assay. *J Virol* 1996;70:6967–6972.
289. Xu B, Yoo S, Guarino LA. Differential transcription of baculovirus late and very late promoters: Fractionation of nuclear extracts by phosphocellulose chromatography. *J Virol* 1995;69:2912–2917.
290. Xu D, Stoltz D. Polydnavirus genome segment families in the ichneumonid parasitoid *Hyposoter fugitivus. J Virol* 1993;67: 1340–1349.
291. Yamao M, Katayama N, Nakazawa H, et al. Gene targeting in the silkworm by use of a baculovirus. *Genes Dev* 1999;13:511–516.
292. Yang S, Miller LK. Activation of baculovirus very late promoters by interaction with very late factor 1. *J Virol* 1999;73:3404–3409.
293. Yoo S, Guarino LA. The *Autographa californica* nuclear polyhedrosis virus ie2 gene encodes transcriptional regulator. *Virology* 1994;202: 746–753.
294. Young JC, MacKinnon EA, Faulkner P. The architecture of the virogenic stroma in isolated nuclei of *Spodoptera frugiperda* cells in vitro infected by *Autographa californica* nuclear polyhedrosis virus. *J Struct Biol* 1993;110:141–153.
295. Zelazny B. Studies on Rhabdionvirus oryctes. I. Effect on larvae of *Oryctes rhinoceros* and inactivation of the virus. *J Invert Pathol* 1972; 20:235–246.

296. Zelazny B. Studies on Rhabdionvirus oryctes II. Effect on adults of *Oryctes rhinoceros. J Invert Pathol* 1973;27:122–131.
297. Zelazny B, Lolong A, Crawford AM. Introduction and field comparison of baculovirus strains against *Oryctes rhinoceros* [*Coleoptera scarabaeidae*] in the Maldives Indian Ocean. *Environ Entomol* 1990; 19:1115–1121.
298. Zhou Q, Krebs JF, Snipas SJ, et al. Interaction of the baculovirus anti-apoptotic protein p35 with caspases: Specificity, kinetics, and characterization of the caspase/p35 complex. *Biochemistry* 1998;37:10757–10765.
299. Zlotnick A, Reddy VS, Dasgupta R, et al. Capsid assembly in a family of animal viruses primes an autoproteolytic maturation that depends on a single aspartic acid residue. *J Biol Chem* 1994;269: 13680–13684.
300. Zoog SJ, Bertin J, Friesen PD. Caspase inhibition by baculovirus P35 requires interaction between the reactive site loop and the beta-sheet core. *J Biol Chem* 1999;274:25995–26002.
301. Zoog SJ, Schiller JJ, Wetter JA, et al. Baculovirus P49 blocks apoptosis by inhibition of P35-insensitive apical caspases. (submitted).

CHAPTER 16

Viruses of Yeasts, Fungi, and Parasitic Microorganisms

Reed B. Wickner

Prions, retroviruses, ds (double-stranded) RNA viruses, ss (single-stranded) RNA viruses, and dsDNA viruses have all been found in simple eukaryote hosts, and the experimental advantages of these systems has made some of these the most thoroughly characterized of their viral classes. This is an overview of these infectious entities and their unique aspects, with some emphasis on recent developments.

One feature common to all the viruses, prions, and retrotransposons (or retroviruses) of yeast and fungi is their wholly intracellular life cycles. These viruses have forsaken the extracellular route of transmission, being passed from cell to cell either vertically or by cytoplasmic mixing, such as occurs in mating, or in hyphal anastomosis (fusion) of filamentous fungi. They resemble, in this regard, the plant cryptoviruses and the intracisternal A type particles (retroelements) and LINEs (retroposons) of mammals. It has been argued that the high frequency of mating and hyphal fusion of fungi in nature makes an extracellular phase dispensible for these viruses, and it is difficult to find strains of *S. cerevisiae* that lack either the L-A or L-BC dsRNA viruses or any of the Ty retrotransposons. Nor is the direct cell-to-cell route of infection completely neglected by mammalian viruses, those of the herpes group and human immunodeficiency virus being prime examples.

However, this mode of transmission means that these viruses must balance the need to spread and propagate against consideration for the viability of their host. Furthermore, the fact that most of these elements are widespread means that the hosts have been selected for the ability to protect themselves. This is clearly seen in the Ty elements, which tend to target sites that can tolerate an insertion. The Ty elements, particularly Ty3, regulate their transcription such that most transposition occurs on mating. This design optimizes the chances of infecting the potentially unoccupied genome of the mating partner. The copy numbers of several of the RNA replicons (L-A dsRNA, L-BC dsRNA, and 20S RNA) are repressed by the host Ski proteins acting in translation (185,226,259,285). Likewise, Ty1 retrotransposition is negatively controlled by the *RTT* genes, which appear to control particle and DNA stability and the structure of the chromatin target (54,138,148,167, 175,219).

Most of the viruses and prions discussed here can best be viewed as selfish RNA or DNA (or selfish protein), but the killer satellite dsRNAs clearly benefit their hosts by allowing them to kill competitors. The [Het-s] prion of *Podospora* is unique among prions described to date in being necessary for a normal cellular function, namely, heterokaryon incompatibility (57).

It is striking that most of the viruses and retroelements discussed use some form of ribosomal frameshifting to make a Gag-Pol fusion protein. This is not surprising for the retroelements, but it was not expected for the dsRNA genomes. Ribosomal frameshifting (in contrast to splicing or RNA editing) provides a mechanism for viruses whose mRNA is their genome to obtain two proteins with overlapping sequence from one mRNA without producing mutant genomes (140). Other translational tricks used include readthrough of stop codons, and internal ribosome entry.

The use of *S. cerevisiae* as a model host for viruses of plants and insects promises to facilitate the understanding of these viruses (141,218), but it will not be dealt with here.

DOUBLE-STRANDED RNA VIRUSES

The fungal dsRNA viruses were first detected in 1948 as "La France" disease of cultivated mushrooms in Pennsylvania, and its study led to the first description of fungal viruses in 1962. The antiviral agents helenine and statolon, discovered in *Penicillium* in the 1950s, later proved to be fungal virus dsRNA that was inducing interferon secretion (reviewed in ref. 31).

The dsRNA viruses are found in many fungal species (Table 1), and include the single-segment *Totiviridae*, the oligosegmented *Partitiviridae*, the potyvirus-like *Hypoviridae* that limit the virulence for chestnut trees of the chestnut blight fungus *Cryphonectria parasitica*, and reoviruses of the same species.

L-A Virus of *S. cerevisiae*, Type Species of the *Totiviridae*

Some strains of *S. cerevisiae* secrete a protein toxin that is lethal to other strains, but to which they themselves are immune (Fig. 1) (182). This "killer character" of some strains is inherited as a non-Mendelian genetic element, and its study led to the discovery of the L-A dsRNA virus and its satellites M_1, M_2, M_{28}, and so on, each M encoding a different toxin-immunity specificity.

L-A Virion Structure

The icosahedral structures of L-A and the *Ustilago* virus P4 are unusual in that they combine T=1 symmetry with 120 coat protein molecules per particle (Fig. 2) (35,41,98). This same symmetry has been found in the cores of all other dsRNA viruses examined, including reovirus, rotavirus, bluetongue virus, aquareovirus, and bacteriophage π6 (see Chapter 17 and Chapter 26; and Chapter 56 in *Fields Virology*, 4th ed.). Because sequence data suggest that dsRNA viruses arose independently from ssRNA viruses (161), rather than one being descended from the other, their common structure suggests that there is something about this structure that is well adapted to the intraviral replication pattern of dsRNA viruses.

The combination of 120 subunits and T=1 icosahedral symmetry implies that individual coat protein monomers can be in either of two environments. This expectation has been verified as subtly different morphology of the nonequivalent Gag protomers (35) (see Fig. 2). The packing of the dsRNA within the particles is less dense than is typical for dsDNA viruses, possibly reflecting the fact (see later) that in both replication and transcription, the genome must translocate sequentially past the RNA-dependent RNA polymerase immobilized on the particle wall, and this requires more space than is required by the static DNA genomes (35). The L-A virions also have 10- to 15-Å pores, which allow entry of nucleotides and exit of (+) strand transcripts but do not allow the dsRNA genome to exit or degradative enzymes to enter (35).

L-A Genome Structure

The L-A (+) strand has two overlapping open reading frames (ORF) (Fig. 3A) (140). They are *gag*, encoding the 76-kd major coat protein, and *pol*, encoding the 100-kd Pol domain of the Gag-Pol fusion protein (111,140). The pol ORF includes the consensus amino acid sequence patterns typical of viral RNA-dependent RNA polymerases. Three *in vitro* single-stranded RNA binding domains have also been localized to Pol (111,223,224), the central one cryptic unless an adjacent inhibitory

TABLE 1. *The dsRNA, ssRNA, and dsDNA viruses of simple eukaryotes*

Virus	Host species	Genome size (kb)	Features (references)
dsRNA viruses			
Totiviridae			One segment, Gag-Pol, T=1 icosahedral particles
L-A	*Saccharomyces cerevisiae*	4.6	Type species
M_1, M_2, M_{28}	*S. cerevisiae*	1.6–1.8	Satellites of L-A; encode killer toxins (244)
L-BC	*S. cerevisiae*	4.6	
Hv190S	*Helminthosporrium victoriae*	4.5	Coat protein phosphorylation (126), internal translational reinitiation
P1-H, P4-H, P6-H	*Ustilago maydis*	2.6–6.1	(160)
*Af*V-S, *Af*V-F	*Aspergillus foetidus*		(32)
*An*V-S, *An*V-S	*A. niger*		(32)
YlV	*Yarrowia lipolytica*		
LRV	*Leishmania braziliensis*	5.28	
GLV	*Giardia lamblia*	6.27	Infectious; transformation
TVV	*Trichomonas vaginalis*	4.6	
GgV-87-1-H	*Gaeumannomyces graminis*		
	Zygosaccharomyces bailii	4.0, 2.9, 1.9	(220) Killer associated
	Eimeria		(239)
	Blastomyces dermatitidis	5.0	(159)
Partitiviridae			
	Atkinsonella hypoxylon	2.2, 2.1, 1.8	(207)
	Penicillium crysogenum		
	P. stoloniferum		
	Agaricus bisporus		
	Rhizoctonia solani	2.2, 2.0	(106)
Hypoviridae			
CHV1-EP713	*Cryphonectria parasitica*		Hypovirulence-assoc. virus
Reoviridae			
	C. parasitica	1 to 3 (11 segs)	Hypovirulence-assoc. virus (91, 211)
ssRNA replicons			
Narnaviridae			
20S RNA (= T dsRNA)	*Saccharomyces cerevisiae*		
23S RNA (= W dsRNA)	*S. cerevisiae*		
NB631 RNA	*Cryphonectria parasitica*		
dsDNA viruses			
PBCV-1 and many others	*Chlorella*	333	(266, 267)

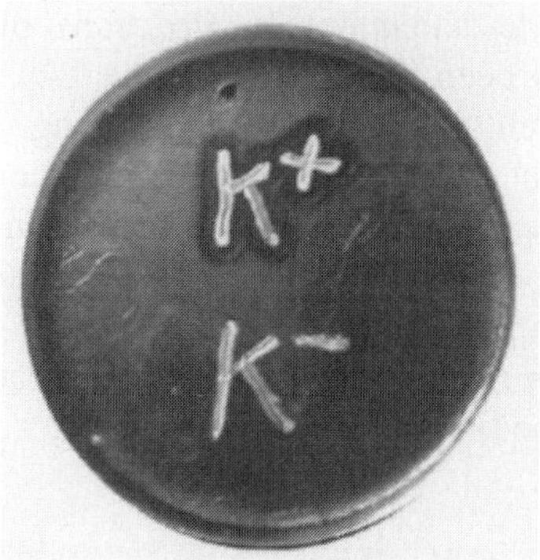

FIG. 1. The killer phenomenon of *S. cerevisiae*. A sensitive strain of yeast was spread as a lawn, and streaks of a killer strain (*above*) or a nonkiller strain (*below*) were applied. After 2 days' incubation, the lawn of the sensitive strain has not grown in a zone around the killer strain. The secreted protein killer toxin, and immunity to the toxin, are encoded by M_1, a satellite dsRNA of the L-A dsRNA virus.

region is deleted (see Fig. 3A). Pol residues 67 to 213 are necessary for packaging of the viral (+) strands (109,224). Neither 5′ cap structure nor 3′ poly(A) has been found on either strand of genomic L-A dsRNA or M_1 dsRNA (30), but there is, at each 3′ end, an uncoded base that can be either A or G (24).

The M dsRNAs each encode, in their 5′ portion, a preprotoxin protein (22,72,178,237) (see Fig. 3B). The M_1 (+) strand has an internal encoded polyA region whose length shows frequent clonal variation, presumably due to transcriptase stuttering (130), and a substantial 3′ region that encodes no protein but contains essential *cis* sites (97,107,124,234,242). As will be detailed later, sites on the L-A and M_1 (+) strands necessary for packaging and (−) strand synthesis have been determined (see Fig. 3), and some limits have been set on the possible transcription signals.

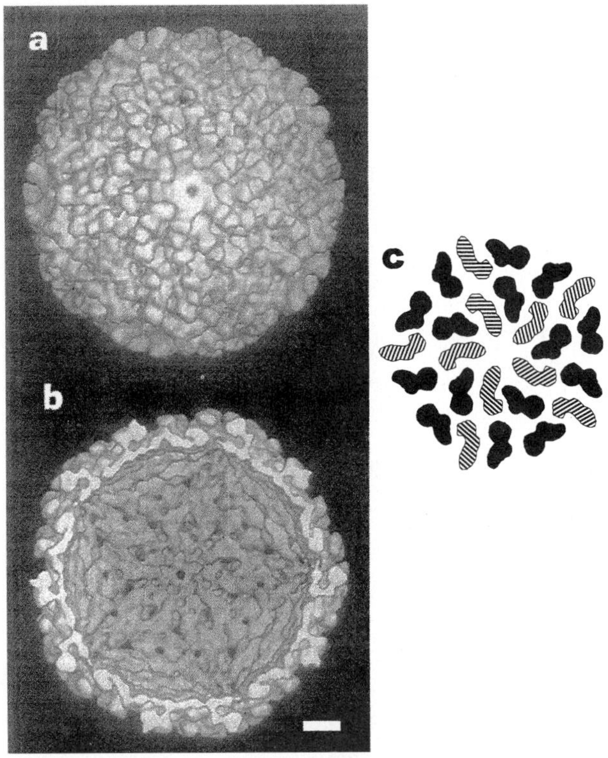

FIG. 2. L-A dsRNA virus capsid reconstruction at 16-Å resolution from cryoelectron microscopy (35). View of the outer (**a**) and inner (**b**) surfaces of the full capsid, viewed along a fivefold axis of symmetry. The internal contents were computationally removed to expose the inner surface (35). Bar = 50 Å. Schematic diagram (**c**) of the arrangement of Gag subunits around the fivefold axis. Note that solid and hatched subunits are identical in primary structure, but occupy distinct, nonequivalent environments (35).

Stages in the Replication Cycle

The L-A replication cycle and the closely related cycle of its satellites are shown in Figure 4 (98,108). L-A dsRNA-containing viral particles synthesize (+) ssRNA in a conservative reaction (108,134), and these new (+) strands are then extruded from the particle (98). There, they serve as mRNA for the production of the Gag and the Gag-Pol fusion proteins. These proteins then assemble with a viral (+) strand to form new particles. The newly assembled viral particles carry out the synthesis of (−) strands on the (+) strand template to form dsRNA and complete the cycle (108).

In addition to their appropriating viral proteins from L-A, the replication cycle of the satellite dsRNAs, M_1, S (deletion mutants of M_1), and X [a 530- basepair (bp) deletion mutant of L-A] are similar to that of L-A itself except that they replicate more than once within the viral particle until it is full (see Fig. 4). Only a single (+) ssRNA is packaged per particle (107), so L-A and M are separately encapsidated. Because the particle capacity is determined by the structure of Gag to be sufficient to accommodate one full-length L-A dsRNA molecule, and the M and X dsRNAs are much smaller, new M or X (+) strand transcripts are often retained within the viral particles, where they are converted to new dsRNA molecules. Then, all new (+) strands are extruded from the now full particle (98,99). This is called the *headful replication mechanism* (in contrast to the headful packaging mechanism of many DNA bacteriophage) (98,99). This implies that extrusion of the transcripts is a mechanical consequence of the head being full, rather than an active process. Both (+) and (−) strands are synthesized within the viral particles, but at different points in the cycle, so the replication is conservative, intraviral, and asynchronous, and it fills the capsid (headful mechanism).

Transcription Reaction ((+) Strand Synthesis)

As in the *Reoviridae*, the transcription reaction for L-A is conservative (108,286), resulting in the overall process of viral replication being conservative (204). However, in *Aspergillus foetidus* slow virus and *Penicillium stoloniferum* slow virus (32), dsRNA transcription is semiconservative. The difference between conservative and semiconservative reactions concerns whether or not there is re-pairing of the template (−) strand with the parental (+) strand that was (in either case) displaced during the synthesis.

A template-dependent *in vitro* transcription reaction method has been developed for the L-A dsRNA virus (113). When L-A dsRNA-containing particles are treated with very low ionic-strength conditions, they rupture, releasing the dsRNA. These opened empty particles can be reisolated free of RNA and carry out a dsRNA template-dependent reaction that is, like the *in vivo* reaction, conservative (113). This reaction is highly template specific, using only L-A, M, and X dsRNAs

FIG. 3. A: Sites and encoded proteins of the L-A (+) strand. The sites responsible for −1 ribosomal frameshifting, (+) ssRNA packaging, and replication are shown. The pseudoknot makes the ribosome pause over the slippery site, where the tRNAs can unpair from the mRNA and re-pair in the −1 frame with correct base pairing of the nonwobble bases. Functional domains in the Pol region are also indicated. 7mGp indicates the cap-binding site at His154 of Gag. **B:** Coding and cis sites of M1 (+) strand. The analogous and homologous processing of the K1 preprotoxin encoded by M1 is compared to that of preproinsulin.

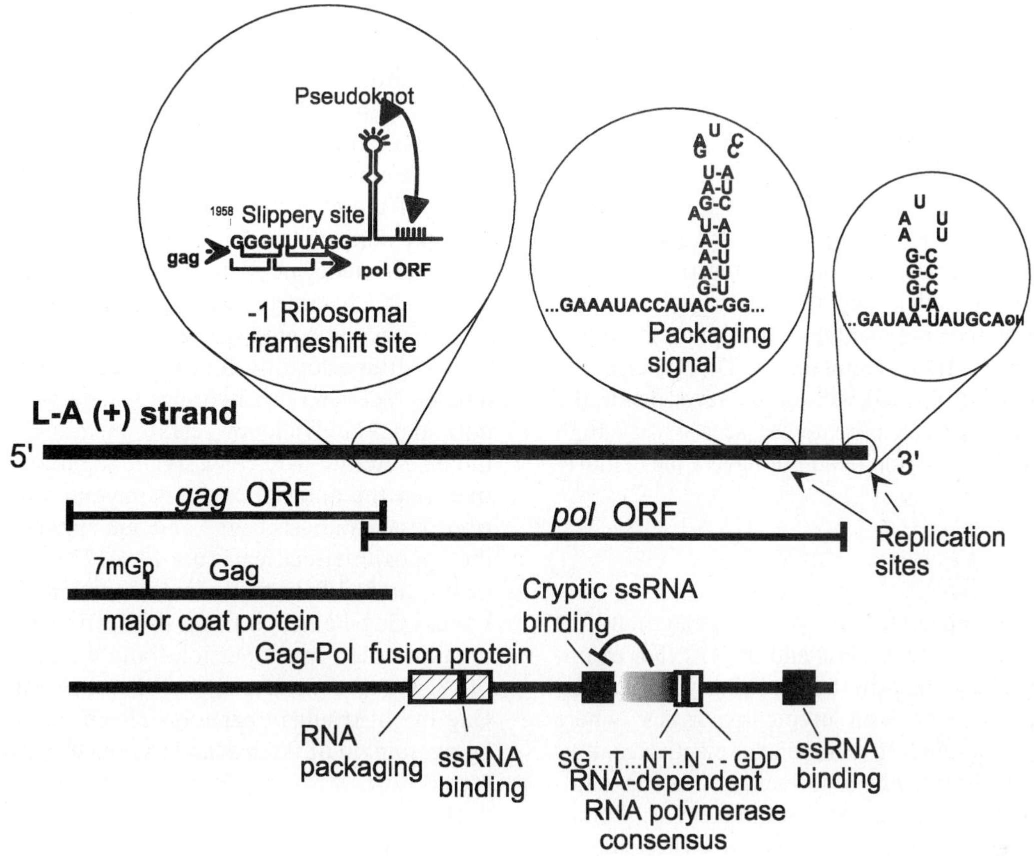
Pseudoknot
1958 Slippery site
GGGUUUAGG
gag
pol ORF
-1 Ribosomal frameshift site
...GAAAUACCAUAC-GG...
Packaging signal
..GAUAA-UAUGCAOH
L-A (+) strand
5'
3'
gag ORF
pol ORF
Replication sites
7mGp
Gag
major coat protein
Cryptic ssRNA binding
Gag-Pol fusion protein
RNA packaging
ssRNA binding
SG...T...NT..N - - GDD
RNA-dependent RNA polymerase consensus
ssRNA binding

A

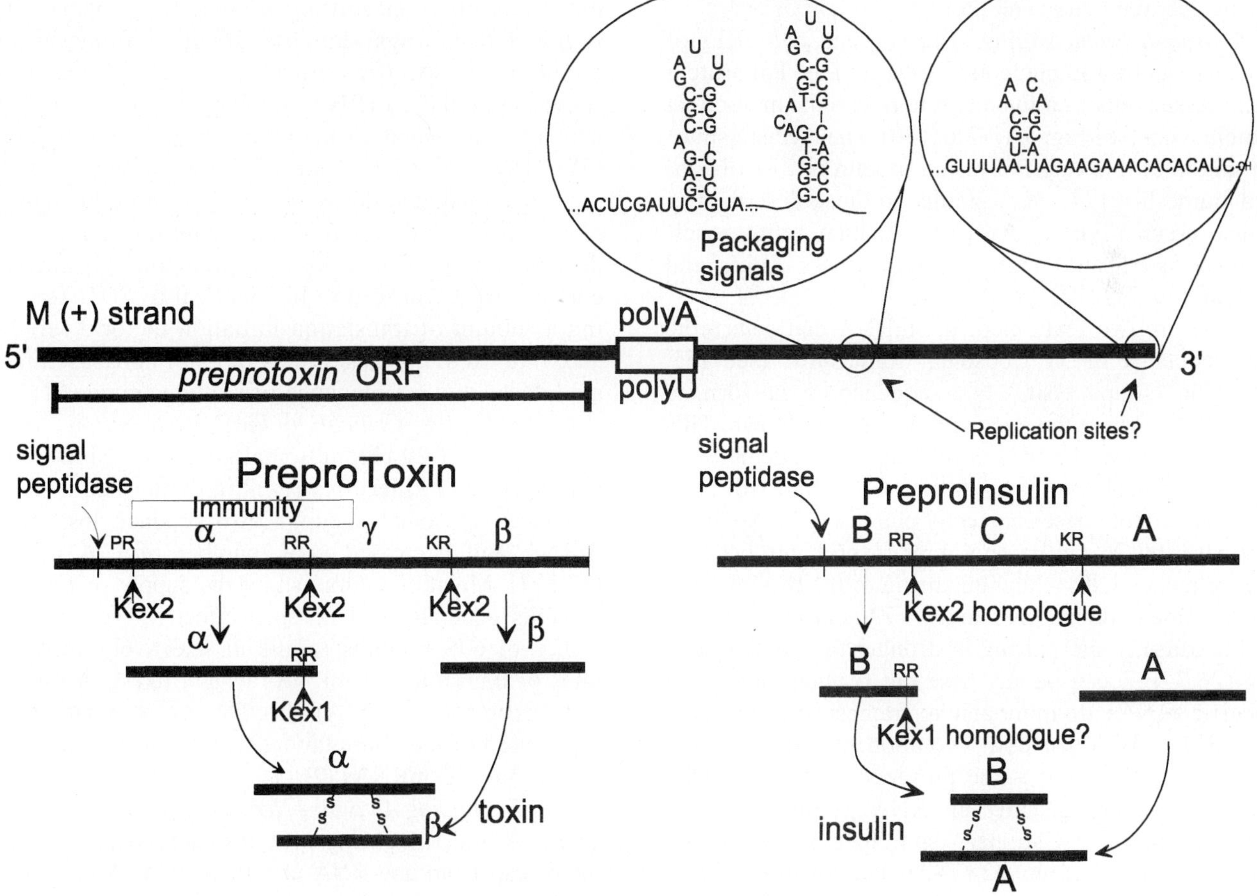
...ACUCGAUUC-GUA...
...GUUUAA-UAGAAGAAACACACAUC-OH
Packaging signals
M (+) strand
5'
polyA
polyU
3'
preprotoxin ORF
Replication sites?
signal peptidase
PreproToxin
Immunity
α γ β
PR RR KR
Kex2 Kex2 Kex2
α β
RR
Kex1
α
toxin
β
signal peptidase
PreproInsulin
B C A
RR KR
Kex2 homologue
B RR A
Kex1 homologue?
B
insulin
A

B

(all physiologic templates), but not L-BC, π6, or rotavirus dsRNAs. Because X dsRNA retains only 25 bp of the end of L-A from which the transcription reaction starts (99), the signal recognized by the transcriptase is most likely within this region, perhaps within the terminal 6 bp that are in common among L-A, M_1, and M_2 (129,258). The template-dependent transcription reaction requires very high concentrations of polyethylene glycol (20%), suggesting that the transcriptase has a low affinity for the dsRNA template (113). Because the dsRNA is normally formed within and stays inside the viral particles, the RNA polymerase sees a very high effective concentration and need not have a particularly high affinity.

Translation

The translation apparatus is a prime battleground for the fight between an RNA virus and its host. For example, interferon acts primarily by blocking viral translation. This can also be seen in picornaviruses, where cleavage of a cap-binding component inactivates host translation (see Chapter 18), or influenza virus cap-stealing and antiinterferon measures (see Chapter 24). Studies of the replication mechanisms of the L-A virus and its satellites have likewise led to the suggestion that translation of viral proteins is the critical event determining the balance between virus and host.

Ribosomal Frameshifting. The *gag* and *pol* ORFs of L-A overlap by 130 nucleotides (nt), and the Pol protein is expressed only as a fusion protein with the major coat protein, Gag (see Fig. 3A) (111,140). The mechanism of formation of this Gag-Pol fusion protein is a −1 ribosomal frameshift (74), very similar to those described in Rous sarcoma virus, many mammalian retroviruses, coronaviruses, and several plant viruses (142, and reviewed in refs. 101,125).

There are two features of the mRNA that determine the frequency of −1 ribosomal frameshifts (see Fig. 3A). The "slippery site" is a sequence of the form X XXY YYZ, where the *gag* reading frame is shown. This sequence allows the tRNAs reading XXY and YYZ to each move back one base on the mRNA and still have their nonwobble bases correctly paired (142). X can be any base, but Y can be only A or U, probably because the frequency with which unpairing of the tRNAs from the 0 frame codons (XXY and YYZ) is also important, and because A site-pairing is stronger than P site-pairing (26,74). Z can be any base but G, suggesting that specific tRNAs are more able to frameshift than others (37,133). The second component determining frameshift efficiency is the presence of a strong secondary structure, usually an RNA pseudoknot, just downstream of the slippery site, to slow ribosomal movement at this point (25,142). The location of this secondary structure is particularly critical (27), and a pseudoknot is far more effective in promoting frameshifting than a simple stem-loop of the same overall melting energy. The pseudoknot, more than the simple stem-loop, should resist melting of the first few bases of the stem, precisely positioning the ribosome with the slippery site in the A and P sites.

The efficiency of −1 frameshifting, and thus the ratio of Gag-Pol fusion protein to Gag protein produced, is critical for viral propagation (76), as is the efficiency of +1 frameshifting for Ty1 retrotransposition frequency (see later). A twofold change away from L-A's normal 1.9% efficiency results in failure to propagate the M_1 satellite dsRNA. L-A propagation is less sensitive, but the antibiotics sparsomycin, which increases ribosomal frameshifting, and anisomycin, which has the opposite effect, can cure L-A (75). The Gag-Pol to Gag ratio is likely to be important for viral assembly. Excess Gag-Pol (high frameshift efficiency) may result in starting too many particles and winding up with too little Gag to complete any of them. In contrast, excess Gag might result in particles closing before the packaging domain of Pol has had a chance to find a viral (+) strand (76).

Host genes affecting the efficiency of −1 frameshifting are called *MOF* (maintenance of frame) (76,77) and are expected to encode ribosomal components or translation factors. The differential effects of specific host mutations on frameshifting at specific slippery sites suggests that drugs similarly affecting frameshifting might target specific viruses (77). *MOF9* has been shown to be the 5S rRNA, showing a role for this 60S subunit component in maintenance of reading frame (78). *MOF4* is *UPF1*, one of the components of the nonsense-mediated decay system (61), and thus Upf1p plays roles in both monitoring reading frame and in the destabilization of mRNAs with premature termination codons. *MOF2* proved to be identical to *SUI1* [encoding a subunit of translation initiation factor 3 (eIF3)], and, like MOF4, it has effects on both nonsense mediated decay and maintenance of reading frame (62).

60S Subunits—Critical to Viral Propagation. Mutations in any of 20 chromosomal genes (called *MAK* for maintenance of killer) that result in diminished levels of free 60S ribosomal subunits also produce loss of M dsRNA and decreased copy number of L-A dsRNA (85,208). Mutations diminishing the supply of free 40S subunits generally had no such effect (208). The deficiency of 60S subunits results in selectively decreased rates of translation of mRNAs which, like L-A mRNA, lack 5′ cap and 3′ poly(A) (85). These *mak* mutations are suppressed by the *ski* mutations that derepress translation of non-poly(A) mRNAs (261).

Gag Decapping Activity—Necessary for M Expression. The L-A and L-BC Gag proteins each covalently bind the 5′ cap from any RNA *in vitro* (17). L-A Gag covalently attaches ^{7m}GMP from the cap to His154 in a reaction that requires only Mg^{2+} (18). Modification of His154 on an L-A cDNA expression clone destroys Gag's ability to covalently bind cap, but it does not prevent the clone's ability to propagate the M_1 satellite virus (18). However, expression of the killer toxin encoded by M_1 is impaired by the His154 mutation. Mutation of the *SKI1/XRN1* gene encoding the 5′ to 3′exoribonuclease, specific for uncapped RNAs and responsible for the major mRNA decay pathway (137), results in restoration of expression of killer toxin in spite of the mutation of His154 of Gag (185). It has been proposed that the virus decaps cellular mRNAs to decoy the Ski1p exoribonuclease from degrading the capless viral mRNA (185).

SKI *Antiviral System Blocks Translation of Viral [Non-poly(A)] mRNA.* The sole essential function of four of the SKI genes of *S. cerevisiae* is the repression of viral copy number, particularly control of M (14,15,222,226, 245,259,285). The SKI proteins repress three unrelated viral systems: L-A and its satellites, L-BC (a dsRNA virus), and the ssRNA replicon called 20S RNA (10,188,259). Detailed studies of the *SKI2* gene suggested that the system acts by limiting translation of viral mRNA (285). Because all of these are cytoplasmic replicons, and none was known to have either 5′ caps or 3′ polyA structures, it was speculated that the *SKI* system recognized the absence of one or both of these structures typical of eukaryotic cellular mRNAs (285). That *SKI2* also represses translation of RNA polymerase I transcripts (probably lacking cap and/or polyA) supports this idea (285).

Electroporation of mRNAs into spheroplasts shows that the Ski2, Ski3, Ski6, Ski7, and Ski8 proteins inhibit the translation of mRNA specifically if it lacks a 3′ polyA structure (13,14,185). Kinetic studies indicate that both the initial rates and the duration of translation are affected by the Ski proteins.

The *SKI2*, *SKI3*, *SKI6*, *SKI7*, and *SKI8* genes have been characterized, and only *SKI6* is essential for growth in the absence of M dsRNA (13,14,189,222, 245,285). Ski2p has helicase motifs, a glycine-arginine-rich domain and it is highly homologous to two mammalian genes (205,285). Ski3p has the TPR an amino acid repeat pattern (222) while Ski8p has a different sequence repeat first identified in β-transducin (189). Ski2p, Ski3p, and Ski8p form a cytoplasmic complex (29). Ski6p is homologous to RNAse PH, a tRNA-processing enzyme (14), and it is part of a nuclear complex of exoribonucleases thought to have a role in rRNA processing (196). Indeed, *ski6* mutants produce abnormal 60S ribosomal subunits (13) and show abnormalities in processing of 5.8S rRNA (13). Ski7p has homology to EF1-α, an elongation factor, suggesting that it is involved in the translation process.

Recently, a yeast homolog of *SKI2* (called *YGR271w* or *SLH1*) has been found whose deletion (*slh1Δ*) depressed L-A copy number as does *ski2Δ* (184). The *ski2Δ slh1Δ* double mutants show dramatically increased L-A, L-BC and M_1 dsRNA copy numbers, but grow normally in the abscence of the L-A and M_1 viruses (238). Remarkably, the *ski2Δ slh1Δ* cells show the same *in vivo* translation kinetics of non-poly(A) mRNA as they do for poly(A)+ mRNA, in spite of the presence of normal amounts of competing poly(A)+ mRNA (238). Thus, the translation apparatus is indifferent to the 3′ poly(A) structure except for the action of the Ski proteins and Slh1p. This suggests that the role of the eukaryote 3′ poly(A), like that of Ski2p and Slh1p, is to allow cells to distinguish their own mRNAs from those of invading viral genomes.

Posttranslational Modification

KEX1, KEX2 *Proteases and Discovery of Prohormone Proteases.* The *kex1* and *kex2* mutants were first isolated because of their inability to produce the "killer" toxin encoded by the M_1 satellite dsRNA (KEX, from killer expression) (282). The *kex2* mutants were noted to have a defect in mating that was specific to cells of the α mating type, and *kex2/kex2* homozygous diploids were defective for sporulation (170). The α-specific mating defect was partially explained by the finding that the cells failed to secrete the α pheromone (170), a peptide that prepares cells of the opposite (**a**) mating type for mating by arresting them in the G1 phase of the cell cycle. The failure to secrete killer toxin and α pheromone was explained by the finding that *KEX2* encodes a protease that cleaves C-terminal to pairs of basic amino acid residues (145), and that *KEX1* encodes a carboxypeptidase that can remove the pair of basic amino acids (55,79). These were the cleavages needed to convert the toxin and α pheromone proproteins to their mature forms (see Fig. 3B).

The specificities of the Kex proteases are the same as those needed to process preproinsulin (see Fig. 3B), preproopiomelanocortin, and other mammalian prohormones, but the enzymes responsible for these maturation cleavages had been elusive. Several genes and enzymes with homology to Kex2p were identified, and evidence that they are involved in these prohormone processing steps is accumulating (reviewed in ref. 246).

There is also evidence that the Kex2p-homologous enzymes are involved in the proteolytic processing of some mammalian viral proteins. Mutant CHO cells resistant to Sindbis virus and Newcastle disease virus were made sensitive by expression of the Kex2p-homolog, mouse furin, or by expression of Kex2p itself (197).

N-*Acetylation of* gag *by Mak3p—Necessary for Assembly. MAK3* is one of the three chromosomal genes known to be necessary for the propagation of the L-A dsRNA virus. Its sequence shows homology with

N-acetyltransferases, particularly with the rimI protein of *Escherichia coli*, which acetylates the N-terminal of ribosomal protein S18 (256). In fact, the L-A Gag protein is normally blocked (presumably acetylated) and is unblocked in a *mak3* mutant host, resulting in failure of viral assembly (257). Mak3p recognizes the N-terminal four amino acid residues of Gag (255), and this signal can be transferred to β-galactosidase, producing *MAK3*-dependent N-terminal acetylation. Like L-A, the major coat proteins of Rous sarcoma virus, tobacco mosaic virus, turnip yellow mosaic virus, alfalfa mosaic virus, and potato X virus are N-terminally acetylated, but the enzymes responsible have not been identified, nor can the role of acetylation for these viruses be examined without altering the primary protein sequence.

Recently, a complex of Mak3p, Mak10p, and Mak31p has been detected (227). Mak10p, Mak31p, and Mak3p are the only three proteins known to be necessary for L-A propagation (16,169,260), and this indicates that Mak10p and Mak31p are also involved in *N*-acetylation of the coat protein. Both *mak3* and *mak10* mutants show slowed growth on glycerol or ethanol, further supporting the idea that their functions are related (73,169,255).

Viral Assembly

The headful replication mechanism implies that the coat protein determines the structure of the head, not the genome. This is typical of isometric viruses, and it has now been confirmed by the finding that expression of the Gag protein alone produces empty particles that are morphologically indistinguishable from normal L-A virions (109). Normal L-A particles have a T=1 icosahedral structure with an asymmetric unit consisting of a dimer of Gag (35; see preceding). Each particle has only one or two Gag-Pol fusion proteins (perhaps as a dimer). The requirement for the Mak3p-catalyzed *N*-acetylation of Gag for assembly suggests that the Mak3/10/31 complex is involved in this process (226).

The existence of a Gag-Pol fusion protein, the ssRNA binding activity of its Pol domain, and the fact that (+) ssRNA is the species encapsidated to form new viral particles, led to a model of assembly and packaging that has been supported by subsequent findings (Fig. 4) (111). The Pol domain of the Gag-Pol fusion protein recognizes and binds to a packaging site on the viral (+) strands. Then (or concomitantly), the Gag domain of the fusion protein associates with the free Gag protein. This leads to encapsidation of a single (+) strand per particle if there is only one Gag-Pol fusion protein (or one dimer) per particle.

In vivo, Pol residues 67 to 213 of the Gag-Pol fusion protein are necessary for packaging of (+) strands, but not for assembly of morphologically normal viral particles (109,224). One of the three single-stranded RNA binding domains of Pol is located within this region and is necessary for the packaging (224) (see Fig. 3A).

The *packaging site* recognized is an internal stem-loop sequence with an A residue bulging from the 5′ side of the stem (see Fig. 3A) (107). This site, located about 400 nt from the 3′ end of the L-A (+) strand, was first identified as necessary for binding of X (+) ssRNA to the opened empty particles (97). Binding requires the stem structure but not the sequence of the stem. In contrast, the sequence of the loop is important. The protruding A residue must be present and must be an A (107). A similar site, similarly located on the M_1 (+) strand, was found (107) by examining the predicted folded structure of the M_1 sequence (124), and another was found by studying sequences involved in exclusion of M_1 (242). Either the L-A (X) or M_1 stem-loops are sufficient for binding, but the addition of 10 bp from the 5′ side of either one improves the binding substantially (107,242). Both the L-A and M_1 sites contain direct repeat sequences whose significance has not yet been determined. A site with the same structure has also been found in a similar location in the M_{28} satellite dsRNA (236).

The L-A and M_1 sites can each serve as a portable packaging signal *in vivo*, directing packaging of heterologous transcripts by L-A virus or by proteins produced from the L-A cDNA clone (107,109). The heterologous transcripts were packaged alone in viral particles, confirming the prediction of the headful replication model that a single (+) strand is initially packaged per particle.

The ratio of Gag-Pol fusion protein to Gag can be altered *in vivo* by adjusting the efficiency of ribosomal frameshifting and, as discussed, this ratio is important for M_1 satellite dsRNA propagation but less so for L-A itself (75,77). Whereas M_1 or X particle assembly can fail in a Gag-poor cell, an L-A (+) strand could be its own supply of Gag that will not be exhausted until completion of the particle makes the L-A (+) strand no longer available to the ribosomes. This form of *cis*-packaging could explain the differential effect of frameshift efficiency on M_1 and L-A propagation.

Replication [(–) Strand Synthesis]

Newly assembled viral particles contain an L-A (+) strand and are capable of converting it to the dsRNA form when supplied with nucleoside triphosphates (108). The particles formed in this reaction have all the properties of mature L-A particles and can carry out the transcription reaction (110).

To study the detailed mechanism of the replication reaction, it was necessary to establish a template-depen-

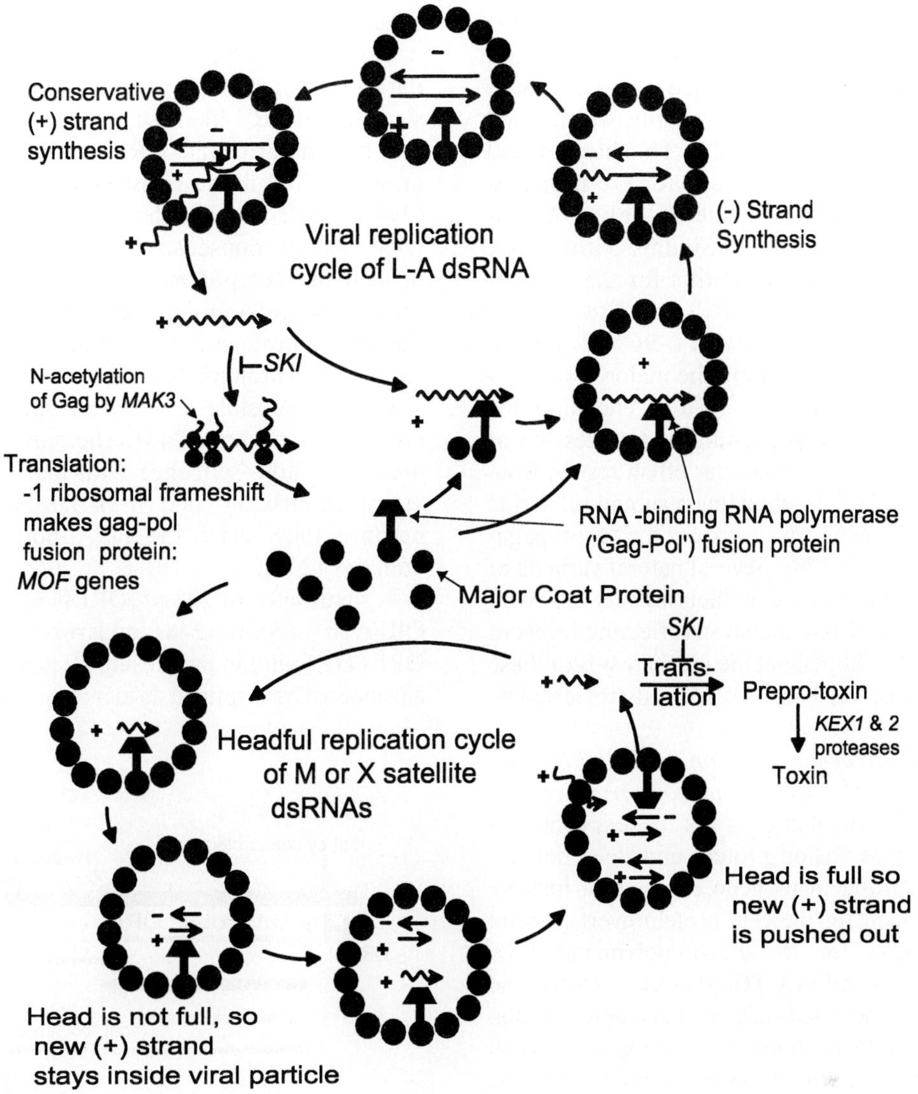

FIG. 4. Replication cycles of L-A virus and its satellite dsRNAs, M and X. The packaging region of the Pol domain of Gag-Pol binds to the packaging site of (+) strands as the Gag domain associates with other Gag molecules. This ensures packaging of viral plus strands (76,111). L-A particles have only one dsRNA molecule per particle. But the smaller M or X dsRNAs replicate within the viral coat until they fill the head (98,99).

dent *in vitro* reaction. The opened empty particles, when supplied with viral (+) strands, Mg^{2+}, nucleoside triphosphates, and a low concentration of polyethylene glycol, carry out (−) strand synthesis to form dsRNA (112). Only L-A, M, or X (+) strand templates are active in this reaction, supporting the notion that it accurately reflects the *in vivo* reaction.

A maximally active template requires both sequences at the 3′ end of the L-A (or X) plus strand and internal sequences (the internal replication enhancer) overlapping the packaging signal (97). The 3′ end of L-A (+) strands has a stem-loop whose structure is necessary for template activity. While the sequence of the loop and that of the 3′ terminal four nucleotides are important, that of the stem is not. In spite of the requirements for these structures and sequences in the context of L-A, the 3′ terminal 33 nucleotides of M_1's (+) strand can substitute for the L-A 3′ end, although there is little or no similarity between the two sequences (see Fig. 3) (97). The internal replication enhancer and the 3′ end site must be bound together for optimal template activity in the replication reaction (114). However, they need not be covalently attached and can simply be hydrogen bonded. This suggests that the RNA polymerase binds first to the internal site and is thus brought close to the 3′ end site where polymerization is to begin.

Because the RNA-dependent RNA polymerase consensus domains defined by Kamer and Argos (147) have since been found in essentially all (+) ssRNA and dsRNA viruses examined, the detailed mutagenesis of the most highly conserved of these regions was carried out using the L-A cDNA clone (225). This has defined the extent of the domains necessary for the propagation of the M_1 satellite dsRNA. Interestingly, homologous regions from Reovirus or Sindbis virus RNA polymerases could partially substitute for that of L-A (225).

Other Factors Affecting L-A, M, and L-BC Replication. Mutation of either *POR1*, encoding the major mitochondrial outer membrane porin, or *NUC1*, encoding the major mitochondrial nuclease, results in derepression of L-A copy number (73,177). A similar effect results from mutation of *scs1/lbc2* (122), encoding a subunit of serine palmitoyltransferase. *MKT1* is necessary for M_2 propagation, but not for M_1 (278,279). Several natural variants of L-A have been described based on their interactions' with *MKT1*, M_2 dsRNA, and *mak* mutations affecting levels of free 60S ribosomal subunits, but the mechanisms of these interactions have not yet been determined (reviewed in ref. 280).

Totiviridae *Using Internal Initiation to Make RNA Pol.* The 190S virus of *Helminthosporium victoriae* (Hv190SV) is a totivirus that does not make a coat protein–RNA polymerase fusion protein and does not use ribosomal frameshifting in its gene expression. Instead, the termination codon for the coat protein overlaps with the initiation codon for the RNA polymerase, the sequence being . . .GGA CAA **TG** AGT G. . . (139). The RNA polymerase is detected only as a separate protein, and it is suggested to be translated by the occasional reinitiation of ribosomes that have just terminated at the end of the coat protein part of the mRNA.

Two viruses of the filamentous fungus *Sphaeropsis sapinea*, a pathogen of pine trees, are closely related to Hv190SV in sequence, and they apparently use the same translation strategy to express their RNA-dependent RNA polymerase (217).

Leishmania dsRNA Viruses

Leishmania is a flagellated protozoan that causes cutaneous, visceral, or mucosal infections of man. *Leishmania* virus (LRV1-1) was first discovered as an RNA species associated with cytoplasmic, 32 nm virus particles (252). A similar virus (LRV1-4) was found in another strain and shown to be associated with an RNA polymerase activity (283). A survey of 71 *Leishmania* isolates showed related viruses present in 12, all of which were *L. braziliensis* or *L. guyanensis* originating in the Amazon basin (128). These species cause cutaneous and mucocutaneous forms of leishmaniasis, but not all such isolates carry the virus, nor is there evidence that the virus affects pathogenicity.

The replication cycle of LRV appears to be quite similar to that of the L-A virus of *S. cerevisiae* (276). The structure of LRV likewise closely resembles L-A (248). The two major ORFs, ORF2 and ORF3, overlap by 71 nt, with ORF3 in the +1 frame relative to ORF2 (Fig. 5) (248). ORF2 encodes the major coat protein (33), and ORF3 has the consensus patterns typical of viral RNA-dependent RNA polymerases. This suggests that a Gag-Pol fusion protein might be made (248), and an *in vitro* translation product of the predicted size (33) is a candidate for this protein. The sequence of the overlap region suggests a possible Ty1-like +1 shift site or a pseudoknot-promoted hop (248). The similarity of the LRV1 *pol* amino acid sequence with that of L-A of *S. cerevisiae* is striking, and it is far beyond that simply because they share the RNA polymerase consensus domains (248).

A small ORF of 228 nt (ORF1) is present upstream of ORF2 in LRV1-1 (248), and two such small upstream ORFs are found in the closely related LRV1-4 (235). The absence of the spliced leader sequence common to all

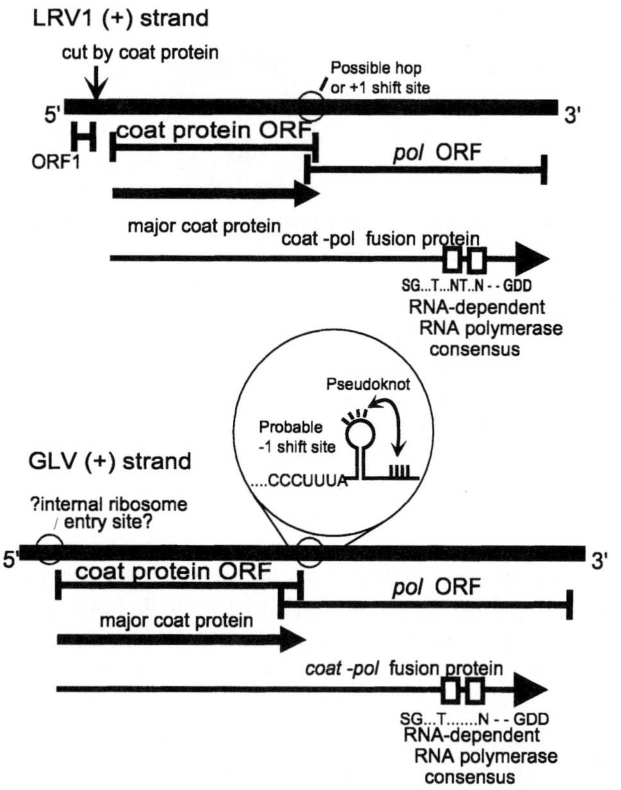

FIG. 5. Genome structure and expression of *Leishmania* virus, LRV1 (248), and the *Giardia* virus, GLV (273). There are several similarities of these viruses to each other and to the *Saccharomyces* virus, L-A, which has led to their classification together as totiviruses.

Leishmania cellular mRNAs suggests that this upstream region may be untranslated.

The capsid protein of LRV has an endonuclease activity that cuts viral (+) strands at GAUC*CG, 320 nt from the 5′ end in LRV1-4 (180). The role of this unique activity is not yet clear.

Giardia lamblia Virus

The Giardiavirus (GLV) is an infectious totivirus, with a single-segment, 6.1 kb double-stranded RNA genome (271). Its host, *Giardia lamblia*, is a primitive eukaryote with two nuclei but no mitochondria, Golgi, or endoplasmic reticulum. This protozoan is a flagellated intestinal parasite of mammals with a wide distribution.

Unlike other known viruses of fungi or parasites discussed here, GLV is found in the culture supernatant and readily infects *G. lamblia* cells. Infected cells contain 36 nm isometric particles composed of a major 100-kd protein and a minor 190-kd protein (194). Purified viral (+) ssRNA can be reintroduced into a virus-free strain by electroporation, and a new infection can be initiated in this way (116). Inserting luciferase within an *in vitro* transcript of a cDNA clone of GLV, replacing most of the Gag ORF, and electroporating the hybrid RNA into GLV-infected *Giardia* trophozoites, resulted in stable expression of luciferase in the recipient cells and the production of viral particles able to transmit luciferase expression to newly infected cells (67).

The structure of the GLV genome (see Fig. 5) (271) has several features in common with other *Totiviridae* and with certain animal viruses. There are two major ORFs: The 5′ ORF encodes the 100-kd major coat protein. The 3′ ORF has the typical RNA-dependent RNA polymerase motifs, and it is expressed only as a fusion protein with the 5′ ORF (271). Thus, expression in GLV resembles that of retroviruses, the *Saccharomyces* L-A virus, and the *Leishmania* dsRNA virus LRV-1 in forming a gag-pol fusion protein. The structure of the 210 nt overlap region of the *gag* and *pol* ORFs strongly suggests that the mechanism of fusion protein formation is by the same −1 ribosomal frameshift as that used by many animal retroviruses and the yeast L-A dsRNA virus. A slippery site C CCU UUA (*gag* frame shown) is followed closely by a predicted pseudoknot, as has been shown to be essential in these systems and in coronaviruses for programmed frameshifting.

The 5′ noncoding region of the GLV genome has seven AUG codons, each followed by a very short reading frame (271). This feature appears to be common among the *Cryphonectria* hypoviruses, LRV1, and GLV. The 5′ and 3′ UTRs are necessary for replication of the luciferase hybrid viruses, but the 5′ 265 nt of the Gag coding region further promotes expression of luciferase in these hybrids without affecting transcript levels, indicating a translational control mechanism (68). The results are consistent with an internal ribosome entry site bypassing the small upstream ORFs.

Trichomonas Virus and Host Phenotypic Variation

Many strains of *Trichomonas vaginalis* carry 33 nm viral particles composed of an 85-kd major coat protein and containing 5.5 kb dsRNA (272). This 5.5 kb dsRNA in fact consists of three distinct dsRNA species that do not cross-hybridize (152). Sequence analyses of two of the species indicate that each has a typical totivirus structure with overlapping 5′ Gag and 3′ Pol ORFs (250). Like the LRV1 totivirus, the Pol ORF is in the +1 frame relative to Gag (250).

Remarkably, the presence of the virus is correlated with a phenotypic variation of the host cells (270). Expression of a major surface antigen switches on and off in cells carrying the virus, but its transcription is always off in virus-free strains (153). Cells often lose the virus on serial passage, and loss of the virus is always accompanied by loss of phenotypic variation (270).

Partitiviridae

The *Partitiviridae* have a bipartite genome with the two segments separately encapsidated in particles containing the proteins encoded by both segments. This group includes viruses of the filamentous fungi *Penicillium*, and *Aspergillus*, and the mushroom *Agaricus*, as well as many other fungi. It also includes a large group of plant cryptoviruses (20,202), whose genome is dsRNA and whose biology is much like that of the systems discussed in detail here.

Atkinsonella hypoxylon *Partitivirus 2H.* This isolate of *Atkinsonella hypoxylon* strain 2H has three dsRNA segments of 2180, 2135, and 1790 nt. Segment 1 encodes an RNA-dependent RNA polymerase, and segment 2 encodes a 74-kd protein that may be the major coat protein (207). The third segment does not appear to encode a protein (207).

VIRUSES REDUCING VIRULENCE OF *Cryphonectria parasitica*

The American chestnut tree was devastated by the accidental introduction, in 1905, of the pathogenic fungus *Cryphonectria parasitica*, along with an oriental variety of the chestnut tree (reviewed in ref. 206). The fungus virtually eliminated the upper parts of the chestnut trees in the eastern United States, but the root systems are not killed and shoots continue to emerge, only to have their growth limited by the reattack of the fungus. *C. parasitica* had a similar effect in Europe, but in the 1950s, the emergence of fungal strains in Italy with markedly reduced virulence to the trees was noted. These "hypovirulent" strains (Fig. 6), later also found in Michigan, could

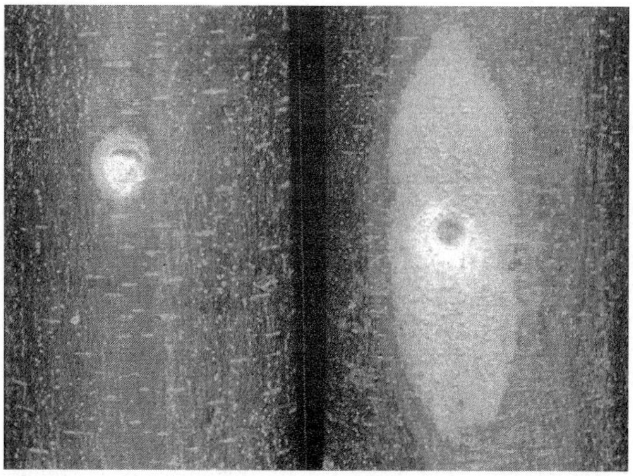

FIG. 6. Virulent (uninfected, *right*) and hypovirulent (virus-infected, *left*) *Cryphonectria parasitica* (chestnut blight fungus) inoculated into chestnut trees. Infection of the fungus by any of several hypoviruses attenuates its virulence toward the trees. (Photo courtesy of Dr. Donald Nuss.)

transmit their hypovirulence by hyphal anastomosis to virulent strains, and this was used successfully for the biologic control of chestnut blight in Europe. Hypovirulent strains also show decreased asexual spore formation, decreased production of laccase (a phenol oxidase possibly involved in pathogenesis), and reduction in pigment formation (reviewed in 206).

The cytoplasmically inherited factor that reduces the pathogenicity of the fungus and produces these hypovirulence-associated traits was identified as any of several apparently unrelated dsRNA replicons found in the hypovirulent strains and not in the virulent strains (6,66,135). Curing the dsRNAs by growth in the presence of cycloheximide was accompanied by the return of virulence (115).

Genome Structure

The most thoroughly studied hypovirulence-producing virus is CHV1-EP713, the L-dsRNA of hypovirulent *C. parasitica* strain EP713, a 12,712-bp molecule whose (+) strand has two long ORFs, ORFA and ORFB (Fig. 7) (240). Each ORF encodes a papain-like cysteine protease in its N-terminal portion that self-cleaves the primary translation products at least once, as shown in Figure 7 (49,241). The presence of related papain-like proteases and helicase domains, as well as RNA-dependent RNA polymerase motifs, has led to the suggestion that L-dsRNA of *C. parasitica* is related to the potyviruses, a group of (+) ssRNA viruses of plants (162).

The ORFA and ORFB overlap by a single nucleotide, with the UAA termination codon of the first overlapping with the AUG codon of the second (240). The mechanism by which ORFB is expressed has not yet been defined, but this structure implies that the mechanism will not involve ribosomal frameshifting or termination codon read-through. Rather, reinitiation is the most likely mechanism. The translation of ORFA also poses an interesting problem, as the 5′ noncoding region contains six short ORFs (240). Whether ribosomes initiate internally as in the case of picornaviruses (see Chapter 18) or use these tiny ORFs for regulatory purposes, as in the GCN4 gene of *S. cerevisiae* (136), is not yet clear.

Virus Replication in Intracellular Vesicles

Unlike other mycoviruses, most of the *C. parasitica* dsRNAs described to date are not associated with virus particles. Rather, they are found in intracellular vesicles (80,131). These vesicles have an RNA polymerase activity that produces both ssRNA and dsRNA (100). Most of the label is incorporated into viral (+) strands (100). This

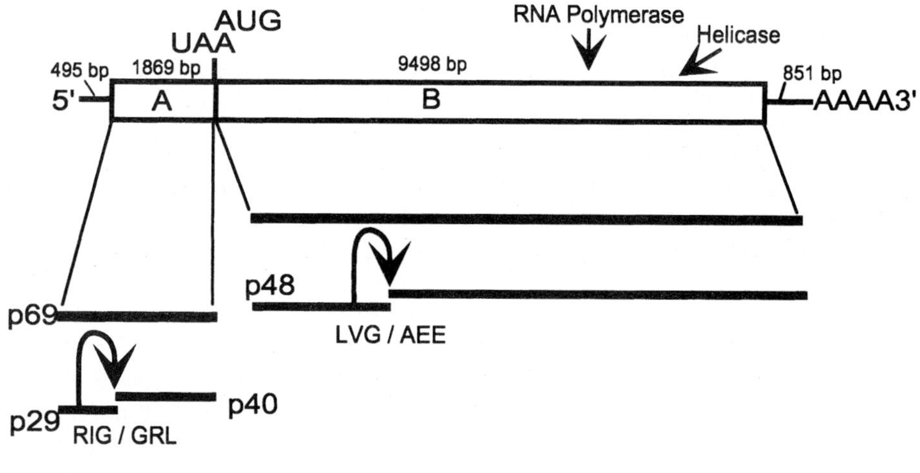

FIG. 7. Coding information and protein processing of the *Cryphonectria parasitica* virus, L. (Adapted from ref. 206, with permission.) The sites of action of the p29 and p48 proteases are indicated. This virus is now designated CHV1-EP713, the type member of the *Hypoviridae*.

is reminiscent of the membrane association of *in vivo* RNA synthesis of many (+) strand RNA viruses, supporting the notion that this virus is not closely related to other fungal viruses.

Virus Induction of Hypovirulence

CHV1-EP713 has very specific effects on certain genes. For example, the laccase gene encodes a phenol oxidase believed to be involved in pathogenesis. Transcription of the laccase gene is repressed by CHV1-EP713 infection (46,228), an effect that can be produced by expression of just the p29 protease encoded by part of ORFA (48). Although p29 is sufficient to alter fungal phenotypes, it is neither necessary nor sufficient to cause hypovirulence (60). Deletion of p29 from the virus results in decreased induction of the hypovirulence-associated traits, but no decrease in hypovirulence itself. Moreover, it is not the protease activity of p29 that produces hypovirulence (60). The symptom-determining domain of p29 has now been localized to the interval Phe25 to Gln73 of p29 (25). The effect of CHV1-EP713 on laccase appears to be transmitted by an influence on the inositol triphosphate–calcium signal transduction system of the fungus, possibly explaining the multiple phenotypic effects of hypovirulence (165).

Cryparin, a hydrophobic cell-surface protein, is also reduced in hypovirulent strains, an effect mediated at transcription (295). Another gene, *Vir2*, was isolated based on its decreased transcription in a hypovirulent strain. Although no effect was seen on virulence itself, deletion of this gene partially mimics some of the hypvirulent-associated traits, with decreased asexual sporulation and fruiting body formation and impaired sexual crossing ability (294). The hypovirulence-associated traits are thus caused by specific effects of viral gene products, rather than by the presence of a replicating dsRNA.

Recently, G protein signaling has been implicated in the induction of hypovirulence by CHV1-EP713. Hypovirus infection leads to decreased expression of the host Giα (α inhibitory subunit of G protein) and a concomitant increase in cAMP levels (40,45). Moreover, disruption of *cpg-1*, the gene for Giα, results (in an uninfected strain) in elevated cAMP levels, total loss of virulence, and the development of the same associated phenotypes seen on virus-induced hypovirulence (118).

Infectious cDNA Clones and Biologic Control of Chestnut Blight

Introduction of complete cDNA clones of L-dsRNA under control of the *C. parasitica* glyceraldehyde-3-phosphate dehydrogenase promoter resulted in both a complete hypovirulence phenotype of the fungus and the launching of the RNA replicon in a form transmissible to other strains (47). In addition to its usefulness in studying the mechanism of the effects of CHV1-EP713 dsRNA on the cell, this infectious cDNA clone method is an important advance in attempts to control chestnut blight. Although artificial inoculation of trees with hypovirulent fungal strains in Europe resulted in spread of the hypovirulence dsRNAs to virulent strains and control of the blight, this approach has not succeeded in the United States. CHV RNA spreads by fusion of the growing fungal cells with other cells, a process called hyphal anastomosis, but not by sexual crosses (4). Hyphal anastomosis requires that strains have identical alleles at several different loci determining compatibility. The number of compatibility groups is apparently much greater in the United States, limiting the spread of the hypovirulence dsRNA.

In contrast, infectious cDNA incorporated into the *C. parasitica* genome, while generating dsRNA replicons, will also naturally spread to other mating and vegetative compatibility groups through sexual transmission (47, 205). It is thus expected to be more effective in the biologic control of chestnut blight than the natural virus, and early results support this expectation (5).

A Reovirus of *Cryphonectria*

Two strains of *C. parasitica* have been found carrying reovirus-like elements (91,211), one of which (C18) is associated with hypovirulence (91). Strains C18 and 9B-2-1 each have 11 dsRNA segments ranging in size from about 1 to about 3 kb and associated with 60 nm virus particles, unlike the vesicles in which the potyvirus-like *Hypoviridae* are found. These 11 segments are present in equimolar amounts and transmission studies show that either all or none of the segments are transmitted, suggesting that they are parts of a single viral genome. Blotting experiments suggest that the C18 and 9B-2-1 genomes are not closely related, but both apparently cause hypovirulence. This system adds new dimensions to the study of both hypovirulence and the *Reoviridae*.

SINGLE-STRANDED RNA REPLICONS

20S RNA

In 1971, a stable species of RNA, intermediate in size between 18S and 25S rRNAs, dubbed 20S RNA, was found to appear specifically in cells exposed to the condition used to induce meiosis and sporulation—namely, when acetate is supplied as the carbon source in the absence of a nitrogen source (146). The ability to produce 20S RNA was then found to be inherited as a non-Mendelian genetic element, distinct from other known elements (123). It was not connected with meiosis, except that the same culture conditions are used to induce both (123). 20S RNA was finally proven to be an independent

RNA replicon whose copy number is inducible in acetate (188). Its sequence shows that its 2,500 nucleotides encode a single 95-kd protein with some similarities to the RNA-dependent RNA polymerases of RNA phages and RNA viruses (190,230). W dsRNA, a minor species inducible by growth at high temperature (277), proved to be the replicative form of 20S RNA (190,230). Electron micrographs of purified 20S RNA showed about 50% circular molecules (188), but biochemical experiments indicate that the RNA itself is not circular (231). Recently, the terminal sequences of 20S RNA were shown to be 5′GGGGC . . . . . . GCCCC-OH3′ (232), suggesting that a circular structure may have been formed by hydrogen bonding.

20S RNA is an apparently naked cytoplasmic replicon with no coat protein (284). The 91-kd RNA polymerase is found bound specifically to the 20S RNA genome (119), and these complexes have RNA polymerase activity—that is, synthesizing 20S RNA and its complementary strand (120). Replication intermediates of 20S RNA include W dsRNA, which is a unit-length molecule, and larger, apparently double-length species (190). Single-stranded molecules of approximately dimer length have also been detected on denaturing gels (190).

23S RNA

T dsRNA was discovered as a minor species of dsRNA easily detected in cells lacking L-A and L-BC, and shown to be, like W dsRNA, an independent replicon inducible by growth of cells at high temperature (277). T is the replicative form of 23S ssRNA (96). 23S RNA has substantial homology with 20S RNA, and likewise appears to encode an RNA-dependent RNA polymerase (96), with which it is associated in extracts (95). All strains known to have T dsRNA also have W dsRNA, but many strains with W lack T (277). Whether T depends on W is not clear.

Control of 20S and 23S RNA Replication

The copy numbers for 20S RNA and 23S RNA are controlled by media conditions, requiring acetate as the carbon source and the absence of a nitrogen source for their 10,000-fold induction (96,146,188,277). Both are also induced by growing cells at 37°, and at least 20S is repressed by the *SKI* system (188,277). The *SKI* effect apparently reflects the absence of 3′ poly(A) on 20S mRNA (see preceding).

The *Cryphonectria parasitica* Mitochondrial Replicon NB631 dsRNA

Polashock and Hillman (216) have described a mitochondrial dsRNA species in *C. parasitica* strain NB631. If one assumes the mitochondrial genetic code (UGA = Trp), then the NB631 dsRNA has a single long ORF that encodes an RNA-dependent RNA polymerase. This RNA polymerase is most closely related to those of 20S and 23S RNAs, and all are more closely related to RNA phage such as Qβ, than to RNA viruses of higher organisms (215,229). The degree of similarity is such that these elements must be very close relatives. Nevertheless, 20S RNA and 23S RNA are primarily ssRNA replicons with small amounts of the dsRNA replicative form found in cells, whereas NB631 has been identified as a dsRNA element.

NB631 dsRNA is transferred by hyphal anastomosis, like other *C. parasitica* RNA replicons, but unlike those, and other viruses of filamentous fungi, it is also efficiently transmitted by meiotic spore formation if the female parent had the virus (215).

A dsRNA in *Rhizoctonia solani* Also Found as Chromosomal DNA

The M_2 dsRNA of the plant pathogen *Rhizoctonia solani* is a 3,750-bp molecule with a single ORF, and with a high similarity to the NB631 dsRNA. Some of the RNA-dependent RNA polymerase motifs are found, and the results indicate that this protein is an RNA-dependent RNA polymerase (RDRP) (164). Remarkably, the same sequences are present in the DNA genome of the fungus, and the original hypovirulent isolate carrying M_2 derives from a virulent strain having the DNA copy but lacking the free dsRNA (164).

RETROVIRUSES (RETROELEMENTS)

Retroviruses, Retrotransposons, Retroposons, and Retrointrons

Retroelements (Table 2) all share their use of reverse transcriptase in their propagation. The retrotransposons (Table 3) of fungi and parasitic microorganisms resemble mammalian retroviruses in all essentials except for their lacking an *env* (envelope) gene and, in part for this reason, are restricted to propagation without leaving the intracellular environment (Fig. 8). Nonetheless, the frequency with which these cells mate in nature is so high that most of these elements are widely distributed in their respective species. The retroposons are one step further removed in that they lack the long terminal repeat (LTR) structure, and their transposition process differs from those of the other groups. These elements resemble the mammalian LINE elements, but they have the advantage of readily detectable transposition and facile host genetics for their study. For example, Tad, of *Neurospora*, can retrotranspose between nuclei of a heterokaryon (156,157).

TABLE 2. *Retrotransposons of simple eukaryotes*

Retrovirus (copy #)	Host species	LTRs	ε (unique)	Group[a]	Reference
Ty1, Ty2 (217, 34)	*Saccharomyces cerevisiae*	δ–334–8 bp	5.2 kb	*copia*	(21)
Ty3 (41)	*S. cerevisiae*	σ–340 bp	4.7	*gypsy*	(132)
Ty4 (32)	*S. cerevisiae*	τ–371 bp	5.6	*copia*	(249) (143)
Ty5 (7)	*S. cerevisiae*	245 bp		*copia*	(269)
Tf1, Tf2	*Schizosaccharomyces pombe*	349–358 bp	4.4	*gypsy*	(172)
DIRS-1	*Dictyostelium discoideum*	ITRs	4.2		(34)
DRE	*D. discoideum*	complex TRs			(183)
Tp1	*Physarum polycephalum*	277 bp	8.3	*copia*	(233)
CfT-1	*Cladosporium fulvum*	427 bp	6.1	*gypsy*	(192)
pCal	*Candida albicans*	280 bp	5.9	*copia*	(191)
CRE1	*Crithidia fasciculata*	—		LINE	(117)
SLACS, CZAR	*Trypanosoma brucei, T. cruzi*	—	6.7	LINE	Site-specific insertion in spliced leader (3)
TOC1	*Chlamydomonas reinhardtii*	217, 237 bp	4.6		(65)
Tad	*Neurospora*	—	7.0	LINE	(156) (157)

[a]Based on amino acid sequence homology and gene order, retrotransposons may be divided into those similar to the *copia* element or the *gypsy* element of *Drosophila* (82). Copy numbers of *S. cerevisiae* retrotransposons in the genome are from ref. 154. LINE-like elements are retroposons, lacking LTRs.
LTR, long terminal repeat.

TABLE 3. *Groups of retroelements*

Element	*env*	LTRs	RT	Examples
Retrovirus	+	+	+	RSV, HIV
Retrotransposon	–	+	+	Ty1–5
Retroposon	–	–	+	LINEs, Tad
Retrointron	–	–	+	intron aI1 of *COX1*

LTR, long terminal repeat; RT, reverse transcriptase; RSV, respiratory syncytial virus; HIV, human immunodeficiency virus.

A group of reverse-transcriptase-encoding introns in mitochondrial DNA of *S. cerevisiae* has also been identified (151). These are introns aI1 and aI2 of the COX1 (cytochrome oxidase subunit I) gene. These introns are capable of retrotransposition both into their normal location and into heterologous locations, both *in vitro* (151) and *in vivo* (199). These retroelements lack LTRs and have only a single ORF. Their properties suggest that introns may have begun as parasitic elements.

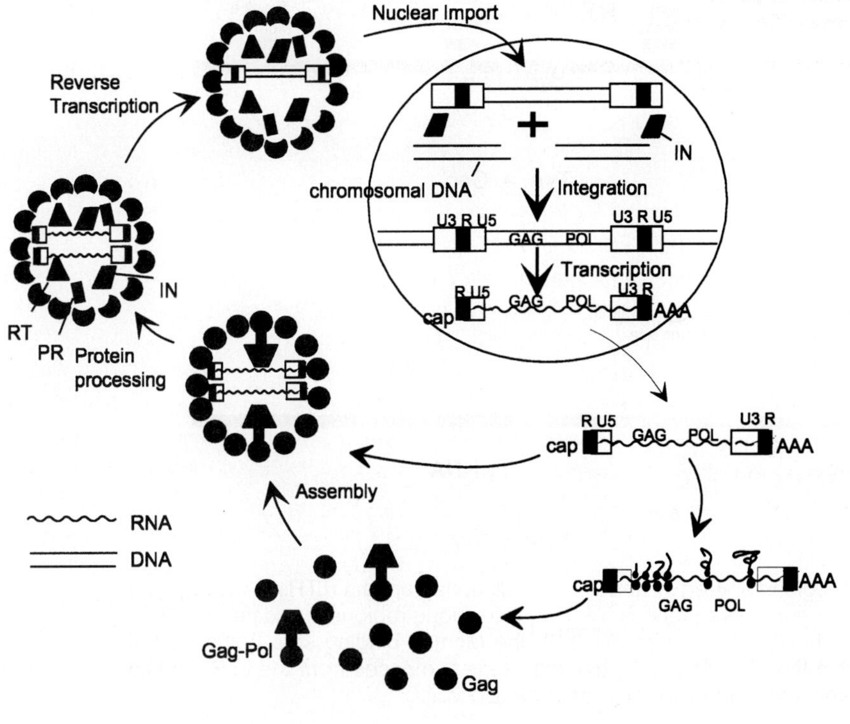

FIG. 8. The Ty replication cycle. It is likely that all retrotransposons follow this cycle.

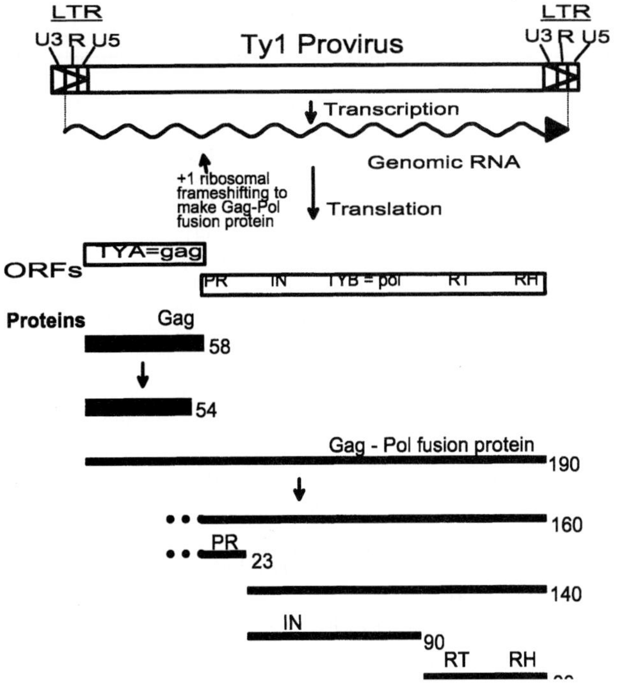

FIG. 9. Genome structure and expression of Ty1. Gag and Gag-Pol are the primary translation products, which are processed by cleavage with the viral protease to form the proteins shown. (Adapted from ref. 121, with permission.)

The retrotransposons are also divided based on amino acid sequence homologies and gene order in the *pol* domain into the *copia*-like and the *gypsy*-like elements. *Copia* and *gypsy* are retroelements of *Drosophila*. Because Ty3 is more similar to gypsy than to Ty1 (132,290), it is likely that Ty3 and Ty1 entered the yeast genomes at different times, and thus that horizontal transfer of these elements does occur.

Structure of Tys and Other Retroelements

The Ty elements of *S. cerevisiae* each have LTRs of 245 to 371 bp, separated by a unique region (called ε) of 4.7 to 5.6 kb (Figs. 9 and 10) (21,51,132). The major Ty RNA transcript begins within the 5′ LTR (at base 241 from the 5′ end in Ty1) and ends at base 289 of the 3′ LTR, 45 bp from the 3′ end of the element (see Fig. 10) (90). This provides the basis for the conventional division of retroviral LTRs into the U3 region (present only at the 3′ end of the Ty RNA, but located at the 5′ end of the LTR), the R region (repeated at both ends of Ty RNA), and the U5 region (present only at the 5′ end of Ty RNA, but at the 3′ end of the LTR).

Ty1 through Ty4 all have two overlapping ORFs, TYA, corresponding to *gag*, and TYB, homologous to the *pol* of mammalian retroviruses. Like mammalian retroviruses and *gypsy*, Ty3 has the gene order protease (PR)–reverse transcriptase (RT)–RNase H (RH)–integrase (IN) in the *pol* ORF (132), whereas Ty1 and Ty2 have the *copia* order PR-IN-RT-RH (51,275).

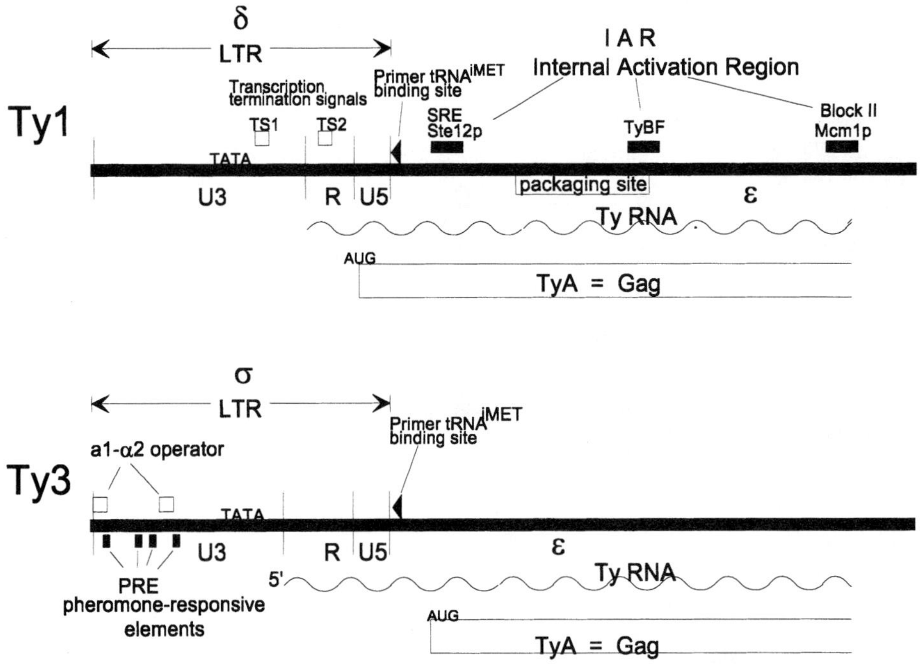

FIG. 10. Structure and functional regions of the Ty1 and Ty3 long terminal repeats (LTRs). Although the LTRs of Ty1 and Ty2 are similar, the control sequences within ε, the unique regions, are different. SRE, Site-responsive element; TyBF, Ty binding factor site; Block II, the Mcm1p binding site. Ty38s control sequences are apparently all within the LTR, its primer binding site is two bases from the LTR, and its Gag protein initiation codon is within the unique region, not in the LTRs.

Replication Cycle of *S. cerevisiae* Ty Elements

The Ty replication cycle resembles that of mammalian retroviruses except that it begins and ends with the integrated form of the genome (see Fig. 8). Ty transcripts made with RNA polymerase II are translated to make the Gag (TYA) and Gag-Pol fusion (TYA-TYB) proteins. These proteins assemble, packaging the Ty RNA to make particles that are homologs of the core particles of retroviruses. The reverse transcriptase and RNase H make a dsDNA copy of the genome, and integrase inserts this into the genome, producing a short repeat of the chromosomal integration site.

Reverse Transcription

The reverse transcriptase and RNase H–homologous domains are present in the Ty1 particles as a 60-kd protein that is produced by proteolytic processing of the 190-kd Gag-Pol fusion protein (see Fig. 9) (121). Isolated Ty1 particles have reverse transcriptase that is active on either the endogenous Ty1 RNA or externally added templates. The Ty particles are also open to externally added enzymes, indicating that they are not impermeable shells but have pores. This porous structure may help explain how pseudogene formation can occur (71).

The mechanism of reverse transcription of Ty RNA is largely the same as that for mammalian retroviruses (but see ref. 166). The primer for reverse transcription is $tRNA_i^{Met}$, with 10 nucleotides of the 3′ acceptor stem complementary to a site on the Ty1 (+) strand just 3′ to the 5′ LTR, called the (–) primer binding site (–PBS) (39). This tRNA is specifically packaged in viral particles (39). Interestingly, although the primer function of the initiator tRNAMet depends on its complementarity with the –PBS, its packaging is independent of this complementarity (39). This indicates that the $tRNA_i^{Met}$ is recognized by some other component of the Ty virus particle, and that it is probably not the acceptor stem of the tRNA that is recognized.

Integration

Ty3 shows a tight specificity for target sites, integrating 16 or 17 bp upstream of the 5′ ends of tRNA coding regions (29,36). The DRE element of *Dictyostelium discoideum* and the spliced leader-specific elements SLACS, CZAR, and CRE1 of trypanosomes have a similar integration target specificity (3,117,183). Other genes transcribed by RNA polymerase III, such as 5S ribosomal RNA and U6 small nuclear RNA, are similarly targets for Ty3 (36). However, no common consensus sequence could be deduced for the insertion sites, suggesting that the integration apparatus was recognizing some aspect of chromatin structure or the RNA polymerase III transcription apparatus itself at these sites. Substitution of four purines with pyrimidines at the site of transcription initiation without moving the promoter did not change the site of Ty3 insertion. Eliminating transcription by destroying the promoter (box B inside the tRNA gene) eliminated target activity. But leaving the original transcription initiation site and Ty3 insertion site intact and moving box A of the promoter to a new site moved the site of transcription initiation and changed the Ty3 insertion site to a comparable position (36). This indicates that the integration apparatus recognizes the transcription apparatus but not the transcription initiation site or the promoter itself.

Other Tys are capable of insertion at many different sites, with Ty1 producing a five-bp duplication of the target DNA (102), but these sites tend to be within 750 bases of a tRNA gene or other RNA polymerase III–transcribed gene (144,154). Ty1 insertions in RNA *pol* II–transcribed genes tend to be in the 5′ part of the *URA3*, *LYS2*, and *CAN1* genes (86,175,201), with control regions targeted far more often than the ORFs. Ty5 specifically targets regions of silent chromatin, such as the telomeric regions or the silent mating type loci (296).

An *in vitro* integration system has been established for Ty1 using Ty1 viral particles produced from an element carrying a copy of the *E. coli supF* gene and, as target, λ DNA from a multiple amber mutant suppressible by *supF* (87,88). Using this system, it has been shown that linear double-stranded DNA substrates carrying the terminal 12 bp at each end of the LTR are sufficient for the integration reaction to occur at normal efficiency (88). There are also no nucleotide requirements. The substrate DNA must have 3′ hydroxyls, suggesting that the reaction involves covalent attachment of these 3′ ends to the target DNA. Unlike mammalian retroviruses, Ty1's IN does not remove two terminal bases in the process of integration (88), probably because in Ty1 the –PBS is immediately adjacent to the U5 part of the LTR. Ty3, however, resembles mammalian retroviruses in this regard (S. Sandmeyer, personal communication).

In fact, the purified IN protein is capable of carrying out an integration model reaction without other components of the viral particle (198). This suggests that it may be sufficient for IN and the reverse transcript to enter the nucleus for integration.

Expression

Control of Transcription

Ty1 transcription is controlled by MAT, the yeast mating type locus. MATa/MATα diploid cells have 20-fold lower Ty1 transcript levels than MATa or MATα haploid cells or MATa/MATa or MATα/MATα diploids (89). Exposure of cells to mating pheromones, a step that immediately precedes mating itself, produces a posttranscriptional blockage of Ty1 transposition (293). Is this a control strategy adopted by Ty1 or imposed by the host, and why?

DNA damage, induced by ultraviolet irradiation or 4-nitroquinoline-1-oxide also induce Ty1 transposition by inducing transcription of the element (24). Is this effect adaptive for Ty1 as a first step in finding a new home, or is it a consequence of a failure of the host anti-Ty system?

Retroelements all must cajole the cellular RNA polymerase II into transcribing their proviral form to make viral RNA. They are constrained, however, to place the controlling sequences inside the limits of the element. While most mammalian retroviruses have enhancers in their LTRs upstream of the start site of transcription, Ty1 and Ty2 elements have major transcriptional control sequences downstream of both the transcript start site and the translation start site, most of them inside the unique region ε (see Fig. 10). Ty1 has two major downstream sites responsible for its haploid-specific transcription: the sterile-responsive element (SRE) binds Ste12p, and another site (block II or PRTF) binds Mcm1p (53,92) (see Fig. 10). Ty2 has one upstream activation site (174), and at least two downstream activation regions, one of which (DAS1) responds to Gcn4p (103,264). Ty2 also has several downstream repression sites (DRS) (104).

Transcription of both Ty3 and Ty5 are, like that of Ty1, much higher in haploid cells than in diploids. Moreover, its transcription and transposition are derepressed by exposure of cells to the mating pheromones (52,150,265). Ty3 transposition is, in fact, induced in mating cells and Ty3 transposing from the genome of one mating partner to that of the other occurs at high rates (158). Ty3 transcription is induced before mating and repressed after mating by mating type control, but the particles synthesized before mating are sufficient to give a burst of transposition from one genome into the other (158). Here, the interpretation of preparation to transpose into the potentially Ty3-free genome of the mating partner seems clear.

In diploid *Saccharomyces* cells, the MATa1-MATα2 protein complex (encoded by the mating type locus) represses haploid-specific cellular genes. The regulation of Ty3 transcription involves two a1-α2 consensus recognition sites, determining mating type repression, and three PRE sequences, determining pheromone responsive expression, all located within the 5′ LTR of the Ty3 element (16,265). An upstream repression sequence (URS) is located at the junction of the 5′ LTR and the adjacent tRNA gene (16). Thus, in contrast to Ty1 and Ty2, most of whose control regions are located within the unique region downstream of the transcription and translation start sites, Ty3's transcription control regions are largely upstream within the U3 region of the LTR (see Fig. 10).

Effect of Ty Insertion on Cellular Genes

Insertion of Ty elements into the control regions of cellular genes can activate, inactivate, or alter the control of the target gene (93,287; reviewed in 21). The Ty insertions often move the normal regulatory sequences 5 kb away from the target gene, eliminating the normal regulation. Insertions of Ty whose 5′ end is close to the 5′ end of the target gene impose the Ty transcriptional control on the target gene. This produces a divergent transcription of the Ty element and the target gene, but both are under mating type control because of the effect of the Ty control region.

Chromosomal Genes Regulating Ty Transcription

Mutant cellular genes which have come under control of Ty1 have been used extensively to investigate the cellular genes affecting the transcription of Ty1 itself (50,288,289). Second-site mutations (suppressors) that restore the normal expression of the target genes have defined a large group of genes, called *SPT*, that include the TATA binding factor TFIID, the genes encoding histones, and many general transcription factors with effects on many genes (e.g., *SNF2*, *SNF5*, *SNF6*, *GAL11*, *SIN1*). In addition, the control of the target genes by mating type and mating pheromones have led to studies of effects of the mating type and pheromone control pathway genes on Ty itself. For example, *STE12* controls Ty1 transcription, as do the genes upstream of *STE12* in the mating type control kinase cascade (93,94).

+1 Ribosomal Frameshifting

Like mammalian retroviruses, Ty elements direct the synthesis of a Gag protein and a Gag-Pol fusion protein (Fig. 11). For reasons that are not yet clear, each of the *Saccharomyces* Ty elements uses +1 ribosomal frameshifting, whereas animal retroviruses all use −1 frameshifting (or readthrough of a terminator) to make Gag-Pol (reviewed in 101,125). As shown by studies of the L-A dsRNA virus, yeast can perform −1 ribosomal frameshifts by the same simultaneous slippage mechanism used by retroviruses.

The mechanisms of the +1 frameshifts in Ty1 or Ty2 (see Fig. 11) and Ty3 all involve the combination of starvation for a rare tRNA and an unusual tRNA able to perform the frameshift (13,105). In the case of Ty1, the slippery site on the mRNA is CUU-AGG-C. The ribosomes are slowed by the AGG codon at the A ribosomal site. This codon is recognized by a $tRNA^{Arg}$ that is present in low abundance in yeast, so it is called a hungry codon. The $tRNA^{Leu}$, located at the P site while the A site is waiting for the AGG codon to be occupied, has as its anticodon UAG, and it is capable of pairing with either the 0 frame CUU codon or the +1 frame codon UUA. When it slips into the +1 frame, the GGC codon can be easily recognized by an abundant $tRNA^{Gly}$ species, and the ribosomes then continue in the +1 pol reading frame to make Gag-Pol fusion protein (13).

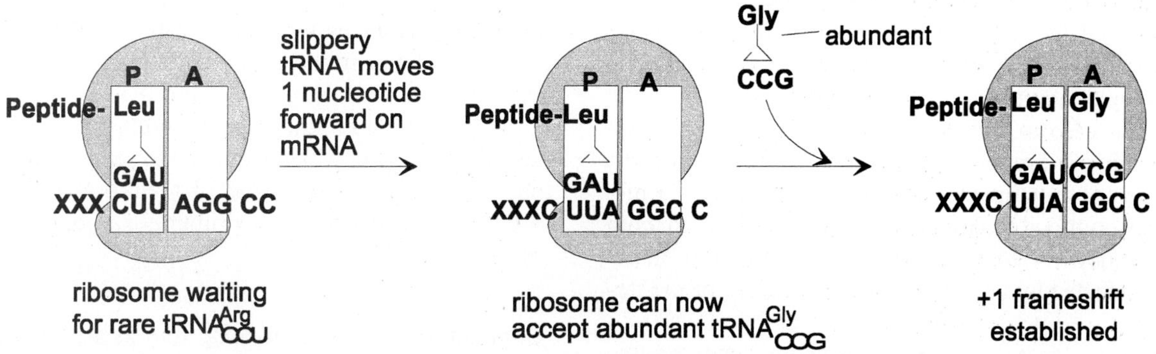

FIG. 11. Mechanism postulated for +1 ribosomal frameshifting of Ty1. (Adapted from ref. 12, with permission.) Ty3 frameshifting involves the new tRNA pairing in the +1 frame without a shift of the peptidyl tRNA as for Ty1 (268).

The efficiency of the Ty1 +1 ribosomal frameshift depends on the scarcity of the $tRNA^{Arg}$ recognizing the AGG codon. Thus, artificially oversupplying this tRNA lowers frameshift efficiency (13) and also lowers transposition frequency (291). Likewise, deletion of the gene for this $tRNA^{Arg}$ increases the efficiency of frameshifting and lowers the frequency of transposition (149). Starvation of cells for spermidine elevates the efficiency of Ty1 +1 ribosomal frameshifting and results in decreased transposition efficiency (8). Like the similar experiments done with the L-A dsRNA virus of *S. cerevisiae*, these results suggest that drugs affecting frameshifting efficiency might be useful as antivirals.

The Ty3 frameshift site is GCG-AGU-U, and, like that of Ty1, it is based on a hungry codon in the ribosomal A site, namely AGU (105). AGU is recognized by a low-abundance $tRNA^{Ser}$, so the ribosome pauses at this point. But the $tRNA^{Ala}{}_{CGC}$ that decodes the GCG codon in the P site cannot slip +1 and re-pair. Rather, it is believed that the valine tRNA simply pairs out of frame (268).

Proteolytic Processing and Phosphorylation

Ty1 Gag is expressed as a primary translation product of about 58 kd, most of which is processed by the Ty1 protease to form the 54-kd major particle protein (1). Gag is phosphorylated (193), and this phosphorylation is increased concomitant with the inhibition of transposition that occurs when cells are treated with mating pheromone (293). After Pol is synthesized as a 190-kd Gag-Pol fusion protein, it is processed through several intermediates to form a 23-kd protease, the 90-kd integrase, and the 60-kd reverse transcriptase–RNase H (see Fig. 9) (121).

Packaging: RNA Sites and Protein Requirements

The Ty1 RNA site determining packaging has been localized to within a 381-nt region between nt 239 and 620 (see Fig. 10) (292). The RNA structure recognized and the parts of TYA or TYA-TYB proteins that recognize this region have not yet been determined.

Debranching Enzyme and Ty1

Mutation of *DBR1*, encoding the enzyme that debranches the lariat structure produced by intron excision by cleaving the 2′-5′ linkage at the branchpoint, results in a ninefold decrease in Ty1 transposition efficiency (38). However, the explanation of this unexpected finding remains unclear.

Host Limitations on Ty Transposition Efficiency

Although normal cells have about 35 chromosomal copies of Ty1, most of which are probably transposition competent (64), transposition is a relatively rare event. Most studies of the mechanism of transposition have used a high-copy plasmid with a GAL1-promoted Ty1 carrying a marker (such as *HIS3*) included in the Ty1 to facilitate detection of transposition (21). When Ty1 transposition is induced with such a plasmid, although Ty1 RNA is increased only a few fold over that derived from the normal chromosomal Ty1 copies, the frequency of transposition increases about 100-fold (63). One point at which transposition is blocked in uninduced cells is at the processing of viral proteins, particularly the PR and IN proteins encoded by TYB (63). Several host genes have been identified whose mutation derepresses Ty1 transposition, analogous to the effect of ski mutations on RNA virus copy number (see preceding).

Mutation of the cellular *rad6* gene, encoding a ubiquitin-conjugating enzyme, increases the frequency of Ty transposition at either *URA3* or *CAN1* (214). This effect was not caused by altered Ty transcript levels, and it was seen even when retrotransposition from a GAL1-promoted Ty1 was studied. The *rad6* mutation is believed to alter chromatin structure by failing to ubiquitinate histones, suggesting that its effect on Ty1 transposition is on the nature of the target. Indeed, Ty1's target-site specificity for gene control regions is apparently eliminated by the *rad6* mutation (148,175).

Another case of target-level regulation of Ty1 retrotransposition is found on mutation of *CAC3*, encoding a subunit of chromatin assembly factor, and *HIR3*, a histone transcription regulation gene (218). Here again, both the frequency of integration and the distribution of insertions is affected by alterations of the structure of the target (138).

Mutation of the *FUS3* mitogen-activated protein kinase (MAP kinase) results in an over 20-fold increased Ty1 transposition frequency (54). Ty1 transcript levels and primary translation products were not affected by *fus3*, but virus particle–associated processing products of TyB and Ty cDNA were each elevated 10-fold or greater in the mutant. The Fus3 kinase is activated by exposure to the mating pheromones via a cascade of kinases, so this explains the inhibition of Ty1 transposition by exposure to mating pheromones (293). Although Fus3 may act indirectly to block Ty1 transposition, several observations suggest a direct action (54). TyA is normally phosphorylated, but it is hyperphosphorylated when cells are treated with α pheromone, which is known to activate Fus3 (293). TyA has several consensus sites for Fus3 phosphorylation.

Also inhibiting Ty1 retrotransposition are components of the nucleotide excision repair/transcription factor TFIIH (167). *SSL2* and *RAD3* encode DNA helicases with roles in both nucleotide excision-repair and in the basal transcription factor TFIIH. Mutants in either of these genes show elevated frequencies of Ty1 retrotransposition without alterations of the distribution of integration sites (167). There is no elevation of Ty1 proteins, but the level of Ty1 cDNA is elevated in either mutant (167). These results indicate that Ssl2p and Rad3p either inhibit reverse transcription or, perhaps more plausibly, destabilize Ty1 cDNA (167).

It is thus apparent that the host has several levels of defense against Ty1 attack: stability of viral particles, stability of cDNA, and structure of the target sites.

Schizosaccharomyces pombe Retroelements

The Tf1 and Tf2 elements of *S. pombe* are unusual in that a single ORF encodes both Gag and Pol (172). From the primary 140-kd translation product, the viral protease cleaves the proteins that form the viral particles (173). In view of the strict requirement for the ratio of Gag to Gag-Pol in Ty1 (149,291) and retroviruses, the assembly process in Tf1 and Tf2 must be significantly different. In log phase cells, the ratio of Gag to IN in particles is close to 1, whereas in stationary cells, it is quite high (7). Selective degradation of the non-Gag protein components alters the ratio after particle formation (7).

The priming mechanism of Tf1 is also unique. Instead of tRNA-priming as for other retrotransposons and retroviruses, Tf1 (–) strand DNA synthesis is primed by the first 11 nucleotides at the 5′ end of the viral RNA, which is complementary to the primer-binding site (171,176). A hairpin is formed, which is nicked to separate the first 11 nucleotides from the 5′ end of the RNA and give it a 3′OH that can serve as a primer for strong-stop DNA synthesis.

Candida albicans Retrotransposon as a Plasmid

Most retrotransposons have minute amounts of cDNA present in normal strains, but that of *C. albicans* (pCal) produces 50 to 100 copies per cell of linear dsDNA in a particular strain of *Candida* (191). pCal is a member of the Ty1/*copia* group found in integrated form in most strains, and the basis for its high free levels is not yet known. pCal is also unique among retrotransposons in that it uses readthrough of a stop codon to make its Gag-Pol fusion, as in murine leukemia virus (191).

Summary of Retroelements

The mating type and pheromone control of Ty transcription is clearly adapted to maximize transposition activity at the time when a potentially unoccupied genome becomes available (mating), and to minimize potential damage to the host, whose health is indispensable for survival. Posttranslational mechanisms, determined by the host, also limit transposition.

Among the many interesting questions about Ty elements are, Why do all Ty's use +1 frameshifting, but mammalian retroviruses use −1 frameshifting or termination readthrough to make their Gag-Pol fusion proteins? How does RNA polymerase II know to stop in the 3′ LTR, but to keep going in the identical sequence in the 5′ LTR? What does Dbr1, the debranching enzyme, do for Ty1? The bewildering array of retroelements continues to amaze.

DNA VIRUSES: *CHLORELLA* VIRUSES

Chlorella is a unicellular eukaryotic alga with a rigid cell wall and a single chloroplast (reviewed in ref. 266). Most *Chlorella* species are free-living, but several, called collectively zoochlorellae, live as endosymbionts (intracellular symbionts) of *Hydra* or *Paramecium*.

An attempt to isolate zoochlorellae free of their *Hydra* or *Paramecium* host often induces multiplication of a virus that grows and kills the zoochlorellae. These viruses are called HVCV (for *Hydra viridis Chlorella* virus) or PBCV (for *Paramecium bursaria Chlorella* virus) (reviewed in refs. 266,267). Hundreds of *Chlorella* viruses have been isolated directly from fresh water and are found throughout the world. They are grown on cultured zoochlorellae and form lytic plaques on agar plates.

Chlorella viruses are large (150 to 230 nm), polyhedral particles containing 5% to 10% lipid. The dsDNA genome of PBCV-1, the best studied *Chlorella* virus, is 333 kb, one of the largest viruses known. PBCV-1 DNA is linear with (a) terminal inverted repeats of 2.2 kb, (b) terminal hairpin structures, and (c) shorter direct repeats within the inverted terminal repeats (245). All three characteristics are in common with the poxviruses, vaccinia virus and African swine fever virus. Some other features are shared with the iridoviruses.

Chlorella virus DNA is heavily methylated, with 5-methylcytosine accounting for as much as 47% of C residues and 6-methyladenine for up to 37% of A residues. Surprisingly, the *Chlorella* viruses encode their own methylases. They also have been found to encode a variety of restriction endonucleases, similar in properties and, in many cases, in specificity to bacterial type II restriction endonucleases. The variety of such methylases and restriction endonucleases has only begun to be explored, but it is clear that a wide variety of specificities will be found (203). The function of these enzymes is completely unclear, and there is evidence against their being required for either degradation of host DNA or exclusion of other co-infecting viruses (reviewed in ref. 203).

It is not surprising to find glycosylated viral proteins, and the 54-kd major capsid protein of PBCV-1 has a carbohydrate component of about 5 kd. What is unexpected is that the virus encodes products that determine the glycosylation of Vp54 (274). Antivirus monoclonal antibodies directed against the carbohydrate moiety of Vp54 were used to select resistant mutants. The resulting virus mutants had altered glycoprotein moieties, but unaltered Vp54 amino acid sequence, indicating that the virus encodes either its own glycosyl transferases or products that control the host enzymes.

The complete sequence of PBCV-1 showed that the 330,742-bp genome encodes enzymes for synthesis of hyaluronic acid, aspartate transcarbamylase (uracil biosynthesis), an EF-3 homolog (translation elongation factor), 10 tRNA genes, genes with self-splicing type I introns, and numerous enzymes involved in nucleic acid metabolism.

Large DNA viruses of marine brown algae have also been described (reviewed in ref. 267).

PRIONS OF *SACCHAROMYCES* AND *PODOSPORA*

The concept of an infectious protein arose in studies of the transmissible spongiform encephalopathies, such as scrapie of sheep, mad cow disease, and Creutzfeldt-Jakob disease of humans (see Chapter 37). Based on genetic evidence (Fig. 12), two non-Mendelian genetic elements of *S. cerevisiae*, [URE3] and [PSI], were identified as

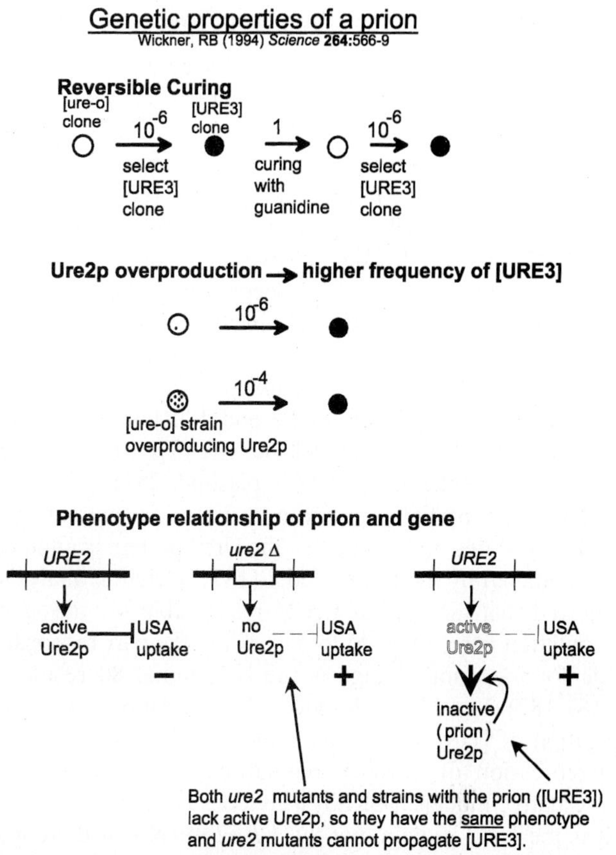

FIG. 12. Three genetic criteria for a prion. These are unusual features, expected of a prion but not of a nucleic acid replicon. (Adapted from ref. 281, with permission.)

prion (infectious protein) forms of Ure2p and Sup35p, respectively (281). This conclusion is supported by extensive further evidence and both appear to be transmissible amyloidoses, a remarkably close parallel to the mammalian disease.

[URE3]—A Transmissible Amyloidosis of Ure2p

In 1971, Lacroute described a non-Mendelian genetic element of *S. cerevisiae* called [URE3], which allowed cells to take up ureidosuccinate in spite of the presence of a rich nitrogen source such as ammonia (163). Ureidosuccinate is normally produced by aspartate transcarbamylase in the uracil biosynthesis pathway, and its uptake from the medium by Dal5p is repressed by ammonium. Chromosomal *ure2* mutants have the same effects as [URE3], but in addition they fail to propagate the [URE3] genetic element (2,281). Ure2p is inhibited by Mks1p (84) and posttranslationally inhibits the transcription activator, Gln3p (56). Gln3p positively regulates many genes in nitrogen metabolism, including *DAL5*, whose product is necessary for ureidosuccinate uptake (195,221):

NH_3—| Mks1p—| Ure2p—| Gln3p → N catabolism genes

Genetic Evidence That [URE3] Is a Prion

Three lines of genetic evidence indicate that [URE3] is actually an altered form of Ure2p that has lost its activity in repressing nitrogen metabolic enzymes through Gln3p but has acquired the ability to convert the normal Ure2p to this altered form (see Fig. 12) (281). First, [URE3] is curable by growth of cells on guanidine HCl, but the curing is reversible in that [URE3] derivatives may again be selected from the cured strain (281). Second, overproduction of Ure2p leads to a 20- to 100-fold increase in the frequency with which [URE3] arises *de novo* (281). Third, the requirement of Ure2p for propagation of [URE3] and the identical phenotypes of *ure2Δ* and [URE3] are easily explained by the prion model, but not if [URE3] were a nucleic acid replicon—a virus or plasmid (281).

Ure2p is partially protease resistant in extracts of [URE3] strains, indicating that the Ure2 protein is altered, as predicted by the prion model (187). Deletion analysis showed that the part of Ure2p responsible for nitrogen regulation is residues 90 to 354, while the part responsible for the prion change is the N-terminal 80 residues (181,187) (Fig. 13A;. Moreover, the generation and propagation of [URE3] was unaffected by the repression or derepression of nitrogen regulation, eliminating some alternative models. [URE3] truly does arise *de novo*, and it is the Ure2 protein, not the *URE2* mRNA or the copy number of the *URE2* gene that induces [URE3] to arise (185).

Amyloid Formation In Vitro *by Ure2p Promoted by the Prion Domain*

Ure2p–green fluorescent protein fusions were found to be aggregated in [URE3] cells, indicating that aggregation is involved in the [URE3] change (83). Recent *in vitro* studies have shown that the Ure2p prion domain synthetic peptide can form amyloid, and that it can direct the conversion of the full-length native Ure2p into amyloid (see Fig. 13B) (253). The product of this reaction can seed further amyloid filament formation *in vitro*, suggesting that the [URE3] phenomenon is a transmissible amyloidosis of yeast (253). It appears that the conversion of Ure2p to amyloid inactivates the protein, and at the same time provides a seed for the further polymerization of newly synthesized Ure2p. It is proposed that the amyloid formed by Ure2p consists of a β-sheet core of the prion domain with the C-terminal nitrogen regulation domain attached as shown in Figure 13C.

[PSI]—A Transmissible Amyloidosis of Sup35p

In 1965, Cox described [PSI], a non-Mendelian genetic element of *S. cerevisiae* that increases the efficiency of nonsense suppression by classical tRNA suppressors (58,59). Like [URE3], [PSI] is reversibly curable, in this

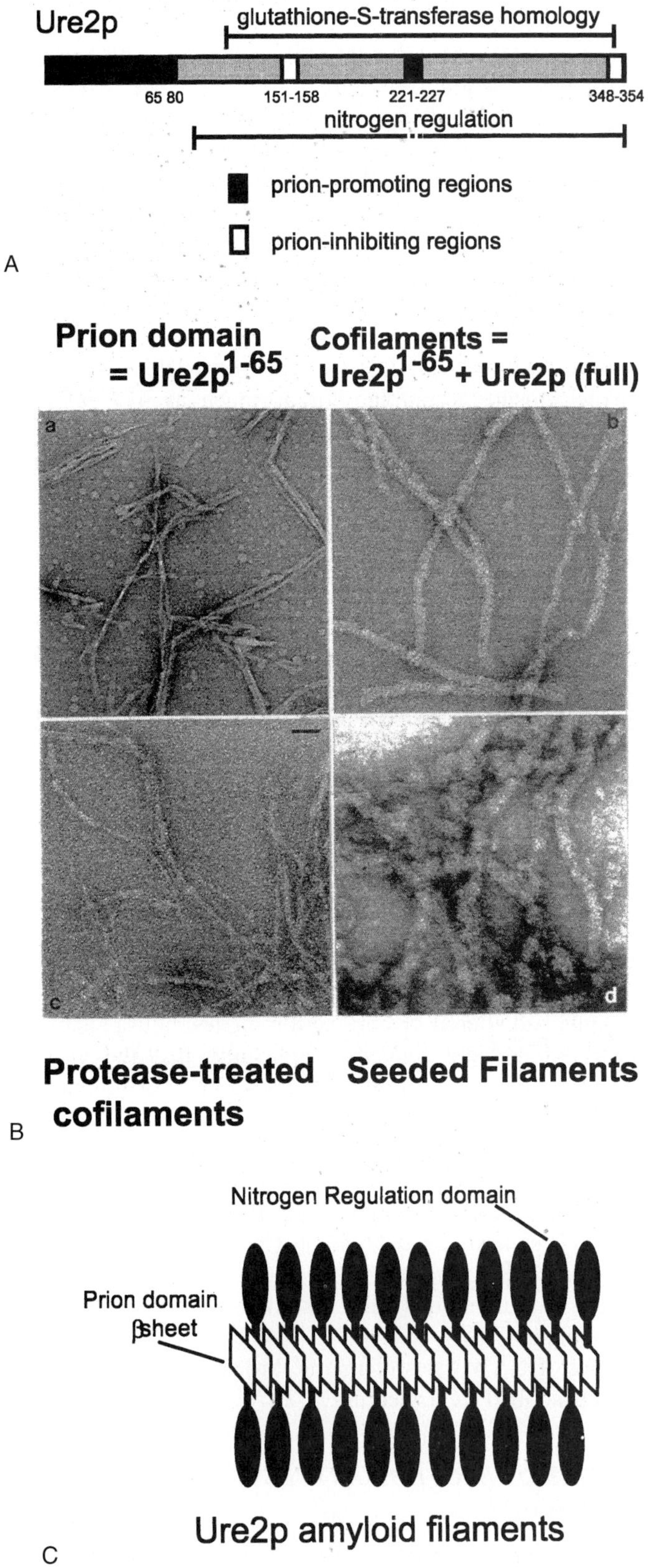

FIG. 13. A: Domains of Ure2p (181,186). **B:** Amyloid formation by Ure2p *in vitro* (253). **C:** Model of Ure2p amyloid structure (253).

case either by guanidine or by high-osmotic-strength media (42,179,243,262). Overexpression of Sup35p increases the frequency with which [PSI] arises by 100-fold (42), like the induction of [URE3] appearance by Ure2p overproduction (see preceding). Finally, the phenotype of [PSI] is like that of *sup35* mutants, and *SUP35* is necessary for propagation of [PSI] (81,252), as *URE2* is necessary for propagation of [URE3]. This logical parallel with [URE3] led to the suggestion that [PSI] is also a prion form of Sup35p (281).

In support of the prion model for [PSI], it was shown that Sup35p is aggregated in [PSI+] strains, but not in [psi−] strains (210,212). Further, it was found that it was the overproduction of the Sup35 protein, not the *SUP35* mRNA or the gene in high copy number, that caused the *de novo* appearance of [PSI] (70).

Chaperone Involvement in [PSI] Propagation

Chernoff found that either overproduction of Hsp104p or deletion of the *HSP104* gene resulted in the inability of cells to propagate [PSI] (Fig. 14) (43,44). This finding is important because it at once supported the prion model for [PSI], it was the first proof of involvement of a chaperone in a prion phenomenon, and it provides a potential pathway to treatment of prion diseases. Because Hsp104 disaggregates denatured proteins *in vivo* (209), overproduction of Hsp104 probably cures [PSI] by disaggregating the aggregated Sup35p (see Fig. 14). Whether deficiency of Hsp104 results in loss of [PSI] because Hsp104 participates in the conversion of the normal to the prion form of Sup35p or because Hsp104 must partially disaggregate the prion form of Sup35p to ensure its segregation to both daughter cells remains unclear.

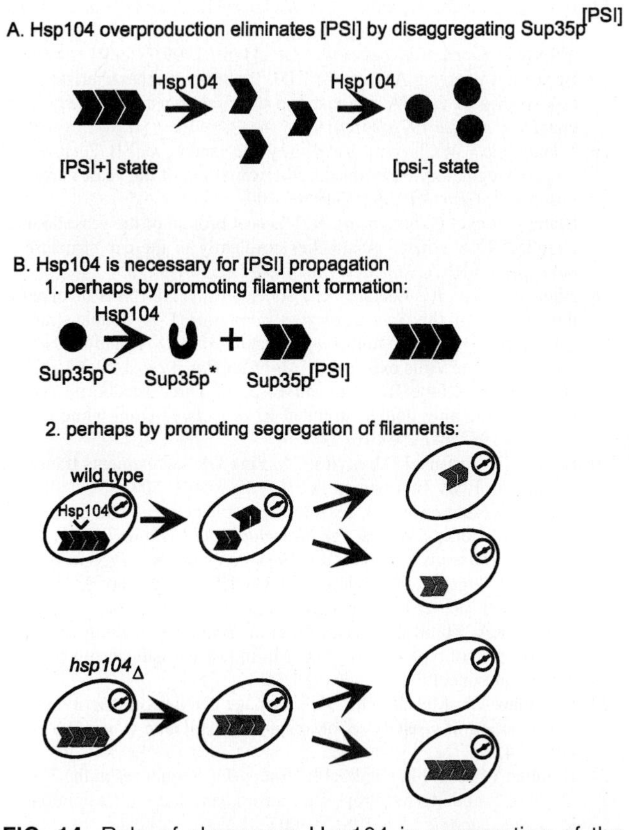

FIG. 14. Role of chaperone Hsp104 in propagation of the [PSI] prion of *S. cerevisiae* (43,44). Overproduction of Hsp104 cures the [PSI] prion by renaturing aggregates of Sup35p. Normal levels of Hsp104 are needed for [PSI] propagation, perhaps because it has a role in catalyzing Sup35p filament (aggregate) formation or in breaking up aggregates to ensure that each daughter cell gets at least one aggregate.

Amyloid Formation by Sup35p **In Vitro**

The *in vitro* aggregation of native soluble Sup35p seeded by the prion form from [PSI+] cells will continue indefinitely as long as fresh native Sup35p is supplied (213). Further, synthetic prion domain peptide spontaneously forms amyloid *in vitro* (155). In addition, the full-length Sup35p, made in *E. coli*, forms β-sheet-rich filaments spontaneously when diluted out of denaturant, a process that can be accelerated specifically by an extract from [PSI+] cells (127).

[Het-s]—A Prion of *Podospora* Responsible for a Normal Function

When two colonies of the same strain of filamentous fungus meet, they fuse their cellular processes (called hyphae) in a process called hyphal anastomosis or vegetative fusion. This allows exchange of cytoplasm and even nuclei and allows cooperation between the colonies in obtaining nutrients. However, a virus initially present in only one colony will spread throughout the other colony, so the process is tightly controlled, requiring identity of the two strains at 6 to 10 special chromosomal loci, called *het* loci in *Podospora anserina*. Fusion of two strains that differ at a *het* locus begins, but it is quickly arrested with death of the few fused hyphae and formation of a barrier to further hyphal fusion. This is called the heterokaryon incompatibility reaction (Fig. 15) (11,229; reviewed in 10).

One of the het genes of Podospora is *het-s*, with alleles *het-s* and *het-S* encoding a 289-residue protein differing at 14 positions (263), although the difference at residue 33 is sufficient to trigger the incompatibility reaction (69).

Rizet found that *het-s* strains could show the incompatibility reaction only if they also carried a non-Mendelian genetic element, called [Het-s] (229). [Het-s] could be "cured" from a male strain by mating, but from the cured strain, [Het-s] cells arose at a frequency of about 10^{-7} (12). This is the *reversible curing* criteria for a prion.

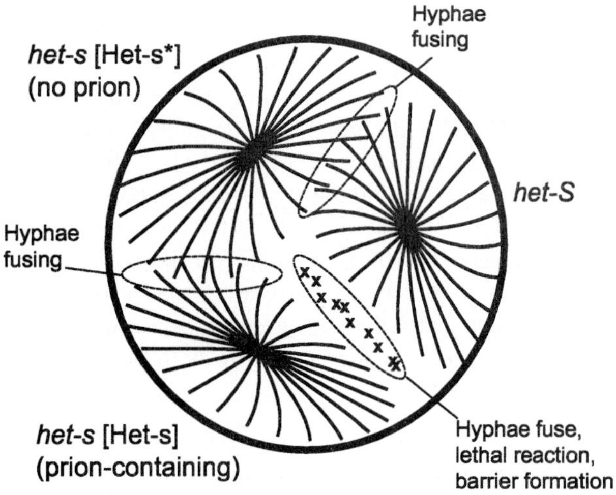

FIG. 15. The [Het-s] prion of *Podospora anserina* is required for heterokaryon incompatibility. (Reprinted from ref. 57, with permission.)

Coustou et al. have made the case that [Het-s] is a prion of the protein encoded by *het-s* (57). They showed that overproduction of the Het-s protein increased the frequency with which [Het-s] arose, and that the Het-s protein is relatively protease resistant in strains carrying [Het-s]. Moreover, deletion of the *het-s* gene makes a cell unable to propagate the [Het-s] non-Mendelian genetic element (57).

Beyond its obvious interest as a new prion, [Het-s] is particularly important because it is the first case in which a prion appears to be responsible for a normal cellular function. Heterokaryon incompatibility is observed in most filamentous fungi, usually controlled by chromosomal genes that have no particularly unusual features. In this case, it requires the [Het-s] prion to be observed. This suggests that other prions may be found responsible for normal cellular functions.

PERSPECTIVE

The discovery of prions of yeast and fungi has resolved the debate over whether prions could exist at all and widened the scope of this concept, showing that it is not unique to a single mammalian protein. The possibility is now open for exploring the mechanisms of amyloid and prion generation and propagation using yeast, and using these systems to devise approaches to the many heretofore intractable amyloid diseases.

REFERENCES

1. Adams SE, Mellor J, Gull K, et al. The functions and relationships of Ty-VLP proteins in yeast reflect those of mammalian retroviral proteins. *Cell* 1987;49:111–119.
2. Aigle M, Lacroute F. Genetical aspects of [URE3], a non-Mendelian, cytoplasmically inherited mutation in yeast. *Molec Gen Genet* 1975; 136:327–335.
3. Aksoy S, Williams S, Chang S, Richards FF. SLACS retrotransposon from *Trypanosoma brucei gambiense* is similar to mammalian LINEs. *Nucleic Acids Res* 1990;18:785–792.
4. Anagnostakis SL. Biological control of chestnut blight. *Science* 1982; 215:466–471.
5. Anagnostakis SL, Chen B, Geletka LM, Nuss DL. Hypovirus transmission to ascospore progeny by field-released transgenic hypovirus strains of *Cryphonectria parasitica. Phytopathology* 1998;88:598–604.
6. Anagnostakis SL, Day PR. Hypovirulence conversion in *Endothia parasitica. Phytopathology* 1979;69:1226–1229.
7. Atwood A, Lin J-H, Levin HL. The retrotransposon Tf1 assembles virus-like particles that contain an excess Gag relative to integrase because of a regulated degradation process. *Mol Cell Biol* 1996;16:338–346.
8. Balasundaram D, Dinman JD, Wickner RB, et al. Spermidine deficiency increases +1 ribosomal frameshifting efficiency and inhibits Ty1 retrotransposition in *Saccharomyces cerevisiae. Proc Natl Acad Sci U S A* 1994;91:172–176.
9. Ball SG, Tirtiaux C, Wickner RB. Genetic control of L-A and L-BC dsRNA copy number in killer systems of *Saccharomyces cerevisiae. Genetics* 1984;107:199–217.
10. Begueret J, Turq B, Clave C. Vegetative incompatibility in filamentous fungi: het genes begin to talk. *Trends Genet* 1994;10:441–446.
11. Beisson-Schecroun J. Incompatibilte cellulaire et interactions nucleo-cytoplasmiques dans les phenomenes de barrage chez *Podospora anserina. Ann Genet* 1962;4:3–50.
12. Belcourt MF, Farabaugh PJ. Ribosomal frameshifting in the yeast retrotransposon Ty: tRNAs induce slippage on a 7 nucleotide minimal site. *Cell* 1990;62:339–352.
13. Benard L, Carroll K, Valle RCP, Wickner RB. Ski6p is a homolog of RNA-processing enzymes that affects translation of non-poly(A) mRNAs and 60S ribosomal subunit biogenesis. *Mol Cell Biol* 1998; 18:2688–2696.
14. Benard L, Carroll K, Valle RCP, Wickner RB. The Ski7 antiviral protein is an EF1-α homolog that blocks expression of non-poly(A) mRNA in *Saccharomyces cerevisiae. J Virol* 1999;73:2893–2900.
15. Bevan EA, Herring AJ, Mitchell DJ. Preliminary characterization of two species of dsRNA in yeast and their relationship to the "killer" character. *Nature* 1973;245:81–86.
16. Bilanchone VW, Claypool JA, Kinsey PT, Sandmeyer SB. Positive and negative regulatory elements control expression of the yeast retrotransposon Ty3. *Genetics* 1993;134:685–700.
17. Blanc A, Goyer C, Sonenberg N. The coat protein of the yeast double-stranded RNA virus L-A attaches covalently to the cap structure of eukaryotic mRNA. *Mol Cell Biol* 1992;12:3390–3398.
18. Blanc A, Ribas JC, Wickner RB, Sonenberg N. His154 is involved in the linkage of the *Saccharomyces cerevisiae* L-A double-stranded RNA virus gag protein to the cap structure of mRNAs and is essential for M_1 satellite virus expression. *Mol Cell Biol* 1994;14:2664–2674.
19. Boccardo G, Milne RG, Luisoni E, et al. Three seedborne cryptic viruses containing double-stranded RNA isolated from white clover. *Virology* 1985;147:29–40.
20. Boeke JD, Garfinkel DJ, Styles CA, Fink GR. Ty elements transpose through an RNA intermediate. *Cell* 1985;40:491–500.
21. Boeke JD, Sandmeyer SB. Yeast transposable elements. In: Broach JR, Pringle JR, Jones EW, eds. *The Molecular and Cellular Biology of the Yeast Saccharomyces cerevisiae: Genome Dynamics, Protein Synthesis and Energetics.* Plainview, NY: Cold Spring Harbor Laboratory Press, 1991;193–261.
22. Bostian KA, Elliott Q, Bussey H, et al. Sequence of the preprotoxin dsRNA gene of type I killer yeast: Multiple processing events produce a two-component toxin. *Cell* 1984;36:741–751.
23. Bradshaw VA, McEntee K. DNA damage activates transcription and transposition of yeast Ty retrotransposons. *Mol Gen Genet* 1989;218: 465–474.
24. Brennan VE, Field L, Cizdziel P, Bruenn JA. Sequences at the 3′ ends of yeast viral dsRNAs: Proposed transcriptase and replicase initiation sites. *Nucleic Acids Res* 1981;9:4007–4021.
25. Brierley I, Dingard P, Inglis SC. Characterization of an efficient coronavirus ribosomal frameshifting signal: Requirement for an RNA pseudoknot. *Cell* 1989;57:537–547.
26. Brierley I, Jenner AJ, Inglis SC. Mutational analysis of the "slippery-sequence" component of a coronavirus ribosomal frameshifting signal. *J Mol Biol* 1992;227:463–479.
27. Brierley I, Rolley NJ, Jenner AJ, Inglis SC. Mutational analysis of the

RNA pseudoknot component of a coronavirus ribosomal frameshifting signal. *J Mol Biol* 1991;220:889–902.
28. Brodeur GM, Sandmeyer SB, Olson MV. Consistent association between sigma elements and tRNA genes. *Proc Natl Acad Sci U S A* 1983;80:3292–3296.
29. Brown JT, Bai X, Johnson AW. The yeast antiviral proteins Ski2p, Ski3p and Ski8p exist as a complex *in vivo*. *RNA* 2000;6:449–457.
30. Bruenn J, Keitz B. The 5′ ends of yeast killer factor RNAs are pppGp. *Nucleic Acids Res* 1976;3:2427–2436.
31. Buck KW. Fungal viruses, double-stranded RNA and interferon induction. In: Lemke PA, ed. *Viruses and Plasmids in Fungi*. New York: Marcel Dekker, 1979;1–42.
32. Buck KW. Replication of double-stranded RNA mycoviruses. In: Lemke PA, ed. *Viruses and Plasmids in Fungi*. New York: Marcel Dekker, 1979;93–160.
33. Cadd TL, Keenan MC, Patterson JL. Detection of *Leishmania* RNA virus 1 proteins. *J Virol* 1993;67:5647–5650.
34. Cappello J, Handelsman K, Lodish HF. Sequence of *Dictyostelium* DIRS-1: An apparent retrotransposon with inverted terminal repeats and an internal circle junction sequence. *Cell* 1985;43: 105–115.
35. Caston JR, Trus BL, Booy FP, et al. Structure of L-A virus: A specialized compartment for the transcription and replication of double-stranded RNA. *J Cell Biol* 1997;138:975–985.
36. Chalker DL, Sandmeyer SB. Ty3 integrates within the region of RNA polymerase II transcription initiation. *Genes Dev* 1992;6:117–128.
37. Chamorro M, Parkin N, Varmus HE. An RNA pseudoknot and an optimal heptameric shift site are required for highly efficient ribosomal frameshifting on a retroviral messenger RNA. *Proc Natl Acad Sci U S A* 1992;89:713–717.
38. Chapman KB, Boeke JD. Isolation and characterization of the gene encoding yeast debranching enzyme. *Cell* 1991;65:483–492.
39. Chapman KB, Bystrom AS, Boeke JD. Initiator methionine tRNA is essential for Ty1 transposition in yeast. *Proc Natl Acad Sci U S A* 1992;89:3236–3240.
40. Chen B, Gao S, Choi GH, Nuss DL. Extensive alteration of fungal gene transcript accumulation and elevatioin of G-protein-regulated cAMP levels by a virulence-attenuating hypovirus. *Proc Natl Acad Sci U S A* 1996;93:7996–8000.
41. Cheng RH, Caston JR, Wang G-J, et al. Fungal virus capsids are cytoplasmic compartments for the replication of double-stranded RNA formed as icosahedral shells of asymmetric Gag dimers. *J Mol Biol* 1994;244:255–258.
42. Chernoff YO, Derkach IL, Inge-Vechtomov SG. Multicopy SUP35 gene induces de-novo appearance of psi-like factors in the yeast *Saccharomyces cerevisiae*. *Curr Genet* 1993;24:268–270.
43. Chernoff YO, Lindquist SL, Ono B-I, et al. Role of the chaperone protein Hsp104 in propagation of the yeast prion-like factor [psi+]. *Science* 1995;268:880–884.
44. Chernoff YO, Ono B-I. Dosage-dependent modifiers of PSI-dependent omnipotent suppression in yeast. In: Brown AJP, Tuite MF, McCarthy JEG, eds. *Protein Synthesis and Targeting in Yeast*. Berlin: Springer-Verlag, 1992;101–107.
45. Choi GH, Chen B, Nuss DL. Virus-mediated or transgenic suppression of a G protein α subunit and attenuation of fungal virulence. *Proc Natl Acad Sci U S A* 1995;92:305–309.
46. Choi GH, Larson TG, Nuss DL. Molecular analysis of the laccase gene from the chestnut blight fungus and selective suppression of its expression in an isogenic hypovirulent strain. *Mol Plant Microbe Interact* 1992;5:119–128.
47. Choi GH, Nuss DL. Hypovirulence of chestnut blight fungus conferred by an infectious viral cDNA. *Science* 1992;257:800–803.
48. Choi GH, Nuss DL. A viral gene confers hypovirulence-associated traits to the chestnut blight fungus. *EMBO J* 1992;11:473–477.
49. Choi GH, Shapira R, Nuss DL. Cotranslational autoproteolysis involved in gene expression from a double-stranded RNA genetic element associated with hypovirulence of the chestnut blight fungus. *Proc Natl Acad Sci U S A* 1991;88:1167–1171.
50. Ciriacy M, Freidel K, Lohning C. Characterization of trans-acting mutations affecting Ty and Ty-mediated transcription in *Saccharomyces cerevisiae*. *Curr Genet* 1991;20:441–448.
51. Clare J, Farabaugh PJ. Nucleotide sequence of a yeast Ty element: Evidence for an unusual mechanism of gene expression. *Proc Natl Acad Sci U S A* 1985;82:2828–2833.
52. Clark DJ, Bilanchone VW, Haywood LJ, et al. A yeast sigma composite element, Ty3, has properties of a retrotransposon. *J Biol Chem* 1988;263:1413–1423.
53. Company M, Errede B. Identification of a Ty1 regulatory sequence responsive to STE7 and STE12. *Mol Cell Biol* 1988;8:2545–2554.
54. Conte D, Barber E, Garfinkel DJ, Curcio MJ. Post-translational regulation of Ty1 retrotransposition by mitogen-activated protein kinase Fus3. *Mol Cell Biol* 1998;18:2502–2513.
55. Cooper A, Bussey H. Characterization of the yeast KEX1 gene product: A carboxypeptidase involved in processing secreted precursor proteins. *Mol Cell Biol* 1989;9:2706–2714.
56. Courchesne WE, Magasanik B. Regulation of nitrogen assimilation in *Saccharomyces cerevisiae*: Roles of the URE2 and GLN3 genes. *J Bacteriol* 1988;170:708–713.
57. Coustou V, Deleu C, Saupe S, Begueret J. The protein product of the *het-s* heterokaryon incompatibility gene of the fungus *Podospora anserina* behaves as a prion analog. *Proc Natl Acad Sci U S A* 1997; 94:9773–9778.
58. Cox BS. PSI, a cytoplasmic suppressor of super-suppressor in yeast. *Heredity* 1965;20:505–521.
59. Cox BS, Tuite MF, McLaughlin CS. The PSI factor of yeast: A problem in inheritance. *Yeast* 1988;4:159–179.
60. Craven MG, Pawlyk DM, Choi GH, Nuss DL. Papain-like protease p29 as a symptom determinant encoded by a hypovirulence-associated virus of the chestnut blight fungus. *J Virol* 1993;67:6513–6521.
61. Cui Y, Dinman JD, Peltz SW. *Mof4-1* is an allele of the *UPF1/IFS2* gene which affects both mRNA turnover and −1 ribosomal frameshifting efficiency. *EMBO J* 1996;15:5726–5736.
62. Cui Y, Gonzalez CI, Kinzy TG, et al. Mutations in the *MOF2/SUI1* gene affect both translation and nonsense-mediated mRNA decay. *RNA* 1999;5:1–12.
63. Curcio MJ, Garfinkel DJ. Posttranslational control of Ty1 retrotransposition occurs at the level of protein processing. *Mol Cell Biol* 1992;12:2813–2825.
64. Curcio MJ, Sanders NJ, Garfinkel DJ. Transcriptional competence and transcription of endogenous Ty elements in *Saccharomyces cerevisiae*: Implications for regulation of transposition. *Mol Cell Biol* 1988;8: 3571–3581.
65. Day A, Rochaix JD. A transposon with an unusual LTR arrangement from *Chlamydomonas reinhardtii* contains an internal tandem array of 76 bp repeats. *Nucleic Acids Res* 1991;19:1259–1266.
66. Day PR, Dodds JA, Elliston JE, et al. Double-stranded RNA in *Endothia parasitica*. *Phytopathology* 1977;67:1393–1396.
67. De-Chao Y, Wang AL, Wang CC. Amplification, expression and packaging of a foreign gene by Giardiavirus in *Giardia lamblia*. *J Virol* 1996;70:8752–8757.
68. De-Chao Y, Wang CC. Identification of *cis*-acting signals in the giardiavirus (GLV) genome required for expression of firefly luciferase in *Giardia lamblia*. *RNA* 1996;2:824–834.
69. Deleu C, Clave C, Begueret J. A single amino acid difference is sufficient to elicit vegetative incompatibility in the fungus *Podospora anserina*. *Genetics* 1993;135:45–52.
70. Derkatch IL, Chernoff YO, Kushnirov VV, et al. Genesis and variability of [PSI] prion factors in *Saccharomyces cerevisiae*. *Genetics* 1996; 144:1375–1386.
71. Derr LK, Strathern JN, Garfinkel DJ. RNA-mediated recombination in *S. cerevisiae*. *Cell* 1991;67:355–364.
72. Dignard D, Whiteway M, Germain D, et al. Expression in yeast of a cDNA copy of the K2 killer toxin gene. *Mol Gen Genet* 1991;227: 127–136.
73. Dihanich M, Van Tuinen E, Lambris JD, Marshallsay B. Accumulation of viruslike particles in a yeast mutant lacking a mitochondrial pore protein. *Mol Cell Biol* 1989;9:1100–1108.
74. Dinman JD, Icho T, Wickner RB. A −1 ribosomal frameshift in a double-stranded RNA virus of yeast forms a gag-pol fusion protein. *Proc Natl Acad Sci U S A* 1991;88:174–178.
75. Dinman JD, Ruiz-Echevarria MJ, Czaplinski K, Peltz SW. Peptidyltransferase inhibitors have antiviral properties by altering programmed −1 ribosomal frameshifting efficiencies: Development of model systems. *Proc Natl Acad Sci U S A* 1997;94:6606–6611.
76. Dinman JD, Wickner RB. Ribosomal frameshifting efficiency and *gag/gag-pol* ratio are critical for yeast M_1 double-stranded RNA virus propagation. *J Virol* 1992;66:3669–3676.
77. Dinman JD, Wickner RB. Translational maintenance of frame:

Mutants of *Saccharomyces cerevisiae* with altered −1 ribosomal frameshifting efficiencies. *Genetics* 1994;136:75–86.
78. Dinman JD, Wickner RB. 5S rRNA is involved in fidelity of translational reading frame. *Genetics* 1995;141:95–105.
79. Dmochowska A, Dignard D, Henning D, et al. Yeast *KEX1* gene encodes a putative protease with a carboxypeptidase B–like function involved in killer toxin and alpha factor precursor processing. *Cell* 1987;50:573–584.
80. Dodds JA. Association of type 1 viral-like dsRNA with club-shaped particles in hypovirulent strains of *Endothia parasitica. Virology* 1980;107:1–12.
81. Doel SM, McCready SJ, Nierras CR, Cox BS. The dominant *PNM2−* mutation which eliminates the [PSI] factor of *Saccharomyces cerevisiae* is the result of a missense mutation in the *SUP35* gene. *Genetics* 1994;137:659–670.
82. Doolittle RF, Feng DF, Johnson MS, McClure MA. Origins and evolutionary relationships of retroviruses. *Q Rev Biol* 1989;64:1–30.
83. Edskes HK, Gray VT, Wickner RB. The [URE3] prion is an aggregated form of Ure2p that can be cured by overexpression of Ure2p fragments. *Proc Natl Acad Sci U S A* 1999;96:1498–1503.
84. Edskes HK, Hanover JA, Wickner RB. Mks1p is a regulator of nitrogen catabolism upstream of Ure2p in *Saccharomyces cerevisiae. Genetics* 1999;153:585–594.
85. Edskes HK, Ohtake Y, Wickner RB. Mak21p of *Saccharomyces cerevisiae*, a homolog of human CAATT-binding protein, is essential for 60S ribosomal subunit biogenesis. *J Biol Chem* 1998;273:28912–28920.
86. Eibel H, Philippsen P. Preferential integration of yeast transposable element Ty into a promoter region. *Nature* 1984;307:386–388.
87. Eichinger DJ, Boeke JD. The DNA intermediate in yeast Ty! element transposition copurifies with virus-like particles: Cell-free Ty1 transposition. *Cell* 1988;54:955–966.
88. Eichinger DJ, Boeke JD. A specific terminal structure is required for Ty1 transposition. *Genes Dev* 1990;4:324–330.
89. Elder RT, John TPS, Stinchcomb DT, Davis RW. Studies on the transposable element Ty1 of yeast. I. RNA homologous to Ty1. *Cold Spring Harb Symp Quant Biol* 1981;45:581–591.
90. Elder RT, Loh EY, Davis RW. RNA from the yeast transposable element Ty1 has both ends in the direct repeats, a structure similar to retrovirus RNA. *Proc Natl Acad Sci U S A* 1983;80:2432–2436.
91. Enebak SA, Hillman BI, MacDonald WL. A hypovirulent isolate of *Cryphonectria parasitica* with multiple, genetically unique dsRNA segments. *Molec Plant Microbe Interact* 1994;7:590–595.
92. Errede B. MCM1 binds to a transcriptional control element in Ty1. *Mol Cell Biol* 1993;13:57–62.
93. Errede B, Cardillo TS, Sherman F, et al. Mating signals control expression of mutations resulting from insertion of a transposable repetitive element adjacent to diverse yeast genes. *Cell* 1980;22: 427–436.
94. Errede B, Cardillo TS, Wever G, Sherman F. Studies on transposable elements in yeast. I. ROAM mutations causing increased expression of yeast genes: Their activation by signals directed toward conjugation functions and their formation by insertion of Ty1 repetitive elements. *Cold Spring Harbor Symp Quant Biol* 1981;45:593–602.
95. Esteban LM, Fujimura T, Garcia-Cuellar M, Esteban R. Association of yeast viral 23S RNA with its putative RNA-dependent RNA polymerase. *J Biol Chem* 1994;269:29771–29777.
96. Esteban LM, Rodriguez CN, Esteban R. T double-stranded RNA (dsRNA) sequence reveals that T and W dsRNAs form a new RNA family in *Saccharomyces cerevisiae*. Identification of 23 S RNA as the single-stranded form of T dsRNA. *J Biol Chem* 1992;267: 10874–10881.
97. Esteban R, Fujimura T, Wickner RB. Internal and terminal cis-acting sites are necessary for in vitro replication of the L-A double-stranded RNA virus of yeast. *EMBO J* 1989;8:947–954.
98. Esteban R, Wickner RB. Three different M_1 RNA-containing viruslike particle types in *Saccharomyces cerevisiae*: In vitro M_1 double-stranded RNA synthesis. *Mol Cell Biol* 1986;6:1552–1561.
99. Esteban R, Wickner RB. A deletion mutant of L-A double-stranded RNA replicates like M_1 double-stranded RNA. *J Virol* 1988;62:1278–1285.
100. Fahima T, Kazmierczak P, Hansen DR, et al. Membrane-associated replication of an unencapsidated double-stranded RNA of the fungus, *Cryphonectria parasitica. Virology* 1993;195:81–89.
101. Farabaugh PJ. Programmed translational frameshifting. *Microbiol Rev* 1996;60:103–134.
102. Farabaugh PJ, Fink GR. Insertion of the eukaryotic transposable element Ty1 creates a 5 base pair duplication. *Nature* 1980;286:352–356.
103. Farabaugh PJ, Liao XB, Belcourt M, et al. Enhancer and silencerlike sites within the transcribed portion of a Ty2 tranposable element of *Saccharomyces cerevisiae. Mol Cell Biol* 1989;9:4824–4834.
104. Farabaugh PJ, Vimaladithan A, Turkel S, et al. Three downstream sites repress transcription of a Ty2 retrotransposon in *Saccharomyces cerevisiae. Mol Cell Biol* 1993;13:2081–2090.
105. Farabaugh PJ, Zhao H, Vimaladithan A. A novel programmed frameshift expresses the POL3 gene of retrotranposon Ty3 of yeast: Frameshifting without tRNA slippage. *Cell* 1993;74:93–103.
106. Finkler A, Ben-Zvi BS, Koltin Y, Barash I. Transcription and in vitro translation of the dsRNA virus isolated from *Rhizoctonia solani. Virus Genes* 1988;1:205–219.
107. Fujimura T, Esteban R, Esteban LM, Wickner RB. Portable encapsidation signal of the L-A double-stranded RNA virus of *S. cerevisiae. Cell* 1990;62:819–828.
108. Fujimura T, Esteban R, Wickner RB. In vitro L-A double-stranded RNA synthesis in virus-like particles from *Saccharomyces cerevisiae. Proc Natl Acad Sci U S A* 1986;83:4433–4437.
109. Fujimura T, Ribas JC, Makhov AM, Wickner RB. Pol of gag-pol fusion protein required for encapsidation of viral RNA of yeast L-A virus. *Nature* 1992;359:746–749.
110. Fujimura T, Wickner RB. L-A double-stranded RNA viruslike particle replication cycle in *Saccharomyces cerevisiae*: Particle maturation in vitro and effects of mak10 and pet18 mutations. *Mol Cell Biol* 1987; 7:420–426.
111. Fujimura T, Wickner RB. Gene overlap results in a viral protein having an RNA binding domain and a major coat protein domain. *Cell* 1988;55:663–671.
112. Fujimura T, Wickner RB. Replicase of L-A virus-like particles of *Saccharomyces cerevisiae*. In vitro conversion of exogenous L-A and M_1 single-stranded RNAs to double-stranded form. *J Biol Chem* 1988; 263:454–460.
113. Fujimura T, Wickner RB. Reconstitution of template-dependent in vitro transcriptase activity of a yeast double-stranded RNA virus. *J Biol Chem* 1989;264:10872–10877.
114. Fujimura T, Wickner RB. Interaction of two *cis* sites with the RNA replicase of the yeast L-A virus. *J Biol Chem* 1992;267:2708–2713.
115. Fulbright DW. Effect of eliminating dsRNA in hypovirulent *Endothia parasitica. Phytopathology* 1984;74:722–724.
116. Furfine ES, Wang CC. Transfection of the *Giardia lamblia* double-stranded RNA virus into *Giardia lamblia* by electroporation of a single-stranded RNA copy of the viral genome. *Mol Cell Biol* 1990; 10:3659–3663.
117. Gabriel A, Yen TJ, Schwartz DC, et al. A rapidly rearranging retrotransposon within the miniexon gene locus of *Crithidia fasciculata. Mol Cell Biol* 1990;10:615–624.
118. Gao S, Nuss DL. Distinct roles for two G-protein α subunits in fungal virulence, morphology and reproduction revealed by targeted gene disruption. *Proc Natl Acad Sci U S A* 1996;93:14122–14127.
119. Garcia-Cuellar MP, Esteban LM, Fujimura T, et al. Yeast viral 20S RNA is associated with its cognate RNA-dependent RNA polymerase. *J Biol Chem* 1995;270:20084–20089.
120. Garcia-Cuellar MP, Esteban R, Fujimura T. RNA-dependent RNA polymerase activity associated with the yeast viral p91/20S RNA ribonucleoprotein complex. *RNA* 1997;3:27–36.
121. Garfinkel DJ, Hedge A-M, Youngren SD, Copeland TD. Proteolytic processing of *pol-TYB* proteins from the yeast retrotransposon Ty1. *J Virol* 1991;65:4573–4581.
122. Garnepudi VR, Zhao C, Beeler T, Dunn T. Serine palmitoyltransferase (*scs1/lcb2*) mutants have elevated copy number of the L-A dsRNA virus. *Yeast* 1997;13:299–304.
123. Garvik B, Haber JE. New cytoplasmic genetic element that controls 20S RNA synthesis during sporulation in yeast. *J Bacteriol* 1978; 134:261–269.
124. Georgopoulos DE, Hannig EM, Leibowitz MJ. Sequence of the M1-2 region of killer virus double-stranded RNA. *Basic Life Sci* 1986; 40:203–213.
125. Gesteland RF, Atkins JF. Recoding: Dynamic reprogramming of translation. *Ann Rev Biochem* 1996;65:741–768.
126. Ghabrial SA, Havens WM. The *Helminthosporium victoriae* 190S mycovirus has two forms distinguishable by capsid protein composition and phosphorylation state. *Virology* 1992;188:657–665.

127. Glover JR, Kowal AS, Shirmer EC, et al. Self-seeded fibers formed by Sup35, the protein determinant of [PSI+], a heritable prion-like factor of *S. cerevisiae*. *Cell* 1997;89:811–819.
128. Guilbride L, Myler PJ, Stuart K. Distribution and sequence divergence of LRV1 viruses among different *Leishmania* species. *Mol Biochem Parisitol* 1992;54:101–104.
129. Hannig EM, Leibowitz MJ. Structure and expression of the M2 genomic segment of a type 2 killer virus of yeast. *Nucleic Acids Res* 1985;13:4379–4400.
130. Hannig EM, Williams TL, Leibowitz MJ. The internal polyadenylate tract of yeast killer virus M_1 double-stranded RNA is variable in length. *Virology* 1986;152:149–158.
131. Hansen DR, Alfen NKV, Gillies K, Powell WA. Naked dsRNA association with hypovirulence in *Endothia parasitica* is packaged in fungal vesicles. *J Gen Virol* 1985;66:2605–2614.
132. Hansen LJ, Chalker DL, Sandmeyer SB. Ty3, a yeast retrotransposon associated with tRNA genes, has homology to animal retroviruses. *Mol Cell Biol* 1988;8:5245–5256.
133. Hatfield D, Levin JG, Rein A, Oroszlan S. Translational suppression in retroviral gene expression. *Adv Vir Res* 1992;41:193–239.
134. Herring AJ, Bevan EA. Yeast virus-like particles possess a capsid-associated single-stranded RNA polymerase. *Nature* 1977;268:464–466.
135. Hillman BI, Fulbright DW, Nuss DL, Alfen NKV. *Hypoviridae.* In: Murphy FA, Faquet CM, Bishop DHL, et al., eds. *Virus Taxonomy.* New York: Springer-Verlag, 1995:515–520.
136. Hinnebusch AG, Liebman SW. Protein synthesis and translational control in *Saccharomyces cerevisiae*. In: Broach JR, Pringle JR, Jones EW, eds. *The Molecular and Cellular Biology of the Yeast Saccharomyces: Genome Dynamics, Protein Synthesis and Energetics,* vol. 1. Cold Spring Harbor, NY: Cold Spring Harbor Press, 1991;627–735.
137. Hsu CL, Stevens A. Yeast cells lacking $5'\rightarrow3'$ exoribonuclease 1 contain mRNA species that are poly(A) deficient and partially lack the $5'$ cap structure. *Mol Cell Biol* 1993;13:4826–4835.
138. Huang H, Hong JY, Burck CL, Liebman SW. Host genes that affect the target-site distribution of the yeast retrotransposon Ty1. *Genetics* 1999;151:1393–1407.
139. Huang S, Ghabrial SA. Organization and expression of the double-stranded RNA genome of *Helminthosporium victoriae* 190S virus, a totivirus infecting a plant pathogenic filamentous fungus. *Proc Natl Acad Sci U S A* 1996;93:12541–12546.
140. Icho T, Wickner RB. The double-stranded RNA genome of yeast virus L-A encodes its own putative RNA polymerase by fusing two open reading frames. *J Biol Chem* 1989;264:6716–6723.
141. Ishikawa M, Diez J, Restrepo-Hartwig M, Ahlquist P. Yeast mutations in multiple complementation groups inhibit brome mosaic virus RNA replication and transcription and perturb regulated expression of the viral polymerase-like gene. *Proc Natl Acad Sci U S A* 1997;94: 13810–13815.
142. Jacks T, Madhani HD, Masiarz FR, Varmus HE. Signals for ribosomal frameshifting in the Rous sarcoma virus gag-pol region. *Cell* 1988; 55:447–458.
143. Janetzky B, Lehle L. Ty4, a new retrotransposon from *Saccharomyces cerevisiae,* flanked by tau-elements. *J Biol Chem* 1992;267: 19798–19805.
144. Ji H, Moore DP, Blomberg MA, et al. Hotspots for unselected Ty1 transposition events on yeast chromosome III are near tRNA genes and LTR sequences. *Cell* 1993;73:1007–1018.
145. Julius D, Brake A, Blair L, et al. Isolation of the putative structural gene for the lysine-arginine–cleaving endopeptidase required for the processing of yeast prepro-alpha factor. *Cell* 1984;36:309–318.
146. Kadowaki K, Halvorson HO. Appearance of a new species of ribonucleic acid during sporulation in *Saccharomyces cerevisiae*. *J Bacteriol* 1971;105:826–830.
147. Kamer G, Argos P. Primary structural comparison of RNA-dependent polymerase from plant, animal and bacterial viruses. *Nucleic Acids Res* 1984;12:7269–7282.
148. Kang XL, Yadao F, Gietz RD, Kunz BA. Elimination of the yeast RAD6 ubiquitin conjugase enhances base-pair transitions and G.C–T.A transversions as well as transposition of the Ty element: Implications for the control of spontaneous mutation. *Genetics* 1992;130:285–294.
149. Kawakami K, Pande S, Faiola B, et al. A rare tRNA-Arg(CCU) that regulates Ty1 element ribosomal frameshifting is essential for Ty1 retrotransposition in *Saccharomyces cerevisiae*. *Genetics* 1993;135: 309–320.
150. Ke N, Irwin PA, Voytas DF. The pheromone response pathway activates transcription of Ty5 retrotransposons located within silent chromatin. *EMBO J* 1997;16:6272–6280.
151. Kennell JC, Moran JV, Perlman PS, et al. Reverse transcriptase activity associated with maturase-encoding group II introns in yeast mitochondria. *Cell* 1993;73:133–146.
152. Khoshnan A, Alderete JF. Multiple double-stranded RNA segments are associated with virus particles infecting *Trichomonas vaginalis. J Virol* 1993;67:6950–6955.
153. Khoshnan A, Alderete JF. *Trichomonas vaginalis* with a double-stranded RNA virus has upregulated levels of phenotypically variable immunogen mRNA. *J Virol* 1994;68:4035–4038.
154. Kim JM, Vanguri S, Boeke JD, et al. Transposable elements and genome organization: A comprehensive survey of retrotransposons revealed by the complete *Saccharomyces cerevisiae* genome sequence. *Genome Res* 1998;8:464–478.
155. King C-Y, Tittmann P, Gross H, et al. Prion-inducing domain 2-114 of yeast Sup35 protein transforms in vitro into amyloid-like filaments. *Proc Natl Acad Sci U S A* 1997;94:6618–6622.
156. Kinsey JA. Tad, a LINE-like transposable element of Neurospora, can transposse between nuclei in heterokaryons. *Genetics* 1990;126: 317–323.
157. Kinsey JA. Transnuclear retrotransposition of the Tad element of *Neurospora. Proc Natl Acad Sci U S A* 1993;90:9384–9387.
158. Kinsey PT, Sandmeyer SB. Ty3 transposes in mating populations of yeast. *Genetics* 1995;139:81–94.
159. Kohno S, Fujimura T, Rulong S, Kwon-Chung KJ. Double-stranded RNA virus in the human pathogenic fungus *Blastomyces dermatitidis. J Virol* 1994;68:7554–7558.
160. Koltin Y. The killer system of *Ustilago maydis*: Secreted polypeptides encoded by viruses. In: Koltin Y, Leibowitz MJ, eds. *Viruses of Fungi and Simple Eukaryotes.* New York: Marcel Dekker, 1988:209–242.
161. Koonin EV. Evolution of double-stranded RNA viruses: A case of polyphyletic origin from different groups of positive-stranded RNA viruses. *Semin Virol* 1992;3:327–339.
162. Koonin EV, Choi GH, Nuss DL, et al. Evidence for common ancestry of a chestnut blight hypovirulence-associated double-stranded RNA and a group of positive-strand RNA plant viruses. *Proc Natl Acad Sci U S A* 1991;88:10647–10651.
163. Lacroute F. Non-Mendelian mutation allowing ureidosuccinic acid uptake in yeast. *J Bacteriol* 1971;106:519–522.
164. Lakshman DK, Jian J, Tavantzis SM. A double-stranded RNA element from a hypovirulent strain of *Rhizoctonia solani* occurs in DNA form and is genetically related to the pentafunctional AROM protein of the shikimate pathway. *Proc Natl Acad Sci U S A* 1998;95:6425–6429.
165. Larson TG, Choi GH, Nuss DL. Regulatory pathways governing modulation of fungal gene expression by a virulence-attenuating mycovirus. *EMBO J* 1992;11:4539–4548.
166. Lauermann V, Boeke JD. Plus strand strong-stop DNA transfer in yeast Ty retrotransposons. *EMBO J* 1997;16:6603–6612.
167. Lee B-S, Lichtenstein CP, Faiola B, et al. Posttranslational inhibition of Ty1 retrotransposition by nucleotide excision repair/transcription factor TFIIH subunits Ssl2p and Rad3p. *Genetics* 1998;148:1743–1761.
168. Lee S-G, Lee I, Kang C, Song K. Identification and characterization of a human cDNA homologous to yeast SKI2. *Genomics* 1994;25: 660–666.
169. Lee Y-J, Wickner RB. MAK10, a glucose-repressible gene necessary for replication of a dsRNA virus of *Saccharomyces cerevisiae*, has T cell receptor α-subunit motifs. *Genetics* 1992;132:87–96.
170. Leibowitz MJ, Wickner RB. A chromosomal gene required for killer plasmid expression, mating, and spore maturation in *Saccharomyces cerevisiae*. *Proc Natl Acad Sci U S A* 1976;73:2061–2065.
171. Levin HL. A novel mechanism of self-primed reverse transcription defines a new family of retroelements. *Mol Cell Biol* 1995;15: 3310–3317.
172. Levin HL, Boeke JD. Demonstration of retrotransposition of the Tf1 element in fission yeast. *EMBO J* 1992;11:1145–1153.
173. Levin HL, Weaver DC, Boeke JD. Novel gene expression mechanism in a fission yeast retroelement: Tf1 proteins are derived from a single primary translation product. *EMBO J* 1993;12:4885–4895.
174. Liao XB, Clare JJ, Farabaugh PJ. The upstream activation site of a Ty2 element of yeast is necessary but not sufficient to promote maximal transcription of the element. *Proc Natl Acad Sci U S A* 1987;84: 8520–8524.

175. Liebman SW, Newman G. A ubiquitin-conjugating enzyme, RAD6, affects the distribution of Ty1 retrotransposon integration positions. *Genetics* 1993;133:499–508.
176. Lin J-H, Levin HL. A complex structure in the mRNA of Tf1 is recognized and cleaved to generate the primer of reverse transcription. *Genes Dev* 1997;11:270–285.
177. Liu Y, Dieckmann CL. Overproduction of yeast virus–like particle coat protein genome in strains deficient in a mitochondrial nuclease. *Mol Cell Biol* 1989;9:3323–3331.
178. Lolle S, Skipper N, Bussey H, Thomas DY. The expression of cDNA clones of yeast M_1 double-stranded RNA in yeast confers both killer and immunity pheonotypes. *EMBO J* 1984;3:1283–1387.
179. Lund PM, Cox BS. Reversion analysis of [psi–] mutations in *Saccharomyces cerevisiae*. *Genet Res* 1981;37:173–182.
180. MacBeth KJ, Patterson JL. Single-site cleavage in the 5′ untranslated region of Leishmaniavirus RNA is mediated by the viral capsid protein. *Proc Natl Acad Sci U S A* 1995;92:8994–8998.
181. Maddelein M-L, Wickner RB. Two prion-inducing regions of Ure2p are non-overlapping. *Mol Cell Biol* 1999;19:4516–4524.
182. Makower M, Bevan EA. The inheritance of a killer character in yeast (*Saccharomyces cerevisiae*). *Proc Int Congr Genet* 1963;11:202.
183. Marschalek R, Hofmann J, Schumann G, et al. Structure of DRE, a retrotransposable element which integrates with position speicificity upstream of *Dictyostelium discoideum* tRNA genes. *Mol Cell Biol* 1992;12:229–239.
184. Martegani E, Vanoiu M, Mauri 1, et al. Identification of gene encoding a putative RNA-helicase, homologous to SKI2, in chromosome VII of Saccharomyces cerevisae. *Yeast* 1997;13:391–397.
185. Masison DC, Blanc A, Ribas JC, et al. Decoying the cap-mRNA degradation system by a dsRNA virus and poly(A)-mRNA surveillance by a yeast antiviral system. *Mol Cell Biol* 1995;15:2763–2771.
186. Masison DC, Maddelein M-L, Wickner RB. The prion model for [URE3] of yeast: Spontaneous generation and requirements for propagation. *Proc Natl Acad Sci U S A* 1997;94:12503–12508.
187. Masison DC, Wickner RB. Prion-inducing domain of yeast Ure2p and protease resistance of Ure2p in prion-containing cells. *Science* 1995; 270:93–95.
188. Matsumoto Y, Fishel R, Wickner RB. Circular single-stranded RNA replicon in *Saccharomyces cerevisiae*. *Proc Natl Acad Sci U S A* 1990;87:7628–7632.
189. Matsumoto Y, Sarkar G, Sommer SS, Wickner RB. A yeast antiviral protein, SKI8, shares a repeated amino acid sequence pattern with beta-subunits of G proteins and several other proteins. *Yeast* 1993;8:43–51.
190. Matsumoto Y, Wickner RB. Yeast 20 S RNA replicon. Replication intermediates and encoded putative RNA polymerase. *J Biol Chem* 1991;266:12779–12783.
191. Matthews GD, Goodwin TJD, Butler MI, et al. pCal, a highly unusual Ty1/*copia* retrotransposon from the pathogenic yeast *Candida albicans*. *J Bacteriol* 1997;179:7118–7128.
192. McHale MT, Roberts IN, Noble SM, et al. CfT-1: An LTR-retrotransposon in *Cladosporium fulvum*, a fungal pathogen of tomato. *Mol Gen Genet* 1992;233:337–347.
193. Mellor M, Fulton AM, Dobson MJ, et al. A retrovirus-like strategy for the expression of a fusion protein encoded by yeast transposon Ty1. *Nature* 1985;313:243–246.
194. Miller RL, Wang AL, Wang CC. Purification and characterization of the *Giardia lamblia* double-stranded RNA virus. *Mol Biochem Parasitol* 1988;28:189–196.
195. Mitchell AP, Magasanik B. Regulation of glutamine-repressible gene products by the GLN3 function in *Saccharomyces cerevisiae*. *Mol Cell Biol* 1984;4:2758–2766.
196. Mitchell P, Petfalski E, Shevchenko A, et al. The exosome, a conserved eukaryotic RNA processing complex containing multiple 3′→5′ exoribonucleases. *Cell* 1997;91:457–466.
197. Moehring JM, Inocencio NM, Robertson BJ, Moehring TJ. Expression of mouse furin in a Chinese hamster cell resistant to *Pseudomonas* exotoxin A and viruses complements the genetic lesion. *J Biol Chem* 1993;268:2590–2594.
198. Moore SP, Garfinkel DJ. Expression and partial purification of enzymatically active recombinant Ty1 integrase in *Saccharomyces cerevisiae*. *Proc Natl Acad Sci U S A* 1994;91:1843–1847.
199. Mueller MW, Allmaier M, Eskes R, Schweyen RJ. Transposition of group II intron aI1 in yeast and invasion of mitochondrial genes at new locations. *Nature* 1993;366:174–176.
200. Munroe D, Jacobson A. Tales of poly(A): A review. *Gene* 1990;91: 151–158.
201. Natsoulis G, Thomas W, Roghmann MC, et al. Ty1 tranposition in *Saccharomyces cerevisiae* is nonrandom. *Genetics* 1989;123:269–279.
202. Natsuaki T, Natsuaki KT, Okuda S, et al. Relationships between the cryptic and temperate viruses of alfalfa, beet and white clover. *Intervirology* 1986;25:69–75.
203. Nelson M, Zhang Y, Van Etten JL. DNA methyltransferases and DNA site-specific endonucleases encoded by *Chlorella* viruses. In: Jost JP, Saluz HP, eds. *DNA Methylation: Molecular Biology and Biological Significance.* Basel: Birkhauser Verlag, 1993:186–211.
204. Newman AM, Elliot SG, McLaughlin CS, et al. Replication of double-stranded RNA of the virus-like particles of *Saccharomyces cerevisiae*. *J Virol* 1981;38:263–271.
205. Nomura N, Miyajima N, Sazuka T, et al. Prediction of the coding sequences of unidentified genes. II. The coding sequences of 40 new genes (KIAA 0041-KIAH 0080) deduced by analysis of randomly sampled cDNA clones from human immature mycloid cell line KG1. *DNA Res* 1994;1:27–35.
206. Nuss DL. Biological control of chestnut blight: An example of virus-mediated attenuation of fungal pathogenesis. *Microbiol Rev* 1992;56: 561–576.
207. Oh C-S, Hillman BI. Genome organization of a partitivirus from the filamentous ascomycete *Atkinsonella hypoxylon*. *J Gen Virol* 1995;76: 1461–1470.
208. Ohtake Y, Wickner RB. Yeast virus propagation depends critically on free 60S ribosomal subunit concentration. *Mol Cell Biol* 1995;15: 2772–2781.
209. Parsell DA, Kowal AS, Singer MA, Lindquist S. Protein disaggregation mediated by heat-shock protein Hsp104. *Nature* 1994;372:475–478.
210. Patino MM, Liu J-J, Glover JR, Lindquist S. Support for the prion hypothesis for inheritance of a phenotypic trait in yeast. *Science* 1996; 273:622–626.
211. Paul CP, Fulbright DW. Double-stranded RNA molecules from Michigan hypovirulent isolates of *Endothia parasitica* vary in size and sequence homology. *Phytopathology* 1988;78:751–755.
212. Paushkin SV, Kushnirov VV, Smirnov VN, Ter-Avanesyan MD. Propagation of the yeast prion-like [*psi*+] determinant is mediated by oligomerization of the *SUP35*-encoded polypeptide chain release factor. *EMBO J* 1996;15:3127–3134.
213. Paushkin SV, Kushnirov VV, Smirnov VN, Ter-Avanesyan MD. *In vitro* propagation of the prion-like state of yeast Sup35 protein. *Science* 1997;277:381–383.
214. Picologlou S, Brown N, Leibman SW. Mutations in *RAD6*, a yeast gene encoding a ubiquitin-conjugating enzyme, stimulate retrotransposition. *Mol Cell Biol* 1990;10:1017–1022.
215. Polashock JJ, Bedker PJ, Hillman BI. Movement of a small mitochondrial double-stranded RNA element of *Cryphonectria parasitica*: Ascospore inheritance and implications for mitochondrial recombination. *Mol Gen Genet* 1997;256:566–571.
216. Polashock JJ, Hillman BI. A small mitochondrial double-stranded (ds) RNA element associated with a hypovirulent strain of the chestnut blight fungus and ancestrally related to yeast cytoplasmic T and W dsRNAs. *Proc Natl Acad Sci U S A* 1994;91:8680–8684.
217. Preisig O, Wingfield BD, Wingfield MJ. Coinfection of a fungal pathogen by two distinct double-stranded RNA viruses. *Virology* 1998;252:399–406.
218. Price BD, Rueckert RR, Ahlquist P. Complete replication of an animal virus and maintenance of expressioin vectors derived from it in *Saccharomyces cerevisiae*. *Proc Natl Acad Sci U S A* 1996;93: 9465–9470.
219. Qian Z, Huang H, Hong JY, et al. Yeast Ty1 retrotransposition is stimulated by a synergistic interaction between mutations in chromatin assembly factor I and histone regulatory proteins. *Mol Cell Biol* 1998;18:4783–4792.
220. Radler F, Herzberger S, Schonig I, Schwarz P. Investigation of a killer strain of *Zygosaccharomyces bailii*. *J Gen Microbiol* 1993;139:495–500.
221. Rai R, Genbauffe F, Lea HZ, Cooper TG. Transcriptional regulation of the DAL5 gene in *Saccharomyces cerevisiae*. *J Bacteriol* 1987;169: 3521–3524.
222. Rhee SK, Icho T, Wickner RB. Structure and nuclear localization signal of the SKI3 antiviral protein of *Saccharomyces cerevisiae*. *Yeast* 1989;5:149–158.
223. Ribas JC, Fujimura T, Wickner RB. A cryptic RNA–binding domain

in the Pol region of the L-A dsRNA virus Gag-Pol fusion protein. *J Virol* 1994;68:6014–6020.

224. Ribas JC, Fujimura T, Wickner RB. Essential RNA binding and packaging domains of the Gag-Pol fusion protein of the L-A double-stranded RNA virus of *Saccharomyces cerevisiae*. *J Biol Chem* 1994; 269:28420–28428.
225. Ribas JC, Wickner RB. RNA-dependent RNA polymerase consensus sequence of the L-A double-stranded RNA virus: Definition of essential domains. *Proc Natl Acad Sci U S A* 1992;89:2185–2189.
226. Ridley SP, Sommer SS, Wickner RB. Superkiller mutations in *Saccharomyces cerevisiae* suppress exclusion of M_2 double-stranded RNA by L-A-HN and confer cold sensitivity in the presence of M and L-A-HN. *Mol Cell Biol* 1984;4:761–770.
227. Rigaut G, Shevchenko A, Rutz B, et al. A generic protein purification method for protein complex characterization and proteome exploration. *Nat Biotech* 1999;17:1030–1032.
228. Rigling D, Alfen NKV. Regulation of laccase biosynthesis in the plant pathogenic fungus *Cryphonectria parasitica* by double-stranded RNA. *J Bacteriol* 1991;173:8000–8003.
229. Rizet G. Les phenomenes de barrage chez *Podospora anserina*: Analyse genetique des barrages entre les souches s et S. *Rev Cytol Biol Veg* 1952;13:51–92.
230. Rodriguez CN, Esteban LM, Esteban R. Molecular cloning and characterization of W double-stranded RNA, a linear molecule present in *Saccharomyces cerevisiae*. Identification of its single-stranded RNA form as 20 S RNA. *J Biol Chem* 1991;266:12772–12778.
231. Rodriguez-Cousino N, Esteban R. Both yeast W double-stranded RNA and its single-stranded form 20S RNA are linear. *Nucleic Acids Res* 1992;20:2761–2766.
232. Rodriguez-Cousino N, Solorzano A, Fujimura T, Esteban R. Yeast positive-strand virus-like RNA replicons. 20S and 23S RNA terminal nucleotide sequences and 3′ end secondary structures resemble those of RNA coliphages. *J Biol Chem* 1998;273:20363–20371.
233. Rothnie HM, McCurrach KJ, Glover LA, Hardman N. Retrotransposon-like nature of Tp1 elements: Implications for the organization of highly repetitive, hypermethylated DNA in the genome of *Physarum polycephalum*. *Nucleic Acids Res* 1991;19:279–286.
234. Russell PJ, Bennett AM, Love Z, Baggott DM. Cloning, sequencing and expression of a full-length cDNA copy of the M_1 double-stranded RNA virus from the yeast, *Saccharomyces cerevisiae*. *Yeast* 1997;13: 829–836.
235. Scheffter S, Widmer G, Patterson JL. Complete sequence of Leishmania RNA virus 1-4 and identification of conserved sequences. *Virology* 1994;199:479–483.
236. Schmitt MJ. Cloning and expression of a cDNA copy of the viral K28 killer toxin gene in yeast. *Mol Gen Genet* 1995;246:236–246.
237. Schmitt MJ, Tipper DJ. Genetic analysis of maintenance and expression of L and M double-stranded RNAs from yeast killer virus K28. *Yeast* 1992;8:373–384.
238. Searfoss AM, Wickner RB. 3′ poly(A) is dispensable for translation. *Proc Natl Acad Sci USA* 2000;97:9133–9137.
239. Sepp T, Entzeroth R, Mertsching J, et al. Novel ribonucleic acid species in *Eimeria nieschilzi* are associated with RNA-dependent RNA polymerase activity. *Parasitol Res* 1991;77:581–584.
240. Shapira R, Choi GH, Nuss DL. Virus-like genetic organization and expression strategy for a double-stranded RNA genetic element assocaited with biological control of chestnut blight. *EMBO J* 1991;10: 731–739.
241. Shapira R, Nuss DL. Gene expression by a hypovirulence-associated virus of the chestnut blight fungus involves two papain-like protease activities. *J Biol Chem* 1991;266:19419–19425.
242. Shen Y, Bruenn JA. RNA structural requirements for RNA binding, replication, and packaging in the yeast double-stranded RNA virus. *Virology* 1993;195:481–491.
243. Singh AC, Helms C, Sherman F. Mutation of the non-Mendelian suppressor [PSI] in yeast by hypertonic media. *Proc Natl Acad Sci U S A* 1979;76:1952–1956.
244. Sommer SS, Wickner RB. Yeast L dsRNA consists of at least three distinct RNAs: Evidence that the non-Mendelian genes [HOK], [NEX] and [EXL] are on one of these dsRNAs. *Cell* 1982;31:429–441.
245. Sommer SS, Wickner RB. Gene disruption indicates that the only essential function of the SKI8 chromosomal gene is to protect *Saccharomyces cerevisiae* from viral cytopathology. *Virology* 1987;157: 252–256.
246. Steiner DF, Smeekens SP, Ohagi S, Chan SJ. The new enzymology of precursor processing endoproteases. *J Biol Chem* 1992;267: 23435–23438.
247. Strasser P, Zhang Y, Rohozinski J, Van Etten JL. The termini of the *Chlorella* virus PBCV-1 genome are identical 2.2 kbp inverted repeats. *Virology* 1991;180:763–769.
248. Stuart KD, Weeks R, Guilbride L, Myler PJ. Molecular organization of *Leishmania* RNA virus 1. *Proc Natl Acad Sci U S A* 1992;89: 8596–8600.
249. Stucka R, Lochmuller H, Feldmann H. Ty4, a novel low-copy number element in *Saccharomyces cerevisiae*: One copy is located in a cluster of Ty elements and tRNA genes. *Nucleic Acids Res* 1989;17:4993–5001.
250. Su HM, Tai JH. Genomic organization and sequence conservation in type I *Trichomonas vaginalis* viruses. *Virology* 1996;222:470–473.
251. Suzuki N, Chen B, Nuss DL. Mapping of a hypovirus p29 protease symptom determinant domain with sequence similarity to potyvirus HC-Pro protease. *J Virol* 1999;73:9478–9484.
252. Tarr PI, Aline RF, Smiley BL, Scholler J, Keithly J, Stuart K. LR1: A candidate RNA virus of *Leishmania*. *Proc Natl Acad Sci U S A* 1988;85:9572–9575.
253. Taylor KL, Cheng N, Williams RW, et al. Prion domain initiation of amyloid formation *in vitro* from native Ure2p. *Science* 1999;283:1339–1343.
254. TerAvanesyan A, Dagkesamanskaya AR, Kushnirov VV, Smirnov VN. The SUP35 omnipotent suppressor gene is involved in the maintenance of the non-Mendelian determinant [psi+] in the yeast *Saccharomyces cerevisiae*. *Genetics* 1994;137:671–676.
255. Tercero JC, Dinman JD, Wickner RB. Yeast MAK3 *N*-acetyltransferase recognizes the N-terminal four amino acids of the major coat protein (gag) of the L-A double-stranded RNA virus. *J Bacteriol* 1993;175:3192–3194.
256. Tercero JC, Riles LE, Wickner RB. Localized mutagenesis and evidence for post-transcriptional regulation of MAK3, a putative *N*-acetyltransferase required for dsRNA virus propagation in *Saccharomyces cerevisiae*. *J Biol Chem* 1992;267:20270–20276.
257. Tercero JC, Wickner RB. *MAK3* encodes an *N*-acetyltransferase whose modification of the L-A gag N-terminus is necessary for virus particle assembly. *J Biol Chem* 1992;267:20277–20281.
258. Thiele DJ, Hannig EM, Leibowitz MJ. Multiple L double-stranded RNA species of *Saccharomyces cerevisiae*: Evidence for separate encapsidation. *Mol Cell Biol* 1984;4:92–100.
259. Toh-e A, Guerry P, Wickner RB. Chromosomal superkiller mutants of *Saccharomyces cerevisiae*. *J Bacteriol* 1978;136:1002–1007.
260. Toh-e A, Sahashi Y. The *PET18* locus of *Saccharomyces cerevisiae*: A complex locus containing multiple genes. *Yeast* 1985;1:159–172.
261. Toh-e A, Wickner RB. "Superkiller" mutations suppress chromosomal mutations affecting double-stranded RNA killer plasmid replication in *Saccharomyces cerevisiae*. *Proc Natl Acad Sci U S A* 1980;77:527–530.
262. Tuite MF, Mundy CR, Cox BS. Agents that cause a high frequency of genetic change from [*psi+*] to [*psi-*] in *Saccharomyces cerevisiae*. *Genetics* 1981;98:691–711.
263. Turcq B, Deleu C, Denayrolles M, Begueret J. Two allelic genes responsible for vegetative incompatibility in the fungus *Podospora anserina* are not essential for cell viability. *Mol Gen Genet* 1991; 288:265–269.
264. Turkel S, Farabaugh PJ. Interspersion of an unusual GCN4 activation site with a complex transcriptional repression site in Ty2 elements of *Saccharomyces cerevisiae*. *Mol Cell Biol* 1993;13:2091–2103.
265. Van Arsdell SW, Stetler GL, Thorner J. The yeast repeated element sigma contains a hormone-inducible promoter. *Mol Cell Biol* 1987; 7:749–759.
266. Van Etten JL, Lane LC, Meints RH. Viruses and viruslike particles of eukaryotic algai. *Microbiol Rev* 1991;55:586–620.
267. Van Etten JL, Meints RH. Giant viruses infecting algae. *Ann Rev Microbiol* 1999;53:447–494.
268. Vimaladithan A, Farabaugh PJ. Special peptidyl-tRNA molecules can promote translational frameshifting without slippage. *Mol Cell Biol* 1994;14:8107–8116.
269. Voytas DF, Boeke JD. Yeast retrotransposon revealed. *Nature* 1992; 358:717.
270. Wang A, Wang CC, Alderete JF. *Trichomonas vaginalis* phenotypic variation occurs only among trichomonads infected with the double-stranded RNA virus. *J Exp Med* 1987;166:142–150.
271. Wang AL, Wang CC. Discovery of a specific double-stranded RNA virus in *Giardia lamblia*. *Mol Biochem Parasitol* 1986;21:269–276.

272. Wang AL, Wang CC. The double-stranded RNA in *Trichomonas vaginalis* may originate from virus-like particles. *Proc Natl Acad Sci U S A* 1986;83:7956–7960.
273. Wang AL, Yang H-M, Shen KA, Wang CC. Giardiavirus double-stranded RNA genome encodes a capsid polypeptide and a gag-pol-like fusion protein by a translational frameshift. *Proc Natl Acad Sci U S A* 1993;90:8595–8589.
274. Wang I-N, Li Y, Que Q, et al. Evidence for virus-encoded glycosylation specificity. *Proc Natl Acad Sci U S A* 1993;90:3840–3844.
275. Warmington JR, Waring RB, Newlon CS, et al. Nucleotide sequence characterization of Ty1-17, a class II transposon from yeast. *Nucleic Acids Res* 1985;13:6679–6693.
276. Weeks R, Aline RF, Myler PJ, Stuart K. LRV1 viral particles in *Leishmania guyanensis* contain double-stranded or single-stranded RNA. *J Virol* 1992;66:1389–1393.
277. Wesolowski M, Wickner RB. Two new double-stranded RNA molecules showing non-mendelian inheritance and heat inducibility in *Saccharomyces cerevisiae. Mol Cell Biol* 1984;4:181–187.
278. Wickner RB. Plasmids controlling exclusion of the K_2 killer double-stranded RNA plasmid of yeast. *Cell* 1980;21:217–226.
279. Wickner RB. Killer systems in *Saccharomyces cerevisiae*: Three distinct modes of exclusion of M2 double-stranded RNA by three species of double-stranded RNA, M1, L-A-E, and L-A-HN. *Mol Cell Biol* 1983;3:654–661.
280. Wickner RB. Yeast RNA virology: The killer systems. In: Broach JR, Pringle JR, Jones EW, eds. *The Molecular and Cellular Biology of the Yeast Saccharomyces: Genome Dynamics, Protein Synthesis, and Energetics.* Plainview, NY: Cold Spring Harbor Laboratory Press, 1991;263–296.
281. Wickner RB. Evidence for a prion analog in *S. cerevisiae*: The [URE3] non-Mendelian genetic element as an altered URE2 protein. *Science* 1994;264:566–569.
282. Wickner RB, Leibowitz MJ. Two chromosomal genes required for killing expression in killer strains of *Saccharomyces cerevisiae. Genetics* 1976;82:429–442.
283. Widmer G, Comeau AM, Furlong DB, et al. Characterization of a RNA virus from the parasite *Leishmania. Proc Natl Acad Sci U S A* 1989;86:5979–5982.
284. Widner WR, Matsumoto Y, Wickner RB. Is 20S RNA naked? *Mol Cell Biol* 1991;11:2905–2908.
285. Widner WR, Wickner RB. Evidence that the *SKI* antiviral system of *Saccharomyces cerevisiae* acts by blocking expression of viral mRNA. *Mol Cell Biol* 1993;13:4331–4341.
286. Williams TL, Leibowitz MJ. Conservative mechanism of the in vitro transcription of killer virus of yeast. *Virology* 1987;158:231–234.
287. Williamson VM, Cox D, Young ET, et al. Characterization of transposable element-associated mutations that alter yeast alcohol dehydrogenase II expression. *Mol Cell Biol* 1983;3:20–31.
288. Winston F. Analysis of *SPT* genes: A genetic approach toward analysis of TFIID, histones, and other transcription factors of yeast. In: McKnight SL, Yamamoto KR, eds. *Transcription Regulation*, vol. 2. Cold Spring Harbor, NY: Cold Spring Harbor Laboratory Press, 1992;1271–1293.
289. Winston F, Chaleff DT, Valent B, Fink GR. Mutations affecting Ty-mediated expression of the HIS4 gene in *Saccharomyces cerevisiae. Genetics* 1984;107:179–197.
290. Xiong Y, Eickbush TH. Origin and evolution of retroelements based upon their reverse transcriptase sequences. *EMBO J* 1990;9:3353–3362.
291. Xu H, Boeke JD. Host genes that influence transposition in yeast: The abundance of a rare tRNA regulates Ty1 transposition frequency. *Proc Natl Acad Sci U S A* 1990;87:8360–8364.
292. Xu H, Boeke JD. Localization of sequences required in *cis* for yeast Ty1 element transposition near the long terminal repeats: Analysis of mini-Ty elemnets. *Mol Cell Biol* 1990;10:2695–2702.
293. Xu H, Boeke JD. Inhibition of Ty1 transposition by mating pheromones in *Saccharomyces cerevisiae. Mol Cell Biol* 1991;11:2736–2743.
294. Zhang L, Churchill ACL, Kazmierczak P, et al. Hypovirulence-associated traits induced by a mycovirus of *Cryphonectria parasitica* are mimicked by targeted inactivation of a host gene. *Mol Cell Biol* 1993;13:7782–7792.
295. Zhang L, Villalon D, Sun Y, et al. Virus-associated down-regulation of the gene encoding cryparin, an abundant cell-surface protein from the chestnut blight fungus, *Cryphonectria parasitica. Gene* 1994;139:59–64.
296. Zou S, Voytas DF. Silent chromatin determines target preference of the *Saccharomyces* retrotransposon Ty5. *Proc Natl Acad Sci U S A* 1997; 94:7412–7416.

CHAPTER 17

Bacteriophages

Allan M. Campbell

HISTORY

Bacterial viruses (generally called bacteriophages or simply phages) were discovered independently by Twort and d'Herelle as filtrable, transmissible agents of bacterial lysis (21,68). Although their relevance to animal and plant viruses was not universally accepted, phages proved so tractable to experimentation that information about their nature was soon forthcoming. For example, their ability to form isolated plaques on bacterial lawns was noted, and d'Herelle correctly attributed the linearity of plaque assays to the self-replicating nature of the phage particles (as expected for a subcellular pathogen) rather than to the cooperative effect of many particles (as expected for a typical poison).

The early hope that phage might be used to combat pathogenic bacteria (either therapeutically or in decontamination of the environment, such as in purifying water supplies) did not materialize at that time, although efforts toward that goal have been renewed (51). Starting in the 1920s, phages were widely used in the typing of bacterial strains of medical interest.

A new era in phage research was initiated in the early 1940s by Max Delbrück, Salvador Luria, and their disciples. Their efforts laid the groundwork for the use of phage in the fundamental experiments of molecular biology, but the work itself is notable for its deemphasis of biochemistry and its focus on basic biologic information relevant to the mechanism of self-replication. The techniques used were simple, mainly microbiologic, and some of the questions investigated had already received indicative answers in the previous two decades. What was new was an emphasis on sharp, incisive answers, quantitative where appropriate, and the development of a few standardized systems.

Conditions were determined for the rapid, reproducible attachment of phage to bacterial cells, allowing synchronous infection of all the cells in a culture, with the resulting "one-step" growth. The effect of varying the ratio of phage to bacteria (multiplicity of infection) was analyzed as a problem in random statistics. It was also shown that infected cells pass through an eclipse phase, where infectious phage is unrecoverable from infected cells, and that infectious particles appear at a later time (3). The ability of one phage to exclude another, and of coinfecting phage to interact productively either genetically (by recombination) or phenotypically (by complementation or phenotypic mixing) or both (as in the production of viable phage from cells multiply infected with radiation-damaged particles) was rigorously documented. Quantitative analysis at a comparable level was introduced into animal virology, with the development of plaque assays on tissue monolayers. Thus, the foundations of modern animal virology (independent of its molecular aspects) go back to the phage work of the 1940s.

Central to the quantitative analysis of phage experiments is the random (Poisson) distribution, which states that, when a mean number s of objects (such as virions) are distributed randomly among containers (such as infected cells), then the fraction of containers with exactly r objects is $Pr = s^r e^{-s}/r!$, where e is the base of natural logarithms (2.718...) and $r! = 1 \times 2 \times ... (r-1)r$, with $0! = 1$. Although s can be any nonnegative number, r is restricted to integral values (a cell cannot be infected with half a virion).

Of particular interest is the zero term $P_0 = e^{-s}$. Thus we expect that, when phage and bacteria are mixed at a ratio of 2:1, the fraction of infected cells should be e^{-2}, or about 0.14. To be exact, this calculation requires that every cell have the same large number of surface sites for viral attachment. Although this is not precisely true, the calculation accords fairly well with experiment.

The distribution also applied to the single burst experiment, where infected cells, before lysis, were diluted and distributed so that each tube received, on average, less than a single cell. For example, with an average number of 0.2 infected cells per tube, the fraction P_0 of sterile tubes is $e^{-0.2}$, or 0.818; the fraction P_1 of tubes with exactly one infected cell is $0.2e^{-0.2}$, or 0.162; the fraction with two infected cells is $0.2^2/2e^{-0.2}$, or 0.0162, and so on. Aside from pipetting errors or confounding factors like cell clumping, this calculation is precise.

Studies of phage genetics started in the 1940s with the construction of recombinational maps (36) and continued in the 1950s with Benzer's analysis of fine structure genetics of the T4*r*II genes (10) and with the discovery and use of conditionally lethal mutations in λ and T4, which allowed dissection of the developmental programs of phages (13,26). The rII work depended conceptually on the prior discovery of phenotypic mixing (54), which showed that when mutants of the same phage co-infect a cell, phage gene products are drawn from a common pool. And the later conditional lethal studies depended on the operational protocol laid out in the rII studies.

Serious phage biochemistry was initiated in the 1930s, when Schlesinger determined that phage particles were about 50% DNA and 50% protein (62). It did not enter into the mainstream of phage work until the 1950s, when Hershey and Chase showed by radiolabeling that the phosphorus (DNA) entered the cell during T2 infection but that most of the sulfur (protein) did not (35). The experiment followed the demonstration of the eclipse phase, and the use of electron microscopy to show that empty phage heads remain attached to the cell envelope and that the DNA of virions could be separated from the protein shell by osmotic shock (2). Concurrently, the enzymology of T4 infection was developed in detail, clearly indicating that the phage was introducing instructions for proteins present neither in the uninfected cell nor in the virion.

It was reported in the 1920s that many bacterial strains harbored phage permanently and secreted it into the medium, so that every culture contained phage. Such strains are called lysogenic. The Luria-Delbrück school initially chose to ignore lysogeny, in part because of the possibility that the phenomenon might be explainable simply by the adherence of extracellular phage particles to the bacterial surface and their occasional detachment from it. Increased rigor was introduced by Lwoff et al. around 1950 in a series of experiments showing first, that when individual cells were allowed to divide and daughter cells separated into different drops of liquid by micromanipulation, both daughters retained the ability to produce phage; second, that an occasional cell lysed and liberated a burst of phage (so that it was unnecessary to postulate secretion by living cells); and third, that certain treatments (such as ultraviolet light or other agents that induce the SOS response) induce mass lysis and phage liberation by all cells of the culture (49). As with infected cells in the eclipse phase, no infectious phage were found when lysogenic cells were artificially disrupted.

Phages capable of producing lysogenic complexes are called temperate, and the noninfectious form in which phage genetic information is transmitted is called prophage. Of the temperate phages, coliphage λ has been studied most intensively, partly because it grows in the K-12 strain of *Escherichia coli*, for which conjugational and transductional mapping were possible by the 1950s. It was soon shown that prophage has a specific location on the bacterial map, and later that its genome is linearly inserted into the continuity of the bacterial chromosome (16,44).

From 1950 onward, the virtues of a simple identifiable genome with rigorous genetics that could be simultaneously introduced into (or induced to replicate in) all the cells of a culture made phage the favored experimental material for many of the classic experiments of molecular biology, such as the demonstration of DNA breakage and joining during genetic recombination, and the proof of the triplet code. In the 1960s, λ, in particular, became the model for study of the genetic hierarchy controlling a simple developmental program. Although the initial investigations on conditionally lethal mutations were pursued in far more depth with T4 than with λ, λ had some inherent advantages: The initiation of the entire program of the lytic cycle from two promoters directly controlled by repressor, the uniformity of the DNA molecules extracted from virions, and the specific probes for different parts of the genome provided by specialized transducing phages and deletions or substitutions (whose locations could be seen via heteroduplex mapping) made the effects of genetic manipulation on molecular events readily interpretable; and the existence of alternative pathways toward lysis or lysogeny added to the interest.

Since 1970, phage work has merged with the rest of biology because artificial cloning allows the application to many systems of the techniques early available for phage. The background data on phage systems, plus their facile manipulation, continue to allow their study at a high level of sophistication.

VIRULENT PHAGES

Like viruses in general, phages can be divided into those with RNA genomes (mostly small and single stranded), those with small DNA genomes (generally less than 10 kilobases, mostly single stranded), and those with medium to large DNA genomes (30 to 200 kb). The last group includes most of the temperate phages, as well as the first virulent phages to be studied intensively.

Large DNA Phages

The classic T coliphages selected for study by the Luria-Delbrück school fall into four groups: T1 (about 50 kb); T2, T4, and T6 (about 170 kb); T3 and T7 (40 kb); and T5 (about 130 kb). The members of a group have similar virion morphology and can produce viable recombinants in mixed infection.

Phage T4

Virion

T4 was the object of many classic experiments. More than 200 T4 genes were identified through mutational studies. The virion contains 43 phage-encoded proteins, of which 16 are located in the head that encapsidates the DNA, and 27 form the tail through which DNA passes into the cell during infection. The head is an elongated T=13 icosahedron with an extra equatorial row of capsomeres. The tail consists of a hollow core (surrounded by a contractile sheath) that terminates in a baseplate to which are attached six fibers. The whole apparatus functions to inject phage DNA into the interior of the cell. The tips of the tail fibers make initial contact with lipopolysaccharide surface receptors on the bacterium. Once the phage is anchored by tail fiber attachment, random motion brings the baseplate into contact with the cell surface. Either this contact or the tail fiber attachment itself triggers conformational changes in the tail: The center of the baseplate opens like a shutter, allowing the tip of the core to pass through, and the sheath contracts, driving the core through the cell envelope, after which DNA is released into the cell. The double-stranded DNA is distinctive in containing hydroxymethylcytosine (HMC) (heavily glucosylated) rather than cytosine. It is cyclically permuted and terminally repetitious—that is, the sequences of various molecules can be represented as ABCDEFGHAB, DEFGHABCDE, GHABCDEFGH, and so on. This is most simply demonstrated by allowing the DNA to separate into single strands and then reannealing with complementary strands from other virions, generating circular duplexes with single-stranded tails (Fig. 1).

DNA Transactions

Infection triggers a massive degradation of cytosine-containing host DNA with subsequent enzymatic conversion of deoxycytosine monophosphate to deoxyhydroxymethylcytosine monophosphate. The phage encodes enzymes that perform these and other conversions of deoxyribonucleotides, which are then used in phage replication. Bidirectional replication is initiated at several origins along the DNA, and elongation is performed by a complex of phage-encoded enzymes, leading- and lagging-strand synthesis proceeding coordinately from a single replication complex. Because there is no mechanism for priming synthesis at the extreme 5′ end of the lagging strand, this first round of replication produces linear molecules with protruding 3′ ends.

Soon after infection, these early replication origins cease to function (because replication there requires priming by RNA made by host RNA polymerase, whose promoter recognition specificity is altered). Late replication initiates at recombination intermediates formed by invasion of 3′ ends into homologous double-stranded DNA. Because of the terminal redundancy, such homologous sequences are available, even in single infection. As replication proceeds, repeated invasions of this kind generate a complex network of intracellular viral DNA, which includes end-to-end concatemers (the preferred packaging substrate for T4). In packaging, empty heads are first assembled, then filled with DNA. Cutting is coordinated with packaging, so that headful lengths are cut to size after the head is filled. The packaging length exceeds the genome length, hence the terminal redundancy. The position of molecular ends along the concatemer is close to random.

This picture of the DNA transactions has genetic consequences; in fact, much of it was inferred from genetic studies that preceded the biochemistry and molecular biology. First, the recombination rate in T4 infection is very high, producing a linkage map thousands of centimorgans in length. It was early noted that this corresponded to about one recombination per replication cycle. Second, the linkage map is circular, as expected if virion DNA has random endpoints. Third, when cells are infected with phages of two different genotypes, some of the progeny particles can carry different information within the terminal duplication; for example, in a mixed infection between T4 and T4*h*, some progeny plaques contain phage of both *h* and *h*+ genotypes. Another mechanism that generates mixed plaques is packaging of heteroduplex DNA recombination intermediates. Both types of heterozygous progeny are demonstrable (65).

Finally, there are genetic implications of headful packaging. If the length of the terminal overlap represents the difference between packaging length (determined by head size) and genome length, then that length should change in a predictable manner if either packaging length or genome length is deliberately altered. The first test was

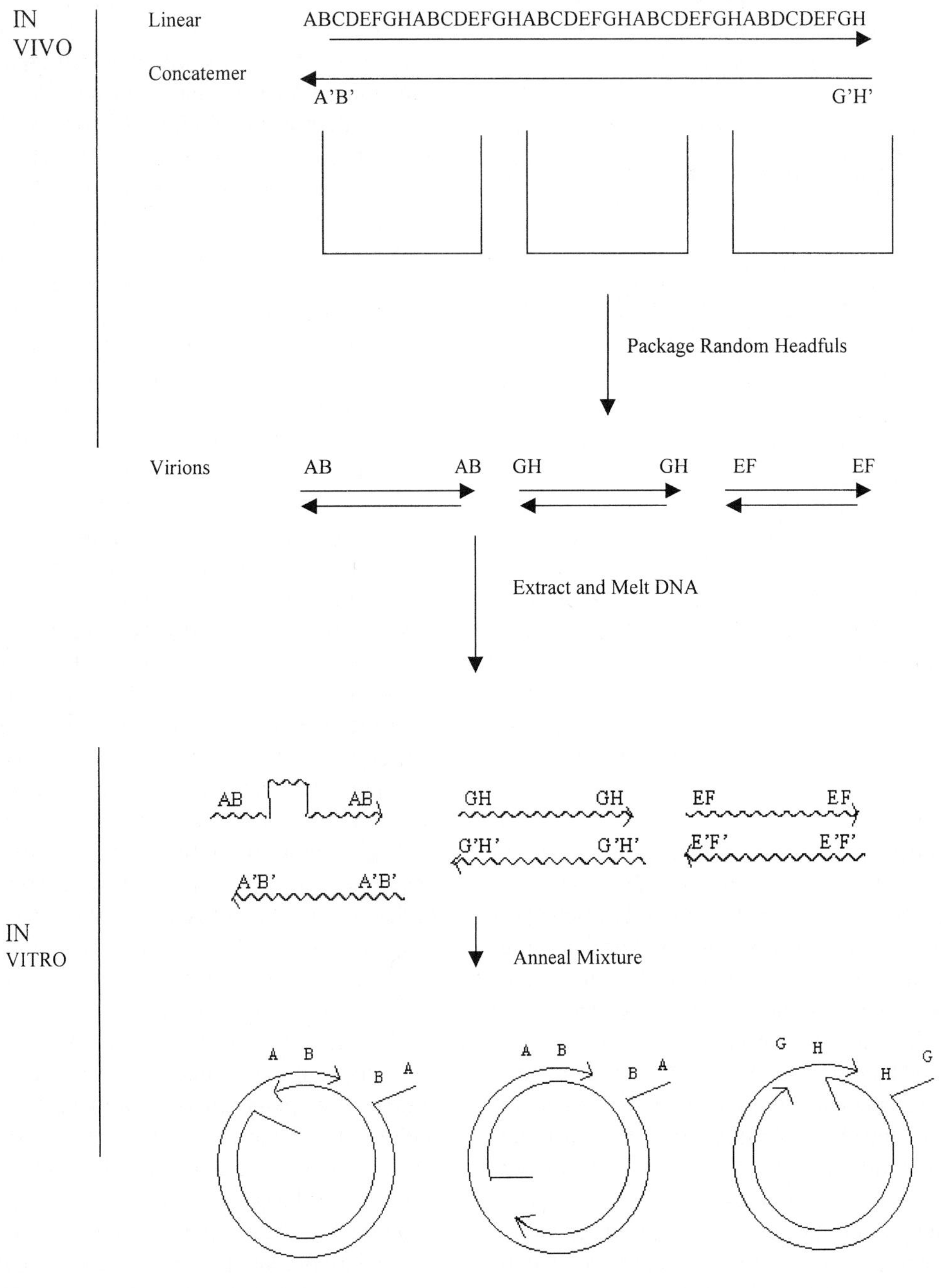

FIG. 1. Genesis (*in vivo*) and demonstration (*in vitro*) of circular permutation of T4. Within infected cells, replication generates a DNA network with linear concatemeric segments. From these, headfuls of DNA, cut randomly, are packaged. Thus DNA extracted from virions has random endpoints. When single strands reassociate, the complementary strands in general have different starting points and thus pair as shown.

to alter genome length with a nonlethal deletion. The prediction that this would increase the length of the terminal overlap (and therefore the fraction of particles heterozygous for any locus in the genome) was fulfilled (67). Later experiments with other phages that use headful packaging, such as P22, showed that increasing the genome length by insertion of extra DNA has the reverse effect of decreasing the terminal overlap.

The opposite experiment, where genome length remains constant but packaging length changes, was accomplished through examination of virions with abnormal morphology. Preparations of T4 contain a small fraction of virions whose heads are isometric rather than elongated, separable from the majority type by ultracentrifugation. Certain treatments (such as phage development in the presence of amino acid analogs) induce formation of giant particles with the same diameter as normal virions but additional rows of capsomeres, approaching helical tubes in shape. Missense mutations in the major capsid protein can increase the proportion of both isometric and giant particles. Both types of abnormal particle inject their DNA into cells. The packaging capacity of isometric particles is about 67% that of normal virions; accordingly, single infection is unproductive, but multiple infection allows a normal cycle through recombination between molecules of less than genome length with random endpoints. Giant particles have longer than normal DNA (up to several genome lengths) and a correspondingly high degree of heterozygosity when coming from mixed infection. They are also highly resistant to ultraviolet light because of complementation and recombination between damaged genomes.

Regulation

The genes whose products are needed for phage DNA synthesis and host DNA breakdown, including those mediating nucleotide metabolism and the seven proteins of the replication complex, are all expressed immediately after infection, being transcribed from promoters recognizable by *E. coli* RNA polymerase with σ70. With time, early synthesis shuts off and other genes that code for virion components and lysis genes are activated. The shutoff of early genes is effected at both the transcriptional and the translational levels. Translational control is sometimes autogenous, as for the DNA polymerase gp43 and the single-stranded binding protein gp32; many other early genes are controlled by a dedicated translational repressor, the product of the *regA* gene, itself an early gene subject to autogenous control (4,71). (In phage work, gp means gene product, not glycoprotein, as elsewhere in this book.)

Transcriptional control operates on three different types of T4 promoters. The early promoters have sequences approximating the consensus for *E. coli* σ70 (with a small but apparently real difference in consensus). Middle promoters require *E. coli* polymerase with σ70, in addition to the T4-specified positive regulators MotA and AsiA (1). Their hallmark is a sequence TGCTT at around −32. Late promoters follow −12 consensus TATAAATA. They are transcribed by *E. coli* holoenzyme, with a phage-coded σ factor (gp55) replacing σ70. In normal infection, late promoter activation requires concurrent DNA replication. *In vitro*, activation can be achieved by nicks or gaps on the nontranscribed strand near the promoter; treatments that create damage *in vivo* can also induce some replication-independent transcription.

In vitro, activation of late transcription by nicks or gaps requires three replication proteins, gp45 and gp44/62, which form a sliding clamp that loads at the nick or gap and moves along the DNA (29). An RNA polymerase-associated protein, gp33, is also required, as well as gp55. Transcription cannot be stimulated by bringing the DNA interruption spatially close to the promoter through catenation of DNA molecules; enhancement is seen only when all signals are on the same DNA double helix, as expected from the sliding clamp model. The exact relationship between these *in vitro* results and the *in vivo* dependence of late transcription on replication is unknown.

Some other ancillary changes during infection may reinforce the temporal sequence but are not essential for it. For example, the α subunit of RNA polymerase becomes adenosine diphosphate (ADP)-ribosylated a few minutes after infection by the action of either of two phage gene products: gp*alt*, which is activated during virion assembly and injected along with the DNA, and gp*mod*. ADP-ribosylation modifies polymerase specificity, but both successful infection and shutoff of host promoters occur in its absence (in *alt*/*mod* double mutants), perhaps because of a multiplicity of functionally overlapping shutoff mechanisms. Shutoff of host transcription is also effected by a T4-encoded transcriptional terminator protein (Alc), which recognizes cytosine-containing DNA.

Thus the chemical marking of phage DNA by HMC is used as a passover signal: Transcription of the host's cytosine (C)-containing DNA is first reduced by the Alc protein (39) and then C-containing DNA is degraded. T4 also has some noteworthy features with no known regulatory role, such as genes that are discontinuous because of intron splicing or ribosomal skipping (8,72).

Assembly

Once late genes are expressed, the stage is set for assembling virions. The T4 virion was the first biologic structure of comparable complexity whose pathways of assembly were worked out, from a combination of physical and genetic knowledge. The major technical factors facilitating the study were, first, the availability of conditionally lethal mutations in genes for individual virion proteins; second, the fact that the final steps of the pathway were readily executed *in vitro* so that reactions in the pathway could be distinguished from irrelevant interactions or side reactions that do not contribute to the yield of functional plaque-forming particles; and third, the facility of operations by then standard in phage work, such as assay for complexes stable to dilution.

The results of these studies suggested several general principles whose rationalization as effective strategies and extension to other phages has been subsequently assessed and updated. One of these is the repeated use of subassembly pathways rather than a single linear pathway. Thus, heads, tails, tail fibers, and soluble protein (gp63) catalyzing tail fiber addition are all made separately. Heads and tails combine first to form complexes that are both visible by electron microscopy and stable to dilution, and finally tail fibers are added to the complex. The tail consists of a baseplate (to which the fibers attach) composed of a central hub surrounded by six wedges. Hub and wedges are made separately, then combined to form the baseplate (Fig. 2). Likewise, in tail fiber assembly, the distal and proximal segments are assembled separately, then combined immediately before addition to the head–tail complex. The most obvious advantage of subassembly pathways is that mistakes in assembly can be rejected for each pathway separately, rather than ruining entire virions.

A second general rule is that linear elements are built from the end in (toward their junction with the rest of the virion). In tail assembly, baseplates are made first, then the core and sheath are added to them. Likewise, wedges are formed by adding different protein units successively, beginning with one of the outermost units, and finishing with the one that interacts with the hub. This strategy ensures that the intermediates of the subassembly pathway cannot compete with the final product for assembly into the virion. The order of assembly of the wedges themselves may be prescribed by allosteric changes on addition to the complex or by the recognition of binding sites that contain elements of more than one of the proteins already present. In fiber addition to head-tail complexes, fibers do not add efficiently to base plates until heads and tails are joined, apparently because the bend in the fibers contacts the head–tail junction and interacts with it. A protein (gp*wac*) in the collar serves this function *in vitro*, although it is not essential for plaque formation *in vivo*. In free virions, fibers are frequently wrapped around the tail sheath, becoming extended only under specific conditions.

The joining of fibers to head–tail complexes attracted attention early because it proceeds by catalysis of a noncovalent interaction. The catalyst (gp63) also functions as an RNA ligase that apparently acts during (but is not essential for) DNA synthesis. Protein catalysis of a one-step noncovalent interaction was novel at the time, and its discovery was too far in advance of later work on chaperonins to have wide impact.

Tail assembly raised the question of length determination. The core and sheath are both formed by polymerization of single protein species. Core assembly is initiated through nucleation on the baseplate, followed by addition of subunits to build the structure. How is the number of subunits counted, so as to ensure the observed uniformity among virions? The answer (better documented for λ than for T4) is by use of a linear measuring stick protein that is embedded within the core and eliminated when assembly is complete (40).

The T4 tail fiber is a bent, linear structure with several specific protein monomers or dimers arranged end to end, terminating in a dimer of gp37. This protein at the tip of the tail fiber is so arranged that its amino acid sequence (and hence its genetic map) is colinear with the fiber axis (7). The specificity for host cell receptors and neutralizing antibodies lies in the distal portion, near the tip, which is also the location of mutations for altered host range.

The pathway of capsid formation in T4 (as for isometric capsids of any virus) is still understood in less depth than

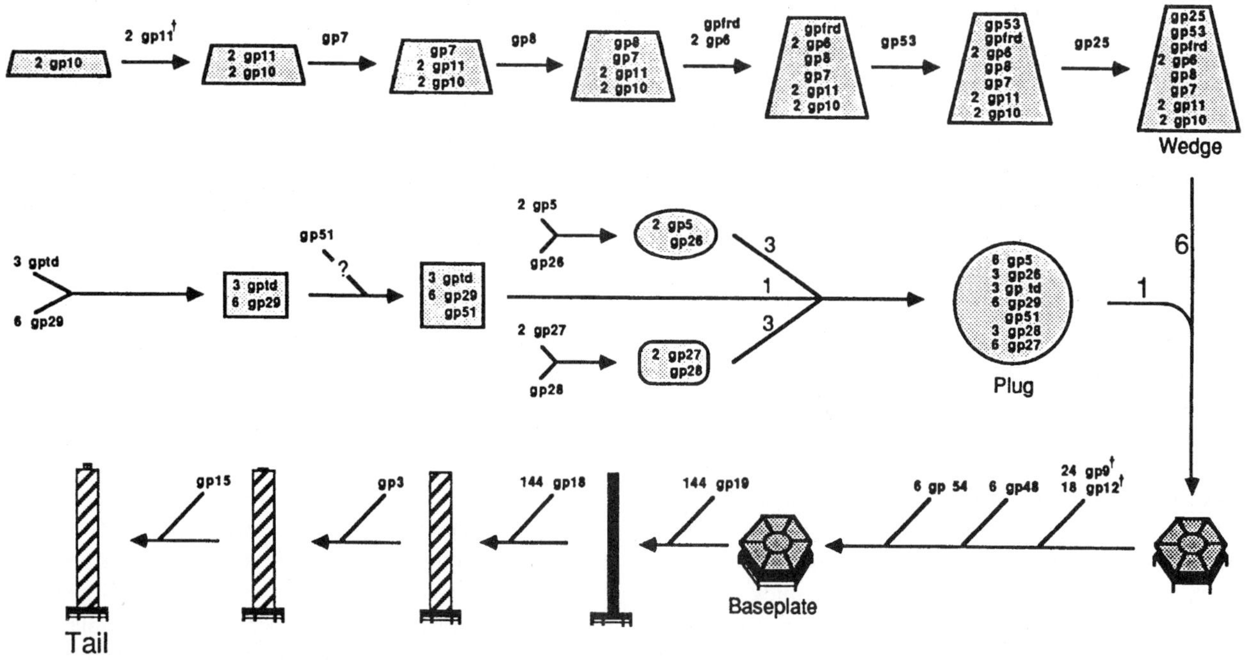

FIG. 2. Assembly pathway of T4 tails. Proteins must be added in the indicated order, except that gp11, gp12, and gp9 (indicated by †) can be added at later times as well. (From ref. 17, with permission.)

tail assembly, but several established features are noteworthy. Some of these are better understood for other phages (λ, P22) and inferred for T4. The capsid is synthesized first, and it is filled with DNA later. This fits with the determination of DNA content by head size, but it is more directly established by the association of capsids assembled early with DNA made late in infection (47). Second, capsids are not built directly into their final form; rather, capsid proteins associate with an internal scaffolding protein, which fills the interior of the prohead and is later extruded through holes in the protein shell, which expands to its final shape before DNA enters. Both scaffolding protein (gp24) and the major head protein (gp23) have a shape-determining role [inferred from the aberrations in shape caused by certain missense mutations (12)]. Probably both proteins are added to the structure concurrently. How these proteins actually determine the elongated icosahedral shape is unknown, and the intermediate states are no better understood than for any other closed lattice. After the prohead expands and assumes a more obviously icosahedral shape, two decoration proteins, gp*hoc* and gp*soc*, are added at regular positions in the lattice; neither protein is essential for formation of functional virions. Third, assembly requires nucleation from one vertex, in which minor capsid proteins, noncapsid proteins, and host chaperonins (*gro*EL) all participate. This unique vertex becomes the portal vertex through which DNA enters the virion and to which the tail later attaches. DNA packaging requires two phage proteins (gp16 and gp17) that probably act at the portal vertex but are not present in the final virion. Protein gp17 has been identified as the endonuclease that cuts the DNA from the concatemer during packaging (11). Another packaging gene, gp49, is needed for processing the DNA substrate. Only linear DNA is packaged, but intracellular T4 DNA becomes highly branched during replication and recombination; gp49 cleaves Holliday junctions and other branched structures, creating packageable lengths of linear DNA (11). Fourth, processing of gp23 takes place concurrently with assembly. Figure 3 presents the general scheme for virion assembly in double-stranded DNA phages.

Lysis

The final stage of the T4 cycle is cellular lysis, releasing virions into the medium. Lysis requires two gene products: a lysozyme (gpe), which attacks the bonds joining *N*-acetylglucosamines in the rigid murein layer, and a holin (gpt), which creates holes in the inner membrane, allowing the lysozyme to reach its substrate. Other genes affect the timing of lysis. The status of gpt as a holin is not fully established and rests largely on analogy to λ gpS (75). In *e t*+ mutants, the cell dies and the membrane potential collapses at the normal time of lysis, whereas in *e*+ *t* mutants, the cell continues to produce lysozyme and intracellular phage long after the normal time of lysis.

It is clearly desirable to coordinate the time of lysis with the rest of the lytic cycle, but no regulatory system serving this function has been identified. The timing of lysis appears to be determined largely by the accumulation of gpt, formed coordinately with other late proteins. One genetic system that regulates time of lysis under certain conditions is the *r*II locus. T4*r* mutants were discovered by their ability to form larger than normal plaques, and the *r*II mutants have the related property of inability to plate on strains expressing the *rex* genes of λ [which provided the selective conditions for Benzer's classical studies on fine structure genetics (9)]. However, their effect on lysis and plaque size is attributable to the absence, in *r*II mutants, of lysis inhibition. When a cell infected with T4*r*+ is superinfected before lysis by another T4 particle, lysis is delayed and intracellular phage development continues, for a period of up to several hours beyond the normal latent period of 24 min. The rIIA and rIIB membrane proteins must mediate this response and must likewise destroy membrane damage inflicted by the λ *rex* system in response to superinfection, but their mechanism of action is unknown.

Phage T7

Each group of T phages has unique properties. This brief account of phage T7 is intended to indicate some major differences from the T4 paradigm. The phage T7 virion contains 39,936 base pairs (bp) of linear double-stranded DNA (completely sequenced). It is terminally redundant (like T4) but not cyclically permuted. The length of the terminal overlap is 160 bp (25). Immediately after infection, host RNA polymerase initiates transcription from a promoter near the left end of the molecule, whose products include an antirestriction factor, a protein kinase that phosphorylates and inactivates *E. coli* RNA polymerase, a new T7-specific RNA polymerase, and a DNA ligase. After a few minutes, T7 polymerase replaces host polymerase and all transcription takes place on the 81% of the genome toward the right end. The first genes transcribed by T7 polymerase (nearer to the left end) include a DNA polymerase and recombination genes. Later, after replication ensues, the late genes encoding virion components and at least one lysis gene are expressed. Late gene expression does not require replication, as it does in T4, and the host polymerase is replaced rather than reprogrammed. Even without inactivation of host polymerase, the T7 RNA polymerase competes so effectively for nucleoside triphosphates that it redirects almost all transcription to T7 promoters, a feature that has been exploited in the design of T7-based expression vectors for DNA cloning.

The first cycle of DNA replication proceeds bidirectionally from a unique origin of the linear monomer. As with T4, concatemers are probably generated through strand invasion of terminal segments into other molecules

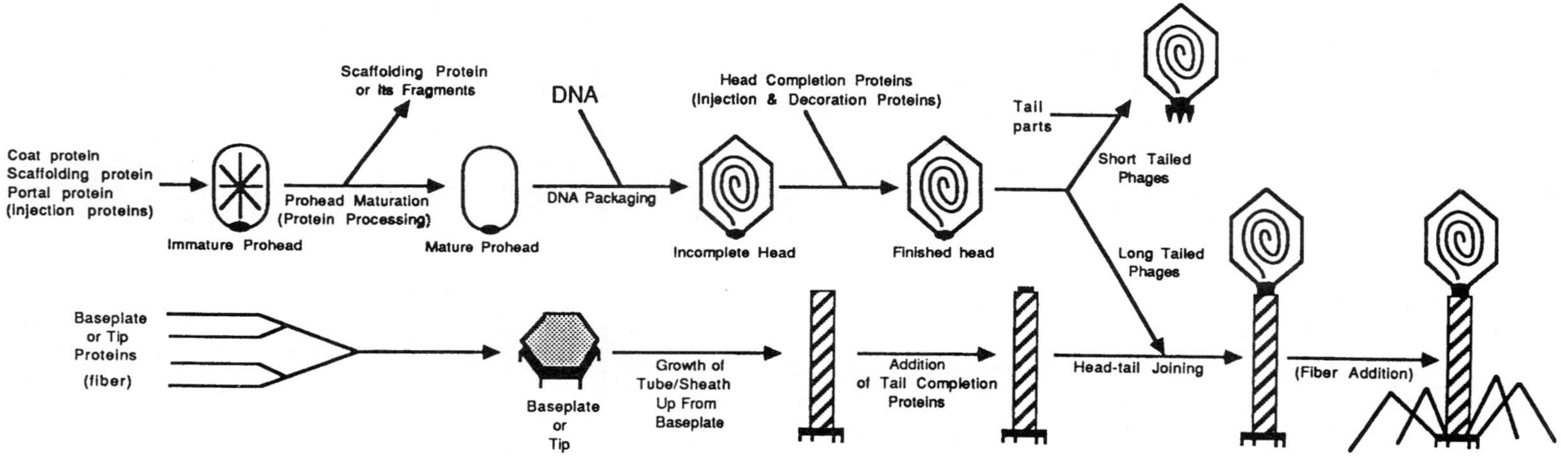

FIG. 3. Generalized assembly pathway for dsDNA phages with tailed virions, such as T4 and λ. (From ref. 17, with permission.)

within the 160-bp terminal repeat. Replication then generates concatemers in which the unique 39,616 viral sequences alternate with single copies of the 160-bp repeat. If complete virion DNA molecules with repeats at both ends were cut and packaged from such concatemers, half of the genomes would lack terminal repeats. It was suggested that T7 might solve the problem by cutting the DNA in opposite strands at the two ends of the repeat, creating protruding 160-base 5′ ends, followed by DNA synthesis to produce flush ends.

The actual solution is apparently more complicated and wasteful. Replication of one strand initiated from a nick near the 160-bp segment proceeds leftward through the 160-bp segment to a reverse repeat beyond the segment. The displaced strand is then nicked at the end of the reverse repeat, which folds back and initiates synthesis rightward through the 160-bp segment. Thus, two copies of the 160-bp segment are present, which can be trimmed to size and packaged (19). Packaging proceeds from right to left processively along the concatemer (66). Because T7 packages the DNA between two specific sites, the amount of DNA per head is not fixed by head size. From study of T7 variants with deletions or duplications, the packaging limits of T7 are about 85% to 103% of normal genome length (F. W. Studier, personal communication).

Small DNA Phages

Some phages package small covalently closed circles of (+) strand genomic DNA in their virions. There are two groups: isometric and filamentous. Although the two groups are not detectably related in sequence and differ in modes of attachment, packaging, and egress, their replication mechanisms are similar.

Isometric Phages

The prototype is $\phi \times 174$. The virion (25 to 35 nm) has an icosahedral T=1 capsid, composed of three polypeptide species: gpF (60 copies), gpG (60 copies), and gpH (12 copies). gpG and gpH are considered spike proteins and can be physically removed without disrupting the integrity of the capsid. The spike proteins are necessary for attachment to cells, and gpH enters the infected cell with the DNA and participates in phage development. Such participation is not essential for all productive infection, because transfection by pure (+) strand DNA from virions leads to some phage production.

Once within the cell, the DNA becomes coated with single-stranded binding protein (Ssb), then begins to replicate. The first cycle [parental single strand → double-stranded replicative form (RF)] is mediated entirely by host enzymes. Transcription by host DNA–dependent RNA polymerase at a unique site near a DNA hairpin provides a primer, which is extended by the host replication complex and then digested away. At completion of the cycle, the new DNA strand is ligated to give a covalently closed circle (the RF). Transcription from RF by host RNA polymerase leads to production of phage proteins, among them a dimeric protein gpA, which works only in *cis* (i.e., an A- mutant cannot be complemented in *trans*, perhaps because the protein binds rapidly and irreversibly to DNA near the site of transcription). Rolling circle replication is initiated when gpA binds to RF at a specific origin site and nicks its parental (+) strand, which is then extended by the action of a host-specified DNA helicase (Rep) followed by the host elongation complex. The displaced 5′ end is not free but remains bound to the growing point through the gpA dimer. The displaced strand is coated with Ssb and remains single stranded (no lagging-strand synthesis). When one genome length of DNA has been synthesized and the growing point comes to the origin, the displaced DNA is cut from the newly synthesized DNA and its ends are ligated, giving a single-stranded circle and a double-stranded (RF) circle, both of which can recycle through further rounds of replication. Thus, a fraction of the (+) strands in infected cells are linear and from monomer to dimer length, whereas both (+) and (–) strands are present as monomer circles.

With time, virion proteins accumulate and form empty proheads, and concurrently a phage-specified DNA-binding protein (gpC) is made. On some of the (+) strands, gpC competes with Ssb for binding to the Rep-gpA complex, and these interact with proheads to become encapsidated into virions. Thus, the DNA is directed toward packaging before it encounters the prohead (5). The replicating pool then ceases to expand as (+) strands are packaged (Fig. 4). The multiplication cycle ends with lysis, mediated by the phage gpE protein. The mode of gpE action is uncertain, but it does not involve either a lysozyme or a holin (75).

Filamentous DNA Phages

The virions of filamentous phages, of which phage fd is the prototype, differ from those of most helical viruses in that the capsid surrounds a DNA molecule that is not linear but circular and therefore is doubled back on itself, although unpaired. The replication cycle of the filamentous DNA phages is similar to that of the isometric phages. Infection is initiated by adsorption of the end of a virion to the terminus of an F-coded pilus, used during bacterial conjugation. The details of DNA entry are obscure. As with $\phi \times 174$, ssDNA formed at late times is coated with a phage-specified DNA-binding protein (gp5) that directs the DNA to packaging rather than to recycling. Packaging is concomitant with egress. The major coat protein (gp8) is embedded in the cell membrane. As phage DNA enters the membrane, gp5 is exchanged for a helical capsid of gp8. Subunits of gp8 are proteolytically processed as they are added to phage

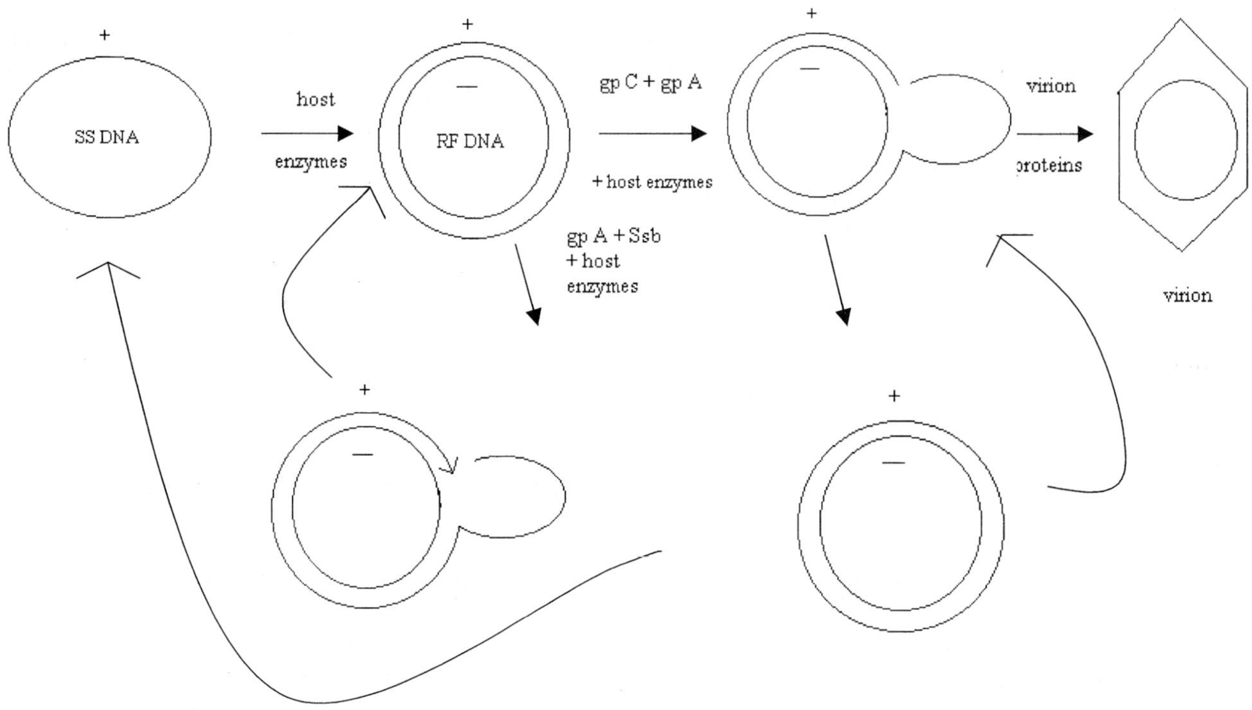

FIG. 4. Replication of ΦX174. The DNA injected from the virion as a closed ring of single-stranded (+) DNA is first replicated by host enzymes to give the supercoiled double-stranded replicating form (RF). Early after infection (*left*), the (+) strand is cleaved by the phage-coded gpA, and rolling circle replication is initiated. One cycle of replication produces one SS and one RF DNA. At late times, interaction with gpC initiates rolling circle replication, but here the SS DNA is packaged into virions. In early replication, SS DNAs are coated with the host single-strand binding protein Ssb; in late replication, they are coated with gpC until packaging.

DNA, and virions are extruded through the cell envelope without loss of cell viability. Except for a few enveloped phages, these are the only phages whose egress does not require lysis.

The filamentous phages (especially M13) are popular as cloning vectors because of their high yields, the absence of a packaging limit, and the single-strandedness of the product. Cloning is generally accomplished through cutting and ligation of RF DNA, followed by transfection. Filamentous phages have also had extensive use in phage display libraries.

RNA Phages

The common RNA phages have isometric T=1 virions, each containing a single linear single-stranded RNA molecule about 4 kb in length, encoding three to four genes and capable of assuming extensive secondary structure. They enter bacterial cells by attachment to the sides of F pili (rather than the ends, as with the filamentous DNA phages). Like the filamentous phages, they are only able to infect bacteria that harbor the F plasmid. The four genes of phage MS2 encode the coat protein (C), an RNA-dependent RNA polymerase (P), a lysin (L), and a fourth protein (A, for assembly) present in one copy per virion. The genes are arranged in the order 5′A-C-(L)-P3′, where the L gene overlaps the 3′ end of C and the 5′ end of P.

In these phages, there is no known distinction between replication and transcription. All RNA copies are full length, and gene expression is controlled at the translational level. Nevertheless, they have developed a program of temporal control exquisitely tailored to their needs. The *A* gene at the 5′ end is available for translation only in nascent RNA that has not yet folded into its most stable secondary configuration, a reasonable strategy for obtaining one copy per virion. The *C* gene, on the other hand, is available for translation at all times. The *P* gene is under a more complex control. Translation of the *C* gene is needed to open the secondary structure that otherwise sequesters the *P* ribosome binding site; but coat protein itself, binding to the RNA upstream of the *P* gene, inhibits polymerase translation. The first control delays the onset of phage replication whenever conditions for protein synthesis are poor; the second means that, as with T4 or T7, synthesis at late times is diverted to virion components (in this case, coat protein), with minimal competition from polymerase synthesis. The *L* gene lacks a ribosome binding site of its own. Lysin synthesis results from reattachment of ribosomes that initiated at the ribosome binding site for *C*, then disengaged as a result of high-frequency frameshifting and reattached at the AUG for L (41). By tying the accumulation of lysin to the rate of coat protein synthesis, this arrangement should help coordinate the time of lysis with the rest of phage development.

In broad outline, the mechanism of RNA synthesis is similar to that of most linear single-stranded RNA viruses. RNA phage replication enjoys the distinction of being the first system in which *in vitro* replication of a nucleic acid was shown to initiate at a specific origin (33). In conjunction with three host proteins (elongation factors Tu and Ts and ribosomal protein S1, all part of the machinery for host protein synthesis), the phage polymerase initiates replication at the 3′ end of a (+) strand. Generally, several subsequent initiations take place at the same end before the first (−) strand is completed. When completed (−) strands dissociate from their (+) strand templates, they are used in a similar manner as templates for (+) strand synthesis.

Because of their small size and rapid mutation rate, RNA phage genomes have been used in studies of *in vitro* evolution, where enzyme is supplied and those RNA molecules structurally capable of the most rapid rate of multiplication are selected (37). The most consistent result was selection for much smaller molecules, which always include the terminal sequences recognized by the polymerase. The results are instructive with respect to the defective interfering particles that accumulate *in vivo* during the high-multiplicity passage of many viruses. In the absence of added template, the replicase can also create short sequences *de novo* and copy them.

TEMPERATE PHAGES

Temperate phages are mostly large (>20 kb) double-stranded DNA viruses. Three prototypes can be distinguished based on their modes of establishment of lysogeny. The first, represented by coliphage λ, inserts DNA into the chromosome at one or a few preferred sites. The second, represented by phage Mu-1, inserts it anywhere in the host chromosome by use of a phage-coded transposase. In the third, represented by phage P1, prophage DNA is not inserted into the chromosome but instead is maintained as a plasmid. Some other phages, such as satellite phage P4, can be maintained either as inserted prophages or as plasmids. The inserted state can be stably maintained only if the phage genes for autonomous replication are repressed, whereas in the plasmid state some viral functions are expressed without killing the cell.

Phage λ

The development of λ has become a paradigm for gene control in developing systems. An infected cell has one of two options: either to lyse and produce viral progeny or to survive as a lysogen. Once a cell is committed to one of these pathways, there are several safeguards to stabilize the decision.

The λ virion is isometric, with a T=7 configuration of capsomeres and a long tail terminating in a single fiber. The virion DNA is a 48,502-bp linear molecule with complementary 12-base 5′ overhangs. Once injected into the cell, the DNA ends pair and are ligated by host ligase to generate a covalently closed circle. Figure 5 shows a genetic map of λ in its circular form.

Commitment

After infection, host RNA polymerase initiates transcription at three promoters: *p*L, *p*R, and *p*R′. The *p*L and *p*R transcripts each contain one gene (*N* and *cro*, respectively). The *p*R′ transcript contains no genes. The Cro protein binds to the operators controlling *p*L and *p*R and represses transcription from them; however, because *cro* itself is transcribed from *p*R, the Cro concentration never reaches a level where repression is complete. The gpN protein is an antiterminator, which allows transcription at *p*L and *p*R to read through ordinary termination signals. The seminal early observations leading to this conclusion were, first, that the λ gene *exo*, which is downstream of *N*, requires for expression both a functional gpN (suppliable in *trans*) and a derepressed *p*L (in *cis*), and second, that terminators of ordinary bacterial operons such as *trp* are read through when placed downstream of *p*L in the presence of gpN (28,48).

Antitermination by gpN is effected by binding to specific RNA sequences (*nut* sites) that are generated early in the transcripts from *p*L and *p*R. The *nut*R RNA includes a binding site (*boxA*) for host protein NusA, and a stem-loop sequence (*boxB*) specific for λ's gpN. NusA (the principal elongation factor for *E. coli* RNA polymerase) is the product of one of the *nus* genes, isolated by screening for mutants with an "*N* undersupply" phenotype, so that even λN^+ behaves like an N^- mutant on *nus* mutants. Various λ-related phages have distinct N specificities determined by the sequence in the *boxB* loop. The gpN–NusA complex bound to *nut* RNA interacts with the RNA polymerase that has passed the *nut* site and is transcribing downstream from it and modifies transcription so that normal termination signals are no longer recognized. The complex N−NusA–RNA polymerase –*nut*^{R} site is stabilized by interaction with other host factors: NusB, NusG, and ribosomal protein S10 (50).

The result of antitermination is that both leftward and rightward transcription proceed beyond the primary terminators (*t*L1 and *t*R1, respectively). The leftward transcript includes several genes whose functions are not essential to either lytic or lysogenic development, although some of them play ancillary roles in DNA replication (*exo*, β) or lysogenization (*cIII*). The rightward

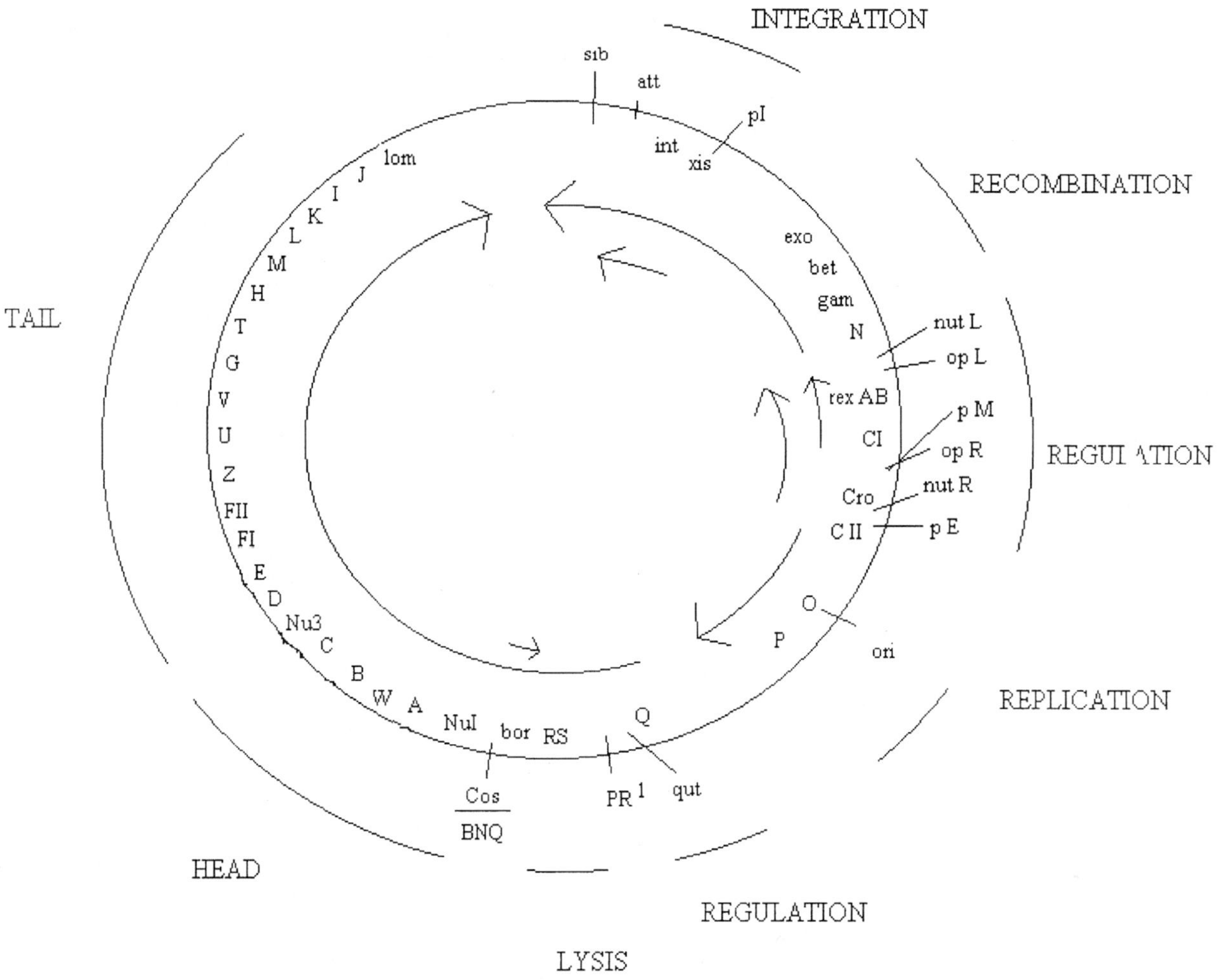

FIG 5. Genetic map of λ in its circular (replicating) form. Genes are shown inside the circle; sites are outside. Transcripts are shown inside the circle. Genes are clustered according to function in the phage life cycle. The *bor* and *lom* genes affect host phenotype in lysogens. Functions of most other phage genes and sites are discussed in the text. Some genes with minor or unknown functions are not shown.

transcript includes *cII* (whose product promotes lysogenization), replication genes *O* and *P*, and gene *Q*, the antiterminating positive regulator of late transcription.

The CII protein is a positive effector of transcription initiating at site pE within *cII* and proceeding leftward beyond *p*R through genes *cI* and *rexAB*. The CI protein (repressor) binds to the same operator sites as Cro and represses transcription from *p*L and *p*R, thus stopping all transcription characteristic of the lytic cycle.

If CII were formed at high concentration in all infected cells, they all should become lysogenic. In fact, among cells under the same ambient conditions, some commit to lysis and others to lysogeny, presumably because of stochastic fluctuations in early molecular events. Mathematical modeling with measured kinetic parameters adequately predicts the observed proportions of cells committed to the two pathways as a function of the phage-to-bacterial ratio (6). The critical biochemical players are CII (which is metabolically unstable because of proteolysis; CIII (which stabilizes CII in a manner dependent on the phage-to-bacterial ratio); and Cro, which accumulates with time and represses synthesis of CII. Cro accumulation thus functions as a developmental clock; when its concentration becomes high, CII decays and the cell is committed to lysis.

In those cells where repression is established, further events are needed to ensure stable lysogeny. First, repressor synthesis must continue in the lysogen so that the lytic cycle functions are shut off permanently. Once repression is established, *p*R transcription stops and CII disappears. Repressor does not disappear as well, because *cI* transcription commences from the maintenance promoter pM immediately to the left of *o*R.

The *o*R and *o*L operators are tripartite, with three binding sites separated by short spacers. Both repressor and Cro recognize these binding sites, but with different relative affinities. Cro binds most tightly to *o*R3 (which represses leftward transcription from *p*M) and less tightly

TABLE 1. *Gene regulation by repressor (R) and Cro (C) at one oR*

Leftward transcription from pM	oR3	oR2	oR1	Rightward transcription from pR
(*cI*←)				(*cro*→)
Low	—	—	—	On
On	—	R	R	Off
Off	R	R	R	Off
Off	C	—	—	On
Off	C	C	—	Off
Off	C	—	C	Off
Off	C	C	C	Off

Source: Adapted from ref. 58, with permission.

to *o*R2 and *o*R1 (repressing rightward transcription from *p*R). Repressor, on the other hand, binds tightly and cooperatively to oR2 and oR1, which both represses transcription from pR and stimulates transcription from pM. At high repressor concentration (unsustainable in the steady state) repressor also binds to oR3 and represses its own synthesis (Table 1). Thus, once a high concentration of repressor is achieved through transcription from pE, repression is self-sustaining (58). The inhibition by Cro of spontaneous initiation at pM reinforces the decision to follow the lytic pathway.

Commitment to lysogeny requires not only repression of lytic cycle genes but also insertion of phage DNA into the host chromosome. Insertion is mediated by the phage-coded integrase (Fig. 6). The structural gene for integrase, *int*, is transcribed from two promoters: the major

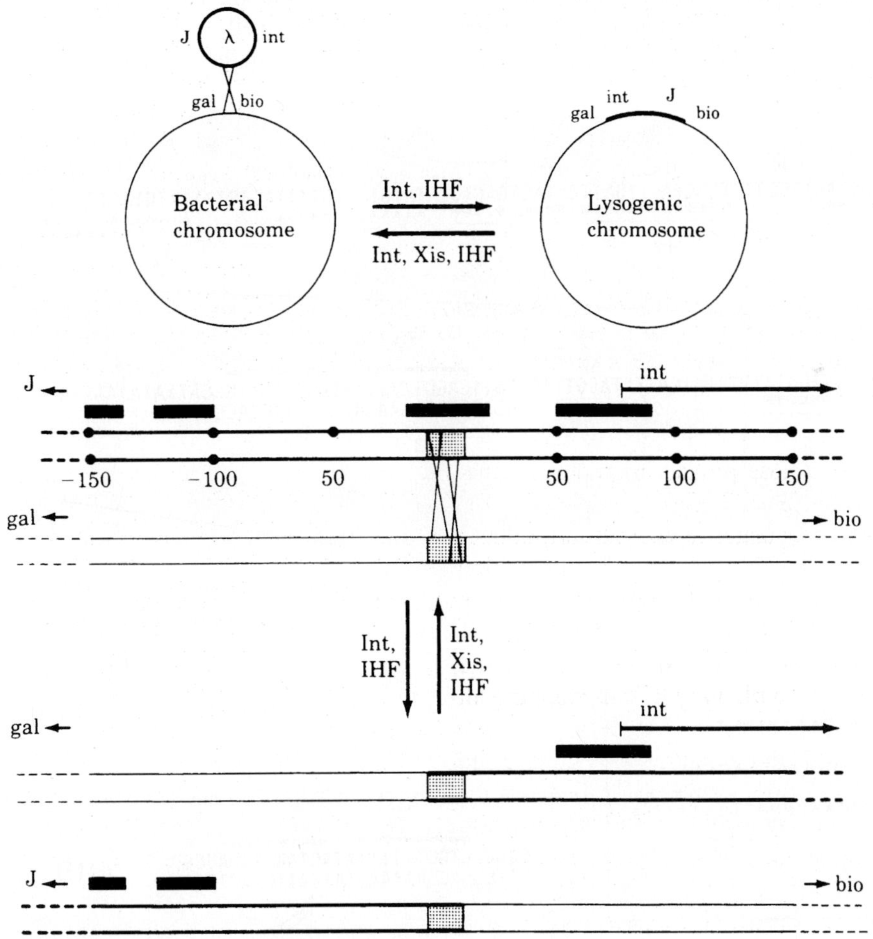

FIG. 6. Insertion of λ DNA into the bacterial chromosome. **Top:** Overall process. **Bottom:** Detail of action at the crossover point. The 15-bp identity between phage and host DNA is *stippled.* The *heavy bars* overlying the phage DNA are Int-binding sites. The 3′ end of the *int* gene overlaps the right site. (Reproduced from ref. 14, with permission.)

leftward promoter *p*L and a CII-activated promoter *p*I. The latter is the important promoter for lysogenization. Its control by CII ensures that insertion occurs in those cells where repression is established.

Integrase promotes reciprocal recombination between sites on phage and host DNA, which inserts the phage DNA into the continuity of the host chromosome. The recombination occurs within a 15-bp sequence that is identical in phage and host. Both *in vivo* and *in vitro*, the minimal length of specific sequence required in the *attB* partner is 21 bp, and that in the *attP* partner is about 240 bp. A linear *attB* molecule functions *in vitro*, but *attP* must be supercoiled for optimal activity.

Integrase has two DNA binding sites. The strong binding sites (in the N-terminal part of the molecule) recognize arm sites, which are located on *attP* at positions –130, –80, +60, +70, and +80 (where 0 is the center of the 15-bp identity) (Fig. 7). Integrase molecules bound to these sites on DNA, bent appropriately by the host-encoded DNA bending integration host factor (IHF) protein, are so positioned that they can bind (in their C-terminal domains) to core sites, which are symmetrically disposed about the crossover point and approach the consensus 5′CAACTTNNT3′. Core sites are present in both *attP* and *attB*. The actual crossover then takes place by an exchange on the left between the "top" strands of the two double helices to create a Holliday junction, and resolution by exchange between the bottom two strands. The nicking site in the top strands is 7 bp to the left of the nicking site in the bottom strands. The process was once imagined to require branch migration of the Holliday junction between the two sites. However, recent data favor strand swapping between nicking and sealing, so that the Holliday structure exists only at the midpoint between the two sites (55). The left-right orientation here is determined by the positions of the arm sites on the *attP* partner, not by the core sequences themselves (41). Host and phage sites are aligned by protein–protein and DNA–protein interaction, and DNA–DNA recognition is restricted to the 7-bp overlap segment where branch migration occurs.

Commitment to lysogeny is further reinforced by a third CII-activated promoter *p*AQ, located within gene *Q* reading leftward. By inhibiting *Q* translation, this antisense transcript apparently minimizes *Q*-promoted late gene transcription characteristic of the lytic cycle.

Lysogeny

Once established, the lysogenic state is quite stable. Lysogenic cells divide to give lysogenic progeny. Lysogeny can break down either through spontaneous

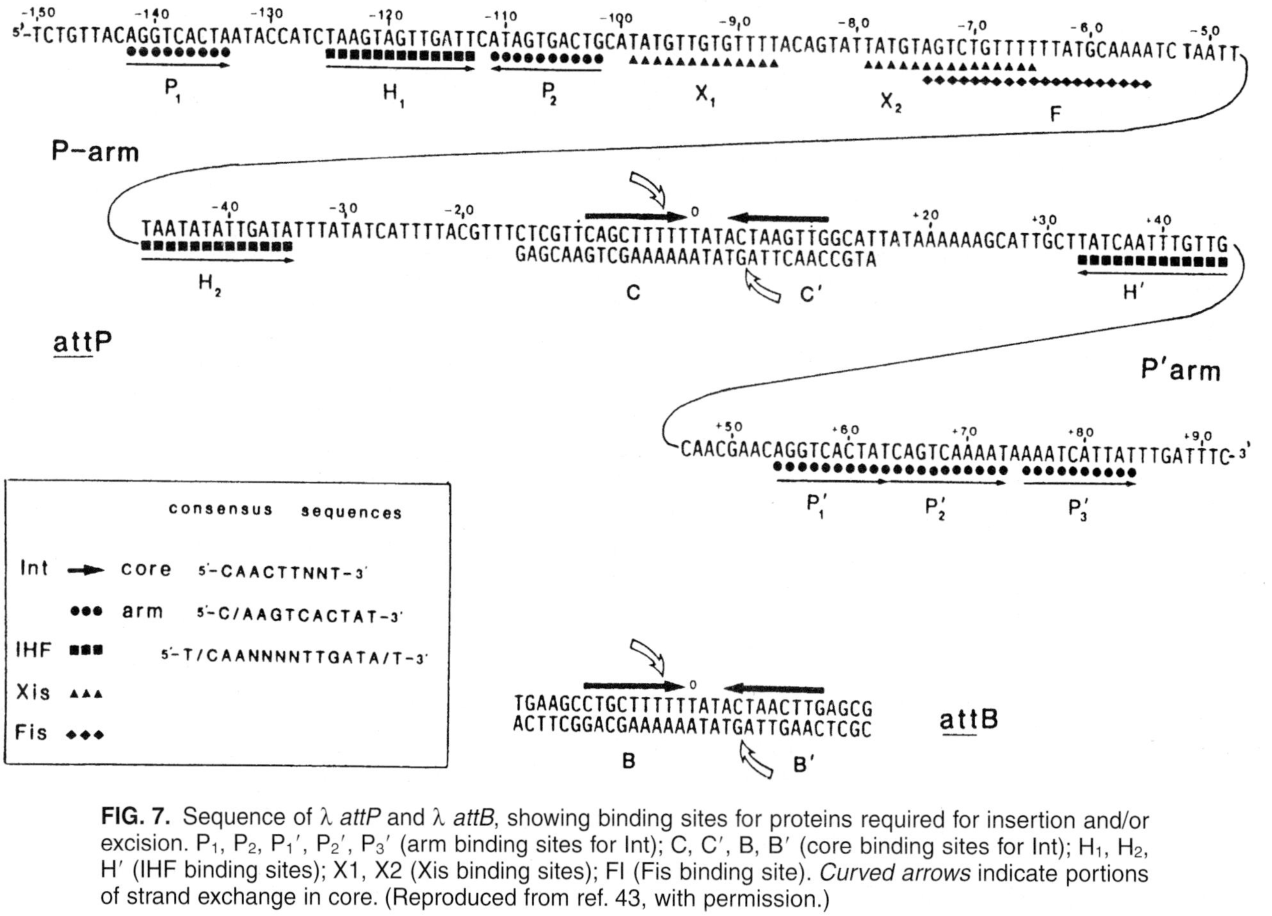

FIG. 7. Sequence of λ *attP* and λ *attB*, showing binding sites for proteins required for insertion and/or excision. P_1, P_2, P_1', P_2', P_3' (arm binding sites for Int); C, C′, B, B′ (core binding sites for Int); H_1, H_2, H′ (IHF binding sites); X1, X2 (Xis binding sites); FI (Fis binding site). *Curved arrows* indicate portions of strand exchange in core. (Reproduced from ref. 43, with permission.)

switching to the lytic cycle (which happens about once every 10^4 cell divisions in an actively growing culture) or by spontaneous loss of prophage with cell survival (which happens less than once every 10^6 cell divisions). As long as repressor is present, *cI* transcription from *p*M continues, and more repressor is made. If repressor concentration rises so high as to saturate *o*R3, then repressor synthesis ceases until it returns to a lower level. Likewise, once the prophage is stably inserted into the chromosome, it remains so; there is a low rate of integrase synthesis from the *p*I promoter (not activated by CII) but essentially no excisionase (a phage-coded protein required for excision, though not for insertion).

Some ancillary factors reinforce this stability. One of these is the need for antitermination by gpN to initiate lytic development. This requirement puts a double lock on the system, because any transcripts made during a momentary unblocking of the operator sites will not get anywhere until the gpN that has been made by the first transcript can extend other transcripts. Because gpN is unstable and accidents should be rare, this will seldom happen. Stabilization of lysogeny is one reason that has been suggested for the use by λ of antitermination (rather than simply mutating the termination sites). Poising the lysis/lysogeny decision to depend on molecular fluctuations may be another reason.

Escape from Lysogeny

About once every 10^4 cell divisions, stability breaks down. Detailed knowledge of what happens in those rare cells is unavailable, but the rate is strongly depressed in *recA*⁻ hosts. This fact suggests that these spontaneous transitions to lytic development have the same primary basis as the mass induction of this transition by exposure to ultraviolet light or other DNA-damaging agents. In that case, the initial event is the activation of the proteolytic activity of RecA protein by products of DNA degradation, such as single-stranded DNA. RecA is not a conventional protease, but it accelerates the specific cleavage of the host LexA protein, which can autocatalyze the same cleavage under extreme conditions. LexA is a repressor for many DNA repair functions, and RecA-promoted LexA cleavage turns these genes on. Like LexA, λ repressor is sensitive to RecA-enhanced autoproteolysis (45).

RecA activation is one means of inducing the switch to lysis in almost all cells of a lysogenic culture. Another method makes use of λ *cIts* mutants, which form a thermolabile repressor. With an appropriate mutant, lysogeny is quite stable at 30°C, but a shift to 43°C rapidly inactivates repressor in all cells. After derepression, transcription initiates from *p*L and *p*R. One early consequence of *p*L transcription is excision of the prophage from the chromosome. Whereas insertion requires only one phage-coded protein, integrase, excision requires a second protein, excisionase, as well. Excisionase is encoded by a gene *xis*, upstream from *int* and overlapping it by 20 bp. The CII-dependent *p*I promoter used during lysogenization lies at the 5′ end of *xis*, and the start site is within *xis* so that the *p*I transcript makes only integrase. From the *p*L transcript, *int* and *xis* are expressed coordinately.

The mechanism of excisionase (Xis) action is not fully understood. Excisionase binds to two specific sites in the left arm of *attR*, bends the DNA, and interacts with integrase; one of the two excisionase molecules can be replaced by a host DNA-bending protein, Fis. Conventional enzymes are pure catalysts, and the nature of the catalysts cannot determine the direction of the reaction. Superficially, excisionase appears to reverse the integrase reaction; however, in excision as in insertion, cutting and resealing on the left precede cutting on the right; therefore, excision is not a true reversal of insertion. What remains unsolved is why integrase alone fails to promote the true reversal.

The *p*L transcript is subject to posttranscriptional control. In infected cells, either before commitment or after commitment to lysis, *int* and *xis* are cotranscribed; however, little integrase is made. This is because of exonucleolytic (3′ → 5′) degradation of the transcript after cleavage by host enzyme RNase III at a site (*sib*) downstream of *att*. This process (retroregulation) prevents untimely or wasteful synthesis of integrase. Retroregulation does not affect *p*L transcripts made from a derepressed prophage, because the *sib* site is at the other end of the prophage. It also does not affect *p*I transcripts, which terminate within *sib* and therefore are resistant to RNase III. Because the *p*L transcript is made by an RNA polymerase molecule operating in the antitermination mode and reading through *sib*, it is degraded; this is another function for antitermination in the λ life cycle. Despite the elegance and apparent utility of the retroregulation mechanism, deletion or mutation of the *sib* site has no observed effect on λ development as normally studied in the laboratory.

The potentiality of controlling insertion and excision differentially provides a rationale for the use of arm sites by λ integrase. Some related site-specific recombinases recognize only core sites, but in those cases there is no recognition of directionality.

When lytic development is induced in a lysogen, a small fraction (about 10^{-5}) of the particles produced result from abnormal excision that follows from breakage and joining of DNA at sites other than the *att* sites. If the excised DNA includes the *cos* sites and is within the packaging limits of the λ virion, it can be packaged and used to infect other cells. Thus, a lysate produced by induction can transfer host genes that lie close to the λ insertion site (such as *gal* or *bio*) into recipient cells. This specialized transduction is a form of natural cloning. The transduced bacterial DNA segment need not replace its homolog in the recipient; instead, the cell becomes lyso-

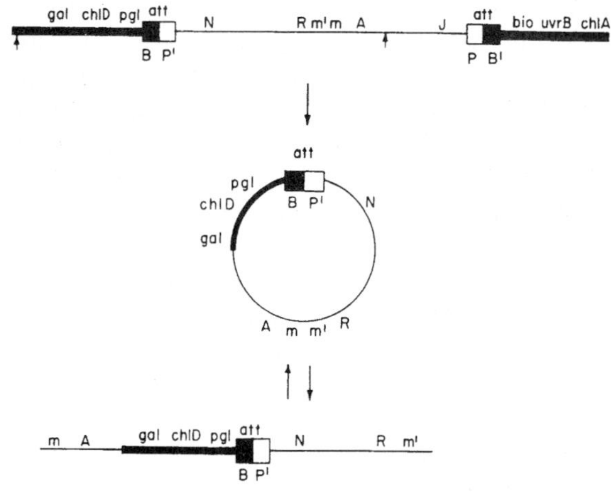

FIG. 8. Genesis of λ *gal* specialized transducing phage. *Arrows* indicate positions of breaking and joining of heterologous DNA in a particular isolate. The m and m′ indicate the ends of mature λ DNA (equivalent to *cos*). (Reproduced from ref. 14, with permission.)

genic for the specialized transducing phage and is diploid for the transduced segment (Figs. 8 and 9).

The genesis of specialized transducing phages may be comparable to the acquisition of oncogenes by retroviruses. Although the mechanisms may differ substantially, specialized transduction has provided a useful model because the entire process can be followed in the laboratory. With retroviruses, until very recently the critical events have generally occurred in nature from progenitors of inferred structure.

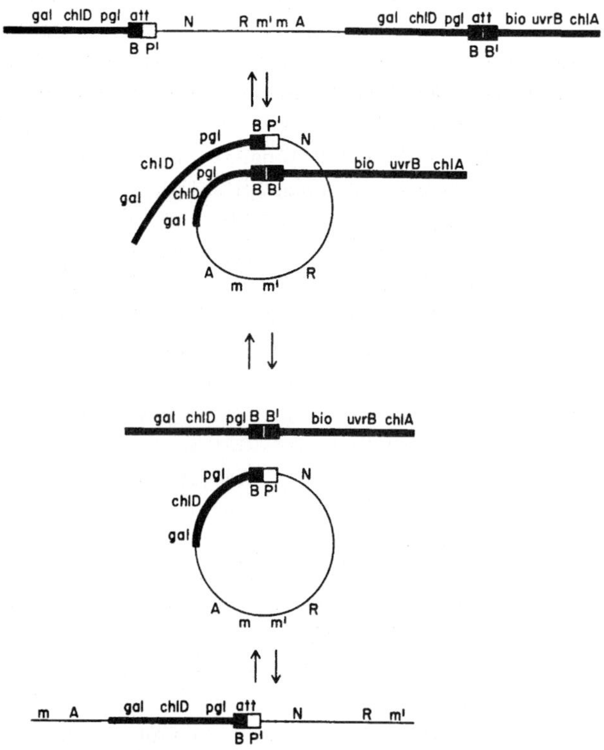

FIG. 9. Lysogenization by λ *gal* (*bottom line*) to produce a heterogenote with two copies of *gal* separated by λ DNA. (Reproduced from ref. 14, with permission.)

Lytic Development

Lytic development can be studied either in infected cells or in derepressed lysogens. Because of the high degree of synchrony obtainable, the method of choice has usually been thermal induction of lysogens carrying *cIts* prophages. The genetic program and its readout are well understood. At early times, most transcription is from *p*L and *p*R. The only protein of the *p*L transcript that is essential for lytic development is gpN. The pR transcript contains three important genes: *O* and *P* (replication) and *Q* (late gene activation). As time proceeds, gpQ accumulates and causes antitermination of the short transcript starting at *p*R′ (downstream from *Q*). The mechanism of antitermination differs from that performed by gpN. The recognition elements for antitermination overlap the promoter. *Q* antitermination also requires a pause site close to the start site. The gpQ binds to the complex of DNA and paused σ70-containing RNA polymerase, and it replaces σ70 in the complex. The gpQ-containing polymerase then transcribes downstream DNA without stopping at ordinary termination signals (60).

At any rate, as gpQ accumulates, transcription of genes for lysis and virion formation becomes increasingly rapid. Concurrently, the rate of transcription from *p*L and *p*R decreases as Cro accumulates, producing an orderly transition from early gene expression to late gene expression.

Bidirectional DNA replication initiates from an origin within gene *O*. The gpO protein recognizes the origin and also recognizes gpP, which in turn recruits the host DnaB helicase into the initiation complex. Disassembly of the initiation complex to leave an elongation complex requires three host heat shock proteins (DnaJ, DnaK, and GrpE). Elongation proceeds, as in the host, by the combined action of DnaB helicase, DnaG primase, and Pol III holoenzyme, the polymerase. Theta-form replication can reproduce monomer circles, but a switch to rolling circle replication occurs in some molecules. λ rolling circle replication (which predominates at late times) differs from that of φX in two major respects. First, the tails are double stranded rather than single stranded because lagging-strand synthesis takes place on the displaced strand. Second, tails can grow to multigenomic lengths rather than stopping when a single genome has been spun off.

Multigenomic tails are the primary substrates for λ packaging. Empty proheads are first assembled, composed mainly of the major capsid protein gpE. Later, DNA enters the prohead, which increases in size and becomes more conspicuously icosahedral, and the smaller decoration protein gpD is added to the shell, with gpD hexamers interspersed among gpE trimers in a T=7 arrangement.

Efficient DNA packaging requires the presence of specific sequences (called *cos*, for cohesive site) at both ends of the packaged genome; hence, multigenomic tails or multimeric circles are good packaging substrates and monomer circles are poor ones. Cutting at *cos* is effected by a heterodimeric protein, terminase, whose subunits are encoded by λ genes *Nul* and *A*. DNA molecules are packaged from left to right so a DNA monomer can be cut from the concatemer at its left end early in packaging and at its right end after the DNA has entered the virion. The *cos* site (about 200 bp in length) has three components: a binding site (*cos*B), recognized by gpNul before the DNA is cut at either end; a nicking site (*cos*N), at which DNA is cut at sites 12 bp apart in the two strands to generate the packaged single-strand overhangs of virion DNA; and a termination site (*cos*Q), required for the final nicking at the right end (20). Packaging is processive. After one genome is packaged, the next genome to the right can be packaged with no requirement for recognition of *cos*B on the second or subsequent genomes (27).

Because λ packages the DNA between two *cos* sites, the amount of DNA per head can be changed by deletions or insertions (as in T7). The packaging limits are from about 79% to 110% of normal λ length. Internal *cos* sites artificially placed within λ at less than or near the lower limit can be packaged uncut, as though scanning for *cos* sites becomes more efficient as the head fills. λ-based *in vitro* packaging systems have been used for efficient delivery of *cos*-containing plasmid-cloning vectors (cosmids) into *E. coli* cells.

Table 2 indicates the packaging limits for some phages described in this chapter. Those with headful packaging are listed with the same upper and lower limits. In fact, there is some random variation around the mean value. Alternative forms with different head sizes, such as the isometric and giant particles of T4 or the λ virions formed by D^- mutants, are not considered.

Genome Organization

The functional clustering of genes on the λ map is notable. Not only do genes acting in a single pathway (head formation, tail formation, replication) lie together on the map, but genes for DNA binding lie close to their target sites, products of adjacent genes in a cluster frequently interact directly, and even within genes determinants are ordered so that they lie close to the elements with which they interact. For example, the *cos*B site is at the end of *cos*, next to the *Nul* gene whose product recognizes *cos*B; *Nul* in turn lies next to *A*, whose product forms the terminase heterodimer with gpNul. In both head and tail clusters, the same tendency is observed, the tail fiber gene *J* being most distal from the head cluster. The *att* site is adjacent to the *int* gene, and *cI* and *cro* are close to their target sites. The N-terminus of gpO recognizes the *ori* site that lies within the 5′ end of *O*, whereas the C-terminus interacts with the product of the adjacent *P* gene. The clustering of major functional groups could increase regulatory efficiency, but the finer orderings may be more related to the disruptive effect of recombination on coevolved functions.

Phage Mu-1 as a Model Transposon

Mu-1 first attracted attention as a phage capable of inducing bacterial mutations at a high rate. The mutations proved to be insertions of Mu-1 into random sites on the host chromosome, disrupting the genes or operons into which it inserted.

Like λ, Mu-1 can follow two alternative developmental pathways, leading on the one hand to a transcriptionally quiescent prophage and on the other to a lytic cycle with replication, packaging, and lysis. In λ, the DNA transactions in these two pathways are distinct. Insertion plays no role in λ replication, which proceeds normally if either the *int* gene or the *att* sites are deleted. With Mu-1, on the other hand, replication and insertion are minor variations of a common pathway, transposition. In Mu-1 replication, transposition happens many times during each cycle of infection, which has made it a system of choice for studying the biochemistry of transposition (compared with most bacterial transposons, which transpose naturally at rates such as 10^{-6} per cell division).

Mu-1 DNA is inserted into host DNA at all stages of its life cycle, even in the virion. When linear DNA from the virion is injected into a cell and the Mu-specific trans-

TABLE 2. *DNA cutting and packaging*

Phage	Packaging substrate	First cut	Second cut	Packaging limits (% of genome)
T4	Concatemer	Random	Headful	102
P22	Concatemer	*pac* site	Headful	109
λ	Concatemer	*cos* site	*cos* site	79–110
T7	Concatemer	Terminal overlap	Terminal repeat	85–103
φX174	Dimer ss of rolling circle	Replication origin	Replication origin	Limited
M13	Dimer ss of rolling circle	Replication origin	Replication origin	Unlimited
Mu-1	Inserted monomer	Near left end	Headful	105
P1	Concatemer	*pac* site	Headful	110

posase is made, the first step in replication is transposition of Mu-1 DNA into the chromosome. Among bacterial transposons, the transposition mechanism may be either replicative (generating transposon copies in both the donor and the target site) or conservative (excising the transposon from the donor and inserting it into the target site). In cells destined to become lysogenic, the initial transposition is conservative rather than replicative. In cells destined to lyse, Mu-1 undergoes repeated rounds of replicative transposition.

The initial steps of replicative and conservative transposition are the same. The 3′ end of the two transposon strands undergo strand transfer reactions with target DNA at positions displaced by five base pairs. Replication then initiates from the recessed 3′ ends of the target DNA. In conservative transposition, the nicked donor DNA adjacent to the transposon is cut in the other strand and digested away; replication fills the gap, and ligation incorporates the parental transposon bodily into the target site (Fig. 10). In replicative transposition, the donor

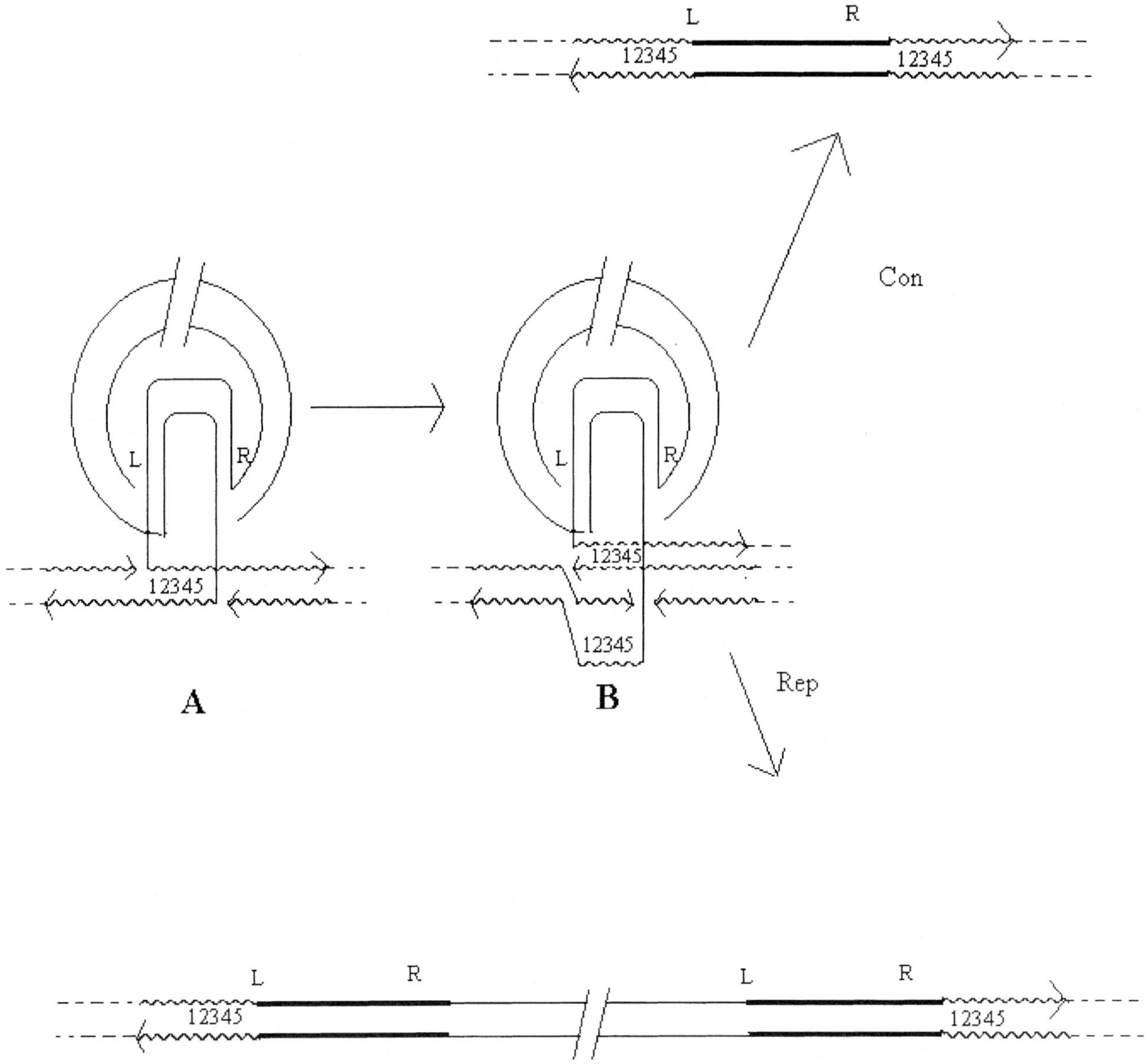

FIG. 10. Transposition of Mu phage. **A:** The stage immediately following strand transfer. **B:** The oligonucleotide sequence (12345) of the target molecule has been replicated. In conservative transposition (Con), the donor DNA is digested away and the Mu DNA is inserted into the target DNA, flanked by a direct oligonucleotide repeat; this is the usual fate of infecting DNA, where the donor is linear DNA (Mu and some flanking host sequence). In replicative transposition (Rep), replication from the 3′ ends shown in (**B**) continues through the Mu, terminating with ligation to the free 5′ end of donor DNA. This is the mechanism of Mu replication in the infected cell, where donor and target DNAs (both circular) are derived from the host chromosome. Mu DNA, with left and right ends indicated; , donor DNA; , target DNA.

strands remain attached to the 5′ transposon ends, and replication proceeds through the transposon with ligation to the free 5′ donor ends at the opposite end of the transposon. This produces two semiconserved transposon copies, each joined to donor DNA at one end and target DNA at the other (52). Replicative transposition from a chromosomal donor produces two inserted copies accompanied by chromosomal rearrangement (inversion or excision); if replicative transposition happened from a linear infecting molecule (unaccompanied by subsequent recombination), it would linearize the chromosome.

In Mu-1 packaging, the left end of the inserted DNA is recognized, and cutting takes place within the flanking DNA, 50 to 150 bp to the left of the left end. Packaging is then by headfuls, and the headful length is longer than the genome length. Therefore, 500 to 3,000 bp of DNA on the right end of the virion molecule is host DNA. Thus virion DNA molecules have random segments of host DNA at their termini. When virion DNA is separated into single strands and reannealed, the host sequences are visibly unpaired when viewed in the electron microscope.

An internal segment of Mu-1 DNA about 3 kb in length is invertible through the action of a phage-coded integrase, so reannealed molecules are sometimes unpaired in this segment as well. The gene for the tail fiber protein spans one boundary of the invertible segments so that two types of tail fibers with different host specificities can be formed, depending on the orientation. Thus, if Mu-1 grown on *E. coli* K-12 encounters an alternative host such as *Citrobacter*, the rare particle that attaches to *Citrobacter* can invade and replicate. The rate of inversion is about 10^{-5} per generation. Certain other phages, such as P1, have related invertible segments.

In lysogens, inserted Mu-1 can occasionally transpose without induction of a full lytic cycle. Thus, inserted Mu-1 behaves in all respects as a bacterial transposon.

Phage P1 as a Model Plasmid

The P1 virion contains about 100 kb of linear double-stranded DNA in an isometric T=16 capsid. As in T4, the DNA is cyclically permuted and terminally redundant. Unlike T4 (but like *Salmonella* phage P22, a relative of λ), processive packaging does not initiate at random but instead at specific *pac* sites. After infection, reciprocal recombination within the terminal overlap creates a circular DNA molecule of about 90 kb. Some of this recombination is mediated by a site-specific recombinase (Cre) whose target site (*lox*) is close to the *pac* site. The Cre–*lox* system has proven useful for generating controlled deletions and rearrangements during development of multicellular eukaryotes.

The cell can now enter either a lytic cycle or a lysogenic cycle. Unlike λ or Mu-1, the lysogenic alternative entails replication of the circular P1 DNA as a plasmid and therefore requires expression of phage-coded replication genes. In lysogens, P1 is maintained at low copy number (about one per chromosome) and has an efficient partitioning mechanism so that both daughters of a dividing cell receive a P1 copy. The mechanism is similar to that used by other stringently controlled low copy number plasmids, such as the fertility factor F, and in some respects to that of the bacterial chromosome. The partitioning mechanism could potentially become ineffective if homologous recombination created a dimeric molecule, which could not pass into both daughter cells; this problem is greatly diminished by the site-specific *lox*–Cre recombination, which rapidly and reversibly equilibrates monomers with dimers. The elements for replication and partitioning (except *lox*–Cre) are localized in 1.5 kb of P1 DNA that can replicate as a plasmid when circularized; it includes a specific replication origin (*oriR*), its cognate replication initiator (*repA*), and a DNA sequence (*incA*) that controls replication by binding and sequestering *repA* (72).

In cells destined to lyse, P1 DNA replication (like that of λ) proceeds in both a theta form and a rolling circle mode, the latter providing the packaging substrate. The replication origin used is distinct from the plasmid origin *oriR*. Rare mistakes lead to occasional packaging of random fragments of host DNA instead of phage DNA. Such fragments are responsible for the generalized transduction of bacterial genes. Generalized transduction at detectable frequencies is observed for most phages that use headful packaging, but not by wild-type λ, probably because in λ both cutting (at both ends) and injection require the specific *cosN* sequence, whereas in P1 or P22 initial cutting at sequences resembling *pac* sites can initiate processive packaging. Mutations that relax the specificity and thereby increase the frequency of transduction have been isolated in both P22 and P1 (63,71).

DEFECTIVE PHAGES AND PHAGELIKE OBJECTS

The fact that Mu-1 can behave as a transposon and P1 as a plasmid underscores some of the commonality between phages and nonviral elements. Transposable elements are common in bacteria, and most of them seem to use a biochemistry similar to that of Mu-1. Most bacterial transposons are smaller than Mu-1, going down to simple insertion sequences a few hundred base pairs long; and typical transposons carry genes affecting conspicuous bacterial traits such as antibiotic resistance (15). Transposition is usually conservative for some elements, replicative for others. Those using replicative transposition frequently resolve the resulting cointegrate structures through use of a site-specific recombinase that acts on a sequence internal to the element. Some transposons integrate and excise by a recombination mechanism similar in some respects to λ insertion (64).

Bacterial plasmids fall into two general groups: elements with small genomes, present in many copies per cell and replicating randomly with respect to the cell division cycle, and larger elements similar in size to phage P1, present in one or a few copies per cell and partitioned regularly at cell division. Conjugative plasmids resemble viruses as autonomous elements capable of infecting cells, but they differ from them in the absence of an extracellular phase.

DNA sequences closely related to those of temperate phages are found in the genomes of many natural bacteria. For example, Southern hybridization of enteric bacteria with λ DNA usually turns up some λ-related sequences (59). Most of these are probably defective prophages: remnants of previous lysogenization that have since lost phage function through deletion or mutation. The K-12 strain of *E. coli* is naturally lysogenic for λ but also harbors four λ-related elements: DLP12, Rac, e14, and Qin. Such elements could in principle be of some value to the host or could even be precursors rather than descendants of complete phages; however, each defective prophage contains an array of genes from different functional clusters of the phage genome, frequently in the same order found in active phages, so that a role as host elements seems contrived. Defective lysogens arise from active lysogens in the laboratory by prophage mutations, and they frequently retain superinfection immunity, SOS-induced lysis, and production of structures resembling phage heads, tails, or complete virions.

Many natural strains liberate (or produce on induction) such phagelike or phage-related particles, which have not been shown to be infectious. Many bacteria also produce proteins (bacteriocins) that are toxic to other strains of the same bacterial species but not to the producing strain. Bacteriocins are sometimes encoded on plasmids and act through diverse mechanisms. Operationally, some phagelike objects qualify as bacteriocins.

For example, many natural strains of *Bacillus subtilis* and several other *Bacillus* species harbor a prophage-like element, phage of *Bacillus subtilis* (PBS), that has been localized on the chromosome. After SOS induction, the cells lyse and liberate many virion-like particles with tails and DNA-filled heads. This is not simply a phage whose sensitive host remains to be discovered, because the large majority of particles contain random segments of host DNA with no significant preference for packaging prophage DNA. Like a bacteriocin, these particles kill other *Bacillus* cells. The producing strain is resistant, at least sometimes because the particles fail to be adsorbed. There are several varieties of PBS, each with a different killing specificity (76).

PBS has some similarity to mutants of generalized transducing phages that have lost (in this case, completely) their extreme preference for initiating packaging at phage-specified *pac* sites. Its wide distribution and the variety of killing specificities suggest that the bacteriocin-like activity confers a selective advantage to the host. Inasmuch as some bacteriocins are single protein molecules, a DNA-filled virion seems an especially clumsy and expensive kind of bacteriocin to have been so successful in evolution.

EVOLUTION AND NATURAL BIOLOGY OF PHAGES

For historical reasons, the coliphages have become workhorses of molecular biology and remain among the most thoroughly understood biologic objects. Phages are found throughout the prokaryotic world in a variety comparable with that of eukaryotic viruses, including enveloped virions with double-stranded RNA genomes (69), linear DNA genomes with protein covalently bound to their 5′ ends (61), and satellite viruses like P4 [which forms virions with the capsid protein of its helper virus P2, induces late gene function from P2 prophage, lysogenizes P2 lysogens using its own integrase but can establish a plasmid state in P2 nonlysogens, and represses its own genes by the use of antisense RNA rather than a protein repressor (45)]. Compared with our knowledge of phage development in infected cells, little is known about their natural ecology or population biology. Some aspects are worthy of note.

Abundance

In some natural environments, phagelike particles are much more numerous than one might suspect from plaque assays on susceptible hosts. In estuaries, concentrations as high as 10^8 have been reported. If most of these are infectious (and they may very well not be), they potentially could play a major role in the natural cycling of the biosphere (31).

Host Defense Mechanisms

Bacteria have evolved mechanisms for phage resistance, and phages have evolved counterstrategies, presumably indicating in some measure the significant impact that phage infection can have. A host defense mechanism unique to prokaryotes is restriction/modification. Restriction enzymes damage DNA that has not undergone chemical modification at specific sites (most frequently methylation) by cleaving it either at those sites or nearby; nonspecific exonucleases then degrade the resulting linear fragments. Cells protect their own DNA from the restriction enzymes they make by modifying it. A phage that escapes restriction becomes modified and is fully infectious on a restricting host in the next cycle; so the strategy can be effective for the host only if the strains sensitive to a given phage have various restriction specificities. A strain with a rare restriction specificity will exclude almost all phage it encounters and will be favored over one with a common specificity; so eventually the rare specificity will become common. The recognition sites for restriction enzymes are frequently symmetrical, even if the cleavage takes place at a variable distance from the recognition site; this allows the modification of either strand to prevent cleavage, which ensures that, during semiconservative replication, a new strand that has not yet been modified is protected from destruction.

Phages have many strategies for avoiding restriction. The first level is a paucity of recognition sequence. Phages of *Bacillus*, where many known restriction enzymes recognize four-base palindromes, have few such palindromes in their DNA; coliphages are deficient in six-base palindromes, which are sites for some of the enzymes they naturally encounter (38). Various phages also have enzymes that destroy 5-adenosylmethionine, a cofactor for restriction (T3), expedite modification of phage DNA before restriction enzymes can cleave (λ), or block recognition sites by wholesale nonspecific DNA modification (T4).

Some restriction enzymes are encoded by chromosomal genes, but many are encoded by phages or plasmids. Many resistance mechanisms contributing to defense of the host may in fact be manifestations of competition between extrachromosomal elements preserving their cellular territories.

One element may exclude others by diverse mechanisms, and in many cases exclusion may be an incidental side effect of the phage life cycle. The repressors of temperate prophages (essential for the internal stability of lysogens) render the lysogens immune to superinfection by phage of the carried type, and this superinfection immunity probably selects for diversification of repressor specificities. Certain phages, such as the ε phages of *Salmonella*, encode enzymes that alter the polysaccharide surface receptors used in phage attachment, so that lysogens not only are immune but also cannot be penetrated by DNA of the same type. The alteration also takes place during the lytic cycle and reduces phage loss from attachment to fragments of cell envelope after lysis. The λ-related phage HKO22 has a variant of the λ*N* gene that competes with λ*N* when λ infects an HKO22 lysogen and causes termination rather than antitermination of early λ transcripts (55). The λ Rex proteins trigger a collapse of membrane potential when a λ lysogen is infected with certain other phages (such as T4 *rII* mutants), preventing the production of viral progeny (57). The Lit protease (encoded by the defective λ-related prophage e14) is activated by the major head protein of T4 to hydrolyze its specific substrate, elongation factor Ef-Tu (30). These last three mechanisms do not protect the infected cell but may protect other cells in a colony by impeding viral replication.

Natural Recombination

Third, the study of natural isolates has provided some perspectives on variation and the recombination among phages in nature. The λ-related (lambdoid) phages are a good example.

The way that phage workers have approached taxonomy differs substantially from the method used by many medical virologists. In medical virology, once a virus such as measles is identified as a disease agent, many isolates from different clinical sources are examined, and those sharing some acceptable degree of similarity to the type virus are classified as measles virus. For epidemiology, some such approach is necessary. Phage workers are not epidemiologists, and their interest in natural variation is relatively recent. Many investigators have been more interested in developing highly defined experimental systems. To that end, each isolate is given its own name. λ refers only to the prophage present in *E. coli* K-12 and its laboratory descendants; K-12 refers to one bacterial isolate, not to other natural strains with similar properties. Workers with a different perspective might have classified all lambdoid phages as natural variants of λ, and the same can be said of other phage groups such as T2, T4, and T6.

The lambdoid phages have a common genetic map and the ability to generate viable hybrids when crossed in the laboratory. They came from various sources (usually from lysogenic bacteria) isolated over the past 70 years from Europe, Asia, and the United States. Genetic variation among the lambdoid phages is apparent from both functional specificity and DNA sequence. For example, phages with at least a dozen repressor specificities have been isolated; where the sequences are known, homologies between heterospecific repressor genes are barely discernible. Phages with different repressors have corresponding differences in their *cro* genes and operator sites.

Lambdoid phages also exhibit major variations in virion structure. Those phages (such as λ) that plate on *E. coli* K-12 have long, flexible tails terminating in a single fiber that attaches to the *malB* chemotaxis protein of the outer membrane. Phages such as P22 (from *Salmonella*) have short, stubby tails and attach to the lipopolysaccharide 0-antigen of smooth strains of *Enterobacteria*, including *E. coli* (22). And in certain phage heads (such as HK97's), morphologically similar to that of λ, the major capsid proteins are covalently joined into multimers that are catenated to create an indissoluble chainmail configuration (24).

If the λ sequence is compared with that of any other lambdoid phage (or, equivalently, if heteroduplexes of the two phages are constructed), the general result is that the sequences match closely in some parts of the genome, whereas homologies are weak or absent in others. This is not because some sequences are highly conserved, because another phage pair shows a different set of matching segments; instead, the whole pattern strongly indicates that it is generated by frequent natural recombination so that in any phage pair, some portions of their genomes are of recent common ancestry. When defective prophages are compared with known lambdoid phages, they likewise are closely related to different phages in different segments. For example, the defective prophage DLP12 has an *int* gene and a partially deleted *xis* gene related to phage P22, followed by segments homologous to λ's *exo* and P/*ren* genes, followed by analogs (*qsr'*) of λ QSR unrelated to any known λ phage, followed by *cos* DNA similar to λ's. Thus, all the lambdoid phages, including the defective prophages, seem to be drawn from a common gene pool.

Among the lambdoid phages, some genes that may serve viral functions have been borrowed from outside the λ pool. Gene 12 of P22 occupies the same position in the genome as λ gene P, but gene 12 is a homolog of the bacterial *dnaB* gene, and λ gpP recruits the host DnaB helicase to participate in phage replication. Wild-type λ has a gene for side tail fibers (*stf*) that facilitate phage attachment. (In the λ commonly used in laboratories, *stf* has been inactivated by a frameshift.) The *stf* gene is closely related to tail fiber genes of other groups of coliphages (32). Most lambdoid phages encode a true lysozyme that hydrolyzes glycosidic bonds; λ makes instead a transglycosylase that attacks the same bonds but has no detectable homology to lysozyme (75). The λ lysozyme may have been appropriated from some external source, as yet unidentified.

Sequence comparisons of a wide variety of phages and prophages indicate that most double-stranded DNA phage genomes are chimeric products of both ongoing and ancient gene exchange (34). Thus, even apparently unrelated phages seem to have occasionally drawn genes from a common pool.

The natural function of genetic recombination is not obvious. In λ, as in sexual eukaryotes, it is clear that recombination has a substantial evolutionary impact. But that does not tell us at what level natural selection acts to preserve recombination as a process, or whether recombination is an accidental byproduct of gene activities selected to function in repair or replication. One classic argument for the value of recombination is that an asexual line deteriorates through accumulation of deleterious mutations, which can be corrected by recombination with other lines that are the wild type for the loci of those particular mutations (53). The first experimental demonstration of this Muller's ratchet effect came from phage ϕ6 (18); corroborative evidence from animal viruses has since appeared (23). Muller's ratchet may be central to the evolution of certain human viruses such as influenza, where the clonally selected epidemic strains are eventually replaced by reassortants with avian viruses.

In their natural ecology, phages exhibit many of the same features observed in eukaryotic viruses, and they will probably find increasing use as model systems.

PHAGE-BORNE GENES FOR BACTERIAL TOXINS AND OTHER PROTEINS AFFECTING HOST PHENOTYPE

In the prototypical temperate phages (λ, Mu), most of the genome (especially genes needed for lytic growth) is strongly down-regulated in the prophage. For this reason, lysogeny is generally not an overt property of a bacterial strain, and many natural bacteria harbor prophages that remain unrecognized unless they show inducible lysis (not seen with all temperate phages) or unless a phage-sensitive bacterial host is available. However, lysogeny by some phages markedly affects host phenotype—a phenomenon known as lysogenic conversion.

Lysogenic conversions frequently entail changes in the bacterial surface, and they sometimes affect the virulence of pathogenic bacteria. Their existence raises the questions of how the relevant genes became phage-associated, what advantage (if any) they confer on the phage, and how expression of the acquired genes is influenced by the phage's biology.

Gene Acquisition

The genesis of transducing phages by abnormal excision (see Fig. 8) is one way that a phage may acquirc host genes. This mode places the acquired genes next to the phage *att* site. Other genes (such as those for antibiotic resistance) may enter the phage genome in transposons. The phage-borne genes for some bacterial toxins (diphtheria, cholera) are adjacent to *att* sites, whereas others, such as Shiga toxin, are not.

Selective Value for the Phage

Some conversions (such as those described earlier by the λ phages of *Salmonella*) may benefit a phage by altering phage receptors on the bacterial surface. Some lambdoid phages have a gene (*nmpC*) with homology and partial functional equivalence to the major *E. coli* outer membrane protein gene *ompC* (whose product is a receptor for many phages). NmpC may replace OmpC, altering the cell's adsorption characteristics. Both these changes affect the antigenic specificity of the lysogen and could influence its ability to survive in a human host.

Phage λ makes two proteins (Bor and Lom) that may increase a lysogen's ability to colonize the human intestine, thereby indirectly expanding the phage's habitat.

Relation to Phage Biology

Most of the genes described previously are expressed in lysogens, using promoters distinct from those that transcribe phage genes. Thus the *bor* gene (see Fig. 5) is transcribed in the opposite direction from the λ late operon in which it is embedded. Transcription of the genes for diphtheria and cholera toxins is controlled by host transcription factors and is responsive to cues such as iron concentration.

Unlike most other temperate phages, the cholera phage (CTXϕ) is a single-stranded filamentous DNA phage similar to M13. Toxin expression from the integrated prophages is controlled by host factors (ToxR and ToxT). However, when phage replication is induced, the excised phage genome makes large amounts of toxin independently of ToxR and ToxT. The genes for Shiga toxin are in a lambdoid phage downstream of pR′ (see Fig. 5). Although they can be expressed in the prophage from an iron-regulated promoter, high-level expression requires induction of the phage lytic cycle with concomitant Q-mediated antitermination. Phage-mediated lysis may also promote the liberation of toxin into the medium (70). Thus the phage lytic cycle may contribute significantly to the pathogenesis of toxin-producing bacteria.

REFERENCES

1. Adelman K, Brody EN, Buckle M. Stimulation of bacteriophage T4 middle transcription by the proteases MutA and AsiA occurs at two distinct steps in the transcription cycle. *Proc Natl Acad Sci USA* 1998; 95:15247–15252.
2. Anderson TF. The reactions of bacterial viruses with their host cells. *Botan Rev* 1949;15:464–505.
3. Anderson TF, Doermann AH. The intracellular growth of bacteriophages II. The growth of T3 studied by sonic disintegration and by T6-cyanide lysis of infected cells. *J Gen Physiol* 1952;35:657–667.
4. Andrake M, Guild N, Hsu T, et al. DNA polymerase of bacteriophage T4 is an autogenous translational repressor. *Proc Natl Acad Sci U S A* 1988;85:7942–7946.
5. Aoyama A, Hamatake RK, Hayashi M. *In vitro* synthesis of bacteriophage ΠX174 by purified components. *Proc Natl Acad Sci U S A* 1983;80:4195–4199.
6. Arkin A, Ross J, McAdams HH. Stochastic kinetic analysis of development pathway bifurcation in phage λ-infected *Escherichia coli* cells. *Genetics* 1998;149:1633–1638.
7. Beckendorf SK. Structure of the distal half of the bacteriophage T4 tail fiber. *J Mol Biol* 1973;73:37–53.
8. Belfort M, Ehrenman K, Chandry PS. Genetic and molecular analysis of RNA splicing in *Escherichia coli. Methods Enzymol* 1990;181: 521–539.
9. Benzer S. The elementary units of heredity. In: McElroy WD, Glass B, eds. *The Chemical Basis of Heredity.* Baltimore: Johns Hopkins Press, 1957:76–93.
10. Benzer S. On the topology of the genetic fine structure. *Proc Natl Acad Sci U S A* 1959;45:1607–1620.
11. Bhattacharyya SP, Rao VB. A novel terminase activity associated with the DNA packaging protein gp17 of bacteriophage T4. *Virology* 1993;196:34–44.
12. Black L, Showe M. Morphogenesis of the T4 head. In: Mathews C, Kutter E, Mosig G, Berget P, eds. *Bacteriophage T4.* Washington, DC: ASM Publications, 1983:219–245.
13. Campbell A. Sensitive mutants of bacteriophage λ. *Virology* 1961;14: 22–32.
14. Campbell A. Genetic structure. In: Hershey AD, ed. *The Bacteriophage Lambda.* Cold Spring Harbor, NY: Cold Spring Harbor Laboratory, 1971:13–44.
15. Campbell A. Transposons and their evolutionary significance. In: Nei M, Koehn RK, eds. *Evolution of Genes and Proteins.* Sunderland, MA: Sinauer, 1983.
16. Campbell AM. Episomes. *Adv Genet* 1962;11:101–146.
17. Casjens S, Hendrix R. Control mechanisms in dsDNA bacteriophage assembly. In: Calendar R, ed. *The Bacteriophages.* New York: Plenum Press, 1988:15–91.
18. Chao L. Fitness of RNA virus decreased by Muller's ratchet. *Nature* 1990;348:454–455.
19. Chung Y-B, Nardone C, Hinkle DC. Bacteriophage T7 packaging. III. A "hairpin" end formed on T7 concatemers may be an intermediate in the primary reaction. *J Mol Biol* 1990;216:939–948.
20. Cue D, Feiss M. A site required for termination of packaging of the phage λ chromosome. *Proc Natl Acad Sci U S A* 1993;90:9290–9294.
21. D'Herelle F. Sur un microbe invisible antagonist des bacilles dysenterique. *Compt Rend Acad Sci* 1917;165:373–375.
22. Dhillon TS, Poon AP, Chan D, Clark AJ. General transducing phages like *Salmonella* phage P22 isolated using a smooth strain of *Eschericha coli* as host. *FEMS Microbiol Lett* 1998;161:129–133.
23. Duarte EA, Clarke DK, Moya A, et al. Many-trillionfold amplification of single RNA virus particles fails to overcome the Muller's ratchet effect. *J Virol* 1993;67:3620–3623.
24. Duda RL. Protein chainmail: Catenated protein in viral capsids. *Cell* 1998;94:55–60.
25. Dunn J, Studier W. Complete nucleotide sequence of bacteriophage T7 DNA and the location of T7 genetic elements. *J Mol Biol* 1983;166: 477–535.
26. Epstein RH, Bolle A, Steinberg CM, et al. Physiological studies of conditional lethal mutants of bacteriophage T4D. *Cold Spring Harb Symp Quant Biol* 1963;28:375–394.
27. Feiss M, Sippy J, Miller G. Processive action of terminase during sequential packaging of bacteriophage λ chromosomes. *J Mol Biol* 1985;186:759–771.
28. Franklin NC. Altered reading of genetic signals fused to the N operon of bacteriophage λ: genetic evidence for modification of polymerase by the protein product of the *N* gene. *J Mol Biol* 1974;89:33–48.
29. Geiduschek EP, Fu T-J, Kassavetes GA, et al. Transcripted activation by a topologically linkable protein: forging a connection between replication and gene activity. *Nucleic Acids Mol Biol* 1997;11:130–135.
30. Gieorgiu T, Yu Y-TN, Ekanwe S, et al. Specific peptide-activated proteolytic cleavage of *Escherichia coli* elongation factor Tu. *Proc Natl Acad Sci U S A* 1998;95:2891–2895.
31. Goyal SM, Gerba CP, Bitton G, eds. *Phage Ecology.* New York: John Wiley & Sons, 1987.
32. Haggard-Ljungquist E, Halling C, Calendar R. DNA sequences of the tail fiber genes of bacteriophage P2: Evidence for horizontal transfer of tail fiber genes among unrelated bacteriophages. *J Bacteriol* 1992;174: 1462–1977.
33. Haruna I, Spiegelman S. Specific template requirements of RNA replicases. *Proc Natl Acad Sci U S A* 1965;54:579–587.
34. Hendrix RW, Smith MCM, Burns RN, et al. Evolutionary relationships among diverse bacteriophages and prophages. All the world's a phage. *Proc Natl Acad Sci U S A* 1999;95:2192–2197.
35. Hershey AD, Chase M. Independent functions of viral protein and nucleic acid in growth of bacteriophage. *J Gen Physiol* 1952;36:31–56.
36. Hershey AD, Rotman R. Linkage among genes controlling inhibition of lysis in a bacterial virus. *Proc Natl Acad Sci U S A* 1948;34:89–96.
37. Kacian DL, Mills DR, Kramer FR, Spiegelman S. A replicating RNA molecule suitable for a detailed analysis of extracellular evolution and replication. *Proc Natl Acad Sci U S A* 1972;69:3038–3042.
38. Karlin S, Burge C, Campbell AM. Statistical analysis of counts and distributions of restriction sites in DNA sequences. *Nucleic Acids Res* 1992;20:1363–1370.
39. Kashlev M, Nudler E, Goldfarb A, et al. Bacteriophage T4 Alc protein: A transcription termination factor sensing local modification of DNA. *Cell* 1993;75:147–154.
40. Katsura I, Hendrix R. Length determination in bacteriophage lambda tails. *Cell* 1984;39:691–698.
41. Kestelein RA, Remaut E, Fiers W, van Duin J. Lysis gene expression of RNA phage MS2 depends on a frameshift during translation of the overlapping coat protein gene. *Nature* 1982;285:35–41.
42. Kitts PA, Nash HA. Homology-dependent interactions in phage site-specific recombination. *Nature* 1987;329:346–348.
43. Landy A. Dynamic, structural and regulatory aspects of λ site-specific recombination. *Annu Rev Biochem* 1989;58:913–949.
44. Lederberg EM, Lederberg J. Genetic studies of lysogenicity in *Escherichia coli. Genetics* 1953;38:51–64.
45. Lindquist BH, Dehó G, Calendar R. Mechanisms of genome propagation and helper exploitation by satellite phage P4. *Microbiol Rev* 193; 57:683–702.
46. Little JW. Mechanism of specific LexA cleavage: Autodigestion and the role of RecA coprotease. *Biochimie* 1991;73:411–422.
47. Luftig RB, Wood WB, Okinawa R. Bacteriophage T4 head morphogenesis. On the nature of gene 49–defective heads and their role as intermediates. *J Mol Biol* 1971;57:553–573.
48. Luzzati D. Regulation of λ exonuclease synthesis: Role of the N gene product and λ repressor. *J Mol Biol* 1970;49:515–519.
49. Lwoff A. Lysogeny. *Bacteriol Rev* 1953;17:269–337.
50. Mason SW, Li J, Greenblatt J. Host factor requirements for processive antitermination of transcription and suppression of pausing by the N protein of bacteriophage lambda. *J Biol Chem* 1992;267:19418–19426.

51. Merril CR, Biswas B, Coulton R, et al. Long-circulating bacteriophage as antibacterial agents. *Proc Natl Acad Sci U S A* 1996;93:3188–3192.
52. Mizuuchi K, Craigie R. Mechanism of bacteriophage Mu transposition. *Annu Rev Genet* 1986;20:385–430.
53. Muller HJ. The relation of recombination to mutational advance. *Mutat Res* 1964;1:2–9.
54. Novick A, Szilard L. Virus strains of identical phenotype but different genotype. *Science* 1951;113:34–35.
55. Nunes-Duby SE, Azaro MA, Landy A. Swapping DNA strands and sensing homology without branch migration in lambda site-specific recombination. *Curr Biol* 1995;5:139–148.
56. Oberto J, Weisberg RA, Gottesman ME. Structure and function of the *nun* gene and the immunity region of the lambdoid phage HK022. *J Mol Biol* 1989;207:675–693.
57. Parma DH, Snyder M, Soboleosh S, et al. The Rex system of bacteriophage λ: Tolerance and altruistic cell death. *Genes Dev* 1992;6:497–510.
58. Ptashne M. *A Genetic Switch.* Cambridge, MA: Cell Press and Blackwell, 1992.
59. Riley M, Anilionis A. Conservation and variation of nucleotide sequences within related bacterial genomes: Enterobacteria. *J Bacteriol* 1980;143:366–376.
60. Roberts JW, Yarnell W, Bartlett E, et al. Antitermination by bacteriophage lambda Q protein. *Cold Spring Harb Symp Quant Biol* 1998;63: 319–325.
61. Salas M. Phages with protein attached to their DNA ends. In: Calendar R, ed. *The Bacteriophages.* New York: Plenum Press, 1988:169–192.
62. Schlesinger M. The Feulgen reaction of the bacteriophage substance. *Nature* 1936;138:508–509.
63. Schmieger H, Backhaus H. The origin of DNA in transducing particles in P22-mutants with increased transduction-frequencies (HT-mutants). *Mol Gen Genet* 1973;120:181–190.
64. Scott JR. Sex and the single circle: Conjugative transposons. *J Bacteriol* 1992;174:6005–6010.
65. Séchaud J, Streisinger G, Emrich J, et al. Chromosome structure in phage T4. II. Terminal redundancy and heterozygosis. *Proc Natl Acad Sci U S A* 1965;54:1333–1339.
66. Son M, Watson RH, Sewer P. The direction and rate of phage T7 DNA packaging *in vitro. Virology* 1993;196:282–289.
67. Streisinger G, Emrich J, Stahl MM. Chromosome structure in phage T4. III. Terminal redundancy and length determination. *Proc Natl Acad Sci U S A* 1967;57:292–295.
68. Twart F. An investigation on the nature of ultramicroscopic viruses. *Lancet* 1915;189:1241–1243.
69. Van Etten JL, Burbank DE, Cuppels PA, et al. Semiconservative replication of double-stranded RNA by a virion-associated RNA polymerase. *J Virol* 1980;33:769–783.
70. Waldor MK. Bacteriophage biology and bacterial virulence. *Trends Microbiol* 1998;6:295–297.
71. Wall JD, Harriman PD. Phage P1 mutants with altered transducing abilities for *Escherichia coli. Virology* 1974;59:532–544.
72. Weiss RB, Huang WM, Dunn DM. A nascent peptide is required for ribosomal bypass of the coding gap in bacteriophage T4 gene 60. *Cell* 1990;62:117–126.
73. Winter RB, Morrissey L, Gauss P, et al. Bacteriophage T4 *regA* protein binds to mRNAs and prevents translation initiation. *Proc Natl Acad Sci U S A* 1987;84:7822–7826.
74. Yarmolinsky MB, Sternberg N. Bacteriophage P1. In: Calendar R, ed. *The Bacteriophages.* New York: Plenum Press, 1988:291–418.
75. Young R. Bacteriophage lysis: Mechanism and regulation. *Microbiol Rev* 1992;56:430–481.
76. Zahler SA. Temperate bacteriophage of *Bacillus subtilis.* In: Calendar R, ed. *The Bacteriophages.* New York: Plenum Press, 1988:559–592.

SECTION II

Specific Virus Families

CHAPTER 18

Picornaviridae: The Viruses and Their Replication

Vincent R. Racaniello

The Picornaviridae are nonenveloped viruses with a single-stranded RNA genome of positive polarity. This virus family contains many important human and animal pathogens, including poliovirus, hepatitis A virus, foot-and-mouth disease virus, and rhinovirus. The name of the virus family was intended to convey the small size of the viruses (pico, a small unit of measurement [10^{-12}]) and the type of nucleic acid that constitutes the viral genome (RNA).

Picornaviruses have played important roles in the development of modern virology. Foot-and-mouth disease virus was the first animal virus to be discovered, by Loeffler and Frosch in 1898 (193). Poliovirus was isolated 10 years later (182), a discovery spurred by the emergence of epidemic poliomyelitis at the turn of the 20th century. Forty years later, the discovery that poliovirus could be propagated in cultured cells led the way to studies of viral replication (84). The plaque assay, an essential method for quantification of viral infectivity, was developed with poliovirus (80). The first RNA-dependent RNA polymerase identified was that of mengovirus (20), a picornavirus, and the synthesis of a precursor polyprotein from which viral proteins are derived by proteolytic processing was first identified in poliovirus-infected cells (297). The first infectious DNA clone of an animal RNA virus was that of poliovirus (259), and the first three-dimensional structures of viruses determined by x-ray crystallography were those of poliovirus (142) and rhinovirus (272). Poliovirus RNA was the first messenger RNA (mRNA) shown to lack a 5′ cap structure (139,231). This observation was subsequently explained by the finding that the genome RNA of poliovirus, and other picornaviruses, is translated by internal ribosome binding (155,244), a process now known to occur on cellular mRNAs (158,195).

Because they cause such serious diseases, poliovirus and foot-and-mouth disease virus have been the best-studied picornaviruses. Research on poliovirus has led to the development of two effective vaccines, and it is likely that poliomyelitis will be eradicated from the globe within the first 5 years of the new millennium. The World Health Organization has established a future goal of cessation of vaccination, at which time all poliovirus stocks must be destroyed. As a result, all research on this virus will cease. Poliovirus is truly a virus with a brilliant past, but with no future.

CLASSIFICATION

The family Picornaviridae consists of six genera: aphthovirus, cardiovirus, enterovirus, hepatovirus, parechovirus, and rhinovirus (Table 1), which all contain viruses that infect vertebrates. Other picornaviruses of

TABLE 1. *Members of the family* Picornaviridae

Genus	Number of serotypes	Type species	Other members
Aphthovirus	7	Foot-and-mouth disease virus O	Foot-and-mouth disease viruses A and C, Asia 1, SAT 1, SAT 2, SAT 3
Cardiovirus	2	Encephalomycarditis virus[a]	Theiler's murine encephalomyelitis virus
Enterovirus	100	Poliovirus 1	Polioviruses 2 and 3
			Bovine enteroviruses 1 and 2
			Human coxsackieviruses A1–A22,[b] and A24
			Human coxsackieviruses B1–B5[c]
			Human echoviruses 1–7,[d] 9,[e] 11–21, 24–27,[f] 29–33
			Human enteroviruses 68–71
			Porcine enteroviruses 1–13
			Simian enteroviruses 1–18
			Vilyuisk human encephalomyelitis virus
Hepatovirus	2	Human hepatitis A virus[g]	Simian hepatitis A virus
Parechovirus	2	Human parechovirus 1	Human parechovirus 2
Rhinovirus	103	Human rhinovirus 1A	Human rhinoviruses 2–100
			Bovine rhinoviruses 1–3

[a]Strains of this virus include mengovirus, Columbia-SK virus, and maus Elberfeld virus.
[b]Coxsackievirus A23 was shown to be echovirus 9.
[c]Swine vesicular disease virus is similar to coxsackievirus B5.
[d]Echovirus 8 was shown to be echovirus 1.
[e]Echovirus 10 was shown to be reovirus 1.
[f]Echovirus 22 and 23 have been moved to a separate genus, Parechovirus, and renamed parechovirus 1 and 2; echovirus 28 was shown to be rhinovirus A1.
[g]Formerly enterovirus 72.
SAT, South African type.

invertebrates, such as cricket paralysis virus and *Drosophila* C virus, have not been assigned a genus.

The aphthoviruses (foot-and-mouth disease virus) infect cloven-footed animals, such as cattle, goats, pigs, and sheep, but rarely infect humans. Seven serotypes of this virus have been identified, and within each serotype are many subtypes. These viruses are highly labile and rapidly lose infectivity at pH values of less than 7.0.

There are two "clusters" of cardioviruses. The encephalomyocarditis-like viruses (encephalomyocarditis virus, Columbia SK virus, maus Elberfeld virus, and mengovirus) are murine viruses but can also infect other hosts, including humans, monkeys, pigs, elephants, and squirrels. The second cluster includes the Theiler's murine encephalomyelitis viruses. Strains such as GDVII cause a disease in mice that resembles poliomyelitis. The TO strains are less virulent and cause a chronic demyelinating disease that resembles multiple sclerosis. Vilyuisk human encephalomyelitis virus, or Vilyuisk virus, originally classified as an enterovirus, was recently transferred to the Theiler's cluster of the cardioviruses. Vilyuisk virus is believe to cause a neurodegenerative disease among the Yakuts people of Siberia and was originally isolated from the cerebrospinal fluid of a patient with a chronic case of encephalomyelitis (191). Nucleotide sequence analysis of Vilyuisk virus RNA indicates that it is a divergent Theiler's virus (258), justifying its transfer to the cardioviruses.

As the name implies, enteroviruses replicate in the alimentary tract, and as might be expected, they are resistant to low pH. This genus includes poliovirus (3 serotypes), coxsackievirus (23 serotypes), echovirus (28 serotypes), human enterovirus (4 serotypes), and many nonhuman enteric viruses. Formerly a member of the enterovirus genus, human hepatitis A virus (1 serotype) has been reclassified into a separate genus, hepatovirus. This reclassification was based on a number of unique properties of the virus, including nucleotide and amino acid sequence dissimilarity with other picornaviruses, replication in cell culture without cytopathic effect, and the existence of only one serotype.

The parechovirus genus contains two serotypes of human parechovirus that were previously classified as echoviruses types 22 and 23. Studies of the nucleotide sequence of the viral genome revealed no greater than 30% amino acid identity with other picornaviruses. In addition, the capsid consists of three, not four, capsid proteins. These and other differences led to the reclassification of these viruses (294).

There are 103 serotypes of rhinoviruses, so named because they replicate in the nasopharynx. These viruses, which are important agents of the common cold, are extremely acid labile.

VIRION STRUCTURE

Physical Properties

Picornavirus virions are spherical in shape with a diameter of about 30 nm (Fig. 1). The particles are simple in that they are composed of a protein shell surrounding the naked RNA genome. The virus particles lack a lipid envelope, and their infectivity is insensitive to organic solvents. Cardioviruses, enteroviruses, hepatoviruses, and parechoviruses are acid stable and retain infectivity at pH values of 3.0 and lower. In contrast, rhinoviruses and aphthoviruses are labile at pH values of less than 6.0. Differences in pH stability are related to the sites of replication of the virus. For example, rhinoviruses and aphthoviruses replicate in the respiratory tract and need not be acid stable. As discussed later, the acid lability of these viruses plays a role in uncoating of the viral genome. Cardioviruses, enteroviruses, hepatoviruses, and parechoviruses pass through the stomach to gain access to the intestine and therefore must be resistant to low pH. The structural basis for the acid lability of foot-and-mouth disease virus is partly understood (see Entry by Endocytosis).

The buoyant densities of picornaviruses are quite different (Table 2). Cardioviruses and enteroviruses have a buoyant density of 1.34 g/mL, that of foot-and-mouth disease virus is 1.45 g/mL, and rhinoviruses have an intermediate value (1.40 g/mL). The reason for the difference lies in the permeability of the viral capsid to cesium. The capsid of poliovirus does not allow cesium to reach the RNA interior; hence, the virus bands at an abnormally light buoyant density (90). In contrast, aphthovirus capsids contain pores that allow cesium to enter (2). The rhinovirus capsid is permeable to cesium, but the presence of polyamines in the capsid interior limits the amount of cesium that may enter, explaining the intermediate value (90).

Ratio of Particles to Infectious Viruses

The ratio of particles to infectious virus is determined by dividing the number of virus particles in a sample (determined by electron microscopy or spectrophotometric measurements) by the plaque titer, yielding the particle-to-plaque forming unit ratio. This ratio is a measurement of the fraction of virus particles that can complete an infectious cycle. The particle-to-plaque forming unit ratio of poliovirus ranges from 30 to 1,000, and that of other picornaviruses is in the same range. The high particle-to-plaque forming unit ratio may be caused by the presence of lethal mutations in the viral genome. This explanation, however, probably does not apply to all picornaviruses; it has been shown that the infectivity of aphthovirus RNA approaches one infectious unit per molecule. An alternative explanation is that all viruses do not successfully complete an infectious cycle because they fail at one of the many steps—attachment, entry, replication, and assembly—that a virus must go through to complete the infectious cycle.

High-Resolution Structure of the Virion

The capsids of picornaviruses are composed of four structural proteins: VP1, VP2, VP3, and VP4. The exception is the parechoviruses, which contain only three capsid polypeptides: VP1, VP2, and VP0, the uncleaved precursor to VP2 + VP4. In the 1960s, Caspar and Klug, elaborating the principles of virus structure, concluded that the best way to build a shell with nonidentical subunits is to arrange the proteins with icosahedral symmetry (51). An icosahedron is a solid composed of 20 triangular faces and 12 vertices (see Fig. 1). The smallest number of subunits that can be used to compose such a solid is 60. The results of x-ray diffraction studies, electron microscopic observations, and biochemical studies of virus particles and their dissociation products led to the hypothesis that the picornavirus capsid contains 60 structural proteins arranged into an icosahedral lattice (274). Our understanding of the structure of picornaviruses took an enormous leap in 1985 when the atomic structures of poliovirus type 1 (142) and human rhinovirus 14 (272) were determined by x-ray crystallography. Since then, the high-resolution structures of many other picornaviruses have been determined.

The basic building block of the picornavirus capsid is the protomer, which contains one copy each of VP1, VP2, VP3, and VP4. The shell is formed by VP1 to VP3, and VP4 lies on its inner surface. VP1, VP2, and VP3 have no sequence homology, yet all three proteins have the same topology: they form an eight-stranded antiparallel β-barrel (also called a β-barrel jelly roll or a Swiss-roll β-barrel) (see Fig. 1). This domain is a wedge-shaped structure made up of two antiparallel β-sheets. One β-sheet forms the wall of the wedge, and the second, which has a bend in the center, forms both a wall and the floor. The wedge shape facilitates the packing of structural units to form a dense, rigid protein shell. Packing of the β-barrel domains is strengthened by a network of protein–protein contacts on the interior of the capsid, particularly around the 5-fold axes. This network, which is formed by the N-terminal extensions of VP1 to VP3 as well as VP4, is essential for the stability of the virion. VP4 is quite different from the other three proteins in that it has an extended conformation. This protein is similar in position and conformation to the NH2-terminal sequences of VP1 and VP3 and functions as a detached NH2-terminal extension of VP2 rather than an independent capsid protein.

The main structural differences among VP1, VP2, and VP3 lie in the loops that connect the β-strands and the N- and C-terminal sequences that extend from the β-barrel domain. These amino acid sequences give each picornavirus its distinct morphology and antigenicity. The C-termini are located on the surface of the virion, and the N-termini are on the interior, indicating that significant rearrangement of the P1 precursor occurs on proteolytic cleavage.

Resolution of the structures of poliovirus and rhinovirus yielded a great surprise: the β-barrel domains were strikingly similar in structure to those of plant viruses whose structures had been solved 5 years earlier,

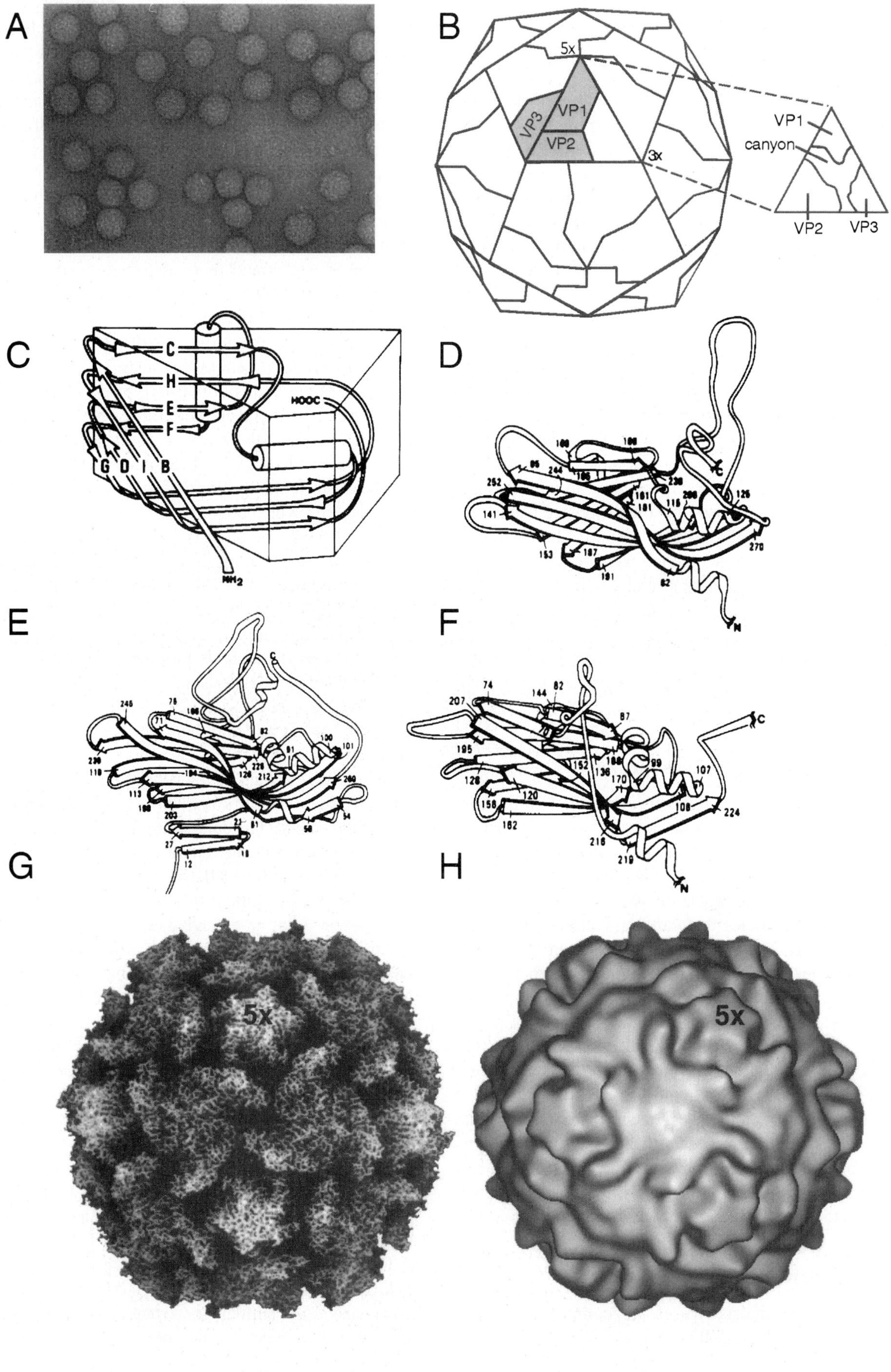
A
B
5x
VP3
VP1
VP2
3x
VP1
canyon
VP2
VP3
C
C
H
E
F
G
D
I
B
HOOC
NH2
D
E
F
G
H
5x
5x

TABLE 2. *Physical properties of some picornaviruses*

Genus	pH stability	Virion buoyant density	Sedimentation coefficient
Aphthovirus	Labile, <7	1.43–1.45	142–146S
Cardiovirus	Stable, 3–9	1.34	160S
Enterovirus	Stable, 3–9	1.34	160S
Hepatovirus	Stable	1.34	160S
Rhinovirus	Labile, <6	1.40	160S

southern bean mosaic virus and tomato bushy stunt virus. Yet the capsid proteins of these viruses bear no sequence homology with those of the picornaviruses. It has since become apparent that similar protein topology is found in the capsid proteins of many plant, insect, and vertebrate positive-stranded RNA viruses as well as in the DNA-containing papovaviruses and adenoviruses. These findings suggest that either the polypeptides evolved from a common ancestor or that the β-barrel domain is one of the few ways to allow proteins to pack to form a sphere.

Surface of the Virion

Resolution of the structures of poliovirus and human rhinovirus revealed that the surfaces of these viruses have a corrugated topography; there is a prominent star-shaped plateau (mesa) at the 5-fold axis of symmetry, surrounded by a deep depression ("canyon") and another protrusion at the 3-fold axis (see Fig. 1). It was originally proposed that the canyon is the receptor binding site, and this hypothesis has been proved for poliovirus and rhinovirus. However, not all picornaviruses have canyons. The surfaces of aphthoviruses and cardioviruses lack canyons and are much smoother in appearance. As discussed later, other features of these viruses serve as receptor-binding sites.

Interior of the Virion

A network formed by the N-termini on the interior of the capsid contributes significantly to its stability. At the 5-fold axis of symmetry, the N-termini of five VP3 molecules form a cylindrically parallel β-sheet. This structure is surrounded by five three-stranded β-sheets formed by the N-termini of VP4 and VP1. The myristate group attached to the N-terminus of VP4 mediates the interaction between these two structures (61). Interactions among pentamers are stabilized by a seven-stranded β-sheet, composed of four β-strands of the VP3 β-barrel and one strand from the N-terminus of VP1 that surround a two-stranded β-sheet made from the N-terminus of VP2 from a neighboring pentamer (86).

An extra 1500 nucleotides can be added to the poliovirus genome and successfully packaged, indicating that the interior of the capsid is not completely full (7). It has been suggested that picornaviral capsids are stabilized by interactions with the RNA genome, based on findings with bean pod mottle virus, which is related to picornaviruses. In this virus, ordered RNA can be observed at the 3-fold axis, and packaging of viral RNA stabilizes subunit interactions (58,188). Unfortunately, little information is available about the arrangement of the RNA genome of picornaviruses because the nucleic acid is usually not visible. Nevertheless, a few nucleotides have been tentatively identified in a similar location in the structures of P3/Sabin and rhinovirus type 14 (18,86). In the atomic structure of poliovirus P2/Lansing, RNA bases have been observed stacking with conserved aromatic residues of VP4 (185). This interaction could play a role in capsid stability or uncoating.

FIG. 1. Structural features of picornaviruses. **A:** Electron micrograph of negatively stained poliovirus, magnification 270,000. (Courtesy of N. Cheng and D. M. Belnap, National Institutes of Health.) **B:** Schematic of the picornavirus capsid, showing the pseudoequivalent packing arrangement of VP1, VP2, and VP3. VP4 is on the interior of the capsid. The biologic protomer (*gray*) is not the same as the icosahedral asymmetric subunit (*triangle expanded at right*). **C:** Diagram of how the eight β-strands of each capsid protein form a wedgelike structure with loops connecting the strands. These loops decorate the surface of the particle and give each subunit distinctive morphology and antigenicity. In many picornaviruses, the neutralizing antigenic sites are located in the BC loops of VP1 and VP3 and in the EF loop of VP2. These loops can accommodate extra amino acids without affecting the framework of the capsid (45). **D to F:** Ribbon diagrams of polioviruses VP1, VP2, and VP3, showing the common β-barrel structure that is also common to many other viral capsid proteins. The N- and C-termini of each capsid protein are separated by almost 50 angstroms. (C-F, adapted form ref. 142, with permission.) **G:** Model of poliovirus type 1, Mahoney, based on x-ray crystallographic structure determined at 2.9 ≈ (142). The model is highlighted by radial depth cuing so that portions of the model farthest from the center are bright. The 5-fold axis of symmetry is marked; it is characterized by a prominent star-shaped mesa. Surrounding the 5-fold axis is the canyon, which is the receptor-binding site. At the 3-fold axis is a propeller-shaped feature. **H:** Model of poliovirus type 1, Mahoney, made by image reconstruction from cryoelectron microscopy data. The resolution is 20 Å. The star-shaped mesa, canyon, and propeller are clearly visible.

The Hydrophobic Pocket

Within the core of VP1, just beneath the canyon floor of many picornaviruses, is a hydrophobic tunnel or pocket. In poliovirus types 1 and 3, the pocket is believed to contain sphingosine (86); an unidentified lipid has been found in human rhinoviruses types 1A and 16, and a C16 fatty acid has been modeled in the pocket of coxsackievirus B3 (127,168,225). In contrast, the pocket of human rhinovirus type 14 is empty (18).

The same hydrophobic pocket is also the binding site for antipicornavirus drugs such as the WIN compounds produced by Sterling-Winthrop (290) as well as similar molecules produced by Schering-Plough (Kenilworth, NJ) and Janssen Pharmaceutica (Titusville, NJ) (13,68). Some of these drugs have been evaluated in clinical trials (1). These hydrophobic, sausage-shaped compounds bind tightly in the hydrophobic tunnel, displacing any lipid that is present. As discussed later, such drugs inhibit either binding or uncoating. Drug-dependent mutants of poliovirus spontaneously lose infectivity at 37°C, probably because they do not contain lipid in the pocket (224).

Myristate

Myristic acid (*n*-tetradecanoic acid) is covalently linked to glycine at the amino-terminus of VP4 of most picornaviruses (61). This residue is an integral part of the viral capsid. The N-termini of VP3 intertwine around the 5-fold axis to form a twisted tube of parallel β-structure (142). The five myristyl groups extend from the N-termini of VP4 and cradle the twisted tube formed by VP3 (61). The myristyl groups interact with amino acid side chains of VP4 and VP3. Mutagenesis of VP4 has revealed a role for myristic acid modification in virus assembly and in the stability of the capsid (14,196–198,220).

Neutralizing Antigenic Sites

As shown in Table 1, there are many different serotypes in the picornavirus family. Although the atomic structures of many picornaviruses have been solved, they provide no insight into why some picornaviruses, such as rhinovirus, occur in so many serotypes, whereas there are only three serotypes of poliovirus. However, serotype is determined by the connecting loops and C-termini of the capsid proteins that decorate the outer surface of the virion. These contain the major neutralization antigenic sites of the virus. Such sites are defined by mutations that confer resistance to neutralization with monoclonal antibodies directed against the viral capsid (213,214,286).

GENOME STRUCTURE AND ORGANIZATION

General Features

The genome of picornaviruses, a single positive-stranded RNA molecule, is infectious because it can be translated on entry into the cell and produce all the viral proteins required for viral replication. The picornavirus genome is unique because it is covalently linked at the 5′ end to a protein called VPg (virion protein, genome linked) (88,184). VPg is covalently joined to the 5′-uridylylate moiety of the viral RNA by an O4-(5′-uridylyl)-tyrosine linkage. All picornavirus genomes are linked to VPg, which varies in length from 22 to 24 amino acid residues. The tyrosine that is linked to the viral RNA is always the third amino acid from the N-terminus. VPg is encoded by a single viral gene in all picornaviruses except the genome of foot-and-mouth disease virus, which encodes three VPg genes (89). VPg is not required for infectivity of poliovirus RNA; if it is removed from viral RNA by treatment with proteinase, the specific infectivity of the viral RNA is not reduced. VPg is not found on viral mRNA that is associated with cellular ribosomes and undergoing translation; these mRNAs contain only uridine 5′-phosphate (pU) at their 5′ ends. The lack of VPg is the only difference between poliovirus virion RNA and mRNA (230,249). VPg is removed from virion RNA by a host protein called *unlinking enzyme* (9). It is not known whether removal of VPg is a prerequisite for association with ribosomes or is a result of that association. Although VPg RNA can be translated in cell-free extracts, it is possible that VPg is rapidly cleaved from the RNA such that only RNAs lacking VPg are translated (112,217,316). VPg is present on nascent RNA chains of the replicative intermediate RNA and on negative-stranded RNAs, which has led to the suggestion that poliovirus RNA synthesis uses VPg as a primer (229,248). The role of VPg in viral RNA synthesis figures prominently in recent models of poliovirus RNA replication and is discussed in subsequent sections.

Nucleotide sequence analysis of many picornavirus RNAs has revealed a common organizational pattern (Fig. 2). The genomes vary in length from 7,209 to 8,450 bases. The 5′-noncoding regions of picornaviruses are long (624 to 1,199 nucleotides) and highly structured (Fig. 3). This region of the genome contains sequences that control genome replication and translation (see Genome Replication and mRNA Synthesis). The 5′-noncoding region contains the internal ribosome entry site (IRES), an element that directs translation of the mRNA by internal ribosome binding. Based on the RNA structure, two major classes of IRES elements have been defined (see Fig. 3). The 5′-untranslated regions of aphthoviruses and cardioviruses contain a poly(C) tract that varies in length among different virus strains (80 to 250 nucleotides in cardioviruses, 100 to 170 nucleotides in aphthoviruses). Among cardioviruses, longer poly(C) length is associated with higher virulence in animals (79,129).

The 3′-noncoding region of picornaviruses is short, ranging in length from 47 nucleotides for human rhinovirus 14 to 125 bases for encephalomyocarditis virus. This region also contains a secondary structure, notably a pseudoknot, that has been implicated in controlling viral

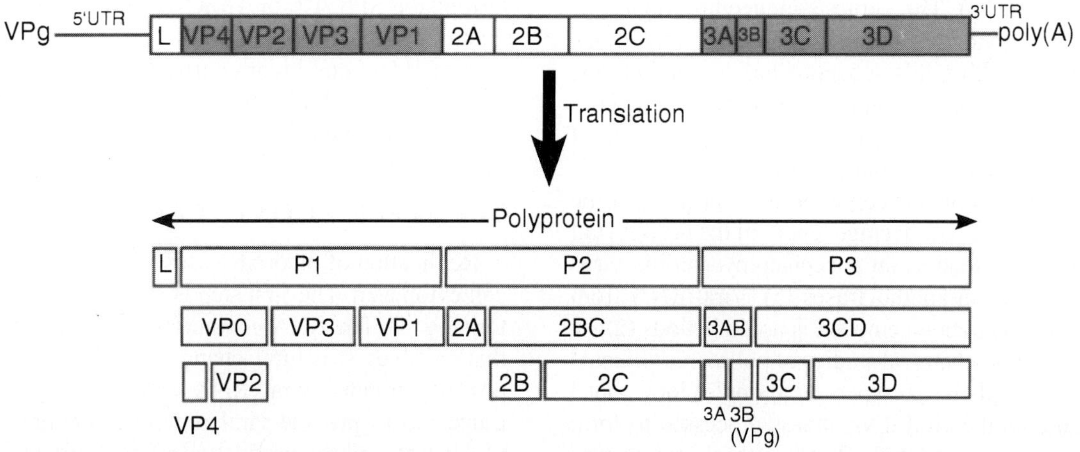

FIG. 2. Organization of the picornavirus genome. **Top:** Diagram of the viral RNA genome, with the genome-linked protein VPg at the 5′ end, the 5′ untranslated region, the protein coding region, the 3′ untranslated region, and the poly(A) tail. L is a leader protein encoded in the genomes of cardioviruses and aphthoviruses but not other picornaviruses. Coding regions for the viral proteins are indicated. **Bottom:** Processing pattern of picornavirus polyprotein. The coding region has been divided into three regions, P1, P2, and P3, which are separated by nascent cleavage by two viral proteinases, 2A and 3C. Intermediate and final cleavage products are indicated. The proteinase responsible for cleavage of VP0 has not been identified. Proteins L and 2A carry out cleavages described in Figure 10. The remaining cleavages are carried out by $3C^{pro}$ and its precursor, $3CD^{pro}$.

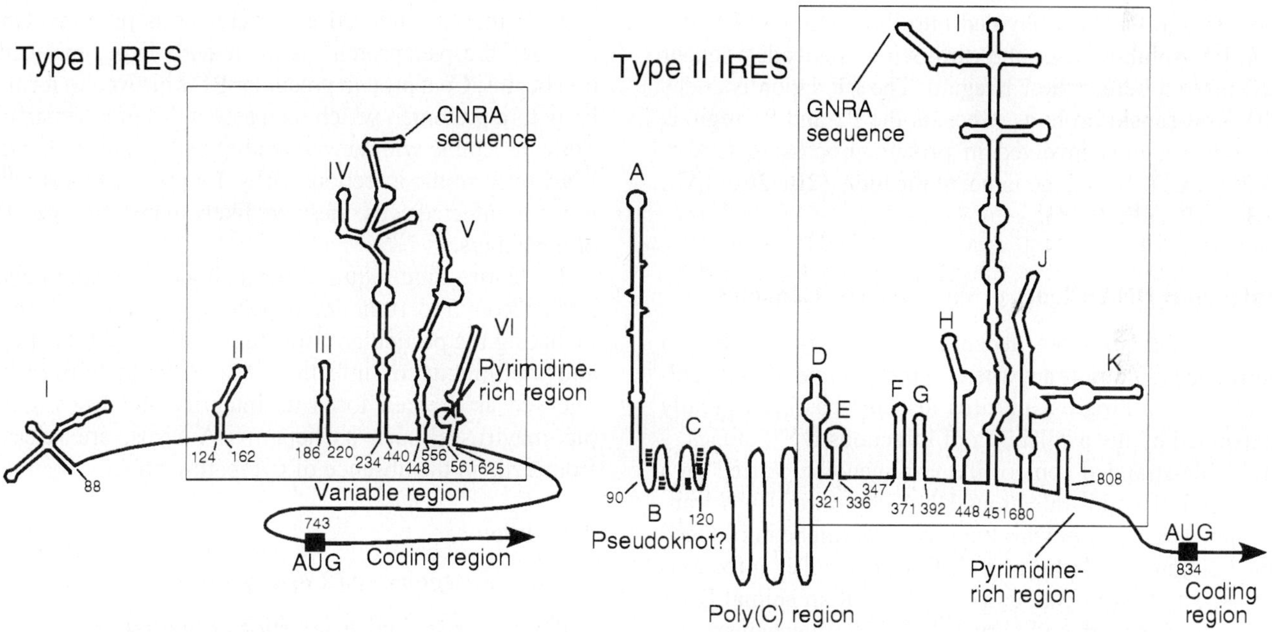

FIG. 3. Two major classes of picornavirus internal ribosome entry site (IRES). **Left:** The 5′ untranslated region of poliovirus. **Right:** The same region from encephalomyocarditis virus. The IRES is indicated by a box. Predicated secondary and tertiary structures (RNA pseudoknots) are labeled. The poliovirus IRES is a type I IRES, also found in the genomes of other enteroviruses and rhinoviruses. The genomes of cardioviruses and aphthoviruses contain a type II IRES. The GNRA loop and pyrimidine-rich region are features that are conserved in both the type I and type II IRES. The IRES of hepatoviruses differs from the type I and type II IRES and probably constitutes a third class. (Adapted from Stewart SR, Semler BL. RNA determinants of picornavirus cap-independent translation initiation. *Semin Virol* 1997;8: 242–255, with permission.)

RNA synthesis (154). The entire 3′-noncoding region of poliovirus and rhinovirus is not required for infectivity, although RNA lacking this sequence has low infectivity, and the resulting viruses replicate poorly (301). Both poliovirus virion RNA and mRNA contain a 3′ stretch of poly(A) (326). Negative-stranded RNA contains a 5′ stretch of poly(U), which is copied to form poly(A) of the positive strand (325). The average length of the poly(A) tail varies from 35 nucleotides in encephalomyocarditis virus to 100 nucleotides in aphthoviruses (5). Viral RNA from which the poly(A) tract is removed is noninfectious (293).

The results of biochemical studies of poliovirus-infected cells had predicted the presence of a single, long, open reading frame on the viral RNA that is processed to form individual viral proteins (297). This hypothesis was proved when the nucleotide sequence of the poliovirus genome was determined, which revealed a single open reading frame in the viral RNA (173,260). A similar strategy, in which a single polyprotein is synthesized, is used by all picornaviruses. The polyprotein is cleaved during translation, so that the full-length product is not observed. Cleavage is carried out by virus-encoded proteinases to yield 11 to 12 final cleavage products. Some of the uncleaved precursors also have functions during replication.

To unify the nomenclature of picornavirus proteins, the polyprotein has been divided into three regions: P1, P2, and P3. Aphthoviruses and cardioviruses encode a leader (L) protein before the P1 region. The P1 region encodes the viral capsid proteins, whereas the P2 and P3 regions encode proteins involved in protein processing ($2A^{pro}$, $3C^{pro}$, $3CD^{pro}$) and genome replication (2B, 2C, 3AB, $3B^{VPg}$, $3CD^{pro}$, $3D^{pol}$).

Infectious DNA Clones of Picornavirus Genomes

Recombinant DNA techniques make it possible to introduce mutations anywhere in the genome of most animal viruses. Progress in virus research has been greatly expanded by the availability of infectious DNA clones—a double-stranded copy of the viral genome carried on a bacterial plasmid. Infectious DNA clones, or RNA transcripts derived by *in vitro* transcription, can be introduced into cultured cells by transfection to recover infectious virus. The first infectious DNA clone of an animal RNA virus was that of poliovirus (259). The mechanism for infectivity of cloned poliovirus DNA is unknown but might result from production of RNA in the nucleus, by cellular DNA-dependent RNA polymerase, from cryptic, promoter-like elements in the plasmid. The initial transcripts produced are longer than poliovirus RNA but can be translated and replicated. The extra sequences must be removed or not copied because viruses produced from cloned DNA have authentic 5′- and 3′-termini.

The infectivity of cloned poliovirus DNA (10^3 plaque-forming units per μg) is much lower than that of genomic RNA (10^6 plaque-forming units per μg). The development of plasmid vectors incorporating promoters for bacteriophage SP6, T7, or T3 RNA polymerase for the production of RNA transcripts *in vitro* enabled the production of infectious picornavirus RNA from cloned DNA (309). Such RNA transcripts have an infectivity approaching that of genomic RNA.

THE REPLICATION CYCLE

Replication of picornaviruses takes place entirely in the cell cytoplasm. The first step is attachment to a cell receptor (Fig. 4). The RNA genome is then uncoated, a process that involves structural changes in the capsid. Once the positive-stranded viral RNA enters the cytoplasm, it is translated to provide viral proteins essential for genome replication and the production of new virus particles. The viral proteins are synthesized from a polyprotein precursor, which is cleaved nascently. Cleavages are carried out mainly by two viral proteinases, $2A^{pro}$ and $3C^{pro}/3CD^{pro}$. Among the proteins that are synthesized are the viral RNA-dependent RNA polymerase and accessory proteins required for genome replication and mRNA synthesis. The first step in genome replication is copying of the input positive-stranded RNA to form a negative-stranded intermediate; this step is followed by the production of additional positive strands. These events occur on small membranous vesicles that are induced by several virus proteins. Once the pool of capsid proteins is sufficiently large, encapsidation begins. Coat protein precursor P1 is cleaved to form an immature protomer, which then assembles into pentamers. These assemble with newly synthesized, positive-stranded RNA to form the infectious virus. Empty capsids are also found in infected cells; these are likely to be a storage form of pentamers.

The entire time required for a single replication cycle ranges from 5 to 10 hours, depending on many variables, including the particular virus, temperature, pH, host cell, and multiplicity of infection. Many picornaviruses are released as the cell loses its integrity and lyses. Other picornaviruses, such as hepatitis A virus, are released from cells in the absence of cytopathic effect.

Attachment

Cellular Receptors and Coreceptors

Picornaviruses initiate infection of cells by first attaching to the host cell membrane through a host cell receptor. The nature of picornavirus receptors remained obscure until 1989, when the receptors for poliovirus and the major group rhinoviruses were identified (121,212,296). Since then, receptors for many other members of this virus family have been identified (Table 3). Examination of picornavirus receptor usage illustrates a number of important points. First, picornaviruses use a wide variety of cell surface molecules for cellular receptors. Second, many picornaviruses share cellular receptors. For example, the cell surface protein CD55 is a receptor for certain coxsackieviruses A and B, echoviruses, and enterovirus 70. Third, for some

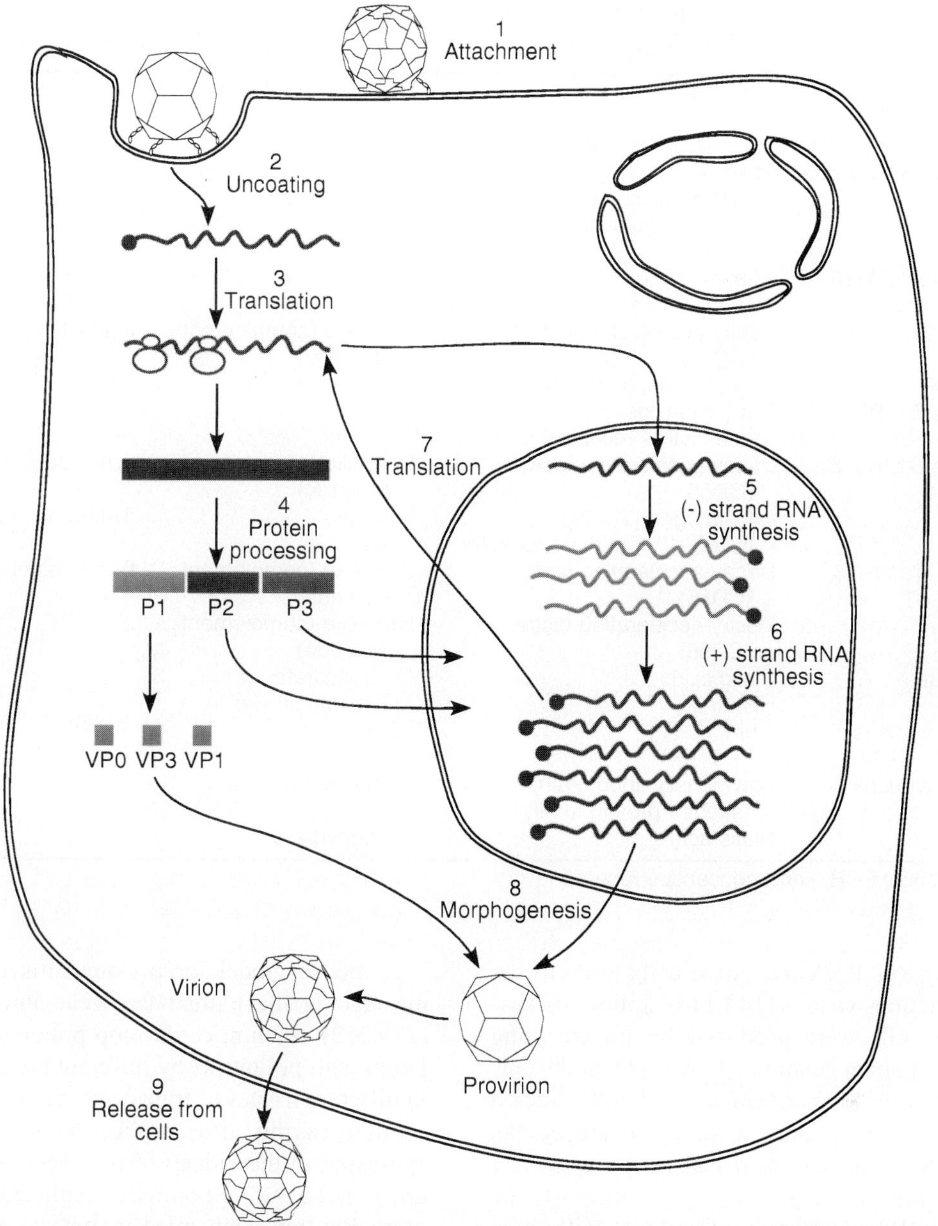

FIG. 4. Overview of the picornavirus replication cycle. Virus binds to a cellular receptor *(1)* and the genome is uncoated *(2)*. VPg is removed from the viral RNA, which is then translated *(3)*. The polyprotein is cleaved nascently to produce individual viral proteins *(4)*. RNA synthesis occurs on membrane vesicles (not drawn to scale in this diagram). Viral (+) strand RNA is copied by the viral RNA polymerase to form full-length (–) strand RNAs *(5)*, which are then copied to produce additional (+) strand RNAs *(6)*. Early in infection, newly synthesized (+) strand RNA is translated to produce additional viral proteins *(7)*. Later in infection, the (+) strands enter the morphogenetic pathway *(8)*. Newly synthesized virus particles are released from the cell by lysis *(9)*.

picornaviruses, a single type of receptor is sufficient for entry of viruses into cells. Viruses in this category include polioviruses and rhinoviruses. For other viruses, a second molecule, or coreceptor, is needed for virus entry into cells. For example, coxsackievirus A21, which attaches to CD55, requires intercellular adhesion molecule 1 (ICAM-1) for entry into cells (283). The precise role of coreceptors in picornavirus entry is not yet known.

One Type of Receptor Molecule for Virus Binding and Entry

The poliovirus receptor (Pvr, CD155) was identified by DNA transformation (212). It was known that mouse cells are not susceptible to poliovirus infection because they lack cellular receptors (208). Mouse cells are permissive to poliovirus replication, however, because intro-

TABLE 3. *Cell receptors for picornaviruses*

Virus	Receptor	Type of receptor	Coreceptor	References
Foot-and-mouth disease virus (cell culture adapted)	Heparan sulfate	Glycosaminoglycan		152
Foot-and-mouth disease virus	$\alpha_v\beta_3$ (Vitronectin receptor)	Integrin		226
Encephalomyocarditis virus	Vcam-1	Ig-like		146
	Sialylated glycophorin A (for hemagglutination only)	Carbohydrate		
Polioviruses 1–3	Pvr	Ig-like		212
Coxsackieviruses A13, A18, A21	Icam-1	Ig-like		64
Coxsackievirus A21	Decay-accelerating factor (CD55)	SCR-like (complement cascade)	Icam=1	283
Coxsackievirus A9	$\alpha_v\beta_3$ (Vitronectin receptor)	Integrin		268
Coxsackieviruses B1–B6	Car (coxsackievirus-adenovirus receptor)	Ig-like		34
Coxsackieviruses B1, B3, B5	Decay-accelerating factor (CD55)	SCR-like (complement cascade)	$\alpha_v\beta_6$-Integrin	4, 282
Echoviruses 1, 8	$\alpha_2\beta_1$-Integrin (Vla-2)	Integrin	β_2-Microglobulin	35, 320
Parechovirus 1	$\alpha_v\beta_1$, $\alpha_v\beta_3$ (Vitronectin receptor)	Integrin		306
Echoviruses 3, 6, 7, 11–13, 20, 21, 24, 29, 33	Decay-accelerating factor (CD55)	SCR-like (complement cascade)	β_2-Microglobulin	33, 257, 319, 320
Enterovirus, 70	Decay-accelerating factor (CD55)	SCR-like (complement cascade)		165
Bovine enterovirus	Sialic acid	Carbohydrate		330
Hepatitis A virus	HAVcr-1	Ig-like, mucin-like		164
Major group rhinoviruses (91 serotypes)	Icam-1	Ig-like		121, 296, 303
Minor group rhinoviruses (10 serotypes)	Low-density lipoprotein receptor protein family	Signaling receptor		141
Rhinovirus 87	Sialic acid	Carbohydrate		307

Ig, immunoglobulin; SCR, short consensus repeat.

duction of poliovirus RNA into these cells leads to the synthesis of infectious viruses (143,144). Poliovirus-susceptible mouse cells were produced by transforming mouse cells with human genomic DNA (211). Such cells were identified using a monoclonal antibody directed against the poliovirus receptor. Cloning of the human poliovirus receptor gene revealed that the receptor is a integral membrane protein and a member of the immunoglobulin (Ig) superfamily of proteins, with three extracellular Ig-like domains (212) (Fig. 5). The first Ig-like domain contains the site that binds poliovirus. This conclusion comes from three different types of experiments. First, cells expressing the first Ig-like domain of Pvr, either alone or as a hybrid with other Ig-like proteins, are susceptible to infection with poliovirus (177, 218,280,281). Second, mutations in the first Ig-like domain of Pvr interfere with poliovirus binding (15,36, 219). Mutations in the C′C" loop, the C-terminus of the D-strand, and the DE and FG loops of Pvr domain 1 cause alterations in virus binding to the receptor. Third, models of the poliovirus–Pvr complex produced from cryoelectron microscopy data indicate that only domain 1 contacts the virus surface (32,136,323) (see Fig. 5). Mutations that affect receptor binding map to the virion–Pvr interface as determined by these structural studies.

A mouse model for poliomyelitis was developed by introducing the human Pvr gene into transgenic mice (179,262). Such mice develop poliomyelitis after inoculation with poliovirus by different routes. Pvr expression in different tissues of transgenic mice is not always sufficient to permit virus replication. For example, Pvr is expressed in the kidney of transgenic mice, but the kidney is not a site of poliovirus replication (263). Furthermore, Pvr transgenic mice are not susceptible to infection by the oral route, the natural route of infection in humans, probably because of a postreceptor block to replication in mouse intestinal cells (332).

Expression of Pvr on cultured cells derived from different animal species leads to susceptibility to poliovirus infection. It therefore seems likely that Pvr is the only molecule required for poliovirus binding and entry. At one time, it was believed that the lymphocyte homing receptor, CD44, might be a coreceptor for poliovirus because a monoclonal antibody against this protein blocks poliovirus binding to cells (284,285). It was subsequently shown that CD44 is not a receptor for poliovirus and is not required for poliovirus infection of cells that express Pvr (43,93). It seems likely that Pvr and CD44 are associated in the cell membrane (94) and that anti-CD44 antibodies block poliovirus attachment by blocking the poliovirus-binding sites on Pvr.

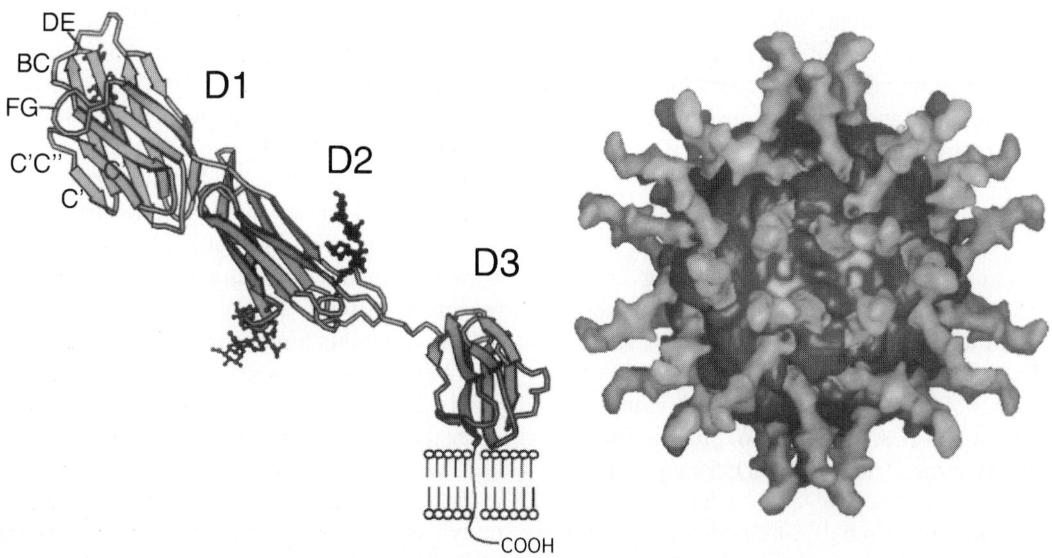

FIG. 5. Interaction of poliovirus with its cellular receptor. **Left:** Model of the poliovirus receptor produced from homology modeling and the density map from cryoelectron microscopy data of a virus-receptor complex (32). Immunoglobulin-like domains are labeled. The receptor contacts the virus only through domain 1; principal loops involved in the contact are labeled. Carbohydrate side chains have been modeled on domains 1 and 2. **Right:** Image reconstruction of poliovirus type 1 and a soluble form of Pvr, lacking the transmembrane and cytoplasmic domains (32). Domain 1 of Pvr binds in the canyon of the virus; no other receptor domains contact the particle. There are 60 receptor binding sites on each viral capsid; the complexes were produced with saturating amounts of Pvr, and all binding sites on the capsid are occupied.

The normal cellular function of Pvr is unknown. Sequence homologs of Pvr have been identified in humans (Prr1/Nectin-1 [81,194]), monkeys (Agm1 and Agm2 [178]), mice (Prr1, Mph/Prr2/Nectin-2, Nectin-3 [218,277]), and rats (pE4 [52]). Only Pvr, Agm1, and Agm2 encode proteins that can function as cell receptors for poliovirus (178,211,218; V. Racaniello, unpublished data, 1999). Pvr, Nectin-1, and Nectin-2 are coreceptors for alphaherpesviruses (102,287,321). Nectin-1 and Nectin-2 are homophilic adhesion proteins that interact with the actin cytoskeleton through a cytoplasmic linker protein called *afadin* (299). Mice lacking the Nectin-2 protein are sterile and produce sperm with cytoskeletal and nuclear defects (42). It is not known whether Pvr is also an adhesion molecule; it lacks the sequence in the cytoplasmic domain that is responsible for binding of Nectin-1 and Nectin-2 to afadin (299).

The cell surface receptor for the major group of human rhinoviruses (about 91 serotypes) was identified using monoclonal antibodies directed against the cellular binding site to isolate the receptor protein from susceptible cells. Amino acid sequence analysis of the purified protein revealed that it is ICAM-1, an integral membrane protein that is also a member of the Ig superfamily of proteins (121,296,303). The normal cellular functions of ICAM-1 are to bind its ligand, lymphocyte function–associated antigen 1 (LFA-1) on the surface of lymphocytes and to promote a wide range of immunologic functions (308). Erythrocytes infected with *Plasmodium falciparum* gain the ability to bind ICAM-1 on endothelial cells, allowing the parasite to become sequestered in tissues. ICAM-1 is expressed on the surfaces of many tissues, including the nasal epithelium, which is the entry site for rhinoviruses.

Mutagenesis of ICAM-1 DNA has revealed that the binding site for rhinovirus is located in the first Ig-like domain (204,261,295). The binding sites for two other known ligands of ICAM-1, LFA-1 and *Plasmodium falciparum*–infected erythrocytes, are also located in the first domain. A model of the rhinovirus–ICAM-1 complex produced from cryoelectron microscopy data, combined with x-ray structures of both components, confirms that only domain 1 of ICAM-1 contacts the virus surface (30, 50,180,236). The residues of ICAM-1 that contact rhinovirus are located in the BC, CD, DE, and FG loops of the first aminoterminal domain. These findings agree with the results of mutational analysis that identify amino acids crucial for virus binding.

A comparison of the structures of virus–receptor complexes of two different picornaviruses reveals significant differences. The orientation of the receptors bound to their viruses are strikingly different. The long axis of ICAM-1 is perpendicular to the capsid surface, whereas Pvr binds at a glancing angle. In addition, the "footprint" of Pvr on poliovirus is significantly larger than that of ICAM-1 on rhinovirus, and the receptor sites on the poliovirus capsid are more exposed. The extra surface area on poliovirus includes the knob of VP3 and the C-terminus of VP1 from the fivefold-related promoter in the southeast corner of the road map describing the contact of Pvr on poliovirus. As discussed later, these differences may account for some of the differences in kinetic and affinity constants between the two virus-receptor complexes.

Receptors and Coreceptors Needed for Infection

Many enteroviruses bind to decay-accelerating factor (DAF, or CD55), a member of the complement cascade (see Table 3). For most of these viruses, however, interaction with CD55 is not sufficient for infection. For example, coxsackievirus A21 binds to CD55, but infection does not occur unless ICAM-1 is also present (283). Some coxsackie B viruses that bind CD55 may require $\alpha_v\beta_6$-integrin as a coreceptor (4), whereas some echoviruses that bind integrin $\alpha_2\beta_1$ or CD55 are believed to require β_2-microglobulin as a coreceptor (320).

Alternative Receptors

Certain viruses bind to different cell surface receptors, depending on the virus isolate or the cell line (see Table 3). Foot-and-mouth disease virus A12 attaches to cells through the integrin $\alpha_v\beta_3$ (226). However, the O strain of foot-and-mouth disease virus, which has been passaged many times in cell culture, cannot bind to $\alpha_v\beta_3$; instead, this virus uses cell surface heparan sulfate (152). The type A12 strain cannot infect cells that do not express $\alpha_v\beta_3$, even when heparan sulfate is present on the cell surface. It is believed that laboratory adaptation of foot-and-mouth disease virus in cultured cells expressing low levels of $\alpha_v\beta_3$ leads to the selection of a virus that binds an alternative receptor.

How Picornaviruses Attach to Cell Receptors

As discussed previously, the capsids of picornaviruses are composed of four proteins arranged with icosahedral symmetry. Among the family members, the capsid proteins are arranged similarly, but the surface architecture varies. These differences account for not only the different serotypes but also the different modes of interaction with cell receptors. For example, the capsids of polioviruses, rhinoviruses, and coxsackieviruses have a groove, or canyon, surrounding each fivefold axis of symmetry. In contrast, cardioviruses and aphthoviruses do not have canyons.

The canyons of poliovirus and rhinovirus have been shown to be the sites of interaction with cell receptors. Mutation of amino acids that line the canyons of poliovirus and rhinovirus can alter the affinity of binding to receptors (65–67,134,189). Models of the interaction of poliovirus and rhinovirus with their cellular receptors have been produced from cryoelectron microscopy and x-ray crystallographic data (30,32,50,136,180,236,323). As discussed previously, these models reveal that only domain 1 of Pvr or ICAM-1 penetrates the canyon of the respective virus. For both rhinovirus and poliovirus, the footprint of the receptor defined by structural models agrees with the results of mutational data. More detail is available about the ICAM-1–rhinovirus interaction because the x-ray crystallographic structure of ICAM-1 has been determined (30,50). This information, however, does not explain why major and minor group rhinoviruses recognize different receptors. Minor group rhinoviruses have no obvious amino acid sequence differences from members of the major group; indeed, the major group rhinoviruses 14 and 16 are more distantly related to each other than to the minor group rhinoviruses 1A and 2.

It was originally believed that the picornavirus canyons were too deep and narrow to allow penetration by antibody molecules, which contain adjacent Ig domains (271). This physical barrier was believed to hide amino acids crucial for receptor binding from the immune system. Structural studies of a rhinovirus–antibody complex, however, revealed that antibody does penetrate deep into the canyon, as does ICAM-1 (289). The shape of the picornavirus canyon is therefore not likely to play a role in concealing virus from the immune system.

Beneath the canyon floor is the hydrophobic pocket that opens at the base of the canyon and extends toward the fivefold axis of symmetry (see The Hydrophobic Pocket, earlier). The pocket appears to be occupied in many picornaviruses with a fatty acid or related compound. Certain antiviral drugs, such as the WIN compounds, displace the lipid and bind tightly within the pocket (290). Binding of such drugs to rhinovirus 14 causes conformational changes in the canyon that prevent attachment to cells (250). In contrast, drug binding to rhinoviruses 1A, 3, and 16 and to poliovirus causes smaller structural changes in the capsid (120,126,140). Inhibition of rhinovirus 16 binding by these compounds is probably not a consequence of altering the receptor binding site, but rather the result of preventing conformational changes required for receptor binding. Such compounds do not inhibit binding of poliovirus, but rather uncoating (209).

The capsids of some picornaviruses, including coxsackievirus A9 and foot-and-mouth disease virus, do not have prominent canyons. These viruses are believed to attach to cell receptors through surface loops. In foot-and-mouth disease virus, an Arg-Gly-Asp sequence in the flexible βG-βH loop of the capsid protein VP1 is recognized by integrin receptors on cells (91). Arg-Gly-Asp–containing peptides block attachment of foot-and-mouth disease virus (28), and alteration of this sequence interferes with virus binding (200). In coxsackievirus A9, the Arg-Gly-Asp sequence is present in a 17–amino acid extension of the C-terminus of VP1 and is also the site of attachment to cell receptors (53,268). Alteration of this sequence does not abolish binding to cells, however, suggesting that the virus can bind to another cell surface receptor (147).

As discussed previously, foot-and-mouth disease virus uses alternative receptors, either integrin or heparan sulfate, depending on the virus isolate. The binding site for heparan sulfate on cell culture–adapted foot-and-mouth disease virus is a shallow depression on the virion surface, where the three major capsid proteins, VP1, VP2 and VP3, are located (96). Binding specificity is controlled by two preformed sulfate-binding sites on the capsid. Residue 56 of VP3 is a critical regulator of receptor recognition. In field isolates of the virus, this amino acid is histidine. Adaptation to cell culture selects for viruses with an arginine at this position, which forms the high-affinity heparan sulfate–binding site.

Kinetics and Affinity of the Virus–Receptor Interaction

The affinity and kinetics of picornaviruses binding to soluble forms of their receptors have been studied by surface plasmon resonance. Such parameters are important because they describe the interaction of virus with receptor, which enables a better understanding of the reaction and its comparison to other systems. There are two classes of receptor-binding sites, with distinct binding affinities, on the capsids of poliovirus and rhinovirus (49, 205,323). The association rates for the two binding classes are 25- and 13-fold higher for the poliovirus–sPvr interaction than for the rhinovirus–sICAM interaction at 20°C. The greater association rate of poliovirus and Pvr may be due, in part, to differences in the extent of contact between virus and receptor (see earlier). In contrast, whereas there are two dissociation rate constants for the poliovirus–Pvr interaction, only one has been reported for the rhinovirus 3–ICAM interaction. The dissociation rates for the poliovirus–sPvr interaction are 1.5-fold and 2.0-fold faster than for the rhinovirus–sICAM interaction, indicating greater instability of the former complex. The affinity constants for the poliovirus–sPvr interaction are 19-fold and 6-fold greater than those reported for the rhinovirus–sICAM-1 complex.

In contrast to the observations with poliovirus and rhinovirus, a single class of binding site was found on echovirus 11 for a soluble form of its receptor, CD55 (183). The affinity of this interaction is at least 4 times lower than either of the binding sites on poliovirus for sPvr. The association rate for the interaction between echovirus 11 and CD55 is faster than that of poliovirus–sPvr and rhinovirus–sICAM-1. One explanation for these findings is that the contact between echovirus 11 and CD55 is more extensive than that of the other two virus-receptor complexes. The binding site for CD55 on echovirus 11 may also be more accessible than those of Pvr and ICAM-1. The dissociation rate for the echovirus–CD55 interaction is at least 97 times faster than that of either the poliovirus–sPvr or the rhinovirus–sICAM-1 interaction. These findings are consistent with a more accessible binding site for CD55 on echovirus 11, compared with the receptor-binding sites on poliovirus and rhinovirus. Atomic interactions between CD55 and echovirus 11 may be weaker than between the other two viruses and their receptors. The faster dissociation rate of the echovirus 11–CD55 complex may be related to the finding that the interaction does not lead to structural changes of the virus particle (257), as occurs with poliovirus and rhinovirus.

Why do poliovirus and rhinovirus have two classes of receptor binding sites? The receptors for both viruses make contacts at two major sites on the virus surface, one in a cleft on the south rim of the canyon, and a second on the side of the mesa on the north rim. These two contact sites may correspond to the two classes of binding sites. Two classes of binding sites may also be a consequence of the structural flexibility exhibited by both viruses, which may cause exposure of different binding sites. Normally internal parts of the poliovirus and rhinovirus capsid proteins have been shown to be transiently displayed on the virion surface, a process called *breathing* (186, 187). As discussed later, the interaction of poliovirus and rhinovirus with their cellular receptors leads to irreversible and more extensive structural changes. In contrast to the findings with poliovirus and rhinovirus, binding of echovirus 11 with CD55 can be described by a simple 1:1 binding model. Such behavior, which would be expected for the interaction of two preformed binding sites, is consistent with the fact that the echovirus–CD55 interaction does not result in detectable structural changes in the capsid (257).

Entry Into Cells

Once picornaviruses have attached to their cellular receptor, the viral capsid must dissociate to release the RNA genome, which must enter the cytoplasm, the site of picornavirus replication. For some picornaviruses, interaction with a cell receptor serves only to concentrate virus on the cell surface; release of the genome is a consequence of low pH or perhaps the activity of a coreceptor. For other picornaviruses, the cell receptor is also an unzipper and initiates conformational changes in the virus that lead to release of the genome.

Formation of a Pore in the Cell Membrane

The interaction of poliovirus with its receptor, Pvr, leads to major structural changes in the virus. The resulting particles, called *altered,* or *A, particles,* contain the viral RNA but have lost the internal capsid protein VP4. In addition, the N-terminus of VP1, which is normally on the interior of the capsid, is on the surface of the A particle (95). This sequence of VP1 is hydrophobic, and as a result, the A particles have an increased affinity for membranes compared with the native virus particle. In one hypothesis for poliovirus entry, receptor binding leads to these conformational changes; the exposed lipophilic N-terminus of VP1 then inserts into the cell membrane, forming a pore through which the viral RNA can travel to the cytoplasm (Fig. 6). The finding that A particles, when added to lipid bilayers, induce the formation of ion channels supports this hypothesis (304). A model of the A particle produced from cryoelectron microscopy provides more insight into uncoating of the poliovirus genome (31). Compared with the native virus, capsid domains in the A particle have moved up to 9 Å, in a process that has been compared to

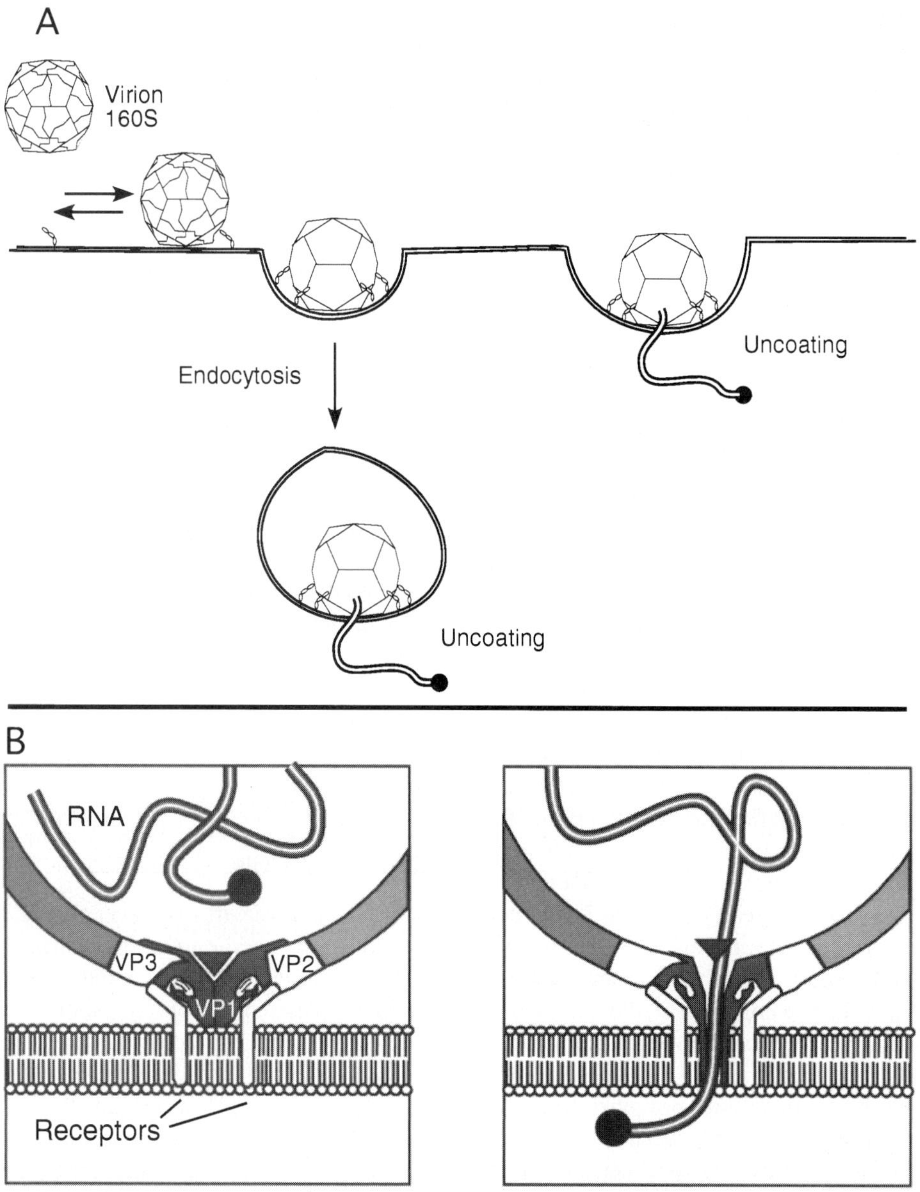

FIG. 6. Model for poliovirus entry into cells. **A:** Overview of poliovirus entry. The 160S native virus particle binds its cellular receptor, Pvr, and at temperatures greater than 33°C, undergoes a receptor-mediated conformational transition, leading to the production of altered *(A)* particles. These particles, which may be entry intermediates, are hydrophobic and have lost capsid protein VP4. The N-terminus of VP1, normally on the interior of the capsid, is translocated to the surface. The viral RNA, shown as a *curved line,* may exit the particle from the plasma membrane or from within endosomes. **B:** Hypothetical mechanism for translocation of poliovirus RNA across the cell membrane. At the left is a cross-section of a virus particle that has just bound Pvr at the cell surface. The viral RNA is in the capsid, and lipid occupies the hydrophobic pocket. Pvr docks on the capsid in the canyon, above the hydrophobic pocket. At right, the capsid has undergone the receptor-mediated conformational change. Docking of the receptor in the canyon leads to loss of the lipid in the hydrophobic pocket, allowing the capsid to undergo conformational changes. The extruded N-termini of VP1 form a pore in the cell membrane through which the viral RNA may pass. The dark triangle is the VP3 β-cylinder, which could move out of the way like a float valve (31).

the movements of Earth's tectonic plates. These movements produce gaps between the capsid subunits, and it is hypothesized that the gaps in the area where VP1, VP2, and VP3 meet could allow the emergence of VP4 and the N-terminus of VP1. In this model, VP4 and the VP1 N-terminus are extruded from the bottom of the canyon and are arranged around the mesa at the fivefold axis of symmetry. There, the five predicted amphipathic helices at the N-termini of VP1 would be in position to insert into the plasma membrane. A pore is formed, and then VP3, which forms a plug blocking the fivefold axis, is moved, allowing the RNA to exit the particle.

The ultimate disposition of VP4 released from the viral capsid is not known, but it is clear that this protein is required for an early stage of cell entry. A virus containing a mutation in VP4 can bind to cells and be converted to A particles, but these are blocked at a subsequent step in virus entry (221). VP4 and VP2 are produced, during virus assembly, from the precursor VP0, which remains uncleaved until RNA encapsidation. Cleavage of VP0 can therefore be viewed as a way of priming the capsid for uncoating because cleavage separates VP4 from VP2.

Although the A particle has biochemical and structural properties consistent with an entry intermediate, its role in entry has been questioned by the results of experiments demonstrating that poliovirus can replicate at 25°C, a temperature at which A particle formation cannot be detected (77). Perhaps the A particle detected at higher temperatures is a stable end product and an exaggerated form of an uncoating intermediate. The uncoating intermediate may be unstable and difficult to detect. However, the A particle is likely to be similar to the uncoating intermediate, and thus warrants further study.

Although it is believed that poliovirus RNA crosses the cell membrane, it is not known whether that event occurs at the plasma membrane or from within endosomes (see Fig. 6). Drugs, such as bafilomycin A1, that block acidification of endosomes through their inhibition of proton transport into the vesicles, do not inhibit poliovirus infection (245). These drugs effectively inhibit infection by viruses that enter the cytoplasm from acidic endosomes, such as influenza virus and Semliki Forest virus. Although it is likely that poliovirus RNA could enter at either the plasma or endosomal membrane, it is clear that endocytosis alone is not sufficient to trigger poliovirus uncoating. For example, antibody-coated poliovirus particles cannot efficiently infect cells expressing Fc receptors, which are efficiently endocytosed (16,199). This finding suggests that Pvr-mediated conformational changes in poliovirus are crucial to the uncoating process.

Entry by Endocytosis

Some picornaviruses, such as foot-and-mouth disease virus and rhinovirus, enter cells by receptor-mediated endocytosis, and uncoating is triggered by acidification of the endosomal, pH-dependent pathway (47,200). Infection of cells by these viruses is inhibited by weak bases and ionophores that block the acidification of endosomes (47,48). Consistent with this mechanism of entry, foot-and-mouth disease virus that has been coated with antibody can bind to and infect cells that express Fc receptors, in contrast to poliovirus (see earlier) (199). The cell receptor for foot-and-mouth disease virus is therefore a "hook": it does not induce uncoating-related changes in the virus particle, but rather serves only to tether the virus to the cell and bring it into the endocytic pathway.

The mechanism by which low pH causes disassembly of the foot-and-mouth disease virus capsid has been illuminated by structural and genetic studies. At a pH of about 6.5, the viral capsid dissociates to pentamers, releasing the viral RNA (315). Examination of the atomic structure of the virus revealed a high density of histidine residues lining the pentamer interface (2). These residues confer stability to the capsid; because the pKa of histidine is 6.8, close to the pH at which the virus dissociates, protonation of the side chains of the histidines might cause electrostatic repulsion, leading to disassembly (70). To test this hypothesis, a histidine residue at position 142 of VP3 was changed to arginine by mutagenesis. The resulting capsids were more stable at low pH than wild-type capsids (83), supporting the proposed role of the histidine residue in acid-catalyzed disassembly.

Regulation of Uncoating by Cellular Molecules

The hydrophobic pocket located below each protomer surface appears to be a critical regulator of the receptor-induced structural transitions of poliovirus. In poliovirus type 1, each pocket is occupied by a natural ligand that is believed to be a molecule of sphingosine (Fig. 7) (86, 324). The capsids of rhinoviruses 1A and 16 each contain lipids that are shorter than sphingosine (167,235), whereas that of coxsackievirus B3 has been modeled as a C16 fatty acid (225). The icosahedral symmetry of the capsid would allow each virion to contain up to 60 lipid molecules. In some picornaviruses, the pockets are apparently empty, such as in rhinovirus types 3 and 14 (18,333).

These lipids are thought contribute to the stability of the native virus particle by locking the capsid in a stable configuration and preventing conformational changes. Removal of the lipid is probably necessary to provide the capsid with sufficient flexibility to undergo the changes that permit the RNA to leave the shell. This hypothesis comes from the study of antiviral drugs, such as the WIN compounds, that displace the lipid and bind tightly in the hydrophobic pocket. These antiviral compounds block breathing of the rhinovirus capsid, the process by which normally internal parts of the capsid proteins are transiently displayed on the virion surface (186). Polioviruses containing bound WIN compounds can bind to cells, but the interaction with Pvr does not result in the production of A particles (92,331). WIN compounds appear to inhibit poliovirus infectivity by preventing Pvr-mediated conformational alterations that are required for uncoating. Additional support for the role of lipids in uncoating comes from the analysis of poliovirus mutants that cannot replicate unless WIN compounds are present (224). Such WIN-dependent mutants spontaneously convert to altered particles at 37°C, in the absence of the cell receptor, probably because of the absence of lipid in the hydrophobic pocket. The lipids can be considered to be switches that determine whether the virus is stable (lipid present) or will uncoat (lipid absent). It is not known what causes the lipid to be released from the capsid. Pvr docks onto the poliovirus capsid just above the hydrophobic pocket (see Fig. 6), which suggests that the interaction of the virus with receptor may initiate structural changes in the virion that lead to the release of the lipid. Incubation of poliovirus with Pvr for short periods at low temperatures appears to result in release of the lipid (32).

Translation of the Viral RNA

Internal Ribosome Binding: The Internal Ribosome Entry Site

Once the picornavirus positive-stranded genomic RNA is released into the cell cytoplasm, it must be translated because it cannot be copied by any cellular RNA polymerase and no viral enzymes are brought into the cell within the viral capsid. Several experimental findings led to the belief that translation of the picornavirus genome was accomplished by an unusual mechanism. The positive-stranded RNA genomes lack 5′-terminal cap structures; although virion RNA is linked to the viral protein VPg, this protein is removed by a cellular "unlinking" enzyme on entry of the RNA into the cell (8). Furthermore, picornavirus genomes are efficiently translated in infected cells despite inhibition of cellular mRNA translation. Determination of the nucleotide sequence of poliovirus positive-stranded RNA revealed a 741-nucleotide 5′-untranslated region that contains seven AUG codons (174,260). Such 5′-noncoding regions, which were subsequently found in other picornaviruses, contain highly ordered RNA structures (265,288). These

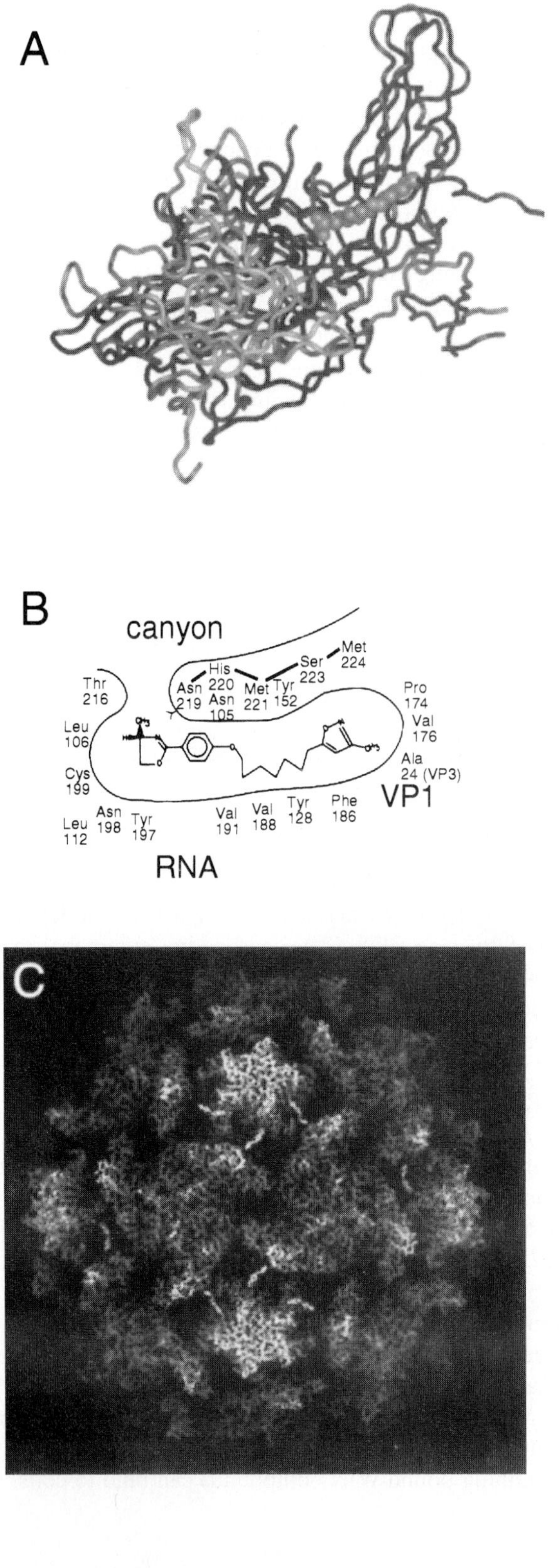

FIG. 7. The hydrophobic pocket in the picornavirus capsid. **A:** Cellular lipid bound in the hydrophobic pocket of poliovirus type 1. Side view of a protomer, consisting of one copy each of VP1, VP2, VP3, and VP4. RNA is below, and the 5-fold axis of symmetry is at the upper right. Gray spheres represent what is believed to be a molecule of sphingosine bound in the hydrophobic pocket. The lipid is just below the canyon floor. **B:** WIN52084 bound in the hydrophobic pocket. These drugs displace the lipid from the pocket, thereby blocking infectivity. **C:** Drug bound in the poliovirus pocket. R78206, a WIN-like compound, bound in the poliovirus capsid. The bound drug is the small white molecule at the base of the canyon. The drug appears to be exposed on the surface but is actually in the hydrophobic pocket. The capsid model is shown in a radial depth-cued representation, in which atoms are colored according to whether they are near the center of the virus (*black*) or far from the center (*white*). Residues at the bottom of the canyon are dark because they are at a position of low radius. The bound drug is not depth cued.

features led to the suggestion that ribosomes do not scan through the picornaviral 5′-untranslated regions, but rather bind to an internal sequence. The 5′-untranslated region of poliovirus positive-stranded RNA was subsequently shown to contain a sequence that promotes translation initiation by internal ribosome binding, or the IRES (Fig. 8).

The picornavirus IRES contains extensive regions of RNA secondary structure that is conserved within the type I (enteroviruses and rhinoviruses) and type II (cardioviruses and aphthoviruses) IRES (see Fig. 3). One sequence motif that is conserved among these two types of IRES is a GNRA sequence (N, any nucleotide; R, purine) in stem-loop IV of the type I IRES and in stem-

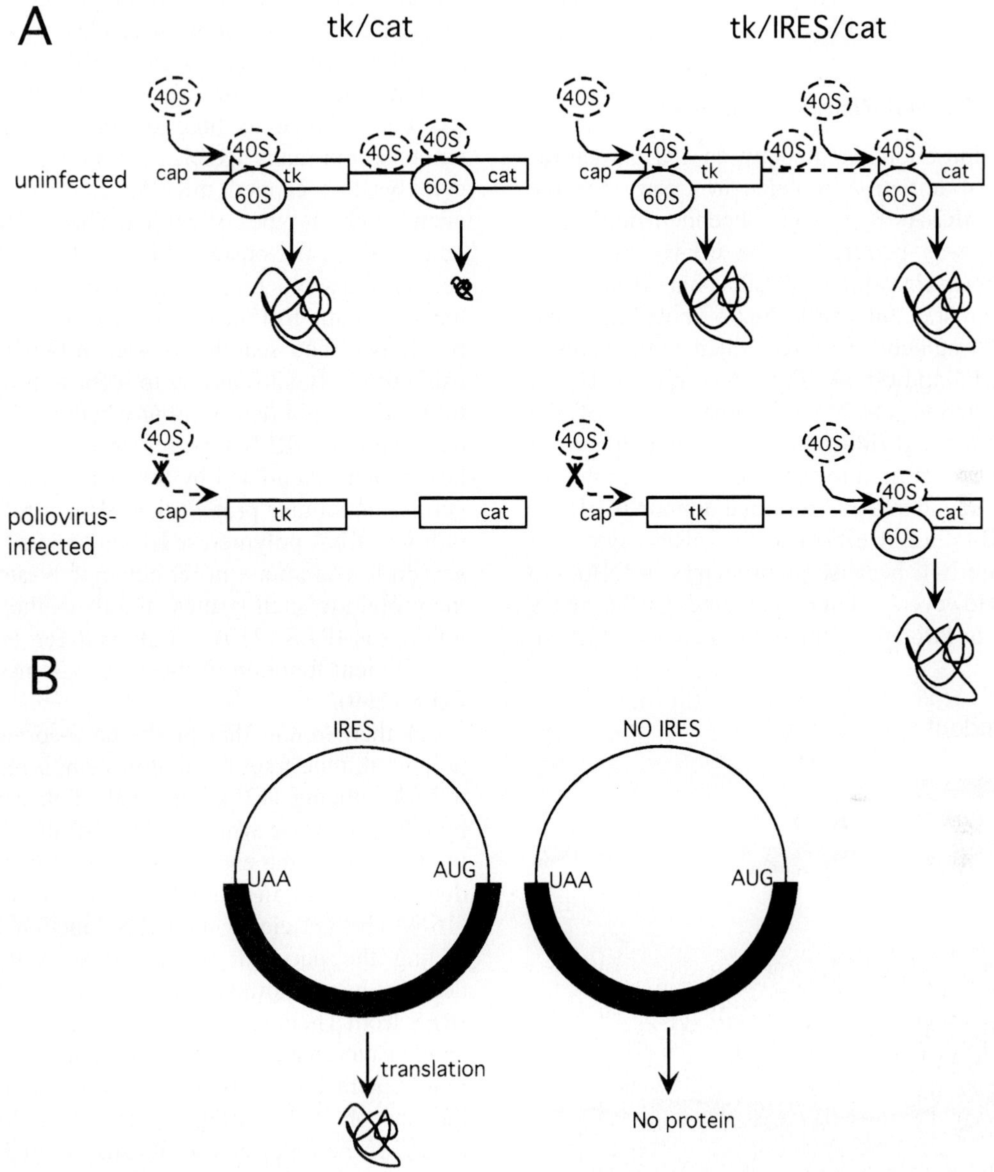

FIG. 8. Discovery of the internal ribosome entry site (IRES). **A:** Bicistronic mRNA assay used to discover the IRES (244). Plasmids were constructed that encode two reporter molecules, thymidine kinase (tk) and chloramphenicol acetyl transferase (cat), separated by an IRES (*solid line*) or a spacer (*dotted line*). After introduction into mammalian cells, the plasmids give rise to mRNAs of the structure shown in the figure. In uninfected cells (*top line*), both reporter molecules can be detected, although cat synthesis is inefficient without an IRES and is probably due to reinitiation. In poliovirus-infected cells, 5′ end–dependent initiation is inhibited, and no proteins are detected without an IRES, demonstrating internal ribosome binding. **B:** Circular mRNA assay for an IRES. Circular mRNAs were constructed and translated *in vitro* in cell extracts. In the absence of an IRES, no protein is observed because 5′-end initiation requires a free 5′-end. Inclusion of an IRES allows protein translation from the circular mRNA, demonstrating internal ribosome binding (56).

loop I of the type II IRES. Another conserved element is an Yn-Xm-AUG motif, in which Yn is a pyrimidine-rich region and Xm is a 15- to 25-nucleotide spacer followed by an AUG codon. In the type II and hepatitis A virus IRES, this codon is the initiator AUG; in the type I IRES, the initiator is located 30 to 150 nucleotides further downstream. Translation initiation through a type 1 IRES involves binding of the 40S ribosomal subunit to the IRES and scanning of the subunit to the AUG initiation codon. The 40S subunit probably binds at the AUG initiation codon of a type II IRES.

Mechanism of Internal Ribosome Binding

Translation initiation directed by an IRES requires the same set of initiation proteins necessary for the translation of mRNAs by 5′ end–dependent initiation. The exception was believed to be eIF4G, which is cleaved in picornavirus-infected cells, inactivating the translation of most cellular mRNAs. We now know that the C-terminal fragment of eIF4G, which contains binding sites for eIF3 and eIF4A (Fig. 9), stimulates IRES-mediated translation (44,234). In one model of the mechanism of internal ribosome binding, the 40S ribosomal subunit is recruited to the IRES through interaction with eIF3 bound to the C-terminal domain of eIF4G (see Fig. 9). Binding of eIF4G to the mRNA does not occur through eIF4E because picornavirus mRNAs are not capped. However, eIF4G may bind to the IRES either directly or through a "linker" protein (see Fig. 9).

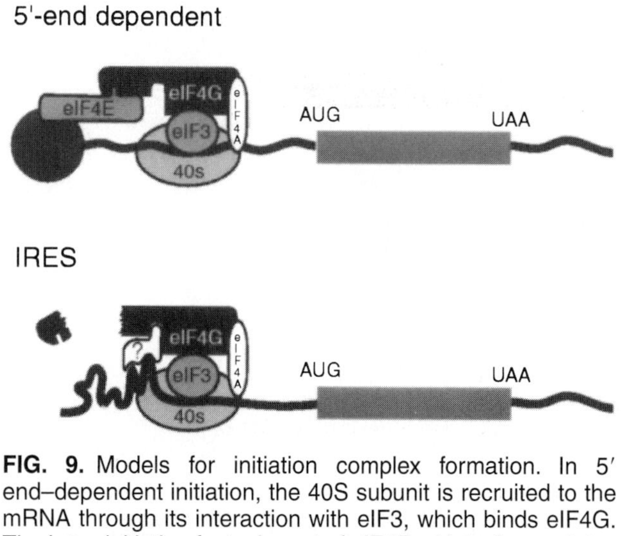

FIG. 9. Models for initiation complex formation. In 5′ end–dependent initiation, the 40S subunit is recruited to the mRNA through its interaction with eIF3, which binds eIF4G. The latter initiation factor is part of eIF4F, which also contains eIF4A, a helicase to unwind RNA secondary structure, and eIF4E, the cap-binding protein. Binding of eIF4E to the cap thus positions eIF4E at the 5′-end and positions the 40S subunit on the mRNA. In IRES-dependent translation, a 5′-end is not required. The eIF3–40S complex is believed to be recruited to the RNA by the interaction of eIF4G with cellular IRES-binding proteins, marked by ?. No such universal IRES-binding protein has been identified.

It has been reported that eIF4G mRNA contains an IRES (100,101), suggesting a mechanism for its synthesis in picornavirus-infected cells, in which 5′ end–dependent translation initiation is inhibited. Stimulation of IRES function by the C-terminal proteolytic fragment of eIF4G may explain the observation that IRES activity is enhanced in cells in which the poliovirus protease $2A^{pro}$ is expressed (131). Protease $2A^{pro}$ is one of the picornaviral proteinases responsible for cleavage of eIF4G. Although the IRES of most picornaviruses functions with cleaved eIF4G, that of hepatitis A virus requires intact eIF4G (41).

Only one IRES, from cricket paralysis virus (322), has been shown to function *in vitro* in wheat germ extracts, and many IRESes function poorly in reticulocyte lysates; capped mRNAs can be translated efficiently in both types of extract. These observations may be explained if ribosome binding to the IRES requires cell proteins other than the canonical translation proteins, perhaps to link the IRES to eIF4G, as discussed previously. The search for such proteins has involved using mobility-shift assays to identify proteins that bind to the IRES and determining whether such proteins are necessary for IRES function in cell-free extracts. One host protein identified by this approach is the autoantigen La, a cellular protein that plays a role in the maturation of RNA polymerase III transcripts (210). It is present in low amounts in reticulocyte lysates; addition of the protein to such lysates stimulates the activity of the poliovirus IRES (210). La autoantigen is also required for efficient function of the encephalomyocarditis virus IRES (169).

Another protein that binds the picornavirus IRES is polypyrimidine tract-binding protein, a regulator of pre-mRNA splicing (138). Removal of this protein from a reticulocyte lysate with an RNA affinity column inhibits the function of the encephalomyocarditis virus IRES but does not affect translation by 5′ end–dependent initiation (161). The deficiency in IRES function is restored by adding the purified protein back to the lysate. The depleted lysate, however, still supports the function of the IRES from Theiler's murine encephalomyocarditis virus, another picornavirus. It was subsequently shown that the requirement for polypyrimidine tract-binding protein by the encephalomyocarditis virus IRES depends on the nature of the reporter and the size of an A-rich bulge in the IRES (162). Polypyrimidine tract–binding protein is required for the function of the IRES of poliovirus and rhinovirus (149).

HeLa cell extracts also contain unr, an RNA-binding protein with five cold-shock domains that is required for IRES function (148). Recombinant unr stimulates the function of the rhinovirus IRES in the reticulocyte lysate and acts synergistically with recombinant polypyrimidine tract–binding protein to stimulate translation mediated by the rhinovirus IRES. However, unr does not augment the stimulation of the poliovirus IRES by polypyrimidine tract–binding protein.

Ribosome-associated poly r(C)–binding proteins bind at multiple sites within the poliovirus IRES (38,98). One binding site for these proteins has been identified within stem-loop IV of the poliovirus IRES (see Fig. 3) (38). Mutations in this region that abolish binding of poly r(C)–binding proteins cause decreased translation *in vitro.* Furthermore, depletion of poly r(C)–binding proteins from HeLa cell translation extracts results in inhibition of poliovirus IRES function (39). When this assay was used to survey a wide range of picornaviral IRES elements, it was found that poly r(C)–binding proteins are required for function of the type I, but not the type II, IRES (318). These results provide the first evidence of a difference in the manner in which the type I and type II IRES function. A second binding site for poly r(C)–binding proteins has been identified within a cloverleaf RNA structure that forms within the first 108 nucleotides of the positive-stranded poliovirus RNA genome (98,239). The interaction of poly r(C)–binding proteins with this part of the RNA has been proposed to regulate whether a positive-stranded RNA molecule is translated or replicated.

From the preceding discussion, it is clear that no single protein has been identified that is essential for the function of every IRES. It is certainly reasonable to propose that certain types of IRES have different requirements for cellular proteins. A different view is that cellular proteins, such as polypyrimidine tract–binding protein, may act as RNA chaperones, maintaining the IRES in a structure that permits it to bind directly to the translational machinery (151). IRESes that do not require such chaperones may fold properly without the need for cellular proteins. In support of this hypothesis, the IRES of hepatitis C virus, a flavivirus, has been shown to bind directly to eIF3 and the ribosomal 40S subunit, without a requirement for eIF4F (246).

Processing of the Viral Polyprotein

Picornavirus proteins are synthesized by the translation of a single, long, open reading frame on the viral positive-stranded RNA genome, followed by cleavage of the polyprotein by virus-encoded proteinases (Fig. 10; see Fig. 2). This strategy allows the synthesis of multiple protein products from a single RNA genome. The polyprotein is not observed in infected cells because it is

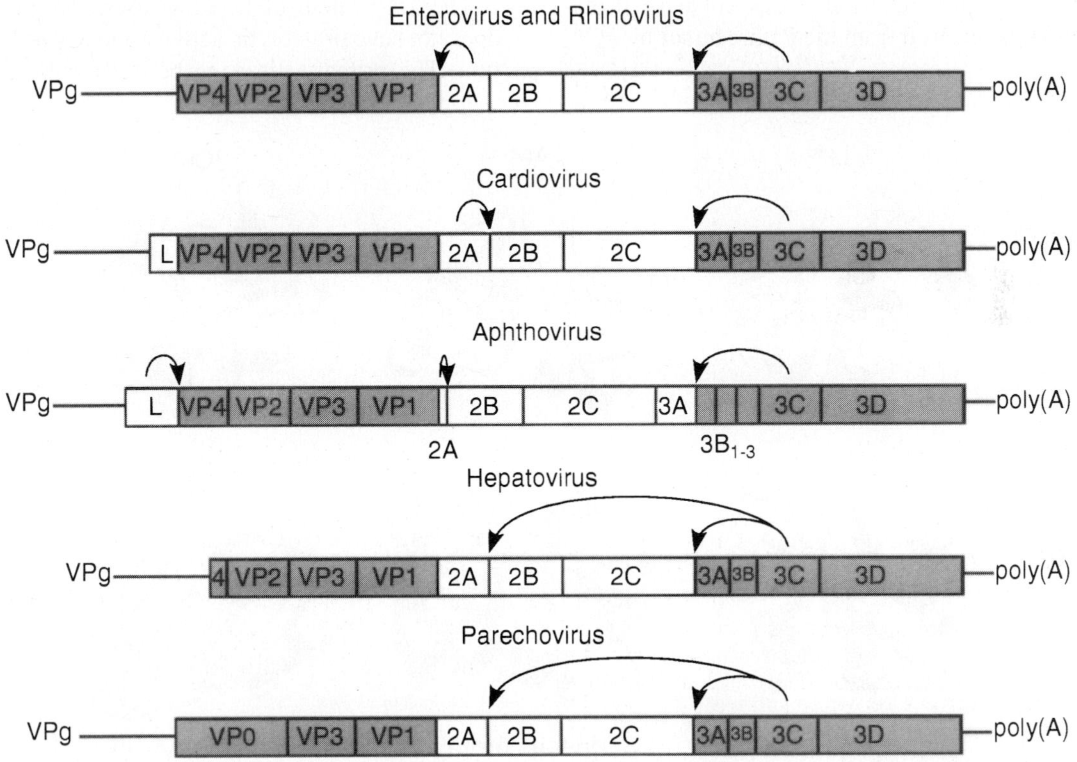

FIG. 10. Primary cleavages of picornavirus polyprotein. In cells infected with enteroviruses and rhinoviruses, nascent P1 is cleaved from P2 by $2A^{pro}$. In cells infected with cardioviruses and aphthoviruses, the P1–P2 junction is cleaved by $3C^{pro}$. The 2A proteins of these viruses are not proteinases, but they cause their own release at the junction with 2B. In all viruses shown, the P2–P3 cleavage is carried out by $3C^{pro}$. In hepatoviruses and parechoviruses, $3C^{pro}$ also carries out primary cleavage at the 2A–2B junction. The L^{pro} proteinase of foot-and-mouth disease virus catalyzes its release from VP4.

processed as soon as the protease coding sequences have been translated. The polyprotein precursor is processed cotranslationally by intramolecular reactions (in *cis*) in what are called primary cleavages, followed by secondary processing in *cis* or in *trans* (intermolecular). Picornavirus genomes encode three proteinases: L^{pro}, $2A^{pro}$, and $3C^{pro}$, which carry out cleavage of the polyprotein.

In contrast to other picornaviruses, the first protein encoded in the genome of cardioviruses and aphthoviruses is the L protein (see Figs. 2 and 10). The L protein of foot-and-mouth disease virus is a proteinase that releases itself from the polyprotein by cleaving between its C-terminus and the N-terminus of VP4. Based on sequence analysis, it was suggested that foot-and-mouth disease virus L^{pro} is related to thiol proteases (118). This prediction was supported by the results of site-directed mutagenesis, which showed that Cys-51 and His-148 are the active-site amino acids (252,266). The atomic structure of L^{pro} reveals that it consists of two domains, with a topology related to that of papain, a thiol proteinase (123) (Fig. 11). The active-site His is located at the top of the central α-helix, and substrate binds in the groove between the two domains (see Fig. 11). Besides releasing itself from the polyprotein, L^{pro} also cleaves the translation initiation factor eIF4G to effect inhibition of cellular translation (73). In cardioviruses, the L protein, which does not have proteolytic activity, is released from the P1 precursor by $3C^{pro}$ (238).

In cells infected with enteroviruses or rhinoviruses, the primary cleavage between P1 and P2 is mediated by $2A^{pro}$. In addition, $2A^{pro}$ cleaves the host cell protein eIF4G (see Cleavage of eIF4G). In the protein precursor of rhinovirus, poliovirus, and some other enteroviruses, the cleavage site for $2A^{pro}$ is between tyrosine and glycine. Other sites cleaved by $2A^{pro}$ include threonine-glycine and phenylalanine-glycine in certain coxsackieviruses and echoviruses. Based on sequence alignments, it was suggested that the structure of $2A^{pro}$ would resemble that of small bacterial chymotrypsin-like proteinases such as *Streptomyces griseus* proteinase A and would possess a catalytic triad consisting of His-20, Asp-38, and an active-site nucleophile of Cys-109 rather than serine (29). The results of site-directed mutagenesis and the resolution of the atomic structure of rhinovirus $2A^{pro}$ confirm that these residues compose the active site and that the fold of $2A^{pro}$ is very similar to that of *S. griseus* proteinase A (247,292,329) (see Fig. 11). However, $2A^{pro}$ differs from all known chymotrypsin-like proteinases in that the N-terminal domain is not a β-barrel, but rather a four-stranded antiparallel β-sheet. Another unusual feature of $2A^{pro}$ is a tightly bound zinc ion located at the beginning of the C-terminal domain. Biochemical and structural studies indicate that zinc is essential for the structure of the enzyme (247,291,317).

The 2A protein of hepatoviruses and parechoviruses does not have proteolytic activity and has no known function. The primary cleavage between the capsid protein

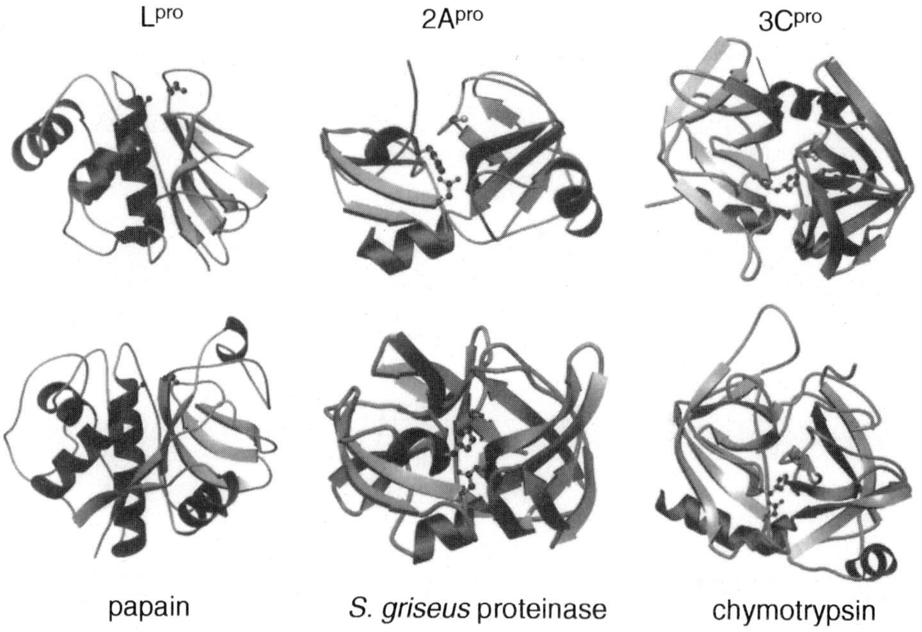

FIG. 11. Three dimensional structures of hepatitis A virus $3C^{pro}$, rhinovirus $2A^{pro}$, and L^{pro} of foot-and-mouth disease virus. Below each is the cellular proteinase that is structurally similar to each viral enzyme. Only the globular domain of L^{pro} is shown because the remaining residues have no counterpart in papain. Catalytic residues are drawn as *balls* and *sticks*. The rhinovirus $2A^{pro}$ structure is a model that was predicted before the crystal structure was solved. (Adapted from Seipelt J, Guarne A, Bergmann E, et al. The structures of piconaviral proteinases. *Virus Res* 1999;62:159–168, with permission.)

precursor and the P2 region of these viruses is carried out by $3C^{pro}$ (see Fig. 10) (157,278,279).

The 2A protein of aphthoviruses and cardioviruses does not have proteolytic activity and is not related to other picornavirus 2A proteins. In cells infected with these viruses, the VP1/2A cleavage is not carried out by 2A, but rather by $3C^{pro}$ (238). Aphthovirus 2A protein is only 18 amino acids in length, yet this protein can catalyze autocleavage at the junction with 2B, even in heterologous polyproteins (275). The 2A protein of cardioviruses is 150 amino acids long, yet only the last 19 amino acids, plus the first amino acid from 2B, proline, are required for cleavage from 2B (76). Mutations within the conserved amino acid sequence Asn-Pro-Gly-Pro, which contains the cleavage site Gly-Pro, disrupt cleavage (238). The mechanism of aphthovirus- and cardiovirus 2A–mediated cleavage is not understood and represents a novel form of peptide bond scission probably involving a single turnover event.

All picornaviruses encode $3C^{pro}$, which carries out a primary cleavage between 2C and 3A (see Fig. 10). In hepatoviruses and parechoviruses, $3C^{pro}$ also cleaves between 2A and 2B (see Fig. 10). Unlike the other picornavirus proteinases, $3C^{pro}$ also carries out secondary cleavages of the P1 and P2 precursors. Poliovirus $3C^{pro}$ cleaves only at the Gln-Gly dipeptide; however, $3C^{pro}$ of other picornaviruses has less strict cleavage specificities and cleaves at other sites, including Gln-Ser, Gln-Ile, Gln-Asn, Gln-Ala, Gln-Thr, and Gln-Val. There are clearly other determinants of cleavage because not all such dipeptides in picornavirus polyproteins are cleaved by $3C^{pro}$. Additional determinants include accessibility of the cleavage site to the enzyme, recognition of secondary and tertiary structures in the substrate by the enzyme, and amino acid sequences surrounding the cleavage site. For example, efficient cleavage of poliovirus Gln-Gly pairs requires an Ala at the P4 position (Gln is residue P1, numbering is toward the N-terminus) (37).

Sequence comparisons with cellular proteinases led to the prediction that $3C^{pro}$ folds similarly to the chymotrypsin-like serine proteinases (29,114–117). The putative catalytic triad was believed to consist of His-40, Asp-71 (aphthoviruses and cardioviruses) or Glu-71 (enteroviruses and rhinoviruses), and Cys-147 as the nucleophilic residue, in contrast to serine in cellular serine proteinases. These predictions have been confirmed by site-directed mutagenesis and by resolution of the atomic structures of rhinovirus, hepatitis A virus, and poliovirus $3C^{pro}$ (55,122,132,166,201,222,247). The viral enzyme folds into two equivalent β-barrels like chymotrypsin (see Fig. 11) but differs in some of the connecting loops, the orientation of the catalytic residues, and in areas needed for transition-state stabilization. The acidic member of the catalytic triad, Glu or Asp, points away from the active-site His and is therefore not believed to assist in catalysis. However, $3C^{pro}$ also binds viral RNA (see Genome Replication and mRNA Synthesis), and this binding site is distal from the active site of the enzyme. The presence of this RNA-binding site imposes evolutionary constraints on $3C^{pro}$ that are not found in other proteinases.

Both $3C^{pro}$ and $2A^{pro}$ are active in the nascent polypeptide and release themselves from the polyprotein by self-cleavage. After the proteinases have been released, they cleave the polyprotein in *trans*. The cascade of processing events varies for different picornaviruses. In cells infected with rhinovirus and enteroviruses, the initial event in the processing cascade is the release of the P1 precursor from the nascent P2–P3 protein by $2A^{pro}$. The activity of $2A^{pro}$ does not depend on whether it is cleaved from the precursor (137), but further processing of P1 by $3CD^{pro}$ does not occur unless $2A^{pro}$ is released from P1 (228,328). Next, $3CD^{pro}$ is released from the P3 precursor by autocatalytic cleavage; it is this proteinase, and not $3C^{pro}$, which carries out secondary cleavage of glutamine-glycine dipeptides in poliovirus P1 (160,327). Both $3C^{pro}$ and $3CD^{pro}$ can process proteins of the P2 and P3 regions. 3D may be required to recognize structural motifs in properly folded P1, allowing efficient processing of the $3C^{pro}$ part of the enzyme. The presence of multiple activities in a single protein is not found among eukaryotic proteinases and is an example of how the coding capacity of small viral genomes can be maximized. Not all picornaviruses require $3CD^{pro}$ to process P1; aphthoviruses, cardioviruses, and hepatoviruses produce $3C^{pro}$ that can cleave P1 without additional viral protein sequence.

An advantage of the polyprotein strategy is that expression can be controlled by the rate and extent of proteolytic processing. Alternative use of cleavage sites can also produce proteins with different activities. For example, because $3CD^{pro}$ is required for processing of the poliovirus capsid protein precursor P1, the extent of capsid protein processing can be controlled by regulating the amount of $3CD^{pro}$ that is produced. Because $3CD^{pro}$ does not possess RNA polymerase activity, some of it must be cleaved to allow RNA replication.

A final processing step occurs during maturation, when VP0 is cleaved to form VP4 and VP2. This event is discussed later.

Genome Replication and mRNA Synthesis

In the 1950s, it was believed that the genome of RNA viruses was replicated by the cellular DNA-dependent RNA polymerase, through an intermediate DNA strand. The replication of RNA viruses was therefore thought to occur entirely in the cell nucleus. In the early 1960s, studies of mengovirus showed that virus infection results in the induction of a cytoplasmic enzyme that can synthesize viral RNA in the presence of actinomycin D (21). This observation suggested that viral genome replication occurred through a virus-specific RNA-dependent RNA polymerase because cellular RNA synthesis is DNA dependent, occurs in the nucleus, and is sensitive to actinomycin D. Shortly thereafter, a similar cytoplasmic, actinomycin D–resistant genome replication system was discovered in poliovirus-infected cells (19). Since then, most studies of picornavirus RNA synthesis have been carried out with poliovirus.

In poliovirus-infected cells, the positive-stranded genome is amplified through a negative-stranded intermediate, resulting in about 50,000 genomes per cell. Three forms of RNA have been identified in the cell: single-stranded RNAs, replicative intermediate (RI), and replicative form (RF). Single-stranded RNA is the most abundant form and is exclusively positive-stranded; free negative strands have never been detected in infected cells. RI is full-length RNA from which six to eight nascent strands are attached. RI is largely of positive polarity with nascent negative strands, although the opposite configuration has been detected. RF is a double-stranded structure, consisting of one full-length copy of the positive and negative strands. Viral RNA synthesis is asymmetric in that the synthesis of positive strands is 25 to 65 times greater than the synthesis of negative strands (106,232).

The Viral RNA-Dependent RNA Polymerase, 3D^{pol}

The first evidence for a viral RNA-dependent RNA polymerase activity came from experiments in which lysates from cells infected with mengovirus or poliovirus were assayed for viral RNA polymerase activity by the incorporation of a radioactive nucleotide into viral RNA (21). Initial experiments demonstrated that the viral RNA polymerase is associated with a cellular membrane fraction, subsequently shown to be smooth membranes, which was called the *RNA replication complex* (109). A major component of the replication complex was a viral protein that migrated at 63,000 daltons on polyacrylamide gels (therefore called p63), which was suggested to be the viral RNA-dependent RNA polymerase. However, other viral and host proteins, including 2BC, 2C, 3AB, and 3C^{pro}, were detected in the RNA replication complexes.

A limitation of this early work was that replication complexes did not respond to the addition of template RNA, but rather copied viral RNA already present in the complex. Therefore, attempts were made to purify a template-dependent enzyme from membrane fractions of infected cells, using a poly(A) template and an oligo(U) primer. A poly(U) polymerase activity was purified from poliovirus-infected cells, which could also copy poliovirus RNA in the presence of an oligo(U) primer. Highly purified preparations contained only p63, the major viral protein found in membranous replication complexes (87,310). This protein is the poliovirus RNA polymerase, now known as 3D^{pol}. In the absence of an oligo(U) primer, 3D^{pol} cannot copy poliovirus RNA. Recombinant 3D^{pol} purified from bacteria or insect cells also requires the presence of an oligo(U) primer to copy poliovirus RNA (227,256). 3D^{pol} is therefore a template- and primer-dependent enzyme that can copy poliovirus RNA. Its molecular weight predicted from the amino acid sequence is 53 kd.

The structures of three of the four types of polymerases, DNA-dependent DNA polymerase, DNA-dependent RNA polymerase, and RNA-dependent DNA polymerase (reverse transcriptase), are characterized by analogy with a right hand, consisting of a palm, fingers, and thumb. The palm domain contains the active site of the enzyme. The first structure of an RNA-dependent RNA polymerase is that of poliovirus 3D^{pol}, which was determined at 2.6 Å resolution by x-ray crystallography (133). The enzyme has the same overall shape as other polymerases, although the fingers and thumb differ (Fig. 12). The palm domain is similar to that of other polymerases and contains four conserved amino acid motifs that are found in other RNA-dependent polymerases. 3D^{pol} also contains a fifth motif between the palm and thumb subdomains, which is found in RNA-dependent but not DNA-dependent polymerases.

In addition to its enzymatic activity, poliovirus 3Dpol is also a cooperative single-stranded RNA-binding protein and can unwind duplex RNA without the need for adenosine triphosphate hydrolysis (59,240). Consistent with these findings, two regions of polymerase–polymerase interaction have been observed in 3D^{pol} protein crystals. The first, called interface I, is extensive and involves more than 23 amino acid side chains on two different surfaces of the protein (Fig. 13). This interaction

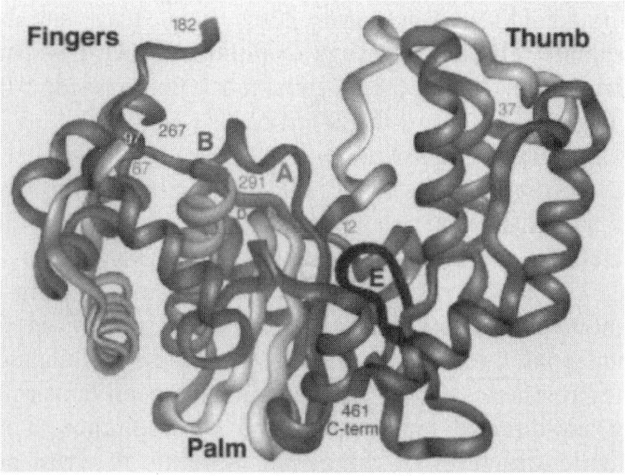

FIG. 12. Three dimensional structure of poliovirus 3D^{pol}. Thumb, palm, and fingers subdomains are labeled. The two white regions have no counterparts in other polymerases. The region connecting these sequences is disordered (amino acids 33 to 66); hence, it is not known whether these residues are connected across the active site (considered unlikely) or whether amino acids 14 to 35 are from a separate molecule. If the latter is correct, such interactions may lead to oligomerization. (Adapted from ref. 133, with permission.)

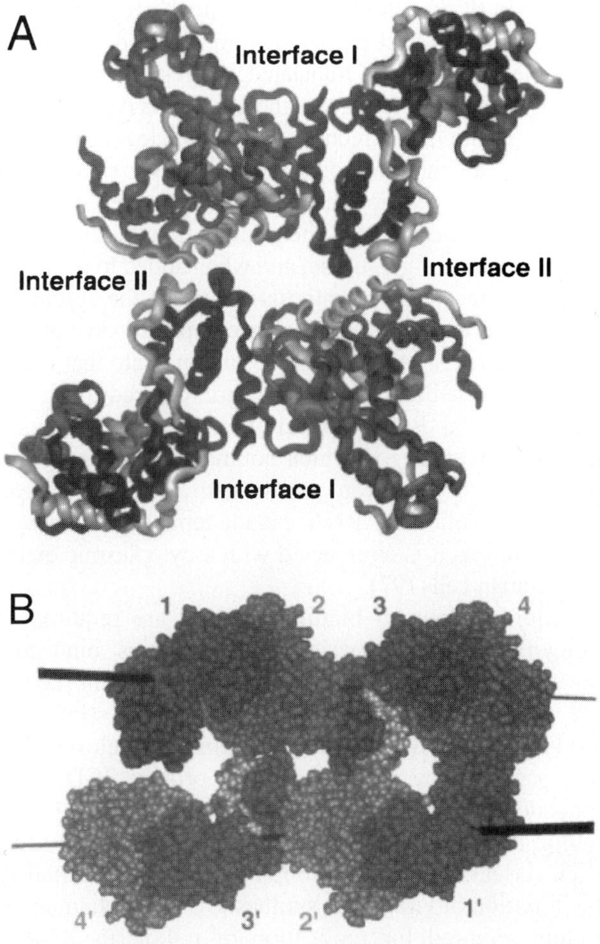

FIG. 13. Interactions among $3D^{pol}$ molecules in protein crystals. **A:** The manner in which four polymerase molecules interact is shown. Interface I, between the front of the thumb subdomain of one molecule and the back of the palm subdomain of another, leads to head-to-tail fibers of the enzyme. Interface II, formed by interactions between the two N-terminal regions of the polymerase (*white*), is a result of contacts between polymerase molecules in neighboring fibers. **B:** Model of how $3D^{pol}$ might oligomerize on RNA. Shown are two fibers formed by interface I interactions. Each fiber contains four polymerase molecules. The two fibers interact across interface II; the axis of each is shown in *black*. (Adapted from ref. 133, with permission.)

occurs in a head-to-tail fashion and results in long fibers of polymerase molecules. When RNA is modeled into the $3D^{pol}$ structure based on the location of DNA in the crystal structure of DNA bound to human immunodeficiency virus type 1 reverse transcriptase, it falls along the fibers formed by interface I interactions. Interface II is formed by N-terminal polypeptide segments, which may lead to a network of polymerase fibers in combination with interactions at interface I. These N-terminal polypeptide segments may originate from different polymerase molecules. The N-terminus of $3D^{pol}$ is required for enzyme activity, which would support the idea that interface II interactions are of functional consequence. The viral nucleoproteins of negative-stranded RNA viruses are also cooperative single-stranded RNA-binding proteins. The function of these proteins is to allow multiple rounds of RNA synthesis by keeping the RNA single stranded and preventing base-pairing between template and product. The single-stranded RNA–binding properties of $3D^{pol}$ may have a similar function in infected cells.

Viral Accessory Proteins

The poliovirus capsid proteins are not required for viral RNA synthesis; the region of the viral genome that encodes these proteins can be deleted without affecting the ability of viral RNA to replicate in cells (163). However, the capsid coding regions of rhinovirus, Theiler's virus, and mengovirus contain a cis-acting RNA sequence required for genome replication (192,206,207). A cis-acting RNA sequence required for RNA replication has also been identified in the poliovirus protein 2C coding region (113). Genetic and biochemical studies implicate most proteins of the P2 and P3 regions of the genome in RNA synthesis.

2A Protein

As discussed previously, $2A^{pro}$ protein is necessary for proteolytic cleavage of the polyprotein. Whether this is the sole requirement for this protein in viral replication was addressed by placing a second IRES element in the poliovirus genome before the $2A^{pro}$ coding region, effectively alleviating the need for the processing activity of the enzyme. Such viruses are viable (216). However, deletion of part of the coding region for $2A^{pro}$ is lethal. These results suggest that $2A^{pro}$ also plays a role in viral RNA replication, although its function in this process is not known.

2B Protein

Mutagenesis of 2B protein of poliovirus and coxsackievirus results in viruses with defects in RNA synthesis (159,311). The C-terminus of 2B contains a hydrophobic region and a conserved putative amphipathic α-helix that appear to be crucial to the function of the protein (312). However, the role of 2B in RNA synthesis is not known. Protein 2B has been shown to induce cell membrane permeability (6,276,313,314), which may play a role in release of virus from cells. Protein 2B is also partly responsible for the proliferation of membranous vesicles in infected cells, which are the sites of viral RNA replication. Because protein 3A has the same effect, it is not clear whether altered membrane proliferation is responsible for the RNA-defective phenotype in 2B mutants.

2C Protein

Mutations responsible for resistance of poliovirus and echovirus to guanidine hydrochloride, which blocks viral

RNA replication, are located in the 2C protein (175,253, 254). This compound has been shown to inhibit specifically the initiation of negative-stranded RNA synthesis and has no effect on initiation of positive-stranded RNA synthesis or on elongation on either strand (25). Protein 2C binds RNA, has nucleoside triphosphatase (NTPase) activity (267) that is inhibited by guanidine (251), and shares amino acid homology with known RNA helicases, proteins encoded by most positive-stranded RNA viruses with large genomes. These enzymes are believed to be necessary to unwind double-stranded RNA structures that form during RNA replication. Purified protein 2C, however, does not have RNA helicase activity (267). Alteration of conserved amino acids within the NTPase domain of 2C results in loss of viral infectivity. 2C may therefore have two functions during viral RNA synthesis: as an NTPase, and directing replication complexes to cell membranes. Expression of 2C leads to the formation of membrane vesicles and may contribute to the formation of the replication complex (60).

3AB Protein

Protein 3AB is believed to anchor VPg in membranes for the priming step of RNA synthesis. The purified protein greatly stimulates $3D^{pol}$ activity *in vitro* (241,255, 264) as well as the proteolytic activity of $3CD^{pro}$ (215). 3AB interacts with $3D^{pol}$ and 3CD in infected cells and with $3D^{pol}$ in the yeast two-hybrid system (145). Mutations in $3D^{pol}$ that disrupt its interaction with 3AB result in viruses with defects in protein processing and viral RNA synthesis (104,105). A complex of 3AB and 3CD also binds the 3′-terminal sequence of poliovirus RNA. 3AB is therefore a stimulatory cofactor for $3D^{pol}$.

Cellular Accessory Proteins

Early studies of poliovirus replication using purified components suggested that a host cell protein is required for copying the viral RNA by $3D^{pol}$ in the absence of an oligo(U) primer (72). Although this protein was never identified, the concept of a host factor required for poliovirus replication endured, largely because there was ample precedent for the participation of host cell components in a viral RNA replicase. The best studied example is the RNA replicase of the bacteriophage Qβ, which is a multisubunit enzyme consisting of a 65-kd virus-encoded protein and three host proteins: ribosomal protein S1 and translation factors EF-Tu and EF-Ts. The 65-kd viral protein has no RNA polymerase activity in the absence of the host factors but has sequence similarity with known RNA-dependent RNA polymerases. A subunit of the translation initiation factor eIF-3 is part of the polymerase from brome mosaic virus. Two different experimental systems have recently been used to provide additional evidence that poliovirus RNA synthesis requires host cell components.

When purified poliovirus RNA is incubated *in vitro* with a cytoplasmic extract prepared from cultured, permissive cells, the viral RNA is translated, the resulting protein is proteolytically processed, and the genome is replicated and assembled into new infectious virus particles (217). When guanidine, an inhibitor of poliovirus RNA synthesis, is included in the reaction, complexes are formed, but elongation cannot occur (25). The preinitiation complexes can be isolated free of guanidine, and when added to new cytoplasmic extracts, RNA synthesis occurs. In the absence of cytoplasmic extract, preinitiation complexes do not synthesize viral RNA (24). These results indicate that one or more soluble cellular components are required for the initiation of viral RNA replication. A similar conclusion derives from studies in which poliovirus RNA is injected into oocytes derived from the African clawed toad, *Xenopus laevis*. Poliovirus RNA cannot replicate in *Xenopus* oocytes unless it is co-injected with a cytoplasmic extract from human cells (97).

Cellular poly r(C)–binding proteins are required for poliovirus RNA synthesis. These proteins bind to a cloverleaf-like secondary structure that forms in the first 108 nucleotides of positive-stranded RNA (Fig. 14). Binding of poly r(C)–binding protein to the cloverleaf is necessary for the binding of viral protein 3CD to the opposite side of the same cloverleaf (10,11,98,239). Formation of a ribonucleoprotein complex composed of the 5′ cloverleaf, 3CD, and a cellular protein is essential for the initiation of viral RNA synthesis (10). The human cell protein required for replication of poliovirus RNA in *Xenopus* oocytes has also been identified as poly r(C)–binding protein (98). A model of how these interactions lead to viral RNA synthesis is shown in Figure 14.

Another candidate for a host protein that is involved in poliovirus RNA synthesis is Sam68 (Src-associated in mitosis, 68 kd), which is associated with $3D^{pol}$ in poliovirus-infected cells (203). Sam68 is normally located in the cell nucleus but becomes redistributed to the cytoplasm during poliovirus infection. Sam68 can also be isolated from infected cells using an antibody directed against viral protein 2C, which is present in membranous RNA replication complexes. These results suggest that Sam68 may have a role in poliovirus RNA synthesis, although no direct experimental support for this hypothesis has emerged.

A Protein-Linked Primer for RNA Synthesis

As discussed previously, poliovirus $3D^{pol}$ is a primer-dependent enzyme that will not copy poliovirus RNA *in vitro* without an oligo(U) primer. The discovery of VPg linked to poliovirus genome RNA, as well as to the 5′ end of newly synthesized positive- and negative-stranded RNAs, suggested that VPg might be involved in the initiation of RNA synthesis. This hypothesis was supported by the finding that both VPg and a uridylylated form of the protein, VPg-pUpU, can be found in infected cells (69). Furthermore, VPg-pUpU can be synthesized *in vitro* in a membrane fraction from poliovirus-infected cells (300). It was also argued that a precursor of VPg, known as 3AB, is likely to participate in the initiation reaction. 3AB is a membrane-bound polypeptide and therefore an ideal candidate to act as a VPg donor in membranous replication complexes. Viruses containing a mutation in 3AB that decreases its hydrophobicity are defective in initiation of RNA synthesis, *in vitro* uridylylation of VPg, and *in vivo* synthesis of positive-stranded viral RNAs (104,105). Because no protein larger than VPg has been detected linked to nascent RNA strands, it is likely that 3AB is rapidly cleaved by the proteinase $3C^{pro}$ to form VPg RNA. Additional evidence that VPg can serve as a primer for poliovirus RNA synthesis comes from experiments in which synthetic VPg is first uridylylated *in vitro,* then added to an *in vitro* polymerase reaction containing a poly(A) template and $3D^{pol}$ (242). The labeled, uridylylated VPg is extended to form poly(U). Thus, poliovirus RNA replication is primed by a genome-linked protein, a mechanism also involved in adenovirus DNA replication. A model for VPg priming of poliovirus RNA synthesis is shown in Figure 15.

The Cellular Site of RNA Synthesis

Messenger RNA and genome synthesis of picornaviruses, like that of most RNA viruses, occurs in the cytoplasm of the cell. Cells infected with poliovirus accumulate small membranous vesicles that are the sites of poliovirus RNA synthesis (109,223). The accumulation of these vesicles is believed to be a result of the inhibition of membrane vesicle transport from the endoplasmic reticulum to the cell surface. Expression of the viral proteins 2B or 3A is sufficient to block the transport of glycoproteins to the cell surface, and it has been suggested that this inhibition leads to the accumulation of vesicles on which viral RNA synthesis occurs (74,75,314). Proteins 2BC and 2C might also contribute to the accumulation of such vesicles because expression of these proteins leads to membrane proliferation in cells (60).

Two other findings indicate the importance of vesicles in viral RNA synthesis. First, poliovirus RNA synthesis is inhibited by cerulenin, an inhibitor of lipid synthesis (124). Viral RNA replication is also inhibited by the fun-

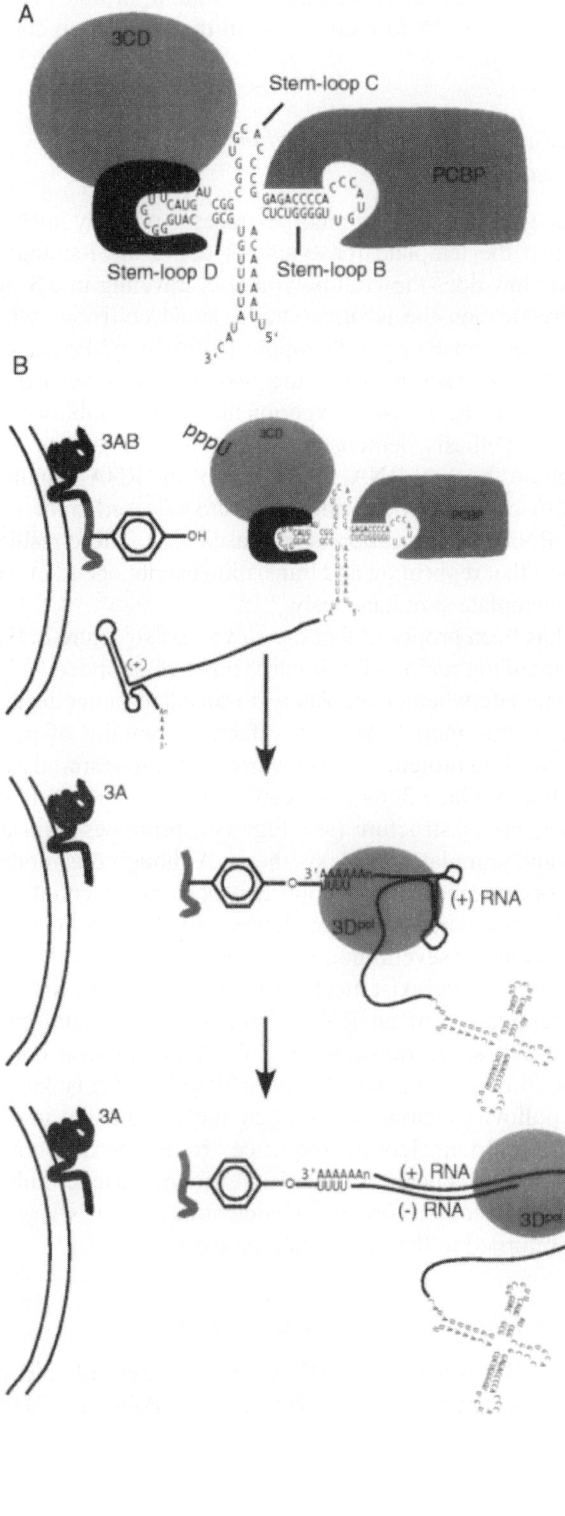

FIG. 14. Model for the synthesis of poliovirus (–) strand RNA. **A:** Schematic of the ribonucleoprotein complex that forms on a cloverleaf-like structure in the first 108 nucleotides of the viral (+) strand RNA. Binding of poly r(C) binding protein to stem-loop B is required for binding of viral 3CD to stem-loop D. This complex is required for synthesis of (+) and (–) strand RNA. **B:** Model for the initiation of (–) strand RNA synthesis. **Top:** the ribonucleoprotein complex has formed around the cloverleaf-like structure on the (+) strand and interacts with membrane-bound 3AB. Middle: 3AB is uridylylated and cleaved to release VPg-pUpU, and 3CD is cleaved to $3C^{pro}$ and $3D^{pol}$. Uridylylation and cleavage are carried out by 3CD. The $3D^{pol}$ then uses VPg-pUpU to prime RNA synthesis at the 3′-end of the viral (+) strand. A pseudoknot in the 3′-untranslated region may facilitate recognition of the 3′-end. **Bottom:** Elongation of a (–) strand RNA. Once this strand is complete, a cloverleaf forms at the 5′-end, leading to formation of another ribonucleoprotein complex and (+) strand RNA synthesis. Thus, many initiation reactions can occur on the original (+) strand RNA while (–) strands are being elongated.

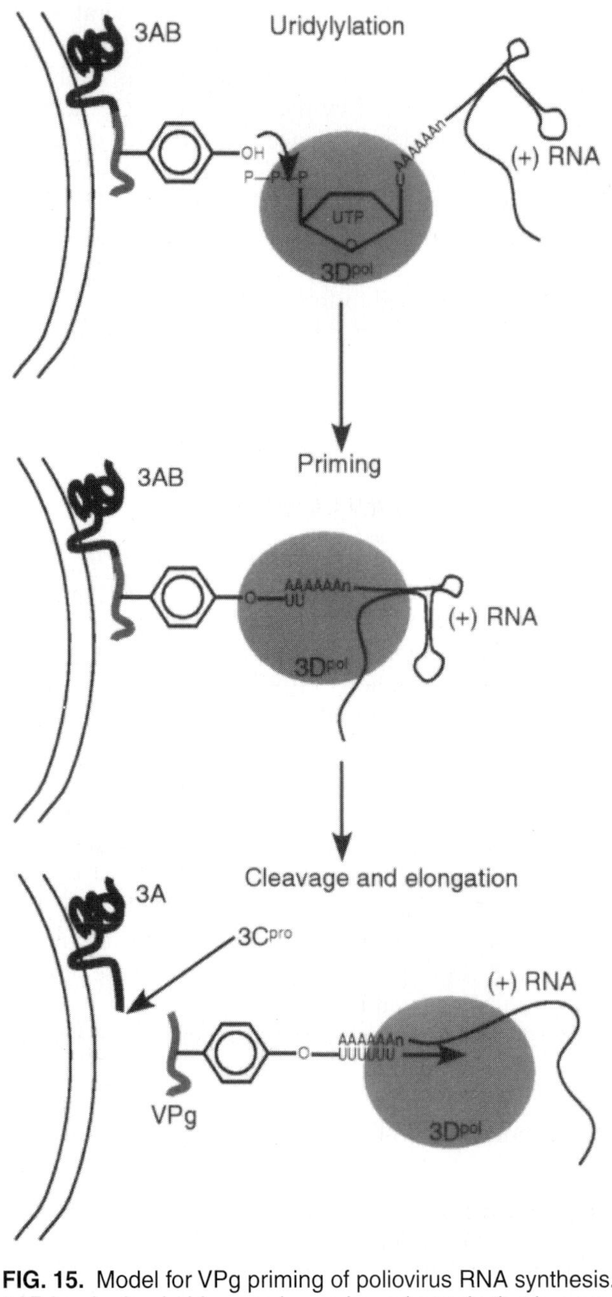

FIG. 15. Model for VPg priming of poliovirus RNA synthesis. 3AB is a hydrophobic, membrane-bound protein that is a precursor of VPg and probably participates in the initiation reaction. Uridylylation of membrane-bound 3AB is carried out by $3D^{pol}$ and is dependent on RNA template. Priming of RNA synthesis by 3AB-pUpU and cleavage to release VPg-pUpU probably occur in rapid succession because no protein larger than VPg linked to nascent RNA strands has been detected.

gal metabolite brefeldin A, which blocks the transport of proteins from the endoplasmic reticulum to the cell surface (150,202). Brefeldin A inhibits protein transport by blocking the movement of membrane vesicles from the endoplasmic reticulum to the Golgi apparatus and among the compartments of the Golgi. In the presence of brefeldin A, membranous vesicles derived from the endoplasmic reticulum do not accumulate in infected cells, leading to an inhibition of viral RNA synthesis. Poliovirus, therefore, appears to produce the membrane vesicles important for its replication by inhibiting an intracellular protein transport pathway. Because poliovirus is nonenveloped, its replication does not require the protein glycosylation and secretion functions of the endoplasmic reticulum and Golgi apparatus.

Two viral proteins, 2C and 3AB, bring the replication complex to membranous vesicles. As discussed previously, 3AB is a hydrophobic protein that anchors the protein primer VPg in the membrane for RNA synthesis. Protein 2C has an RNA-binding domain, which might anchor viral RNA to membranes in the replication complexes (82).

Translation and Replication of the Same RNA Molecule

The genomic RNA of picornaviruses is not only mRNA but also the template for synthesis of negative-stranded RNA. How does the viral polymerase, traveling in a 3′ to 5′ direction on the positive strand, avoid collisions with ribosomes translating in the opposite direction? Perhaps a mechanism exists to avoid the two processes occurring simultaneously. *In vitro* experiments using inhibitors of protein synthesis demonstrate that when ribosomes are frozen on the viral RNA, replication of the RNA is inhibited. In contrast, when ribosomes are released from the viral RNA, its replication is increased (26). These results suggest that replication and translation cannot occur on the same template simultaneously.

It has been proposed that the cloverleaf structure in the 5′-noncoding region of poliovirus positive-stranded RNA can regulate whether the RNA is translated or replicated (99). In this model, early in infection, binding of poly r(C)–binding protein to the cloverleaf structure stimulates translation. Once 3CD has been synthesized, it binds to the cloverleaf structure (see Fig. 14), represses translation, and stimulates RNA synthesis. Although this model has some experimental support, it does not account for the fact that viral RNA translation and RNA replication both occur for several hours in infected cells.

Whether there exist mechanisms to regulate translation and replication of an RNA, there is experimental evidence that some ribosome and RNA polymerase collisions do occur. This conclusion is based on the isolation of a poliovirus variant whose genome contains an insertion of a 15 nucleotide sequence from 28S ribosomal RNA (54). Apparently, the RNA polymerase collided with a ribosome, copied 15 nucleotides of rRNA, and then returned to the viral RNA template.

Discrimination of Viral and Cellular RNA

The RNA-dependent RNA polymerases of picornaviruses are template-specific enzymes. Poliovirus $3D^{pol}$

copies only viral RNAs, not cellular mRNAs, in infected cells. However, the purified enzyme will copy any polyadenylated RNA if provided with an oligo(U) primer. This observation has led to the suggestion that template specificity probably resides in the interaction of replication proteins with sequence elements in the viral RNA. The 3′-noncoding region of the viral positive-stranded RNA contains an RNA pseudoknot conserved among picornaviruses that is believed to play a role in the specificity of copying by $3D^{pol}$ (154). Disruption of the pseudoknot by mutagenesis produces viruses that have impaired RNA synthesis, indicating the importance of the structure in the synthesis of negative-stranded RNA. $3D^{pol}$ or 3CD cannot bind to the 3′ end of poliovirus RNA unless 3AB is present. Thus, the 3AB–$3D^{pol}$ complex may determine the specificity of binding to the 3′ pseudoknot. Despite experimental results that underscore the importance of the pseudoknot in RNA synthesis, polioviruses from which the entire 3′-noncoding region of the viral RNA has been removed are able to replicate, albeit inefficiently (301). It seems likely that there are other primary determinants of template selection by the polymerase, such as cis-acting RNA sequences within the coding region and membrane association of the RNA polymerase, which would lead to increased local concentrations of essential components. Template specificity may also be conferred by the position of the $3D^{pol}$ gene at the very 3′ end of the viral RNA; translation places the polymerase at the 3′ end of the genome, ready for initiation. Early in infection, the pseudoknot structure might facilitate template selection when few polymerase molecules are available and membrane association has not yet provided highly concentrated areas of replication components.

A cloverleaf-like structure that forms in the 5′-noncoding region also plays an important role in template specificity. The finding that a mutation in a cloverleaf-like structure in the 5′-noncoding region that affects RNA synthesis could be complemented by a suppressor mutation in 3C led to the suggestion that $3C^{pro}$ might bind the cloverleaf and play a role in viral RNA replication (12). It was subsequently found that 3CD binds the cloverleaf structure in the positive strand, together with a cellular protein, now known to be poly r(C)–binding protein, that is required for complex formation (see later) (10,11,239). The RNA-binding domain of 3CD is contained within the 3C portion of the protein, on the opposite face of the molecule from the site involved in proteolysis. Mutations within this domain abolish complex formation and RNA replication without affecting viral protein processing. 3CD, therefore, plays an important role in viral RNA synthesis by participating in formation of a ribonucleoprotein complex at the 5′ end of the positive-stranded RNA. A role for these interactions in viral RNA replication is suggested in the model in Figure 14.

Recombination

Recombination, the exchange of nucleotide sequences among different genome RNA molecules, was first discovered in cells infected with poliovirus, and was subsequently found to occur with other positive- and negative-stranded RNA viruses. The frequency of recombination, which is calculated by dividing the yield of recombinant virus by the sum of the yields of parental viruses, can be relatively high. In one study of poliovirus and foot-and-mouth disease virus, the recombination frequency was 0.9%, leading to the estimation that 10% to 20% of the viral genomes recombine in one growth cycle. When poliovirus recombination is studied by quantitative polymerase chain reaction, obviating the necessity to select for viable viruses, the recombination frequency for marker loci 600 nucleotides apart was 2×10^{-3}, which is similar to estimates obtained using selectable markers (156). RNA recombination also occurs in natural infections. For example, intertypic recombinants among the three serotypes of Sabin poliovirus vaccine strains are readily isolated from the intestines of vaccinees; some recombinants contain sequences from all three serotypes (46). The significance of these recombinants is unknown, but it has been suggested that such viruses are selected for their improved ability to replicate in the human alimentary tract compared with the parental viruses.

Poliovirus recombination mainly occurs between nucleotide sequences of the two parental genome RNA strands that have a high percentage of nucleotide identity and is called base pairing dependent (Fig. 16). RNA recombination is believed to be coupled with the process of genome RNA replication: it occurs by template switch-

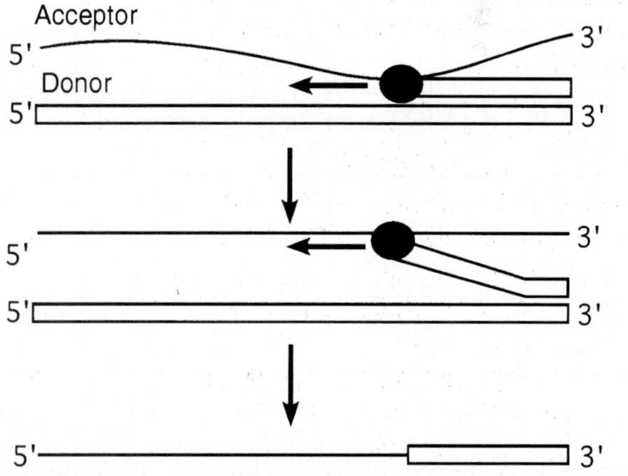

FIG. 16. RNA recombination. Schematic diagram of RNA recombination in picornavirus-infected cells by template switching, or copy-choice. Two parental genomes, the acceptor and donor, are shown as a *line* and *box.* The RNA polymerase, a *black oval,* is shown copying the 3′ end of donor RNA and switching to the acceptor genome (middle). As a result of this template switch, the recombinant RNA shown at the bottom is formed.

ing during negative strand synthesis, as first demonstrated in poliovirus-infected cells (172). The RNA polymerase first copies the 3′ end of one parental positive strand, then switches templates and continues synthesis at the corresponding position on a second parental positive strand (see Fig. 16). Template switching in poliovirus-infected cells occurs predominantly during negative strand synthesis because the concentration of positive-strand acceptors for template switching is 25- to 65-fold higher than that of negative-strand acceptors. This template-switching mechanism of recombination is also known as *copy-choice.* A prediction of the copy-choice mechanism is that recombination frequencies should be lower between different poliovirus serotypes, a prediction that has been verified experimentally. For example, recombination between poliovirus types 1 and 2 occurs about 100 times less frequently than among type 1 polioviruses (the different poliovirus serotypes differ by about 15% in their nucleotide sequences) (170). The cause of template switching is not known, but it might be triggered by pausing of the polymerase during chain elongation.

Assembly of Virus Particles

Morphogenesis of picornaviruses has been studied extensively because the 60-subunit capsid is relatively simple and the assembly intermediates can be readily detected in infected cells (Fig. 17). During the synthesis of the P1 protein, the capsid protein precursor, the central β-barrel domains form, and intramolecular interactions among the surfaces of these domains leads to formation of the structural units. Once P1 is released from the 2A protein, the VP0–VP3 and VP3–VP1 bonds are cleaved by proteinase 3CD^{pro}. These cleavage sites are located in flexible regions between the β-barrels; there is considerable movement of the aminotermini and carboxyltermini after cleavage, but the contacts between β-barrels are not disturbed (142). In the mature capsid, the carboxyltermini of VP1, VP2, and VP3 are on the outer surface of the capsid, whereas the aminotermini are on the interior, where they participate in an extensive network of interactions among protomers. This process produces the first assembly intermediate in the poliovirus pathway, the 5S protomer, the immature structural unit consisting of one copy each of VP0, VP3, and VP1. Five protomers then assemble to form a pentamer, which sediments at 14S. Cleavage of P1 is probably required for assembly of the pentamer (237). This conclusion is supported by examination of the virion structure. The β-cylinder at the fivefold axis of symmetry is formed from the N-termini of neighboring VP3 molecules; the cylinder is surrounded by a bundle composed of the aminotermini of VP0 and VP1. For these interactions to occur, proteolytic cleavage of the capsid proteins must occur to allow movement of the aminotermini.

Pentamers are important intermediates in the assembly of all picornaviruses (40,269). They can self-assemble *in vitro* or *in vivo* into 80S empty capsids; in one model of assembly, newly synthesized viral RNA is inserted into these particles to form the provirion (153), in which the capsid protein VP0 remains uncleaved. This assembly model would seemingly require an opening in the empty capsid through which the RNA can enter. Examination of the high-resolution x-ray crystallographic structure of these particles does not provide evidence for such an opening (27). This finding does not exclude this morphogenetic pathway because the pore might be dynamic and not observed in the crystals. In an alternative morphogenesis pathway, 4S pentamers assemble with virion RNA to form provirions. In this model, for which there is some experimental support (233), the empty capsids

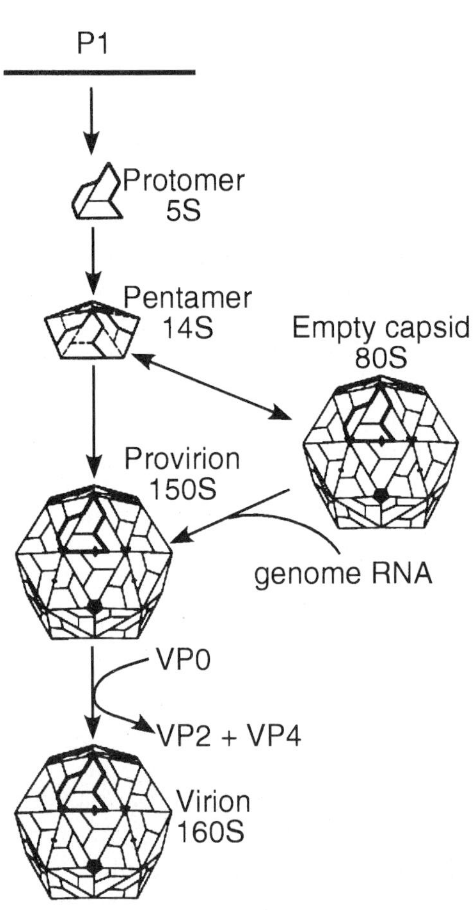

FIG. 17. Morphogenesis of picornaviruses. The capsid protein precursor, P1, folds nascently, is cleaved from P2, and then is further cleaved to VP0 + VP3 + VP1 by 3CD^{pro}. Protomers (5S) self-assemble into 14S pentamers, and pentamers assemble into 80S empty capsids. In one model of encapsidation, RNA is threaded into the empty capsid, producing a 150S provirion in which VP0 is uncleaved. Another possibility is that pentamers assemble around the RNA genome and that empty capsids are storage depots for pentamers. Cleavage of VP0 is the final morphogenetic step that produces the infectious 160S virion. The proteinase responsible for the cleavage of VP0 is unknown. (Adapted from Hellen CUT, Wimmer E. *Human enterovirus infections.* Washington, DC: ASM Press, DC, 1995, with permission.)

found in infected cells serve as storage depots for 14S pentamers.

The final morphogenetic step involves cleavage of most of the VP0 molecules to VP4 + VP2. The proteinase that carries out this final maturation cleavage has not been identified. The VP0 scissile bond is located on the interior of empty capsids and mature virions and is inaccessible to viral or cellular proteinases. The presence of a conserved serine in VP2 near one of the cleaved termini of VP2 led to a model that cleavage occurs by a novel autocatalytic serine protease-like mechanism in which basic viral RNA groups serve as proton abstracters during the cleavage reaction (17). However, replacement of ser-10 does not impair VP0 cleavage (135). More recently, it has been suggested that a conserved histidine in VP2 may be involved in catalysis, together with the viral RNA (27,71).

The structure of the 80S particle reveals differences in the network formed by the N-terminal extensions of the capsid proteins on the inner surface of the shell, compared with the native virion (27). In empty capsids, VP4 and the entire N-terminal extensions of VP1 and VP2 are disordered, and many stabilizing interactions that are present in the mature virion are not present. Thus, cleavage of VP0 establishes the ordered N-terminal network, an interlocking seven-stranded β-sheet formed by residues from adjacent pentamers. This network results in an increase in particle stability and the acquisition of infectivity.

The picornavirus encapsidation process is highly specific, resulting in packaging of only positive-stranded RNA, and not viral mRNA, negative-stranded viral RNA, or any cellular RNA (230,232). VPg is probably not an encapsidation signal because VPg-containing negative-stranded RNA is not packaged. The coupling of encapsidation to viral RNA synthesis may explain the selective packaging of viral positive-stranded RNA. In infected cells, newly synthesized RNA is packaged into virions within 5 minutes, whereas incorporation of capsid proteins in virions requires at least 20 minutes (22). The pool of viral RNA available for packaging is therefore small, whereas the pool of capsid proteins is large. If capsid formation is inhibited with *p*-fluorophenylalanine, the accumulated RNA cannot be packaged after removal of the inhibitor (130). These results suggest that packaging of the viral genome is linked to RNA synthesis, and would explain why only RNAs containing VPg are encapsidated.

During its synthesis, the P1 capsid protein precursor is linked to myristic acid at the aminoterminal glycine residue of VP4 that is exposed after removal of the initiation Met residue (61). The myristate groups, which form part of a network of interactions between subunits that form when protomers assemble into pentamers, cluster around the fivefold axis of symmetry and stabilize the β-cylinder that is made by the aminotermini of five copies of VP3. Mutagenesis indicates that the myristate group plays a role in stabilizing pentamers and therefore virions (14,196–198,220).

Effects of Viral Multiplication on the Host Cell

Inhibition of 5′ End–Dependent mRNA Translation

Cleavage of eIF4G

In cultured mammalian cells, poliovirus infection results in inhibition of cellular protein synthesis. By 2 hours after infection, polyribosomes are disrupted, and translation of nearly all cellular mRNAs stops and is replaced by viral mRNA translation (Fig. 18). Poliovirus

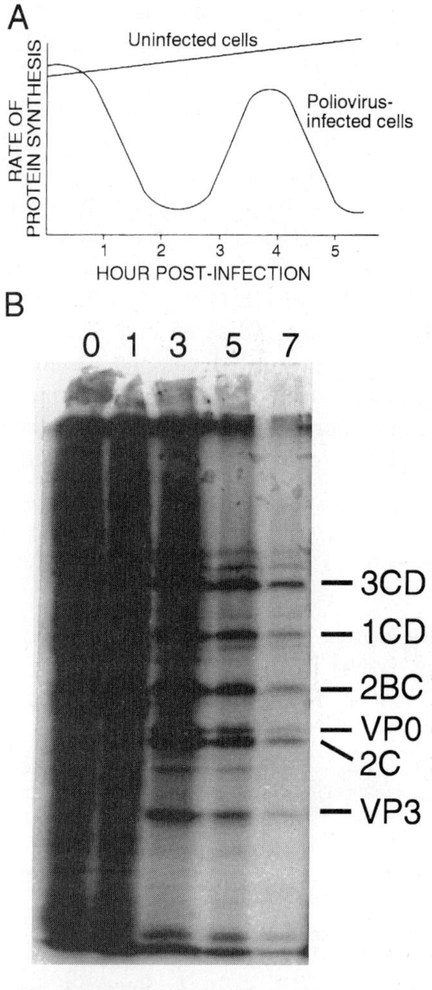

FIG. 18. Inhibition of cellular translation in cells infected with poliovirus. **A:** Protein synthesis in poliovirus-infected and uninfected cells at different times after infection. Poliovirus infection results in inhibition of host cell translation beginning about 1 hour after infection. The increase in translation beginning 3 hours after infection is due to the synthesis of viral proteins. **B:** Polyacrylamide gel showing inhibition of cellular translation. At different times after infection (indicated at the top of each lane), cells were incubated with ^{35}S-methionine for 15 minutes; the cell extracts were then fractionated on an SDS-polyacrylamide gel. By 5 hours after infection, host translation is markedly inhibited and replaced by the synthesis of viral proteins, identified at the right.

mRNA, but not capped mRNAs, can be translated in extracts from infected cells. In such extracts, one translation initiation factor, eIF4F, has been inactivated by cleavage of the eIF4GI/II component (85,270,305). Cleavage of eIF4G prevents eIF4F from recruiting 40S ribosomal subunits to capped mRNAs because it releases the N-terminal domain of eIF4G, which binds eIF4E, which in turn binds the 5′ cap of cellular mRNAs (Fig. 19). The synthesis of poliovirus proteins is not affected because the viral RNA is translated by internal ribosome binding, a process that does not require eIF4E. However, optimal function of the IRES does require the C-terminal fragment of eIF4G, which, as discussed previously, is necessary to anchor 40S ribosomal subunits to the IRES. Cleavage of eIF4G by picornaviruses inhibits cell translation and is also a strategy for stimulating IRES-dependent translation. Although both eIF4GI and eIF4GII are cleaved in poliovirus- and rhinovirus-infected cells, the kinetics of shutoff of host translation correlates with cleavage of eIF4GII and not eIF4GI (119,298).

Both forms of eIF4G are cleaved by protease 2A^{pro} of poliovirus and rhinovirus (119,298). *In vitro* cleavage of eIF4G by purified 2A^{pro} of rhinovirus is inefficient unless eIF4G is bound to eIF4E (128). This finding indicates that eIF4G is not cleaved as an individual polypeptide, but rather as part of the eIF4F complex. Binding of eIF4E to eIF4G may induce conformational changes in eIF4G that make it a more efficient substrate for the protease. Poliovirus 2A^{pro} efficiently cleaves eIF4GI, but not eIF4GII, consistent with the differential cleavage of these proteins during virus infection (119). Cleavage of eIF4G in cells infected with foot-and-mouth disease virus is carried out by the L^{pro} protein. The cleavage sites in eIF4G for the two proteinases are different: L^{pro} cleaves between Gly-479 and Arg-480, whereas 2A^{pro} cleaves between Arg-486 and Gly-487 (171,181).

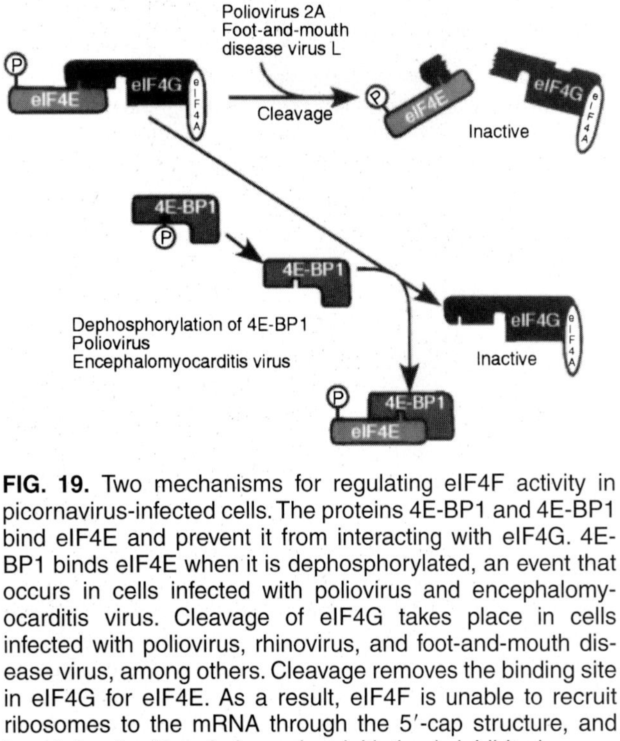

FIG. 19. Two mechanisms for regulating eIF4F activity in picornavirus-infected cells. The proteins 4E-BP1 and 4E-BP1 bind eIF4E and prevent it from interacting with eIF4G. 4E-BP1 binds eIF4E when it is dephosphorylated, an event that occurs in cells infected with poliovirus and encephalomyocarditis virus. Cleavage of eIF4G takes place in cells infected with poliovirus, rhinovirus, and foot-and-mouth disease virus, among others. Cleavage removes the binding site in eIF4G for eIF4E. As a result, eIF4F is unable to recruit ribosomes to the mRNA through the 5′-cap structure, and translation by 5′ end–dependent initiation is inhibited.

Modulation of eIF4E Activity

Two related low-molecular-weight cell proteins, 4E-BP1 and 4E-BP2, bind to eIF4E and inhibit translation by 5′ end–dependent scanning, but not by internal ribosome entry (see Fig. 19) (243). 4E-BP1 is identical to a protein called PHAS-I (phosphorylated heat- and acid-stable protein regulated by insulin), which was previously known to be an important phosphorylation substrate in cells treated with insulin and growth factors (190). Phosphorylation of 4E-BP1 *in vitro* blocks its association with eIF4E. Binding of either 4E-BP1 or 4E-BP2 to eIF4E does not prevent it from interacting with the 5′ cap but does inhibit binding to eIF4G. Consequently, active eIF4F is not formed. eIF4G and the 4E-BPs have a common sequence motif that binds eIF4E. Treatment of cells with hormones and growth factors leads to the phosphorylation of 4E-BP1 and its release from eIF4E. Those mRNAs with extensive secondary structure in the 5′-untranslated region, which are translated poorly, are preferentially sensitive to the phosphorylation state of 4E-BP1. As expected, translation by internal ribosome binding is not affected when 4E-BP1 is dephosphorylated. The nature of the signaling pathway through which binding of extracellular ligands leads to phosphorylation of 4E-BPs has not yet been elucidated (107).

Infection with several picornaviruses causes alteration of the phosphorylation state of 4E-BP1 and 4E-BP2 (see Fig. 19). Infection of cells with encephalomyocarditis virus causes inhibition of cellular translation, but in contrast to the shutoff that occurs in poliovirus-infected cells, shutoff cellular protein synthesis occurs late in infection and is not mediated by cleavage of eIF4G. Infection with encephalomyocarditis virus induces dephosphorylation of 4E-BP1, which then binds eIF4E to prevent it from forming eIF4F (108). Translation of cellular mRNAs is inhibited, but that of the viral RNA is not inhibited because it contains an IRES. Dephosphorylation of 4E-BP1 also occurs late in cells infected with poliovirus, but this event does not coincide with inhibition of cellular translation, which occurs earlier in infection (108).

Inhibition of Cellular RNA Synthesis

Infection of cells with picornaviruses leads to a rapid inhibition of host cell RNA synthesis catalyzed by all three classes of DNA-dependent RNA polymerase. RNA polymerases I, II, and III from poliovirus-infected cells are enzymatically active, suggesting that accessory proteins may be the target of transcriptional inhibition. Studies of *in vitro* systems have demonstrated the inhibition of specific transcription factors required by each of the three RNA polymerases. The RNA polymerase factor TFIID, which is a multiprotein complex, is inactivated in poliovirus-infected cells (176). This inactivation appears to be due, at least in part, to cleavage of a subunit of TFIID, the TATA-binding protein, by protease $3C^{pro}$ (63). A pol III DNA-binding transcription factor, TFIIC, is also cleaved and inactivated by $3C^{pro}$ (62). The target of $3C^{pro}$ is the α subunit of TFIIIC, which contacts the pol III promoter. An unidentified pol I transcription factor is cleaved by $3C^{pro}$, resulting in inhibition of pol I transcription in infected cells (273).

Cytopathic Effects

When cells are productively infected with poliovirus, they develop the characteristic morphologic changes known as *cytopathic effects.* These include condensation of chromatin, nuclear blebbing, proliferation of membranous vesicles, changes in membrane permeability, leakage of intracellular components, and shriveling of the entire cell. The cause of cytopathic effects is unknown. One hypothesis is that leakage of lysosomal contents is partly responsible (125). Although cellular RNA, protein, and DNA synthesis are inhibited during the first few hours of infection, they cannot account for cytopathic effects.

When poliovirus reproduction is hindered by certain drugs or other restrictive conditions, cell death occurs through induction of apoptosis (302). Although certain manifestations of cytopathic effects and apoptosis are similar, such as chromatin condensation and nuclear deformation, the pathways leading to their induction differ (3). During productive infections of cultured cells with poliovirus, apoptosis is blocked by a virus-encoded inhibitor (302). However, viral replication and central nervous system injury in mice infected with poliovirus are associated with apoptosis (110). Expression in cells of poliovirus protein 2A or 3C leads to induction of apoptosis (23,111). The viral inhibitor of apoptosis has not been identified. The ability of different strains of Theiler's murine encephalomyelitis virus to induce apoptosis may be a determinant of disease. The TO strain of Theiler's virus, which causes a persistent demyelinating disease in mice, encodes an additional protein, L* (57). This protein is produced by initiation from an AUG that is 13 nucleotides downstream from the initiator AUG of the polyprotein, in a different reading frame. In contrast, nondemyelinating strains of the virus, such as GDVII, do not encode L*. It was subsequently found that L* has antiapoptotic properties in macrophages and is critical for virus persistence (103). The ability of L* to inhibit apoptosis may be a key factor in determining whether infection of mice results in acute disease or persistence and demyelination.

PERSPECTIVES

Since the isolation of poliovirus in 1908, research on the virus has waxed and waned. With each lull in activity, questions were raised about whether it was productive to continue research on the virus. Each time, new technologies emerged that allowed the field to advance and become active once again. With global eradication of poliomyelitis looming on the horizon, research on poliovirus is as vibrant as ever. Many questions remain about nearly every stage of the replicative cycle, and an unprecedented array of experimental techniques and reagents are available to address them. We are on the verge of understanding the dynamics of the virion as it binds to the receptor and releases its nucleic acid. Why has poliovirus selected its particular receptor? Does the interaction lead to intracellular signaling that is beneficial for the virus? How is the genome extruded from the virus particle? Does the mechanism of RNA synthesis in infected cells resemble that which occurs *in vitro?* Why does RNA synthesis occur on membranes, and how is translation and replication regulated so that the processes do not collide? What other host proteins are involved in RNA synthesis, and what are their roles? How does the viral RNA enter the virion, and what causes the dramatic reorganization of the interior during the final stages of maturation? The study of poliovirus provides a unique opportunity to address fundamental questions in virology. However, we may not be able to answer these and many other interesting questions before the time comes to destroy all stocks of poliovirus, as part of the polio eradication effort (78). Fortunately, the same questions apply to other members of the Picornaviridae, and it is anticipated that research activity on these viruses will rapidly intensify in the next few years. Although future versions of this chapter may not contain as much information about poliovirus, the lessons we have learned will not be forgotten.

REFERENCES

1. Abdel-Rahman SM, Kearns GL. Single oral dose escalation pharmacokinetics of pleconaril (VP 63843) capsules in adults. *J Clin Pharmacol* 1999;39:613–618.
2. Acharya R, Fry E, Stuart D, et al. The three-dimensional structure of foot-and-mouth disease virus at 2.9 Å resolution. *Nature* 1989;337:709–716.
3. Agol VI, Belov GA, Bienz K, et al. Two types of death of poliovirus-infected cells: Caspase involvement in the apoptosis but not cytopathic effect. *Virology* 1998;252:343–353.
4. Agrez MV, Shafren DR, Gu X, et al. Integrin alpha v beta 6 enhances coxsackievirus B1 lytic infection of human colon cancer cells. *Virology* 1997;239:71–77.
5. Ahlquist P, Kaesberg P. Determination of the length distribution of poly(A) at the 3′ terminus of the virion RNAs of EMC virus, poliovirus, rhinovirus, RAV-61 and CPMV and of mouse globin mRNA. *Nucleic Acids Res* 1979;7:1195–1204.

6. Aldabe R, Barco A, Carrasco L. Membrane permeabilization by poliovirus proteins 2B and 2BC. *J Biol Chem* 1996;271: 23134–23137.
7. Alexander L, Lu HH, Wimmer E. Polioviruses containing picornavirus type 1 and/or type 2 internal ribosomal entry site elements: Genetic hybrids and the expression of a foreign gene. *Proc Natl Acad Sci U S A* 1994;91:1406–1410.
8. Ambros V, Baltimore D. Purification and properties of a HeLa cell enzyme able to remove the 5′-terminal protein from poliovirus RNA. *J Biol Chem* 1980;255:6739–6744.
9. Ambros V, Pettersson RF, Baltimore D. An enzymatic activity in uninfected cells that cleaves the linkage between poliovirion RNA and the 5′ terminal protein. *Cell* 1978;15:1439–1446.
10. Andino R, Rieckhof GE, Achacoso PL, Baltimore D. Poliovirus RNA synthesis utilizes an RNP complex formed around the 5′-end of viral RNA. *EMBO J* 1993;12:3587–3598.
11. Andino R, Rieckhof GE, Baltimore D. A functional ribonucleoprotein complex forms around the 5′ end of poliovirus RNA. *Cell* 1990; 63:369–380.
12. Andino R, Rieckhof GE, Trono D, Baltimore D. Substitutions in the protease (3Cpro) gene of poliovirus can suppress a mutation in the 5′ noncoding region. *J Virol* 1990;64:607–612.
13. Andries K, Dewindt B, Snoeks J, et al. Two groups of rhinoviruses revealed by a panel of antiviral compounds present sequence divergence and differential pathogenicity. *J Virol* 1990;64:1117–1123.
14. Ansardi DC, Luo M, Morrow CD. Mutations in the poliovirus P1 capsid precursor at arginine residues VP4-ARG34, VP3-ARG223, and VP1-ARG129 affect virus assembly and encapsidation of genomic RNA. *Virology* 1994;199:20–34.
15. Aoki J, Koike S, Ise I, et al. Amino acid residues on human poliovirus receptor involved in interaction with poliovirus. *J Biol Chem* 1994; 269:8431–8438.
16. Arita M, Horie H, Nomoto A. Interaction of poliovirus with its receptor affords a high level of infectivity to the virion in poliovirus infections mediated by the Fc receptor. *J Virol* 1999;73:1066–1074.
17. Arnold E, Luo M, Vriend G, et al. Implications of the picornavirus capsid structure for polyprotein processing. *Proc Natl Acad Sci U S A* 1987;84:21–25.
18. Arnold E, Rossmann MG. Analysis of the structure of a common cold virus, human rhinovirus 14, refined at a resolution of 3.0 A. *J Mol Biol* 1990;211:763–801.
19. Baltimore D, Eggers HJ, Franklin RM, Tamm I. Poliovirus-induced RNA polymerase and the effects of virus-specific inhibitors on its production. *Proc Natl Acad Sci U S A* 1963;49:843–849.
20. Baltimore D, Franklin RM. A new ribonucleic acid polymerase appearing after mengovirus infection of L-cells. *J Biol Chem* 1963; 238:3395–3400.
21. Baltimore D, Franklin RM. Properties of the mengovirus and poliovirus RNA polymerases. *Cold Spring Harbor Symp Quant Biol* 1963;28:105–108.
22. Baltimore D, Girard M, Darnell JE. Aspects of the synthesis of poliovirus RNA and the formation of virus particles. *Virology* 1966; 29:179–189.
23. Barco A, Feduchi E, Carrasco L. Poliovirus protease $3C^{pro}$ kills cells by apoptosis. *Virology* 2000;266:352–360.
24. Barton DJ, Black EP, Flanegan JB. Complete replication of poliovirus in vitro: Preinitiation RNA replication complexes require soluble cellular factors for the synthesis of VPg-linked RNA. *J Virol* 1995;69: 5516–5527.
25. Barton DJ, Flanegan JB. Synchronous replication of poliovirus RNA: Initiation of negative-strand RNA synthesis requires the guanidine-inhibited activity of protein 2C. *J Virol* 1997;71:8482–8489.
26. Barton DJ, Morasco BJ, Flanegan JB. Translating ribosomes inhibit poliovirus negative-strand RNA synthesis. *J Virol* 1999;73: 10104–10112.
27. Basavappa R, Syed R, Flore O, et al. Role and mechanism of the maturation cleavage of VP0 in poliovirus assembly: Structure of the empty capsid assembly intermediate at 2.9 Å resolution. *Protein Sci* 1994;3:1651–1669.
28. Baxt B, Becker Y. The effect of peptides containing the arginine-glycine-aspartic acid sequence on the adsorption of foot-and-mouth disease virus to tissue culture cells. *Virus Genes* 1990;4:73–83.
29. Bazan JF, Fletterick RJ. Viral cysteine proteases are homologous to the trypsin-like family of serine proteases: Structural and functional implications. *Proc Natl Acad Sci U S A* 1988;85:7872–7876.
30. Bella J, Kolatkar PR, Marlor CW, et al. The structure of the two amino-terminal domains of human ICAM-1 suggests how it functions as a rhinovirus receptor and as an LFA-1 integrin ligand. *Proc Natl Acad Sci U S A* 1998;95:4140–4145.
31. Belnap DM, Filman DJ, Trus BL, et al. Molecular tectonic model of virus structural transitions: The putative cell entry states of poliovirus. *J Virol* 2000;74:1342–1354.
32. Belnap DM, McDermott BM Jr, Filman DJ, et al. Three-dimensional structure of poliovirus receptor bound to poliovirus. *Proc Natl Acad Sci U S A* 2000;97:73–78.
33. Bergelson JM, Chan M, Solomon KR, et al. Decay-accelerating factor (CD55), a glycosylphosphatidylinositol-anchored complement regulatory protein, is a receptor for several echoviruses. *Proc Natl Acad Sci U S A* 1994;91:6245–6249.
34. Bergelson JM, Cunningham JA, Droguett G, et al. Isolation of a common receptor for Coxsackie B viruses and adenoviruses 2 and 5. *Science* 1997;275:1320–1323.
35. Bergelson JM, Shepley MP, Chan BM, et al. Identification of the integrin VLA-2 as a receptor for echovirus 1. *Science* 1992;255: 1718–1720.
36. Bernhardt G, Harber J, Zibert A, et al. The poliovirus receptor: Identification of domains and amino acid residues critical for virus binding. *Virology* 1994;203:344–356.
37. Blair WS, Semler BL. Role for the P4 amino acid residue in substrate utilization by the poliovirus 3CD proteinase. *J Virol* 1991;65: 6111–6123.
38. Blyn LB, Swiderek KM, Richards O, et al. Poly(rC) binding protein 2 binds to stem-loop IV of the poliovirus RNA 5′ noncoding region: Identification by automated liquid chromatography-tandem mass spectrometry. *Proc Natl Acad Sci U S A* 1996;93:11115–11120.
39. Blyn LB, Towner JS, Semler BL, Ehrenfeld E. Requirement of poly(rC) binding protein 2 for translation of poliovirus RNA. *J Virol* 1997;71:6243–6246.
40. Boege U, Ko DS, Scraba DG. Toward an in vitro system for picornavirus assembly: Purification of mengovirus 14S capsid precursor particles. *J Virol* 1986;57:275–284.
41. Borman AM, Kean KM. Intact eukaryotic initiation factor 4G is required for hepatitis A virus internal initiation of translation. *Virology* 1997;237:129–136.
42. Bouchard MJ, Dong Y, McDermott BM Jr, et al. Defects in nuclear and cytoskeletal morphology and mitochondrial localization in spermatozoa of mice lacking nectin-2, a component of cell-cell adherens junctions. *Mol Cell Biol* 2000;20:2865–2873.
43. Bouchard MJ, Racaniello VR. CD44 is not required for poliovirus replication. *J Virol* 1997;71:2793–2798.
44. Buckley B, Ehrenfeld E. The cap-binding protein complex in uninfected and poliovirus-infected HeLa cells. *J Biol Chem* 1987;262: 13599–13606.
45. Burke KL, Almond JW, Evans DJ. Antigen chimeras of poliovirus. *Prog Med Virol* 1991;38:56–68.
46. Cammack N, Phillips A, Dunn G, et al. Intertypic genomic rearrangements of poliovirus strains in vaccinees. *Virology* 1988;167:507–514.
47. Carrillo EC, Giachetti C, Campos RH. Effect of lysosomotropic agents on the foot-and-mouth disease virus replication. *Virology* 1984;135:542–545.
48. Carrillo EC, Giachetti C, Campos RH. Early steps in FMDV replication: Further analysis of the effects of chloroquine. *Virology* 1985; 147:118–125.
49. Casasnovas JM, Springer TA. Kinetics and thermodynamics of virus binding to receptor: Studies with rhinovirus, intercellular adhesion molecule-1 (ICAM-1), and surface plasmon resonance. *J Biol Chem* 1995;270:13216–13224.
50. Casasnovas JM, Stehle T, Liu JH, et al. A dimeric crystal structure for the N-terminal two domains of intercellular adhesion molecule-1. *Proc Natl Acad Sci U S A* 1998;95:4134–4139.
51. Caspar DL, Klug A. Physical principles in the construction of regular viruses. *Cold Spring Harbor Symp Quant Biol* 1962;27:1–22.
52. Chadeneau C, LeMoullac B, Denis MG. A novel member of the immunoglobulin gene superfamily expressed in rat carcinoma cell lines. *J Biol Chem* 1994;269:15601–15605.
53. Chang KH, Day C, Walker J, et al. The nucleotide sequences of wild-type coxsackievirus A9 strains imply that an RGD motif in VP1 is functionally significant. *J Gen Virol* 1992;73:621–626.
54. Charini WA, Todd S, Gutman GA, Semler BL. Transduction of a human RNA sequence by poliovirus. *J Virol* 1994;68:6547–6552.

55. Cheah KC, Leong LE, Porter AG. Site-directed mutagenesis suggests close functional relationship between a human rhinovirus 3C cysteine protease and cellular trypsin-like serine proteases. *J Biol Chem* 1990; 265:7180–7187.
56. Chen C, Sarnow P. Initiation of protein synthesis by the eukaryotic translational apparatus on circular RNAs. *Science* 1995;268:415–417.
57. Chen HH, Kong WP, Zhang L, et al. A picornaviral protein synthesized out of frame with the polyprotein plays a key role in a virus-induced immune-mediated demyelinating disease. *Nat Med* 1995;1: 927–931.
58. Chen ZG, Stauffacher C, Li Y, et al. Protein-RNA interactions in an icosahedral virus at 3.0 Å resolution. *Science* 1989;245:154–159.
59. Cho MW, Richards OC, Dmitrieva TM, et al. RNA duplex unwinding activity of poliovirus RNA-dependent RNA polymerase $3D^{pol}$. *J Virol* 1993;67:3010–3018.
60. Cho MW, Teterina N, Egger D, et al. Membrane rearrangement and vesicle induction by recombinant poliovirus 2C and 2BC in human cells. *Virology* 1994;202:129–145.
61. Chow M, Newman JF, Filman D, et al. Myristylation of picornavirus capsid protein VP4 and its structural significance. *Nature* 1987;327: 482–486.
62. Clark ME, Hümmerle T, Wimmer E, Dasgupta A. Poliovirus proteinase 3C converts an active form of transcription factor IIIC to an inactive form: A mechanism for inhibition of host cell polymerase III transcription by poliovirus. *EMBO J* 1991;10:2941–2947.
63. Clark ME, Lieberman PM, Berk AJ, Dasgupta A. Direct cleavage of human TATA-binding protein by poliovirus protease 3C in vivo and in vitro. *Mol Cell Biol* 1993;13:1232–1237.
64. Colonno RJ, Callahan PL, Long WJ. Isolation of a monoclonal antibody that blocks attachment of the major group of human rhinoviruses. *J Virol* 1986;57:7–12.
65. Colonno RJ, Condra JH, Mizutani S, et al. Evidence for the direct involvement of the rhinovirus canyon in receptor binding. *Proc Natl Acad Sci U S A* 1988;85:5449–5453.
66. Colston E, Racaniello VR. Soluble receptor-resistant poliovirus mutants identify surface and internal capsid residues that control interaction with the cell receptor. *EMBO J* 1994;13:5855–5862.
67. Colston EM, Racaniello VR. Poliovirus variants selected on mutant receptor-expressing cells identify capsid residues that expand receptor recognition. *J Virol* 1995;69:4823–4829.
68. Cox S, Buontempo PJ, Wright-Minogue J, et al. Antipicornavirus activity of SCH 47802 and analogs: In vitro and in vivo studies. *Antiviral Res* 1996;32:71–79.
69. Crawford NM, Baltimore D. Genome-linked protein VPg of poliovirus is present as free VPg and VPg-pUpU in poliovirus-infected cells. *Proc Natl Acad Sci U S A* 1983;80:7452–7455.
70. Curry S, Abrams CC, Fry E, et al. Viral RNA modulates the acid sensitivity of foot-and-mouth disease virus capsids. *J Virol* 1995;69: 430–438.
71. Curry S, Fry E, Blakemore W, et al. Dissecting the roles of VP0 cleavage and RNA packaging in picornavirus capsid stabilization: The structure of empty capsids of foot-and-mouth disease virus. *J Virol* 1997;71:9743–9752.
72. Dasgupta A, Zabel P, Baltimore D. Dependence of the activity of the poliovirus replicase on a host cell protein. *Cell* 1980;19:423–429.
73. Devaney MA, Vakharia VN, Lloyd RE, et al. Leader protein of foot-and-mouth disease virus is required for cleavage of the p220 component of the cap-binding protein complex. *J Virol* 1988;62:4407–4409.
74. Doedens JR, Giddings TH Jr, Kirkegaard K. Inhibition of endoplasmic reticulum-to-Golgi traffic by poliovirus protein 3A: Genetic and ultrastructural analysis. *J Virol* 1997;71:9054–9064.
75. Doedens JR, Kirkegaard K. Inhibition of cellular protein secretion by poliovirus proteins 2B and 3A. *EMBO J* 1995;14:894–907.
76. Donnelly ML, Gani D, Flint M, et al. The cleavage activities of aphthovirus and cardiovirus 2A proteins. *J Gen Virol* 1997;78:13–21.
77. Dove AW, Racaniello VR. Cold-adapted poliovirus mutants bypass a postentry replication block. *J Virol* 1997;71:4728–4735.
78. Dowdle WR, Birmingham ME. The biologic principles of poliovirus eradication. *J Infect Dis* 1997;175[Suppl 1]:S286–S292.
79. Duke GM, Osorio JE, Palmenberg AC. Attenuation of Mengo virus through genetic engineering of the 5′ noncoding poly(C) tract. *Nature* 1990;343:474–476.
80. Dulbecco R. Production of plaques in monolayer tissue cultures by single particles of an animal virus. *Proc Natl Acad Sci U S A* 1952;38: 747–752.
81. Eberle F, Dubreuil P, Mattei MG, et al. The human PRR2 gene, related to the human poliovirus receptor gene (PVR), is the true homolog of the murine MPH gene. *Gene* 1995;159:267–272.
82. Echeverri AC, Dasgupta A. Amino terminal regions of poliovirus 2C protein mediate membrane binding. *Virology* 1995;208:540–553.
83. Ellard FM, Drew J, Blakemore WE, et al. Evidence for the role of His-142 of protein 1C in the acid-induced disassembly of foot-and-mouth disease virus capsids. *J Gen Virol* 1999;80:1911–1918.
84. Enders JF, Weller TH, Robbins FC. Cultivation of the Lansing strain of poliomyelitis virus in cultures of various human embryonic tissues. *Science* 1949;109:85–87.
85. Etchison D, Milburn SC, Edery I, et al. Inhibition of HeLa cell protein synthesis following poliovirus infection correlates with the proteolysis of a 220,000-dalton polypeptide associated with eucaryotic initiation factor 3 and a cap binding protein complex. *J Biol Chem* 1982; 257:14806–14810.
86. Filman DJ, Syed R, Chow M, et al. Structural factors that control conformational transitions and serotype specificity in type 3 poliovirus. *EMBO J* 1989;8:1567–1579.
87. Flanegan JB, Baltimore D. Poliovirus-specific primer-dependent RNA polymerase able to copy poly(A). *Proc Natl Acad Sci U S A* 1977;74: 3677–3680.
88. Flanegan JB, Petterson RF, Ambros V, et al. Covalent linkage of a protein to a defined nucleotide sequence at the 5′-terminus of virion and replicative intermediate RNAs of poliovirus. *Proc Natl Acad Sci U S A* 1977;74:961–965.
89. Forss S, Schaller H. A tandem repeat gene in a picornavirus. *Nucleic Acids Res* 1982;10:6441–6450.
90. Fout GS, Medappa KC, Mapoles JE, Rueckert RR. Radiochemical determination of polyamines in poliovirus and human rhinovirus 14. *J Biol Chem* 1984;259:3639–3643.
91. Fox G, Parry NR, Barnett PV, et al. The cell attachment site on foot-and-mouth disease virus includes the amino acid sequence RGD (arginine-glycine-aspartic acid). *J Gen Virol* 1989;70:625–637.
92. Fox MP, Otto MJ, McKinlay MA. Prevention of rhinovirus and poliovirus uncoating by WIN 51711, a new antiviral drug. *Antimicrob Agents Chemother* 1986;30:110–116.
93. Freistadt MS, Eberle KE. CD44 is not required for poliovirus replication in cultured cells and does not limit replication in monocytes. *Virology* 1996;224:542–547.
94. Freistadt MS, Eberle KE. Physical association between CD155 and CD44 in human monocytes. *Mol Immunol* 1997;34:1247–1257.
95. Fricks CE, Hogle JM. Cell-induced conformational change in poliovirus: Externalization of the amino terminus of VP1 is responsible for liposome binding. *J Virol* 1990;64:1934–1945.
96. Fry EE, Lea SM, Jackson T, et al. The structure and function of a foot-and-mouth disease virus-oligosaccharide receptor complex. *EMBO J* 1999;18:543–554.
97. Gamarnik AV, Andino R. Replication of poliovirus in Xenopus oocytes requires two human factors. *EMBO J* 1996;15:5988–5998.
98. Gamarnik AV, Andino R. Two functional complexes formed by KH domain containing proteins with the 5′ noncoding region of poliovirus RNA. *RNA* 1997;3:882–892.
99. Gamarnik AV, Andino R. Switch from translation to RNA replication in a positive-stranded RNA virus. *Genes Dev* 1998;12:2293–2304.
100. Gan W, Celle ML, Rhoads RE. Functional characterization of the internal ribosome entry site of eIF4G mRNA. *J Biol Chem* 1998;273: 5006–5012.
101. Gan W, Rhoads RE. Internal initiation of translation directed by the 5′-untranslated region of the mRNA for eIF4G, a factor involved in the picornavirus-induced switch from cap-dependent to internal initiation. *J Biol Chem* 1996;271:623–626.
102. Geraghty RJ, Krummenacher C, Cohen GH, et al. Entry of alphaherpesviruses mediated by poliovirus receptor-related protein 1 and poliovirus receptor. *Science* 1998;280:1618–1620.
103. Ghadge GD, Ma L, Sato S, et al. A protein critical for a Theiler's virus-induced immune system-mediated demyelinating disease has a cell type-specific antiapoptotic effect and a key role in virus persistence. *J Virol* 1998;72:8605–8612.
104. Giachetti C, Hwang S-S, Semler BL. cis-Acting lesions targeted to the hydrophobic domain of a poliovirus membrane protein involved in RNA replication. *J Virol* 1992;66:6045–6057.
105. Giachetti C, Semler BL. Molecular genetic analysis of poliovirus RNA replication by mutagenesis of a VPg precursor polypeptide. In: Brinton MA, Heinz FX, eds. *New aspects of positive-strand RNA*

viruses. Washington, DC: American Society for Microbiology, 1990: 83–93.
106. Giachetti C, Semler BL. Role of a viral membrane polypeptide in strand-specific initiation of poliovirus RNA synthesis. *J Virol* 1991; 65:2647–2654.
107. Gingras AC, Kennedy SG, O'Leary MA, et al. 4E-BP1, a repressor of mRNA translation, is phosphorylated and inactivated by the Akt(PKB) signaling pathway. *Genes Dev* 1998;12:502–513.
108. Gingras AC, Svitkin Y, Belsham GJ, et al. Activation of the translational suppressor 4E-BP1 following infection with encephalomyocarditis virus and poliovirus. *Proc Natl Acad Sci U S A* 1996;93: 5578–5583.
109. Girard M, Baltimore D, Darnell JE. The poliovirus replicaiton complex: Sites for synthesis of poliovirus RNA. *J Mol Biol* 1967;24: 59–74.
110. Girard S, Couderc T, Destombes J, et al. Poliovirus induces apoptosis in the mouse central nervous system. *J Virol* 1999;73:6066–6072.
111. Goldstaub D, Gradi A, Bercovitch Z, et al. Poliovirus 2A protease induces apoptotic cell death. *Mol Cell Biol* 2000;20:1271–1277.
112. Golini F, Semler BL, Dorner AJ, Wimmer E. Protein-linked RNA of poliovirus is competent to form an initiation complex of translation in vitro. *Nature* 1980;287:600–603.
113. Goodfellow I, Chaudhry Y, Richardson A, et al. Identification of a cis-acting replication element within the poliovirus coding region. *J Virol* 2000;74:4590–4600.
114. Gorbalenya AE, Blinov VM, Donchenko AP. Poliovirus-encoded proteinase 3C: A possible evolutionary link between cellular serine and cysteine proteinase families. *FEBS Lett* 1986;194:253–257.
115. Gorbalenya AE, Donchenko AP, Blinov VM, Koonin EV. Cysteine proteases of positive strand RNA viruses and chymotrypsin-like serine proteases: A distinct protein superfamily with a common structural fold. *FEBS Lett* 1989;243:103–114.
116. Gorbalenya AE, Donchenko AP, Koonin EV, Blinov VM. N-terminal domains of putative helicases of flavi- and pestiviruses may be serine proteases. *Nucleic Acids Res* 1989;17:3889–3897.
117. Gorbalenya AE, Koonin EV, Blinov VM, Donchenko AP. Sobemovirus genome appears to encode a serine protease related to cysteine proteases of picornaviruses. *FEBS Lett* 1988;236:287–290.
118. Gorbalenya AE, Koonin EV, Lai MM. Putative papain-related thiol proteases of positive-strand RNA viruses: Identification of rubi- and aphthovirus proteases and delineation of a novel conserved domain associated with proteases of rubi-, alpha- and coronaviruses. *FEBS Lett* 1991;288:201–205.
119. Gradi A, Svitkin YV, Imataka H, Sonenberg N. Proteolysis of human eukaryotic translation initiation factor eIF4GII, but not eIF4GI, coincides with the shutoff of host protein synthesis after poliovirus infection. *Proc Natl Acad Sci U S A* 1998;95:11089–11094.
120. Grant RA, Hiremath CN, Filman DJ, et al. Structures of poliovirus complexes with anti-viral drugs: Implications for viral stability and drug design. *Curr Biol* 1994;4:784–797.
121. Greve JM, Davis G, Meyer AM, et al. The major human rhinovirus receptor is ICAM-1. *Cell* 1989;56:839–847.
122. Grubman MJ, Zellner M, Bablanian G, et al. Identification of the active-site residues of the 3C proteinase of foot-and-mouth disease virus. *Virology* 1995;213:581–589.
123. Guarne A, Tormo J, Kirchweger R, et al. Structure of the foot-and-mouth disease virus leader protease: A papain-like fold adapted for self-processing and eIF4G recognition. *EMBO J* 1998;17:7469–7479.
124. Guinea R, Carrasco L. Phospholipid biosynthesis and poliovirus genome replication, two coupled phenomena. *EMBO J* 1990;9: 2011–2016.
125. Guskey LE, Smith PC, Wolff DA. Patterns of cytopathology and lysosomal enzyme release in poliovirus-infected HEp-2 cells treated with either 2-(alpha-hydroxybenzyl)-benzimidazole or guanidine HCl. *J Gen Virol* 1970;6:151–161.
126. Hadfield AT, Diana GD, Rossmann MG. Analysis of three structurally related antiviral compounds in complex with human rhinovirus 16. *Proc Natl Acad Sci U S A* 1999;96:14730–14735.
127. Hadfield AT, Lee W, Zhao R, et al. The refined structure of human rhinovirus 16 at 2.15 A resolution: Implications for the viral life cycle. *Structure* 1997;5:427–441.
128. Haghighat A, Svitkin Y, Novoa I, et al. The eIF4G-eIF4E complex is the target for direct cleavage by the rhinovirus 2A proteinase. *J Virol* 1996;70:8444–8450.
129. Hahn H, Palmenberg AC. Encephalomyocarditis viruses with short poly(C) tracts are more virulent than their mengovirus counterparts. *J Virol* 1995;69:2697–2699.
130. Halperen S, Eggers HJ, Tamm I. Evidence for uncoupled synthesis of viral RNA and viral capsids. *Virology* 1964;24:36–46.
131. Hambidge SJ, Sarnow P. Translational enhancement of the poliovirus 5′ noncoding region mediated by virus-encoded polypeptide 2A. *Proc Natl Acad Sci U S A* 1992;89:10272–10276.
132. Hammerle T, Hellen CU, Wimmer E. Site-directed mutagenesis of the putative catalytic triad of poliovirus 3C proteinase. *J Biol Chem* 1991; 266:5412–5416.
133. Hansen JL, Long AM, Schultz SC. Structure of the RNA-dependent RNA polymerase of poliovirus. *Structure* 1997;5:1109–1122.
134. Harber J, Bernhardt G, Lu H-H, et al. Canyon rim residues, including antigenic determinants, modulate serotype-specific binding of polioviruses to mutants of the poliovirus receptor. *Virology* 1995;214: 559–570.
135. Harber JJ, Bradley J, Anderson CW, Wimmer E. Catalysis of poliovirus VP0 maturation cleavage is not mediated by serine 10 of VP2. *J Virol* 1991;65:326–334.
136. He Y, Bowman VD, Mueller S, et al. Interaction of the poliovirus receptor with poliovirus. *Proc Natl Acad Sci U S A* 2000;97:79–84.
137. Hellen CU, Facke M, Krausslich HG, et al. Characterization of poliovirus 2A proteinase by mutational analysis: Residues required for autocatalytic activity are essential for induction of cleavage of eukaryotic initiation factor 4F polypeptide p220. *J Virol* 1991;65: 4226–4231.
138. Hellen CU, Witherell GW, Schmid M, et al. A cytoplasmic 57-kDa protein that is required for translation of picornavirus RNA by internal ribosomal entry is identical to the nuclear pyrimidine tract-binding protein. *Proc Natl Acad Sci U S A* 1993;90:7642–7646.
139. Hewlett MJ, Rose JK, Baltimore D. 5′-Terminal structure of poliovirus polyribosomal RNA is pUp. *Proc Natl Acad Sci U S A* 1976;73:327–330.
140. Hiremath CN, Grant RA, Filman DJ, Hogle JM. The binding of the anti-viral drug WIN51711 to the Sabin strain of type 3 poliovirus: Structural comparison with drug binding to rhinovirus 14. *Acta Crystallogr* Section D 1994;D51:473–489.
141. Hofer F, Gruenberger M, Kowalski H, et al. Members of the low density lipoprotein receptor family mediate cell entry of a minor-group common cold virus. *Proc Natl Acad Sci U S A* 1994;91:1839–1842.
142. Hogle JM, Chow M, Filman DJ. Three-dimensional structure of poliovirus at 2.9 Å resolution. *Science* 1985;229:1358–1365.
143. Holland JJ, McLaren JC, Syverton JT. The mammalian cell virus relationship. III. Production of infectious poliovirus by non-primate cells exposed to poliovirus ribonucleic acid. *Proc Soc Exp Biol Med* 1959; 100:843–845.
144. Holland JJ, McLaren JC, Syverton JT. The mammalian cell virus relationship. IV. Infection of naturally insusceptible cells with enterovirus ribonucleic acid. *J Exp Med* 1959;110:65–80.
145. Hope DA, Diamond SE, Kirkegaard K. Genetic dissection of interaction between poliovirus 3D polymerase and viral protein 3AB. *J Virol* 1997;71:9490–9498.
146. Huber SA. VCAM-1 is a receptor for encephalomyocarditis virus on murine vascular endothelial cells. *J Virol* 1994;68:3453–3458.
147. Hughes PJ, Horsnell C, Hyypia T, Stanway G. The coxsackievirus A9 RGD motif is not essential for virus viability. *J Virol* 1995;69: 8035–8040.
148. Hunt SL, Hsuan JJ, Totty N, Jackson RJ. unr, A cellular cytoplasmic RNA-binding protein with five cold-shock domains, is required for internal initiation of translation of human rhinovirus RNA. *Genes Dev* 1999;13:437–448.
149. Hunt SL, Jackson RJ. Polypyrimidine-tract binding protein (PTB) is necessary, but not sufficient, for efficient internal initiation of translation of human rhinovirus-2 RNA. *RNA* 1999;5:344–359.
150. Irurzun A, Perez L, Carrasco L. Involvement of membrane traffic in the replication of poliovirus genomes: Effects of brefeldin A. *Virology* 1992;191:166–175.
151. Jackson RJ, Hunt SL, Reynolds JE, Kaminski A. Cap-dependent and cap-independent translation: Operational distinctions and mechanistic interpretations. *Curr Top Microbiol Immunol* 1995;203:1–29.
152. Jackson T, Ellard FM, Ghazaleh RA, et al. Efficient infection of cells in culture by type O foot-and-mouth disease virus requires binding to cell surface heparan sulfate. *J Virol* 1996;70:5282–5287.

153. Jacobson MF, Baltimore D. Morphogenesis of poliovirus. I. Association of the viral RNA with coat protein. *J Mol Biol* 1968;3:369–378.
154. Jacobson SJ, Konings DA, Sarnow P. Biochemical and genetic evidence for a pseudoknot structure at the 3′ terminus of the poliovirus RNA genome and its role in viral RNA amplification. *J Virol* 1993;67:2961–2971.
155. Jang SK, Krausslich H-G, Nicklin MJH, et al. A segment of the 5′ nontranslated region of encephalomyocarditis virus RNA directs internal entry of ribosomes during in vitro translation. *J Virol* 1988; 62:2636–2643.
156. Jarvis TC, Kirkegaard K. Poliovirus RNA recombination: Mechanistic studies in the absence of selection. *EMBO J* 1992;11:3135–3145.
157. Jia XY, Summers DF, Ehrenfeld E. Primary cleavage of the HAV capsid protein precursor in the middle of the proposed 2A coding region. *Virology* 1993;193:515–519.
158. Johannes G, Carter MS, Eisen MB, et al. Identification of eukaryotic mRNAs that are translated at reduced cap binding complex eIF4F concentrations using a cDNA microarray. *Proc Natl Acad Sci U S A* 1999;96:13118–13123.
159. Johnson KL, Sarnow P. Three poliovirus 2B mutants exhibit noncomplementable defects in viral RNA amplification and display dosage-dependent dominance over wild-type poliovirus. *J Virol* 1991;65: 4341–4349.
160. Jore J, De Geus B, Jackson RJ, et al. Poliovirus protein 3CD is the active protease for processing of the precursor protein P1 in vitro. *J Gen Virol* 1988;69:1627–1636.
161. Kaminski A, Hunt SL, Patton JG, Jackson RJ. Direct evidence that polypyrimidine tract binding protein (PTB) is essential for internal initiation of translation of encephalomyocarditis virus RNA. *RNA* 1995;1:924–938.
162. Kaminski A, Jackson RJ. The polypyrimidine tract binding protein (PTB) requirement for internal initiation of translation of cardiovirus RNAs is conditional rather than absolute. *RNA* 1998;4:626–638.
163. Kaplan G, Racaniello VR. Construction and characterization of poliovirus subgenomic replicons. *J Virol* 1988;62:1687–1696.
164. Kaplan G, Totsuka A, Thompson P, et al. Identification of a surface glycoprotein on African green monkey kidney cells as a receptor for hepatitis A virus. *EMBO J* 1996;15:4282–4296.
165. Karnauchow TM, Tolson DL, Harrison BA, et al. The HeLa cell receptor for enterovirus 70 is decay-accelerating factor (CD55). *J Virol* 1996;70:5143–5152.
166. Kean KM, Teterina NL, Marc D, Girard M. Analysis of putative active site residues of the poliovirus 3C protease. *Virology* 1991;181: 609–619.
167. Kim KH, Willingmann P, Gong ZX, et al. A comparison of the anti-rhinoviral drug binding pocket in HRV14 and HRV1A. *J Mol Biol* 1993;230:206–227.
168. Kim SS, Smith TJ, Chapman MS, et al. Crystal structure of human rhinovirus serotype 1A (HRV1A). *J Mol Biol* 1989;210:91–111.
169. Kim YK, Jang SK. La protein is required for efficient translation driven by encephalomyocarditis virus internal ribosomal entry site. *J Gen Virol* 1999;80:3159–3166.
170. King AM. Preferred sites of recombination in poliovirus RNA: An analysis of 40 intertypic cross-over sequences. *Nucleic Acids Res* 1988;16:11705–11723.
171. Kirchweger R, Ziegler E, Lamphear BJ, et al. Foot-and-mouth disease virus leader proteinase: Purification of the Lb form and determination of its cleavage site on eIF-4 gamma. *J Virol* 1994;68:5677–5684.
172. Kirkegaard K, Baltimore D. The mechanism of RNA recombination in poliovirus. *Cell* 1986;47:433–443.
173. Kitamura N, Semler BL, Rothberg PG, et al. Primary structure, gene organization and polypeptide expression of poliovirus RNA. *Nature* 1981;291:547–553.
174. Kitamura N, Semler BL, Rothberg PG, et al. Primary structure, gene organization and polypeptide expression of poliovirus RNA. *Nature* 1981;291:547–553.
175. Klein M, Hadaschik D, Zimmermann H, et al. The picornavirus replication inhibitors HBB and guanidine in the echovirus-9 system: The significance of viral protein 2C. *J Gen Virol* 2000;81:895–901.
176. Kliewer S, Dasgupta A. An RNA polymerase II transcription factor inactivated in poliovirus-infected cells copurified with transcription factor TFIID. *Mol Cell Biol* 1988;8:3175–3182.
177. Koike S, Ise I, Nomoto A. Functional domains of the poliovirus receptor. *Proc Natl Acad Sci U S A* 1991;88:4104–4108.
178. Koike S, Ise I, Sato Y, et al. A second gene for the African green monkey poliovirus receptor that has no putative N-glycosylation site in the functional N-terminal immunoglobulin-like domain. *J Virol* 1992; 66:7059–7066.
179. Koike S, Taya C, Kurata T, et al. Transgenic mice susceptible to poliovirus. *Proc Natl Acad Sci U S A* 1991;88:951–955.
180. Kolatkar PR, Bella J, Olson NH, et al. Structural studies of two rhinovirus serotypes complexed with fragments of their cellular receptor. *EMBO J* 1999;18:6249–6259.
181. Lamphear BJ, Yan R, Yang F, et al. Mapping the cleavage site in protein synthesis initiation factor eIF-4 gamma of the 2A proteases from human Coxsackievirus and rhinovirus. *J Biol Chem* 1993;268: 19200–19203.
182. Landsteiner K, Popper E. Mikroscopische prúparate von einem menschlichen und zwei affentückermarker. *Wein Klin Wschr* 1908;21: 1930.
183. Lea SM, Powell RM, McKee T, et al. Determination of the affinity and kinetic constants for the interaction between the human virus echovirus 11 and its cellular receptor, CD55. *J Biol Chem* 1998;273: 30443–30447.
184. Lee YF, Nomoto A, Detjen BM, Wimmer E. A protein covalently linked to poliovirus genome RNA. *Proc Natl Acad Sci U S A* 1977; 74:59–63.
185. Lentz KN, Smith AD, Geisler SC, et al. Structure of poliovirus type 2 Lansing complexed with antiviral agent SCH48973: Comparison of the structural and biological properties of three poliovirus serotypes. *Structure* 1997;5:961–978.
186. Lewis JK, Bothner B, Smith TJ, Siuzdak G. Antiviral agent blocks breathing of the common cold virus. *Proc Natl Acad Sci U S A* 1998; 95:6774–6778.
187. Li Q, Yafal AG, Lee YM, et al. Poliovirus neutralization by antibodies to internal epitopes of VP4 and VP1 results from reversible exposure of these sequences at physiological temperature. *J Virol* 1994;68: 3965–3970.
188. Li T, Chen Z, Johnson JE, Thomas GJ Jr. Conformations, interactions, and thermostabilities of RNA and proteins in bean pod mottle virus: Investigation of solution and crystal structures by laser Raman spectroscopy. *Biochemistry* 1992;31:6673–6682.
189. Liao S, Racaniello V. Allele-specific adaptation of poliovirus VP1 B-C loop variants to mutant cell receptors. *J Virol* 1997;71:9770–9777.
190. Lin TA, Kong X, Haystead TA, et al. PHAS-I as a link between mitogen-activated protein kinase and translation initiation. *Science* 1994; 266:653–656.
191. Lipton HL, Friedmann A, Sethi P, Crowther JR. Characterization of Vilyuisk virus as a picornavirus. *J Med Virol* 1983;12:195–203.
192. Lobert PE, Escriou N, Ruelle J, Michiels T. A coding RNA sequence acts as a replication signal in cardioviruses. *Proc Natl Acad Sci U S A* 1999;96:11560–11565.
193. Loeffler F, Frosch P. Report of the Commission for Research on foot-and-mouth disease. In: Hahon N, ed. *Selected papers on virology.* Englewood Cliffs, NJ: Prentice-Hall, 1964:64–68.
194. Lopez M, Eberlé F, Mattei MG, et al. Complementary DNA characterization and chromosomal localization of a human gene related to the poliovirus receptor-encoding gene. *Gene* 1995;155:261–265.
195. Macejak DG, Sarnow P. Internal initiation of translation mediated by the 5′ leader of a cellular mRNA. *Nature* 1991;353:90–94.
196. Marc D, Drugeon G, Haenni AL, et al. Role of myristoylation of poliovirus capsid protein VP4 as determined by site-directed mutagenesis of its N-terminal sequence. *EMBO J* 1989;8:2661–2668.
197. Marc D, Girard M, van der Werf S. A Gly to Ala substitution in poliovirus capsid protein VP0 blocks its myristoylation and prevents viral assembly. *J Gen Virol* 1991;72:1151–1157.
198. Marc D, Masson G, Girard M, van der Werf S. Lack of myristoylation of poliovirus capsid polypeptide VP0 prevents the formation of virions or results in the assembly of noninfectious virus particles. *J Virol* 1990;64:4099–4107.
199. Mason PW, Baxt B, Brown F, et al. Antibody-complexed foot-and-mouth disease virus, but not poliovirus, can infect normally insusceptible cells via the Fc receptor. *Virology* 1993;192:568–577.
200. Mason PW, Rieder E, Baxt B. RGD sequence of foot-and-mouth disease virus is essential for infecting cells via the natural receptor but can be bypassed by an antibody-dependent enhancement pathway. *Proc Natl Acad Sci U S A* 1994;91:1932–1936.
201. Matthews DA, Smith WW, Ferre RA, et al. Structure of human rhi-

novirus 3C protease reveals a trypsin-like polypeptide fold, RNA-binding site, and means for cleaving precursor polyprotein. *Cell* 1994; 77:761–771.
202. Maynell LA, Kirkegaard K, Klymkowsky MW. Inhibition of poliovirus RNA synthesis by brefeldin A. *J Virol* 1992;66:1985–1994.
203. McBride AE, Schlegel A, Kirkegaard K. Human protein Sam68 relocalization and interaction with poliovirus RNA polymerase in infected cells. *Proc Natl Acad Sci U S A* 1996;93:2296–2301.
204. McClelland A, deBear J, Yost SC, et al. Identification of monoclonal antibody epitopes and critical residues for rhinovirus binding in domain 1 of ICAM-1. *Proc Natl Acad Sci U S A* 1991;88:7993–7997.
205. McDermott BM Jr, Rux AH, Eisenberg RJ, et al. Two distinct binding affinities of poliovirus for its cellular receptor. *J Biol Chem* 2000; 275:23089–23096.
206. McKnight KL, Lemon SM. Capsid coding sequence is required for efficient replication of human rhinovirus 14 RNA. *J Virol* 1996;70: 1941–1952.
207. McKnight KL, Lemon SM. The rhinovirus type 14 genome contains an internally located RNA structure that is required for viral replication. *RNA* 1998;4:1569–1584.
208. McLaren LC, Holland JJ, Syverton JT. The mammalian cell-virus relationship. I. Attachment of poliovirus to cultivated cells of primate and non-primate origin. *J Exp Med* 1959;109:475–485.
209. McSharry JJ, Caliguiri LA, Eggers HJ. Inhibition of uncoating of poliovirus by arildone, a new antiviral drug. *Virology* 1979;97: 307–315.
210. Meerovitch K, Svitkin YV, Lee HS, et al. La autoantigen enhances and corrects aberrant translation of poliovirus RNA in reticulocyte lysate. *J Virol* 1993;67:3798–3807.
211. Mendelsohn C, Johnson B, Lionetti KA, et al. Transformation of a human poliovirus receptor gene into mouse cells. *Proc Natl Acad Sci U S A* 1986;83:7845–7849.
212. Mendelsohn CL, Wimmer E, Racaniello VR. Cellular receptor for poliovirus: Molecular cloning, nucleotide sequence, and expression of a new member of the immunoglobulin superfamily. *Cell* 1989;56: 855–865.
213. Minor PD, Ferguson M, Evans DM, et al. Antigenic structure of polioviruses of serotypes 1, 2 and 3. *J Gen Virol* 1986;67:1283–1291.
214. Minor PD, Schild GC, Bootman J, et al. Location and primary structure of a major antigenic site for poliovirus neutralization. *Nature* 1983;301:674–679.
215. Molla A, Harris KS, Paul AV, et al. Stimulation of poliovirus proteinase $3C^{pro}$-related proteolysis by the genome-linked protein VPg and its precursor 3AB. *J Biol Chem* 1994;269:27015–27020.
216. Molla A, Paul AV, Schmid M, et al. Studies on dicistronic polioviruses implicate viral proteinase $2A^{pro}$ in RNA replication. *Virology* 1993; 196:739–747.
217. Molla A, Paul AV, Wimmer E. Cell-free, de novo synthesis of poliovirus. *Science* 1991;254:1647–1651.
218. Morrison ME, Racaniello VR. Molecular cloning and expression of a murine homolog of the human poliovirus receptor gene. *J Virol* 1992; 66:2807–2813.
219. Morrison ME, Yuan-Jing H, Wien MW, et al. Homolog scanning mutagenesis reveals poliovirus receptor residues important for virus binding and replication. *J Virol* 1994;68:2578–2588.
220. Moscufo N, Chow M. Myristate-protein interactions in poliovirus: Interactions of VP4 threonine 28 contribute to the structural conformation of assembly intermediates and the stability of assembled virions. *J Virol* 1992;66:6849–6857.
221. Moscufo N, Yafal AG, Rogove A, et al. A mutation in VP4 defines a new step in the late stages of cell entry by poliovirus. *J Virol* 1993; 67:5075–5078.
222. Mosimann SC, Cherney MM, Sia S, et al. Refined X-ray crystallographic structure of the poliovirus 3C gene product. *J Mol Biol* 1997; 273:1032–1047.
223. Mosser AG, Caliguiri LA, Tamm I. Incorporation of lipid precursors into cytoplasmic membranes of poliovirus-infected HeLa cells. *Virology* 1972;47:39–47.
224. Mosser AG, Rueckert RR. WIN 51711-dependent mutants of poliovirus type 3: Evidence that virions decay after release from cells unless drug is present. *J Virol* 1993;67:1246–1254.
225. Muckelbauer JK, Kremer M, Minor I, et al. The structure of coxsackievirus B3 at 3.5 Å resolution. *Structure* 1995;3:653–667.
226. Neff S, Sa-Carvalho D, Rieder E, et al. Foot-and-mouth disease virus virulent for cattle utilizes the integrin $\alpha_v\beta_3$ as its receptor. *J Virol* 1998;72:3587–3594.
227. Neufeld KL, Richards OC, Ehrenfeld E. Purification, characterization and comparison of poliovirus RNA polymerase from native and recombinant sources. *J Biol Chem* 1991;266:24212–24219.
228. Nicklin MJ, Krausslich HG, Toyoda H, et al. Poliovirus polypeptide precursors: Expression in vitro and processing by exogenous 3C and 2A proteinases. *Proc Natl Acad Sci U S A* 1987;84:4002–4006.
229. Nomoto A, Detjen B, Pozzatti R, Wimmer E. The location of the polio genome protein in viral RNAs and its implication for RNA synthesis. *Nature* 1977;268:208–213.
230. Nomoto A, Kitamura N, Golini F, Wimmer E. The 5′-terminal structures of poliovirion RNA and poliovirus mRNA differ only in the genome-linked protein VPg. *Proc Natl Acad Sci U S A* 1977;74: 5345–5349.
231. Nomoto A, Lee YF, Wimmer E. The 5′ end of poliovirus mRNA is not capped with m7G(5′)ppp(5′)np. *Proc Natl Acad Sci U S A* 1976;73: 375–380.
232. Novak JE, Kirkegaard K. Improved method for detecting poliovirus negative strands used to demonstrate specificity of positive-strand encapsidation and the ratio of positive to negative strands in infected cells. *J Virol* 1991;65:3384–3387.
233. Nugent CI, Kirkegaard K. RNA binding properties of poliovirus subviral particles. *J Virol* 1995;69:13–22.
234. Ohlmann T, Rau M, Morley SJ, Pain VM. Proteolytic cleavage of initiation factor eIF-4 gamma in the reticulocyte lysate inhibits translation of capped mRNAs but enhances that of uncapped mRNAs. *Nucleic Acids Res* 1995;23:334–340.
235. Oliveira MA, Zhao R, Lee WM, et al. The structure of human rhinovirus 16. *Structure* 1993;1:51–68.
236. Olson NH, Kolatkar PR, Oliveira MA, et al. Structure of a human rhinovirus complexed with its receptor molecule. *Proc Natl Acad Sci U S A* 1993;90:507–511.
237. Palmenberg AC. In vitro synthesis and assembly of picornaviral capsid intermediate structures. *J Virol* 1982;44:900–906.
238. Palmenberg AC, Parks GD, Hall DJ, et al. Proteolytic processing of the cardioviral P2 region: Primary 2A/2B cleavage in clone-derived precursors. *Virology* 1992;190:754–762.
239. Parsley TB, Towner JS, Blyn LB, et al. Poly (rC) binding protein 2 forms a ternary complex with the 5′-terminal sequences of poliovirus RNA and the viral 3CD proteinase. *RNA* 1997;3:1124–1134.
240. Pata JD, Schultz SC, Kirkegaard K. Functional oligomerization of poliovirus RNA-dependent RNA polymerase. *RNA* 1995;1:466–477.
241. Paul AV, Cao X, Harris KS, et al. Studies with poliovirus polymerase $3D^{pol}$: Stimulation of poly(U) synthesis in vitro by purified poliovirus protein 3AB. *J Biol Chem* 1994;269:29173–29181.
242. Paul AV, van Boom JH, Filippov D, Wimmer E. Protein-primed RNA synthesis by purified poliovirus RNA polymerase. *Nature* 1998;393: 280–284.
243. Pause A, Belsham GJ, Gingras AC, et al. Insulin-dependent stimulation of protein synthesis by phosphorylation of a regulator of 5′-cap function. *Nature* 1994;371:762–767.
244. Pelletier J, Sonenberg N. Internal initiation of translation of eukaryotic mRNA directed by a sequence derived from poliovirus RNA. *Nature* 1988;334:320–325.
245. Perez L, Carrasco L. Entry of poliovirus into cells does not require a low-pH step. *J Virol* 1993;67:4543–4548.
246. Pestova TV, Shatsky IN, Fletcher SP, et al. A prokaryotic-like mode of cytoplasmic eukaryotic ribosome binding to the initiation codon during internal translation initiation of hepatitis C and classical swine fever virus RNAs. *Genes Dev* 1998;12:67–83.
247. Petersen JF, Cherney MM, Liebig HD, et al. The structure of the 2A proteinase from a common cold virus: A proteinase responsible for the shut-off of host-cell protein synthesis. *EMBO J* 1999;18:5463–5475.
248. Pettersson RF, Ambros V, Baltimore D. Identification of a protein linked to nascent poliovirus RNA and to the polyuridylic acid of negative-strand RNA. *J Virol* 1978;27:357–365.
249. Pettersson RF, Flanegan JB, Rose JK, Baltimore D. 5′-Terminal nucleotide sequences of polio virus polyribosomal RNA and virion RNA are identical. *Nature* 1977;268:270–272.
250. Pevear DC, Fancher MJ, Felock PJ, et al. Conformational change in the floor of the human rhinovirus canyon blocks adsorption to HeLa cell receptors. *J Virol* 1989;63:2002–2007.
251. Pfister T, Wimmer E. Characterization of the nucleoside triphos-

phatase activity of poliovirus protein 2C reveals a mechanism by which guanidine inhibits poliovirus replication. *J Biol Chem* 1999; 274:6992–7001.
252. Piccone ME, Zellner M, Kumosinski TF, et al. Identification of the active-site residues of the L proteinase of foot-and-mouth disease virus. *J Virol* 1995;69:4950–4956.
253. Pincus SE, Diamond DC, Emini EA, Wimmer E. Guanidine-selected mutants of poliovirus: Mapping of point mutations to polypeptide 2C. *J Virol* 1986;57:638–646.
254. Pincus SE, Wimmer E. Production of guanidine-resistant and -dependent poliovirus mutants from cloned cDNA: Mutations in polypeptide 2C are directly responsible for altered guanidine sensitivity. *J Virol* 1986;60:793–796.
255. Plotch SJ, Palant O. Poliovirus protein 3AB forms a complex with and stimulates the activity of the viral RNA polymerase, $3D^{pol}$. *J Virol* 1995;69:7169–7179.
256. Plotch SJ, Palant O, Gluzman Y. Purification and properties of poliovirus RNA polymerase expressed in *Escherichia coli*. *J Virol* 1989;63:216–225.
257. Powell RM, Ward T, Evans DJ, Almond JW. Interaction between echovirus 7 and its receptor, decay-accelerating factor (CD55): Evidence for a secondary cellular factor in A-particle formation. *J Virol* 1997;71:9306–9312.
258. Pritchard AE, Strom T, Lipton HL. Nucleotide sequence identifies Vilyuisk virus as a divergent Theiler's virus. *Virology* 1992;191: 469–472.
259. Racaniello VR, Baltimore D. Cloned poliovirus complementary DNA is infectious in mammalian cells. *Science* 1981;214:916–919.
260. Racaniello VR, Baltimore D. Molecular cloning of poliovirus cDNA and determination of the complete nucleotide sequence of the viral genome. *Proc Natl Acad Sci U S A* 1981;78:4887–4891.
261. Register RB, Uncapher CR, Naylor AM, et al. Human-murine chimeras of ICAM-1 identify amino acid residues critical for rhinovirus and antibody binding. *J Virol* 1991;65:6589–6596.
262. Ren R, Costantini FC, Gorgacz EJ, et al. Transgenic mice expressing a human poliovirus receptor: A new model for poliomyelitis. *Cell* 1990;63:353–362.
263. Ren R, Racaniello V. Human poliovirus receptor gene expression and poliovirus tissue tropism in transgenic mice. *J Virol* 1992;66:296–304.
264. Richards OC, Ehrenfeld E. Effects of poliovirus 3AB protein on 3D polymerase-catalyzed reaction. *J Biol Chem* 1998;273:12832–12840.
265. Rivera V, Welsh J, Maizel JJ. Comparative sequence analysis of the 5′-noncoding region of the enteroviruses and rhinoviruses. *Virology* 1988;165:42–50.
266. Roberts PJ, Belsham GJ. Identification of critical amino acids within the foot-and-mouth disease virus leader protein, a cysteine protease. *Virology* 1995;213:140–146.
267. Rodriguez PL, Carrasco L. Poliovirus protein 2C has ATPase and GTPase activities. *J Biol Chem* 1993;268:8105–8110.
268. Roivainen M, Hyypia T, Piirainen L, et al. RGD-dependent entry of coxsackievirus A9 into host cells and its bypass after cleavage of VP1 protein by intestinal proteases. *J Virol* 1991;65:4735–4740.
269. Rombaut B, Vrijsen R, Boeye A. New evidence for the precursor role of 14 S subunits in poliovirus morphogenesis. *Virology* 1990;177: 411–414.
270. Rose JK, Trachsel H, Leong K, Baltimore D. Inhibition of translation by poliovirus: Inactivation of a specific initiation factor. *Proc Natl Acad Sci U S A* 1978;75:2732–2736.
271. Rossmann MG. The canyon hypothesis: Hiding the host cell receptor attachment site on a viral surface from immune surveillance. *J Biol Chem* 1989;264:14587–14590.
272. Rossmann MG, Arnold E, Erickson JW, et al. Structure of a human common cold virus and functional relationship to other picornaviruses. *Nature* 1985;317:145–153.
273. Rubinstein SJ, Hammerle T, Wimmer E, Dasgupta A. Infection of HeLa cells with poliovirus results in modification of a complex that binds to the rRNA promoter. *J Virol* 1992;66:3062–3068.
274. Rueckert RR, Dunker AK, Stoltzfus CM. The structure of mouse-Elberfeld virus: A model. *Proc Natl Acad Sci U S A* 1969;62:912–919.
275. Ryan MD, Drew J. Foot-and-mouth disease virus 2A oligopeptide mediated cleavage of an artificial polyprotein. *EMBO J* 1994;13: 928–933.
276. Sandoval IV, Carrasco L. Poliovirus infection and expression of the poliovirus protein 2B provoke the disassembly of the Golgi complex, the organelle target for the antipoliovirus drug Ro-090179. *J Virol* 1997;71:4679–4693.
277. Satoh-Horikawa K, Nakanishi H, Takahashi K, et al. Nectin-3, a new member of immunoglobulin-like cell adhesion molecules that shows homophilic and heterophilic cell-cell adhesion activities. *J Biol Chem* 2000;275:10291–10299.
278. Schultheiss T, Emerson SU, Purcell RH, Gauss-Muller V. Polyprotein processing in echovirus 22: A first assessment. *Biochem Biophys Res Commun* 1995;217:1120–1127.
279. Schultheiss T, Kusov YY, Gauss-Muller V. Proteinase 3C of hepatitis A virus (HAV) cleaves the HAV polyprotein P2-P3 at all sites including VP1/2A and 2A/2B. *Virology* 1994;198:275–281.
280. Selinka H-C, Zibert A, Wimmer E. Poliovirus can enter and infect mammalian cells by way of an intercellular adhesion molecule 1 pathway. *Proc Natl Acad Sci U S A* 1991;88:3598–3602.
281. Selinka H-C, Zibert A, Wimmer E. A chimeric poliovirus/CD4 receptor confers susceptibility to poliovirus on mouse cells. *J Virol* 1992;66:2523–2526.
282. Shafren DR, Bates RC, Agrez MV, et al. Coxsackieviruses B1, B3, and B5 use decay accelerating factor as a receptor for cell attachment. *J Virol* 1995;69:3873–3877.
283. Shafren DR, Dorahy DJ, Ingham RA, et al. Coxsackievirus A21 binds to decay-accelerating factor but requires intercellular adhesion molecule 1 for cell entry. *J Virol* 1997;71:4736–4743.
284. Shepley MP, Racaniello VR. A monoclonal antibody that blocks poliovirus attachment recognizes the lymphocyte homing receptor CD44. *J Virol* 1994;68:1301–1308.
285. Shepley MP, Sherry B, Weiner HL. Monoclonal antibody identification of a 100-kDa membrane protein in HeLa cells and human spinal cord involved in poliovirus attachment. *Proc Natl Acad Sci U S A* 1988;85:7743–7747.
286. Sherry B, Mosser AG, Colonno RJ, Rueckert RR. Use of monoclonal antibodies to identify four neutralization immunogens on a common cold picornavirus, human rhinovirus 14. *J Virol* 1986;57:246–257.
287. Shukla D, Rowe CL, Dong Y, et al. The murine homolog (Mph) of human herpesvirus entry protein B (HveB) mediates entry of pseudorabies virus but not herpes simplex virus types 1 and 2. *J Virol* 1999;73:4493–4497.
288. Skinner MA, Racaniello VR, Dunn G, et al. A new model for the secondary structure of the 5′ noncoding RNA of poliovirus is supported by biochemical and genetic data which also show that RNA secondary structure is important to neurovirulence. *J Mol Biol* 1989;207: 379–392.
289. Smith TJ, Chase ES, Schmidt TJ, et al. Neutralizing antibody to human rhinovirus 14 penetrates the receptor-binding canyon. *Nature* 1996;383:350–354.
290. Smith TJ, Kremer MJ, Luo M, et al. The site of attachment in human rhinovirus 14 for antiviral agents that inhibit uncoating. *Science* 1986; 233:1286–1293.
291. Sommergruber W, Casari G, Fessl F, et al. The 2A proteinase of human rhinovirus is a zinc containing enzyme. *Virology* 1994;204:815–818.
292. Sommergruber W, Seipelt J, Fessl F, et al. Mutational analyses support a model for the HRV2 2A proteinase. *Virology* 1997;234:203–214.
293. Spector DH, Baltimore D. Requirement of 3′-terminal polyadenylic acid for the infectivity of poliovirus RNA. *Proc Natl Acad Sci U S A* 1974;71:2983–2987.
294. Stanway G, Hyypia T. Parechoviruses. *J Virol* 1999;73:5249–5254.
295. Staunton DE, Dustin ML, Erickson HP, Springer TA. The arrangement of the immunoglobulin-like domains of ICAM-1 and the binding sites for LFA-1 and rhinovirus. *Cell* 1990;61:243–254.
296. Staunton DE, Merluzzi VJ, Rothlein R, et al. A cell adhesion molecule, ICAM-1, is the major surface receptor for rhinoviruses. *Cell* 1989;56:849–853.
297. Summers DF, Maizel JV. Evidence for large precursor proteins in poliovirus synthesis. *Proc Natl Acad Sci U S A* 1968;59:966–971.
298. Svitkin YV, Gradi A, Imataka H, et al. Eukaryotic initiation factor 4GII (eIF4GII), but not eIF4GI, cleavage correlates with inhibition of host cell protein synthesis after human rhinovirus infection. *J Virol* 1999;73:3467–3472.
299. Takahashi K, Nakanishi H, Miyahara M, et al. Nectin/PRR: An immunoglobulin-like cell adhesion molecule recruited to cadherin-based adherens junctions through interaction with Afadin, a PDZ domain-containing protein. *J Cell Biol* 1999;145:539–549.
300. Takegami T, Kuhn RJ, Anderson CW, Wimmer E. Membrane-depen-

dent uridylylation of the genome-linked protein VPg of poliovirus. *Proc Natl Acad Sci U S A* 1983;80:7447–7451.
301. Todd S, Towner JS, Brown DM, Semler BL. Replication-competent picornaviruses with complete genomic RNA 3′ noncoding region deletions. *J Virol* 1997;71:8868–8874.
302. Tolskaya EA, Romanova LI, Kolesnikova MS, et al. Apoptosis-inducing and apoptosis-preventing functions of poliovirus. *J Virol* 1995;69: 1181–1189.
303. Tomassini JE, Graham D, DeWitt CM, et al. cDNA cloning reveals that the major group rhinovirus receptor on HeLa cells is intercellular adhesion molecule 1. *Proc Natl Acad Sci U S A* 1989;86:4907–4911.
304. Tosteson MT, Chow M. Characterization of the ion channels formed by poliovirus in planar lipid membranes. *J Virol* 1997;71:507–511.
305. Trachsel H, Sonenberg N, Shatkin AJ, et al. Purification of a factor that restores translation of vesicular stomatitis virus mRNA in extracts from poliovirus-infected HeLa cells. *Proc Natl Acad Sci U S A* 1980; 77:770–774.
306. Triantafilou K, Triantafilou M, Takada Y, Fernandez N. Human parechovirus 1 utilizes integrins $\alpha_v\beta_3$ and $\alpha_v\beta_1$ as receptors. *J Virol* 2000; 74:5856–5862.
307. Uncapher CR, DeWitt CM, Colonno RJ. The major and minor group receptor families contain all but one human rhinovirus serotype. *Virology* 1991;180:814–817.
308. van de Stolpe A, van der Saag PT. Intercellular adhesion molecule-1. *J Mol Med* 1996;74:13–33.
309. van der Werf S, Bradley J, Wimmer E, et al. Synthesis of infectious poliovirus RNA by purified T7 RNA polymerase. *Proc Natl Acad Sci U S A* 1986;83:2330–2334.
310. Van Dyke TA, Flanegan JB. Identification of poliovirus polypeptide p63 as a soluble RNA-dependent RNA polymerase. *J Virol* 1980;35: 732–740.
311. van Kuppeveld FJ, Galama JM, Zoll J, Melchers WJ. Genetic analysis of a hydrophobic domain of coxsackie B3 virus protein 2B: A moderate degree of hydrophobicity is required for a cis-acting function in viral RNA synthesis. *J Virol* 1995;69:7782–7790.
312. van Kuppeveld FJ, Galama JM, Zoll J, et al. Coxsackie B3 virus protein 2B contains cationic amphipathic helix that is required for viral RNA replication. *J Virol* 1996;70:3876–3886.
313. van Kuppeveld FJ, Hoenderop JG, Smeets RL, et al. Coxsackievirus protein 2B modifies endoplasmic reticulum membrane and plasma membrane permeability and facilitates virus release. *EMBO J* 1997; 16:3519–3532.
314. van Kuppeveld FJ, Melchers WJ, Kirkegaard K, Doedens JR. Structure-function analysis of coxsackie B3 virus protein 2B. *Virology* 1997;227:111–118.
315. van Vlijmen HW, Curry S, Schaefer M, Karplus M. Titration calculations of foot-and-mouth disease virus capsids and their stabilities as a function of pH. *J Mol Biol* 1998;275:295–308.
316. Villa-Komaroff L, Guttman N, Baltimore D, Lodishi HF. Complete translation of poliovirus RNA in a eukaryotic cell-free system. *Proc Natl Acad Sci U S A* 1975;72:4157–4161.
317. Voss T, Meyer R, Sommergruber W. Spectroscopic characterization of rhinoviral protease 2A: Zn is essential for the structural integrity. *Protein Sci* 1995;4:2526–2531.
318. Walter BL, Nguyen JH, Ehrenfeld E, Semler BL. Differential utilization of poly(rC) binding protein 2 in translation directed by picornavirus IRES elements. *RNA* 1999;5:1570–1585.
319. Ward T, Pipkin PA, Clarkson NA, et al. Decay-accelerating factor CD55 is identified as the receptor for echovirus 7 using CELICS, a rapid immuno-focal cloning method. *EMBO J* 1994;13:5070–5074.
320. Ward T, Powell RM, Pipkin PA, et al. Role for β-microglobulin in echovirus infection of rhabdomyosarcoma cells. *J Virol* 1998;72: 5360–5365.
321. Warner MS, Geraghty RJ, Martinez WM, et al. A cell surface protein with herpesvirus entry activity (HveB) confers susceptibility to infection by mutants of herpes simplex virus type 1, herpes simplex virus type 2, and pseudorabies virus. *Virology* 1998;246:179–189.
322. Wilson JE, Powell MJ, Hoover SE, Sarnow P. Naturally occurring dicistronic cricket paralysis virus RNA is regulated by two internal ribosome entry sites. *Mol Cell Biol* 2000;20:4990–4999.
323. Xing L, Tjarnlund K, Lindqvist B, et al. Distinct cellular receptor interactions in poliovirus and rhinoviruses. *EMBO J* 2000;19: 1207–1216.
324. Yeates TO, Jacobson DH, Martin A, et al. Three-dimensional structure of a mouse-adapted type 2/type 1 poliovirus chimera. *EMBO J* 1991; 10:2331–2341.
325. Yogo Y, Teng MH, Wimmer E. Poly(U) in poliovirus minus RNA is 5′-terminal. *Biochem Biophys Res Commun* 1974;61:1101–1109.
326. Yogo Y, Wimmer E. Polyadenylic acid at the 3′-terminus of poliovirus RNA. *Proc Natl Acad Sci U S A* 1972;69:1877–1882.
327. Ypma-Wong MF, Dewalt PG, Johnson VH, et al. Protein 3CD is the major poliovirus proteinase responsible for cleavage of the P1 capsid precursor. *Virology* 1988;166:265–270.
328. Ypma-Wong MF, Semler BL. In vitro molecular genetics as a tool for determining the differential cleavage specificities of the poliovirus 3C proteinase. *Nucleic Acids Res* 1987;15:2069–2088.
329. Yu SF, Lloyd RE. Identification of essential amino acid residues in the functional activity of poliovirus 2A protease. *Virology* 1991;182: 615–625.
330. Zajac I, Crowell R. Location and regeneration of enterovius receptors of HeLa cells. *J Bacteriol* 1965;89:1097–1100.
331. Zeichhardt H, Otto MJ, McKinlay MA, et al. Inhibition of poliovirus uncoating by disoxaril (WIN 51711). *Virology* 1987;160:281–285.
332. Zhang S, Racaniello VR. Expression of PVR in intestinal epithelial cells is not sufficient to permit poliovirus replication in the mouse gut. *J Virol* 1997;71:4915–4920.
333. Zhao R, Pevear DC, Kremer MJ, et al. Human rhinovirus 3 at 3.0 Å resolution. *Structure* 1996;4:1205–1220.

CHAPTER 19

Togaviridae: The Viruses and Their Replication

Sondra Schlesinger and Milton J. Schlesinger

TOGAVIRUSES

The *Togaviridae* were among the first well-characterized viruses containing a lipid envelope. Initially this family included a wide spectrum of viruses associated with different diseases (166). The relatively early recognition that they had a "coat" led to their being classified as Togaviruses (from the Latin *toga,* a Roman mantle or cloak). Many of the original members are now in different families, and the *Togaviridae* consists of only two genera: alphaviruses and rubivirus. Both are small, lipid-enveloped, spherical particles with a single-stranded positive RNA genome ranging in size from 9.7 for rubivirus to 11.8 kilobases for alphaviruses. Members of the alphavirus genus are grouped on the basis of genome homologies. In amino acid sequence, they share a minimum identity of about 60% in the nonstructural proteins and 40% in the structural proteins. From recent taxonomic data, the alphaviruses consist of 22 separate species, based on a combination of antigenic relationships and on divergence in genome sequence of greater than 23% and amino acid sequence of greater than 10% in the E1 gene (240). A phylogenetic relationship has been estimated based on the nsP1, nsp4, and E1 genes (240), and seven antigenic complexes can be grouped by serologic cross-reactivity (240). This number may increase, as salmon pancreas disease virus also appears to be a member of this genus (252).

The type-specific member of the alphaviruses is Sindbis virus, whose structure and replication have been studied in great detail. In addition, both Sindbis and Semliki Forest viruses have provided valuable models for examining the synthesis, posttranslational modifications, and localization of membrane glycoproteins. Most of the information presented in this chapter was obtained by studies with these two viruses, although other alphaviruses are beginning to contribute to our knowledge of the replication strategy and diversity of this genus.

Rubella virus, the sole member thus far of the rubivirus genus, is well known for its ability to cause disease in humans. Alphaviruses and rubella virus share many features, which originally suggested that they evolved from a common ancestor. A more detailed scrutiny of homologies, however, makes it difficult to propose a straightforward evolutionary relatedness.

Virion Structure

The dominant feature of alphavirus structure is a T=4 icosahedral nucleocapsid surrounded by a lipid envelope embedded with glycoprotein components also arranged in a T=4 icosahedral lattice. A clear picture of the organization of protein and lipid in the virion emerged from low-angle x-ray scattering (74), from negatively stained electron micrographs, and most recently from images obtained by cryoelectron microscopy (see later). Virions are about 70 nm in diameter, and the core or nucleocapsid is 40 nm in diameter. The molecular weight of the virion is about 52×10^6, with a density of 1.22 g/cc. The RNA genome is encapsidated in an icosahedral protein shell composed of a single species of protein (the capsid protein of 30–33 kd) and enveloped by a lipid bilayer derived from the host-cell plasma membrane. Lipid accounts for 30% of the dry weight of virions and is enriched in cholesterol and sphingolipid. Image reconstruction from cryoelectron micrographs has led to low-resolution structures for Semliki Forest, Sindbis, and Ross River viruses (25,45,58,157,158,213). These images (Fig. 1) reveal an arrangement of glycoprotein spikes distributed as 80 trimers, which project about 100 Å from the outer surface and are located at the local and strict three-fold axis of the icosahedral lattice. Each trimer contains three heterodimers consisting of the two viral glycoproteins E1 and E2. The heterodimers appear intertwined but flare out in a triangular, flower-like shape to form distinct bilobed petals. The most distal portion of the lobes contains domains of the E2 glycoprotein, which have epitopes recognized by monoclonal antibodies, and images with Fab fragments attached to either Sindbis or Ross River virus E2 have been obtained from cryoelectron micrographs (213). Each spike has a hollow cavity in its center, and the glycoproteins splay out to form a protein shell or skirt covering most of the outer surface of the membrane bilayer. Small holes in this shell appear at the two-fold and five-fold axis and at the base of each spike. Each spike is anchored in the membrane by three pairs of transmembrane domains, and each third of a trimeric spike interacts at the inner leaflet of the membrane with a different hexamer or pentamer of the nucleocapsid. Protein mass that is found immediately underlying the membrane is believed to represent the 33-amino-acid cytoplasmic domain of the E2 glycoprotein, which forms a binding site for nucleocapsids during the assembly process. A cryoelectron micrograph image of a mutant of Sindbis virus defective in cleavage of the precursor (PE2) to E2 and a small peptide, E3, revealed that the amino-terminus of PE2 is positioned as a bulge in the heterodimer localized midway between the center of the trimer and the tip of the spike (158). Analysis of a similar type of mutant of Semliki Forest virus indicated that the PE2 form of the trimer was a more open arrangement of spikes when compared with the wild-type virus, and the E3, which is retained in the virion, is positioned at the distal portion of the mature spike (45).

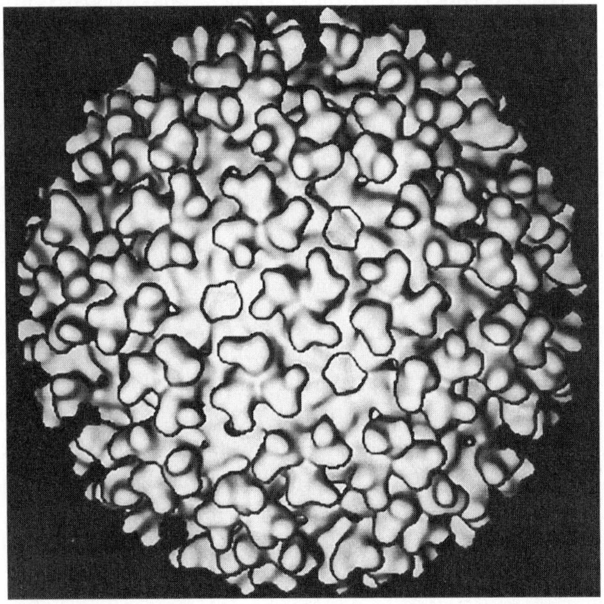

FIG. 1. Image reconstruction from cryoelectron micrographs of Ross River virus. The view is down the three-fold axis and shows the outer surface composed of flower-like projections of the E1/E2 heterodimers arranged as trimers and the interconnective portions that form a shell of protein. Very little of the lipid envelope is visible through three small openings of this shell. The resolution is about 20 Å. Courtesy of R.J. Kuhn, Purdue University, West Lafayette, IN.

The alphavirus nucleocapsid consists of 240 copies of the capsid protein (25,26,58,157,159). The Sindbis virus capsid protein was crystallized, and the atomic structure of the C-terminal half determined by x-ray diffraction to a resolution of 3 Å (Fig. 2) (26,224). Amino acids from positions 114 of the capsid sequence to the carboxy terminus at amino acid 264 were traced. The monomer fold was like mammalian serine proteases of the chymotrypsin family and closely related to the bacterial serine proteinases such as α-lytic proteinase, a result consistent with previous observations that alphavirus capsid proteins are autoproteases (5,68,132). The chain is folded into two Greek key β-barrel domains with the C- terminal tryptophan located between the domains and occupying the active proteinase site. The structure of the latter reveals the catalytic triad of serine, histidine, and aspartate (conserved among the serine proteinases) surrounding a hydrophobic pocket occupied by the tryptophan, which is the substrate for cleavage of the capsid from the nascent polypeptide (26,224). After cleavage, further catalytic activity is prevented by the tryptophan in the substrate-binding pocket. A structure of the Semliki Forest virus capsid protein, purified from virions, has been determined from crystals that diffracted to a resolution of 3 Å (28). The carboxyl-terminal 149 residues are folded like those of the Sindbis virus capsid in a chymotrypsin-like serine proteinase; however, a hydrophobic surface pocket that is occupied by amino acids from a neighboring molecule in the Sindbis virus capsid structure and may function as a binding site during assembly is empty. Several alphavirus capsid proteins have been produced as recombinant proteins in *Escherichia coli,* and the structure of the Sindbis virus capsid protein has been extended to residue 106, based on crystals that diffracted to a resolution of 2 Å (99).

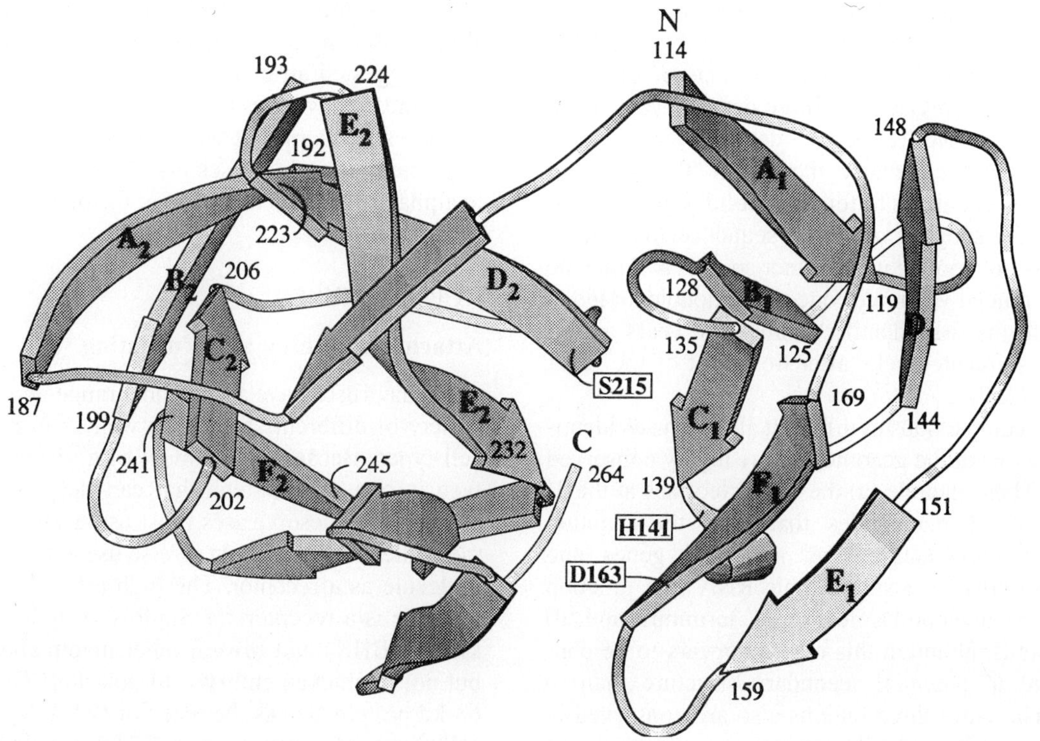

FIG. 2. Schematic drawing of the polypeptide chain of Sindbis virus capsid protein with secondary structure nomenclature based on x-ray diffraction analysis. The structure has since been extended toward the amino terminus to amino acid 106 (27). The catalytic triad of the active site serine-proteinase are in boxes. This picture was taken from Choi et al. (26), with permission, and was provided by M.G. Rossmann, Purdue University, West Lafayette, IN.

Genome Structure and Organization

The overall organization of the genomes of alphaviruses and rubella virus is shown in Fig. 3, where similarities and distinctions between them are noted. The genomes are arranged in two modules: the 5′ two thirds codes for the nonstructural proteins (nsPs) required for transcription and replication of the RNA, and the 3′ one third codes for the structural proteins. The 5′ terminus is capped with a 7-methylguanosine, and the 3′ terminus is polyadenylated. During replication, a discrete subgenomic mRNA species, identical in sequence to the 3′ ter-

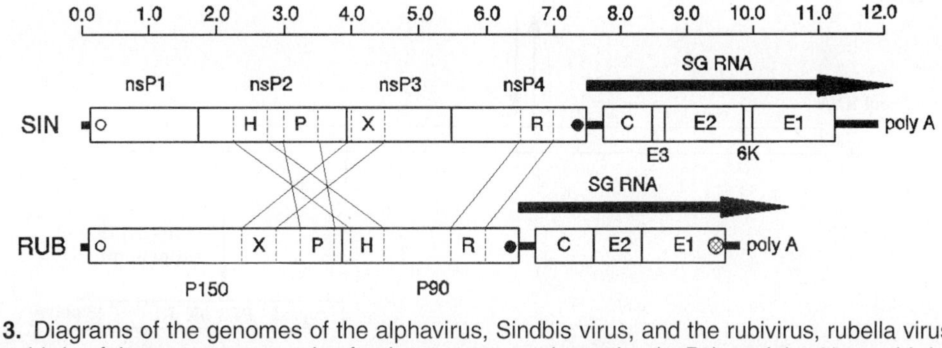

FIG. 3. Diagrams of the genomes of the alphavirus, Sindbis virus, and the rubivirus, rubella virus. The 5′ two thirds of these genomes codes for the nonstructural proteins (nsPs), and the 3′ one third codes for the structural proteins, translated from subgenomic (SG) RNAs. Untranslated regions are designated by *black lines*, and open reading frames, by *open boxes*. Designations are for individual proteins, which are processed from precursors. The scale at the top of the figure is in kilobases. The *open circles* near the 5′ termini and the *closed circles* at the start of the subgenomic RNAs indicate conserved sequences in the alphavirus and rubella virus genomes. The location of the amino acid motifs for helicases (*H*), replicases (*R*) and cysteine proteases (*P*) are indicated. See text for more details. *X*, A small region of homology between the deduced amino acid sequences in the Sindbis virus nsP3 and the nsP of rubella virus. This figure was adapted from refs. 35 and 49, with permission, and was provided by T. Frey, Georgia State University, Atlanta, GA.

minal one third of the genomic RNA, is synthesized (see also Fig. 4). This RNA also is capped and polyadenylated and serves as the mRNA for the synthesis of the viral structural proteins [reviewed in more detail in (219)]. An additional virus-specific RNA, detected in Sindbis virus–infected cells, contains the 5′ two thirds of the genome; the 3′ end maps to four nucleotides upstream of the start of the subgenomic RNA sequence. Its role in replication is not known; it is a minor species and may be the single-stranded version of one of the double-stranded replicative forms first identified almost 30 years ago in Sindbis virus–infected cells after treatment of the RNA with RNase (257).

Sequence comparisons of different alphaviruses identified four regions of the genome that are highly conserved (149–151). These include (a) the 19 nucleotides at the 3′ terminus, (b) 21 nucleotides that span the junction between the nonstructural and structural genes and include the start of the subgenomic RNA (the junction region), (c) 51 nucleotides near the 5′ terminus, and (d) the 5′ terminus, although this region appears to be conserved more in potential secondary structure than in sequence. The latter three regions also are conserved in rubella virus (35), and all four regions appear to be involved in the regulation of viral RNA synthesis. Sequence analyses also revealed similarities in the genome organization and in the sequences of the nonstructural proteins of alphaviruses and a number of plant viruses, some of which are quite distinct from alphaviruses in their overall structure [reviewed in (219)]. This suggested an evolutionary relatedness between the plant and alphaviruses and led to the definition of a Sindbis-like superfamily. It was this type of comparison that suggested that rubiviruses may be more distantly related to alphaviruses than are some of the plant viruses (35,49).

ALPHAVIRUSES

Attachment, Entry, and Uncoating

Alphaviruses have a wide host range and replicate in a variety of different species, as well as in many different cell types. Because attachment of a virion to a cell surface is one of the steps that can define host range, it seemed that these viruses must use a variety of different molecules for attachment or else use a ubiquitous surface molecule as a receptor. The high-affinity 67-kd laminin receptor is a receptor for Sindbis virus in baby hamster kidney (BHK) and several other mammalian cells (236) but not in chicken embryo fibroblasts (CEF), in which a 63-kd protein acts as the receptor (237). Mouse neuronal cells have other receptors: a 74-kd protein was detected on neuroblastoma cells that are loosely adherent, and a 110-kd protein was identified on firmly adherent cells (227). Recent studies have shown that heparan sulfate is an effective cell-surface ligand for binding of Sindbis

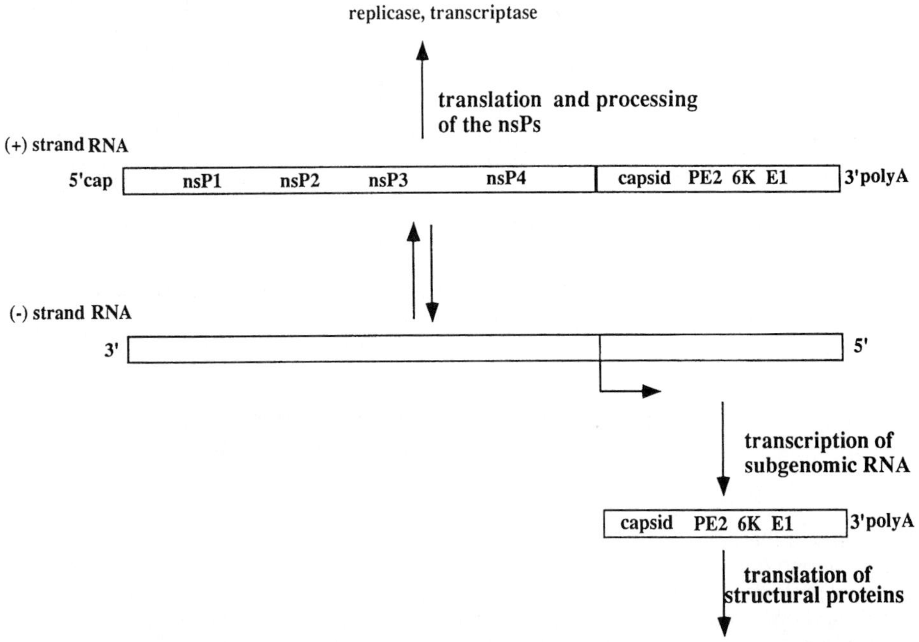

FIG. 4. Replication and transcription of alphavirus RNA. The first two thirds of the (+) strand genomic RNA serves as the mRNA for translation of the nsPs, which are eventually processed into four proteins (see text and Fig. 5). The (–) strand complementary strand is the template for the synthesis of both new genomic RNAs and the subgenomic 26S RNA, which codes for the structural proteins. The 5′ terminus of the (–) strand has a polyU stretch that is assumed to be the template for the polyA tract at the 3′ terminus of the genomic and subgenomic RNAs.

virus to mammalian cells (19,90). A Chinese hamster ovary cell line selected for resistance to Sindbis virus infection is deficient in expression of sulfated glycosaminoglycans, heparan sulfate, and chondroitin sulfate (83). A strain of Sindbis virus composed of a consensus sequence derived from natural isolates does not bind to heparan sulfate; variants that do bind are rapidly selected by growth on cultured BHK cells (90). Thus heparan sulfate–like molecules may not function as natural receptors for Sindbis viruses, and high-affinity binding of laboratory strains to this ligand appears to be a consequence of cultured-cell adaptation. Non–heparan-binding strains of Sindbis virus are more virulent in animals (90).

The viral glycoprotein E2 is the protein that interacts with these receptors. Antibodies directed primarily against the E2 protein neutralize viral infectivity, and amino acid changes in the E2 protein can affect both the efficiency of binding of the virus to neural cells and virulence in mice (81,105,199,226). Convincing evidence for the importance of E2 in binding virus to the cell surface came from experiments in which Sindbis virus mutants unable to bind to CEF were altered in the E2 protein (39).

Attachment of Sindbis virus to cells leads to the exposure on both glycoproteins of new transitional epitopes, which are indicative of conformational changes (46,135). These epitopes were detected also when purified virus was treated with heat, reducing agents, or low pH (134). Some of these changes may involve reduction of critical disulfide bonds in the glycoproteins, which may disrupt protein–protein associations in the envelope and be important for disassembly of the particle (1,7,8). Disulfide bond exchange had been proposed as a mechanism for allowing entry of virus at neutral pH at the cell surface, but further studies with both Semliki Forest and Sindbis virus failed to show significant inhibition of virus infection in the presence of thiol-blocking reagents (65).

In most cells, alphaviruses gain entry to the cell via the endocytic pathway, which normally functions for uptake of receptor–ligand complexes (33,128). Bound virus accumulates in coated pits, which are endocytosed to form coated vesicles. These vesicles are subsequently uncoated to form acidified endosomes, providing conditions that trigger fusion of the virus membrane with the vesicle membrane. The mechanism of receptor-mediated endocytosis for alphavirus penetration into cultured cells is supported by many studies, which include (a) the inability of bound Sindbis virus to effect antibody-mediated, complement-dependent cell lysis, indicating a rapid loss of virus glycoprotein from the cell surface (44); (b) the ability of lysosomotropic amines, which raise the pH of endocytic vesicles, to inhibit initiation of virus replication, demonstrating that acidified vesicles are required for early virus-replication events; (c) a requirement for a low pH (5–6) for fusogenic activity by Sindbis and Semliki Forest virus glycoproteins (230,254–256); (d) a block in fusion by concanamycin, a selective inhibitor of vacuolar proton–adenosine triphosphatase (ATPase) (80); and (e) the detection of virus in coated vesicles immediately after uptake from the cell surface, as revealed by electron micrographs of virus entry (256). Alternative pathways not involving acidified endosomes may exist, as a Chinese hamster ovary cell mutant defective in the endosome acidification was able to replicate Sindbis virus (41).

Studies with Semliki Forest and Sindbis viruses have demonstrated that the low-pH environment of the endosome leads to a dissociation of the E1/E2 heterodimer and a concomitant trimerization of the E1 subunits, which acquire new epitopes and become trypsin resistant (212,233,234). These alterations suggest that the E1 trimer is the fusion-active form of the protein, with a structure possibly analogous to the low pH–induced structure of the influenza virus HA2 protein (22,209). A highly conserved, hydrophobic sequence in the Semliki Forest virus E1 protein about 80 amino acids from the amino terminus is postulated to function as a fusion peptide, and mutations in this sequence shift the pH threshold for fusion to lower pH values (87), or block E1 homotrimer formation (89). Mutations in PE2 that prevent its cleavage to E2 also can affect fusion by controlling the formation and dissociation of the E1/E2 dimer (65,87).

Fusion of Semliki Forest and Sindbis viruses also requires the presence of cholesterol and sphingolipid in the target membrane (121,144,163,212). Dependence of Semliki Forest and Sindbis viruses on membrane cholesterol could be relieved by mutations in the E1 glycoprotein (121,231). One of these mutants, noted as srf-3, in which Pro^{226} in E1 was changed to Ser, was less dependent on cholesterol for trimer formation of E1 but retained the requirements for low-pH activation and sphingolipid exhibited by the wild-type virus (88).

Fusion leads to release of the nucleocapsid into the cytoplasm and must be followed by an uncoating event to permit the RNA to become accessible to ribosomes for initiation of translation. Several reports, based on *in vivo* and *in vitro* experiments, suggested that the binding of the nucleocapsid to ribosomes triggers the uncoating process (205,229,245,247,249,250). The capsid protein itself appears to have a ribosome-binding site between amino acids 94 and 106 of the capsid sequence (251), which is in the same region of the protein that interacts with viral RNA during encapsidation (64,152).

Transcription, Translation, and Replication of the Genome

The genomic RNA serves as the messenger RNA for translation of the viral nonstructural proteins and as a template for the synthesis of the complementary minus strand. The minus strand, in turn, provides the template for the synthesis of both new genomic RNA and subgenomic RNA [Fig. 4; for a more detailed review, see (219)]. Translation of the virion RNA is initiated at a single AUG near the 5′ terminus of the RNA and proceeds uninterrupted for two thirds of the mRNA until encountering three termination codons located just downstream of the start of the sequences corresponding to the subgenomic RNA. The polyprotein is cleaved to four distinct polypeptides designated nsP1, nsP2, nsP3, and nsP4, according to their order in the genome. The protease responsible for these cleavages is encoded in sequences at the C-terminal domain of nsP2 (34,73,216). The genomes of Sindbis virus and several other alphaviruses have an opal termination codon a few codons before the nsP4 gene, and nsP4 is produced by read-through of the opal codon followed by proteolytic cleavage (218). Mutagenesis of the opal codon to one that encodes an amino acid or to the other two translation-termination codons adversely affects viral replication at low multiplicities of infection (109). An opal codon at this position in the genome of alphaviruses is common but not universal, and no termination codon exists at this position in Semliki Forest or O'Nyong-nyong virus genomes (217).

A number of activities must be carried out by the nsPs in their role as replicative enzymes. The isolation, characterization, and mapping of temperature-sensitive (*ts*) mutants defective in viral RNA synthesis at the nonpermissive temperature provided initial clues to identify the functions of each of the polypeptides (17,18,69,71). The RNA^- *ts* mutants fell into four complementation groups, which have been correlated with specific nsPs. The individual functions were predicted by gene-sequence homologies with known proteins [reviewed in (219)]. These include domains that are conserved among the alphavirus-like superfamily in three of the four nsPs. The nsP1 protein contains a methyltransferase domain; the amino terminal region of nsP2 contains nucleotide-triphosphate binding motifs homologous to those found in bacterial helicases (see Fig. 3); and nsP4 has a GDD motif present in a number of viral RNA polymerases.

The predictions based on sequence homologies are being confirmed by functional tests. nsP1 has both guanine-7-methyltransferase and guanyltransferase activities (4,136,193). Mutagenic studies have defined amino acids essential for these activities (3,235). nsP1 also has been implicated in the synthesis of minus strand RNA (71,238). The protein is palmitoylated, and mutagenesis of the conserved cysteine residues, Cys^{418}, Cys^{419}, and Cys^{420}, to alanine prevented the addition of palmitate and decreased the ability of nsP1 to bind to membranes (93). This protein appears to be involved in the association of the alphavirus replicase to membranes (4). Expression of nsP1 in cultured cells using a vaccinia virus expression system induced filopodia and rearrangement of actin filaments (94). These effects, also observed in virus-infected cells, indicate that nsP1 can affect the cytoskeleton.

nsP2 is involved in the regulation of minus strand RNA synthesis (189) and in the initiation of subgenomic RNA synthesis (222). As mentioned earlier, it also functions in proteolytic processing of the nsPs (34,73,216). The Semliki Forest virus nsp2, expressed in and purified from *E. coli,* is an RNA helicase (66). About half of the Sindbis and Semliki Forest virus nsP2 is associated with the nuclear fraction in virus-infected BHK cells, although its function there is not known (12,160). A pentapeptide in the carboxy-terminal region of the Semliki Forest virus nsP2 is required for nuclear localization (177). A mutant of Semliki Forest virus, in which the Arg^{649} of the nuclear localization signal (P^{648}RRV) in nsP2 was converted to Asp, was distinguished from the parental virus by two criteria: inhibition of host DNA synthesis was less than that seen in cells infected with the parental virus, and even more striking, its pathogenicity in mice was greatly diminished (176). Studies with Sindbis virus and Sindbis virus replicons (self-replicating genomes that lack the structural protein genes) have shown that mutations in nsP2, and specifically in Pro^{726}, can lead to a significant reduction in viral RNA synthesis and permit the establishment of persistent infections in cultured BHK cells (38,50).

nsP3 does not have sequence motifs found in other RNA virus genomes, and its function remains unknown. It is phosphorylated (108,161), and mutants in this gene define an additional complementation group (96). nsP4 has been identified as the viral polymerase. Mutations in this gene affect the synthesis of all viral RNAs, and *in vitro* studies of Sindbis virus–infected cells establish nsP4 as the viral polymerase (13,69,100,188). All of the sequenced alphaviruses have a tyrosine at the amino terminus of nsP4. Shirako and Strauss (204) made a series of mutations to alter this amino acid and found that viable viruses were obtained only when the N-terminus was an aromatic amino acid or histidine.

Replication and transcription of alphavirus RNAs occur on cellular membranes (12,57). Studies with Sindbis virus have defined the proteolytic processing scheme for the nsPs and have led to an elegant model for the regulation of viral RNA synthesis. Proteolytic processing has been analyzed by translation of mRNAs *in vitro* (32, 73), by expression of nsP genes in a vaccinia virus transient expression system (101–103), and by expression in cultured cells of Sindbis virus genomic RNAs containing site-directed mutations in the nsP genes (202,203). Each of these has provided important information for the proposed scheme illustrated in Fig. 5. The Sindbis virus nsPs are initially translated as two polyproteins, P123 and P1234, depending on whether the in-frame opal termination codon is suppressed. Cleavage of the latter at the 3/4 site occurs rapidly to form the complex P123 and nsP4, which is postulated to initiate minus-strand synthesis. Evidence for this is based on the result that nsP4 plus a P123, which is cleavage defective, but not a cleavage-

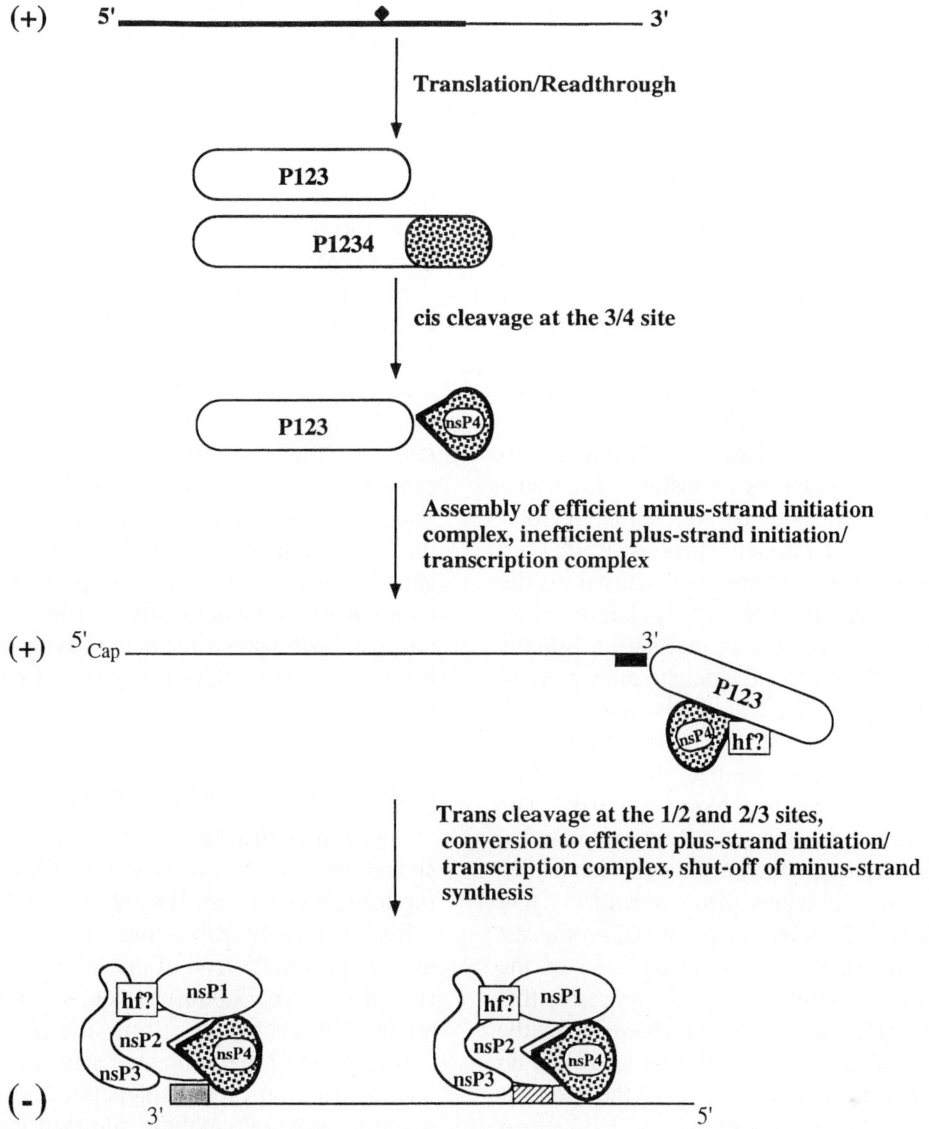

FIG. 5. A model for the temporal regulation of minus- and plus-strand RNA synthesis. The protein complex that initiates (–) strand RNA synthesis is composed of P123 and nsP4. This complex is also able to synthesize (+) strands, but inefficiently. Efficient synthesis of (+) strand genomic and subgenomic RNAs occurs after trans-cleavage at the 1/2 and 2/3 sites of the polyprotein; the latter cleavage results in the shut-off of (–) strand synthesis. Host factors (hf) are most likely involved in these reactions. From ref. 103, with permission, and provided by Drs. J. Lemm and C.M. Rice, Washington University, St. Louis, MO.

defective P1234, can function efficiently in the synthesis of minus-strand RNAs (101–103,203). In the vaccinia expression system that leads to high levels of the nsPs, both plus- and minus-strand RNAs were synthesized, although minus stands were synthesized preferentially. In addition, in the vaccinia virus system, functional replication complexes were not formed when the nsPs were expressed as individual polypeptides or as different combinations of individual nsPs (101,102). The most convincing argument for a role for P123 in the synthesis of minus strands is based on studies in which the Asn^{614} of nsP2 was changed to Asp (103,216). This mutation leads to more efficient processing of P123 *in vitro,* but RNAs containing this mutation do not give rise to viable Sindbis virus in transfection assays (216). With the vaccinia virus expression system, minus-strand RNA synthesis could not be detected when this mutation was present in P123, but it was restored when the mutation was inserted into a P123 protein that was also cleavage defective (103).

This model explains some aspects of the regulation of alphavirus RNA synthesis, in particular, the low level of minus strands synthesized by the replication complexes, the continued requirement for protein synthesis for production of minus strands, and the cessation of minus-strand synthesis several hours after infection (190,191). *In vitro* translation studies show that processing of P123 occurs in trans and, in infected cells, the accumulation of P123 should accelerate its cleavage, leading to cessation of minus-strand synthesis. The partially and fully processed complexes carry out plus-strand RNA synthesis, which continues throughout the infection cycle. Not all of the earlier studies can be explained by this model, and there are mutations in both nsP4 and in nsP2 that permit continued synthesis of minus strands, even after cleavage of the proteins has occurred (188,189).

Attempts to study alphavirus RNA replication in cell-free extracts had been hindered by an inability to initiate viral RNA synthesis. Extracts prepared from alphavirus-infected cells would elongate endogenous RNA, but added templates were not functional (13). Based on the studies described earlier (and see Fig. 5), Lemm et al. (100) established an *in vitro* system that uses a Sindbis virus RNA template to initiate and elongate minus-strand RNAs. Extracts were prepared from cells infected with vaccinia virus recombinants: one expressing an nsP123 that had a defective protease so that the polyprotein would not be cleaved, and the other expressing nsP4. The addition of a plus-strand Sindbis virus RNA template led to the synthesis of the complementary minus stand. Furthermore, membrane fractions from extracts that expressed only the 123 polyprotein could synthesize genome-length minus-strand RNAs on addition of the appropriate template and solubilized nsP4, indicating that this system can be used to purify and characterize the nsP4 polymerase. In these studies, nsP4 by itself had no detectable polymerase activity. None of the extracts tested was able to synthesize plus strands.

The four conserved sequences, noted earlier, in the alphavirus genome were presumed to be replicase-binding sites and to function as promoter elements. Strauss et al. carried out extensive mutagenesis on three of these regions in the Sindbis virus genome: the 3′ nontranslated region (91), the 51 nucleotides located between nucleotides 155 and 205 (143), and the 5′ nontranslated 44 nucleotides (142). They show an important role for these sequences, as most of the mutations affect viral growth, frequently in a host cell–dependent manner, with strikingly different effects in chicken embryo fibroblasts and mosquito cells. These results support the contention that host proteins are involved in alphavirus RNA replication.

The fourth conserved region of the alphavirus genome surrounds the start of the subgenomic RNA. The minimal promoter region contains 19 nucleotides upstream and 5 nucleotides downstream of the start site for transcription of the subgenomic RNA, which coincides with the conserved region (107). Promoter activity is enhanced, however, when additional sequences in this region are included in the RNA (107,173). Additional studies of this promoter were carried out by the construction of Sindbis virus derivatives with two subgenomic RNA promoters: the wild-type promoter which was used for expression of the structural protein genes, and a second promoter, which was placed upstream of the chloramphenicol acetyltransferase gene and was subjected to modifications (173). Minimal promoters from other alphaviruses, but not from rubella virus, could be used by the Sindbis virus nonstructural proteins (77).

A role for host-cell proteins in alphavirus RNA synthesis was inferred from observations made in both vertebrate and invertebrate cells [reviewed in (219)]. Gel-retardation assays have been used to identify potential candidates (154,155) and led to the isolation from mosquito cells of a 50-kd protein that has a high affinity for the 3′ terminus of the Sindbis virus minus-RNA strand and the identification of this protein as the mosquito homolog of the La autoantigen (156). The human La protein has been shown to interact with several other viral RNAs, suggesting that it may have a central role in viral RNA replication.

Expression of Virus Structural Protein Genes

Alphavirus structural proteins are translated from the subgenomic RNA early (2–3 hours after infection) in the replication cycle, probably as soon as the subgenomic mRNA is formed. Ribosomes initiate translation at a single site near the 5′ end of this RNA and proceed uninterrupted for some 3,000 nucleotides to a termination site about 300 nucleotides from the 3′ poly A terminus [reviewed in (219)]. The first sequences to be translated encode the viral capsid polypeptide, which folds to form a serine–protease catalytic site (see Fig. 2) that cleaves the capsid from the nascent polyprotein at a tryptophan–serine bond. Substitution of the C-terminal tryptophan by alanine, arginine, or phenylalanine showed that only tryptophan is an effective autoproteolytic substrate (210). Continued translation of the mRNA produces a signal sequence that facilitates translocation of the remaining polypeptide into the lumen of the endoplasmic reticulum (Fig. 6). As the protein emerges into this vesicle, it is modified by covalent attachment of oligosaccharides (201) and, later, by proteolytic cleavages carried out by host-cell signalase (110). The final products of translation are the capsid, two large (~45 kd) type I transmembrane glycoproteins, noted p62 or PE2 and E1, and a small (6 kd) membrane-embedded protein; the topology of these three membrane-bound proteins is shown in Fig. 7. Much of the data supporting this model derive from (a) assignments of domains with 22 hydrophobic amino acids in the sequences of the p62, 6K, and E1 as either signal- or stop-transfer sequences that span the membrane (see Fig. 6); (b) expression of cDNA constructs of

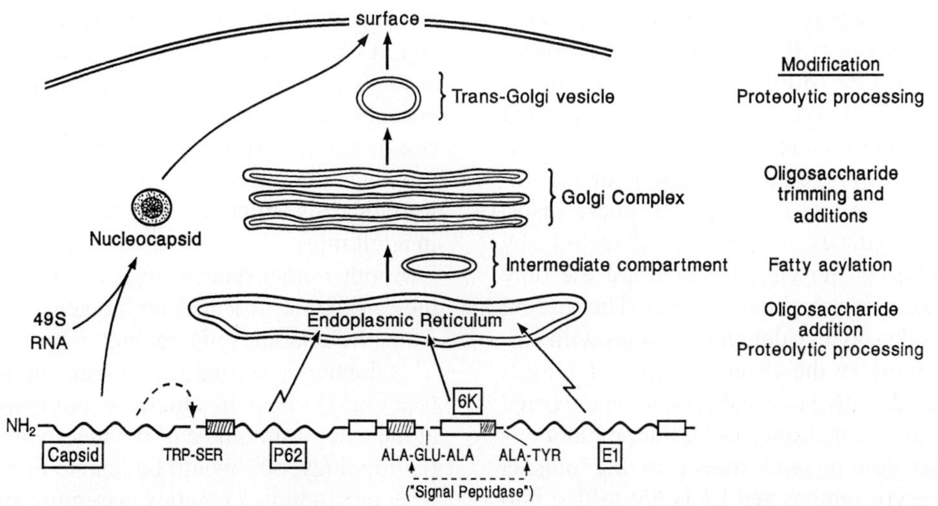

FIG. 6. Processing and modifications of the Sindbis virus structural proteins. Capsid is released co-translationally by autoproteolysis and assembles to encapsidate the 49S genomic RNA. The p62, 6K, and E1 proteins are modified during transport to the cell surface. Signal sequence, *shaded rectangle*; hydrophobic sequences, *open rectangle*.

Semliki Forest virus subgenomic RNA under the control of a heterologous promoter or expression of the Semliki Forest virus RNA genome, which show that the carboxy termini of either p62 or the 6-kd protein can function as a signal sequence for E1 (110,131); and (c) a change in the localization of the E2 carboxyl terminus to the inner leaflet of the bilayer during its transport to the cell surface (113). The p62, E1, and 6K proteins appear to move as a cohort through the secretory vesicles from their site of synthesis on the endoplasmic reticulum to their ultimate location at the plasma membrane of the cell (see Fig. 6). This process takes about 30 minutes at physiologic temperatures and leads to several posttranslational modifications. Among these are the trimming of and additions to the three oligosaccharides on Sindbis virus p62 and to the two on E1. Cellular enzymes localized to various compartments of the secretory system carry out these modifications in a manner resembling that found for cellular proteins destined for the plasma membrane or secretion to the extracellular fluid. Thus the precise composition of the oligosaccharides on the virus is dependent on the host cell in which the virus replicates (86).

A heterodimer of p62 and E1 forms very shortly after synthesis of the latter, and association is more effective

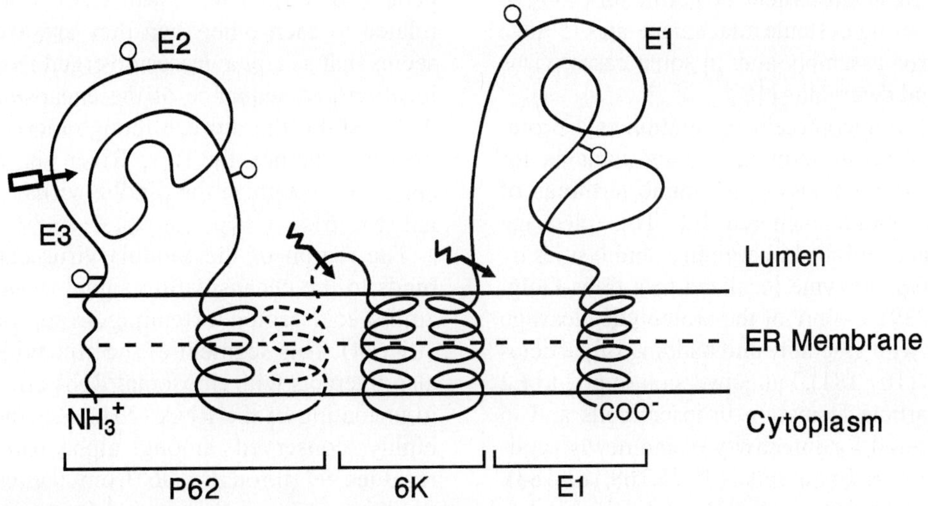

FIG. 7. Topology of the Sindbis virus p62 and E1 glycoproteins and the 6K protein in the endoplasmic reticulum membrane. The *dashed* part of p62 is removed from its transmembrane configuration and binds to the inner face of the lipid bilayer during transport to the cell surface. Host cell signalase activity, ⤳; host cell furin-type protease, ▭→. Refer to text for detail.

when both proteins are expressed from the same genome instead of different RNAs (11). The folding of these proteins requires the formation of intrachain disulfide bonds and has been shown to involve a transient covalent interaction between the nascent and newly synthesized E1 and PE2 and the host-cell chaperones, protein disulfide isomerase and Erp57 (139). These disulfide-bonded intermediates could be detected by radioactive labeling, as the viral proteins are the only ones being synthesized in the infected cells. The folding pathway also includes noncovalent interactions with calnexin and calreticulin. In the absence of p62, E1 folds into disulfide-linked aggregates and fails to be exported from the endoplasmic reticulum (6,21), but p62 alone is capable of proper folding and transit to the plasma membrane. The newly synthesized E1 is not folded into its thermodynamically stable state but becomes trapped in a metastable conformation through the chaperone-like activity of p62 (6,36). The heterodimer complex trimerizes while still in the endoplasmic reticulum and is relatively stable to low-pH exposure. Continuous chaperoning by p62 and its proteolytically modified E2 maintains E1 in this metastable state in the virion spikes until low pH dissociates the dimers and leads to trimers of thermodynamically stable E1. The latter are distinguishable by new epitopes and rearrangement of disulfide bonds (140,197).

Palmitate acylation occurs at three sites on the Sindbis virus p62, four sites on the 6K protein, and one site on E1 during transport of the proteins after they have exited from the endoplasmic reticulum and before entrance into the Golgi complex [see Fig. 6 and (14,124,198)]. Cysteines oriented to the cytoplasmic face of the lipid bilayer are the sites of fatty acylation. The role of these fatty acids in glycoprotein function is unknown, but they probably affect interactions of the proteins with the lipid bilayer. Blocking their attachment by cerulenin (194) or by mutationally altering cysteine attachment sites (59,82) interferes with virus assembly and, in some cases, virus stability to heat and detergents (182).

A critical step in glycoprotein maturation is a proteolytic cleavage in p62 to form E3, which contains for Sindbis virus 64 amino acids of the amino terminus of p62, and the membrane-anchored E2. This cleavage occurs at a sequence enriched in arginines and lysines by a host cell furin-type enzyme localized to a trans-Golgi vesicle (138,186,239). Failure of the proteolytic cleavage does not interfere with assembly and budding of particles in vertebrate cells (167,181), but conversion of p62 to E2 is essential for particle formation in insect cells and in most cases is required for infectivity of the newly replicated particles in vertebrate cells (39,75,168,181,184). The failure of an alphavirus containing p62–E1 spikes to replicate in a cell may be due to the inability of the E1 to undergo the low pH–induced conformation required for its fusogenic activity (116,117). One variant of Sindbis virus, which has an uncleaved p62, contains an additional suppressor mutation in the E2 protein and is as infectious as the wild-type virus (76). A strain of Venezuelan equine encephalitis virus that was blocked in P62 cleavage gave rise to viable revertants containing suppressor mutations in either E2 or E1 (31). The E1 revertant grew normally in BHK cells but poorly in insect cells and was attenuated in adult mice.

Another important change occurs in the topology of the carboxy-terminal 33 amino acids of p62 as it transits from the endoplasmic reticulum to the Golgi vesicles. This domain is shifted from a transmembrane orientation (see Fig. 7) to one in which most of these amino acids are at the cytoplasmic face of the membrane (113). In its initial topology, p62 would be unable to bind nucleocapsid, thus precluding premature assembly of particles at the endoplasmic reticulum membranes.

Assembly of Nucleocapsids and Enveloped Virions

The assembly of nucleocapsids includes both oligomerization of the capsid protein and selection of the genomic RNA for encapsidation. Although the subgenomic RNA is present in molar excess, it is the genomic RNA that is packaged into nucleocapsids and virions. The first evidence that selectivity was due to a packaging or encapsidation signal in the 5′ region of the genome was the identification in the Sindbis virus genome of a 132-nucleotide fragment extending from nucleotide 945 to 1,076 in the nsP1 gene that interacts specifically with the capsid protein in binding assays and increases the encapsidation of an RNA in infected cells (56,241,242). Specificity appears to lie in the structure rather than in the sequence of the oligonucleotide (241). In contrast, the encapsidation signals for both Ross River and Semliki Forest virus are in the nsP2 gene (56,253). These two viruses are more closely related to each other than they are to Sindbis virus. It seems that as alphaviruses diverged from each other, the location and sequence of the encapsidation signal also diverged. Furthermore, although there could be similarities in structure, the Ross River virus capsid does not appear to recognize the Sindbis virus encapsidation signal (51,56).

The region of the Sindbis virus capsid protein that binds to the encapsidation signal is embedded in a 32-amino-acid region extending from amino acids 76 to 107 (64). This segment of the alphavirus capsid protein also interacts with ribosomal RNA and may be involved in uncoating of the RNA (251). Residues 97 to 106 are highly conserved among alphaviruses. Deletion of residues 97 through 106 from the capsid protein of Sindbis virus did not significantly inhibit particle assembly but reduced infectious titers more than 100-fold (152). Most of the particles contained the subgenomic RNA instead of the virus genome supporting the conclusion that these amino acids are important in packaging specificity.

Loss of discrimination in encapsidation also was observed with a Sindbis virus recombinant in which the capsid gene was replaced with the Ross River capsid gene (51). Furthermore, a deletion of amino acids 65 to 109 from this capsid protein did not reduce particle production, but they were almost completely devoid of viral genome RNA (51). This deletion eliminated most of the basic residues in the peptide chain and indicated that capsid–capsid interactions can occur in the absence of nucleic acid binding. The ability to form empty particles by removal of positively charged residues in the protein was first observed with icosahedral plant viruses (43,215).

Another exception to the strong selection of genomic over subgenomic RNA for encapsidation was described with Auravirus. This alphavirus packages both RNAs, although the ratio of genomic to subgenomic RNA is three- to 10-fold higher in virions than in infected cells (180). This result originally suggested that Auravirus subgenomic RNA contained an encapsidation signal; however, it is more likely that an encapsidation signal in the genomic RNA is not so efficient as that in other alphaviruses, resulting in less specificity in packaging. It appears that specific interactions between an RNA and an alphavirus capsid protein will favor encapsidation of that RNA, but in their absence, the capsid protein will interact with and package those RNAs that are most abundant.

In vitro assembly of nucleocapsids was carried out initially with capsid protein purified from virus (246,250), but recombinant capsid proteins expressed in *E. coli* have been used more recently (223). Both studies demonstrated that assembly can occur with a variety of nucleic acids, but in competition experiments, Sindbis virus RNA is preferentially packaged (196,223). Sindbis capsid proteins that lack the first 19 amino acids can assemble into nucleocapsids, but those deleted in the first 31 amino acids do not assemble by themselves (223). These and those missing the first 80 amino acids can be incorporated into nucleocapsids in the presence of competent capsid proteins. In mixed reactions with Sindbis and Ross River virus capsid proteins, only homologous nucleocapsids were detected (223).

The Sindbis capsid protein starting at amino acid 106 was crystallized, and the x-ray structure analysis showed that the amino terminal residues 108–111 of one chain associate with an adjacent molecule and that these residues bind into a hydrophobic pocket of the neighboring molecule (27). This finding, taken together with their mutational studies, led Lee et al. (99) to propose that residues 108 to 110 are important in the interactions between capsid monomers and also in the binding between the nucleocapsid and the C-terminal tail of the E2 glycoprotein (99).

The final stages in the replication of alphaviruses occur when nucleocapsids interact with the host-cell plasma membrane at sites occupied by viral transmembrane glycoproteins. This nucleation event leads to binding of additional virus glycoproteins and a bending of the membrane around the nucleocapsid until the bilayers meet and fuse to release the enveloped particle (20,62). Electron micrographs graphically illustrate this process (Fig. 8). Budding of alphaviruses requires the presence of both nucleocapsids and the heterodimeric complex of virus-encoded glycoproteins (10,220,263); however, mutations in the capsid protein that prevent the accumulation of stable nucleocapsids in the cytoplasm do not decrease the efficiency of Semliki Forest virus budding (48,211). This suggests that capsid–capsid interactions are stabilized by binding of spikes to the capsid protein, and in some cases, nucleocapsid assembly may occur concomitant with virus budding. The specific molecular interactions between alphavirus nucleocapsids and spike glycoproteins have not been identified; however, a motif at the carboxy terminus of E2 that is within a hydrophobic sequence localized to the cytoplasmic face of the membrane bilayer is essential for assembly. A tyrosine and a leucine residue near the amino-terminal portion of

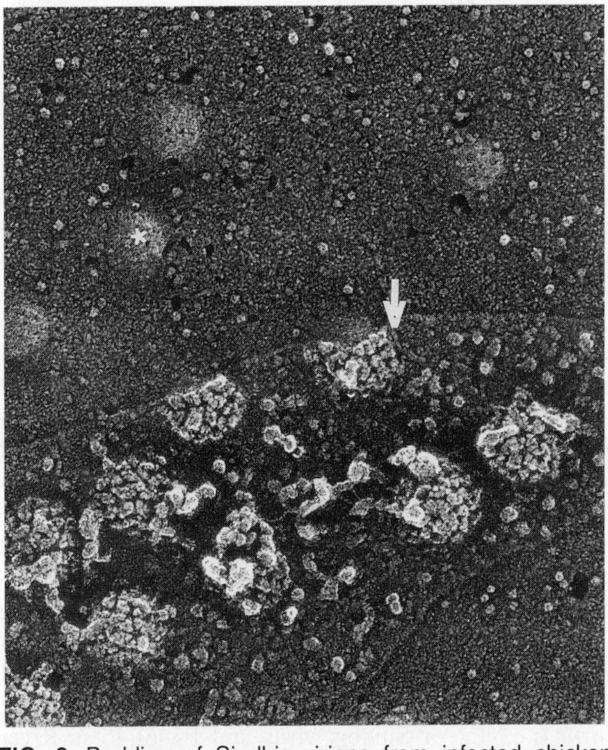

FIG. 8. Budding of Sindbis virions from infected chicken embryo fibroblasts. Cells were quick frozen and freeze fractured. The electron micrograph shows the fracture across the surface membrane of the cell (*white arrow*). On the bottom is the outer surface of the cell with clusters of virus glycoproteins at sites of budding. On the top is the inner leaflet of the surface lipid bilayer with viral nucleocapsids bound to the inner cytoplasmic side of the membrane. Sample preparation for electron microscopy was carried out by Dr. J. Heuser, Washington University School of Medicine, St. Louis, MO.

this sequence are highly conserved among the alphaviruses and are postulated to bind in a hydrophobic pocket containing a tyrosine and a tryptophan on the surface of the nucleocapsid (98,99,211). On association of E2 with the nucleocapsid, this pocket is hypothesized to undergo a conformational change that destabilizes and activates the core for eventual disassembly after virus entry into a host cell (98).

A number of studies using site-directed mutations in the E2 cytoplasmic domain and the capsid protein (60,82, 97,153,211) provided further evidence for an interaction between the E2 cytoplasmic tail and the nucleocapsid, and mutations in the Sindbis virus capsid gene can partially suppress mutations in the E2 cytoplasmic domain that inhibit assembly (183). Capsid–E2 binding specificity also was demonstrated by experiments in which the gene for the Sindbis virus capsid protein was embedded in the Ross River virus genome (120). Virion particle production was greatly reduced with this chimera, but could be increased when seven amino acids of the Sindbis virus E2 cytoplasmic sequence were substituted for Ross River virus sequences. These results supported earlier studies in which a very hydrophobic six-amino-acid peptide corresponding to a conserved sequence within the E2 carboxy-terminal domain were shown to inhibit selectively Sindbis and Semliki Forest virus assembly and budding (30). Similar kinds of peptides with sequences identical to those in the E2 carboxyl terminus of Semliki Forest virus were reported to bind capsids (133). Not all chimeras, however, are defective; those in which the capsid protein gene was derived from either Semliki Forest virus or Ross River virus with the remaining genes from Sindbis virus assembled infectious virus at normal levels (51,214).

Effective budding also requires lateral interactions among the glycoprotein heterodimers, leading to trimeric and higher oligomeric forms such as the pentameric and hexameric structures that are positioned around the two-fold and five-fold axes of the virion. Hexagonal arrays of spikes were detected when membranes from Sindbis virions were examined by electron microscopy (232). These larger forms of the heterodimer would lead to polyvalent binding of the nucleocapsid to the E2 cytoplasmic ligands and could provide the force for membrane bending (62). Their formation also precludes insertion of host-cell proteins into the virus envelope. Defects in one of the glycoproteins (42) or its substitution by a chimeric form (i.e., E2 of Sindbis virus and E1 of Ross River virus) can interfere with the oligomerization process and decrease the amounts of secreted virus (262). In the latter case, heterodimers were formed, but no binding of nucleocapsids occurred at the plasma membrane. A series of suppressor mutations (five in Sindbis virus E2 and two in Ross River virus E1) increase progeny virus formation (260). The two adaptive changes in E1 were located adjacent to the membrane anchor domain of this protein. Based on cryoelectron microscopic reconstructions of Ross River virus (25), this region is part of the stalk that forms the spikes on the surface of the virion and consists of three entwined heterodimers; thus the mutations could affect trimer formation. Abnormal, multicored particles are released from cells infected with a Sindbis virus mutant containing the substitution of valine for alanine at position 344 in the E2 protein, and this phenotype can be partially corrected by a second, compensatory mutation in E1 (219).

The small, hydrophobic, fatty acylated membrane-associated 6K protein plays an important but still undefined role in alphavirus assembly and budding. Mutations in the 6K gene affect virus formation both quantitatively and qualitatively. Single-site mutations can lead to enhanced production of aberrant particles that contain multiple nucleocapsid cores, and a Semliki Forest virus mutant that totally lacks the 6K gene is highly defective in virus budding in BHK cells but much less so in insect cells (112,118). In the deletion mutant grown in BHK cells, virus cores align along the plasma membrane, and glycoproteins are not altered in their maturation and translocation. The 6K protein also interacts specifically with the E1/PE2 heterodimer, as shown by studies with a chimeric virus genome containing Sindbis virus glycoprotein sequences but a Ross River virus 6K virus sequence. This chimera was highly defective both in virus formation and in conformational changes occurring during maturation of the E1 glycoprotein (262). Mutations in the 6K Sindbis virus gene can be suppressed by mutations in the E2 glycoprotein, indicating a role for this protein in glycoprotein oligomerization during virus assembly (81). Because of its lipophilic properties, the 6K protein has been postulated to influence the selection of lipids that interact with the transmembrane domains of the glycoproteins, which, in turn, affect the deformability of the bilayer required for the extreme curvature that occurs as budding proceeds (20).

In most infected vertebrate cells, the plasma membrane is the site of alphavirus assembly; however, budding of Semliki Forest virus is selective in polarized epithelial cells, occurring only at the basal lateral surface (178,179) and, in cultured rat hippocampal neurons, this virus is secreted exclusively from membranes of the dendrites (37). In insect cells, budding occurs intracellularly, and virus-loaded vesicles are later disgorged to the extracellular fluid (137). In general, the lipid composition of alphaviruses closely resembles that of the membrane of the host cell (104). The ratio of cholesterol to phospholipid, however, is much higher in the membrane of alphaviruses than in the cellular membranes (175), and this may explain why Semliki Forest and Sindbis virus budding requires the presence of cholesterol in exiting the host-cell membrane (121,126). Virus membranes also are much more densely packed with protein and have a greater curvature than do the corresponding cellular membranes; thus their membranes are less fluid than are cellular membranes (200).

Alphaviruses as Vectors for the Expression of Heterologous Proteins

Sindbis virus, Semliki Forest virus, and Venezuelan equine encephalitis virus have all been genetically engineered to express heterologous proteins. Several different types of vectors have been described; the most versatile are those in which a heterologous gene replaces the structural protein genes (111,172,258). These vectors are self-replicating (replicons) but are not packaged and released from cells as virion particles. They can be complemented by defective "helper" RNAs that provide the structural proteins and allow replicons to be assembled into particles under conditions in which the helper itself is not packaged (15,111,172). Such particles are infectious but self-limiting, as they produce nsPs as well as genomic and subgenomic RNAs but, in the absence of structural proteins, do not form new particles.

Studies with replicons lacking the structural proteins led to the discovery of a translational enhancer in the viral subgenomic mRNA within the coding region of the capsid (54,208). The sequences that function as an enhancer are located about 25 nucleotides downstream of the AUG start codon and form a hairpin-like structure (55). Translation is stimulated about 10-fold, but only in infected cells (54,207). The existence and importance of this enhancer was clearly demonstrated for replicons derived from Sindbis and Semliki Forest virus but not for those from Venezuelan equine encephalitis virus (55,172).

A second type of expression vector contains two subgenomic RNA promoters; one controls the synthesis of the subgenomic mRNA that codes for the viral structural proteins, and the other controls the synthesis of the subgenomic RNA that codes for the heterologous protein (52). These vectors produce infectious virus particles able to spread throughout a culture.

Alphavirus vectors are being used for production of proteins in a variety of eukaryotic cells and have provided a useful tool for studies of protein expression and modification (52,63,122,195). They also are being developed as vaccines; for example, replicons expressing heterologous viral antigens, packaged into infectious particles or as DNA plasmids, have been introduced into animals. Initial studies in mice with DNA plasmids have been promising, as they induce an immune response at much lower doses than do conventional DNA plasmids.

A completely different approach to the use of alphaviruses as vectors had been to insert heterologous amino acid sequences into the viral structural proteins in such a way that the virus is still viable, but the heterologous epitope is expressed and can function as an immunogen. London et al. (119) made random insertions of an epitope from Rift Valley Fever virus into the structural protein genes of Sindbis virus. They then selected viable viruses containing the insert and found not only that the insertions were tolerated but also that the chimeric Sindbis virus could be used as a vaccine to make mice resistant to infection by Rift Valley Fever virus. Those initial studies and the subsequent isolation of Sindbis virus mutants that were defective in their ability to bind to vertebrate cells (39) served as a foundation for Ohno et al. (145), who devised a strategy to target Sindbis vector particles to specific cell types. They inserted the immunoglobulin G (IgG)-binding domain of protein A into the PE2 glycoprotein. This allowed them to target these Sindbis virus replicon particles to a particular cell type by adding monoclonal antibodies against a surface marker on those cells.

Recombination

Based on sequence comparisons, at least one alphavirus, western equine encephalitis virus, arose by recombination between eastern equine encephalitis virus and a Sindbis-like virus (67). Recombination also has been observed between replicons and defective helper RNAs. The latter events may arise more frequently than those between two virus genomes because crossovers do not have to be precise. Sequence analysis of these recombinant RNAs demonstrated that crossovers occurred within the defective modules (244). Recombinational events giving rise to infectious virion RNAs could create deletions, rearrangements, or insertions, as long as they occurred outside of each functional module (172,244).

More-detailed studies have been undertaken in efforts to define the mechanism and requirements for recombination (72,78,174). Surprisingly, recombination was detected with Sindbis virus RNA molecules that were unable to replicate because of deletions at the 5′ or 3′ terminus. Recombination events observed in laboratory studies usually take place under conditions in which high concentrations of RNAs are mixed together. Although these events are probably less likely to occur under conditions of natural infection, they do indicate that exchange between RNA molecules may play a role in the evolution of RNA viruses.

Effects of Alphavirus Infection on the Host Cell

Infection of vertebrate cells by most alphaviruses leads to inhibition of host-cell protein synthesis and cell death. Mechanisms that have been proposed for shut-off of host-cell protein synthesis include inhibition of host factors required for protein synthesis, with preferential translation of viral mRNAs, changes in the ionic environment of infected cells, which favors translation of viral RNAs, and direct inhibition by capsid protein [reviewed in (219)]. Infection of BHK cells with Sindbis virus replicons showed that inhibition of host-cell protein synthesis occurs at essentially the same rate under conditions in which no structural proteins or no viral subgenomic mRNA is synthesized (53). These data provide strong evidence that the structural proteins are not involved in mechanisms that inhibit host protein synthesis. Synthesis of the viral glycoproteins, however, leads to a much more rapid appearance of cytopathic effects than is seen in their absence (53). Furthermore, as mentioned later and in more detail (in Chapter 30 in *Fields Virology*, 4th ed.), differences in the viral glycoprotein E2 can greatly affect how the cell responds to infection.

Cell death in alphavirus-infected vertebrate cells occurs by apoptosis (106,192), but in mosquito cells, the mechanism appears to be different and may more closely resemble necrosis (85). Infection of many *Aedes albopictus* (mosquito) cell clones leads to persistent infection (16), although it also may be cytopathic (84,187,225). In those cell cultures in which a persistent infection is established, the production of virus is comparable to that observed in most vertebrate cells during the first 24 hours, but then decreases several orders of magnitude during the persistent infection phase. The mechanism leading to persistence in mosquito cell lines is not known, although there have been reports that cells infected with Sindbis virus produce an antiviral factor, and intracellular factors appear to restrict virus production (84).

It has been possible to establish persistent infections in some vertebrate cells. Two different types have been described. In one, essentially all of the cells are infected, but the synthesis of virus-specific RNA and protein in each cell is greatly reduced. This type of persistent infection was established in BHK cells by using defective interfering particles (243). The defective RNAs interfere with the replication of the genomic RNAs, leading to inhibition of viral RNA replication and virus production. The virus itself underwent a genetic change, converting it to a much less cytopathic mutant that was itself able to cause persistent infections in BHK cells. Several mutations were identified, but only one that converted the Pro^{726} to Ser in the nsP2 protein was able to confer this phenotype on the virus (38). The decrease in cytopathic effects also was correlated with an eight- to 10-fold decrease in viral RNA synthesis.

A completely different approach to establishing this type of persistent infection in BHK cells was undertaken by using Sindbis virus replicons that express a gene (the *pac* gene) that codes for an enzyme that destroys puromycin. In the presence of puromycin, only cells that could eliminate this compound would survive, and only those cells that contained a Sindbis virus replicon that was not cytopathic could survive its replication and transcription, which would be required to express the *pac* gene. This selection procedure led to the isolation of several noncytopathic replicons (50). The one that has been analyzed in most detail has a single mutation, which led to the change of a single amino acid (Pro^{726} to Leu) in nsP2, the same amino acid that was changed in the Sindbis virus mutant isolated from the persistent infection. The identification of several mutations in the nsP2 gene that lead to persistent infections and the localization of nsP2 in the nucleus suggest that this protein may have some as yet undefined functions affecting host-cell survival (176). These noncytopathic replicons are now being used as expression vectors in BHK cells (2).

A second type of persistent infection that has been described is one in which most of the cells are not infected, but the virus continues to persist because of a small fraction of cells that are susceptible and maintain the virus. In this case, the titer per culture is low, but those cells that do get infected may produce normal levels of virus and do not survive. An early example was the establishment of a persistent infection of mouse L929 cells by Semliki Forest virus. Only 1% to 20% of these cells expressed virus-specific antigens, and induction of interferon was the major factor in permitting the L cells to survive infection (130).

More recently the expression of other cellular genes has been shown to cause a significant decrease in virus replication and may lead to a persistent infection. The human MxA protein is a member of a family of guanosine triphosphatases (GTPases). When it was expressed in the human cell line Hep-2, the cells became almost completely resistant to infection by Semliki Forest virus: only 1% of the cells showed evidence of infection, but the virus was eventually cleared from the culture (95). Persistent infections by Sindbis virus and Semliki Forest virus could be established in a rat prostate carcinoma cell line (AT-3 cells) expressing the human *bcl-2* gene (106,192). The bcl-2 protein is a well-established antiapoptotic agent. In these cells, virus replication is severely restricted, with titers 10- to 100-fold lower in the AT-3 *bcl-2*–expressing cells than in the controls (192, 228). As in the previous examples, only a small fraction of the AT-3 cells produced virus-specific antigens, indicating that the low titers were due to only a small number of the cells being productively infected. Further studies with Sindbis virus led to the discovery that the ability to establish this type of persistent infection was dependent on the strain used and was correlated with a single amino acid in the E2 glycoprotein (228) [and see Chapter 30 in *Fields Virology*, 4th ed.].

Another restriction on Sindbis virus replication has been observed in mouse cells and is dependent on the class I major histocompatibility complex (MHC) haplotype. Sindbis virus replication was more than 100-fold higher in mouse cells that express the $H\text{-}2^k$ haplotype than in cells expressing the $H\text{-}2^d$ haplotype. The difference does not appear to be at binding or entry, but at the level of viral RNA synthesis (70). This difference also depends on the strain of Sindbis virus and specifically on the E2 glycoprotein.

RUBIVIRUSES

Rubella virus has long existed in the shadow of the alphaviruses. In the early studies of structure and replication of Togaviruses, it seemed that rubella virus was very similar to alphaviruses, but perhaps its replication was not so robust. This picture is gradually changing as we learn more about rubella virus—the properties of this virus and its interactions with its host cell have some special features. One major difference is the limited host range of rubella virus: it is found only in humans and does not grow in insect cells. Furthermore rubella virus grows slowly and to low titers in cultured vertebrate cells. Infection is much less cytopathic than that observed with alphaviruses, and persistent infections are readily established [reviewed in (49)]. It has been established that cell death in infected Vero cells occurs by apoptosis and involves a p53-dependent pathway (129,171). Chapter 31 in *Fields Virology*, 4th ed. describes these viruses in more detail.

Virion Structure and Entry

Rubella virions closely resemble alphaviruses in general morphology and physical characteristics; however, virion preparations are much more pleomorphic, and little is known about the icosahedral lattices and distribution of the glycoproteins on the virion surface. Two type 1 membrane glycoproteins form spikes projecting from the lipid membrane envelope; they are noted as E1 (282 amino acids) and E2 (481 amino acids) and are postulated to form heterodimers [reviewed in (49)]. Virion cores are similar to but somewhat smaller than alphavirus nucleocapsids and contain multiple copies of a single capsid protein about 290 to 300 amino acids in length that are present in virions as disulfide-linked dimers. The amino-terminal portion of the capsid is like that of the alphaviruses, enriched in arginines and containing a binding site for the genomic 40S RNA (115). Binding assays identified a 29-nucleotide region (nucleotides 347–375) in the rubella virus genome as the sequence required for specific interaction of RNA with the capsid protein. Studies to determine if this sequence is essential for or enhances encapsidation of the RNA have not yet been done.

In cultured Vero cells, rubella virus infection but not transfection of RNA was inhibited by lysosomotropic agents (162); thus this virus appears to enter the cell by receptor-mediated endocytosis and after membrane fusion in an acidified endosome delivers its RNA to the infected cell cytoplasm.

Transcription, Translation, and Replication of the Genome

The replication of rubella virus does follow the same strategy as that of alphaviruses: the genomic RNA is first translated to produce the nonstructural proteins that are required for the synthesis of the complementary minus-strand RNA, the genomic RNA, and the subgenomic RNA [reviewed in (49)]. The subgenomic RNA is the mRNA for the viral structural proteins. Amino acid sequence homologies between rubella virus and the alphaviruses exist only within the nsPs (see Fig. 3), but proteolytic processing of the rubella virus nsP is distinct from that of alphaviruses. The 5′ two thirds of the rubella virus genome is translated to a polyprotein of 240 kd that is posttranslationally cleaved into two polypeptides, one 150 and the other 90 kd. Region-specific antibodies located the 150-kd protein at the amino terminus, and the 90-kd protein at the carboxyl terminus of the polyprotein (47). Mutation of the cysteine at residue 1151 led to the accumulation of the largest protein at the expense of the two smaller proteins, providing evidence that the larger protein was the precursor of the smaller and that the cysteine was essential for protease activity (127). The protease responsible for cleavage is located at the C-terminus of p150 and is a papain-type cysteine protease. It requires divalent cations, contains zinc binding domains required for activity, and functions both in cis and trans (114,261). A histidine at position 1273 also is critical for activity. The site of cleavage is a gly-gly-gly sequence at positions 1299 through 1301 (23).

The first cDNA clone of rubella virus able to be transcribed into infectious RNA was derived from a strain (w-Therien) that forms opaque plaques on Vero cells. cDNA fragments obtained from a different strain (f-Therien) of rubella virus that gives clear plaques were used to replace equivalent segments in the clone (169). A swap of the 3′ half of the genome led to an increase in specific infectivity, but the exchange of the 5′ fragments resulted in clear plaques. The exchange of a region near the most 5′ terminal fragment had the strongest effect on cytopathogenicity. The more cytopathic viruses produced more nonstructural proteins, and because the levels of the viral RNA species were similar, this result suggests that the amounts of the rubella virus nonstructural proteins can affect cell killing.

The 3′-terminal 305 nucleotides of rubella RNA has four stem–loop structures, two of which (SL1 and SL2) are located in the coding region of the E1 glycoprotein gene and two in the 59-nucleotide untranslated region. Nakhashi et al. (141) first showed by UV light–induced covalent cross-linking and gel-retardation assays that the 3′ terminus of the genomic plus-strand RNA bound three cellular proteins of molecular masses 61, 63, and 68 kd. The 61-kd protein was identified as calreticulin, a calcium-binding protein usually found in the endoplasmic reticulum of eukaryotic cells (206). SL2 is the binding site for calreticulin, and binding is localized to the N-terminal domain of the protein (9). Site-directed mutagenesis of SL2 led to loss of binding of calreticulin, in particular for those mutations that destabilized the stem structure (24). Decreased binding of calreticulin did not correlate with inhibition of virus growth. Although this suggests that calreticulin binding is not required for virus viability, it was proposed that local intracellular concentrations of the protein might be high enough to allow binding to occur. Alternatively, the binding of calreticulin may have some role in human infections in which innate and immune responses can affect virus replication.

Extensive mutagenesis of SL3 and SL4 indicated that most of these regions were required for virus replication. In addition, further studies demonstrated the formation of three RNA–protein complexes with the 3′ untranslated region, and UV cross-linking detected host proteins with molecular masses of 120, 80, 66, 55, 48, and 36 kd bound to this region of the RNA (24).

A very detailed mutagenesis analysis also was carried out for the 5′ terminus of rubella virus RNA (170). Although many of these mutations had an effect on virus growth, most were not lethal. Mutations that were lethal included all of those that removed the two As at nucleotides 2 and 3, either by mutation or by deletion. Two cellular proteins, one 59 and the other 52 kd, when bound to the 5′ terminus, were immunoprecipitated with a Ro-type human polyclonal serum obtained from patients with autoimmune disorders (164,165). A subset of sera recognized the La autoantigen or both the La and Ro autoantigens. The La autoantigen binds to the 5′ stem–loop of rubella virus genomic RNA with relatively high specificity both *in vivo* and *in vitro* and affects the expression of the RNA (40). It is not yet possible to interpret the significance of the binding of these proteins to rubella virus RNA. The finding that these proteins are autoantigens has led to the speculations that their involvement in infection may lead to the arthritic symptoms associated with rubella virus infections. As mentioned previously, the La autoantigen is now implicated in the replication of a number of different RNA viruses, but how it is involved remains to be discovered.

Some headway on rubella viral RNA replication is being made. Virus replication complexes in Vero-infected cells have been localized to vacuoles of endolysosomal origin and tubular membranes with antibodies directed against the p150 replicase (92). Colocalization of lysosomal markers with double-stranded RNA antibodies was found by confocal microscopy, supporting the proposal that replication occurred on virus-modified lysosomes (125).

Synthesis of Structural Proteins and Virus Assembly

Translation of the rubella subgenomic mRNA produces a polyprotein that is proteolytically processed by a pathway different from that of the alphaviruses (29,146–148). The rubella virus capsid protein lacks an autoprotease activity. Stretches of 23 and 20 hydrophobic amino acids precede the amino termini of the E2 and E1 glycoproteins and act as signals for the translocation of the glycoproteins into the lumen of the endoplasmic reticulum. Cleavages between the capsid and E2 and between E2 and E1 are catalyzed by the host-cell signalase. After cleavage, the E2 signal sequence remains attached to the capsid protein, which becomes anchored to the membrane (79,221). The latter interaction is probably important in targeting the assembly of the virus nucleocapsid to intracellular membranes. There is no small hydrophobic "linker" protein between the two glycoproteins nor is there a precursor form of E2.

The two rubella virus glycoproteins resemble those of the alphaviruses in name, but their structure and synthesis are distinct [(29,146–148) and reviewed in (49)]. Both rubella virus glycoproteins contain N-linked oligosaccharides, and E2 also contains O-linked glycans (123,185). These proteins are retained in the Golgi organelle, and only a small fraction reach the plasma membrane. The transmembrane domain of E2 has a Golgi retention signal in contrast to E1, which contains a retention signal for the endoplasmic reticulum in its transmembrane and cytoplasmic domain. The latter is overridden in the heterodimer, but both are required for virus particles to be secreted from infected cells (61). Site-directed mutagenesis studies indicate that a 29-amino-acid sequence in E1 may be the fusion peptide for the heterodimer complex of this virus (259). The accumulation of the viral glycoproteins in the Golgi complex may explain why virus assembly appears to occur mainly at this site. Nucleocapsids of rubella virus become visible only during the budding process and apparently do not assemble independent of an association with the glycoproteins.

PERSPECTIVES

Togaviruses and, in particular, alphaviruses are among the best-characterized RNA enveloped viruses. This chapter has documented much of our knowledge of the structure and replication of these viruses, but many questions remain unanswered. Progress on determining the three-dimensional structure of the virus continues to be made by using cryoelectron microscopy, and a structure for the E1 glycoprotein is being determined (248). These and other structural studies should provide a clearer picture of assembly and disassembly of these viruses. In the last few years, several functions of the individual alphavirus nonstructural proteins have been identified, but little progress has been made on how these proteins work in concert to replicate and transcribe viral RNA. Proteolytic cleavage of the nsP complex plays an essential role in the regulation of viral RNA synthesis, but the details have not yet been worked out. It will be important to learn if this type of regulation extends to the synthesis of rubella virus RNAs. Several different host-cell proteins that bind to viral RNAs have been identified, but there are no models for how these proteins might be involved in viral RNA synthesis. The ability to initiate alphavirus RNA synthesis in cellular extracts represents an important first step in uncovering the details of viral RNA synthesis (100).

There is at least one unsolved puzzle that stems from studies on the requirements for alphavirus RNA synthesis in cultured cells. Studies with both Sindbis and Semliki Forest virus replicons have demonstrated that viral RNA replication and the shut-off of host-cell protein synthesis occur in the absence of any of the viral structural proteins. Based on those results, it would seem that neither the viral glycoproteins nor the capsid protein plays a role in viral RNA replication nor in the inhibition of host-cell protein synthesis. In contrast, several publications proposed that the Sindbis virus glycoproteins are involved in regulating viral RNA synthesis. Relatively few changes in these viral glycoproteins can lead to extensive differences in the outcome of infection, as was reported for a rat prostate carcinoma cell line expressing *bcl-2* (228) and for mouse cells depending on their class I MHC molecules (70). In these examples, as for Semliki Forest virus in Hep-2 cells expressing the human MxA protein (95), the block in replication occurs at a very early step, but it has not yet been established to be a direct inhibition of viral RNA synthesis. One explanation to resolve this apparent discrepancy would be that the interaction of certain alphavirus glycoproteins with cellular membranes can interfere with the binding of the nsP complex to these membranes; this and other alternatives should be explored. An important future goal will be to correlate these observations in cultured cells with pathogenesis in humans and animals.

REFERENCES

1. Abell BA, Brown DT. Sindbis virus membrane fusion is mediated by reduction of glycoprotein disulfide bridges at the cell surface. *J Virol* 1993;67:5496–5501.
2. Agapov EV, Frolov I, Lindenbach BD, et al. Noncytopathic Sindbis virus RNA vectors for heterologous gene expression. *Proc Natl Acad Sci U S A* 1998;95:12989–12994.
3. Ahola T, Laakkonen P, Vihinen H, et al. Critical residues of Semliki Forest virus RNA capping enzyme involved in methyltransferase and guanylyltransferase-like activities. *J Virol* 1997;71:392–397.
4. Ahola T, Lampio A, Auvinen P, et al. Semliki Forest virus mRNA capping enzyme requires association with anionic membrane phospholipids for activity. *EMBO J* 1999;18:3164–3172.
5. Aliperti G, Schlesinger MJ. Evidence for an autoprotease of Sindbis virus capsid protein. *Virology* 1978;90:366–369.
6. Andersson H, Barth BU, Ekstrom M, et al. Oligomerization-dependent folding of the membrane fusion protein of Semliki Forest virus. *J Virol* 1997;71:9654–9663.
7. Anthony RP, Brown DT. Protein-protein interactions in an alphavirus membrane. *J Virol* 1991;65:1187–1194.
8. Anthony RP, Paredes AM, Brown DT. Disulfide bonds are essential for the stability of the Sindbis virus envelope. *Virology* 1992;190: 330–336.
9. Atreya CD, Singh NK, Nakhasi HL. The rubella virus RNA binding activity of human calreticulin is localized to the N-terminal domain. *J Virol* 1995;69:3848–3851.
10. Barth BU, Garoff H. The nucleocapsid-binding spike subunit E2 of Semliki Forest virus requires complex formation with the E1 subunit for activity. *J Virol* 1997;71:7857–7865.
11. Barth BU, Wahlberg JM, Garoff H. The oligomerization reaction of the Semliki Forest virus membrane protein subunits. *J Cell Biol* 1995; 128:283–291.
12. Barton DJ, Sawicki S, Sawicki DL. Solubilization and immunoprecipitation of alphavirus replication complexes. *J Virol* 1991;65: 1496–1506.
13. Barton DJ, Sawicki SG, Sawicki DL. Demonstration in vitro of temperature-sensitive elongation of RNA in Sindbis virus mutant ts6. *J Virol* 1988;62:3597–3602.
14. Bonatti S, Migliaccio G, Simons K. Palmitylation of viral membrane glycoproteins takes place after exit from the endoplasmic reticulum. *J Biol Chem* 1989;264:12590–12595.
15. Bredenbeek PJ, Frolov I, Rice CM, et al. Sindbis virus expression vectors: Packaging of RNA replicons by using defective helper RNAs. *J Virol* 1993;67:6439–6446.
16. Brown DT, Condreay LD. Replication of alphaviruses in mosquito cells. In: Schlesinger S, Schlesinger MJ, eds. *The Togaviridae and Flaviviridae.* New York: Plenum Press, 1986:171–207.
17. Burge BW, Pfefferkorn ER. Complementation between temperature-sensitive mutants of Sindbis virus. *Virology* 1966;30:214–223.
18. Burge BW, Pfefferkorn ER. Isolation and characterization of conditional-lethal mutants of Sindbis virus. *Virology* 1966;30:204–213.
19. Byrnes AP, Griffin DE. Binding of Sindbis virus to cell surface heparan sulfate. *J Virol* 1998;72:7349–7356.
20. Cadd TL, Skoging U, Liljestrom P. Budding of enveloped viruses from the plasma membrane. *Bioessays* 1997;19:993–1000.
21. Carleton M, Lee H, Mulvey M, et al. Role of glycoprotein PE2 in formation and maturation of the Sindbis virus spike. *J Virol* 1997;71: 1558–1566.
22. Carr CM, Kim PS. A spring-loaded mechanism for the conformational change of influenza hemagglutinin. *Cell* 1993;73:823–832.
23. Chen JP, Strauss JH, Strauss EG, et al. Characterization of the rubella virus nonstructural protease domain and its cleavage site. *J Virol* 1996;70:4707–4713.
24. Chen MH, Frey TK. Mutagenic analysis of the 3′ cis-acting elements of the rubella virus genome. *J Virol* 1999;73:3386–3403.
25. Cheng RH, Kuhn RJ, Olson NH, et al. Nucleocapsid and glycoprotein organization in an enveloped virus. *Cell* 1995;80:621–630.
26. Choi H-K, Tong L, Minor W, et al. Structure of Sindbis virus core protein reveals a chymotrypsin like serine protease and the organization of the virion. *Nature* 1991;354:37–43.
27. Choi HK, Lee S, Zhang YP, et al. Structural analysis of Sindbis virus capsid mutants involving assembly and catalysis. *J Mol Biol* 1996; 262:151–167.
28. Choi HK, Lu G, Lee S, et al. Structure of Semliki Forest virus core protein. *Proteins* 1997;27:345–359.
29. Clarke DM, Loo TW, Hui I, et al. Nucleotide sequence and in vitro expression of rubella virus 24S subgenomic messenger RNA encoding the structural proteins E1, E2 and C. *Nucleic Acids Res* 1987;15: 3041–3057.
30. Collier NC, Adams SP, Weingarten H, et al. Inhibition of enveloped RNA virus formation by peptides corresponding to glycoprotein sequences. *Antiviral Chem Chemother* 1992;3:31–36.
31. Davis NL, Brown KW, Greenwald GF, et al. Attenuated mutants of Venezuelan equine encephalitis virus containing lethal mutations in the PE2 cleavage signal combined with a second-site suppressor mutation in E1. *Virology* 1995;212:102–110.
32. de Groot RJ, Hardy WR, Shirako Y, et al. Cleavage-site preferences of Sindbis virus polyproteins containing the non-structural proteinase: Evidence for temporal regulation of polyprotein processing in vivo. *EMBO J* 1990;9:2631–2638.
33. DeTulleo L, Kirchhausen T. The clathrin endocytic pathway in viral infection. *EMBO J* 1998;17:4585–4593.
34. Ding M, Schlesinger MJ. Evidence that Sindbis virus nsP2 is an autoprotease which processes the virus nonstructural polyprotein. *Virology* 1989;171:280–284.
35. Dominguez G, Wang C-Y, Frey TK. Sequence of the genome RNA of rubella virus: Evidence for genetic rearrangement during Togavirus evolution. *Virology* 1990;177:225–238.
36. Doms RW, Lamb RA, Rose JK, et al. Folding and assembly of viral membrane proteins. *Virology* 1993;193:545–562.
37. Dotti CG, Kartenbeck J, Simons K. Polarized distribution of the viral glycoproteins of vesicular stomatitis, fowl plague and Semliki Forest viruses in hippocampal neurons in culture: A light and electron microscopy study. *Brain Res* 1993;610:141–147.
38. Dryga SA, Dryga OA, Schlesinger S. Identification of mutations in a

Sindbis virus variant able to establish persistent infection in BHK cells: The importance of a mutation in the nsP2 gene. *Virology* 1997; 228:74–83.
39. Dubuisson J, Rice CM. Sindbis virus attachment: Isolation and characterization of mutants with impaired binding to vertebrate cells. *J Virol* 1993;67:3363–3374.
40. Duncan RC, Nakhasi HL. La autoantigen binding to a 5′ cis-element of rubella virus RNA correlates with element function in vivo. *Gene* 1997;201:137–149.
41. Edwards J, Brown DT. Sindbis virus infection of a Chinese hamster ovary cell mutant defective in the acidification of endosomes. *Virology* 1991;182:28–33.
42. Ekstrom M, Liljestrom P, Garoff H. Membrane protein lateral interactions control Semliki Forest virus budding. *EMBO J* 1994;13: 1058–1064.
43. Erickson JW, Rossmann MG. Assembly and crystallization of a T=1 icosahedral particle from trypsinized southern bean mosaic virus coat protein. *Virology* 1982;116:128–136.
44. Fan DP, Sefton BM. The entry into host cells of Sindbis virus, vesicular stomatitis virus and Sendai virus. *Cell* 1978;15:985–992.
45. Ferlenghi I, Gowen B, de Haas F, et al. The first step: Activation of the Semliki Forest virus spike protein precursor causes a localized conformational change in the trimeric spike. *J Mol Biol* 1998;283:71–81.
46. Flynn DC, Meyer WJ, Mackenzie JMJ, et al. A conformational change in Sindbis virus glycoproteins E1 and E2 is detected at the plasma membrane as a consequence of early virus-cell interaction. *J Virol* 1990;64:3643–3653.
47. Forng R-Y, Frey TK. Identification of the rubella virus nonstructural proteins. *Virology* 1995;206:843–853.
48. Forsell K, Griffiths G, Garoff H. Preformed cytoplasmic nucleocapsids are not necessary for alphavirus budding. *EMBO J* 1996;15: 6495–6505.
49. Frey TK. Molecular biology of rubella virus. *Adv Virus Res* 1994;44: 69–160.
50. Frolov I, Agapov E, Hoffman TA Jr, et al. Selection of RNA replicons capable of persistent noncytopathic replication in mammalian cells. *J Virol* 1999;73:3854–3865.
51. Frolov I, Frolova E, Schlesinger S. Sindbis virus replicons and Sindbis virus: Assembly of chimeras and of particles deficient in virus RNA. *J Virol* 1997;71:2819–2829.
52. Frolov I, Hoffman TA, Pragai BM, et al. Alphavirus-based expression vectors: Strategies and applications. *Proc Natl Acad Sci U S A* 1996; 93:11371–11377.
53. Frolov I, Schlesinger S. Comparison of the effects of Sindbis virus and Sindbis virus replicons on host cell protein synthesis and cytopathogenicity in BHK cells. *J Virol* 1994;68:1721–1727.
54. Frolov I, Schlesinger S. Translation of Sindbis virus mRNA: Effects of sequences downstream of the initiating codon. *J Virol* 1994;68: 8111–8117.
55. Frolov I, Schlesinger S. Translation of Sindbis virus mRNA: Analysis of sequences downstream of the initiating AUG codon that enhance translation. *J Virol* 1996;70:1182–1190.
56. Frolova E, Frolov I, Schlesinger S. Packaging signals in alphaviruses. *J Virol* 1997;71:248–258.
57. Froshauer S, Kartenbeck J, Helenius A. Alphavirus RNA replication is located on the cytoplasmic surface of endosomes and lysosomes. *J Cell Biol* 1988;107:2075–2086.
58. Fuller SD, Berriman JA, Butcher SJ, et al. Low pH induces swiveling of the glycoprotein heterodimers in the Semliki Forest virus spike complex. *Cell* 1995;81:715–725.
59. Gaedigk-Nitschko K, Ding M, Levy MA, et al. Site-directed mutations in the Sindbis virus 6K protein reveal sites for fatty acylation and the underacylated protein affects virus release and virion structure. *Virology* 1990;175:282–291.
60. Gaedigk-Nitschko K, Schlesinger MJ. Site-directed mutations in Sindbis virus E2 glycoprotein's cytoplasmic domain and the 6K protein lead to similar defects in virus assembly and budding. *Virology* 1991;183:206–214.
61. Garbutt M, Law LM, Chan H, et al. Role of rubella virus glycoprotein domains in assembly of virus-like particles. *J Virol* 1999;73: 3524–3533.
62. Garoff H, Hewson R, Opstelten DJE. Virus maturation by budding. *Microbiol Mol Biol Rev* 1998;62:1171–1190.
63. Garoff H, Li KJ. Recent advances in gene expression using alphavirus vectors. *Curr Opin Biotechnol* 1998;9:464–469.
64. Geigenmüller-Gnirke U, Nitschko H, Schlesinger S. Deletion analysis of the capsid protein of Sindbis virus: Identification of the RNA binding region. *J Virol* 1993;67:1620–1626.
65. Glomb-Reinmund S, Kielian M. The role of low pH and disulfide shuffling in the entry and fusion of Semliki Forest virus and Sindbis virus. *Virology* 1998;248:372–381.
66. Gomez de Cedron M, Ehsani N, Mikkola ML, et al. RNA helicase activity of Semliki Forest virus replicase protein NSP2. *FEBS Lett* 1999;448:19–22.
67. Hahn CS, Lustig S, Strauss EG, et al. Western equine encephalitis virus is a recombinant virus. *Proc Natl Acad Sci U S A* 1988;85: 5997–6001.
68. Hahn CS, Strauss EG, Strauss JH. Sequence analysis of three Sindbis virus mutants temperature-sensitive in the capsid protein autoproteinase. *Proc Natl Acad Sci U S A* 1985;82:4648–4652.
69. Hahn YS, Grakoui A, Rice CM, et al. Mapping of RNA^- temperature-sensitive mutants of Sindbis virus: Complementation group F mutants have lesions in nsP4. *J Virol* 1989;63:1194–1202.
70. Hahn YS, Guanzon A, Rice CM, et al. Class I MHC molecule-mediated inhibition of Sindbis virus replication. *J Immunol* 1999;162: 69–77.
71. Hahn YS, Strauss EG, Strauss JH. Mapping of RNA^- temperature-sensitive mutants of Sindbis virus: Assignment of complementation groups A, B, and G to nonstructural proteins. *J Virol* 1989;63: 3142–3150.
72. Hajjou M, Hill KR, Subramaniam SV, et al. Nonhomologous RNA-RNA recombination events at the 3′ nontranslated region of the Sindbis virus genome: Hot spots and utilization of nonviral sequences. *J Virol* 1996;70:5153–5164.
73. Hardy WR, Strauss JH. Processing the nonstructural polyproteins of Sindbis virus: Nonstructural proteinase is in the C-terminal half of nsP2 and functions both in cis and in trans. *J Virol* 1989;63: 4653–4664.
74. Harrison SC, David A, Jumblatt J, et al. Lipid and protein organization in Sindbis virus. *J Mol Biol* 1971;60:533–538.
75. Heidner HW, Knott TA, Johnston RE. Differential processing of Sindbis virus glycoprotein PE2 in cultured vertebrate and arthropod cells. *J Virol* 1996;70:2069–2073.
76. Heidner HW, McKnight KL, Davis NL, et al. Lethality of PE2 incorporation into Sindbis virus can be suppressed by second-site mutations in E3 and E2: Pleiotropic effects of PE2 incorporation on replication in cultured vertebrate cells, mosquito cells, and neonatal mice. *J Virol* 1994;68:2683–2692.
77. Hertz JM, Huang HV. Utilization of heterologous alphavirus junction sequences as promoters by Sindbis virus. *J Virol* 1992;66:857–864.
78. Hill KR, Hajjou M, Hu JY, et al. RNA-RNA recombination in Sindbis virus: roles of the 3′ conserved motif, poly(A) tail, and nonviral sequences of template RNAs in polymerase recognition and template switching. *J Virol* 1997;71:2693–2704.
79. Hobman TC, Gillam S. In vitro and in vivo expression of rubella virus E2 glycoprotein: The signal peptide is located in the C-terminal region of capsid protein. *Virology* 1989;173:241–250.
80. Irurzun A, Nieva JL, Carrasco L. Entry of Semliki forest virus into cells: Effects of concanamycin A and nigericin on viral membrane fusion and infection. *Virology* 1997;227:488–492.
81. Ivanova L, Lustig S, Schlesinger MJ. A pseudo-revertant of a Sindbis virus 6K protein mutant, which corrects for aberrant particle formation, contains two new mutations that map to the ectodomain of the E2 glycoprotein. *Virology* 1995;206:1027–1034.
82. Ivanova L, Schlesinger MJ. Site-directed mutations in the Sindbis virus E2 glycoprotein identify palmitoylation sites and affect virus budding. *J Virol* 1993;67:2546–2551.
83. Jan JT, Byrnes AP, Griffin DE. Characterization of a Chinese hamster ovary cell line developed by retroviral insertional mutagenesis that is resistant to Sindbis virus infection. *J Virol* 1999;73:4919–4924.
84. Karpf AR, Blake JM, Brown DT. Characterization of the infection of *Aedes albopictus* cell clones by Sindbis virus. *Virus Res* 1997;50: 1–13.
85. Karpf AR, Brown DT. Comparison of Sindbis virus-induced pathology in mosquito and vertebrate cell cultures. *Virology* 1998;240: 193–201.
86. Keegstra K, Sefton B, Burke D. Sindbis virus glycoproteins: Effect of the host cell on the oligosaccharides. *J Virol* 1975;16:613–620.
87. Kielian M. Membrane fusion and the alphavirus life cycle. *Adv Virus Res* 1995;45:113–151.

88. Kielian M, Chatterjee PK, Gibbons DL, et al. Specific roles for lipids in virus fusion and exit: Examples from the alphaviruses. *Subcell Biochem* 2000;34:405–455.
89. Kielian M, Klimjack MR, Ghosh S, et al. Mechanisms of mutations inhibiting fusion and infection by Semliki Forest virus. *J Cell Biol* 1996;134:863–872.
90. Klimstra WB, Ryman KD, Johnston RE. Adaptation of Sindbis virus to BHK cells selects for use of heparan sulfate as an attachment receptor. *J Virol* 1998;72:7357–7366.
91. Kuhn RJ, Hong Z, Strauss JH. Mutagenesis of the 3′ nontranslated region of Sindbis virus RNA. *J Virol* 1990;64:1465–1476.
92. Kujala P, Ahola T, Ehsani N, et al. Intracellular distribution of rubella virus nonstructural protein P150. *J Virol* 1999;73:7805–7811.
93. Laakkonen P, Ahola T, Kaariainen L. The effects of palmitoylation on membrane association of Semliki forest virus RNA capping enzyme. *J Biol Chem* 1996;271:28567–28571.
94. Laakkonen P, Auvinen P, Kujala P, et al. Alphavirus replicase protein NSP1 induces filopodia and rearrangement of actin filaments. *J Virol* 1998;72:10265–10269.
95. Landis H, Simon-Jodicke A, Kloti A, et al. Human MxA protein confers resistance to Semliki Forest virus and inhibits the amplification of a Semliki Forest virus-based replicon in the absence of viral structural proteins. *J Virol* 1998;72:1516–1522.
96. LaStarza MW, Lemm JA, Rice CM. Genetic analysis of the nsP3 region of Sindbis virus: Evidence for roles in minus-strand and subgenomic RNA synthesis. *J Virol* 1994;68:5781–5791.
97. Lee H, Brown DT. Mutations in an exposed domain of Sindbis virus capsid protein result in the production of noninfectious virions and morphological variants. *Virology* 1994;202:390–400.
98. Lee S, Kuhn RJ, Rossmann MG. Probing the potential glycoprotein binding site of Sindbis virus capsid protein with dioxane and model building. *Proteins* 1998;33:311–317.
99. Lee S, Owen KE, Choi HK, et al. Identification of a protein binding site on the surface of the alphavirus nucleocapsid and its implication in virus assembly. *Structure* 1996;4:531–541.
100. Lemm JA, Bergqvist A, Read CM, et al. Template-dependent initiation of Sindbis virus RNA replication in vitro. *J Virol* 1998;72:6546–6553.
101. Lemm JA, Rice CM. Assembly of functional Sindbis virus RNA replication complexes: Requirement for coexpression of P123 and P34. *J Virol* 1993;67:1905–1915.
102. Lemm JA, Rice CM. Roles of nonstructural polyproteins and cleavage products in regulating Sindbis virus RNA replication and transcription. *J Virol* 1993;67:1916–1926.
103. Lemm JA, Rumenapf T, Strauss EG, et al. Polypeptide requirements for assembly of functional Sindbis virus replication complexes: A model for the temporal regulation of minus- and plus-strand RNA synthesis. *EMBO J* 1994;13:2925–2934.
104. Lenard J. Lipids of alphaviruses. In: Schlesinger RW, ed. *The Togaviruses.* New York: Academic Press, 1980:335–341.
105. Levine B, Griffin DE. Molecular analysis of neurovirulent strains of Sindbis virus that evolve during persistent infection of SCID mice. *J Virol* 1993;67:6872–6875.
106. Levine B, Huang Q, Isaacs JT, et al. Conversion of lytic to persistent alphavirus infection by the *bcl-2* cellular oncogene. *Nature* 1993;361: 739–742.
107. Levis R, Schlesinger S, Huang HV. Promoter for Sindbis virus RNA-dependent subgenomic RNA transcription. *J Virol* 1990;64:1726–1733.
108. Li G, La Starza MW, Hardy WR, et al. Phosphorylation of Sindbis virus nsP3 in vivo and in vitro. *Virology* 1990;179:416–427.
109. Li G, Rice CM. Mutagenesis of the in-frame opal termination codon preceding nsP4 of Sindbis virus: Studies of translational readthrough and its effect on viral replication. *J Virol* 1989;63:1326–1337.
110. Liljeström P, Garoff H. Internally located cleavable signal sequences direct the formation of Semliki Forest virus membrane proteins from a polyprotein precursor. *J Virol* 1991;65:147–154.
111. Liljeström P, Garoff H. A new generation of animal cell expression vectors based on the Semliki Forest virus replicon. *Biotechnology* 1991;9:1356–1361.
112. Liljeström P, Lusa S, Huylebroeck D, et al. In vitro mutagenesis of a full-length cDNA clone of Semliki Forest virus: The small 6,000-molecular-weight membrane protein modulates virus release. *J Virol* 1991;65:4107–4113.
113. Liu N, Brown DT. Transient translocation of the cytoplasmic (endo) domain of a type I membrane glycoprotein into cellular membranes. *J Cell Biol* 1993;120:877–883.
114. Liu X, Ropp SL, Jackson RJ, et al. The rubella virus nonstructural protease requires divalent cations for activity and functions in trans. *J Virol* 1998;72:4463–4466.
115. Liu Z, Yang D, Qiu Z, et al. Identification of domains in rubella virus genomic RNA and capsid protein necessary for specific interaction. *J Virol* 1996;70:2184–2190.
116. Lobigs M, Garoff H. Fusion function of the Semliki Forest virus spike is activated by proteolytic cleavage of the envelope glycoprotein precursor p62. *J Virol* 1990;64:1233–1240.
117. Lobigs M, Wahlberg JM, Garoff H. Spike protein oligomerization control of Semliki Forest virus fusion. *J Virol* 1990;64:5214–5218.
118. Loewy A, Smyth J, von Bonsdorff CH, et al. The 6-kilodalton membrane protein of Semliki Forest virus is involved in the budding process. *J Virol* 1995;69:469–475.
119. London SD, Schmaljohn AL, Dalrymple JM, et al. Infectious enveloped RNA virus antigenic chimeras. *Proc Natl Acad Sci U S A* 1991;89:207–211.
120. Lopez S, Yao J-S, Kuhn RJ, et al. Nucleocapsid-glycoprotein interactions required for assembly of alphaviruses. *J Virol* 1994;68: 1316–1323.
121. Lu YE, Cassese T, Kielian M. The cholesterol requirement for Sindbis virus entry and exit and characterization of a spike protein region involved in cholesterol dependence. *J Virol* 1999;73:4272–4278.
122. Lundstrom K. Alphaviruses as expression vectors. *Curr Opin Biotechnol* 1997;8:578–582.
123. Lundström ML, Mauraccher CA, Tingle AJ. Characterization of carbohydrates linked to rubella virus glycoprotein E2. *J Gen Virol* 1991;72:843–850.
124. Magee AI, Koyama AH, Malfer C, et al. Release of fatty acids from virus glycoproteins by hydroxylamine. *Biochim Biophys Acta* 1984; 798:156–166.
125. Magliano D, Marshall JA, Bowden DS, et al. Rubella virus replication complexes are virus-modified lysosomes. *Virology* 1998;240:57–63.
126. Marquardt MT, Phalen T, Kielian M. Cholesterol is required in the exit pathway of Semliki Forest virus. *J Cell Biol* 1993;123:57–65.
127. Marr LD, Wang C-Y, Frey TK. Expression of the rubella virus nonstructural protein ORF and demonstration of proteolytic processing. *Virology* 1994;198:586–592.
128. Marsh M, Helenius A. Virus entry into animal cells. *Adv Virus Res* 1989;36:107–151.
129. Megyeri K, Berencsi K, Halazonetis TD, et al. Involvement of a p53-dependent pathway in rubella virus-induced apoptosis. *Virology* 1999;259:74–84.
130. Meinkoth J, Kennedy SI. Semliki forest virus persistence in mouse L929 cells. *Virology* 1980;100:141–155.
131. Melancon P, Garoff H. Reinitiation of translocation in the Semliki Forest virus structural polyprotein: Identification of the signal for the E1 glycoprotein. *EMBO J* 1986;5:1551–1560.
132. Melancon P, Garoff H. Processing of the Semliki Forest virus structural polyprotein: Role of the capsid protease. *J Virol* 1987;61: 1301–1309.
133. Metsikko K, Garoff H. Oligomers of the cytoplasmic domain of the p62/E2 membrane protein of Semliki Forest virus bind to the nucleocapsid in vitro. *J Virol* 1990;64:4678–4683.
134. Meyer WJ, Gidwitz S, Ayers VK, et al. Conformational alteration of Sindbis virion glycoproteins induced by heat, reducing agents, or low pH. *J Virol* 1992;66:3504–3513.
135. Meyer WJ, Johnston RE. Structural rearrangement of infecting Sindbis virions at the cell surface: Mapping of newly accessible epitopes. *J Virol* 1993;67:5117–5125.
136. Mi S, Durbin R, Huang HV, et al. Association of the Sindbis virus RNA methyltransferase activity with the nonstructural protein nsP1. *Virology* 1989;1770:385–391.
137. Miller ML, Brown DT. Morphogenesis of Sindbis virus in three subclones of *Aedes albopictus* (mosquito) cells. *J Virol* 1992;66: 4180–4190.
138. Moehring JM, Inocencio NM, Robertson BJ, et al. Expression of mouse furin in a Chinese hamster cell resistant to *Pseudomonas* exotoxin A and viruses complements the genetic lesion. *J Biol Chem* 1993;268:2590–2594.
139. Molinari M, Helenius A. Glycoproteins form mixed disulphides with oxidoreductases during folding in living cells. *Nature* 1999;402:90–93.
140. Mulvey M, Brown DT. Formation and rearrangement of disulfide bonds during maturation of the Sindbis virus E1 glycoprotein. *J Virol* 1994;68:805–812.

141. Nakhasi HL, Rouault TA, Haile DJ, et al. Specific high-affinity binding of host cell proteins to the 3′ region of rubella virus RNA. *New Biol* 1990;2:255–264.
142. Niesters HGM, Strauss JH. Defined mutations in the 5′ nontranslated sequence of Sindbis virus RNA. *J Virol* 1990;64:4162–4168.
143. Niesters HGM, Strauss JH. Mutagenesis of the conserved 51-nucleotide region of Sindbis virus. *J Virol* 1990;64:1639–1647.
144. Nieva JL, Bron R, Corver J, et al. Membrane fusion of Semliki Forest virus requires sphingolipids in the target membrane. *EMBO J* 1994; 13:2797–2804.
145. Ohno K, Sawai K, Iijima Y, et al. Cell-specific targeting of Sindbis virus vectors displaying IgG-binding domains of protein A. *Nat Biotechnol* 1997;15:763–767.
146. Oker-Blom C. The gene order for rubella virus structural proteins is NH_2-C-E2-E1-COOH. *J Virol* 1984;51:354–358.
147. Oker-Blom C, Kalkkinen N, Kääriäinen L, et al. Rubella virus contains one capsid protein and three envelope glycoproteins, E1, E2a, and E2b. *J Virol* 1983;46:964–973.
148. Oker-Blom C, Ulmanen I, Kääriäinen L, et al. Rubella virus 40S genome specifies a 24S subgenomic mRNA that codes for a precursor to structural proteins. *J Virol* 1984;49:403–408.
149. Ou J-H, Rice CM, Dalgarno L, et al. Sequence studies of several alphavirus genomic RNAs in the region containing the start of the subgenomic RNA. *Proc Natl Acad Sci U S A* 1982;79:5235–5239.
150. Ou J-H, Strauss EG, Strauss JH. Comparative studies of the 3′-terminal sequences of several alphavirus RNAs. *Virology* 1981;109: 281–289.
151. Ou J-H, Strauss EG, Strauss JH. The 5′-terminal sequences of the genomic RNAs of several alphaviruses. *J Mol Biol* 1983;168:1–15.
152. Owen KE, Kuhn RJ. Identification of a region in the Sindbis virus nucleocapsid protein that is involved in specificity of RNA encapsidation. *J Virol* 1996;70:2757–2763.
153. Owen KE, Kuhn RJ. Alphavirus budding is dependent on the interaction between the nucleocapsid and hydrophobic amino acids on the cytoplasmic domain of the E2 envelope glycoprotein. *Virology* 1997; 230:187–196.
154. Pardigon N, Lenches E, Strauss JH. Multiple binding sites for cellular proteins in the 3′ end of Sindbis alphavirus minus-sense RNA. *J Virol* 1993;67:5003–5011.
155. Pardigon N, Strauss JH. Cellular proteins bind to the 3′ end of Sindbis virus minus-strand RNA. *J Virol* 1992;66:1007–1015.
156. Pardigon N, Strauss JH. Mosquito homolog of the La autoantigen binds to Sindbis virus RNA. *J Virol* 1996;70:1173–1181.
157. Paredes AM, Brown DT, Rothnagel R, et al. Three-dimensional structure of a membrane-containing virus. *Proc Natl Acad Sci U S A* 1993; 90:9095–9099.
158. Paredes AM, Heidner H, Thuman-Commike P, et al. Structural localization of the E3 glycoprotein in attenuated Sindbis virus mutants. *J Virol* 1998;72:1534–1541.
159. Paredes AM, Simon MN, Brown DT. The mass of the Sindbis virus nucleocapsid suggests it has T=4 icosahedral symmetry. *Virology* 1992;187:329–332.
160. Peränen J, Rikkonen M, Liljeström P, et al. Nuclear localization of the Semliki Forest virus-specific nonstructural protein nsP2. *J Virol* 1990; 64:1888–1896.
161. Peränen J, Takkinen K, Kalkkinen N, et al. Semliki Forest virus-specific non-structural protein nsP3 is a phosphoprotein. *J Gen Virol* 1988;69:2165–2178.
162. Petruzziello R, Orsi N, Macchia S, et al. Pathway of rubella virus infectious entry into Vero cells. *J Gen Virol* 1996;77:303–308.
163. Phalen T, Kielian M. Cholesterol is required for infection by Semliki Forest virus. *J Cell Biol* 1991;112:615–623.
164. Pogue GP, Cao X-Q, Singh NK, et al. 5′ Sequences of rubella virus RNA stimulate translation of chimeric RNAs and specifically interact with two host-encoded proteins. *J Virol* 1993;67:7106–7117.
165. Pogue GP, Hofmann J, Duncan R, et al. Autoantigens interact with cis-acting elements of rubella virus RNA. *J Virol* 1996;70:6269–6277.
166. Porterfield JS. Comparative and historical aspects of the Togaviridae and Flaviviridae. In: Schlesinger S, Schlesinger MJ, eds. *The Togaviridae and Flaviviridae.* New York: Plenum Press, 1986:1–19.
167. Presley JF, Brown DT. The proteolytic cleavage of PE2 to envelope glycoprotein E2 is not strictly required for the maturation of Sindbis virus. *J Virol* 1989;63:1975–1980.
168. Presley JF, Polo JM, Johnston RE, et al. Proteolytic processing of the Sindbis virus membrane protein precursor PE2 is nonessential for growth in vertebrate cells but is required for efficient growth in invertebrate cells. *J Virol* 1991;65:1905–1909.
169. Pugachev KV, Abernathy ES, Frey TK. Improvement of the specific infectivity of the rubella virus (RUB) infectious clone: Determinants of cytopathogenicity induced by RUB map to the nonstructural proteins. *J Virol* 1997;71:562–568.
170. Pugachev KV, Frey TK. Effects of defined mutations in the 5′ non-translated region of rubella virus genomic RNA on virus viability and macromolecule synthesis. *J Virol* 1998;72:641–650.
171. Pugachev KV, Frey TK. Rubella virus induces apoptosis in culture cells. *Virology* 1998;250:359–370.
172. Pushko P, Parker M, Ludwig GV, et al. Replicon-helper systems from attenuated Venezuelan equine encephalitis virus: Expression of heterologous genes in vitro and immunization against heterologous pathogens in vivo. *Virology* 1997;239:389–401.
173. Raju R, Huang HV. Analysis of Sindbis virus promoter recognition in vivo, using novel vectors with two subgenomic mRNA promoters. *J Virol* 1991;65:2531–2510.
174. Raju R, Subramaniam SV, Hajjou M. Genesis of Sindbis virus by in vivo recombination of nonreplicative RNA precursors. *J Virol* 1995; 69:7391–7401.
175. Renkonen O, Kääriäinen L, Simons K, et al. The lipid composition of Semliki Forest virus and of plasma membranes of the host cells. *Virology* 1971;46:318–326.
176. Rikkonen M. Functional significance of the nuclear-targeting and NTP-binding motifs of Semliki Forest virus nonstructural protein nsP2. *Virology* 1996;218:352–361.
177. Rikkonen M, Peränen J, Kääriäinen L. Nuclear and nucleolar targeting signals of Semliki Forest virus nonstructural protein nsP2. *Virology* 1992;189:462–473.
178. Rodriguez BE, Sabatini DD. Asymmetric budding of viruses in epithelial monlayers: A model system for study of epithelial polarity. *Proc Natl Acad Sci U S A* 1978;75:5071–5075.
179. Roman LM, Garoff H. Alteration of the cytoplasmic domain of the membrane-spanning glycoprotein p62 of Semliki Forest virus does not affect its polar distribution in established lines of Madin-Darby canine kidney cells. *J Cell Biol* 1986;103:2607–2618.
180. Rümenapf T, Strauss EG, Strauss JH. Subgenomic mRNA of Aura alphavirus is packaged. *J Virol* 1994;68:56–62.
181. Russell DL, Dalrymple JM, Johnston RE. Sindbis virus mutations which coordinately affect glycoprotein processing, penetration and virulence in mice. *J Virol* 1989;63:1619–1629.
182. Ryan C, Ivanova L, Schlesinger MJ. Effects of site-directed mutations of transmembrane cysteines in Sindbis virus E1 and E2 glycoproteins on palmitylation and virus replication. *Virology* 1998;249:62–67.
183. Ryan C, Ivanova L, Schlesinger MJ. Mutations in the Sindbis virus capsid gene can partially suppress mutations in the cytoplasmic domain of the virus E2 glycoprotein spike. *Virology* 1998;243: 380–387.
184. Salminen A, Wahlberg JM, Lobigs M, et al. Membrane fusion process of Semliki Forest virus II: Cleavage-dependent reorganization of the spike protein complex controls virus entry. *J Cell Biol* 1992;116: 349–357.
185. Sanchez A, Frey TK. Vaccinia-vectored expression of the rubella virus structural proteins and characterization of the E1 and E2 glycosidic linkages. *Virology* 1991;183:636–646.
186. Sariola M, Saraste J, Kuismanen E. Communication of post-Golgi elements with early endocytic pathway: Regulation of endoproteolytic cleavage of Semliki Forest virus p62 precursor. *J Cell Sci* 1995;108: 2465–2475.
187. Sarver N, Stollar V. Sindbis virus-induced cytopathic effect in clones of *Aedes albopictus* (Singh) cells. *Virology* 1977;80:390–400.
188. Sawicki DL, Barkhimer DB, Sawicki SG, et al. Temperature sensitive shut-off of alphavirus minus strand RNA synthesis maps to a non-structural protein nsP4. *Virology* 1990;174:43–52.
189. Sawicki DL, Sawicki SG. A second nonstructural protein functions in the regulation of alphavirus negative-strand RNA synthesis. *J Virol* 1993;67:3605–3610.
190. Sawicki DL, Sawicki SG, Keränen S, et al. Specific Sindbis virus coded functions for minus strand RNA synthesis. *J Virol* 1981;39: 348–358.

191. Sawicki SG, Sawicki DL, Kääriäinen L, et al. A Sindbis virus mutant temperature-sensitive in the regulation of minus-strand RNA synthesis. *Virology* 1981;115:161–172.
192. Scallan MF, Allsopp TE, Fazakerley JK. bcl-2 acts early to restrict Semliki Forest virus replication and delays virus-induced programmed cell death. *J Virol* 1997;71:1583–1590.
193. Scheidel LM, Stollar V. Mutations that confer resistance to mycophenolic acid and ribavirin on Sindbis virus map to the nonstructural protein nsP1. *Virology* 1991;181:490–499.
194. Schlesinger MJ, Malfer C. Cerulenin blocks fatty acid acylation of glycoproteins and inhibits vesicular stomatitis and Sindbis virus particle formation. *J Biol Chem* 1982;257:9887–9890.
195. Schlesinger S, Dubensky TW. Alphavirus vectors for gene expression and vaccines. *Curr Opin Biotechnol* 1999;10:434–439.
196. Schlesinger S, Weiss B, Nitschko H. Sindbis virus RNAs bind the viral capsid protein specifically and are preferentially encapsidated. In: Brinton MA, Heinz FX, eds. *New aspects of positive-strand RNA viruses*. Washington, DC: American Society for Microbiology, 1990: 237–244.
197. Schmaljohn AL, Kokuban KM, Cole GA. Protective monoclonal antibodies define maturational and pH-dependent antigenic changes in Sindbis virus E1 glycoprotein. *Virology* 1983;130:144–154.
198. Schmidt MFG, Schlesinger MJ. Relation of fatty acid attachment to the translation and maturation of vesicular stomatitis and Sindbis virus membrane glycoproteins. *J Biol Chem* 1980;255:3334–3339.
199. Schoepp RJ, Johnston RE. Directed mutagenesis of a Sindbis virus pathogenesis site. *Virology* 1993;193:149–159.
200. Sefton B, Gaffney BJ. Effect of the viral proteins on the fluidity of the membrane lipids in Sindbis virus. *J Mol Biol* 1974;90:343–358.
201. Sefton BM. Immediate glycosylation of Sindbis virus membrane proteins. *Cell* 1977;10:659–668.
202. Shirako Y, Strauss JH. Cleavage between nsP1 and nsP2 initiates the processing pathway of Sindbis virus nonstructural polyprotein P123. *Virology* 1990;177:54–64.
203. Shirako Y, Strauss JH. Regulation of Sindbis virus RNA replication: Uncleaved P123 and nsP4 function in minus strand RNA synthesis whereas cleaved products from P123 are required for efficient plus strand RNA synthesis. *J Virol* 1994;68:1874–1885.
204. Shirako Y, Strauss JH. Requirement for an aromatic amino acid or histidine at the N terminus of Sindbis virus RNA polymerase. *J Virol* 1998;72:2310–2315.
205. Singh I, Helenius A. Role of ribosomes in Semliki Forest virus nucleocapsid uncoating. *J Virol* 1992;66:7049–7058.
206. Singh NK, Atreya CD, Nakhasi HL. Identification of calreticulin as a rubella virus RNA binding protein. *Proc Natl Acad Sci U S A* 1994;91:12770–12774.
207. Sjoberg EM, Garoff H. The translation-enhancing region of the Semliki Forest virus subgenome is only functional in the virus-infected cell. *J Gen Virol* 1996;77:1323–1327.
208. Sjoberg EM, Suomalainen M, Garoff H. A significantly improved Semliki Forest virus expression system based on translation enhancer segments from the viral capsid gene. *Biotechnol N Y* 1994;12: 1127–1131.
209. Skehel JJ, Wiley DC. Coiled coils in both intracellular vesicle and viral membrane fusion. *Cell* 1998;95:871–874.
210. Skoging U, Liljestrom P. Role of the C-terminal tryptophan residue for the structure-function of the alphavirus capsid protein. *J Mol Biol* 1998;279:865–872.
211. Skoging U, Vihinen M, Nilsson L, et al. Aromatic interactions define the binding of the alphavirus spike to its nucleocapsid. *Structure* 1996;4:519–529.
212. Smit JM, Bittman R, Wilschut J. Low-pH-dependent fusion of Sindbis virus with receptor-free cholesterol- and sphingolipid-containing liposomes. *J Virol* 1999;73:8476–8484.
213. Smith TJ, Cheng RH, Olson NH, et al. Putative receptor binding sites on alphaviruses as visualized by cryoelectron microscopy. *Proc Natl Acad Sci U S A* 1995;92:10648–10652.
214. Smyth J, Suomalainen M, Garoff H. Efficient multiplication of a Semliki Forest virus chimera containing Sindbis virus spikes. *J Virol* 1997; 71:818–823.
215. Sorger PK, Stockley PG, Harrison SC. Structure and assembly of turnip crinkle virus II. Mechanism of reassembly in vitro. *J Mol Biol* 1986;191:639–658.
216. Strauss EG, De Groot RJ, Levinson R, et al. Identification of the active site residues in the nsP2 proteinases of Sindbis virus. *Virology* 1992;191:932–940.
217. Strauss EG, Levinson R, Rice CM, et al. Nonstructural proteins nsP3 and nsP4 of Ross River and O'Nyong-nyong viruses: Sequence and comparison with those of other alphaviruses. *Virology* 1988;164: 265–274.
218. Strauss EG, Rice CM, Strauss JH. Sequence coding for the alphavirus nonstructural proteins is interrupted by an opal termination codon. *Proc Natl Acad Sci U S A* 1983;80:5271–5275.
219. Strauss JH, Strauss EG. The alphaviruses: gene expression, replication, and evolution. *Microbiol Rev* 1994;58:491–562.
220. Suomalainen M, Garoff H. Alphavirus spike-nucleocapsid interaction and network antibodies. *J Virol* 1992;66:5106–5109.
221. Suomalainen M, Garoff H, Baron MD. The E2 signal sequence of rubella virus remains part of the capsid protein and confers membrane association in vitro. *J Virol* 1990;64:5500–5509.
222. Suopanki J, Sawicki DL, Sawicki SG, et al. Regulation of alphavirus 26S mRNA transcription by replicase component nsP2. *J Gen Virol* 1998;79:309–319.
223. Tellinghuisen TL, Hamburger AE, Fisher BR, et al. In vitro assembly of alphavirus cores by using nucleocapsid protein expressed in *Escherichia coli*. *J Virol* 1999;73:5309–5319.
224. Tong L, Wengler G, Rossmann MG. Refined structure of Sindbis virus core protein and comparison with other chymotrypsin-like serine proteinase structures. *J Mol Biol* 1993;230:228–247.
225. Tooker P, Kennedy SI. Semliki Forest virus multiplication in clones of *Aedes albopictus* cells. *J Virol* 1981;37:589–600.
226. Tucker PC, Griffin DE. Mechanism of altered Sindbis virus neurovirulence associated with a single-amino-acid change in the E2 glycoprotein. *J Virol* 1991;65:1551–1557.
227. Ubol S, Griffin D. Identification of a putative alphavirus receptor on mouse neural cells. *J Virol* 1991;65:6913–6921.
228. Ubol S, Tucker PC, Griffin DE, et al. Neurovirulent strains of Alphavirus induce apoptosis in bcl-2-expressing cells: Role of a single amino acid change in the E2 glycoprotein. *Proc Natl Acad Sci U S A* 1994;91:5202–5206.
229. Ulmanen I, Söderlund H, Kääriäinen L. Semliki Forest virus capsid protein associates with the 60S ribosomal subunit in infected cells. *J Virol* 1976;20:203–210.
230. Vaananen P, Kääriäinen L. Fusion and haemolysis of erythrocytes caused by three togaviruses; Semliki Forest, Sindbis and rubella. *J Gen Virol* 1980;46:467–475.
231. Vashishtha M, Phalen T, Marquardt MT, et al. A single point mutation controls the cholesterol dependence of Semliki Forest virus entry and exit. *J Cell Biol* 1998;140:91–99.
232. von Bonsdorff CH, Harrison SC. Hexagonal glycoprotein arrays from Sindbis virus membranes. *J Virol* 1978;28:578–583.
233. Wahlberg JM, Bron R, Wilschut J, et al. Membrane fusion of Semliki Forest virus involves homotrimers of the fusion protein. *J Virol* 1992; 66:7309–7318.
234. Wahlberg JM, Garoff H. Membrane fusion process of Semliki Forest virus I: Low pH-induced rearrangement in spike protein quaternary structure precedes virus penetration into cells. *J Cell Biol* 1992;116: 339–348.
235. Wang HL, O'Rear J, Stollar V. Mutagenesis of the Sindbis virus nsP1 protein: Effects on methyltransferase activity and viral infectivity. *Virology* 1996;217:527–531.
236. Wang K-S, Kuhn RJ, Strauss EG, et al. High-affinity laminin receptor is a receptor for Sindbis virus in mammalian cells. *J Virol* 1992;66: 4992–5001.
237. Wang K-S, Schmaljohn AL, Kuhn RJ, et al. Antiidiotypic antibodies as probes for the Sindbis virus receptor. *Virology* 1991;181:694–702.
238. Wang Y-F, Sawicki SG, Sawicki DL. Sindbis nsP1 functions in negative-strand RNA synthesis. *J Virol* 1991;65:985–988.
239. Watson DG, Moehring JM, Moehring TJ. A mutant CHO-K1 strain with resistance to *Pseudomonas* exotoxin A and alphaviruses fails to cleave Sindbis virus glycoprotein PE2. *J Virol* 1991;65:2332–2339.
240. Weaver SC, Dalgarno L, Frey TK, et al. Family Togaviridae. In: van Regenmortel MV, Fauguet CM, Bishop DHI, et al., eds. Virus taxonomy: Seventh report of the International Committee on Taxonomy of Viruses. San Diego, CA: Academic Press, 2000:879–889.
241. Weiss B, Geigenmüller-Gnirke U, Schlesinger S. Interactions between

Sindbis virus RNAs and a 68 amino acid derivative of the viral capsid protein further define the capsid binding site. *Nucleic Acids Res* 1994; 22:780–786.
242. Weiss B, Nitschko H, Ghattas I, et al. Evidence for specificity in the encapsidation of Sindbis virus RNAs. *J Virol* 1989;63:5310–5318.
243. Weiss B, Rosenthal R, Schlesinger S. Establishment and maintenance of persistent infection by Sindbis virus in BHK cells. *J Virol* 1980;33: 463–474.
244. Weiss BG, Schlesinger S. Recombination between Sindbis virus RNAs. *J Virol* 1991;65:4017–4025.
245. Wengler G. The mode of assembly of alphavirus cores implies a mechanism for the disassembly of the cores in the early stages of infection. *Arch Virol* 1987;94:1–14.
246. Wengler G, Boege U, Wengler G, et al. The core protein of the alphavirus Sindbis virus assembles into core-like nucleoproteins with the viral genome RNA and with other single-stranded nucleic acids in vitro. *Virology* 1982;118:401–410.
247. Wengler G, Gros C. Analyses of the role of structural changes in the regulation of uncoating and assembly of alphavirus cores. *Virology* 1996;222:123–132.
248. Wengler G, Rey FA. The isolation of the ectodomain of the alphavirus E1 protein as a soluble hemagglutinin and its crystallization. *Virology* 1999;257:472–482.
249. Wengler G, Wengler G. Identification of a transfer of viral core protein to cellular ribosomes during the early stages of alphavirus infection. *Virology* 1984;134:435–442.
250. Wengler G, Wengler G, Boege U, et al. Establishment and analysis of a system which allows assembly and disassembly of alphavirus core-like particles under physiological conditions in vitro. *Virology* 1984; 132:401–410.
251. Wengler G, Würkner D, Wengler G. Identification of a sequence element in the alphavirus core protein which mediates interaction of cores with ribosomes and the disassembly of cores. *Virology* 1992;191:880–888.
252. Weston JH, Welsh MD, McLoughlin MF, et al. Salmon pancreas disease virus, an alphavirus infecting farmed Atlantic salmon, *Salmo salar* L. *Virology* 1999;256:188–195.
253. White CL, Thomson M, Dimmock NJ. Deletion analysis of a defective interfering Semliki Forest virus RNA genome defines a region in the nsP2 sequence that is required for efficient packaging of the genome into virus particles. *J Virol* 1998;72:4320–4326.
254. White J, Helenius A. pH-Dependent fusion between the Semliki Forest virus membrane and liposomes. *Proc Natl Acad Sci U S A* 1980; 77:3273–3277.
255. White J, Kartenbeck J, Helenius A. Fusion of Semliki Forest virus with the plasma membrane can be induced by low pH. *J Cell Biol* 1980;87:264–272.
256. White J, Matlin K, Helenius A. Cell fusion by Semliki Forest, influenza, vesicular stomatitis viruses. *J Cell Biol* 1981;89:674–679.
257. Wielgosz MM, Huang HV. A novel viral RNA species in Sindbis virus-infected cells. *J Virol* 1997;71:9108–9117.
258. Xiong C, Levis R, Shen P, et al. Sindbis virus: An efficient, broad host range vector for gene expression in animal cells. *Science* 1989;243: 1188–1191.
259. Yang D, Hwang D, Qiu Z, et al. Effects of mutations in the rubella virus E1 glycoprotein on E1-E2 interaction and membrane fusion activity. *J Virol* 1998;72:8747–8755.
260. Yao J, Strauss EG, Strauss JH. Molecular genetic study of the interaction of Sindbis virus E2 with Ross River virus E1 for virus budding. *J Virol* 1998;72:1418–1423.
261. Yao J, Yang D, Chong P, et al. Proteolytic processing of rubella virus nonstructural proteins. *Virology* 1998;246:74–82.
262. Yao JS, Strauss EG, Strauss JH. Interactions between PE2, E1, and 6K required for assembly of alphaviruses studied with chimeric viruses. *J Virol* 1996;70:7910–7920.
263. Zhao H, Garoff H. Role of cell surface spikes in alphavirus budding. *J Virol* 1992;66:7089–7095.

CHAPTER 20

Flaviviridae: The Viruses and Their Replication

Brett D. Lindenbach and Charles M. Rice

At the dawn of human virus research, nearly one century ago, Walter Reed demonstrated that the disease known as yellow fever could be experimentally transferred via the filtered serum of an infected individual (565) and that this infectious agent was transmitted to man by mosquitoes (566). The discovery of this viral pathogen eventually led to the derivation of a live-attenuated strain that has been effectively used for human vaccination for over 60 years (452,664,701). It is now appreciated that yellow fever virus (YF) is but one representative of a large family of related positive-strand RNA viruses, the *Flaviviridae* (from the Latin *flavus*, yellow). This family currently consists of three genera: the flaviviruses, the pestiviruses (from the Latin *pestis*, plague), and the hepaciviruses (from the Greek *hepar*, *hepatos*, liver) (177,761). In addition to these genera, a group of unassigned viruses, the GB agents, are awaiting formal classification within the family. As detailed later, members of this family exhibit diverse biologic properties and a lack of serologic cross-reactivity, although they share similarities in virion morphology, genome organization, and presumed RNA replication strategy. The increasing significance of *Flaviviridae* as human and animal pathogens (Chapters 33 and 34 in *Fields Virology*, 4th ed.) emphasizes that their study remains no less pertinent than in Reed's time.

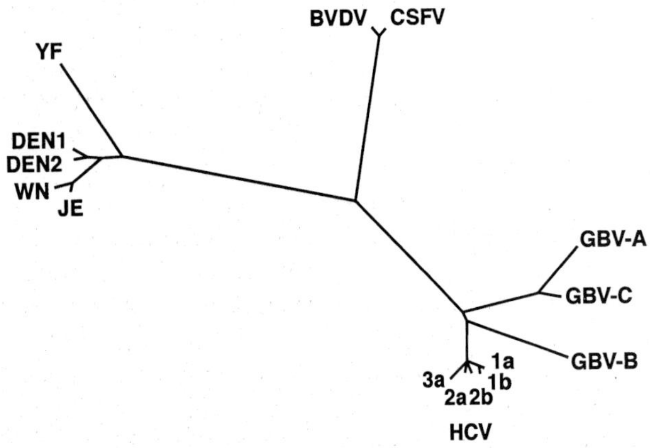

FIG. 1. The *Flaviviridae.* Phylogenetic tree based on parsimony analysis of NS3 helicase regions. Shown are members of the *Flavivirus* genus: yellow fever virus (*YF*), dengue-1 (*DEN-1*), dengue-2 (*DEN-2*), West Nile virus (*WN*), and Japanese encephalitis (*JE*); the *Pestivirus* genus: bovine viral diarrhea virus (*BVDV*) and classical swine fever (*CSFV*); several hepacivirus (*HCV*) isolates; and the unclassified viruses GBV-A, GBV-B, and GBV-C. (Figure adapted from ref. 640, with permission.)

The flaviviruses and pestiviruses were formerly considered to be members of the family *Togaviridae*, based on traditional methods of virus classification. However, through the study of viral genes, virus structure, and the viral replication cycle, it became apparent that these viruses represented an evolutionarily distinct group, and they have been subsequently reclassified as a separate virus family, the *Flaviviridae* (761). The diversity of viruses within the *Flaviviridae* is partially illustrated in Figure 1 and Table 1. Comparative sequence analysis has permitted classification of positive-stranded RNA viruses based on inferred evolutionary relationships. The *Flaviviridae* are members of the positive-strand virus supergroup 2, bearing distant similarity in their RNA-dependent RNA polymerases (RdRps) to coliphages and the plant-infecting carmo-, tombus-, diantho-, and subgroup I luteoviruses (345). The *Flaviviridae* are the only member of polymerase supergroup 2 to also encode RNA helicases, although members of polymerase supergroup 1 contain similar helicases. Thus this family of viruses is likely to exhibit a unique mode of genome replication.

FAMILY CHARACTERISTICS AND REPLICATION CYCLE

Common features believed to be shared by the three genera and highlights of the replication cycle are diagrammed in Figure 2. Our understanding of these steps is far from complete and the current view is based largely on studies with flaviviruses. Modifications are likely as more information becomes available, particularly for hepatitis C virus (HCV) and the pestiviruses. Enveloped virions are composed of a lipid bilayer with two or more species of envelope (E) proteins surrounding a nucleocapsid that consists of a single-stranded positive-sense genome RNA complexed with multiple copies of a small, basic capsid (C) protein.

Binding and uptake are believed to involve receptor-mediated endocytosis via cellular receptors specific for viral envelope proteins. Fusion of the virion envelope with cellular membranes delivers the nucleocapsid to the cytoplasm, where translation of the genome RNA occurs. The organization of the genome RNA is similar for all genera. All known viral proteins are produced as part of a single long polyprotein of more than 3,000 amino acids that is cleaved by a combination of host and viral proteases. The structural proteins are encoded in the N-terminal portion of the polyprotein, with the nonstructural proteins in the remainder. Sequence motifs characteristic of a serine protease, RNA helicase, and an RdRp are found in similar locations in the polyproteins of all three genera (444). The cleavage products containing these regions are believed to form the enzymatic components of the RNA replicase. RNA replication occurs in cytoplasmic replication complexes that are associated with perinuclear membranes, and it occurs via synthesis of a genome-length minus-strand RNA intermediate. RNA synthesis is resistant to actinomycin D, an inhibitor of DNA-dependent RNA polymerases. Progeny virions are thought to assemble by budding through intracellular membranes into cytoplasmic vesicles. These vesicles follow the host secretory pathway, fuse with the plasma membrane, and release mature virions into the extracellular compartment.

THE FLAVIVIRUSES

Background and Classification

The flavivirus genus consists of nearly 80 viruses, many of which are arthropod-borne human pathogens. Flaviviruses cause a variety of diseases including fevers, encephalitis, and hemorrhagic fevers (Chapter 33 in *Fields Virology*, 4th ed.). Entities of major global concern include dengue fever with its associated dengue hemorrhagic fever (DHF) and shock syndrome (DSS) (reviewed in refs. 219, 234, and 584), Japanese encephalitis (451), and yellow fever (reviewed in ref. 709). Other flaviviruses of regional or endemic concern include Kyasanur Forest disease, Murray Valley encephalitis (MVE), St. Louis encephalitis, tick-borne encephalitis (TBE), and West Nile (WN) viruses. Decreases in mosquito control efforts during the latter part of the 20th century, coupled with societal factors such as increased transportation and dense urbanization, have contributed to the reemergence of flaviviruses such as dengue (DEN) in South and Central America (453, 480). In 1999, WN virus was isolated

TABLE 1. *Members of the* Flaviviridae

Flaviviruses Antigenic Group (#,[a] vector[b])	Type members
Tick-borne encephalitis (12, T)	Central European encephalitis (TBE-W) Far Eastern encephalitis (TBE-FE)
Rio Bravo (6, T[c])	Rio Bravo
Japanese encephalitis (10, M)	Japanese encephalitis (JE) Kunjin (KUN) Murray Valley encephalitis (MVE) St. Louis encephalitis (SLE) West Nile (WN)
Tyuleniy (3, T)	Tyuleniy
Ntaya (5, M[c])	Ntaya
Uganda S (4, M)	Uganda S
Dengue (4, M)	Dengue type 1 (DEN-1) Dengue type 2 (DEN-2) Dengue type 3 (DEN-3) Dengue type 4 (DEN-4)
Modoc (5, U)	Modoc
Ungrouped (17, M[c])	Yellow fever (YF)
Pestiviruses Species	Type member
Bovine viral diarrhea virus 1 (BVDV-1)	BVDV strain NADL
Bovine viral diarrhea virus 2 (BVDV-2)	BVDV strain 890
Hog cholera or classical swine fever virus (CSFV[d])	CSFV Alfort/187
Border disease virus (BDV)	BDV BD31
Hepaciviruses Species	Type member
Hepatitis C virus (HCV)[e]	HCV-1
Unassigned[f] Group	Type member
GB virus-A-like viruses	GB virus-A (GBV-A)
GB virus-B	GB virus-B (GBV-B)
GB virus-C	GB virus-C (GBV-C, HGV[g])

[a]Number of recognized members in each antigenic group (from ref. 86, with permission).

[b]Arthropod vectors: T, tick; M, mosquito; U, unidentified or no vector.

[c]Arthropod vectors for some members of these groups have not been identified. The ungrouped flaviviruses include mosquito- and tick-transmitted viruses as well as some with no known vector.

[d]In the pestivirus literature, HCV has been a common abbreviation for hog cholera virus. More recent publications and this chapter use CSFV to avoid confusion with the human hepatitis C viruses.

[e]The hepatitis C viruses include a large number of isolates, which can be divided into six major genotypes and over 100 subtypes on the basis of genetic divergence (for example, see refs. 81, 582, 636).

[f]Several animal and human viruses most closely related to HCV have recently been described (see ref. 638 for review). These viruses have been tentatively assigned to the *Flaviviridae* based on their genomic organization and genetic similarity to recognized members of the family.

[g]GBV-C and hepatitis G virus (HGV) refer to the same viral agent (386, 640). Currently, it is unclear if this prevalent human virus is associated with clinical disease.

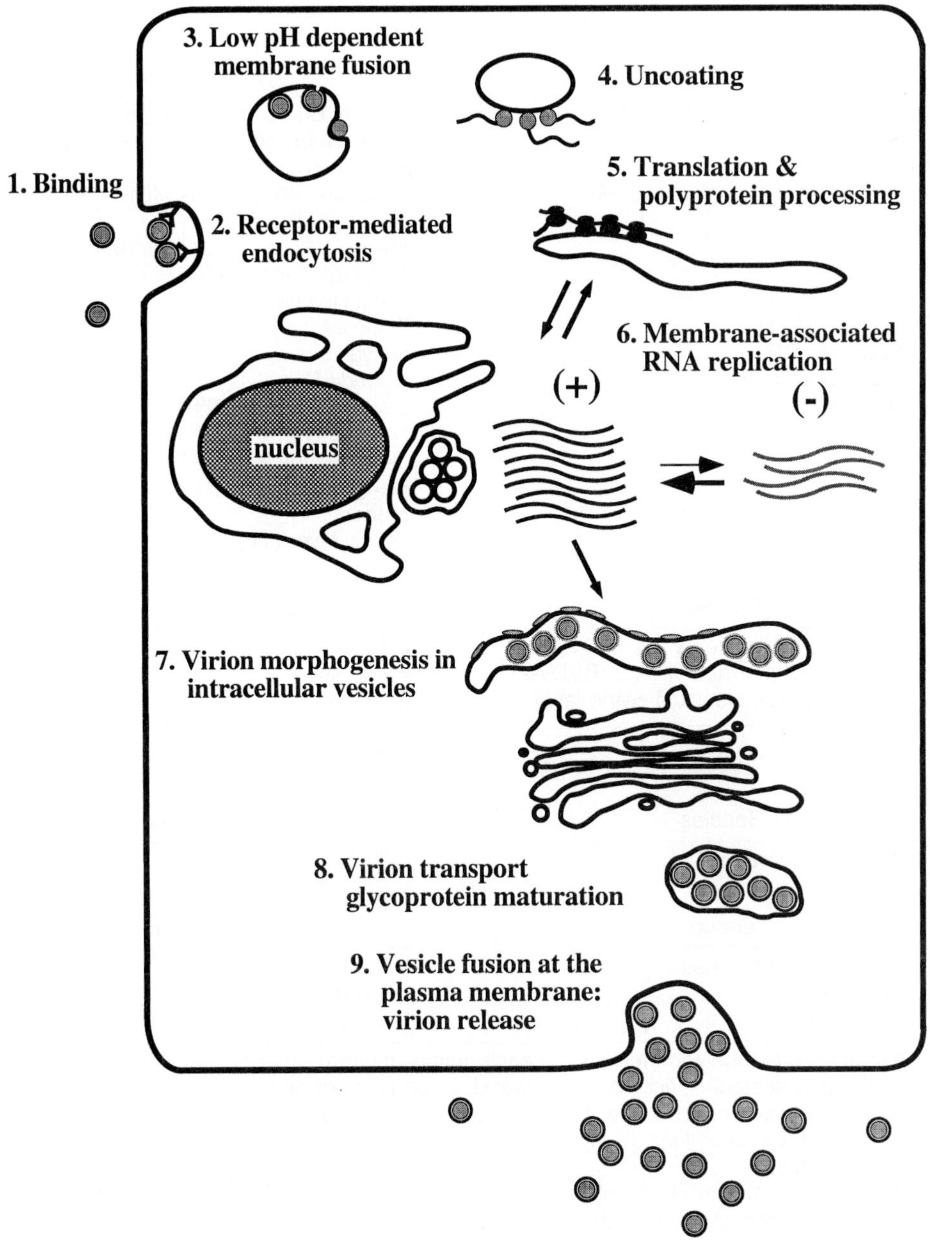

FIG. 2. Life cycle of the *Flaviviridae*. See the text for further details.

for the first time in the western hemisphere during an outbreak in New York City that was responsible for several human cases of encephalitis, including four deaths (17,22,358).

Vaccination is available for YF, using the live-attenuated 17D strain, and for TBE and Japanese encephalitis (JE) using inactivated virus (253). Efforts to derive live-attenuated strains of other flaviviruses have met with only limited success. Development of effective DEN vaccines that exhibit cross-protection, thought to be important for preventing subsequent dengue-associated immunopathogenesis (see later), are proving to be particularly challenging. The ability to genetically manipulate flaviviruses, described later, is being used to develop novel approaches to vaccine design (65,95,223,224,408,526). One promising candidate live-attenuated vaccine is a chimeric flavivirus created by replacing the structural glycoproteins of YF-17D with those of JE (95,224,454, 455). A similar approach to create a vaccine against DEN-2 is under investigation (223).

Viruses within the genus are categorized into antigenic complexes and subcomplexes based on classical serologic criteria (85,86) or into clusters, clades, and species, according to molecular phylogenetics (349,807). These latter methods have permitted the classification of viruses such as YF, which lacks close relatives. Mosquito-

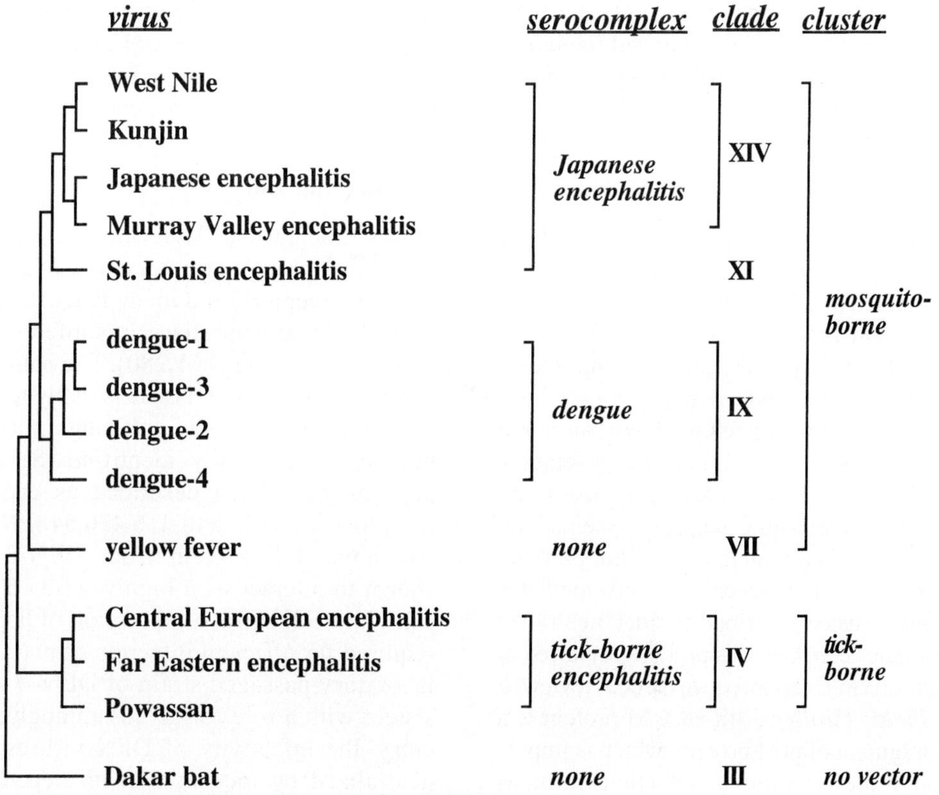

FIG. 3. Organization of the *Flavivirus* genus. The dendrogram on the *left* shows the relationships of selected flaviviruses based on a recent phylogenetic analysis (349). Evolutionary distance is not represented in this figure. The serologic and phylogenetic classifications of these viruses are indicated to the *right*.

borne and tick-borne flaviviruses, although quite distinct, appear to have evolved via a common ancestral line that diverged from non-vector-borne viruses (i.e., those for which no arthropod vectors are known) (349,807). The salient features of flavivirus taxonomy are illustrated in Figure 3, with emphasis given to viruses that are mentioned in this chapter. Two additional points should be clarified with regard to this genus organization. First, the trivial name tick-borne encephalitis virus is commonly applied to both Central European encephalitis virus and Far Eastern encephalitis virus, although they clearly represent distinct viruses with differences in vector species, geographical distribution, and sequence relatedness (153). In addition, because of the high mutation rate of RNA viruses, it is expected that each flavivirus exists as a complex, interrelated population of quasi-species (Chapter 13 in *Fields Virology*, 4th ed.). Recent evidence for intertypic recombination among DEN viruses hints at the unrealized diversity potentially lurking within flavivirus populations (774).

Experimental Systems

Flaviviruses can be cultured in whole animals such as chick embryos, suckling mouse brain, and mosquitoes, as well as in primary or established cell lines of mammalian, avian, or insect origin. In vertebrate cells, dramatic cytopathic and ultrastructural effects can occur, including vacuolation and proliferation of intracellular membranes (472); infection is commonly cytocidal, although some vertebrate cell types do not show these effects and become chronically infected. Even during the peak of virus production, a major inhibition of host macromolecular synthesis is not observed (68,713,759,760). Arthropod cells in culture may demonstrate cytopathic effects, most frequently manifested as cell fusion and syncytia formation (reviewed in refs. 68, 663, and 712). However, infection of mosquito cells is often noncytopathic, and persistent infections can be established (476). Mosquitoes remain chronically infected for life and produce extremely high levels of infectious virus particles in the salivary glands.

The life cycle of flaviviruses is increasingly understood at the molecular genetic level, and complete genome sequences exist for at least one member of each taxonomic group (see, for example, refs. 232, 248, 322, 412, and 573). Furthermore, flaviviruses can be recovered from cells containing RNA transcripts of viral cDNAs, allowing flavivirus biology to be probed with reverse genetics (213,218,281,310,322,331,354,366,410, 527,572,665). Such reverse genetic systems are also being exploited to express foreign genes (323,726), to provide stable genetic stocks for live-attenuated flavivirus vaccines (331,572), and to assist in the design of novel vaccine strategies (65,95,223,224,408,526).

Structure and Physical Properties of the Virion

Flavivirus particles appear to be spherical, 40 to 60 nm in diameter, containing an electron dense core (about 30 nm diameter) surrounded by a lipid bilayer (Fig. 4A) (472). Mature virions sediment between 170 and 210S, have a buoyant density of 1.19 to 1.23 g/mL, and are composed of 6% RNA, 66% protein, 9% carbohydrate, and 17% lipid (592,712). Because of the lipid envelope, flaviviruses are readily inactivated by organic solvents and detergents (592). Three viral proteins are associated with virions: the E (envelope), M (membrane), and C (capsid) proteins. The E protein is the major surface protein of the viral particle, probably interacts with viral receptors, and mediates virus–cell membrane fusion. Antibodies that neutralize virus infectivity usually recognize this protein (reviewed in ref. 253), and mutations in E can affect virulence (reviewed in Chapter 33 in *Fields Virology*, 4th ed.). M protein is a small proteolytic fragment of prM protein, which is important for maturation of the virus into an infectious form, as described later. Discrete nucleocapsids, composed of C protein and genomic RNA (120 to 140S, buoyant density 1.30 to 1.31 g/mL), can be isolated after solubilization of the envelope with nonionic detergents (592).

Binding and Entry

It is thought that flaviviruses attach to the surface of host cells through an interaction of E protein with one or more receptors, and many E-reactive antibodies have been shown to neutralize virus infectivity by interfering with virus binding (251,280). The patterning of receptor expression in animal tissues is likely to contribute to flavivirus tropism *in vivo*, although such receptors have not been specifically identified. Several cell surface proteins have been described as candidate flavivirus receptors (47,329,346,416,470,548,596). In addition, recombinant E protein from DEN-2 virus has been shown to interact with highly sulfated glycosaminoglycans, and cell surface expression of heparan sulfate was required for efficient infection of mammalian cells by a laboratory-passaged strain of DEN-2 virus (107). Consistent with a role for glycosaminoglycans in flavivirus entry, the infectivity of DEN viruses can be partially neutralized by incubation with heparin or highly sul-

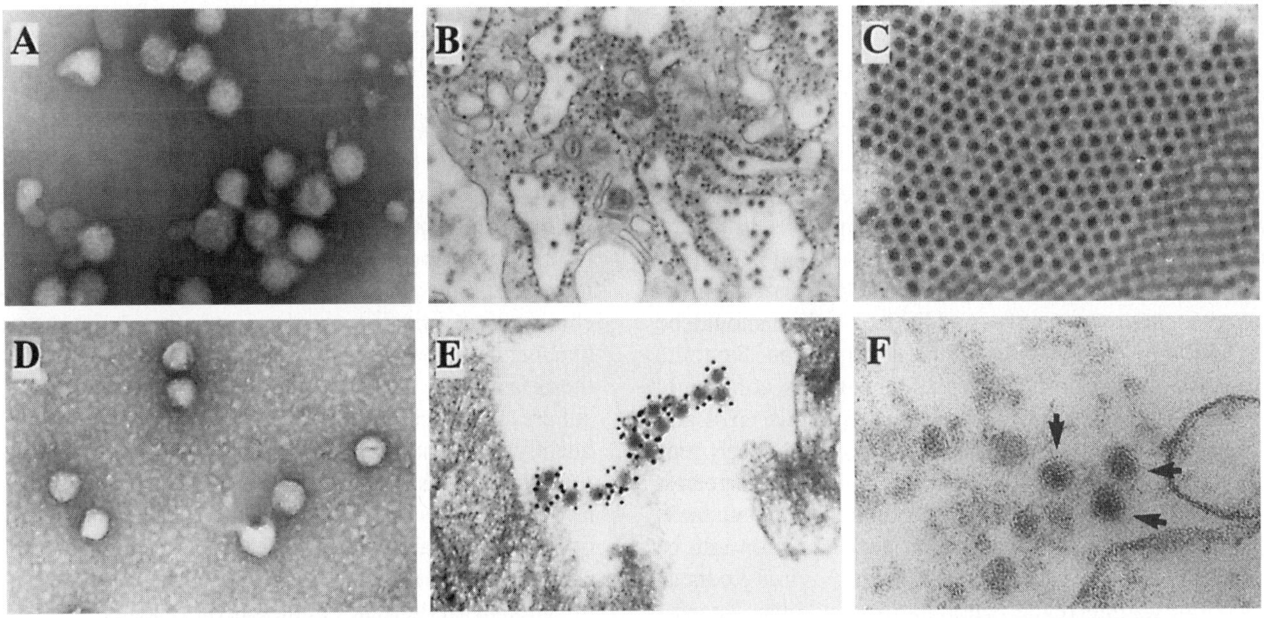

FIG. 4. Electron micrographs of virions and infected cells. **A:** Purified St. Louis encephalitis (SLE) virus negatively stained with ammonium molybdate (472). Surface projections appear as a very thin, indistinct layer. (Courtesy of Dr. Frederick A. Murphy.) **B:** Thin section of a BHK-21 cell at 48 hours after infection showing SLE virions in the cisternae of the endoplasmic reticulum (765). (Courtesy of Frederick A. Murphy, Sylvia G. Whitfield, and A. K. Harrison.) **C:** Para-crystalline array of SLE virus in a *Culex pipiens* mosquito salivary gland cell 25 days after blood-meal-feeding on an infected suckling mouse. (Courtesy of Sylvia G. Whitfield, Frederick A. Murphy, and W. Daniel Sudia.) **D:** Classical swine fever virus (CSFV) virions negatively stained with uranyl acetate. (Courtesy of Dr. Frank Weiland.) **E:** Ultrathin section of STE cells infected with CSFV and immunostained with E^{rns}-specific monoclonal antibody (MAb) 24/16 and colloidal gold. Bar = 100 nm. (From ref. 746, with permission.) **F:** Thin section showing virus-like particles (*arrows*) in HPBALL cells harvested 14 days after infection with HCV (632). Particles measured approximately 50 nm in diameter. (Courtesy of Dr. Yokho Shimizu.)

fated heparan (107,280). An additional mechanism of flavivirus binding, typically referred to as antibody-dependent enhancement (ADE), has been demonstrated for a number of flaviviruses cultured *in vitro* (236–238,388,509–511,520,616). ADE involves the increased binding of virus opsinized with subneutralizing concentrations of flavivirus-reactive antibodies to cells expressing immunoglobulin Fc receptors (509,616). It has been hypothesized that this mechanism might occur *in vivo* and, by altering tissue tropism, could contribute to the enhanced pathogenesis frequently observed in secondary infections by other DEN types (reviewed in refs. 234, 235, and 584).

After binding, it is generally believed that virions are taken up by receptor-mediated endocytosis (192,292,481, 487), although direct fusion at the plasma membrane has also been observed (244,245). Ultrastructural studies have localized single virions and virion aggregates to clathrin-coated pits on the cell surface, and uptake of virus particles into coated vesicles rapidly follows attachment (192,194). Virions are later found in uncoated prelysosomal vesicles, where an acid-catalyzed membrane fusion is thought to release the nucleocapsid into the cytoplasm (192,194,254,481). Consistent with this, a conformational change in the viral E protein, which probably exposes a fusogenic domain (567; and see later), occurs at low pH (11,221,254,330,583,611,659). Acid pH can promote fusion of virions with liposomal membranes *in vitro* or at the plasma membrane of cultured cells (193,194,222,330,550,667), although in the latter case this mode of entry does not lead to productive infection (194,330). Following entry and fusion, nucleocapsids are presumably disassembled, genomic RNA is translated, and RNA is initiated.

Genome Structure

The genome of flaviviruses consists of a single-stranded RNA about 11 kilobases (kb) in length. This RNA contains a 5′ cap ($m^7G5'ppp5'A$) at the 5′ end and lacks a polyadenylate tail (756). Genomic RNA is the messenger RNA for translation of a single long open reading frame (ORF) as a large polyprotein, as described later. Surrounding the ORF are 5′ and 3′ noncoding regions (NCRs) of around 100 nucleotides (nt) and 400 to 700 nt, respectively. These regions contain conserved sequences and predicted RNA structures that are likely to serve as cis-acting elements directing the processes of genome amplification, translation, or packaging. Although it is not yet feasible to directly study the structures of flavivirus RNAs *in vivo*, the ability of RNA to adapt alternative foldings could regulate these competing processes (231,538).

The 5′ NCR sequence is poorly conserved between flaviviruses, but it appears to contain common secondary structural elements that influence the translation of flavivirus genomes (69,84,231). However, the most significant function of the 5′ NCR probably resides in its reverse complement, the 3′ NCR of viral minus strands, which forms the site for initiation of plus-strand synthesis. Deletions engineered into the 5′ NCR of DEN-4 were shown to have dramatic effects on the ability to recover live viruses, but they do not correlate with the translational efficiency of the mutant genomes (84). Interestingly, one of the resultant mutants exhibited a limited host-range growth phenotype, suggesting potential interactions of this region (or its reverse complement) with host-specific factors. In keeping with this, cellular proteins were shown to bind specifically to a terminal stem-loop in the 3′ NCR of WN virus minus strand (627).

The 3′ NCR of the flavivirus genome, which presumably functions as a promoter for minus-strand synthesis, exhibits a great deal of sequence divergence and size heterogeneity. Nevertheless, computational analyses have revealed features that are common to all flaviviruses or that are conserved within specific taxonomic groups, and that tend to cluster in a region proximal to the 3′ end (538,552,735,739). RNA folding predictions based on thermodynamic considerations, covariation analyses, and biochemical probing support the existence of a 90- to 120-nt stem-loop structure at the 3′ terminus of all flavivirus genomes, with the potential to form a pseudoknot involving an adjacent stem-loop (70,206,231,411,412, 538,552,573,627,666,677,751,811). Several lines of evidence suggest a functional role for this structure in viral RNA replication. Mutations engineered within the 3′ terminal stem-loop of the genome of DEN-2 virus greatly affected the ability to recover live viruses, and one of the recovered viruses exhibited a host restricted-growth phenotype (808). Several cellular proteins bind to this region of WN virus RNA, including the phosphorylated form of translation elongation factor 1α (49,50). Furthermore, viral replicase proteins NS3 and NS5 have been shown to bind to the terminal stem-loop RNA *in vitro* (103,133). The conserved portion of the 3′ NCR also contains consensus sequences (CS1 and CS2) that are retained among all mosquito-borne flaviviruses, one of which has the potential to base-pair with a conserved region in the 5′ region of the ORF, suggesting that cyclization of flavivirus genomes is possible (231). A DEN-4 genome engineered to contain a deletion in CS1 indicates that this element is required for virus viability (429). Complementarity in the proposed cyclization sequences was recently shown to be required for efficient RdRP activity *in vitro*, although the upstream element could be supplied in trans (803). Similarly, stretches of conserved RNA sequence and potential cyclization sequences are also found in the genome RNAs of tick-borne flaviviruses (412,413,415). Other regions in the 3′ NCR, which may be dispensable for virus replication in culture, nevertheless appear to be important determinants for growth in mammalian hosts, and further analysis of such regions is likely to contribute greater insight into flavivirus pathogenesis and vaccine development (414,429,537).

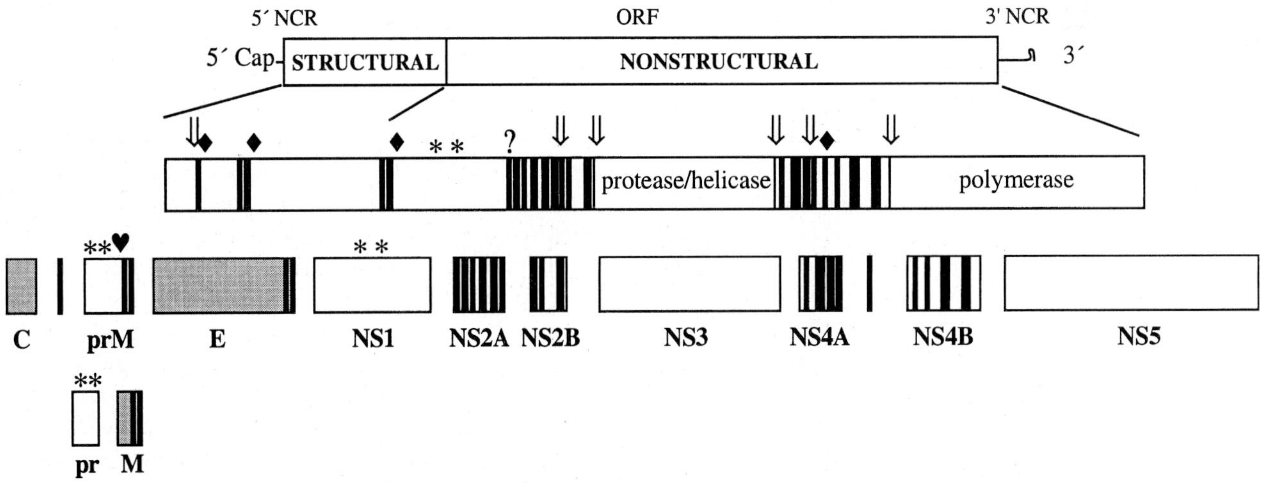

FIG. 5. Translation and processing of the flavivirus polyprotein. At the top is depicted the viral genome with the structural and nonstructural protein coding regions, the 5′ cap, and the 5′ and 3′ NCRs indicated. Boxes below the genome indicate precursors and mature proteins generated by the proteolytic processing cascade. Mature structural proteins are indicated by *shaded boxes* and the nonstructural proteins and structural protein precursors by *open boxes.* Contiguous stretches of uncharged amino acids are shown by *black bars. Asterisks* denote proteins with N-linked glycans but do not necessarily indicate the position or number of sites utilized. Cleavage sites for host signalase (♦), the viral serine protease (↓), furin or other Golgi-localized protease (♥), or unknown proteases (**?**) are indicated.

Translation and Proteolytic Processing

The flavivirus genome is translated as a large polyprotein that is processed co- and posttranslationally by cellular proteases and a virally encoded serine protease (described later) into at least 10 discrete products. As depicted in Figure 5, the N-terminal one quarter of the polyprotein encodes the structural proteins, and the remainder contains the nonstructural (NS) proteins, in the following order: C-prM-E-NS1-NS2A-NS3-NS4A-NS4B-NS5 (573). Based on the deduced hydrophobicity of the viral proteins, their predicted membrane topology is illustrated in Figure 6. This model is supported by experimental data (89,757), although the transmembrane regions have not been well defined.

Features of the Structural Proteins

The C Protein

C protein (about 11 kd) is highly basic (55,573,711), consistent with its proposed role in forming a ribonucleoprotein complex with packaged genomic RNA. Basic residues are concentrated at the N- and C-termini of C, and they probably act cooperatively to specifically bind genomic RNA (323). The central portion of C contains a hydrophobic domain that interacts with cellular membranes and may play a role in virion assembly (418). The nascent C protein (anchC) contains a C-terminal hydrophobic domain (491) that acts as a signal sequence for translocation of prM into the lumen of the endoplas-

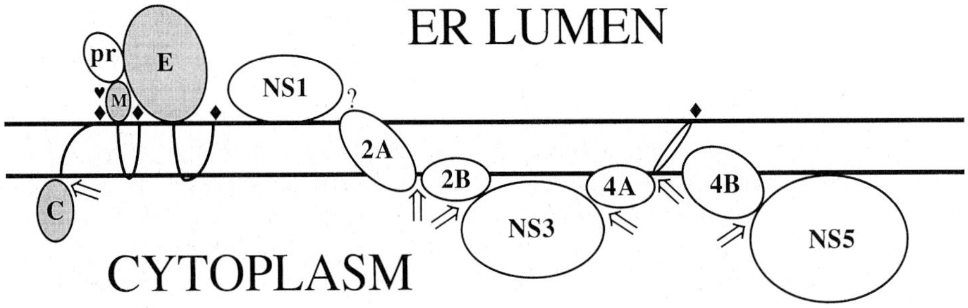

FIG. 6. Membrane topology of flavivirus proteins. The proposed orientation of the flavivirus polyprotein cleavage products with respect to the ER membrane is shown. The proteins are drawn to scale (areas are proportional to the number of amino acids) and arranged in order (left to right) of their appearance in the polyprotein. Mature structural proteins are *shaded* and C-terminal membrane-spanning segments of M and E are indicated. Cleavage sites for host signalase (♦), the viral serine protease (↓), furin or other Golgi-localized protease (♥), or unknown proteases (**?**) are indicated.

mic reticulum (ER). Mature C protein is generated by viral serine protease cleavage at a site upstream of this hydrophobic domain (16,395,785).

The prM Protein

The N-terminus of prM (about 26 kd) is generated in the ER by host signal peptidase. This processing event appears to require prior processing of anchC by the cytoplasmic viral serine protease (16,395,788), although the temporal order of these cleavages has been questioned (787,788). However, in support of this model, signalase cleavage at this site can be made viral protease-independent by cleaving anchC with another protease (660) or by improving the context of the signalase cleavage site (366,661). Interestingly, improvement of the prM signalase cleavage context was shown to be lethal for YF virion production (366). Thus, the availability of viral protease activity may regulate structural protein processing, and therefore virion assembly, over the course of an infection. During the egress of virions through the secretory pathway, prM is cleaved by the trans-Golgi resident enzyme furin (653), to form the structural protein M (about 8 kd) and the N-terminal "pr" segment, which is secreted into the extracellular medium (474). The N-terminal "pr" segment is predominantly hydrophilic and contains one to three N-linked glycosylation sites (93) and six conserved cysteine residues, all of which participate in intramolecular disulfide bridges (492). The structural protein M, located in the C-terminal portion of prM, is present in mature virions and contains a shortened ectodomain (about 41 amino acids) followed by two potential membrane-spanning domains. Antibodies to prM can mediate protective immunity (316), perhaps by neutralization of released virions that contain some uncleaved prM (see later).

The E Protein

E protein (about 50 kd) is a type I membrane protein, containing adjacent transmembrane domains in the C-terminus that serve to anchor this protein to the membrane and as the signal sequence for NS1 translocation (573). E protein contains 12 highly conserved Cys residues that form intramolecular disulfide bonds (492), and it is often glycosylated (93,768).

The three-dimensional structure of TBE E protein was determined by x-ray crystallography of a soluble tryptic fragment obtained from purified virions (Fig. 7) (567). These data indicate that E protein is divided into three structural domains and forms head-to-tail homodimeric rods that are thought to lie parallel to the virion surface in

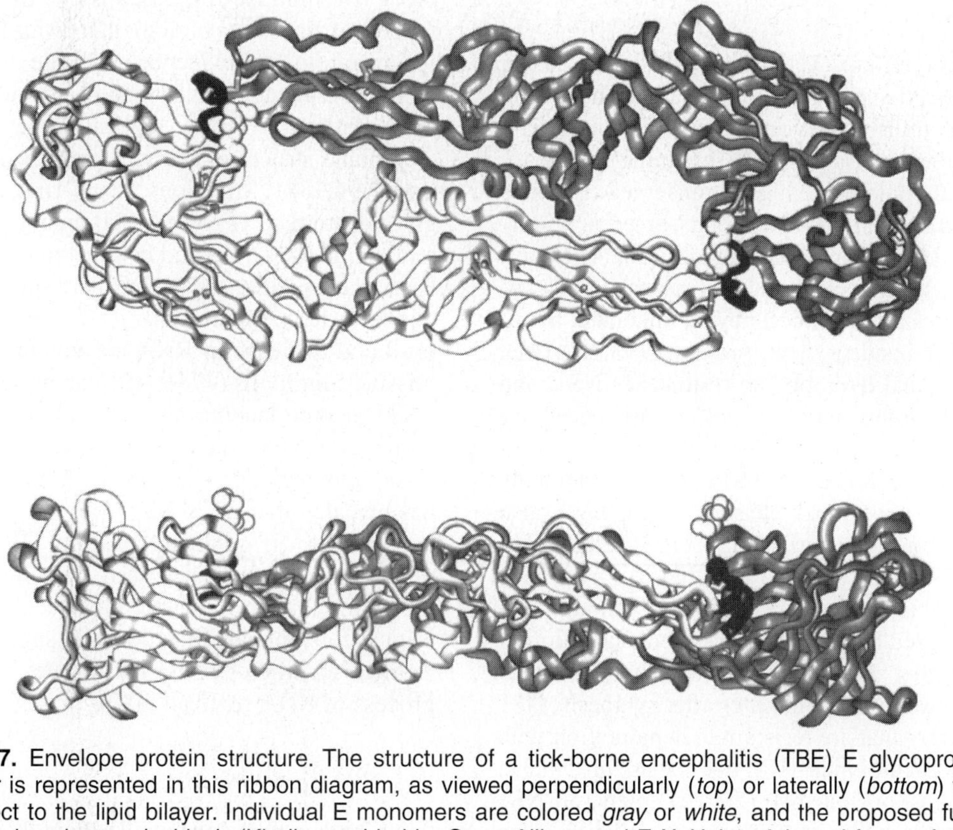

FIG. 7. Envelope protein structure. The structure of a tick-borne encephalitis (TBE) E glycoprotein dimer is represented in this ribbon diagram, as viewed perpendicularly (*top*) or laterally (*bottom*) with respect to the lipid bilayer. Individual E monomers are colored *gray* or *white*, and the proposed fusogenic domains are in *black*. (Kindly provided by Steve Allison and F. X. Heinz. Adapted from ref. 567, with permission.)

a meshlike network. This structural model provides a framework for understanding the molecular basis of E protein interactions. Structural regions of the ectodomain contain putative receptor binding sites (107,567), a potential fusogenic domain (567), contact sites for E homodimer formation (567), a region involved in prM–E interaction (12), and the trigger for low-pH-induced rearrangement (659). E protein homodimers disassociate at low pH, and each monomer reassociates with two adjacent E proteins, perhaps around a three-fold axis of symmetry at the stalk, to form trimeric complexes (11,254, 659). E trimers are thought to extend outward from the virion surface, presumably exposing the hydrophobic fusogenic domains. The stem-anchor region of E, for which structure was not determined, contains determinants for E trimer formation and for stabilization of prM-E heterodimers (12,741). Mutations in the putative receptor binding site in the TBE E protein gave rise to viruses with attenuated growth in culture and reduced virulence in mice (409). For some mosquito-borne flaviviruses, a similar region of E protein contains a putative integrin-binding motif Arg-Gly-Asp. Mutation of this sequence in E of MVE virus produced viruses with decreased entry kinetics, increased reliance on glycosaminoglycans for entry, and attenuated virulence (366).

Features of the Nonstructural Proteins

The NS1 Protein

The NS1 glycoprotein (M_r of about 46 kd) exists in cell-associated, cell-surface, or extracellular nonvirion forms. NS1 is translocated into the ER lumen and released from the C-terminus of E by signal peptidase (161,571,757). It contains 12 highly conserved cysteines that form intramolecular disulfide bonds, and it is rapidly glycosylated on two or three Asn residues (367,419,646). NS1 is cleaved from its downstream neighbor, NS2A, around 10 minutes after synthesis by an unknown, membrane-bound, ER-resident host protease (93,160,161). The eight C-terminal hydrophobic residues of NS1, and more than 140 amino acids of NS2A, are necessary determinants of this cleavage (93,160,272,517). Truncated and elongated forms of NS1, which presumably contain alternate C-terminal cleavage sites, have also been described for some viruses (53,419). In addition, murine cells persistently infected with JE virus have been found to produce truncated forms of NS1, although this appears to be caused by an uncharacterized adaptation of the host cells rather than by alterations within the viral genome (104). Twenty to 40 minutes after synthesis, NS1 forms homodimers that are resistant to denaturation with 6M urea or 5M guanidinium-HCl, but that are unstable at high temperatures or low pH (769). Dimers of NS1 exhibit a partially hydrophobic nature, pelleting with membranes and fractionating equally into the aqueous and detergent phases upon extraction with Triton X-114 (769). A point mutation has been identified in Kunjin NS1 that destabilizes NS1 dimers and confers a replication defect on the virus (233), indicating a functional role for NS1 dimerization. NS1 appears to be peripherally associated with membranes, as it does not contain any putative transmembrane domains or known lipid modifications, and it can be released from membranes by sodium carbonate (pH 11.5), 8M urea, or 5M guandinium-HCl (161,757).

NS1 is slowly secreted from mammalian cells and is not secreted from mosquito cells (419,530,770). During secretion, one of the N-linked glycans is modified to contain complex sugars (367,419,477,540), and three NS1 dimers come together into a soluble hexameric form (132,170).

NS1 was first characterized as the soluble (non-virion-associated) complement-fixing (SCF) antigen present in the sera and tissues of experimentally infected animals (63). It is now understood that the extracellular forms of NS1 strongly elicit humoral immune responses, and immunization with purified or recombinant NS1 can be protective (159,297,383,546,617,706). Furthermore, protective immunity can be passively transferred with antibodies against NS1, apparently by their ability to direct complement-mediated lysis of infected cells via interaction with the cell-surface-associated form of NS1 (255, 618,619). The secretion of a viral NS protein that elicits protective immune responses is one of the more curious aspects of flavivirus biology that await further inquiry.

Several lines of evidence implicate NS1 in the process of RNA replication. NS1 has been found to co-localize with markers of RNA replication in association with membrane structures that are presumed sites of replication (404,764). Mutations at the first or both N-linked glycosylation sites of NS1 dramatically impair virus replication (477,539) and demonstrate a decrease in viral RNA accumulation (477). Furthermore, a YF mutant containing a temperature-sensitive lesion in NS1 showed a profound decrease in RNA accumulation under nonpermissive conditions (478). NS1 can be supplied in trans to a YF genome lacking a functional NS1 gene, and RNA replication is blocked at a very early stage in the absence of complementing NS1 (384). Further genetic analysis has revealed that DEN NS1 does not productively interact with the YF replicase in trans (385). This block in replication can be suppressed by a mutation in NS4A, indicating that an interaction between NS1 and NS4A is critical for replicase function and suggesting a potential mechanism whereby NS1 participates in the cytoplasmic process of RNA replication (385).

The NS2A and NS2B Proteins

NS2A is a relatively small (about 22 kd), hydrophobic protein of unknown function. Cleavage of NS1-2A occurs in the ER, as previously mentioned, whereas the C-terminus is generated via cleavage at the NS2A/2B junction by the cytoplasmic serine protease, indicating that this protein must be membrane spanning. An alternative cleavage within YF NS2A can also be utilized by the viral protease, leading to a C-terminally truncated form of this protein that is about 2 kd smaller in mass (92,483). Mutations that block cleavage at either site are lethal for some aspect of YF replication (483). NS2A has been localized to presumed sites of RNA replication, and *in vitro* studies with a recombinant glutathione-S-transferase-KUN NS2A fusion protein suggest that this protein binds to NS3 and NS5, as well as to RNA transcripts of the 3′ NCR (405). Thus, this protein might function in recruitment of RNA templates to the membrane-bound replicase.

NS2B is a small (about 14 kd) membrane-associated protein containing two hydrophobic domains surrounding a conserved hydrophilic region (573,757). It forms a complex with NS3 and is a required cofactor for the serine protease function of NS3 (20,90,94,162,299). Deletion analysis indicates that a 40-amino-acid region in the central conserved domain of NS2B is required for NS2B-3 protease activity, and mutations in the central conserved domain that destabilize interaction with NS3 abolish protease activity (94,121,146,162,299).

The NS3 Protein

NS3 is a large (about 70 kd) cytoplasmic protein that associates with membranes via its interaction with NS2B (20,94,121). NS3 contains several enzymatic activities that implicate this protein in polyprotein processing and RNA replication.

The N-terminal one third of NS3 contains homology to trypsin-like serine proteases (34,35,198), an enzymatic activity that has been confirmed by deletion analysis (97,163,534,752) and by site-directed mutagenesis of the residues comprising the proposed catalytic triad (YF NS3 residues His-53, Asp-77, and Ser-138) (97,541,722,752, 810) or the substrate-binding pocket (533,722). Mutations in NS3 that abolish protease activity also prevent the recovery of viable mutant viruses, substantiating a crucial role for this enzyme in the virus life cycle (94). Expression of the N-terminal 167 to 181 residues of NS3, together with NS2B, is sufficient to form the active protease (90,373). The NS2B-3 protease cleaves in both cis and trans configurations, and it mediates cleavages at the NS2A/NS2B, NS2B/NS3, NS3/NS4A, and NS4B/NS5 junctions, as well as cleavages that generate the C-termini of mature C (16,786) and NS4A (377), and minor cleavages within NS2A (483) and NS3 (20,700). Alignment of known cleavage sites and mutation of these residues have been used to characterize the substrate specificity of this enzyme. These data indicate that the NS2B-3 protease preferentially cleaves after pairs of basic residues and before an amino acid with a small side chain (94,96, 378,483). However, some nonconservative mutations at these sites are tolerated, and several canonical dibasic cleavage motifs within the polyprotein are apparently not utilized, suggesting that contextual information contributes to cleavage site selection. The structure of a recombinant DEN-2 NS3 protease domain, in the absence of cofactor NS2B, has recently been resolved to 2.1 Å by using x-ray crystallography (475). This model exhibits structural similarities to other serine proteases including the NS3-4A protease of HCV (described later), provides a framework for the interpretation of NS3 mutagenesis studies, and suggests that NS2B could contribute to substrate binding specificity (475).

The C-terminal three quarters of NS3, which slightly overlaps the serine protease domain (373), has been implicated in RNA replication. This region has significant homology to RNA helicases containing the motif Asp-Glu-Ala-(Asp/His) (199). These enzymes utilize the energy of nucleoside triphosphate (NTP) hydrolysis to power RNA unwinding (302). RNA-stimulated NTPase activity has been demonstrated for full-length and N-terminally truncated NS3 (373,744,754). Recently, DEN-2 NS3 has been shown to contain an NTP-dependent RNA unwinding activity, consistent with the function of NS3 as an RNA helicase (373). The precise role of an RNA helicase is not known for flaviviruses (302), but it may help to dissociate nascent RNA strands from their template during RNA replication, or perhaps unwind secondary structures involved in template recognition or initiation of RNA synthesis. In this regard, NS3 was shown to bind to a region of the 3′ NCR containing the terminal stem-loop, in association with NS5 (103,133). A minor truncated form of NS3 has been described that apparently results from recognition of a cryptic NS2B-3 protease cleavage site within the helicase domain of NS3 (20, 541,700). The biologic consequences of this alternative processing event are not well understood, although it may serve to disrupt the helicase function of NS3. In addition to the NTPase/RNA helicase activity of NS3, the C-terminal region of this protein also contains an RNA triphosphatase activity, which is distinct from the NTPase activity (755). This enzyme is likely to be involved in modifying the 5′ end of the genome in preparation for 5′ cap addition by a guanylyltransferase activity.

NS4A and NS4B

NS4A and NS4B are relatively small (about 16 kd and 27 kd, respectively) hydrophobic proteins that are membrane associated (377,405,762). Based on its subcellular distribution (405) and interaction with NS1 (385), NS4A appears to function in RNA replication, perhaps by anchoring replicase components to cellular membranes. NS4B also localizes to presumed sites of RNA replication, but it also appears to be dispersed throughout cytoplasmic membranes, and possibly the nucleus (762).

The N-terminus of NS4A is generated by the NS2B-3 protease (394), whereas the C-terminus of NS4A contains a transmembrane domain that serves to translocate NS4B into the ER. The NS2B-3 protease cleaves at a site within NS4A, just upstream of this signal sequence, and mutations that block this cleavage also block subsequent signal peptidase cleavage in the ER lumen to generate the N-terminus of NS4B (377,533). This unusual coordinated processing scheme, which is strikingly similar to processing at the C–prM junction, might serve to regulate replicase function. Furthermore, unprocessed NS3-4A and NS4A-4B have been detected in flavivirus-infected cells (93,394,533), suggesting that polyprotein cleavage in this region may be inefficient or controlled in additional ways. NS4B is posttranslationally modified to a form that appears to be about 2 kd smaller than the nascent protein, although the nature of this modification is unknown (93,533).

NS5

NS5, the largest (about 103 kd) and most conserved flavivirus protein, contains sequence homology to RdRPs of other positive-strand RNA viruses, including the invariant Gly-Asp-Asp (GDD) motif common to these enzymes (573). Purified recombinant NS5 exhibits RdRP activity in primer extension reactions (681), and NS5 protein has been found to fractionate with RdRP activity in infected cell extracts (116). NS5 also shares homology with methyltransferase enzymes involved in RNA cap formation and is thus probably involved in methylation of the 5′ RNA cap structure (344). Site-directed mutagenesis has confirmed that motifs implicated in polymerase and methyltransferase activities are essential for virus replication, and that the functions of NS5 can be supplied in trans (318–321). NS5 can be phosphorylated by an unknown cellular Ser/Thr kinase (311,466,561), a feature that is also conserved in the NS5A proteins of the pestiviruses and HCVs (see later). The role of NS5 phosphorylation remains obscure, but it may regulate the interaction of NS5 and NS3 (311), or a subcellular redistribution of NS5 into the cell nucleus (176,311).

RNA Replication

Following translation and processing of the viral proteins, a viral replicase is assembled from NS proteins, the viral RNA, and presumably some host factors. The replicase associates with membranes, probably through interactions involving the small hydrophobic NS proteins. Replication begins with the synthesis of a genome-length minus-strand RNA, which then serves as a template for the synthesis of additional plus-strand RNAs. The first round of minus-strand accumulation has been detected just over 3 hours after infection (384). Viral RNA synthesis appears to be asymmetric *in vivo*, with a plus-strand accumulation more than 10 times greater than that of minus strands (120,477). Viral minus strands appear to accumulate even late after infection and have been isolated exclusively in double-stranded forms (120,756). Flavivirus replication can be followed *in vivo* by metabolic labeling of virus-specific RNAs in the presence of actinomycin D, an inhibitor of DNA-dependent RNA polymerases. Three major species of labeled flavivirus RNAs have been described, one type sedimenting at 40S, another at 20S, and a heterogeneous population at 20S to 28S (120,756). 40S RNA is sensitive to RNase treatment and is identical to virion-associated RNA, consistent with its being genomic RNA (756). 20S RNA, frequently termed the replicative form (RF), is likely to be a transiently stable duplex of viral plus- and minus-strand RNAs based on RNase resistance and conversion to an RNase sensitive form that comigrates with 40S RNA by heat denaturation (756). The 20S to 28S RNAs are partially sensitive to RNase treatment and are described as replicative intermediate (RI) RNAs that most likely contain duplex regions and recently synthesized plus-strand RNAs displaced by nascent strands undergoing elongation (117,120). Pulse-chase analyses indicate that RF and RI RNAs are precursors to the 40S (genomic) RNA (117,120). This mode of replication, with minus strands serving as templates for the production of multiple plus strands, can be described as semiconservative and asymmetric (117).

RdRP activity has been studied *in vitro* by using crude cytoplasmic preparations of infected cells, and similar RNA forms have been demonstrated in these reactions (31,115,117,214–216,803). However, these *in vitro* systems appear to involve chain elongation rather than *de novo* initiation, and the complete process of flavivirus RNA replication has not yet been fully reconstructed in an *in vitro* model. Physical characterization of these preparations indicates that flavivirus RdRP activity cosediments with dense membrane fractions enriched for several NS proteins and membrane structures morphologically similar to those found in virus-infected cells (116). RdRP activity has also been retained after solubilization in various detergents (116,214), although an intact flavivirus replicase has not yet been purified.

Membrane Reorganization and the Compartmentalization of Flavivirus Replication

Several studies have described ultrastructural changes in membranes of flavivirus-infected cells, predominately in the perinuclear region. In general, the earliest event is the proliferation of ER membranes (473,486), followed by the appearance of smooth membrane structures around the time of early logarithmic virus production. Smooth membrane structures are small clusters of vesicles containing electron-dense material within the lumen of smooth ER (87,363,473,486,488). These structures continue to accumulate during later times of infection, when they become adjacent to newly formed convoluted membranes. Convoluted membranes appear to be contiguous with the ER as randomly folded membranes or highly ordered structures that are sometimes described as paracrystalline arrays (363,473). All of these membrane alterations are concentrated in densely sedimenting membrane fractions from Kunjin-infected cells that are enriched for RdRP activity along with viral proteins NS2A, NS2B, NS3, NS4A, NS4B, and possibly NS1 (116). With the improved preservation of cellular membranes afforded by cryosectioning, Mackenzie et al. (404) demonstrated the appearance of vesicle packets, clusters of vesicles (each 100 to 200 nm in diameter) bound by a smooth membrane, during late times of infection. It seems likely that vesicle packets are related to or identical with smooth membrane structures, and they are often associated with smooth ER or Golgi-like membranes undergoing a morphologic process of wrapping. Such structures are also enriched for markers of the trans-Golgi (403).

The subcellular sites of RNA replication have been probed by metabolic labeling of nascent RNAs (64,662,763), by immunolabeling with sera reactive to double-stranded RNA, which presumably recognizes RF and RI RNAs (404,405,763,764), and by *in situ* hybridization (212). Apart from one report of nuclear replication (64), all investigations concur that viral RNAs accumulate in association with cytoplasmic membranes in the perinuclear region of mammalian cells and, in particular, with vesicle packets (404). NS1, NS2A, NS3, and NS4A have all been shown to localize to vesicle packets (404,405,764). Thus, it appears that along with double-stranded RNA, proteins implicated in RNA replication associate with vesicle packets. In contrast, the components of the viral serine protease, NS2B and NS3, colocalize with convoluted membranes (764). The membrane reorganization that occurs in infected cells might therefore give rise to adjacent, but distinct subcellular structures where viral polyprotein processing or RNA replication take place. It should however be emphasized that vesicle packets have been described only at late times after infection compared to the onset of RNA replication, and the sites of early RNA synthesis have not been defined. Furthermore, much remains to be learned about how interactions among NS proteins (103,133,311,385, 405), between NS proteins and viral RNA (103,133,405), and between viral RNA and host factors (49,50,627) combine to form an active replicase.

Assembly and Release of Virus Particles

Ultrastructural studies indicate that virion morphogenesis occurs in association with intracellular membranes (reviewed in ref. 472). Electron microscopic studies of flavivirus-infected cells have consistently demonstrated morphologically mature virions within the lumen of a compartment believed to be the ER (142,246,247,292, 333,363,404,424,473,485,497,650,651,740). In many studies, virions appear to accumulate within disorderly arrays of membrane-bound vesicles (see Fig. 4B). Budding intermediates and clearly distinguishable cytoplasmic nucleocapsids have not been frequently observed, suggesting that the process of assembly is rapid. Nascent virions are believed to be transported by bulk flow through the secretory pathway to the cell surface, where exocytosis occurs. Budding of virions at the plasma membrane has been occasionally observed (246,424,497, 650), and it does not appear to be a major mechanism for virion formation. These ultrastructural observations, together with studies on structural protein biosynthesis, oligomer formation, and the properties of intracellular and released virions, suggest the following model for virion assembly and maturation: The highly basic C protein interacts with viral genomic RNA in the cytoplasm to form a nucleocapsid precursor. The orientation of C, prM, and E with respect to the ER membrane would suggest that nucleocapsids acquire an envelope by budding into the ER lumen. Cosynthesis of E and prM is necessary for proper folding of E (341). These proteins have been shown to be associated as detergent-stable heterodimers (11,12,254,741,753) that can form higher-order structures, which may represent virion-associated lattices (741).

Later stages in virion maturation include glycan modification of E (for some viruses) and prM by trimming and terminal addition (93,419,491), implying that virions move through an exocytosis pathway similar to that used for synthesis of host plasma membrane glycoproteins. Although differences in the efficiency of prM cleavage have been noted (474,741), this cleavage generally distinguishes released virus from intracellular virus particles (626). Intracellular M-containing virions have not been detected, suggesting that prM cleavage occurs just prior to release of mature virions. This cleavage can be inhibited by elevating the pH in intracellular compartments (254,550,626), consistent with catalysis by furin (254, 550). Although inhibition of prM cleavage does not impair virus release, studies on prM-containing particles suggest that this cleavage is required to generate highly infectious virus (11,220,254,551,626,653,753). As seen for the alphavirus structural proteins (729–731, and see Chapter 19), experimental data suggest that flaviviruses use oligomerization and prM cleavage to regulate the activation of E-protein-mediated fusion activity. The current hypothesis is that the function of prM in the prM–E heterodimer is to prevent E from undergoing an acid-catalyzed conformational change during transit of immature virions through an acidic intracellular compartment (220,222,254,550,753). Upon cleavage of prM and release of mature virus, the E–M interaction is destabilized (753). The differences in intracellular and extracel-

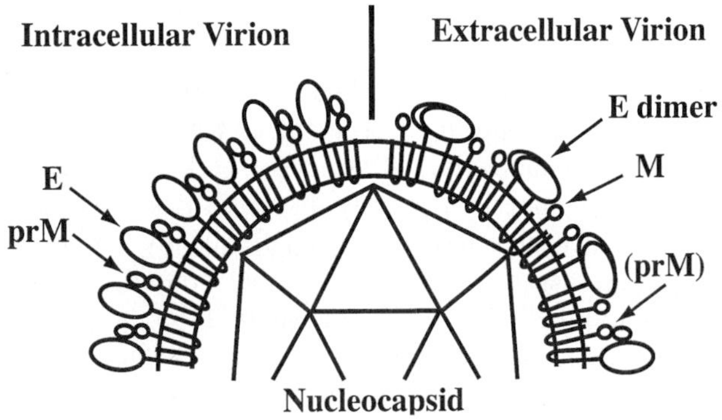

FIG. 8. Envelope proteins of intracellular and extracellular flavivirus virions. (Adapted from ref. 91, with permission.)

lular virions are illustrated in Figure 8. The hemagglutination activity exhibited by flaviviruses, which depends on low pH, probably results from activation of the fusogenic activity of E protein.

In addition to mature virions, slowly sedimenting (70S) noninfectious particles, which are also capable of agglutinating red blood cells at acid pH (called SHA, for slowly sedimenting hemagglutinin; for review, see ref. 592), are released from flavivirus-infected cells. SHA particles appear as 14-nm doughnut-like structures and are composed of E and M, with variable amounts of prM (592). Recent studies have shown that expression of prM and E is sufficient for release of SHA-like particles (11,341,420). These particles, which are fusogenic, provide an excellent model system for examining the functions of E and prM (12,611), and they show promise as immunogens that elicit protective immunity (128,342, 343,420,524).

Generation of Defective Flaviviruses and the Involvement of Host Resistance Genes

Defective-interfering (DI) particles have been valuable tools for the study of RNA virus replication, and DIs can contribute to viral pathogenesis *in vivo*. For some virus families, strongly interfering DI particles, containing truncated and rearranged genomic RNAs, are easily generated by high-multiplicity passage. These RNAs contain cis-acting sequences necessary for replication and packaging but do not encode a complete or functional set of viral proteins, and therefore they need a helper virus to supply these functions in trans. In the case of flaviviruses, although DI particles have been observed in persistently infected vertebrate cell cultures, strongly interfering DIs are not readily obtained under these conditions or during serial high-multiplicity passaging (68). Several potential explanations exist for this observation, including the possibility that, under the conditions tested, most of the virus-specified components of the replication machinery are required in cis. In this regard, some viral replicase components can be supplied in trans (151,266,318–321, 384), whereas several Kunjin virus nonstructural genes or their gene products are apparently required in cis (321). It is unclear whether this latter observation is the result of defects at the protein or RNA level. One group has recently described DI genomes in Vero cells persistently infected with MVE virus (357). Characterization of these RNA species indicated that they contain in-frame deletions of 2.3 to 2.6 kb in the prM, E, and NS1 genes. It is unlikely that the truncated NS1 is functional, and it is most likely complemented in trans, although it may contribute to interference. Of the few flavivirus DIs that have been characterized, all contain in-frame deletions, suggesting that selective pressure maintains the downstream ORF for the translation of one or more NS proteins in cis.

A system in which DIs appear to be readily generated has been studied in some detail (reviewed in ref. 68). Investigations into the heritable susceptibility of mice to YF infection (608) led to the discovery that multiple dominant alleles at a single locus on chromosome 5 can confer resistance to flaviviruses (67,598–601,719,720). Flaviviruses can replicate in resistant mice, but the spread of infection is slower, with significantly lower peak viremias (10^3- to 10^4-fold) than in susceptible mice. In primary fibroblasts from resistant mice, viral RNA synthesis was reduced, lower titers of infectious virions were released, and a high proportion of DIs were found even after a single growth cycle (67). Analyses of viral RNAs in the brains of infected mice suggest a block in RNA replication but do not necessarily support the existence of DI particles in this system (721). Nevertheless, these results indicate that a specific, but as yet unidentified, host gene can have dramatic effects on flavivirus RNA synthesis. Interestingly, RNA–protein complexes involving the 3′ NCR of the viral minus strand were found to be less stable in cell extracts prepared from a flavivirus-resistant mouse strain (627).

THE HEPATITIS C VIRUSES

Background and Classification

Following the development of diagnostic tests for hepatitis A and B viruses, an additional agent, which could be experimentally transmitted to chimpanzees (14,265,671), became recognized as the major cause of transfusion-acquired hepatitis. The causative agent, previously designated non-A, non-B hepatitis, and now referred to as hepatitis C virus, was identified in 1989 through expression cloning of cDNAs derived from the serum of an experimentally infected animal (113). Recognition of this pathogen led to the development of diagnostic tests for screening blood supplies, which dramatically decreased the incidence of posttransfusion hepatitis. Nevertheless, about 170 million people, roughly 3% of the human population, are infected with

HCV (19), and virus transmission remains a significant public health concern. The most notable feature of HCV infections is that they typically persist, often lasting for decades, with more than 70% of cases progressing to chronic hepatitis, a condition that predisposes patients to developing chronic active hepatitis, cirrhosis of the liver, and hepatocellular carcinoma (Chapter 34 in *Fields Virology*, 4th ed.). In addition to the sequelae resulting from chronic liver infection, HCV has been associated with other human diseases. Of nearly 30 such associations, which include a number of autoimmune diseases, the linkage between HCV infection and mixed type II cryoglobulinemia is the most striking. This disease is characterized by symptoms ranging from palpable purpura and fatigue, to life-threatening vasculitis of vital organs, such as the kidneys (2). Treatment for HCV typically involves the use of interferon-α, with or without ribavirin, although poor response to these treatments is not uncommon. The considerable diversity among HCV isolates, the emergence of genetic variants in chronically infected individuals, and the low level of protective immunity elicited after HCV infection present major challenges to the development of more effective therapies and vaccines. HCV is extremely refractile to growth in culture and there are currently no good animal models of this disease outside the chimpanzee. Despite these obstacles, intense scientific scrutiny over the past decade has yielded an astonishing wealth of information about this virus and its components. Much has been learned about the enzymology of viral replication proteins, and high-resolution crystallographic analyses have provided structural information for approximately 40% of the HCV genome and more than half of the nonstructural region. Understanding the biologic roles of these proteins is likely to come from recent progress in efficient initiation of HCV RNA replication in culture.

HCV is the sole member of the *Hepacivirus* genus (582). Hepaciviruses share some common features with the pestiviruses including genome organization, limited sequence relatedness, and a similar mechanism of translational control. HCV exhibits even greater similarity to the recently described GB agents, but there are also some important differences such as the potential to encode an obvious capsid protein. Within the *Hepacivirus* genus, numerous isolates of HCV are currently grouped into six major genotypes and several subtypes based on phylogenetic analysis of complete genome sequences or subgenomic fragments (81,636), although this taxonomic scheme appears to be inadequate for fully describing the diversity of recent HCV isolates, particularly those from Southeast Asia (582). It remains unclear whether there is a correlation between HCV genotype and disease severity or clinical outcome, although patients with genotype 1 viruses are clearly less responsive to treatment with antivirals (see ref. 457 and references therein).

Experimental Systems

Progress toward an understanding of HCV molecular biology has been hampered by its limited replication in cell culture and the lack of small animal models. Most of the early work, aimed at defining the physical properties of the virus and pathogenesis induced during acute and chronic infection, involved clinical samples from patients with posttransfusion hepatitis and chronic liver disease, or from experimental infection of chimpanzees (734). In chimpanzees, HCV RNA is detected in the serum as early as 3 days after inoculation and typically increases to 10^5 to 10^7 HCV RNA molecules per milliliter during the acute phase. Little evidence of hepatocellular damage is seen despite these high levels of viremia. Two to 3 months after infection, inflammatory infiltrates are seen in the liver, with areas of focal necrosis and release of enzymes such as alanine amino transferase (ALT) into circulation. This acute hepatitis coincides with the emergence of HCV-specific cellular immune responses and the appearance of HCV-specific antibodies in many (but not all) cases. In humans, acute hepatitis with overt clinical disease is seen in only about 25% of those infected. Circulating virus becomes undetectable and is apparently spontaneously cleared in 20% to 30% of cases (15). In chimpanzees, the rate of acute resolved infection may be somewhat higher (32). Chronic infections predominate, with only rare instances of clearance without treatment with interferon alone or in combination with ribavirin. Although HCV was originally thought to replicate poorly *in vivo*, recent models based on measuring viral loads after interferon therapy (356,484) or plasmapheresis (549) suggest a production rate of about 10^{12} virions per day and a virion half-life of 2 to 3 hours.

Since 1997, the availability of functional cDNA clones and infectious transcribed RNAs have allowed studies in the chimpanzee model to define the importance of viral replication determinants and to follow the evolution of the virus and host immune responses in acute-resolving versus chronic infections. For example, it has been shown that the HCV-encoded enzymes and conserved RNA elements in the 3′ NCR are essential (340,792) and that extensive variation in the glycoproteins or elsewhere are not required to establish chronic infection (406). Subunit vaccination studies (112) have provided evidence for protective immunity and encourage efforts to develop HCV vaccines for health care workers and other high-risk groups.

In contrast to the chimpanzee model, efforts to develop small-animal models for HCV infection have met with only limited success (202). One model, an irradiated beige/nude/X-linked immunodeficient (BNX) mouse reconstituted with bone marrow from mice with severe combined immunodeficiency disease (SCID), and engrafted with human liver tissue, supported limited HBV and HCV replication (189). Similarly, immunodeficient mice engrafted with human hepatocytes under the kidney capsule and maintained long term by stimulation of the hepatocyte growth factor receptor allow HBV and HDV replication but have not been shown to be permissive for HCV (496). Other murine models for HBV (73) or woodchuck hepatitis virus (516) may ultimately succeed for HCV, but further work is needed. A single report indicates that a Chinese subspecies of the tupaia or tree shrew, *Tupaia belangeri chinensis*, is susceptible to HCV infection (778). These animals have not achieved widespread use, as they are outbred, caught in the wild, and difficult to maintain and breed in captivity, and HCV infection in them is sporadic even in immunocompromised animals.

Because of their remarkable contribution to the study of HBV pathogenesis (109), transgenic mice with liver-directed expression of HCV proteins have also been created. Thus far, the establishment of a transgenic mouse line that can launch replication-competent HCV RNAs or produce infectious virus particles has not been reported. Mice expressing the HCV capsid protein (also referred to as core or C protein), the structural region or even the entire HCV polyprotein have been derived. Interestingly, at least one line expressing the HCV C protein develops lipid droplets in hepatocytes (i.e., steatosis) and progresses to hepatocellular carcinoma (464,465). This could be related to HCV-associated disease in humans and C-protein-induced lipid droplet formation (25) and transformation (98,300,554,714) in cell cultures. However, studies with other transgenic mice have not confirmed these C-protein-associated effects (317,503,733). Transgenic mice expressing the HCV structural region have been reported to develop spontaneous focal infiltration of lymphocytes and hepatocyte necrosis, and they were more sensitive to liver cell damage induced by injection of anti-Fas antibody (267). In other cases, no pathology was noted (317,336). The Cre/loxP system can be used for activation of HCV transgenes in hepatocytes; it provides an elegant approach for studying the effects of HCV proteins on hepatocyte function and the role of HCV-specific immune responses in pathogenesis (732, 733).

Most cell culture studies of HCV have utilized transient transfection protocols or infection with recombinant viruses designed to express HCV proteins. Although such experiments have provided useful information, they may not mimic the situation in HCV-infected hepatocytes. For more than two decades, attempts have been made to propagate the non-A, non-B agent, and later HCV, in various cell cultures. In the postgenomic era of HCV research, when viral RNA can be measured qualitatively and quantitatively, much more has been published on this subject. Continuous hepatoma, B-cell and T-cell lines, primary hepatocytes from humans and chimpanzees, and peripheral blood mononuclear cells (PBMC) have all been reported to support HCV replication (see ref. 29 for review). HCV replication is usually defined by strand-specific reverse transcriptase polymerase chain reaction (RT-PCR) detection of minus-strand RNA. Unfortunately, this technique has been generally unreliable because of false priming during the RT step (225,359,597). Furthermore, accumulation of minus-strand RNA does not necessarily reflect complete replication as opposed to arrest after a single round of minus-strand synthesis. Immunofluorescent detection of HCV antigens, *in situ* hybridization, selection of variant sequences during culture, infection of naive cells or a chimpanzee with cell culture supernate, electron microscopy, inhibition by interferon-α, antisense oligonucleotides, and HCV-specific ribozymes have all been used as indicators of HCV replication in cell culture. Unfortunately, none of the culture systems reported to date have been robust enough to permit classical virologic, biochemical, or genetic dissection of the HCV replication cycle.

One problem that has plagued (and perhaps confused) cell culture infection studies is the limited availability of standardized inocula. As described later, the physical properties of circulating HCV RNA and the specific infectivity of different isolates (RNA molecules per chimpanzee infectious dose, or CID) are highly variable. The best sources of infectious material are acute-phase human or chimpanzee sera that have been titrated for infectivity in chimpanzees. Recently, several laboratories have been making such inocula (often derived from infectious cDNA clones) for each of the major HCV genotypes and subtypes (see ref. 79, and later).

Human hepatitis viruses have been notoriously difficult to grow in cell culture. This presumably results from defects at one or multiple steps of the replication cycle. For positive-strand RNA viruses such as HCV, transfection with infectious RNA can circumvent the entry steps, allowing translation and initiation of RNA replication in permissive cells. Full-length cDNA clones of HCV have been constructed for genotypes 1a, 1b, and 2a and the infectivity of transcribed RNAs validated by intrahepatic inoculation of chimpanzees (36,337,790,791,793). Despite this, attempts to initiate replication by transfection of the same RNAs into cell cultures have not met with success. Such experiments are complicated by a high background of transfected RNA that can persist for months, depending on cell type. Two reports have claimed productive replication after transfection with transcribed RNAs (134,799). These results remain unconfirmed, and it is worth noting that neither study used transcripts containing the correct 3′ NCR. This sequence is the most highly conserved RNA element in the HCV genome, and it was later shown to be required for replication *in vivo* (see later).

A breakthrough for the field was reported in 1999 by Lohmann et al. (397). Based on results for the pestiviruses (43), these investigators engineered bicistronic subgenomic HCV replicons in which the neomycin resistance gene replaced the majority of the HCV structural region and the internal ribosome entry site (IRES) from the encephalomyocarditis virus (EMCV) was used to drive translation of the HCV replicase (beginning with either NS2 or NS3). At low frequency, G418-resistant colonies could be selected that harbored persistently replicating HCV RNAs at a copy number of 500 to 5,000 plus-strand RNAs per cell. More recently, adaptive mutations in the NS5A protein have been identified that allow efficient initiation of HCV RNA replication in as many as 10% of transfected hepatoma cells (51). Thus far, this system has been established for only a single genotype 1b HCV isolate and is restricted to Huh7 cells, a human hepatoma line. Despite this limited host range, we now have a powerful genetic system that should also enhance efforts to identify specific inhibitors of HCV RNA replication. A major gap in our experimental arsenal continues to be the lack of systems that support efficient replication of full-length genome RNAs, particle assembly, and release of infectious virus.

Structure and Physical Properties of the Virion

The size of the infectious virus, based on filtration experiments, is between 30 and 80 nm (62,250,806). HCV particles isolated from pooled human plasma (675), present in hepatocytes from infected chimpanzees, and produced in cell culture (303,535,625,631) have been tentatively visualized by electron microscopy (see Fig. 4F). Initial measurements of the buoyant density of infectious material in sucrose yielded a range of values, with the majority present in a low density pool of less than 1.1 g/mL (60). Subsequent studies have used RT-PCR to detect HCV-specific RNA as an indirect measure of potentially infectious virus present in sera from chronically infected humans or experimentally infected chimpanzees. From these studies, it has become clear that considerable heterogeneity exists between different clinical samples, and that many factors can affect the behavior of particles containing HCV RNA (261,704,745). Such factors include association with immunoglobulins (261,745) or low-density lipoprotein (704,705,745) that may be influenced by genotype (479). In highly infectious acute-phase chimpanzee serum, HCV-specific RNA is usually detected in fractions of low buoyant density (1.03 to 1.1 g/mL) (88,261). In other samples, the presence of HCV antibodies and formation of immune complexes correlate with particles of higher density and lower infectivity (261). Treatment of particles with chloroform, which inactivates infectivity (61,166), or with nonionic detergents, produces RNA-containing particles of higher density (1.17 to 1.25 g/mL) believed to represent HCV nucleocapsids (261,307,446) of about 33 nm (675). The virion protein composition has not been determined, but putative HCV structural proteins include a basic C protein and two membrane glycoproteins, E1 and E2 (see later).

Binding and Entry

For the reasons just stated (lack of standardized infectious stocks, heterogeneous physical properties of virions, and poor infection in cell culture), these steps in the HCV replication cycle have been difficult to study. Even in the infection systems reported, there has been no systematic determination of basic parameters such as optimal adsorption conditions, or requirement for internalization or acidification. Interestingly, it has been shown that bovine and human lactoferrin can block infectivity of HCV in cell culture (288), presumably by binding to virus particles via the E2 glycoprotein (798).

Candidate receptors include the tetraspanin CD81 and the low-density lipoprotein receptor (LDLR). CD81 binds the ectodomain of the E2 glycoprotein and, to a lesser extent, HCV RNA-containing material from infectious plasma (523). The determinants in CD81 responsible for E2 binding reside in the large extracellular loop (LEL), a domain that exhibits species-specific heterogeneity. Specific amino acids in the LEL, important for binding to human and chimpanzee CD81 but not to that of African green monkey, have been mapped (256). However, this initial match between E2–CD81 binding and HCV species tropism is not absolute, as HCV E2 binds even more avidly to tamarin CD81 even though these animals are probably not permissive hosts (10,431). CD81 is expressed on most cell types, including B and T cells, making it unlikely that it is the sole determinant of HCV hepatotropism. Interaction between HCV E2 and CD81-containing signalling complexes on B cells has been postulated to play a role in modulating B-cell activation. This is of interest given the association of HCV with extrahepatic B-cell disorders such as mixed type II cryoglobulinemia and possibly non-Hodgkins B-cell lymphoma (for review, see ref. 570). LDLR has been attractive as a candidate HCV receptor since the discovery of the association between infectious HCV and low-density lipoprotein (LDL) or very low density lipoprotein (VLDL) (3,456,704,705). Coating of virions with serum lipoproteins during their secretion from hepatocytes or after release into circulation could shield the virus from neutralizing antibodies and provide a mechanism for binding and entry that is independent of the HCV glycoproteins. Recent studies indicate that HCV RNA-containing particles can be endocytosed via the LDLR in cell culture (3). What is not clear from the experiments thus far is whether either of these interactions (with CD81 or LDLR) actually leads to productive infection.

In lieu of an efficient infectivity assay, surrogate approaches have been employed. One report utilized vesicular stomatitis virus pseudotypes incorporating cell surface expressed chimeric forms of the HCV glycoproteins (353). Particles expressing either E1 or E2 demonstrated low levels of infectivity that could be neutralized by polyclonal antibodies produced in chimpanzees that had been immunized with candidate glycoprotein subunit vaccines. Because the two HCV glycoproteins are believed to assemble as heterodimers and mature in the ER (see later), it is unclear if the infectivity being measured in this assay reflects the function of these proteins in the native HCV particle. More recently, a cell–cell fusion assay has been described that requires cell surface expression of both HCV glycoproteins, exhibits low-pH enhanced fusion, and shows some selectivity for certain hepatoma lines (678). Experiments using this system suggest that expression of human CD81 is not sufficient for fusion and that other cell surface proteins and glycosaminoglycans are important.

Genome Structure

The HCV genome is about 9.6 kb in length, considerably shorter than that of flaviviruses. Based on characterization of the HCV translation strategy, and the absence of sequences corresponding to the presumed methyltransferase and RNA triphosphatase enzymes of flaviviruses, it is expected that the HCV genome does not include a 5′ cap structure. The 5′ NCR is a highly conserved RNA sequence element, about 341 nt in length, that biochemical probing and computer modeling indicate is folded into a complex structure consisting of four major domains and a

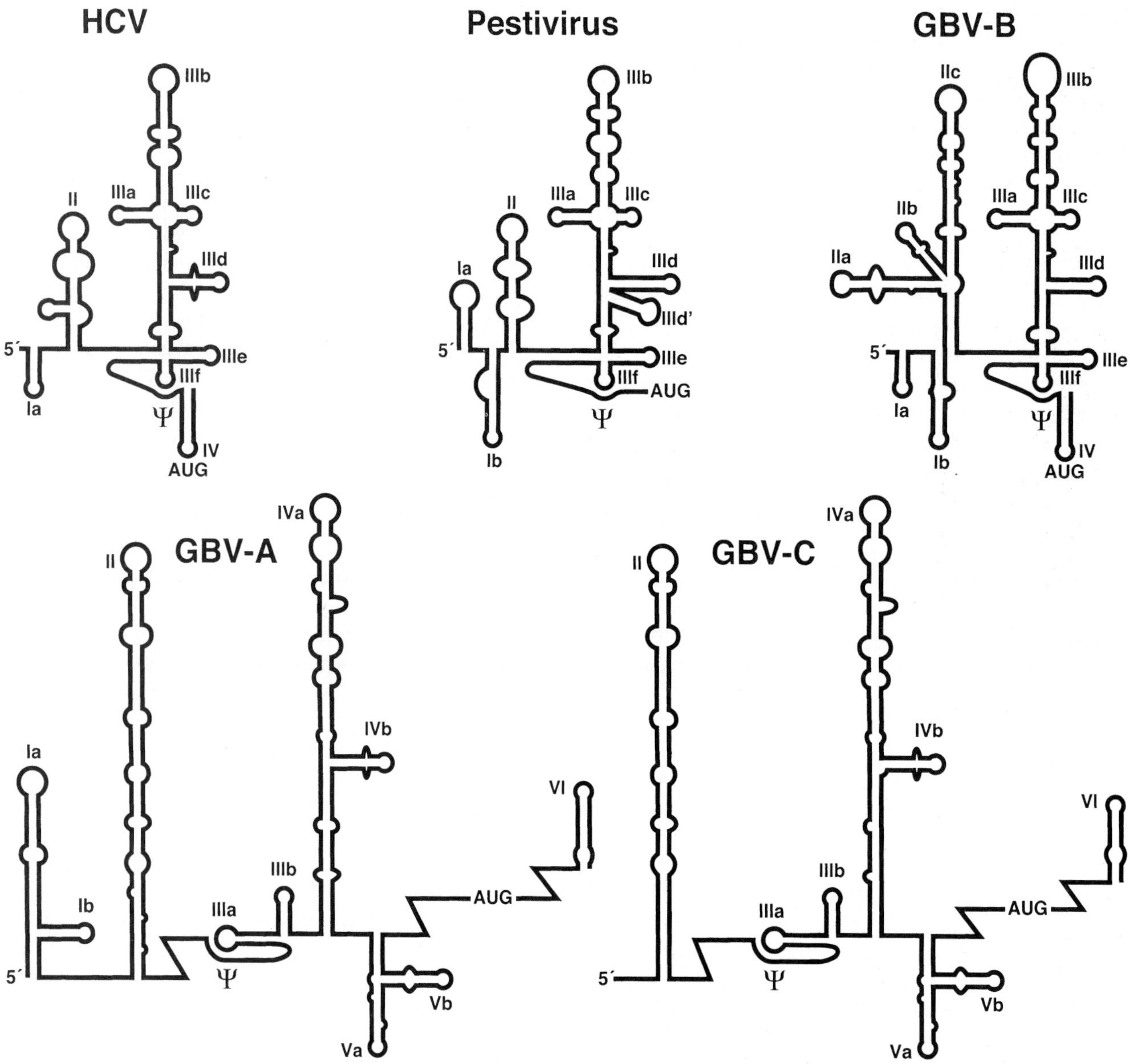

FIG. 9. Predicted secondary structures of pestivirus, hepatitis C virus (HCV), and GB virus internal ribosome entry site (IRES) elements. Model for the secondary and tertiary structures within the 5′ NCRs of HCV, pestiviruses, GB virus A (*GBV-A*), B (*GBV-B*), and C (*GBV-C*). The polyprotein initiation site is indicated by AUG. Major structural domains are labeled *I to VI*. Predicted hairpin loops are indicated by *letters*, and pseudoknots are emphasized with a Ψ symbol. The models are based on computer-assisted folding and mutational analysis. (Courtesy of R. Rijnbrand and S. Lemon. For reviews see ref. 581.)

pseudoknot (Fig. 9) (72,270,645,738). The 5′ NCR probably contains the reverse complement of the information that is read by the replication machinery (i.e., from the 3′ end of viral minus strands) to direct plus-strand RNA initiation. As described later, the 5′ NCR also functions as an IRES to direct cap-independent translation of a single large ORF of about 3,011 codons. The 3′ NCR was initially thought to terminate in polyadenosine (239) or polyuridine (101,106,249,312,498–500,676,685,742,782). However, the previously mentioned studies could not exclude false-priming as a source of these findings. Improved methods for cloning 3′ ends of RNAs later revealed that the HCV 3′ NCR actually consists of a short (about 40-nt) variable domain and a polyuridine/polypyrimidine tract, followed by a highly conserved 98-nt sequence (339,683,684,783). The latter two regions were shown to be essential for recovery of infectious HCV in chimpanzees (340,792). Biochemical probing has not fully resolved the secondary structure of the conserved 98-nt element, although the 3′-most 45-nt sequence has been shown to form a stable stem-loop (52). The HCV 3′ NCR has been shown to interact with several cellular proteins including polypyrimidine tract binding (PTB) protein (197,295,715), which may contribute to the enhanced translational efficiency observed for RNAs containing a 5′ IRES element and the HCV 3′ NCR (296), as well as glyceraldehyde-3-phosphate dehydrogenase (519), and ubiquitous cellular proteins of 87 and 130 kd (289).

Translation and Proteolytic Processing

As mentioned before, the 5′ NCR of HCV has been shown to have IRES activity, directing cap-independent initiation in a number of translation systems (182,270, 287,401,569,578,716,737). The secondary structure of the HCV 5′ NCR (see Fig. 9) provides a framework for understanding the function of the HCV IRES. Although it is unclear whether the approximately 109 5′-proximal nucleotides are necessary for IRES function (568,716), deletion of stem-loop I seems to have a positive effect on translation (270,578,800). The AUG codon used for initiation is precisely defined at a position within stem-loop IV (568,580), the stability of which affects IRES activity (268). The 3′ boundary of the IRES is unclear, with conflicting reports concluding that sequences downstream of the initiation AUG are necessary (270,401,569) or that sequences lacking a complete stem-loop IV are sufficient (716,737). A pseudoknot formed by base-pairing of stem-loop IIIf to a region just upstream of stem-loop IV has been shown to be critical for IRES function (736, and see ref. 581 for further discussion). Interestingly, biochemical reconstitution of internal ribosomal entry for both hepacivirus and pestivirus IRES elements indicated that ribosomal 40S subunits and translational initiation factor eIF3 directly bind to discrete IRES regions, thereby bypassing the need for canonical translation initiation factors eIF4A, eIF4B, and eIF4F (514,515,642). Additional cellular factors that have been shown to bind the HCV IRES, typically enhancing translation, include PTB (8,304), La antigen (9), heterogeneous nuclear ribonucleoprotein L (230), and proteins of 25, 87, and 120 kd (184,797). Furthermore, IRES activity may also involve interaction with one or more cell cycle–specific factors (269).

The organization and processing of the HCV polyprotein is shown in Figure 10. Ten major polypeptides are produced by co- or posttranslational cleavage of the polyprotein and are arranged in the order NH_2-C-E1-E2-p7-NS2-NS3-NS4A-NS4B-NS5A-NS5B-COOH (203–205,379). Cleavages within the structural region (C/E1, E1/E2, and E2/p7) and at the p7/NS2 junction are thought to be mediated by the ER resident cellular signal peptidase, based on the hydrophobicity of regions just upstream of these cleavage sites (258,379,448,449,623), the dependence of cleavage on the presence of membranes (258,282,379,448,449, 602,603) and signal-recognition particles (602,603), and mutagenesis of cleavage sites into suboptimal substrates for signal peptidase (448,449). An additional cleavage event probably removes the E1 signal sequence to produce mature C protein (282,602), although the responsible enzyme has not been definitively identified. Processing at the E2/p7 junction is incomplete, leading to accumulation

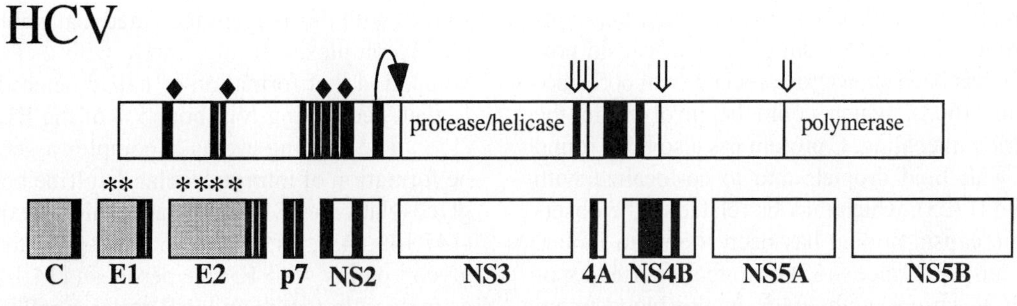

FIG. 10. Organization and processing of the HCV polyprotein. *Shading* and *symbols* identifying proteolytic cleavages are the same as described in Figure 3, except that the *curved arrow* indicates the autocatalytic cleavage at the NS2-3 site catalyzed by the NS2-3 autoprotease.

of E2–p7 (379,448,623). Cleavages in the nonstructural region of the polyprotein are mediated by two virus encoded proteases: the zinc-stimulated NS2-3 autoprotease, which cleaves at the NS2/3 junction (204,259), or the NS3 serine protease (26,152,203,259,407,707), which utilizes NS4A as a cofactor for efficient processing at the 3/4A, 4A/4B, 4B/5A, and 5A/5B sites (27,157,380,688).

Features of the Structural Proteins

The C Protein

C is a highly conserved basic protein, appearing as 19- and 21-kd forms (82,205,241,282,390,391,461,553,602, 670,796). The slower-migrating minor form is believed to result from signalase cleavage at only the C/E1 junction, whereas the faster-migrating "mature" form results from cleavage at a second site near residue 173, as discussed before. C protein associates with membranes, particularly the cytoplasmic surface of the ER (99,241,258,326,461, 553,602,670). A minor 16-kd truncated form of C has also been reported by one group (391,392). In terms of HCV particle assembly, binding of C to the HCV 5′ NCR (284,686) has been demonstrated, although nonspecific binding of RNA to C has also been reported (284,602). Multimerization of C, another likely step in the assembly process, has also been observed and requires the N-terminal 115 amino acids of C (423,490). Interaction of C with E1, but not with E2, has been suggested by coprecipitation experiments (393).

Nuclear localization of C, particularly truncated forms lacking C-terminal hydrophobic sequences, has also been reported (99,390,391,553,629,670,796). However, nuclear localization of the intact C protein remains controversial (25,82,461,462,602). Several functions have been proposed for nuclear forms of C protein, including the modulation of cellular gene transcription (555,558,559), repression of transcription from the human immunodeficiency virus 1 (HIV-1) long terminal repeat sequences (649), and the suppression of hepatitis B virus (HBV) transcription and replication in Huh-7 cells (629). This latter effect may be regulated by phosphorylation of C protein at Ser-99 and Ser-116 (628). However, expression of C protein in mice does not appear to inhibit transgene-initiated HBV replication (503). Several additional functions have been proposed for cytoplasmic forms of capsid protein. C protein has been shown to associate with 60S ribosomal subunits (602), which could be involved in the process of virion uncoating. C protein has also been found to associate with lipid droplets and to co-localize with apolipoprotein II (25), which may be related to the observation that the capsid protein has been shown to induce steatosis in transgenic mice (465) or to the reported association of HCV virions with lipids in the bloodstream (704,705). C protein also interacts with the lymphotoxin β receptor (102,422) and tumor necrosis factor receptor 1 (TNFR-1) (815), two members of the TNFR family of cytokine receptors. Interaction with these signalling pathways could be involved in modulating the effectiveness of host antiviral immune responses. In addition, these observations may be related to correlations between C protein expression and cellular sensitivity to apoptosis, although conflicting effects have been reported (102,556,557,585, 815). The C protein has also been reported to transform primary rat embryo fibroblasts (REF) in cooperation with Ras (554) or an immortalized REF cell line called Rat-1 (98). In one study, capsid protein expression in transgenic mice induced hepatocellular carcinoma (464), although such tumors were not reported in other studies of transgenic mice expressing C protein (317,503,733). Thus, although the capsid protein has been the subject of much research, additional work is needed to determine the significance of these observations with respect to specific steps of the viral life cycle and HCV pathogenesis.

Envelope Glycoproteins

HCV E1 and E2, glycoproteins containing type I C-terminal transmembrane anchors, are heavily modified by N-linked glycosylation (205,258,275,283,290,335,336, 360,372,425,426,443,489,547,593,623,648). Based on the extent and type of glycosylation (148,257,360,547, 593,623,648), protection from protease digestion (258, 393), and association with the ER-resident proteins calnexin (114,149), calreticulin (114), immunoglobulin heavy-chain binding protein (BiP) (114), and protein disulfide isomerase (138), E1 and E2 have been shown to be retained within the lumen of the ER. Signals for ER retention have been mapped to the transmembrane domains of both glycoproteins (122,123,150,172). E1 folds slowly and noncovalently interacts with the membrane-proximal domain of E2 to form what are believed to be native heterodimers (123,138,148,149,205,360,426, 443,547). In addition, disulfide-linked aggregates of E1 and E2 have been described (148,205). A valuable tool for studying HCV glycoprotein maturation has been a conformation-sensitive monoclonal antibody, H2, with specificity for noncovalently associated E1E2 heterodimers, which are protease resistant and have been released from the ER chaperone calnexin (138). Kinetic studies with this reagent indicated that stable noncovalent E1E2 complexes form slowly, with a $T_{1/2}$ of about 2 hours, and that formation of native heterodimers is inefficient, accounting for about 5% of the E1E2 complexes (138). The limiting events in complex assembly appear to be formation of intramolecular disulfide bonds in E1 and glycosylation of E1, steps that require coexpression of E2 (147,149,443), as well as productive interaction of the glycoproteins with ER chaperones (114,149,443). Interestingly, calreticulin and BiP preferentially associate with aggregates of misfolded proteins, whereas calnexin is associated with newly synthesized glycoproteins, oxidized monomeric forms, and noncovalent heterodimers (114,149). Overexpression of these three chaperones (using vaccinia virus), either individually or in combination, does not increase the efficiency of productive E1E2 folding (114), suggesting that other unidentified chaperones and folding enzymes may be limiting for proper HCV glycoprotein folding.

As viral glycoproteins, E1 and E2 must have critical interactions with host molecules. It has been noted that E1 residues 264 to 290 bear similarity to suspected or known fusion peptides from flavivirus and paramyxovirus glycoproteins and may perform an analogous function during HCV entry (173). As mentioned, the ectodomain of E2 was shown to bind to the human tetraspanin-family cell surface membrane protein CD81 (523), an interaction that appears to involve a conformationally sensitive region of E2 (171,173) and an extracellular subdomain of CD81 (171,256). This interaction may play a key role in HCV binding and entry, but direct demonstration of this is lacking. In addition, interaction of CD81 with soluble forms of E2 was shown to have antiproliferative effects on lymphocytes (171). The N-terminal portion of E2 contains a hypervariable region (HVR1) (351,493) that is likely to reflect adaptation of the virus to the host immune response and selection of immune escape variants (164,165,315,622,633,750). Indeed, E2 HVR1 has been shown to be a target for neutralizing antibodies (257,314,749,750). Nonetheless, recent work has shown that HVR1 is not essential for replication or chronic infection in chimpanzees, although deletion of this sequence debilitates the virus (175). In addition, expression of E2 has been shown to inhibit the function of the interferon-inducible double-stranded-RNA-activated protein kinase PKR (699), although it is unclear how the proposed interaction involving the E2 ectodomain with cytoplasmic PKR actually occurs.

Features of the Nonstructural Proteins

p7 and NS2

No function is known for the small hydrophobic p7 protein, which is thought to be inefficiently released from the C terminus of E2 by signal peptidase (379,448,449, 623). By analogy with pestivirus p7 (154), HCV p7 and E2–p7 are probably not associated with virions, although an efficient cell culture system is needed to test this.

NS2 (about 23 kd) contains a predicted cysteine protease domain (200), which interacts with the immediately downstream 180 amino acids of NS3 to form the NS2/3 autoprotease that cleaves at the NS2/3 junction (204,259). NS2/3 protease activity is necessary for the *in vivo* infectivity of full-length HCV genomes (340). However, NS2 is dispensable for RNA replication of subgenomic HCV replicons in culture (51,397), and no function is known for NS2 other than in NS2–3 cleavage. NS2/3 activity, which is distinct from the serine protease activity of NS3, is stimulated *in vitro* by addition of microsomal membranes (204,603), various detergents (522), and Zn^{2+} (259). The former two reagents probably allow for proper conformation of the moderately hydrophobic NS2. It is unclear whether Zn^{2+} plays a catalytic or structural role in 2–3 processing. Interestingly, crystallographic (328,400,789) and biochemical (135,658) analyses have identified a site for tetrahedral coordination of Zn^{2+} (HCV polyprotein residues Cys-1123, Cys-1125, Cys-1171, and His-1175) in the region of NS3 required for NS2–3 protease activity, and suggested that this Zn^{2+} ion plays an essential structural role in the NS3 serine protease domain. Consistent with a role for this Zn^{2+} ion in both types of processing, mutations at Cys-1123, Cys-1125, and Cys-1171 inhibit NS2–3 cleavage as well as downstream cleavages catalyzed by the serine protease (259). Mutation of His-1175 has a less dramatic effect (204,259,658), perhaps because this residue indirectly interacts with Zn^{2+} via an H_2O molecule. Although cleavage at the 2/3 site is thought to occur by an autocatalytic mechanism, bimolecular cleavage has been shown to occur, albeit inefficiently, with functional NS2 and/or NS3 protease subunits when coexpressed with substrates containing mutations in either NS2 or NS3 (but not both) that inactivate the NS2–3 protease (204,562). Requirement for a functional NS2 or NS3 region in cis suggests that the overall conformation of NS2/3 may play a role in orienting the NS2/3 cleavage site. In support of this model, mutagenesis of the P5 to P3′ positions at the NS2/3 cleavage site indicated that conformation is a more important determinant for cleavage than primary sequence (263,562).

The NS3 Protein

Like the flavivirus NS3 protein, HCV NS3 (about 70 kd) encodes a serine protease domain in the N-terminal one third of the protein, and an NTPase/helicase domain in the C-terminal two thirds. The serine protease is responsible for cleavage at the NS3/4A, NS4A/4B, NS4B/5A, and NS5A/5B sites (26,152,203,205,259,407,707), and it is required for infectivity of HCV genomes *in vivo* (340). Cleavage at the NS3/4A site occurs in cis, whereas trans cleavage can occur at downstream sites (27,380,689,707). Analysis of cleavage products has revealed that these cleavage sites are highly conserved and conform to the sequence (Asp/Glu)XXXX(Cys/Thr)(Ser/Ala) (152,203, 525). As shown by site-directed mutagenesis and molecular modeling, the P1 residue appears to be an important determinant for cleavage efficiency except at the NS3/4A autocleavage site (28,338,370,525). NS4A is a cofactor for serine protease activity, critical for all serine protease-dependent cleavages except NS5A/5B, although this cleavage can be stimulated by NS4A (27,157,380,690). Cofactor activity requires stable complex formation between

NS3 and NS4A (30,158,381,607), an interaction that also serves to stabilize NS3 and anchor it to cellular membranes (260,690,773).

The structure of the NS3 serine protease domain alone (400), or in complex with an NS4A-derived cofactor (328,789) has been determined by x-ray crystallography. The HCV serine protease structure is similar to other members of the trypsin superfamily, with active site residues and a substrate binding pocket located in a cleft separating two β-barrel domains. Unique to the HCV enzyme, the NS4A cofactor forms an integral part of this structure, interacting with the extreme N-terminal residues of NS3 to form two antiparallel β strands not found in trypsin and altering the geometry of the catalytic site (328,789). These data also reveal an important structural role of the coordinated Zn^{2+} ion for proper folding of the serine protease domain (328,400), a result that is supported by biochemical studies (135,658). Within the predicted substrate-binding pocket, Phe-1180 probably interacts with the conserved Cys residues present in the P1 position of the 4A/4B, 4B/5A, and 5A/5B sites (328,400,525,789). Based on the interaction of NS3 and NS4A, protein engineering studies have created single-chain NS3–NS4A fusion proteins (scNS3–NS4A) with full serine protease activity (144,274,504,692). The structure of full-length NS3 with NS4A cofactor was determined by x-ray crystallography of one scNS3–NS4A (Fig. 11) (795). Folding of the protease and helicase domains of this molecule resembles that of each individual domain (the helicase domain is described later), separated by a single flexible loop (795). Interestingly, the C-terminus of NS3 interacts with the protease active site in a manner consistent with a protease:product (795). Since NS3/4A cleavage occurs autocatalytically, this model provides a unique glimpse at polyprotein cis processing and suggests structural rearrangements that are needed for subsequent trans processing events (795).

HCV NS3 is a member of the Asp-Glu-Cys-His (DECH) subfamily of DEAD-box helicases. The NTPase/helicase activities of NS3 have been demonstrated for recombinant full-length NS3 (188,271,352,463) or the C-terminal two thirds of NS3 (252,301,325,531,669,674). Like the flavivirus enzyme, HCV NS3 ATPase activity is stimulated by single-stranded nucleic acids (227,228,271, 301,305,463,531,669,674). NS3 unwinds RNA and DNA homo- and heteroduplexes in a 3′ to 5′ direction (674), and this requires Mg^{2+} or Mn^{2+} and ATP, suggesting that helicase activity is coupled to ATP hydrolysis (301,463,

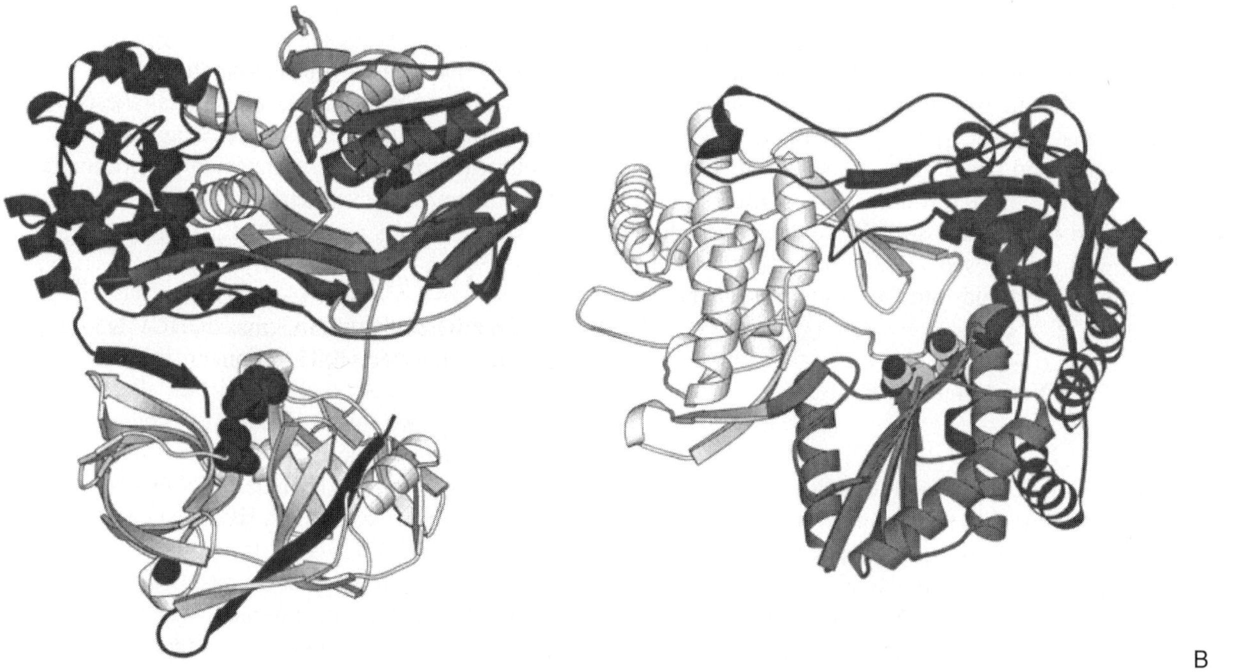

A B

FIG. 11. Structures of enzymatic components of the HCV replicase. **A:** The β-barrels of the HCV protease and three subdomains of the helicase are colored from *white to black* along the polypeptide chain. The NS3 protease catalytic triad, the solvent-exposed protease-associated zinc, and a phosphate ion in the helicase NTP binding site are indicated by *dark spheres*, and NS4A is represented by a *black strand.* **B:** The HCV NS5 RNA-dependent RNA (RdRP) polymerase exhibits a globular shape, unique among known polymerase structures. Nevertheless, this viral enzyme retains the typical polymerase subdomain organization consisting of fingers, palm, and thumb subdomains shown in *black, gray,* and *white,* respectively. Catalytic residues within the canonical RdRP GDD motif are shown as space-filling *spheres.* In both diagrams, ribbons follow the polypeptide fold and reveal locations of sheets and helices. [Courtesy of N. Yao, C. Lesburg, and P. Weber (see refs. 371 and 795).]

531). However, other NTPs and dNTPs can substitute for ATP in this reaction (301,464), and ATP is not required for RNA binding (188). The crystal structure of the HCV NS3 helicase domain has been determined to a resolution of 2.1 to 2.3 Å in the presence (327) or absence (110,794) of a bound oligonucleotide. These data all reveal three well-defined structural domains surrounding a central axis and separated by distinct clefts (110,327,794). The first two domains, which contain all of the conserved NTPase/helicase motifs, each contain a parallel, six-stranded β sheet surrounded by a number of α helices. However, domain 1 contains a seventh, antiparallel β strand, and domain 2 contains an additional pair of antiparallel β strands that extend into the vicinity of domain 3, which is completely α helical. The catalytic site is located in domain 1 near the cleft that separates it from domain 2. RNA substrate binds in the cleft that separates domains 1 and 2 from domain 3, with the 5′ end near domain 2 (327). Although the precise role of RNA helicases in replication is unknown, mutations in NS3 that disrupt helicase activity ablate HCV infectivity *in vivo* (340).

In addition to its roles in HCV polyprotein processing and RNA replication, several other functions have been proposed for NS3. Cyclic AMP–dependent protein kinase (PKA)-dependent phosphorylation was inhibited by synthetic peptides corresponding to a region of HCV NS3 that exhibits similarity to a PKA inhibitor protein and a PKA autophosphorylation site (56–58). Furthermore, a truncated NS3 protein containing this region was able to interact with the catalytic subunit of PKA and inhibited its forskolin-stimulated nuclear translocation and PKA-catalyzed phosphorylation (57). The serine protease domain of NS3 has been found to have weak transforming activity in NIH-3T3 cells (595) and can suppress actinomycin D–induced apoptosis (180). It is unclear whether these effects may be related to an observed subcellular co-localization of NS3 and the cellular tumor suppressor gene product p53 (294,471).

NS4A and NS4B

The 54-residue NS4A protein (about 8 kd) contains a hydrophobic N-terminal domain followed by a highly charged region. The serine protease cofactor activity of NS4A (see preceding) is contained within a 12-amino-acid region in the central portion of NS4A (30,381,630, 690,708). NS4A also associates with membranes (690, 773), probably through the hydrophobic N-terminal region, and interacts with other replicase components (293,382). NS4B (about 30 kd) is a hydrophobic protein of unknown function.

NS5A

NS5A is a hydrophilic but membrane-associated protein that exists in at least two forms with apparent molecular masses of 56 and 58 kd. Although these forms were originally thought to be the product of alternative proteolysis (260), it is now clear that they result from differential phosphorylation (306,691). NS5A phosphorylation occurs mostly on serine residues and, to a lesser extent, on threonine (306,564). The "basal" phosphorylation site (or sites) of HCV-J NS5A, which is thought to occur for both p56 and p58, has been mapped by serial deletion to the region downstream of polyprotein residue 2350 (690). p58 is "hyperphosphorylated" at additional sites that remain unmodified in the p56 form. Deletion analyses suggest that these hyperphosphorylation sites reside in a conserved, central region of the polyprotein that extends from residue 2200 to residue 2250 (690). Site-directed mutagenesis of the nine conserved serines in this region tentatively identified these sites of p58 phosphorylation as Ser-2197, Ser-2201, and Ser-2204 (690). For an HCV genotype 1a isolate, a major site of *in vitro* and *in vivo* phosphorylation has been mapped to NS5A residue Ser-2321. However, this serine residue is not conserved among the different HCV genotypes (563). For the HCV-J isolate, NS4A associates with NS5A (21) and enhances p58 production and, by inference, hyperphosphorylation at the upstream sites (306,691). However, this effect of NS4A seems to be isolate specific (262) and more recent studies suggest that multiple determinants, including all of the upstream NS proteins, influence NS5A phosphorylation when the protein is expressed in the context of an HCV NS polyprotein (334,389,482).

The kinase responsible for NS5A phosphorylation is thought to be of cellular origin, since (a) NS5A contains no recognizable kinase motifs, (b) phosphorylation of NS5A expressed transiently in cultured cells occurs in the absence of other viral proteins (564,691), and (c) phosphorylation of NS5A expressed in *E. coli* depends on the addition of eukaryotic cell extracts (285,563). Although the identity of the NS5A kinase is not known, biochemical properties of an NS5A-associated kinase activity with similarities to the kinase responsible for NS5A phosphorylation *in vivo* have already been characterized. This NS5A-associated kinase is active *in vitro* over a broad pH range, has an apparent preference for $MnCl_2$ over $MgCl_2$, and is inhibited strongly by $CaCl_2$ at concentrations over 0.5 mM (564). Furthermore, specific inhibitors of PKA and protein kinase C have little or no effect on NS5A phosphorylation *in vitro* or *in vivo*. However, both types of NS5A phosphorylation are inhibited by olomoucine, an inhibitor of certain proline-directed kinases. The resistance of NS5A phosphorylation to treatment with a specific PKA inhibitor casts some doubt on the suggestion that PKA is the major effector of NS5A phosphorylation (285). Although the preference of the NS5A-associated kinase for Mn^{2+} over Mg^{2+} is somewhat unusual among serine/threonine kinases, as is its inhibition by Ca^{2+}, the NS5A and NS5 proteins of bovine viral diarrhea virus (BVDV) and YF, respectively, associate with a kinase that has similar properties (561). More work is needed to determine the role of NS5A and NS5A phosphorylation in viral replication.

Analysis of full-length genome sequences for three HCV genotype 1b isolates obtained from different Japanese patients before and after interferon therapy found mutations clustered primarily in E2 HVR1 and the C-terminal half of NS5A (155). Further analysis suggested that the amino acid sequence from polyprotein position 2209 to 2248 in NS5A correlated with the effectiveness of interferon treatment in these and other Japanese patients infected with genotype 1b. Consequently, this stretch of amino acids was designated the interferon sensitivity–determining region (ISDR) (155,156). Although confirmed by most other groups working with Japanese patients infected with genotype 1b, 2a, or 2b HCV strains, this correlation was substantially weaker or lacking in patients infected with genotype 1a strains or European patients infected with strains of genotype 1b, 2b, or 3a (see ref. 508 for review).

In any case, following up on this possible link between NS5A and response to interferon, NS5A was found to interact with and inhibit the interferon-stimulated, double-stranded-RNA-dependent kinase PKR (187). PKR is a major effector of the host antiviral defense pathway that represses translation by phosphorylating the α subunit of the translation initiation factor eIF2. Evidence suggests that HCV NS5A interacts with PKR and inhibits dimerization that is required for PKR activation (185). The region of NS5A implicated in this interaction with PKR includes the ISDR as well as downstream sequences. Several studies have shown that cells expressing NS5A can partially resist the antiviral effects of interferon (186,505,528,647). Somewhat surprisingly, such effects can be observed in the absence of the ISDR (528) and occur independently of the PKR-eIF2 pathway in the context of the complete HCV polyprotein (178). Interestingly, mutations that allow more efficient initiation of HCV subgenomic replicon replication in cell culture cluster in NS5A in the region just upstream of the ISDR and include a 47-amino-acid deletion that encompasses the ISDR (51). These data suggest that NS5A plays an active role in RNA replication and that the ISDR is not essential in cell culture. In addition, deletion of the ISDR does not appear to increase the sensitivity of HCV RNA replication to interferon α in this system (51), consistent with previous observations (528).

N-terminally truncated forms of NS5A fused to the DNA-binding domain of the *Saccharomyces cerevisiae* Gal4 protein activate transcription of reporter genes under the control of promoters containing Gal4 binding sites (119,313,687). This trans-activating ability has been linked to ISDR sequences that may be associated with increased interferon sensitivity (181). The physiologic relevance of these findings is questionable, because the full-length NS5A protein lacks this trans-activating ability and has a cytoplasmic localization. However, NS5A does contain a sequence in its C-terminal region that has the potential to function as a nuclear localization signal (286), raising the possibility that proteolytic removal of the N-terminal region of NS5A (417,463) could result in its transport to the nucleus and activation of the transcription of certain cellular genes. Indeed, recent work has provided evidence for caspase-mediated cleavages in NS5A that liberate a nuclear form whose ability to function as a transcriptional activator is regulated by PKA (606).

In addition to these features, NS5A interacts with several cellular proteins. These include growth-factor-receptor-bound protein-2 adaptor protein, an interaction that can perturb mitogenic signalling (682); a SNARE-like protein, hVAP-33, that is ER and Golgi associated and may participate in intracellular membrane trafficking (717); a novel cellular transcription factor SRCAP (190); and human karyopherin beta3, a protein that may participate in nuclear trafficking of RNAs and proteins (118). The role of these interactions in HCV replication or in virus-induced modulation of host cell function remains to be established.

NS5B

NS5B (about 68 kd) is a hydrophilic protein containing the GDD motif common to RdRPs. As expected, mutation of the polymerase active sites destroy the *in vivo* infectivity of HCV genomes (340) and replication of HCV subgenomes in culture (51,397). RdRP activity has been demonstrated *in vitro* for recombinant NS5B (7,44,396,784,805), although these reactions do not show specificity for HCV templates. DNA or RNA oligonucleotide primers can be extended by the NS5B RdRP on homopolymeric templates or cellular RNAs (6,7, 44,396,784). RNAs terminating with the HCV 3′ NCR, which contains a stable 3′ hairpin (see preceding), can also be utilized as self-priming templates for RNA extension by NS5B (44,396). *De novo*, primer-independent initiation of RNA synthesis has recently been demonstrated in RdRP assays, usually by increasing concentrations of the initiating nucleotide (402,494,814). The more reliable of these studies (402,814) included templates that were chemically blocked at the 3′ end and therefore unable to function as primers. Biochemical characterization of RdRP activity reveals a requirement for the divalent cations Mn^{2+} or Mg^{2+}, but not Zn^{2+} (6,44,167,396,402, 784,805), near neutral pH (7,44,396,784), and low (i.e., 100-mM) concentrations of salt (399,784). The rate of elongation on a genome-length HCV RNA template was estimated to be 150 to 200 nucleotides per minute at 22°C (399,494), and it was independent of NS5B concentration (399), indicating that NS5B is highly processive. Terminal nucleotidyl transferase activity was reported in one preparation of NS5B purified from insect cells (44).

However, several other purified NS5B preparations were apparently free of this activity (7,784,805), suggesting that it is more likely to be due to a copurifying cellular enzyme than an inherent property of NS5B (396).

The hydrophobic C-terminal 21 amino acids can be deleted from NS5B to produce soluble, fully active RdRP (167,396,402,784). This finding greatly enabled several high-resolution structural determinations of NS5B by x-ray crystallography (4,66,371). NS5B bears structural similarity to other polymerases, adopting a "right hand" conformation with a palm subdomain containing active site residues, and discernible fingers and thumb subdomains (see Fig. 11). However, extensive interactions between the fingers and thumb subdomains serve to fully encircle the NS5B active site. Despite the absence of substrate in these experiments, this resembles the closed conformation described for other polymerases (66), suggesting that NS5B may not undergo the typical conformational rotation upon template–primer binding (298, 374). Residues thought to be involved in metal ion coordination, substrate binding, and nucleotide discrimination are spatially organized as for HIV-1 reverse transcriptase (4,66,371). Another notable feature of NS5B is a unique β-loop projecting from the thumb subdomain that probably interacts with the template–primer and could affect NS5B fidelity and/or processivity (4,66,371). The thumb subdomain also contains structural similarity to "armadillo" repeats, which could be involved in mediating protein–protein interactions within the replicase complex (66).

The C-terminal hydrophobic domain of NS5B mediates association with perinuclear membranes, the presumed site of HCV RNA replication (784), and includes determinants for interaction with NS5A (784). Although NS5B binds RNAs nonspecifically, it does show some preference for RNAs containing the HCV 3′ NCR (108,495). NS5B has also been shown to directly interact with NS3 and NS4A (293), which in turn have been shown to form complexes with NS4B and NS5A (21,382). It is likely, yet unproven, that these interactions are important for assembly of a functional HCV RNA replication complex.

RNA Replication

As in other *Flaviviridae*, RNA replication in HCV is likely to occur in association with perinuclear membranes and involve the combined actions of the viral polymerase, helicase, other viral nonstructural proteins, and presumably some host factors (260,293,334,382,482). Because of the lack of an efficient cell culture system, the events of HCV RNA replication are only poorly understood. Detection of viral plus- and minus-strand RNAs in infectious culture systems or clinical samples have been limited to RT-PCR amplification. The most reliable of these methods are designed to eliminate false priming and ensure strand specificity during reverse transcription (225,359). Characterization of HCV subgenomes efficiently replicating in culture by RT-PCR or Northern blot reveals that subgenomes accumulate to 50 to 5,000 copies per cell in these systems (51,397), and that minus strands are 5- to 10-fold less abundant than plus strands (397), which is in agreement with the plus-to-minus-strand ratio observed in infected hepatocytes (359). It has not yet been determined whether viral minus strands can be isolated as RIs or in duplex RFs.

Assembly and Release of Virus Particles

In the absence of an efficient system for culturing HCV, much of what we know about HCV virion assembly comes from heterologous expression studies. Although packaging signals of the HCV genome are not yet characterized, C protein has been shown to interact with stem-loop IIId of the 5′ NCR (634,686). Furthermore, homotypic interactions of C protein (423,490) could be relevant to the formation of viral nucleocapsids. Based on the ER retention of viral glycoproteins E1 and E2, it seems likely that nucleocapsid precursors bud into the ER to acquire a lipid envelope and native heterodimers of the viral glycoproteins, then pass through the host secretory pathway and are released at the cell surface. Formation of virus-like particles (VLPs) by expression of the HCV structural proteins has met with limited success. Presumably nonenveloped (about 30 nm) and enveloped (about 45 nm) VLPs containing C protein were observed in HeLa G cells expressing the full-length HCV coding region via the vaccinia virus-T7 system (447). Enveloped VLPs containing HCV RNA were also observed in insect cells expressing the HCV 5′ NCR and structural region via a recombinant baculovirus (33). These VLPs were observed in intracellular vesicles late in infection (at 72 to 96 hr) but were not secreted and could be released only after mild detergent treatment and sonication. One study indicated that extracellular HCV particles partially purified from human plasma do contain complex N-linked glycans, suggestive of transit through the secretory pathway, although these carbohydrate moieties were not shown to be specifically associated with E1 or E2 (604).

Association of Hepatitis C Virus with HCC

A significant fraction of chronically infected patients slowly progress from chronic active hepatitis to cirrhosis and then to hepato-cellular carcinoma (HCC) (see refs. 54 and 635 and references therein). The mean onset for development of primary HCC has been estimated to be 20 to 30 years (332,594). Studies have identified both positive- and negative-strand HCV RNA in tumorous tissue from some but not all patients. The slow onset and the apparent association with preexisting cirrhosis suggest that HCV may not directly cause HCC but rather predisposes the organ to carcinogenic events. However, these observations do not exclude the possibility that expression of particular HCV gene products in chronically infected cells might contribute to carcinogenesis. In this regard, expression of C (98,300,554,714), NS3 (595), NS4B (501), and NS5A (186,191) in certain cell cultures can lead to anchorage-independent growth, enhanced formation of colonies in soft agar, and induction of tumor formation in immunodeficient mice. As mentioned earlier, some transgenic mouse lines expressing the C protein develop hepatocellular carcinoma similar in appearance to the human cancer (464). However, the relevance of these observations to the association between HCV and HCC in humans remains to be established.

THE PESTIVIRUSES

Background and Classification

Pestiviruses are animal pathogens of major economic importance, particularly in the livestock industry. They include the type member, bovine viral diarrhea virus, as well as classical swine fever virus (CSFV), formerly known as hog cholera virus, and border disease virus (BDV) of sheep (536). Based on comparative studies, two distinct species of BVDV have recently been identified, BVDV-1 and BVDV-2 (39,42,513,576). Newly described pestiviruses further indicate that additional diversity exists within this genus (39,724). Within the *Flaviviridae*, pestiviruses show greater similarity in genome structure and translation to the hepaciviruses than do the flaviviruses. For this reason, pestivirus research has received increased attention in the search for surrogate model systems to understand the less tractable hepaciviruses.

Pestiviruses are responsible for a spectrum of diseases within their natural hosts (reviewed in ref. 702). CSFV, typically transmitted oronasally, leads to acute or chronic hemorrhagic syndromes with significant mortality. Ruminant pestiviruses, on the other hand, usually cause inapparent or mild symptoms in adult animals. A notable exception is BVDV-2, which is associated with a severe acute hemorrhagic condition in calves (130,513,560, 576). In addition, congenital transmission of pestiviruses can cause fetal death and acute syndromes of the newborn, or it can lead to persistent infection of the offspring in a carrier state. Persistently infected ruminants can be susceptible to a rare but fatal mucosal disease (MD) later in life. Interestingly, development of MD correlates with viral genome alterations that affect the outcome of viral infection on host cells in culture. Recent efforts in pestivirus research have revealed interesting and novel features of these virus–host interactions. Although live attenuated strains and inactivated virus preparations are available for vaccination against CSFV and BVDV (450), there is a need for improved pestivirus vaccines. Insights into pestivirus biology are also being applied to the design of such tools (18,59,77,131,243,588,725,766).

Experimental Systems

In infected animal hosts, viral antigens and infectious virus can be detected in a variety of tissue types including epithelial cells at the site of entry, endothelial cells, lymphoreticular cells, and macrophages. In persistently infected animals, BVDV can be detected in most tissues including PBMC, the gastrointestinal tract, and neurons. Primary and continuous cell lines from natural host species are usually permissive for pestivirus replication in cell culture, although considerable differences in replication efficiencies have been noted (273,588). Highly permissive cell lines have been described for propagation of CSFV (458,588). Infection of permissive tissue culture cells is usually noncytopathic; however, variants of the ruminant pestiviruses capable of causing cytopathic effects can be isolated from animals with mucosal disease. Based on this cell culture phenotype, pestivirus isolates are referred to as either noncytopathogenic (ncp) or cytopathogenic (cp) biotypes.

Complete genome sequences have been determined for a number of pestiviruses (40,71,126,137,139,432,437, 459,460,574,575,586). This has led to the construction of reverse genetic systems (347,430,437,442,459,586,727) that are being used to probe mechanisms of pestivirus replication and the molecular basis of cytopathogenesis and virulence.

Structure and Physical Properties of the Virion

Pestiviruses have been difficult to purify because of modest growth in cell culture, inefficient release from infected cells, and association with cellular debris (362). Identification of efficient culture systems has facilitated visualization of virus particles by electron microscopy (450,746) (see Fig. 4D,E) and the characterization of the structural components of the virion (703). The spherical particles are 40 to 60 nm in diameter and enveloped, and they contain an electron-dense inner core with a diameter of about 30 nm (273). Pestivirus virions band at a buoyant density of 1.134 g/mL in sucrose and are inactivated by heat, organic solvents, and detergents (588). Unlike flaviviruses, which are rapidly inactivated by low pH, pestiviruses can survive over a relatively broad pH range (376). The chemical composition of highly purified preparations of pestivirus particles has not been determined, but in addition to the genome RNA and lipid bilayer, four structural proteins are present. These proteins include capsid protein, C, and three envelope glycoproteins E^{rns} (for ribonuclease, soluble), E1, and E2 (591,703).

Binding and Entry

Based on examples from other viruses, the binding and entry of pestiviruses is likely to be a multistep process involving initial attachment of virions, interaction with specific receptor(s), internalization, and membrane fusion. Specific cell surface receptors for pestiviruses have not been fully characterized. One candidate receptor is a pair of proteins, with apparent relative masses of 60 kd and 93 kd, which are recognized by three monoclonal antibodies capable of blocking infection of several BVDV-1 strains (613). Another potential receptor is a 50-kd cell surface protein identified by using an antiidiotypic antiserum (directed against E2-specific antibodies) that can block binding of BVDV-1 to bovine cells (445,780,781). It has been shown that recombinant E2 and E^{rns} can bind independently to cell surfaces (277). E2 adsorption competitively inhibits infection with homotypic and heterotypic pestiviruses, whereas inhibition by E^{rns} demonstrates virus specificity and requires large amounts of E^{rns} (277). This latter point may be explained by a high receptor density, which correlates with the observed binding of E^{rns} to cell surface glycosaminoglycans (291). Additional information regarding the entry process may come from further characterization of a mutant bovine kidney cell line that is resistant to infection by several pestiviruses but is capable of supporting their replication following RNA transfection or chemically induced virus–cell fusion (174). This cell line was also found to be deficient in expression of the LDLR, a factor putatively involved in hepacivirus binding and entry, and antibodies against this receptor inhibited infection of bovine cells with BVDV-1 (3).

Genome Structure

The pestivirus genome consists of a single-stranded RNA of about 12.3 kb in length (71,126,137,139,432, 460). As discussed later, larger and smaller genome RNAs containing duplications, deletions, and other rearrangements have been found for most cytopathic pestiviruses. The long ORF of about 4,000 codons is flanked by a 5′ NCR of 372 to 385 nucleotides, and a 3′ NCR of 229 to 273 nucleotides (71,126). The 5′ terminus does not appear to contain a cap structure (71,140). Construction of chimeric BVDV genomes containing 5′ NCRs of HCV or EMCV revealed that two 5′-terminal stem-loop structures in the BVDV genome (domains Ia and Ib in Fig. 9) are important for efficient RNA replication, and that the minimal 5′ cis-acting replication element consists of only the terminal tetranucleotide, 5′-GUAU (179). Pestivirus genome RNAs do not contain 3′ poly(A) (126,432,458) but appear to terminate with a short poly(C) tract. The 3′ NCR consists of a variable region near the end of the ORF, followed by a conserved region (140,804). Structural probing revealed that the conserved region forms two hairpins separated by a single-stranded region, and mutational analysis indicated that the terminal hairpin and single-stranded region contain important primary and secondary structural elements that probably function in cis to direct minus-strand initiation (804).

Translation and Proteolytic Processing

Cap-independent translational initiation of the pestivirus genome is mediated by a 5′ IRES element that bears structural and functional similarity to the HCV IRES (see Fig. 9) (72,140,529,579). Structure–function studies have demonstrated that domain I is dispensable for IRES activity, that domains II and III contain structures critical for function, that the 3′ end of the IRES may extend into the ORF, and that a pseudoknot formed from base-pairing of loop IIIf to a region just upstream of the translational start site is necessary for IRES activity (111,529,579). As for hepaciviruses, the pestivirus IRES has been shown to bind ribosomal 40S subunits independent from translation initiation factors eIF4A, eIF4B, and eIF4F (514,515,642). Pestivirus proteins are translated from genomic RNA as a single large polyprotein, which is processed into individual viral proteins (458,543,587). The current model of pestivirus polyprotein processing comes mainly from analysis of virus-infected cells (5, 125,127,591) and expression of pestivirus polyproteins using the vaccinia or baculovirus systems (348,518,590, 591,693,771,779). Cleavage products have been localized in the polyprotein using region-specific antisera (125, 656) and proteolytic processing sites within the polyprotein have been determined by protein sequencing (154, 348,591,655,693,779). The order of the cleavage products in the BVDV-NADL polyprotein is NH_2-N^{pro}-C-E^{rns}-E1-E2-p7-NS2-NS3-NS4A-NS4B-NS5A-NS5B-COOH (Fig. 12) (125,127,439).

Unlike other *Flaviviridae*, the first pestivirus protein encoded in the long ORF is a nonstructural protein, N^{pro}. This autoprotease is responsible for cleavage at the N^{pro}/C site (655,703,771). Processing in the pestivirus structural region appears to be mediated by at least two additional proteases. Although some of the cleavages are slightly delayed, host signal peptidase is believed to cleave at the C/E^{rns} and E1/E2 sites and the site generating the C terminus of E2 (591). The E^{rns}-E1 polyprotein (gp62) is converted slowly to the mature products by an unknown mechanism (591). E1 and E2 are believed to be anchored in the lipid bilayer via C-terminal membrane segments, and some E^{rns} remains associated with the virion via noncovalent interactions that have not been defined (591). A small hydrophobic protein, p7, is produced by signal peptidase, although incomplete processing at the E2/p7 site is observed leading to accumulation of uncleaved E2/p7 (154,242). The pestivirus NS3 protein contains the viral serine protease domain and is responsible for processing

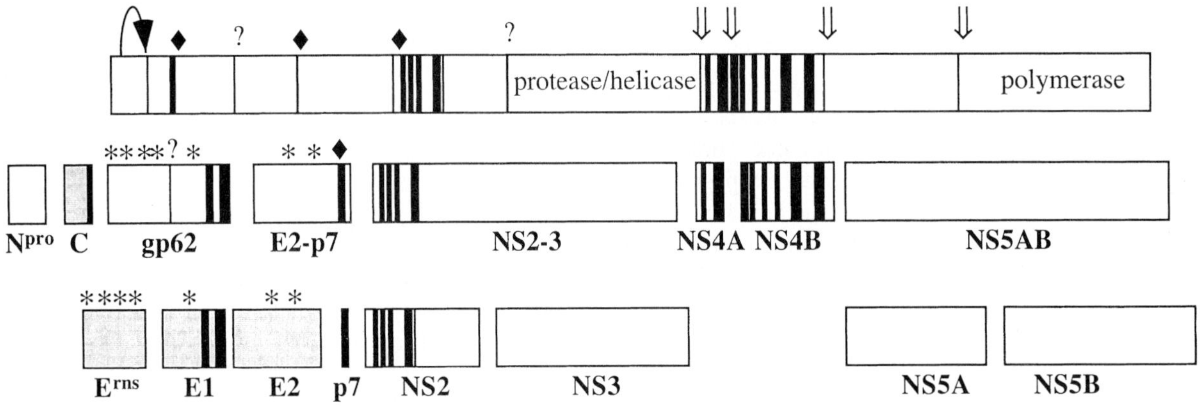

FIG. 12. Processing of the pestivirus polyprotein. *Shading* and *symbols* identifying proteolytic cleavages for the cpBVDV NADL strain are the same as those described in Figure 3, except that the proposed autocatalytic cleavage releasing the N-terminal nonstructural protein N^{pro} from the pestivirus polyprotein (see refs. 655 and 771) is indicated by a *curved arrow.*

at four downstream nonstructural cleavage sites to generate NS4A, NS4B, NS5A, and NS5B (see Fig. 12) (693,771,779). Differences in NS2–3 processing are observed between pestivirus isolates (see ref. 42 and citations therein). Isolates of ncpBVDV do not process NS2-3, whereas those of BDV are able to cleave NS2–3 inefficiently, producing NS3. For CSFV and cpBVDV biotypes, NS2–3 cleavage is efficient but incomplete so that both NS2–3 and NS3 are observed. In the case of the cpBVDV biotypes, the cleavage generating the NS3 N-terminus is produced via several different mechanisms involving RNA recombinational events (detailed later). Enzymes responsible for cleavage at the NS2/3 site in the CSFV and BDV polyproteins have not been elucidated.

Features of Pestivirus Proteins

The N^{pro} Autoprotease

As mentioned earlier, the first protein in the pestivirus polyprotein, the N^{pro} autoprotease (655,771), is a nonstructural protein (703). This enzyme cleaves at its C-terminal sequence Cys↓Ser, which is conserved among pestiviruses (655). Site-directed mutagenesis has identified residues Glu-22, His-49, and Cys-69 as being important for catalysis, and it has been suggested that N^{pro} may be an unusual subtilisin-like cysteine protease (589). Autoproteolysis is the only known function of N^{pro}, and cellular ubiquitin, which directs appropriate C-terminal cleavage by ubiquitin C-terminal hydrolase, can functionally substitute for N^{pro} in replication-competent genomes (43,694,710). Furthermore, N^{pro} is dispensable for autonomous RNA replication in engineered and spontaneously derived subgenomes (43,467,694,710).

Pestivirus Structural Proteins

N^{pro} is followed by the virion nucleocapsid protein C, a conserved, highly basic, 14-kd polypeptide consisting of 21% Lys with a net charge of +12. The C terminus of the virion C protein has not been defined, and it is unknown if it retains the hydrophobic segment postulated to serve as the signal sequence initiating translocation of E^{rns} into the ER lumen.

The E^{rns} glycoprotein (gp44/48, formerly known as E0), is heavily glycosylated at seven to nine potential N-linked glycosylation sites, and it forms disulfide-linked homodimers (703). This protein does not contain a potential membrane-spanning domain and is found noncovalently associated with released virus particles or secreted into the culture medium (591,746,748). Recombinant E^{rns} binds strongly to the surface of cells, probably via interaction with glycosaminoglycans, and it can inhibit infection in a virus-specific manner (291,748). Interestingly, E^{rns} has been shown to possess an unusual ribonuclease activity with specificity for uridine residues (276,620, 767). Glycosylation and dimer formation are not required for this activity (767). Although the function of E^{rns} ribonuclease activity is not yet clear, it appears to be important for some aspect of the virus life cycle. Antibodies that inhibit ribonuclease activity also tend to neutralize virus infectivity (767), and mutations in E^{rns} that destroy ribonuclease activity give rise to viruses that may be more cytopathic in culture but are attenuated *in vivo*

(278,435). In addition, recombinant E^{rns} appears to be toxic to lymphocytes *in vitro* (76), perhaps contributing to the marked leukopenia seen in natural infections (668). Although cytotoxicity is a feature of other soluble ribonucleases (reviewed in ref. 612), it is unclear whether the ribonuclease activity of E^{rns} is related to its toxicity.

Both E1 (gp33) and E2 (gp55) are predicted to be integral membrane proteins and contain two to three, and four to six N-linked glycosylation sites, respectively (see ref. 747). E1 and E2 are associated as disulfide-linked heterodimers that form slowly (591); E2 is also present in homodimers (703,747). As mentioned before, recombinant CSFV E2 can bind to cells and block infection of CSFV and BVDV, suggesting that a common E2 receptor is utilized by these pestiviruses for binding and entry (277). Although the precise roles of the viral glycoproteins in virus assembly and entry remain to be defined, monoclonal antibodies to E^{rns} (746) or E2 (145,506,723, 747,758) can neutralize virus infectivity, and both antigens can elicit protective immunity (279,590,725).

Pestivirus Nonstructural Proteins

Following the virion structural proteins, the first nonstructural protein is p7, and it consists of a central charged region separating hydrophobic termini (154). The role of this small protein is unknown, but it appears to be required for production of infectious virus (242) but not RNA replication (43). Like the hepacivirus protein, pestivirus p7 is inefficiently cleaved from E2, probably via signal peptidase (154,379). Uncleaved E2–p7 is not required for replication in cell culture (242) and both E2–p7 and p7 appear to remain cell associated and do not copurify with virus particles (154).

The NS2 protein (about 54 kd) is present as the N-terminal portion of NS2–3 (about 125 kd) and is found as a mature cleavage product only for some cpBVDV strains (ref. 441 and citations therein). As detailed later, NS2/3 cleavage in cpBVDV can be regulated by several alterations in the NS2 coding region, including genome rearrangements and insertion of cellular sequences. The precise role of NS2 in NS2–3 processing is unclear, and the function of NS2 is largely unknown. Reconstruction of DI-like subgenomes that lack NS2 indicate that it is dispensable for autonomous RNA replication (43,467, 694). However, a correlation between the efficiency of NS2–3 cleavage and the levels of RNA replication has been noted (347,430). NS2 also appears to contain a segment with homology to zinc-finger motifs present in some DNA binding proteins (136).

As for all members of the *Flaviviridae*, the pestivirus NS3 contains an N-terminal serine protease domain (34,91,198,772) followed by motifs characteristic of RNA helicases (199). Uncleaved NS2–3 must be capable of functioning in pestivirus replication, as this protein is not processed in cells infected with ncpBVDV strains. NS3 protease activity (and probably NS2–3 protease activity) requires NS4A as a protein cofactor (779). From cleavage site mapping and comparative analysis, the serine protease was shown to cleave between Leu and small uncharged amino acids L↓(S/A/N) (693,779). Most substitutions of the serine nucleophile eliminate processing at these sites (771,779) and destroy virus infectivity (779). Surprisingly, however, enzymatic activity was retained in mutants containing threonine at this position (695). Additional mutations that disable serine protease activity confirm its essential role in virus viability (207). The NS3 protein of BVDV has been purified and shown to possess RNA helicase (743) and RNA-stimulated NTPase (680) activities. Site-directed mutagenesis of the conserved helicase and NTPase motifs inhibited or destroyed these activities and viral replication coordinately (207,217).

The hydrophobic NS4A and NS4B proteins are similar in size, composition, and hydropathic properties to the NS4A and NS4B proteins of other family members. The only known function of these proteins is the serine protease cofactor activity of NS4A (771,779). As for HCV, cofactor activity involves interaction of a central domain of NS4A with the N-terminal region of NS3 (695).

The remaining two proteins, NS5A (about 58 kd) and NS5B (about 75 kd), are present as mature cleavage products as well as an uncleaved form, NS5AB (about 133 kd) (125,127). Neither protein contains the motifs postulated to be involved in methyltransferase or RNA triphosphatase activities, consistent with the lack of a 5′ RNA cap structure on pestivirus genomes. Little is known about the function of NS5A. This protein was found to be phosphorylated by a cellular serine/threonine kinase with properties similar to enzymes that phosphorylate flavivirus NS5 and hepacivirus NS5A (561). NS5B contains motifs characteristic of RdRPs (124,126). The RNA polymerase activity of recombinant NS5B has been characterized *in vitro* and found to extend template-primed RNAs into double-stranded "copy-back" products (355, 398,657,812) or to catalyze *de novo* initiation from short synthetic RNA or DNA templates (308,355). Polymerase activity is particularly responsive to GTP concentration, most likely because of a strong preference for initiation with guanylate (308,398).

RNA Replication

Analysis of pestivirus RNA replication is still at an early stage, although this process appears to be similar to that of flaviviruses. Minus- and plus-strand RNAs have been detected from 4 to 6 hours after infection, followed by the asymmetric accumulation of additional minus- and excess plus-strand RNAs (196). Accumulation of genome-length intracellular pestivirus RNAs, which comigrate with virion RNA, generally follows the time course of infectious virus release, maximal virus titers being achieved about 12 to 24 hours after infection

(196,458,542). Double-stranded RF RNAs and partial duplex RI RNAs, containing about six nascent strands, have been tentatively identified (195,196,542). The role of these RNA isoforms in replication remains to be elucidated.

As described later, there is good evidence that nonhomologous recombination can occur within pestivirus RNAs, and between pestivirus RNAs and host cellular RNAs (reviewed in ref. 441). Although the details of these recombination events are unknown, a likely mechanism is via copy-choice template recruitment during minus-strand synthesis, which is consistent with the coding orientation of cellular inserts. Given the frequency of pestivirus–cellular RNA recombinants compared to other positive-strand viruses, this is an interesting and potentially unusual characteristic of the pestivirus replicase.

Assembly and Release of Virus Particles

Other than the features of the virion structural proteins described before, little information is available on the assembly and release of pestiviruses from infected cells. Pestivirus structural proteins are not found at the plasma membrane (209,748). Electron microscopic examination of virus-infected cells (46,208) suggests that pestiviruses mature in intracellular vesicles and are released by exocytosis. Formation of infectious BVDV-1 particles can be blocked by ER α-glucosidase inhibitors, presumably via misfolding of the viral envelope glycoproteins (816). A substantial fraction of infectious virus remains cell associated and some can be released from infected cells by successive freeze-thaw cycles (361,458). Interestingly, E^{rns} and E2 have been immunolocalized on isolated virus particles by electron microscopy, but E2 was not seen in particles undergoing secretion (or perhaps reattachment) at the cell surface (748). This suggests that E2 may be conformationally inaccessible to antibodies prior to a delayed maturation process.

Pathogenesis of MD and the Generation of Cytopathogenic Pestiviruses via RNA Recombination

Mucosal disease is the most severe outcome of BVDV infection and is usually fatal (reviewed in refs. 23, 74, 75, 441, and 702). This disease can occur when a fetus is infected *in utero* with an ncpBVDV strain. If infection with ncpBVDV occurs between 80 and 100 days of gestation, animals may become tolerized to BVDV antigens and remain persistently infected for life. In the case of a persistently infected animal exhibiting MD, both cp and ncp biotypes of BVDV can be isolated (427). The close serologic relatedness of ncp–cp pairs isolated from an MD-affected animal led to the suggestion that cpBVDV might arise from ncpBVDV by a rare mutational event. Molecular characterization of a number of these ncp–cp pairs has verified this hypothesis and led to the remarkable discovery that some cpBVDV biotypes are generated via RNA recombination (211,434,438,439,698). In every case studied thus far, these rare events led to the production of NS3 (in addition to NS2–3), which is thought to be responsible for cpBVDV cytopathogenicity in cell culture and the pathogenesis of MD in the immunotolerant animal. Although less well characterized, a similar mucosal syndrome correlating with viral cytopathogenicity exists for BDV. Cytopathic CSFV strains have been described but do not seem to correlate with a particular disease state.

Sequence analysis of several independent cpBVDV isolates has revealed some common genome rearrangements resulting from RNA recombination (reviewed in ref. 441), and a few representative genome structures are illustrated in Figure 13. In the case of the Osloss and NADL strains, an in-frame insertion of cellular sequences is found in the NS2 gene (434,438). The Osloss insertion encodes a host ubiquitin monomer, which presumably directs cleavage at the ubiquitin/NS3 junction by the cellular enzyme ubiquitin C-terminal hydrolase. This role for the ubiquitin insertion has been confirmed for another cpBVDV with a similar genome rearrangement (697). The host sequence found in the NADL strain corresponds to a 270-nt portion of a bovine mRNA whose gene product has not been characterized (434). Deletion of this insertion from a cloned BVDV-NADL genome gave rise to a virus that did not produce NS3, was noncytopathic in culture, and exhibited reduced levels of RNA replication (430). Similar insertions of this same host gene have also been found to correlate with NS3 production and cytopathogenicity in two cpBDV isolates (37). Interestingly, a much smaller insertion is found in the NS2 gene of cpBVDV strain CP7, which contains a 27-nt duplication from an upstream region of the NS2 gene in an alternate reading frame (696). This insertion also leads to the production of NS3 (696) and a virus that is cytopathic in culture (437).

The CP1 and Pe515 cpBVDV strains contain large duplications encompassing the NS3 coding region and insertions of either ubiquitin sequences (438,439) or a duplicated copy of the N^{pro} autoprotease (439), respectively. Genome rearrangements with duplicated viral sequences flanking ubiquitin insertion sites have also been noted (545), which probably result from multiple independent recombination events (441). Additional cellular gene insertions have also been found in the context of genomic duplications, and they correlate with NS3 production and cytopathogenicity. These include the SMT3B ubiquitin homolog (544), a ribosomal S27a–ubiquitin gene fusion (41), and light chain 3 of microtubule-associated proteins 1A and 1B (436).

Several cpBVDV-1, cpBVDV-2, and cpCSFV strains consist of a paired DI particle and an ncp helper virus (38,350,440,698,710). An example of a cpBVDV-1 DI is represented by CP9, which contains a precise deletion of

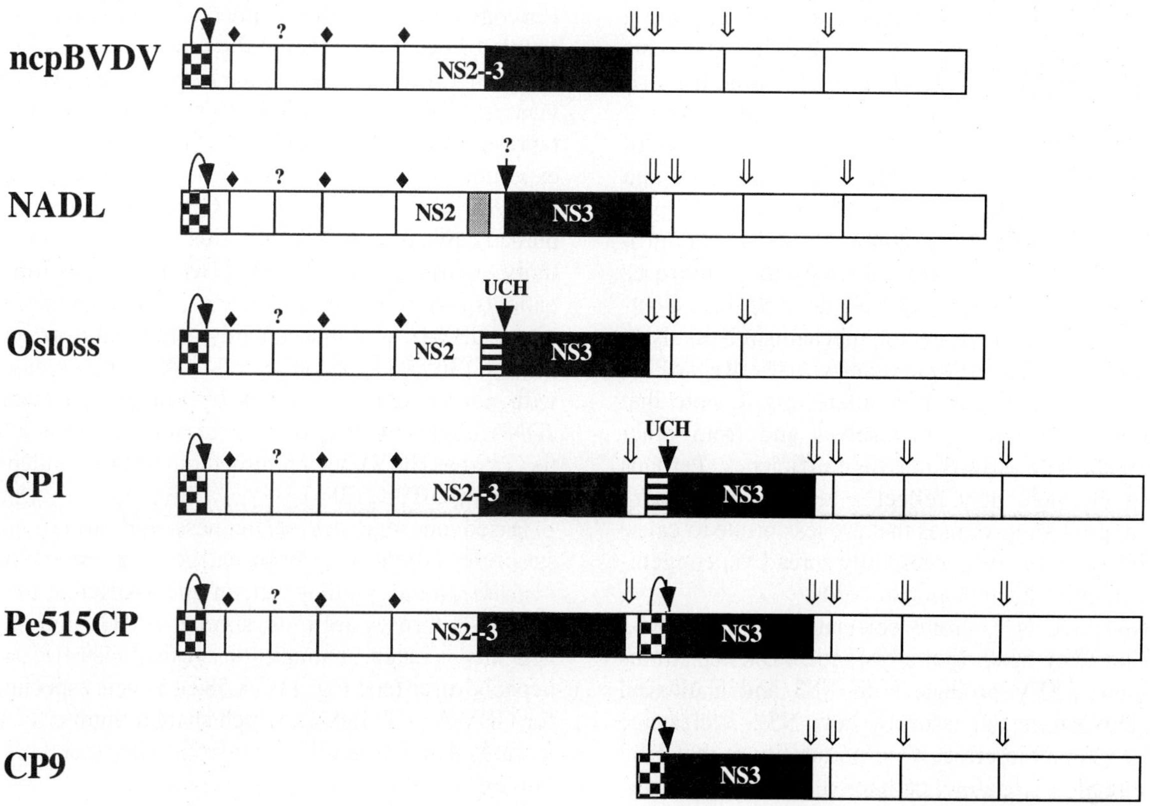

FIG. 13. Genome rearrangements associated with the generation of cytopathogenic bovine viral diarrhea virus (cpBVDV). The *top* diagram indicates the polyprotein of a typical ncpBVDV isolate. *Below*, the polyproteins encoded by five different cpBVDV isolates generated by RNA recombination are shown: NADL (432,433), Osloss (433), CP1 (438), Pe515CP (439), and CP9 (698). For all of the cpBVDV isolates, these polyprotein structures allow the production of both NS2-3 and NS3. In-frame insertions of host sequences are present in NADL (*shaded region*), Osloss (*striped region*), and CP1 (*striped region*). The enzyme responsible for NS3 production in the NADL strain is unknown, but the inserted ubiquitin sequences in Osloss and CP1 provide sites for processing by host ubiquitin C-terminal hydrolase (UCH) (697). For Pe515CP and the CP9 defective-interfering (DI) RNA, the N^{pro} autoprotease (*checkered box*) mediates the cleavage producing the NS3 N-terminus. The nomenclature and organization of the cleavage products and the symbols for the normal processing enzymes are defined in Figures 3 and 10. The location of NS3 *(filled region)* is emphasized.

the C-E^{rns}-E1-E2-p7-NS2 genes resulting in an in-frame fusion of N^{pro} and NS3 (698). Such subgenomes are capable of autonomous replication, express NS3, and induce cytopathic effects within cells (43,467,694). Pestivirus DIs interfere with the replication of helper viruses, which presumably provide packaging functions in trans.

Despite myriad ways that cp pestiviruses can be generated via RNA recombination, a few cpBVDV strains have been described that lack known genome alterations (136,210,512,545). For one such cp strain, BVDV-Oregon, NS2–3 cleavage was shown to be dependent on sequence information contained within NS2 and the first 66 amino acids of NS3 (348). Introduction of this NS2 gene into a heterologous ncpBVDV-1 genome led to NS2–3 processing and cytopathogenicity (347). Surprisingly, a relatively few amino acid changes in NS2 could account for this difference in cleavage efficiency. Nevertheless, due to the lack of an ncp counterpart, it can only be surmised that this strain had been derived by accumulated point mutations in the NS2 region.

Clearly, the unifying feature of cp pestiviruses is the production of NS3. As stated before, except for rearrangements that juxtapose ubiquitin or N^{pro} with NS3, the identity of the protease(s) responsible for NS2–3 cleavage in other cpBVDV strains, as well as in ncpCSFV and ncpBDV, is unknown. Involvement of the NS3 serine protease activity in NS2–3 cleavage has been excluded via mutagenesis or deletion in several cpBVDV polyproteins (348,436,696,779). One possibility is that foreign gene insertions in NS2 might signal a cellular protease to cleave at the NS2/3 junction, perhaps by inducing a conformation within NS2 similar to the NS2 proteins from ncpBDV, ncpCSFV, or BVDV-Oregon, which all cleave NS2–3 despite the absence of genome alterations. Alternatively, such changes might activate a latent or cryptic protease activity encoded by NS2. This could explain how the BVDV-Oregon NS2 gene is sufficient to direct NS2–3 cleavage, as well as explain NS2–3 cleavage in ncpCSFV and ncpBDV despite the absence of genome rearrangements. Further, in this regard, HCV and GBV-C (see the next section, The GB Viruses) NS2 proteins contain the catalytic residues of NS2–3 autoproteases, although there is scant homology to pestiviruses in this region. Thus if pestivirus NS2 does perform a catalytic role in NS2–3 cleavage, the mechanism is likely to be different from that of these other viruses. Regardless of the mechanistic details, it is interesting to note that pestiviruses differ among themselves and from other family members in NS2–3 cleavage efficiency. Perhaps inefficient cleavage may reflect a recent evolutionary adaptation, producing viruses that are less prone to cause disease but nevertheless successfully spread via congenital routes in domesticated animal herds.

Whereas there is a strong correlation between NS3 production and cytopathogenicity of cpBVDV, ncp strains of BDV and CSFV produce both NS3 and uncleaved NS2–3. This raises the issue of how NS2–3 cleavage leads to a cytopathic effect. One possibility is that NS3 may be directly cytopathic, perhaps involving the serine protease activity. Pestivirus cytopathology proceeds via apoptosis (264,621,809), a cell death pathway involving cellular protease effectors (reviewed in ref. 324). According to this model, the relative abundance of NS3 would determine its effect within a host cell. In this regard, cpBDV and cpCSFV seem to express increased amounts of NS3 (37,42,440). Alternatively, it has been noted that cpBVDV exhibits an increased efficiency of RNA replication compared with paired ncp viruses (347,430). Thus, NS2–3 cleavage might directly result in enhanced RNA replication, and a byproduct of this process could be responsible for cytopathogenicity. In this regard, enhanced levels of RI and RF RNA forms could activate the double-stranded RNA-activated kinase PKR, a known inducer of apoptosis (24,141,652). A larger question is how cytopathic effects on the cellular level lead to MD in infected animals. Increased cell death could directly contribute to tissue injury and induce inflammation. There is also evidence that animals with MD show increased numbers of infected cells (375), perhaps because of increased replication of cpBVDV. In addition, cpBVDV might exhibit differences in tropism that could contribute to disease (375).

THE GB VIRUSES

Discovery, Distribution, and Origin

In the early 1990s, a residual number of hepatitis cases were still not attributable to HAV, HBV, HCV, or the recently described hepatitis E virus (Chapter 89 in *Fields Virology*, 4th ed.). Efforts aimed at identifying additional agents of hepatitis revealed three novel viruses that have been tentatively assigned to the *Flaviviridae*. Two of these viruses, GBV-A and GBV-B, were cloned via subtractive representational methods from the serum of a tamarin experimentally infected with a hepatitis agent originally derived from a human patient, GB (641). Although some human cases of non-A–E hepatitis showed serologic reactivity to GBV-A and GBV-B, RT-PCR analysis from these patients failed to detect either virus. Rather, a third related virus, GBV-C, was subsequently identified from one such patient (365,640). Cloning of novel viruses associated with non-A, non-B hepatitis by immunoscreening of a cDNA library identified an agent, initially termed hepatitis G virus (HGV), which turned out to be an independent isolate of GBV-C (386).

Based on sequence relatedness and overall genome structure, GBVs have been categorized within the *Flaviviridae*, although they remain unclassified at the genus level. GB viruses are most similar to HCV but phylogenetically distant enough to resist classification as hepaciviruses (see Fig. 1) (78,582). This is especially true for GBV-A and GBV-C, which share a number of unique features that distinguish them from other members of the family.

The inability to detect GBV-A or GBV-B in human samples led to investigations into their origins. Interestingly, GBV-A has been detected in several species of New World monkeys in the absence of experimental infection or overt disease (78,100,364,615). Viral sequences isolated from within a single primate species were highly related, whereas sequences isolated from separate species showed greater divergence, indicating that GBV-As are indigenous monkey viruses that have adapted to their hosts over extended periods of time (78,100,364,615). These results, and observations made during early cross-challenge experiments, provide support for the view that the original GBV-A isolate may have been acquired during passage of the GB agent in tamarins (78,502). The distribution of GBV-B in nature is unknown, as the only source of this virus is the original tamarin-passaged GB serum used to identify GBV-A and GBV-B.

Since its initial discovery, GBV-C has been found to be surprisingly common, with viral RNA detected in about 1% to 4% of healthy human volunteer blood donors (168,421,654,775). Phylogenetic analysis of GBV-C sequences has been complicated by an apparent bias against synonymous substitution in some parts of the genome, leading to differences in inferred relationships depending on the subgenomic regions under comparison (309,521,728). The molecular basis for this bias is unclear; it may involve evolutionary constraints imposed by RNA secondary structures (637) or cryptic ORFs (507,643). Nevertheless, standardization of results has been achieved through the use of an appropriate molecular timepiece, such as the 5′ NCR, the E2 gene, or complete genome sequences. These results indicate that variation among GBV-C isolates occurs in distinct genotypes that reflect their geographical distribution (183, 387,469,643,644). GBV-C RNA has also been detected in the serum of wild chimpanzees (1) and chimpanzees infected with a putative hepatitis agent (48). Chimpanzee-infecting GBV-Cs were found to be more closely related to each other than to human-infecting GBV-Cs, suggesting coevolution of these viruses with their hosts (1,48,100).

Genome Structure and Expression

Complete or nearly complete genome sequences have been determined for a number of GBVs, and functional full-length infectious clones have been assembled for GBV-B (80) and GBV-C (777). Like the other family members, the GBV genomes encode a single long ORF containing structural protein genes [(C)-E1-E2] in the 5′ one third, followed by nonstructural protein genes (NS2-NS3-NS4A-NS4B-NS5A-NS45B) in the remainder (365,468). The 5′ NCR of GBV-B contains 445 nucleotides, which is about 30% larger than the HCV 5′ NCR, but it has significant similarity in primary and presumed secondary structure to the HCV 5′ NCR (see Fig. 11) (268,468). In contrast, GBV-A and GBV-C have 5′ NCRs of 508 to 593 nucleotides that share about 50% identity to each other and can be folded into similar structures (see Fig. 11), but that do not resemble the 5′ NCRs of HCV or GBV-B (639). The long 5′ NCRs of all three GBVs contain multiple initiator AUG codons, and initiation of polyprotein translation is thought to be dependent on IRES activities, which have been demonstrated for all three GBV 5′ NCRs (201,577,639). The GBV-B 3′ NCR is 361 nucleotides in length, containing a short poly(U) stretch 30 nucleotides downstream of the stop codon, followed by 309 nucleotides of unique sequence (80,609). Although this region of the GBV-B genome does not contain sequence homology with HCV, the 3′ 47 nucleotides of GBV-B is predicted to fold into a structure very similar to SL-I at the 3′ end of the HCV genome (80,609). The 3′ NCRs of GBV-A and GBV-C are highly conserved only within these virus groups, although a short 17-nucleotide stretch is also well conserved among all GBVs (609).

The relationships among GBVs and between HCV are also reflected in the organization of structural proteins. Like HCV, GBV-B encodes a basic capsid protein followed by two envelope glycoproteins. The genomes for GBV-A and GBV-C also contain E1 and E2 glycoproteins, but they lack any obvious capsid-like protein (386,468). *In vitro* translation of RNAs containing the GBV-A or GBV-C 5′ NCR localized the translational start site to a conserved AUG immediately upstream of the E1 coding region (639). However, it has been observed that GBV-C-infected humans generate antibody responses against a small basic peptide that can be translated from an in-frame upstream AUG, suggesting that such a protein is expressed *in vivo* (777). Alternative explanations for the lack of a capsid-like protein include the possibilities that GBV-A and GBV-C might usurp a capsid-like protein of the host cell or a co-infecting virus, or that additional GBV proteins may be involved. In this regard, a region of the GBV-C NS5A gene exhibiting a bias against synonymous substitution has been noted to potentially encode a small basic protein (10 kd, pI 11.5) in an alternate reading frame (507). Furthermore, it remains possible that GBV-A and GBV-C virions might lack a distinct nucleocapsid. However, biophysical characterization of GBV-C particles indicate that GBV-C RNA can be found in low-density (1.07 g/mL) and intermediate-density (about 1.18 g/mL) fractions on a variety of density gradients (428,605,777). Pretreatment with detergents or organic solvents to remove membranes shifts the peak of viral RNA to a higher-density form that may represent nucleocapsids that have recently been visualized by electron microscopy (776).

The nonstructural proteins of GBVs show the greatest similarity to HCV, and the boundaries of cognate NS2, NS3, NS4A, NS4B, NS5A, and NS5B proteins have been proposed (365,468). Catalytic residues of the HCV NS2-3 autoprotease are conserved among GBV NS2 proteins (365,468), and this enzymatic activity has been described for GBV-C (45). Similarly, active sites of the HCV NS3 serine protease are retained in NS3 of GBVs. Biochemical characterization of the GBV-B serine protease activity indicates that it shares substrate specificity with the HCV enzyme and requires the virus-specific cofactor NS4A (83,610). The C-terminal region of GBV NS3 proteins retain the similarity to supergroup 2 RNA helicases that is common to the *Flaviviridae* (365,468), and NTP-dependent RNA unwinding activity has been demonstrated for NS3 proteins of GBV-B and GBV-C (229,813). NS5B contains similarity to the supergroup 2 RNA polymerases (365,468,641).

Association with Disease?

GBV-A has not been shown to cause disease in nonhuman primates, whereas GBV-B causes hepatitis in experimentally infected tamarins (80,614). As described before, although both of these viruses were thought to be derived from a source of human hepatitis, it appears that GBV-A had been acquired during primate passage and GBV-B has been isolated only from tamarin-passaged GB material. Attempts to identify a GBV in the original GB clinical sample have failed, most likely because of degradation during storage (614).

Human infection with GBV-C is well documented, although direct association of this virus with human disease has proven to be elusive (reviewed in ref. 638). Epidemiologic evidence suggests that it is primarily blood-borne, although other modes of transmission appear possible (105,169,240,624,654). These risk factors overlap with those of HBV and HCV, and the frequency of coinfections with GBV-C and other viruses have complicated etiologic determinations (13,386). It appears that a majority of GBV-C infections are subclinical, with only mild symptoms that typically resolve with the appearance of anti-E2 antibody (143,226,368,369,672,673). Viral persistence seems to occur in about 5% to 10% of GBV-C infections (226,421). A few studies have implicated GBV-C in acute and chronic non-A–E hepatitis (168), fulminant hepatitis (679,801,802), or other liver disease (129). However, recent work suggests that GBV-C is a lymphotropic virus (718). Clearly, more work needs to be done to establish the clinical significance of GBV-C and related viruses.

SUMMARY AND QUESTIONS

Although much has been learned about the general life cycle of the *Flaviviridae*, it is quite complex, and large gaps in our knowledge exist for every step. The ongoing development of improved genetic and biochemical tools to study these viruses will certainly enable a more complete picture of their biology. Recent progress has been made in identifying host cell surface molecules that could be involved in binding and entry of viruses, although the details of such interactions, and how these control virus tropism and infection *in vivo*, is largely unknown. The general strategies of genome translation and polyprotein processing have been elucidated. Yet details such as the proteolytic processing mechanism of the flavivirus NS1-2A or pestivirus NS2-3 polypeptides need to be resolved. More effort is needed to understand the functional significance of polyprotein processing events for RNA replication, virus–host interaction, and virion formation. Furthermore, it is not understood how the competing processes of genome translation and genome replication are regulated for this virus family. New insights have emerged regarding the enzymology of some viral nonstructural proteins, as well as the identity of a few host proteins that most likely contribute to genome replication. However, the role of several nonstructural proteins in this process are unknown. More description is needed for how all these components, together with viral RNA, combine to produce a functional replicase. As for all positive-strand RNA viruses, the role of membranes in the process of RNA replication remains a mystery. It is interesting that phosphorylation of polypeptides upstream of the polymerase seems to be a conserved feature within the family. Identification of the relevant kinase(s) should allow the significance of this posttranslational modification to be addressed. Nearly all of what we know about virus–cell interaction for HCV has come from the study of heterologous systems, which have suggested important roles for HCV-specific gene products in interferon sensitivity and the development of HCC. The emergence of improved systems for studying HCV in culture will permit all of this work to be reevaluated, and moreover, it will undoubtedly reveal unexpected and novel aspects of HCV biology. Our understanding of virion formation is still at an early stage, and it is not yet clear how structural proteins combine to form nascent virions, where this process occurs, and whether packaging is temporally regulated within the replication cycle. The lack of obvious capsid proteins for GBV-A and GBV-C raises the questions of whether these virions actually contain nucleocapsids and, if so, what the identity of the capsid proteins is. It is fascinating that pestiviruses encode a ribonuclease within the extracellular domain of an envelope glycoprotein, although the biologic role of this activity remains to be clarified. Also, what is the role of the secreted flavivirus NS1 protein? Why does production of NS3 by cpBVDV correlate with cytopathogenicity and fatal MD? Are GBVs involved in human disease? What mechanisms are involved in the establishment and maintenance of chronic infections by pestiviruses and HCVs? Answers to these and other pressing questions should reveal the unique aspects to the replication of this evolutionarily distinct family of viruses. This will provide information useful for the development of effective immunization and therapeutic strategies to control diseases caused by these diverse and important pathogens. Clearly, the most exciting period of research into the *Flaviviridae* lies ahead.

REFERENCES

1. Adams NJ, Prescott LE, Jarvis LM, et al. Detection in chimpanzees of a novel flavivirus related to GB virus-C/hepatitis G virus. *J Gen Virol* 1998;79:1871–1877.
2. Agnello V. Mixed cryoglobulinemia and other extrahepatic manifestations of hepatitis C virus infection. In: Liang TJ, Hoofnagle JH, eds. *Hepatitis C.* San Diego: Academic Press, 2000:295–314.
3. Agnello V, Abel G, Elfahal M, Knight GB, Zhang Q-X. Hepatitis C virus and other *Flaviviridae* viruses enter cells via low density lipoprotein receptor. *Proc Natl Acad Sci U S A* 1999;96:12766–12771.
4. Ago H, Adachi T, Yoshida A, et al. Crystal structure of the RNA-dependent RNA polymerase of hepatitis C virus. *Structure Fold Des* 1999;7:1417–1426.
5. Akkina RK. Pestivirus bovine viral diarrhea virus polypeptides: Identification of new precursor proteins and alternative cleavage pathways. *Virus Res* 1991;19:67–81.
6. Al RH, Xie Y, Wang Y, Hagedorn CH. Expression of recombinant hepatitis C virus non-structural protein 5B in *Escherichia coli*. *Virus Res* 1998;53:141–149.
7. Al RH, Xie Y, Wang Y, et al. Expression of recombinant hepatitis C virus NS5B. *Nucleic Acids Symp Ser* 1997;36:197–199.
8. Ali N, Siddiqui A. Interaction of polypyrimidine tract-binding protein with the 5′ noncoding region of the hepatitis C virus RNA genome and its functional requirement in internal initiation of translation. *J Virol* 1995;69:6367–6375.
9. Ali N, Siddiqui A. The La antigen binds 5′ noncoding region of the hepatitis C virus RNA in the context of the initiator AUG codon and stimulates internal ribosome entry site-mediated translation. *Proc Natl Acad Sci U S A* 1997;94:2249–2254.
10. Allander T, Forns X, Emerson SU, et al. Hepatitis C virus envelope protein E2 binds CD81 of tamarins. *Virology* 2000;277:358–367.
11. Allison SL, Schalich J, Stiasny K, et al. Oligomeric rearrangement of tick-borne encephalitis virus envelope proteins induced by an acidic pH. *J Virol* 1995;69:695–700.

12. Allison SL, Stiasny K, Stadler K, et al. Mapping of functional elements in the stem-anchor region of tick-borne encephalitis virus envelope protein E. *J Virol* 1999;73:5605–5612.
13. Alter HJ. The cloning and clinical implications of HGV and HGBV-C [editorial; comment]. *N Engl J Med* 1996;334:1536–1537.
14. Alter HJ, Purcell RH, Holland PV, Popper H. Transmissible agent in non-A, non-B hepatitis. *Lancet* 1978;1:459–463.
15. Alter HJ, Seeff LB. Recovery, persistence and sequelae in hepatitis C virus infection: A perspective on the long-term outcome. *Semin Liver Dis* 2000;20:17–25.
16. Amberg SM, Nestorowicz A, McCourt DW, Rice CM. NS2B-3 proteinase-mediated processing in the yellow fever virus structural region: *In vitro* and *in vivo* studies. *J Virol* 1994;68:3794–3802.
17. Anderson JF, Andreadis TG, Vossbrinck CR, et al. Isolation of West Nile virus from mosquitoes, crows, and a Cooper's hawk in Connecticut. *Science* 1999;286:2331–2333.
18. Andrew ME, Morrissy CJ, Lenghaus C, et al. Protection of pigs against classical swine fever with DNA-delivered gp55. *Vaccine* 2000; 18:1932–1938.
19. Anonymous. World Health Organization—Hepatitis C: Global prevalence. *Wkly Epidemiol Rec* 1997;72:341–344.
20. Arias CF, Preugschat F, Strauss JH. Dengue 2 virus NS2B and NS3 form a stable complex that can cleave NS3 within the helicase domain. *Virology* 1993;193:888–899.
21. Asabe S-I, Tanji Y, Satoh S, et al. The N-terminal region of hepatitis C virus-encoded NS5A is important for NS4A-dependent phosphorylation. *J Virol* 1997;71:790–796.
22. Asnis D, Conetta R, Waldman G, et al. Outbreak of West Nile-like Viral Encephalitis—New York, 1999. *MMWR Morb Mortal Wkly Rep* 1999;48:845–849.
23. Baker JC. Bovine viral diarrhea virus: A review. *J Am Vet Med Assoc* 1987;190:1449–1458.
24. Balachandran S, Kim CN, Yeh WC, et al. Activation of the dsRNA-dependent protein kinase, PKR, induces apoptosis through FADD-mediated death signaling. *EMBO J* 1998;17:6888–6902.
25. Barba G, Harper F, Harada T, et al. Hepatitis C virus core protein shows a cytoplasmic localization and associates to cellular lipid storage droplets. *Proc Natl Acad Sci U S A* 1997;94:1200–1205.
26. Bartenschlager R, Ahlborn-Laake L, Mous J, Jacobsen H. Nonstructural protein 3 of the hepatitis C virus encodes a serine-type proteinase required for cleavage at the NS3/4 and NS4/5 junctions. *J Virol* 1993; 67:3835–3844.
27. Bartenschlager R, Ahlborn-Laake L, Mous J, Jacobsen H. Kinetic and structural analyses of hepatitis C virus polyprotein processing. *J Virol* 1994;68:5045–5055.
28. Bartenschlager R, Ahlborn-Laake L, Yasargil K, et al. Substrate determinants for cleavage in cis and in trans by the hepatitis C virus NS3 proteinase. *J Virol* 1995;69:198–205.
29. Bartenschlager R, Lohmann V. Replication of hepatitis C virus. *J Gen Virology* 2000;81:1631–1648.
30. Bartenschlager R, Lohmann V, Wilkinson T, Koch JO. Complex formation between the NS3 serine-type proteinase of the hepatitis C virus and NS4A and its importance for polyprotein maturation. *J Virol* 1995;69:7519–7528.
31. Bartholomeusz AI, Wright PJ. Synthesis of dengue virus RNA *in vitro*: Initiation and the involvement of proteins NS3 and NS5. *Arch Virol* 1993;128:111–121.
32. Bassett SE, Brasky KM, Lanford RE. Analysis of hepatitis C virus-inoculated chimpanzees reveals unexpected clinical profiles. *J Virol* 1998;72:2589–2599.
33. Baumert TF, Ito S, Wong DT, Liang TJ. Hepatitis C virus structural proteins assemble into viruslike particles in insect cells. *J Virol* 1998;72:3827–3836.
34. Bazan JF, Fletterick RJ. Detection of a trypsin-like serine protease domain in flaviviruses and pestiviruses. *Virology* 1989;171:637–639.
35. Bazan JF, Fletterick RJ. Structural and catalytic models of trypsin-like viral proteases. *Semin Virol* 1990;1:311–322.
36. Beard MR, Abell G, Honda M, et al. An infectious molecular clone of a Japanese genotype 1b hepatitis C virus. *Hepatology* 1999;30: 316–324.
37. Becher P, Meyers G, Shannon AD, Thiel H-J. Cytopathogenicity of border disease virus is correlated with integration of cellular sequences into the viral genome. *J Virol* 1996;70:2992–2998.
38. Becher P, Orlich M, Konig M, Thiel HJ. Nonhomologous RNA recombination in bovine viral diarrhea virus: Molecular characterization of a variety of subgenomic RNAs isolated during an outbreak of fatal mucosal disease. *J Virol* 1999;73:5646–5653.
39. Becher P, Orlich M, Kosmidou A, et al. Genetic diversity of pestiviruses: Identification of novel groups and implications for classification. *Virology* 1999;262:64–71.
40. Becher P, Orlich M, Thiel H-J. Complete genomic sequence of border disease virus, a pestivirus from sheep. *J Virol* 1998;72:5165–5173.
41. Becher P, Orlich M, Thiel HJ. Ribosomal S27a coding sequences upstream of ubiquitin coding sequences in the genome of a pestivirus. *J Virol* 1998;72:8697–8704.
42. Becher P, Shannon AD, Tautz N, Thiel H-J. Molecular characterization of border disease virus, a pestivirus from sheep. *Virology* 1994;198: 542–551.
43. Behrens S-E, Grassmann CW, Thiel H-J, et al. Characterization of an autonomous subgenomic pestivirus RNA replicon. *J Virol* 1998;72: 2364–2372.
44. Behrens SE, Tomei L, DeFrancesco R. Identification and properties of the RNA-dependent RNA polymerase of hepatitis C virus. *EMBO J* 1996;15:12–22.
45. Belyaev AS, Chong S, Novikov A, et al. Hepatitis G virus encodes protease activities which can effect processing of the virus putative nonstructural proteins. *J Virol* 1998;72:868–872.
46. Bielefeldt Ohmann H, Bloch B. Electron microscopic studies of bovine viral diarrhea virus in tissues of diseased calves and in cell cultures. *Arch Virol* 1982;71:57–74.
47. Bielefeldt-Ohmann H. Analysis of antibody-independent binding of dengue viruses and dengue virus envelope protein to human myelomonocytic cells and B lymphocytes. *Virus Res* 1998;57:63–79.
48. Birkenmeyer LG, Desai SM, Muerhoff AS, et al. Isolation of a GB virus-related genome from a chimpanzee. *J Med Virol* 1998;56:44–51.
49. Blackwell JL, Brinton MA. BHK cell proteins that bind to the 3′ stem-loop structure of the West Nile virus genome RNA. *J Virol* 1995;69: 5650–5658.
50. Blackwell JL, Brinton MA. Translation elongation factor-1 alpha interacts with the 3′ stem-loop region of West Nile virus genomic RNA. *J Virol* 1997;71:6433–6444.
51. Blight KJ, Kolykhalov AA, Rice CM. Efficient initiation of HCV RNA replication in cell culture. *Science* 2000;290:1972–1974.
52. Blight KJ, Rice CM. Secondary structure determination of the conserved 98-base sequence at the 3′ terminus of hepatitis C virus genome RNA. *J Virol* 1997;71:7345–7352.
53. Blitvich BJ, Scanlon D, Shiell BJ, et al. Identification and analysis of truncated and elongated species of the flavivirus NS1 protein. *Virus Res* 1999;60:67–79.
54. Blum HE. Does hepatitis C virus cause hepatocellular carcinoma? *Hepatology* 1994;19:251–255.
55. Boege U, Heinz FX, Wengler G, Kunz C. Amino acid compositions and amino-terminal sequences of the structural proteins of a flavivirus, European tick-borne encephalitis virus. *Virology* 1983;126: 651–657.
56. Borowski P, Heiland M, Oehlmann K, et al. Non-structural protein 3 of hepatitis C virus inhibits phosphorylation mediated by cAMP-dependent protein kinase. *Eur J Biochem* 1996;237:611–618.
57. Borowski P, Oehlmann K, Heiland M, Laufs R. Nonstructural protein 3 of hepatitis C virus blocks the distribution of the free catalytic subunit of cyclic AMP-dependent protein kinase. *J Virol* 1997;71: 2838–2843.
58. Borowski P, zur Wiesch JS, Resch K, et al. Protein kinase C recognizes the protein kinase A-binding motif of nonstructural protein 3 of hepatitis C virus. *J Biol Chem* 1999;274:30722–30728.
59. Bouma A, de Smit AJ, de Kluijver EP, et al. Efficacy and stability of a subunit vaccine based on glycoprotein E2 of classical swine fever virus. *Vet Microbiol* 1999;66:101–114.
60. Bradley D, McCaustland K, Krawczynski K, et al. Hepatitis C virus: Buoyant density of the factor VIII-derived isolate in sucrose. *J Med Virol* 1991;34:206–208.
61. Bradley DW, Maynard JE, Popper H, et al. Posttransfusion non-A, non-B hepatitis: Physicochemical properties of two distinct agents. *J Infect Dis* 1983;148:254–265.
62. Bradley DW, McCaustland KA, Cook EH, et al. Posttransfusion non-A, non-B hepatitis in Chimpanzees: Physicochemical evidence that the tubule-forming agent is a small, enveloped virus. *Gastroenterology* 1985;88:773–779.

63. Brandt WE, Chiewslip D, Harris DL, Russell PK. Partial purification and characterization of a dengue virus soluble complement-fixing antigen. *J Immunol* 1970;105:1565–1568.
64. Brawner IA, Trousdale MD, Trent DW. Cellular localization of Saint Louis encephalitis virus replication. *Acta Virol* 1979;23:284–294.
65. Bray M, Men R, Lai CJ. Monkeys immunized with intertypic chimeric dengue viruses are protected against wild-type virus challenge. *J Virol* 1996;70:4162–4166.
66. Bressanelli S, Tomei L, Roussel A, et al. Crystal structure of the RNA-dependent RNA polymerase of hepatitis C virus. *Proc Natl Acad Sci U S A* 1999;96:13034–13039.
67. Brinton MA. Analysis of extracellular West Nile virus particles produced by cell cultures from genetically resistant and susceptible mice indicates enhanced amplification of defective interfering particles by resistant cultures. *J Virol* 1983;46:860–870.
68. Brinton MA. Replication of flaviviruses. In: Schlesinger S, Schlesinger MJ, eds. *The Togaviridae and Flaviviridae.* New York: Plenum Press, 1986:327–365.
69. Brinton MA, Dispoto JH. Sequence and secondary structure analysis of the 5′-terminal region of flavivirus genome RNA. *Virology* 1988;162:290–299.
70. Brinton MA, Fernandez AV, Amato J. The 3′-nucleotides of flavivirus genomic RNA form a conserved secondary structure. *Virology* 1986; 153:113–121.
71. Brock KV, Deng R, Riblet SM. Nucleotide sequencing of 5′ and 3′ termini of bovine viral diarrhea virus by RNA ligation and PCR. *J Virol Methods* 1992;38:39–46.
72. Brown EA, Zhang H, Ping LH, Lemon SM. Secondary structure of the 5′ nontranslated regions of hepatitis C virus and pestivirus genomic RNAs. *Nucleic Acids Res* 1992;20:5041–5045.
73. Brown JJ, Parashar B, Moshage H, et al. A long-term hepatitis B viremia model generated by transplanting nontumorigenic immortalized human hepatocytes in Rag-2-deficient mice. *Hepatology* 2000; 31:173–181.
74. Brownlie J. Pathogenesis of mucosal disease and molecular aspects of bovine virus diarrhoea virus. *Vet Microbiol* 1990;23:371–382.
75. Brownlie J, Clarke MC. Experimental and spontaneous mucosal disease of cattle: A validation of Koch's postulates in the definition of pathogenesis. *Intervirology* 1993;35:51–59.
76. Bruschke CJ, Hulst MM, Moormann RJ, et al. Glycoprotein E^{rns} of pestiviruses induces apoptosis in lymphocytes of several species. *J Virol* 1997;71:6692–6696.
77. Bruschke CJ, van Oirschot JT, van Rijn PA. An experimental multivalent bovine virus diarrhea virus E2 subunit vaccine and two experimental conventionally inactivated vaccines induce partial fetal protection in sheep. *Vaccine* 1999;17:1983–1991.
78. Bukh J, Apgar CL. Five new or recently discovered (GBV-A) virus species are indigenous to New World monkeys and may constitute a separate genus of the *Flaviviridae*. *Virology* 1997;229:429–436.
79. Bukh J, Apgar CL, Engle R, et al. Experimental infection of chimpanzees with hepatitis C virus of genotype 5a: Genetic analysis of the virus and generation of a standardized challenge pool. *J Infect Dis* 1998;178:1193–1197.
80. Bukh J, Apgar CL, Yanagi M. Toward a surrogate model for hepatitis C virus: An infectious molecular clone of the GB virus-B hepatitis agent. *Virology* 1999;262:470–478.
81. Bukh J, Miller RH, Purcell RH. Genetic heterogeneity of hepatitis C virus: Quasispecies and genotypes. *Semin Liver Dis* 1995;15:41–63.
82. Buratti E, Baralle FE, Tisminetzky SG. Localization of the different hepatitis C virus core gene products expressed in COS-1 cells. *Cell Mol Biol (Noisy-le-grand)* 1998;44:505–512.
83. Butkiewicz N, Yao N, Zhong W, et al. Virus-specific cofactor requirement and chimeric hepatitis C virus/GB virus B nonstructural protein 3. *J Virol* 2000;74:4291–4301.
84. Cahour A, Pletnev A, Vazielle FM, et al. Growth-restricted dengue virus mutants containing deletions in the 5′ noncoding region of the RNA genome. *Virology* 1995;207:68–76.
85. Calisher CH. Antigenic classification and taxonomy of flaviviruses (family *Flaviviridae*) emphasizing a universal system for the taxonomy of viruses causing tick-borne encephalitis [see comments]. *Acta Virol* 1988;32:469–478.
86. Calisher CH, Karabatsos N, Dalrymple JM, et al. Antigenic relationships between flaviviruses as determined by cross-neutralization tests with polyclonal antisera. *J Gen Virol* 1989;70:37–43.
87. Cardiff RD, Russ SB, Brandt WE, Russell PK. Cytological localization of dengue-2 antigens: An immunological study with ultrastructural correlation. *Infect Immun* 1973;7:809–816.
88. Carrick RJ, Schlauder GG, Peterson DA, Mushahwar IK. Examination of the buoyant density of hepatitis C virus by the polymerase chain reaction. *J Virol Methods* 1992;39:279–289.
89. Cauchi MR, Henchal EA, Wright PJ. The sensitivity of cell-associated dengue virus proteins to trypsin and the detection of trypsin-resistant fragments of the nonstructural protein NS1. *Virology* 1991;180: 659–667.
90. Chambers TJ, Grakoui A, Rice CM. Processing of the yellow fever virus nonstructural polyprotein: A catalytically active NS3 proteinase domain and NS2B are required for cleavages at dibasic sites. *J Virol* 1991;65:6042–6050.
91. Chambers TJ, Hahn CS, Galler R, Rice CM. Flavivirus genome organization, expression, and replication. *Annu Rev Microbiol* 1990;44: 649–688.
92. Chambers TJ, McCourt DW, Rice CM. Yellow fever virus proteins NS2A, NS2B, and NS4B: Identification and partial N-terminal amino acid sequence analysis. *Virology* 1989;169:100–109.
93. Chambers TJ, McCourt DW, Rice CM. Production of yellow fever virus proteins in infected cells: Identification of discrete polyprotein species and analysis of cleavage kinetics using region-specific polyclonal antisera. *Virology* 1990;177:159–174.
94. Chambers TJ, Nestorowicz A, Amberg SM, Rice CM. Mutagenesis of the yellow fever virus NS2B protein: Effects on proteolytic processing, NS2B-NS3 complex formation, and viral replication. *J Virol* 1993;67:6797–6807.
95. Chambers TJ, Nestorowicz A, Mason PW, Rice CM. Yellow fever/Japanese encephalitis chimeric viruses: Construction and biological properties. *J Virol* 1999;73:3095–3101.
96. Chambers TJ, Nestorowicz A, Rice CM. Mutagenesis of the yellow fever virus NS2B/3 cleavage site: Determinants of cleavage site specificity and effects on polyprotein processing and viral replication. *J Virol* 1995;69:1600–1605.
97. Chambers TJ, Weir RC, Grakoui A, et al. Evidence that the N-terminal domain of nonstructural protein NS3 from yellow fever virus is a serine protease responsible for site-specific cleavages in the viral polyprotein. *Proc Natl Acad Sci U S A* 1990;87:8898–8902.
98. Chang J, Yang S-H, Cho Y-G, et al. Hepatitis C virus core from two different genotypes has an oncogenic potential but is not sufficient for transforming primary rat embryo fibroblasts in cooperation with the H-*ras* oncogene. *J Virol* 1998;72:3060–3065.
99. Chang SC, Yen J-H, Kang H-Y, et al. Nuclear localization signals in the core protein of hepatitis C virus. *Biochem Biophys Res Comm* 1994;205:1284–1290.
100. Charrel RN, De Micco P, de Lamballerie X. Phylogenetic analysis of GB viruses A and C: Evidence for cospeciation between virus isolates and their primate hosts. *J Gen Virol* 1999;80:2329–2335.
101. Chayama K, Tsubota A, Koida I, et al. Nucleotide sequence of hepatitis C virus (type 3b) isolated from a Japanese patient with chronic hepatitis C. *J Gen Virol* 1994;75:3623–3628.
102. Chen C-M, You L-R, Hwang L-H, Lee Y-H. Direct interaction of hepatitis C virus core protein with the cellular lymphotoxin-b receptor. *J Virol* 1997;71:9417–9426.
103. Chen CJ, Kuo MD, Chien LJ, et al. RNA-protein interactions: Involvement of NS3, NS5, and 3′ noncoding regions of Japanese encephalitis virus genomic RNA. *J Virol* 1997;71:3466–3473.
104. Chen LK, Liao CL, Lin CG, et al. Persistence of Japanese encephalitis virus is associated with abnormal expression of the nonstructural protein NS1 in host cells. *Virology* 1996;217:220–229.
105. Chen M, Sonnerborg A, Johansson B, Sallberg M. Detection of hepatitis G virus (GB virus C) RNA in human saliva. *J Clin Microbiol* 1997;35:973–975.
106. Chen P-J, Lin M-H, Tai K-F, et al. The Taiwanese hepatitis C virus genome: Sequence determination and mapping the 5′ termini of viral genomic and antigenomic RNA. *Virology* 1992;188:102–113.
107. Chen Y, Maguire T, Hileman RE, et al. Dengue virus infectivity depends on envelope protein binding to target cell heparan sulfate [see comments]. *Nat Med* 1997;3:866–871.
108. Cheng JC, Chang MF, Chang SC. Specific interaction between the hepatitis C virus NS5B RNA polymerase and the 3′ end of the viral RNA. *J Virol* 1999;73:7044–7049.
109. Chisari FV. Hepatitis B virus transgenic mice: Models of viral

immunobiology and pathogenesis. *Curr Top Microbiol Immunol* 1996; 206:149–173.

110. Cho HS, Ha NC, Kang LW, et al. Crystal structure of RNA helicase from genotype 1b hepatitis C virus. A feasible mechanism of unwinding duplex RNA. *J Biol Chem* 1998;273:15045–15052.
111. Chon SK, Perez DR, Donis RO. Genetic analysis of the internal ribosome entry segment of bovine viral diarrhea virus. *Virology* 1998;251: 370–382.
112. Choo Q-L, Kuo G, Ralston R, et al. Vaccination of chimpanzees against infection by the hepatitis C virus. *Proc Natl Acad Sci U S A* 1994;91:1294–1298.
113. Choo Q-L, Kuo G, Weiner AJ, et al. Isolation of a cDNA clone derived from a blood-borne non-A, non-B viral hepatitis genome. *Science* 1989;244:359–362.
114. Chookhi A, Ung S, Wychowski C, Dubuisson J. Involvement of endoplasmic reticulum chaperones in the folding of hepatitis C virus glycoproteins. *J Virol* 1998;72:3851–3858.
115. Chu PW, Westaway EG. Characterization of Kunjin virus RNA-dependent RNA polymerase: Reinitiation of synthesis *in vitro*. *Virology* 1987;157:330–337.
116. Chu PW, Westaway EG. Molecular and ultrastructural analysis of heavy membrane fractions associated with the replication of Kunjin virus RNA. *Arch Virol* 1992;125:177–191.
117. Chu PWG, Westaway EG. Replication strategy of Kunjin virus: Evidence for recycling role of replicative form RNA as template in semiconservative and asymmetric replication. *Virology* 1985;140:68–79.
118. Chung KM, Lee J, Kim JE, et al. Nonstructural protein 5A of hepatitis C virus inhibits the function of karyopherin beta3. *J Virol* 2000;74:5233–5241.
119. Chung KM, Song OK, Jang SK. Hepatitis C virus nonstructural protein 5A contains potential transcriptional activator domains. *Mol Cells* 1997;7:661–667.
120. Cleaves GR, Ryan TE, Schlesinger RW. Identification and characterization of type 2 dengue virus replicative intermediate and replicative form RNAs. *Virology* 1981;111:73–83.
121. Clum S, Ebner KE, Padmanabhan R. Cotranslational membrane insertion of the serine proteinase precursor NS2B-NS3(Pro) of dengue virus type 2 is required for efficient *in vitro* processing and is mediated through the hydrophobic regions of NS2B. *J Biol Chem* 1997; 272:30715–30723.
122. Cocquerel L, Duvet S, Meunier J-C, et al. The transmembrane domain of hepatitis C virus glycoprotein E1 is a signal for static retention in the endoplasmic reticulum. *J Virol* 1999;73:2641–2649.
123. Cocquerel L, Meunier J-C, Pillez A, et al. A retention signal necessary and sufficient for endoplasmic reticulum localization maps to the transmembrane domain of hepatitis C virus glycoprotein E2. *J Virol* 1998;72:2183–2191.
124. Collett MS, Anderson DK, Retzel E. Comparisons of the pestivirus bovine viral diarrhoea virus with members of the flaviviridae. *J Gen Virol* 1988;69:2637–2643.
125. Collett MS, Larson R, Belzer SK, Retzel E. Proteins encoded by bovine viral diarrhea virus: The genomic organization of a pestivirus. *Virology* 1988;165:200–208.
126. Collett MS, Larson R, Gold C, et al. Molecular cloning and nucleotide sequence of the pestivirus bovine viral diarrhea virus. *Virology* 1988; 165:191–199.
127. Collett MS, Wiskerchen MA, Welniak E, Belzer SK. Bovine viral diarrhea virus genomic organization. *Arch Virol Suppl* 1991;3:19–27.
128. Colombage G, Hall R, Pavy M, Lobigs M. DNA-based and alphavirus-vectored immunisation with prM and E proteins elicits long-lived and protective immunity against the flavivirus, Murray Valley encephalitis virus. *Virology* 1998;250:151–163.
129. Colombatto P, Randone A, Civitico G, et al. Hepatitis G virus RNA in the serum of patients with elevated gamma glutamyl transpeptidase and alkaline phosphatase: A specific liver disease? [corrected] [published erratum appears in *J Viral Hepat* 1997;4:143]. *J Viral Hepat* 1996;3:301–306.
130. Corapi WV, French TW, Dubovi EJ. Severe thrombocytopenia in young calves experimentally infected with noncytopathic bovine viral diarrhea virus. *J Virol* 1989;63:3934–3943.
131. Cortese VS, Grooms DL, Ellis J, et al. Protection of pregnant cattle and their fetuses against infection with bovine viral diarrhea virus type 1 by use of a modified-live virus vaccine. *Am J Vet Res* 1998;59: 1409–1413.
132. Crooks AJ, Lee JM, Easterbrook LM, et al. The NS1 protein of tick-borne encephalitis virus forms multimeric species upon secretion from the host cell. *J Gen Virol* 1994;75:3453–3460.
133. Cui T, Sugrue RJ, Xu Q, et al. Recombinant dengue virus type 1 NS3 protein exhibits specific viral RNA binding and NTPase activity regulated by the NS5 protein. *Virology* 1998;246:409–417.
134. Dash S, Halim A-B, Tsuji H, et al. Transfection of HepG2 cells with infectious hepatitis C virus genome. *Am J Pathol* 1997;151:363–373.
135. De Francesco R, Urbani A, Nardi MC, et al. A zinc binding site in viral serine proteinases. *Biochemistry* 1996;35:13282–13287.
136. De Moerlooze L, Desport M, Renard A, et al. The coding region for the 54-kd protein of several pestiviruses lacks host insertions but reveals a "zinc finger-like" domain. *Virology* 1990;177:812–815.
137. De Moerlooze L, Lecomte C, Brown-Shimmer S, et al. Nucleotide sequence of the bovine viral diarrhoea virus Osloss strain: Comparison with related viruses and identification of specific DNA probes in the 5′ untranslated region. *J Gen Virol* 1993;74:1433–1438.
138. Deleersnyder V, Pillez A, Wychowski C, et al. Formation of native hepatitis C virus glycoprotein complexes. *J Virol* 1997;71:697–704.
139. Deng R, Brock KV. Molecular cloning and nucleotide sequence of a pestivirus genome, noncytopathic bovine viral diarrhea virus strain SD-1. *Virology* 1992;191:867–869.
140. Deng R, Brock KV. 5′ and 3′ untranslated regions of pestivirus genome: Primary and secondary structure analyses. *Nucleic Acids Res* 1993;21:1949–1957.
141. Der SD, Yang YL, Weissmann C, Williams BR. A double-stranded RNA-activated protein kinase-dependent pathway mediating stress-induced apoptosis. *Proc Natl Acad Sci U S A* 1997;94:3279–3283.
142. Deubel V, Digoutte J-P, Mattei X, Pandare D. Morphogenesis of yellow fever virus in *Aedes aegypti* cultured cells. II. An ultrastructural study. *Am J Trop Med Hyg* 1981;30:1071–1077.
143. Dille BJ, Surowy TK, Gutierrez RA, et al. An ELISA for detection of antibodies to the E2 protein of GB virus C. *J Infect Dis* 1997;175: 458–461.
144. Dimasi N, Pasquo A, Martin F, et al. Engineering, characterization and phage display of hepatitis C virus NS3 protease and NS4A cofactor peptide as a single-chain protein. *Protein Eng* 1998;11:1257–1265.
145. Donis RO, Corapi W, Dubovi EJ. Neutralizing monoclonal antibodies to bovine viral diarrhoea virus bind to the 56K to 58K glycoprotein. *J Gen Virol* 1988;69:77–86.
146. Droll DA, Kirishna Murthy HM, Chambers TJ. Yellow fever virus NS2B-3 protease: Charged-to-alanine mutagenesis and deletion analysis define regions important for protease complex formation and function. *Virology* 2000;275:335–347.
147. Dubuisson J, Duvet S, Meunier JC, et al. Glycosylation of the hepatitis C virus envelope protein E1 is dependent on the presence of a downstream sequence on the viral polyprotein. *J Biol Chem* 2000; 275:30605–30609.
148. Dubuisson J, Hsu HH, Cheung RC, et al. Formation and intracellular localization of hepatitis C virus envelope glycoprotein complexes expressed by recombinant vaccinia and Sindbis viruses. *J Virol* 1994;68:6147–6160.
149. Dubuisson J, Rice CM. Hepatitis C virus glycoprotein folding: Disulfide bond formation and association with calnexin. *J Virol* 1996;70: 778–786.
150. Duvet S, Cocquerel L, Pillez A, et al. Hepatitis C virus glycoprotein complex localization in the endoplasmic reticulum involves a determinant for retention and not retrieval. *J Biol Chem* 1998;273: 32088–32095.
151. Eastman PS, Blair CD. Temperature-sensitive mutants of Japanese encephalitis virus. *J Virol* 1985;55:611–616.
152. Eckart MR, Selby M, Masiarz F, et al. The hepatitis C virus encodes a serine protease involved in processing of the putative nonstructural proteins from the viral polyprotein precursor. *Biochem Biophys Res Commun* 1993;192:399–406.
153. Ecker M, Allison SL, Meixner T, Heinz FX. Sequence analysis and genetic classification of tick-borne encephalitis viruses from Europe and Asia. *J Gen Virol* 1999;80:179–185.
154. Elbers K, Tautz N, Becher P, et al. Processing in the pestivirus E2-NS2 region: Identification of proteins p7 and E2p7. *J Virol* 1996;70: 4131–4135.
155. Enomoto N, Sakuma I, Asahina Y, et al. Comparison of full-length sequences of interferon-sensitive and resistant hepatitis C virus 1b. *J Clin Invest* 1995;96:224–230.

156. Enomoto N, Sakuma I, Asahina Y, et al. Mutations in the nonstructural protein 5A gene and response to interferon in patients with chronic hepatitis C virus 1b infection. *N Engl J Med* 1996;334:77–81.
157. Failla C, Tomei L, DeFrancesco R. Both NS3 and NS4A are required for proteolytic processing of hepatitis C virus nonstructural proteins. *J Virol* 1994;68:3753–3760.
158. Failla C, Tomei L, DeFrancesco R. An amino-terminal domain of the hepatitis C virus NS3 protease is essential for interaction with NS4A. *J Virol* 1995;69:1769–1777.
159. Falgout B, Bray M, Schlesinger JJ, Lai CJ. Immunization of mice with recombinant vaccinia virus expressing authentic dengue virus nonstructural protein NS1 protects against lethal dengue virus encephalitis. *J Virol* 1990;64:4356–4363.
160. Falgout B, Chanock R, Lai C-J. Proper processing of dengue virus nonstructural glycoprotein NS1 requires the N-terminal hydrophobic signal sequence and the downstream nonstructural protein NS2a. *J Virol* 1989;63:1852–1860.
161. Falgout B, Markoff L. Evidence that flavivirus NS1-NS2A cleavage is mediated by a membrane-bound host protease in the endoplasmic reticulum. *J Virol* 1995;69:7232–7243.
162. Falgout B, Miller RH, Lai C-J. Deletion analysis of Dengue virus type 4 nonstructural protein NS2B: Identification of a domain required for NS2B-NS3 proteinase activity. *J Virol* 1993;67:2034–2042.
163. Falgout B, Pethel M, Zhang Y-M, Lai C-J. Both nonstructural proteins NS2B and NS3 are required for the proteolytic processing of Dengue virus nonstructural proteins. *J Virol* 1991;65:2467–2475.
164. Farci P, Alter HJ, Wong DC, et al. Prevention of hepatitis C virus infection in chimpanzees after antibody-mediated *in vitro* neutralization. *Proc Natl Acad Sci U S A* 1994;91:7792–7796.
165. Farci P, Shimoda A, Wong D, et al. Prevention of hepatitis C virus infection in chimpanzees by hyperimmune serum against the hypervariable region 1 of the envelope 2 protein. *Proc Natl Acad Sci U S A* 1996;93:15394–15399.
166. Feinstone SM, Mihalik KB, Kamimura T, et al. Inactivation of hepatitis B virus and non-A, non-B hepatitis by chloroform. *Infect Immun* 1983;41:816–821.
167. Ferrari E, Wright-Minogue J, Fang JW, et al. Characterization of soluble hepatitis C virus RNA-dependent RNA polymerase expressed in *Escherichia coli*. *J Virol* 1999;73:1649–1654.
168. Fiordalisi G, Zanella I, Mantero G, et al. High prevalence of GB virus C infection in a group of Italian patients with hepatitis of unknown etiology. *J Infect Dis* 1996;174:181–183.
169. Fischler B, Lara C, Chen M, et al. Genetic evidence for mother-to-infant transmission of hepatitis G virus. *J Infect Dis* 1997;176:281–285.
170. Flamand M, Megret F, Mathieu M, et al. Dengue virus type 1 nonstructural glycoprotein NS1 is secreted from mammalian cells as a soluble hexamer in a glycosylation-dependent fashion. *J Virol* 1999;73:6104–6110.
171. Flint M, Maidens C, Loomis-Price LD, et al. Characterization of hepatitis C virus E2 glycoprotein interaction with a putative cellular receptor, CD81. *J Virol* 1999;73:6235–6244.
172. Flint M, McKeating JA. The C-terminal region of the hepatitis C virus E1 glycoprotein confers localization within the endoplasmic reticulum. *J Gen Virol* 1999;80:1943–1947.
173. Flint M, Thomas JM, Maidens CM, et al. Functional analysis of cell surface-expressed hepatitis C virus E2 glycoprotein. *J Virol* 1999;73:6782–6790.
174. Flores EF, Kreutz LC, Donis RO. Swine and ruminant pestiviruses require the same cellular factor to enter bovine cells. *J Gen Virol* 1996;77:1295–1303.
175. Forns X, Thimme R, Govindarajan S, et al. Hepatitis C virus lacking the hypervariable region 1 of the second envelope glycoprotein is infectious and causes acute resolving or persistent infection in chimpanzees. *Proc Natl Acad Sci U S A* 2000;97:13318–13323.
176. Forwood JK, Brooks A, Briggs LJ, et al. The 37-amino-acid interdomain of dengue virus NS5 protein contains a functional NLS and inhibitory CK2 site. *Biochem Biophys Res Commun* 1999;257:731–737.
177. Francki RIB, Fauquet CM, Knudson DL, Brown F. Classification and nomenclature of viruses: Fifth report of the international committee on taxonomy of viruses. *Arch Virol Suppl* 1991;2:223.
178. Francois C, Duverlie G, Rebouillat D, et al. Expression of hepatitis C virus proteins interferes with the antiviral action of interferon independently of PKR-mediated control of protein synthesis. *J Virol* 2000;74:5587–5596.
179. Frolov I, McBride MS, Rice CM. cis-acting RNA elements required for replication of bovine viral diarrhea virus-hepatitis C virus 5′ nontranslated region chimeras. *RNA* 1998;4:1418–1435.
180. Fujita T, Ishido S, Muramatsu S, et al. Suppression of actinomycin D-induced apoptosis by the NS3 protein of hepatitis C virus. *Biochem Biophys Res Commun* 1996;229:825–831.
181. Fukuma T, Enomoto N, Marumo F, Sato C. Mutations in the interferon-sensitivity determining region of hepatitis C virus and transcriptional activity of the nonstructural region 5A protein. *Hepatology* 1998;28:1147–1153.
182. Fukushi S, Katayama K, Kurihara C, et al. Complete 5′ noncoding region is necessary for the efficient internal initiation of hepatitis C virus RNA. *Biochem Biophys Res Commun* 1994;199:425–432.
183. Fukushi S, Kurihara C, Ishiyama N, et al. Nucleotide sequence of the 5′ noncoding region of hepatitis G virus isolated from Japanese patients: Comparison with reported isolates. *Biochem Biophys Res Commun* 1996;226:314–318.
184. Fukushi S, Kurihara C, Ishiyama N, et al. The sequence element of the internal ribosome entry site and a 25-kilodalton cellular protein contribute to efficient internal initiation of translation of hepatitis C virus RNA. *J Virol* 1997;71:1662–1666.
185. Gale M Jr, Blakely CM, Kwieciszewski B, et al. Control of PKR protein kinase by hepatitis C virus nonstructural 5A protein: Molecular mechanisms of kinase regulation. *Mol Cell Biol* 1998;18:5208–5218.
186. Gale M Jr, Kwieciszewski B, Dossett M, et al. Antiapoptotic and oncogenic potentials of hepatitis C virus are linked to interferon resistance by viral repression of the PKR protein kinase. *J Virol* 1999;73:6506–6516.
187. Gale MJ Jr, Korth MJ, Tang NM, et al. Evidence that hepatitis C virus resistance to interferon is mediated through repression of the PKR protein kinase by the nonstructural 5A protein. *Virology* 1997;230:217–227.
188. Gallinari P, Brennan D, Nardi C, et al. Multiple enzymatic activities associated with recombinant NS3 protein of hepatitis C virus. *J Virol* 1998;72:6758–6769.
189. Galun E, Burakova T, Ketzinel M, et al. Hepatitis C virus viremia in SCID→BNX mouse chimera. *J Infect Dis* 1995;172:25–30.
190. Ghosh AK, Majumder M, Steele R, et al. Hepatitis C virus NS5A protein modulates transcription through a novel cellular transcription factor SRCAP. *J Biol Chem* 2000;275:7184–7188.
191. Ghosh AK, Steele R, Meyer K, et al. Hepatitis C virus NS5A protein modulates cell cycle regulatory genes and promotes cell growth. *J Gen Virol* 1999;80:1179–1183.
192. Gollins SW, Porterfield JS. Flavivirus infection enhancement in macrophages: An electron microscopic study of viral cellular entry. *J Gen Virol* 1985;66:1969–1982.
193. Gollins SW, Porterfield JS. pH-dependent fusion between the flavivirus West Nile and liposomal model membranes. *J Gen Virol* 1986;67:157–166.
194. Gollins SW, Porterfield JS. The uncoating and infectivity of the flavivirus West Nile on interaction with cells: Effects of pH and ammonium chloride. *J Gen Virol* 1986;67:1941–1950.
195. Gong Y, Shannon A, Westaway EG, Gowans EJ. The replicative intermediate molecule of bovine viral diarrhoea virus contains multiple nascent strands. *Arch Virol* 1998;143:399–404.
196. Gong Y, Trowbridge R, Macnaughton TB, et al. Characterization of RNA synthesis during a one-step growth curve and of the replication mechanism of bovine viral diarrhoea virus. *J Gen Virol* 1996;2729–2736.
197. Gontarek RR, Gutshall LL, Herold KM, et al. hnRNP C and polypyrimidine tract-binding protein specifically interact with the pyrimidine-rich region within the 3′NTR of the HCV RNA genome. *Nucleic Acids Res* 1999;27:1457–1463.
198. Gorbalenya AE, Donchenko AP, Koonin EV, Blinov VM. N-terminal domains of putative helicases of flavi- and pestiviruses may be serine proteases. *Nucleic Acids Res* 1989;17:3889–3897.
199. Gorbalenya AE, Koonin EV, Donchenko AP, Blinov VM. Two related superfamilies of putative helicases involved in replication, recombination, repair and expression of DNA and RNA genomes. *Nucleic Acids Res* 1989;17:4713–4729.
200. Gorbalenya AE, Snijder EJ. Viral cysteine proteinases. *Perspect Drug Disc Des* 1996;6:64–86.
201. Grace K, Gartland M, Karayiannis P, et al. The 5′ untranslated region of GB virus B shows functional similarity to the internal ribosome entry site of hepatitis C virus. *J Gen Virol* 1999;80:2337–2341.

202. Grakoui A, Hanson HL, Rice CM. Bad time for Bonzo? Experimental models of HCV infection, replication and pathogenesis. *Hepatology* 2001 (in press).
203. Grakoui A, McCourt DW, Wychowski C, et al. Characterization of the hepatitis C virus-encoded serine proteinase: Determination of proteinase-dependent polyprotein cleavage sites. *J Virol* 1993;67: 2832–2843.
204. Grakoui A, McCourt DW, Wychowski C, et al. A second hepatitis C virus-encoded proteinase. *Proc Natl Acad Sci U S A* 1993;90: 10583–10587.
205. Grakoui A, Wychowski C, Lin C, et al. Expression and identification of hepatitis C virus polyprotein cleavage products. *J Virol* 1993;67: 1385–1395.
206. Grange T, Bouloy M, Girard M. Stable secondary structure at the 3′ end of the genome of yellow fever virus (17D vaccine strain). *FEBS Lett* 1985;188:159–163.
207. Grassmann CW, Isken O, Behrens SE. Assignment of the multifunctional NS3 protein of bovine viral diarrhea virus during RNA replication: An *in vivo* and *in vitro* study. *J Virol* 1999;73:9196–9205.
208. Gray EW, Nettleton PF. The ultrastructure of cell cultures infected with border disease and bovine virus diarrhoea viruses. *J Gen Virol* 1987;68:2339–2346.
209. Greiser-Wilke I, Dittmar KE, Liess B, Moennig V. Immunofluorescence studies of biotype-specific expression of bovine viral diarrhoea virus epitopes in infected cells. *J Gen Virol* 1991;72:2015–2019.
210. Greiser-Wilke I, Dittmar KE, Liess B, Moennig V. Heterogeneous expression of the non-structural protein p80/p125 in cells infected with different pestiviruses. *J Gen Virol* 1992;73:47–52.
211. Greiser-Wilke I, Haas L, Dittmar K, et al. RNA insertions and gene duplications in the nonstructural protein p125 region of pestivirus strains and isolates *in vitro* and *in vivo*. *Virology* 1993;193:977–980.
212. Grief C, Galler R, Cortes LM, Barth OM. Intracellular localisation of dengue-2 RNA in mosquito cell culture using electron microscopic in situ hybridisation. *Arch Virol* 1997;142:2347–2357.
213. Gritsun TS, Gould EA. Infectious transcripts of tick-borne encephalitis virus, generated in days by RT-PCR. *Virology* 1995;214:611–618.
214. Grun JB, Brinton MA. Characterization of West Nile virus RNA-dependent RNA polymerase and cellular terminal adenylyl and uridylyl transferase in cell-free extracts. *J Virol* 1986;60:1113–1124.
215. Grun JB, Brinton MA. Dissociation of NS5 from cell fractions containing West Nile virus-specific polymerase activity. *J Virol* 1987;61: 3641–3644.
216. Grun JB, Brinton MA. Separation of functional West Nile virus replication complexes from intracellular membrane fragments. *J Gen Virol* 1988;69:3121–3127.
217. Gu B, Liu C, Lin-Goerke J, et al. The RNA helicase and nucleotide triphosphatase activities of the bovine viral diarrhea virus NS3 protein are essential for viral replication. *J Virol* 2000;74:1794–1800.
218. Gualano RC, Pryor MJ, Cauchi MR, et al. Identification of a major determinant of mouse neurovirulence of dengue virus type 2 using stably cloned genomic-length cDNA. *J Gen Virol* 1998;79:437–446.
219. Gubler DJ, Meltzer M. Impact of dengue/dengue hemorrhagic fever on the developing world. *Adv Virus Res* 1999;53:35–70.
220. Guirakhoo F, Bolin RA, Roehrig JT. The Murray Valley encephalitis virus prM protein confers acid resistance to virus particles and alters the expression of epitopes within the R2 domain of E glycoprotein. *Virology* 1992;191:921–931.
221. Guirakhoo F, Heinz FX, Kunz C. Epitope model of tick-borne encephalitis virus envelope glycoprotein E: Analysis of structural properties, role of carbohydrate side chain, and conformational changes occurring at acidic pH. *Virology* 1989;169:90–99.
222. Guirakhoo F, Heinz FX, Mandl CW, et al. Fusion activity of flaviviruses: Comparison of mature and immature (prM-containing) tick-borne encephalitis virions. *J Gen Virol* 1991;72:1323–1329.
223. Guirakhoo F, Weltzin R, Chambers TJ, et al. Recombinant chimeric yellow fever-dengue type 2 virus is immunogenic and protective in nonhuman primates. *J Virol* 2000;74:5477–5485.
224. Guirakhoo F, Zhang ZX, Chambers TJ, et al. Immunogenicity, genetic stability, and protective efficacy of a recombinant, chimeric yellow fever-Japanese encephalitis virus (ChimeriVax-JE) as a live, attenuated vaccine candidate against Japanese encephalitis. *Virology* 1999; 257:363–372.
225. Gunji T, Kato N, Hijikata M, et al. Specific detection of positive and negative stranded hepatitis C viral RNA using chemical RNA modification. *Arch Virol* 1994;134:293–302.
226. Gutierrez RA, Dawson GJ, Knigge MF, et al. Seroprevalence of GB virus C and persistence of RNA and antibody. *J Med Virol* 1997;53:167–173.
227. Gwack Y, Kim DW, Han JH, Choe J. Characterization of RNA binding activity and RNA helicase activity of the hepatitis C virus NS3 protein. *Biochem Biophys Res Commun* 1996;225:654–659.
228. Gwack Y, Kim DW, Han JH, Choe J. DNA helicase activity of the hepatitis C virus nonstructural protein 3. *Eur J Biochem* 1997;250: 47–54.
229. Gwack Y, Yoo H, Song I, et al. RNA-stimulated ATPase and RNA helicase activities and RNA binding domain of hepatitis G virus nonstructural protein 3. *J Virol* 1999;73:2909–2915.
230. Hahm B, Kim YK, Kim JH, et al. Heterogeneous nuclear ribonucleoprotein L interacts with the 3′ border of the internal ribosomal entry site of hepatitis C virus. *J Virol* 1998;72:8782–8788.
231. Hahn CS, Hahn YS, Rice CM, et al. Conserved elements in the 3′ untranslated region of flavivirus RNAs and potential cyclization sequences. *J Mol Biol* 1987;198:33–41.
232. Hahn YS, Galler R, Hunkapiller T, et al. Nucleotide sequence of dengue 2 RNA and comparison of the encoded proteins with those of other flaviviruses. *Virology* 1988;162:167–180.
233. Hall RA, Khromykh AA, Mackenzie JM, et al. Loss of dimerisation of the nonstructural protein NS1 of Kunjin virus delays viral replication and reduces virulence in mice, but still allows secretion of NS1. *Virology* 1999;264:66–75.
234. Halstead SB. Pathogenesis of dengue: Challenges to molecular biology. *Science* 1988;239:476–481.
235. Halstead SB. Antibody, macrophages, dengue virus infection, shock, and hemorrhage: A pathogenetic cascade. *Rev Infect Dis* 1989;11 (suppl 4):S830–839.
236. Halstead SB, O'Rourke EJ. Antibody-enhanced dengue virus infection in primate leukocytes. *Nature* 1977;265:739–741.
237. Halstead SB, O'Rourke EJ. Dengue viruses and mononuclear phagocytes. I. Infection enhancement by non-neutralizing antibody. *J Exp Med* 1977;146:201–217.
238. Halstead SB, O'Rourke EJ, Allison AC. Dengue viruses and mononuclear phagocytes. II. Identity of blood and tissue leukocytes supporting *in vitro* infection. *J Exp Med* 1977;146:218–229.
239. Han JH, Shyamala V, Richman KH, et al. Characterization of the terminal regions of hepatitis C viral RNA: Indentification of conserved sequences in the 5′ untranslated region and poly(A) tails at the 3′ end. *Proc Natl Acad Sci U S A* 1991;88:1711–1715.
240. Handa A, Jubran RF, Dickstein B, et al. GB virus C/hepatitis G virus infection is frequent in American children and young adults. *Clin Infect Dis* 2000;30:569–571.
241. Harada S, Watanabe Y, Takeuchi K, et al. Expression of processed core protein of hepatitis C virus in mammalian cells. *J Virol* 1991;65: 3015–3021.
242. Harada T, Tautz N, Thiel HJ. E2-p7 region of the bovine viral diarrhea virus polyprotein: Processing and functional studies. *J Virol* 2000;74: 9498–9506.
243. Harpin S, Hurley DJ, Mbikay M, et al. Vaccination of cattle with a DNA plasmid encoding the bovine viral diarrhoea virus major glycoprotein E2. *J Gen Virol* 1999;80:3137–3144.
244. Hase T, Summers PL, Cohen WH. A comparative study of entry modes into C6/36 cells by Semliki Forest and Japanese encephalitis viruses. *Arch Virol* 1989;108:101–114.
245. Hase T, Summers PL, Eckels KH. Flavivirus entry into cultured mosquito cells and human peripheral blood monocytes. *Arch Virol* 1989; 104:129–143.
246. Hase T, Summers PL, Eckels KH, Baze WB. An electron and immunoelectron microscopic study of dengue-2 virus infection of cultured mosquito cells: Maturation events. *Arch Virol* 1987;92:273–291.
247. Hase T, Summers PL, Eckels KH, Baze WB. Maturation process of Japanese encephalitis virus in cultured mosquito cells *in vitro* and mouse brain cells *in vivo*. *Arch Virol* 1987;96:135–151.
248. Hashimoto H, Nomoto A, Watanabe K, et al. Molecular cloning and complete nucleotide sequence of the genome of Japanese encephalitis virus Beijing-1 strain. *Virus Genes* 1988;1:305–317.
249. Hayashi N, Higashi H, Kaminaka K, et al. Molecular cloning and heterogeneity of the human hepatitis C virus (HCV) genome. *J Hepatol* 1993;17(suppl. 3):S94–107.
250. He LF, Alling D, Popkin T, et al. Determining the size of non-A, non-B hepatitis by filtration. *J Infect Dis* 1987;156:636–640.
251. He RT, Innis BL, Nisalak A, et al. Antibodies that block virus attachment to Vero cells are a major component of the human neutralizing

antibody response against dengue virus type 2. *J Med Virol* 1995;45: 451–461.
252. Heilek GM, Peterson MG. A point mutation abolishes the helicase but not the nucleoside triphosphatase activity of hepatitis C virus NS3 protein. *J Virol* 1997;71:6264–6266.
253. Heinz FX. Epitope mapping of flavivirus glycoproteins. *Adv Virus Res* 1986;31:103–168.
254. Heinz FX, Stiasny K, Puschner-Auer G, et al. Structural changes and functional control of the tick-borne encephalitis virus glycoprotein E by the heterodimeric association with protein prM. *Virology* 1994; 198:109–117.
255. Henchal EA, Henchal LS, Schlesinger JJ. Synergistic interactions of anti-NS1 monoclonal antibodies protect passively immunized mice from lethal challenge with dengue 2 virus. *J Gen Virol* 1988;69: 2101–2107.
256. Higginbottom A, Quinn ER, Kuo CC, et al. Identification of amino acid residues in CD81 critical for interaction with hepatitis C virus envelope glycoprotein E2. *J Virol* 2000;74:3642–3649.
257. Hijikata M, Kato N, Ootsuyama Y, et al. Hypervariable regions in the putative glycoprotein of hepatitis C virus. *Biochem Biophys Res Commun* 1991;175:220–228.
258. Hijikata M, Kato N, Ootsuyama Y, et al. Gene mapping of the putative structural region of the hepatitis C virus genome by *in vitro* processing analysis. *Proc Natl Acad Sci U S A* 1991;88:5547–5551.
259. Hijikata M, Mizushima H, Akagi T, et al. Two distinct proteinase activities required for the processing of a putative nonstructural precursor protein of hepatitis C virus. *J Virol* 1993;67:4665–4675.
260. Hijikata M, Mizushima H, Tanji Y, et al. Proteolytic processing and membrane association of putative nonstructural proteins of hepatitis C virus. *Proc Natl Acad Sci U S A* 1993;90:10773–10777.
261. Hijikata M, Shimizu YK, Kato H, et al. Equilibrium centrifugation studies of hepatitis C virus: Evidence for circulating immune complexes. *J Virol* 1993;67:1953–1958.
262. Hirota M, Satoh S, Asabe S, et al. Phosphorylation of nonstructural 5A protein of hepatitis C virus: HCV group-specific hyperphosphorylation. *Virology* 1999;257:130–137.
263. Hirowatari Y, Hijikata M, Tanji Y, et al. Two proteinase activities in HCV polypeptide expressed in insect cells using baculovirus vector. *Arch Virol* 1993;133:349–356.
264. Hoff HS, Donis RO. Induction of apoptosis and cleavage of poly (ADP-ribose) polymerase by cytopathic bovine viral diarrhea virus infection. *Virus Res* 1997;49:101–113.
265. Hollinger FB, Gitnick G, Aach RD, et al. Non-A, non-B hepatitis transmission in chimpanzees: A project of the transfusion-transmitted viruses study group. *Intervirology* 1978;10:60–68.
266. Hollingshead PG, Brawner TA, Fleming TP. St. Louis encephalitis virus temperature-sensitive mutants. I. Induction, isolation, and preliminary characterization. *Arch Virol* 1983;75:171–179.
267. Honda A, Arai Y, Hirota N, et al. Hepatitis C virus structural proteins induce liver cell injury in transgenic mice. *J Med Virol* 1999;59:281–289.
268. Honda M, Brown EA, Lemon SM. Stability of a stem-loop involving the initiator AUG controls the efficiency of internal initiation of translation on hepatitis C virus RNA. *RNA* 1996;2:955–968.
269. Honda M, Kaneko S, Matsushita E, et al. Cell cycle regulation of hepatitis C virus internal ribosome entry site-directed translation. *Gastroenterology* 2000;118:152–162.
270. Honda M, Ping LH, Rijnbrand RC, et al. Structural requirements for initiation of translation by internal ribosome entry within genome-length hepatitis C virus RNA. *Virology* 1996;222:31–42.
271. Hong Z, Ferrari E, Wright-Minogue J, et al. Enzymatic characterization of hepatitis C virus NS3/4A complexes expressed in mammalian cells by using the herpes simplex virus amplicon system. *J Virol* 1996; 70:4261–4268.
272. Hori H, Lai C-J. Cleavage of dengue virus NS1-NS2A requires an octapeptide sequence at the C terminus of NS1. *J Virol* 1990;64: 4573–4577.
273. Horzinek MC. *Non-Arthropod-Borne Togaviruses*. London: Academic Press, 1981.
274. Howe AY, Chase R, Taremi SS, et al. A novel recombinant single-chain hepatitis C virus NS3-NS4A protein with improved helicase activity. *Protein Sci* 1999;8:1332–1341.
275. Hsu HH, Donets M, Greenberg HB, Feinstone SM. Characterization of hepatitis C virus structural proteins with a recombinant baculovirus expression system. *Hepatology* 1993;17:763–771.
276. Hulst MM, Himes G, Newbigin E, Moorman RJM. Glycoprotein E2 of classical swine fever virus: Expression in insect cells and identification as a ribonuclease. *Virology* 1994;200:558–565.
277. Hulst MM, Moormann RJ. Inhibition of pestivirus infection in cell culture by envelope proteins E(rns) and E2 of classical swine fever virus: E(rns) and E2 interact with different receptors. *J Gen Virol* 1997;78:2779–2787.
278. Hulst MM, Panoto FE, Hoekman A, et al. Inactivation of the RNase activity of glycoprotein E^{rns} results in a cytopathogenic virus. *J Virol* 1998;72:151–157.
279. Hulst MM, Westra DF, Wensvoort G, Moormann RJ. Glycoprotein E1 of hog cholera virus expressed in insect cells protects swine from hog cholera. *J Virol* 1993;67:5435–5442.
280. Hung SL, Lee PL, Chen HW, et al. Analysis of the steps involved in Dengue virus entry into host cells. *Virology* 1999;257:156–167.
281. Hurrelbrink RJ, Nestorowicz A, McMinn PC. Characterization of infectious Murray Valley encephalitis virus derived from a stably cloned genome-length cDNA. *J Gen Virol* 1999;80:3115–3125.
282. Hüssy P, Langen H, Mous J, Jacobsen H. Hepatitis C virus core protein: Carboxy-terminal boundaries of two processed species suggest cleavage by a signal peptide peptidase. *Virology* 1996;224:93–104.
283. Hüssy P, Schmid G, Mous J, Jacobsen H. Purification and *in vitro*-phospholabeling of secretory envelope proteins E1 and E2 of hepatitis C virus expressed in insect cells. *Virus Res* 1996;45: 45–57.
284. Hwang SB, Lo S-Y, Ou J-H, Lai MMC. Detection of cellular proteins and viral core protein interacting with the 5′ untranslated region of hepatitis C virus RNA. *J Biomed Sci* 1995;2:227–236.
285. Ide Y, Tanimoto A, Sasaguri Y, Padmanabhan R. Hepatitis C virus NS5A protein is phosphorylated *in vitro* by a stably bound protein kinase from HeLa cells and by cAMP-dependent protein kinase A-a catalytic subunit. *Gene* 1997;201:151–158.
286. Ide Y, Zhang L, Chen M, et al. Characterization of the nuclear localization signal and subcellular distribution of hepatitis C virus nonstructural protein NS5A. *Gene* 1996;182:203–211.
287. Iizuka N, Najita L, Franzusoff A, Sarnow P. Cap-dependent and cap-independent translation by internal initiation of mRNAs in cell extracts prepared from *Saccharomyces cerevisiae. Mol Cell Biol* 1994; 14:7322–7330.
288. Ikeda M, Sugiyama K, Tanaka T, et al. Lactoferrin markedly inhibits hepatitis C virus infection in cultured human hepatocytes. *Biochem Biophys Res Commun* 1998;245:549–553.
289. Inoue Y, Miyazaki M, Ohashi R, et al. Ubiquitous presence of cellular proteins that specifically bind to the 3′ terminal region of hepatitis C virus. *Biochem Biophys Res Commun* 1998;245:198–203.
290. Inudoh M, Nyunoya H, Tanaka T, et al. Antigenicity of hepatitis C virus envelope proteins expressed in Chinese hamster ovary cells. *Vaccine* 1996;14:1590–1596.
291. Iqbal M, Flick-Smith H, McCauley JW. Interactions of bovine viral diarrhoea virus glycoprotein E(rns) with cell surface glycosaminoglycans. *J Gen Virol* 2000;81:451–459.
292. Ishak R, Tovey DG, Howard CR. Morphogenesis of yellow fever virus 17D in infected cell cultures. *J Gen Virol* 1988;69:325–335.
293. Ishido S, Fujita T, Hotta H. Complex formation of NS5B with NS3 and NS4A proteins of hepatitis C virus. *Biochem Biophys Res Commun* 1998;244:35–40.
294. Ishido S, Muramatsu S, Fujita T, et al. Wild-type, but not mutant-type, p53 enhances nuclear accumulation of the NS3 protein of hepatitis C virus. *Biochem Biophys Res Commun* 1997;230:431–436.
295. Ito T, Lai MMC. Determination of the secondary structure of and cellular protein binding to the 3′-untranslated region of the hepatitis C virus RNA genome. *J Virol* 1997;71:8698–8706.
296. Ito T, Tahara SM, Lai MMC. The 3′-untranslated region of hepatitis C virus RNA enhances translation from an internal ribosomal entry site. *J Virol* 1998;72:8789–8796.
297. Jacobs SC, Stephenson JR, Wilkinson GW. High-level expression of the tick-borne encephalitis virus NS1 protein by using an adenovirus-based vector: Protection elicited in a murine model. *J Virol* 1992;66: 2086–2095.
298. Jäger J, Smerdon SJ, Wang J, et al. Comparison of three different crystal forms shows HIV-1 reverse transcriptase displays an internal swivel motion. *Structure* 1994;2:869–876.
299. Jan LR, Yang CS, Trent DW, et al. Processing of Japanese encephalitis virus non-structural proteins: NS2B-NS3 complex and heterologous proteases. *J Gen Virol* 1995;76:573–580.
300. Jin DY, Wang HL, Zhou Y, et al. Hepatitis C virus core protein-

induced loss of LZIP function correlates with cellular transformation. *EMBO J* 2000;19:729–740.
301. Jin L, Peterson DL. Expression, isolation, and characterization of the hepatitis C virus ATPase/RNA helicase. *Arch Biochem Biophys* 1995; 323:47–53.
302. Kadare G, Haenni AL. Virus-encoded RNA helicases. *J Virol* 1997;71: 2583–2590.
303. Kaito M, Watanabe S, Tsukiyama-Kohara K, et al. Hepatitis C virus particle detected by immunoelectron microscopic study. *J Gen Virol* 1994;75:1755–1760.
304. Kaminski A, Hunt SL, Patton JG, Jackson RJ. Direct evidence that polypyrimidine tract binding protein (PTB) is essential for internal initiation of translation of encephalomyocarditis virus RNA. *RNA* 1995;1:924–938.
305. Kanai A, Tanabe K, Kohara M. Poly(U) binding activity of hepatitis C virus NS3 protein, a putative RNA helicase. *FEBS Lett* 1995;376: 221–224.
306. Kaneko T, Tanji Y, Satoh S, et al. Production of two phosphoproteins from the NS5A region of the hepatitis C viral genome. *Biochem Biophys Res Commun* 1994;205:320–326.
307. Kanto T, Hayashi N, Takehara T, et al. Buoyant density of hepatitis C virus recovered from infected hosts: Two different features in sucrose equilibrium density-gradient centrifugation related to degree of liver inflammation. *Hepatology* 1994;19:296–302.
308. Kao CC, Del Vecchio AM, Zhong W. De novo initiation of RNA synthesis by a recombinant flaviviridae RNA-dependent RNA polymerase. *Virology* 1999;253:1–7.
309. Kao JH, Chen PJ, Hsiang SC, et al. Phylogenetic analysis of GB virus C: Comparison of isolates from Africa, North America, and Taiwan. *J Infect Dis* 1996;174:410–413.
310. Kapoor M, Zhang L, Mohan PM, Padmanabhan R. Synthesis and characterization of an infectious dengue virus type-2 RNA genome (New Guinea C strain). *Gene* 1995;162:175–180.
311. Kapoor M, Zhang L, Ramachandra M, et al. Association between NS3 and NS5 proteins of dengue virus type 2 in the putative RNA replicase is linked to differential phosphorylation of NS5. *J Biol Chem* 1995; 270:19100–19106.
312. Kato N, Hijikata M, Ootsuyama Y, et al. Molecular cloning of the human hepatitis C virus genome from Japanese patients with non-A, non-B hepatitis. *Proc Natl Acad Sci U S A* 1990;87:9524–9528.
313. Kato N, Lan K-H, Ono-Nita SK, et al. Hepatitis C virus nonstructural region 5A protein is a potent transcriptional activator. *J Virol* 1997;71: 8856–8859.
314. Kato N, Ootsuyama Y, Ohkoshi S, et al. Characterization of hypervariable regions in the putative envelope protein of hepatitis C virus. *Biochem Biophys Res Commun* 1992;189:119–127.
315. Kato N, Sekiya H, Ootsuyama Y, et al. Humoral immune response to hypervariable region 1 of the putative envelope glycoprotein (gp70) of hepatitis C virus. *J Virol* 1993;67:3923–3930.
316. Kaufman BM, Summers PL, Dubois DR, et al. Monoclonal antibodies for dengue virus prM glycoprotein protect mice against lethal dengue infection. *Am J Trop Med Hyg* 1989;41:576–580.
317. Kawamura T, Furusaka A, Koziel MJ, et al. Transgenic expression of hepatitis C virus structural proteins in the mouse. *Hepatology* 1997; 25:1014–1021.
318. Khromykh AA, Kenney MT, Westaway EG. trans-Complementation of flavivirus RNA polymerase gene NS5 by using Kunjin virus replicon-expressing BHK cells. *J Virol* 1998;72:7270–7279.
319. Khromykh AA, Sedlak PL, Guyatt KJ, et al. Efficient trans-complementation of the flavivirus kunjin NS5 protein but not of the NS1 protein requires its coexpression with other components of the viral replicase. *J Virol* 1999;73:10272–10280.
320. Khromykh AA, Sedlak PL, Westaway EG. trans-Complementation analysis of the flavivirus Kunjin ns5 gene reveals an essential role for translation of its N-terminal half in RNA replication. *J Virol* 1999;73: 9247–9255.
321. Khromykh AA, Sedlak PL, Westaway EG. cis- and trans-acting elements in flavivirus RNA replication. *J Virol* 2000;74:3253–3263.
322. Khromykh AA, Westaway EG. Completion of Kunjin virus RNA sequence and recovery of an infectious RNA transcribed from stably cloned full-length cDNA. *J Virol* 1994;68:4580–4588.
323. Khromykh AA, Westaway EG. Subgenomic replicons of the flavivirus Kunjin: Construction and applications. *J Virol* 1997;71:1497–1505.
324. Kidd VJ. Proteolytic activities that mediate apoptosis. *Annu Rev Physiol* 1998;60:533–573.
325. Kim DW, Gwack Y, Han JH, Choe J. C-terminal domain of the hepatitis C virus NS3 protein contains an RNA helicase activity. *Biochem Biophys Res Commun* 1995;215:160–166.
326. Kim DW, Suzuki R, Harada T, et al. Trans-suppression of gene expression by hepatitis C viral core protein. *Jpn J Med Sci Biol* 1994;47: 211–220.
327. Kim JL, Morgenstern KA, Griffith JP, et al. Hepatitis C virus NS3 RNA helicase domain with a bound oligonucleotide: The crystal structure provides insights into the mode of unwinding. *Structure* 1998;6:89–100.
328. Kim JL, Morgenstern KA, Lin C, et al. Crystal structure of the hepatitis C virus NS3 protease domain complexed with a synthetic NS4A cofactor peptide. *Cell* 1996;87:343–355.
329. Kimura T, Kimura-Kuroda J, Nagashima K, Yasui K. Analysis of virus-cell binding characteristics on the determination of Japanese encephalitis virus susceptibility. *Arch Virol* 1994;139:239–251.
330. Kimura T, Ohyama A. Association between the pH-dependent conformational change of West Nile flavivirus E protein and virus-mediated membrane fusion. *J Gen Virol* 1988;69:1247–1254.
331. Kinney RM, Butrapet S, Chang GJ, et al. Construction of infectious cDNA clones for dengue 2 virus: Strain 16681 and its attenuated vaccine derivative, strain PDK-53. *Virology* 1997;230:300–308.
332. Kiyosawa K, Sodeyama T, Tanaka E, et al. Interrelationship of blood transfusion, non-A, non-B hepatitis and hepatocellular carcinoma: Analysis by detection of antibody to hepatitis C virus. *Hepatology* 1990;12:671–675.
333. Ko KK, Igarashi A, Fukai K. Electron microscopic observation on *Aedes albopictus* cells infected with dengue viruses. *Arch Virol* 1979; 62:41–52.
334. Koch JO, Bartenschlager R. Modulation of hepatitis C virus NS5A hyperphosphorylation by nonstructural proteins NS3, NS4A, and NS4B. *J Virol* 1999;73:7138–7146.
335. Kohara M, Tsukiyama-Kohara K, Maki N, et al. Expression and characterization of glycoprotein gp35 of hepatitis C virus using recombinant vaccinia virus. *J Gen Virol* 1992;73:2313–2318.
336. Koike K, Moriya K, Ishibashi K, et al. Expression of hepatitis C virus envelope proteins in transgenic mice. *J Gen Virol* 1995;76:3031–3038.
337. Kolykhalov AA, Agapov EV, Blight KJ, et al. Transmission of hepatitis C by intrahepatic inoculation with transcribed RNA. *Science* 1997; 277:570–574.
338. Kolykhalov AA, Agapov EV, Rice CM. Specificity of the hepatitis C virus serine proteinase: Effects of substitutions at the 3/4A, 4A/4B, 4B/5A, and 5A/5B cleavage sites on polyprotein processing. *J Virol* 1994;68:7525–7533.
339. Kolykhalov AA, Feinstone SM, Rice CM. Identification of a highly conserved sequence element at the 3′ terminus of hepatitis C virus genome RNA. *J Virol* 1996;70:3363–3371.
340. Kolykhalov AA, Mihalik K, Feinstone SM, Rice CM. Hepatitis C virus-encoded enzymatic activities and conserved RNA elements in the 3′ nontranslated region are essential for virus replication *in vivo*. *J Virol* 2000;74:2046–2051.
341. Konishi E, Mason PW. Proper maturation of the Japanese encephalitis virus envelope glycoprotein requires cosynthesis with the premembrane protein. *J Virol* 1993;67:1672–1675.
342. Konishi E, Pincus S, Paoletti E, et al. Mice immunized with a subviral particle containing the Japanese encephalitis virus prM/M and E proteins are protected from lethal JEV infection. *Virology* 1992;188:714–720.
343. Konishi E, Yamaoka M, Khin Sane W, et al. Induction of protective immunity against Japanese encephalitis in mice by immunization with a plasmid encoding Japanese encephalitis virus premembrane and envelope genes. *J Virol* 1998;72:4925–4930.
344. Koonin EV. Computer-assisted identification of a putative methyltransferase domain in NS5 protein of flaviviruses and lambda 2 protein of reovirus. *J Gen Virol* 1993;74:733–740.
345. Koonin EV, Dolja VV. Evolution and taxonomy of positive-strand RNA viruses: Implications of comparative analysis of amino acid sequences [published erratum appears in *Crit Rev Biochem Mol Biol* 1993;28:546]. *Crit Rev Biochem Mol Biol* 1993;28:375–430.
346. Kopecky J, Grubhoffer L, Kovar V, et al. A putative host cell receptor for tick-borne encephalitis virus identified by anti-idiotypic antibodies and virus affinoblotting. *Intervirology* 1999;42:9–16.
347. Kümmerer BM, Meyers G. Correlation between point mutations in NS2 and the viability and cytopathogenicity of bovine viral diarrhea virus strain Oregon analyzed with an infectious cDNA clone. *J Virol* 2000;74:390–400.

348. Kümmerer BM, Stoll D, Meyers G. Bovine viral diarrhea virus strain Oregon: A novel mechanism for processing of NS2-3 based on point mutations. *J Virol* 1998;72:4127–4138.
349. Kuno G, Chang GJ, Tsuchiya KR, et al. Phylogeny of the genus *Flavivirus*. *J Virol* 1998;72:73–83.
350. Kupfermann H, Thiel H-J, Dubovi EJ, Meyers G. Bovine viral diarrhea virus: Characterization of a cytopathogenic defective interfering particle with two internal deletions. *J Virol* 1996;70:8175–8181.
351. Kurosaki M, Enomoto N, Marumo F, Sato C. Rapid sequence variation of the hypervariable region of hepatitis C virus during the course of chronic infection. *Hepatology* 1993;18:1293–1299.
352. Kyono K, Miyashiro M, Taguchi I. Detection of hepatitis C virus helicase activity using the scintillation proximity assay system. *Anal Biochem* 1998;257:120–126.
353. Lagging LM, Meyer K, Owens RJ, Ray R. Functional role of hepatitis C virus chimeric glycoproteins in the infectivity of pseudotyped virus. *J Virol* 1998;72:3539–3546.
354. Lai C-J, Zhao B, Hori H, Bray M. Infectious RNA transcribed from stably cloned full-length cDNA of dengue type 4 virus. *Proc Natl Acad Sci U S A* 1991;88:5139–5143.
355. Lai VC, Kao CC, Ferrari E, et al. Mutational analysis of bovine viral diarrhea virus RNA-dependent RNA polymerase. *J Virol* 1999;73: 10129–10136.
356. Lam NP, Neumann AU, Gretch DR, et al. Dose-dependent acute clearance of hepatitis C genotype 1 virus with interferon alfa. *Hepatology* 1997;26:226–231.
357. Lancaster MU, Hodgetts SI, Mackenzie JS, Urosevic N. Characterization of defective viral RNA produced during persistent infection of Vero cells with Murray Valley encephalitis virus. *J Virol* 1998;72: 2474–2482.
358. Lanciotti RS, Roehrig JT, Deubel V, et al. Origin of the West Nile virus responsible for an outbreak of encephalitis in the northeastern United States. *Science* 1999;286:2333–2337.
359. Lanford RE, Chavez D, Chisari FV, Sureau C. Lack of detection of negative-strand hepatitis C virus RNA in peripheral blood mononuclear cells and other extrahepatic tissues by the highly strand-specific rTth reverse transcriptase PCR. *J Virol* 1995;69:8079–8083.
360. Lanford RE, Notvall L, Chavez D, et al. Analysis of hepatitis C virus capsid, E1, and E2/NS1 proteins expressed in insect cells. *Virology* 1993;197:225–235.
361. Laude H. Improved method for the purification of hog cholera virus. *Arch Virol* 1977;54:41–51.
362. Laude H. Hog cholera virus: Art and facts. *Ann Rech Vet* 1987;18: 127–138.
363. Leary K, Blair CD. Sequential events in the morphogenesis of Japanese encephalitis virus. *J Ultrastruct Res* 1980;72:123–129.
364. Leary TP, Desai SM, Yamaguchi J, et al. Species-specific variants of GB virus A in captive monkeys [published erratum appears in *J Virol* 1997;71:8953]. *J Virol* 1996;70:9028–9030.
365. Leary TP, Muerhoff AS, Simons JN, et al. Sequence and genomic organization of GBV-C: A novel member of the *Flaviviridae* associated with human non-A-E hepatitis. *J Med Virol* 1996;48:60–67.
366. Lee E, Stocks CE, Amberg SM, et al. Mutagenesis of the signal sequence of yellow fever virus prM protein: Enhancement of signalase cleavage *in vitro* is lethal for virus production. *J Virol* 2000; 74:24–32.
367. Lee JM, Crooks AJ, Stephenson JR. The synthesis and maturation of a non-structural extracellular antigen from tick-borne encephalitis virus and its relationship to the intracellular NS1 protein. *J Gen Virol* 1989;70:335–343.
368. Lefrere JJ, Loiseau P, Maury J, et al. Natural history of GBV-C/hepatitis G virus infection through the follow-up of GBV-C/hepatitis G virus-infected blood donors and recipients studied by RNA polymerase chain reaction and anti-E2 serology. *Blood* 1997;90: 3776–3780.
369. Lefrere JJ, Roudot-Thoraval F, Morand-Joubert L, et al. Prevalence of GB virus type C/hepatitis G virus RNA and of anti-E2 in individuals at high or low risk for blood-borne or sexually transmitted viruses: Evidence of sexual and parenteral transmission. *Transfusion* 1999;39: 83–94.
370. Leinbach SS, Bhat RA, Xia S-M, et al. Substrate specificity of the NS3 serine proteinase of hepatitis C virus as determined by mutagenesis at the NS3/NS4A junction. *Virology* 1994;204:163–169.
371. Lesburg CA, Cable MB, Ferrari E, et al. Crystal structure of the RNA-dependent RNA polymerase from hepatitis C virus reveals a fully encircled active site. *Nat Struct Biol* 1999;6:937–943.
372. Lesniewski R, Okasinski G, Carrick R, et al. Antibody to hepatitis C virus second envelope (HCV-E2) glycoprotein: A new marker of HCV infection closely associated with viremia. *J Med Virol* 1995;45: 415–422.
373. Li H, Clum S, You S, et al. The serine protease and RNA-stimulated nucleoside triphosphatase and RNA helicase functional domains of dengue virus type 2 NS3 converge within a region of 20 amino acids. *J Virol* 1999;73:3108–3116.
374. Li Y, Korolev S, Waksman G. Crystal structures of open and closed forms of binary and ternary complexes of the large fragment of *Thermus aquaticus* DNA polymerase I: Structural basis for nucleotide incorporation. *EMBO J* 1998;17:7514–7525.
375. Liebler EM, Waschbusch J, Pohlenz JF, et al. Distribution of antigen of noncytopathogenic and cytopathogenic bovine virus diarrhea virus biotypes in the intestinal tract of calves following experimental production of mucosal disease. *Arch Virol Suppl* 1991;3:109–124.
376. Liess B. Hog cholera. In: *A World Geography of Epidemiology and Control*. London: Academic Press, 1981:627–650.
377. Lin C, Amberg SM, Chambers TJ, Rice CM. Cleavage at a novel site in the NS4A region by the yellow fever virus NS2B-3 proteinase is a prerequisite for processing at the downstream 4A/4B signalase site. *J Virol* 1993;67:2327–2335.
378. Lin C, Chambers TJ, Rice CM. Mutagenesis of conserved residues at the yellow fever virus 3/4A and 4B/5 dibasic cleavage sites: Effects on cleavage efficiency and polyprotein processing. *Virology* 1993;192: 596–604.
379. Lin C, Lindenbach BD, Prágai B, et al. Processing of the hepatitis C virus E2-NS2 region: Identification of p7 and two distinct E2-specific products with different C termini. *J Virol* 1994;68:5063–5073.
380. Lin C, Prágai B, Grakoui A, et al. Hepatitis C virus NS3 serine proteinase: Trans-cleavage requirements and processing kinetics. *J Virol* 1994;68:8147–8157.
381. Lin C, Thomson JA, Rice CM. A central region in the hepatitis C virus NS4A protein allows formation of an active NS3-NS4A serine proteinase complex *in vivo* and *in vitro*. *J Virol* 1995;69:4373–4380.
382. Lin C, Wu JW, Hsiao K, Su MS. The hepatitis C virus NS4A protein: Interactions with the NS4B and NS5A proteins. *J Virol* 1997;71: 6465–6471.
383. Lin YL, Chen LK, Liao CL, et al. DNA immunization with Japanese encephalitis virus nonstructural protein NS1 elicits protective immunity in mice. *J Virol* 1998;72:191–200.
384. Lindenbach BD, Rice CM. trans-Complementation of yellow fever virus NS1 reveals a role in early RNA replication. *J Virol* 1997;71: 9608–9617.
385. Lindenbach BD, Rice CM. Genetic interaction of flavivirus nonstructural proteins NS1 and NS4A as a determinant of replicase function. *J Virol* 1999;73:4611–4621.
386. Linnen J, Wages J, Zhangkeck ZY, et al. Molecular cloning and disease association of hepatitis G virus: A transfusion-transmissible agent. *Science* 1996;271:505–508.
387. Linnen JM, Fung K, Fry KE, et al. Sequence variation and phylogenetic analysis of the 5′ terminus of hepatitis G virus. *J Viral Hepat* 1997;4:293–302.
388. Liprandi F, Walder R. Replication of virulent and attenuated strains of yellow fever virus in human monocytes and macrophage-like cells (U937). *Arch Virol* 1983;76:51–61.
389. Liu Q, Bhat RA, Prince AM, Zhang P. The hepatitis C virus NS2 protein generated by NS2-3 autocleavage is required for NS5A phosphorylation. *Biochem Biophys Res Commun* 1999;254:572–577.
390. Liu Q, Tackney C, Bhat RA, et al. Regulated processing of hepatitis C virus core protein is linked to subcellular localization. *J Virol* 1997;71: 657–662.
391. Lo S-Y, Masiarz F, Hwang SB, et al. Differential subcellular localization of hepatitis C virus core gene products. *Virology* 1995;213:455–461.
392. Lo S-Y, Selby M, Tong M, Ou J-H. Comparative studies of the core gene products of two different hepatitis C virus isolates: Two alternative forms determined by a single amino acid substitution. *Virology* 1994;199:124–131.
393. Lo S-Y, Selby MJ, Ou J-H. Interaction between hepatitis C virus core protein and E1 envelope protein. *J Virol* 1996;70:5177–5182.
394. Lobigs M. Proteolytic processing of a Murray Valley encephalitis virus non-structural polyprotein segment containing the viral pro-

teinase: Accumulation of a NS3-4A precursor which requires mature NS3 for efficient processing. *J Gen Virol* 1992;73:2305–2312.

395. Lobigs M. Flavivirus premembrane protein cleavage and spike heterodimer secretion requires the function of the viral proteinase NS3. *Proc Natl Acad Sci U S A* 1993;90:6218–6222.
396. Lohmann V, Körner F, Herian U, Bartenschlager R. Biochemical properties of hepatitis C virus NS5B RNA-dependent RNA polymerase and identification of amino acid sequence motifs essential for enzymatic activity. *J Virol* 1997;71:8416–8428.
397. Lohmann V, Korner F, Koch JO, et al. Replication of subgenomic hepatitis C virus RNAs in a hepatoma cell line. *Science* 1999;285: 110–113.
398. Lohmann V, Overton H, Bartenschlager R. Selective stimulation of hepatitis C virus and pestivirus NS5B RNA polymerase activity by GTP. *J Biol Chem* 1999;274:10807–10815.
399. Lohmann V, Roos A, Korner F, et al. Biochemical and kinetic analyses of NS5B RNA-dependent RNA polymerase of the hepatitis C virus. *Virology* 1998;249:108–118.
400. Love RA, Parge H, Wickersham JA, et al. The crystal structure of hepatitis C virus NS3 proteinase reveals a trypsin-like fold and a structural zinc binding site. *Cell* 1996;87:331–342.
401. Lu HH, Wimmer E. Poliovirus chimeras replicating under the translational control of genetic elements of hepatitis C virus reveal unusual properties of the internal ribosomal entry site of hepatitis C virus. *Proc Natl Acad Sci U S A* 1996;93:1412–1417.
402. Luo G, Hamatake RK, Mathis DM, et al. De novo initiation of RNA synthesis by the RNA-dependent RNA polymerase (NS5B) of hepatitis C virus. *J Virol* 2000;74:851–863.
403. Mackenzie JM, Jones MK, Westaway EG. Markers for trans-Golgi membranes and the intermediate compartment localize to induced membranes with distinct replication functions in flavivirus-infected cells. *J Virol* 1999;73:9555–9567.
404. Mackenzie JM, Jones MK, Young PR. Immunolocalization of the dengue virus nonstructural glycoprotein NS1 suggests a role in viral RNA replication. *Virology* 1996;220:232–240.
405. Mackenzie JM, Khromykh AA, Jones MK, Westaway EG. Subcellular localization and some biochemical properties of the flavivirus Kunjin nonstructural proteins NS2A and NS4A. *Virology* 1998;245:203–215.
406. Major ME, Mihalik K, Fernandez J, et al. Long term follow-up of chimpanzees inoculated with the first infectious clone for hepatitis C virus. *J Virol* 1999;73:3317–3325.
407. Manabe S, Fuke I, Tanishita O, et al. Production of nonstructural proteins of hepatitis C virus requires a putative viral protease encoded by NS3. *Virology* 1994;198:636–644.
408. Mandl CW, Aberle JH, Aberle SW, et al. *In vitro*-synthesized infectious RNA as an attenuated live vaccine in a flavivirus model [see comments]. *Nat Med* 1998;4:1438–1440.
409. Mandl CW, Allison SL, Holzmann H, et al. Attenuation of tick-borne encephalitis virus by structure-based site-specific mutagenesis of a putative flavivirus receptor binding site. *J Virol* 2000;74:9601–9609.
410. Mandl CW, Ecker M, Holzmann H, et al. Infectious cDNA clones of tick-borne encephalitis virus European subtype prototypic strain Neudoerfl and high virulence strain Hypr. *J Gen Virol* 1997;78:1049–1057.
411. Mandl CW, Heinz FX, Puchhammer-Stöckl E, Kunz C. Sequencing the termini of capped viral RNA by 5′-3′ ligation and PCR. *Biotechniques* 1991;10:486.
412. Mandl CW, Heinz FX, Stöckl E, Kunz C. Genome sequence of tick-borne encephalitis virus (Western subtype) and comparative analysis of nonstructural proteins with other flaviviruses. *Virology* 1989;173: 291–301.
413. Mandl CW, Holzmann H, Kunz C, Heinz FX. Complete genomic sequence of Powassan virus: Evaluation of genetic elements in tick-borne versus mosquito-borne flaviviruses. *Virology* 1993;194:173–184.
414. Mandl CW, Holzmann H, Meixner T, et al. Spontaneous and engineered deletions in the 3′ noncoding region of tick-borne encephalitis virus: Construction of highly attenuated mutants of a flavivirus. *J Virol* 1998;72:2132–2140.
415. Mandl CW, Kunz C, Heinz FX. Presence of poly(A) in a flavivirus: Significant differences between the 3′ noncoding regions of the genomic RNAs of tick-borne encephalitis virus strains. *J Virol* 1991; 65:4070–4077.
416. Marianneau P, Megret F, Olivier R, et al. Dengue 1 virus binding to human hepatoma HepG2 and simian Vero cell surfaces differs. *J Gen Virol* 1996;77:2547–2554.
417. Markland W, Petrillo RA, Fitzgibbon M, et al. Purification and characterization of the NS3 serine protease domain of hepatitis C virus expressed in *Saccharomyces cerevisiae. J Gen Virol* 1997;78:39–43.
418. Markoff L, Falgout B, Chang A. A conserved internal hydrophobic domain mediates the stable membrane integration of the dengue virus capsid protein. *Virology* 1997;233:105–117.
419. Mason PW. Maturation of Japanese encephalitis virus glycoproteins produced by infected mammalian and mosquito cells. *Virology* 1989; 169:354–364.
420. Mason PW, Pincus S, Fournier MJ, et al. Japanese encephalitis virus-vaccinia recombinants produce particulate forms of the structural membrane proteins and induce high levels of protection against lethal JEV infection. *Virology* 1991;180:294–305.
421. Masuko K, Mitsui T, Iwano K, et al. Infection with hepatitis GB virus C in patients on maintenance hemodialysis [see comments]. *N Engl J Med* 1996;334:1485–1490.
422. Matsumoto M, Hsieh T-Y, Zhu N, et al. Hepatitis C virus core protein interacts with the cytoplasmic tail of lymphotoxin-β receptor. *J Virol* 1997;71:1301–1309.
423. Matsumoto M, Hwang SB, Jeng K-S, et al. Homotypic interaction and multimerization of hepatitis C virus core protein. *Virology* 1996;218: 43–51.
424. Matsumura T, Shiraki K, Sashitaka T, Hotta S. Morphogenesis of dengue-1 virus in cultures of a human leukemic leukocyte line (J-111). *Microbiol Immunol* 1977;21:329–334.
425. Matsuura Y, Harada S, Suzuki R, et al. Expression of processed envelope protein of hepatitis C virus in mammalian and insect cells. *J Virol* 1992;66:1425–1431.
426. Matsuura Y, Suzuki T, Suzuki R, et al. Processing of E1 and E2 glycoproteins of hepatitis C virus expressed in mammalian and insect cells. *Virology* 1994;205:141–150.
427. McClurkin AW, Bolin SR, Coria MF. Isolation of cytopathic and noncytopathic bovine viral diarrhea virus from the spleen of cattle acutely and chronically affected with bovine viral diarrhea. *J Am Vet Med Assoc* 1985;186:568–569.
428. Melvin SL, Dawson GJ, Carrick RJ, et al. Biophysical characterization of GB virus C from human plasma. *J Virol Methods* 1998;71:147–157.
429. Men R, Bray M, Clark D, et al. Dengue type 4 virus mutants containing deletion in the 3′ noncoding region of the RNA genome: Analysis of growth restriction in cell culture and altered viremia pattern and immunogenicity in rhesus monkeys. *J Virol* 1996;70:3930–3937.
430. Mendez E, Ruggli N, Collett MS, Rice CM. Infectious bovine viral diarrhea virus (strain NADL) RNA from stable cDNA clones: A cellular insert determines NS3 production and viral cytopathogenicity. *J Virol* 1998;72:4737–4745.
431. Meola A, Sbardellati A, Bruni Ercole B, et al. Binding of hepatitis C virus E2 glycoprotein to CD81 does not correlate with species permissiveness to infection. *J Virol* 2000;74:5933–5938.
432. Meyers G, Rümenapf T, Thiel H-J. Molecular cloning and nucleotide sequence of the genome of hog cholera virus. *Virology* 1989;171: 555–567.
433. Meyers G, Rümenapf T, Thiel H-J. Ubiquitin in a togavirus [letter]. *Nature* 1989;341:491.
434. Meyers G, Rümenapf T, Thiel H-J. Insertion of ubiquitin-coding sequence in the RNA genome of a togavirus. In: Brinton MA, Heinz FX, eds. *New Aspects of Positive Strand RNA Viruses.* Washington, DC: American Society for Microbiology, 1990:25–29.
435. Meyers G, Saalmuller A, Buttner M. Mutations abrogating the RNase activity in glycoprotein E(rns) of the pestivirus classical swine fever virus lead to virus attenuation. *J Virol* 1999;73:10224–10235.
436. Meyers G, Stoll D, Gunn M. Insertion of a sequence encoding light chain 3 of microtubule-associated proteins 1A and 1B in a pestivirus genome: Connection with virus cytopathogenicity and induction of lethal disease in cattle. *J Virol* 1998;72:4139–4148.
437. Meyers G, Tautz N, Becher P, et al. Recovery of cytopathogenic and noncytopathogenic bovine viral diarrhea viruses from cDNA constructs. *J Virol* 1996;70:8606–8613.
438. Meyers G, Tautz N, Dubovi EJ, Thiel H-J. Viral cytopathogenicity correlated with integration of ubiquitin-coding sequences. *Virology* 1991; 180:602–616.
439. Meyers G, Tautz N, Stark R, et al. Rearrangement of viral sequences in cytopathogenic pestiviruses. *Virology* 1992;191:368–386.
440. Meyers G, Thiel H-J. Cytopathogenicity of classical swine fever virus caused by defective interfering particles. *J Virol* 1995;69:3683–3689.

441. Meyers G, Thiel H-J. Molecular characterization of pestiviruses. *Adv Virus Res* 1996;47:53–118.
442. Meyers G, Thiel H-J, Rumenapf T. Classical swine fever virus: Recovery of infectious viruses from cDNA constructs and generation of recombinant cytopathogenic defective interfering particles. *J Virol* 1996;70:1588–1595.
443. Michalak JP, Wychowski C, Choukhi A, et al. Characterization of truncated forms of the hepatitis C virus glycoproteins. *J Gen Virol* 1997;78:2299–2306.
444. Miller RH, Purcell RH. Hepatitis C virus shares amino acid sequence similarity with pestiviruses and flaviviruses as well as members of two plant virus supergroups. *Proc Natl Acad Sci U S A* 1990;87:2057–2061.
445. Minocha HC, Xue W, Reddy JR. A 50 kDa membrane protein from bovine kidney cells is a putative receptor for bovine viral diarrhea virus (BVDV). *Adv Exp Med Biol* 1997;412:145–148.
446. Miyamoto H, Okamoto H, Sato K, et al. Extraordinarily low density of hepatitis C virus estimated by sucrose density centrifugation and polymerase chain reaction. *J Gen Virol* 1992;73:715–718.
447. Mizuno M, Yamada G, Tanaka T, et al. Virion-like structures in HeLa G cells transfected with the full-length sequence of the hepatitis C virus genome. *Gastroenterology* 1995;109:1933–1940.
448. Mizushima H, Hijikata H, Asabe S-I, et al. Two hepatitis C virus glycoprotein E2 products with different C termini. *J Virol* 1994;68:6215–6222.
449. Mizushima H, Hijikata M, Tanji Y, et al. Analysis of N-terminal processing of hepatitis C virus nonstructural protein 2. *J Virol* 1994;68:2731–2734.
450. Moennig V, Plagemann PG. The pestiviruses. *Adv Virus Res* 1992;41:53–98.
451. Monath TP. Japanese encephalitis—A plague of the Orient. *N Engl J Med* 1988;319:641–643.
452. Monath TP. Yellow fever: Victor, Victoria? Conqueror, conquest? Epidemics and research in the last forty years and prospects for the future. *Am J Trop Med Hyg* 1991;45:1–43.
453. Monath TP. Dengue: The risk to developed and developing countries. *Proc Natl Acad Sci U S A* 1994;91:2395–2400.
454. Monath TP, Levenbook I, Soike K, et al. Chimeric yellow fever virus 17D-Japanese encephalitis virus vaccine: Dose-response effectiveness and extended safety testing in rhesus monkeys. *J Virol* 2000;74:1742–1751.
455. Monath TP, Soike K, Levenbook I, et al. Recombinant, chimaeric live, attenuated vaccine (ChimeriVax) incorporating the envelope genes of Japanese encephalitis (SA14-14-2) virus and the capsid and nonstructural genes of yellow fever (17D) virus is safe, immunogenic and protective in non-human primates. *Vaccine* 1999;17:1869–1882.
456. Monazahian M, Bohme I, Bonk S, et al. Low density lipoprotein receptor as a candidate receptor for hepatitis C virus. *J Med Virol* 1999;57:223–229.
457. Mondelli MU, Silini E. Clincal significance of hepatitis C genotypes. *J Hepatol* 1999;31:65–70.
458. Moormann RJ, Hulst MM. Hog cholera virus: Identification and characterization of the viral RNA and the virus-specific RNA synthesized in infected swine kidney cells. *Virus Res* 1988;11:281–291.
459. Moormann RJ, van Gennip HG, Miedema GK, et al. Infectious RNA transcribed from an engineered full-length cDNA template of the genome of a pestivirus. *J Virol* 1996;70:763–770.
460. Moormann RJ, Warmerdam PA, van der Meer B, et al. Molecular cloning and nucleotide sequence of hog cholera virus strain Brescia and mapping of the genomic region encoding envelope protein E1. *Virology* 1990;177:184–198.
461. Moradpour D, Englert C, Wakita T, Wands JR. Characterization of cell lines allowing tightly regulated expression of hepatitis C virus core protein. *Virology* 1996;222:51–63.
462. Moradpour D, Wakita T, Wands JR, Blum HE. Tightly regulated expression of the entire hepatitis C virus structural region in continuous human cell lines. *Biochem Biophys Res Commun* 1998;246:920–924.
463. Morgenstern KA, Landro JA, Hsiao K, et al. Polynucleotide modulation of the protease, nucleoside triphosphatase, and helicase activities of a hepatitis C virus NS3-NS4A complex isolated from transfected COS cells. *J Virol* 1997;71:3767–3775.
464. Moriya K, Fujie H, Shintani Y, et al. The core protein of hepatitis C virus induces hepatocellular carcinoma in transgenic mice. *Nat Med* 1998;4:1065–1067.
465. Moriya K, Yotsuyanagi Y, Shintani Y, et al. Hepatitis C virus core protein induces hepatic steatosis in transgenic mice. *J Gen Virol* 1997;78:1527–1531.
466. Morozova OV, Tsekhanovskaya NA, Maksimova TG, et al. Phosphorylation of tick-borne encephalitis virus NS5 protein. *Virus Res* 1997;49:9–15.
467. Moser C, Stettler P, Tratschin JD, Hofmann MA. Cytopathogenic and noncytopathogenic RNA replicons of classical swine fever virus. *J Virol* 1999;73:7787–7794.
468. Muerhoff AS, Leary TP, Simons JN, et al. Genomic organization of GB viruses A and B: Two new members of the *Flaviviridae* associated with GB agent hepatitis. *J Virol* 1995;69:5621–5630.
469. Muerhoff AS, Smith DB, Leary TP, et al. Identification of GB virus C variants by phylogenetic analysis of 5′-untranslated and coding region sequences [published erratum appears in *J Virol* 1997;71:8952]. *J Virol* 1997;71:6501–6508.
470. Munoz ML, Cisneros A, Cruz J, et al. Putative dengue virus receptors from mosquito cells. *FEMS Microbiol Lett* 1998;168:251–258.
471. Muramatsu S, Ishido S, Fujita T, et al. Nuclear localization of the NS3 protein of hepatitis C virus and factors affecting the localization. *J Virol* 1997;71:4954–4961.
472. Murphy FA. Togavirus morphology and morphogenesis. In: Schlesinger RW, eds. *The Togaviruses: Biology, Structure, Replication.* New York: Academic Press, 1980:241–316.
473. Murphy FA, Harrison AK, Gary GW Jr, et al. St. Louis encephalitis virus infection in mice. Electron microscopic studies of central nervous system. *Lab Invest* 1968;19:652–662.
474. Murray JM, Aaskov JG, Wright PJ. Processing of the dengue virus type 2 proteins prM and C-prM. *J Gen Virol* 1993;74:175–182.
475. Murthy HM, Clum S, Padmanabhan R. Dengue virus NS3 serine protease. Crystal structure and insights into interaction of the active site with substrates by molecular modeling and structural analysis of mutational effects. *J Biol Chem* 1999;274:5573–5580.
476. Mussgay M, Enzmann P-J, Horzinek MC, Weiland E. Growth cycle of arboviruses in vertebrate and arthropod cells. *Prog Med Virol* 1975;19:258–323.
477. Muylaert IR, Galler RG, Rice CM. Mutagenesis of the N-linked glycosylation sites of the yellow fever virus NS1 protein: Effects on virus replication and mouse neurovirulence. *Virology* 1996;222:159–168.
478. Muylaert IR, Galler RG, Rice CM. Genetic analysis of yellow fever virus NS1 protein: Identification of a temperature-sensitive mutation which blocks RNA accumulation. *J Virol* 1997;71:291–298.
479. Nagasaka A, Hige S, Matsushima T, et al. Differential flotation centrifugation study of hepatitis C virus and response to interferon therapy. *J Med Virol* 1997;52:190–194.
480. Nathanson N. Emergence of new viral infections: Implications for the blood supply. *Biologicals* 1998;26:77–84.
481. Nawa M. Effects of bafilomycin A1 on Japanese encephalitis virus in C6/36 mosquito cells. *Arch Virol* 1998;143:1555–1568.
482. Neddermann P, Clementi A, De Francesco R. Hyperphosphorylation of the hepatitis C virus NS5A protein requires an active NS3 protease, NS4A, NS4B, and NS5A encoded on the same polyprotein. *J Virol* 1999;73:9984–9991.
483. Nestorowicz A, Chambers TJ, Rice CM. Mutagenesis of the yellow fever virus NS2A/2B cleavage site: Effects on proteolytic processing, viral replication and evidence for alternative processing of the NS2A protein. *Virology* 1994;199:114–123.
484. Neumann AU, Lam NP, Dahari H, et al. Hepatitis C viral dynamics *in vivo* and the antiviral efficacy of interferon-alpha therapy. *Science* 1998;282:103–107.
485. Ng ML. Ultrastructural studies of Kunjin virus-infected *Aedes albopictus* cells. *J Gen Virol* 1987;68:577–582.
486. Ng ML, Hong SS. Flavivirus infection: Essential ultrastructural changes and association of Kunjin virus NS3 protein with microtubules. *Arch Virol* 1989;106:103–120.
487. Ng ML, Lau LC. Possible involvement of receptors in the entry of Kunjin virus into Vero cells. *Arch Virol* 1988;100:199–211.
488. Ng ML, Yeong FM, Tan SH. Cryosubstitution technique reveals new morphology of flavivirus-induced structures. *J Virol Methods* 1994;49:305–314.
489. Nishihara T, Nozaki C, Nakatake H, et al. Secretion and purification of hepatitis C virus NS1 glycoprotein produced by recombinant baculovirus-infected insect cells. *Gene* 1993;129:207–214.
490. Nolandt O, Kern V, Muller H, et al. Analysis of hepatitis C virus core protein interaction domains. *J Gen Virol* 1997;78:1331–1340.

491. Nowak T, Färber PM, Wengler G, Wengler G. Analyses of the terminal sequences of West Nile virus structural proteins and of the *in vitro* translation of these proteins allow the proposal of a complete scheme of the proteolytic cleavages involved in their synthesis. *Virology* 1989; 169:365–376.
492. Nowak T, Wengler G. Analysis of disulfides present in the membrane proteins of the West Nile flavivirus. *Virology* 1987;156:127–137.
493. Ogata N, Alter HJ, Miller RH, Purcell RH. Nucleotide sequence and mutation rate of the H strain of hepatitis C virus. *Proc Natl Acad Sci U S A* 1991;88:3392–3396.
494. Oh JW, Ito T, Lai MM. A recombinant hepatitis C virus RNA-dependent RNA polymerase capable of copying the full-length viral RNA. *J Virol* 1999;73:7694–7702.
495. Oh JW, Sheu GT, Lai MM. Template requirement and initiation site selection by hepatitis C virus polymerase on a minimal viral RNA template. *J Biol Chem* 2000;275:17710–17717.
496. Ohashi K, Marion PL, Nakai H, et al. Sustained survival of human hepatocytes in mice: A model for *in vivo* infection with human hepatitis B and hepatitis delta viruses. *Nat Med* 2000;6:337–341.
497. Ohyama A, Ito T, Tanimura E, et al. Electron microscopic observation of the budding maturation of group B arboviruses. *Microbiol Immunol* 1977;21:535–538.
498. Okamoto H, Kojima M, Sakamoto M, et al. The entire nucleotide sequence and classification of a hepatitis C virus isolate of a novel genotype from an Indonesian patient with chronic liver disease. *J Gen Virol* 1994;75:629–635.
499. Okamoto H, Kurai K, Okada S-I, et al. Full-length sequence of a hepatitis C virus genome having poor homology to reported isolates: Comparative study of four distinct genotypes. *Virology* 1992;188: 331–341.
500. Okamoto H, Okada S, Sugiyama Y, et al. Nucleotide sequence of the genomic RNA of hepatitis C virus isolated from a human carrier: Comparison with reported isolates for conserved and divergent regions. *J Gen Virol* 1991;72:2697–2704.
501. Park JS, Yang JM, Min MK. Hepatitis C virus nonstructural protein NS4B transforms NIH3T3 cells in cooperation with the Ha-ras oncogene. *Biochem Biophys Res Commun* 2000;267:581–587.
502. Parks WP, Melnick JL. Attempted isolation of hepatitis viruses in marmosets. *J Infect Dis* 1969;120:539–547.
503. Pasquinelli C, Shoenberger JM, Chung J, et al. Hepatitis C virus core and E2 protein expression in transgenic mice. *Hepatology* 1997;25: 719–727.
504. Pasquo A, Nardi MC, Dimasi N, et al. Rational design and functional expression of a constitutively active single-chain NS4A-NS3 proteinase. *Fold Des* 1998;3:433–441.
505. Paterson M, Laxton CD, Thomas HC, et al. Hepatitis C virus NS5A protein inhibits interferon antiviral activity, but the effects do not correlate with clinical response. *Gastroenterology* 1999;117: 1187–1197.
506. Paton DJ, Lowings JP, Barrett AD. Epitope mapping of the gp53 envelope protein of bovine viral diarrhea virus. *Virology* 1992;190: 763–772.
507. Pavesi A. Detection of signature sequences in overlapping genes and prediction of a novel overlapping gene in hepatitis G virus. *J Mol Evol* 2000;50:284–295.
508. Pawlotsky JM. Hepatitis C virus (HCV) NS5A protein: Role in HCV replication and resistance to interferon-alpha. *J Viral Hepat* 1999;6 (suppl 1):47–48.
509. Peiris JS, Porterfield JS. Antibody-mediated enhancement of Flavivirus replication in macrophage-like cell lines. *Nature* 1979;282: 509–511.
510. Peiris JS, Porterfield JS. Antibody-dependent enhancement of plaque formation on cell lines of macrophage origin—A sensitive assay for antiviral antibody. *J Gen Virol* 1981;57:119–125.
511. Peiris JS, Porterfield JS. Antibody-dependent plaque enhancement: Its antigenic specificity in relation to Togaviridae. *J Gen Virol* 1982;58: 291–296.
512. Pellerin C, Moir S, Lecomte J, Tijssen P. Comparison of the p125 coding region of bovine viral diarrhea viruses. *Vet Microbiol* 1995;45: 45–57.
513. Pellerin C, van den Hurk J, Lecomte J, Tussen P. Identification of a new group of bovine viral diarrhea virus strains associated with severe outbreaks and high mortalities. *Virology* 1994;203:260–268.
514. Pestova TV, Hellen CU. Internal initiation of translation of bovine viral diarrhea virus RNA. *Virology* 1999;258:249–256.
515. Pestova TV, Shatsky IN, Fletcher SP, et al. A prokaryotic-like mode of cytoplasmic eukaryotic ribosome binding to the initiation codon during internal translation initiation of hepatitis C and classical swine fever virus RNAs. *Genes Dev* 1998;12:67–83.
516. Peterson J, Dandri M, Gupta S, Rogler CE. Liver repopulation with xenogenic hepatocytes in B and T cell-deficient mice leads to chronic hepadnavirus infection and clonal growth of hepatocellular carcinoma. *Proc Natl Acad Sci U S A* 1998;95:310–315.
517. Pethel M, Falgout B, Lai C-J. Mutational analysis of the octapeptide sequence motif at the NS1-NS2A cleavage junction of dengue type 4 virus. *J Virol* 1992;66:7225–7231.
518. Petric M, Yolken RH, Dubovi EJ, et al. Baculovirus expression of pestivirus non-structural proteins. *J Gen Virol* 1992;73:1867–1871.
519. Petrik J, Parker H, Alexander GJ. Human hepatic glyceraldehyde-3-phosphate dehydrogenase binds to the poly(U) tract of the 3′ non-coding region of hepatitis C virus genomic RNA. *J Gen Virol* 1999;80: 3109–3113.
520. Phillpotts RJ, Stephenson JR, Porterfield JS. Antibody-dependent enhancement of tick-borne encephalitis virus infectivity. *J Gen Virol* 1985;66:1831–1837.
521. Pickering JM, Thomas HC, Karayiannis P. Genetic diversity between hepatitis G virus isolates: Analysis of nucleotide variation in the NS-3 and putative "core" peptide genes. *J Gen Virol* 1997;78:53–60.
522. Pieroni L, Santolini E, Fipaldini C, et al. *In vitro* study of the NS2-3 protease of hepatitis C virus. *J Virol* 1997;71:6373–6380.
523. Pileri P, Uematsu Y, Compagnoli S, et al. Binding of hepatitis C virus to CD81. *Science* 1998;282:938–941.
524. Pincus S, Mason PW, Konishi E, et al. Recombinant vaccinia virus producing the prM and E proteins of yellow fever virus protects mice from lethal yellow fever encephalitis. *Virology* 1992;187:290–297.
525. Pizzi E, Tramontano A, Tomei L, et al. Molecular-model of the specificity pocket of the hepatitis C virus protease: Implications for substrate recognition. *Proc Natl Acad Sci U S A* 1994;91:888–892.
526. Pletnev AG, Men R. Attenuation of the Langat tick-borne flavivirus by chimerization with mosquito-borne flavivirus dengue type 4. *Proc Natl Acad Sci U S A* 1998;95:1746–1751.
527. Polo S, Ketner G, Levis R, Falgout B. Infectious RNA transcripts from full-length dengue virus type 2 cDNA clones made in yeast. *J Virol* 1997;71:5366–5374.
528. Polyak SJ, Paschal DM, McArdle S, et al. Characterization of the effects of hepatitis C virus nonstructural 5A protein expression in human cell lines and on interferon-sensitive virus replication. *Hepatology* 1999;29:1262–1271.
529. Poole TL, Wang C, Popp RA, et al. Pestivirus translation initiation occurs by internal ribosome entry. *Virology* 1995;206:750–754.
530. Post PR, Carvalho R, Galler R. Glycosylation and secretion of yellow fever virus nonstructural protein NS1. *Virus Res* 1991;18:291–302.
531. Preugschat F, Averett DR, Clarke BE, Porter DJT. A steady-state and pre-steady-state kinetic analysis of the NTPase activity associated with the hepatitis C virus NS3 helicase domain. *J Biol Chem* 1996; 271:24449–24457.
532. Preugschat F, Lenches EM, Strauss JH. Flavivirus enzyme-substrate interactions studied with chimeric proteinases: Identification of an intragenic locus important for substrate recognition. *J Virol* 1991;65: 4749–4758.
533. Preugschat F, Strauss JH. Processing of nonstructural proteins NS4A and NS4B of dengue 2 virus *in vitro* and *in vivo*. *Virology* 1991;185: 689–697.
534. Preugschat F, Yao C-W, Strauss JH. *In vitro* processing of dengue virus type 2 nonstructural proteins NS2A, NS2B, and NS3. *J Virol* 1990;64:4364–4374.
535. Prince AM, Huima-Byron T, Parker TS, Levine DM. Visualization of hepatitis C virions and putative defective interfering particles isolated from low-density lipoproteins. *J Viral Hepat* 1996;3:11–17.
536. Pringle CR. Virus taxonomy—1999. The universal system of virus taxonomy, updated to include the new proposals ratified by the International Committee on Taxonomy of Viruses during 1998 [news] [published erratum appears in *Arch Virol* 1999;144:1667]. *Arch Virol* 1999;144:421–429.
537. Proutski V, Gaunt MW, Gould EA, Holmes EC. Secondary structure of the 3′-untranslated region of yellow fever virus: Implications for virulence, attenuation and vaccine development. *J Gen Virol* 1997;78:1543–1549.
538. Proutski V, Gould EA, Holmes EC. Secondary structure of the 3′ untranslated region of flaviviruses: Similarities and differences. *Nucleic Acids Res* 1997;25:1194–1202.

539. Pryor MJ, Gualano RC, Lin B, et al. Growth restriction of dengue virus type 2 by site-specific mutagenesis of virus-encoded glycoproteins. *J Gen Virol* 1998;79:2631–2639.
540. Pryor MJ, Wright PJ. Glycosylation mutants of dengue virus NS1 protein. *J Gen Virol* 1994;75:1183–1187.
541. Pugachev KV, Nomokonova NY, Dobrikova EY, Wolf YI. Site-directed mutagenesis of the tick-borne encephalitis virus NS3 gene reveals the putative serine protease domain of the NS3 protein. *FEBS Lett* 1993;328:115–118.
542. Purchio AF, Larson R, Collett MS. Characterization of virus-specific RNA synthesized in bovine cells infected with bovine viral diarrhea virus. *J Virol* 1983;48:320–324.
543. Purchio AF, Larson R, Torborg LL, Collett MS. Cell-free translation of bovine viral diarrhea virus RNA. *J Virol* 1984;52:973–975.
544. Qi F, Ridpath JF, Berry ES. Insertion of a bovine SMT3B gene in NS4B and duplication of NS3 in a bovine viral diarrhea virus genome correlate with the cytopathogenicity of the virus. *Virus Res* 1998;57: 1–9.
545. Qi F, Ridpath JF, Lewis T, et al. Analysis of the bovine viral diarrhea virus genome for possible cellular insertions. *Virology* 1992;189: 285–292.
546. Qu X, Chen W, Maguire T, Austin F. Immunoreactivity and protective effects in mice of a recombinant dengue 2 Tonga virus NS1 protein produced in a baculovirus expression system. *J Gen Virol* 1993;74: 89–97.
547. Ralston R, Thudium K, Berger K, et al. Characterization of hepatitis C virus envelope glycoprotein complexes expressed by recombinant vaccinia viruses. *J Virol* 1993;67:6753–6761.
548. Ramos-Castaneda J, Imbert JL, Barron BL, Ramos C. A 65-kDa trypsin-sensible membrane cell protein as a possible receptor for dengue virus in cultured neuroblastoma cells. *J Neurovirol* 1997;3: 435–440.
549. Ramratnam B, Bonhoeffer S, Binley J, et al. Rapid production and clearance of HIV-1 and hepatitis C virus assessed by large volume plasma apheresis. *Lancet* 1999;354:1782–1785.
550. Randolph VB, Stollar V. Low pH-induced cell fusion in flavivirus-infected *Aedes albopictus* cell cultures. *J Gen Virol* 1990;71: 1845–1850.
551. Randolph VB, Winkler G, Stollar V. Acidotropic amines inhibit proteolytic processing of flavivirus prM protein. *Virology* 1990;174: 450–458.
552. Rauscher S, Flamm C, Mandl CW, et al. Secondary structure of the 3′-noncoding region of flavivirus genomes: Comparative analysis of base pairing probabilities. *RNA* 1997;3:779–791.
553. Ravaggi A, Natoli G, Primi D, et al. Intracellular localization of full-length and truncated hepatitis C virus core protein expressed in mammalian cells. *J Hepatol* 1994;20:833–836.
554. Ray RB, Lagging LM, Meyer K, Ray R. Hepatitis C virus core protein cooperates with *ras* and transforms primary rat embryo fibroblasts to tumorigenic phenotype. *J Virol* 1996;70:4438–4443.
555. Ray RB, Lagging LM, Meyer K, et al. Transcriptional regulation of cellular and viral promoters by the hepatitis C virus core protein. *Virus Res* 1995;37:209–220.
556. Ray RB, Meyer K, Ray R. Suppression of apoptotic cell death by hepatitis C virus core protein. *Virology* 1996;226:176–182.
557. Ray RB, Meyer K, Steele R, et al. Inhibition of tumor necrosis factor (TNF-α)-mediated apoptosis by hepatitis C virus core protein. *J Biol Chem* 1998;273:2256–2259.
558. Ray RB, Steele R, Meyer K, Ray R. Transcriptional repression of p53 promoter by hepatitis C virus core protein. *J Biol Chem* 1997;272: 10983–10986.
559. Ray RB, Steele R, Meyer K, Ray R. Hepatitis C virus core protein represses p21WAF1/Cip1/Sid1 promoter activity. *Gene* 1998;208: 331–336.
560. Rebhun WC, French TW, Perdrizet JA, et al. Thrombocytopenia associated with acute bovine virus diarrhea infection in cattle. *J Vet Intern Med* 1989;3:42–46.
561. Reed KE, Gorbalenya AE, Rice CM. The NS5A/NS5 proteins of viruses from three genera of the family *Flaviviridae* are phosphorylated by associated serine/threonine kinases. *J Virol* 1998;72: 6199–6206.
562. Reed KE, Grakoui A, Rice CM. The hepatitis C virus NS2-3 autoproteinase: Cleavage site mutagenesis and requirements for bimolecular cleavage. *J Virol* 1995;69:4127–4136.
563. Reed KE, Rice CM. Identification of the major phosphorylation site of the hepatitis C virus H strain NS5A protein as serine 2321. *J Biol Chem* 1999;274:28011–28018.
564. Reed KE, Xu J, Rice CM. Phosphorylation of the hepatitis C virus NS5A protein *in vitro* and *in vivo*: Properties of the NS5A-associated kinase. *J Virol* 1997;71:7187–7197.
565. Reed W, Carroll J. The etiology of yellow fever. A supplemental note. *Am Med* 1902;3:301–305.
566. Reed W, Carroll J, Agramonte A. The etiology of yellow fever. An additional note. *JAMA* 1901;36:431–440.
567. Rey F, Heinz FX, Mandl C, et al. Crystal structure of the envelope glycoprotein E from tick borne encephalitis virus. *Nature* 1995;375: 291–298.
568. Reynolds JE, Kaminski A, Carroll AR, et al. Internal initiation of translation of hepatitis C virus RNA: The ribosome entry site is at the authentic initiation codon. *RNA* 1996;2:867–878.
569. Reynolds JE, Kaminski A, Kettinen HJ, et al. Unique features of internal initiation of hepatitis C virus RNA translation. *EMBO J* 1995;14: 6010–6020.
570. Rice CM. Is CD81 the key to hepatitis C virus entry? *Hepatology* 1999;29:990–992.
571. Rice CM, Aebersold R, Teplow DB, et al. Partial N-terminal amino acid sequences of three nonstructural proteins of two flaviviruses. *Virology* 1986;151:1–9.
572. Rice CM, Grakoui A, Galler R, Chambers TJ. Transcription of infectious yellow fever virus RNA from full-length cDNA templates produced by *in vitro* ligation. *New Biol* 1989;1:285–296.
573. Rice CM, Lenches EM, Eddy SR, et al. Nucleotide sequence of yellow fever virus: Implications for flavivirus gene expression and evolution. *Science* 1985;229:726–733.
574. Ridpath JF, Bolin SR. The genomic sequence of a virulent bovine viral diarrhea virus (BVDV) from the type 2 genotype: Detection of a large genomic insertion in a noncytopathic BVDV. *Virology* 1995;212: 39–46.
575. Ridpath JF, Bolin SR. Comparison of the complete genomic sequence of the border disease virus, BD31, to other pestiviruses. *Virus Res* 1997;50:237–243.
576. Ridpath JF, Bolin SR, Dubovi EJ. Segregation of bovine viral diarrhea virus into genotypes. *Virology* 1994;205:66–74.
577. Rijnbrand R, Abell G, Lemon SM. Mutational analysis of the GB virus B internal ribosome entry site. *J Virol* 2000;74:773–783.
578. Rijnbrand R, Bredenbeek PJ, van der Straaten T, et al. Almost the entire 5′ non-translated region of hepatitis C virus is required for cap-independent translation. *FEBS Lett* 1995;365:115–119.
579. Rijnbrand R, van der Straaten T, van Rijn PA, et al. Internal entry of ribosomes is directed by the 5′ noncoding region of classical swine fever virus and is dependent on the presence of an RNA pseudoknot upstream of the initiation codon. *J Virol* 1997;71:451–457.
580. Rijnbrand RC, Abbink TE, Haasnoot PC, et al. The influence of AUG codons in the hepatitis C virus 5′ nontranslated region on translation and mapping of the translation initiation window. *Virology* 1996;226: 47–56.
581. Rijnbrand RCA, Lemon SM. Internal ribosome entry site-mediated translation in hepatitis C virus replication. In: Hagedorn C, Rice CM, eds. *Hepatitis C Virus*. Berlin: Springer-Verlag, 2000:85–116.
582. Robertson B, Myers G, Howard C, et al. Classification, nomenclature, and database development for hepatitis C virus (HCV) and related viruses: Proposals for standardization. International Committee on Virus Taxonomy [news]. *Arch Virol* 1998;143:2493–503.
583. Roehrig JT, Johnson AJ, Hunt AR, et al. Antibodies to dengue 2 virus E-glycoprotein synthetic peptides identify antigenic conformation. *Virology* 1990;177:668–675.
584. Rothman AL, Ennis FA. Immunopathogenesis of Dengue hemorrhagic fever. *Virology* 1999;257:1–6.
585. Ruggieri A, Harada T, Matsuura Y, Miyamura T. Sensitization to Fas-mediated apoptosis by hepatitis C virus core protein. *Virology* 1997; 229:68–76.
586. Ruggli N, Tratschin JD, Mittelholzer C, Hofmann MA. Nucleotide sequence of classical swine fever virus strain Alfort/187 and transcription of infectious RNA from stably cloned full-length cDNA. *J Virol* 1996;70:3478–3487.
587. Rümenapf T, Meyers G, Stark R, Thiel H-J. Hog cholera virus—Characterization of specific antiserum and identification of cDNA clones. *Virology* 1989;171:18–27.

588. Rümenapf T, Meyers G, Stark R, Thiel H-J. Molecular characterization of hog cholera virus. *Arch Virol Suppl* 1991;3:7–18.
589. Rümenapf T, Stark R, Heimann M, Thiel H-J. N-terminal protease of pestiviruses: Identification of putative catalytic residues by site-directed mutagenesis. *J Virol* 1998;72:2544–2547.
590. Rümenapf T, Stark R, Meyers G, Thiel H-J. Structural proteins of hog cholera virus expressed by vaccinia virus: Further characterization and induction of protective immunity. *J Virol* 1991;65:589–597.
591. Rümenapf T, Unger G, Strauss JH, Thiel H-J. Processing of the envelope glycoproteins of pestiviruses. *J Virol* 1993;67:3288–3294.
592. Russell PK, Brandt WE, Dalrymple JM. Chemical and antigenic structure of flaviviruses. In: Schlesinger RW, eds. *The Togaviruses: Biology, Structure, Replication.* New York: Academic Press, 1980: 503–529.
593. Ryu W-S, Choi D-Y, Yang J-Y, et al. Characterization of the putative E2 envelope glycoprotein of hepatitis C virus expressed in stably transformed Chinese hamster ovary cells. *Mol Cells* 1995;5:563–568.
594. Saito I, Miyamura T, Ohbayashi A, et al. Hepatitis C virus infection is associated with the development of hepatocellular carcinoma. *Proc Natl Acad Sci U S A* 1990;87:6547–6549.
595. Sakamuro D, Furukawa T, Takegami T. Hepatitis C virus nonstructural protein NS3 transforms NIH 3T3 cells. *J Virol* 1995;69:3893–3896.
596. Salas-Benito JS, del Angel RM. Identification of two surface proteins from C6/36 cells that bind dengue type 4 virus. *J Virol* 1997;71: 7246–7252.
597. Sangar DV, Carroll AR. A tale of two strands: Reverse-transcriptase polymerase chain reaction detection of hepatitis C virus replication. *Hepatology* 1998;28:1173–1176.
598. Sangster MY, Heliams DB, MacKenzie JS, Shellam GR. Genetic studies of flavivirus resistance in inbred strains derived from wild mice: Evidence for a new resistance allele at the flavivirus resistance locus (Flv). *J Virol* 1993;67:340–347.
599. Sangster MY, Mackenzie JS, Shellam GR. Genetically determined resistance to flavivirus infection in wild *Mus musculus domesticus* and other taxonomic groups in the genus *Mus. Arch Virol* 1998;143: 697–715.
600. Sangster MY, Shellam GR. Genetically controlled resistance to flaviviruses within the house mouse complex of species. *Curr Top Microbiol Immunol* 1986;127:313–318.
601. Sangster MY, Urosevic N, Mansfield JP, et al. Mapping the Flv locus controlling resistance to flaviviruses on mouse chromosome 5. *J Virol* 1994;68:448–452.
602. Santolini E, Migliaccio G, La Monica N. Biosynthesis and biochemical properties of the hepatitis C virus core protein. *J Virol* 1994;68: 3631–3641.
603. Santolini E, Pacini L, Fipaldini C, et al. The NS2 protein of hepatitis C virus is a transmembrane polypeptide. *J Virol* 1995;69:7461–7471.
604. Sato K, Okamoto H, Aihara S, et al. Demonstration of sugar moiety on the surface of hepatitis C virions recovered from the circulation of infected humans. *Virology* 1993;196:354–357.
605. Sato K, Tanaka T, Okamoto H, et al. Association of circulating hepatitis G virus with lipoproteins for a lack of binding with antibodies. *Biochem Biophys Res Commun* 1996;229:719–725.
606. Satoh S, Hirota M, Noguchi T, et al. Cleavage of hepatitis C virus nonstructural protein 5A by a caspase-like protease(s) in mammalian cells. *Virology* 2000;270:476–487.
607. Satoh S, Tanji Y, Hijikata M, et al. The N-terminal region of hepatitis C virus nonstructural protein 3 (NS3) is essential for stable complex formation with NS4A. *J Virol* 1995;69:4255–4260.
608. Sawyer WA, Lloyd W. The use of mice in tests of immunity against yellow fever. *J Exp Med* 1931;54:533–555.
609. Sbardellati A, Scarselli E, Tomei L, et al. Identification of a novel sequence at the 3′ end of the GB virus B genome. *J Virol* 1999;73: 10546–10550.
610. Scarselli E, Urbani A, Sbardellati A, et al. GB virus B and hepatitis C virus NS3 serine proteases share substrate specificity. *J Virol* 1997;71: 4985–4989.
611. Schalich J, Allison SL, Stiasny K, et al. Recombinant subviral particles from tick-borne encephalitis virus are fusogenic and provide a model system for studying flavivirus envelope glycoprotein functions. *J Virol* 1996;70:4549–4557.
612. Schein CH. From housekeeper to microsurgeon: The diagnostic and therapeutic potential of ribonucleases [published erratum appears in *Nat Biotechnol* 1997;15:927]. *Nat Biotechnol* 1997;15:529–536.
613. Schelp C, Greiser-Wilke I, Wolf G, et al. Identification of cell membrane proteins linked to susceptibility to bovine viral diarrhoea virus infection. *Arch Virol* 1995;140:1997–2009.
614. Schlauder GG, Dawson GJ, Simons JN, et al. Molecular and serologic analysis in the transmission of the GB hepatitis agents. *J Med Virol* 1995;46:81–90.
615. Schlauder GG, Pilot-Matias TJ, Gabriel GS, et al. Origin of GB-hepatitis viruses [letter; comment]. *Lancet* 1995;346:447–448.
616. Schlesinger JJ, Brandriss MW. 17D yellow fever virus infection of P388D1 cells mediated by monoclonal antibodies: Properties of the macrophage Fc receptor. *J Gen Virol* 1983;64:1255–1262.
617. Schlesinger JJ, Brandriss MW, Cropp CB, Monath TP. Protection against yellow fever in monkeys by immunization with yellow fever virus nonstructural protein NS1. *J Virol* 1986;60:1153–1155.
618. Schlesinger JJ, Brandriss MW, Walsh EE. Protection against 17D yellow fever encephalitis in mice by passive transfer of monoclonal antibodies to the nonstructural glycoprotein gp48 and by active immunization with gp48. *J Immunol* 1985;135:2805–2809.
619. Schlesinger JJ, Foltzer M, Chapman S. The Fc portion of antibody to yellow fever virus NS1 is a determinant of protection against YF encephalitis in mice. *Virology* 1993;192:132–141.
620. Schneider R, Unger G, Stark R, et al. Identification of a structural glycoprotein of an RNA virus as a ribonuclease. *Science* 1993;261: 1169–1171.
621. Schweizer M, Peterhans E. Oxidative stress in cells infected with bovine viral diarrhoea virus: A crucial step in the induction of apoptosis. *J Gen Virol* 1999;80:1147–1155.
622. Sekiya H, Kato N, Ootsuyama Y, et al. Genetic alterations of the putative envelope proteins encoding region of the hepatitis C virus in the progression to relapsed phase from acute hepatitis: Humoral immune response to hypervariable region 1. *Int J Cancer* 1994;57: 664–670.
623. Selby MJ, Glazer E, Masiarz F, Houghton M. Complex processing and protein:protein interactions in the E2:NS2 region of HCV. *Virology* 1994;204:114–122.
624. Semprini AE, Persico T, Thiers V, et al. Absence of hepatitis C virus and detection of hepatitis G virus/GB virus C RNA sequences in the semen of infected men. *J Infect Dis* 1998;177:848–854.
625. Serafino A, Valli MB, Alessandrini A, et al. Ultrastructural observations of viral particles within hepatitis C virus-infected human B lymphoblastoid cell line. *Res Virol* 1997;148:153–159.
626. Shapiro D, Brandt WE, Russell PK. Change involving a viral membrane glycoprotein during morphogenesis of group B arboviruses. *Virology* 1972;50:906–911.
627. Shi PY, Li W, Brinton MA. Cell proteins bind specifically to West Nile virus minus-strand 3′ stem-loop RNA. *J Virol* 1996;70:6278–6287.
628. Shih C-M, Chen C-M, Chen S-Y, Lee Y-HW. Modulation of the trans-suppression activity of hepatitis C virus core protein by phosphorylation. *J Virol* 1995;69:1160–1171.
629. Shih CM, Lo SJ, Miyamura T, et al. Suppression of hepatitis B virus expression and replication by hepatitis C virus core protein in HuH-7 cells. *J Virol* 1993;67:5823–5832.
630. Shimizu Y, Yamaji K, Masuho Y, et al. Identification of the sequence on NS4A required for enhanced cleavage of the NS5A/5B site by hepatitis C virus NS3 protease. *J Virol* 1996;70:127–132.
631. Shimizu Y, Yoshikura H. Multicycle infection of hepatitis C virus in cell culture and inhibition by alpha and beta interferons. *J Virol* 1994; 68:8406–8408.
632. Shimizu YK, Feinstone SM, Kohara M, et al. Hepatitis C virus: Detection of intracellular virus particles by electron microscopy. *Hepatology* 1996;23:205–209.
633. Shimizu YK, Igarashi H, Kiyohara T, et al. A hyperimmune serum against a synthetic peptide corresponding to the hypervariable region 1 of hepatitis C virus can prevent viral infection in cell cultures. *Virology* 1996;223:409–412.
634. Shimoike T, Mimori S, Tani H, et al. Interaction of hepatitis C virus core protein with viral sense RNA and suppression of its translation. *J Virol* 1999;73:9718–9725.
635. Shimotohno K. Hepatocellular carcinoma in Japan and its linkage to infection with hepatitis C virus. *Semin Virol* 1993;4:305–312.
636. Simmonds P. Variability of hepatitis C virus genome. *Curr Stud Hematol Blood Transfus* 1994;61:12–35.
637. Simmonds P, Smith DB. Structural constraints on RNA virus evolution. *J Virol* 1999;73:5787–5794.

638. Simons JN, Desai SM, Mushahwar IK. The GB viruses. *Curr Top Microbiol Immunol* 2000;242:341–375.
639. Simons JN, Desai SM, Schultz DE, et al. Translation initiation in GB viruses A and C: Evidence for internal ribosome entry and implications for genome organization. *J Virol* 1996;70:6126–6135.
640. Simons JN, Leary TP, Dawson GJ, et al. Isolation of novel virus-like sequences associated with human hepatitis. *Nat Med* 1995;1:564–569.
641. Simons JN, Pilotmatias TJ, Leary TP, et al. Identification of two flavivirus-like genomes in the GB hepatitis agent. *Proc Natl Acad Sci U S A* 1995;92:3401–3405.
642. Sizova DV, Kolupaeva VG, Pestova TV, et al. Specific interaction of eukaryotic translation initiation factor 3 with the 5′ nontranslated regions of hepatitis C virus and classical swine fever virus RNAs. *J Virol* 1998;72:4775–4782.
643. Smith DB, Basaras M, Frost S, et al. Phylogenetic analysis of GBV-C/hepatitis G virus. *J Gen Virol* 2000;81:769–780.
644. Smith DB, Cuceanu N, Davidson F, et al. Discrimination of hepatitis G virus/GBV-C geographical variants by analysis of the 5′ non-coding region. *J Gen Virol* 1997;78:1533–1542.
645. Smith DB, Mellor J, Jarvis LM, and Group TIHCS. Variation of the hepatitis C virus 5′ non-coding region: Implications for secondary structure, virus detection and typing. *J Gen Virol* 1995;76:1749–1761.
646. Smith GW, Wright PJ. Synthesis of proteins and glycoproteins in dengue type 2 virus-infected Vero and *Aedes albopictus* cells. *J Gen Virol* 1985;66:559–571.
647. Song J, Fujii M, Wang F, et al. The NS5A protein of hepatitis C virus partially inhibits the antiviral activity of interferon. *J Gen Virol* 1999; 80:879–886.
648. Spaete RR, Alexander D, Rugroden ME, et al. Characterization of the hepatitis E2/NS1 gene product expressed in mammalian cells. *Virology* 1992;188:819–830.
649. Srinivas RV, Ray RB, Meyer K, Ray R. Hepatitis C virus core protein inhibits human immunodeficiency virus type 1 replication. *Virus Res* 1996;45:87–92.
650. Sriurairatna S, Bhamarapravati N. Replication of dengue-2 virus in *Aedes albopictus* mosquitoes. *Am J Trop Med Hyg* 1977;26:1199–1205.
651. Sriurairatna S, Bhamarapravati N, Phalavadhtana O. Dengue virus infection of mice: Morphology and morphogenesis of dengue type 2 virus in suckling mouse neurones. *Infect Immun* 1973;8:1017–1028.
652. Srivastava SP, Kumar KU, Kaufman RJ. Phosphorylation of eukaryotic translation initiation factor 2 mediates apoptosis in response to activation of the double-stranded RNA-dependent protein kinase. *J Biol Chem* 1998;273:2416–2423.
653. Stadler K, Allison SL, Schalich J, Heinz FX. Proteolytic activation of tick-borne encephalitis virus by furin. *J Virol* 1997;71:8475–8481.
654. Stark K, Bienzle U, Hess G, et al. Detection of the hepatitis G virus genome among injecting drug users, homosexual and bisexual men, and blood donors. *J Infect Dis* 1996;174:1320–1323.
655. Stark R, Meyers G, Rümenapf T, Thiel H-J. Processing of pestivirus polyprotein: Cleavage site between autoprotease and nucleocapsid protein of classical swine fever virus. *J Virol* 1993;67:7088–7095.
656. Stark R, Rümenapf T, Meyers G, Thiel H-J. Genomic localization of hog cholera virus glycoproteins. *Virology* 1990;174:286–289.
657. Steffens S, Thiel HJ, Behrens SE. The RNA-dependent RNA polymerases of different members of the family *Flaviviridae* exhibit similar properties *in vitro*. *J Gen Virol* 1999;80:2583–2590.
658. Stempniak M, Hostomska Z, Nodes BR, Hostomsky Z. The NS3 proteinase domain of hepatitis C virus is a zinc-containing enzyme. *J Virol* 1997;71:2881–2886.
659. Stiasny K, Allison SL, Marchler-Bauer A, et al. Structural requirements for low-pH-induced rearrangements in the envelope glycoprotein of tick-borne encephalitis virus. *J Virol* 1996;70:8142–8147.
660. Stocks CE, Lobigs M. Posttranslational signal peptidase cleavage at the flavivirus C-prM junction *in vitro*. *J Virol* 1995;69:8123–8126.
661. Stocks CE, Lobigs M. Signal peptidase cleavage at the flavivirus C-prM junction: Dependence on the viral NS2B-3 protease for efficient processing requires determinants in C, the signal peptide, and prM. *J Virol* 1998;72:2141–2149.
662. Stohlman SA, Wisseman CL Jr, Eylar OR, Silverman DJ. Dengue virus-induced modifications of host cell membranes. *J Virol* 1975;16: 1017–1026.
663. Stollar V. Togaviruses in cultured arthropod cells. In: Schlesinger RW, ed. *The Togaviruses—Biology, Structure, Replication*. New York: Academic Press, 1980:584–621.
664. Strode GK. *Yellow fever*. New York: McGraw-Hill, 1951.
665. Sumiyoshi H, Hoke CH, Trent DW. Infectious Japanese encephalitis virus RNA can be synthesized from *in vitro*–ligated cDNA templates. *J Virol* 1992;66:5425–5431.
666. Sumiyoshi H, Mori C, Fuke I, et al. Complete nucleotide sequence of the Japanese encephalitis virus genome RNA. *Virology* 1987;161: 497–510.
667. Summers PL, Cohen WH, Ruiz MM, et al. Flaviviruses can mediate fusion from without in *Aedes albopictus* mosquito cell cultures. *Virus Res* 1989;12:383–392.
668. Susa M, Konig M, Saalmuller A, et al. Pathogenesis of classical swine fever: B-lymphocyte deficiency caused by hog cholera virus. *J Virol* 1992;66:1171–1175.
669. Suzich JA, Tamura JK, Palmer-Hill F, et al. Hepatitis C virus NS3 protein polynucleotide-stimulated nucleoside triphosphatase and comparison with the related pestivirus and flavivirus enzymes. *J Virol* 1993; 67:6152–6158.
670. Suzuki R, Matsuura Y, Susuki T, et al. Nuclear localization of the truncated hepatitis C virus core protein with its hydrophobic C terminus deleted. *J Gen Virol* 1995;76:53–61.
671. Tabor E, Garety RJ, Drucker JA, et al. Transmission of non-A, non-B hepatitis from man to chimpanzee. *Lancet* 1978;1:463–466.
672. Tacke M, Kiyosawa K, Stark K, et al. Detection of antibodies to a putative hepatitis G virus envelope protein [see comments] [published erratum appears in *Lancet* 1997;349:736]. *Lancet* 1997;349:318–320.
673. Tacke M, Schmolke S, Schlueter V, et al. Humoral immune response to the E2 protein of hepatitis G virus is associated with long-term recovery from infection and reveals a high frequency of hepatitis G virus exposure among healthy blood donors. *Hepatology* 1997;26: 1626–1633.
674. Tai C-L, Chi W-K, Chen D-S, Hwang L-H. The helicase activity associated with hepatitis C virus nonstructural protein 3 (NS3). *J Virol* 1996;70:8477–8484.
675. Takahashi K, Kishimoto S, Yoshizawa H, et al. p26 protein and 33-nm particle associated with nucleocapsid of hepatitis C virus recovered from the circulation of infected hosts. *Virology* 1992;191:431–434.
676. Takamizawa A, Mori C, Fuke I, et al. Structure and organization of the hepatitis C virus genome isolated from human carriers. *J Virol* 1991; 65:1105–1113.
677. Takegami T, Washizu M, Yasui K. Nucleotide sequence at the 3′ end of Japanese encephalitis virus genome RNA. *Virology* 1986;152: 483–486.
678. Takikawa S, Ishii K, Aizaki H, et al. Cell fusion activity of hepatitis C virus envelope proteins. *J Virol* 2000;74:5066–5074.
679. Tameda Y, Kosaka Y, Tagawa S, et al. Infection with GB virus C (GBV-C) in patients with fulminant hepatitis. *J Hepatol* 1996;25: 842–847.
680. Tamura JK, Warrener P, Collett MS. RNA-stimulated NTPase activity associated with the p80 protein of the pestivirus bovine viral diarrhea virus. *Virology* 1993;193:1–10.
681. Tan BH, Fu J, Sugrue RJ, et al. Recombinant dengue type 1 virus NS5 protein expressed in *Escherichia coli* exhibits RNA-dependent RNA polymerase activity. *Virology* 1996;216:317–325.
682. Tan S-L, Nakao H, He Y, et al. NS5A, a non-structural protein of hepatitis C virus, binds growth factor receptor-bound protein 2 adaptor protein in a src homology 3 domain/ligand-dependent manner and perturbs mitogenic signaling. *Proc Natl Acad Sci U S A* 1999;96: 5533–5538.
683. Tanaka T, Kato N, Cho M-J, Shimotohno K. A novel sequence found at the 3′ terminus of hepatitis C virus genome. *Biochem Biophys Res Commun* 1995;215:744–749.
684. Tanaka T, Kato N, Cho M-J, et al. Structure of the 3′ terminus of the hepatitis C virus genome. *J Virol* 1996;70:3307–3312.
685. Tanaka T, Kato N, Nakagawa M, et al. Molecular cloning of hepatitis C virus genome from a single Japanese carrier: Sequence variation within the same individual and among infected individuals. *Virus Res* 1992;23:39–53.
686. Tanaka Y, Shimoike T, Ishii K, et al. Selective binding of hepatitis C virus core protein to synthetic oligonucleotides corresponding to the 5′ untranslated region of the viral genome. *Virology* 2000;270:229–236.
687. Tanimoto A, Ide Y, Arima N, et al. The amino terminal deletion mutants of hepatitis C virus nonstructural protein NS5A function as transcriptional activators in yeast. *Biochem Biophys Res Commun* 1997;236:360–364.

688. Tanji Y, Hijikata M, Hirowatari Y, Shimotohno K. Hepatitis C virus polyprotein processing: Kinetics and mutagenic analysis of serine proteinase-dependent cleavage. *J Virol* 1994;68:8418–8422.
689. Tanji Y, Hijikata M, Hirowatari Y, Shimotohno K. Identification of the domain required for trans-cleavage activity of hepatitis C viral serine proteinase. *Gene* 1994;145:215–219.
690. Tanji Y, Hijikata M, Satoh S, et al. Hepatitis C virus-encoded nonstructural protein NS4A has versatile functions in viral protein processing. *J Virol* 1995;69:1575–1581.
691. Tanji Y, Kaneko T, Satoh S, Shimotohno K. Phosphorylation of hepatitis C virus-encoded nonstructural protein NS5A. *J Virol* 1995;69:3980–3986.
692. Taremi SS, Beyer B, Maher M, et al. Construction, expression, and characterization of a novel fully activated recombinant single-chain hepatitis C virus protease. *Protein Sci* 1998;7:2143–2149.
693. Tautz N, Elbers K, Stoll D, et al. Serine protease of pestiviruses: Determination of cleavage sites. *J Virol* 1997;71:5415–5422.
694. Tautz N, Harada T, Kaiser A, et al. Establishment and characterization of cytopathogenic and noncytopathogenic pestivirus replicons. *J Virol* 1999;73:9422–9432.
695. Tautz N, Kaiser A, Thiel HJ. NS3 serine protease of bovine viral diarrhea virus: Characterization of active site residues, NS4A cofactor domain, and protease-cofactor interactions. *Virology* 2000;273:351–363.
696. Tautz N, Meyers G, Stark R, et al. Cytopathogenicity of a pestivirus correlates with a 27-nucleotide insertion. *J Virol* 1996;70:7851–7858.
697. Tautz N, Meyers G, Thiel H-J. Processing of poly-ubiquitin in the polyprotein of an RNA virus. *Virology* 1993;197:74–85.
698. Tautz N, Thiel H-J, Dubovi EJ, Meyers G. Pathogenesis of mucosal disease: A cytopathogenic pestivirus generated by an internal deletion. *J Virol* 1994;68:3289–3297.
699. Taylor DR, Shi ST, Romano PR, et al. Inhibition of the interferon-inducible protein kinase PKR by HCV E2 protein [see comments]. *Science* 1999;285:107–110.
700. Teo KF, Wright PJ. Internal proteolysis of the NS3 protein specified by dengue virus 2. *J Gen Virol* 1997;78:337–341.
701. Theiler M, Smith HH. Use of yellow fever virus modified by *in vitro* cultivation for human immunization. *J Exp Med* 1937;65:787–800.
702. Thiel H-J, Plagemann PGW, Moennig V. Pestiviruses. In: Fields BN, Knipe DM, Howley PM, eds. *Fields Virology.* New York: Raven Press, 1996:1059–1073.
703. Thiel H-J, Stark R, Weiland E, et al. Hog cholera virus: Molecular composition of virions from a pestivirus. *J Virol* 1991;65:4705–4712.
704. Thomssen R, Bonk S, Propfe C, et al. Association of hepatitis C virus in human sera with beta-lipoprotein. *Med Microbiol Immunol* 1992; 181:293–300.
705. Thomssen R, Bonk S, Thiele A. Density heterogeneities of hepatitis C virus in human sera due to the binding of beta-lipoproteins and immunoglobulins. *Med Microbiol Immunol* 1993;182:329–334.
706. Timofeev AV, Ozherelkov SV, Pronin AV, et al. Immunological basis for protection in a murine model of tick-borne encephalitis by a recombinant adenovirus carrying the gene encoding the NS1 nonstructural protein. *J Gen Virol* 1998;79:689–695.
707. Tomei L, Failla C, Santolini E, et al. NS3 is a serine protease required for processing of hepatitis C virus polyprotein. *J Virol* 1993;67: 4017–4026.
708. Tomei L, Failla C, Vitale RL, et al. A central hydrophobic domain of the hepatitis C virus NS4A protein is necessary and sufficient for the activation of the NS3 protease. *J Gen Virol* 1996;77:1065–1070.
709. Tomori O. Impact of yellow fever on the developing world. *Adv Virus Res* 1999;53:5–34.
710. Tratschin JD, Moser C, Ruggli N, Hofmann MA. Classical swine fever virus leader proteinase N^{pro} is not required for viral replication in cell culture. *J Virol* 1998;72:7681–7684.
711. Trent DW. Antigenic characterization of flavivirus structural proteins separated by isoelectric focusing. *J Virol* 1977;22:608–618.
712. Trent DW, Naeve CW. Biochemistry and replication. In: Monath T, ed. *St. Louis Encephalitis.* Washington, DC: American Public Health Association, 1980:159–199.
713. Trent DW, Swensen CC, Qureshi AA. Synthesis of Saint Louis encephalitis virus ribonucleic acid in BHK-21-13 cells. *J Virol* 1969; 3:385–394.
714. Tsuchihara K, Hijikata M, Fukuda K, et al. Hepatitis C virus core protein regulates cell growth and signal transduction pathway transmitting growth stimuli. *Virology* 1999;258:100–107.
715. Tsuchihara K, Tanaka T, Hijikata M, et al. Specific interaction of polypyrimidine tract-binding protein with the extreme 3′-terminal structure of the hepatitis C virus genome, the 3′X. *J Virol* 1997;71: 6720–6726.
716. Tsukiyama-Kohara K, Iizuka N, Kohara M, Nomoto A. Internal ribosome entry site within hepatitis C virus RNA. *J Virol* 1992;66: 1476–1483.
717. Tu H, Gao L, Shi ST, et al. Hepatitis C virus RNA polymerase and NS5A complex with a SNARE-like protein. *Virology* 1999;263:30–41.
718. Tucker TJ, Smuts HE, Knobel GD, et al. Evidence that GBV-C/hepatitis G virus is primarily at lymphotropic virus. *J Viral Hepat* 2000;61: 52–58.
719. Urosevic N, Mansfield JP, Mackenzie JS, Shellam GR. Low resolution mapping around the flavivirus resistance locus (Flv) on mouse chromosome 5. *Mamm Genome* 1995;6:454–458.
720. Urosevic N, Silvia OJ, Sangster MY, et al. Development and characterization of new flavivirus-resistant mouse strains bearing Flv(r)-like and Flv(mr) alleles from wild or wild-derived mice. *J Gen Virol* 1999;80:897–906.
721. Urosevic N, van Maanen M, Mansfield JP, et al. Molecular characterization of virus-specific RNA produced in the brains of flavivirus-susceptible and -resistant mice after challenge with Murray Valley encephalitis virus. *J Gen Virol* 1997;78:23–29.
722. Valle RP, Falgout B. Mutagenesis of the NS3 protease of dengue virus type 2. *J Virol* 1998;72:624–632.
723. van Rijn PA, van Gennip HG, de Meijer EJ, Moormann RJ. Epitope mapping of envelope glycoprotein E1 of hog cholera virus strain Brescia. *J Gen Virol* 1993;74:2053–2060.
724. van Rijn PA, van Gennip HG, Leendertse CH, et al. Subdivision of the pestivirus genus based on envelope glycoprotein E2. *Virology* 1997; 237:337–348.
725. van Zijl M, Wensvoort G, de Kluyver E, et al. Live attenuated pseudorabies virus expressing envelope glycoprotein E1 of hog cholera virus protects swine against both pseudorabies and hog cholera. *J Virol* 1991;65:2761–2765.
726. Varnavski AN, Khromykh AA. Noncytopathic flavivirus replicon RNA-based system for expression and delivery of heterologous genes. *Virology* 1999;255:366–375.
727. Vassilev VB, Collett MS, Donis RO. Authentic and chimeric full-length genomic cDNA clones of bovine viral diarrhea virus that yield infectious transcripts. *J Virol* 1997;71:471–478.
728. Viazov S, Riffelmann M, Khoudyakov Y, et al. Genetic heterogeneity of hepatitis G virus isolates from different parts of the world. *J Gen Virol* 1997;78:577–581.
729. Wahlberg JM, Boere WAM, Garoff H. The heterodimeric association between the membrane proteins of Semliki Forest virus changes its sensitivity to low pH during virus maturation. *J Virol* 1989;63: 4991–4997.
730. Wahlberg JM, Bron R, Wilschut J, Garoff H. Membrane fusion of Semliki Forest virus involves homotrimers of the fusion protein. *J Virol* 1992;66:7309–7318.
731. Wahlberg JM, Garoff H. Membrane fusion process of Semliki Forest virus I: Low pH–induced rearrangement in spike protein quaternary structure precedes virus penetration into cells. *J Cell Biol* 1992;116:339–348.
732. Wakita T, Katsume A, Kato J, et al. Possible role of cytotoxic T cells in acute liver injury in hepatitis C virus cDNA transgenic mice mediated by Cre/loxP system. *J Med Virol* 2000;62:308–317.
733. Wakita T, Taya C, Katsume A, et al. Efficient conditional transgene expression in hepatitis C virus cDNA transgenic mice mediated by the Cre/loxP system. *J Biol Chem* 1998;273:9001–9006.
734. Walker CM. Comparative features of hepatitis C virus infection in humans and chimpanzees. *Springer Semin Immunopathol* 1997;19: 85–98.
735. Wallner G, Mandl CW, Kunz C, Heinz FX. The flavivirus 3′-noncoding region: Extensive size heterogeneity independent of evolutionary relationships among strains of tick-borne encephalitis virus. *Virology* 1995;213:169–178.
736. Wang C, Le SY, Ali N, Siddiqui A. An RNA pseudoknot is an essential structural element of the internal ribosome entry site located within the hepatitis C virus 5′ noncoding region. *RNA* 1995;1:526–537.
737. Wang C, Sarnow P, Siddiqui A. Translation of human hepatitis C virus RNA in cultured cells is mediated by an internal ribosome-binding mechanism. *J Virol* 1993;67:3338–3344.

738. Wang C, Siddiqui A. Structure and function of the hepatitis C virus internal ribosome entry site. *Curr Top Microbiol Immunol* 1995;203: 99–115.
739. Wang E, Weaver SC, Shope RE, et al. Genetic variation in yellow fever virus: Duplication in the 3′ noncoding region of strains from Africa. *Virology* 1996;225:274–281.
740. Wang JJ, Liao CL, Yang CI, et al. Localizations of NS3 and E proteins in mouse brain infected with mutant strain of Japanese encephalitis virus. *Arch Virol* 1998;143:2353–2369.
741. Wang S, He R, Anderson R. PrM- and cell-binding domains of the dengue virus E protein. *J Virol* 1999;73:2547–2551.
742. Wang Y, Okamoto H, Tsuda F, et al. Prevalence, genotypes, and an isolate (HC-C2) of hepatitis C virus in Chinese patients with liver disease. *J Med Virol* 1993;40:254–260.
743. Warrener P, Collett MS. Pestivirus NS3 (p80) protein possesses RNA helicase activity. *J Virol* 1995;69:1720–1726.
744. Warrener P, Tamura JK, Collett MS. An RNA-stimulated NTPase activity associated with yellow fever virus NS3 protein expressed in bacteria. *J Virol* 1993;67:989–996.
745. Watson JP, Bevitt DJ, Spickett GP, et al. Hepatitis C virus density heterogeneity and viral titre in acute and chronic infection: A comparison of immunodeficient and immunocompetent patients. *J Hepatol* 1996;25:599–607.
746. Weiland E, Ahl R, Stark R, et al. A second envelope glycoprotein mediates neutralization of a pestivirus, hog cholera virus. *J Virol* 1992;66:3677–3682.
747. Weiland E, Stark R, Haas B, et al. Pestivirus glycoprotein which induces neutralizing antibodies form part of a disulfide-linked heterodimer. *J Virol* 1990;64:3563–3569.
748. Weiland F, Weiland E, Unger G, et al. Localization of pestiviral envelope proteins E(rns) and E2 at the cell surface and on isolated particles. *J Gen Virol* 1999;80:1157–1165.
749. Weiner AJ, Brauer MJ, Rosenblatt J, et al. Variable and hypervariable domains are found in the regions of HCV corresponding to the flavivirus envelope and NS1 proteins and the pestivirus envelope glycoproteins. *Virology* 1991;180:842–848.
750. Weiner AJ, Geysen HM, Christopherson C, et al. Evidence for immune selection of hepatitis C virus (HCV) putative envelope glycoprotein variants: Potential role in chronic HCV infections. *Proc Natl Acad Sci U S A* 1992;89:3468–3472.
751. Wengler G, Castle E. Analysis of structural properties which possibly are characteristics for the 3′-terminal sequences of the genome RNA of flaviviruses. *J Gen Virol* 1986;67:1183–1188.
752. Wengler G, Czaya G, Färber PM, Hegemann JH. *In vitro* synthesis of West Nile virus proteins indicates that the amino-terminal segment of the NS3 protein contains the active centre of the protease which cleaves the viral polyprotein after multiple basic amino acids. *J Gen Virol* 1991;72:851–858.
753. Wengler G, Wengler G. Cell-associated West Nile flavivirus is covered with E+pre-M protein heterodimers which are destroyed and reorganized by proteolytic cleavage during virus release. *J Virol* 1989;63: 2521–2526.
754. Wengler G, Wengler G. The carboxy-terminal part of the NS3 protein of the West Nile flavivirus can be isolated as a soluble protein after proteolytic cleavage and represents an RNA-stimulated NTPase. *Virology* 1991;184:707–715.
755. Wengler G, Wengler G. The NS 3 nonstructural protein of flaviviruses contains an RNA triphosphatase activity. *Virology* 1993;197:265–273.
756. Wengler G, Wengler G, Gross HJ. Studies on virus-specific nucleic acids synthesized in vertebrate and mosquito cells infected with flaviviruses. *Virology* 1978;89:423–437.
757. Wengler G, Wengler G, Nowak T, Castle E. Description of a procedure which allows isolation of viral nonstructural proteins from BHK vertebrate cells infected with the West Nile flavivirus in a state which allows their direct chemical characterization. *Virology* 1990;177:795–801.
758. Wensvoort G. Topographical and functional mapping of epitopes on hog cholera virus with monoclonal antibodies. *J Gen Virol* 1989;70: 2865–2876.
759. Westaway EG. Replication of flaviviruses. In: Schlesinger RW, ed. *The Togaviruses: Biology, Structure, Replication.* New York: Academic Press, 1980:531–581.
760. Westaway EG. Flavivirus replication strategy. *Adv Virus Res* 1987;33: 45–90.
761. Westaway EG, Brinton MA, Gaidamovich SY, et al. *Flaviviridae. Intervirology* 1985;24:183–192.
762. Westaway EG, Khromykh AA, Kenney MT, et al. Proteins C and NS4B of the flavivirus Kunjin translocate independently into the nucleus. *Virology* 1997;234:31–41.
763. Westaway EG, Khromykh AA, Mackenzie JM. Nascent flavivirus RNA colocalized in situ with double-stranded RNA in stable replication complexes. *Virology* 1999;258:108–117.
764. Westaway EG, Mackenzie JM, Kenney MT, et al. Ultrastructure of Kunjin virus-infected cells: Colocalization of NS1 and NS3 with double-stranded RNA, and of NS2B with NS3, in virus-induced membrane structures. *J Virol* 1997;71:6650–6661.
765. Whitfield SG, Murphy FA, Sudia WD. St. Louis encephalitis virus: An ultrastructural study of infection in a mosquito vector. *Virology* 1973;56:70–87.
766. Widjojoatmodjo MN, van Gennip HG, Bouma A, et al. Classical swine fever virus E(rns) deletion mutants: Trans-complementation and potential use as nontransmissible, modified, live-attenuated marker vaccines. *J Virol* 2000;74:2973–2980.
767. Windisch JM, Schneider R, Stark R, et al. RNase of classical swine fever virus: Biochemical characterization and inhibition by virus-neutralizing monoclonal antibodies. *J Virol* 1996;70:352–358.
768. Winkler G, Heinz FX, Kunz C. Studies on the glycosylation of flavivirus E proteins and the role of carbohydrate in antigenic structure. *Virology* 1987;159:237–243.
769. Winkler G, Maxwell SE, Ruemmler C, Stollar V. Newly synthesized dengue-2 virus nonstructural protein NS1 is a soluble protein but becomes partially hydrophobic and membrane-associated after dimerization. *Virology* 1989;171:302–305.
770. Winkler G, Randolph VB, Cleaves GR, et al. Evidence that the mature form of the flavivirus nonstructural protein NS1 is a dimer. *Virology* 1988;162:187–196.
771. Wiskerchen M, Belzer SK, Collett MS. Pestivirus gene expression: The first protein product of the bovine viral diarrhea virus large open reading frame, p20, possesses proteolytic activity. *J Virol* 1991;65: 4508–4514.
772. Wiskerchen M, Collett MS. Pestivirus gene expression: Protein p80 of bovine viral diarrhea virus is a proteinase involved in polyprotein processing. *Virology* 1991;184:341–350.
773. Wölk B, Sansonno D, Kräusslich H-G, et al. Subcellular localization, stability and trans-cleavage of hepatitis C virus NS3-4A complex expressed in tetracyclin-regulated cell lines. *J Virol* 2000;74: 2293–2304.
774. Worobey M, Rambaut A, Holmes EC. Widespread intra-serotype recombination in natural populations of dengue virus. *Proc Natl Acad Sci U S A* 1999;96:7352–7357.
775. Wu RR, Mizokami M, Cao K, et al. GB virus C/hepatitis G virus infection in southern China. *J Infect Dis* 1997;175:168–171.
776. Xiang J, Daniels KJ, Soll DR, et al. Visualization and characterization of GB-virus-C particles: Evidence for a nucleocapsid. *J Viral Hepat* 1999;6(Suppl 1):16–22.
777. Xiang J, Klinzman D, McLinden J, et al. Characterization of hepatitis G virus (GB-C virus) particles: Evidence for a nucleocapsid and expression of sequences upstream of the E1 protein. *J Virol* 1998;72: 2738–2744.
778. Xie ZC, Riezu-Boj JI, Lasarte JJ, et al. Transmission of hepatitis C virus infection to tree shrews. *Virology* 1998;244:513–520.
779. Xu J, Mendez E, Caron PR, et al. Bovine viral diarrhea virus NS3 serine proteinase: Polyprotein cleavage sites, cofactor requirements, and molecular model of an enzyme essential for pestivirus replication. *J Virol* 1997;71:5312–5322.
780. Xue W, Minocha HC. Identification of the cell surface receptor for bovine viral diarrhoea virus by using anti-idiotypic antibodies. *J Gen Virol* 1993;74:73–79.
781. Xue W, Zhang S, Minocha HC. Characterization of a putative receptor protein for bovine viral diarrhea virus. *Vet Microbiol* 1997;57: 105–118.
782. Yamada N, Tanihara K, Mizokami M, et al. Full-length sequence of the genome of hepatitis C virus type 3a: Comparative study with different genotypes. *J Gen Virol* 1994;75:3279–3284.
783. Yamada N, Tanihara K, Takada A, et al. Genetic organization and diversity of the 3′ noncoding region of the hepatitis C virus genome. *Virology* 1996;223:255–261.

784. Yamashita T, Kaneko S, Shirota Y, et al. RNA-dependent RNA polymerase activity of the soluble recombinant hepatitis C virus NS5B protein truncated at the C-terminal region. *J Biol Chem* 1998;273: 15479–15486.
785. Yamshchikov VF, Compans RW. Regulation of the late events in flavivirus protein processing and maturation. *Virology* 1993;192:38–51.
786. Yamshchikov VF, Compans RW. Processing of the intracellular form of the West Nile virus capsid protein by the viral NS2B-NS3 protease: An *in vitro* study. *J Virol* 1994;68:5765–5771.
787. Yamshchikov VF, Compans RW. Formation of the flavivirus envelope: Role of the viral NS2B-NS3 protease. *J Virol* 1995;69:1995–2003.
788. Yamshchikov VF, Trent DW, Compans RW. Upregulation of signalase processing and induction of prM-E secretion by the flavivirus NS2B-NS3 protease: Roles of protease components. *J Virol* 1997;71: 4364–4371.
789. Yan Y, Li Y, Munshi S, et al. Complex of NS3 protease and NS4A peptide of BK strain hepatitis C virus: A 2.2 Å resolution structure in a hexagonal crystal form. *Protein Sci* 1998;7:837–847.
790. Yanagi M, Purcell RH, Emerson SU, Bukh J. Transcripts from a single full-length cDNA clone of hepatitis C virus are infectious when directly transfected into the liver of a chimpanzee. *Proc Natl Acad Sci U S A* 1997;94:8738–8743.
791. Yanagi M, Purcell RH, Emerson SU, Bukh J. Hepatitis C virus: An infectious molecular clone of a second major genotype (2a) and lack of viability of intertypic 1a and 2a chimeras. *Virology* 1999;262: 250–263.
792. Yanagi M, St. Claire M, Emerson SU, et al. *In vivo* analysis of the 3′ untranslated region of the hepatitis C virus after *in vitro* mutagenesis of an infectious cDNA clone. *Proc Natl Acad Sci U S A* 1999;96: 2291–2295.
793. Yanagi M, St. Claire M, Shapiro M, et al. Transcripts of a chimeric cDNA clone of hepatitis C virus genotype 1b are infectious *in vivo*. *Virology* 1998;244:161–172.
794. Yao N, Hesson T, Cable M, et al. Structure of the hepatitis C virus RNA helicase domain. *Nat Struct Biol* 1997;4:463–467.
795. Yao N, Reichert P, Taremi SS, et al. Molecular views of viral polyprotein processing revealed by the crystal structure of the hepatitis C virus bifunctional protease-helicase. *Structure Fold Des* 1999;7: 1353–1363.
796. Yasui K, Wakita T, Tsukiyama-Kohara K, et al. The native form and maturation process of hepatitis C virus core protein. *J Virol* 1998;72: 6048–6055.
797. Yen J-H, Chang SC, Hu C-R, et al. Cellular proteins specifically bind to the 5′-noncoding region of hepatitis C virus RNA. *Virology* 1995; 208:723–732.
798. Yi M, Kaneko S, Yu DY, Murakami S. Hepatitis C virus envelope proteins bind lactoferrin. *J Virol* 1997;71:5997–6002.
799. Yoo BJ, Selby M, Choe J, et al. Transfection of a differentiated human hepatoma cell line (Huh7) with *in vitro*-transcribed hepatitis C virus (HCV) RNA and establishment of a long-term culture persistently infected with HCV. *J Virol* 1995;69:32–38.
800. Yoo BJ, Spaete RR, Geballe AP, et al. 5′ end-dependent translation initiation of hepatitis C viral RNA and the presence of putative positive and negative translational control elements within the 5′ untranslated region. *Virology* 1992;191:889–899.
801. Yoshiba M, Inoue K, Sekiyama K. Hepatitis GB virus C [letter]. *N Engl J Med* 1996;335:1392–1393.
802. Yoshiba M, Okamoto H, Mishiro S. Detection of the GBV-C hepatitis virus genome in serum from patients with fulminant hepatitis of unknown aetiology [see comments]. *Lancet* 1995;346:1131–1132.
803. You S, Padmanabhan R. A novel *in vitro* replication system for dengue virus. Initiation of RNA synthesis at the 3′-end of exogenous viral RNA templates requires 5′- and 3′-terminal complementary sequence motifs of the viral RNA. *J Biol Chem* 1999;274:33714–33722.
804. Yu H, Grassmann CW, Behrens SE. Sequence and structural elements at the 3′ terminus of bovine viral diarrhea virus genomic RNA: Functional role during RNA replication. *J Virol* 1999;73:3638–3648.
805. Yuan Z-H, Kumar U, Thomas HC, et al. Expression, purification, and partial characterization of HCV RNA polymerase. *Biochem Biophys Res Commun* 1997;232:231–235.
806. Yuasa T, Ishikawa G, Manabe S, et al. The particle size of hepatitis C virus estimated by filtration through microporous regenerated cellulose fibre. *J Gen Virol* 1991;72:2021–2024.
807. Zanotto PM, Gould EA, Gao GF, et al. Population dynamics of flaviviruses revealed by molecular phylogenies [see comments]. *Proc Natl Acad Sci U S A* 1996;93:548–553.
808. Zeng L, Falgout B, Markoff L. Identification of specific nucleotide sequences within the conserved 3′-SL in the dengue type 2 virus genome required for replication. *J Virol* 1998;72:7510–7522.
809. Zhang G, Aldridge S, Clarke MC, McCauley JW. Cell death induced by cytopathic bovine viral diarrhoea virus is mediated by apoptosis. *J Gen Virol* 1996;77:1677–1681.
810. Zhang L, Mohan PM, Padmanabhan R. Processing and localization of dengue virus type 2 polyprotein precursor NS3-NS4A-NS4B-NS5. *J Virol* 1992;66:7549–7554.
811. Zhao B, Mackow E, Buckler-White A, et al. Cloning full length dengue 4 viral DNA sequences: Analysis of genes coding for structural proteins. *Virology* 1986;155:77–88.
812. Zhong W, Gutshall LL, Del Vecchio AM. Identification and characterization of an RNA-dependent RNA polymerase activity within the nonstructural protein 5B region of bovine viral diarrhea virus. *J Virol* 1998;72:9365–9369.
813. Zhong W, Ingravallo P, Wright-Minogue J, et al. Nucleoside triphosphatase and RNA helicase activities associated with GB virus B nonstructural protein 3. *Virology* 1999;261:216–226.
814. Zhong W, Uss AS, Ferrari E, et al. De novo initiation of RNA synthesis by hepatitis C virus nonstructural protein 5B polymerase. *J Virol* 2000;74:2017–2022.
815. Zhu N, Khoshnan A, Schneider R, et al. Hepatitis C virus core protein binds to the cytoplasmic domain of tumor necrosis factor (TNF) receptor 1 and enhances TNF-induced apoptosis. *J Virol* 1998;72:3691–3697.
816. Zitzmann N, Mehta AS, Carrouee S, et al. Imino sugars inhibit the formation and secretion of bovine viral diarrhea virus, a pestivirus model of hepatitis C virus: Implications for the development of broad spectrum anti-hepatitis virus agents. *Proc Natl Acad Sci U S A* 1999;96: 11878–11882.

CHAPTER 21

Coronaviridae: The Viruses and Their Replication

Michael M. C. Lai and Kathryn V. Holmes

CLASSIFICATION

Coronaviruses, a genus in the family *Coronaviridae*, are large, enveloped, positive-stranded RNA viruses that cause highly prevalent diseases in humans and domestic animals (Table 1). They have the largest genomes of all RNA viruses and replicate by a unique mechanism, which results in a high frequency of recombination. Virions mature by budding at intracellular membranes, and infection with some coronaviruses induces cell fusion.

Coronaviruses were first recognized as a distinct virus group by their characteristic virion morphology in negatively stained preparations (1,36) (Fig. 1). The viral envelopes are studded with long, petal-shaped spikes, giving coronaviruses the appearance of a crown (Latin, *corona*), and the nucleocapsids are long, flexible helices. Other characteristics that define Coronaviridae include the 3′-coterminal, nested-set structure of the mRNAs, unique RNA transcription strategy, genome organization, nucleotide sequence homology, and the properties of their structural proteins (36,138). The Coronaviridae family includes two genera, coronavirus and torovirus, which share many features of genome organization and replication strategy but have different virion morphology and genome lengths. The Coronaviridae, together with the Arteriviridae family, are classified in the order Nidovirales, whose member viruses share a unique feature: they all synthesize a nested set of multiple subgenomic mRNAs (34). Toroviruses and all members of the Arteriviridae family infect only animals. This chapter discusses coronaviruses exclusively.

Coronaviruses can be divided into three serologically distinct groups (see Table 1). Within each serogroup, the viruses are classified according to their natural hosts, nucleotide sequences, and serologic relationships. Most coronaviruses naturally infect only one animal species or, at most, a limited number of closely related species. Virus replication *in vivo* can be either disseminated, causing systemic infections, or restricted to a few cell types, often the epithelial cells of the respiratory or enteric tracts and macrophages, causing localized infections (see Table 1). Nucleotide sequences of the entire genomes of several coronaviruses, including avian infectious bronchitis virus (IBV), murine hepatitis virus (MHV), human coronavirus 229E (HCoV-229E), and porcine transmissible gastroenteritis virus (TGEV), confirm the similarity of the genome organization of these different coronaviruses (28, 72,94,95,144).

TABLE 1. *Serotypes, natural hosts, and diseases of coronavirus*

Antigenic group	Virus	Host	Respiratory infection	Enteric infection	Hepatitis	Neurologic infection	Other[a]
I	HCoV-229E	Human	X			?	
	TGEV, PRCoV	Pig	X	X			X
	CCoV	Dog		X			
	FECoV	Cat		X			
	FIPV	Cat	X	X	X	X	X
	RbCoV	Rabbit		X			X
II	HCoV-OC43	Human	X	?		?	
	MHV	Mouse	X	X	X	X	
	SDAV	Rat					X
	HEV	Pig	X	X		X	
	BCoV	Cow	X	X			
	TCoV	Turkey	X	X			
III	IBV	Chicken	X		X		X
	TCoV	Turkey	X	X			

[a]Other diseases caused by coronaviruses include infectious peritonitis, immunologic disorders, runting, nephritis, pancreatitis, parotitis, myocarditis, and sialodacryoadenitis.

HCoV-229E, human respiratory coronavirus; TGEV, porcine transmissible gastroenteritis virus; PRCoV, porcine respiratory coronavirus; CCoV, canine coronavirus; FECoV, feline enteric coronavirus; FIPV, feline infectious peritonitis virus; RbCoV, rabbit coronavirus; HCoV-OC43, human respiratory coronavirus; MHV, murine hepatitis virus; SDAV, sialodacryoadenitis virus; HEV, porcine hemagglutinating encephalomyelitis virus; BCoV, bovine coronavirus; IBV, avian infectious bronchitis virus; TCoV, turkey coronavirus.

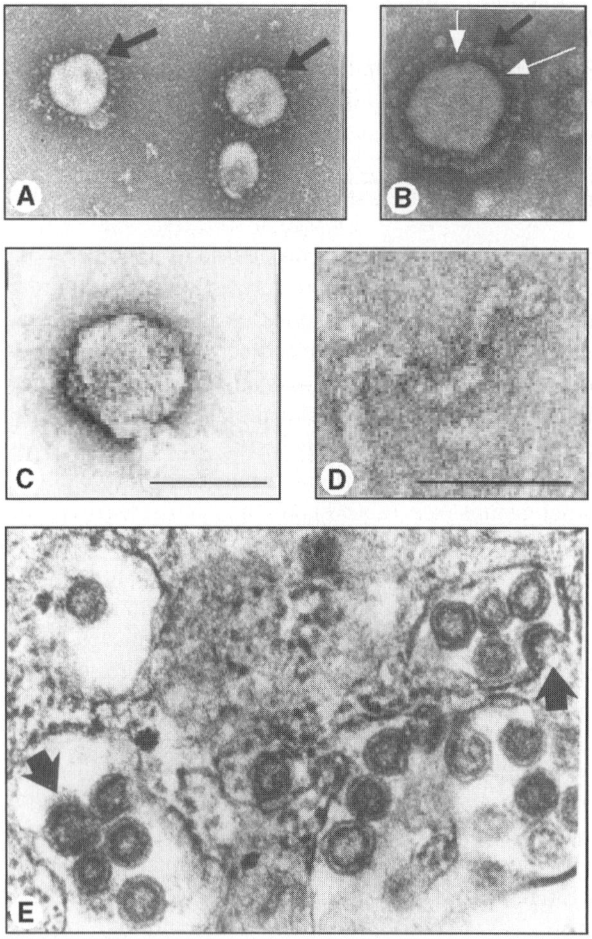

FIG. 1. Morphology of coronaviruses. Human respiratory coronavirus HCoV-OC43 (original magnification, ×90,000) **(A)** and turkey enteric coronavirus TCoV **(B)** in negatively stained preparations. The large, petal-shaped spikes (*black arrows*), composed of the S glycoprotein, seen on the envelopes of both viruses distinguish coronaviruses from other enveloped viruses. Some coronaviruses also exhibit a fringe of shorter spikes composed of the hemagglutinin-esterase (HE) glycoprotein (*white arrows*). **C:** Internal core of porcine transmissible gastroenteritis virus (TGEV). The core was obtained after removal of envelope by treatment with NP-40 and appears to have a spherical symmetry. **D:** Helical nucleocapsid released from the TGEV core structure by Triton X-100 treatment. *Bar:* 70 nm. **E:** Human cell infected with human respiratory coronavirus HCoV-229E. Spherical virions are seen budding at membranes of the ER and in smooth-walled vesicles (*arrows*). The electron-dense helical nucleocapsid is visible as slender, flexible tubules within the virions. The virus particles of some coronaviruses may mature further into electron-dense particles (215) (original magnification, ×60,000). (**B** courtesy of Peter Tijssen; **C and D** courtesy of Luis Enjuanes.)

VIRION MORPHOLOGY AND STRUCTURE

The structure of coronavirus virions is diagrammed in Figure 2. The virions are spherical enveloped particles about 100 to 120 nm in diameter. Inside the virion is a single-stranded, positive-sense genomic RNA 27 to 32 kb in size, the largest of all RNA virus genomes (28,72,94, 138,144). The RNA genome associates with the N (nucleocapsid) phosphoprotein (50–60 kd) to form a long, flexible, helical nucleocapsid (175,254). When released from the virus particles, the nucleocapsids appear as extended tubular strands 14 to 16 nm in diameter (211,254) (see Fig. 1, panel **D**). Recent studies showed that in at least two coronaviruses (TGEV and MHV), the helical nucleocapsid is enclosed within an "internal core structure," 65 nm in diameter, that is spherical, and possibly icosahedral, in form. The core is composed of M (membrane) glycoprotein (and probably N protein as well). It can be released from virions by NP-40 treatment (211) (see Fig. 1, panel **C**). The virus core is enclosed by a lipoprotein envelope, which is formed during virus budding from intracellular membranes (91,201,264). Two types of prominent spikes line the outside of the virion. The long spikes (20 nm), which consist of the S (spike) glycoprotein, are present on all coronaviruses; the short spikes, which consist of the HE (hemagglutinin-esterase) glycoprotein, are present in only some coronaviruses (see Fig. 1, panels **A** and **B**). The envelope also contains the M glycoprotein, which spans the lipid bilayer three times (171–173); thus, the M protein is apparently a component of both the internal core structure and the envelope. The

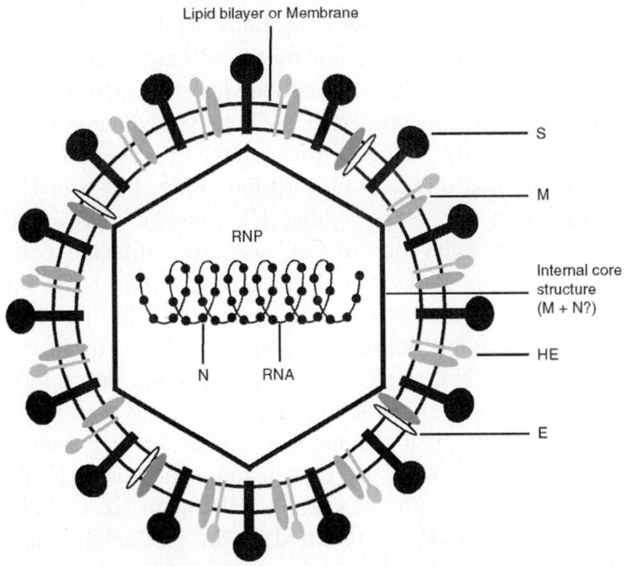

FIG. 2. Model of coronavirus structure: a schematic diagram of virion structure. S, spike glycoprotein; M, membrane glycoprotein; E, small envelope protein; HE, hemagglutinin-esterase glycoprotein; N, nucleocapsid phosphoprotein; ICS, internal core-shell composed of M glycoprotein; NC, nucleocapsid.

envelope also contains an E (envelope) protein, which is present in much smaller amounts than the other viral envelope proteins (87,271,295).

Structural Proteins

The S glycoprotein forms the large, petal-shaped spikes on the surface of the virion. This heavily glycosylated protein has a molecular mass of about 150 to 180 kd. S can be divided into three structural domains (from N- to C-terminus): a large external domain that is further divided into two subdomains, S1 and S2; a transmembrane domain; and a short carboxylterminal cytoplasmic domain. The S1 subdomain includes the N-terminal half of the molecule and forms the globular portion of the spikes. It contains sequences that are responsible for binding to specific receptors on the membranes of susceptible cells. S1 sequences are variable, containing various degrees of deletion and substitutions in different coronavirus strains or isolates. Mutations in S1 sequences have been associated with altered antigenicity and pathogenicity of the virus (74,99). In contrast, S2 sequences are more conserved. S2 is acylated and contains two heptad repeat motifs that suggest a coiled-coil structure (53,167). Indeed, evidence suggests that the mature S protein forms an oligomer, most likely a trimer (58). Thus, S2 subdomain probably constitutes the stalk of the viral spike. In most MHV strains and in bovine coronavirus (BCoV), the 180-kd S protein is cleaved during or after virus maturation by a cellular protease to yield the S1 and S2 proteins that remain noncovalently associated in the viral spikes. The extent of S cleavage varies among different coronaviruses and also depends on the host cell types (81,253). The cleavage of S into S1 and S2 may enhance the cell fusion activity or viral infectivity (89,255), but even uncleaved S protein can mediate cell–cell fusion and fusion of the viral envelope with host cell membranes, though at a lower efficiency (26,245,259). The S proteins of coronaviruses in group I are not cleaved; even so, some of these viruses, such as feline infectious peritonitis virus (FIPV), can induce cell–cell fusion (54).

The S glycoprotein has several important biologic functions (Table 2). Monoclonal antibodies against S can neutralize virus infectivity (47,77), consistent with the observation that S protein binds to cellular receptors (86,128). The receptor-binding domain of the S protein of MHV is localized within the N-terminal 330 amino acids of the S1 domain (257). Consequently, the amino acid sequences of the S1 domain can determine the target cell specificity of coronaviruses in animals (99,219).

S protein also induces fusion of the viral envelope with host cell membranes and, sometimes, cell–cell fusion. Expression of coronavirus S protein alone can induce fusion of receptor-bearing cells (54,259,294). The membrane fusion activity is most likely conferred by the internal hydrophobic sequences within the S2 (167). However,

TABLE 2. *Properties and functions of coronavirus structural proteins*

Nucleocapsid phosphoprotein **N**	Binds to viral RNA Forms nucleocapsid Elicits cell-mediated immunity
Membrane glycoprotein **M** (formerly **E1**)	An integral membrane protein on the Golgi Determines virus-budding site Triggers virus particle assembly Interacts with viral nucleocapsid Forms the shell of internal viral core (of TGEV and MHV) Induces α-interferon
Envelope (Small membrane) protein **E** (formerly **sM**)	Triggers virus particle assembly Associated with viral envelope May cause apoptosis
Spike glycoprotein **S** (formerly **E2**)	Forms large spikes on virion surfaces Binds to specific cellular receptors Induces fusion of viral envelope with cell membranes (plasma membrane or endosomal membrane) May induce cell–cell fusion Binds Fc fragment of immunoglobulin (MHV and TGEV) Binds 9-O-acetylated neuraminic acid or *N*-glycolylneuraminic acid Induces neutralizing antibody Elicits cell-mediated immunity
Hemagglutinin-esterase glycoprotein **HE** (formerly **E3**)	Forms small spikes on the virion surface of some coronaviruses Binds to 9-O-acetylated neuraminic acid Causes hemagglutination May cause hemadsorption Esterase cleaves acetyl groups from 9-O-acetyl neuraminic acid

TGEV, porcine transmissible gastroenteritis virus; MHV, mouse hepatitis virus.

the fusion activity can be affected by sequences at multiple sites in the S2 as well as S1 (84,217).

Several other biologic activities have been associated with the S protein (see Table 2). The presence of MHV S protein on the plasma membrane of infected cells makes the cells susceptible to B-cell–mediated cytotoxicity (108,280), and the S glycoproteins of several coronaviruses share a similar sequence with the Fcγ receptor for immunoglobulin (Ig), enabling the S protein to bind to the Fc fragment of IgG (198). This molecular mimicry may play a role in viral pathogenesis. The S proteins of BCoV and HCoV-OC43 can also bind 9-*O*-acetylated neuraminic acid-containing glycans and possess a hemagglutinating activity (227–229). This binding may be involved in the first step of virus infection for these viruses. Thus, S is a large, multifunctional protein that plays a central role in the biology and pathogenesis of coronavirus infections.

The HE glycoprotein is found on the virions of some group II coronaviruses and turkey coronavirus (TCoV) (group III) as a disulfide-linked dimer of a 65- to 70-kd protein that forms short spikes on the virions (see Figs. 1 and 2) (104,117,129,231). The presence or absence of this protein is highly variable even among group II coronaviruses, and its structure is frequently mutated or completely deleted during serial virus passaging in culture (288), suggesting that the HE protein is not essential for viral replication. Interestingly, the HE protein of coronavirus shares about 30% amino acid sequence similarity with the hemagglutinin protein of influenza C virus and may have been derived by a recombination between an HE mRNA of influenza C virus and the genomic RNA of an ancestral coronavirus (168). Like the S proteins of BCoV and HCoV-OC43, HE protein of various coronaviruses binds 9-*O*-acetylated neuraminic acid residues (229,231,274) and likely contributes to the hemagglutination and hemadsorption activities of coronaviruses. As the name implies, HE has an acetylesterase activity that cleaves acetyl groups from 9-*O*-acetylated neuraminic acid (274,290), thereby preventing or reversing the hemagglutination or hemadsorption induced by S or HE. These properties suggest that HE may be involved in either virus entry or virus release from infected cells. Indeed, some monoclonal antibodies against HE of BCoV can neutralize virus infectivity (64). In this virus, HE may mediate initial adsorption of the virus to cell membranes, but subsequent steps of virus entry most likely require the interaction of the S protein with a specific receptor, in a mechanism similar to that seen in other coronaviruses. This conclusion is supported by the finding that infection of murine cells by an HE-containing strain of MHV is inhibited by the monoclonal antibodies against the cellular receptor (83) or the viral S protein, despite the presence of HE protein in the virion (77). Thus, HE appears to be a "luxury" protein and is not absolutely necessary for virus infection in culture. Nevertheless, the presence of HE in a virus may alter its pathogenicity in animals (287).

The M glycoprotein differs from other coronavirus glycoproteins in that only a short aminoterminal domain of M is exposed on the exterior of the viral envelope. This domain is followed by a triple-membrane–spanning domain, an α-helical domain, and a large carboxylterminal domain inside the viral envelope (7,163,171,217). In some coronaviruses, such as TGEV, the carboxylterminus of the M protein is exposed on the virion surface (212). Glycosylation of the aminoterminal domain is O-linked for MHV and N-linked for IBV and TGEV (65,106,142,197). Monoclonal antibodies against the external domain of M neutralize viral infectivity, but only in the presence of complement (47). M proteins of some coronaviruses can induce interferon-α (43). The M proteins are targeted to the Golgi apparatus and not transported to the plasma membrane (172,173,258). In TGEV and MHV virions, the M glycoprotein is present not only in the viral envelope but also in the internal core structure (211).

An additional small envelope protein (E, formerly called sM), which is 9 to 12 kd, was recently shown to be associated with the viral envelope (87,159,295). Both E and M proteins are required for budding of virions (see Assembly and Release of Virions) (27,271). The topology and abundance of the E protein in the viral envelope have not been precisely determined.

The nucleocapsid protein, N, is a phosphoprotein of 50 to 60 kd that interacts with viral genomic RNA to form the viral nucleocapsid. N has three relatively conserved structural domains, including an RNA-binding domain in the middle (187) that binds to the leader sequence of viral RNA (249). N protein in the viral nucleocapsid further interacts with M (254), leading to the formation of virus particles. N may also play a role in viral RNA synthesis, as suggested by a study in which an antibody directed against N inhibited an *in vitro* coronavirus RNA polymerase reaction (49). N protein also binds to cellular membranes and phospholipids (5), a property that may help to facilitate both virus assembly and formation of RNA replication complexes.

Coronaviruses, like other positive-stranded RNA viruses, do not incorporate RNA-dependent RNA polymerase into mature virions. Protein kinase activity is present in purified virions, but it is not yet clear whether it is a viral or cellular enzyme (240).

Viral Genome

The genomes of several coronaviruses are illustrated in Figure 3. Coronavirus genomic RNAs are capped, polyadenylated, positive-stranded RNAs of 27 to 32 kb in length. They can function as mRNAs, and the purified genomic RNA is infectious (164,226). At the 5′ end of the genome is a sequence of 65 to 98 nucleotides, termed the *leader RNA,* that is also present at the 5′ ends of all subgenomic mRNAs (139,238,243). An untranslated region (UTR) of 200 to 400 nucleotides follows this leader

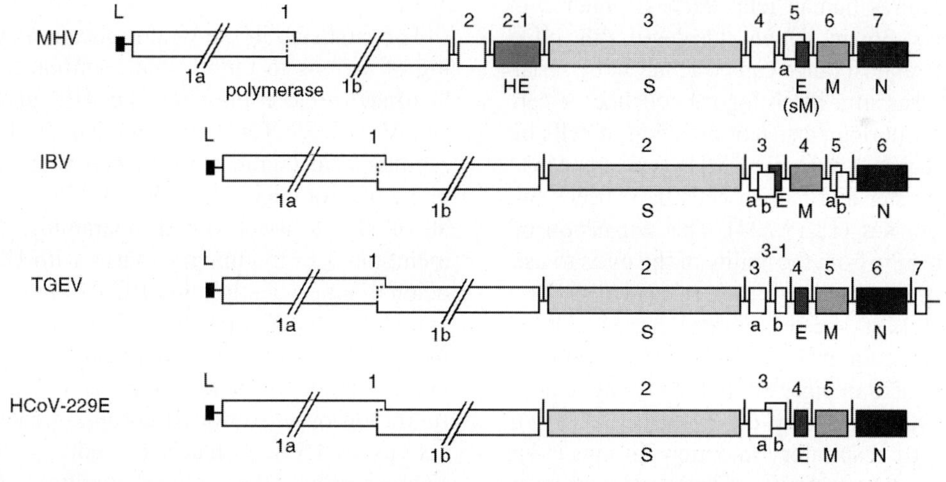

FIG. 3. Genomic organization of coronaviruses. The structures of four coronavirus genomic RNAs, for which complete sequences are available, are shown. The sizes of the genes are drawn about to scale, except for gene 1. The murine hepatitis virus (MHV) genome is 31.2 kb, and its gene 1 is 22 kb. The genomes for avian infectious bronchitis virus (IBV), porcine transmissible gastroenteritis virus (TGEV), and human respiratory coronavirus (HCoV)–229E are 27.6, 28.5, and 27.2 kb, respectively. The 5′ end consists of a cap and a 65- to 98-base long leader sequence (L). *Shaded boxes* represent open reading frames (ORFs) encoding structural proteins; *unshaded boxes* encode nonstructural proteins. The *vertical lines* represent intergenic sequences (IG). The area between two IGs represents one gene; the separate ORFs within each gene are translated from a single mRNA species. Note the variations in the number, sequences, and locations of the ORFs encoding the nonstructural proteins. Coronavirus genomes are polyadenylated at the 3′ end.

sequence. At the 3′ end of the RNA genome is another UTR of 200 to 500 nucleotides, followed by poly(A) of variable length. The sequences of both the 3′- and 5′-UTR are important for RNA replication and transcription. The remaining genomic sequence includes 7 to 10 open reading frames (ORFs). Gene 1, which comprises two thirds of the genome from the 5′ end, is about 20 to 22 kb in length. It consists of two overlapping ORFs (1a and 1b). These ORFs are translated into a polyprotein, which is the precursor of viral polymerase. The order of the genes encoding the polymerase (*Pol*) and the four structural proteins that are present in all coronaviruses is 5′-*Pol*-S-E-M-N-3′. These genes are interspersed with several ORFs encoding various nonstructural proteins and the HE glycoprotein, which differ markedly among coronaviruses in number, nucleotide sequence, gene order, and method of expression (138) (see Fig. 3). The functions of most of the nonstructural protein gene products are unknown; some are absent in genomes of some coronaviruses (232,291). The marked variability of coronavirus genome structure may be the result of RNA recombination.

GROWTH OF CORONAVIRUSES

Most coronaviruses infect only the cells of their natural host species and a few closely related species. Some coronavirus strains may infect a wider range of cells under certain experimental conditions; for example, intracerebral inoculation of some MHV strains into owls and African green monkeys can result in central nervous system infection (33,192). Primary isolation of human respiratory coronaviruses often requires human fetal tracheal organ cultures (see Chapter 36 in *Fields Virology*, 4th ed.). Expansion of the viral host range can be achieved by serial passaging of the virus in a heterologous cell line or can occur spontaneously during persistent infection of cells of the natural host species. A variety of MHV variants capable of infecting hamster and human cells have been isolated by these processes (18,19,224). This expansion of host ranges often results from the ability of the virus to use an expanded repertoire of receptor molecules (18).

In their natural host species, coronaviruses exhibit marked tissue tropism; for example, TGEV causes mainly gastrointestinal diseases in pigs, whereas a closely related virus strain, porcine respiratory coronavirus (PRCoV), causes predominantly respiratory infections in pigs (51). The species and tissue specificity of the virus is at least partially determined by the nature and distribution of cellular receptor molecules and by sequence variations in the viral S glycoprotein (219).

Coronavirus replication takes place in the cytoplasm of infected cells and can occur in enucleated cells, although at a low efficiency (29,281). However, actinomycin D has been reported to inhibit the replication of some coronaviruses in some cell lines (67,73,148). Thus, the possible role of the nucleus in coronavirus replication is still debatable. Infectious coronaviruses can be isolated from culture fluids and from infected cells disrupted by freezing and thawing. Infectivity of MHV virions is fairly stable at pH 6.0, but the virus is rapidly inactivated at a mildly alkaline pH (256). Coronaviruses can cause either cytocidal or persistent infections of cells in culture and in animal infections, depending on the virus strain and the host cell. In cytocidal coronavirus infections, cells may form multinucleated syncytia, lyse, or both. Plaques on infected cell cultures can be visualized by cell lysis, fusion, neutral red staining, or, in the case of BCoV, hemadsorption. Persistent HCoV-229E infection can be established in some human cell lines, producing virus for weeks without cytopathic effects or cell death (39). After an acute lytic infection, many coronaviruses establish persistently infected carrier cultures with minimal cytopathic effects; these cultures are resistant to superinfection by the wild-type virus (39,50,89,105).

Coronaviruses and their replication *in vitro* and *in vivo* can be detected by sensitive immunoassays with various monoclonal antibodies, nucleic acid hybridization, and reverse transcription–polymerase chain reaction (RT-PCR) as well as by plaque assay, immunofluorescence, and, in some cases, hemadsorption (34,48,193).

CORONAVIRUS REPLICATION

The major events in the coronavirus replicative cycle are summarized in Figure 4.

Attachment

The first step in the viral replication cycle is the binding of virions to the plasma membranes of target cells. Coronaviruses containing the HE glycoprotein (e.g., BCoV, HCoV-OC43) may bind to 9-*O*-acetylated neuraminic acid (sialic acid), a common moiety on membrane macromolecules (229,231,275). Enzymatic removal of the 9-*O*-acetylated neuraminic acid from cell membranes or treatment of virus with HE-specific monoclonal antibodies inhibits BCoV infection but does not completely block it (63,64,229), suggesting that the binding of HE to 9-*O*-acetylated neuraminic acid residues is necessary for, or at least can facilitate, virus infection. Inhibition by diisopropylfluorophosphate of the esterase activity of HE also markedly reduces BCoV infectivity (274); however, the esterase activity is likely involved in virus release rather than in virus entry because the newly synthesized virions may be trapped by the neuraminic acid residues on cell surface molecules and require esterase for virus release. In any case, virus binding to neuraminic acid residues may not be a crucial step for virus infection because many coronaviruses do not bind sialic acids. Furthermore, because sialic acid is a common cell surface carbohydrate and the tissue tropism of coronaviruses is restricted, this HE-sialic acid binding

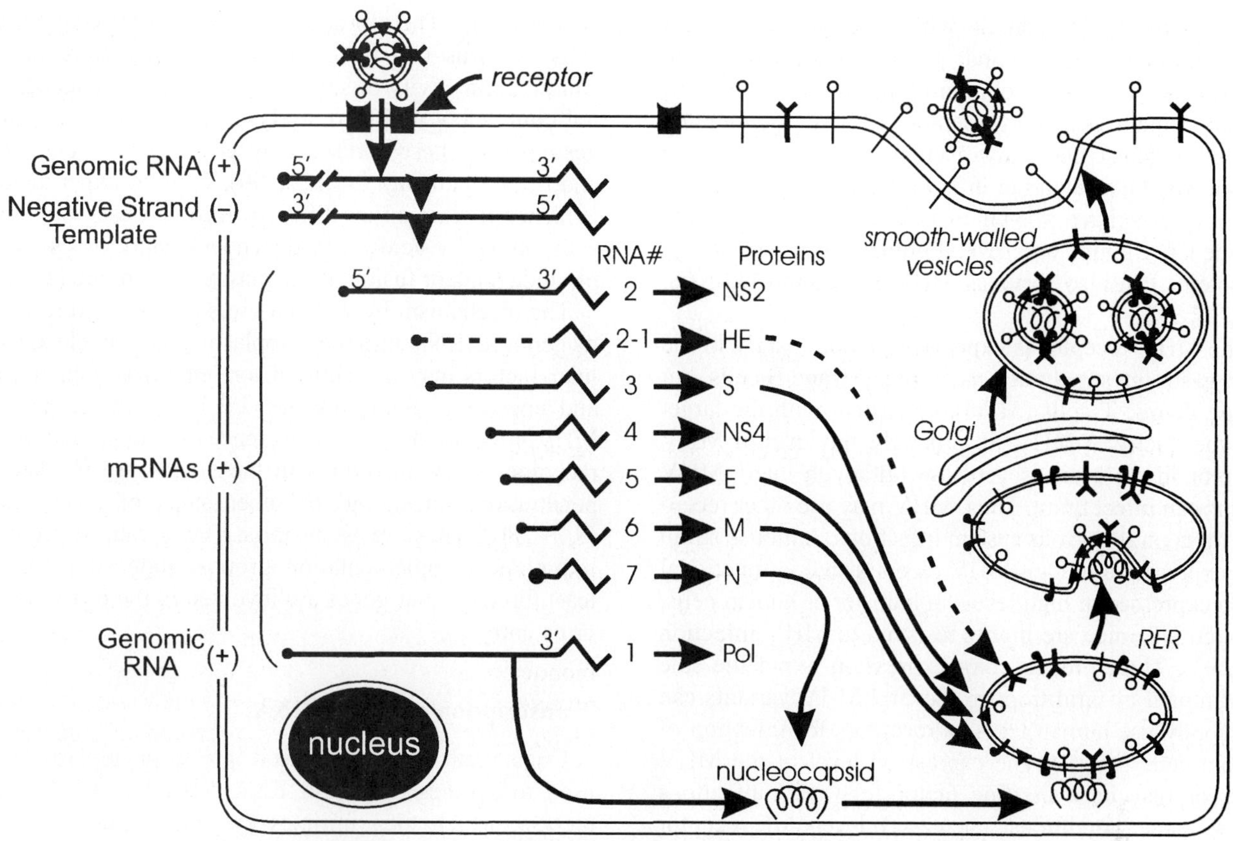

FIG. 4. Coronavirus replication cycle. Virions bind to the plasma membrane by interaction of the spikes with specific receptor glycoproteins or glycans. Penetration occurs by S protein–mediated fusion of the viral envelope with the plasma membrane or endosomal membranes. The gene 1 of viral genomic RNA is translated into a polyprotein, which is cotranslationally or posttranslationally processed to yield an RNA-dependent RNA polymerase (Pol) and other proteins involved in viral RNA synthesis. The Pol products use the genomic RNA as a template to synthesize negative-stranded RNAs, which are, in turn, used to synthesize genomic RNA and subgenomic mRNAs. The mRNAs in infected cells consist of an overlapping nested set of 3′ coterminal RNAs containing a common leader RNA sequence at the 5′ end. The mechanism of subgenomic mRNA synthesis has not been established (see Fig. 5). With a few exceptions, each mRNA is translated to yield only the protein encoded by the 5′ most open reading frame of the mRNA. These proteins include structural proteins N, M, E, S, and HE and several non-structural proteins. The N protein and newly synthesized genomic RNA assemble in the cytoplasm to form helical nucleocapsids. The membrane glycoprotein M is inserted in endoplasmic reticulum (ER) and anchored in the Golgi apparatus. Nucleocapsid (N plus genomic RNA) probably first binds to M protein at the budding compartment that lies between the RER and the Golgi. Similarly, E protein is also transported through the ER to the Golgi, where E and M proteins interact to trigger the budding of virions, enclosing the nucleocapsid. The S and HE glycoproteins are also translated on membrane-bound polysomes, inserted into the RER, and transported to the Golgi complex. These proteins are cotranslationally glycosylated, then trimerized and transported through the Golgi apparatus, where they undergo further modifications and, in some coronaviruses, are cleaved into two subunits, S1 and S2. During transport, some S and HE proteins associate with M protein and are incorporated into the maturing virus particles. Excess S and HE proteins that are not incorporated into virions are transported to the plasma membrane, where they may participate in cell–cell fusion or hemadsorption, respectively. Virions are apparently released by exocytosis-like fusion of smooth-walled, virion-containing vesicles with the plasma membrane. Virions may remain adsorbed to the plasma membranes of infected cells. The entire cycle of coronavirus replication takes place in the cytoplasm.

may not be sufficient to determine viral tropism. Recent studies have shown that the S protein of TGEV binds *N*-glycolyl neuraminic acid, whereas S protein of PRCoV, which is related to TGEV but causes primarily respiratory infections, does not, raising the possibility that this binding may contribute to the enterotropism of TGEV (230).

The main determinant of viral tropism is likely the binding of the S protein to a specific receptor glycoprotein on the cell surface. Receptors have been identified for several coronaviruses. The MHV receptor is a murine biliary glycoprotein belonging to the carcinoembryonic antigen (CEA) family in the Ig superfamily (69,283). It has an extracellular domain with four Ig-like loops, a transmembrane region, and a short intracytoplasmic domain. The viral S glycoprotein binds to the N-terminal Ig-like domain of MHV receptors (70). A monoclonal antibody against the receptor blocks MHV infection in murine cell culture and in infant mice (203,238). Subsequent studies have shown that other members of the murine CEA family and several human CEA-related glycoproteins can also serve as MHV receptors (44,45,68, 194,292,293).

The MHV receptor is expressed predominantly in the liver, gastrointestinal tract, macrophages, and B cells, but not on thymic T cells (51,88), consistent with the target cell specificity of MHV. Surprisingly, the level of MHV receptor in the brain is very low, although many MHV strains can infect brain. Thus, MHV may use other receptors for central nervous system infections. A mouse strain SJL expresses a mutant MHV receptor that is functional when expressed at high levels in hamster or human cells, and yet SJL mice are highly resistant to MHV infection (68,293). Therefore, receptor expression is not the sole determinant of viral tropism. Several MHV variants can efficiently use human CEA as receptors for infection of human cells (18,19). The expression level of the MHV receptor may be a limiting factor for MHV infections under some conditions; increased levels of receptor expression can enhance the susceptibility of the cells to MHV infection (46,220). It is interesting to note that MHV infects polarized epithelial cells through only the apical, not the basolateral, surface (214), consistent with the MHV receptor expression pattern in respiratory and enteric epithelium in mice (88).

HCoV-229E, TGEV, FIPV, and probably canine coronaviruses (CCoV) use the cell membrane–bound metalloprotease, aminopeptidase N (APN), of their respective host species (23,57,285), rather than CEA-like molecules, as a receptor. APN is widely distributed on many cell types, including respiratory and enteric epithelial cells and neuronal and glial cells (131). Some monoclonal antibodies against porcine or human APN block the binding of TGEV or HCoV-229E virions to their target cells (57,285). However, the protease activity of APN is not necessary for the receptor function; inhibitors of APN and mutations of APN that abrogate the enzymatic activity do not block virus infection (57,283).

Penetration and Uncoating

After virus binds to a specific receptor, it enters the cell, a step that involves fusion of the viral envelope with either the plasma membrane or the endosomal membranes. MHV, BCoV, and IBV exhibit a neutral or slightly alkaline pH optimum for induction of cell–cell fusion (149,204,256,279), suggesting that these viruses may cause fusion of the viral envelope with the plasma membrane at the normal physiological pH of the extracellular environment. Therefore, these viruses probably enter cells by virus–cell fusion at the plasma membrane. In contrast, infectivity of some MHV strains is reduced, but not completely inhibited, by lysosomotropic drugs, suggesting that these viruses may enter cells through the endosomal pathway (84,127,190). Current experimental evidence indicates that different coronaviruses can enter cells either by acidic pH–dependent endocytosis or by pH-independent fusion at the plasma membrane (124).

The mechanism by which a virus uncoats and releases its genomic RNA into the cytoplasm is not yet clear. Cellular factors may be required for both virus penetration and uncoating. Some murine cell lines are resistant to MHV infection despite the presence of a functional MHV receptor; MHV infections in these cells are blocked at penetration, uncoating, or other steps of virus entry (8,79,286). These resistant mouse cells can be grouped into three complementation groups, suggesting that at least three cellular genes are involved in the processes of virus entry (8).

Transcription of Viral mRNA

Once viral RNA is released into the cytoplasm, it is used to synthesize a viral RNA-dependent RNA polymerase, which then initiates the transcription of viral mRNAs. Coronaviruses synthesize multiple subgenomic mRNAs, each of which translates one or, occasionally, more than one protein. There is a subgenomic mRNA for the expression of every viral gene except gene 1, which is expressed from the genomic RNA. Five to seven subgenomic mRNAs are synthesized in infected cells, depending on the coronavirus strain or isolate. These viral mRNAs are represented by numbers in order of decreasing size (138); mRNAs discovered after these numbers were assigned are denoted by a hyphen and a second number (e.g., mRNA 2-1) (37). The mRNAs form a nested set with a common 3′ end and poly(A) (see Fig. 4). Although each mRNA, except the smallest, contains two or more ORFs, only the 5′-most ORF is translated, with minor exceptions, as noted later. Thus, these mRNAs are functionally monocistronic.

A characteristic feature of coronavirus subgenomic mRNAs is the presence at their 5′ end of a leader sequence, 65 to 98 bases long, that is identical to the sequence at the 5′ end of the genomic RNA (139,238, 243). This leader sequence is not found elsewhere in the genome; however, the sequence between each gene, termed the *intergenic sequence* (16) (Fig. 5; see also Fig. 3), or transcription-associated sequence (TAS) (100) shares a sequence homology of 7 to 18 nucleotides with the 3′ end of the leader (238). The core sequence of the intergenic sequence for MHV is UCUAAAC or a variant of it (112), whereas the 3′ end of the leader consists of several tandem repeats of UCUAA. Sequence comparison of viral genomic and mRNAs suggests that subge-

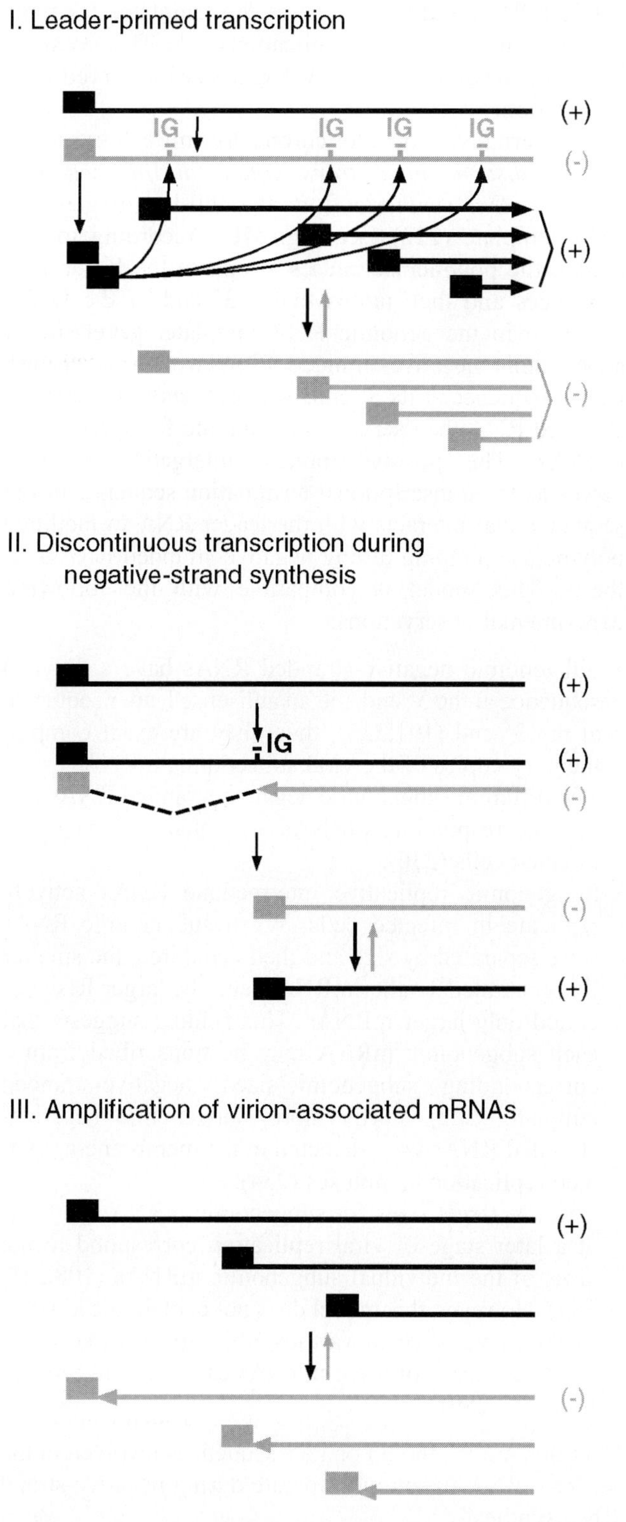

FIG. 5. Proposed models of coronavirus mRNA transcription (see text). *Solid lines* represent positive-stranded RNA; *dashed lines* represent negative-stranded RNA. *Boxes* represent the leader RNA or antileader. *Arrowheads* indicate the direction of transcription.

nomic mRNAs are derived by juxtaposition of the leader sequence to the mRNAs through the UCUAA repeat sequence (238). The mechanism of joining these two RNA elements is discussed later in this section.

The viral genomic RNA is first transcribed into negative-stranded RNA, which is then used as the template for synthesis of mRNAs and genomic RNA. Studies have shown that both genomic- and subgenomic-sized negative-stranded RNAs are present in relative ratios comparable to those of the corresponding positive-stranded genomic and subgenomic mRNAs (222,235,236). All the negative-stranded RNAs were in double-stranded form; no free negative-stranded RNA was detected (210,221, 222). The mechanism of synthesis and the functions of the subgenomic- and genomic-length negative-stranded RNAs are subjects of controversy. There are several models to explain how the subgenomic mRNAs are synthesized so that the leader RNA is fused to the mRNAs (see Fig. 5). Several pieces of experimental data are relevant to the formulation of these models: ultraviolet (UV) light transcriptional mapping studies (108,248,289) indicate that the UV target sizes of subgenomic mRNAs are roughly equivalent to the physical sizes of the individual mRNAs, suggesting that they are transcribed independently. Early in infection, the UV target sizes of the subgenomic mRNAs are equivalent to that of the genomic RNA (176,288), indicating that synthesis of a genomic-sized RNA is a prerequisite for subgenomic mRNA transcription. The difference in UV target size between the early and late stages of viral infection suggests that different mechanisms of RNA synthesis may operate at different stages of the viral replication cycle. Furthermore, in cells simultaneously infected with two different MHV strains, as much as half of the mRNAs may contain a leader sequence derived from one strain and coding sequences from the other strain (184), indicating that the leader sequence can be freely exchanged during transcription. This observation has been reproduced using a defective-interfering (DI) RNA vector system (see later), in which most of the DI-derived subgenomic mRNAs contain a leader sequence derived from the helper viral RNA molecule (109,297). Therefore, all models of coronavirus transcription include a discontinuous transcription process by which the leader sequence and mRNA sequences are derived from two different RNA molecules (109,297).

The first model for coronavirus mRNA synthesis involves *leader-primed transcription* (135) (see Fig. 5**I**). According to this model, discontinuous transcription occurs during positive-stranded RNA synthesis. The genomic RNA is first transcribed into a full-length negative-stranded RNA. Transcription of the leader RNA begins at the 3′ end of the full-length, negative-stranded template RNA and terminates at the end of the leader sequence. The leader dissociates from the template, possibly with the polymerase, and subsequently binds to any intergenic sequence on the negative-stranded template and serves as the primer for mRNA transcription, resulting in an mRNA that contains a leader RNA fused to the mRNA. Several pieces of evidence are consistent with this model:

- MHV-infected cells contain free leader RNAs ranging in size from 50 to 90 nucleotides (16); however, free leader RNAs were not found in BCoV-infected cells (42).
- Leader RNAs transcribed from two different MHV strains in the same cell can be randomly joined to mRNAs from either strain (184).
- In an *in vitro* transcription system using lysates derived from MHV-infected cells, exogenously added leader RNA can be incorporated into subgenomic mRNAs (10).
- Studies using a DI RNA vector system showed that the appearance of full-length, genomic-sized negative-stranded RNA precedes the appearance of subgenomic negative-stranded RNA and subgenomic positive-strand mRNAs (4). Furthermore, the appearance of subgenomic mRNAs preceded the synthesis of subgenomic negative-stranded RNA, suggesting that the subgenomic mRNAs are most likely synthesized from the genomic-sized negative-stranded RNA template, at least early in infection. The subgenomic negative-stranded RNA could be generated from amplification of the subgenomic mRNA (4). However, the possible differences in the relative sensitivity for detection of the different RNA species in this study have not been rigorously excluded.

According to this transcription model, the IG or TAS sequences serve as promoters for mRNA transcription. In the case of MHV, these sequences include a minimal core promoter sequence of seven nucleotides (UCUAAAC) (111,178). When this seven-nucleotide sequence is inserted into the DI RNA and expressed in the MHV-infected cells, a subgenomic mRNA is transcribed from this intergenic sequence site (179). The transcribed MHV mRNA contains a leader sequence derived from the 5′ end of the same RNA molecule (in *cis*) or a different RNA molecule (in *trans*) (297). Fusion of the leader RNA occurs within the UCUAAAC sequence. Additional sequences neighboring these seven nucleotides may also contribute to the joining of these two RNA regions (267).

The intergenic sequences preceding the various ORFs show some variability. Certain mRNAs, such as MHV mRNA 2-1, can be transcribed only when the leader RNA sequence (particularly its 3′ end) and the intergenic sequence preceding the gene (i.e., HE gene) are compatible (133), suggesting that the interaction between the leader RNA and intergenic sequence regulates mRNA transcription. Deletion or mutation of the leader RNA abolishes or severely reduces mRNA transcription (152,297). According to this model, the subgenomic negative-stranded RNAs are synthesized from the subgenomic mRNA and may serve as the templates for transcription later in the viral replication cycle. This possibility would account for the UV target sizes observed later in infection.

An alternative model for coronavirus mRNA transcription is *discontinuous transcription during negative-stranded RNA synthesis* from the full-length genomic RNA template (222) (see Fig. 5**II**). According to this model, the polymerase pauses at one of the IG or TAS sequences and then jumps to the 3′ end of the leader sequence in the genomic RNA template, generating a subgenomic negative-stranded RNA with an antisense leader sequence at its 3′ end. This subgenomic negative-stranded RNA then serves as a template for synthesis of mRNAs. The positive-stranded intergenic sequence serves as the transcriptional termination sequence or the sequence that interacts with the leader RNA to facilitate polymerase jumping during negative-stranded RNA synthesis. This model is compatible with the following experimental observations:

- Subgenomic negative-stranded RNAs have a poly(U) sequence at the 5′ end and an antisense leader sequence at the 3′ end (101,235); thus, they are exact complementary copies of the viral subgenomic mRNAs.
- The different subgenomic negative-stranded RNAs and their corresponding mRNAs are equally abundant in infected cells (236).
- Subgenomic replicative intermediate RNAs actively replicate in infected cells. When subgenomic RNAs were separated by size and then denatured, the smaller RIs generated smaller mRNAs, and the larger RIs generated only larger mRNAs. This finding suggests that each subgenomic mRNA may be transcribed from a corresponding subgenomic-sized, negative-stranded template (222). Furthermore, subgenomic negative-stranded RNAs were detected in the membrane-associated replication complexes (234).
- The UV target sizes for subgenomic mRNA synthesis at a later stage of viral replication correspond to the sizes of the individual subgenomic mRNAs (108,248, 289). However, this model does not explain the kinetics of the appearance of various RNA species (4) or the UV target sizes of these mRNAs early in viral replication (176,289).

In this model, the IG or TAS sequences involved in the leader-mRNA fusion will operate during negative-strand RNA synthesis.

A third model (see Fig. 5**III**) is based on the finding that subgenomic mRNAs are incorporated into virions of some coronaviruses, including BCoV, TGEV, and IBV (103,236,298), along with the full-length genomic RNA. This model proposes that, after virus entry, the subgenomic mRNAs associated with the incoming virions are used directly as templates for the synthesis of subgenomic negative-stranded RNAs, which, in turn, serve as templates for the synthesis of additional subgenomic mRNAs (232,233). This model is not compatible with the discontinuous nature of coronavirus RNA synthesis. Furthermore, not all coronaviruses have been found to contain virion-associated subgenomic mRNAs. Coronavirus positive-stranded mRNAs cannot be amplified when transfected into infected cells (41,152).Nevertheless, it is possible that this model may operate at some stages of the viral replication cycle for some coronaviruses.

Data available at this time cannot unequivocally establish or exclude any of these models. The difficulty in differentiating these models is partially due to the fact that subgenomic negative-stranded RNAs can be copied from subgenomic mRNAs and vice versa because the subgenomic RNAs contain the complete cis-acting signals for negative-stranded RNA synthesis (155). So far, the synthesis of the subgenomic mRNAs and the synthesis of subgenomic negative-stranded RNAs have not been uncoupled in infected cells under any experimental conditions. Therefore, it is difficult to determine experimentally which subgenomic RNA species, positive- or negative-sense, comes first. Furthermore, most of the studies were performed late in infection when both positive- and negative-stranded subgenomic RNAs were already present and presumably could be further copied from each other. It is possible that elements from each of these models may operate at various stages of the viral life cycle. Comparative information about RNA transcription mechanisms in other related viruses, such as toroviruses and arteriviruses, may help to elucidate coronavirus RNA transcription because they have smaller RNA genomes and polymerase genes (59,242); furthermore, infectious viral complementary DNA (cDNA) or its transcripts are available for arteriviruses (269,270). However, there are no leader sequences on torovirus subgenomic mRNAs, and coronavirus replication has a high frequency of leader switching that is not seen in arterivirus replication.

Coronavirus RNA synthesis takes place on membranous structures associated with the endoplasmic reticulum (ER), Golgi complex, or late endosomes, depending on the cell types (61,237,265). Most of the gene 1 proteins are associated with the newly synthesized viral RNA. This observation is consistent with the finding that MHV temperature-sensitive mutants with defects in gene 1 can be classified into five complementation groups, all of which are defective in viral RNA synthesis (15). Anti-N antibody has been shown to inhibit MHV RNA synthesis *in vitro,* suggesting that N protein is involved in RNA transcription (49). Host components may also be involved in viral RNA synthesis (150,151).

In addition to the leader RNA and intergenic sequences, several other RNA elements, including the 3′ end of the viral genome (155,156), are involved in the regulation of coronavirus mRNA transcription. About 55 nucleotides at the 3′ end of the genomic RNA and the poly(A) sequence are required for the initiation of negative-stranded RNA synthesis (155); in contrast, the presence of the entire 3′-UTR region (305 nucleotides) is necessary for mRNA transcription (156). The difference in the lengths of the 3′ end sequences required for negative-stranded RNA and mRNA synthesis suggests that most of the 3′ end cis-acting sequence is involved in the synthesis of positive-stranded RNA. Thus, the 3′ end of viral RNA (or 5′ end of negative-stranded RNA) likely interacts with the leader or intergenic sequence to regulate mRNA transcription.

Replication of Genomic RNA

The viral genomic-sized RNA in the infected cell consists of two components: the mRNA encoding gene 1 products (5%) and the genomic RNA to be packaged into nucleocapsids and virions (95%) (210,244). Unlike the discontinuous synthesis of subgenomic mRNA, the production of genomic RNA presumably requires uninterrupted synthesis using a full-length, negative-stranded template. Therefore, the mechanism of genomic RNA replication conceivably differs from that of subgenomic mRNA transcription. It has been shown, however, that some genomic-sized RNAs of MHV may be synthesized by discontinuous transcription, that is, fusion of the leader sequence to a UUUAUAAAC sequence immediately downstream of the leader RNA, thereby creating a genomic-sized RNA with a small deletion (296). This mechanism has also been demonstrated in DI RNA replication. During MHV DI RNA replication, the leader sequence of the DI RNA can be rapidly replaced by that of the helper virus RNA (181), suggesting that MHV RNA replication involves a free leader RNA (of either positive or negative sense), similar to the discontinuous transcription of subgenomic mRNAs. In addition, the leader sequence of MHV RNA genome undergoes rapid evolution in the number of UCUAA repeats at the 3′ end of the leader (180). These UCUAA sequences are also hot spots of RNA recombination, possibly as a result of discontinuous synthesis (116). Therefore, the replication of genomic RNA appears to occur by discontinuous synthesis involving a leader RNA as well.

Studies of MHV DI RNA have also revealed information regarding the minimum cis-acting signals for coronavirus genomic RNA replication. Replication of the MHV DI RNA requires sequences of about 400 to 800 nucleotides at both the 3′ and 5′ ends of the genomic RNA and an internal replication signal of about 135 nucleotides (119,154). However, other DI RNAs of MHV and BCoV do not require this internal sequence for replication (41,169). This difference is likely due to differences in the secondary structure of the RNA genomes between different viral strains (120). The lengths of the cis-acting signals for RNA replication at both ends of the viral RNA differ slightly from those required for mRNA transcription (152,154,156). Additionally, the 3′ end cis-acting signal for genomic RNA replication (154) is longer than that required for negative-stranded RNA synthesis (155), again suggesting long-range interactions between the two ends of the genomic RNA during RNA replication.

Translation of Viral Proteins

Although all but the smallest coronavirus mRNAs contain multiple ORFs, only the 5′-most ORF of each mRNA is generally translated by a cap-dependent ribosomal scanning mechanism (see Fig. 4). Most of the structural proteins, including S, M, N and HE, are translated from separate mRNAs by this mechanism. Because each of the coronavirus mRNAs contains a 5′ leader sequence, which enhances translation in virus-infected cell lysates (260), virus-specific mRNAs may be preferentially translated in the face of translational shutoff in the infected cells. Other viral proteins are translated by other distinct mechanisms (see Fig. 3). First, the mRNA 1 of all coronaviruses contains two large overlapping ORFs that are translated into one polyprotein by a ribosomal frameshifting mechanism (28,30,72,94,144). Translation of this gene, however, is initiated by the conventional cap-dependent translation mechanism. Second, in several coronavirus mRNAs, it is the second or third ORF that is most efficiently translated. For example, the E protein is translated from the second ORF of MHV mRNA 5 and the third ORF of IBV mRNA 3. These ORFs are preceded by an internal ribosomal entry site sequence that allows ribosomes to bypass the upstream ORFs and translate the downstream ORF by a cap-independent translation mechanism (161,262). Some of the upstream ORFs are also translated, but the translational efficiency and functional significance of these proteins are not clear. Third, several other mRNAs contain two overlapping ORFs, both of which are translated by unknown mechanisms. For example, mRNA 5 of IBV contains two ORFs that are both translated *in vitro* and *in vivo* (160), and an internal ORF (termed I) within the N genes of MHV and BCoV is translated *in vivo* (75,233).

Processing and Intracellular Transport of Viral Proteins

Polymerase Precursor Polyprotein 1a and 1b

Polyprotein 1a and 1b is presumably the first and only viral protein synthesized from the incoming viral genome because it is required for viral RNA synthesis. (Other viral proteins are translated from subgenomic mRNAs.) Once viral RNA synthesis begins, more gene 1 protein products are translated from the newly synthesized genomic RNA. The primary gene product (from ORF 1a and 1b), which is predicted to be nearly 700 to 800 kd, is cotranslationally or posttranslationally processed into multiple proteins by its own proteases. ORF 1a contains at least two protease domains: a papain-like cysteine protease (PLP) and a chymotrypsin-picornavirus 3C–like protease (3CLp) (90,144). In some viruses (e.g., MHV, HCoV-229E, and TGEV), there are two copies of the PLP domain, PLP1 and PLP2. PLP and 3CLp cleave the polyprotein into multiple proteins through a complex series of processing intermediates, some of which have not been unequivocally identified. In MHV, PLP1 is responsible for cleaving the aminoterminal proteins p28 and p65 from the polyprotein (11,12,24,60,62) (Fig. 6). The remaining portion of the polyprotein (including both ORF 1a and ORF 1b) is most likely processed by 3CLp (157,162,299,300). 3CLp itself is cleaved from the polyprotein by its own autoprotease activity into a protein of 27 kd, which has both trans- and cis-acting proteolytic activities (158,165,166,299). The 3CLp-mediated cleavage sites were predicted by computer analysis to be mostly at Q/S or Q/A sites (90,144); many of these have been confirmed by experimental analysis. A 100-kd protein from ORF 1b is thought to contain the polymerase domain (92,157), although the polymerase activity has not been directly demonstrated. A genetic complementation group thought to be responsible for mRNA transcription has been mapped to the coding region for this protein (223). A 67-kd protein has been shown to include the helicase domain (61). Many of these proteins and possibly their processing intermediates are colocalized with the newly synthesized viral RNA and, thus, are presumably present in the RNA replication complex, which is associated with the membranous structures in the infected cells (61,237,265). PLP2 has recently been shown to cleave at the upstream border of MP1 domain (112).

S Protein

The S protein is cotranslationally inserted into the rough endoplasmic reticulum (RER) and glycosylated with N-linked glycans. The protein is linked by multiple intramolecular disulfide bonds to form a complex structure and then oligomerized into homotrimers (58,199). Transportation of the S protein to the Golgi complex is accompanied by trimming of high mannose oligosaccharides and the addition of terminal sugars to form mature glycans. The S2 domain undergoes fatty acylation, probably on cysteine residues (225,255). Cleavage of S into S1 and S2 occurs after the conversion of glycans from simple to complex forms (272), either in the Golgi complex or extracellularly. Typically, the cleavage site is flanked by several basic amino acids (38,170); coronavirus S proteins that lack these residues, such as those of HCoV-229E or FIPV, are not cleaved. Most of the S protein accumulates in the Golgi of infected cells, where it participates in virus particle assembly; however, some S

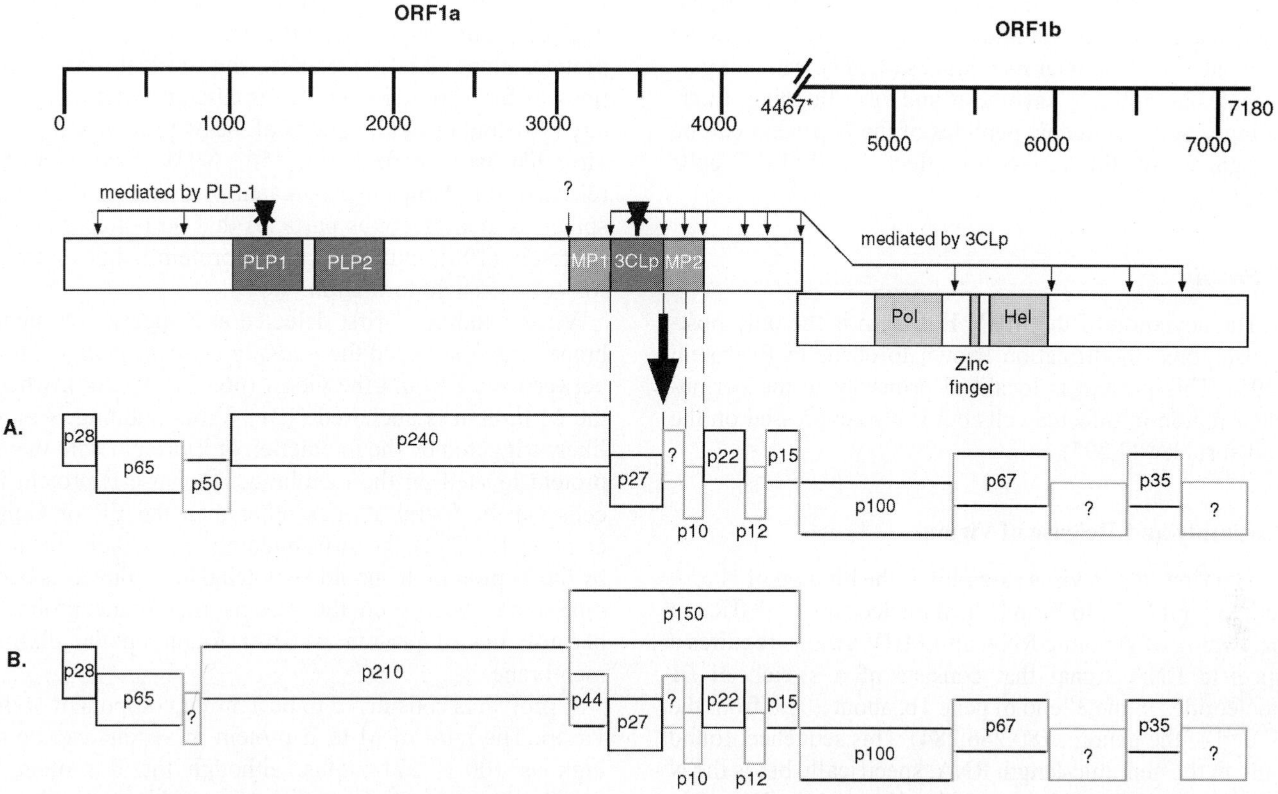

FIG. 6. Presumptive proteolytic products of the murine hepatitis virus (MHV) gene 1 (polymerase). Unlike the structural proteins of coronaviruses, which are each encoded by a separate mRNA, the proteins composing RNA-dependent RNA polymerases are formed by virus-encoded proteolytic processing of a precursor polyprotein. Open reading frames (ORFs) 1a and 1b are translated into a polyprotein by a ribosomal frame-shifting mechanism. The predicted and confirmed functional domains of ORF 1a and 1b are indicated. Two versions of the presumptive proteolytic processing pathways are shown. The *dashed lines* represent the unconfirmed products or cleavage sites. The full-length primary translation product and intermediates are not shown. The functions of most of these peptides are not yet known. PLP1, PLP2, papain-like cysteine protease 1 and 2; 3CLp, poliovirus 3C-like protease; Pol, predicted polymerase; Hel, predicted helicase; MP, membrane-binding domain. (Courtesy of Susan C. Baker and Mark Denison.)

oligomers are transported to the plasma membrane, where it may mediate cell–cell fusion (91,272).

M Protein

The M protein is synthesized on membrane-bound polysomes and inserted into the ER membranes by an internal signal sequence (215). M protein is highly hydrophobic and spans the membrane three times (7,216). In IBV and TGEV, the aminoterminal domain of the M protein, which is located on the luminal side of the ER, is cotranslationally glycosylated with N-linked glycans (247); however, the corresponding domain in MHV is posttranslationally glycosylated by O-linked glycans in the Golgi apparatus (106,196,197). The mature M protein accumulates in the Golgi apparatus, but unlike S, it is not transported to the plasma membrane. The nature of the membrane-targeting sequence in the M proteins of different coronaviruses is variable (163,171).

HE Protein

The HE protein is cotranslationally glycosylated by N-linked glycans in the RER and forms disulfide-linked dimers of 165 to 170 kd (104,117,290). It is transported to the Golgi, where the N-linked glycans are converted to the complex form (290) and incorporated into the envelope of budding virus particles. HE protein that is not incorporated into budding virions is transported to the plasma membrane and expressed on the cell surface (117).

N Protein

The N protein is translated on free polysomes and rapidly phosphorylated on serine residues in the cytosol

(247), but the extent of phosphorylation and its functional significance are not yet known. Some N protein may be associated with cellular membranes (4,247), where it participates in viral RNA synthesis and virus budding. Interestingly, some antigenic peptides of the N protein can be recognized on the surface of infected cells by T cells (25,251,277).

E Protein

The acylation of the MHV E protein is the only posttranslational modification known to occur in E protein (295). This protein is localized primarily in the perinuclear region in infected cells but is also expressed on the cell surface (87,295).

Assembly and Release of Virions

The first step in virus assembly is the binding of N protein to viral RNA to form helical nucleocapsids. Efficient packaging of genomic RNA into MHV virions requires a specific RNA signal that consists of a stretch of 61 nucleotides in the 3′ end of gene 1b, about 20 kb from the 5′ end of the genome (80,266,284). This sequence, found only in the genomic-length RNA, specifically binds the N protein (188). Thus, the interaction between the N protein and this packaging signal is likely the initial step of nucleocapsid formation. BCoV, TGEV, and IBV virions also package small amounts of all subgenomic mRNAs, which do not contain this packaging signal (103,235, 236,298). These virion-associated mRNAs have been postulated to serve as templates for amplification of the subgenomic mRNAs for these viruses (237). Even DI RNAs without a typical packaging signal can be incorporated into virions, albeit inefficiently (40,182). The packaging of subgenomic mRNAs and these DI RNAs into virions may be mediated by the binding of N protein to the leader sequences of these RNAs (249).

Once the nucleocapsid is formed, it interacts with the M protein at the cellular membranes (254), most likely the ER or the Golgi complex. Studies have shown that the N protein by itself cannot be packaged into virions; it can be enveloped only together with the viral RNA (27,271), suggesting either that M protein interacts directly with the viral RNA or that the viral RNA–N protein interaction induces a conformational change in the N protein, enabling it to interact with the M protein. This interaction may lead to the formation of the spherical internal core shell surrounding the nucleocapsid (211) and, at the same time, enable the nucleocapsid to be packaged into budding virus particles, which are formed on the membranes of the ER and Golgi.

Although the interaction of the nucleocapsid with M protein likely triggers the packaging of the nucleocapsid into virions, the formation of virus particles cannot occur without an additional viral protein, the E protein. In fact, formation of virus-like particles, which do not have nucleocapsids, can occur in the presence of the M and E proteins alone (27,271). Studies showed that most mutations of the E protein resulted in altered virus morphology (76), and most alterations of the M protein abrogated virus-like particle formation (56). MHV virions can be released from tunicamycin-treated, virus-infected cells as spikeless, noninfectious particles that do not contain the S protein (106), indicating that S protein is not essential for virus particle formation.

Virus budding is first detected at a specialized membrane structure called the *budding compartment,* located between the ER and the Golgi (66,121,263,264), where the M protein is anchored (121). Virus budding is most likely triggered by the interaction of E protein with the M protein located on the membrane. Because E protein in cells can be found at sites other than the ER or Golgi complex (86,292), the virus budding site is likely dictated by the M protein. It should be noted that coronavirus budding never occurs on the plasma membrane probably because the M protein is never found on the plasma membrane.

E protein is considered to be a minor component of the virion. The ratio of M to E protein in virions can be as high as 100:1 (271); thus, although the E protein is required for the initiation of virus assembly and budding, it may serve only as a scaffolding protein that is not an essential part of the mature virion. The expression of E protein induces curvature of the M-containing intracellular membrane (271); thus, E protein may be involved in the pinching off of the budding virions into the budding compartment.

The S and HE proteins are incorporated into virions through their interactions with M protein. The formation of S–M and HE–M complexes occurs in the pre-Golgi complex (195,200). These two complexes then form an S–M–HE ternary complex before the glycoproteins undergo trimming of their sugar chains (197). Thus, the processing of virion-associated glycoproteins most likely occurs as virions pass through the Golgi. After budding, virus particles may undergo further morphologic changes within the Golgi, resulting in the appearance of mature virus particles with a compact, electron-dense internal core, as they reach the secretory vesicles (213,218). Virions accumulate in large, smooth-walled vesicles, which eventually fuse with the plasma membrane to release virus into extracellular space (91). Virus release is restricted to certain areas of cells; for example, MHV-A59 virions are released from the basolateral surface of certain polarized murine cells (214). The mechanism of release site restriction is unknown.

Effects on Host Cells

Coronavirus-induced cytopathic effects vary with the virus strain and the host cell. Infection with certain coronaviruses, such as MHV, BCoV, IBV or FIPV, induces cell fusion in culture and in infected tissues. Even those coronaviruses that cause little or no cell fusion induce rounding and lysis of cells (84,89). The mechanisms of coronavirus-induced cytopathic effects are poorly understood. Some MHV strains are known to inhibit translation of cellular proteins (98,239) and cause selective inhibition of transcription of some cellular genes (132). Infected cells may undergo fragmentation and rearrangement of the Golgi apparatus late in infection (143). TGEV and some MHV strains may also induce apoptosis in some cell types, which may be mediated by the E protein (3,22,71). A combination of these virus-induced effects may contribute to the cytopathic effects observed in host cells late in infection.

Persistent coronavirus infection occurs readily in cell culture. Generally, after the initial cytocidal infection, carrier cultures arise, in which only a fraction of the cells produce infectious virus at any time, and virus production continues for months (89,105,140). Cells in persistently infected cultures are resistant to superinfection with wild-type virus, and various replication-defective mutants are frequently selected from these cultures (84,89,102,105, 252). These mutant viruses may modulate virus dissemination in culture. Virus persistence in culture may also be due to the selection of coronavirus-resistant cells, whereby only a small number of cells remain susceptible to coronavirus infections, thus limiting the extent of viral dissemination (103,174,220). Both viral and cellular evolutions likely contribute to the maintenance of persistent infections. In fact, the virus and host cells often coevolve during persistent infection, resulting in the selection of both resistant cells and virus mutants with an expanded host range (46,224). HCoV-229E has been demonstrated to establish persistent infection in human oligodendrocyte and glial cell lines (6).

Although most coronavirus infections in animals are acute and self-limited, persistent coronavirus infection *in vivo* can occur in immunocompromised hosts, such as nude or newborn mice (20,21,209,261,278). Some temperature-sensitive or monoclonal antibody neutralization-escape mutants of MHV are particularly prone to cause persistent infection in animals (32,78,122). Persistency also has been noted in natural infections of feline enteric coronavirus (FECoV) in cats (96). In such cases, FECoV may undergo serial evolution, forming a distinct virus quasi-species in each cat. These chronic FECoV carriers would be resistant to superinfection (96).

CORONAVIRUS GENETICS

Virus Mutants

Like most RNA viruses, coronaviruses are thought to mutate at a high frequency because of the high error frequencies of RNA polymerases (246). However, in one case in which the entire MHV genome was sequenced after repeated passages of the virus in culture, surprisingly few mutations were detected (146). Nevertheless, multiple types of mutants have been isolated.

Temperature-sensitive (ts) MHV mutants have been classified into at least seven complementation groups (145), five of which are RNA negative, that is, they cannot synthesize RNA at the nonpermissive temperature (145,223). All of the RNA-negative mutations have been mapped to locations within gene 1 (15), suggesting that at least five separate functions of gene 1 products are required for viral RNA synthesis. Several complementation groups of RNA-positive mutants replicate viral RNA at the nonpermissive temperature but show altered cytopathic effects or fail to produce infectious virions (15, 145). The RNA-positive mutants have defects in the genes encoding the S or N structural proteins (123,188, 205). Some ts mutants differ in virulence from wild-type virus in animal infections. For example, although the wild-type JHM strain of MHV causes acute encephalitis in mice, some of its ts mutants cause a subacute demyelinating disease (93,125).

Deletion mutants also occur frequently. Many natural MHV strains have deletions of up to 200 amino acids in a hypervariable region of the S protein and show altered biologic properties *in vivo* (14,85,203). The most striking example of the biologic importance of deletion mutations is the emergence of PRCoV from TGEV. TGEV causes epizootic enteric infections in pigs. In the early 1980s, PRCoV emerged in Europe as a new virus that caused widespread epizootic respiratory infections in pigs (141). Nucleotide sequence comparison of the two viruses showed that PRCoV was a derivative of TGEV with a large deletion within the S protein (31,202,281). Similar PRCoV strains have emerged independently in the United States as deletion mutants in the S gene of TGEV (9,141). FIPV most likely arose from deletion mutations of FECoV in a similar manner (273).

RNA Recombination

A unique feature of coronavirus genetics is a high frequency of RNA recombination, particularly in MHV (136). Although nonsegmented genomes of RNA viruses generally exhibit very low or undetectable recombination frequencies, the recombination frequencies for the entire coronavirus genome have been calculated to be as high as 25% (15). RNA recombinants were first isolated during co-infection with different ts mutants of MHV at the nonpermissive temperature (137). Additional recombinants were isolated using selectable genetic markers such as neutralization-escape mutants and strains that differ in cell fusion activity (113,115,116,181). To date, RNA recombination has been demonstrated for MHV, TGEV, and IBV, both in tissue culture and in experimental and natural animal infections (13,114,126,276).

The high frequency of RNA recombination in coronaviruses is probably the result of the unique mechanism of coronavirus RNA synthesis, which involves discontinuous transcription and polymerase jumping (136). It is possible that the viral polymerase associated with the incomplete nascent RNAs dissociates from its template at a random point and switches to a homologous site on a different RNA template to complete RNA synthesis by a copy-choice mechanism (14,136).

RNA recombination is an important mechanism in the natural evolution of coronaviruses. For example, new strains of IBV in poultry flocks are the result of natural recombination between different field strains (34,110, 131,276). RNA recombination may also play a role in the evolution of different coronavirus species. For example, a reversal in the order of the M gene and gene 5 on the IBV and MHV genomes (see Fig. 3) may have occurred because of homologous recombination at consensus intergenic regions between the two genes in a progenitor of one of the viruses. Recombination may also explain the acquisition of the HE gene from an mRNA of influenza C virus by a progenitor of the group II coronaviruses (168). Some biotypes of FECoV appear to have arisen by recombination between FECoV and canine coronavirus (97).

RNA recombination has been developed into a potent genetic tool to introduce desired RNA sequences into coronavirus genomes. Cells are transfected with a DI RNA containing RNA sequences with desired mutations and then infected with a ts mutant that has a defect in the N gene. Recombination can take place between the DI RNA and the viral RNA at any homologous site; some of the resulting wild-type viruses may incorporate the part of a DI RNA sequence that contains the introduced RNA sequences and can be selected by using the appropriate selection markers (123,130,147,188,205). This approach, termed *targeted RNA recombination* (123), is an important tool for genetic manipulation of coronaviruses because full-length infectious cDNA clones of coronavirus genomic RNA are not yet available for most coronaviruses.

Defective-Interfering RNA

When a coronavirus such as MHV is passaged at a high multiplicity of infection, new RNA species smaller than the genomic RNA emerge (185). These are DI RNAs, which can replicate only in the presence of a helper virus and may interfere with the replication of the helper virus. DI RNAs have been detected for MHV, IBV, and TGEV during viral replication in cell culture (185,189,207). Three different types of DI RNAs have been demonstrated (177). The first type, typified by the DIssE RNA (177) of MHV, replicates efficiently but is not packaged efficiently into virions. However, small amounts of this DI RNA can be nonspecifically incorporated into virions; thus, it can be maintained and amplified during serial virus passages in culture (182). The second type, typified by the DIssF RNA (177) of MHV, contains a packaging signal that enables it to be incorporated into virions efficiently (186,266). The third type, typified by the DIssA RNA (177) of MHV, is not a true DI RNA because it has retained the ability to replicate. It contains small deletions at multiple sites, is nearly the size of the viral genomic RNA, encodes a functional polymerase, and can replicate even in the absence of a helper virus (118,182). All of the DI RNAs contain both the 5′ and 3′ ends of the viral genome, which include the cis-acting signals for RNA replication. Most of them also contain an ORF encoding a protein that is fused from different viral proteins (183). The presence of an ORF, which may or may not encode functional viral proteins, may enhance the fitness of the DI RNA during evolution (55,119,153), although the ORF or its protein product is not necessary for RNA replication (153,208).

During serial passages of viruses in cell culture, the original DI RNAs frequently disappear, and new ones of different sizes are generated (177). The continuous evolution of DI RNAs is often due to recombination between the original DI RNA and the RNA of helper virus (82). DI RNAs with a longer ORF have a selective advantage over those with a shorter ORF, contributing to the evolution of DI RNA (119,268). DI RNAs have not been detected during natural coronavirus infections; thus, their biologic significance in coronavirus infection is not clear.

CONCLUSIONS

Coronaviruses are unique among RNA viruses in many aspects of their viral structure and replication. They are characterized by exceptionally large RNA genomes, nested subgenomic mRNAs, discontinuous transcription mechanism, high-frequency RNA recombination, and the unusually large number of gene products associated with RNA synthesis. Coronavirus RNA incorporates two different gene expression strategies: polyprotein processing for gene 1 and one–gene–to–one–mRNA expression for the other genes, probably a reflection of their unusual evolutionary origin. Many questions regarding the coronavirus replication cycle remain unresolved, including the mechanism of mRNA transcription, the functions of gene 1 proteins and other nonstructural proteins, and the mechanisms of virus entry and assembly. Recent findings suggest that the structure of virions and the role of cellular factors in viral replication need to be reevaluated.

Coronavirus research has been hampered by the lack of infectious cDNA or RNA transcripts, so that standard reverse genetics approaches are inapplicable. Construction of a functional full-length genomic cDNA has been difficult because of the large size of the coronavirus RNA genome. Only recently did the construction of an infectious coronavirus cDNA (for TGEV) succeed (2). Such infectious recombinant genomes will undoubtedly facilitate the coronavirus research. In addition, studies of the related but less complex toroviruses and arteriviruses should also further enhance our understanding of the exceptionally complex coronavirus replication cycle.

REFERENCES

1. Almeida JD, Berry DM, Cunningham CH, et al. Coronaviruses. *Nature* 1968;220:650.
2. Almazán F, González JM, Pénzes Z, et al. Engineering the largest RNA virus genome as an infectious bacterial artificial chromosome. *Proc Natl Acad Sci USA* 2000;97:5516–5521.
3. An S, Chen C-J, Yu X, et al. Induction of apoptosis in murine coronavirus-infected cultured cells and demonstration of E protein as an apoptosis inducer. *J Virol* 1999;73:7853–7859.
4. An S, Maeda A, Makino S. Coronavirus transcription early in infection. *J Virol* 1998;72:8517–8524.
5. Anderson R, Wong F. Membrane and phospholipid binding by murine coronaviral nucleocapsid N protein. *Virology* 1993;194:224–232.
6. Arbour N, Ekande S, Cote G, et al. Persistent infection of human oligodendrocytic and neuroglial cell lines by human coronavirus 229E. *J Virol* 1999;73:3326–3337.
7. Armstrong J, Niemann H, Smeekens S, et al. Sequence and topology of a model intracellular membrane protein, E1 glycoprotein, from a coronavirus. *Nature* (London) 1984;308:751–752.
8. Asanaka M, Lai MMC. Cell fusion studies identified multiple cellular factors involved in mouse hepatitis virus entry. *Virology* 1993;197: 732–741.
9. Bae I, Jackwood DJ, Benfield DA, et al. Differentiation of transmissible gastroenteritis virus from porcine respiratory coronavirus and other antigenically related coronaviruses by using cDNA probes specific for the 5′ region of the S glycoprotein gene. *J Clin Microbiol* 1991;29:215–218.
10. Baker SC, Lai MM-C. An in vitro system for the leader-primed transcription of coronavirus mRNAs. *EMBO J* 1990;9:4173–4179.
11. Baker SC, Shieh C-K, Soe LH, et al. Identification of a domain required for the autoproteolytic cleavage of murine coronavirus gene A polyprotein. *J Virol* 1989;63:3693–3699.
12. Baker SC, Yokomori K, Dong S, et al. Identification of the catalytic sites of a papain-like cystein proteinase of murine coronavirus. *J Virol* 1993;67:6056–6063.
13. Ballesteros ML, Sanchez CM, Enjuanes L. Two amino acid changes at the N-terminus of transmissible gastroenteritis coronavirus spike protein result in the loss of enteric tropism. *Virology* 1997;227:378–388.
14. Banner LR, Keck JG, Lai MM-C. A clustering of RNA recombination sites adjacent to a hypervariable region of the peplomer gene of murine coronavirus. *Virology* 1990;175:548–555.
15. Baric RS, Fu K, Schaad MC, Stohlman SA. Establishing a genetic recombination map for murine coronavirus strain A59 complementation groups. *Virology* 1990;177:646–656.
16. Baric RS, Shieh C-K, Stohlman SA, Lai MMC. Analysis of intracellular small RNAs of mouse hepatitis virus: evidence for discontinuous transcription. *Virology* 1987;156:342–354.
17. Baric RS, Stohlman SA, Razavi MK, Lai MMC. Characterization of leader-related small RNAs in coronavirus-infected cells: Further evidence for leader-primed mechanism of transcription. *Virus Res* 1985; 3:19–33.
18. Baric RS, Sullivan E, Hensley L, et al. Persistent infection promotes cross-species transmissibility of mouse hepatitis virus. *J Virol* 1999;73:638–649.
19. Baric RS, Yount B, Hensley L, et al. Episodic evolution mediates interspecies transfer of a murine coronavirus. *J Virol* 1997;71: 1946–1955.
20. Barthold SW. Mouse hepatitis virus biology and epizootiology. In: Bhatt PN, Jacoby RO, Morse HC III, New AE, eds. *Viral and mycoplasmal infections of laboratory rodents:* Effects on biomedical research. Orlando, FL: Academic Press, 1986:571–601.
21. Barthold SW, Smith AL, Lord PF, et al. Epizootic coronaviral typhlocolitis in suckling mice. *Lab Anim Sci* 1982;32:376–383.
22. Belyavsky M, Belyavskaya E, Levy GA, Leibowitz JL. Coronavirus MHV-3-induced apoptosis in macrophages. *Virology* 1998;250: 41–49.
23. Benbacer L, Kut E, Besnardeau L, et al. Interspecies aminopeptidase-N chimeras reveal species-specific receptor recognition by canine coronavirus, feline infectious peritonitis virus, and transmissible gastroenteritis virus. *J Virol* 1997;71:734–737.
24. Bonilla PJ, Hughes SA, Weiss SR. Characterization of a second cleavage site and demonstration of activity in trans by the papain-like proteinase of the murine coronavirus mouse hepatitis virus strain A59. *J Virol* 1997;71:900–909.
25. Boots AM, Van Lierop MJ, Kusters JG, et al. MHV class II-restricted T-cell hybridomas recognizing the nucleocapsid protein of avian coronavirus IBV. *Immunology* 1991;72:10–14.
26. Bos ECW, Heijnen L, Luytjes W, Spaan WJM. Mutational analysis of the murine coronavirus spike protein: Effect on cell-to-cell fusion. *Virology* 1995;214:453–463.
27. Bos ECW, Luytjes W, van der Meulen H, et al. The production of recombinant infectious DI-particles of a murine coronavirus in the absence of helper virus. *Virology* 1996;218:52–60.
28. Boursnell MEG, Brown TDK, Foulds IJ, et al. Completion of the sequence of the genome of the coronavirus avian infectious bronchitis virus. *J Gen Virol* 1987;68:57–77.
29. Brayton PR, Ganges RG, Stohlman SA. Host cell nuclear function and murine hepatitis virus replication. *J Gen Virol* 1981;56:457–460.
30. Brierley I, Jenner AJ, Inglis SC. Mutational analysis of the "slippery-sequence" component of a coronavirus ribosomal frameshifting signal. *J Mol Biol* 1992;227:463–479.
31. Britton P, Mawditt KL, Page KW. The cloning and sequencing of the virion protein genes from a British isolate of porcine respiratory coronavirus: Comparison with transmissible gastroenteritis virus genes. *Virus Res* 1991;21:181–198.
32. Buchmeier MJ, Dalziel RG, Koolen MJM. Coronavirus-induced CNS disease: A model for virus-induced CNS disease–a model for virus-induced demyelination. *J Neuroimmunol* 1988;20:111–116.
33. Cabirac GF, Soike KF, Zhang JY, et al. Entry of coronavirus into primate CNS following peripheral infection. *Microb Pathog* 1994;16: 349–357.
34. Cavanagh D. Recent advances in avian virology. *Br Vet J* 1992;48: 199–222.
35. Cavanagh D. Nidovirales: A new order comprising Coronaviridae and Arteriviridae. *Arch Virol* 1997;142:629–233.
36. Cavanagh D, Brian DA, Brinton MA, et al. Coronaviridae. In: Murphy FA, Fauquet CM, Bishop DHL, et al., eds. *Virus taxonomy.* Sixth Report of the International Committee on Taxonomy of Viruses. Vienna: Springer-Verlag, 1995:407–411.
37. Cavanagh D, Brian DA, Enjuanes L, et al. Recommendations of the Coronavirus Study Group for the nomenclature of the structural proteins, mRNAs and genes of coronaviruses. *Virology* 1990;176: 306–307.
38. Cavanagh D, Davis PJ, Pappin DJC, et al. Coronavirus IBV: Partial amino terminal sequencing of the spike polypeptide S2 identifies the sequence Arg-Arg-Phe-Arg-Arg at the cleavage site of the spike precurser propolypeptide of IBV strains Beaudette and M41. *Virus Res* 1986;4:133–143.
39. Chaloner-Larsson G, Johnson-Lussenburg CM. Establishment and maintenance of a persistent infection of L132 cells by human coronavirus strain 229E. *Arch Virol* 1981;69:117–129.
40. Chang RY, Brian DA. Cis requirement for N-specific protein sequence in bovine coronavirus defective interfering RNA replication. *J Virol* 1996;70:2201–2207.
41. Chang RY, Hofman MA, Sethna PB, Brian DA. A cis-acting function for the coronavirus leader in defective-interfering RNA replication. *J Virol* 1994;68:8223–8231.
42. Chang RY, Krishnan R, Brian DA. The UCUAAAC promoter motif is not required for high-frequency leader recombination in bovine coronavirus defective interfering RNA. *J Virol* 1996;70:2720–2729.
43. Charley B, Laude H. Induction of alpha interferon by transmissible gastroenteritis coronavirus: Role of transmembrane glycoprotein E1. *J Virol* 1988;62:8–11.
44. Chen DS, Asanaka M, Chen FS, et al. Human carcinoembryonic antigen and biliary glycoprotein can serve as mouse hepatitis virus receptors. *J Virol* 1997;71:1688–1691.
45. Chen DS, Asanaka M, Yokomori K, et al. A pregnancy-specific glycoprotein is expressed in the brain and serves as a receptor for mouse hepatitis virus. *Proc Natl Acad Sci U S A* 1995;92:12095–12099.
46. Chen W, Baric RS. Molecular anatomy of mouse hepatitis virus per-

sistence: Coevolution of increased host cell resistance and virus virulence. *J Virol* 1996;70:3947–3960.
47. Collins AR, Knobler RL, Powell H, Buchmeier MJ. Monoclonal antibodies to murine hepatitis virus-4 (strain JHM) define the viral glycoprotein responsible for attachment and cell-cell fusion. *Virology* 1982;119:358–371.
48. Collisson EW, Li JZ, Sneed LW, et al. Detection of avian infectious bronchitis viral infection using in situ hybridization and recombinant DNA. *Vet Microbiol* 1990;24:261–271.
49. Compton SR, Rogers DB, Holmes KV, et al. In vitro replication of mouse hepatitis virus strain A59. *J Virol* 1987;61:1814–1820.
50. Coulter-Mackie MB, Flintoff WF, Dales S. In vivo and in vitro models of demyelinating disease X: A schwannoma-L-2 somatic cell hybrid persistently yielding high titres of mouse hepatitis virus strain JHM. *Virus Res* 1984;1:477–487.
51. Coutelier JP, Godfraind C, Dveksler GS, et al. B lymphocyte and macrophage expression of carcinoembryonic antigen-related adhesion molecules that serve as receptors for murine coronavirus. *Eur J Immunol* 1994;24:1383–1390.
52. Cox E, Pensaert MB, Callebaut P, van Deun K. Intestinal replication of a respiratory coronavirus closely related antigenically to the enteric transmissible gastroenteritis virus. *Vet Microbiol* 1990;23:237–243.
53. de Groot RJ, Luytjes W, Horzinek MC, et al. Evidence for a coiled-coil structure in the spike proteins of coronaviruses. *J Mol Biol* 1987; 196:963–966.
54. de Groot RJ, Van Leen RW, Dalderup MJM, et al. Stably expressed FIPV peplomer protein induces cell fusion and elicits neutralizing antibodies in mice. *Virology* 1989;171:493–502.
55. de Groot RM, van der Most RG, Spaan WJM. The fitness of defective interfering murine coronavirus DI-a and its derivatives is decreased by nonsense and frameshift mutations. *J Virol* 1992;66:5898–5905.
56. de Haan CAM, Kuo L, Masters PS, et al. Coronavirus particle assembly: Primary structure requirements of the membrane protein. *J Virol* 1998;72:6838–6850.
57. Delmas B, Gelfi JL, Haridon R, et al. Aminopeptidase N is a major receptor for the entero-pathogenic coronavirus TGEV. *Nature* 1992; 357:417–420.
58. Delmas B, Laude H. Assembly of coronavirus spike protein into trimers and its role in epitope expression. *J Virol* 1990;64:5367–5375.
59. den Boon JA, Snijder EJ, Chirnside ED, et al. Equine arteritis virus is not a togavirus but belongs to the coronaviruslike superfamily. *J Virol* 1991;65:2910–2920.
60. Denison MR, Hughes SA, Weiss SR. Identification and characterization of a 65-kDa protein processed from the gene 1 polyprotein of the murine coronavirus MHV-A59. *Virology* 1995;207:316–320.
61. Denison MR, Spaan WJM, van der Meer Y, et al. The putative helicase of the coronavirus mouse hepatitis virus is processed from the replicase gene polyprotein and localizes in complexes that are active in viral RNA synthesis. *J Virol* 1999;73:6862–6871.
62. Denison MR, Zoltick PW, Hughes SA, et al. Intracellular processing of the N-terminal ORF 1a proteins of the coronavirus MHV-A59 requires multiple proteolytic events. *Virology* 1992;189:274–284.
63. Deregt D, Babiuk LA. Monoclonal antibodies to bovine coronavirus: Characteristics and topographical mapping of neutralizing epitopes on the E2 and E3 glycoproteins. *Virology* 1987;161:410–420.
64. Deregt D, Gifford GA, Khalid Ijaz M, et al. Monoclonal antibodies to bovine coronavirus glycoproteins E2 and E3: Demonstration of in vivo neutralizing activity. *J Gen Virol* 1989;70:993–998.
65. Deregt D, Sabara M, Babiuk LA. Structural proteins of bovine coronavirus and their intracellular processing. *J Gen Virol* 1987;68: 2863–2877.
66. Dubois-Dalcq ME, Doller EW, Haspel MV, Holmes KV. Cell tropism and expression of mouse hepatitis viruses (MHV) in mouse spinal cord cultures. *Virology* 1982;119:317–331.
67. Dupuy JM, Lamontagne L. Genetically-determined sensitivity to MHV3 infections is expressed in vitro in lymphoid cells and macrophages. *Adv Exp Med Biol* 1987;218:455–463.
68. Dveksler GS, Dieffenbach CW, Cardellichio CB, et al. Several members of the mouse carcinoembryonic antigen-related glycoprotein family are functional receptors for the coronavirus mouse hepatitis virus-A59. *J Virol* 1993;67:1–8.
69. Dveksler GS, Pensiero MN, Cardellichio CB, et al. Cloning of the mouse hepatitis virus (MHV) receptor: Expression in human and hamster cell lines confers susceptibility to MHV. *J Virol* 1991;65:6881–6891.
70. Dveksler GS, Pensiero MN, Dieffenbach CW, et al. Mouse hepatitis virus strain A59 and blocking antireceptor monoclonal antibody bind to the N-terminal domain of cellular receptor. *Proc Natl Acad Sci U S A* 1993;90:1716–1720.
71. Eleouet J-F, Chilmonczyk S, Besnardeau L, Laude H. Transmissible gastroenteritis coronavirus induces programmed cell death in infected cells through a caspase-dependent pathway. *J Virol* 1998;72:4918–4924.
72. Eleouet J-F, Rasschaert D, Lambert P, et al. Complete sequence (20 kilobases) of the polyprotein-encoding gene 1 of transmissible gastroenteritis virus. *Virology* 1995;206:817–822.
73. Evans MR, Simpson RW. The coronavirus avian infectious bronchitis virus requires the cell nucleus and host transcriptional factors. *Virology* 1980;105:582–591.
74. Fazakerley JK, Parker SE, Bloom F, Buchmeier MJ. The V5A13.1 envelope glycoprotein deletion mutant of mouse hepatitis virus type-4 is neuroattenuated by its reduced rate of spread in the central nervous system. *Virology* 1992;187:178–188.
75. Fischer F, Peng D, Hingley ST, et al. The internal open reading frame within the nucleocapsid gene of mouse hepatitis virus encodes a structural protein that is not essential for viral replication. *J Virol* 1997;71: 996–1003.
76. Fischer F, Stegen CF, Masters PS, Samsonoff WA. Analysis of constructed E gene mutants of mouse hepatitis virus confirms a pivotal role for E protein in coronavirus assembly. *J Virol* 1998;72: 7885–7894.
77. Fleming JO, Stohlman SA, Harmon RC, et al. Antigenic relationship of murine coronaviruses: Analysis using monoclonal antibodies to JHM (MHV-4) virus. *Virology* 1983;131:296–307.
78. Fleming JO, Trousdale MD, El-Zaatari FAK, et al. Pathogenicity of antigenic variants of murine coronavirus JHM selected with monoclonal antibodies. *J Virol* 1986;58:869–875.
79. Flintoff WF. Replication of murine coronaviruses in somatic cell hybrids between murine fibroblasts and rat schwannoma cells. *Virology* 1984;134:450–459.
80. Fosmire JA, Hwang K, Makino S. Identification and characterization of a coronavirus packaging signal. *J Virol* 1992;66:3522–3530.
81. Frana MF, Behnke JN, Sturman LS, Holmes KV. Proteolytic cleavage of the E2 glycoprotein of murine coronavirus: Host-dependent differences in proteolytic cleavage and cell fusion. *J Virol* 1985;56:912–920.
82. Furuya T, Macnaughton TB, La Monica N, Lai MMC. Natural evolution of coronavirus defective-interfering RNA involves RNA recombination. *Virology* 1993;194:408–413.
83. Gagneten S, Gout O, Dubois-Dalcq M, et al. Interaction of mouse hepatitis virus (MHV) spike glycoprotein with receptor glycoprotein MHVR is required for infection with an MHV strain that expresses the hemagglutinin-esterase glycoprotein. *J Virol* 1995;69:889–895.
84. Gallagher TM, Escarmis C, Buchmeier MJ. Alteration of the pH dependence of coronavirus-induced cell fusion: Effect of mutations in the spike glycoprotein. *J Virol* 1991;65:1916–1928.
85. Gallagher TM, Parker SE, Buchmeier MJ. Neutralization-resistant variants of a neurotropic coronavirus are generated by deletions within the amino-terminal half of the spike glycoprotein. *J Virol* 1990;64:731–741.
86. Godet M, Grosclaude J, Delmas B, Laude H. Major receptor-binding and neutralization determinants are located within the same domain of the transmissible gastroenteritis virus (coronavirus) spike protein. *J Virol* 1994;68:8008–8016.
87. Godet M, L'Haridon R, Vautherot J-F, Laude H. TGEV coronavirus ORF4 encodes a membrane protein that is incorporated into virions. *Virology* 1992;188:666–675.
88. Godfraind C, Langreth SG, Cardellichio CB, et al. Tissue and cellular distribution of an adhesion molecule in the carcinoembryonic antigen family that serves as a receptor for mouse hepatitis virus. *Lab Invest* 1995;73:615–627.
89. Gombold JL, Hingley ST, Weiss SR. Fusion-defective mutants of mouse hepatitis virus A59 contain a mutation in the spike protein cleavage signal. *J Virol* 1993;67:4504–4512.
90. Gorbalenya AE, Koonin EV, Donchencko AP, Blinov VM. Coronavirus genome: Prediction of putative functional domains in the non-structural polyprotein by comparative amino acid sequence analysis. *Nucleic Acids Res* 1989;17:4847–4861.
91. Griffiths G, Rottier PJM. Cell biology of viruses that assemble along the biosynthetic pathway. *Semin Cell Biol* 1992;3:367–381.
92. Grotzinger C, Heusipp G, Ziebuhr J, et al. Characterization of a 105-

kDa polypeptide encoded in gene 1 of the human coronavirus HCV 229E. *Virology* 1996;222:227–235.
93. Haspel MV, Lampert PW, Oldstone MBA. Temperature-sensitive mutants of mouse hepatitis virus produce a high incidence of demyelination. *Proc Natl Acad Sci U S A* 1978;75:4033–4036.
94. Herold J, Raabe T, Schelle-Prinz B, Siddell SG. Nucleotide sequence of the human coronavirus 229E RNA polymerase locus. *Virology* 1993;195:680–691.
95. Herold J, Raabe T, Siddell SG. Molecular analysis of the human coronavirus (strain 229E) genome. *Arch Virol Suppl* 1993;7:63–74.
96. Herrewegh AA, Mahler M, Hedrich HJ, et al. Persistence and evolution of feline coronavirus in a closed cat-breeding colony. *Virology* 1997;234:349–363.
97. Herrewegh AAPM, Smeenk I, Horzinek MC, et al. Feline coronavirus type II strains 79-1683 and 79-1146 originate from a double recombination between feline coronavirus type I and canine coronavirus. *J Virol* 1998;72:4508–4514.
98. Hilton A, Mizzen L, MacIntyre G, et al. Translational control in murine hepatitis virus infection. *J Gen Virol* 1986;67:923–932.
99. Hingley ST, Gombold JL, Lavi E, Weiss SR. MHV-A59 fusion mutants are attenuated and display altered hepatotropism. *Virology* 1994;200:1–10.
100. Hiscox JA, Mawditt KL, Cavanagh D, et al. Investigation of the control of coronavirus subgenomic mRNA transcription by using T7-generated negative-sense RNA transcripts. *J Virol* 1995;69:6219–6227.
101. Hofmann MA, Brian DA. The 5′-end of coronavirus minus-strand RNAs contains a short poly(U) tract. *J Virol* 1991;65:6331–6333.
102. Hofmann MA, Senanayake SD, Brian DA. A translation-attenuating intraleader open reading frame is selected on coronavirus mRNAs during persistent infection. *Proc Natl Acad Sci U S A* 1993;90: 11733–11737.
103. Hofmann MA, Sethna PB, Brian DA. Bovine coronavirus mRNA replication continues throughout persistent infection in cell culture. *J Virol* 1990;64:4108–4114.
104. Hogue BG, Kienzle TE, Brian DA. Synthesis and processing of the bovine enteric coronavirus haemagglutinin protein. *J Gen Virol* 1989; 70:345–352.
105. Holmes KV, Behnke JN. Evolution of a coronavirus during persistent infection in vitro. *Adv Exp Med Biol* 1981;142:287–299.
106. Holmes KV, Doller EW, Sturman LS. Tunicamycin-resistant glycosylation of coronavirus glycoprotein: Demonstration of a novel type of viral glycoprotein. *Virology* 1981;115:334–344.
107. Holmes KV, Welsh RM, Haspel MV. Natural cytotoxicity against mouse hepatitis virus-infected target cells. *J Immunol* 1986;136: 1446–1453.
108. Jacobs L, Spaan WJM, Horzinek MC, van der Zeijst BAM. Synthesis of subgenomic mRNA's of mouse hepatitis virus is initiated independently: Evidence from UV transcription mapping. *J Virol* 1981;39:401–406.
109. Jeong YS, Makino S. Evidence for coronavirus discontinuous transcription. *J Virol* 1994;68:2615–2623.
110. Jia W, Karaca K, Parrish CR, Naqi SA. A novel variant of avian infectious bronchitis virus resulting from recombination among three different strains. *Arch Virol* 1995;140:259–271.
111. Joo M, Makino S. Mutagenic analysis of the coronavirus intergenic consensus sequence. *J Virol* 1992;66:6330–6337.
112. Kanjanahaluethai A, Baker SC. Identification of mouse hepatitis virus papain-like proteinase 2 activity. *J Virol* 2000;74:7911–7921.
113. Keck JG, Makino S, Soe LH, et al. RNA recombination of coronavirus. *Adv Exp Med Biol* 1987;218:99–107.
114. Keck JG, Matsushima GK, Makino S, et al. In vivo RNA-RNA recombination of coronavirus in mouse brain. *J Virol* 1988;62:1810–1813.
115. Keck JG, Soe LH, Makino S, et al. RNA recombination of murine coronaviruses: recombination between fusion-positive MHV-A59 and fusion-negative MHV-2. *J Virol* 1988;62:1989–1998.
116. Keck JG, Stohlman SA, Soe LH, et al. Multiple recombination sites at the 5′-end of murine coronavirus RNA. *Virology* 1987;156:331–341.
117. Kienzle TE, Abraham S, Hogue BG, Brian DA. Structure and orientation of expressed bovine coronavirus hemagglutinin-esterase protein. *J Virol* 1990;64:1834–1838.
118. Kim KH, Makino S. Two murine coronavirus genes suffice for viral RNA synthesis. *J Virol* 1995;69:2313–2321.
119. Kim Y-N, Lai MMC, Makino S. Generation and selection of coronavirus defective interfering RNA with large open reading frame by RNA recombination and possible editing. *Virology* 1993;194:244–253.
120. Kim Y-N, Makino S. Characterization of a murine coronavirus defective interfering RNA internal cis-acting replication signal. *J Virol* 1995;69:4963–4971.
121. Klumperman J, Locker JK, Meijer A, et al. Coronavirus M proteins accumulate in the Golgi complex beyond the site of virion budding. *J Virol* 1994;68:6523–6534.
122. Knobler RL, Lampert PW, Oldstone MB. Virus persistence and recurring demyelination produced by a temperature-sensitive mutant of MHV-4. *Nature* 1982;298:279–280.
123. Koetzner CA, Parker MM, Ricard CS, et al. Repair and mutagenesis of the genome of a deletion mutant of the coronavirus mouse hepatitis virus by targeted RNA recombination. *J Virol* 1992;66:1841–1848.
124. Kooi C, Cervin M, Anderson R. Differentiation of acid-pH-dependent and -nondependent entry pathways for mouse hepatitis virus. *Virology* 1991;180:108–119.
125. Koolen MJM, Osterhaus ADME, van Steenis G, et al. Temperature-sensitive mutants of mouse hepatitis virus strain A59: Isolation, characterization and neuropathogenic properties. *Virology* 1983;125: 393–402.
126. Kottier SA, Cavanagh D, Britton P. Experimental evidence of recombination in coronavirus infectious bronchitis virus. *Virology* 1995; 213:569–580.
127. Krzystyniak K, Dupuy JM. Entry of mouse hepatitis virus 3 into cells. *J Gen Virol* 1984;65:227–231.
128. Kubo H, Yamada YK, Taguchi F. Localization of neutralizing epitopes and the receptor-binding site within the amino-terminal 330 amino acids of the murine coronavirus spike protein. *J Virol* 1994;68:5403–5410.
129. Kunkel F, Herrler G. Structural and functional analysis of the surface protein of human coronavirus OC43. *Virology* 1993;195:195–202.
130. Kuo L, Godeke GJ, Raamsman MJ, et al. Retargeting of coronavirus by substitution of the spike glycoprotein ectodomain: Crossing the host cell species barrier. *J Virol* 2000;74:1393–1406.
131. Kusters JG, Niesters HGM, Lenstra JA, et al. Phylogeny of antigenic variants of avian coronavirus IBV. *Virology* 1989;169:217–221.
132. Kyuwa S, Cohen M, Nelson G, et al. Modulation of cellular macromolecular synthesis by coronavirus: Implication for pathogenesis. *J Virol* 1994;68:6815–6819.
133. La Monica N, Yokomori K, Lai MMC. Coronavirus mRNA synthesis: Identification of novel transcription initiation signals which are differentially regulated by different leader sequences. *Virology* 1992; 188:402–407.
134. Lachance C, Arbour N, Cashman NR, Talbot PJ. Involvement of aminopeptidase N (CD13) in infection of human neural cells by human coronavirus 229E. *J Virol* 1998;72:6511–6519.
135. Lai MMC. Coronavirus leader RNA-primed transcription: An alternative mechanism to RNA splicing. *BioEssays* 1986;5:257–260.
136. Lai MMC. RNA recombination in animal and plant viruses. *Microbiol Rev* 1992;56:61–79.
137. Lai MMC, Baric RS, Makino S, et al. Recombination between nonsegmented RNA genomes of murine coronaviruses. *J Virol* 1985;56: 449–456.
138. Lai MMC, Cavanagh D. The molecular biology of coronaviruses. In: Maramorosch K, Murphy FA, Shatkin A, eds. *Advances in virus research.* New York: Academic Press, 1997:1–100.
139. Lai MMC, Patton CD, Baric RS, Stohlman SA. Presence of leader sequences in the mRNA of mouse hepatitis virus. *J Virol* 1983;46: 1027–1033.
140. Lamontagne LM, Dupuy JM. Persistent infection with mouse hepatitis virus 3 in mouse lymphoid cell lines. *Infect Immunol* 1984;44: 716–723.
141. Laude H. Porcine respiratory coronavirus: molecular features and virus-host interactions. *Vet Res* 1993;24:125–150.
142. Laude H, Rasschaert D, Huet JC. Sequence and N-terminal processing of the transmembrane protein E1 of the coronavirus transmissible gastroenteritis virus. *J Gen Virol* 1987;68:1687–1693.
143. Lavi E, Wang Q, Weiss SR, Gonatas NK. Syncytia formation induced by coronavirus infection is associated with fragmentation and rearrangement of the Golgi apparatus. *Virology* 1996;221:325–334.
144. Lee H-J, Shieh C-K, Gorbalenya AE, et al. The complete sequence (22 kilobases) of murine coronavirus gene 1 encoding the putative proteases and RNA polymerase. *Virology* 1991;180:567–582.
145. Leibowitz JL, DeVries JR, Haspel MV. Genetic analysis of murine hepatitis virus strain JHM. *J Virol* 1982;42:1080–1087.
146. Leparc-Goffart I, Hingley ST, Chua MM, et al. Altered pathogenesis

of a mutant of the murine coronavirus MHV-A59 is associated with a Q159L amino acid substitution in the spike protein. *Virology* 1997;239:1–10.
147. Leparc-Goffart I, Hingley ST, Chua MM, et al. Targeted recombination within the spike gene of murine coronavirus mouse hepatitis virus A59: Q159 is a determinant of hepatotropism. *J Virol* 1998;72: 9628–9636.
148. Lewis EL, Harbour DA, Beringer JE, Grinsted J. Differential in vitro inhibition of feline enteric coronavirus and feline infectious peritonitis virus by actinomycin D. *J Gen Virol* 1992;73:3285–3288.
149. Li D, Cavanagh D. Coronavirus IBV-induced membrane fusion occurs at near-neutral pH. *Arch Virol* 1992;122:307–316.
150. Li H-P, Huang P, Park S, Lai MMC. Polypyrimidine tract-binding protein binds to the leader RNA of mouse hepatitis virus and serves as a regulator of viral transcription. *J Virol* 1999;73:772–777.
151. Li H-P, Zhang X, Duncan R, et al. Heterogeneous nuclear ribonucleoprotein A1 binds to the transcription-regulatory region of mouse hepatitis virus RNA. *Proc Natl Acad Sci U S A* 1997;94:9544–9549.
152. Liao C-L, Lai MMC. Requirement of the 5′-end genomic sequence as an upstream cis-acting element for coronavirus subgenomic mRNA transcription. *J Virol* 1994;68:4727–4737.
153. Liao C-L, Lai MMC. A cis-acting viral protein is not required for the replication of a coronavirus defective-interfering RNA. *Virology* 1995;209:428–436.
154. Lin Y-J, Lai MMC. Deletion mapping of a mouse hepatitis virus defective interfering RNA reveals the requirement of an internal and discontiguous sequence for replication. *J Virol* 1993;67:6110–6118.
155. Lin Y-J, Liao C-L, Lai MMC. Identification of the cis-acting signal for minus-strand RNA synthesis of a murine coronavirus: Implications for the role of minus-strand RNA in RNA replication and transcription. *J Virol* 1994;68:8131–8140.
156. Lin Y-J, Zhang X, Wu R-C, Lai MMC. The 3′ untranslated region of coronavirus RNA is required for subgenomic mRNA transcription from a defective interfering RNA. *J Virol* 1996;70:7236–7240.
157. Liu DX, Brierley I, Tibbles KW, Brown TDK. A 100-kilodalton polypeptide encoded by open reading frame (ORF) 1b of the coronavirus infectious bronchitis virus is processed by ORF 1a products. *J Virol* 1994;68:5772–5780.
158. Liu DX, Brown TDK. Characterisation and mutational analysis of an ORF 1a-encoding proteinase domain responsible for pr oteolytic processing of the infectious bronchitis virus 1a/1b polyprotein. *Virology* 1995;209:420–427.
159. Liu DX, Cavanagh D, Green P, Inglis SC. A polycistronic mRNA specified by the coronavirus infectious bronchitis virus. *Virology* 1991;184:531–544.
160. Liu DX, Inglis SC. Identification of two new polypeptides encoded by mRNA5 of the coronavirus infectious bronchitis virus. *Virology* 1992; 186:342–347.
161. Liu DX, Inglis SC. Internal entry of ribosomes on a tricistronic mRNA encoded by infectious bronchitis virus [published erratum appears in *J Virol* 1992;66:6840]. *J Virol* 1992;66:6143–6154.
162. Liu DX, Shen S, Xu HY, Wang SF. Proteolytic mapping of the coronavirus infectious bronchitis virus 1b polyprotein: Evidence for the presence of four cleavage sites of the 3C-like proteinase and identification of two novel cleavage products. *Virology* 1998;246:288–299.
163. Locker JK, Rose JK, Horzinek MC, Rottier PJM. Membrane assembly of the triple-spanning coronavirus M protein: Individual transmembrane domains show preferred orientation. *J Biol Chem* 1992; 267:21911–21918.
164. Lomniczi B. Biological properties of avian coronavirus RNA. *J Gen Virol* 1977;36:531–533.
165. Lu XT, Lu YQ, Denison MR. Intracellular and in vitro-translated 27-kDa proteins contain the 3C-like proteinase activity of the coronavirus MHV-A59. *Virology* 1996;222:375–382.
166. Lu YQ, Lu XT, Denison MR. Identification and characterization of a serine-like proteinase of the murine coronavirus MHV-A59. *J Virol* 1995;69:3554–3559.
167. Luo Z, Weiss S. Roles in cell-to-cell fusion of two conserved hydrophobic regions in the murine coronavirus spike protein. *Virology* 1998;244:483–494.
168. Luytjes W, Bredenbeek PJ, Noten AFH, et al. Sequence of mouse hepatitis virus A59 mRNA 2: Indications for RNA-recombination between coronavirus and influenza C virus. *Virology* 1988;166: 415–422.
169. Luytjes W, Gerritsma H, Spaan WJM. Replication of synthetic defective interfering RNAs derived from coronavirus mouse hepatitis virus-A59. *Virology* 1996;216:174–183.
170. Luytjes W, Sturman LS, Bredenbeek PJ, et al. Primary structure of the glycoprotein E2 of coronavirus MHV-A59 and identification of the trypsin cleavage site. *Virology* 1987;161:479–487.
171. Machamer CE, Grim MG, Esquela A, et al. Retention of a cis Golgi protein requires polar residues on one face of a predicted a-helix in the transmembrane domain. *Mol Biol Cell* 1993;4:695–704.
172. Machamer CE, Mentone SA, Rose JK, Farquhar MG. The E1 glycoprotein of an avian coronavirus is targeted to the cis Golgi complex. *Proc Natl Acad Sci U S A* 1990;87:6944–6948.
173. Machamer CE, Rose JK. A specific transmembrane domain of a coronavirus E1 glycoprotein is required for its retention in the Golgi region. *J Cell Biol* 1987;105:1205–1214.
174. MacIntyre G, Wong F, Anderson R. A model for persistent murine coronavirus infection involving maintenance via cytopathically infected cell centres. *J Gen Virol* 1989;70:763–768.
175. Macnaughton MR, Davies HA, Nermut MV. Ribonucleoprotein-like structures from coronavirus particles. *J Gen Virol* 1978;39:545–549.
176. Maeda A, An S, Makino S. Importance of coronavirus negative-strand genomic RNA synthesis prior to subgenomic RNA transcription. *Virus Res* 1998;57:35–42.
177. Makino S, Fujioka N, Fujiwara K. Structure of the intracellular defective viral RNAs of defective interfering particles of mouse hepatitis virus. *J Virol* 1985;54:329–336.
178. Makino S, Joo M. Effect of intergenic consensus sequence flanking sequences on coronavirus transcription. *J Virol* 1993;67:3304–3311.
179. Makino S, Joo M, Makino JK. A system for study of coronavirus mRNA synthesis: A regulated, expressed subgenomic defective-interfering RNA results from intergenic site insertion. *J Virol* 1991;65: 6031–6041.
180. Makino S, Lai MMC. Evolution of the 5′-end of genomic RNA of murine coronaviruses during passages in vitro. *Virology* 1989;169: 227–232.
181. Makino S, Lai MMC. High-frequency leader sequence switching during coronavirus defective-interfering RNA replication. *J Virol* 1989; 63:5285–5292.
182. Makino S, Shieh C-K, Keck JG, Lai MMC. Defective interfering particles of murine coronavirus: Mechanism of synthesis of defective viral RNAs. *Virology* 1988;163:104–111.
183. Makino S, Shieh C-K, Soe LH, et al. Primary structure and translation of a defective-interfering RNA of murine coronavirus. *Virology* 1988; 166:550–560.
184. Makino S, Stohlman SA, Lai MMC. Leader sequences of murine coronavirus mRNAs can be freely reassorted: Evidence for the role of free leader RNA in transcription. *Proc Natl Acad Sci U S A* 1986; 83:4204–4208.
185. Makino S, Taguchi F, Fujiwara K. Defective interfering particles of mouse hepatitis virus. *Virology* 1984;133:9–17.
186. Makino S, Yokomori K, Lai MMC. Analysis of efficiently packaged defective-interfering RNAs of murine coronavirus: Localization of a possible RNA-packaging signal. *J Virol* 1990;64:6045–6053.
187. Masters PS. Localization of an RNA-binding domain in the nucleocapsid protein of the coronavirus mouse hepatitis virus. *Arch Virol* 1992;125:141–160.
188. Masters PS, Koetzner CA, Kerr CA, Heo Y. Optimization of targeted RNA recombination and mapping of a novel nucleocapsid gene mutation in the coronavirus mouse hepatitis virus. *J Virol* 1994;68:328–337.
189. Mendez A, Smerdou C, Izeta A, et al. Molecular characterization of transmissible gastroenteritis coronavirus defective interfering genomes: Packaging and heterogeneity. *Virology* 1996;217:495–507.
190. Mizzen L, Hilton A, Cheley S, Anderson R. Attenuation of murine coronavirus infection by ammonium chloride. *Virology* 1985;142: 378–388.
191. Molenkamp R, Spaan WJM. Identification of a specific interaction between the coronavirus mouse hepatitis virus A59 nucleocapsid protein and packaging signal. *Virology* 1997;239:78–86.
192. Murray RS, Cai G-Y, Hoel K, et al. Coronavirus infects and causes demyelination in primate central nervous system. *Virology* 1992;188: 274–284.
193. Myint S, Siddell S, Tyrrell D. Detection of human coronavirus 229E in nasal washings using RNA: RNA hybridisation. *J Med Virol* 1989; 29:70–73.

194. Nedellec P, Dveksler GS, Daniels E, et al. Bgp2, a new member of the carcinoembryonic antigen-related gene family, encodes an alternative receptor for mouse hepatitis virus. *J Virol* 1994;68:4525–4537.
195. Nguyen V-P, Hogue BG. Protein interactions during coronavirus assembly. *J Virol* 1997;71:9278–9284.
196. Niemann H, Boschek B, Evans D, et al. Post-translational glycosylation of coronavirus glycoprotein E1: Inhibition by monensin. *EMBO J* 1982;1:1499–1504.
197. Niemann H, Geyer R, Klenk HD, et al. The carbohydrates of mouse hepatitis virus (MHV) A59: Structures of the O-glycosidically linked oligosaccharides of glycoprotein E1. *EMBO J* 1984;3:665–670.
198. Oleszak EL, Perlman S, Leibowitz JL. MHV S peplomer protein expressed by a recombinant vaccinia virus vector exhibits IgG Fc-receptor activity. *Virology* 1992;186:122–132.
199. Opstelten DJE, de Groote P, Horzinek MC, et al. Disulfide bonds in folding and transport of mouse hepatitis coronavirus glycoproteins. *J Virol* 1993;67:7394–7401.
200. Opstelten DJE, Raamsman MJB, Wolfs K, et al. Envelope glycoprotein interactions in coronavirus assembly. *J Cell Biol* 1995;131: 339–349.
201. Oshiro LS. Coronaviruses. In: Dalton AJ, Haguenau F, eds. *Ultrastructure of animal viruses and bacteriophages:* An atlas. New York: Academic Press, 1973:331–343.
202. Page KW, Mawditt KL, Britton P. Sequence comparison of the 5′ end of mRNA 3 from transmissible gastroenteritis virus and porcine respiratory coronavirus. *J Gen Virol* 1991;72:579–587.
203. Parker SE, Gallagher TM, Buchmeier MJ. Sequence analysis reveals extensive polymorphism and evidence of deletions within the E2 glycoprotein gene of several strains of murine hepatitis virus. *Virology* 1989;173:664–673.
204. Payne HR, Storz J. Analysis of cell fusion induced by bovine coronavirus infection. *Arch Virol* 1988;103:27–33.
205. Peng D, Koetzner CA, Masters PS. Analysis of second-site revertants of a murine coronavirus nucleocapsid protein deletion mutant and construction of nucleocapsid protein mutants by targeted RNA recombination. *J Virol* 1995;69:3449–3457.
206. Pensiero MN, Dveksler GS, Cardellichio CB, et al. Binding of the coronavirus mouse hepatitis virus A59 to its receptor expressed from a recombinant vaccinia virus depends on posttranslational processing of the receptor glycoprotein. *J Virol* 1992;66:4028–4039.
207. Penzes Z, Tibbles K, Shaw K, et al. Characterization of a replicating and packaged defective RNA of avian coronavirus infectious bronchitis virus. *Virology* 1994;203:286–293.
208. Penzes Z, Wroe C, Brown TDK, et al. Replication and packaging of coronavirus infectious bronchitis virus defective RNAs lacking a long open reading frame. *J Virol* 1996;70:8660–8668.
209. Perlman S, Jacobsen G, Moore S. Regional localization of virus in the central nervous system of mice persistently infected with murine coronavirus JHM. *Virology* 1988;166:328–338.
210. Perlman S, Ries D, Bolger E, et al. MHV nucleocapsid synthesis in the presence of cyclohexamide and accumulation of negative-strand MHV RNA. *Virus Res* 1986;6:261–272.
211. Risco C, Anton IM, Enjuanes L, Carrascosa JL. The transmissible gastroenteritis coronavirus contains a spherical core shell consisting of M and N proteins. *J Virol* 1996;70:4773–4777.
212. Risco C, Anton IM, Sune C, et al. Membrane protein molecules of transmissible gastroenteritis coronavirus also expose the carboxy-terminal region on the external surface of the virion. *J Virol* 1995;69: 5269–5277.
213. Risco C, Muntion M, Enjuanes L, Carrascosa JL. Two types of virus-related particles are found during transmissible gastroenteritis virus morphogenesis. *J Virol* 1998;72:4022–4031.
214. Rossen JWA, Voorhout WF, Horzinek MC, et al. MHV-A59 enters polarized murine epithelial cells through the apical surface but is released basolaterally. *Virology* 1995;210:54–66.
215. Rottier P, Armstrong J, Meyer DI. Signal recognition particle-dependent insertion of coronavirus E1, an intracellular membrane glycoprotein. *J Biol Chem* 1985;260:4648–4652.
216. Rottier PJM, Welling GW, Welling-Wester S, et al. Predicted membrane topology of the coronavirus protein E1. *Biochemistry* 1986;25: 1335–1339.
217. Routledge E, Stauber R, Pfleiderer M, Siddell SG. Analysis of murine coronavirus surface glycoprotein functions by using monoclonal antibodies. *J Virol* 1991;65:254–262.
218. Salanueva IJ, Carrascosa JL, Risco C. Structural maturation of the transmissible gastroenteritis coronavirus. *J Virol* 1999;73:7952–7964.
219. Sanchez CM, Izeta A, Sanchez-Morgado JM, et al. Targeted recombination demonstrates that the spike gene of transmissible gastroenteritis coronavirus is a determinant of its enteric tropism and virulence. *J Virol* 1999;73:7607–7618.
220. Sawicki SG, Lu JH, Holmes KV. Persistent infection of cultured cells with mouse hepatitis virus (MHV) results from epigenetic expression of the MHV receptor. *J Virol* 1995;69:5535–5543.
221. Sawicki SG, Sawicki DL. Coronavirus minus-strand RNA synthesis and effect of cycloheximide on coronavirus RNA synthesis. *J Virol* 1986;57:328–334.
222. Sawicki SG, Sawicki DL. Coronavirus transcription: Subgenomic mouse hepatitis virus replicative intermediates function in RNA synthesis. *J Virol* 1990;64:1050–1056.
223. Schaad MC, Stohlman SA, Egbert J, et al. Genetics of mouse hepatitis virus transcription: Identification of cistrons which may function in positive and negative strand RNA synthesis. *Virology* 1990;177: 634–645.
224. Schickli JH, Zelus BD, Wentworth DE, et al. The murine coronavirus mouse hepatitis virus strain A59 from persistently infected murine cells exhibits an extended host range. *J Virol* 1997;71:9499–9507.
225. Schmidt MFG. Acylation of viral spike glycoproteins: A feature of enveloped RNA viruses. *Virology* 1982;116:327–338.
226. Schochetman G, Stevens RH, Simpson RW. Presence of infectious polyadenylated RNA in the coronavirus avian bronchitis virus. *Virology* 1977;77:772–782.
227. Schultze B, Cavanagh D, Herrler G. Neuraminidase treatment of avian infectious bronchitis coronavirus reveals a hemagglutinating activity that is dependent on sialic acid-containing receptors on erythrocytes. *Virology* 1992;189:792–794.
228. Schultze B, Gross HJ, Brossmer R, Herrler G. The S protein of bovine coronavirus is a hemagglutinin recognizing 9-O-acetylated sialic acid as a receptor determinant. *J Virol* 1991;65:6232–6237.
229. Schultze B, Herrler G. Bovine coronavirus uses N-acetyl-9-O-acetylneuraminic acid as a receptor determinant to initiate the infection of cultured cells. *J Gen Virol* 1992;73:901–906.
230. Schultze B, Krempl C, Ballesteros ML, et al. Transmissible gastroenteritis coronavirus, but not the related porcine respiratory coronavirus, has a sialic acid (N-glycolylneuraminic acid) binding activity. *J Virol* 1996;70:5634–5637.
231. Schultze B, Wahn K, Klenk H-D, Herrler G. Isolated HE-protein from hemagglutinating encephalomyelitis virus and bovine coronavirus has receptor-destroying and receptor-binding activity. *Virology* 1991;180: 221–228.
232. Schwarz B, Routledge E, Siddell SG. Murine coronavirus nonstructural protein ns2 is not essential for virus replication in transformed cells. *J Virol* 1990;64:4784–4791.
233. Senanayake SD, Hofmann MA, Maki JL, Brian DA. The nucleocapsid protein gene of bovine coronavirus is bicistronic. *J Virol* 1992;66: 5277–5283.
234. Sethna PB, Brian DA. Coronavirus genomic and subgenomic minus-strand RNAs copartition in membrane-protected replication complexes. *J Virol* 1997;71:7744–7749.
235. Sethna PB, Hofmann MA, Brian DA. Minus-strand copies of replicating coronavirus mRNAs contain antileaders. *J Virol* 1991;65:320–325.
236. Sethna PB, Hung SL, Brian DA. Coronavirus subgenomic minus-strand RNAs and the potential for mRNA replicons. *Proc Natl Acad Sci U S A* 1989;86:5626–5630.
237. Shi ST, Schiller JJ, Kanjanahaluethai A, et al. Colocalization and membrane association of murine hepatitis virus gene 1 products and de novo-synthesized viral RNA in infected cells. *J Virol* 1999;73: 5957–5969.
238. Shieh C-K, Soe LH, Makino S, et al. The 5′-end sequence of the murine coronavirus genome: Implications for multiple fusion sites in leader-primed transcription. *Virology* 1987;156:321–330.
239. Siddell S, Wege H, Barthel A, ter Meulen V. Coronavirus JHM: Intracellular protein synthesis. *J Gen Virol* 1980;53:145–155.
240. Siddell SG, Barthel A, ter Meulen V. Coronavirus JHM: A virion-associated protein kinase. *J Gen Virol* 1981;52:235–243.
241. Smith AL, Cardellichio CB, Winograd DF, et al. Monoclonal antibody to the receptor for murine coronavirus MHV-A59 inhibits viral replication in vivo. *J Infect Dis* 1991;163:879–882.
242. Snijder EJ, den Boon JA, Horzinek MC, Spaan WJM. Comparison of

the genome organization of toro- and coronaviruses: evidence for two nonhomologous RNA recombination events during Berne virus evolution. *Virology* 1991;180:448–452.

243. Spaan W, Delius H, Skinner M, et al. Coronavirus mRNA synthesis involves fusion of non-contiguous sequences. *EMBO J* 1983;2: 1839–1844.
244. Spaan WJM, Rottier PJM, Horzinek MC, van der Zeijst BAM. Isolation and identification of virus-specific mRNA in cells infected with mouse hepatitis virus (MHV-A59). *Virology* 1981;108:424–434.
245. Stauber R, Pfleiderer M, Siddell S. Proteolytic cleavage of the murine coronavirus surface glycoprotein is not required for fusion activity. *J Gen Virol* 1993;74:183–191.
246. Steinhauer DA, Holland JJ. Direct method for quantitation of extreme polymerase error frequencies at selected single base sites in viral RNA. *J Virol* 1986;57:219–228.
247. Stern DF, Sefton BM. Coronavirus proteins: Structure and function of the oligosaccharides of the avian infectious bronchitis glycoproteins. *J Virol* 1982;44:804–812.
248. Stern DF, Sefton BM. Synthesis of coronavirus mRNAs: Kinetics of inactivation of infectious bronchitis virus RNA synthesis by UV light. *J Virol* 1982;42:755–759.
249. Stohlman SA, Baric RS, Nelson GN, et al. Specific interaction between coronavirus leader RNA and nucleocapsid protein. *J Virol* 1988;62:4288–4295.
250. Stohlman SA, Fleming JO, Patton CD, Lai MMC. Synthesis and subcellular localization of the murine coronavirus necleocapsid protein. *Virology* 1983;130:527–532.
251. Stohlman SA, Kyuwa S, Polo JM, et al. Characterization of mouse hepatitis virus-specific cytotoxic T cells derived from the central nervous system of mice infected with the JHM strain. *J Virol* 1993;67: 7050–7059.
252. Stohlman SA, Sakaguchi AY, Weiner LP. Characterization of the cold-sensitive murine hepatitis virus mutants rescued from latently infected cells by cell fusion. *Virology* 1979;98:448–455.
253. Storz J, Zhang XM, Rott R. Comparison of hemagglutinating, receptor-destroying, and acetylesterase activities of avirulent and virulent bovine coronavirus strains. *Arch Virol* 1992;125:193–204.
254. Sturman LS, Holmes KV, Behnke J. Isolation of coronavirus envelope glycoproteins and interaction with the viral nucleocapsid. *J Virol* 1980;33:449–462.
255. Sturman LS, Ricard CS, Holmes KV. Proteolytic cleavage of the E2 glycoprotein of murine coronavirus: Activation of cell fusing activity of virions by trypsin and separation of two different 90K cleavage fragments. *J Virol* 1985;56:904–911.
256. Sturman LS, Ricard CS, Holmes KV. Conformational change of the coronavirus peplomer glycoprotein at pH 8.0 and 37°C correlates with virus aggregation and virus-induced cell fusion. *J Virol* 1990;64: 3042–3050.
257. Suzuki H, Taguchi F. Analysis of receptor-binding site of murine coronavirus spike protein. *J Virol* 1996;70:2632–2636.
258. Swift AM, Machamer CE. A Golgi retention signal in a membrane-spanning domain of coronavirus E1 protein. *J Cell Biol* 1991;115: 19–30.
259. Taguchi F. Fusion formation by the uncleaved spike protein of murine coronavirus JHMV variant cl-2. *J Virol* 1993;67:1195–1202.
260. Tahara SM, Dietlin TA, Bergmann CC, et al. Coronavirus translational regulation: Leader affects mRNA efficiency. *Virology* 1994;202: 621–630.
261. Tamura T, Taguchi F, Ueda K, Fujiwara K. Persistent infection with mouse hepatitis virus of low virulence in nude mice. *Microbiol Immunol* 1977;21:683–691.
262. Thiel V, Siddell SG. Internal ribosome entry in the coding region of murine hepatitis virus mRNA 5. *J Gen Virol* 1994;75:3041–3046.
263. Tooze J, Tooze S, Warren G. Replication of coronavirus MHV-A59 in sac-cells: Determination of the first site of budding of progeny virions. *Eur J Cell Biol* 1984;33:281–293.
264. Tooze J, Tooze SA. Infection of AtT20 murine pituitary tumour cells by mouse hepatitis virus strain A59: Virus budding is restricted to the Golgi region. *Eur J Cell Biol* 1985;37:203–212.
265. van der Meer Y, Snijder EJ, Dobbe JC, et al. Localization of mouse hepatitis virus nonstructural proteins and RNA synthesis indicates a role for late endosomes in viral replication. *J Virol* 1999;73: 7641–7657.
266. van der Most RG, Bredenbeek PJ, Spaan WJM. A domain at the 3′ end of the polymerase gene is essential for encapsidation of coronavirus defective interfering RNAs. *J Virol* 1991;65:3219–3226.
267. van der Most RG, de Groot RJ, Spaan WJM. Subgenomic RNA synthesis directed by a synthetic defective interfering RNA of mouse hepatitis virus: A study of coronavirus transcription initiation. *J Virol* 1994;68:3656–3666.
268. van der Most RG, Heijnen L, Spaan WJM, de Groot RJ. Homologous RNA recombination allows efficient introduction of site-specific mutations into the genome of coronavirus MHV-A59 via synthetic co-replicating RNAs. *Nucleic Acids Res* 1992;20:3375–3381.
269. van Marle G, van Dinten LC, Spaan WJ, et al. Characterization of an equine arteritis virus replicase mutant defective in subgenomic mRNA synthesis. *J Virol* 1999;73:5274–5281.
270. vanDinten LC, den Boon JA, Wassenaar ALM, et al. An infectious arterivirus cDNA clone: Identification of a replicase point mutation that abolishes discontinuous mRNA transcription. *Proc Natl Acad Sci U S A* 1997;94:991–996.
271. Vennema H, Godeke GJ, Rossen JWA, et al. Nucleocapsid-independent assembly of coronavirus-like particles by co-expression of viral envelope protein genes. *EMBO J* 1996;15:2020–2028.
272. Vennema H, Heijnen L, Zijderveld A, et al. Intracellular transport of recombinant coronavirus spike proteins: Implications for virus assembly. *J Virol* 1990;64:339–346.
273. Vennema H, Poland A, Foley J, Pedersen NC. Feline infectious peritonitis viruses arise by mutation from endemic feline enteric coronaviruses. *Virology* 1998;243:150–157.
274. Vlasak R, Luytjes W, Lieder J, et al. The E3 protein of bovine coronavirus is a receptor-destroying enzyme with acetyltransferase activity. *J Virol* 1988;62:4686–4690.
275. Vlasak R, Luytjes W, Spaan W, Palese P. Human and bovine coronaviruses recognize sialic acid-containing receptors similar to those of influenza C viruses. *Proc Natl Acad Sci U S A* 1988;85:4526–4529.
276. Wang L, Junker D, Collison EW. Evidence of natural recombination within the S1 gene of the infectious bronchitis virus. *Virology* 1993; 192:710–716.
277. Wege H, Schliephake A, Korner H, et al. An immunodominant CD4+ T cell site on the nucleocapsid protein of murine coronavirus contributes to protection against encephalomyelitis. *J Gen Virol* 1993;74: 1287–1294.
278. Wege H, Siddell SG, ter Meulen V. The biology and pathogenesis of coronaviruses. *Curr Top Microbiol Immunol* 1982;99:165–200.
279. Weismiller DG, Sturman LS, Buchmeier MJ, et al. Monoclonal antibodies to the peplomer glycoprotein of coronavirus mouse hepatitis virus identify two subunits and detect a conformational change in the subunit released under mild alkaline conditions. *J Virol* 1990;64: 3051–3055.
280. Welsh RM, Haspel MV, Parker DC, Holmes KV. Natural cytotoxicity against mouse hepatitis virus-infected cells. II. A cytotoxic effector cell with a B lymphocyte phenotype. *J Immunol* 1986;136: 1454–1460.
281. Wesley RD, Woods RD, Cheung AK. Genetic analysis of porcine respiratory coronavirus, an attenuated variant of transmissible gastroenteritis virus. *J Virol* 1991;65:3369–3373.
282. Wilhelmsen KC, Leibowitz JL, Bond CW, Robb JA. The replication of murine coronaviruses in enucleated cells. *Virology* 1981;110: 225–230.
283. Williams RK, Jiang GS, Holmes KV. Receptor for mouse hepatitis virus is a member of the carcinoembryonic antigen family of glycoproteins. *Proc Natl Acad Sci U S A* 1991;88:5533–5536.
284. Woo K, Joo M, Narayanan K, et al. Murine coronavirus packaging signal confers packaging to nonviral RNA. *J Virol* 1997;71:824–827.
285. Yeager CL, Ashumn RA, Williams RK, et al. Human aminopeptidase N is a receptor for human coronavirus 229E. *Nature* 1992;357: 420–422.
286. Yokomori K, Asanaka M, Stohlman SA, Lai MMC. A spike protein-dependent cellular factor other than the viral receptor is required for mouse hepatitis virus entry. *Virology* 1993;196:45–56.
287. Yokomori K, Baker SC, Stohlman SA, Lai MMC. Hemagglutinin-esterase-specific monoclonal antibodies alter the neuropathogenicity of mouse hepatitis virus. *J Virol* 1992;66:2865–2874.
288. Yokomori K, Banner LR, Lai MMC. Heterogeneity of gene expression of hemagglutinin-esterase (HE) protein of murine coronaviruses. *Virology* 1991;183:647–657.
289. Yokomori K, Banner LR, Lai MMC. Coronavirus mRNA transcription:

UV light transcriptional mapping studies suggest an early requirement for a genomic-length template. *J Virol* 1992;66:4671–4678.

290. Yokomori K, La Monica N, Makino S, et al. Biosynthesis, structure, and biological activities of envelope protein gp65 of murine coronavirus. *Virology* 1989;173:683–691.
291. Yokomori K, Lai MMC. Mouse hepatitis virus S RNA sequence reveals that nonstructural proteins NS4 and NS5a are not essential for murine coronavirus replication. *J Virol* 1991;65:5605–5608.
292. Yokomori K, Lai MMC. Mouse hepatitis virus utilizes two carcinoembryonic antigens as alternative receptors. *J Virol* 1992;66: 6194–6199.
293. Yokomori K, Lai MMC. The receptor for mouse hepatitis virus in the resistant mouse strain SJL is functional: Implications for the requirement of a second factor for viral infection. *J Virol* 1992;66: 6931–6938.
294. Yoo DW, Parker MD, Babiuk LA. The S2 subunit of the spike glycoprotein of bovine coronavirus mediates membrane fusion in insect cells. *Virology* 1991;180:395–399.
295. Yu X, Bi W, Weiss SR, Leibowitz JL. Mouse hepatitis virus gene 5b protein is a new virion envelope protein. *Virology* 1994;202: 1018–1023.
296. Zhang X, Lai MMC. A 5′-proximal RNA sequence of murine coronavirus as a potential initiation site for genomic-length mRNA transcription. *J Virol* 1996;70:705–711.
297. Zhang X, Liao C-L, Lai MMC. Coronavirus leader RNA regulates and initiates subgenomic mRNA transcription, both in trans and in cis. *J Virol* 1994;68:4738–4746.
298. Zhao X, Shaw K, Cavanagh D. Presence of subgenomic mRNAs in virions of coronavirus IBV. *Virology* 1993;196:172–178.
299. Ziebuhr J, Herold J, Siddell SG. Characterization of a human coronavirus (strain 229E) 3C-like proteinase activity. *J Virol* 1995;69: 4331–4338.
300. Ziebuhr J, Siddell SG. Processing of the human coronavirus 229E replicase polyproteins by the virus-encoded 3C-like proteinase: Identification of proteolytic products and cleavage sites common to pp1a and pp1ab. *J Virol* 1999;73:177–185.

CHAPTER 22

Rhabdoviridae: The Viruses and Their Replication

John K. Rose and Michael A. Whitt

The *Rhabdoviridae* are enveloped RNA viruses that are the simplest of all the nonsegmented negative-stranded RNA viruses classified in the large order of Mononegavirales. The genetic organization of rhabdoviruses is similar to that of the larger *Paramyxoviridae* and *Filoviridae* of the same order, and many aspects of rhabdovirus transcription and replication are similar as well. Because the genomes are in the negative (noncoding) sense, all of these viruses must carry an RNA-dependent RNA polymerase in the virion. The first such polymerase was identified in a rhabdovirus (8). Soon after infection when the viral genome is released into the cell, the RNA-dependent polymerase transcribes the genome to make subgenomic viral mRNAs that are translated to make viral proteins. Viral genome replication requires ongoing viral protein synthesis and results in synthesis of full-length copies of the antigenome followed by synthesis of full-length genomes that are subsequently packaged to form progeny virions.

CLASSIFICATION

Viruses of the family *Rhabdoviridae* are widely distributed in nature, where they infect vertebrates and invertebrates as well as many species of plants. The rhabdoviruses that cause rabies and economically important diseases of fish appear to have life cycles confined to vertebrate species. All other rhabdoviruses are thought to be transmitted to vertebrates and plants by infected arthropods, which may be the original hosts from which all rhabdoviruses evolved. Shope and Tesh (191) have provided an excellent review of the ecology and classification of rhabdoviruses that infect vertebrates. Characteristically, all rhabdoviruses have a wide host range, although many have adapted to grow in specific hosts and at their particular ambient temperatures.

In addition to numerous plant rhabdoviruses (85), more than 70 rhabdoviruses of vertebrates have been identified and classified. The viruses of the family *Rhab-*

doviridae known to infect mammals, including humans, have been classified into two genera: the *Vesiculovirus* genus, whose name is derived from vesicular stomatitis virus (VSV); and the *Lyssavirus* genus, otherwise known as the rabies and rabies-like viruses. The well characterized viruses of these two genera are listed in Table 1, which was adapted from the review by Shope and Tesh (191), with modification based on Bilsel and colleagues (17). Unlike vertebrate rhabdoviruses that replicate in the cytoplasm, the related *Bornaviridae* replicate in the nucleus (as do plant rhabdoviruses) and are now classified as a separate virus family.

Among the animal rhabdoviruses, many of those belonging to the genus *Vesiculovirus* infect biting insects. At least some of these insects can transmit the viruses to animals, and insect transmission may explain the seasonal nature of the disease. The list of insect vectors that may transmit vesiculoviruses to animals includes blackflies, sandflies, and mosquitoes. Evidence for insect-to-animal transmission has been reviewed in detail recently (112). The VSVs found commonly in the Western Hemisphere are divided into two distinct serotypes, called *New Jersey* and *Indiana,* and these share about 50% amino acid sequence identity in their glycoproteins (60,174). Detailed subclassification of the viruses within these serotypes has been described based on extensive nucleotide sequence analysis (17,18,143). In addition, these studies noted a remarkable genetic stability of the viruses over many years of natural infection in particular geographic locations, despite the well-known high rate of mutation of VSV and other RNA viruses passaged in tissue culture (197).

TABLE 1. *Members of two major rhabdovirus genera*

Virus	Source of virus in nature
Vesiculovirus (VSV) genus	
VSV—New Jersey	Mammals, mosquitoes, midges, blackflies, houseflies
VSV—Indiana	Mammals, mosquitoes, sandflies
VSV—Indiana 2 (Cocal)	Mammals, mosquitoes, mites
VSV—Indiana 3 (Alagoas)	Mammals, sandflies
Jurona	Mosquitoes
Carajas	Sandflies
Maraba	Sandflies
Piry	Mammals
Calchaqui	Mosquitoes
Yug Bogdanovac	Sandflies
Isfahan	Sandflies, ticks
Chandipura	Mammals, sandflies
Perinet	Mosquitoes, sandflies
Porton-S	Mosquitoes
Lyssavirus genus	
Rabies	Dogs, cats, wild carnivores, bats, cattle, humans
Lagos bat	Bats
Mokola	Shrews, humans, dogs, cats
Duvenhave	Humans, bats
Duvenhage	Humans, bats
Obodhiang	*Mansonia* mosquitoes
Kotonkan	*Culicoides* mosquitoes

Adapted from refs. 17 and 191, with permission.

The New Jersey and Indiana serotypes of VSV infect insects and mammals (see Table 1) and cause the economically important disease called *vesicular stomatitis* in cattle, horses, and swine. The disease, which has been thoroughly and recently reviewed (112), is characterized by vesicular lesions of the tongue, gums, teats, and hooves, and its symptoms resemble those of foot-and-mouth disease. Infected animals recover from VSV infections within about 2 weeks. Vesicular stomatitis is enzootic in Mexico, Central America, and northern South America, and small-scale outbreaks occur relatively frequently in the southwestern United States. Other serotypes of VSV, such as Chandipura and Isfahan, are found outside the Western Hemisphere in India and Iran and have also been associated with vesicular disease in domestic animals (226). The Chandipura glycoprotein sequence shares about 40% amino acid sequence identity with either the Indiana or the New Jersey glycoproteins (129). In contrast, the glycoprotein of the distantly related rabies virus shares only about 20% amino acid sequence identity with the VSV G protein (173).

VSV infection has been observed in people exposed to infected animals or inadvertently exposed in the laboratory (49,88). Infection in humans can result in influenza-like symptoms lasting a few days or in vesicular lesions of the mouth, but infection may often be asymptomatic. A very high percentage of humans living in rural areas where VSV infection of animals is common (eg, rural Panama) have high titers of antibody to VSV (207), but VSV infection is not normally associated with human disease in these areas. The pathogenesis of the rabies viruses is quite distinct from that of the vesiculoviruses and is described thoroughly in Chapter 39 in *Fields Virology*, 4th ed.

VIRION STRUCTURE

Rhabdovirus virions are composed of an external membrane derived from the cell in which the virus grew and an internal ribonucleoprotein core (Fig. 1). The single viral glycoprotein spans the membrane once and forms an array of about 400 trimeric spikes that extend from the viral membrane. The glycoprotein spikes are clearly visible in the electron micrograph of bullet-shaped VSV particles, shown in Figure 2. About 1,800 molecules of the viral matrix (M) protein are inside the viral envelope between the membrane and the nucleocapsid core. This core contains the single negative strand of genomic RNA, which ranges from about 11 to 12 kb in length in different rhabdoviruses. The bullet-shaped particles, 180 nm long and 75 nm wide, are typical of all rhabdoviruses, except certain plant rhabdoviruses that are bacilliform in shape and almost twice the length (85).

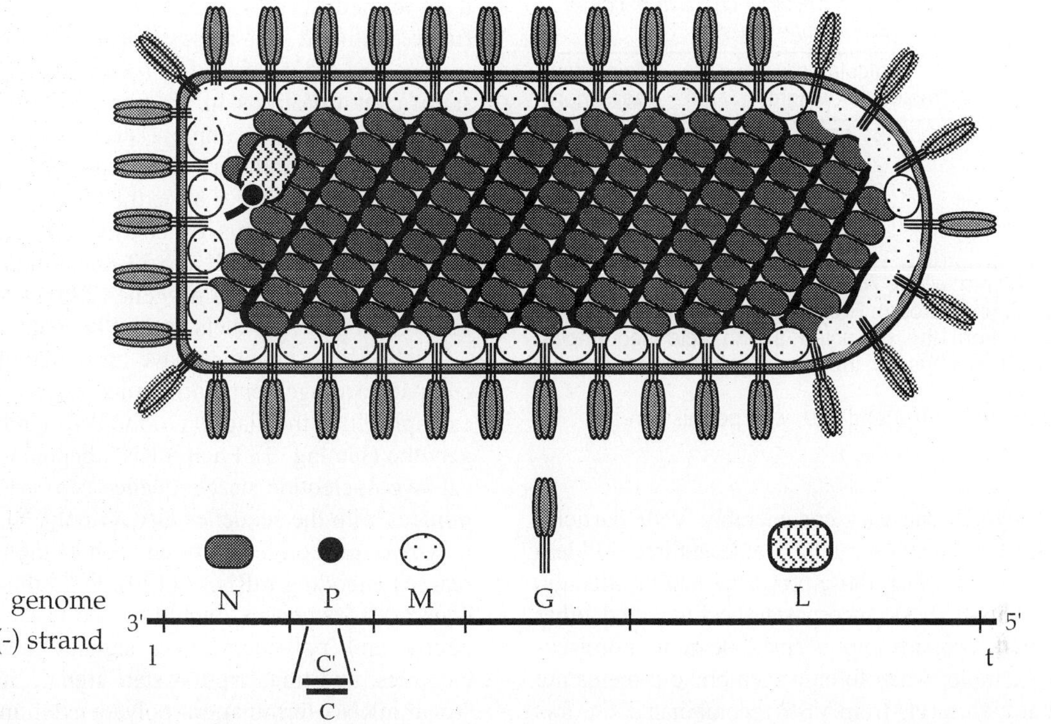

FIG. 1. Schematic representation of vesicular stomatitis virus (VSV) showing the two major structural components: the nucleocapsid (RNP) core, which contains single-stranded RNA tightly encased in the major N protein and the minor polymerase proteins L and P; and the membrane bilayer containing the transmembrane glycoprotein (*G*) and the peripheral matrix (*M*) protein, which adheres to the inner membrane surface and binds to the RNP core. Shown below is the gene order of the VSV genome with symbols representing the expressed proteins. The region of the P gene encoding the C proteins is indicated. (Modified from a drawing by Dr. Randall Owens.)

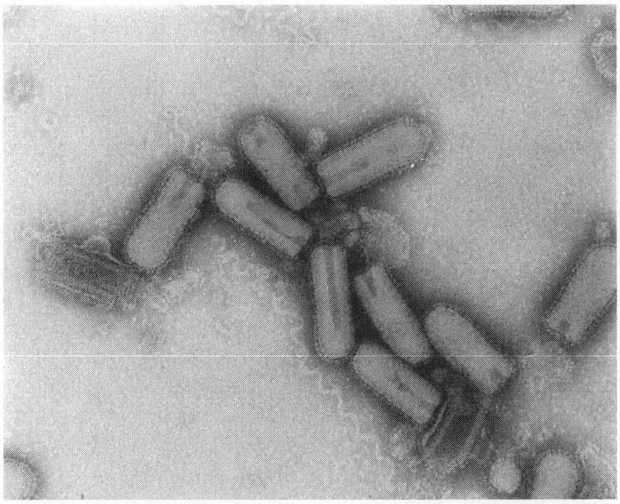

FIG. 2. Electron micrograph of vesicular stomatitis virus (VSV), negatively stained with phosphotungstic acid. Disrupted virions show the helical nucleocapsid core. The surface of intact virions shows protruding glycoprotein spikes.

The genomic RNA is in a tight complex with about 1,200 molecules of nucleocapsid protein that are arranged like beads on a string along the RNA, with each N protein molecule covering about nine nucleotides. This ribonucleoprotein complex is coiled into a tightly packed helix of about 35 turns within the virion. This helix is clearly visible in the two disrupted particles seen in Figure 2, and extended nucleocapsids from disrupted particles are visible as well. The viral RNA-dependent RNA polymerase, composed of the L and P proteins, is associated with the nucleocapsid core, and L and P proteins are present in about 50 and 500 molecules per virion, respectively. The gene order for VSV is diagrammed in Figure 1, with symbols for the structural proteins encoded by each of the genes. As discussed in detail later, separate mRNAs corresponding to each gene are transcribed sequentially beginning at the 3′ end of the genomic RNA. Even during transcription and replication of full-length genomes, the genome and antigenome RNAs remain in a tight complex with the N protein.

Table 2 lists the molecular weights of VSV (Indiana serotype) proteins, predicted from the gene sequences, the number of molecules of each found per virion, and the physical characteristics of virus particles. The protein composition of the particles is constant except for the glyco-

TABLE 2. *Composition and physical characteristics of vesicular stomatitis virus*[a]

Proteins	Calculated molecular weight[b]	Molecules per virion
N	47,355	1,258
P (NS)	29,878	466
M	26,064	1,826
G	63,416	1,205
L	240,707	50

[a]Length, 180 nm; width, 75 nm; S_{20w}, 660 Svedbergs; density, 1.16 g/mL (in sucrose); RNA length, 11,161 nucleotides.
[b]Calculated from the predicted amino acid sequences, including 6,000 daltons for the two N-linked glycans on G protein.
Adapted from refs. 169 and 209, with permission.

protein (G), which can vary considerably. VSV particles produced early in infection can have at least three-fold less G protein per virion than those produced late in infection (116). In addition, VSV incorporates cellular and other viral membrane proteins into its envelope quite promiscuously. For example, when foreign membrane proteins are expressed at high levels from VSV recombinants, the foreign proteins can represent as much as 25% of the total protein in the VSV envelope (182). These studies emphasize the imprecise nature of VSV membrane assembly.

GENOME STRUCTURE AND ENCODED PROTEINS

Rhabdovirus genomes contain a minimum of five genes in the order 3′ N-P-M-G-L 5′, as shown for the VSV Indiana genome in Figure 3. In VSV, two small proteins termed C and C′ are encoded in a second reading frame within P, but these appear specific to vesiculoviruses and are not found in lyssaviruses. There are also significant variations in the genome structure of other rhabdoviruses. For example, fish rhabdoviruses generally have an extra small gene between G and L (100), plant rhabdoviruses can have an extra gene between P and M (72), and sigma virus of *Drosophila* has three genes between N and G as well as a 33-nucleotide overlap of the G gene with the preceding gene (206). The functions of these extra gene products are not known.

Rhabdovirus genomes have an extremely simple and compact arrangement with little wasted space. This is exemplified in the diagram of the VSV (Indiana serotype) genome (see Fig. 3). Each mRNA begins with the identical five nucleotide start sequence cap-AACAG, and terminates with the sequence UAUG-poly(A), and there are only two nucleotides between each of the genomic RNA regions encoding mRNAs (170). Only the very minimal conserved sequences, including the transcription termination and polyadenylation signals, intergenic dinucleotides, and transcription start signals, are required to signal mRNA termination, polyadenylation, and reinitiation of the subsequent transcript (183). The 5′- and 3′-noncoding regions on the mRNAs are typically short, although there are some virus-specific exceptions. The leader and trailer regions preceding and following the sequences complementary to the mRNAs are also short. Presumably, the genetic selection favoring rapid replication has prevented accumulation of extra sequences that would slow genome replication.

In light of this conservation of genome size in the rhabdoviruses, it is interesting to note that VSV can replicate

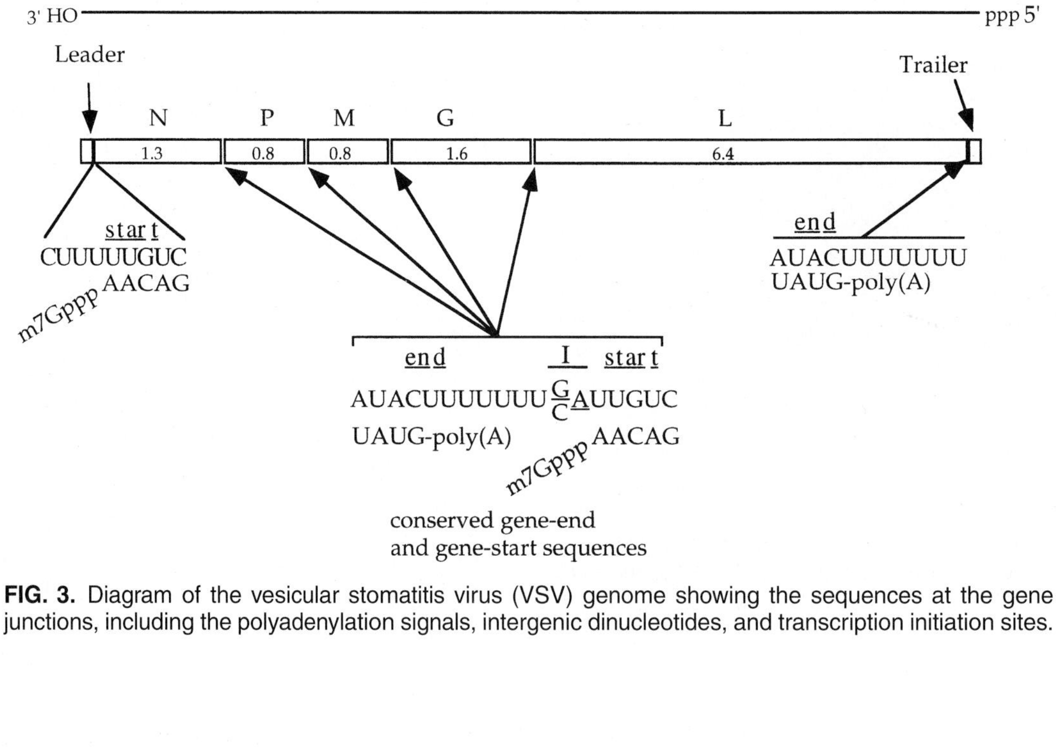

FIG. 3. Diagram of the vesicular stomatitis virus (VSV) genome showing the sequences at the gene junctions, including the polyadenylation signals, intergenic dinucleotides, and transcription initiation sites.

its genome and assemble virus particles efficiently even when large additions are made to the genome. As discussed under Molecular Genetics of Rhabdoviruses, the reverse genetic system for VSV, first established by Lawson and associates (102), has allowed expression of foreign genes within the VSV genome when appropriate transcription start and stop sequences are included (183). Many VSV recombinants have been made that express extra genes. The addition of single genes of less than 2,000 nucleotides in length generally has little effect on VSV growth in tissue culture or on pathogenesis in mice (98,165,166,182,183), whereas the addition of two extra genes totaling 4,200 nucleotides, a 40% increase in genome size, decreased virus titers only about three-fold (68). Because the helical nature of the VSV nucleocapsid does not put major constraints on virus length, virus particles can grow longer without large effects on viral replication or packaging. The increase in particle length is as expected when particles are imaged by electron microscopy (182).

Nucleocapsid Protein (N)

The rhabdovirus nucleocapsid protein serves the critical function of tightly packaging the RNA genome into a RNase-resistant core that is the template for both transcription and replication. From the length of the VSV Indiana genome and the number of N protein molecules per virion (see Table 2), each N protein molecule would cover about 9 nucleotides of RNA. This N protein–RNA complex interacts with the P–L polymerase complex during transcription and replication, and with the M protein during nucleocapsid condensation, membrane binding, and budding. As discussed under Genome Replication, the VSV N protein recognizes specific packaging sequences in the 5′ ends of both the genomic and antigenomic RNA, and the level of VSV N protein is thought to regulate the switch from transcription to replication.

Relatively little is known about the domain structure of the nucleocapsid protein, but deletion of the five C-terminal amino acids abolishes RNA-binding activity, and certain point mutations in this sequence can also prevent RNA binding (37). Other studies indicate that this domain of N protein is required for N–P protein interactions (204). The formation of N–P complexes is important for preventing N protein aggregation (40), which occurs when N protein is expressed at high levels in the absence of other viral proteins (76).

P Gene and Encoded Proteins (P and C)

The VSV P protein, or phosphoprotein, in combination with the L protein, forms the viral transcriptase–replicase complex (47). The P protein of VSV is an acidic protein of 265 amino acids (numbers from P of the Indiana serotype) (59) and is found in various phosphorylated forms in cells and virions. Sequence comparison studies have defined a domain structure for VSV P protein (18). It has an acidic N-terminal domain of 150 amino acids containing phosphorylation sites, followed by a highly variable region from residues 150 to 210 called the *hinge.* Domain II, also containing phosphorylation sites, spans from residues 210 to 244. Domain II is followed by a basic C-terminal domain III consisting of 21 amino acids. P protein is phosphorylated by casein kinase II on serine and threonine residues located in the N-terminal acidic domain (12), and, as discussed in the transcription section below, this phosphorylation is required to generate polymerase activity (11). The P protein forms trimers after phosphorylation, and only after trimerization is it able to bind the L protein and the N–RNA complex to form the active transcriptase (61). Binding of L protein also stabilizes the P trimer (61). The active polymerase complex is therefore an L–P3–N–RNA complex.

Recent studies have implicated phosphorylation of sites in domain II in regulation of P protein function during replication (81). It was suggested in that study and in an earlier study (33) that differential phosphorylation might regulate the switch from transcription to replication. As discussed under Genome Replication, differential phosphorylation may result in the formation of two distinct polymerase complexes: one that functions as a transcriptase and another that functions as a replicase (151). The P protein of Sendai virus and the P proteins of other *Paramyxoviridae* are also phosphorylated, and phosphorylation has been implicated in controlling P protein function. In a recent study, however, the major phosphorylation sites were eliminated from the Sendai P protein by mutagenesis of the gene. Replacement of the wild-type gene with the mutated gene in virus had no measurable effect on Sendai virus transcription or replication, and the mutant virus showed normal pathogenesis in animals (77). Although the paramyxovirus and rhabdovirus P proteins are highly divergent in sequence, these results suggest caution in interpretation of *in vitro* studies of rhabdovirus P protein mutants until the effects of the mutations are analyzed using reverse genetics of infectious virus.

In addition to encoding the P protein component of the viral polymerase, the VSV *P* gene encodes two small basic proteins of 55 and 65 amino acids from a second reading frame. This reading frame is presumably accessed by ribosomal scanning and initiation at the second and third AUGs in the P mRNA (see Fig. 1). Expression of these proteins, called C and C′, was first identified in cells infected with the New Jersey serotype of VSV (196), but similar proteins are also made by the VSV Indiana serotype (99).

Potential functions of the VSV C proteins were investigated by incorporating a mutated *P* gene eliminating C protein expression into infectious VSV. A stop codon was incorporated into the C and C′ coding sequence in such a way that the P protein sequence was unchanged (99). Virus that no longer expressed C proteins showed growth kinetics identical to wild-type virus. The amounts of viral mRNAs and proteins synthesized and incorporated into virions were indistinguishable for mutant and wild-type viruses, and the kinetics of host protein synthesis shutoff were also identical for both (99). Although the C and C′ proteins are dispensable for VSV growth in tissue culture, they are known to be conserved in all vesiculoviruses (196) and thus may play a role in viral pathogenesis or transmission by insect vectors. Studies on pathogenesis of C negative mutants in mice showed that they were no less pathogenic than the parental virus (A. Roberts and J. Rose, unpublished results). Pathogenesis in normal host animals, such as cattle, or replication in insects has not yet been examined.

Large Protein (L)

The first complete rhabdovirus *L* gene sequence was determined by Schubert for the VSV Indiana serotype (188), and since that time, numerous rhabdovirus *L* genes have been sequenced. All of these proteins consist of more than 2,100 amino acids in a single polypeptide chain. As discussed previously, the complex of L and P proteins constitutes the active RNA polymerase that copies the N–RNA template to produce mRNA, or complete antigenomes and genomes. The large size reflects the multifunctional nature of these proteins in transcription, replication, mRNA capping (2), methylation of 5′ cap structures (74), polyadenylation (189), and replication of the viral RNA.

The domains of rhabdovirus L proteins involved in the multiple enzymatic activities have not been clearly mapped except for a potential methyltransferase domain (74). Rhabdoviruses and paramyxovirus L proteins all contain a highly conserved GDN motif (155), which is a variant of the GDD motif found in positive-stranded RNA virus polymerases. Mutations within this core motif in the VSV polymerase block transcription activity *in vitro,* and a mutant GDD retains partial activity (194). Mutations in the GDN sequence of rabies L protein abolish both transcription and replication activities in a minigenome replication system (184).

The addition of poly(A) to rhabdovirus mRNAs is thought to result from repetitive copying by the polymerase of the U7 sequence found at the end of each gene (189). Mutations in L protein of VSV are known to cause aberrant polyadenylation of mRNAs and are consistent with a role for L in this process (79,80). In addition, a compound, *S*-adenosyl homocysteine, which blocks methylation of cap structures, also promotes synthesis of extremely long poly(A) on VSV mRNAs (175). This effect presumably reflects interference with normally coordinated functions of the polymerase.

There is also recent evidence that the VSV polymerase requires cellular translational elongation factors EF-1α, -1β, and -1γ to be fully active (38). These proteins had not previously been identified as components of the VSV virion, perhaps because they are present only at very low levels. A precise stoichiometry of these factors relative to L protein needs to be determined in virions because the virion polymerase is active in generation of all viral mRNAs without addition of host factors (140).

Glycoprotein (G)

All rhabdoviruses encode a membrane glycoprotein consisting of about 500 amino acids in a single polypeptide chain. The VSV envelope contains about 1,200 molecules of this single transmembrane G protein that form 400 trimeric spikes (42,97) arranged in a coat on the virion membrane (see Figs. 1 and 2). The VSV G protein (Indiana) is synthesized as a precursor of 511 amino acids (174), from which an N-terminal signal sequence of 16 amino acids is cleaved after the protein is inserted into the endoplasmic reticulum (ER) (115). The VSV G protein is a typical type I membrane glycoprotein, with most of the amino acids exposed on the virion surface (Fig. 4). There are two sites of N-linked glycosylation, and both

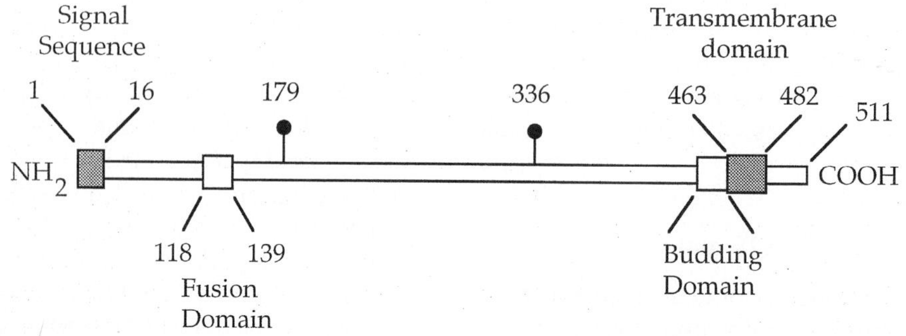

FIG. 4. Schematic of the vesicular stomatitis virus (VSV) glycoprotein illustrating the functional domains.

glycans are processed to the complex type (159). A hydrophobic domain of 20 amino acids spans the membrane, and a 29–amino acid cytoplasmic domain extends into the virion. A single molecule of palmitate is esterified to a cysteine residue in the cytoplasmic domain of some rhabdovirus G proteins (171,180), but the function of the palmitate is unclear because a mutant G protein lacking palmitate has normal membrane fusion activity, assembles normally into virions (224), and reconstitutes fully infectious virus (L. Buonocore and J. Rose, unpublished data).

The VSV G protein has served as an important model for many studies on protein folding, assembly, and transport to the cell surface (43). Immediately after synthesis and before the correct disulfide bonds are formed, G protein associates with a molecular chaperone in the ER called *BiP* (GRP78), which assists in protein folding (125). Correctly folded monomers are released from BiP within about 3 minutes after synthesis, and these then assemble into trimers in about 7 minutes before leaving the ER. A second molecular chaperone, calnexin, recognizes monoglucosylated oligosaccharides on VSV G protein and is bound and released from VSV G with kinetics that are slightly delayed compared with those of BiP, suggesting sequential action of these two chaperones (69). Transport of G protein to the Golgi occurs within about 15 minutes, and protein appears on the cell surface after about 30 minutes (16).

Mutations in all three domains of the VSV G protein that affect transport from the ER have been analyzed in detail. Mutations in the extracellular domain typically prevent correct folding of G monomers and induce aggregation with BiP protein before trimerization (44). When VSV G protein monomers have severe folding defects, for example, because of an absence of glycosylation sites, they are found in large, disulfide-bonded aggregates that remain permanently bound to BiP protein in the ER (44,126,127,154). Mutations in the transmembrane domain can also affect transport by inducing aggregation and preventing transport, whereas mutations in the cytoplasmic domain that reduce the transport rate do not appear to affect the folding of the extracellular domain (44,172). These results indicate that the cytoplasmic tail of the glycoprotein contains a signal that accelerates protein exit from the ER, perhaps by signaling concentration of the protein at sites of vesicle budding from the ER. Detailed mapping of the cytoplasmic tail has implicated a diacidic signal Asp-X-Glu, where X represents any amino acid in accelerating export (144). Further studies have shown that this transport signal extends to a Y-X-X-aliphatic motif in the cytoplasmic tail (190). The VSV G cytoplasmic tail is required for sorting to the basolateral membrane of polarized MDCK cells (158), and the same signal (Y-X-X-aliphatic) that is involved in promoting G protein export from the ER is also involved in sorting to the basolateral membrane (210). Basolateral sorting of VSV G protein is presumably important for systemic spread of the virus, as occurs during natural infections of livestock.

VSV G protein trimers are not tightly associated, but instead are in a constant and rapid equilibrium with monomeric subunits in the ER (235) and at the cell surface (234), or when examined in solution after solubilization with detergent (124). Once assembled into virions, it is likely that a trimeric or higher-order G protein structure is stabilized by lateral interactions among trimers on the virion surface and by interactions with the internal virion components.

VSV G protein undergoes a conformational change at pH values below about 6.1, and this conformational change stabilizes the trimer (42). The low pH-induced conformational change presumably exposes a hydrophobic domain that can insert into a target membrane and mediate membrane fusion (52,163). A linear hydrophobic domain typical of fusion domains in other viral fusion proteins is not obvious in the VSV G protein sequence, although the N-terminus is somewhat hydrophobic. Initial studies with small hydrophobic peptides corresponding to the N-terminus of the mature VSV G protein showed that these could mediate hemolysis, and it was suggested that hemolysis might be equated with membrane fusion activity (178). However, a change in the peptide sequence that abolished hemolysis had no effect on fusion activity when introduced at the N-terminus of the VSV G protein (228). These results indicate that the hemolysis assay employing peptides is not always relevant to membrane fusion, but they do not rule out a direct role for the N-terminus in the membrane fusion process.

Studies with mutants of the VSV G protein have implicated the involvement of other domains in the fusion process. A site for N-linked glycosylation introduced at amino acid 117 completely abolished the membrane fusion activity of G protein without blocking folding, transport to the cell surface, or incorporation into virions (225). The proximity of this mutation to a sequence of 19 uncharged amino acids (amino acids 118 to 136) suggested that this domain might be involved in fusion. Analysis of linker insertion mutants that failed to induce cell fusion identified the same site as well as two other distant sites in G protein that affected membrane fusion (114). Additional studies pointed to the importance of amino acids 118 to 136 because mutations in this region either abolish fusion or affect the pH threshold for fusion (54,55,236). A hydrophobic photolabeling technique identified a peptide from residues 59 to 221 of VSV G protein interacting with the hydrophobic membrane core (45). Because this region encompasses residues 118 to 136, the result also provides support for the role of the 118 to 136 domain in membrane insertion during fusion. A region in a similar position in rabies virus G protein (residues 103 to 179) was identified using the same probe (45).

Matrix Protein (M)

The matrix (M) protein is the smallest and most abundant protein in the rhabdovirus virion. Despite its small size, M protein has many functions. VSV M protein plays critical roles in condensation of nucleocapsids during virus assembly, in disruption of the cytoskeleton, and in inhibition of host functions as described in the sections that follow. It also has an intrinsic ability to cause budding of vesicles from cells when expressed alone (89), a property that is probably important in natural budding and appears related to the presence of proline-rich motif that binds to WW domains of cellular proteins (71). A fraction of VSV M protein is associated with membranes in infected cells; most is cytoplasmic (30,31,131,231) whereas the rest of M protein is located in the nucleus of infected cells (123). Because of M protein association with the plasma membrane and with nucleocapsids, it has been proposed that M acts as a bridge between the viral envelope and the nucleocapsid (see Fig. 1). Recent studies of rabies virus support this location for its M protein (136), but other studies of VSV suggest that M protein may form a cigar-shaped internal structure, which has been proposed to form a scaffold around which the nucleocapsid is wound (9,10). It seems highly improbable that M protein could occupy different positions in rabies and VSV, but this issue awaits resolution with more definitive analytical techniques. A report that M protein can stabilize G protein trimers *in vitro* (119) and that membranes from cells expressing M protein bind nucleocapsids (30) also supports the idea that M bridges the gap between the nucleocapsid and the G protein. The VSV M protein is highly basic and does not contain hydrophobic domains that are sufficient to act as membrane spans. However, the amino terminus of VSV M may be membrane associated because it can be labeled with a hydrophobic photoaffinity probe (108).

The VSV M protein is phosphorylated on serine and threonine residues between amino acids 20 and 35, but the assembly functions of M protein are not disrupted when the major sites of phosphorylation are disrupted (92), and the function of phosphorylation, if any, remains to be determined.

STAGES OF REPLICATION

The replication and assembly of members of the *Rhabdoviridae* family can be divided into distinct stages as depicted in Figure 5. Although many of these events occur simultaneously in an infected cell, it is convenient to consider the process of infection as a linear series of events that proceeds in the following order: adsorption, entry and uncoating, transcription, replication, assembly, and budding.

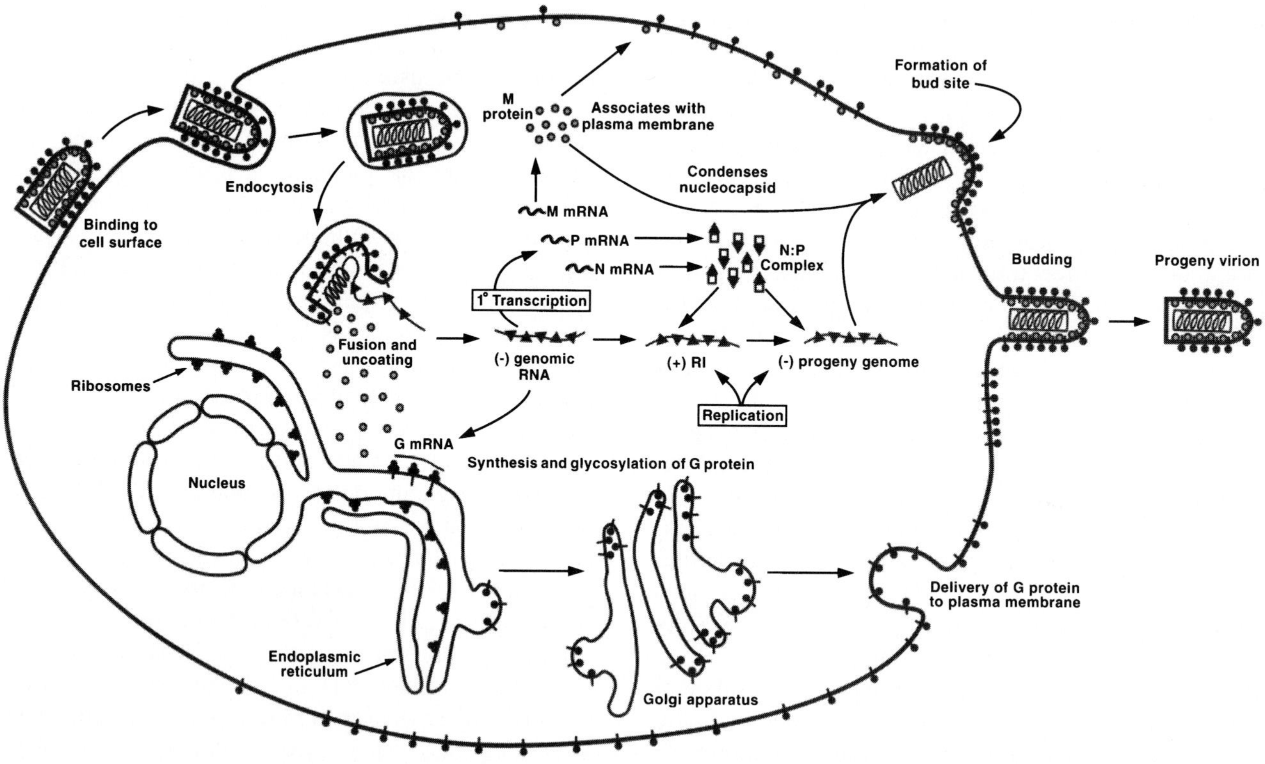

FIG. 5. Diagram of the life cycle of a rhabdovirus.

Adsorption

Rhabdoviral infection is initiated by attachment of virus to a receptor on the host cell surface. The receptors for the attachment of rhabdoviruses have been difficult to identify because of the generally broad host range and the binding properties of rhabdovirus particles. Virus adsorption is inefficient and difficult to quantitate for viruses in this family. For example, VSV binding is pH dependent, and maximal binding occurs between pH 6.5 and 6.0 (56,130); yet even at the optimal pH, binding fails to reach equilibrium (130). Furthermore, when virus is prebound at 4°C, only a limited amount of virus is internalized when cells are warmed to 37°C (130). However, virus infectivity can be increased more than 20-fold when virus is adsorbed at pH 6.3 versus when virus is bound at neutral pH (56). The pH dependence of binding correlates well with pH-induced conformational changes in the G protein (56), suggesting that the receptor-binding site in the envelope protein becomes exposed during the transition from the neutral to the acid conformation.

Kinetic analysis of VSV binding to Vero cells suggested that two separate sites (saturable and unsaturable) exist for attachment of VSV (179). To identify the saturable binding component, Vero cell membranes were disrupted with the dialyzable, nonionic detergent octyl-D-glucopyranoside. When analyzed in a competitive binding assay, the extract specifically inhibited the saturable, high-affinity binding of 35S-methionine–labeled VSV to Vero cells (177). The binding inhibitor was resistant to protease and neuraminidase but was inactivated by phospholipase C, suggesting it was a phospholipid. Of all phospholipids tested, only phosphatidylserine totally inhibited the high-affinity binding of VSV to Vero cells and also inhibited VSV plaque formation by 80% to 90% but did not block herpesvirus plaque formation (177). Based on these results, it is thought that phosphatidylserine may be one of the VSV receptors, at least on Vero cells. The identification of phospholipid binding domains in other rhabdovirus glycoproteins supports this idea and suggests that phosphatidylserine binding is a common feature of rhabdovirus envelope proteins (48).

The receptor for rabies virus has been controversial, and recent evidence indicates that several different receptors can be used. Sequence similarities between a region in the rabies glycoprotein and snake venom neurotoxins initially led to the hypothesis that the nicotinic acetylcholine receptor (AChR) is a receptor for rabies virus (109), and evidence supporting this has been obtained (62,70). Infection of cell lines that lack AChR, however, indicated that other molecules must also be used by rabies virus for entry (160). Recently, two additional receptors for rabies virus entry were identified. Using a random-primed cDNA expression library constructed from neuroblastoma cell (NG108) mRNA, the murine low-affinity nerve-growth factor receptor was identified as a functional receptor for street rabies virus (212). In a separate study, it was shown that the neural cell adhesion molecule can also serve as a receptor for the CVS (challenge virus standard) strain of rabies virus both in cultured cells and in mice (211).

Entry and Uncoating

After binding, the virions are endocytosed through a clathrin-dependent pathway typical of receptor-mediated endocytosis (130). Subsequent reductions in the pH of the endocytic compartment eventually trigger a membrane fusion reaction between the envelope of the endocytosed virion and the endosomal membrane. This fusion event is catalyzed by the G protein and results in the release of the ribonucleoprotein (RNP) core into the host cell cytoplasm (130). Either concomitant with membrane fusion or immediately after, M protein dissociates from the RNP core (164). The combined processes of membrane fusion and M protein dissociation constitute the uncoating event for rhabdoviruses. The trigger for M protein dissociation from RNPs is not known.

Transcription

The first synthetic event that occurs after uncoating of RNPs is transcription of viral-specific mRNAs by the L–P3 polymerase complex brought into the cell by the virion. Primary transcription occurs in the absence of protein synthesis, unlike genome replication, which requires newly synthesized N and P proteins and ongoing translation (41). The template for VSV transcription is the genome RNA complexed with the N protein in a ribonuclease-resistant form. As discussed previously, both the L and P proteins are required for polymerase activity (47). The P protein does not possess any known enzymatic activity, but instead acts as an accessory factor that may modify the activity of L protein through the phosphorylation status of P. The importance of P protein phosphorylation for transcription has been studied most extensively for VSV. Phosphorylation of serine and threonine residues in the N-terminal domain I of P protein by casein kinase II converts P to a transcription-competent state using an *in vitro* transcription assay (12). Although the absolute requirement for P protein phosphorylation in transcription has been questioned (195), studies using a transcriptionally active VSV mini-genome expressed from plasmid DNA support the conclusion that phosphorylation is required for transcription *in vivo* (151). The additional negative charge of the phosphates presumably induces conformational changes and results in the formation of P protein trimers that bind to L protein to constitute the active polymerase (61). There is also a recent report that the L protein of VSV requires cellular translational elongation factors EF-1α, -1β, and -1γ to be fully active in an *in vitro* transcription assay (38), indicating that host factors may also contribute to the activity of the polymerase.

Transcription begins at the exact 3′ end of the genome, where the polymerase first synthesizes a small 47-nucleotide RNA called the *leader*. Each of the five mRNAs encoding the viral proteins is then synthesized in the order it appears from the 3′ end of the genome. The leader is neither capped nor polyadenylated, but it is encapsidated once sufficient quantities of the N protein, in the form of N–P complexes, are synthesized.

Sequential transcription of VSV genes was first shown indirectly through the effect of increasing doses of ultraviolet (UV) irradiation on synthesis of the individual transcripts detected in a coupled transcription-translation system (7) and also by direct analysis of the transcripts separated by electrophoresis (1). Sequential transcription was also demonstrated directly by nucleic acid hybridization of sequences synthesized *in vitro* or by detection of specific oligonucleotides from the 5′ ends of the mRNAs (83,84). The latter studies were inconsistent with independent initiation of mRNA synthesis on each gene because the synthesis of 5′ mRNA sequences was dependent on transcription of the preceding mRNA. Studies involving reconstitution of purified nucleocapsid template with solubilized transcriptase showed that only leader RNA sequences are made initially and that mRNA oligonucleotides appear only after full-length leader has been synthesized (46). Thus, the VSV polymerase is not free to initiate transcription independently on each gene, and sequential transcription appears as a result of an obligatory entrance of all polymerases at the leader gene.

In vitro transcription studies also demonstrated that the VSV polymerase pauses for 1 to 2 minutes at each gene junction and then reinitiates synthesis on the downstream gene with only 70% to 80% frequency (83). The pause time may represent, at least in part, time required to copy repetitively the U7 sequence to generate the poly(A) on each mRNA.

Transcriptional attenuation is a common feature of nonsegmented negative-stranded RNA viruses, and this phenomenon results in a gradient of mRNA synthesis such that the N message is the most abundant in infected cells and the L message is the least abundant (83,214). Therefore, VSV transcription is both sequential and polar. The polarity of transcription is an inherent property of the polymerase, and attenuation results from events that occur when the polymerase interacts with cis-acting signals at each gene junction. Extra foreign genes inserted into VSV are subject to and exert the same 20% to 30% attenuation effect (98,167,183), and when VSV's own genes are rearranged, there is still a 20% to 30% attenuation at each gene junction regardless of gene order (6,217).

The mechanism leading to the generation of individual transcripts during a rhabdoviral infection is not completely understood, but there is strong evidence supporting a start and stop model for rhabdoviral transcription. In this model, the polymerase initiates transcription at the 3′ end of the genome and then terminates transcription at the leader–*N* gene junction. The polymerase then reinitiates at the conserved start site 3′ UUGUC . . . . 5′ of the *N* gene, and sequential transcription ensues. There is evidence from a VSV mutant called *polR* that the polymerase can initiate internally at the *N* gene start site (32), but this seems to be a unique property of the *polR* mutant that results from a mutation in the N protein, and once the leader–*N* gene junction is traversed, subsequent transcription occurs by the start and stop mechanism.

The use of transcriptionally active VSV mini-genomes (described later under Molecular Genetics of Rhabdoviruses) has allowed the dissection of cis-acting signals that are important for transcript initiation, capping and methylation, and polyadenylation and termination. Using a dicistronic mini-genome system, it was found that the first three nucleotides of the conserved 3′ UUGUC . . . . 5′ start sequence (complementary to the cap-AACAG at the beginning of each mRNA) were the most important for VSV gene expression. The U at position 1 and G at position 3 were absolutely required for transcript accumulation in infected cells, whereas the second position could be a pyrimidine, although U was preferred (201). Remarkably, mutations at the second position and substituting a C for a U at the first position did not prevent initiation per se, but instead affected modifications at the 5′ end of the mRNA as well as polymerase processivity (203). Because the polymerase is responsible for addition of the 5′-7mGpppG cap, the conserved sequences at the beginning of each gene appear to contain separate but overlapping signals for capping and for transcript initiation. Thus, transcript initiation and 5′ end modification (presumably capping) are linked, yet separable, events.

The mechanism by which VSV transcripts are capped has not yet been defined, but because the entire VSV life cycle is carried out in the cytoplasm of the cell, it is thought that the host nuclear enzymes are not involved. Analysis of the cap structure found on VSV transcripts revealed that both the α and β phosphates of the 5′–5′ triphosphate linkage of the guanosine cap are contributed by a guanosine diphosphate (GDP) donor (2). Therefore, the addition of the 5′–5′ guanosine cap cannot be mediated by a covalent nucleotidyl transfer reaction with guanosine monophosphate (GMP) as occurs during typical eukaryotic capping. Available evidence indicates that the polymerase complex mediates the capping reaction because mRNAs generated during *in vitro* transcription reactions with detergent solubilized purified virions are efficiently capped (2). Although the L protein does share some sequence homology to nucleotide binding proteins, it shows no homology to covalent nucleotidyl transferases (192), and there have been no mutations identified in L protein that affect capping. However, viruses that are deficient in methyltransferase activity have been isolated, and the defect has been mapped to L protein (74).

Recently, it was suggested that the GTP- and GDP-binding properties of the α subunit of EF-1 associated with L protein may play a role in the VSV capping reaction (38). It is possible that other host proteins may associate with L to mediate transcript capping, but as mentioned previously (L protein section), these must be found on only a fraction of the polymerase complexes found in virions.

After transcript elongation, the polymerase encounters the conserved stop-polyadenylation signal consisting of 3′-AUAC(U7)-5′. Two events can occur once the polymerase reaches this sequence. For most transcripts, the polymerase pauses and reiteratively copies, or "stutters," over the seven uridinylate residues to produce a poly(A) tail about 150 nucleotides in length before terminating. Occasionally, the stop-polyadenylation signal is ignored, and transcription continues past the intergenic region and through the next gene, generating a read-through transcript that becomes polyadenylated at the downstream stop-polyadenylation site (75). Studies to define the stop-polyadenylation signal revealed that reducing the length of the U7 tract, even by one nucleotide, or changing the C of the preceding 3′-AUAC(U7)-5′ to any other nucleotide prevents termination and causes exclusive read-through transcription at the mutated gene junction (13).

After polyadenylation, the polymerase scans through the intergenic dinucleotide in a nontranscriptive mode until the next transcription start sequence is encountered (14,201,202). The attenuation of expression observed for downstream genes presumably results from some of the polymerases dissociating from the template after polyadenylation or during the transition from polyadenylation and termination to reinitiation at adjacent downstream gene.

Genome Replication

During transcription, the VSV polymerase responds to signals that result in the synthesis of the leader RNA and individual mRNAs. In contrast, during replication, the polymerase must ignore these signals and synthesize genome-length positive-stranded RNA. This RNA is then replicated to form the genomic negative-stranded RNA. Unlike transcription, VSV replication requires ongoing translation, particularly of viral N and P proteins. This was found initially because inhibition of protein synthesis by cyclohexamide would prevent RNA replication but not transcription (41). The original concept that the N protein alone is sufficient for replication of VSV RNPs has been superseded by evidence that ongoing synthesis of both N and P proteins, complexed in a 1:1 molar ratio, is far more efficient for supporting viral replication *in vitro* (152). The basis for this requirement was initially explained by a widely accepted model for negative-stranded virus replication, which also accounted for the switch from transcription to replication. In this model, encapsidation of leader RNA by newly synthesized N protein (22) causes an antitermination event that signals the polymerase to begin processive RNA synthesis such that the signals for mRNA initiation and termination are ignored (3,21). Therefore, once sufficient quantities of N protein (or more appropriately, N–P complexes) have accumulated, there is a switch from primarily discontinuous mRNA transcription to the synthesis of genome-length, positive-sense replicative intermediates (RI). The RI, like the genome, must also be fully encapsidated to serve as a template for the synthesis of progeny negative-sense genomes. This model is attractive because immediately after virus entry, transcription would be favored over replication. At later times, when the concentration of N protein increases, replication would be favored.

More recently, a modification of this model has been developed that suggests that transcriptase and replicase are two different complexes, each with a unique composition. The two-polymerase model arose from studies using P protein mutants that were defective in transcription but that could support efficient replication of VSV defective interfering (DI) RNAs (39,151). The P protein mutants either had substitutions in the conserved C-terminal basic residues and could bind N protein but did not interact efficiently with L protein (39), or were defective in domain I phosphorylation (151). Because phosphorylation is required for P protein oligomerization, transcriptional activation, and interaction with L protein, the transcriptase would be composed of an L–P3 complex, whereas the replicase would consist of an L–(N–P) complex in which P protein is not phosphorylated. Regulation of P protein phosphorylation and ongoing viral protein synthesis would therefore affect the formation of the two different complexes at different times after infection.

Encapsidation of the genome and antigenome by N protein is intimately tied to and essential for virus replication. Encapsidation occurs as the genomic RNA is synthesized rather than after synthesis is complete, which fits well with the antitermination model described previously for the switch from transcription to replication. It was recognized early that the RNA encapsidation signal must reside in the 5′-terminal sequences of the genome (the trailer region) and the antigenome (the leader) because the leader RNA, the RI, and progeny genomes are the only virus-specific products that are encapsidated (3,21,110). Sequence comparisons between different serotypes of VSV revealed that 14 of the 18 terminal nucleotides of the genome are highly conserved. From this observation, it was postulated that five adenine residues repeated at every third position from the 5′ end of either the genomic or antigenomic RNA are important for the selective encapsidation of these RNAs (21,23). *In vitro* encapsidation reactions using synthetic RNAs containing the 19 terminal nucleotides of VSV and either purified N protein or N protein synthesized *in vitro* (36,141) supports this hypothesis. More recent studies using subgenomic replicons have confirmed that the 5′-

terminal residues of the genome are critical for efficient encapsidation (151); however, it appears that sequences beyond the first 19 nucleotides, yet within the 5′ terminal trailer region, are also important and greatly affect the efficiency of the process (221).

For rabies virus, leader encapsidation may also be regulated by the phosphorylation status of N protein. Unlike the VSV N protein, which is not phosphorylated, rabies N is phosphorylated on serine residues, and the unphosphorylated form of N protein binds more tightly to leader RNA *in vitro* (230).

One of the challenges in understanding rhabdovirus replication is that two distinct events must occur sequentially: first, production of a complete positive RNA strand complementary to the entire parental template, followed by production of complete negative-stranded (progeny) RNAs. There is also a significant asymmetry in the amount of positive-sense RI to negative-sense genome that is made in infected cells. For both rabies and VSV, the genome is about 20- to 50-fold more abundant than the RI. The basis for this asymmetry appears to result solely from the activity of the promoter sequences found at the 3′ end of the genome or RI.

It had long been assumed that sequences at the extreme 3′ end of the genomic and antigenomic RNA were important for polymerase binding and that the complementary sequences found at the 5′ ends were required for encapsidation by N protein. Recently, specific sequences have been identified that play a role in regulating the balance between transcription of mRNAs, which are not encapsidated by N protein, and replication of the genome and antigenome, which are encapsidated. Using deletion analysis and cDNA-derived model subgenomic RNAs based on a naturally occurring defective-interfering virus of VSV, Pattnaik and colleagues have shown that the signals necessary for both replication and encapsidation are present within the 5′-terminal 36 nucleotides and the 3′-terminal 51 nucleotides (149). This result confirms the long-standing hypothesis that the promoter for polymerase binding is contained within the terminal sequences of the genome. A subsequent study further delineated the minimal replication signal as being the 3′-terminal 24 nucleotides of the trailer complement; however, the sequence of the next 20 nucleotides, specifically those found at the 3′ end of the positive-sense RI, serves as a specific enhancer of replication (113). Therefore, sequences at the 3′ end of the antigenome of wild-type VSV provide the basis for differential (enhanced) replication of the genome over the antigenome in infected cells. Similarly, distinct elements in leader region have been identified that are important for transcription but that are not required for replication (221).

In an elegant demonstration of the power of reverse genetics, Finke and Conzelmann constructed an ambisense rabies virus genome that contained identical, transcriptionally active (genomic) promoters at the genomic and antigenomic termini and that transcribed a foreign gene from the antigenomic RNA. Analysis of replication products revealed that the ratio of genome to antigenome was 1:1 in infected cells, indicating that promoter strength was primarily responsible for maintaining the balance of genome to RI. This study also showed that packaging of rabies genomic or antigenomic RNPs into virions is random and depends only on the ratio of the RNPs in infected cells. For wild-type rabies virus, genomic and RI RNPs were present in cells at a ratio of 49:1 and were incorporated into virions at the same ratio. In contrast, the ambisense mutant genomic and antigenomic RNAs were packaged equally into virions.

Although the ratio of genome to antigenome is primarily affected by sequence-specific elements in the antigenomic promoter, there is evidence that other factors may also contribute to the replication efficiency of rhabdovirus genomes. For example, it has been suggested that the extent of terminal complementarity can also affect whether the template (in this case, a defective interfering RNA) predominantly directs transcription or replication (218). Thus, replication may also be regulated by interactions between the ends of the genome. These authors suggested that there is communication between the ends of rhabdoviral genomes through base pairing and that this somehow affects replication efficiency (218).

Assembly and Budding

The process of rhabdovirus assembly can be divided into three distinct phases: (a) encapsidation of newly replicated genomic RNA by N protein, (b) simultaneous condensation of the ribonucleocapsid core by M protein and association with the plasma membrane, and (c) particle envelopment and release. The first step, encapsidation, occurs in the cytoplasm and results when nascent genomic RNA associates with newly synthesized N, P, and L proteins to form RNP complexes. These are often referred to as *nucleocapsids* or *RNP cores.* Because RNA encapsidation is required for RNA replication and transcription, this step was described in the preceding section.

After encapsidation, the RNP complex associates with the plasma membrane and condenses into a tightly coiled structure called a *skeleton* before release from the cell. Numerous studies have demonstrated that the matrix protein is responsible for both of these events (10,64,93, 121,122,136). Thus, M protein plays a critical role in virus assembly and budding. Most of our understanding of RNP condensation is derived from *in vitro* studies in which RNP cores are isolated from detergent solubilized virions in high salt buffers, which results in the release of M protein in a process somewhat analogous to virus uncoating after membrane fusion. RNPs isolated under these conditions appear as loosely coiled, extended filaments and are transcriptionally active. The process can be reversed by the addition of purified M protein to the extended RNP cores in low ionic strength buffers, which results in RNP condensation and the formation of skeleton-like structures similar to those seen within virions (142). The addition of M protein to RNPs also inhibits VSV transcription *in vitro* (29); therefore, the reversible nature of RNP condensation by M protein is thought to be critical for virus infectivity (121).

Condensation of RNP cores provides an explanation for the inhibitory activity of M protein, but it also poses a dilemma. How can viral transcription levels remain high when the cytoplasm of infected cells contain high concentrations of RNP cores and M protein? One explanation is that RNP condensation does not occur until the RNP cores associate with the inner leaflet of the plasma membrane just before budding (131,147); therefore, RNP condensation is a highly regulated process. The demonstration that 10% to 20% of M protein associates with the inner leaflet of the plasma membrane (30) and that the membrane-associated fraction can bind nucleocapsids partially stripped of M protein (31) provided an explanation for the regulated assembly of RNPs at the cell surface. However, recent evidence suggests that an additional priming event is needed because neither cytoplasmic nor membrane-associated M protein can bind to RNPs that are completely free of residual M protein (51). The priming event may involve the formation of specific M protein complexes (63) or may require modification of the RNP core by host factors (51). The topology of M protein with respect to the RNP core during RNP condensation has been a topic of debate and was discussed previously.

After RNP condensation, rhabdovirus particles are released from infected cells by budding from the cell surface. During budding, the condensed core becomes enclosed within a membrane envelope that, for VSV, has about 1,200 molecules of virally encoded G protein and smaller amounts of normal cellular membrane proteins. Early models of rhabdovirus assembly postulated that the incorporation of G protein into virions results from specific interactions between the cytoplasmic tail of G protein and components of the condensed RNP core (139,193). Evidence supporting this model came from studies showing that G proteins with truncated cytoplasmic tails were not efficiently incorporated into virions (223) and that the addition of the G tail was necessary for the incorporation of heterologous viral glycoproteins into virus particles (133,148). G protein, however, is not needed for VSV or rabies budding, although it greatly enhances budding efficiency (96, 134,185,205). Cells infected with recombinant viruses recovered from plasmids in which the G gene was deleted produced noninfectious particles with the characteristic bullet-shaped morphology of rhabdoviruses. Therefore, interactions between G protein and the condensed RNP core are not required to initiate the budding process, although they enhance its efficiency 10- to 30-fold.

Studies to define a role of the G protein cytoplasmic tail in virus assembly have revealed that rabies virus and VSV have distinct requirements. Except in one case in which the cytoplasmic tail of a heterologous protein contained a sequence that greatly reduced incorporation of the glycoprotein into VSV particles (87,148), appending the cytoplasmic tail of VSV G protein to heterologous proteins does not increase virus budding or glycoprotein incorporation (90,168,182). Similarly, the recovery of infectious VSV containing G proteins with truncated cytoplasmic tails or chimeric G proteins with foreign cytoplasmic sequences indicated that a short cytoplasmic domain is important for efficient virus budding but that the specific amino acid sequence in that domain was not important (181). In contrast, the assembly of foreign glycoproteins into rabies virus appears highly dependent on the rabies G cytoplasmic tail (132,133), although infectious rabies virus can be recovered when the entire cytoplasmic domain is deleted (134). The basis for this difference between rabies virus and VSV is not known, but it may reflect a fundamental difference in the way that the M–RNP core interacts or organizes the G protein spikes in the viral envelope.

In comparison with the role of G protein in virus budding, mutation or deletion of the M gene has a much more drastic effect on virus assembly. Temperature-sensitive M protein mutants of VSV produce very low levels of spherical or pleomorphic-shaped particles at the restrictive temperature (122). Similarly, a recombinant rabies virus lacking the M gene produces about 10^5 fewer particles than the wild-type virus, and these particles have a filamentous morphology (136). Complementation with the wild-type M protein expressed from plasmids increases virus budding (136) and converts both the VSV and rabies M mutants to the typical bullet-shaped morphology of rhabdoviruses (122,136). The observation that transient expression of M protein, in the absence of other viral proteins, causes membrane evagination and the release of small membrane-enclosed vesicles (89) supports the idea that M protein has an intrinsic budding activity. Such an activity is reminiscent of the ability of retrovirus Gag proteins, when expressed alone, to produce virus-like particles, and it has been proposed that rhabdovirus M proteins and retrovirus MA proteins may be structurally and functionally similar (107). The recent demonstration that a highly conserved motif (PPxY) in the N-terminus of rhabdovirus M proteins can functionally substitute for the late-domain (L domain) of an avian retrovirus gag protein provides support for this hypothesis (35). Point mutations in the PPxY motif of VSV M protein do not affect membrane localization but significantly reduce both M-dependent vesicle budding (71) as well as the amount of virus released from infected cells (86). Retrovirus L domains function in the last step of virus budding, namely membrane fission and virus release (227). Therefore, the PPxY motif in rhabdovirus M proteins may also be involved in virus release but not RNP condensation or the initiation of virus budding. Thus, high-level virus production results from the concerted action of both the M and G proteins, and only when M protein is absent do rhabdoviruses fail to assemble.

Although far from complete, the available data support a model of assembly in which nucleocapsids bind to regions of the plasma membrane enriched in both M and G proteins. Once nucleocapsids bind to these regions, RNP condensation occurs, and formation of the bud site is initiated. In VSV, specific interactions between the cytoplasmic tail of G protein and the condensed RNP core appear not to be required, although a short cytoplasmic tail of G may insert into a pocket on the condensed core and promote a specific arrangement of G trimers in the viral membrane (181).

VSV buds preferentially from the basolateral surface of polarized epithelial cells (25), a property that is likely important in systemic spread of the virus in infected animals. The sorting of VSV G protein to the basolateral domain of polarized cells independent of other VSV proteins (65,199) and the presence of a dominant basolateral sorting signal in VSV G (210) could explain the preferential polarized release of VSV from the basolateral surface. There is also evidence for independent polarized sorting of M protein to the basolateral membrane (15), but signals in M protein involved in the sorting have not yet been identified.

Because specific sequences in the transmembrane and cytoplasmic domains of VSV G are not required for efficient budding, it seemed likely that G protein sequences important for driving efficient budding would reside in the ectodomain. The recent identification of a "budding domain" in the membrane-proximal region of the G ectodomain provides support for this hypothesis (168). The mechanism by which this domain acts to enhance budding is not understood. It could act to promote association of large arrays of G protein, which would induce membrane curvature at the bud site, or it could have more indirect effects on modifying the local lipid environment to promote interactions with areas of the membrane containing M–RNP complexes. The final step in virus budding requires a membrane fission event that results in release of the virus from the host cell. Little is known about how this occurs, but it has been suggested that the PPxY motif in M protein facilitates virus release through the recruitment of host factors that contain WW domains (35,71).

The use of reverse genetic systems has greatly advanced our understanding of protein domains involved in rhabdovirus assembly, but there are still many questions that remain unanswered. For example, little is known about the contribution that host factors play in virus assembly and release. A complete understanding of the roles of individual viral proteins and of potential host factors involved in virus budding will likely require detailed structural information on the individual components as well as sophisticated biochemical assays to measure directly protein–protein and protein–lipid interactions.

Production of Defective Interfering Particles

As with many other viruses, passage of rhabdoviruses in tissue culture leads to accumulation of defective interfering viruses called DI particles. These particles have a normal VSV protein composition but have truncated RNA genomes lacking some or all of the viral structural protein genes and therefore they can only propagate in cells co-infected with parental virus. The DI particles out-replicate parental virus and rapidly accumulate to higher levels than parental virus during passage at high multiplicity. Elimination of DI particles from virus cultures can be accomplished by low-multiplicity infection and repetitive isolation of virus from single plaques. DI particles can also be separated from the parental virus based on velocity of sedimentation on sucrose gradients. Perrault (153) has provided an excellent review of the DI particle structure and formation.

Typical types of VSV DI particles are illustrated in Figure 6. The most common type of DI particle contains RNAs with complementary terminal sequences that rapidly self-anneal to form short stems or longer snap-back structures after the template-associated N protein is removed. These DIs lack the 3′ leader sequence (Le) used to initiate transcription of the viral genes and replication of the antigenomic RNA. These DIs have a strong replicative advantage over standard genomes. Because of the self-complementary nature of the DI genome ends, replication of either strand initiates on the complement of the 5′ trailer sequence (Tr′). This is the same sequence that serves as the promoter for synthesis of VSV genomic RNA and is a stronger promoter than the 3′ leader sequence (Le), which initiates synthesis of antigenomic RNA. This difference in relative promoter strengths discussed in the preceding section on genome replication would explain the excess synthesis of genomic RNA relative to antigenomic RNA in infected cells. DI RNAs that retain both ends of standard genome at their termini are less common and do not compete as well against the standard genome, probably because they, like the standard genome, are involved in transcription as well as replication and do not have as strong a promoter for their positive-stranded RNA replication.

Generation of DI RNA molecules from a standard virus is believed to occur after a viral polymerase with

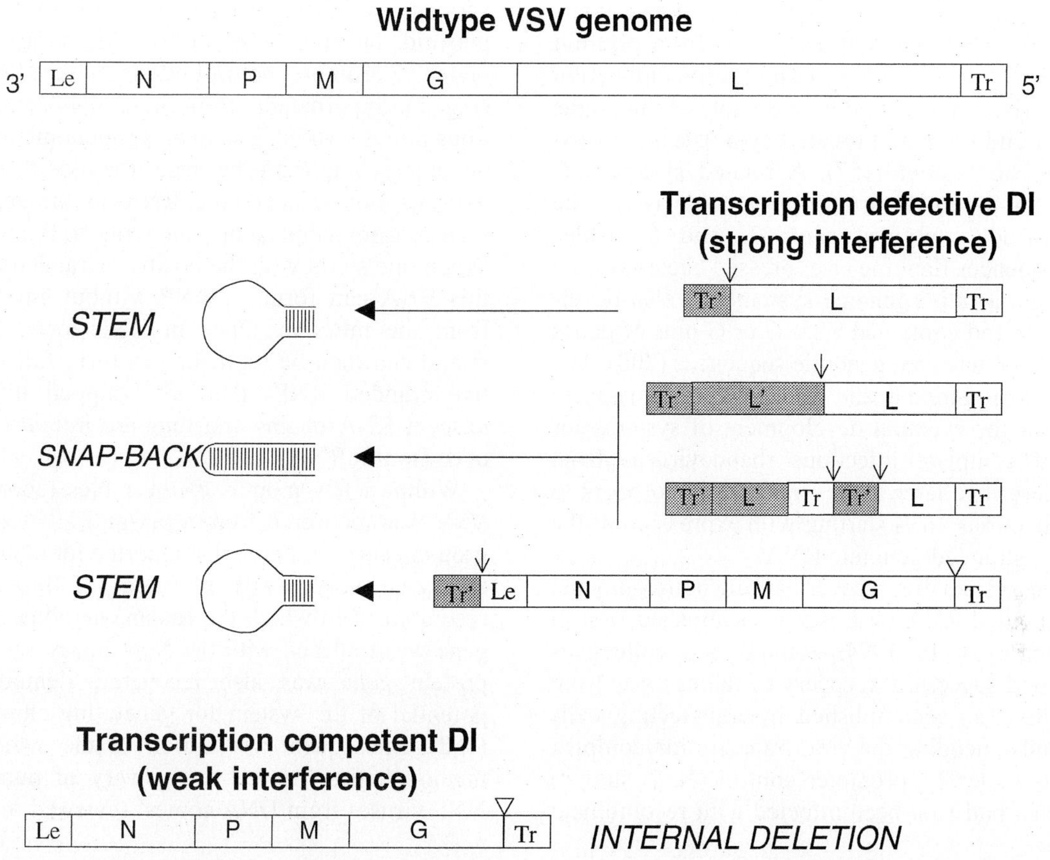

FIG. 6. Schematic representation of different classes of rhabdovirus DI particles. (Courtesy of Dr. J. Perrault, San Diego State University.)

its attached nascent RNA chain dissociates from its template and resumes synthesis at a new site either on its own nascent chain or on a different template molecule (153). Generation of the first two types of DIs illustrated in Figure 6 could occur by a single switch (*arrow* indicates switch site) of the polymerase to copy its own nascent chain. Other, more complex types of DIs can result from multiple polymerase switches, including switches to downstream sites on a template to generate internal deletions (*triangles* in Fig. 6). Multiple switch events are possible, and DIs with more extensive genome rearrangements have been reported (146,176).

MOLECULAR GENETICS OF RHABDOVIRUSES

The ability to perform precise molecular genetic analysis of rhabdoviruses required the development of systems for recovering infectious viruses from DNA copies. Recovery of rhabdoviruses and other nonsegmented negative-stranded RNA viruses (NNS viruses) from DNA presented a unique problem because neither their genomic nor their antigenomic RNAs serve as mRNAs, and neither can be used directly to recover infectious virus. This contrasts with the positive-stranded RNA viruses in which the genomic RNA transcribed from DNA can be used to initiate infection. The minimal infectious unit for the NNS RNA viruses is the genomic RNA complexed with nucleocapsid and RNA polymerase proteins in a RNP complex. Because the NNS RNA viruses have genomes that are quite large (11 to 18 kb), it has not been possible to assemble their RNAs into infectious RNPs *in vitro,* an approach that did work earlier to introduce individual RNA segments into influenza virus (118).

Recovery of Infectious Rabies and Vesicular Stomatitis Virus from Plasmid DNA

Before the recovery of complete, infectious negative-stranded RNA viruses from DNA, several laboratories developed systems that allowed replication of small, defective negative-stranded RNA genomes or RNA mini-genomes that were derived from DNA copies. The RNA mini-genome constructs contained one or more genes flanked by short 3′ and 5′ sequences derived from the natural virus genome and containing the signals required for replication (reviewed in reference 167). The first such system for VSV employed a defective interfering particle RNA that was expressed from plasmid DNA (150). The VSV proteins required for replication of this RNA (N, P, and L) and for assembly of infectious particles (M and G) were provided by a vaccinia virus-based expression system (57). A related system was developed for a rabies virus mini-genome (34). The rabies construct contained short 3′ and 5′ rabies genomic sequences flanking an expressed bacterial gene (*CAT*). A similar mini-genome system was also developed for VSV and contained VSV *G* or *G* plus *M* genes flanked by VSV terminal genomic sequences (200). The replicating mini-genome and DI RNA systems were important for the eventual development of systems for recovery of complete infectious rhabdoviruses from DNA. As described later, however, they did not work to generate infectious virus starting with expression of the the negative-stranded genomic RNA.

The basic system for recovery of all nonsegmented negative-stranded RNA viruses was established first in the rhabdoviruses. In 1994, Schnell and colleagues (186) reported successful recovery of rabies virus from cDNAs. This was accomplished by transfecting cells with plasmids encoding the viral transcription complex components under T7 promoter control (N, L, and P) into cells that had first been infected with recombinant vaccinia expressing T7 polymerase (57). In addition, a plasmid encoding the full-length viral antigenome under T7 promoter control was transfected into the cells (Fig. 7). Supernatants from these cells contained infectious rabies viruses. Use of an antigenome instead of the genome is important because it avoids the problem of hybridization of genomic RNA to the mRNAs transcribed from the plasmids encoding N, P, and L proteins. When one starts with the positive-stranded antigenome, this RNA can form an RNP without any interference from the mRNAs. Once in RNP form, the positive strand can then be replicated to form full-length negative-stranded RNPs that are wrapped into RNPs as nascent RNA chains and thus are immune to interference from mRNAs.

Within a few months of the rabies report, infectious VSV was recovered from a plasmid DNA copy using a protocol very similar to that reported for rabies (102), and this was subsequently repeated (220). An infectious recombinant in which the Indiana serotype glycoprotein gene was replaced with the New Jersey serotype glycoprotein gene was also recovered, demonstrating the potential of the system for generating chimeric viruses (102). Subsequent application of the same or similar methodologies has led to recovery of numerous other NNS viruses from DNA copies (reviewed in 167).

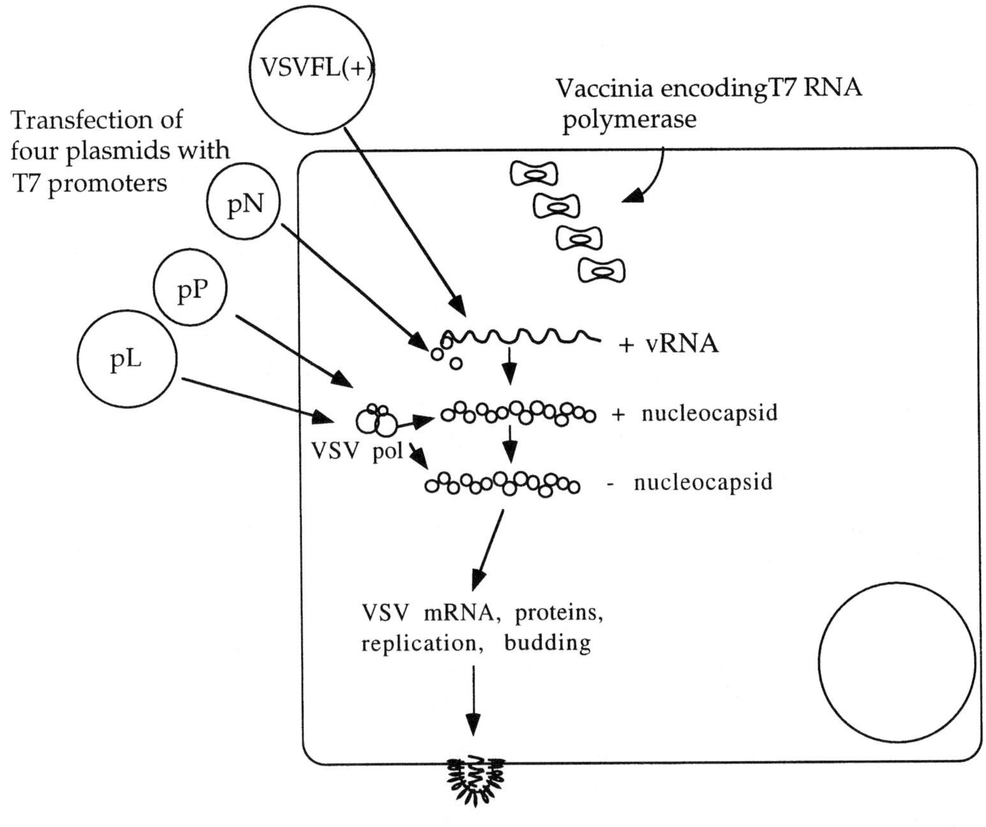

FIG. 7. Diagram of the system for recovery of rhabdoviruses from plasmid DNA.

Rhabdoviruses as Gene Expression, Vaccine, and Targeting Vectors

As described previously, the reverse genetic systems for rhabdoviruses have been crucial to dissecting numerous aspects of virus replication and assembly. Additional foreign genes can be introduced into recombinant rhabdoviruses, and foreign gene expression is generally stable (135,183). In VSV vectors, the expressed proteins can represent as much as 5% of the total cell protein 7 hours after infection (167,183).

The potential of recombinant VSVs as vaccine vectors was shown in a study in which a VSV recombinant expressing an influenza hemagglutinin gene was used in mice. A single intranasal inoculation with as little as 10 plaque-forming units induces a potent and protective immune response to influenza (166). VSV vectors have also been attenuated through mutations in the cytoplasmic tail of VSV G protein such that there is little or no pathogenesis even in 6-week-old mice (165), yet strong and protective immune responses are still generated. Ongoing studies of VSV vectors in rhesus macaques indicate a lack of pathogenesis and induction of strong cellular and humoral immune responses to encoded HIV envelope protein (J. Rose and colleagues, unpublished observations). These studies indicate that VSV may have potential as a vaccine vector in humans.

Other studies have illustrated the potential of recombinant VSVs as targeting vectors. A recombinant virus lacking its glycoprotein gene but encoding instead the human immunodeficiency virus (HIV) receptor and coreceptor was shown to incorporate both foreign glycoproteins into its coat. Furthermore, this virus could specifically target, infect, and kill HIV-infected cells *in vitro* (185). Related studies performed with rabies virus pseudotypes also suggested the potential of rabies as a targeting vector (133).

The potential of rhabdovirus recombinants as surrogate viruses for viruses that are dangerous or impossible to grow was illustrated by a recent study in which the VSV glycoprotein gene was replaced with an HIV envelope gene. In addition, a gene encoding green fluorescent protein was included (24). This virus infects cells using the HIV receptor and coreceptor and can be used as a fast and convenient assay for HIV neutralization. In another strategy, investigators have used a virus lacking G protein but encoding green fluorescent protein (GFP) to generate pseudotyped virus containing the envelope glycoprotein of Ebola virus. The pseudotypes allowed the identification of cell surface determinants important for Ebola virus infection (205) and resulted in the identification of a putative fusion domain in the Ebola glycoprotein (82) without the need to work under BSL-4 containment conditions. The promiscuous nature of VSV assembly that allows for extensive incorporation of foreign proteins into the envelope suggests that numerous similar applications are possible.

Given the extensive progress with reverse genetics of rhabdoviruses made recently, we can expect to see many new applications of this exciting technology in the years to come.

MOLECULAR BASIS OF PATHOGENESIS

General Aspects

Despite the similarities in structure between the lyssaviruses and vesiculoviruses, the former generally cause a relatively slow and progressive disease, and the latter cause acute disease that is eliminated rapidly by host immune responses. The pathogenesis of rabies virus is addressed in a subsequent chapter, and the veterinary aspects of vesiculovirus pathogenesis have been thoroughly and recently reviewed (112).

The basis for VSV pathogenesis appears intimately tied to the replication potential of the virus. For example, a mutation truncating the VSV G cytoplasmic domain from 29 amino acids to 9 amino acids reduces the virus yield only two-fold in tissue culture (181) but nearly eliminates pathogenesis in a mouse model (165). Complete elimination of the cytoplasmic domain reduces the virus yields about 10-fold (181) and completely eliminates pathogenesis in the mouse model while still allowing replication sufficient to induce strong immune responses (165). Similar results have been obtained using rearranged VSV genomes in which reduction in virus yield in culture correlates with reduced pathogenesis in animals (217). Rapid production of new virions is probably crucial to virus spread before immune responses result in virus clearance. In an infected animal, in which virus replication is likely an exponential process initially, even two-fold differences in final virus yield per cell in tissue culture are rapidly amplified to much greater differences in virus load in an animal.

Almost all vertebrate cells tested and many invertebrate cells are susceptible to VSV infection. The replication of VSV can vary widely in different cell types, and infectious virus yields also vary, but little is known of the molecular basis for this variation. For example, VSV yields in baby hamster kidney cells (BHK-21) are about 100,000 particles per cell, of which about 10% can be infectious. Optimal VSV titers obtained in BHK cells range from 10^9 to 10^{10} per milliliter of medium. In contrast, VSV yields in HeLa cells are typically less than 5% of those obtained in BHK cells. The human lymphoblastoid cell line Raji is infected by VSV, but the viral RNA synthesis is low, and the VSV particles produced have an abnormal protein composition with only low levels of matrix protein (145,219). Rabbit corneal cells are infected by VSV but produce less than one infectious particle per cell. Co-infection with vaccinia virus reverses the block to VSV replication through an unknown mechanism (208). In *Drosophila* melanogaster cells, VSV establishes a persistent, noncytopathic infection, and virus titers are low (229). This may be due in part to a deficiency of VSV G protein in the viral particles that are produced (229).

At high multiplicities of infection in BHK cells, VSV cytopathic effects (cell rounding) can be evident 1 to 2 hours after infection. At lower multiplicity, the cytopathic effects may not be evident for 4 to 5 hours in BHK cells. In other cell types in which VSV replication is less robust, cytopathic effects often require longer to become evident.

The cell rounding effects of VSV appear to be due largely to expression of the VSV M protein. M protein expression alone in cells causes rounding and detachment by rapidly depolymerizing actin as well as tubulin and vimentin. This causes the breakdown of stress fibers, microtubules, and intermediate filaments (20,120,137, 231). The VSV glycoprotein is also toxic to cells when expressed in large quantities, although stable cell lines can be made constitutively expressing low levels of G protein (53,158). The mechanism of toxicity of VSV G protein is not known, but it may involve a low level of membrane fusion activity even at neutral pH.

Inhibition of Cellular Protein Synthesis

VSV infection results in substantial inhibition of cellular protein synthesis within 3 to 4 hours after infection when the VSV proteins are the major proteins synthesized by the infected cells. When total poly(A)-positive mRNAs are purified from infected cells and translated *in vitro* in reticulocyte lysates, the mRNAs encode predominantly the VSV proteins, suggesting a major change in the ratio of viral mRNAs to host mRNAs in the infected cells (95). Lodish and Porter (117) carried out a study that suggested a competition mechanism for the inhibition of cellular mRNA translation. They found that the total amount of translatable mRNA in cells increased about three-fold after infection owing to substantial viral mRNA synthesis, and they suggested that inhibition of cellular protein synthesis could be explained at least in part by competition for ribosomes by the large excess of viral mRNAs. Based on analysis of polysome size, the efficiency of initiation of translation on cellular and viral mRNAs was found to be about the same in infected cells, but cellular ribosomes were distributed among more mRNAs after infection (117). A subsequent study (187) challenged this purely passive shutoff mechanism because severe limitation of VSV transcription did not substantially reduce the inhibition of host mRNA translation. However, a specific mechanism that discriminates between cellular mRNAs and viral mRNAs has not been identified. The fact that host mRNAs expressed from VSV recombinants are translated with efficiencies similar to viral mRNAs (98,182,183) suggests a lack of discrimination based on mRNA sequence alone, unless the selective specificity is present solely within the minimal 5′- or 3′-terminal nucleotides required on each mRNA as part of the VSV transcription initiation or termination signals.

Inhibition of Cellular Transcription, mRNA Transport, and DNA Synthesis

VSV infection results in inhibition of host cell mRNA synthesis and expression, and even a low level of the VSV matrix protein is sufficient for this inhibition (19). The mechanism of inhibition appears to result at least in part from inactivation of the transcription factor TFIID (233). In addition to having direct effects on host transcription, the VSV matrix protein blocks transport of mRNAs from the nucleus (73). This study showed that M protein interferes with transport that is dependent on the nuclear guanosine triphosphatase Ran-TC4 and its associated factors.

Other studies suggested a role for the VSV leader RNA in inhibition of RNA synthesis. VSV transcription is known to be required for inhibition of cellular RNA synthesis (216). Because the VSV leader RNA is transcribed first from the VSV genome, its transcription is most resistant to inactivation by UV light. Virions exposed to high doses of UV are still able to synthesize leader RNA and inhibit cellular mRNA synthesis (66), suggesting a role of the leader in this inhibition. *In vitro* transcription experiments using oligodeoxynucleotides having sequences homologous to leader RNA also supported a role for the leader in inhibition of transcription (67). However, other experiments showing a requirement for protein synthesis in inhibition of host RNA synthesis are not consistent with leader RNA alone being responsible for the inhibition of host RNA synthesis (156). The interpretation of the UV inactivation experiments was questioned by Whitaker-Dowling and Youngner (222), who showed that the doses of UV used to implicate leader RNA were sufficient to cause direct damage (cleavage) of VSV virion proteins.

The same types of UV inactivation experiments that implicated leader in inhibition of RNA synthesis also implicated leader in inhibition of cellular DNA synthesis. The mechanism of the inhibition is not known, but studies performed in an *in vitro* system for adenovirus replication showed that oligodeoxynucleotides corresponding in sequence to the VSV leader RNA could inhibit adenovirus DNA replication (162). The VSV leader is know to be rapidly transported into the cell nucleus after infection (101), a property consistent with a role in inhibition of both DNA replication and DNA-dependent transcription.

IMMUNE RESPONSES

There has been relatively little research on immunity to VSV in natural host animals, such as cattle, in which the virus infects epithelial cells and causes vesicular lesions.

The virus is cleared effectively by the immune system, but the types of immune responses required for clearance have not been studied in the natural hosts. Interestingly, the immunity to VSV after natural infection in cattle is not long-lived, and the same strain of VSV appears to be able to infect cattle in subsequent years, despite the presence of extremely high serum neutralizing antibody titers to the infecting strain (213). The mechanism of reinfection does not involve genetic drift in the virus glycoprotein as the sequence is unchanged in the reinfecting virus. There is also evidence that some VSV genomic RNA but not mRNA sequences can persist in experimentally infected cows after infectious virus has been cleared, but the mechanism of this persistence is not known (111).

Most studies of immunity to VSV have been performed in more tractable mouse systems, and the pathogenesis in laboratory mice is quite different from that in the natural host animals. When inoculated intranasally in some mouse strains, such as Balb/c or C57BL/6, VSV can infect the brain and cause a lethal encephalitis (78,161). VSV has also been found to replicate in the lungs of Balb/c mice after intranasal inoculation (165, 166). Other routes of infection in mice, such as the intraperitioneal route, can induce immunity to VSV without significant pathogenesis, even when high titers of virus are inoculated. High and protective levels of antibodies to VSV persist in mice and diminish only two- to four-fold even 2 years after infection (165).

Role of Interferons

In VSV infection, as in infection with many other pathogens, interferons (IFNs) provide a critical front line of defense. Although VSV isolates differ in their ability to induce IFN (128), VSV replication is extremely sensitive to IFN action. The IFN response in mice slows the spread of VSV infection until an antibody response can completely control the infection. The importance of the IFN response was shown in IFN-α- and IFN-β-receptor–deficient mice (198). Infection of these mice results in rapid, disseminated VSV replication in multiple organs, and the mice die within a few days. Other studies with mice deficient in the JAK-STAT IFN signaling pathway have also revealed extreme sensitivity to VSV infection (138).

Roles of Antibody and Cytotoxic T Cells

The relative importance of antibody and cytotoxic T cells in immunity to viral infection varies depending on the virus and host in question. Antibody is a crucial component of immunity to VSV in mice. All neutralizing antibodies to VSV recognize the single exposed transmembrane glycoprotein G (94). Studies in IFN-receptor–deficient mice showed that passively transferred antibody to VSV G protected these mice efficiently against systemic infection (198). In contrast, passively transferred VSV-specific T cells were unable to protect these mice. The relative unimportance of T cells in immunity to VSV has also been shown in experiments involving mice lacking CD8+ T cells. These mice are as resistant to VSV as control mice with normal levels of CD8+ cells T cells (58). However, T-cell responses, although insufficient on their own, can protect from VSV-induced disease in an immunocompetent mouse. This was shown in experiments in which a T-cell response to purified VSV nucleocapsid protein protected mice from a normally lethal VSV infection (4).

Neutralization

Infection of mice by VSV induces a rapid production of neutralizing immunoglobulin M (IgM) antibody, which occurs independently of T-cell help, followed by appearance of neutralizing IgG antibodies that are dependent on T-cell help for their production (106). The ability of VSV to induce IgM independent of T-cell help appears to be related to the presence of G protein in a dense array on the viral surface (5).

The molecular requirements for antibody-mediated neutralization of VSV *in vitro* and protection against lethal disease *in vivo* have been studied in detail using a monovalent single-chain antibody and antibody fragments generated from VSV-neutralizing antibodies (91, 103,104). These experiments demonstrate that neutralization of VSV and protection against disease do not require Fc-mediated mechanisms and that antibody cross-linking is not crucial for protection. Although the mechanism by which antibodies neutralize VSV has not been studied, it probably requires antibody physically shielding most VSV G spikes on the virion and thereby blocking attachment and fusion. This is likely because in rabies virus neutralization, the number of antibody molecules required for complete neutralization of a virion is at least half the number of viral glycoprotein spikes (50). Multiple epitopes binding neutralizing monoclonal antibodies have been described for the G proteins from the Indiana and New Jersey serotypes of VSV (26,105,215)

T-Cell Epitopes

Early studies in mice revealed that epitopes in both the VSV N and G proteins are recognized by cytotoxic T cells (157,232). The VSV Indiana nucleocapsid protein contains an immunodominant H-2 Kb epitope binding class I major histocompatibility complex in C57BL/6 (B6) mice. This peptide, N52-59 (RGYVYQGL), was among the first viral cytotoxic T-lymphocyte epitopes to be identified and sequenced (191). Subsequent studies have shown class II major histocompatibility complex restricted epitopes recognized by cytolytic T cells in Balb/c mice (27). The helper T-cell epitopes in the G protein have been analyzed with a complete panel of overlapping synthetic peptides. Three different helper T-cell epitopes in C57BL/6 mice and two in BALB/c mice were defined in VSV G (Indiana) (28).

REFERENCES

1. Abraham G, Banerjee AK. Sequential transcription of the genes of vesicular stomatitis virus. *Proc Natl Acad Sci U S A* 1976;73: 1504–1508.
2. Abraham G, Rhodes DP, Banerjee AK. The 5′ terminal structure of the methylated mRNA synthesized in vitro by vesicular stomatitis virus. *Cell* 1975;5:51–58.
3. Arnheiter H, Davis NL, Wertz G, et al. Role of the nucleocapsid protein in regulating vesicular stomatitis virus RNA synthesis. *Cell* 1985; 41:259–267.
4. Bachmann MF, Hengartner H, Zinkernagel RM. Immunization with recombinant protein: Conditions for cytotoxic T cell and/or antibody induction. *Med Microbiol Immunol* (Berl) 1994;183:315–324.
5. Bachmann MF, Hengartner H, Zinkernagel RM. T helper cell-independent neutralizing B cell response against vesicular stomatitis virus: Role of antigen patterns in B cell induction? *Eur J Immunol* 1995;25: 3445–3451.
6. Ball LA, Pringle CR, Flanagan B, et al. Phenotypic consequences of rearranging the P, M, and G genes of vesicular stomatitis virus. *J Virol* 1999;73:4705–4712.
7. Ball LA, White CN. Order of transcription of genes of vesicular stomatitis virus. *Proc Natl Acad Sci U S A* 1976;73:442–446.
8. Baltimore D, Huang AS, Stampfer M. Ribonucleic acid synthesis of vesicular stomatitis virus, II. An RNA polymerase in the virion. *Proc Natl Acad Sci U S A* 1970;66:572–576.
9. Barge A, Gagnon J, Chaffotte A, et al. Rod-like shape of vesicular stomatitis virus matrix protein. *Virology* 1996;219:465–470.
10. Barge A, Gaudin Y, Coulon P, Ruigrok RW. Vesicular stomatitis virus M protein may be inside the ribonucleocapsid coil. *J Virol* 1993;67: 7246–7253.
11. Barik S, Banerjee AK. Cloning and expression of the vesicular stomatitis virus phosphoprotein gene in Escherichia coli: Analysis of phosphorylation status versus transcriptional activity. *J Virol* 1991;65: 1719–1726.
12. Barik S, Banerjee AK. Phosphorylation by cellular casein kinase II is essential for transcriptional activity of vesicular stomatitis virus phosphoprotein P. *Proc Natl Acad Sci U S A* 1992;89:6570–6574.
13. Barr JN, Whelan SP, Wertz GW. cis-Acting signals involved in termination of vesicular stomatitis virus mRNA synthesis include the conserved AUAC and the U7 signal for polyadenylation. *J Virol* 1997;71: 8718–8725.
14. Barr JN, Whelan SP, Wertz GW. Role of the intergenic dinucleotide in vesicular stomatitis virus RNA transcription. *J Virol* 1997;71:1794–1801.
15. Bergmann JE, Fusco PJ. The M protein of vesicular stomatitis virus associates specifically with the basolateral membranes of polarized epithelial cells independently of the G protein. *J Cell Biol* 1988;107: 1707–1715.
16. Bergmann JE, Tokuyasu KT, Singer SJ. Passage of an integral membrane protein, the vesicular stomatitis virus glycoprotein, through the Golgi apparatus en route to the plasma membrane. *Proc Natl Acad Sci U S A* 1981;78:1746–1750.
17. Bilsel PA, Nichol ST. Polymerase errors accumulating during natural evolution of the glycoprotein gene of vesicular stomatitis virus Indiana serotype isolates. *J Virol* 1990;64:4873–4883.
18. Bilsel PA, Rowe JE, Fitch WM, Nichol ST. Phosphoprotein and nucleocapsid protein evolution of vesicular stomatitis virus New Jersey. *J Virol* 1990;64:2498–2504.
19. Black BL, Lyles DS. Vesicular stomatitis virus matrix protein inhibits host cell-directed transcription of target genes in vivo. *J Virol* 1992; 66:4058–4064.
20. Blondel D, Harmison GG, Schubert M. Role of matrix protein in cytopathogenesis of vesicular stomatitis virus. *J Virol* 1990;64: 1716–1725.
21. Blumberg BM, Giorgi C, Kolakofsky D. N protein of vesicular stomatitis virus selectively encapsidates leader RNA in vitro. *Cell* 1983;32: 559–567.
22. Blumberg BM, Kolakofsky D. An analytical review of defective infections of vesicular stomatitis virus. *J Gen Virol* 1983;64:1839–1847.
23. Blumberg BM, Leppert M, Kolakofsky D. Interaction of VSV leader RNA and nucleocapsid protein may control VSV genome replication. *Cell* 1981;23:837–845.
24. Boritz E, Gerlach J, Johnson JE, Rose JK. Replication-competent rhabdoviruses with human immunodeficiency virus type 1 coats and green fluorescent protein: Entry by a pH-independent pathway. *J Virol* 1999;73:6937–6945.
25. Boulan ER, Sabatini DD. Asymmetric budding of viruses in epithelial monlayers: A model system for study of epithelial polarity. *Proc Natl Acad Sci U S A* 1978;75:5071–5075.
26. Bricker BJ, Snyder RM, Fox JW, et al. Monoclonal antibodies to the glycoprotein of vesicular stomatitis virus (New Jersey serotype): A method for preliminary mapping of epitopes. *Virology* 1987;161:533–540.
27. Browning M, Reiss CS, Huang AS. The soluble viral glycoprotein of vesicular stomatitis virus efficiently sensitizes target cells for lysis by CD4+ T lymphocytes. *J Virol* 1990;64:3810–3816.
28. Burkhart C, Freer G, Castro R, et al. Characterization of T-helper epitopes of the glycoprotein of vesicular stomatitis virus. *J Virol* 1994; 68:1573–1580.
29. Carroll AR, Wagner RR. Role of the membrane (M) protein in endogenous inhibition of in vitro transcription of vesicular stomatitis virus. *J Virol* 1979;29:134–142.
30. Chong LD, Rose JK. Membrane association of functional vesicular stomatitis virus matrix protein in vivo. *J Virol* 1993;67:407–414.
31. Chong LD, Rose JK. Interactions of normal and mutant vesicular stomatitis virus matrix proteins with the plasma membrane and nucleocapsids. *J Virol* 1994;68:441–447.
32. Chuang JL, Perrault J. Initiation of vesicular stomatitis virus mutant polR1 transcription internally at the N gene in vitro. *J Virol* 1997; 71:1466–1475.
33. Clinton GM, Burge BW, Huang AS. Effects of phosphorylation and pH on the association of NS protein with vesicular stomatitis virus cores. *J Virol* 1978;27:340–346.
34. Conzelmann KK, Schnell M. Rescue of synthetic genomic RNA analogs of rabies virus by plasmid-encoded proteins. *J Virol* 1994;68: 713–719.
35. Craven RC, Harty RN, Paragas J, et al. Late domain function identified in the vesicular stomatitis virus M protein by use of rhabdovirus-retrovirus chimeras. *J Virol* 1999;73:3359–3365.
36. Das T, Banerjee AK. Role of the phosphoprotein (P) in the encapsidation of presynthesized and de novo synthesized vesicular stomatitis virus RNA by the nucleocapsid protein N in vitro. *Cell Mol Biol* 1992; 38:17–26.
37. Das T, Chakrabarti BK, Chattopadhyay D, Banerjee AK. Carboxy-terminal five amino acids of the nucleocapsid protein of vesicular stomatitis virus are required for encapsidation and replication of genome RNA. *Virology* 1999;259:219–227.
38. Das T, Mathur M, Gupta AK, et al. RNA polymerase of vesicular stomatitis virus specifically associates with translation elongation factor-1 alphabetagamma for its activity. *Proc Natl Acad Sci U S A* 1998; 95:1449–1454.
39. Das T, Pattnaik AK, Takacs AM, et al. Basic amino acid residues at the carboxy-terminal eleven amino acid region of the phosphoprotein (P) are required for transcription but not for replication of vesicular stomatitis virus genome RNA. *Virology* 1997;238:103–114.
40. Davis NL, Arnheiter H, Wertz GW. Vesicular stomatitis virus N and NS proteins form multiple complexes. *J Virol* 1986;59:751–754.
41. Davis NL, Wertz GW. Synthesis of vesicular stomatitis virus negative-strand RNA in vitro: Dependence on viral protein synthesis. *J Virol* 1982;41:821–832.
42. Doms RW, Keller DS, Helenius A, Balch WE. Role for adenosine triphosphate in regulating the assembly and transport of vesicular stomatitis virus G protein trimers. *J Cell Biol* 1987;105:1957–1969.
43. Doms RW, Lamb RA, Rose JK, Helenius A. Folding and assembly of viral membrane proteins. *Virology* 1993;193:545–562.
44. Doms RW, Ruusala A, Machamer C, et al. Differential effects of mutations in three domains on folding, quaternary structure, and intracellular transport of vesicular stomatitis virus G protein. *J Cell Biol* 1988;107:89–99.
45. Durrer P, Gaudin Y, Ruigrok RW, et al. Photolabeling identifies a putative fusion domain in the envelope glycoprotein of rabies and vesicular stomatitis viruses. *J Biol Chem* 1995;270:17575–17581.

46. Emerson SU. Reconstitution studies detect a single polymerase entry site on the vesicular stomatitis virus genome. *Cell* 1982;31:635–642.
47. Emerson SU, Yu Y. Both NS and L proteins are required for in vitro RNA synthesis by vesicular stomatitis virus. *J Virol* 1975;15:1348–1356.
48. Estepa A, Coll JM. Pepscan mapping and fusion-related properties of the major phosphatidylserine-binding domain of the glycoprotein of viral hemorrhagic septicemia virus, a salmonid rhabdovirus. *Virology* 1996;216:60–70.
49. Fields BN, Hawkins K. Human infection with the virus of vesicular stomatitis during an epizootic. *N Engl J Med* 1967;277:989–994.
50. Flamand A, Raux H, Gaudin Y, Ruigrok RW. Mechanisms of rabies virus neutralization. *Virology* 1993;194:302–313.
51. Flood EA, Lyles DS. Assembly of nucleocapsids with cytosolic and membrane-derived matrix proteins of vesicular stomatitis virus. *Virology* 1999;261:295–308.
52. Florkiewicz RZ, Rose JK. A cell line expressing vesicular stomatitis virus glycoprotein fuses at low pH. *Science* 1984;225:721–723.
53. Florkiewicz RZ, Smith A, Bergmann JE, Rose JK. Isolation of stable mouse cell lines that express cell surface and secreted forms of the vesicular stomatitis virus glycoprotein. *J Cell Biol* 1983;97:1381–1388.
54. Fredericksen BL, Whitt MA. Vesicular stomatitis virus glycoprotein mutations that affect membrane fusion activity and abolish virus infectivity. *J Virol* 1995;69:1435–1443.
55. Fredericksen BL, Whitt MA. Mutations at two conserved acidic amino acids in the glycoprotein of vesicular stomatitis virus affect pH-dependent conformational changes and reduce the pH threshold for membrane fusion. *Virology* 1996;217:49–57.
56. Fredericksen BL, Whitt MA. Attenuation of recombinant vesicular stomatitis viruses encoding mutant glycoproteins demonstrate a critical role for maintaining a high pH threshold for membrane fusion in viral fitness. *Virology* 1998;240:349–358.
57. Fuerst TR, Earl PL, Moss B. Use of a hybrid vaccinia virus-T7 RNA polymerase system for expression of target genes. *Mol Cell Biol* 1987; 7:2538–2544.
58. Fung-Leung WP, Schilham MW, Rahemtulla A, et al. CD8 is needed for development of cytotoxic T cells but not helper T cells. *Cell* 1991; 65:443–449.
59. Gallione CJ, Greene JR, Iverson LE, Rose JK. Nucleotide sequences of the mRNA's encoding the vesicular stomatitis virus N and NS proteins. *J Virol* 1981;39:529–535.
60. Gallione CJ, Rose JK. Nucleotide sequence of a cDNA clone encoding the entire glycoprotein from the New Jersey serotype of vesicular stomatitis virus. *J Virol* 1983;46:162–169.
61. Gao Y, Greenfield NJ, Cleverley DZ, Lenard J. The transcriptional form of the phosphoprotein of vesicular stomatitis virus is a trimer: Structure and stability. *Biochemistry* 1996;35:14569–14573.
62. Gastka M, Horvath J, Lentz TL. Rabies virus binding to the nicotinic acetylcholine receptor alpha subunit demonstrated by virus overlay protein binding assay. *J Gen Virol* 1996;77:2437–2440.
63. Gaudin Y, Barge A, Ebel C, Ruigrok RWH. Aggregation of VSV M protein is reversible and mediated by nucleation sites: Implication for viral assembly. *Virology* 1995;206:28–37.
64. Gaudin Y, Tuffereau C, Segretain D, et al. Reversible conformational changes and fusion activity of rabies virus glycoprotein. *J Virol* 1991; 65:4853–4859.
65. Gottlieb TA, Gonzalez A, Rizzolo L, et al. Sorting and endocytosis of viral glycoproteins in transfected polarized epithelial cells. *J Cell Biol* 1986;102:1242–1255.
66. Grinnell BW, Wagner RR. Comparative inhibition of cellular transcription by vesicular stomatitis virus serotypes New Jersey and Indiana: Role of each viral leader RNA. *J Virol* 1983;48:88–101.
67. Grinnell BW, Wagner RR. Nucleotide sequence and secondary structure of VSV leader RNA and homologous DNA involved in inhibition of DNA-dependent transcription. *Cell* 1984;36:533–543.
68. Haglund K, Forman J, Kräusslich H-G, Rose J. Expression of human immunodeficiency virus type 1 Gag protein precursor and envelope proteins from a vesicular stomatitis virus recombinant: High-level production of virus-like particles containing HIV envelope. *Virology* 2000;268:112–121.
69. Hammond C, Helenius A. Folding of VSV G protein: Sequential interaction with BiP and calnexin. *Science* 1994;266:456–458.
70. Hanham CA, Zhao F, Tignor GH. Evidence from the anti-idiotypic network that the acetylcholine receptor is a rabies virus receptor. *J Virol* 1993;67:530–542.
71. Harty RN, Paragas J, Sudol M, Palese P. A proline-rich motif within the matrix protein of vesicular stomatitis virus and rabies virus interacts with WW domains of cellular proteins: Implications for viral budding. *J Virol* 1999;73:2921–2929.
72. Heaton LA, Hillman BI, Hunter BG, et al. Physical map of the genome of sonchus yellow net virus, a plant rhabdovirus with six genes and conserved gene junction sequences. *Proc Natl Acad Sci U S A* 1989;86:8665–8668.
73. Her LS, Lund E, Dahlberg JE. Inhibition of Ran guanosine triphosphatase-dependent nuclear transport by the matrix protein of vesicular stomatitis virus. *Science* 1997;276:1845–1848.
74. Hercyk N, Horikami SM, Moyer SA. The vesicular stomatitis virus L protein possesses the mRNA methyltransferase activities. *Virology* 1988;163:222–225.
75. Herman RC, Schubert M, Keene JD, Lazzarini RA. Polycistronic vesicular stomatitis virus RNA transcripts. *Proc Natl Acad Sci U S A* 1980;77:4662–4665.
76. Howard M, Wertz G. Vesicular stomatitis virus RNA replication: A role for the NS protein. *J Gen Virol* 1989;70:2683–2694.
77. Hu C, Kato A, Bowman MC, et al. Role of primary constitutive phosphorylation of sendai virus P and V proteins in viral replication and pathogenesis [In Process Citation]. *Virology* 1999;263:195–208.
78. Huneycutt BS, Bi Z, Aoki CJ, Reiss CS. Central neuropathogenesis of vesicular stomatitis virus infection of immunodeficient mice. *J Virol* 1993;67:6698–6706.
79. Hunt DM. Vesicular stomatitis virus mutant with altered polyadenylic acid polymerase activity in vitro. *J Virol* 1983;46:788–799.
80. Hunt DM, Hutchinson KL. Amino acid changes in the L polymerase protein of vesicular stomatitis virus which confer aberrant polyadenylation and temperature-sensitive phenotypes. *Virology* 1993;193:786–793.
81. Hwang LN, Englund N, Das T, et al. Optimal replication activity of vesicular stomatitis virus RNA polymerase requires phosphorylation of a residue(s) at carboxy-terminal domain II of its accessory subunit, phosphoprotein P. *J Virol* 1999;73:5613–5620.
82. Ito H, Watanabe S, Sanchez A, et al. Mutational analysis of the putative fusion domain of Ebola virus glycoprotein. *J Virol* 1999;73: 8907–8912.
83. Iverson LE, Rose JK. Localized attenuation and discontinuous synthesis during vesicular stomatitis virus transcription. *Cell* 1981;23:477–484.
84. Iverson LE, Rose JK. Sequential synthesis of 5′-proximal vesicular stomatitis virus mRNA sequences. *J Virol* 1982;44:356–365.
85. Jackson A, Francki R, Zuidema D. Biology, structure, and replication of plant rhabdoviruses. In: Wagner R, ed. *The rhabdoviruses.* New York: Plenum, 1987:427–508.
86. Jayakar H, Whitt MA. Mutations in the PPXY motif of VSVmatrix protein reduce virus budding and delay cytopathic effects. *J Virol* 2000;74:9818–9827.
87. Johnson JE, Rodgers W, Rose JK. A plasma membrane localization signal in the HIV-1 envelope cytoplasmic domain prevents localization at sites of vesicular stomatitis virus budding and incorporation into VSV virions. *Virology* 1998;251:244–252.
88. Johnson KM, Vogel JE, Peralta PH. Clinical and serological response to laboratory-acquired human infection by Indiana type vesicular stomatitis virus (VSV). *Am J Trop Med Hyg* 1966;15:244–246.
89. Justice PA, Sun W, Li Y, et al. Membrane vesiculation function and exocytosis of wild-type and mutant matrix proteins of vesicular stomatitis virus. *J Virol* 1995;69:3156–3160.
90. Kahn JS, Schnell MJ, Buonocore L, Rose JK. Recombinant vesicular stomatitis virus expressing respiratory syncytial virus (RSV) glycoproteins: RSV fusion protein can mediate infection and cell fusion. *Virology* 1999;254:81–91.
91. Kalinke U, Krebber A, Krebber C, et al. Monovalent single-chain Fv fragments and bivalent miniantibodies bound to vesicular stomatitis virus protect against lethal infection. *Eur J Immunol* 1996;26: 2801–2806.
92. Kaptur PE, McKenzie MO, Wertz GW, Lyles DS. Assembly functions of vesicular stomatitis virus matrix protein are not disrupted by mutations at major sites of phosphorylation. *Virology* 1995;206:894–903.
93. Kaptur PE, Rhodes RB, Lyles DS. Sequences of the vesicular stomatitis virus matrix protein involved in binding to nucleocapsids. *J Virol* 1991;65:1057–1065.
94. Kelley JM, Emerson SU, Wagner RR. The glycoprotein of vesicular stomatitis virus is the antigen that gives rise to and reacts with neutralizing antibody. *J Virol* 1972;10:1231–1235.

95. Knipe D, Rose JK, Lodish HF. Translation of individual species of vesicular stomatitis viral mRNA. *J Virol* 1975;15:1004–1011.
96. Knipe DM, Baltimore D, Lodish HF. Maturation of viral proteins in cells infected with temperature-sensitive mutants of vesicular stomatitis virus. *J Virol* 1977;21:1149–1158.
97. Kreis TE, Lodish HF. Oligomerization is essential for transport of vesicular stomatitis viral glycoprotein to the cell surface. *Cell* 1986; 46:929–937.
98. Kretzschmar E, Buonocore L, Schnell MJ, Rose JK. High-efficiency incorporation of functional influenza virus glycoproteins into recombinant vesicular stomatitis viruses. *J Virol* 1997;71:5982–5989.
99. Kretzschmar E, Peluso R, Schnell MJ, et al. Normal replication of vesicular stomatitis virus without C proteins. *Virology* 1996;216:309–316.
100. Kurath G, Ahern KG, Pearson GD, Leong JC. Molecular cloning of the six mRNA species of infectious hematopoietic necrosis virus, a fish rhabdovirus, and gene order determination by R-loop mapping. *J Virol* 1985;53:469–476.
101. Kurilla MG, Piwnica-Worms H, Keene JD. Rapid and transient localization of the leader RNA of vesicular stomatitis virus in the nuclei of infected cells. *Proc Natl Acad Sci U S A* 1982;79:5240–5244.
102. Lawson ND, Stillman EA, Whitt MA, Rose JK. Recombinant vesicular stomatitis viruses from DNA. *Proc Natl Acad Sci U S A* 1995; 92:4477–4481.
103. Lefrancois L, Lyles DS. The interaction of antibody with the major surface glycoprotein of vesicular stomatitis virus. I. Analysis of neutralizing epitopes with monoclonal antibodies. *Virology* 1982;121: 157–167.
104. Lefrancois L, Lyles DS. The interaction of antibody with the major surface glycoprotein of vesicular stomatitis virus. II. Monoclonal antibodies of nonneutralizing and cross-reactive epitopes of Indiana and New Jersey serotypes. *Virology* 1982;121:168–174.
105. Lefrancois L, Lyles DS. Antigenic determinants of vesicular stomatitis virus: Analysis with antigenic variants. *J Immunol* 1983;130:394–398.
106. Leist TP, Cobbold SP, Waldmann H, et al. Functional analysis of T lymphocyte subsets in antiviral host defense. *J Immunol* 1987;138: 2278–2281.
107. Lenard J. Negative-strand virus M and retrovirus MA proteins: All in a family? *Virology* 1996;216:289–298.
108. Lenard J, Vanderoef R. Localization of the membrane-associated region of vesicular stomatitis virus M protein at the N terminus, using the hydrophobic, photoreactive probe 125I-TID. *J Virol* 1990;64: 3486–3491.
109. Lentz TL, Burrage TG, Smith AL, et al. Is the acetylcholine receptor a rabies virus receptor? *Science* 1982;215:182–184.
110. Leppert M, Rittenhouse L, Perrault J, et al. Plus and minus strand leader RNAs in negative strand virus-infected cells. *Cell* 1979;18: 735–747.
111. Letchworth GJ, Barrera JC, Fishel JR, Rodriguez L. Vesicular stomatitis New Jersey virus RNA persists in cattle following convalescence. *Virology* 1996;219:480–484.
112. Letchworth GJ, Rodriguez LL, Del cbarrera J. Vesicular stomatitis. *Vet J* 1999;157:239–260.
113. Li T, Pattnaik AK. Replication signals in the genome of vesicular stomatitis virus and its defective interfering particles: Identification of a sequence element that enhances DI RNA replication. *Virology* 1997; 232:248–259.
114. Li Y, Drone C, Sat E, Ghosh HP. Mutational analysis of the vesicular stomatitis virus glycoprotein G for membrane fusion domains. *J Virol* 1993;67:4070–4077.
115. Lingappa VR, Katz FN, Lodish HF, Blobel G. A signal sequence for the insertion of a transmembrane glycoprotein: Similarities to the signals of secretory proteins in primary structure and function. *J Biol Chem* 1978;253:8667–8670.
116. Lodish HF, Porter M. Heterogeneity of vesicular stomatitis virus particles: Implications for virion assembly. *J Virol* 1980;33:52–58.
117. Lodish HF, Porter M. Translational control of protein synthesis after infection by vesicular stomatitis virus. *J Virol* 1980;36:719–733.
118. Luytjes W, Krystal M, Enami M, et al. Amplification, expression, and packaging of foreign gene by influenza virus. *Cell* 1989;59:1107–1113.
119. Lyles DS, McKenzie M, Parce JW. Subunit interactions of vesicular stomatitis virus envelope glycoprotein stabilized by binding to viral matrix protein. *J Virol* 1992;66:349–358.
120. Lyles DS, McKenzie MO. Activity of vesicular stomatitis virus M protein mutants in cell rounding is correlated with the ability to inhibit host gene expression and is not correlated with virus assembly function. *Virology* 1997;229:77–89.
121. Lyles DS, McKenzie MO. Reversible and irreversible steps in assembly and disassembly and vesicular stomatitis virus: Equilibria and kinetics of dissociation of nucleocapsid-M protein complexes assembled in vivo. *Biochemistry* 1998;37:439–450.
122. Lyles DS, McKenzie MO, Daptur PE, et al. Complementation of M gene mutants of vesicular stomatitis virus by plasmid-derived M protein converts spherical extracellular particles into native bullet shapes. *Virology* 1996;217:76–87.
123. Lyles DS, Puddington L, McCreedy BJ Jr. Vesicular stomatitis virus M protein in the nuclei of infected cells. *J Virol* 1988;62:4387–4392.
124. Lyles DS, Varela VA, Parce JW. Dynamic nature of the quaternary structure of the vesicular stomatitis virus envelope glycoprotein. *Biochemistry* 1990;29:2442–2449.
125. Machamer CE, Doms RW, Bole DG, et al. Heavy chain binding protein recognizes incompletely disulfide-bonded forms of vesicular stomatitis virus G protein. *J Biol Chem* 1990;265:6879–6883.
126. Machamer CE, Rose JK. Influence of new glycosylation sites on expression of the vesicular stomatitis virus G protein at the plasma membrane. *J Biol Chem* 1988;263:5948–5954.
127. Machamer CE, Rose JK. Vesicular stomatitis virus G proteins with altered glycosylation sites display temperature-sensitive intracellular transport and are subject to aberrant intermolecular disulfide bonding. *J Biol Chem* 1988;263:5955–5960.
128. Marcus PI, Rodriguez LL, Sekellick MJ. Interferon induction as a quasispecies marker of vesicular stomatitis virus populations. *J Virol* 1998;72:542–549.
129. Masters PS, Bhella RS, Butcher M, et al. Structure and expression of the glycoprotein gene of Chandipura virus [published erratum appears in *Virology* 1990;174(2):630]. *Virology* 1989;171:285–290.
130. Matlin KS, Reggio H, Helenius A, Simons K. Pathway of vesicular stomatitis virus entry leading to infection. *J Mol Biol* 1982;156: 609–631.
131. McCreedy BJ Jr, Lyles DS. Distribution of M protein and nucleocapsid protein of vesicular stomatitis virus in infected cell plasma membranes. *Virus Res* 1989;14:189–205.
132. Mebatsion T, Conzelmann KK. Specific infection of CD4+ target cells by recombinant rabies virus pseudotypes carrying the HIV-1 envelope spike protein. *Proc Natl Acad Sci U S A* 1996;93:11366–11370.
133. Mebatsion T, Finke S, Weiland F, Conzelmann K-K. A CXCR4/CD4 pseudotype rhabdovirus that selectively infects HIV-1 envelope protein-expressing cells. *Cell* 1997;90:841–847.
134. Mebatsion T, Konig M, Conzelmann K-K. Budding of rabies virus particles in the absence of the spike glycoprotein. *Cell* 1996;84:941–951.
135. Mebatsion T, Schnell MJ, Cox JH, et al. Highly stable expression of a foreign gene from rabies virus vectors. *Proc Natl Acad Sci U S A* 1996;93:7310–7314.
136. Mebatsion T, Weiland F, Conzelmann KK. Matrix protein of rabies virus is responsible for the assembly and budding of bullet-shaped particles and interacts with the transmembrane spike glycoprotein G. *J Virol* 1999;73:242–250.
137. Melki R, Gaudin Y, Blondel D. Interaction between tubulin and the viral matrix protein of vesicular stomatitis virus: Possible implications in the viral cytopathic effect. *Virology* 1994;202:339–347.
138. Meraz MA, White JM, Sheehan KC, et al. Targeted disruption of the Stat1 gene in mice reveals unexpected physiologic specificity in the JAK-STAT signaling pathway. *Cell* 1996;84:431–442.
139. Metsikko K, Simons K. The budding mechanism of spikeless vesicular stomatitis virus particles. *EMBO J* 1986;5:1913–1920.
140. Moyer SA, Banerjee AK. Messenger RNA species synthesized in vitro by the virion-associated RNA polymerase of vesicular stomatitis virus. *Cell* 1975;4:37–43.
141. Moyer SA, Smallwood-Kentro S, Haddad A, Prevec L. Assembly and transcription of synthetic vesicular stomatitis virus nucleocapsids. *J Virol* 1991;65:2170–2178.
142. Newcomb WW, Brown JC. Role of the vesicular stomatitis virus matrix protein in maintaining the viral nucleocapsid in the condensed form found in native virions. *J Virol* 1981;39:295–299.
143. Nichol ST, Rowe JE, Fitch WM. Glycoprotein evolution of vesicular stomatitis virus New Jersey. *Virology* 1989;168:281–291.
144. Nishimura N, Balch WE. A di-acidic signal required for selective export from the endoplasmic reticulum. *Science* 1997;277:556–558.
145. Nowakowski M, Bloom BR, Ehrenfeld E, Summers DF. Restricted

replication of vesicular stomatitis virus in human lymphoblastoid cells. *J Virol* 1973;12:1272–1278.
146. O'Hara PJ, Nichol ST, Horodyski FM, Holland JJ. Vesicular stomatitis virus defective interfering particles can contain extensive genomic sequence rearrangements and base substitutions. *Cell* 1984;36:915–924.
147. Odenwald WF, Arnheiter H, Dubois-Dalcq M, Lazzarini RA. Stereo images of vesicular stomatitis virus assembly. *J Virol* 1986;57:922–932.
148. Owens RJ, Rose JK. Cytoplasmic domain requirement for incorporation of a foreign envelope protein into vesicular stomatitis virus. *J Virol* 1993;67:360–365.
149. Pattnaik AK, Ball LA, LeGrone A, Wertz GW. The termini of VSV DI particle RNAs are sufficient to signal RNA encapsidation, replication, and budding to generate infectious particles. *Virology* 1995;206: 760–764.
150. Pattnaik AK, Ball LA, LeGrone AW, Wertz GW. Infectious defective interfering particles of VSV from transcripts of a cDNA clone. *Cell* 1992;69:1011–1020.
151. Pattnaik AK, Hwang L, Li T, et al. Phosphorylation within the amino-terminal acidic domain I of the phosphoprotein of vesicular stomatitis virus is required for transcription but not for replication. *J Virol* 1997;71:8167–8175.
152. Peluso RW, Moyer SA. Viral proteins required for the in vitro replication of vesicular stomatitis virus defective interfering particle genome RNA. *Virology* 1988;162:369–376.
153. Perrault J. Origin and replication of defective interfering particles. *Curr Top Microbiol Immunol* 1981;93:151–207.
154. Pitta AM, Rose JK, Machamer CE. A single-amino-acid substitution eliminates the stringent carbohydrate requirement for intracellular transport of a viral glycoprotein. *J Virol* 1989;63:3801–3809.
155. Poch O, Blumberg BM, Bougueleret L, Tordo N. Sequence comparison of five polymerases (L proteins) of unsegmented negative-strand RNA viruses: Theoretical assignment of functional domains. *J Gen Virol* 1990;71:1153–1162.
156. Poirot MK, Schnitzlein WM, Reichmann ME. The requirement of protein synthesis for VSV inhibition of host cell RNA synthesis. *Virology* 1985;140:91–101.
157. Puddington L, Bevan MJ, Rose JK, Lefrancois L. N protein is the predominant antigen recognized by vesicular stomatitis virus-specific cytotoxic T cells. *J Virol* 1986;60:708–717.
158. Puddington L, Woodgett C, Rose JK. Replacement of the cytoplasmic domain alters sorting of a viral glycoprotein in polarized cells. *Proc Natl Acad Sci U S A* 1987;84:2756–2760.
159. Reading CL, Penhoet EE, Ballou CE. Carbohydrate structure of vesicular stomatitis virus glycoprotein. *J Biol Chem* 1978;253:5600–5612.
160. Reagan KJ, Wunner WH. Rabies virus interaction with various cell lines is independent of the acetylcholine receptor. *Arch Virol* 1985; 84:277–282.
161. Reiss CS, Plakhov IV, Komatsu T. Viral replication in olfactory receptor neurons and entry into the olfactory bulb and brain. *Ann N Y Acad Sci* 1998;855:751–761.
162. Remenick J, Kenny MK, McGowan JJ. Inhibition of adenovirus DNA replication by vesicular stomatitis virus leader RNA. *J Virol* 1988; 62:1286–1292.
163. Riedel H, Kondor-Koch C, Garoff H. Cell surface expression of fusogenic vesicular stomatitis virus G protein from cloned cDNA. *EMBO J* 1984;3:1477–1483.
164. Rigaut KD, Birk DE, Lenard J. Intracellular distribution of input vesicular stomatitis virus proteins after uncoating. *J Virol* 1991;65: 2622–2628.
165. Roberts A, Buonocore L, Price R, et al. Attenuated vesicular stomatitis viruses as vaccine vectors. *J Virol* 1999;73:3723–3732.
166. Roberts A, Kretzschmar E, Perkins AS, et al. Vaccination with a recombinant vesicular stomatitis virus expressing an influenza virus hemagglutinin provides complete protection from influenza virus challenge. *J Virol* 1998;72:4704–4711.
167. Roberts A, Rose JK. Recovery of negative-strand RNA viruses from plasmid DNAs: A positive approach revitalizes a negative field. *Virology* 1998;247:1–6.
168. Robison CS, Whitt MA. The membrane-proximal stem region of vesicular stomatitis virus G protein confers efficient virus assembly. *J Virol* 2000;74:2239–2246.
169. Rose J, Schubert M. Rhabdovirus genomes and their products. In: Wagner RR, ed. *The rhabdoviruses.* New York: Plenum, 1987: 129–166.
170. Rose JK. Complete intergenic and flanking gene sequences from the genome of vesicular stomatitis virus. *Cell* 1980;19:415–421.
171. Rose JK, Adams GA, Gallione CJ. The presence of cysteine in the cytoplasmic domain of the vesicular stomatitis virus glycoprotein is required for palmitate addition. *Proc Natl Acad Sci U S A* 1984; 81:2050–2054.
172. Rose JK, Bergmann JE. Altered cytoplasmic domains affect intracellular transport of the vesicular stomatitis virus glycoprotein. *Cell* 1983;34:513–524.
173. Rose JK, Doolittle RF, Anilionis A, et al. Homology between the glycoproteins of vesicular stomatitis virus and rabies virus. *J Virol* 1982; 43:361–364.
174. Rose JK, Gallione CJ. Nucleotide sequences of the mRNA's encoding the vesicular stomatitis virus G and M proteins determined from cDNA clones containing the complete coding regions. *J Virol* 1981; 39:519–528.
175. Rose JK, Lodish HF, Brock ML. Giant heterogeneous polyadenylic acid on vesicular stomatitis virus mRNA synthesized in vitro in the presence of S-adenosylhomocysteine. *J Virol* 1977;21:683–693.
176. Rud EW, Banerjee AK, Kang CY. Defective interfering particles of VSVNJ (Ogden), generated by heat treatment, contain multiple internal genomic deletions. *Virology* 1986;155:61–76.
177. Schlegel R, Tralka TS, Willingham MC, Pastan I. Inhibition of VSV binding and infectivity by phosphatidylserine: Is phosphatidylserine a VSV-binding site? *Cell* 1983;32:639–646.
178. Schlegel R, Wade M. Biologically active peptides of the vesicular stomatitis virus glycoprotein. *J Virol* 1985;53:319–323.
179. Schlegel R, Willingham MC, Pastan IH. Saturable binding sites for vesicular stomatitis virus on the surface of Vero cells. *J Virol* 1982; 43:871–875.
180. Schmidt MF, Schlesinger MJ. Fatty acid binding to vesicular stomatitis virus glycoprotein: A new type of post-translational modification of the viral glycoprotein. *Cell* 1979;17:813–819.
181. Schnell MJ, Buonocore L, Boritz E, et al. Requirement for a non-specific glycoprotein cytoplasmic domain sequence to drive efficient budding of vesicular stomatitis virus. *EMBO J* 1998;17:1289–1296.
182. Schnell MJ, Buonocore L, Kretzschmar E, et al. Foreign glycoproteins expressed from recombinant vesicular stomatitis viruses are incorporated efficiently into virus particles. *Proc Natl Acad Sci U S A* 1996; 93:11359–11365.
183. Schnell MJ, Buonocore L, Whitt MA, Rose JK. The minimal conserved transcription stop-start signal promotes stable expression of a foreign gene in vesicular stomatitis virus. *J Virol* 1996;70:2318–2323.
184. Schnell MJ, Conzelmann KK. Polymerase activity of in vitro mutated rabies virus L protein. *Virology* 1995;214:522–530.
185. Schnell MJ, Johnson JE, Buonocore L, Rose JK. Construction of a novel virus that targets HIV-1-infected cells and controls HIV-1 infection. *Cell* 1997;90:849–857.
186. Schnell MJ, Mebatsion T, Conzelmann KK. Infectious rabies viruses from cloned cDNA. *EMBO J* 1994;13:4195–4203.
187. Schnitzlein WM, O'Banion MK, Poirot MK, Reichmann ME. Effect of intracellular vesicular stomatitis virus mRNA concentration on the inhibition of host cell protein synthesis. *J Virol* 1983;45:206–214.
188. Schubert M, Harmison GG, Meier E. Primary structure of the vesicular stomatitis virus polymerase (L) gene: Evidence for a high frequency of mutations. *J Virol* 1984;51:505–514.
189. Schubert M, Keene JD, Herman RC, Lazzarini RA. Site of the vesicular stomatitis virus genome specifying polyadenylation at the end of the L gene mRNA. *J Virol* 1980;34:550–559.
190. Sevier CS, Weisz OA, Davis M, Machamer CE. Efficient export of the vesicular stomatitis virus G protein from the endoplasmic reticulum requires a signal in the cytoplasmic tail that includes both tyrosine-based and di-acidic motifs. *Mol Biol Cell* 2000;11:13–22.
191. Shope R, Tesh R. The ecology of rhabdoviruses that infect vertebrates. In Wagner R, ed. *The rhabdoviruses.* New York: Plenum, 1987:509–534.
192. Shuman S. A proposed mechanism of mRNA synthesis and capping by vesicular stomatitis virus. *Virology* 1997;227:1–6.
193. Simons K, Garoff H. The budding mechanisms of enveloped animal viruses. *J Gen Virol* 1980;50:1–21.
194. Sleat DE, Banerjee AK. Transcriptional activity and mutational analysis of recombinant vesicular stomatitis virus RNA polymerase. *J Virol* 1993;67:1334–1339.
195. Spadafora D, Canter DM, Jackson RL, Perrault J. Constitutive phosphorylation of the vesicular stomatitis virus P protein modulates poly-

merase complex formation but is not essential for transcription or replication. *J Virol* 1996;70:4538–4548.
196. Spiropoulou CF, Nichol ST. A small highly basic protein is encoded in overlapping frame within the P gene of vesicular stomatitis virus. *J Virol* 1993;67:3103–3110.
197. Steinhauer DA, de la Torre JC, Holland JJ. High nucleotide substitution error frequencies in clonal pools of vesicular stomatitis virus. *J Virol* 1989;63:2063–2071.
198. Steinhoff U, Muller U, Schertler A, et al. Antiviral protection by vesicular stomatitis virus-specific antibodies in alpha/beta interferon receptor-deficient mice. *J Virol* 1995;69:2153–2158.
199. Stephens EB, Compans RW, Earl P, Moss B. Surface expression of viral glycoproteins is polarized in epithelial cells infected with recombinant vaccinia viral vectors. *EMBO J* 1986;5:237–245.
200. Stillman EA, Rose JK, Whitt MA. Replication and amplification of novel vesicular stomatitis virus minigenomes encoding viral structural proteins. *J Virol* 1995;69:2946–2953.
201. Stillman EA, Whitt MA. Mutational analyses of the intergenic dinucleotide and the transcriptional start sequence of vesicular stomatitis virus (VSV) define sequences required for efficient termination and initiation of VSV transcripts. *J Virol* 1997;71:2127–2137.
202. Stillman EA, Whitt MA. The length and sequence composition of vesicular stomatitis virus intergenic regions affect mRNA levels and the site of transcript initiation. *J Virol* 1998;72:5565–5572.
203. Stillman EA, Whitt MA. Transcript initiation and 5′-end modifications are separable events during vesicular stomatitis virus transcription. *J Virol* 1999;73:7199–7209.
204. Takacs AM, Das T, Banerjee AK. Mapping of interacting domains between the nucleocapsid protein and the phosphoprotein of vesicular stomatitis virus by using a two-hybrid system. *Proc Natl Acad Sci U S A* 1993;90:10375–10379.
205. Takada A, Robison C, Goto H, et al. A novel system for functional analysis of Ebola virus glycoprotein. *Proc Natl Acad Sci U S A* 1997; 94:14764–14769.
206. Teninges D, Bras F, Dezelee S. Genome organization of the sigma rhabdovirus: Six genes and a gene overlap. *Virology* 1993;193:1018–1023.
207. Tesh RB, Peralta PH, Johnson KM. Ecologic studies of vesicular stomatitis virus. I. Prevalence of infection among animals and humans living in an area of endemic VSV activity. *Am J Epidemiol* 1969;90: 255–261.
208. Thacore HR, Youngner JS. Abortive infection of a rabbit cornea cell line by vesicular stomatitis virus: Conversion to productive infection by superinfection with vaccinia virus. *J Virol* 1975;16:322–329.
209. Thomas D, Newcomb WW, Brown JC, et al. Mass and molecular composition of vesicular stomatitis virus: A scanning transmission electron microscopy analysis. *J Virol* 1985;54:598–607.
210. Thomas DC, Brewer CB, Roth MG. Vesicular stomatitis virus glycoprotein contains a dominant cytoplasmic basolateral sorting signal critically dependent upon a tyrosine. *J Biol Chem* 1993;268:3313–3320.
211. Thoulouze MI, Lafage M, Schachner M, et al. The neural cell adhesion molecule is a receptor for rabies virus. *J Virol* 1998;72:7181–7190.
212. Tuffereau C, Benejean J, Alfonso AM, et al. Neuronal cell surface molecules mediate specific binding to rabies virus glycoprotein expressed by a recombinant baculovirus on the surfaces of lepidopteran cells. *J Virol* 1998;72:1085–1091.
213. Vernon SD, Rodriguez LL, Letchworth GJ. Vesicular stomatitis New Jersey virus glycoprotein gene sequence and neutralizing epitope stability in an enzootic focus. *Virology* 1990;177:209–215.
214. Villareal LP, Breindl M, Holland JJ. Determination of molar ratios of vesicular stomatitis virus induced RNA species in BHK21 cells. *Biochemistry* 1976;15:1663–1667.
215. Volk WA, Synder RM, Benjamin DC, Wagner RR. Monoclonal antibodies to the glycoprotein of vesicular stomatitis virus: Comparative neutralizing activity. *J Virol* 1982;42:220–227.
216. Weck PK, Wagner RR. Transcription of vesicular stomatitis virus is required to shut off cellular RNA synthesis. *J Virol* 1979;30:410–413.
217. Wertz GW, Perepelitsa VP, Ball LA. Gene rearrangement attenuates expression and lethality of a nonsegmented negative strand RNA virus. *Proc Natl Acad Sci U S A* 1998;95:3501–3506.
218. Wertz GW, Whelan S, LeGrone A, Ball LA. Extent of terminal complementarity modulates the balance between transcription and replication of vesicular stomatitis virus RNA. *Proc Natl Acad Sci U S A* 1994;91:8587–8591.
219. Wethers JA, Johnson GP, Schumacher CL, Herman RC. Nonpermissive infection of lymphoblastoid cells by vesicular stomatitis virus. II. Effect on viral morphogenesis. *Virus Res* 1985;2:345–358.
220. Whelan SP, Ball LA, Barr JN, Wertz GT. Efficient recovery of infectious vesicular stomatitis virus entirely from cDNA clones. *Proc Natl Acad Sci U S A* 1995;92:8388–8392.
221. Whelan SPJ, Wertz GW. Regulation of RNA synthesis by the genomic termini of vesicular stomatitis virus: Identification of distinct sequences essential for transcription but not replication. *J Virol* 1999; 73:297–306.
222. Whitaker-Dowling P, Youngner JS. Alteration of vesicular stomatitis virus L and NS proteins by uv irradiation: Implications for the mechanism of host cell shut-off. *Virology* 1988;164:171–175.
223. Whitt MA, Chong L, Rose JK. Glycoprotein cytoplasmic domain sequences required for rescue of a vesicular stomatitis virus glycoprotein mutant. *J Virol* 1989;63:3569–3578.
224. Whitt MA, Rose JK. Fatty acid acylation is not required for membrane fusion activity or glycoprotein assembly into VSV virions. *Virology* 1991;185:875–878.
225. Whitt MA, Zagouras P, Crise B, Rose JK. A fusion-defective mutant of the vesicular stomatitis virus glycoprotein. *J Virol* 1990;64:4907–4913.
226. Wilks CR, House JA. Susceptibility of various animals to the vesiculoviruses Isfahan and Chandipura. *J Hyg* (Lond) 1986;97: 359–368.
227. Wills JW, Cameron CE, Wilson CB, et al. An assembly domain of the Rous sarcoma virus Gag protein required late in budding. *J Virol* 1994;68:6605–6618.
228. Woodgett C, Rose JK. Amino-terminal mutation of the vesicular stomatitis virus glycoprotein does not affect its fusion activity. *J Virol* 1986;59:486–489.
229. Wyers F, Richard-Molard C, Blondel D, Dezelee S. Vesicular stomatitis virus growth in *Drosophila melanogaster* cells: G protein deficiency. *J Virol* 1980;33:411–422.
230. Yang J, Koprowski H, Dietzschold B, Fu ZF. Phosphorylation of rabies virus nucleoprotein regulates viral RNA transcription and replication by modulating leader RNA encapsidation. *J Virol* 1999;73: 1661–1664.
231. Ye Z, Sun W, Suryanarayana K, et al. Membrane-binding domains and cytopathogenesis of the matrix protein of vesicular stomatitis virus. *J Virol* 1994;68:7386–7396.
232. Yewdell JW, Bennink JR, Mackett M, et al. Recognition of cloned vesicular stomatitis virus internal and external gene products by cytotoxic T lymphocytes. *J Exp Med* 1986;163:1529–1538.
233. Yuan H, Yoza BK, Lyles DS. Inhibition of host RNA polymerase II-dependent transcription by vesicular stomatitis virus results from inactivation of TFIID. *Virology* 1998;251:383–392.
234. Zagouras P, Rose JK. Dynamic equilibrium between vesicular stomatitis virus glycoprotein monomers and trimers in the Golgi and at the cell surface. *J Virol* 1993;67:7533–7538.
235. Zagouras P, Ruusala A, Rose JK. Dissociation and reassociation of oligomeric viral glycoprotein subunits in the endoplasmic reticulum. *J Virol* 1991;65:1976–1984.
236. Zhang L, Ghosh HP. Characterization of the putative fusogenic domain in vesicular stomatitis virus glycoprotein G. *J Virol* 1994;68: 2186–2193.

CHAPTER 23

Paramyxoviridae: The Viruses and Their Replication

Robert A. Lamb and Daniel Kolakofsky

The *Paramyxoviridae* include some of the great and ubiquitous disease-causing viruses of humans and animals, including one of the most infectious viruses known (measles), some of the most prevalent viruses known (measles, respiratory syncytial, parainfluenza viruses, and mumps virus), a virus that has been targeted by the World Health Organization for eradication (measles), viruses that have a major economic impact on poultry and animal rearing (Newcastle disease and rinderpest), and some newly discovered viruses and diseases (pinniped morbilliviruses, Hendra virus, and Nipah virus). The *Paramyxoviridae* are enveloped, negative-stranded RNA viruses that have special relationships to two other families of negative-strand RNA viruses, namely the *Orthomyxoviridae* (for the biologic properties of the envelope glycoproteins) and the *Rhabdoviridae* (for the similarity of organization of the nonsegmented genome and its expression). The *Paramyxoviridae* are defined by having a protein (F) that causes viral–cell membrane fusion at neutral pH. The genomic RNA of all negative-strand RNA viruses has to serve two functions: first as a template for synthesis of mRNAs, and second as a template for synthesis of the antigenome (+) strand. Negative-strand RNA viruses encode and package their own RNA polymerase (RNAP), but mRNAs are synthesized only after the virus has been uncoated in the infected cell. Viral replication occurs after synthesis of the mRNAs and requires the continuous synthesis of viral proteins. The newly synthesized antigenome (+) strand serves as the template for further copies of the (–) strand genomic RNA.

CLASSIFICATION

The family *Paramyxoviridae* has been reclassified in 2000 by the International Committee on the Taxonomy of Viruses into two subfamilies, the *Paramyxovirinae* and the *Pneumovirinae. Paramyxovirinae* contains three genera, Respirovirus, Rubulavirus, and Morbillivirus. *Pneumovirinae* contains the genera Pneumovirus and Metapneumovirus. The new classification is based on morphologic criteria, the organization of the genome, the biologic activities of the proteins, and the sequence relationship of the encoded proteins, now that most of the genome sequences have been obtained. The recently isolated Hendra virus, from horses and humans in Australia, Nipah virus, from pigs and humans in Malaysia, and a tree shrew (*Tupaia*) Paramyxovirus are presently unclassified members of the *Paramyxovirinae.* Newcastle disease virus (NDV) and other avian paramyxoviruses have been included in the Rubulavirus genus, primarily because of their nonconserved intergenic junctions and lack of a C-protein open reading frame (ORF), hallmarks specific to the Rubulavirus genus (see later, and Fig. 6). However, the organization of the NDV P gene and its mRNA editing profile resemble those found for species of the genera Morbillivirus and Respirovirus, but not for other species in the genus Rubulavirus. Thus, further consideration of the appropriate taxonomy of NDV and avian paramyxoviruses is required.

The morphologic distinguishing feature among enveloped viruses for the subfamily *Paramyxovirinae* is the size and shape of the nucleocapsids (diameter of 18 nm, 1 μm in length, a pitch of 5.5 nm), which have a left-handed helical symmetry. The biologic criteria are (a) antigenic cross-reactivity between members of a genus and (b) the presence (Respirovirus and Rubulavirus) or absence (Morbillivirus) of neuraminidase activity. In addition, the different coding potentials of the P genes are considered and there is the presence of an extra gene (SH) in some rubulaviruses. The pneumoviruses can be distinguished from *Paramyxovirinae* morphologically, as they contain narrower nucleocapsids. In addition, the *Pneumovirinae* have major differences in the number of encoded proteins and an attachment protein that is very different from that of *Paramyxovirinae.* Examples of members of the three genera are shown in Table 1, and a phylogenetic majority-rule-consensus tree based on a combined cluster alignment of the nucleocapsid and phosphoprotein amino acid sequences is shown in Figure 1.

TABLE 1. *Examples of members of the family* Paramyxoviridae

Family *Paramyxoviridae*
Subfamily *Paramyxovirinae*
Genus Respirovirus
Sendai virus (mouse parainfluenza virus type 1)
Human parainfluenza virus types 1 and 3 (hPIV1/3)
Bovine parainfluenza virus type 3 (bPIV3)
Genus Rubulavirus
Simian virus 5 (canine parainfluenza virus type 2)
Mumps virus
Newcastle disease virus (avian paramyxovirus 1) (NDV)
Human parainfluenza virus types 2, 4a, and 4b (hPIV2/4a/4b)
Genus Morbillivirus
Measles virus
Dolphin Morbillivirus
Canine distemper virus
Peste-des-petits-ruminants virus
Phocine distemper virus
Rinderpest virus
Subfamily *Pneumovirinae*
Genus Pneumovirus
Human respiratory syncytial virus (hRSV)
Bovine respiratory syncytial virus (bRSV)
Pneumonia virus of mice
Genus Metapneumovirus
Avian pneumovirus (formerly called turkey rhinotracheitis virus)
Unclassified paramyxoviruses
Tupaia Paramyxovirus
Hendra virus
Nipah virus

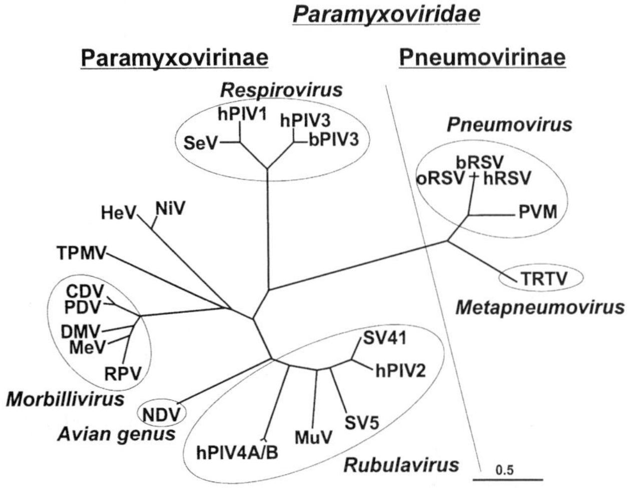

FIG. 1. Evolutionary relationships of the *Paramyxoviridae.* Phylogenetic majority-rule consensus tree of the family *Paramyxoviridae* based on a combined cluster alignment of the nucleocapsid and phosphoprotein amino acid sequences of selected family members. Branch lengths represent relative phylogenetic distances according to maximum likelihood estimates based on the Dayhoff PAM matrix. Bootstrap support is 100% for all branching points, with the only exceptions being Hev (98%) and TPMV (77%). The following Paramyxovirus species are included in the cluster alignment (GenBank/EMBL/SwissProt accession numbers are given in parentheses): HeV (Hendra virus) (AF017149); TPMV (Tupaia Paramyxovirus) (AF079780); CDV (canine distemper virus) (P04865, P06940); PDV (phocine distemper virus) (P35944, P35939); DMV (dolphin Morbillivirus) (X75961, Z47758); MeV (measles virus) (Z66517); RPV (rinderpest virus) (Q03332, Q03335); NDV (Newcastle disease virus) (Z30084, Q06427); hPIV-4A (human parainfluenza virus 4A) (P17240, P22044); hPIV-4B (human parainfluenza virus 4B) (P17241, P21738); MuV (Mumps virus) (P21277, P19717); SV5 (simian parainfluenza virus 5) (AF052755); hPIV-2 (human parainfluenza virus 2) (P21737, P23056); SV41 (simian parainfluenza virus 41) (P27018, S60813); SeV (Sendai virus) (P04858, P04860); hPIV-1 (human parainfluenza virus 1) (P24304, P28054); hPIV-3 (human parainfluenza virus 3) (P06159, P06162); bPIV-3 (bovine parainfluenza virus 3) (P06161, P06163): oRSV (ovine respiratory syncytial virus) (Q83957, Q83956); bRSV (bovine respiratory syncytial virus) (P22677, P33454); hRSV (human respiratory syncytial virus) (P03418, P03421); PVM (pneumonia virus of mice) (P26589, U096449); TRTV (turkey rhinotracheitis virus) (U39295, U22110). Although not yet approved by the International Committee for the Taxonomy of Viruses, there is a wealth of data to suggest it is appropriate to remove NDV from the genus Rubulavirus and to designate it as belonging to a new avian genus of the *Paramyxoviridae.* (Adapted from ref. 276, with permission).

STRUCTURE AND REPLICATION STRATEGY OF THE *PARAMYXOVIRIDAE*

Paramyxoviruses contain nonsegmented, single-stranded RNA genomes of negative polarity, and they replicate entirely in the cytoplasm. Their genomes are 15 to 19 kB in length, and the genomes contain six to ten tandemly linked genes. A lipid envelope containing two surface glycoproteins (F and HN, or H or G), which mediate the entry and exit of the virus from its host cell, surrounds the virions. Inside the envelope lies a helical nucleocapsid core containing the RNA genome and the nucleocapsid (N), phospho- (P), and large (L) proteins, which initiate intracellular virus replication. Residing between the envelope and the core lies the viral matrix (M) protein that is important in virion architecture and that is released from the core during virus entry. In addition to the genes encoding structural proteins, paramyxoviruses contain "accessory" genes, which are found mostly as additional transcriptional units interspersed with the tandemly linked invariant genes. For the *Paramyxovirinae*, the accessory genes are found mostly as ORFs that overlap within the P gene transcriptional unit.

Intracellular replication of paramyxoviruses begins with the viral RNA-dependent RNAP (minimally, a homotetramer of P and a single L protein) transcribing the N-encapsidated genome RNA (N:RNA) into 5′ capped and 3′ polyadenylated mRNAs. The viral RNAP (vRNAP) begins all RNA synthesis at the 3′ end of the genome, and it transcribes the genes into mRNAs in a sequential (and polar) manner by terminating and reinitiating at each of the gene junctions. The junctions consist of a gene-end sequence, at which polyadenylation occurs by the reiterative copying of four to seven uridylates (followed by release of the mRNA), a short nontranscribed intergenic region, and a gene-start sequence that specifies capping as well as mRNA initiation. The RNAP occasionally fails to reinitiate the downstream mRNA at each junction, leading to the loss of transcription of further-downstream genes, and hence there is a gradient of mRNA synthesis that is inversely proportional to the distance of the gene from the 3′ end of the genome. After primary transcription and translation, when sufficient amounts of unassembled N protein are present, viral RNA synthesis becomes coupled to the concomitant encapsidation of the nascent (+) RNA chain. Under these conditions, vRNAP ignores all the junctions (and editing sites), to produce an exact complementary antigenome chain, in a fully assembled nucleocapsid.

Virion Structure

The *Paramyxoviridae* contain a lipid bilayer envelope that is derived from the plasma membrane of the host cell in which the virus is grown (reviewed in ref. 43). *Paramyxoviridae* are generally spherical and 150 to 350 nm in diameter, but they can be pleiomorphic, and filamentous forms can be observed. Inserted into the envelope are glycoprotein spikes that extend about 8 to 12 nm from the surface of the membrane and that can be readily visualized by electron microscopy (EM). Inside the viral membrane is the nucleocapsid core (sometimes called the ribonucleoprotein core), which contains the 15,000- to 19,000-nucleotide, single-stranded RNA genome. Figure 2 is a highly stylized schematic diagram of the virions. F and HN are actually trimers and tetramers, respectively. No attempt has been made to represent the real abundance of F, HN, SH, or N subunits in the virion. The pleiomorphic nature of virion particles under EM is illustrated in Figure 3, and a comparison of the RNPs of influenza virus, rabies virus, and Sendai virus is shown in Figure 4.

The helical nucleocapsid, rather than the free genome RNA, is the template for all RNA synthesis. For Sendai virus, each nucleocapsid is composed of about 2,600 N, 300 P, and 50 L proteins (164). The N protein and genome RNA together form a core structure, to which the P and L proteins are attached. This nucleocapsid core is remarkably stable, as it withstands the high salt and gravity forces of cesium chloride density gradient centrifugation. By EM, the P and L proteins of nucleocapsids are not observed; they can be visualized only with the aid of antibodies (224). Holonucleocapsids (N:RNA plus P and L) have the capacity to transcribe mRNAs *in vitro*, presumably mimicking primary transcription in infected cells, and they are thought to be the minimal unit of infectivity.

When negatively stained preparations of Paramyxovirus nucleocapsids are viewed by EM, the most tightly coiled forms resemble the Tobamovirus tobacco mosaic virus (TMV)—that is, a relatively rigid coiled rod 18 nm in diameter, with a central hollow core of 4 nm and a helical pitch of about 5 nm (51,52,89). Unlike TMV, however, in which the nucleocapsid must disassemble so that its (+) RNA genome can function as a template, Paramyxovirus nucleocapsids function without disassembling; as far as we know, these nucleocapsids never disassemble naturally. This remarkable property is undoubtedly associated with the finding that, unlike TMV, these nucleocapsids are not rigid, although they become more rigid on trypsin treatment (194).

Sendai virus nucleocapsids exist in several distinct morphologic states at normal salt concentration (79, 113,114). The most prevalent form in negatively stained preparations is the most tightly coiled one, with a helical pitch of 5.3 nm. Two other forms, one with a slightly larger pitch of 6.8 nm, and another with a much larger pitch of 37.5 nm, have also been noted. The fact that no structures of intermediate pitch have been found indicates that these are distinct states. It is thought that the template is copied without dissociation of N protein from the nucleocapsid, and the uncoiling of the nucleocapsid may be necessary for the polymerase to gain access to the RNA bases. It is possible that the viral

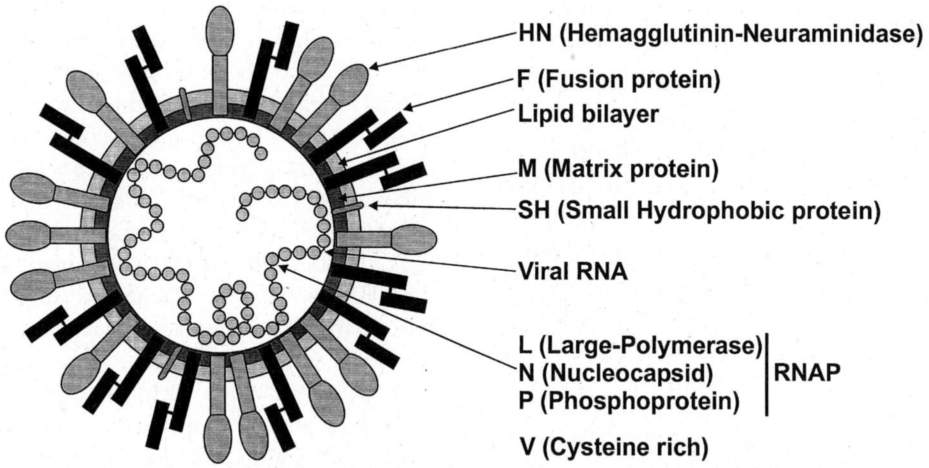

FIG. 2. Schematic diagram of a Paramyxovirus (not drawn to scale). The lipid bilayer is shown as the *gray concentric circle*, and underlying the lipid bilayer is the viral matrix protein shown as a *black concentric circle.* Inserted through the viral membrane are the hemagglutinin-neuraminidase (*HN*) attachment glycoprotein, and the (*F*) fusion glycoprotein. The relative abundance of HN and F is not illustrated by the diagram. The small integral membrane protein, SH, is found only in some rubulaviruses, such as SV5. The HN protein is thought to have a stalk region and a globular head, and the F protein consists of two sulfide-linked chains, F_1 and F_2. The HN protein is a tetramer and the F protein a trimer. Inside the virus is the negative-stranded virion RNA, which is encapsidated with the nucleocapsid protein (*N*). Associated with the nucleocapsid are the L and P proteins, and together this complex has RNA-dependent RNA transcriptase activity. For the rubulaviruses, the cysteine-rich protein V is found as an internal component of the virion, whereas for other members of the family, the V protein is found only in virus-infected cells. The nature of possible interactions between the cytoplasmic tails of the glycoprotein spikes and the matrix protein, and the interactions between the matrix protein and the nucleocapsid have not been fully elucidated and no attempt has been made to illustrate them.

polymerase traverses the nucleocapsid template by uncoiling the helix in front of it and recoiling it once the polymerase has passed a given position, much the same as cellular RNAP generates its template "bubble" in traversing dsDNA.

As expected, the diameter of the nucleocapsid decreases as the pitch increases and the nucleocapsid lengthens, and for Sendai virus the diameter is 3.5 nm less for the 6.8-nm form than for the 5.3-nm-pitch form. These latter values are very similar to those of Pneumovirus nucleocapsids, which also have a pitch of 7 nm. As discussed earlier, these differences in nucleocapsid morphology are used to distinguish the different *Paramyxoviridae*, but they probably relate mainly to the form that predominates in negatively stained preparations.

THE *PARAMYXOVIRIDAE* GENOMES AND THEIR ENCODED PROTEINS

Today we know the complete genome sequence for almost all members of the *Paramyxoviridae*, including Sendai virus, human parainfluenza virus 3 (hPIV-3), simian virus 5 (SV5), mumps virus, measles virus, canine distemper virus (CDV), and respiratory syncytial virus (RSV). (They are obtainable from the Web, at http://www.ncbi.nlm.nih.gov.) The 15,000- to 19,000-nucleotide genomic RNA contains a 3′ extracistronic region of about 50 nucleotides, known as the leader, and a 5′ extracistronic region of 50 to 161 nucleotides, known as the trailer [or the (–) leader]. These control regions are essential for transcription and replication, and they flank the six genes (seven for certain rubulaviruses and eight to ten for pneumoviruses) (note that by the convention used for paramyxoviruses, the term *gene* refers to the genome sequence encoding a single mRNA, even if that mRNA contains more than one ORF and encodes more than one protein). The coding capacity of the genome of *Paramyxovirinae* is extended by the use of overlapping ORFs in the P gene. The gene order of a representative member of each subfamily is shown in Figure 5. At the beginning and end of each gene are conserved transcriptional control sequences that are copied into mRNA. Between the

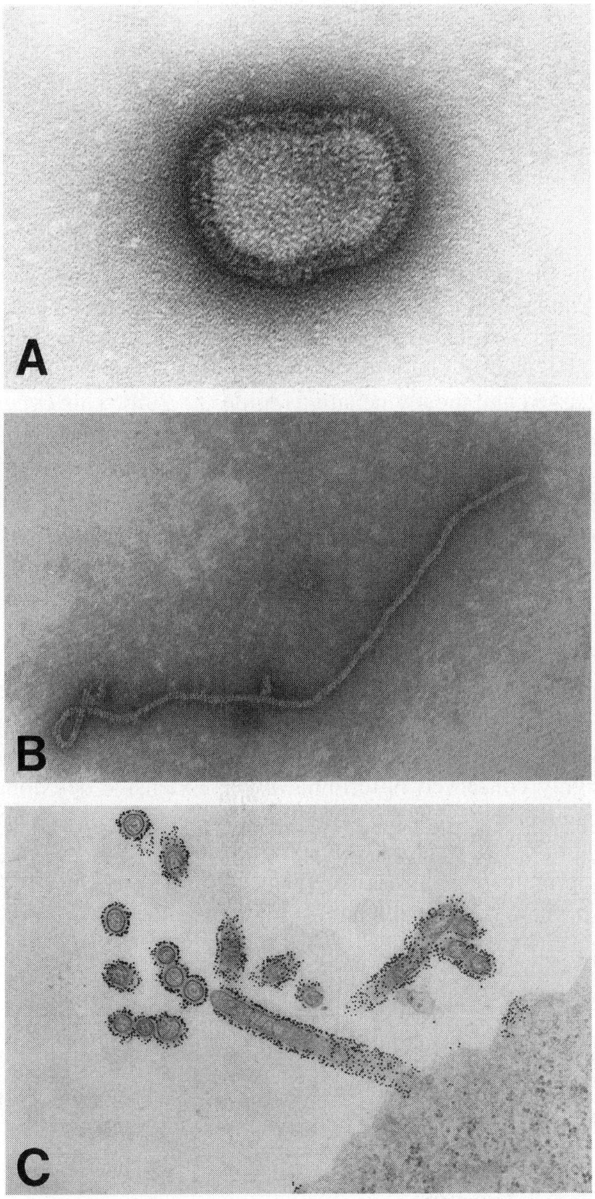

FIG. 3. Ultrastructure of SV5 virions revealed by negative staining. **A:** Negatively stained SV5 particle. The glycoprotein spikes on intact 150- to 300-nm virus particles can be observed (×226,280). **B:** Negatively stained SV5 nucleocapsid (×74,570). **C:** Budding SV5 virions particles from the surface of CV-1 cells. Colloidal gold staining of HN is shown (×24,700) (Micrographs courtesy of George Leser, Northwestern University).

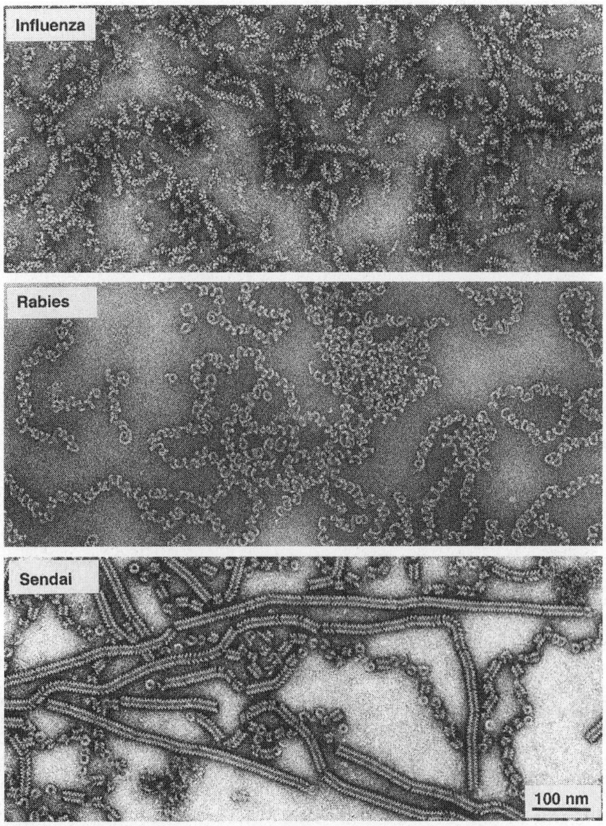

FIG. 4. Nucleocapsids of negative-strand RNA viruses. Electron micrographs of the nucleocapsids of three negative-strand RNA viruses, negatively stained with 1% sodium silicotungstate. *Top:* Ribonucleoprotein particles of influenza virus with a stoichiometry of 24 nucleotides per NP monomer. *Middle:* Nucleocapsids of rabies virus with a stoichiometry of nine nucleotides per N monomer. *Bottom:* Nucleocapsids of Sendai virus with a stoichiometry of six nucleotides per N monomer. All micrographs have the same magnification (bar = 100 nm). (Micrographs courtesy of Rob Ruigrok, European Molecular Biology Laboratory, Grenoble, France.)

gene boundaries are intergenic regions (Fig. 6). These are precisely three nucleotides long for the respiroviruses and morbilliviruses but are quite variable in length for the rubulaviruses (1 to 47 nucleotides) and pneumoviruses (1 to 56 nucleotides) (see Fig. 6).

The Nucleocapsid Protein

The nucleocapsid (N) protein serves several functions in virus replication, including encapsidation of the genome RNA into an RNase-resistant nucleocapsid (the template for RNA synthesis), association with the P-L polymerase during transcription and replication, and, most likely, interaction with the M protein during virus assembly. The intracellular concentration of unassembled N is also thought to be a major factor controlling the relative rates of transcription and replication from the genome templates, by analogy to studies made on the Rhabdovirus vesicular stomatitis virus (VSV) (13,14).

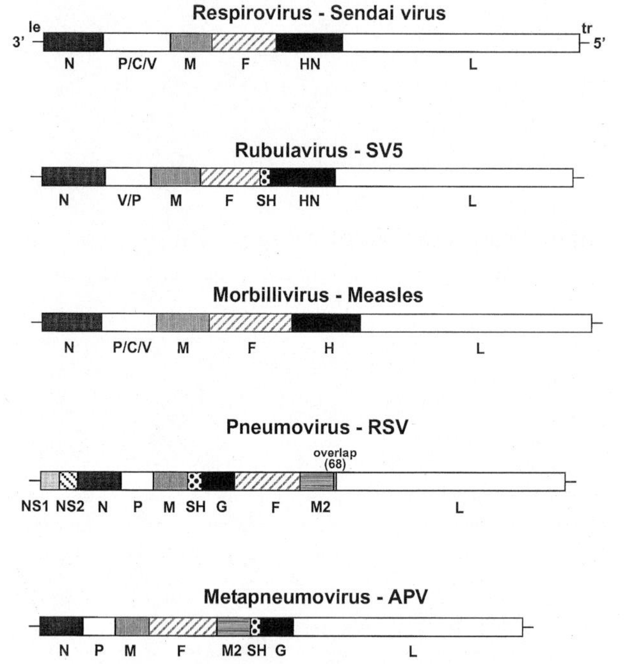

FIG. 5. Genetic map of a typical member of each genus of the *Paramyxoviridae*. The gene size is drawn to scale. Gene boundaries are shown by *vertical lines*. The hRSV L gene transcription overlaps that of the M2 gene by 68 nucleotides, and the bRSV overlap is 67 nucleotides, whereas PMV and APV do not have an overlap.

The nucleotide sequence of the N gene of paramyxoviruses predicts that the N proteins range from 489 to 553 amino acids [molecular weight ratio (M_r) 53,167 to 57,896], and, unexpectedly for a protein that interacts with RNA, the protein has a net charge of −7 to −12, with the exception of mumps virus (+2). A comparison of these protein sequences, coupled with data obtained from protease digestions of nucleocapsids, suggests that N contains two domains. The N-terminal 80% of the protein of about 500 residues is relatively well conserved among related viruses, whereas the C-terminal 20% is poorly conserved, although this domain always contains a highly charged and mostly negative region (58,208). This hypervariable C-terminus appears to be a tail extending from the surface of a globular N-terminal body, because the C-terminal sequences of the SV5 and Sendai virus N protein in nucleocapsids are hypersensitive to trypsin digestion, leaving a 48-kd N-terminal core (53,114,194). However, the overall structure of the nucleocapsid seen by EM, and the resistance of the genomic RNA within this structure to nuclease attack are mostly unchanged by trypsin treatment (151). These data indicate that the determinants for the helical nature of the nucleocapsid, as well as the RNA binding domains, must lie within the highly conserved N-terminal body. Extensive deletional analysis indicates the N-terminal region of Sendai virus N protein is required for nucleocapsid assembly (18). For N proteins, an invariant sequence F-X4-Y-X4-S-Y-A-M-G (where X is any residue) is found near the middle of the

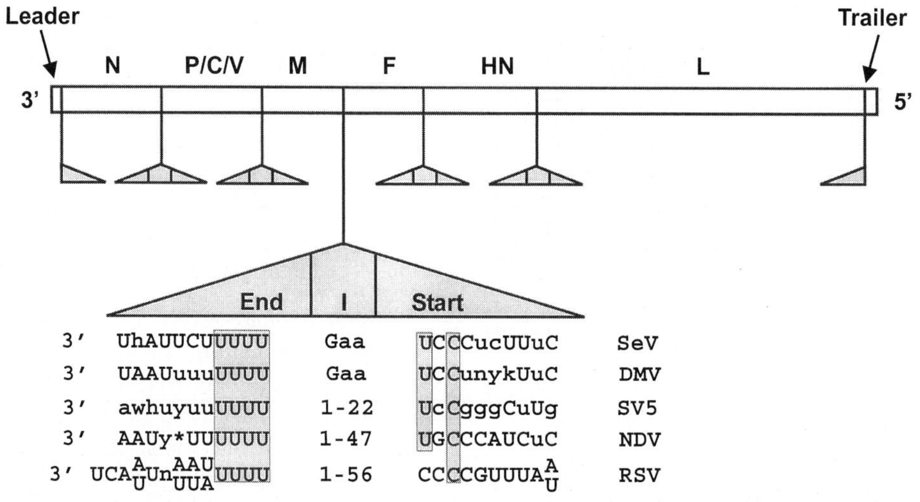

FIG. 6. Schematic diagram of a Paramyxovirus genome and the transcription end, intercistronic, and transcriptional start sequences. The positions of the extragenic 3′-terminal leader region and the 5′-terminal trailer region are shown. The conserved transcription regulatory sequences at the gene boundaries are indicated. These are sometimes known as E (end), I (intergenic), and S (start) sequences. The junctional sequences of representative viruses of each group, as (–) RNA, are shown. Nucleotides that are strictly conserved at each viral junctions are shown as *capital letters*; those that are mostly conserved (four of six junctions or better) are shown in *lower-case letters.* Other letters are used for less conservation. *, includes nucleotide deletions.

protein in a region predicted to be hydrophobic, and it could be involved in N:N contacts during assembly (190), but the presence of several conserved aromatic residues also suggests that it may be involved in RNA binding. In any event, N does not appear to be a classic RNA binding protein, in that it does not contain any previously recognized RNA-binding motifs, nor does N interact with RNAs after transfer of the N protein to nitrocellulose membranes and probing with RNA (Northwestern blots). The C-terminal tail, on the other hand, contains most of the N-protein phosphorylation sites and antigenic sites (133,239).

The structure–function relationship of the Sendai virus N protein was examined using a cDNA-encoded genome of a defective-interfering (DI) particle, whose intracellular replication was directed by N, P, and L protein expressed from cotransfected cDNAs (58) (see later section, Molecularly Engineered Genetics). The entire C-terminal tail of N was found to be dispensable for assembling an encapsidated, complementary copy of the template, whereas deletions anywhere within the N-terminal body of the protein eliminated this activity. Thus, the C-terminal tail is not essential for assembling the nascent chain and helping the polymerase to ignore the junctions. However, templates that were themselves assembled with tailless N proteins were unable to act as templates for new rounds of genome replication. The highly charged domain of the C-terminal tail appears to be essential for this function, as deletions downstream of this domain have little or no effect. The precise template function of the N-protein C-terminal tail is unclear, but it may be required for the transition between helical states, as nucleocapsids with tailless N protein appear more rigid in electron micrographs (194). The tail, moreover, appears to mediate P-protein binding to nucleocapsids, as binding of antibodies specific to the C-terminal tail leads to the release of the normally tightly bound P proteins, both for Sendai virus and hPIV-1 (239). Whether P binds directly to this C-terminal tail domain is unclear, but if so, it could participate in the helical transitions thought necessary for template function.

The P Gene and Its Encoded Proteins

For the *Paramyxovirinae*, the P gene represents an extraordinary example of a virus compacting as much genetic information as possible into a small gene. The P gene gives rise to a plethora of polypeptides by means of using overlapping reading frames on a single mRNA transcript, by a remarkable process of transcription known as RNA editing, or pseudotemplated addition of nucleotides. The consequence of the addition of pseudotemplated nucleotides to an mRNA is that there is a shift of a translational reading frame into an alternative reading frame, and hence a new protein is translated (Table 2). In this chapter, it will be considered that the P genes of the *Paramyxovirinae* are composed of a series of modules that are combined in various ways via mRNA editing, or as additional modules expressed via unusual translational initiation (16,59,103,169). An illogical sequence of letters (C, C′, D, I, P, V, W, X, Y1, Y2, and Z) has been used to name the various Paramyxovirus P gene products. However, based on some new biochemical data and some limited functional data for Sendai virus, a new nomenclature system is being introduced in this chapter, to describe the different P modules encoded by the P gene.

All viruses of the *Paramyxovirinae* (with the notable exception of hPIV-1) contain an editing site, at which G residues are inserted into the P mRNA in a programmed manner during its synthesis (Fig. 7, the dotted vertical line) (35,215,274,281). The number of G residues inserted varies between the different viruses and appears to be matched to the organization of their alternate ORFs. The editing site separates each P gene into two segments, and it generates three different mRNAs in which the three

TABLE 2. *Examples of expressible P gene open reading frames*

		Ribosomal choice				mRNA editing		
Paramyxovirus	Host	P	V	C′	C	D	V	P
Sendai	Mouse	+	–	+	+	–	+	–
hPIV1	Human	+	–	+	+	–	–	–
bPIV3	Cattle	+	–	–	+	+	+	–
hPIV3	Human	+	–	–	+	+	(+)	–
Mumps	Human	–	+	–	–	–	–	+
SV5	Dog	–	+	–	–	–	–	+
hPIV2 and hPIV4	Human	–	+	–	–	–	–	+
NDV	Fowl	+	–	–	–	–	+	–
Measles	Human	+	–	–	+	–	+	–
Canine distemper	Dog	+	–	–	+	–	+	–
Rinderpest	Cattle	+	–	–	+	–	+	–
Phocine distemper	Seals	+	–	–	+	–	+	–

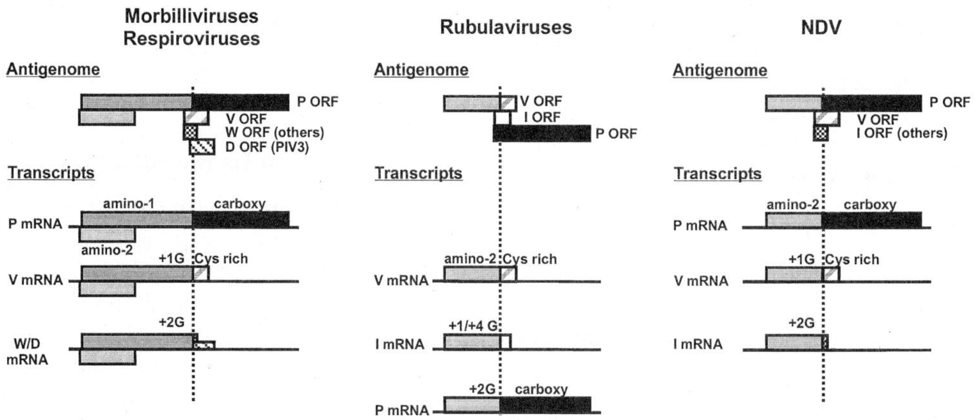

FIG. 7. Schematic diagram of the P gene of representative paramyxoviruses. For the respiroviruses and morbilliviruses, the mRNA for the P protein is transcribed faithfully (unedited) from the viral genome. Transcriptional RNA editing with the addition of one G nucleotide at the editing site produces an mRNA that encodes the V protein. Addition of two G nucleotides at the editing site produces an mRNA that encodes the W or D proteins (depending on the virus). The P mRNAs of the respiroviruses and morbilliviruses also contain the P-amino 2 (C protein) ORF at the 5′ end of the mRNA independent of editing status (*light shading*). The unedited version of the Rubulavirus "P" mRNA encodes the V protein (*light shading*); the addition of two G nucleotides produces the P mRNA and the addition of one G produces the I mRNA. NDV follows the Respirovirus and Morbillivirus pattern, and its unedited mRNA is translated to yield the P protein, and RNA editing produces the V mRNA. The cysteine-rich domain of the V protein is indicated by *cross-hatching.* The RNA editing site, at which nontemplated nucleotides are added to the mRNAs is indicated by the *vertical dotted line.* As described in the text, the P gene is translated into a series of proteins that are thought to consist of a series of modules. P-amino 1 (*medium shading*) and P-amino 2 (*light shading*) are two modules upstream of the RNA editing site, and P-carboxy (*black shading*) is the P module downstream of the RNA editing site. Some sequence relatedness and limited functional studies have led to the speculation that P-amino 2 (C ORF) of Respirovirus is functionally related to the N-terminal module of the Rubulavirus P and V proteins. Thus, the P-amino 1 module is unique to the respiroviruses and morbilliviruses.

possible reading frames downstream of the editing site are fused to a unique upstream ORF (see Fig. 7). These mRNAs are translated into three polypeptides with a common N-terminal segment and different C-terminal segments, called P, V, and W/D/I. In respiroviruses and morbilliviruses, additional P-gene complexity is provided by the presence of two (overlapping) ORFs (designated P-amino 1 and P-amino 2) upstream of the editing site, only one of which (P-amino 1) extends to the editing site. For Sendai virus and hPIV-1, the ORF that terminates before the editing site (P-amino 2, or C ORF) can also code for a nested set of up to four polypeptides, because of the use of four ribosomal initiation sites. For rubulaviruses, there is a single ORF upstream of the editing site (designated P-amino 2), which may be the counterpart of the respiroviruses and morbilliviruses C genes (see later). The mechanisms of expression of the protein products derived from the P gene are described later.

The Phosphoprotein

The P protein is the only P gene product that is essential for viral RNA synthesis (61), and it is involved in all its aspects. The Sendai virus P protein was first characterized as a homotrimer, but more recent biochemical evidence indicates the protein contains a coiled-coil domain that is tetrameric, and the entire protein is expected to be a tetramer (270). P protein is an essential component of the vRNAP and the nascent chain assembly complex (129), and additional P protein is also required during RNA synthesis (55). Although the L protein is thought to contain all vRNAP catalytic activities (222), L binds to the N:RNA template via the P proteins (129). This interaction between P and L requires a domain in P that maps to the C-terminal end of the coiled-coil oligomerization regions (Fig. 8) (62,238). This very C-terminal domain of P, which binds to the N:RNA, is predicted to form an α-helical bundle. These domains (all downstream of the editing site) that fall in the region called P-carboxy are essential for viral RNA synthesis. For Sendai virus, the P-carboxy region is also sufficient for RNA synthesis, as this protein fragment by itself (residues 325 to 568) can substitute for intact P protein in all aspects of mRNA synthesis (55,63). Thus, the P-carboxy region represents the polymerase (pol) cofactor module. This region is relatively well conserved in predicted secondary structure for all viruses of the *Paramyxovirinae*, and all P proteins carry this essential module as the C-terminal segment of a fusion protein; this module is never naturally expressed by itself. For respiroviruses, morbilliviruses, and NDV,

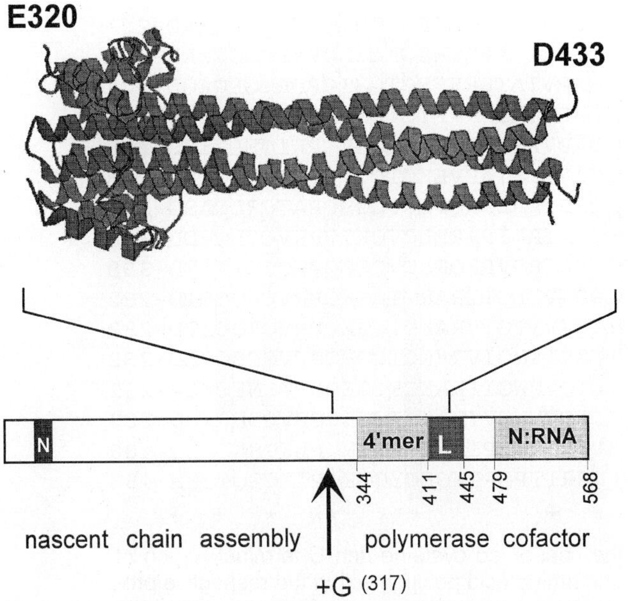

FIG. 8. Structure and function of the Sendai virus P protein. The P protein is shown below as a *horizontal bar.* Its known functional domains—namely, chaperoning unassembled N protein during the nascent chain assembly step of genome replication (N), self-assembly as a tetramer (4-mer), L protein binding site (L), and N:RNA binding site (N:RNA)—as determined by deletion analysis and discussed in the text, are indicated. Numbers refer to amino acid positions. The G insertion site (or editing site) in codon 317 used during mRNA synthesis, which separates the nascent chain assembly and polymerase cofactor domains of the P protein, is indicated. The core of the P protein homotetramer, a coiled coil of four parallel α-helices buttressed at their N-terminal ends by four short α-helical bundles (from E320 to D433), determined by x-ray crystallography (courtesy of Tabourieh and coworkers, EMBL, Grenoble, France, unpublished), is shown at the top of the figure.

the P-carboxy pol-cofactor module is translated from the unedited mRNA (see Fig. 7); for the viruses in the genus Rubulavirus, the P-carboxy pol-cofactor module is translated from an mRNA with a 2G insertion (see Fig. 7). Although little is known about the RSV P protein, it too is predicted to contain a coiled-coil domain, and it interacts with itself in a yeast two-hybrid system (256). P protein oligomerization thus appears to be a general property of this virus family.

For genome replication, in which RNA synthesis and assembly into nucleocapsids are coupled, at least for Sendai virus, one additional P-protein domain near the N-terminus (defined by deletion of residues 33 to 41) is also required (62). This domain apparently chaperones unassembled N protein during nascent chain assembly (assembly module), as the substrate for genome assembly is a P-N complex (129). The rest of the Sendai virus P protein is apparently dispensable for (unregulated) genome RNA synthesis and assembly, as a P protein in which residues 78 to 324 have been deleted is still quite active for mini-genome replication in transfected cells (62). The remaining P gene accessory proteins, like residues 78 to 324 of the Sendai virus P protein, are not required for the basic process of replicating viral genomes and expressing their mRNAs. Nevertheless, most of the accessory proteins play a role in regulating viral RNA synthesis, and/or in countering host cell defenses to viral infection. The properties and functions of the individual protein modules translated from the P gene are described next.

P Gene Modules (ORFs) Downstream of the Editing Site

Cysteine-Rich V ORF

The V ORF is found in the middle of the P gene of all three genera, and the V protein is expressed by all morbilliviruses and rubulaviruses, but only by some of the respiroviruses. In Sendai virus (281), bPIV-3 (219), the morbilliviruses (35), and NDV (258), the cysteine-rich V ORF is translated from an mRNA with a single G insertion, whereas in rubulaviruses the V protein is translated from the unedited mRNA (211,274). In either case, the resulting fusion protein is called V. The C-terminal portion of the V ORF is by far the best conserved of all the various P gene ORFs (Fig. 9), even though the V ORF is absent in hPIV-1 (184) and may not be expressed in hPIV-3 (76,93), both respiroviruses. There are seven perfectly conserved cysteine residues, and this domain binds two atoms of Zn^{2+} (176,212). The V domains of several (though not all) viruses specifically interact with the large subunit of the cellular damage-specific DNA-binding protein (UV-DDB) (175), but the consequences of this interaction and the function of V protein cysteine-rich domain remain to be elucidated. Like the P-carboxy pol-cofactor module, the cysteine-rich V ORF is found only as the C-terminal segment of a fusion protein; this module is never expressed by itself.

The W/D/I ORF

The W/D ORF of respiroviruses and morbilliviruses is expressed from mRNAs with two inserted G residues (see Fig. 7). For most of these viruses, the insertion of two G residues into the mRNA is relatively rare and the ORF is closed by a stop codon shortly after the editing site. In these cases, it is referred to as the W ORF, and the ensuing P-amino-W fusion protein is called the W protein. The W ORF appears to serve mainly to truncate the P protein, producing essentially the N-terminal P-amino 1 assembly module of the P protein by itself. Despite the low abundance of +2G mRNAs in Sendai virus–infected cells (about 10% of the total P mRNA), the Sendai virus W protein can be easily detected (57). In two closely related respiroviruses (b-PIV-3 and hPIV-3) (92,243), the

```
SV5     169-GFHRREYSIGWVGDEVKVTEWCNPSCSPITAAARRFECTCHQCPVTCSECERD-221
MuV     168-GGHRREWSLSWVQGEVRVFEWCNPICSPITAAARFHSCKCGNCPAKCDQCERD-220
SV41    172-GRHRREWSIAWVGDEVKVYEWCNPTCAPVTATDRKFSCTCGTCPDRCGECEGD-224
HPIV2   172-GNHRREWSIAWVGDQVKVFEWCNPRCAPVTASARKFTCTCGSCPSICGECEGD-224
HPIV4A  176-PRHRREYSISWVNGRTTISEWCNPCCAPVKSTASVEKCTCGRCPKICELCIRD-228
HPIV4B  176-PRHRREHSISWVNGRTTISEWCNPCCAPVKSIASVEKCTCGRCPKICELCIRD-228
NDV     175-PGHRREHSISWTMGGVTTISWCNPSCSPIRAEPRQYSCTCGSCPATCRLCASD-227
SeV     316-KGHRREHIIYERDGYIVDESWCNPVCSRIRIIPRRELCVCKTCPKVCKLCRDD-368
BPIV3   346-RGHRREHSIYREGDYIITESWCNPICSKIRPVPRQESCVCGECPKQCGYCIED-398
MeV     230-KGHRREISLIWDGDRVFIDRWCNPMCSKVTLGTIRARCTCGECPRVCEQCRTD-282
RPV     230-KGHRREIDLIWNDGRVFIDRWCNPTCSKVTVGTVRAKCICGECPRVCEQCITD-282
DMV     230-KGHRREISLIWDGDRVFIDRWCNPTCSRIKMGIVRVKCTCGECPPVCDECRED-282
CDV     230-KGHRREVSLTWNGDSCWIDKWCNPICTQVNWGIIRAKCFCGECPPTCNECKDD-282
PDV     230-KGHRREVSLTWNDDRCWIDKWCNPICTQVNWGVIRAKCICGECPPVCDDCKDD-282
TPMV    228-KGHRREYSMVWSNDGVFIESWCNPMCARIRPLPIREICVCGRCPLKCSKCLLD-280
HeV     404-KGHRREVSICWDGRRAWVEEWCNPVCSRITPQPRKQECYCGECPTECSQCCHE-456
              ****  +           **** *  +        * *  **  *  *  +
```

FIG. 9. Multiple amino acid sequence alignment of the conserved cysteine-rich C-terminal region of selected Paramyxovirus V proteins. *Numbers* indicate the amino acid position within the respective proteins. Conserved amino acid residues are shown in *boldface letters*, two areas of exceptionally high conservation are *boxed*, and the positions of the seven conserved cysteine residues are *shaded*. *Asterisks* and *plus symbols* below the alignment indicate identical and similar amino acid residues, respectively. The amino acid sequences of the Paramyxovirus species used in the alignment were from the P gene sequences indicated in Figure 1. (Adapted from ref. 276, with permission.)

+2 ORF extends for 131 amino acids from the editing site (and is called D), and +2G mRNAs are not rare in h/bPIV-3-infected cells [it has been observed that mRNAs with one to six inserted G residues are almost equally abundant (93,219)]. The encoded P-amino 1-D fusion protein is called the D protein. The Rubulavirus protein in which the single upstream ORF (P-amino 2) is fused to the third possible (+1/+4) downstream ORF is also found in Rubulavirus-infected cells, and it is called I (119,211). However, because of constraints of the Rubulavirus mRNA editing mechanism, a single G is rarely inserted at this editing site, and the I protein is expressed from a +4G mRNA (211,274). Thus, the Rubulavirus P, V, and W/D/I proteins contain the N-terminal module of the P-ORF (P-amino 2), fused to, respectively, the P polymerase cofactor module (P-carboxy), the V ORF, and the W/D/I ORF (depending on the virus) in the remaining reading frame.

P Gene Modules (ORFs) Upstream of the Editing Site

Two types of P gene ORF are found upstream of the editing site, P-amino 1 and P-amino 2. The rationale for this nomenclature is based on the available data, and on speculation that P-amino 2 of Sendai virus (formerly called the nest set of proteins C′, C, Y1, and Y2) have biochemical and sequence relationships to the N-terminal domain of the P protein of the rubulaviruses. Some limited data pertaining to the proteins of Sendai virus and SV5 involved in the interferon response to these viruses, also support the notion that the P-amino 2 domain of Sendai virus and the N-terminal P domain of SV5 are related in that they interact with different parts of the interferon-signalling pathway (see later). The P-amino 1 domain that is found only in respiroviruses and morbilliviruses is longer than P-amino 2 and is acidic in nature. P-amino 2, which is encoded by all P genes of the *Paramyxovirinae*, is shorter than P-amino 1 and is basic in nature.

P-Amino 1 Module

Unlike the downstream P-carboxy pol-cofactor module and the cysteine-rich V ORF module, whose conservation is evident across the entire virus subfamily, the ORF(s) upstream of the editing site are conserved only within each genus and can be very different between genera. For respiroviruses and morbilliviruses, the longer ORF (P-amino 1, with about 300 amino acids) that is fused to the downstream modules is relatively poorly conserved between genera, but they are all acidic in nature (pI of about 5.5). For Sendai virus, P-amino 1 contains a short region near the N-terminus (defined by deletion analysis) that is required to chaperone unassembled N protein as a P-N complex during the nascent chain assembly step of genome replication (62) (see Fig. 8). P-amino 1 also contains most of the serine and threonine phosphorylation sites of the P protein (23). The one or two major sites of each protein (and the respective kinases that catalyze the phosphorylation) are known for several viruses (66,136). For the respiroviruses, mutational analysis at these sites, within the context of an infectious cDNA and recovery of viable virus, has so far not been informative (134).

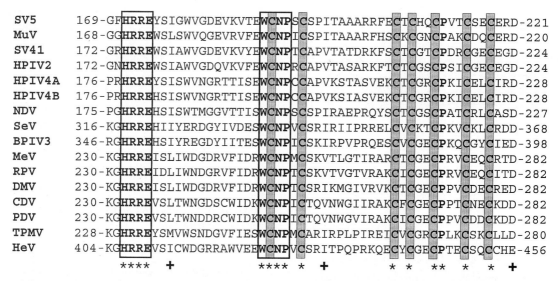

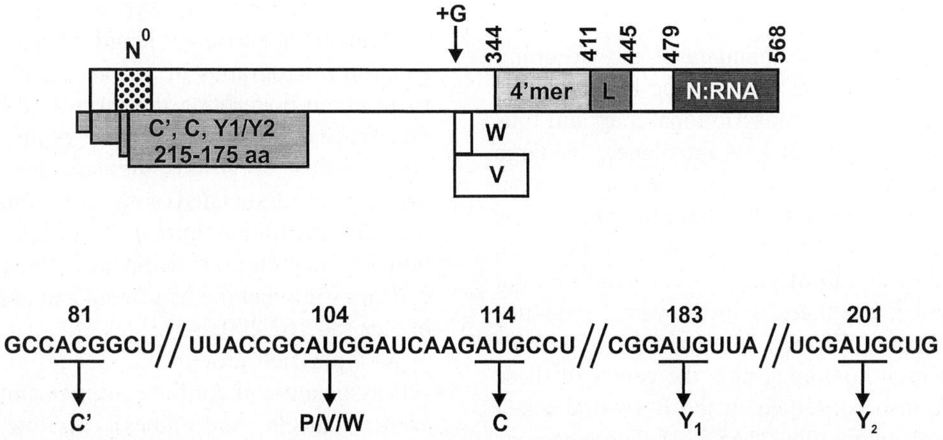

FIG. 10. Representation of the Sendai virus P mRNA to illustrate the use of multiple initiation codons. The nucleotide sequences surrounding the initiation codons for C′, P, C, Y_1, and Y_2, all of which are derived from the C ORF, are indicated. The various functional domains of the P protein are also indicated. Note that the Y_1 and Y_2 initiation sites overlap the N assembly domain of P. The AUG codon at position 104 also starts the V and W proteins in the edited P gene mRNAs. All the initiation codons (the ACG for C8), except for the first one, are in a suboptimal context for initiation.

P-Amino 2, Including the C ORFs

As discussed earlier, two of the criteria used for considering the single Rubulavirus ORF (P-amino 2) with the C ORF of respiroviruses and morbilliviruses is that they are both about 170 amino acids and are basic (pI of about 10.5) and show a small degree of sequence relatedness. For respiroviruses and morbilliviruses, the C ORF overlaps the P-amino 1 module, and it is accessed by translational choice (Fig. 10). Morbilliviruses express one C protein (10) as do the newly isolated Hendra virus (301), Nipah virus (105a), and tree shrew Morbillivirus (276), whereas the respiroviruses, such as Sendai virus and hPIV-1, express four C-like proteins (C′, C, Y1, and Y2) (60,99). The C protein ORFs of the respiroviruses and morbilliviruses are found at the same relative location on the P gene, and when their sequences are aligned there is clear conservation within each genus, but there is little conservation between these two genera. Although the NDV (avian Paramyxovirus) P gene does not contain a separate P-amino 2 ORF, the N-terminal domain of its P protein (before the editing site) is similar in size and overall charge to the P-amino 2 module and thus it may be a functional counterpart of the P-amino 2 (C) module. Similarly, for the rubulaviruses parts of the sequence of the V/P protein, shared N-terminal domain (P-amino 2) can be aligned with the Respirovirus P-amino 2 (C) protein sequence but not the Morbillivirus P-amino 2 (C) protein sequence (Fig. 11). Consistent with the different nature of the P protein N-terminal segments, the Respirovirus and Morbillivirus V proteins (P-amino 1 + V ORFs) are not found associated with viral nucleocapsids intracellularly or in virus particles (57,252), in contrast to the Rubulavirus V proteins (P-amino 2 + V ORFs), which are associated with intracellular nucleocapsids and found in virions (212,284). The various P-amino 2 ORFs may well serve different functions that are genus specific. Assuming that the various Paramyxovirus P proteins are functionally equivalent (N assembly module + pol-cofactor), the N assembly module would be contained within the P-amino 2 ORF of the Rubulavirus and NDV P protein.

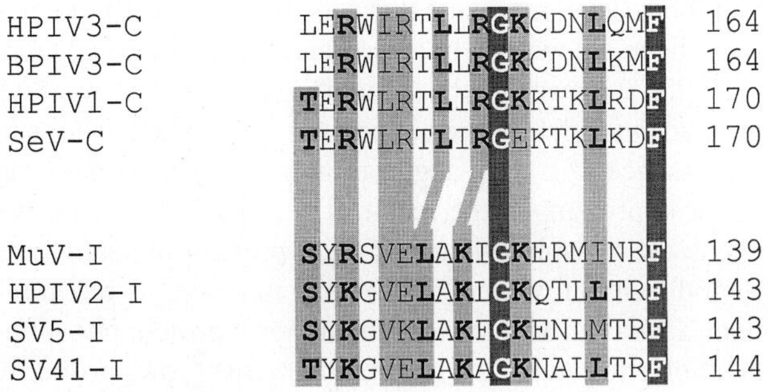
HPIV3-C LERWIRTLLRGKCDNLQMF 164
BPIV3-C LERWIRTLLRGKCDNLKMF 164
HPIV1-C TERWLRTLIRGKKTKLRDF 170
SeV-C TERWLRTLIRGEKTKLKDF 170
MuV-I SYRSVELAKIGKERMINRF 139
HPIV2-I SYKGVELAKIGKQTLLTRF 143
SV5-I SYKGVKLAKFGKENLMTRF 143
SV41-I TYKGVELAKAGKNALLTRF 144

FIG. 11. A short stretch of sequence relatedness between the Respirovirus C proteins and P-amino 2 ORF of the Rubulavirus V/P/I proteins. Amino acid sequence relatedness of a region of the C proteins of hPIV-3, bPIV-3, hPIV-1, and Sendai virus (SeV) with the V/P/I proteins of mumps virus (MuV), hPIV-2, SV5, and SV41. The position of the phenylalanine whose mutation to serine in Sendai virus and hPIV-3 attenuates virulence, is shown on the *right.* Residues that are conserved by amino acid assignment and spacing within the segment are indicated by *black boxes*: residues that are semiconserved by assignment or spacing are indicated by *gray boxes.*

The Large Protein

The L protein is the least abundant of the structural proteins (about 50 copies per virion). The L gene is the most promoter-distal in the transcriptional map and thus the last to be transcribed. Its low abundance, its large size, and its localization to transcriptionally active viral cores suggested that it might be the viral polymerase. The L genes of most paramyxoviruses have now been sequenced and they are all of very similar length (about 2,200 amino acids), but there is little overall sequence homology outside the subfamily. There are, however, five short regions of high homology near the center of these proteins that are also conserved in the RNA-dependent RNAPs of other virus families (145,222). These regions are thought to represent structural features of a common, ancestral polymerase "fold" (222). Mutational analysis of the highly conserved residues of these homology regions indicates that these regions are essential for RNAP activity (257).

The P and L proteins form a complex, and both proteins are required for polymerase activity with N:RNA templates (61,105,129). The precise composition of the viral polymerase is unclear, but transcriptionally active nucleocapsids contain five to ten P proteins per L protein, and this complex can make mRNA *in vitro*, which is capped at its 5′ end and also contains a poly(A) tail at the 3′ end. Polyadenylation is thought to result from polymerase stuttering on a short stretch of U residues, but the capping step requires both guanylyl and methyl transferase activities. These latter activities are thought to be provided by the L protein, by analogy to VSV (see Chapter 22), and because similar reactions have not been described for cellular enzymes that operate in the cytoplasm. The Sendai virus L protein purified from virions was also found to phosphorylate the N and P proteins, and it has been suggested that L is the kinase (80) that has long been known to be associated with the viral core (160,235). However, the Sendai virus P and V proteins are phosphorylated when expressed in transfected cells in the absence of L (64), suggesting that phosphate addition to these proteins is the result of cellular kinases. In any event, the phosphorylation of these proteins appears to be a modification without an obvious function, as recombinant Sendai virus that lacks the major P protein phosphorylation site can be rescued and this virus grows normally both in tissue culture and in mice (134).

The Matrix Protein

The Paramyxovirus matrix (M) protein is the most abundant protein in the virion. The nucleotide sequence of the M gene and predicted amino acid sequence of many paramyxoviruses indicate that these proteins contain 341 to 375 residues (M_r about 38,500 to 42,500), are quite basic proteins (net charge at neutral pH of +14 to +17), and are somewhat hydrophobic, although there are no domains of sufficient length to span a lipid bilayer. In electron micrographs of virions, an electron-dense layer is observed underlying the viral lipid bilayer and this is thought to represent the location of this protein. Fractionation studies of virions indicate that the M protein is peripherally associated with membranes and is not an intrinsic membrane protein. Reconstitution studies of purified M protein, and fractionation studies of infected cells indicate that the M protein can associate with membranes (84,162,200,245).

As a purified protein, the Sendai virus M protein can self-associate and form two-dimensional paracrystalline arrays (sheets and tubes) in low salt conditions (6,115,120), and there is a paracrystalline array of identical periodicity at the inner surface of the plasma membrane of infected cells when examined by EM after freeze-fracture (6). In addition, the M protein is also associated with nucleocapsids (261,299). The M protein probably contains amphipathic α-helices that insert themselves into the inner leaflet of the lipid bilayer, to coat this surface and organize its contacts with the helical nucleocapsid (15). Evidence that the M protein of Sendai virus interacts specifically with membranes expressing individually the F and HN glycoproteins has also been obtained, which implies that there is an interaction of the F and HN cytoplasmic tails with the M protein (246). Furthermore, genetically engineered recombinant measles virus and SV5 that lack glycoprotein cytoplasmic tails show a subcellular redistribution of the matrix protein (33,251). Thus, the M protein is considered to be the central organizer of viral morphogenesis, interacting with the cytoplasmic tails of the integral membrane proteins, the lipid bilayer, and the nucleocapsids. The self-association of M and its contact with the nucleocapsid may be the driving force in forming a budding virus particle (217). The relative abundance of basic residues in the M protein may reflect their importance in ionic interactions with the acidic N proteins.

Consistent with its central role in virus budding, M is often inactivated in persistent Paramyxovirus infections where budding fails to occur. For example, in subacute sclerosing panencephalitis (SSPE), a rare, progressive, and invariably fatal persistent measles virus infection of the brain, the M protein is either absent for a variety of reasons (reviewed in ref. 34) or, when present, is not associated with budding structures *in vivo* and is unable to bind to viral nucleocapsids *in vitro* (124,125). Although a genetically engineered recombinant measles virus that lacks an M protein has been obtained (32), it produces a four-log lower titer of released infectious particles than wild-type virus and remains mostly cell associated. Therefore it is reasonable to conclude that the M protein does play a very important function in virus assembly. Moreover, in model systems of persistent Sendai virus infection in culture in which the normally lytic infection is converted to a persistent one using DI particles, the change from a lytic to a persistent infection correlates mainly with M protein instability and an absence of budding structures (236).

The M protein of several paramyxoviruses is phosphorylated. For Sendai virus, a large proportion of the M protein is phosphorylated yet the M protein found in virions is not phosphorylated (163). However, a Sendai virus could be rescued from an infectious cDNA in which the single phosphorylation site in Sendai virus M protein had been eliminated (241). This M protein phosphorylation-minus mutant did not show an altered phenotype from wild-type virus in either cultured cells or mice. For the Rhabdovirus VSV, there is clear evidence that the VSV M protein that is associated with the RNP structure inhibits viral transcription (see Chapter 22). For *Paramyxovirinae*, there is no evidence that association of RNPs with M protein shuts down RNA synthesis in preparation for virus assembly, and this function may be carried out by another viral protein, such as the C protein.

Envelope Glycoproteins

All *Paramyxoviridae* possess two integral membrane proteins, and some rubulaviruses and all pneumoviruses encode a third integral membrane protein (Figs. 12 and 13). One glycoprotein (HN, H, or G) is involved in cell attachment and the other glycoprotein (F) in mediating pH-independent fusion of the viral envelope with the plasma membrane of the host cell. The assignment of specific biologic activities to individual glycoproteins was originally made on the basis of purification and reconstitution studies, mainly for the Sendai virus and SV5 proteins (248,250). For the respiroviruses and rubulaviruses, the attachment glycoprotein binds to cellular sialic acid–containing receptors, and these can be glycoproteins or glycolipids. The binding is probably of fairly low affinity but of sufficiently high avidity that these viruses agglutinate erythrocytes (hemagglutination). The attachment proteins of respiroviruses and rubulaviruses also have neuraminidase activity, and the proteins have been designated hemagglutinin-neuraminidase (HN). The Morbillivirus attachment protein (H) can cause agglutination of primate erythrocytes but lacks detectable neuraminidase or esterase activity. The restricted host range of measles virus for primate cells made it unlikely that sialic acid was the primary receptor for measles virus. It has been found that measles virus has a specific cellular receptor, the complement-binding protein known as either the membrane cofactor protein (MCP) or CD46 (74,201). The Pneumovirus RSV does not cause detectable hemagglutination, and the cellular

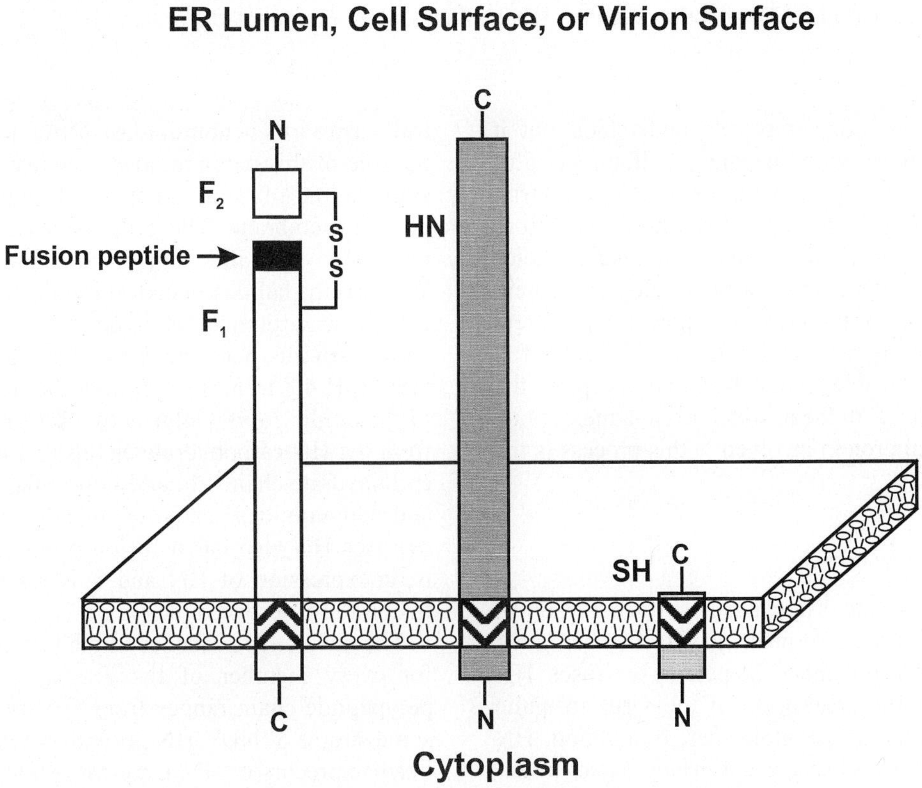

FIG. 12. Schematic diagram showing the orientation of Paramyxovirus integral membrane proteins. The F and HN protein orientations are shown. In *Paramyxovirnae*, only SV5 and mumps have an SH gene.

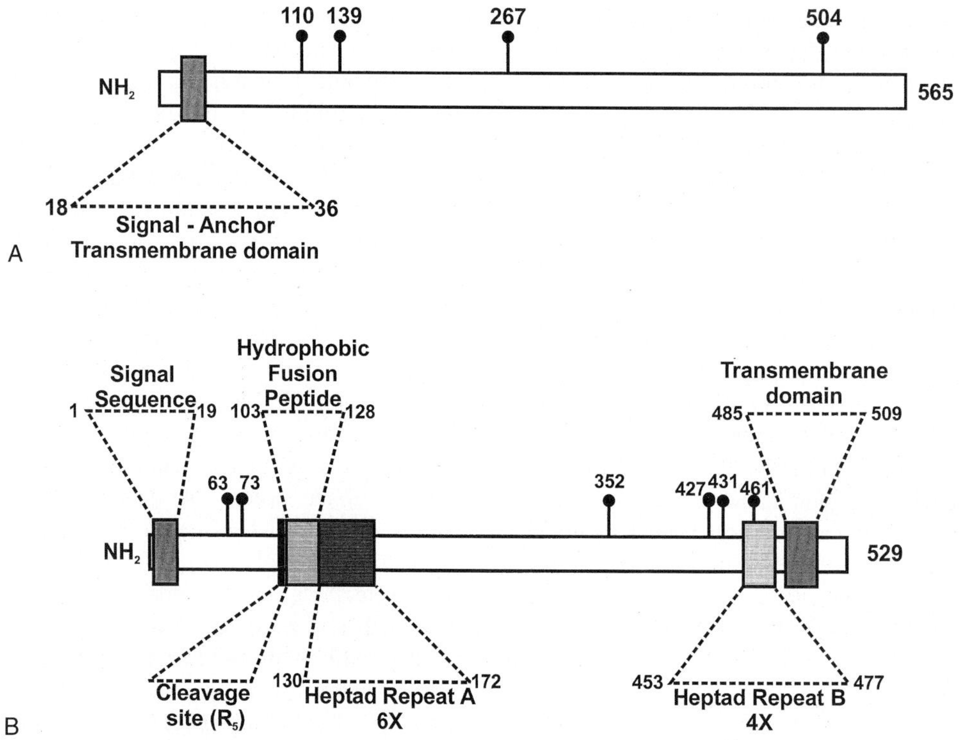

FIG. 13. Schematic diagram to show important domains and features of the Paramyxovirus glycoproteins. **A:** Hemagglutinin-neuraminidase attachment protein (based on the predicted sequence of the SV5 HN gene (121). The signal anchor transmembrane domain and the sites used for addition of N-linked carbohydrate (lollipops) (202) are indicated. **B:** Fusion protein (based on the predicted sequence of the SV5 F gene). The position of the signal sequence, the transmembrane domain, the cleavage site, the hydrophobic fusion peptide, and the heptad repeats A and B are indicated. The sites used for addition of N-linked carbohydrate (lollipops) (7) are indicated. R5 indicates the five arginine residues site for cleavage-activation. The heptad repeats A (six heptads) and B (four heptads) are shown.

receptor for RSV is not completely understood but it involves interactions with heparan sulfate, a glucosaminoglycan that is part of the extracellular matrix. Interestingly, the G protein of RSV can be deleted from the viral genome (146), and Sendai virus-like particles devoid of HN can infect cells via the asialoglycoprotein receptor (173). Both of these cases suggest the F protein may have a binding activity. After attachment of a *Paramyxoviridae* particle to the host-cell receptor, the viral envelope fuses with the host-cell plasma membrane, and the major viral protein involved in this process is the F glycoprotein.

Attachment Protein

The Respirovirus and Rubulavirus surface glycoprotein HN is a multifunctional protein as well as being the major antigenic determinant of the paramyxoviruses. HN is responsible for the adsorption of the virus to sialic acid–containing cell-surface molecules. In addition, HN mediates enzymatic cleavage of sialic acid (neuraminidase activity) from the surface of virions and the surface of infected cells. By analogy to the role of influenza virus neuraminidase (NA), it seems likely that the role of this neuraminidase activity is to prevent self-aggregation of viral particles during budding at the plasma membrane. These dual activities of HN can be modulated by halide ion concentration and pH (186). Whereas the halide ion concentration and pH of the extracellular environment is optimal for hemagglutination, Paramyxovirus neuraminidases have an acidic pH optimum (pH 4.8 to 5.5) suggesting that neuraminidase acts in the acidic *trans* Golgi network to remove sialic acid from the HN carbohydrate chains and from the F protein carbohydrate chains. In addition to the hemagglutinating and neuraminidase activities of HN, for most paramyxoviruses HN also has a fusion promoting activity—that is, coexpression of HN and F is required for cell–cell fusion to be observed (see later).

The nucleotide sequence of the HN gene is now known for every member of the *Paramyxovirinae*. The HN polypeptide chain ranges from 565 to 582 residues. For some strains of NDV, HN is synthesized as a biologically inactive precursor (HN_0), and 90 residues from the C-terminus are removed to activate the molecule (199,200). A schematic diagram of important features of the HN amino acid sequence is shown in Figure 13. The HN proteins are type II integral membrane proteins that span the membrane once. The HN protein contains a single hydrophobic domain, located close to the N-terminus, that acts as a combined signal and anchorage domain, targeting the nascent chain as it emerges from the ribosome to the membrane of the endoplasmic reticulum (ER) and ensuring the translocation of the polypeptide chain across the membrane, bringing about the stable anchoring of the protein in the lipid bilayer. This orientation of HN (see Fig. 12) is analogous to that of the influenza virus NA. Interestingly, all of the cellular enzymes that are resident in compartments of the exocytic pathway and that use carbohydrates as substrates are type II integral membrane proteins, suggesting evolution of all carbohydrate-modifying enzymes from a common progenitor.

The HN glycoproteins contain from four to six sites for the addition of N-linked carbohydrate chains. For the SV5 HN molecule, it has been shown that four sites are used (202). The Paramyxovirus HN glycoproteins have conserved cysteine, proline, and glycine residues between related paramyxoviruses, strongly suggesting a similarity of protein structure. HN forms an oligomer consisting of disulfide-linked homodimers that form a noncovalently linked tetramer. The oligomeric form of HN has been examined in detail by using bifunctional cross-linking reagents and sucrose density gradient analysis (179,193,203,237,275). Sendai virus HN molecules that were proteolytically removed from the surface of virions (at residue 131) retain enzymatic activity and with EM appeared as box-shaped molecules (10 × 10 nm) consisting of four subunits with fourfold symmetry (275). For the Paramyxovirus HN protein, the type II membrane orientation, the presence of a protease-accessible stalk that is not essential for enzymatic activity, and the existence of a tetrameric oligomeric form all parallel influenza virus NA. In addition, Paramyxovirus HN proteins contain a conserved sequence N-R-K-S-K-S that is similar to the known sialic acid binding site of influenza virus NA (280; reviewed in ref. 192). Computer modelling studies predicted that HN will have a β-sheet propeller motif similar to NA of influenza virus (50,166), and the recently obtained atomic structure of NDV HN bears out these predictions (54) (Fig. 14).

For years, it was a matter of debate as to whether HN molecules contain combined or separate active sites for hemagglutinating and neuraminidase activities. Some evidence has been interpreted to indicate a single site that binds sialic acid tightly (hemagglutination) but hydrolyses the molecule slowly (neuraminidase) (249), whereas studies with temperature-sensitive mutants and monoclonal antibody inhibition of activities had been interpreted to suggest there are separate sites for the two activities (223,225). However, analysis of the atomic structure of the NDV HN protein suggests the presence of only a single sialic binding site (54).

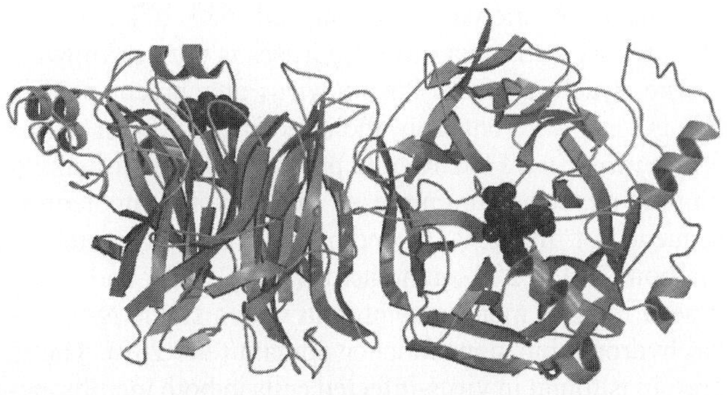

FIG. 14. The hemagglutinin-neuraminidase three-dimensional structure. Protease released, purified NDV HN was crystallized in the presence of the general sialidase/neuraminidase inhibitor 2-deoxy-2,3-dehydro-N-acetyl neuraminic acid (Neu5ac2n, or DANA). In the crystal, the molecule exists as a dimer whose parts are arranged such that the active sites are roughly at 90° to one another. The picture therefore shows a top and side view of each other monomer. The fold of each monomer is the characteristic β-propeller found in other neuraminidases, such as that of influenza virus. DANA is shown bound to the molecule. Structural studies have shown that the sialic acid binding (hemagglutinin) and sialic acid hydrolysis (neuraminidase) sites occupy the same location on the molecule. A structural difference was observed in HN crystallized alone or in complex with the receptor, suggesting a possible mechanism for transmission of a conformational change upon sialic acid binding that could trigger fusion through interactions of HN with the fusion protein. (Figure of the three-dimensional structure of the NDV HN provided by Susan Crennell, Toru Takimoto, Allen Portner, and Garry Taylor.)

The SV5 HN protein, upon being transported to the cell surface, is rapidly internalized by the clathrin-mediated endocytosis pathway (171). The signal for internalization is unusual as it is not located in the cytoplasmic tail but rather at the boundary of the transmembrane (TM) domain and the ectodomain (172). The reason for the internalization of SV5 HN, a process seemingly in conflict with virus assembly, is not known.

The Morbillivirus attachment protein (H) has extensive sequence relatedness and similarity with the HN glycoprotein of respiroviruses and rubulaviruses (reviewed in ref. 192). However, as discussed previously, the Morbillivirus H glycoprotein lacks detectable neuraminidase activity. Measles virus infection is restricted to cells derived from higher primates, and this observation eventually led to identification of the measles virus cellular receptor molecule as CD46, a complement cofactor (74,201), The measles virus receptor CD46 is a low-abundance cell surface protein, and in measles virus–infected cells the expression of CD46 is down-regulated. Therefore, CD46 is unlikely to cause virus aggregation during virus budding. Thus, measles virus, and morbilliviruses in general, may not need a neuraminidase activity in the manner in which other paramyxoviruses need a neuraminidase activity to act as a receptor-destroying enzyme to free the virus from the cell surface. The receptor for CDV and other morbilliviruses is not yet known.

The structure of the Pneumovirus attachment protein (G) is very different from the attachment protein of the *Paramyxovirinae*. The RSV G protein has neither hemagglutinating nor neuraminidase activity. The nucleotide sequence of the RSV G gene predicts that the protein is of about 289 to 299 amino acids (M_r 32,587), and it is a type II integral membrane protein with a single N-terminal hydrophobic signal/anchor domain (247,289). The G protein is found in virus-infected cells in both membrane-bound and proteolytically cleaved soluble forms. The distinguishing feature of the RSV G protein is the extent of its carbohydrate modification. On SDS polyacrylamide gel electrophoresis, the protein migrates with an apparent M_r of about 84,000 to 90,000, and the dramatic increase in molecular weight over that predicted for the polypeptide chain is because 8 to 12 kd is caused by the addition of N-linked carbohydrate (four potential addition sites) and 40 to 50 kd is caused by the addition of O-linked glycosylation (77 potential acceptor serine or threonine residues; 30% of total residues) (44,290, and references therein). Quite remarkably, it appears the RSV G protein is not essential for virus assembly or growth in tissue culture or animals, but it does confer a growth advantage. A virus that had been extensively passaged in cells was found to contain a spontaneous deletion of the G and SH genes (146), yet the virus replicated in Vero cells. In addition, the G gene has been deleted from recombinant virus recovered from an infectious cDNA clone (see Chapter 45 in *Fields Virology*, 4th ed.). These finding suggest that RSV has an alternative mechanism for attachment to cells that does not involve G protein.

Fusion Protein

The Paramyxovirus fusion (F) proteins mediate viral penetration by fusion between the virion envelope and the host cell plasma membrane, and this fusion event occurs at neutral pH. The consequence of the fusion reaction is that the nucleocapsid is delivered to the cytoplasm. Later in infection, the F proteins expressed at the plasma membrane of infected cells can mediate fusion with neighboring cells to form syncytia (giant cell formation), a cytopathic effect that can lead to tissue necrosis *in vivo* and might also be a mechanism of virus spread.

Paramyxovirus fusion proteins are synthesized as an inactive precursor (F_0) that is cleaved by a host-cell protease. This releases the new N-terminus of F_1, thus forming the biologically active protein consisting of the disulfide-linked chains F_1 and F_2 (128,250). The Paramyxovirus F genes encode 540 to 580 residues (see Fig. 13). The F proteins are type I integral membrane proteins, which span the membrane once and contain at their N-terminus a cleavable signal sequence that targets the nascent polypeptide chain synthesis to the membrane of the ER. At their C-termini, a hydrophobic stop-transfer domain (a TM domain) anchors the protein in the membrane, leaving a short cytoplasmic tail (about 20 to 40 residues). Comparison of the amino acid sequences of Paramyxovirus F proteins (reviewed in ref. 192) does not show overall major regions of sequence identity, but the similar placement of cysteine, glycine, and proline residues together with the overall hydrophobicity of the F proteins suggests a similar structure for all F proteins. The Respirovirus and Rubulavirus F_2 and F_1 subunits are glycosylated and there are a total of three to six potential sites for the addition of N-linked carbohydrate. For SV5 F protein, it is known that all four potential sites for addition of N-linked carbohydrate are used (7). The Morbillivirus F protein contains three sites in the F_2 subunit for N-linked carbohydrate addition, and all three sites are used, and there are no sites in F_1 for N-linked carbohydrate addition (2).

Protein sequencing studies of the F protein and nucleotide sequencing studies of the F genes have indicated that the N-terminal 25 residues of F_1 (fusion peptide) are extensively hydrophobic and this region of the F protein is highly conserved among F proteins of the *Paramyxovirinae* (up to 90% identity) (Fig. 15). The Paramyxovirus fusion peptides are thought to intercalate into target membranes, initiating the fusion process, and evidence for direct insertion into bilayers has been obtained using hydrophobic photoaffinity labeling probes (204). It has also been shown that the fusion peptides are sufficiently hydrophobic that they can act as a TM anchor domain to convert a formerly soluble protein to a membrane-bound form (210). The invariant nature of many of the residues of the fusion peptide between Paramyxovirus F proteins suggests a role more complex than preservation of hydrophobic residues required for a membrane-intercalating domain; neither signal sequences nor membrane anchorage domains show sequence conservation beyond their hydrophobic nature. It has been noted that if the fusion peptide is assumed to be an α-helix, then the invariant residues are located on one face of the helix (255). Interestingly, in a study on the conserved residues of the fusion peptide when the glycine residues at position 3, 7, or 12 were changed to alanine, and the altered F proteins expressed, a dramatic increase in syncytium formation was observed (130). Thus, the invariant amino acids in the fusion peptide may preserve a balance between high fusion activity and successful viral replication, as high fusion activity is deleterious to cell viability.

The fusion proteins of several widely disparate viruses share several important common features. The Paramyxovirus F protein, the human and simian immunodeficiency virus (HIV and SIV) gp160, Ebola virus GP, and influenza virus hemagglutinin (HA) protein all form homotrimers (26,39,85,237,296) that must be proteolytically cleaved to be biologically active (144,153,250). The resulting TM domain–containing subunits (Paramyx-

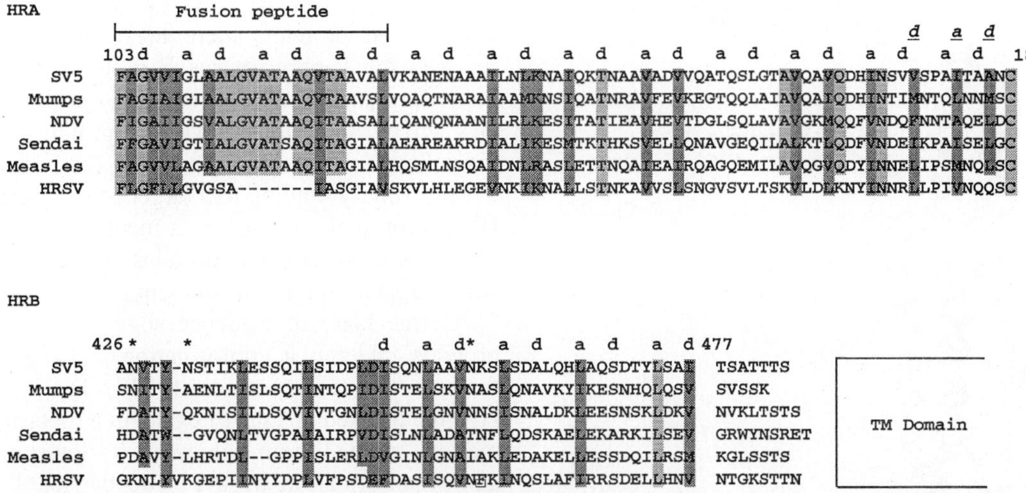

FIG. 15. Sequence alignment of the fusion peptide and the heptad repeats HRA and HRB of the SV5 F protein with that of other paramyxoviruses. Conserved residues among members of the *Paramyxovirinae* (i.e., not including hRSV) are *shaded light gray* and residues with similar properties (hydrophobic or charged) are *shaded dark gray.* Those residues that are also conserved in HRSV, which is evolutionarily distant from other paramyxoviruses, are indicated in the HRSV sequence with the appropriate shading. Letters immediately above the sequence indicate the predicted hydrophobic heptad repeat a and *d* residues. The predicted heptad is incorrect for residues 175 to 184, and the observed *a* and *d* residues in the atomic structure (see Fig. 16) are indicated above the predicted repeat and underlined. *Asterisks* indicate N-linked carbohydrate sites for the SV5 F protein. The SV5 sequence is numbered. NDV, Newcastle disease virus; HRSV, human respiratory syncytial virus. (Adapted from ref. 8, with permission.).

ovirus F, F_1; HIV gp160, gp41; Ebola GP, GP2; influenza HA, HA_2), contain a hydrophobic fusion peptide at the new N-termini, which has been shown to insert into the target membrane during the fusion process (4,65,104, 118). Additionally, two 4-3 heptad repeat regions are present in each of these fusion proteins, one near the fusion peptide and one in close proximity to the TM domain (20,38). These regions are thought to be important in the fusion reaction, as mutations within these domains frequently lead to a fusion-deficient phenotype (29,42,240, 254), and peptides corresponding to these regions have been demonstrated to block the fusion process (139,142, 165,177,196,229,293,294,297,300).

The atomic structure of uncleaved and cleaved influenza virus HA are known (40,296). However, this is not the case for the intact glycoproteins HIV-1/SIV gp160, Ebola virus GP, or the Paramyxovirus F protein. However, biochemical, EM, nuclear magnetic resonance, and x-ray crystallographic analyses of most of HA_2 (22), portions of HIV-1/SIV gp41 (12,25,39,177,264,286,287), a portion of a retrovirus Env-TM domain (85), and most of Ebola virus GP2 (178,285) indicate that their heptad repeat regions show considerable similarity in that they all form trimeric coiled coils, with the N-terminal heptad repeat forming an interior, trimeric coiled coil surrounded by three antiparallel helices. This structure has been suggested to represent the final, most stable form of the protein, present either during or subsequent to membrane fusion, with peptide inhibitors most likely functioning by preventing formation of this core (12,177).

The Paramyxovirus F protein membrane proximal subunit (F_1) differs from that of HA_2, gp41, Env-TM, and GP2 because its ectodomain is much larger in size (383 residues versus 120 to 185 residues). F_1 contains two heptad repeat regions, one (HRA) adjacent to the fusion peptide and the other (HRB) adjacent to the TM domain (see Fig. 13). In contrast to the HA_2, gp41, Env-TM, and GP2 just described, where heptad repeats are separated only by small spacer regions, in paramyxoviruses about 250 residues separate the heptad repeat regions. Nonetheless, biochemical and EM analysis indicated that the Paramyxovirus heptad repeat peptides form a rod-shaped structure approximately 96 Å in length. Peptides (N-1) derived from HRA form a three-stranded α-helical coiled coil around which three peptides (C-1) derived from HRB are packed in an antiparallel manner. The N-terminus of N-1 and the C-terminus of C-1 are localized to the same end of the rod, placing the fusion peptides and TM domains close together (77,142). These biochemical data were confirmed by solving the crystal structure of the SV5 F_1 N-1/C-1 complex to 1.4 Å resolution (8). The 64 amino acids of N-1 fold into an 18-turn α-helix stretching the entire length of the coiled coil. The C-terminal 25 residues of C-1 form a seven-turn amphipathic α-helix, whereas amino acids 440 to 450 form an extended chain (Figs. 16 and 17).

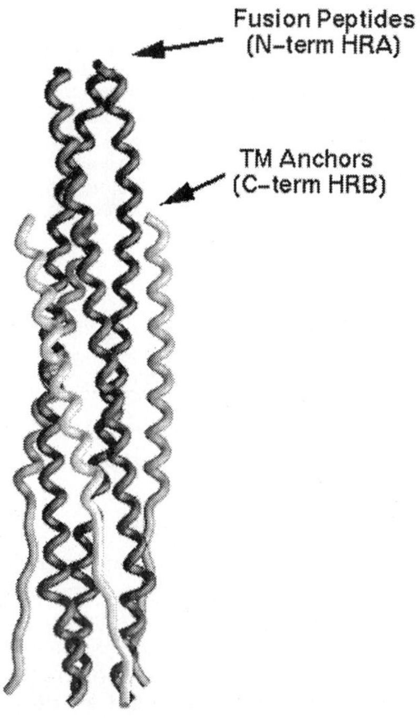

FIG. 16. The SV5 F1 core trimer structure. The complete SV5 F1 core trimer is shown. The central HRA (N-1) trimeric coiled coil is shown in *dark gray* and the buttressing antiparallel HRB (C-1) helices are shown in *light gray.* (Adapted from ref. 8, with permission.)

Despite the similarity of core structure among these viral fusion proteins, there are important differences between the Paramyxovirus F proteins and other viral fusion proteins. Unlike influenza virus HA protein and HIV gp160, the Paramyxovirus F protein does not provide the primary binding role for the virus: Paramyxovirus primary binding to a target cell is mediated by the HN glycoprotein. However, as mentioned before, at least two *Paramyxoviridae* F proteins, those of Sendai and RSVs, appear to have attachment activity.

A large body of evidence suggests that viral fusion proteins undergo a conformational change to become fusion active (reviewed in ref. 117). For influenza virus HA, the cleaved HA (296) exists in a metastable conformation, trapped from achieving its lower-energy fusogenic conformation by a kinetic barrier. During virus uncoating in endosomes, the low pH environment of the endosomal lumen triggers a conformational change in HA, in which two separate α-helical regions in HA_2 (296) rearrange to form a single triple-stranded coiled coil (22,41). After this conformational change, the fusion peptide is relocated by about 100 Å to one end of the rod-shaped coiled coil (22): the basis of the "spring-loaded mechanism" of fusion (30). For HIV-1 gp120/gp41 and retrovirus Env-SU+Env-TM, binding to the viral receptor may induce the conformational change to release the

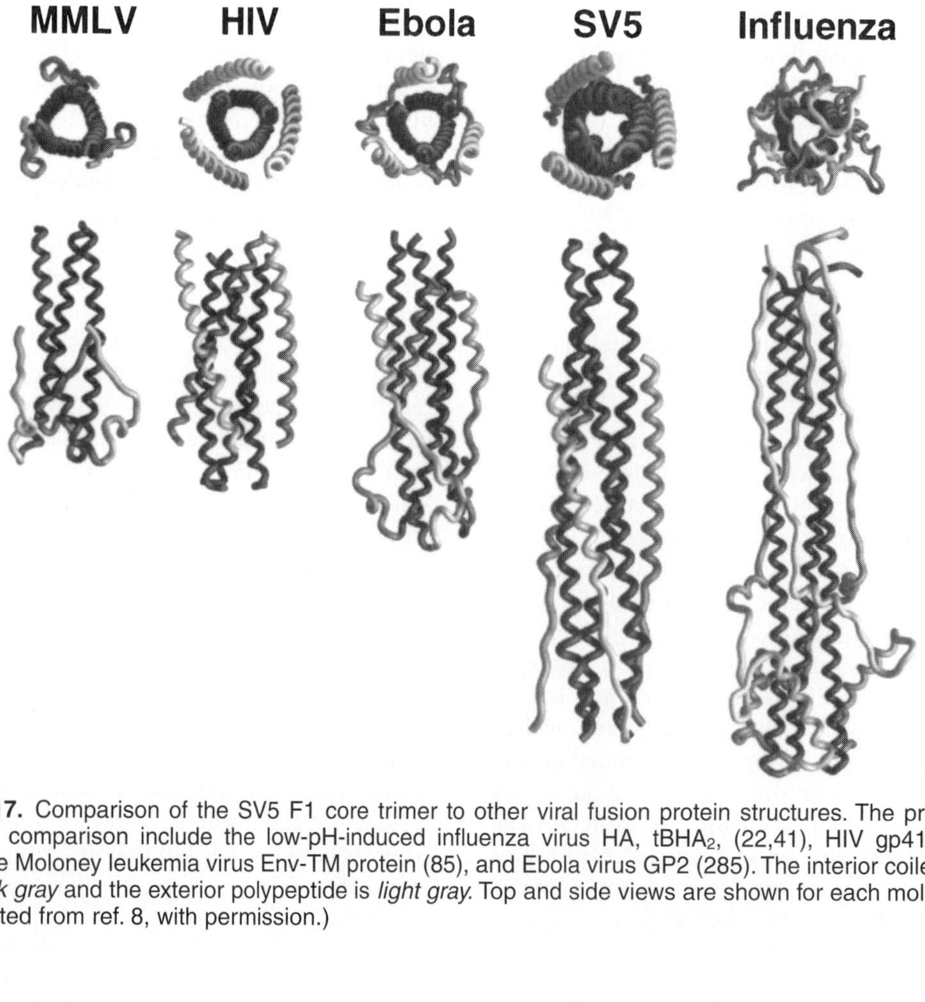

FIG. 17. Comparison of the SV5 F1 core trimer to other viral fusion protein structures. The proteins under comparison include the low-pH-induced influenza virus HA, $tBHA_2$, (22,41), HIV gp41 (39), murine Moloney leukemia virus Env-TM protein (85), and Ebola virus GP2 (285). The interior coiled coil is *dark gray* and the exterior polypeptide is *light gray.* Top and side views are shown for each molecule. (Adapted from ref. 8, with permission.)

fusion peptide (65,91,189). The trigger for the putative conformational changes of Paramyxovirus F proteins is unknown, although as described later for many paramyxoviruses there is a requirement for HN in mediating the fusion reaction (reviewed in ref. 161).

Although the Paramyxovirus F protein is the principal viral glycoprotein involved in virus–cell and cell–cell fusion, the emerging picture indicates the presence of a complex biologic machine. The SV5, measles virus, or RSV F cDNAs when expressed in mammalian cells cause syncytium formation (1,2,131,143,206,209,214), although it is important to note it is likely that many more cells express the F protein than are found in multinucleated cells (209). However, for many other paramyxoviruses including NDV, hPIV-2, hPIV-3, bPIV-3, mumps virus, and CDV (37,78,131,135,191,242,271,295,298) coexpression of F and HN (H for the morbilliviruses) is required for syncytium formation. Furthermore, there is a requirement that the homologous (i.e., of the same virus) HN, and not a heterologous HN, be coexpressed in the same cell (131,135, 253). Thus, it has been suggested that a type-specific interaction occurs between the HN and F protein that is necessary for fusion to occur (135,161,253). A great deal of effort has been spent to map the regions of F and HN that interact. Mutations have been identified in the HN globular domain (68,188), stalk region (253,260,302), and TM anchor (17,185) that decrease or abolish fusogenic activity with no effect on receptor recognition. Analysis of the fusion-promoting activity of chimeric HN molecules derived from different paramyxoviruses suggests that both the TM domain (with much of the stalk region) and parts of the globular head impart F specificity (70,265,278). Coimmunoprecipitation assays also indicate that F and HN can exist in a complex (259,298), and that for hPIV-3, F and HN undergo antibody-induced co-capping indicative of protein complex formation (298). Perhaps most intriguingly, a point mutation was found in the NDV HN globular head that abolishes both its receptor recognition and neuraminidase activity, and that also abolishes its ability to interact with F in coimmunoprecipitation assays (69). These latter data suggest that HN interacts with F only after binding its receptor.

A model that would rationalize the involvement of HN (or H) in fusion promotion is one in which the hypothesized conformational change in F to release the fusion peptide is highly regulated. For those *Paramyxovirinae* that require HN (or H) and F to be coexpressed to observe fusion, the first step would be the binding of HN (or H) to its receptor. On binding ligand, the HN (or H) protein would undergo its own conformational change, which in turn could trigger a conformational change in F to release the fusion peptide. In this way, F and HN operate as a coupled molecular scaffold to release and direct the fusion peptide to the target membrane (reviewed in ref. 161). Examination of mutants of SV5 F protein that require coexpression of HN to mediate fusion indicates that the HN function for F protein triggering can be supplanted by providing energy from raising the temperature, suggesting that the F–HN interaction provides energy to convert cleaved F from a metastable form to a fusogenic form (213).

Cleavage Activation

As discussed, the precursor F_0 molecule is biologically inactive and cleavage of F_0 to the disulfide linked subunits F_1 and F_2 activates the protein, rendering the molecule fusion-active and permitting viral infectivity. Thus, cleavage of F_0 is a candidate to be a key determinant for infectivity and pathogenicity, and for certain viruses this appears to be the case. Proteolytic activation of F_0 involves the sequential action of two enzymes, the host protease that cleaves at the carboxyl side of an arginine residue, and a host carboxypeptidase that removes the basic residues. The *Paramyxoviridae* can be divided into two groups: those that have F proteins with multiple basic residues at the cleavage site and those with F proteins that have a single basic residue at the cleavage site (Table 3). Cleavage of F proteins containing multiple basic residues at the cleavage site occurs intracellularly during transport of the protein through the *trans* Golgi network.

Furin is a cellular protease localized to the *trans* Golgi network, and its sequence specificity for cleavage is R-X-K/R-R. The available evidence suggests that furin, a subtilisin-like endoprotease, is the (or one of the) protease(s) that cleaves F proteins intracellularly (207; reviewed in ref. 153).

Paramyxoviruses that have F proteins with single basic residues in the cleavage site (e.g., Sendai virus) are not usually cleaved when grown in tissue culture and, thus, only a single cycle of growth is obtained. However, the F_0 precursor that is expressed at the cell surface and incorporated into released virions can be cleavage-activated by the addition of exogenous protease (250), leading to multiple rounds of replication.

TABLE 3. *Amino acid sequences upstream of the F protein cleavage site of some members of the* Paramyxoviridae

Sendai virus	G - V - P - Q - S - R ↓
hPIV1	D - N - P - Q - S - R ↓
hPIV3	D - P - **R** - T - **K** - **R** ↓
SV5	T - R - **R** - R - **R** - **R** ↓
Mumps	S - R - **R** - H - **K** - **R** ↓
NDV (virulent strain)	G - R - **R** - Q - **R/K** - **R** ↓
NDV (avirulent strain)	G/E - G - K/R - Q - G/S - R ↓
Measles	S - R - **R** - H - **K** - **R** ↓
RS V	K - K - **R** - K - **R** - **R** ↓

Consensus sequence for furin protease cleavage is

R - X - **R/K** - **R** ↓

Data from Hosaka et al. (125).

Purification of a protease from the allantoic fluid of embryonated chicken eggs has indicated that the endoprotease responsible for Sendai virus activation is homologous to the blood clotting factor Xa, a member of the prothrombin family (100,102). A protease with a similar substrate specificity is secreted from Clara cells of the bronchial epithelium in rats and mice, and this enzyme is probably responsible for activating paramyxoviruses in the respiratory tract. For NDV, the nature of the cleavage site correlates with virulence of the virus. Those strains with multiple basic residues in the F_0 cleavage site are virulent and readily disseminate through the host, whereas those strains with F_0 molecules having single basic residues are avirulent and tend to be restricted to the respiratory tract where the necessary secreted protease can be found (199).

Other Envelope Proteins

The rubulaviruses SV5 and mumps virus both contain a small gene located between F and HN, designated SH (122,123). The SV5 SH protein is a 44-residue, type II integral membrane protein that is expressed at the plasma membrane and is packaged in virions (see Fig. 12). The functional role of SH in the replicative cycle of SV5 is unknown, and in tissue culture cells it can be deleted from an infectious cDNA and recombinant SV5 recovered (111). For mumps virus, although an mRNA transcript derived from the SH gene has been detected (81,82), identification of the SH protein was accomplished only recently (262).

Members of the *Pneumovirinae* also encode an SH protein. The RSV SH protein contains 64 amino acids and is expressed at the plasma membrane of RSV-infected cells as a type II integral membrane protein, and it is packaged in virions (49,205). In RSV-infected cells, four SH-related polypeptide species have been identified: The M_r 4,800 species is thought to result from the initiation of protein synthesis at an internal AUG codon; the M_r 7,500 species is unglycosylated SH; the M_r 13,000 to 15,000 species is SH containing one high mannose N-linked carbohydrate chain; and the M_r 21,000 to 30,000 species is generated by the addition of polylactosaminoglycan to the N-linked carbohydrate chain (3,205). The SH gene was found to be deleted spontaneously from a virus passaged extensively *in vitro* (146), and it has been deleted from recombinant RSV (21) with only minor alterations in virus growth properties in tissue culture cells, or in the respiratory tract of mice or chimpanzees. Thus, the role of the SH protein in the RSV life cycle is not understood.

Pneumovirus M2 Gene

The RSV M2 gene contains two partially overlapping ORFs, designated M2-1 and M2-2, which give rise to two proteins, M2-1 (194 amino acids) and M2-2 (90 amino acids), respectively (47). The mechanism for translating the M2-2 ORF is not clear, but it may involve a ribosomal stop-restart mechanism analogous to that used for synthesis of the influenza B virus BM2 protein (132) (see Chapter 24). The M2-1 protein is an essential transcriptional elongation factor (45,87), and in its absence the polymerase does not transcribe beyond the NS1 and NS2 genes (87). The M2-1 gene also increases RNAP processivity across the gene junctions, attenuating transcriptional termination (87,106,107). The M2-2 gene is not essential for RSV growth, as it can be deleted from a recombinant RSV (11,140). However, the ΔM2-2 virus grows slowly in tissue culture and there is an increase in transcription and decrease in RNA replication (11,140), suggesting that M2-2 protein is involved in regulating transcription and RNA replication.

Pneumovirus NS1 and NS2 Genes

The RSV NS1 (139 amino acids) and NS2 (124 amino acids) are considered to be nonstructural proteins, although the difficulty in purifying virions from contaminating infected-cell debris for this poorly growing virus makes this assignment provisional. Neither protein is thought to be essential for virus growth in cultured cells or in chimpanzees, as the genes can be deleted from a recombinant RSV, but growth *in vitro* and *in vivo* is reduced substantially (19,273,292). In a minireplicon system, when NS1 was expressed, it was inhibitory to both transcription and replication (5), and expression of NS2 at high levels had a small inhibitory effect on transcription and replication (272). Thus, the role of these accessory proteins in the RSV life cycle remains to be fully understood.

STAGES OF REPLICATION

As far as is known, all aspects of the replication of *Paramyxoviridae* take place in the cytoplasm. An overview of the life cycle of the virus is shown schematically in Figure 18, and a diagram indicating the differences between transcription and replication is shown in Figure 19. Unlike in influenza viruses, mRNA synthesis in *Paramyxoviridae* is insensitive to DNA-intercalating drugs such as actinomycin D (reviewed in ref. 43), and the *Paramyxoviridae* can replicate in enucleated cells (221). In cell culture, single-cycle growth curves are generally of 14 to 30 hours duration, but they can be as short as 10 hours for virulent strains of NDV. The effect of viral replication on host macromolecular synthesis is quite variable, ranging from almost complete shutoff late in infection for NDV, to no obvious effect with SV5.

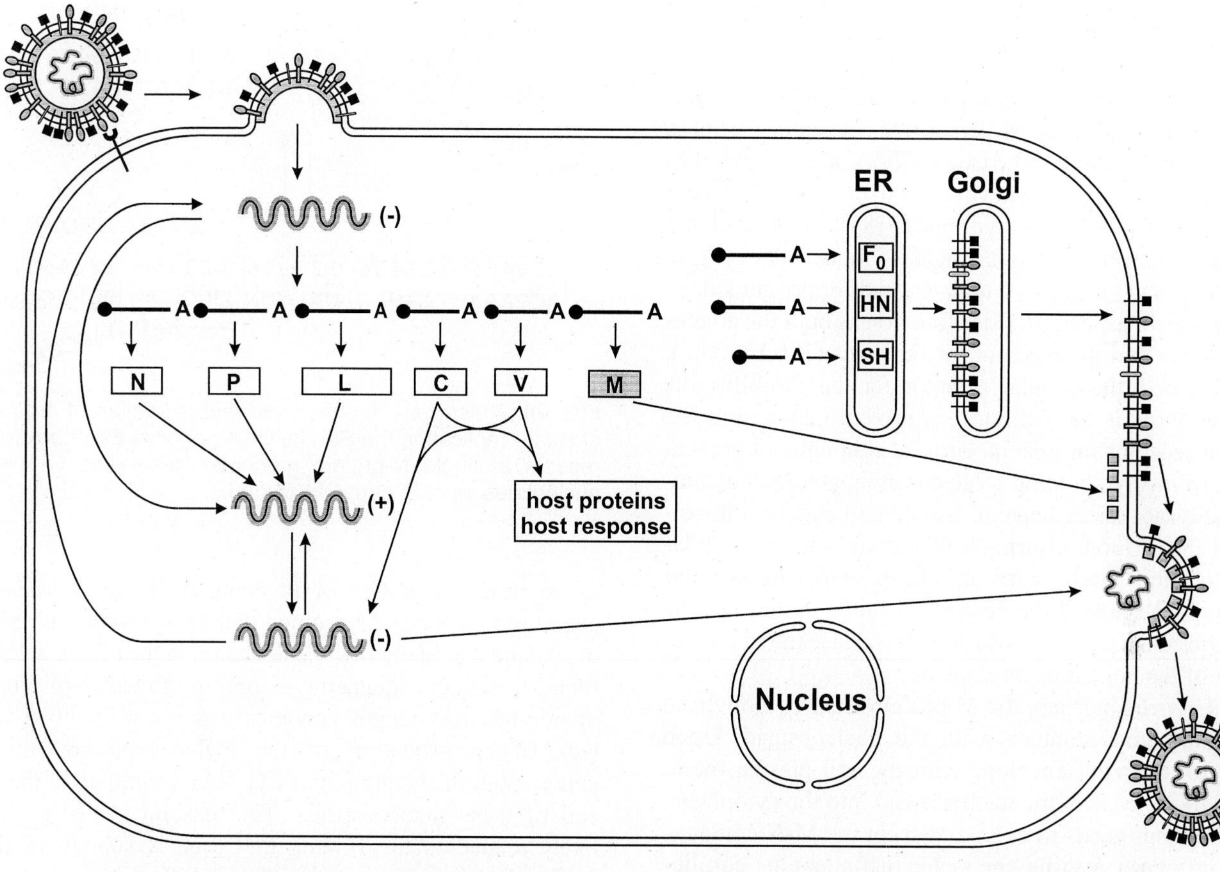

FIG. 18. Schematic representation of the life cycle of a Paramyxovirus. See text for details of the viral life cycle. The gradient of decreasing molar abundance of the mRNAs from N to L resulting from polar transcription is not illustrated [the 5′ mRNA cap is indicated with a *filled circle* and 3′ poly(A) tail by *(A)*]. Also not illustrated are the relative abundances of genomic nucleocapsid and antigenomic nucleocapsid (indicated with *wavy gray lines*, – and +, respectively). Secondary transcription by newly made genomic nucleocapsids also is not illustrated.

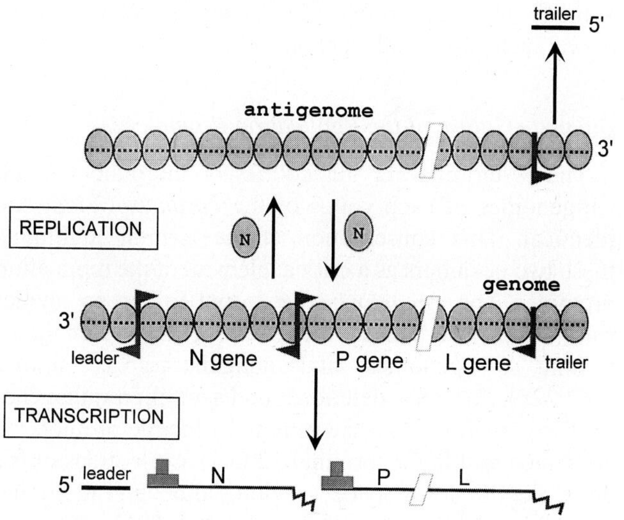

FIG. 19. Paramyxovirus RNA synthesis. Viral nucleocapsids, the templates for RNA synthesis, are shown as a linear array of N subunits (*ovals*), with *short vertical lines* and *arrowheads* indicating the gene junctions. The viral polymerase (P-L) transcribes the genome template, starting at its 3′ end, to generate the (+) leader RNA and the successive capped (*boxes*) and polyadenylated (*squiggly line*) mRNAs, by stopping and restarting at each junction. Once these primary transcripts have generated sufficient viral proteins, unassembled N (as a P-N complex) begins to assemble the nascent leader chain, and the coordinate assembly and synthesis of the RNA causes the polymerase to ignore the junctions, yielding the antigenome nucleocapsid. In this capacity, P acts as a chaperone to deliver N to the nascent RNA. The P-L polymerase can also initiate RNA synthesis at the 3′ end of the antigenome in the absence of sufficient P-N, but only a (–) leader RNA (representing the 5′ trailer of genome RNA) is made in this case. Note that genomic and antigenomic RNAs never appear as naked RNAs.

Virus Adsorption and Entry

For the respiroviruses and rubulaviruses, it has long been accepted that molecules containing sialic acid (sialoglycoconjugates) serve as cell surface receptors. This is based on the fact that sialidase of *Vibrio cholerae* acted as a "receptor-destroying enzyme" and protected the host cell from infection (reviewed in ref. 181). Sialic acid, the acyl derivative of neuraminic acid, is found both on glycoproteins and on lipids (sialoglycolipids or gangliosides). For Sendai virus, gangliosides function as both the attachment factor and the receptor for the virus (180,182,183). As described, the cellular receptor for the Morbillivirus measles virus is the cell surface protein CD46, and the cellular receptor for pneumoviruses, although not proven, seems to involve binding to glycosaminoglycans containing the disaccharide heparan sulfate and chondroitin sulfate B (88). Upon adsorption of the virus to the cellular receptor, the viral membrane fuses with the cellular plasma membrane at the neutral pH found at the cell surface, the consequence of which is the release into the cytoplasm of the helical nucleocapsids.

In the virus particle, the M protein shell is thought to make numerous contacts with the nucleocapsid. Upon fusion of the viral envelope with the cell plasma membrane and release of the nucleocapsid into the cytoplasm, a mechanism needs to exist to disrupt the M-N contacts. With influenza A virus, the factor that alters the equilibrium between self-assembly and disassembly is thought to be the difference in pH between the acidic uncoating compartment (endosomes) and the assembly site (plasma membrane). The driving force for Paramyxovirus uncoating is not known.

Viral RNA Synthesis

Viral Transcription (mRNA Synthesis)

All viral RNA synthesis begins at the very 3′ end of the genome, and the cis-acting promoter sequences serve the dual function of initiating leader RNAs and antigenomes. The vRNAP for mRNA synthesis first has to transcribe the leader RNA before beginning mRNA synthesis at the N gene start signal (see Fig. 19). The recent discovery of two unexpected properties of the *Paramyxovirinae* has provided information on how vRNAP interacts with the genome 3′ end to initiate RNA synthesis.

Requirement for Hexamer Genome Length for Efficient Genome Replication: The "Rule of Six"

Efficient replication of model mini-genomes in transfected cells requires that their total length be a multiple of six (Fig. 20) (27). For every Respirovirus or Rubulavirus examined to date using a mini-genome replication assay, RNA replication has been found to be much more efficient when the artificial genome was designed to be a multiple of six nucleotides. Out of 11 complete *Paramyxovirinae* genomic sequences determined to date, six were multiples of six, and it is likely that the deviation in the others will be found to reflect sequencing errors. Inefficient replication of non-hexamer-length genomes was not a result of the lack of encapsidation of the cDNA-expressed mini-genome but of the inability of vRNAP to initiate at the 3′ end of these nucleocapsids. This hexamer rule is most likely related to the finding that each N subunit of the nucleocapsid is associated with precisely six nucleotides (79). The association of N monomers with nucleotide hexamers presumably begins with the first nucleotide at the 5′ end of the nascent chain, and it continues by assembling six nucleotides at a time until the 3′ end is reached, maintaining a precise hexamer arrangement (see Fig. 20). The efficiency of the 3′-end promoter then presumably depends on the position of the cis-acting sequences relative to the N subunits, and this is determined by the total number of nucleotides in the genome chain.

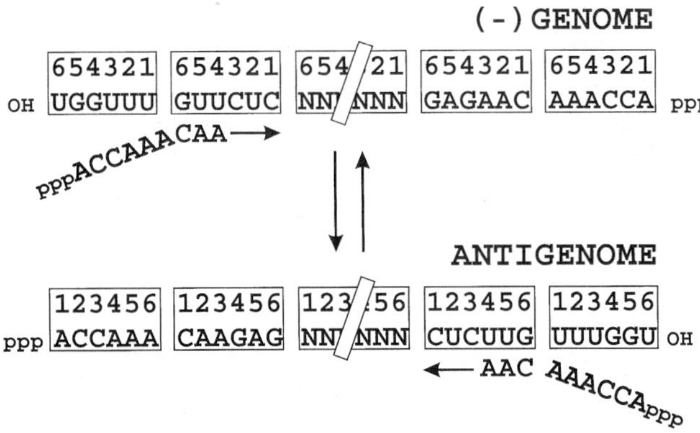

FIG. 20. Rule of six. A schematic representation of the rule of six for replicating the Sendai virus genome. Each *box* represents a single N-protein monomer associated with six nucleotides. ppp, 5′ end; OH, 3′ end.

Bipartite Nature of the Replication Promoter

The 3′-terminal 12 nucleotides of the genomes and antigenomes of each genus of the *Paramyxovirinae* are identical. This conservation at the termini highlights these two hexamers as a critical element of the replication promoter. The *Pneumovirinae* do not follow an integer rule (244); nevertheless, the extent of identity at the 3′ termini of genomes and antigenomes is similar (187,228). For RSV, deletional and saturation mutagenesis has confirmed that the minimal genomic promoter is contained within the terminal 12 to 15 nucleotides of the 44-nucleotide-long leader region, although additional sequences downstream also enhanced RNA synthesis (see Chapter 45 in *Fields Virology*, 4th ed.). For the *Paramyxovirinae*, it has not been possible to examine the limits of the replication promoters by deletion analysis (see later). Instead, sequence exchanges were made between the genomic and antigenomic promoters, which determines the relative replication efficiency of model mini-genomes (28). In this way, sequences that extended 30 nucleotides from the 3′ end were found to affect Sendai virus replication efficiency.

Although sequences beyond the first 30 nucleotides of the Sendai virus genomic and antigenomic promoters could be exchanged freely (269), the deletion of any nucleotides downstream of the promoters, even if the hexamer rule was not violated, was highly deleterious (220, 268). Similar results were found at the antigenomic promoter of SV5, where again sequence exchanges, but not deletions, downstream of the conserved 3′-end element were permitted (197). This suggested that a second promoter element lay downstream of the end element, and that the spacing between the two elements was critical for promoter function. This internal promoter element has been identified for both Sendai virus (268) and SV5 (197,198), and it consists of a single template C, or a 3′-GC dinucleotide, respectively, repeated three times with an internal spacing of precisely six nucleotides in the 13th, 14th, and 15th hexamer from the 3′ end. The position of the two promoter elements is shown in Figure 21 in the context of the proposed structure of the Sendai virus nucleocapsid. As each turn of the nucleocapsid helix contains 13 N subunits, each associated with precisely six nucleotides (79), the terminal and internal promoter elements are aligned on the same face of the helix. Both promoter elements can then simultaneously interact with vRNAP to initiate RNA synthesis at the 3′ end of the nucleocapsid. Morbilliviruses contain the same internal promoter element as respiroviruses, and all the members of the *Paramyxovirinae* probably contain bipartite replication promoters. In contrast, pneumoviruses do not appear to contain bipartite promoters, as RSV-based mini-genomes require only about 40 nucleotides from each genome end for efficient replication (see Chapter 45 in *Fields Virology*, 4th ed.).

Primary Transcription

Early in virus infection, before the primary translation products have accumulated (or in the presence of drugs that inhibit protein synthesis at any stage of the infection), vRNAP is restricted to the production of leader RNAs and mRNAs. A leader RNA termination site has not been demonstrated by mutational analysis for any nonsegmented negative-strand RNA virus, and vRNAP that has initiated at the genome 3′ end and reads through the leader–N junction may simply become nonprocessive and release its nascent chain heterogeneously within the N gene.

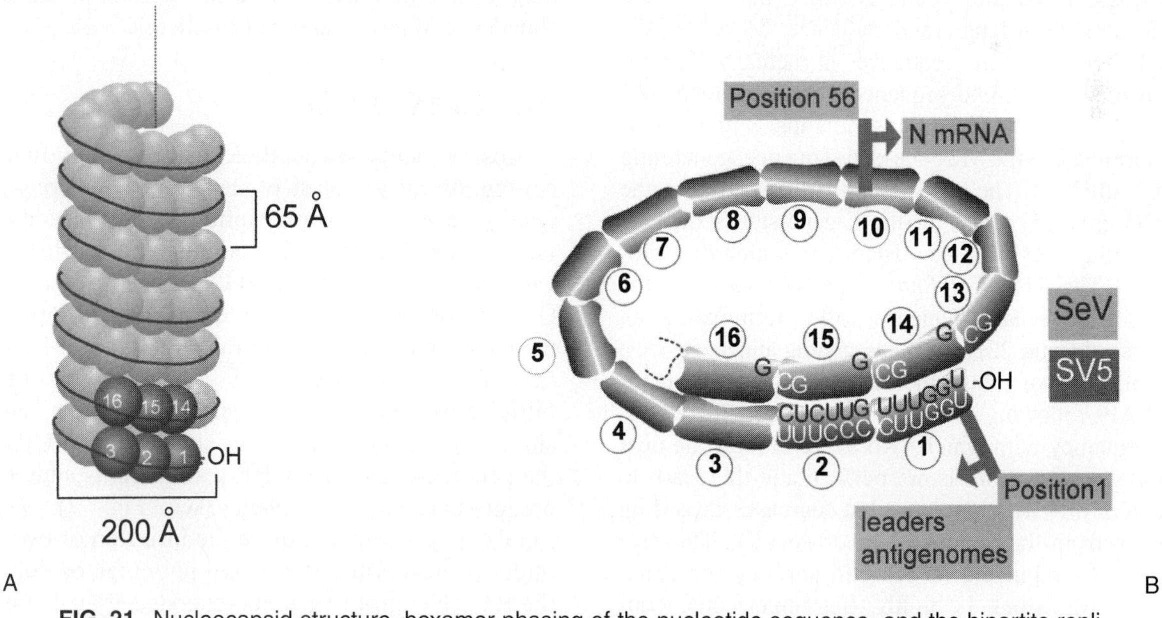

FIG. 21. Nucleocapsid structure, hexamer phasing of the nucleotide sequence, and the bipartite replication promoters of the *Paramyxovirinae*. **A:** A model of the Sendai virus nucleocapsid as an assembly of single N-protein subunits (*shaded spheres*), in the form of a left-handed helix with 13 subunits per turn, a pitch of 65 Å, and a hollow central core of 50 Å in diameter. The numbers refer to the position of each N subunit from the RNA 3′ end. **B:** Expanded view of the first 16 N-protein subunits (drawn as *rounded rectangles*, numbered from the RNA 3′ end) of the genome nucleocapsid. Positions refer to the nucleotide sequence relative to the RNA 3′ (OH) end. The invariant elements of the bipartite genomic and antigenomic promoters of Sendai virus and SV5 are shown relative to the N subunits; each subunit contains precisely six nucleotides. The start sites for the leader RNA, antigenome RNA, and N mRNA are indicated with *arrows*. Note that both elements of the bipartite replication promoter are found on the same face of the helix, whereas N mRNA synthesis starts on the opposite face of the helix.

N mRNAs are invariably initiated opposite the second nucleotide of the 10th hexamer (see Fig. 21, genome map position 56) for the *Paramyxovirinae* (157). More than 90% of vRNAP that have initiated the Sendai virus N mRNA (and capped its 5′ end) go on to finish the N mRNA (283). The processivity of this vRNAP during mRNA synthesis (transcription) is thus quite different from that which has initiated at the genome 3′ end and reads through the leader–N junction in the process of RNA replication, which depends on concurrent assembly of the nascent chain for processivity. The vRNAP that has (re)initiated at position 56 in the process of transcription also responds to the cis-acting gene-end sequence at high frequency (see later), whereas during RNA replication these signals are ignored. mRNA 3′ end formation and polyadenylation occurs by vRNAP reiteratively copying a short run of template uridylylates (four to seven long) within the gene-end sequence (see Fig. 6). This process leads to termination and release of the mRNA, and vRNAP is then free to move on to the next gene-start site and to reinitiate the next mRNA.

Initiation of a downstream mRNA depends on termination of the upstream mRNA consistent with a single vRNAP entry site at the genome 3′ end. For respiroviruses and morbilliviruses, the next gene-start sequence is separated from the gene-end sequence by precisely three conserved nucleotides (3′GAA; see Fig. 6). In contrast, for rubulaviruses, NDV, and pneumoviruses, the intergenic region is variable in length and sequence. Moreover, for RSV the L gene-start sequence is actually located upstream of the gene-end sequence of the upstream M2 gene (48). Thus, 90% of the transcripts that initiate the L mRNA terminate at the M2 gene-end sequence, generating aborted L mRNAs. The vRNAP is then free to scan the N:RNA in either direction for the L gene-start sequence, much as cellular RNAPs scan dsDNA in search of a promoter (86). The RNAP of *Rhabdoviridae* also scans the N:RNA for gene-start sequences after terminating an mRNA (see Chapter 22), and this scanning appears to be a general property of nonsegmented negative-strand RNA virus RNAPs following release of a completed mRNA.

The frequency with which vRNAP reinitiates the next mRNA at gene junctions is not perfect, and this leads to a gradient of mRNA abundance that decreases according to distance from the genome 3′ end (36,127). This frequency can be regulated (at least in part) by the gene-start sequence, which is highly, but imperfectly, conserved. Reducing reinitiation at one junction leads to a coordinate reduction in the expression of all the downstream genes. Failure to terminate at a gene-end sequence, in contrast, leads to di- (or tri-) cistronic mRNAs in which only the upstream cistron is normally translated, because of the usual requirement that a eukaryotic ORF initiate near a 5′ mRNA end. However, vRNAP that reads through a junction is spared falloff because of inefficient reinitiation. There are numerous examples of paramyxoviruses that specifically down-regulate the expression of particular genes, especially the F gene, by generating di-cistronic M-F mRNAs. In several cases, readthrough of this junction is associated with deviations from the consensus gene-end sequence; the most extreme example being the complete lack of an apparent gene-end signal in the M-F junction of SV41. For SV5, whose M gene-end sequence (3′-A**G**UUUCU$_4$) deviates from the consensus at a single position and contains the shortest U run (3′-A**A**NUUCU$_{4-7}$), lengthening the U run was without effect. However, converting the **G** five positions upstream of the U run to **A** restored vRNAP response to this gene-end sequence and prevented readthrough of this junction. However, analysis of genetically engineered recombinant Sendai virus and SV5, in which the gene termination, intercistronic region, and gene-start [EIS (see Fig. 6)] were switched for other EIS sequences, suggests that the simple model of transcriptional attenuation from the genome 3′ end is not the only factor determining mRNA accumulation, particularly from the L mRNA (110,147).

RSV gene-end sequences are more diverse than their gene-start sequences (see Fig. 6). They operate at variable efficiency (see Chapter 45 in *Fields Virology*, 4th ed.). This may be relevant to RSV infections, as the M2-1 protein not only increases vRNAP processivity between junctions during transcription, it also promotes readthrough of the junctions. M2-1 may play a role in fine-tuning the relative abundance of mono- and dicistronic mRNAs.

P Gene mRNA Editing

Most Paramyxovirus P genes contain a functional editing site at the start of the internal, overlapping V ORF (see Fig. 7). Transcription yields, in addition to faithful (unedited) mRNA, edited versions that contain variable numbers of inserted G residues. The number of G insertions that occur for each virus group mirrors their requirements to switch between the in-frame and *trans*-frame downstream ORFs (see Fig. 7). For the morbilliviruses, respiroviruses, and NDV, which require a single nucleotide insertion to shift to the V ORF from the genome-encoded P ORF, a single G is added as the predominant editing event (see Fig. 7). For the rubulaviruses, which require the insertion of two nucleotides to access the P-carboxy pol-cofactor domain of the P ORF from the genome-encoded V ORF, insertion of two Gs constitutes a high proportion of editing events. For bPIV-3 and hPIV-3, where both the V and D ORFs overlap the middle of the genome-encoded P ORF, one to six G residues are added at roughly equal frequency so that mRNAs encoding all three overlapping ORFs are transcribed.

As the paramyxoviruses replicate in the cytoplasm, they must provide enzymes for all aspects of their mRNA synthesis. Paramyxovirus vRNAPs polyadenylate their

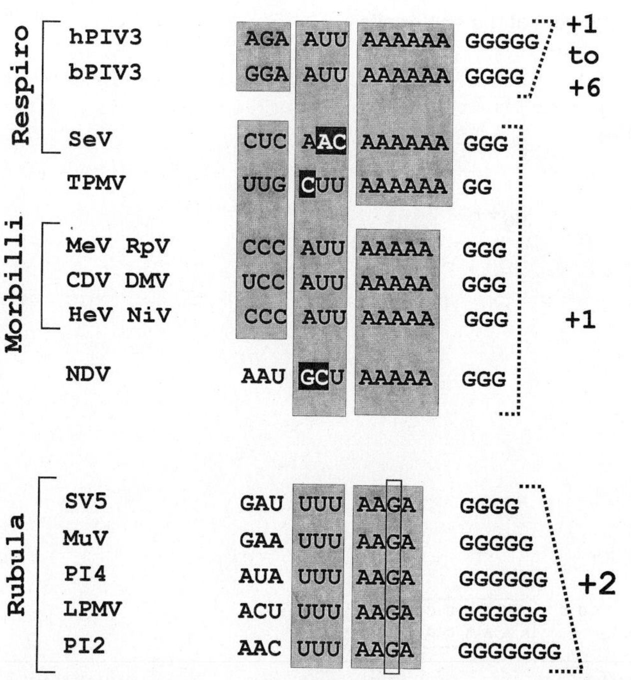

FIG. 22. Sequence relationships at the Paramyxovirus P gene editing sites. The sequences are written as (+) RNA, 5′ to 3′, and are grouped into the three current genera of the *Paramyxovirinae* except for NDV. Spaces have been introduced to emphasize the different elements of the sequence, and *shaded boxes* indicate sequence conservation. The short G run, which is expanded during mRNA editing, is shown on the right, together with the pattern of G insertions that occurs for each group. Note that the A run preceding the G run may be the only part of this cis-acting sequence that is strictly conserved according to genus. Also note that the second A residue upstream of the Rubulavirus G run is replaced by a G (highlighted with *rectangle*), which is thought to account for why most rubulaviruses insert a minimum of two G residues when stuttering begins (282).

mRNAs by stuttering on a short run of template U residues (four to seven nucleotides long) at the end of each gene. By analogy to the polyadenylation mechanism, it was suggested that the G insertions at the specific site in the P gene (Fig. 22) would occur similarly by pseudotemplated transcription (35,138,274,281), and there is now strong experimental evidence that the insertions occur cotranscriptionally, by a stuttering mechanism (108,109,282). This mechanism of pseudotemplated transcription, outlined in Figure 23, would apply as well to mRNA polyadenylation if the mRNA–template hybrid is reduced to four base pairs (108).

Genome Replication

The (−) genome replicates via a full-length complementary copy called the antigenome, which, like the genome, is found only in assembled form. Compared to *Rhabdoviridae*, there are considerable amounts of antigenomes in Paramyxovirus-infected cells (10% to 40% of genome-sized RNAs for Sendai virus). Antigenomes can also represent 5% to 20% of the genome-sized RNAs in virus particles, as discrimination against antigenome nucleocapsids is poor during virus assembly (155,156,231). However, they contain no ORFs of any note and no mRNAs are known to be transcribed from them. The sole function of antigenomes is thought to be as an intermediate in genome replication, although the short trailer RNAs expressed from the antigenome 3′ ends (see Fig. 19) may also play a role in preventing the host cell from undergoing programmed cell death (98).

A schematic diagram of the essential differences between transcription and replication is shown in Figure 19. After translation of the primary transcripts and accumulation of the viral proteins, antigenome synthesis begins. Here, ostensibly the same vRNAP (until then engaged solely in mRNA synthesis) copies the same template, but it now ignores all the junctional signals (and editing sites) and synthesizes an exact, complementary copy. Transcription and replication were first distinguished by finding that, when infected cells are treated with drugs that inhibit protein synthesis, mRNA synthesis continued normally but genome synthesis was lost very quickly (232). As genome synthesis and encapsidation appear to occur concomitantly, this requirement for ongoing protein synthesis has been associated with the continued supply of unassembled N necessary for genome encapsidation. The manner in which the coupling of genome assembly and synthesis leads to vRNAP ignoring the gene junctions and editing signals remains unclear (reviewed in ref. 158).

This coupling of genome assembly and synthesis also leads to a self-regulatory system for controlling the relative levels of transcription and replication. For VSV, the site for the initiation of antigenome encapsidation has been mapped to the first 14 nucleotides of the leader sequence, and for paramyxoviruses a similar situation appears to apply. In measles virus–infected cells, a rare polyadenylated transcript representing the leader and N gene sequences fused together is found, but only as a nucleocapsid, whereas the N mRNA is found only in a nonassembled form (31). As the leader sequences contain the encapsidation site, the leader must be separated from the body of the first mRNA (by termination and reinitiation at the first junction) to prevent the first mRNA from ending up in an assembled and untranslatable form. The proposed self-regulatory mechanism would then be quite straightforward; when unassembled N is limiting, vRNAP is preferentially engaged in mRNA synthesis, raising the intracellular levels of all the viral proteins, including unassembled N. When unassembled N levels are sufficient, some vRNAP would be switched to replication, thereby lowering the levels of unassembled N, as each initiation of encapsidation would commit about 2,600 N monomers to finish the assembled genome chain (154). The rare measles virus leader-N mRNA (31),

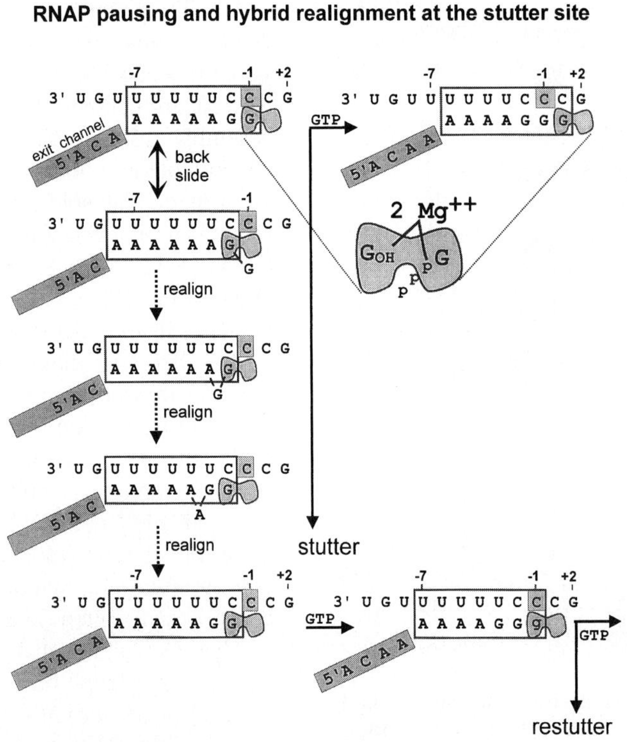

FIG. 23. A competitive kinetic model for Sendai virus RNAP stuttering elongation. The template and mRNA chains of the transcription elongation complex (TEC) at the editing site are shown schematically. The putative seven base-pair hybrid between the polypyrimidine tract of the (–) genome (top strand) and the polypurine run of the nascent mRNA chain (bottom strand) when the TEC is at the editing site is *boxed.* The NTP binding site (position +1) is empty. The nascent mRNA upstream (*left*) of the hybrid is proposed to enter an exit channel (*boxed in gray*) before reaching the surface of the RNAP, and this limits the length of the hybrid as TEC proceeds. The exit channel is thought to contain 10 nucleotides. The bipartite active site, in which the nascent mRNA 3′ end (position –1) and the NTP α-phosphate are coordinated via two Mg^{++} ions is highlighted in *gray.* The TEC at the *top left* is at the editing site (middle template C, *boxed in gray*) and has just incorporated a strictly templated G (position –1). The TEC at the unique editing site presumably pauses because of backsliding of RNAP by one position along both the template and the mRNA chains, undoing the last base pair (bp) of the hybrid (and removing the mRNA 3′ end from the active site) and reforming one bp upstream. RNAP at pause sites is envisaged as oscillating between the inactive backtracked alignment (*second line*) and the active alignment (*top line*). If a strictly templated GMP is the next nucleotide incorporated, RNAP moves past the unique stutter site and resumes normal elongation (*top right*). Alternatively, realignment of the hybrid also repositions the mRNA 3′ end in the active site. Hybrid realignment when RNAP is in the backtracked state is initiated when the unpaired 3′G re-pairs with C-2 (*third line*), causing the penultimate G to bulge out. Realignment is completed on translocation of the single nucleotide bulge to the upstream side of the hybrid (*fourth line*), reforming a seven-bp hybrid that is nearly as stable as its predecessor (*fifth line*). The mRNA 3′ G is now correctly repositioned in the active site, and nucleotide addition at this point leads to a single pseudotemplated G insertion, or stutter (lower-case g, *bottom right*). Having stuttered once, the transcription complex is back to where it started and has the same choices (second branchpoint, *bottom right*). Escape from stuttering occurs when TEC moves to a template position where hybrid realignment (stuttering) is no longer favored. Numbers above the genome sequence always indicate positions relative to the mRNA 3′ end at the start of the stutter (*top left*, position –1).

described previously, was presumably made by vRNAP that began the synthesis of an antigenome nucleocapsid but nevertheless polyadenylated and terminated the chain at the second junction. The assembly and synthesis steps can then sometimes become uncoupled, possibly because assembly of the nascent chain does not keep pace with vRNAP movement as it approaches a junction. Whether the level of unassembled N is the only mechanism that controls the relative levels of Sendai virus transcription versus RNA replication remains unclear. For RSV, however, there is increasing evidence that other viral gene products (e.g., the M2-2 protein) may also play a role (see preceding and Chapter 45 in *Fields Virology*, 4th ed.).

Genome synthesis from antigenome templates is thought to take place in a fashion similar to that of antigenome synthesis, in that the promoter at the 3′ end of the antigenome is also always "on," and short trailer [also called (–) leader] RNAs are made from this region independently of ongoing protein synthesis (see Fig. 19). However, in contrast to synthesis from genome templates, there are no reinitiation sites on the antigenome template, so termination of the trailer RNAs in the absence of sufficient unassembled N protein serves only to recycle vRNAP. Under conditions of sufficient intracellular concentrations of unassembled N (and perhaps other viral proteins), encapsidation of the nascent trailer chain would quickly begin and this would prevent termination and lead to the synthesis on an encapsidated minus-strand genome.

Virion Assembly and Release

Like all other events in the life cycle of replication of paramyxoviruses, the intracellular site of nucleocapsid assembly is the cytoplasm. The nucleocapsids are thought to be assembled in two steps: first, association of free N subunits with the genome or template RNA to form the helical RNP structure, and second, the association of the P-L protein complex (152). By analogy to the mechanism of assembly of TMV nucleocapsid, which uses a defined nucleation site for the association of the first coat protein subunit with the RNA, and the observation that the Paramyxovirus mRNAs are not encapsidated (in contrast to antigenomes), it has been assumed that the (+) leader (5′ end of the antigenome) and (–) trailer (5′ end of the genome) regions contain specific sequences for initiating encapsidation (14).

The assembly of the second part of the virus, the envelope, is at the cell surface. In polarized epithelial cells, the *Paramyxovirinae* bud only from the apical surface. The viral integral membrane proteins are synthesized in the ER and undergo a step-wise conformational maturation before transport through the secretory pathway. The mechanisms of viral glycoprotein folding, oligomeric assembly, and sorting have been extensively characterized. Folding and conformational maturation of glycoproteins are not spontaneous events that occur in the cell. Rather, they are assisted by numerous folding enzymes and molecular chaperones. Viral integral membrane proteins, particularly HA and NA of influenza A virus, the G protein of VSV, and the HN protein of SV5 and Sendai virus, have been used extensively as paradigms of cellular glycoproteins, and much of the current understanding of the process occurring in the exocytotic pathway has been learned from studying these proteins (reviewed in refs. 73, 116). Only correctly folded and assembled proteins are generally transported out of the ER. In the Golgi apparatus, the carbohydrate chains may be modified from the high-mannose to the complex form, and for those F proteins with multiple basic cleavage sites, cleavage occurs in the trans Golgi network. Finally, the glycoproteins are transported to the plasma membrane.

The mechanism by which the virus particle is assembled at the plasma membrane is unknown. As discussed, the viral M proteins are thought to play a major role in bringing the assembled ribonucleoprotein core to the appropriate patch on the plasma membrane to form a budding virion (Fig. 24). The protein–protein interactions involved in assembling a virion presumably must be specific, as cellular membrane proteins are largely excluded from the virions. It is presumed that the glycoprotein cytoplasmic tails make important contacts with the M protein, which, in turn, associates with the nucleocapsid. Genetically engineered recombinant measles virus and

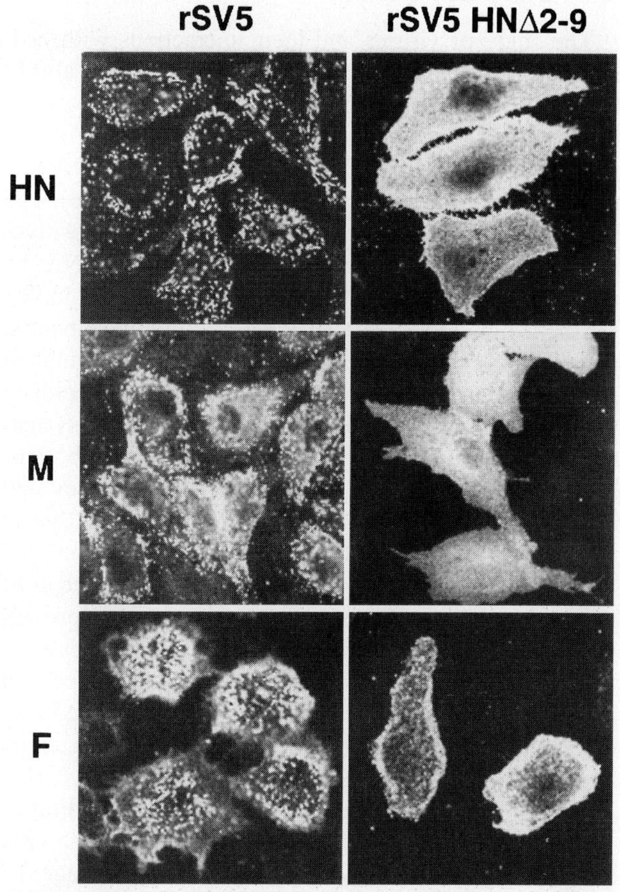

FIG. 24. Altered localization of viral proteins in cells infected with recombinant SV5 expressing an HN protein with a truncated cytoplasmic tail. In wild-type recombinant SV5 (rSV5)-infected cells, HN was found in highly localized patches on the cell surface, and it is likely that these patches are the sites of budding virus. In contrast, in cells infected with rSV5 HNΔ2–9, a recombinant SV5 lacking residues two to nine of the HN cytoplasmic tail, a striking redistribution of the HN staining pattern was observed, with HN being distributed all across the cell surface. Concomitant with the altered HN staining pattern in cells infected with rSV5 HNΔ2–9, a redistribution of the M protein straining pattern was observed. The similarity of HN and M staining patterns suggests that targeting of M protein into presumptive budding sites at the cell surface depends on the presence of an HN cytoplasmic tail. (Adapted from ref. 251, with permission.)

SV5 that lack glycoprotein cytoplasmic tails are defective in assembly and there is a relocalization of the subcellular distribution of the matrix protein (33,251). For Sendai virus HN protein, the cytoplasmic tail sequence SYWST has been shown to be important for incorporation into virions (263). Those *Paramyxovirinae* that have neuraminidase activity contain glycoproteins that lack sialic modification of their carbohydrate chains, and it is thought that the HN neuraminidase activity serves the same purpose as NA in influenza virus, to prevent self-binding and to prevent reattachment to the infected cell.

MOLECULARLY ENGINEERED GENETICS (REVERSE GENETICS)

The study of viruses and their interactions with host cells and organisms has benefited greatly from the ability to engineer specific mutations into viral genomes, a technique known as reverse genetics (288). For RNA viruses, genome manipulation of the positive-sense RNA bacteriophage Qβ was the first to be performed (90,266). The negative-stranded RNA viruses, in contrast to positive-sense RNA viruses, require that the virion RNA be assembled into an active transcriptase–replicase complex for the genome to initiate virus replication. Nonetheless, techniques to manipulate the genomes of nonsegmented negative-strand RNA viruses have now been developed (reviewed in ref. 230). The development of the system originally proved quite frustrating. A number of laboratories studying a number of different rhabdoviruses and paramyxoviruses, worked over a period of several years to establish the methods of reconstructing functional nucleocapsids from transfected cells. The concept of replicating mini-genomes using support plasmids providing N, P, and L proteins in *trans* was key to the development of the technology. This culminated in the successful recovery of infectious rabies virus in 1994, followed several months later by VSV, and several months later by Sendai, hRSV, and measles virus.

Rabies virus was rescued when plasmids encoding L, P, and N protein, as well as a plasmid containing the viral antigenome, all under control of the bacteriophage T7 RNA polymerase promoter, were transfected into cells infected with a recombinant vaccinia virus expressing the bacteriophage T7 RNA polymerase protein (vac-T7). For example, the following viruses have been rescued: VSV (170,291), measles virus (227), hRSV (45,141), Sendai virus (97,150,174), rinderpest virus (9), hPIV-3 (75,126), SV5 (112), NDV (218,233), and bRSV (19). A schematic diagram showing the general scheme for rescue is illustrated for SV5 in Figure 25. Some refinements to the original technique have been made, such as the use of stably transfected cell lines expressing the bacteriophage T7 RNA polymerase (in lieu of vac-T7 infection), or one or more of the viral proteins required for genome replication (19,227).

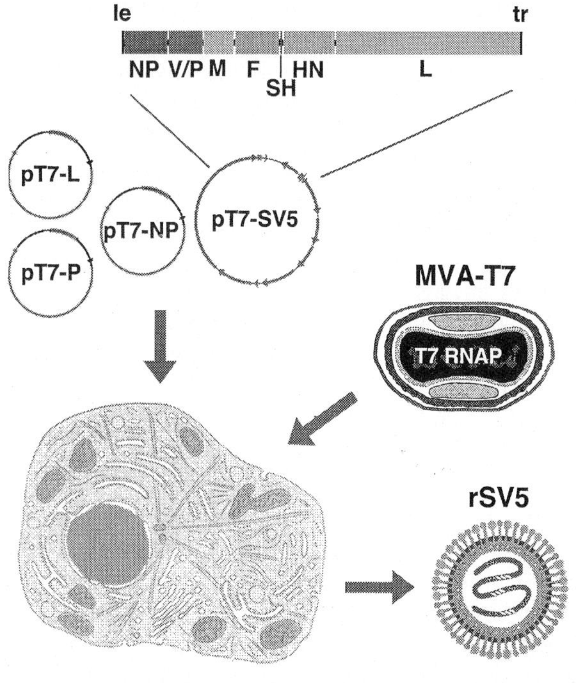

FIG. 25. Schematic diagram for generating infectious SV5 from cloned cDNA. Nonsegmented negative-strand virus rescue involves the transfection of plasmids encoding the viral P, N, and L proteins (and sometimes other viral proteins, depending on the virus), as well as the viral antigenome, all under control of the T7 promoter. The bacteriophage T7 RNA polymerase is provided either by infection with a vaccinia virus expressing T7 polymerase (in this case, modified vaccinia virus Ankara, MVA-T7) or by transfecting into cell lines that stably express the protein. pT7-SV5 contains a complete copy of the SV5 genome (15,246 nucleotides) and is flanked at one end by a bacteriophage T7 RNA polymerase (T7 RNAP) promoter and at the other end by a hepatitis delta virus ribozyme and T7 transcriptional terminator. The plasmids pT7-L, pT7-P, and pT7-N each contain the cDNA for the SV5 L, P, and N proteins, respectively, under the control of T7 RNAP promoters, such that mRNA transcripts encoding L, P, and N can be transcribed using T7 RNAP. A549 cells (a human cell line that is permissive for SV5 and can be efficiently transfected) were infected with MVA-T7 and transfected with pT7-SV5 and the three support plasmids pT7-L, pT7-P, and pT7-N. (Adapted from ref. 112, with permission.)

VIRAL ACCESSORY GENES AND THEIR INTERACTIONS WITH THE HOST

In all studies on reconstituting intracellular virus replication in transfected cells from model mini-genomes, only the P (as defined above), L, and N proteins were found to be strictly required to initiate genome expression and amplification. However, for RSV, coexpression of the M2-1 protein increases vRNAP processivity during transcription (46,87,107). For all the other accessory proteins, their initial coexpression was either without effect or it inhibited mini-genome replication. For the Sendai virus C protein, inhibition of replication was so severe that C coexpression from the P-protein support plasmid had to be suppressed to recover infectious virus (24). Despite these neutral or negative effects on genome replication and expression in transfected cells, reverse genetics has shown that the accessory genes also exert positive effects during natural infections of cells in culture, or in animals as a result of interaction with the host, such as countering the interferon system (see later).

Respirovirus and Morbillivirus V, W, and D Proteins

Infectious measles virus or Sendai virus engineered to have inactive editing sites (i.e., by introduction of mutations at the editing site, so that these viruses cannot express their V and W proteins) are viable, and they grow in cell culture slightly more rapidly than wild-type virus (67,148,252), consistent with an inhibitory role for V and W in genome amplification (56). However, an important step toward understanding the role of the V protein in the Sendai virus life cycle was made when it was found that, although the Sendai virus–edit minus mutant grew perfectly well in cell culture, it was avirulent for mice (148). In contrast to wild-type virus, Sendai virus–edit minus could not sustain its infection of the respiratory tract and was quickly cleared from the animal. Given that mice could restrict Sendai virus–edit minus replication so quickly, it was suggested that V functioned to counteract some aspect of the animal's innate immune system (148).

To examine whether this avirulence was caused by the loss of V, or W, or both proteins, Sendai virus–Vstop mutant, in which the V ORF is closed and expresses a W-like protein in place of V, was characterized (67,149). In 3-week-old outbred mice, Sendai virus–Vstop was almost as attenuated for virulence as Sendai virus–edit minus. In inbred mice, however, Sendai virus–Vstop was almost as virulent as wild-type Sendai virus, whereas Sendai virus–edit minus remained avirulent. Thus, the W protein can mostly replace the V protein for counteracting host defenses in the inbred mouse strain. The W protein, however, cannot replace the V protein in the more robust outbred animals, where the cysteine-rich domain of the V protein is clearly required for virulence. The finding that the cysteine-rich domain of V protein is not essential for virulence in some mice may be relevant for hPIV-1, which does not contain a V ORF or an editing site (184). The hPIV-1 may express low levels of a W-like protein by other means, such as ribosomal frameshifting. For hPIV-3, two or more (depending on the strain) stop codons are present between the editing site and the almost perfectly conserved cysteine-rich domain, and a V-like protein has not been demonstrated biochemically in hPIV-3 infections. Nevertheless, the introduction of stop codons in both the V and D ORFs simultaneously (but not individually) attenuated hPIV-3 replication *in vivo* (76). Thus, a hPIV-3 V-like protein may be expressed at low levels after all, by some mechanism other than editing, and may contribute to viral virulence along with the D protein.

Measles virus–edit minus mutant is also attenuated compared to wild-type virus in mice with severe combined immunodeficiency disease (SCID) that have been engrafted with human thymocyte/liver as a substrate for measles virus replication. Measles virus–edit minus mutant also grows to lower titers in the lungs of cotton rats (277,279). Measles virus–edit minus is also slightly less virulent in transgenic mice that express the human CD46 receptor (195,216). Thus, Morbillivirus V/W proteins may also function in countering host defenses. On the other hand, rubulaviruses that cannot express their V protein have not been reported. It may be that the Rubulavirus V protein has a significant role in intracellular virus replication. Precisely what aspect of innate immunity the V, W, or D proteins affect remains unclear. Neither natural killer cells nor the interferon system seems to be involved for Sendai virus (96,101).

C Proteins and Rubulavirus V Proteins

Measles viruses that cannot express their single C protein are viable, and they replicate in cell culture in a manner similar to wild-type viruses (226). The hPIV-3 also expresses a single C protein, but hPIV-3-C-minus growth is clearly restricted in cell culture (76). Sendai virus, in contrast, expresses four "C" proteins (C′, C, Y_1, and Y_2), and recombinant Sendai virus (rSeV), which cannot express any of their C proteins, is at the limit of recovery from DNA and grows to titers that are four logs lower than wild-type virus (159,167). The number of expressed C proteins, and their relative importance for the intracellular replication of each virus, is thus quite different, with the caveat that the "wild-type" measles virus is a cell culture–adapted mutant.

The Sendai virus C′ and C proteins (but not Y_1 and Y_2) are promoter-specific inhibitors of viral RNA synthesis (24,267). Consistent with this, infections with rSeV that cannot express C′ or C individually (by mutating their ribosomal start codons) accumulate more viral RNAs than wild-type rSeV infection, and cytopathic effects are seen earlier (167). However, the simultaneous absence of both C′ and C paradoxically delays viral RNA accumulation and cytopathic effects, and these viruses form "pinhole" plaques. Thus, in addition to their negative effects on viral RNA synthesis (which apparently operate later in infection when these essentially nonstructural proteins have accumulated), C′ and C apparently also provide a positive function without which the onset of viral RNA accumulation intracellularly is delayed. This positive function of C is not seen when a recombinant Sendai virus infection is launched from plasmids in transfected cells. Here, the early events in the infectious process have been bypassed (by jump-starting viral replication from DNA), and only the later inhibitory effects are detected.

Presumably either C′ or C (but not Y_1 or Y_2) can supply this early required function in cell culture infections. Viruses unable to express either C′ or C individually would have this function provided by the remaining protein and would not show a debilitated phenotype.

Mutation of residue phenylalanine 170 of the Sendai virus C protein to serine (by classic or reverse genetics) strongly reduces virulence in mice. The C protein F170S mutation was discovered as one of two mutations (the other in the L gene) in a highly virulent virus strain (Sendai virus strain M; LD_{50} of 40) that became avirulent (Sendai virus variant MVC; LD_{50} of >800,000) on adaptation to LLC-MK2 cells (137). Recombinant Sendai virus carrying the C protein F170S mutation in an otherwise wild-type background is also avirulent in mice (95), and introduction of this mutation into hPIV-3 (C protein F164S) similarly attenuated virulence *in vivo* (76). Although rSeV-C protein F170S was avirulent, it grew normally in the mouse respiratory tract at first. However, like Sendai virus–edit minus, virus was then quickly cleared. The rapidity of the antiviral response in immunologically naive mice again suggested that some aspect of innate immunity is involved. One such function has recently been identified. Infection of interferon (IFN)-competent cells with Sendai virus, or SV5, does not induce an IFN-mediated antiviral state. These infections do not affect the secretion of IFN but somehow interfere with its receptor-mediated signaling, as they prevent added IFN from inducing an antiviral state (71,96). For Sendai virus, the C gene is clearly involved, as Sendai virus-C protein F170S infection does not interdict IFN signaling (96), and C protein expression independent of virus infection prevents added IFN from activating IFN-responsive promoters (94). Consistent with this latter finding, Sendai virus-(C-minus) infection was avirulent, whereas Sendai virus-(C′-minus) was found to be as virulent for mice as wild-type virus, even though this virus overexpresses Y_1 and Y_2. Thus, the AUG_{114}-initiated C protein is specifically required for virulence in mice, or to interfere with IFN signaling (96,168). For SV5, however, it is the V protein that functions to interdict IFN signaling (71), and the SV5 V protein interferes with IFN signalling by causing the proteasomal degradation of the transcription factor, STAT-1 (72). Given that the IFN system is the first line of defense against viral infections, it is possible that the Morbillivirus C proteins (83,195,216) or one of the Pneumovirus accessory proteins, also functions to counteract the IFN-mediated cellular antiviral response.

REFERENCES

1. Alkhatib G, Richardson C, Shen SH. Intracellular processing, glycosylation, and cell-surface expression of the measles virus fusion protein (F) encoded by a recombinant adenovirus. *Virology* 1990;175: 262–270.
2. Alkhatib G, Shen S-H, Briedis D, et al. Functional analysis of N-linked glycosylation mutants of the measles virus fusion protein synthesized by recombinant vaccinia virus vectors. *J Virol* 1994;68: 1522–1531.
3. Anderson K, King AM, Lerch RA, Wertz GW. Polylactosaminoglycan modification of the respiratory syncytial virus small hydrophobic (SH) protein: A conserved feature among human and bovine respiratory syncytial viruses. *Virology* 1992;191:417–430.
4. Asano K, Asano A. Why is a specific amino acid sequence of F glycoprotein required for the membrane fusion reaction between envelope of HVJ (Sendai virus) and target cell membranes? *Biochem Int* 1985;10:115–122.
5. Atreya PL, Peeples ME, Collins PL. The NS1 protein of human respiratory syncytial virus is a potent inhibitor of minigenome transcription and RNA replication. *J Virol* 1998;72:1452–1461.
6. Bachi T. Intramembrane structural differentiation in Sendai virus maturation. *Virology* 1980;106:41–49.
7. Bagai S, Lamb RA. Individual roles of N-linked oligosaccharide chains in intracellular transport of the Paramyxovirus SV5 fusion protein. *Virology* 1995;209:250–256.
8. Baker KA, Dutch RE, Lamb RA, Jardetzky TS. Structural basis for Paramyxovirus-mediated membrane fusion. *Mol Cell* 1999;3: 309–319.
9. Baron MD, Barrett T. Rescue of rinderpest virus from cloned cDNA. *J Virol* 1997;71:1265–1271.
10. Bellini WJ, Englund G, Rozenblatt S, et al. Measles virus P gene codes for two proteins. *J Virol* 1985;53:908–919.
11. Bermingham A, Collins PL. The M2-2 protein of human respiratory syncytial virus is a regulatory factor involved in the balance between RNA replication and transcription. *Proc Natl Acad Sci U S A* 1999;96: 11259–11264.
12. Blacklow SC, Lu M, Kim PS. A trimeric subdomain of the simian immunodeficiency virus envelope glycoprotein. *Biochemistry* 1995; 34:14956–14962.
13. Blumberg BM, Kolakofsky D. Intracellular vesicular stomatitis virus leader RNAs are found in nucleocapsid structures. *J Virol* 1981;40: 568–576.
14. Blumberg BM, Leppert M, Kolakofsky D. Interaction of VSV leader RNA and nucleocapsid protein may control VSV genome replication. *Cell* 1981;23:837–845.
15. Blumberg BM, Rose K, Simona MG, et al. Analysis of the Sendai virus M gene and protein. *J Virol* 1984;52:656–663.
16. Boeck R, Curran J, Matsuoka Y, et al. The parainfluenza virus type 1 P/C gene uses a very efficient GUG codon to start its C protein. *J Virol* 1992;66:1765–1768.
17. Bousse T, Takimoto T, Gorman WL, et al. Regions on the hemagglutinin-neuraminidase proteins of human parainfluenza virus type-1 and Sendai virus important for membrane fusion. *Virology* 1994;204: 506–514.
18. Buchholz CJ, Spehner D, Drillien R, et al. The conserved N-terminal region of Sendai virus nucleocapsid protein NP is required for nucleocapsid assembly. *J Virol* 1993;67:5803–5812.
19. Buchholz UJ, Finke S, Conzelmann KK. Generation of bovine respiratory syncytial virus (BRSV) from cDNA: BRSV NS2 is not essential for virus replication in tissue culture, and the human RSV leader region acts as a functional BRSV genome promoter. *J Virol* 1999;73: 251–259.
20. Buckland R, Malvoisin E, Beauverger P, Wild F. A leucine zipper structure present in the measles virus fusion protein is not required for its tetramerization but is essential for fusion. *J Gen Virol* 1992;73: 1703–1707.
21. Bukreyev A, Whitehead SS, Murphy BR, Collins PL. Recombinant respiratory syncytial virus from which the entire SH gene has been deleted grows efficiently in cell culture and exhibits site-specific attenuation in the respiratory tract of the mouse. *J Virol* 1997;71: 8973–8982.
22. Bullough PA, Hughson FM, Skehel JJ, Wiley DC. Structure of influenza haemagglutinin at the pH of membrane fusion. *Nature* 1994; 371:37–43.
23. Byrappa S, Pan YB, Gupta KC. Sendai virus P protein is constitutively phosphorylated at serine249: High phosphorylation potential of the P protein. *Virology* 1996;216:228–234.
24. Cadd T, Garcin D, Tapparel C, et al. The Sendai Paramyxovirus accessory C proteins inhibit viral genome amplification in a promoter-specific fashion. *J Virol* 1996;70:5067–5074.

25. Caffrey M, Cai M, Kaufman J, et al. Three-dimensional solution structure of the 44 kDa ectodomain of SIV gp41. *EMBO J* 1998;17: 4572–4584.
26. Calain P, Roux L. Generation of measles virus defective interfering particles and their presence in a preparation of attenuated live-virus vaccine. *J Virol* 1988;62:2859–2866.
27. Calain P, Roux L. The rule of six, a basic feature for efficient replication of Sendai virus defective interfering RNA. *J Virol* 1993;67: 4822–4830.
28. Calain P, Roux L. Functional characterisation of the genomic and antigenomic promoters of Sendai virus. *Virology* 1995;212:163–173.
29. Cao J, Bergeron L, Helseth E, et al. Effects of amino acid changes in the extracellular domain of the human immunodeficiency virus type 1 gp41 envelope glycoprotein. *J Virol* 1993;67:2747–2755.
30. Carr CM, Kim PS. A spring-loaded mechanism for the conformational change of influenza hemagglutinin. *Cell* 1993;73:823–832.
31. Castaneda SJ, Wong TC. Leader sequence distinguishes between translatable and encapsidated measles virus RNAs. *J Virol* 1990;64: 222–230.
32. Cathomen T, Mrkic B, Spehner D, et al. A matrix-less measles virus is infectious and elicits extensive cell fusion: Consequences for propagation in the brain. *EMBO J* 1998;17:3899–3908.
33. Cathomen T, Naim HY, Cattaneo R. Measles viruses with altered envelope protein cytoplasmic tails gain cell fusion competence. *J Virol* 1998;72:1224–1234.
34. Cattaneo R, Billeter MA. Mutations and A/I hypermutations in measles virus persistent infections. *Curr Top Microbiol Immunol* 1992;176:63–74.
35. Cattaneo R, Kaelin K, Baezko K, Billeter MA. Measles virus editing provides an additional cysteine-rich protein. *Cell* 1989;56:759–764.
36. Cattaneo R, Rebmann G, Schmid A, et al. Altered transcription of a defective measles virus genome derived from a diseased human brain. *EMBO J* 1987;6:681–688.
37. Cattaneo R, Rose JK. Cell fusion by the envelope glycoproteins of persistent measles viruses which cause lethal human brain disease. *J Virol* 1993;67:1493–1502.
38. Chambers P, Pringle CR, Easton AJ. Heptad repeat sequences are located adjacent to hydrophobic regions in several types of virus fusion glycoproteins. *J Gen Virol* 1990;71:3075–3080.
39. Chan DC, Fass D, Berger JM, Kim PS. Core structure of gp41 from the HIV envelope glycoprotein. *Cell* 1997;89:263–273.
40. Chen J, Lee KH, Steinhauer DA, et al. Structure of the hemagglutinin precursor cleavage site, a determinant of influenza pathogenicity and the origin of the labile conformation. *Cell* 1998;95:409–417.
41. Chen J, Skehel JJ, Wiley DC. N- and C-terminal residues combine in the fusion-pH influenza hemagglutinin HA_2 subunit to form an N cap that terminates the triple-stranded coiled coil. *Proc Natl Acad Sci U S A* 1999;96:8967–8972.
42. Chen SS-L, Lee C-N, Lee W-R, et al. Mutational analysis of the leucine zipper-like motif of the human immunodeficiency virus type 1 envelope transmembrane glycoprotein. *J Virol* 1993;67:3615–3619.
43. Choppin PW, Compans RW. Reproduction of paramyxoviruses. In: Fraenkel-Conrat H, Wagner RR, eds. *Comprehensive Virology*, vol. 4. New York: Plenum Press, 1975:95–178.
44. Collins PL, ed. *The Molecular Biology of Human Respiratory Syncytial Virus (RSV) of the Genus Pneumovirus.* New York: Plenum Press, 1991.
45. Collins PL, Hill MG, Camargo E, et al. Production of infectious human respiratory syncytial virus from cloned cDNA confirms an essential role for the transcription elongation factor from the 5′ proximal open reading frame of the M2 mRNA in gene expression and provides a capability for vaccine development. *Proc Natl Acad Sci U S A* 1995;92:11563–11567.
46. Collins PL, Hill MG, Cristina J, Grosfeld H. Transcription elongation factor of respiratory syncytial virus, a nonsegmented negative-strand RNA virus. *Proc Natl Acad Sci U S A* 1996;93:81–85.
47. Collins PL, Hill MG, Johnson PR. The two open reading frames of the 22K mRNA of human respiratory syncytial virus: Sequence comparison of antigenic subgroups A and B and expression *in vitro*. *J Gen Virol* 1990;71:3015–3020.
48. Collins PL, Olmsted RA, Spriggs MK, et al. Gene overlap and site-specific attenuation of transcription of the viral polymerase L gene of human respiratory syncytial virus. *Proc Natl Acad Sci U S A* 1987;84: 5134–5138.
49. Collins PL, Wertz GW. The 1A protein gene of human respiratory syncytial virus: Nucleotide sequence of the mRNA and a related polycistronic transcript. *Virology* 1985;141:283–291.
50. Colman PM, Hoyne PA, Lawrence MC. Sequence and structure alignment of Paramyxovirus hemagglutinin-neuraminidase with influenza virus neuraminidase. *J Virol* 1993;67:2972–2980.
51. Compans RW, Choppin PW. Isolation and properties of the helical nucleocapsid of the parainfluenza virus SV5. *Proc Natl Acad Sci U S A* 1967;57:949–956.
52. Compans RW, Choppin PW. The length of the helical nucleocapsid of Newcastle disease virus. *Virology* 1967;33:344–346.
53. Compans RW, Mountcastle WE, Choppin PW. The sense of the helix of Paramyxovirus nucleocapsids. *J Mol Biol* 1972;65:167–169.
54. Crenell S, Takimoto T, Porter A, Taylor G. Crystal structure of the multifactional paramyxovirus hemagglutinin-neuraminidase. *Nat Struct Biol* 2000;7:1068–1074.
55. Curran J. Reexamination of the Sendai virus P protein domains required for RNA synthesis: A possible supplemental role for the P protein. *Virology* 1996;221:130–140.
56. Curran J, Boeck R, Kolakofsky D. The Sendai virus P gene expresses both an essential protein and an inhibitor of RNA synthesis by shuffling modules via mRNA editing. *EMBO J* 1991;10:3079–3085.
57. Curran J, de Melo M, Moyer S, Kolakofsky D. Characterization of the Sendai virus V protein with an anti-peptide antiserum. *Virology* 1991;184:108–116.
58. Curran J, Homann H, Buchholz C, et al. The hypervariable C-terminal tail of the Sendai Paramyxovirus nucleocapsid protein is required for template function but not for RNA encapsidation. *J Virol* 1993;67: 4358–4364.
59. Curran J, Kolakofsky D. Ribosomal initiation from an ACG codon in the Sendai virus P/C mRNA. *EMBO J* 1988;7:245–251.
60. Curran J, Kolakofsky D. Scanning independent ribosomal initiation of the Sendai virus Y proteins *in vitro* and *in vivo*. *EMBO J* 1989;8:521–526.
61. Curran J, Marq JB, Kolakofsky D. The Sendai virus nonstructural C proteins specifically inhibit viral mRNA synthesis. *Virology* 1992; 189:647–656.
62. Curran J, Marq J-B, Kolakofsky D. An N-terminal domain of the Sendai Paramyxovirus P protein acts as a chaperone for the NP protein during the nascent chain assembly step of genome replication. *J Virol* 1995;69:849–855.
63. Curran J, Pelet T, Kolakofsky D. An acidic activation-like domain of the Sendai virus P protein is required for RNA synthesis and encapsidation. *Virology* 1994;202:875–884.
64. Curran JA, Kolakofsky D. Rescue of a Sendai virus DI genome by other parainfluenza viruses: Implications for genome replication. *Virology* 1991;182:168–176.
65. Damico RL, Crane J, Bates P. Receptor-triggered membrane association of a model retroviral glycoprotein. *Proc Natl Acad Sci U S A* 1998;95:2580–2585.
66. De BP, Gupta S, Banerjee AK. Cellular protein kinase C isoform zeta regulates human parainfluenza virus type 3 replication. *Proc Natl Acad Sci U S A* 1995;92:5204–5208.
67. Delenda C, Taylor G, Hausmann S, et al. Sendai viruses with altered P, V, and W protein expression. *Virology* 1998;242:327–337.
68. Deng R, Wang Z, Glickman RL, Iorio RM. Glycosylation within an antigenic site on the HN glycoprotein of Newcastle disease virus interferes with its role in the promotion of membrane function. *Virology* 1994;204:17–26.
69. Deng R, Wang Z, Mahon PJ, et al. Mutations in the Newcastle disease virus hemagglutinin-neuraminidase protein that interfere with its ability to interact with the homologous F protein in the promotion of fusion. *Virology* 1999;253:43–54.
70. Deng R, Wang Z, Mirza AM, Iorio RM. Localization of a domain on the Paramyxovirus attachment protein required for the promotion of cellular fusion by its homologous fusion protein spike. *Virology* 1995;209:457–469.
71. Didcock L, Young DF, Goodbourn S, Randall RE. Sendai virus and simian virus 5 block activation of interferon- responsive genes: Importance for virus pathogenesis. *J Virol* 1999;73:3125–3133.
72. Didcock L, Young DF, Goodbourn S, Randall RE. The V protein of simian virus 5 inhibits interferon signalling by targeting STAT1 for proteasome-mediated degradation. *J Virol* 1999;73:9928–9933.
73. Doms RW, Lamb RA, Rose JK, Helenius A. Folding and assembly of viral membrane proteins. *Virology* 1993;193:545–562.

74. Dorig RE, Marcil A, Chopra A, Richardson CD. The human CD46 molecule is a receptor for measles virus (Edmonston strain). *Cell* 1993;75:295–305.
75. Durbin AP, Hall SL, Siew JW, et al. Recovery of infectious human parainfluenza virus type 3 from cDNA. *Virology* 1997;235:323–332.
76. Durbin AP, McAuliffe JM, Collins PL, Murphy BR. Mutations in the C, D, and V open reading frames of human parainfluenza virus type 3 attenuate replication in rodents and primates. *Virology* 1999;261: 319–330.
77. Dutch RE, Leser GP, Lamb RA. Paramyxovirus fusion protein: Characterization of the core trimer, a rod-shaped complex with helices in antiparallel orientation. *Virology* 1999;254:147–159.
78. Ebata SN, Cote MJ, Kang CY, Dimock K. The fusion and hemagglutinin-neuraminidase glycoproteins of human parainfluenza virus 3 are both required for fusion. *Virology* 1991;183:437–441.
79. Egelman EH, Wu SS, Amrein M, et al. The Sendai virus nucleocapsid exists in at least four different helical states. *J Virol* 1989;63:2233–2243.
80. Einberger H, Mertz R, Hofschneider PH, Neubert WJ. Purification, renaturation and reconstituted protein kinase activity of the Sendai virus large (L) protein: L protein phosphorylates the NP and P proteins *in vitro*. *J Virol* 1990;64:4274–4280.
81. Elango N, Kovamees J, Varsanyi TM, Norrby E. mRNA sequence and deduced amino acid sequence of the mumps virus small hydrophobic protein gene. *J Virol* 1989;63:1413–1415.
82. Elliott GD, Afzal MA, Martin SJ, Rima BK. Nucleotide sequence of the matrix, fusion, and putative SH protein genes of mumps virus and their deduced amino acid sequences. *Virus Res* 1989;12:61–75.
83. Escoffier C, Manie S, Vincent S, et al. Nonstructural C protein is required for efficient measles virus replication in human peripheral blood cells. *J Virol* 1999;73:1695–1698.
84. Faaberg KS, Peeples ME. Association of soluble matrix protein of Newcastle disease virus with liposomes is independent of ionic conditions. *Virology* 1988;166:123–132.
85. Fass D, Harrison SC, Kim PS. Retrovirus envelope domain at 1.7 Å resolution. *Nat Struct Biol* 1996;3:465–469.
86. Fearns R, Collins PL. Model for polymerase access to the overlapped L gene of respiratory syncytial virus. *J Virol* 1999;73:388–397.
87. Fearns R, Collins PL. Role of the M2-1 transcription anti-termination protein of respiratory syncytial virus in sequential transcription. *J Virol* 1999;73:5852–5864.
88. Feldman SA, Hendry RM, Beeler JA. Identification of a linear heparin binding domain for human respiratory syncytial virus attachment glycoprotein G. *J Virol* 1999;73:6610–6617.
89. Finch JT, Gibbs AJ. Observations on the structure of the nucleocapsids of some paramyxoviruses. *J Gen Virol* 1970;6:141–150.
90. Flavell RA, Sabo DL, Bandle EF, Weissmann C. Site-directed mutagenesis: Generation of an extracistronic mutation in bacteriophage Q? *J Mol Biol* 1974;89:255–272.
91. Furuta RA, Wild CT, Weng Y, Weiss CD. Capture of an early fusion-active conformation of HIV-1 gp41. *Nat Struct Biol* 1998;5:276–279.
92. Galinski MS, Mink MA, Pons MW. Molecular cloning and sequence analysis of the human parainfluenza 3 virus gene encoding the L protein. *Virology* 1988;165:499–510.
93. Galinski MS, Troy RM, Banerjee AK. RNA editing in the phosphoprotein gene of the human parainfluenza virus type 3. *Virology* 1992;186:543–550.
94. Garcin D, Curran J, Kolakofsky D. Sendai virus C proteins must interact directly with cellular components to interfere with interferon action. *J Virol* 2000;74:8823–8830.
95. Garcin D, Itoh M, Kolakofsky D. A point mutation in the Sendai virus accessory C proteins attenuated virulence for mice, but not virus growth in cell culture. *Virology* 1997;238:424–431.
96. Garcin D, Latorre P, Kolakofsky D. Sendai virus C proteins counteract the interferon-mediated induction of an antiviral state. *J Virol* 1999;73:6559–6665.
97. Garcin D, Pelet T, Calain P, et al. A highly recombinogenic system for the recovery of infectious Sendai Paramyxovirus from cDNA: Generation of a novel copy-back nondefective interfering virus. *EMBO J* 1995;14:6087–6094.
98. Garcin D, Taylor G, Tanebayashi K, et al. The short Sendai virus leader region controls induction of programmed cell death. *Virology* 1998;243:340–353.
99. Giorgi C, Blumberg BM, Kolakofsky D. Sendai virus contains overlapping genes expressed from a single mRNA. *Cell* 1983;35:829–836.
100. Gotoh B, Ogasawara T, Toyoda T, et al. An endoprotease homologous to the blood clotting factor X as a determinant of viral tropism in chick embryo. *EMBO J* 1990;9:4189–4195.
101. Gotoh B, Takeuchi K, Komatsu T, et al. Knockout of the Sendai virus C gene eliminates the viral ability to prevent the interferon-alpha/beta mediated responses. *FEBS Lett* 1999;459:205–210.
102. Gotoh B, Yamauchi F, Ogasawara T, Nagai Y. Isolation of factor Xa from chick embryo as the amniotic endoprotease responsible for Paramyxovirus activation. *FEBS Lett* 1992;296:274–278.
103. Gupta KC, Patwardhan S. ACG, the initiator codon for a Sendai virus protein. *J Biol Chem* 1988;263:8553–8556.
104. Hacker D, Raju R, Kolakofsky D. La Crosse virus nucleocapsid protein controls its own synthesis in mosquito cells by encapsidating its mRNA. *J Virol* 1989;63:5166–5174.
105. Hamaguchi M, Yoshida T, Nishikawa K, et al. Transcriptive complex of Newcastle disease virus. I. Both L and P proteins are required to constitute an active complex. *Virology* 1983;128:105–117.
105a. Harcourt BH, Tamin A, Ksiazek TG, et al. Molecular characterization of Nipah virus, a newly emergent paramyxovirus. *Virology* 2000;271: 334–349.
106. Hardy RW, Harmon SB, Wertz GW. Diverse gene junctions of respiratory syncytial virus modulate the efficiency of transcription termination and respond differently to M2-mediated antitermination. *J Virol* 1999;73:170–176.
107. Hardy RW, Wertz GW. The product of the respiratory syncytial virus M2 gene ORF1 enhances readthrough of intergenic junctions during viral transcription. *J Virol* 1998;72:520–526.
108. Hausmann S, Garcin D, Delenda C, Kolakofsky D. The versatility of Paramyxovirus RNA polymerase stuttering. *J Virol* 1999;73: 5568–5576.
109. Hausmann S, Garcin D, Morel AS, Kolakofsky D. Two nucleotides immediately upstream of the essential A6G3 slippery sequence modulate the pattern of G insertions during Sendai virus mRNA editing. *J Virol* 1999;73:343–351.
110. He B, Lamb RA. Effect of inserting Paramyxovirus simian virus 5 gene junctions at the HN/L gene junction: Analysis of accumulation of mRNAs transcribed from rescued viable viruses. *J Virol* 1999;73: 6228–6234.
111. He B, Leser GP, Paterson RG, Lamb RA. The Paramyxovirus SV5 small hydrophobic (SH) protein is not essential for virus growth in tissue culture cells. *Virology* 1998;250:30–40.
112. He B, Paterson RG, Ward CD, Lamb RA. Recovery of infectious SV5 from cloned DNA and expression of a foreign gene. *Virology* 1997;237:249–260.
113. Heggeness MH, Scheid A, Choppin PW. Conformation of the helical nucleocapsids of paramyxoviruses and vesicular stomatitis virus: Reversible coiling and uncoiling induced by changes in salt concentration. *Proc Natl Acad Sci U S A* 1980;77:2631–2635.
114. Heggeness MH, Scheid A, Choppin PW. The relationship of conformational changes in the Sendai virus nucleocapsid to proteolytic cleavage of the NP polypeptide. *Virology* 1981;114:555–562.
115. Heggeness MH, Smith PR, Choppin PW. *In vitro* assembly of the nonglycosylated membrane protein (M) of Sendai virus. *Proc Natl Acad Sci U S A* 1982;79:6232–6236.
116. Helenius A. How N-linked oligosaccharides affect glycoprotein folding in the endoplasmic reticulum. *Mol Biol Cell* 1994;5:253–265.
117. Hernandez LD, Hoffman LR, Wolfsberg TG, White JM. Virus-cell and cell-cell fusion. *Annu Rev* 1996;12:627–661.
118. Hernandez LD, Peters RJ, Delos SE, et al. Activation of a retroviral membrane fusion protein: Soluble receptor-induced liposome binding of the ALSV envelope glycoprotein. *J Cell Biol* 1997;139:1455–1464.
119. Herrler G, Compans RW. Synthesis of mumps virus polypeptides in infected Vero cells. *Virology* 1982;119:430–438.
120. Hewitt JA. Studies on the subunit composition of the M-protein of Sendai virus. *FEBS Lett* 1977;81:395–398.
121. Hiebert SW, Paterson RG, Lamb RA. Hemagglutinin-neuraminidase protein of the Paramyxovirus simian virus 5: Nucleotide sequence of the mRNA predicts an N-terminal membrane anchor. *J Virol* 1985;54:1–6.
122. Hiebert SW, Paterson RG, Lamb RA. Identification and predicted sequence of a previously unrecognized small hydrophobic protein, SH, of the Paramyxovirus simian virus 5. *J Virol* 1985;55:744–751.
123. Hiebert SW, Richardson CD, Lamb RA. Cell surface expression and orientation in membranes of the 44 amino acid SH protein of simian virus 5. *J Virol* 1988;62:2347–2357.

124. Hirano A, Ayata M, Wang AH, Wong TC. Functional analysis of matrix proteins expressed from cloned genes of measles virus variants that cause subacute sclerosing panencephalitis reveals a common defect in nucleocapsid binding. *J Virol* 1993;67:1848–1853.
125. Hirano A, Wang AH, Gombart AF, Wong TC. The matrix proteins of neurovirulent subacute sclerosing panencephalitis virus and its acute measles virus progenitor are functionally different. *Proc Natl Acad Sci U S A* 1992;89:8745–8749.
126. Hoffman MA, Banerjee AK. An infectious clone of human parainfluenza virus type 3. *J Virol* 1997;71:4272–4277.
127. Homann HE, Hofschneider PH, Neubert WJ. Sendai virus expression in lytically and persistently infected cells. *Virology* 1990;177:131–140.
128. Homma M, Tamagawa S. Restoration of the fusion activity of L cell-borne Sendai virus by trypsin. *J Gen Virol* 1973;19:423–426.
129. Horikami SM, Curran J, Kolakofsky D, Moyer SA. Complexes of Sendai virus NP-P and P-L proteins are required for defective interfering particle genome replication *in vitro*. *J Virol* 1992;66: 4901–4908.
130. Horvath CM, Lamb RA. Studies on the fusion peptide of a Paramyxovirus fusion glycoprotein: Roles of conserved residues in cell fusion. *J Virol* 1992;66:2443–2455.
131. Horvath CM, Paterson RG, Shaughnessy MA, et al. Biological activity of Paramyxovirus fusion proteins: Factors influencing formation of syncytia. *J Virol* 1992;66:4564–4569.
132. Horvath CM, Williams MA, Lamb RA. Eukaryotic coupled translation of tandem cistrons: Identification of the influenza B virus BM2 polypeptide. *EMBO J* 1990;9:2639–2647.
133. Hsu C-H, Kingsbury DW. Topography of phosphate residues in Sendai virus proteins. *Virology* 1982;120:225–234.
134. Hu CJ, Kato A, Bowman MC, et al. Role of primary constitutive phosphorylation of Sendai virus P and V proteins in viral replication and pathogenesis. *Virology* 1999;263:195–208.
135. Hu X, Ray R, Compans RW. Functional interactions between the fusion protein and hemagglutinin-neuraminidase of human parainfluenza viruses. *J Virol* 1992;66:1528–1534.
136. Huntley CC, De BP, Banerjee AK. Phosphorylation of Sendai virus phosphoprotein by cellular protein kinase C zeta. *J Biol Chem* 1997;272:16578–16584.
137. Itoh M, Isegawa Y, Hotta H, Homma M. Isolation of an avirulent mutant of Sendai virus with two amino acid mutations from a highly virulent field strain through adaptation to LLC- MK2 cells. *J Gen Virol* 1997;78:3207–3215.
138. Jacques JP, Kolakofsky D. Pseudo-templated transcription in prokaryotic and eukaryotic organisms. *Genes Dev* 1991;5:707–713.
139. Jiang S, Lin K, Strick N, Neurath AR. Inhibition of HIV-1 infection by a fusion domain binding peptide from the HIV-1 envelope glycoprotein GP41. *Biochem Biophys Res Common* 1993;195:533–538.
140. Jin H, Cheng X, Zhou HZ, et al. Respiratory syncytial virus that lacks open reading frame 2 of the M2 gene (M2-2) has altered growth characteristics and is attenuated in rodents. *J Virol* 2000;74:74–82.
141. Jin H, Clarke D, Zhou HZ-Y, et al. Recombinant human respiratory syncytial virus (RSV) from cDNA and construction of subgroup A and B chimeric RSV. *Virology* 1998;251:206–214.
142. Joshi SB, Dutch RE, Lamb RA. A core trimer of the Paramyxovirus fusion protein: Parallels to influenza virus hemagglutinin and HIV-1 gp41. *Virology* 1998;248:20–34.
143. Kahn JS, Schnell MJ, Buonocore L, Rose JK. Recombinant vesicular stomatitis virus expressing respiratory syncytial virus (RSV) glycoproteins: RSV fusion protein can mediate infection and cell fusion. *Virology* 1999;254:81–91.
144. Kalderon D, Roberts BL, Richardson WD, Smith AE. A short amino acid sequence able to specify nuclear location. *Cell* 1984;39:499–509.
145. Kamer G, Argos P. Primary structural comparison of RNA-dependent polymerases from plant, animal, and bacterial viruses. *Nucleic Acids Res* 1984;12:7169–7282.
146. Karron RA, Buonagurio DA, Georgiu AF, et al. Respiratory syncytial virus (RSV) SH and G proteins are not essential for viral replication *in vitro*: Clinical evaluation and molecular characterization of a cold-passaged, attenuated RSV subgroup B mutant. *Proc Natl Acad Sci U S A* 1997;94:13961–13966.
147. Kato A, Kiyotani K, Hasan MK, et al. Sendai virus gene start signals are not equivalent in reinitiation capacity: Moderation at the fusion protein gene. *J Virol* 1999;73:9237–9246.
148. Kato A, Kiyotani K, Sakai Y, et al. The Paramyxovirus, Sendai virus, V protein encodes a luxury function required for viral pathogenesis. *EMBO J* 1997;16:578–587.
149. Kato A, Kiyotani K, Sakai Y, et al. Importance of the cysteine-rich carboxyl-terminal half of V protein for Sendai virus pathogenesis. *J Virol* 1997;71:7266–7272.
150. Kato A, Sakai Y, Shioda T, et al. Initiation of Sendai virus multiplication from transfected cDNA or RNA with negative or positive sense. *Genes Cells* 1996;1:569–579.
151. Kingsbury DW, Darlington RW. Isolation and properties of Newcastle disease virus nucleocapsid. *J Virol* 1968;2:248–255.
152. Kingsbury DW, Hsu CH, Murti KG. Intracellular metabolism of Sendai virus nucleocapsids. *Virology* 1978;91:86–94.
153. Klenk H-D, Garten W. Host cell proteases controlling virus pathogenicity. *Trends Microbiol* 1994;2:39–43.
154. Kolakofsky D, Blumberg BM. *A model for the control of non-segmented negative strand viruses genome replication*. Presented at Virus Persistence Symposium 33, Society for General Microbiology. Cambridge: Cambridge University Press, 1982:203–213.
155. Kolakofsky D, Bruschi A. Antigenomes in Sendai virions and Sendai virus-infected cells. *Virology* 1975;66:185–191.
156. Kolakofsky D, de la Tour EB, Bruschi A. Self-annealing of Sendai virus RNA. *J Virol* 1974;14:33–39.
157. Kolakofsky D, Pelet T, Garin D, et al. Paramyxovirus RNA synthesis and the requirement for hexamer genome length: The rule of six revisited. *J Virol* 1998;72:891–899.
158. Kolakofsky D, Vidal S, Curran J. Paramyxovirus RNA synthesis and P gene expression. In: Kingsbury DW, ed. *The Paramyxoviruses*. New York: Plenum Press, 1991:215–233.
159. Kurotani A, Kiyotani K, Kato A, et al. Sendai virus C proteins are categorically nonessential gene products but silencing their expression severly impairs viral replication and pathogenesis. *Genes Cells* 1998; 3:111–124.
160. Lamb RA. The phosphorylation of Sendai virus proteins by a virus particle-associated protein kinase. *J Gen Virol* 1975;26:249–263.
161. Lamb RA. Paramyxovirus fusion: A hypothesis for changes. *Virology* 1993;197:1–11.
162. Lamb RA, Choppin PW. The synthesis of Sendai virus polypeptides in infected cells. II. Intracellular distribution of polypeptides. *Virology* 1977;81:371–381.
163. Lamb RA, Choppin PW. The synthesis of Sendai virus polypeptides in infected cells. III. Phosphorylation of polypeptides. *Virology* 1977;81:382–397.
164. Lamb RA, Mahy BW, Choppin PW. The synthesis of Sendai virus polypeptides in infected cells. *Virology* 1976;69:116–131.
165. Lambert DM, Barney S, Lambert AL, et al. Peptides from conserved regions of Paramyxovirus fusion (F) proteins are potent inhibitors of viral fusion. *Proc Natl Acad Sci U S A* 1996;93:2186–2191.
166. Langedijk JPM, Daus FJ, van Oirschot JT. Sequence and structure alignment of *Paramyxoviridae* attachment proteins and discovery of enzymatic activity for a Morbillivirus hemagglutinin. *J Virol* 1997;71: 6155–6167.
167. Latorre P, Cadd T, Itoh M, et al. The various Sendai virus C proteins are not functionally equivalent and exert both positive and negative effects on viral RNA accumulation during the course of infection. *J Virol* 1998;72:5984–5993.
168. Latorre P, Cadd T, Itoh M, et al. The various Sendai virus C proteins are not functionally equivalent and exert both positive and negative effects on viral RNA accumulation during the course of infection. *J Virol* 1999;72:5984–5993.
169. Latorre P, Kolakofsky D, Curran J. Sendai virus Y proteins are initiated by a ribosomal shunt. *Mol Cell Biol* 1999;18:5021–5031.
170. Lawson N, Stillman E, Whitt M, Rose J. Recombinant vesicular stomatitis viruses from DNA. *Proc Natl Acad Sci U S A* 1995;92: 4471–4481.
171. Leser GP, Ector KJ, Lamb RA. The Paramyxovirus simian virus 5 hemagglutinin-neuraminidase glycoprotein, but not the fusion glycoprotein, is internalized via coated pits and enters the endocytic pathway. *Mol Biol Cell* 1996;7:155–172.
172. Leser GP, Ector KJ, Ng DT, et al. The signal for clathrin-mediated endocytosis of the Paramyxovirus SV5 HN protein resides at the transmembrane domain-ectodomain boundary region. *Virology* 1999;262:79– 92.
173. Leyrer S, Bitzer M, Lauer U, et al. Sendai virus-like particles devoid of haemagglutinin-neuraminidase protein infect cells via the human asialoglycoprotein receptor. *J Gen Virol* 1998;79:683–687.

174. Leyrer S, Neubert WJ, Sedlmeier R. Rapid and efficient recovery of Sendai virus from cDNA: Factors influencing recombinant virus rescue. *J Virol Methods* 1998;75:47–58.
175. Lin GY, Paterson RG, Richardson CD, Lamb RA. The V protein of the Paramyxovirus SV5 interacts with damage-specific DNA binding protein. *Virology* 1998;249:189–200.
176. Liston P, Briedis DJ. Measles virus V protein binds zinc. *Virology* 1994;198:399–404.
177. Lu M, Blacklow SC, Kim PS. A trimeric structural domain of the HIV-1 transmembrane glycoprotein. *Nat Struct Biol* 1995;2:1075–1082.
178. Malashkevich VN, Schneider BJ, McNally ML, et al. Core structure of the envelope glycoprotein GP2 from Ebola virus at 1.9-A resolution. *Proc Natl Acad Sci U S A* 1999;96:2662–2667.
179. Markwell MA, Fox CF. Protein-protein interactions within paramyxoviruses identified by native disulfide bonding or reversible chemical cross-linking. *J Virol* 1980;33:152–166.
180. Markwell MA, Portner A, Schwartz AL. An alternative route of infection for viruses: Entry by means of the asialoglycoprotein receptor of a Sendai virus mutant lacking its attachment protein. *Proc Natl Acad Sci U S A* 1985;82:978–982.
181. Markwell MAK. New frontiers opened by the exploration of host cell receptors. In: Kingsbury DW, ed. *The Paramyxoviruses.* New York: Plenum Press, 1991:407–425.
182. Markwell MAK, Fredman P, Svennerholm L. Specific gangliosides are receptors for Sendai virus. *Adv Exp Biol* 1984;174:369–379.
183. Markwell MAK, Moss J, Hom BE, et al. Expression of gangliosides as receptors at the cell surface controls infection of NCTC 2071 cells by Sendai virus. *Virology* 1986;155:356–364.
184. Matsuoka Y, Curran J, Pelet T, et al. The P gene of human parainfluenza virus type 1 encodes P and C proteins but not a cysteine-rich V protein. *J Virol* 1991;65:3406–3410.
185. McGinnes L, Sergel T, Morrison T. Mutations in the transmembrane domain of the HN protein of Newcastle disease virus affect the structure and activity of the protein. *Virology* 1993;196:101–110.
186. Merz DC, Prehm P, Scheid A, Choppin PW. Inhibition of the neuraminidase of paramyxoviruses by halide ions: A possible means of modulating the two activities of the HN protein. *Virology* 1981;112:296–305.
187. Mink MA, Stec DS, Collins PL. Nucleotide sequences of the 3′ leader and 5′ trailer regions of human respiratory syncytial virus genomic RNA. *Virology* 1991;185:615–624.
188. Mirza AM, Deng R, Iorio RM. Site-directed mutagenesis of a conserved hexapeptide in the Paramyxovirus hemagglutinin-neuraminidae glycoprotein: Effects on antigenic structure and function. *J Virol* 1994;68:5093–5099.
189. Moore JP, McKeating JA, Weiss RA, Sattentau QJ. Dissociation of gp120 from HIV-1 virions induced by soluble CD4. *Science* 1990;250: 1130–1142.
190. Morgan EM, Re GG, Kingsbury DW. Complete sequence of the Sendai virus NP gene from a cloned insert. *Virology* 1984;135: 279–287.
191. Morrison T, McQuain C, McGinnes L. Complementation between avirulent Newcastle disease virus and a fusion protein gene expressed from a retrovirus vector: Requirements for membrane fusion. *J Virol* 1991;65:813–822.
192. Morrison T, Portner A. Structure, function, and intracellular processing of the glycoproteins of *Paramyxoviridae*. In: Kingsbury DW, ed. *The Paramyxoviruses.* New York: Plenum Press, 1991:347–382.
193. Morrison TG, McQuain C, O'Connell KF, McGinnes LW. Mature, cell-associated HN protein of Newcastle disease virus exists in two forms differentiated by posttranslational modifications. *Virus Res* 1990;15:113–133.
194. Mountcastle WE, Compans RW, Lackland H, Choppin PW. Proteolytic cleavage of subunits of the nucleocapsid of the Paramyxovirus simian virus 5. *J Virol* 1974;14:1253–1261.
195. Mrkic B, Odermatt B, Klein MA, et al. Lymphatic dissemination and comparative pathology of recombinant measles viruses in genetically modified mice. *J Virol* 2000;74:1364–1372.
196. Munoz-Barroso I, Durell S, Sakaguchi K, et al. Dilation of the human immunodeficiency virus-1 envelope glycoprotein fusion pore revealed by the inhibitory action of a synthetic peptide from gp41. *J Cell Biol* 1998;140:315–323.
197. Murphy SK, Ito Y, Parks GD. A functional antigenomic promoter for the Paramyxovirus simian virus 5 requires proper spacing between an essential internal segment and the 3′ terminus. *J Virol* 1998;72:10–19.
198. Murphy SK, Parks GD. RNA replication for the Paramyxovirus simian virus 5 requries an internal repeated (CGNNNN) sequence motif. *J Virol* 1999;73:805–809.
199. Nagai Y, Klenk H-D. Activation of precursors to both glycoproteins of Newcastle disease virus by proteolytic cleavage. *Virology* 1977; 77:125–134.
200. Nagai Y, Ogura H, Klenk H-D. Studies on the assembly of the envelope of Newcastle disease virus. *Virology* 1976;69:523–538.
201. Naniche D, Varior-Krishnan G, Cervoni F, et al. Human membrane cofactor protein (CD46) acts as a cellular receptor for measles virus. *J Virol* 1993;67:6025–6032.
202. Ng DT, Hiebert SW, Lamb RA. Different roles of individual N-linked oligosaccharide chains in folding, assembly, and transport of the simian virus 5 hemagglutinin-neuraminidase. *Mol Cell Biol* 1990;10: 1989–2001.
203. Ng DT, Randall RE, Lamb RA. Intracellular maturation and transport of the SV5 type II glycoprotein hemagglutinin-neuraminidase: Specific and transient association with GRP78-BiP in the endoplasmic reticulum and extensive internalization from the cell surface. *J Cell Biol* 1989;109:3273–3289.
204. Novick SL, Hoekstra D. Membrane penetration of Sendai virus glycoproteins during the early stage of fusion with liposomes as determined by hydrophobic affinity labeling. *Proc Natl Acad Sci U S A* 1988;85:7433–7437.
205. Olmsted RA, Collins PL. The 1A protein of respiratory syncytial virus is an integral membrane protein present as multiple, structurally distinct species. *J Virol* 1989;63:2019–2029.
206. Olmsted RA, Elango N, Prince GA, et al. Expression of the F glycoprotein of respiratory syncytial virus by a recombinant vaccinia virus: Comparison of the individual contributions of the F and G glycoproteins to host immunity. *Proc Natl Acad Sci U S A* 1986;83:7462–7466.
207. Ortmann D, Ohuchi M, Angliker H, et al. Proteolytic cleavage of wild type and mutants of the F protein of human parainfluenza virus type 3 by two subtilisin-like endoproteases, furin and KEX2. *J Virol* 1994;68:2772–2776.
208. Parks GD, Ward CD, Lamb RA. Molecular cloning of the NP and L genes of simian virus 5: Identification of highly conserved domains in Paramyxovirus NP and L proteins. *Virus Res* 1992;22:259–279.
209. Paterson RG, Hiebert SW, Lamb RA. Expression at the cell surface of biologically active fusion and hemagglutinin-neuraminidase proteins of the Paramyxovirus simian virus 5 from cloned cDNA. *Proc Natl Acad Sci U S A* 1985;82:7520–7524.
210. Paterson RG, Lamb RA. Ability of the hydrophobic fusion-related external domain of a Paramyxovirus F protein to act as a membrane anchor. *Cell* 1987;48:441–452.
211. Paterson RG, Lamb RA. RNA editing by G-nucleotide insertion in mumps virus P-gene mRNA transcripts. *J Virol* 1990;64:4137–4145.
212. Paterson RG, Leser GP, Shaughnessy MA, Lamb RA. The Paramyxovirus SV5 V protein binds two atoms of zinc and is a structural component of virions. *Virology* 1995;208:121–131.
213. Paterson RG, Russell CJ, Lamb RA. Fusion protein of the Paramyxovirus SV5: Destabilizing and stabilizing mutants of fusion activation. *Virology* 2000;270:17–30.
214. Paterson RG, Shaughnessy MA, Lamb RA. Analysis of the relationship between cleavability of a Paramyxovirus fusion protein and length of the connecting peptide. *J Virol* 1989;63:1293–1301.
215. Paterson RG, Thomas SM, Lamb RA. Specific nontemplated nucleotide addition to a simian virus 5 mRNA: Prediction of a common mechanism by which unrecognized hybrid P-cysteine-rich proteins are encoded by Paramyxovirus "P" genes. In: Kolakofsky D, Mahy BWJ, eds. *Genetics and Pathogenicity of Negative Strand Viruses.* London: Elsevier, 1989:232–245.
216. Patterson JB, Thomas D, Lewicki H, et al. V and C proteins of measles virus function as virulence factors *in vivo. Virology* 2000;267:80–89.
217. Peeples ME. Paramyxovirus M proteins: Pulling it all together and taking it on the road. In: Kingsbury DW, ed. *The Paramyxoviruses.* New York: Plenum Press, 1991:427–456.
218. Peeters BP, de Leeuw OS, Koch G, Gielkens AL. Rescue of Newcastle disease virus from cloned cDNA: Evidence that cleavability of the fusion protein is a major determinant for virulence. *J Virol* 1999;73: 5001–5009.
219. Pelet T, Curran J, Kolakofsky D. The P gene of bovine parainfluenza virus 3 expresses all three reading frames from a single mRNA editing site. *EMBO J* 1991;10:443–448.

220. Pelet T, Delenda C, Gubbay O, et al. Partial characterization of a Sendai virus replication promoter and the rule of six. *Virology* 1996; 224:405–414.
221. Pennington TH, Pringle CR. Negative strand viruses in enucleate cells. In: Mahy BWJ, Barry RD, eds. *Negative Strand Viruses and the Host Cell.* New York: Academic Press, 1978:457–464.
222. Poch O, Blumberg BM, Bougueleret L, Tordo N. Sequence comparison of five polymerases (L proteins) of unsegmented negative-strand RNA viruses: Theoretical assignment of functional domains. *J Gen Virol* 1990;71:1153–1162.
223. Portner A. The HN glycoprotein of Sendai virus: Analysis of site(s) involved in hemagglutinating and neuraminidase activities. *Virology* 1981;115:375–384.
224. Portner A, Murti KG, Morgan EM, Kingsbury DW. Antibodies against Sendai virus L protein: Distribution of the protein in nucleocapsids revealed by immunoelectron microscopy. *Virology* 1988;163: 236–239.
225. Portner A, Scroggs RA, Marx PS, Kingsbury DW. A temperature-sensitive mutant of Sendai virus with an altered hemagglutinin-neuraminidase polypeptide: Consequences for virus assembly and cytopathology. *Virology* 1975;67:179–187.
226. Radecke F, Billeter MA. The nonstructural C protein is not essential for multiplication of Edmonston B strain measles virus in cultured cells. *Virology* 1996;217:418–421.
227. Radecke F, Spielhofer P, Schneider H, et al. Rescue of measles viruses from cloned DNA. *EMBO J* 1995;14:5773–5784.
228. Randhawa JS, Marriott AC, Pringle CR, Easton AJ. Rescue of synthetic minireplicons establishes the absence of the NS1 and NS2 genes from avian Pneumovirus. *J Virol* 1997;71:9849–9854.
229. Rapaport D, Ovadia M, Shai Y. A synthetic peptide corresponding to a conserved heptad repeat domain is a potent inhibitor of Sendai virus-cell fusion: An emerging similarity with functional domains of other viruses. *EMBO J* 1995;14:5524–5531.
230. Roberts A, Rose JK. Recovery of negative-strand RNA viruses from plasmid DNAs: A positive approach revitalizes a negative field. *Virology* 1998;247:1–6.
231. Robinson WS. Self-annealing of subgroup 2 myxovirus RNAs. *Nature* 1970;225:944–945.
232. Robinson WS. Sendai virus RNA synthesis and nucleocapsid formation in the presence of cycloheximide. *Virology* 1971;44:494–502.
233. Romer-Oberdorfer A, Mundt E, Mebatsion T, et al. Generation of recombinant lentogenic Newcastle disease virus from cDNA. *J Gen Virol* 1999;80:2987–2995.
234. Deleted in page proofs .
235. Roux L, Kolakofsky D. Protein kinase associated with Sendai virions. *J Virol* 1974;13:545–547.
236. Roux L, Waldvogel FA. Instability of the viral M protein in BHK-21 cells persistently infected with Sendai virus. *Cell* 1982;28:293–302.
237. Russell R, Paterson RG, Lamb RA. Studies with cross-linking reagents on the oligomeric form of the Paramyxovirus fusion protein. *Virology* 1994;199:160–168.
238. Ryan KW, Portner A. Separate domains of Sendai virus P protein are required for binding to viral nucleocapsids. *Virology* 1990;174: 515–521.
239. Ryan KW, Portner A, Murti KG. Antibodies to Paramyxovirus nucleoproteins define regions important for immunogenicity and nucleocapsid assembly. *Virology* 1993;193:376–384.
240. Sagara J, Tsukita S, Yonemura S, et al. Cellular actin-binding ezrin-radixin-moesin (ERM) family proteins are incorporated into the rabies virion and closely associated with viral envelope proteins in the cell. *Virology* 1995;206:485–494.
241. Sakaguchi T, Kiyotani K, Kato A, et al. Phosphorylation of the Sendai virus M protein is not essential for virus replication either *in vitro* or *in vivo. Virology* 1997;235:360–366.
242. Sakai Y, Shibuta H. Syncytium formation by recombinant vaccinia viruses carrying bovine parainfluenza 3 virus envelope protein genes. *J Virol* 1989;63:3661–3668.
243. Sakai Y, Suzu S, Shioda T, Shibuta H. Nucleotide sequence of the bovine parainfluenza 3 virus genome: Its 3′ end and the genes of NP, P, C and M proteins. *Nucleic Acids Res* 1987;15:2927–2944.
244. Samal SK, Collins PL. RNA replication by a respiratory syncytial virus RNA analog does not obey the rule of six and retains a nonviral trinucleotide extension at the leader end. *J Virol* 1996;70:5075–5082.
245. Sanderson CM, McQueen NL, Nayak DP. Sendai virus assembly: M protein binds to viral glycoproteins in transit through the secretory pathway. *J Virol* 1993;67:651–663.
246. Sanderson CM, Wu H-H, Nayak DP. Sendai virus M protein binds independently to either the F or the HN glycoprotein *in vivo. J Virol* 1993;68:69–76.
247. Satake M, Coligan JE, Elango N, et al. Respiratory syncytial virus envelope glycoprotein (G) has a novel structure. *Nucleic Acids Res* 1985;13:7795–7812.
248. Scheid A, Caliguiri LA, Compans RW, Choppin PW. Isolation of Paramyxovirus glycoproteins. Association of both hemagglutinating and neuraminidase activities with the larger SV5 glycoprotein. *Virology* 1972;50:640–652.
249. Scheid A, Choppin PW. The hemagglutinating and neuraminidase protein of a Paramyxovirus: Interaction with neuraminic acid in affinity chromatography. *Virology* 1974;62:125–133.
250. Scheid A, Choppin PW. Identification of biological activities of Paramyxovirus glycoproteins. Activation of cell fusion, hemolysis, and infectivity of proteolytic cleavage of an inactive precursor protein of Sendai virus. *Virology* 1974;57:475–490.
251. Schmitt AP, He B, Lamb RA. Involvement of the cytoplasmic domain of the hemagglutinin-neuraminidase protein in assembly of the Paramyxovirus simian virus 5. *J Virol* 1999;73:8703–87812.
252. Schneider H, Kaelin K, Billeter MA. Recombinant measles viruses defective for RNA editing and V protein synthesis are viable in cultured cells. *Virology* 1997;227:314–322.
253. Sergel T, McGinnes LW, Peeples ME, Morrison TG. The attachment function of the Newcastle disease virus hemagglutinin-neuraminidase protein can be separated from fusion promotion by mutation. *Virology* 1993;193:717–726.
254. Sergel-German T, McQuain C, Morrison T. Mutations in the fusion peptide and heptad repeat regions of the Newcastle disease virus fusion protein block fusion. *J Virol* 1994;68:7654–7658.
255. Server AC, Smith JA, Waxham MN, et al. Purification and amino-terminal protein sequence analysis of the mumps virus fusion protein. *Virology* 1985;144:373–383.
256. Slack MS, Easton AJ. Characterization of the interaction of the human respiratory syncytial virus phosphoprotein and nucleocapsid protein using the two-hybrid system. *Virus Res* 1998;55:167–176.
257. Smallwood S, Easson CD, Feller JA, et al. Mutations in conserved domain II of the large (L) subunit of the Sendai virus RNA polymerase abolish RNA synthesis. *Virology* 1999;262:375–383.
258. Steward M, Vipond IB, Millar NS, Emmerson PT. RNA editing in Newcastle disease virus. *J Gen Virol* 1993;74:2539–2547.
259. Stone-Hulslander J, Morrison TG. Detection of an interaction between the HN and F proteins in Newcastle disease virus-infected cells. *J Virol* 1997;71:6287–6295.
260. Stone-Hulslander J, Morrison TG. Mutational analysis of heptad repeats in the membraneproximal region of Newcastle disease virus HN protein. *J Virol* 1999;73:3630–3637.
261. Stricker R, Mottet G, Roux L. The Sendai virus matrix protein appears to be recruited in the cytoplasm by the viral nucleocapsid to function in viral assembly and budding. *J Gen Virol* 1994;75:1031–1042.
262. Takeuchi K, Tanabayashi K, Hishiyama M, et al. Variation of nucleotide sequences and transcription of the SH gene among mumps virus strains. *Virology* 1991;181:364–366.
263. Takimoto T, Bousse T, Coronel EC, et al. Cytoplasmic domain of Sendai virus HN protein contains a specific sequence required for its incorporation into virions. *J Virol* 1998;72:9747–9754.
264. Tan K, Liu J-H, Wang J-H, et al. Atomic structure of a thermostable subdomain of HIV-1 gp41. *Proc Natl Acad Sci U S A* 1997;94: 12303–12308.
265. Tanabayashi K, Compans RW. Functional interaction of Paramyxovirus glycoproteins: Identification of a domain in Sendai virus HN which promotes cell fusion. *J Virol* 1996;70:6112–6118.
266. Taniguchi T, Palmieri M, Weissman C. Qβ DNA-containing hybrid plasmids giving rise to Qβ phage formation in the bacterial host. *Nature* 1978;274:2293–2298.
267. Tapparel C, Hausmann S, Pelet T, et al. Inhibition of Sendai virus genome replication due to promoter-increased selectivity: A possible role for the accessory C proteins. *J Virol* 1997;71:9588–9599.
268. Tapparel C, Maruice D, Roux L. The activity of Sendai virus genomic and antigenomic promoters requires a second element past the leader template regions: A motif (GNNNNN)3 is essential for replication. *J Virol* 1998;72:3117–3128.

269. Tapparel C, Roux L. The efficiency of Sendai virus genome replication: The importance of the RNA primary sequence independent of terminal complementarity. *Virology* 1996;225:163–171.
270. Tarbouriech N, Curran J, Ebel C, et al. On the domain structure and the polymerization state of the sendai virus P protein. *Virology* 2000;266:99–109.
271. Taylor J, Pincus S, Tartaglia J, et al. Vaccinia virus recombinants expressing either the measles virus fusion or hemagglutinin glycoprotein protect dogs against canine distemper virus challenge. *J Virol* 1991;65:4263–4274.
272. Teng MN, Collins PL. Identification of the respiratory syncytial virus proteins required for formation and passage of helper-dependent infectious particles. *J Virol* 1998;72:5707–5716.
273. Teng MN, Collins PL. Altered growth characteristics of recombinant respiratory syncytial viruses which do not produce NS2 protein. *J Virol* 1999;73:466–473.
274. Thomas SM, Lamb RA, Paterson RG. Two mRNAs that differ by two nontemplated nucleotides encode the amino coterminal proteins P and V of the Paramyxovirus SV5. *Cell* 1988;54:891–902.
275. Thompson SD, Laver WG, Murti KG, Portner A. Isolation of a biologically active soluble form of the hemagglutinin-neuraminidase protein of Sendai virus. *J Virol* 1988;62:4653–4660.
276. Tidona CA, Kurz HW, Gelderblom HR, Darai G. Isolation and molecular characterization of a novel cytopathogenic Paramyxovirus from tree shrews. *Virology* 1999;258:425–434.
277. Tober C, Seufert M, Schneider H, et al. Expression of measles virus V protein is associated with pathogenicity and control of viral RNA synthesis. *J Virol* 1998;72:8124–8132.
278. Tsurodome M, Kawano M, Yuasa T, etal. Identification of regions on the hemagglutinin-neuraminidase protein of human parainfluenza virus type 2 important for promoting cell fusion. *Virology* 1995;213: 190–203.
279. Valsamakis A, Schneider H, Auwaerter PG, et al. Recombinant measles viruses with mutations in the C, V, or F gene have altered growth phenotypes *in vivo*. *J Virol* 1998;72:7754–7761.
280. Varghese JN, Laver WG, Colman PM. Structure of the influenza virus glycoprotein antigen neuraminidase at 2.9 Å resolution. *Nature* 1983; 303:35–40.
281. Vidal S, Curran J, Kolakofsky D. Editing of the Sendai virus P/C mRNA by G insertion occurs during mRNA synthesis via a virus-encoded activity. *J Virol* 1990;64:239–246.
282. Vidal S, Curran J, Kolakofsky D. A stuttering model for Paramyxovirus P mRNA editing. *EMBO J* 1990;9:2017–2022.
283. Vidal S, Kolakofsky D. Modified model for the switch from Sendai virus transcription to replication. *J Virol* 1989;63:1951–1958.
284. Watanabe N, Kawano M, Tsurudome M, et al. Binding of the V proteins to the nucleocapsid proteins of human parainfluenza type 2 virus. *Med Microbiol Immunol (Berl)* 1996;185:89–94.
285. Weissenhorn W, Carfi A, Lee K-H, et al. Crystal structure of the Ebola virus membrane fusion subunit, GP2, from the envelope glycoprotein ectodomain. *Mol Cell* 1998;2:605–616.
286. Weissenhorn W, Dessen A, Harrison SC, et al. Atomic structure of the ectodomain from HIV-1 gp41. *Nature* 1997;387:426–430.
287. Weissenhorn W, Wharton SA, Calder LJ, et al. The ectodomain of HIV-1 env subunit gp41 forms a soluble, α-helical, rod-like oligomer in the absence of gp120 and the N-terminal fusion peptide. *EMBO J* 1996;15:1507–1514.
288. Weissmann C. Reversed genetics. A new approach to the elucidation of structure-function relationships. *Trends Biochem Sci* 1978;3: N109–N111.
289. Wertz GW, Collins PL, Huang Y, et al. Nucleotide sequence of the G protein gene of human respiratory syncytial virus reveals an unusual type of viral membrane protein. *Proc Natl Acad Sci U S A* 1985;82: 4075–4079.
290. Wertz GW, Krieger M, Ball LA. Structure and cell surface maturation of the attachment glycoprotein of human respiratory syncytial virus in a cell line deficient in O glycosylation. *J Virol* 1989;63:4767–4776.
291. Whelan SP, Ball LA, Barr JN, Wertz GT. Efficient recovery of infectious vesicular stomatitis virus entirely from cDNA clones. *Proc Natl Acad Sci U S A* 1995;92:8388–8392.
292. Whitehead SS, Bukreyev A, Teng MN, et al. Recombinant respiratory syncytial virus bearing a deletion of either the NS2 or SH gene is attenuated in chimpanzees. *J Virol* 1999;73:3438–3442.
293. Wild C, Oas T, McDanal C, et al. A synthetic peptide inhibitor of human immunodeficiency virus replication: Correlation between solution structure and viral inhibition. *Proc Natl Acad Sci U S A* 1992; 89:10537–10541.
294. Wild CT, Shugars DC, Greenwell TK, et al. Peptides corresponding to a predictive α-helical domain of human immunodeficiency virus type 1 gp41 are potent inhibitors of virus infection. *Proc Natl Acad Sci U S A* 1994;91:9770–9774.
295. Wild TF, Malvoisin E, Buckland R. Measles virus: Both the haemagglutinin and fusion glycoproteins are required for fusion. *J Gen Virol* 1991;72:439–442.
296. Wilson IA, Skehel JJ, Wiley DC. Structure of the haemagglutinin membrane glycoprotein of influenza virus at 3 Å resolution. *Nature* 1981;289:366–375.
297. Yao Q, Compans RW. Peptides corresponding to the heptad repeat sequence of human parainfluenza virus fusion protein are potent inhibitors of virus infection. *Virology* 1996;223:103–112.
298. Yao Q, Hu X, Compans RW. Association of the parainfluenza virus fusion and hemagglutinin-neuraminidase glycoproteins on cell surfaces. *J Virol* 1997;71:650–656.
299. Yoshida T, Nakayama Y, Nagura H, et al. Inhibition of the assembly of Newcastle disease virus by monensin. *Virus Res* 1986;4:179–195.
300. Young JK, Hicks RP, Wright GE, Morrison TG. Analysis of a peptide inhibitor of Paramyxovirus (NDV) fusion using biological assays, NMR, and molecular modeling. *Virology* 1997;238:291–304.
301. Yu M, Hansson E, Langedijk JP, et al. The attachment protein of Hendra virus has high structural similarity but limited primary sequence homology compared with viruses in the genus Paramyxovirus. *Virology* 1998;251:227–233.
302. Yuasa T, Kawano M, Tabata N, et al. A cell fusion-inhibiting monoclonal antibody binds to the presumed stalk domain of the human parainfluenza type 2 virus hemagglutinin-neuraminidase protein. *Virology* 1995;206:1117–1125.

CHAPTER 24

Orthomyxoviridae: The Viruses and Their Replication

Robert A. Lamb and Robert M. Krug

The *Orthomyxoviridae* are enveloped viruses with a segmented single-stranded RNA genome that has been termed "*negative stranded*" because the viral messenger RNAs (mRNAs) are transcribed from the viral RNA segments; by convention, mRNA is positive stranded. The genomic RNA of negative-stranded RNA viruses has to serve two functions: first as a template for synthesis of mRNAs and second as a template for synthesis of the antigenome positive strand. Negative-stranded RNA viruses encode and package their own RNA-dependent RNA transcriptase, but mRNAs are only synthesized once the virus has been uncoated in the infected cell. Viral replication occurs after synthesis of the mRNAs and requires synthesis of viral proteins. The newly synthesized antigenome positive strand (for influenza virus, often termed *template RNA* or *complementary RNA* [cRNA]) serves as the template for further copies of the negative-stranded genomic RNA.

Among the RNA viruses, influenza virus is special in that all of its RNA synthesis—transcription and replication—takes place in the nucleus of the infected cell. The nucleus provides the environment for the synthesis of influenza virus mRNAs by an unusual process: initiation requires m^7GpppX^m-containing capped primers that are generated from a subset of host cell RNAs by an influenza virus–encoded cap-dependent endonuclease. In addition to stealing the capped 5′ end of host mRNAs, influenza virus uses another aspect of the host cell nuclear function, namely the splicing machinery. The mRNAs synthesized by influenza virus and by one other virus, bornavirus (see Chapter 517 in *Fields Virology*, 4th ed.), provide the only known examples of splicing of RNA that is not transcribed from DNA by RNA polymerase II.

In recent years, a remarkable catalog of mechanisms has been identified by which eukaryotic cells have expanded their genome-coding capacity beyond the linear array of nucleotide sequences usually thought to encode a protein. Such coding strategies create diversity by increasing the number of proteins encoded and, in addition, provide a means by which the expression of these proteins can be regulated. Eukaryotic viruses have usually provided the prototypic example of molecular mechanisms that serve to maximize coding potentials. Indeed, the compactness of the viral genome may be an important factor contributing to the success of a virus as a cellular parasite. The influenza viruses provide some remarkable examples of genome diversity: spliced mRNAs and overlapping reading frames, bicistronic mRNAs and overlapping reading frames, and coupled translation of tandem cistrons. The variety of mechanisms used for the synthesis of proteins by influenza virus provides a paradigm of successful exploitation of a genome.

CLASSIFICATION

The family *Orthomyxoviridae* (from the Greek *orthos,* meaning "standard, correct," and *myxa*, meaning "mucus") contains four genera as defined in the seventh report of the International Committee for the Taxonomy of Viruses: influenza A, B, and C viruses, and thogotovirus (sometimes called influenza D viruses). Influenza viruses were named *Orthomyxoviridae* because of their ability to bind to mucus (hemagglutination) and to distinguish them from another family of enveloped negative-stranded RNA viruses (*Paramyxoviridae*). Influenza is from the Italian form of Latin *influentia*, meaning "epidemic," originally used because epidemics were thought to be due to astrological or other occult influences.

The influenza A, B, and C viruses can be distinguished on the basis of antigenic differences between their nucleocapsid (NP) and matrix (M) proteins. Influenza A viruses are further divided into subtypes based on the antigenic nature of their hemagglutinin (HA) and neuraminidase (NA) glycoproteins. Other important characteristics that distinguish influenza A, B, and C viruses are as follows:

1. Influenza A viruses infect naturally a wide variety of avian species, humans, and several other mammalian species, including swine and horses. Influenza B virus appears to infect naturally only humans, and influenza C virus has been isolated mainly from humans but also from swine in China.
2. The surface glycoproteins of influenza A viruses (HA and NA) exhibit much greater amino acid sequence variability than their counterparts in the influenza B viruses. Influenza C virus has only a single multifunctional glycoprotein, the hemagglutinin-esterase-fusion protein (HEF).
3. As discussed later, there are morphologic features that distinguish influenza A and B viruses from influenza C viruses.
4. Although influenza A, B, and C viruses possess similar proteins, each virus type has distinct mechanisms for encoding proteins.
5. Influenza A and B viruses each contain eight distinct RNA segments, whereas influenza C viruses contain seven RNA segments.

Little is known about the genus *Thogotovirus,* which comprises tickborne viruses that are structural and genetically related to influenza A, B, and C viruses (190) and contain a single glycoprotein (218). Because of space limitations and the need to discuss basic principles, these viruses are not considered further.

VIRION STRUCTURE

The *Orthomyxoviridae* are composed of about 1% RNA, 70% protein, 20% lipid, and 5% to 8% carbohydrate (reviewed in 51). The lipid envelope of influenza viruses is derived from the plasma membrane of the host cell in which the virus is grown (reviewed in 51). Influenza A and B virions are morphologically indistinguishable, whereas influenza C virions can be distinguished from the other genera because the glycoprotein spike is organized into orderly hexagonal arrays (51). Influenza A or B virions grown in eggs or in tissue culture cells have a fairly regular appearance in the electron microscope, with particles that are 80 to 120 nm in diameter. In contrast, virus strains isolated from humans or animals and propagated by single passage in culture exhibit greater heterogeneity and pleomorphism. The morphologic characteristics of influenza A viruses are a genetic trait (153) but also depend on the cell type in which the virus is grown (285). Although the genes that specify spherical morphology have not be identified, the trait segregates independently of the HA and NA proteins (155).

The most striking feature of the influenza A virion is a layer of about 500 spikes radiating outward (10 to 14 nm) from the lipid envelope. These spikes are of two types: rod-shaped spikes of HA and mushroom-shaped spikes of NA. The ratio of HA to NA varies but is usually 4:1 to 5:1. Influenza A, B, and C viruses also encode another integral membrane protein, the M_2, NB, and CM2 proteins, respectively. Biochemical evidence indicates these proteins are only present in a few copies in virions (13,24,337,395). The viral matrix protein (M_1) is thought to underlie the lipid bilayer and to associate with the ribonucleoprotein core of the virus. M_1 is the most abundant virion protein (Table 1). There is no evidence for the existence of a stable lipid-free "core" structure other than the ribonucleoprotein (RNP).

Inside the virus, observable by thin-sectioning of virus or by disrupting particles, are the RNP structures, which can be separated into different size classes (68) and contain eight different segments of single-stranded RNA. (Fig. 1 presents a schematic diagram of virion, and Fig. 2 shows electron microscopy photographs). The RNPs have

TABLE 1. *Influenza A virus genome RNA segments and coding assignments*

Segment	Length[a] (nucleotides)	mRNA length (nucleotides)[b]	Encoded polypeptide	Nascent polypeptide length[c] (aa)	Mol. wt. predicted	Approx. no. molecules per virion	Remarks
1	2,341	2,320	PB2	759	85,700	30–60	M^7-GpppX^m N^m (cap) recognition of host cell RNA; component of RNA transcriptase complex
2	2,341	2,320	PB1	757	86,500	30–60	Endonuclease activity; catalyzes nucleotide addition; component of RNA transcriptase, and replication complex
3	2,233	2,211	PA	716	84,200	30–60	Component of RNA transcriptase and replicase complex; function unknown
4	1,778	1,757	HA	566	61,468[d]	500	Major surface glycoprotein; trimer; receptor (sialic acid) binding; proteolytic cleavage activation; low-pH–induced conformational change and fusion activity; major antigenic determinant
5	1,565	1,540	NP	498	56,101	1000	Monomer binds to RNA to form coiled ribonucleoprotein; involved in switch from mRNA to template RNA synthesis and in virion RNA synthesis
6	1,413	1,392	NA	454	50,087[d]	100	Surface glycoprotein; neuraminidase activity; tetramer; antigenic determinant
7	1,027	1,005	M_1	252	27,801	3000	Major protein of virion, underlies lipid bilayer; interacts with RNPs and NS_2
		315	M_2	97	11,010	20–60	Integral membrane protein; ion channel activity essential for virus uncoating; channel inhibited by amantadine
		276	?	? (9)	—	—	Spliced mRNA sequence predicts that 9–amino acid peptide could be made
8	890	868	NS_1	230	26,815	—	High abundance, nonstructural protein in cytoplasm and nucleus; inhibits celluar pre-mRNA 3′ end cleavage and polyadenylation; inhibits pre-mRNA splicing; sequesters dsRNA from PKR kinase reducing interferon response
		395	NS_2	121	14,216	130–200	Minor component of virions; cytoplasmic and nuclear location; interacts with M_1 and involved in nuclear export of RNPs

[a]For A/PR/8/34 strain.
[b]Deduced from RNA sequence, excluding poly(A) tract.
[c]Determined by nucleotide sequence analysis and protein sequencing.
[d]Contribution of carbohydrate makes observed mol. wt. larger.

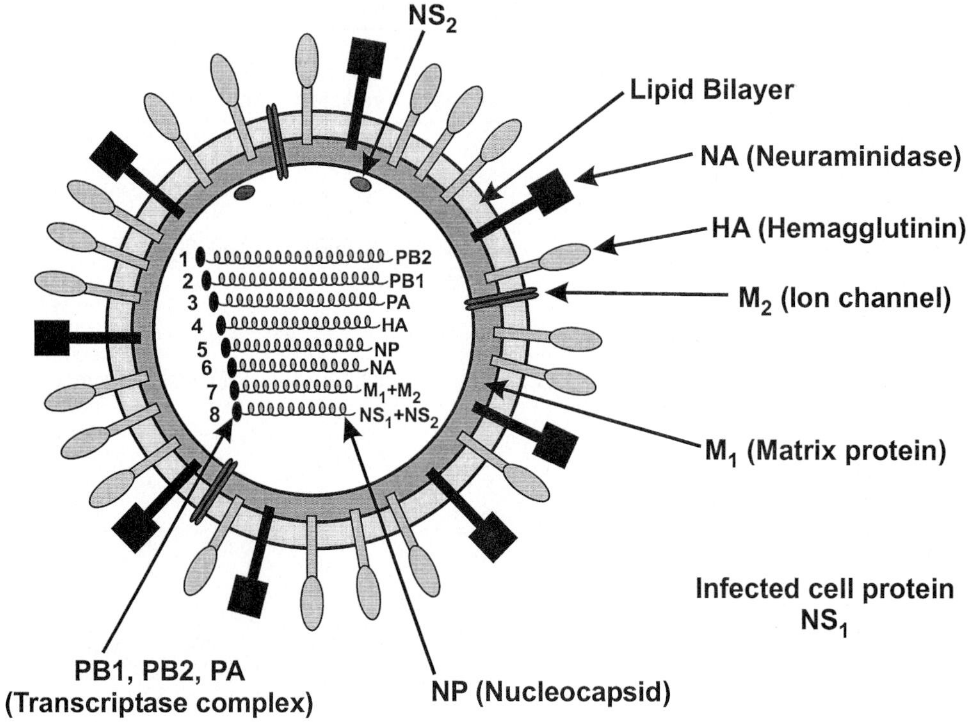

FIG. 1. A schematic diagram of the structure of the influenza A virus particle. Three types of integral membrane protein —hemagglutinin (HA), neuraminidase (NA), and small amounts of the M_2 ion channel protein—are inserted through the lipid bilayer of the viral membrane. The virion matrix protein M_1 is thought to underlie the lipid bilayer but also to interact with the helical ribonucleoproteins (RNPs). Within the envelope are eight segments of single-stranded genome RNA (ranging from 2341 to 890 nucleotides) contained in the form of an RNP. Associated with the RNPs are small amounts of the transcriptase complex, consisting of the proteins PB1, PB2, and PA. The coding assignments of the eight RNA segments are also illustrated. RNA segments 7 and 8 each code for more than one protein (M_1 and M_2, and NS_1 and NS_2, respectively). NS_1 is found only in infected cells and is not thought to be a structural component of the virus, but small amounts of NS_2 are present in purified virions.

the appearance of flexible rods (272); depending on the salt concentration during sample preparation or method of staining, the flexibility of the RNPs appears to vary (52,109,272). The RNP strands often exhibit loops on one end and a periodicity of alternating major and minor grooves, suggesting that the structure is formed by a strand that is folded back on itself and then coiled on itself to form a type of twin-stranded helix. Larger helical structures, interpreted to be formed by the orderly aggregation of the smaller segments, have occasionally been seen in partially disrupted virions (5,220). These structures might represent ordered complexes of the eight separate RNPs.

The RNPs consist of four protein species and RNA. NP is the predominant protein subunit of the nucleocapsid and coats the RNA: about 20 nucleotides per NP subunit. Associated with the RNPs is the RNA-dependent RNA polymerase complex consisting of the three P (polymerase) proteins, PB1, PB2, and PA, which are present at only 30 to 60 copies per virion (133,176). The RNA in the RNP complex remains sensitive to digestion by RNAase, and the RNA can be displaced by polyvinylsulfate (reviewed in 171). This suggests that the structure of the influenza virus RNP is very different from that of the RNAase-insensitive *Paramyxoviridae* RNP (see Chapter 23). The polymerase proteins in the RNP complex carry out the cap-binding, endonuclease, RNA synthesis and polyadenylation reactions described later (194,265–268).

The NS_2 protein (named as the second protein encoded by RNA segment 8) is present at 130 to 200 molecules per virion and forms an association with the M_1 protein (282,388), which is thought to be an essential interaction in the virus life cycle for export of the RNP complex from the nucleus (236) (see later). It has been suggested that NS_2 be renamed NEP for nuclear export protein (236).

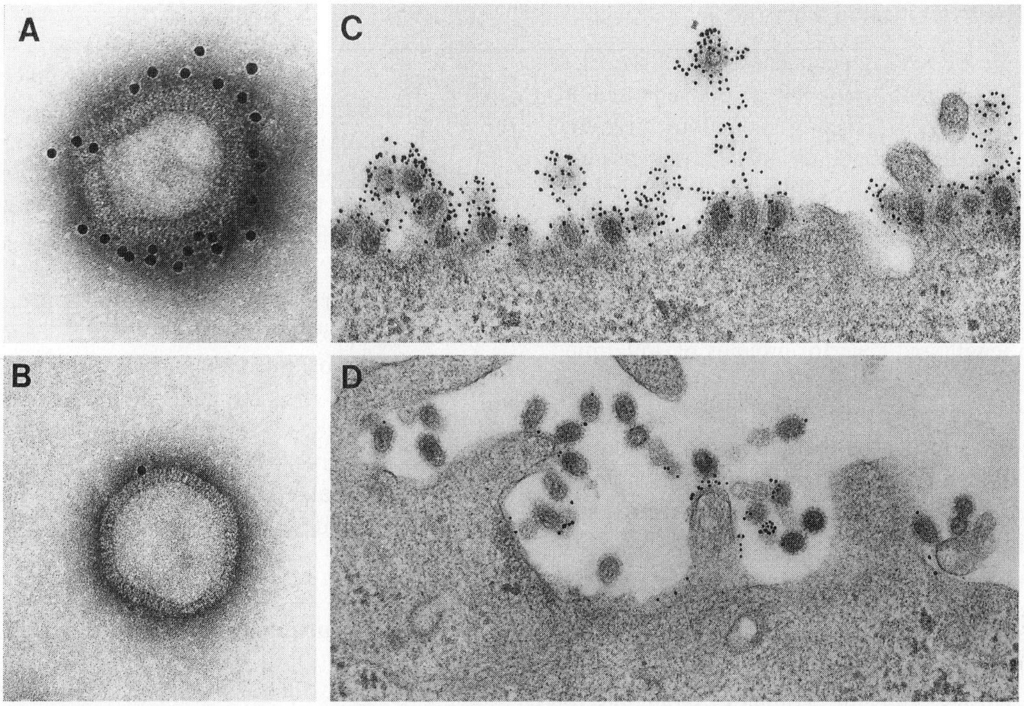

FIG. 2. Electron micrographs of purified influenza virus virions and virions budding from the surface of MDCK cells. **A:** Influenza A/Udorn/72 virus negatively stained with hemagglutinin (HA) decorated with 10-nm gold. **B:** Influenza A/Udorn/72 virus negatively stained with M_2 decorated with 10-nm gold. **A** and **B,** Final magnification ×227,500. **C:** Thin section of an influenza A/Udorn/72 virus-infected MDCK cell with HA decorated with 10-nm gold. **D:** Thin section of an influenza A/Udorn/72 virus–infected MDCK cell with HA decorated with 10-nm gold. **C** and **D,** Final magnification ×58,000. (Data from George Leser, Northwestern University.)

INFLUENZA VIRUS GENOME ORGANIZATION AND ENCODED PROTEINS

Influenza A and B viruses each contain eight segments of single-stranded RNA (ssRNA), and influenza C viruses contain seven segments of ssRNA (influenza C viruses lack an *NA* gene). The early evidence for a segmented genome of influenza viruses has been extensively reviewed (172). The major step forward in understanding the structure of the influenza virus genome came from the electrophoretic separation of the virion RNAs on polyacrylamide gels (10,214,246,247,271,283,284). The assignment of specific RNA segments to virus polypeptides was made in three ways:

1. One method depended on the apparent differences between strains in the electrophoretic mobility of the RNA segments on polyacrylamide gels and the ability to distinguish proteins between strains, either by immunologic methods for HA and NA or by differences in the gel mobility of polypeptides. Reassortants were prepared between two parental strains, with comparisons made of the mobilities of the RNA segments and polypeptides between the parental types and each recombinant. From the analyses, gene assignments were made (reviewed in 244).
2. A hybridization strategy was dependent on base-sequence homologies between corresponding RNA segments of different strains and temperature-sensitive (ts) mutants (302).
3. A direct method of hybrid arrest of translation of individual influenza virus mRNAs using purified vRNA segments (173,174).

The gene assignment for influenza A virus is as follows: RNA segment 1 codes for PB2, 2 for PB1, 3 for PA, 4 for HA, 5 for NP, 6 for NA, 7 for M_1 and M_2, and 8 for NS_1 and NS_2 (see Table 1). The complete nucleotide sequence of influenza A virus PR/8/34, and many RNA segments of other subtypes, was obtained by 1982 (reviewed in 171); today, the complete sequence of many influenza A and B viruses and one influenza C virus has been obtained. The PR/8/34 strain of influenza A virus contains 13,588 nucleotides. In this chapter, for space considerations, no attempt has been made to cite the original publication of the several hundred influenza virus nucleotide sequences obtained and deposited in the EMBL/GenBank database.

The Polymerase Proteins and Their Genes

The three largest RNA segments encode the PB1, PB2, and PA proteins (apparent M_r 96,000, 87,000, and 85,000, respectively) (133,176). Because of anomalous migration of influenza virus RNA segments on gels, the proteins encoded by RNA segments 1 and 3 from different subtypes are different. Therefore, the proteins are named after their behavior on isoelectric focusing gels: two P proteins were found to be basic (PB1 and PB2) and one acidic (PA) (125,343,383). RNA segments 1 and 2 are both 2,341 nucleotides in length and code for proteins of 759 amino acids (PB2) and 757 amino acids (PB1), respectively; PB1 and PB2 are basic proteins at pH 6.5, with a net charge of +28. Because the sizes of the two polypeptides PB1 and PB2 are very similar, the ability to separate them on polyacrylamide gel electrophoresis must be due to factors such as differential binding of SDS. RNA segment 3 is 2,233 nucleotides in length and codes for a protein of 716 amino acids that has a charge of −13.5 at pH 6.5. The three P proteins form a complex in the cytoplasm and nucleus of cells that is largely resistant to disruption by normal immunoprecipitation buffers and the complex sediments on sucrose gradients at 11S to 22S (63). After synthesis in the cytoplasm, the P proteins are transported to the nucleus, possibly as a complex. However, expression of the individual P proteins from cDNA has shown that each P protein migrates to the nucleus and each contains a karyophilic signal (1,139,324). A description of the known functions of the PB2, PB1, and PA proteins in RNA synthesis is presented later.

Influenza B and C viruses also encode three P proteins that show extensive sequence identity and homology to those of influenza A virus, and it is presumed these proteins have similar roles and properties such as those of influenza A virus.

The Nucleocapsid Protein and Its Gene

NP is the major structural protein that interacts with the RNA segments to form RNP. NP is also one of the type-specific antigens; that is, it is distinct for each of influenza A, B, and C viruses. NP is also the major target of cross-reactive cytotoxic T lymphocytes generated against all influenza virus subtypes in mice and humans (reviewed in 391). It is encoded by RNA segment 5 of influenza A virus and is 1,565 nucleotides in length. NP contains 498 amino acids with a predicted M_r of 56,101, and the protein is rich in arginine residues and has a net positive charge of +14 at pH 6.5 (384). Unlike what might be expected for a protein that interacts with the acidic phosphate residues of RNA, however, there are no clusters of basic residues. This implies that many regions of the NP molecule may contribute to RNA bindings. After synthesis in the cytoplasm, NP molecules are transported to the nucleus. Nuclear targeting of NP is an intrinsic property of the protein (199,295). Two nuclear localization signals (NLS) have been localized to NP: residues 198 to 216 (360) and residues 1 to 38 (230,355). Thus, NP may interact with several members of the importin family, soluble protein receptors involved in nuclear import. NP residues 327 to 345, originally thought to be an NLS (59), are now thought to be cytoplasmic retention signal (64). Late in virus-infected cells, NP of influenza A virus is cleaved from a 56-kd protein to a 53-kd protein by a cellular caspase, but it is not known whether NP cleavage is merely a marker for the onset of apoptosis in infected cells or has a specific function in virus–host interaction (400).

Influenza B virus NP contains 560 amino acids and is 47% homologous to influenza A virus NP, and the influenza C virus NP protein contains 565 amino acids and has several regions of homology with the NP of influenza A and B viruses (reviewed in 171).

The Hemagglutinin Protein and Its Gene

Introduction

The hemagglutinin was originally named because of the ability of the virus to agglutinate erythrocytes (116,213) by attachment to specific sialic acid–containing receptors. HA has three known roles during the influenza virus replicative cycle:

1. HA binds to sialic acid–containing receptors on the cell surface, bringing about the attachment of a virus particle to the cell.
2. HA is responsible for penetration of the virus into the cell cytoplasm by mediating the fusion of the membrane of the endocytosed virus particle with the endosomal membrane, the consequence of which is the viral nucleocapsids are released into the cytoplasm.
3. HA is the major antigen of the virus against which neutralizing antibodies are produced, and influenza virus epidemics are associated with changes in its antigenic structure.

HA is encoded by RNA segment 4 and is synthesized on membrane-bound ribososmes and translocated into the lumen of the endoplasmic reticulum (ER) of infected cells as a single polypeptide HA_0 (M_r about 76,000). The HA spike glycoprotein is a homotrimer (375,380) of noncovalently linked monomers. Each HA polypeptide chain (H3 subtype) consists of an ectodomain of 512 residues, a carboxyl-terminal proximal transmembrane domain of 27 residues, and a cytoplasmic tail of 10 residues (347). HA is cotranslationally modified by the addition of up to seven oligosaccharide chains added to the ectodomain, and three palmitate residues are added via a thioether linkage to the three C-terminal proximal cysteine residues (223,224, 301). Depending on the virus strain, host cell type, and growth conditions, HA exists either in an uncleaved precursor form (HA_0) or in a cleaved form consisting of two disulfide-linked chains (HA_1, M_r about 47,000; and HA_2, M_r about 29,000). Cleavage is a prerequisite for the virus to be infectious and hence is a crucial determinant in pathogenicity and in the spread of infection (reviewed in 329). The newly liberated N-terminus of HA_2 (fusion peptide) is hydrophobic, is highly conserved among HAs of different influenza virus strains, and is an essential participant in HA fusion activity.

RNA Segment 4: Gene Structure and Hemagglutinin Amino Acid Sequence

The first gene of influenza virus to have its nucleotide sequence determined was HA (274). Since then, the nucleotide sequence of RNA segment 4 of all 15 known HA antigenic subtypes and many variants within a subtype have been determined. RNA segment 4 ranges from 1,742 to 1,778 nucleotides and encodes a polypeptide of 562 to 566 residues. The HA_1 chain is from 319 to 326 residues, and HA_2 is from 221 to 222 residues. Depending on the HA subtype, the number of residues lost on proteolytic cleavage between HA_1 and HA_2 ranges from one to six residues. The deduced amino acid sequence of the influenza B/Lee/40 HA has 24% homology to HA_1 and 39% homology to HA_2 of A/PR/8/34, suggesting a close evolutionary relationship between influenza A and B virus HAs (169,170).

Three-Dimensional Structure of Hemagglutinin

Although intact HA "spikes" can be isolated from purified influenza virions and infected cells by detergent solubilization of membranes, when the detergent is removed, the hydrophobic transmembrane domains aggregate and HA "rosettes" form. However, bromelain treatment of virus releases an antigenically and structurally intact trimeric ectodomain of HA (BHA), which is water soluble and contains all of HA_1 and the first 175 of the 221 residues of HA_2 (23,376). BHA of influenza virus A/Aichi/68 H3 subtype crystallized, and from x-ray diffraction data, the three-dimensional structure of both cleaved and uncleaved HA was determined (39,376,380) (Fig. 3).

HA_0 and cleaved $HA_1 + HA_2$ are superimposable in structure except for 19 residues, in a sequence bracketing the cleavage site. The HA trimer extends 135 Å from the membrane and is composed of two predominant regions: (1) a long fibrous stem extending 76 Å from the membrane, which forms a triple-stranded coiled-coil of α-helices and is derived from HA_2 residues; and (2) the globular head of the molecule, which is derived from HA_1 residues and consists predominantly of an antiparallel β-sheet (see Fig. 3). In uncleaved HA_0, eight residues that immediately surround the cleavage site, including five hydrophobic residues of HA_2, project away from the molecules into aqueous solvent. HA_0 contains a deep cavity, which is partially filled by the C-terminus of HA_1 and which swings out of the way on cleavage. This permits filling of the cavity by residues 1 to 10 of the hydrophobic fusion peptide (the newly generated N-terminus of HA_2). Cleaved HA contains the fusion peptides buried in the subunit interfaces of the stem of the trimer (see Fig. 3) and is presumed to exist in a metastable form. Uncleaved HA cannot undergo the low-pH–induced refolding events associated with HA-mediated membrane fusion. It is not known whether it is the positioning of the fusion peptide in the cavity that sets the trigger or whether the covalent bond that links HA_1 to HA_2 restricts the movement of the fusion peptide. However, the localized structural rearrangement on cleavage causes nonpolar residues of the fusion peptide to bury ionizable residues located in the cavity, residues that have been implicated in the low-pH–induced refolding event (39).

The HA receptor-binding site is a pocket located on each subunit at the distal end of the molecule (see Fig. 3). The pocket is inaccessible to antibody, and the residues forming the pocket (Tyr-98, Trp-153, His-183, Glu-190, Leu-194) are largely conserved among subtypes (380; reviewed in 321 and 370). Confirmation that the pocket is the receptor-binding site was obtained by isolating HAs with single–amino acid substitutions at residue 226 that conveyed an altered specificity for sialic acid linked to galactose by either α2,6 or α2,3 linkages (288,367). Because the receptor-binding specificities differ among human trachea (α2,6), avian intestine (α2,3), and pig tracheae (α2,3 and α2,6) (134), the number of types of HA molecules that can transfer successfully from one species to another may be restricted.

The three-dimensional structure of HA indicates that five of the six carbohydrate chains on HA_1 and one carbohydrate chain on HA_2 lie on the lateral surface. The only exception is one carbohydrate chain on HA_1, which appears to stabilize the oligomeric contacts between globular units at the top of the structure (380). Although there is no known required function for carbohydrate on the native HA molecule, addition of carbohydrate is needed for the correct folding of HA in the ER (reviewed in 66).

Five antigenic sites have been mapped on the three-dimensional structure of HA by determining the location of amino acid changes in HAs of natural influenza virus isolates and in HAs of antigenic variants selected by growth in the presence of monoclonal antibodies (376). The regions of antigenic variation cover much of the surface of the globular head of HA, including residues around the antibody-inaccessible receptor-binding pocket. Monoclonal antibodies to each of the five antigenic sites neutralize the infectivity of the virus.

The Low-pH–Induced Hemagglutinin Conformational Change

Exposure of HA to low pH (299,371) triggers a progression of irreversible conformational changes that ultimately

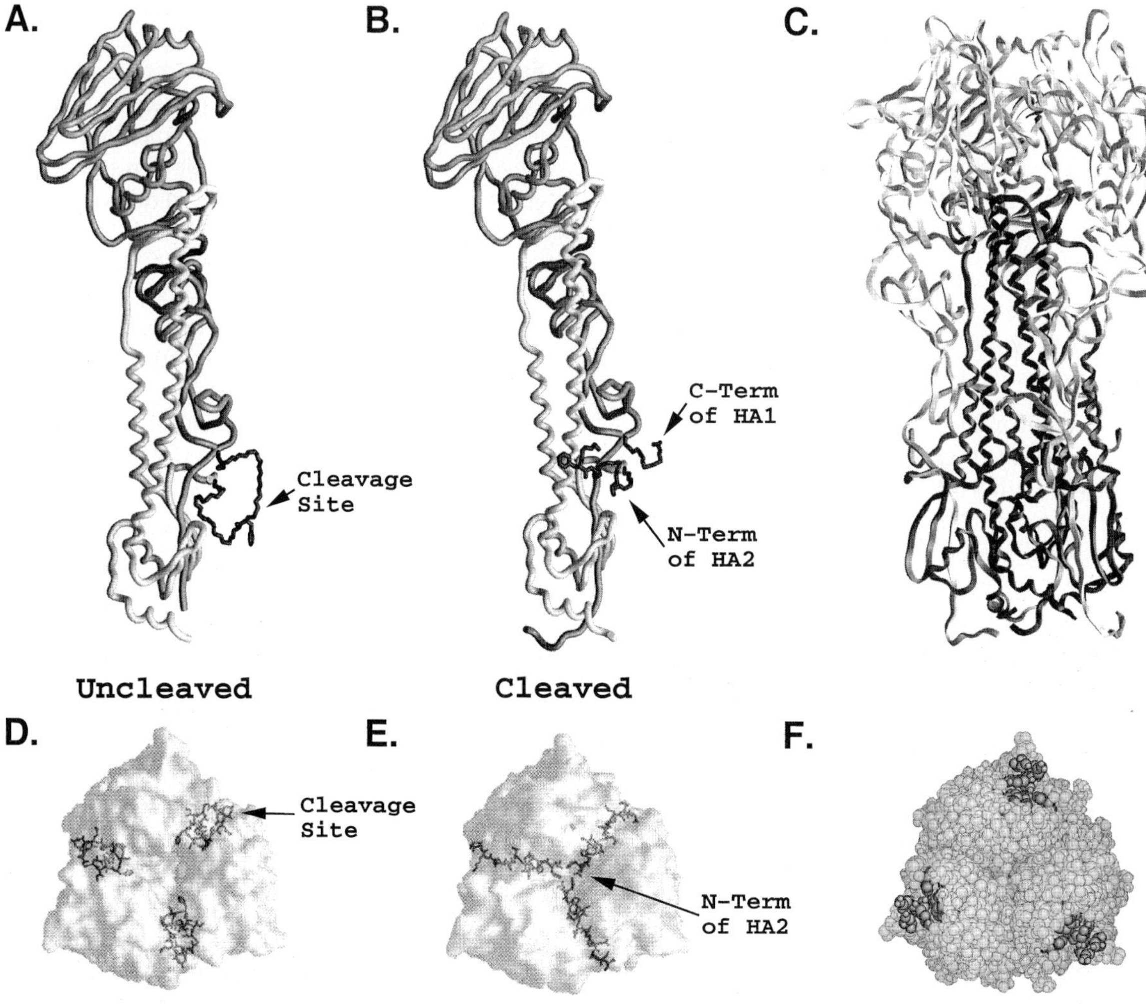

FIG. 3. Schematic diagram of the three-dimensional structure of the uncleaved hemagglutinin (HA) trimer and the cleaved HA trimer as determined from x-ray diffraction data. **A:** Side view of uncleaved HA monomer. **B:** Side view of cleaved HA monomer. **C:** Side view of cleaved HA trimer. **D:** Top down view of uncleaved HA trimer. **E:** Top down view of cleaved HA trimer. For **D** and **E,** shown in *dark gray* are the residues of the C-terminus of HA_1 and the N-terminus of HA_2 that change their position on cleavage. Note that the fusion peptide on cleavage becomes burried in the interior of the trimer. **F:** Top down view of the HA trimer. The residues that make contact with the HA receptor, sialic acid, are shown in *dark gray.* This figure was produced using Protein Data Bank (http://www.rcsb.org/pdb/) coordinate files 1HGF, 1HA0 and 1HGG.

lead to fusion of the viral and cellular membranes. The low pH found in endosomal compartments is the physiologically relevant trigger to release the hydrophobic fusion peptides. However, heat and urea treatments can also induce this change (36,293). Thus, native (pH neutral) cleaved HA is considered to be in a metastable state, and the low-pH–induced form is in a more stable form.

The HA low-pH–induced conformational change, in which HA_1 remains largely unchanged but HA_2 undergoes a refolding event, has been studied extensively. Low pH treatment of HA makes the protein susceptible to digestion by several proteases (58,65,318), and the single disulfide bond that links the HA_1 and HA_2 subunits becomes exposed (97). Furthermore, new antigenic epitopes are revealed with the concomitant loss of others (57,363,372). Despite these changes, x-ray crystallographic analysis indicated that the monomeric HA_1 globular head is virtually unaltered in structure after low-pH treatment (15). Nonetheless, rational engineering of cysteine residues into the head of HA_1 indicates that partial dissociation of the most distal region of the trimer occurs (90).

The x-ray crystallographic structure of proteolytic fragments of the low-pH–induced form of HA has been determined (33,40) (Fig. 4). In part, the structure fits with a model predicted for the low-pH–induced form (37). The x-ray structure shows that a protein refolding event occurs in which the fusion peptide is relocated more than 100 Å toward the target membrane (see Fig. 4). This refolding can be seen by comparison of the neutral-pH form with the low-pH–induced form. In the neutral-pH form, HA_2 residues 76 to 126 form a long α-helix, residues 56 to 75 form an extended loop, and residues 38 to 55 form a short α-helix (380). In comparison, in the low-pH–induced conformation, HA_2 residues 40 to 105 form a triple-stranded α-helical coiled-coil extending 100 Å. The N-terminal coiled-coil is terminated by a four-residue (HA_2 residues 34 to 37), threefold annular N cap structure that prevents the α-helix from propagating further toward the fusion peptide. Residues 106 to 112, which in the neutral structure are α-helical, uncoil to form an extended loop; the membrane proximal region of HA_2 swings up to pack against the long coiled-coil, running antiparallel to the N-terminal α-helix, packing in the groove between α-helices in the coiled-coil (see Fig. 4). The N- and C-terminal residues of HA_2 form an extensive set of interactions that fix the N-terminal and C-terminal residues of the molecule together at one extreme end of a thermally stable rodlike structure (33,40). The refolding event that moves the fusion peptide toward the target membrane is an essential step in bringing the two bilayers together. The mechanism by which two bilayers of two opposing membranes are fused together is not known, but some important observations have been made:

1. The conformational change in HA has to occur at the right time and in the right place because premature release of the HA fusion peptide causes oligomers to aggregate (294; reviewed in 319), and the refolding of HA_2 to its final and energetically most stable form is irreversible (40).
2. The fusion peptide can intercalate into lipid bilayers (reviewed in 30).
3. Several trimers are required to form a competent fusion pore (72).

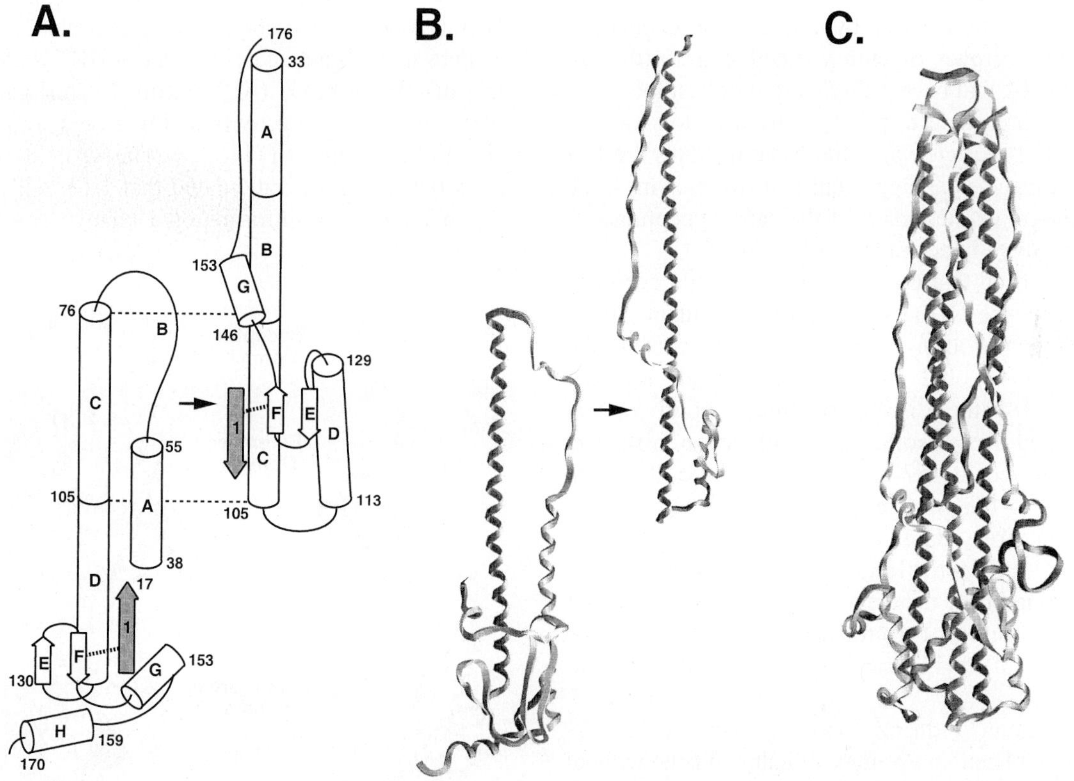

FIG. 4. The three-dimensional structure of the influenza virus HA after low-pH-induced protein refolding. **A:** Schematic diagram drawn from analysis of the x-ray crystallographic data of a proteolytic fragment of HA ($TBHA_2$) in the low pH-induced conformation. Only a monomer is shown. The long α-helix, extending 100 Å from near the proteolytic cleavage site at HA_2 residue 38 to HA_2 residue 105, participates in forming a triple-stranded coiled-coil in the trimer. In addition, the membrane-proximal portion of HA_2 swings up to pack against this long coiled-coil; residues HA_2 106 to 112, helical in the neutral pH structure, form an extended loop. (Redrawn from data of refs. 33 and 40). **B:** The atomic structure of a proteolytic fragment of the low-pH–induced form of HA_2 monomer. **C:** The atomic structure of a proteolytic fragment of the low-pH–induced form of HA_2 trimer. (This figure was produced using coordinate files available from Protein Data Bank coordinate file 1HTM and http://crystal.harvard.edu/wiley/coordinate_files.html.)

4. HA requires its transmembrane domain for complete fusion to occur. A genetically engineered HA anchored to membranes with a glycosyl phosphatidylinositol anchor promotes hemifusion but not complete fusion (150).
5. It has been hypothesized that the free energy released on refolding of HA_2 may be used in the process of membrane fusion (40).

Cleavage Activation of Hemagglutinin and Its Correlation with Pathogenicity

As discussed previously, cleavage of the HA_0 precursor to HA_1 and HA_2 is a prerequisite for the conformational change to the low pH form and hence is a prerequisite for virus infectivity (158,187). Those HAs that contain the sequence R-X-K/R-R in the connecting peptide are cleaved intracellularly by furin, a protease resident in the trans-Golgi network (TGN) (330; reviewed in 157). Those HAs with a single arginine residue in the connecting peptide (including all three known antigenic subtypes of human influenza) are not cleaved when grown in tissue culture cells (except for strain A/WSN/33; see later), but these HAs can be cleaved by addition of exogenous trypsin. When grown in embryonated eggs, influenza viruses with HA that have a single arginine residue at the cleavage site are cleaved, probably by a factor Xa–like protease (93). After cleavage, the basic residues are lost from the cleavage site, suggesting that two enzymes, the protease and an exopeptidase of the carboxypeptidase B type, are involved in activation of HA (67,87).

It was proposed that the cleavage site would correlate with the virulence of the virus and that virulent strains would contain the furin recognition motif, whereas the avirulent strains would contain only a single arginine residue (18,148); there is experimental support for this notion derived from work done with avian influenza viruses (reviewed in 157 and 329). However, there are complexities to this simple correlation: some avirulent H5 influenza virus strains have a furin recognition site. These avirulent H5 virus HAs contain an oligosaccharide chain positioned near the cleavage site, which is thought to alter accessibility of a protease to the cleavage site, whereas the virulent H5 virus HAs lack this oligosaccharide (146,147).

Among human influenza viruses, only A/WSN/33 (H1N1) can replicate in a variety of cultured cells without addition of trypsin (44), and genetic studies indicate that WSN NA is essential for WSN HA cleavage (303). It has been determined that WSN NA binds and sequesters the serum protease precursor plasminogen (92), a protease previously implicated in HA cleavage in tissue culture cells (189). Presumably, the binding of plasminogen by NA leads to a higher local concentration of the protease precursor. The structural basis for WSN NA binding plasminogen is thought to be the presence of a C-terminal lysine residue, and the absence of an oligosaccharide side chain found on all other N1 subtype NA molecules (92,196).

Influenza C Virus Glycoprotein, HEF

Influenza C virus contains only a single glycoprotein that has three activities: hemagglutinin, esterase, and fusion (HEF). The HEF protein has receptor-binding activity for 9-*O*-acetyl-*N*-acetylneuraminic acid, a fusion activity, and a receptor-destroying activity, which is a neuraminate-*O*-acetyl esterase (and not a neuraminidase) (113,348). The atomic structure of a protease-released form of HEF has been determined (289) (Fig. 5). Although HEF and HA have only about 12% sequence identity, the overall structure and details of the protein folds are quite similar. HEF is a polypeptide of 655 residues and consists of three domains: (1) an elongated stem active in membrane fusion that is closely related to the structure of HA_2 of influenza A virus, (2) a receptor-destroying esterase domain, and (3) a receptor-binding domain. The receptor-binding domain is inserted into a loop of the (esterase) domain, and the esterase domain is inserted into a loop in the stem. The esterase domain of HEF is related in structure to the esterase of *Streptomyces scabies* and a brain acetylhydrolase. HEF is cleaved by a trypsin-like protease (with a concomitant gain of low-pH–induced fusion activity and infectivity) to two disulfide-linked subunits (111,239). The structure of HEF is such that it can be anticipated that HEF will undergo a low-pH–induced conformational change similar to that

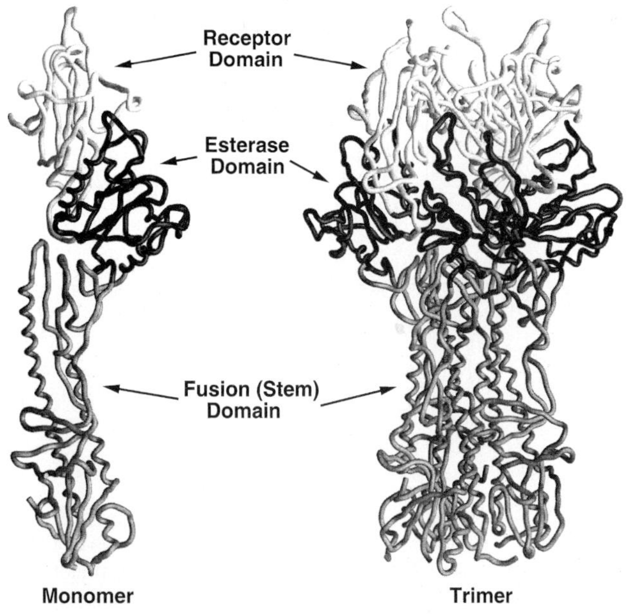

FIG. 5. The structure of the influenza C virus HEF glycoprotein. (**Left:** monomer. **Right:** trimer. Fusion, esterase, and receptor domains are indicated. (This figure was derived from atomic coordinates available from http://crystal.harvard.edu/wiley/coordinate_files.html.)

known to occur for HA. The principal difference is that, unlike HA, the hydrophobic fusion peptide of HEF is not at the immediate N-terminus but instead is located six residues from the N-terminus of HEF. The hydrophobic fusion peptide tucks into the trimer, and the six N-terminal residues of HEF loop back out.

At one time, it was thought possible that intracellular transport of HEF might require the expression of a second viral protein. However, expression of biologically active HEF of influenza C virus strains C/Ann Arbor/1/50 and C/Taylor/1223/47 indicated their cell surface expression did not require coexpression of another viral protein (257).

The Neuraminidase and Its Gene

Introduction

The NA integral membrane protein is the second subtype-specific glycoprotein of influenza A and B viruses. The NA is a homotetramer (M_r about 220,000) containing a head domain that is enzymatically active and a stalk region that is attached to the membrane. NA is important both for its biologic activity in removing sialic acid from glycoproteins and as a major antigenic determinant that undergoes antigenic variation. Neuraminidase (acylneuraminyl hydrolase, EC 3.2.1.18) catalyzes the cleavage of the α-ketosidic linkage between a terminal sialic acid and an adjacent D-galactose or D-galactosamine (94). The role of NA in the influenza virus life cycle is still unclear. Influenza viruses containing a ts mutation in NA aggregate at the surface of infected cells at the nonpermissive temperature, suggesting that one function of NA is the removal of sialic acid from HA, NA, and the cell surface (248). NA may also permit transport of the virus through the mucin layer present in the respiratory tract, enabling the virus to find its way to the target epithelial cells. Some avian neuraminidases (N1–3, N5–9; N4 not tested) also have a receptor binding site that causes hemagglutination, although the role of this receptor binding function in the influenza virus life cycle is not clear (103,160,186).

RNA Segment 6: Gene Structure and NA Amino Acid Sequence

The nucleotide sequence of all nine NA subtypes has been obtained (reviewed in 47 and 171). For the A/PR/8/34 subtype, RNA segment 6 is 1,413 nucleotides in length and encodes a polypeptide of 453 residues. The NA polypeptide contains only one hydrophobic domain sufficient to span a lipid bilayer, which is located near its N-terminus (residues 7 to 35). This domain acts as a combined uncleaved signal and anchor domain that both targets NA to the membrane of the ER and brings about its stable attachment in the membrane. Thus, NA is oriented with its N-terminus in the cytoplasm, and it is a prototype class II integral membrane protein (Fig. 6). There are five sites for the potential addition of N-linked carbohydrate.

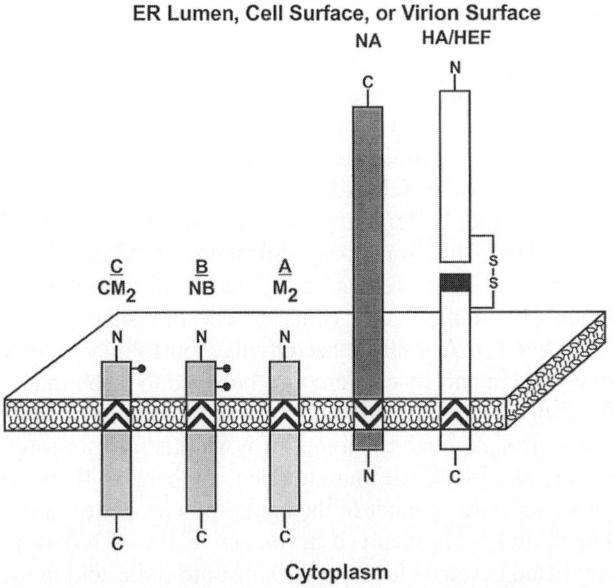

FIG. 6. Schematic representation of the orientation of the influenza A, B and C virus integral membrane proteins HA (HEF), NA, M_2, NB, and CM2.

Comparison of NA sequences among the nine subtypes of influenza A virus and influenza B virus reveals varying degrees of homology for the cytoplasmic tail, transmembrane (TM) domain, stalk, the head overall, and the catalytic active site. The cytoplasmic tail N-Met-Asn-Pro-Asn-Gly-Lys is conserved among influenza A subtypes (perhaps for a role in viral assembly; see later) but not between type A and B viruses. The TM domains of the A virus subtypes and B viruses share only the common property of hydrophobicity and not sequence homology. The stalks show a great deal of variability even between influenza A virus subtypes both in amino acid sequence and in length (62 to 82 residues, and the A/WS/33 stalk is 24 residues). The head domain shows extensive homology (42% to 57%) between influenza A virus subtypes and some homology (29%) between the type A and B viruses.

Influenza B virus RNA segment 6, in addition to containing the open reading frame (ORF) which encodes NA (466 residues), contains a second ORF of 100 residues (NB) that overlaps the NA reading frame by 292 nucleotides (309). The initiation codon used to initiate NA is the second AUG initiation codon from the 5′ end of the mRNA. The NB initiation codon is the first AUG codon from the 5′ end of the mRNA, and it is separated from the second AUG codon by 4 nucleotides (309). NB and NA proteins accumulate in virus-infected cells in a 0.6:1 ratio, suggesting that about 60% of ribosome preinitiation complexes scanning the NB/NA mRNA do not initiate protein synthesis at the first AUG codon but continue scanning to the second downstream AUG codon (378).

Three-Dimensional Structure of Neuraminidase

NA molecules lacking their TM domain and part of the stalk region can be obtained by pronase digestion. The isolated heads of the molecules retain enzymatic activity and antigenic properties. The protease-released neuraminidases of A/Tokyo/3/67, A/RI/5+/57, A/Tern/Australia/75, and B/Beijing/87, among others, have been crystallized, and from x-ray diffraction data, the three-dimensional structure has been determined to high resolution (19,34,48,49,345) (Fig. 7). The box-shaped head (100 Å × 100 Å × 60 Å) has circular fourfold symmetry stabilized in part by calcium ions believed to be bound on the fourfold axis of symmetry among a cluster of eight acidic groups. Each monomer of NA folds into six topographically identical, four-stranded, antiparallel β-sheets arranged in the manner of the blades of a propeller (345). The amino acids involved in the active site of NA were identified based on locating the substrate sialic acid in the molecule and obtaining an electron density difference map (49). The substrate-binding site was identified as a large pocket on the surface of each subunit rimmed by charged residues and consisting of nine acidic and six basic residues that are conserved between influenza A and B viruses. Mutagenesis of these conserved residues indicate that changes in these sites result in a loss of enzymatic activity (193).

The HA activity reported for the N9 subtype of NA is associated with a second sialic acid (Neu5Ac)-binding site on the surface of NA separate from the enzyme active site (362). The x-ray structure of a complex of Neu5Ac with N9 NA indicates Neu5Ac binds in the second site in the chair conformation in a similar way to which Neu5Ac binds to HA (344).

In a manner analogous to that done for HA, antigenic sites were mapped on NA by analysis of changes in naturally existing strains and in variants selected with monoclonal antibodies. Four antigenic sites were identified in influenza A virus NA, each consisting of multiple epitopes (364), and these cluster into the distal surface loops that connect the various strands of β-sheet. Note that antibodies to NA are not neutralizing but rather inhibit plaque size enlargement when incorporated into the overlay medium (154).

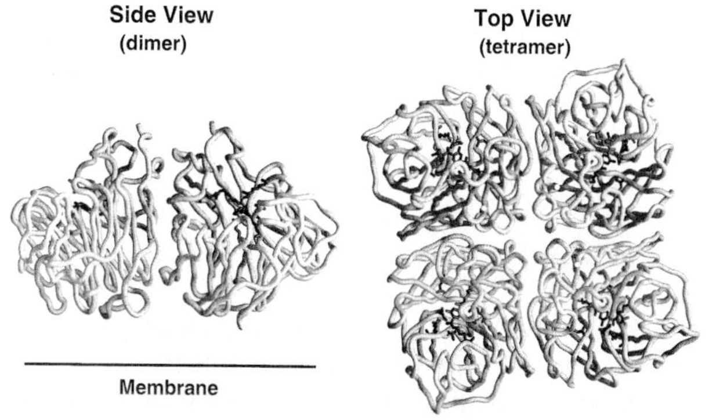

FIG. 7. Structure of the influenza A virus neuraminidase. **Left:** Side view of NA dimer. **Right:** Top down view of NA tetramer. (This figure was produced using Protein Data Bank coordinate file 7NN9.)

The Influenza B Virus NB Glycoprotein

The NB ORF on influenza B virus RNA segment 6 encodes the NB glycoprotein (Fig. 8). NB is an integral membrane protein that is abundantly expressed at the plasma membrane of influenza B virus–infected cells (308), and genetic and biochemical data have indicated that NB is oriented in membranes with an 18-residue N-terminal ectodomain, a 22-residue TM domain, and a 60-residue cytoplasmic tail (377). NB lacks a cleavable signal sequence but instead contains a single hydrophobic domain that is thought both to target NB to membranes and to anchor NB in a stable manner. The N-terminal ectodomain of NB contains two N-linked carbohydrate chains attached to residues 3 and 7 (377). These carbohydrate chains are further modified by the addition of a number of repeating units of galactose β1→4-*N*-acetylglucosamine β1→3 (Gal β1→4-GlcNAc β1→3) attached to a (mannose)$_3$ (GlcNAc)$_2$ core oligosaccharide, known as *polylactosaminoglycan modification* (377,379). Originally, NB was thought to be lacking from virions, but recent analysis of virions, after endo-β-galactosidase digestion to remove polylactosaminoglycan, suggests that NB is a component of virions present at about 100 copies per virion (13,24). The function of NB in the influenza virus life cycle is not known. The influenza B virus NB glycoprotein has the same uncommon membrane orientation (type III integral membrane protein) as the influenza A virus M_2 protein encoded by RNA segment 7 (see later and Fig. 6). The influenza A virus M_2 protein has ion channel activity, but influenza B virus lacks a direct M_2 counterpart. However, because the replication strategies of the influenza type A and B viruses are similar, there has been considerable speculation that the influenza B virus NB protein may have ion channel activity (reviewed in 184). NB has been expressed in bacteria and the purified NB protein incorporated into planar bilayers. Electrophysiologic recordings from these preparations indicated an ion channel activity (335). However, the lack of a selective inhibitor makes it difficult to assign definitively an ion channel activity to NB.

RNA Segment 7 of Influenza Virus

Introduction

RNA segment 7 of influenza A virus encodes two known proteins, the matrix protein M_1, which lies inside the lipid envelope and constitutes the most abundant polypeptide in the virion, and the M_2 protein, which is a

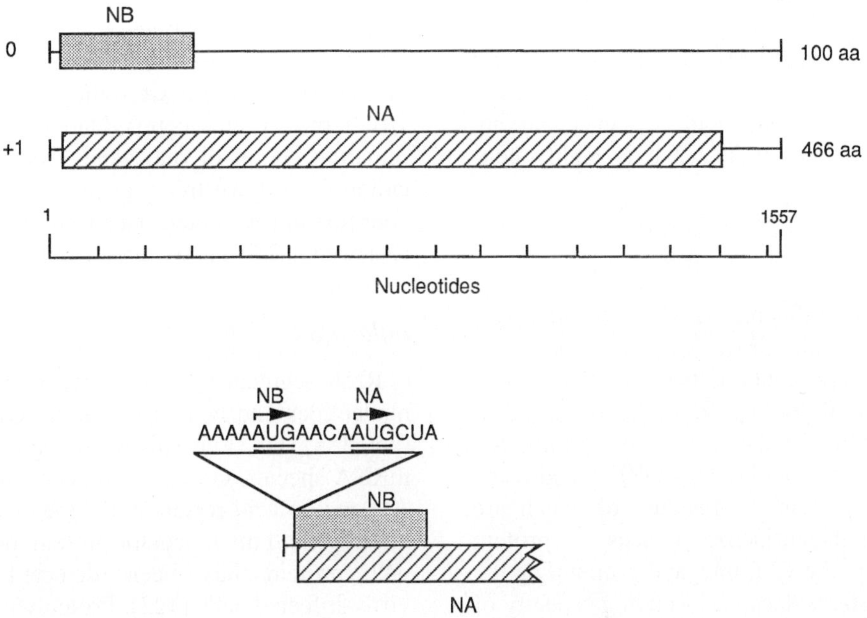

FIG. 8. Schematic representation of open reading frames (ORFs) in influenza B virus RNA segment 6. The NB and NA overlapping reading frames are shown. **Lower section:** Nucleotide sequences surrounding the AUG codons used to initiate the synthesis of NB and NA glycoproteins. (Drawn from data in ref. 308, with permission.)

minor component of virions and has ion channel activity. Three mRNA transcripts have been identified that are derived from influenza A virus RNA segment 7: a colinear transcript encoding M_1 protein, a spliced mRNA encoding the M_2 protein, and an alternatively spliced mRNA ($mRNA_3$), which has the potential to encode a 9–amino acid peptide, but it has not been identified in virus-infected cells. Influenza B virus RNA segment 7 encodes two polypeptides using tandem cistrons: the matrix protein M_1 and the 109-residue BM_2 protein of unknown function. The equivalent RNA segment in influenza C virus (RNA segment 6) is transcribed into a colinear mRNA that encodes the p42 protein. A portion of the colinear transcripts are spliced to form the mRNA encoding the matrix protein. The p42 precursor protein is translated from the colinear mRNA and subsequently processed to yield p31 and CM2 proteins.

RNA Segment 7 Gene Structure and Encoded Proteins

Influenza A Virus

RNA segment 7 of influenza A virus encodes two known proteins, M_1 and M_2. The gene is 1,027 nucleotides in chain length and has one large ORF of 252 residues that encodes the M_1 protein (2,180,382) (Fig. 9). A colinear transcript mRNA encodes the M_1 protein, whereas the M_2 protein is encoded by a spliced mRNA (183). The M_2 mRNA contains a 51-nucleotide virus-specific leader sequence, a 689-nucleotide intron, and a 271-nucleotide [excluding poly(A) tail] body region. The leader sequence of the M_2 mRNA body region encodes 88 residues in the +1 reading frame and overlaps the M_1 protein by 14 residues. A second, alternatively spliced mRNA ($mRNA_3$) has also been identified; it has a 5′ leader sequence of 11 virus-specific nucleotides and shares the same 3′ splice site as the M_2 mRNA. No evidence has been obtained to indicate that $mRNA_3$ is trans-

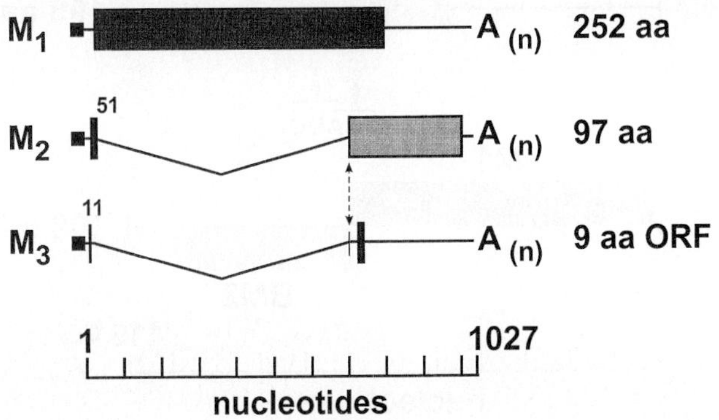

FIG. 9. Schematic diagram of the influenza A virus M_1, M_2, and $mRNA_3$ and their coding regions. Thin lines at the 5′- and 3′-termini of the mRNAs represent untranslated regions. *Shaded* or *hatched areas* represent coding regions in 0 or +1 reading frames, respectively. The introns are shown by the V-shaped lines. Rectangles at 5′ ends of the mRNAs represent heterogeneous nucleotides derived from cellular RNAs that are covalently linked to viral sequences. No evidence has yet been obtained that $mRNA_3$ is translated *in vivo.* (Adapted from ref. 182, with permission.)

lated, but if it is, it would yield a 9-residue peptide identical to the C-terminus of the M_1 protein (183).

The M_1 protein contains 252 residues (M_r, 27,801) and is a type-specific antigen of influenza virus, and comparison of its predicted amino acid sequence among influenza A virus subtypes indicates it is highly conserved (reviewed in 171).

Influenza B Virus

RNA segment 7 of influenza B virus encodes two known proteins, M_1 and BM_2. The gene is 1,191 nucleotides in length and contains two ORFs (Fig. 10). The first ORF in the 0 reading frame begins at AUG codon nucleotides 25 to 27 and continues to a termination codon at nucleotides 769 to 771. This ORF encodes the 248–amino acid M_1 protein, 63 residues of which are identical to those of the influenza A virus M_1 protein (27). A second ORF in the +2 frame, and overlapping the M_1 protein ORF by 86 residues, has a coding capacity of 195 residues and is designated BM_2 (27,126). A polypeptide, BM_2, derived from the BM_2 ORF, was identified in cells infected with influenza B virus by using an antisera generated to a β-galactosidase–BM_2 ORF fusion protein (126). The BM_2 protein appears to be a soluble and cytoplasmically located protein of unknown function. A mutational analysis indicates that the BM_2 protein initiation codon overlaps with the termination codon of the M_1 protein in a translational stop-and-start pentanucleotide

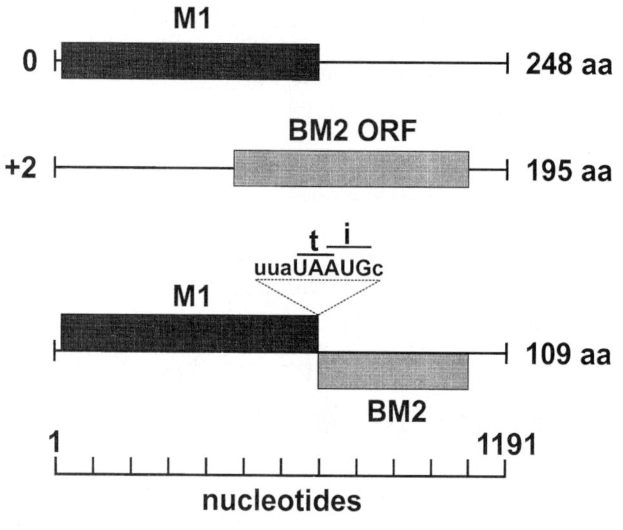

FIG. 10. Schematic representation of the open reading frames (ORFs) in influenza B virus RNA segment 7. **Top two lines:** The ORF encoding the M_1 protein contains 248 residues, and the BM_2 ORF consists of 195 residues (27). **Third line:** the extent of the BM_2 ORF used to translate the BM_2 protein found in influenza B virus–infected cells. The pentanucleotide at which M_1 translation termination (*t; UAA*) and BM_2 translation initiation (*i; AUG*) is shown in capital letters. (Data from ref. 126, with permission).

UAAUG, and that expression of the BM_2 protein requires termination of M_1 synthesis adjacent to the 5′ end of the BM_2 coding region; thus, termination of translation and the reinitiation event are tightly coupled (126) (see Fig. 10). In prokaryotes, coupled tandem cistrons with the termination codon of one gene overlapping the initiation codon for a downstream gene is a common situation for coordinating regulated bacterial genes (e.g., *trp* operon; reviewed in 234); however, it is uncommon in eukaryotes.

Influenza C Virus

RNA segment 6 of influenza C virus contains 1,180 nucleotides and contains a single ORF of 374 residues (259,386) (Fig. 11). This RNA segment gives rise to two mRNA species. One is a colinear mRNA that contains a 374–amino acid residue ORF (seg 6 ORF) that is translated to yield the precursor protein, p42. Synthesis of the p42 protein has been detected in influenza C virus–infected cells (122). Proteolytic cleavage of p42 at an internal signal peptidase cleavage site gives rise to the p31 and CM2 proteins (124,259). The second mRNA species that results from splicing of the colinear mRNA (386) encodes the matrix (CM1) protein, consisting of the N-terminal 242 residues of the seg 6 ORF followed by a stop codon introduced through mRNA splicing. The N-terminal product of p42 cleavage, p31, is identical in amino acid sequence to the CM1 protein except for the presence of 17 amino acids at its C-terminus that are mostly hydrophobic. The p31 protein binds tightly to lipid membranes with properties more like those of the integral membrane protein CM2 than those of the peripheral membrane protein CM1, and it is rapidly degraded in virus-infected cells (259,260).

The influenza C virus CM2 protein is a small glycosylated integral membrane protein (115 residues) that spans the membrane once. The CM2 protein forms disulfide-linked dimers and tetramers and is oriented in membranes in a NoutCin orientation. CM2 contains a single site for N-linked carbohydrate addition, which is frequently further modified with lactosaminoglycans. The CM2 protein is abundantly expressed at the cell surface of virus-infected and cDNA-transfected cells and is incorporated into influenza C virions (123,258) (see Fig. 6).

The Matrix Protein

It is now virtually dogma that the matrix protein underlies the viral lipid envelope and provides rigidity to the membrane. In addition, it is widely believed that the M_1 protein interacts with the cytoplasmic tails of the HA, NA, and M_2 proteins and also interacts with the RNP. However, experimental evidence for these very plausible interactions has been difficult to obtain. Solubility properties of purified M_1 protein (i.e., soluble in chloroform-

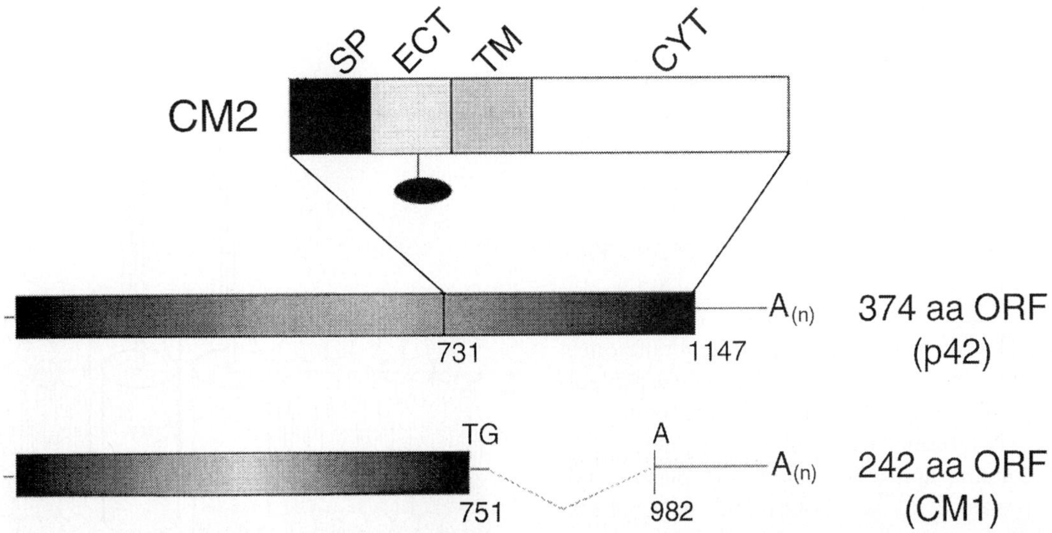

FIG. 11. The CM2 glycoprotein is a translation product of the full-length, colinear mRNA derived from influenza C virus RNA segment 6. Schematic diagram depicting the mRNAs derived from influenza C virus RNA segment 6 and their encoded proteins. The CM2 protein is processed from p42, and CM2 has been shown to contain a cleaved signal peptide (*SP*), an amino-terminal extracellular domain (*Ect*) modified by addition of N-linked carbohydrate (*black oval*), a hydrophobic transmembrane domain (*TM*), and an intracellular cytoplasmic tail (*Cyt*). (Data from ref. 259, with permission.)

methanol and 0.5 M KCl) are consistent with the protein being a peripheral membrane protein. An interaction between M_1 and lipid has been shown *in vivo* using light-activated cross-linking and *in vitro* using purified M_1 protein and liposomes (reviewed in 171). Contacts between the M_1 protein and the RNPs are suggested by finding that purified RNPs often contain M_1 protein; and by using immunoelectron microscopy, it has been found that the RNPs are heavily labeled with M_1 antibody (221). Purified M_1 protein inhibits transcription *in vitro* (390,402), and if M_1 protein is not dissociated from the RNPs *in vivo,* the RNPs fail to be transported to the nucleus (208). At late times after infection, transport of the M_1 protein into the nucleus is required for exit of the newly assembled RNPs from the nucleus (208) (see later). An interaction between the M_1 protein and RNA has been demonstrated by using filter-binding assays and blotting procedures (351,390). An NLS has been mapped to residues 101 to 105 (RKLKR) (389).

The x-ray crystal structure of the N-terminal portion of the M_1 protein (residues 2 to 158) at low pH has been determined (304) (Fig. 12). Under these conditions the M_1 protein fragment forms a dimer related by a noncrystallographic twofold axis at pH 4.0. Each monomer consists of nine α-helices, eight loop regions, and no β-strands (304). A highly positively charged region (10 residues from each monomer) on the dimer surface is well positioned to bind RNA, whereas the hydrophobic surface opposite the RNA-binding region is hypothesized to be involved in membrane interactions. It is possible that the hydrophobic surface could be buried or exposed after a conformational change (304). The M_1 protein contains a zinc-binding motif (Cys-Cys-His-His type, residues 148 to 162 of influenza virus A/PR/8/34 M_1 protein). However, the x-ray crystallographic structure indicates this sequence does not form a functional zinc finger (304).

An interaction between M_1 and the M_2 protein has been suggested based on the observation that virus growth restriction by anti-M_2 antibodies can be overcome by mutations in M_1 (394) (see later). Finally, an interaction has been observed between M_1 and the NS_2 protein found in purified virions (388).

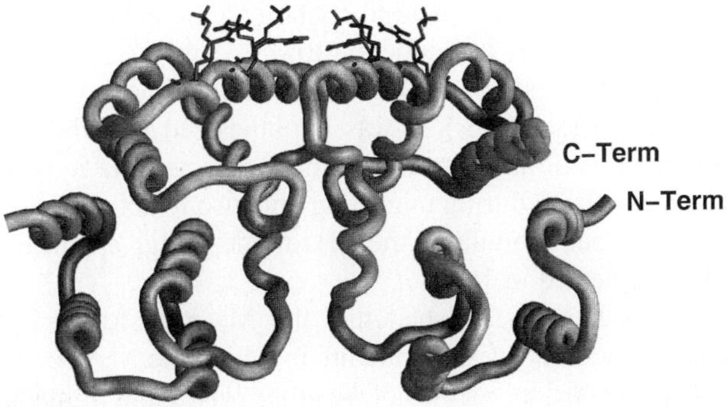

FIG. 12. Three-dimensional structure of the influenza A virus matrix protein. The structure shown is a dimer of M_1 residues 1 to 158. The 9 helical regions in each monomer are clearly visible, and the 10 positively charged residues at the top of the structure that are thought to interact with RNA are shown. (This figure was produced using Protein Data Bank coordinate file 1AA7.)

The M_2 Protein and Its Ion Channel Activity

As discussed previously, the M_2 integral membrane protein (97 amino acids) is encoded by a spliced mRNA derived from genome RNA segment 7 (173,183). The M_2 protein is abundantly expressed at the plasma membrane of virus-infected cells but is greatly underrepresented in virions because only a few (on average, 20 to 60) molecules are incorporated into virus particles (185,395,396). In polarized cells, the M_2 protein is expressed at the apical cell surface (128), the surface at which influenza virus particles bud. The M_2 protein spans the membrane once; by using domain-specific antibodies and specific proteolysis, it has been shown that M_2 protein is orientated such that it has 24 N-terminal extracellular residues, a 19-residue TM domain, and a 54-residue cytoplasmic tail (185). The presence of an N-terminal extracellular domain in the absence of a cleavable signal sequence indicates that the M_2 protein is a model type III integral membrane protein that is dependent on the signal recognition particle for cotranslational insertion into the ER membrane (130) (see Fig. 6). The M_2 protein cytoplasmic domain is posttranslationally modified by phosphorylation on a serine (residue 64) (119) and palmitoylation on cysteine (residue 50) (119,333,346), but neither posttranslational modification is required for the function of the M_2 ion channel (38,119,340).

The native form of the M_2 protein is minimally a homotetramer consisting of either a pair of disulfide-linked dimers or disulfide-linked tetramers (9,117,298,334) that form a left-handed four-helix bundle with an interhelix tilt of 20 to 30 degrees (161,262) (Fig. 13).

The M_2 protein TM domain was deduced to be the target of the anti–influenza virus drug amantadine. Amantadine (1-aminoadamantane hydrochloride) displays a specific anti–influenza A virus action (60) and has been used in the prophylaxis and treatment of influenza A virus infections (reviewed in 243). Mutants that were resistant to amantadine were found to contain amino acid changes in the M_2 protein TM domain (108).

From studies on the effect of amantadine on virus replication (see later), it was hypothesized that the M_2 protein functions as an ion channel that permits ions to enter the virion during uncoating and also to act as an ion channel that modulates the pH of the Golgi apparatus (334; reviewed in 104).

It has been established that the M_2 protein has ion channel activity by experiments in which the M_2 protein was expressed in oocytes of *Xenopus laevis* and in mammalian cells, and measuring membrane currents. This M_2 ion channel activity is blocked by amantadine and is regulated by changes in pH. The channel is activated at the lowered pH found in endosomes and the TGN (43,118,263,352–354). The ion selectivity of the M_2 ion channel activity indicated the M_2 channel is highly specific for H^+ ions (43,219).

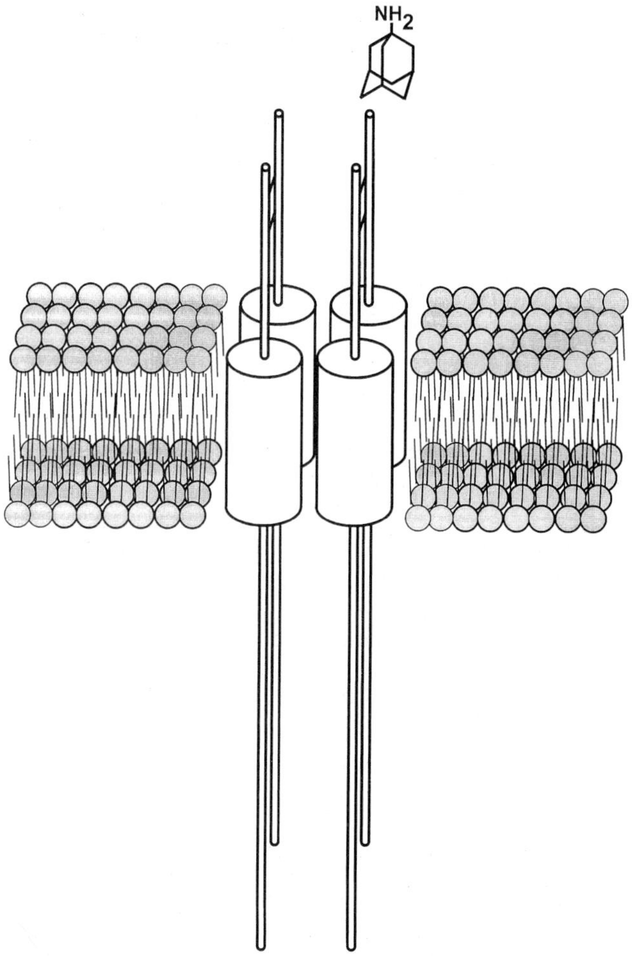

FIG. 13. Schematic diagram of the influenza virus M_2 protein ion channel in a membrane. The influenza virus M_2 protein is a disulfide-linked homotetramer with each chain consisting of 97 amino acid residues with 24 residues exposed extracellularly, a 19-residue transmembrane domain, and a 54-residue cytoplasmic tail. The disulfide bonds can form between the same subunit partners, as shown; otherwise, after the first bond is made, the second disulfide can link to another partner to form the fully disulfide-linked tetramer. The M_2 protein has a pH-activated ion channel activity that conducts protons. The channel is specifically blocked by the antiviral drug amantadine hydrochloride. The pore of the channel has been shown to be the transmembrane domain of the M_2 protein. The ion channel activity is essential for the uncoating of influenza virus in endosomal compartments in the infected cell. (Drawn from data in ref. 185, with permission.)

RNA Segment 8 of Influenza Virus: Unspliced and Spliced mRNAs Encode the NS_1 and NS_2 Proteins

RNA segment 8 of influenza A and B viruses and the smallest RNA segment of influenza C virus (RNA 7) encode two proteins, NS_1 and NS_2. NS_1 is encoded by a colinear mRNA transcript, whereas NS_2 is encoded by a spliced mRNA. The finding of a spliced NS_2 mRNA was the first evidence for splicing with an RNA virus that does not use a DNA intermediate in its replication.

RNA Segment 8 Gene Structure and Encoded Proteins

RNA segment 8 of influenza A virus is 890 nucleotides in length and contains a large ORF encoding the NS_1 protein (M_r about 26,000), ranging from 202 to 237 residues depending on the virus. In addition to the NS_1 protein, genetic and biochemical evidence has shown that RNA segment 8 encodes a second protein, NS_2 (M_r about 14,000) and that NS_2 is translated from a small mRNA (350 nucleotides) (131,132,174,177,178). Nucleotide sequencing studies indicated that the NS_1 mRNA is unspliced, directly encoding the NS_1 protein, whereas the NS_2 mRNA contains a 473-nucleotide intron. NS_1 and NS_2 share a 56-nucleotide leader sequence that contains the AUG codon used for initiation of protein synthesis. Consequently, the NS_1 and NS_2 proteins share 9 N-terminal amino acids before the intron; translation of the body of the NS_2 mRNA then continues in the +1 ORF, which overlaps the NS_1 frame by 70 residues (181). The arrangement of the NS_1 and NS_2 mRNAs and their ORFs is shown in Figure 14.

RNA segment 8 of influenza B virus is 1,096 nucleotides in length and contains a large ORF of 281 residues encoding NS_1 (281 residues; M_r, 32,026). An analogous arrangement of unspliced and spliced mRNA transcripts is found to encode NS_1 and NS_2, as described previously for influenza A virus. The NS_2 mRNA has a 5′ leader sequence of 75 nucleotides, which is shared with the NS_1 mRNA, and contains the AUG codon used for initiation of protein synthesis, such that 10 N-terminal residues are shared between NS_1 and NS_2. The 350-nucleotide body region of the NS_2 mRNA encodes in the +1 reading frame 112 residues, overlapping the NS_1 ORF by 52 residues (25,26).

RNA segment 7 of influenza C virus (the equivalent of RNA segment 8 for influenza A and B viruses) contains 934 nucleotides. The NS_1 protein contains 286 residues (225). The NS_2 protein (122 residues) is encoded by a spliced mRNA: 62 N-terminal residues are shared by NS_1 and NS_2, and after the splice junction, translation continues in the +1 ORF for 59 residues. The second ORF of influenza virus RNA segment 7 is completely overlapped by that of the NS_1 protein (226).

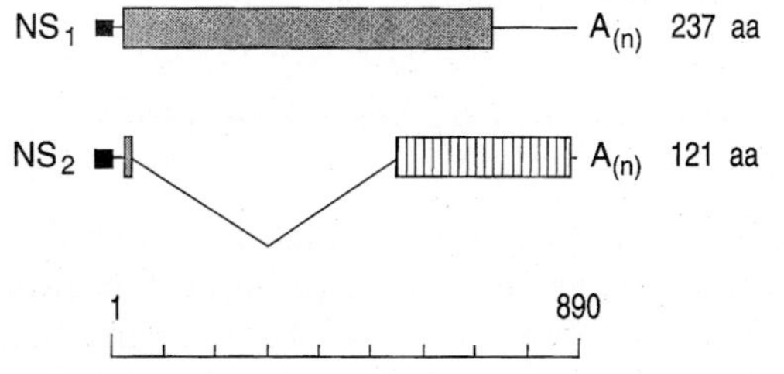

FIG. 14. Model for the arrangement of the influenza A virus NS_1 and NS_2 mRNAs and their coding regions. Thin lines at the 5′- and 3′-termini of the mRNAs represent untranslated regions. *Shaded* or *hatched areas* represent coding regions in 0 or +1 reading frames, respectively. The intron is shown by the *V-shaped line.* Rectangles at the 5′ ends of the mRNAs represent heterogeneous nucleotides derived from cellular RNAs that are covalently linked to viral sequences. (Adapted from ref. 177, with permission.)

The NS_1 Protein

The NS_1 protein (M_r about 26,000) is expressed in large amounts in influenza virus–infected, cells but it has not been detected in virions, hence the designation NS for *nonstructural* (166,188,317). NS_1 is found in infected cells in the nucleus and is associated with polysomes (50,166,168,188). The NLS within NS_1 has been mapped, and it has been found that the protein contains two separate signals (residues 34 to 38 and within residues 203 to 237) (99). The NS_1 protein also contains a nuclear export signal (NES), a short leucine-rich sequence that mediates the nuclear export of proteins (reviewed in 91). The NS_1 NES has been mapped to residues 138 to 147 (198).

Where the NS_1 and NS_2 ORFs overlap (in NS_1 proteins of 237 residues), the amino acid sequences indicate that NS_2 is conserved at the expense of NS_1 (reviewed in 171). These observations support the original suggestion (385) that NS_1 and NS_2 may have been colinear on the vRNA but not overlapping and that read-through of a termination codon at the C-terminus of NS_1 allowed the NS_1 protein to become longer.

NS_1 protein is a multifunctional protein, and many of its functions in the influenza virus life cycle have been determined as described later.

The NS_2 Protein

The NS_2 protein (M_r about 11,000), originally thought to be nonstructural, is now known to exist in virions (130 to 200 molecules on average) and to form an association with the M_1 protein (282,388). The subcellular localization of NS_2 has been indicated to be nuclear (98) and cytoplasmic (324). The NS_2 protein has an NES sequence, and its role in the export of RNPs out of the nucleus is discussed later.

STAGES OF REPLICATION OF INFLUENZA VIRUSES

Virus Adsorption, Entry, and Uncoating

Influenza viruses bind to sialic acid residues present on cell surface glycoproteins or glycolipids through the receptor-binding site in the distal tip of the HA molecules (see Three-Dimensional Structure of Hemagglutinin, earlier). Different influenza viruses have different specificities for sialic acid linked to galactose by α2,3 or α2,6 linkages, and this is dependent on specific residues in the HA receptor-binding pocket (367) (see Fig. 3). Carbohydrate chains of avian intestine contain predominantly sialic acid linked to galactose by α2,3 linkages, pig trachea contain sialic acid linked to galactose by α2,3 and α2,6 linkages, and human trachea carbohydrate chains contain predominantly sialic acid linked to galactose by α2,6 linkages (134). The specificity of HA for sialic acid in α2,3 or α2,6 linkages to galactose is a key determinant in restricting the transfer of influenza virus directly from avian species to humans without mutations in the HA sialic acid–binding site occurring (see Chapter 47 in *Fields Virology*, 4th ed.). Although the interaction of HA with sialic acid is of fairly low affinity, a high avidity of the virus for cell surfaces is probably achieved by multiple low-affinity interactions.

Influenza viruses enter cells by receptor-mediated endocytosis, the high-capacity endocytic activity by which components of the medium are internalized in clathrin-coated membrane-bound vesicles, formed by invagination of specialized coated-pit domains of the plasma membrane. After internalization, the clathrin coat is removed, and vesicles fuse with endosomes (a series of organelles of increasingly acidic pH), beginning with mildly acidic primary endosomes and progressing to late endosomes. The acidification of endosomes is brought about by H^+-ATPases. The uncoating of influenza virions in endosomes is dependent on the acidic pH of this compartment, and agents such as acidotropic weak bases (ammonium chloride, chloroquine) and carboxylic ionophores (monesin and nigericin) raise the pH of endosomes and block influenza virus uncoating (211). However, these acidotropic weak bases do not have a specific anti–influenza virus effect: raising the intraluminal pH of endosomes blocks the uncoating of most viruses that enter cells by the endocytic pathway (reviewed in 207). For the influenza virus RNPs to penetrate into the cytosol, they have to cross the membrane of the virion and that of endosomes. This is accomplished by HA-mediated fusion of the viral membrane with the cellular membrane (see The Low-pH–Induced Hemagglutinin Conformational Change, earlier) (Figs. 15 and 16). The precise time and location of penetration depends on the pH dependence of the transition of HA to its low-pH–induced form. For human strains such as A/Japan/305/57, the transition to the HA low-pH form occurs at pH 5.3, which is found in late endosomes and occurs with a half-life of 20 to 35 minutes after virus entry (328).

Studies with the antiviral drug amantadine led to the hypothesis that the M_2 ion channel activity is essential for the uncoating process. For all influenza A virus strains, the amantadine block to viral replication occurs at an early stage in the virus life cycle between the steps of virus penetration and uncoating (32,320). In the presence of the drug, the influenza virus M_1 protein fails to dissociate from the RNPs, and transport of the RNPs to the nucleus is blocked (208). Once a virion particle has been endocytosed, the low-pH–activated ion channel activity of the virion-associated M_2 protein (118,263,354) permits the flow of ions from the endosome to the virion interior, to disrupt protein–protein interactions and free the RNPs from the M_1 protein (see Fig. 16) (reviewed in 104, 110, and 179). Support for this idea comes from detergent solubilization studies that demonstrate that the interaction between M_1 and the RNPs can be disrupted by mildly acidic pH (397,399). An attractive feature of this hypothesis for virus uncoating is that the low pH of endosomes where uncoating occurs, in contrast to the neutral pH at the plasma membrane where assembly occurs, would push the equilibrium of the disassembly–assembly process in favor of uncoating. Another consequence of the M_2 protein ion channel activity in virions during the uncoating process may be to prepare HA for the fusion process. It has been found that fusion of influenza virus with liposomes is slowed in the presence of amantadine, and it was suggested that intraviral low pH facilitates influenza virus fusion, possibly by weakening interactions of the cytoplasmic tail of HA with the M_1 protein or RNPs (28,369).

Microinjection and immunoelectron microscopy experiments indicate that the RNPs enter the nucleus through the nuclear pore as an intact RNP after the M_1 protein has been dissociated from the RNP. All four proteins that are in the RNP (NP, PB1, PB2, and PA) contain NLS, and the RNPs are actively transported into the nucleus (reviewed in 374). The M_1 protein that has dissociated from the RNP, or newly synthesized M_1 protein, may enter the nucleus by passive diffusion because it is below the 50-kd cutoff for energy-dependent selective nuclear uptake mechanisms, but as discussed previously, a putative NLS in the M_1 protein has been identified. An examination of the fate of the proteins of the infecting virion indicates that whereas HA is degraded in lysosomes (half-life, 120 minutes), more than 30% to 35% of M_1 and NP persists for many hours (209).

Messenger RNA Synthesis and Replication of Virion RNA

Distinctive Feature of Influenza Virus mRNA Synthesis

Unlike other RNA viruses, influenza virus mRNA synthesis has a unique dependence on host cell nuclear function. One early observation was that α-amanatin, at concentrations that specifically inhibit the cellular DNA-dependent RNA polymerase II, inhibits influenza virus mRNA synthesis in infected cells, but not the virus mRNA synthesis that is catalyzed *in vitro* by the virion-associated transcriptase (175,205,325).

The discovery of the role of this host nuclear function came from studies of the virion-associated polymerase (reviewed in 163). The important observation was that this enzyme is incapable of initiating viral mRNA syn-

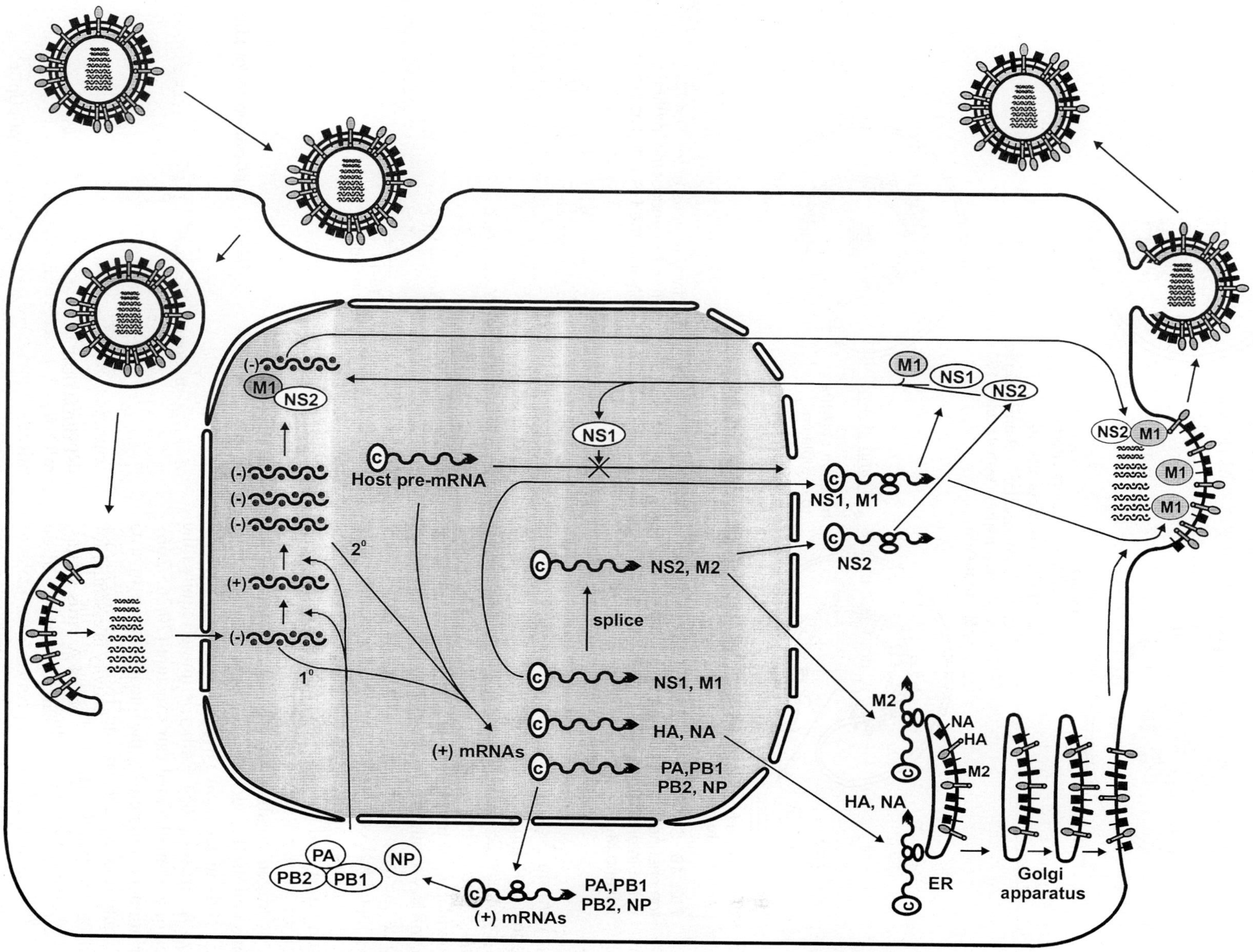

FIG. 15. Schematic diagram of the life cycle of influenza virus. See text for details of the model.

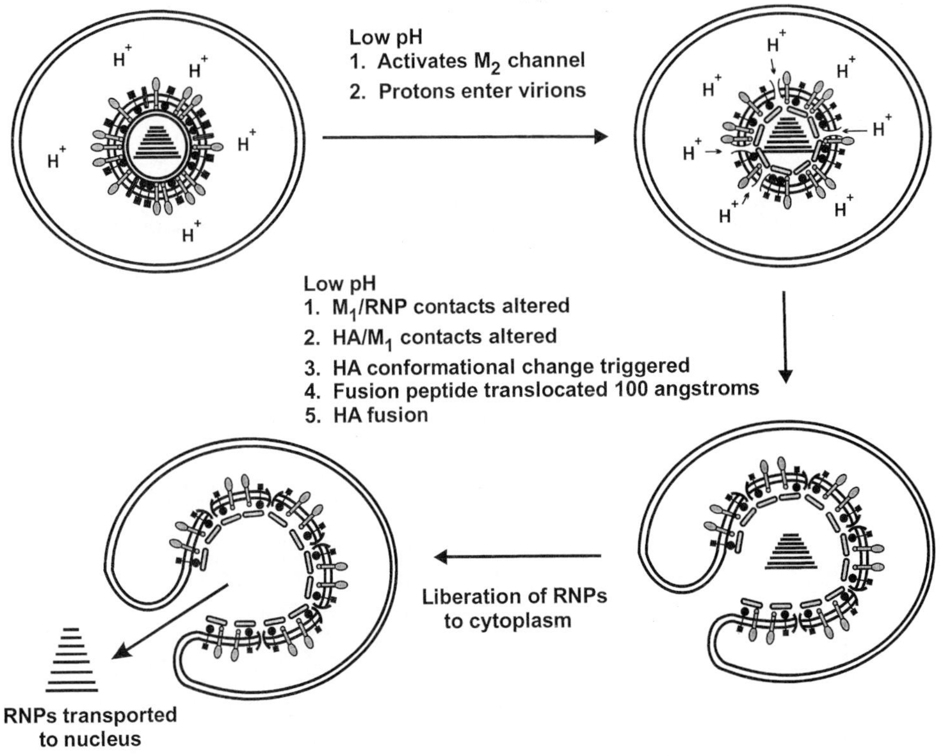

FIG. 16. Schematic diagram of the proposed role of the M_2 ion channel activity in virus entry. The M_2 ion channel activity is thought to facilitate the flow of protons from the lumen of the endosome into the virion interior, bringing about dissociation of protein–protein interactions between the HA cytoplasmic tail and M_1, M_1, and lipid or RNPs and M_1 from the RNPs.

thesis *in vitro* unless a primer is supplied. The primers are capped (m^7GpppX^m-containing) RNA fragments derived by cleavage of host cell RNA polymerase II transcripts. Hence, influenza virus scavenges host cell RNA polymerase II transcripts to supply the primers for its own mRNA synthesis. A cap-dependent endonuclease that is intrinsic to the influenza virus polymerase cleaves capped RNAs 10 to 13 nucleotides from their 5′ ends, preferentially at a purine residue (266) (Fig. 17). The resulting capped fragments serve as primers for the initiation of viral mRNA synthesis. Priming does not require hydrogen bonding between the capped primer fragments and the 12-nucleotide sequence that is found at the 3′ ends of all eight virion (vRNA) segments of influenza A viruses (165). Rather, priming requires the presence of a 5′-methylated cap structure (20,265,266). Transcription is initiated by the incorporation of a G residue onto the 3′ end of the resulting fragments, directed by the penultimate C residue of the vRNAs (20,21,114,164,265,266). This process has been called *cap snatching*.

Overview of mRNA Synthesis and Virion RNA Replication

Most of our knowledge concerning influenza virus gene expression and RNA replication has been gained

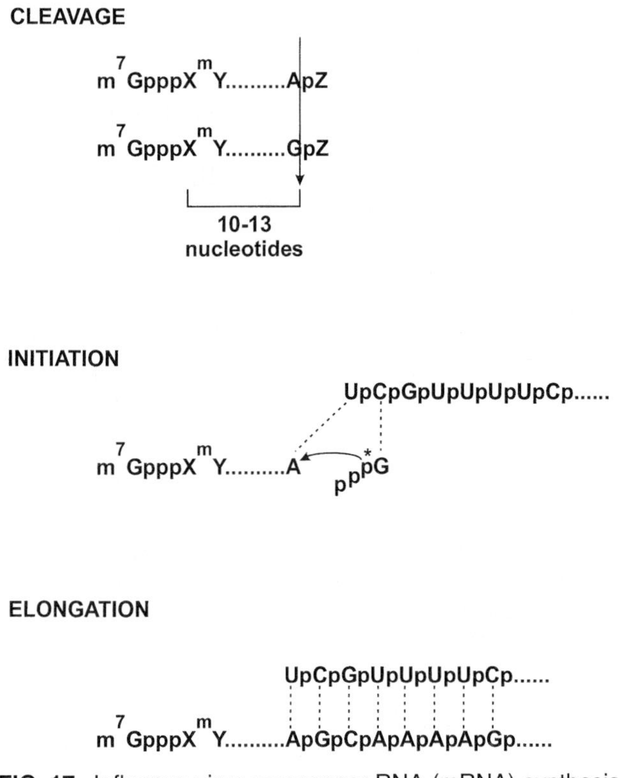

FIG. 17. Influenza virus messenger RNA (mRNA) synthesis requires initiation by capped RNA primers cleaved from cellular nuclear RNAs (see text for details).

from studying influenza A viruses. After priming with 5′ capped host-derived mRNA fragments, the mRNA chains are elongated, copying the template up to a point at which a stretch of uridine residues is reached, 15 to 22 nucleotides before the 5′ ends of the vRNAs. At this uridine (u) stretch, which ranges in length from 4 to 7 residues in the vRNA segments, transcription terminates, and polyadenylate residues [poly(A)] are added to the mRNAs (105,286) (Fig. 18). Termination occurs apparently as a result of stuttering or reiterative copying of the stretch of U residues, thereby adding a poly(A) tail to the 3′ ends of the viral mRNAs (203,273,286). For replication to occur, an alternative type of transcription is required that results in the production of full-length copies of the vRNAs. The full-length transcripts, or *template RNAs,* are initiated without a primer and are not terminated at the poly(A) site used during mRNA synthesis (105–107). The second step in replication is the copying of the template RNAs into vRNAs (163). This synthesis also occurs without a primer because the vRNAs contain 5′ triphosphorylated ends (393). The three types of virus-specific RNAs—mRNAs, template RNAs, and vRNAs—are all synthesized in the nucleus (305,306,323). In the nucleus, the viral mRNAs undergo at least some of the same processing steps as cellular RNA precursors. Internal adenosine residues of influenza virus mRNAs are methylated (167,227), and two of the viral mRNAs are spliced.

Viral mRNA Synthesis

The initial information about the mechanism of viral mRNA synthesis was obtained from *in vitro* studies of the polymerase complex isolated from virions by detergent disruption. The nucleocapsids consist of the individual vRNAs associated with four viral proteins: the NP protein and the three P proteins (PB1, PB2, and PA) (133,343). The P proteins catalyze viral mRNA synthesis, and some of their roles were determined by analyses of the *in vitro* reaction catalyzed by virion nucleocapsids. By using ultraviolet (UV) light–induced cross-linking, it was shown that the three P proteins exist in the form of a complex and that the PB2 protein in this complex recognizes and binds to the cap of the primer RNA (16,22, 343). Cap recognition by PB2 was verified by analysis of the *in vitro* transcription activity of the nucleocapsids derived from PB2 ts mutants (342). The UV–cross-linking experiments also indicated that the PB1 protein most likely catalyzes nucleotide addition (22). No specific role for PA in viral mRNA synthesis has been found.

New insights into the mechanism of mRNA synthesis have been provided by experiments in which viral polymerase complexes are formed using recombinant gene expression, specifically vaccinia virus vectors encoding the three P proteins. When cells are co-infected with three vaccinia viruses encoding the PB2, PB1, and PA proteins, the polymerase complexes that are assembled are inactive in all *in vitro* assays designed to measure the various activities of the polymerase. The polymerase complexes acquire cap-binding and endonuclease activities only when influenza vRNA is present (45,100,194,341). First, binding of the common 5′-terminal sequence of the vRNA segments (AGUAGAAACAAG) activates the capped RNA-binding activity of the PB2 protein. Subsequent binding of the common 3′ terminal sequence of the vRNA segments (UCGU/CUUUCGUCC) activates endonuclease activity, thereby enabling the polymerase complex to catalyze capped RNA-primed mRNA synthesis. Consequently, vRNA molecules function not only as templates for mRNA synthesis but also as essential cofactors that activate the catalytic functions of the poly-

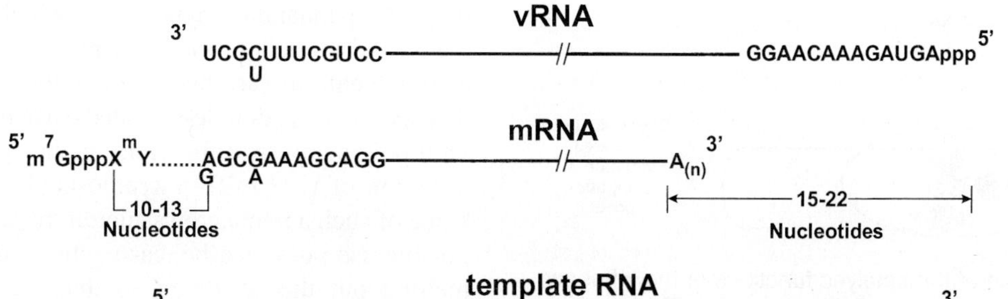

FIG. 18. Schematic diagram to illustrate the differences between influenza virus virion RNA (vRNA) segments, mRNAs, and full-length cRNA or template RNA. The conserved 12 nucleotides at the 3′ end and 13 nucleotides at the 5′ end of each influenza A virus vRNA segment are indicated. The mRNAs contain an m^7GpppN^m cap structure and, on average, 10 to 13 nucleotides derived from a subset of host cell RNAs (see Fig. 17 and text). Polyadenylation of the mRNAs occurs at a site 15 to 22 nucleotides before the 5′ end of the vRNA segment. The template RNA contains at its 5′-terminus pppA, and it is a complete copy of the vRNA segment. Depending on the RNA segment, there is a U/A or C/G at position 4.

merase that produce capped RNA primers. By means of this control mechanism, the production of primers is activated only when the template for viral mRNA synthesis, namely vRNA, is present.

By using these recombinant polymerase complexes, the sequences of five active sites of the viral polymerase have been identified (194,194a) (Fig. 19). As indicated previously, in the absence of vRNA, the complex of the three P proteins is enzymatically inactive. However, the PB1 subunit of these complexes contains a functional binding site for the 5′-terminal sequence of vRNA. This binding site is composed of an amino acid sequence that is centered around two essential arginine residues at positions 571 and 572. This amino acid sequence, which is conserved in all sequenced influenza A virus PB1 proteins, does not exhibit significant homology to any sequence in the database.

As a result of binding the 5′-terminal sequence of vRNA, two new functions of the polymerase are activated:

1. An allosteric change occurs in PB2 to activate the cap-binding activity (45,100,194,194a,341), and the region of PB2 important in the process is a tryptophan-rich domain, thought to be analogous to the cap-binding domain in the eIF4E translation initiation factor (206,212).
2. An allosteric change occurs in PB1 to activate the RNA-binding activity specific for the 3′-terminal sequence of vRNA. The region of PB1 involved in this activity is located in a sequence 300 amino acids distant from the PB1 sequence that binds the 5′-terminal sequence of vRNA (194).

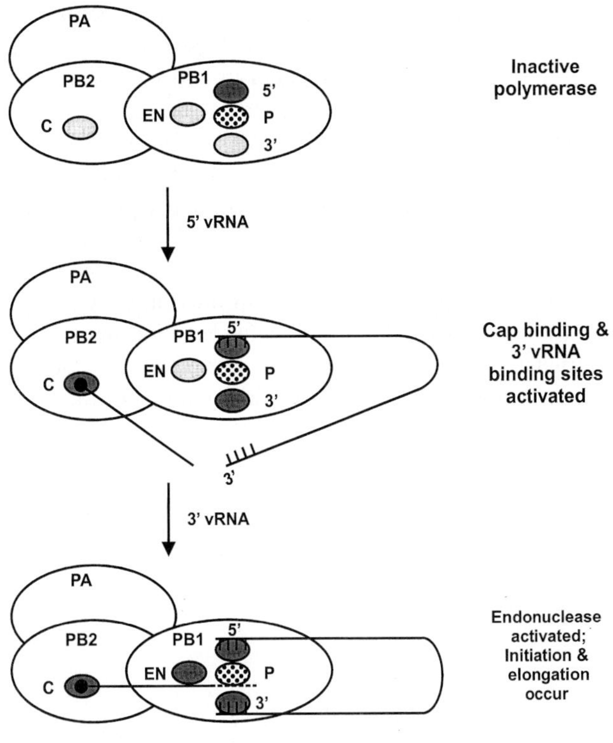

FIG. 19. Activation of the catalytic functions of the influenza virus polymerase by specific vRNA sequences. This model is described in the text. 5′, the binding site for the 5′ end of vRNA; 3′, the binding site for the 3′ end of vRNA; C, the binding site for capped RNA; EN, endonuclease active site; P, polymerase active site. *Light gray* denotes an inactive site, and *dark gray* denotes an active site. The P site is shown with interior dots because it is not known whether it is constitutively active or requires activation. The 5′ cap structure of the capped RNA is denoted by a *black circle.* (Modified from ref. 194, with permission.)

When the 3′-terminal sequence of vRNA subsequently binds to PB1, a second allosteric alteration causes the activation of the enzymatic activity that endonucleolytically cleaves capped mRNAs 10 to 13 nucleotides from their 5′ end sequences (45,100,194,341). The endonuclease active site, which is in the PB1 protein subunit, contains at least three essential acidic amino acids, comparable to the active sites of other enzymes that cut polynucleotides to produce 3′-OH ends, including RNase H and polynucleotidyl transferases, such as retroviral integrases and bacteriophage Mμ transposase (387).

The capped RNA fragments that are produced by the endonuclease serve as primers for the initiation of viral mRNA synthesis. Nucleotide addition is catalyzed by the PB1 protein, which contains the four conserved sequence motifs of RNA-dependent RNA polymerases (14,269). Mutagenesis experiments established that a core sequence of one of these motifs, namely the SDD sequence at amino acids 444 to 446 of the PB1 protein, is part of the active site for nucleotide addition (14). Thus, the PB1 protein plays a central role in the catalytic activity of the viral polymerase, both in the activation of the enzyme activities that produce capped RNA primers and in the subsequent catalysis of RNA chain elongation.

A key feature of this system is the requirement that the 5′ and 3′ ends of vRNA bind to the PB1 protein sequentially as ssRNA sequences that are not hydrogen-bonded to each other. These results are not consistent with the original "panhandle" hypothesis, which postulated that the 5′ and 3′ ends of vRNA, which exhibit considerable complementarity, are hydrogen-bonded to each and that this extensively double-stranded structure binds to the viral polymerase and functions as the "promoter" for the initiation of viral mRNA synthesis (120,127). The existence of such a panhandle structure requires that the viral polymerase possess a helicase activity that is capable of melting out this structure so that the polymerase can access and copy the bases at the 3′ end of the vRNA. However, when the 5′ and 3′ ends of vRNA are in the form of a hydrogen-bonded structure, the addition of this RNA species to the functional polymerase complexes formed using vaccinia virus vectors does not activate either cap-binding or endonuclease activity (341), indicating that these polymerase complexes lack the requisite helicase activity. Other experiments have also led to modifications of the original "panhandle" model; for example, in the "RNA-fork" model, most of the 5′- and 3′-terminal bases are not hydrogen-bonded to each other (81). Finally, biochemical experiments have shown that the 5′ and 3′ ends of vRNA molecules in the activated nucleocapsids that are isolated from influenza virions are not juxtaposed unless the polymerase is present (159).

The model for the initiation and subsequent elongation of influenza virus mRNA chains suggests a mechanism for the polyadenylation and termination of synthesis that occur before the 5′ end of the vRNA is reached (Fig. 20). It can be postulated that the specific binding of the 5′ end of vRNA to the PB1 subunit of the polymerase persists throughout mRNA synthesis. Consequently, the vRNAs

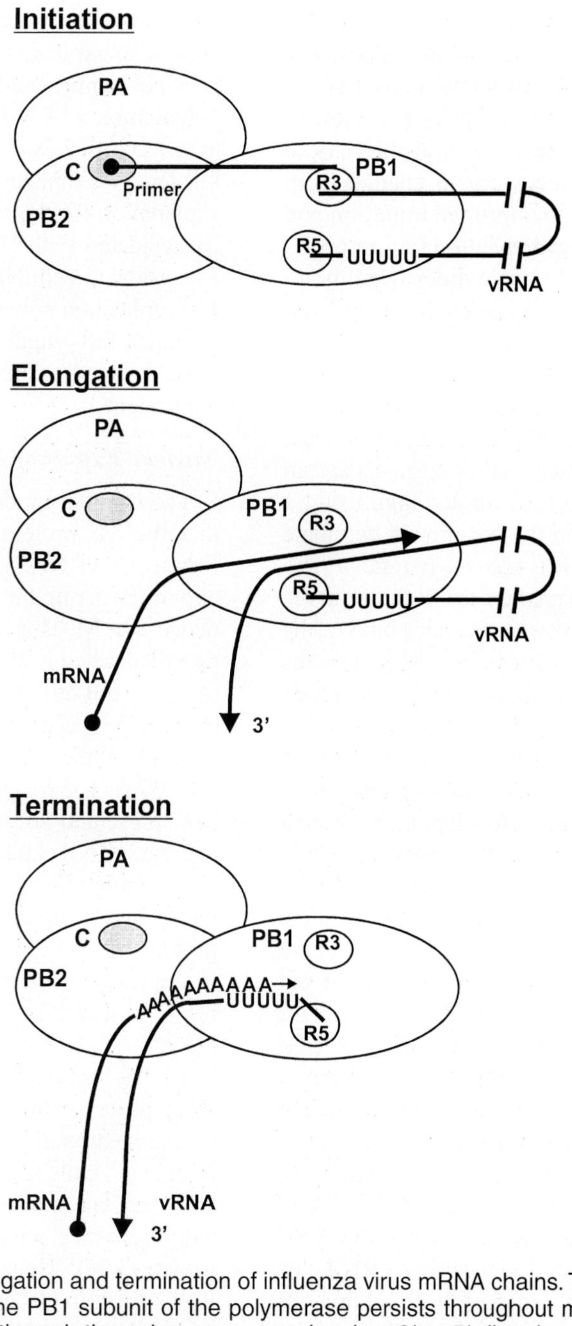

FIG. 20. Model for the elongation and termination of influenza virus mRNA chains. The specific binding of the 5′ end of vRNA to the PB1 subunit of the polymerase persists throughout mRNA synthesis, so that the vRNA is threaded through the polymerase complex, in a 3′ to 5′ direction, during mRNA synthesis. R3 and R5 are the sites on PB1 to which the 3′ and 5′ ends of the vRNA bind. As a consequence of binding both the 3′ and 5′ ends of the RNAS, the polymerase itself acts as a physical barrier to continuation of mRNA synthesis, resulting in the reiterative copying of the 5- to 7-U residues that is adjacent to the polymerase-binding site, followed by termination.

would be threaded through the polymerase complex, in a 3′ to 5′ direction, during mRNA synthesis. Eventually, the polymerase itself would act as a physical barrier to continuation of mRNA synthesis through its site of attachment. This block would result in the reiterative copying of the stretch of U residues in the vRNA template that is adjacent to the polymerase-binding site, thereby producing the poly(A) sequence followed by termination.

Replication of Virion RNA

Replication of virion RNA occurs in two steps: the synthesis of template RNAs, the full-length copies of the vRNAs; and the copying of template RNAs into vRNAs (163). To switch from the synthesis of viral mRNAs to that of template RNAs, it is necessary to change from capped RNA-primed initiation to unprimed initiation and to prevent termination and polyadenylation (antitermination) at the poly(A) site, 15 to 22 nucleotides from the 5′ ends of the vRNA templates, that is used during viral mRNA synthesis.

Antitermination requires NP proteins that are not associated with nucleocapsids (11), and this antitermination activity is found in the soluble fraction of infected cell nuclear extracts and can be specifically depleted using an antiserum directed against the NP protein (11). In addition, using a virus containing a ts mutation in the NP protein, template RNA, but not mRNA synthesis, is ts both *in vivo* and *in vitro* (215,306). The most likely explanation for these results is that the nonnucleocapsid NP protein molecules bind to the common 5′ ends of the nascent transcripts (11). It seems possible that as additional NP protein molecules are added to the elongating RNAs, they bind to the sequence of 4 to 7 A residues in the mRNA that are copied from the stretch of U residues in the vRNA template. As a consequence, this mRNA sequence is prevented from slipping backward along the vRNA template, and reiterative copying of the stretch of U residues in the vRNA template would be blocked. Supporting data for this hypothesis are awaited, however, and it is not clear how this process would eliminate the physical barrier to the copying of the 5′ ends of the vRNAs caused by the polymerase itself. This mechanism predicts that the number of NP protein molecules in infected cells regulates the levels of mRNA synthesis versus genome RNA replication because full-length template RNAs are synthesized only when NP protein molecules are present.

The next step in replication, copying the full-length template RNAs to produce negative-stranded vRNAs, also requires the addition of NP protein molecules to the elongating RNA molecules (306). No vRNA-sense RNAs of discrete sizes are made in the absence of these soluble NP molecules, indicating that elongation of vRNA chains most likely ceases at any time at which NP is not available. Consequently, the newly synthesized vRNAs are in the form of nucleocapsids that can be readily packaged into progeny virus particles.

As noted previously, the switch from mRNA synthesis to the synthesis of full-length template RNAs requires that the polymerase switch from capped RNA-primed initiation to unprimed initiation. The biochemical process by which this occurs is not known, but one hypothesis for this change in initiation is that the form of the polymerase that carries out vRNA replication differs from the one that carries out mRNA synthesis (163). According to this hypothesis, the mRNA synthesis polymerase produces only subgenomic, polyadenylated mRNAs, even in the presence of NP protein molecules. This polymerase requires the PB2 cap-binding protein to produce capped RNA primers, but apparently does not require the PA protein. In contrast, the replication polymerase, which is present only in infected cells and not in virus particles, requires NP protein molecules to produce full-length template and vRNA strands. This provides an explanation for the fact that vRNA and template RNA are encapsidated with NP subunits, whereas mRNAs are not encapsidated with NP subunits (105,270; reviewed in 163). The replication polymerase initiates the unprimed synthesis of either full-length template RNAs or vRNAs, and presumably requires the PA protein, but not the PB2 cap-binding protein.

Nuclear Export of Ribonucleoproteins

The original model for vRNP nuclear export proposed that the M_1 protein promoted vRNP nuclear export by forming a vRNP-M_1 complex in the nucleus (209) with export occurring through the NES on M_1. Confirming evidence that M_1 is a mediator of vRNP nuclear export was provided when it was found that expressed M_1 can induce the export of nuclear-trapped vRNPs (31). However, vRNP export can occur even when the vast majority of M_1 is trapped in the nucleus by altered hyperphosphorylation (281,373). The M_1 protein lacks an NES, and evidence has been presented that the NES is provided by the NS_2 protein and that vRNP export is mediated by a vRNP-M_1-NS_2 protein complex (236,358) (Fig. 21). The NES in the NS_2 protein would overcome the NLS sequences in the NP and P proteins, a phenomenon that has been observed in other examples of nuclear export (91). The NS_2 protein, which has been shown to bind to the M1 protein (358), contains a leucine-rich region at residues 97 to 105, which is a putative NES for interacting with an exportin, a family of cellular proteins that mediate nuclear export (236); and microinjection of anti-NS^2 antiserum inhibits vRNP export in infected cells (236). There is also the possibility that the NLS sequences in the NP and P proteins are overidden by a different mechanism mediated by the tight binding of NP to actin (64). Thus, in the life cycle of influenza virus, RNPs from input virions are transported into the nucleus, where their transcription and replication occurs, and new RNPs are transported back from the nucleus to the cytoplasm. Thus, knowledge of the switch required for nuclear import and nuclear export of the RNPs is crucial to understanding viral replication.

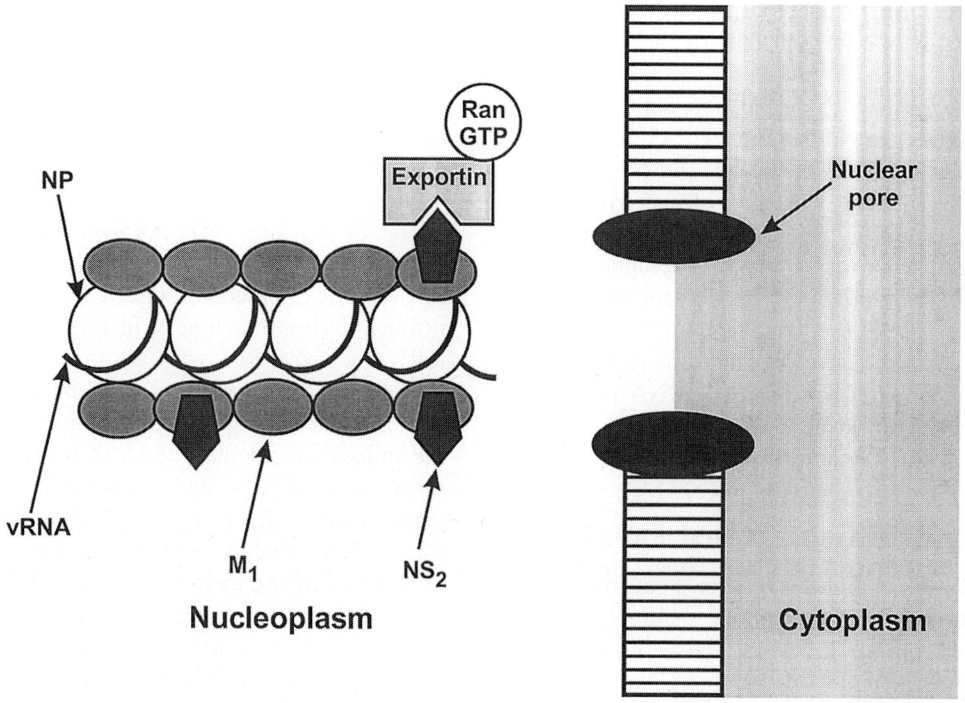

FIG. 21. An M_1-NS_2 protein complex mediates the nuclear export of vRNA-containing nucleocapsids. The current model for export of vRNPs from the nucleus is shown. A nuclear export signal in NS_2 interacts with a member of the cellular exportin family of proteins. The exportin is most likely associated in a complex with RAN-GTP protein to mediate export of the RNP–M_1–NS_2 protein complex from the nucleus. (Modified from ref. 236, with permission.)

Regulation of Viral Gene Expression in Infected Cells

Influenza virus infection can be divided into an early and late phase of gene expression. However, unlike DNA viruses, in which specific patterns of transcription occur before and after DNA replication, the phases of influenza virus gene expression entail quantitative changes of transcription of individual RNA segments as opposed to qualitative changes (176,305,316).

During the early phase, the synthesis of specific vRNAs, viral mRNAs, and viral proteins are coupled (106,305,323). The first event detected after primary transcription is the synthesis of template RNAs, presumably copied off the parental vRNAs. About equimolar amounts of each of the template RNAs are made. The peak rate of template RNA synthesis occurs early and then sharply declines. Specific template RNAs are then selectively transcribed into vRNAs. Specifically, the NS and NP vRNAs are preferentially synthesized early, whereas the synthesis of M segment vRNA is delayed. The rate of synthesis of a particular vRNA correlates with, and therefore most likely determines, the rate of synthesis of the corresponding mRNA and of its encoded protein. The NS_1 and NP mRNAs and proteins are preferentially synthesized at early times, whereas the synthesis of the M_1 mRNA and protein are delayed. Thus, the control of viral protein synthesis during the early phase is predominantly a direct consequence of the regulation of vRNA synthesis, that is, the selective copying of specific template RNAs into vRNAs.

During the late phase, the relationships between the syntheses of vRNAs, viral mRNAs, and viral proteins change dramatically (305). The synthesis of all the viral mRNAs reaches its peak rate at the beginning of the late phase, and the rate of synthesis of all the mRNAs then decreases precipitously. In contrast, the rate of synthesis of all the vRNAs remains at or near maximum during the second phase. Thus, vRNA and viral mRNA synthesis are not coupled during the second phase. In addition, viral mRNA and protein synthesis are not coupled because the synthesis of all the viral proteins continues at maximum levels during the second phase. Previously synthesized viral mRNAs undoubtedly direct viral protein synthesis during the second phase. The pattern of protein synthesis during the second phase differs from that in the first phase. During the second phase, two structural proteins, M_1 and HA, which are poorly synthesized in the first phase, are synthesized at high rates along with the other structural proteins.

As discussed previously, the synthesis of all three types of virus-specific RNAs occurs in the nucleus (163). The template RNAs, which are synthesized only at early times, remain in the nucleus to direct vRNA synthesis throughout infection (305). In contrast, the vRNAs, which are in the form of nucleocapsids, are efficiently exported to the cytoplasm, particularly at later times (73,306).

A significant part of the replication control system established by influenza virus in infected cells is directed at the preferential synthesis of the NP and NS_1 proteins early and at delaying the synthesis of the M_1 protein (306). The NP protein is synthesized early presumably because it is needed for the synthesis of template RNAs and vRNAs. The NS_1 protein is needed for other early functions (as discussed later). It is likely that the synthesis of the M_1 protein is delayed because this protein stops the transcription of vRNA into viral mRNA (402) and functions in the transport of vRNA-containing nucleocapsids from the nucleus to the cytoplasm (208).

Posttranscriptional Processing of Viral mRNAs

Most pre-mRNAs in higher eukaryotes contain introns that must be precisely removed to generate functional mRNAs (reviewed in 307). Several conserved sequence elements have been found in all introns: 5′ splice site, 3′ splice site, and the branch site. In mammalian systems, an additional requirement is a polypyrimidine tract, which lies between the branch site and 3′ splice site. Influenza virus exploits the host nuclear machinery that splices cellular pre-mRNAs. As discussed previously, in influenza A virus–infected cells, two full-length viral mRNAs, the NS_1 and M_1 mRNAs (encoding the influenza A virus NS_1 protein [NS_{1A}] and the M_1 protein, respectively) are spliced by the cellular splicing machinery in the nucleus to form smaller viral mRNAs that encode two other proteins, NS_2 and M_2, respectively. Whereas the entirety of the population of cellular pre-mRNA molecules is usually spliced, only a portion of the influenza viral precursor NS_1 and M_1 mRNA molecules are spliced, and both the unspliced and spliced viral mRNAs are exported to the cytoplasm (163). Incomplete splicing and nuclear export of unspliced viral pre-mRNAs is not restricted to influenza virus; it also occurs in cells infected with retroviruses, both "simple" retroviruses (such as avian and murine leukemia viruses) and "complex" retroviruses (*Lentiviridae,* which include human immunodeficiency virus type 1) (see Chapter 28).

Regulated Splicing of Viral NS_1 and M_1 mRNAs

In influenza A virus–infected cells, splicing is regulated such that the steady-state amount of the spliced mRNAs is only about 10% of that of the unspliced mRNAs (177,180). It is likely that the extent of splicing of NS_1 (or M_1) mRNA is determined by competition between the splicing rate and the rate of nuclear export of NS_1 (or M_1) mRNA.

The rate of splicing of NS_1 mRNA in influenza virus–infected cells appears to be controlled solely by cis-acting sequences in NS_1 mRNA itself. This conclusion stems from the observation that the rate of splicing of NS_1 mRNA encoded in an adenovirus recombinant is not significantly different from the splicing rate of NS_1 mRNA in influenza virus–infected cells (4 hours after infection) (3).

In contrast to the rate of splicing, the rate of nuclear export of NS_1 mRNA is not intrinsic to the NS_1 mRNA sequence, but rather varies depending on whether the NS_1 mRNA is expressed through a DNA vector or through influenza virus machinery in infected cells. When NS_1 mRNA is expressed with an adenovirus vector (3), its nuclear export is totally blocked because NS_1 mRNA is committed to the splicing pathway (in accordance with the splicesome retention theory). In contrast, in influenza virus–infected cells, nuclear export of NS_1 mRNA is efficient, and the rate of splicing of NS_1 mRNA largely, if not totally, determines the extent of splicing. It is not known how the nuclear export of unspliced NS_1 mRNA is facilitated in influenza virus–infected cells. Viral proteins do not appear to be required for the facilitated nuclear export of unspliced NS_1 mRNA (4).

Control of the Alternative Splicing of M_1 mRNA by Both Viral and Cellular Proteins

The splicing of M_1 mRNA of influenza A virus is complicated by the use of alternative 5′ splice sites (183,312) (Fig. 22; see Fig. 10). When the 5′ splice site at position 11 (the first virus-coded nucleotide at the 5′ end of the mRNA is assigned position number 1) is used, mRNA3 is produced. The mRNA3 5′ splice site, CAG\GUAGAU, fits the consensus sequence for 5′ splice sites (C/AAAG\GUA/GAGU) closely. By contrast, the 5′ splice site for the M_2 mRNA (at position 51), AAC\GUAUGU, does not fit the consensus as well because there is a C rather than a G at the 3′ end of the 5′ exon. The common 3′ splice site, G7G(A)4(U)3GCAG\G, deviates from the consensus (U/CnNC/UAG\G) in that it does not contain an immediately adjacent polypyrimidine tract. When the M_1 gene is expressed in uninfected cells using a transient transfection DNA vector, only the strong mRNA3 5′ splice site and not the weaker M_2 5′ splice site is used (4,182). This raised the question of how the M_2 mRNA 5′ splice site and the mRNA3 5′ splice site are used in influenza virus–infected cells.

It has been shown that the alternative splicing of influenza viral M_1 mRNA is controlled by both viral and cellular proteins (310,312) (see Fig. 22). The weaker M_2 5′ splice site of M_1 mRNA is not used in infected cells at early times of infection because of the presence of the stronger mRNA3 5′ splice site. The switch to the M_2 5′ splice site occurs at later times in infected cells because the viral polymerase complex binds to a sequence near the 5′ end of M_1 mRNA, thereby blocking the mRNA3 5′

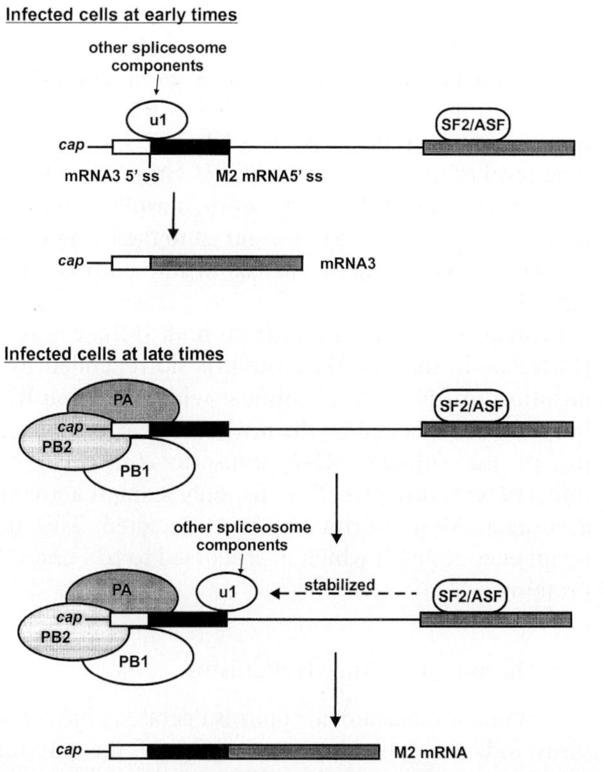

FIG. 22. Mechanism by which the viral polymerase complex and the cellular SF2/ASF splicing factor control the alternative splicing of influenza virus M_1 mRNA. See text for details of the mechanism. (Redrawn from ref. 310, with permission.)

splice site (312). The polymerase complex binds to the sequence (AGCAAAAGCAGG), which is the complement of the first 12 nucleotides found at the 3′ end of each of the virion RNA segments, and it is located immediately 3′ to the 5′ terminal 10 to 13 nucleotides that are "snatched" from host cell RNAs during viral mRNA synthesis. As a result of this binding, the polymerase protein complex acquires cap-binding activity, thereby enhancing the binding of the polymerase complex to the capped M_1 mRNA. As the cap-binding activity of the polymerase complex is also activated by the common 3′-terminal sequence during the initiation of viral mRNA synthesis (as discussed previously), it is likely that the 5′-viral mRNA sequence and the 3′-terminal sequence of vRNA bind to the same site on the PB1 subunit even though these two RNA sequences differ at 4 out of the 12 positions. Thus, the production of M_2 mRNA is delayed until sufficient amounts of the polymerase complex are synthesized, so that the time course of synthesis and assembly of functional polymerase complexes controls the time at which the M_2 5′ splice site can be used in infected cells.

Although the binding of the viral polymerase to the 5′ end of the M_1 mRNA causes the M_2 5′ splice site to be the only available 5′ splice site in the M_1 mRNA molecule, the weak M_2 5′ splice site is poorly used unless the cellular SF2/ASF splicing factor is present (310). SF2/ASF is an SR protein, a member of a family of proteins containing a domain rich in serine and arginine and functioning in both alternative and constitutive splicing (83,162). The SF2/ASF protein binds specifically to a purine-rich sequence, called a *splicing enhancer sequence,* in the 3′ exon of M_1 mRNA, and this binding, through a series of protein–protein interactions, results in the activation of the M_2 5′ splice site (310) (see Fig. 22). Consequently, the control of the alternative splicing of influenza viral M_1 mRNA involves the viral polymerase complex, which determines the time at which the M_2 5′ splice site can be activated in infected cells, and the cellular splicing factor SF2/ASF, which controls this activation. The latter function is totally dependent on the former function: SF2/ASF does not activate the M_2 5′ splice site of M_1 mRNA when the mRNA3 5′ splice site is unblocked. As a consequence of this alternative splicing mechanism, influenza virus has ceded the control of the level of expression of one of its gene products, the M_2 ion channel protein, to a cellular nuclear protein, the SF2/ASF splicing factor. Nonetheless, most of the M_1 mRNA molecules are not spliced, and these M_1 mRNA molecules are transported to the cytoplasm to direct the synthesis of the M_1 protein.

Viral mRNAs Are Not Cannabilized for Their 5′ Caps

The viral polymerase exhibits selectivity by "snatching" caps from cellular pre-mRNAs, but not viral mRNAs (163). This selectivity is essential because if the 5′ ends of viral mRNAs were also cleaved and used as primers, net synthesis of viral mRNAs would not occur. The mechanism for the selectivity emerged from studying the mechanism of alternative splicing of the viral M_1 mRNA, when it was found that the viral polymerase complex binds to the specific sequence 5′ AGCAAAAGCAGG 3′ found in all mRNAs that is complementary to nucleotides 1 to 12 of the 3′ end of each vRNA segment. This polymerase binding also serves a common function: selective protection of the 5′ ends of viral mRNAs, but not cellular pre-mRNAs, from endonucleolytic cleavage catalyzed by the polymerase complex (311). Thus, the three influenza virus P proteins carry out two disparate, opposing functions: the endonucleolytic cleavage of all capped mRNAs, and the selective protection of viral mRNAs, but not cellular pre-mRNAs, against this cleavage (311). The acquisition of these two very different functions stems from the fact that the complex of the three P proteins lacks any detectable activity in the absence of specific vRNA sequences (45,100,194,341) (Fig. 23; see Fig. 22). Influenza virus mRNAs lack the sequence complementary to the 5′ end of vRNA; therefore, mRNAs can activate only cap-binding activity and not the endonuclease activity.

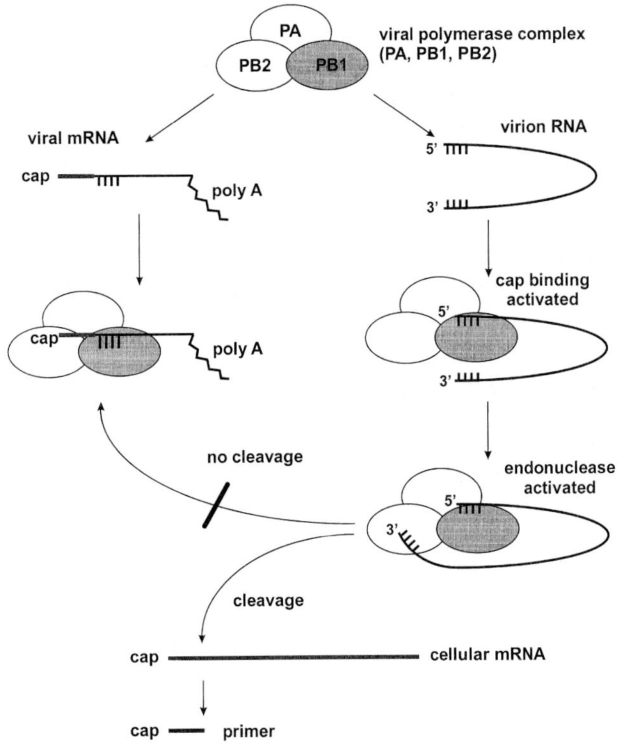

FIG. 23. The influenza viral P protein complex carries out two disparate, opposing functions. The viral P protein complex lacks any detectable activity in the absence of a specific RNA sequence. One specific RNA sequence to which it binds is the 5′-terminal AGUAGAAACAAG sequence present on all eight virion RNA segments. As a result of this binding, the viral P protein complex acquires cap-binding activity. Subsequent binding of the 3′ end of the virion RNA results in the acquisition of cap-dependent endonuclease and transcriptase activities. The other specific sequence to which it binds is the AGCAAAAGCAGG sequence that is found both in viral template RNAs, where it is located at the 5′ ends (not shown), and in viral mRNAs, where it is located immediately 3′ to the 5′ sequence "snatched" from host cell–capped RNAs (shown). As a result of the latter binding, the 5′ ends of viral mRNAs are protected against cleavage by the viral cap-dependent endonuclease. In contrast, the 5′ ends of host cell mRNAs are not protected and are cleaved by the viral endonuclease. (Redrawn from ref. 311, with permission.)

Splicing in Cells Infected with Influenza B and C Viruses

Splicing also occurs in cells infected with influenza B and C viruses. As with influenza A virus, the NS_1 mRNA of influenza B virus is spliced to form a smaller NS_2 mRNA (25). Both the ORF and the intron of the NS_1 mRNA of influenza virus B/Lee/40 are larger than those of the NS_1 mRNA of influenza virus A/Udorn/72; the sizes of the NS_2 mRNAs of the two virus strains are similar. The 5′ splice site, GAG\GUGGGU, of the NS_1 mRNA of influenza B virus fits the consensus sequence closely, whereas the 3′ splice site, GAUCGGACAG\U, deviates from the consensus sequence in two ways: (a) absence of a pyrimidine tract immediately upstream of the 39-terminal AG of the intron; and (b) presence of a U rather than a G at the 5′ end of the 3′ exon. The extent of splicing of the influenza B virus NS_1 mRNA is regulated like that of the influenza A virus NS_1 mRNA; the steady-state level of the spliced influenza B virus NS_2 mRNA is only about 5% to 10% of that of the unspliced influenza B virus NS_1 mRNA (25). In contrast to the M_1 mRNA of influenza A virus, the M_1 mRNA of influenza B virus is not spliced.

Influenza C virus differs from both influenza A and B viruses in that its M_1 protein is not encoded by an unspliced mRNA that is colinear with the virion RNA, but rather is encoded by the mRNA that arises by splicing of the colinear RNA transcript (386). In cells infected with influenza C virus, only a small amount of a colinear M transcript has been detected. This transcript encodes p42, which is processed to p31 and CM2 proteins.

Translational Control Mechanisms

Two major translational controls operate in influenza A virus–infected cells: (a) suppression of the interferon (IFN)-induced block against all protein synthesis, thereby ensuring the efficient translation of virus-specific proteins in infected cells (141,163); and (b) shutoff of the translation of cellular mRNAs, resulting in the selective translation of viral mRNAs (163,176,188,316,317).

Unless a virus-specific defense mechanism were established, overall translation in influenza virus–infected cells would be inhibited because of the production of virus-specific RNA molecules that contain double-stranded regions. The potential for the formation of such double-stranded RNA (dsRNA) molecules stems from the presence of both positive-sense and negative-sense RNAs that are synthesized in the nucleus during infection (163). These viral dsRNA molecules would activate the cellular kinase PKR (141). This dsRNA-activated kinase is expressed constitutively in eukaryotic cells at low levels, and its synthesis is substantially induced by IFN (141,210). Because virus-specific dsRNA also induces IFN (reviewed in 141), increased levels of PKR would be expected to be present in influenza virus–infected cells, and it has been shown that PKR is initially activated during infection (141). Continued activation of PKR would lead to a global shutdown of protein synthesis because activated PKR phosphorylates the α-subunit of the initiation factor eIF-2 (141,210). This initiation factor forms the ternary complex (eIF-2) · g GTP · (met-tRNAi) that binds to the initiating 40S ribosomal subunit before mRNA is bound (135). Phosphorylation of the α-subunit of eIF-2 prevents the recycling of eIF-2–g GDP to form the functional form of eIF-2, eIF-2-GTP (reviewed in 296). Recycling has been shown to be catalyzed by the factor eIF-2B, which is trapped in an inactive complex with eIF-2-GDP when the α-subunit of eIF-2 is phosphorylated (reviewed in 296). Without this recycling of eIF-2 by eIF-2B, protein synthesis initiation is effectively blocked.

Influenza virus mounts a two-pronged attack against the action of PKR. The virus-specific NS_1 protein binds to, and hence sequesters, viral dsRNA molecules, thereby blocking the activation of PKR (102,202). In addition, a 58-kd cellular protein that inhibits PKR function is activated in influenza virus–infected cells (191,192). The experimental evidence indicates that this 58-kd cellular protein interacts directly with PKR, and that influenza virus activates the inhibitory activity of the 58-kd protein by dissociating it from its own natural inhibitor.

In contrast, the mechanism by which viral mRNAs are selectively translated over cellular mRNAs in infected cells is poorly understood. One of the key elements in the shutoff of host cell protein synthesis takes place in the nucleus of infected cells: newly synthesized cellular pre-mRNAs are degraded (143). This degradation is probably initiated by the cleavage of the 5′ ends of cellular pre-mRNAs transcripts by the viral cap-dependent endonuclease (163). The resulting decapped RNAs would be more susceptible to degradation by cellular nucleases, as it has been shown that the 5′ cap structure stabilizes RNAs against nucleolytic degradation both *in vivo* and in cell extracts (6). This degradation is probably significantly enhanced by the action of the viral NS_1 protein, which blocks the nuclear export of cellular mRNAs (as discussed later). As a consequence, the mRNAs in the cytoplasm of influenza virus–infected cells are composed of cellular mRNAs synthesized before infection ("old cellular mRNAs") and viral mRNAs synthesized after infection ("new viral mRNAs"). Nonetheless, high levels of these old cellular mRNAs are found in the cytoplasm of infected cells (143). These cellular mRNAs are stable and also functional, as assayed by their efficient translation in reticulocyte extracts *in vitro* (143). Consequently, the shutoff of host cell protein synthesis, which is complete by about 3 hours after infection in several cell lines, probably does not result from the degradation or modification of cytoplasmic old cellular mRNAs. Based on the polysome distribution of several representative cellular mRNAs in uninfected and infected cells, it has been concluded that both the initiation and the elongation step in the translation of old cellular mRNAs are blocked in infected cells (142).

A molecular mechanism for a selective block against the elongation of cellular, but not viral, proteins has not been established. However, selectivity at initiation is probably due at least in part to the fact that influenza viral mRNAs are efficient initiators of translation (79,142,143). Other possible mechanisms for the selective translational initiation of viral over cellular mRNAs include the following:

1. The inhibition of the activation and activity of PKR may be partial, rather than complete (142,163). Under such conditions, the translation of viral mRNAs would be favored over the translation of cellular mRNAs because influenza viral mRNAs are better initiators of translation (142,143).
2. The NS_1 protein may bind to the 5′-untranslated regions (5′-UTRs) of viral mRNAs, thereby causing, in a manner unknown, the selective translation of these mRNAs (61,74,251). However, no binding of the NS_1 protein to the 5′-UTR in full-length viral mRNAs has been detected (278). Nonetheless, the NS_1 protein may play a role in translation in infected cells because the NS_1 protein appears to be associated with the polysomes of virus-infected cells (50, 78,166).
3. Cellular proteins function in the selective translation of influenza virus mRNAs in infected cells. It has been reported that: (a) the cellular RNA-binding protein GRSF-1 specifically binds to the 5′-UTRs of viral mRNAs (252); and (b) the human homologue of the Stauffen protein, which binds to dsRNA, interacts with the NS_1 protein that is associated with polysomes in infected cells (78).
4. One or more cellular protein initiation factors may be modified in influenza virus–infected cells (79), a strategy employed by some other viruses to ensure that their mRNAs are selectively translated (89).

Roles of the NS1 Protein

The nonstructural protein NS_1 of influenza A virus (NS_{1A} protein) was first identified in 1971 (188), but only recently have its multiple functions in the influenza virus life cycle become evident. The observation that provided the initial insight into these functions was that the NS_{1A} protein inhibits the nuclear export of poly(A)-containing mRNAs in transient transfection experiments (4,82,275). Subsequent experiments established that the NS_{1A} protein is a posttranscriptional regulator that has several activities.

Functional Domains of the NS_{1A} Protein

Two major functional domains of the 237–amino acid NS_{1A} protein have been identified. The first is a sequence near the N-terminus that constitutes the RNA-binding domain. The NS_{1A} protein binds with similar dissociation constants to three RNAs: poly(A), a specific stem-bulge in U6 snRNA, and dsRNA (202,278,279). This domain is also required for dimerization of the NS_{1A} protein, the state in which it exists both *in vivo* and *in vitro* (229).

Structural analysis of the RNA-binding domain of the NS_{1A} protein was facilitated by the demonstration that a fragment of the NS1 protein containing the first 73 N-terminal residues (NS_{1A} residues 1 to 73) possesses all the RNA-binding and dimerization activities of the full-length protein (276). Both nuclear magnetic resonance imaging and x-ray crystallography studies demonstrated that the dimeric NS_{1A} residues 1 to 73 RNA-binding domain in the absence of RNA adopts a novel six-helical chain fold (42,200) (Fig. 24). Mutagenesis studies demonstrated that any alanine replacement that causes disruption of the dimer also leads to the loss of RNA-binding activity, indicating that the dimer structure is essential for RNA-binding. Surprisingly, only one amino acid side chain is absolutely required for RNA-binding without significantly affecting dimerization, namely, the arginine side chain at position 38, which is in the second helix of each monomer (see Fig. 24). This result indicates that this arginine side chain probably interacts directly with the RNA target. This interaction is primarily electrostatic because replacement of this arginine with lysine had no effect on RNA binding. A second basic amino acid, the lysine at position 41, which is also in helix 2 (see Fig. 24), makes a strong contribution to the affinity of binding.

It has been proposed that helix 2 and helix 2′, which are antiparallel and next to each other in the dimer conformation, constitute the interaction face between the NS_{1A} RNA-binding domain and its RNA targets (42).

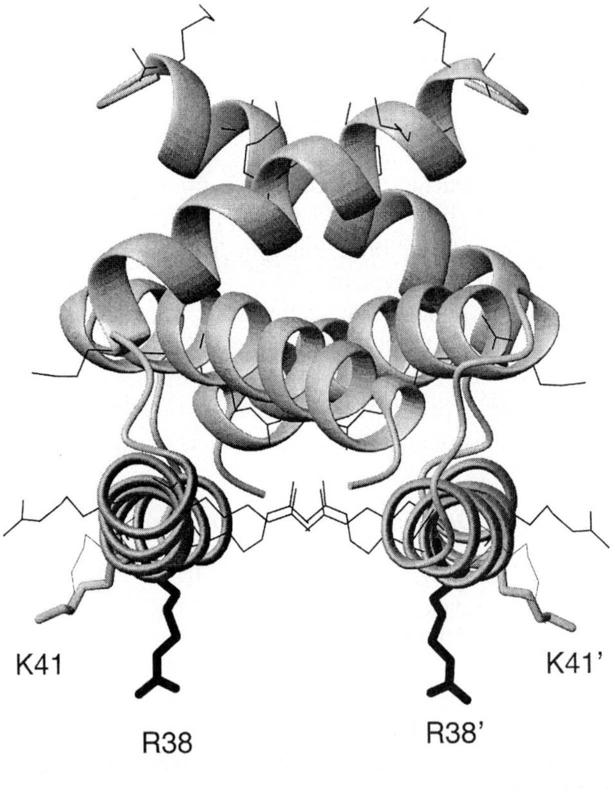

FIG. 24. The three-dimensional structure of the RNA-binding domain of the NS_{1A} protein. The four basic amino acids (R38, R38′, K41, K41′), which are required for, or strongly enhance, RNA-binding are shown. All the other solvent-exposed basic amino acids are shown in stick diagram format. (Redrawn from data in refs. 42 and 357, with permission.)

This puts the NS_{1A} protein in the small group of proteins that bind to their specific RNA targets through one or more α-helices rather than by β-sheets. The dimeric six-helical NS_{1A} RNA-binding domain almost certainly does not bind in the major groove of a dsRNA target. Rather, at least one basic amino acid (arginine 38, arginine 38′), in each of the antiparallel helices 2 and 2′ (see Fig. 24), probably contacts the negatively charged phosphate backbone of dsRNA. Consequently, the dimer structure serves to position arginine 38 on helix 2 so that it is a specific distance (16.5 Å) from the corresponding arginine 38′ on helix 2′. This distance is close to that (17 Å) found between the antiparallel phosphodiester backbones surrounding the minor groove of dsRNA. Presumably, the NS_{1A} RNA-binding domain recognizes a comparable type of dsRNA conformation when it binds to all its specific RNA targets.

The second functional domain, which is located in the C-terminal half of the molecule, is not required for RNA binding but is required for the inhibition of the nuclear export of poly(A)-containing mRNAs (275). Although mutagenesis originally identified the amino acid sequence from 134 to 161 as the effector domain (275), it is likely that the effector domain extends from amino acid 74 (at the end of the RNA-binding domain) to amino acid 237, the carboxyl-terminal amino acid. This domain was presumed to be an effector domain that interacts with host nuclear proteins to inhibit nuclear RNA export (see later). On the basis of current information, it can be concluded that all naturally occurring influenza A viruses encode an NS_{1A} protein that contains an effector domain. At one time, it was thought that one naturally occurring influenza virus, A/Turkey/Oregon/71, encoded an NS_{1A} protein lacking the C-terminal sequence containing the effector domain (235). It has since been established, however, that naturally occurring A/Turkey/Oregon/71 virus encodes a full-length NS_{1A} protein, indicating that the previously characterized virus isolate was probably generated during multiple passages in the laboratory (331).

The NS_{1A} Protein Interferes with the Cellular Machinery that Produces the 3′ Ends of Cellular mRNAs

The effector domain of the NS_{1A} protein interacts functionally with two essential proteins of the mammalian pre-mRNA 3′ end processing machinery: the human 30-kd subunit of the cleavage and polyadenylation specificity factor (CPSF) (228); and poly(A)-binding protein II (PABII) (41). Many of the functions of these two cellular proteins have been established (Fig. 25). The CPSF factor binds to the AAUAAA poly(A) signal located about 15 to 30 nucleotides upstream of the cleavage site in pre-mRNAs and is required for both cleavage and polyadenylation of pre-mRNAs (350). The 30-kd subunit is one of the two subunits of CPSF that has been impli-

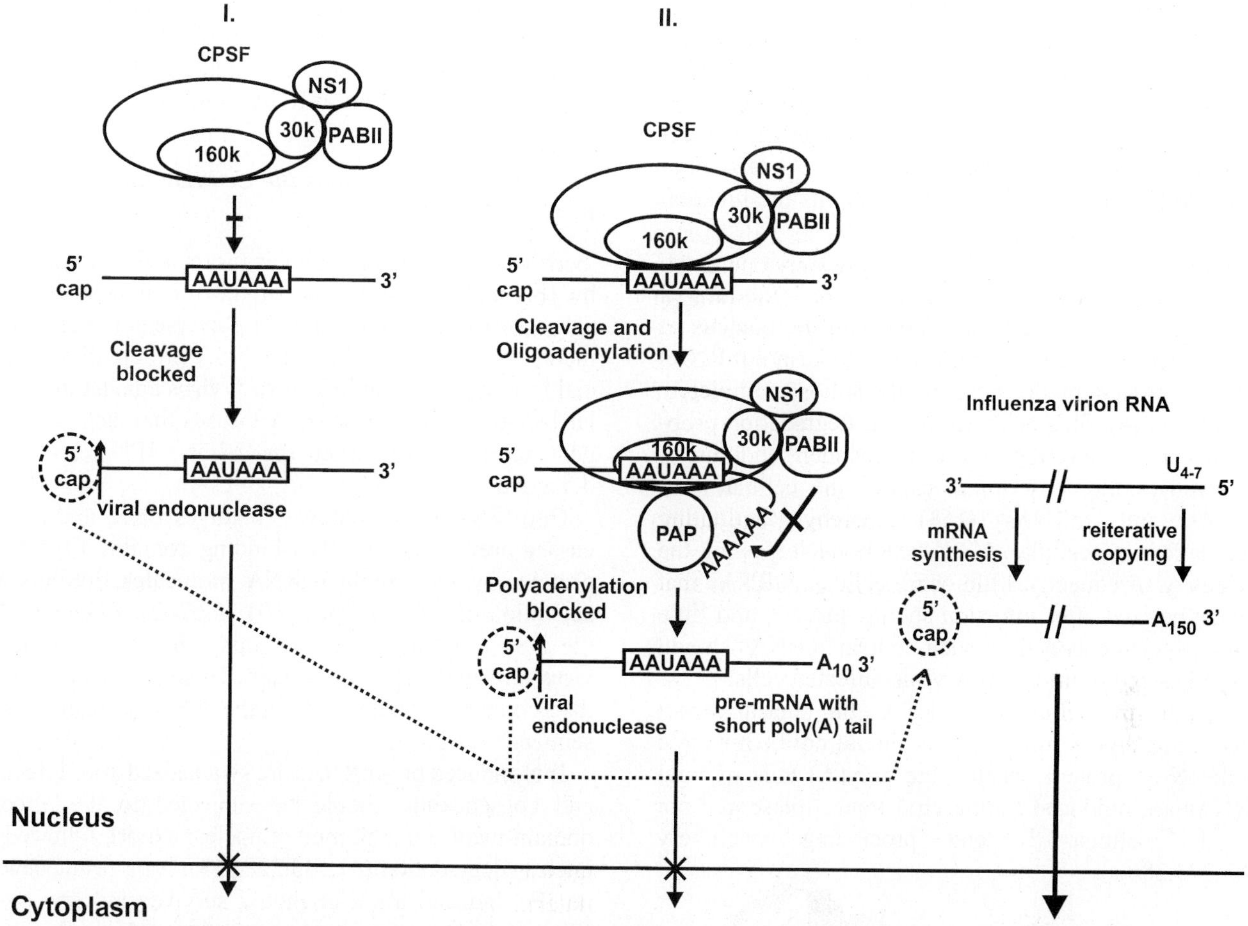

FIG. 25. Proposed two-pronged mechanism by which the NS_1 protein of influenza A virus inhibits the cellular 3′ end processing system in infected cells. *Pathway I:* The binding of the NS_1 protein (and PABII) to the 30-kd subunit of cleavage and polyadenylation specificity factor (CPSF) blocks the binding of CPSF to the AAUAAA sequence of some cellular pre-mRNA molecules, thereby blocking 3′ cleavage of these pre-mRNAs. The uncleaved pre-mRNAs remain in the nucleus. *Pathway II:* CPSF binds to the AAUAAA sequence of other cellular pre-mRNA molecules, despite the binding of the NS_1 protein and PABII to the 30-kd CPSF subunit. A short poly(A) sequence is then added to these cleaved pre-mRNAs by PAP in a CPSF-dependent reaction. Subsequent elongation of the short poly(A) sequence is blocked by the binding of the NS_1 protein to PABII, resulting in the nuclear accumulation of cleaved pre-mRNAs containing short poly(A) tails. In both pathways, an individual NS_{1A} protein forms a complex with both PABII and the 30-kd subunit of CPSF. In this complex, the two cellular 3′-processing proteins, 30-kd CPSF and PABII, also bind directly to each other. The presence of PABII in the 3′-processing complexes that are formed before 3′ cleavage probably results from the binding of PABII to the NS_{1A} protein because PABII has not been found in 3′ cleavage complexes formed *in vitro* in the absence of the NS_{1A} protein. Both species of the cellular pre-mRNAs that are sequestered in the nucleus are cleaved by the virion cap-dependent endonuclease to produce the primers required for viral mRNA synthesis. The 3′-terminal poly(A) sequence on viral mRNAs is produced by the viral transcriptase, which reiteratively copies a stretch of 4 to 7 U in the virion RNA templates. The poly(A)-containing viral mRNAs are exported from the nucleus. (Redrawn from refs. 41 and 228, with permission).

cated in the specific binding to the AAUAAA polyadenylation signal (88,149). In contrast, the PABII protein functions after 3′ cleavage of the cellular pre-mRNA, and is required for the processive elongation of poly(A) chains catalyzed by the cellular poly(A) polymerase (reviewed in 350). In the absence of PABII, poly(A) polymerase adds only short poly(A) tails to the 3′ cleaved pre-mRNA.

Binding of the influenza virus NS_{1A} protein through its effector domain to the 30-kd CPSF subunit dramatically inhibits CPSF function and hence inhibits the 3′ end cleavage and polyadenylation of the cellular pre-mRNAs that are synthesized after infection (see Fig. 25, pathway I) (228). Indeed, influenza viruses that contain ts mutations in the NS_{1A} protein coding sequence inhibit 3′ cleavage of cellular pre-mRNAs at the permissive, but not at the nonpermissive, temperature (313). Nonetheless, 3′ cleavage of some cellular pre-mRNAs still occurs in virus-infected cells, followed by the addition of short poly(A) tails catalyzed by the cellular poly(A) polymerase (see Fig. 25, pathway II) (41). The subsequent processive elongation of these short poly(A) tails does not occur because the NS_{1A} protein inhibits the function of the cellular PABII protein (41).

Both the cellular pre-mRNAs that do not undergo cleavage and those that contain short (about 12 nucleotides) poly(A) tails accumulate in the nucleus of infected cell. The newly synthesized cellular pre-mRNAs that are trapped in the nucleus are almost completely degraded (144). This efficient nuclear degradation probably occurs because the viral cap-dependent endonuclease removes the 5′ terminal cap of the cellular pre-mRNAs and mRNAs (163), thereby facilitating degradation by cellular 5′-3′ exoribonucleases in the nucleus. Consequently, little or no cellular mRNAs that are synthesized after infection should survive, and little or no proteins encoded by such cellular mRNAs should be synthesized in influenza A virus–infected cells.

In contrast to cellular pre-mRNAs, the nuclear export of viral mRNAs in infected cells should not be hindered by the NS_{1A} protein because the poly(A) tails of viral mRNAs are produced by the viral transcriptase and not by the cellular 3′ end processing machinery (203,273,286).

The NS_{1A} Protein Inhibits the Splicing of Pre-mRNAs

By using transfection experiments, it was established that the NS_{1A} protein inhibits the splicing of cellular pre-mRNAs *in vivo* (82,201) and that purified recombinant NS_{1A} protein inhibits pre-mRNA splicing *in vitro,* catalyzed by nuclear extracts from uninfected cells (201,279). Splicing inhibition *in vitro* is mediated by the binding of the NS_{1A} protein to a specific stem-bulge in U6 snRNA (279), an snRNA that plays a central role in the splicing most of the cellular pre-mRNAs (307). In contrast, splicing inhibition *in vivo* requires the effector domain as well as the RNA-binding domain of the NS_{1A} protein (201).

However, it has not yet been conclusively established that the NS_{1A} protein inhibits the splicing of cellular pre-mRNAs in virus-infected cells. Any such inhibition is obscured by the rapid degradation of cellular pre-mRNAs that occurs in the nucleus of infected cells (143,163). The only evidence for the NS_{1A} protein-mediated inhibition of cellular pre-mRNA splicing in infected cells is that the NS_{1A} protein synthesized during virus infection is specifically associated with U6 snRNA molecules (202). Several important questions about the presumed inhibition of the splicing of cellular pre-mRNAs in virus-infected cells have not yet been addressed. Thus, it is not known how the NS_{1A} protein-mediated inhibition of pre-mRNA splicing would benefit virus gene expression and how the splicing of the viral M_1 and NS_1 mRNAs by the cellular splicing machinery could take place in the face of an overall inhibition of pre-mRNA splicing.

The NS_{1A} Protein Inhibits the Cellular Interferon Response

The several hundred cellular proteins that are induced by IFN-α/β constitute one of the initial host defenses against virus infection (62,327). Reverse genetics experiments have established that the NS_{1A} protein plays a crucial role in protecting influenza A virus against the cellular IFN response: influenza A viruses that lack the NS_{1A} gene replicate only when the cellular IFN response is defective (84).

One IFN-induced pathway involves PKR, and as discussed previously, the RNA-binding domain of the NS_{1A} protein, by binding to dsRNA molecules, inhibits the activation of PKR *in vitro* (101,102,202). Evidence that the NS_{1A} protein carries out this function in influenza virus–infected cells was obtained using mutant viruses that contain ts mutations in the NS_{1A} protein coding sequence (102).

IFN-induced pre-mRNAs are synthesized after infection and consequently should be subjected to the effector domain-mediated inhibition of nuclear export, followed by nuclear degradation (41,143,228,313). As a result, few or no IFN-induced mRNAs should survive, and few or no IFN-induced proteins should be synthesized in influenza A virus–infected cells. Consistent with such a role of the effector domain, laboratory-generated viruses that lack deletions of the effector domain fail to protect the virus against IFN (70). Only in Vero cells, which are defective in IFN production, do these mutant viruses grow as well as wild-type virus in tissue culture. The efficiency of replication of these mutant viruses in MDCK cells, which produce IFN, is inversely correlated with the length of the effector domain of the encoded NS_{1A} protein, and these viruses are attenuated in wild-type mice that produce IFN.

A Latent Nuclear Export Signal in the Effector Domain of the NS_{1A} Protein

An amino acid sequence in the effector domain of the NS_{1A} protein (amino acids 134 to 147) has the same spacing of hydrophobic residues (leucines) as other proven NES sequences (reviewed in 91). When this short NS_{1A} sequence is linked to a heterologous protein, it functions as an NES; that is, it transports the heterologous protein from the nucleus to the cytoplasm (198).

In uninfected cells that are transfected with the NS_{1A} gene, however, the NES of the NS_{1A} protein does not function. In contrast, in influenza virus–infected cells, the NES of a fraction of the wild-type NS_{1A} protein molecules is activated, and a substantial amount of the NS_{1A}

protein is found in the cytoplasm. The mechanism by which the NES of the NS_{1A} protein is activated in infected cells has not yet been established. In addition, the functions of the NS_{1A} protein molecules that are exported to the cytoplasm of virus-infected cells have not been identified. Several possibilities have been suggested. For example, the binding of dsRNA by the NS_{1A} protein to inhibit the activation of the PKR kinase, a cytoplasmic enzyme, could occur in the cytoplasm (102,202). Furthermore, as discussed previously, NS_{1A} protein molecules in the cytoplasm may also play other roles in the translation of viral mRNAs.

Comparison of the NS_{1A} Protein with the Influenza B Virus NS_1 Protein (NS_{1B} Protein)

The NS_{1A} and NS_{1B} proteins share little sequence homology, and NS_{1B} proteins are usually larger than NS_{1A} proteins (26). For example, the NS_{1B} protein encoded by B/Lee/40 virus is 281 amino acids long, whereas the NS_{1A} protein encoded by A/Udorn/72 is only 237 amino acids long. However, the NS_{1B} protein binds to the same specific RNA targets as the NS_{1A} protein (356). In addition, as is the case with the NS_{1A} protein, an N-terminal fragment of the NS_{1B} protein possesses all the RNA-binding and dimerization activities of the full-length protein and is largely α-helical (356). The NS_{1B} fragment is 93 amino acids long, and is thus about 20 amino acids longer than the functional N-terminal fragment of the NS_{1A} protein. A reasonable alignment between the two N-terminal fragments that perfectly aligns helix 2 and 2′ can be made (357). Thus, influenza B viruses probably encodes an NS_{1B} proteins with a N-terminal, six-helical RNA-binding domain similar to that of the NS_{1A} protein.

In contrast to the RNA-binding and dimerization domain, the effector domain of the NS_{1A} protein is not conserved in the NS_{1B} protein (356). Thus, unlike the NS_{1A} protein, the NS_{1B} protein does not inhibit either the nuclear export of cellular mRNAs or the splicing of cellular pre-mRNAs (356). Consequently, these effector domain functions are not needed for the propagation of influenza B viruses in nature, and the function of the large C-terminal region of NS_{1B} proteins is not known. All naturally occurring influenza B viruses encode an NS_{1B} protein with such a large C-terminal region (235). This fundamental difference between NS_{1A} and NS_{1B} proteins probably contributes to the different biologic properties of influenza A and B viruses.

Viral Assembly and Release

Intracellular Transport of the Integral Membrane Proteins

The influenza virus integral membrane proteins HA, HEF, NA, M_2, and NB are synthesized on membrane-bound ribosomes and are translocated across the membrane of the ER in a signal recognition particle (SRP)-dependent manner (71,130). For HA, the N-terminal signal sequence is cleaved in the ER by signal peptidase: NA, M_2, and NB do not contain cleavable signal sequences. N-linked carbohydrate chains are transferred to HA, NA, NB, and CM2 (M_2 is not glycosylated) *en bloc* from a dolicyl lipid carrier, and trimming of terminal glucose residues from mannose-rich oligosaccharides occurs in the ER. The HA and NA have been used as prototypes from which much of what we know about the process of folding and oligomerization of an integral membrane protein has been learned. For HA, a large body of data indicates that there is a step-wise conformational maturation of the protein with independent folding of specific domains in the HA monomer, followed by trimerization and the completion of folding to the pH neutral form of HA (reviewed in 66). Once correctly folded and assembled, proteins are transported out of the ER to the Golgi apparatus. There, oligosaccharide chains may be further processed to the complex form. For influenza virus A/Aichi/68 HA, five carbohydrate chains are in the complex form, and two are in the high mannose form (359). HA and NA lack terminal sialic acid on their complex carbohydrate chains in influenza virus–infected cells, presumably because of the action of the viral NA (8,156). Palmitoylation of the three C-terminal proximal cysteine residues of HA (two in the cytoplasmic tail and one in the presumed TM domain) and palmitoylation of the M_2 protein cytoplasmic tail residue 50 (119,333,346) are thought to occur in the cis-Golgi complex. In HAs containing a furin cleavage site, cleavage activation occurs in the TGN (330).

In polarized epithelial cells, influenza viruses assemble and bud at the apical surface of cells (287,290), and it has been shown that HA (influenza A virus), HEF, NA (influenza A virus), M_2, and CM2, when expressed alone from cDNAs in polarized cells, are transported to the apical surface (128,140,291,398). Thus, apical transport is an intrinsic property of these proteins.

The last step in intracellular transport is the expression of the proteins at the plasma membrane. Although HA appears to be diffusely distributed over the surface, M_2, NA, and the influenza C virus HEF glycoprotein appear to cluster in patches (53,54,112,128,140,185,395,396). At the present time, the significance of this cell surface distribution is not known.

Role of M_2 Ion Channel Activity on Maturation of Hemagglutinin in the trans-Golgi Network

Amantadine has a second late effect during the replication of avian influenza virus A/chicken/Germany/34 (H7N1) fowl plague virus (FPV) Rostock. A premature conformational change occurs in its HA in the TGN during the transport of HA to the cell surface (95,96,332; (reviewed in 179). This form of HA is indistinguishable from the low-pH–induced form of HA. Several experiments indicate that the M_2 ion channel activity also functions in the TGN and associated transport vesicles, where it regulates intracompartmental pH and as a result keeps the pH above the threshold at which the FPV Rostock HA conformational change occurs (238,297,332,339; reviewed in 104,179). Consequently, in the presence of amantadine, the low-pH–induced conformational change occurs, and the resulting extrusion of the fusion peptide at the wrong time and in the wrong subcellular compartment results in the aggregation of HA molecules; hence, budding is greatly reduced (292). However, it is clear that the avian influenza virus FPV Rostock, even for an influenza virus with an HA that is cleaved intracellularly, is an exceptional case in requiring a functional M_2 protein ion channel activity in the TGN. Other viruses that also contain an H7 HA do not share such a requirement because their pH of transition to the low-pH–induced form is lower (96).

The Budding Process

Influenza viruses can be observed to bud from the plasma membrane of infected cells morphologically (reviewed in 51) (see Fig. 2). Electron microscopic observations suggest that the precursor to the envelope of a budding virion is a patch of cell membrane containing viral envelope proteins (reviewed in 51). Host cell membrane proteins appear to be excluded from virions. In addition, among virus-encoded proteins, there must be a positive selection or a rejection process. The ratio of M_2 to HA at the plasma membrane is about 1:4, whereas in the virus, it is 1:25 (185,395).

Interactions between the cytoplasmic tails of the viral integral membrane proteins and the internal proteins of the virion likely provide the necessary molecular information for formation of the budding particle. The 10- to 11-residue HA C-terminal cytoplasmic tail and the six residues constituting the predicted NA cytoplasmic tail are highly conserved among the HA and NA subtypes (47,233). Given the mutation rate of the influenza virus RNA genome, this sequence conservation suggests an important function for the HA and NA cytoplasmic tails. To elucidate such a function, reverse genetics procedures were used to generate influenza viruses that lack either the cytoplasmic tail of HA (136,138) or the cytoplasmic tail of NA (86,217) or both cytoplasmic tails (137). Based on observation of properties of these mutant viruses, a model was proposed in which, for the normal budding of influenza virus, the requirements of the HA and NA cytoplasmic tail interactions with an internal component of the virion (most likely the M_1 protein) are so crucial for normal budding that these two cytoplasmic tail interactions are redundant (137). When both cytoplasmic tails are eliminated, the virions possessed greatly altered morphology (137).

The M_1 and M_2 proteins may also form crucial interactions during virus assembly and budding. It has been found that a monoclonal antibody (14C2) with specificity for the M_2 ectodomain restricts the size of plaque growth of a variety of influenza A virus strains (395). This M_2 antibody reduces the level of cell surface expression of M_2 and reduces the level of influenza virus particle formation in a single cycle of infection (129). Furthermore, this M_2 antibody also reduces the level of filamentous particle formation (285). When variant viruses resistant to the antibody were isolated, they were found to have compensating changes in the cytoplasmic tail of M_2 as well as in the N-terminal domain of the M_1 protein (394). These variant viruses resistant to the antibody retain the filamentous particle phenotype (285). Thus, the evidence suggests important roles for the putative M_1 and M_2 interactions in virus assembly.

The positive selection or exclusion process for inclusion of viral integral membrane proteins into virus particles may be affected by the organization of the lipids in the plasma membrane. It was long thought that the lipids of the plasma membrane functioned mainly as a solvent for membrane proteins (the fluid mosaic model) (315). However, more recently, this view has been refined to include lateral organization resulting from preferential packaging of sphingolipids and cholesterol into moving "platforms," or "rafts," in which specific membrane proteins become incorporated (29,314). Rafts can incorporate specific proteins, including many, but not all, glycophosphatidylinositol-anchored proteins and N-terminally myristoylated and palmitoylated cytoplasmic proteins (216; reviewed in 314). Rafts also incorporate some integral membrane proteins. HA and NA enter cholesterol-sphingomyelin–rich raft domains, and it is becoming increasing clear that the rafts are the site of assembly of budding virions at the plasma membrane (300,398). The M_1 protein also associates with these rafts, but this association is decreased in cells infected with viruses lacking both the HA and NA cytoplasmic tails (398). In contrast, the M_2 ion channel protein is largely excluded from rafts (398), thereby providing an explanation for the low amount of M_2 protein in virions as compared with HA (185,395). However, some M_2 is included into virions, and for the positive inclusion of M_2 into virions, it has been suggested that the extracellular domain of M_2 is required (250).

The mechanism by which the bud pinches off from the plasma membrane is not known. For retroviruses, there is a role for monoubiquitination of Gag in the budding process (255), and it is known that monoubiquitination of some receptor protein promotes their internalization and down-regulation (115). Thus, for retroviruses, budding involves cellular machinery, and this is also likely to be the case for influenza virus. To release fully formed influenza virions from the cell surface, the action of the viral NA is thought to be needed because in the absence of NA activity, sialic acid present on the carbohydrate chains of HA and cell surface molecules causes the virus to aggregate to itself and the cell surface through the HA sialic acid receptor–binding pocket (248).

Packaging a Segmented Genome

Production of an infectious influenza virus particle requires incorporation of at least one copy of the eight genomic segments. Nevertheless, random packaging cannot be distinguished from a selective mechanism for inclusion of a full complement of genomic RNAs. A random packaging mechanism in which any eight RNA segments of the genome are incorporated into virions would generate a maximum of 1 infectious particle for every 400 assembled ($8!/8^8$), a number within the range of noninfectious to infectious particles found in virion preparations. If 12 segments can be randomly packaged, 10% of virions would contain one copy of each of the eight segments (77).

A selective mechanism for incorporation of one copy of each RNA segment exists for the three segments of dsRNA of phage $\phi 6$. The positive strand of each segment is packaged before synthesis of the complementary negative strands within particles. The particle-to-plaque forming unit ratio is close to 1, indicating that essentially all particles contain a complete complement of genome segments. Such precise packaging appears to be due to the serial (sequential) dependence of packaging of the positive-stranded RNA segments with the smallest segment entering first, followed by the medium dsRNA segment and then the largest dsRNA segment (277).

For influenza virus, particles containing more than eight RNA segments (77) and less than eight RNA segments (208) have been obtained consistent with random packaging. However, the specific interference with packaging of wild-type RNA segment 1, but of no other genome segment, by an internally deleted defective RNA segment 1, argues strongly for a specific mechanism of packaging, at least for RNA segment 1 (69,237).

GENETICS OF INFLUENZA VIRUSES

RNA Segment Reassortment

Influenza type A, B, and C viruses can form reassortants *in vivo* between members of the homotypic virus type but not between types. The emergence of new pandemic strains of influenza A virus usually results from such a reassortment. The consequence of this reassortment is the appearance of a new virus subtype containing a novel HA or NA that is immunologically distinct from those of the previous circulating strain. In the 20th century, there was the appearance of "Spanish" influenza in 1918 and 1919, with an HA related to those of swine viruses or H1 subtype viruses. Viruses of this subtype circulated until 1957, when viruses of the H2N2 subtype (Asian strains) were isolated. The H2 subtype HA has little or no cross-reactivity with the H1 HA. In addition to containing an H2 HA, the Asian strains had a new NA (N2). For 11 years, the H2N2 strains of influenza virus spread and changed until the next pandemic in 1968 with the introduction of a new H3 subtype (Hong Kong strains). In 1976, an H1N1 virus reemerged, and in 1997 and 1998, in Hong Kong, a virulent avian H5 virus crossed the species barrier from birds to humans (see Chapter 47 in *Fields Virology*, 4th ed.). The extensive changes in the HA or NA that lead to new subtypes of human influenza viruses are known as *antigenic shifts* (reviewed in 152 and 366) (see Chapter 47 in *Fields Virology*, 4th ed.). These drastic antigenic changes come about from the reassortment of previously circulating human viruses and influenza viruses of animal origin. There is a great deal of evidence for the reassortment of RNA segments between human and animal viruses *in vivo* (365) and among human viruses in nature (392). It has been established that the A/Hong Kong/68 H3N2 virus contains the NA and all genes encoding internal proteins, except that for PB1, from an Asian (H2N2) strain; the genes for HA and PB1 are thought to be derived from a strain that is closely related to Eurasian avian viruses and A/equine/Miami/63 (H3N8 viruses) (145).

Theoretically, it might be expected that *in vivo,* the eight RNA segments of influenza A virus could give rise to 256 possible reassortants. However, a random segregation does not occur because certain viral proteins apparently need their matched strain-specific cognate protein. Nowhere is this more clearly demonstrated than with the requirement of the A/chicken/Germany/34 (H7N1) fowl plague virus Rostock HA (encoded by RNA segment 4), which always cosegregates with its cognate M_2 protein (encoded by RNA segment 7) (95,96).

RNA Mutations

Minor changes in antigenic character of influenza viruses occur as a result of the accumulation of amino acid changes due to mutation; of principal importance are changes in HA and NA. This process is known as *antigenic drift* and occurs with influenza A, B, and C viruses (reviewed in 152 and 366) (see Chapter 47 in *Fields Virology*, 4th ed.). However, influenza A viruses show a high number of substitutions accumulating in a sequential pattern with time, whereas influenza C viruses isolated decades apart show much lesser degrees of variability (reviewed in 322). The mutation rate for the H3 HA (HA_1 domain) has been estimated to be 6.7×10^{-3} substitutions per site per year. The observation that the nucleotide substitutions in HA were found predominantly in HA_1 suggests that many substitutions may be selected for by the immune pressure (322 and references therein).

Many studies have been performed to analyze the rate of mutation of RNA viruses in tissue culture. Recent calculations, which take into consideration many artifacts of earlier studies, indicate the influenza virus mutation rate at 1.5×10^{-5} mutations per nucleotide per infectious cycle (253). However, although the influenza virus mutation rate is high compared with mammalian DNA genomes (10^{-8} to 10^{-11} per incorporated nucleotide), the mutation rate of influenza A virus is not markedly different from that of other RNA viruses (reviewed in 322).

RNA Recombination

RNA recombination is the joining of two separate RNA chains by crossing-over or copy-choice mechanisms. Historically for influenza virus, the term *RNA recombination* has been used to mean RNA segment reassortment. Unlike the situation with the positive-stranded RNA viruses, the *Coronaviridae* and *Picornaviridae* (see Chapters 18 and 21), in which RNA recombination occurs at high frequency, until recently, recombination had not been measured for influenza viruses. However, natural examples of RNA recombination have been found when HAs were identified that contain at the HA_1/HA_2 cleavage site either an insertion of 54 nucleotides derived from host 28S ribosomal RNA (151,242) or 60 nucleotides derived from the NP gene (241). In addition, using molecular genetic techniques (see later), RNA recombination within an RNA segment has been shown to occur (12).

Molecularly Engineered Genetics (Reverse Genetics)

The study of viruses and their interactions with host cells and organisms has benefited greatly from the ability to engineer specific mutations into viral genomes, a technique known as *reverse genetics* (368). The negative-stranded RNA viruses present a difficult problem because the virion RNA is assembled with an active transcriptase complex for the genome to initiate replication.

The finding that it was possible to isolate an active polymerase complex from influenza virus RNP cores by using CsCl-glycerol gradient centrifugation (121) made it possible to transcribe *in vitro* short synthetic RNA molecules containing the influenza virus 5′- and 3′-terminal nucleotide sequences (254). It was then shown that an artificial gene construct containing the 5′- and 3′-terminal nucleotide sequences flanking a chloramphenicol acetyltransferase (CAT) reporter gene could be replicated *in vivo* in cells infected with a "helper" virus. The artificial CAT gene was replicated and packaged into virions, and it could be passaged several times in cells (204). These important experiments made it possible to introduce mutations into the influenza virus genome (75). This technology was later improved by finding that the efficiency of isolating a virus containing a foreign gene is enhanced if the transcription of the synthetic RNA is performed in the presence of the influenza virus RNA polymerase complex (76) (Fig. 26). The application of a strong selection pressure against the helper virus is

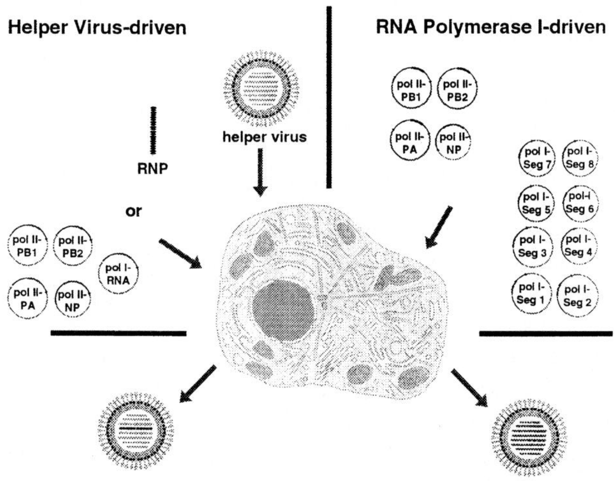

FIG. 26. Influenza virus reverse genetics. The initial replacement of individual RNA segments of influenza virus involved either the *in vitro* reconstitution of vRNPs or *in vivo* assembly of vRNPs after transfection of a cell with plasmids that use pol II promoters driving the expression of the PA, PB1, PB2, and NP proteins, and pol I promoters and terminators controlling viral genome synthesis. Influenza virus rescue entirely from plasmid DNA involves the transfection of plasmids encoding each of the eight RNA segments (under control of the pol I promoter and terminator), four of the proteins that make up the polymerase complex (under control of the pol II promoter) and is aided by, but does not require, the other five viral structural proteins. (Redrawn from ref. 257, with permission.)

needed to isolate progeny virus containing the plasmid DNA-derived RNA segment, and for this reason, the method has been used mainly for analysis of the surface proteins of the virus, because of strong antibody-dependent selection procedures. Several important discoveries pertaining to individual influenza virus proteins, as well as demonstrating the use of influenza virus to serve as a viral expression vector, have been obtained by application of this reverse genetics technology (7,12,85,195,197, 222,245,249,261,280,326,401; reviewed in 231 and 256).

Recently, two very similar systems have been established in which helper influenza virus is not needed, making it possible to manipulate every gene in the influenza virus genome (see Fig. 26) (80,232,264). In one system, the host cell is conscripted into making the vRNPs using specific properties of the cellular DNA-dependent RNA polymerase I (pol I) promoter and transcription terminator sequences. The essence of the system is that pol I transcription and termination signals permit the production of artificial influenza virus RNA segments with the same 5′- and 3′-termini as authentic vRNAs. Eight plasmids encoding each of the influenza virus genomic RNA segments under the control of the the pol I promoter and terminator are transfected into cells together with four plasmids encoding the polymerase complex proteins and NP cDNAs under control of an RNA polymerase type II (pol II) promoter (232). In the other system a pol I promoter and aribozyme are used (80,264).

MEANS OF CONTROLLING INFLUENZA VIRUS

Influenza virus causes widespread human disease. In a typical year, influenza virus afflicts 10% -20% of the U.S. population, causing up to 40,000 deaths. During pandemics, a much greater loss of life occurs. The 1918 pandemic was the worse of those pandemic: at least 20 million people died worldwide, many of whom were young adults in the prime of life (56). The reason for the high pathogenicity of this particular virus strain has not yet been ascertained (361). The potential for the reemergence of a highly pathogenic influenza virus strain is exemplified by the sudden appearance of a lethal virus in Hong Kong in 1997, which killed 6 of the 18 infected individuals (46). This virus was transmitted from birds to humans, contrary to the long-held dogma that such a transmission was not possible because the viral receptors on avian cells differ from those on human cells. The spread of infection was controlled because the entire live bird market population in Hong Kong was sacrificed and because the virus did not develop the ability to spread from humans to humans. Usually, influenza virus is readily transmitted from humans to humans by aerosol. For these and other reasons, influenza virus is now considered a dangerous threat as a reemerging viral disease (240).

A detailed description of the means of controlling future influenza virus epidemics is beyond the scope of this chapter. Many reviews of this subject have been published elsewhere (see 35 and 55). Here, we outline a few salient features of the currently employed means of control.

The primary means of controlling influenza virus epidemics at the present time is vaccination (55). The vaccine, which is made up of formaldehyde-fixed virus (killed) or surface glycoproteins (split), has to be reformulated each year because, as discussed previously in this chapter, the viral HA, the protein that elicits the primary neutralizing immune response, usually undergoes changes that render the previous year's vaccine ineffective against the new strain. Each year, the new vaccine takes about 6 months to produce, which is clearly too long to control a fast-moving epidemic. In addition, the 1997 Hong Kong virus demonstrated another difficulty, namely, that it could not be grown in embryonated eggs because it was so pathogenic that it killed the embryos before high levels of virus were produced (338).

In contrast to vaccines, antivirals can be rapidly employed to combat an epidemic, and the efficacy of antiviral therapy against influenza virus has been greatly enhanced because the virus can now be detected at an early time of infection using rapid diagnostic tests (55). Several approaches have been employed to identify compounds that specifically inhibit influenza virus replication. The antiviral drug amantadine (rimantadine) (Fig. 27) exemplifies a compound that was identified by a mass screening empirical approach. As discussed previously, amantadine only inhibits influenza A virus because its target site of action is the M_2 ion channel protein. These drugs have other limitations: they are effective against some, but not all, strains of influenza A viruses; virus mutants that are resistant to these drugs rapidly emerge; and these drugs cause undesirable side effects (e.g., anxiety, lightheadedness, seizures) (55,381).

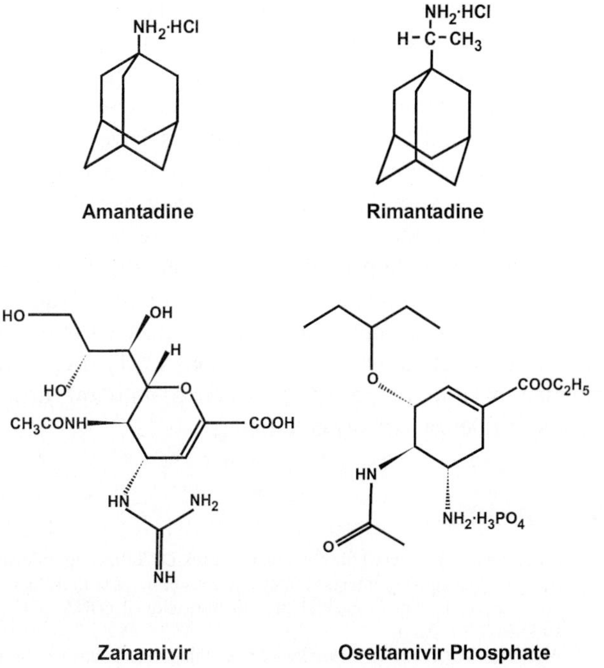

FIG. 27. Influenza virus antiviral compounds. The structures of amantadine, rimantadine (Flumadine), zamanivir (Relenza), and oseltamivir phosphate (Tamiflu) are shown.

Another approach, rational drug design, has been used to devise inhibitors of NA. As discussed previously, the sialic acid–binding site on NA was identified as a large pocket on the surface of each of the four subunits (49). The pocket is lined by amino acids that are invariant in all influenza A and B viruses that have been characterized. The crystal structure indicated that there should be an empty cavity in this pocket when sialic acid is in the pocket, which led to the prediction that substitution of the 4-hydroxyl group of sialic acid with an amino or guanidinyl group would increase the binding interaction of the resulting compound (349). X-ray crystallography confirmed this prediction. Two compounds (4-amino or 4-guanidino 2-deoxy-2,3-didehydro-D-*N*-acetylneuraminic acid) were synthesized, and they were found to be extremely effective inhibitors of NA of both influenza A and B viruses, and these compounds were orders of magnitude less active against an array of nonviral neuraminidases. These compounds, particularly the 4-guanidino derivative (Zanamivir or Relenza; see Fig. 27), inhibit influenza virus plaque formation and virus replication in ferrets (349). This drug has to be administered by nasal spray, and similar rational drug design resulted in another NA inhibitor that can be administered orally, GS4104 (Oseltamivir or Tamiflu) (336; see Fig. 27). Viruses resistant to these NA inhibitors have occurred infrequently *in vitro,* and many appear to map to HA (17,336). However, in the first year of their use (the 1999 to 2000 winter), these two new drugs were not as effective as had been hoped: they shortened the length of influenza virus symptoms by only about 1 day and did not decrease serious complications of influenza virus infections (e.g., pneumonia, hospitalization) (381). Research directed at developing more effective antiviral drugs against influenza virus is continuing.

REFERENCES

1. Akkina RK, Chambers TM, Londo DR, Nayak DP. Intracellular localization of the viral polymerase proteins in cells infected with influenza virus and cells expressing PB1 protein from cloned cDNA. *J Virol* 1987;61:2217–2224.
2. Allen H, McCauley J, Waterfield M, Gething MJ. Influenza virus RNA segment 7 has the coding capacity for two polypeptides. *Virology* 1980;107:548–551.
3. Alonso-Caplen FV, Krug RM. Regulation of the extent of splicing of influenza virus NS1 mRNA: Role of the rates of splicing and of the nucleocytoplasmic transport of NS1 mRNA. *Mol Cell Biol* 1991; 11:1092–1098.
4. Alonso-Caplen FV, Nemeroff ME, Qiu Y, Krug RM. Nucleocytoplasmic transport: The influenza virus NS1 protein regulates the transport of spliced NS2 mRNA and its precursor NS1 mRNA. *Genes Dev* 1992;6:255–267.
5. Apostolov K, Flewett TH. Internal structure of influenza virus. *Virology* 1965;26:506–508.
6. Banerjee AK. 5′-Terminal cap structure in eukaryotic messenger ribonucleic acids. *Microbiol Rev* 1980;44:175–205.
7. Barclay WS, Palese P. Influenza B viruses with site-specific mutations introduced into the HA gene. *J Virol* 1995;69:1275–1279.
8. Basak S, Tomana M, Compans RW. Sialic acid is incorporated into influenza hemagglutinin glycoproteins in the absence of viral neuraminidase. *Virus Res* 1985;2:61–68.
9. Bauer CM, Pinto LH, Cross TA, Lamb RA. The influenza virus M_2 ion channel protein: Probing the structure of the transmembrane domain in intact cells by using engineered disulfide cross-linking. *Virology* 1999;254:196–209.
10. Bean WJ Jr, Simpson RW. Transcriptase activity and genome composition of defective influenza virus. *J Virol* 1976;18:365–369.
11. Beaton AR, Krug RM. Transcription antitermination during influenza viral template RNA synthesis requires the nucleocapsid protein and the absence of a 5′ capped end. *Proc Natl Acad Sci U S A* 1986;83: 6282–6286.
12. Bergmann M, Garcia-Sastre A, Palese P. Transfection-mediated recombination of influenza A virus. *J Virol* 1992;66:7576–7580.
13. Betakova T, Nermut MV, Hay AJ. The NB protein is an integral component of the membrane of influenza B virus. *J Gen Virol* 1996;77: 2689–2694.
14. Biswas SK, Nayak DP. Mutational analysis of the conserved motifs of influenza A virus polymerase basic protein 1. *J Virol* 1994;68: 1819–1826.
15. Bizebard T, Gigant B, Rigolet P, et al. Structure of influenza virus haemagglutinin complexed with a neutralizing antibody. *Nature* 1995; 376:92–94.
16. Blaas D, Patzelt E, Kuechler E. Cap-recognizing protein of influenza virus. *Virology* 1982;116:339–348.
17. Blick TJ, Sahasrabudhe A, McDonald M, et al. The interaction of neuraminidase and hemagglutinin mutations in influenza virus in resistance to 4-guanidino-Neu5Ac2en. *Virology* 1998;246:95–103.
18. Bosch F, Orlich M, Klenk H-D, Rott R. The structure of the hemagglutinin, a determinant for the pathogenicity of influenza viruses. *Virology* 1979;95:197–207.
19. Bossart-Whitaker P, Carson M, Babu YS, et al. Three-dimensional structure of influenza A N9 neuraminidase and its complex with the inhibitor 2-deoxy 2, 3-dehydro-N-acetyl neuraminic acid. *J Mol Biol* 1993;232:1069–1083.
20. Bouloy M, Morgan MA, Shatkin AJ, Krug RM. Cap and internal nucleotides of reovirus mRNA primers are incorporated into influenza viral complementary RNA during transcription in vitro. *J Virol* 1979; 32:895–904.
21. Bouloy M, Plotch SJ, Krug RM. Globin mRNAs are primers for the transcription of influenza viral RNA in vitro. *Proc Natl Acad Sci U S A* 1978;75:4886–4890.
22. Braam J, Ulmanen I, Krug RM. Molecular model of a eucaryotic transcription complex: Functions and movements of influenza P proteins during capped RNA-primed transcription. *Cell* 1983;34:609–618.
23. Brand CM, Skehel JJ. Crystalline antigen from the influenza virus envelope. *Nature* 1972;238:145–147.
24. Brassard DL, Leser GP, Lamb RA. Influenza B virus NB glycoprotein is a component of virions. *Virology* 1996;220:350–360.
25. Briedis DJ, Lamb RA. Influenza B virus genome: Sequences and structural organization of RNA segment 8 and the mRNAs coding for the NS1 and NS2 proteins. *J Virol* 1982;42:186–193.
26. Briedis DJ, Lamb RA, Choppin PW. Influenza B virus RNA segment 8 codes for two nonstructural proteins. *Virology* 1981;112:417–425.
27. Briedis DJ, Lamb RA, Choppin PW. Sequence of RNA segment 7 of the influenza B virus genome: Partial amino acid homology between the membrane proteins (M1) of influenza A and B viruses and conservation of a second open reading frame. *Virology* 1982;116:581–588.
28. Bron R, Kendal AP, Klenk H-D, Wilschut J. Role of the M2 protein in influenza virus membrane fusion: Effects of amantadine and monensin on fusion kinetics. *Virology* 1993;195:808–811.
29. Brown DA, Rose JK. Sorting of GPI-anchored proteins to glycolipid-enriched membrane subdomains during transport to the apical cell surface. *Cell* 1992;68:533–544.
30. Brunner J, Tsurudome M. Fusion protein membrane interactions as studied by hydrophobic photolabeling, In: Bentz J ed. *Viral fusion mechanisms.* Boca Raton, FL: CRC Press, 1993:104–123.
31. Bui M, Wills EG, Helenius A, Whittaker GR. Role of the influenza virus M1 protein in nuclear export of viral ribonucleoproteins. *J Virol* 2000;74:1781–1786.
32. Bukrinskaya AG, Vorkunova NK, Kornilayeva GV, et al. Influenza virus uncoating in infected cells and effects of rimantadine. *J Gen Virol* 1982;60:49–59.
33. Bullough PA, Hughson FM, Skehel JJ, Wiley DC. Structure of influenza haemagglutinin at the pH of membrane fusion. *Nature* 1994; 371:37–43.
34. Burmeister WP, Ruigrok RWH, Cusack S. The 2.2 Å resolution crystal structure of influenza B neuraminidase and its complex with sialic acid. *EMBO J* 1992;11:49–56.
35. Calfee DP, Hayden FG. New approaches to influenza chemotherapy. Neuraminidase inhibitors. *Drugs* 1998;56:537–553.
36. Carr CM, Chaudhry C, Kim PS. Influenza hemagglutinin is spring-loaded by a metastable native conformation. *Proc Natl Acad Sci U S A* 1997;94:14306–14313.
37. Carr CM, Kim PS. A spring-loaded mechanism for the conformational change of influenza hemagglutinin. *Cell* 1993;73:823–832.
38. Castrucci MR, Hughes M, Calzoletti L, et al. The cysteine residues of the M2 protein are not required for influenza A virus replication. *Virology* 1997;238:128–134.
39. Chen J, Lee KH, Steinhauer DA, et al. Structure of the hemagglutinin precursor cleavage site, a determinant of influenza pathogenicity and the origin of the labile conformation. *Cell* 1998;95:409–417.
40. Chen J, Skehel JJ, Wiley DC. N- and C-terminal residues combine in the fusion-pH influenza hemagglutinin HA2 subunit to form an N cap that terminates the triple-stranded coiled coil. *Proc Natl Acad Sci U S A* 1999;96:8967–8972.
41. Chen Z, Li Y, Krug RM. Influenza A virus NS1 protein targets poly(A)-binding protein II of the cellular 3′ end processing machinery. *EMBO J* 1999;18:2273–2283.
42. Chien CY, Tejero R, Huang Y, et al. A novel RNA-binding motif in influenza A virus non-structural protein 1. *Nat Struct Biol* 1997;4: 891–895.
43. Chizhmakov IV, Geraghty FM, Ogden DC, et al. Selective proton per-

meability and pH regulation of the influenza virus M2 channel expressed in mouse erythroleukaemia cells. *J Physiol* 1996;494: 329–336.
44. Choppin PW. Replication of influenza virus in a continuous cell line: High yield of infective virsu from cells inoculated at high multiplicity. *Virology* 1969;39:130–134.
45. Cianci C, Tiley L, Krystal M. Differential activation of the influenza virus polymerase via template RNA binding. *J Virol* 1995;69: 3995–3999.
46. Class EC, Osterhaus AD, van Beek R, et al. Human influenza A H5N1 virus related to a highly pathogenic avian influenza virus. *Lancet* 1998;351:472–477.
47. Colman PM. Neuraminidase: Enzyme and antigen, In: Krug RM, ed. *The influenza viruses.* New York: Plenum Press, 1989:175–218.
48. Colman PM, Laver WG, Varghese JN, et al. Three-dimensional structure of a complex of antibody with influenza virus neuraminidase. *Nature* 1987;326:358–363.
49. Colman PM, Varghese JN, Laver WG. Structure of the catalytic and antigenic sites in influenza virus neuraminidase. *Nature* 1983;303: 41–44.
50. Compans RW. Influenza virus proteins. II. Association with components of the cytoplasm. *Virology* 1973;51:56–70.
51. Compans RW, Choppin PW. Reproduction of myxoviruses. In: Fraenkel-Conrat H, Wagner RR, ed. *Comprehensive virology*, vol. IV. New York: Plenum Press, 1975:179–252.
52. Compans RW, Content J, Duesberg PH. Structure of the ribonucleoprotein of influenza virus. *J Virol* 1972;10:795–800.
53. Compans RW, Dimmock NJ. An electron microscopic study of single-cycle infection of chick embryo fibroblasts by influenza virus. *Virology* 1969;39:499–515.
54. Compans RW, Dimmock NJ, Meier-Ewert H. Effect of antibody to neuraminidase on the maturation and hemagglutinating activity of an influenza A2 virus. *J Virol* 1969;4:528–534.
55. Cox NJ, Subbarao K. Influenza. *Lancet* 1999;354:1277–1282.
56. Crosby AW. *America's forgotten pandemic:* The influenza of 1919. Cambridge, UK: Cambridge University Press, 1990.
57. Daniels RS, Douglas AR, Skehel JJ, Wiley DC. Analyses of the antigenicity of influenza haemagglutinin at the pH optimum for virus-mediated membrane fusion. *J Gen Virol* 1983;64:1657–1662.
58. Daniels RS, Downie JC, Hay AJ, et al. Fusion mutants of the influenza virus hemagglutinin glycoprotein. *Cell* 1985;40:431–439.
59. Davey J, Dimmock NJ, Colman A. Identification of the sequence responsible for the nuclear accumulation of the influenza virus nucleoprotein in Xenopus oocytes. *Cell* 1985;40:667–675.
60. Davies WL, Grunert RR, Haff RF, et al. Antiviral activity of 1-adamantanamine (amantadine). *Science* 1964;144:862–863.
61. de la Luna S, Fortes PA, Beloso A, Ortin J. Influenza virus NS1 protein enhances the rate of translation initiation of viral mRNAs. *J Virol* 1995;69:2427–2433.
62. Der SD, Zhou A, Williams BR, Silverman RH. Identification of genes differentially regulated by interferon alpha, beta, or gamma using oligonucleotide arrays. *Proc Natl Acad Sci U S A* 1998;95: 15623–15628.
63. Detjen BM, St. Angelo C, Katze MG, Krug RM. The three influenza virus polymerase (P) proteins not associated with viral nucleocapsids in the infected cell are in the form of a complex. *J Virol* 1987;61: 16–22.
64. Digard P, Elton D, Bishop K, et al. Modulation of nuclear localization of the influenza virus nucleoprotein through interaction with actin filaments. *J Virol* 1999;73:2222–2231.
65. Doms RW, Helenius A, White J. Membrane fusion activity of the influenza virus hemagglutinin: The low pH-induced conformational change. *J Biol Chem* 1985;260:2973–2981.
66. Doms RW, Lamb RA, Rose JK, Helenius A. Folding and assembly of viral membrane proteins. *Virology* 1993;193:545–562.
67. Dopheide TA, Ward CW. The carboxyl-terminal sequence of the heavy chain of a Hong Kong influenza hemagglutinin. *Eur J Biochem* 1978; 85:393–398.
68. Duesberg P. Distinct subunits of the ribonucleoprotein of influenza virus. *J Mol Biol* 1969;42:485–499.
69. Duhaut SD, McCauley JW. Defective RNAs inhibit the assembly of influenza virus genome segments in a segment-specific manner. *Virology* 1996;216:326–337.
70. Egorov A, Brandt S, Sereinig S, et al. Transfectant influenza A viruses with long deletions in the NS1 protein grow efficiently in Vero cells. *J Virol* 1998;72:6437–6441.
71. Elder KT, Bye JM, Skehel JJ, et al. *In vitro* synthesis, glycosylation, and membrane insertion of influenza virus haemagglutinin. *Virology* 1979;95:343–350.
72. Ellens H, Bentz J, Mason D, et al. Fusion of influenza hemagglutinin-expressing fibroblasts with glycophorin-bearing liposomes: Role of hemagglutinin surface density. *Biochemistry* 1990;29:9697–9707.
73. Enami K, Qiao Y, Fukuda R, Enami M. An influenza virus temperature-sensitive mutant defective in the nuclear-cytoplasmic transport of the negative-sense viral RNAs. *Virology* 1993;194:822–827.
74. Enami K, Sato TA, Nakada S, Enami M. Influenza virus NS1 protein stimulates translation of the M1 protein. *J Virol* 1994;68:1432–1437.
75. Enami M, Luytjes W, Krystal M, Palese P. Introduction of site-specific mutations into the genome of influenza virus. *Proc Natl Acad Sci U S A* 1990;87:3802–3805.
76. Enami M, Palese P. High-efficiency formation of influenza virus transfectants. *J Virol* 1991;65:2711–2713.
77. Enami M, Sharma G, Benham C, Palese P. An influenza virus containing nine different RNA segments. *Virology* 1991;185:291–298.
78. Falcon AM, Fortes P, Marion RM, et al. Interaction of influenza virus NS1 protein and the human homologue of Staufen *in vitro* and *in vivo. Nucleic Acids Res* 1999;27:2241–2247.
79. Feigenblum D, Schneider RJ. Modification of eukaryotic initiation factor 4F during infection by influenza virus. *J Virol* 1993;67: 3027–3035.
80. Fodor E, Devenish L, Engelhardt OG, et al. Rescue of influenza A virus from recombinant DNA. *J Virol* 1999;73:9679–9682.
81. Fodor E, Pritlove DC, Brownlee GG. Characterization of the RNA-fork model of virion RNA in the initiation of transcription in influenza A virus. *J Virol* 1995;69:4012–4019.
82. Fortes P, Beloso A, Ortin J. Influenza virus NS1 protein inhibits pre-mRNA splicing and blocks mRNA nucleocytoplasmic transport. *EMBO J* 1994;13:704–712.
83. Fu XD. Specific commitment of different pre-mRNAs to splicing by single SR proteins. *Nature* 1993;365:82–85.
84. Garcia-Sastre A, Egorov A, Matassov D, et al. Influenza A virus lacking the NS1 gene replicates in interferon-deficient systems. *Virology* 1998;252:324–330.
85. Garcia-Sastre A, Muster T, Barclay WS, et al. Use of a mammalian internal ribosomal entry site element for expression of a foreign protein by a transfectant influenza virus. *J Virol* 1994;68:6254–6261.
86. Garcia-Sastre A, Palese P. The cytoplasmic tail of the neuraminidase protein of influenza A virus does not play an important role in the packaging of this protein into viral envelopes. *Virus Res* 1995;37: 37–47.
87. Garten W, Klenk H-D. Characterization of the carboxypeptidase involved in the proteolytic cleavage of the influenza haemagglutinin. *Intervirology* 1983;20:181–189.
88. Gilmartin GM, Nevins JR. Molecular analyses of two poly(A) site-processing factors that determine the recognition and efficiency of cleavage of the pre-mRNA. *Mol Cell Biol* 1991;11:2432–2438.
89. Gingras AC, Sonenberg N. Adenovirus infection inactivates the translational inhibitors 4E-BP1 and 4E-BP2. *Virology* 1997;237:182–186.
90. Godley L, Pfeifer J, Steinhauer D, et al. Introduction of intersubunit disulfide bonds in the membrane-distal region of the influenza hemagglutinin abolishes membrane fusion activity. *Cell* 1992;68:635–645.
91. Gorlich D, Mattaj IW. Nucleocytoplasmic transport. *Science* 1996; 271:1513–1518.
92. Goto H, Kawaoka Y. A novel mechanism for the acquisition of virulence by a human influenza A virus. *Proc Natl Acad Sci U S A* 1998; 95:10224–10228.
93. Gotoh B, Ogasawara T, Toyoda T, et al. An endoprotease homologous to the blood clotting factor X as a determinant of viral tropism in chick embryo. *EMBO J* 1990;9:4189–4195.
94. Gottschalk A. The specific enzyme of influenza virus and Vibrio cholerae. *Biochim Biophys Acta* 1957;23:645–646.
95. Grambas S, Bennett MS, Hay AJ. Influence of amantadine resistance mutations on the pH regulatory function of the M2 protein of influenza A viruses. *Virology* 1992;191:541–549.
96. Grambas S, Hay AJ. Maturation of influenza A virus hemagglutinin: Estimates of the pH encountered during transport and its regulation by the M2 protein. *Virology* 1992;190:11–18.
97. Graves PN, Schulman JL, Young JF, Palese P. Preparation of influenza

virus subviral particles lacking the HA1 subunit of hemagglutinin: Unmasking of cross-reactive HA2 determinants. *Virology* 1983;126: 106–116.

98. Greenspan D, Krystal M, Nakada S, et al. Expression of influenza virus NS2 nonstructural protein in bacteria and localization of NS2 in infected eucaryotic cells. *J Virol* 1985;54:833–843.
99. Greenspan D, Palese P, Krystal M. Two nuclear location signals in the influenza virus NS1 nonstructural protein. *J Virol* 1988;62:3020–3026.
100. Hagen M, Chung TD, Butcher JA, Krystal M. Recombinant influenza virus polymerase: Requirement of both 5′ and 3′ viral ends for endonuclease activity. *J Virol* 1994;68:1509–1515.
101. Hatada E, Fukuda R. Binding of influenza A virus NS1 protein to ds RNA in vitro. *J Gen Virol* 1992;73:3325–3329.
102. Hatada E, Saito S, Fukuda R. Mutant influenza viruses with a defective NS1 protein cannot block the activation of PKR in infected cells. *J Virol* 1999;73:2425–2433.
103. Hausmann J, Kretzschmar E, Garten W, Klenk HD. N1 neuraminidase of influenza virus A/FPV/Rostock/34 has haemadsorbing activity. *J Gen Virol* 1995;76:1719–28.
104. Hay AJ. The action of adamantanamines against influenza A viruses: Inhibition of the M2 ion channel protein. *Semin Virol* 1992;3:21–30.
105. Hay AJ, Abraham G, Skehel JJ, et al. Influenza virus messenger RNAs are incomplete transcripts of the genome RNAs. *Nucleic Acids Res* 1977;4:4197–4209.
106. Hay AJ, Lomniczi B, Bellamy AR, Skehel JJ. Transcription of the influenza virus genome. *Virology* 1977;83:337–355.
107. Hay AJ, Skehel JJ, McCauley J. Characterization of influenza virus RNA complete transcripts. *Virology* 1982;116:517–522.
108. Hay AJ, Wolstenholme AJ, Skehel JJ, Smith MH. The molecular basis of the specific anti-influenza action of amantadine. *EMBO J* 1985; 4:3021–3024.
109. Heggeness MH, Smith PR, Ulmanen I, et al. Studies on the helical nucleocapsid of influenza virus. *Virology* 1982;118:466–470.
110. Helenius A. Unpacking the incoming influenza virus. *Cell* 1992;69: 577–578.
111. Herrler G, Compans RW, Meier-Ewert H. A precursor glycoprotein in influenza C virus. *Virology* 1979;99:49–56.
112. Herrler G, Nagele A, Meier-Ewert H, et al. Isolation and structural analysis of influenza C virion glycoproteins. *Virology* 1981;113: 439–451.
113. Herrler G, Rott R, Klenk H-D, et al. The receptor-destroying enzyme of influenza C virus is neuraminate-O-acetyl esterase. *EMBO J* 1985;4:2711–2720.
114. Herz C, Stavnezer E, Krug RM, Gurney T Jr. Influenza virus, an RNA virus, synthesizes its messenger RNA in the nucleus of infected cells. *Cell* 1981;26:391–400.
115. Hicke L. Gettin' down with ubiquitin: Turning off cell-surface receptors, transporters and channels. *Trends Cell Biol* 1999;9:107–112.
116. Hirst GK. Agglutination of red cells by allantoic fluid of chick embryos infected with influenza virus. *Science* 1941;94:22–23.
117. Holsinger LJ, Lamb RA. Influenza virus M2 integral membrane protein is a homotetramer stabilized by formation of disulfide bonds. *Virology* 1991;183:32–43.
118. Holsinger LJ, Nichani D, Pinto LH, Lamb RA. Influenza A virus M_2 ion channel protein: A structure-function analysis. *J Virol* 1994;68: 1551–1563.
119. Holsinger LJ, Shaughnessy MA, Micko A, et al. Analysis of the post-translational modifications of the influenza virus M2 protein. *J Virol* 1995;69:1219–1225.
120. Honda A, Ueda K, Nagata K, Ishihama A. Identification of the RNA polymerase binding site on genome RNA of the influenza virus. *J Biochem* (Tokyo) 1987;102:1241–1249.
121. Honda A, Ueda K, Nagata K, Ishihama A. RNA polmerase of influenza virus: Role of NP on RNA chain elongation. *J Biochem* (Tokyo) 1988;104:1021–1026.
122. Hongo S, Gao P, Sugawara K, et al. Identification of a 374 amino acid protein encoded by RNA segment 6 of influenza C virus. *J Gen Virol* 1998;79:2207–2213.
123. Hongo S, Sugawara K, Muraki Y, et al. Characterization of a second protein (CM2) encoded by RNA segment 6 of influenza C virus. *J Virol* 1997;71:2786–2792.
124. Hongo S, Sugawara K, Muraki Y, et al. Influenza C virus CM2 protein is produced from a 374-amino-acid protein (P42) by signal peptidase cleavage. *J Virol* 1999;73:46–50.
125. Horisberger MA. The large P proteins of influenza A viruses are composed of one acidic and two basic polypeptides. *Virology* 1980;107: 302–305.
126. Horvath CM, Williams MA, Lamb RA. Eukaryotic coupled translation of tandem cistrons: Identification of the influenza B virus BM2 polypeptide. *EMBO J* 1990;9:2639–2647.
127. Hsu MT, Parvin JD, Gupta S, et al. Genomic RNAs of influenza viruses are held in a circular conformation in virions and in infected cells by a terminal panhandle. *Proc Natl Acad Sci U S A* 1987;84: 8140–8144.
128. Hughey PG, Compans RW, Zebedee SL, Lamb RA. Expression of the influenza A virus M2 protein is restricted to apical surfaces of polarized epithelial cells. *J Virol* 1992;66:5542–5552.
129. Hughey PG, Roberts PC, Holsinger LJ, et al. Effects of antibody to the influenza A virus M2 protein on M2 surface expression and virus assembly. *Virology* 1995;212:411–421.
130. Hull JD, Gilmore R, Lamb RA. Integration of a small integral membrane protein, M2, of influenza virus into the endoplasmic reticulum: Analysis of the internal signal-anchor domain of a protein with an ectoplasmic NH2 terminus. *J Cell Biol* 1988;106:1489–1498.
131. Inglis SC, Almond JW. An influenza virus gene encoding two different proteins. *Phil Trans R Soc Lond* 1980;288:375–381.
132. Inglis SC, Barrett T, Brown CM, Almond JW. The smallest genome RNA segment of influenza virus contains two genes that may overlap. *Proc Natl Acad Sci U S A* 1979;76:3790–3794.
133. Inglis SC, Lamb RA, Carroll AR, Mahy BWJ. Polypeptides specified by the influenza virus genome. I. Evidence for eight distinct gene products specified by fowl plague virus. *Virology* 1976;74:489–503.
134. Ito T, Couceiro JNSS, Kelm S, et al. Molecular basis for the generation in pigs of influenza A viruses with pandemic potential. *J Virol* 1998;72:7367–7373.
135. Jagus R, Anderson WF, Safer B. The regulation of initiation of mammalian protein synthesis. *Prog Nucleic Acid Res* 1981;25:127–185.
136. Jin H, Leser G, Lamb RA. The influenza virus hemagglutinin cytoplasmic tail is not essential for virus assembly or infectivity. *EMBO J* 1994;13:5504–5515.
137. Jin H, Leser GP, Zhang J, Lamb RA. Influenza virus hemagglutinin and neuraminidase cytoplasmic tails control particle shape. *EMBO J* 1997;16:1236–1247.
138. Jin H, Subbarao K, Bagai S, et al. Palmitylation of the influenza virus hemagglutinin (H3) is not essential for virus assembly or infectivity. *J Virol* 1996;70:1406–1414.
139. Jones IM, Reay PA, Philpott KL. Nuclear location of all three influenza polymerase proteins and a nuclear signal in polymerase PB2. *EMBO J* 1986;5:2371–2376.
140. Jones LV, Compans RW, Davis AR, et al. Surface expression of influenza virus neuraminidase, an amino-terminally anchored viral membrane glycoprotein, in polarized epithelial cells. *Mol Cell Biol* 1985;5:2181–2189.
141. Katze MG. The war against the interferon-induced dsRNA activated protein kinase: Can viruses win? *J Interferon Res* 1992;12:241–248.
142. Katze MG, De Corato D, Krug RM. Cellular mRNA translation is blocked at both initiation and elongation after infection by influenza virus or adenovirus. *J Virol* 1986;60:1027–1039.
143. Katze MG, Krug RM. The metabolism of RNA polymerase II transcripts in influenza virus-infected cells. *Mol Cell Biol* 1984;4: 2198–2206.
144. Katze MG, Krug RM. Translational control in influenza virus-infected cells. *Enzyme* 1990;44:265–277.
145. Kawaoka Y, Krauss S, Webster RG. Avian-to-human transmission of the PB1 gene of influenza A viruses in the 1957 and 1968 pandemics. *J Virol* 1989;63:4603–4608.
146. Kawaoka Y, Naeve CW, Webster RG. Is virulence of H5N2 influenza viruses in chickens associated with loss of carbohydrate from the hemagglutinin. *Virology* 1984;139:303–316.
147. Kawaoka Y, Webster RG. Interplay between carbohydrate in the stalk and the length of the connecting peptide determines the cleavability of influenza virus hemagglutinin. *J Virol* 1989;63:3296–3300.
148. Kawaoka Y, Webster RG. Sequence requirements for cleavage activation of influenza virus hemagglutinin expressed in mammalian cells. *Proc Natl Acad Sci U S A* 1988;85:324–328.
149. Keller W, Minvielle-Sebastia L. A comparison of mammalian and yeast pre-mRNA 3′-end processing. *Curr Opin Cell Biol* 1997;9: 329–336.

150. Kemble GW, Danieli T, White JM. Lipid-anchored influenza hemagglutinin promotes hemifusion, not complete fusion. *Cell* 1994;76:383–391.
151. Khatchikian D, Orlich M, Rott R. Increased viral pathogenicity after insertion of a 28S ribosomal RNA sequence into the hemagglutinin gene of an influenza virus. *Nature* 1989;340:156–157.
152. Kilbourne ED. *Influenza.* New York: Plenum, 1987.
153. Kilbourne ED. Influenza virus genetics. *Prog Med Virol* 1963;5:79–126.
154. Kilbourne ED, Laver WG, Schulman JL, Webster RG. Antiviral activity of antiserum specific for an influenza virus neuraminidase. *J Virol* 1968;2:281–288.
155. Kilbourne ED, Schulman JL, Schild GC, et al. Correlated studies of a recombinant influenza-virus vaccine. I. Derivation and characterization of virus and vaccine. *J Infect Dis* 1971;124:449–462.
156. Klenk H-D, Compans RW, Choppin WP. An electron microscopic study of the presence or absence of neuraminic acid in enveloped viruses. *Virology* 1970;42:1158–1162.
157. Klenk H-D, Garten W. Host cell proteases controlling virus pathogenicity. *Trends Microbiol* 1994;2:39–43.
158. Klenk H-D, Rott R, Orlich M, Blodorn J. Activation of influenza A viruses by trypsin treatment. *Virology* 1975;68:426–439.
159. Klumpp K, Ruigrok RWH, Baudin F. Roles of the influenza virus polymerase and nucleoprotein in forming a functional RNP structure. *EMBO J* 1997;16:1248–1257.
160. Kobasa D, Rodgers ME, Wells K, Kawaoka Y. Neuraminidase hemadsorption activity, conserved in avian influenza A viruses, does not influence viral replication in ducks. *J Virol* 1997;71:6706–6713.
161. Kovacs FA, Denny JK, Song Z, et al. Helix tilt of the M2 transmembrane peptide from influenza A virus: An intrinsic property. *J Mol Biol* 2000;295:117–125.
162. Krainer AR, Mayeda A, Kozak D, Binns G. Functional expression of cloned human splicing factor SF2: Homology to RNA-binding proteins, U1-70K, and Drosophila splicing regulators. *Cell* 1991;66:383–398.
163. Krug RM, Alonso-Caplen FV, Julkunen I, Katze MG. Expression and replication of the influenza virus genome. In: Krug RM, ed. *The influenza viruses.* New York: Plenum, 1989:89–152.
164. Krug RM, Broni B, Bouloy M. Are the 5′ ends of influenza viral mRNAs synthesized in vivo donated by host mRNAs. *Cell* 1979;18:329–334.
165. Krug RM, Broni BA, LaFiandra AJ, et al. Priming and inhibitory activities of RNAs for the influenza viral transcriptase do not require base pairing with the virion template RNA. *Proc Natl Acad Sci U S A* 1980;77:5874–5878.
166. Krug RM, Etkind PR. Cytoplasmic and nuclear virus-specific proteins in influenza virus-infected MDCK cells. *Virology* 1973;56:334–348.
167. Krug RM, Morgan MA, Shatkin AJ. Influenza viral mRNA contains internal N6-methyladenosine and 5′-terminal 7-methylguanosine in cap structures. *J Virol* 1976;20:45–53.
168. Krug RM, Soeiro R. Studies on the intranuclear localization of influenza virus-specific proteins. *Virology* 1975;64:378–387.
169. Krystal M, Elliott RM, Benz EW Jr, et al. Evolution of influenza A and B viruses: Conservation of structural features in the hemagglutinin genes. *Proc Natl Acad Sci U S A* 1982;79:4800–4804.
170. Krystal M, Young JF, Palese P, et al. Sequential mutations in hemagglutinins of influenza B virus isolates: Definition of antigenic domains. *Proc Natl Acad Sci U S A* 1983;80:4527–4531.
171. Lamb RA. Genes and proteins of the influenza viruses, In: Krug RM, ed. *The influenza viruses.* New York: Plenum, 1989:1–87.
172. Lamb RA, Choppin PW. The gene structure and replication of influenza virus. *Annu Rev Biochem* 1983;52:467–506.
173. Lamb RA, Choppin PW. Identification of a second protein (M2) encoded by RNA segment 7 of influenza virus. *Virology* 1981;112:729–737.
174. Lamb RA, Choppin PW. Segment 8 of the influenza virus genome is unique in coding for two polypeptides. *Proc Natl Acad Sci U S A* 1979;76:4908–4912.
175. Lamb RA, Choppin PW. Synthesis of influenza virus polypeptides in cells resistant to alpha-amanitin: Evidence for the involvement of cellular RNA polymerase II in virus replication. *J Virol* 1977;23:816–819.
176. Lamb RA, Choppin PW. Synthesis of influenza virus proteins in infected cells: Translation of viral polypeptides, including three P polypeptides, from RNA produced by primary transcription. *Virology* 1976;74:504–519.
177. Lamb RA, Choppin PW, Chanock RM, Lai C-J. Mapping of the two overlapping genes for polypeptides NS1 and NS2 on RNA segment 8 of influenza virus genome. *Proc Natl Acad Sci U S A* 1980;77:1857–1861.
178. Lamb RA, Etkind PR, Choppin PW. Evidence for a ninth influenza viral polypeptide. *Virology* 1978;91:60–78.
179. Lamb RA, Holsinger LJ, Pinto LH. The influenza A virus M_2 ion channel protein and its role in the influenza virus life cycle, In: Wimmer E, ed. *Receptor-mediated virus entry into cells.* Cold Spring Harbor, NY: Cold Spring Harbor Press, 1994:303–321.
180. Lamb RA, Lai C-J. Conservation of the influenza virus membrane protein (M_1) amino acid sequence and an open reading frame of RNA segment 7 encoding a second protein (M_2) in H1N1 and H3N2 strains. *Virology* 1981;112:746–751.
181. Lamb RA, Lai C-J. Sequence of interrupted and uninterrupted mRNAs and cloned DNA coding for the two overlapping nonstructural proteins of influenza virus. *Cell* 1980;21:475–485.
182. Lamb RA, Lai C-J. Spliced and unspliced messenger RNAs synthesized from cloned influenza virus M DNA in an SV40 vector: Expression of the influenza virus membrane protein (M1). *Virology* 1982;123:237–256.
183. Lamb RA, Lai C-J, Choppin PW. Sequences of mRNAs derived from genome RNA segment 7 of influenza virus: Colinear and interrupted mRNAs code for overlapping proteins. *Proc Natl Acad Sci U S A* 1981;78:4170–4174.
184. Lamb RA, Pinto LH. Do Vpu and Vpr of human immunodeficiency virus type 1 and NB of influenza B virus have ion channel activities in the viral life cycles. *Virology* 1997;229:1–11.
185. Lamb RA, Zebedee SL, Richardson CD. Influenza virus M2 protein is an integral membrane protein expressed on the infected-cell surface. *Cell* 1985;40:627–633.
186. Laver WG, Colman PM, Webster RG, et al. Influenza virus neuraminidase with hemagglutinin activity. *Virology* 1984;137:314–323.
187. Lazarowitz SG, Choppin PW. Enhancement of the infectivity of influenza A and B viruses by proteolytic cleavage of the hemagglutinin polypeptide. *Virology* 1975;68:440–454.
188. Lazarowitz SG, Compans RW, Choppin PW. Influenza virus structural and nonstructural proteins in infected cells and their plasma membranes. *Virology* 1971;46:830–843.
189. Lazarowitz SG, Goldberg AR, Choppin PW. Proteolytic cleavage by plasmin of the HA polypeptide of influenza virus: Host cell activation of serum plasminogen. *Virology* 1973;56:172–180.
190. Leahy MB, Dessens JT, Weber F, et al. The fourth genus in the Orthomyxoviridae: sequence analyses of two Thogoto virus polymerase proteins and comparison with influenza viruses. *Virus Res* 1997;50:215–224.
191. Lee TG, Tomita J, Hovanessian AG, Katze G. Characterization and regulation of the 58,000-dalton cellular inhibitor of the interferon-induced, dsRNA-activated protein kinase. *J Biol Chem* 1992;267:14238–14243.
192. Lee TG, Tomita J, Hovanessian AG, Katze MG. Purification and partial characterization of a cellular inhibitor of the interferon-induced protein kinase of Mr 68,000 from influenza virus-infected cells. *Proc Natl Acad Sci U S A* 1990;87:6208–6212.
193. Lentz MR, Webster RG, Air GM. Site-directed mutation of the active site of influenza neuraminidase and implications for the catalytic mechanism. *Biochemistry* 1987;26:5321–5358.
194. Li M-L, Ramirez BC, Krug RM. RNA-dependent activation of primer RNA production by influenza virus polymerase: Different regions of the same protein subunit constitute the two required RNA-binding sites. *EMBO J* 1998;17:5844–5852.
194a. Li M-L, Rao P, Krug RM. The active sites of the influenza cap-dependent endonuclease are on different polymerase subunits. *EMBO J* 2001; in press.
195. Li S, Polonis V, Isobe H, et al. Chimeric influenza virus induces neutralizing antibodies and cytotoxic T cells against human immunodeficiency virus type 1. *J Virol* 1993;67:6659–6666.
196. Li S, Schulman J, Itamura S, Palese P. Glycosylation of neuraminidase determines the neurovirulence of influenza A/WSN/33 virus. *J Virol* 1993;67:6667–6673.
197. Li S, Schulman JL, Moran T, et al. Influenza A virus transfectants with chimeric hemagglutinin containing epitopes from different subtypes. *J Virol* 1992;66:399–404.
198. Li Y, Yamakita Y, Krug RM. Regulation of a nuclear export signal by

an adjacent inhibitory sequence: The effector domain of the influenza virus NS1 protein. *Proc Natl Acad Sci U S A* 1998;95:4864–4869.
199. Lin BC, Lai CJ. The influenza virus nucleoprotein synthesized from cloned DNA in a simian virus 40 vector is detected in the nucleus. *J Virol* 1983;45:434–438.
200. Liu J, Lynch PA, Chien CY, et al. Crystal structure of the unique RNA-binding domain of the influenza virus NS1 protein. *Nat Struct Biol* 1997;4:896–899.
201. Lu Y, Qian X-Y, Krug RM. The influenza virus NS1 protein: A novel inhibitor of pre-mRNA splicing. *Genes Dev* 1994;8:1817–1828.
202. Lu Y, Wambach M, Katze MG, Krug RM. Binding of the influenza virus NS1 protein to double-stranded RNA inhibits the activation of the protein kinase that phosphorylates the eIF-2 translation initiation factor. *Virology* 1995;214:222–228.
203. Luo G, Luytjes W, Enami M, Palese P. The polyadenylation signal of influenza virus RNA involves a stretch of uridines followed by the RNA duplex of the panhandle structure. *J Virol* 1991;65:2861–2867.
204. Luytjes W, Krystal M, Enami M, et al. Amplification, expression and packaging of a foreign gene by influenza virus. *Cell* 1989;58: 1107–1113.
205. Mahy BWJ, Hastie ND, Armstrong SJ. Inhibition of influenza virus replication by α-amantinin: Mode of action. *Proc Natl Acad Sci U S A* 1972;69:1421–1424.
206. Marcotrigiano J, Gingras AC, Sonenberg N, Burley SK. Cocrystal structure of the messenger RNA 5′ cap-binding protein (eIF4E) bound to 7-methyl-GDP. *Cell* 1997;89:951–961.
207. Marsh M, Helenius A. Virus entry into animal cells. *Adv Virus Res* 1989;36:107–151.
208. Martin K, Helenius A. Nuclear transport of influenza virus ribonucleoproteins: The viral matrix protein (M1) promotes export and inhibits import. *Cell* 1991;67:117–130.
209. Martin K, Helenius A. Transport of incoming influenza virus nucleocapsids into the nucleus. *J Virol* 1991;65:232–244.
210. Mathews MC. Viral evasion of cellular defense mechanisms: Regulation of the protein kinase DAI by RNA effectors. *Semin Virol* 1993; 4:247–257.
211. Matlin KS, Reggio H, Helenius A, Simons K. The entry of enveloped viruses into an epithelial cell line. *Prog Clin Biol Res* 1982;91: 599–611.
212. Matsuo H, Li H, McGuire AM, et al. Structure of translation factor eIF4E bound to m7GDP and interaction with 4E-binding protein. *Nat Struct Biol* 1997;4:717–724.
213. McClelland L, Hare R. The adsorption of influenza virus by red cells and a new in vitro method of measuring antibodies for influenza virus. *Can J Public Health* 1941;32:530–538.
214. McGeoch D, Fellner P, Newton C. Influenza virus genome consists of eight distinct RNA species. *Proc Natl Acad Sci U S A* 1976;73: 3045–3049.
215. Medcalf L, Poole E, Elton D, Digard P. Temperature-sensitive lesions in two influenza A viruses defective for replicative transcription disrupt RNA binding by the nucleoprotein. *J Virol* 1999;73:7349–7356.
216. Melkonian KA, Ostermeyer AG, Chen JZ, et al. Role of lipid modifications in targeting proteins to detergent-resistant membrane rafts. Many raft proteins are acylated, while few are prenylated. *J Biol Chem* 1999;274:3910–3917.
217. Mitnaul LJ, Castrucci MR, Murti KG, Kawaoka Y. The cytoplasmic tail of influenza A virus neuraminidase (NA) affects NA incorporation into virions, virion morphology, and virulence in mice but is not essential for virus replication. *J Virol* 1996;70:873–879.
218. Morse MA, Marriott AC, Nuttall PA. The glycoprotein of Thogoto virus (a tick-borne orthomyxo-like virus) is related to the baculovirus glycoprotein GP64. *Virology* 1992;186:640–646.
219. Mould JA, Li H-C, Dudlak CS, et al. Mechanism for proton conduction of the M(2) ion channel of influenza A virus. *J Biol Chem* 2000;275:8592–8599.
220. Murti KG, Bean WJ Jr, Webster RG. Helical ribonucleoproteins of influenza virus: An electron microscope analysis. *Virology* 1980;104: 224–229.
221. Murti KG, Brown PS, Bean WJ Jr, Webster RG. Composition of the helical internal components of influenza virus as revealed by immunogold labeling/electron microscopy. *Virology* 1992;186: 294–299.
222. Muster T, Subbarao EK, Enami M, et al. An influenza A virus containing influenza B virus 5′ and 3′ noncoding regions on the neuraminidase gene is attenuated in mice. *Proc Natl Acad Sci U S A* 1991; 88:5177–5181.
223. Naeve CW, Williams D. Fatty acids on the A/Japan/305/57 influenza virus hemagglutinin have a role in membrane fusion. *EMBO J* 1990; 9:3857–3866.
224. Naim HY, Roth MG. Basis for selective incorporation of glycoproteins into the influenza virus envelope. *J Virol* 1993;67:4831–4841.
225. Nakada S, Graves PN, Desselberger U, et al. Influenza C virus RNA 7 codes for a nonstructural protein. *J Virol* 1985;56:221–226.
226. Nakada S, Graves PN, Palese P. The influenza C virus NS gene: Evidence for a spliced mRNA and a second NS gene product (NS2 protein). *Virus Res* 1986;4:263–273.
227. Narayan P, Ayers DF, Rottman FM, et al. Unequal distribution of N6-methyladenosine in influenza virus mRNAs. *Mol Cell Biol* 1987;7: 1572–1575.
228. Nemeroff ME, Barabino SM, Li Y, et al. Influenza virus NS1 protein interacts with the cellular 30kDa subunit of CPSF and inhibits 3′ end formation of cellular pre-mRNAs. *Mol Cell* 1998;1:991–1000.
229. Nemeroff ME, Qian X-Y, Krug RM. The influenza virus NS1 protein forms multimers in vitro and in vivo. *Virology* 1995;212:422–428.
230. Neumann G, Castrucci MR, Kawaoka Y. Nuclear import and export of influenza virus nucleoprotein. *J Virol* 1997;71:9690–9700.
231. Neumann G, Kawaoka Y. Genetic engineering of influenza and other negative-strand RNA viruses containing segmented genomes. *Adv Virus Res* 1999;53:265–300.
232. Neumann G, Watanabe T, Ito H, et al. Generation of influenza A viruses entirely from cloned cDNAs. *Proc Natl Acad Sci U S A* 1999; 96:9345–9350.
233. Nobusawa E, Aoyama T, Kato H, et al. Comparison of complete amino acid sequences and receptor-binding properties among 13 serotypes of hemagglutinin of influenza A viruses. *Virology* 1991;182:475–485.
234. Normark S, Bergstrom S, Edlund T, et al. Overlapping genes. *Annu Rev Genet* 1983;17:499–525.
235. Norton GP, Tanaka T, Tobita K, et al. Infectious influenza A and B virus variants with long carboxyl terminal deletions in the NS1 polypeptides. *Virology* 1987;156:204–213.
236. O'Neill RE, Talon J, Palese P. The influenza virus NEP (NS2 protein) mediates the nuclear export of viral ribonucleoproteins. *EMBO J* 1998;17:288–296.
237. Odagiri T, Tashiro M. Segment-specific noncoding sequences of the influenza virus genome RNA are involved in the specific competition between defective interfering RNA and its progenitor RNA segment at the virion assembly step. *J Virol* 1997;71:2138–2145.
238. Ohuchi M, Cramer A, Vey M, et al. Rescue of vector-expressed fowl plague virus hemagglutinin in biologically active form by acidotropic agents and coexpressed M2 protein. *J Virol* 1994;68:920–926.
239. Ohuchi M, Ohuchi R, Mifune K. Demonstration of hemolytic and fusion activities of influenza C virus. *J Virol* 1982;42:1076–1079.
240. Oldstone MBA, Levine AJ. Virology in the next millenium. *Cell* 2000;100:139–142.
241. Orlich M, Gottwald H, Rott R. Nonhomologous recombination between the HA gene and the NP gene of an influenza virus. *Virology* 1994;204:462–465.
242. Orlich M, Khatchikian D, Teigler A, Rott R. Structural variation occuring in the hemagglutinin of influenza virus A/turkey/Oregon/71 during adaptation to different cell types. *Virology* 1990;176: 531–538.
243. Oxford JS, Galbraith A. Antiviral activity of amantadine: A review of laboratory and clinical data. *Pharmacol Ther* 1980;11:181–262.
244. Palese P. The genes of influenza virus. *Cell* 1977;10:1–10.
245. Palese P. Genetic engineering of infectious negative-strand RNA viruses. *Trends Microbiol* 1995;3:123–125.
246. Palese P, Schulman JL. Differences in RNA patterns of influenza A viruses. *J Virol* 1976;17:876–884.
247. Palese P, Schulman JL. Mapping of the influenza virus genome: Identification of the hemagglutinin and the neuraminidase genes. *Proc Natl Acad Sci U S A* 1976;73:2142–2146.
248. Palese P, Tobita K, Ueda M, Compans RW. Characterization of temperature sensitive influenza virus mutants defective in neuraminidase. *Virology* 1974;61:397–410.
249. Palese P, Zheng H, Engelhardt OG, et al. Negative-strand RNA viruses: Genetic engineering and applications. *Proc Natl Acad Sci U S A* 1996;93:11354–11358.
250. Park EK, Castrucci MR, Portner A, Kawaoka Y. The M2 ectodomain

is important for its incorporation into influenza A virions. *J Virol* 1998;72:2449–2455.
251. Park YW, Katze MG. Translational control by influenza virus: Identification of cis-acting sequences and trans-acting factors which may regulate selective viral mRNA translation. *J Biol Chem* 1995;270: 28433–28439.
252. Park YW, Wilusz J, Katze MG. Regulation of eukaryotic protein synthesis: Selective influenza viral mRNA translation is mediated by the cellular RNA-binding protein GRSF-1. *Proc Natl Acad Sci U S A* 1999;96:6694–6699.
253. Parvin JD, Moscona A, Pan WT, et al. Measurement of the mutation rates of animal viruses: Influenza A virus and poliovirus type 1. *J Virol* 1986;59:377–383.
254. Parvin JD, Palese P, Honda A, et al. Promoter analysis of influenza virus RNA polymerase. *J Virol* 1989;63:5142–5152.
255. Patnaik A, Chau V, Wills JW. Ubiquitin is part of the retrovirus budding machinery. *Proc Natl Acad Sci U S A* 2000;97:13069–13074.
256. Pekosz A, He B, Lamb RA. Reverse genetics of negative-strand RNA viruses: Closing the circle. *Proc Natl Acad Sci U S A* 1999;96: 8804–8806.
257. Pekosz A, Lamb RA. Cell surface expression of biologically active influenza C virus HEF glycoprotein expressed from cDNA. *J Virol* 1999;73:8808–8812.
258. Pekosz A, Lamb RA. The CM2 protein of influenza C virus is an oligomeric integral membrane glycoprotein structurally analogous to influenza A virus M2 and influenza B virus NB proteins. *Virology* 1997;237:439–51.
259. Pekosz A, Lamb RA. Influenza C virus CM2 integral membrane glycoprotein is produced from a polypeptide precursor by cleavage of an internal signal sequence. *Proc Natl Acad Sci U S A* 1998;95:13233–13238.
260. Pekosz A, Lamb RA. Membrane insertion, processing and degradation of the p42, p31 and CM2 proteins encoded by RNA segment six of influenza C virus. *J Virol* 2000;74:10480–10488.
261. Percy N, Barclay WS, Garcia-Sastre A, Palese P. Expression of a foreign protein by influenza A virus. *J Virol* 1994;68:4486–4492.
262. Pinto LH, Dieckmann GR, Gandhi CS, et al. A functionally defined model for the M2 proton channel of influenza A virus suggests a mechanism for its ion selectivity. *Proc Natl Acad Sci U S A* 1997; 94:11301–11306.
263. Pinto LH, Holsinger LJ, Lamb RA. Influenza virus M2 protein has ion channel activity. *Cell* 1992;69:517–528.
264. Pleschka S, Jaskunas SR, Engelhardt OG, et al. A plasmid-based reverse genetics system for influenza A virus. *J Virol* 1996;70: 4188–4192.
265. Plotch SJ, Bouloy M, Krug RM. Transfer of 5′-terminal cap of globin mRNA to influenza viral complementary RNA during transcription in vitro. *Proc Natl Acad Sci U S A* 1979;76:1618–1622.
266. Plotch SJ, Bouloy M, Ulmanen I, Krug RM. A unique cap(m7Gpp-pXm)-dependent influenza virion endonuclease cleaves capped RNAs to generate the primers that initiate viral RNA transcription. *Cell* 1981;23:847–858.
267. Plotch SJ, Krug RM. Influenza virion transcriptase: Synthesis *in vitro* of large, polyadenylic acid-containing complementary RNA. *J Virol* 1977;21:24–34.
268. Plotch SJ, Krug RM. Segments of influenza virus complementary RNA synthesized in vitro. *J Virol* 1978;25:579–586.
269. Poch O, Sauvaget I, Delarue M, Tordo N. Identification of four conserved motifs among the RNA-dependent polymerase encoding elements. *EMBO J* 1989;8:3867–3874.
270. Pons MW. Isolation of influenza virus ribonucleoprotein from infected cells. Demonstration of the presence of negative-stranded RNA in viral RNP. *Virology* 1971;46:149–160.
271. Pons MW. A re-examination of influenza single-and double-stranded RNAs by gel electrophoresis. *Virology* 1976;69:789–792.
272. Pons MW, Schulze IT, Hirst GK, Hauser R. Isolation and characterization of the ribonucleoprotein of influenza virus. *Virology* 1969;39: 250–259.
273. Poon LL, Pritlove DC, Fodor EE, Brownlee GG. Direct evidence that the poly(A) tail of influenza virus mRNA is synthesized by reiterative copying of a U tract in the virion RNA template. *J Virol* 1999;73: 3473–3476.
274. Porter AG, Barber C, Carey NH, et al. Complete nucleotide sequence of an influenza virus haemagglutinin gene from cloned DNA. *Nature* 1979;282:471–477.
275. Qian X-Y, Alonso-Caplen F, Krug RM. Two functional domains of the influenza virus NS1 protein are required for regulation of nuclear export of mRNA. *J Virol* 1994;68:2433–2441.
276. Qian XY, Chien CY, Lu Y, et al. An amino-terminal polypeptide fragment of the influenza virus NS1 protein possesses specific RNA-binding activity and largely helical backbone structure. *RNA* 1995;1: 948–956.
277. Qiao X, Qiao J, Mindich L. Stoichiometric packaging of the three genomic segments of double-stranded RNA bacteriophage ϕ6. *Proc Natl Acad Sci U S A* 1997;94:4074–4079.
278. Qiu Y, Krug RM. The influenza virus NS1 protein is a poly A-binding protein that inhibits the nuclear export of mRNAs containing poly A. *J Virol* 1994;68:2425–2432.
279. Qiu Y, Nemeroff M, Krug RM. The influenza virus NS1 protein binds to a specific region in human U6 snRNA and inhibits U6-U2 and U6-U4 snRNA interactions during splicing. *RNA* 1995;1:304–316.
280. Restifo NP, Surman DR, Zheng H, et al. Transfectant influenza A viruses are effective recombinant immunogens in the treatment of experimental cancer. *Virology* 1998;249:89–97.
281. Rey O, Nayak DP. Nuclear retention of M1 protein in a temperature-sensitive mutant of influenza (A/WSN/33) virus does not affect nuclear export of viral ribonucleoproteins. *J Virol* 1992;66: 5815–5824.
282. Richardson JC, Akkina RK. NS2 protein of influenza virus is found in purified virus and phosphorylated in infected cells. *Arch Virol* 1991; 116:69–80.
283. Ritchey MB, Palese P, Kilbourne ED. RNAs of influenza A, B, and C viruses. *J Virol* 1976;18:738–744.
284. Ritchey MB, Palese P, Schulman JL. Mapping of the influenza virus genome. III. Identification of genes coding for nucleoprotein, membrane protein, and nonstructural protein. *J Virol* 1976;20:307–313.
285. Roberts PC, Lamb RA, Compans RW. The M1 and M2 proteins of influenza A virus are important determinants in filamentous particle formation. *Virology* 1998;240:127–137.
286. Robertson JS, Schubert M, Lazzarini RA. Polyadenylation sites for influenza mRNA. *J Virol* 1981;38:157–163.
287. Rodriguez-Boulan E, Sabatini DD. Asymmetric budding of viruses in epithelial monolayers: A model system for study of epithelial polarity. *Proc Natl Acad Sci U S A* 1978;75:5071–5075.
288. Rogers GN, Paulson JC, Daniels RS, et al. Single amino acid substitutions in influenza haemagglutinin change receptor binding specificity. *Nature* 1983;304:76–78.
289. Rosenthal PB, Zhang X, Formanowski F, et al. Structure of the haemagglutinin-esterase-fusion glycoprotein of influenza C virus. *Nature* 1998;396:92–96.
290. Roth MG, Fitzpatrick JP, Compans RW. Polarity of influenza and vesicular stomatitis virus maturation MDCK cells: Lack of a requirement for glycosylation of viral glycoproteins. *Proc Natl Acad Sci U S A* 1979;76:6430–6434.
291. Roth MG, Gundersen D, Patil N, Rodriguez-Boulan E. The large external domain is sufficient for the correct sorting of secreted or chimeric influenza virus hemagglutinins in polarized monkey kidney cells. *J Cell Biol* 1987;104:769–782.
292. Ruigrok RWH, Hirst EMA, Hay AJ. The specific inhibition of influenza A virus maturation by amantadine: An electron microscopic examination. *J Gen Virol* 1991;72:191–194.
293. Ruigrok RWH, Martin SR, Wharton SA, et al. Conformational changes in the hemagglutinin of influenza virus which accompany heat-induced fusion of virus with liposomes. *Virology* 1986;155: 484–497.
294. Ruigrok RWH, Wrigley NG, Calder LJ, et al. Electron microscopy of the low pH structure of influenza virus hemagglutinin. *EMBO J* 1986;5:4149.
295. Ryan KW, Mackow ER, Chanock RM, Lai C-J. Functional expression of influenza A viral nucleoprotein in cells transformed with cloned DNA. *Virology* 1986;154:144–154.
296. Safer B. 2B or not 2B: Regulation of the catalytic utilization of eIF-2. *Cell* 1983;33:7–8.
297. Sakaguchi T, Leser GP, Lamb RA. The ion channel activity of the influenza virus M2 protein affects transport through the Golgi apparatus. *J Cell Biol* 1996;133:733–747.
298. Sakaguchi T, Tu Q, Pinto LH, Lamb RA. The active oligomeric state of the minimalistic influenza virus M2 ion channel is a tetramer. *Proc Natl Acad Sci U S A* 1997;94:5000–5004.

299. Sato SB, Kawasaki K, Ohnishi S-I. Haemolytic activity of influenza virus haemagglutinin glycoproteins activated in mildly acidic environments. *Proc Natl Acad Sci U S A* 1983;80:3153–3157.
300. Scheiffele P, Rietveld A, Wilk T, Simons K. Influenza viruses select ordered lipid domains during budding from the plasma membrane. *J Biol Chem* 1999;274:2038–2044.
301. Schmidt MFG. Acylation of viral spike glycoproteins: A feature of enveloped RNA viruses. *Virology* 1982;116:327–338.
302. Scholtissek C, Harms E, Rohde W, et al. Correlation between RNA fragments of fowl plague virus and their corresponding gene functions. *Virology* 1976;74:332–344.
303. Schulman JL, Palese P. Virulence factors of influenza A viruses: WSN virus neuraminidase required for plaque production in MDBK cells. *J Virol* 1977;24:170–176.
304. Sha B, Luo M. Structure of a bifunctional membrane-RNA binding protein, influenza virus matrix protein M1. *Nat Struct Biol* 1997;4: 239–244.
305. Shapiro GI, Gurney T Jr, Krug RM. Influenza virus gene expression: Control mechanisms at early and late times of infection and nuclear-cytoplasmic transport of virus-specific RNAs. *J Virol* 1987;61: 764–773.
306. Shapiro GI, Krug RM. Influenza virus RNA replication in vitro: Synthesis of viral template RNAs and virion RNAs in the absence of an added primer. *J Virol* 1988;62:2285–2290.
307. Sharp PA. Split genes and RNA splicing. *Cell* 1994;77:805–815.
308. Shaw MW, Choppin PW, Lamb RA. A previously unrecognized influenza B virus glycoprotein from a bicistronic mRNA that also encodes the viral neuraminidase. *Proc Natl Acad Sci U S A* 1983;80: 4879–4883.
309. Shaw MW, Lamb RA, Erickson BW, et al. Complete nucleotide sequence of the neuraminidase gene of influenza B virus. *Proc Natl Acad Sci U S A* 1982;79:6817–6821.
310. Shih SR, Krug RM. Novel exploitation of a nuclear function by influenza virus: The cellular SF2/ASF splicing factor controls the amount of the essential viral M2 ion channel protein in infected cells. *EMBO J* 1996;15:5415–5427.
311. Shih SR, Krug RM. Surprising function of the three influenza viral polymerase proteins: Selective protection of viral mRNAs against the cap-snatching reaction catalyzed by the same polymerase proteins. *Virology* 1996;226:430–435.
312. Shih SR, Nemeroff ME, Krug RM. The choice of alternative 5′ splice sites in influenza virus M1 mRNA is regulated by the viral polymerase complex. *Proc Natl Acad Sci U S A* 1995;92:6324–6328.
313. Shimizu K, Iguchi A, Gomyou R, Ono Y. Influenza virus inhibits cleavage of the HSP70 pre-mRNAs at the polyadenylation site. *Virology* 1999;254:213–219.
314. Simons K, Ikonen E. Functional rafts in cell membranes. *Nature* 1997;387:569–572.
315. Singer SJ, Nicolson GL. The fluid mosaic model of the structure of cell membranes. *Science* 1972;175:720–731.
316. Skehel JJ. Early polypeptide synthesis in influenza virus-infected cells. *Virology* 1973;56:394–399.
317. Skehel JJ. Polypeptide synthesis in influenza virus-infected cells. *Virology* 1972;49:23–36.
318. Skehel JJ, Bayley PM, Brown EB, et al. Changes in the conformation of influenza virus hemagglutinin at the pH optimum of virus-mediated membrane fusion. *Proc Natl Acad Sci U S A* 1982;79:968–972.
319. Skehel JJ, Bizebard T, Bullough PA, et al. Membrane fusion by influenza hemagglutinin. *Cold Spring Harb Symp Quant Biol* 1995; 60:573–580.
320. Skehel JJ, Hay AJ, Armstrong JA. On the mechanism of inhibition of influenza virus replication by amantadine hydrochloride. *J Gen Virol* 1978;38:97–110.
321. Skehel JJ, Wiley DC. Receptor binding and membrane fusion in virus entry: The influenza hemagglutinin. *Annu Rev Biochem* 2000;69: 531–569.
322. Smith FL, Palese P. Variation in influenza virus genes: Epidemiology, pathogenic, and evolutionary consequences. In: Krug RM, ed. *The influenza viruses.* New York: Plenum, 1989.
323. Smith GL, Hay AJ. Replication of the influenza virus genome. *Virology* 1982;118:96–108.
324. Smith GL, Levin JZ, Palese P, Moss B. Synthesis and cellular location of the ten influenza polypeptides individually expressed by recombinant vaccinia viruses. *Virology* 1987;160:336–345.
325. Spooner LLR, Barry RD. Participation of DNA-dependent RNA polymerase 2 in replication of influenza viruses. *Nature* 1977;268: 650–652.
326. Staczek J, Gilleland HE Jr, Gilleland LB, et al. A chimeric influenza virus expressing an epitope of outer membrane protein F of Pseudomonas aeruginosa affords protection against challenge with P. aeruginosa in a murine model of chronic pulmonary infection. *Infect Immun* 1998;66:3990–3994.
327. Stark GR, Kerr IM, Williams BR, et al. How cells respond to interferons. *Annu Rev Biochem* 1998;67:227–264.
328. Stegmann T, Morselt HWM, Scholma J, Wilschut J. Fusion of influenza virus in an intracellular acidic compartment measured by fluorescence dequenching. *Biochim Biophys Acta* 1987;904:165–170.
329. Steinhauer DA. Role of hemagglutinin cleavage for the pathogenicity of influenza virus. *Virology* 1999;258:1–20.
330. Stieneke-Grober A, Vey M, Angliker H, et al. Influenza virus hemagglutinin with multibasic cleavage site is activated by furin, a subtilisin-like endoprotease. *EMBO J* 1992;11:2407–2414.
331. Suarez DL, Perdue ML. Multiple alignment comparison of the nonstructural genes of influenza A viruses. *Virus Res* 1998;54:59–69.
332. Sugrue RJ, Bahadur G, Zambon MC, et al. Specific structural alteration of the influenza haemagglutinin by amantadine. *EMBO J* 1990;9:3469–3476.
333. Sugrue RJ, Belshe RB, Hay AJ. Palmitoylation of the influenza A virus M2 protein. *Virology* 1990;179:51–56.
334. Sugrue RJ, Hay AJ. Structural characteristics of the M2 protein of the influenza A viruses: Evidence that it forms a tetrameric channel. *Virology* 1991;180:617–624.
335. Sunstrom NA, Premkumar LS, Premkumar A, et al. Ion channels formed by NB, an influenza B virus protein. *J Membr Biol* 1996;150: 127–132.
336. Tai CY, Escarpe PA, Sidwell RW, et al. Characterization of human influenza virus variants selected in vitro in the presence of the neuraminidase inhibitor GS 4071. *Antimicrob Agents Chemother* 1998; 42:3234–3241.
337. Taka Y, Hongo S, Muraki Y, et al. Phosphorylation of influenza C virus CM2 protein. *Virus Res* 1998;58:65–72.
338. Takada A, Kuboki N, Okazaki K, et al. A virulent avian influenza virus as a vaccine strain against a potential human pandemic. *J Virol* 1999;73:8303–8307.
339. Takeuchi K, Lamb RA. Influenza virus M_2 protein ion channel activity stabilizes the native form of fowl plague virus hemagglutinin during intracellular transport. *J Virol* 1994;68:911–919.
340. Thomas JM, Stevens MP, Percy N, Barclay WS. Phosphorylation of the M2 protein of influenza A virus is not essential for virus viability. *Virology* 1998;252:54–64.
341. Tiley LS, Hagen M, Matthews JT, Krystal M. Sequence-specific binding of the influenza virus RNA polymerase to sequences located at the 5′ ends of the viral RNAs. *J Virol* 1994;68:5108–5116.
342. Ulmanen I, Broni BA, Krug RM. Influenza virus temperature-sensitive cap(m7GpppNm)-dependent endonuclease. *J Virol* 1983;45:27–35.
343. Ulmanen I, Broni BA, Krug RM. Role of two of the influenza virus core P proteins in recognizing cap 1 structures (m7GpppNm) on RNAs and in initiating viral RNA transcription. *Proc Natl Acad Sci U S A* 1981;78:7355–7359.
344. Varghese JN, Colman PM, van Donkelaar A, et al. Structural evidence for a second sialic acid binding site in avian influenza virus neuraminidases. *Proc Natl Acad Sci U S A* 1997;94:11808–11812.
345. Varghese JN, Laver WG, Colman PM. Structure of the influenza virus glycoprotein antigen neuraminidase at 2.9 Å resolution. *Nature* 1983; 303:35–40.
346. Veit M, Klenk H-D, Kendal A, Rott R. The M2 protein of influenza A virus is acylated. *Virology* 1991;184:227–234.
347. Verhoeyen M, Fang R, Min Jou W, et al. Antigenic drift between the haemagglutinin of the Hong Kong influenza strains A/Aichi/2/68 and A/Victoria/3/75. *Nature* 1980;286:771–776.
348. Vlasak R, Krystal M, Nacht M, Palese P. The influenza C virus glycoprotein (HE) exhibits receptor-binding (hemagglutinin) and receptor-destroying (esterase) activities. *Virology* 1987;160:419–425.
349. von Itzstein M, Wu WY, Kok GB, et al. Rational design of potent sialidase-based inhibitors of influenza virus replication. *Nature* 1993; 363:418–423.
350. Wahle E, Keller W. The biochemistry of polyadenylation. *Trends Biochem Sci* 1996;21:247–250.
351. Wakefield L, Brownlee GG. RNA-binding properties of influenza A virus matrix protein M1. *Nucleic Acids Res* 1989;17:8569–8580.

352. Wang C, Lamb RA, Pinto LH. Activation of the M2 ion channel of influenza virus: A role for the transmembrane domain histidine residue. *Biophys J* 1995;69:1363–1371.
353. Wang C, Lamb RA, Pinto LH. Direct measurement of the influenza A virus M2 protein ion channel activity in mammalian cells. *Virology* 1994;205:133–140.
354. Wang C, Takeuchi K, Pinto LH, Lamb RA. Ion channel activity of influenza A virus M2 protein: Characterization of the amantadine block. *J Virol* 1993;67:5585–5594.
355. Wang P, Palese P, O'Neill RE. The NPI-1/NPI-3 (karyopherin α) binding site on the influenza A virus nucleoprotein NP is a nonconventional nuclear localization signal. *J Virol* 1997;71:1850–1856.
356. Wang W, Krug RM. The RNA binding and effector domains of the viral NS1 protein are conserved to different extents among influenza A and B viruses. *Virology* 1996;223:41–50.
357. Wang W, Riedel K, Lynch P, et al. RNA binding by the novel helical domain of the influenza virus NS1 protein requires its dimer structure and a small number of specific basic amino acids. *RNA* 1999;5: 195–205.
358. Ward AC, Castelli LA, Lucantoni AC, et al. Expression and analysis of the NS2 protein of influenza A virus. *Arch Virol* 1995;140: 2067–2073.
359. Ward CW, Dopheide TAA. The Hong Kong (H3) hemagglutinin: Complete amino acid sequence and oligosaccharide distribution for the heavy chain of A/Memphis/102/72, In: Laver G, Air G, ed. *Structure and variation in influenza virus.* New York: Elsevier/North-Holland, 1980:27–38.
360. Weber F, Kochs G, Gruber S, Haller O. A classical bipartite nuclear localization signal on Thogoto and influenza A virus nucleoproteins. *Virology* 1998;250:9–18.
361. Webster RG. 1918 Spanish influenza: The secrets remain elusive. *Proc Natl Acad Sci U S A* 1999;96:1164–1166.
362. Webster RG, Air GM, Metzger DW, et al. Antigenic structure and variation in an influenza virus N9 neuraminidase. *J Virol* 1987;61: 2910–2916.
363. Webster RG, Brown LE, Jackson DC. Changes in the antigenicity of the hemagglutinin molecule of H3 influenza virus at acidic pH. *Virology* 1983;126:587–599.
364. Webster RG, Brown LE, Laver WG. Antigenic and biological characterization of influenza virus neuraminidase (N2) with monoclonal antibodies. *Virology* 1984;135:30–42.
365. Webster RG, Laver WG. Antigenic variation in influenza virus: Biology and chemistry. *Prog Med Virol* 1971;13:271–338.
366. Webster RG, Laver WG, Air GM, Schild GC. Molecular mechanisms of variation in influenza viruses. *Nature* 1982;296:115–121.
367. Weis W, Brown JH, Cusack S, et al. Structure of the influenza virus haemagglutinin complexed with its receptor, sialic acid. *Nature* 1988;333:426–431.
368. Weissmann C. Reversed genetics: A new approach to the elucidation of structure-function relationships. *Trends Biochem Sci* 1978;3: N109–N111.
369. Wharton SA, Belshe RB, Skehel JJ, Hay AJ. Role of virion M2 protein in influenza virus uncoating: Specific reduction in the rate of membrane fusion between virus and liposomes by amantadine. *J Gen Virol* 1994;75:945–948.
370. Wharton SA, Weis W, Skehel JJ, Wiley DC. Structure, function, and antigenicity of the hemagglutinin of influenza virus, In: Krug RM, ed. *The influenza viruses.* New York: Plenum, 1989:153–173.
371. White J, Matlin K, Helenius A. Cell fusion by Semliki Forest, influenza, and vesicular stomatitis viruses. *J Cell Biol* 1981;89:674–679.
372. White JM, Wilson IA. Anti-peptide antibodies detect steps in a protein conformational change: Low-pH activation of the influenza virus hemagglutinin. *J Cell Biol* 1987;105:2887–2896.
373. Whittaker G, Kemler I, Helenius A. Hyperphosphorylation of mutant influenza virus matrix protein, M1, causes its retention in the nucleus. *J Virol* 1995;69:439–445.
374. Whittaker GR, Helenius A. Nuclear import and export of viruses and virus genomes. *Virology* 1998;246:1–23.
375. Wiley DC, Skehel JJ. Crystallization and x-ray diffraction studies on the haemagglutinin glycoprotein from the membrane of influenza virus. *J Mol Biol* 1977;112:343–347.
376. Wiley DC, Wilson IA, Skehel JJ. Structural identification of the antibody-binding sites of Hong Kong influenza haemagglutinin and their involvement in antigenic variation. *Nature* 1981;289:373–378.
377. Williams MA, Lamb RA. Determination of the orientation of an integral membrane protein and sites of glycosylation by oligonucleotide-directed mutagenesis: Influenza B virus NB glycoprotein lacks a cleavable signal sequence and has an extracellular NH2-terminal region. *Mol Cell Biol* 1986;6:4317–4328.
378. Williams MA, Lamb RA. Effect of mutations and deletions in a bicistronic mRNA on the synthesis of influenza B virus NB and NA glycoproteins. *J Virol* 1989;63:28–35.
379. Williams MA, Lamb RA. Polylactosaminoglycan modification of a small integral membrane glycoprotein, influenza B virus NB. *Mol Cell Biol* 1988;8:1186–1196.
380. Wilson IA, Skehel JJ, Wiley DC. Structure of the haemagglutinin membrane glycoprotein of influenza virus at 3 Å resolution. *Nature* 1981;289:366–373.
381. Winquist AG, Fukuda K, Bridges CB, Cox NJ. Neuraminidase inhibitors for treatment of influenza A and B infections. *MMWR CDC Surveill Summ* 1999;48:1–9.
382. Winter G, Fields S. Cloning of influenza cDNA into M13: The sequence of the RNA segment encoding the A/PR/8/34 matrix protein. *Nucleic Acids Res* 1980;8:1965–1974.
383. Winter G, Fields S. Nucleotide sequence of human influenza A/PR/8/34 segment 2. *Nucleic Acids Res* 1982;10:2135–2143.
384. Winter G, Fields S. The structure of the gene encoding the nucleoprotein of human influenza virus A/PR/8/34. *Virology* 1981;114:423–428.
385. Winter G, Fields S, Gait MJ, Brownlee GG. The use of synthetic oligodeoxynucleotide primers in cloning and sequencing segment 8 of influenza virus (A/PR/8/34). *Nucleic Acids Res* 1981;9:237–245.
386. Yamashita M, Krystal M, Palese P. Evidence that the matrix protein of influenza C virus is coded for by a spliced mRNA. *J Virol* 1988;62: 3348–3355.
387. Yang W, Steitz TA. Recombining the structures of HIV integrase, RuvC and RNase H. *Structure* 1995;3:131–134.
388. Yasuda J, Nakada S, Kato A, et al. Molecular assembly of influenza virus: Association of the NS2 protein with virion matrix. *Virology* 1993;196:249–255.
389. Ye Z, Robinson D, Wagner RR. Nucleus-targeting domain of the matrix protein (M1) of influenza virus. *J Virol* 1995;69:1964–1970.
390. Ye ZP, Baylor NW, Wagner RR. Transcription-inhibition and RNA-binding domains of influenza A virus matrix protein mapped with anti-idiotypic antibodies and synthetic peptides. *J Virol* 1989;63: 3586–3594.
391. Yewdell JW, Hackett CJ. Specificity and function of T lymphocytes induced by influenza A viruses, In: Krug RM, ed. *The influenza viruses.* New York: Plenum, 1989:361–429.
392. Young JF, Palese P. Evolution of human influenza A viruses in nature: Recombination contributes to genetic variation of H1N1 strains. *Proc Natl Acad Sci U S A* 1979;76:6547–6551.
393. Young RJ, Content J. 5′-Terminus of influenza virus RNA. *Nature* 1971;230:140–142.
394. Zebedee SL, Lamb RA. Growth restriction of influenza A virus by M_2 protein antibody is genetically linked to the M1 protein. *Proc Natl Acad Sci U S A* 1989;86:1061–1065.
395. Zebedee SL, Lamb RA. Influenza A virus M2 protein: Monoclonal antibody restriction of virus growth and detection of M_2 in virions. *J Virol* 1988;62:2762–2772.
396. Zebedee SL, Richardson CD, Lamb RA. Characterization of the influenza virus M_2 integral membrane protein and expression at the infected-cell surface from cloned cDNA. *J Virol* 1985;56:502–511.
397. Zhang J, Lamb RA. Characterization of the membrane association of the influenza virus matrix protein in living cells. *Virology* 1996;225: 255–266.
398. Zhang J, Pekosz A, Lamb RA. Influenza virus assembly and lipid raft microdomains: A role for the cytoplasmic tails of the spike glycoproteins. *J Virol* 2000;74:4634–4644.
399. Zhirnov OP. Isolation of matrix protein M1 from influenza viruses by acid-dependent extraction with nonionic detergent. *Virology* 1992; 186:324–330.
400. Zhirnov OP, Konakova TE, Garten W, Klenk H. Caspase-dependent N-terminal cleavage of influenza virus nucleocapsid protein in infected cells. *J Virol* 1999;73:10158–10163.
401. Zurcher T, Luo G, Palese P. Mutations at palmitylation sites of the influenza virus hemagglutinin affect virus formation. *J Virol* 1994;68: 5748–5754.
402. Zvonarjev AY, Ghendon YZ. Influence of membrane (M) protein on influenza A virus virion transcriptase activity in vitro and its susceptibility to rimantadine. *J Virol* 1980;33:583–586.

CHAPTER 25

Bunyaviridae: The Viruses and Their Replication

Connie S. Schmaljohn and Jay W. Hooper

CLASSIFICATION

The family *Bunyaviridae* was established in 1975 to encompass a large group of arthropod-borne viruses sharing morphologic, morphogenic, and antigenic properties (55). The family currently contains four genera of animal-infecting viruses (*Bunyavirus, Hantavirus, Nairovirus,* and *Phlebovirus* genera) and one genus of plant-infecting viruses (*Tospovirus* genus). Most viruses in the family were isolated from or are transmitted by arthropods, primarily mosquitoes, ticks, sand flies, or thrips. Hantaviruses are exceptions; these viruses are rodent borne and are transmitted in aerosolized rodent excreta.

Viruses in the family *Bunyaviridae* were classified historically based on their antigenic relationships. Serogroups were identified that contain viruses related by their reactivity in any serologic test. Bunyaviruses, phleboviruses, and nairoviruses were further divided into complexes of closely related members of a serogroup. Genetic characterization of newly discovered viruses has largely circumvented serologic classification methods, particularly for the hantaviruses, which are very difficult to isolate and propagate in cell cultures.

Efforts to classify viruses as species resulted in a revision in the catalogue of viruses in the family *Bunyaviridae.* The most recent report from the International Committee on the Taxonomy of Viruses lists 47 species (and four tentative species) in the *Bunyavirus* genus, 22 species in the *Hantavirus* genus, seven species in the *Nairovirus* genus, nine species in the *Phlebovirus* genus (and 16 ungrouped viruses), and eight species in the *Tospovirus* genus (and five tentative species) (169). In addition, seven groups (19 viruses) and 21 ungrouped viruses are probable members of the family, but have not been characterized molecularly or antigenically. Because classification criteria vary among the genera, as well as among virus families, it is certain that the taxonomy of the family *Bunyaviridae* will continue to evolve.

VIRION STRUCTURE

Morphology

Virions are spherical, 80 to 120 nm in diameter, and display surface glycoprotein projections of 5 to 10 nm, which are embedded in a lipid bilayered envelope approximately 5- to 7-nm thick (Fig. 1A). Electron microscopy and biochemical studies of the bunyavirus La Crosse virus suggest that there are 270 to 1,400 glycoprotein spikes per virion (76,137). The spikes are generally thought to consist of heterodimers of the viral glycoproteins, G1 and G2; however, one study suggested that homodimers make up the minimal surface unit of the

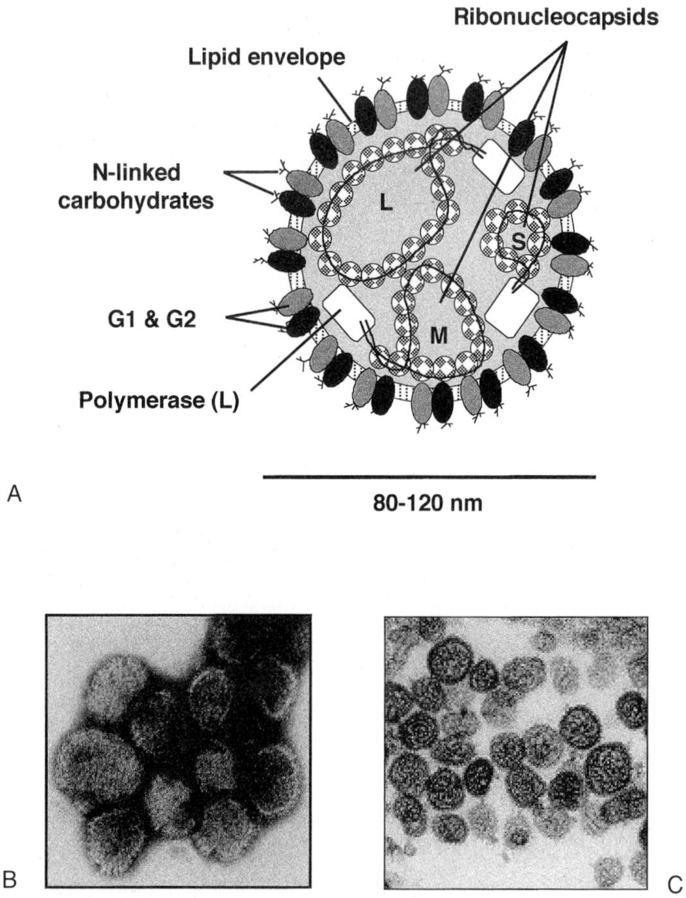

FIG. 1. Morphology of *Bunyaviridae* virions. **A:** Schematic cross section of virus. The three RNA genome segments (S, M, and L) are complexed with nucleocapsid protein to form ribonucleocapsid structures. The nucleocapsids and RNA-dependent RNA polymerase are packaged within a lipid envelope that contains the viral glycoproteins, G1 and G2. Note that there is no matrix protein. **B:** Electron micrograph of glutaraldehyde-fixed, negatively stained Hantaan virions (*Hantavirus* genus). The morphologic units on the surface form a grid-like pattern. As described in the text, viruses in other genera have varying characteristic surface structures. **C:** Thin-section electron micrograph of Puumala virus (*Hantavirus* genus). The interior of the virions has a filamentous or coiled-bead appearance, presumably due to the presence of the ribonucleocapsids. Micrographs courtesy of T. Geisbert, K. Kuhl, and J.E. White, U.S. Army Medical Research Institute of Infectious Diseases, Frederick, MD.

phlebovirus, Uukuniemi virus (176). Studies have not been conducted to exclude the presence of homodimers for other viruses in the family. The glycoproteins interact to form surface morphologic units that vary among viruses in different genera. Viruses in the *Phlebovirus* genus (e.g., Rift Valley fever, Punta Toro, sandfly fever Sicilian, and Uukuniemi viruses) have round, closely packed morphologic units, approximately 10 to 11 nm in diameter, with central cavities approximately 5 nm in diameter (49,120,194). Negative staining of glutaraldehyde-fixed particles, as well as freeze-etching techniques, demonstrated that the surface units of Uukuniemi virus are penton-hexon clusters arranged in a T=12, P=3 icosahedral surface lattice with hexon–hexon distances estimated at 12.5 to 16 nm for stained viral particles and 17 nm for freeze-etched samples (213).

The surface structure of viruses in the *Hantavirus* genus (e.g., Hantaan virus) also are distinctly ordered and have a unique square grid-like appearance (see Fig. 1B) (124,221). In contrast, virions in the *Bunyavirus* genus (e.g., Anhembi, La Crosse, and Bunyamwera viruses) have surfaces covered with knob-like morphologic units with no detectable order (120,204). Similarly, no obvious order was found for the small surface structures with central cavities observed on viruses in the *Nairovirus* genus (e.g., Crimean Congo hemorrhagic fever, Qalyub, and Dugbe viruses) (17,120).

The appearance of viruses in the *Tospovirus* genus (e.g., tomato spotted wilt and impatiens necrotic spot viruses) has been likened to that of the nairoviruses (128). Other than the presence of glycoprotein projections, which are observed as a fringe on negatively stained virions, distinctive surface structure has not been noted for these viruses (98).

The interior of virions, as observed by thin-section electron microscopy, has a filamentous or coiled bead appearance, presumably due to the presence of the ribonucleocapsids (see Fig. 1C) (41,63,79).

Biochemical and Biophysical Properties

The composition and structure of virions has been inferred from biochemical and morphologic studies. An overall chemical content of 2% RNA, 58% protein, 33% lipid, and 7% carbohydrate was estimated for Uukuniemi virus (139). Sedimentation coefficients of virions range from 400 to 500 S, and their buoyant densities in sucrose are 1.16 to 1.18 g/cc, and in CsCl, 1.20 to 1.21 g/cc. Treatment with lipid solvents or nonionic detergents removes the viral envelope and results in loss of infectivity for arthropods and mammals (121,128,139). For plants, the envelope is not required for infectivity, as demonstrated in studies with tomato spotted wilt virus, for which repeated mechanical passage among plants resulted in a defective virus that was unable to produce enveloped particles but was able to infect and replicate in plant cells (170). These studies provide indirect evidence that the L polymerase protein remains associated with ribonucleocapsids and is active despite the absence of intact virions.

GENOME STRUCTURE AND ORGANIZATION

Viral Genome

Virions contain three single-stranded RNA genome segments designated large (L), medium (M), and small

(S). All three gene segments of a virus have the same complementary nucleotides at their 3′ and 5′ termini. The terminal nucleotide sequences are highly conserved among viruses within a genus, but differ from those of viruses in other genera (Table 1). Base-pairing of the terminal nucleotides is predicted to form stable panhandle structures and noncovalently closed circular RNAs. Direct support for base-pairing comes from electron microscopy of RNA extracted from virions, in which three sizes of circular RNAs were evident (77).

The RNA segments are complexed with N to form individual L, M, and S nucleocapsids, which appear to be helical (138). Nucleocapsids released by nonionic detergent treatment of virions often also appear as circular structures in electron micrographs, suggesting that the complementary RNAs can base-pair even when complexed with protein in an estimated ratio of 4% RNA:96% protein (137,157,165). This hypothesis is supported by data showing cross-linking of the ends of nucleocapsid-enclosed RNAs by treatment with psoralens, which are photoreactive, nucleic acid, cross-linking agents (165).

At least one each of the L, M, and S ribonucleocapsids must be contained in a virion for infectivity; however, equal numbers of nucleocapsids may not always be packaged in mature virions, as suggested by various reports of equimolar or nonequimolar ratios of L, M, and S RNAs (16,81,207). Unequal complements of the ribonucleocapsids may contribute to the size differences of virions observed by electron microscopy (204).

In addition to ribonucleocapsids containing virion sense RNA (vRNA), certain viruses in the *Phlebovirus* and *Tospovirus* genera encapsidate small amounts of complementary sense RNA (cRNA) of their ambisense genes (i.e., S, but not M for Uukuniemi virus, and both M and S for tomato spotted wilt virus) (102,191). For the bunyavirus, La Crosse virus, S segment cRNA was detected in virions synthesized in insect cells, but not in mammalian cells (165). The significance of this finding, if any, is not known.

Coding Strategies of Viral Genes

Both similarities and noteworthy differences in the coding strategies of viruses in the family *Bunyaviridae* are known. Viruses in each genus encode all structural proteins (N, G1, G2, and L) in virus cRNA. Nonstructural proteins are encoded in the M segment cRNA of phleboviruses and bunyaviruses and in the S segment cRNA of bunyaviruses. In addition, phleboviruses encode a nonstructural protein in their S segment vRNA, and tospoviruses encode nonstructural proteins in both their M and S segment vRNAs. Therefore bunyaviruses, hantaviruses, and nairoviruses use strictly negative-sense coding strategies, but phleboviruses and tospoviruses use ambisense coding strategies (Fig. 3).

S Segment Strategies

Viruses in the *Bunyavirus* genus have smaller S segments than those of viruses in other genera (Fig. 2A). Two polypeptides, N and NSs, are encoded in overlapping reading frames in cRNA (15). The presence of NSs in virus-infected cells was demonstrated for several members of the genus (46). Only one S segment mRNA species can be found in bunyavirus-infected cells (26); therefore N and NSs likely are generated by ribosomal recognition of start codons in both reading frames.

TABLE 1. *Terminal nucleotide sequences of the S, M, and L genome segments of representative members of the family Bunyaviridae*

Genus Virus	Consensus S, M, L terminal nucleotides	Gene sizes (accession no.) S	M	L
Bunyavirus				
Bunyamwera	3′ UCAUCACAUG— 5′ AGUAGUGUGC—	961 (D00353)	4458 (M11852)	6875 (X14383)
Hantavirus				
Hantaan	3′ AUCAUCAUCUG— 5′ UAGUAGUAUGC—	1696 (M14626)	3616 (M14627)	6533 (X55901)
Nairovirus				
Dugbe	3′ AGAGUUUCU— 5′ UCUCAAAGA—	1712 (M25150)	4888 (M94133)	12255 (U15018)
Phlebovirus				
Rift Valley fever	3′ UGUGUUUC— 5′ ACACAAAG—	1690 (X53771)	3885 (M11157)	6404 (X56464)
Tospovirus				
Tomato spotted wilt	3′UCUCGUUA— 5′ AGAGCAAU—	2916 (D00645)	4821 (S48091)	8897 (D10066)

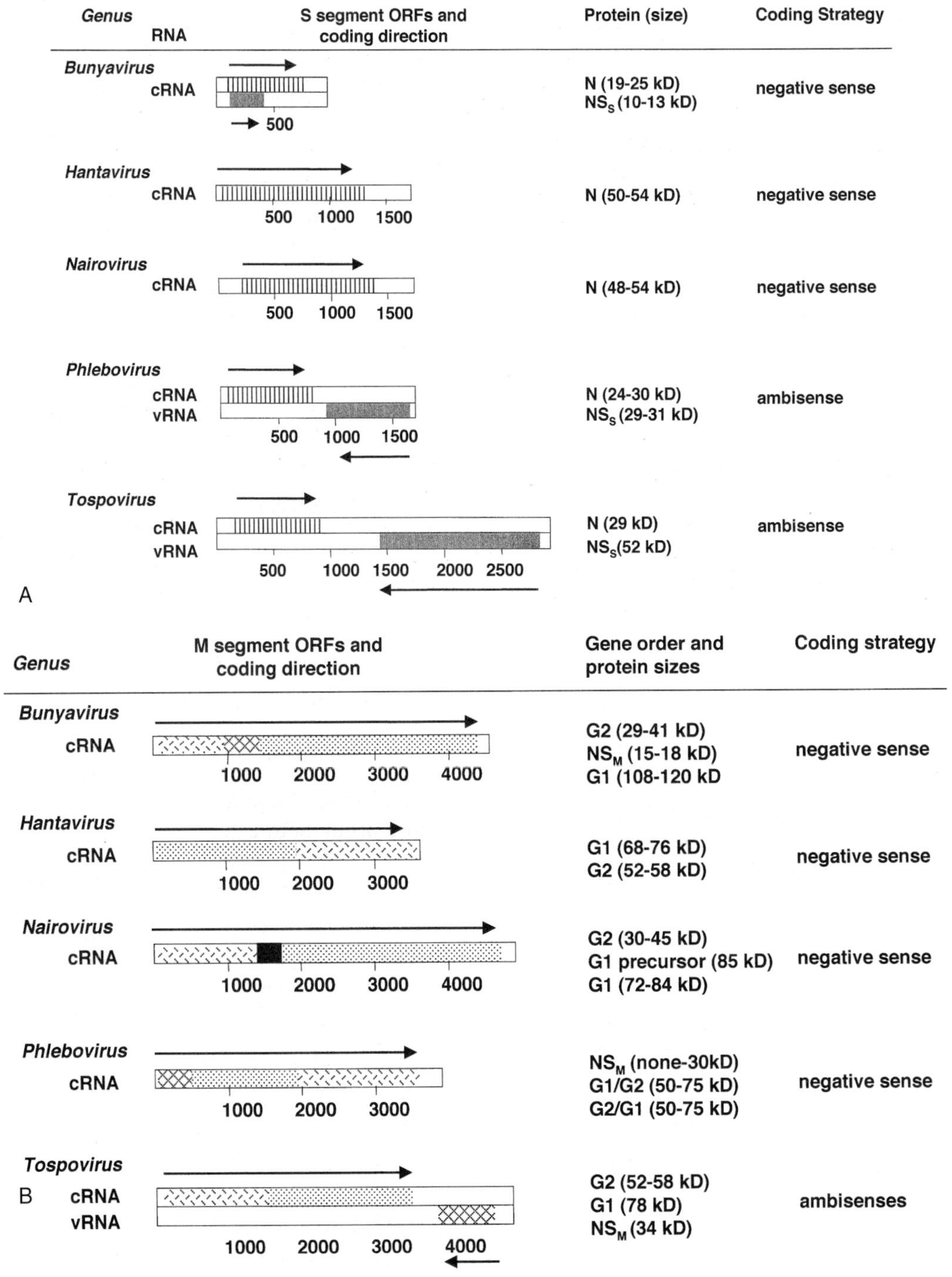

FIG. 2. Genomic structure and coding strategies of viruses in the family *Bunyaviridae.* All members of this family have a genome that consists of three single-stranded RNA segments (S, M, and L) that have either a negative-sense or ambisense coding strategy. Numbers of nucleotides for the L, M, and S segments listed below the boxes, which represent relative sizes of the gene segments and show regions encoding the viral proteins. **A:** S-segment coding strategies. Hantaviruses and nairoviruses use negative-sense coding to express a single protein, N from their virion complementary-sense RNA (cRNA). Bunyaviruses also use negative-sense coding but express two proteins, N and NSs, from overlapping open reading frames (ORFs) of cRNA. Phleboviruses and tospoviruses use ambisense coding to express two proteins, N and NSs, from separate, subgenomic mRNAs. Lines, N coding regions; solid, NSs coding regions. **B:** M segment coding strategies. Bunyaviruses, hantaviruses, nairoviruses, and phleboviruses all use negative-sense coding to express two surface glycoproteins, G1 and G2, from a single ORF of cRNA. Bunyaviruses and phleboviruses encode an additional nonstructural protein, NSm, in the same ORF. M segment products are processed from a precursor polyprotein by cotranslational cleavage. Tospoviruses generate two subgenomic messages and use ambisense coding to express G1 and G2, from an ORF in cRNA, and NSm, from an ORF in vRNA. *Dots*, G1 and G2; *cross-hatch*, NSm coding regions; *solid*, G1 precursor region of nairoviruses.

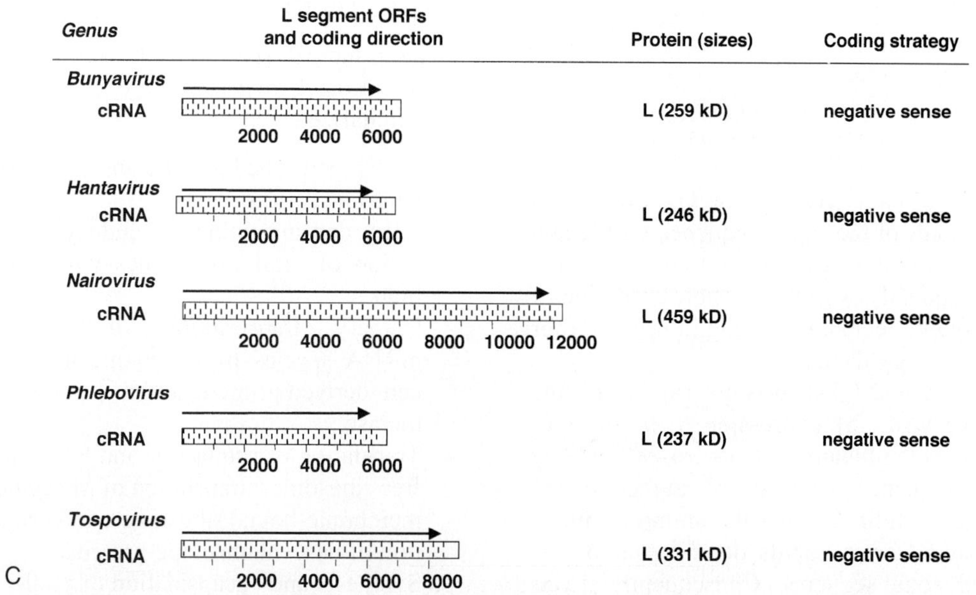

FIG. 2. *Continued.* **C:** L segment. All viruses in the family use negative-sense coding to express the L protein, which is the RNA-dependent RNA polymerase, from an ORF in cRNA. Vertical dashes, L coding region.

Hantaviruses and nairoviruses encode larger nucleocapsid proteins than do viruses in other genera, but are not known to encode NSs proteins (see Fig. 2A) (117,187,217). Although some hantaviruses (e.g., Sin Nombre, Puumala, and Prospect Hill viruses) have an overlapping reading frame with N that has a coding potential of approximately 6 kd, NSs proteins have not been detected in hantavirus-infected cells (141,195,197). Only one S segment mRNA, similar in size to the coding region for N, was identified in hantavirus- or nairovirus-infected cells, indicating that transcription termination occurs shortly after the translation stop codon (81,186,216). Certain hantaviruses (e.g., Sin Nombre virus) have long 3′ noncoding regions (>700 nt) containing numerous repeated sequences. These repeats may result from polymerase slippage on the vRNA template (195).

The ambisense coding strategy of the S segments of phleboviruses and tospoviruses produces N from a subgenomic mRNA that is complementary to vRNA, and NSs from a subgenomic mRNA of the same polarity as vRNA (see Fig. 2A) (37,82). Evidence that the mRNA for NSs is copied from cRNA (after genome replication) comes from time-course studies. For the phlebovirus Uukuniemi virus, N was detected at 4 to 6 hours after infection, whereas NSs did not appear until 8 hours after infection (192,205). Likewise, the mRNA for NSs of the tospovirus, tomato spotted wilt virus, was detected in infected plant cells 15 hours later than for N (196). In addition, studies with the phlebovirus, Punta Toro virus, demonstrated that protein synthesis inhibitors arrest production of NSs mRNA, but not N mRNA (84). These results suggest that protein synthesis must occur before the NSs mRNA can be made. The requirement for protein synthesis is probably related to the need for an adequate supply of newly formed N to encapsidate nascent cRNA, which in turn is then available as a transcription template for NSs mRNA (see transcription section later).

M Segment Strategies

The M segment encodes the two envelope glycoproteins, G1 and G2, in a single open reading frame (ORF) of cRNA. Some viruses encode NSm proteins, and others do not. Except for the tospoviruses, which use an ambisense strategy to generate NSm from a subgenomic mRNA, a single mRNA, nearly equivalent in size to the cRNA ORF, has been detected in virus-infected cells (30,86,118,186). The G1 and G2 gene order varies between genera and even among viruses of a single genus; however, these discrepancies are due to nomenclature anomalies rather than to functional differences. That is, the G1 and G2 designations refer to the electrophoretic migration of the envelope proteins, with G1 being the more slowly migrating band on an sodium dodecylsulfate (SDS)-polyacrylamide gel.

Bunyaviruses have a cRNA M segment gene order of 5′-G2-NSm-G1-3′ (see Fig. 2B) (53). The synthesis of NSm in bunyavirus-infected cells was confirmed by immune-precipitation with antisera to viruses or to synthetic peptides representing amino acids predicted from the NSm coding region (53,56,134).

Hantaviruses have a M segment cRNA gene order of 5′-G1-G2-3′ (188). Immune-precipitation with antisera to peptides representing predicted G1 or G2 amino acids showed that the carboxyl terminus of G1 extends to within 17 amino acids of the signal sequence for G2 and that the carboxyl terminus of G2 extends to the end of the ORF (188). Consequently, with the possible exception of a very short intergenic region, no coding information for a NSm polypeptide is available.

A gene order of 5′-G2-G1-3′ was determined for the nairovirus, Dugbe virus, by expression of portions of the genes with recombinant baculoviruses and by amino-terminal sequence analysis of authentic G1 (116). These studies indicated that the amino terminus of G1 was about 50 amino acids downstream of the nearest predicted signal sequence. Consequently, it was postulated that G1 arises by proteolytic processing of a precursor protein (116). Further studies are needed to confirm this finding and to determine if additional nonstructural proteins are encoded in the nairovirus M segment.

The M segment gene order and the coding strategy varies among viruses in the *Phlebovirus* genus. The tick-borne phleboviruses (e.g., Uukuniemi virus) encode only G1 and G2 proteins (178) in cRNA, whereas the mosquito- and sandfly-vectored phleboviruses also have coding information for a NSm protein. For Rift Valley fever virus, the cRNA gene order is 5′-NSm-G2-G1-3′ (32). The gene order for Punta Toro virus is 5′-NSm-G1-G2-3′, but the reversed order has no significance, as indicated at the beginning of this section. The NSm protein of Rift Valley fever virus, but not that of Punta Toro virus, could be detected in virus-infected cells (83,93).

Like the S segments, the M segments of tospoviruses use an ambisense coding strategy. The cRNA has a gene order of 5′-G2-G1-3′, and the vRNA encodes NSm (108). There are separate, subgenomic messages for the G1–G2 precursor and for NSm (101,108). NSm is readily detected in infected plants and is the only M segment nonstructural protein in the *Bunyaviridae* family to have a defined role (i.e., it is a movement protein, as discussed later).

L Segment Strategies

A conventional negative-sense coding strategy was found for all L segments of viruses in the family *Bunyaviridae.* For each L segment described thus far, there are fewer than 200 nucleotides of total noncoding information, and there is no evidence for additional coding regions in either the cRNA or vRNA (36,47,130,131,183, 210).

STAGES OF REPLICATION

The principal stages of the replication process for viruses in the *Bunyaviridae* are illustrated in Fig. 3 and are summarized.

1. Attachment, mediated by an interaction of viral proteins and host receptors.
2. Entry and uncoating, by endocytosis of virions and fusion of viral membranes with endosomal membranes.
3. Primary transcription of viral-complementary mRNA species from genome templates using host cell–derived primers, and the virion-associated polymerase.
4. Translation of primary L and S segment mRNAs by free ribosomes, translation of M segment mRNAs by membrane-bound ribosomes, and primary glycosylation of nascent envelope proteins.
5. Synthesis and encapsidation of viral-complementary RNA to serve as templates for genomic RNA or, in some cases, for subgenomic mRNA.
6. Genome replication.
7. Secondary transcription of mRNA from newly synthesized genomes and of ambisense mRNAs from cRNA.
8. Continued translation and RNA replication.
9. Morphogenesis, including accumulation of G1 and G2 in the Golgi, terminal glycosylation, and acquisition of modified host membranes, generally by budding into the Golgi cisternae.
10. Fusion of cytoplasmic vesicles with the plasma membrane and release of mature virions.

Attachment and Entry

Viral Attachment Proteins and Cellular Receptors

The mechanisms by which members of the family *Bunyaviridae* gain access to the host cell's cytoplasm appear similar to those reported for many other enveloped viruses. The first step involves an interaction between cell-surface receptors and viral attachment proteins, G1 and/or G2. The functions of G1 and G2 during attachment and entry may vary among the genera. For the bunyavirus, LaCrosse virus, it was suggested that G1 might be used for attachment to mammalian cells, whereas G2 might be used for attachment to mosquito cells (113). However, studies involving proteolytic digestion of virions or incubation of virions with glycoprotein-specific antibodies implicated G1 as the attachment protein for mammalian cells, mosquito cells, and mosquitoes (67,71,75,96,148,201). For viruses in other genera, little is known concerning the use of G1 or G2 for attachment. The presence of neutralizing and hemagglutination-inhibiting sites on both the G1 and G2 proteins of the phleboviruses, Rift Valley fever (94), and Punta Toro

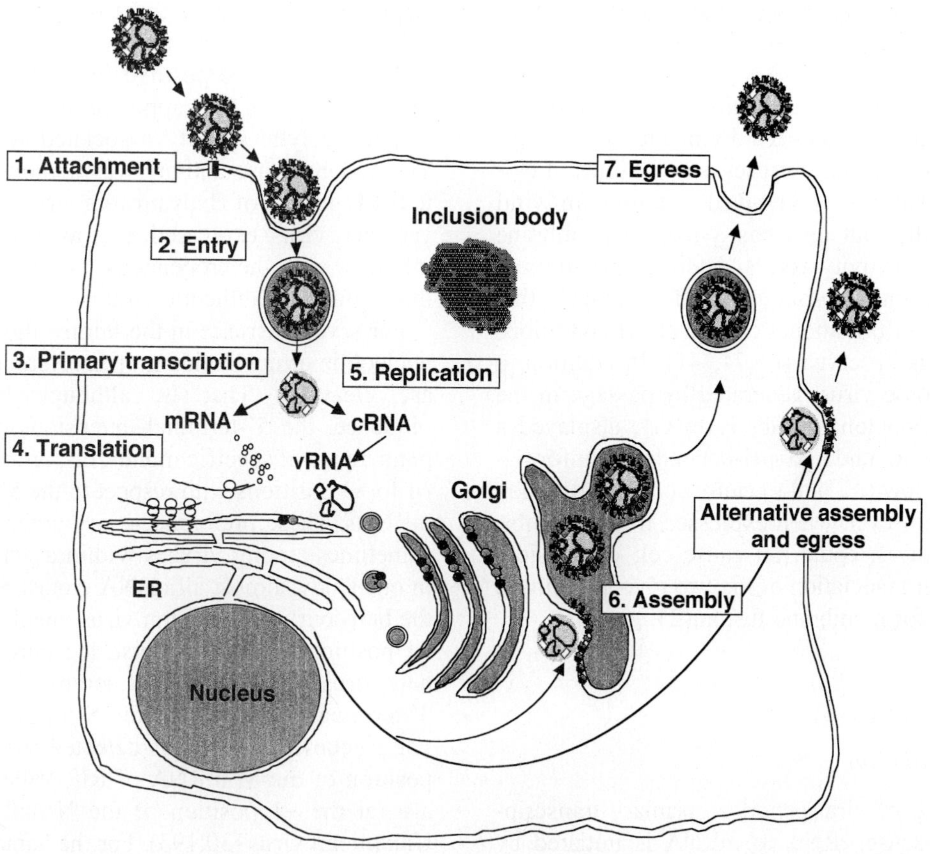

FIG. 3. Replication cycle of viruses in the family *Bunyaviridae.* Steps in the replication cycle are numbered as follows: *1*, attachment of virions to cell-surface receptors; *2*, entry via receptor-mediated endocytosis followed by membrane fusion, allowing viral ribonucleocapsids and RNA-dependent RNA polymerase access to the cytoplasm; *3*, primary transcription; *4*, translation of viral proteins; *5*, replication of vRNA via a cRNA intermediate; *6*, assembly of virions at the Golgi or plasma membrane; *7*, egress by budding into the Golgi followed by exocytosis, or budding through the plasma membrane. For several members of the family, inclusion bodies are found in the cytoplasm. *ER*, endoplasmic reticulum; *black and white boxes*, receptor; *open circles*, N; *shaded circles*, G1 and G2

(159) viruses, and on those of the hantavirus Hantaan virus (9,35), suggest that both proteins may be involved in attachment, either directly or because of conformational requirements.

Host-cell receptors have not been identified for most viruses in the family; however, β_3 integrins, which are surface proteins found on endothelial cells and platelets, were found to facilitate cellular entry of some pathogenic hantaviruses (59,60). Evidence for this comes from studies in which cells were rendered resistant to hantavirus infection by pretreating them with vitronectin, the physiologic ligand of β_3 integrins, or with β_3 integrin–specific antibodies. Consistent with these findings, stably transformed CHO cells expressing β_3 integrins supported hantavirus infections, whereas normal CHO cells did not. A nonpathogenic hantavirus, Prospect Hill virus, was found to use β_1 integrins rather than β_3 integrins, suggesting a role for viral receptors in determining virulence (60). Whether integrins are involved in virion attachment, or a postattachment entry event, has not been determined.

Entry of the Viral Genome into the Host Cytoplasm

Shortly after attachment, viruses in the *Phlebovirus* and *Nairovirus* genera were observed in phagocytic vacuoles (49,181). This finding suggests a mode of viral entry similar to that first described for alphaviruses in which the virus is endocytosed in coated vesicles (119). Acidification of the endosomes is thought to promote a conformational change in G1 and/or G2 that facilitates fusion of the viral and cell membranes, allowing the viral genome and polymerase access to the cytoplasm. Consistent with this, treating cells with ammonium chloride to prevent acidification of endosomes inhibited infection by the bunyavirus, California encephalitis virus, or the phlebovirus, Uukuniemi virus (74,176). Additional indirect support for membrane fusion as a mode of entry came from experiments demonstrating the ability of viruses in the family to mediate syncytia formation at low pH (10,64–66,86).

Whether one or both of the envelope proteins are necessary for viral entry has not been defined for most members of the family. For bunyaviruses, several lines of evidence indicate that G1 is involved not only in viral attachment to cells, but also has a role in membrane fusion. Protease sensitivity assays, detergent partitioning experiments, and antibody-binding studies, suggest that G1 undergoes a conformational change at pH conditions in which fusion is observed (65,74,147). In addition, a mutant of La Crosse virus, generated by passage in the presence of a monoclonal antibody to G1, displayed a reduced capacity to undergo pH-dependent conformational changes at low pH, and to cause cell-to-cell fusion (65). G1 alone, however, when expressed from recombinant vaccinia viruses, could not cause cell–cell fusion, suggesting that an association of the two glycoproteins is probably needed for membrane fusion (23,86).

Primary Transcription

Transcription Initiation

After uncoating of viral genomes, primary transcription of negative-sense vRNA to mRNA is initiated by interaction of the virion-associated polymerase (L) and the three viral RNA templates (18,167). Only ribonucleocapsids, not free RNA, can serve as transcription templates, as demonstrated in studies with expressed phlebovirus and bunyavirus L and N proteins. In these studies, transcription depended on the presence of both proteins and was unaffected by the presence of other viral proteins (43,112).

Like influenza viruses, viruses in the family *Bunyaviridae* prime mRNA synthesis with capped oligonucleotides that are scavenged from host mRNAs. Unlike influenza viruses, which take primers from newly synthesized mRNAs in the host cell's nucleus (85), members of the *Bunyaviridae* family use primers cleaved from cytoplasmic host-cell mRNAs. A result of this mode of mRNA transcription is the presence of 5′ terminal extensions of approximately 10 to 20 heterogeneous nucleotides that are not found in vRNA (14). Studies using anti-cap antibodies to immunoselect mRNAs (73) provided direct proof for the presence of caps on the scavenged primers and substantiated earlier, indirect findings that showed stimulation of La Crosse virus transcription by methylated cap analogs such as m^7GpppAm, or naturally capped RNAs (144). Further evidence for capped extensions of mRNAs was provided by a study with the tospovirus, tomato spotted wilt virus, in which plants were coinfected with the tospovirus and with a positive-strand RNA virus (alfalfa mosaic virus). The tospovirus acquired 5′ mRNA extensions with nucleotide sequences that matched those of the other virus. Presumably, these extensions retained the cap structures normally found on the positive-strand RNA viral messages (42). Cleavage of the capped primers is accomplished by endonucleolytic activity associated with virions (144). The endonuclease activity was demonstrated to localize to the L protein of Bunyamwera virus in studies in which vaccinia virus–expressed L was shown to transcribe mRNAs with heterogeneous extensions analogous to those found on authentic viral mRNAs (90).

For several viruses in the family, there appears to be a nucleotide or nucleotide motif preference for endonuclease cleavage. That is, although heterogeneous in sequence, the 5′-terminal extensions often have a preponderance of specific mono-, di-, or trinucleotides at the −1 to −3 positions with respect to the 5′ terminus of their mRNAs. These preferences vary among the genera, and sometimes among viruses within a genus. For example, in one study, almost all cDNA clones of the S mRNA of the bunyavirus, Germiston virus, displayed U or G at the −1 position (19). In contrast, the bunyavirus, snowshoe hare virus, was found most commonly to have A as the 3′-terminal nucleotide of the S mRNA extensions (52). For phleboviruses, C was detected most often at the −1 position of the M mRNA of Rift Valley fever virus and also at the −1 position of the N and NSs mRNAs of Uukuniemi virus (30,193). For the hantaviruses, Hantaan and Sin Nombre viruses, the preferred −1 nucleotide was G (38,81), and for the nairovirus, Dugbe virus, C was most common (91). Examination of terminal nucleotides of 20 clones of N mRNAs of tomato spotted wilt virus revealed no base preference at the endonucleolytic cleavage site (209); however, a preference for A was observed in studies in which oligonucleotides were acquired from messages of another plant virus (42). A selective preference for an entire primer sequence was observed with La Crosse virus in persistently infected mosquitoes. In both embryonating and dormant eggs, specific, but different, 5′-extensions were observed on the majority of mRNAs (39). It was not determined whether the paucity of heterogeneous sequences related to poor availability of diverse host mRNAs, or to a preference by La Crosse virus for certain mRNAs as a source of primers.

A preferred primer sequence, or a favored nucleotide at the site of cleavage, might imply that a restricted or specific subset of host mRNAs is used for generating transcription primers, perhaps because of a need for limited base pairing with the viral genome. In one study, the 3′-terminal nucleotides of the scavenged host primers often were similar to the 5′-terminal viral nucleotides (91). It was proposed that after transcription of two or three nucleotides of the nascent mRNA, the viral polymerase might slip backward on the template before further elongation, resulting in a partial reiteration of the 5′-terminal sequence. This mechanism would explain findings with the bunyavirus, Germiston virus, which had an insertion of U or GU between the primer and viral sequences (211). Likewise, the mechanism could explain the finding that Bunyamwera virus mRNAs, which were synthesized by vaccinia virus–expressed L protein, had insertions of GU or AGU (90). Polymerase slippage also was suggested to be a possible reason for the AG insertions observed in a few mRNAs of the tospovirus, tomato spotted wilt virus (42).

An extension of this concept, termed "prime and realign," was proposed for mRNA transcription of hantaviruses (58). According to this model, priming by host oligonucleotides with a terminal G residue would initiate transcription by aligning at the third nucleotide of the viral RNA template (C residue). After synthesis of a few oligonucleotides, the nascent RNA could realign by slipping backward two nucleotides on the repeated terminal sequences (AUCAUCAUC) (see Table 1), such that the G becomes the first nucleotide of the nontemplated 5′ extensions. The frequent deletion of one or two of the triplet repeats in hantaviral mRNA supports this sort of slippage mechanism and suggests that sometimes the initial priming might start at the C residue of the third triplet in the conserved sequence rather than at the C of the second triplet (58). A prime-and-realign model also was postulated for transcription of hantaviral vRNA and cRNA, except that transcription would initiate with pppG alignment at the third nucleotide (C residue) of the template RNA. After synthesis of several nucleotides, polymerase slipping would realign the nascent RNA such that the initial priming G residue would overhang the template. It was further theorized that nucleolytic activity of the L protein might remove the overhanging G, leaving a monophosphorylated U residue at the nascent 5′ end. The presence of the monophosphorylated U on Hantaan virus RNA was experimentally demonstrated (58).

Indirect evidence suggesting that a prime-and-realign method of initiation is used by phleboviruses was obtained by using a reconstituted transcription system to study the polymerase recognition sequence at the 3′ termini of the ambisense S segment RNA of Rift Valley fever virus. In those studies, mutational analysis of the terminal nucleotides revealed that the first 13 nucleotides are required for polymerase recognition, but that one of the two terminal dinucleotides (UGUG) could be removed without deleterious effects on transcription (161). These data also suggested that realignment is not a prerequisite for transcription initiation.

Host Factors

Beyond the need for host-derived primers for initiating mRNA synthesis, little is known about the role that host factors might play in viral replication. Although transcriptional host factors have not been identified, they cannot presently be excluded. Whereas inhibitors of host-cell protein synthesis, such as cycloheximide and puromycin, have been found to have no effect on primary transcription in other negative-strand RNA virus families (e.g., *Orthomyxoviridae, Rhabdoviridae,* and *Paramyxoviridae*), conflicting data exist on their effects on viruses in the *Bunyaviridae* family. Early reports indicated that the bunyaviruses, Bunyamwera and Akabane viruses, were sensitive to cycloheximide (1) and that either no or greatly reduced amounts of S mRNA could be detected in La Crosse bunyavirus–infected cell cultures treated with cycloheximide or puromycin (145,162). In addition, La Crosse virion–associated polymerase produced only incomplete transcripts *in vitro* unless rabbit reticulocyte lysates were added to provide a coupled transcription–translation system. In the coupled system, drugs that inhibit protein synthesis also inhibited full-length mRNA synthesis and resulted in the reappearance of the incomplete transcripts (13,163). This led to a hypothesis that translation of the nascent bunyavirus S mRNA is required to prevent premature termination of primary transcription products and that the nascent chain may be interacting with its template to cause premature termination. Such a translation requirement was postulated to be similar to that observed in certain bacterial systems, whereby ribosomes prevent RNA–RNA interaction and thus premature termination (163).

For the bunyavirus, Germiston virus, although S segment mRNA was inhibited in cell culture by either anisomycin or cycloheximide, full-length S transcripts could be obtained in an *in vitro* transcription system without added translational capabilities (61). Further studies, however, revealed that these full-length transcripts were obtained only under conditions of increased temperature, and that premature termination products were obtained under more usual transcription conditions. Adding of reticulocyte lysate improved transcription significantly and restored the ability for full-length transcription to occur (211).

The mechanism of the inhibition of transcription by proteinase inhibitors was more clearly defined for Germiston virus, in that adding the translation inhibitors cycloheximide, puromycin, or anisomycin, but not edeine, inhibited transcription. Because edeine inhibits translation by preventing the 40S and 60S ribosomal subunits from complexing, but still allows the 40S subunit to scan the transcript, the need for ongoing protein synthesis was postulated to be at the level of ribosome scanning, and to be independent of the need for actual translation (211). These data are consistent with an earlier hypothesis that scanning ribosomes prevent premature termination by preventing base-pairing between the template RNA and the transcript, which would cause the polymerase to halt and terminate prematurely. This theory is based on the finding that if inosine was substituted for guanosine in the *in vitro* transcription reaction, thus destabilizing base pairing, less premature termination was observed (13).

Results conflicting with these findings were obtained with the bunyavirus, snowshoe hare virus, in that strand-specific cDNA probes were able to detect full-length S segment mRNA (but not vRNA) readily in the presence of puromycin or cycloheximide (52). These results suggest that primary transcription depends neither on ongoing host protein synthesis nor on ribosomal scanning. A similar finding was obtained with La Crosse virus transcription in mosquito cells, in that translation inhibitors had no effect on transcription, suggesting that host-cell factors may influence the ability of the viral polymerase to function in the presence of such inhibitors (166). At present, it is unclear whether the variations reported in transcriptional requirements for viruses in this genus are due to differences in their transcriptional properties or to differences in the sensitivities of methods used.

Transcription Termination

Differences between vRNA and mRNA are found, not only at their 5′-termini but also at their 3′-termini. For gene segments with simple negative-sense coding, mRNAs are truncated at the 3′-termini by approximately 100 nucleotides as compared with cRNA (19,20,30,52, 145,146,158,164). Potential transcription-termination sites have been proposed for the S segments of the bunyaviruses La Crosse (145) and snowshoe hare viruses (51,52) at or near the genomic sequence, 3′-G/CUU-UUU, which is similar to other negative-strand RNA viral transcription termination–polyadenylation signals (72, 174). U-rich regions also were observed at putative transcription-termination sites for the M and S segments of the bunyavirus Germiston virus (3′-AUGUUUUUGUU and 3′-GGGGUUUGUU, respectively) (19) and the M mRNA of hantaviruses (81). Despite these findings, there is little evidence to suggest that the mRNAs of viruses in the family *Bunyaviridae* are polyadenylated (146,158, 205). Moreover, transcription-termination sites without the homopolymeric U5 or U6 tract have been proposed for numerous gene segments of viruses in the family. For example, a C-rich motif was proposed as the site of termination for the S mRNA of Sin Nombre virus (CCCAC CC) (81), and purine-rich regions have been suggested as termination sites for the S and M segment mRNAs of snowshoe hare virus (5′-GGUGGGGGGUGGGG and 5′-GGUGGGGGGUGGGG, respectively), (51) and the M segments of the phleboviruses Rift Valley fever and Punta Toro viruses (5′-UGGGGUGGUGGGGU and 5′-GGUGAGAGUGUAGAAAG, respectively) (30). If these sequences are involved in transcription termination, the mechanism by which they are recognized will require further study.

Interestingly, the polymerase protein of Bunyamwera virus, expressed with a recombinant vaccinia virus, was able to transcribe virion-derived nucleocapsids, and some of the S transcripts terminated at the authentic transcription-termination site, but most did not (90). These results suggest that an additional factor(s), of either viral or cellular origin, may be required for consistent transcription termination. Likewise, in studies with the bunyavirus, Germiston virus, transcription termination was abolished if the drug edeine was included in reaction mixtures. Two suggested mechanisms to explain these findings were proposed. One possibility is that transcription termination involves an interaction between the transcriptase and a newly synthesized viral protein, such as NSs. This could not be a familial characteristic, however, because hantaviruses and nairoviruses do not encode NSs proteins. A second possibility is that the abnormal presence of scanning 40S ribosomes might mask the transcription-termination site (90,211).

The mechanism of transcription termination of the ambisense genes of phleboviruses and tospoviruses may differ from negative-sense genes, and is likely to involve RNA secondary structure. The transcription-termination sites for both the N and NSs mRNAs of Punta Toro virus were mapped by hybridizing a series of synthetic oligonucleotides corresponding to vRNA or cRNA to the messages. The results indicated that the 3′ termini of both mRNAs are within 40 nucleotides of one another (50). Computer analysis of the intergenic region and the sequences encoding the 3′ termini of the messages revealed a long, inverted complementary sequence that could potentially form a hairpin structure.

Similar stable hairpin structures are predicted to occur in the intergenic regions of the S and M segments of tospoviruses (37,104,108). For the S segment of the phlebovirus Uukuniemi virus, although there is a noncoding region of 70 nucleotides between the N and NSs genes, hybridization studies demonstrated that the 3′ ends of the subgenomic messages overlap one another by about 100 nucleotides. Thus the 3′ end of the NSs mRNA extends into the coding region of N, and the 3′ end of the N mRNA terminates just before the coding sequences for N. A short palindromic sequence in the intergenic region (including the 3′ ends of each mRNA) was predicted to allow formation of an A/U-rich hairpin structure (193). Similar (but shorter), energetically favored structures have been identified in intergenic regions of the S segments of the arenaviruses, Pichinde and lymphocytic choriomeningitis viruses, which also use ambisense coding (175). For the *Bunyaviridae,* such structures could affect transcription termination only if they can form while the genome is complexed with N, and there is no direct evidence that this occurs.

In addition to secondary structure, particular sequences or motifs also may play a role in transcription termination of ambisense mRNAs. Comparing the S-segment sequences of several phleboviruses revealed the presence of G-rich regions and similar sequence motifs in the intergenic regions of Rift Valley fever, Toscana and sandfly fever Sicilian viruses, but not for Punta Toro or

Uukuniemi viruses (62). Currently, there is no conclusive evidence that either of these mechanisms (i.e., secondary structure or gene sequence) is important for transcription termination with viruses in this family.

Genome Replication

For negative-strand viruses, the change from primary transcription to replication requires a switch from mRNA synthesis to synthesis of full-length cRNA templates and then vRNA. For viruses in the family *Bunyaviridae,* the polymerase protein, acting either alone or in concert with undefined viral or cellular factors, must first function as a cap-dependent endonuclease to generate a primer for transcription of a nonencapsidated, subgenomic mRNA. At some point, the polymerase must switch to a process of independently initiating transcription at the precise 3′ end of the template to produce a full-length transcript. The processes involved in making that switch from primary transcription to genome replication have not been defined completely for any member of the family. Presumably, some viral or host factor is required to signal a suppression of the transcription-termination signal responsible for generation of truncated mRNA. There is no question that genome replication and subsequent secondary transcription are prevented by translational inhibitors such as cycloheximide. These results indicate that continuous protein synthesis is required for replication of the genome. Although not proven, it is likely that synthesis of N is required for genome replication, as described for other negative-strand RNA viruses such as the rhabdovirus, vesicular stomatitis virus, and the paramyxovirus, Sendai virus (see Chapters 22 and 23). For these viruses, encapsidation by N seems to serve as an antitermination signal, thus allowing full-length genome synthesis. It was suggested that the vesicular stomatitis virus NS protein also is involved and acts to control the availability of N (78). A similar mechanism appears plausible for viruses in the family *Bunyaviridae,* whereby N would function to regulate replication and might be tempered by the presence of nonstructural proteins, where they exist. A model for genome transcription and replication based on information presented earlier, and modified slightly from that proposed by Simons (190), is presented in Fig. 4.

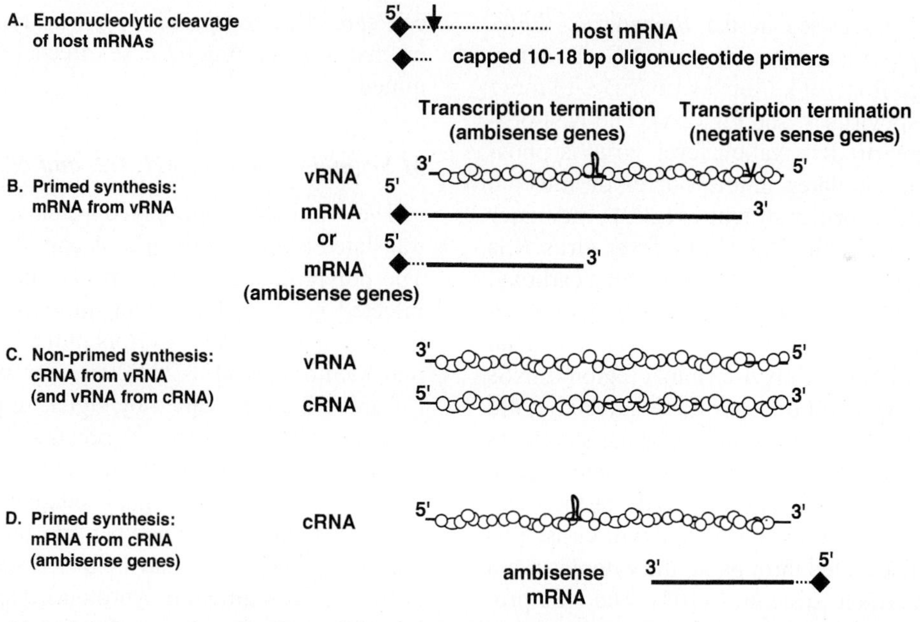

FIG. 4. Transcription and replication of RNA (*Bunyaviridae* family viruses). **A:** Transcription of viral mRNA is preceded by endonucleolytic cleavage of host mRNA caps and adjacent oligonucleotides (*solid diamond*) by viral polymerase (cap snatching). **B:** The capped oligonucleotides prime transcription of viral mRNA from the virion-encapsidated RNAs (vRNAs). Negative-sense genes are copied to yield mRNAs nearly as long as the vRNA template. Ambisense genes (S segments of phleboviruses and tospoviruses, and M segments of tospoviruses) are copied to yield mRNAs complementary to the 3′ portion of the vRNA template. A hairpin structure (*hairpin shape*) is believed to be involved in transcription termination of ambisense genes. An undefined transcription termination signal (*V*) is found near the 5′ end of the vRNA template for negative-sense gene segments. **C:** Replication involves primer-independent synthesis of complementary RNA (cRNA) from vRNA templates followed by primer-independent synthesis of progeny vRNA from cRNA templates. **D:** For viruses that use ambisense coding strategies to express nonstructural proteins (NSs of phleboviruses and tospoviruses and NSm of tospoviruses), the cRNA also serves as template for mRNA synthesis. As in primary transcription, capped, host-derived oligonucleotides prime synthesis of the ambisense mRNAs, and transcription termination occurs at a predicted hairpin structure.

Translation and Processing of Viral Proteins

Viral polypeptides are synthesized shortly after infection, with S and L mRNAs translated on free ribosomes, and M mRNAs translated on membrane-bound ribosomes. Expression products vary among the genera, and even within a genus.

S Segment Products: N and NSs

The N proteins of viruses in the family range in size from approximately 19 kd for bunyaviruses to 54 kd for hantaviruses and nairoviruses (see Fig. 2A). Posttranslational modifications to N have not been described. Few studies have characterized interactions of N and viral RNA. Biochemical analysis of RNA binding by N of Hantaan virus suggested that specific recognition of vRNA by N occurs in the terminal, noncoding regions of vRNA (189). For Hantaan and Puumala viruses, it was suggested that the carboxyl-terminal portion of N is needed for nucleic acid binding (68). In contrast, both amino-terminal and carboxyl-terminal portions of N of the tospovirus, tomato spotted wilt virus, were postulated to bind to RNA (172).

In addition to N, viruses in the *Bunyavirus, Phlebovirus*, and *Tospovirus* genera produce NSs proteins. Sizes of NSs range from 10 kd for bunyaviruses to more than 50 kd for tospoviruses (see Fig. 2A). The NSs protein of the phlebovirus Rift Valley fever virus is phosphorylated and accumulates in the nuclei of infected cells, where it forms fibrillar structures (200). The major phosphorylation sites of the Rift Valley fever virus NSs were mapped to serine residues located near the carboxyl terminus of the protein (100). Expression studies revealed that fibrils could form in the absence of other viral proteins; however, if the carboxyl-terminal region of NSs was removed, NSs was still transported to nuclei, but did not coalesce into fibrils (224). Similar fibrillar structures of NSs were observed for some strains of tomato spotted wilt virus, but the structures appeared only in the cytoplasm. For other strains of tomato spotted wilt virus, NSs was found to be distributed throughout the cytoplasm but did not form discernible structures (103). The NSs protein of the phlebovirus Uukuniemi virus was also found to be distributed throughout the cytoplasm. This protein was not phosphorylated but did associate specifically with the 40S ribosomal subunit (192). The significance of this association, if any, was not determined.

The characteristics and functions of NSs are not well defined, and there is no evidence that NSs proteins serve the same function for viruses in different genera. Comparing the deduced amino acid sequences of NSs for five different phleboviruses revealed homologies of only 17% to 30% (62). However, comparison of the NSs gene sequences for a number of strains of a single phlebovirus, Rift Valley fever virus, showed that certain areas were highly conserved (182). These data suggest that there may be a strong evolutionary pressure to maintain distinct portions of the NSs for individual viruses, but that the remainder of the protein can diverge without affecting the function of NSs.

For phleboviruses and tospoviruses, it is unlikely that NSs is involved in early stages of replication because their ambisense mRNAs are produced only after vRNA has been copied to cRNA; therefore, NSs appears later in infection than the structural proteins. Consequently, it is likely that NSs is involved in late stages of replication, in morphogenesis, or in the spread of newly formed viruses. Consistent with this, a mutant of the phlebovirus Rift Valley fever virus, with an in-frame deletion of about 70% of the coding information for NSs, was found to replicate in Vero and mosquito cells, but not in human lung diploid cells. In addition, the deleted virus was avirulent in mice and hamsters, as compared with wild-type virus (132). These data suggest a role for the phlebovirus NSs in host range and perhaps in virus dissemination. Similarly, disruption of the coding sequences of NSs in a genetically engineered Bunyamwera virus resulted in a mutant virus that produced smaller plaques, displayed reduced shutoff of host-cell protein synthesis, and showed poorer cell-to-cell spread as compared with wild-type virus (22). The mechanism resulting in these effects remains to be determined.

M Segment Products: G1, G2, and NSm

The viral envelope glycoproteins, G1 and G2, are translated from a single mRNA complementary to vRNA. The polyprotein precursor of G1 and G2 is not seen in infected cells, and has been observed only by *in vitro* translation of RNA transcripts in the absence of microsomal membranes (178,202,205). For most viruses, both G1 and G2 are preceded by signal sequences; therefore, cleavage of the polyprotein precursor is likely mediated by host signalase (54). The nairovirus, Dugbe virus, differs in that there is no signal sequence immediately preceding G1 (the second polypeptide encoded in the ORF); therefore, this protein may be processed from a precursor (116). All M segment polyproteins display variable numbers of predicted transmembrane regions, and a hydrophobic sequence at the carboxyl terminus, indicative of a membrane anchor region. Thus the M segment translation products of viruses in the family *Bunyaviridae* are typical class 1 membrane proteins, with the amino terminus exposed on the surface of the virion and the carboxyl terminus anchored in the membrane.

M segment gene products have a cysteine content of approximately 4% to 7% (32,83,101,108,110,116,188). For related viruses, the positions of the cysteine residues in the polyprotein are highly conserved, suggesting that extensive disulfide-bridge formation may occur and that the positions may be crucial for determining correct polypeptide folding. The secondary structure of the proteins also is involved in immunogenicity, as indicated by the finding that neutralizing or protective epitopes are often nonlinear (11,215).

The nonstructural protein, NSm, produced by phleboviruses and bunyaviruses, is translated from the same mRNA as G1 and G2, whereas that of tospoviruses comes from an ambisense mRNA. There is no known functional equivalence of NSm proteins of viruses in different genera. Hantaviruses and nairoviruses produce no known M segment products except for G1 and G2 (116,188). However, because nairovirus-infected cells display several viral polypeptides of unknown origin (25,116,219), it is possible that additional precursor–product relationships may still be uncovered. In contrast, some viruses in the *Phlebovirus* and *Bunyavirus* genera produce NSm from the same M segment mRNA as G1 and G2. The NSm protein of bunyaviruses is encoded between the G1 and G2 proteins (53,134). Its hydropathy profile suggests that it is a membrane-bound protein, and expression studies demonstrated that it localizes to the Golgi along with G1 and G2 (134). Although a function for this protein has not been identified, it was suggested that it might be involved in facilitating virion assembly in the Golgi (134).

For the phlebovirus, Rift Valley fever virus, a NSm of approximately 14 kd is cleaved from the amino terminus of the polyprotein translation product. Sequence studies revealed five in-frame translation-initiation codons upstream of the amino-terminus of G2. Mutational analysis of those codons indicated that the first four can be used efficiently to translate G2 and G1. NSm was found to originate from the second ATG, and a 78-kd polypeptide, representing uncleaved NSm and G2, was translated from the first ATG (92,203). Pulse-chase experiments revealed no precursor–product relationship between the 78- and 14-kd proteins; thus it appears that use of the first and second ATGs, respectively, is what dictates generation of these proteins (31). Both the 14-kd NSm and the 78-kd polypeptide are found in abundance in Rift Valley fever virus–infected cells, (32,92,202), suggesting that they might play a role in replication or morphogenesis.

An even larger NSm (~30 kd) is cleaved from the amino terminus of the M segment polyprotein of the phlebovirus, Punta Toro virus. *In vitro* expression studies indicated that both envelope glycoproteins could be produced in the absence of the NSm coding region (123), but other studies to evaluate the use of the 13 potential translation-initiation codons present in the NSm coding information have not been reported. No homology between the NSm proteins of Punta Toro and Rift Valley fever viruses was apparent (83).

In contrast to Punta Toro and Rift Valley fever phleboviruses, the tick-borne phlebovirus, Uukuniemi virus, does not produce an NSm. The first (and only) initiation codon preceding sequences of the envelope glycoproteins is located 17 amino acids upstream of the amino terminus of G1 (178); hence the G1 protein of Uukuniemi virus appears to be analogous to the 78-kd NSm–G2 fusion product produced by Rift Valley fever virus (although there is no obvious sequence homology of these predicted products). Until a function can be assigned to NSm, it is impossible to determine whether Uukuniemi virus replicates in the absence of such a function or accomplishes whatever function is required without removal of a portion of the amino terminus of G1.

Unlike all other viruses in the family, the NSm protein of tospoviruses is translated from an ambisense mRNA (101). It is also the only NSm protein in the family to have an assigned function. By subcellular fractionation of infected plants, or in thin-section immunoelectron microscopy studies, the NSm of tomato spotted wilt virus was found to be present in cell wall–containing fractions or associated with aggregates of nucleocapsids and with the plasmodesmata (101). Expression of the NSm protein in plant cells or insect cells revealed that the protein first appeared near the cell surface and later as tubular structures protruding from the cell surface. In infected leaf tissues, the tubules were observed only in the plasmodesmata (198). These data were interpreted to indicate that the tospovirus NSm protein is involved in cell-to-cell movement of the nonenveloped ribonucleocapsid structures across the cell walls in infected plants.

All G1 and G2 proteins examined to date possess asparagine-linked oligosaccharides. Two broad classes of asparagine-linked oligosaccharides, complex or high-mannose (simple), generally are found on mature glycoproteins (reviewed in 111). Often both types are attached to the same polypeptide chain. As described for the hemagglutinin protein of influenza virus, as well as other glycoproteins (reviewed in 99,105), for oligosaccharides to evolve from the high-mannose type to the complex type, they are normally transported through the Golgi, where mannose residues are trimmed and terminal residues added. Examination of the oligosaccharides attached to the G1 and G2 proteins of Uukuniemi virus in infected cells revealed that G2 has mostly high-mannose glycans, whereas G1 contains both complex and a novel intermediate-type oligosaccharide (152). Similar results were obtained with the bunyaviruses Inkoo and La Crosse viruses (115,152), whereas the glycoproteins of Hantaan virus were found to be mostly of the high-mannose type (8,180,185). These findings indicate that the proteins are incompletely processed through the Golgi. This is likely related to retention of G1 and G2 in the Golgi, where assembly and release occur.

Between four and nine potential glycosylation sites were identified in the deduced amino acid sequences of the G1 and G2 proteins of viruses in the family (32,53,70, 83,101,108,110,178,188). The number of sites actually used in mature virion proteins has not been defined for all viruses; however, G2 of the phlebovirus Rift Valley fever virus was demonstrated to be glycosylated at its single available site and at least three of four possible G1 sites (92). Examination of glycosylated tryptic oligopeptides of the envelope glycoproteins of several bunyaviruses suggested that all three potential glycosylation sites on G2 are used and at least one of two sites on G1 (214). The single glycosylation site available in the G2 protein of Hantaan virus is used, and this site is conserved among numerous other hantaviruses (7,185). Potential N-linked sites also were identified in the NSm proteins of phleboviruses and tospoviruses, and at least for Rift Valley fever virus, are used to some extent (31,92). The NSm of Bunyamwera was found not to be glycosylated (110).

L Segment Product: L Polymerase Protein

The L proteins of viruses in the family *Bunyaviridae* range in size from about 237 kd for phleboviruses to 459 kd for nairoviruses (see Fig. 2C). This huge difference in protein sizes might reflect varying functional activities of the enzymes, but as yet, there are no data to support this. There are no known processing or posttranslational modifications to the L proteins (208). Comparing the deduced amino acid sequence of the L proteins of viruses in the family *Bunyaviridae* revealed several conserved motifs commonly associated with RNA polymerases (69,131, 160,173). In addition, two novel regions, found at the amino terminus of the L protein of the phlebovirus Rift Valley fever virus, were shown to be conserved only in the polymerases of viruses in the *Bunyaviridae* and *Arenaviridae* families (131).

The function of the L protein as the viral polymerase was confirmed by using L protein expressed from vaccinia virus recombinants to transcribe authentic bunyavirus ribonucleocapsid templates (89). Endonuclease activity also was demonstrated, *in vitro,* with expressed Bunyamwera virus L protein, providing evidence that the L protein is responsible for generating the capped primers needed for transcription (90)

Transport of Viral Proteins, Assembly, and Release

One of the earliest notable features found to distinguish members of the family *Bunyaviridae* from other negative-strand RNA viruses was that virions are formed intracellularly by a budding process at smooth-surface vesicles in the Golgi (Fig. 5A) (16,114,133,212). The plant-infecting members of the family, the tospoviruses, also appear to assemble in the Golgi; however, it was suggested that instead of budding, there is a coalescence of Golgi membranes around the ribonucleocapsids (95). Although most members of the family examined have been found to mature in the Golgi, budding at membranes other than those associated with the Golgi also has been reported for some viruses. The hantaviruses, Sin Nombre and Black Creek Canal viruses, were shown to bud preferentially from the plasma membrane of infected cells

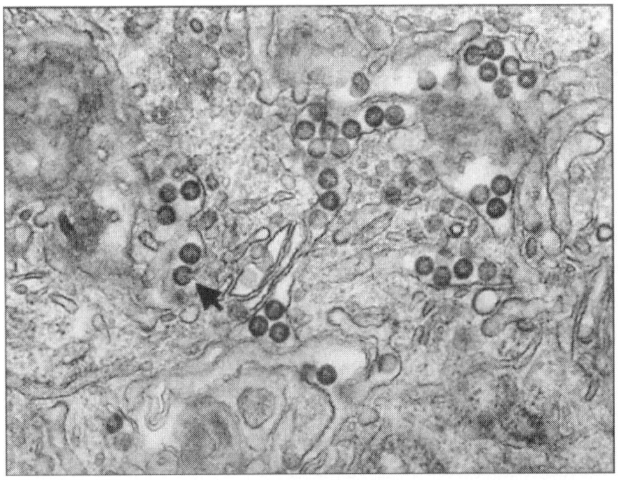
A

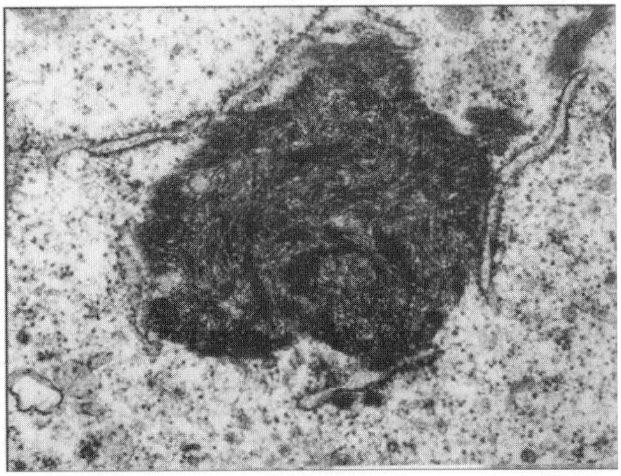
B

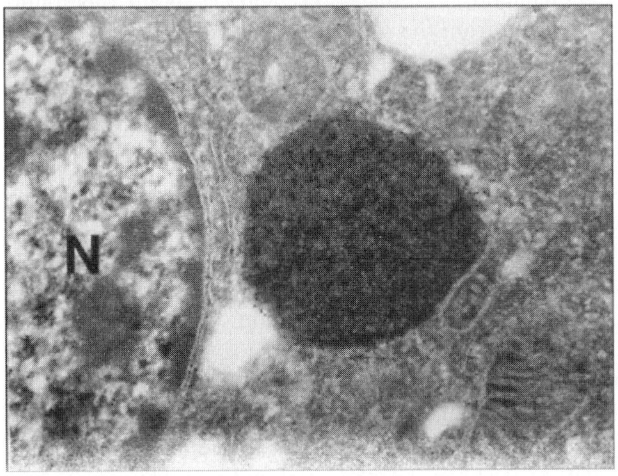

C

FIG. 5. Thin-section micrographs showing virions and cytoplasmic inclusion bodies found in cells infected with viruses in the family *Bunyaviridae.* **A:** Rift Valley fever virus (*Phlebovirus* genus) in the Golgi cisternae of primary rat hepatocytes (3). *Arrow,* A particle budding through Golgi membranes. Magnification ×54,000. **B:** Inclusions found in the brains of rats infected with Seoul virus (*Hantavirus* genus). Magnification ×53,000. **C:** Immunoelectron micrograph of Seoul virus inclusion bodies reacted with antibodies to the nucleocapsid protein. *N,* Nucleus. Magnification ×65,000. Micrographs courtesy of T. Geisbert, U.S. Army Medical Research Institute of Infectious Diseases, Frederick, MD.

(63,168). Similarly, the phlebovirus, Rift Valley fever virus, was found to bud from the plasma membrane as well as in the Golgi of primary rat hepatocytes (3). Because Rift Valley fever virus is a hepatotropic virus and can cause liver necrosis and death in animals, these results raise questions of possible differences in morphogenesis in target versus nontarget cell types that might affect pathogenesis and/or immune defense. The reason(s) for maturation of viruses in the family *Bunyaviridae* in the Golgi complex as opposed to the more usual mode of viral morphogenesis (budding at the plasma membrane) are not known completely; however, important clues have been obtained by studying the viral proteins' transport to and retention in the Golgi.

Golgi Targeting and Retention

Expression of M gene segments of representative phleboviruses, hantaviruses, and bunyaviruses demonstrated that G1 and G2 are targeted to the Golgi in the absence of other viral components (29,123,134,151,180,218). When expressed individually, the first glycoprotein of the M segment ORF (i.e., encoded in the 5′ portion of the M segment) was able to exit the endoplasmic reticulum (ER), but the second glycoprotein remained in the ER (23,107,122,125,150,177). These data indicate that the signal for Golgi transport resides in the first protein encoded in the M segment ORF and that dimerization of G1 and G2 in the ER is necessary for efficient transport of the downstream product.

The Golgi complex actually consists of several subcompartments, including the cis-, medial, and trans-Golgi (reviewed in 126). The exact location in the Golgi where the viral glycoproteins accumulate has not been conclusively determined. By using the fungal antibacterial reagent, brefeldin A, which inhibits transport of proteins out of the ER and causes a redistribution of the Golgi component to the ER, the glycoproteins of the phlebovirus Punta Toro virus were found to be localized in the cis/medial Golgi membranes (27). Similar redistribution of G1 and G2 from the Golgi to the ER were observed after brefeldin A treatment of cells infected with vaccinia virus recombinants expressing the M segment of Bunyamwera virus (134). Immunohistochemical and electron-microscopy studies of Uukuniemi virus demonstrated that budding may begin as early as pre-Golgi intermediate compartment and that virus budding continues in the Golgi stack (88). Similar studies are needed to determine if localization is the same for viruses in other genera.

The mechanism by which G1 and G2 are arrested in the Golgi is not completely known. To map the Golgi targeting and retention signal(s) of phleboviruses, a series of deleted and chimeric genes were constructed and their expression products examined for Golgi targeting and retention. The cytoplasmic tail of the first glycoprotein encoded in the M cRNA was found to contain the targeting signal (4,5,122). For Uukuniemi virus, the minimal transport signal was a 30-amino-acid peptide within the cytoplasmic tail (5). Similar expression studies with M2 segment constructs of Hantaan virus also demonstrated that the cytoplasmic tail of the upstream glycoprotein was needed for exit of the proteins from the ER. Although G2 did not have a targeting signal, results suggested that it might contribute to retention in the Golgi (6).

The NSm proteins are not known to play a role in transport or Golgi retention. For representative phleboviruses and bunyaviruses, expression of G1 and G2 in the absence of NSm had no effect on their transport to the Golgi (23,107,123,134,218). However, when the entire M segments were expressed, NSm colocalized to the Golgi with G1 and G2, suggesting an interaction of these proteins before their exit from the ER.

Kinetics of Transport

Examination of the types and amounts of oligosaccharides attached to viral proteins has been used to assess transit of the proteins through the Golgi compartments. For example, shortly after primary glycosylation of nascent proteins at the ER, oligosaccharides are susceptible to cleavage by endoglycosidase H (endo-H), an enzyme that cleaves only high-mannose residues. Later, after removal of glucose residues at the rough ER, migration of the glycoproteins to the smooth ER and Golgi, trimming of residues, and attachment of peripheral sugars, the oligosaccharides are no longer susceptible to endo-H cleavage. This acquired resistance to endo-H therefore generally indicates that the proteins have been processed through the Golgi. The time required to convert between endo-H susceptibility and resistance correlates with the time needed for protein transport from the ER to the Golgi.

For the phlebovirus, Punta Toro virus, heterodimerization occurred between newly synthesized G1 and G2 within 3 minutes after protein synthesis, and the dimers were found to be linked by disulfide bonds. The dimeric G1/G2 proteins were observed both during transport and after accumulation in the Golgi complex (27). For another phlebovirus, Uukuniemi virus, it was found that the transport of G1 and G2 from their site of synthesis on the rough ER through the Golgi occurred at an estimated 2 to 3 times slower rate than that of most viral membrane glycoproteins destined to be transported to the plasma membrane (57). That is, endo-H resistance was achieved at 45 and 90 to 150 minutes for G1 and G2 of Uukuniemi virus (106), compared with 15 to 20 minutes for the hemagglutinin protein of influenza virus or the G protein of vesicular stomatitis virus (33,40,199). The finding that Uukuniemi virus G1 and G2 have different transport kinetics (i.e., G1 is incorporated into virions 20 minutes faster than G2) suggests that the dimers may arise from different precursor proteins, possibly because faster-folding G1 can not dimerize with slower-folding G2 until G2 has reached its correct conformation (223). In this same study, the G1 and G2 proteins of Uukuniemi virus were found to exit the ER quickly, but did not enter the Golgi for 15 to 20 minutes. The investigators interpreted these findings as indicating that the G1 and G2 proteins may dimerize in an intermediate compartment between the ER and Golgi (223).

Assembly and Release

Unlike most other negative-strand RNA viruses, members of the *Bunyaviridae* do not have a matrix (M) protein to link the integral viral envelope proteins and their nucleocapsids and to act as the nucleating step for assembly. The absence of M protein suggests a direct interaction between the ribonucleocapsids, which accumulate on the cytoplasmic side of vesicular membranes, and viral envelope proteins, which are displayed on the luminal side. Electron microscopy of cells infected with the phleboviruses, Punta Toro or Karimbad viruses, revealed that ribonucleocapsids and spike structures (i.e., viral envelope glycoproteins) were present only in regions of Golgi membranes where budding appeared to be occurring, and not on adjacent areas of the same membrane, suggesting a transmembranal interaction of N with G1 or G2 (194).

The signal directing the ribonucleocapsids to the budding compartment is not known. Excess ribonucleocapsids of hantaviruses (see Fig. 5B and C) tospoviruses, and nairoviruses were found to accumulate in large cytoplasmic inclusions, suggesting that only ribonucleocapsids that interact with the envelope proteins are transported to the Golgi (17,63,80,97,129,206). It is likely that the transmembrane domains of G1 or G2 that are exposed on the cytoplasmic face of the membrane are involved in this interaction. Candidate transmembrane regions have been predicted from hydropathic characteristics of derived amino acid sequences representing the envelope proteins of all members of the *Bunyaviridae* examined to date. Direct examination of the phlebovirus, Karimabad virus, by enzymatic digestion of exposed proteins embedded in intracellular membranes, demonstrated that approximately 12% of G1 and/or G2 was exposed on the cytoplasmic face of membranes in infected cells and was accessible to digestion. A large protease-resistant fragment was identified, which was presumably sequestered in the membrane in a manner that rendered it safe from enzymatic digestion (194). These enzyme-resistant fragments may therefore represent transmembrane regions of proteins, which could provide the interaction between ribonucleocapsids and the cellular membranes required for envelopment. For Uukuniemi virus, the cytoplasmic tail of G1, which is at least 70 residues long, may be a logical candidate for interaction with the nucleocapsids (156,178). Similar cytoplasmic tails also are predicted for other members of the family.

After budding into the Golgi cisternae, virions apparently are transported to the cell surface within vesicles analogous to those in the secretory pathway. The release of virus from infected cells presumably occurs when the virus-containing vesicles fuse with the cellular plasma membrane (i.e., by normal exocytosis). Numerous viruses in the family have been observed late in infection within vesicles or in the process of exocytosis by electron microscopy (41,181,194). In polarized cells, the phleboviruses, Rift Valley fever and Punta Toro viruses, were found to be released primarily from the basolateral surface, whereas the hantavirus, Black Creek Canal virus, was released from the apical surface (3,28,168). Such polarized release of viruses might be important for disseminating virus during natural infection to produce a systemic disease (28).

The assembly and release of tospoviruses may differ from those processes of other viruses in the family. A model was proposed in which Golgi membranes with integral viral envelope proteins wrap around ribonucleocapsids. These particles may then fuse with each other or with ER membranes to release single enveloped particles into the cisternae (95). Mature virions accumulated within the ER cisternae likely remain there until ingested by thrips. Release of tospoviruses from insect cells probably occurs via secretory exocytosis similar to that of animal-infecting members of the family (222).

EFFECTS OF VIRAL REPLICATION ON HOST CELLS

The cytopathic effects observed in cultured cells infected with members of the family *Bunyaviridae* vary widely, depending on both the virus and the type of host cell studied. Viruses in all genera except the *Hantavirus* genus are capable of alternately replicating in vertebrates (or plants for tospoviruses) and arthropods and generally are cytolytic for their vertebrate/plant hosts but cause little or no cytopathogenicity in their invertebrate hosts (12,87,114,222). Some viruses display a very narrow host range, especially for arthropod vectors. Although the reason for this has not been defined completely, studies on La Crosse variant and revertant viruses suggested that the specificity was related to G1, probably at the level of viral attachment to susceptible cells (201). In natural infections of mammals, viruses are often targeted to a particular organ or cell type. For example, bunyaviruses such as La Crosse virus appear to be neurotropic (142); the phlebovirus, Rift Valley fever virus, is primarily hepatotropic (2,3,44,153,154); and the hantavirus, Hantaan virus, persists in rodent lungs (109). It will be interesting to determine whether this targeting is due solely to host-cell receptors or to other factors such as differences in effects on host-cell metabolism in targeted cell types versus the unnatural situation in cultured vertebrate cell lines.

Effects on Host-Cell Metabolism

In vertebrate cells, bunyaviruses and some phleboviruses were found to cause a reduction in host-cell protein synthesis, which became more prominent as the infection progressed. For example, by 5 hours after infection, Bunyamwera virus–infected cells showed reduced levels of host protein synthesis, and by 7 hours, there was almost no synthesis (149). Similar results were obtained in La Crosse virus–infected cells (115). Rift Valley fever virus–infected cells displayed reduced host protein synthesis, which gradually became more pronounced from 4 to 20 hours after infection (140). In contrast, a reduction in host protein synthesis did not occur, even late in infection, with another phlebovirus, Uukuniemi virus, or with the nairovirus Dugbe virus (25,155,205), both of which are transmitted by ticks rather than mosquitoes. Host protein synthesis was slightly inhibited, however, in a *Xenopus laevis* (frog) cell line infected with the tick-borne nairovirus, Clo Mor, or the phlebovirus, St. Abb's head (220). Hantaviruses not only cause no detectable reduction in host macromolecular synthesis (45,184), but they also routinely establish persistent, noncytolytic infections in susceptible mammalian host cells, a finding consistent with their nonpathogenic persistence in their natural rodent hosts (109).

The mechanism of host protein shutoff has not been determined; however, recent studies with Bunyamwera virus derived from cDNA indicated that mutations introduced into the NSs coding region drastically reduced the shutoff of host protein synthesis (21,22). Whether this is a direct consequence of eliminating NSs or a secondary effect remains to be determined. It is noteworthy that some of the viruses that do not shut off host protein synthesis do not produce an NSs protein (e.g., hantaviruses and nairoviruses) and/or do not produce NSm proteins (e.g., Uukuniemi and hantaviruses).

The arthropod-borne members of the family, like most other arboviruses, cause little detectable cytopathology in mosquito cell cultures, and viral persistence is readily established (24,48,135,136,179). Unlike cultured vertebrate cells, mosquito cells infected with the bunyavirus, Marituba virus, displayed no reduction in host macromolecular synthesis; thus viral infection apparently does not drastically interfere with normal cellular processes (24). One suggested reason for this is that, in arthropod cells, excess viral proteins do not accumulate in the cells but rather are more efficiently processed into mature virions (135). Another possibility is that viral transcriptase may be less active in arthropod cells than in mammalian cells and that the endonuclease activity of the polymerase (which is used to acquire transcriptional primers) is detrimental to host-cell messages. A reduced level of activity of the viral transcriptase would, therefore, produce less damage to host-cell messages and consequently to protein synthesis (179).

Persistence, both in insect and mammalian cells, can be mediated by defective interfering (DI) viruses. Conventional DI particles, which displayed deletions only in L, were described for Bunyamwera virus. The defect in L was found to be a single internal deletion, amounting to 72% to 77% of the L RNA segment (143). Defective L RNA segments and resultant DI particles also were reported for the bunyavirus, Germiston virus (34), and for the tospovirus, tomato spotted wilt virus (170,171). The tospovirus deletions, which were generated by repeated high-multiplicity passage, amounted to 60% to 80% of the L segment (171). Interestingly, the L deletions identified both in the tomato spotted wilt and Bunyamwera DI particles were in-frame, thus allowing translation of truncated L polypeptides (143,171). The significance of this finding is not known, but conservation of the terminal sequences and the observed encapsidation of these shortened L segments suggest that they may retain all signals necessary for replication, transcription, and translation, and might be able to interfere at several steps in the replication process.

Persistent infections of viruses in the family have also been described that do not involve typical DI particles. For Bunyamwera virus, temperature sensitive and plaque morphology mutants were recovered from persistent infections of mosquito cells (48,135). These carrier cultures were found to be resistant to superinfection with homologous virus. In addition, virus released from the cultures inhibited infection of normal mosquito cells by standard virus (48). No evidence for deleted RNAs was obtained; thus classic DI particles were apparently not involved (48,179). For the hantavirus, Seoul virus, persistence in mammalian cell cultures was found to be related to short deletions in the conserved terminal regions of the gene segments, particularly the 5′ end of the L segment (127). It will be interesting to determine if similar deletions occur in rodents persistently infected with hantaviruses.

CONCLUSION

The family *Bunyaviridae,* a large and widely diverse group of viruses, is divided into five genera based on molecular properties and serologic relationships among its members. Viruses in different genera display common morphologic, biochemical, and genetic attributes, yet have unique replicative properties. All viruses have three-segmented, single-stranded RNA genomes and encode their N, G1/G2, and L proteins in the S, M, and L genome segments, respectively. Viruses in this family generally display an unusual Golgi-associated morphogenesis and usually acquire their envelopes by budding into intracytoplasmic vacuoles. Recent advances in the molecular biology of viruses, including the development of *in vitro* replication systems and infectious clones, should allow rapid progress in furthering our understanding of these viruses. Among the unresolved questions to be answered are the following: Can the polymerase carry out all of the replication functions by itself, or are cellular factors involved? What dictates the switch in polymerase function from primer-dependent mRNA synthesis to primer-independent cRNA synthesis? What are the functions of the nonstructural proteins encoded in the S and M segments of some viruses? What are the protein–protein and protein–nucleic acid interactions? How do virions assemble to include a full complement of the genome segments? What factors permit viral persistence? It is likely that the answers to these questions will differ for the many diverse viruses in this family.

REFERENCES

1. Abraham G, Pattnaik A. Early RNA synthesis in Bunyamwera virus-infected cells. *J Gen Virol* 1983;64:1277–1290.
2. Anderson G, Slone T, Peters C. Pathogenesis of Rift Valley fever virus (RVFV) in inbred rats. *Microb Pathog* 1987;283–293.
3. Anderson G, Smith J. Immunoelectron microscopy of Rift Valley morphogenesis in primary rat hepatocytes. *Virology* 1987;161:91–100.
4. Andersson AM, Melin L, Bean A, et al. A retention signal necessary and sufficient for Golgi localization. *J Virol* 1997;71:4717–4727.
5. Andersson AM, Pettersson RF. Targeting of a short peptide derived from the cytoplasmic tail of the G1 membrane glycoprotein of Uukuniemi virus (*Bunyaviridae*) to the Golgi complex. *J Virol* 1998;72: 9585–9596.
6. Anheir B, Lober C, Lindow S, et al. Intracellular maturation of Hantaan virus glycoproteins. In: *Abstracts XIth International Congress of Virology.* Sydney, Australia: 1999:291.
7. Antic D, Kang C, Spik K, et al. Comparison of the deduced gene products of the L, M and S genome segments of hantaviruses. *Virus Res* 1992;24:35–46.
8. Antic D, Wright K, Kang C. Maturation of Hantaan virus glycoproteins G1 and G2. *Virology* 1992;189:324–328.
9. Arikawa J, Schmaljohn A, Schmaljohn C, et al. Characterization of Hantaan virus envelope glycoprotein antigenic determinants by monoclonal antibodies. *J Gen Virol* 1989;70:615–624.
10. Arikawa J, Takashima I, Hashimoto N. Cell fusion by haemorrhagic fever with renal syndrome (HFRS) viruses and its application for titration of virus infectivity and neutralizing antibody. *Arch Virol* 1985;86:303–313.
11. Battles J, Dalrymple J. Genetic variation among geographic isolates of Rift Valley Fever virus. *Am J Trop Med Hyg* 1988;39:617–631.
12. Beaty B, Calisher C. *Bunyaviridae*—natural history. *Curr Top Microbiol Immunol* 1991;169:27–78.
13. Bellocq C, Raju R, Patterson J, et al. Translational requirement of La Crosse virus S-mRNA synthesis: In vitro studies. *J Virol* 1987;61: 87–95.
14. Bishop D, Gay M, Matsuoko Y. Nonviral heterogeneous sequences are present at the 5′ ends of one species of snowshoe hare bunyavirus S complementary RNA. *Nucleic Acids Res* 1983;11:6409–6419.
15. Bishop D, Gould K, Akashi H, et al. The complete sequence and coding content of snowshoe hare bunyavirus small (S) viral RNA species. *Nucleic Acids Res* 1982;10:3703–3713.
16. Bishop D, Shope R. *Bunyaviridae. Comp Virol* 1979;14:1–156.
17. Booth T, Gould E, Nuttall P. Structure and morphogenesis of Dugbe virus (*Bunyaviridae*, Nairovirus) studied by immunogold electron microscopy of ultrathin cryosections. *Virus Res* 1991;21:199–212.
18. Bouloy M, Hannoun C. Studies on lumbo virus replication I. RNA-dependent RNA polymerase associated with virions. *Virology* 1976; 69:258–264.
19. Bouloy M, Pardigon N, Vialat P, et al. Characterization of the 5′ and 3′ ends of viral messenger RNAs Isolated from BHK21 cells infected with Germiston virus (Bunyavirus). *Virology* 1990;175:50–58.
20. Bouloy M, Vialat M, Girard M, et al. A transcript from the S segment of the Germiston bunyavirus is uncapped and codes for the nucleoprotein and a nonstructural protein. *J Virol* 1984;49:717–723.
21. Bridgen A, Elliott RM. Rescue of a segmented negative-strand RNA virus entirely from cloned complementary DNAs. *Proc Natl Acad Sci U S A* 1996;93:15400–15404.
22. Bridgen A, Fazakerley J, Elliott R. Generation of a Bunyamwera virus NSs minus mutant by reverse genetics. *XIth International Congress of Virology.* Sydney, Australia: 1999:8.
23. Bupp K, Stillmock K, Gonzalez-Scarano F. Analysis of the intracellular transport properties of recombinant La Crosse virus glycoproteins. *Virology* 1996;220:485–490.
24. Carvalho M, Frugulhetti I, Rebello M. Marituba (*Bunyaviridae*) virus replication in cultured *Aedes albopictus* cells and in L-A9 cells. *Arch Virol* 1986;90:325–335.
25. Cash P. Polypeptide synthesis of dugbe virus, a member of the Nairovirus genus of the *Bunyaviridae. J Gen Virol* 1985;66:141–148.
26. Cash P, Vezza A, Gentsch J, et al. Genome complexities of the three mRNA species of snowshoe hare bunyavirus and in vitro translation of S mRNA to viral N polypeptide. *J Virol* 1979;31:685–694.
27. Chen S, Compans R. Oligomerization, transport, and Golgi retention of Punta Toro virus glycoproteins. *J Virol* 1991;65:5902–5909.
28. Chen S, Matsuoka Y, Compans R. Assembly and polarized release of Punta Toro virus and effects of brefeldin A. *J Virol* 1991;65: 1427–1439.
29. Chen S, Matsuoka Y, Compans R. Golgi complex localization of the Punta Toro virus G2 protein requires its association with the G1 protein. *Virology* 1991;183:351–365.
30. Collett MS. Messenger RNA of the M segment RNA of Rift Valley fever virus. *Virology* 1986;151:151–156.
31. Collett MS, Kakach L, Suzich JA, et al. Gene products and expression strategy of the M segment of the phlebovirus Rift Valley fever virus. In: Mahy B, Kolakofsky D, eds. *Genetics and pathogenicity of negative strand viruses.* Amsterdam: Elsevier Biomedical Press, 1988: 49–57.
32. Collett MS, Purchio AF, Keegan K, et al. Complete nucleotide sequence of the M RNA segment of Rift Valley fever virus. *Virology* 1985;144:228–245.
33. Copeland CS, Zimmer KP, Wagner KR, et al. Folding, trimerization and transport are sequential events in the biogenesis of influenza virus hemagglutinin. *Cell* 1988;53:197–209.
34. Cunningham C, Szilagyi JF. Viral RNAs synthesized in cells infected with Germiston bunyavirus. *Virology* 1987;157:431–439.
35. Dantas JR, Okuno Y, Asada H, et al. Characterization of glycoproteins of virus causing hemorrhagic fever with renal syndrome (HFRS) using monoclonal antibodies. *Virology* 1986;151:379–384.
36. de Haan P, Kormelink R, de Oliveira RR, et al. Tomato spotted wilt virus L RNA encodes a putative RNA polymerase. *J Gen Virol* 1991; 72:2207–2216.
37. de Haan P, Wagemakers L, Peters D, et al. The S RNA segment of tomato spotted wilt virus has an ambisense character. *J Gen Virol* 1990;71:1001–1007.
38. Dobbs M, Kang CY. Hantaan virus mRNAs contain non-viral 5′ end sequences and lack poly(A) at the 3′ end. In: *Abstracts, IXth International Congress of Virology.* 1993:44.
39. Dobie DK, Blair CD, Chandler LJ, et al. Analysis of LaCrosse virus S mRNA 5′ termini in infected mosquito cells and *Aedes triseriatus* mosquitoes. *J Virol* 1997;71:4395–4399.
40. Doms RW, Keller DS, Helenius A, et al. Role for adenosine triphosphate in regulating the assembly and transport of vesicular stomatitis virus G protein trimers. *J Cell Biol* 1987;105:1957–1969.
41. Donets MA, Chumakov MP, Korolev MB, et al. Physicochemical characteristics, morphology and morphogenesis of virions of the causative agent of Crimean hemorrhagic fever. *Intervirology* 1977;8: 294–308.
42. Duijsings D, Kormelink R, Goldbach R. Alfalfa mosaic virus RNAs serve as cap donors for tomato spotted wilt virus transcription during coinfection of *Nicotiana benthamiana. J Virol* 1999;73:5172–5175.
43. Dunn EF, Pritlove DC, Jin H, et al, Transcription of a recombinant bunyavirus RNA template by transiently expressed bunyavirus proteins. *Virology* 1995;211:133–143.
44. Easterday BC. Rift Valley Fever. *Adv Vet Sci* 1965;10:65–127.
45. Elliott LH, Kiley MP, McCormick JB. Hantaan virus: Identification of virion proteins. *J Gen Virol* 1984;65:1285–1293.
46. Elliott RM. Identification of nonstructural proteins encoded by viruses of the Bunyamwera serogroup (family *Bunyaviridae*). *Virology* 1985;143:119–126.

47. Elliott RM. Nucleotide sequence analysis of the large (L) genomic RNA segment of Bunyamwera virus, the prototype of the family *Bunyaviridae*. *Virology* 1989;173:426–436.
48. Elliott RM, Wilkie ML. Persistent infection of *Aedes albopictus* C6/36 cells by Bunyamwera virus. *Virology* 1986;150:21–32.
49. Ellis DS, Shirodaria PV, Fleming E, et al. Morphology and development of Rift Valley fever virus in Vero cell cultures. *J Med Virol* 1988; 24:161–174.
50. Emery VC. Characterization of Punta Toro S mRNA species and identification of an inverted complementary sequence in the intergenic region of Punta Toro phlebovirus ambisense S RNA that is involved in mRNA transcription termination. *Virology* 1987;156:1–11.
51. Eshita Y, Bishop DH. The complete sequence of the M RNA of snowshoe hare bunyavirus reveals the presence of internal hydrophobic domains in the viral glycoprotein. *Virology* 1984;137:227–240.
52. Eshita Y, Ericson B, Romanowski V, et al. Analyses of the mRNA transcription processes of snowshoe hare bunyavirus S and M RNA species. *J Virol* 1985;55:681–689.
53. Fazakerley JK, Gonzalez-Scarano F, Strickler J, et al. Organization of the middle RNA segment of snowshoe hare Bunyavirus. *Virology* 1988;167:422–432.
54. Fazakerley JK, Ross AM. Computer analysis suggests a role for signal sequences in processing polyproteins of enveloped RNA viruses and as a mechanism of viral fusion. *Virus Genes* 1989;2:223–239.
55. Fenner R. The classification and nomenclature of viruses. *Intervirology* 1975;6:1–12.
56. Fuller F, Bishop DHL. Identification of virus-coded nonstructural polypeptides in Bunyavirus-infected cells. *J Virol* 1982;41:643–648.
57. Gahmberg N, Kuismanen E, Keranen S, et al. Uukuniemi virus glycoproteins accumulate in and cause morphological changes of the Golgi complex in the absence of virus maturation. *J Virol* 1986;57:899–906.
58. Garcin D, Lezzi M, Dobbs M, et al. The 5′ ends of Hantaan virus (*Bunyaviridae*) RNAs suggest a prime-and-realign mechanism for the initiation of RNA synthesis. *J Virol* 1995;69:5754–5762.
59. Gavrilovskaya IN, Brown EJ, Ginsberg MH, et al. Cellular entry of hantaviruses which cause hemorrhagic fever with renal syndrome is mediated by beta3 integrins. *J Virol* 1999;73:3951–3599.
60. Gavrilovskaya IN, Shepley M, Shaw R, et al. Beta3 integrins mediate the cellular entry of hantaviruses that cause respiratory failure. *Proc Natl Acad Sci U S A* 1998;95:7074–7079.
61. Gerbaud S, Vialat P, Pardigon N, et al. The S segment of the Germiston virus RNA genome can code for three proteins. *Virus Res* 1987;8: 1–13.
62. Giorgi C, Accardi L, Nicoletti L, et al. Sequences and coding strategies of the S RNAs of Toscana and Rift Valley fever viruses compared to those of Punta Toro, Sicilian sandfly fever, and Uukuniemi viruses. *Virology* 1991;180:738–753.
63. Goldsmith CS, Elliott LH, Peters CJ, et al. Ultrastructural characteristics of Sin Nombre virus, causative agent of hantavirus pulmonary syndrome. *Arch Virol* 1995;140:2107–2122.
64. Gonzalez-Scarano F. La Crosse virus G1 glycoprotein undergoes a conformational change at the pH of fusion. *Virology* 1985;140: 209–216.
65. Gonzalez-Scarano F, Janssen RS, Najjar JA, et al. An avirulent G1 glycoprotein variant of La Crosse bunyavirus with defective fusion function. *J Virol* 1985;54:757–763.
66. Gonzalez-Scarano F, Pobjecky N, Nathanson N. La Crosse bunyavirus can mediate pH-dependent fusion from without. *Virology* 1984;132: 222–225.
67. Gonzalez-Scarano F, Shope RE, et al. Characterization of monoclonal antibodies against the G1 and N proteins of La Crosse and Tahyna, two California serogroup bunyaviruses. *Virology* 1982;120:42–53.
68. Gott P, Stohwasser R, Schnitzer P, et al. RNA binding of recombinant nucleocapsid proteins of hantaviruses. *Virology* 1993;194: 332–337.
69. Gowda S, Satyanarayana T, Naidu RA, et al. Characterization of the large (L) RNA of peanut bud necrosis tospovirus. *Arch Virol* 1998; 143:2381–2390.
70. Grady LJ, Sanders ML, Campbell WP. The sequence of the M RNA of an isolate of La Crosse virus. *J Gen Virol* 1987;68:3057–3071.
71. Grady LJ, Srihongse S, Grayson MA, et al. Monoclonal antibodies against La Crosse virus. *J Gen Virol* 1983;64:1699–1704.
72. Gupta KC, Kingsbury DW. Conserved polyadenylation signals in two negative-strand RNA virus families. *Virology* 1982;120:518–523.
73. Hacker D. Anti-mRNAS in La Crosse bunyavirus-infected cells. *J Virol* 1990;64:5051–5057.
74. Hacker JK, Hardy JL. Adsorptive endocytosis of California encephalitis virus into mosquito and mammalian cells: A role for G1. *Virology* 1997;235:40–47.
75. Hacker JK, Volkman LE, Hardy JL. Requirement for the G1 protein of California encephalitis virus in infection in vitro and in vivo. *Virology* 1995;206:945–953.
76. Hewlett MJ, Chiu W. Virion structure. In: Kolakofsky D, ed. *Current topics in microbiology and immunology*. New York: Springer Verlag, 1991:79–90.
77. Hewlett MJ, Pettersson RF, Baltimore D. Circular forms of Uukuniemi virion RNA: An electron microscopic study. *J Virol* 1977;21: 1085–1093.
78. Howard M, Davis N, Patton J, et al. Roles of vesicular stomatitis virus (VSV) N and NS proteins in viral RNA replication. In: Mahy B, Kolakofsky D, eds. *The biology of negative strand viruses*. Amsterdam: Elsevier Science Publishers, 1987:134–149.
79. Hung T, Chou ZY, Zhao TX, et al. Morphology and morphogenesis of viruses of hemorrhagic fever with renal syndrome (HFRS). I. Some peculiar aspects of the morphogenesis of various strains of HFRS virus. *Intervirology* 1985;23:97–108.
80. Hung T, Xia SM, Chan ZY, et al. Morphology and morphogenesis of viruses of hemorrhagic fever with renal syndrome. II. Inclusion bodies—ultrastructural markers of hantavirus-infected cells. *Intervirology* 1987;27:45–52.
81. Hutchinson KL, Peters CJ, Nichol ST. Sin Nombre virus mRNA synthesis. *Virology* 1996;224:139–149.
82. Ihara T, Akashi H, Bishop DH. Novel coding strategy (ambisense genomic RNA) revealed by sequence analyses of Punta Toro phlebovirus S RNA. *Virology* 1984;136:293–306.
83. Ihara T, Dalrymple JM, Bishop DHL. Complete sequences of the glycoprotein and M RNA of Punta Toro phlebovirus compared to those of Rift Valley fever virus. *Virology* 1985;144:246–259.
84. Ihara T, Matsuura Y, Bishop DH. Analyses of the mRNA transcription processes of Punta Toro phlebovirus (*Bunyaviridae*). *Virology* 1985; 147:317–325.
85. Ishihama A, Nagata K. Viral RNA polymerases. *CRC Crit Rev Biochem* 1988;23:27–76.
86. Jacoby D, Cooke C, Prabakaran I, et al. Expression of the La Crosse M segment proteins in a recombinant vaccinia expression system mediates pH-dependent cellular fusion. *Virology* 1993;193:993–996.
87. James WS, Millican D. Host-adaptive antigenic variation in bunyaviruses. *J Gen Virol* 1986;67:2803–2806.
88. Jantti J, Hilden P, Ronka H, et al. Immunocytochemical analysis of Uukuniemi virus budding compartments: Role of the intermediate compartment and the Golgi stack in virus maturation. *J Virol* 1997;71: 1162–1172.
89. Jin H, Elliott RM. Expression of functional Bunyamwera virus L protein by recombinant vaccinia viruses. *J Virol* 1991;65:4182–4189.
90. Jin H, Elliott RM. Characterization of Bunyamwera virus S RNA that is transcribed and replicated by the L protein expressed from recombinant vaccinia virus. *J Virol* 1993;67:1396–1404.
91. Jin H, Elliott RM. Non-viral sequences at the 5′ ends of Dugbe nairovirus S mRNAs. *J Gen Virol* 1993;74:2293–2297.
92. Kakach LT, Suzich JA, Collett MS. Rift Valley fever virus M segment: Phlebovirus expression strategy and protein glycosylation. *Virology* 1989;170:505–510.
93. Kakach LT, Wasmoen TL, Collett MS. Rift Valley fever virus M segment: Use of recombinant vaccinia viruses to study phlebovirus gene expression. *J Virol* 1988;62:826–833.
94. Keegan K, Collett MS. Use of bacterial expression cloning to define the amino acid sequencing of antigenic determinants on the G2 glycoprotein of Rift Valley fever virus. *J Virol* 1986;58:263–270.
95. Kikkert M, Van Lent J, Storms M, et al. Tomato spotted wilt virus particle morphogenesis in plant cells. *J Virol* 1999;73:2288–2297.
96. Kingsford L, Ishizawa LD, Hill DW. Biological activities of monoclonal antibodies reactive with antigenic sites mapped on the G1 glycoprotein of La Crosse virus. *Virology* 1983;90:443–455.
97. Kitajima EW, De Avila AC, De OResende R, et al. Comparative cytological and immunogold labelling studies on different isolates of tomato spotted wilt virus. *J Submicrosc Cytol Pathol* 1992;24: 1–4.
98. Kitajima EW, Resende RD, de Avila AC, et al. Immuno-electron

microscopical detection of tomato spotted wilt virus and its nucleocapsids in crude plant extracts. *J Virol Methods* 1992;38:313–322.
99. Klenk HD, Rott R. Cotranslational and posttranslational processing processing of viral glycoproteins. *Curr Top Microbiol Immunol* 1980; 90:19–48.
100. Kohl A, di Bartolo V, Bouloy M. The Rift Valley fever virus nonstructural protein NSs is phosphorylated at serine residues located in casein kinase II consensus motifs in the carboxy-terminus. *Virology* 1999; 263:517–525.
101. Kormelink R, de Haan P, Meurs C, et al. The nucleotide sequence of the M RNA segment of tomato spotted wilt virus, a bunyavirus with two ambisense RNA segments. *J Gen Virol* 1992;73:2795–2804.
102. Kormelink R, de Haan P, Peters D, et al. Viral RNA synthesis in tomato spotted wilt virus-infected *Nicotiana rustica* plants. *J Gen Virol* 1992;73:687–693.
103. Kormelink R, Kitajima EW, De Haan P, et al. The nonstructural protein (NSs) encoded by the ambisense S RNA segment of tomato spotted wilt virus is associated with fibrous structures in infected plant cells. *Virology* 1991;181:459–468.
104. Kormelink R, Van Poelwijk F, Peters D, et al. Non-viral heterogeneous sequences at the 5′ ends of tomato spotted wilt virus mRNAs. *J Gen Virol* 1992;73:2125–2128.
105. Kornfeld R, Kornfeld S. Assembly of asparagine-linked oligosaccharides. *Annu Rev Biochem* 1985;54:631–664.
106. Kuismanen E. Posttranslational processing of Uukuniemi virus glycoproteins G1 and G2. *J Virol* 1984;51:806–812.
107. Lappin DF, Nakitare GW, Palfreyman JW, et al. Localization of Bunyamwera bunyavirus G1 glycoprotein to the Golgi requires association with G2 but not with NSm. *J Gen Virol* 1994;75:3441–3451.
108. Law MD, Speck J, Moyer JW. The M RNA of impatiens necrotic spot tospovirus (*Bunyaviridae*) has an ambisense genomic organization. *Virology* 1992;188:732–741.
109. Lee HW, Lee PW, Baek LJ, et al. Intraspecific transmission of Hantaan virus, etiologic agent of Korean hemorrhagic fever, in the rodent *Apodemus agrarius*. *Am J Trop Med Hyg* 1981;30:1106–1112.
110. Lees JF, Pringle CR, Elliot RM. Nucleotide sequence of the Bunyamwera virus M RNA segment: Conservation of structural features in the bunyavirus glycoprotein gene product. *Virology* 1986;148:1–14.
111. Lennarz WJ, ed. *The biochemistry of glycoproteins and proteoglycans*. New York: Plenum Press, 1980.
112. Lopez N, Muller R, Prehaud C, et al. The L protein of Rift Valley fever virus can rescue viral ribonucleoproteins and transcribe synthetic genome-like RNA molecules. *J Virol* 1995;69:3972–3979.
113. Ludwig GV, Israel BA, Christensen BM, et al. Role of La Crosse virus glycoproteins in attachment of virus to host cells. *Virology* 1991;181: 564–571.
114. Lyons MJ, Heyduk J. Aspects of the developmental morphology of California encephalitis virus in cultured vertebrate and arthropod cells and in mouse brain. *Virology* 1973;54:37–52.
115. Madoff DH, Lenard J. A membrane glycoprotein that accumulates intracellularly: Cellular processing of the large glycoprotein of La Crosse virus. *Cell* 1982;28:821–829.
116. Marriott AC, el Ghorr AA, Nuttall PA, et al. Dugbe nairovirus M RNA: Nucleotide sequence and coding strategy. *Virology* 1992;190: 606–615.
117. Marriott AC, Nuttall PA. Comparison of the S RNA segments and nucleoprotein sequences of Crimean-Congo hemorrhagic fever, Hazara, and Dugbe viruses. *Virology* 1992;189:795–799.
118. Marriott AC, Nuttall PA. Molecular biology of nairoviruses. In: Elliott RM, ed. *The* Bunyaviridae. New York: Plenum Press, 1996:91–104.
119. Marsh M, Helenius A. Adsorptive endocytosis of Semliki Forest virus. *J Mol Biol* 1980;142:439–454.
120. Martin ML, Regnery HL, Sasso DR, et al. Distinction between *Bunyaviridae* genera by surface structure and comparison with Hantaan virus using negative stain electron microscopy. *Arch Virol* 1985;86: 17–28.
121. Mathews REF. Fourth report of the International Committee on Taxonomy of Viruses. *Intervirology* 1982;17:1–200.
122. Matsuoka Y, Chen SY, Compans RW. A signal for Golgi retention in the bunyavirus G1 glycoprotein. *J Biol Chem* 1994;269:22565–22573.
123. Matsuoka Y, Ihara T, Bishop DH, et al. Intracellular accumulation of Punta Toro virus glycoproteins expressed from cloned cDNA. *Virology* 1988;167:251–260.
124. McCormick JB, Palmer EL, Sasso DR, et al. Morphological identification of the agent of Korean haemorrhagic fever (Hantaan virus) as a member of the *Bunyaviridae*. *Lancet* 1982;1:765–767.
125. Melin L, Persson R, Andersson A, Bergstrom A, et al. The membrane glycoprotein G1 of Uukuniemi virus contains a signal for localization to the Golgi complex. *Virus Res* 1995;36:49–66.
126. Mellman I, Simons K. The Golgi complex: In vitro vertas? *Cell* 1992; 68:829–840.
127. Meyer BJ, Schmaljohn C. The accumulation of terminally deleted RNAs may play a role in hantavirus persistence. *J Virol* 2000;74: 1321–1331.
128. Milne RG, Francki RI. Should tomato spotted wilt virus be considered as a possible member of the family *Bunyaviridae? Intervirology* 1984; 22:72–76.
129. Mori F, Kobayashi K, Itakura C, Arikawa J, et al. Pathological studies on central nervous tissues of rats infected with *Rattus* serotype hantavirus (SR-11 strain). *Zentralbl Veterinarmed [B]* 1991;38:665–672.
130. Muller R, Argentini C, Bouloy M, et al. Completion of the genome sequence of Rift Valley fever phlebovirus indicates that the L RNA is negative sense or ambisense and codes for a putative transcriptase-replicase. *Nucleic Acids Res* 1991;19:5433.
131. Müller R, Poch O, Delarue M, et al. Rift Valley fever virus L segment: Correction of the sequence and possible functional role of newly identified regions conserved in RNA-dependent polymerases. *J Gen Virol* 1994;75:1345–1352.
132. Müller R, Saluzzo JF, Lopez N, et al. Characterization of clone 13, a naturally attenuated avirulent isolate of Rift Valley fever virus, which is altered in the small segment. *Am J Trop Med Hyg* 1995;53:405–411.
133. Murphy FA, Harrison AK, Whitfield SG. Morphologic and morphogenetic similarities of Bunyamwera serological supergroup viruses and several other arthropod-borne viruses. *Intervirology* 1973;1: 297–316.
134. Nakitare GW, Elliott RM. Expression of the Bunyamwera virus M genome segment and intracellular localization of NSm. *Virology* 1993;195:511–520.
135. Newton SE, Short NJ, Dalgarno L. Bunyamwera virus replication in cultured *Aedes albopictus* (mosquito) cells: Establishment of a persistent viral infection. *J Virol* 1981;38:1015–1024.
136. Nicoletti L, Verani P. Growth of Phlebovirus Toscana in a mosquito (*Aedes pseudoscutellaris*) cell line (AP-61): Establishment of a persistent infection. *Arch Virol* 1985;85:35–45.
137. Obijeski JF, Bishop DH, Murphy FA, et al. Structural proteins of La Crosse virus. *J Virol* 1976;19:985–997.
138. Obijeski JF, Bishop DH, Palmer EL, et al. Segmented genome and nucleocapsid of La Crosse virus. *J Virol* 1976;20:664–675.
139. Obijeski JF, Murphy FA. *Bunyaviridae: Recent biochemical developments.* J *Gen Virol* 1977;37:1–14.
140. Parker MD, Smith JF, Dalrymple JM. Rift Valley fever virus intracellular RNA: a functional analysis. In: Compans R, Bishop D, eds. *Segmented negative strand viruses.* Orlando: Academic Press, 1984: 21–28.
141. Parrington MA, Kang CY. Nucleotide sequence analysis of the S genomic segment of Prospect Hill virus: comparison with the prototype Hantavirus. *Virology* 1990;175:167–175.
142. Parsonson I, McPhee DA. Bunyavirus pathogenesis. *Adv Virus Res* 1985;30:279–316.
143. Patel AH, Elliott RM. Characterization of Bunyamwera virus defective interfering particles. *J Gen Virol* 1992;73:389–396.
144. Patterson JL, Holloway B, Kolakofsky D. La Crosse virions contain a primer-stimulated RNA polymerase and a methylated cap-dependent endonuclease. *J Virol* 1984;52:215–222.
145. Patterson JL, Kolakofsky D. Characterization of La Crosse virus small-genome segment transcripts. *J Virol* 1984;49:680–685.
146. Pattnaik AK, Abraham G. Identification of four complementary RNA species in Akabane virus-infected cells. *J Virol* 1983;47:452–462.
147. Pekosz A, Gonzalez-Scarano F. The extracellular domain of La Crosse virus G1 forms oligomers and undergoes pH-dependent conformational changes. *Virology* 1996;225:243–247.
148. Pekosz A, Griot C, Nathanson N, et al. Tropism of bunyaviruses: evidence for a G1 glycoprotein-mediated entry pathway common to the California serogroup. *Virology* 1995;214:339–348.
149. Pennington TH, Pringle CR, McCrae MA. Bunyamwera virus-induced polypeptide synthesis. *J Virol* 1977;24:397–400.
150. Pensiero MN, Hay J. The Hantaan virus M-segment glycoproteins G1 and G2 can be expressed independently. *J Virol* 1992;66:1907–1914.

151. Pensiero MN, Jennings GB, Schmaljohn CS, et al. Expression of the Hantaan virus M genome segment by using a vaccinia virus recombinant. *J Virol* 1988;62:696–702.
152. Pesonen M, Kuismanen E, Pettersson RF. Monosaccharide sequence of protein-bound glycans of Uukuniemi virus. *J Virol* 1982;41:390–400.
153. Peters CJ, Jones D, Trotter R, et al. Experimental Rift Valley fever in rhesus macaques. *Arch Virol* 1988;99:31–44.
154. Peters CJ, Liu CT, Anderson GW Jr, et al. Pathogenesis of viral hemorrhagic fevers: Rift Valley fever and Lassa fever contrasted. *Rev Infect Dis* 1989;11:S743–S749.
155. Pettersson RF. Effect of Uukuniemi virus infection on host cell macromolecule synthesis. *Med Biol* 1974;52:90–97.
156. Pettersson RF. Protein localization and virus assembly at intracellular membranes. *Curr Top Microbiol Immunol* 1991;170:67–106.
157. Pettersson RF, Bonsdorf CH. Ribonucleoproteins of Uukuniemi virus are circular. *J Virol* 1975;15:386–392.
158. Pettersson RF, Kuismanen E, Rauonnholm R, et al. mRNAs of Uukuniemi virus, a bunyavirus. In: Becker Y, ed. *Viral messenger RNA transcription, processing, splicing, and molecular structure.* Boston: Nijhoff Publishing, 1985:283–300.
159. Pifat DY, Osterling MC, Smith JF. Antigenic analysis of Punta Toro virus and identification of protective determinants with monoclonal antibodies. *Virology* 1988;167:442–450.
160. Poch O, Sauvaget I, Delarue M, et al. Identification of four conserved motifs among the RNA-dependent polymerase encoding elements. *EMBO J* 1989;8:3867–3875.
161. Prehaud C, Lopez N, Blok MJ, et al. Analysis of the 3′ terminal sequence recognized by the Rift Valley fever virus transcription complex in its ambisense S segment. *Virology* 1997;227:189–197.
162. Raju R, Kolakofsky D. Inhibitors of protein synthesis inhibit both LaCrosse virus S-mRNA and S genome syntheses in vivo. *Virus Res* 1986;5:1–9.
163. Raju R, Kolakofsky D. Translational requirement of La Crosse virus S-mRNA synthesis. *J Virol* 1987;63:122–128.
164. Raju R, Kolakofsky D. Unusual transcripts in La Crosse virus-infected cells and the site for nucleocapsid assembly. *J Virol* 1987;61:667–672.
165. Raju R, Kolakofsky D. The ends of La Crosse virus genome and antigenome RNAs within nucleocapsids are base paired. *J Virol* 1989;63:122–128.
166. Raju R, Raju L, Kolakofsky D. The translational requirement for complete La Crosse virus mRNA synthesis is cell-type dependent. *J Virol* 1989;63:5159–5165.
167. Ranki M, Pettersson RF. Uukuneimi virus contains an RNA polymerase. *J Virol* 1975;16:1420–1425.
168. Ravkov EV, Nichol ST, Compans RW. Polarized entry and release in epithelial cells of Black Creek Canal. *J Virol* 1997;71:1147–1154.
169. Regenmortel V, Fauquet CM, Bishop DHL, et al. Virus taxonomy. In: *Seventh report of the International Committee on Taxonomy of Viruses.* Vienna: Springer-Verlag, 2000.
170. Resende R de O, de Haan P, de Avila AC, et al. Generation of envelope and defective interfering RNA mutants of tomato spotted wilt virus by mechanical passage. *J Gen Virol* 1991;72:2375–2383.
171. Resende R de O, de Haan P, van de Vossen E, et al. Defective interfering L RNA segments of tomato spotted wilt virus retain both virus genome termini and have extensive internal deletions. *J Gen Virol* 1992;73:2509–2516.
172. Richmond KE, Chenault K, Sherwood JL, et al. Characterization of the nucleic acid binding properties of tomato spotted wilt virus nucleocapsid protein. *Virology* 1998;248:6–11.
173. Roberts A, Rossier C, Kolakofsky D, et al. Completion of the La Crosse virus genome sequence and genetic comparisons of the L proteins of the *Bunyaviridae. Virology* 1995;206:742–745.
174. Robertson JS, Schubert M, Lazzarini RA. Polyadenylation sites for influenza virus mRNA. *J Virol* 1981;38:157–163.
175. Romanowski V, Bishop DHL. Conserved sequences and coding of two strains of lymphocylic choriomeningitis virus (WE and ARM) and Pichinde arenavirus. *Virus Res* 1985;2:35–51.
176. Rönka H, Hilden P, Von Bonsdorff CH, et al. Homodimeric association of the spike glycoproteins G1 and G2 of Uukuniemi virus. *Virology* 1995;211:241–250.
177. Rönnholm R. Localization to the Golgi complex of Uukuniemi virus glycoproteins G1 and G2 expressed from cloned cDNAs. *J Virol* 1992;66:4525–4531.
178. Rönnholm R, Pettersson RF. Complete nucleotide sequence of the M RNA segment of Uukuniemi virus encoding the membrane glycoproteins G1 and G2. *Virology* 1987;160:191–202.
179. Rossier C, Raju R, Kolakofsky D. La Crosse virus gene expression in mammalian and mosquito cells. *Virology* 1988;165:539–548.
180. Ruusala A, Persson R, Schmaljohn CS, et al. Coexpression of the membrane glycoproteins G1 and G2 of Hantaan virus is required for targeting to the Golgi complex. *Virology* 1992;186:53–64.
181. Rwambo PM, Shaw MK, Rurangirwa FR, et al. Ultrastructural studies on the replication and morphogenesis of Nairobi sheep disease virus, a nairovirus. *Arch Virol* 1996;141:1479–1492.
182. Sall AA, de AZPM, Zeller HG, et al. Variability of the NS(S) protein among Rift Valley fever virus isolates. *J Gen Virol* 1997;78:2853–2858.
183. Schmaljohn CS. Nucleotide sequence of the L genome segment of Hantaan virus. *Nucleic Acids Res* 1990;18:6728.
184. Schmaljohn CS, Dalrymple JM. Biochemical characterization of Hantaan virus. In: Compans RW, Bishop DHL, eds. *Segmented negative strand viruses.* New York: Elsevier, 1984;117–124.
185. Schmaljohn CS, Hasty SE, Rasmussen L, et al. Hantaan virus replication: effects of monensin, tunicamycin and endoglycosidases on the structural glycoproteins. *J Gen Virol* 1986;67:707–717.
186. Schmaljohn CS, Jennings GB, Dalrymple JM. Identification of Hantaan virus messenger RNA species. In: Mahy B, Kolakofsky D, eds. *The biology of negative strand viruses.* Amsterdam: Elsevier, 1987:116–121.
187. Schmaljohn CS, Jennings GB, Hay J, et al. Coding strategy of the S genome of Hantaan virus. *Virology* 1986;155:633–643.
188. Schmaljohn CS, Schmaljohn AL, Dalrymple JM. Hantaan virus M RNA: Coding strategy, nucleotide sequence, and gene order. *Virology* 1987;157:31–39.
189. Severson WE, Partin L, Schmaljohn CS, et al. Characterization of the Hantaan N protein-ribonucleic acid interaction. *J Biol Chem* 1999;274:33732–33739.
190. Simons JF. *Exploring the molecular biology of Uukuniemi virus: Studies on the S segment, its mRNAs and protein products and the L segment.* Stockholm, Sweden: Ludwig Institute for Cancer Research, Stockholm Branch and Department of Physiological Chemistry, Karolinska Institute, 1992.
191. Simons JF, Hellman U, Pettersson RF. Uukuniemi virus S RNA segment: Ambisense coding strategy, packaging of complementary strands into virions, and homology to members of the genus Phlebovirus. *J Virol* 1990;64:247–255.
192. Simons JF, Persson R, Pettersson RF. Association of the nonstructural protein NSs of Uukuniemi virus with the 40S ribosomal subunit. *J Virol* 1992;66:4233–4241.
193. Simons JF, Pettersson RF. Host-derived 5′ ends and overlapping complementary 3′ ends of the two mRNAs transcribed from the ambisense S segment of Uukuniemi virus. *J Virol* 1991;65:4741–4748.
194. Smith JF, Pifat DY. Morphogenesis of sandfly viruses (*Bunyaviridae* family). *Virology* 1982;121:61–81.
195. Spiropoulou CF, Morzunov S, Feldmann H, et al. Genome structure and variability of a virus causing hantavirus pulmonary syndrome. *Virology* 1994;200:715–723.
196. Steinecke P, Heinze C, Oehmen E, et al. Early events of tomato spotted wilt transcription and replication in protoplasts. *New Microbiol* 1998;21:263–268.
197. Stohwasser R, Giebel LB, Zoller L, et al. Molecular characterization of the RNA S segment of nephropathia epidemica virus strain Hällnas B1. *Virology* 1990;174:79–86.
198. Storms MM, Kormelink R, Peters D, et al. The nonstructural NSm protein of tomato spotted wilt virus induces tubular structures in plant and insect cells. *Virology* 1995;214:485–493.
199. Strous GJAM, Lodish HF. Intracellular transport of secretory and membrane proteins in hepatoma cells infected with vesicular stomatitis virus. *Cell* 1980;22:709–717.
200. Struthers JK, Swanepoel R. Identification of a major non-structural protein in the nuclei of Rift Valley fever virus-infected cells. *J Gen Virol* 1982;60:381–384.
201. Sundin DR, Beaty BJ, Nathanson N, et al. A G1 glycoprotein epitope of La Crosse virus: A determinant of infection of *Aedes triseriatus. Science* 1987;235:591–593.
202. Suzich JA, Collett MS. Rift Valley fever virus M segment: Cell-free transcription and translation of virus-complementary RNA. *Virology* 1988;164:478–486.

203. Suzich JA, Kakach LT, Collett MS. Expression strategy of a phlebovirus: Biogenesis of proteins from the Rift Valley fever virus M segment. *J Virol* 1990;64:1549–1555.
204. Talmon Y, Prasad BV, Clerx JP, et al. Electron microscopy of vitrified-hydrated La Crosse virus. *J Virol* 1987;61:2319–2321.
205. Ulmanen I, Seppala P, Pettersson RF. In vitro translation of Uukuniemi virus-specific RNAs: Identification of a nonstructural protein and a precursor to the membrane glycoproteins. *J Virol* 1981;37:72–79.
206. Urban LA, Huang PY, Moyer JW. Cytoplasmic inclusions in cells infected with isolates of L and I serogroups of tomato spotted wilt virus. *Phytopathology* 1991;81:525–529.
207. Urquidi V, Bishop DHL. Non-random reassortment between the tripartite RNA genomes of La Crosse and snowshoe hare viruses. *J Gen Virol* 1992;73:2255–2265.
208. van Poelwijk F, Boye K, Oosterling R, et al. Detection of the L protein of tomato spotted wilt virus. *Virology* 1993;197:468–470.
209. van Poelwijk F, Kolkman J, Goldbach R. Sequence analysis of the 5′ ends of tomato spotted wilt virus N mRNAs. *Arch Virol* 1996;141:177–184.
210. van Poelwijk F, Prins M, Goldbach R. Completion of the impatiens necrotic spot virus genome sequence and genetic comparison of the L proteins within the family *Bunyaviridae*. *J Gen Virol* 1997;78:543–546.
211. Vialat P, Bouloy M. Germiston virus transcriptase requires active 40S ribosomal subunits and utilizes capped cellular RNAs. *J Virol* 1992;66:685–693.
212. von Bonsdorff C-H, Saikku P, Oker-Blom N. Electron microscopy study on development of Uukuniemi virus. *Acta Virol* 1970;14:109–114.
213. von Bonsdorff CH, Pettersson R. Surface structure of Uukuniemi virus. *J Virol* 1975;16:1296–1307.
214. Vorndam AV, Trent DW. Oligosaccharides of the California encephalitis viruses. *Virology* 1979;95:1–7.
215. Wang MW, Pennock DG, Spik KW, et al. Epitope mapping studies with neutralizing and non-neutralizing monoclonal antibodies to the G1 and G2 envelope glycoproteins of Hantaan virus. *Virology* 1993;197:757–766.
216. Ward VK, Marriott AC, el Ghorr AA, et al. Coding strategy of the S RNA segment of Dugbe virus (Nairovirus; *Bunyaviridae*). *Virology* 1990;175:518–524.
217. Ward VK, Marriott AC, Polyzoni T, et al. Expression of the nucleocapsid protein of Dugbe virus and antigenic cross-reactions with other nairoviruses. *Virus Res* 1992;24:223–229.
218. Wasmoen TL, Kakach LT, Collett MS. Rift Valley fever virus M segment: Cellular localization of M segment-encoded proteins. *Virology* 1988;166:275–280.
219. Watret GE, Elliott RM. The proteins and RNAs specified by Clo Mor virus, a Scottish nairovirus. *J Gen Virol* 1985;66:2513–2516.
220. Watret GE, Pringle CR, Elliot RM. Synthesis of bunyavirus-specific proteins in a continuous cell line (ETC-2) derived from *Xenopus laevis*. *J Gen Virol* 1985;66:473–482.
221. White JD, Shirey FG, French GR, et al. Hantaan virus, etiological agent of Korean haemorrhagic fever, has *Bunyaviridae*-like morphology. *Lancet* 1982;1:768–771.
222. Wijkamp I, van Lent J, Kormelink R, et al. Multiplication of tomato spotted wilt virus in its insect vector, *Frankliniella occidentalis*. *J Gen Virol* 1993;74:341–349.
223. Wikstrom L, Persson R, Pettersson RF. Intracellular transport of the G1 and G2 membrane glycoproteins of Uukuniemi virus. In: Kolakosky D, Mahy B, eds. *Genetics and pathogenicity of negative strand viruses*. Amsterdam: Elsevier, 1989:33–41.
224. Yadani FZ, Kohl A, Prehaud C, et al. The carboxy-terminal acidic domain of Rift Valley fever virus NSs protein is essential for the formation of filamentous structures but not for the nuclear localization of the protein. *J Virol* 1999;73:5018–5025.

CHAPTER 26

Reoviruses and Their Replication

Max L. Nibert and Leslie A. Schiff

Viruses with double-stranded RNA (dsRNA) genomes illustrate the potency of evolution at exploiting credible strategies for genome organization and replication. The dsRNA viruses include several human pathogens, most notably the human rotaviruses and Colorado tick fever virus, and numerous pathogens of other organisms including mammals, birds, fish, insects, and plants. In addition, studies of the dsRNA viruses have contributed a number of fundamental concepts to the fields of virology and molecular biology. To name some examples, we draw from work on the nonfusogenic mammalian orthoreoviruses (reoviruses), which are the primary focus of this chapter. Reoviruses provided one of the first systems for *in vitro* studies of RNA synthesis (52,426,445) and evidence for the 5′ cap structure on eukaryotic mRNAs, its mechanism of synthesis, and its importance in mRNA translation (165). Early evidence for the consensus sequence for translation initiation in eukaryotic mRNAs was also obtained from work on reoviruses (249). The use of reassortant genetics to identify allelic differences in reovirus genome segments that segregate with phenotypic differences between reovirus strains (416), demonstrated the value of genetic approaches to virology at a time when such approaches were not yet developed for many other animal viruses. Moreover, several of these early genetic studies with reoviruses concerned the basis of viral pathogenesis and yielded some of the first evidence for the role of animal virus receptor-binding proteins in tropism and/or virulence (494). Studies with reoviruses also provided early evidence for the role of M cells in viral penetration of the mucosal barrier during entry into an animal host (512).

CLASSIFICATION

dsRNA Viruses

Viruses with dsRNA genomes are currently grouped into six families: *Reoviridae*, *Birnaviridae*, *Totiviridae*, *Partitiviridae*, *Hypoviridae*, and *Cystoviridae* (Table 1). Viruses in only two of these families, *Reoviridae* and *Birnaviridae*, are known to infect vertebrates, and those in only one, *Reoviridae*, are known to infect mammals. The six families are distinguished by their genome organizations, protein coding strategies, virion structures, and other differences, in addition to host range. They are sufficiently different in their RNA polymerase sequences, for example, to have earned speculation that at least some arose from different plus-strand RNA virus ancestors (241). Certain structural features are nonetheless shared across family lines and beg explanations in evolutionary terms. For example, the outer capsid layer of *Reoviridae*, the single capsid layer of *Birnaviridae*, and the outer capsid layer of *Cystoviridae* are all arranged with T=13 (laevo) symmetry (63,71,310), which is not seen elsewhere in the virus world. Similarly, the inner capsid layer of *Reoviridae*, the single capsid layer of *Totiviridae*, and the inner capsid layer of *Cystoviridae* are arranged with a form of T=1 symmetry in which the icosahedral asymmetric unit is defined by an asymmetric dimer of the major capsid protein (71,79,378), also not in other viruses.

The *Reoviridae* Family

Of the six dsRNA virus families, *Reoviridae* is the largest and most diverse in terms of the host range of its members (see Table 1). The genomes of these viruses comprise 10, 11, or 12 segments of dsRNA, each encoding one to three proteins (usually one) on only one of the complementary strands. Their mature virions have characteristic sizes (60 to 85 nm, excluding the extended fiber proteins that project from the surfaces of some members), no lipid envelope, and proteins arranged in concentric layers that generally reflect icosahedral symmetry. A distinguishing feature of their replication cycles, also found in dsRNA viruses in other families, is synthesis of viral mRNAs by virally encoded enzymes within the icosahedral particles.

Despite these similarities, viruses in the nine recognized genera of this family (see Table 1) exhibit substantial genetic, biochemical, structural, and biologic differences. Regions of significant sequence similarity across genus lines are few and of limited size, and thus evolutionary connections among the genera remain a matter of speculation (but see later for a recent exception concerning the genera *Orthoreovirus* and *Aquareovirus*). Ongoing exchanges of genetic material between genera, such as genome segment reassortment, appear unlikely given the extent of differences. Viruses in a subset of the genera (see Table 1) have a turret-like protein projecting outwardly from the innermost capsid layer and surrounding the fivefold axes of their particles, which suggests a division of the family into turreted and nonturreted groups (206).

The *Orthoreovirus* Genus

The *Orthoreovirus* genus includes the prototype members of the *Reoviridae* family, the nonfusogenic mammalian orthoreoviruses, which are the primary focus of this and Chapter 53 in *Fields Virology*, 4th ed. Fusogenic

TABLE 1. *dsRNA viruses*

Family	No. of Genera	No. of Genome segments	Hosts
Reoviridae	9	10–12	
Turreted[a]			
Orthoreovirus		10	Mammals, birds, reptiles
Aquareovirus		11	Fish, molluscs
Cypovirus		10	Insects
Fijivirus		10	Plants, insectsb
Oryzavirus		10	Plants, insects[b]
Nonturreted[a]			
Rotavirus		11	Mammals, birds
Orbivirus		10	Mammals, birds, arthropods[b]
Coltivirus		12	Mammals, arthropods[b]
Phytoreovirus		12	Plants, insects[b]
Birnaviridae	3	2	Birds, fish, insects
Totiviridae	3	1–4	Fungi, protozoa
Partitiviridae	4	2–4	Fungi, plants
Hypoviridae	1	1	Fungi
Cystoviridae	1	3	Bacteria

[a]Proposed division based on presence or absence of turret-like protein projecting around fivefold axes from innermost capsid layer (206).

[b]Serve as vectors for transmission to other hosts.

orthoreovirus isolates from mammals, birds, and reptiles are discussed as well, but in a more limited fashion. Designation of the latter isolates as fusogenic reflects their capacity to cause infected cells to fuse together into large multinucleated syncytia. This is an unusual property for nonenveloped viruses, which lack a classical fusion glycoprotein. The mechanism and functional roles of syncytia formation in the life cycles of these viruses is the subject of active investigation (139,307,340) but seems to involve a fusion-associated small transmembrane (FAST) protein encoded by each (438).

Viral isolates were first assigned to the *Orthoreovirus* genus based on similar traits, including a genome comprising 10 segments of dsRNA, the size and morphology of particles by electron microscopy, the number and arrangement of structural proteins within particles, and serologic reactivities. More recently, nucleotide sequences derived from the viral RNAs have confirmed the appropriateness of grouping these isolates, both nonfusogenic and fusogenic, within the same genus. The capacity of related isolates of these viruses to reassort their genome segments upon co-infection of cells, giving rise to infectious reassortant progeny viruses, plays an important role in their evolution (87,189,235). It also suggests a practical approach for designating species of virus within the genus: If particular isolates can reassort genome segments to produce infectious reassortant progeny, then they can be said to belong to the same species (134). Reassortment among nonfusogenic mammalian isolates and also among avian isolates has been demonstrated (373,409), but reassortment between these two groups has not. No reassortment has been reported for the fusogenic mammalian or reptilian isolates.

The name reovirus involves an acronym for respiratory and enteric orphan (397), reflecting that the initial isolates came from human respiratory and enteric tracts but were not associated with any serious human disease. With the isolation and characterization of other dsRNA viruses and the adoption of a standard virus classification scheme, this acronym was retained for the encompassing family of dsRNA viruses, *Reoviridae*, all members of which could then be called reoviruses. As a consequence, the prefix ortho- was added to the name of the initial isolates (orthoreoviruses) and their genus (*Orthoreovirus*) to distinguish them from other members of the family. Despite these formal changes in nomenclature, the orthoreoviruses are still commonly referred to as reoviruses.

Nonfusogenic Mammalian Orthoreoviruses

The nonfusogenic mammalian orthoreoviruses are ubiquitous agents (349) that infect and can be isolated from a wide variety of mammalian species including humans (390,459). Some recent studies have described new isolates from humans, pigs, dogs, and cats (162,189, 222,240,316). There is little evidence for restrictions to the range of mammalian species in which a given isolate can replicate. Nonfusogenic mammalian orthoreoviruses can also be isolated from a variety of fresh- and saltwater sources (297,331), consistent with their pervasiveness and predominantly enteric route of infection. Although association with serious human disease is rare, sporadic cases suggest this can occur (222). In addition, although still debated (461), some data suggest that these viruses are a common cause of extrahepatic biliary atresia and other types of cholestatic liver disease in human infants (122,474). A recent survey of human sera collected in Germany showed that 54% and 15% contained reovirus-specific IgG and IgA antibodies, respectively, indicating frequent human infections (412). Chapter 53 in *Fields Virology*, 4th ed. contains a current review of these viruses as agents of disease and tools for studies of viral pathogenesis. Some basic properties of the nonfusogenic mammalian orthoreoviruses are listed in Table 2.

Three distinct serotypes of nonfusogenic mammalian orthoreoviruses are identified by neutralization and hemagglutination-inhibition tests (390,397,459). An isolate from a healthy child is the prototype for reovirus type 1 (type 1 Lang); an isolate from a child with diarrhea is the prototype for reovirus type 2 (type 2 Jones); and isolates from a child with diarrhea (type 3 Dearing) and a child with an upper respiratory illness (type 3 Abney) are prototypes for reovirus type 3 (375,391,397). Although these prototypes are studied most extensively, other isolates from all three serotypes have been studied as well (209). Further discussions of the basis and significance of serotype, and its relationship to the evolution of these viruses, are found later. According to nucleotide sequences, the nonfusogenic mammalian isolates constitute one distinct phylogenetic group (species) within the *Orthoreovirus* genus (134), consistent with their capacity for genome segment reassortment.

Avian Orthoreoviruses

The avian orthoreoviruses remain less well characterized at the molecular level than the nonfusogenic mammalian isolates. They can be isolated from both domestic and wild birds, in which they can cause a variety of diseases including tenosynovitis (arthritis), a gastrointestinal maladsorption syndrome, and runting. The avian orthoreoviruses are divided into five or more serotypes by neutralization tests (501). Most avian orthoreoviruses promote the formation of multinucleated syncytia within infected cultures and are thus said to be fusogenic. Unlike the nonfusogenic mammalian orthoreoviruses, they lack the capacity to agglutinate red blood cells (340) and thus may lack the capacity to bind the cellular carbohydrate receptors that have been implicated in hemagglutination by the nonfusogenic mammalian orthoreoviruses (see later). Some isolates can be adapted for growth in mam-

TABLE 2. *Properties of Nonfusogenic Mammalian Reoviruses*

Genome	Double-stranded RNA 10 gene segments in three size classes (L, M, S) Total size ~23,500 base pairs Gene segments encode either one or two proteins each. Gene segments are transcribed into full-length mRNAs. Plus strands of gene segments have 5′ caps. Nontranslated regions at segment termini are short. Gene segments can undergo reassortment between virus strains.
Particles	Spherical, with icosahedral (5:3:2) symmetry Nonenveloped Total diameter ~85 nm (excluding σ1 fibers) Two concentric protein capsids: outer capsid subunits in T = 13 lattice, arrangement of inner capsid subunits in T = 1 8 structural proteins: 4 proteins in outer capsid [λ2, μ1 (mostly as cleavage fragments μ1N and μ1C), σ1, and σ3] and 4 proteins in inner capsid (λ1, λ3, μ2, and σ2) Subviral particles (ISVPs and cores) can be generated from fully intact particles (virions) by controlled proteolysis. Cell-attachment protein σ1 can extend from the virion and ISVP surface as a long fiber. Protein λ2 forms pentamers that protrude from the core surface.
Replication	Fully cytoplasmic Sialic acid can serve as cell surface receptor for recognition by cell-attachment protein σ1. Proteolytic processing of outer capsid proteins σ3 and μ1/μ1C is essential to infection and can occur either extracellularly or in endo/lysosomes. Uncoating of parent particles is incomplete: genomic dsRNA does not exit particles to enter the cytoplasm. Transcription and capping of viral mRNAs occur within particles and are mediated by particle-associated enzymes. Segment assortment and packaging involves mRNAs. Minus-strand synthesis occurs within assembling particles. Mature virions are inefficiently released from infected cells by lysis.

malian cells (340,501) or will grow in mammalian cells under certain conditions (285). The particle forms and proteins of mammalian and avian orthoreoviruses have several features and properties in common (133,291, 292). Recent sequence determinations for the small (S) genome segments of several avian orthoreovirus isolates showed that they constitute at least one other distinct phylogenetic group (species) within the *Orthoreovirus* genus (134), consistent with their capacity for genome segment reassortment.

Other Orthoreoviruses

Nelson Bay virus (NBV), an orthoreovirus isolate from an Australian flying fox, exhibits characteristics intermediate between the more classical mammalian and avian isolates. In particular, although it was isolated from a mammal and replicates in mammalian cell culture, it induces syncytia formation in those cultures and is thus fusogenic like the avian orthoreoviruses (171,508). A recent orthoreovirus isolate from a baboon research colony in Texas (designated baboon reovirus, or BRV) (262) exhibits properties similar to those of NBV, including replication and syncytia formation in mammalian cell culture, but it is distinguishable in certain respects (138). Nucleotide sequences determined for the S genome segments of these viruses indicate that the fusogenic viruses NBV and BRV represent two additional phylogenetic groups within the *Orthoreovirus* genus, distinct from both the nonfusogenic mammalian virus group and the fusogenic avian virus group (134). Fusogenic virus isolates from snakes have also been assigned to this genus (256,481), but identification of their relationships to the four defined phylogenetic groups awaits nucleotide sequence determinations. Recent evidence from structure determinations (338) and nucleotide sequences (149) suggests that most or all of the fusogenic viruses with 11 genome segments currently grouped in the genus *Aquareovirus* share significant homology with orthoreoviruses and may warrant grouping within the same genus.

The remainder of this chapter is devoted to a description of the nonfusogenic mammalian orthoreoviruses, which are henceforth called reoviruses for simplicity. When mentioned for comparison, other viruses are explicitly identified.

THE GENOME

Physical Characteristics

Double-Stranded

An observation that the viral inclusions in reovirus-infected cells stain orthochromatically green with acridine orange provided the first evidence that the genomic

RNA is double stranded (188). Physicochemical properties and nuclease sensitivities of the virion RNA, including resistance to the single-strand-specific nuclease S1, are consistent with its double-stranded nature (39,187, 334,420). Moreover, S1 resistance suggests that the plus and minus strands of the genomic dsRNA are fully collinear and complementary (334). The base composition of the genome indicates both G/C and A/U ratios of one, again suggesting that the genome contains two complementary strands (39,187). X-ray diffraction studies of the isolated genomic dsRNA indicate that it adopts a classical A-form duplex structure, constituting a right-handed double helix with about 10 base pairs per turn, a 30-Å pitch (3-Å translation per base pair), and nucleotides oriented at 75° to 80° to the long axis (15). Other physical characteristics of the dsRNA genome as it is found within virus particles are discussed later.

Segments and Nomenclature

The dsRNA genome of reoviruses is routinely isolated from virus particles in the form of discrete segments. Early evidence from electron microscopy, sedimentation, and chromatography showed that these segments are divided among large (L), medium (M), and small (S) size classes (36,141,185,477,488). Separation on polyacrylamide gel electrophoresis provided the first evidence for 10 discrete segments: three large (L1, L2, L3), three medium (M1, M2, M3), and four small (S1, S2, S3, S4) (428,489). Both electron microscopy and quantitation of 3′ hydroxyl groups demonstrated that the 10 isolated genome segments are linear and have two free ends (141,185,312,477). In addition to the different sizes, early evidence that each of the 10 segments is unique included that neither denatured segments from the different size classes nor plus-strand RNAs transcribed from them can cross-hybridize (39,488,489). Many subsequent studies, including sequence determinations and *in vitro* protein translations, have confirmed that reoviruses contain 10 distinct genome segments.

Because they are commonly isolated as discrete units, the 10 genome segments are thought to take this form within reovirus particles. Nevertheless, reports of longer-than-segment-length dsRNA molecules released from reovirus particles under certain conditions (141,185,190, 233) might indicate that the genome segments are linked end to end within particles, either noncovalently or through a covalent interaction that is usually broken when the particles are disrupted. Relevance of the form of the genome segments within particles to plus-strand RNA synthesis is discussed later.

As mentioned earlier, the 10 genome segments are routinely distinguishable on polyacrylamide gels, and purified virions contain equimolar quantities of the 10 species (428). Homologous segments from different isolates commonly exhibit differences in their electrophoretic mobilities (370), despite having the same or very similar sequence lengths. The numbering scheme standardly used for the genome segments within each size class reflects the relative migrations in Tris-acetate polyacrylamide gels of the segments from isolate type 3 Dearing (419). Once the segments' protein-coding capacities were determined (302,332), this numbering scheme became meaningfully applicable to all isolates. For example, the genome segment that encodes the core turret protein λ2 is always designated to be L2, because that is the case for type 3 Dearing using the standard gel systems. It is important to recognize, however, that with changes in gel system, the order of genome segments within each size class can change; for example, the medium segments of type 3 Dearing migrate in the order M1-M2-M3 in Tris-acetate gels, but M2-M1-M3 in Tris-glycine gels (373). In addition, homologous genome segments from different isolates can show different orders of migration; for example, the small segments of type 3 Dearing migrate in the order S1-S2-S3-S4, but those of type 1 Lang migrate in the order S1-S2-S4-S3 (373). Last, different genome segments from the same size class can comigrate in certain cases, giving the appearance of nine or fewer segments.

The fact that reoviruses have segmented genomes has important biological and experimental consequences because of the phenomenon of genome segment reassortment. Differences in the electrophoretic migration of genome segments from two parental viruses used for coinfection provide a simple means for determining the parental origin of each genome segment in a reassortant virus (332,373,419). Differences in electrophoretic migration of the viral proteins and restriction fragment length polymorphisms defined using DNA copies of the genome segments have also been used in confirming the genotypes of reassortant viruses (346).

Modifications Including the 5′ Cap

Each reovirus genome segment has an identical blocking group at the 5′ end of its plus strand: a dimethylated cap 1 structure like that formed on cellular mRNA precursors by cell nuclear enzymes (91,166, 313) (Fig. 1). In the case of the reovirus plus-strand RNAs, how-

```
   m7   m2′
    \     \
5′  GpppGpCpUpA------pUpCpApUpC-OH  3′
         :  :  :  :           :  :  :  :  :
3′   HO-CpGpApUp------ApGpUpApGpp   5′
```

FIG. 1. Conserved features of reovirus dsRNA genome segment termini. Both plus (*top*) and minus (*bottom*) strands are shown. Nucleosides are shown in *bold. Dashes* in strand interiors indicate nucleotides that vary in number and sequence from segment to segment. *Colons* represent base-pairing.

ever, the cap is formed by viral enzymes within viral particles (165,168). The cap is important for efficient protein translation from the free plus-strand RNAs (61,333) because of recognition by cellular translation initiation factor eIF-4E, and it enhances the stability of the free plus-strand RNAs by protecting them from 5′ exonucleases (164). In the reovirus life cycle, the cap may also be important for packaging into viral particles and/or minus-strand synthesis, because plus-strand RNAs either lacking a 5′ cap or containing a 5′ cap 2 structure (with a third methyl group added by a cell cytoplasmic enzyme) are found in large amounts in reovirus-infected cells but are not found in viral particles (121,166,313).

The 5′ end of each genomic minus strand is thought to be an unblocked diphosphate (25,91) (see Fig. 1); however, the resistance of this terminus to labeling with polynucleotide kinase provides some evidence for blockage by an unknown structure (313). The presence of a diphosphate at the minus-strand 5′ end, and not a triphosphate as would be initially present following minus-strand synthesis from nucleoside triphosphate precursors, probably reflects the activity of an RNA triphosphate phosphohydrolase within reovirus particles (25,91). As stated earlier, both 3′ termini of each genomic dsRNA segment take the form of unblocked hydroxyl groups (312) (see Fig. 1). Other modifications to the genomic ribonucleotides, such as methylation or deamination, have not been demonstrated.

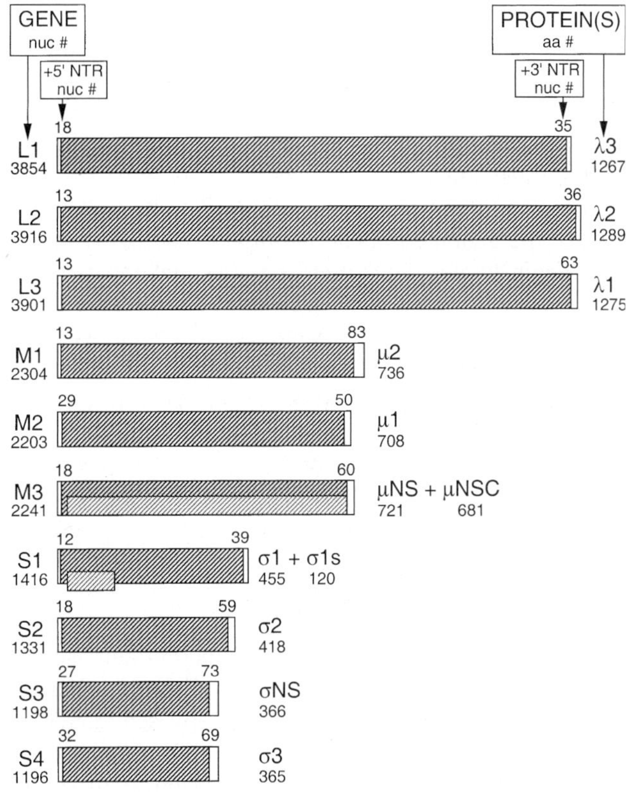

FIG. 2. Coding strategies of the 10 genome segments of reovirus type 3 Dearing. Segments are drawn approximately to scale and are oriented so that left-to-right corresponds to 5′-to-3′ for the protein-coding plus strands. The segment names and lengths in nucleotides (*nuc #*) are listed at *left.* The portion of each segment encompassed by protein-coding sequences is *hatched.* Short nontranslated regions (*NTR*) at the ends of each segment remain unshaded, and the lengths of these regions in nucleotides (*nuc #*) are designated above. Names of encoded proteins and their lengths in amino acids (*aa #*) are listed at *right.* The S1 segment encodes two proteins as shown: The σ1s protein (*offset, lighter hatching*) initiates at a second initiator codon in a different reading frame from σ1 (*darker hatching*). A second protein, μNSC (*lighter hatching*) also arises from the M3 segment, but it is thought to initiate at a second initiator codon in the same reading frame as μNS (*darker hatching*).

Sequence-Based Features

Sequence Determinations

Initial sequence determinations were of terminal regions of the reovirus genome segments and mRNAs (12,170). Subsequent full-length determinations were made directly from genome-derived RNA strands using reverse transcriptase as the sequencing enzyme (31,120), from one or more cloned DNA copies of the segments (26,77,189,213, 235,335,414,503,505,506), or from DNA copies of the segments obtained by reverse transcriptase-polymerase chain reaction (RT-PCR) without subsequent cloning (198,303). A complete genome sequence has been determined for prototype isolate type 3 Dearing and encompasses a total of about 23,500 bp (506). Lengths of the individual genome segments from this isolate range from 3,916 bp for L2, to 1,196 bp for S4 (Fig. 2). Nearly complete genome sequences have also been determined for prototype isolates type 1 Lang and type 2 Jones. The lengths of individual genome segments of type 1 Lang and type 2 Jones are either identical or very similar (give or take four nucleotides) to those of type 3 Dearing, except for the S1 genome segment, which encodes the serotype-determining and receptor-binding protein σ1 and has lengths of 1,463, 1,440, and 1,416 bp in type 1 Lang, type 2 Jones, and type 3 Dearing, respectively. Several genes from other reovirus isolates have been sequenced as well.

Protein-Coding Strategies and Nomenclature

Proteins encoded by the 10 reovirus genome segments can be resolved by electrophoresis on different types of sodium dodecyl sulfate (SDS)-polyacrylamide gels (30,93,100,105,370,449,531). Twelve primary translation products are currently known, with eight genome segments coding for one protein each, and two coding for two each (see Fig. 2). Eight of the 12 proteins (λ1, λ2, λ3, μ1, μ2, σ1, σ2, and σ3) are structural—that is, present within mature reovirus particles—whereas four (μNS, μNSC, σNS, and σ1s) are nonstructural and are thought to mediate functions during the intracellular steps in reovirus replication. Genetic analyses with reassortant viruses (332) and *in vitro* translation of isolated mRNAs (302) were used to determine which proteins are encoded by each of the gene segments.

The names of the reovirus proteins include Greek letter designations for proteins of large (λ), medium (μ), and small (σ) size classes. Each protein is encoded by a genome segment of the corresponding size class. However, the numbering scheme does not always correspond between proteins and their encoding genome segments. For example, although the second most slowly migrating genome segment L2 encodes the second most slowly migrating protein λ2 in the standard gels, the third most slowly migrating genome segment L3 encodes the most slowly migrating protein λ1 (see Fig. 2). There are several reasons for these discrepancies, including (a) that the numbers were first assigned to the proteins of reovirus type 3 Dearing according to their relative electrophoretic migrations in a standard phosphate-urea gel system (449) before the protein-coding capacities of the genome segments were determined, and (b) that the two low-copy structural proteins λ3 and μ2, as well as the four nonstructural proteins, were identified and named later than the others. In addition, the names of some proteins have been changed over time; for example, nonstructural protein μNS was originally called μ0 (531). Nevertheless, the protein names and their attribution to particular genome segments are now standardly defined as in Figure 2.

Each reovirus genome segment is transcribed end to end by enzymes within viral transcriptase particles to yield full-length, plus-strand copies that serve as mRNAs. Each mRNA includes one long open reading frame (ORF) that spans almost the whole length of the plus-strand sequence. In each case, this long ORF encodes a predicted protein that approximates the size of the larger protein attributed to that segment (see Fig. 2). In addition, the long ORF in each plus strand begins with an AUG that is protected from RNase degradation upon the binding of ribosomes (249). Reovirus translation is generally consistent with the scanning model for eukaryotic translation initiation. The AUG at the beginning of the long ORF in each plus strand is thus almost always the 5′-most AUG in the RNA sequence and is consistently located within an excellent to reasonable context for translation initiation according to the eukaryotic consensus (248). Some of the differences in translational efficiency among the reovirus plus-strand RNAs (169) may be attributable to differences in approximating this consensus, although other determinants are probably also important (see later). The S1 genome segment is unique in encoding a second protein product, σ1s, in a separate but overlapping ORF from the larger product σ1 (145,218,404). The initiation codon for σ1s translation is the first out-of-frame AUG within the σ1 ORF (29,78,328,335). The start codons for the σ1 and σ1s ORFs are separately protected from RNase degradation upon binding of ribosomes (246). The M3 gene segment also encodes a second protein, μNSC, but in this case translation appears to start from the second or third in-frame AUG within the same ORF as μNS (303,503). Important sequence determinants for translation from these downstream start codons in S1 and M3 remain to be fully defined (see later). Additional small ORFs are found in all reovirus genes, but evidence for their translation in cells is lacking. There is also no evidence that proteins are translated from the minus RNA strands of reovirus, consistent with the fact that free minus strands are not released into the cytoplasm as part of the replication cycle (410).

Terminal Nontranslated Regions

Nontranslated regions at the 5′ and 3′ ends of the reovirus plus strands (outside the boundaries of the long ORF in each) represent only a small part of the genome (see Fig. 2). The lengths of the 5′ nontranslated regions range from 12 (S1 and L2 genome segments from certain isolates) to 32 (S4 genome segment) nucleotides. As shown for other eukaryotic mRNAs, such variations in length of the 5′ nontranslated regions in the reovirus plus strands may affect their relative translational efficiencies (385). The 3′ nontranslated regions range from 32 (L1 genome segment) to 80 (M1 genome segment from certain isolates) nucleotides. Among homologous genome segments from different isolates, lengths of the nontranslated sequences are often, but not always, conserved (135,303).

The plus strands of all genome segments analyzed to date contain the extreme 5′ tetranucleotide 5′-GCUA and the extreme 3′ pentanucleotide UCAUC-3′ (12) (see Fig. 1). In addition, longer regions of sequences near the ends of the genome segments, extending through the nontranslated regions and into the protein-coding regions, are often less variable between isolates than more internal sequences (87,189,235). Sequences near the 5′ and 3′ ends of the reovirus plus strands also show a propensity to form base pairs in RNA secondary structure predictions, suggesting that these regions may interact in the free plus strands to form panhandle-like structures that may be important for RNA functions (87,274,526). Though a minimal portion of the genome, the nontranslated regions are likely to include sequences important for RNA packaging, recognition by the viral RNA polymerase for initiating plus- and minus-strand synthesis, and translational efficiency; however, the exact sequences that fulfill these functions have yet to be delimited for reoviruses.

PARTICLES

Virions and Partially Uncoated Derivatives

The mature reovirus virion contains all eight viral structural proteins (Fig. 3), but it is not known to contain any of the viral nonstructural proteins or any cellular pro-

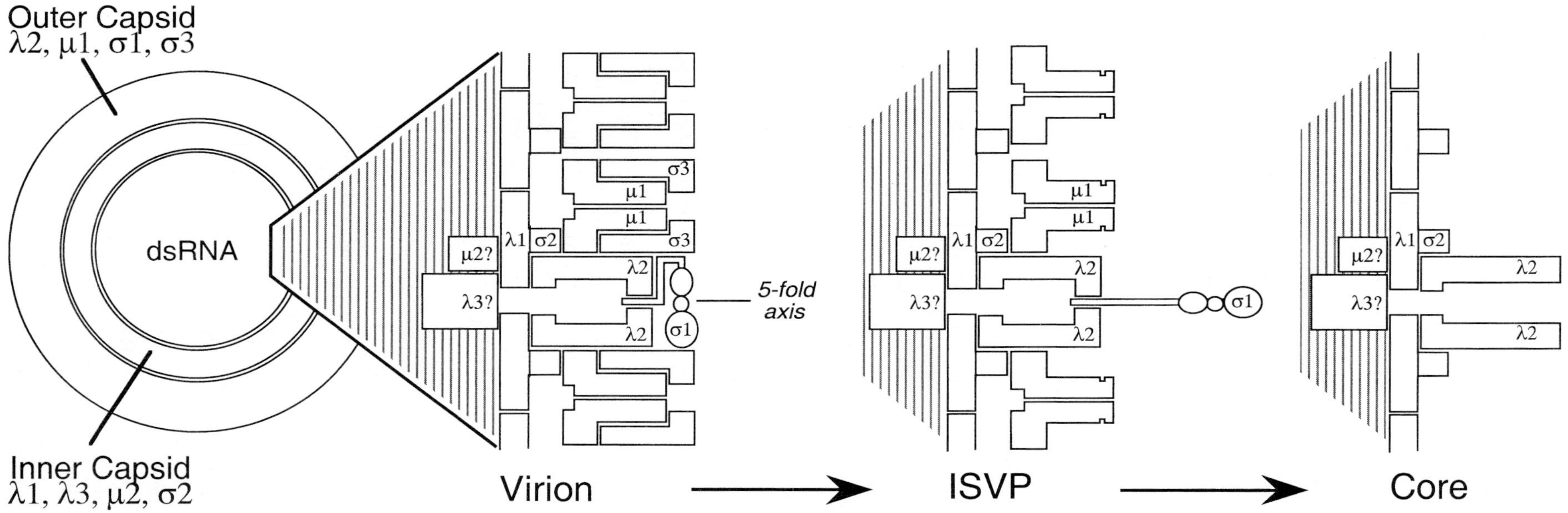

FIG. 3. Diagrams of reovirus structural elements. The two concentric capsids and centrally located dsRNA genome in reovirus virions are drawn in cross-section at *left.* Proteins in the outer capsid and inner capsid are designated. A wedge of the virion capsids, encompassing an axis of fivefold symmetry (labeled), is drawn in greater detail and shows approximate locations and interactions between reovirus proteins (labeled) as currently understood. Positions of open or potential channels through the outer capsid at axes of fivefold (P1) or sixfold (P2 and P3) symmetry are indicated (nomenclature from ref. 310). The position and interaction indicated for the λ3 and μ2 proteins are hypothetical. The position of the nonextended σ1 protein in virions is also hypothetical. Comparable wedges from a reovirus infectious subvirion particle (ISVP) and core are shown at *right* and reveal the loss and change in conformation of outer capsid proteins in these particle forms. The ISVP is distinguished by absence of the σ3 protein, by an endoproteolytically cleaved μ1 protein (*notching*), and by a conformationally altered (extended) σ1 protein. The core is distinguished by additional absence of the μ1 and σ1 proteins and by a conformationally altered λ2 protein. The conformational change in λ2 and loss of σ1 have opened a channel through the λ2 "turret" that protrudes from the core surface.

teins. The virion is the predominant form of particle released from infected cells in culture or animals or after artificial disruption of infected cell cultures in the laboratory. Virions can readily undergo partial uncoating to yield two distinct types of subvirion particles: infectious (or intermediate) subvirion particles (ISVPs) (51,223, 425) and cores (298,426,449). These subvirion particles differ in protein content, in the conformation of certain proteins, and in other physicochemical and biological properties (Table 3, and see Fig. 3). The primary difference between ISVPs and virions is the lack of one outer capsid protein, σ3, in ISVPs. The primary difference between cores and virions is the lack, in cores, of three outer capsid proteins: σ3, σ1, and μ1. ISVPs and cores can be routinely generated by treating virions with purified proteases *in vitro*. ISVPs and cores, or particles similar to these forms, also occur naturally in the course of infection and play specific roles in both early and later stages of reovirus replication (see later section). Some authors have discussed "subviral particles" (SVPs), in which case they are usually describing ISVP-like particles (16,84,440,443).

A representative study in which all three of the preceding particle types were compared by negative-stain electron microscopy indicated diameters of 73 nm for virions, 64 nm for ISVPs, and 51 nm for cores (51). Diameters obtained from cryoelectron micrographs, in which shrinkage artifacts common to negative staining (200) are minimal, were 85, 80, and 60 nm for virions (excluding the σ1 fiber), ISVPs (excluding the σ1 fiber), and cores (excluding the λ2 turrets), respectively (131,310). The latter values concur with those obtained by low-angle x-ray diffraction (199). Virions, ISVPs, and cores exhibit distinct morphologies in negative-stain electron micrographs (51,109,163,238,278,298,309,449,478). Virions appear roughly spheroidal, with smooth perimeters, except for flattened areas that are apparent in certain orientations. Few details of subunit arrangement are apparent in negatively stained virions. ISVPs appear even more spheroidal than virions; furthermore, regions of their perimeters often have a saw-toothed appearance suggesting structural subunits (μ1 protein). Long fibers (σ1 protein) are sometimes seen extending from the surfaces of virions and ISVPs (163). Negatively stained cores are more distinctive in that they have prominent turrets (λ2 protein) protruding from their surfaces.

Radial and Axial Distributions of Proteins Within Particles

Observations from negative-stain electron micrographs first defined reovirus virions as icosahedrally symmetrical objects comprising two radially concentric, separable protein shells (inner capsid and outer capsid) surrounding the centrally condensed RNA genome (109,278,298, 478). The description of two radially differentiated protein layers within reovirus virions was supported by data from dynamic light scattering (200) and low-angle x-ray diffraction (199). The latter studies also showed the outer capsid to be substantially thicker than the inner capsid and to have a higher water content. Some of these early studies suggested axial differentiation of proteins within

TABLE 3. *Characteristics of common reovirus particle forms*

Feature or property	Virion	ISVP	Core
Buoyant density in CsCl (g/cm^3)	1.36	1.38	1.43
Sedimentation value (S)	730	630	470
Molecular weight (MDa)			
From diffusion coefficient	130	ND	52
Estimated from components	127	103	49
Particles per mL at 1 OD_{260} (× 10^{12})	2.1	2.7	4.4
Diameter (nm)			
Negative-stain electron microscopy	73	64	51
Cryoelectron microscopy	85	80	60
Low-angle x-ray diffraction	83	ND	60
Outer capsid proteins			
σ3	Present	Absent (degraded)	Absent (degraded)
σ1	Present	Present as conformer (extended)	Absent (eluted)
μ1/μ1 C	Present	Present as μ1δ/δ + φ fragments	Absent (degraded)
λ2	Present	Present	Present as conformer
Inner capsid proteins	Present	Present	Present
10 dsRNA gene segments	Present	Present	Present
Oligonucleotides	Present	Variable	Absent
Infectivity after attachment to cell surface	High	High	Low
Interactions with membrane bilayers	No	Yes	No
Transcription-related activities			
Initiation and capping	Yes	Yes	Yes
Elongation	No	No	Yes

reovirus particles as well, in that the protruding turrets of λ2 protein were seen surrounding the fivefold axes in cores (298,426,449,500) and, somewhat later, the projecting fibers of σ1 protein were seen to extend from the fivefold axes in certain virions and ISVPs (22,161,163). Evidence for extrusion of the viral plus-strand transcripts from the fivefold axes of actively transcribing cores supported the notion of axial differentiation of proteins and their associated functions (27,516).

Components of Viral Particles

Early studies used negative-stain electron microscopy to describe the precise arrangements of proteins and their symmetry relationships within the reovirus capsids. These studies, although accurate in several details for the outer capsid (238,309), were largely superseded by ones using cryoelectron microscopy and three-dimensional image analysis (130,131,310). An analysis of the structure of cores at 3.6 Å resolution using x-ray crystallography has recently defined the inner capsid structure in much greater detail (378). Information about each structural protein, in addition to that immediately following, can be found in the Proteins section.

Core Components

T=1 Core Shell

The core shell (inner shell in virions) is formed by 120 copies of the λ1 protein. The λ1 subunits are arranged with T=1 symmetry, with a parallel dimer of λ1 composing the asymmetric unit. Five of these asymmetric units, containing a total of 10 λ1 subunits, surround each icosahedral fivefold axis in the core. Twelve of these decameric units of λ1 then interact to form the complete core shell. This shell is flat and thin but approximately continuous, being permeated by small, radially directed channels at only a few positions including the fivefold axes (378). Such channels are seemingly required to allow entrance of ribonucleoside triphosphates and exit of newly synthesized mRNAs during transcription by cores (see later). The two λ1 subunits per asymmetric unit have similar, but nonidentical, structures, which allows them to pack tightly within the decamers and intact shell. Five copies of λ1 from each decamer approach the fivefold axis and interact with each other around it. The other five copies of λ1 from each decamer approach the five surrounding threefold axes and interact with the homologous copies of λ1 from adjacent decamers in the shell. An N-terminal region of λ1 was not fully visualized in core crystals, but the portions of it that were visualized are located internal to the main core shell, they assume an extended conformation, and appear attributable to the copies of λ1 that approach the threefold axes (378). Thus, an N-terminal region (240 amino acids) of the copies of λ1 that approach the fivefold axes remains to be placed in the core structure.

Internal Transcriptase Complexes

A proteinaceous structure internal to the λ1 shell has been visualized to date only at lower resolution by cryoelectron microscopy and x-ray crystallography (130,378). This structure has a flower-like appearance and projects below the shell by 65 Å (central stalk) to 80 Å (surrounding petals) at each of the 12 fivefold axes. Biochemical evidence suggests that it, or other poorly visualized internal structures, are formed in whole or part by an N-terminal region of λ1 and the two low copy number core proteins λ3 (12 copies) and μ2 (12 to 24 copies) (130). Functions assigned to these proteins through other studies (see later) have led to the proposal that these complexes represent the viral transcriptase complexes, which transcribe the genomic dsRNA segments into mRNAs (see later). Additional work is needed to define the structures of these complexes in more detail.

External Turrets and Nodules

Sitting directly atop the λ1 shell are two other core proteins: λ2 and σ2. A pentamer of λ2 forms each of the 12 characteristic turret-like structures or "spikes" that project by more than 100 Å above the λ1 shell on the core surface, surrounding the fivefold axes (a total of 60 λ2 subunits per particle). The individual monomers of λ2 within each pentamer are identical and exhibit an extended, multidomain structure (378). Each monomer spirals around the fivefold axis, enclosing a large solvent cavity within the center of the turret and giving the turret walls an interlocking structure. Three domains in each monomer, including the one λ2 domain that contacts λ1, represent enzymes involved in mRNA capping (see later). The catalytic pockets of these enzymatic domains face into the central cavity of each pentameric turret. A channel through the base of the turret connects the fivefold channel through the λ1 shell (see earlier) with the turret cavity and is very likely important for the movement of nascent transcripts. The opening at the top of the λ2 turret exhibits variable diameter in different visualizations of cores, as determined by different orientations of a series of outermost, apparently nonenzymatic, flaplike domains of λ2 (131,281,310,378). A more closed conformation of these flaps may be important for retaining nascent transcripts inside the turret for capping (378), whereas a more open conformation may be important for release of the transcripts after capping is complete (27,378,516). Specific mechanisms for regulating these conformational changes remain unknown. In virions and ISVPs, however, the flaps uniformly adopt a more closed conformation (130,131,310). The closed conformation may be important for the capacity of λ2 to bind the σ1 fiber protein at the fivefold axes (see later).

Monomers of σ2 form the 150 ovoid nodules that sit atop the λ1 shell and decorate the core surface at the twofold axes and surrounding the threefold and fivefold axes (131,310,378). Each of the 60 copies surrounding the fivefold axes makes a minor contact with one λ2 subunit. The 60 near-fivefold and 60 near-threefold copies of σ2 have similar, but nonidentical, structures, allowing them to make distinct contacts with the underlying λ1 molecules. The 30 twofold copies of σ2 were only partially resolved at high resolution in the crystal structure of cores, because they can adopt either of two equivalent, twofold symmetrical orientations at each of these positions. Each twofold copy of σ2 appears to make minor contacts with surrounding near-fivefold and near-threefold copies of the protein. Because each σ2 copy appears to make contacts with λ1 across subunit boundaries within the λ1 shell, σ2 is proposed to serve as a stabilizing clamp for that shell (378).

Although they are core proteins and thus classically identified as components of the inner capsid, proteins λ2 and σ2 occupy structural positions that are clearly distinct from those of the core shell protein λ1. They sit atop the λ1 shell, at radial positions between the core shell and the T=13 outer shell (see later). In fact, the extended conformation of λ2 allows it to extend upward into the outer capsid lattice and to occupy positions within the outer lattice surrounding each fivefold axis (see later). Thus, it is possible to describe σ2 and the bottom, λ1-binding domain of λ2 (see earlier) as forming an incomplete, intermediate protein layer in reovirus particles, which separates the T=1 core shell and T=13 outer shell and is probably important for interactions between them. By extending up into the outer shell, λ2 may be especially important for holding the two shells together.

Outer Capsid

T=13 Outer Shell

The reovirus outer capsid layer has been analyzed using a number of different styles of electron microscopy. The results of these studies agree that the outer shell has subunits arranged in a skewed, T=13 (laevo) lattice (131,238,309,310). The lattice is formed primarily by 600 molecules of protein μ1. The stoichiometry of μ1 fails to account for 180 of the expected 780 (13 × 60) subunits in a classical T=13 structure. The remaining positions are occupied instead by 60 molecules of protein λ2, which substitute for μ1 around each fivefold axis such that one molecule of λ2 occupies three of the μ1 subunit positions. This lattice exhibits a very similar structure in virions and ISVPs, except that in virions the σ3 protein is also present (see later).

The μ1 protein appears to be organized in trimeric complexes within virions and ISVPs (131,238,309). The trimers are most apparent at higher axial radii in ISVPs, where adjacent trimers make contact across local twofold axes (131). At lower radii, other intertrimer contacts are seen, giving μ1 a structure that interlocks across the outer capsid. Because the μ1 network is substituted around each fivefold axis by λ2, not all μ1 subunits are in identical positions. The copies of μ1 adjacent to λ2 appear to contact that protein directly. Only some of the 600 μ1 subunits appear to be in proper position to contact the σ2 nodules projecting from the surface of the core.

The mass of μ1 and σ3 is arranged around large solvent channels that pass axially through the outer capsid (131,310). Two different types of channels are present because of substitution by λ2 around the fivefold axes. The two channel types are designated P2 and P3 and range in diameter from 2.5 to 11 nm at different axial radii in ISVPs. Each P2 channel is partially blocked by a λ2 subunit. The diameters of both P2 and P3 channels are decreased at higher radii in virions by the presence of σ3 (see later). The purpose of these channels is not known, but they may be required for conformational changes in μ1 involved in membrane penetration (see later).

An observation that the μ1 and σ3 proteins bind to each other in solution (83,260,437,471) is reflected in intimate contacts between these proteins within the virion outer capsid (131). Difference maps between images of virions and ISVPs permit densities to be attributed specifically to σ3 and suggest that each σ3 subunit is elongated in an axial direction. The σ3 subunits project 34 Å above the outer extent of μ1 and look like "fingers" on the virion surface (131,310). Each copy of σ3 appears to contact as many as three adjacent μ1 subunits and may in this way serve to stabilize the outer capsid structure. Six and four subunits of σ3 are placed around the perimeters of the P3 and P2 channels, respectively, and appear to contact each other side to side to form complete and partial hexamers. Because of the presence of λ2, not all σ3 subunits are in identical positions. One of the σ3 copies adjacent to each λ2 subunit appears to contact that protein directly.

The arrangement of μ1 in virions and ISVPs exhibits only minor differences (131,219), despite the fact that μ1 has undergone an additional endoproteolytic cleavage in ISVPs. Thus, the major difference between these two particle types is the loss of 600 σ3 subunits without a major perturbation of underlying structures in the outer capsid or core regions. This observation contributes to an interpretation that the primary contacts within the outer shell are made among subunits of μ1 and λ2, while σ3 effectively decorates this lattice. However, only μ1 in complex with σ3 appears to be competent for assembly into the outer shell (83,437).

Extending Fibers

In negatively stained images of some virions and ISVPs, σ1 is seen as a long fiber that projects out more than 40 nm from the particle surface (131,163). The spacing of these fibers suggests location at the fivefold axes, as does work with antibodies indicating that σ1 and λ2 are in close proximity within virions (202,260). Small portions from near the base of the σ1 fiber are all that is standardly visualized by cryoelectron microscopy and three-dimensional reconstruction of virions and ISVPs (130,131,310), probably because of the flexible nature of these fibers. The placement of σ1 atop λ2 is further supported by a recent study demonstrating the absence of σ1-attributed density in a cryoelectron microscopy reconstruction of cores that have been "recoated" *in vitro* with the μ1 and σ3 proteins, but not σ1 (83). The σ1 fibers seen extending from particles in raw micrographs (131,163) have a head-and-tail morphology, with the head distal to the particle-bound end. The extreme base of the tail is proposed to interact with λ2, at a binding site created by five λ2 subunits. Because each σ1 fiber most likely represents a homotrimer of that protein (see later), binding of σ1 to λ2 appears to involve a three-to-five symmetry mismatch. Some evidence suggests that σ1 can also assume a less extended conformation in virions (131,163), but the nature of this alternative conformation remains undefined. Different conformations of σ1 may be important for its roles in mediating binding to cell surface receptors (see later). The σ1 protein appears to be lost from cores by elution following conformational changes in the outermost flaplike domains of λ2 (131).

RNA Components

Centrally Condensed dsRNA

Low-angle x-ray diffraction, cryoelectron microscopy, and x-ray crystallography all indicate that the genomic dsRNA is found in reovirus particles within a central sphere, about 49 nm in diameter, and that it is well ordered so that adjacent helices are locally parallel and separated by distances of 25 to 27 Å (131,199,378). Regions of local disorder in the parallel packing scheme are expected to permit the RNA to pack into the available space. Given the measured interhelix distances and the size of the 10 genome segments, calculations indicate that the central cavity should provide just enough room to accommodate the total genome (341). Thus, large quantities of protein are unlikely to be bound to the packaged dsRNA, consistent with other observations. An additional conclusion is that random packaging of more than 10 segments per particle is an unlikely explanation for the high ratio of particles to plaque-forming units (pfu) in reoviruses. The arrangement of the genomic dsRNA has relevance to the mechanism of reovirus transcription (see later). The dispositions of the segment ends are unknown, but the end containing the 3′ end of the minus strand is expected to be bound by the RNA polymerase to permit efficient onset of transcription upon entry of the particle into cells.

Oligonucleotides

About 25% of the RNA in purified virions is in the form of small, single-stranded oligonucleotides (37, 427), which can be grouped into two major classes (34). Quantities can vary widely with conditions of virus growth, including temperature (253), as well as between virions obtained from the same purification (150). About 70% of the oligonucleotides (~2,000 copies per virion) terminate with a 5′GC(U)(A) and are two to nine residues long (35,38,348). The conserved 5′ sequences suggest that these are the products of abortive transcription. They are often termed initiator oligonucleotides, and those packaged into virions are generated in the final stages of morphogenesis (38,151). Oligoadenylates constitute a second major class of oligonucleotides, which are two to 20 residues long and present in about 850 copies per virion (34,348,462). Like the initiator oligonucleotides, they appear to result from an alternative activity of the viral transcriptase and are also generated in the final stages of morphogenesis (532). Whereas virions contain both classes of oligonucleotides, cores lack them (73,151,223,425,449). Whether oligonucleotides are present in ISVPs is controversial (84,223,425). Their exact locations within virions remain unknown (199). Functions of the oligonucleotides are also unknown, but there is evidence that they are not required for infectivity (73,151).

Molecular Weights

Molecular weights for virions and cores of reovirus type 3 Dearing were determined from diffusion coefficients to be 129.5 and 52.3 megadaltons (MDa), respectively (150). The total weight of the genomic RNA is calculated to be 15.1 MDa from sequences of the 10 genome segments of this isolate. Oligonucleotides are estimated to contribute another 5 MDa to the weight of virions (348). Thus, proteins are expected to contribute roughly 109 and 37 MDa (85% and 70% of totals) to the molecular weights of virions and cores, respectively. These weights correspond well with those obtained by calculation from sequence-predicted masses of the proteins and current estimates for their copy numbers in particles (see Table 3). Similar estimates can be made for ISVPs (see Table 3). For these calculations, it was assumed that the proteins in virions are full length, given the lack of evidence for loss of mass by protein cleavage, and good correlations between molecular weights calculated from sequences and those estimated from gels. The crystal structure for the reovirus core indicates that the assembled forms of λ2 and σ2 are indeed full length (except for lacking their initiator methionines), and that the assembled form of λ1 extends to its sequence-predicted C terminus (the N terminus of λ1 was not well visualized in the crystal structure) (378).

Purification of Particles and Their Infectivities

Murine L929 cells are commonly used for plaque assay and for growing virions for purification. For purification, virions are released from cells by sonication and then dissociated from other components by treatment with deoxycholate and extraction with freon (39,128,163,223420,449) or a newer freon substitute (308). Final purification of virions is commonly achieved by centrifugation through a cesium chloride (CsCl) gradient. Values for sedimentation and buoyant density of reovirus particles are shown in Table 3 (51,150,163,449). Banded virions are dialyzed into buffer (often 150mM NaCl, 10mM $MgCl_2$, 10mM Tris, pH 7.5) for storage at 4°C, where they can remain stable and infectious for extended periods. An average yield from this procedure is 1×10^{13} virions (~about 1.8 mg) per 1×10^{8} cells. The equivalence 1 OD_{260} = 185 μg protein per mL = 2.1×10^{12} virions per mL is routinely used for estimating the concentration of purified virions (449).

Chymotrypsin is most commonly used to convert virions to ISVPs or cores *in vitro* (51,163,223,344,425,426, 449,454,467). At fixed conditions (buffer, enzyme concentration, temperature, time of treatment), the concentration of virions included in the mixture determines whether ISVPs or cores are obtained as products (51,54,57,60, 163,223). The particular conditions yielding one or the other particle form can vary between isolates (101,127, 223). ISVPs or cores generated by this treatment can be purified by centrifugation through CsCl gradients. Purified ISVPs are commonly stored in the same buffer as virions, but a different buffer (1M NaCl, 100mM MgCl2, 20mM HEPES, pH 8.0) was found to maintain cores in a nonaggregated state (101). Comparisons of protein quantities in virions and subvirion particles suggest the following equivalences: 1 OD_{260} = 2.7×10^{12} ISVPs per mL and 1 OD_{260} = 4.4×10^{12} cores per mL (100).

When purified virions are tested for infectivity by plaque assay in L cells, a particle-to-pfu ratio of from 50:1 to 500:1 is commonly obtained (14,144,226,467). The basis for this high ratio is unknown; it could reflect either that defective particles are present in the preparations or that productive infection involves a complex process that only a statistically determined subset of infectious particles can routinely complete. In a few studies, a ratio approaching 1:1 between particles and infectious units has been reported; however, these studies included special circumstances such as protease activation of viral particles and measurement of infectious units by a fluorescent focus assay (454). In general, the efficiency of infection is mildly enhanced in preparations of ISVPs, and reduced by several orders of magnitude in preparations of cores. An exception to the enhanced infectivity of ISVPs is seen with isolates type 3 Dearing and type 3 clone 31, which have a σ1 cell-attachment protein that is sensitive to protease cleavage during the generation of ISVPs and that exhibits an associated loss in infectivity (85,342).

Other Types of Icosahedral Reovirus Particles

Top Component Particles

"Empty" virions, which contain markedly reduced quantities of dsRNA gene segments and oligonucleotides, account for a large proportion of the particles purified from reovirus-infected cells (380,449). Their buoyant density is 1.29 g/cm^3, lower than that of full virions and consistent with their lack of RNA (150,163, 255,449); thus, they migrate above full virions in CsCl gradients and are called top component particles. Both their protein content and morphology are very similar to those of full virions, except that negative stains can enter their central cavity (449,500). Protease treatments of empty virions can be used to generate empty ISVPs and empty cores (130,277,449,500). Empty particles have been used in studies that address the function of reovirus proteins (196,277,416) and have provided evidence for the inwardly protruding transcriptase complexes within reovirus particles (130). The derivation of empty virions is unknown; however, they are unlikely to be precursors of full virions during morphogenesis (226). Methods for increasing the relative yields of empty virions from infected cells have been described (255).

Particle Assembly Intermediates from Infected Cells

Isolation of particles from infected cells can provide insight into reovirus assembly and other aspects of replication. Gradient fractionation of assembly intermediates from infected cells tentatively identified distinct particle populations engaged in minus-strand RNA synthesis (replicase particles) and plus-strand RNA synthesis (transcriptase particles) (323). The latter particles were found to represent cores that are associated with variable amounts of the nonstructural protein μNS (323,532). Particles obtained from infections with temperature-sensitive (ts) or other assembly-restricted mutants are useful for identifying putative assembly intermediates that accumulate behind the restrictive block. Core-like particles that accumulate at nonpermissive temperature with ts group B and G mutants provide evidence for generation of the core as a central intermediate in virion morphogenesis (322). Similarly, particles containing core proteins λ1, λ3, and σ2, but lacking other core components, have been shown to accumulate at nonpermissive temperature with one L2-segment ts mutant and have been proposed to suggest a role for this particle type in core assembly (204).

Particles Assembled In Whole or In Part from Recombinant Proteins

Coexpression of subsets of recombinant reovirus core proteins in HeLa cells using vaccinia virus vectors has resulted in production of empty core-like particles containing the following proteins: λ1 and σ2; λ1, λ2, and σ2; λ1, λ3, and σ2; and λ1, λ2, λ3, and σ2 (513). The minimal protein complement for core-like particle assembly in this system thus appears to be λ1 and σ2. These findings provide evidence for packaging of λ3 independently of λ2. Additional assemblies of core protein μ2, outer capsid proteins, or viral RNA in this type of system have not yet been reported.

ISVPs and cores, generated from virions by *in vitro* protease treatment and then purified, can serve as platforms for *in vitro* assembly of the missing outer capsid proteins. This process, recently termed recoating (219), was first indicated by the binding to ISVPs of σ3 from infected cells (16). A subsequent study using *in vitro* translated, recombinant σ3 demonstrated its feasibility for more controlled studies (430). The recent study demonstrates that approximately full levels of baculovirus-expressed recombinant σ3 can be bound to ISVPs *in vitro*, yielding recoated particles that are very similar to virions in a large number of structural and biological properties (219). The recoating approach has also been extended to cores, to which baculovirus-expressed recombinant μ1 and σ3 proteins, or μ1, σ3, and σ1 proteins, can be bound (83,151). The utility of this general approach lies not only in its capacity to address the structure and assembly of the reovirus outer capsid but also in the fact that the resulting particles demonstrate infectivity properties attributable to the *in vitro* assembled proteins (see later). Another variation to this approach involves the binding of nonstructural protein μNS to cores (66), yielding particles that appear to mimic transcriptase particles isolated from infected cells (323).

PROTEINS

The eight species of viral proteins in mature reovirus virions (structural proteins) have particle-based functions that are critical to initiation of infection and synthesis of the capped viral mRNAs (Table 4). These same proteins may also play regulatory or other "nonstructural" roles within the infected cell. General characteristics and functions of these proteins are discussed later. The five core proteins (λ1, λ2, λ3, μ2, and σ2) are described first, followed by descriptions of the three additional proteins in the virion outer capsid (μ1, σ1, and σ3). Examination of proteins in reovirus-infected cells initially revealed two other virally encoded proteins that are not present in mature virions (nonstructural proteins) and that are now called μNS and σNS (531). A smaller form of μNS, called μNSC, is also found in infected cells (260). Nucleotide sequencing (29,78,246,328,335) plus *in vitro* translation of viral mRNAs and comparison with proteins from reovirus-infected cells (80,145,218,404) identified an additional nonstructural protein, σ1s (227), encoded by the second ORF in the S1 genome segment. All four nonstructural proteins are discussed in detail later (see Table 4).

Structural Proteins in the Core

λ1

The λ1 protein (142 kd, 1,275 amino acids) is the primary constituent of the core shell (296,500,513) and is present in 120 copies per particle (100,378). In recombi-

TABLE 4. *Reovirus proteins*

Encoding segment	Protein	Mass (kd)	Copy no. per virion	Location in virions	Presence in particle forms[a]	Function or property
L1	λ3	142	12	Inner capsid	V, I, C	RNA-dependent RNA polymerase
L2	λ2	145	60	Outer capsid, core spike	V, I, C	Guanylyltransferase, methyltransferases
L3	λ1	143	120	Inner capsid	V, I, C	Binds RNA, Zn metalloprotein, NTPase?, RNA helicase?, RNA triphosphatase?
M1	μ2	83	20	Inner capsid	V, I, C	Binds RNA, NTPase?
M2	μ1	76	600	Outer capsid	V, I	N-myristoylated, cleaved into fragments, role in penetration, role in transcriptase activation
M3	μNS	80	0	Nonstructural	—	Binds core, role in secondary transcription, probable role in RNA assortment or replication
	μNSC	75	0	Nonstructural	—	Unknown
S1	σ1	49	36	Outer capsid	V, I	Cell-attachment protein, hemagglutinin, primary serotype determinant
	σ1s	14	0	Nonstructural	—	Dispensable in cell culture
S2	σ2	47	150	Inner capsid	V, I, C	Binds dsRNA
S3	σNS	41	0	Nonstructural	—	Binds ssRNA, probable role in RNA assortment or replication
S4	σ3	41	600	Outer capsid	V	Sensitive to protease degradation, binds dsRNA, zinc metalloprotein, effects on translation

[a]V, virion; I, ISVP; C, core.

nant form, it requires coexpression with core nodule protein σ2 to assemble into icosahedral particles (513). Recombinant λ1 was also shown to interact with core turret protein λ2 and low-copy core protein λ3 (460). In native particles, λ1 has extensive contacts with σ2 and λ2 (378), and it is thought to interact with one or both of the low-copy-number core proteins, λ3 and μ2, as well (130,378). An N-terminal region of λ1 was proposed to project into the core interior based on its protease sensitivity in top component particles (130) and to be more hydrophilic and flexible than the rest of the protein based on sequence analyses (198). This N-terminal region was not fully visualized in core crystals, but the portions of it that were visualized are located internal to the main core shell and assume an extended conformation (378). The λ1 sequence contains a conserved CCHH zinc-finger motif near the junction between this N-terminal region and the rest of the protein (26,198), and λ1 was shown to bind Zn^{2+} in a blotting assay (407) and in core crystals (378). The role of the zinc finger remains unknown.

Functions of the λ1 protein are only partly understood. Recent reassortant analyses showed that the L3 genome segment encoding λ1 contributes to determining differences in the NTPase activities of cores (354,355), consistent with the presence of nucleotide-binding motifs near the λ1 N-terminus (26,44,354). Moreover, recent studies with partially purified recombinant λ1 protein showed it to possess not only NTPase activity but also RNA triphosphate phosphohydrolase and helicase activities (44,45). These findings tentatively assign λ1 to mediating the first step in mRNA capping by reovirus particles as well as to mediating RNA duplex unwinding during one or more step in reovirus plus- and/or minus-strand RNA synthesis. A conformational change in λ1 during transcription by cores was previously noted (366). Consistent with its RNA-directed enzymatic activities, the λ1 protein was shown to have an RNA binding activity (both ssRNA and dsRNA, but ssRNA preferred) that is not specific for reovirus RNA and is mediated by sequences near the N-terminus of λ1, not including the zinc finger (46,263,407). In another reassortant analysis, the L3 genome segment was shown to be a genetic determinant of isolate-dependent differences in viral yields in L cells (295).

σ2

The σ2 protein (47 kd, 418 amino acids) interacts with λ1 to form the core shell (296,500,513). Initial estimates suggested 120 or 180 σ2 copies per particle (100,449), but the recently determined core crystal structure showed that σ2 forms 150 nodule-like features that reside fully external to λ1 on the core surface (378). In addition to binding to λ1, 60 copies of σ2 in cores share a small region of interaction with λ2 (378). Furthermore, it appears likely that σ2, and not λ1 as previously inferred (306), binds to the base of major outer capsid protein μ1 in virions and plays a role in anchoring it in the particle (378).

The functions of σ2 remain poorly understood. The σ2 protein shows weak affinity for dsRNA (120,407), but the significance of this finding appears uncertain given the external location of σ2 in cores (378). In recombinant form, σ2 must be coexpressed with core shell protein λ1 for assembly of icosahedral particles to occur (513). A ts mutant whose lesion maps to the S2 genome segment encoding σ2 (373) fails to assemble particles or to synthesize dsRNA at nonpermissive temperature, suggesting a role for σ2 in one or more steps in replicase particle assembly, including RNA selection or replication (99,104,160,216,296). Selection and characterization of ts^+ revertants from this mutant showed the reversion events to be exclusively intragenic and to involve true reversion at σ2 residue 383 in all instances (99). In reassortant analyses, the S2 genome segment encoding σ2 was shown to be a genetic determinant of isolate-dependent differences in the induction of interferon α/β in cultured murine cardiac myocytes (436).

λ2

Pentamers of the λ2 protein (144 kd, 1,288 to 1,289 amino acids) form the turret-like projections that surround the fivefold axes of cores (367,500), providing a total of 60 λ2 subunits per particle (100,131,367,378). There is evidence for λ2 interactions with each of the other seven structural proteins: λ1, λ3, μ2, and σ2 in cores and μ1, σ3, and σ1 in the outer capsid of virions (83,131,202,204,306,310,378,460,500). However, the evidence for λ2 interactions with low-copy core proteins λ3 and μ2 within particles remains weak or indirect, and these interactions now seem less likely given the recent core crystal structure showing that λ2 sits fully atop the λ1 shell (378). A λ2 fragment lacking about 15 kd can represent more than 10% of the λ2 molecules in certain preparations of virions (100,260), but the significance of this fragment is unknown. It may represent cleavage and loss of a C-terminal region of λ2, as recently shown to occur *in vitro* after exposing cores to mild heat and protease (281).

The λ2 protein plays important roles in particle assembly. Some ts mutants whose lesions map to the L2 genome segment encoding λ2 (332) synthesize dsRNA and form core-like particles, but not whole virions, at nonpermissive temperature, suggesting a role for λ2 in outer capsid assembly (160,322). A small C-terminal region of λ2 appears to constitute the binding site for σ1 after a larger C-terminal portion of λ2 undergoes a structural rearrangement from its position in cores (83,131, 281,378). Another ts mutant whose lesion maps to L2 was shown to accumulate core-like particles that are deficient in λ2, the low-copy core protein μ2, and the genomic dsRNA segments at nonpermissive temperature

(204). The characteristics of these particles suggest a role for λ2 in replicase particle assembly (including RNA selection, replication, and packaging) as well as in outer capsid assembly (204). Also suggesting a role for λ2 in RNA replication or packaging was a genetic study with reassortant viruses showing that the L2 genome segment determines an isolate-dependent difference in the generation of genome segment deletions and defective interfering (DI) stocks during serial passage of reoviruses at high multiplicity of infection (MOI) (67).

The λ2 protein also mediates enzymatic activities in 5′ capping of the reovirus mRNAs. A series of studies with native and recombinant λ2 confirmed that it mediates the RNA guanylyltransferase activity in mRNA capping (93,152,279,280,286,424). Reovirus cores incubated with [α-^{32}P] GTP form covalent λ2–GMP complexes, consistent with this activity (93,152,281,424). An early study localized the GMP linkage to lysine 226 in the N-terminal half of λ2 (152), but a more recent study contested that finding and proposed lysine 190 as the linkage site (279). The latter study also showed that an N-terminal 42-kd region of recombinant λ2 is sufficient for guanylyltransferase activity. The crystal structure of reovirus cores revealed that this region constitutes an independent domain that also provides the contacts to λ1 and σ2 in cores (378).

Evidence that λ2 mediates one or both of the methyltransferase activities in mRNA capping, for which S-adenosyl-L-methionine (SAM) is the methyl donor (422), remains more indirect, as recombinant λ2 has not yet been shown to mediate these activities (279,286). This lack of activity by recombinant λ2 may reflect that it is monomeric whereas only the pentameric form of λ2 in cores may be active at methyl transfer (279,286,378). Evidence for the methyltransferase activity of λ2 includes that it is the only core protein labeled by 8-azido-SAM (414), that it includes a small central region of sequence with similarity to the SAM-binding motif of other viral and cellular methyltransferases (242), and that both λ2 in cores and recombinant λ2 bind to SAM in an ultraviolet (UV) cross-linking assay via a central region of sequence that overlaps the previously identified SAM-binding motif (242,280). Most recently, the core crystal structure revealed that a site in each of two separate domains formed by a large central region of λ2 sequence can bind to S-adenosyl-L-homocysteine, the product of methyl transfer from SAM, suggesting that these two domains represent the two capping methyltransferases (378). Which domain represents the 7-N-methyl-transferase and which the 2′-O-methyltransferase remain undefined, but the domain formed by the more C-terminal sequences, and including the previously identified SAM-binding site (242,280), is proposed to be the 2′-O-methyltransferase (378). A small region of λ2 sequence that approximates the A element of a GTP-binding motif (414) may constitute part of the RNA 5′-end binding site of one of the methyltransferases (the proposed 2′-O-methyltransferase) (378).

Conformational changes in an external portion of the λ2 turret formed by C-terminal sequences of λ2 are known to occur during generation of cores, resulting in an increase in the diameter of a channel through the top of the turret (130,131). This conformational change may be important for allowing or regulating transcript capping and release from cores (27,378,516). It may also be important for allowing σ1 loss during viral entry (83,131). The mechanism of this conformational change in λ2 and its probable regulation by other viral proteins remain poorly characterized.

In other reassortant analyses, the L2 genome segment encoding λ2 has been shown to be a genetic determinant of isolate-dependent differences in the crystallization of core particles (101), growth in enteric tissues of newborn mice after intragastric inoculation (49), transmission between newborn mice (237), growth and injury in different organs of mice with severe combined immunodeficiency disease (SCID) (194), induction of myocarditis in newborn mice (433), and induction of interferon α/β and sensitivity of viral growth to interferon α/β in cultured murine cardiac myocytes (436).

λ3

λ3 (142 kd, 1,267 amino acids) is a low-copy core protein (62,105,215), estimated to be present in only 12 copies per particle, or one copy per icosahedral fivefold axis (100). It has not been definitively localized within particles, but it was shown to be a component of the core shell that is not exposed to the core exterior (76). It is thought to be a constituent of the protein complexes that project into the interior of reovirus particles near the fivefold axes (130,378). Recombinant λ3 was shown to interact with core shell protein λ1 and core turret protein λ2 (460). It is suspected to interact with those same two proteins, and perhaps also with the other low-copy core protein μ2, within particles (130,194,433).

The functions of λ3 appear to relate to its role as a component of the reovirus RNA polymerase. A ts mutant whose lesion maps to the L1 genome segment encoding λ3 (373) is severely reduced for dsRNA synthesis (104, 216) and forms empty particles at nonpermissive temperature (160), suggesting a role for λ3 in one or more steps in replicase particle assembly including RNA selection or replication. An early reassortant study indicated that the L1 genome segment determines an isolate-dependent difference in the pH optimum of core transcription, suggesting that λ3 may be the viral transcriptase (127). A more recent reassortant study showed that L1 contributes to determining a difference in the amounts of transcripts produced by cores, consistent with the previous suggestion (519). A central portion of the deduced amino acid sequence of λ3 includes sequence motifs common to the catalytic regions of RNA polymerases (69,241,243,326). Furthermore, recombinant, purified λ3 demonstrates poly(C)-dependent poly(G) polymerase activity *in vitro* (460). These findings suggest that λ3 represents the catalytic subunit of the reovirus RNA-dependent RNA polymerase, which is likely to mediate both plus- and minus-strand RNA synthesis within reovirus particles. The L1 genome segment encoding λ3 was also shown to be a genetic determinant of isolate-dependent differences in growth in L cells and cultured mouse heart cells (295), growth in MDCK cells (383), induction of myocarditis in newborn mice (433), and growth and injury in different organs of SCID mice (194).

μ2

μ2 (83 to 84 kd, 736 amino acids) is another low-copy core protein, estimated to be present in about 20 copies per particle (100). It has not been definitively localized within particles but is thought to reside near the fivefold axes, either interior to (130,378) or within (204) the core shell and possibly contributing to the protein complexes that project into the interior of reovirus particles near the fivefold axes (130,378). It has not been demonstrated to interact with any other reovirus protein, but it was proposed to interact with the core turret protein λ2 (204), the other low-copy core protein λ3 (130,194,433), and perhaps with the core shell protein λ1 as well (130,378).

The functions of μ2 are only partly understood. Temperature-sensitive mutants with a lesion in the M1 genome segment encoding μ2 fail to synthesize dsRNA at nonpermissive temperature, suggesting a role for μ2 in one or more steps in replicase particle assembly, including RNA selection or replication (99,503). Constitutive expression of μ2 in L cells allows complementation of one of these ts mutants (527). Recombinant μ2 protein was recently shown to have an RNA-binding activity (both ssRNA and dsRNA) that is not specific for reovirus RNA (65). Recent reassortant analyses showed that the M1 genome segment encoding μ2 determines a difference in the temperature optimum of core transcription (519) and contributes to determining differences in the amounts of transcripts produced by cores (519) and the NTPase activities of cores (355). Together, these findings suggest that μ2 represents a cofactor or second subunit of the reovirus RNA polymerase. The M1 genome segment was also shown to be a genetic determinant of isolate-dependent differences in plaque size and extent of cytopathic effect in L cells (318); growth in cultured murine cardiac myocytes and bovine aortic endothelial cells (294,295); growth in MDCK cells (383); induction of myocarditis in newborn mice (433,434), levels of viral RNA synthesis, induction of interferon α/β and sensitivity of viral growth to interferon α/β in cultured murine cardiac myocytes (432,436); and growth and injury in different organs of SCID mice (194). It was hypothesized that the role of μ2 protein as a determinant of viral cytopathology may explain its low level of translation *in vivo* (388), but a higher level of μ2 expression by reovirus type 1 Lang versus type 3 Dearing was recently demonstrated (527). Most recently, μ2 was suggested to play a role in determining the rate of viral inclusion formation in reovirus-infected cells (299).

More Structural Proteins in the Outer Capsid

μ1

The μ1 protein (76 kd, 708 amino acids), together with σ3, forms the bulk of the virion outer capsid (449). It is present in virions in 600 copies, in the form of 1:1 complexes with σ3 (100,220,260). It also interacts with core proteins λ2 and σ2 in virions (131,306,378). The μ1 protein is modified by addition of a myristoyl (C_{14} saturated fatty acyl) group to its N-terminus following loss of the initiator methionine (347) (Fig. 4). In virions, most μ1 appears to occur as a 72-kd fragment, μ1C, that is generated from μ1 by proteolytic cleavage (530). N-terminal sequencing localizes this cleavage between residues 42 and 43 in μ1 (220,364), indicating that μ1C is a C-terminal fragment of μ1 (see Fig. 4). The cleavage of μ1 to μ1C also yields a 4.2-kd myristoylated N-terminal fragment, μ1N, that is retained in particles in stoichiometric amounts (347) and is quite likely the same virion component identified as component viii in earlier studies (449). The capacity of μ1 to undergo this cleavage is sensitive to the residues surrounding the μ1N–μ1C junction, and these residues are also important for determining μ1 interactions with σ3 (471). Based on sequence similarity

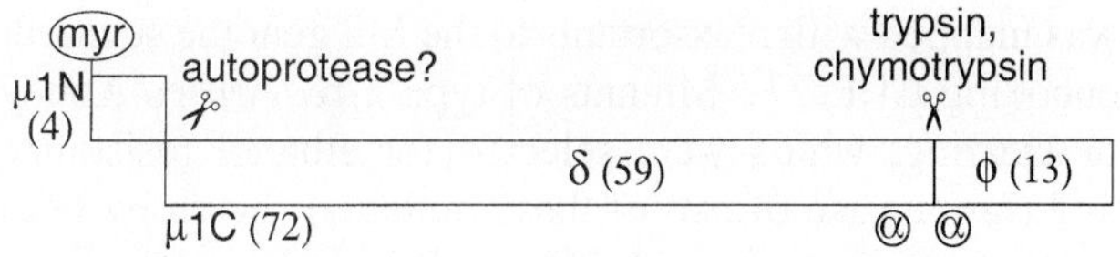

FIG. 4. Outer capsid protein μ1. Most (95%) of the μ1 protein (76 kd) in virions undergoes an assembly-related cleavage (*scissors*) into small amino-terminal and large carboxyl-terminal fragments designated μ1N (4 kd, as indicated) and μ1C (72 kd), respectively. An autoprotease activity appears to be involved in this cleavagen. The μ1N fragment (like uncleaved μ1) is modified by an amide-linked myristoyl group (*myr*), probably at its extreme amino terminus. When ISVPs are generated by the action of exogenous proteases, such as trypsin or chymotrypsin, on virion proteins, the μ1C fragment undergoes additional cleavage (*scissors*) nearer its carboxyl terminus. The products are large amino-terminal and small carboxyl-terminal fragments designated δ (59 kd) and ϕ (13 kd), respectively. The δ–ϕ cleavage junction is flanked by predicted long amphipathic α-helices (α) which are proposed to play a role in membrane interaction and penetration by reoviruses. The small amount of uncleaved μ1 protein in virions is also cleaved during generation of ISVPs to produce fragments μ1δ [μ1N + δ] and ϕ.

to the VP4–VP2 autolytic cleavage junction in the VP0 protein of enteroviruses, cleavage at the μ1N–μ1C junction is thought to be autolytic as well (347). A small amount of μ1 in virions (commonly ≤5%) appears to remain uncleaved, similar to the VP0 protein of enteroviruses. Genetic studies have implicated μ1 in determining isolate-dependent differences in the sensitivity of virions and ISVPs to inactivation with ethanol, phenol, and heat (129,208,497).

In the cytoplasm of infected cells, 90% of free M2-encoded protein is μ1, whereas 95% of the protein complexed with σ3 has been cleaved to μ1C (260). This finding suggests that the μ1N–μ1C cleavage is linked to formation of the μ1–σ3 complex. This hypothesis is further supported by studies with ts mutant viruses and mutant σ3 and μ1 molecules expressed in transfected cells (43,471). For example, μ1 expressed from an M2 genome segment that lacks the signal for myristoylation neither forms complexes with σ3 nor undergoes cleavage to μ1C (471). Several lines of evidence suggest that when σ3 and μ1 interact, both proteins undergo conformational changes that influence their functions in viral entry and assembly, respectively (430,437). μ1 interaction with σ3 also inhibits the dsRNA binding activity of the latter and thereby interferes with its translational effects, suggesting a regulatory function for μ1 prior to its assembly onto particles (471,521). Complexes of μ1 and σ3 are almost certainly the form of these proteins that is assembled onto cores in generating mature virions (83,260,430,437).

Several lines of evidence now indicate that a primary function of particle-bound μ1 is in penetration of the cellular membrane barrier during entry into cells at the onset of infection. A genetic difference in the capacity of ISVPs of reovirus isolates type 1 Lang and type 3 Abney to permeabilize membranes, causing ^{51}Cr release from L cells, was mapped with reassortants to the M2 genome segment encoding μ1 (277). Mutants of type 3 reoviruses Abney or Dearing, which were selected for ethanol resistance and (in the case of two of these mutants) shown by both reassortant analysis and M2 nucleotide sequencing to harbor resistance mutations in their μ1 proteins (208,497), show correlative changes in ISVP-mediated ^{51}Cr release and thermostability consistent with an effect of μ1-determined particle stability on membrane permeabilization (208). Certain μ1-specific monoclonal antibodies can block ISVP-mediated ^{51}Cr release from L cells at a postattachment step (207) and can also block virion-initiated infections of L cells at a step following both attachment and proteolytic processing (483). When assembled at nonpermissive temperature, virions of ts mutant A279 and also of reassortants containing the M2 genome segment of this mutant show a defect in entry into L cells characterized by accumulation of infecting particles within lysosomes (203). The strong hemolytic activity of ISVP-like particles derived from recoated core particles lacking σ1, compared with the negligible hemolytic activity of cores, implicates μ1 in this form of membrane premeabilization as well (83). A role for the N-terminal myristoyl group on μ1/μ1N in membrane penetration was proposed (347) but remains unproven. Binding of alkyl sulfate detergents to virions, with an associated block to μ1 cleavage at the δ–ϕ junction by exogenous proteases (see later), was proposed to reflect an early, reversible step in membrane binding by μ1 during entry (82).

Another function of particle-bound μ1 appears to be in regulation of the particle-bound RNA transcriptase. An isolate-dependent difference in the conditions required for conversion of virions to cores, with associated activation of the transcriptase, was mapped with reassortants to the M2 genome segment encoding μ1 (127). Biochemical studies suggest an association between loss or rearrangement of μ1 and transcriptase activation (127,146), although the precise mechanism of this effect remains undefined. The structural changes in μ1 involved in transcriptase activation may be important for membrane penetration as well.

Despite marked sequence conservation among the M2 genome segments from different reovirus isolates (208,220,505), genetic analyses with reassortant viruses have associated M2 with a number of isolate-dependent differences in viral phenotypes, including the several described earlier. In addition, the reduced neurovirulence of reovirus type 3 clone 8 after intracerebral inoculation into newborn mice was shown to be determined by its M2 genome segment (210). Interference between reovirus isolates upon co-infection of L cells was shown to be genetically determined by the M2 genome segment and to involve steps in infection following uncoating (392,394). Polymorphisms in the M2 genome segment were also linked to isolate-dependent differences in reovirus-induced apoptosis and the inhibition of DNA synthesis in cultured cells (383,475).

The μ1 and μ1C proteins undergo a distinct proteolytic cleavage near their shared C-terminus after exposure to proteases in vitro (51,220,223,344,425), within endocytic compartments of cultured cells early in infection (59,82,84,440,467), and within the intestinal lumen of newborn mice after peroral inoculation (28,50). This cleavage, which occurs after residue Tyr-581 with chymotrypsin and after residues Arg-584 with trypsin, generates a large (59 to 60 kd), acidic, N-terminal fragment named μ1δ when derived from μ1, or δ when derived from μ1C, as well as a small (12 to 13 kd), basic, C-terminal fragment named ϕ (344) (see Fig 4). The μ1δ/δ and ϕ fragments remain bound to ISVPs in stoichiometric amounts (344). The C-terminal cleavage of μ1/μ1C was previously proposed to be required for the penetration of cell membranes during viral entry (344), but the normal infectivity and hemolytic activity of ISVP-like particles in which little or no cleavage at the δ–ϕ junction has occurred strongly suggest that this is not the case (82,83).

Thus, at present, the biological significance of the δ–ϕ cleavage remains unknown. A small number of μ1/μ1C molecules remain uncleaved at the δ–ϕ junction in most or all preparations of ISVPs (100,344).

Several studies suggest that a fraction of μ1 and its fragments in virions undergo modifications in addition to myristoylation. It was reported that 2% to 4% of μ1C molecules in virions are O-glycosylated on serine or threonine residues (250). Evidence was also presented for the presence of one or more phosphoserine residues per molecule of μ1C in virions (251). It was further shown that several of the μ1C and component viii (μ1N) molecules in virions are both polyadenylated and ADP-ribosylated (75). Although cryo-electron microscopy reconstructions indicate that the μ1 protein in virions and ISVPs is centered in trimeric clusters (131), other data suggest that it is linked into disulfide-bonded dimers (211) through cysteine 679 in the ϕ portion of μ1 (220). The role(s) of this disulfide bond in assembly or infection remains unknown.

σ3

The σ3 protein (41 kd, 365 amino acids), together with μ1, forms the bulk of the virion outer capsid (449), where it interacts with proteins λ2 and μ1 and perhaps also with σ1 (131,163,261,306,310,482). It is present in virions in 600 copies and in the form of 1:1 complexes with μ1 (100,220,260). Genetic studies with reassortant viruses implicated σ3 in determining differences in the sensitivity of virions to inactivation with heat and SDS (129). In addition, by recoating ISVPs with recombinant σ3 *in vitro*, the thermostability of those particles can be increased to approximately that of virions (219). Thus, σ3 may play a role in stabilizing virions for survival in environments outside cells (345).

Balancing its stabilizing effects, the σ3 protein must be removed from virions, by proteolysis in the natural setting, for infection of cells to proceed beyond the steps of receptor binding and endocytic uptake and trafficking (19,219,467,483,499). Within cells, σ3 proteolysis is thought to occur within endocytic vacuoles, preceding penetration of viral particles into the cytoplasm, and to be predominantly mediated by acidic cysteine proteases of lysosomal origin (19,20,244,442,467). Genetic studies indicate that mutations in the S4 genome segment encoding σ3 play a critical role in the establishment and/or maintenance of persistent reovirus infections, and that this effect at least partly involves mutations in σ3 that enhance its sensitivity to proteolysis during entry into cells (6,19,499,511). Proteolytic removal of σ3 from reovirus particles also occurs in the lumen of the small intestine during infection of newborn mice by the enteric route (28,50) and may be required for infection to proceed by that route in some cases (28), possibly by allowing viral particles to attach to M cells, through which they can be translocated across the epithelial barrier (10). Proteolysis of σ3 is most likely mediated by alkaline proteases of pancreatic origin in the enteric system (28,50). A protease-sensitive region centrally located within the σ3 sequence has been described (407), and additional C-terminal sequences have been identified to influence the rate at which σ3 is cleaved by both acidic and alkaline proteases (219,499).

In addition to its functions before and during viral entry, σ3 plays an important role in outer capsid assembly. A ts mutant whose lesion maps to the S4 genome segment encoding σ3 accumulates dsRNA-containing core-like particles at the nonpermissive temperature (110,322, 437). Biochemical studies with this mutant suggest that, at the nonpermissive temperature, σ3 is misfolded such that it cannot interact with μ1 (283); thus it appears that σ3 may be required to interact with and promote a conformational change in μ1 that enables these proteins to assemble onto core particles (437). The interaction between σ3 and μ1 also causes a conformational change in σ3 that renders it more susceptible to proteolysis (430), consistent with the requirement for σ3 proteolysis during viral entry. Other evidence suggests that σ3 may have a function early in particle assembly or RNA selection, replication, or packaging involving its association with the reovirus mRNAs soon after they are synthesized in infected cells and its continued association with these nucleoprotein complexes through the process of minus-strand synthesis and the consequent generation and selection of the 10 genomic dsRNA molecules (13). A role for σ3 in RNA selection or packaging is also suggested by recent evidence that mutations in σ3 are needed to permit mixing of genome segments from different reovirus isolates within certain reassortants (386).

Biochemical studies reveal that σ3 binds dsRNA in a sequence-independent manner (211), and a dsRNA-binding activity has been localized to a C-terminal fragment of σ3 (311,407). This C-terminal fragment contains two copies of a basic amino acid motif that has been proposed to contribute to dsRNA binding (115,282,311,485). The capacity of σ3 to bind dsRNA is inhibited by association with μ1 and enhanced when certain N-terminal sequences of σ3 are either removed by proteolysis or mutated (43,311,407,431,471,485, 521). The positive effect of these N-terminal mutations in σ3 is thought to occur through a reduction in μ1 binding to σ3 and/or a reduction in steric hindrance to dsRNA binding provided by interactions between different σ3 regions. Emerging evidence suggests that the dsRNA-binding activity of σ3 is important for its function in translational control within infected cells (see later section).

The σ3 protein occurs as a zinc metalloprotein in virions (407), and σ3 binds Zn^{2+} in biochemical assays (283, 407). A zinc-finger motif is found in an N-terminal portion of σ3 (407). Current evidence indicates that this zinc finger includes a CCHC motif (283) similar to that found in retrovirus nucleocapsid proteins. The coordination of Zn^{2+} appears to play a structural role in σ3, because mutations in the coordinating residues eliminate the capacity of σ3 to bind to μ1 (431) and decrease its stability *in vitro* (431) and in cells (283). There is no evidence to support an association between the Zn^{2+}- and dsRNA-binding activities of σ3.

In most infected cells, σ3 is localized to the cytoplasm and becomes concentrated in perinuclear regions where viral assembly takes place (408). However, in transfected cells and following infection with some reovirus isolates, σ3 has been shown to localize to the nucleus (408,520). Nuclear localization of σ3 is inhibited by mutations that destroy dsRNA binding and also by coexpression with μ1 (520). To date, no function has been ascribed to nuclear σ3.

An early genetic study with reassortant viruses indicated that the S4 genome segment encoding σ3 determines an isolate-dependent difference in inhibition of cellular RNA and protein synthesis (417). A recent study provided evidence that such differences in effects on translation of cellular mRNAs may be based in genetically determined differences in σ3 localization within cells, with σ3 proteins that are more broadly distributed in the cytoplasm providing greater sparing of cellular mRNA translation, possibly by blocking activation of the interferon-induced and dsRNA-activated protein kinase PKR (408). The differences in localization may be attributable to differences in σ3–μ1 affinity between isolates (408). Other studies suggest roles for σ3 in the regulation of viral transcription (16) and translation. The σ3 protein was found to be enriched in the translation initiation factor fraction of eukaryotic cells expressing a cloned S4 genome segment (264) and was suggested to stimulate the translation of late (uncapped) viral mRNAs within infected cells (265,266). Several studies found that expression of σ3 can stimulate expression of reporter genes (178,275,282,290,413,471,521). It was hypothesized that the effect of σ3 on translation relates to its capacity to bind dsRNA and thereby sequester the activator of PKR, which phosphorylates eIF2α and inhibits translation initiation (214,275,463,521). This hypothesis is supported by the observation that σ3 can substitute for the analogous dsRNA binding activity of vaccinia virus protein E3L (32).

σ1

According to current estimates, the σ1 protein (49 to 51 kd, 455 to 470 amino acids) is present in no more than 36 copies per virion outer capsid, or one σ1 trimer per icosahedral vertex (100,465). In purified virions, some of the σ1 trimers may be lost, yielding particles with fewer than one per vertex (257). A minimum of three σ1 trimers per particle was found to be required for full infectivity (257). Earlier interpretations that σ1 takes the form of a dimer or tetramer (22,29,30,161,343) appear to have been in error. The σ1 protein interacts with λ2 and perhaps also with σ3 in the virion outer capsid (131,163,202,261, 306,310,482). It may be capable of adopting two very different conformations, one in which it extends as an elongated fiber from the particle surface and another in which it is more folded or retracted (22,131,161,163,345).

Sequence analyses yielded a model in which residues in the N-terminal third of σ1 adopt an α-helical coiled-coil structure (29,163,343). Two-dimensional reconstructions from electron micrographs of σ1 fibers later revealed significant substructure within the tail region (161). Related work identified repeats of hydrophobic residues within a central portion of σ1 sequences and suggested that different morphologic regions in the tail result from sequences assuming distinct supersecondary structures: alternating regions of α-helical coiled-coil and β-sheet motifs (161,343) (Fig. 5). The head appears to be formed by sequences in the C-terminal third of σ1 and to have a more complex globular structure (29,136, 161,163,343,473).

Numerous studies have implicated σ1 as the reovirus cell-attachment protein (14,22,124,144,261,293,363,470, 490–492,517) and the protein against which serotype-specific neutralizing antibodies are directed (22,70,293, 363,457,482,493,517). Sequencing of S1 genes from neutralization-resistant mutants identified two residues in the C-terminal third of type 3 Dearing σ1 that influence neutralization by the monoclonal antibody G5 (31). Evidence that these mutants exhibit altered tropisms within the murine brain (234,455,456) led to a hypothesis that the C-terminal head region of σ1 mediates receptor binding. Sequence similarities between type 3 Dearing σ1 and an antiidiotypic monoclonal antibody directed against G5 identified other residues in the C-terminal third of σ1 that may serve as receptor contacts (68,509). Other work based on the antiidiotypic antibody has identified candidate cellular receptors for this region of σ1 (see later section). In contemporary work, a C-terminal proteolytic fragment of σ1 and deletion mutants that retain a large C-terminal portion of σ1 were found to retain L-cell binding activity (136,336,473,518). Deletion and site-directed mutagenesis within a C-terminal portion of σ1 indicate that the extreme C-terminus and other conserved amino acids in this region contribute to the structure and function of the head domain (136,473).

The σ1 protein also serves as the viral hemagglutinin (22,30,70,293,495,517). Hemagglutination by type 3 reovirus isolates involves binding of σ1 to sialic acid residues on the erythrocyte surface (14,175,362), large amounts of which are attached to the major erythrocyte surface protein glycophorin A (361). Strong evidence now indicates that the region of type 3 σ1 that mediates glycophorin A binding and hemagglutination is distinct from the region that mediates L-cell binding. Early such evidence came from monoclonal antibodies that identify distinct σ1 epitopes involved in neutralization and

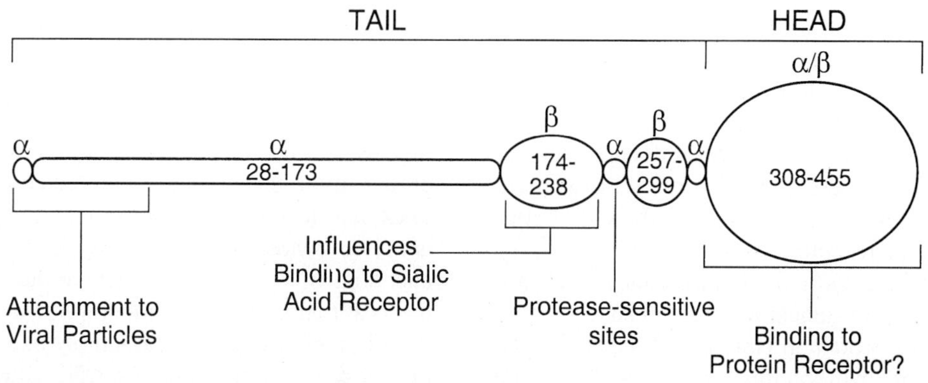

FIG. 5. Cell-attachment protein σ1. Trimers of the reovirus σ1 protein can be isolated from viral particles as extended fibers characterized by tail and head domains as shown. Distinct regions within the tail are proposed to be formed by sequences that assume α-helical coiled-coil and cross-β-sheet super-secondary structures as labeled [sequences assigned to the larger tail regions and head in σ1 proteins from type 3 (*T3*) reovirus strains are indicated by position number]. Properties or activities associated with different regions of the type 3 σ1 proteins are indicated.

hemagglutination inhibition (70,457). Findings with deletion mutants (336) and proteolytic fragments (518) of type 3 Dearing σ1 provided additional evidence that glycophorin A and L-cell binding are separable functions of this protein, most likely mediated by different protein regions. Analysis of deduced σ1 sequences from 11 type 3 isolates that differ in capacity to agglutinate erythrocytes and bind glycophorin A subsequently provided evidence that a small central region in the σ1 tail, characterized by β-sheet motifs, is involved in these properties (118). These findings were supported by studies on growth in murine erythroleukemia (MEL) cells, which indicate that growth in MEL cells is dependent on virus binding to sialylated receptors on the cell surface, that certain type 3 isolates defective for sialic acid binding (118) are also defective for growth in MEL cells, that these isolates can undergo selection for sialic acid binding and growth in MEL cells by serial passage in those cells, and that this selection involves genetic changes in the S1 genome segment resulting in amino acid changes in the central β-sheet region of the σ1 tail that was previously implicated in sialic acid binding (see Fig. 5) (88,396). Recent work using chimeric and truncated recombinant σ1 proteins concur with this localization (86). Binding to sialic acid appears not to be involved in hemagglutination or attachment to other cells by type 1 and type 2 reoviruses (118,360), but the alternative moieties that are bound by these isolates remain to be identified. The fact that neutralization and hemagglutination inhibition epitopes overlap in the type 1 Lang σ1 protein suggests that the separation of protein and carbohydrate receptor binding functions indicated for type 3 σ1 proteins may not hold true for type 1 σ1 proteins (70,457). In addition, a more distal region of the σ1 tail, closer to the head in primary sequence and putative structure, was recently implicated in hemagglutination by type 1 Lang σ1 by using chimeric and truncated recombinant σ1 proteins (86).

A flexible "neck" region has been described to separate the fibrous tail from the globular head of σ1 (137). It has been recognized for some time that this region of isolated native or recombinant type 3 Dearing σ1 protein is sensitive to proteolysis (22,136,137,465,518). Sequences that influence or impart this sensitivity have now been identified, as have the sites for proteolysis by intestinal serine proteases (85,137). The mechanism for protease sensitivity is proposed to involve disruption of α-helical coiled-coil structure within a limited region of the σ1 tail (85). The sensitivity of type 3 Dearing σ1 to proteolysis by intestinal proteases and the consequent reduction in infectivity provides a logical mechanistic explanation for the reduced capacity of reovirus type 3 Dearing to infect mice by the enteric route (85,342). In addition, because the protease-sensitive region is found between the σ1 head and the sialic binding region in the tail (85,137), findings with ISVPs containing protease-cleaved type 3 Dearing σ1 provide further evidence for the separation of the two receptor binding activities within two different regions of the protein (342).

The long α-helical coiled-coil tail region of σ1 may allow for projection of the more distal receptor binding regions away from the particle for better accessibility for binding to those receptors. A recent study indicated that engagement of receptors on cells via the C-terminal regions of σ1 leads to reversible conformational changes in more N-terminal tail regions of σ1, as well as in other capsid proteins, suggesting that conformational changes in the σ1 tail may be important for relaying information about receptor binding to other capsid proteins as part of the entry process (156). Consistent with this hypothesis is the finding that certain mutations in the long α-helical region of the σ1 tail that are selected during persistent infections can reduce σ1 oligomer stability and have effects on reovirus entry (511). Recent evidence suggests that σ1 sequences near the base of the σ1 tail (including residues 36 and 54) mediate a glycosyl hydrolase activity, which may be important for reovirus infections in the mammalian intestine by permitting hydrolysis of soluble or surface-bound mucin proteins and thereby better access to cell surface receptors (47).

Sequences near the extreme N-terminus of σ1 are thought to form a virus-attachment region that anchors this protein to the λ2 protein in viral particles (see Fig. 5). A small region of hydrophobic amino acids at the extreme N-terminus was first predicted to fulfill this function through a coupling of sequence analysis and electron microscopy (22,161,163,343). Subsequent work with C-terminally truncated recombinant σ1 proteins demonstrated that residues between positions 3 and 34 (of reovirus type 3 Dearing σ1) are required for virion anchoring (270,284).

A number of studies indicate that σ1 folds into its native conformation via a multistep process that provides a useful model for folding of an oligomeric fiber protein (259). Monomers of σ1 do not bind to cells and they exhibit extreme protease sensitivity, indicating the importance of oligomerization for σ1 structure and function (268). Folding of σ1 involves two distinct trimerization events. An N-terminal region of σ1, which includes a portion of the predicted long α-helical coiled coil, possesses a capacity to undergo oligomerization independently of other sequences (23,136,269,271,473). N-terminal trimerization occurs co-translationally and does not require ATP or cellular chaperone proteins HSP70 and HSP90 (181,182,267,271). In contrast, trimerization of C-terminal σ1 sequences is a posttranslational event that requires ATP and both of those chaperones (181,182,267,271). Additional maturation events in both N- and C-terminal regions are required to generate the final σ1 structure (271).

A wide variety of phenotypic differences among reovirus isolates have been mapped to the S1 genome segment by reassortant analyses, and many of these have been proposed to relate to the function of σ1 as the reovirus cell-attachment protein. Recent examples include studies that have implicated S1/σ1 as a genetic determinant of phenotypic differences in inhibition of cellular DNA synthesis in L cells (416,475), induction of apoptosis in L cells (475,476) and MDCK cells (383), efficiency of infection of cultured murine cardiac myocytes (432), induction of biliary atresia in newborn mice (510), growth and injury in different organs of SCID mice (194), viral growth and neutrophil response in a rat model for reovirus-induced pneumonia (325), and the capacity of viral mutants selected during persistent infections to grow in the presence of ammonium chloride as well as in mutant cells that have been cured of persistent infection (499,511).

Nonstructural Proteins

σNS

The σNS protein (41 kd, 366 amino acids) is predicted to have a high α-helical content (381,504) but a low propensity to form α-helical coiled coils (303). It appears to exist as a small oligomer in free solution (179,183). A ts mutant whose lesion maps to the S3 genome segment encoding σNS (373) is severely reduced in dsRNA synthesis at nonpermissive temperature, suggesting a role for σNS in replicase particle assembly including RNA selection or replication (104,216). σNS shows strong affinity for ssRNA, including, but not specific for, the reovirus mRNAs (179,180,183,184,211,382,458). It binds poorly to dsRNA (180,211,382). Binding to ssRNA is cooperative and can lead to displacement of short DNA oligonucleotides from RNA–DNA hybrids (180). A small region of sequence at the extreme N-terminus of σNS is important for ssRNA binding (179). Complexes containing σNS and ssRNA can be readily isolated from infected cells and resolved on columns or gradients (179,183,184 211,458). According to immunoprecipitation studies with protein-specific antibodies, σNS binds to the reovirus mRNAs shortly after they are synthesized in infected cells, and it remains bound in these complexes, along with other viral proteins, through the process of minus-strand synthesis and the consequent generation and selection of the 10 genomic dsRNA molecules (13). Thus, σNS appears likely to play one or more important roles in the selection, replication, and/or packaging of reovirus RNA for the assembly of progeny particles. A possible role in translation was also acknowledged (179). 15–19S complexes obtained from infected cells and containing σNS and ssRNA were reported to have poly(C)-dependent poly(G) polymerase activity (184); however, that activity was also demonstrated for purified reovirus λ3 protein (460) and has not been demonstrated for purified σNS (179,382), suggesting that the activity in 15–19S complexes (184) was caused by contaminating λ3.

μNS and μNSC

Although first thought to be a cleavage product of μNS (80 kd, 721 amino acids) (260), μNSC appears instead to be formed by alternative translation initiation at the second or third AUG in the M3 mRNA, in the same ORF as μNS (303,503). μNS and μNSC are thus likely to share the same sequences except for an extra 4 to 5 kd of sequence at the N-terminus of μNS. Possible functional differences between μNS and μNSC have not been addressed. A C-terminal portion of μNS/μNSC is predicted to have a high α-helical content and similarity with myosins (503), as well as a propensity to form α-helical coiled coils (303). It appears to take the form of a small oligomer in free solution (66). The μNS protein has been shown to associate with the cytoskeleton in infected cells, to which it may anchor other viral components during replication or assembly (319). According to immunoprecipitation studies with protein-specific antibodies, μNS and/or μNSC binds to reovirus mRNAs shortly after the RNAs are synthesized in infected cells and before the RNAs associate with other viral proteins (13). In addition, μNS and/or μNSC remains bound in these complexes, along with other viral proteins, through the process of minus-strand synthesis and the consequent generation and selection of the 10 genomic dsRNA molecules (13). Thus, μNS and/or μNSC appears likely to play one or more important role in the replication, selection, and/or packaging of reovirus RNA for the assembly of progeny particles. One reassortant study showed that the M3 genome segment encoding μNS/μNSC determines an isolate-dependent difference in the specific genome segments that undergo deletion during serial passage of viruses at high MOI, consistent with a role in RNA replication or packaging (67). Other studies found that μNS is a component of rapidly sedimenting particle assembly intermediates that can be isolated from reovirus-infected cells (323,322,532). Although disputed by subsequent work (446), one of these studies (323) provided evidence that μNS is a major component of the secondary transcriptase particles that produce most (95%) of the viral mRNAs within reovirus-infected cells (see later section). Recent evidence that recombinant μNS protein can bind to cores in large amounts *in vitro*, but does not inhibit their transcriptional and capping activities, is consistent with the original evidence of Morgan and Zweerink (323) and suggests that μNS may play a role in transcript production and outer capsid assembly within infected cells (66).

σ1s

The σ1s protein (14 to 15 kd, 119 to 125 amino acids) is highly variable between reovirus isolates, even within the same serotype (78,117,135). It is strongly basic, and an N-terminal cluster of basic residues is its most conserved feature. A role for this basic protein in binding to nucleic acid was proposed (218), and localization of σ1s to both cytoplasm and nucleus was noted (40,384). As a second translation product derived from the S1 genome segment, σ1s might be responsible for some of the differences in biologic properties that have been mapped to S1 and tentatively attributed to the other protein derived from this segment, the cell-attachment protein σ1 (see earlier section). When expressed to high levels in uninfected mammalian cells, recombinant σ1s does not affect cellular DNA synthesis or cause cytopathic effects; however, when expressed to high levels in cells that have also been infected with certain reovirus isolates, recombinant σ1s potentiates the viral inhibition of cellular DNA synthesis and the cytopathic effects of infection as well (147). These findings suggest a role for σ1s in reovirus effects on host cells. Recent evidence for a reovirus mutant having a stop codon early in the σ1s ORF indicates that this protein is dispensable for reovirus growth in L and MDCK cells as well as for induction of apoptosis in L cells (384). Whether it is required for replication in certain cells or performs some other function related to growth and/or spread in host animals remains to be determined. The σ1s protein has alternatively been called p14 (80), σ1bNS (328), σs (404), and σ1NS (40).

GENETICS

Mutants

Mutants Obtained by Selection, Screen, or Passage

Temperature-Sensitive Mutants

Reovirus ts mutants were classically defined by their reduced capacity to replicate at 39°C as opposed to 31°C (159). Recent studies indicate that 40°C is a more effective temperature for distinguishing certain ts mutants (102,203). Temperature-sensitive mutants from 7 of the 10 genetic groups (genome segments) of reovirus type 3 Dearing were first isolated after chemical mutagenesis with nitrous acid (groups B, D, and E), nitroso-guanidine (groups C, F, and G), or proflavin (group A) (159,212). Mutants from the other three groups were isolated from type 3 Dearing stocks subjected to serial passage at high MOI (group H) or from persistently infected cultures (groups I and J) (3,4,8). All groups but F were assigned to discrete genome segments by reassortant analyses (332,368,369,373). The prototype group F isolate was assigned to the M3 segment based on its capacity to complement ts mutants from the other groups (369). A recent study failed to confirm the original findings for the prototype isolates of groups F, H, and J (99), indicating that these isolates cannot fulfill their initial promise of providing isolated ts lesions in the M3, M1, and S1 genome segments, respectively. The same and another recent study nonetheless described a new set of ts mutants (99,102), one of which has been shown to represent a new prototype isolate for ts group H (M1 segment) (99). To date, sequencing studies have identified nucleotide and amino acid changes in mutants from groups C (102,507), E (504), G (110), and H (99). Temperature-sensitive mutants in groups A, B, C, D, E, G, and H have been analyzed extensively with respect to their morphologic, biochemical, and biologic properties (discussed at other places in this chapter).

Suppressor Mutants

Reversion of ts mutants to the ts^+ phenotype might occur through a change in the same gene, either at the site of the original mutation (true reversion) or at a second site (intragenic suppression). Alternatively, mutation in a second gene might suppress the defect produced by the original mutation (extragenic suppression). A recent study found that one reovirus ts mutant (tsC447, with a lesion in the S2 genome segment encoding core nodule protein σ2) undergoes true reversion exclusively (102); nevertheless, a number of revertants of other reovirus ts mutants result from extragenic suppression (371,372, 374). A commonly described mechanism for extragenic suppression involves mutation in a gene product that interacts directly with the original ts product. Interactions between reovirus protein pairs μ1-σ3, μ1-λ1, and λ2-σ1 were inferred in this manner (221,306).

Deletion Mutants and Defective Stocks

Some reovirus isolates accumulate deletion mutants during serial passage at high MOI (5,67,356,358,411). Genome segments L1 and L3 are most commonly deleted, but L2 and M1 deletions are also seen. A series of deleted M1 segments were analyzed and found to lack internal sequence regions (525). Based on the smallest deleted M1 segments, the minimum sizes for retained 5′- and 3′-terminal regions of the plus strand were 132 to 135 and 182 to 185 bases, respectively, suggesting that these regions contain the essential signals for RNA synthesis and packaging. One genetic study compared isolates type 1 Lang and type 3 Dearing, which differ in their capacity to accumulate deletion mutants (67). This study showed that the L2 genome segment determines whether or not deletions accumulate, and that the M3 genome segment determines in which segments the deletions occur. The L2 and M3 gene products λ2 and μNS/μNSC may play a role in synthesis or packaging of reovirus RNA such that they influence the generation or amplification of deletion mutants.

Some reovirus stocks that have been serially passed at high MOI can be classified as DI stocks (3,5–7,67,119, 356,358,411). The traits of defective stocks include the presence of deletion mutants, the capacity to interfere with growth of wild-type (wt) virus (see later), and the capacity to establish persistent infections. The role of deletion mutants in the latter two properties is unclear, because defective stocks contain a variety of mutants, including a high frequency of tsG (S4 genome segment) mutants (3,5), some of which are known to mediate interference (3,81). Given that the nondeleted genome segments in defective stocks are normal with respect to transcription and reassortment, it was suggested that interference and facilitation of persistent infections are linked to specific mutations in nondeleted segments such as S4, rather than to the deleted ones (5,6,67).

Neutralization-Resistant Mutants

Neutralizing monoclonal antibodies directed against the cell-attachment protein σ1 were used to select neutralization-resistant mutants of isolate type 3 Dearing, and changes in the mutants were localized to two residues in the C-terminal third of σ1 (31,456). The mutants were found to be altered in their pathogenic behaviors within newborn mice (234,455,456), possibly because their mutations fall in or near a receptor-binding region of σ1.

Inactivation-Resistant Mutants

Physicochemical agents (e.g., heat or ethanol) can cause large reductions in reovirus infectivity, and differences between isolates in their sensitivities to these agents can be attributed to specific genome segments by reassortant analyses (128,129). One such difference in ethanol sensitivity was genetically mapped to the M2 genome segment (129). Ethanol-resistant mutants were subsequently isolated in which relevant mutations were also localized to M2, within a 200-amino-acid central region of the encoded major outer capsid protein μ1 (208,497). These mutants exhibit increased thermostability and a decreased capacity to permeabilize cells as detected by release of ^{51}Cr (208), a marker for membrane rupture during viral entry (56,277). Thus, mutants selected with physicochemical agents may be used to study the structure and function of reovirus particles, as well as to define the mechanisms of inactivation by these agents.

Other Mutants

Other types of reovirus mutants obtained after passage in cells or animals, with or without a defined mechanism for selection, have been described. These include small-plaque mutants (7), cold-sensitive mutants (8), mutants selected during persistent infections in L cells and genetically mapped to the S1 and S4 genome segments (119,499,511), mutants selected for binding to sialic-acid-containing receptors by growth in MEL cells and genetically mapped to the S1 genome segment (88), and mutants with altered organ tropism and virulence obtained after passage in mice and genetically mapped to several genome segments including M1 and S1 (193,194,434,435). A particularly fortuitous mutant is one of those selected for growth in MEL cells which, in addition to having a mutation in S1 that affects the sialic binding activity of σ1, has a second mutation in S1 that introduces a stop codon near the beginning of the σ1s-encoding ORF (88). This mutant was used to show that expression of σ1s is dispensable for reovirus replication and induction of apoptosis in L and MDCK cells (384).

Genetically Engineered Mutants or Mutations

It has been demonstrated that reovirus mRNAs can be infectious after transfection into cells (386,389), and this infectious RNA system has been used to construct a double ts mutant using virally produced RNAs obtained from two different single ts mutants (387). Despite the clear promise of this approach for genetic engineering of reoviruses, it has not yet been modified to allow the efficient recovery of infectious particles containing genome segments derived from cloned and mutated DNA copies. As a result, genetic engineering with reoviruses has been largely restricted to studies in which isolated mutant gene products have been analyzed for activity *in vitro* or in transfected cells. In a recent study, recombinant μ2 protein constitutively expressed in L cells was shown to complement the growth of a tsH mutant (a lesion in the M1 genome segment encoding low-copy core protein μ2) at nonpermissive temperature (527). This offers a new genetic approach for identifying sequence determinants of μ2 function and promises to be applicable to other reovirus gene products as well. In addition, a series of recent reports have demonstrated that genetically engineered reovirus outer capsid proteins μ1, σ1, and σ3 can be bound to the surfaces of subvirion particles (ISVPs or cores), regenerating virion-like particles that are infectious (83,151,219). This offers another new genetic approach for identifying sequence determinants of μ1, σ1, and σ3 functions during the entry phase of productive infection.

Interactions Between Viruses

Reassortment

Reassortment of genome segments between reoviruses occurs not only in cultured cells but also in mice (496). Sequencing studies indicate that reassortment in nature is a major determinant of reovirus evolution (see later). Reassortment was first demonstrated in two-factor crosses (157,159). L cells were co-infected with two ts mutants at permissive temperature, and reassortants were detected by assaying for ts^+ progeny at nonpermissive temperature. If a cross between two ts mutants did not produce ts^+ reassortants, the mutants were considered to have lesions in the same genome segment. On the other hand, if a cross between two ts mutants resulted in ts^+ reassortants, the mutants were considered to have lesions in different genome segments. In this way, the available ts mutants were separated into five different genetic groups (157). The discovery of electrophoretic differences for protein μ1/μ1C in certain ts mutants provided an additional marker (μ+ versus μ–, to indicate wt versus faster mobility) that could be used in genetic crosses to evaluate reassortment (106). Three-factor crosses were performed using this mobility marker in combination with the ts phenotype and confirmed that reovirus genome segments behave as discrete genetic elements during reassortment (107). In subsequent experiments, ts mutants representing the five remaining genetic groups were identified, and separate co-infections involving one ts mutant and one wt isolate were used in reassortant analyses to assign each ts group to a particular genome segment (see earlier section). Reassortment of genome segments between wt isolates, irrespective of serotype, has been subsequently demonstrated in numerous studies.

If reassortment of genome segments from two co-infected isolates were a random process, then almost all of the progeny from the co-infection should be reassortants [1,022 of 1,024 (2^{10}) possible combinations of genome segments from the two parents]. In practice, however, a much lower frequency of reassortants has been seen among co-infection progeny [3% to 20% in one series of crosses (159)]. A variety of factors could contribute to reovirus reassortment's exhibiting such deviation from randomness, including that not all genome segments or their protein products from two isolates can be productively paired without accommodating mutations. Supportive data in this regard came from a statistical study of 83 reassortants derived from reoviruses type 1 Lang and type 3 Dearing. These reassortants showed significant deviations from randomness for the distributions of parental alleles in certain of the possible pairings of the 10 genome segments (346). Possibly reflecting the same or a similar phenomenon is evidence that reovirus reassortants commonly contain mutations in the S4 genome segment, suggesting that such mutations may be necessary to improve the fitness of certain reassortants for independent replication (228,229,386).

Complementation and Interference

Complementation refers to interactions of viral gene products in co-infected cells that result in enhanced yield of one or both parental viruses without a change in genotype. Interference refers to the capacity of certain viruses to decrease the yield of other viruses upon co- or superinfection. Although reassortants were readily identified after co-infections with reovirus ts mutants, enhanced yields of progeny at the nonpermissive temperature were often not observed (157,159). This lack of complementation was explained by the phenomenon of interference. Temperature-sensitive mutants from groups A, B, C, and G were found to interfere with the growth of wt virus, whereas those from groups D and E were not (81). Genetic crosses established that interference is a dominant trait. The degree of interference with the growth of wt virus can be substantial (50% or more), and it increases if the MOI of the interfering ts mutant is increased (81). Significant complementation occurs only if both parental ts mutants are noninterfering (81,216). Interference with growth of wt virus is also a property of defective high-passage stocks, which may reflect the frequent presence of interfering group G ts mutants (3,5).

The molecular basis of interference with reoviruses remains poorly defined in most cases. It was suggested that interfering ts mutants encode mutant proteins that become incorporated into progeny virions and reduce their infectivity (5). In support of this model, one study identified dominant-negative mutations in σ1 that interfere with the capacity of wt σ1 to assemble into functional oligomers (271). Mutant proteins from interfering ts mutants may act similarly to interfere with assembly and function of reovirus protein complexes. Recent studies on the mechanism of interference during co-infections with certain pairs of wt reoviruses revealed that interference occurs by 8 to 10 hours after infection, after viral entry and uncoating but before or during accumulation of newly synthesized dsRNA (392,394). These results are consistent with a model in which interference occurs at the stage of progeny particle assembly (394). Genetic evidence from one of these studies identifies the M2 genome segment (which encodes major outer capsid protein μ1) as the primary determinant of interference in this system (392).

Other Types of Interactions

There is no evidence for recombination between either homologous or heterologous reovirus genome segments. Reoviruses can undergo multiplicity reactivation after inactivation with genome-damaging agents like ultraviolet radiation (300), probably reflecting the capacity of viruses to reassort mRNAs produced from nondamaged genome segments. There is recent evidence for phenotypic mixing of proteins within progeny virions assembled during co-infections with pairs of reovirus isolates that have distinguishable properties attributable to those proteins (393). A recent study found no evidence for super-infection exclusion during temporally asynchronous infections of cultured cells with pairs of reovirus ts mutants, which may have significance for the evolution of reoviruses in nature by allowing co-infection and reassortment even when different viruses infect cells at different times (236).

Naturally Occurring Variation

Exploitation for Genetic Studies

Reovirus isolates obtained from nature commonly exhibit qualitative or quantitative differences in phenotypes of biological interest. Substantial progress in attributing these phenotypic differences to individual genome segments, and thus presumably to specific sequence differences between the two parental alleles of these segments, has come from the generation and characterization of reassortant viruses derived from the two parents. Early studies used this approach to identify the S1 segment as the primary determinant of a difference between reoviruses type 1 Lang and type 3 Dearing in tropism and virulence for newborn mice after intracranial inoculation (492,494). Numerous subsequent studies, involving these and other isolates, have succeeded in attributing other phenotypic differences to single genome segments (127,210,237,354,417,434). In other cases, reassortant analysis has attributed the phenotypic difference to more than one genome segment at a time, indicating that genetic differences in two or more viral components are involved (49,194,355,433,499,519).

The availability of reovirus genome sequences has permitted another type of study that takes advantage of naturally occurring variation among isolates. In this approach, the protein sequences deduced from individual genome segments of different isolates are compared in an effort to link specific, variable sequences with a phenotypic difference that is known to be linked to these segments. In successful applications of this approach, a small variable region in the cell-attachment protein σ1 was implicated in the failure of σ1 from four type 3 isolates to bind sialylated proteins on the erythrocyte surface (118), and a single variable amino acid in σ1 was implicated in the susceptibility of σ1 from two other type 3 isolates to undergo cleavage by intestinal proteases (85). In each of these cases, additional studies have confirmed the reliability of the original conclusions (85,88). Other applications have been reported for studies of the λ1 and σ3 proteins (198,235).

Evolution of Reoviruses

Although useful for scoring reassortants, electrophoretic mobility differences between homologous genome segments and proteins of different reovirus isolates are not generally meaningful for classification (209,370). Nucleotide and deduced amino acid sequences provide the most reliable information for understanding reovirus evolution (241). Sequences are available for all 10 genome segments of the prototype isolates type 1 Lang, type 2 Jones, and type 3 Dearing. Except for the serotype-determining S1 segment, homologous segments from the prototypes are similar at the level of 70.6–97.8% and 80.0–99.3% identity in pairwise comparisons of nucleotide and deduced amino acid sequences, respectively. For every gene but S1, the type 2 Jones sequence is most distinct, which led to a suggestion that it diverged from a common ancestor prior to type 1 Lang and type Dearing (506).

The σ1-encoding S1 genome segments of reoviruses exhibit the greatest extent of variability among the 10 segments. The variability includes differences in length, the need for multiple gaps to align deduced σ1 sequences, and reduced sequence similarity (only 26% to 49% identity in σ1 sequences in pair wise comparisons) (135,343). Among the three prototype isolates, the type 3 Dearing S1 sequence is most divergent. On the other hand, examination of S1 genes from a set of 11 type 3 isolates revealed no differences in length or need for gaps to optimize σ1 alignments, and sequence divergence similar to that between prototypes for other genome segments was seen (86% to 99% identity in pair wise comparisons of deduced σ1 protein sequences) (117). In sum, these findings suggest that three versions of the S1 genome segment, corresponding to the three serotypes, arose from progenitors at different times in the past and have diverged at a rate similar to that of other segments since those times.

Reassortment of genome segments between viruses is another important force in reovirus evolution. Variable rates of change in third codon bases seen for different genome segments from type 1 Lang and type 3 Dearing suggest that the segments in these two isolates were combined by reassortment after having had distinct evolutionary histories (506). A study of S2 genome segment sequences from 11 type 1 and type 3 isolates was the first to show convincingly that a segment other than S1 has diverged independently of the serotype of isolate from which it was obtained for sequencing (87). Subsequent studies have yielded similar findings for L2, S3, and S4 genome segment sequences from multiple type 1, type 2, and type 3 isolates and also showed topological differences in the phylogenetic trees drawn for these and S2 sequences obtained from the same isolates (87,189,235). These findings indicate that each of these genome segments has had an evolutionary history distinct from those of many or all of the other segments with which it is combined in the current isolates, consistent with ongoing reassortment of segments in nature. The same studies also showed that evolution of the genome segments is independent of host of origin. Despite this strong evidence for evolution at the level of individual genome segments, one study has shown evidence for the existence of coevolving sets of reovirus proteins (482) and another has shown evidence for nonrandom segregation of segments during generation of reassortants in the laboratory, indicating bias for or against certain RNA or protein pairings (346). The significance of these possible biases on the evolution of reoviruses in nature remains uncertain.

REPLICATION CYCLE

A diagram of the reovirus replication cycle is shown in Figure 6. Subsequent sections of this chapter discuss details of the depicted events, but a brief description follows here. The first step in reovirus infection is attachment of the virion (or ISVP) to receptor molecules on the cell surface. Following *attachment*, virion particles are taken up from the cell surface by receptor-mediated *endocytosis* and delivered into vacuoles resembling endosomes and lysosomes. Within these vacuoles, reovirus outer capsid proteins undergo specific proteolytic cleavages, which are acid dependent and represent an essential step in the infection process. In some situations, ISVPs are generated by *extracellular proteolysis*, and the entry of such particles is acid independent and may not require endocytosis. The mechanism by which reoviruses interact with and penetrate the vacuolar or plasma membrane barrier is unknown, but it appears to depend on preceding *proteolysis*, as only the ISVP form exhibits *membrane interaction* in available assays. Coincident with or following *penetration*, a derivative of the ISVP (perhaps a core particle as shown in Fig. 6) becomes transcriptionally active and begins synthesis of the 10 capped viral mRNAs. These products of *primary transcription* are used for the translation of viral proteins by the cellular *protein synthesis* machinery. In addition, the early transcripts associate with newly made viral proteins to form progeny RNA *assortment* complexes. Within subsequently derived replicase particles, each of the 10 packaged plus strands serves as a template for *minus-strand synthesis*. Viral mRNAs are also transcribed by progeny subviral particles (*secondary transcription*), which have a unique protein composition. These "late" transcripts serve as the primary templates for viral protein synthesis later in infection. The final steps of virion *capsid assembly* are not well defined but may involve the addition of preformed complexes of outer capsid proteins to core-like particles. Mature virions undergo an inefficient process of *release* from infected cells following cell lysis.

Early Steps in Replication: Entry into Cells and Production of Primary Transcripts

Attachment to Cell Surface Receptors

Numerous studies have investigated the attachment of reoviruses to erythrocytes and other cells, some of which are capable of undergoing productive infection. Most studies have utilized cells *in vitro* (see later), but some have investigated the binding of reoviruses to different cells within host animals. These studies generally indicate that defined receptor moieties, exposed on the cell surface, are responsible for binding reovirus particles via specific interactions with the viral hemagglutinin and cell-attachment protein σ1. Attachment to surface receptors is considered a required first step in the productive infection of cells. Interactions of cell surface proteins with other reovirus proteins, contributing to attachment or subsequent steps in infection, remain possible but undefined.

Hemagglutination

Hemagglutination has been used as a convenient assay to study the attachment capabilities of reovirus particles. Isolates from all three serotypes agglutinate human type O erythrocytes, but only type 3 isolates agglutinate bovine red cells. This difference between strains type 1 Lang and type 3 Dearing was mapped to their S1 genes, implicating the encoded structural protein σ1 as the reovirus hemagglutinin (495). Hemagglutination can also be mediated by purified σ1, and biochemical and molecular genetic studies have suggested that a central region

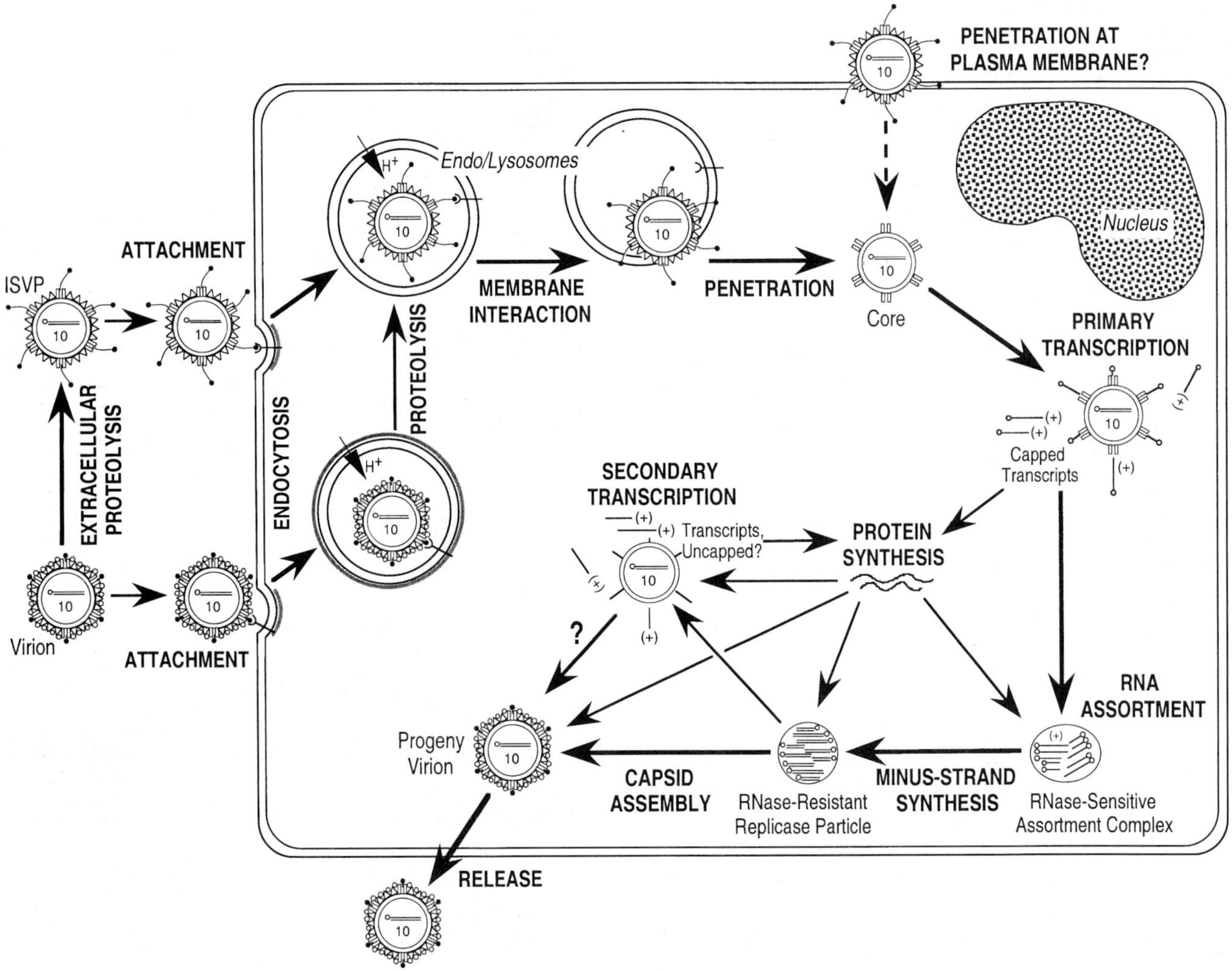

FIG. 6. Reovirus replication cycle. See text for detailed explanation. The primary steps in replication are labeled in *bold capital letters.* Virions, ISVPs, and cores, as well as other assembly-related particle forms are indicated. Capped plus-stranded RNAs—as part of the 10 dsRNA genome segments, as cytoplasmic transcripts, and as assortment elements—are indicated (*5′-terminal open circles* represent caps). Uptake from the cell surface is shown to involve receptor-mediated endocytosis, with viral particles sequentially associated with clathrin-coated pits, clathrin-coated vesicles, endosomes, and lysosomes (the last three compartments are acidic as shown). The roles played by individual reovirus proteins are not indicated here.

of sequences in type 3 σ1 proteins is involved in this activity (see earlier section).

A decrease in hemagglutination is commonly noted after erythrocytes are treated with periodate or proteases, suggesting that one or more glycoproteins on the red cell surface serves as the receptor for virus binding prior to agglutination (14,421). There is strong evidence, including the sensitivity of hemagglutination to treatment of red cells with neuraminidase and to treatment of virions with sialoglycoproteins, that sialic (N-acetylneuraminic) acid residues are essential components of the erythrocyte receptor for type 3 reoviruses (14,88,175,361). Glycophorin A is the primary sialoglycoprotein found on human erythrocytes and is capable, in purified form, of binding to the σ1 proteins of type 3 Dearing and other type 3 strains (118,336, 361, 482,518); thus, glycophorin A was specifically proposed to represent the erythrocyte receptor for type 3 reoviruses (361).

Hemagglutination by type 1 and type 2 reoviruses has been studied less thoroughly than that by type 3 isolates, but it does have some different characteristics. Unlike type 3 Dearing and some other type 3 strains, reovirus type 1 Lang is deficient in binding to sialoglycoproteins, including glycophorin A, as determined by its S1 gene (118,360). The erythrocyte receptor for type 1 and type 2 reoviruses remains undefined.

Attachment to Other Cells

Studies of reovirus attachment have been performed with a variety of cultured cells, utilizing different virus strains and techniques of analysis. Attachment to L cells by strain type 3 Dearing appears to be mediated by one or more populations of saturable receptors. Estimates for the number of attachment sites per cell range between 1×10^4 and 5×10^5, and the receptors exhibit a dissociation constant for virus binding of 0.25 to 13 nM (9,14,144,173, 406). Maximal attachment is generally achieved after 30 to 90 minutes regardless of temperature (14,144,173). Studies in other cell types or with strain type 1 Lang have provided similar estimates for the copy numbers and dissociation constants of receptors (9,144,173,288,406,479). Competition experiments have disputed whether type 3 Dearing and type 1 Lang bind to the same (261) or different (9,144,490) receptors on L cells; a recent study argues for one receptor being shared by these two strains, plus a second being restricted to type 3 Dearing (9). There is general agreement that attachment is mediated primarily or exclusively by the σ1 protein.

The nature of the L-cell receptor(s) for reovirus type 3 Dearing is well studied but remains incompletely defined (reviewed in ref. 405). There is generally consistent evidence for involvement of a sialoglycoprotein based on the decreased virus-binding capacity of L cells treated with proteases, periodate, neuraminidase, or particular lectins (14,173,174,395). The capacity of type 3 Dearing virions or σ1 protein molecules to bind L cells is similarly decreased in the presence of sialoglycoproteins (174,360, 361,509), gangliosides (14), or free sugars that contain α-linked sialic acid residues (362). The latter observations have been used to argue that the L-cell receptor, like the erythrocyte receptor described earlier, includes sialic acid. One study suggested that the α-anomer of sialic acid is the minimal receptor determinant required for reovirus (type 3 Dearing) recognition (362). Correlation between the capacity of certain type 3 strains to bind glycophorin and their capacity to bind and productively infect MEL cells (88,396) is consistent with a model in which binding to sialic acid is critically important for infection of at least some cells.

Other data suggest that one or more specific proteins, perhaps sialylated glycoproteins, can serve as cell surface receptors for type 3 Dearing. Initial data in this regard were acquired using an antiidiotype approach (reviewed in ref. 158). Antibodies were raised against the anti-σ1 monoclonal antibody G5, which blocks the binding of type 3 Dearing to cells and thereby neutralizes its infectivity. These preparations of G5-specific antibodies, as well as similarly derived monoclonal antibodies, exhibited behaviors predicted for antiidiotypic antibodies: They were capable of blocking the binding of type 3 Dearing to cells, presumably by mimicking within their own structures a portion of the attachment site on σ1 and thus binding to σ1-specific receptors on the cell surface (68,339,509). A monoclonal antiidiotypic antibody was subsequently used to identify a 67-kd membrane glycoprotein, having notable structural similarity to the β-adrenergic receptor, as a probable receptor for reovirus type 3 Dearing (94). Subsequent studies have provided mixed support for this hypothesis (89,90,125,406), and it currently seems unlikely that this protein represents the sole or even primary receptor for reoviruses on many cells. Other reports describe receptors for reovirus type 3 Dearing that include the epidermal growth factor (EGF) receptor (469), a 54-kd protein on endothelial cells recognized by both type 3 Dearing and type 1 Lang (479), and multiple sialoglycoproteins on L and human erythroleukemia cells (89). Reports describing specific receptors for reovirus type 1 Lang are less frequent but include a 47-kd protein from mouse intestinal epithelial cells (490) and undefined moieties on Caco-2 cells (9) and mouse ependymal cells (339).

Whether sialic acid or another protein element(s) alone is sufficient to mediate reovirus attachment to cells resulting in productive infection remains in question. A two-step mechanism involving initial binding to sialic acid and subsequent interaction with a specific protein receptor has been suggested (362). Available data suggest that differences in receptors are likely to exist between cell types and between reovirus serotypes or strains. It may also be important to distinguish attachment that leads to productive infection from attachment that is nonproductive. The capacity of attachment to lead to virus uptake from the cell surface by endocytosis may be an important distinguishing feature in this case (89,395). The importance of multivalent attachment via two or more of the σ1 oligomers present in viral particles remains undefined. Differences in the attachment process for virions and ISVPs are also unknown.

Endocytic Uptake and Proteolytic Activation

Thin-section electron micrographs of cells soon after infection reveal reovirus particles associated with clathrin-coated pits or vesicles at or near the plasma membrane, suggesting that uptake from the cell surface can occur by receptor-mediated endocytosis (56,59,395,467) (see Fig. 6). Particles are subsequently observed within vacuoles resembling endosomes and lysosomes (56,59,177,395,442, 467). Treatment with colchicine and nocodazole does not inhibit endocytosis, but it does inhibit the movement of these virus-containing vacuoles toward perinuclear regions, suggesting that vacuole translocation occurs along microtubules (177). Only some of the proteins to which reovirus particles bind on the cell surface may be capable of signaling endocytic uptake (89,395).

Experiments with radiolabeled virions provide evidence for proteolysis of viral proteins within hydrolytic compartments of the endocytic pathway (late endosomes or lysosomes), starting 20 to 30 minutes after infection at 37°C (442,443,467). The proteolytic cleavages are notable in that they involve only certain outer capsid components. Specifically, degradation of protein σ3 and conversion of protein μ1C to its stable cleavage product δ are observed, generating particles very similar to ISVPs that result from *in vitro* proteolysis (59,84,344,440,467). The reproducibility of these limited cleavages suggested that the generation of ISVP-like particles by proteolysis within lysosomes may be a required step in reovirus infection.

More direct evidence for proteolytic activation as a required step in infection arose from an observation that infection is inhibited by the weak base ammonium chloride, which raises the pH within endosomes and lysosomes (72). Later experiments revealed that an early step in infections initiated by virions, but not ISVPs, is inhibited by this agent (50,119,287,467). In addition, the extent of inhibition was found to correlate with the extent to which cleavages of proteins σ3 and μ1C in infecting virions are blocked. It was suggested that, by raising the pH within endosomes and lysosomes, ammonium chloride inhibits the activity of acidic proteases within those compartments and blocks the generation of ISVPs. ISVPs may resist the block to infection by ammonium chloride because they have undergone proteolysis *in vitro* and thus no longer contain an acid-dependent step in their replication cycle (467). Proteolysis appears to activate reovirus particles for the next steps in infection, membrane interaction and penetration (see later).

In certain settings, proteolytic activation of virions occurs outside cells, before attachment and endocytosis (see Fig. 6). When newborn mice are perorally inoculated with virions, proteolysis to generate ISVPs occurs within the lumen of the small intestine and is probably mediated by pancreatic serine proteases (28,50). Extracellularly generated ISVPs are apparently required to initiate infection of mouse tissues by that route (10,28), but the basis for this requirement is unknown. ISVPs generated *in vitro* may have the capacity to bypass endocytic uptake and to penetrate into the cytoplasm directly through the plasma membrane (see later).

Interaction with and Penetration of Cell Membranes

As with other nonenveloped viruses, the mechanism by which reoviruses cross the membrane barrier during entry into cells (see Fig. 6) remains poorly defined. Three assays have demonstrated a direct interaction between reovirus particles and lipid bilayers. One involves the capacity of particles to effect the release of ^{51}Cr from preloaded L cells (56,277). Another revealed the capacity of particles to induce conductance through artificial planar bilayers (472). Finally, reovirus particles can mediate lysis of erythrocytes, resulting in the release of hemoglobin (82,83,219). Membrane interaction in all these assays is restricted to ISVPs: Virions and cores did not exhibit the activity. Moreover, the membrane interactions did not require acid pH. These findings are consistent with a model in which ISVPs are required intermediates in the process of reovirus entry into cells and in which the acid-dependent step in reovirus entry (the one inhibited by ammonium chloride) is proteolytic activation rather than membrane interaction (277,345,467,472).

Available data implicate the outer capsid protein μ1, which covers most of the surface of ISVPs, in mediating direct interactions with membranes. A strain difference in the capacity of ISVPs to mediate ^{51}Cr release from L cells was mapped to the M2 gene, which encodes μ1 (277). Changes in the ^{51}Cr release phenotype have been associated with certain μ1 mutations (208). Studies with recoated cores indicate that the μ1 protein is the only additional outer capsid protein that must be present in those particles for erythrocyte lysis to proceed (83). Features of the μ1 protein noted to be consistent with a role in membrane interaction include the modification of it and its amino-terminal fragment μ1N with a myristoyl group (347), and the presence of a predicted pair of long, amphipathic α-helices flanking the cleavage junction between the μ1δ/δ and ϕ fragments of μ1/μ1C that are found in ISVPs (344). A conformational change in μ1 is expected to precede reovirus-membrane interaction according to one model (277,344,345). The relative importance to membrane interaction of σ3 degradation and μ1/μ1C cleavage into fragments μ1δ/δ and ϕ remains somewhat unclear (20); however, some data indicate that the μ1/μ1C cleavage into μ1δ/δ and ϕ is dispensable (82,83).

Direct interaction of viral components with a cell membrane is expected to be one step in a process that gives reovirus particles access to the cytoplasm, where there are substrates for transcribing and capping the viral mRNAs and ribosomes for translating them (see Fig. 6). As nonenveloped viruses, reoviruses cannot use fusion as a general mechanism for this process, and little is known about the steps that follow membrane interaction and permit reovirus components to penetrate into the cytoplasm. Suggested possibilities are that membrane interaction results in local disruption of the bilayer such that virus enters the cytoplasm directly through a large breach, or that a more precise, pore-like structure is formed by viral proteins within the membrane, through which viral components enter the cytoplasm (56,59,344,345,472).

A current model (see Fig. 6) suggests that when ISVP-like particles are generated from virions by proteolytic activation within late endosomes or lysosomes, membrane interaction and penetration are most likely to occur within and from those vacuoles (56,59,345,467). When ISVPs are generated *in vitro*, however, they may be capable of penetrating directly through the plasma membrane, prior to endocytosis (see Fig. 6) (56,59,277), although other work suggests that ISVPs also undergo endocytic uptake and sequestration into vacuoles prior to penetration (467). Whether penetration through plasma membrane by extracellularly generated ISVPs occurs routinely during reovirus infections remains to be determined.

Plus-Strand RNA Synthesis (Transcription)

Notable features of reovirus transcription include the stability and productivity of the transcriptase and its encasement within icosahedral particles (24,52,127,230, 272,426,445). A common system for *in vitro* transcription includes reovirus cores, ribonucleoside triphosphates, and an ATP-regenerating source. The products of transcription are single-stranded RNAs, which are released from the transcribing particle (24,27). Reovirus transcription is conservative and asymmetric (24,272,445). Ten distinct transcripts have been identified, which by hybridization and sequencing (247,301) represent full-length copies of the 10 genomic plus strands. Except for abortive initiation (see later), there is no evidence that any of the gene segments give rise to less-than-full-length transcripts as part of the viral replication strategy.

If appropriate substrates are provided, transcripts produced by purified reovirus particles *in vitro* can undergo capping and methylation at their 5′ ends, indicating that the capping enzymes are also present within the particles (see later). Capping imparts increased stability to reovirus mRNAs (164) and increases the efficiency with which many mRNAs are translated within eukaryotic cells (424). Reovirus transcripts are not polyadenylated: their 3′ ends are fully complementary to the 5′ ends of the genomic minus strands that serve as templates for their synthesis.

Transcriptase Activation

Early studies showed that the virion-associated transcriptase can be activated by heat (52) or by treatment with proteases such as chymotrypsin (426). For protease treatments yielding cores as end products, transcriptase activation was correlated with loss of protein μ1 from particles (55,127,223). In addition, a strain difference in the treatment conditions needed to generate cores and activate transcription was mapped to the M2 gene, which encodes μ1 (127). A number of parameters (e.g., the concentration and nature of monovalent cations, divalent cations, proteases, and viral particles) were found to affect whether transcriptase activation occurs during protease treatments, in general correlating with whether cores were produced (51,54,55,60,127,223).

Although some studies suggest that ISVPs are transcriptionally active (16,84,425,440), others indicate that the transcriptase is latent in ISVPs but can be activated under certain conditions without additional proteolysis (54,55,58,146,403). One study correlated the switch-on of transcriptase activity in ISVPs with a change in the μ1δ fragment of μ1 (146). From these studies, a model was proposed in which virions undergo transcriptase activation via two steps (55,59,146,345). The first step requires proteolysis and produces ISVPs. The second step is protease independent, produces transcriptionally active particles, and may be linked to penetration during entry into cells.

Although virions cannot make full-length transcripts, they have been reported to synthesize short oligonucleotides when given appropriate substrates (151,515). This important finding suggests that the transcriptase is constitutively active in virions but capable of limited or no elongation. Capping enzymes are also active in virions (74,231,515); thus, transcriptase activation must primarily involve relief of a block to elongation. The nature of this block is unknown, but it may relate to movement of the dsRNA templates (151,226,424). Changes in the outer capsid are essential for activation (see earlier), implying that interactions between outer and inner capsid proteins may produce the elongation block. One study suggested that structural changes in the core occur at the onset of transcription (366), and it may be that these changes are required for elongation but are inhibited by the outer capsid proteins in virions and ISVPs. A conformational change in λ2 (131) may be important for transcriptase activation in that it opens a fivefold channel through which the substrates or products of transcription may be required to pass.

Initiator oligonucleotides are the major transcription products produced *in vitro* by both virions and cores, even though cores can at low frequency elongate these into full-length transcripts (151,514,522). This and other findings indicate that the onset of elongation is the rate-limiting step in reovirus transcription (230,514,515,522). Three phases of transcriptase activity are thus suggested: efficient, repetitive initiation yielding large amounts of initiator oligonucleotides, an inefficient onset to the elongation process, and elongation yielding smaller amounts of full-length transcripts (515).

Primary Transcription Within Cells

Two phases of transcription by reoviruses are known to occur within infected cells, based on the derivation of the transcribing particle. Primary transcription is mediated by particles derived by partial uncoating of infecting particles (59,84,440,442,443). It results in production of capped transcripts that serve both as mRNAs for translation and as templates for minus-strand synthesis within progeny particles. Primary transcripts are detected by 2 hours after infection, reach a maximum at 6 to 8 hours, and decrease to undetectable levels by 12 hours (224,442,530). Secondary transcription is mediated by particles assembled from newly synthesized RNA and protein molecules and is the source of 95% of the transcripts produced during infection (216,523). Secondary transcripts have been reported to remain uncapped, but this has been disputed (see later section).

Primary transcription may be subject to regulation within cells, but some authors have disputed these findings as well (224,441,530). Transcripts from four "pre-early" genome segments (L1, M3, S3, and S4) have been reported to be preferentially synthesized during the first several hours of infection (357,451,489). Moreover, transcription from the six other genes was suggested to require new protein synthesis because it is blocked with cycloheximide (258,425,489). One hypothesis is that a cellular repressor prevents transcription of the six later genes and that a protein encoded by a pre-early gene interferes with its activity (258,357,523).

The nature of the primary transcriptase particle remains in question; however, because of their transcriptional activity *in vitro*, cores are assigned this role in one model (see Fig. 6). In one study, transcriptionally active particles derived from input particles were isolated from infected cells and were shown to have the characteristics of cores, perhaps indicating that additional uncoating occurs in association with or subsequent to penetration (59). Because proteinase K was used to separate the particles from cell debris in this study, however, degradation of outer capsid components may have occurred before the particles were characterized (523). Other studies suggest that the primary transcriptase particle is more similar to an ISVP, in that it still contains the μ1 protein (16,84,425, 440,443).

The intracellular site of primary transcription also remains undetermined. Thin-section electron micrographs have been reported to show small numbers of core-like particles free within the cytoplasm of newly infected cells (49,59), suggesting that the primary transcriptase particle is introduced fully into the cytoplasm (see Fig. 6). In fact, most reovirus particles in such micrographs are located within endocytic vacuoles (59,442, 467). Although these may be particles that have not yet succeeded in initiating infection, they might also represent the primary transcriptase particles. Thus, another model was proposed in which the primary transcriptase particle remains within a vacuole but inserts its λ2 pentamers through the membrane so that mRNAs can be extruded into the cytoplasm (467).

Discrete Enzyme Activities in Reovirus Transcription and mRNA Capping

Each of the steps in reovirus transcription and mRNA capping (Fig. 7) (167) is mediated by an enzyme present in cores and encoded by a viral genome segment. The 5′ cap of reovirus transcripts includes a 7-N-methyl guanosine linked by three phosphate groups to the 5′-terminal, template-encoded guanosine present in all reovirus mRNAs (153,165). The 5′-terminal, template-encoded guanosine is 2′-O-methylated (153,165). The next residue in all reovirus mRNAs is cytidine, which can also undergo 2′-O-methylation, but by a cellular cytoplasmic methyltransferase (121). Reovirus capping activities can be uncoupled from transcription and readily function when exogenous substrates, including preformed oligonucleotides and reovirus mRNAs in some cases, are incubated with viral particles (168,321,337).

RNA Polymerase

Early work failed to associate polymerase activity with any individual reovirus proteins after disruption of cores (226,230,500). The transcriptase (dsRNA-dependent

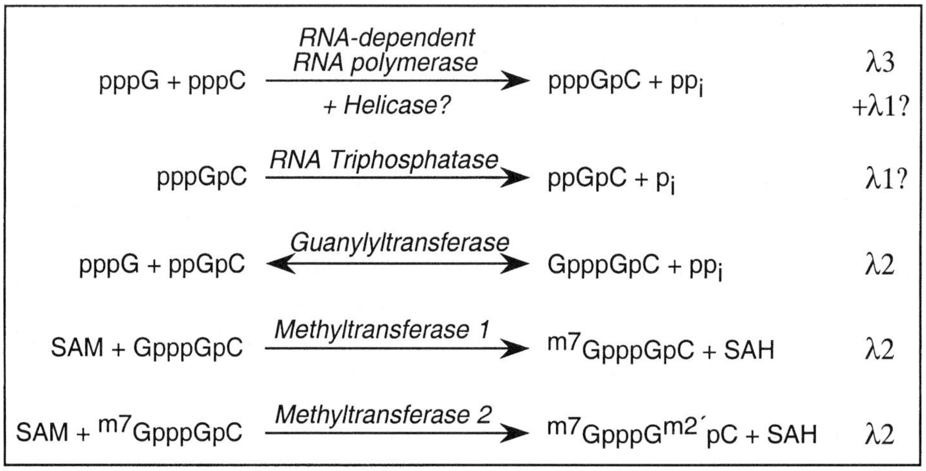

FIG. 7. Enzymatic activities in transcription and capping by reoviruses. Polymerization of nucleoside triphosphates (shown here for the first nucleotide pair) as specified by a genomic dsRNA template is mediated by the dsRNA-dependent RNA polymerase. The RNA triphosphatase generates a nucleosidyl diphosphate at the 5′ end of the nascent mRNA and sets the stage for formation of the dimethylated 5′ cap by sequential actions of the guanylyltransferase and methyltransferases. The role of an independent helicase in reovirus transcription is proposed but not proven. Individual reovirus proteins proven or suspected to mediate each activity are indicated at *right*. SAM, S-adenosyl methionine; SAH, S-adenosyl homocysteine.

RNA polymerase) was later suggested to be formed by portions of both core proteins λ1 and λ2 because of their apparent labeling by pyridoxal phosphate during transcription (320,321). Recent work indicates that the minor core protein λ3 is likely to be the catalytic subunit of the transcriptase (69,127,243,326,460). A limited spectrum of activity [poly(C)-dependent poly(G) polymerase] has been reported for λ3 expressed in isolation, which probably indicates that other core proteins are needed to form the complete transcriptase (460). The λ3 protein is also likely to be a primary component of the ssRNA-dependent RNA polymerase that operates during minus-strand synthesis. Sequences in reovirus RNAs that are specifically recognized by the polymerase (e.g., initiation sites) have yet to be defined.

RNA Helicase

The double-stranded nature of the reovirus genome necessitates an RNA duplex unwinding activity for transcription to proceed. This activity might be inherent in the polymerase but also may be localized to another core protein and take the form of a classical RNA helicase (44,354,355,460). One report suggested that the antiviral drug ribavirin inhibits reovirus replication by interfering with helicase activity (376). Some recent evidence suggests that helicase activity may be associated with core shell protein λ1 (44,354).

RNA Triphosphatase

An RNA triphosphatase (RNA triphosphate phosphohydrolase) initiates formation of the 5′ cap on reovirus mRNAs by releasing inorganic phosphate from the originally triphosphorylated 5′ end of the transcript, thereby yielding a 5′ diphosphate group (see Fig. 7). An NTPase nucleoside triphosphatase has been found in reovirus virions and cores (53,231,354,355) and may represent this enzyme. Recent work with recombinant λ1 protein indicates that it has such an activity, suggesting that it performs this function during 5′ cap generation by reovirus particles (45).

RNA Guanylyltransferase

An N-terminal domain of protein λ2 has been defined as the reovirus guanylyltransferase (280,378). Its enzymatic mechanism includes formation of a covalent λ2–GMP intermediate, probably at lysine 190, using GTP as substrate (93,152,279,423). The GMP is subsequently transferred to the 5′ diphosphate of reovirus mRNAs (see Fig. 7). The guanylyltransferase is promiscuous in its specificity for GMP-acceptors in that PP_i, GDP, GTP, and both ppG- and ppA-terminated oligonucleotides work as substrates (93,167). A GTP-dependent, pyrophosphate exchange activity associated with cores (484) represents guanylylation plus its reverse reaction. After methylation, transcript termini become resistant to pyrophosphate exchange (167); thus, reversibility of guanylylation may be required to ensure that proper 5′GpppG caps are formed on transcripts to act as substrates for methylation (see later).

RNA Methyltransferases

Final proof is lacking for the protein that mediates methyltransferase activities to modify the 5′-terminal guanosines of reovirus mRNAs (see Fig. 7), but a role for λ2 is strongly indicated by the presence of two methylase-like domains identified in the crystal structure of core-bound λ2 (378). SAM serves as methyl group donor for these reactions yielding S-adenosyl homocysteine (SAH) as a by-product (154,167). Indeed, SAH was found to bind both methylase-like domains of λ2 in core crystals (378), and one of these regions was found to undergo cross-linking to radiolabeled SAM in other experiments (280). The 5′-terminal structure of reovirus mRNAs is specifically recognized by the methyltransferase(s), as GpppG and GpppGC can act as methyl acceptors but GppG, GppppG, and GpppGA cannot (424).

Organization and Mechanism of the Transcription Machinery

The sequential action of enzymes that synthesize reovirus mRNAs implies a precise structural organization within the core. Some studies suggest that capping of nascent mRNAs occurs when they are only 2 to 15 nucleotides long (167,321), in which case the transcriptase and capping enzymes must be close together. Because preformed oligonucleotides and reovirus mRNAs can be capped by cores (168,321,337), the capping enzymes must be accessible to external solvent; however, antibodies have not been found to inhibit any transcription-related activity (424).

Transcription-related enzymes may be located in complexes near the fivefold axes of reovirus particles. Electron micrographs of transcribing cores suggest that mRNAs are released through the λ2 spikes that protrude upward around the fivefold axes of cores (27,500). This idea is supported by reconstructed images from cryoelectron microscopy showing a channel through the λ2 pentamer that is open in cores (131,310). The low copy number in which λ3 is found in cores (about 12 copies) has also been used to argue that it is located near the fivefold axes.

Each of the 10 reovirus gene segments may represent an independent transcriptional unit. Both *in vitro* and in cells later in infection, transcripts from the 10 segments are produced at rates that are approximately proportional to the reciprocals of their lengths (24,225,445,489,530). Given that transcript elongation is the rate-limiting step in transcription (see later), this finding suggests a model for transcription in which each of the 10 genes is transcribed independently, and not as part of a linked array (225,226,424). A feature of this model is that it involves at least 10 transcriptases within the reovirus core (445). Electron micrographs of transcribing cores with multiple mRNAs being simultaneously extruded around the particle perimeter support this idea (27). Both moving transcriptase and moving template models for reovirus transcription have been proposed (226,424,515). Experiments in which transcription was inhibited by cross-linking genomic dsRNA are consistent with both these models (337,424); however, the moving template model is generally accepted. According to this model, a set of transcription-related enzymes is fixed near the base of each λ2 spike within the core. It is proposed that the entire length of each dsRNA gene segment moves past the fixed transcriptase and that the nascent mRNA is directed past the capping enzymes and out the λ2 spike (378,516). The liquid crystalline state of the packaged genomic dsRNA (131,199) may permit it the freedom of movement required by this model.

Later Steps in Replication: Amplification of Viral Products and Assembly of Progeny Virions

Translation of Viral mRNAs

Shortly after the onset of infection, there is a gradual increase in synthesis of reovirus proteins and a decrease in synthesis of cellular proteins (186,417). Newly synthesized viral proteins are detected by 2 hours after infection, and by 10 hours most of the proteins synthesized in the infected cell are viral in origin (530). The capacity of viral mRNA to associate with ribosomes may be a host-range determinant, as certain avian reoviruses can enter mammalian cells and transcribe their early mRNAs yet fail to initiate protein synthesis (42,285). The mechanism by which viral protein synthesis comes to predominate in infected cells is not well understood.

In addition to regulation of translation of viral versus cellular mRNAs, translation of the different reovirus transcripts is regulated. Reovirus mRNAs differ in translation frequency by as much as 30-fold (225). Because the different genome segments are transcribed at variable rates, inversely proportional to segment length, and because the transcripts appear to have similar stabilities, differences in the amounts of each viral mRNA provide one source of variability in the amounts of each protein that are synthesized (258,530). A second source of variability is in the translation frequency of the different mRNAs. Such variability has been found in both infected cells and *in vitro* translation systems (17,169,191,273,304,305,530,531). Nucleotide sequences of reovirus mRNAs at the −3 and +4 positions flanking the initiator AUG contribute to differing translation efficiencies *in vitro* (245); however, other nucleotide positions may influence the efficiency of translation of these mRNAs *in vivo* (41,329,385). Because the 5′ nontranslated regions of the reovirus mRNAs are short (12 to 32 bases), this length may also contribute to translation rate; for example, the two reovirus proteins made in largest quantities—μ1 and σ3—have the longest 5′ nontranslated regions. For the S1 mRNA, from which two unrelated proteins are translated, it was proposed that translation rates are regulated at the level of polypeptide elongation (41,126,148). The observation that the M1 mRNA is translated much less efficiently *in vivo* than *in vitro* has suggested that its translation may be influenced by negative regulatory factors in cells (388). Reovirus mRNAs also may differ in capacity to compete for components of the translation machinery (64,285,377). Several studies suggest that levels of translation may be affected by the influence of different viral mRNAs on negative regulators of translation, such as the dsRNA-activated protein kinase (41,48,400).

Assortment and Packaging of the 10 Viral mRNAs

The mechanism ensuring that 10 unique dsRNA segments are assembled into each newly formed virion remains unknown. Pieces of evidence that the reovirus genes are assorted selectively are that a particle-to-pfu ratio as low as 1 has been reported (454), and that the central cavity of reovirus particles is not large enough to accommodate many more than the 10 unique segments (131,199,341). It is generally accepted that assortment of the 10 segments occurs at the level of the reovirus mRNAs, and that minus-strand synthesis to generate dsRNA occurs later, within a nascent viral particle (486, 528,529) (see later and Fig. 6). It has been suggested that assortment and minus-strand synthesis may be more intimately linked than previously interpreted (13).

Assortment is likely to involve signals that identify an RNA as viral and not cellular, as well as signals that specify each of the 10 segments as unique. The relevance of either RNA–protein or RNA–RNA interactions to this process is unclear. All 10 reovirus gene segments contain short conserved regions at the 5′ and 3′ ends of their plus and minus strands, but it is not known if these sequences play any role in packaging. Sequences near the termini of some reovirus ssRNAs may interact in a panhandle-like structure, which may be important for packaging (87, 274,526). Analysis of mutants containing internal deletions of their M1 genes identified sequences within 130 to 190 nucleotides of the 5′ and 3′ termini that contain the minimum required signals for packaging (525). The plus strand of each genomic segment contains a 5′ cap identical to that on mRNAs made by primary transcriptase particles (166), so the cap might serve as a packaging signal as well.

One early study hypothesized that σNS plays a role in mRNA assortment and packaging because of its capacity to bind ssRNA (211). Protein assemblies, containing primarily σNS and apparently capable of binding to selected regions of reovirus mRNAs, were subsequently isolated from infected cells, consistent with the idea that this protein plays a significant role in the earliest stages of particle assembly (183,184,458). In a more recent study, protein-specific antisera were used to precipitate protein–RNA complexes from infected cells in an attempt to identify components of the assorting particle (13). This work suggested that σNS, as well as μNS and σ3, associate with individual reovirus mRNAs to form small nucleoprotein complexes soon after transcription, but that μNS or σ3 (not σNS) binds to the mRNAs first. Recent evidence that σNS binds to ssRNA with positive cooperativity and demonstrates an ATP-independent, duplex-unwinding activity is consistent with a role for this protein in packaging and/or minus-strand synthesis (179,180).

Minus-Strand Synthesis: The Replicase Reaction

Each packaged plus strand serves as a template for synthesis of one minus-strand copy, which remains base-paired to the plus strand after synthesis and thereby regenerates the genomic dsRNA (1,398,399,410,528). Minus-strand synthesis proceeds from an initiation point at the extreme 3′ end of each template, and once the minus strand is synthesized, it remains within the nascent progeny particle. The viral replicase catalyzes a single round of minus-strand synthesis. Initiation of minus-strand synthesis, but not elongation, appears to depend on continuing protein synthesis (489), but this effect remains poorly understood.

Although preparations of replicase particles are often heterogeneous and include particles with transcriptase activity (323,398,487,529), it seems likely that these two activities are associated with discrete types of particles (323). Particles with replicase activity have a buoyant density similar to that of virions, are morphologically indistinct, and contain the viral core proteins with reduced amounts of λ2 and other outer capsid proteins relative to virions (323,529). The replicase activity associated with nascent particles is susceptible to RNase, but once minus-strand synthesis is complete, the particles become RNase-resistant (1). Recent work suggests that λ3 acts as the ssRNA-dependent dsRNA polymerase of reoviruses (460), but the roles of other proteins in minus-strand synthesis remain undefined. At end of minus-strand synthesis, RNA polymerase is positioned to jump strands and begin plus-strand synthesis using the minus strand as template.

Secondary Transcription

Secondary transcription is defined as that mediated by newly assembled subviral particles within infected cells. These particles must be derived from those with replicase activity, and they are distinguishable by sedimentation behavior, by the presence of a full complement of dsRNA, by the presence of variable amounts of protein μNS, and by reduced amounts of λ2 and the other outer capsid proteins (323,447,532). The appearance of "late" viral mRNAs represents transcription by progeny subviral particles (secondary transcriptase particles) (323, 447,524,529). According to some studies, these secondary transcriptase particles contain latent capping enzymes and produce uncapped mRNAs (447,523,524). These uncapped viral mRNAs are proposed to be translated preferentially at later times in infection. Late viral transcripts begin to appear at 4 to 6 hours after infection, reach maximum amounts (greatly exceeding the quantity of primary transcripts) at 12 hours, and subsequently decrease (252,448,489,523). Whether they serve only for translation into proteins or whether they may also be packaged into progeny particles and serve as templates for minus-strand synthesis remains controversial (157, 324,410,523). The recent evidence that recombinant μNS protein can bind to cores without inhibiting their transcription and capping activities, while at the same time blocking outer capsid assembly, is consistent with a model in which μNS serves to increase the production of capped transcripts within infected cells (66). It is not known if particles that engage in secondary transcription can go on to form mature virions (see Fig. 6).

Assembly of the Viral Capsids

A great deal remains to be understood about the protein and nucleoprotein complexes involved in assembling the inner and outer capsids in reovirus particles (see Fig. 6). The earliest reovirus particles may be ones that contain reovirus mRNAs primarily in complex with σ3 and the nonstructural proteins μNS and σNS (13,183). The next particle along the assembly pathway is described to lack nonstructural proteins, to include both inner and outer capsid proteins, and to be RNase sensitive (1,323). These "replicase particles" contain an ssRNA-dependent dsRNA polymerase activity and appear to be engaged in minus-strand synthesis (323). With the completion of minus-strand synthesis, the replicase particles become RNase resistant, probably reflecting the occurrence of structural rearrangements within the particle (1,523). Additional copies of the outer capsid proteins may be added to form complete virion particles (323,532). A final step in morphogenesis is synthesis of the virion-associated oligonucleotides, which appears to occur as the viral transcriptase undergoes inhibition during outer capsid assembly (16,38,151,347,439,532).

Many of the reovirus structural proteins exhibit some degree of self-assembly, in the absence of viral RNA or a full complement of viral proteins. For example, cells coexpressing the major inner capsid proteins λ1 and σ2 form particles that are morphologically similar to core shells (513). When λ2 and λ3 are coexpressed with λ1 and σ2, they are incorporated into particles as well, the former creating spikes that project from the inner capsid surface as expected (513). Other findings suggest that λ1 and σ2 may self-assemble into oligomers (dimers or trimers) before or after interacting in larger assemblies (102,131). The λ2 protein, however, does not form pentamers in the absence of other proteins (286). The exact order in which these proteins come together to form nascent infectious particles, and the roles of RNA and the minor core protein μ2 in this process, are unknown.

Assembly of the outer capsid is also poorly understood. The major outer capsid proteins σ3 and μ1 bind together in solution to form hetero-oligomers (131,211, 260,471,530). Whether the σ3-associated cleavage of μ1 into fragments μ1N and μ1C (260,347,471) is required for assembly is unknown. The fact that a mutant with a ts lesion in S4 (which encodes σ3) results in the accumulation of core-like particles as assembly intermediates (160,322) may suggest that preformed complexes of μ1 and σ3 are required to bind to nascent particles. Similar observations with a ts mutant in L2 (which encodes λ2) may suggest a role for λ2 in initiating the binding of these complexes to particles (160,322,368). Recently developed systems for recoating reovirus cores with recombinant outer capsid proteins have provided additional evidence that preformed complexes of μ1 and σ3 are required for assembly into particles and that the assembly of μ1 and σ3 can occur independently of σ1 (83,151). A significant body of work has addressed the self-assembly of σ1 oligomers. Sequences near the amino terminus of σ1 are likely to mediate its interactions with λ2 within virions (22,131,161,163,270,284,343).

Release from Cells

There is little or no evidence for a specific mechanism such as membrane budding or vesicular transport by which reovirus particles might be released from infected cells in the absence of cytolysis. Thus, release of newly assembled reovirus virions is thought to follow cell death and the associated breakdown of the plasma membrane. Recent evidence indicates that apoptosis is an important mechanism of reovirus-induced cell death in the case of type 3 reovirus isolates (114,383,475,476).

EFFECTS ON THE HOST CELL

Viral Factories and Interactions with the Cytoskeleton

Reovirus-infected cells develop cytoplasmic inclusions that are not bound by cellular membranes (11,188,379). Inclusions first appear as phase-dense granules scattered in the cytoplasm, but these move toward the nucleus and increase in size as infection progresses (160,379,415, 453). Viral factories contain dsRNA (188,444), viral polypeptides (109,160,299,379,453), and both complete and incomplete particles (18,109,160,379), but they do not contain ribosomes (415). Particles are often found in crystalline arrays. The characteristics and temporal development of viral factories can vary with growth conditions and virus strain (160,299). The μ2 proteins of reoviruses type 1 Lang and type 3 Dearing appear to be the primary determinant of a difference in the rate of inclusion formation observed with these two strains (299). A mechanistic description of the viral factories as "organelles" for reovirus replication and assembly remains in its infancy.

Immunocytochemical studies reveal progressive disruption and reorganization of the vimentin (intermediate) filament network in reovirus-infected fibroblasts (415). Vimentin filaments are specifically incorporated into viral factories and may play a direct role in replication (109,415,418). The nonstructural protein μNS may associate with vimentin filaments to anchor structures involved in viral assembly to the network (319). Disruption or reorganization of intermediate filaments may cause changes in cell shape that typify the cytopathic effect of reovirus infection and may contribute to cell injury (415,418).

Immunocytochemical studies reveal little change in the distribution of microtubules and microfilaments within reovirus-infected cells (415). In addition, experiments with microtubule-disrupting agents suggest that intact microtubules are not required for productive reovirus infection in cultured cells (18,108,452). Microtubules extend directly through viral factories (18,108,109,160, 415,453), nevertheless, and there is evidence to suggest that proteins σ1 (18) and μNS (319) may each associate with them. Other studies implicate microtubules in the transport of reovirus particles within endocytic vacuoles early in infection (177).

Inhibition of Cellular DNA Synthesis and Induction of Apoptosis

One consequence of reovirus infection can be the inhibition of cellular DNA synthesis (142,186,416,475). Inhibition of DNA synthesis is detected 8 to 12 hours after infection of L cells with type 3 strains (142,186,416,475), occurs more rapidly as the MOI is increased (429), and has been suggested to involve a G1/S transition block (103,143,195,197). Inhibition of L-cell DNA synthesis also occurs with UV-inactivated virions, but not with cores or empty virions (196,255,416,429). In an early genetic study, the basis for a strain difference in inhibition by both live and UV-inactivated virions of T1L and T3D was mapped to the S1 genome segment (416), which encodes both the cell-attachment protein σ1 and the nonstructural protein σ1s. Genetic studies indicate that S1 is also the primary determinant of strain-specific differences in the induction of apoptosis (383,475,476). Like inhibition of cellular DNA synthesis, apoptosis can be induced by UV-inactivated, replication-incompetent virions and it can be blocked by antibodies directed against the cell-attachment protein σ1 (476).

The observation that both strain-specific differences in DNA synthesis inhibition and apoptosis induction segregate with the S1 genome segment suggested that these two processes might occur through related pathways. Recent studies do not support this hypothesis. Studies using a σ1s-deficient reovirus strain demonstrate that reovirus induces cell cycle arrest at the G2/M transition, that this effect requires the nonstructural protein σ1s, and that it occurs in the absence of apoptosis (365). Current efforts are focused on understanding the cellular pathways that are involved in reovirus-induced apoptosis *in vitro* and *in vivo*. Evidence suggests that induction involves cellular proteases including calpains (114) and caspase 8 (92), is blocked by Bcl-2 overexpression (383), is dependent on NF-κB activation (98), and involves the TRAIL-receptor binding pathway (92). More work is needed to establish the relationships among the various molecules implicated to date in reovirus-induced apoptosis.

Given the fact that not all reovirus strains induce apoptosis to high levels, the importance of this process in reovirus replication and disease induction remains somewhat uncertain. Neither is it clear if any reovirus-encoded molecules function to block apoptosis. The results of several studies support the notion that reovirus-induced apoptosis does not negatively impact viral growth (383) and does not depend on efficient viral replication (114). However, virus-induced apoptosis may play a significant role in pathogenesis, as one recent study revealed a correlation between areas of viral growth in the central nervous system (CNS) and apoptosis within those tissues (359).

Effects on Cellular RNA and Protein Synthesis

Reovirus infection can also result in the inhibition of cellular RNA and/or protein synthesis (186,252,276, 417,530). Viral replication is required for this effect; moreover, inhibition is MOI dependent, suggesting that increasing amounts of viral products have increasing effects (417). In one case, a strain difference in the inhibition of cellular RNA and protein synthesis was mapped to the S4 genome segment, which encodes the σ3 protein (417). This result was initially interpreted as evidence that σ3 plays a direct role in the mechanism of translational inhibition, but more recent studies suggest that σ3 functions to block an inhibitory signal in infected cells (408). Some cell lines support reovirus infection yet are resistant to inhibition of cellular protein synthesis (112, 123,317).

The molecular mechanism(s) that result in protein synthesis inhibition in reovirus-infected cells have yet to be determined, but several lines of indirect evidence suggest that σ3 may influence the level of translation by regulating the activation of the interferon-induced, dsRNA-activated protein kinase, PKR. Activation of the dsRNA-activated protein kinase results in phosphorylation of eIF-2α and inhibition of translation initiation. *In vitro* studies, and others in heterologous viral systems, indicate that σ3 can down-regulate PKR by sequestering its dsRNA activator (32,214,275,521). The ability to interfere with PKR activation is consistent with the finding that expression of σ3 in transfected cells can stimulate translation from a reporter gene (178,290,413,471,521).

As yet, we do not understand the molecular basis for reovirus strain-specific effects on cellular protein synthesis. The σ3 molecules from strains with distinct phenotypes are highly homologous in regions proposed to mediate dsRNA binding (115,235). Several pieces of evidence are consistent with a model in which strain differences in σ3–μ1 affinity determine the amount of free σ3 available to bind dsRNA and block PKR activation (178,214,275,408,471,521). The finding that σ3 is localized throughout the cytoplasm in cells in which cellular translation is not inhibited, but is localized to perinuclear viral factories in cells in which cellular translation is inhibited, provides support for a model in which σ3 down-regulates the dsRNA-activated protein kinase locally, typically sparing viral but not cellular protein synthesis from the inhibitory activity of PKR (408).

There is some controversial evidence that late in reovirus infection there is a switch to cap-independent translation. There are reports that late reovirus transcripts may lack a 5′ cap (446,524), and some studies suggest that reovirus infection induces a modification of the cell translation machinery such that uncapped mRNAs are preferentially translated over capped (cellular) mRNAs (447,448). In one study, extracts from reovirus-infected cells were shown not to support translation of capped mRNAs (450). It has been speculated that a cellular protein required for capped mRNA synthesis may be inactivated in these infected cells (523). To date, however, there is no evidence that either EIF-4G or EIF-4E, translation factors that are known to be modified or inactivated in other virus-infected cells, are inactivated in reovirus-infected cells (140,239). Other studies imply that infection does not result in modification of the existing translation machinery but instead induces a factor that stimulates translation of uncapped mRNAs (266); moreover, protein σ3 can apparently function as such a factor *in vitro* (264,265). Reports in conflict with the preceding ones indicate that reovirus-infected cells can translate capped and uncapped mRNAs with equal efficiency (123,330), suggesting a hypothesis that the preferential translation of reovirus mRNAs in infected cells is mediated by mRNA competition for a limiting translation factor (64,285,377). The reasons for discrepancies between studies are unclear; they may reflect the complexity of mechanisms that contribute to regulation of translation in reovirus-infected cells.

Interferon Induction

Reoviruses can induce infected cells to express interferon (205,254,418,436). With ts mutants, interferon induction correlates with yields of infectious virus but not with amounts of viral dsRNA, ssRNA, or protein made in infected cells (254). Using myocarditic and nonmyocarditic reovirus strains, one genetic study mapped the viral determinants of interferon induction to the M1, S2, and L2 genome segments encoding core proteins μ2, σ2, and λ2, respectively (436). A subset of these segments determines myocarditic potential and mRNA levels in infected cardiac myocyte cultures (432). These results suggest that levels of viral mRNA may determine the extent of interferon induction.

It is generally accepted that the genomic dsRNA of reoviruses can serve as a potent inducer of interferon during infection (205,254,289). The reovirus replication cycle, throughout which the genome remains encased within a protein capsid, may have evolved in part to prevent the genomic dsRNA from inducing a florid interferon response. Regions of dsRNA formed within particular reovirus mRNAs (for example the S1 mRNA) (48) might also play a role in interferon induction. The induction of interferon β in certain cell types in response to reovirus infection was recently shown to depend on interferon regulatory factor 3 (353).

Treatment with UV has been used to study interferon induction by reoviruses (205,254). Interferon induction by viral particles is far more resistant to UV inactivation than is infectivity. UV-treated reoviruses induce interferon more rapidly than occurs during productive infection, suggesting that a different mechanism is involved. A range of UV doses was found to increase the potency of strain T3D as an interferon inducer; in addition, UV treatment turned one ts mutant (tsC447) into an extremely potent inducer, even at nonpermissive temperature. It was proposed that UV treatment destabilizes the viral core so that genomic dsRNA from input particles escapes into the cytoplasm (205).

Interferons may inhibit reovirus replication by a variety of mechanisms. In general, interferon α/β appears to block the translation of early reovirus mRNAs (502). As discussed earlier, interferon-induced expression of the eIF-2α kinase, PKR, may explain the inhibition of viral protein synthesis in some reovirus-infected cells (113, 192,350,401); however, interferon γ is a poor inducer of this kinase and decreases the yield of progeny virions without having a major effect on viral protein synthesis (176,402). In other studies, cells treated with interferon α/β were found to contain an 2′,5′-oligo(A)-dependent endoribonuclease (RNase L) that cleaves reovirus mRNAs and may facilitate the antiviral state (21,314,315, 351); however, whether an endoribonuclease contributes to inhibiting the translation of reovirus mRNAs within cells in which the dsRNA-activated protein kinase has been proposed to function remains controversial (314, 315,352). Reovirus strains can differ in the extent to which their replication is inhibited by interferon (217). Several studies have demonstrated that reovirus can replicate efficiently in interferon-treated cells despite activation of antiviral effector enzymes (111,155).

Effects on Other Functions in Differentiated Cells

Some studies have identified reovirus effects on differentiated cells. In MDCK (polarized epithelial) cells, reoviruses produced persistent infections characterized by failure to form tight junctions, reduced EGF receptor expression, and increased expression of the adhesion molecule VCAM (317). In 3T3 (primary fibroblast) cells, reoviruses also produced persistent infections, characterized in this case by decreased expression of EGF receptors and increased expression of insulin receptors (480). Thus, reovirus persistence in a variety of differentiated cells can significantly alter cellular functions, including some involved in cellular growth control.

A number of interesting early studies demonstrated that transformed cells are more susceptible to reovirus-induced cytolysis than are untransformed cells (132,201). Until recently, there were few clues to explain the molecular basis of these observations. Evidence now suggests the involvement of the EGF receptor-linked signal transduction pathway in the efficiency of reovirus infection in differentiated cells (464,466). More recent studies demonstrate that activation of the *ras* signalling pathway (an event downstream of EGF receptor activation) renders cells susceptible to reovirus infection, and it has been suggested that a component of the *ras* pathway might function to down-regulate PKR, thereby promoting translation of reovirus mRNAs and thus viral replication (463).

Other studies investigated how interactions between the reovirus cell-attachment protein and its cell surface receptor(s) affect functions in differentiated cells. In optic nerve glial cultures, ligand binding to the reovirus type 3 receptor stimulated expression of galactocerebroside and myelin basic protein (96,97). Ligand binding to the type 3 receptor in rats also caused changes in oligodendrocyte function resulting in altered myelin expression (95). In another study, interaction of reovirus with thyroid follicular epithelial cells caused induction of major histocompatibility complex (MHC) class II molecules (172). Because this occurred even in the absence of viral replication, reovirus attachment to cell surface receptors may be sufficient to affect the expression of cellular proteins, probably through receptor-linked signaling pathways.

Persistent Infections

Although commonly causing the death of cells in which they replicate (lytic), reoviruses can produce nonlytic, persistent infections in a variety of cultured cells (2,4,6–8,33,67,112,116,119,132,317,463,468,480,498). Continuous maintenance of persistently infected cultures for months or even years is possible. Reoviruses have not yet been reported to persist in host mammals in the natural world, but recent studies have shown evidence for delayed clearance or chronic infection in laboratory mice. One of these studies involved infection of normal mice with reoviruses selected during persistent infections in L cells and showed delayed clearance from the CNS (327). The other studies involved infection of SCID mice with wt reoviruses and showed selection of organ-specific variants during the course of the chronic infection (193,194). Mechanistic relationships between these chronic infections in animals and persistent infections in culture remain undefined. Persistent infections in cultured cells by reoviruses appear best described as carrier cultures (2,7,116,119,498) and have been proposed to involve two distinguishable phases, establishment and maintenance. Certain aspects of reovirus–cell interaction (e.g., proteolytic uncoating during viral entry) appear to influence both phases of persistent infection, however, suggesting that the two phases may not be as mechanistically separable as first proposed.

Establishment

Viral characteristics can influence the establishment of persistent reovirus infections. Establishment of persistently infected L cells can be facilitated with defective stocks obtained by serially passing viruses at high MOI (6,7,67,119). Defective stocks contain a variety of mutants (see earlier section) including some that favor the establishment of persistent infections (6). Wild-type isolates can differ in their capacities to establish persistent infections in L cells after undergoing serial passage at high MOI. In the case of reoviruses type 1 Lang and type 3 Dearing, this difference is determined by their L2 genome segments (67). A current model links the L2 gene product λ2 to the generation or amplification of different mutants within defective stocks, including those that favor the establishment of persistent infection, but the mechanism of λ2 activity in this regard remains unknown.

Cellular characteristics can also influence the establishment of persistent reovirus infections. Wild-type reoviruses can establish persistent infections in several differentiated cell lines (33,112,116,132,317,468,480, 498). The basis for an apparent relationship between cell differentiation and establishment of persistent infection remains unclear, but the resistance of some cells to reovirus-induced inhibition of cellular macromolecular synthesis has been proposed to play a role (112,132). The resistance of some cells to reovirus-induced apoptosis, or other mechanisms of killing, may also be involved. Other evidence suggests that some differentiated cells may favor the establishment of persistent infection by restricting reovirus disassembly as part of the entry process (498). Consistent with the latter proposal is evidence that persistent infections in L cells can be established using wt reoviruses if the cells are treated with ammonium chloride, which interferes with viral entry, during the first few days of infection (72).

Maintenance

A variety of viral mutants accumulate in cultures during persistent reovirus infections. Some of these mutants may play no role in the maintenance of persistence but reflect that reoviruses undergo extensive genetic changes during long-term persistent culture (4,6–8). On the other hand, cell lines cured of persistent reovirus infection by passing with neutralizing antibodies (PI cells) are found to support reduced growth of wt reoviruses relative to viruses isolated from persistently infected cultures (PI viruses) (2,119,232). This finding argues that both viruses and cells undergo mutation during the maintenance of persistent infection, and the complementary nature of the effects of these mutations on viral growth suggests that a process of virus–cell coevolution is a characteristic feature of the maintenance phase (2,119, 232). Current evidence suggests that at least an element of this coevolution is based on steps in reovirus entry, with PI cells evolving to resist one or more steps in viral entry, and PI viruses evolving to evade these cellular counter-measures (119).

Specific Mutations Involved in Persistence

Mutant S4 genome segments from defective stocks (3) appear to play a critical role in the establishment of persistent reovirus infections in L cells (6). Because persistent infection appears to require that cellular injury be attenuated, it was proposed (6) that these mutations in S4 might be required for attentuating the shut-off of host RNA and protein synthesis characteristic of most reovirus infections (417) or for enabling PI viruses to interfere with the growth of wt, lytic virus (5,81). Although the S4 gene product, σ3, can influence the activation state of interferon-induced enzymes (214), interferon does not appear to play a protective role in persistent reovirus infection of at least one cell line (111).

More recent evidence suggests that mutations in the S4 genome segment are selected during the maintenance phase of persistent infection in L cells, as part of the virus–cell coevolution described earlier. Mutations in S4 determine the capacity of certain PI viruses to replicate in cells that have been cured of persistent infection (511). In addition, the S4 mutations in these and other PI viruses have been found to facilitate the proteolytic cleavage of the encoded outer capsid protein σ3 (499). Interestingly, a recent study revealed that cured cells have a defect in the maturation of cathepsin L, a lysosomal cysteine protease that may be responsible for virion uncoating in L cells (20). These results provide support for the model in which viral mutations that increase the efficiency of disassembly enable reovirus to maintain a persistent infection in cells that have evolved to restrict this step. These findings lend support to the hypothesis that reovirus persistence in L cells involves a carrier culture in which continuing transmission of virus between cells by an extracellular route is required for maintenance (119).

Mutations in the S1 genome segment appear also to be selected during the maintenance phase of persistent infections in L cells and can determine the capacity of certain PI viruses to replicate in cells that have been cured of persistent infection, independently of any mutations in S4 (232,511). In these and certain other PI viruses, the mutations in S1 are linked to decreased stability of the σ1 (receptor binding protein) oligomer and its decreased capacity to mediate sialic-acid-dependent hemagglutination (511). The decrease in σ1 oligomer stability in these viruses has been proposed to play a determinative role in the maintenance of persistent infections (511), but further work is needed to clarify the relative roles of S1 and S4 mutations in this regard.

REFERENCES

1. Acs G, Klett H, Schonberg M, et al. Mechanism of reovirus double-stranded ribonucleic acid synthesis *in vivo* and *in vitro*. *J Virol* 1971;8:684–689.
2. Ahmed R, Canning WM, Kauffman RS, et al. Role of the host cell in persistent viral infection: Coevolution of L cells and reovirus during persistent infection. *Cell* 1981;25:325–332.
3. Ahmed R, Chakraborty PR, Fields BN. Genetic variation during lytic reovirus infection: High-passage stocks of wild-type reovirus contain temperature-sensitive mutants. *J Virol* 1980;34:285–287.
4. Ahmed R, Chakraborty PR, Graham AF, et al. Genetic variation during persistent reovirus infection: Presence of extragenically suppressed temperature-sensitive lesions in wild-type virus isolated from persistently infected cells. *J Virol* 1980;34:383–389.
5. Ahmed R, Fields BN. Reassortment of genome segments between reovirus defective interfering particles and infectious virus: Construction of temperature-sensitive and attenuated viruses by rescue of mutations from DI particles. *Virology* 1981;111:351–363.
6. Ahmed R, Fields BN. Role of the S4 gene in the establishment of persistent reovirus infection in L cells. *Cell* 1982;28:605–612.
7. Ahmed R, Graham AF. Persistent infections in L cells with temperature-sensitive mutants of reovirus. *J Virol* 1977;23:250–262.
8. Ahmed R, Kauffman RS, Fields BN. Genetic variation during persistent reovirus infection: Isolation of cold-sensitive and temperature-sensitive mutants from persistently infected L cells. *Virology* 1983;131:71–78.
9. Ambler L, Mackay M. Reovirus 1 and 3 bind and internalise at the apical surface of intestinal epithelial cells. *Virology* 1991;184:162–169.
10. Amerongen HM, Wilson GA, Fields BN, Neutra MR. Proteolytic processing of reovirus is required for adherence to intestinal M cells. *J Virol* 1994;68:8428–8432.
11. Anderson N, Doane FW. An electron-microscope study of reovirus type 2 in L cells. *J Pathol Bacteriol* 1966;92:433–439.
12. Antczak JB, Chmelo R, Pickup DJ, Joklik WK. Sequence at both termini of the 10 genes of reovirus serotype 3 (strain Dearing). *Virology* 1982;121:307–319.
13. Antczak JB, Joklik WK. Reovirus genome segment assortment into progeny genomes studied by the use of monoclonal antibodies directed against reovirus proteins. *Virology* 1992;187:760–776.
14. Armstrong G, Paul R, Lee P. Studies on reovirus receptors of L cells: Virus binding characteristics and comparison with reovirus receptors of erythrocytes. *Virology* 1984;138:37–48.
15. Arnott S, Wilkins MH, Fuller W, Langridge R. Molecular and crystal structures of double-helical RNA. II. Determination and comparison of diffracted intensities for the alpha and beta crystalline forms of reovirus RNA and their interpretation in terms of groups of three RNA molecules. *J Mol Biol* 1967;27:525–533.
16. Astell C, Silverstein SC, Levin DH, Acs G. Regulation of the reovirus RNA transcriptase by a viral capsomere protein. *Virology* 1972;48:648–654.
17. Atwater JA, Munemitsu SM, Samuel CE. Biosynthesis of reovirus-specified polypeptides. Efficiency of expression of cDNAs of the reovirus S1 and S4 genes in transfected animal cells differs at the level of translation. *Virology* 1987;159:350–357.
18. Babiss LE, Luftig RB, Weatherbee JA, et al. Reovirus serotypes 1 and 3 differ in their *in vitro* association with microtubules. *J Virol* 1979;30:863–874.
19. Baer GS, Dermody TS. Mutations in reovirus outer-capsid protein σ3 selected during persistent infections of L cells confer resistance to protease inhibitor E64. *J Virol* 1997;71:4921–4928.
20. Baer GS, Ebert DH, Chung CJ, et al. Mutant cells selected during persistent reovirus infection do not express mature cathepsin L and do not support reovirus disassembly. *J Virol* 1999;73:9532–9543.
21. Baglioni C, De Benedetti A, Williams GJ. Cleavage of nascent reovirus mRNA by localized activation of the 2′-5′-oligoadenylate-dependent endoribonuclease. *J Virol* 1984;52:865–871.
22. Banerjea AC, Brechling KA, Ray CA, et al. High-level synthesis of biologically active reovirus protein σ1 in a mammalian expression vector system. *Virology* 1988;167:601–612.
23. Banerjea AC, Joklik WK. Reovirus protein σ1 translated *in vitro*, as well as truncated derivatives of it that lack up to two-thirds of its C-terminal portion, exists as two major tetrameric molecular species that differ in electrophoretic mobility. *Virology* 1990;179:460–462.
24. Banerjee AK, Shatkin AJ. Transcription *in vitro* by reovirus-associated ribonucleic acid-dependent polymerase. *J Virol* 1970;6:1–11.
25. Banerjee AK, Shatkin AJ. Guanosine-5′-diphosphate at the 5′ termini of reovirus RNA: Evidence for a segmented genome within the virion. *J Mol Biol* 1971;61:643–653.
26. Bartlett JA, Joklik WK. The sequence of the reovirus serotype 3 L3 genome segment which encodes the major core protein λ1. *Virology* 1988;167:31–37.
27. Bartlett NM, Gillies SC, Bullivant S, Bellamy AR. Electron microscopy study of reovirus reaction cores. *J Virol* 1974;14:315–326.
28. Bass DM, Bodkin D, Dambrauskas R, et al. Intraluminal proteolytic activation plays an important role in replication of type 1 reovirus in the intestines of neonatal mice. *J Virol* 1990;64:1830–1833.
29. Bassel-Duby R, Jayasuriya A, Chatterjee D, et al. Sequence of the reovirus haemagglutinin predicts a coiled-coil structure. *Nature* 1985;315:421–423.
30. Bassel-Duby R, Nibert ML, Homcy CJ, et al. Evidence that the σ1 protein of reovirus serotype 3 is a multimer. *J Virol* 1987;61:1834–1841.
31. Bassel-Duby R, Spriggs DR, Tyler KL, Fields BN. Identification of attenuating mutations on the reovirus type 3 S1 double-stranded RNA segment with a rapid sequencing technique. *J Virol* 1986;60:64–67.
32. Beattie E, Denzler KL, Tartaglia J, et al. Reversal of the interferon-sensitive phenotype of a vaccinia virus lacking E3L by expression of the reovirus S4 gene. *J Virol* 1995;69:499–505.
33. Bell TM, Ross MG. Persistent latent infection of human embryonic cells with reovirus type 3. *Nature* 1966;212:412–414.
34. Bellamy AR, Hole LV. Single-stranded oligonucleotides from reovirus type 3. *Virology* 1970;40:808–819.
35. Bellamy AR, Hole LV, Baguley BC. Isolation of the trinucleotide pppGpCpU from reovirus. *Virology* 1970;42:415–420.
36. Bellamy AR, Joklik WK. Studies on reovirus RNA. II. Characterization of reovirus messenger RNA and of the genome RNA segments from which it is transcribed. *J Mol Biol* 1967;29:19–26.
37. Bellamy AR, Joklik WK. Studies on the A-rich RNA of reovirus. *Proc Natl Acad Sci U S A* 1967;58:1389–1395.
38. Bellamy AR, Nichols JL, Joklik WK. Nucleotide sequences of reovirus oligonucleotides: Evidence for abortive RNA synthesis during virus maturation. *Nature* 1972;238:49–51.
39. Bellamy AR, Shapiro L, August JT, Joklik WK. Studies on reovirus

RNA. I. Characterization of reovirus genome RNA. *J Mol Biol* 1967; 29:1–17.
40. Belli BA, Samuel CE. Biosynthesis of reovirus-specified polypeptides: Expression of reovirus S1-encoded σ1NS protein in transfected and infected cells as measured with serotype specific polyclonal antibody. *Virology* 1991;185:698–709.
41. Belli BA, Samuel CE. Biosynthesis of reovirus-specified polypeptides: Identification of regions of the bicistronic reovirus S1 mRNA that affect the efficiency of translation in animal cells. *Virology* 1993; 193:16–27.
42. Benavente J, Shatkin AJ. Avian reovirus mRNAs are nonfunctional in infected mouse cells: Translational basis for virus host-range restriction. *Proc Natl Acad Sci U S A* 1988;85:4257–4261.
43. Bergeron J, Mabrouk T, Garzon S, Lemay G. Characterization of the thermosensitive ts453 reovirus mutant: Increased dsRNA binding of σ3 protein correlates with interferon resistance. *Virology* 1998;246: 199–210.
44. Bisaillon M, Bergeron J, Lemay G. Characterization of the nucleoside triphosphate phosphohydrolase and helicase activities of the reovirus λ1 protein. *J Biol Chem* 1997;272:18298–18303.
45. Bisaillon M, Lemay G. Characterization of the reovirus λ1 protein RNA 5′-triphosphatase activity. *J Biol Chem* 1997;272:29954–29957.
46. Bisaillon M, Lemay G. Molecular dissection of the reovirus λ1 protein nucleic acids binding site. *Virus Res* 1997;51:231–237.
47. Bisaillon M, Senechal S, Bernier L, Lemay G. A glycosyl hydrolase activity of mammalian reovirus σ1 protein can contribute to viral infection through a mucus layer. *J Mol Biol* 1999;286:759–773.
48. Bischoff JR, Samuel CE. Mechanism of interferon action. Activation of the human P1/eIF-2 alpha protein kinase by individual reovirus s-class mRNAs: S1 mRNA is a potent activator relative to s4 mRNA. *Virology* 1989;172:106–115.
49. Bodkin DK, Fields BN. Growth and survival of reovirus in intestinal tissue: Role of the L2 and S1 genes. *J Virol* 1989;63:1188–1193.
50. Bodkin DK, Nibert ML, Fields BN. Proteolytic digestion of reovirus in the intestinal lumens of neonatal mice. *J Virol* 1989;63:4676–4681.
51. Borsa J, Copps TP, Sargent MD, et al. New intermediate subviral particles in the *in vitro* uncoating of reovirus virions by chymotrypsin. *J Virol* 1973;11:552–564.
52. Borsa J, Graham AF. Reovirus: RNA polymerase activity in purified virions. *Biochem Biophys Res Commun* 1968;33:895–901.
53. Borsa J, Grover J, Chapman JD. Presence of nucleoside triphosphate phosphohydrolase activity in purified virions of reovirus. *J Virol* 1970;6:295–302.
54. Borsa J, Long DG, Copps TP, et al. Reovirus transcriptase activation *in vitro*: Further studies on the facilitation phenomenon. *Intervirology* 1974;3:15–35.
55. Borsa J, Long DG, Sargent MD, et al. Reovirus transcriptase activation *in vitro*: Involvement of an endogenous uncoating activity in the second stage of the process. *Intervirology* 1974;4:171–188.
56. Borsa J, Morash BD, Sargent MD, et al. Two modes of entry of reovirus particles into L cells. *J Gen Virol* 1979;45:161–170.
57. Borsa J, Sargent MD, Copps TP, et al. Specific monovalent cation effects on modification of reovirus infectivity by chymotrypsin digestion *in vitro*. *J Virol* 1973;11:1017–1019.
58. Borsa J, Sargent MD, Ewing DD, Einspenner M. Perturbation of the switch-on of transcriptase activity in intermediate subviral particles from reovirus. *Journal of Cellular Physiology* 1982;112:10–18.
59. Borsa J, Sargent MD, Lievaart PA, Copps TP. Reovirus: Evidence for a second step in the intracellular uncoating and transcriptase activation process. *Virology* 1981;111:191–200.
60. Borsa J, Sargent MD, Long DG, Chapman JD. Extraordinary effects of specific monovalent cations on activation of reovirus transcriptase by chymotrypsin *in vitro*. *J Virol* 1973;11:207–217.
61. Both GW, Furuichi Y, Muthukrishnan S, Shatkin AJ. Ribosome binding to reovirus mRNA in protein synthesis requires 5′ terminal 7-methylguanosine. *Cell* 1975;6:185–195.
62. Both GW, Lavi S, Shatkin AJ. Synthesis of all the gene products of the reovirus genome *in vivo* and *in vitro*. *Cell* 1975;4:173–180.
63. Bottcher B, Kiselev N, Stel'Mashchuk V, et al. Three-dimensional structure of infectious bursal disease virus determined by electron cryomicroscopy. *J Virol* 1997;71:325–330.
64. Brendler T, Godefroy-Colburn T, Yu S, Thach RE. The role of mRNA competition in regulating translation. III. Comparison of *in vitro* and *in vivo* results. *J Biol Chem* 1981;256:11755–11761.
65. Brentano L, Noah DL, Brown EG, Sherry B. The reovirus protein μ2, encoded by the M1 gene, is an RNA-binding protein. *J Virol* 1998;72:8354–8357.
66. Broering T, McCutcheon A, Centonze V, Nibert M. Reovirus nonstructural protein μNS binds to reovirus cores, but does not inhibit their transcription activity. *J Virol* 2000;74:5516–5524.
67. Brown EG, Nibert ML, Fields BN. The L2 gene of reovirus serotype 3 controls the capacity to interfere, accumulate deletions, and establish persistent infection. In: Compans RW, Bishop DHL, eds. *Double-Stranded RNA Viruses*. New York: Elsevier Biomedical, 1983: 275–288.
68. Bruck C, Co MS, Slaoui M, et al. Nucleic acid sequence of an internal image-bearing monoclonal anti-idiotype and its comparison to the sequence of the external antigen. *Proc Natl Acad Sci U S A* 1986;83: 6578–6582.
69. Bruenn JA. Relationships among the positive strand and double-stranded RNA viruses as viewed through their RNA-dependent RNA polymerases. *Nucleic Acids Res* 1991;19:217–226.
70. Burstin SJ, Spriggs DR, Fields BN. Evidence for functional domains on the reovirus type 3 hemagglutinin. *Virology* 1982;117:146–155.
71. Butcher S, Dokland T, Ojala P, et al. Intermediates in the assembly pathway of the double-stranded RNA virus ϕ6. *EMBO J* 1997;16: 4477–4487.
72. Canning WM, Fields BN. Ammonium chloride prevents lytic growth of reovirus and helps to establish persistent infection in mouse L cells. *Science* 1983;219:987–988.
73. Carter C, Stoltzfus CM, Banerjee AK, Shatkin AJ. Origin of reovirus oligo(A). *J Virol* 1974;13:1331–1337.
74. Carter CA. Methylation of reovirus oligonucleotides *in vivo* and *in vitro*. *Virology* 1977;80:249–259.
75. Carter CA, Lin BY, Metlay M. Polyadenylylation of reovirus proteins. Analysis of the RNA bound to structural proteins. *J Biol Chem* 1980; 255:6479–6485.
76. Cashdollar LW. Characterization and structural localization of the reovirus λ3 protein. *Res Virol* 1994;145:277–285.
77. Cashdollar LW, Chmelo R, Esparza J, et al. Molecular cloning of the complete genome of reovirus serotype 3. *Virology* 1984;133:191–196.
78. Cashdollar LW, Chmelo RA, Wiener JR, Joklik WK. Sequences of the S1 genes of the three serotypes of reovirus. *Proc Natl Acad Sci U S A* 1985;82:24–28.
79. Caston J, Trus B, Booy F, et al. Structure of L-A virus: A specialized compartment for the transcription and replication of double-stranded RNA. *J Cell Biol* 1997;138:975–985.
80. Ceruzzi M, Shatkin AJ. Expression of reovirus p14 in bacteria and identification in the cytoplasm of infected mouse L cells. *Virology* 1986;153:35–45.
81. Chakraborty PR, Ahmed R, Fields BN. Genetics of reovirus: The relationship of interference to complementation and reassortment of temperature-sensitive mutants at nonpermissive temperature. *Virology* 1979;94:119–127.
82. Chandran K, Nibert ML. Protease cleavage of reovirus capsid protein μ1/μ1C is blocked by alkyl sulfate detergents, yielding a new type of infectious subvirion particle. *J Virol* 1998;72:467–475.
83. Chandran K, Walker SB, Chen Y, et al. *In vitro* recoating of reovirus cores with baculovirus-expressed outer-capsid proteins μ1 and σ3. *J Virol* 1999;73:3941–3950.
84. Chang C-T, Zweerink HJ. Fate of parental reovirus in infected cell. *Virology* 1971;46:544–555.
85. Chappell JD, Barton ES, Smith TH, et al. Cleavage susceptibility of reovirus attachment protein σ1 during proteolytic disassembly of virions is determined by a sequence polymorphism in the σ1 neck. *J Virol* 1998;72:8205–8213.
86. Chappell JD, Duong JL, Wright BW, Dermody TS. Identification of carbohydrate-binding domains in the attachment proteins of type 1 and type 3 reoviruses. *J Virol* 2000;74:8472–8479.
87. Chappell JD, Goral MI, Rodgers SE, et al. Sequence diversity within the reovirus S2 gene: Reovirus genes reassort in nature and their termini are predicted to form a panhandle motif. *J Virol* 1994;68:750–756.
88. Chappell JD, Gunn VL, Wetzel JD, et al. Mutations in type 3 reovirus that determine binding to sialic acid are contained in the fibrous tail domain of viral attachment protein σ1. *J Virol* 1997;71:1834–1841.
89. Choi AH. Internalization of virus binding proteins during entry of reovirus into K562 erythroleukemia cells. *Virology* 1994;200: 301–306.

90. Choi AH, Lee PW. Does the beta-adrenergic receptor function as a reovirus receptor? *Virology* 1988;163:191–197.
91. Chow N-L, Shatkin AJ. Blocked and unblocked 5 termini in reovirus genome RNA. *J Virol* 1975;15:1057–1064.
92. Clarke P, Meintzer SM, Gibson S, et al. Reovirus-induced apoptosis is mediated by TRAIL. *J Virol* 2000;74:8135–8139.
93. Cleveland DR, Zarbl H, Millward S. Reovirus guanylyltransferase is L2 gene product λ2. *J Virol* 1986;60:307–311.
94. Co MS, Gaulton GN, Tominaga A, et al. Structural similarities between the mammalian beta-adrenergic and reovirus type 3 receptors. *Proc Natl Acad Sci U S A* 1985;82:5315–5318.
95. Cohen JA, Sergott RC, Williams WV, et al. *In vivo* modulation of oligodendrocyte function by an anti-receptor antibody. *Pathobiology* 1992;60:151–156.
96. Cohen JA, Williams WV, Geller HM, Greene MI. Anti-reovirus receptor antibody accelerates expression of the optic nerve oligodendrocyte developmental program. *Proc Natl Acad Sci U S A* 1991;88:1266–1270.
97. Cohen JA, Williams WV, Weiner DB, et al. Ligand binding to the cell surface receptor for reovirus type 3 stimulates galactocerebroside expression by developing oligodendrocytes. *Proc Natl Acad Sci U S A* 1990;87:4922–4926.
98. Connolly JL, Rodgers SE, Clarke P, et al. Reovirus-induced apoptosis requires activation of transcription factor NF-kappaB. *J Virol* 2000;74:2981–2989.
99. Coombs KM. Identification and characterization of a double-stranded RNA reovirus temperature-sensitive mutant defective in minor core protein μ2. *J Virol* 1996;70:4237–4245.
100. Coombs KM. Stoichiometry of reovirus structural proteins in virus, ISVP, and core particles. *Virology* 1998;243:218–228.
101. Coombs KM, Fields BN, Harrison SC. Crystallization of the reovirus type 3 Dearing core. Crystal packing is determined by the λ2 protein. *J Mol Biol* 1990;215:1–5.
102. Coombs KM, Mak SC, Petrycky-Cox LD. Studies of the major reovirus core protein σ2: Reversion of the assembly-defective mutant tsC447 is an intragenic process and involves back mutation of Asp-383 to Asn. *J Virol* 1994;68:177–186.
103. Cox DC, Shaw JE. Inhibition of the initiation of cellular DNA synthesis after reovirus infection. *J Virol* 1974;13:760–761.
104. Cross RK, Fields BN. Temperature-sensitive mutants of reovirus type 3: Studies on the synthesis of viral RNA. *Virology* 1972;50:799–809.
105. Cross RK, Fields BN. Reovirus-specific polypeptides: Analysis using discontinuous gel electrophoresis. *J Virol* 1976;19:162–173.
106. Cross RK, Fields BN. Temperature-sensitive mutants of reovirus type 3: Evidence for aberrant μ1 and μ2 polypeptide species. *J Virol* 1976;19:174–179.
107. Cross RK, Fields BN. Use of an aberrant polypeptide as a marker in three-factor crosses: Further evidence for independent reassortment as the mechanism of recombination between temperature-sensitive mutants of reovirus type 3. *Virology* 1976;74:345–362.
108. Dales S. Association between the spindle apparatus and reovirus. *Proc Natl Acad Sci U S A* 1963;50:268–275.
109. Dales S, Gomatos P, Hsu KC. The uptake and development of reovirus in strain L cells followed with labelled viral ribonucleic acid and ferritin-antibody conjugates. *Virology* 1965;25:193–211.
110. Danis C, Garzon S, Lemay G. Further characterization of the ts453 mutant of mammalian orthoreovirus serotype 3 and nucleotide sequence of the mutated S4 gene. *Virology* 1992;190:494–498.
111. Danis C, Mabrouk T, Faure M, Lemay G. Interferon has no protective effect during acute or persistent reovirus infection of mouse SC1 fibroblasts. *Virus Res* 1997;51:139–149.
112. Danis C, Mabrouk T, Garzon S, Lemay G. Establishment of persistent reovirus infection in SC1 cells: Absence of protein synthesis inhibition and increased level of double-stranded RNA-activated protein kinase. *Virus Res* 1993;27:253–265.
113. De Benedetti A, Williams GJ, Baglioni C. Inhibition of binding to initiation complexes of nascent reovirus mRNA by double-stranded RNA-dependent protein kinase. *J Virol* 1985;54:408–413.
114. Debiasi RL, Squier MK, Pike B, et al. Reovirus-induced apoptosis is preceded by increased cellular calpain activity and is blocked by calpain inhibitors. *J Virol* 1999;73:695–701.
115. Denzler KL, Jacobs BL. Site-directed mutagenic analysis of reovirus σ3 protein binding to dsRNA. *Virology* 1994;204:190–199.
116. Dermody TS, Chappell JD, Hofler JG, et al. Eradication of persistent reovirus infection from a B-cell hybridoma. *Virology* 1995;212:272–276.
117. Dermody TS, Nibert ML, Bassel-Duby R, Fields BN. Sequence diversity in S1 genes and S1 translation products of 11 serotype 3 reovirus strains. *J Virol* 1990;64:4842–4850.
118. Dermody TS, Nibert ML, Bassel-Duby R, Fields BN. A σ1 region important for hemagglutination by serotype 3 reovirus strains. *J Virol* 1990;64:5173–5176.
119. Dermody TS, Nibert ML, Wetzel JD, et al. Cells and viruses with mutations affecting viral entry are selected during persistent infections of L cells with mammalian reoviruses. *J Virol* 1993;67:2055–2063.
120. Dermody TS, Schiff LA, Nibert ML, et al. The S2 gene nucleotide sequences of prototype strains of the three reovirus serotypes: Characterization of reovirus core protein σ2. *J Virol* 1991;65:5721–5731.
121. Desrosiers RC, Sen GC, Lengyel P. Difference in 5′ terminal structure between the mRNA and the double-stranded virion RNA of reovirus. *Biochem Biophys Res Commun* 1976;73:32–39.
122. Dessanti A, Massarelli G, Piga MT, et al. Biliary, anorectal and esophageal atresia: A new entity? *Tohoku J Exp Med* 1997;181:49–55.
123. Detjen BM, Walden WE, Thach RE. Translational specificity in reovirus-infected mouse fibroblasts. *J Biol Chem* 1982;257:9855–9860.
124. Dichter MA, Weiner HL. Infection of neuronal cell cultures with reovirus mimics *in vitro* patterns of neurotropism. *Ann Neurol* 1984;16:603–610.
125. Donta ST, Shanley JD. Reovirus type 3 binds to antagonist domains of the beta-adrenergic receptor. *J Virol* 1990;64:639–641.
126. Doohan JP, Samuel CE. Biosynthesis of reovirus-specified polypeptides: Ribosome pausing during the translation of reovirus S1 mRNA. *Virology* 1992;186:409–425.
127. Drayna D, Fields BN. Activation and characterization of the reovirus transcriptase: Genetic analysis. *J Virol* 1982;41:110–118.
128. Drayna D, Fields BN. Biochemical studies on the mechanism of chemical and physical inactivation of reovirus. *J Gen Virol* 1982;63:161–170.
129. Drayna D, Fields BN. Genetic studies on the mechanism of chemical and physical inactivation of reovirus. *J Gen Virol* 1982;63:149–159.
130. Dryden KA, Farsetta DL, Wang G, et al. Internal structures containing transcriptase-related proteins in top component particles of mammalian orthoreovirus. *Virology* 1998;245:33–46.
131. Dryden KA, Wang G, Yeager M, et al. Early steps in reovirus infection are associated with dramatic changes in supramolecular structure and protein conformation: Analysis of virions and subviral particles by cryoelectron microscopy and image reconstruction. *J Cell Biol* 1993;122:1023–1041.
132. Duncan MR, Stanish SM, Cox DC. Differential sensitivity of normal and transformed human cells to reovirus infection. *J Virol* 1978;28:444–449.
133. Duncan R. The low pH-dependent entry of avian reovirus is accompanied by two specific cleavages of the major outer capsid protein μ2C. *Virology* 1996;219:179–189.
134. Duncan R. Extensive sequence divergence and phylogenetic relationships between the fusogenic and nonfusogenic orthoreoviruses: A species proposal. *Virology* 1999;260:316–328.
135. Duncan R, Horne D, Cashdollar LW, et al. Identification of conserved domains in the cell attachment proteins of the three serotypes of reovirus. *Virology* 1990;174:399–409.
136. Duncan R, Horne D, Strong JE, et al. Conformational and functional analysis of the carboxyl-terminal globular head of the reovirus cell attachment protein. *Virology* 1991;182:810–819.
137. Duncan R, Lee PW. Localization of two protease-sensitive regions separating distinct domains in the reovirus cell-attachment protein σ1. *Virology* 1994;203:149–152.
138. Duncan R, Murphy FA, Mirkovic RR. Characterization of a novel syncytium-inducing baboon reovirus. *Virology* 1995;212:752–756.
139. Duncan R, Sullivan K. Characterization of two avian reoviruses that exhibit strain-specific quantitative differences in their syncytium-inducing and pathogenic capabilities. *Virology* 1998;250:263–272.
140. Duncan RF. Protein synthesis initiation factor modifications during viral infections: Implications for translational control. *Electrophoresis* 1990;11:219–227.
141. Dunnebacke TH, Kleinschmidt AK. Ribonucleic acid from reovirus as seen in protein monolayers by electron microscopy. *Z Naturforsch B* 1967;22:159–164.

142. Ensminger WD, Tamm I. Cellular DNA and protein synthesis in reovirus-infected L cells. *Virology* 1969;39:357–360.
143. Ensminger WD, Tamm I. The step in cellular DNA synthesis blocked by reovirus infection. *Virology* 1969;39:935–938.
144. Epstein RL, Powers ML, Rogart RB, Weiner HL. Binding of ^{125}I-labeled reovirus to cell surface receptors. *Virology* 1984;133:46–55.
145. Ernst H, Shatkin AJ. Reovirus hemagglutinin mRNA codes for two polypeptides in overlapping reading frames. *Proc Natl Acad Sci U S A* 1985;82:48–52.
146. Ewing DD, Sargent MD, Borsa J. Switch-on of transcriptase function in reovirus: Analysis of polypeptide changes using 2-D gels. *Virology* 1985;144:448–456.
147. Fajardo E, Shatkin AJ. Expression of the two reovirus S1 gene products in transfected mammalian cells. *Virology* 1990;178:223–231.
148. Fajardo JE, Shatkin AJ. Effects of elongation on the translation of a reovirus bicistronic mRNA. *Enzyme* 1990;44:235–243.
149. Fang Q, Attoui H, Biagini JF, et al. Sequence of genome segments 1, 2, and 3 of the grass carp reovirus (genus *Aquareovirus*, family *Reoviridae*). *Biochem Biophys Res Communun* 2000;274:762–766.
150. Farrell JA, Harvey JD, Bellamy AR. Biophysical studies of reovirus type 3. I. The molecular weight of reovirus and reovirus cores. *Virology* 1974;62:145–153.
151. Farsetta DL, Chandran K, Nibert ML. Transcriptional activities of reovirus RNA polymerase in recoated cores. Initiation and elongation are regulated by separate mechanisms. *J Biol Chem* 2000;275: 39693–39701.
152. Fausnaugh J, Shatkin AJ. Active site localization in a viral mRNA capping enzyme. *J Biol Chem* 1990;265:7669–7672.
153. Faust M, Hastings KE, Millward S. m7G5′ppp5′GmptCpUp at the 5′ terminus of reovirus messenger RNA. *Nucleic Acids Res* 1975;2: 1329–1343.
154. Faust M, Millward S. *In vitro* methylation of nascent reovirus mRNA by a virion-associated methyl transferase. *Nucleic Acids Res* 1974;1:1739–1752.
155. Feduchi E, Esteban M, Carrasco L. Reovirus type 3 synthesizes proteins in interferon-treated HeLa cells without reversing the antiviral state. *Virology* 1988;164:420–426.
156. Fernandes J, Tang D, Leone G, Lee PW. Binding of reovirus to receptor leads to conformational changes in viral capsid proteins that are reversible upon virus detachment. *J Biol Chem* 1994;269: 17043–17047.
157. Fields BN. Temperature-sensitive mutants of reovirus type 3 features of genetic recombination. *Virology* 1971;46:142–148.
158. Fields BN, Greene MI. Genetic and molecular mechanisms of viral pathogenesis: Implications for prevention and treatment. *Nature* 1982; 300:19–23.
159. Fields BN, Joklik WK. Isolation and preliminary genetic and biochemical characterization of temperature-sensitive mutants of reovirus. *Virology* 1969;37:335–342.
160. Fields BN, Raine CS, Baum SG. Temperature-sensitive mutants of reovirus type 3: Defects in viral maturation as studied by immunofluorescence and electron microscopy. *Virology* 1971;43:569–578.
161. Fraser RD, Furlong DB, Trus BL, et al. Molecular structure of the cell-attachment protein of reovirus: Correlation of computer-processed electron micrographs with sequence-based predictions. *J Virol* 1990; 64:2990–3000.
162. Fukutomi T, Sanekata T, Akashi H. Isolation of reovirus type 2 from diarrheal feces of pigs. *J Vet Med Sci* 1996;58:555–557.
163. Furlong DB, Nibert ML, Fields BN. σ1 protein of mammalian reoviruses extends from the surfaces of viral particles. *J Virol* 1988; 62:246–256.
164. Furuichi Y, LaFiandra A, Shatkin AJ. 5′-Terminal structure and mRNA stability. *Nature* 1977;266:235–239.
165. Furuichi Y, Morgan M, Muthukrishnan S, Shatkin AJ. Reovirus messenger RNA contains a methylated, blocked 5′-terminal structure: m-7G(5′)ppp(5′)G-MpCp-. *Proc Natl Acad Sci U S A* 1975;72:362–366.
166. Furuichi Y, Muthukrishnan S, Shatkin AJ. 5′-Terminal m-7G(5′) ppp(5′)G-m-p *in vivo*: Identification in reovirus genome RNA. *Proc Natl Acad Sci U S A* 1975;72:742–745.
167. Furuichi Y, Muthukrishnan S, Tomasz J, Shatkin AJ. Mechanism of formation of reovirus mRNA 5′-terminal blocked and methylated sequence, m7GpppGmpC. *J Biol Chem* 1976;251:5043–5053.
168. Furuichi Y, Shatkin AJ. 5′-termini of reovirus mRNA: Ability of viral cores to form caps post-transcriptionally. *Virology* 1977;77:566–578.
169. Gaillard RK Jr, Joklik WK. The relative translation efficiencies of reovirus messenger RNAs. *Virology* 1985;147:336–348.
170. Gaillard RK, Li JK, Keene JD, Joklik WK. The sequence at the termini of four genes of the three reovirus serotypes. *Virology* 1982;121: 320–326.
171. Gard G, Compans RW. Structure and cytopathic effects of Nelson Bay virus. *J Virol* 1970;6:100–106.
172. Gaulton GN, Stein ME, Safko B, Stadecker MJ. Direct induction of Ia antigen on murine thyroid-derived epithelial cells by reovirus. *J Immunol* 1989;142:3821–3825.
173. Gentsch JR, Hatfield JW. Saturable attachment sites for type 3 mammalian reovirus on murine L cells and human HeLa cells. *Virus Res* 1984;1:401–414.
174. Gentsch JR, Pacitti AF. Effect of neuraminidase treatment of cells and effect of soluble glycoproteins on type 3 reovirus attachment to murine L cells. *J Virol* 1985;56:356–364.
175. Gentsch JR, Pacitti AF. Differential interaction of reovirus type 3 with sialylated receptor components on animal cells. *Virology* 1987;161: 245–248.
176. George CX, Samuel CE. Mechanism of interferon action. Expression of reovirus S3 gene in transfected COS cells and subsequent inhibition at the level of protein synthesis by type I but not by type II interferon. *Virology* 1988;166:573–582.
177. Georgi A, Mottola-Hartshorn C, Warner A, et al. Detection of individual fluorescently labeled reovirions in living cells. *Proc Natl Acad Sci U S A* 1990;87:6579–6583.
178. Giantini M, Shatkin AJ. Stimulation of chloramphenicol acetyltransferase mRNA translation by reovirus capsid polypeptide σ3 in cotransfected COS cells. *J Virol* 1989;63:2415–2421.
179. Gillian AL, Nibert ML. Amino terminus of reovirus nonstructural protein σNS is important for ssRNA binding and nucleoprotein complex formation. *Virology* 1998;240:1–11.
180. Gillian AL, Schmechel SC, Livny J, et al. Reovirus nonstructural protein σNS binds in multiple copies to single-stranded RNA and shares properties with single-stranded DNA binding proteins. *J Virol* 2000; 74:5939–5948.
181. Gilmore R, Coffey MC, Lee PW. Active participation of Hsp90 in the biogenesis of the trimeric reovirus cell attachment protein σ1. *J Biol Chem* 1998;273:15227–15233.
182. Gilmore R, Coffey MC, Leone G, et al. Co-translational trimerization of the reovirus cell attachment protein. *EMBO J* 1996;15:2651–2658.
183. Gomatos PJ, Prakash O, Stamatos NM. Small reovirus particle composed solely of sigma NS with specificity for binding different nucleic acids. *J Virol* 1981;39:115–124.
184. Gomatos PJ, Stamatos NM, Sarkar NH. Small reovirus-specific particle with polycytidylate-dependent RNA polymerase activity. *J Virol* 1980;36:556–565.
185. Gomatos PJ, Stoeckenius W. Electron microscope studies on reovirus RNA. *Proc Natl Acad Sci U S A* 1964;52:1449–1455.
186. Gomatos PJ, Tamm I. Macromolecular synthesis in reovirus-infected L cells. *Biochim Biophys Acta* 1963;72:651–653.
187. Gomatos PJ, Tamm I. The secondary structure of reovirus RNA. *Proc Natl Acad Sci U S A* 1963;49:707–714.
188. Gomatos PJ, Tamm I, Dales S, Franklin RM. Reovirus type 3: Physical characteristics and interactions with L cells. *Virology* 1962;17: 441–454.
189. Goral MI, Mochow-Grundy M, Dermody TS. Sequence diversity within the reovirus S3 gene: Reoviruses evolve independently of host species, geographic locale, and date of isolation. *Virology* 1996;216: 265–271.
190. Granboulan N, Niveleau A. Etude au microscope electronique du RNA de reovirus. *J Microsc (Paris)* 1967;6:23–30.
191. Graziadei WD, Roy D, Konigsberg W, Lengyel P. Translation of reovirus messenger ribonucleic acids synthesized *in vitro* into reovirus proteins in a mouse L cell extract. *Arch Biochem Biophys* 1973;158: 266–275.
192. Gupta SL, Holmes SL, Mehra LL. Interferon action against reovirus: Activation of interferon-induced protein kinase in mouse L929 cells upon reovirus infection. *Virology* 1982;120:495–499.
193. Haller BL, Barkon ML, Li XY, et al. Brain- and intestine-specific variants of reovirus serotype 3 strain Dearing are selected during chronic infection of severe combined immunodeficient mice. *J Virol* 1995;69:3933–3937.
194. Haller BL, Barkon ML, Vogler GP, Virgin HW IV. Genetic mapping of

reovirus virulence and organ tropism in severe combined immunodeficient mice: Organ-specific virulence genes. *J Virol* 1995;69:357–364.
195. Hand R, Ensminger WD, Tamm I. Cellular DNA replication in infections with cytocidal RNA viruses. *Virology* 1971;44:527–536.
196. Hand R, Tamm I. Reovirus: Effect of noninfective viral components on cellular deoxyribonucleic acid synthesis. *J Virol* 1973;11:223–231.
197. Hand R, Tamm I. Initiation of DNA replication in mammalian cells and its inhibition by reovirus infection. *J Mol Biol* 1974;82:175–183.
198. Harrison SJ, Farsetta DL, Kim J, et al. Mammalian reovirus L3 gene sequences and evidence for a distinct amino-terminal region of the λ1 protein. *Virology* 1999;258:54–64.
199. Harvey JD, Bellamy AR, Earnshaw WC, Schutt C. Biophysical studies of reovirus type 3. IV. Low-angle x-ray diffraction studies. *Virology* 1981;112:240–249.
200. Harvey JD, Farrell JA, Bellamy AR. Biophysical studies of reovirus type 3. II. Properties of the hydrated particle. *Virology* 1974;62:154–160.
201. Hashiro G, Loh PC, Yau JT. The preferential cytotoxicity of reovirus for certain transformed cell lines. *Arch Virol* 1977;54:307–315.
202. Hayes EC, Lee PWK, Miller SE, Joklik WK. The interaction of a series of hybridoma IgGs with reovirus particles. Demonstration that the core protein λ2 is exposed on the particle surface. *Virology* 1981;108:147–155.
203. Hazelton PR, Coombs KM. The reovirus mutant tsA279 has temperature-sensitive lesions in the M2 and L2 genes: The M2 gene is associated with decreased viral protein production and blockade in transmembrane transport. *Virology* 1995;207:46–58.
204. Hazelton PR, Coombs KM. The reovirus mutant tsA279 L2 gene is associated with generation of a spikeless core particle: Implications for capsid assembly. *J Virol* 1999;73:2298–2308.
205. Henderson DR, Joklik WK. The mechanism of interferon induction by UV-irradiated reovirus. *Virology* 1978;91:389–406.
206. Hill C, Booth T, Prasad B, et al. The structure of a cypovirus and the functional organization of dsRNA viruses. *Nature Structural Biology* 1999;6:565–568.
207. Hooper JW, Fields BN. Monoclonal antibodies to reovirus σ1 and μ1 proteins inhibit chromium release from mouse L cells. *J Virol* 1996;70:672–677.
208. Hooper JW, Fields BN. Role of the μ1 protein in reovirus stability and capacity to cause chromium release from host cells. *J Virol* 1996;70:459–467.
209. Hrdy DB, Rosen L, Fields BN. Polymorphism of the migration of double-stranded RNA genome segments of reovirus isolates from humans, cattle, and mice. *J Virol* 1979;31:104–111.
210. Hrdy DB, Rubin DH, Fields BN. Molecular basis of reovirus neurovirulence: Role of the M2 gene in avirulence. *Proc Natl Acad Sci U S A* 1982;79:1298–1302.
211. Huismans H, Joklik WK. Reovirus-coded polypeptides in infected cells: Isolation of two native monomeric polypeptides with affinity for single-stranded and double-stranded RNA, respectively. *Virology* 1976;70:411–424.
212. Ikegami N, Gomatos PJ. Temperature-sensitive conditional-lethal mutants of reovirus 3. I. Isolation and characterization. *Virology* 1968;36:447–458.
213. Imai M, Richardson MA, Ikegami N, et al. Molecular cloning of double-stranded RNA virus genomes. *Proc Natl Acad Sci U S A* 1983;80:373–377.
214. Imani F, Jacobs BL. Inhibitory activity for the interferon-induced protein kinase is associated with the reovirus serotype 1 σ3 protein. *Proc Natl Acad Sci U S A* 1988;85:7887–7891.
215. Ito Y, Joklik WK. Temperature-sensitive mutants of reovirus. 3. Evidence that mutants of group D ("RNA-negative") are structural polypeptide mutants. *Virology* 1972;50:282–286.
216. Ito Y, Joklik WK. Temperature-sensitive mutants of reovirus. I. Patterns of gene expression by mutants of groups C, D, and E. *Virology* 1972;50:189–201.
217. Jacobs BL, Ferguson RE. The Lang strain of reovirus serotype 1 and the Dearing strain of reovirus serotype 3 differ in their sensitivities to beta interferon. *J Virol* 1991;65:5102–5104.
218. Jacobs BL, Samuel CE. Biosynthesis of reovirus-specified polypeptides: The reovirus s1 mRNA encodes two primary translation products. *Virology* 1985;143:63–74.
219. Jané-Valbuena J, Nibert ML, Spencer SM, et al. Reovirus virion-like particles obtained by recoating infectious subvirion particles with baculovirus-expressed σ3 protein: An approach for analyzing σ3 functions during virus entry. *J Virol* 1999;73:2963–2973.
220. Jayasuriya AK, Nibert ML, Fields BN. Complete nucleotide sequence of the M2 gene segment of reovirus type 3 dearing and analysis of its protein product μ1. *Virology* 1988;163:591–602.
221. Jayasuriya AKA. *Molecular Characterization of the Reovirus M2 Gene.* Cambridge, MA: Harvard University, 1991.
222. Johansson PJ, Sveger T, Ahlfors K, et al. Reovirus type 1 associated with meningitis. *Scand J Infect Dis* 1996;28:117–120.
223. Joklik WK. Studies on the effect of chymotrypsin on reovirions. *Virology* 1972;49:700–715.
224. Joklik WK. Reproduction of reoviridae. In: Fraenkel-Conrat H, Wagner RR, eds. *Comprehensive Virology.* New York: Plenum Press, 1974:231–334.
225. Joklik WK. Structure and function of the reovirus genome. *Microbiol Rev* 1981;45:483–501.
226. Joklik WK. The reovirus particle. In: Joklik WK, ed. *The Reoviridae.* New York: Plenum Press, 1983:9–78.
227. Joklik WK. Recent progress in reovirus research. *Annu Rev Genet* 1985;19:537–575.
228. Joklik WK, Roner MR. What reassorts when reovirus genome segments reassort? *J Biol Chem* 1995;270:4181–4184.
229. Joklik WK, Roner MR. Molecular recognition in the assembly of the segmented reovirus genome. *Prog Nucleic Acid Res Mol Biol* 1996;53:249–281.
230. Kapuler AM. An extraordinary temperature dependence of the reovirus transcriptase. *Biochemistry* 1970;9:4453–4457.
231. Kapuler AM, Mendelsohn N, Klett H, Acs G. Four base-specific nucleoside 5′-triphosphatases in the subviral core of reovirus. *Nature* 1970;225:1209–1213.
232. Kauffman RS, Ahmed R, Fields BN. Selection of a mutant S1 gene during reovirus persistent infection of L cells: Role in maintenance of the persistent state. *Virology* 1983;131:79–87.
233. Kavenoff R, Talcove D, Mudd JA. Genome-sized RNA from reovirus particles. *Proc Natl Acad Sci U S A* 1975;72:4317–4321.
234. Kaye KM, Spriggs DR, Bassel-Duby R, et al. Genetic basis for altered pathogenesis of an immune-selected antigenic variant of reovirus type 3 (Dearing). *J Virol* 1986;59:90–97.
235. Kedl R, Schmechel S, Schiff L. Comparative sequence analysis of the reovirus S4 genes from 13 serotype 1 and serotype 3 field isolates. *J Virol* 1995;69:552–559.
236. Keirstead ND, Coombs KM. Absence of superinfection exclusion during asynchronous reovirus infections of mouse, monkey, and human cell lines. *Virus Res* 1998;54:225–235.
237. Keroack M, Fields BN. Viral shedding and transmission between hosts determined by reovirus L2 gene. *Science* 1986;232:1635–1638.
238. Khaustov VI, Korolev MB, Reingold VN. The structure of the capsid inner layer of reoviruses. Brief report. *Arch Virol* 1987;93:163–167.
239. Kleijn M, Vrins CLJ, Voorma HO, Thomas AAM. Phosphorylation state of the cap-binding protein eIF4E during viral infection. *Virology* 1996;217:486–494.
240. Kokubu T, Takahashi T, Takamura K, et al. Isolation of reovirus type 3 from dogs with diarrhea. *J Vet Med Sci* 1993;55:453–454.
241. Koonin EV. Evolution of double-stranded RNA viruses: A case for polyphyletic origin from different groups of positive-stranded RNA viruses. *Semin Virol* 1992;3:327–340.
242. Koonin EV. Computer-assisted identification of a putative methyltransferase domain in NS5 protein of flaviviruses and λ2 protein of reovirus. *J Gen Virol* 1993;74:733–740.
243. Koonin EV, Gorbalenya AE, Chumakov KM. Tentative identification of RNA-dependent RNA polymerases of dsRNA viruses and their relationship to positive strand RNA viral polymerases. *FEBS Lett* 1989;252:42–46.
244. Kothandaraman S, Hebert MC, Raines RT, Nibert ML. No role for pepstatin-A-sensitive acidic proteinases in reovirus infections of L or MDCK cells. *Virology* 1998;251:264–272.
245. Kozak M. Possible role of flanking nucleotides in recognition of the AUG initiator codon by eukaryotic ribosomes. *Nucleic Acids Res* 1981;9:5233–5252.
246. Kozak M. Analysis of ribosome binding sites from the s1 message of reovirus. Initiation at the first and second AUG codons. *J Mol Biol* 1982;156:807–820.

247. Kozak M. Sequences of ribosome binding sites from the large size class of reovirus mRNA. *J Virol* 1982;42:467–473.
248. Kozak M. Recognition of AUG and alternative initiator codons is augmented by G in position +4 but is not generally affected by the nucleotides in positions +5 and +6. *EMBO J* 1997;16:2482–2492.
249. Kozak M, Shatkin AJ. Identification of features in 5′ terminal fragments from reovirus mRNA which are important for ribosome binding. *Cell* 1978;13:201–212.
250. Krystal G, Perrault J, Graham AF. Evidence for a glycoprotein in reovirus. *Virology* 1976;72:308–321.
251. Krystal G, Winn P, Millward S, Sakuma S. Evidence for phosphoproteins in reovirus. *Virology* 1975;64:505–512.
252. Kudo H, Graham AF. Selective inhibition of reovirus induced RNA in L cells. *Biochem Biophys Res Commun* 1966;24:150–155.
253. Lai KC, Bellamy AR. Factors affecting the amount of oligonucleotides in reovirus particles. *Virology* 1971;45:821–823.
254. Lai MH, Joklik WK. The induction of interferon by temperature-sensitive mutants of reovirus, UV-irradiated reovirus, and subviral reovirus particles. *Virology* 1973;51:191–204.
255. Lai MH, Werenne JJ, Joklik WK. The preparation of reovirus top component and its effect on host DNA and protein synthesis. *Virology* 1973;54:237–244.
256. Lamirande EW, Nichols DK, Owens JW, et al. Isolation and experimental transmission of a reovirus pathogenic in ratsnakes (*Elaphe* species). *Virus Res* 1999;63:135–141.
257. Larson SM, Antczak JB, Joklik WK. Reovirus exists in the form of 13 particle species that differ in their content of protein σ1. *Virology* 1994;201:303–311.
258. Lau RY, Van Alstyne D, Berckmans R, Graham AF. Synthesis of reovirus-specific polypeptides in cells pretreated with cycloheximide. *J Virol* 1975;16:470–478.
259. Lee PWK. Reovirus protein σ1: From cell attachment to protein oligomerization and folding mechanisms. *Bioessays* 1994;16:199–206.
260. Lee PWK, Hayes EC, Joklik WK. Characterization of anti-reovirus immunoglobulins secreted by cloned hybridoma cell lines. *Virology* 1981;108:134–146.
261. Lee PWK, Hayes EC, Joklik WK. Protein σ1 is the reovirus cell attachment protein. *Virology* 1981;108:156–163.
262. Leland MM, Hubbard GB, Sentmore HT III, et al. Outbreak of *Orthoreovirus*-induced meningoencephalomyelitis in baboons. *Comp Med* 2000;50:199–205.
263. Lemay G, Danis C. Reovirus λ1 protein: Affinity for double-stranded nucleic acids by a small amino-terminal region of the protein independent from the zinc finger motif. *J Gen Virol* 1994;75:3261–3266.
264. Lemay G, Millward S. Expression of the cloned S4 gene of reovirus serotype 3 in transformed eucaryotic cells: Enrichment of the viral protein in the crude initiation factor fraction. *Virus Res* 1986;6:133–140.
265. Lemieux R, Lemay G, Millward S. The viral protein σ3 participates in translation of late viral mRNA in reovirus-infected L cells. *J Virol* 1987;61:2472–2479.
266. Lemieux R, Zarbl H, Millward S. mRNA discrimination in extracts from uninfected and reovirus-infected L-cells. *J Virol* 1984;51:215–222.
267. Leone G, Coffey MC, Gilmore R, et al. C-terminal trimerization, but not N-terminal trimerization, of the reovirus cell attachment protein is a posttranslational and Hsp70/ATP-dependent process. *J Biol Chem* 1996;271:8466–8471.
268. Leone G, Duncan R, Lee PWK. Trimerization of the reovirus cell attachment protein (sigma-I) induces conformational changes in sigma-I necessary for its cell-binding function. *Virology* 1991;184:758–761.
269. Leone G, Duncan R, Mah DCW, et al. The amino-terminal heptad repeat region of reovirus cell attachment protein σ1 is responsible for σ1 oligomer stability and possesses intrinsic oligomerization function. *Virology* 1991;182:336–345.
270. Leone G, Mah DCW, Lee PWK. The incorporation of reovirus cell attachment protein σ1 into virions requires the amino terminal hydrophobic tail and the adjacent heptad repeat region. *Virology* 1991;182:346–350.
271. Leone G, Maybaum L, Lee PW. The reovirus cell attachment protein possesses two independently active trimerization domains: Basis of dominant negative effects. *Cell* 1992;71:479–488.
272. Levin DH, Mendelsohn N, Schonberg M, et al. Properties of RNA transcriptase in reovirus subviral particles. *Proc Natl Acad Sci U S A* 1970;66:890–897.
273. Levin KH, Samuel CE. Biosynthesis of reovirus-specified polypeptides. Purification and characterization of the small-sized class mRNAs of reovirus type 3: Coding assignments and translational efficiencies. *Virology* 1980;106:1–13.
274. Li JK, Keene JD, Scheible PP, Joklik WK. Nature of the 3′-terminal sequences of the plus and minus strands of the S1 gene of reovirus serotypes 1, 2 and 3. *Virology* 1980;105:41–51.
275. Lloyd RM, Shatkin AJ. Translational stimulation by reovirus polypeptide σ3: Substitution for VAI RNA and inhibition of phosphorylation of the alpha subunit of eukaryotic initiation factor 2. *J Virol* 1992;66:6878–6884.
276. Loh PC, Soergel M. Macromolecular synthesis in cells infected with reovirus type 2 and the effect of ARA-C. *Nature* 1967;214:622–623.
277. Lucia-Jandris P, Hooper JW, Fields BN. Reovirus M2 gene is associated with chromium release from mouse L cells. *J Virol* 1993;67:5339–5345.
278. Luftig RB, Kilham SS, Hay AJ, et al. An ultrastructural study of virions and cores of reovirus type 3. *Virology* 1972;48:170–181.
279. Luongo C, Reinisch KM, Harrison SC, Nibert ML. Identification of the guanylyltransferase region and active site in reovirus mRNA capping protein λ2. *J Biol Chem* 2000;275:2804–2810.
280. Luongo CL, Contreras CM, Farsetta DL, Nibert ML. Binding site for S-adenosyl-L-methionine in a central region of mammalian reovirus λ2 protein. Evidence for activities in mRNA cap methylation. *J Biol Chem* 1998;273:23773–23780.
281. Luongo CL, Dryden KA, Farsetta DL, et al. Localization of a C-terminal region of λ2 protein in reovirus cores. *J Virol* 1997;71:8035–8040.
282. Mabrouk T, Danis C, Lemay G. Two basic motifs of reovirus σ3 protein are involved in double-stranded RNA binding. *Biochem Cell Biol* 1995;73:137–145.
283. Mabrouk T, Lemay G. The sequence similarity of reovirus σ3 protein to picornaviral proteases is unrelated to its role in μ1 viral protein cleavage. *Virology* 1994;202:615–620.
284. Mah DCW, Leone G, Jankowski JM, Lee PWK. The amino-terminal quarter of reovirus cell attachment protein σ1 possesses intrinsic virion-anchoring function. *Virology* 1990;179:95–103.
285. Mallo M, Martinez-Costas J, Benavente J. The stimulatory effect of actinomycin D on avian reovirus replication in L cells suggests that translational competition dictates the fate of the infection. *J Virol* 1991;65:5506–5512.
286. Mao ZX, Joklik WK. Isolation and enzymatic characterization of protein λ2, the reovirus guanylyltransferase. *Virology* 1991;185:377–386.
287. Maratos-Flier E, Goodman MJ, Murray AH, Kahn CR. Ammonium inhibits processing and cytotoxicity of reovirus, a nonenveloped virus. *J Clin Invest* 1986;78:1003–1007.
288. Maratos-Flier E, Kahn CR, Spriggs DR, Fields BN. Specific plasma membrane receptors for reovirus on rat pituitary cells in culture. *J Clin Invest* 1983;72:617–621.
289. Marcus PI. Interferon induction by viruses: One molecule of dsRNA as the threshold for interferon induction. *Interferon* 1983;5:116–180.
290. Martin PE, McCrae MA. Analysis of the stimulation of reporter gene expression by the σ3 protein of reovirus in co-transfected cells. *J Gen Virol* 1993;74:1055–1062.
291. Martinez-Costas J, Grande A, Varela R, et al. Protein architecture of avian reovirus S1133 and identification of the cell attachment protein. *J Virol* 1997;71:59–64.
292. Martinez-Costas J, Varela R, Benavente J. Endogenous enzymatic activities of the avian reovirus S1133: Identification of the viral capping enzyme. *Virology* 1995;206:1017–1026.
293. Masri S, Nagata L, Mah D, Lee P. Functional expression in *Escherichia coli* of cloned reovirus S1 gene encoding the viral cell attachment protein σ1. *Virology* 1986;149:83–90.
294. Matoba Y, Colucci WS, Fields BN, Smith TW. The reovirus M1 gene determines the relative capacity of growth of reovirus in cultured bovine aortic endothelial cells. *J Clin Invest* 1993;92:2883–2888.
295. Matoba Y, Sherry B, Fields BN, Smith TW. Identification of the viral genes responsible for growth of strains of reovirus in cultured mouse heart cells. *J Clin Invest* 1991;87:1628–1633.
296. Matsuhisa T, Joklik WK. Temperature-sensitive mutants of reovirus. V. Studies on the nature of the temperature-sensitive lesion of the group C mutant ts447. *Virology* 1974;60:380–389.

297. Matsuura K, Ishikura M, Nakayama T, et al. Ecological studies on reovirus pollution of rivers in Toyama Prefecture. II. Molecular epidemiological study of reoviruses isolated from river water. *Microbiol Immunol* 1993;37:305–310.
298. Mayor HD, Jamison RM, Jordan LE, Mitchell MV. Reoviruses. II. Structure and composition of the virion. *J Bacteriol* 1965;89:1548–1556.
299. Mbisa JL, Becker MM, Zou S, et al. Reovirus μ2 protein determines strain-specific differences in the rate of viral inclusion formation in L929 cells. *Virology* 2000;272:16–26.
300. McClain ME, Spendlove RS. Multiplicity reactivation of reovirus particles after exposure to ultraviolet light. *J Bacteriol* 1966;92:1422–1429.
301. McCrae MA. Terminal structure of reovirus RNAs. *J Gen Virol* 1981;55:393–403.
302. McCrae MA, Joklik WK. The nature of the polypeptide encoded by each of the 10 double-stranded RNA segments of reovirus type 3. *Virology* 1978;89:578–593.
303. McCutcheon AM, Broering TJ, Nibert ML. Mammalian reovirus M3 gene sequences and conservation of coiled-coil motifs near the carboxyl terminus of the μNS protein. *Virology* 1999;264:16–24.
304. McDowell MJ, Joklik WK. An *in vitro* protein synthesizing system from mouse L fibroblasts infected with reovirus. *Virology* 1971;45:724–733.
305. McDowell MJ, Joklik WK, Villa-Komaroff L, Lodish HF. Translation of reovirus messenger RNAs synthetesized *in vitro* into reovirus polypeptides by several mammalian cell-free extracts. *Proc Natl Acad Sci U S A* 1972;69:2649–2653.
306. McPhillips TH, Ramig RF. Extragenic suppression of temperature-sensitive phenotype in reovirus: Mapping suppressor mutations. *Virology* 1984;135:428–439.
307. Meanger J, Wickramasinghe R, Enriquez CE, Wilcox GE. Association between the sigma C protein of avian reovirus and virus-induced fusion of cells. *Arch Virol* 1999;144:193–197.
308. Mendez II, Hermann LL, Hazelton PR, Coombs KM. A comparative analysis of freon substitutes in the purification of reovirus and calicivirus. *J Virol Methods* 2000;90:59–67.
309. Metcalf P. The symmetry of the reovirus outer shell. *J Ultrastruct Res* 1982;78:292–301.
310. Metcalf P, Cyrklaff M, Adrian M. The three-dimensional structure of reovirus obtained by cryo-electron microscopy. *EMBO J* 1991;10:3129–3136.
311. Miller JE, Samuel CE. Proteolytic cleavage of the reovirus σ3 protein results in enhanced double-stranded RNA-binding activity: Identification of a repeated basic amino acid motif within the C-terminal binding region. *J Virol* 1992;66:5347–5356.
312. Millward S, Graham AF. Structural studies on reovirus: Discontinuities in the genome. *Proc Natl Acad Sci U S A* 1970;65:422–429.
313. Miura K, Watanabe K, Sugiura M, Shatkin AJ. The 5′-terminal nucleotide sequences of the double-stranded RNA of human reovirus. *Proc Natl Acad Sci U S A* 1974;71:3979–3983.
314. Miyamoto NG, Jacobs BL, Samuel CE. Mechanism of interferon action. Effect of double-stranded RNA and the 5′-O-monophosphate form of 2′,5′-oligoadenylate on the inhibition of reovirus mRNA translation *in vitro*. *J Biol Chem* 1983;258:15232–15237.
315. Miyamoto NG, Samuel CE. Mechanism of interferon action. Interferon-mediated inhibition of reovirus mRNA translation in the absence of detectable mRNA degradation but in the presence of protein phosphorylation. *Virology* 1980;107:461–475.
316. Mochizuki M, Tamazumi T, Kawanishi A, et al. Serotype 2 reoviruses from the feces of cats with and without diarrhea. *J Vet Med Sci* 1992;54:963–968.
317. Montgomery LB, Kao CY, Verdin E, et al. Infection of a polarized epithelial cell line with wild-type reovirus leads to virus persistence and altered cellular function. *J Gen Virol* 1991;72:2939–2946.
318. Moody MD, Joklik WK. The function of reovirus proteins during the reovirus multiplication cycle: Analysis using monoreassortants. *Virology* 1989;173:437–446.
319. Mora M, Partin K, Bhatia M, et al. Association of reovirus proteins with the structural matrix of infected cells. *Virology* 1987;159:265–277.
320. Morgan EM, Kingsbury DW. Pyridoxal phosphate as a probe of reovirus transcriptase. *Biochemistry* 1980;19:484–489.
321. Morgan EM, Kingsbury DW. Reovirus enzymes that modify messenger RNA are inhibited by perturbation of the lambda proteins. *Virology* 1981;113:565–572.
322. Morgan EM, Zweerink HJ. Reovirus morphogenesis. Corelike particles in cells infected at 39 degrees with wild-type reovirus and temperature-sensitive mutants of groups B and G. *Virology* 1974;59:556–565.
323. Morgan EM, Zweerink HJ. Characterization of transcriptase and replicase particles isolated from reovirus-infected cells. *Virology* 1975;68:455–466.
324. Morgan EM, Zweerink HJ. Characterization of the double-stranded RNA in replicase particles in reovirus-infected cells. *Virology* 1977;77:421–423.
325. Morin MJ, Warner A, Fields BN. Reovirus infection in rat lungs as a model to study the pathogenesis of viral pneumonia. *J Virol* 1996;70:541–548.
326. Morozov SY. A possible relationship of reovirus putative RNA polymerase to polymerases of positive-strand RNA viruses. *Nucleic Acids Res* 1989;17:5394.
327. Morrison LA, Fields BN, Dermody TS. Prolonged replication in the mouse central nervous system of reoviruses isolated from persistently infected cell cultures. *J Virol* 1993;67:3019–3026.
328. Munemitsu SM, Atwater JA, Samuel CE. Biosynthesis of reovirus-specified polypeptides. Molecular cDNA cloning and nucleotide sequence of the reovirus serotype 1 Lang strain bicistronic s1 mRNA which encodes the minor capsid polypeptide σ1a and the nonstructural polypeptide σ1bNS. *Biochem Biophys Res Commun* 1986;140:508–514.
329. Munemitsu SM, Samuel CE. Biosynthesis of reovirus-specified polypeptides: Effect of point mutation of the sequences flanking the 5′-proximal AUG initiator codons of the reovirus S1 and S4 genes on the efficiency of mRNA translation. *Virology* 1988;163:643–646.
330. Munoz A, Alonso MA, Carrasco L. The regulation of translation in reovirus-infected cells. *J Gen Virol* 1985;66:2161–2170.
331. Muscillo M, Carducci A, Larosa G, et al. Enteric virus detection in Adriatic seawater by cell culture, polymerase chain reaction and polyacrylamide gel electrophoresis. *Water Res* 1997;31:1980–1984.
332. Mustoe TA, Ramig RF, Sharpe AH, Fields BN. A genetic map of reovirus. III. Assignment of the double-stranded RNA-positive mutant groups A, B, and G to genome segments. *Virology* 1978;85:545–556.
333. Muthukrishnan S, Both GW, Furuichi Y, Shatkin AJ. 5′-Terminal 7-methylguanosine in eukaryotic mRNA is required for translation. *Nature* 1975;255:33–37.
334. Muthukrishnan S, Shatkin AJ. Reovirus genome RNA segments: Resistance to S-1 nuclease. *Virology* 1975;64:96–105.
335. Nagata L, Masri S, Mah D, Lee P. Molecular cloning and sequencing of the reovirus (serotype 3) S1 gene which encodes the viral cell attachment protein σ1. *Nucleic Acids Res* 1984;12:8699–8710.
336. Nagata L, Masri S, Pon R, Lee P. Analysis of functional domains on reovirus cell attachment protein σ1 using cloned S1 gene deletion mutants. *Virology* 1987;160:162–168.
337. Nakashima K, LaFiandra AJ, Shatkin AJ. Differential dependence of reovirus-associated enzyme activities on genome RNA as determined by psoralen photosensitivity. *J Biol Chem* 1979;254:8007–8014.
338. Nason EL, Samal SK, Prasad BVV. Trypsin-induced structural transformation in aquareovirus. *J Virol* 2000;74:6546–6555.
339. Nepom JT, Weiner HL, Dichter MA, et al. Identification of a hemagglutinin-specific idiotype associated with reovirus recognition shared by lymphoid and neural cells. *J Exp Med* 1982;155:155–167.
340. Ni Y, Ramig RF. Characterization of avian reovirus-induced cell fusion: The role of viral structural proteins. *Virology* 1993;194:705–714.
341. Nibert ML. Structure of mammalian orthoreovirus particles. *Curr Top Microbiol Immunol* 1998;238(I):1–30.
342. Nibert ML, Chappell JD, Dermody TS. Infectious subvirion particles of reovirus type 3 Dearing exhibit a loss in infectivity and contain a cleaved σ1 protein. *J Virol* 1995;69:5057–5067.
343. Nibert ML, Dermody TS, Fields BN. Structure of the reovirus cell-attachment protein: A model for the domain organization of σ1. *J Virol* 1990;64:2976–2989.
344. Nibert ML, Fields BN. A carboxy-terminal fragment of protein μ1/μ1C is present in infectious subvirion particles of mammalian reoviruses and is proposed to have a role in penetration. *J Virol* 1992;-66:6408–6418.
345. Nibert ML, Furlong DB, Fields BN. Mechanisms of viral pathogene-

sis. Distinct forms of reoviruses and their roles during replication in cells and host. *J Clin Invest* 1991;88:727–734.
346. Nibert ML, Margraf RL, Coombs KM. Nonrandom segregation of parental alleles in reovirus reassortants. *J Virol* 1996;70:7295–7300.
347. Nibert ML, Schiff LA, Fields BN. Mammalian reoviruses contain a myristoylated structural protein. *J Virol* 1991;65:1960–1967.
348. Nichols JL, Bellamy AR, Joklik WK. Identification of the nucleotide sequences of the oligonucleotides present in reovirions. *Virology* 1972;49:562–572.
349. Nicklas W, Kraft V, Meyer B. Contamination of transplantable tumors, cell lines, and monoclonal antibodies with rodent viruses. *Lab Anim Sci* 1993;43:296–300.
350. Nilsen TW, Maroney PA, Baglioni C. Inhibition of protein synthesis in reovirus-infected HeLa cells with elevated levels of interferon-induced protein kinase activity. *J Biol Chem* 1982;257:14593–14596.
351. Nilsen TW, Maroney PA, Baglioni C. Synthesis of (2′-5′)oligoadenylate and activation of an endoribonuclease in interferon-treated HeLa cells infected with reovirus. *J Virol* 1982;42:1039–1045.
352. Nilsen TW, Maroney PA, Baglioni C. Maintenance of protein synthesis in spite of mRNA breakdown in interferon-treated HeLa cells infected with reovirus. *Mol Cell Biol* 1983;3:64–69.
353. Noah DL, Blum MA, Sherry B. Interferon regulatory factor 3 is required for viral induction of beta interferon in primary cardiac myocyte cultures. *J Virol* 1999;73:10208–10213.
354. Noble S, Nibert ML. Characterization of an ATPase activity in reovirus cores and its genetic association with core-shell protein λ1. *J Virol* 1997;71:2182–2191.
355. Noble S, Nibert ML. Core protein μ2 is a second determinant of nucleoside triphosphatase activities by reovirus cores. *J Virol* 1997; 71:7728–7735.
356. Nonoyama M, Graham AF. Appearance of defective virions in clones of reovirus. *J Virol* 1970;6:693–694.
357. Nonoyama M, Millward S, Graham AF. Control of transcription of the reovirus genome. *Nucleic Acids Res* 1974;1:373–385.
358. Nonoyama M, Watanabe Y, Graham AF. Defective virions of reovirus. *J Virol* 1970;6:226–236.
359. Oberhaus SM, Smith RL, Clayton GH, et al. Reovirus infection and tissue injury in the mouse central nervous system are associated with apoptosis. *J Virol* 1997;71:2100–2106.
360. Pacitti AF, Gentsch JR. Inhibition of reovirus type 3 binding to host cells by sialylated glycoproteins is mediated through the viral attachment protein. *J Virol* 1987;61:1407–1415.
361. Paul R, Lee P. Glycophorin is the reovirus receptor on human erythrocytes. *Virology* 1987;159:94–101.
362. Paul RW, Choi AHC, Lee PWK. The alpha-anomeric form of sialic acid is the minimal receptor determinant recognized by reovirus. *Virology* 1989;172:382–385.
363. Pelletier J, Nicholson R, Bassel-Duby R, et al. Expression of reovirus type 3 (Dearing) σ1 and σs polypeptides in *Escherichia coli. J Gen Virol* 1987;68:135–145.
364. Pett DM, Vanaman TC, Joklik WK. Studies on the amino and carboxyl terminal amino acid sequences of reovirus capsid polypeptides. *Virology* 1973;52:174–186.
365. Poggioli GJ, Keefer C, Connolly JL, et al. Reovirus-induced G(2)/M cell cycle arrest requires σ1s and occurs in the absence of apoptosis. *J Virol* 2000;74:9562–9570.
366. Powell KF, Harvey JD, Bellamy AR. Reovirus RNA transcriptase: Evidence for a conformational change during activation of the core particle. *Virology* 1984;137:1–8.
367. Ralph SJ, Harvey JD, Bellamy AR. Subunit structure of the reovirus spike. *J Virol* 1980;36:894–896.
368. Ramig R, Fields BN. Genetics of reovirus. In: Joklik WK, ed. *The Reoviridae*. New York: Plenum Press, 1983:197–228.
369. Ramig RF, Ahmed R, Fields BN. A genetic map of reovirus: Assignment of the newly defined mutant groups H, I, and J to genome segments. *Virology* 1983;125:299–313.
370. Ramig RF, Cross RK, Fields BN. Genome RNAs and polypeptides of reovirus serotypes 1, 2, and 3. *J Virol* 1977;22:726–733.
371. Ramig RF, Fields BN. Method for rapidly screening revertants of reovirus temperature-sensitive mutants for extragenic suppression. *Virology* 1977;81:170–173.
372. Ramig RF, Fields BN. Revertants of temperature-sensitive mutants of reovirus: Evidence for frequent extragenic suppression. *Virology* 1979;92:155–167.
373. Ramig RF, Mustoe TA, Sharpe AH, Fields BN. A genetic map of reovirus. II. Assignment of the double-stranded RNA-negative mutant groups C, D, and E to genome segments. *Virology* 1978;85:531–534.
374. Ramig RF, White RM, Fields BN. Suppression of the temperature-sensitive phenotype of a mutant of reovirus type 3. *Science* 1977;195:406–407.
375. Ramos-Alvarez M, Sabin AB. Enteropathogenic viruses and bacteria. Role in summer diarrheal diseases of infancy and early childhood. *JAMA* 1958;167:147–156.
376. Rankin JT Jr, Eppes SB, Antczak JB, Joklik WK. Studies on the mechanism of the antiviral activity of ribavirin against reovirus. *Virology* 1989;168:147–158.
377. Ray BK, Brendler TG, Adya S, et al. Role of mRNA competition in regulating translation: Further characterization of mRNA discriminatory initiation factors. *Proc Natl Acad Sci U S A* 1983;80:663–667.
378. Reinisch KM, Nibert ML, Harrison SC. Structure of the reovirus core at 3.6 Å resolution. *Nature* 2000;404:960–967.
379. Rhim JS, Jordan LE, Mayor HD. Cytochemical, fluorescent-antibody and electron microscopic studies on the growth of reovirus (ECHO 10) in tissue culture. *Virology* 1962;17:342–355.
380. Rhim JS, Smith KO, Melnick JL. Complete and coreless forms of reovirus (ECHO 10): Ratio of number of virus particles to infective units in the one-step growth cycle. *Virology* 1961;15:428–435.
381. Richardson MA, Furuichi Y. Nucleotide sequence of reovirus genome segment S3, encoding non-structural protein sigma NS. *Nucleic Acids Res* 1983;11:6399–6408.
382. Richardson MA, Furuichi Y. Synthesis in *Escherichia coli* of the reovirus nonstructural protein sigma NS. *J Virol* 1985;56:527–533.
383. Rodgers SE, Barton ES, Oberhaus SM, et al. Reovirus-induced apoptosis of MDCK cells is not linked to viral yield and is blocked by Bcl-2. *J Virol* 1997;71:2540–2546.
384. Rodgers SE, Connolly JL, Chappell JD, Dermody TS. Reovirus growth in cell culture does not require the full complement of viral proteins: Identification of a σ1s-null mutant. *J Virol* 1998;72: 8597–8604.
385. Roner MR, Gaillard RK Jr, Joklik WK. Control of reovirus messenger RNA translation efficiency by the regions upstream of initiation codons. *Virology* 1989;168:292–301.
386. Roner MR, Lin PN, Nepluev I, et al. Identification of signals required for the insertion of heterologous genome segments into the reovirus genome. *Proc Natl Acad Sci U S A* 1995;92:12362–12366.
387. Roner MR, Nepliouev I, Sherry B, Joklik WK. Construction and characterization of a reovirus double temperature-sensitive mutant. *Proc Natl Acad Sci U S A* 1997;94:6826–6830.
388. Roner MR, Roner LA, Joklik WK. Translation of reovirus RNA species m1 can initiate at either of the first two in-frame initiation codons. *Proc Natl Acad Sci U S A* 1993;90:8947–8951.
389. Roner MR, Sutphin LA, Joklik WK. Reovirus RNA is infectious. *Virology* 1990;179:845–852.
390. Rosen L. Reoviruses in animals other than man. *Ann N Y Acad Sci* 1962;101:461–465.
391. Rosen L, Hovis JF, Mastrota FM, et al. Observations on a newly recognized virus (Abney) of the reovirus family. *Am J Hyg* 1960;71: 258–265.
392. Rozinov MN, Fields BN. Interference following mixed infection of reovirus isolates is linked to the M2 gene. *J Virol* 1994;68:6667–6671.
393. Rozinov MN, Fields BN. Evidence for phenotypic mixing with reovirus in cell culture. *Virology* 1996;215:207–210.
394. Rozinov MN, Fields BN. Interference of reovirus strains occurs between the stages of uncoating and dsRNA accumulation. *J Gen Virol* 1996;77:1425–1429.
395. Rubin DH, Weiner DB, Dworkin C, et al. Receptor utilization by reovirus type 3: Distinct binding sites on thymoma and fibroblast cell lines result in differential compartmentalization of virions. *Microb Pathog* 1992;12:351–365.
396. Rubin DH, Wetzel JD, Williams WV, et al. Binding of type 3 reovirus by a domain of the σ1 protein important for hemagglutination leads to infection of murine erythroleukemia cells. *J Clin Invest* 1992;90: 2536–2542.
397. Sabin AB. Reoviruses. *Science* 1959;130:1387–1389.
398. Sakuma S, Watanabe Y. Unilateral synthesis of reovirus double-stranded ribonucleic acid by a cell-free replicase system. *J Virol* 1971;8:190–196.
399. Sakuma S, Watanabe Y. Reovirus replicase-directed synthesis of double-stranded ribonucleic acid. *J Virol* 1972;10:628–638.

400. Samuel CE, Brody MS. Biosynthesis of reovirus-specified polypeptides. 2-Aminopurine increases the efficiency of translation of reovirus s1 mRNA but not s4 mRNA in transfected cells. *Virology* 1990;176:106–113.
401. Samuel CE, Duncan R, Knutson GS, Hershey JW. Mechanism of interferon action. Increased phosphorylation of protein synthesis initiation factor eIF-2 alpha in interferon-treated, reovirus-infected mouse L929 fibroblasts *in vitro* and *in vivo*. *J Biol Chem* 1984;259: 13451–13457.
402. Samuel CE, Knutson GS. Mechanism of interferon action: Human leukocyte and immune interferons regulate the expression of different genes and induce different antiviral states in human amnion U cells. *Virology* 1983;130:474–484.
403. Sargent MD, Borsa J. Effects of calcium and magnesium on the switch-on of transcriptase function in reovirus *in vitro*. *Can J Biochem Cell Biol* 1984;62:162–169.
404. Sarkar G, Pelletier J, Bassel-Duby R, et al. Identification of a new polypeptide coded by reovirus gene S1. *J Virol* 1985;54:720–725.
405. Sauve GJ, Saragovi HU, Greene MI. Reovirus receptors. *Adv Virus Res* 1993;42:325–341.
406. Sawutz DG, Bassel-Duby R, Homcy CJ. High affinity binding of reovirus type 3 to cells that lack beta adrenergic receptor activity. *Life Sci* 1987;40:399–406.
407. Schiff LA, Nibert ML, Co MS, et al. Distinct binding sites for zinc and double-stranded RNA in the reovirus outer capsid protein σ3. *Mol Cell Biol* 1988;8:273–283.
408. Schmechel S, Chute M, Skinner P, et al. Preferential translation of reovirus mRNA by a σ3-dependent mechanism. *Virology* 1997;232: 62–73.
409. Schnitzer T. Protein coding assignment of the S genes of the avian reovirus S1133. *Virology* 1985;141:167–170.
410. Schonberg M, Silverstein SC, Levin DH, Acs G. Asynchronous synthesis of the complementary strands of the reovirus genome. *Proc Natl Acad Sci U S A* 1971;68:505–508.
411. Schuerch AR, Matsuhisa T, Joklik WK. Temperature-sensitive mutants of reovirus. VI. Mutant ts 447 and ts 556 particles that lack either one or two genome RNA segments. *Intervirology* 1974;3:36–46.
412. Selb B, Weber B. A study of human reovirus IgG and IgA antibodies by ELISA and western blot. *J Virol Methods* 1994;47:15–25.
413. Seliger LS, Giantini M, Shatkin AJ. Translational effects and sequence comparisons of the three serotypes of the reovirus S4 gene. *Virology* 1992;187:202–210.
414. Seliger LS, Zheng K, Shatkin AJ. Complete nucleotide sequence of reovirus L2 gene and deduced amino acid sequence of viral mRNA guanylyltransferase. *J Biol Chem* 1987;262:16289–16293.
415. Sharpe AH, Chen LB, Fields BN. The interaction of mammalian reoviruses with the cytoskeleton of monkey kidney CV-1 cells. *Virology* 1982;120:399–411.
416. Sharpe AH, Fields BN. Reovirus inhibition of cellular DNA synthesis: Role of the S1 gene. *J Virol* 1981;38:389–392.
417. Sharpe AH, Fields BN. Reovirus inhibition of cellular RNA and protein synthesis: Role of the S4 gene. *Virology* 1982;122:381–391.
418. Sharpe AH, Fields BN. Pathogenesis of viral infections. Basic concepts derived from the reovirus model. *N Engl J Med* 1985;312: 486–497.
419. Sharpe AH, Ramig RF, Mustoe TA, Fields BN. A genetic map of reovirus. 1. Correlation of genome RNAs between serotypes 1, 2, and 3. *Virology* 1978;84:63–74.
420. Shatkin AJ. Inactivity of purified reovirus RNA as a template for *E. coli* polymerases *in vitro*. *Proc Natl Acad Sci U S A* 1965;54:1721–1728.
421. Shatkin AJ. Viruses containing double-stranded RNA. In: Fraenkel-Conrat H, ed. *Molecular Basis of Virology*. New York: Reinhold Book, 1968:351–392.
422. Shatkin AJ. Methylated messenger RNA synthesis *in vitro* by purified reovirus. *Proc Natl Acad Sci U S A* 1974;71:3204–3207.
423. Shatkin AJ, Furuichi Y, LaFiandra AJ, Yamakawa M. Initiation of mRNA synthesis and 5′-terminal modification of reovirus transcripts. In: Compans RW, Bishop DHL, eds. *Double-stranded RNA Viruses*. New York: Elsevier, 1983:43–54.
424. Shatkin AJ, Kozak M. Biochemical aspects of reovirus transcription and translation. In: Joklik WK, ed. *The Reoviridae*. New York: Plenum Press, 1983:79–106.
425. Shatkin AJ, LaFiandra AJ. Transcription by infectious subviral particles of reovirus. *J Virol* 1972;10:698–706.
426. Shatkin AJ, Sipe JD. RNA polymerase activity in purified reoviruses. *Proc Natl Acad Sci U S A* 1968;61:1462–1469.
427. Shatkin AJ, Sipe JD. Single-stranded adenine-rich RNA from purified reoviruses. *Proc Natl Acad Sci U S A* 1968;59:246–253.
428. Shatkin AJ, Sipe JD, Loh P. Separation of ten reovirus genome segments by polyacrylamide gel electrophoresis. *J Virol* 1968;2:986–991.
429. Shaw JE, Cox DC. Early inhibition of cellular DNA synthesis by high multiplicities of infectious and UV-inactivated Reovirus. *J Virol* 1973;12:704–710.
430. Shepard DA, Ehnstrom JG, Schiff LA. Association of reovirus outer capsid proteins σ3 and μ1 causes a conformational change that renders σ3 protease sensitive. *J Virol* 1995;69:8180–8184.
431. Shepard DA, Ehnstrom JG, Skinner PJ, Schiff LA. Mutations in the zinc-binding motif of the reovirus capsid protein σ3 eliminate its ability to associate with capsid protein μ1. *J Virol* 1996;70:2065–2068.
432. Sherry B, Baty CJ, Blum MA. Reovirus-induced acute myocarditis in mice correlates with viral RNA synthesis rather than generation of infectious virus in cardiac myocytes. *J Virol* 1996;70:6709–6715.
433. Sherry B, Blum MA. Multiple viral core proteins are determinants of reovirus-induced acute myocarditis. *J Virol* 1994;68:8461–8465.
434. Sherry B, Fields BN. The reovirus M1 gene, encoding a viral core protein, is associated with the myocarditic phenotype of a reovirus variant. *J Virol* 1989;63:4850–4856.
435. Sherry B, Schoen FJ, Wenske E, Fields BN. Derivation and characterization of an efficiently myocarditic reovirus variant. *J Virol* 1989;63: 4840–4849.
436. Sherry B, Torres J, Blum MA. Reovirus induction of and sensitivity to beta interferon in cardiac myocyte cultures correlate with induction of myocarditis and are determined by viral core proteins. *J Virol* 1998;72: 1314–1323.
437. Shing M, Coombs KM. Assembly of the reovirus outer capsid requires μ1/σ3 interactions which are prevented by misfolded σ3 protein in temperature-sensitive mutant tsG453. *Virus Res* 1996;46:19–29.
438. Shmulevitz M, Duncan R. A new class of fusion-associated small transmembrane (FAST) proteins encoded by the nonenveloped fusogenic reoviruses. *EMBO J* 2000;19:902–912.
439. Silverstein SC, Astell C, Christman J, et al. Synthesis of reovirus oligo adenylic acid *in vivo* and *in vitro*. *J Virol* 1974;13:740–752.
440. Silverstein SC, Astell C, Levin DH, et al. The mechanisms of reovirus uncoating and gene activation *in vivo*. *Virology* 1972;47:797–806.
441. Silverstein SC, Christman JK, Acs G. The reovirus replicative cycle. *Annu Rev Biochem* 1976;45:375–408.
442. Silverstein SC, Dales S. The penetration of reovirus RNA and initiation of its genetic function in L-strain fibroblasts. *J Cell Biol* 1968;36: 197–230.
443. Silverstein SC, Schonberg M, Levin DH, Acs G. The reovirus replicative cycle: Conservation of parental RNA and protein. *Proc Natl Acad Sci U S A* 1970;67:275–281.
444. Silverstein SC, Schur PH. Immunofluorescent localization of double-stranded RNA in reovirus-infected cells. *Virology* 1970;41:564–566.
445. Skehel JJ, Joklik WK. Studies on the *in vitro* transcription of reovirus RNA catalyzed by reovirus cores. *Virology* 1969;39:822–831.
446. Skup D, Millward S. mRNA capping enzymes are masked in reovirus progeny subviral particles. *J Virol* 1980;34:490–496.
447. Skup D, Millward S. Reovirus-induced modification of cap-dependent translation in infected L cells. *Proc Natl Acad Sci U S A* 1980;77: 152–156.
448. Skup D, Zarbl H, Millward S. Regulation of translation in L-cells infected with reovirus. *J Mol Biol* 1981;151:35–55.
449. Smith RE, Zweerink HJ, Joklik WK. Polypeptide components of virions, top component and cores of reovirus type 3. *Virology* 1969;39: 791–810.
450. Sonenberg N, Skup D, Trachsel H, Millward S. *In vitro* translation in reovirus- and poliovirus-infected cell extracts. Effects of anti-cap binding protein monoclonal antibody. *J Biol Chem* 1981;256:4138–4141.
451. Spandidos DA, Krystal G, Graham AF. Regulated transcription of the genomes of defective virions and temperature-sensitive mutants of reovirus. *J Virol* 1976;18:7–19.
452. Spendlove RS, Lennette EH, Chin JN, Knight CO. Effect of antimitotic agents on intracellular reovirus antigen. *Cancer Res* 1964;24: 1826–1833.
453. Spendlove RS, Lennette EH, Knight CO, Chin JH. Development of viral antigen and infectious virus on HeLa cells infected with reovirus. *J Immunol* 1963;90:548–553.

454. Spendlove RS, McClain ME, Lennette EH. Enhancement of reovirus infectivity by extracellular removal or alteration of the virus capsid by proteolytic enzymes. *J Gen Virol* 1970;8:83–94.
455. Spriggs DR, Bronson RT, Fields BN. Hemagglutinin variants of reovirus type 3 have altered central nervous system tropism. *Science* 1983;220:505–507.
456. Spriggs DR, Fields BN. Attenuated reovirus type 3 strains generated by selection of haemagglutinin antigenic variants. *Nature* 1982;297: 68–70.
457. Spriggs DR, Kaye K, Fields BN. Topological analysis of the reovirus type 3 hemagglutinin. *Virology* 1983;127:220–224.
458. Stamatos NM, Gomatos PJ. Binding to selected regions of reovirus mRNAs by a nonstructural reovirus protein. *Proc Natl Acad Sci U S A* 1982;79:3457–3461.
459. Stanley NF. Reoviruses. *Br Med Bull* 1967;23:150–154.
460. Starnes MC, Joklik WK. Reovirus protein λ3 is a poly(C)-dependent poly(G) polymerase. *Virology* 1993;193:356–366.
461. Steele MI, Marshall CM, Lloyd RE, Randolph VE. Reovirus 3 not detected by reverse transcriptase-mediated polymerase chain reaction analysis of preserved tissue from infants with cholestatic liver disease. *Hepatology* 1995;21:697–702.
462. Stoltzfus CM, Banerjee AK. Two oligonucleotide classes of single-stranded ribopolymers in reovirus A-rich RNA. *Arch Biochem Biophys* 1972;152:733–743.
463. Strong JE, Coffey MC, Tang D, et al. The molecular basis of viral oncolysis: Usurpation of the Ras signaling pathway by reovirus. *EMBO J* 1998;17:3351–3362.
464. Strong JE, Lee PWK. The v-*erbB* oncogene confers enhanced cellular susceptibility to reovirus infection. *J Virol* 1996;70:612–616.
465. Strong JE, Leone G, Duncan R, et al. Biochemical and biophysical characterization of the reovirus cell attachment protein σ1: Evidence that it is a homotrimer. *Virology* 1991;184:23–32.
466. Strong JE, Tang D, Lee PWK. Evidence that the epidermal growth factor receptor on host cells confers reovirus infection efficiency. *Virology* 1993;197:405–411.
467. Sturzenbecker LJ, Nibert M, Furlong D, Fields BN. Intracellular digestion of reovirus particles requires a low pH and is an essential step in the viral infectious cycle. *J Virol* 1987;61:2351–2361.
468. Taber R, Alexander V, Whitford W. Persistent reovirus infection of CHO cells resulting in virus resistance. *J Virol* 1976;17:513–524.
469. Tang D, Strong JE, Lee PW. Recognition of the epidermal growth factor receptor by reovirus. *Virology* 1993;197:412–414.
470. Tardieu M, Weiner HL. Viral receptors on isolated murine and human ependymal cells. *Science* 1982;215:419–421.
471. Tillotson L, Shatkin AJ. Reovirus polypeptide σ3 and N-terminal myristoylation of polypeptide μ1 are required for site-specific cleavage to μ1C in transfected cells. *J Virol* 1992;66:2180–2186.
472. Tosteson MT, Nibert ML, Fields BN. Ion channels induced in lipid bilayers by subvirion particles of the nonenveloped mammalian reoviruses. *Proc Natl Acad Sci U S A* 1993;90:10549–10552.
473. Turner DL, Duncan R, Lee PW. Site-directed mutagenesis of the C-terminal portion of reovirus protein σ1: Evidence for a conformation-dependent receptor binding domain. *Virology* 1992;186:219–227.
474. Tyler KL, Sokol RJ, Oberhaus SM, et al. Detection of reovirus RNA in hepatobiliary tissues from patients with extrahepatic biliary atresia and choledochal cysts. *Hepatology* 1998;27:1475–1482.
475. Tyler KL, Squier MK, Brown AL, et al. Linkage between reovirus-induced apoptosis and inhibition of cellular DNA synthesis: Role of the S1 and M2 genes. *J Virol* 1996;70:7984–7991.
476. Tyler KL, Squier MK, Rodgers SE, et al. Differences in the capacity of reovirus strains to induce apoptosis are determined by the viral attachment protein σ1. *J Virol* 1995;69:6972–6979.
477. Vasquez C, Kleinschmidt AK. Electron microscopy of RNA strands released from individual reovirus particles. *J Mol Biol* 1968;34: 137–147.
478. Vasquez C, Tournier P. The morphology of reovirus. *Virology* 1962; 17:503–510.
479. Verdin EM, King GL, Maratos-Flier E. Characterization of a common high-affinity receptor for reovirus serotypes 1 and 3 on endothelial cells. *J Virol* 1989;63:1318–1325.
480. Verdin EM, Maratos-Flier E, Carpentier JL, Kahn CR. Persistent infection with a nontransforming RNA virus leads to impaired growth factor receptors and response. *J Cell Physiol* 1986;128:457–465.
481. Vieler E, Baumgartner W, Herbst W, Kohler G. Characterization of a reovirus isolate from a rattle snake, *Crotalus viridis*, with neurological dysfunction. *Arch Virol* 1994;138:341–344.
482. Virgin HW IV, Mann MA, Fields BN, Tyler KL. Monoclonal antibodies to reovirus reveal structure/function relationships between capsid proteins and genetics of susceptibility to antibody action. *J Virol* 1991;65:6772–6781.
483. Virgin HW IV, Mann MA, Tyler KL. Protective antibodies inhibit reovirus internalization and uncoating by intracellular proteases. *J Virol* 1994;68:6719–6729.
484. Wachsman JT, Levin DH, Acs G. Ribonucleoside triphosphate-dependent pyrophosphate exchange of reovirus cores. *J Virol* 1970;6: 563–565.
485. Wang Q, Bergeron J, Mabrouk T, Lemay G. Site-directed mutagenesis of the double-stranded RNA binding domain of bacterially expressed σ3 reovirus protein. *Virus Res* 1996;41:141–151.
486. Ward RL, Shatkin AJ. Association of reovirus mRNA with viral proteins: A possible mechanism for linking the genome segments. *Arch Biochem Biophys* 1972;152:378–384.
487. Watanabe Y, Gauntt CJ, Graham AF. Reovirus-induced ribonucleic acid polymerase. *J Virol* 1968;2:869–877.
488. Watanabe Y, Graham AF. Structural units of reovirus ribonucleic acid and their possible functional significance. *J Virol* 1967;1:665–677.
489. Watanabe Y, Millward S, Graham AF. Regulation of transcription of the reovirus genome. *J Mol Biol* 1968;36:107–123.
490. Weiner DB, Girard K, Williams WV, et al. Reovirus type 1 and type 3 differ in their binding to isolated intestinal epithelial cells. *Microb Pathog* 1988;5:29–40.
491. Weiner HL, Ault KA, Fields BN. Interaction of reovirus with cell surface receptors. I. Murine and human lymphocytes have a receptor for the hemagglutinin of reovirus type 3. *J Immunol* 1980;124: 2143–2148.
492. Weiner HL, Drayna D, Averill DR Jr, Fields BN. Molecular basis of reovirus virulence: Role of the S1 gene. *Proc Natl Acad Sci U S A* 1977;74:5744–5748.
493. Weiner HL, Fields BN. Neutralization of reovirus: The gene responsible for the neutralization antigen. *J Exp Med* 1977;146:1305–1310.
494. Weiner HL, Powers ML, Fields BN. Absolute linkage of virulence and central nervous system cell tropism of reoviruses to viral hemagglutinin. *J Infect Dis* 1980;141:609–616.
495. Weiner HL, Ramig RF, Mustoe TA, Fields BN. Identification of the gene coding for the hemagglutinin of reovirus. *Virology* 1978;86: 581–584.
496. Wenske EA, Chanock SJ, Krata L, Fields BN. Genetic reassortment of mammalian reoviruses in mice. *J Virol* 1985;56:613–616.
497. Wessner DR, Fields BN. Isolation and genetic characterization of ethanol-resistant reovirus mutants. *J Virol* 1993;67:2442–2447.
498. Wetzel JD, Chappell JD, Fogo AB, Dermody TS. Efficiency of viral entry determines the capacity of murine erythroleukemia cells to support persistent infections by mammalian reoviruses. *J Virol* 1997; 71:299–306.
499. Wetzel JD, Wilson GJ, Baer GS, et al. Reovirus variants selected during persistent infections of L cells contain mutations in the viral S1 and S4 genes and are altered in viral disassembly. *J Virol* 1997;71:1362–1369.
500. White CK, Zweerink HJ. Studies on the structure of reovirus cores: Selective removal of polypeptide λ2. *Virology* 1976;70:171–180.
501. Wickramasinghe R, Meanger J, Enriquez C, Wilcox G. Avian reovirus proteins associated with neutralization of virus infectivity. *Virology* 1993;194:688–696.
502. Wiebe ME, Joklik TW. The mechanism of inhibition of reovirus replication by interferon. *Virology* 1975;66:229–240.
503. Wiener JR, Bartlett JA, Joklik WK. The sequences of reovirus serotype 3 genome segments M1 and M3 encoding the minor protein μ2 and the major nonstructural protein μNS, respectively. *Virology* 1989;169:293–304.
504. Wiener JR, Joklik WK. Comparison of the reovirus serotype 1, 2, and 3 S3 genome segments encoding the nonstructural protein sigma NS. *Virology* 1987;161:332–339.
505. Wiener JR, Joklik WK. Evolution of reovirus genes: A comparison of serotype 1, 2, and 3 M2 genome segments, which encode the major structural capsid protein μ1C. *Virology* 1988;163:603–613.
506. Wiener JR, Joklik WK. The sequences of the reovirus serotype 1, 2, and 3 L1 genome segments and analysis of the mode of divergence of the reovirus serotypes. *Virology* 1989;169:194–203.
507. Wiener JR, McLaughlin T, Joklik WK. The sequences of the S2

genome segments of reovirus serotype 3 and of the dsRNA-negative mutant ts447. *Virology* 1989;170:340–341.
508. Wilcox GE, Compans RW. Cell fusion induced by Nelson Bay virus. *Virology* 1982;123:312–322.
509. Williams WV, Kieber Emmons T, Weiner DB, et al. Contact residues and predicted structure of the reovirus type 3-receptor interaction. *J Biol Chem* 1991;266:9241–9250.
510. Wilson GA, Morrison LA, Fields BN. Association of the reovirus S1 gene with serotype 3-induced biliary atresia in mice. *J Virol* 1994; 68:6458–6465.
511. Wilson GJ, Wetzel JD, Puryear W, et al. Persistent reovirus infections of L cells select mutations in viral attachment protein σ1 that alter oligomer stability. *J Virol* 1996;70:6598–6606.
512. Wolf JL, Rubin DH, Finberg R, et al. Intestinal M cells: A pathway for entry of reovirus into the host. *Science* 1981;212:471–472.
513. Xu P, Miller SE, Joklik WK. Generation of reovirus core-like particles in cells infected with hybrid vaccinia viruses that express genome segments L1, L2, L3, and S2. *Virology* 1993;197:726–731.
514. Yamakawa M, Furuichi Y, Nakashima K, et al. Excess synthesis of viral mRNA 5-terminal oligonucleotides by reovirus transcriptase. *J Biol Chem* 1981;256:6507–6514.
515. Yamakawa M, Furuichi Y, Shatkin AJ. Reovirus transcriptase and capping enzymes are active in intact virions. *Virology* 1982;118:157–168.
516. Yeager M, Weiner S, Coombs KM. Transcriptionally active reovirus core particles visualized by electron cryo-microscopy and image reconstruction. *Biophys J* 1996;70:A116.
517. Yeung M, Gill M, Alibhai S, et al. Purification and characterization of the reovirus cell attachment protein σ1. *Virology* 1987;156:377–385.
518. Yeung M, Lim D, Duncan R, et al. The cell attachment proteins of type 1 and type 3 reovirus are differentially susceptible to trypsin and chymotrypsin. *Virology* 1989;170:62–70.
519. Yin P, Cheang M, Coombs KM. The M1 gene is associated with differences in the temperature optimum of the transcriptase activity in reovirus core particles. *J Virol* 1996;70:1223–1227.
520. Yue Z, Shatkin AJ. Regulated, stable expression and nuclear presence of retrovirus double-stranded RNA-binding protein σ3 in HeLa cells. *J Virol* 1996;70:3497–3501.
521. Yue Z, Shatkin AJ. Double-stranded RNA-dependent protein kinase (PKR) is regulated by reovirus structural proteins. *Virology* 1997;234: 364–371.
522. Zarbl H, Hastings KE, Millward S. Reovirus core particles synthesize capped oligonucleotides as a result of abortive transcription. *Arch Biochem Biophys* 1980;202:348–360.
523. Zarbl H, Millward S. The reovirus multiplication cycle. In: Joklik WK, ed. *The Reoviridae*. New York: Plenum Press, 1983:107–196.
524. Zarbl H, Skup D, Millward S. Reovirus progeny subviral particles synthesize uncapped mRNA. *J Virol* 1980;34:497–505.
525. Zou S, Brown EG. Identification of sequence elements containing signals for replication and encapsidation of the reovirus M1 genome segment. *Virology* 1992;186:377–388.
526. Zou S, Brown EG. Nucleotide sequence comparison of the M1 genome segment of reovirus type 1 Lang and type 3 Dearing. *Virus Res* 1992;22:159–164.
527. Zou S, Brown EG. Stable expression of the reovirus μ2 protein in mouse L cells complements the growth of a reovirus ts mutant with a defect in its M1 gene. *Virology* 1996;217:42–48.
528. Zweerink HJ. Multiple forms of SS leads to DS RNA polymerase activity in reovirus-infected cells. *Nature* 1974;247:313–315.
529. Zweerink HJ, Ito Y, Matsuhisa T. Synthesis of reovirus double-stranded RNA within virionlike particles. *Virology* 1972;50: 349–358.
530. Zweerink HJ, Joklik WK. Studies on the intracellular synthesis of reovirus-specified proteins. *Virology* 1970;41:501–518.
531. Zweerink HJ, McDowell MJ, Joklik WK. Essential and nonessential noncapsid reovirus proteins. *Virology* 1971;45:716–723.
532. Zweerink HJ, Morgan EM, Skyler JS. Reovirus morphogenesis: Characterization of subviral particles in infected cells. *Virology* 1976;73: 442–453.

CHAPTER 27

Retroviridae: The Retroviruses and Their Replication

Stephen P. Goff

The retrovirus family, the *Retroviridae*, consists of a large and diverse group of viruses found in all vertebrates. These viruses replicate through an extraordinary and unique life cycle, differentiating them sharply from other viruses. The virion particles generally contain a genomic RNA, but upon entry into the host cell, this RNA is reverse transcribed into a DNA form of the genome that is integrated into the host chromosomal DNA. The integrated form of the viral DNA, the provirus, then serves as the template for the formation of viral RNAs and proteins that assemble progeny virions. These features of life cycle—especially the reverse flow of genetic information from RNA to DNA, and the establishment of the DNA in an integrated form in the host genome—are the defining hallmarks of the retroviruses. This life cycle also accounts for many of their diverse biologic activities. The creation of the proviral DNA confers on the viruses a powerful ability to (a) maintain a persistent infection despite a host immune response, and (b) enter the germ line, permitting the vertical transmission of virus.

The retroviruses have played a unique role in the history of molecular biology. They have attracted attention on several grounds.

- Biochemistry: The viral replication enzymes, including the reverse transcriptase (RT) and integrase (IN), are extraordinarily useful tools in manipulating nucleic acids *in vitro* and *in vivo*. Through the preparation of cDNAs, RT has been crucial for studies of mRNA synthesis and gene regulation.
- Pathogenicity: Retroviruses are known as major pathogens affecting nearly all vertebrates. Human immunodeficiency virus type 1 (HIV-1), the agent of the acquired immunodeficiency disease syndrome (AIDS) pandemic, will probably cause more human death and suffering than all but a handful of pathogens in recorded history.
- Markers of evolutionary history: The insertion of a provirus into the germ line provides a Mendelian tag that marks an event at a particular time in evolution. The inheritance of that tag can then be used to follow speciation, migrations, and divergence of species.
- Insertional activation of oncogenes: The integration of retroviral DNA is inherently mutagenic, and retrovirus replication thus causes gross alterations of host genes. When insertions lead to tumor formation, the locations serve to identify new oncogenes.
- Transduction: Retroviruses can acquire host sequences in the formation of acutely transforming genomes. The identity, structure, and expression of these genes has provided much of our current knowledge of the routes by which normal growth control can be subverted by genetic alterations.
- Gene delivery vectors: The structure of transforming viruses provided a model for the use of retroviruses to deliver therapeutic genes efficiently and cleanly into cells. Retroviruses now serve as major tools in the medical black bag of gene therapists.

This chapter will describe the replication and molecular biology of the retroviruses, concentrating on the most broadly conserved aspects of the life cycle. Because of the magnitude of the retroviral literature, citations here cannot be comprehensive, and referencing has been selective and concentrated on more recent publications. The distinctive features of the human retroviruses, especially the lentiviruses and spumaviruses, will be addressed in much more detail in *Fields Virology*, 4th ed. A comprehensive review of retroviral biology [*Retroviruses* (130)] has recently been published and should be consulted for additional details of almost all aspects of their replication.

TAXONOMIC CLASSIFICATION

The retroviruses were originally classified by the morphology of the virion core as visualized in the electron microscope. Examples of the appearance of the virions in these micrographs are presented in Figure 1. The virion particles are spherical and surrounded by an envelope consisting of a lipid membrane bilayer. The surface is studded by projections of an envelope glycoprotein. There is a spherical layer of protein under the membrane, and an internal nucleocapsid (or nucleoid) whose shape varies from virus to virus. The shape and position of the nucleocapsid core was historically used as the major classifying feature of the retroviral genera. A-type viruses were defined as those forming intracellular structures with a characteristic morphology, a thick shell with a hollow, electron-lucent center. These particles are now appreciated as representing an immature capsid on route toward the formation of other structures. This term is thus no longer in use to denote a virus classification, although it is used to describe the structures formed by some virus-related intracellular retrotransposons (the intracisternal A-type particles, or IAPs) (400,444). B-type viruses show a round but eccentrically positioned inner core. C-type viruses assemble at the plasma membrane and contain a central, symmetrically placed, spherical inner core. The D-type viruses assemble in the cytoplasm, via an A-type intermediate, and on budding they exhibit a distinctive cylindrical core.

These older classifications have been useful in partially defining the various genera of the family *Retroviridae*, but the number of genera has now been increased on the basis of new criteria. The genera have recently been formalized and given new names by the International Committee on Taxonomy of Viruses. The alpharetroviruses, betaretroviruses, and gammaretroviruses are considered "simple" retroviruses, whereas the deltaretroviruses, epsilonretroviruses, lentiviruses, and spumaviruses are considered "complex." The simple viruses encode only the Gag, Pro, Pol, and Env gene products; the complex viruses encode these same gene products but also an array of small regulatory proteins with a range of functions. The properties of the viruses belonging to each of these genera will be summarized briefly here. Representative members of each genus are listed in Table 1.

Alpharetroviruses

The alpharetroviruses are simple retroviruses characterized by a C-type morphology, and are typified by the avian leukemia viruses (ALV). The genome contains *gag*, *pro*, *pol*, and *env* genes, with no additional known genes; *pro* is at the 3′ end of *gag* and in the same reading frame. The tRNA primer is tRNATrp. The viruses are widespread in many avian host species. The ALV members are classified into 10 subgroups (termed A through J) by their distinct receptor utilization. The first four subgroups represent exogenous viruses of chickens; the subgroup E includes a family of endogenous chicken viruses; and subgroups F and G include endogenous viruses of pheasants.

Betaretroviruses

The betaretroviruses are simple retroviruses characterized by either a B-type morphology, with a round eccentric core, or a D-type morphology, with a cylindrical core. The best-known examples are the mouse mammary tumor virus (MMTV) and the Mason-Pfizer monkey virus (MPMV). Assembly occurs in the cytoplasm via an A-type intermediate, and the completed immature particle is then transported to the plasma membrane and budded. The genomes contain *gag*, *pro*, *pol*, and *env* genes, and the *gag*, *pro*, and *pol* genes are all in different reading frames. The genome of MMTV contains an additional gene termed the *sag* gene, for superantigen. The viruses also contain a dUTPase region as part of the *pro* open reading frame (ORF) (204). The tRNA primer is tRNALys-3 or tRNALys-1,2. There are both exogenous and endogenous viruses in this genus. Examples are found in mice, primates, and sheep.

Gammaretroviruses

The gammaretroviruses are simple viruses characterized by a C-type morphology. This genus has the largest number of members known, including the murine leukemia viruses (MuLVs), the feline leukemia viruses (FeLVs), and the gibbon ape leukemia virus (GALV). The genome contains only *gag*, *pro*, *pol*, and *env* genes; the *gag*, *pro*, and *pol* sequences are in the same reading frame, and the Gag-Pro-Pol protein is expressed by translational readthrough of a stop codon at the end of *gag*. The genome primer is tRNAPro or tRNAGlu (132,514). The murine viruses are divided into subgroups by their distinct receptor utilization. Many exogenous and endogenous viruses are found in diverse mammals, and examples have been isolated from reptiles and birds.

Deltaretroviruses

The deltaretroviruses are complex viruses characterized by a C-type morphology. The most famous examples are the human T-lymphotropic viruses (HTLVs) and the bovine leukemia virus (BLV). The genome contains *gag*, *pro*, *pol*, and *env* genes; the *gag*, *pro*, and *pol* genes are present in three different reading frames, and expression of the Gag-Pro-Pol protein requires two successive frameshifts. In addition, the genomes contain regulatory genes termed *rex* and *tax* that are expressed from an alternatively spliced mRNA. These gene products control the synthesis and processing of the viral RNAs. The tRNA primer is tRNAPro. No closely related endogenous viruses are known, and the exogenous viruses are only rarely found in a few mammals.

Epsilonretroviruses

The epsilonretroviruses are complex viruses characterized by a C-type morphology. The prototype is the walleye dermal sarcoma virus (469). The genomes contain *gag*, *pro*, *pol*, and *env* genes; the *gag*, *pro*, and *pol* genes are in the same reading frame. They also contain one to three additional genes termed *orfs A, B,* and *C*. The *orfA*-gene is a viral homolog of the host cyclin D gene and so may regulate the cell cycle (410). The viruses use tRNAHis or Arg as the primer. The only known examples are exogenous viruses in fish and reptiles.

Lentiviruses

The lentiviruses are complex viruses characterized by a unique virion morphology, with cylindrical or conical

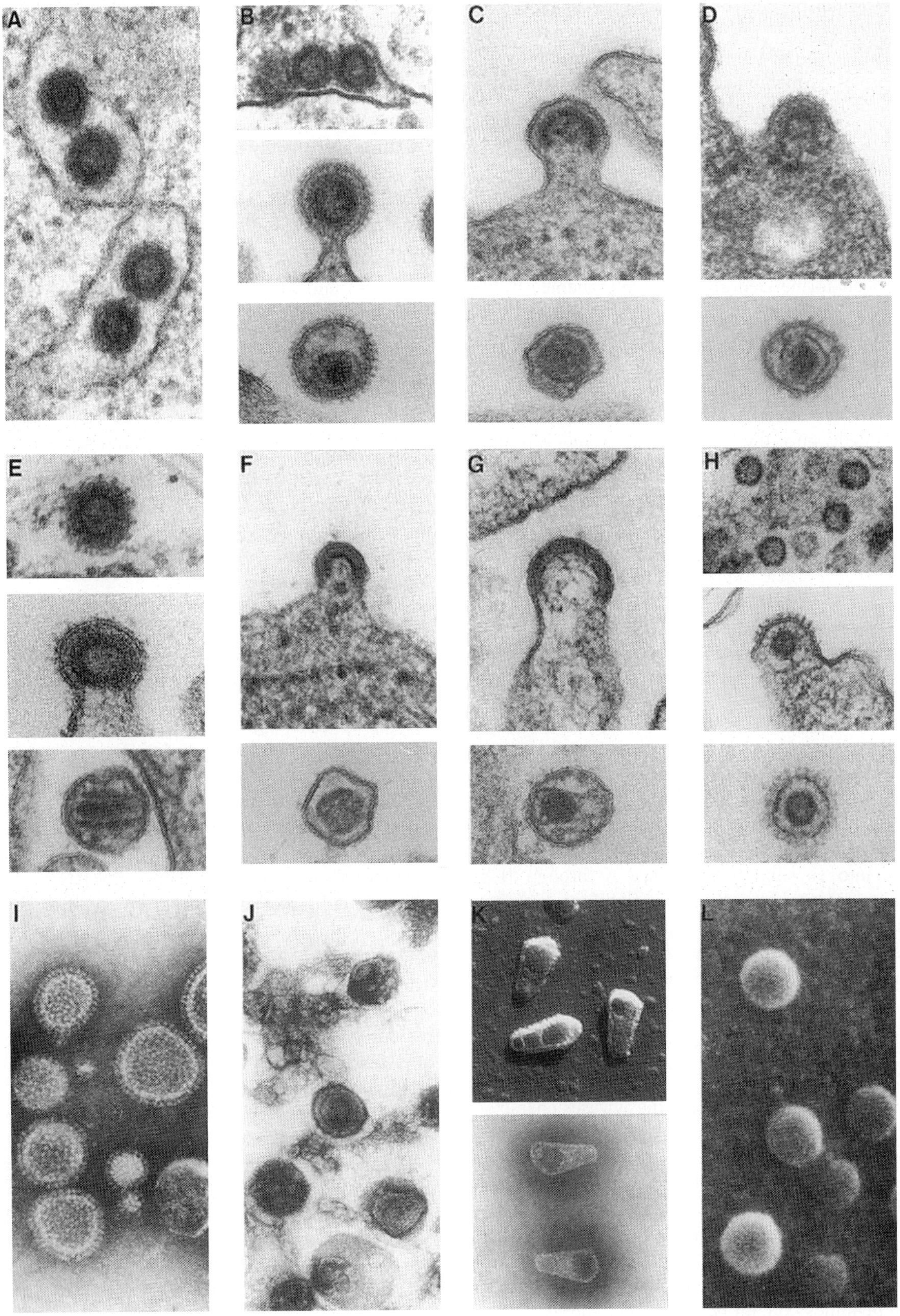

TABLE 1. *Retrovirus genera*

New name	Examples	Morphology
Alpharetrovirus	Avian leukosis virus (ALV) Rous sarcoma virus (RSV)	C-type
Betaretrovirus	Mouse mammary tumor virus (MMTV) Mason-Pfizer monkey virus (MPMV) Jaagsiekte sheep retrovirus (JSRV)	B-, D-type
Gammaretrovirus	Murine leukemia viruses (MuLV) Feline leukemia virus (FeLV) Gibbon ape leukemia virus (GaLV) Reticuloendotheliosis virus (RevT)	C-type
Deltaretrovirus	Human T-lymphotropic virus (HTLV)-1, -2 Bovine leukemia virus (BLV) Simian T-lymphotropic virus (STLV)-1, -2, -3	—
Epsilonretrovirus	Walleye dermal sarcoma virus Walleye epidermal hyperplasia virus 1	—
Lentivirus	Human immunodeficiency virus type 1 (HIV-1) HIV-2 Simian immunodeficiency virus (SIV) Equine infectious anemia virus (EIAV) Feline immunodeficiency virus (FIV) Caprine arthritis encephalitis virus (CAEV) Visna/maedi virus	Rod/cone core
Spumavirus	Human foamy virus (HFV)	Immature

cores. The most important example is HIV-1, but nonprimate viruses in the genus include the caprine arthritis encephalitis virus (CAEV) and visna virus. The genomes express *gag*, *pro*, *pol*, and *env* genes; *gag* is in one reading frame, and *pro-pol* in another. A single frameshift is used to express Gag-Pro-Pol. The Pol region of the nonprimate lentiviruses includes a domain for deoxyuridine triphosphatase (dUTPase). A number of accessory genes are also expressed. In HIV-1, these genes are *vif*, *vpr*, *vpu*, *tat*, *rev*, and *nef*; these genes control transcription, RNA processing, virion assembly, host gene expression, and a number of other replication functions (150). The tRNA primer is tRNALys1,2. A large number of exogenous viruses in this genus have been found in diverse mammals, but the only endogenous sequences are relatively distant from these viruses.

Spumaviruses

The spumaviruses are complex viruses with a unique virion morphology, containing prominent spikes on the surface and a central but uncondensed core. The prototype example is the human foamy virus (HFV). The virion is assembled in the cytoplasm and budded into the endoplasmic reticulum (ER) and the plasma membrane. There is probably only a single cleavage of the

FIG. 1. Electron micrographs of representative virion particles. The diameters of all the particles are approximately 100 nm. **Panel A:** Type A particles. Intracisternal A particles in the endoplasmic reticulum. **Panel B:** Betaretrovirus. Mouse mammary tumor virus (MMTV), type B morphology (*top*, intracytoplasmic particles; *middle*, budding particles; *bottom*, mature extracellular particles). **Panel C:** Gammaretrovirus. Murine leukemia virus (MLV) type C morphology (*top*, budding; *bottom*, mature extracellular particles). **Panel D:** Alpharetrovirus. Avian leukosis virus, type C morphology (*top*, budding; *bottom*, mature extracellular particles). **Panel E:** Betaretrovirus. Mason Pfizer monkey virus (MPMV), type D morphology (*top*, intracytoplasmic A-type particles; *middle*, budding; *bottom*, mature extracellular particles). **Panel F:** Deltaretrovirus. Bovine leukemia virus (BLV) (*top*, budding; *bottom*, mature extracellular particles). **Panel G:** Lentivirus. Bovine immunodeficiency virus (*top*, budding; *bottom*, mature extracellular particles). **Panel H:** Spumavirus. Bovine syncytial virus (*top*, intracytoplasmic particles; *middle*, budding; *bottom*, mature extracellular particles). **Panel I:** Betaretrovirus. Mouse mammary tumor virus, type B morphology, visualized by negative staining with phosphotungstic acid. **Panel J:** Gammaretrovirus, visualized as pseudoreplica stained with uranyl acetate. **Panel K:** Lentivirus. Purified cone-shaped cores of equine infectious anemia virus (*top*, cores visualized by shadow casting technique; *bottom*, cores visualized by negative staining with phosphotungstic acid). **Panel L:** Budding retroviral particles visualized by scanning electron microscopy. (Micrographs are courtesy of Dr. Matthew Gonda and reproduced from ref. 708, with permission.)

Gag protein near the C-terminus (797), and no major change in morphology during maturation. The genomes express *gag*, *pro*, *pol*, and *env* genes, and also at least two accessory genes known as *tas/bel-1*, and *bet* (242,483). The *tas* gene encodes a transcriptional trans-activator. Unique features are the separate expression of the Pol protein from a spliced mRNA and the presence of large amounts of reverse transcribed DNA in the virion (493). The genome contains a second transcriptional start site near the 3′ end of the *env* gene. The tRNA primer is tRNALys1,2. A number of exogenous viruses have been found in diverse mammals, and distantly related sequences are present as endogenous elements in the human genome (141).

Evolutionary Relationships

The sequences of the various retroviral genomes have been compared and used to determine the relatedness of any pair (475). A number of phylogenetic trees can be constructed using *gag*, *pro*, *pol*, or *env* genes, and in most aspects these trees are similar. A tree based on comparisons of the *pol* gene (Fig. 2) shows the clustering of viruses within each of the main genera. However, it is important to realize that a phylogenetic tree is not necessarily identical to an evolutionary history, and that the history that led to the formation of the known genera is not necessarily simple. It is noteworthy that there is no obvious clustering of all the simple viruses into a group apart from all the complex viruses. Thus, complex viruses probably arose from the simple ones more than once, with many evolving through the independent acquisition of separate genes.

The retroviruses are related to viruses of other families. The retroviral RTs show close sequence similarity to the polymerases of the hepadnaviruses and the caulimoviruses, which also replicate by reverse transcription. The retroviruses also show extensive similarity in both *gag* and *pol* gene sequences to the retrotransposons, endogenous mobile elements with long terminal repeats (LTRs), and to retroposons, elements without LTRs. Retroviral RTs show more distant similarity to the group II mitochondrial introns; to the retrons, elements in myxobacteria and rare isolates of *Escherichia coli*; and to telomerase, an RT responsible for maintenance of the chromosomal termini in eukaryotes; and they show a slight similarity to the DNA polymerases of viruses and hosts (474).

Transforming Viruses

During the replication of any retrovirus, replication-defective variants can arise through deletion or recombination events. Such mutants or variants can be propagated as a mixed virus culture along with the wild-type parent. In these mixtures of two genomes, the replication-competent parent acts as a helper virus to provide the missing replication functions in *trans* for the replication-defective transforming virus. In extremely rare events, the genomes of a replication-competent virus can acquire novel host sequences that provide significant new biologic activities to the virus. If the new gene product is mitogenic or anti-apoptotic for the host cell, or in more subtle ways alters the growth of the cell, the recombinant may become a potent oncogenic virus. A large number of such transducing viruses have been isolated and characterized as derivatives

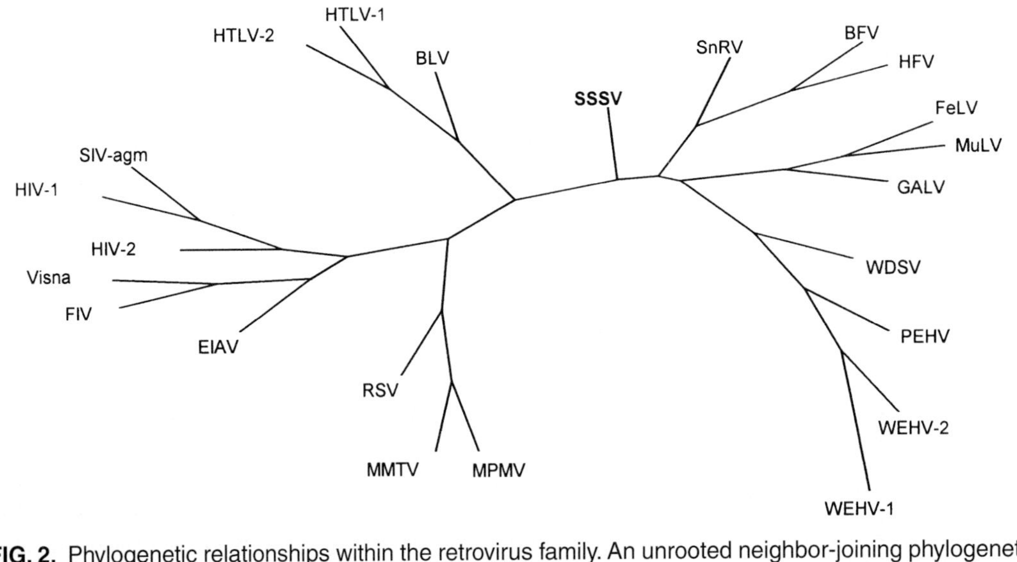

FIG. 2. Phylogenetic relationships within the retrovirus family. An unrooted neighbor-joining phylogenetic tree, constructed with the PHYLIP package based on an alignment of the amino acid residues of reverse transcriptase genes of several retroviruses (777). (Provided courtesy of S. Quackenbush and J. Casey.)

TABLE 2. *Examples of acute transforming retroviruses*

Parental virus	Transforming virus	Transduced gene
Avian leukosis virus (ALV)	Rous sarcoma virus	c-*src*
	Avian myeloblastosis virus	c-*myb*
	Avian erythroblastosis virus	c-*erbA,B*
	Avian myelocytomatosis virus 29	c-*myc*
	Avian sarcoma virus CT10	c-*crk*
	Fujinami sarcoma virus	c-*fps*
	Y73 avian sarcoma virus	c-*yes*
	Avian sarcoma virus 17	c-*jun*
Moloney Murine leukemia virus (MuLV)	Abelson MuLV	c-*abl*
	Harvey sarcoma virus	H-*ras*
	Kirsten sarcoma virus	Ki-*ras*
	Moloney murine sarcoma virus	c-*mos*
	FBJ murine sarcoma virus	c-*fos*
	3611-MSV	c-*raf*
Feline leukemia virus	Synder-Theilen feline sarcoma virus	c-*fes*
	Gardner-Arnstein feline sarcoma virus	c-*fes*
	McDonough feline sarcoma virus	c-*fms*
Simian sarcoma-associated virus	Wooly monkey sarcoma virus	c-*sis*

of one or another of the replication-competent parent viruses. In each case, the morphology and host range of the virus is determined by the helper virus that provides the replication functions to the defective genome. A partial listing of the most intensively studied of these viruses is presented in Table 2.

VIRION STRUCTURE

Retrovirus virions are initially assembled and released from infected cells as immature particles containing unprocessed Gag and Gag-Pol precursors of the proteins that eventually make up the mature virus. The immature virion morphology is spherical, with a characteristic electron-lucent center. The virions have been described as a protein vesicle, to suggest some fluidity in the interactions between the individual Gag proteins that make up the particle. At maturation, the precursor proteins are cleaved, and the structure and morphology of the virion changes drastically (784). The mature retrovirus particle is a spherical structure, roughly 100 nm in diameter. The size of the virions in a given preparation is not highly homogeneous but rather varies over a fairly wide range, suggesting that a discrete, highly ordered structure may not exist. After processing of the Gag precursor during virion maturation, the capsid (CA) protein collapses to form a more ordered paracrystalline core, but even then the overall diameter of the virion is heterogeneous and suggestive of considerable disorder. The virions exhibit a buoyant density in sucrose in the range of 1.16 to 1.18 g/mL. The sedimentation rate of the particles is typically about 600 S. The virions are sensitive to heat, detergent, and formaldehyde.

Virion Proteins

The stoichiometry of the various viral gene products in the virion are not very firmly established, but estimates suggest that about 1,500 to perhaps 2,000 Gag precursors are present per particle. After processing, all cleavage products are thought to be retained, suggesting equimolar presence of these proteins in the mature virions. The levels of the Pol proteins are typically about 1/10 to 1/20 of the Gag proteins, corresponding to about 100 to 200 molecules per virion. The levels of the Env proteins are quite variable among the viruses. For the gammaretroviruses, the levels of Env are close to that of Gag; perhaps 1,200 monomers, or 400 trimers, are present per virion. For the lentiviruses, the levels of Env per virion are much lower, possibly as low as 10 trimers per virion.

Nomenclature

The cleavage of Gag, Pol, and Env precursors forms the products in the mature infectious virions. These proteins are named by convention by a two-letter code: MA for matrix or membrane-associated protein, CA for capsid, NC for nucleocapsid, PR for protease, DU for dUTPase, RT for reverse transcriptase, IN for integrase, SU for surface protein, and TM for transmembrane protein (416). The localization of these proteins in the mature virion is not known with great precision, but a highly schematic version of the generic retrovirion can be drawn (Fig. 3).

Arrangement of Virion Components

The genomic RNA is highly condensed in the virion by its association with the nucleocapsid protein, NC. The complex is contained within a protein core largely composed of the CA protein, another *gag* gene product. The shape of the core differs among the various retroviral genera, and indeed it is a distinguishing feature of each genus. In most of the viruses, the core is roughly spheri-

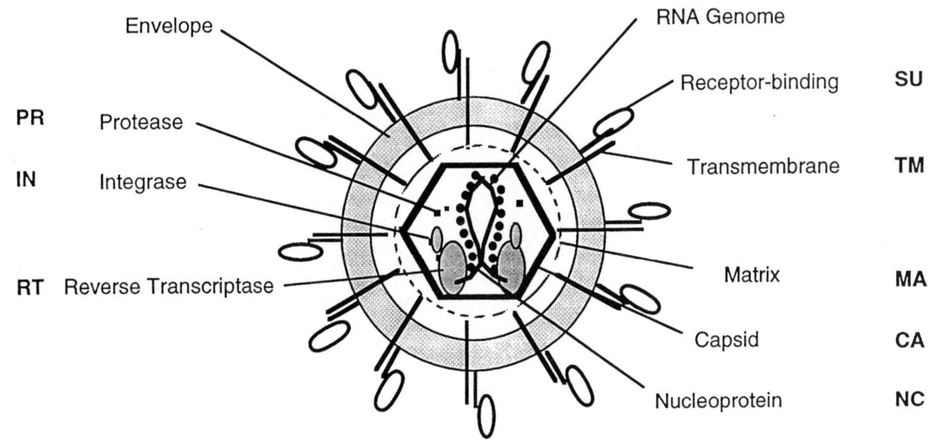

FIG. 3. Generalized retrovirion structure and components. A highly schematic view of the arrangement of viral gene products within the virion particle. The two-letter nomenclature for each protein is indicated.

cal, but in some cases it is either conical or cylindrical. In all the viruses, the core is surrounded by a roughly spherical shell consisting of MA, which in turn is surrounded by the lipid bilayer of the virion envelope. The virion membrane contains the envelope glycoprotein, with the TM subunit present as a single-pass transmembrane protein anchor, and the SU subunit as an entirely extravirion protein bound to TM. The envelope proteins for those viruses examined closely have been found to reside in the membrane as trimers.

ORGANIZATION OF THE RNA GENOME

The viral genome is a dimer of linear, positive-sense, single-stranded RNA, with each monomer 7 to 13 kilobases (kb) in size. The viral genomic RNA is present as a homodimer of two identical sequences, and thus the virions are functionally diploid. The dimer is maintained by interactions between the two 5′ ends of the RNAs in a self-complementary region termed the dimer linkage structure (DLS). The RNA genome is generated by normal host transcriptional machinery and thus exhibits many of the features of normal mRNA. The RNA is capped at the 5′ end, using the common $_{m7}G5'ppp5'G_{m}p$ structure; and it contains a string of poly(A) sequences, about 200 long, at the 3′ end.

A number of sequence blocks are so important that they have been named to facilitate descriptions of their functions in the life cycle (Fig. 4). These key sequences are clustered at the termini of the RNA. A short sequence, the R (for repeated) region, is so called because it is present twice in the RNA: once immediately after the cap at the 5′ end and again at the 3′ end, just before the poly(A) tail. Downstream of the 5′ R lies another sequence, termed U5 for unique 5′ sequence, which includes one of the *att* sites required for proviral integration. The U5 region is followed by the primer binding site (pbs), an 18-nt sequence at which a host tRNA is hybridized to the genome and the site of initiation of minus-strand DNA synthesis.

The region downstream from the pbs often contains the major signals for the encapsidation of the viral RNA into the virion particle, in sequences called the Psi element. The region also often contains a major splice donor site for the formation of subgenomic mRNAs. The bulk of the RNA sequences that follow are coding regions for the viral proteins. The genomes of all the replication-competent retroviruses contain at a minimum three large genes, or ORFs: from 5′ to 3′ along the genome, the genes are termed *gag*, for group-specific antigen; *pol*, for polymerase; and *env*, for envelope. The three genes in the simple retroviruses occupy nearly all the available space in the center of the genome.

Downstream of the genes lies a short polypurine tract (ppt), a run of at least nine A and G residues. The ppt is the site of initiation of the plus-strand DNA. The ppt is

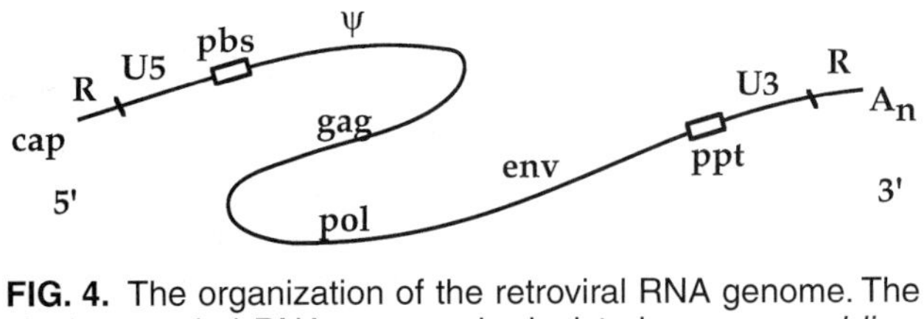

FIG. 4. The organization of the retroviral RNA genome. The single-stranded RNA genome is depicted as a *curved line.* From 5′ to 3′ along the RNA, the features include a 5′ cap structure; *R*, a sequence block repeated at both 5′ and 3′ ends; *U5*, a unique 5′ sequence block; *pbs*, the primer binding site and site of initiation of minus-strand DNA synthesis; *Y*, the major recognition site for the packaging of the viral RNA into the virion particle; the *gag*, *pol*, and *env* genes; *ppt*, the polypurine tract and site of initiation of the plus-strand DNA synthesis; *U3*, a unique 3′ sequence block; the second copy of the R sequence; and finally, a 3′ poly(A) sequence.

TABLE 3. *Size of sequence blocks in various retroviral RNAs (nt)*

Virus (example)	U3	R	U5
Alpharetrovirus (ALV)	150–250	18–21	80
Betaretrovirus (MMTV)	1200	15	120
Gammaretrovirus (MLV)	450	60	75
Deltaretrovirus (HTLV)	250–350	120–240	100–200
Lentivirus (HIV-1)	450	100	60–80
Spumavirus (HFV)	800	200	150

followed by a sequence block termed U3 for unique 3′ sequence; this region contains a number of key cis-acting elements for viral gene expression, and one of the *att* sites required for DNA integration. The U3 abuts the 3′ copy of the R region, which is followed by the poly(A) tail. As we shall see, the R, U5, U3, pbs, and ppt sequences all play important roles in reverse transcription. The lengths of these sequence blocks in various retroviruses are summarized in Table 3.

OVERVIEW OF THE LIFE CYCLE

The retroviruses replicate through a complex life cycle. A short summary of the steps of the cycle is as follows (a schematic view is shown in Fig. 5):

- Receptor binding and membrane fusion
- Internalization and uncoating
- Reverse transcription of the RNA genome to form double-stranded linear DNA
- Nuclear entry of the DNA
- Integration of the linear DNA to form the provirus
- Transcription of the provirus to form viral RNAs
- Splicing and nuclear export of the RNAs
- Translation of the RNAs to form precursor proteins
- Assembly of the virion and packaging of the viral RNA genome
- Budding and release of the virions
- Proteolytic processing of the precursors and maturation of the virions

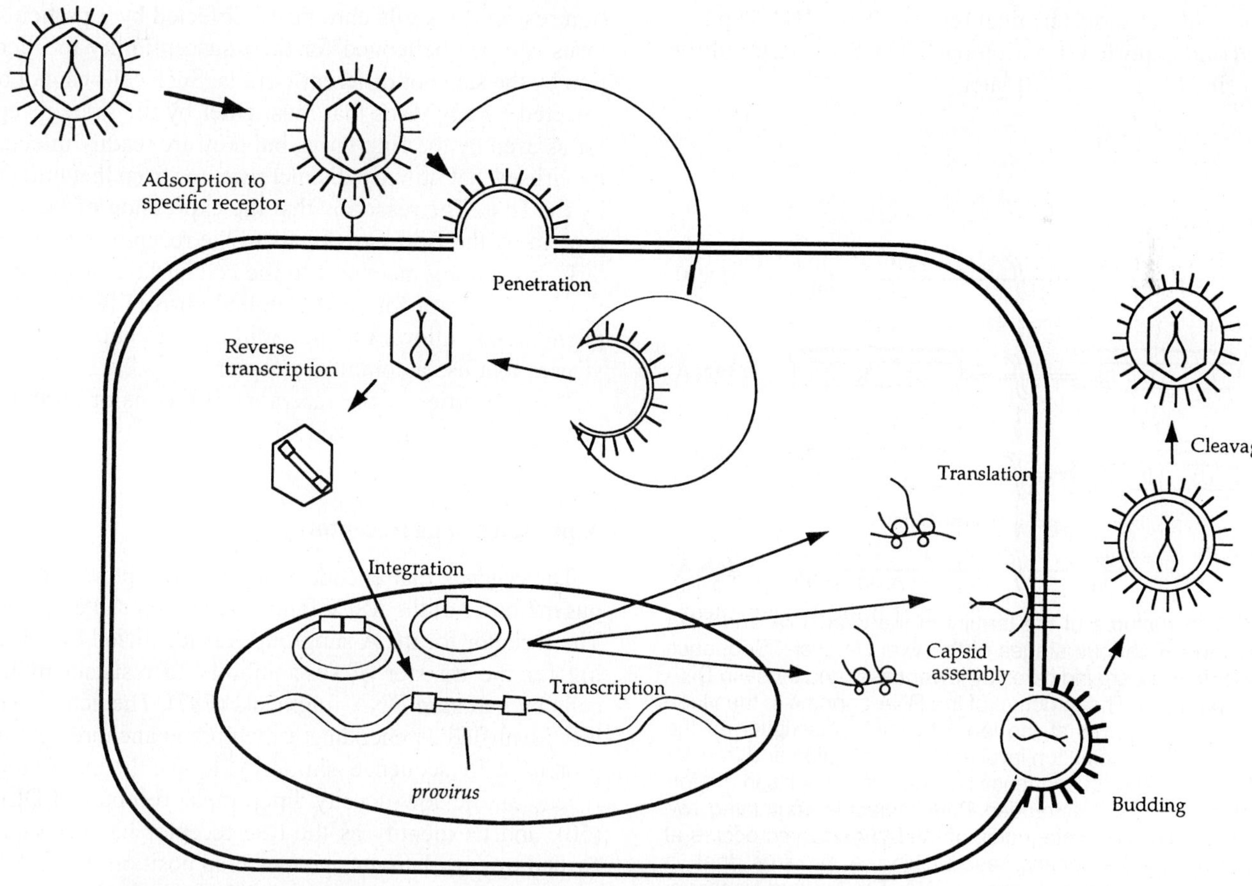

FIG. 5. A schematic view of the retrovirus life cycle. The major steps in the replication of a typical retrovirus are indicated, including those in the early phase of the life cycle, extending from the infecting virion (*top left*) to the formation of the integrated provirus, and those in the late phase of the life cycle, extending from the provirus to the formation of mature progeny virus (*right*).

Changes in the Viral Genome

A quick perusal of this list reveals that the life cycle begins with an RNA genome, passes through an intracellular DNA intermediate, and is completed with a return to an RNA form in the progeny virus particle. An overview of the structures of the genome at various times in this cycle is presented in Figure 6. The RNA genome of the virion contains short terminal repeats (the R region) at its termini. During reverse transcription, as we shall see later, sequence blocks termed U5 and U3 are duplicated, so that the resulting double-stranded DNA is longer at both ends than the RNA template. This DNA thus contains LTRs (consisting of sequence blocks U3, R, and U5) at both ends. The next step is the integration of the DNA to form the provirus; the integrated provirus is collinear with the preintegrative DNA, and it retains the LTRs [except for one or two base pairs (bps) lost during the course of integration]. Finally, the DNA is forward transcribed by the RNA polymerase II system to produce the progeny RNA genome. Transcription is initiated at the U3-R boundary of the 5′ LTR, and the transcripts are processed and polyadenylated at the R-U5 boundary of the 3′ LTR, recreating the exact structure of the input RNA, complete with its short terminal repeats. This RNA is packaged and exported in virion particles. Each step will be described in more detail later.

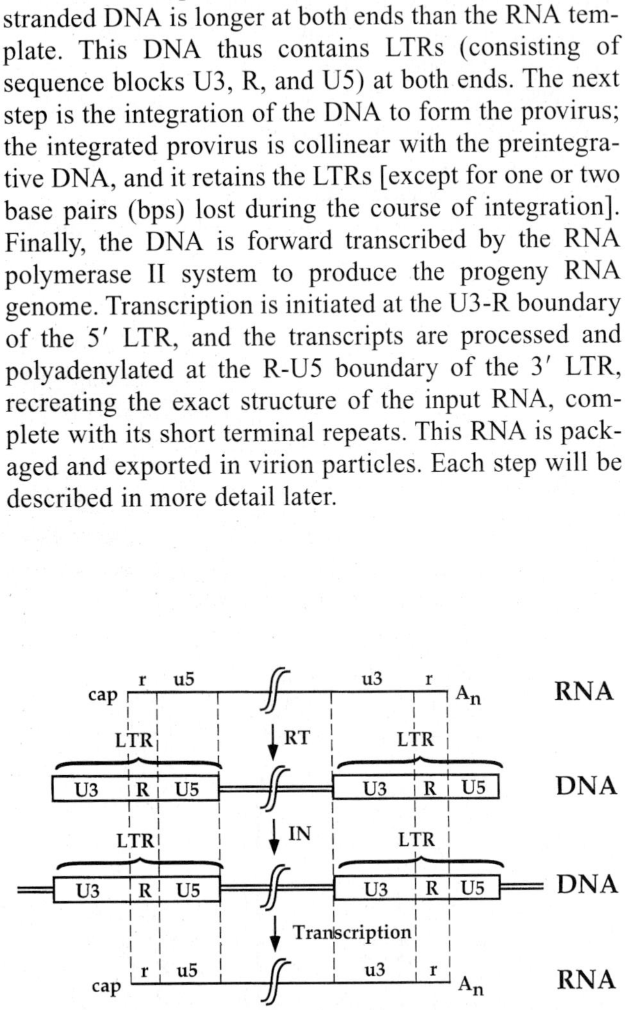

FIG. 6. Structures of the termini of the viral RNA and DNA genomes at various stages of the viral life cycle. Sequence blocks in RNA are indicated by lower case, and those in DNA by upper case. The structure of the RNA genome in the virion particle is indicated at the top. Reverse transcription of the RNA soon after infection involves the duplication and translocation of u5 and u3 sequence blocks, and it results in the formation of a double-stranded DNA molecule containing two terminal LTRs. The integration of the DNA genome occurs at the terminal sequences, establishing a provirus that is collinear with the preintegrative DNA. The forward transcription of the provirus is initiated at the U3/R border in the provirus; the resulting RNAs are cleaved and polyadenylated at the r/u5 border, recreating a viral RNA genome (*bottom*) identical to the infecting RNA.

THE VIRUS RECEPTORS

To enter a cell and initiate infection, all retroviruses require an interaction between a cell surface molecule—a receptor—and the envelope protein on the virion surface. The interactions are complex, involving an initial binding, drastic conformational changes in the envelope protein, an induced fusion of the viral and cellular membranes, and the internalization of the virion core into the cytoplasm. The SU subunit of Env is thought to make the major initial contacts with the receptor, and the TM subunit is thought to be most important for membrane fusion. The reorganization of the two lipid bilayers—one on the virion and one on the cell—to join them and evert the core into the cell is a remarkable process. The details of these complex processes are not understood for any retrovirus, and the whole Env protein is likely to be involved in efficient entry. However, there is a great deal of information about the identity and structures of the receptors used by various retroviruses. It is apparent that these viruses utilize an extraordinarily diverse set of cell surface molecules as receptors (see refs. 60 and 754 for reviews).

An important tool in the analysis of receptor utilization is the phenomenon of virus interference, or superinfection resistance. Cells chronically infected by a particular virus can be challenged for their susceptibility to infection by the same or different viruses. Such cells cannot be infected by any virus that must enter by the same receptor as used by the first virus, but they are readily infected by viruses that utilize a distinct receptor from that utilized by the first. The reason is that the expression of the Env protein by the first virus binds to the receptor intracellularly, preventing its export to the cell surface or its function as a receptor for newly applied virus (148,369). The phenomenon allows for the rapid classification of those viruses that use a common receptor.

The properties of the receptors of the major retroviral genera will be summarized later.

Alpharetrovirus Receptors

Three genes that encode functional receptors for various members of the ASLV family have been characterized. The receptor for the A subgroup was identified by selecting for the transfer of susceptibility to resistant mouse cells by genomic DNA fragments (787). The active gene was identified as encoding a membrane-anchored glycoprotein with sequence similarity to the ligand-binding repeat of the low-density lipoprotein receptor (LDLR) (50), and its identity as the true receptor has been confirmed by correlating its genetic map position with the *tv-a* locus (49). A soluble form of the receptor binds virus and blocks its infectivity (135). Functional versions of the protein can be anchored into the membrane either by a transmembrane segment or by a glycosylphosphaticlylinosital (GPI) anchor, and the receptor can even be fused to a foreign membrane protein, the epidermal growth factor (EGF) receptor, to permit efficient virus entry (667). The key determinants of the receptor for virus recognition and utilization have been identified (627).

The *tv-b* locus, encoding the receptor for both the B and D subgroups of the ALV, was similarly cloned and shown to encode a protein termed CAR1, unrelated to *tv-a* but with sequence similarity to the receptors for tumor necrosis factor (TNF) and the Fas death receptors (95). The intracellular portion of the molecule contains the sequence of a "death domain," present on other cytotoxic receptors, and can trigger the apoptotic death of the cell upon ligand binding. This response is likely to mediate the toxic effects of the cytopathic ASLVs. However, non-cytopathic viruses seem also able to bind and trigger the same receptors, and so the basis for the distinct effects of the two virus classes remains uncertain.

The *tv-e* locus is present in turkey but not chicken, and it allows infection by the subgroup E viruses. The gene was cloned by its sequence similarity to the chicken *tv-b* locus (5). The cloned gene product was shown to confer susceptibility to subgroup E but not B viruses, and to allow binding of subgroup E envelopes to the cell surface.

Betaretrovirus Receptors

A receptor for MMTV has been identified by gene transfer of cDNA libraries (278). The gene product allows cells to bind virus, and it allows infection by pseudotypes carrying the MMTV envelope. A second receptor for the betaretroviruses was also recently identified. The type D simian viruses, including MPMV and SRV-1, -2, -4, and -5, show cross-interference with three type C viruses: feline endogenous virus (RD114), baboon endogenous virus (BaEV), and avian reticuloendotheliosis virus (REV), suggesting that they all utilize a common cell surface receptor. Gene transfer of a human cDNA library into nonpermissive mouse cells was used to identify a gene that conferred susceptibility to infection by RD114 (694). The cDNA encoded a protein of 541 amino acids nearly identical to the previously cloned human Na^+-dependent neutral-amino-acid transporter named Bo (371,596). Consistent with this similarity, expression of the RD114 receptor in NIH 3T3 cells resulted in enhanced cellular uptake of L-^{3}H-alanine and L-^{3}H-glutamine.

Gammaretrovirus Receptors

A total of four receptors have been characterized for various subgroups of the MuLVs and their relatives, although there are others not yet identified (488). The ecotropic murine viruses are the most studied of this group, including the Moloney MuLV (MMLV), Friend MuLV, and Rauscher MuLV, as well as endogenous viruses from the AKR mouse, the AKR MuLV (AKV). The ecotropic receptor used by all these viruses is expressed on all strains of laboratory and wild mice of the species *Mus musculus*, mapping to the Rec1 locus on chromosome 5; a functional receptor is also expressed by rats. The ecotropic receptor was identified by gene transfer to nonpermissive human cells, selecting for susceptibility to MuLV infection (13). The gene encodes a membrane glycoprotein of 67 kd containing a total of 14 membrane-spanning domains; critical portions have been identified by mutational analyses. The corresponding human gene is highly homologous, but it cannot serve as a functional receptor by virtue of a small number of amino acid changes in the third extracellular loop of the protein. Other subtle mutations in this region of the receptor of other strains of mouse and of other rodents can cause varying changes in the susceptibility of the cell to infection by different ecotropic viruses (12,197). The SU subunit of the envelope protein binds to the receptor *in vitro* using a relatively small pocket region (162). The normal function of the protein has been identified as a transporter or permease for cationic, basic amino acids (379). The receptor, termed mCAT-1, was shown to be identical to y+, the previously characterized transporter in mammalian cells. The gene for mCAT-1 is now known as *Atrc1*. There is no strong evidence for a coreceptor or for any additional molecules besides the receptor being required; however, it has been noted that the infectivity of various cell lines does not correlate with the levels of receptor (747). Thus, it is possible that other molecules may modulate virus utilization of the receptor.

The amphotropic receptor is utilized by a group of MuLVs derived from wild mice and able to infect a wide range of mammalian species, including humans. The receptor was cloned by selection for susceptibility to virus infection after transfection of cDNA libraries into nonpermissive Chinese hamster ovary (CHO) cells (195, 490), and by its homology to the gene for the previously identified GALV receptor (734). The gene, known variously as *Ram1* or GLVR2 or rPiT-2, encodes a 652-amino-acid protein that functions as a sodium-dependent phosphate symporter (368). The protein is predicted to contain 10 membrane-spanning domains, and residues in extracellular loops 2 and 4 have been shown important for virus entry (418,446). The synthesis and stability of the receptor is regulated by phosphate levels, and its down-regulation by virus infection results in substantial reduction in phosphate uptake by cells.

The receptor utilized in common by the GALV, the simian sarcoma–associated helper virus, and the FeLV subgroup B (698) is widely expressed in many mammals, including primates, cat, dog, mink, rabbit, and rat (but not mouse), as well as in some avian species. The human receptor, termed GLVR1 or hPiT-1, was cloned by gene transfer into nonpermissive mouse cells (346,517). The sequence of the gene predicts the existence of 10 membrane-spanning segments, and a large third intracellular loop. The protein shows similarity to that of a *Neurospora* phosphate permease gene, pho4+, and has been shown directly to serve as a sodium-dependent phosphate symporter (368,521). Specific amino acid changes introduced into the fourth extracellular loop can block FeLV-B and simian sarcoma–associated virus (SSAV) infection without affecting GALV, suggesting that these various viruses interact in slightly different ways with the receptor. GALV cannot use the human amphotropic receptor GLVR2, but a single amino acid change in the receptor will permit its use (198).

The xenotropic MuLVs are viruses present as proviruses in the mouse germline but unable to infect inbred mouse cells. These viruses can infect some wild mice and mice of other species, as well as other mammals. The polytropic MuLVs are also endogenous viruses with a wide host range that includes many mammalian species. These viruses are often detected by the appearance of portions of the envelope sequences in recombinant polytropic viruses called mink cell focus-forming (MCF) viruses that arise during the replication of ecotropic viruses in mice. These MCF viruses can infect a wider range of cells than the parental viruses and can accelerate the course of leukemogenesis induced in mice by the ecotropic viruses. Xenotropic and polytropic MuLVs cross-interfere to various extents in nonmurine species and in wild Asian mice, suggesting that they might use a common receptor for infection. The mouse receptor for the polytropic viruses was cloned by gene transfer and was identified with the *Rmc1* gene (783). The human xenotropic receptor was cloned similarly (51,693). The human xenotropic receptor mediates infection by both the xenotropic and the polytropic viruses, whereas the homologous protein of inbred mice mediates only polytropic MuLV infections. The gene encodes a membrane protein related to the yeast Syg1p protein (suppressor of yeast G alpha deletion). Its function is unknown, but its multiple membrane-spanning segments and its sequence suggest that it may act as a G-coupled receptor.

Very recently, the isolation of a distinct receptor utilized by the subgroup C FeLVs (FeLV-C) for entry into heterologous cells (590). The cDNA recovered was predicted to encode a protein with 12 membrane-spanning domains with significant sequence similarity to the D-glucarate transporters of bacteria and nematodes. The binding of virus to this receptor may be responsible for the pathogenicity, a block in erythroid differentiation.

Additional receptors for other gammaretroviruses are known to exist. Three newly characterized porcine endogenous retroviruses (PERV-A, -B, and -C) have been tested in interference assays with each other and with murine viruses using the known receptors, and all three apparently utilize distinct and novel receptors (697). The identity of these molecules is presently unknown.

Deltaretrovirus Receptors

The receptors for the delta-retroviruses are not well characterized yet. A candidate gene has been identified as a possible receptor for BLV (526,579). A determinant of the HTLV-1 receptor has been mapped to human chromosome 17 (671).

Lentivirus Receptors

The first receptor identified for any retrovirus was the CD4 molecule, established as essential for infection by HIV-1 (153,385,451). Soluble forms of CD4 can bind to virions and inhibit infection; in some strains of virus, CD4 induces release or shedding of the SU subunit from the virion. However, other strains are quite resistant to inhibition by soluble CD4. CD4 is an important surface protein on T cells, and with few exceptions it serves to define the helper subset of T cells. CD4 is also expressed at significant levels on dendritic cells, on macrophages, and on certain cells in the brain, which may be related astrocytes rather than cells of neural origin. The limited distribution of expression of CD4 accounts well for the tropism of HIV-1, largely restricted to helper T cells and macrophages. There may be other routes of entry utilized at lower efficiency: Antibody to virus, for example, can promote virus entry into cells by the Fc receptor (696).

Early work established, however, that although CD4 was sufficient to mediate virus binding to a cell surface, it was not sufficient to mediate virus infection and entry. For example, rodent cells and other cells of nonprimate origin could not be successfully infected by HIV-1 even if they were engineered to express human CD4. Searches for genes that would render such cells sensitive to virus infection ultimately led to the identification of various members of the chemokine receptor family, notably CCR5 and CXCR4, as coreceptors that were needed to mediate the postbinding step of membrane fusion and virus entry (194,233,268,660). The regions of the human coreceptors that are needed for virus entry have been identified (186,268,593,659), although, surprisingly, some HIV-1 isolates can utilize the murine CXCR4 (551). Antibodies to the coreceptor as well as the natural ligand for these molecules, the chemokines themselves, can block virus entry. Variants of simian immunodeficiency virus (SIV) and HIV-1 have been identified that are CD4-independent, needing only a chemokine receptor for infection; these viruses suggest that a chemokine receptor might have been the primary receptor for a primordial virus. A further proof of the importance of the chemokine receptor is the existence of a mutant allele of the gene encoding CCR5 in the human population, a 32-bp deletion, that confers dramatic virus resistance to homozygous individuals. More discussion of the roles of CD4 and the coreceptors in virus entry will be presented in the following Chapter 28 in this ed. on HIV-1.

PENETRATION AND UNCOATING

Once virus particles have bound to the receptor, the virion and host membranes fuse together, and the virion core is delivered into the cytoplasm of the infected cell. For most retroviruses, the processes of fusion and entry are thought to be pH independent; that is, they are not dependent on an endosomal acidification step to induce a pH-dependent change in the conformation of the envelope (see, e.g., refs. 467, 476, and 677). Thus, fusion can occur at the cell surface. However, there may be exceptions; early tests suggested that the ecotropic MuLVs could be inhibited from infection of some cells by drugs that block the acidification (476). This property has been mapped to the TM portion of the envelope protein (515).

It is not known whether specific uncoating steps are required before reverse transcription can begin. It is clear that the processing of the Gag precursor to the mature Gag proteins is required; immature virions are uninfectious and cannot initiate reverse transcription, and mutants that prevent particular cleavages of the Gag protein are similarly blocked. A large number of mutant viruses with other alterations in the *gag* gene have been shown to be defective in early steps of infection, before reverse transcription, but the functions of Gag proteins at this stage remain uncertain. Some of these mutations affect CA, suggesting that a mutant core may not properly open or allow the initiation of reverse transcription. Other mutations lie in NC (280), suggesting that the nucleic acid itself is bound inappropriately by the mutant protein, or again, is not properly unfolded for reverse transcription. There are also indications that host factors are important in these early stages (263). In the case of HIV-1, the host protein cyclophilin is required for the efficient initiation of reverse transcription, and Gag mutants that do not package cyclophilin cannot initiate reverse transcription (90). A plausible role for this protein is to facilitate virion disassembly. Recently, inhibitors have been used to demonstrate a role of the cytoskeleton in virus entry, and furthermore to suggest that viruses may utilize different entry pathways in different cell lines (384). Biochemical analyses of these early events are made difficult by the presence of large numbers of defective particles that are probably not on the infectious pathway and that tend to obscure the properties of the rare particles that are on this pathway.

REVERSE TRANSCRIPTION

The reverse transcription of the viral RNA genome into a double-stranded DNA form is the defining hallmark of the retroviruses and the step from which these viruses derive their name. The course of reverse transcription is complex and highly ordered, involving the initiation of DNA synthesis at precise positions, and translocations of DNA intermediates that result in duplication of sequence blocks in the final product (reviewed in refs. 271 and 708). The major steps in the reaction are relatively well established, largely through the analysis of reactions carried out *in vitro* in purified virion particles (the so-called endogenous reaction).

Reverse transcription normally begins soon after entry of the virion core into the cytoplasm of the infected cell. The reaction takes place in a large complex, roughly resembling the virion core, and containing Gag proteins including NC, RT, IN, and the viral RNA (87). The signal that triggers the onset of DNA synthesis is not known, although it may be as simple as the exposure of the viral core to the relatively high levels of deoxyribonucleotides present in the cytoplasm. This notion is consistent with the observation that simply stripping or permeabilizing the virion membrane with detergents in the presence of deoxyribonucleotides is sufficient to induce DNA synthesis. This may also be at least part of the explanation for the difficulty HIV has in completing reverse transcription and infection in quiescent cells (794). In some cells, notably cells arrested by starvation, triphosphate levels may be low and limiting for RT, so that addition of exogenous nucleosides can stimulate viral DNA synthesis (286).

It has been recently appreciated that DNA synthesis can be initiated "prematurely" during virion assembly and release, such that virion preparations can be shown to contain small amounts of the early DNA intermediates, such as minus-strand strong-stop DNA (437,718,795,804). In most cases, the levels of these DNAs are very low, indicating that only a very small minority of the virion particles have carried out any significant synthesis. However, some circumstances affecting the rate of production and release of virions may enhance this synthesis (183). In addition, in some particular retroviruses, notably the spumaviruses, substantial DNA synthesis may occur during assembly, such that the major form of the genome found in mature virions is a partially or even completely reverse transcribed DNA molecule (493,790). These viruses thus resemble the hepadnaviruses more closely than the conventional retroviruses in the relative timing of assembly and reverse transcription.

Steps in Reverse Transcription of the Retroviral Genome

The course of reverse transcription is complex. The reaction can be broken down into a series of discrete steps (271), as presented in Figure 7.

Formation of Minus-Strand Strong-Stop DNA

The process of reverse transcription is initiated from the paired 3′ OH of a primer tRNA annealed to the viral RNA genome at a complementary sequence termed the pbs.

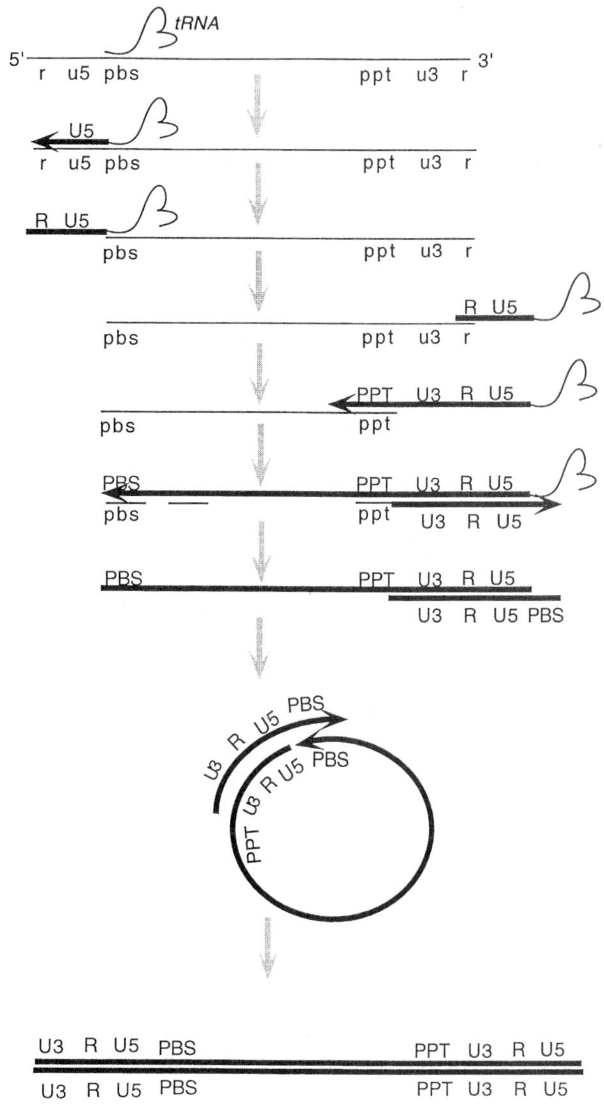

FIG. 7. The reverse transcription of the retroviral genome. *Thin lines* represent RNA; *thick lines* represent DNA. See text for details. Drawing courtesy of A. Telesnitsky.

DNA is first synthesized from this primer, using the plus-strand RNA genome as template, to form minus-strand DNA sequences. Synthesis occurs toward the 5′ end of the RNA to generate U5 and R sequences. The intermediate formed in this step is termed minus-strand strong-stop DNA. The primer tRNA remains attached to its 5′ end.

First Translocation

The next step involves the translocation, or "jump," of the strong-stop DNA from the 5′ to the 3′ end of the genome. This translocation requires the degradation of those 5′ RNA sequences that were placed in RNA:DNA hybrid form by the formation of strong-stop DNA. The degradation is mediated by the RNase H activity of RT; mutants with altered RNase H activity do not mediate the translocation (71,702). This step exposes the single-stranded DNA and facilitates its annealing to the R sequences at the 3′ end of the genome. Normally, a full-length strong-stop DNA, synthesized by copying to the 5′ cap of the RNA, performs the translocation (404), although incomplete molecules can jump at low efficiency. Specific sequences or structures in or near the R region are required for efficient jumping (14,716). The NC protein may facilitate the transfer step. Although there have been reports that jumping is always in *trans,* from one RNA template to the other RNA in the virion, the best evidence is that minus-strand strong-stop jumping goes randomly to either RNA (788).

Long Minus-Strand DNA Synthesis

The annealing of minus-strand strong-stop DNA recreates a suitable primer-template structure for DNA synthesis, and RT can now continue to elongate the minus-strand strong-stop DNA to form long minus-strand products. Synthesis ends in the vicinity of the pbs. As the genome enters RNA:DNA hybrid form, the RNA becomes susceptible to RNase H action and is degraded.

Initiation of Plus-Strand DNA Synthesis

The primer for plus-strand synthesis is created by the digestion of the genomic RNA by RNase H. A particular short, purine-rich sequence near the 3′ end of the genome, the ppt, is relatively resistant to the activity of RNase H. The oligonucleotide remains hybridized to the minus-strand DNA and serves as the primer for synthesis of the plus-strand DNA, using the minus-strand DNA as template. Sequences upstream of the ppt, an AT-rich region called the T-box, are also important for proper priming (333,621). The primer, once it has served to initiate DNA synthesis, is quickly removed from the DNA, presumably by RNase H action. Synthesis proceeds toward the 5′ end of the minus strand, first copying the U3, R, and U5 sequences, and then extending to copy a portion of the primer tRNA still present at its 5′ end. Elongation stops at a modified base normally found at position 19 of the tRNA. The resulting intermediate is termed plus-strand strong-stop DNA.

In some viruses, secondary plus-strand initiation sites are used. There may be multiple RNA primers generated from the RNA genome by the nuclease action of RNase H that can initiate DNA synthesis at dispersed heterogeneous sites. In the case of the lentiviruses and spumaviruses, a second copy of the ppt sequence near the center of the genome is used at high efficiency and is important for proper completion of reverse transcription (112).

Removal of tRNA

In the next step, the primer tRNA at the 5′ end of the minus-strand DNA is removed by RNase H. Its removal may occur in two stages, with an initial cleavage near the RNA–DNA junction and a second one within the tRNA. The cleavage need not occur exactly at the RNA–DNA junction, and a single ribonucleotide base (A) is normally left on the 5′ terminus of the minus strand (588,646,664, 758) without affecting subsequent processes. The sequence of bases near the junction can significantly modulate the cleavage by RNase H (663). Recent experiments indicate that the posttranscriptional modifications present in the natural tRNA may be important for proper recognition by RT and for plus-strand strong-stop translocation (37).

The Second Translocation

The removal of the tRNA exposes the 3′ end of the plus-strand strong-stop DNA to permit its pairing with the 3′ end of the minus-strand DNA. The sequences anneal via the shared pbs sequences. This annealing forms a circular intermediate, with both 3′ termini in a suitable structure for elongation.

Completion of Both Strands

Both strands are now elongated. The final extension of the minus-strand DNA is coupled to displacement of the plus-strand strong-stop DNA from the 5′ end of the minus strand; as minus-strand elongation occurs, the plus-strand strong stop is peeled away and transferred to the 3′ end of the minus strand. At the end of this elongation, the circle is opened up into a linear DNA. The plus strands are all extended, and displacement synthesis may occur to remove short DNAs and make longer plus-strand DNAs (372). Any internally primed plus-strand DNAs may be prevented from participating in strong-stop translocation simply by kinetics; the normal plus-strand strong-stop DNA may simply form first, and elongation to transfer it to the minus strand may occur before it could be displaced by any plus-strand elongation (88). Finally, the plus-strand strong-stop DNA is extended to complete the plus strand.

When multiple plus-strand initiation events occur, the completed plus strand will consist of adjacent fragments and so contain nicks or discontinuities. Displacement synthesis by an upstream fragment can slowly displace downstream RNAs and DNAs, leading to longer plus strands (372). However, some nicks or gaps may persist in the final double-stranded product. These breaks may be at heterogeneous positions, although strong sites of plus-strand initiation, such as the one at the central ppt of lentiviruses, can lead to specific sites for such discontinuities. Sequences near the central ppt of the lentiviruses cause termination of synthesis during elongation from upstream primers, thus ensuring the maintenance of a discontinuity at this site (113). This site retains a partially displaced sequence or overlap of a few nucleotides—99 nt in the case of HIV-1. The structure has been shown to persist even to the time of integration of the DNA into the cell. Host DNA repair processes ultimately correct all such discontinuities.

Although most of the viral DNA is made in the cytoplasm, it may not always be completed in the cytoplasm. For some viruses, completion of the two DNA strands may occur only after entry into the nucleus (415). Specific mutants with alterations in the Cys-His residues of the NC protein show an interesting phenotype: the formation of linear DNA with heterogeneous and truncated ends (282). These experiments suggest that NC plays a role in the completion, or the stabilization of the ends, of the viral DNA.

A key consequence of the two translocation events that occur during reverse transcription is the duplication of sequences—duplication of U5 during minus-strand strong-stop DNA translocation, and of U3 during plus-strand strong-stop DNA translocation. The resulting DNA contains two LTRs that are assembled during reverse transcription. Each LTR consists of the sequence blocks U3-R-U5. The positions of the LTR edges—the left edge of U3 and the right edge of U5—are determined by the sites of initiation of DNA synthesis for the two DNA strands. Thus, the terminal sequences of the complete DNA molecule are also determined by these sites of initiation. These sequences for most viruses are perfect or imperfect inverted repeats, and they serve an important role during integration of the DNA (see later).

Biochemistry and Structure of Reverse Transcriptase

The enzyme that mediates the complex series of events outlined above is RT, one of the most famous of the viral polymerases (44, and reviewed in ref. 661). All RTs contain two separate activities present in two separate domains: a DNA polymerase able to incorporate deoxyribonucleotides on either an RNA or a DNA template, and an RNase H activity able to degrade RNA only in duplex form. These two activities are responsible for the various steps of reverse transcription. Two distinct domains of the enzyme contain these two activities: an aminoterminal domain contains the DNA polymerase, and a carboxyterminal domain contains the RNase H activity (700). Whereas isolated domains can be shown to exhibit either one of the two activities separately, an intact enzyme is required for full activity and specificity. However, the two functions can be provided by two mutant RT molecules so long as they are co-incorporated into a single virion (707).

DNA Polymerase

The DNA polymerase activity is similar to that of all host and viral DNA polymerases in requiring a primer, which can be either RNA or DNA, and a template, which can also be either RNA or DNA. RTs incorporate dXTPs to a growing 3′ OH end with release of inorganic pyrophosphate (PPi), and they require divalent cations, usually Mg^{2+}. The primer must contain a 3′ OH end that is paired with the template. RTs cannot perform nick-translation reactions, but they can efficiently perform strand displacement synthesis. The only fundamental way in which RTs are unusual among the DNA polymerases is that they exhibit comparable specific activity on either DNA or RNA templates.

RTs are readily obtained from purified virion particles, and they can be even more easily prepared as recombinant proteins expressed in bacteria. RTs are relatively slow DNA polymerases, under standard conditions incorporating only 1 to 100 nucleotides per second, depending on the template. Further, they exhibit poor processivity, and tend to release primer-template frequently *in vitro*. The enzyme must then rebind to the substrate to continue synthesis. Secondary structures in RNA templates can strongly enhance the pausing of RT and its tendency to release from the template (298). The enzyme also exhibits low fidelity, and although the values of the error rate vary widely with the primer (533), template (374,378), and type of assay, the misincorporation rate of most RTs under physiologic conditions is on the order of 10^{-4} errors per base incorporated. This rate suggests that during replication there would be approximately one mutation per genome per reverse transcription cycle. Indeed, the mutation rate observed *in vivo* is roughly consistent with this high error rate (101,184,380,496,654), although fidelity *in vivo* may be somewhat better than *in vitro* (461). Drug-resistant variants that do not incorporate chain-terminating analogs are often found to exhibit higher fidelity, perhaps because they require a more precise fit for the correct incoming triphosphate to allow for discrimination against the analog. A wide range of types of mutations are created by RT errors, and both the type and the frequency of appearance of each type of mutation exhibit a complex dependence on sequences and structures in the template (54,553,554).

RTs do not generally exhibit a proofreading nuclease activity (52), and misincorporated bases are not removed efficiently by most RTs as they are by host DNA polymerases. Very recently, however, mutants of the HIV-1 RT resistant to azidothymidine (AZT) have been shown to exhibit an enhanced ability to remove the incorporated AZT moiety at the 3′ end through a pyrophosphorolysis reaction (486). Thus, it is possible for RT to remove some such analogs and rescue a terminated chain for continued elongation.

RNase H

The RNase H of RT is an endonuclease that releases oligonucleotides with a 3′ OH and a 5′ PO_4. This property allows the products of RNase H action to serve as primers for initiation of DNA synthesis by the DNA polymerase function of RT. There is an obligate requirement that the RNA be in duplex form, normally an RNA–DNA hybrid. However, retroviral RTs are also able to degrade RNA–RNA duplexes (57,70), an activity termed RNaseH* (318). The RNase H enzyme is capable of acting on the RNA of a template in concert with the polymerase as it moves along a nucleic acid, and as it does so its active site is located about 17 to 18 bp behind the growing 3′ end (279). RNase H can also act independently of polymerization. All RNase H activity requires a divalent cation.

Subunit Structures

RT is incorporated into the virion particle during assembly in the form of a large Gag-Pol precursor (see later), and it is released by proteolytic processing of the precursor during virion maturation. Different viruses make somewhat different cleavages in the precursor, and thus the RTs exhibit several different subunit structures (see later). In the gammaretroviruses, RT is a simple monomer in solution, corresponding only to the aminoterminal DNA polymerase and the carboxyterminal RNase H domains. These two domains can be expressed separately, and the isolated proteins exhibit their respective activities (700), although the specificity of the RNase H is affected by this separation. There is some evidence, however, that while bound to the substrate and carrying out DNA synthesis, this RT may act as a dimer (706). In the avian viruses, the RT is present as an αβ heterodimer, composed of a smaller α subunit containing the DNA polymerase and RNase H domains, and a larger β subunit containing these two domains but also retaining the IN domain. In the lentiviruses, RT is again a heterodimer with a larger subunit (p66) containing the DNA polymerase and RNase H domains, and a smaller subunit (p51) lacking RNase H. The properties of the different enzymes as DNA polymerases are very similar in spite of these different subunit structures, and so the significance of these various compositions for RT function is unclear.

Crystal Structures

The three-dimensional structures of a number of RTs have been determined by x-ray crystallographic studies. Structures of the unliganded HIV-1 RT (320,622), RT bound to nonnucleoside RT inhibitors (160,174,391, 605), RT bound to an RNA pseudoknot inhibitor (343), and RT bound to a duplex oligonucleotide (28,324,341, 342), as well as the isolated RNase H domain (163), have all been reported. The two subunits are folded quite differently, so the overall structure is highly asymmetric. The structure of the p66 is similar to that of a right hand, with fingers, palm, and thumb domains all named on the basis of their position in the structure (Fig. 8). The nucleic acid lies in the grip of the hand, held by the fingers and thumb. The YXDD motif present

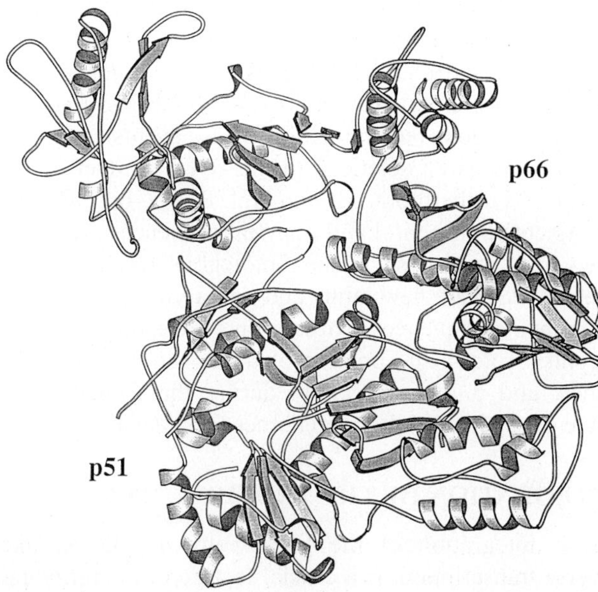

FIG. 8. A ribbon diagram of the heterodimeric reverse transcriptase of HIV-1, showing the p66 (*top*) and p51 (*bottom*) subunits. The molecule is arranged in the conventional orientation to show its similarity to the human right hand, palm up. The image was generated by Hans-Erik G. Aronson (Department of Biochemistry and Molecular Biophysics, Columbia University) using MOLSCRIPT (396). The HIV RT coordinates used to draw the image were retrieved as file 1VRT.pdb from the Research Collaboratory for Structural Bioinformatics (RCSB) Protein Data Bank (PDB) (http://www.rcsb.org/pdb). HIV RT secondary structural elements were defined according to the header (HELIX and SHEET records) of the coordinate file. The structure as solved was originally a complex of RT and the inhibitor nevirapine (604).

at the active site for the DNA polymerase lies at the base of the palm. The RNase H domain is attached to the hand at the wrist. The p51 subunit, while made up of the same domains as the aminoterminal part of p66, is folded differently and lies under the hand, not making direct contact with the nucleic acid and so not thought to participate in the chemistry. The structure of p66 with and without a liganded nucleic acid is quite different, with the thumb domain flexing to allow substrate binding. Theoretical considerations suggest the thumb may move during elongation (41). A structure of the fingers and palm subdomain of the MMLV RT at very high resolution (269) has also been determined.

Inhibitors

RT is a major target of antiviral drugs useful in the treatment of retroviral diseases such as AIDS. All such drugs used to date are inhibitors of the DNA polymerase activity of RT, and they fall into two classes: nucleoside analog inhibitors (chain terminators) and nonnucleoside RT inhibitors (NNRTIs). The nucleoside analogs are typically precursors and need to be activated by phosphorylation to the triphosphate form. These are then incorporated by RT into the growing chain, and they serve to block further elongation. Examples include AZT, ddC, ddI, d4T, and 3TC. The NNRTIs are a group of compounds that are structurally diverse but nevertheless interact with a common binding pocket in RT to prevent its normal activity (724). There are indications that the binding may inhibit the enzyme's flexibility. For both classes of inhibitors, monotherapy with a single drug selects for drug-resistant variants that quickly predominate in the virus population, and for each drug, a pattern of mutations has been identified that serves to indicate the appearance of drug resistance (411). In many cases, these mutations alter the binding site for the nucleoside or NNRTI such that the drug cannot bind and so cannot inhibit the enzyme. In the case of AZT, however, the mutations do not prevent the binding and incorporation of AZT-triphosphate into the growing chain but rather seem to activate a reverse reaction in which the AZT nucleotide is removed from the chain, subsequently permitting normal elongation (486). Combination therapy, typically involving the simultaneous treatment with three different drugs, can suppress virus replication to such an extent that variants resistant to all the drugs do not appear, at least for months or years.

RECOMBINATION

The process of reverse transcription could in principle take place using a single template RNA molecule. In fact, however, retrovirions contain two copies of the RNA genome copackaged into one particle, and the course of reverse transcription typically makes use of both RNAs (322,686). Recombination occurs between homologous sequences in the two RNAs (170,562), and it happens normally at a surprisingly high frequency, perhaps once per replication event per genome on average (799). Normally the two RNAs in a virion are identical, so that homologous recombination events are invisible and without consequence. When the two RNAs are distinct, however, as when they derive from two viruses or viral strains, the result is a very high frequency of recombination between them among the resulting proviral DNAs. Thus, physical markers and genetic markers recombine rapidly whenever the two genomes are copackaged into one virion and so are coextant during a single round of reverse transcription. The frequency is highly dependent on the sequence and structure of the RNA in the region undergoing recombination (19). Similar recombination does not occur at high frequency when cells are co-infected simultaneously with two separate virus preparations, suggesting that each virus particle performs its own reverse transcription reaction in the cytoplasm in *cis*, and does not freely exchange RNAs with other reactions happening in the same cell.

Models for Recombination

Two mechanisms can provide for recombination between two genomes. In one, the copy choice model, recombination occurs during minus-strand synthesis. As RT proceeds along an RNA, it has the potential to carry out a template switch in which an incomplete DNA copied from one template serves to prime further elongation on the other RNA molecule (447,561). Pausing may enhance this transfer, and structural features in the RNA may act as hot spots for such recombination. A break in an RNA genome, which may be encountered often, would cause a "forced copy choice"; transfer to the other RNA would rescue an otherwise dead virus, and this may represent the major evolutionary basis for high-frequency recombination in the viruses. The RNase H activity of RT may help release an incomplete DNA and so promote its serving as primer on the new template, and NC may also facilitate the reaction (510).

In the other model, the strand-displacement assimilation model, recombination may occur during plus-strand synthesis. When multiple plus-strand fragments are elongating on the minus-strand template, strand displacement can expose the 5′ end of such fragments. If a second minus-strand DNA has been synthesized, these can then pair with this other minus-strand DNA to form a bridged "H" structure as intermediates; further synthesis and repair would lead to the transfer of sequences to the new DNA (353). These H structures are visible in electron micrographs of the nucleic acids from reverse transcription reactions. However, it is not clear how often this mechanism is used. The general inefficiency of reverse transcription dictates that two minus-strand DNAs may not always be available in one virion to permit this latter process, so it may be infrequent.

When a recombination event occurs, there is a nonrandom increase in the probability that another recombination will occur nearby—a phenomenon called negative interference (20,323). This suggests that RT or the genomes may become recombination prone at specific times. When multiple recombination events occur, the resulting DNA is a patchwork of the sequences derived from the two input RNAs.

The translocation of the strong-stop DNAs provides a special opportunity for recombination between the two viral genomes. When the minus-strand strong-stop DNA is formed, it has the potential to translocate from the 5′ end of its template to the 3′ end of either RNA molecule; although this event has been reported to occur strictly in *cis*, or strictly in *trans*, it most likely occurs randomly. Similarly, when plus-strand strong-stop DNA is formed, it too could in principle translocate to the 3′ of either minus strand. However, this translocation seems most often to occur in *cis*, perhaps simply because the frequency with which two long minus-strand DNAs are formed, and so are available to serve as acceptors, is low.

Recombination between two RNAs during reverse transcription can also occur between nonhomologous sites at lower frequency. Reconstructions suggest that these events are perhaps 100 to 1,000 times less frequent than homologous recombination. These events can result in duplications or deletions in the DNA product of the reaction. Furthermore, if nonviral RNAs or chimeric RNAs containing viral and nonviral sequences are packaged into virions, such nonhomologous recombination events can create new joints and link a viral sequence to the nonviral sequences. These events are thought to play a central role in the process of transduction of cellular genes, and most importantly during the formation of acute oncogenic retroviral genomes (see later).

INTEGRATION OF THE PROVIRAL DNA

The integration of the linear retroviral DNA, like reverse transcription, is a crucial feature of the retroviral life cycle. Integration is required for efficient replication of most retroviruses; mutants that are unable to integrate do not establish a spreading infection. The orderly and efficient integration of viral DNA is also unique to the retroviruses. Although infection by some DNA viruses can result in the integration of viral DNA fragments into the host genome at low efficiency, these events are not the result of specific viral functions. Further, the establishment of the integrated provirus is responsible for much of retroviral biology. It accounts for the ability of the viruses to persist in the infected cell, for their ability to permanently enter the germline, and for the mutagenic and oncogenic activities of the leukemia viruses.

Once the provirus is established, the DNA is permanently incorporated into the genome of the infected cell. There is no mechanism by which it can be efficiently eliminated. At very low frequencies, homologous recombination between the two LTRs can delete most of the provirus, but even here a single ("solo") LTR remains (736). As the host cell divides, the provirus is transmitted to daughter cells as a new Mendelian locus. Thus, it is likely to persist in the cell for its normal life span, and to convert the cell permanently to a chronic producer of progeny virus.

Unintegrated DNA Forms

The product of the reverse transcription reaction, as outlined earlier, is a full-length double-stranded linear DNA version of the genome, flanked at each end by copies of the LTR. The next step is the movement of the DNA into the nucleus, and the appearance two new DNA forms: closed circular molecules containing either one or two tandem copies of the LTR (Fig. 9). A small amount of the one-LTR circle may be formed during reverse transcription (see preceding), but the bulk is thought to be formed by homologous recombination between the two

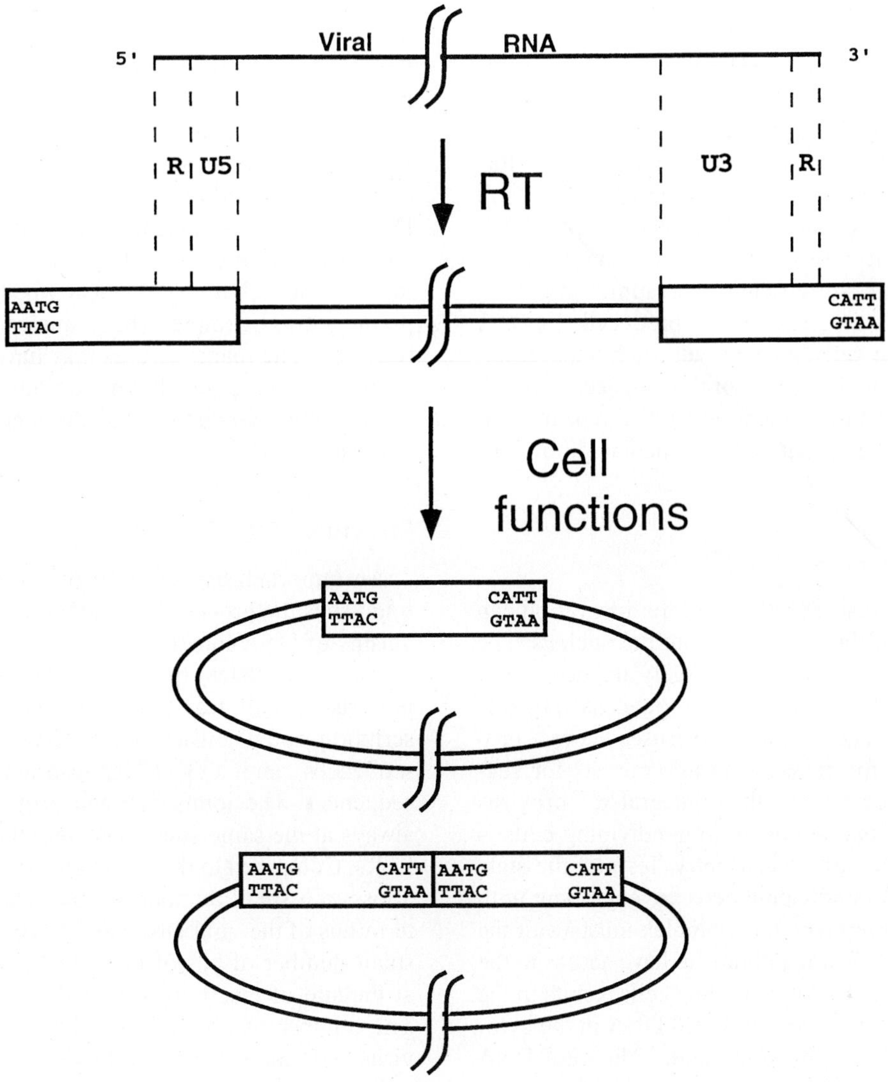

FIG. 9. Unintegrated DNA structures formed after retroviral infection. The incoming RNA genome (*top*) is converted by RT to a double-stranded linear DNA containing two LTRs (*boxes*) in the cytoplasm. The termini of the DNA consist of short inverted repeats and always contain a conserved CA dinucleotide near the 3′ ends; the 3′ terminal sequences of the MLVs (CATT) are shown. The linear DNA is then localized to the nucleus, and two circular double-stranded DNAs are formed: a circle containing one LTR, and a circle containing two tandem LTRs. The LTR–LTR junction contains a unique inverted repeat sequence.

LTRs of the linear DNA. Little is known about the requirements for the formation of circles, although recently, mutants with alterations in portions of the MuLV Gag p12 protein have been shown to be blocked after synthesis of the linear DNA and before formation of circles (793). The tandem two-LTR circles are apparently formed by the blunt-end ligation of the termini of the linear DNA. This event creates a unique sequence, termed the LTR–LTR junction, that is often used as a hallmark of nuclear entry of the viral DNA. The joints are often imperfect, with loss of nucleotides from one or both termini at the joint (664,758). There are also some circles that arise by autointegration of the ends of the linear DNA into internal sites, forming DNAs with deletions or inversions (658); these circles are generally nonfunctional in terms of generating progeny virus.

Because three distinct unintegrated DNA forms coexist in the nucleus, it was uncertain for many years which form might serve as the precursor for establishment of the integrated provirus. In spite of prejudices based on such precedents as phage lambda, it is now clear that circles are not efficient substrates in the integration reaction (206,427), and that the immediate precursor for the integration reaction is the linear duplex DNA. The circles are apparently dead-end products of a side reaction, formed by host enzymes acting on linear DNAs that have failed to integrate. There are settings and cell types in which unintegrated viral DNAs are observed to accumulate to high levels; various tissues in human HIV disease show considerable circular DNAs. While this DNA may reflect some unusual processing of the DNA, much of it is probably formed simply by massive infection occurring shortly before the DNA is harvested (620).

The unintegrated DNA is not a good substrate for forward transcription (636), perhaps because it is still retained in a complex that is poorly accessible to RNA polymerase. Mutant viruses that cannot integrate are unable to establish an efficient spreading infection, although low levels of virus can be produced (649). A very small subset of cells infected with such integration-defective mutants do integrate viral sequences through nonviral means, creating oligomeric tandem repeats similar to those formed after naked DNA-mediated transformation (294).

Entry into the Nucleus

A key step that must take place before integration can occur is the entry of the viral DNA into the nucleus. The mechanisms of nuclear entry are largely unknown, but there are probably at least two distinct routes used by different retroviruses. The simple retroviruses show a profound requirement for passage through mitosis for successful establishment of the integrated provirus (420,489,624,735), and the block in nondividing cells is at or close to the step of nuclear entry. Tests of the state of the viral DNA in nondividing cells are consistent with the notion that the preintegration complex must await the breakdown of the nuclear membrane to have access to the cellular DNA. Infection of nondividing cells results in the accumulation of linear double-stranded DNA in the cytoplasm, and no further signs of infection. The viral DNA will persist in the cell for some time, and if the cell is stimulated to undergo division, the viral DNA will integrate and infection will proceed. However, the DNA loses its capacity to become activated in this way fairly rapidly (23,489). The restriction is quantitatively very significant, and it profoundly limits the utility of simple retroviral vectors for gene therapy.

In contrast, the lentiviruses and spumaviruses are able to successfully infect nondividing cells, and thus there must be an active transport of the viral DNA through an intact nuclear membrane (100,419,635,752). This capability has made lentiviruses very attractive as gene delivery vectors for gene therapy applications. The molecular basis for this capability is a subject of great controversy. The lentiviral MA and Vpr proteins have been argued as essential for the infection of nondividing cells (257,507, 513,743), and the phosphorylation of MA has been argued as necessary to promote dissociation from the membrane and allow nuclear import (99,106,258,259). These findings have not been universally confirmed (247,248,392), however, and the role of MA in these steps is uncertain. Similarly, it has been shown that the Vpr protein is present in the preintegration complex and can bind to nucleoporin components that may mediate nuclear import. However, here too universal support for this model has not been forthcoming. DNA structures present at the second internal copy of the ppt have also been suggested as important for infection of nondividing cells (798). Another attractive model is that the IN protein might be involved in the nuclear import of the complex. IN itself contains nuclear localization signals (257,401), and these can function to target ectopically expressed IN to the nucleus, but it is not clear whether this is related to preintegration complex (PIC) nuclear import or nuclear retention. The foamy viruses may have a distinctive route of nuclear entry involving microtubular transport and centrosomal association, but the mechanism is not well understood (635).

Structure of the Provirus

An important aspect of retroviral integration that distinguishes the process from nonviral or other viral mechanisms of DNA integration is the fact that the insertions create a consistent provirus structure. The integrated provirus is collinear with the product of reverse transcription, and it consists of a 5′ LTR, the intervening viral sequences, and a 3′ LTR, inserted cleanly into host sequences. The joints between host and viral DNA are always at the same sites, very near the edges of the viral LTRs. Compared to the unintegrated linear DNA, there is a loss of a small number of bps, usually two, from each terminus of the viral DNA; and there is a duplication of a small number of bps of host DNA initially present once at the site of insertion that flank the provirus (Fig. 10). The number of bps duplicated is characteristic of each virus and ranges from four to six.

Biochemistry of Integration

The actual integration of the viral DNA into a target is mediated *in vivo* by the viral IN protein (540,591,649), which is brought into the cell inside the virion and acts to insert the linear DNA into the host chromosome. Some IN functions have been studied by analysis of viral DNA formed *in vivo* (630). Most of our understanding of IN function, however, has been obtained through analysis of *in vitro* integration reactions, first using complexes extracted from infected cells (96,256), and later using recombinant IN protein. The reaction proceeds in two steps: 3′ end processing and strand transfer. A schematic view of these reactions is shown in Figure 11.

3′-End Processing

In the first step, the two terminal nucleotides at the 3′ ends of the blunt-ended linear DNA are removed by the IN to produce recessed 3′ ends and correspondingly protruding 5′ ends. This cleavage occurs endonucleolytically at a highly conserved CA sequence, and it releases a din-

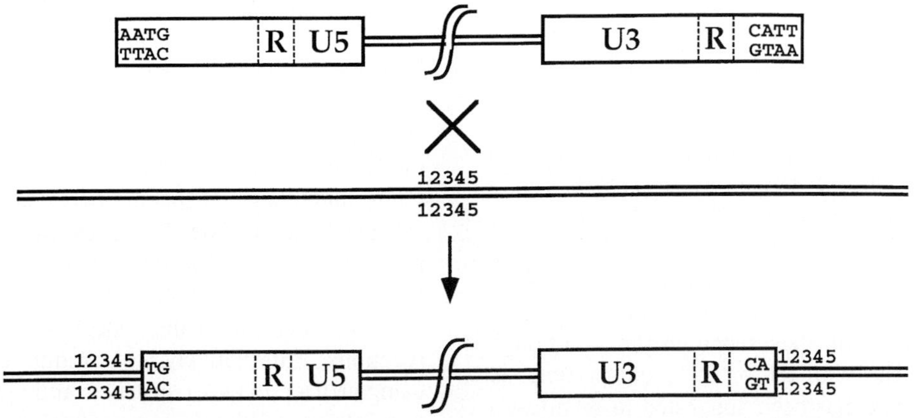

FIG. 10. Integration of the viral DNA to form the provirus. The precursor for the formation of the provirus is a linear double-stranded DNA containing two LTRs (boxes) and with inverted repeat sequences at the termini. The target site in the host DNA is indicated by the arbitrary sequence block denoted 12345. Integration occurs by joining the 38 CA dinucleotides near the termini to the target DNA. The reaction is associated with loss of two bps at the termini of the viral DNA, and with duplication of a small number of bps (five shown here) initially present only once in the target DNA.

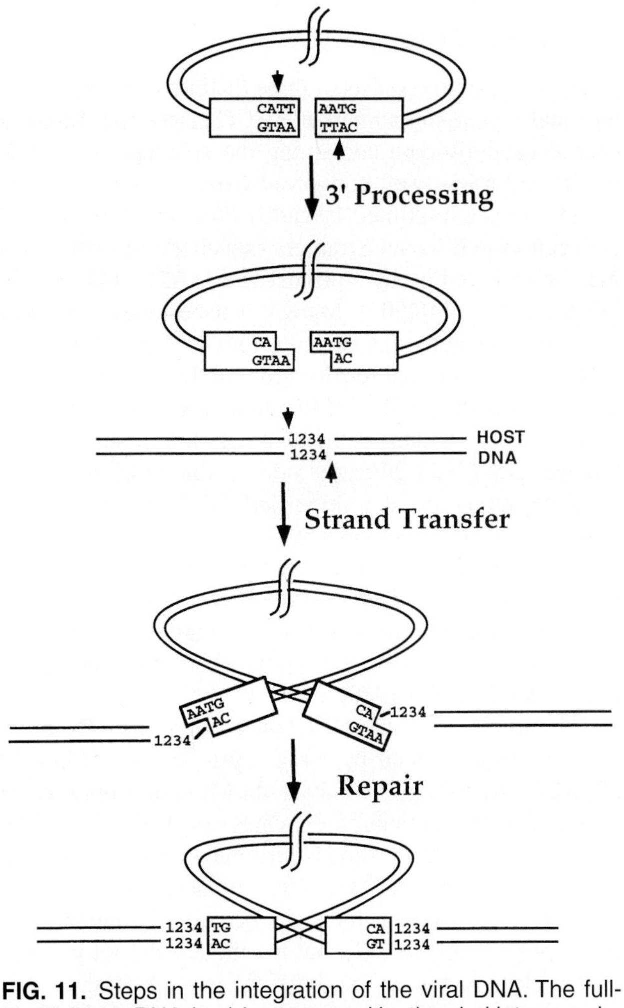

FIG. 11. Steps in the integration of the viral DNA. The full-length linear DNA (*top*) is processed by the viral integrase by the endonucleolytic removal of dinucleotides at the 3′ termini. The resulting DNA is then used in a strand transfer reaction in which the 3′ OH ends make staggered breaks in the two strands of the target site DNA. The resulting gapped intermediate is presumably repaired by host enzymes.

ucleotide. For most viruses, the terminal sequence is such that a TT dinucleotide is released, although this rule has exceptions. The ends do not remain covalently bound to protein, and the energy of the hydrolyzed phosphodiester bond is not retained.

Strand Transfer

In the second step, the 3′ OH ends created by processing are used in a strand transfer reaction to attack the phosphodiester bonds of the target DNA (256). The attack occurs by an Sn2-type reaction, with inversion of the phosphorus center as detected with chiral labeling of the phosphate (213). The formation of the new phosphodiester bond between the viral end and the host DNA displaces one of the phosphodiester bonds in the host DNA, leaving a nick. The protruding 5′ end of the viral DNA is not joined to the host DNA by IN. The reaction is a direct transesterification, and so no ATP or other energy source is required. Mutational studies strongly suggest that the two activities—processing and joining—utilize the same active site residues. In fact the two steps involve similar chemistry: 3′-end processing is an attack on DNA by a hydroxyl residue of water, while joining is an attack on DNA by a 3′ hydroxyl residue of another DNA. It should be noted that other hydroxyl residues can participate; alcohols such as glycerol can be utilized (740), and the 3′ OH of a DNA can even attack a phosphodiester bond on the same DNA, forming a cyclic product (213).

Disintegration

The IN protein exhibits a third enzymatic activity *in vitro*: a reversal of the integration reaction known as disintegration (118). This activity releases DNA from a branched structure and seals the nick at the site of the branch. The significance of the activity *in vivo* is uncertain.

Target Site Duplication

In a wild-type virus, when the two ends are joined to the two strands of the target DNA, the two sites of attack are staggered by a few bps. After the joining, the resulting structure contains short gaps in the host DNA and unpaired bases from each 5′ end of the viral DNA. The 5′ ends of the viral DNA are not joined to host DNA by any known activities of IN. However, the 5′ ends are very quickly repaired *in vivo*, almost as quickly as the initial integration reaction (623). These discontinuities are presumed to be repaired by the host repair enzymes, although it is possible that the viral RT or IN could participate. Indeed, the IN protein has been suggested to manifest a DNA polymerase activity that might fill in the gaps. The processing and filling in the gaps creates a short duplication of sequence that was present only once at the target site; these duplications flank the integrated provirus. The number of bases duplicated is characteristic of each virus. Thus, the murine and feline viruses cause a four-bp duplication; HIV-1 causes a five-bp duplication; and the avian viruses cause a six-bp duplication.

Viral *att* Sites

The sequences at the termini of the viral DNA, the *att* sites, are recognized by the viral IN protein and are important for end processing and joining (103,125,131, 739). These terminal sequences are imperfect inverted repeats. The most conserved residues are a CA dinucleotide pair that lies near the 3′ terminus and determines the site of 3′ processing. Although these bases are absolutely conserved among all the retroviruses, and among many transposable elements, small changes can be tolerated, and mutants can utilize TA or CG relatively well (134). Sequences upstream from the CA for perhaps 10 to 12 bp are needed for efficient integration, but these sequences are different for different viruses, with no indication of broadly conserved sequence motifs. Since the two termini of any given virus are somewhat different, they usually show differential efficiency of utilization in various assays (472). The fact that two distinct ends are bound together in a complex may be important for the concerted integration of these ends into the target (744).

The sequence-specific binding to the *att* site is probably performed by the core domain of IN (367). The nonspecific DNA binding activity of IN has made it difficult to detect sequence-specific binding to these regions, although under some conditions preferential binding to the authentic sequences can be demonstrated (217). A demonstration that an IN mutation can compensate for a mutation in the DNA termini provides nice evidence for the delicate interaction between IN and the DNA termini (188).

Both 3′-processing and strand-transfer reactions are concerted reactions *in vivo*. The processing step occurs simultaneously at both termini of the viral DNA and requires the correct sequences at both termini. Thus, a mutation altering the sequence at one end of the viral DNA blocks the processing reaction at both ends (504). This result suggests strongly that the reaction requires both termini to be loaded into a complex before hydrolysis proceeds. Similarly, the strand transfer reaction normally occurs so that both ends are joined to the target DNA, and at a fixed spacing between the two sites along the DNA helix. The 3′-processing and strand-transfer reactions can both be carried out *in vitro* using native PICs, extracted from recently infected cells, and these reactions reconstruct the concerted nature of the *in vivo* reactions. Alternatively, integration can be performed using artificial DNA constructs and recombinant IN protein. However, these systems typically mediate only a half-reaction—that is, the uncoupled processing of one viral terminus and its joining into a single target DNA. Recent efforts have led to the identification of conditions and factors that can mediate formation of a complex and enhance concerted joining (8,240,745). Once such a protein–nucleic acid complex is formed, it is quite stable.

Structure of the Integrase

The IN protein consists of three distinct domains: an N-terminal region containing an HHCC zinc-finger motif; a central catalytic core containing the so-called D,D-35-E motif; and a less well conserved C-terminal region. The IN protein is a multimer: It readily dimerizes, and at high concentration it forms tetramers as well. All three regions may be involved in the multimerization of IN (21) and in DNA binding (448,503). Many of the residues important for enzymatic activities have been identified by mutagenesis. The most crucial residues for catalysis are the acidic amino acids in the D,D-35-E motif, a highly conserved array of three residues in the core region of many INs and transposases (403). Mutants indicate that both the N-and the C-terminus are also important for function. Surprisingly, pairs of IN mutants with alterations in different regions of the molecule can complement to restore normal function (212,732). The separate N-terminal domain can even complement a nonoverlapping fragment, suggesting that these domains can still coassemble into a functional oligomeric complex (780).

The structures of the HIV-1 and avian virus IN cores have been determined by x-ray crystallography (98,192, 275,452), revealing a compact dimer with similarity to prokaryotic recombination enzymes and RNase H (781). The structures of the N- and C-terminal domains have been determined by nuclear magnetic resonance (NMR) (105, 199,200,433). The structures can be partially merged into a complete molecule (22), but the models do not yet provide a clear picture of the binding sites for viral or host DNAs or the mechanism of the reaction. Indeed, the likely active sites are not located at positions in the dimeric molecule that could mediate concerted integration of two termini into a single target DNA. Cross-linking studies have helped the development of some models for the interaction of IN with DNA (309). We note that the avian IN is phosphorylated at a carboxyterminal serine (316), but the significance of this modification is not clear.

Preintegration Complex

IN does not normally act alone, and a large complex of proteins and nucleic acid is responsible for mediating the formation of the provirus *in vivo* (87,115,224). The nature and components of the PIC, or intasome, are not known in any detail for either the simple or the complex viruses. The PIC of the simple viruses seems to contain CA, RT, and IN, but other viral proteins may be present (87). Many of these proteins probably stay with the DNA even after entry into the nucleus (617). The PICs of the complex viruses do not contain detectable CA but instead contain MA, NC, Vpr, RT, and IN (492). Thus, the PICs of these viruses may be very different, consistent with their very distinctive ability to infect nondividing cells. Normal PICs apparently contain a large structure covering the two ends of the DNA, and perhaps holding them in proximity. The formation of this structure, detected as a footprint in a modified nuclease sensitivity assay (750), requires both IN and the correct sequences at the termini of the DNA (751).

Host Proteins and Integration

A number of host proteins have been recently identified as potentially involved in the establishment of the provirus. One such protein, Ini1, was recovered in a yeast two-hybrid screen as interacting with the HIV-1 IN protein (356). This protein binds to IN and can enhance its activity *in vitro*. Ini1 is the human homolog of the yeast Snf5 protein, a component of the SNF/SWI complex involved in chromatin remodeling, and the interaction of IN with this complex raises the possibility of several contributions it may make to the course of integration. Ini1 is not present in the virion but associates with the PIC in the early phase of the life cycle. Another such protein is BAF-1, a low-molecular-weight protein recovered from the MuLV PIC for its ability to inhibit autointegration of the LTR edges into internal sites in the viral DNA (413,414). By inhibiting this reaction, BAF-1 can enhance normal integration into target DNAs in trans. The structure of BAF-1 has been recently determined by NMR, leading to models for its ability to bind and condense DNA (104). Other proteins include the high mobility group (HMG) proteins, important in transcriptional regulation at many promoters and found to dramatically stimulate concerted integration of the two LTRs into a target DNA *in vitro* (311); and HMG I(Y), similarly important in forming protein complexes on promoters, and stimulating both overall and concerted integration *in vitro* (223,421). The viral NC protein also exhibits similar activity (109). The relative importance of these and other proteins in modifying the integration reaction remains uncertain.

Recently, the integration of retroviral DNA has been shown to activate an apoptotic program in cells deficient in the DNA-stimulated protein kinase (DNA-PK), an enzyme implicated in the DNA damage response and required for the proper rearrangement of immunoglobulin gene and T-cell receptor gene segments in lymphocyte precursors (156). Although it is not clear whether DNA-PK plays any direct role in integration, the enzyme must be involved in sensing the products of active IN and responding to the damage. Its absence leads to substantial cell death in cells exposed to an active IN.

Distribution of Integration Sites

An important issue affecting the ability of the retroviruses to create mutations is the distribution of integration sites in the host genome. Proviruses are probably inserted at nearly random locations in the genome, with no or little sequence specificity, and thus have the opportunity to create mutations in any gene. Various studies, however, have suggested some deviations from a completely random distribution. Some potential targets for insertional mutagenesis seem to be less often disrupted after infection than predicted for truly random distribution of integration sites (383), suggesting that there may be "cold spots." There may be some modest preference for transcriptionally active genes (498,643), for DNase I hypersensitive sites (625,738), or for open or accessible chromatin, but other studies have not detected such biases. Similarly, there have been reports of highly preferred integration sites or hot spots (655), but these observations have not been reproducibly confirmed (770). DNA in chromatin, such as simian virus 40 (SV40) DNA covered with nucleosomes, is a good substrate for integration *in vitro* (584), so nucleosomes probably do not need to be removed to allow efficient targeting; the presence of nucleosomes can, however, induce a 10-bp periodicity onto the pattern of integration, presumably reflecting the accessibility of the outside of the DNA helix to the PIC. DNA bound by other more sequence-specific binding proteins can be protected from integration (586). Heterochromatic satellite repeat DNAs seem to be disfavored sites of integration (110). The sites that are selected can have profound position effects on the ability of the provirus to be expressed, with some sites silent and some expressed at high levels, but on average the transcription of proviruses arising by natural infection is more efficient than when the same DNA is introduced artificially by transfection (331).

EXPRESSION OF VIRAL RNAS

The integration of the provirus signals a dramatic change in the life style of the retroviruses: It marks the end of the early phase of the life cycle and the beginning of the late phase. The early phase is driven by viral enzymes performing abnormal events such as reverse transcription and DNA integration, whereas the late phase is mediated by host enzymes performing such relatively normal processes as transcription and translation. This late phase of gene expression may begin immediately with the synthesis of viral RNAs and proteins, and the assembly of progeny virions (see Fig. 12 for an overview). For many viruses, the transcriptional promoters that drive this expression are constitutively active and cause the production of virions in a relatively unregulated way. In other viruses, the activity of the promoter may be regulated, either by viral or host factors. This section will review the basic phenomena of proviral gene expression and mention briefly the regulation exhibited by the complex retroviruses.

Overview of Viral RNA Synthesis

The synthesis of viral RNA from the viral DNA leads to the formation of a long primary transcript, which is then processed and may be spliced to form a small number of stable transcripts. The U3 region of the LTR contains a promoter recognized by the RNA polymerase II system, and these sequences direct the initiation of transcription starting at the U3-R border. Cellular machinery then caps the 5′ end of the RNA with $_{m7}G5'ppp5'G_{m}p$. The first G residue after the cap is a templated base in the provirus. Transcription proceeds through the genome, and continues through the 3′ LTR and into the downstream flanking host DNA. Finally, the RNA is cleaved and polyadenylated at the R-U5 border of the 3′ LTR, generating a complete, unspliced viral genomic RNA suitable for incorporation into the virion particle. Most genomes contain an AAUAAA sequence acting as the signal for this 3′ processing. The sequence normally lies in the R region (159), but the complete sequence needed for recognition can be complex, lying upstream or downstream (78,171,730), and it may even be discontinuous, brought together by RNA folding to create the functional signal (6,46). The exact site of polyadenylation is not critical for virus replication; mutants in which the polyadenylation signal is inactivated generate longer RNAs that extend into downstream flanking sequences (800), and these RNAs are quite efficiently able to mediate normal replication (689). A subset of the RNA is spliced to give rise to one or more subgenomic RNAs. The patterns of spliced mRNAs can be simple or exceedingly complex. Both the unspliced and the spliced RNAs are then exported from the nucleus for translation.

Initiation of Transcription

The efficiency of initiation of transcription at the 5′ LTR is the major determinant of the levels of viral RNA formed in the cell. The promoter in the LTR is typically a very potent one, and the levels of viral RNA are often constitutively high. However, the cell type, the physiologic state, and the integration site (10,229) can all result in substantial variation in the efficiency of transcription. In some viruses, the promoter is not constitutively active but depends on the activity of specific transcription factors such as the glucocorticoid receptors.

Positive Regulatory Elements in U3

The transcriptional elements in the U3 region of the simple viruses contain both core promoter sequences and enhancers. The core promoters contain a TATA box, bound by TFIIB; a CCAAT box, bound by CEBP (633); and sometimes an initiator sequence near the U3-R border. The U3 regions of even closely related retroviruses are very diverse and can evolve rapidly during viral replication. The enhancers are similar to those found in many host promoters, in that they contain multiple short sequence motifs, arranged in very close packing; often there are tandemly repeated copies of some of these motifs. These short sequences are the binding sites for a large number of host factors that regulate transcription (e.g., see ref. 674). Different cells and cell types will make use of distinct arrays of these factors to mediate transcription from a given viral LTR (284,287,505,606). The factors are not simply additive but may interact in complex ways on particular viral sequences.

Examples of the identity and distribution of known binding motifs in a few LTRs are shown in Figure 13. A partial list of these factors used by various retrovirus LTRs includes Sp1; USF-1; the Ets family of factors, which includes more than 20 members in vertebrates; the core-binding factor (CBF), consisting of an a-b heterodimer; nuclear factor 1 (NF1); and a mammalian type C retrovirus enhancer factor (MCREF-1). Specific viruses often contain recognition sites for other, more specific positive regulatory factors. Major examples of such factors include the glucocorticoid receptors, driving expression of the MMTV genome (25,140), and to a much lesser extent, other MuLVs; NF-κB, important for expression from the HIV-1 LTR in certain cell types (122,628); the GATA factors for Cas-BR-E and other viruses (47); and the myb protein (161). Evidence has recently been obtained that the STAT factors, DNA binding proteins normally activated the Janus kinases (Jaks) may also be important for MMTV transcription (589).

Negative Regulatory Elements

A number of negative regulatory factors that reduce viral expression have been identified. Embryonic carcinoma cells, and true embryonic cells, are the best-characterized examples of cell types that strongly represses LTR-mediated transcription through expression of negative regulatory

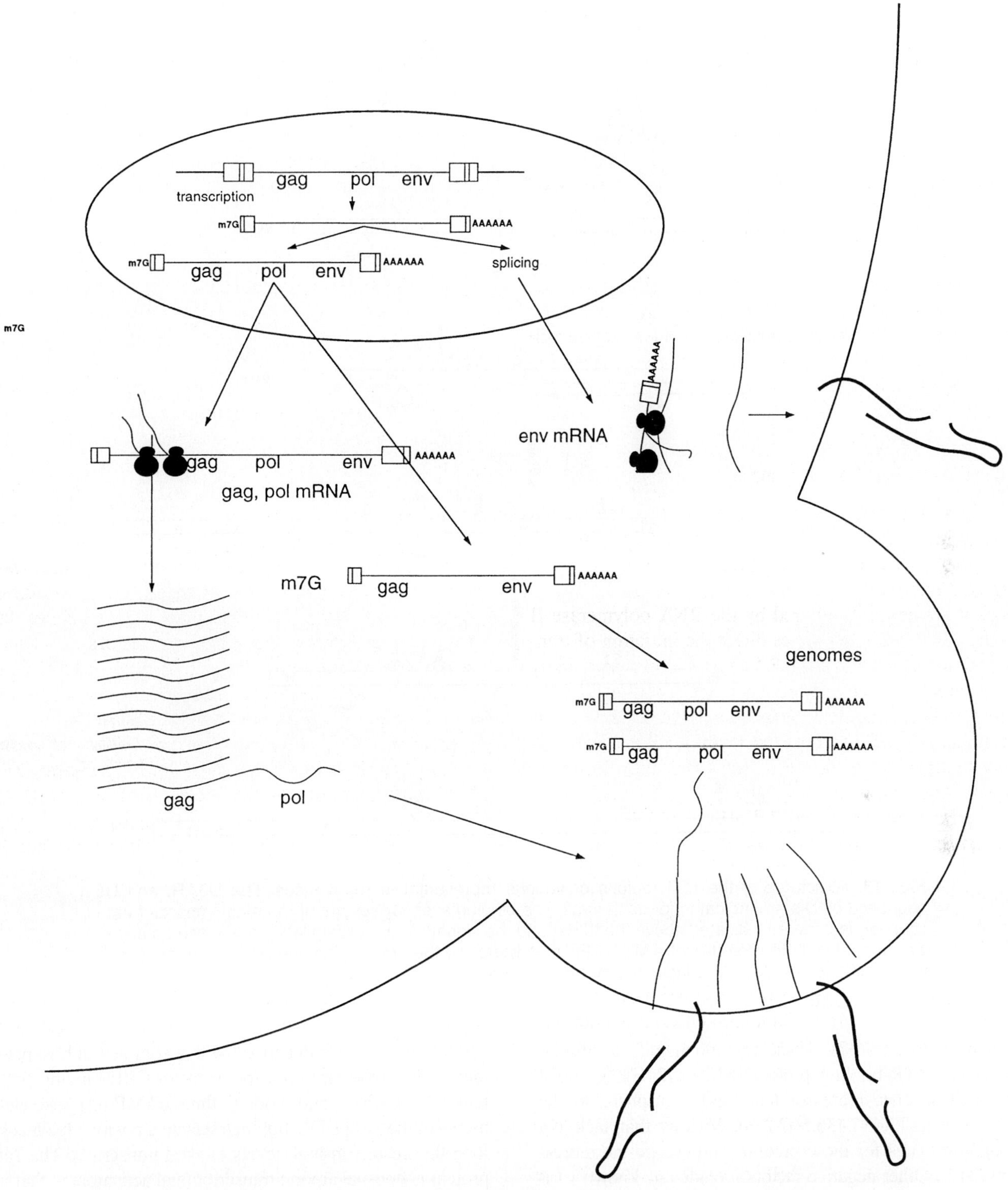

FIG. 12. The late stages of the retroviral life cycle. The integrated provirus is used as the template (*top*) for the expression of viral RNAs. A subset of the transcripts are spliced, and the unspliced and spliced mRNAs are exported to the cytoplasm. The unspliced RNA is used to make Gag and Gag-Pol proteins and also serves as the genome; spliced mRNA is used to make Env proteins. The proteins and RNA associate under the membrane to form the budding progeny virion.

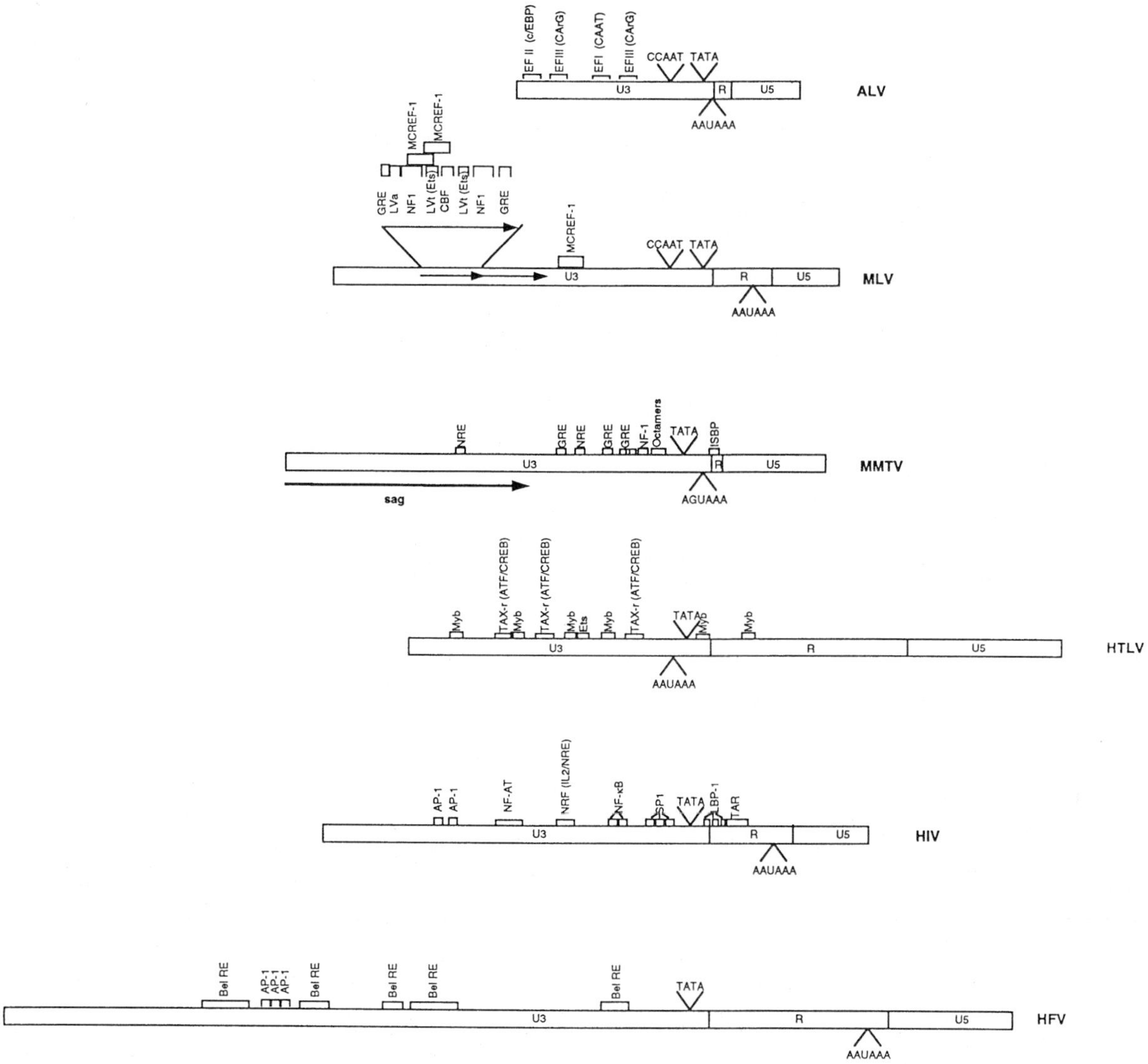

FIG. 13. Structures of the LTR regions of various representative retroviruses. The U3, R, and U5 sequence blocks are indicated for each virus. The binding sites for several of the most important transcription factors are indicated above the LTRs, and the signals for polyadenylation are indicated below. The imperfect direct repeats in the MLV LTR are indicated by the *arrows.* The open reading frame (ORF) for the *sag* gene of MMTV is indicated by the *bold arrow.*

proteins (237,373,737). These factors include a cellular embryonal LTR-binding protein (ELP) (721,722); and a stem-cell specific repressor that binds, curiously, to the tRNA pbs (373,435,436,567,778). Viruses that lack the recognition sites for these proteins can escape the repression (310). Other negative factors include one known variously as UCRBP, NF-E1, or YY1 (241); and others less well characterized (111).

Trans-acting Viral Regulatory Factors

The complex retroviruses encode an array of small regulatory proteins that can activate transcription from the viral LTR in trans. Examples of these transactivators include the HTLV-1 Tax protein (168) and the HIV-1 Tat protein (149). The Tax protein acts in concert with a complex of host proteins, the activating transcription factor/CRE-binding protein (ATF/CREB), and binds to three cAMP response elements in the viral LTR. Tax thus sets up a positive feedback loop that results in high levels of viral transcripts. The Tat protein is unusual among transcriptional activators in that it binds to a structure in the 5′ end of nascent viral RNA (175,652), rather than to DNA. Tat binds to a bulged hairpin structure, the TAR element, and recruits a pair of host proteins, cyclinT/cdk9, to the RNA. These proteins enhance the ability of RNA polymerase to elongate beyond the LTR and down the genome with high processivity, probably by phosphorylation of the C-terminal repeat domain (CTD) of the polymerase. Again, the result is a strong positive feedback loop that results in high levels of viral RNA. (For more detailed discussion of *tat* function, see Chapter 28 and refs. 149 and 150).

Beginning and Ending the RNA

Because there are two identical LTRs in the provirus, it is possible that transcription can be initiated at both the 5′ LTR and the 3′ LTR. However, the 5′ LTR is generally much more efficiently utilized than the 3′ LTR (306). One possible mechanism is promoter interference, in which the upstream promoter being active suppresses the utilization of the downstream promoter (151). It is possible that elements near the 3′ LTR may restrict use of the downstream LTR, so that generally transcripts initiating at the 5′ LTR predominate. These restraints may be lost in tumors, in which transcription from the 3′ LTR can be significantly enhanced (76). Similarly, since there are two LTRs, transcripts might be subject to 3′-end processing at either the 5′ LTR or the 3′ LTR. For those viruses with a long R region, there are signals for RNA cleavage and polyadenylation at both ends of the RNA, and so these events could occur at both 5′ and 3′ sites. However, it is likely that sequences near the 5′ end of the RNA (or the lack of sequences) restrict processing at the 5′ LTR. The RNA that begins at the 5′ LTR is so short when the site for cleavage is reached (the length of the R region) that structural constraints may limit its recognition by the processing enzymes (337). Finally, there may be signals promoting this recognition that are present only at the 3′ sequences. Thus, most of the RNAs formed extend from the 5′ LTR to the 3′ LTR (306). There is at least one exception to this rule: The foamy viruses include a second internal promoter required for the formation of the Tas and Bet regulatory proteins (429,430,482). The separate promoter for formation of these proteins presumably reflects a need for their temporally ordered and regulated synthesis.

RNA Processing

The full-length transcript of the retroviral genome is directed into several pathways. A portion of the transcripts is exported directly from the nucleus and serves as the genome to be packaged into the progeny virion particle, assembling either at the plasma membrane or in the cytoplasm. Another portion with identical structure is also exported and used for translation to form the Gag and Gag-Pol polyproteins. It is not yet clear if these two subsets are truly distinct, whether there can be interchange between the pools, or whether there is a single pool of such molecules used for both purposes. It has been proposed that the translated mRNAs are selectively packaged in *cis* (370). A third portion is spliced to yield subgenomic mRNAs. For the simple retroviruses, there is a single spliced mRNA encoding the Env glycoprotein. For the complex viruses, there can be multiple alternatively spliced mRNAs, encoding both Env and an array of auxiliary proteins (150,619). Examples of the complicated array of mRNAs that are formed for both simple and complex viruses are shown in Figure 14. The protein products of these multiply spliced mRNAs will be discussed in later chapters.

The splicing and subsequent export from the nucleus of only a portion of an initially transcribed RNA is an

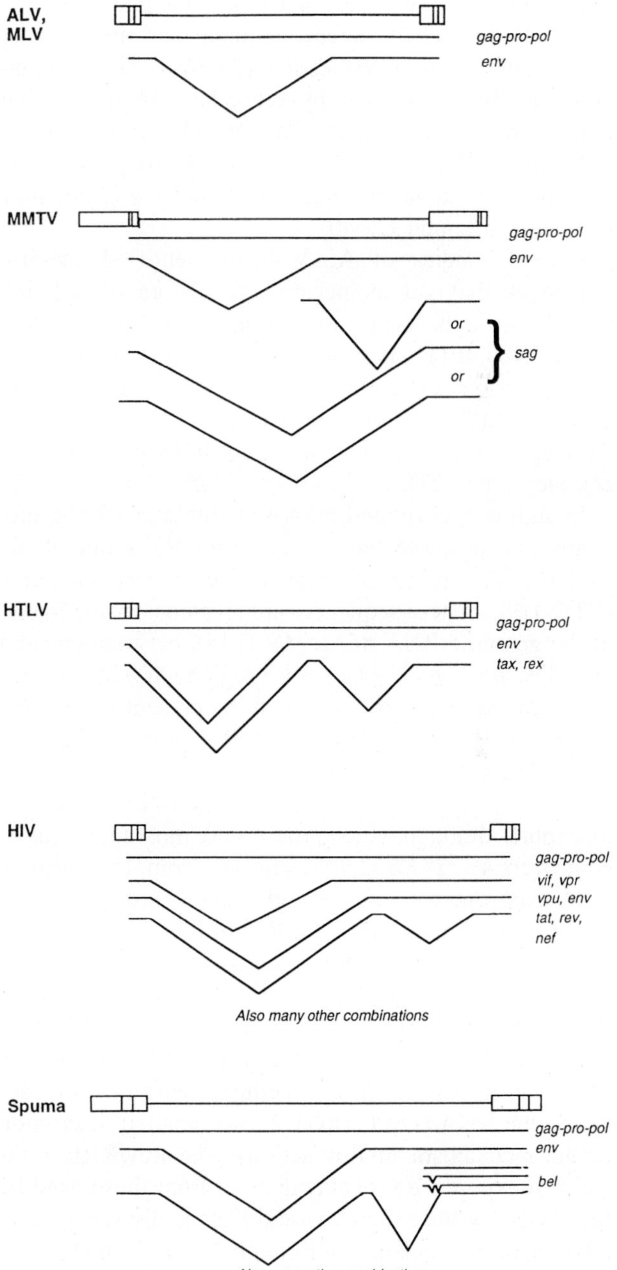

FIG. 14. Splicing patterns of representative retroviral RNAs. All retroviruses direct the synthesis of an unspliced RNA transcript, as well as a variable array of subgenomic mRNAs. Examples of the splicing patterns of the mRNAs of various retroviruses are show. The complex viruses such as HIV-1 also encode a larger array of mRNAs containing various combinations of exons.

extraordinary process; normally, splicing goes to completion, and only then is the mRNA exported. The export of a precursor mRNA is prevented until splicing is complete. At least three aspects of the retroviral genome may promote the export of unspliced mRNAs. First, the splice sites of the viral RNA may have quite poor overall efficiency of utilization by the splicing machinery in the cell (365). Indeed, the sequences at the splice donor and acceptor regions are often poor matches to the consensus sequences for splice sites, and mutations that make the sites better matches increase splicing and are actually deleterious to virus replication (31,364). These mutations can be suppressed by secondary mutations that reduce splicing efficiency. The overall folding of the RNA may affect the efficiency of splicing, and thus sequences at some distance, as in the *gag* gene, may modulate splicing (32,680).

Second, studies of ASLV have identified specific sequences that act as negative regulators of splicing (NRS) through their interaction with host factors (17,137,480,481). These elements can be important for the expression of transduced genes in some viruses (666). Similar signals may exist in other viruses; mutations in the Gag region of MuLV can affect RNA processing in complex ways (27).

In addition, unspliced mRNAs contain *cis*-acting elements that promote the export of the RNA out of the nucleus, the so-called constitutive export elements (CTEs) (92). These sequences are located near the 3′ end of the genomic RNA of MPMV (216), between *env* and the LTR, and possibly in similar regions of ASLV (520). CTE function of the MuLVs may be present in the Gag region (382), or possibly in the R region of the LTR (719). The CTE is recognized by one or more host proteins that assemble a complex onto the RNA to mediate its export, although which proteins are most important is controversial (293,552,703). In the complex viruses, RNA export is regulated through complex interactions of both *trans*-acting proteins, the Rex or Rev gene products, and *cis*-acting sites, the Rev-responsive elements (RREs) that promote RNA export and the *cis*-acting repressive sequences (CRS) elements that prevent it (127,152,154, 173,208,230,313,455–457). A key aspect of this process is the recruitment of Crm1, a cellular nuclear export factor, to the RNA (see Chapter 28 for detailed discussion of the mechanism of Rev action). The Rev/RRE pathways of export are probably distinct from those used by the CTEs, because the two are differentially sensitive to a competitive block acting through Crm1 (77,634).

Viral RNAs are subject to other modifications common to cellular mRNAs. Like cellular mRNAs, the N6 position on specific A residues can be methylated (357), and other sites can be modified by double-stranded RNA adenosine deaminase (295). The significance of these modifications is uncertain.

TRANSLATION AND PROTEIN PROCESSING

All retroviral genomes, at a minimum, contain ORFs designated the *gag*, *pro*, *pol*, and *env* genes. These genes are expressed by complex mechanisms to form precursor proteins, which are then processed during and after virion assembly to form the mature, infectious virus particle. The expression of the various proteins as large precursors that are subsequently cleaved provides several advantages: It allows for many proteins to be made from one ORF, it ensures that the proteins are made at proper ratios, and it allows many proteins to be targeted to the virion during assembly as a single entity. The *gag*, *pro*, and *pol* genes are expressed in a complex way from the full-length unspliced mRNA. The arrangement of these genes, and especially the way *pro* is expressed, are different in different viruses. A summary of the arrangement of the ORFs of various viruses is shown in Figure 15.

Gag Gene Expression

The *gag* gene is present at the 5′ proximal position on all retroviral genomes. A full-length mRNA, identical in sequence to the genomic RNA, is translated in the cytoplasm to form a Gag precursor protein, in the 50- to 80-kd range. Translation begins with an AUG initiator codon and proceeds to a terminator codon at the 3′ end of the ORF. The viral RNA typically contains a relatively long 5′ untranslated region (UTR), and it has been uncertain whether ribosomes could scan from the 5′ cap to the start codon for Gag translation. These 5′ RNA sequences are predicted to contain stable secondary structures that would inhibit scanning. Furthermore, the long 5′ UTRs often contain AUG codons in contexts that are favorable for translation, that are not in frame with the *gag* ORF, and that presumably would inhibit successful translation of Gag (178). Recent experiments suggest that for the MuLVs, an internal ribosome entry site (IRES) is present near the start of the *gag* ORF and is used to initiate translation in a cap-independent mechanism (63,729). Thus, at least in these viruses, ribosomes can bind directly near the *gag* gene and do not need to scan the mRNA. However, other viruses, such as HIV-1, may not use such sequences (487).

Some retroviruses encode an additional Gag protein besides the major product. This Gag protein is longer than the major product and derives from translational initiation at a nonconventional CUG codon upstream from the initiating AUG codon. Translation beginning at this codon first forms an N-terminal leader sequence and then proceeds in the same reading frame through the normal AUG and the rest of the Gag protein. Thus, where the proteins overlap, their sequences are identical. The leader sequence contains a functional signal peptide directing the translation machinery to the ER, and specifying that the Gag protein be cotranslationally inserted into the

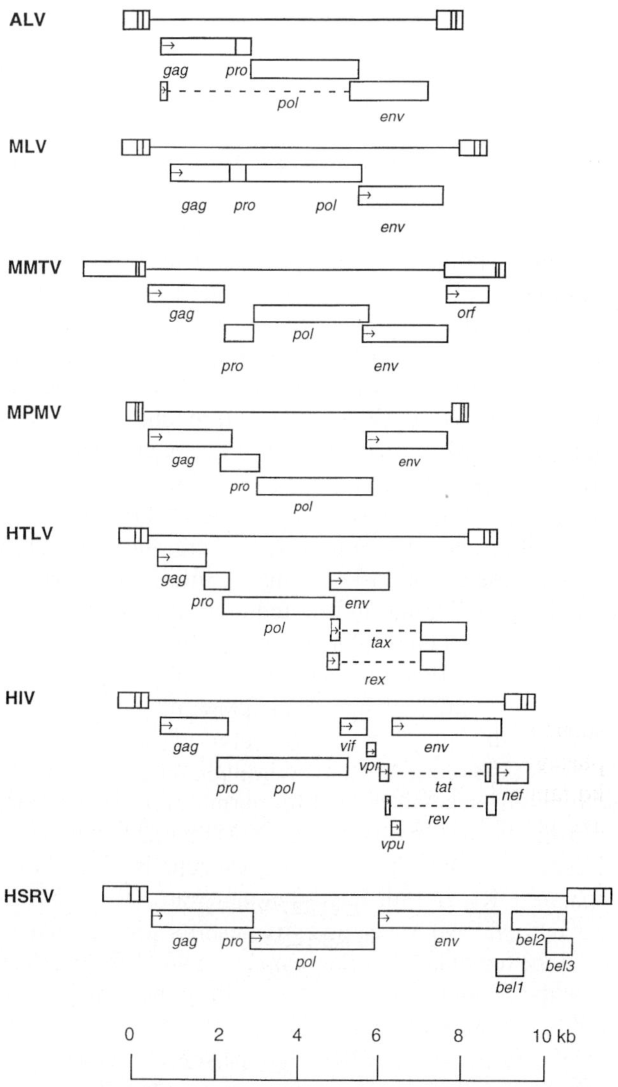

FIG. 15. Arrangements of the ORFs encoded by various retroviruses. The major ORFs of each virus are indicated by the *open boxes.* ORFs in the same reading frame are in the same line, and ORFs in different frames are on different lines. Translational starts are indicated by the *small arrows.* Spliced introns are indicated by the *dashed lines.*

secretory pathway. The Gag become glycosylated at several sites, is transported via the Golgi to the cell surface, and persists for some time as a membrane-bound glycoprotein, with the carboxyl-terminal domain exposed on the cell surface (570). The protein is processed into several fragments and has a relatively short half-life. The function of the protein is uncertain. It is not required for virus replication, and mutant viruses lacking the protein show no gross defects (648). The glycosylated Gag is a prominent immunogen in infected animals, however, and it may thereby or in some other way modulate the replication and the leukemogenicity of the viruses (139). The neuropathogenesis associated with some of the MuLVs may depend on sequences in glycosylated Gag (255,580).

The major Gag product is often modified by the addition of myristic acid, a relatively rare 14-carbon fatty acid, to the penultimate aminoterminal residue, a glycine (304). The addition is mediated by a myristyl CoA transferase that cotranslationally transfers myristate from a myristyl CoA donor to the amino group of the glycine residue, forming an amide bond. The fatty acid is important for the membrane localization and binding of the Gag precursor, increasing the hydrophobicity of the aminoterminal domain. Mutant Gags in which the glycine is altered are not modified, and these Gags do not associate with membrane properly and do not aggregate to form virions (97,285,599). It should be noted that although myristate is important, it is not sufficient for membrane targeting; hydrophobic residues in the MA domain are also required. Furthermore, basic residues further downstream in the MA of some viruses form a patch of positive charge that may interact with negatively charged phospholipids in the membrane.

An aminoterminal myristate is not found on the Gags of bovine immunodeficiency-like virus (BIV), equine infectious anemia virus (EIAV), visna, or ASLV. For the avian retroviruses, the aminoterminus is not myristylated but rather acetylated. The Gag protein of these viruses is apparently sufficiently hydrophobic to be targeted to the membrane without the fatty acid in avian cells, although, curiously, not in mammalian cells. Alteration of the avian Gag to allow its myristylation permits virion assembly in mammalian cells (765) and does not block its function in avian cells (215).

Pro Gene Expression

The relative position of the *pro* gene on retroviral genomes is always similar—in between *gag* and *pol.* However, the *pro* gene is expressed in very different ways in different viruses. Sometimes it is fused in frame onto the 3′ end of *gag*, sometimes it is fused to the 5′ end of *pol*, and sometimes it is present as a separate reading frame. These various patterns have led to considerable confusion in the literature; sometimes *pro* is considered a portion of *gag*, or sometimes of *pol*. Because of these different patterns of expression, it is best to consider this ORF as a separate gene.

The various arrangements of the *pro* gene and its mode of expression are as follows. For the alpharetroviruses, *gag* and *pro* are fused and expressed as a single protein; *pol* is in a different reading frame, and a frameshift is used to express the Gag-Pro-Pol polyprotein. For the beta- and deltaretroviruses, *gag*, *pro*, and *pol* are all in different frames, and successive frameshifts are used to express Gag-Pro and Gag-Pro-Pol polyproteins. For the gamma- and epsilonretroviruses, *gag* and a *pro-pol* fusion are in the same reading frame and separated by a stop codon, and translational readthrough is used to make Gag-Pro-Pol. For the lentiviruses, *gag* and a *pro-pol* fusion are in different reading frames, and frameshifting is used to make Gag-Pro-Pol. Finally, for the spumaviruses, *pro* is fused to *pol*, and the Pro-Pol protein is expressed without Gag, from a spliced mRNA. More will be said about these varied mechanisms of expression in the following section.

Pol Gene Expression

The *pol* gene encodes several proteins needed at lower levels for the replication of the virus, including the RT and IN enzymes. The *pol* ORF is not expressed as a separate protein in most retroviruses, but rather is expressed as a part of a larger Gag-Pro-Pol fusion protein. The Gag-Pro-Pol protein must be made at the correct abundance, in proportion to the amount of Gag protein, for efficient assembly of infectious virus; expression of only Gag-Pro-Pol does not result in virion assembly (231,548). The formation of this protein is mediated by either one of two mechanisms, depending on the virus.

Translational Readthrough

In the gamma- and epsilonretroviruses, the Gag and Pro-Pol ORFs are in the same reading frame and are separated by a single UAG stop codon at the boundary between Gag and Pro-Pol. The translation of Gag-Pro-Pol in these viruses occurs by translational readthrough—that is, by suppression of termination—at the UAG stop codon (786). Most of the time, translation of the RNA results simply in the formation of the Gag protein. But approximately 5% to 10% of the time, ribosomes translating the RNA do not terminate at the UAG codon but instead utilize a normal aminoacyl tRNA, usually a glutamine tRNA, to insert an amino acid at the position of the stop codon. Translation then continues, in frame, through the entire long *pro-pol* ORF, resulting in the formation of a long Gag-Pro-Pol precursor protein. The high-level suppression of termination is specified by a specific structure in the RNA immediately downstream of the UAG stop codon (314,539). The precise features of this structure that are required for suppression are not completely known, but they include a purine-rich sequence immediately downstream of the stop codon, and a pseudoknot formed from the next 60 or so nucleotides (11,232,236,273,766,767). The structure may slow translation, and it may also in some other way alter the balance between termination, which requires binding of termination factors eRF-1 and eRF-3 by the ribosome, as opposed to incorporation of an amino acid, which requires misreading of the codon by an aminoacyl tRNA. No changes in the tRNA pool occur during infection (234). The signals in the RNA can operate to mediate suppression of both UAA and UGA termination codons as well (235).

Translational Frameshifting

In the alpharetroviruses and lentiviruses, the *gag* and *pol* ORFs lie in different reading frames, and the formation of the Gag-Pro-Pol fusion is mediated by a translational frameshift mechanism (340). Most of the time, translation again results in the simple formation of the Gag protein. But approximately 10% of the time, as the translation approaches a specific site near the end of the *gag* ORF, the ribosome slips back one nucleotide (a −1 frameshift) and proceeds onward in the new reading frame. The ribosome passes through the stop codon out of frame and so continues to synthesize protein using the codons of the *pol* ORF. As for readthrough, the determinants of frameshifting lie in the RNA sequence and structure near the site of the event (338,462,550,769). The requirements for frameshifting include a "slippery site," a string of homopolymeric bases where the frameshift occurs; these are oligo-U or oligo-A in different viruses. In addition, the frameshifting requires either a very large and near-perfect hairpin or stem-loop structure; or a large pseudoknot structure, similar to those used in readthrough, although apparently containing a distinctive bend at the junction of the two paired sequences (117,187,358,653). As for readthrough, the proper frameshifting efficiency is crucial for normal virus replication.

In the betaretroviruses (e.g., MMTV) and deltaretroviruses (e.g., BLV, HTLV-1), the *pro* gene is present as a separate ORF, in a different reading frame from that of *gag* or *pol*. Two successive frameshifts are utilized to make the long Gag-Pro-Pol fusion protein (339,497,508). Near the 3′ end of the *gag* ORF, ribosomes carry out a first (−1) frameshift and continue into the pro ORF; near the 3′ end of the pro ORF, they perform a second (−1) frameshift and continue on into the *pol* ORF. These two frameshifts occur at extremely high frequencies—as much as 30% of the time that the ribosome transits through each site—so that the overall frequency of formation of the Gag-Pro-Pol protein is perhaps 10% that of formation of Gag.

Separate Pol Expression

The spumaviruses are unique among the retroviruses in that the synthesis of the Pol protein is not mediated by the formation of a Gag-Pol fusion protein. Instead, a separate subgenomic spliced mRNA (352) is translated directly to form a separate Pro-Pol protein (214,428). This protein must be directed to the assembling virion by distinct domains rather than by the Gag portion of a Gag-Pol fusion.

Env Gene Expression

In all retroviruses, the *env* gene is expressed from a distinct subgenomic mRNA. The *env* message is a singly spliced mRNA, in which a 5′ leader is joined to the coding region of *env*. Thus, the bulk of the *gag* and *pol* genes are removed as an intron from the mRNA. The resulting message is exported to the cytoplasm and translated from a conventional AUG initiator codon. In the alpharetroviruses, the AUG is actually the same one used for Gag translation; it lies in the leader, and the splicing brings this AUG and the first six codons into frame with the *env* coding region. The first translated amino acids constitute a hydrophobic signal peptide, and they direct the nascent protein to the rough ER. The leader is removed by a cellular protease (the signal protease) in the ER, and the protein is heavily glycosylated by transfer of oligosaccharide from a dolichol carrier to asparagine residues on Env. These residues lie in the conventional Asn-X-Ser/Thr motifs recognized by the modification enzymes. Near the end of the cotranslational insertion of Env into the ER, a highly hydrophobic sequence acts as a stop transfer signal to anchor the protein in the membrane. The remaining C-terminal portion of the protein stays on the cytoplasmic side of the membrane.

Before the Env proteins are transported to the cell surface, they are folded and oligomerized in the ER. The formation of oligomers is required for stable expression of the protein, and it is sensitive to overall conformation; many mutants of Env show defects in oligomerization (723). There is considerable controversy about the oligomeric state of the Env protein in different viruses and at different times during their transport (193,201,202,573,753). The most-studied envelope proteins (ASLV and HIV-1) may pass through dimeric or tetrameric intermediates, but the nature of these intermediates is not clear. Although some laboratories disagree (see e.g., refs. 193, 479, 642, and 713), ultimately these envelopes probably form trimers in the mature virus (202,441). The folding of the protein is presumably catalyzed by chaperone proteins in the ER, and the formation of disulfide bonds between various pairs of cysteine residues is similarly catalyzed by disulfide interchange enzymes.

The Env protein is then exported to the Golgi, and it is cleaved by furin proteases to form the separate SU and TM subunits. This cleavage is essential for the normal function of the Env protein. The cleavage occurs at a dibasic pair of amino acids (177), and it produces a hydrophobic N-terminus for the TM protein that is required to mediate fusion of the viral and host membranes during virus entry. In the Golgi, the sugar residues are modified by the sequential removal of mannose residues and addition of N-acetyl glucosamine and other sugars to many of the oligosaccharide. O-linked glycosylation and sulfation of Env glycoproteins have also been documented (572,656). The pathway by which Env is transported to the cell surface is not fully understood, but presumably host vesicular transport systems are utilized. There is evidence that clathrin adaptor complexes interact with the cytoplasmic tail of Env and direct its movement to the plasma membrane (64). The protein typically becomes a prominent cell surface protein on the infected cell.

In polarized epithelial cells, Env proteins are often restricted to the basolateral surface of the cell (534). This localization is mediated by a tyrosine-based motif, Yxxπ, present in the cytoplasmic tail of Env (x, any amino acid; π, hydrophobic residue) (432,535). Remarkably, this targeting of Env can redirect the budding of Gag proteins to this surface.

Other Viral Gene Products

The complex retroviruses express a number of small proteins with a range of functions. The proteins are translated from subgenomic mRNAs, usually resulting from multiple splicing events that join a 5′ LTR to a number of small exons encoding the protein. These gene products will be discussed in greater detail in later chapters, but a short summary follows (see refs. 149, 150, 290, 485, and 577 for reviews).

Deltaretroviruses

Tax

The Tax gene product is a positive regulator of transcription from the viral LTR. Tax functions in association with the ATF/CREB by binding to three cAMP response elements in the viral LTR. Tax also plays a role in transformation, perhaps through E2F-1 activation or through effects on the cell cycle.

Rex

The Rex gene product facilitates the export of unspliced and singly spliced viral mRNAs from the nucleus. Its action is probably similar to that of the lentiviral Rev protein.

Epsilonretroviruses

ORF A

The ORF A product of the piscine retroviruses is a cyclin D homolog that functions as a cyclin in yeast (410). The function of the protein in virus replication or tumor formation is uncertain.

ORFs b and c

The function of these ORFs is unknown.

Lentiviruses

Tat

The Tat protein is a potent transactivator of transcription from the viral LTR. The protein acts by binding to a hairpin structure, the TAR element, encoded in the R region of nascent viral RNA, and recruiting host factors cyclinT and Cdk9 to the RNA. Tat does not increase the rate of RNA polymerase II initiation but seems to enhance its processivity or elongation, perhaps by phosphorylation of the CTD of pol II.

Rev

The Rev protein mediates the export of the unspliced and singly spliced viral RNAs from the nucleus, thus permitting the expression of the Gag, Pol, and Env gene products. Rev binds to the RRE present in the HIV-1 *env* gene, and by interacting with the importin Crm1, it acts to export the viral RNAs through the nuclear pore.

Nef

The Nef protein is a multifunctional protein not essential for replication in some cells in culture, but important for replication *in vivo*. Nef-defective viruses do not induce high-level viremia in infected animals, and progression to disease is delayed or prevented (376). Nef down-regulates the CD4 receptor from the cell surface, facilitating virus release, probably by bridging CD4 to adapter proteins (APs) (569). Nef also down-regulates MHC class I levels, thereby inhibiting the cytotoxic T-lymphocyte–mediated lysis of HIV-1–infected cells. Finally, Nef may enhance virion assembly and release through unknown mechanisms.

Vpr

The Vpr protein, as noted later, is packaged at high levels into virion particles through an interaction with the p6 domain of Gag (39,651). Vpr may facilitate the import of the PIC into the nucleus in nondividing cells. Vpr also causes a strong cell cycle arrest in the G2 stage of the cell cycle, perhaps through an indirect inhibition of Cdc25 phosphatase activity.

Vif

The Vif protein is expressed at high levels in the cytoplasm, and it is packaged into virion particles of both homologous and heterologous viruses. Vif enhances infectivity of virus produced in certain nonpermissive cells, perhaps by blocking the action of a cell-specific inhibitor.

Vpu

The Vpu gene product, found only in HIV-1, is a membrane protein that enhances virion production and also mediates the degradation of CD4 by the ubiquitin-conjugating pathway (644,762).

Spumaviruses

Tas

The Tas (or Bel1) protein is a transactivator of transcription from the viral LTR, acting at sequences near the 5′ end of the genome. Its mechanism of action may be similar to that of the lentiviral Tat protein.

Bet, Bel2, and Bel3

The functions of the *bet* (and the overlapping *bel2*) and the *bel3* genes are unknown, although there is some evidence that the Bel3 protein may be a negative regulator of replication.

VIRION ASSEMBLY

As the Gag, Gag-Pro-Pol, and Env proteins are synthesized, they come together to form progeny virions (reviewed in refs. 246, 330, 637, 691, and 764). The assembly of the retrovirus particle is driven primarily by the Gag precursor protein. Gag is required for the formation of a virion, and indeed it is sufficient to mediate the assembly and release of a "bald" particle—lacking infectivity and the "hair" of the Env protein. The Gag protein that is responsible for assembly is the uncleaved Gag precursor. This form of the protein is thus targeted for assembly and export—the "way out" of the cell. Once the Gag proteins are processed, changes in virion structure can occur to promote entry—the "way in" to the next cell.

There are two major routes by which the various retroviruses assemble their virions.

Assembly of C-type Virions

For most of the retroviruses, those with the C-type morphology, assembly occurs at the plasma membrane; in these cases, the Gag precursor protein is targeted to the cytoplasmic face of the plasma membrane by hydrophobic sequences, by basic residues, and sometimes by a myristic acid moiety (304) present at the aminoterminus. It is not clear if monomeric or dimeric or higher-order structures of Gag are transported to the membrane to begin assembly. The Gag proteins then aggregate, presumably by side-to-side contacts, and create a patch under the membrane. As the patch of protein grows, curvature is induced in the membrane, causing the nascent virus to bud outward. The bud eventually grows to a complete sphere, attached to the cell by a narrow stalk. The stalk is then pinched off, the virion is released, and the host membrane is sealed. The various steps are depicted in Figure 16.

Assembly of B- and D-type Virions

In the alternative lifestyle of the viruses with B- and D-type morphology, the betaretroviruses and the spumaviruses assemble in the cytoplasm and are subsequently transported to the plasma membrane for envelopment and release (610). These two pathways would seem relatively distinct, and one might suppose that the

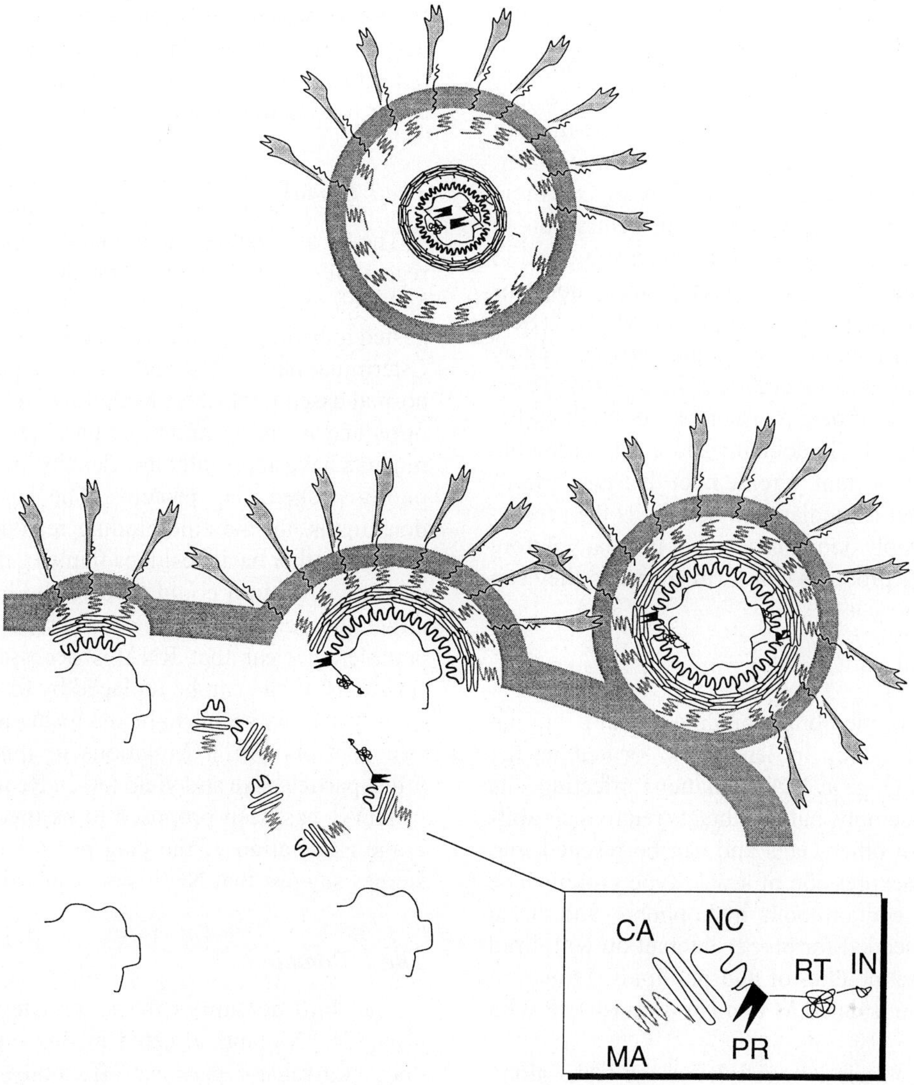

FIG. 16. A schematic diagram of the process of virion assembly. The Gag precursor, containing the MA, CA, and NC domains, and the Gag-Pol precursor, containing the MA, CA, NC, PR, RT, and IN domains (see *blowup*), are transported to the inner leaflet of the plasma membrane. The proteins bind the viral genomic RNA (*thin line*). Curvature is induced in the membrane as the virion grows, and the roughly spherical particle is finally pinched off and released from the cell. The virion proteins are reorganized upon processing by the viral protease to form the mature, infectious virus (*top*).

two groups of viruses would have evolved very different requirements for assembly, and that the details of the Gag-Gag interactions would be different. But these two mechanisms are not so far apart. Indeed, a single amino acid substitution in the MA protein of MPMV can change the morphogenetic pathway of the virus from a cytoplasmic site of assembly to a membrane site of assembly (612). Thus, the main difference may be the timing of exposure of determinants for membrane transport: In the C-types, such a determinant might be constitutively available, whereas for the B- and D-types, the determinant may not be exposed until assembly occurs. For both mechanisms, the nascent virions consist of a spherical particle surrounded by a lipid bilayer, which is pinched off from the cell and then released into the extracellular space.

Assembly of Intracisternal A-type Particles

There is a third route by which retroviral-like particles can assemble, although it is not known to be important for any infectious agent. The endogenous retroviral elements known as IAPs direct the synthesis of virus-like particles with an immature morphology in the cytoplasm of cells expressing these elements. The particles are budded into the lumen of the ER and are not released efficiently outside the cell. These steps may be most closely related to the formation of hepatitis B virions.

Gag and Virion Assembly

For most retroviruses, the expression of the Gag precursor is sufficient to mediate virion assembly and release, earning the protein the name, the particle-making machine. [An exception to this rule is the foamy viruses, which also require the presence of the Env glycoprotein for efficient budding (568).] Because of its central role in virion assembly, the Gag proteins have been subjected to intense mutational analyses to define the domains required for various steps in the process (296,764). Surprisingly, small portions of Gag, containing only a few critical regions, can still assemble virions (746). Three domains seem to be crucial: a membrane-binding (M) domain; an interaction (I) domain; and a late assembly (L) domain. It is important to remember that the form of the Gag protein that is mediating assembly is the precursor; thus, the assembly domains need not lie neatly within any of the cleavage products that form later, and they can span cleavage sites.

The M Domain

The M domain, or membrane-binding domain, ranging from 30 to 90 residues in length, is located at the aminoterminus of Gag, in MA. Mutations affecting this domain abolish assembly, but M mutants retain their ability to interact with other Gags and can be rescued into particles by the coexpression of a wild-type protein. The region seems to contain both hydrophobic and basic residues that are needed for proper interaction with lipid and with the acidic moieties of phospholipids. Structural information for the isolated M domain is consistent with this role (478).

For many retroviruses, myristylation of Gag, along with specific residues in MA, is required for membrane binding. This interaction with membrane, in turn, is important for virion assembly of the C-type viruses, and for their proper subsequent Gag processing (645). Mutational studies have led to the notion of a "myristyl switch," in which the myristic acid is exposed to mediate plasma membrane binding during virion assembly, but then can be sequestered in the compact globular core of MA after Gag processing (524,536,672,803). Although this region is generally considered important for virion assembly, surprisingly, much of the Rous sarcoma virus (RSV) MA (511), and the entire HIV-1 MA domain (597) can be deleted from Gag without preventing assembly, so long as a functional membrane binding signal is retained. In the latter case, there are some effects on assembly: Virions are budded indiscriminately into both intracellular membranes as well as at the cell surface. The aminoterminal sequences of Gag can be replaced with a heterologous membrane binding signal, such as that present at the aminoterminus of the Src kinase. It should be noted that the interaction of Gag with membrane is not required for assembly of the B- or D-type viruses per se. For these viruses, mutations in the myristate addition signals do not affect the cytoplasmic assembly of the virions, but rather block the transport of the assembled particles to the plasma membrane (611).

The I Domain

The I, or interaction, domain is defined as a major region of Gag-Gag interaction, largely contained in the NC region. Although the major I domain has been suggested to lie in NC, some analyses have suggested that the C-terminal half of CA and NC are equally important for normal assembly (1,85). Mutations in the I domain block or reduce assembly, and those particles produced by these mutants have aberrantly low density, indicating fewer and poorly packed Gag proteins. The key feature of the I domains is not the zinc-binding residues of the Cys-His box, but rather basic residues flanking the boxes (89). The assembly function could involve the binding of RNA—either the genomic RNA or other RNAs—but it is not completely clear that RNA is necessary. The assembly functions of NC can be replaced by foreign proteins, and the key activity seems to be the formation of protein–protein contacts (801). Mutations in this region can also affect particle size and yield (397). Recently, the I domain of HIV-1 has been proposed to be involved in the membrane association of the Gag precursor (640), but other studies suggest that NC is not required (523).

The L Domain

The third domain is the L, or late assembly, domain (763,776). Mutants affected in this function fail to produce and release particles efficiently, and although the mutant Gag proteins form spherical structures, they accumulate under the membrane and do not progress normally. The buds remain tethered to the cell surface by a membrane stalk, suggesting that the function of the L domain is to mediate virus–cell separation. Recently, the domain has been shown to also be important in determining the size of the virion: The structures formed by L domain mutants are often large and heterogeneous in diameter (264). L domains lie at different locations in the Gag proteins of different viruses. In ASLV, MPMV, and the MuLVs, the L domain lies in the aminoterminal third of the protein and its critical residues are the PPPY motif. In HIV-1, the domain lies in p6, at the C terminus, and instead contains the motif PTAP. Remarkably, many of these L domain motifs are interchangeable among the various retroviruses and show a substantial position independence for their function (544). It is likely that these motifs represent the binding site for some protein important for the late stages of budding, and indeed the PPPY motif has been identified as the recognition sequence for the WW-domain family of proteins, including the Yes-associated protein YAP, NEDD45, and many others (265). Recently, the L domain of the EIAV Gag has been shown to associate with a cellular adapter protein, AP-2, which could mediate transport or localization steps (587). Which of these (or other proteins that may interact with the L domain) are most crucial for virion release remains uncertain. A curious additional link between two of these proteins is provided by the observation that both HIV-1 p6 and the MuLV p12 proteins are modified by the addition of ubiquitin at low levels (529). It is possible that a PPPY-binding host protein is responsible for this modification.

Virion Assembly *In Vitro*

Recently, Gag proteins and fragments of Gag have been shown competent to assemble *in vitro* to form various structures that more or less closely resemble virion cores (196,386,638,673). The CA-NC portions of ASLV and HIV-1 expressed as recombinant proteins can assemble to form particles or long hollow tubes; the formation of these structures is dramatically enhanced by the addition of RNA, and the length of the tubes is determined by the length of the RNA (108). Larger Gag fragments that include more aminoterminal regions can assemble into spherical particles (292), and this assembly is stimulated by RNA and host cell extracts (107). Although HIV-1 Gag interacts with cyclophilin A *in vitro* and *in vivo*, addition of cyclophilin A to assembly reactions has only little effect (288). HIV-1 Gag CA-NC fragments can assemble into conical structures (262), with a pitch that falls into discrete values. Image reconstruction of these cones has allowed the formation of a model for the packing of the protein into hexagonal arrays. Virus-like particles have also been formed with the Gag proteins of MPMV in cell-free protein synthesis systems.

Virion Size

The number of Gag proteins per virion particle is estimated to be in the range of 1,200 to 1,800, although this number may vary somewhat from virus to virus. The number of Gag-Pol proteins is roughly 10 to 20 times lower, approximately 100 to 200 per virion. It is unlikely that these proteins form a completely homogeneous, ordered crystalline array, but rather they may form a "protein micelle" that is somewhat fluid like a lipid micelle. The diameter of even wild-type virus preparations is not tightly homogeneous but shows a distribution that suggests some flexibility in the structures during assembly. However, the average size of the particle is determined by the Gag protein, and mutants with alterations in Gag often show abnormal or excessively heterogeneous diameters (397). Mutations in the CA domain commonly show this phenotype. Thus, CA-CA contact may play a role in determining the angle between Gags during their packing into a spherical shape. The heterogeneity of virions has frustrated efforts to determine the detailed structure, although chemical cross-linking has provided some clues (297).

Gag proteins of one virus are sometimes able to interact with the Gags of another virus to coassemble and form mixed virion particles. Various mutants with alterations in the Gag proteins of the MuLVs can coassemble into particles that show phenotypes of both parental Gags (361,598). Viruses of very different genera can even form mixed particles in some cases (59). The physical interactions between Gags can be monitored in other assay systems as well (243,442).

Incorporation of Other Proteins into Assembling Virions

During assembly, other proteins are incorporated into the particle by contacts to Gag; these include Gag-Pol, Env, and auxiliary proteins encoded by the complex viruses. The Gag-Pol precursor is thought to be incorporated into the assembling bud by virtue of the Gag protein present at the aminoterminus. Gag to Gag-Pol contacts can in some cases lead to the incorporation of mutants of Gag-Pol that do not retain the myristate modification to the aminoterminus (549), suggesting that the interaction is quite strong. Gag fusions to foreign proteins can be similarly incorporated into particles formed by Gag (351); this process can even be used to target antiviral proteins into virions. Consistent with this notion, many mutations that block assembly of Gag, when tested in the context of Gag-Pol, are found have similar effects on the incorporation of Gag-Pol (146,650). However, some mutations in HIV-1 Gag have also been identified that specifically affect the incorporation of Gag-Pol, suggesting that Gag-Pol utilizes some distinctive contacts not important for Gag-Gag interactions (662). Further, in the spumaviruses, Pol is incorporated without an appended Gag region, suggesting that distinct interactions must be utilized for its incorporation (214).

The Env protein is thought to be concentrated at the sites of budding and incorporated into the virions by virtue of contacts between the cytoplasmic tail of Env and the aminoterminal portion of Gag. These interactions have been difficult to document directly, although there is some biochemical evidence (143) and cross-linking studies (267) in support of these contacts. Genetics has provided good evidence for this interaction. Selected mutants of MA show defects in Env incorporation (181,250,791), and some mutants of the cytoplasmic tail of TM are not efficiently incorporated (792). In addition, Env proteins that are specifically directed to the basolateral surface of polarized epithelial cells can redirect the sites of budding of Gag from a nonspecific assembly on both membranes to the exclusive assembly at basolateral membranes (432,535), and they can similarly redirect Gag in neurons (749). Finally, mutants and revertants of these mutants with second-site suppressors in the binding partner have provided strong evidence for these interactions (249,250). However, it should be noted that the envelope proteins of viruses very distant from retroviruses, including vesicular stomatitis virus (VSV) and influenza, can be functionally incorporated into retrovirus particles without any obvious sequence similarity in their cytoplasmic tails. Furthermore, truncating the tail of ASLV Env does not prevent its incorporation or function (563). Thus, there may be mechanisms to direct Env proteins to assembling virions without these specific contacts to Gag—a default pathway, or a pathway using other interactions. Indeed, other distinct parts of Gag, including the p6 region of HIV-1 Gag, have been implicated in Env incorporation (528).

The HIV-1 protein Vpr is efficiently incorporated into assembling virions at very high levels, approaching equimolarity with Gag. This incorporation requires the presence of the p6 domain of Gag (651) and may be mediated by a direct interaction (39). The binding can be used to direct foreign proteins into the particle; a fusion between Vpr and a foreign protein will be targeted to virions. Furthermore, Vpr can be used to direct separately expressed versions of RT or IN to particles in a functional form, to complement mutations in the RT or IN domains of the Gag-Pol fusion (402).

Host Proteins in the Virion

A number of host proteins have been shown to be present inside the virion particle; in most cases, the significance of the protein is unknown. Prominent among the virion-associated factors are a number of cytoskeletal proteins. These include actin (33,512,530,760) and various members of the Ezrin-Radixin-Moesin (ERM) family, specifically ezrin, moesin, and cofilin (530). The Gag, and especially the nucleocapsid protein of HIV-1 have been shown to directly bind to actin (426,609,760), perhaps offering a mechanism for its incorporation into the particle. A complication in analyzing virion-associated proteins is that virion preparations tend to be contaminated with substantial amounts of microvesicles, entities released by cells that exhibit a density and size very similar to that of virions, and containing an array of host proteins (66).

The virions of HIV-1 contain substantial levels of cyclophilin A, a proline isomerase of uncertain function but implicated in protein folding and signal transduction (244,443,712). The incorporation of cyclophilin A is not required for assembly, but it is important for efficient entry of HIV-1 into newly infected cells, before the process of reverse transcription is initiated (90). Its exact role is uncertain. Several other proteins have also been found in virions: a translational elongation factor, eIF-1a (121), and a protein known as H03 (408), with similarity to histidyl tRNA synthetase, are additional examples.

Host proteins may also be attracted into virion cores by mechanisms other than Gag. Recently, the host uracil DNA glycosidase, responsible for removing uracil bases from DNA, was shown to be incorporated into virions by contacts to IN (761). Another protein, the RNA transporter staufen, was shown to be incorporated into virions, probably through contact to viral RNA (502).

There are also substantial levels of host proteins in the virion envelope. The mechanism of incorporation of these proteins into the virion is not clear, and in most cases again the significance is uncertain. However, one such molecule, major histocompatability complex (MHC) class I, is present at levels approaching those of the Env protein and can be functionally significant, in that xenogeneic antibodies targeted to MHC can neutralize the infectivity of viruses such as HIV-1 (33,34).

RNA PACKAGING

The RNA genome is incorporated by virtue of interactions between specific RNA sequences near the 5′ end of the genome, termed the packaging or Psi sequences, and specific residues in the NC domain of Gag (see refs. 30 and 61). Both partners in this interaction have been intensively studied.

Gag Sequences Important for Packaging

The Gag precursor is probably the form of the protein that is responsible for packaging the RNA (519), and the NC portion of the precursor plays the largest role. Mutations affecting the NC protein often reduce the incorporation of the genomic RNA into the virion particle (see ref. 61 for review). The most crucial sequences are the Cys-His boxes, short sequence blocks resembling zinc fingers and containing the motif Cys-X2-Cys-X4-His-X4-Cys, but basic residues elsewhere in the NC molecule are also important (319,578). The NC protein of various viruses contains either one or two copies of the Cys-His box. When two copies are present, they are not equivalent or interchangeable, suggesting that they mediate distinct interactions with RNA (281). Some viral cores can cross-package heterologous viral RNAs, suggesting good binding to the heterologous Psi region, and sometimes there is a strong preference for the homologous RNA. Exchanging the NC domains between viruses can sometimes transfer the preferential selectivity of a Gag protein for its cognate RNA, although the specificity of these hybrid Gags is often poor, and in some cases other sequences in Gag can determine the preference for RNA packaging by chimeric Gags.

RNA Sequences Important for Packaging

The packaging or Psi regions on the viral RNA genome that are recognized for incorporation are quite distinct in nucleic acid sequence among the various viruses. The key Psi regions lie near the 5′ end of the RNA, generally between the LTR and Gag. However, other regions of the genome can affect RNA packaging, including sequences upstream in R and in U5, downstream in Gag coding regions, and even near the 3′ end of the genome. In the case of ALSV, a region of 270 nt is necessary and sufficient to mediate the packaging of a foreign RNA (29,45,366). In the case of the MuLVs, sequences that are at least partially sufficient to mediate packaging have been similarly identified (3). These Psi regions are relatively autonomous; Psi can be moved to ectopic positions in the genome with at least some retention of function (459).

The various Psi sequences have been predicted or shown to form a number of stem-loops, often containing GACG in the loops. Reversion analysis of mutants with alterations in these loops confirms the importance of the stem-loop structure (182). Mutational studies show that several such loops may incrementally contribute to the efficiency of packaging of the RNA, although one or two are often found to be most important (238,501). Recently, one of the stem-loop structures of the HIV-1 Psi was replaced by a completely foreign sequence that was selected on the basis of its binding activity with NC; the resulting RNA was efficiently packaged and utilized for replication, strongly suggesting that the binding to Gag is the key function of Psi (124). A structure of the HIV-1 NC bound to one such stem-loop has been resolved by NMR, revealing specific contacts between both hydrophobic and basic residues of NC and nucleotides in the stem-loop of the RNA (165).

Dimerization of the Viral Genome

Mature virions contain a dimeric RNA that is highly condensed into a stable, compactly folded structure referred to as the 70S dimer on the basis of its sedimentation rate. Packaging of RNA is associated with the dimerization of the RNA, but it is not completely clear whether the genome is present as a dimer before it is incorporated into virions or is incorporated as a monomer and then dimerized after its incorporation. However, some ASLV mutants suggest that monomeric RNA can be packaged under some circumstances (527), implying that dimerization may follow packaging. There are specific sequences in the RNA, termed dimerization or dimer linkage structures (DLS), that are required for RNA dimerization *in vitro*, and for the formation of the dimeric virion RNA *in vivo*. These DLS elements are in close proximity or even intermingled with sequences required for packaging of the RNA, often making it difficult to determine their separate contributions to these processes. The dimerization of viral RNAs can be induced *in vitro*, and it is stimulated by the addition of NC or the Gag precursor. However, it is uncertain to what extent these reactions reflect dimerization *in vivo*.

The viral RNA in newly budded virions is present as an unstable dimer, dissociated by heat at relatively low temperatures, and it becomes condensed to a more stable dimer during virion maturation (254). This condensation requires the proteolytic processing of Gag (252) and may be mediated by the free NC upon its release from the precursor. A model for the process of dimerization, the "kissing loop" model, suggests that duplex formation between two RNAs is initiated between loops on the two RNAs and propagates outward through the stems to form a more stable duplex. It is possible, but by no means certain, that such changes in the duplex regions could account for the change in thermal stability upon maturation.

Many cells contain vast arrays of endogenous proviruses and retrovirus-like elements, a subset of which can be expressed constitutively or under various conditions of stress to produce large amounts of genomic RNA. If such a cell is infected by an exogenous virus or has been engineered by expression constructs to produce virions, the particles will incorporate the endogenous RNAs along with the viral RNA (65,556). The endogenous retroviral RNAs, notably the VL30 RNAs of rodents, contain highly efficient Psi sequences (484,717), presumably because they were selected to compete with the homologous genomes of exogenous viruses for packaging.

Virions also contain a number of host RNAs of uncertain significance. There are substantial levels of 7S RNA, a low-molecular-weight RNA thought to function in host RNA splicing (116). In addition, there are low levels of host mRNA. Particles released without efficient packaging of the viral genome (as are produced by Psi-mutant genomes) may carry enhanced levels of host RNAs, and various mutants with alterations in NC can show selective enhancement of both endogenous viral and host RNAs (484). A variant avian leukosis virus (ALV), SE21Q1b, packages unusually high levels of host RNA (260,425) and is capable of transducing these host sequences into new cells by reverse transcription (445). This phenotype of high-efficiency transduction is associated with an unusually high level of proviral expression and particle production rather than any specific alteration in a viral protein (18).

Incorporation of tRNA Primer

A key aspect of RNA packaging is the incorporation of a host tRNA along with the genome to serve as the initiating primer for minus-strand DNA synthesis (for review, see ref. 453). Virions contain a substantial pool of free tRNA, perhaps 50 to 100 copies per particle. The bulk of these tRNAs are not associated with the genomic RNA and are present in virions that lack the genome. In some viruses, these tRNAs are largely representative of the pool of tRNAs in the cell, whereas in others they are highly enriched for the tRNAs needed for priming DNA synthesis, although even here many other tRNAs are present. Viruses prepared without the Pol proteins do not show this enrichment, suggesting that Pol, and most probably the RT protein, are responsible for bringing these tRNAs into the virion (566). In accord with this notion, the RT of ASLV has been shown to preferentially bind tRNATrp from a mixture of tRNAs, accounting for its enrichment in the virion (538). Similarly, HIV-1 RT preferentially binds tRNALys3, and the interaction domain has been shown to at least include the anticodon loop of the tRNA. However, no similar preference for the natural primer tRNAPro has been detected for the MuLV RT. It may be significant that the MuLVs have been shown to be able to utilize a range of different primer tRNAs when only the complementary sequence in the genome (the pbs) is altered to promote their use.

tRNA Primer Placement

A very small subset of the incorporated tRNAs—two per virion—are annealed to the pbs, an 18-nt sequence near the 5′ end of the genome with perfect complementarity to the 3′ sequences of a specific primer tRNA. The pbs sequences are, as one would expect, essential for normal reverse transcription of the virus (613). The sequence of the pbs can determine the primer tRNA that is utilized (789), but changes in the pbs tend to revert back to the wild type (759), suggesting that alternate tRNAs do not function well. An interesting aspect of reverse transcription provides an efficient mechanism for this reversion: The use of the original tRNA even once during replication will convert the pbs back to the original sequence, because the tRNA itself is the template for the DNA copy of the pbs. Other sequence blocks of the tRNA are also paired with complementary sequences in R and U5 to form a large, complex structure required for proper tRNA primer placement and utilization (7,126,205,328,334). These other sequences are presumably responsible for the selectivity for the natural tRNA primer. In the alpharetroviruses, *pol* gene products are required to mediate the placement of the tRNA on the genome, but in the gammaretroviruses, *pol* is not required (253). The Gag precursor, and especially the NC domain, are thought to play a major role in promoting the annealing of the tRNA to the genome. Although NC can promote annealing of complementary RNAs and DNAs *in vitro*, its role and the mechanism by which it may act *in vivo* remain uncertain.

PROTEIN PROCESSING AND VIRION MATURATION

As retrovirions are budded from the cell surface, the Gag and Gag-Pro-Pol precursor proteins are proteolytically cleaved to release the smaller proteins present in the infectious virions (for review, see ref. 741). The cleavage of Gag and Gag-Pro-Pol is mediated by the viral protease PR, which is expressed either in Gag, Gag-Pol, or Gag-Pro-Pol fusion proteins. Thus, PR is responsible for cleaving itself out of a precursor protein and then making a number of other cleavages in these proteins.

Activation of the Protease

The processing of Gag and Gag-Pro-Pol precursors is intimately linked to assembly and budding, and it is controlled so that the precursors are not cleaved until they are assembled. It is not certain how PR is regulated during assembly to begin cleaving its substrates. The structure of PR has revealed that the active enzyme is a homodimer (see later), and thus its activation could be promoted by dimerization of the Gag or Gag-Pro-Pol precursor associated with assembly. As the virions form, one could imagine the high concentrations of the protein generating an active PR that would begin to cleave Gag and Gag-Pro-Pol, and that would release the mature PR dimer as well. However, for the betaretroviruses such as MPMV, this mechanism cannot explain the delay in processing. For these viruses, assembly occurs in the cytoplasm and should result in the establishment of a high concentration of Gag-Pro-Pol at that time. Yet cleavage does not begin in the cytoplasm, but rather is restrained until budding and export of the preformed virion particle. Thus, other unknown mechanisms, perhaps coupled to membrane association, must be responsible. Similar conclusions were reached from analysis of IAP virions, in which assembly in various intracellular locations did not result in processing—membrane association was required (755).

Various domains of Gag have been suggested to inhibit PR (266), and conformational changes could relieve this inhibition. In the alpharetroviruses, a cleavage at the NC-PR boundary is required to release active PR, so activating this cleavage could serve as a trigger (102). Similar cleavages at the p6*-PR boundary are important for full activation of the HIV-1 PR (711). Another possibility is the activation of the PR by a drop in the pH associated with virion release. It should be noted that the overexpression of PR in many artificial settings, both in bacteria and in animal cells, as a Gag-PR fusion or alone, can result in formation of highly active enzyme (24). The high-level expression of PR is often toxic for cells, presumably because of its inappropriate action on many host proteins.

Protease Structure and Function

The retroviral proteases are aspartyl proteases with clear sequence similarity to members of the cellular family of aspartyl proteases (362,434,742). The three-dimensional structure of many proteases, including those from ALSV, HIV-1, HIV-2, SIV, feline immunodeficiency virus (FIV), and EIAV, have been determined by x-ray crystallography (406,409,491,509,582,616,748,772). The viral enzymes are small, typically containing about 100 amino acids, and are homodimers as isolated from virions. Each subunit contributes to the active site a single aspartate residue, lying in a loop near the center of the molecule. There is a long cleft at the interface between the subunits where the substrate lies; there are pockets to interact with each of the side chains of the substrate, conferring specificity to the enzyme. Each subunit has a flap consisting of an antiparallel sheet with a b-turn that covers the cleft, and this flap moves out of the way to permit the binding of the substrate into the active site.

Retroviral proteases have a complex specificity for substrate peptides (560). The enzyme makes contact with approximately seven or eight side chains on the substrate and thus can select its cleavage sites on the basis of at least these amino acids. The cleavage sites tend to be within hydrophobic sequences and yet must lie in accessible and extended conformations. Some analyses of the various sites in Gag and Gag-Pol that are recognized by PR suggest that either one of two sequence motifs constitutes a consensus site: One set has an aromatic residue or proline flanking the cleavage site, and the other set has aliphatic residues at these positions. Mutational analyses have allowed further definition of the residues on PR that make specific contacts to the substrate.

Protease Inhibitors

Studies of mutant viruses lacking PR demonstrated that the protease is essential for virus replication. Viruses lacking a functional PR can still express Gag and Gag-Pol precursors, and they can mediate the assembly and release of immature virion particles. Thus, PR is not required for the process of virion assembly per se. However, these particles are noninfectious and are blocked at an early step prior to the initiation of reverse transcription (147,363,390). Because of its essential role in virus infectivity, PR was appreciated early in the course of the AIDS epidemic as an attractive target for antiviral therapy. A number of molecules have been generated that can bind and inhibit PR, including peptide mimetics with uncleavable, nonsessile bonds at the cleavage site (158,494). Some are transition state analogs, and may have inhibition constants (K_i) in the nanomolar or subnanomolar range. These inhibitors have been extremely effective antiviral agents, and because they target a distinct enzyme and a distinct step in the life cycle from the RT inhibitors, they have been particularly effective in combination with earlier drugs targeted at RT. The combination of three drugs that include a protease inhibitor is now the standard of treatment for AIDS, and such highly active antiretroviral therapy (HAART) can keep virus loads below detectable levels in some patients for many years. Ultimately, however, point mutations in PR that confer resistance to the drugs can arise (210), allowing some virus replication in spite of therapy.

Processing of the Gag Precursor

During and after release from the cell, the Gag precursor is cleaved by the protease into a series of products present at equimolar levels in the virion. The number and size of the products vary considerably among the various viruses; the spumaretroviral Gag is exceptional in undergoing the fewest cleavages. A summary of the Gag products of some representative viruses is shown in Table 4. There are many features of these products common to most of the retroviruses.

The Matrix Protein

Beginning at the aminoterminus, most Gags are processed to form a membrane-associated or matrix protein (MA). The MA protein is thought to remain bound to the inner face of the membrane as a peripheral membrane protein, and it can be cross-linked to lipid. MA may make contacts with the cytoplasmic tail of the envelope protein. When the precursor Gag is myristylated at the aminoterminus, the corresponding MA protein retains that myristate and so is presumably bound tightly into the mem-

TABLE 4. *Virion proteins found in mature particles of various retroviruses*

Protein	ALV	MLV	MMTV	MPMV	HTLV-1	HIV	HFV
MA	p19	p15	p10	p10	p19/15	p17	—
?	p10	p12	p21	p24	—	—	—
CA	p27	p30	p27	p27	p24	p24	p33
NC	p12	p10	p14	p14	p12	p7	—
DU	—	—	p30	—	p15	—	—
PR	p15	p14	p13	?	p14	p14	p10
RT	αβ	p80	?	?	?	p66/51	p80
IN	pp32	p46	?	?	?	p31	p40
SU	gp85	gp70	gp52	gp70	gp60	gp120	gp130
TM	gp37	p15E	gp36	gp22	gp30	gp40	gp48

ALV, avian leukemia virus; MLV, murine leukemia virus; MMTV, mouse mammary tumor virus; MPMV, Mason-Pfizer monkey virus; HTLV-1, human T-lymphotropic virus type 1; HIV, human immunodeficiency virus; HFV, human foamy virus.

Proteins: MA, matrix; CA, capsid; NC, nucleocapsid; DU, deoxyuridine triphosphatase; PR, protease; RT, reverse transcriptase; IN, integrase; SU, surface; TM, transmembrane.

brane. The compact structure of the MPMV MA protein has been elucidated by NMR (136,473). The MA proteins of HIV-1 and SIV have been shown to form trimers in crystallization studies (56,595) and can contribute to the ability of a larger Gag precursor to form trimers in solution (500). The protein can form extended sheets of trimers, with a large opening in the network. If similar structures were to form in a sphere, the surface could have openings into which the envelope tail may fit.

The Capsid Protein

Gag proteins are cleaved to generate a large product serving as the major capsid protein (CA) in the virion core. The CA protein is relatively well conserved among Gags and contains the only highly conserved motif among Gags, the major homology region (MHR). The function of this motif remains uncertain; although mutations in the region affect virion assembly in some viruses (145,458,685), it is not absolutely required for this process, as the entire CA domain of ASLV can be deleted without blocking assembly. CA is thought to form the shell of the condensed inner core of the mature virus, and thus it makes either a spherical, a cylindrical, or a conical structure, depending on the virion morphology. The protein has proved difficult to crystallize, and the structure of the complete protein is uncertain (495), but the structures of both the N-terminal and C-terminal fragments of the HIV-1 CA have been determined (261,272). Very recently, the analogous structures of the RSV capsid (393) and of the EIAV CA protein (345) have been determined and used to model a structure of the virion core. The CA protein can form dimers in solution, and recombinant proteins containing CA, or CA plus NC, can assemble to form higher-order structures consisting of either tubes, spheres, or, in the case of HIV-1, cones (262). CA has also been studied after tethering sheets of the protein to membrane (48). Image reconstruction of electron micrographs, coupled to the subdomain structures, have led to models for the packing of CA to form these large assemblies. The major CA-CA contacts must form after processing during the condensation of the virion core, and they may be very different from any contacts that exist in the immature virion particle (211).

The Nucleocapsid Protein

All Gag proteins except for those of the spumaviruses are cleaved to produce a nucleocapsid protein, NC, located near the carboxyl terminus of the precursor. NC proteins are small, highly basic proteins containing one or two copies of the Cys-His motif, Cys-X2-Cys-X4-His-X4-Cys. These sequences bind a single Zn^{2+} ion avidly, and they fold around the ion into a characteristic structure that is smaller and rather different from the better-known zinc-finger structure. The structures of NC proteins in solution have been studied by NMR, which revealed a tightly folded knuckle with disordered flanking sequences (389,499). The interaction with zinc results in the incorporation of substantial levels of Zn^{2+} into all retrovirus virion particles (67).

The NC protein in virions is closely associated with the viral RNA, probably coating the entire RNA molecule; the stoichiometry of binding is such that each NC molecule can bind to about six nucleotides of RNA. NC proteins bind nonspecifically to heteropolymeric single-stranded nucleic acid with moderate affinity (728). However, NCs also exhibit specificity. Tests of binding to nucleic acids of defined sequence have shown that NCs bind poorly to poly(A), and most tightly to nucleic acids containing GT dinucleotides, especially alternating (GT)n polymers (239). In addition, NC has been shown to exhibit sequence-specific binding activity *in vitro* for nucleic acids containing the Psi region, required for packaging of the viral RNA (62,123). The interaction can also be assayed in reconstructed systems in yeast via the so-called three-hybrid method (40,412). This binding presumably reflects at least some aspect of its role in packaging the genome. A specific complex of the HIV-1 NC with a stem-loop derived from Psi has been studied by NMR, and the resulting structure shows a number of specific contacts between hydrophobic residues of NC and bases in the four-nucleotide loop, and between basic residues and specific phosphates in the stem and loop (165).

NC proteins change the base-pairing properties of nucleic acids and thus can have profound effects on the kinetics and thermodynamics of annealing (166,720). Under various conditions *in vitro*, NC can stimulate the dimerization of RNAs, and duplex formation between tRNA and its complementary sequences at the pbs (81). Thus, NC can help promote primer tRNA placement during virion assembly (603). NC can also help melt out secondary structures, and it may facilitate the movement of RT along the template during reverse transcription (775). In addition, it is clear that NC can bind to double-stranded nucleic acid, and thus it is probably retained on the viral DNA after its synthesis by RT. NC mutants have been found that affect the course of DNA synthesis or DNA stability during the early stages of virus infection, suggesting a role in the processing of the DNA and protection of DNA from degradation (282,699). Finally, NC has been shown to promote the concerted integration of the two termini of the viral DNA into a target sequence (see earlier, and ref. 109).

An important class of inhibitors of virus infectivity and replication that act by targeting the NC protein has been identified (615,725). These compounds, disulfide-substituted benzamides (DIBAs), eject the zinc ion from NC and cross-link the cysteines via disulfide bonds. Virions treated with these compounds are potently inactivated without disrupting the virion structure, and the course of virion assembly in infected cells is similarly blocked

(531,601,629,727). Drug-resistant variants are not readily recovered.

Other Gag Products

Some retroviral Gag proteins, including those of the alpha-, beta-, and gammaretroviruses, contain one or more poorly conserved domains of 10 to 24 kd lying between MA and CA. The functions of these proteins is unclear. The ASLV p2 protein, the MuLV p12 protein, and the MPMV p24 protein contain a PPPY motif that plays an important role in late stages of virion assembly (see earlier). The MuLV p12 protein has also been shown to play a role in the early stages of infection (146,793).

In the lentiviruses, a p6 domain is present at the carboxyl terminus. The role of p6 is unclear, although it contains the L domain and thus may be important in virion release; it also is required to mediate the incorporation of Vpr into virion particles, perhaps by providing a direct docking site. Proteins can be targeted to virions by generating Vpr-X fusions, which are incorporated into lentiviral virions in a p6-dependent manner.

Processing of the Gag-Pro-Pol Precursor

At the same time that the Gag precursors are cleaved during virion maturation, the Pro and Pol region of the Gag-Pro-Pol precursor is also cleaved, giving rise to the PR, RT, and IN products. The Pro and Pol–containing precursors of different viruses are cleaved in diverse patterns (Fig. 17). In the gammaretroviruses, the Pol region is processed by complete digestion to form PR, RT, and IN (321,701). In the alpharetroviruses, the Pol region is cleaved to produce a heterodimeric RT with a larger β subunit and a smaller α subunit. The larger β subunit contains both RT and IN domains. It is not clear whether the IN domain in the context of this subunit performs an important function, although it is responsible for a weak nuclease activity associated with RT (277). A portion of the Pol precursor undergoes an additional cleavage to produce the α subunit of RT, an aminoterminal fragment of the β subunit, and the separate IN protein. In the lentiviruses, Pol is processed to give rise to PR, a heterodimeric RT, and IN. However, the RT of these viruses is not identical to the heterodimeric RT of the alpharetroviruses. Here, the IN domain is fully removed from RT. One RT subunit remains intact (for HIV-1, this is the p66 subunit), and the other subunit undergoes an additional cleavage to remove a carboxyl-terminal domain (to form the p51 subunit). The functional significance of the different subunit structures of these various RTs is unclear, as they all perform a very similar set of reactions during virus replication. The processing of Pol precursors may be associated with the activation of the DNA polymerase of RT. In the alpharetroviruses, the immature Gag-Pol protein has very low DNA polymerase activity, and its maturation results in a large increase in activity (144,679). However, the immature Gag-Pol protein of MuLV and HIV-1 has high DNA polymerase activity, and there is only a very modest increase upon maturation (147).

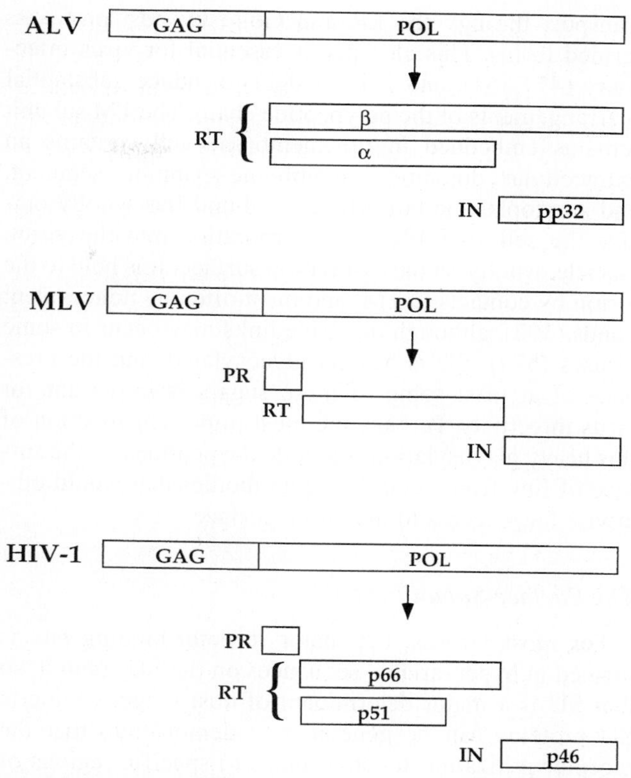

FIG. 17. Cleavage patterns during the processing of the Gag-Pol fusion proteins of various retroviruses. The structure of the mature cleavage products found in the virion particles are shown aligned with their location in the precursor.

The Gag-Pro-Pol precursor of the betaretroviruses and the nonprimate lentiviruses is also processed to produce the dUTPase protein, DU. In the betaretroviruses, the *pro* ORF encodes both DU and PR; in the nonprimate lentiviruses, the enzyme is encoded in the *pol* ORF, and DU lies in between RT and IN in the polyprotein. This enzyme acts to reduce the levels of dUTP that could otherwise be incorporated into viral DNA. Mutants of FIV lacking the function indeed show increased rates of mutation during replication (417), and similar mutants of CAEV tend to accumulate G-to-A substitution mutations (726), presumably as a result of incorporation of deoxyuridine (dU) residues that are subsequently read as deoxythymidine (dT). The FIV enzyme has been crystallized, and the structure of the protein has been determined by x-ray diffraction (583).

Processing of the Env Precursor

The major proteolytic cleavage of the Env protein to form the SU and TM subunits is performed during its transport through the ER and Golgi by host proteases termed furins. This cleavage is essential for virus infectivity (477,564), and it is thought to induce substantial rearrangements of the polypeptide chain. The TM subunit remains embedded in the membrane and contains an extracellular domain, a membrane-spanning segment, and a cytoplasmic tail. The SU subunit lies wholly outside the cell, and after its incorporation into the virion particle, wholly on the extravirion surface. It is held to the virion by contacts to TM, and most often by noncovalent bonds (302), although disulfide links may occur in some viruses (574). SU is heavily glycosylated, and the presence of at least some of these sugars is important for virus infectivity. Perhaps the most important function of this heavy glycosylation is to hide the peptides on the surface of Env from neutralizing antibodies that would otherwise have access to the virion surface.

The Surface Subunit (SU)

For most viruses, the major receptor-binding site is located in hypervariable sequences on the SU subunit, so that SU is a major determinant of host range. Chimeric SU proteins can be generated to demonstrate that the receptor utilization function maps to specific regions of the protein. The key regions of the avian Env proteins have been similarly defined by selecting for changes in host range *in vivo*; these studies show that very small changes can result in the use of new receptors (704). The structures of two SU proteins have been recently determined at high resolution: a fragment of MuLV SU (225), and a fragment of the HIV-1 SU bound to its receptor CD4 (405,618). These structures suggest that the receptors make contacts to the envelope in shallow pockets that may not be readily bound by antibodies.

The Transmembrane Subunit (TM)

The TM subunit contains the so-called fusion peptide at its aminoterminus, and TM is thought to play the major role in fusion of the virion and host membrane (167,251,303,308,639). Many TM mutations are defective for membrane fusion (189,805). However, mutations blocking fusion can lie in SU as well (796). The entire Env protein probably acts as a unified machine to mediate fusion, with complex interactions between the subunits (155), and with major movements of the subunits during the process of fusion. The fusion peptide of TM may simply insert into the host membrane, or it may make contacts to proteins. The major contacts for oligomer formation of Env are thought to lie in TM (203); isolated TM proteins form trimers in solution (227) and in crystals (225,226,387,454). The trimer is held together by a modified leucine zipper motif that bridges the monomers via hydrophobic interactions. This zipper region is crucial for virus infectivity (422,594,757).

It is possible to separate the two major functions of the Env protein onto two different molecules that cooperate to mediate these steps. Thus, the receptor binding function can be mediated by one Env protein, and the membrane fusion function can be mediated by another Env. This is apparent in the ability of two Env proteins to complement in mixed oligomers (602,802). It is also demonstrated by the ability of a wild-type Env to provide the membrane fusion function for a chimeric Env that on its own can mediate only cell surface binding.

The TM subunit of the MuLVs undergoes a second cleavage during virion assembly (359) that is mediated by the viral protease, PR. This step removes a short sequence called p2E, or the R peptide, from the carboxyl terminus of TM (289). The cleavage step may require presentation of the tail to the protease, or some conformational change in the tail, that is mediated by Gag proteins; alterations in the MA or p12 Gag proteins can modulate the cleavage of TM (377,793). Astonishingly, the cleavage is necessary to activate the fusogenic activity of the envelope protein and thus for virus entry (94,600). Mutants in which the tail is truncated at the site of cleavage are constitutively activated for fusion, and these viruses induce dramatic syncytia in receptor-positive cells. Mutants in which the tail is not removed are inhibited for fusion, and particular residues can be shown to be required (779). How the cytoplasmic tail inhibits the fusogenic activity of Env is very much unclear.

In a similar way, the cytoplasmic tails of the TM of MPMV (670) and EIAV (614) are processed by the protease. In the case of MPMV, the presence of the intact tail is necessary for efficient incorporation of Env into the virion. The majority of the retroviruses, however, do not carry out cleavage of TM, and for these viruses an intact tail is needed for infectivity (190). The replication of some viruses in host cells of foreign species can select for alterations and truncations of the TM tails (388,614,657). The selective advantage conferred by this truncation is not well understood, although various aspects of Env function seem to be enhanced by this truncation (806).

Morphologic Changes upon Virion Maturation

The maturation of retrovirus particles is a complex process that is required for the formation of an infectious virus. The particles that are initially assembled either at the plasma membrane (by most retroviruses) or in the cytoplasm (by the betaretroviruses) have a characteristic immature morphology: The particles are round and stain with an electron-dense ring and a relatively electron-lucent center. After release from the cell, the morphology changes to a more condensed structure, with a central core largely detached from the surrounding envelope. In the alpha-, gamma-, and deltaretroviruses, the core is spherical and concentric with the envelope; in the betaretroviruses, the core is spherical but eccentrically placed within the envelope; in the lentiviruses, the core is cylindrical or conical, with thin connections to the surrounding shell. In the spumaviruses, the morphology does not change dramatically after assembly.

Mutant viruses lacking the protease show little change in morphology. Thus, cleavage of Gag and Gag-Pol is required for the restructuring of the virion into the mature form (363). The changes in morphology visible in electron micrographs are probably associated with major rearrangements of the Gag proteins. Indeed, the physical properties of the virus change dramatically upon maturation. Whereas the immature core is quite stable to nonionic detergents and harsh conditions, the mature virion core is relatively labile. This change may reflect the inability of the immature virion, and the acquired ability of the mature virion, to uncoat upon infection of new cells and initiate reverse transcription.

RETROVIRAL DISEASES

The Varied Effects of Retroviral Infection

Retroviruses cause an extremely wide range of responses in infected animal hosts. The discussion of retroviral pathogenesis will begin with a little-appreciated but important point: Retroviruses in general are surprisingly benign. The vast majority of the replication-competent retroviruses are not cytopathic, and the infection of cells causes remarkably little impact on their replication or physiology. The morphology, the control of cell division, and the doubling time of cells in culture are not significantly changed after infection. Once a chronic infection is established, only a relatively small amount of the cellular metabolism is committed to virus expression: Typically, a small percentage of the cellular mRNA and protein is viral, and so the cell can perform its normal functions and survive for its normal lifespan. Indeed, animals show few acute affects upon infection. The animals do become viremic, and a vigorous immune response is often mounted that can reduce the levels of virus production. However, infected mice or birds may live relatively normal lives for many months or years, and so it is appropriate to consider the viruses as relatively benign parasites. It is noteworthy that the virus is not eliminated but only suppressed by the immune response, and low-level viremia usually persists in infected animals for life.

Retroviruses often do, however, cause disease. The chronic viremia of the replication-competent retroviruses is tantamount to high-level mutagenesis of the infected cells, for each infection event is associated with a proviral insertion that constitutes a mutation. Eventually, the odds are that a cell will suffer an insertion that alters the normal control of cell division or cell survival, and abnormal proliferation of this cell results in tumorigenesis. Many retroviruses cause disease in this way, including the so-called slow leukemia viruses and agents such as MMTV. A few retroviruses, however, are more pathogenic: A small minority of the retroviruses are directly cytopathic, and many of the infected cells are killed. These agents can thus destroy the infected tissues and directly impair their function. These include the cytopathic avian viruses and, probably, the AIDS virus, HIV-1. Finally, a special class of retroviruses exists, the so-called acute transforming viruses, that can induce a rapid tumor formation. These viruses were among the first filterable oncogenic agents ever discovered, and their dramatic effects were a major motivation for the intense study of all the tumor viruses throughout the 20th century. We now understand that these agents are transducing viruses; the replication of retroviruses allows recombination events between viral and host sequences that move genes onto the viral genome. These viruses carry and express host genes at inappropriate levels, in inappropriate cells, and often with drastic alterations in gene structure. If the gene product so expressed by the virus is mitogenic or antiapoptotic, the result can be a potent alteration in the physiology of the infected cell. These acute transforming viruses can thus initiate a highly aggressive tumor very efficiently and with minimal latency, because each infection of a cell has the high potential to initiate an oncogenic transformation event. Most often, the acquisition of the host gene comes with a loss of a viral gene essential for its replication; as a result, these viruses are often replication-defective and depend on a helper virus, usually a replication-competent leukemia virus, for their transmission to new cells. Each of these various classes of pathogenic viruses will be discussed in turn.

Diseases Caused by the Replication-Competent Retroviruses

The typical pathology of many of the simple replication-competent retroviruses is the development of leukemia or lymphoma after a very long latency. For this reason, these agents are often called the slow leukemia viruses. Examples are found in rodents, including the many MuLVs, and in birds, including the avian leukemia-leukosis viruses. The symptoms eventually begin with a lymphoid hyperplasia (681), which may be directly attributed to the immune response; not all the affected cells are infected, and the proliferating cells may be stimulated by cytokines that are released in response to the infection (93). These cells may include a preleukemic state of partially transformed cells (164). There may be some cell killing resulting from enhanced apoptosis in these early times (82), although the mechanism of the apoptosis and the relationship to tumorigenesis is unclear. A subset of these expanding cells progress to frank leukemia, which ultimately can be fatal in susceptible animals. These observations strongly suggest that leukemogenesis is a multistep phenomenon, and it is also likely that the virus plays a role in more than one of these steps (221). The cell type transformed by the virus can be very narrowly defined, or more broadly variable, but will depend strongly on viral determinants. For example, the ASLV group of viruses typically cause a bursal or B-cell lymphoma in birds; the MMLV causes a T-cell leukemia; the Friend helper MuLV causes an erythroleukemia; MMTV causes a mammary epithelial tumor.

In some species and settings, the infecting virus is the proximal agent of disease; such is the case with infection of rats by the MMLV. However, the course of leukemogenesis in mice and other animals is often associated with the appearance of recombinant retroviruses derived from the parental infecting virus and endogenous sequences present in the germline (114,218,471). The recombinant viruses are often the true or proximal pathogens. These viruses are heterogeneous in structure and phenotype, but most contain substitutions of the *env* gene and LTR that confer novel properties to the initial virus (172). Some of the viruses arising in mice can be detected through an expanded host range, as an ecotropic virus acquires *env* sequences that allow infection through the xenotropic or dual-tropic receptors; these viruses are the MCF viruses (312). The range of cell types and the replication ability of the input virus can be expanded by recombination to significantly enhance the incidence of leukemia and shorten the latency period to disease. The donor sequences for these recombination events are not all universally present in a given species but are highly variable from strain to strain (16,407,592). The presence or absence of suitable endogenous proviruses in the germline that provide the sequences needed for recombination can control the severity and course of disease.

Leukemogenesis by Insertional Activation

The most common mechanism of action of the replication-competent viruses in initiating tumors is termed proviral insertional mutagenesis, and it leads to the activation of endogenous proto-oncogenes (300,516,559). During replication in the infected animal, an enormous number of cells are infected and so acquire new proviral DNA insertions at near-random sites. Each of these insertions constitutes a somatic mutation, and thus retrovirus infection can be thought of as similar to a massive exposure to a potent mutagen. The vast majority of the insertions are harmless, causing no significant change in host gene expression, and the majority of those that do disrupt genes simply create a recessive mutation at one allele out of two present in the cell, again causing no significant change in the overall pattern of gene expression. But very rarely, a provirus insertion can create a dominant-acting mutation that profoundly alters the physiology of the cell. When a provirus integrates near a gene that controls growth and so alters its expression, the cell may proliferate and ultimately form a clonal tumor in which all cells contain the provirus integrated at the same site.

A large number of cellular genes have been identified as potential targets for insertional activation in retrovirus-induced tumors. Among the most notable are an array of transcription factors, including *c-myc, N-myc, c-myb, Fli1, Fli2, Ets1 (Tpl1), Evi1 (Fim3), Bmi1 (Flvi2),* and *Spi1* (PU.1); a number of secreted growth factors, such as *Wnt1 (Int1), Wnt3 (Int4), Int2 (Fgf3),* and *Fgf8;* growth factor receptors, including *c-erbB, Int3 (Notch4), Mis6 (Notch1), c-fms (Fim2),* the prolactin receptor, and Fit1; and genes implicated in intracellular signal transduction pathways, such as the serine/threonine kinases *Pim1* and *Pim2.* Many of these genes are also known to be involved in or implicated in tumorigenesis in other settings, either when transduced on retroviral genomes or when activated by more conventional mutations. However, a number of the proto-oncogenes have only been identified by virtue of their having served as target sites during tumorigenesis by leukemia viruses, and thus this route has made important contributions to our list of known proto-oncogenes. Many of these genes would not have been obvious candidates to control cell division or transform cells, such as the translation initiation factor eIF3 (35).

The patterns of activation of these proto-oncogenes by retroviral insertion are quite varied. At least four distinct mechanisms have been observed (Fig. 18).

1. Promoter insertion. The provirus may insert upstream of the gene or within the gene, and in the same transcriptional orientation as the gene. Transcription beginning in the 3′ LTR reads into the gene and results in high-level expression of a transcript with R-U5 sequences at the 5′ end. The resulting transcripts may be similar to the natural transcripts, but they may be longer or truncated relative to the normal mRNAs.
2. Enhancer insertion. The provirus may insert either upstream or downstream of the gene, and in either orientation relative to the gene. The insertion brings the powerful transcriptional enhancers present in the U3 regions of the two LTRs into close proximity of the gene, and so activates the endogenous promoter elements. Although the levels are inappropriately high, the structure of the resulting transcript is normal.
3. Posttranscriptional stimulation of expression. The provirus may insert downstream of the coding region and stabilize the formation of an mRNA. The provirus may provide a polyadenylation signal that enhances the formation of stable transcripts, or the insertion may remove RNA destabilization signals in the 3′ UTR that would normally mediate the rapid turnover of the RNA. These mechanisms can result in inappropriately high steady-state levels of the mRNA and protein products.
4. Readthrough transcription. The provirus inserts upstream or in the gene, but transcription initiates in the 5′ LTR, reads through the provirus, and continues into the gene. The formation of such transcripts is

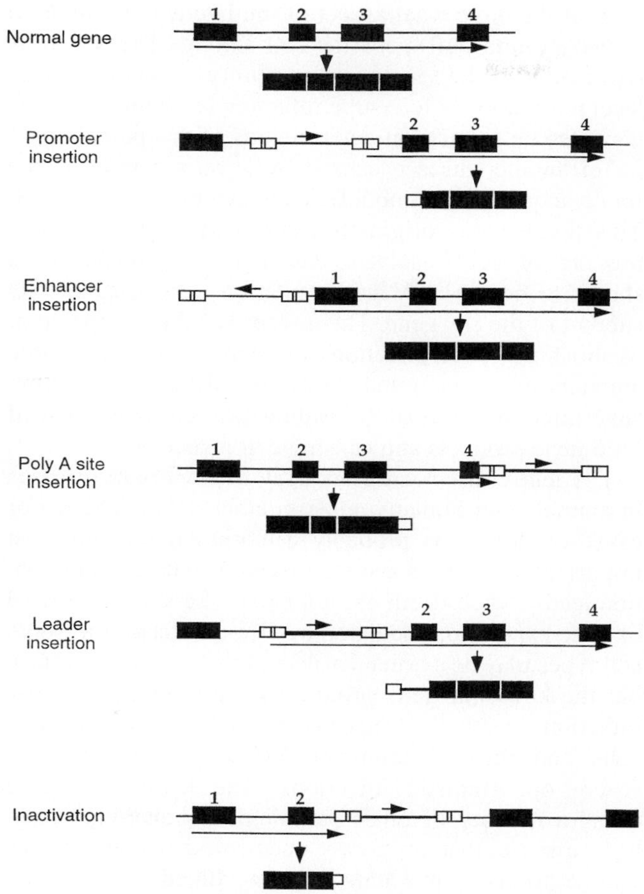

FIG. 18. Genetic alterations in target gene expression induced by retroviral insertional mutagenesis. Various changes in normal gene expression that have been observed upon insertion of retroviral DNA are diagrammed. A target gene containing four exons is used in these examples (*top*). *Promoter insertion:* Insertion of the provirus in the same transcriptional orientation in the first intron is shown to result in the formation of a new mRNA initiated in the 3′ LTR and extending into the downstream exons. *Enhancer insertion:* Insertion upstream of the gene, in this case in reverse orientation, is shown enhancing the expression from the natural promoter. *Poly(A) site insertion:* Insertion at the 3′ end of the gene in the forward orientation is shown providing a poly(A) addition signal and thereby increasing the levels of a prematurely truncated mRNA. *Leader insertion:* Insertion of the provirus in the same transcriptional orientation is shown to result in the formation of an RNA initiating in the 5′ LTR, extending through the provirus and into downstream exons. Splicing results in the retention of only the viral leader on the chimeric mRNA. *Inactivation:* Insertion is shown causing premature end formation of the mRNA, resulting in the formation of an inactive fragment.

often enhanced by mutations in the provirus, such as loss of the 3′ LTR. The transcripts may be spliced aberrantly in complex patterns.

Insertional activation of a proto-oncogene by a provirus is not sufficient on its own to fully transform a cell but represents only one step in a progression to a frank leukemia or tumor. Other mutations are usually required; these mutations can be point mutations in other proto-oncogenes or loss of function mutations of tumor suppressor genes. In some retroviral tumors, more than one oncogene can be activated by insertion of separate proviruses. Similarly, an acute transforming genome is usually not sufficient to transform a cell in one step, and additional mutations must arise. In some tumors induced by a replication-defective transforming virus, the helper virus may provide such mutations by its own insertional activation event (576).

Gene inactivation, as opposed to gene activation, is also an important event in some tumors. Retrovirus insertion can frequently disrupt gene expression to effectively produce a null or hypomorphic mutation (see Fig. 18). These mutations are normally silent, as a second allele would be expected to continue to express a functional gene product. However, if the host animal is already heterozygous due to an inherited germline mutation in one allele, or if the insertional inactivation is coupled to a loss of the other allele by other means, the net result can be homozygous loss of function. When the target gene is a tumor suppressor, the consequence is the promotion of tumorigenesis.

Viral Determinants of Pathogenicity

Several viral genes and sequences can affect the incidence and severity of retroviral disease. The viral LTR contains the most important determinants of leukemogenicity and of the cell tropism for transformation. The enhancer and promoter elements of the LTR are responsible for proto-oncogene activation, and their relative transcriptional activity thus controls the transforming ability of many viruses (220,222,276,335). If these elements are strongly tissue or cell type specific, the virus will be most competent for transformation of those cells in which the LTR is most active. A variety of viruses show profound tropisms for transformation that are controlled in this way (36,84,438,541). For example, the promoter of the MMLV is most active in T cells, and the virus shows strong tropism for the formation of T-cell leukemias. The Friend helper virus LTR contains an enhancer that is most active in erythroid cells, and the virus is correspondingly highly tropic for erythroid cells (86). The promoter of MMTV contains glucocorticoid response elements that provide high-level expression only in cells with high levels of the glucocorticoid receptor and only when exposed to glucocorticoids; as a result, MMTV is specific for mammary tumors (291). Variant betaretroviruses, such as the thymotropic DMBA-LV virus, show selectivity for T cells that is probably attributable to changes in the LTR (42). Determinants of leukemogenicity have also been mapped to *gag*, *pol*, and *env* genes, although in most cases it is not clear what aspects of their functions are required. It may be that vigorous replication *in vivo* is the simple key feature of a highly transforming leukemia virus. There may also be trans-acting functions encoded by the leukemia viruses that modulate expression of specific host genes (219,283). The MuLV and FeLV LTRs encode short RNAs that can trans-activate host genes, apparently through activation of an AP-1-like activity (270).

Other aspects of infection, distinct from the genetic makeup of the virus or host, can modulate the pathology associated with infection. For example, the route of entry of the virus can affect the disease course (55). Presumably, the route can determine the initial cell types infected and the route of virus spread.

Other Retroviral Diseases

Cytopathic Viruses

Some viruses show distinctive pathogenicity mediated by specific gene products. Cas-Br-E MLV is a well-studied murine virus that induces a hind-limb paralysis with significant neuronal loss in the absence of an inflammatory response (581). Both neurons and glial cells accumulate vacuoles. The virus targets endothelial cells and microglial cells (450) in the brain, and it is likely that the infection of the microglial cells is most crucial to disease induction. Infection may impair or block the neuronal support function of these cells, resulting in loss of neurons, although the mechanism of neuronal cell death is unclear. It is possible that the expression of the Env protein is toxic. The major determinant of pathogenicity is in the SU subunit of the Env protein (449,542). A number of other MuLVs, such as the ts1 mutant of the MMLV TB strain (774), can cause neurologic symptoms, including hind-limb paralysis and spongiform encephalomyelopathy (69), and in these cases too the SU protein is thought to be important (692). TR1.3, a Friend-related MuLV, is a neuropathogenic virus that induces fusion of capillary endothelial cells, leading to a hemorrhagic stroke syndrome (545). The crucial determinant in the virus is a tryptophan residue at position 102 of the SU protein (120,546). In some viruses the LTR is also likely to play a role in disease induction (169,543), perhaps by determining the level of expression and the ability to spread efficiently and access the primary target cell.

A number of the ASLV group of viruses are cytopathic (756) and can cause an acute wasting disease characterized by poor growth, anemia, and immunosuppression associated with atrophy of the bursa and thymus (607). The disease probably reflects the ability of these viruses to lyse infected cells (375,756). Recently, the isolation of the ALV receptor for the subgroup B viruses and its identification as a member of the TNF receptor family suggests the possibility that the binding of Env to the receptor is directly triggering an apoptotic response. The cytopathic and the noncytopathic viruses both seem to be able to trigger similar responses, however, so that it is not clear at this time what aspect of the interaction might be necessary and sufficient for cell killing. The vigorous replication of the virus, and an ability to mediate high-level reinfection before superinfection resistance appears, may also be significant determinants of cytopathology.

Yet another disease caused by a variant virus is the feline acquired immunodeficiency syndrome, or FAIDS. This disease was originally associated with a complex mixture of FeLV isolates. The agent responsible was shown to be an FeLV with mutations affecting the SU subunit of the *env* gene. The mutant FeLV is incapable of establishing superinfection resistance, and so large amounts of unintegrated viral DNA accumulate during superinfection, ultimately leading to high expression of viral gene products and causing cell lysis.

The lentiviruses cause an array of important diseases in animals and humans, most notably AIDS. The major cause of disease is probably cell killing, but the most important target cells and the mechanism by which infection leads to cell death are not clear. The very high level of gene expression mediated by HIV-1 infection in some cell types may be a crucial aspect of the cell killing (668), but the key viral gene products remain obscure. HIV-1 infection eventually leads to depletion of CD4-positive cells and thus to immunodeficiency, culminating in severe opportunistic infections. The lentiviruses also cause a number of other pathologies, including neurologic disease, that are poorly understood. These diseases will be discussed in *Fields Virology*, 4th ed.

Stimulation of Host Cell Proliferation

MMTVs lead to the formation of mammary tumors through the insertional activation of a number of proto-oncogenes. However, unlike other simple retroviruses, MMTVs carry an additional gene termed *sag*, for superantigen, that is important for disease induction (see ref. 129 for review). Sag proteins bind to MHC class II molecules in regions that are common to molecules with many different binding specificities, and so they can activate as many as 10% of all T cells. The *sag* gene is located in the U3 region of the MMTV LTR and encodes a low-abundance glycosylated membrane protein (91). The protein must be proteolytically processed for proper export to the cell surface (547). Importantly, expression of a functional Sag protein by MMTV is required to establish infection in an animal. The virus is normally transmitted in mother's milk to newborn mice, infects B cells in the Peyer's patch, and induces a vigorous Sag-mediated stimulation of T cells. There follows a B-cell response that provides a large pool of susceptible B cells for the virus (26), and it is these cells that then carry the virus to the mammary gland. The infection of the mammary epithelial cells ultimately leads to transformation of these cells by insertional activation. This pattern of viral spread through one intermediate cell type, ultimately leading to disease in another cell type, is a paradigm for complex viral pathologies, such as that exhibited by polioviruses.

The *sag* gene of MMTV was also appreciated as acting as a host gene important in disease progression when a number of mouse genes, termed Mls for minor lymphocyte-stimulating antigen, were shown to map to endogenous MMTV proviruses, and were ultimately identified as the *sag* genes. The expression of Mls results in the clonal deletion of many T cells in mice carrying the gene (2). Thus, mice carrying endogenous proviruses will often lose T cells needed for virus replication, and so will be resistant to exogenous MMTV disease.

A number of other viruses carry variants of the normal replication genes that cause specific pathologies in the infected host. One spleen focus-forming virus, SFFV-P, causes a severe polycythemia; infection leads to a massive expansion of erythroid precursors (BFU-E and CFU-E) and a concomitant loss of mature red cells. This agent consists of a complex of a replication-defective variant and a Friend MuLV helper virus to propagate it. The defective genomes carry a mutant *env* gene encoding a shorter SU molecule, termed gp55, that no longer functions to mediate virus entry. However, gp55 can bind directly to the erythropoietin receptor (EpoR) and stimulate the mitogenic and differentiative responses normally triggered by ligand binding to the receptor. This activity allows the virus to infect these dividing pre-erythroid cells, and the continued expression of the envelope protein in these cells promotes their factor-independent growth and expansion in an autocrine loop (632). Ultimately, a frank erythroleukemia results and may be associated with proviral activation of proto-oncogenes occurring as a result of the continuing infections. It is clear that the *env* gene of the virus is sufficient to cause the disease (773). A very similar virus, the SFFV-A, causes a severe splenomegaly and anemia. This virus is closely related to SFFV-P and also activates the EpoR to expand immature cells. Variation in the envelope between these two strains alters the target cell and the consequences of its expansion (354,631). It should be noted that this mitogenic activity of gp55 is not a completely novel property of the deleted Env. The parental F-MuLV helper Env protein has a weak ability to bind and send mitogenic signals through the EpoR, presumably resulting in expansion of EpoR-positive cells. This increase in target cell number is presumably able to enhance virus spread and so serves as a positively selected trait for the virus. Other Env proteins, including those of the MCF viruses, may activate the interleukin 2 (IL-2) receptor.

Another replication-defective variant, the murine acquired immune deficiency syndrome or MAIDS virus, causes a relatively acute hyperproliferation of B-lineage cells in infected mice (38,327,381). There is a subsequent proliferation of macrophages and CD4+ T cells. The expansion of these cells displaces many other cell types, including T cells, and the animals eventually show a significantly defective immune response. The mechanism of the immunodeficiency is not fully clear, and there is some indication that an antigen-driven stimulation leads to an anergic state. However the immunosuppression occurs, the disease is in reality a lymphoproliferative disorder and is quite distinct from human AIDS in its pathology. The causative agent is again a replication-defective variant carried by a replication-competent helper virus (326). The defective genome encodes a mutant Gag precursor in which the central portion, including the p12 region, is replaced by a foreign Gag derived from endogenous retrovirus sequences (325,398,399). The altered Gag has been shown to interact with the c-Abl protein, a tyrosine kinase first identified as the transduced oncogene of the Abelson MuLV, in that virus expressed as a Gag-Abl fusion protein. Thus, the MAIDS virus seems to act by forming a noncovalent interaction with the c-Abl protein as an approximate mimic of the Gag-Abl protein formed by transduction on the Abelson virus (191).

An ovine disease has recently attracted attention as a potential model for human lung cancer. Sheep pulmonary adenomatosis (SPA) is a contagious bronchiolo-alveolar carcinoma of sheep associated with an exogenous type D/B retrovirus, Jaagsiekte sheep retrovirus (JSRV) (785). The etiology of the disease is unclear, although the epithelial tumor cells are sites of large amounts of viral DNA (537).

Two of the epsilonretroviruses, the piscine (fish) retroviruses, cause a dermal sarcoma that shows a remarkable seasonal appearance and regression. The mechanism of transformation of cells by the virus is not totally clear, but it seems to reflect the activity of a cyclin D homolog encoded by the viral genome. This gene, the *ORF a* gene, may induce inappropriate entry of the cells into cycle by activation of a cyclin-dependent kinase (cdk).

Host Determinants of Retroviral Disease

A number of genes have been identified that determine sensitivity or resistance to retroviral diseases. Some of these genes act at the level of virus replication, directly controlling the ability of the virus to spread. The Fv1 locus is a good example of a gene that acts in a cell-autonomous way to restrict the replication of various MuLVs (348). Fv1 was identified in the early 1970s as mediating resistance to leukemogenesis by the Friend MuLV (424,571). Two naturally occurring alleles provide resistance: the $Fv1^b$ allele (in Balb/c mice) allows replication of B-tropic viruses but blocks N-tropic viruses, whereas the $Fv1^n$ allele (in NIH Swiss mice) allows replication of N-tropic viruses but blocks B-tropic viruses. Resistance is dominant in heterozygous animals. The tropism of the MuLVs can be characterized by their ability to replicate in cells of particular genotypes: N-tropic viruses grow only on $Fv1^{nn}$ cells, B-tropic viruses grow only on $FV1^{bb}$ cells, and NB-tropic viruses grow on both. The determinants of viral tropism lie in the *gag* gene and affect a small sequence of the CA protein (83,315,532,626). The block to infection in resistant cells is at an interesting stage: largely, it occurs after reverse transcription and before nuclear entry and provirus integration (349,350,782). Curiously, the block to integration that is observed for a particular virus and cell combination *in vivo* is lost when the PIC is extracted and tested for its ability to integrate *in vitro* (585). Recently, the Fv1 gene was cloned and identified as a unique member of an endogenous retrovirus gene family, showing similarity to the *gag* genes of the human endogenous retrovirus (HERV)-L family (68). This family is widely distributed in mammals (58). The two alleles differ by a few point mutations and a different carboxyl-terminal region. Thus, the intracellular expression of this variant Gag protein can somehow interact with the incoming viral DNA and its associated CA protein to block infection. Another gene in this series has an even simpler mode of action: The Fv4 gene (687) restricts virus replication by blocking the receptor. The Fv4 locus is a defective endogenous provirus that encodes an Env protein fragment; the product down-regulates the receptor and renders mice resistant to infection by exogenous viruses (332,394).

A large set of those genes that affect sensitivity to viral disease modify the availability of target cells for virus growth, or the immune response to virus infection, and therefore indirectly control the levels of viremia. The Fv2 gene is an example of such a gene (423). Virus susceptibility is dominant over virus resistance at this locus. The virus-susceptible allele encodes a truncated form of the stem-cell kinase receptor (Stk) that promotes virus-induced erythroleukemia (565); expansion of the Fv2s-expressing cells may provide increased cells for virus replication. The $Fv2^{rr}$ homozygous mice are resistant because of a limited expansion of BFU-E clones and a reduced ability of the Friend MuLV to find sensitive targets (79,688). Finally, mutations in certain genes can sensitize or predispose organisms to oncogenic transformation by retroviruses. Because transformation is almost always a multistep process, mutations in one of the genes in a transforming pathway can increase the frequency with which a virus-mediated loss of another gene becomes manifest as a frank tumor. Thus, knock-out mutations of such tumor suppressors as the p53 or p73 genes can sensitize to transformation by a number of oncogenic retroviruses (53,714). Similarly, a preexisting transgene such as a regulated version of the *myc* oncogene, Eμ-Myc, can predispose particular cells expressing the gene to insertional activation of other proto-oncogenes in viremic animals (733). New integration sites that would not normally be detected in wild-type mice are often utilized in such mice.

ACUTE TRANSFORMING RETROVIRUSES: TRANSDUCTION OF CELLULAR PROTO-ONCOGENES

There exist more potent transforming retroviruses than the slow leukemia viruses, and these can initiate rapid tumor formation with a quickly fatal outcome. These viruses are recombinant transducing viruses that have acquired portions of cellular genes that are responsible for the transforming activity. The prototype of these viruses is the Rous sarcoma virus, which carries a transforming version of the c-*src* gene. In the exceptional case of RSV, the viral replication functions, including the coding regions for the Gag, Pol, and Env proteins, are all intact so that the resulting transducing genome is replication competent. In nearly all other cases, the acquisition of the transforming gene from the host has occurred with a loss of one or more of the viral replication functions, so that the resulting virus is replication defective. However, these genomes retain all the cis-acting elements needed for their replication, and thus can be transmitted from one cell to another by a replication-competent helper virus. The concerted replication of two viral genomes in a complex—a replication-competent helper virus and a replication-defective acute transforming virus—is a common feature of most of the transforming viruses.

Transforming viral genomes exhibit a range of different structures, but they have some features in common. Those segments required in cis for viral replication are always retained: The LTRs, the pbs, and the ppt are present because they are required for reverse transcription and forward transcription. The RNA packaging signals are retained. Many of the regions required in trans are often deleted, since these functions can be provided by the helper, and are replaced with the host sequences. The host gene may be expressed separately, or, more often, it is fused to Gag, Pol, or Env sequences to form a fusion protein.

The formation of a transducing virus is thought to involve a complex series of events that results in the acquisition of the coding regions of a host gene by the replication-competent parental virus (690). Several models have been proposed to account for the observed structures, including DNA-based events (e.g., see ref. 647) but more often RNA-based events (summarized in ref. 716). The most commonly accepted model includes the following steps (Fig. 19):

- The process begins with the insertion of a provirus upstream of the gene to be transduced. An insertion in the middle of a gene can initiate the transduction of the downstream portion of that gene.
- Next, readthrough transcription beginning in the 5′ LTR generates a large RNA containing viral sequences fused to downstream sequences. This event can be enhanced by lesions in the 3′ LTR that prevent normal RNA processing and polyadenylation at this site. Alternatively, a deletion in the DNA could fuse the 5′ half of the provirus to downstream sequences, again leading to the expression of a fusion RNA.
- In either mechanism, the chimeric RNA can be spliced and is then packaged into virions along with the RNA of a helper virus (307,689).

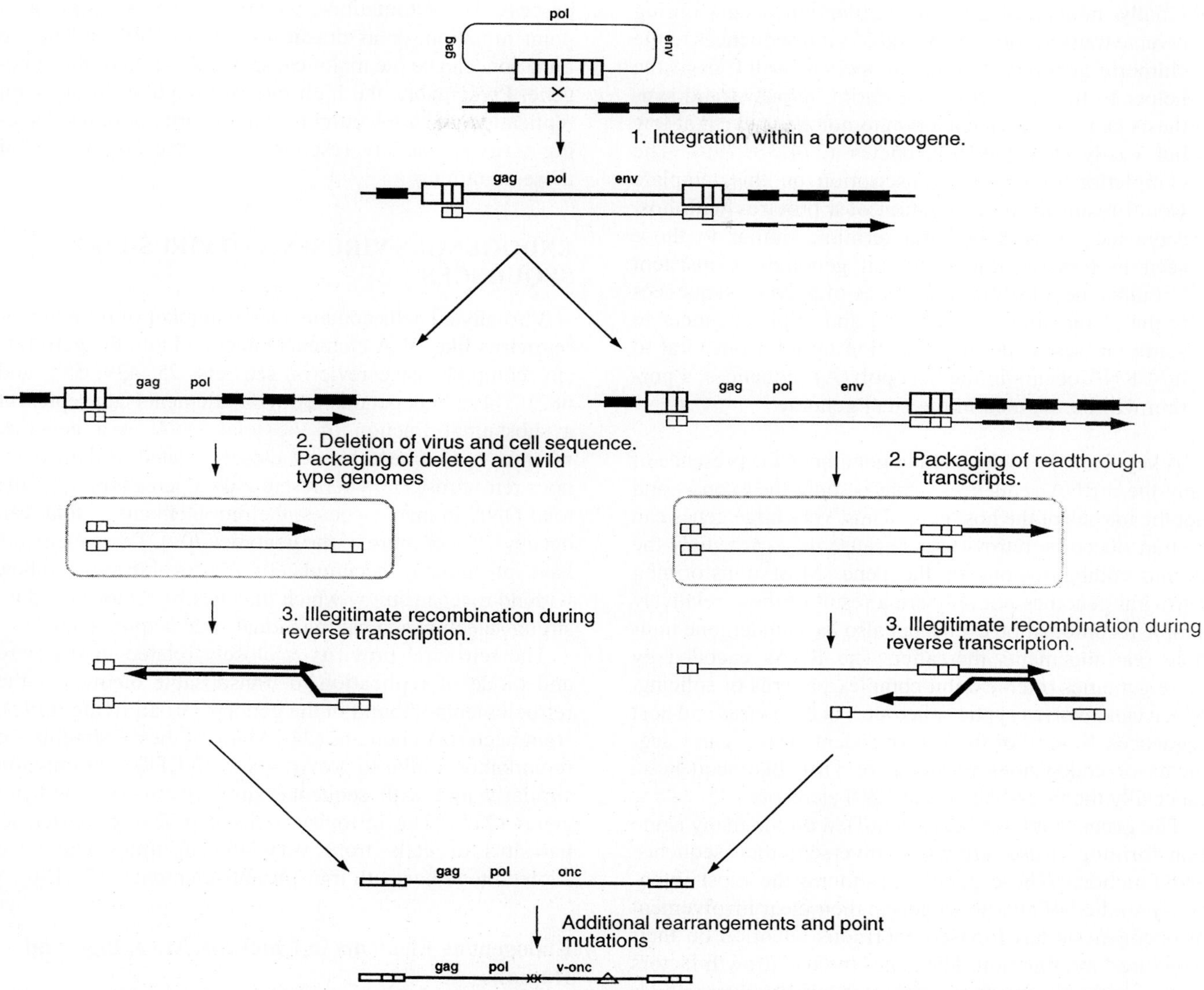

FIG. 19. Two pathways for the acquisition of host oncogenes by a replication-competent retroviruses in the formation of an acute transforming genome. Integration is shown establishing a provirus within a proto-oncogene in the same transcriptional orientation (*top*). Either of two processes then occurs. In one mechanism (*left*), a deletion of the chromosomal DNA fuses the 5′ half of the provirus to the downstream portion of the gene. The fused DNA then encodes a fused RNA, which may be spliced and packaged into virion particles along with wild-type helper RNA. During reverse transcription, RT switches from the helper to the fusion RNA to append the 3′ portion of the helper onto the hybrid RNA. The completed reverse-transcribed DNA is integrated and transmitted thereafter as a replication-defective viral genome. In the other mechanism (*right*), a readthrough RNA extending from the 5′ LTR through the provirus and into the downstream portion of the gene is formed. The RNA is packaged into virion particles along with wild-type helper RNA. During reverse transcription, RT switches from helper to host and back to helper RNAs to form the hybrid genome. As before, the completed reverse transcribed DNA is integrated and transmitted thereafter as a replication-defective viral genome. In either scenario, the transducing genome may undergo additional rearrangements and mutations under selective pressure for more efficient transforming activity and transmission.

- Finally, nonhomologous recombination occurs during reverse transcription to append 3′ viral sequences to the chimeric genome. A template switch by RT from the helper to the chimeric RNA during minus-strand synthesis can mediate such a nonhomologous event at low but easily detected frequencies (274,710,799). The completion of reverse transcription on this template would result in the generation of a provirus with host sequences flanked by viral termini, similar to those seen in transforming retroviral genomes. Consistent with this model is the appearance of poly(A) sequences at the 3′ junction between host and viral sequences in some viruses; if the translocation by RT from viral to host RNA occurs in the host poly(A) sequences, a portion will be retained in the final genome.

A key feature of the resulting genome is the presence of only the mRNA sequences—that is, only the exons—and not the introns of the host gene. Thus, very large genes can be transduced by retroviruses because they carry only the exonic coding regions of the gene. Most transforming retroviral genomes not only are a result of these relatively simple recombination events but also have undergone multiple rearrangements thereafter. The RNAs encoded by these genomes often exhibit complex patterns of splicing, which can involve cryptic splice sites in both virus and host sequences. Several of the known rodent viruses carry segments of endogenous retroviral or virus-like sequences, especially the virus-like 30S (VL30) elements.

The genes that have been identified on the many acute transforming viruses are wildly diverse in their sequence and functions. These genes are among the most intensively studied of all known genes; their clear involvement in oncogenesis has focused enormous attention on their structures and function. The genes include growth factors (v-*Sis*); growth factor receptors (v-*erbB*); intracellular tyrosine kinases (v-*src*, v-*fps*, v-*fes*, v-*abl*), members of the G protein family (H-*ras*, Ki-*ras*); transcription factors (v-*myc*, v-*erbA*); and many others. The genes are now appreciated as playing major roles in mitogenic signalling pathways, in the control of the cell cycle, and in antiapoptotic pathways that act to limit cell survival. There is no indication that all such genes have been identified, and it is likely that new transforming viruses will continue to provide new examples of genes that can be activated by transduction to initiate tumor formation.

The acquisition of these genes, as noted earlier, is often associated with fusion of the coding region to Gag, Pol, or Env sequences. Thus, the expression of the oncogene results in a fusion protein that may exhibit dramatically altered biochemical activity, intracellular localization, or stability. These changes are often a key aspect of the activation of the normal function of the proto-oncogene to create the fully transforming viral oncogene. In other cases, or in addition to these alterations, there may be specific mutations that arise during or after the transduction process. These mutations, which may be as simple as a point mutation, or as drastic as a frameshift or deletion mutation, can be the major cause of activation of the oncogene. Presumably, the high rate of mutation during viral replication and a selection for tumor formation in enhancing virus spread are responsible for the appearance of these mutations.

ENDOGENOUS VIRUSES AND VIRUS-LIKE SEQUENCES

Virtually all cells contain a large number of retroviral or retrovirus-like DNA elements integrated into the germline (for comprehensive reviews, see refs. 75, 439, 558, and 682). These endogenous retroviral elements can represent a substantial fraction of the total DNA in a genome; whereas the sequences most closely related to the exogenous retroviruses may represent only a percent or so of the total DNA in many species, the retroelements in total can occupy 10% or more of the genome (709). These elements have presumably accumulated over evolutionary times, with no mechanism by which they can be removed and no strong selection against individuals that acquire them.

The retroviral provirus is closely related in structure and mode of replication to transposable elements—the retroelements—found in the genomes of all living things, from bacteria to humans (74). Many of these elements are remarkably similar to proviruses, with LTRs that function similarly and with sequence similarity to *gag* and *pol* genes (715). The retroviruses have probably existed as parasites of cells from very ancient times and have evolved together with transposable elements (179,180).

Endogenous Elements in Chickens, Mice, Pigs, and Humans

Endogenous retroviruses have been characterized for many avian species. Large numbers of sequences have been characterized in chickens and other birds (329) and can be grouped into at least four families. The ALV-related elements were among the first to be discovered, including the replication-competent provirus RAV-0. Most of the other family members are replication defective and lack *env* sequences. The newer families of such viruses continue to be characterized (665).

There is a vast literature describing the endogenous retrovirus sequences in inbred mice (58,80,138,336,395, 683). At least eight families have been described, although only four have been studied in detail. The VL30 (for virus-like 30S) elements are present in the genome at a copy number of perhaps 100 to 200 (4); these elements encode a 30S RNA that is packaged efficiently into the virion particles of exogenous viruses and so contaminates most virion RNAs. They presumably represent a parasitic RNA that spreads by exploiting exogenous viruses. Second, the IAP elements are present at a level of about 1,000 to 2,000 copies in the genome (444,518,525). These elements can express intracellular particles containing RT, but the particles are budded into the ER and not released from cells. Most lack *env* genes and so cannot form infectious particles. However, a few members do contain *env* sequences (608). Some IAPs can transpose intracellularly at low frequencies (301). Third, there are a small number of proviruses (0 to 4 per genome) closely related to MMTV that encode functional B-type viruses. Fourth, there are proviruses related to the exogenous MuLVs, present at 50 to 100 copies per genome (683). These proviruses are all very similar to one another, but they can be divided (according to their similarity to exogenous viruses that utilize particular receptors) into four groups: the ecotropic, xenotropic, polytropic, and modified polytropic. The distribution of these sequences among different murine species and subspecies can help reveal their evolution and spread. For example, xenotropic MLV-related proviruses are present only in *M. musculus* subspecies, whereas polytropic MLV-related proviruses are found in both *M. musculus* and *M. spretus*. Replication-competent members of the family are found in many, but not all, inbred mice (128). (For reviews of the properties of the murine endogenous retrovirus genomes, see refs. 245 and 344).

Recently, the potential to use pig organs or cells in xenotransplantation into humans has raised considerable interest in the presence of endogenous retroviral elements in the pig (522,684). Although viruses can be rescued from porcine cells (9), and although these viruses can infect human cells quite efficiently (557,768), preliminary studies suggest they are not easily transmitted to humans in transplant settings (305,555). There remains a real possibility for their transfer to humans, however, and the consequences could be significant.

Retroviral elements are also abundant in the human genome (73,439,463,468). These elements are collectively termed HERVs, and subgroups are denoted by a letter indicating the amino acid specificity of the tRNA primer. Most are defective, but a very small number of these elements are still actively transcribed in somatic cells and are capable of transposition to new sites (176). The distribution of the HERV-K family in various primates has been surveyed to help build evolutionary trees of these species (347,678). There are also provirus families distantly related to the lentiviruses (317); some have the potential to encode rev-like elements that could, in principle, be pathogenic (440). A detailed review of the HERVs is presented in Chapter 62 in *Fields Virology*, 4th ed.

Properties of the Endogenous Provirus-like Elements

The distribution of elements in a given strain is relatively stable over the course of a few generations. Thus, most individuals in an inbred population show a constant, characteristic pattern of endogenous elements. The rate of loss of a given provirus is very low, and the appearance of new proviruses is rare in most animals. However, the pattern is quite different in different species, and even in different strains of animals, suggesting that rearrangements happen often over longer evolutionary times. It is known that new copies can appear at higher frequency if newborn females are viremic (431,675). Thus, early infection of germ cells can introduce new proviruses into the germline. This route can even be used to create mutations *de novo* in laboratory mice at reasonable frequencies.

Most endogenous proviruses are transcriptionally silent; the DNA is often heavily methylated and so repressed. These may reflect the mechanisms by which the transcription of many exogenous viruses are repressed *in vivo*. Expression of many of the endogenous viral RNAs is induced by agents causing DNA damage, such as ultraviolet light and bromodeoxyuridine, and the expression of others is stimulated by glucocorticoids (207). The IAPs are often induced during the differentiation of various cell types (695), and even more often in immortalized tumor cell lines.

The bulk of the endogenous retroviruses are fossil DNAs, grossly defective, and no longer capable of encoding proteins; the ORFs contain numerous stop codons and frameshifts that would preclude the formation of any functional viral gene products. However, these elements can often give rise to RNAs, and these RNAs can be packaged efficiently by virions encoded by exogenous viruses and thus can give rise to new proviruses. Furthermore, these copackaged RNAs can then recombine with the exogenous viral RNAs and so contribute small sequence blocks to these viruses, potentially altering the host range and replication properties of the virus. The continuous contribution of endogenous sequences to virus evolution is a fact that needs to be considered whenever genetic selections are imposed on a virus. In addition, a few of the elements are functional and can transpose intracellularly (705) or even give rise to replication-competent viruses. Even when viruses are induced from the elements, however, the viruses are most often not highly pathogenic for the host in which they reside. Thus, many of the inducible elements in the mouse are xenotropic and cannot spread in the animal; and those that can, do not cause an acute disease. The LTRs of the endogenous elements are often quite weak as transcriptional promoters as compared to those of exogenous viruses. This may reflect selections against highly pathogenic agents either before or after their introduction into the germline.

The creation of a new provirus in the germline by necessity creates a mutation, and although most such insertions probably have no significant effect, occasionally deleterious germline mutations occur. A number of ancient, "spontaneous" mutations, upon analysis, have been found to have been caused by a proviral insertion. These include such classic mutations as the rd1 allele, which causes a slow retinal degeneration, and which includes an insertion affecting the beta subunit of the retinal cGMP phosphodiesterase; the hr mutation, which causes a hairless phenotype; the dilute coat-color allele d; and a mutation termed Slp (for sex-limited protein) in the C4 complement gene, in which an insertion of a viral LTR renders the gene androgen responsive.

Many of the endogenous elements may be positively selected in their host species. This may be the result of advantageous mutations that are created by the insertion, or antiviral effects mediated by the gene products encoded by the endogenous proviruses. The Fv1 and Fv4 genes are examples of such elements. These virus-like elements confer resistance to exogenous viruses and so may serve to protect the host from leukemia induced by infection. The MMTV *sag* gene, if present on an endogenous provirus, acts to delete T cells that would respond to the superantigen; thus, subsequent infection by an exogenous MMTV cannot use *sag* to induce a proliferation of cells needed for its vigorous replication. Thus, the inherited provirus protects the host from MMTV disease.

RETROVIRAL VECTORS, PACKAGING LINES, AND GENE THERAPY

The structure and mechanism of transmission of the naturally arising replication-defective transforming viral genomes provide a clear model for the directed use of retroviruses to mediate gene transfer. Retroviral vectors that mimic the structure of the transforming viruses can readily be generated, and these vectors can be engineered to carry the cDNA sequences of virtually any gene. These genomes can then be propagated with wild-type virus as helper. However, it is also possible to generate helper-free preparations of particles that transduce the vector genome via the early steps of the life cycle, without delivering the helper genome, thereby preventing subsequent spread of the vector. These helper-free particles are generated in packaging cell lines: cells engineered to express the *gag*, *pol*, and *env* genes but not expressing packageable helper viral RNAs. The first such lines simply carried a provirus lacking the Psi site, the RNA packaging signal (460). These cells produce virions deficient in the helper genome, and introducing a Psi+ vector construct into these cells results in the encapsidation and release of the vector RNA into those particles. These particles can then be harvested and used to deliver the vector and its gene into susceptible cells. It is also possible to generate transducing virus preparations by transiently transfecting cells with DNAs that encode the helper functions and DNAs that encode the vector. This approach is preferable in instances where the viral gene products are toxic and therefore difficult to express stably in a packaging cell line.

A limitation of these packaging systems is that small amounts of the Psi-minus helper RNA are encapsidated along with the vector. Endogenous retroviral genomes, such as VL30 RNAs (4), are also encapsidated efficiently, and recombination events between these RNAs during reverse transcription can recreate a replication-competent virus (556,641). These events are probably similar to recombinational repair of mutations in genomes that occur during growth in cell culture (132,133,470). This issue has raised considerable fears that gene therapy vectors intended for therapeutic use could initiate a viremia, and perhaps a viral leukemia, in patients. More elaborate cell lines, in which the *gag*, *pol*, or *env* genes are expressed via separate RNAs, can reduce the frequency with which such recombination events occur to very low levels (142,157,465,466).

Retrovirus particles transducing a desirable gene can be directed to target cells through the use of many distinct envelope proteins. This method is possible because retrovirus particles can readily form pseudotypes; that is, they can incorporate and use the envelope proteins of a wide array of different viruses (209,299,676,771). The wide range of pseudotypes that can be formed presumably reflects the flexibility of the core–envelope interaction. The host range can be further expanded or restricted by the engineering of envelopes with new binding specificities (731). Chimeric envelope molecules have been particularly popular tools in targeting virions to new receptors (119,360,464,669). Another approach is to engineer animals that express a foreign receptor in a tissue-specific manner, and deliver genes with a virus envelope that recognizes only the transgenic receptor (228). The envelope–receptor interaction can even be reversed: It is possible to express a particular virus receptor molecule on the virion surface, and thereby to target the virus to those cells expressing the corresponding viral envelope (43).

A major limitation of early retroviral gene therapy efforts is the inability of most helper viruses to mediate the infection and transduction of nondividing cells. The major block is during the early stages of infection, when there is a strong requirement for cell division for infection by most viruses (624). However, the lentiviruses have the ability to infect nondividing cells, and thus gene therapy based on lentiviral packaging systems could overcome this limitation (for review, see ref. 15). Recent efforts have substantiated these expectations: Delivery to nondividing neurons, and to poorly dividing primary lymphocyte cultures, has been demonstrated with vectors based on HIV-1 (72,185,355,506,507) as well as FIV (575).

PERSPECTIVES

The study of retroviruses has led to a detailed characterization of many steps of virus replication but also to important fundamental discoveries concerning host physiology and genetics. The viruses have served as entrés into such phenomena as cell surface receptors, cell division, DNA synthesis, the cell cycle, mechanisms of gene expression, and intracellular transport. The value of focusing on retrovirus functions in unraveling cellular functions is clear: These agents have evolved over huge periods of time to exploit key aspects of the cell, and we should make use of their success to help identify those aspects. There is every reason to believe that their continued study will yet reveal new aspects of cell physiology.

REFERENCES

1. Accola MA, Hoglund S, Gottlinger HG. A putative alpha-helical structure which overlaps the capsid-p2 boundary in the human immunodeficiency virus type 1 Gag precursor is crucial for viral particle assembly. *J Virol* 1998;72:2072–2078.
2. Acha-Orbea H, Shakhov AN, Scarpellino L, et al. Clonal deletion of Vβ14-bearing T cells in mice transgenic for mammary tumour virus. *Nature* 1991;250:207–211.
3. Adam MA, Miller AD. Identification of a signal in a murine retrovirus that is sufficient for packaging of nonretroviral RNA into virions. *J Virol* 1988;62:3802–3806.
4. Adams SE, Rathjen PD, Stanway CA, et al. Complete nucleotide sequence of a mouse VL30 retro-element. *Mol Cell Biol* 1988;8:2989–2998.
5. Adkins HB, Brojatsch J, Naughton J, et al. Identification of a cellular receptor for subgroup E avian leukosis virus. *Proc Natl Acad Sci U S A* 1997;94:11617–11622.
6. Ahmed YF, Gilmartin GM, Hanly SM, et al. The HTLV-1 rex response element mediates a novel form of mRNA polyadenylation. *Cell* 1991;64:727–738.
7. Aiyar A, Cobrinik D, Ge Z, et al. Interaction between retroviral U5 RNA and the TψC loop of the tRNATrp primer is required for efficient initiation of reverse transcription. *J Virol* 1992;66:24604–2472.
8. Aiyar A, Hindmarsh P, Skalka AM, Leis J. Concerted integration of linear retroviral DNA by the avian sarcoma virus integrase *in vitro*: Dependence on both long terminal repeat termini. *J Virol* 1996;70:3571–3580.
9. Akiyoshi DE, Denaro M, Zhu H, et al. Identification of a full-length cDNA for an endogenous retrovirus of miniature swine. *J Virol* 1998;72:4503–4507.
10. Akroyd J, Fincham VJ, Green AR, et al. Transcription of Rous sarcoma proviruses in rat cells is determined by chromosomal position effects that fluctuate and can operate over long distances. *Oncogene* 1987;1:347–355.
11. Alam SL, Wills NM, Ingram JA, et al. Structural studies of the RNA pseudoknot required for readthrough of the gag-termination codon of murine leukemia virus. *J Mol Biol* 1999;288:837–852.
12. Albritton LM, Kim JW, Tseng L, Cunningham JM. Envelope-binding domain in the cationic amino acid transporter determines the host range of ecotropic murine retroviruses. *J Virol* 1993;67:2091–2096.
13. Albritton LM, Tseng L, Scadden D, Cunningham JM. A putative murine ecotropic retrovirus receptor gene encodes a multiple membrane-spanning protein and confers susceptibility to virus infection. *Cell* 1989;57:659–666.
14. Allain B, Rascle JB, de Rocquigny H, et al. CIS elements and trans-acting factors required for minus strand DNA transfer during reverse transcription of the genomic RNA of murine leukemia virus. *J Mol Biol* 1998;277:225–235.
15. Amado RG, Chen ISY. Lentiviral vectors-the promise of gene therapy within reach? *Science* 1999;285:674–676.
16. Amanuma H, Laigret F, Nishi M, et al. Identification of putative endogenous proviral templates for progenitor mink cells focus-forming (MCF) MuLV-related RNAs. *Virology* 1988;164:556–561.
17. Amendt BA, Simpson SB, Stoltzfus CM. Inhibition of RNA splicing at the Rous sarcoma virus src 3′ splice site is mediated by an interaction between a negative cis element and a chicken embryo fibroblast nuclear factor. *J Virol* 1995;69:5068–5076.
18. Anderson DJ, Stone J, Lum R, Linial ML. The packaging phenotype of the SE21Q1b provirus is related to high proviral expression and not trans-acting factors. *J Virol* 1995;69:7319–7323.
19. Anderson JA, Bowman EH, Hu WS. Retroviral recombination rates do not increase linearly with marker distance and are limited by the size of the recombining subpopulation. *J Virol* 1998;72:1195–1202.
20. Anderson JA, Teufel RJ 2nd, Yin PD, Hu WS. Correlated template-switching events during minus-strand DNA synthesis: A mechanism for high negative interference during retroviral recombination. *J Virol* 1998;72:1186–1194.
21. Andrake MD, Skalka AM. Multimerization determinants reside in both the catalytic core and C terminus of avian sarcoma virus integrase. *J Biol Chem* 1995;270:29299–29306.
22. Andrake MD, Skalka AM. Retroviral integrase: Putting the pieces together. *J Biol Chem* 1996;271:19633–19636.
23. Andreadis ST, Brott D, Fuller AO, Palsson BO. Moloney murine leukemia virus-derived retroviral vectors decay intracellularly with a half-life in the range of 5.5 to 7.5 hours. *J Virol* 1997;71:7541–7548.
24. Arad G, Bar-Meir R, Almog N, et al. Avian sarcoma leukemia virus protease linked to the adjacent Gag polyprotein is enzymatically active. *Virology* 1995;214:439–444.
25. Archer TK, Lefebvre P, Wolford RG, Hager GL. Transcription factor loading on the MMTV promoter: A bimodal mechanism for promoter activation. *Science* 1992;255:1573–1576.
26. Ardavin C, Martin P, Ferrero I, et al. B cell response after MMTV infection: Extrafollicular plasmablasts represent the main infected population and can transmit viral infection. *J Immunol* 1999;162:2538–2545.
27. Armentano D, Yu S-F, Kantoff PW, et al. Effect of internal viral sequences on the utility of retroviral vectors. *J Virol* 1987;61:1647–1650.
28. Arnold E, Jacobo-Molina A, Nanni RG, et al. Structure of HIV-1 reverse transcriptase/DNA complex at 7 Å resolution showing active site locations. *Nature* 1992;357:85–89.
29. Aronoff R, Hajjar AM, Linial ML. Avian retroviral RNA encapsidation: Reexamination of functional 5′ RNA sequences and the role of nucleocapsid cys-his motifs. *J Virol* 1993;67:178–188.
30. Aronoff R, Linial M. Specificity of retroviral RNA packaging. *J Virol* 1991;65:71–80.
31. Arrigo S, Beemon K. Regulation of Rous sarcoma virus RNA splicing and stability. *Mol Cell Biol* 1988;18:4858–4867.
32. Arrigo S, Yun M, Beemon K. Cis-acting regulatory elements within *gag* genes of avian retroviruses. *Mol Cell Biol* 1987;7:388–392.
33. Arthur LO, Bess JWJ, Sowder RCI, et al. Cellular proteins bound to immunodeficiency viruses: Implications for pathogenesis for vaccines. *Science* 1992;258:1935–1938.
34. Arthur LO, Pyle SW, Nara PL, et al. Serological responses in chimpanzees inoculated with human immunodeficiency virus glycoprotein (gp120) subunit vaccine. *Proc Natl Acad Sci U S A* 1987;84:8583–8587.
35. Asano K, Merrick WC, Hershey JW. The translation initiation factor eIF3-p48 subunit is encoded by int-6, a site of frequent integration by the mouse mammary tumor virus genome. *J Biol Chem* 1997;272:23477–23480.
36. Athas GB, Choi B, Prabhu S, et al. Genetic determinants of feline leukemia virus-induced multicentric lymphomas. *Virology* 1995;214:431–438.
37. Auxilien S, Keith G, Le Grice SF, Darlix JL. Role of post-transcriptional modifications of primer tRNALys,3 in the fidelity and efficacy of plus strand DNA transfer during HIV-1 reverse transcription. *J Biol Chem* 1999;274:4412–4420.
38. Aziz DC, Hanna Z, Jolicoeur P. Severe immunodeficiency disease induced by a defective murine leukaemia virus. *Nature* 1989;338:505–508.
39. Bachand F, Yao XJ, Hrimech M, et al. Incorporation of Vpr into human immunodeficiency virus type 1 requires a direct interaction with the p6 domain of the p55 gag precursor. *J Biol Chem* 1999;274:9083–9091.
40. Bacharach E, Goff SP. Binding of the human immunodeficiency virus type 1 Gag protein to the viral RNA encapsidation signal in the yeast three-hybrid system. *J Virol* 1998;72:6944–6949.
41. Bahar I, Erman B, Jernigan RL, et al. Collective motions in HIV-1 reverse transcriptase: Examination of flexibility and enzyme function. *J Mol Biol* 1999;285:1023–1037.
42. Ball JK, Arthur LO, Dekaban G. The involvement of a type-B retrovirus in the induction of thymic lymphomas. *Virology* 1985;140:159–172.
43. Balliet JW, Bates P. Efficient infection mediated by viral receptors incorporated into retroviral particles. *J Virol* 1998;72:671–676.
44. Baltimore D. RNA-dependent DNA polymerase in virions of RNA tumour viruses. *Nature* 1970;226:1209–1211.
45. Banks JD, Yeo A, Green K, et al. A minimal avian retroviral packaging sequence has a complex structure. *J Virol* 1998;72:6190–6194.
46. Bar-Shira A, Panet A, Honigman A. An RNA secondary structure juxtaposes two remote genetic signals for human T-cell leukemia virus type I RNA 3′-end processing. *J Virol* 1991;65:5165–5173.

47. Barat C, Rassart E. Members of the GATA family of transcription factors bind to the U3 region of Cas-Br-E and graffi retroviruses and transactivate their expression. *J Virol* 1998;72:5579–5588.
48. Barklis E, McDermott J, Wilkens S, et al. Structural analysis of membrane-bound retrovirus capsid proteins. *EMBO J* 1997;16:1199–1213.
49. Bates P, Rong L, Varmus HE, et al. Genetic mapping of the cloned subgroup A avian sarcoma and leukosis virus receptor gene to the TVA locus. *J Virol* 1998;72:2505–2508.
50. Bates P, Young JA, Varmus HE. A receptor for subgroup A Rous sarcoma virus is related to the low density lipoprotein receptor. *Cell* 1993;74:1043–1051.
51. Battini JL, Rasko JE, Miller AD. A human cell-surface receptor for xenotropic and polytropic murine leukemia viruses: Possible role in G protein-coupled signal transduction. *Proc Natl Acad Sci U S A* 1999; 96:1385–1390.
52. Battula N, Loeb LA. On the fidelity of DNA replication. Lack of exodeoxyribonuclease activity and error-correcting function in avian myeloblastosis virus DNA polymerase. *J Biol Chem* 1976;251:982–986.
53. Baxter EW, Blyth K, Donehower LA, et al. Moloney murine leukemia virus-induced lymphomas in p53-deficient mice: Overlapping pathways in tumor development? *J Virol* 1996;70:2095–2100.
54. Bebenek K, Abbotts J, Wilson SH, Kunkel TA. Error-prone polymerization by HIV-1 reverse transcriptase. Contribution of template-primer misalignment, miscoding, and termination probability to mutational hot spots. *J Biol Chem* 1993;268:10324–10334.
55. Belli B, Fan H. The leukemogenic potential of an enhancer variant of Moloney murine leukemia virus varies with the route of inoculation. *J Virol* 1994;68:6883–6889.
56. Belyaev AS, Stuart D, Sutton G, Roy P. Crystallization and preliminary x-ray investigation of recombinant simian immunodeficiency virus matrix protein. *J Mol Biol* 1994;241:744–746.
57. Ben-Artzi H, Zeelon E, Gorecki M, Panet A. Double-stranded RNA-dependent RNase activity associated with human immunodeficiency virus type 1 reverse transcriptase. *Proc Natl Acad Sci U S A* 1992; 89:927–931.
58. Benit L, Lallemand JB, Casella JF, et al. ERV-L elements: A family of endogenous retrovirus-like elements active throughout the evolution of mammals. *J Virol* 1999;73:3301–3308.
59. Bennett RP, Wills JW. Conditions for copackaging rous sarcoma virus and murine leukemia virus Gag proteins during retroviral budding. *J Virol* 1999;73:2045–2051.
60. Berger EA, Murphy PM, Farber JM. Chemokine receptors as HIV-1 coreceptors: Roles in viral entry, tropism, and disease. *Annu Rev Immunol* 1999;17:657–700.
61. Berkowitz R, Fisher J, Goff SP. RNA packaging. *Curr Top Microbiol Immunol* 1996;214:177–218.
62. Berkowitz RD, Luban J, Goff SP. Specific binding of human immunodeficiency virus type 1 gag polyprotein and nucleocapsid protein to viral RNAs detected by RNA mobility shift assays. *J Virol* 1993; 67:7190–7200.
63. Berlioz C, Darlix JL. An internal ribosomal entry mechanism promotes translation of murine leukemia virus gag polyprotein precursors. *J Virol* 1995;69:2214–2222.
64. Berlioz-Torrent C, Shacklett BL, Erdtmann L, et al. Interactions of the cytoplasmic domains of human and simian retroviral transmembrane proteins with components of the clathrin adaptor complexes modulate intracellular and cell surface expression of envelope glycoproteins. *J Virol* 1999;73:1350–1361.
65. Besmer P, Olshevsky U, Baltimore D, et al. Virus-like 30S RNA in mouse cells. *J Virol* 1979;29:1168–1176.
66. Bess JW Jr, Gorelick RJ, Bosche WJ, et al. Microvesicles are a source of contaminating cellular proteins found in purified HIV-1 preparations. *Virology* 1997;230:134–144.
67. Bess JW Jr, Powell PJ, Issaq HJ, et al. Tightly bound zinc in human immunodeficiency virus type 1, human T-cell leukemia virus type I, and other retroviruses. *J Virol* 1992;66:840–847.
68. Best S, Le Tissier P, Towers G, Stoye JP. Positional cloning of the mouse retrovirus restriction gene Fv1. *Nature* 1996;382:826–829.
69. Bilello JA, Pitts OM, Hoffman PM. Characterization of a progressive neurodegenerative disease induced by a temperature-sensitive Moloney murine leukemia virus infection. *J Virol* 1986;59:234–241.
70. Blain SW, Goff SP. Nuclease activities of Moloney murine leukemia virus reverse transcriptase: Mutants with altered substrate specificities. *J Biol Chem* 1993;268:23585–23592.
71. Blain SW, Goff SP. Effects on DNA synthesis and translocation caused by mutations in the RNase H domain of Moloney murine leukemia virus reverse transcriptase. *J Virol* 1995;69:4440–4452.
72. Blomer U, Naldini L, Kafri T, et al. Highly efficient and sustained gene transfer in adult neurons with a lentivirus vector. *J Virol* 1997;71: 6641–6649.
73. Blond JL, Beseme F, Duret L, et al. Molecular characterization and placental expression of HERV-W, a new human endogenous retrovirus family. *J Virol* 1999;73:1175–1185.
74. Boeke JD, Garfinkel DJ, Styles CA, Fink GR. Ty elements transpose through an RNA intermediate. *Cell* 1985;40:491–500.
75. Boeke JD, Stoye JP. Retrotransposons, endogenous retroviruses, and the evolution of retroelements. In: Coffin JM, Hughes SH, Varmus HE, eds. *Retroviruses*. Cold Spring Harbor, NY: Cold Spring Harbor Press, 1997:343–436.
76. Boerkoel CF, Kung H-J. Transcriptional interaction between retroviral long terminal repeats (LTRs): Mechanism of 5′ LTR suppression and 3′ LTR promoter activation of c-myc in avian B-cell lymphomas. *J Virol* 1992;66:4814–4823.
77. Bogerd HP, Echarri A, Ross TM, Cullen BR. Inhibition of human immunodeficiency virus Rev and human T-cell leukemia virus Rex function, but not Mason-Pfizer monkey virus constitutive transport element activity, by a mutant human nucleoporin targeted to Crm1. *J Virol* 1998;72:8627–8635.
78. Bohnlein S, Hauber J, Cullen BR. Identification of a U5-specific sequence required for efficient polyadenylation within the human immunodeficiency virus long terminal repeat. *J Virol* 1989;63:421–424.
79. Bondurant MC, Koury MJ, Krantz SB. The Fv-2 gene controls induction of erythroid burst formation by Friend virus infection *in vitro*: Studies of growth regulators and viral replication. *J Gen Virol* 1985; 66:83–96.
80. Bonham L, Wolgamot G, Miller AD. Molecular cloning of *Mus dunni* endogenous virus: An unusual retrovirus in a new murine viral interference group with a wide host range. *J Virol* 1997;71:4663–4670.
81. Bonnet-Mathoniere B, Girard PM, Muriaux D, Paoletti J. Nucleocapsid protein 10 activates dimerization of the RNA of Moloney murine leukaemia virus *in vitro*. *Eur J Biochem* 1996;238:129–135.
82. Bonzon C, Fan H. Moloney murine leukemia virus-induced preleukemic thymic atrophy and enhanced thymocyte apoptosis correlate with disease pathogenicity. *J Virol* 1999;73:2434–2441.
83. Boone LR, Glover PL, Innes CL, et al. Fv-1 N- and B-tropism-specific sequences in murine leukemia virus and related endogenous proviral genomes. *J Virol* 1988;62:2644–2650.
84. Boral AL, Okenquist SA, Lenz J. Identification of the SL3-3 virus enhancer core as a T-lymphoma cell-specific element. *J Virol* 1988; 63:76–84.
85. Borsetti A, Ohagen A, Gottlinger HG. The C-terminal half of the human immunodeficiency virus type 1 Gag precursor is sufficient for efficient particle assembly. *J Virol* 1998;72:9313–9317.
86. Bosze Z, Thiesen H-J, Charnay P. A transcriptional enhancer with specificity for erythroid cells is located in the long terminal repeat of the Friend murine leukemia virus. *EMBO J* 1986;5:1615–1624.
87. Bowerman B, Brown PO, Bishop JM, Varmus HE. A nucleoprotein complex mediates the integration of retroviral DNA. *Genes Dev* 1989; 3:469–478.
88. Bowman EH, Pathak VK, Hu WS. Efficient initiation and strand transfer of polypurine tract-primed plus-strand DNA prevent strand transfer of internally initiated plus-strand DNA. *J Virol* 1996;70:1687–1694.
89. Bowzard JB, Bennett RP, Krishna NK, et al. Importance of basic residues in the nucleocapsid sequence for retrovirus Gag assembly and complementation rescue. *J Virol* 1998;72:9034–9044.
90. Braaten D, Franke EK, Luban J. Cyclophilin A is required for an early step in the life cycle of human immunodeficiency virus type 1 before the initiation of reverse transcription. *J Virol* 1996;70:3551–3560.
91. Brandt-Carlson C, Butel JS. Detection and characterization of a glycoprotein encoded by the mouse mammary tumor virus long terminal repeat gene. *J Virol* 1991;65:6051–6060.
92. Bray M, Prasad S, Dubay JW, et al. A small element from the Mason-Pfizer monkey virus genome makes human immunodeficiency virus type 1 expression and replication Rev-independent. *Proc Natl Acad Sci U S A* 1994;91:1256–1260.
93. Brightman BK, Davis BR, Fan H. Preleukemic hematopoietic hyperplasia induced by Moloney murine leukemia virus is an indirect consequence of viral infection. *J Virol* 1990;64:4582–4584.

94. Brody BA, Rhee SS, Hunter E. Postassembly cleavage of a retroviral glycoprotein cytoplasmic domain removes a necessary incorporation signal and activates fusion activity. *J Virol* 1994;68:4620–4627.
95. Brojatsch J, Naughton J, Rolls MM, et al. CAR1, a TNFR-related protein, is a cellular receptor for cytopathic avian leukosis-sarcoma viruses and mediates apoptosis. *Cell* 1996;87:845–855.
96. Brown PO, Bowerman B, Varmus HE, Bishop JM. Correct integration of retroviral DNA *in vitro*. *Cell* 1987;49:347–356.
97. Bryant M, Ratner L. Myristoylation-dependent replication and assembly of human immunodeficiency virus 1. *Proc Natl Acad Sci U S A* 1990;87:523–527.
98. Bujacz G, Jaskolski M, Alexandratos J, et al. High-resolution structure of the catalytic domain of avian sarcoma virus integrase. *J Mol Biol* 1995;253:333–346.
99. Bukrinskaya AG, Ghorpade A, Heinzinger NK, et al. Phosphorylation-dependent human immunodeficiency virus type 1 infection and nuclear targeting of viral DNA. *Proc Natl Acad Sci U S A* 1996;93: 367–371.
100. Bukrinsky MI, Sharova N, Dempsey MP, et al. Active nuclear import of human immunodeficiency virus type 1 preintegration complexes. *Proc Natl Acad Sci U S A* 1992;89:6580–6584.
101. Burns DP, Temin HM. High rates of frameshift mutations within homo-oligomeric runs during a single cycle of retroviral replication. *J Virol* 1994;68:4196–4203.
102. Burstein H, Bizub D, Kotler M, et al. Processing of avian retroviral gag polyprotein precursors is blocked by a mutation at the NC-PR cleavage site. *J Virol* 1992;66:1781–1785.
103. Bushman FD, Craigie R. Sequence requirements for integration of Moloney murine leukemia virus DNA *in vitro*. *J Virol* 1990;64: 5645–5648.
104. Cai M, Huang Y, Zheng R, et al. Solution structure of the cellular factor BAF responsible for protecting retroviral DNA from autointegration. *Nat Struct Biol* 1998;5:903–909.
105. Cai M, Zheng R, Caffrey M, et al. Solution structure of the N-terminal zinc binding domain of HIV-1 integrase. *Nat Struct Biol* 1997;4: 567–577.
106. Camaur D, Gallay P, Swingler S, Trono D. Human immunodeficiency virus matrix tyrosine phosphorylation: Characterization of the kinase and its substrate requirements. *J Virol* 1997;71:6834–6841.
107. Campbell S, Rein A. *In vitro* assembly properties of human immunodeficiency virus type 1 Gag protein lacking the p6 domain. *J Virol* 1999;73:2270–2279.
108. Campbell S, Vogt VM. Self-assembly *in vitro* of purified CA-NC proteins from Rous sarcoma virus and human immunodeficiency virus type 1. *J Virol* 1995;69:6487–6497.
109. Carteau S, Gorelick RJ, Bushman FD. Coupled integration of human immunodeficiency virus type 1 cDNA ends by purified integrase in vitro: Stimulation by the viral nucleocapsid protein. *J Virol* 1999;73:6670–6679.
110. Carteau S, Hoffmann C, Bushman F. Chromosome structure and human immunodeficiency virus type 1 cDNA integration: Centromeric alphoid repeats are a disfavored target. *J Virol* 1998;72: 4005–4014.
111. Ch'ang L-Y, Yang WK, Myer FE, Yang D-M. Negative regulatory element associated with potentially functional promoter and enhancer elements in the long terminal repeats of endogenous murine leukemia virus-related proviral sequences. *J Virol* 1989;63:2746–2757.
112. Charneau P, Alizon M, Clavel F. A second origin of DNA plus-strand synthesis is required for optimal human immunodeficiency virus replication. *J Virol* 1992;66:2814–2820.
113. Charneau P, Mirambeau G, Roux P, et al. HIV-1 reverse transcription. A termination step at the center of the genome. *J Mol Biol* 1994; 241:651–662.
114. Chattopadhyay SK, Cloyd MW, Linemeyer DL, et al. Cellular origin and role of mink cell focus-forming viruses in murine thymic lymphomas. *Nature* 1982;295:25–31.
115. Chen H, Wei SQ, Engelman A. Multiple integrase functions are required to form the native structure of the human immunodeficiency virus type I intasome. *J Biol Chem* 1999;274:17358–17364.
116. Chen P-J, Cywinski A, Taylor JM. Reverse transcription of 7S L RNA by an avian retrovirus. *J Virol* 1985;54:278–284.
117. Chen X, Kang H, Shen LX, et al. A characteristic bent conformation of RNA pseudoknots promotes −1 frameshifting during translation of retroviral RNA. *J Mol Biol* 1996;260:479–483.
118. Chow SA, Vincent KA, Ellison V, Brown PO. Reversal of integration and DNA splicing mediated by integrase of human immunodeficiency virus. *Science* 1992;255:723–726.
119. Chu TH, Martinez I, Sheay WC, Dornburg R. Cell targeting with retroviral vector particles containing antibody-envelope fusion proteins. *Gene Ther* 1994;1:292–299.
120. Chung M, Kizhatil K, Albritton LM, Gaulton GN. Induction of syncytia by neuropathogenic murine leukemia viruses depend on receptor density, host cell determinants, and the intrinsic fusion potential of envelope protein. *J Virol* 1999;73:9377–9385.
121. Cimarelli A, Luban J. Translation elongation factor 1-alpha interacts specifically with the human immunodeficiency virus type 1 Gag polyprotein. *J Virol* 1999;73:5388–5401.
122. Clark L, Matthews JR, Hay RT. Interaction of enhancer-binding protein EBPI (NF-κB) with the human immunodeficiency virus type 1 enhancer. *J Virol* 1990;64:1335–1344.
123. Clever J, Sassetti C, Parslow TG. RNA secondary structure and binding sites for *gag* gene products in the 5′ packaging signal of human immunodeficiency virus type 1. *J Virol* 1995;69:2101–2109.
124. Clever JL, Taplitz RA, Lochrie MA, et al. A heterologous high-affinity RNA ligand for human immunodeficiency virus Gag protein has RNA packaging activity. *J Virol* 2000;74:541–546.
125. Cobrinik D, Katz R, Terry R, et al. Avian sarcoma and leukosis virus pol-endonuclease recognition of the tandem long terminal repeat junction: Minimum site required for cleavage is also required for viral growth. *J Virol* 1987;61:1999–2008.
126. Cobrinik D, Soskey L, Leis J. A retroviral RNA secondary structure required for efficient initiation of reverse transcription. *J Virol* 1988; 62:3622–3630.
127. Cochrane AW, Chen C-H, Rosen CA. Specific interaction of the human immunodeficiency virus Rev protein with a structured region in the *env* mRNA. *Proc Natl Acad Sci U S A* 1990;87:1198–1202.
128. Coffin JM. Endogenous viruses. In: Weiss RA, Teich NM, Varmus HE, Coffin JM, eds. *RNA Tumor Viruses*. Cold Spring Harbor, NY: Cold Spring Harbor Laboratory, 1982:1109–1204.
129. Coffin JM. Superantigens and endogenous retroviruses: A confluence of puzzles. *Science* 1992;255:411–413.
130. Coffin JM, Hughes SH, Varmus HE, eds. *Retroviruses*. Cold Spring Harbor, NY: Cold Spring Harbor Press, 1997.
131. Colicelli J, Goff SP. Mutants and pseudorevertants of Moloney murine leukemia virus with alterations at the integration site. *Cell* 1985;42: 573–580.
132. Colicelli J, Goff SP. Isolation of a recombinant murine leukemia virus utilizing a new primer tRNA. *J Virol* 1986;57:37–45.
133. Colicelli J, Goff SP. Identification of endogenous retroviral sequences as potential donors for recombinational repair of mutant retroviruses: Positions of crossover points. *Virology* 1987;160:518–522.
134. Colicelli J, Goff SP. Sequence and spacing requirements of a retrovirus integration site. *J Mol Biol* 1988;199:47–59.
135. Connolly L, Zingler K, Young JA. A soluble form of a receptor for subgroup A avian leukosis and sarcoma viruses (ALSV-A) blocks infection and binds directly to ALSV-A. *J Virol* 1994;68:2760–2764.
136. Conte MR, Klikova M, Hunter E, et al. The three-dimensional solution structure of the matrix protein from the type D retrovirus, the Mason-Pfizer monkey virus, and implications for the morphology of retroviral assembly. *EMBO J* 1997;16:5819–5826.
137. Cook CR, McNally MT. Characterization of an RNP complex that assembles on the Rous sarcoma virus negative regulator of splicing element. *Nucleic Acids Res* 1996;24:4962–4968.
138. Copeland NG, Hutchinson KW, Jenkins. NA. Excision of the DBA ecotropic provirus in dilute coat-color revertants of mice occurs by homologous recombination involving the viral LTRs. *Cell* 1983;33: 379–387.
139. Corbin A, Prats AC, Darlix JL, Sitbon M. A nonstructural gag-encoded glycoprotein precursor is necessary for efficient spreading and pathogenesis of murine leukemia viruses. *J Virol* 1994;68: 3857–3867.
140. Cordingley MG, Riegel AT, Hager GL. Steroid-dependent interaction of transcription factors with the inducible promoter of mouse mammary tumor virus *in vivo*. *Cell* 1987;48:261–270.
141. Cordonnier A, Casella JF, Heidmann T. Isolation of novel human endogenous retrovirus-like elements with foamy virus-related pol sequence. *J Virol* 1995;69:5890–5897.
142. Coset F-L, Legras C, Chebloune Y, et al. A new avian leukosis virus-

based packaging cell line that uses two separate transcomplementing helper genomes. *J Virol* 1990;64:1070–1078.
143. Cosson P. Direct interaction between the envelope and matrix proteins of HIV-1. *EMBO J* 1996;15:5783–5788.
144. Craven RC, Bennett RP, Wills JW. Role of the avian retroviral protease in the activation of reverse transcriptase during virion assembly. *J Virol* 1991;65:6205–6217.
145. Craven RC, Leure-duPree AE, Weldon RA Jr, Wills JW. Genetic analysis of the major homology region of the Rous sarcoma virus Gag protein. *J Virol* 1995;69:4213–4227.
146. Crawford S, Goff SP. Mutations in gag proteins p12 and p15 of Moloney murine leukemia virus block early stages of infection. *J Virol* 1984;49:909–917.
147. Crawford S, Goff SP. A deletion mutation in the 5′ part of the *pol* gene of Moloney murine leukemia virus blocks proteolytic processing of the gag and pol polyproteins. *J Virol* 1985;53:899–907.
148. Crise B, Buonocore L, Rose JK. CD4 is retained in the endoplasmic reticulum by the human immunodeficiency virus type 1 glycoprotein precursor. *J Virol* 1990;64:5585–5593.
149. Cullen BR. HIV-1 auxiliary proteins: Making connections in a dying cell. *Cell* 1998;93:685–692.
150. Cullen BR, Greene WC. Functions of the auxiliary gene products of the human immunodeficiency virus type 1. *Virology* 1990;178:1–5.
151. Cullen BR, Lomedico PT, Ju G. Transcriptional interference in avian retroviruses: Implications for the promoter insertion model of leukemogenesis. *Nature* 1984;307:241–244.
152. Daefler S, Klotman ME, Wong-Staal F. Trans-activating rev protein of the human immunodeficiency virus 1 interacts directly and specifically with its target RNA. *Proc Natl Acad Sci U S A* 1990;87: 4571–4575.
153. Dalgleish AG, Beverly PCL, Clapham PR, et al. The CD4 (T4) antigen is an essential component of the receptor for the AIDS retrovirus. *Nature* 1984;312:763–767.
154. Daly TJ, Cook KS, Gray GS, et al. Specific binding of HIV-1 recombinant Rev protein to the Rev-responsive element *in vitro*. *Nature* 1989;342:816–819.
155. Damico RL, Crane J, Bates P. Receptor-triggered membrane association of a model retroviral glycoprotein. *Proc Natl Acad Sci U S A* 1998;95:2580–2585.
156. Daniel R, Katz RA, Skalka AM. A role for DNA-PK in retroviral DNA integration. *Science* 1999;284:644–647.
157. Danos O, Mulligan RC. Safe and efficient generation of recombinant retroviruses with amphotropic and ecotropic host ranges. *Proc Natl Acad Sci U S A* 1988;85:6460–6464.
158. Darke PL, Huff JR. HIV protease as an inhibitor target for the treatment of AIDS. *Adv Pharmacol* 1994;25:399–454.
159. Das AT, Klaver B, Berkhout B. A hairpin structure in the R region of the human immunodeficiency virus type 1 RNA genome is instrumental in polyadenylation site selection. *J Virol* 1999;73:81–91.
160. Das K, Ding J, Hsiou Y, et al. Crystal structures of 8-Cl and 9-Cl TIBO complexed with wild-type HIV-1 RT and 8-Cl TIBO complexed with the Tyr181Cys HIV-1 RT drug-resistant mutant. *J Mol Biol* 1996; 264:1085–1100.
161. Dasgupta P, Saikumar P, Reddy CD, Reddy EP. Myb protein binds to human immunodeficiency virus 1 long terminal repeat (LTR) sequences and transactivates LTR-mediated transcription. *Proc Natl Acad Sci U S A* 1990;87:8090–8094.
162. Davey RA, Zuo Y, Cunningham JM. Identification of a receptor-binding pocket on the envelope protein of friend murine leukemia virus. *J Virol* 1999;73:3758–3763.
163. Davies JFI, Hostomska Z, Hostomsky Z, et al. Crystal structure of the ribonuclease H domain of HIV-1 reverse transcriptase. *Science* 1991; 252:88–95.
164. Davis BR, Brightman BK, Chandy KG, Fan H. Characterization of a preleukemic state induced by Moloney murine leukemia virus: Evidence for two infection events during leukemogenesis. *Proc Natl Acad Sci U S A* 1987;84:4875–4879.
165. De Guzman RN, Wu ZR, Stalling CC, et al. Structure of the HIV-1 nucleocapsid protein bound to the SL3 psi-RNA recognition element. *Science* 1998;279:384–388.
166. De Rocquigny H, Gabus C, Vincent A, et al. Viral RNA annealing activities of human immunodeficiency virus type 1 nucleocapsid protein require only peptide domains outside the zinc fingers. *Proc Natl Acad Sci U S A* 1992;89:6472–6476.
167. Denesvre C, Sonigo P, Corbin A, et al. Influence of transmembrane domains on the fusogenic abilities of human and murine leukemia retrovirus envelopes. *J Virol* 1995;69:4149–4157.
168. Derse D. Bovine leukemia virus transcription is controlled by a virus-encoded trans-acting factor and by cis-acting response elements. *J Virol* 1987;61:2462–2471.
169. DesGroseillers L, Rassart E, Robitaille Y, Jolicoeur P. Retrovirus-induced spongiform encephalopathy: The 3′-end long terminal repeat-containing viral sequences influence the incidence of the disease and the specificity of the neurological syndrome. *Proc Natl Acad Sci U S A* 1985;82:8818–8822.
170. DeStefano J, Ghosh J, Prasad B, Raja A. High fidelity of internal strand transfer catalyzed by human immunodeficiency virus reverse transcriptase. *J Biol Chem* 1998;273:1483–1489.
171. DeZazzo JD, Kilpatrick JE, Imperiale MJ. Involvement of long terminal repeat U3 sequences overlapping the transcription control region in human immunodeficiency virus type 1 mRNA 3′ end formation. *Mol Cell Biol* 1991;11:1624–1630.
172. DiFronzo NL, Holland CA. Sequence-specific and/or stereospecific constraints of the U3 enhancer elements of MCF 247-W are important for pathogenicity. *J Virol* 1999;73:234–241.
173. Dillon PJ, Nelbock P, Perkins A, Rosen CA. Function of the human immunodeficiency virus types 1 and 2 rev proteins is dependent on their ability to interact with a structured region present in *env* gene mRNA. *J Virol* 1990;64:4428–4437.
174. Ding J, Das K, Tantillo C, et al. Structure of HIV-1 reverse transcriptase in a complex with the non-nucleoside inhibitor alpha-APA R 95845 at 2.8 A resolution. *Structure* 1995;3:365–379.
175. Dingwall C, Ernberg I, Gait MJ, et al. HIV-1 tat protein stimulates transcription by binding to a U-rich bulge in the stem of the TAR RNA structure. *EMBO J* 1990;9:4145–4154.
176. Dombroski BA, Mathias SL, Nanthakumar E, et al. Isolation of an active human transposable element. *Science* 1991;254:1805–1807.
177. Dong J, Dubay JW, Perez LG, Hunter E. Mutations within the proteolytic cleavage site of the Rous sarcoma virus glycoprotein define a requirement for dibasic residues for intracellular cleavage. *J Virol* 1992;66:865–874.
178. Donze O, Damay P, Spahr PF. The first and third uORFs in RSV leader RNA are efficiently translated: Implications for translational regulation and viral RNA packaging. *Nucleic Acids Res* 1995;23:861–868.
179. Doolittle RF, Feng D-F. Tracing the origin of retroviruses. *Curr Top Microbiol Immunol* 1992;176:195–212.
180. Doolittle RF, Feng D-F, Johnson MS, McClure MA. Origins and evolutionary relationships of retroviruses. *Quart Rev Biol* 1989;64:1–30.
181. Dorfman T, Mammano F, Haseltine WA, Gottlinger HG. Role of the matrix protein in the virion association of the human immunodeficiency virus type 1 envelope glycoprotein. *J Virol* 1994;68:1689–1696.
182. Doria-Rose NA, Vogt VM. *In vivo* selection of Rous sarcoma virus mutants with randomized sequences in the packaging signal. *J Virol* 1998;72:8073–8082.
183. Dornadula G, Zhang H, Shetty S, Pomerantz RJ. HIV-1 virions produced from replicating peripheral blood lymphocytes are more infectious than those from nonproliferating macrophages due to higher levels of intravirion reverse transcripts: Implications for pathogenesis and transmission. *Virology* 1999;253:10–16.
184. Dougherty JP, Temin HM. Determination of the rate of base-pair substitution and insertion mutations in retrovirus replication. *J Virol* 1988;62:2817–2822.
185. Douglas J, Kelly P, Evans JT, Garcia JV. Efficient transduction of human lymphocytes and CD34+ cells via human immunodeficiency virus-based gene transfer vectors. *Hum Gene Ther* 1999;10:935–945.
186. Dragic T, Trkola A, Lin SW, et al. Amino-terminal substitutions in the CCR5 coreceptor impair gp120 binding and human immunodeficiency virus type 1 entry. *J Virol* 1998;72:279–285.
187. Du Z, Holland JA, Hansen MR, et al. Base-pairings within the RNA pseudoknot associated with the simian retrovirus-1 gag-pro frameshift site. *J Mol Biol* 1997;270:464–470.
188. Du Z, Ilyinskii PO, Lally K, et al. A mutation in integrase can compensate for mutations in the simian immunodeficiency virus att site. *J Virol* 1997;71:8124–8132.
189. Dubay JW, Roberts SJ, Brody B, Hunter E. Mutations in the leucine zipper of the human immunodeficiency virus type 1 transmembrane glycoprotein affect fusion and infectivity. *J Virol* 1992;66:4748–4756.
190. Dubay JW, Roberts SJ, Hahn BH, Hunter E. Truncation of the human

immunodeficiency virus type 1 transmembrane glycoprotein cytoplasmic domain blocks virus infectivity. *J Virol* 1992;66:6641–6648.
191. Dupraz P, Rebai N, Klein SJ, et al. The murine AIDS virus Gag precursor protein binds to the SH3 domain of c-Abl. *J Virol* 1997;71:2615–2620.
192. Dyda F, Hickman AB, Jenkins TM, et al. Crystal structure of the catalytic domain of HIV-1 integrase: Similarity to other polynucleotidyl transferases. *Science* 1994;266:1981–1986.
193. Earl PL, Doms RW, Moss B. Oligomeric structure of the human immunodeficiency virus type 1 envelope glycoprotein. *Proc Natl Acad Sci U S A* 1990;87:648–652.
194. Edinger AL, Hoffman TL, Sharron M, et al. An orphan seven-transmembrane domain receptor expressed widely in the brain functions as a coreceptor for human immunodeficiency virus type 1 and simian immunodeficiency virus. *J Virol* 1998;72:7934–7940.
195. Eglitis MA, Kadan MJ, Wonilowicz E, Gould L. Introduction of human genomic sequences renders CHO-K1 cells susceptible to infection by amphotropic retroviruses. *J Virol* 1993;67:1100–1104.
196. Ehrlich LS, Agresta BE, Carter CA. Assembly of recombinant human immunodeficiency virus type 1 capsid protein *in vitro*. *J Virol* 1992;66:4874–4883.
197. Eiden MV, Farrell K, Wilson CA. Glycosylation-dependent inactivation of the ecotropic murine leukemia virus receptor. *J Virol* 1994;68:626–631.
198. Eiden MV, Farrell KB, Wilson CA. Substitution of a single amino acid residue is sufficient to allow the human amphotropic murine leukemia virus receptor to also function as a gibbon ape leukemia virus receptor. *J Virol* 1996;70:1080–1085.
199. Eijkelenboom AP, Lutzke RA, Boelens R, et al. The DNA-binding domain of HIV-1 integrase has an SH3-like fold. *Nat Struct Biol* 1995;2:807–810.
200. Eijkelenboom AP, van den Ent FM, Vos A, et al. The solution structure of the amino-terminal HHCC domain of HIV-2 integrase: A three-helix bundle stabilized by zinc. *Curr Biol* 1997;7:739–746.
201. Einfeld D. Maturation and assembly of retroviral glycoproteins. *Curr Top Microbiol Immunol* 1996;214:133–176.
202. Einfeld D, Hunter E. Oligomeric structure of a prototype retrovirus glycoprotein. *Proc Natl Acad Sci U S A* 1988;85:8688–8692.
203. Einfeld DA, Hunter E. Mutational analysis of the oligomer assembly domain in the transmembrane subunit of the Rous sarcoma virus glycoprotein. *J Virol* 1997;71:2383–2389.
204. Elder JH, Lerner DL, Hasselkus-Light CS, et al. Distinct subsets of retroviruses encode dUTPase. *J Virol* 1992;66:1791–1794.
205. Elgavish T, VanLoock MS, Harvey SC. Exploring three-dimensional structures of the HIV-1 RNA/tRNALys3 initiation complex. *J Mol Biol* 1999;285:449–453.
206. Ellis J, Bernstein A. Retrovirus vectors containing an internal attachment site: Evidence that circles are not intermediates to murine retrovirus integration. *J Virol* 1989;63:2844–2846.
207. Emanoil-Ravier R, Mercier G, Canivet M, et al. Dexamethasone stimulates expression of transposable type A intracisternal retroviruslike genes in mouse (*Mus musculus*) cells. *J Virol* 1988;62:3867–3869.
208. Emerman M, Vazeux R, Peden K. The rev gene product of the human immunodeficiency virus affects envelope-specific RNA localization. *Cell* 1989;57:1155–1165.
209. Emi N, Friedmann T, Yee J-K. Pseudotype formation of murine leukemia virus with the G protein of vesicular stomatitis virus. *J Virol* 1991;65:1202–1207.
210. Emini EA, Schleif WA, Deutsch P, Condra JH. *In vivo* selection of HIV-1 variants with reduced susceptibility to the protease inhibitor L-735,524 and related compounds. *Adv Exp Med Biol* 1996;394:327–331.
211. Endrich MM, Gehrig P, Gehring H. Maturation-induced conformational changes of HIV-1 capsid protein and identification of two high affinity sites for cyclophilins in the C-terminal domain. *J Biol Chem* 1999;274:5326–5332.
212. Engelman A, Bushman FD, Craigie R. Identification of discrete functional domains of HIV-1 integrase and their organization within an active multimeric complex. *EMBO J* 1993;12:3269–3275.
213. Engelman A, Mizuuchi K, Craigie R. HIV-1 DNA integration: Mechanism of viral DNA cleavage and DNA strand transfer. *Cell* 1991;67:1211–1222.
214. Enssle J, Jordan I, Mauer B, Rethwilm A. Foamy virus reverse transcriptase is expressed independently from the Gag protein. *Proc Natl Acad Sci U S A* 1996;93:4137–4141.
215. Erdie CR, Wills JW. Myristylation of Rous sarcoma virus gag protein does not prevent replication in avian cells. *J Virol* 1990;64:5204–5208.
216. Ernst RK, Bray M, Rekosh D, Hammarskjold ML. Secondary structure and mutational analysis of the Mason-Pfizer monkey virus RNA constitutive transport element. *RNA* 1997;3:210–222.
217. Esposito D, Craigie R. Sequence specificity of viral end DNA binding by HIV-1 integrase reveals critical regions for protein-DNA interaction. *EMBO J* 1998;17:5832–5843.
218. Evans LH, Cloyd MW. Generation of mink cell focus-forming viruses by Friend murine leukemia virus: Recombination with specific endogenous proviral sequences. *J Virol* 1984;49:772–781.
219. Faller DV, Weng H, Graves DT, Choi SY. Moloney murine leukemia virus long terminal repeat activates monocyte chemotactic protein-1 protein expression and chemotactic activity. *J Cell Physiol* 1997;172:240–252.
220. Fan H. Influences of the long terminal repeats on retrovirus pathogenicity. *Sem Virol* 1990;1:165–174.
221. Fan H. Leukemogenesis by Moloney murine leukemia virus: A multistep process. *Trends Microbiol* 1997;5:74–82.
222. Fan H, Chute H, Chao E, Pattengale PK. Leukemogenicity of Moloney murine leukemia viruses carrying polyoma enhancer sequences in the long terminal repeat is dependent on the nature of the inserted polyoma sequences. *Virology* 1988;166:58–65.
223. Farnet CM, Bushman FD. HIV-1 cDNA integration: Requirement of HMG I(Y) protein for function of preintegration complexes *in vitro*. *Cell* 1997;88:483–492.
224. Farnet CM, Haseltine WA. Determination of viral proteins present in the human immunodeficiency virus type 1 preintegration complex. *J Virol* 1991;65:1910–1915.
225. Fass D, Davey RA, Hamson CA, et al. Structure of a murine leukemia virus receptor-binding glycoprotein at 2.0 angstrom resolution. *Science* 1997;277:1662–1666.
226. Fass D, Harrison SC, Kim PS. Retrovirus envelope domain at 1.7 angstrom resolution. *Nat Struct Biol* 1996;3:465–469.
227. Fass D, Kim PS. Dissection of a retrovirus envelope protein reveals structural similarity to influenza hemagglutinin. *Curr Biol* 1995;5:1377–1383.
228. Federspiel MJ, Bates P, Young JA, et al. A system for tissue-specific gene targeting: Transgenic mice susceptible to subgroup A avian leukosis virus-based retroviral vectors. *Proc Natl Acad Sci U S A* 1994;91:11241–11245.
229. Feinstein SC, Ross SR, Yamamoto KR. Chromosomal position effects determine transcriptional potential of integrated mammary tumor virus DNA. *J Mol Biol* 1982;156:549–566.
230. Felber BK, Hadzopoulou-Cladaras M, Cladaras C, et al. Rev protein of human immunodeficiency virus 1 affects the stability and transport of the viral mRNA. *Proc Natl Acad Sci U S A* 1989;86:1495–1499.
231. Felsenstein KM, Goff SP. Expression of the gag-pol fusion protein of Moloney murine leukemia virus without gag protein does not induce virion formation or proteolytic processing. *J Virol* 1988;62:2179–2182.
232. Felsenstein KM, Goff SP. Mutational analysis of the gag-pol junction of Moloney murine leukemia virus: Requirements for expression of the gag-pol fusion protein. *J Virol* 1992;66:6601–6608.
233. Feng Y, Broder CC, Kennedy PE, Berger EA. HIV-1 entry cofactor: Functional cDNA cloning of a seven-transmembrane, G protein-coupled receptor. *Science* 1996;272:872–877.
234. Feng Y-X, Hatfield DL, Rein A, Levin JG. Translational readthrough of the murine leukemia virus *gag* gene amber codon does not require virus-induced alteration of tRNA. *J Virol* 1989;63:2405–2410.
235. Feng Y-X, Levin JG, Hatfield DL, et al. Suppression of UAA and UGA termination codons in mutant murine leukemia viruses. *J Virol* 1989;63:2870–2873.
236. Feng Y-X, Yan H, Rein A, Levin JG. Bipartite signal for read-through suppression in murine leukemia virus mRNA: An eight-nucleotide purine-rich sequence immediately downstream of the gag termination codon followed by an RNA pseudoknot. *J Virol* 1992;66:5127–5132.
237. Feuer G, Taketo M, Hanecak RC, Fan H. Two blocks in Moloney murine leukemia virus expression in undifferentiated F9 embryonal carcinoma cells as determined by transient expression assays. *J Virol* 1989;63:2317–2324.
238. Fisher J, Goff SP. Mutational analysis of stem-loops in the RNA packaging signal of the Moloney murine leukemia virus. *Virology* 1998;244:133–145.
239. Fisher RJ, Rein A, Fivash M, et al. Sequence-specific binding of

human immunodeficiency virus type 1 nucleocapsid protein to short oligonucleotides. *J Virol* 1998;72:1902–1909.
240. Fitzgerald ML, Vora AC, Zeh WG, Grandgenett DP. Concerted integration of viral DNA termini by purified avian myeloblastosis virus integrase. *J Virol* 1992;66:6257–6263.
241. Flanagan JR, Becker KG, Ennist DL, et al. Cloning of a negative transcription factor that binds to the upstream conserved region of Moloney murine leukemia virus. *Mol Cell Biol* 1992;12:38–44.
242. Flugel RM, Rethwilm A, Maurer B, Darai G. Nucleotide sequence of the *env* gene and its flanking regions of the human spumaretrovirus reveals two novel genes. *EMBO J* 1987;6:2077–2084.
243. Franke EK, Yuan HE, Bossolt KL, et al. Specificity and sequence requirements for interactions between various retroviral Gag proteins. *J Virol* 1994;68:5300–5305.
244. Franke EK, Yuan HE, Luban J. Specific incorporation of cyclophilin A into HIV-1 virions. *Nature* 1994;372:359–362.
245. Frankel WN, Stoye JP, Taylor BA, Coffin JM. A linkage map of endogenous murine leukemia proviruses. *Genetics* 1990;124:221–236.
246. Freed EO. HIV-1 gag proteins: Diverse functions in the virus life cycle. *Virology* 1998;251:1–15.
247. Freed EO, Englund G, Maldarelli F, Martin MA. Phosphorylation of residue 131 of HIV-1 matrix is not required for macrophage infection. *Cell* 1997;88:171–173.
248. Freed EO, Englund G, Martin MA. Role of the basic domain of human immunodeficiency virus type 1 matrix in macrophage infection. *J Virol* 1995;69:3949–3954.
249. Freed EO, Martin MA. Virion incorporation of envelope glycoproteins with long but not short cytoplasmic tails is blocked by specific, single amino acid substitutions in the human immunodeficiency virus type 1 matrix. *J Virol* 1995;69:1984–1989.
250. Freed EO, Martin MA. Domains of the human immunodeficiency virus type 1 matrix and gp41 cytoplasmic tail required for envelope incorporation into virions. *J Virol* 1996;70:341–51.
251. Freed EO, Myers DJ, Risser R. Characterization of the fusion domain of the human immunodeficiency virus type1 envelope glycoprotein gp41. *Proc Natl Acad Sci U S A* 1990;87:4650–4654.
252. Fu W, Gorelick RJ, Rein A. Characterization of human immunodeficiency virus type 1 dimeric RNA from wild-type and protease-defective virions. *J Virol* 1994;68:5013–5018.
253. Fu W, Ortiz-Conde BA, Gorelick RJ, et al. Placement of tRNA primer on the primer-binding site requires *pol* gene expression in avian but not murine retroviruses. *J Virol* 1997;71:6940–6946.
254. Fu W, Rein A. Maturation of dimeric viral RNA of Moloney murine leukemia virus. *J Virol* 1993;67:5443–5449.
255. Fujisawa R, McAtee FJ, Wehrly K, Portis JL. The neuroinvasiveness of a murine retrovirus is influenced by a dileucine-containing sequence in the cytoplasmic tail of glycosylated Gag. *J Virol* 1998;72:5619–5625.
256. Fujiwara T, Mizuuchi K. Retroviral DNA integration: Structure of an integration intermediate. *Cell* 1988;54:497–504.
257. Gallay P, Hope T, Chin D, Trono D. HIV-1 infection of nondividing cells through the recognition of integrase by the importin/karyopherin pathway. *Proc Natl Acad Sci U S A* 1997;94:9825–9830.
258. Gallay P, Swingler S, Aiken C, Trono D. HIV-1 infection of nondividing cells: C-terminal tyrosine phosphorylation of the viral matrix protein is a key regulator. *Cell* 1995;80:379–388.
259. Gallay P, Swingler S, Song J, et al. HIV nuclear import is governed by the phosphotyrosine-mediated binding of matrix to the core domain of integrase. *Cell* 1995;83:569–576.
260. Gallis B, Linial M, Eisenmann R. An avian oncovirus mutant deficient in genomic RNA: Characterization of the packaged RNA as cellular messenger RNA. *Virology* 1979;94:146–161.
261. Gamble TR, Yoo S, Vajdos FF, et al. Structure of the carboxyl-terminal dimerization domain of the HIV-1 capsid protein. *Science* 1997;278:849–853.
262. Ganser BK, Li S, Klishko VY, et al. Assembly and analysis of conical models for the HIV-1 core. *Science* 1999;283:80–83.
263. Gao G, Goff SP. Somatic cell mutants resistant to retrovirus replication: Intracellular blocks during the early stages of infection. *Mol Biol Cell* 1999;10:1705–1717.
264. Garnier L, Parent LJ, Rovinski B, et al. Identification of retroviral late domains as determinants of particle size. *J Virol* 1999;73:2309–2320.
265. Garnier L, Wills JW, Verderame MF, Sudol M. WW domains and retrovirus budding. *Nature* 1996;381:744–745.
266. Gatlin J, Arrigo SJ, Schmidt MG. Regulation of intracellular human immunodeficiency virus type-1 protease activity. *Virology* 1998;244:87–96.
267. Gebhardt A, Bosch JV, Ziemiecki A, Friis RR. Rous sarcoma virus p19 and gp35 can be chemically crosslinked to high molecular weight complexes. *J Mol Biol* 1984;174:297–317.
268. Genoud S, Kajumo F, Guo Y, et al. CCR5-Mediated human immunodeficiency virus entry depends on an amino-terminal gp120-binding site and on the conformational integrity of all four extracellular domains. *J Virol* 1999;73:1645–1648.
269. Georgiadis MM, Jessen SM, Ogata CM, et al. Mechanistic implications from the structure of a catalytic fragment of Moloney murine leukemia virus reverse transcriptase. *Structure* 1995;3:879–892.
270. Ghosh SK, Faller DV. Feline leukemia virus long terminal repeat activates collagenase IV gene expression through AP-1. *J Virol* 1999;73:4931–4940.
271. Gilboa E, Mitra SW, Goff S, Baltimore D. A detailed model of reverse transcription and tests of crucial aspects. *Cell* 1979;18:93–100.
272. Gitti RK, Lee BM, Walker J, et al. Structure of the amino-terminal core domain of the HIV-1 capsid protein. *Science* 1996;273:231–235.
273. Gluick TC, Wills NM, Gesteland RF, Draper DE. Folding of an mRNA pseudoknot required for stop codon readthrough: Effects of mono- and divalent ions on stability. *Biochemistry* 1997;36:16173–16186.
274. Goldfarb MP, Weinberg RA. Generation of novel, biologically active Harvey sarcoma viruses via apparent illegitimate recombination. *J Virol* 1981;38:136–150.
275. Goldgur Y, Dyda F, Hickman AB, et al. Three new structures of the core domain of HIV-1 integrase: An active site that binds magnesium. *Proc Natl Acad Sci U S A* 1998;95:9150–9154.
276. Golemis E, Li Y, Fredrickson TN, et al. Distinct segments within the enhancer region collaborate to specify the type of leukemia induced by nondefective Friend and Moloney viruses. *J Virol* 1988;63:328–337.
277. Golomb M, Grandgenett DP. Endonuclease activity of purified RNA directed DNA polymerase from AMV. *J Biol Chem* 1979;254:1606–1613.
278. Golovkina TV, Dzuris J, van den Hoogen B, et al. A novel membrane protein is a mouse mammary tumor virus receptor. *J Virol* 1998;72:3066–3071.
279. Gopalakrishnan V, Peliska JA, Benkovic SJ. Human immunodeficiency virus type 1 reverse transcriptase: Spatial and temporal relationshp between the polymerase and RNase H activities. *Proc Natl Acad Sci U S A* 1992;89:10763–10767.
280. Gorelick RJ, Benveniste RE, Gagliardi TD, et al. Nucleocapsid protein zinc-finger mutants of simian immunodeficiency virus strain mne produce virions that are replication defective *in vitro* and *in vivo*. *Virology* 1999;253:259–270.
281. Gorelick RJ, Chabot DJ, Rein A, et al. The two zinc fingers in the human immunodeficiency virus type 1 nucleocapsid protein are not functionally equivalent. *J Virol* 1993;67:4027–4036.
282. Gorelick RJ, Fu W, Gagliardi TD, et al. Characterization of the block in replication of nucleocapsid protein zinc finger mutants from Moloney murine leukemia virus. *J Virol* 1999;73:8185–8195.
283. Gorska-Flipot I, Huang M, Cantin M, et al. U3 long terminal repeat-mediated induction of intracellular immunity by a murine retrovirus: A novel model of latency for retroviruses. *J Virol* 1992;66:7201–7210.
284. Gorska-Flipot I, Jolicoeur P. DNA-binding proteins that interact with the long terminal repeat of radiation leukemia virus. *J Virol* 1990;64:1566–1572.
285. Gottlinger HG, Sodroski JG, Haseltine WA. Role of capsid precursor processing and myristoylation in morphogenesis and infectivity of human immunodeficiency virus type 1. *Proc Natl Acad Sci U S A* 1989;86:5781–5785.
286. Goulaouic H, Subra F, Mouscadet JF, et al. Exogenous nucleosides promote the completion of MoMLV DNA synthesis in G0-arrested Balb c/3T3 fibroblasts. *Virology* 1994;200:87–97.
287. Granger SW, Fan H. *In vivo* footprinting of the enhancer sequences in the upstream long terminal repeat of Moloney murine leukemia virus: Differential binding of nuclear factors in different cell types. *J Virol* 1998;72:8961–8970.
288. Grattinger M, Hohenberg H, Thomas D, et al. *In vitro* assembly properties of wild-type and cyclophilin-binding defective human immunodeficiency virus capsid proteins in the presence and absence of cyclophilin A. *Virology* 1999;257:247–260.
289. Green N, Shinnick TM, Witte O, et al. Sequence-specific antibodies

show that maturation of Moloney leukemia virus envelope polyprotein involves removal of a COOH-terminal peptide. *Proc Natl Acad Sci U S A* 1981;78:6023–6027.
290. Green PL, Chen IS. Regulation of human T cell leukemia virus expression. *FASEB J* 1990;4:169–175.
291. Grimm SL, Nordeen SK. Mouse mammary tumor virus sequences responsible for activating cellular oncogenes. *J Virol* 1998;72: 9428–9435.
292. Gross I, Hohenberg H, Huckhagel C, Krausslich HG. N-terminal extension of human immunodeficiency virus capsid protein converts the *in vitro* assembly phenotype from tubular to spherical particles. *J Virol* 1998;72:4798–4810.
293. Gruter P, Tabernero C, von Kobbe C, et al. TAP, the human homolog of Mex67p, mediates CTE-dependent RNA export from the nucleus. *Mol Cell* 1998;1:649–659.
294. Hagino-Yamagishi K, Donehower LA, Varmus HE. Retroviral DNA integrated during infection by an integration-deficient mutant of murine leukemia virus is oligomeric. *J Virol* 1987;61:1964–1971.
295. Hajjar AM, Linial ML. Modification of retroviral RNA by double-stranded RNA adenosine deaminase. *J Virol* 1995;69:5878–5882.
296. Hansen M, Jelinek L, Whiting S, Barklis E. Transport and assembly of gag proteins into Moloney murine leukemia virus. *J Virol* 1990;64: 5306–5316.
297. Hansen MS, Barklis E. Structural interactions between retroviral Gag proteins examined by cysteine cross-linking. *J Virol* 1995;69: 1150–1159.
298. Harrison GP, Mayo MS, Hunter E, Lever AM. Pausing of reverse transcriptase on retroviral RNA templates is influenced by secondary structures both 5′ and 3′ of the catalytic site. *Nucleic Acids Res* 1998; 26:3433–3442.
299. Hatziioannou T, Valsesia-Wittmann S, Russell SJ, Cosset FL. Incorporation of fowl plague virus hemagglutinin into murine leukemia virus particles and analysis of the infectivity of the pseudotyped retroviruses. *J Virol* 1998;72:5313–5317.
300. Hayward WS, Neel BG, Astrin SM. Activation of a cellular *onc* gene by promoter insertion in ALV-induced lymphomas. *Nature* 1981;290: 475–480.
301. Heidmann O, Heidmann T. Retrotranposition of a mouse IAP sequence tagged with an indicator gene. *Cell* 1991;64:159–170.
302. Helseth E, Olshevsky U, Furman C, Sodroski J. Human immunodeficiency virus type 1 gp120 envelope glycoprotein regions important for association with the gp41 transmembrane glycoprotein. *J Virol* 1991; 65:2119–2123.
303. Helseth E, Oshevsky U, Gabuzda D, et al. Changes in the transmembrane region of the human immunodeficiency virus type 1 gp41 envelope glycoprotein affect membrane fusion. *J Virol* 1990;64:6314–6318.
304. Henderson LE, Krutzsch HC, Oroszlan S. Myristyl amino-terminal acylation of murine retrovirus proteins: An unusual post-translational protein modification. *Proc Natl Acad Sci U S A* 1983;80:339–343.
305. Heneine W, Tibell A, Switzer WM, et al. No evidence of infection with porcine endogenous retrovirus in recipients of porcine islet-cell xenografts. *Lancet* 1998;352:695–699.
306. Herman SA, Coffin JM. Differential transcription from the long terminal repeats of integrated avian leukosis virus DNA. *J Virol* 1986;60:497–505.
307. Herman SA, Coffin JM. Efficient packaging of readthrough RNA in ALV: Implications for oncogene transduction. *Science* 1987;236: 845–848.
308. Hernandez LD, White JM. Mutational analysis of the candidate internal fusion peptide of the avian leukosis and sarcoma virus subgroup A envelope glycoprotein. *J Virol* 1998;72:3259–3267.
309. Heuer TS, Brown PO. Photo-cross-linking studies suggest a model for the architecture of an active human immunodeficiency virus type 1 integrase-DNA complex. *Biochemistry* 1998;37:6667–6678.
310. Hilberg F, Stocking C, Ostertag W, Grez M. Functional analysis of a retroviral host-range mutant: Altered long terminal repeat sequences allow expression in embryonal carcinoma cells. *Proc Natl Acad Sci U S A* 1987;84:5232–5236.
311. Hindmarsh P, Ridky T, Reeves R, et al. HMG protein family members stimulate human immunodeficiency virus type 1 and avian sarcoma virus concerted DNA integration *in vitro*. *J Virol* 1999;73:2994–3003.
312. Holland CA, Wozney J, Hopkins N. Nucleotide sequence of the gp70 gene of murine retrovirus MCF 247. *J Virol* 1983;47:413–420.
313. Holland SM, Ahmad N, Maitra RK, et al. Human immunodeficiency virus rev protein recognizes a target sequence in rev-responsive element RNA within the context of RNA secondary structure. *J Virol* 1990;64:5966–5975.
314. Honigman A, Wolf D, Yaish S, et al. *Cis* acting RNA sequences control the gag-pol translation readthreough in murine leukemia virus. *Virology* 1991;183:313–319.
315. Hopkins N, Schindler J, Hynes R. Six NB-tropic murine leukemia viruses derived from a B-tropic virus of BALB/c have altered p30. *J Virol* 1977;21:309–318.
316. Horton R, Mumm S, Grandgenett DP. Avian retrovirus pp32 DNA endonuclease is phosphorylated on Ser in the carboxyl-terminal region. *J Virol* 1988;62:2067–2075.
317. Horwitz MS, Boyce-Jacino MT, Faras AJ. Novel human endogenous sequences related to human immunodeficiency virus type 1. *J Virol* 1992;66:2170–2179.
318. Hostomsky Z, Hughes SH, Goff SP, Le Grice SF. Redesignation of the RNase D activity associated with retroviral reverse transcriptase as RNase H. *J Virol* 1994;68:1970–1971.
319. Housset V, de Rocquigny H, Roques BP, Darlix J-L. Basic amino acids flanking the zinc finger of Moloney murine leukemia virus nucleocapsid protein NCp10 are critical for virus infectivity. *J Virol* 1993;67:2537–2545.
320. Hsiou Y, Ding J, Das K, et al. Structure of unliganded HIV-1 reverse transcriptase at 2.7 Å resolution: Implications of conformational changes for polymerization and inhibition mechanisms. *Structure* 1996;4:853–860.
321. Hu SC, Court DL, Zweig M, Levin JG. Murine leukemia virus *pol* gene products: Analysis with antisera generated against reverse transcriptase and endonuclease fusion proteins expressed in *Escherichia coli*. *J Virol* 1986;60:267–274.
322. Hu W-S, Temin HM. Retroviral recombination and reverse transcription. *Science* 1990;250:1227–1233.
323. Hu WS, Bowman EH, Delviks KA, Pathak VK. Homologous recombination occurs in a distinct retroviral subpopulation and exhibits high negative interference. *J Virol* 1997;71:6028–6036.
324. Huang H, Chopra R, Verdine GL, Harrison SC. Structure of a covalently trapped catalytic complex of HIV-1 reverse transcriptase: Implications for drug resistance. *Science* 1998;282:1669–1675.
325. Huang M, Jolicoeur P. Characterization of the gag/fusion protein encoded by the defective duplan retrovirus inducing murine acquired immunodeficiency syndrome. *J Virol* 1990;64:5764–5772.
326. Huang M, Simard C, Jolicoeur P. Immunodeficiency and clonal growth of target cells induced by helper-free defective retrovirus. *Science* 1989;246:1614–1617.
327. Huang M, Simard C, Kay DG, Jolicoeur P. The majority of cells infected with the defective murine AIDS virus belong to the B-cell lineage. *J Virol* 1991;65:6562–6571.
328. Huang Y, Khorchid A, Gabor J, et al. The role of nucleocapsid and U5 stem/A-rich loop sequences in tRNA(3Lys) genomic placement and initiation of reverse transcription in human immunodeficiency virus type 1. *J Virol* 1998;72:3907–3915.
329. Humphries EH, Danhof ML, Hlozanek I. Characterization of endogenous viral loci in five lines of white leghorn chickens. *Virology* 1984;135:125–138.
330. Hunter E. Macromolecular interactions in the assembly of HIV and other retroviruses. *Semin Virol* 1994;5:71–83.
331. Hwang JV, Gilboa E. Expression of genes introduced into cells by retroviral infection is more efficient than that of genes introduced into cells by DNA transfection. *J Virol* 1984;50:417–424.
332. Ikeda H, Sugimura H. Fv-4 resistance gene: A truncated endogenous murine leukemia virus with ecotropic interference properties. *J Virol* 1989;63:5405–5412.
333. Ilyinskii PO, Desrosiers RC. Identification of a sequence element immediately upstream of the polypurine tract that is essential for replication of simian immunodeficiency virus. *EMBO J* 1998;17:3766–3774.
334. Isel C, Westhof E, Massire C, et al. Structural basis for the specificity of the initiation of HIV-1 reverse transcription. *EMBO J* 1999;18: 1038–1048.
335. Ishimoto A, Takimoto M, Adachi A, et al. Sequences responsible for erythroid and lymphoid leukemia in the long terminal repeats of Friend-mink cell focus-forming and Moloney murine leukemia viruses. *J Virol* 1987;61:1861–1866.
336. Itin A, Keshet E. A novel retroviruslike family in mouse DNA. *J Virol* 1986;59:301–307.

337. Iwasaki K, Temin HM. The efficiency of RNA 3′ end formation is determined by the distance between the cap site and the poly(A) site in spleen necrosis virus. *Genes Dev* 1990;4:2299–2307.
338. Jacks T, Madhani HD, Masiarz FR, Varmus HE. Signals for ribosomal frameshifting in the Rous sarcoma virus gag-pol region. *Cell* 1988; 55:447–458.
339. Jacks T, Townsley K, Varmus HE, Majors J. Two efficient ribosomal frameshifing events are required for synthesis of mouse mammary tumor virus gag-related polyproteins. *Proc Natl Acad Sci U S A* 1987;84:4298–4302.
340. Jacks T, Varmus HE. Expression of the Rous sarcoma virus *pol* gene by ribosomal frameshifting. *Science* 1985;230:1237–1242.
341. Jacobo-Molina A, Clark ADJ, Williams RL, et al. Crystals of a ternary complex of human immunodeficiency virus type 1 reverse transcriptase with a monoclonal antibody fab fragment and double-stranded DNA diffract x-rays to a 3.5-Å resolution. *Proc Natl Acad Sci U S A* 1991;88:10895–10899.
342. Jacobo-Molina A, Ding J, Nanni RG, et al. Crystal structure of human immunodeficiency virus type 1 reverse transcriptase complexed with double-stranded DNA at 3.0 Å resolution shows bent DNA. *Proc Natl Acad Sci U S A* 1993;90:6320–6324.
343. Jaeger J, Restle T, Steitz TA. The structure of HIV-1 reverse transcriptase complexed with an RNA pseudoknot inhibitor. *EMBO J* 1998;17:4535–4542.
344. Jenkins NA, Copeland NG, Taylor BA, Lee BK. Organization, distribution and stability of endogenous ecotropic murine leukemia virus DNA in chromosomes of Mus musculus. *J Virol* 1982;43:26–36.
345. Jin Z, Jin L, Peterson DL, Lawson CL. Model for lentivirus capsid core assembly based on crystal dimers of EIAV p26. *J Mol Biol* 1999;286:83–93.
346. Johann SV, Gibbons JJ, O'Hara B. GLVR1, a receptor for gibbon ape leukemia virus, is homologous to a phosphate permease of *Neurospora crassa* and is expressed at high levels in the brain and thymus. *J Virol* 1992;66:1635–1640.
347. Johnson WE, Coffin JM. Contructing primate phylogenies from ancient retrovirus sequences. *Proc Natl Acad Sci U S A* 1999;96: 10254–10260.
348. Jolicoeur P. The Fv-1 gene of the mouse and its control of murine leukemia virus replication. *Curr Top Microbiol Immunol* 1979;86: 67–122.
349. Jolicoeur P, Baltimore D. Effect of Fv-1 gene product on proviral DNA formation and integration in cells infected with murine leukemia viruses. *Proc Natl Acad Sci U S A* 1976;73:2236–2240.
350. Jolicoeur P, Rassart E. Effect of Fv-1 gene product on synthesis of linear and supercoiled viral DNA in cells infected with murine leukemia virus. *J Virol* 1980;33:183–195.
351. Jones TA, Blaug G, Hansen M, Barklis E. Assembly of gag-b-galactosidase proteins into retrovirus particles. *J Virol* 1990;64:2265–2279.
352. Jordan I, Enssle J, Guttler E, et al. Expression of human foamy virus reverse transcriptase involves a spliced pol mRNA. *Virology* 1996;224:314–319.
353. Junghans RP, Boone LR, Skalka AM. Retroviral DNA H structures: Displacement-assimilation model of recombination. *Cell* 1982;30:53–62.
354. Kabat D. Molecular biology of Friend viral erythroleukemia. *Curr Top Microbiol Immunol* 1989;148:1–42.
355. Kafri T, van Praag H, Ouyang L, et al. A packaging cell line for lentivirus vectors. *J Virol* 1999;73:576–584.
356. Kalpana GV, Marmon S, Wang W, et al. Binding and stimulation of HIV-1 integrase by a human homolog of yeast transcription factor SNF5. *Science* 1994;266:2002–2006.
357. Kane SE, Beemon K. Precise localization of m6A in Rous sarcoma virus RNA reveals clustering of methylation sites: Implications for RNA processing. *Mol Cell Biol* 1985;5:2298–2306.
358. Kang H, Tinoco I Jr. A mutant RNA pseudoknot that promotes ribosomal frameshifting in mouse mammary tumor virus. *Nucleic Acids Res* 1997;25:1943–1949.
359. Karshin WL, Arcement LJ, Naso RB, Arlinghaus RB. Common precursor for Rauscher leukemia virus gp69/71, p15(E), and p12(E). *J Virol* 1977;23:787–798.
360. Kasahara N, Dozy AM, Kan YW. Tissue-specific targeting of retroviral vectors through ligand-receptor interactions. *Science* 1994;266: 1373–1376.
361. Kashmiri SVS, Rein A, Bassin RH, et al. Donation of N- or B-tropic phenotype to NB-tropic murine leukemia virus during mixed infections. *J Virol* 1977;22:626–633.
362. Katoh I, Ikawa Y, Yoshinaka Y. Retrovirus protease characterized by a dimeric aspartic proteinase. *J Virol* 1989;63:2226–2232.
363. Katoh I, Yoshinaka Y, Rein A, et al. Murine leukemia virus maturation: Protease region required for conversion from "immature" to "mature" core form and for virus infectivity. *Virology* 1985;145:280–292.
364. Katz RA, Kotler M, Skalka AM. Cis-acting intron mutations that affect the efficiency of avian retroviral RNA splicing: Implications for mechanisms of control. *J Virol* 1988;62:2686–2695.
365. Katz RA, Skalka AM. Control of retroviral RNA splicing through maintenance of suboptimal processing signals. *Mol Cell Biol* 1990; 10:696–704.
366. Katz RA, Terry RW, Skalka AM. A conserved cis-acting sequence in the 5′ leader of avian sarcoma virus RNA is required for packaging. *J Virol* 1986;59:163–167.
367. Katzman M, Sudol M. Mapping viral DNA specificity to the central region of integrase by using functional human immunodeficiency virus type 1/visna virus chimeric proteins. *J Virol* 1998;72:1744–1753.
368. Kavanaugh MP, Miller DG, Zhang W, et al. Cell-surface receptors for gibbon ape leukemia virus and amphotropic murine retrovirus are inducible sodium-dependent phosphate symporters. *Proc Natl Acad Sci U S A* 1994;91:7071–7075.
369. Kawamura I, Koga Y, Oh-hori N, et al. Depletion of the surface CD4 molecule by the envelope protein of human immunodeficiency virus expressed in a human CD4+. *J Virol* 1989;63:3748–3754.
370. Kaye JF, Lever AM. Human immunodeficiency virus types 1 and 2 differ in the predominant mechanism used for selection of genomic RNA for encapsidation. *J Virol* 1999;73:3023–3031.
371. Kekuda R, Prasad PR, Fei YJ, et al. Cloning of the sodium-dependent, broad-scope, neutral amino acid transporter Bo from a human placental choriocarcinoma cell line. *J Biol Chem* 1996;271:18657–18661.
372. Kelleher CD, Champoux JJ. Characterization of RNA strand displacement synthesis by Moloney murine leukemia virus reverse transcriptase. *J Biol Chem* 1998;273:9976–9986.
373. Kempler GF, Berwin B, Nanassy O, Barklis E. Characterization of the Moloney murine leukemia virus stem cell-specific repressor binding sites. *Virology* 1993;193:690–699.
374. Kerr SG, Anderson KS. RNA dependent DNA replication fidelity of HIV-1 reverse transcriptase: Evidence of discrimination between DNA and RNA substrates. *Biochemistry* 1997;36:14056–14063.
375. Keshet E, Temin HM. Cell killing by spleen necrosis virus is correlated with a transient accumulation of spleen necrosis virus DNA. *J Virol* 1979;31:376–388.
376. Kestler HWI, Ringler DJ, Mori K, et al. Importance of the *nef* gene for maintenance of high virus loads and for development of AIDS. *Cell* 1991;65:651–662.
377. Kiernan RE, Freed EO. Cleavage of the murine leukemia virus transmembrane *env* protein by human immunodeficiency virus type 1 protease: Transdominant inhibition by matrix mutations. *J Virol* 1998; 72:9621–9627.
378. Kim B, Hathaway TR, Loeb LA. Fidelity of mutant HIV-1 reverse transcriptases: Interaction with the single-stranded template influences the accuracy of DNA synthesis. *Biochemistry* 1998;37:5831–5839.
379. Kim JW, Closs EI, Albritton LM, Cunningham JM. Transport of cationic amino acids by the mouse ecotropic retrovirus receptor. *Nature* 1991;352:725–728.
380. Kim T, Mudry RA Jr, Rexrode CA 2nd, Pathak VK. Retroviral mutation rates and A-to-G hypermutations during different stages of retroviral replication. *J Virol* 1996;70:7594–7602.
381. Kim WK, Tang Y, Kenny JJ, et al. In murine AIDS, B cells are early targets of defective virus and are required for efficient infection and expression of defective virus in T cells and macrophages. *J Virol* 1994;68:6767–6769.
382. King JA, Bridger JM, Gounari F, et al. The extended packaging sequence of MoMLV contains a constitutive mRNA nuclear export function. *FEBS Lett* 1998;434:367–371.
383. King W, Patel MD, Lobel LI, et al. Insertion mutagenesis of embryonal carcinoma cells by retroviruses. *Science* 1985;228:554–558.
384. Kizhatil K, Albritton LM. Requirements for different components of the host cell cytoskeleton distinguish ecotropic murine leukemia virus entry via endocytosis from entry via surface fusion. *J Virol* 1997; 71:7145–7156.
385. Klatzman D, Champagne E, Chamaret S, et al. T-lymphocyte T4 mol-

ecule behaves as the receptor for human retrovirus LAV. *Nature* 1984;312:767–768.

386. Klikova M, Rhee SS, Hunter E, Ruml T. Efficient *in vivo* and *in vitro* assembly of retroviral capsids from Gag precursor proteins expressed in bacteria. *J Virol* 1995;69:1093–1098.
387. Kobe B, Center RJ, Kemp BE, Poumbourios P. Crystal structure of human T cell leukemia virus type 1 gp21 ectodomain crystallized as a maltose-binding protein chimera reveals structural evolution of retroviral transmembrane proteins. *Proc Natl Acad Sci U S A* 1999;96: 4319–4324.
388. Kodama T, Wooley DP, Naidu YM, et al. Significance of premature stop codons in *env* of simian immunodeficiency virus. *J Virol* 1989; 63:4709–4714.
389. Kodera Y, Sato K, Tsukahara T, et al. High-resolution solution NMR structure of the minimal active domain of the human immunodeficiency virus type-2 nucleocapsid protein. *Biochemistry* 1998;37:17704–17713.
390. Kohl NE, Emini EA, Schleif WA, et al. Active human immunodeficiency virus protease is required for viral infectivity. *Proc Natl Acad Sci U S A* 1988;85:4686–4690.
391. Kohlstaedt LA, Wang J, Friedman JM, et al. Crystal structure at 3.5Å resolution of HIV-1 reverse transcriptase complexed with an inhibitor. *Science* 1992;256:1783–1790.
392. Kootstra NA, Schuitemaker H. Phenotype of HIV-1 lacking a functional nuclear localization signal in matrix protein of gag and Vpr is comparable to wild-type HIV-1 in primary macrophages. *Virology* 1999;253:170–180.
393. Kovari LC, Momany CA, Miyagi F, et al. Crystals of Rous sarcoma virus capsid protein show a helical arrangement of protein subunits. *Virology* 1997;238:79–84.
394. Kozak CA, Gromet NJ, Ikeda H, Buckler CE. A unique sequence related to the ecotropic murine leukemia virus is associated with the Fv-4 restriction gene. *Proc Natl Acad Sci U S A* 1984;81:834–837.
395. Kozak CA, O'Neill RR. Diverse wild mouse origins of xenotropic, mink-cell focus-forming, and two types of ecotropic proviral genes. *J Virol* 1987;61:3082–3088.
396. Kraulis PJ. MOLSCRIPT: A program to produce both detailed and schematic plots of protein structures. *J Appl Crystallogr* 1991;24: 946–950.
397. Krishna NK, Campbell S, Vogt VM, Wills JW. Genetic determinants of Rous sarcoma virus particle size. *J Virol* 1998;72:564–577.
398. Kubo Y, Kakimi K, Higo K, et al. Possible origin of murine AIDS (MAIDS) virus: Conversion of an endogenous retroviral p12gag sequence to a MAIDS-inducing sequence by frameshift mutations. *J Virol* 1996;70:6405–6409.
399. Kubo Y, Kakimi K, Higo K, et al. The p15gag and p12gag regions are both necessary for the pathogenicity of the murine AIDS virus. *J Virol* 1994;68:5532–5537.
400. Kuff EL, Leuders KK. The intracisternal A-particle gene family: Structure and functional aspects. *Adv Cancer Res* 1988;51:183–276.
401. Kukolj G, Katz RA, Skalka AM. Characterization of the nuclear localization signal in the avian sarcoma virus integrase. *Gene* 1998;223: 157–163.
402. Kulkosky J, BouHamdan M, Geist A, Pomerantz RJ. A novel Vpr peptide interactor fused to integrase (IN) restores integration activity to IN-defective HIV-1 virions. *Virology* 1999;255:77–85.
403. Kulkosky J, Jones KS, Katz RA, et al. Residues critical for retroviral integrative recombination in a region that is highly conserved among retroviral/retrotransposon integrases and bacterial insertion sequences transposases. *Mol Cell Biol* 1992;12:2331–2338.
404. Kulpa D, Topping R, Telesnitsky A. Determination of the site of first strand transfer during Moloney murine leukemia virus reverse transcription and identification of strand transfer-associated reverse transcriptase errors. *EMBO J* 1997;16:856–865.
405. Kwong PD, Wyatt R, Robinson J, et al. Structure of an HIV gp120 envelope glycoprotein in complex with the CD4 receptor and a neutralizing human antibody. *Nature* 1998;393:648–659.
406. Laco GS, Schalk-Hihi C, Lubkowski J, et al. Crystal structures of the inactive D30N mutant of feline immunodeficiency virus protease complexed with a substrate and an inhibitor. *Biochemistry* 1997;36: 10696–10708.
407. Laigret F, Repaske R, Boulukos K, et al. Potential progenitor sequences of mink cell focus-forming (MCF) murine leukemia viruses: Ecotropic, xenotropic, and MCF-related viral RNAs are detected concurrently in thymus tissues of AKR mice. *J Virol* 1988;62:376–386.
408. Lama J, Trono D. Human immunodeficiency virus type 1 matrix protein interacts with cellular protein HO3. *J Virol* 1998;72:1671–1676.
409. Lapatto R, Blundell T, Hemmings A, et al. X-ray analysis of HIV-1 proteinase at 2.7 Å resolution confirms structural homology among retroviral enzymes. *Nature* 1989;342:299–302.
410. LaPierre LA, Casey JW, Holzschu DL. Walleye retroviruses associated with skin tumors and hyperplasias encode cyclin D homologs. *J Virol* 1998;72:8765–8771.
411. Larder BA, Kemp SD. Multiple mutations in HIV-1 reverse transcriptase confer high-level resistance to zidovudine (AZT). *Science* 1989;246:1155–1158.
412. Lee E, Yeo A, Kraemer B, et al. The Gag domains required for avian retroviral RNA encapsidation determined by using two independent assays. *J Virol* 1999;73:6282–6292.
413. Lee MS, Craigie R. Protection of retroviral DNA from autointegration: Involvement of a cellular factor. *Proc Natl Acad Sci U S A* 1994;91:9823–9827.
414. Lee MS, Craigie R. A previously unidentified host protein protects retroviral DNA from autointegration. *Proc Natl Acad Sci U S A* 1998;95:1528–1533.
415. Lee YMH, Coffin JM. Relationship of avian retrovirus DNA synthesis to integration *in vitro*. *Mol Cell Biol* 1991;11:1419–1430.
416. Leis J, Baltimore D, Bishop JM, et al. Standardized and simplified nomenclature for proteins common to all retroviruses. *J Virol* 1988;62:1808–1809.
417. Lerner DL, Wagaman PC, Phillips TR, et al. Increased mutation frequency of feline immunodeficiency virus lacking functional deoxyuridine-triphosphatase. *Proc Natl Acad Sci U S A* 1995;92: 7480–7484.
418. Leverett BD, Farrell KB, Eiden MV, Wilson CA. Entry of amphotropic murine leukemia virus is influenced by residues in the putative second extracellular domain of its receptor, Pit2. *J Virol* 1998;72:4956–4961.
419. Lewis P, Hensel M, Emerman M. Human immunodeficiency virus infection of cells arrested in the cell cycle. *EMBO J* 1992;11:3053–3058.
420. Lewis PF, Emerman M. Passage through mitosis is required for oncoretroviruses but not for the human immunodeficiency virus. *J Virol* 1994;68:510–516.
421. Li L, Farnet CM, Anderson WF, Bushman FD. Modulation of activity of Moloney murine leukemia virus preintegration complexes by host factors *in vitro*. *J Virol* 1998;72:2125–2131.
422. Li X, McDermott B, Yuan B, Goff SP. Homomeric interactions between transmembrane proteins of Moloney murine leukemia virus. *J Virol* 1996;70:1266–1270.
423. Lilly F. Fv-2: Identification and location of a second gene governing the spleen focus repsonse to Friend leukemia virus in mice. *J Natl Cancer Inst* 1970;45:163–169.
424. Lilly F, Pincus T. Genetic control of murine viral leukemogenesis. *Adv Cancer Res* 1973;17:231–277.
425. Linial M, Medeiros E, Hayward WS. An avian oncovirus mutant (SE 21Q1b) deficient in genomic RNA: Biological and biochemical characterization. *Cell* 1978;15:1371–1381.
426. Liu B, Dai R, Tian CJ, et al. Interaction of the human immunodeficiency virus type 1 nucleocapsid with actin. *J Virol* 1999;73: 2901–2908.
427. Lobel LI, Murphy JE, Goff SP. The palindromic LTR-LTR junction of Moloney murine leukemia virus is not an efficient substrate for proviral integration. *J Virol* 1989;63:2629–2637.
428. Lochelt M, Flugel RM. The human foamy virus *pol* gene is expressed as a Pro-Pol polyprotein and not as a Gag-Pol fusion protein. *J Virol* 1996;70:1033–1040.
429. Lochelt M, Flugel RM, Aboud M. The human foamy virus internal promoter directs the expression of the functional Bel 1 transactivator and Bet protein early after infection. *J Virol* 1994;68:638–645.
430. Lochelt M, Yu SF, Linial ML, Flugel RM. The human foamy virus internal promoter is required for efficient gene expression and infectivity. *Virology* 1995;206:601–610.
431. Lock LF, Keshet E, Gilbert DJ, et al. Studies of the mechanism of spontaneous germline ecotropic provirus acquisition in mice. *EMBO J* 1988;7:4169–4177.
432. Lodge R, Gottlinger H, Gabuzda D, et al. The intracytoplasmic domain of gp41 mediates polarized budding of human immunodeficiency virus type 1 in MDCK cells. *J Virol* 1994;68:4857–4861.
433. Lodi PJ, Ernst JA, Kuszewski J, et al. Solution structure of the DNA binding domain of HIV-1 integrase. *Biochemistry* 1995;34:9826–9833.

434. Loeb DD, Hutchinson III CA, Edgell MH, et al. Mutational analysis of human immunodeficiency virus type 1 protease suggests functional homology with aspartic proteinases. *J Virol* 1989;63:111–121.
435. Loh TP, Sievert LL, Scott RW. Negative regulation of retrovirus expression in embryonal carcinoma cells mediated by an intragenic domain. *J Virol* 1988;62:4086–4095.
436. Loh TP, Sievert LL, Scott RW. Evidence for a stem-cell-specific repressor of Moloney murine leukemia virus expression in embryonal carcinoma cells. *Mol Cell Biol* 1990;10:4045–4057.
437. Lori F, di Marzo Veronese F, DeVico AL, et al. Viral DNA carried by human immunodeficiency virus type 1 virions. *J Virol* 1992;66:5067–5074.
438. LoSardo JE, Boral AL, Lenz J. Relative importance of elements within the SL3-3 virus enhancer for T-cell specificity. *J Virol* 1990;64:1756–1763.
439. Lower R, Lower J, Kurth R. The viruses in all of us: Characteristics and biological significance of human endogenous retrovirus sequences. *Proc Natl Acad Sci U S A* 1996;93:5177–5184.
440. Lower R, Tonjes RR, Korbmacher C, et al. Identification of a Rev-related protein by analysis of spliced transcripts of the human endogenous retroviruses HTDV/HERV-K. *J Virol* 1995;69:141–149.
441. Lu M, Blacklow SC, Kim PS. A trimeric structural domain of the HIV-1 transmembrane glycoprotein. *Nat Struct Biol* 1995;2:1075–1082.
442. Luban J, Alin KB, Bossolt KL, et al. Genetic assay for multimerization of retroviral gag polyproteins. *J Virol* 1992;66:5157–5160.
443. Luban J, Bossolt KA, Franke EK, et al. Human immunodeficiency virus type 1 gag protein binds to cyclophilins A and B. *Cell* 1993;73:1067–1078.
444. Lueders KK, Kuff EL. Sequences associated with intracisternal A particles are repeated in the mouse genome. *Cell* 1977;12:963–972.
445. Lum R, Linial ML. Retrotransposition of nonviral RNAs in an avian packaging cell line. *J Virol* 1998;72:4057–4064.
446. Lundorf MD, Pedersen FS, O'Hara B, Pedersen L. Amphotropic murine leukemia virus entry is determined by specific combinations of residues from receptor loops 2 and 4. *J Virol* 1999;73:3169–3175.
447. Luo G, Taylor J. Template switching by reverse transcriptase during DNA synthesis. *J Virol* 1990;64:4321–4328.
448. Lutzke RA, Plasterk RH. Structure-based mutational analysis of the C-terminal DNA-binding domain of human immunodeficiency virus type 1 integrase: Critical residues for protein oligomerization and DNA binding. *J Virol* 1998;72:4841–4848.
449. Lynch WP, Brown WJ, Spangrude GJ, Portis JL. Microglial infection by a neurovirulent murine retrovirus results in defective processing of envelope protein and intracellular budding of virus particles. *J Virol* 1994;68:3401–3409.
450. Lynch WP, Snyder EY, Qualtiere L, et al. Late virus replication events in microglia are required for neurovirulent retrovirus-induced spongiform neurodegeneration: Evidence from neural progenitor-derived chimeric mouse brains. *J Virol* 1996;70:8896–8907.
451. Maddon PJ, Dalgleish AG, McDougal JS, et al. The T4 gene encodes the AIDS virus receptor and is expressed in the immune system and the brain. *Cell* 1986;47:333–348.
452. Maignan S, Guilloteau JP, Zhou-Liu Q, et al. Crystal structures of the catalytic domain of HIV-1 integrase free and complexed with its metal cofactor: High level of similarity of the active site with other viral integrases. *J Mol Biol* 1998;282:359–368.
453. Mak J, Kleiman L. Primer tRNAs for reverse transcription. *J Virol* 1997;71:8087–8095.
454. Malashkevich VN, Chan DC, Chutkowski CT, Kim PS. Crystal structure of the simian immunodeficiency virus (SIV) gp41 core: Conserved helical interactions underlie the broad inhibitory activity of gp41 peptides. *Proc Natl Acad Sci U S A* 1998;95:9134–9139.
455. Malim MH, Hauber J, Le S-Y, et al. The HIV-1 rev trans-activator acts through a structured target sequence to activate nuclear export of unspliced viral mRNA. *Nature* 1989;338:254–257.
456. Malim MH, McCarn DF, Tiley LS, Cullen BR. Mutational definitition of the human immunodeficiency virus type 1 rev activation domain. *J Virol* 1991;65:4248–4254.
457. Malim MH, Tiley LS, McCarn DF, et al. HIV-1 structural gene expression requires binding of the Rev trans-activator to its RNA target. *Cell* 1990;60:675–683.
458. Mammano F, Ohagen A, Hoglund S, Gottlinger HG. Role of the major homology region of human immunodeficiency virus type 1 in virion morphogenesis. *J Virol* 1994;68:4927–4936.
459. Mann R, Baltimore D. Varying the position of a retrovirus packaging sequence results in the encapsidation of both unspliced and spliced RNAs. *J Virol* 1985;54:401–407.
460. Mann RS, Mulligan RC, Baltimore D. Construction of a retrovirus packaging mutant and its use to produce helper-free defective retrovirus. *Cell* 1983;32:871–879.
461. Mansky LM, Temin HM. Lower *in vivo* mutation rate of human immunodeficiency virus type 1 than that predicted from the fidelity of purified reverse transcriptase. *J Virol* 1995;69:5087–5094.
462. Marczinke B, Fisher R, Vidakovic M, et al. Secondary structure and mutational analysis of the ribosomal frameshift signal of rous sarcoma virus. *J Mol Biol* 1998;284:205–225.
463. Mariani-Costantini R, Horn TM, Callahan R. Ancestry of a human endogenous retrovirus family. *J Virol* 1989;63:4982–4985.
464. Marin M, Noel D, Valsesia-Wittman S, et al. Targeted infection of human cells via major histocompatibility complex class I molecules by Moloney murine leukemia virus-derived viruses displaying single-chain antibody fragment-envelope fusion proteins. *J Virol* 1996;70:2957–2962.
465. Markowitz D, Goff S, Bank A. Construction and use of a safe and efficient amphotropic packaging cell line. *Virology* 1988;167:400–406.
466. Markowitz D, Goff S, Bank A. A safe packaging line for gene transfer: Separating viral genes on two different plasmids. *J Virol* 1988;62:1120–1124.
467. Marsh M, Helenius A. Virus entry into animal cells. *Adv Virus Res* 1989;36:107–151.
468. Martin J, Herniou E, Cook J, et al. Human endogenous retrovirus type I-related viruses have an apparently widespread distribution within vertebrates. *J Virol* 1997;71:437–443.
469. Martineau D, Bowser PR, Renshaw RR, Casey JW. Molecular characterization of a unique retrovirus associated with a fish tumor. *J Virol* 1992;66:596–599.
470. Martinelli SC, Goff SP. Rapid reversion of a deletion mutation in Moloney murine leukemia virus by recombination with a closely related endogenous provirus. *Virology* 1990;174:135–144.
471. Martinez I, Dornburg R. Mapping of receptor binding domains in the envelope protein of spleen necrosis virus. *J Virol* 1995;69:4339–4346.
472. Masuda T, Kuroda MJ, Harada S. Specific and independent recognition of U3 and U5 att sites by human immunodeficiency virus type 1 integrase *in vivo*. *J Virol* 1998;72:8396–8402.
473. Matthews S, Mikhailov M, Burny A, Roy P. The solution structure of the bovine leukaemia virus matrix protein and similarity with lentiviral matrix proteins. *EMBO J* 1996;15:3267–3274.
474. McClure MA. Evolutionary history of reverse transcriptase. In: Skalka AM, Goff SP, eds. *Reverse Transcriptase*. Cold Spring Harbor, NY: Cold Spring Harbor Press, 1993:425–444.
475. McClure MA, Johnson MS, Feng D-F, Doolittle RF. Sequence comparisons of retroviral proteins: Relative rates of change and general phylogeny. *Proc Natl Acad Sci U S A* 1988;85:2469–2473.
476. McClure MO, Sommerfelt MA, Marsh M, Weiss RA. The pH independence of mammalian retrovirus infection. *J Gen Virol* 1990;71:767–773.
477. McCune JM, Rabin LB, Feinberg MB, et al. Endoproteolytic cleavage of gp160 is required for activation of human immunodeficiency virus. *Cell* 1988;53:55–67.
478. McDonnell JM, Fushman D, Cahill SM, et al. Solution structure and dynamics of the bioactive retroviral M domain from Rous sarcoma virus. *J Mol Biol* 1998;279:921–928.
479. McInerney TL, El Ahmar W, Kemp BE, Poumbourios P. Mutation-directed chemical cross-linking of human immunodeficiency virus type 1 gp41 oligomers. *J Virol* 1998;72:1523–1533.
480. McNally LM, McNally MT. U1 small nuclear ribonucleoprotein and splicing inhibition by the rous sarcoma virus negative regulator of splicing element. *J Virol* 1999;73:2385–2393.
481. McNally MT, Beemon K. Intronic sequences and 3′ splice sites control Rous sarcoma virus RNA splicing. *J Virol* 1992;66:6–11.
482. Mergia A. Simian foamy virus type 1 contains a second promoter located at the 3′ end of the *env* gene. *Virology* 1994;199:219–222.
483. Mergia A, Shaw KES, Pratt-Lowe E, et al. Identification of the simian foamy virus transcriptional transactivator gene (*taf*). *J Virol* 1991;65:2903–2909.
484. Meric C, Goff SP. Characterization of Moloney murine leukemia virus mutants with single-amino-acid substitutions in the cys-his box of the nucleocapsid protein. *J Virol* 1989;63:1558–1568.

485. Mesnard JM, Devaux C. Multiple control levels of cell proliferation by human T-cell leukemia virus type 1 tax protein. *Virology* 1999; 257:277–284.
486. Meyer PR, Matsuura SE, So AG, Scott WA. Unblocking of chain-terminated primer by HIV-1 reverse transcriptase through a nucleotide-dependent mechanism. *Proc Natl Acad Sci U S A* 1998;95: 13471–13476.
487. Miele G, Mouland A, Harrison GP, et al. The human immunodeficiency virus type 1 5′ packaging signal structure affects translation but does not function as an internal ribosome entry site structure. *J Virol* 1996;70:944–951.
488. Miller AD, Wolgamot G. Murine retroviruses use at least six different receptors for entry into Mus dunni cells. *J Virol* 1997;71:4531–4535.
489. Miller DG, Adam MA, Miller AD. Gene transfer by retrovirus vectors occurs only in cells that are actively replicating at the time of infection. *Mol Cell Biol* 1990;10:4239–4242.
490. Miller DG, Edwards RH, Miller AD. Cloning of the cellular receptor for amphotropic murine retroviruses reveals homology to that for gibbon ape leukemia virus. *Proc Natl Acad Sci U S A* 1994;91:78–82.
491. Miller M, Jaskolski M, Mohana Rao JK, et al. Crystal structure of a retroviral protease proves relationship to aspartic protease family. *Nature* 1989;337:576–579.
492. Miller MD, Farnet CM, Bushman FD. Human immunodeficiency virus type 1 preintegration complexes: Studies of organization and composition. *J Virol* 1997;71:5382–5390.
493. Moebes A, Enssle J, Bieniasz PD, et al. Human foamy virus reverse transcription that occurs late in the viral replication cycle. *J Virol* 1997;71:7305–7311.
494. Molla A, Granneman GR, Sun E, Kempf DJ. Recent developments in HIV protease inhibitor therapy. *Antiviral Res* 1998;39:1–23.
495. Momany C, Kovari LC, Prongay AJ, et al. Crystal structure of dimeric HIV-1 capsid protein. *Nat Struct Biol* 1996;3:763–770.
496. Monk RJ, Malik FG, Stokesberry D, Evans LH. Direct determination of the point mutation rate of a murine retrovirus. *J Virol* 1992;66: 3683–3689.
497. Moore R, Dixon M, Smith R, et al. Complete nucleotide sequence of a milk-transmitted mouse mammary tumor virus: Two frameshift suppression events are required for translation of gag and pol. *J Virol* 1987;61:480–490.
498. Mooslehner K, Karls U, Harbers K. Retroviral integration sites in transgenic Mov mice frequently map in the vicinity of transcribed DNA regions. *J Virol* 1990;64:3056–3058.
499. Morellet N, Jullian N, Derocquingny H, et al. Determination of the structure of the nucleocapsid protein NCp7 from the human immunodeficiency virus type-1 by H-1 NMR. *EMBO J* 1992;11:3059–3065.
500. Morikawa Y, Zhang WH, Hockley DJ, et al. Detection of a trimeric human immunodeficiency virus type 1 Gag intermediate is dependent on sequences in the matrix protein, p17. *J Virol* 1998;72:7659–7663.
501. Mougel M, Zhang Y, Barklis E. Cis-active structural motifs involved in specific encapsidation of Moloney murine leukemia virus RNA. *J Virol* 1996;70:5043–5050.
502. Mouland AJ, Mercier J, Luo M, et al. Human staufen is incorporated into HIV-1 particles and is implicated in genomic RNA encapsidation. (Personal communication, 1999.)
503. Mumm SR, Grandgenett DP. Defining nucleic acid-binding properties of avian retrovirus integrase by deletion analysis. *J Virol* 1991;65: 1160–1167.
504. Murphy JE, Goff SP. A mutation at one end of Moloney murine leukemia virus DNA blocks cleavage of both ends by the viral integrase *in vivo*. *J Virol* 1992;66:5092–5095.
505. Nabel GJ, Rice SA, Knipe DM, Baltimore D. Alternative mechanisms for activation of human immunodeficiency virus enhancer in T cells. *Science* 1988;239:1299–1302.
506. Naldini L, Blomer U, Gage FH, et al. Efficient transfer, integration, and sustained long-term expression of the transgene in adult rat brains injected with a lentiviral vector. *Proc Natl Acad Sci U S A* 1996;93: 11382–11388.
507. Naldini L, Blomer U, Gallay P, et al. *In vivo* gene delivery and stable transduction of nondividing cells by a lentiviral vector. *Science* 1996;272:263–267.
508. Nam SH, Copeland TD, Hatanaka M, Oroszlan S. Characterization of ribosomal frameshifting for expression of *pol* gene products of human T-cell leukemia virus type 1. *J Virol* 1993;67:196–203.
509. Navia MA, Fitzgerald PMD, McKeever BM, et al. Three-dimensional structure of aspartyl protease from human immunodeficiency virus HIV-1. *Nature* 1989;337:615–620.
510. Negroni M, Buc H. Recombination during reverse transcription: An evaluation of the role of the nucleocapsid protein. *J Mol Biol* 1999; 286:15–31.
511. Nelle TD, Wills JW. A large region within the Rous sarcoma virus matrix protein is dispensable for budding and infectivity. *J Virol* 1996; 70:2269–2276.
512. Nermut MV, Wallengren K, Pager J. Localization of actin in Moloney murine leukemia virus by immunoelectron microscopy. *Virology* 1999;260:23–34.
513. Nie Z, Bergeron D, Subbramanian RA, et al. The putative alpha helix 2 of human immunodeficiency virus type 1 Vpr contains a determinant which is responsible for the nuclear translocation of proviral DNA in growth-arrested cells. *J Virol* 1998;72:4104–4115.
514. Nikbakht KN, Ou C-y, Boone LR, et al. Nucleotide sequence analysis of endogenous murine leukemia virus-related proviral clones reveals primer-binding sites for glutamine tRNA. *J Virol* 1985;54:889–893.
515. Nussbaum O, Roop A, Anderson WF. Sequences determining the pH dependence of viral entry are distinct from the host range-determining region of the murine ecotropic and amphotropic retrovirus envelope proteins. *J Virol* 1993;67:7402–7405.
516. Nusse R. The activation of cellular oncogenes by retroviral insertion. *Trends Genet* 1986;2:244–247.
517. O'Hara B, Johann SV, Klinger HP, et al. Characterization of a human gene conferring sensitivity to infection by gibbon ape leukemia virus. *Cell Growth Differ* 1990;1:119–127.
518. Obata MM, Khan AS. Structure, distribution and expression of an ancient murine endogneous retroviruslike DNA family. *J Virol* 1988;62:4381–4386.
519. Oertle S, Spahr P-F. Role of the gag polyprotein precursor in packaging and maturation of Rous sarcoma virus genomic RNA. *J Virol* 1990;64:5757–5763.
520. Ogert RA, Lee LH, Beemon KL. Avian retroviral RNA element promotes unspliced RNA accumulation in the cytoplasm. *J Virol* 1996; 70:3834–3843.
521. Olah Z, Lehel C, Anderson WB, et al. The cellular receptor for gibbon ape leukemia virus is a novel high affinity sodium-dependent phosphate transporter. *J Biol Chem* 1994;269:25426–25431.
522. Onions D, Hart D, Mahoney C, et al. Endogenous retroviruses and the safety of porcine xenotransplantation. *Trends Microbiol* 1998;6: 430–431.
523. Ono A, Demirov D, Freed EO. Relationship between human immunodeficiency virus type 1 Gag multimerization and membrane binding. *J Virol* 2000;74:5142–5150.
524. Ono A, Freed EO. Binding of human immunodeficiency virus type 1 Gag to membrane: Role of the matrix amino terminus. *J Virol* 1999;73:4136–4144.
525. Ono M, Cole MD, White AT, Huang RCC. Sequence organization of cloned intracisternal A particle genes. *Cell* 1980;21:465–473.
526. Orlik O, Ban J, Hlavaty J, et al. Polyclonal bovine sera but not virus-neutralizing monoclonal antibodies block bovine leukemia virus (BLV) gp51 binding to recombinant BLV receptor BLVRcp1. *J Virol* 1997;71:3263–3267.
527. Ortiz-Conde BA, Hughes SH. Studies of the genomic RNA of leukosis viruses: Implications for RNA dimerization. *J Virol* 1999;73: 7165–7174.
528. Ott DE, Chertova EN, Busch LK, et al. Mutational analysis of the hydrophobic tail of the human immunodeficiency virus type 1 p6(Gag) protein produces a mutant that fails to package its envelope protein. *J Virol* 1999;73:19–28.
529. Ott DE, Coren LV, Copeland TD, et al. Ubiquitin is covalently attached to the p6Gag proteins of human immunodeficiency virus type 1 and simian immunodeficiency virus and to the p12Gag protein of Moloney murine leukemia virus. *J Virol* 1998;72:2962–2968.
530. Ott DE, Coren LV, Kane BP, et al. Cytoskeletal proteins inside human immunodeficiency virus type 1 virions. *J Virol* 1996;70:7734–7743.
531. Ott DE, Hewes SM, Alvord WG, et al. Inhibition of Friend virus replication by a compound that reacts with the nucleocapsid zinc finger: Anti-retroviral effect demonstrated *in vivo*. *Virology* 1998;243:283–292.
532. Ou C-Y, Boone LR, Koh CK, et al. Nucleotide sequences of gag-pol regions that determine the Fv-1 host range property of BALB/c N-tropic and B-tropic murine leukemia viruses. *J Virol* 1983;48:779–784.
533. Oude Essink BB, Berkhout B. The fidelity of reverse transcription dif-

fers in reactions primed with RNA versus DNA primers. *J Biomed Sci* 1999;6:121–132.
534. Owens RJ, Compans RW. Expression of the human immunodeficiency virus envelope glycoprotein is restricted to basolateral surfaces of polarized epithelial cells. *J Virol* 1989;63:978–982.
535. Owens RJ, Dubay JW, Hunter E, Compans RW. Human immunodeficiency virus envelope protein determines the site of virus release in polarized epithelial cells. *Proc Natl Acad Sci U S A* 1991;88: 3987–3991.
536. Paillart JC, Gottlinger HG. Opposing effects of human immunodeficiency virus type 1 matrix mutations support a myristyl switch model of gag membrane targeting. *J Virol* 1999;73:2604–2612.
537. Palmarini M, Dewar P, De las Heras M, et al. Epithelial tumour cells in the lungs of sheep with pulmonary adenomatosis are major sites of replication for Jaagsiekte retrovirus. *J Gen Virol* 1995;76:2731–2737.
538. Panet A, Haseltine WA, Baltimore D, et al. Specific binding of tryptophan transfer RNA to avian myeloblastosis virus RNA-dependent DNA polymerase (reverse transcriptase). *Proc Natl Acad Sci U S A* 1975;72:2535–2539.
539. Panganiban AT. Retroviral *gag* gene amber codon suppression is caused by an intrinsic cis-acting component of the viral mRNA. *J Virol* 1988;62:3574–3580.
540. Panganiban AT, Temin HM. The retrovirus *pol* gene encodes a product required for DNA integration: Identification of a retrovirus int locus. *Proc Natl Acad Sci U S A* 1984;81:7885–7889.
541. Pantginis J, Beaty RM, Levy LS, Lenz J. The feline leukemia virus long terminal repeat contains a potent genetic determinant of T-cell lymphomagenicity. *J Virol* 1997;71:9786–9791.
542. Paquette Y, Hanna Z, Savard P, et al. Retrovirus-induced murine motor neuron disease: Mapping the determinant of spongiform degeneration within the envelope gene. *Proc Natl Acad Sci U S A* 1989;86: 3896–3900.
543. Paquette Y, Kay DG, Rassart E, et al. Substitution of the U3 long terminal repeat region of the neurotropic Cas-Br-E retrovirus affects its disease-inducing potential. *J Virol* 1990;64:3742–3752.
544. Parent LJ, Bennett RP, Craven RC, et al. Positionally independent and exchangeable late budding functions of the Rous sarcoma virus and human immunodeficiency virus Gag proteins. *J Virol* 1995;69: 5455–5460.
545. Park BH, Lavi E, Gaulton GN. Intracerebral hemorrhages and infarction induced by a murine leukemia virus is influenced by host determinants within endothelial cells. *Virology* 1994;203:393–396.
546. Park BH, Matuschke B, Lavi E, Gaulton GN. A point mutation in the *env* gene of a murine leukemia virus induces syncytium formation and neurologic disease. *J Virol* 1994;68:7516–7524.
547. Park CG, Jung MY, Choi Y, Winslow GM. Proteolytic processing is required for viral superantigen activity. *J Exp Med* 1995;181: 1899–1904.
548. Park J, Morrow CD. Overexpression of the gag-pol precursor from human immunodeficiency virus type 1 proviral genomes results in efficient proteolytic processing in the absence of virion production. *J Virol* 1991;65:5111–5117.
549. Park J, Morrow CD. The nonmyristylated Pr160gag-pol polyprotein of human immunodeficiency virus type 1 interacts with Pr55gag and is incorporated into viruslike particles. *J Virol* 1992;66:6304–6313.
550. Parkin NT, Chamorro M, Varmus HE. Human immunodeficiency virus type 1 gag-pol frameshifting is dependent on downstream mRNA secondary structure: Demonstration by expression *in vivo*. *J Virol* 1992;66:5147–5151.
551. Parolin C, Borsetti A, Choe H, et al. Use of murine CXCR-4 as a second receptor by some T-cell-tropic human immunodeficiency viruses. *J Virol* 1998;72:1652–1656.
552. Pasquinelli AE, Ernst RK, Lund E, et al. The constitutive transport element (CTE) of Mason-Pfizer monkey virus (MPMV) accesses a cellular mRNA export pathway. *EMBO J* 1997;16:7500–7510.
553. Pathak VK, Temin HM. Broad spectrum of *in vivo* forward mutations, hypermutations and mutational hotspots in a retroviral shuttle vector after a single replication cycle: Deletions and deletions with insertions. *Proc Natl Acad Sci U S A* 1990;87:6024–6028.
554. Pathak VK, Temin HM. 5-azacytidine and RNA secondary structure increase the retrovirus mutation rate. *J Virol* 1992;66:3093–3100.
555. Patience C, Patton GS, Takeuchi Y, et al. No evidence of pig DNA or retroviral infection in patients with short-term extracorporeal connection to pig kidneys. *Lancet* 1998;352:699–701.
556. Patience C, Takeuchi Y, Cosset FL, Weiss RA. Packaging of endogenous retroviral sequences in retroviral vectors produced by murine and human packaging cells. *J Virol* 1998;72:2671–2676.
557. Patience C, Takeuchi Y, Weiss RA. Infection of human cells by an endogenous retrovirus of pigs. *Nat Med* 1997;3:282–286.
558. Patience C, Wilkinson DA, Weiss RA. Our retroviral heritage. *Trends Genet* 1997;13:116–120.
559. Payne GS, Courtneidge SA, Crittenden LB, et al. Analysis of avian leukosis virus DNA and RNA in bursal tumours: Viral gene expression is not required for maintenance of the tumor state. *Cell* 1981;23: 311–322.
560. Pearl LH, Taylor WR. Sequence specificity of retroviral proteases. *Nature* 1987;328:482–483.
561. Peliska JA, Benkovic SJ. Mechanism of DNA strand transfer reactions catalyzed by HIV-1 reverse transcriptase. *Science* 1992;258:1112–1118.
562. Peliska JA, Benkovic SJ. Fidelity of *in vitro* DNA strand transfer reactions catalyzed by HIV-1 reverse transcriptase. *Biochemistry* 1994;33: 3890–3895.
563. Perez LG, Davis GL, Hunter E. Mutants of the Rous sarcoma virus envelope glycoprotein that lack the transmembrane anchor and cytoplasmic domains: Analysis of intracellular transport and assembly into virions. *J Virol* 1987;61:2981–2988.
564. Perez LG, Hunter E. Mutations within proeolytic cleavage site of the Rous sarcoma virus glycoprotein that block processing to gp85 and gp37. *J Virol* 1987;61:1609–1614.
565. Persons DA, Paulson RF, Loyd MR, et al. Fv2 encodes a truncated form of the Stk receptor tyrosine kinase. *Nat Genet* 1999;23:159–165.
566. Peters GG, Hu J. Reverse transcriptase as the major determinant for selective packaging of tRNA's into avian sarcoma virus particles. *J Virol* 1980;36:692–700.
567. Petersen R, Kempler G, Barklis E. A stem-cell specific silencer in the primer-binding site of a retrovirus. *Mol Cell Biol* 1991;11:1214–1221.
568. Pietschmann T, Heinkelein M, Heldmann M, et al. Foamy virus capsids require the cognate envelope protein for particle export. *J Virol* 1999;73:2613–2621.
569. Piguet V, Gu F, Foti M, et al. Nef-induced CD4 degradation: A diacidic-based motif in Nef functions as a lysosomal targeting signal through the binding of beta-COP in endosomes. *Cell* 1999;97:63–73.
570. Pillemer EA, Kooistra DA, Witte ON, Weissman IL. Monoclonal antibody to the amino-terminal L sequence of murine leukemia virus glycosylated gag poly proteins demonstrates their unusual orientation in the cell membrane. *J Virol* 1986;57:413–421.
571. Pincus T, Hartley JW, Rowe WP. A major genetic locus affecting resistance to infection with murine leukemia viruses. IV. Dose-response relationships in Fv-1 sensitive and resistant cell cultures. *Virology* 1975;65:333–342.
572. Pinter A, Honnen WJ. O-linked glycosylation of retroviral envelope gene products. *J Virol* 1988;62:1016–1021.
573. Pinter A, Honnen WJ, Tilley SA, et al. Oligomeric structure of gp41, the transmembrane protein of human immunodeficiency virus type 1. *J Virol* 1989;63:2674–2679.
574. Pinter A, Kopelman R, Li Z, et al. Localization of the labile disulfide bond between SU and TM of the murine leukemia virus envelope protein complex to a highly conserved CWLC motif in SU that resembles the active-site sequence of thiol-disulfide exchange enzymes. *J Virol* 1997;71:8073–8077.
575. Poeschla EM, Wong-Staal F, Looney DJ. Efficient transduction of nondividing human cells by feline immunodeficiency virus lentiviral vectors. *Nat Med* 1998;4:354–357.
576. Poirier Y, Kozak C, Jolicoeur P. Identification of a common helper provirus integration site in Abelson murine leukemia virus-induced lymphoma DNA. *J Virol* 1988;62:3985–3992.
577. Pollard VW, Malim MH. The HIV-1 Rev protein. *Annu Rev Microbiol* 1998;52:491–532.
578. Poon DT, Wu J, Aldovini A. Charged amino acid residues of human immunodeficiency virus type 1 nucleocapsid p7 protein involved in RNA packaging and infectivity. *J Virol* 1996;70:6607–6616.
579. Popescu CP, Boscher J, Hayes HC, et al. Chromosomal localization of the BLV receptor candidate gene in cattle, sheep, and goat. *Cytogenet Cell Genet* 1995;69:50–52.
580. Portis JL, Fujisawa R, McAtee FJ. The glycosylated gag protein of MuLV is a determinant of neuroinvasiveness: Analysis of second site revertants of a mutant MuLV lacking expression of this protein. *Virology* 1996;226:384–392.
581. Portis JL, Lynch WP. Dissecting the determinants of neuropathogenesis of the murine oncornaviruses. *Virology* 1998;247:127–136.

582. Powell DJ, Bur D, Wlodawer A, et al. The aspartic proteinase from equine infectious anaemia virus. *Adv Exp Med Biol* 1998;436:41–45.
583. Prasad GS, Stura EA, McRee DE, et al. Crystal structure of dUTP pyrophosphatase from feline immunodeficiency virus. *Protein Sci* 1996;5:2429–2437.
584. Pryciak PM, Sil A, Varmus HE. Retroviral integration into minichromosomes *in vitro*. *EMBO J* 1992;11:291–303.
585. Pryciak PM, Varmus HE. Fv-1 restriction and its effects on murine leukemia virus integration *in vivo* and *in vitro*. *J Virol* 1992;66:5959–5966.
586. Pryciak PM, Varmus HE. Nucleosomes, DNA-binding proteins, and DNA sequence modulate retroviral integration target site selection. *Cell* 1992;69:769–780.
587. Puffer BA, Watkins SC, Montelaro RC. Equine infectious anemia virus Gag polyprotein late domain specifically recruits cellular AP-2 adapter protein complexes during virion assembly. *J Virol* 1998;72:10218–10221.
588. Pullen KA, Ishimoto LK, Champoux JJ. Incomplete removal of the RNA primer for minus-strand DNA synthesis by human immunodeficiency virus type 1 reverse transcriptase. *J Virol* 1992;66:367–373.
589. Qin W, Golovkina TV, Peng T, et al. Mammary gland expression of mouse mammary tumor virus is regulated by a novel element in the long terminal repeat. *J Virol* 1999;73:368–376.
590. Quigley JG, Burns CC, Anderson MM, et al. Cloning of the cellular receptor for feline leukemia virus subgroup C (FeLV-C), a retrovirus that induces red cell aplasia. *Blood* 2000;95:1093–1099.
591. Quinn TP, Grandgenett DP. Genetic evidence that the avian retrovirus DNA endonuclease domain of pol is necessary for viral integration. *J Virol* 1988;62:2307–2312.
592. Quint W, Boelens W, Wezenbeek PV, et al. Generation of AKR mink cell focus-forming viruses: A conserved single-copy xenotropic-like proviruses provides recombinant long terminal repeat sequences. *J Virol* 1984;50:432–438.
593. Rabut GE, Konner JA, Kajumo F, et al. Alanine substitutions of polar and nonpolar residues in the amino-terminal domain of CCR5 differently impair entry of macrophage- and dualtropic isolates of human immunodeficiency virus type 1. *J Virol* 1998;72:3464–3468.
594. Ramsdale EE, Kingsman SM, Kingsman AJ. The "putative" leucine zipper region of murine leukemia virus transmembrane protein (P15e) is essential for viral infectivity. *Virology* 1996;220:100–108.
595. Rao Z, Belyaev AS, Fry E, et al. Crystal structure of SIV matrix antigen and implications for virus assembly. *Nature* 1995;378:743–747.
596. Rasko JE, Battini JL, Gottschalk RJ, et al. The RD114/simian type D retrovirus receptor is a neutral amino acid transporter. *Proc Natl Acad Sci U S A* 1999;96:2129–2134.
597. Reil H, Bukovsky AA, Gelderblom HR, Gottlinger HG. Efficient HIV-1 replication can occur in the absence of the viral matrix protein. *EMBO J* 1998;17:2699–2708.
598. Rein A, Kashmiri SV, Bassin RH, et al. Phenotypic mixing between N- and B-tropic murine leukemia viruses: Infectious particles with dual sensitivity to Fv-1 restriction. *Cell* 1976;7:373–379.
599. Rein A, McClure MR, Rice NR, et al. Myristylation site in Pr65gag is essential for virus particle formation by Moloney murine leukemia virus. *Proc Natl Acad Sci U S A* 1986;83:7246–7250.
600. Rein A, Mirro J, Haynes JG, et al. Function of the cytoplasmic domain of a retroviral transmembrane protein: p15E-p2E cleavage activates the membrane fusion capability of the murine leukemia virus Env protein. *J Virol* 1994;68:1773–1781.
601. Rein A, Ott DE, Mirro J, et al. Inactivation of murine leukemia virus by compounds that react with the zinc finger in the viral nucleocapsid protein. *J Virol* 1996;70:4966–4972.
602. Rein A, Yang C, Haynes JA, et al. Evidence for cooperation between murine leukemia virus Env molecules in mixed oligomers. *J Virol* 1998;72:3432–3435.
603. Remy E, de Rocquigny H, Petitjean P, et al. The annealing of tRNA3Lys to human immunodeficiency virus type 1 primer binding site is critically dependent on the NCp7 zinc fingers structure. *J Biol Chem* 1998;273:4819–4822.
604. Ren J, Esnouf R, Garman E, et al. High resolution structures of HIV-1 RT from four RT-inhibitor complexes. *Nat Struct Biol* 1995;2:293–302.
605. Ren J, Esnouf RM, Hopkins AL, et al. Crystal structures of HIV-1 reverse transcriptase in complex with carboxanilide derivatives. *Biochemistry* 1998;37:14394–14403.
606. Renjifo B, Speck NA, Winandy S, et al. cis-acting elements in the U3 region of a simian immunodeficiency virus. *J Virol* 1990;64:3130–3134.
607. Resnick-Roguel N, Burstein H, Hamburger J, et al. Cytocidal effect caused by the envelope glycoprotein of a newly isolated avian hemangioma-inducing retrovirus. *J Virol* 1989;63:4325–4330.
608. Reuss FU, Schaller HC. cDNA sequence and genomic characterization of intracisternal A-particle-related retroviral elements containing an envelope gene. *J Virol* 1991;65:5702–5709.
609. Rey O, Canon J, Krogstad P. HIV-1 Gag protein associates with F-actin present in microfilaments. *Virology* 1996;220:530–534.
610. Rhee SS, Hui H, Hunter E. Preassembled capsids of type D retroviruses contain a signal sufficient for targeting specifically to the plasma membrane. *J Virol* 1990;64:3844–3852.
611. Rhee SS, Huner E. Myristylation is required for intracellular transport but not for assembly of D-type retrovirus capsids. *J Virol* 1987;61:1045–1053.
612. Rhee SS, Hunter E. A single amino acid substitution within the matrix protein of a type D retrovirus converts its morphogenesis to that of a type C retrovirus. *Cell* 1990;63:77–86.
613. Rhim H, Park J, Morrow CD. Deletions in the tRNALys primer-binding site of human immunodeficiency virus type 1 identify essential regions for reverse transcription. *J Virol* 1991;65:4555–4564.
614. Rice NR, Henderson LE, Sowder RC, et al. Synthesis and processing of the transmembrane envelope protein of equine infectious anemia virus. *J Virol* 1990;64:3770–3778.
615. Rice WG, Schaeffer CA, Harten B, et al. Inhibition of HIV-1 infectivity by zinc-ejecting aromatic C-nitroso compounds. *Nature* 1993;361:473–475.
616. Ringhofer S, Kallen J, Dutzler R, et al. X-ray structure and conformational dynamics of the HIV-1 protease in complex with the inhibitor SDZ283-910: Agreement of time-resolved spectroscopy and molecular dynamics simulations. *J Mol Biol* 1999;286:1147–1159.
617. Risco C, Menendez-Arias L, Copeland TD, et al. Intracellular transport of the murine leukemia virus during acute infection of NIH 3T3 cells: Nuclear import of nucleocapsid protein and integrase. *J Cell Sci* 1995;108:3039–3050.
618. Rizzuto CD, Wyatt R, Hernandez-Ramos N, et al. A conserved HIV gp120 glycoprotein structure involved in chemokine receptor binding. *Science* 1998;280:1949–1953.
619. Robert-Guroff M, Popovic M, Gartner S, et al. Structure and expression of tat-, rev-, and nef-specific transcripts of human immunodeficiency virus type 1 in infected lymphocytes and macrophages. *J Virol* 1990;64:3391–3398.
620. Robinson HL, Zinkus DM. Accumulation of human immunodeficiency virus type 1 DNA in T cells: Result of multiple infection events. *J Virol* 1990;64:4836–4841.
621. Robson ND, Telesnitsky A. Effects of 3′ untranslated region mutations on plus-strand priming during moloney murine leukemia virus replication. *J Virol* 1999;73:948–957.
622. Rodgers DW, Gamblin SJ, Harris BA, et al. The structure of unliganded reverse transcriptase from the human immunodeficiency virus type 1. *Proc Natl Acad Sci U S A* 1995;92:1222–1226.
623. Roe T, Chow SA, Brown PO. 3′-end processing and kinetics of 5′-end joining during retroviral integration *in vivo*. *J Virol* 1997;71:1334–1340.
624. Roe T, Reynolds TC, Yu G, Brown PO. Integration of murine leukemia virus DNA depends on mitosis. *EMBO J* 1993;12:2099–2108.
625. Rohdewohld H, Weiher H, Reik W, et al. Retrovirus integration and chromatin structure: Moloney murine leukemia proviral integration sites map near DNase I-hypersensitive sites. *J Virol* 1987;61:336–343.
626. Rommelaere J, Donis-Keller H, Hopkins N. RNA sequencing provides evidence for allelism of determinants of the N-, B-, or NB-tropism of murine leukemia viruses. *Cell* 1979;16:43–50.
627. Rong L, Gendron K, Strohl B, et al. Characterization of determinants for envelope binding and infection in tva, the subgroup A avian sarcoma and leukosis virus receptor. *J Virol* 1998;72:4552–4559.
628. Ross EK, Buckler-White AJ, Rabson AB, et al. Contribution of NF-κB and Sp1 binding motifs to the replicative capacity of human immunodeficiency virus type 1: Distinct patterns of viral growth are determined by T-cell types. *J Virol* 1991;65:4350–4358.
629. Rossio JL, Esser MT, Suryanarayana K, et al. Inactivation of human immunodeficiency virus type 1 infectivity with preservation of conformational and functional integrity of virion surface proteins. *J Virol* 1998;72:7992–8001.
630. Roth MJ, Schwartzberg PL, Goff SP. Structure of the termini of DNA intermediates in the integration of retroviral DNA: Dependence on IN function and terminal DNA sequence. *Cell* 1989;58:47–54.
631. Ruscetti S, Wolff L. Biological and biochemical differences between

variants of spleen focus-forming virus can be localized to a region containing the 3′ end of the envelope gene. *J Virol* 1985;56:717–722.
632. Ruscetti SK, Janesch NJ, Charaborti A, et al. Friend spleen focus-forming virus induces factor independence in an erythropoietin-dependent erythroleukemia cell line. *J Virol* 1990;64:1057–1062.
633. Ryden TA, Beemon K. Avian retroviral long terminal repeats bind CCAAT/enhancer-binding protein. *Mol Cell Biol* 1989;9:1155–1164.
634. Saavedra C, Felber B, Izaurralde E. The simian retrovirus-1 constitutive transport element, unlike the HIV-1 RRE, uses factors required for cellular mRNA export. *Curr Biol* 1997;7:619–628.
635. Saib A, Puvion-Dutilleul F, Schmid M, et al. Nuclear targeting of incoming human foamy virus Gag proteins involves a centriolar step. *J Virol* 1997;71:1155–1161.
636. Sakai H, Kawamura M, Sakuragi J-I, et al. Integration is essential for efficient gene expression of human immunodeficiency virus type 1. *J Virol* 1993;67:1169–1174.
637. Sakalian M, Hunter E. Molecular events in the assembly of retrovirus particles. *Adv Exp Med Biol* 1998;440:329–339.
638. Sakalian M, Parker SD, Weldon RA Jr, Hunter E. Synthesis and assembly of retrovirus Gag precursors into immature capsids *in vitro*. *J Virol* 1996;70:3706–3715.
639. Salzwedel K, West JT, Hunter E. A conserved tryptophan-rich motif in the membrane-proximal region of the human immunodeficiency virus type 1 gp41 ectodomain is important for Env-mediated fusion and virus infectivity. *J Virol* 1999;73:2469–2480.
640. Sandefur S, Varthakavi V, Spearman P. The I domain is required for efficient plasma membrane binding of human immunodeficiency virus type 1 Pr55Gag. *J Virol* 1998;72:2723–2732.
641. Scarpa M, Cournoyer D, Muzny DM, et al. Characterization of recombinant helper retroviruses from Moloney-based vectors in ecotropic and emphotropic packaging cell lines. *Virology* 1991;180:849–852.
642. Schawaller M, Smith GE, Skehel JJ, Wiley DC. Studies with crosslinking reagents on the oligomeric structure of the env glycoprotein of HIV. *Virology* 1989;172:367–369.
643. Scherdin U, Rhodes K, Breindl M. Transcriptionally active genome regions are preferred targets for retrovirus integration. *J Virol* 1990; 64:907–912.
644. Schubert U, Anton LC, Bacik I, et al. CD4 glycoprotein degradation induced by human immunodeficiency virus type 1 Vpu protein requires the function of proteasomes and the ubiquitin-conjugating pathway. *J Virol* 1998;72:2280–2288.
645. Schultz AM, Rein A. Unmyristylated Moloney murine leukemia virus Pr65gag is excluded from virus assembly and maturation events. *J Virol* 1989;63:2370–2372.
646. Schultz SJ, Whiting SH, Champoux JJ. Cleavage specificities of Moloney murine leukemia virus RNase H implicated in the second strand transfer during reverse transcription. *J Biol Chem* 1995;270: 24135–24145.
647. Schwartz JR, Duesberg S, Duesberg PH. DNA recombination is sufficient for retroviral transduction. *Proc Natl Acad Sci U S A* 1995;92:2460–2464.
648. Schwartzberg P, Colicelli J, Goff SP. Deletion mutants of Moloney murine leukemia virus which lack glycosylated gag protein are replication competent. *J Virol* 1983;46:538–546.
649. Schwartzberg P, Colicelli J, Goff SP. Construction and analysis of deletion mutations in the *pol* gene of Moloney murine leukemia virus: A new viral function required for productive infection. *Cell* 1984;37: 1043–1052.
650. Schwartzberg P, Colicelli J, Gordon ML, Goff SP. Mutations in the *gag* gene of Moloney murine leukemia virus: Effects on production of virions and reverse transcriptase. *J Virol* 1984;49:918–924.
651. Selig L, Pages JC, Tanchou V, et al. Interaction with the p6 domain of the gag precursor mediates incorporation into virions of Vpr and Vpx proteins from primate lentiviruses. *J Virol* 1999;73:592–600.
652. Sharp PA, Marciniak RA. HIV TAR: An RNA enhancer? *Cell* 1989; 59:229–230.
653. Shen LX, Tinoco I Jr. The structure of an RNA pseudoknot that causes efficient frameshifting in mouse mammary tumor virus. *J Mol Biol* 1995;247:963–978.
654. Shields A, Witte WN, Rothenberg E, Baltimore D. High frequency of aberrant expression of Moloney murine leukemia virus in clonal infections. *Cell* 1978;14:601–609.
655. Shih C-C, Stoye JP, Coffin JM. Highly preferred targets for retrovirus integration. *Cell* 1988;53:531–537.
656. Shilatifard A, Merkle RK, Helland DE, et al. Complex-type N-linked oligosaccharides of gp120 from human immunodeficiency virus type 1 contain sulfated N-acetylglucsamine. *J Virol* 1993;67:943–952.
657. Shimizu H, Hasebe F, Tsuchie H, et al. Analysis of a human immunodeficiency virus type 1 isolate carrying a truncated transmembrane glycoprotein. *Virology* 1992;189:534–546.
658. Shoemaker CS, Goff S, Gilboa E, et al. Structure of a cloned circular Moloney murine leukemia virus molecule containing an inverted segment: Implications for retrovirus integration. *Proc Natl Acad Sci U S A* 1980;77:3932–3936.
659. Siciliano SJ, Kuhmann SE, Weng Y, et al. A critical site in the core of the CCR5 chemokine receptor required for binding and infectivity of human immunodeficiency virus type 1. *J Biol Chem* 1999;274:1905–1913.
660. Simmons G, Reeves JD, McKnight A, et al. CXCR4 as a functional coreceptor for human immunodeficiency virus type 1 infection of primary macrophages. *J Virol* 1998;72:8453–8457.
661. Skalka AM, Goff SP. *Reverse Transcriptase*. Cold Spring Harbor, NY: Cold Spring Harbor Press, 1993.
662. Smith AJ, Srinivasakumar N, Hammarskjold M-L, Rekosh D. Requirements for incorporation of Pr160gag-pol from human immunodeficiency virus type 1 into virus-like particles. *J Virol* 1993;67:2266–2275.
663. Smith CM, Leon O, Smith JS, Roth MJ. Sequence requirements for removal of tRNA by an isolated human immunodeficiency virus type 1 RNase H domain. *J Virol* 1998;72:6805–6812.
664. Smith JS, Kim S, Roth MJ. Analysis of long terminal repeat circle junctions of human immunodeficiency virus type 1. *J Virol* 1990;64: 6286–6290.
665. Smith LM, Toye AA, Howes K, et al. Novel endogenous retroviral sequences in the chicken genome closely related to HPRS-103 (subgroup J) avian leukosis virus. *J Gen Virol* 1999;80:261–268.
666. Smith MR, Smith RE, Dunkel I, et al. Genetic determinant of rapid-onset B-cell lymphoma by avian leukosis virus. *J Virol* 1997;71:6534–6540.
667. Snitkovsky S, Young JA. Cell-specific viral targeting mediated by a soluble retroviral receptor-ligand fusion protein. *Proc Natl Acad Sci U S A* 1998;95:7063–7068.
668. Somasundaran M, Robinson HL. Unexpectedly high levels of HIV-1 RNA and protein synthesis in a cytocidal infection. *Science* 1988;242:1554–1557.
669. Somia NV, Zoppe M, Verma IM. Generation of targeted retroviral vectors by using single-chain variable fragment: An approach to *in vivo* gene delivery. *Proc Natl Acad Sci U S A* 1995;92:7570–7574.
670. Sommerfelt MA, Petteway SRJ, Dreyer GB, Hunter E. Effect of retroviral proteinase inhibitors on Mason-Pfizer monkey virus maturation and transmembrane glycoprotein cleavage. *J Virol* 1992;66:4220–4227.
671. Sommerfelt MA, Williams BP, Clapham PR, et al. Human T cell leukemia viruses use a receptor determined by human chromosome 17. *Science* 1988;242:1557–1559.
672. Spearman P, Horton R, Ratner L, Kuli-Zade I. Membrane binding of human immunodeficiency virus type 1 matrix protein *in vivo* supports a conformational myristyl switch mechanism. *J Virol* 1997;71: 6582–6592.
673. Spearman P, Ratner L. Human immunodeficiency virus type 1 capsid formation in reticulocyte lysates. *J Virol* 1996;70:8187–8194.
674. Speck NA, Baltimore D. Six distinct nuclear factors interact with the 75-base-pair repeat of the Moloney murine leukemia virus enhancer. *Mol Cell Biol* 1987;7:1101–1110.
675. Spence SE, Gilbert DJ, Swing DA, et al. Spontaneous germ line virus infection and retroviral insertional mutagenesis in eighteen transgenic Srev lines of mice. *Mol Cell Biol* 1989;9:177–184.
676. Spiegel M, Bitzer M, Schenk A, et al. Pseudotype formation of Moloney murine leukemia virus with Sendai virus glycoprotein F. *J Virol* 1998;72:5296–5302.
677. Stein BS, Gowda SD, Lifson JD, Pennhallow RC, Bensch KG, Engelman EG. pH-independent HIV entry into CD4-positive T cells via virus envelope fusion to the plasma membrane. *Cell* 1987;49:659–669.
678. Steinhuber S, Brack M, Hunsmann G, et al. Distribution of human endogenous retrovirus HERV-K genomes in humans and different primates. *Hum Genet* 1995;96:188–192.
679. Stewart L, Vogt VM. Trans-acting viral protease is necessary and sufficient for activation of avian leukosis virus reverse transcriptase. *J Virol* 1991;65:6218–6231.
680. Stoltzfus CM, Fogarty CJ. Multiple regions in the Rous sarcoma virus *src* gene intron act in cis to affect the accumulation of unspliced RNA. *J Virol* 1989;63:1669–1676.

681. Storch TG, Arnstein GP, Manohar V, et al. Proliferation of infected lymphoid precursors before Moloney murine leukemia virus-induced T-cell lymphoma. *J Natl Cancer Inst* 1985;74:137–143.
682. Stoye JP, Coffin JM. Endogenous viruses. In: Weiss RA, Teich NM, Varmus HE, Coffin JM, eds. *RNA Tumor Viruses.* Cold Spring Harbor, NY: Cold Spring Harbor Laboratory, 1985:357–404 (2/supplements and appendixes).
683. Stoye JP, Coffin JM. The four classes of endogenous murine leukemia virus: Structural relationships and potential for recombination. *J Virol* 1987;61:2659–2669.
684. Stoye JP, Le Tissier P, Takeuchi Y, et al. Endogenous retroviruses: A potential problem for xenotransplantation? *Ann N Y Acad Sci* 1998; 862:67–74.
685. Strambio-de-Castilla C, Hunter E. Mutational analysis of the major homology region of Mason-Pfizer monkey virus by use of saturation mutagenesis. *J Virol* 1992;66:7021–7032.
686. Stuhlmann H, Berg P. Homologous recombination of copackaged retrovirus RNAs during reverse transcription. *J Virol* 1992;66:2378–2388.
687. Suzuki S. Fv-4, a new gene affecting the splenomegaly induction by Friend leukemia virus. *J Exp Med* 1975;45:473–478.
688. Suzuki S, Axelrad AA. Fv-2 locus controls the proportion of erythropoietic progenitor cells (BFU-E) synthesizing DNA in normal mice. *Cell* 1980;19:225–236.
689. Swain A, Coffin JM. Polyadenylation at correct sites in genome RNA is not required for retrovirus replication or genome encapsidation. *J Virol* 1989;63:3301–3306.
690. Swain A, Coffin JM. Mechanism of transduction by retroviruses. *Science* 1992;255:841–845.
691. Swanstrom R, Wills JW. Synthesis, assembly, and processing of viral proteins. In: Coffin JM, Hughes SH, Varmus HE, eds. *Retroviruses*. Cold Spring Harbor, NY: Cold Spring Harbor Press, 1997:263–334.
692. Szurek PF, Yuen PH, Ball JK, Wong PKY. A Val-25-to-Ile substitution in the envelope precursor polyprotein, pPr80env, is responsible for the temperature sensitivity, inefficient processing of gPr80env, and neurovirulence of ts1, a mutant of Moloney murine leukemia virus TB. *J Virol* 1990;64:467–475.
693. Tailor CS, Nouri A, Lee CG, et al. Cloning and characterization of a cell surface receptor for xenotropic and polytropic murine leukemia viruses. *Proc Natl Acad Sci U S A* 1999;96:927–932.
694. Tailor CS, Nouri A, Zhao Y, et al. A sodium-dependent neutral-amino-acid transporter mediates infections of feline and baboon endogenous retroviruses and simian type D retroviruses. *J Virol* 1999;73:4470–4474.
695. Takayama Y, O'Mara M-A, Spilsbury K, et al. Stage-specific expression of intracisternal A-particle sequences in murine myelomonocytic leukemia cell lines and normal myelomonocytic differentiation. *J Virol* 1991;65:2149–2154.
696. Takeda A, Tuazon CU, Ennis FA. Antibody-enhanced infection by HIV-1 via Fc receptor-mediated entry. *Science* 1988;242:580–583.
697. Takeuchi Y, Patience C, Magre S, et al. Host range and interference studies of three classes of pig endogenous retrovirus. *J Virol* 1998;72: 9986–9991.
698. Takeuchi Y, Vile RG, Simpson G, et al. Feline leukemia virus subgroup B uses the same cell surface receptor as gibbon ape leukemia virus. *J Virol* 1992;66:1219–1222.
699. Tanchou V, Decimo D, Pechoux C, et al. Role of the N-terminal zinc finger of human immunodeficiency virus type 1 nucleocapsid protein in virus structure and replication. *J Virol* 1998;72:4442–4447.
700. Tanese N, Goff SP. Domain structure of the Moloney murine leukemia virus reverse transcriptase: Mutational analysis and separate expression of the DNA polymerase and RNase H activities. *Proc Natl Acad Sci U S A* 1988;85:1777–1781.
701. Tanese N, Roth MJ, Goff SP. Analysis of retroviral *pol* gene products with antisera raised against fusion proteins produced in Escherichia coli. *J Virol* 1986;59:328–340.
702. Tanese N, Telesnitsky A, Goff SP. Abortive reverse transcription by mutants of Moloney murine leukemia virus deficient in the reverse transcriptase-associated RNase H function. *J Virol* 1991;65: 4387–4397.
703. Tang H, Gaietta GM, Fischer WH, et al. A cellular cofactor for the constitutive transport element of type D retrovirus. *Science* 1997;276: 1412–1415.
704. Taplitz RA, Coffin JM. Selection of an avian retrovirus mutant with extended receptor usage. *J Virol* 1997;71:7814–7819.
705. Tchenio T, Heidmann T. High-frequency intracellular transposition of a defective mammalian provirus detected by an in situ colorimetric assay. *J Virol* 1992;66:1571–1578.
706. Telesnitsky A, Goff SP. RNase H domain mutations affect the interaction between Moloney murine leukemia virus reverse transcriptase and its primer-template. *Proc Natl Acad Sci U S A* 1993;90:1276–1280.
707. Telesnitsky A, Goff SP. Two defective forms of reverse transcriptase can complement to restore retroviral infectivity. *EMBO J* 1993;12: 4433–4438.
708. Telesnitsky A, Goff SP. Reverse transcription and the generation of retroviral DNA. In: Coffin JM, Hughes SH, Varmus HE, eds. *Retroviruses*. Cold Spring Harbor, NY: Cold Spring Harbor Press, 1997:121–160.
709. Temin HM. Reverse transcription in the eukaryotic genome: Retroviruses, pararetroviruses, retro transposons, and retrotranscripts. *Mol Biol Evol* 1985;6:455–468.
710. Temin HM, Zhang J. 3′ junctions of oncogene-virus sequences and the mechanisms for formation of highly oncogenic retroviruses. *J Virol* 1993;67:1747–1751.
711. Tessmer U, Krausslich HG. Cleavage of human immunodeficiency virus type 1 proteinase from the N-terminally adjacent p6* protein is essential for efficient Gag polyprotein processing and viral infectivity. *J Virol* 1998;72:3459–3463.
712. Thali M, Bukovsky A, Kondo E, et al. Functional association of cyclophilin A with HIV-1 virions. *Nature* 1994;372:363–365.
713. Thomas DJ, Wall JS, Hainfield JF, et al. gp160, the envelope glycoprotein of human immunodeficiency virus type 1, is a dimer of 125-kilodalton subunits stabilized through interactions between their gp41 domains. *J Virol* 1991;65:3797–3803.
714. Thome KC, Radfar A, Rosenberg N. Mutation of Tp53 contributes to the malignant phenotype of Abelson virus-transformed lymphoid cells. *J Virol* 1997;71:8149–8156.
715. Toh H, Ono M, Miyata T. Retroviral gag and DNA endonuclease coding sequences in IgE-binding factor gene. *Nature* 1985;318:388–389.
716. Topping R, Demoitie MA, Shin NH, Telesnitsky A. Cis-acting elements required for strong stop acceptor template selection during Moloney murine leukemia virus reverse transcription. *J Mol Biol* 1998;281:1–15.
717. Torrent C, Gabus C, Darlix JL. A small and efficient dimerization/packaging signal of rat VL30 RNA and its use in murine leukemia virus-VL30-derived vectors for gene transfer. *J Virol* 1994;68:661–667.
718. Trono D. Partial reverse transcripts in virions from human immunodeficiency and murine leukemia viruses. *J Virol* 1992;66:4893–4900.
719. Trubetskoy AM, Okenquist SA, Lenz J. R region sequences in the long terminal repeat of a murine retrovirus specifically increase expression of unspliced RNAs. *J Virol* 1999;73:3477–3483.
720. Tsuchihashi Z, Brown PO. DNA strand exchange and selective DNA annealing promoted by the human immunodeficiency virus type 1 nucleocapsid protein. *J Virol* 1994;68:5863–5870.
721. Tsukiyama T, Niwa O, Yokoro K. Mechanism of suppression of the long terminal repeat of Moloney leukemia virus in mouse embryonal carcinoma cells. *Mol Cell Biol* 1989;9:4670–4676.
722. Tsukiyama T, Niwa O, Yokoro K. Characterization of the negative regulatory element of the 5′ noncoding region of Moloney murine leukemia virus in mouse embryonal carcinoma cells. *Virology* 1990; 177:772–776.
723. Tucker SP, Srinivas RV, Compans RW. Molecular domains involved in oligomerization of the Friend murine leukemia virus envelope glycoprotein. *Virology* 1991;185:710–720.
724. Tucker TJ, Lumma WC, Culberson JC. Development of nonnucleoside HIV reverse transcriptase inhibitors. *Methods Enzymol* 1996;275: 440–472.
725. Tummino PJ, Scholten JD, Harvey PJ, et al. The *in vitro* ejection of zinc from human immunodeficiency virus (HIV) type 1 nucleocapsid protein by disulfide benzamides with cellular anti-HIV activity. *Proc Natl Acad Sci U S A* 1996;93:969–973.
726. Turelli P, Guiguen F, Mornex JF, et al. dUTPase-minus caprine arthritis-encephalitis virus is attenuated for pathogenesis and accumulates G-to-A substitutions. *J Virol* 1997;71:4522–4530.
727. Turpin JA, Terpening SJ, Schaeffer CA, et al. Inhibitors of human immunodeficiency virus type 1 zinc fingers prevent normal processing of gag precursors and result in the release of noninfectious virus particles. *J Virol* 1996;70:6180–6189.
728. Urbaneja MA, Kane BP, Johnson DG, et al. Binding properties of the human immunodeficiency virus type 1 nucleocapsid protein p7 to a model RNA: Elucidation of the structural determinants for function. *J Mol Biol* 1999;287:59–75.

729. Vagner S, Waysbort A, Marenda M, et al. Alternative translation initiation of the Moloney murine leukemia virus mRNA controlled by internal ribosome entry involving the p57/PTB splicing factor. *J Biol Chem* 1995;270:20376–20383.
730. Valsamakis A, Zeichner S, Carswell S, Alwine JC. The human immunodeficiency virus type 1 polyadenylation signal: A 3′ long terminal repeat element upstream of the AAUAAA necessary for efficient polyadenylation. *Proc Natl Acad Sci U S A* 1991;88:2108–2112.
731. Valsesia-Wittmann S, Drynda A, Deleage G, et al. Modifications in the binding domain of avian retrovirus envelope protein to redirect the host range of retroviral vectors. *J Virol* 1994;68:4609–4619.
732. van Gent DC, Vink C, Groeneger AA, Plasterk RH. Complementation between HIV integrase proteins mutated in different domains. *EMBO J* 1993;12:3261–3267.
733. van Lohulzen M, Verbeek S, Scheijen B, et al. Identification of cooperating oncogenes in Eμ-myc transgenic mice by provirus tagging. *Cell* 1991;65:737–752.
734. van Zeijl M, Johann SV, Closs E, et al. A human amphotropic retrovirus receptor is a second member of the gibbon ape leukemia virus receptor family. *Proc Natl Acad Sci U S A* 1994;91:1168–1172.
735. Varmus HE, Padgett T, Heasley S, et al. Cellular functions are required for the synthesis and integration of avian sarcoma virus-specific DNA. *Cell* 1977;11:307–319.
736. Varmus HE, Quintrell NE, Ortiz S. Retroviruses as mutagens: Insertion and excision of a non-transforming provirus alters expression of a resident transforming provirus. *Cell* 1981;25:23–26.
737. Vernet M, Cebrian J. Cis-acting elements that mediate the negative regulation of Moloney murine leukemia virus in mouse early embryos. *J Virol* 1996;70:5630–5633.
738. Vijaya S, Steffen DL, Robinson HL. Acceptor sites for retroviral integrations map near DNase I-hypersensitive sites in chromatin. *J Virol* 1986;60:683–692.
739. Vink C, van Gent DC, Elgersma Y, Plasterk RHA. Human immunodeficiency virus integrase protein requires a subterminal position of its viral DNA recognition sequence for efficient cleavage. *J Virol* 1991;65:4636–4644.
740. Vink C, Yeheskiely E, van der Marel GA, et al. Site-specific hydrolysis and alcoholysis of human immunodeficiency virus DNA termini mediated by the viral integrase protein. *Nucleic Acids Res* 1991;19:6691–6698.
741. Vogt VM. Proteolytic processing and particle maturation. *Curr Top Microbiol Immunol* 1996;214:95–131.
742. von der Helm K, Seelmeier S, Kisselev A, Nitschko H. Identification, purification, and cell culture assays of retroviral proteases. *Methods Enzymol* 1994;241:89–104.
743. von Schwedler U, Kornbluth RS, Trono D. The nuclear localization signal of the matrix protein of human immunodeficiency virus type 1 allows the establishment of infection in macrophages and quiescent T lymphocytes. *Proc Natl Acad Sci U S A* 1994;91:6992–6996.
744. Vora AC, Chiu R, McCord M, et al. Avian retrovirus U3 and U5 DNA inverted repeats. Role Of nonsymmetrical nucleotides in promoting full-site integration by purified virion and bacterial recombinant integrases. *J Biol Chem* 1997;272:23938–23945.
745. Vora AC, Grandgenett DP. Assembly and catalytic properties of retrovirus integrase-DNA complexes capable of efficiently performing concerted integration. *J Virol* 1995;69:7483–7488.
746. Wang CT, Lai HY, Li JJ. Analysis of minimal human immunodeficiency virus type 1 gag coding sequences capable of virus-like particle assembly and release. *J Virol* 1998;72:7950–7959.
747. Wang H, Paul R, Burgeson RE, et al. Plasma membrane receptors for ecotropic murine retroviruses require a limiting accessory factor. *J Virol* 1991;65:6468–6477.
748. Weber IT, Miller M, Jaskolski M, et al. Molecular modeling of the HIV-1 protease and its substrate binding site. *Science* 1989;243:928–931.
749. Weclewicz K, Ekstrom M, Kristensson K, Garoff H. Specific interactions between retrovirus Env and Gag proteins in rat neurons. *J Virol* 1998;72:2832–2845.
750. Wei SQ, Mizuuchi K, Craigie R. A large nucleoprotein assembly at the ends of the viral DNA mediates retroviral DNA integration. *EMBO J* 1997;16:7511–7520.
751. Wei SQ, Mizuuchi K, Craigie R. Footprints on the viral DNA ends in moloney murine leukemia virus preintegration complexes reflect a specific association with integrase. *Proc Natl Acad Sci U S A* 1998;95:10535–10540.
752. Weinberg JB, Matthews TJ, Cullen BR, Malim MH. Productive human immunodeficiency virus type 1 (HIV-1) infection of nonproliferating human monocytes. *J Exp Med* 1991;174:1477–1482.
753. Weiss CD, Levy JA, White JM. Oligomeric organization of gp120 on infectious human immunodeficiency virus type 1 particles. *J Virol* 1990;64:5674–5677.
754. Weiss RA, Tailor CS. Retrovirus receptors. *Cell* 1995;82:531–533.
755. Welker R, Janetzko A, Krausslich HG. Plasma membrane targeting of chimeric intracisternal A-type particle polyproteins leads to particle release and specific activation of the viral proteinase. *J Virol* 1997;71:5209–5217.
756. Weller SK, Temin HM. Cell killing by avian leukosis viruses. *J Virol* 1981;39:713–721.
757. Weng Y, Weiss CD. Mutational analysis of residues in the coiled-coil domain of human immunodeficiency virus type 1 transmembrane protein gp41. *J Virol* 1998;72:9676–9682.
758. Whitcomb JM, Kumar R, Hughes SH. Sequence of the circle junction of human immunodeficiency virus type 1: Implications for reverse transcription and integration. *J Virol* 1990;64:4903–4906.
759. Whitcomb JM, Ortiz-Conde BA, Hughes SH. Replication of avian leukosis viruses with mutations at the primer binding site: Use of alternative tRNAs as primers. *J Virol* 1995;69:6228–6238.
760. Wilk T, Gowen B, Fuller SD. Actin associates with the nucleocapsid domain of the human immunodeficiency virus Gag polyprotein. *J Virol* 1999;73:1931–1940.
761. Willetts KE, Rey F, Agostini I, et al. DNA repair enzyme uracil DNA glycosylase is specifically incorporated into human immunodeficiency virus type 1 viral particles through a Vpr-independent mechanism. *J Virol* 1999;73:1682–1688.
762. Willey RL, Maldarelli F, Martin MA, Strebel K. Human immunodeficiency virus type 1 Vpu protein regulates the formation of intracellular gp160-CD4 complexes. *J Virol* 1992;66:226–234.
763. Wills JW, Cameron CE, Wilson CB, et al. An assembly domain of the Rous sarcoma virus Gag protein required late in budding. *J Virol* 1994;68:6605–6618.
764. Wills JW, Craven RC. Form, function and use of retroviral gag proteins. *AIDS* 1991;5:639–654.
765. Wills JW, Craven RC, Achacoso JA. Creation and expression of myristylated forms of Rous sarcoma virus gag protein in mammalian cells. *J Virol* 1989;63:4331–4343.
766. Wills NM, Gesteland RF, Atkins JF. Evidence that a downstream pseudoknot is required for translational read-through of the Moloney murine leukemia virus gag stop codon. *Proc Natl Acad Sci U S A* 1991;88:6991–6995.
767. Wills NM, Gesteland RF, Atkins JF. Pseudoknot-dependent read-through of retroviral gag termination codons: Importance of sequences in the spacer and loop 2. *EMBO J* 1994;13:4137–4144.
768. Wilson CA, Wong S, Muller J, et al. Type C retrovirus released from porcine primary peripheral blood mononuclear cells infects human cells. *J Virol* 1998;72:3082–3087.
769. Wilson W, Braddock M, Adams SE, et al. HIV expression strategies: Ribosomal frameshifting is directed by a short sequence in both mammalian and yeast systems. *Cell* 1988;55:1159–1169.
770. Withers-Ward ES, Kitamura Y, Barnes JP, Coffin JM. Distribution of targets for avian retrovirus DNA integration *in vivo*. *Genes Dev* 1994;8:1473–1487.
771. Witte ON, Baltimore D. Mechanism of formation of pseudotypes between vesicular stomatitis virus and murine leukemia virus. *Cell* 1977;11:505–511.
772. Wlodawer A, Miller M, Jaskolski M, et al. Conserved folding in retroviral proteases: Crystal structure of a synthetic HIV-1 protease. *Science* 1989;245:616–621.
773. Wolff L, Ruscetti S. The spleen focus-forming virus (SFFV) envelope gene, when introduced into mice in the absence of other SFFV genes, induces acute erythroleukemia. *J Virol* 1988;62:2158–2163.
774. Wong PKY, Knupp C, Yuen PH, et al. ts1, a paralytogenic mutant of Moloney murine leukemia virus TB, has an enhanced ability to replicate in the central nervous system and primary nerve cell culture. *J Virol* 1985;55:760–767.
775. Wu W, Henderson LE, Copeland TD, et al. Human immunodeficiency virus type 1 nucleocapsid protein reduces reverse transcriptase pausing at a secondary structure near the murine leukemia virus polypurine tract. *J Virol* 1996;70:7132–7142.
776. Xiang Y, Cameron CE, Wills JW, Leis J. Fine mapping and character-

ization of the Rous sarcoma virus Pr76gag late assembly domain. *J Virol* 1996;70:5695–5700.
777. Xiong Y, Eickbush TH. Origin and evolution of retroelements based on their reverse transcriptase sequences. *EMBO J.* 1990;9: 3353–3362.
778. Yamauchi M, Freitag B, Khan C, et al. Stem cell factor binding to retrovirus primer binding site silencers. *J Virol* 1995;69:1142–1149.
779. Yang C, Compans RW. Analysis of the murine leukemia virus R peptide: Delineation of the molecular determinants which are important for its fusion inhibition activity. *J Virol* 1997;71:8490–8496.
780. Yang F, Leon O, Greenfield NJ, Roth MJ. Functional interactions of the HHCC domain of moloney murine leukemia virus integrase revealed by nonoverlapping complementation and zinc-dependent dimerization. *J Virol* 1999;73:1809–1817.
781. Yang W, Steitz TA. Recombining the structures of HIV integrase, RuvC and RNase H. *Structure* 1995;3:131–134.
782. Yang WK, Kiggins JO, Yang DM, et al. Synthesis and circularization of N- and B-tropic retroviral DNA in Fv-1 permissive and restrictive mouse cells. *Proc Natl Acad Sci U S A* 1980;77:2994–2998.
783. Yang YL, Guo L, Xu S, et al. Receptors for polytropic and xenotropic mouse leukaemia viruses encoded by a single gene at Rmc1. *Nat Genet* 1999;21:216–219.
784. Yeager M, Wilson-Kubalek EM, Weiner SG, et al. Supramolecular organization of immature and mature murine leukemia virus revealed by electron cryo-microscopy: Implications for retroviral assembly mechanisms. *Proc Natl Acad Sci U S A* 1998;95:7299–7304.
785. York DF, Vigne R, Verwoerd DW, Querat G. Nucleotide sequence of the Jaagsiekte retrovirus, an exogenous and endogenous type D and B retrovirus of sheep and goats. *J Virol* 1992;66:4930–4939.
786. Yoshinaka Y, Katoh I, Copeland TD, Oroszlan SJ. Murine leukemia virus protease is encoded by the gag-pol gene and is synthesized through suppression of an amber termination codon. *Proc Natl Acad Sci U S A* 1985;82:1618–1622.
787. Young JAT, Bates P, Varmus HE. Isolation of a chicken gene that confers suscpetibility to infection by subgroup A avian leukosis and sarcoma viruses. *J Virol* 1993;67:1811–1816.
788. Yu H, Jetzt AE, Ron Y, et al. The nature of human immunodeficiency virus type 1 strand transfers. *J Biol Chem* 1998;273:28384–28391.
789. Yu Q, Morrow CD. Complementarity between 3′ terminal nucleotides of tRNA and primer binding site is a major determinant for selection of the tRNA primer used for initiation of HIV-1 reverse transcription. *Virology* 1999;254:160–168.
790. Yu SF, Sullivan MD, Linial ML. Evidence that the human foamy virus genome is DNA. *J Virol* 1999;73:1565–1572.
791. Yu X, Yuan X, Matsuda Z, et al. The matrix protein of human immunodeficiency virus type 1 is required for incorporation of viral envelope protein into mature virions. *J Virol* 1992;66:4966–4971.
792. Yu X, Yuan X, McLane MF, et al. Mutations in the cytoplasmic domain of human immunodeficiency virus type 1 transmembrane protein impair the incorporation of env proteins into mature virions. *J Virol* 1993;67:213–221.
793. Yuan B, Li X, Goff SP. Mutations altering the Moloney murine leukemia virus p12 Gag protein affect virion production and early events of the virus life cycle. *EMBO J* 1999;18:4700–4710.
794. Zack JA, Arrigo SJ, Weitsman SR, et al. HIV-entry into quiescent primary lymphocytes: Molecular analysis reveals a labile, latent viral structure. *Cell* 1990;61:213–222.
795. Zack JA, Haislip AM, Krogstad P, Chen ISY. Incompletely reverse-transcribed human immunodeficiency virus type 1 genomes in quiescent cells can function as intermediates in the retroviral life cycle. *J Virol* 1992;66:1717–1725.
796. Zavorotinskaya T, Albritton LM. Suppression of a fusion defect by second site mutations in the ecotropic murine leukemia virus surface protein. *J Virol* 1999;73:5034–5042.
797. Zemba M, Wilk T, Rutten T, et al. The carboxy-terminal p3Gag domain of the human foamy virus Gag precursor is required for efficient virus infectivity. *Virology* 1998;247:7–13.
798. Zennou V, Petit C, Guetard D, et al. HIV-1 genome nuclear import is mediated by a central DNA flap. *Cell* 2000;101:173–185.
799. Zhang J, Temin HM. Rate and mechanism of nonhomologous recombination during a single cycle of retroviral replication. *Science* 1993; 259:234–238.
800. Zhang QY, Clausen PA, Yatsula BA, et al. Mutation of polyadenylation signals generates murine retroviruses that produce fused virus-cell RNA transcripts at high frequency. *Virology* 1998;241:80–93.
801. Zhang Y, Qian H, Love Z, Barklis E. Analysis of the assembly function of the human immunodeficiency virus type 1 gag protein nucleocapsid domain. *J Virol* 1998;72:1782–1789.
802. Zhao Y, Lee S, Anderson WF. Functional interactions between monomers of the retroviral envelope protein complex. *J Virol* 1997;71: 6967–6972.
803. Zhou W, Resh MD. Differential membrane binding of the human immunodeficiency virus type 1 matrix protein. *J Virol* 1996;70: 8540–8548.
804. Zhu J, Cunningham JM. Minus-strand DNA is present within murine type C ecotropic retroviruses prior to infection. *J Virol* 1993;67: 2385–2388.
805. Zhu NL, Cannon PM, Chen D, Anderson WF. Mutational analysis of the fusion peptide of Moloney murine leukemia virus transmembrane protein p15E. *J Virol* 1998;72:1632–1639.
806. Zingler K, Littmann DR. Truncation of the cytoplasmic domain of the simian immunodeficiency virus envelope glycoprotein increases env incorporation into particles and fusogenicity and infectivity. *J Virol* 1993;67:2824–2831.

CHAPTER 28

HIVs and Their Replication

Eric O. Freed and Malcolm A. Martin

In the late 1970s and early 1980s, previously healthy patients with symptoms of immunologic dysfunction sought advice and treatment from physicians in the United States and Europe. This new and unusual syndrome was characterized by generalized lymphadenopathy, opportunistic infections (typically *Pneumocystis carinii* pneumonia, but also *Toxoplasma gondii* encephalitis, cytomegalovirus-associated retinitis, and cryptococcal meningitis), and a variety of unusual cancers (non-Hodgkin's lymphoma and Kaposi's sarcoma). A common accompanying laboratory finding in affected individuals was marked depletion of the CD4+ T-lymphocyte subset in the peripheral blood. The disease was first brought to the attention of the general medical community in June 1981, when the Centers for Disease Control described five California men with severe immunodeficiency in the *Morbidity and Mortality Weekly Report* (79). This notification was followed by several reports describing male homosexuals and intravenous drug users with impaired immune systems and T lymphocytes that responded poorly to antigen and mitogen stimulation in functional assays. Within several months, it became clear that a similar immunodeficiency disease was also affecting other groups, including hemophiliacs, blood transfusion recipients, recent Haitian immigrants, and, most significantly, sexual partners and/or children of members of the various risk groups.

The emerging epidemiologic pattern suggested that the new disease was transmitted by a novel pathogen in contaminated blood or following sexual intercourse with an affected individual. Between late 1981 and early 1983, numerous microorganisms were proposed as possible etiologic agents for the acquired immunodeficiency syndrome, or AIDS, as the disease was soon called. The presence of lymphadenopathy in many affected individuals was reminiscent of the clinical course associated with several different human viral pathogens, and it focused attention on virus families known to infect cells of the immune system. A strong case was made for members of the human herpesviruses, particularly cytomegaloviruses (CMVs), which were frequently isolated from AIDS patients and known to replicate efficiently in human lymphocytes (514). Others favored a retroviral etiology based on the presence of antibodies purported to react with human T-cell leukemia virus type-I (HTLV-I), and/or the actual isolation of HTLV-I from AIDS patients (166,216).

In 1983, scientists at the Pasteur Institute recovered an agent from the lymph nodes of an asymptomatic individual who presented with generalized lymphadenopathy of unknown origin (21). During its replication in cultured cells, the lymphadenopathy-associated virus, or LAV as it was subsequently named, released high titers of progeny virions that contained magnesium-dependent reverse transcriptase activity and exhibited electron microscopic

(EM) features typical of retroviruses. However, unlike the commonly studied retroviruses of diverse vertebrate origin such as the avian leukosis viruses (ALVs) and the murine and feline leukemia viruses (MuLV, FLV), LAV was highly cytopathic in human peripheral blood mononuclear cells (PBMC), specifically killing the CD4+ T-lymphocyte subset in the cell cultures (441). Gallo and colleagues at the National Institutes of Health subsequently reported the isolation of retroviruses from AIDS patients, which they named HTLV-III to distinguish them from the noncytopathic HTLV-I, and obtained the first convincing serologic evidence linking exposure to LAV-like retroviruses and immunodeficient individuals from the various groups at risk (507,551). Contemporaneously, Levy and associates (371) recovered a similar retrovirus from both AIDS patients and healthy individuals from the various risk groups, which they named the AIDS-associated retrovirus (ARV). This latter report suggested that the newly discovered human pathogen could induce both asymptomatic and symptomatic infections. The new retrovirus, associated with AIDS in the United States, Europe, and central Africa and exhibiting morphologic and genetic characteristics typical of the *Lentivirus* genus, was named human immunodeficiency virus, or HIV (102) (and subsequently HIV-1). In 1986, a related, but immunologically distinct and less pathogenic human retrovirus (now called HIV-2), was recovered from individuals residing in several west African countries such as Senegal, Ivory Coast, and Guinea-Bissau (97).

CLASSIFICATION OF THE HUMAN IMMUNODEFICIENCY VIRUSES

One of the first features the Pasteur Institute group noted about HIV-1 was its particle-associated reverse transcriptase, a property that placed the new agent in the retrovirus family. This was consistent with EM analyses of particles released from infected cell cultures, which revealed 100- to 120-µm enveloped virions, similar in size and morphology to previously studied retroviruses. The mature HIV-1 particles contained a cone-shaped cylindrical core or nucleoid reminiscent of that previously described for visna virus (Fig. 1A) (242,441). The cloning and sequencing of proviral DNA, initially purified from productively infected cultures of T-lympho-

A

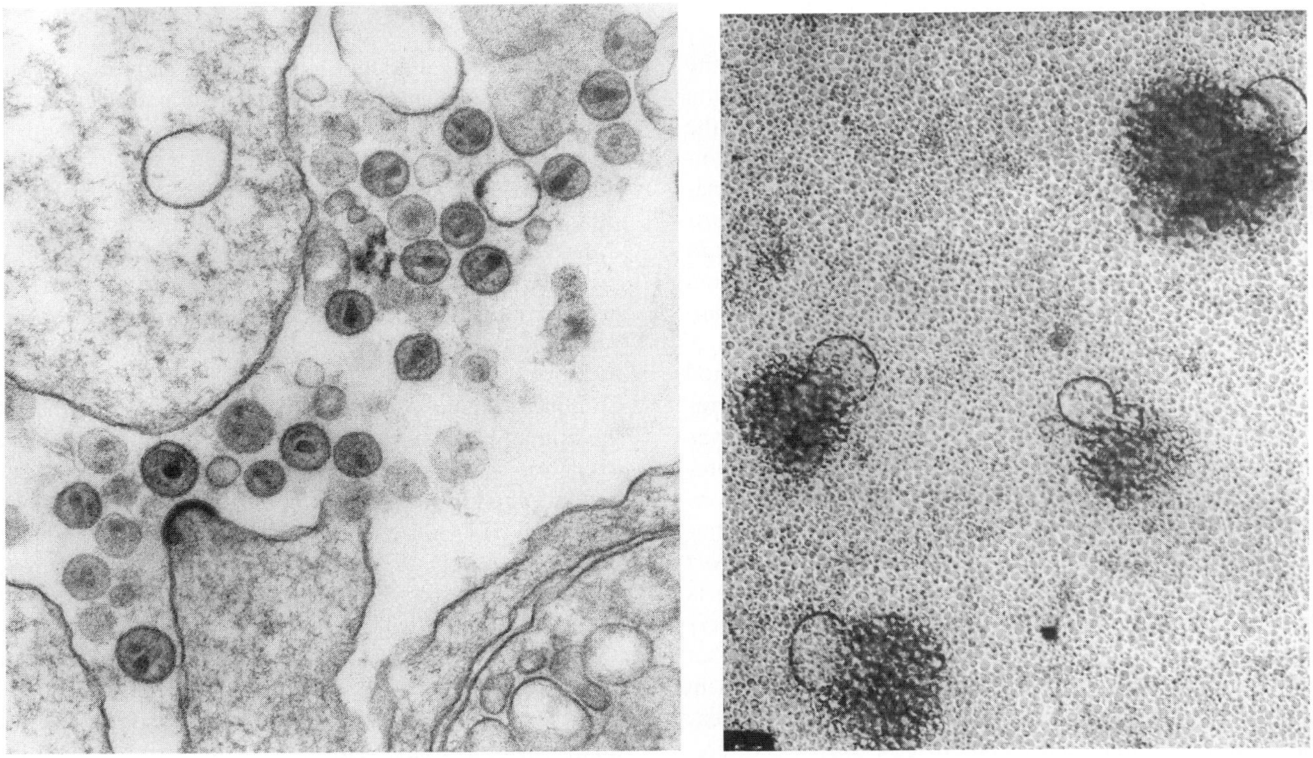

B

FIG. 1. Primate lentiviruses have a distinct morphology and can induce syncytia during productive infections. **A:** Electron micrograph showing a single HIV-1 particle in the process of budding from an infected cultured human PBMC, and several mature virions containing the characteristic conical/bullet-shaped nucleoid (×100,000). (Photomicrograph kindly provided by Dr. Jan Orenstein.) **B:** Typical ballooning syncytia induced by primate lentiviruses as visualized by inverted light microscopy at the time of peak virus production.

cytes/T-cell leukemia lines (T-cell lines), indicated that HIV-1 not only possessed a genomic organization related to other replication-competent retroviruses but placed it, taxonomically, in the *Lentivirus* genus (517,648). This relationship is shown diagrammatically in Figure 1 of Chapter 27. As their name suggests, lentiviruses were known to cause slow, unremitting disease in sheep, horses, and cattle, and to target various lineages of hematopoietic cells, particularly lymphocytes and differentiated macrophages.

Following the isolation, molecular cloning, and initial classification of HIV-1, several genetically distinct primate lentiviruses were discovered and their phylogenetic relationships to HIV-1 were ascertained. For example, viruses isolated from captive macaques or feral monkey species in Africa were shown to possess particle morphologies and genomic organizations similar to those of HIV-1. Because inoculation of Asian macaque species, such as rhesus monkeys, with these newly discovered agents frequently induced an AIDS-like illness, these viruses were named simian immunodeficiency virus (SIV) to distinguish them from the human viruses, HIV-1 and HIV-2.

The phylogenetic relationships of the human lentiviruses are shown in Figure 2; the detailed genetic interrelationships of all members of the *Lentivirus* genus are presented in Figure 2 of Chapter 61 in *Fields Virology*, 4th ed. HIV-2 is more closely related to SIV_{smm} (285), a virus isolated from sooty mangabey monkeys in the wild, than to HIV-1. It is currently believed that HIV-2 represents a zoonotic transmission of SIV_{smm} to man (224). A series of lentiviral isolates from captive chimpanzees, designated SIV_{cpz}, are close genetic relatives of HIV-1. Unlike the other SIVs, which are endemic to African monkeys, the SIV_{cpz} genome contains a *vpu* gene (see below), also present in HIV-1 (298).

It was originally thought that HIV-1, like previously studied replication-competent retroviruses (e.g., MuLVs, ALVs, HTLVs), would be genetically homogeneous. However, as proviral DNAs corresponding to HIV-1 isolates from Europe, North America, and Africa became available

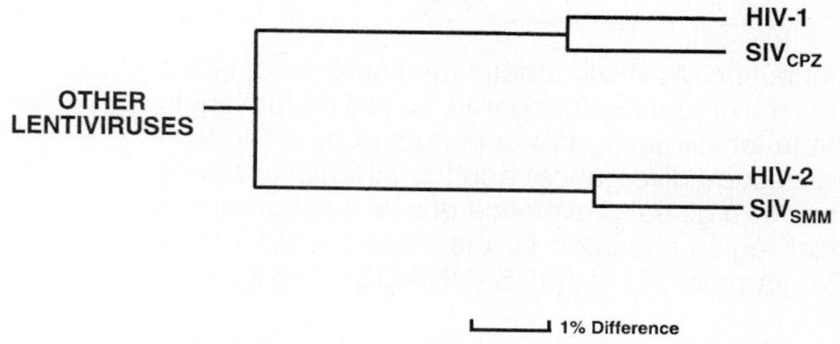

FIG. 2. Phylogenetic relationships of HIV-1 and HIV-2 based on identity of *pol* gene sequences. SIV_{cpz} and SIV_{smm} are subhuman primate lentiviruses recovered from a chimpanzee and sooty mangabey monkey, respectively. (Adapted from ref. 454, with permission.)

and were compared, initially by restriction enzyme digestion, their extensive genetic heterogeneity became apparent (28). No two HIV-1 isolates were identical. When subjected to nucleotide sequence analysis, even HIV-1 samples recovered from a single individual exhibited significant heterology (545). Some of the nucleotide changes (nonsynonymous) resulted in amino acid substitutions, whereas others (synonymous) did not alter the protein sequence. Although nucleotide changes were distributed throughout the HIV-1 genome, the greatest variability occurred in the *env* gene when either intra- or interpatient virus specimens were compared. Hypervariable regions (designated V_1 to V_5), present in the gp120 envelope coding sequences, were sandwiched between relatively conserved (C_1 to C_5) sequences (see Fig. 27 for their locations) (596,666). The term *quasi-species* was subsequently coined to describe the heterogeneous and changing populations of virus present in an HIV-1-infected individual (435). Despite the heterologous nature of different HIV-1 isolates and, in particular, their envelope glycoproteins, a highly conserved and immunodominant domain, located within the gp41 envelope protein, still elicited antibody in infected individuals, which was reactive with (and diagnostic for) HIV-1 samples of diverse geographic origin (238).

The earliest phylogenetic analyses of HIV-1 isolates focused on samples from Europe/North America and Africa; discrete clusters of viruses were identified from these two areas of the world. Distinct genetic subtypes or clades of HIV-1 were subsequently defined and classified into three groups: M (major); O (outlier); and N (non-M or O) (Fig. 3A). The M group of HIV-1, which includes over 95% of the global virus isolates, consists of at least eight discrete clades (A, B, C, D, F, G, H, and J), based on the sequence of complete viral genomes (384,453,673). Members of HIV-1 group O have been recovered from individuals living in Cameroon, Gabon, and Equatorial Guinea; their genomes share less than 50% identity in nucleotide sequence with group M viruses (604). The more recently discovered group N HIV-1 strains have been identified in infected Cameroonians, fail to react serologically in standard whole-virus enzyme-linked immunosorbent assay (ELISA), yet are readily detectable by conventional Western blot analysis (580).

Most current knowledge about HIV-1 genetic variation comes from studies of group M viruses of diverse geographic origin (383,384,604). Data collected during the past decade indicate that the HIV-1 population present within an infected individual can vary from 6% to 10% in nucleotide sequence. HIV-1 isolates within a clade may exhibit nucleotide distances of 15% in *gag* and up to 30% in gp120 coding sequences. Interclade genetic variation may range between 30% and 40% depending on the gene analyzed. HIV-1-like isolates from chimpanzees (SIV_{cpz}) are positioned at two locations in the maximum likelihood tree shown in Figure 3A. $SIV_{cpz\text{-}ant}$ is not closely related to any of the three HIV-1 groups, whereas $SIV_{cpz\text{-}}$

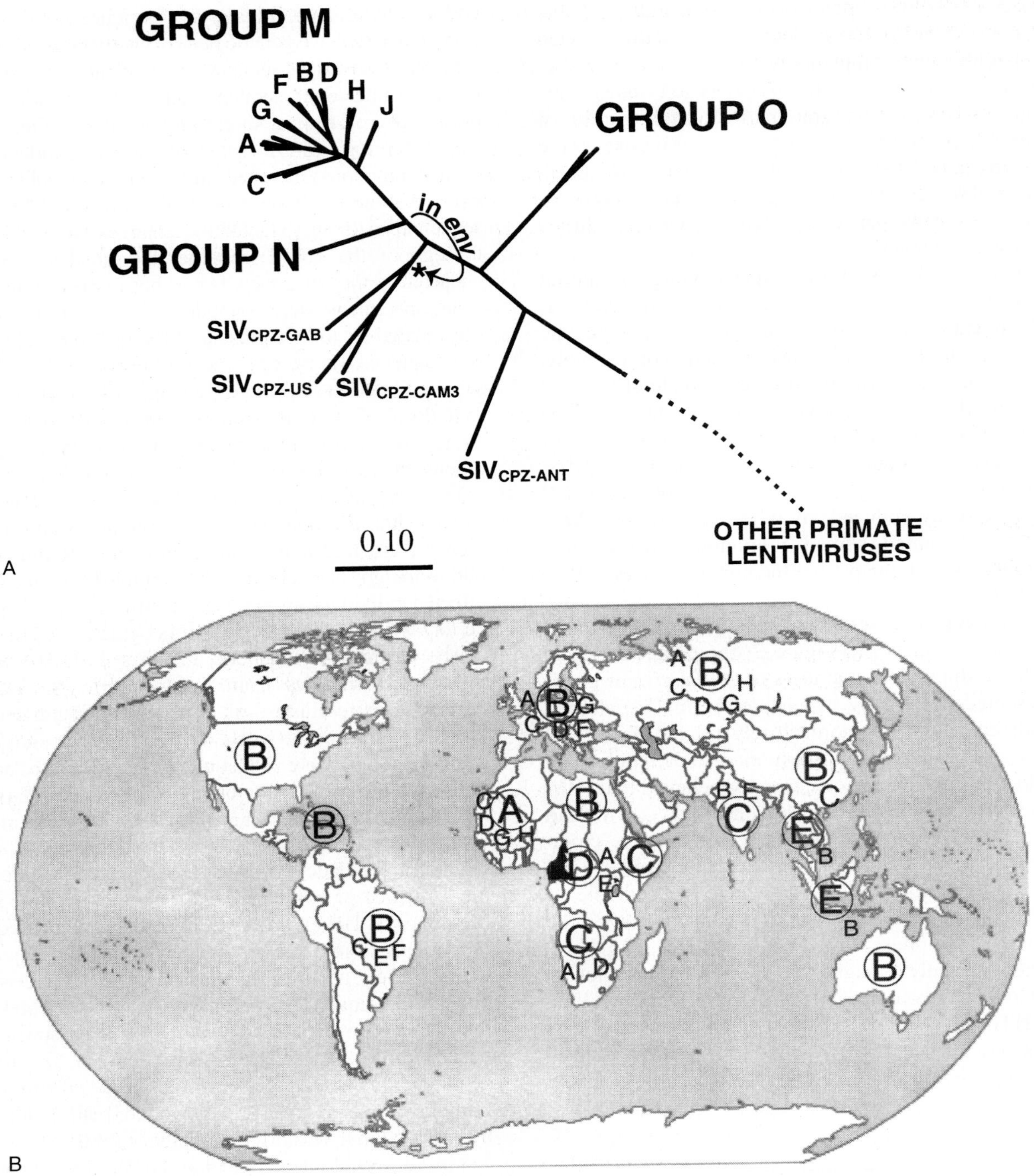

FIG. 3. HIV-1 genetic subtypes and their worldwide distribution. **A:** Phylogenetic relationships of HIV-1 groups M, N, and O with four different SIV_{cpz} isolates. This maximum likelihood tree, based on full-length *pol* gene sequences (115,344) from the indicated primate lentiviruses, was constructed by Bette Korber. The *bar* indicates a genetic distance of 0.1 (10% nucleotide divergence) and the *asterisk* positions group N HIV-1 isolates based on *env* sequences. **B:** The 1998 global prevalence of HIV-1 subgroups is shown with the predominant clade in each geographical region indicated by the *large circled letters.* Based on data collected by the Joint United Nations Programme on HIV/AIDS (UNAIDS). The location of Cameroon on the west coast of Africa is *shaded.*

gab, $SIV_{cpz\text{-}us}$, and $SIV_{cpz\text{-}cam3}$ cluster between group N and group O isolates, based on *pol* gene sequences (115,261).

All of the HIV-1 group M subtypes can be found in Africa (Fig. 3B). Clade A viruses are genetically the most divergent (362) and were the most common HIV-1 subtype in Africa early in the epidemic. With the rapid spread of HIV-1 to southern Africa during the mid to late 1990s, clade C viruses have become the dominant subtype and now account for 48% of HIV-1 infections worldwide (465). Clade B viruses, the most intensively studied HIV-1 subtype, remain the most prevalent isolates in Europe and North America. It should be emphasized, however, that in the context of the different HIV-1 clades, there has been no demonstrated association between antigenic serotypes and HIV-1 genetic subtypes (711).

Approximately 1% to 6% of the HIV-1 isolates in Cameroon are members of group O (424). A somewhat variable immunodominant gp41 region accounts for a 20% failure rate in identifying HIV-1 group O infected individuals by ELISA assays, capable of detecting virtually all persons exposed to HIV-1 group M isolates. Interestingly, unlike group M viruses, group O strains do not require cyclophilin A for biologic activity (see the Gag protein section later) (52).

High rates of genetic recombination are a hallmark of retroviruses. It was initially believed that simultaneous infections by genetically diverse virus strains were not likely to be established in individuals at risk for HIV-1. By 1995, however, it became apparent that a significant fraction of the HIV-1 group M global diversity included interclade viral recombinants. It is now appreciated that HIV-1 recombinants will be found in geographic areas such as Africa, South America, and Southeast Asia, where multiple HIV-1 subtypes coexist and may account for more than 10% of circulating HIV-1 strains (222). Molecularly, the genomes of these recombinant viruses resemble patchwork mosaics, with juxtaposed diverse HIV-1 subtype segments, reflecting the multiple crossover events contributing to their generation. Most HIV-1 recombinants have arisen in Africa and a majority contain segments originally derived from clade A viruses. In Thailand, for example, the composition of the predominant circulating strain consists of a clade A *gag* plus *pol* gene segment and a clade E *env* gene (76). Because the clade E *env* gene in Thai HIV-1 strains is closely related to the clade E *env* present in virus isolates from the Central African Republic, it is believed that the original recombination event occurred in Africa, with the subsequent introduction of a descendent virus into Thailand (223). Interestingly, no full-length HIV-1 subtype E isolate (i.e., with subtype E *gag*, *pol*, and *env* genes) has been reported to date.

Recombination very likely occurred during the evolution of the three HIV-1-related chimpanzee isolates ($SIV_{cpz\text{-}gab}$, $SIV_{cpz\text{-}us}$, and $SIV_{cpz\text{-}cam3}$) based on their different tree locations when *pol* and *env* genes are used to establish phylogenetic relationships (see asterisk, Fig. 3A). When *env* sequences are used, these nonhuman lentiviruses cluster with group N HIV-1 isolates, whereas they map between groups N and O on the basis of their *pol* genes. This discordance points to an ancestral recombinational event between this group of SIV_{cpz} and group M HIV-1 strains (221). An intergroup (groups M and O) recombinant virus has recently been described (496), but no recombination between HIV-1 and HIV-2 has been reported, although mixed *in vivo* infections involving the latter are known to occur (254).

The origin of HIV-1 as a human pathogen remains an unsolved enigma of the AIDS epidemic. As noted earlier, HIV-2 appears to have been transmitted to man from SIV_{smm}-infected sooty mangabeys, which are endemic to west Africa, the same geographical region where HIV-2 is prevalent (224). Previous studies have shown that distinct phylogenetic lineages of SIV_{agm} are associated with different substrains of African green monkeys, each with nonoverlapping geographical ranges (447). This type of association implies exogenous infections hundreds of thousands of years ago and subsequent virus–host coevolution. In this regard, three of the four HIV-1-like viruses recovered from chimpanzees ($SIV_{cpz\text{-}gab}$, $SIV_{cpz\text{-}us}$, and $SIV_{cpz\text{-}cam3}$) were isolated from the central African *Pan troglodytes troglodytes* chimpanzee substrain, whereas the fourth ($SIV_{cpz\text{-}ant}$) was recovered from a completely different chimpanzee lineage, *P. t. schweinfurthii*, whose natural range is in eastern Africa (221). HIV-1 phylogenetic relationships based on *pol* genes (see Fig. 3A) indicate that not only do the viruses recovered from *P. t. troglodytes* subspecies cluster with the three main HIV-1 groups but also their *env* genes are very closely related to the group N virus strains. In contrast, the *P. t. schweinfurthii*–associated virus, $SIV_{cpz\text{-}ant}$, is the outlier, mapping to a highly divergent phylogenetic lineage. These results imply that, as in the case of SIV_{agm} and African green monkeys, host-dependent HIV-1 diversification occurred in discrete chimpanzee substrains. Given the fact that the natural range of *P. t. troglodytes* overlaps geographically with the region in Africa (Cameroon/Gabon) where all three HIV-1 groups are endemic, it seems likely that this chimpanzee subspecies is the source of a zoonosis to humans. A survey of HIV-1 prevalence in feral chimpanzees and in humans living in the same locale will be needed to verify this association.

GENOMIC ORGANIZATION OF THE HUMAN IMMUNODEFICIENCY VIRUSES

The nucleotide sequencing of the original HIV-1 isolates revealed an unexpected result. In contrast to prototypical retroviruses such as ALV and MuLV, whose genomes contain only three genes that encode the three groups of structural proteins [group-specific antigen (*gag*), polymerase (*pol*), and envelope (*env*)], the HIV-1 genome included several additional and overlapping open reading frames (ORFs) of unknown function (Fig. 4).

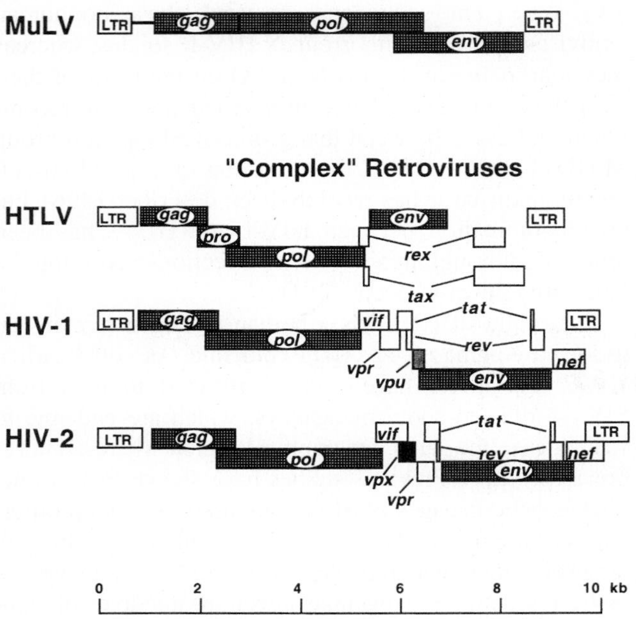

FIG. 4. Genomic organization of simple and complex retroviruses. The genes of Moloney murine leukemia virus (MuLV), HTLV-I, HIV-1 and HIV-2 are depicted as they are arranged in their respective proviral DNAs. The sizes of the different proviral DNAs are shown in proportion to the 9.7-kb HIV provirus.

Although an extra ORF, now known to encode a superantigen, had been previously identified within the 3′ long terminal repeat (LTR) of mouse mammary tumor virus proviral DNA (136), the existence of additional, functionally important retroviral genes was generally unappreciated until the discovery and genomic analysis of HTLV-I (270). The sequencing of HTLV-I proviral DNA revealed the presence of three short, overlapping ORFs, located between the *env* gene and the 3′ LTR. One of these encoded a regulator of transcription, the Tax protein. Not only did HIV-1 and HIV-2 contain multiple additional ORFs, but superficially, their genomic organizations appeared to be identical. However, further analyses demonstrated that HIV-1 contains the distinguishing *vpu* gene (107,602), and HIV-2 encodes the unique *vpx* (321) gene product (see Fig. 4).

As is the case for all replication-competent retroviruses, the three primary HIV-1 translation products, all encoding structural proteins, are initially synthesized as polyprotein precursors, which are subsequently processed by viral or cellular proteases into mature particle-associated proteins (Fig. 5). The 55-kd Gag precursor $Pr55^{Gag}$ is cleaved into the matrix (MA), capsid (CA), nucleocapsid (NC), and p6 proteins. Autocatalysis of the 160-kd Gag-Pol polyprotein, $Pr160^{Gag\text{-}Pol}$, gives rise to the protease (PR), the heterodimeric reverse transcriptase (RT), and the integrase (IN) proteins, whereas proteolytic digestion by a cellular enzyme(s) converts the glycosylated 160-kd Env precursor gp160 to the gp120 surface (SU) and gp41 transmembrane (TM) cleavage products. The remaining six HIV-1-encoded proteins (Vif, Vpr, Tat, Rev, Vpu, and Nef) are the primary translation products of spliced mRNAs.

HIV-1 and HIV-2 have incorporated multiple sequence elements into their genomic RNAs that are required for the balanced and coordinated production of progeny virions. Most of these so-called cis-acting RNA elements (Fig. 6) are present in other retroviral genomes, but a few

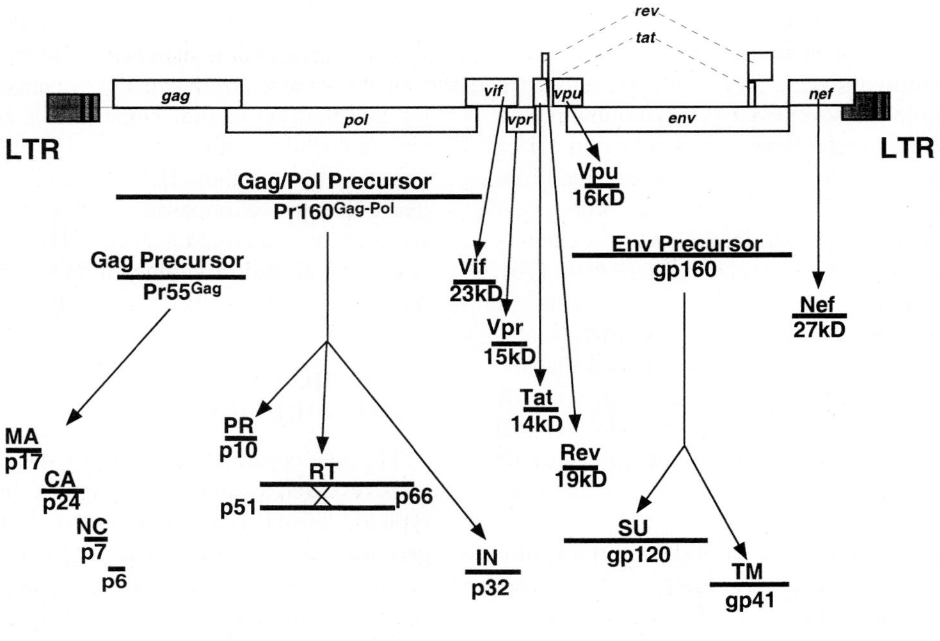

FIG. 5. HIV-encoded proteins. The location of the HIV genes, the sizes of primary translation products (in some cases polyproteins), and the processed mature viral proteins are indicated.

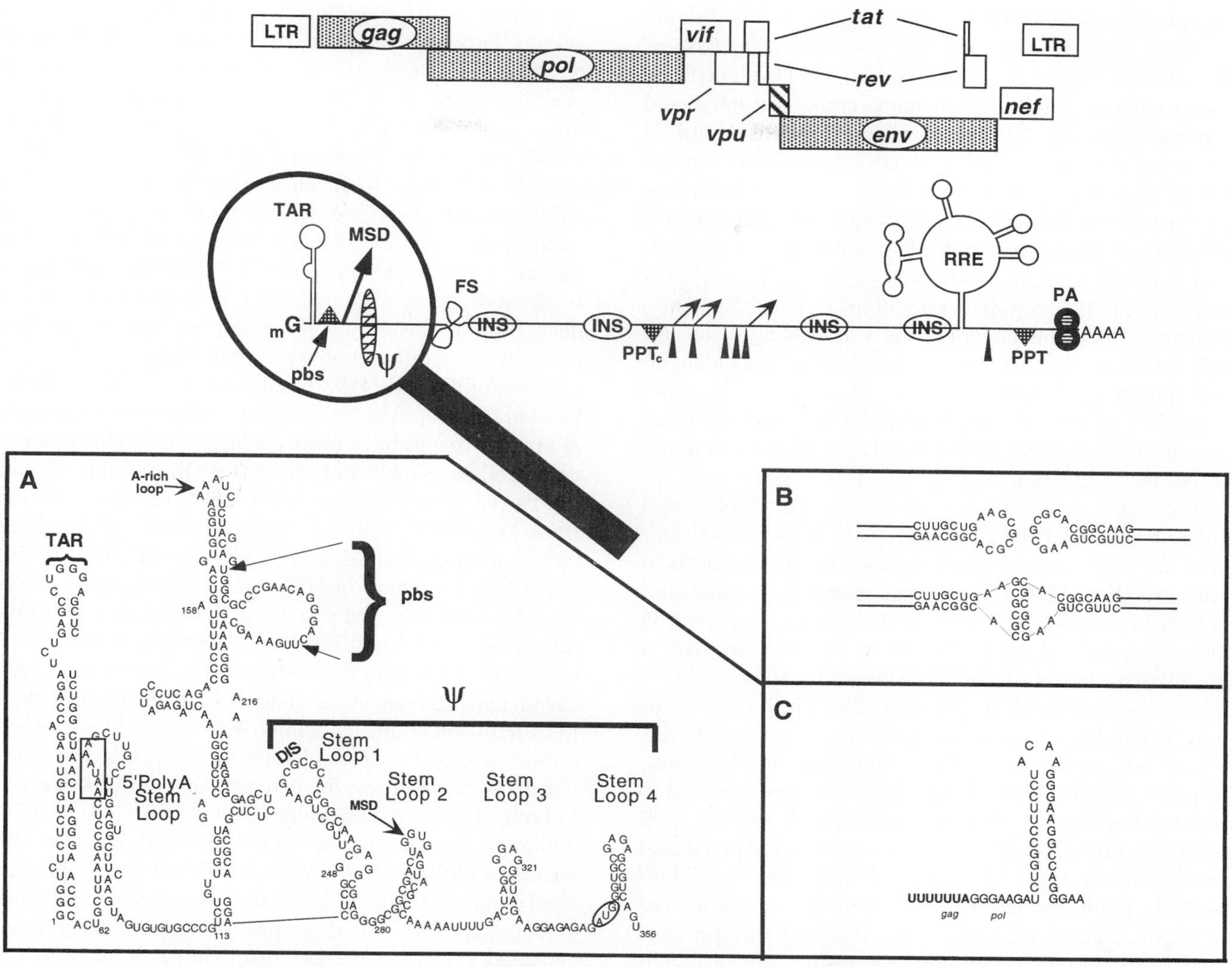

FIG. 6. Cis-acting elements present in the HIV-1 genome. Elements associated with HIV-1 genomic RNA include the methyl capped terminal G residue at the 5′ terminus of viral RNA (*mG*); the Tat-responsive stem-bulge-loop structure (*TAR*); the binding site for the tRNA^{Lys} primer (*pbs*); the major splice donor (*MSD*); the major RNA packaging site (ψ); the frameshifting motif (*FS*); RNA instability/nuclear retention elements (*INS*); the central polypurine tract (*PPTc*); splice acceptors (*arrowheads*); internal splice donors (*small arrows*); the Rev-responsive element (*RRE*); the canonical 3′ polypurine tract (*PPT*); and the polyadenylation signal (*PA*). **A:** The putative secondary structure at the 5′ terminus of HIV-1 mRNAs. The positions of the TAR stem-loop, the poly(A) stem-loop and the boxed poly(A) addition signal, the pbs, the dimerization initiation sequence (*DIS*), the major splice donor (*MSD*), and the translation initiation AUG codon for Gag are indicated. (Adapted from ref. 98, with permission.) **B:** The self-complementary DIS sequences, located at the crown of stem-loop 1, participate in the formation of "kissing loop" intermediates, an initial step in the RNA dimerization reaction. **C:** RNA stem-loop structure downstream of the UUUUUUA HIV-1 frameshifting sequence.

are unique to the primate lentiviruses. The tRNA^{Lys} primer binding site (pbs), the major splice donor sequence (MSD), the encapsidation element (ψ), and an RNA dimerization initiation sequence (DIS), are all located within the 5′-terminal 400 nt (nucleotides) of the HIV-1 genome. In addition to the pbs, the HIV-1 genome contains other elements that help stabilize the encapsidated tRNA^{Lys3} primer. These include an A-rich region located upstream of the pbs, which binds the anticodon loop of the tRNA primer, and a series of complex structural U5 motifs (301,319,374). Furthermore, the Pr55^{Gag} precursor polyprotein appears to play the role of chaperone by catalyzing the annealing of the primer tRNA to the pbs/U5 region during virus assembly (178), a subject discussed in further detail in the Gag section of this chapter. The principal packaging signal for HIV-1 genomic RNA consists of three stem-loop structures, SL1, SL3, and SL4 (Fig. 6, inset A), which span the MSD (99,425). Elements located

(a) at the 5′ terminus of the genome (231), (b) within the so-called poly(A) stem-loop (125), and (c) at the base of the TAR stem (98) are also required for efficient RNA encapsidation. The DIS contains complementary and exposed sequences (GCGCGC in Fig. 6, insets A and B) located at the crown of SL1. It participates in the formation of viral RNA dimers, which are recruited into progeny particles by first forming "kissing loop" intermediates (35,484). Although two polyadenylation signals are present in HIV-1 genomic RNA, only the 3′ AAUAAA hexameric motif directs poly(A) addition. A polyadenylation enhancer, situated upstream of the 3′ polyadenylation signal, stabilizes the binding of the cleavage-polyadenylation-specifying factor to the AAUAAA hexamer (236,631), whereas the upstream poly(A) stem-loop structure has been reported to block poly(A) addition at the 5′ end of the viral RNA (124).

The HIV-1 genome is unique in having a novel central polypurine tract (PPT) in addition to a traditional U3-proximal PPT, both of which are used for the synthesis of plus-strand viral DNA (81). The genomic RNA also contains a heptameric U UUU UUA shift sequence within the *gag* gene, which functions in conjunction with a downstream hairpin (see Fig. 6, inset C) to mediate −1 translational frameshifting (305). The viral RNA folds into two additional complex structures (TAR and RRE), which are involved in RNA synthesis and transport, respectively. The TAR element has also been reported to be required for the efficient initiation of reverse transcription (268). Multiple inhibitory sequences (designated INS in Fig. 6), associated with the instability/nuclear retention of HIV transcripts, are scattered throughout genes encoding Gag, Pol, and Env proteins (403,535). Finally, although adenosine deoxyribonucleotide (A) is not strictly considered a cis-acting element, it is worth noting that HIV-1 genomic RNA contains a significantly higher A content (approximately 39%) than mammalian DNA; this bias contributes to an unusual codon usage (34).

THE BIOLOGY OF HIV INFECTIONS

A quintessential property of HIV-1 and the other primate lentiviruses is to sequentially use CD4 and a second cellular receptor during entry into susceptible cells, a subject discussed more extensively in the section dealing with the envelope glycoproteins. Consequently, the main cellular targets for HIV-1 are the CD4+ T-helper/inducer subset of lymphocytes, CD4+ cells of macrophage lineage, and some populations of dendritic cells. Because HIV-1 infections *in vivo* are limited to humans and chimpanzees and no tractable animal model for HIV-1 currently exists, our current understanding about virus replication derives primarily from retrospective analyses of clinical specimens collected from seropositive individuals and a voluminous body of work examining virus infections in tissue culture systems. The very earliest studies indicated that mitogen-activated human PBMC were the cells of choice for isolating virus from infected persons. Some early HIV-1 isolates were also able to infect continuous CD4+ T leukemia cell lines such as CEM, Jurkat, Hut 78, and the HTLV-I-containing MT-2 and MT-4. Human T-cell lines were clearly more logistically tractable than PBMC, and their use greatly facilitated molecular and genetic studies of HIV-1. Most human T-cell lines released large quantities of virions while undergoing a typical cytopathic infection and cell death, but a few (e.g., H9 cells) became persistently infected and exhibited only minimal cytopathic effects.

Many of the early HIV-1 isolates were classified on the basis of their replicative, cytopathic, and tropic properties. A majority of primary virus isolates, which characteristically replicate slowly and generate small amounts of progeny particles, were labeled "slow/low" to distinguish them from "rapid/high" HIV-1 strains, which exhibit faster infection kinetics and release high titers of virions (179). Some HIV-1 primary isolates, frequently those recovered from symptomatic individuals, induced syncytia formation following co-cultivation of virus-producing PBMC with MT-2 cells (see Fig. 1B) (343). These isolates were designated SI (syncytium-inducing) to distinguish them from non-syncytium-inducing (NSI) strains. Tropism was a third property used to classify HIV-1 primary isolates. For many retroviruses, the determinants of tropism reside in both the external envelope glycoprotein and the LTR. Although changes in the LTR may modulate the efficiency of replication in a variety of T-cell types, the principal determinant of HIV host range resides in the SU Env glycoprotein. All HIV-1 strains can productively infect activated PBMC; some are also able to replicate in cultures of monocyte-derived macrophage (MDM) and have been classified as macrophage- or M-tropic (112). Virus isolated from individuals shortly after they have been infected with HIV-1 are frequently M-tropic (533). Other isolates, often obtained late in the disease course, can establish infections in continuous human CD4+ T-cell lines but not in MDM, and they have been designated T-cell-line or TCL-tropic. Subsequent studies reported primary HIV-1 isolates able to infect both MDM and T-cell lines; such strains have been classified as dual tropic (111). Although exceptions exist, M-tropic isolates, in general, are NSI and "slow/low," whereas TCL-tropic strains are frequently SI and exhibit the "rapid/high" replication phenotype. Forced passage of some primary isolates in continuous CD4+ human cell lines has resulted in T-cell-line adapted (TCLA) HIV-1 strains, which possess altered tropic properties and increased sensitivity to neutralizing antibodies and soluble CD4 (606). In molecular clones corresponding to one of the original TCLA strains, HIV-1_{IIIB}, which had been extensively propagated in Hut 78 cells, the reading frames for the *vpr*, *vpu*, and *nef* genes are not open, suggesting that these three genes are not required for efficient replication in certain human T-cell lines. This is discussed in greater detail in the section dealing with accessory proteins.

The discovery that α and β chemokine receptors function as coreceptors for virus fusion and entry into susceptible CD4+ cells (92,134,177) has led to a revised classification scheme for HIV-1 (Table 1). Isolates can now be grouped on the basis of chemokine receptor utilization in fusion assays in which HIV-1 gp120 and CD4+ coreceptor proteins are expressed in separate cells (43). As indicated in Table 1, HIV-1 isolates using the CXCR4 receptor [now designated X4 viruses (30)] are usually TCL-tropic SI strains, whereas those exclusively utilizing the CCR5 receptor (R5 viruses) are predominantly M-tropic and NSI. The dual-tropic R5/X4 strains, which may comprise the majority of patient isolates and exhibit a continuum of tropic phenotypes, are frequently SI (579). However, because the expression levels of chemokine receptor, CD4, or gp120 may be unphysiologically high in fusion assays for assessing coreceptor usage, the classification of a particular gp120 based on these criteria may not accurately predict coreceptor utilization during actual spreading virus infections of PBMC, T-cell lines, and MDM (91).

The exclusive use of tissue culture systems to classify HIV-1 isolates and to define their replicative phenotypes clearly fails to address a myriad of biologic issues attending viral infections in exposed humans. For example, *in vivo*, most T lymphocytes circulating in the blood or present in lymphoid tissues are resting in the G_0 phase of the cell cycle; potential tissue macrophage targets exist as nondividing cells in G_1 (263). Early studies demonstrated that resting human PBMC do not support productive HIV infections unless they are stimulated with mitogens and propagated in the presence of interleukin (IL)-2 (430). This could reflect the extremely small pool sizes of ribonucleotides, deoxyribonucleotide triphosphates, and ATP in quiescent T lymphocytes (467). Although it is still unclear whether the reverse transcription or the integration step of the HIV-1 replication cycle is dysfunctional in unstimulated T lymphocytes, there is general agreement that no viral proteins or progeny virions are produced (598,696). Activation of resting PBMC up to 14 days following an initial abortive infection is still able to resurrect a productive infection (696).

Growth factors, cytokines, and antigens are physiologic activators of T lymphocytes *in vivo*. Antigen-mediated activation of the T-cell receptor leads to increased expression of several regulatory factors and the transition of lymphocytes from the G_0 resting state to the G_1 phase of the cell cycle. Co-stimulation of CD28 results in increased production of IL-2, surface expression of the IL-2 receptor, and progression through G_1, S, and mitosis. The absence of a co-stimulatory signal, however, leads to the unresponsive anergic state and arrest at the G_1a/G_1b transition point of the cell cycle (235). G_1a cells have a 2N DNA content, produce higher levels of RNA than G_0 cells, but are not committed to progress to S phase; in G_1b, cellular RNA levels are equivalent to those present in S phase and cells pass through the G_1/S checkpoint. Cell-cycle studies have shown that progression into G_1b is required to achieve productive HIV-1 infections of circulating CD4+ T lymphocytes (345). Incubation of resting T lymphocytes with IL-2, IL-4, IL7, or IL-15, in the absence of other stimuli, has also been reported to confer susceptibility to HIV-1 (630).

One of the most prominent and earliest recognized clinical features of AIDS is the selective depletion of CD4+ T cells, a property that correlates with tropism of HIV-1 and its cytopathicity for this lymphocyte subset in tissue culture infections. More detailed studies, primarily using X4 HIV-1 strains, indicated that memory CD4+ cells, rather than naive CD4+ T cells, were preferentially infected and killed (96,557). However, selective loss of CD4+ memory cells is not commonly observed in HIV-1 seropositive individuals. More recent work, employing CD3/CD28 co-stimulation to activate CD4+ T lymphocytes, has confirmed the greater susceptibility of memory cells to X4 viruses but it has also shown that naive but not memory CD4+ cells are infectable by R5 strains of HIV-1 (528). When lymphocytes from HIV-1-infected individuals were, in fact, examined, integrated proviral DNA was detected and virus could be recovered from both memory and naive CD4+ T cells with no evidence of selective chemokine coreceptor usage for either lymphocyte subset (478).

In addition to quiescent CD4+ T lymphocytes, nondividing pleuripotent hematopoietic stem cells (HSC) in G_0 have attracted considerable attention as targets for HIV-1, in the context of both natural infections and development of HIV-1 vectors for gene therapy. HSC are a subset of CD34-positive bone marrow cells that express CD4; some HSC also produce functional cell-surface CXCR4 and CCR5 proteins (571). Unfortunately, conflicting

TABLE 1. *Tropic and biologic properties of HIV-1 isolates*

Chemokine coreceptor used	PBMC replication	Macrophage replication	T-cell-line replication	Replicative phenotype	Synctium-inducing phenotype
X4	+	–	+	Rapid/high	++
R5	+	+	–	Slow/low	–
R5/X4	+	+	+	Rapid/high	+

PBMC, peripheral blood mononuclear cells.

results have been obtained about their susceptibility to HIV-1, most likely reflecting (a) the criteria used for selecting G_0 HSC and not more mature progenitor cells, (b) the purity of the fractionated HSC, and (c) the transduction/infection protocol employed (571,629).

Dendritic cells (DCs) are antigen-presenting cells that capture, transport, and present antigens to CD4+ and CD8+ T lymphocytes. They include Langerhans cells in skin, follicular DCs in germinal centers, interdigitating DCs in T-cell areas of lymph nodes, interstitial DCs in intestinal and genital mucosa, and circulating, blood-derived DCs. It is currently thought that DCs associated with mucosal surfaces may represent the first line of defense against sexually transmitted HIV-1, transporting recently inoculated virus particles from portals of entry to secondary lymphoid organs. Nonetheless, productive HIV-1 infections of different types of purified DCs have been difficult to demonstrate *in vitro* (71), although vigorous virus replication is observed when DCs are first pulsed with virus and then cocultivated with CD4+ T lymphocytes (627). Interestingly, the infectious virions released from such cell conjugates bear T-cell-, not DC-, specific surface proteins acquired during the budding process, implying that a complete virus replicative cycle occurs in the T lymphocyte and that DCs may, in fact, be refractory to HIV-1 infection (189). It has recently been reported that DCs express a C-type lectin (named DC-specific ICAM-3-grabbing nonintegrin, or DC-SIGN) that "captures" HIV by binding to virion-associated gp120 and transmits the virus to T cells expressing CD4 and the appropriate chemokine coreceptor (232). Intriguingly, the virus bound to dendritic cells via DC-SIGN retains infectivity even on long-term culture (>4 days), suggesting that the dendritic cells are able to sequester or "protect" bound virions from degradation. These findings have significant implications for the transmission and dissemination of HIV *in vivo* and may present a novel target for antiviral therapy.

Virtually all lentiviruses have retained the capacity to replicate in nonproliferating, terminally differentiated tissue macrophages. Thus, unlike the oncoretroviruses, which require mitosis and dissolution of the nuclear membrane to complete a cycle of replication, HIV-1 is able to productively infect these G_1- (not G_0-) arrested cells. This property, thought to be mediated by one or more of the viral-encoded proteins, requires that the HIV-1 preintegration complex be translocated through intact nuclear pores. *In vitro*, differentiation of blood-derived monocytes is required for vigorous replication by M-tropic viral strains (562). As is the case for productive infections of T lymphocytes, HIV-1 replication in MDM requires integration of the reverse transcript (163), but only minimal cytopathicity has been reported and morphologically mature virus particles may accumulate intracellularly within intracytoplasmic vacuoles (477).

A variety of approaches have been used to measure the kinetics of HIV-1 infections in cell cultures and to determine the intrinsic infectivity of a virus stock. For example, the end-point dilution of a virus preparation (ID_{50}) is commonly reported as the amount of inoculum having a 50% probability of initiating an infection during a defined observation period. For many commonly used cell-free HIV-1 stocks, the number of physical particles released from 10^6 virus-producing cells in 1 mL of medium can be more than 10^9 physical particles or approximately 10^3 virions per cell (138,429). Such culture supernates will typically contain 10^5 to 10^6 tissue culture ID_{50} (or $TCID_{50}$) per mL. These values will vary depending on the cell type (PBMC versus T-cell line) used and the virus source (primary versus TCLA isolate), but the time required for one complete cycle of HIV-1 infection *in vitro* is usually 3 to 4 days. It is worth noting that the particle-to-infectivity ratio for HIV-1 calculated from these values is quite low (10^{-3} to 10^{-4}). In contrast, the infectivity of virus-producing cells, as measured in co-culture systems, is approximately 10^2 to 10^3 times higher than the infectivity of all of the cell-free particles present in the culture supernate from the same infected cells (138). Taken together, these data suggest that, like many other retroviruses, HIV-1 relies on cell-to-cell transmission for dissemination of virus *in vivo*. Certainly the high density and proximity of virus-infected cells in lymphoid tissue would favor this mode of virus spread.

Although HIV-1 causes the selective loss of cultured CD4+ cells and induces depletion of the same T-lymphocyte subset in virus-infected individuals, the mechanisms responsible for this cytopathic effect are still unknown. Cell death is currently thought to occur by either necrosis or apoptosis, processes that can be distinguished morphologically and biochemically. Direct cell killing by HIV-1 in tissue culture systems can occur as a consequence of single-cell lysis or syncytium formation and is frequently associated with the presence or expression of the viral envelope glycoproteins (74,339). Apoptosis of T lymphocytes, characterized morphologically by nuclear condensation and DNA fragmentation and the absence of an inflammatory response *in vivo*, has been observed in lymph node biopsies from HIV-1-infected individuals (451). It has also been reported that cultured PBMC from HIV-1 seropositive persons undergo spontaneous apoptosis at higher rates than cells from uninfected individuals (255). A critical issue, pertaining specifically to apoptosis, is whether HIV-1 and related primate lentiviruses kill only cells they infect or indirectly cause the death of uninfected bystander cells including CD8+ T lymphocytes. Although many studies have shown that HIV-1-infected cells undergo apoptotic death, the use of reporter virus systems indicates that in cultures of purified T lymphocytes, infected CD4+ cells, not bystander cells, undergo apoptosis (219). The specific apoptotic pathway responsible for cell killing in HIV-1-infected cells has not yet been elucidated.

HIV-1 ANIMAL MODELS

Chimpanzees

Because HIV-1 establishes infections only in humans and chimpanzees and, with rare exceptions (464), induces disease only in humans, multiple questions about the biology of HIV-1 and the capacity of this virus to induce immunodeficiency remain unanswered. These include (a) the mechanism(s) underlying the transient depletion of CD4+ cells that occurs immediately following exposure to the virus; (b) the functional reversibility of this initial CD4+ T cell loss; (c) the pathogenic process(es) leading to the gradual destruction or aberrant functioning of the immune system despite the rapid and nearly complete elimination of the virus from the blood after the acute infection; (d) the irreversible loss of CD4 positive T lymphocytes which accompanies clinical progression to disease onset; (e) the contribution, if any, of specific HIV-1 phenotypes (SI versus NSI; T-cell-line tropic versus macrophage tropic) to virus transmission and disease progression; and (f) the biologic role of "auxiliary" viral genes such as *vpr*, *vif*, and *nef* during the establishment of the initial infection and its subsequent spread to other sites in the body.

In the search for an HIV-1 animal model during the very early phase of the AIDS epidemic, cell suspensions from virus-infected individuals were inoculated into a variety of animals including nonhuman primates, but only chimpanzees consistently became infected. It was later shown that chimpanzees could be reliably infected with relatively low doses of HIV-1 (13), but no longstanding impairment to the immune system was observed. Like the acute infection in man, a primary HIV-1 infection of chimpanzees is characterized by a brief period, lasting several weeks, during which virus can be readily recovered. Unlike in humans, however, the primary HIV-1 infection in chimpanzees is usually asymptomatic, and virus is infrequently recovered from the plasma of inoculated animals (209). Antibodies directed against several of the viral proteins can be detected within several weeks of inoculation, and a rapid decline of the virus load, typically measured by the number of PBMCs needed for HIV-1 isolation or containing viral DNA, is commonly observed. In most instances, virus isolation from persistently infected chimpanzees becomes intermittent after resolution of the primary infection (13,234).

The absence of virus-induced immunodeficiency in any of the more than 150 chimpanzees inoculated with HIV-1 led to a variety of hypotheses to explain the failure of the infection to progress to clinical disease. These included (a) the predominant use of clade B T-cell-line tropic virus isolates; (b) the generally poor replicative capacity/cytopathicity of HIV-1 in chimpanzee PBMC; (c) a failure of HIV-1 to induce apoptosis of CD4+ chimpanzee cells; and (d) the ability of the chimpanzee to mount a potent, long-lived protective response to HIV-1, similar to that reported for SIV-infected (and asymptomatic) sooty mangabeys, the natural host of SIV_{smm}. One chimpanzee, however, did develop high virus loads and a CD4+ T-lymphocyte depletion to the 100 cell/μL range nearly 10 years after documented exposure to two different virus strains ($HIV\text{-}1_{SF2}$ and $HIV\text{-}1_{LAV\text{-}1b}$) (464). These laboratory findings were associated with a nonregenerative anemia, chronic intermittent diarrhea, and the presence of opportunistic microorganisms (e.g., *Blastocytis hominis*, *Balantidium coli*, and *Cryptosporidium*). The transfusion of whole blood from this animal to a second chimpanzee resulted in extremely high plasma viral RNA loads ($>1\times10^7$ copies/mL) and a rapid decline of CD4+ T cells. Biologic and molecular analyses of the HIV-1 recovered from the two affected animals revealed (a) an augmented replication phenotype in chimpanzee PBMC/macrophages, and (b) that the pathogenic variant which had emerged was very likely a recombinant between the original $HIV\text{-}1_{SF2}$ and $HIV\text{-}1_{LAV\text{-}1b}$ input viruses (452).

The failure of chimpanzees to develop disease in a timely fashion following inoculation of tissue culture–adapted or patient-derived virus isolates coupled with their endangered species status has greatly dampened enthusiasm for their use as an animal model of HIV-1–induced immunodeficiency.

Transgenic Mice

When it became apparent, in the late 1980s, that HIV-1 infections could be established only in chimpanzees and humans, potentially more tractable and novel rodent systems were developed to model specific steps of *in vivo* HIV-1 infections. In one approach, transgenic mice, containing varying portions (individual viral genes/cis-acting elements up to the entire HIV-1 genome) of molecularly cloned viral DNA were constructed. Because HIV-1 transgenic mice contain copies of proviral DNA in every cell, they represent *in vivo* systems for modeling the postintegration phase of the virus life cycle. They provide a means for assessing possible deleterious effects of HIV-1–encoded proteins *in vivo* and for monitoring the mammalian responses to different viral gene products.

The earliest and simplest DNA constructs introduced into mice consisted of the HIV-1 LTR linked to a reporter gene [most commonly, chloramphenicol acetyltransferase (CAT)]. Animals bearing the viral promoter/enhancer of transcription usually expressed extremely low levels of CAT activity in specific tissues (skin, eye lens, lymph nodes, spleen, and thymus) (365). It was also reported (641) that HIV-1 LTR-directed expression of the viral *tat* gene induced dermal lesions in mice with features of Kaposi's sarcoma, although this result has not been independently confirmed. Animals harboring copies of full-length and potentially infectious HIV-1 DNA were also constructed and initially maintained in a biosafety level 4 (BL4) facility (367). In these transgenic mice, HIV-1 LTR-directed expression was barely detectable in 23 of 25 founder animals. In one of the two instances of high-level HIV-1 gene activity, heterozygous offspring, generated from a mosaic founder female, exhibited a spontaneous and fatal disease syndrome characterized by severe runting/growth retardation; splenomegaly; lymphadenopathy; dry, scaly skin; and perivascular pulmonary lymphoid infiltrates (367). The second transgenic line, also carrying a complete copy of the HIV-1 genome, has been used to assess the effect of opportunistic microorganisms on the expression of the HIV-1 transgene. Interestingly, *Toxoplasma gondii* or *Mycobacterium avium* infections of these transgenic mice resulted in marked elevations of HIV-1 RNA synthesis in multiple lymphoid tissues (142,230). In both cases, splenic macrophages represented a major target of increased HIV-1 expression.

To overcome the intrinsically low levels of HIV-1 LTR-directed expression in rodents, transgenic mice have also been generated that carry viral genes under the control of cell- or tissue-specific promoters. Mice harboring a transgene consisting of the mouse mammary tumor virus LTR-driving HIV-1 structural genes synthesized substantial amounts of HIV-1 Gag and Pol proteins in mammary and salivary glands, but no associated disease was observed (314). In another study, central nervous system disease developed in mice carrying HIV-1 gp120 coding sequences linked to the murine fibrillary acid protein promoter (621).

Several independent transgenic mouse lines have also been constructed to assess the *in vivo* function(s) of the Nef protein. These included animals in which *nef* expression was directed to T cells by using promoter/enhancers for the δ subunit of the mouse CD3 gene (586), the human CD2 gene (54), and the mouse TCR β gene (375). Altered T-cell activation, CD4+ T-cell down-regulation, and immunologic dysfunction, respectively, were observed in these three lines of transgenic animals. More recently, transgenic mice bearing a complete copy of HIV-1 coding sequences, directed by a chimeric (human–mouse) CD4 promoter/enhancer, were constructed. These animals spontaneously developed muscle wasting, weight loss, severe depletion of lymphocytes from lymphoid organs, diarrhea, and death within 2 to 4 weeks of birth. When individual or combinations of HIV-1 genes within the full-length viral transgene were inactivated, only those animals expressing a functional *nef* gene exhibited the same debilitating clinical syndrome (266). Thus, targeting HIV-1 Nef synthesis to mouse CD4+ cells, in the absence of a spreading viral infection or the expression of other HIV-1 gene products, was sufficient to elicit a disease with some of the characteristics of human AIDS.

Severe Combined Immunodeficient Mice

In addition to their use for investigations of human immune responses, severe combined immunodeficient (SCID) mice, engrafted with human cells, have been used as a small animal model for HIV-1. In one protocol, 10^7 to 10^8 human PBMC are implanted intraperitoneally to create SCID-hu-PBMC animals (445). Human CD8+ T cells in these animals tend to remain in the peritoneal cavity, whereas the CD4+ T lymphocytes migrate to lymphoid tissue; both human T-cell subsets may persist for up to 6 months. The HIV-1-susceptible CD4+ T cells in SCID-hu-PBMC animals represent a population of mature, activated memory cells, functionally similar to those present in adult humans. In a modification of the SCID-hu-PBMC model, PBMC from HIV-1-infected individuals have been implanted into mice and the induction of virus from the transferred cells monitored.

In the second SCID mouse system used for HIV-1 studies (SCID-hu-thy/liv), fragments of human fetal thymus and fetal liver are engrafted under the renal capsule (457). The implanted organs increase in size for several months with CD4+/CD8+ double-positive T-lymphocytes predominating in the differentiating engrafted thymus. The SCID-hu-thy/liv system therefore models the fetal/neonatal human thymus and is relevant for studies of maternal–fetal virus transmission and pediatric HIV-1 infections.

In both SCID-hu systems, HIV-1 infections peak 3 to 4 weeks after inoculation and lead to variable (partial to complete) depletion of CD4+ T cells, depending primarily on the replication phenotype of the virus used (7,446). Any T-cell replacement that occurs is caused by proliferation of the implanted human cells. In general, both macrophage and T-cell tropic HIV-1 strains or primary viral isolates exhibiting rapid infection kinetics are more pathogenic in both SCID-hu mouse systems than more slowly replicating virus strains (311). Although the engrafted human tissue possesses demonstrable functional immunologic activity (299,426), the inoculation of HIV-1 fails to elicit a primary immune response in infected animals. Thus both of the SCID-hu systems model uncontrolled HIV-1 infections characterized by moderate to profound CD4+ T-cell depletions and no humoral or cellular responses to the virus. In some experiments, virus-specific antibodies and cytotoxic T lymphocytes have been adoptively transferred to SCID-hu-PBMC mice prior to virus challenge (489,632).

SIV–HIV Chimeric Viruses

A nonhuman primate lentivirus, initially isolated from a captive rhesus monkey in the mid 1980s, was shown to induce an AIDS-like disease following inoculation of Asian macaques (123,368). As noted earlier, these SIVs establish asymptomatic chronic infections in their natural hosts, different species of African monkeys. The SIV genomic organization, while similar to that of HIV-1, can be distinguished by the presence of the *vpx* and the absence of the *vpu* genes (Fig. 7). When it became apparent that humans and chimpanzees were the only mammalian species that

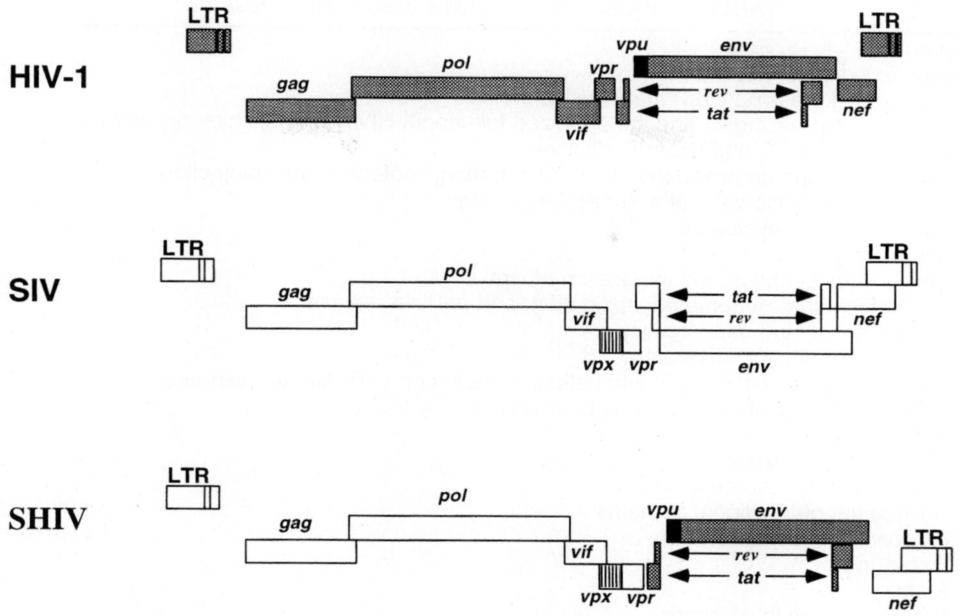

FIG. 7. Genomic organization of HIV-1, SIV, and SHIV lentiviruses. The *vpu* gene of HIV-1 and the *vpx* gene of SIV are highlighted. Some SHIV constructs contain an HIV-1–SIV chimeric *vpr* gene.

could be reliably infected by HIV-1, attention turned to the SIV–Asian macaque model with the idea of constructing chimeric SIV–HIV viruses (SHIVs) capable of infecting small, nonendangered, nonhuman primates. The earliest versions of SHIVs contained 3 to 4 kilobases (kb) of HIV-1 sequences, including the *tat*, *rev*, *vpu*, *env*, and, in some instances, portions of *vpr* and *nef* genes, which were inserted into the genetic backbone of SIV_{mac239} (see Fig. 7). The first generation of SHIVs successfully established chronic infections and elicited immunologic responses in inoculated macaques, but the virus did not replicate to high levels or cause clinical disease (372,573). Nonetheless, subsequent serial animal-to-animal transfers of blood, lymphoid cells, and/or bone marrow resulted in the emergence of pathogenic SHIV strains containing alterations affecting gp120-coding sequences (313,521). In contrast to SIV_{mac239} and HIV-1, which, on average, will induce immunodeficiency in 1 and 10 years following infection of macaque monkeys or man, respectively, some of the highly pathogenic SHIVs cause an unremitting and irreversible depletion of CD4+ T cells within 3 to 4 weeks of inoculation and death due to AIDS in 3 to 4 months. Because they possess and express the HIV-1 *env* gene, these new versions of SHIVs provide a disease endpoint for monitoring the effectiveness of HIV-1 envelope-based vaccine strategies.

THE MOLECULAR BIOLOGY OF HIV-1 REPLICATION

Overview

More than 10,000 papers have been published on HIV-1 since its discovery as the cause of AIDS in 1984. A dizzying array of biochemical, genetic, and immunologic techniques, and biologic systems have been used to study the structure and function of HIV-1-encoded proteins and the host cell mechanisms that regulate virus replication. In addition to the production of HIV-1 proteins in bacterial, yeast, and insect cells, much of this effort has involved transfections of mammalian cells with vectors expressing individual viral proteins or cloned HIV-1 proviral DNA (Table 2). Transfection experiments have been important for elucidating (a) the intracellular location and trafficking of viral proteins, (b) the interaction of HIV-1 proteins with other viral or cellular proteins, (c) the binding of viral and cellular proteins to cis-acting elements associated with the viral genome or proviral DNA, (d) the fusion/entry steps of the virus life cycle, and (e) the assembly and release of progeny virions. In a majority of instances, the cells used for these transfection studies have been both CD4 negative and of nonhematopoietic origin, and they include HeLa, COS, and 293T.

Transfection experiments are to be distinguished from HIV-1 infections, which are characterized by particle-mediated cell entry, in conjunction with the use of one or more surface receptors, and the spread of progeny virions through the culture, in successive cycles of replication. Thus, infections provide an opportunity to integrate the function(s) of an individual viral-encoded protein (or even a subdomain thereof) into the entire HIV-1 replicative cycle. For many studies, single-cycle infections, involving defective HIV-1 genomes, pseudotyped with a heterologous envelope protein, have been used to obtain answers to specific questions, even though the newly produced virus particles are incapable of sustaining a virus

TABLE 2. *Experimental systems used in HIV-1 research*

Transfections

- *Reagents/techniques*
  1. Plasmids expressing individual HIV-1 proteins
  2. Plasmids expressing wt and mutagenized full-length HIV-1 DNAs; chimeric viral DNAs
  3. HeLa, COS, 293T, and $CD4^+$ T-cell lines
  4. Calcium phosphate precipitation, electroporation, lipofection, microinjection
  5. Antibodies specific for viral and cellular proteins
- *Functions/processes evaluated*
  1. Virus entry
  2. Reverse transcription and integration of viral DNA
  3. Virion assembly, genome encapsidation, and particle release
  4. Regulation of viral gene activity
     - *Cis*-acting RNA and DNA elements
     - Effect of wt and mutant viral and cellular proteins on LTR-directed expression
  5. Post transcriptional modifications of viral RNA
     - Splicing
     - Nuclear import/export
  6. Viral protein characterization
     - Delineation of functional domains
     - Intracellular localization
     - Trafficking
     - Stability
  7. Protein–protein interactions
     - Viral–viral
     - Viral–cellular
  8. Effect on/of cellular functions
     - Expression of surface receptors/molecules
     - Activation status/signal transduction
     - Cytopathicity
  9. Production of wt and mutagenized virus stocks

Infections

- *Reagents*
  1. Viruses
     - Wt and mutagenized HIV
     - Chimeric viruses
     - Pseudotyped virions
  2. Cells
     - Primary (PBMC/MDM)
     - Continuous human T cell lines (CEM, SupT1, Jurkat, H9)
     - Continuous human monocytoid cell lines (U937)
     - $CD4^+$ cell lines containing an HIV-1 inducible reporter gene
     - Cell lines expressing CD4 and chemokine coreceptors (GHOST, HOS)
  3. Human serum
- *Functions/processes evaluated*
  1. The contribution of individual HIV genes during spreading virus infections in tissue cultures or in inoculated animals
  2. Events occurring during a discrete phase of productive HIV-1 infections or a single replication cycle
  3. Virus isolation/determination of biologic phenotype
  4. Production of virus stocks
  5. Neutralization of virus infections

In vitro systems

- *Reagents*
  1. Nuclear extracts; purified transcription factors, DNA templates, antibodies
  2. Purified viral (wt and mutagenized) proteins and RNAs
- *Functions/processes evaluated*
  1. Regulation, synthesis, and processing of viral RNA
  2. Virion assembly
  3. Structural analyses
     - X-ray diffraction/NMR analyses of viral and relevant cellular proteins
     - *Cis*-acting RNA elements

HIV, human immunodeficiency virus; wt, wild-type; PBMC, peripheral blood mononuclear cells; MDM, monocyte-derived macrophage; NMR, nuclear magnetic resonance; LTR, long terminal repeat.

infection. It is worth keeping in mind that although transfection experiments and *in vitro* studies such as the yeast two-hybrid system have yielded invaluable information about the function and interacting cellular partners of HIV-1-encoded proteins, the results obtained must always be verified in assays that monitor spreading viral infections.

The HIV-1 replicative cycle (Fig. 8) begins with adsorption of virus particles to CD4 molecules on the surface of susceptible cells. While binding of virions to CD4 is essential for HIV infectivity, their subsequent interaction with a coreceptor, one of which are now known to be the seven membrane-spanning CC or CXC families of chemokine receptors, is required for membrane fusion and entry (92,134,145,177). Although multiple chemokine receptors exhibit activity in fusion/entry assays with HIV-1 gp120 (see the Env section below), the two most important are CXCR4 (previously called fusin, or LESTR) and CCR5. Unlike other enveloped viruses, which utilize receptor-mediated endocytosis to enter

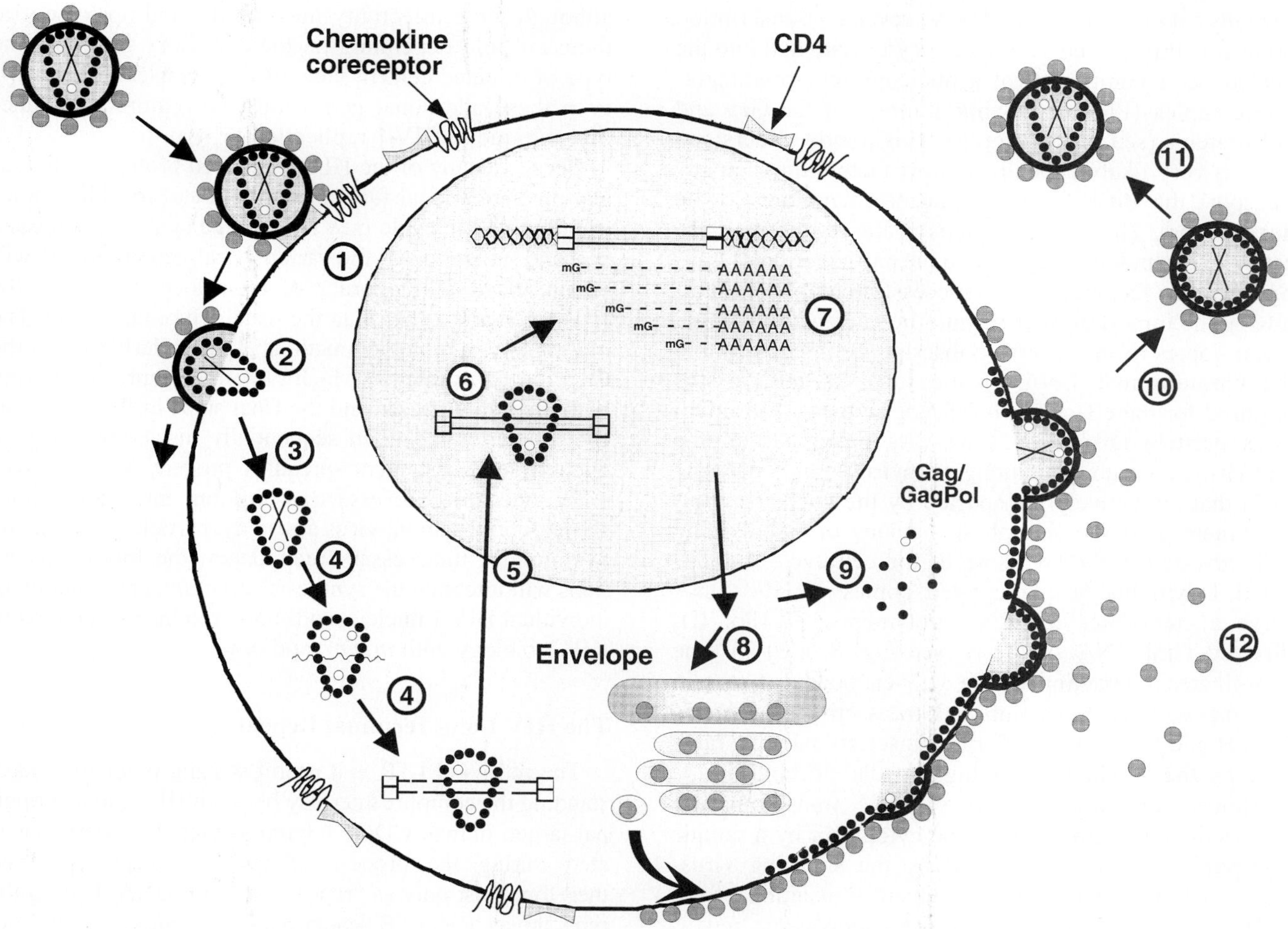

FIG. 8. The HIV-1 replication cycle. Productive HIV-1 infections begin with the adsorption of cell-free virions to cells and their interactions with both the CD4 and chemokine receptors (*step 1*). In the case of HIV, virus entry (*step 2*) is a pH-independent process that occurs following the fusion of viral and cellular membranes and results in the partial uncoating (*step 3*) of incoming virions. Reverse transcription occurs within subviral particles in the cytoplasm of infected cells (*step 4*), and the double-stranded DNA product is transported to the nucleus (*step 5*), where integration into chromosomal DNA (*step 6*) is mediated by the virus-encoded integrase (*open circles*), a component of a subviral preintegration complex. The integrated viral DNA serves as a template for DNA-dependent RNA polymerase (*Pol II*) and leads to the production of mRNAs (*step 7*) that are translated into viral proteins in the cytoplasm of infected cells. Envelope (*step 8*) and Gag plus Gag/Pol (*step 9*) polyproteins are transported via independent pathways to the plasma membrane, where progeny virus particles begin "budding" from cells and are released as immature particles (*step 10*). Subsequent proteolysis by the virion-encoded protease generates mature particles (*step 11*) containing a characteristic condensed core. Non-virion-associated gp 120 envelope protein is also released from cells (*step 12*).

cells, HIV-1 and most other retroviruses directly fuse with the plasma membrane of a susceptible cell. Following entry, subviral particles are partially uncoated in the cytoplasm and initiate the reverse transcription of their viral RNA genomes (see Fig. 8, steps 2 to 4). Investigations of these early events in the virus life cycle have been greatly hampered by the very high (>100:1) retrovirus particle-to-infectivity ratios noted earlier. Thus, simply monitoring the fate of tagged viral proteins during the entry and uncoating steps is unlikely to provide useful information about the composition and trafficking of biologically active virions.

As is the case for other retroelements (51,58,206), the partially double-stranded DNA reverse transcription product is transported through the cytoplasm and into the nucleus as a component of a nucleoprotein–preintegration complex (PIC) containing a subset of the Gag and Pol proteins (see Fig. 8, step 5). This poorly understood process very likely depends on host factors that actively transport the PICs from the plasma membrane to the nuclear pore. These "early" steps in the retrovirus replication cycle undoubtedly require the participation of multiple cellular factors for their successful completion. Following the import of the PIC into the nucleus, full length linear copies of the reverse transcript are integrated into the chromosomal DNA of the infected cell, a step required for the efficient viral RNA synthesis and infectious particle production (568). As noted earlier, the lentiviruses are unique among retroviruses in generating PICs that are actively transported by the nuclear import machinery into the interphase nucleus of nondividing cells arrested in the G_1 phase of the cell cycle. In activated T lymphocytes, integrated copies of HIV DNA serve as templates for RNA polymerase II (Pol II)-directed viral RNA synthesis (see Fig. 8, step 7). The coordinated interaction of the HIV-encoded Tat protein and the cellular transcriptional transactivator proteins NF-κB and Sp1 with the Pol II transcriptional apparatus ensures the production of high levels of viral RNA. Unspliced or partially spliced HIV transcripts are exported from the nucleus to the cytoplasm by a unique transport mechanism mediated by the shuttling virus-encoded Rev protein. The subsequent translation of the gp160 Env precursor occurs in the endoplasmic reticulum, whereas the Gag and Gag-Pol polyproteins are synthesized on free cytoplasmic ribosomes, and they are transported via independent pathways to the plasma membrane (see Fig. 8, steps 8 and 9). The Gag and Gag-Pol polyproteins, in association with dimers of genomic RNA, condense at the plasma membrane to form an electron-dense "bud" (see Fig. 1) that gives rise to a spherical immature particle containing the mature TM and SU envelope glycoproteins. Proteolytic processing of the Gag and Pol proteins by the HIV PR during or immediately after particle release generates the cone-shaped nucleoid characteristic of mature HIV virions (see Fig. 8, steps 10 and 11).

Thus HIV-1 uses the same replicative strategy as the so-called simple retroviruses, which encode only the Gag, Pol, and Env proteins. However, during its evolution, HIV-1 acquired six additional genes to carry out functions that are performed by cellular proteins that are either (a) already present in the cells infected by the simple retroviruses or (b) uniquely required for virus replication, transmission, and survival in hematopoietic cells targeted by the primate lentiviruses. Some of the HIV-1 accessory proteins (Vif, Vpr, Vpu, and Nef) are not required for replication in certain human T-cell lines, although virus infectivity may be affected up to several thousand-fold depending on the accessory gene and the type of infected cell. In view of their conservation, however, these additional genes must be required for functions unique to HIV-1 replication *in vivo*.

Because many of the HIV-1-encoded proteins individually mediate critical functions at both early and late times in the virus life cycle (see Fig. 8), the synthesis, processing, and utilization of the various viral gene products will be presented in the order of their location within the HIV-1 genome rather than the usual temporal format. The multiplicity of biologic functions is particularly true for the Gag and Env proteins, which play important roles during both the initial phases and the final steps of the infectious cycle. Thus, rather than sequentially discussing the production and subsequent spread of progeny virions (virus entry, uncoating, reverse transcription, integration, transcription, translation, virus assembly, particle release), and to minimize unnecessary redundancy, the following sections will integrate the synthesis, structure, and function of individual HIV-1 nucleic acids and proteins in a context of HIV-1 biology both *in vitro* and *in vivo*.

The HIV Long Terminal Repeat

The retroviral LTR is a useful starting point for understanding the complex interplay between HIV and its principal target, human CD4+ T lymphocytes. LTRs are generated during the process of reverse transcription and therefore exist only as "repeats" in viral DNA. During the replicative cycle, LTR sequences serve a multitude of functions in the context of both proviral DNA and genomic RNA (Fig. 9). DNA and RNA sequences, mapping to the R region of the LTR, participate in one of the early steps of reverse transcription by forming intermolecular DNA–RNA hybrid "bridges" linking the newly synthesized DNA strand ("minus" polarity) with the 3′ end of the same or a different genomic RNA template ("plus" polarity). During the integration step of the virus life cycle, LTR elements (*att* sequences) located at the termini of full-length linear viral DNA molecules mediate their insertion into the chromosomal DNA of host cells (109). Other LTR

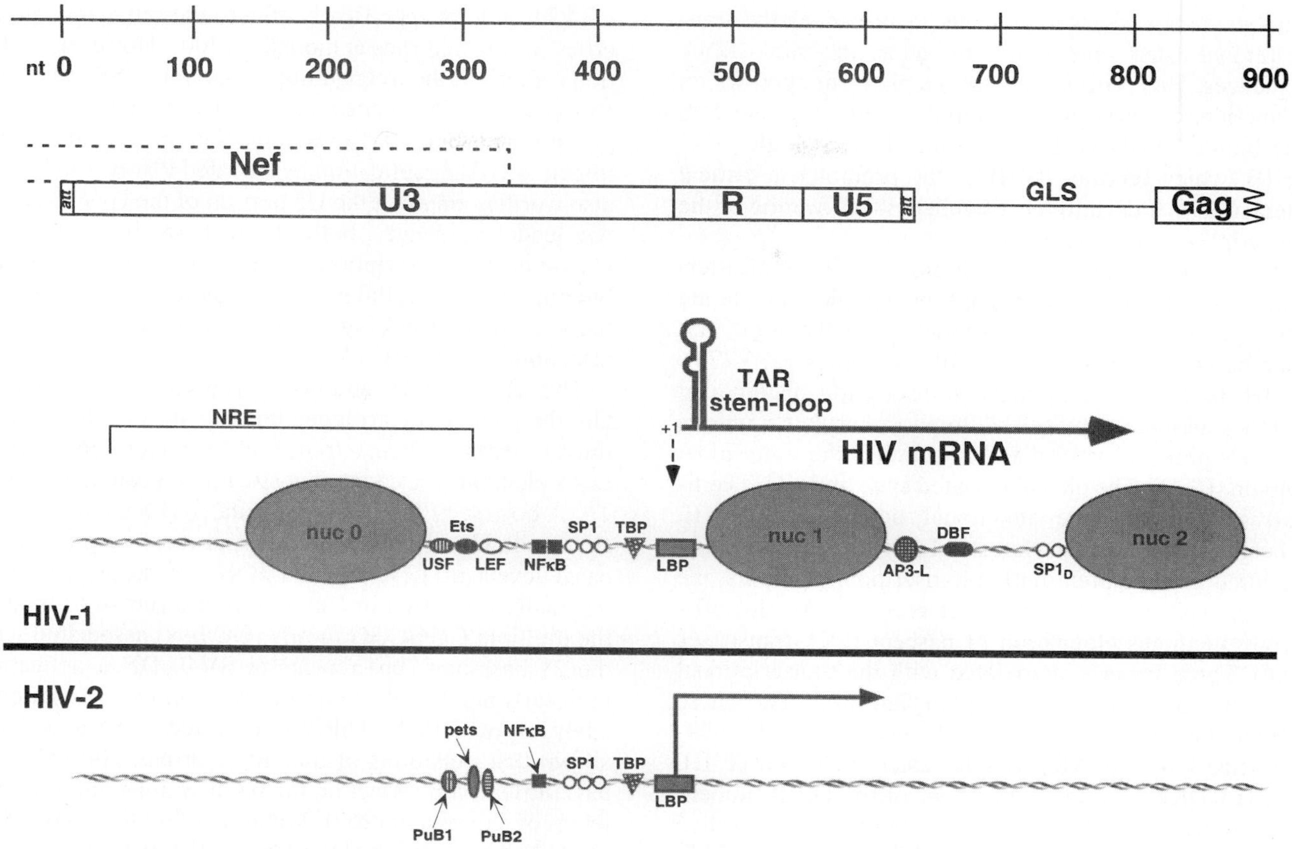

FIG. 9. Structure of the HIV-1 long terminal repeat (LTR). The HIV-1 LTR is a duplicated 630+ bp element located at the termini of integrated proviral DNA and has been divided into three functional subregions. The R (repeat) domain is defined as a 96-bp-nt repeat present at the 3′ and 5′ termini of HIV-1 genomic RNA and all viral mRNAs; U5 is an 84-nt segment located immediately 3′ to the R region; and U3 is a 454-nt segment situated immediately 5′ to R. The region of *nef* gene overlapping U3 and the position of LTR terminal *att* sequences (in the context of full-length viral DNA) are shown at the *top.* The 5′ LTR and adjacent *gag* leader sequence (GLS) are aligned with the subdivided LTR (*middle*) to indicate functionally important binding sites for transcriptional regulatory proteins. For HIV-1, the "enhancer" domain contains three Sp1 binding elements and two NF-κB binding motifs. The transcription start site is located at map position +1, which is defined as the border between U3 and R. The NRE contains binding sites for USF and the Ets proteins. Sequence motifs that interact with the TATA binding protein (TBP), the leader binding protein (LBP), the LEF, AP3-like (AP3-L), the DBF-1, and two downstream Sp1 elements ($SP1_D$) are shown. The position of nucleosomes nuc0, nuc1, and nuc2 are indicated. An HIV-1 RNA transcript, which is initiated at the first nucleotide within the R region (designated +1) and contains the TAR element near its 5′ terminus, is also shown. For HIV-2 (*bottom*), the unique binding sites for the PuB1, pets, and PuB2 transcriptional factors are indicated.

sequences, located in the context of U5 RNA sequences, have been shown to contribute to the packaging of progeny HIV-1 RNA genomes during virus assembly (637).

In the context of integrated viral DNA, the major function of the retroviral LTR is the regulation of viral RNA synthesis. The HIV-1 transcriptional promoter and adjacent regulatory elements, both of which are involved in recruiting the RNA Pol II holoenzyme to the start site of viral RNA synthesis, are located within the U3 region and function in the context of the 5′ LTR (see Fig. 9). In primate lentiviruses, the *nef* ORF overlaps 60% to 70% of the U3 region, directly contributing to the relatively large size (400 to 500 nt) of the HIV-1 U3 compared to other retroviruses. Nef coding sequences of HIV-1, in fact, extend into the 5′ 331 of the 454-nt U3 region (see Fig. 9). The polyadenylation signal (AATAAA) and polyadenylation addition site are also located in the R region but, as noted previously, are active only as components of the 3′ LTR.

Like other eukaryotic cellular promoters, the integrated HIV LTR contains several elements that facilitate the loading of Pol II on the DNA template. The initial recognition of the HIV promoter requires the participation of several general transcription factors (GTFs), including TFIID, which specifically binds to the TATA element, located –29 to –24 nts upstream of the transcriptional start site, and to adjacent viral DNA sequences. This process generates a platform upon which a functional transcriptional complex can be assembled. The bound TFIID is then recognized by a single GTF, TFIIB, which recruits Pol II to the promoter, a critical interaction that definitively establishes the location of the transcription start site (373).

Another GTF (TFIIH), which modifies Pol II allosterically and allows the transcription complex to initiate RNA polymerization and "escape" from the promoter, must be incorporated into the Pol II complex (385,470). TFIIH is a multicomponent transcription factor that includes a kinase activity able to phosphorylate a unique region within the largest Pol II subunit, the C-terminal domain (CTD). The phosphorylated state of the CTD critically determines the functional activity of Pol II. Whereas hypophosphorylated Pol II (Pol IIa) is readily recruited into the preinitiation transcription complex, the hyperphosphorylated form of the enzyme (Pol IIo) efficiently mediates elongation of nascent RNA transcripts (466). Three kinases, associated with the transcriptional apparatus, are known to phosphorylate the CTD. These include (a) the CDK7/cyclin H subunits of the cdk-activating kinase (CAK) complex associated with TFIIH, (b) the CDK8/cyclin C component of the Pol II holoenzyme, and (c) the CDK9/cyclin T subunits of the positive transcription elongation factor b (P-TEFb). Hyperphosphorylation of the CTD induces conformational changes in Pol II that allow the transcription complex to clear the promoter and begin elongating nascent RNA molecules.

In eukaryotic cells, regulatory transcriptional factors, which bind to DNA elements near the promoter, modulate the basal rate of RNA synthesis in response to physiologic cues. These regulatory factors function in a combinatorial fashion via protein–protein interactions to recruit GTFs, as well as the Pol II enzyme itself, to the promoter. This results in the more frequent assembly of stable transcription complexes that are able to readily escape the promoter and generate full-length primary transcripts. As is the case for other eukaryotic cellular promoter/enhancers, the HIV LTR contains its own ensemble of DNA elements to which transcriptional regulatory factors bind (see Fig. 9). Some of these were identified by mutagenesis of LTR-driven reporter gene constructs in transfection experiments, some were found as a result of gel-retardation or DNA footprinting studies, and others were discovered from searches of nucleotide sequence databases. Although early studies of HIV LTR-directed expression of reporter genes suggested that a large domain (–410 to –157) within U3, designated the negative regulatory element (NRE), might "silence" viral gene activity (534), there is little convincing evidence that the NRE plays a significant role during virus replication. Furthermore, mutations located in the region of the SIV *nef* gene that overlaps the NRE segment of the U3 LTR did not specifically affect viral replicative properties in infected rhesus monkeys (300). However, mutations altering the recognition sites for USF, Ets, and LEF-1 (572,575), which are located in the promoter-proximal portion of the *nef* overlap of U3, markedly impaired HIV-1 replication in activated PBMC (332). It is also worth noting that the U5 portion of the HIV LTR and *gag* leader sequences, both of which are situated *downstream* of the transcription start site, also contain cognate binding sites for cellular factors (see Fig. 9) that potentially regulate RNA synthesis during productive viral infections (see later).

The LTRs of HIV and other primate lentiviruses contain three tandemly arranged binding sites for the constitutively expressed Sp1 transcription factor (267); these DNA elements are situated upstream of a canonical Pol II TATA box (see Fig. 9). The Sp1 and TATA elements constitute the HIV-1 core promoter and must be present for basal levels of LTR-directed RNA synthesis. Sp1 was originally identified in HeLa cells and shown to bind to the multiple GGGCGG motifs (GC box) associated with the 21 base-pair (bp) repeats in SV40 DNA, activating both early and late SV40 transcription *in vitro*. Functional analyses of HIV-LTR-driven reporter constructs have shown that mutations of individual or pairs of Sp1 sites have little, if any, effect on the basal or Tat-transactivated levels of expression (267). Mutation of all three HIV Sp1 sites, however, markedly reduced the response to the HIV-1-encoded Tat transactivating protein (32,267). In the context of virus infections, the role of the Sp1 elements is cell type dependent (366,536). Mutations that functionally inactivate all three Sp1 motifs eliminated detectable replication in Jurkat cells, delayed progeny virus production in CEM and H9 cells, and had little effect on infectivity in activated PBMC.

Adjacent to the Sp1 binding sites, the two tandem recognition sites for the NF-κB/Rel family of transcription factors constitute an activatable enhancer for HIV-1 LTR-directed expression (see Fig. 9) (455). Although the LTRs of HIV-2 and SIV retain the triplicated Sp1 motifs, they contain only a single NF-κB binding site. NF-κB is a member of a large family of cellular transcription factors, which include the c-Rel protein of chickens and the dorsal gene product of *Drosophila*, a regulator of pattern development in embryos. Selected members of this NF-κB/Rel gene family are shown diagrammatically in Figure 10. Several contain a highly conserved N-terminal Rel homology domain (RHD), approximately 300 residues in size, that includes DNA binding and dimerization regions and a nuclear localization signal (NLS). A conserved protein kinase A site is present in several but not all RHDs. The p65/Rel A protein contains a potent transcription activation domain located downstream from its RHD. The p50 protein is derived from the p105 precursor, which contains a glycine-rich hinge linked to an ankyrin repeat domain; the p65/Rel A protein, in contrast,

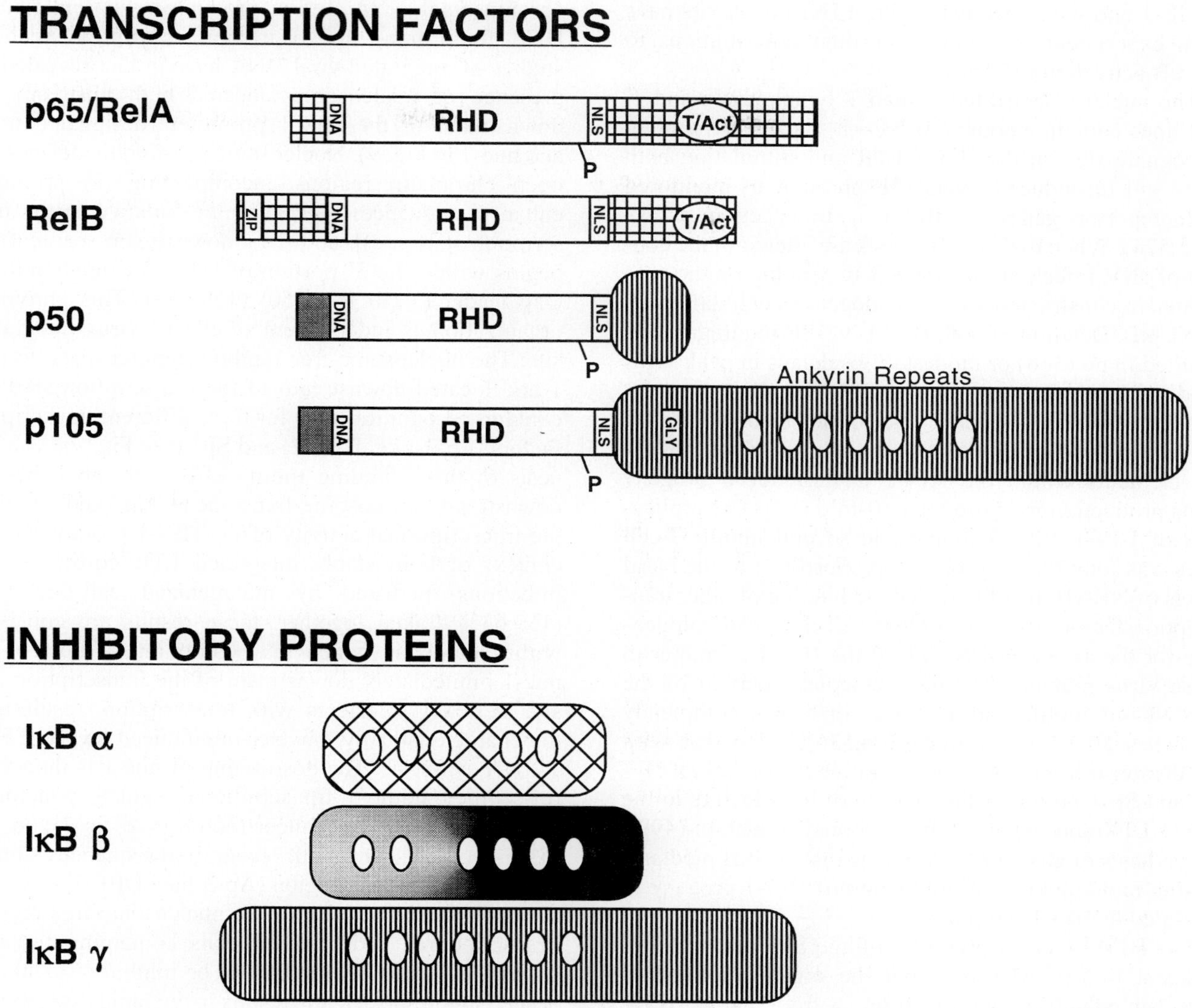

FIG. 10. NF-κB transcriptional regulatory proteins and IkB inhibitors. The NF-κB/Rel family of transcriptional factors shown may contain a Rel homology domain (*RHD*), DNA binding motifs (*DNA*), a leucine zipper (*ZIP*), a nuclear localization signal (*NLS*), a glycine hinge (*GLY*), a transactivation domain (*T/Act*), and a protein kinase A phosphorylation site (*P*). The ankyrin repeats are indicated by the *white ovals.*

is a primary translation product. The inhibitory IκB proteins all contain multiple 30- to 34-amino-acid ankyrin motifs, which provide the interface for binding to various species of NF-κB.

NF-κB "binding activity" was originally identified as the p50-p65/Rel A heterodimer, the most abundant and functionally active form of NF-κB in human T cells (17). Because the various members of the c-Rel family are able to form dimeric NF-κB molecules, a heterogeneous population of homo- and heterodimers with different functional specificities could potentially bind to the two NF-κB sites present in the HIV-1 LTR. NF-κB functional activity is controlled by its intracellular location. In the cytoplasm, NF-κB dimers are complexed to IκB proteins or other Rel family members containing ankyrin repeats, such as the unprocessed p105 protein (see Fig. 10), and cannot be imported into the nucleus (326). The binding of IκBα to the RHD of the p65 subunit of heterodimeric NF-κB results in its sequestration in the cytoplasm due, perhaps, to a masking of the p65 NLS (26). Nearly all of the T lymphocytes encountered by HIV-1 *in vivo* will be quiescent and lack NF-κB binding activity. Activation of mammalian T cells results in the phosphorylation of the bound IκB, the rapid degradation of IκB via the ubiquitin pathway, and the translocation of NF-κB into the nucleus where it can activate multiple eukaryotic genes (326,485). Convergent signal transducing pathways associated with T-cell activation, including those initiated at the IL-1 and tissue necrosis factor (TNF) receptors have been experimentally studied for their contributions to NF-κB activation (75,540).

The nuclei of activated human T lymphocytes and T-cell lines contain amounts of NF-κB capable of binding to cognate sites in the HIV-1 LTR and stimulating both basal and Tat-induced levels of expression, as monitored with reporter genes in transient transfection assays (455,574). When the NF-κB motifs are altered in the context of HIV, infectivity is affected, depending on the type of mutant constructed and the endogenous cellular levels of NF-κB. Deletion of both HIV-1 NF-κB binding motifs resulted in no (366) or modest (536) delays in peak virus production in activated human PBMC, whereas point mutations affecting specific nucleotides involved in NF-κB recognition but not the spatial organization of the NF-κB elements within the HIV-1 LTR, reduced progeny virus production by more than 10-fold (83). The replication of HIV-1 NF-κB mutants in several human T-cell lines was found to be inversely proportional to the basal levels of NF-κB. It is likely that the binding of other transcription factors present in these cell lines can compensate for the absence of NF-κB at the HIV-1 promoter in these virus mutants. The simultaneous mutation of the two NF-κB motifs and all three Sp-1 sites completely abolishes HIV-1 replication (366,536), consistent with the demonstration that the cooperative interaction of NF-κB and Sp-1 promotes the binding of both factors to the HIV-1 LTR and induces transcriptional activation (499). A synthesis of all of these results is that NF-κB mediates a more rapid and robust production of HIV-1 progeny in activated human T lymphocytes.

The HIV-2 LTR also contains three Sp1 binding sites adjacent to its TATA box, but the organization of its upstream enhancer region is different from that of HIV-1 (see Fig. 9). This portion of the HIV-2 U3 LTR contains only a single functional NF-κB motif as well as three other binding sites (PuB1, PuB2, and pets) not present in the HIV-1 LTR (415). The purine-rich PuB1 and PuB2 sequences are recognized by members of the Ets family of proto-oncogenes (mainly Elf-1) and the human autoantigen DEK binds to the pets site (203,361). Thus, while activation of HIV-1 LTR-directed expression following T-cell activation is mediated primarily through the binding of NF-κB to its two cognate sites, induction of HIV-2 gene expression depends on a different set of cellular transactivators.

Most of what is currently known about regulated HIV gene expression comes from experiments in which naked DNA was transiently transfected into mammalian cells. In eukaryotic cells, however, the interactions of transcriptional regulatory proteins with their cognate cis-acting elements is further modulated by the packaging of DNA into chromatin. This is clearly the case for HIV-1 proviral DNA, which becomes stably integrated into host cell chromosomal DNA during productive viral infections. DNA footprinting and restriction enzyme accessibility studies of integrated viral DNA have in fact revealed the presence of nucleosomes located both upstream and downstream of the HIV-1 promoter (designated nuc-0 and nuc-1 in Fig. 9). Nucleosome positioning defines two open chromatin regions encompassing (a) promoter/enhancer sequences [–250 to +11 (relative to the transcription start site)], and (b) a downstream segment that begins within the 3′ portion of U5 and extends into the Gag leader (+150 to +250) (159,635). This chromatin organization is independent of the provirus integration site. The nucleosome-free region promoter-distal to nuc-1 and located downstream of the transcription start site contains recognition sites for three different transcription factors: Ap-3-like, DBF-1, and Sp1 (see Fig. 9). Mutagenesis of these binding motifs effectively abolishes the downstream nucleosome-free zone and markedly inhibits the transcriptional activity of the HIV-1 promoter in the context of both stably integrated LTR constructs and infections mediated by mutagenized cell-free virus (159,633). Taken together, these results are consistent with a model in which the positioning of nucleosome nuc-1 immediately downstream of the transcription start site sterically interferes with transcription, resulting in the characteristically low basal/uninduced levels of HIV-1 RNA synthesis. The positioning of nuc-1 is thought to reflect the binding of transcriptional regulatory factors to upstream promoter/enhancer motifs (viz. Sp 1 and NF-κB sites) and downstream recognition sequences situated in the U5/Gag leader region (Ap-3-like, DBF-1, and Sp1), a combination that creates two nucleosome-free regions. Transcriptional activation of cells containing the integrated HIV-1 LTR with TNF-α or inhibitors of histone deacetylation specifically results in the rapid disruption of nucleosome nuc-1 and generates a 500-bp open chromatin region (635,636). It is not presently known whether the chromatin associated with the HIV-1 template must be remodeled prior to the initiation of transcription or is an inevitable consequence of the RNA synthetic process.

Proteins encoded by several heterologous animal viruses have been reported to transactivate the HIV LTR. Although this effect has been touted by some as indicating that these agents contribute to disease progression, the co-infection of individual human T cells by HIV-1 and other viruses has been difficult to document. On the basis of tropism for CD4+ human mononuclear cells, viruses capable of directly or indirectly transactivating the HIV LTR would include HTLV-I, human CMV (HCMV), human herpes virus type 6 (HHV6), and possibly human adenoviruses (460). In the case of HTLV-I, it has been proposed that elevated levels of NF-κB induced by the viral-encoded Tax protein (18) activate HIV replication by binding to the two NF-κB motifs in its LTR.

HIV-Encoded Regulatory Proteins

Tat

Although the mechanism underlying Tat transactivation of HIV LTR-directed expression was hotly debated for several years, it is now generally agreed that Tat increases the steady-state levels of viral RNA several hundred fold by directing the formation of a more processive Pol II transcription complex in virus-infected cells. Tat is an indispensable viral protein; when the *tat* gene of an infectious molecular proviral clone of HIV is mutagenized, no detectable progeny virions are produced as monitored in either transfection or infectivity assays (128,182). HIV-1 Tat is a nuclear protein containing 101 amino acid residues encoded by two exons (Fig. 11). A shorter 72-amino-acid, "one-exon" HIV-1 Tat protein possesses all the transcriptional activating properties of full-length Tat, as measured in tissue culture infections or in LTR-driven reporter gene experiments. The termination codon following the first Tat exon is highly conserved among diverse HIV-1 isolates, suggesting that the "one-exon" and "two-exon" Tat proteins mediate different functions during productive viral infections *in vivo*.

As previously noted, RNA synthesis in eukaryotic cells is usually modulated by transcription activator proteins, which bind to DNA motifs located *upstream* of their respective promoters and recruit GTFs and the Pol II holoenzyme to the transcription initiation complex. Visna virus, another member of the *Lentivirus* genus, in fact encodes a DNA-binding Tat protein, which binds to Ap-1 sites located in its LTR (283). In contrast, the immediate target of all primate lentiviral Tat transactivating proteins are sequences situated *downstream* of the start site for viral RNA synthesis (534). This unusually situated transactivation response region, or TAR element, also differs from typical binding sites for Pol II transactivators because it is inactive when present (a) in an inverted orientation, (b) 5′ to the promoter, or (c) downstream of the transcription termination site (i.e., in the U5 region of the 3′ LTR) (309). These unusual properties were subsequently reconciled when it was demonstrated that TAR did not function as a DNA recognition site but as an RNA element (33).

The HIV-1 TAR encompasses the 5′-terminal 59 nts of *all* viral RNAs and folds into a stable stem-loop structure (see Fig. 11, middle). It was subsequently shown that the minimal TAR element (mapping between bases +19 and +43) contains three critical components: a base-paired stem, a trinucleotide bulge (containing the sequence UCU at positions +23 to +25), and a hexanucleotide G-rich loop (176). Interestingly, the HIV-2 TAR forms a double stem-loop structure, each arm of which possesses a dinucleotide bulge and the hexanucleotide G-rich loop (see Fig. 11) (160). Sequences located in both the hexanucleotide loop and the bulge of the HIV-1 TAR are required for Tat function. *In vitro*, purified preparations of Tat bind to TAR RNA with high affinity and moderate specificity (140). HIV-1 Tat binds to both wild-type or "loop" mutants of TAR but *not* to TAR elements containing alterations affecting the bulge region (139,542). Modification of the invariant "bulge" U_{+23} nucleotide and elimination of the base pairs immediately above and below the bulge (see Fig. 11) significantly reduce the binding of Tat to TAR (650). Nuclear magnetic resonance (NMR) studies have shown that the binding of a large Tat peptide to TAR causes the major groove in the RNA duplex to widen, thereby generating multiple points of contact between Arg residues in the Tat-binding domain with critical nucleotides (e.g., U_{+23}) and several phosphate groups comprising the TAR backbone (1). This distortion of the TAR structure also brings the loop and bulge regions into close proximity, which could facilitate the interactions of proteins binding to both of these TAR domains.

The functional organization of the HIV-1 Tat protein has been deduced from TAR binding and transcriptional activation experiments using both wild-type and mutagenized derivatives of the Tat protein. The tripartite Tat activation (or effector) domain encompasses the amino-terminal 48 residues, which include (a) a string of highly acidic amino acids (residues 1 to 21), (b) a Cys-rich region (seven invariant, six of which are required for function) between positions 22 and 37, and (c) a hydrophobic core segment (amino acids 38 to 48), which is highly conserved among different HIV isolates (see Fig. 11). The activation domain is critical for recruiting an essential cellular cofactor to TAR; mutations affecting this region of the Tat protein drastically reduce or eliminate transactivation activity (543). The RNA binding domain of Tat has been mapped to a Lys/Arg-rich region between residues 49 and 57 (see Fig. 11); peptides from this Tat segment bind to the TAR bulge region as well as to a few base pairs surrounding the bulge, but with somewhat less affinity and specificity than do purified preparations of Tat protein (116). A nuclear/nucleolar localization signal ($_{48}$Gly-Arg-Lys-Lys-Arg$_{52}$) also overlaps the RNA-binding region of Tat.

At first glance, the functional organization of HIV-1 Tat is highly reminiscent of many other transcriptional regulatory proteins, which contain modular nucleic acid binding and activation domains. However, a growing body of work has revealed that Tat/TAR interactions are more complex *in vivo* and involve the participation of several cellular cofactors. This became apparent from experiments showing that the Arg-rich domain of the Tat protein did not function as an independent RNA-binding module *in vivo*. These experiments indicated three things: (a) The targeting of heterologous fusion proteins to TAR required *both* the RNA binding and activation regions of Tat (392). (b) The RNA binding domain of Tat failed to

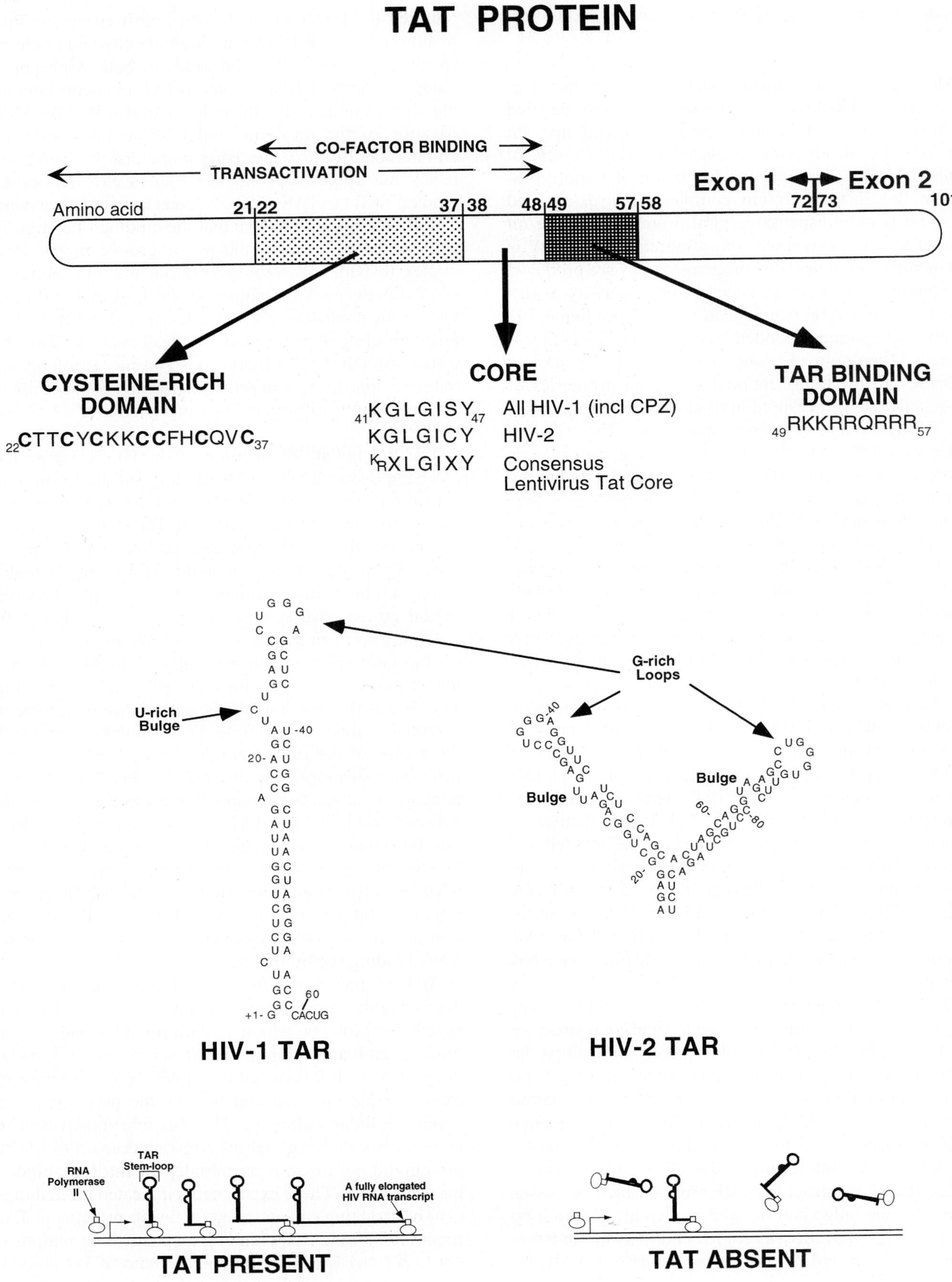
TAT PROTEIN
CO-FACTOR BINDING
TRANSACTIVATION
Exon 1
Exon 2
Amino acid
21 22
37 38
48 49
57 58
72 73
101
CYSTEINE-RICH DOMAIN
22CTTCYCKKCCFHCQVC37
CORE
41KGLGISY47 All HIV-1 (incl CPZ)
KGLGICY HIV-2
KRXLGIXY Consensus Lentivirus Tat Core
TAR BINDING DOMAIN
49RKKRRQRRR57
G-rich Loops
U-rich Bulge
Bulge
Bulge
HIV-1 TAR
HIV-2 TAR
RNA Polymerase II
TAR Stem-loop
A fully elongated HIV RNA transcript
TAT PRESENT
TAT ABSENT

function as a transdominant negative inhibitor of wild-type Tat, as did analogous domains from other RNA binding proteins such as HIV Rev (see later). This result implied that the Tat RNA binding region was neither autonomous nor able to form functional Tat/TAR interactions *in vivo* (398). (c) Wild-type TAR, but not mutant TAR decoys containing changes limited to the G-rich loop, rendered CEM cells resistant to HIV infection (605). The failure of excess Tat protein to relieve the blockade induced by wild-type TAR decoys suggested that at least one loop-binding cellular cofactor, present in limiting amounts, was required for functional Tat/TAR interaction *in vivo*.

Other studies demonstrated that Tat chimeric proteins, which could be targeted to the promoter via heterologous (non-TAR) RNA binding sites, also exhibited high levels of transactivation (569,620). This implied that, if necessary, Tat could function in the absence of TAR and recruit cellular factor(s) to the transcription complex. It was also reported that inefficient Tat transactivation in rodent cells (269) could be overcome if Tat was delivered to the promoter using a surrogate RNA binding site (9). This latter result indicated that a cellular cofactor required for Tat transactivation was indeed present in rodent cells but could not be recruited to or bind TAR. Collectively, these findings are consistent with a model in which Tat uses its transactivation domain to recruit a cellular cofactor (or cofactors) to TAR; in such a scenario, Tat would bind to the TAR bulge and the cofactor(s) to the TAR loop.

The hallmark of HIV LTR-directed RNA synthesis in the absence of Tat is the accumulation of prematurely and randomly terminated transcripts, which are converted to longer RNA species when Tat is expressed (see Fig. 11, bottom). This Tat-deficient phenotype has been observed in *in vitro* transcription experiments, following transient transfection of LTR-driven reporter gene constructs, and in cells harboring integrated HIV proviruses with mutated *tat* genes (173,355,622). Because Tat expression markedly stimulated transcriptional elongation in many of these experimental systems, attention shifted to the possible involvement of the CTD of Pol II, which, as noted earlier, is hyperphosphorylated in highly processive transcription complexes. This line of reasoning was also consistent with the reported inhibition of Tat-stimulated transcription by the adenosine analog DRB, which blocks Pol II–mediated elongation *in vitro* and *in vivo* by inactivating protein kinases (53). The demonstrated requirement of the Pol II CTD for Tat-mediated transactivation of viral RNA synthesis also supported such a model (487,682).

Reports describing the specific interaction of HIV-2 Tat [or just the effector domain of HIV-1 Tat (residues 1 to 48)] with a cellular kinase linked many of these disparate findings and provided the first mechanistic clues about Tat function (280,281). The novel enzymatic activity identified, initially named Tat-associated kinase or TAK, was able to phosphorylate the CTD of Pol II. Contemporaneous studies evaluating Tat-stimulated Pol II processivity in cell-free systems suggested that Tat interacted with components of the TFIIH complex to enhance transcriptional elongation and raised the possibility that TAK might be a TFIIH-associated kinase (227,487). However, it was subsequently shown that Tat binds with high affinity to a Pol II CTD kinase complex (710) related to the *Drosophila* multicomponent P-TEFb mentioned previously, which is catalytically independent of TFIIH (418,497). Moreover, Tat interaction with TFIIH is weak and not dependent on the integrity of its activation domain (84). P-TEFb shares no subunits in common with the TFIIH elongation factor complex, and it regulates the transition from abortive to fully processive transcriptional elongation (417). Additional experimentation revealed that TAK hyperphosphorylated the CTD of Pol II, independent of TFIIH (and its associated CDK7 kinase), and was more sensitive to DRB inhibition than was CDK7 (279,417,418). A recent study indicated that TFIIH activity is not required for HIV-1-mediated transcriptional elongation (84).

The Tat-related kinase component in human P-TEFb was subsequently identified to be PITALRE, a 42-kd CDC2-related kinase. When antibodies directed against PITALRE (now named CDK9) were used to deplete the kinase in nuclear extracts, the residual activity for Tat-simulated RNA chain elongation was reduced nearly 100-fold (498,710). Tat activity could be restored by adding purified P-TEFb to the cell-free system. Furthermore, the identification of novel Tat inhibitors, which specifically abolished CDK9 activity *in vivo* and *in vitro*, coupled with the demonstrated dominant negative effects of a CDK9 mutant on Tat transactivation (409,710), provided strong evidence that CDK9 was intimately involved in regulating Tat function. Taken together, these results suggested that TAK and P-TEFb were functionally indistinguishable transcription factors, sharing the common CTD kinase activity, CDK9. The subsequently demonstrated identity of the cloned catalytic subunit of P-TEFb and the kinase subunit of TAK provided conclusive evidence for this idea (681,710).

Although, as noted previously, earlier studies had shown that TAK/P-TEFb interacted with the activation

FIG. 11. Tat and its TAR response element. Schematic representation of the HIV-1 Tat protein (*top*) with the cysteine-rich activation, core, and TAR-binding domains indicated. The stem-bulge-loop configurations of HIV-1 and HIV-2 TAR elements are shown in the *middle*; the release of prematurely terminated HIV-1 transcriptional complexes from the DNA template in the absence of Tat is depicted at the *bottom*.

domain of HIV-1 Tat, the CDK9 catalytic subunit itself failed to bind to Tat in *in vitro* assays. Equally perplexing was the identification of the TAK/P-TEFb kinase activity in nuclear extracts migrating not as the 42-kd CDK9 but as a 110-kd complex (682). This suggested the existence of a possible cyclin-related partner for CDK9, which might provide substrate specificity. These unresolved issues were clarified with the isolation of the "missing link"—an 87-kd protein from nuclear extracts, which bound to wild-type HIV-1 Tat but not to a mutant Tat protein containing a nonfunctional activation domain (651). The sequence of a cDNA clone encoding the 87-kd protein revealed the presence of an amino-terminal cyclin box that was nearly 40% identical to human cyclin C. The new protein, initially named cyclin T (because it bound to Tat), is encoded by a gene mapping to human chromosome 12. The CDK9 family of kinases are now known to interact with cyclin regulatory subunits, many of which have been cloned and characterized (497). Several human cyclins (T1, T2a, and T2b) can functionally partner CDK9, greatly increasing its kinase activity (498); of these, only cyclin T1 is able to directly bind to the HIV-1 Tat activation domain and is a component of P-TEFb (651).

The binding of Tat to TAR has traditionally been the centerpiece of models for Tat-mediated transactivation. Following the identification of CDK9/cyclinT1 as cellular cofactors of Tat, attention turned to determining how they interacted with Tat, TAR, and the cellular transcriptional machinery. A large body of work revealed the following information: (a) CDK9 and cyclin T1 are components of the large human P-TEFb transcription complex that promotes RNA chain elongation. (b) CDK9/cyclin T1 is present in the nucleus (possibly also the cytoplasm) of eukaryotic cells as an assembled heterodimer, and its recruitment into the Pol II complex is associated with highly processive transcriptional activity. (c) Recombinant cyclin T1 directly binds to the effector domain of wild-type Tat but not to Tat proteins containing mutations affecting this region. This is consistent with the reported interaction of Tat and purified human P-TEFb in the absence of TAR (681,710). (d) The binding of Tat to TAR RNA is markedly enhanced in the presence of cyclin T1. Several reports have, in fact, shown that the Tat/cyclin T1 heterodimer has greater affinity for TAR than does either Tat or cyclin T1 alone (39,225,651). As expected, the interaction of Tat with purified P-TEFb greatly increased the affinity of Tat for TAR (706). (e) The Tat–cyclin T1 complex will bind only to TAR RNA in which both the loop and the bulge are intact, whereas Tat alone requires only the trinucleotide bulge for stable TAR interaction. These results suggest that multiple pair-wise interactions are involved in stabilizing the binding of Tat to TAR: (a) Tat with P-TEFb, (b) Tat with the TAR bulge, (c) cyclin T1 with the TAR loop, and (d) the TAR bulge/TAR loop with Tat/P-TEFb.

As noted earlier, Tat transactivation of HIV-1 LTR-driven gene expression is quite low in rodent cells but can be greatly augmented in rodent somatic cell hybrids containing human chromosome 12 (269). This defect can also be corrected by overexpressing human cyclin T in rodent cells, which results in enhanced Tat transactivation of the HIV-1 LTR to levels measured in human cells (651). Recent studies have shown that the murine homolog of human cyclin T is able to bind to HIV-1 Tat, but the resulting Tat/murine cyclin T heterodimer is not efficiently recruited to TAR (204,225). Substitution of a single amino acid residue in murine cyclin T with its human analog (Tyr to Cys at residue 260) also restores Tat activity in rodent cells (39,225). Thus, the extremely weak Tat transactivation in rodent cells is not caused by a failure to form the Tat/cyclin T heterodimer; rather, the cross-species heterodimer that does form is apparently unable to bind to TAR and deliver P-TEFb to a poorly processive transcription complex.

A model of HIV Tat transactivation is shown in Figure 12. Tat interacts, via its activation domain, with the cyclin T1 subunit of cyclin T1/CDK9, a component of the P-TEFb elongation complex present in the nuclei of virus-infected cells. The binding of human P-TEFb to Tat most likely induces a conformational change in the structure of Tat, which alters its affinity and specificity for binding to TAR RNA. Thus, the function of Tat is to recruit the critical P-TEFb elongation factor to a promoter-proximal location where it can hyperphosphorylate the Pol II CTD, thereby stimulating transcriptional processivity. It is worth noting that expression of both CDK9 and cyclin T1 increases following activation of resting PBMC with phytohemagglutinin (PHA), phorbol myristic acid (PMA) plus ionomycin, anti-CD3 antibody plus IL-2, or antibodies to both anti-CD3 and the CD28 receptor (278). Thus T-cell activation increases steady-state levels of both NF-κB as well as the two cellular cofactors of Tat, resulting in high levels of HIV-1 LTR-directed gene activity.

Possible extracellular roles for Tat have been suggested from studies showing that Tat is taken up by cultured cells, enters the nucleus, and transactivates genes linked to the HIV LTR (191). Tat purified from *Escherichia coli* has also been reported to inhibit antigen-induced, but not mitogen-induced, proliferation of PBMC (639). In a similar vein, it has been reported that low concentrations of Tat modestly stimulate the growth of cultured Kaposi sarcoma cells from patients with AIDS (164). The significance of these extracellular Tat activities in HIV-infected individuals is currently unclear.

Rev

Like other primary RNA transcripts synthesized in eukaryotic cells, HIV pre-mRNAs undergo a series of modifications (capping, 3′-end cleavage, polyadenylation, and splicing) prior to their export to the cytoplasm. Retroviruses utilize the cellular posttranscriptional pro-

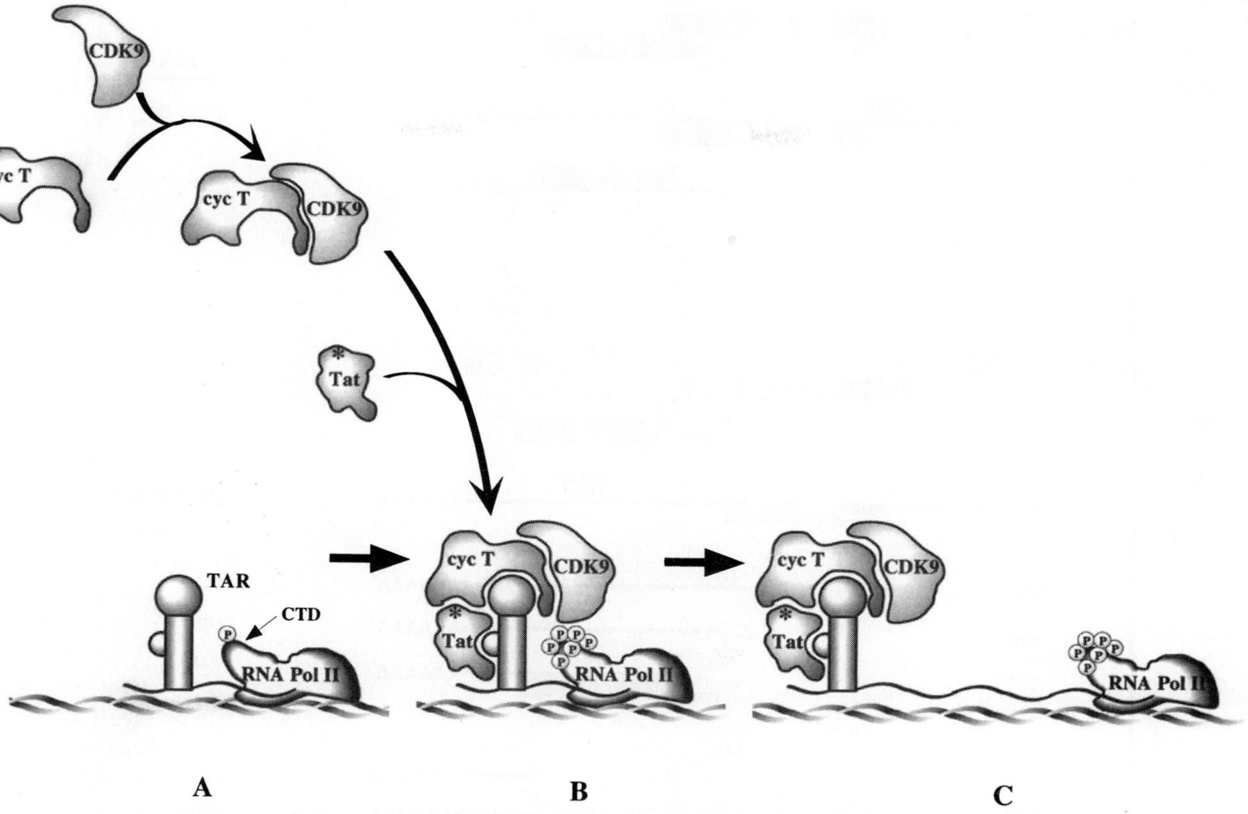

FIG. 12. Tat promotes the phosphorylation of the carboxy terminal domain (*CTD*) of RNA Pol II. **A:** In the absence of Tat binding to TAR, the processivity of the RNA Pol II complex is inefficient. **B:** When the activation domain (*) of Tat interacts with the cyclin T (*cyc T*)/CDK9 complex, the conformation of Tat changes and its affinity and specificity for TAR RNA increases. **C:** By recruiting cyc T and CDK9 (the TAK complex) to a promoter proximal location, Tat mediates the hyperphosphorylation of the CTD and promoter clearance (elongation) of transcriptional complex. (Drawing kindly provided by Dr. Michael Cho.)

cessing machinery to carry out these functions. With few exceptions, introns present in nascent cellular mRNAs must be removed prior to their export from the nucleus, presumably to prevent their translation into nonfunctional proteins. This requirement poses an obvious problem for retroviruses such as HIV, which must export a variety of intron-containing mRNAs into the cytoplasm (e.g., the unspliced 9.2-kbp primary transcript for encapsidation into progeny virions and production of Gag and Pol proteins, as well as several other partially spliced mRNAs such as those encoding Env, Vif, and Vpr proteins). In part, retroviruses have solved the requirement for the removal of all intronic sequences from pre-mRNAs prior to nuclear export by incorporating suboptimal splice sites into their genomes. These sites are inefficiently processed by splicing factors, resulting in the accumulation of unspliced viral RNAs in the nucleus. The nuclear export of intron-containing retroviral RNAs may be additionally impeded as a result of their interaction/retention with the cellular splicing apparatus (456).

All retroviruses must splice their primary RNA transcripts to generate *env* mRNAs, eliminating upstream *gag* and *pol* sequences in the process. For simple retroviruses such as the ALVs and MuLVs, this is the only splicing reaction that the viral pre-mRNA undergoes (Fig. 13, top). In contrast, the splicing of HIV RNA is far more complex because of the presence of both constitutive and alternatively used splice-donor and splice-acceptor motifs scattered through its genomic RNA. Three general classes of HIV mRNAs have been identified in productively infected cells: (a) unspliced genomic RNA, which serves as the mRNA for synthesis of Gag and Pol proteins; (b) partially spliced RNAs, approximately 4.3 to 5.5 kb in size, which are translated into Vif, Vpr, Vpu, and Env proteins; and (c) multiply or completely spliced viral mRNAs, ranging from 1.7 to 2.0 kb in size, which encode the Tat, Rev, and Nef proteins (see Fig. 13, bottom). The first two classes of viral mRNA contain several spliceable introns yet are efficiently exported from the nucleus into the cytoplasm.

Analyses of viral mRNAs by RT polymerase chain reaction (RT-PCR) have revealed the existence of more than 30 different HIV transcripts in virus-producing cells (513,566). These mRNAs are generated as a consequence

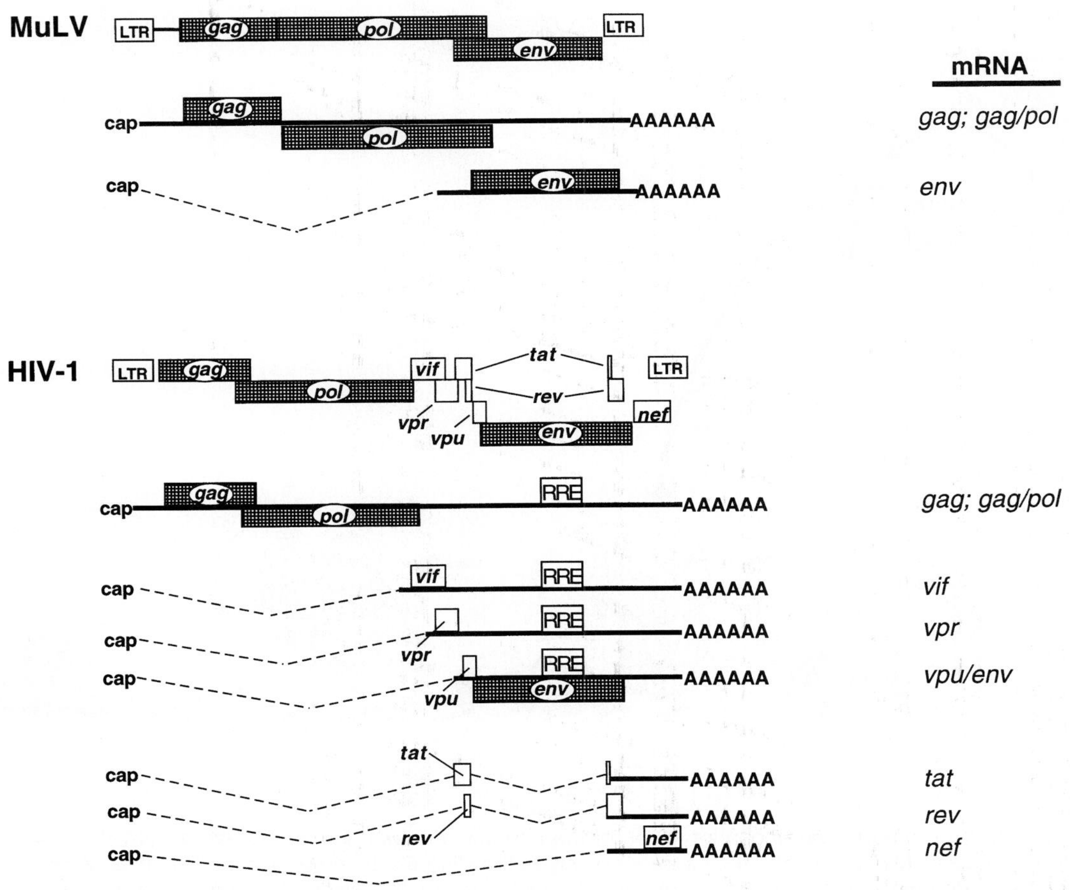

FIG. 13. Retrovirus splicing patterns. In contrast to murine leukemia virus (MuLV), which generates only two discrete mRNA species (the unspliced *gag/pol* and the singly spliced *env*), HIV-1 produces several alternatively spliced mRNAs ranging from the unspliced *gag/pol* to the multiply spliced *tat, rev*, and *nef* RNA transcripts. The genomic organization of the proviral DNA, the location of protein coding sequences, and the position of the Rev-responsive element (*RRE*) in intron-containing mRNAs encoding viral structural proteins are indicated. The *dashed lines* connect the major splice donor to a downstream splice acceptor; alternative forms of *tat, rev, vpu/env*, and *nef* mRNAs, some of which contain short upstream noncoding exons, are not shown.

of alternative selection of the five splice donors (sd) and the more than 10 splice acceptors (sa) embedded in the viral genome (some of which are shown at the top of Fig. 14). Variable usage of this ensemble of splicing signals gives rise to several sets of distinct, closely related RNAs that serve as alternative templates for translation into the same protein. For example, 12 different *rev*, 5 different *nef*, 8 different *tat*, and 16 different *env* mRNAs have been identified (513). This HIV mRNA diversity is caused, in part, by the variable inclusion of two upstream 50- and 74-nt noncoding exons (generated from sa2/sd2 and sa3a/sd3, respectively; Fig. 14) in many of these spliced RNA species. The functional significance of multiple spliced mRNAs encoding the same viral protein, their relative abundance, and the hierarchy of HIV splice site usage are not presently understood.

Complex retroviruses, such as HIV, have dealt with the restriction to the nuclear export of unspliced and incompletely spliced transcripts by incorporating a novel reading frame, encoding the Rev (which stands for regulator of expression of viral proteins) protein, into their genomes. In the absence of Rev, the unspliced *gag/pol* and the partially spliced *vif, vpr*, and *vpu/env* mRNAs fail to accumulate in the cytoplasm, thereby rendering the Rev mutant virus replication incompetent (174,264,588).

HIV-1 Rev is a 19-kd, predominantly nucleolar phosphoprotein containing 116 amino acid residues. Like Tat, Rev is encoded by two exons and contains two functional regions: (a) an Arg-rich domain that mediates RNA binding and nuclear localization, which is flanked by sequences that facilitate Rev multimerization; and (b) a hydrophobic segment, located between residues 73 and 84, that contains several Leu residues, now known to promote nuclear export (see Fig. 15, top) (404,406,407,698). Mutation of any one of three critical Leu residues (at position 78, 81, or 83) within this domain eliminates Rev

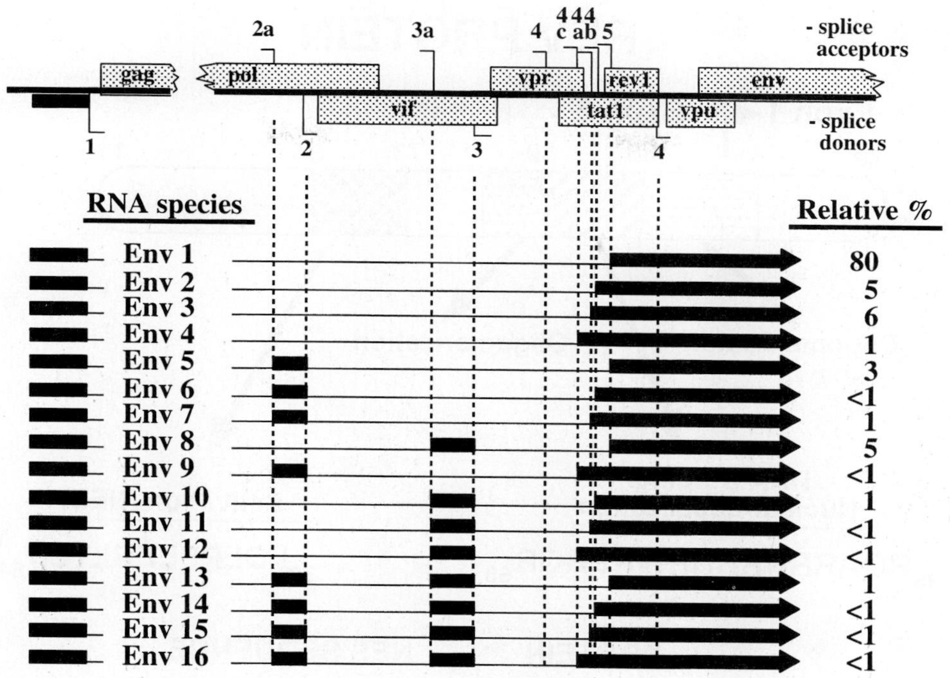

FIG. 14. Structure and relative abundance of differentially spliced HIV-1 *env* mRNAs. For each RNA species, the *dark bars* and associated 3′ *arrows* represent exons included in the spliced transcript as determined by semiquantitative PCR analysis. The relative proportion of each mRNA is indicated at the right.

activity. Unlike those of *tat*, both coding exons of *rev* are required for function (546).

The HIV Rev protein regulates the expression and utilization of viral transcripts by binding to a cis-acting target, the Rev response element (RRE), present in all unspliced and partially spliced viral mRNAs (see Fig. 13). The RRE, located in a 250-nt segment spanning the junction between gp120 and gp41 coding sequences of the *env* gene, is a complex RNA structure containing multiple stem-loops branching from a large central bubble (174,405,535) (see Fig. 15, bottom). The RRE must be present *within* a Rev-responsive transcript and in the *sense* orientation for Rev responsiveness. Nuclease protection, chemical modification, and mutagenesis studies indicate that Rev specifically interacts with a 60+ nt portion of the RRE, designated stem-loop II (see Fig. 15) (129,288,407). This region of the RRE binds to Rev even when isolated from the complete RRE structure, and it mediates Rev responsiveness in functional assays (294). The determinants for high-affinity binding of Rev to RRE reside in the central purine-rich "bubble" in stem-loop II; this bubble contains unusual G:G and G:A base pairs that distort the duplex RNA structure and widen the major groove to accommodate the Rev protein (22, 289,407). NMR analyses have shown that an alpha helical, Arg-rich, 17-residue peptide, from the RNA binding domain of Rev, burrows deep into the major groove of a stem-loop II oligonucleotide, stabilizing the non-Watson-Crick base pairs through specific interactions involving the Arg side chains (23). It is now believed that Rev initially makes high-affinity contact with nucleotides in the RRE loop II bubble as a monomer, thereby generating a nucleation point for the multimerization of additional Rev molecules through cooperative protein–protein and protein–RNA interactions (698,700). The functionally complete RRE is most likely 350 nt in size, and an individual element may accommodate eight or more Rev molecules (410). Although not yet developed into usable antiviral agents, some aminoglycosides are able to block the binding of HIV Rev to its RRE target and inhibit the production of progeny virions (699).

Mutations affecting either the RNA binding or the Leu-rich activation domains of the Rev protein result in loss of function. For example, activation domain mutants are able to bind to the RRE but are functionally inactive. They interfere with the transactivation mediated by wild-type Rev, exerting a trans-dominant effect in assays for Rev function (404). Rev also possesses the unique property of continuously shuttling between the nucleus and the cytoplasm (434). Mutations affecting the Rev activation domain abolish the shuttling and restrict Rev to the nucleus. Multimerization-defective Rev mutants can still bind to the high-affinity RRE site but are unable to form oligomeric complexes (399).

Although the total amount of viral RNA in cells infected with wild-type or Rev-deficient HIV mutants is

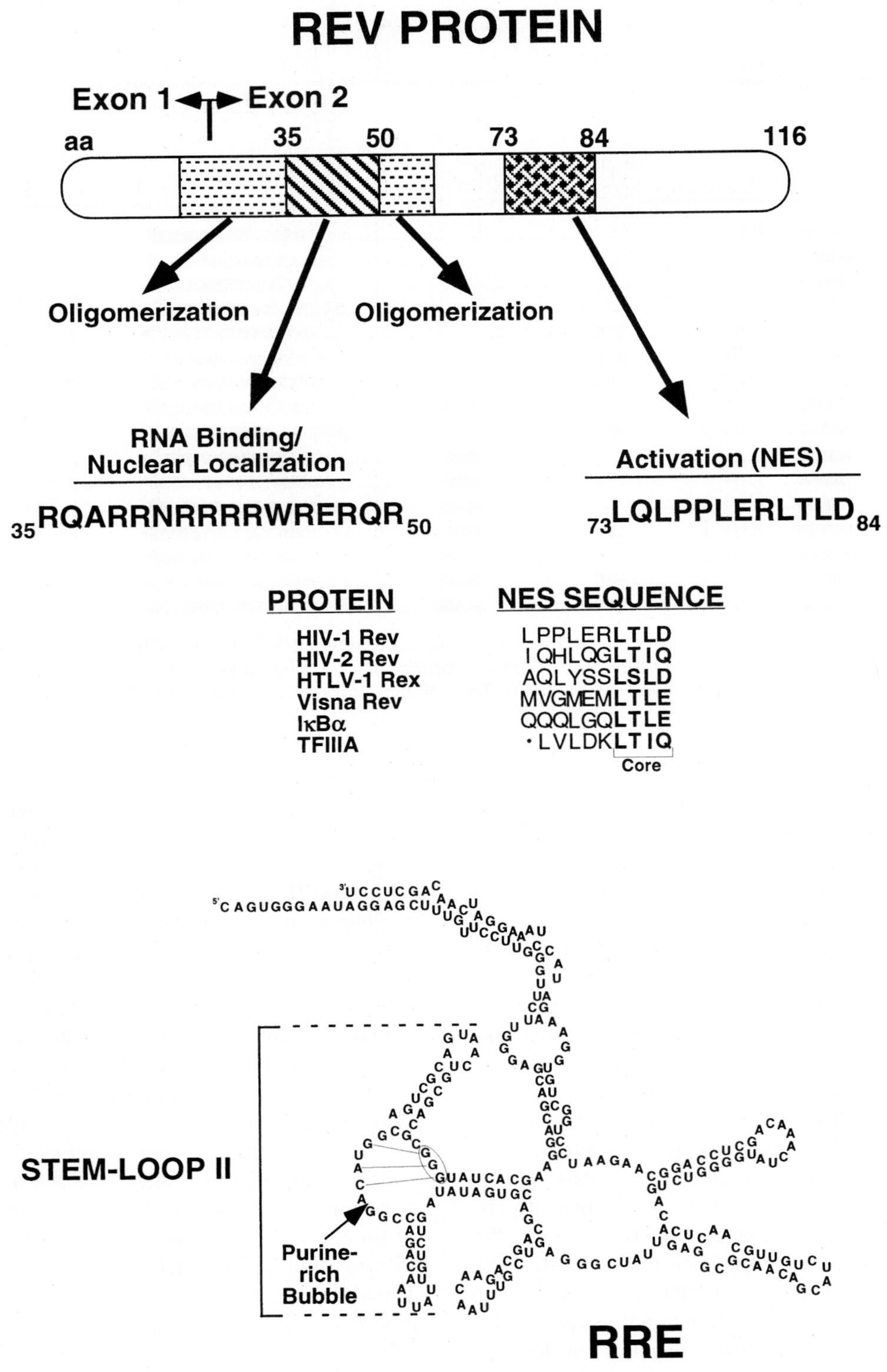

FIG. 15. Rev and its response element, the RRE. A schematic representation of the HIV-1 Rev protein with its RNA-binding, activation, and oligomerization domains is shown at the top. The amino acid sequence of the leucine-rich nuclear export signal (*NES*) present in retroviral Rev/Rex proteins and two cellular proteins are also shown. The core tetramer motif, LxLy, where y is usually a charged residue and x is highly variable, is indicated. The structure of the RRE is presented at the *bottom* with the high-affinity target of HIV-1 Rev (*stem-loop II*) shown. The "bulged" G residues in stem-loop II able to form noncanonical purine–purine base pairs are *circled.*

quite similar, *gag-pol*, *env*, *vif*, and *vpr* mRNAs are either absent or markedly underrepresented in the cytoplasm of cells infected with Rev mutants compared to the relatively normal levels of multiply spliced *tat*, *rev*, and *nef* transcripts in the same cellular compartment (174,405, 588). This pattern of RNA expression initially led to a plethora of proposed posttranscriptional functions mediated by Rev, including (a) the regulation of splicing, (b) nuclear to cytoplasmic transport, (c) RNA stabilization, and (d) stimulating the translation of RRE-containing HIV RNAs. As noted earlier, the HIV-1 genome contains multiple sequence motifs, located in *gag*, *pol*, and *env* genes (and designated INS in Fig. 6), which contribute to a requirement for Rev. These cis-acting AU-rich elements markedly impair the expression of fused reporter genes by impeding RNA transport to the cytoplasm and/or decreasing RNA stability (403,535). It is quite likely that cellular proteins bind to these inhibitory sequences, contributing to the nuclear retention and the intrinsic instability of intron-containing viral RNAs. Rev is able to reverse these effects, provided that an RRE is present in such transcripts.

Careful analyses of HIV RNA expression patterns in different cellular compartments indicated that the ratios of unspliced (or partially spliced) to completely spliced viral transcripts in the nucleus did *not* change in the presence or absence of Rev (174,405). Rather, as noted previously, the hallmark of insufficient Rev expression was a superabundance of the 1.7- to 2.0-kb, completely spliced RNAs. and greatly reduced or no detectable RRE-containing mRNAs *only* in the cytoplasm. Because splicing of viral RNA in the nucleus was not affected by the absence of Rev, attention shifted to the role that Rev might have on HIV RNA transport.

The first unambiguous demonstration that Rev could promote the nuclear export of intron-containing viral RNA came from experiments in which purified Rev protein and RRE-containing RNA molecules were microinjected into cell nuclei (180,656). These studies showed that the RRE-containing unspliced RNA substrates were transported from the nucleus into the cytoplasm only in the presence of Rev. Interestingly, the excised exon (containing the RRE element), derived from those transcripts that did undergo splicing, was also detected in the cytoplasm, indicating that Rev was able to mediate nuclear export *without* inhibiting RNA splicing (181). Other microinjection studies revealed that the Leu-rich Rev activation domain was indeed a nuclear export signal (NES) because, when fused to bovine serum albumin (BSA), it promoted the transport of NES/BSA molecules into the cytoplasm (180,656). In contrast, NES/BSA fusion proteins containing a mutated, nonfunctional Leu-rich Rev domain remained in the nucleus. The nuclear export mediated by the Rev NES was also shown to be energy dependent and was blocked by high concentrations of NES/BSA, a result that implied that the amounts of intracellular nucleus-to-cytoplasm transporting proteins were limiting. Surprisingly, the nuclear export of 5S rRNA and spliceosomal U small nuclear (sn)RNAs, but not Pol II–derived cellular mRNAs, were also inhibited when high concentrations of NES/BSA conjugates were microinjected. In this regard, a growing list of viral and cellular proteins involved in RNA metabolism and signal transduction have been shown to contain a Rev-like, Leu-rich NES (see Fig. 15, middle), which mediates the transport of a variety of substrates from the nucleus to the cytoplasm (303,423). Taken together, these results are consistent with a model in which the Rev effector domain functions as a NES, directing RRE-containing viral RNAs to the cytoplasm via a pathway used by some cellular mRNAs.

The bi-directional passage of proteins between the nucleus and cytoplasm occurs through the nuclear pore complex (NPC) and depends on the presence of NLS and NES transport signals. The NPC is an extremely large (over 100 megadaltons) gated structure composed of 50 to 100 different proteins, called nucleoporins, only a few of which have been characterized (168,603). One class of nucleoporins, thought to directly participate in nuclear-cytoplasmic transport, contains Phe-Gly (FG) repeat domains and are located primarily at the periphery of the NPC. Proteins destined to be imported into the nucleus (e.g., bearing a typical basic-type NLS) initially associate with a member of a growing family of transport "receptors" in the cytoplasm. The first receptor of this type discovered, importin-β, shares structural features and interacting partners with other family members and is considered to be the prototypical transporter. Proteins bearing the basic-type NLS usually begin the import process by first binding to a related transport protein, importin-α. Importin-α serves as a bridge, linking the NLS-containing substrate to importin-β. However, in contrast to most other proteins that carry a classic NLS, Rev appears to bind directly to importin-β, and this heterodimeric complex is transported to the NPC where the importin-β subunit successively binds to and dissociates from the resident nucleoporins, translocating the Rev substrate through the pore and into the nucleoplasm (148).

It is now known that the reverse process, nuclear export, utilizes transport receptors that are also members of the importin-β family. The most well studied of these is named CRM1 (for chromosome region maintenance 1), or exportin 1 (184,595). Studies of HIV-1 Rev and related viral and cellular proteins bearing Leu-rich NES motifs (see Fig. 15) have led to the discovery and established the functions of many proteins involved in nuclear export. A critical experiment linking the Rev NES mechanistically to the nuclear export machinery was the demonstration that the antibiotic leptomycin B (LMB) blocked the nuclear export of Rev-dependent RNAs in HeLa cells and human PBMC (672). A follow-up study, using microinjected *Xenopus* oocytes, indicated that LMB inhibited the nuclear-to-cytoplasmic transport of both the Rev protein and several UsnRNAs (184). Completely unrelated experiments, examining the antimicrobial effects of LMB in yeast, had mapped LMB resistance to the antibiotic to the CRM1 gene (463), an observation reported prior to the time when the role of CRM1 in nuclear export was appreciated. Additional experiments demonstrating that LMB binds directly to *in vitro* translated CRM1 and that overexpression of CRM1 eliminates the LMB blockade of Rev NES-mediated nuclear export suggested that Crm 1 might be the long-sought "export receptor" for proteins containing the Leu-rich NES. This conclusion was also supported by studies showing that CRM1 shuttled between the nucleus and cytoplasm and interacted with the FG repeats present in nucleoporin proteins (184,461,595).

The small GTPase molecule, Ran (41), also plays a central role in nuclear-cytoplasmic transport and is intimately involved in the Rev-mediated nuclear export of intron-containing HIV-1 pre-mRNAs. Ran is a guanine nucleotide-containing enzyme that provides both the energy and the directionality cues for nuclear import and export. Intracellularly, Ran cycles between two forms, RanGTP and RanGDP, which are concentrated primarily in the nucleus and cytoplasm, respectively (304). The specificity of Ran activity in nuclear transport is regulated by the nature of the bound nucleotide. Several cellular proteins are able to modulate the nucleotide-bound state of Ran and, therefore, contribute to the asymmetric distribution of the two Ran forms (42). One of these, the chromatin-associated regulator of chromosomal condensation 1, or RCC1, stimulates the replacement of GDP with GTP when Ran is in the nucleus. On the other hand, two other factors, Ran GTPase activating protein 1 (Ran GAP1) and Ran binding protein 1 (Ran BP1) both augment Ran activity in the cytoplasm by promoting the hydrolysis of the Ran-associated GTP. The net effect of these interactions is the maintenance of the observed RanGTP/RanGDP intracellular gradient required for nuclear import and export functions.

The complete Rev nuclear transport cycle and its critical interacting partners are shown in Figure 16. During the early, postintegration phase of the virus life cycle, the HIV-1 mRNAs transported to the cytoplasm consist almost entirely of intronless, multiply spliced transcripts encoding the Tat, Rev, and Nef proteins. As noted earlier, Rev uses its NLS to bind directly to importin-β in the cytoplasm and is translocated through the nuclear pore as a Rev/importin-β heterodimer. When the complex reaches the nucleus, the binding of RanGTP triggers the Rev/importin-β heterodimer to dissociate and release the Rev subunit. In the nucleoplasm, Rev initiates its role as a nuclear exporter by binding to the high-affinity site on stem-loop II of RRE-containing HIV-1 pre-mRNAs and then multimerizes via cooperative protein–protein and protein–RNA interactions over the entire length of the RRE. When Rev oligomerizes on the RRE, its NES elements become aligned on the outside of an enlarging protein–RNA complex and are available to interact with other proteins (275). Although CRM1 is able to directly bind to Rev (14,184,207), this interaction is nonspecific because it does not require an intact NES and is unaffected by the antibiotic LMB. Instead, to form a functional complex, the multimerized Rev/RRE must interact with CRM1 in the presence of Ran in its GTP bound form. The formation of this complex (RRE/Rev/CRM1/RanGTP) is (a) blocked by the antibiotic LMB, (b) sensitive to Rev NES mutations, and (c) dissociated when RanGTP is hydrolyzed to the RanGDP state (14). The most likely scenario linking all available data is that the entry of RanGTP into a preexisting Rev/CRM1 heterodimer converts it into a functional export complex. This is supported by the results of *in vitro* protease protection experiments showing that the addition of RanGTP further stabilizes the Rev–CRM1 complex, making it more resistant to enzymatic digestion (14). Once a functional REV export complex is formed, it is transported to the NPC where the CRM1 subunit interacts with nucleoporins (185), translocating the entire complex into the cytoplasm. There, in the presence of Ran GAP1 and Ran BP1, the RanGTP component of the export complex is converted to the RanGDP form and the complex disassembles (245,462). Rev is released along with its unspliced and partially spliced HIV-1 RNA "cargo," allowing the latter to be incorporated into progeny virions or be translated into viral proteins. It should be noted that microinjection studies utilizing *Xenopus* oocytes have shown that the export of Rev-responsive RNAs is blocked in the presence of a RanGTP mutant unable to undergo GTP hydrolysis (336). Rev therefore enables lentiviral intron-containing RNAs to elude the cellular splicing machinery and to be transported to the cytoplasm via an export pathway not used by most cellular mRNAs.

It is also worth noting that a constitutive transport element (CTE), isolated from the genomes of type D retroviruses such as Mason-Pfizer monkey virus (MPMV) and simian retrovirus-1, can functionally substitute for the Rev protein and facilitate the nuclear export of unspliced or partially spliced HIV RNAs (55,712). CTEs are likely to be present in the genomes of simple retroviruses that do not encode their own Rev-like transactivating proteins and presumably bind to cellular factors that mediate nucleocytoplasmic transport (433,469,585). One such candidate is the human TAP protein, which binds to CTE loop sequences and mediates nuclear export of CTE-containing RNAs, as monitored in the *Xenopus* oocyte system (256). Microinjection of the MPMV CTE blocks mRNA but not Rev/NES or tRNA nuclear export, suggesting that in *Xenopus* cells, at least, CTE-containing substrates and cellular mRNAs use a nucleus-to-cytoplasm transport system different from that employed by Rev (490).

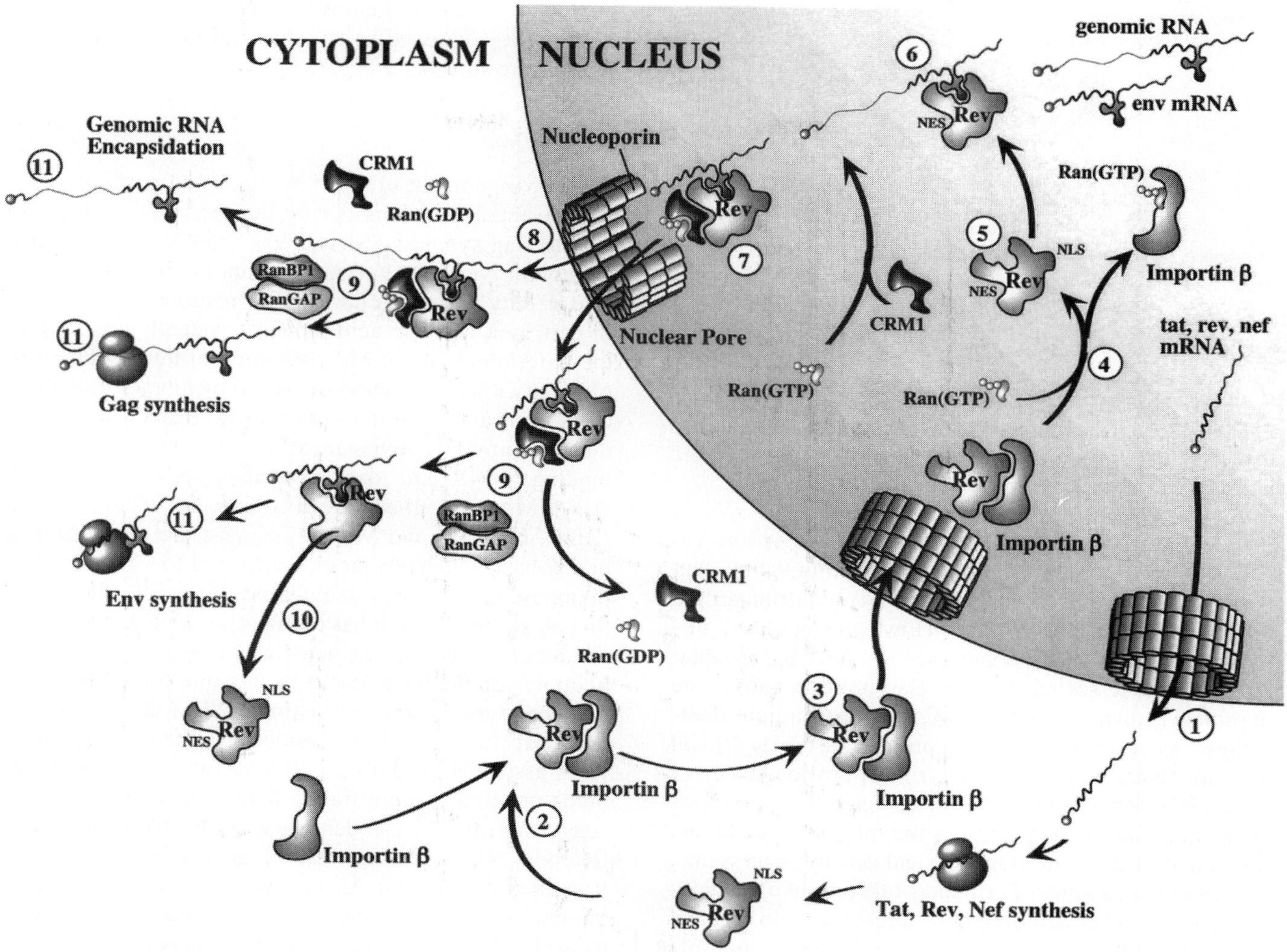

FIG. 16. Rev nuclear export pathway. Intronless multiply spliced HIV-1 mRNAs (*tat*, *rev*, and *nef*) use a Rev-independent pathway to exit the nucleus (*1*). Using its nuclear localization signal (NLS), newly synthesized Rev protein binds to importin β (*2*) and the resulting heterodimer (*3*) is translocated through the nuclear pore. In the nucleus, Rev/ importin β dissociation is mediated by Ran(GTP) (*4*) and the free Rev protein binds (*5*) to RRE-containing viral pre-mRNAs (*6*). The Rev/RRE RNA complex is converted to a functional export structure following the addition of CRM1 and Ran(GTP) (*7*) and is transported through the nuclear pore (*8*). In the cytoplasm, RanBP1/RanGAP mediate the conversion of Ran(GTP) in the export complex to Ran(GDP) (*9*), which then disassembles. Following the release of Rev from intron-containing HIV-1 transcripts (*10*), the full-length viral RNA may be encapsidated into progeny virions or, as is the case for the partially spliced mRNAs, may be translated into viral proteins (*11*). (Drawing kindly provided by Dr. Michael Cho.)

Gag

The Gag proteins of HIV, like those of other retroviruses, are necessary and sufficient for the formation of noninfectious, virus-like particles. Retroviral Gag proteins are generally synthesized as polyprotein precursors; the HIV-1 Gag precursor has been named, based on its apparent molecular mass, $Pr55^{Gag}$. As noted previously, the mRNA for $Pr55^{Gag}$ is the unspliced 9.2-kb transcript (Figs. 5 and 13) that requires Rev for its expression in the cytoplasm. When the *pol* ORF is present, the viral protease (PR) cleaves $Pr55^{Gag}$ during or shortly after budding from the cell to generate the mature Gag proteins p17 (MA), p24 (CA), p7 (NC), and p6 (see Fig. 5). Two spacer peptides are also cleaved out of the Gag precursor: p2, located between CA and NC, and p1, situated between NC and p6. In the virion, MA is localized immediately inside the lipid bilayer of the viral envelope, CA forms the outer portion of the cone-shaped core structure in the center of the particle, and NC is present in the core in a ribonucleoprotein complex with the viral RNA genome (Fig. 17). The location of p6 in the virion remains to be precisely defined. Retroviral Gag proteins perform several principal functions during virus assembly, including

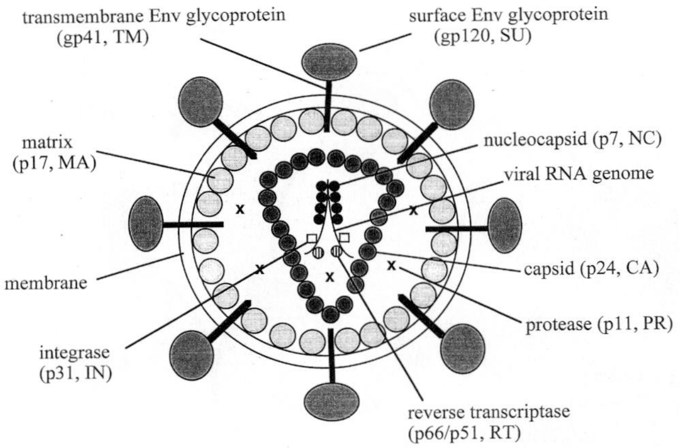

FIG. 17. Schematic representation of a mature HIV-1 virion. (Adapted from ref. 192, with permission.)

(a) forming the structural framework of the virion, (b) encapsidating the viral genome, (c) targeting the nascent particle for export from the cell, and (d) acquiring a lipid bilayer and associated envelope (Env) glycoproteins during particle release (for review, see ref. 192, and Chapter 8). These processes require that Gag proteins participate in protein–protein, protein–RNA, and protein–lipid interactions. As described later, Gag proteins also play critical roles in the early stages of the virus replication cycle.

The HIV $Pr55^{Gag}$ precursor oligomerizes following its translation and is targeted to the plasma membrane, where particles of sufficient size and density to be visible by EM are assembled. Formation of virus-like particles by $Pr55^{Gag}$ is a self-assembly process, with critical Gag–Gag interactions taking place between multiple domains along the Gag precursor. The assembly of virus-like particles does not require the participation of genomic RNA (although the presence of nucleic acid appears to be essential), *pol*-encoded enzymes, or Env glycoproteins, but the production of infectious virions requires the encapsidation of the viral RNA genome and the incorporation of the Env glycoproteins and the Gag-Pol polyprotein precursor $Pr160^{Gag\text{-}Pol}$. Processing of the Gag and Gag-Pol precursor proteins by PR concomitant with budding results in a major structural and morphologic rearrangement, referred to as maturation, during which the core condenses into the cone-shaped structure characteristic of the mature HIV particle (see Fig. 1A). Disruption of this maturation process abolishes virus infectivity.

Detailed NMR and x-ray crystallographic data have provided significant insights into the structure–function relationship of HIV-1 MA, CA, and NC (see later). It remains to be seen, however, to what extent the structures of the mature Gag proteins will reflect those of the corresponding domains of $Pr55^{Gag}$. In some instances, for example at the N-terminus of CA, major refolding accompanies PR-mediated $Pr55^{Gag}$ cleavage. We can hope that future technologic advances will allow this issue to be addressed as structures of larger portions of $Pr55^{Gag}$ are solved.

Matrix Domain

The MA domain of $Pr55^{Gag}$ (Fig. 18A) performs several essential functions during the viral life cycle. Following Gag synthesis, MA directs $Pr55^{Gag}$ to the plasma membrane via a multipartite membrane binding signal. The affinity of the MA domain for membrane is provided in part by a myristic acid moiety covalently attached to the N-terminal Gly of MA. Mutation of this residue significantly impairs binding of Gag to membrane and abolishes virus assembly in most systems. Sequences in MA downstream of the myristate also contribute to membrane binding. NMR and x-ray crystallographic analyses of HIV-1 MA [as well as MA of SIV, bovine leukosis virus (BLV), HTLV-II, and MPMV] suggest that residues in a highly basic patch cluster on the face of MA predicted to juxtapose the plasma membrane (Fig. 19) (422; for review, see ref. 114). It has been proposed that these basic residues interact with the negatively charged acidic phospholipids on the inner leaflet of the lipid bilayer, thereby stabilizing membrane interactions (277,422,708). Mutations affecting these basic residues can be detrimental to virus assembly (194,695,707). The finding that $Pr55^{Gag}$ binds membrane more tightly than MA itself led to the suggestion that MA undergoes a conformational switch following Gag cleavage that triggers its partial release from membrane (708). An analogous switch in membrane binding potential has been described in detail for the retinal rod sensor protein recoverin, which upon binding calcium undergoes a conformation change, referred to as a "myristyl switch," that exposes the myristate moiety and induces membrane binding. A prediction of this model is that mutations in MA downstream of the myristylation consensus signal might increase or decrease Gag membrane binding, perhaps by altering MA conformation; indeed, such mutations have been reported (330,474, 483,593). The ability of MA to partially dissociate from membrane after PR-mediated Gag cleavage would in theory allow it to participate in post-entry steps in virus replication (see later).

The mechanism by which Gag traffics specifically to the plasma membrane rather than to intracellular membranes is still under investigation. Deletion of a large portion of MA (169), as well as single amino acid changes between MA residues 84 and 88 (202,476), cause virus assembly to be redirected to cytoplasmic compartments. Thus, MA appears to contain determinants not only of membrane binding, but, more specifically, of plasma membrane targeting. A role for MA in targeting is supported by the finding that substitution of MA with a heterologous membrane binding signal results in promiscuous assembly both at the plasma membrane and at

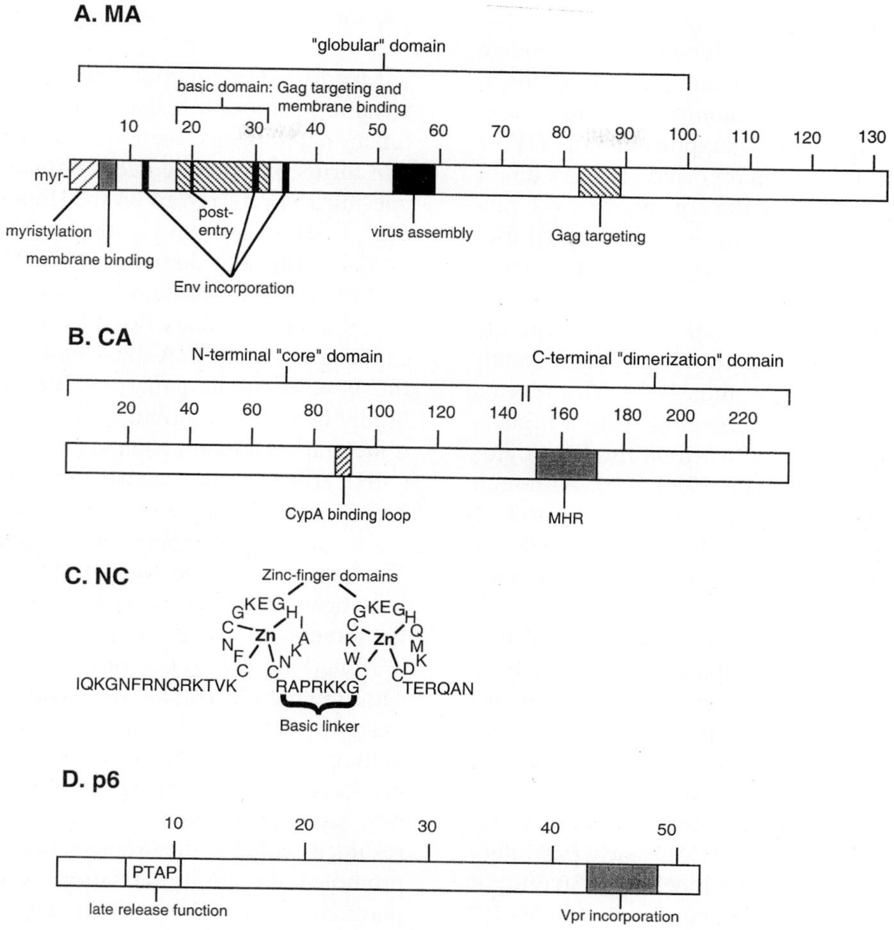

FIG. 18. Linear organization of the major HIV-1 Gag proteins. *Panel A*, matrix (MA); *panel B*, capsid (CA); *panel C*, nucleocapsid (NC); *panel D*, p6. Amino acid positions are indicated, as are major functional domains. (Adapted from ref. 192, with permission.)

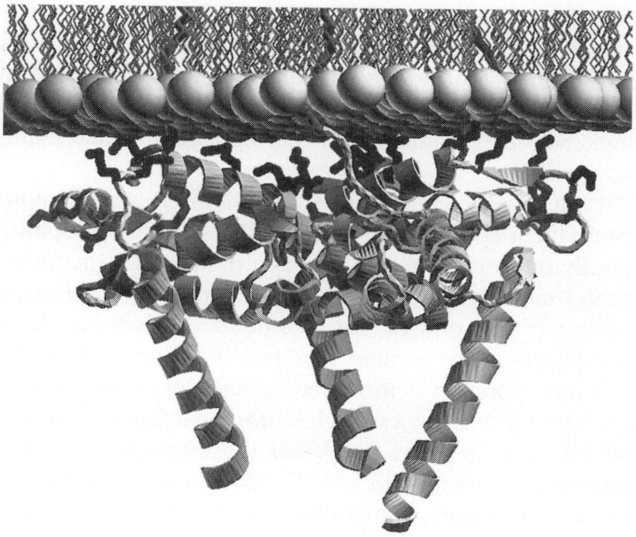

FIG. 19. Structure of a MA trimer bound to membrane. At the *top* is depicted the lipid bilayer; myristate moieties are shown embedded in the bilayer. The helical C-terminal tail of MA is shown projecting away from the globular core. (Reprinted from ref. 284, with permission.)

intracellular sites (520). That a substitution in the MA highly basic domain corrected the mistargeting induced by a residue-86 mutation (475) supports the notion that the basic domain may be a determinant not only of membrane binding but also of plasma membrane targeting. This hypothesis is consistent with the finding that a basic domain deletion appeared to cause a defect in Gag transport (695), and that more subtle mutations in this region retargeted virus assembly to an intracellular site (476).

After Gag binds the plasma membrane, it assembles into particles that bud from the cell. During budding, the viral Env glycoproteins are incorporated into the nascent virions. MA plays a crucial role in this process; small deletions, insertions, and specific point mutations in MA block Env incorporation without perturbing virus assembly. Interestingly, the block to Env incorporation imposed by MA mutations can be reversed by pseudotyping virions with heterologous Env glycoproteins containing short cytoplasmic tails, or by removing sequences within the long cytoplasmic tail of the HIV-1 TM glycoprotein gp41 (196,197,408). These results imply that a specific interaction takes place between MA and gp41, or that MA has evolved to accommodate the long gp41 cytoplasmic tail. Although a direct interaction has been difficult to demonstrate in virus-infected cells, *in vitro* data supporting an HIV-1 MA–gp41 interaction have been reported (117). A direct interaction is also suggested by the ability of HIV-1 Env to induce basolateral Gag budding in polarized epithelial cells (380), and by the recent finding that a single amino acid substitution in MA reversed the Env incorporation defect imposed by a small deletion near the center of the gp41 cytoplasmic tail (448). X-ray crystallographic analysis of both SIV and HIV-1 MA reveals that MA may form trimers that assemble into a higher-order lattice containing holes into which the long cytoplasmic tail of gp41 could insert (284,516). Although this hypothesis provides an appealing model for Env incorporation that is consistent with mutational analyses, the biologic relevance of MA trimerization is currently unclear.

In addition to its function in virus assembly and Env incorporation, it has also been proposed that MA plays a role early in the virus life cycle after Env-induced membrane fusion. Early postfusion steps, which are collectively referred to as uncoating, are poorly understood, and it is not clear mechanistically how MA functions in this process. Nevertheless, it has been reported that mutations in MA impair the synthesis of viral DNA early postinfection, suggesting an early post-entry block (78,330,690). It has also been observed that MA mutants with this "early" defect display impaired endogenous RT activity and increased Gag membrane binding (330). A correlation between increased MA membrane binding and a post-entry defect is consistent with the hypothesis that an inability of MA to disengage from the lipid bilayer after membrane fusion results in an uncoating defect and destabilization of the subviral complex in which reverse transcription takes place (330).

Lentiviruses, including HIV-1, are unique among retroviruses in their ability to infect nondividing cells. It has been proposed that the basic domain of MA, discussed earlier in the context of membrane binding, plays a role in translocating the viral preintegration complex to the nucleus (63,274,645). It was also reported that phosphorylation of a Tyr residue at the C-terminus of MA is required for infectivity in fully differentiated (nondividing) macrophages (214). However, certain key aspects of these studies have been questioned (62,186,193–195, 520). Currently, it appears that Vpr (see section on Vpr) and perhaps IN (213), but not MA, play the dominant role in transporting the preintegration complex to the nucleus. It has also recently been proposed that a central DNA "flap" that is a product of lentiviral reverse transcription (see section on reverse transcription) may promote nuclear import of the viral preintegration complex (701).

Capsid Domain

Like MA, CA functions in both early and late steps in virus replication. CA is composed of two structural and functional domains: the N-terminal two-thirds of the protein forms the so-called core domain, and the C-terminal one-third is referred to as the dimerization domain (see Fig. 18B). NMR and x-ray crystallographic data are available for both domains (217,237,440), but the structure of the entire protein has not yet been resolved. The core domain (residues 1 to 146) is highly helical, with an exposed, cyclophilin A–binding loop (217, and see later); the C-terminal domain (residues 148 to 231) is also highly helical and globular (218). The N-terminus of the dimerization domain contains the major homology region (MHR) (668), which, apart from the zinc-finger motifs in NC, is the only sequence in Gag that displays significant amino acid identity between divergent retrovirus genera. The structures of the N- and C-terminal domains of CA have been combined to create a hypothetical structure for the intact CA (Fig. 20) (218,674).

Mutations within CA produce a range of phenotypes: Those in the C-terminal, dimerization domain often elicit assembly defects, whereas changes in the N-terminal core domain generally do not affect the efficiency of virus production, but rather can inhibit proper virion maturation after release and severely impair infectivity. These results have led to the proposal that the C-terminus of CA promotes Gag multimerization, whereas the N-terminus plays a role in core condensation and morphogenesis. Mutations in the MHR disrupt virus assembly, maturation, and infectivity. Structural analysis of the dimerization domain revealed that MHR residues form a network of intramolecular hydrogen bonds that stabilize the structure of the entire domain (218). Residues 146 to 151 appear to promote the creation of a high-affinity CA interface, which, in conjunction with a more N-terminal β-hairpin interface, is postulated to drive the formation of higher-order CA interactions during assembly and maturation (218).

Using the yeast two-hybrid system, it was demonstrated that HIV-1 Gag binds members of the cyclophilin family of proteins, which function in the cell as peptidyl-prolyl cis-trans isomerases (389). Further investigation indicated that one of these proteins, cyclophilin A, is specifically incorporated into HIV-1 virions (190,618); this incorporation is mediated by an interaction between cyclophilin A and a Pro-rich region near CA amino acid 90 (190). It is noteworthy that the Gag–cyclophilin A interaction is unique to HIV-1; HIV-2 and SIV Gag proteins neither bind cyclophilins nor incorporate them into virions. Treatment of HIV-1-infected cells with cyclosporin A or its analogs, or mutation of CA residues that participate in the CA–cyclophilin A interaction, block the incorporation of cyclophilin A into virions and reduce virus infectivity. Mutant or drug-treated virions, which

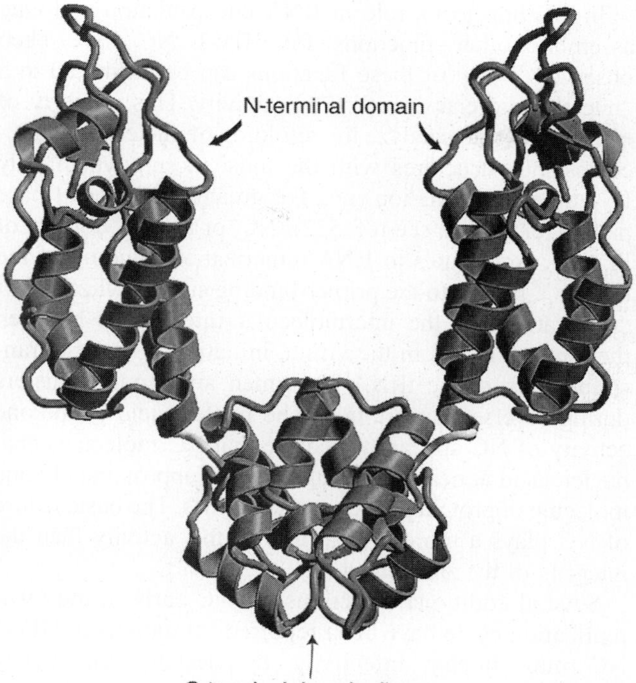

FIG. 20. Model of an HIV-1 CA dimer. The N-terminal core domain is shown at the *top*; the C-terminal dimerization domain is depicted at the *bottom*. The two domains are connected by CA residues 146 and 147. (Reprinted from ref. 674, with permission.)

are impaired for cyclophilin A incorporation, are defective at an early step in the virus life cycle, apparently after membrane fusion but before the initiation of reverse transcription. The mechanism by which cyclophilin A incorporation enhances infectivity is currently unclear. The N-terminal domain of CA forms planar strips between which cyclophilin A intercalates at a Gag-to-cyclophilin A ratio of approximately 10:1; it has been proposed that cyclophilin A might destabilize CA-CA interactions, thereby promoting efficient uncoating after virus entry (217). Alternatively, cyclophilin A in the virion may function as a chaperone during maturation by promoting proper CA refolding and by minimizing unfavorable CA aggregation after Gag processing (250,658).

Several studies have reported that HIV-1 CA, when expressed *in vitro*, is capable of assembling into tubular or spherical particles (157,647). CA-NC fusion proteins form tubes *in vitro* at protein concentrations lower than those required to assemble into similar structures with CA alone; in the case of CA-NC, tube formation appears to depend on the presence of RNA (72). Interestingly, adding as few as four residues of MA to the N-terminus of CA converts *in vitro* particle assembly from tubes to spheres (647). This observation led to the hypothesis that PR-mediated processing at the MA-CA junction causes a major refolding of the CA N-terminus, and that this structural rearrangement plays a key role in promoting the morphologic changes that occur during core condensation. Recently, it was reported that core-like cones can be assembled *in vitro* using CA-NC fusion proteins and RNA; these cones are organized in a manner reminiscent of the fullerene structures formed by elemental carbon (220).

Nucleocapsid Domain

The third major domain synthesized as part of the Gag precursor is the NC (see Fig. 18C). A principal function of NC involves the specific encapsidation of full-length, unspliced (genomic) RNA into virions, although, as is the case with the other Gag proteins, NC serves multiple roles during the virus life cycle. With the exception of the spumaretroviruses, all retroviral NC proteins contain one or two zinc-finger motifs. Unlike most cellular zinc-finger domains, those of retroviruses are of the CCHC type (Cys-X_2-Cys-X_4-His-X_4-Cys). HIV-1 NC contains two zinc-finger motifs, which bind zinc tightly both *in vitro* and in virions (38,591). NMR data indicate that the two HIV-1 NC zinc fingers are brought together into a central globular domain by a highly basic linker domain (see Fig. 18C), which appears to be very flexible (443,608). Mutations that abrogate zinc binding abolish genome encapsidation and virus infectivity. Other mutations within the zinc-finger domains increase the level of spliced versus unspliced viral RNA encapsidated into virions. NC also contains two clusters of basic residues flanking the first zinc finger; mutations in these sequences impair the binding of NC to RNA *in vitro* and RNA encapsidation into virions. NC engages in both sequence-specific and sequence-nonspecific interactions with nucleic acid; in general, the sequence-specific interactions involve the zinc fingers in conjunction with the basic residues, whereas nonspecific interactions are driven largely by the highly basic nature of NC. The specificity of HIV genome encapsidation results from an interaction between NC and an approximately 120-nt sequence located between the 5′ LTR and the Gag initiation codon. This sequence, variously known as the packaging signal, encapsidation element, or ψ-site, folds into a series of four stem-loops (see Fig. 6; for review on RNA encapsidation, see ref. 36). It appears that this secondary structure, rather than the primary nucleotide sequence itself, confers RNA encapsidation specificity. The structure of the HIV-1 NC protein complexed with stem-loop 3 of the ψ-site was determined by NMR spectroscopy (Fig. 21) (130); this structure indicates the involvement of both basic and zinc-finger residues in the NC–ψ interaction. In addition to this specific interaction with the ψ-site, NC may coat the viral RNA in the mature virus particle.

Many HIV-1 NC mutations cause defects in virus assembly and release. This observation suggests a role for NC in Gag multimerization, a function mapping largely to the N-terminal basic domain, rather than the zinc fin-

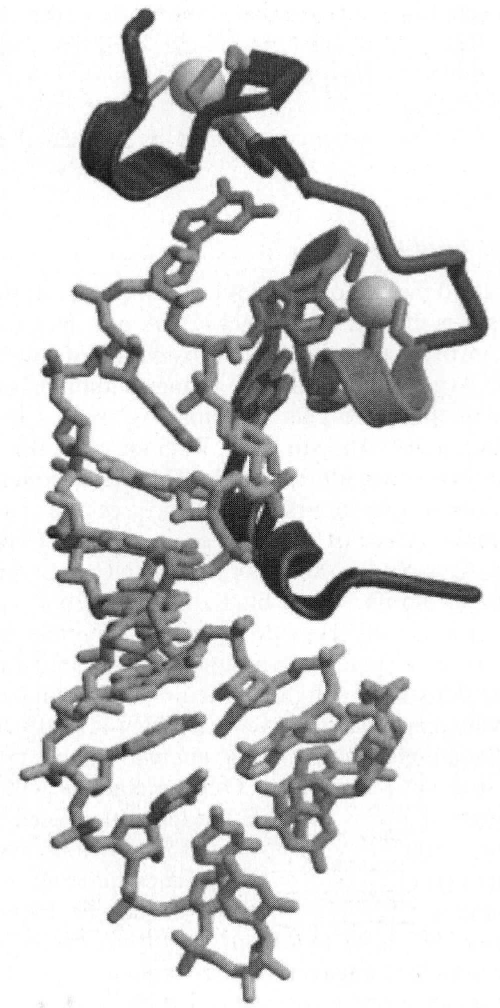

FIG. 21. Complex between NC and stem-loop 3 (SL3) of the HIV-1 packaging signal. The two zinc ions coordinated by the zinc-finger domains are shown as gray balls. (Reprinted from ref. 628, with permission.)

gers. NC appears to play a role in the tight packing of Gag in virions, leading to the production of particles with a density characteristic of retroviral particles (29). It is suspected that NC-RNA interactions are critical for promoting Gag multimerization; according to this model, RNA provides a template along which molecules of Pr55^{Gag} can align and pack. Binding between the NC domain of Pr55^{Gag} and components of the host cell cytoskeleton (F-actin in particular) may also facilitate Gag assembly and transport (376,524,660). It has been proposed that NC plays an important role in binding of HIV-1 Gag to membrane (503,550). However, using membrane flotation centrifugation methods, which effectively distinguish membrane-bound from non-membrane-bound protein, it was determined that a truncated Gag molecule containing only MA and the N-terminal domain of CA exhibited steady-state membrane binding properties comparable to those of Pr55^{Gag} (473).

In addition to its role in RNA encapsidation and Gag assembly, other functions for HIV-1 NC have been observed. Many of these functions can be attributed to a "nucleic acid chaperone" (282) activity. This property of NC enables it to catalyze the refolding of nucleic acid molecules into structures with the most thermodynamically favorable conformation (i.e., the greatest number of base pairs) (for review, see ref. 522). NC, or the NC domain of Pr55^{Gag}, contributes to RNA dimerization, binding of the tRNA^{Lys3} primer to the primer-binding site, stabilization or "maturation" of the intermolecular interactions between the dimeric RNAs in the virion, initiation of reverse transcription from the tRNA^{Lys3} primer, and strand transfers during reverse transcription. The nucleic acid chaperone activity of NC appears to require that NC molecules coat nucleic acid at near-saturating levels of approximately one molecule of protein per seven nucleotides. The basic nature of NC plays a more critical role in this activity than the integrity of the zinc fingers (522).

Several additional functions for NC early in the virus replication cycle have been reported. Mutations in HIV-1 NC may impair infectivity by destabilizing newly reverse-transcribed viral DNA (37). Studies performed with MuLV demonstrated that changing the single CCHC zinc-finger motif to CCCC or CCHH had no effect on zinc binding, tRNA incorporation, RNA encapsidation, or RNA maturation but profoundly impaired virus infectivity (243). Detailed examination of viral DNA in mutant-infected cells revealed that full-length, circular DNA products were formed inefficiently and that a variety of mutations (deletions and insertions) were present at the DNA ends (243). Such aberrations, if present at the ends of linear DNAs, would render these DNAs unsuitable for integration. Similar mutations in the N-terminal zinc finger of the HIV-1 NC have been reported; these changes resulted in defects late in reverse transcription, leading to a lack of circular DNA production (612). It has also been reported that NC stimulates "coupled joining" (wherein both ends of the viral genome integrate into a target DNA) in *in vitro* integration reactions (77) (see section on integrase). Mutations in the NC zinc fingers modulated this stimulatory effect (77).

Because NC participates in multiple steps in the virus life cycle, and because the retroviral CCHC-type zinc-finger motif is relatively rare among cellular proteins, NC presents an attractive target for antivirals. Promising anti-NC compounds attack the sulfurs on the zinc-coordinating Cys residues and cause zinc to be "ejected" from the zinc fingers (526,527). These compounds effectively inhibit virus replication in culture without significant cytotoxicity. Fourteen compounds that demonstrated anti-NC activity *in vitro* were tested for their effect on MuLV replication *in vivo*. One of these compounds, Aldrithiol-2 (2,2′-dithiopyridine), delayed the onset of MuLV-induced disease and reduced virus loads in infected mice (480). Such compounds could also in theory be used to render stocks of HIV particles noninfectious for use in vaccine studies (538).

p6 Protein

In addition to the MA, CA, and NC proteins, retroviral *gag* genes encode a variety of additional ORFs that are generally unique to a particular genus of retrovirus (for review, see ref. 668). HIV-1 encodes a Pro-rich, 6-kd protein, known as p6, at the C-terminus of $Pr55^{Gag}$ (see Fig. 18D). Mutation of p6, specifically within a highly conserved Pro-Thr-Ala-Pro (PTAP) motif, blocks a late step in virus assembly such that virions accumulate at the plasma membrane but fail to release efficiently (248,293). Interestingly, mutation of PR largely reverses this defect (293), suggesting a functional interplay between p6 and PR function, and perhaps explaining why some groups, using Gag-only expression systems, failed to detect a requirement for p6 in virus production. p6 also functions to direct the incorporation of Vpr and Vpx into virions (494,678).

In addition to HIV-1 p6, domains encoded by other retroviral Gag proteins serve analogous "late" roles in virus release. These include p2b of Rous sarcoma virus (667), pp16 of MPMV (685), p9 of equine infectious anemia virus (EIAV) (511), and p12 MuLV (693). Interestingly, at least in certain cases, these late domains can function independently of their position in Gag and can be exchanged from one retrovirus to another (488). These late domain proteins all contain motifs that have been implicated in protein–protein interactions: Pro-X-X-Pro in HIV-1 p6; Pro-Pro-Pro-Tyr in RSV p2b, MPMV pp16, and MuLV p12; and Tyr-X-X-Leu in EIAV p9 (228). It has been proposed that these proteins interact with host cell plasma membrane proteins to facilitate the final release step during virus budding (228). Indeed, p2b of RSV binds proteins containing so-called WW motifs (228), and EIAV p9 has been reported to interact with the AP-2 adapter protein complex (512). Recent evidence implicates the host ubiquitination machinery in the function of retroviral late domains (642a).

Pol

Downstream of *gag* lies the most highly conserved region of the HIV genome, the *pol* gene, which encodes three enzymes: PR, RT, and IN (see Fig. 5). RT and IN are required, respectively, for reverse transcription of the viral RNA genome to a double-stranded DNA copy, and for the integration of the viral DNA into the host cell chromosome. PR plays a critical role late in the life cycle by mediating the production of mature, infectious virions. The *pol* gene products are derived by enzymatic cleavage of a 160-kd Gag-Pol fusion protein, referred to as $Pr160^{Gag\text{-}Pol}$. This fusion protein is produced by ribosomal frameshifting during translation of $Pr55^{Gag}$ (see Figs. 5 and 6C). The frame-shifting mechanism for Gag-Pol expression, also utilized by many other retroviruses, ensures that the *pol*-derived proteins are expressed at a low level, approximately 5% to 10% that of Gag. Like $Pr55^{Gag}$, the N-terminus of $Pr160^{Gag\text{-}Pol}$ is myristylated and targeted to the plasma membrane.

Protease

Early pulse-chase studies performed with avian retroviruses clearly indicated that retroviral Gag proteins are initially synthesized as polyprotein precursors that are cleaved to generate smaller products (643,644). Subsequent studies demonstrated that the processing function is provided by a viral rather than a cellular enzyme, and that proteolytic digestion of the Gag and Gag-Pol precursors is essential for virus infectivity (120,323). Sequence analysis of retroviral PRs indicated that they are related to cellular "aspartic" proteases such as pepsin and renin (for review, see ref. 126). Like these cellular enzymes, retroviral PRs use two apposed Asp residues at the active site to coordinate a water molecule that catalyzes the hydrolysis of a peptide bond in the target protein. Unlike the cellular aspartic proteases, which function as pseudodimers (using two folds within the same molecule to generate the active site), retroviral PRs function as true dimers. X-ray crystallographic data from HIV-1 PR (352,458,671) indicate that the two monomers are held together in part by a four-stranded antiparallel β-sheet derived from both N- and C-terminal ends of each monomer (Fig. 22). The substrate binding site is located within a cleft formed between the two monomers. Like their cellular homologs, the HIV PR dimer contains flexible "flaps" that overhang the binding site and may stabilize the substrate within the cleft; the active-site Asp residues lie in the center of the dimer. Interestingly, although some limited amino acid homology is observed surrounding active-site residues, the primary sequences of retroviral PRs are highly divergent, yet their structures are remarkably similar.

The first cleavage events catalyzed by retroviral PRs during or immediately after virion release from the cell serve to liberate PR from the Gag-Pol precursor. It is still unclear whether this initial cleavage event takes place in cis (intramolecularly) or in trans (intermolecularly); in either case, following the release of PR from the Gag-Pol precursor, the dimeric enzyme cleaves a number of sites in both Gag and Gag-Pol (see Fig. 5). The efficiency with which PR cleaves the individual target sites in Gag and Gag-Pol varies widely and is influenced by two major factors: the amino acid sequence at the site of cleavage, and the context (i.e., the degree of exposure or accessibility) of the cleavage site. The proteolytic processing of model proteins and substrate analogs by the HIV-1 PR indicates that the binding cleft can accommodate a peptide of approximately seven residues in length, and synthetic peptides of this size are cleaved *in vitro* (40).

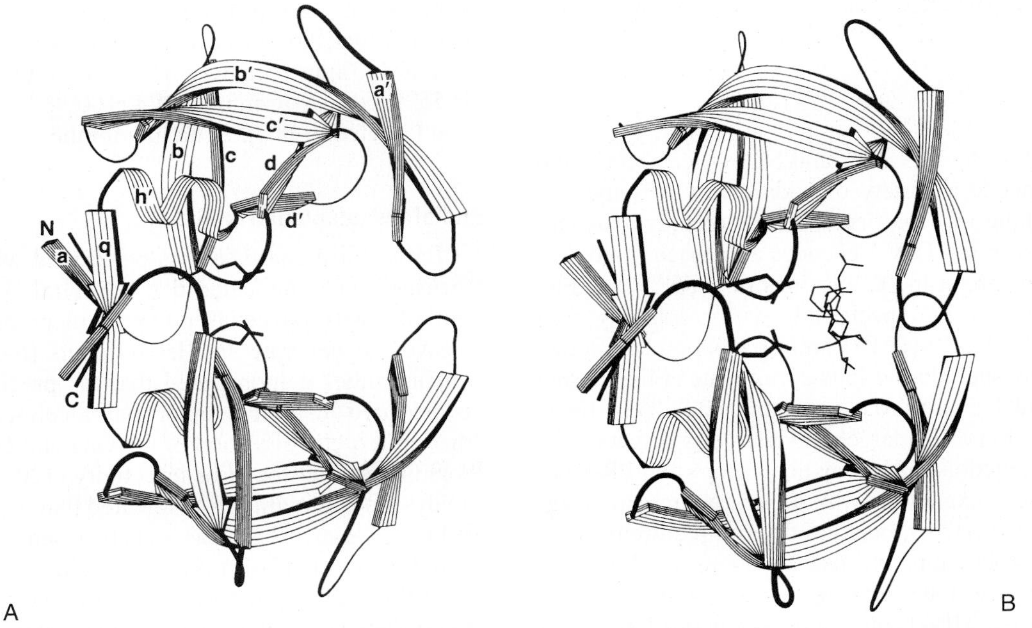

FIG. 22. Structure of the HIV-1 PR dimer uncomplexed (**A**) or complexed (**B**) with the PR inhibitor Ro-31-8558. The following domains are indicated in the first half of the molecule: β-strands *a* (residues 1 to 4), *b* (residues 9 to 15), *c*, and *d* (residues 30 to 35). The active-site residues are at positions 25 to 27. The second half of the molecule is structurally related to the first half, with the following domains indicated: β-strands *a′* (residues 43 to 49), *b′* (residues 52 to 66), *c′* (69 to 78), *d′* (83 to 85), and helix *h′* (86 to 94). The inner portion of the dimer interface is formed by β-strand *q* (residues 95 to 99). (Reprinted from ref. 670, with permission.)

Although a number of studies have attempted to define a consensus target sequence for HIV-1 PR, the rules governing which sites can be cleaved are fairly loose. As a consequence of the relatively divergent PR target sequences present in Gag, and the varying efficiencies with which these sites serve as substrates for PR activity, Gag cleavage takes place as an ordered, step-wise cascade. Processing at the amino terminus of NC is the most rapid *in vitro*, whereas the cleavage converting p25 to p24 CA is the slowest. Mutations in Gag that disrupt the ordered nature of PR-mediated processing severely disrupt virus assembly or subsequent maturation. Furthermore, HIV-1 mutants engineered to synthesize a linked PR dimer (i.e., a duplicated PR-coding region) exhibit rapid, premature processing of Gag and Gag-Pol polyproteins and a block in virus production (349).

PR appears to be most active during the budding process just prior to particle release from the cell (320). PR cleavage of the Gag and Gag-Pol precursors leads to a dramatic change in virion morphology, a process known as maturation. Immature retroviral particles (for example, those produced in the presence of PR inhibitors or an inactive PR) appear doughnut-shaped by EM. In contrast, mature virions contain condensed cores, which in the case of the lentiviruses are cone-shaped (Fig. 1A). Cryo-EM studies have suggested that in immature virions, Gag precursors are aligned in a rodlike fashion like spokes on a wheel, with the N-terminal MA domain associated with the viral lipid and the C-terminus projecting inwards toward the center of the virion (208,686). According to this model, cleavage of Gag by PR releases CA, NC, and p6 from their attachment (via MA) to the lipid and allows CA to form a shell around the NC–RNA complex. One would predict that numerous conformational changes take place within the Gag proteins upon cleavage that allow this structural reorganization to take place. In one case, a major, cleavage-induced refolding has been characterized (see section on CA); however, much remains to be learned about the molecular details of core condensation.

It is clear that premature Gag and Gag-Pol cleavage is severely detrimental to virus assembly. Thus, the activation of PR must be tightly controlled to prevent significant processing prior to the completion of assembly. It is not yet understood how premature PR activation is prevented. One model proposes that the concentration of Gag and Gag-Pol precursor proteins plays the key role in PR activation; sufficiently high concentrations are not achieved until assembly has taken place. This model fails to account for the fact that type B/D retroviruses assemble in the cytoplasm, yet the particles that form maintain an unprocessed, immature state until budding and release have occurred. It has also been suggested that the plasma membrane may provide an environment uniquely compatible with Gag/Gag-Pol processing and virion maturation. However, MA mutations have been described that redirect assembly to the Golgi apparatus or Golgi-derived vesicles; the resulting redirected virus particles can undergo Gag processing and maturation at the intracellular site (202,476). In the case of HIV-1 PR, but not all retroviral PRs, some Gag cleavage can occur in the absence of membrane binding. This point is illustrated by the observation that mutations that block Gag myristylation, and consequently impair membrane binding, do not fully block Gag processing (249). The assembly of high-molecular-weight Gag complexes in the absence of, or prior to, membrane binding (360) suggests that processing of non-membrane-bound Gag may still take place within a large, multimeric Gag/Gag-Pol complex.

HIV-1 PR activity is not limited to cleavage of the Gag and Gag-Pol precursors. Nef is a substrate for PR cleavage, although the implications for Nef function remain unclear (see section on Nef). The cytoplasmic domains of some retroviral Env proteins (e.g., MuLV and MPMV) are also cleaved by PR; in such cases, the cleavage event is essential for Env function (515,523,590). Although no evidence exists that HIV PR cleaves the cytoplasmic tail of gp41, it efficiently cleaves the cytoplasmic domain of the MuLV TM Env protein in HIV-1 virions pseudotyped by MuLV Env (329). The finding that PR-mediated processing of the MuLV TM can be blocked by HIV-1 MA mutations (329) has implications for the use of HIV-based vectors pseudotyped with MuLV Env. In addition to cleavage of viral proteins, PR has been reported to act on a number of cellular proteins (for review, see ref. 642). The role of such events in virus replication and virus-induced cytotoxicity has not been fully elucidated.

Compounds that inhibit HIV-1 PR function have proven to be the most effective antiviral drugs presently available. The development of PR inhibitors represents a classic example of structure-based drug design; detailed knowledge of the topology of the substrate binding site, the enzyme–substrate interaction, and the chemistry of the cleavage reaction enabled investigators to synthesize a large number of inhibitors that potently inhibit PR in culture at nanomolar concentrations. The earliest PR inhibitors were small oligopeptide derivatives that mimicked PR target sequences but contained nonhydrolizable groups (e.g., hydroxyethylenes, hydroxyethylamines, and dihydroxyethylenes) at the P1 and P1′ positions flanking the scissile bond that PR would normally cleave. The early, peptide-based inhibitors were subsequently modified to improve stability and bioavailability, and the structure of the PR active site was used to design novel inhibitory compounds (670). When PR inhibitors are used to treat HIV-infected patients, virus loads decline precipitously, but drug-resistant variants soon emerge. Sequencing of the PR coding region of drug-resistant variants often reveals consistent changes. For example, saquinavir escape mutants frequently contain changes at PR residue 48 and/or 90 (308); ritonavir resistance is often associated with mutations at PR residue 82 (439). The initial changes that confer drug resistance generally result in only partial resistance and may be accompanied by decreased "fitness" (i.e., impaired PR function relative to wild type in the absence of drug) (121). With time, however, additional changes take place within PR that increase resistance and improve fitness. The same secondary mutations are often observed during escape from different PR inhibitors; these changes increase resistance and allow adaptation to the original drug-resistance-conferring mutation. Unfortunately, mutations that arise in the presence of one inhibitor frequently induce at least partial resistance to others (113), a phenomenon known as cross-resistance. In addition to changes in PR, mutations that affect the natural PR targets (i.e., the Gag and Pol cleavage sites) have also been observed (149). Whereas monotherapy with PR inhibitors generally leads to rapid resistance, longer-lasting benefits are achieved with so-called triple therapy (also known as highly active antiretroviral therapy, or HAART), in which a PR inhibitor (e.g., indinavir or saquinavir) is combined with two RT inhibitors (e.g., AZT and 3TC).

Reverse Transcriptase

By definition, retroviruses possess the ability to convert their single-stranded RNA genomes into double-stranded DNA during the early stages of the infection process (20,615). The enzyme that catalyzes this reaction is RT, in conjunction with its associated RNaseH activity. Retroviral RTs have three enzymatic activities: (a) RNA-directed DNA polymerization (for minus-strand DNA synthesis), (b) RNaseH activity (for the degradation of the tRNA primer and genomic RNA present in DNA–RNA hybrid intermediates), and (c) DNA-directed DNA polymerization (for second- or plus-strand DNA synthesis).

The retroviral genome is packaged in the virion as two copies of single-stranded RNA. The two RNAs, which are identical or at least highly homologous, are held together in part by a sequence near their 5′ ends known as the dimer initiation signal (see Fig. 6). Although each retroviral particle carries two strands of RNA, it appears that only one provirus is formed per virion (291). Retroviruses are therefore referred to as pseudodiploid. As with other DNA polymerase reactions, reverse transcription is dependent on the 3′-OH group of a primer to initiate polymerization. Retroviruses employ specific tRNAs for this function—$tRNA^{Lys3}$ in the case of HIV-1. The mechanism of tRNA selection and placement on the template is complex, involving interactions with RT and NC as well as with the 18-nt pbs near the 5′ end of the viral genome. Although the interaction between $tRNA^{Lys3}$ and the HIV-1 genomic RNA involves primarily the tRNA 3′ end and the pbs, more extensive base pairing between these two RNAs has been proposed (301).

Reverse transcription of the retroviral RNA genome to a double-stranded DNA copy proceeds via a series of steps that are outlined briefly later. (For a more detailed description of this process, refer to recent reviews in refs. 246 and 613; and see Chapter 27.)

1. Minus-strand DNA synthesis is initiated from the 3′-OH of the tRNA bound to the pbs. DNA synthesis then proceeds to the 5′ end of the genome.

2. RNaseH digests the RNA portion of the newly formed RNA/DNA hybrid, releasing the resulting short, single-stranded DNA fragment (known as the minus-strand strong-stop DNA).

3. The minus-strand strong-stop DNA is transferred to the 3′ end of the genome where it hybridizes by virtue of a short region of homology (the "repeated" or R region) present at both 5′ and 3′ ends of the RNA genome. Whether this first strand transfer is intermolecular, intramolecular, or both has been the subject of some debate.

4. Minus-strand synthesis, accompanied by partial degradation of the RNA in the resulting RNA–DNA hybrid by RNaseH, continues to the pbs at the 5′ end of the genome.

5. Fragments of RNA that were not removed by RNaseH serve as primers for plus-strand synthesis. The major site of such priming occurs at the PPT; however, residual RNA fragments that remain hybridized to regions outside the PPT can also be used for priming plus-strand synthesis. In the case of HIV-1, one such region, known as the central PPT, appears to be particularly important in this regard (81).

6. RNaseH removes the tRNA that initially served as the primer for minus-strand synthesis. This exposes the pbs at the 3′ end of the plus-strand DNA, allowing the plus-strand DNA to transfer (this is the second-strand transfer) and hybridize with the homologous region at the 3′ end of the minus-strand DNA.

7. Plus- and minus-strand syntheses proceed to completion. Plus-strand synthesis terminates at the end of the minus strand and, for HIV, at a sequence known as the central termination signal (CTS) (82). The position of the central PPT upstream of the CTS results in the displacement of approximately 100 nt of plus-strand DNA and the formation of a triplex DNA structure. Interestingly, it has been suggested recently that this triplex, or "flap" structure may play a role in nuclear import of the viral preintegration complex (701). The final product of reverse transcription is a double-stranded DNA molecule capable of serving as the substrate for integration. Some discontinuities may remain in the final product; these can be resolved following integration (436).

In addition to serving an essential function in the virus life cycle, the enzymatic activity of RT is routinely used in the laboratory to quantitatively monitor levels of virus present in the supernate of infected cultures and to elucidate details of replication at the molecular level. Two types of assays are most commonly employed to measure RT activity. In the "exogenous" assay, virions are disrupted with detergent and the presence of RT is detected by its ability to extend a short oligonucleotide primer (e.g., oligo-dT) using an exogenously provided template [e.g., poly-r(A)] and a radiolabeled deoxynucleoside triphosphate (dNTP) (e.g., α-[^{32}P]TTP). In the "endogenous" reaction, virions are gently disrupted with a mild detergent treatment and provided with dNTPs (one of which is generally radiolabeled), and RT activity is monitored using the viral RNA genome as a template. Depending on the assay conditions, endogenous reactions result in the synthesis of discreet reverse transcription products (e.g., minus-strand strong-stop DNA) or a continuum of DNA species. The endogenous assay is less efficient than the exogenous assay, but because it measures the activity of RT in a relatively native complex, it more closely mimics the conditions of reverse transcription in an infected cell. These assays monitor RT activity in a cell-free setting. Although a limited amount of reverse transcription can take place in the virion under physiologic conditions (382,626), the overwhelming majority of DNA synthesis does not occur until after entry into the target cell. Thus, the detection of postinfection viral DNA synthesis by polymerase chain reaction (PCR) provides the most reliable method for detecting entry and post-entry steps in the virus replication cycle. As mentioned elsewhere in this chapter, PCR amplification of viral DNA after infection has been used extensively to study defects imposed by mutations in Gag, Env, and accessory proteins.

The mature HIV-1 RT holoenzyme is a heterodimer of 66 and 51 kd subunits. The 51-kd subunit (p51) is derived from the 66-kd (p66) subunit by proteolytic removal of the C-terminal 15-kd RNaseH domain of p66 by PR (see Fig. 5). The structure of HIV-1 RT has been determined by x-ray crystallography in a number of studies. The enzyme was crystallized in several contexts: (a) complexed with the nonnucleoside inhibitor nevirapine (340), (b) bound to a short DNA duplex and the Fab portion of an anti-RT antibody (11,306,307), (c) unbound to DNA or inhibitor (165,532), and, most recently, (d) covalently linked to a complex of primer/template, and dNTP (292). The crystal structure of HIV-1 RT reveals a highly asymmetric folding in which the orientations of the p66 and p51 subunits differ substantially. The p66 subunit can be visualized as a right hand, with the polymerase active site within the palm, and a deep template-binding cleft formed by the palm, fingers, and thumb subdomains (11,307) (Fig. 23). The polymerase domain is linked to RNaseH by the connection subdomain. The active site, located in the palm, contains three critical Asp residues (110, 185, and 186) in close proximity, and two coordinated Mg^{2+} ions (Fig. 24). Mutation of these Asp residues abolishes RT polymerizing activity. The orientation of the three active-site Asp residues is similar to that observed in other DNA polymerases (e.g., the Klenow fragment of

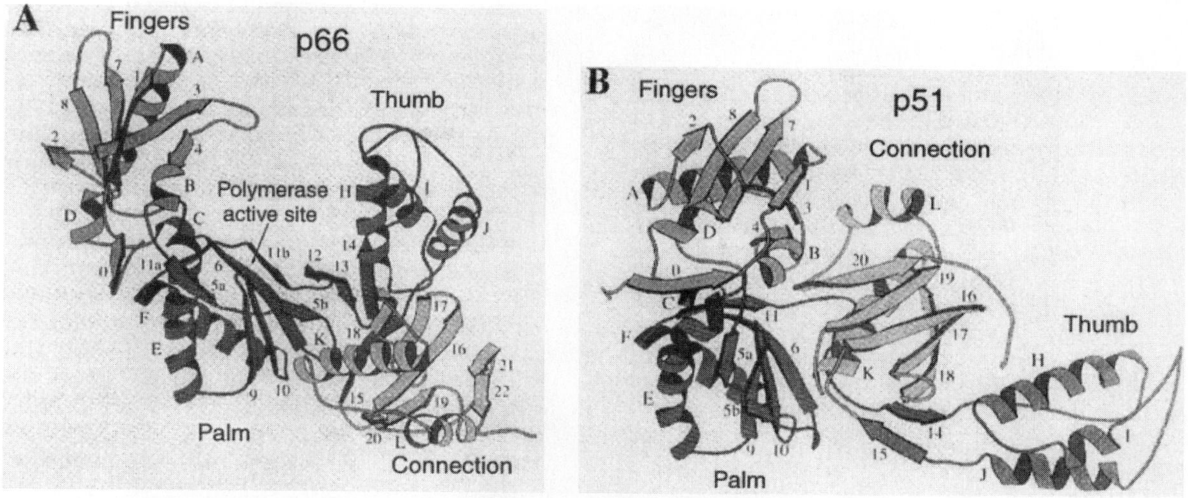

FIG. 23. Ribbon diagrams of the p66 (**A**) and p51 (**B**) RT subunits. Fingers, palm, thumb, and connection domains are shown. (Reprinted from ref. 307, with permission.)

E. coli DNA polI) (10). The p51 subunit appears to be rigid and does not form a polymerizing cleft; Asp 110, 185, and 186 of this subunit are buried within the molecule. Approximately 18 base pairs of the primer–template duplex lie in the nucleic acid binding cleft, stretching from the polymerase active site to the RNaseH domain.

In the RT-primer–template-dNTP structure (292) (see Fig. 24), the presence of a dideoxynucleotide at the 3′ end of the primer allows visualization of the catalytic complex trapped just prior to attack on the incoming dNTP. This structure has been particularly informative regarding the orientation of RT with respect to the primer–template, and the location of mutations that confer resistance to RT inhibitors (see later). Comparison with previously obtained structures (see, e.g., ref. 307) suggests a model whereby the fingers close in to trap the template and dNTP prior to nucleophilic attack of the 3′-OH of the primer on the incoming dNTP. After the addition of the incoming dNTP to the growing chain, it has been proposed that the fingers adopt a more open configuration, thereby releasing the pyrophosphate and enabling RT to bind the next dNTP (292). The structure of the HIV-1 RNaseH has also been determined by x-ray crystallography; this domain displays a global folding similar to that of *E. coli* RNase H (127).

The high rate of variation among HIV populations poses one of the fundamental challenges to effectively controlling this pathogen (for reviews, see refs. 412, 491, and 509). Variation in a retroviral population is influenced by several factors, including the mutation rate per replication cycle, the replication rate (i.e., number of cycles of virus replication per unit time) and the fixation rate (determined by the selective advantage or disadvantage conferred by a particular mutation) (104,105). High mutation rates are largely a consequence of the error-prone nature of RT, which lacks an exonucleolytic proofreading activity, and frequent template switching during reverse transcription (614). Cell-free error rates for purified RTs have been determined (24,510,530), as have *in vivo* retrovirus mutation rates (147,413,492,493). The cell-free error rate measured for HIV-1 RT is more than 10-fold higher than the mutation rate, suggesting that the *in vitro* reaction lacks factor(s) that increase fidelity (413). The total HIV-1 *in vivo* mutation rate (a composite of substitutions, frameshifts, simple deletions, and deletions with insertions) was measured at 3×10^{-5} per cycle of replication (413). Using similar methods, *in vivo* mutation rates of other retroviruses (e.g., spleen necrosis virus, MuLV, and BLV) were observed to be between 2-fold and 10-fold lower than that of HIV-1 (412).

As discussed earlier, retroviral particles contain two copies of single-stranded RNA. The requirement for template switching during reverse transcription appears to have selected for a low affinity between RT and template (614). As a result, template switches occur frequently during reverse transcription (491). Intramolecular jumps lead to mutations (e.g., deletions, insertions, and duplications), whereas intermolecular jumps generate recombinants.

Two general models have been suggested to explain recombination during reverse transcription. The first, which is operative during minus-strand synthesis, is referred as forced copy-choice (103). The second, which applies during plus-strand synthesis, has been named strand displacement-assimilation (317). The forced copy-choice model proposes that when RT encounters a break in the template RNA it jumps to the copackaged RNA and resumes DNA synthesis. This model has been refined more recently with the suggestion that jumps during minus-strand synthesis can occur in the absence of strand

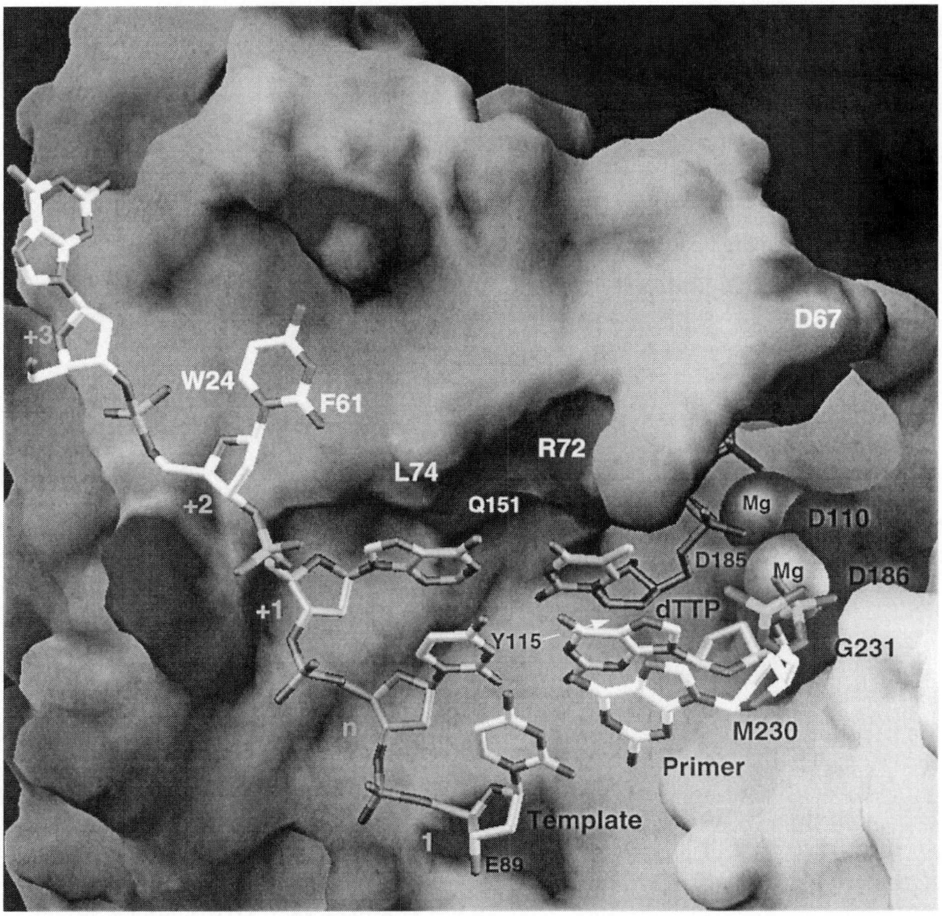

FIG. 24. Active site of a covalently trapped HIV-1 RT catalytic complex. The deoxynucleoside triphosphate (dNTP) pocket is presented, with fingers at the *upper left*, palm in the *center*, and thumb at the *lower right.* The triphosphate of the incoming dNTP is coordinated by residues 65, 72, 113, and 114, and two Mg^{+2} ions. The three active-site Asp residues (110, 185, and 186) are shown. A dideoxynucleotide chain terminator at the 3′ end of the primer traps the complex prior to attack of the incoming dNTP. (Reprinted from ref. 292, with permission.)

breaks (315). According to the strand displacement-assimilation model, the recombination process begins with the displacement of one fragment of internally initiated plus-strand DNA by another plus-strand transcript. The displaced fragment then binds, at a transient gap, to the complementary region of the minus-strand DNA derived from reverse transcription of the copackaged RNA. This intermediate is then resolved, most likely by cellular enzymes, to generate a recombinant double-stranded DNA copy of the viral genome (317). The impact of high rates of recombination on HIV populations is substantial; as noted earlier, 5% to 10% of sequenced virus isolates have been reported to be intersubtype recombinants (531), and recombinants comprise the predominant strains currently circulating in certain parts of the world. Recombination also provides a mechanism for the rapid generation of multiple-drug-resistant HIV variants. It should be noted that rates of mutation and recombination during reverse transcription can be affected by a variety of viral and cellular factors. Imbalances in the dNTP pools in the infected cell can increase the rate of mutation and template switching (316,421,634), and the fidelity of reverse transcription and frequency of recombination can be influenced by the composition of the large macromolecular complex in which reverse transcription takes place. For example, it has been reported that Vpr increases fidelity (411) and that NC promotes recombination (459).

RT has long been a target in the search for antiviral compounds. A number of RT inhibitors have been developed, including the nucleoside analogs [e.g., 3′-azido-3′-deoxythymidine (AZT or zidovudine), 2′-deoxy-3′-thiacytidine (3TC or lamivudine), 2′,3′-dideoxyinosine (ddI or didanosine), and 2′,3′-dideoxycytidine (ddC or zalcitabine)] and the nonnucleoside inhibitors (e.g., nevirapine and delavirdine). The nucleoside analogs act as chain terminators, whereas the nonnucleoside compounds inhibit DNA polymerization by binding a small hydrophobic pocket near the RT active site, thereby inducing an allosteric change at the active site (340). Unfortunately, resistance to these compounds develops rapidly in patients, probably reflecting the fact that resistant variants exist even before the initiation of therapy (105). As is the case for mutations that allow escape from PR inhibitors (see earlier), some changes in RT provide drug resistance whereas others appear to be adaptations to resistance-conferring mutations or function to increase levels of drug resistance. Analysis of the location of resistance mutations in the RT structure has provided important insights into the mechanism of resistance and should be useful in designing additional inhibitors that delay the appearance of escape mutants or effectively combat drug-resistant strains.

Integrase

A distinguishing feature of retrovirus replication is the insertion of a DNA copy of the viral genome into the host cell chromosome following reverse transcription. The integrated viral DNA (the provirus) serves as the template for the synthesis of viral RNAs and is maintained as part of the host cell genome for the lifetime of the infected cell. Retroviral mutants deficient in the ability to integrate generally fail to establish a productive infection.

The integration of viral DNA is catalyzed by integrase, a 32-kd protein generated by PR-mediated cleavage of the C-terminal portion of the HIV-1 Gag-Pol polyprotein (see Fig. 5). The steps in the integration process were originally elucidated in studies using MuLV (59,206), but these findings apply to HIV as well. In all retroviral systems, integration proceeds in the same series of steps (Fig. 25):

1. IN removes two to three nucleotides from the initially blunt 3′ termini of both strands of full-length, linear viral DNA, generating a preintegration substrate with 3′-recessed ends (3′-end processing). This reaction can take place in the cytoplasm of the infected cell.
2. In the nucleus, IN catalyzes a staggered cleavage of the cellular target. Selection of the host DNA target site by IN is essentially sequence independent. The 3′ recessed ends of viral DNA are joined to the 5′ "overhanging" termini of the cleaved cellular DNA (strand transfer).
3. Cellular repair machinery, perhaps in conjunction with IN, fills the gaps, thereby completing the integration process (59,206,539). The integrated HIV provirus is flanked by a 5-bp direct repeat and terminates with the dinucleotides 5′-TG and CA-3′. The direct repeat results from the duplication of cellular target sequences.

Our understanding of the chemistry of the retroviral integration reaction has been greatly assisted by the development of *in vitro* integration assays. Purified IN, expressed in *E. coli*, can carry out 3′-end processing and strand transfer reactions *in vitro* when combined with short synthetic oligonucleotides that mimic the viral DNA ends and a divalent metal ion (Mg^{2+} or Mn^{2+}) (119,324). Using such systems, IN also catalyzes a reaction, known as disintegration, which in essence is the strand transfer reaction in reverse (93). The predominant product in *in vitro* assays using purified HIV-1 IN is a single end joined to one strand of the target, rather than the more physiologically relevant product in which both ends are integrated into the target. To obtain the integration of both ends with high efficiency requires additional proteins as part of a high-molecular-weight complex (see later), or, at a minimum, the presence of NC (77).

Retroviral IN proteins are composed of three structurally and functionally distinct domains: an N-terminal, zinc-finger-containing domain, a core domain, and a relatively nonconserved C-terminal domain (Fig. 26). Because of its low solubility, it has not yet been possible to crystallize the entire 288-amino-acid HIV-1 IN protein. However, the structure of all three domains has been solved independently by x-ray crystallography or NMR methods. The crystal structure of the core domain of the avian sarcoma virus IN has also been determined (60). The N-terminal domain (residues 1 to 55), whose structure was solved by NMR spectroscopy (68), is composed of four helices with a zinc coordinated by amino acids His-12, His-16, Cys-40, and Cys-43. The structure of the N-terminal domain is reminiscent of helical DNA binding proteins that contain a so-called helix-turn-helix motif; however, in the HIV-1 structure this motif contributes to dimer formation. Initially, poor solubility hampered efforts to solve the structure of the core domain. However, attempts at crystallography were successful (153) when it was observed that a Phe-to-Lys change at IN residue 185 greatly increased solubility without disrupting *in vitro* catalytic activity. Each monomer of the HIV-1 IN core domain (IN residues 50 to 212) is composed of a five-stranded β-sheet flanked by helices; this structure bears striking resemblance to other polynucleotidyl transferases including RNaseH and the bacteriophage MuA transposase (153,525). Three highly conserved residues are found in analogous positions in other polynucleotidyl transferases; in HIV-1 IN these are Asp-64, Asp-116 and Glu-152, the so-called D,D-35-E motif (see Fig. 26). Mutations at these positions block HIV IN function both *in vivo* and *in vitro*. The close proximity of these three amino acids in the crystal structure of both avian sarcoma virus (60) and HIV-1 (153) core domains supports the hypothesis that these residues play a central role in catalysis of the polynucleotidyl transfer reaction that is at the heart of the integration process. The C-terminal domain, whose structure has been solved by NMR methods (158,381), adopts a five-stranded β-barrel folding topology reminiscent of a Src homology 3 (SH3) domain. Recently, the x-ray structures of SIV and Rous sarcoma virus IN protein fragments encompassing both the core and C-terminal domains have been solved (89,683).

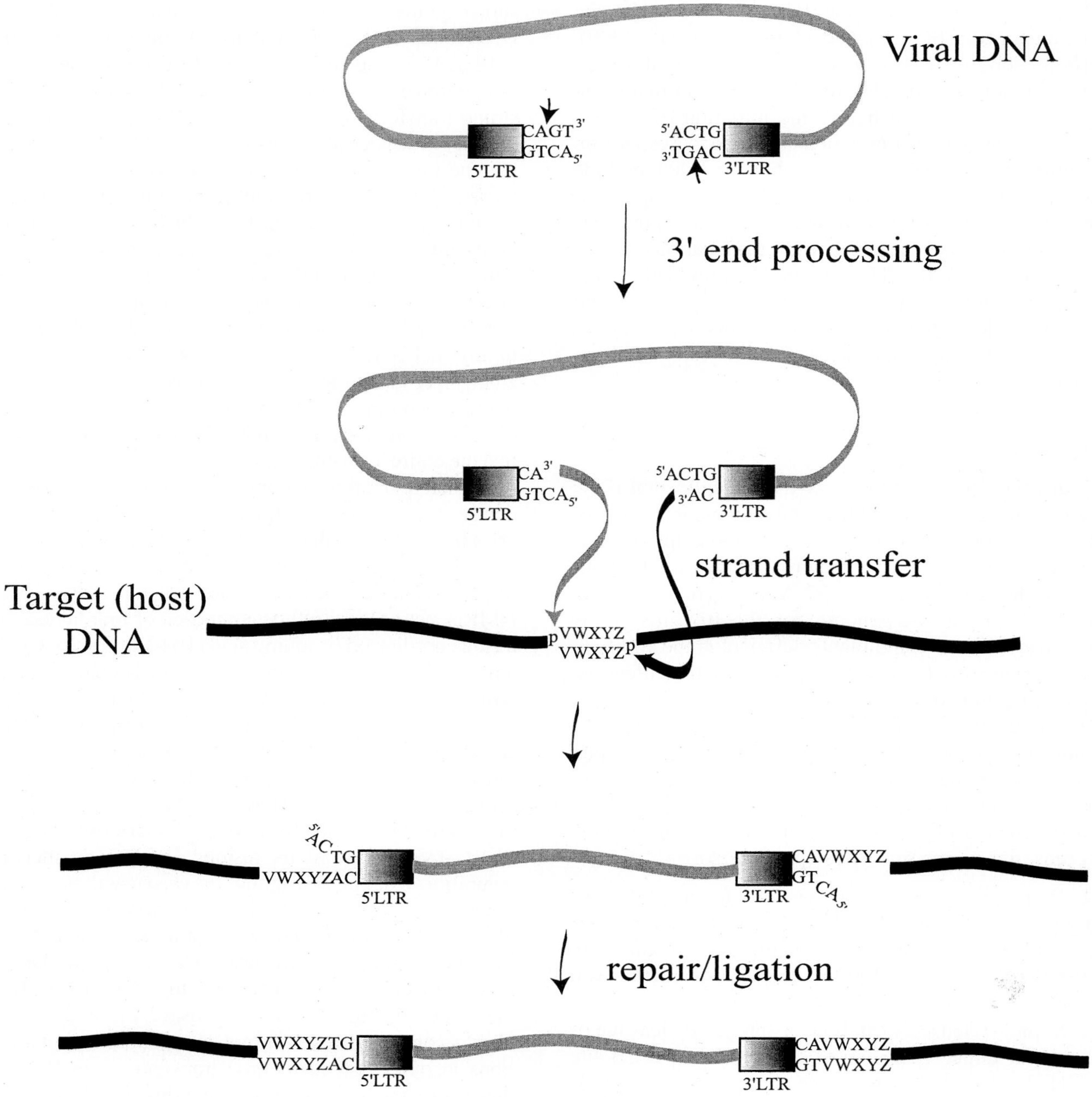

FIG. 25. Schematic depiction of the integration process. Details are provided in the text.

Although it is clear that the core domain of IN plays the central role in catalysis, the functions of the N-terminal and C-terminal domains are less clear. The core domain alone can catalyze the disintegration reaction (66); however, the finding that mutations in the zinc-finger domain disrupt IN tetramerization and catalytic activity suggest a role for this region in stabilizing overall IN structure and promoting the formation of higher-order IN multimers (705). The C-terminal domain is required for both 3′-end processing and integration reactions. Unlike the core domain, which binds DNA only in the presence of a divalent metal ion, the C-terminal domain exhibits strong, and nonspecific, DNA binding even in the absence of metal ion (162). The non-sequence-specific nucleic acid binding properties of the C-terminal domain has led to the suggestion that this region of IN may contribute to the ability of IN to remain associated with the viral genome during reverse transcription (57). It has also been proposed that basic sequences near the junction of the core and C-terminal domains of IN contribute to the nuclear import of the viral preintegration complex (213) (see later).

During reverse transcription and transport of viral DNA to the nucleus, the viral nucleic acid remains asso-

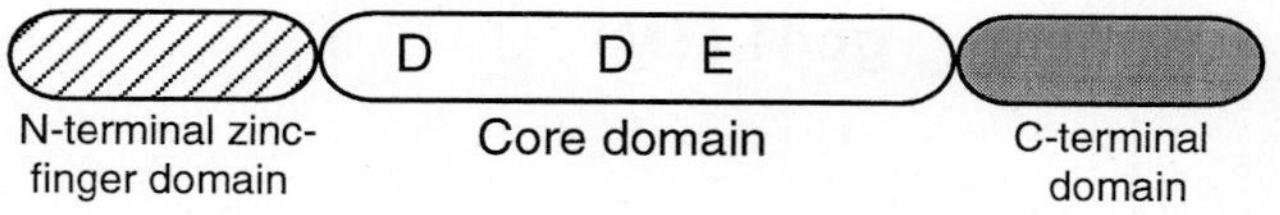

FIG. 26. Schematic representation of an IN monomer. The three structural domains are shown. The catalytic triad of Asp-64, Asp-116, and Glu-152 is represented as D-D-E.

ciated with a high-molecular-weight PIC composed of both viral and cellular proteins (51,58). Lentiviruses are unique among retroviruses in that the host cell does not have to pass through mitosis for productive infection to occur. The lentiviral PIC must therefore contain determinants that facilitate its transport to, and across, the nuclear membrane. As mentioned earlier, although purified IN can catalyze single-ended integration *in vitro*, such events would be dead-end reactions in an infected cell and would fail to produce an integrated provirus. Additional viral proteins are required for the concerted two-ended reactions *in vitro* that mimic the physiologic integration process. In addition to RT and IN, MA, Vpr, and NC have been reported to be present in HIV-1 PICs, whereas CA is absent (64,214,215). The nonhistone chromosomal protein HMG I(Y) also cofractionates with HIV-1 PICs (171) and the human homolog of the yeast protein SNF5 (referred to as IN interactor 1, or INI1) stimulates HIV-1 IN activity *in vitro* (318). The latter protein, which functions as a transcriptional activator, was postulated to promote integration by targeting viral DNA to transcriptionally active regions of the host chromosome (318). Of particular interest is a host-derived protein that prevents suicidal autointegration events (i.e., reactions in which the DNA ends integrate into internal sites within the same viral DNA molecule). This so-called barrier-to-autointegration (BAF) protein was originally identified by its ability to protect MuLV from autointegration (358) and was subsequently proposed to play a similar role for HIV-1 (85). An additional level of complexity is suggested by footprinting studies demonstrating that the ends of the viral DNA are organized into a large complex composed of both viral and cellular proteins (86,652). These complexes have been termed intasomes to distinguish them from the larger PIC.

The development of *in vitro* assays that faithfully reproduce aspects of the integration reaction provide powerful tools with which to screen for agents that block this critical step in HIV replication. Because PICs catalyze reactions that more faithfully reproduce authentic integration, and because they contain additional viral and cellular proteins, they will prove more useful than purified IN in identifying compounds that exhibit antiintegration activity *in vivo*. Several classes of agents inhibit IN function *in vitro*; these include polyanions, nucleotide analogs, and DNA binding compounds (170). Most of these agents are fairly nonspecific in their mode of action, and many compounds that block activity of purified IN are not inhibitory in assays using purified PICs (172). However, certain compounds, such as the dicaffeoylquinic acids, inhibit integration both *in vitro* and in infected cells and appear to be relatively selective for retroviral IN proteins relative to other DNA modifying enzymes and phosphoryltransferases (709). Recently, diketo acid inhibitors have also been shown to be specific and potent inhibitors of the IN-mediated strand transfer reaction (271).

Env

The HIV Env glycoproteins play a major role in the virus life cycle. They contain the determinants that interact with the CD4 receptor and coreceptor, and they catalyze the fusion reaction between the lipid bilayer of the viral envelope and the host cell plasma membrane. In addition, the HIV Env glycoproteins contain epitopes that elicit immune responses that are important from both diagnostic and vaccine development perspectives.

Biosynthesis and Transport

The HIV Env glycoprotein is synthesized from the singly spliced 4.3-kb Vpu/Env bicistronic mRNA (see Figs. 5, 13, and 14); translation occurs on ribosomes associated with the rough endoplasmic reticulum (ER). The 160-kd polyprotein precursor (gp160) is an integral membrane protein that is anchored to cell membranes by a hydrophobic stop-transfer signal in the domain destined to be the mature TM Env glycoprotein, gp41 (Fig. 27). The gp160 is cotranslationally glycosylated, rapidly associates with the host chaperone BiP/GRP78, forms disulfide bonds, and undergoes oligomerization in the ER (154,662). The predominant oligomeric form appears to be a trimer, although dimers and tetramers are also observed. The gp160 is transported to the Golgi, where, like other retroviral envelope precursor proteins, it is proteolytically cleaved by cellular enzymes to the mature SU glycoprotein gp120 and TM glycoprotein gp41 (see Fig. 27). The cellular enzyme responsible for cleavage of retroviral Env precursors following a highly conserved Lys/Arg-X-Lys/Arg-Arg motif is furin or a furin-like protease (262), although other enzymes may also catalyze gp160 processing. Cleavage of gp160 is required for Env-induced fusion activity and virus infectivity (199,427). Subsequent to gp160 cleavage, gp120 and gp41 form a noncovalent association that is critical for transport of the Env complex from the Golgi to the cell surface. The gp120–gp41 interaction is fairly weak, and a substantial amount of gp120 is shed from the surface of Env-expressing cells.

The HIV Env glycoprotein complex, in particular the SU (gp120) domain, is very heavily glycosylated; approximately half the molecular mass of gp160 is composed of

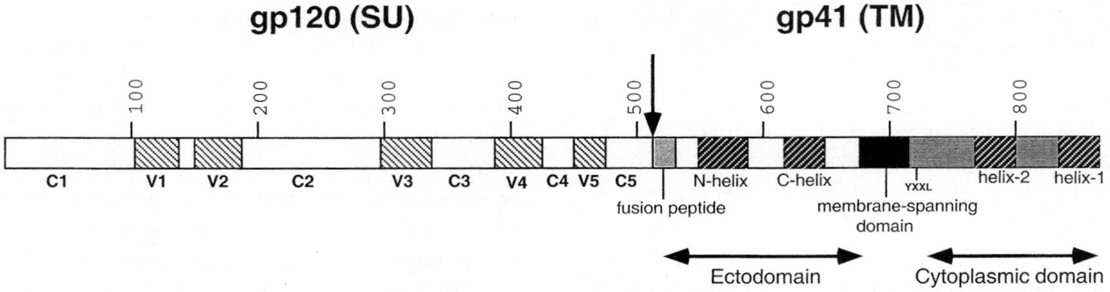

FIG. 27. Linear representation of the HIV-1 Env glycoprotein. The *arrow* indicates the site of gp160 cleavage to gp120 and gp41. In gp120, *cross-hatched areas* represent variable domains (V_1 to V_5) and *open boxes* depict conserved sequences (C_1 to C_5). In the gp41 ectodomain, several domains are indicated: the N-terminal fusion peptide, and the two ectodomain helices (N- and C-helix). The membrane-spanning domain is represented by a *black box.* In the gp41 cytoplasmic domain, the Tyr-X-X-Leu (YXXL) endocytosis motif and two predicted helical domains (helix-1 and -2) are shown. Amino acid numbers are indicated.

oligosaccharide side chains. During transport of Env from its site of synthesis in the ER to the plasma membrane, many of the side chains are modified by the addition of complex sugars. The numerous oligosaccharide side chains form what could be imagined as a sugar cloud obscuring much of gp120 from host immune recognition. As shown in Figure 27, gp120 contains interspersed conserved (C_1 to C_5) and variable (V_1 to V_5) domains. The Cys residues present in the gp120s of different isolates are highly conserved and form disulfide bonds that link the first four variable regions in large loops (364).

Following its arrival at the cell surface, the gp120–gp41 complex is rapidly internalized. Several studies have demonstrated that a Tyr-X-X-Leu sequence in the gp41 cytoplasmic tail (approximately five residues from the membrane-spanning domain) (see Fig. 27) is at least partially responsible for this rapid internalization (351, 541). Analogous motifs are also present in the TM Env proteins of HIV-2, SIV, and several other retroviruses. Tyr-based motifs are known to mediate endocytosis of cellular plasma membrane proteins by binding the μ2 chain of clathrin-associated AP-2 complexes (472), and such interactions have been observed with the HIV-1 and SIV gp41 cytoplasmic domains (44,471). It is currently unclear why retroviral Env glycoproteins would evolve a mechanism to promote rapid internalization, although such a strategy could help evade the host immune response and limit Env-induced cytopathicity. Interestingly, it has been reported that $Pr55^{Gag}$ suppresses HIV-1 Env internalization, perhaps by masking the gp41 endocytosis signals (156). By preventing rapid Env internalization in the presence of Gag, Env incorporation into budding particles might be enhanced.

Env Incorporation into Virions

The mechanism by which the Env glycoproteins are incorporated into budding virus particles remains incompletely characterized. Several lines of evidence suggest that HIV-1 Env glycoproteins are actively recruited into virions via direct interactions between Env and MA:

1. Mutations in the HIV-1 MA can block HIV-1 Env incorporation (146,196,197,691); this incorporation defect can be reversed by pseudotyping virions with heterologous Env glycoproteins or by removing the gp41 cytoplasmic tail (196,197,408).
2. HIV-1 Env directs basolateral budding of Gag in polarized epithelial cells (380,481).
3. A direct binding between HIV-1 MA and peptides derived from the gp41 cytoplasmic tail was reportedly detected *in vitro* (117).
4. A single amino acid change in MA reverses an Env-incorporation defect caused by a small deletion in the gp41 cytoplasmic tail (448).

Some evidence, however, supports a more passive mode of Env incorporation. Heterologous Env proteins [e.g., those of MuLV, HTLV, and vesicular stomatitis virus (VSV)] can be incorporated into HIV-1 virions, and some studies observed that most or all of the cytoplasmic tail of HIV-1 can be removed without blocking Env incorporation. A model that is consistent with currently available data would propose that Env incorporation (and the incorporation of multiple cellular membrane proteins) can occur, in some cases, in the absence of an interaction with Gag; however, the incorporation of full-length HIV-1 Env requires a specific interaction between the gp41 cytoplasmic tail and MA. The effect of gp41 cytoplasmic tail truncation was observed to be strongly cell-type dependent (197); recent characterization of this phenomenon revealed that whereas Env complexes lacking the gp41 cytoplasmic tail could be incorporated into virions produced in certain cell lines (e.g., HeLa, MT-4), in most cell lines and cell types, including primary human PBMC and macrophages, such truncations blocked Env incorporation (449). Thus, it is clear that the gp41 cytoplasmic tail plays a crucial role in Env incorporation. The cell-type dependence of this function suggests the involvement of host cell factors.

In addition to the viral Env glycoproteins, HIV-1 virions incorporate substantial levels of a number of cellular surface proteins. These include the histocompatibility leukocyte antigens class I and II (HLA I and II) and the cell adhesion molecules CD44, LFA-I, and ICAM-1 (for review, see ref. 479). The mode of incorporation of these host-derived proteins, and the significance of their incorporation to HIV biology, are not fully understood.

Tissue Tropism

Distinct HIV/SIV isolates display a striking pattern of selective tropism for subsets of CD4+ cells. As noted earlier, many laboratory-adapted isolates (e.g., HIV-1_{IIIB}, HIV-1_{LAI} or HIV-$1_{SF\text{-}2}$) readily infect activated human PBLs and T-cell lines but cannot replicate efficiently in primary human monocyte-derived macrophages, which are major *in vivo* HIV/SIV targets in the brain, spinal cord, lung, and lymph nodes. In contrast, the host range of macrophage-tropic (M-tropic) strains of HIV, isolated from asymptomatic individuals, is usually limited to PBLs and cells of the monocyte/macrophage lineage; continuous T-cell lines are usually refractory to infection by these isolates. Over time, the virus present in an infected individual gradually changes and cytopathic isolates capable of inducing syncytia and infecting PBLs and T-cell lines become more prevalent. In fact, the evolution of isolates from primarily M-tropic to T-cell-line (TCL-) tropic may play a major role in disease progression (616). The determinants of M- versus TCL-tropism reside primarily in the V_3 loop of gp120; however, amino acids located in the V_1/V_2 domain may be required for full infectivity of recombinant viruses. Observations indicating that isolates of primate lentiviruses displayed selective tropism for distinct populations of CD4+ cells are consistent with the idea that molecules in addition to CD4 are required for HIV Env-induced fusion and entry; this hypothesis was confirmed by the discovery of the HIV/SIV coreceptors (see later).

Membrane Fusion

A primary function of viral Env glycoproteins is to promote a membrane fusion reaction between the lipid bilayers of the viral envelope and host cell membranes. This membrane fusion event enables the viral core to gain entry into the host cell cytoplasm. A number of regions in both gp120 and gp41 have been implicated, directly or indirectly, in Env-mediated membrane fusion. Studies of the HA_2 hemagglutinin protein of the orthomyxoviruses and the F protein of the paramyxoviruses indicated that a highly hydrophobic domain at the N-terminus of these proteins, referred to as the fusion peptide, plays a critical role in membrane fusion (657). Mutational analyses demonstrated that an analogous domain was located at the N-terminus of the HIV-1 (200), HIV-2 (198), and SIV (46) TM glycoproteins (see Fig. 27). Nonhydrophobic substitutions within this region of gp41 greatly reduced or blocked syncytium formation and resulted in the production of noninfectious progeny virions.

C-terminal to the gp41 fusion peptide are two amphipathic helical domains (see Fig. 27) which play a central role in membrane fusion. Mutations in the N-terminal helix (referred to as the N-helix), which contains a Leu zipper-like heptad repeat motif, impair infectivity and membrane fusion activity (73,88,152), and peptides derived from these sequences exhibit potent antiviral activity in culture (659). The structure of the ectodomain of HIV-1 and SIV gp41, the two helical motifs in particular, has been the focus of structural analyses in recent years (67,80,611,653). Structures were determined by x-ray crystallography or NMR spectroscopy either for fusion proteins containing the helical domains, a mixture of peptides derived from the N- and C-helices, or in the case of the SIV structure (67), the intact gp41 ectodomain sequence from residue 27 to 149. These studies obtained fundamentally similar trimeric structures, in which the two helical domains pack in an antiparallel fashion to generate a six-helix bundle (Fig. 28). The N-helices form a coiled-coil in the center of the bundle, with the C-helices packing into hydrophobic grooves on the outside.

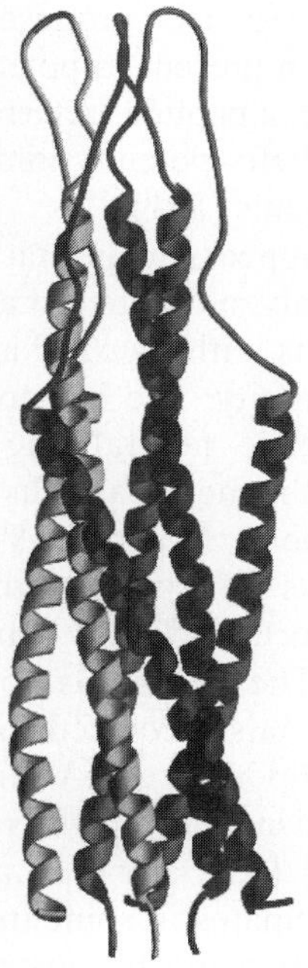

FIG. 28. Trimeric structure of SIV gp41 ectodomain residues 27 to 149. The N-terminal helices are located on the inside of the six-helix bundle; the C-terminal helices pack into hydrophobic grooves on the outside. (Reprinted from ref. 67, with permission.)

Peptides corresponding to the helical domains presumably inhibit fusion (and virus infectivity) by interacting with their complementary binding partner on gp41 and preventing gp41 itself from adopting the six-helix bundle structure. Binding studies using native HIV-1 Env indicated that gp41 could interact with C-helix-derived peptide only after CD4 binding (211). These results, which extend previous observations of CD4-induced conformational changes in the gp41 ectodomain (552), suggest that the N- and C-helices undergo conformational changes (exposure) following CD4 binding, and that these rearrangements are required for membrane fusion (211). In certain respects, the gp41 ectodomain structure bears a strong resemblance to that of the fusion-competent (low-pH-induced) form of influenza HA_2 (65), although in the latter case the N-helices are outside, not inside, the bundle. Structures for both "resting" and fusion-competent forms of influenza HA_2 have been solved. Upon activation of the resting state by low pH, a dramatic conformational change takes place that causes the fusion peptide to move from the center to the end of the trimer, where it can insert into the target membrane. The similarity between the HIV/SIV gp41 and influenza HA_2 ectodomain structures raises the intriguing possibility (80,611,653) that HIV and SIV Envs trigger membrane fusion by the same "spring-loaded" mechanism proposed for influenza (65). However, as only one structure has been determined for HIV/SIV, strong inferences concerning the rearrangements that ultimately trigger membrane fusion may be somewhat premature. An alternative fusion model that does not require major conformational changes in the gp41 core structure has been proposed (67). In any case, the gp41 ectodomain presents a potential target for drug intervention; indeed, a peptide (referred to as T20) corresponding to the C-helix potently inhibits HIV-1 replication in infected patients (331).

Whereas gp41 appears to interact directly with the lipid bilayer to catalyze the membrane fusion reaction, a variety of domains within gp120 are involved in activating Env fusogenicity. The V_3 loop of gp120, which elicits isolate-specific neutralizing antibodies, is an essential player in the membrane fusion reaction. Mutations throughout the V_3 loop of HIV-1 block syncytium formation and virus infectivity without perturbing the processing, transport, and CD4 binding properties of gp120 (201,482). The analogous domain of the HIV-2 Env glycoprotein is also required for fusion and infectivity (198). The importance of V_3 in membrane fusion appears to be a consequence of its role in gp120–coreceptor interactions (see later). In addition to V_3, the V_1/V_2 region participates in some manner in the fusion reaction, as illustrated by the observations that mutations in these variable loops impair fusion (607) and antibodies that bind this region can neutralize virus infectivity (210,431).

CD4 Binding

CD4, the major cell-surface receptor for SIV/HIV, was the first retroviral receptor protein identified (for review, see ref. 48). CD4 is a 55-kd member of the immunoglobulin (Ig) superfamily; it is composed of a highly charged cytoplasmic domain, a single hydrophobic membrane-spanning domain, and four distinct extracellular domains D1 to D4 (397). CD4 normally functions to stabilize the interaction between the T-cell receptor on the surface of T lymphocytes and class II major histocompatibility complex (MHC II) molecules on the surface of antigen-presenting cells. CD4 also recruits $p56^{lck}$ to the T-cell receptor. The high-affinity CD4 binding site for gp120 has been localized to a small segment of the N-terminal extracellular domain, analogous to the second complementarity-determining region (CDR-2) loop of an immunoglobulin light chain variable domain. The cytoplasmic domain of CD4 is not required for its viral receptor function, and mutations that disrupt CD4 internalization do not block HIV entry (25,396). CD4 binding determinants in Env map to the C_3 and C_4 domains of gp120, although a more discontinuous, conformation-dependent domain is clearly involved in high-affinity gp120–CD4 binding. CD4 binding serves not only to promote virion attachment to the target cell but also to induce conformational changes in gp120 and gp41 that are required to activate Env fusogenicity (552,619).

The recent crystallization of a gp120 "core" domain (an unglycosylated gp120 derivative lacking the V_1/V_2 and V_3 loops and the N- and C-termini) complexed with fragments of CD4 and a neutralizing antibody has further refined our understanding of the gp120–CD4 interaction (350,679). The core structure reveals two major domains (referred to as the inner and outer domains) connected by a so-called bridging sheet (Fig. 29). The latter is composed of a four-stranded, antiparallel β-sheet derived from sequences in the V_1/V_2 stem and portions of C_4. Of particular significance is the observation that the CD4 binding site in gp120 (which includes parts of the outer domain and the bridging sheet) is deeply recessed and predicted to be flanked by heavily glycosylated variable regions (350,679). A CD4 residue (Phe-43), shown previously to be critical for gp120 binding, occupies the opening of the CD4-binding cavity while many of the gp120 amino acids important for CD4 binding line the opening of the cavity. A number of the interatomic contacts between gp120 and CD4 are clearly resolved in this structure (350).

The HIV-1 Env glycoprotein binds CD4 not only during the early phase of infection, but also during the transport of gp160 to the cell surface (290). As a consequence of this intracellular association, CD4 is downmodulated from the cell surface, and Env-expressing cells are partially resistant to further infection (47,597). This process,

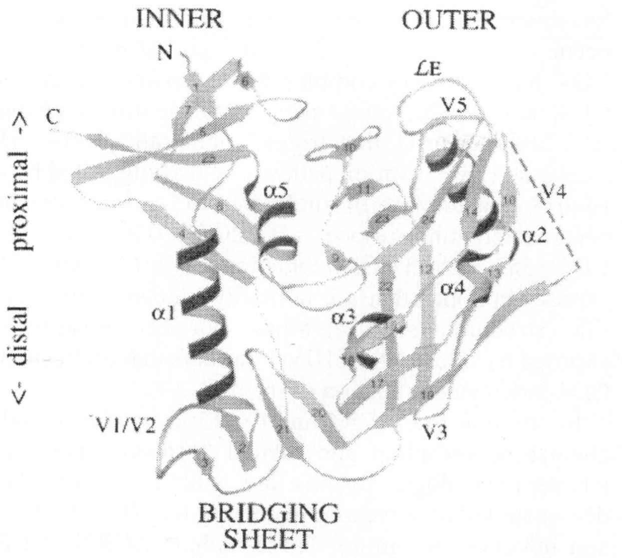

FIG. 29. Ribbon diagram of the gp120 core. In this orientation, the viral membrane would be at the top, the target cell membrane at the bottom. The inner and outer domains are connected by a four-stranded β-bridging sheet. The remnants of variable loops V_1/V_2, V_3, V_4, and V_5 are shown. (Reprinted from ref. 350, with permission.)

known as superinfection interference, was described many years ago for avian retroviruses (544). In the case of HIV-1, the accessory protein Vpu degrades the CD4 component of gp160–CD4 complexes in the ER, thereby releasing Env for transport to the cell surface (see section on Vpu).

The identification of CD4 as the primary receptor for HIV raised the hope that soluble forms of CD4 (sCD4) might display antiviral activity. Indeed, sCD4 can effectively inhibit syncytium formation and HIV infectivity in tissue culture systems primarily by inducing gp120 shedding (442). Unfortunately, this strong inhibitory effect is generally limited to laboratory-adapted isolates. Primary virus strains are neutralized poorly by sCD4, and sCD4 therapy of HIV-infected individuals has little if any impact on the levels of p24 antigenemia or viremia (122).

Coreceptor Interactions

Soon after the identification of CD4 as the major HIV/SIV receptor, it was recognized that this protein is not sufficient for HIV-induced membrane fusion and virus entry. Mouse cells expressing human CD4 were not infectable (395), whereas CD4+ mouse–human cell hybrids could be induced to fuse upon expression of HIV-1 Env (56,150). Furthermore, as mentioned earlier, different HIV-1 isolates often infected only a subset of CD4+ cells. These observations suggested that, in concert with CD4, secondary receptor(s), or coreceptor(s), expressed on human cells functioned in the membrane fusion process. For more than a decade, the identity of potential HIV coreceptors remained elusive. Then, in a remarkably short period of time, a number of studies demonstrated that members of the G protein–coupled receptor superfamily of seven-transmembrane domain proteins provided the long-sought coreceptor function. By screening a human library for cDNAs that could confer on nonhuman cells the ability to fuse with HIV-1 Env-expressing cells, the α-chemokine receptor CXCR4 (originally designated fusin) was identified as the primary coreceptor for TCL-tropic isolates of HIV-1 (177). A separate line of investigation was stimulated by the observation that several β-chemokines produced by CD8+ T-cells (i.e., RANTES, MIP-1α, and MIP-1β) could suppress infection by M-tropic strains of HIV-1, HIV-2, and SIV (100). This finding simultaneously led a number of investigators to test whether the cell-surface proteins that bound these molecules, the β-chemokine receptors, could function as HIV-1 coreceptors. The results indicated that the β-chemokine receptor CCR-5 could, in fact, render CD4+ nonhuman cells permissive for infection by M-tropic isolates of HIV-1 (8,92,134). In recognition of the importance of coreceptors in determining HIV tropism, a nomenclature scheme was devised based on coreceptor usage; isolates (generally M-tropic) that utilized CCR5 were denoted R5 isolates, strains (generally TCL-tropic) that preferentially used CXCR4 were named X4 viruses, and dual-tropic strains that utilized both CCR5 and CXCR4 were denoted R5X4 isolates (30).

In the last several years, numerous additional studies have refined our understanding of coreceptor activity and function. Some of the more important findings are described here. (For further information, refer to more detailed reviews in refs. 31 and 143).

1. It is clear that, depending on the virus isolate, multiple sequences in the N-terminal domain and extracellular loops of CCR5 and CXCR4 can influence coreceptor function, and that the gp120–coreceptor interaction is complex.
2. Signaling through the chemokine receptors is not required for their virus coreceptor function (15).
3. Certain isolates of HIV-1, HIV-2, and SIV use coreceptors in a CD4-independent manner (i.e., as primary receptors) (161,419,508). In fact, the designation of the chemokine receptors as coreceptors may be a misnomer; the observation of CD4-independent HIV/SIV infection, together with the finding that feline immunodeficiency viruses utilize the chemokine receptors but not CD4 (661) suggest that the use of chemokine receptors in lentiviral infection may have predated the involvement of CD4.
4. Direct interactions between coreceptor and gp120 have been detected. This interaction is greatly stimulated by, or is dependent on, the presence of CD4

(353,625,676). Association between CD4 and CCR5 in the absence of gp120 has also been reported (680).

Several domains within gp120 directly or indirectly function in Env/coreceptor interactions. Consistent with its influence on HIV-1 tropism, the V_3 loop plays a major role: Single amino acid changes or deletions in V_3 shift or impair coreceptor usage (92,101), V_3 peptides reportedly interact with CXCR4 (547), antibodies to V_3 block gp120–CCR5 binding (625,676), and an HIV-1 variant that escaped the CXCR4 inhibitor AMD3100 contains substitutions within and in close proximity to the V_3 loop (131) . The V_1/V_2 region also helps determine coreceptor usage (537). In addition to the involvement of variable regions in coreceptor interaction, highly conserved portions of gp120 that are exposed upon CD4 binding appear to interact with coreceptor. The binding of antibodies whose epitopes are revealed upon CD4 exposure can block gp120–CCR5 interaction; these epitopes include residues within the gp120 bridging sheet (350,679). By analyzing a number of Env mutants, a highly conserved structure adjacent to V_3 was recognized as playing a major role in CCR5 binding (529).

A generalized scheme for coreceptor utilization is presented in Table 1. TCL-tropic (X4) isolates infect T-cell lines via CXCR4; M-tropic (R5) strains infect macrophages via CCR5. Dual-tropic (R5X4) isolates can utilize either CCR5 or CXCR4 and can therefore infect both T-cell lines and macrophages. Because primary lymphocytes express both CCR5 and CXCR4, they are infectable by X4, R5, and R5X4 isolates. Although this simple model explains many aspects of coreceptor utilization, it fails to account for certain observations. In particular, the details of coreceptor utilization in macrophages remain to be fully elucidated. Some R5 strains do not efficiently infect primary macrophages (90,141), and β-chemokines, which block CCR5, do not always inhibit HIV infection in macrophages (444,556). Furthermore, macrophages have been reported to express relatively high levels of CXCR4 and yet generally (with some exceptions—e.g., see refs. 578 and 688) cannot be efficiently infected with X4 isolates. Several models have been proposed to explain this latter observation, including (a) X4 strains enter macrophages but are blocked at a post-entry step (555), (b) higher-order CD4–CXCR4–gp120 interactions required for membrane fusion do not take place efficiently in macrophages (137,354), and (c) CCR5 out-competes CXCR4 for binding to CD4, thereby rendering CXCR4 nonfunctional as a coreceptor in macrophages (359). Intriguingly, some dual-tropic isolates are reportedly able to use CXCR4 to infect macrophages that lack CCR5 (687); it thus appears that dual-tropism may arise not only from the ability to utilize both CCR5 and CXCR4 but also from the ability to use CXCR4 on macrophages (687).

The observation that CD4 induces conformational changes in gp120 that enhance interaction with coreceptors suggests that events leading up to membrane fusion occur sequentially (Fig. 30). First gp120 interacts with CD4, then a ternary complex forms between coreceptor, CD4, and gp120, and finally conformational changes take place in gp41 that trigger membrane fusion. This step-wise Env activation pathway is also suggested by the finding that binding of antibodies to the putative coreceptor interacting surface of gp120 (350) is enhanced by CD4 (553,619). Thus, interaction of gp120 with CD4 exposes epitopes that are normally hidden in the native Env structure; such epitopes can be constitutively exposed by selecting for HIV-1 variants that replicate in a CD4-independent fashion (286,341).

In addition to CXCR4 and CCR5, a number of other chemokine receptors and related "orphans" (receptors whose physiologic ligands are unknown) have been demonstrated to serve as coreceptors for HIV/SIV fusion and infection in culture. These include CCR2b, CCR3, CCR8, APJ, Bonzo (STRL33), BOB (GPR15), and US28 (for review, see ref. 31). The significance of this diverse array of potential coreceptors is currently unclear. Many of the studies that defined the ability of HIV/SIV to utilize these alternative coreceptors employed cell culture systems in which very high levels of coreceptor and CD4 were expressed, and membrane fusion or infectivity could be detected with great sensitivity. Evaluation of coreceptor usage of numerous primary isolates has led some investigators to conclude that CCR5 and CXCR4 are likely to account for most if not all coreceptor activity *in vivo* (702,703). However, the possibility remains that in certain tissues alternative coreceptors may play some role. For example, CCR3 has been implicated in HIV-1 infection of microglial cells (272), and the prevalence of APJ expression in the central nervous system has led to the suggestion that this orphan receptor may perform a role in neuropathogenesis of HIV infection (155).

Certain individuals, despite persistent high-risk behavior, remain HIV-1 uninfected (495). The discovery of CCR5, CXCR4, and related molecules as HIV coreceptors raised the possibility that these individuals might have inherited mutant coreceptor alleles. In some instances, this turned out to be the case. The most clear-cut example of this phenomenon involves a CCR5 allele that is relatively common in Caucasian populations. This mutant allele, referred to as CCR5/Δ32, contains a 32-base-pair deletion and encodes a truncated protein that is not efficiently expressed at the cell surface and cannot function as an HIV-1 coreceptor (133,295,379,549). Homozygotes for CCR5/Δ32 are only very rarely infected with HIV-1, highlighting the protective benefits of inheriting this allele. Some limited evidence suggests that CCR5/Δ32 heterozygosity may confer some protective benefits in slowing disease progression (133,379, 549). Since the identification of the CCR5/Δ32 mutation, other inherited polymorphisms in the CCR5 coding region or its regulatory sequences have been reported to

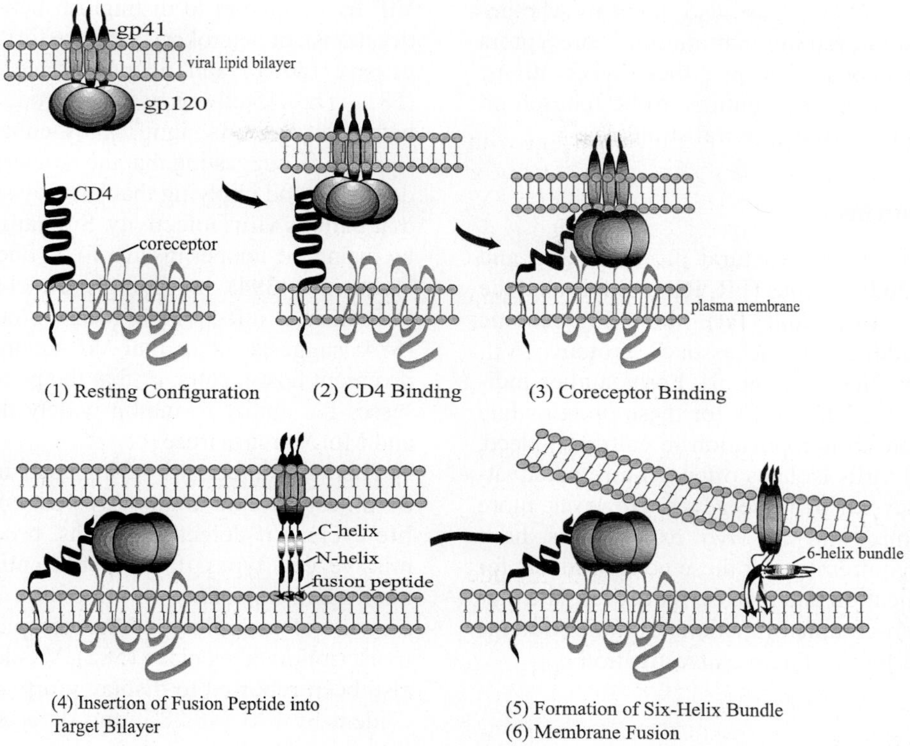

FIG. 30. Schematic representation of the steps leading to membrane fusion. In the resting configuration, the Env glycoprotein complex is in its native state (*1*). CD4 binding (*2*) induces conformation changes in Env that facilitate coreceptor binding (*3*). Following the formation of a ternary gp120/CD4/coreceptor complex, gp41 adopts a hypothetical conformation that allows the fusion peptide to insert into the target lipid bilayer (*4*). The formation of the gp41 six-helix bundle (which involves antiparallel interactions between the gp41 N- and C-helices) (*5*) brings the viral and cellular membranes together and membrane fusion takes place (*6*).

influence HIV-1 transmission or HIV-induced disease progression (420,428). A CCR2 mutation known as CCR2-64I has also been associated with a delay in disease progression, perhaps because of its linkage with the CCR5 gene regulatory region (346,587). It should be emphasized that mutations in genes for currently recognized coreceptors appear to be present in only a minority of multiply exposed, uninfected individuals, suggesting the existence of other mechanisms of protection from HIV infection. One such mechanism associated with altered infectability or disease progression involves the regulation of expression of the chemokines themselves. Analysis of a large number of hemophiliacs exposed to HIV-1-contaminated factor VIII (697) and 100 subjects participating in a Multicenter AIDS Cohort study group (229) revealed that protection correlated with high levels of β-chemokine production. Additionally, a mutation in the regulatory region of the CCR5 ligand RANTES (377), and a single nucleotide polymorphism in the 3′ untranslated region of the mRNA encoding the CXCR4 ligand (SDF-1) (669) were reportedly associated with a delay in disease progression.

The identification of HIV coreceptors presents novel opportunities for antiviral therapy. A derivative of RANTES was synthesized by modifying its N-terminus with aminooxypentane. This molecule, known as (AOP)-RANTES does not induce chemotaxis but potently inhibits infection by a variety of HIV-1 isolates (577). Several low-molecular-weight compounds, including the bicyclam AMD3100 (144) and the polyphemusin analog T22 (450), potently block entry via CXCR4. A chemokine agonist encoded by human herpesvirus 8 (Kaposi's sarcoma–associated virus) was reported to inhibit virus entry through CCR3, CCR5, and CXCR4 (337). In addition to chemokine derivatives and low-molecular-weight coreceptor inhibitors, antibodies against coreceptors have displayed antiviral properties (432,677). Some concern about potential undesirable side effects of treatment with anti-coreceptor agents is warranted; although no observable negative consequences of CCR5 deletion are evident among individuals homozygous for the CCR5/Δ32 mutation, CXCR4 knock-out mice display a range of severe defects including abnormal hematopoiesis, cerebral development, and gastrointestinal tract vascularization (610,713). It is also unclear whether effective therapy would require that multiple coreceptors be targeted simultaneously. Despite these reservations, much effort will undoubtedly continue to be focused on developing coreceptor-based antiviral strategies.

The Accessory Proteins

In addition to the viral structural proteins (Gag and Env), the *pol*-encoded enzymes (PR, RT, and IN), and the regulatory proteins (Rev and Tat), the HIV genome encodes several additional "accessory" proteins: Vif, Vpu, Vpr, Vpx, and Nef (see Fig. 5). Early studies indicated that disruption of the ORFs for these proteins had little or no effect on virus replication in culture; indeed, laboratory-adapted virus isolates often acquire inactivating mutations in several of these genes. However, more recent tissue culture and *in vivo* experiments have revealed a strong requirement for these gene products for efficient virus replication and disease induction. The elucidation of the often-complex functions of these proteins continues to be the focus of active investigation.

Vif

The *vif* (virus infectivity factor) gene is located near the middle of the HIV genome, overlapping with *pol* and *vpr*. The presence of *vif* is a highly conserved feature among lentiviruses; a *vif* product is encoded by all lentiviruses except EIAV (325). Early reports indicated that Vif is not required for efficient virus assembly or release but is necessary for the generation of fully infectious virions (589,600). In subsequent studies, it became apparent that the phenotype of *vif*-defective mutants is strikingly cell-type dependent, and that this phenotype is imposed by the cell in which virus is produced (212). Thus, certain cell lines (e.g., 293T, HeLa, COS, SupT1, CEM-SS, and Jurkat) are "permissive" for *vif*-defective mutants, whereas others, including primary lymphocytes, monocyte-derived macrophages, and some T-cell lines, are "nonpermissive." This observation suggests that host-cell factors in the virus-producing cell play a role in Vif function. Such a role was highlighted by studies in which the activity of different primate lentiviral Vif proteins was evaluated in cells of both human and nonhuman primate origin (584). The infectivity of HIV-1, HIV-2, and SIV_{agm} could be enhanced by HIV-1 Vif when these viruses were expressed in human cells. In contrast, although SIV_{agm} Vif could modulate infectivity of SIV_{agm} produced in African green monkey cells, it was inactive when expressed in human cells.

The important role of the producer cell in Vif function implies either that Vif-permissive cells express a factor that substitutes for Vif, or that nonpermissive cells contain a factor that suppresses virus replication in the absence of Vif. In an attempt to distinguish between these possibilities, transient heterokaryons were formed between Vif-permissive (293T) and nonpermissive (HUT78) cell lines (581). The infectivity of virus produced by the resulting heterokaryons was significantly enhanced by the expression of Vif, suggesting that the nonpermissive phenotype is dominant and implying that Vif may suppress a host factor that inhibits virus infectivity. Similar results were obtained by fusing the nonpermissive T-cell line H9 with permissive HeLa cells (394). Intriguingly, the observation that HIV-1 Vif enhances infectivity of MuLV produced in human cells (584) suggests either that Vif suppresses the activity of divergent host factors, or that the putative host factor possesses the ability to inhibit widely divergent (i.e., HIV-1 and MuLV) retroviruses.

The Vif^- defect, while imposed in the producer cell, becomes apparent at an early post-entry step in the virus life cycle. Vif-defective virions, produced from nonpermissive cell types, fail to efficiently reverse-transcribe their genomes following infection (592,646), perhaps as a result of instability of the complex in which reverse transcription takes place (582). Vif-defective virions have also been reported to display morphologic abnormalities evident by EM (45,287) and defects in endogenous RT activity (241). Some investigators reported that Vif mutation causes a defect in Gag processing, such that Vif^- virions contain increased levels of the Gag precursor $Pr55^{Gag}$ (45,576). An effect of Vif on Gag processing has also been observed *in vitro* (347). However, detailed analyses of Vif^- virions obtained from nonpermissive cells failed to reveal any effect of Vif mutation on viral protein composition (50,188,468).

Several groups have detected the presence of small amounts of Vif in virions (70,188,322,378,583). It is currently not clear whether virion incorporation is necessary for the ability of Vif to enhance virus infectivity, or whether its incorporation is nonspecific and not linked to function. Several studies have raised doubts about the relevance of virion incorporation:

1. Vif is incorporated into MuLV particles (70), suggesting that the incorporation of Vif into virions does not require a specific interaction with other virion components.
2. Using cells that express variable levels of Vif, it was observed that the amount of Vif incorporated into virions is influenced by the levels of Vif expressed by the virus-producing cell, and that the resulting variations in the amount of virion-associated Vif have no effect on virus infectivity (583).
3. At least in some cell culture systems, virus preparations may be contaminated with Vif-containing microvesicles, raising the possibility that even the low levels of virion-associated Vif observed in previous studies may represent an overestimate of the amount actually present in virus particles (135).

Vpr

The *vpr* gene, which overlaps with *vif* at its 5′ end (see Fig. 5), encodes a 14-kd, 96-amino-acid protein that is incorporated at high levels into virus particles (106,694). The incorporation of Vpr into virions appears to be mediated through an interaction with a $(Leu-X-X)_4$ motif near the C-terminus of the $p6^{Gag}$ protein (342,387,494). Vpr contains two predicted helical motifs, one near the N-terminus, the other near the middle of the protein, and a C-terminal Arg-rich domain. Vpr has been predicted to dimerize via residues in the helical domains (563,704). The presence of Vpr is highly conserved among primate lentiviruses. Although Vpr has little influence on HIV replication kinetics in proliferating PBMC or T-cell lines in culture, in nondividing monocyte-derived macrophages its effects are more substantial. Three major functions for Vpr have been proposed: (a) stimulation of gene expression driven by the HIV LTR, (b) transport of the viral preintegration complex to the nucleus during the early stages of the infection process, and (c) arrest of infected cells in the G_2 phase of the cell cycle.

Early studies of HIV-1 Vpr reported that Vpr weakly transactivated expression from the HIV-1 LTR (106). More recent experiments have confirmed this activity and suggest that it may be mediated via interactions between Vpr, Sp1 (554,649), TFIIB (2,334), and TFIID (334). The ability of Vpr to stimulate transcription may be linked to its cell-cycle arrest function (see later).

High levels of virion incorporation suggest a role for Vpr early in the virus life cycle prior to *de novo* gene expression. The observations that deletion of Vpr significantly reduces virus replication in terminally differentiated, nondividing, monocyte-derived macrophages (19), that the HIV-1 preintegration complex contains Vpr (215,274), and that Vpr localizes to the nucleus in HIV-infected or Vpr-expressing cells (388), suggested that Vpr might participate in the nuclear import of the HIV preintegration complex. As discussed previously, this nuclear import capability enables HIV to infect nondividing cells, including monocyte-derived macrophages. Initially, it appeared that MA might play the key role in nuclear import (see section on MA); subsequent studies, however, suggested that MA either has no role or is a relatively minor player in the process compared with Vpr and perhaps IN and a DNA triplex (or flap) structure resulting from lentiviral reverse transcription (see earlier). A number of recent studies have attempted to further define the role Vpr plays in nuclear localization. Mutational analyses have suggested that residues involved in nuclear localization are located at a variety of positions in Vpr, and that the protein lacks a canonical basic-type NLS, such as those found in karyophilic proteins—for example, SV40 large T antigen or nucleoplasmin (for reviews, see refs. 244 and 245). In some cases, Vpr mutations that disrupt nuclear localization may do so by inducing global protein misfolding or instability, complicating the precise mapping of determinants involved in nuclear import. As noted earlier, in the classical basic-type NLS pathway, the importin α (karyopherin α) component of the importin α/β heterodimer binds NLS-containing proteins, whereas the importin β (karyopherin β) component functions in part to mediate docking to the nucleoporins to mediate translocation through the nuclear pore complex (see Fig. 16). This pathway can be blocked by peptides containing the SV40 large T antigen NLS. Other distinct nuclear transport pathways exist, and the process by which cytoplasmic proteins and macromolecular structures destined for the nucleus traffic to the nuclear membrane, associate with components of the nuclear pore complex, and translocate through the nuclear pore is only partially understood. Thus it is perhaps not surprising that no clear consensus exists concerning the mechanism by which Vpr promotes nuclear localization. Divergent observations are in part a result of different experimental systems used to monitor localization, and, perhaps more importantly, due to the fact that some studies assessed the nuclear import of Vpr itself, whereas others followed the fate of a variety of Vpr fusion proteins or HIV-1 PICs containing or lacking Vpr. The diversity of findings is reflected in the results of several recent studies:

1. The observation that Vpr-mediated nuclear localization is not blocked by an SV40 large T antigen NLS suggested that Vpr functions independently of the importin pathway.
2. Based on data using purified PICs either containing or lacking Vpr, it was proposed that Vpr interacts with importin α and increases its affinity for proteins containing basic-type NLSs; it was suggested that Vpr interacts with importin α at a site distinct from that used by either a basic-type NLS or importin β (505,506). This model proposes that Vpr acts to stimulate importin α/β-dependent nuclear import (505,506). Interaction of Vpr with importin α was also reported in a study examining the localization of Vpr itself in both human and yeast cells (640).
3. The analysis of the nuclear transport properties of Vpr fused with heterologous proteins suggested that Vpr interacts directly with nucleoporins (187).
4. The import of Vpr to the nucleus was analyzed using an *in vitro* nuclear transport assay; it was concluded that Vpr contains two independent NLSs that utilize two different nuclear transport pathways, both of which are distinct from the importin α/β pathway (312).

The third major function widely described for Vpr is its ability to arrest cells in the G_2 phase of the cell cycle. Cell-cycle arrest reportedly occurs within hours of infection and is not blocked by antiviral agents, suggesting that it is initiated by the Vpr carried into the cell on virus particles (504). Several studies have indicated that G_2 arrest is linked to inhibition by Vpr of the activity of the $p34^{cdc2}$-cyclin B kinase complex (273,518), perhaps via an interaction with the host protein MOV34 (401). Although the biologic implications of Vpr-induced cell-cycle arrest remain unclear, it has been proposed that increased HIV-LTR-driven transcription in the G_2 phase of the cell cycle could provide a rationale for the evolution of a Vpr cell-cycle arrest function (175,239). This Vpr-induced enhancement of LTR-driven transcription is reportedly mediated by the p300 transcriptional coactivator (175). The nuclear import and cell-cycle arrest functions appear to involve distinct domains in Vpr, as mutations have been reported that disrupt one function but leave the other intact (400). The ability of Vpr to induce cell-cycle arrest not only in primate cells but also in yeast (393) underscores the involvement of highly conserved cellular factors in this phenomenon.

In addition to the properties described earlier, a number of additional functions for Vpr have been described. These include the ability to induce differentiation of rhabdomyosarcoma cells (369), trigger or suppress apoptosis (16,599), interact with the glucocorticoid receptor (519), kill cells by forming ion channels (502), activate HIV gene expression via a transcellular mechanism (370), and reduce mutation rates during reverse transcription (411). The interrelatedness of these diverse functions, and their implications for virus replication and pathogenesis *in vivo*, remain to be characterized.

Vpx

Members of the HIV-2/SIV_{sm}/SIV_{mac} lineage of primate lentiviruses carry an additional gene known as *vpx*. Because of the high degree of relatedness between the *vpr* and *vpx* genes, it was initially proposed that *vpx* was created by a *vpr* gene duplication event after the HIV-2/SIV_{sm}/SIV_{mac} lineage diverged from other primate lentiviruses (623). More recently, it was argued that *vpx* likely arose by acquisition of the SIV_{agm} *vpr* gene by nonhomologous (570) or homologous (624) recombination.

Like Vpr, Vpx is incorporated at high levels in virus particles, also via an interaction with the C-terminus of Gag (276,328,678). Interestingly, in the HIV-2/SIV_{sm}/SIV_{mac} viruses, two of the major functions of HIV-1 Vpr seem to be shared between Vpx and Vpr: Vpx is required for efficient infection of nondividing cells (692), whereas Vpr induces cell cycle arrest but has no role in nuclear targeting (183).

Vpu

A distinguishing feature of the HIV-1 lineage of primate lentiviruses is the presence of the *vpu* gene (see Fig. 4); it is absent from HIV-2 and all SIVs examined to date, with the exception of the closely HIV-1-related SIV_{cpz} (107,298,602). Vpu is a multimeric, 81-amino-acid, integral membrane phosphoprotein containing an N-terminal transmembrane anchor sequence and an approximately 50-amino-acid cytoplasmic domain (402). Three α-helical domains have been predicted: one in the transmembrane sequence (residues 6 to 29), the others in the cytoplasmic domain (residues 32 to 51 and 57 to 72) (675). The sites of phosphorylation have been mapped to two Ser residues at positions 52 and 56 (560). Vpu is translated from a *vpu-env* bicistronic mRNA (567) and is synthesized at intracellular levels comparable to Gag in virus-infected cells. It has not been detected in virus particles. Two principal functions for Vpu have been described: enhancement of virus release and degradation of CD4.

Early studies observed that HIV-1 clones lacking a functional *vpu* gene displayed a pronounced defect in virus particle production (601,602,617). The absence of the Vpu gene product had no discernible effect on the processing or transport of Gag proteins but caused virus particles to be retained at the plasma membrane and in intracellular vesicles (338). The mechanism by which Vpu enhances particle release remains poorly understood; however, a number of observations have been made regarding this property.

1. Enhancement of virus release is independent of Env or CD4 (233,684).
2. Vpu can increase virus production of highly divergent retroviruses (e.g., MuLV, visna, and HIV-2), even though these viruses do not carry a *vpu* gene (247).
3. The N-terminal transmembrane domain appears to be largely responsible for stimulating virus release (558).
4. This function of Vpu does not require phosphorylation (561) but may rely on the ability of Vpu to form cation-selective ion channels (167,559).
5. It was reported that a member of the tetratricopeptide repeat protein family interacts with HIV-1 Gag and suppresses virus release. The ability of Vpu to also interact with this protein and diminish its association with Gag could contribute to the ability of Vpu to enhance virus release (69).

The mechanism by which Vpu induces CD4 degradation has been characterized more completely than its ability to stimulate virus particle release. Vpu directly binds the cytoplasmic tail of CD4 in the ER; residues in the cytoplasmic domain of Vpu, and Vpu phosphorylation, are critical for this process (49,87,363,561,638,663). The degradation of CD4 by Vpu appears to liberate the Env glycoprotein precursor gp160 from its interaction with CD4, thereby enabling Env to continue its transport to the cell surface (664,665). The presence of Env is not required for CD4 degradation (87,665). Progress has been made recently in elucidating the strategy used by Vpu to induce CD4 degradation: Vpu simultaneously interacts with CD4 and with a protein known as h-βTrCP via WD repeat elements present in the latter protein. The ternary CD4/Vpu/h-βTrCP complexes, which can be detected by coimmunoprecipitation, are then targeted for ubiquitin-mediated proteolysis via interaction between the cellular factor Skp1 and an "F box" motif on the h-βTrCP component of the ternary complex (414). Consistent with this model, inhibition of proteosome activity blocks Vpu-mediated CD4 degradation (205).

Nef

The *nef* gene, present only in primate lentiviruses, overlaps with the 3′ LTR and encodes a 27-kd membrane-associated phosphoprotein (see Fig. 5). Membrane binding, mediated by a covalently attached myristic acid moiety and a cluster of N-terminal basic residues (654), is critical for Nef function. Nef is synthesized at high levels from the first mRNA transcript detected after infection. Although Nef was originally labeled a "negative factor" because of reports that it down-regulated virus replication by suppressing transcription from the HIV LTR (3,390), it is now clear that in cultured cells Nef expression either has no effect on virus spread or modestly enhances replication kinetics. The NMR structure of the Nef "core" domain (lacking the N-terminus) has been determined (257,258), and x-ray crystal or NMR structures of the Nef core have been solved for the protein in a complex with Src homology 3 (SH3) domains (12,357) or with the cytoplasmic tail of CD4 (259). In general, the overall folding of Nef is similar to that of helix-turn-helix DNA binding proteins; it contains an unstructured N-terminus, followed by a poly-Pro type II helix (which contains the SH3 binding motif Pro-X-X-Pro), several α-and 3_{10} helices, and a five-stranded antiparallel β-sheet. Residues 150 to 180 form a disordered loop. Interestingly, the binding between Nef and proteins containing SH3 domains (e.g., the Hck Tyr kinase) involves not only the consensus SH3-binding motif (Pro-X-X-Pro) but also discontiguous residues downstream of the poly-Pro type II helix (257).

Several distinct functions for Nef have been widely reported: (a) down-regulation of CD4 and MHC I expression from the cell surface, (b) enhancement of virus infectivity, and (c) modulation of cellular activation pathways. In contrast to the situation in HIV-1-infected cultures, where the role of Nef in virus replication is relatively difficult to measure, Nef appears to be critical for maintaining the high virus loads that are a prerequisite for disease induction *in vivo*. It is currently unclear which of the many activities attributed to Nef in tissue culture are required for its functions *in vivo*.

Like the HIV-1 Env and Vpu proteins, Nef possesses the capacity to down-regulate cell-surface expression of CD4 (226,260). Nef-induced CD4 down-regulation proceeds in a step-wise fashion:

1. Nef interacts with a di-Leu-based motif in the cytoplasmic domain of CD4 (5) and then associates with adapter protein (AP) complexes in clathrin-coated pits to promote rapid CD4 internalization. CD4 endocytosis probably results from a direct interaction between Nef and the μ2 subunit of the AP-2 complex (251,356,500) and perhaps the catalytic subunit of the vacuolar ATPase (386).
2. In the endosome, Nef connects CD4 with the β-subunit of COP I coatomers (β-COP), thereby targeting CD4 for degradation in the lysosome (27,501). Nef may also stimulate CD4 internalization by dissociating CD4 from $p56^{lck}$, which binds the CD4 cytoplasmic tail and normally inhibits CD4 endocytosis (333).

In addition to reducing cell-surface CD4 expression, Nef has been reported to down-regulate MHC I molecule expression (565). In contrast to CD4 down-regulation, which involves a di-Leu-based endocytosis signal in the CD4 cytoplasmic tail, MHC I degradation requires the presence of a Tyr-based motif (356). Cell-surface down-regulation of MHC I by Nef may be accomplished not only by increased rates of protein endocytosis from the cell surface but also as a consequence of reduced trafficking from the trans-Golgi network to the plasma membrane (252,356). Intriguingly, MHC I down-regulation may limit the ability of cytotoxic T lymphocytes (CTLs) to recognize and eliminate virus-infected cells, thus providing HIV and SIV with a mechanism for partially evading at least one component of the host immune response (110). Removing MHC I molecules from the cell surface exposes infected cells to attack by natural killer (NK) cells (689); HIV-1 may avoid this latter problem by not down-regulating those class I molecules (HLA-C and HLA-E) responsible for protection from NK cell lysis (108).

In single-cycle assays, Nef modestly stimulates virus infectivity (95,240,438,594). This function appears to be manifested at an early step in the virus life cycle, since *nef*-deleted mutants fail to efficiently reverse-transcribe their genomes after infection (6,94,564). Mutations in the Pro-X-X-Pro motif, which have no effect on CD4 down-regulation, impair Nef-mediated enhancement of infectivity (240,548), although this phenotype may in part reflect effects of the mutations on protein stability (118). Interestingly, the infectivity defect observed with nef^{-} virus can be partially suppressed by pseudotyping with the vesicular stomatitis virus G glycoprotein (VSV-G) (4). VSV-G directs entry via fusion in a low pH endosome following endocytosis, whereas HIV-1 Env mediates entry via direct fusion at the plasma membrane. This observation implies that the role Nef plays early after entry depends on the route of HIV-1 entry. At this time, however, the mechanism by which Nef enhances virus infectivity remains to be elucidated. It is also unclear to what extent this relatively modest effect contributes to the strong requirement for Nef *in vivo*.

Deletion of the *nef* gene has a profound effect in the SIV/rhesus macaque animal model system. Monkeys inoculated with *nef*-deleted virus develop high-level antibody responses but produce no detectable circulating virus (327); these results indicate that Nef plays a critical role in initiating and sustaining SIV infection *in vivo*. Nef has also been proposed to play a major role in pathogenesis in HIV-1–infected humans. This hypothesis stems in part from the findings of some (132,335), but not others (296,297), that virus isolates derived from individuals who progress to disease slowly harbor *nef* mutations. Nef has been shown to be required for HIV-1 replication and pathogenicity in SCID mice containing human fetal thymus and liver implants (310), and transgenic mice expressing Nef in CD4+ T cells and in cells of the monocytic lineage develop a variety of AIDS-like pathologies (265,266).

A number of studies have suggested that HIV and SIV Nef influence cellular signal transduction pathways and affect the activation state (in either a positive or a negative sense) of Nef-expressing cells (for review, see ref. 416). This area of research remains highly controversial, perhaps owing to differences in the cell culture systems used in various studies, to the inherent complexities of cellular signaling pathways, and to potential differences in the mode of action of SIV versus HIV-1 Nef. As mentioned earlier, HIV and SIV Nef contain a highly conserved consensus binding site for the SH3 domain of Src-family Tyr kinases (Pro-X-X-Pro). Nef has been reported to interact with a Ser/Thr (p21-activated or PAK) kinase and Src-family kinases (e.g., Lyn, Hck, and Lck) and modulate their catalytic activities. As cellular kinases are intimately involved in signaling pathways, such interactions may play a critical role in Nef function. The identification of a naturally occurring mutant SIV *nef* allele has provided some clues into Nef function. A strain of SIV_{mac} known as SIV_{pbj14} induces a rapidly fatal disease in infected macaques characterized by marked T-lymphocyte proliferation, retrafficking of T cells to the gastrointestinal tract, and unremitting diarrhea. In culture, SIV_{pbj14} causes extensive T-lymphocyte activation and displays the unusual property of being able to replicate efficiently in resting PBMC (151). These features are the result of an Arg-to-Tyr mutation that creates a sequence reminiscent of an immunoreceptor tyrosine-based activation motif (ITAM). ITAMs, present in the cytoplasmic tails of T-cell and B-cell receptors, are essential for lymphocyte activation, and the putative ITAM of the SIV_{pbj14} Nef protein appears to activate T-cell signaling (391). Despite the usefulness of the SIV system in understanding Nef function, particularly *in vivo*, caution should be used in extrapolating SIV data to HIV-1 in light of differences observed for SIV versus HIV-1 Nef activities in culture (for example, see ref. 253). In addition to potential direct effects of Nef on stimulating T-cell activation, a recent study demonstrated that Nef expression in macrophages induces the expression and release of the β-chemokines MIP-1α and MIP-1β, which in turn activate resting T lymphocytes (609). Such an effect could help explain the positive effect of Nef on HIV-1 replication *in vivo*.

It has been reported by several groups that Nef is incorporated into virions. Interestingly, as a result of viral PR-mediated cleavage, much of the HIV-1 Nef in virus particles is smaller than the full-length protein detected in infected cells (61,486,655). However, as is the case for Vif, it is not clear what, if any, function is served by virion incorporation, particularly since HIV-1 Nef is incorporated with equivalent efficiency into HIV-1 and MuLV virions (61). The significance of PR-mediated Nef cleavage also remains undefined. In fact, preventing Nef cleavage does not alter its ability to stimulate virus infectivity (437). Recent results suggest that Nef localizes to the viral core (348).

A summary of the major proposed functions of the HIV-1 accessory proteins is presented in Table 3.

TABLE 3. *HIV/SIV accessory proteins*

Protein	Major proposed functions	Comments
Vif	Enhancement of virus infectivity	Phenotype producer cell-dependent Incorporated at low levels in virions
Vpr	Cell cycle arrest Nuclear import	Incorporated at high levels in virions
Vpx	Nuclear import	Incorporated at high levels in virions Present in HIV-2/SIV_{sm}/SIV_{mac} only
Vpu	Increased particle release CD4 degradation	Not detected in virions Present in HIV-1 only
Nef	CD4 and MHC I down-regulation Enhancement of virus infectivity Increased virus load *in vivo* Altered cellular activation pathways	Incorporated at low levels in virions

MHC, major histocompatibility complex; HIV, human immunodeficiency virus; SIV, simian immunodeficiency complex.

REFERENCES

1. Aboul-ela F, Karn J, Varani G. The structure of the human immunodeficiency virus type-1 TAR RNA reveals principles of RNA recognition by Tat protein. *J Mol Biol* 1995;253:313–332.
2. Agostini I, Navarro JM, Rey F, et al. The human immunodeficiency virus type 1 Vpr transactivator: Cooperation with promoter-bound activator domains and binding to TFIIB. *J Mol Biol* 1996;261:599–606.
3. Ahmad N, Venkatesan S. Nef protein of HIV-1 is a transcriptional repressor of HIV-1 LTR [published erratum appears in *Science* 1988;242:242]. *Science* 1988;241:1481–1485.
4. Aiken C. Pseudotyping human immunodeficiency virus type 1 (HIV-1) by the glycoprotein of vesicular stomatitis virus targets HIV-1 entry to an endocytic pathway and suppresses both the requirement for Nef and the sensitivity to cyclosporin A. *J Virol* 1997;71:5871–5877.
5. Aiken C, Konner J, Landau NR, et al. Nef induces CD4 endocytosis: Requirement for a critical dileucine motif in the membrane-proximal CD4 cytoplasmic domain. *Cell* 1994;76:853–864.
6. Aiken C, Trono D. Nef stimulates human immunodeficiency virus type 1 proviral DNA synthesis. *J Virol* 1995;69:5048–5056.
7. Aldrovandi GM, Feuer G, Gao L, et al. The SCID-hu mouse as a model for HIV-1 infection. *Nature* 1993;363:732–736.
8. Alkhatib G, Combadiere C, Broder CC, et al. CC CKR5: A RANTES, MIP-1a MIP-1b receptor as a fusion cofactor for macrophage-tropic HIV-1. *Science* 1996;272:1955–1958.
9. Alonso A, Derse D, Peterlin BM. Human chromosome 12 is required for optimal interactions between Tat and TAR of human immunodeficiency virus type 1 in rodent cells. *J Virol* 1992;66:4617–4621.
10. Arnold E, Ding J, Hughes SH, et al. Structures of DNA and RNA polymerases and their interactions with nucleic acid substrates. *Curr Opin Struct Biol* 1995;5:27–38.
11. Arnold E, Jacobo-Molina A, Nanni RG, et al. Structure of HIV-1 reverse transcriptase/DNA complex at 7 Å resolution showing active site locations. *Nature* 1992;357:85–89.
12. Arold S, Franken P, Strub MP, et al. The crystal structure of HIV-1 Nef protein bound to the Fyn kinase SH3 domain suggests a role for this complex in altered T cell receptor signaling. *Structure* 1997;5:1361–1372.
13. Arthur LO, Bess JW Jr, Waters DJ, et al. Challenge of chimpanzees (*Pan troglodytes*) immunized with human immunodeficiency virus envelope glycoprotein gp120. *J Virol* 1989;63:5046–5053.
14. Askjaer P, Jensen TH, Nilsson J, et al. The specificity of the CRM1-Rev nuclear export signal interaction is mediated by RanGTP. *J Biol Chem* 1998;273:33414–33422.
15. Atchison RE, Gosling J, Monteclaro FS, et al. Multiple extracellular elements of CCR5 and HIV-1 entry: Dissociation from response to chemokines. *Science* 1996;274:1924–1926.
16. Ayyavoo V, Mahboubi A, Mahalingam S, et al. HIV-1 Vpr suppresses immune activation and apoptosis through regulation of nuclear factor kappa B. *Nat Med* 1997;3:1117–1123.
17. Baeuerle PA, Baltimore D. A 65-kD subunit of active NF-κB is required for inhibition of NF-κB by IκB. *Genes Dev* 1989;3:1689–1698.
18. Ballard DW, Böhnlein E, Lowenthal JW, et al. HTLV-I tax induces cellular proteins that activate the κB element in the IL-2 receptor α gene. *Science* 1988;241:1652–1655.
19. Balliet JW, Kolson DL, Eiger G, et al. Distinct effects in primary macrophages and lymphocytes of the human immunodeficiency virus type 1 accessory genes *vpr*, *vpu*, and *nef*: Mutational analysis of a primary HIV-1 isolate. *Virology* 1994;200:623–631.
20. Baltimore D. RNA-dependent DNA polymerase in virions of RNA tumour viruses. *Nature* 1970;226:1209–1211.
21. Barré-Sinoussi F, Chermann JC, Rey F, et al. Isolation of a T-lymphotropic retrovirus from a patient at risk for acquired immune deficiency syndrome (AIDS). *Science* 1983;220:868–871.
22. Bartel DP, Zapp ML, Green MR, et al. HIV-1 Rev regulation involves recognition of non-Watson-Crick base pairs in viral RNA. *Cell* 1991;67:529–536.
23. Battiste JL, Mao H, Rao NS, et al. α helix-RNA major groove recognition in an HIV-1 rev peptide-RRE RNA complex. *Science* 1996;273:1547–1551.
24. Bebenek K, Abbotts J, Roberts JD, et al. Specificity and mechanism of error-prone replication by human immunodeficiency virus-1 reverse transcriptase. *J Biol Chem* 1989;264:16948–16956.
25. Bedinger P, Moriarty A, von Borstel RC II, et al. Internalization of the human immunodeficiency virus does not require the cytoplasmic domain of CD4. *Nature* 1988;334:162–165.
26. Beg AA, Ruben SM, Scheinman RI, et al. I kappa B interacts with the nuclear localization sequences of the subunits of NF-kappa B: A mechanism for cytoplasmic retention [published erratum appears in *Genes Dev* 1992 Dec;6:2664–2665]. *Genes Dev* 1992;6:1899–1913.
27. Benichou S, Bomsel M, Bodeus M, et al. Physical interaction of the HIV-1 Nef protein with beta-COP, a component of non-clathrin-coated vesicles essential for membrane traffic. *J Biol Chem* 1994;269:30073–30076.
28. Benn S, Rutledge R, Folks T, et al. Genomic heterogeneity of AIDS retroviral isolates from North America and Zaire. *Science* 1985;230:949–951.
29. Bennett RP, Nelle TD, Wills JW. Functional chimeras of the Rous sarcoma virus and human immunodeficiency virus gag proteins. *J Virol* 1993;67:6487–6498.
30. Berger EA, Doms RW, Fenyo EM, et al. A new classification for HIV-1 [letter]. *Nature* 1998;391:240.
31. Berger EA, Murphy PM, Farber JM. Chemokine receptors as HIV-1 coreceptors: Roles in viral entry, tropism, and disease. *Annu Rev Immunol* 1999;17:657–700.
32. Berkhout B, Jeang K-T. Functional roles for the TATA promoter and enhancers in basal and Tat-induced expression of the human immunodeficiency virus type 1 long terminal repeat. *J Virol* 1992;66:139–149.
33. Berkhout B, Silverman RH, Jeang K-T. Tat trans-activates the human immunodeficiency virus through a nascent RNA target. *Cell* 1989;59:273–282.
34. Berkhout B, van Hemert FJ. The unusual nucleotide content of the HIV RNA genome results in a biased amino acid composition of HIV proteins. *Nucleic Acids Res* 1994;22:1705–1711.
35. Berkhout B, van Wamel JL. Role of the DIS hairpin in replication of human immunodeficiency virus type 1. *J Virol* 1996;70:6723–6732.
36. Berkowitz R, Fisher J, Goff SP. RNA packaging. *Curr Top Microbiol Immunol* 1996;214:177–218.
37. Berthoux L, Pechoux C, Ottmann M, et al. Mutations in the N-terminal domain of human immunodeficiency virus type 1 nucleocapsid protein affect virion core structure and proviral DNA synthesis. *J Virol* 1997;71:6973–6981.
38. Bess JW Jr, Powell PJ, Issaq HJ, et al. Tightly bound zinc in human immunodeficiency virus type 1, human T-cell leukemia virus type I, and other retroviruses. *J Virol* 1992;66:840–847.
39. Bieniasz PD, Grdina TA, Bogerd HP, et al. Recruitment of a protein complex containing Tat and cyclin T1 to TAR governs the species specificity of HIV-1 Tat. *EMBO J* 1998;17:7056–7065.
40. Billich S, Knoop M-T, Hansen J, et al. Synthetic peptides as substrates and inhibitors of human immune deficiency virus-1 protease. *J Biol Chem* 1988;263:17905–17908.
41. Bischoff FR, Ponstingl H. Mitotic regulator protein RCC1 is complexed with a nuclear *ras*-related polypeptide. *Proc Natl Acad Sci U S A* 1991;88:10830–10834.
42. Bischoff FR, Ponstingl H. Catalysis of guanine nucleotide exchange of Ran by RCC1 and stimulation of hydrolysis of Ran-bound GTP by Ran-GAP1. *Methods Enzymol* 1995;257:135–144.
43. Bjorndal A, Deng H, Jansson M, et al. Coreceptor usage of primary human immunodeficiency virus type 1 isolates varies according to biological phenotype. *J Virol* 1997;71:7478–7487.
44. Boge M, Wyss S, Bonifacino JS, et al. A membrane-proximal tyrosine-based signal mediates internalization of the HIV-1 envelope glycoprotein via interaction with the AP-2 clathrin adaptor. *J Biol Chem* 1998;273:15773–15778.
45. Borman AM, Quillent C, Charneau P, et al. Human immunodeficiency virus type 1 Vif$^-$ mutant particles from restrictive cells: Role of Vif in correct particle assembly and infectivity. *J Virol* 1995;69:2058–2067.
46. Bosch ML, Earl PL, Fargnoli K, et al. Identification of the fusion peptide of primate immunodeficiency viruses. *Science* 1989;244:694–697.
47. Bour S, Boulerice F, Wainberg MA. Inhibition of gp160 and CD4 maturation in U937 cells after both defective and productive infections by human immunodeficiency virus type 1. *J Virol* 1991;65:6387–6396.
48. Bour S, Geleziunas R, Wainberg MA. The human immunodeficiency virus type 1 (HIV-1) CD4 receptor and its central role in promotion of HIV-1 infection. *Microbiol Rev* 1995;59:63–93.
49. Bour S, Schubert U, Strebel K. The human immunodeficiency virus

type 1 Vpu protein specifically binds to the cytoplasmic domain of CD4: Implications for the mechanism of degradation. *J Virol* 1995;69: 1510–1520.
50. Bouyac M, Rey F, Nascimbeni M, et al. Phenotypically Vif⁻ human immunodeficiency virus type 1 is produced by chronically infected restrictive cells. *J Virol* 1997;71:2473–2477.
51. Bowerman B, Brown PO, Bishop JM, et al. A nucleoprotein complex mediates the integration of retroviral DNA. *Genes Dev* 1989;3: 469–478.
52. Braaten D, Franke EK, Luban J. Cyclophilin A is required for the replication of group M human immunodeficiency virus type 1 (HIV-1) and simian immunodeficiency virus SIV(CPZ)GAB but not group O HIV-1 or other primate immunodeficiency viruses. *J Virol* 1996;70:4220–4227.
53. Braddock M, Thorburn AM, Kingsman AJ, et al. Blocking of Tat-dependent HIV-1 RNA modification by an inhibitor of RNA polymerase II processivity. *Nature* 1991;350:439–441.
54. Brady HJ, Pennington DJ, Miles CG, et al. CD4 cell surface downregulation in HIV-1 Nef transgenic mice is a consequence of intracellular sequestration. *EMBO J* 1993;12:4923–4932.
55. Bray M, Prasad S, Dubay JW, et al. A small element from the Mason-Pfizer monkey virus genome makes human immunodeficiency virus type 1 expression and replication Rev-independent. *Proc Natl Acad Sci U S A* 1994;91:1256–1260.
56. Broder CC, Dimitrov DS, Blumenthal R, et al. The block to HIV-1 envelope glycoprotein-mediated membrane fusion in animal cells expressing human CD4 can be overcome by a human cell component(s). *Virology* 1993;193:483–491.
57. Brown PO. Integration. In: Coffin JM, Hughes SH, Varmus HE, eds. *Retroviruses.* Cold Spring Harbor, NY: Cold Spring Harbor Laboratory Press, 1997:161–203.
58. Brown PO, Bowerman B, Varmus HE, et al. Correct integration of retroviral DNA in vitro. *Cell* 1987;49:347–356.
59. Brown PO, Bowerman B, Varmus HE, et al. Retroviral integration: Structure of the initial covalent product and its precursor, and a role for the viral IN protein. *Proc Natl Acad Sci U S A* 1989;86:2525–2529.
60. Bujacz G, Jaskolski M, Alexandratos J, et al. High-resolution structure of the catalytic domain of avian sarcoma virus integrase. *J Mol Biol* 1995;253:333–346.
61. Bukovsky AA, Dorfman T, Weimann A, et al. Nef association with human immunodeficiency virus type 1 virions and cleavage by the viral protease. *J Virol* 1997;71:1013–1018.
62. Bukrinskaya AG, Ghorpade A, Heinzinger NK, et al. Phosphorylation-dependent human immunodeficiency virus type 1 infection and nuclear targeting of viral DNA. *Proc Natl Acad Sci U S A* 1996;93: 367–371.
63. Bukrinsky MI, Haggerty S, Dempsey MP, et al. A nuclear localization signal within HIV-1 matrix protein that governs infection of non-dividing cells. *Nature* 1993;365:666–669.
64. Bukrinsky MI, Sharova N, McDonald TL, et al. Association of integrase, matrix, and reverse transcriptase antigens of human immunodeficiency virus type 1 with viral nucleic acids following acute infection. *Proc Natl Acad Sci U S A* 1993;90:6125–6129.
65. Bullough PA, Hughson FM, Skehel JJ, et al. Structure of influenza haemagglutinin at the pH of membrane fusion. *Nature* 1994;371: 37–43.
66. Bushman FD, Engelman A, Palmer I, et al. Domains of the integrase protein of human immunodeficiency virus type 1 responsible for polynucleotidyl transfer and zinc binding. *Proc Natl Acad Sci U S A* 1993;90:3428–3432.
67. Caffrey M, Cai M, Kaufman J, et al. Three-dimensional solution structure of the 44 kDa ectodomain of SIV gp41. *EMBO J* 1998;17: 4572–4584.
68. Cai M, Zheng R, Caffrey M, et al. Solution structure of the N-terminal zinc binding domain of HIV-1 integrase. *Nat Struct Biol* 1997;4: 567–577.
69. Callahan MA, Handley MA, Lee YH, et al. Functional interaction of human immunodeficiency virus type 1 Vpu and Gag with a novel member of the tetratricopeptide repeat protein family [published erratum appears in *J Virol* 1998;72:8461]. *J Virol* 1998;72:5189–5197.
70. Camaur D, Trono D. Characterization of human immunodeficiency virus type 1 Vif particle incorporation. *J Virol* 1996;70:6106–6111.
71. Cameron P, Pope M, Granelli-Piperno A, et al. Dendritic cells and the replication of HIV-1. *J Leukoc Biol* 1996;59:158–171.
72. Campbell S, Vogt VM. Self-assembly in vitro of purified CA-NC proteins from Rous sarcoma virus and human immunodeficiency virus type 1. *J Virol* 1995;69:6487–6497.
73. Cao J, Bergeron L, Helseth E, et al. Effects of amino acid changes in the extracellular domain of the human immunodeficiency virus type 1 gp41 envelope glycoprotein. *J Virol* 1993;67:2747–2755.
74. Cao J, Park IW, Cooper A, et al. Molecular determinants of acute single-cell lysis by human immunodeficiency virus type 1. *J Virol* 1996; 70:1340–1354.
75. Cao Z, Henzel WJ, Gao X. IRAK: A kinase associated with the interleukin-1 receptor. *Science* 1996;271:1128–1131.
76. Carr JK, Salminen MO, Koch C, et al. Full-length sequence and mosaic structure of a human immunodeficiency virus type 1 isolate from Thailand. *J Virol* 1996;70:5935–5943.
77. Carteau S, Gorelick RJ, Bushman FD. Coupled integration of human immunodeficiency virus type 1 cDNA ends by purified integrase in vitro: Stimulation by the viral nucleocapsid protein. *J Virol* 1999; 73:6670–6679.
78. Casella CR, Raffini LJ, Panganiban AT. Pleiotropic mutations in the HIV-1 matrix protein that affect diverse steps in replication. *Virology* 1997;228:294–306.
79. CDC. *Pneumocystis* pneumonia—Los Angeles. *MMWR Morb Mortal Wkly Rep* 1981;30:250–252.
80. Chan DC, Fass D, Berger JM, et al. Core structure of gp41 from the HIV envelope glycoprotein. *Cell* 1997;89:263–273.
81. Charneau P, Alizon M, Clavel F. A second origin of DNA plus-strand synthesis is required for optimal human immunodeficiency virus replication. *J Virol* 1992;66:2814–2820.
82. Charneau P, Mirambeau G, Roux P, et al. HIV-1 reverse transcription. A termination step at the center of the genome. *J Mol Biol* 1994;241:651–662.
83. Chen BK, Feinberg MB, Baltimore D. The κB sites in the human immunodeficiency virus type 1 long terminal repeat enhance virus replication yet are not absolutely required for viral growth. *J Virol* 1997;71:5495–5504.
84. Chen D, Zhou Q. Tat activates human immunodeficiency virus type 1 transcriptional elongation independent of TFIIH kinase. *Mol Cell Biol* 1999;19:2863–2871.
85. Chen H, Engelman A. The barrier-to-autointegration protein is a host factor for HIV type 1 integration. *Proc Natl Acad Sci U S A* 1998;95: 15270–15274.
86. Chen H, Wei SQ, Engelman A. Multiple integrase functions are required to form the native structure of the human immunodeficiency virus type I intasome. *J Biol Chem* 1999;274:17358–17364.
87. Chen MY, Maldarelli F, Karczewski MK, et al. Human immunodeficiency virus type 1 Vpu protein induces degradation of CD4 in vitro: The cytoplasmic domain of CD4 contributes to Vpu sensitivity. *J Virol* 1993;67:3877–3884.
88. Chen SS, Lee CN, Lee WR, et al. Mutational analysis of the leucine zipper-like motif of the human immunodeficiency virus type 1 envelope transmembrane glycoprotein. *J Virol* 1993;67:3615–3619.
89. Chen Z, Yan Y, Munshi S, et al. X-ray structure of simian immunodeficiency virus integrase containing the core and C-terminal domain (residues 50-293)—An initial glance of the viral DNA binding platform. *J Mol Biol* 2000;296:521–533.
90. Cheng-Mayer C, Liu R, Landau NR, et al. Macrophage tropism of human immunodeficiency virus type 1 and utilization of the CC-CKR5 coreceptor. *J Virol* 1997;71:1657–1661.
91. Cho MW, Lee MK, Carney MC, et al. Identification of determinants on a dualtropic human immunodeficiency virus type 1 envelope glycoprotein that confer usage of CXCR4. *J Virol* 1998;72:2509–2515.
92. Choe H, Farzan M, Sun Y, et al. The β-chemokine receptors CCR3 and CCR5 facilitate infection by primary HIV-1 isolates. *Cell* 1996;85: 1135–1148.
93. Chow SA, Vincent KA, Ellison V, et al. Reversal of integration and DNA splicing mediated by integrase of human immunodeficiency virus. *Science* 1992;255:723–726.
94. Chowers MY, Pandori MW, Spina CA, et al. The growth advantage conferred by HIV-1 nef is determined at the level of viral DNA formation and is independent of CD4 downregulation. *Virology* 1995; 212:451–457.
95. Chowers MY, Spina CA, Kwoh TJ, et al. Optimal infectivity in vitro of human immunodeficiency virus type 1 requires an intact *nef* gene. *J Virol* 1994;68:2906–2914.
96. Chun TW, Chadwick K, Margolick J, et al. Differential susceptibility of naive and memory CD4+ T cells to the cytopathic effects of infec-

tion with human immunodeficiency virus type 1 strain LAI. *J Virol* 1997;71:4436–4444.
97. Clavel F, Guétard D, Brun-Vézinet F, et al. Isolation of a new human retrovirus from West African patients with AIDS. *Science* 1986;233: 343–346.
98. Clever JL, Eckstein DA, Parslow TG. Genetic dissociation of the encapsidation and reverse transcription functions in the 5′ R region of human immunodeficiency virus type 1. *J Virol* 1999;73:101–109.
99. Clever JL, Parslow TG. Mutant human immunodeficiency virus type 1 genomes with defects in RNA dimerization or encapsidation. *J Virol* 1997;71:3407–3414.
100. Cocchi F, DeVico AL, Garzino-Demo A, et al. Identification of RANTES, MIP-1α, and MIP-1β as the major HIV-suppressive factors produced by CD8+ T cells. *Science* 1995;270:1811–1815.
101. Cocchi F, DeVico AL, Garzino-Demo A, et al. The V3 domain of the HIV-1 gp120 envelope glycoprotein is critical for chemokine-mediated blockade of infection. *Nat Med* 1996;2:1244–1247.
102. Coffin J, Haase A, Levy JA, et al. Human immunodeficiency viruses [letter]. *Science* 1986;232:697.
103. Coffin JM. Structure, replication, and recombination of retrovirus genomes: Some unifying hypotheses. *J Gen Virol* 1979;42:1–26.
104. Coffin JM. Genetic diversity and evolution of retroviruses. *Curr Top Microbiol Immunol* 1992;176:143–164.
105. Coffin JM. HIV population dynamics in vivo: Implications for genetic variation, pathogenesis, and therapy. *Science* 1995;267:483–489.
106. Cohen EA, Dehni G, Sodroski JG, et al. Human immunodeficiency virus vpr product is a virion-associated regulatory protein. *J Virol* 1990;64:3097–3099.
107. Cohen EA, Terwilliger EF, Sodroski JG, et al. Identification of a protein encoded by the *vpu* gene of HIV-1. *Nature* 1988;334:532–534.
108. Cohen GB, Gandhi RT, Davis DM, et al. The selective downregulation of class I major histocompatibility complex proteins by HIV-1 protects HIV-infected cells from NK cells. *Immunity* 1999;10:661–671.
109. Colicelli J, Goff SP. Mutants and pseudorevertants of Moloney murine leukemia virus with alterations at the integration site. *Cell* 1985;42: 573–580.
110. Collins KL, Chen BK, Kalams SA, et al. HIV-1 Nef protein protects infected primary cells against killing by cytotoxic T lymphocytes. *Nature* 1998;391:397–401.
111. Collman R, Balliet JW, Gregory SA, et al. An infectious molecular clone of an unusual macrophage-tropic and highly cytopathic strain of human immunodeficiency virus type 1. *J Virol* 1992;66:7517–7521.
112. Collman R, Hassan NF, Walker R, et al. Infection of monocyte-derived macrophages with human immunodeficiency virus type 1 (HIV-1). Monocyte-tropic and lymphocyte-tropic strains of HIV-1 show distinctive patterns of replication in a panel of cell types. *J Exp Med* 1989;170:1149–1163.
113. Condra JH, Schleif WA, Blahy OM, et al. In vivo emergence of HIV-1 variants resistant to multiple protease inhibitors. *Nature* 1995; 374:569–571.
114. Conte MR, Matthews S. Retroviral matrix proteins: A structural perspective. *Virology* 1998;246:191–198.
115. Corbet S, Muller-Trutwin MC, Versmisse P, et al. *env* sequences of simian immunodeficiency viruses from chimpanzees in Cameroon are strongly related to those of human immunodeficiency virus group N from the same geographic area. *J Virol* 2000;74:529–534.
116. Cordingley MG, LaFemina RL, Callahan PL, et al. Sequence-specific interaction of Tat protein and Tat peptides with the transactivation-responsive sequence element of human immunodeficiency virus type 1 in vitro. *Proc Natl Acad Sci U S A* 1990;87:8985–8989.
117. Cosson P. Direct interaction between the envelope and matrix proteins of HIV-1. *EMBO J* 1996;15:5783–5788.
118. Craig HM, Pandori MW, Riggs NL, et al. Analysis of the SH3-binding region of HIV-1 *nef*: Partial functional defects introduced by mutations in the polyproline helix and the hydrophobic pocket. *Virology* 1999;262:55–63.
119. Craigie R, Fujiwara T, Bushman F. The IN protein of Moloney murine leukemia virus processes the viral DNA ends and accomplishes their integration in vitro. *Cell* 1990;62:829–837.
120. Crawford S, Goff SP. A deletion mutation in the 5′ part of the *pol* gene of Moloney murine leukemia virus blocks proteolytic processing of the *gag* and *pol* polyproteins. *J Virol* 1985;53:899–907.
121. Croteau G, Doyon L, Thibeault D, et al. Impaired fitness of human immunodeficiency virus type 1 variants with high-level resistance to protease inhibitors. *J Virol* 1997;71:1089–1096.
122. Daar ES, Li XL, Moudgil T, et al. High concentrations of recombinant soluble CD4 are required to neutralize primary human immunodeficiency virus type 1 isolates. *Proc Natl Acad Sci U S A* 1990;87: 6574–6578.
123. Daniel MD, Letvin NL, King NW, et al. Isolation of T-cell tropic HTLV-III-like retrovirus from macaques. *Science* 1985;228:1201–1204.
124. Das AT, Klaver B, Berkhout B. A hairpin structure in the R region of the human immunodeficiency virus type 1 RNA genome is instrumental in polyadenylation site selection. *J Virol* 1999;73:81–91.
125. Das AT, Klaver B, Klasens BI, et al. A conserved hairpin motif in the R-U5 region of the human immunodeficiency virus type 1 RNA genome is essential for replication. *J Virol* 1997;71:2346–2356.
126. Davies DR. The structure and function of the aspartic proteinases. *Annu Rev Biophys Biophys Chem* 1990;19:189–215.
127. Davies JF II, Hostomska Z, Hostomsky Z, et al. Crystal structure of the ribonuclease H domain of HIV-1 reverse transcriptase. *Science* 1991;252:88–95.
128. Dayton AI, Sodroski JG, Rosen CA, et al. The trans-activator gene of the human T cell lymphotropic virus type III is required for replication. *Cell* 1986;44:941–947.
129. Dayton ET, Powell DM, Dayton AI. Functional analysis of CAR, the target sequence for the Rev protein of HIV-1. *Science* 1989;246: 1625–1629.
130. De Guzman RN, Wu ZR, Stalling CC, et al. Structure of the HIV-1 nucleocapsid protein bound to the SL3 ψ-RNA recognition element. *Science* 1998;279:384–388.
131. de Vreese K, Kofler-Mongold V, Leutgeb C, et al. The molecular target of bicyclams, potent inhibitors of human immunodeficiency virus replication. *J Virol* 1996;70:689–696.
132. Deacon NJ, Tsykin A, Solomon A, et al. Genomic structure of an attenuated quasi species of HIV-1 from a blood transfusion donor and recipients. *Science* 1995;270:988–991.
133. Dean M, Carrington M, Winkler C, et al. Genetic restriction of HIV-1 infection and progression to AIDS by a deletion allele of the CKR5 structural gene [published erratum appears in *Science* 1996;274: 1069]. *Science* 1996;273:1856–1862.
134. Deng H, Liu R, Ellmeier W, et al. Identification of a major co-receptor for primary isolates of HIV-1. *Nature* 1996;381:661–666.
135. Dettenhofer M, Yu XF. Highly purified human immunodeficiency virus type 1 reveals a virtual absence of Vif in virions. *J Virol* 1999;73: 1460–1467.
136. Dickson C, Peters G. Protein-coding potential of mouse mammary tumor virus genome RNA as examined by in vitro translation. *J Virol* 1981;37:36–47.
137. Dimitrov DS, Norwood D, Stantchev TS, et al. A mechanism of resistance to HIV-1 entry: Inefficient interactions of CXCR4 with CD4 and gp120 in macrophages. *Virology* 1999;259:1–6.
138. Dimitrov DS, Willey RL, Sato H, et al. Quantitation of human immunodeficiency virus type 1 infection kinetics. *J Virol* 1993;67:2182–2190.
139. Dingwall C, Ernberg I, Gait MJ, et al. Human immunodeficiency virus 1 *tat* protein binds trans-activation-responsive region (TAR) RNA *in vitro*. *Proc Natl Acad Sci U S A* 1989;86:6925–6929.
140. Dingwall C, Ernberg I, Gait MJ, et al. HIV-1 tat protein stimulates transcription by binding to a U-rich bulge in the stem of the TAR RNA structure. *EMBO J* 1990;9:4145–4153.
141. Dittmar MT, McKnight A, Simmons G, et al. HIV-1 tropism and co-receptor use [letter]. *Nature* 1997;385:495–496.
142. Doherty TM, Chougnet C, Schito M, et al. Infection of HIV-1 transgenic mice with *Mycobacterium avium* induces the expression of infectious virus selectively from a Mac-1-positive host cell population. *J Immunol* 1999;163:1506–1515.
143. Doms RW, Peiper SC. Unwelcomed guests with master keys: How HIV uses chemokine receptors for cellular entry. *Virology* 1997;235:179–190.
144. Donzella GA, Schols D, Lin SW, et al. AMD3100, a small molecule inhibitor of HIV-1 entry via the CXCR4 co-receptor. *Nat Med* 1998;4: 72–77.
145. Doranz BJ, Rucker J, Yi Y, et al. A dual-tropic primary HIV-1 isolate that uses fusin and the β-chemokine receptors CKR-5, CKR-3, and CKR-2b as fusion cofactors. *Cell* 1996;85:1149–1158.
146. Dorfman T, Mammano F, Haseltine WA, et al. Role of the matrix protein in the virion association of the human immunodeficiency virus type 1 envelope glycoprotein. *J Virol* 1994;68:1689–1696.
147. Dougherty JP, Temin HM. Determination of the rate of base-pair substitution and insertion mutations in retrovirus replication. *J Virol* 1988;62:2817–2822.

148. Doye V, Hurt E. From nucleoporins to nuclear pore complexes. *Curr Opin Cell Biol* 1997;9:401–411.
149. Doyon L, Croteau G, Thibeault D, et al. Second locus involved in human immunodeficiency virus type 1 resistance to protease inhibitors. *J Virol* 1996;70:3763–3769.
150. Dragic T, Charneau P, Clavel F, et al. Complementation of murine cells for human immunodeficiency virus envelope/CD4-mediated fusion in human/murine heterokaryons. *J Virol* 1992;66:4794–4802.
151. Du Z, Lang SM, Sasseville VG, et al. Identification of a *nef* allele that causes lymphocyte activation and acute disease in macaque monkeys. *Cell* 1995;82:665–674.
152. Dubay JW, Roberts SJ, Brody B, et al. Mutations in the leucine zipper of the human immunodeficiency virus type 1 transmembrane glycoprotein affect fusion and infectivity. *J Virol* 1992;66:4748–4756.
153. Dyda F, Hickman AB, Jenkins TM, et al. Crystal structure of the catalytic domain of HIV-1 integrase: Similarity to other polynucleotidyl transferases. *Science* 1994;266:1981–1986.
154. Earl PL, Moss B, Doms RW. Folding, interaction with GRP78-BiP, assembly, and transport of the human immunodeficiency virus type 1 envelope protein. *J Virol* 1991;65:2047–2055.
155. Edinger AL, Hoffman TL, Sharron M, et al. An orphan seven-transmembrane domain receptor expressed widely in the brain functions as a coreceptor for human immunodeficiency virus type 1 and simian immunodeficiency virus. *J Virol* 1998;72:7934–7940.
156. Egan MA, Carruth LM, Rowell JF, et al. Human immunodeficiency virus type 1 envelope protein endocytosis mediated by a highly conserved intrinsic internalization signal in the cytoplasmic domain of gp41 is suppressed in the presence of the $Pr55^{gag}$ precursor protein. *J Virol* 1996;70:6547–6556.
157. Ehrlich LS, Agresta BE, Carter CA. Assembly of recombinant human immunodeficiency virus type 1 capsid protein in vitro. *J Virol* 1992; 66:4874–4883.
158. Eijkelenboom AP, Lutzke RA, Boelens R, et al. The DNA-binding domain of HIV-1 integrase has an SH3-like fold. *Nat Struct Biol* 1995; 2:807–810.
159. El Kharroubi A, Martin MA. *cis*-acting sequences located downstream of the human immunodeficiency virus type 1 promoter affect its chromatin structure and transcriptional activity. *Mol Cell Biol* 1996;16:2958–2966.
160. Emerman M, Guyader M, Montagnier L, et al. The specificity of the human immunodeficiency virus type 2 transactivator is different from that of human immunodeficiency virus type 1. *EMBO J* 1987;6: 3755–3760.
161. Endres MJ, Clapham PR, Marsh M, et al. CD4-independent infection by HIV-2 is mediated by fusin/CXCR4. *Cell* 1996;87:745–756.
162. Engelman A, Hickman AB, Craigie R. The core and carboxyl-terminal domains of the integrase protein of human immunodeficiency virus type 1 each contribute to nonspecific DNA binding. *J Virol* 1994;68:5911–5917.
163. Englund G, Theodore TS, Freed EO, et al. Integration is required for productive infection of monocyte-derived macrophages by human immunodeficiency virus type 1. *J Virol* 1995;69:3216–3219.
164. Ensoli B, Barillari G, Salahuddin SZ, et al. Tat protein of HIV-1 stimulates growth of cells derived from Kaposi's sarcoma lesions of AIDS patients. *Nature* 1990;345:84–86.
165. Esnouf R, Ren J, Ross C, et al. Mechanism of inhibition of HIV-1 reverse transcriptase by non-nucleoside inhibitors. *Nat Struct Biol* 1995;2:303–308.
166. Essex M, McLane MF, Lee TH, et al. Antibodies to cell membrane antigens associated with human T-cell leukemia virus in patients with AIDS. *Science* 1983;220:859–862.
167. Ewart GD, Sutherland T, Gage PW, et al. The Vpu protein of human immunodeficiency virus type 1 forms cation-selective ion channels. *J Virol* 1996;70:7108–7115.
168. Fabre E, Hurt E. Yeast genetics to dissect the nuclear pore complex and nucleocytoplasmic trafficking. *Annu Rev Genet* 1997;31:277–313.
169. Facke M, Janetzko A, Shoeman RL, et al. A large deletion in the matrix domain of the human immunodeficiency virus *gag* gene redirects virus particle assembly from the plasma membrane to the endoplasmic reticulum. *J Virol* 1993;67:4972–4980.
170. Farnet CM, Bushman FD. HIV cDNA integration: Molecular biology and inhibitor development. *AIDS* 1996;10:S3–11.
171. Farnet CM, Bushman FD. HIV-1 cDNA integration: Requirement of HMG I(Y) protein for function of preintegration complexes in vitro. *Cell* 1997;88:483–492.
172. Farnet CM, Wang B, Lipford JR, et al. Differential inhibition of HIV-1 preintegration complexes and purified integrase protein by small molecules. *Proc Natl Acad Sci U S A* 1996;93:9742–9747.
173. Feinberg MB, Baltimore D, Frankel AD. The role of Tat in the human immunodeficiency virus life cycle indicates a primary effect on transcriptional elongation. *Proc Natl Acad Sci U S A* 1991;88:4045–4049.
174. Felber BK, Hadzopoulou-Cladaras M, Cladaras C, et al. Rev protein of human immunodeficiency virus type 1 affects the stability and transport of the viral mRNA. *Proc Natl Acad Sci U S A* 1989;86:1495–1499.
175. Felzien LK, Woffendin C, Hottiger MO, et al. HIV transcriptional activation by the accessory protein, VPR, is mediated by the p300 co-activator. *Proc Natl Acad Sci U S A* 1998;95:5281–5286.
176. Feng S, Holland EC. HIV-1 *tat trans*-activation requires the loop sequence within *tar*. *Nature* 1988;334:165–167.
177. Feng Y, Broder CC, Kennedy PE, et al. HIV-1 entry cofactor: Functional cDNA cloning of a seven-transmembrane, G protein-coupled receptor. *Science* 1996;272:872–877.
178. Feng YX, Campbell S, Harvin D, et al. The human immunodeficiency virus type 1 Gag polyprotein has nucleic acid chaperone activity: Possible role in dimerization of genomic RNA and placement of tRNA on the primer binding site. *J Virol* 1999;73:4251–4256.
179. Fenyö EM, Morfeldt-Månson L, Chiodi F, et al. Distinct replicative and cytopathic characteristics of human immunodeficiency virus isolates. *J Virol* 1988;62:4414–4419.
180. Fischer U, Huber J, Boelens WC, et al. The HIV-1 Rev activation domain is a nuclear export signal that accesses an export pathway used by specific cellular RNAs. *Cell* 1995;82:475–483.
181. Fischer U, Meyer S, Teufel M, et al. Evidence that HIV-1 Rev directly promotes the nuclear export of unspliced RNA. *EMBO J* 1994;13: 4105–4112.
182. Fisher AG, Feinberg MB, Josephs SF, et al. The *trans*-activator gene of HTLV-III is essential for virus replication. *Nature* 1986;320:367–371.
183. Fletcher TM III, Brichacek B, Sharova N, et al. Nuclear import and cell cycle arrest functions of the HIV-1 Vpr protein are encoded by two separate genes in HIV-2/SIV(SM). *EMBO J* 1996;15:6155–6165.
184. Fornerod M, Ohno M, Yoshida M, et al. CRM1 is an export receptor for leucine-rich nuclear export signals. *Cell* 1997;90:1051–1060.
185. Fornerod M, van Deursen J, van Baal S, et al. The human homologue of yeast CRM1 is in a dynamic subcomplex with CAN/Nup214 and a novel nuclear pore component Nup88. *EMBO J* 1997;16:807–816.
186. Fouchier RA, Meyer BE, Simon JH, et al. HIV-1 infection of non-dividing cells: Evidence that the amino-terminal basic region of the viral matrix protein is important for Gag processing but not for post-entry nuclear import. *EMBO J* 1997;16:4531–4539.
187. Fouchier RA, Meyer BE, Simon JH, et al. Interaction of the human immunodeficiency virus type 1 Vpr protein with the nuclear pore complex. *J Virol* 1998;72:6004–6013.
188. Fouchier RA, Simon JH, Jaffe AB, et al. Human immunodeficiency virus type 1 Vif does not influence expression or virion incorporation of *gag-*, *pol-*, and *env*-encoded proteins. *J Virol* 1996;70:8263–8269.
189. Frank I, Kacani L, Stoiber H, et al. Human immunodeficiency virus type 1 derived from cocultures of immature dendritic cells with autologous T cells carries T-cell-specific molecules on its surface and is highly infectious. *J Virol* 1999;73:3449–3454.
190. Franke EK, Yuan HE, Luban J. Specific incorporation of cyclophilin A into HIV-1 virions. *Nature* 1994;372:359–362.
191. Frankel AD, Pabo CO. Cellular uptake of the Tat protein from human immunodeficiency virus. *Cell* 1988;55:1189–1193.
192. Freed EO. HIV-1 Gag proteins: Diverse functions in the virus life cycle. *Virology* 1998;251:1–15.
193. Freed EO, Englund G, Maldarelli F, et al. Phosphorylation of residue 131 of HIV-1 matrix is not required for macrophage infection. *Cell* 1997;88:171–173; discussion 173–174.
194. Freed EO, Englund G, Martin MA. Role of the basic domain of human immunodeficiency virus type 1 matrix in macrophage infection. *J Virol* 1995;69:3949–3954.
195. Freed EO, Martin MA. HIV-1 infection of non-dividing cells [letter; comment]. *Nature* 1994;369:107–108.
196. Freed EO, Martin MA. Virion incorporation of envelope glycoproteins with long but not short cytoplasmic tails is blocked by specific, single amino acid substitutions in the human immunodeficiency virus type 1 matrix. *J Virol* 1995;69:1984–1989.
197. Freed EO, Martin MA. Domains of the human immunodeficiency virus type 1 matrix and gp41 cytoplasmic tail required for envelope incorporation into virions. *J Virol* 1996;70:341–351.

198. Freed EO, Myers DJ. Identification and characterization of fusion and processing domains of the human immunodeficiency virus type 2 envelope glycoprotein. *J Virol* 1992;66:5472–5478.
199. Freed EO, Myers DJ, Risser R. Mutational analysis of the cleavage sequence of the human immunodeficiency virus type 1 envelope glycoprotein precursor gp160. *J Virol* 1989;63:4670–4675.
200. Freed EO, Myers DJ, Risser R. Characterization of the fusion domain of the human immunodeficiency virus type 1 envelope glycoprotein gp41. *Proc Natl Acad Sci U S A* 1990;87:4650–4654.
201. Freed EO, Myers DJ, Risser R. Identification of the principal neutralizing determinant of human immunodeficiency virus type 1 as a fusion domain. *J Virol* 1991;65:190–194.
202. Freed EO, Orenstein JM, Buckler-White AJ, et al. Single amino acid changes in the human immunodeficiency virus type 1 matrix protein block virus particle production. *J Virol* 1994;68:5311–5320.
203. Fu GK, Grosveld G, Markovitz DM. DEK, an autoantigen involved in a chromosomal translocation in acute myelogenous leukemia, binds to the HIV-2 enhancer. *Proc Natl Acad Sci U S A* 1997;94:1811–1815.
204. Fujinaga K, Taube R, Wimmer J, et al. Interactions between human cyclin T, Tat, and the transactivation response element (TAR) are disrupted by a cysteine to tyrosine substitution found in mouse cyclin T. *Proc Natl Acad Sci U S A* 1999;96:1285–1290.
205. Fujita K, Omura S, Silver J. Rapid degradation of CD4 in cells expressing human immunodeficiency virus type 1 Env and Vpu is blocked by proteasome inhibitors. *J Gen Virol* 1997;78:619–625.
206. Fujiwara T, Mizuuchi K. Retroviral DNA integration: Structure of an integration intermediate. *Cell* 1988;54:497–504.
207. Fukuda M, Asano S, Nakamura T, et al. CRM1 is responsible for intracellular transport mediated by the nuclear export signal. *Nature* 1997;390:308–311.
208. Fuller SD, Wilk T, Gowen BE, et al. Cryo-electron microscopy reveals ordered domains in the immature HIV-1 particle. *Curr Biol* 1997;7:729–738.
209. Fultz PN, McClure HM, Swenson RB, et al. Persistent infection of chimpanzees with human T-lymphotropic virus type III/lymphadenopathy-associated virus: A potential model for acquired immunodeficiency syndrome. *J Virol* 1986;58:116–124.
210. Fung MS, Sun CR, Gordon WL, et al. Identification and characterization of a neutralization site within the second variable region of human immunodeficiency virus type 1 gp120. *J Virol* 1992;66:848–856.
211. Furuta RA, Wild CT, Weng Y, et al. Capture of an early fusion-active conformation of HIV-1 gp41 [published erratum appears in *Nat Struct Biol* 1998;5:612]. *Nat Struct Biol* 1998;5:276–279.
212. Gabuzda DH, Lawrence K, Langhoff E, et al. Role of *vif* in replication of human immunodeficiency virus type 1 in CD4$^+$ T lymphocytes. *J Virol* 1992;66:6489–6495.
213. Gallay P, Hope T, Chin D, et al. HIV-1 infection of nondividing cells through the recognition of integrase by the importin/karyopherin pathway. *Proc Natl Acad Sci U S A* 1997;94:9825–9830.
214. Gallay P, Swingler S, Aiken C, et al. HIV-1 infection of nondividing cells: C-terminal tyrosine phosphorylation of the viral matrix protein is a key regulator. *Cell* 1995;80:379–388.
215. Gallay P, Swingler S, Song J, et al. HIV nuclear import is governed by the phosphotyrosine-mediated binding of matrix to the core domain of integrase. *Cell* 1995;83:569–576.
216. Gallo RC, Sarin PS, Gelmann EP, et al. Isolation of human T-cell leukemia virus in acquired immune deficiency syndrome (AIDS). *Science* 1983;220:865–867.
217. Gamble TR, Vajdos FF, Yoo S, et al. Crystal structure of human cyclophilin A bound to the amino-terminal domain of HIV-1 capsid. *Cell* 1996;87:1285–1294.
218. Gamble TR, Yoo S, Vajdos FF, et al. Structure of the carboxyl-terminal dimerization domain of the HIV-1 capsid protein. *Science* 1997;278:849–853.
219. Gandhi RT, Chen BK, Straus SE, et al. HIV-1 directly kills CD4$^+$ T cells by a Fas-independent mechanism. *J Exp Med* 1998;187:1113–1122.
220. Ganser BK, Li S, Klishko VY, et al. Assembly and analysis of conical models for the HIV-1 core. *Science* 1999;283:80–83.
221. Gao F, Bailes E, Robertson DL, et al. Origin of HIV-1 in the chimpanzee *Pan troglodytes troglodytes*. *Nature* 1999;397:436–441.
222. Gao F, Robertson DL, Carruthers CD, et al. A comprehensive panel of near-full-length clones and reference sequences for non-subtype B isolates of human immunodeficiency virus type 1. *J Virol* 1998;72:5680–5698.
223. Gao F, Robertson DL, Morrison SG, et al. The heterosexual human immunodeficiency virus type 1 epidemic in Thailand is caused by an intersubtype (A/E) recombinant of African origin. *J Virol* 1996;70:7013–7029.
224. Gao F, Yue L, White AT, et al. Human infection by genetically diverse SIV_{SM}-related HIV-2 in West Africa. *Nature* 1992;358:495–499.
225. Garber ME, Wei P, KewalRamani VN, et al. The interaction between HIV-1 Tat and human cyclin T1 requires zinc and a critical cysteine residue that is not conserved in the murine CycT1 protein. *Genes Dev* 1998;12:3512–3527.
226. Garcia JV, Miller AD. Serine phosphorylation-independent downregulation of cell-surface CD4 by *nef*. *Nature* 1991;350:508–511.
227. Garcia-Martinez LF, Mavankal G, Neveu JM, et al. Purification of a Tat-associated kinase reveals a TFIIH complex that modulates HIV-1 transcription. *EMBO J* 1997;16:2836–2850.
228. Garnier L, Wills JW, Verderame MF, et al. WW domains and retrovirus budding [letter]. *Nature* 1996;381:744–745.
229. Garzino-Demo A, Moss RB, Margolick JB, et al. Spontaneous and antigen-induced production of HIV-inhibitory β-chemokines are associated with AIDS-free status. *Proc Natl Acad Sci U S A* 1999;96:11986–11991.
230. Gazzinelli RT, Sher A, Cheever A, et al. Infection of human immunodeficiency virus 1 transgenic mice with *Toxoplasma gondii* stimulates proviral transcription in macrophages in vivo. *J Exp Med* 1996;183:1645–1655.
231. Geigenmuller U, Linial ML. Specific binding of human immunodeficiency virus type 1 (HIV-1) Gag-derived proteins to a 5′ HIV-1 genomic RNA sequence. *J Virol* 1996;70:667–671.
232. Geijtenbeek TB, Kwon DS, Torensma R, et al. DC-SIGN, a dendritic cell-specific HIV-1-binding protein that enhances trans-infection of T cells. *Cell* 2000;100:587–597.
233. Geraghty RJ, Panganiban AT. Human immunodeficiency virus type 1 Vpu has a CD4- and an envelope glycoprotein-independent function. *J Virol* 1993;67:4190–4194.
234. Gibbs CJ Jr, Peters R, Gravell M, et al. Observations after human immunodeficiency virus immunization and challenge of human immunodeficiency virus seropositive and seronegative chimpanzees. *Proc Natl Acad Sci U S A* 1991;88:3348–3352.
235. Gilbert KM, Weigle WO. Th1 cell anergy and blockade in G1a phase of the cell cycle. *J Immunol* 1993;151:1245–1254.
236. Gilmartin GM, Fleming ES, Oetjen J, et al. CPSF recognition of an HIV-1 mRNA 3′-processing enhancer: Multiple sequence contacts involved in poly(A) site definition. *Genes Dev* 1995;9:72–83.
237. Gitti RK, Lee BM, Walker J, et al. Structure of the amino-terminal core domain of the HIV-1 capsid protein. *Science* 1996;273:231–235.
238. Gnann JW Jr, Nelson JA, Oldstone MBA. Fine mapping of an immunodominant domain in the transmembrane glycoprotein of human immunodeficiency virus. *J Virol* 1987;61:2639–2641.
239. Goh WC, Rogel ME, Kinsey CM, et al. HIV-1 Vpr increases viral expression by manipulation of the cell cycle: A mechanism for selection of Vpr in vivo. *Nat Med* 1998;4:65–71.
240. Goldsmith MA, Warmerdam MT, Atchison RE, et al. Dissociation of the CD4 downregulation and viral infectivity enhancement functions of human immunodeficiency virus type 1 Nef. *J Virol* 1995;69:4112–4121.
241. Goncalves J, Korin Y, Zack J, et al. Role of Vif in human immunodeficiency virus type 1 reverse transcription. *J Virol* 1996;70:8701–8709.
242. Gonda MA, Wong-Staal F, Gallo RC, et al. Sequence homology and morphologic similarity of HTLV-III and visna virus, a pathogenic lentivirus. *Science* 1985;227:173–177.
243. Gorelick RJ, Fu W, Gagliardi TD, et al. Characterization of the block in replication of nucleocapsid protein zinc finger mutants from Moloney murine leukemia virus. *J Virol* 1999;73:8185–8195.
244. Gorlich D. Transport into and out of the cell nucleus. *EMBO J* 1998;17:2721–2727.
245. Gorlich D, Mattaj IW. Nucleocytoplasmic transport. *Science* 1996;271:1513–1518.
246. Gotte M, Li X, Wainberg MA. HIV-1 reverse transcription: A brief overview focused on structure-function relationships among molecules involved in initiation of the reaction. *Arch Biochem Biophys* 1999;365:199–210.
247. Gottlinger HG, Dorfman T, Cohen EA, et al. Vpu protein of human immunodeficiency virus type 1 enhances the release of capsids produced by *gag* gene constructs of widely divergent retroviruses. *Proc Natl Acad Sci U S A* 1993;90:7381–7385.

248. Gottlinger HG, Dorfman T, Sodroski JG, et al. Effect of mutations affecting the p6 gag protein on human immunodeficiency virus particle release. *Proc Natl Acad Sci U S A* 1991;88:3195–3199.
249. Göttlinger HG, Sodroski JG, Haseltine WA. Role of capsid precursor processing and myristoylation in morphogenesis and infectivity of human immunodeficiency virus type 1. *Proc Natl Acad Sci U S A* 1989;86:5781–5785.
250. Grattinger M, Hohenberg H, Thomas D, et al. In vitro assembly properties of wild-type and cyclophilin-binding defective human immunodeficiency virus capsid proteins in the presence and absence of cyclophilin A. *Virology* 1999;257:247–260.
251. Greenberg ME, Bronson S, Lock M, et al. Co-localization of HIV-1 Nef with the AP-2 adaptor protein complex correlates with Nef-induced CD4 down-regulation. *EMBO J* 1997;16:6964–6976.
252. Greenberg ME, Iafrate AJ, Skowronski J. The SH3 domain-binding surface and an acidic motif in HIV-1 Nef regulate trafficking of class I MHC complexes. *EMBO J* 1998;17:2777–2789.
253. Greenway AL, Dutartre H, Allen K, et al. Simian immunodeficiency virus and human immunodeficiency virus type 1 nef proteins show distinct patterns and mechanisms of Src kinase activation. *J Virol* 1999;73:6152–6158.
254. Grez M, Dietrich U, Balfe P, et al. Genetic analysis of human immunodeficiency virus type 1 and 2 (HIV-1 and HIV-2) mixed infections in India reveals a recent spread of HIV-1 and HIV-2 from a single ancestor for each of these viruses. *J Virol* 1994;68:2161–2168.
255. Groux H, Torpier G, Monte D, et al. Activation-induced death by apoptosis in CD4+ T cells from human immunodeficiency virus-infected asymptomatic individuals. *J Exp Med* 1992;175:331–340.
256. Gruter P, Tabernero C, von Kobbe C, et al. TAP, the human homolog of Mex67p, mediates CTE-dependent RNA export from the nucleus. *Mol Cell* 1998;1:649–659.
257. Grzesiek S, Bax A, Clore GM, et al. The solution structure of HIV-1 Nef reveals an unexpected fold and permits delineation of the binding surface for the SH3 domain of Hck tyrosine protein kinase. *Nat Struct Biol* 1996;3:340–345.
258. Grzesiek S, Bax A, Hu JS, et al. Refined solution structure and backbone dynamics of HIV-1 Nef. *Protein Sci* 1997;6:1248–1263.
259. Grzesiek S, Stahl SJ, Wingfield PT, et al. The CD4 determinant for downregulation by HIV-1 Nef directly binds to Nef. Mapping of the Nef binding surface by NMR. *Biochemistry* 1996;35:10256–10261.
260. Guy B, Kieny MP, Riviere Y, et al. HIV F/3′ *orf* encodes a phosphorylated GTP-binding protein resembling an oncogene product. *Nature* 1987;330:266–269.
261. Hahn BH, Shaw GM, De Cock KM, et al. AIDS as a zoonosis: Scientific and public health implications. *Science* 2000;287:607–614.
262. Hallenberger S, Bosch V, Angliker H, et al. Inhibition of furin-mediated cleavage activation of HIV-1 glycoprotein gp160. *Nature* 1992; 360:358–361.
263. Hamilton JA, Vairo G, Cocks BG. Inhibition of S-phase progression in macrophages is linked to G1/S-phase suppression of DNA synthesis genes. *J Immunol* 1992;148:4028–4035.
264. Hammarskjöld M-L, Heimer J, Hammarskjöld B, et al. Regulation of human immunodeficiency virus *env* expression by the *rev* gene product. *J Virol* 1989;63:1959–1966.
265. Hanna Z, Kay DG, Cool M, et al. Transgenic mice expressing human immunodeficiency virus type 1 in immune cells develop a severe AIDS-like disease. *J Virol* 1998;72:121–132.
266. Hanna Z, Kay DG, Rebai N, et al. Nef harbors a major determinant of pathogenicity for an AIDS-like disease induced by HIV-1 in transgenic mice. *Cell* 1998;95:163–175.
267. Harrich D, Garcia J, Wu F, et al. Role of SP1-binding domains in *in vivo* transcriptional regulation of the human immunodeficiency virus type 1 long terminal repeat. *J Virol* 1989;63:2585–2591.
268. Harrich D, Ulich C, Gaynor RB. A critical role for the TAR element in promoting efficient human immunodeficiency virus type 1 reverse transcription. *J Virol* 1996;70:4017–4027.
269. Hart CE, Ou C-Y, Galphin JC, et al. Human chromosome 12 is required for elevated HIV-1 expression in human-hamster hybrid cells. *Science* 1989;246:488–491.
270. Haseltine WA, Sodroski J, Patarca R, et al. Structure of 3′ terminal region of type II human T lymphotropic virus: Evidence for new coding region. *Science* 1984;225:419–421.
271. Hazuda DJ, Felock P, Witmer M, et al. Inhibitors of strand transfer that prevent integration and inhibit HIV-1 replication in cells. *Science* 2000;287:646–650.
272. He J, Chen Y, Farzan M, et al. CCR3 and CCR5 are co-receptors for HIV-1 infection of microglia. *Nature* 1997;385:645–649.
273. He J, Choe S, Walker R, et al. Human immunodeficiency virus type 1 viral protein R (Vpr) arrests cells in the G2 phase of the cell cycle by inhibiting p34cdc2 activity. *J Virol* 1995;69:6705–6711.
274. Heinzinger NK, Bukinsky MI, Haggerty SA, et al. The Vpr protein of human immunodeficiency virus type 1 influences nuclear localization of viral nucleic acids in nondividing host cells. *Proc Natl Acad Sci U S A* 1994;91:7311–7315.
275. Henderson BR, Percipalle P. Interactions between HIV Rev and nuclear import and export factors: The Rev nuclear localisation signal mediates specific binding to human importin-β. *J Mol Biol* 1997;274: 693–707.
276. Henderson LE, Sowder RC, Copeland TD, et al. Isolation and characterization of a novel protein (X-ORF product) from SIV and HIV-2. *Science* 1988;241:199–201.
277. Hermida-Matsumoto L, Resh MD. Human immunodeficiency virus type 1 protease triggers a myristoyl switch that modulates membrane binding of $Pr55^{gag}$ and p17MA. *J Virol* 1999;73:1902–1908.
278. Herrmann CH, Carroll RG, Wei P, et al. Tat-associated kinase, TAK, activity is regulated by distinct mechanisms in peripheral blood lymphocytes and promonocytic cell lines. *J Virol* 1998;72:9881–9888.
279. Herrmann CH, Gold MO, Rice AP. Viral transactivators specifically target distinct cellular protein kinases that phosphorylate the RNA polymerase II C-terminal domain. *Nucleic Acids Res* 1996;24:501–508.
280. Herrmann CH, Rice AP. Specific interaction of the human immunodeficiency virus Tat proteins with a cellular protein kinase. *Virology* 1993;197:601–608.
281. Herrmann CH, Rice AP. Lentivirus Tat proteins specifically associate with a cellular protein kinase, TAK, that hyperphosphorylates the carboxyl-terminal domain of the large subunit of RNA polymerase II: Candidate for a Tat cofactor. *J Virol* 1995;69:1612–1620.
282. Herschlag D. RNA chaperones and the RNA folding problem. *J Biol Chem* 1995;270:20871–20874.
283. Hess JL, Small JA, Clements JE. Sequences in the visna virus long terminal repeat that control transcriptional activity and respond to viral trans-activation: Involvement of AP-1 sites in basal activity and trans-activation. *J Virol* 1989;63:3001–3015.
284. Hill CP, Worthylake D, Bancroft DP, et al. Crystal structures of the trimeric human immunodeficiency virus type 1 matrix protein: Implications for membrane association and assembly. *Proc Natl Acad Sci U S A* 1996;93:3099–3104.
285. Hirsch VM, Olmsted RA, Murphey-Corb M, et al. An African primate lentivirus (SIV_{sm}) closely related to HIV-2. *Nature* 1989;339: 389–392.
286. Hoffman TL, LaBranche CC, Zhang W, et al. Stable exposure of the coreceptor-binding site in a CD4-independent HIV-1 envelope protein. *Proc Natl Acad Sci U S A* 1999;96:6359–6364.
287. Hoglund S, Ohagen A, Lawrence K, et al. Role of vif during packing of the core of HIV-1. *Virology* 1994;201:349–355.
288. Holland SM, Ahmad N, Maitra RK, et al. Human immunodeficiency virus Rev protein recognizes a target sequence in Rev-responsive element RNA within the context of RNA secondary structure [published erratum appears in *J Virol* 1992;66:1288]. *J Virol* 1990;64:5966–5975.
289. Holland SM, Chavez M, Gerstberger S, et al. A specific sequence with a bulged guanosine residue(s) in a stem-bulge-stem structure of Rev-responsive element RNA is required for *trans* activation by human immunodeficiency virus type 1 Rev. *J Virol* 1992;66:3699–3706.
290. Hoxie JA, Alpers JD, Rackowski JL, et al. Alterations in T4 (CD4) protein and mRNA synthesis in cells infected with HIV. *Science* 1986; 234:1123–1127.
291. Hu WS, Temin HM. Genetic consequences of packaging two RNA genomes in one retroviral particle: Pseudodiploidy and high rate of genetic recombination. *Proc Natl Acad Sci U S A* 1990;87:1556–1560.
292. Huang H, Chopra R, Verdine GL, et al. Structure of a covalently trapped catalytic complex of HIV-1 reverse transcriptase: Implications for drug resistance. *Science* 1998;282:1669–1675.
293. Huang M, Orenstein JM, Martin MA, et al. $p6^{Gag}$ is required for particle production from full-length human immunodeficiency virus type 1 molecular clones expressing protease. *J Virol* 1995;69:6810–6818.
294. Huang X, Hope TJ, Bond BL, et al. Minimal Rev-response element for type 1 human immunodeficiency virus. *J Virol* 1991;65:2131–2134.
295. Huang Y, Paxton WA, Wolinsky SM, et al. The role of a mutant CCR5 allele in HIV-1 transmission and disease progression. *Nat Med* 1996; 2:1240–1243.

296. Huang Y, Zhang L, Ho DD. Biological characterization of nef in long-term survivors of human immunodeficiency virus type 1 infection. *J Virol* 1995;69:8142–8146.
297. Huang Y, Zhang L, Ho DD. Characterization of nef sequences in long-term survivors of human immunodeficiency virus type 1 infection. *J Virol* 1995;69:93–100.
298. Huet T, Cheynier R, Meyerhans A, et al. Genetic organization of a chimpanzee lentivirus related to HIV-1. *Nature* 1990;345:356–359.
299. Ifversen P, Martensson C, Danielsson L, et al. Induction of primary antigen-specific immune reponses in SCID-hu-PBL by coupled T-B epitopes. *Immunology* 1995;84:111–116.
300. Ilyinskii PO, Daniel MD, Simon MA, et al. The role of upstream U3 sequences in the pathogenesis of simian immunodeficiency virus-induced AIDS in rhesus monkeys. *J Virol* 1994;68:5933–5944.
301. Isel C, Ehresmann C, Keith G, et al. Initiation of reverse transcription of HIV-1: Secondary structure of the HIV-1 RNA/tRNA(3Lys) (template/primer). *J Mol Biol* 1995;247:236–250.
302. Isel C, Westhof E, Massire C, et al. Structural basis for the specificity of the initiation of HIV-1 reverse transcription. *EMBO J* 1999;18: 1038–1048.
303. Izaurralde E, Adam S. Transport of macromolecules between the nucleus and the cytoplasm. *RNA* 1998;4:351–364.
304. Izaurralde E, Kutay U, von Kobbe C, et al. The asymmetric distribution of the constituents of the Ran system is essential for transport into and out of the nucleus. *EMBO J* 1997;16:6535–6547.
305. Jacks T, Power MD, Masiarz FR, et al. Characterization of ribosomal frameshifting in HIV-1 *gag-pol* expression. *Nature* 1988;331: 280–283.
306. Jacobo-Molina A, Clark AD Jr, Williams RL, et al. Crystals of a ternary complex of human immunodeficiency virus type 1 reverse transcriptase with a monoclonal antibody Fab fragment and double-stranded DNA diffract x-rays to 3.5-Å resolution. *Proc Natl Acad Sci U S A* 1991;88:10895–10899.
307. Jacobo-Molina A, Ding J, Nanni RG, et al. Crystal structure of human immunodeficiency virus type 1 reverse transcriptase complexed with double-stranded DNA at 3.0 Å resolution shows bent DNA. *Proc Natl Acad Sci U S A* 1993;90:6320–6324.
308. Jacobsen H, Hanggi M, Ott M, et al. In vivo resistance to a human immunodeficiency virus type 1 proteinase inhibitor: Mutations, kinetics, and frequencies. *J Infect Dis* 1996;173:1379–1387.
309. Jakobovits A, Smith DH, Jakobovits EB, et al. A discrete element 3′ of human immunodeficiency virus 1 (HIV-1) and HIV-2 mRNA initiation sites mediates transcriptional activation by an HIV *trans* activator. *Mol Cell Biol* 1988;8:2555–2561.
310. Jamieson BD, Aldrovandi GM, Planelles V, et al. Requirement of human immunodeficiency virus type 1 nef for in vivo replication and pathogenicity. *J Virol* 1994;68:3478–3485.
311. Jamieson BD, Pang S, Aldrovandi GM, et al. In vivo pathogenic properties of two clonal human immunodeficiency virus type 1 isolates. *J Virol* 1995;69:6259–6264.
312. Jenkins Y, McEntee M, Weis K, et al. Characterization of HIV-1 vpr nuclear import: Analysis of signals and pathways. *J Cell Biol* 1998; 143:875–885.
313. Joag SV, Li Z, Foresman L, et al. Chimeric simian/human immunodeficiency virus that causes progressive loss of CD4+ T cells and AIDS in pig-tailed macaques. *J Virol* 1996;70:3189–3197.
314. Jolicoeur P, Laperriere A, Beaulieu N. Efficient production of human immunodeficiency virus proteins in transgenic mice. *J Virol* 1992;66: 3904–3908.
315. Julias JG, Hash D, Pathak VK. E^- vectors: Development of novel self-inactivating and self-activating retroviral vectors for safer gene therapy. *J Virol* 1995;69:6839–6846.
316. Julias JG, Pathak VK. Deoxyribonucleoside triphosphate pool imbalances in vivo are associated with an increased retroviral mutation rate. *J Virol* 1998;72:7941–7949.
317. Junghans RP, Boone LR, Skalka AM. Retroviral DNA H structures: Displacement-assimilation model of recombination. *Cell* 1982;30: 53–62.
318. Kalpana GV, Marmon S, Wang W, et al. Binding and stimulation of HIV-1 integrase by a human homolog of yeast transcription factor SNF5. *Science* 1994;266:2002–2006.
319. Kang SM, Morrow CD. Genetic analysis of a unique human immunodeficiency virus type 1 (HIV-1) with a primer binding site complementary to tRNAMet supports a role for U5-PBS stem-loop RNA structures in initiation of HIV-1 reverse transcription. *J Virol* 1999;73:1818–1827.
320. Kaplan AH, Manchester M, Swanstrom R. The activity of the protease of human immunodeficiency virus type 1 is initiated at the membrane of infected cells before the release of viral proteins and is required for release to occur with maximum efficiency. *J Virol* 1994;68:6782–6786.
321. Kappes JC, Morrow CD, Lee S-W, et al. Identification of a novel retroviral gene unique to human immunodeficiency virus type 2 and simian immunodeficiency virus SIV_{MAC}. *J Virol* 1988;62:3501–3505.
322. Karczewski MK, Strebel K. Cytoskeleton association and virion incorporation of the human immunodeficiency virus type 1 Vif protein. *J Virol* 1996;70:494–507.
323. Katoh I, Yoshinaka Y, Rein A, et al. Murine leukemia virus maturation: Protease region required for conversion from "immature" to "mature" core form and for virus infectivity. *Virology* 1985;145:280–292.
324. Katz RA, Merkel G, Kulkosky J, et al. The avian retroviral IN protein is both necessary and sufficient for integrative recombination in vitro. *Cell* 1990;63:87–95.
325. Kawakami T, Sherman L, Dahlberg J, et al. Nucleotide sequence analysis of equine infectious anemia virus proviral DNA. *Virology* 1987;158:300–312.
326. Kerr LD, Inoue J-I, Davis N, et al. The rel-associated pp40 protein prevents DNA binding of Rel and NF-κB: Relationship with IκBβ and regulation by phosphorylation. *Genes Dev* 1991;5:1464–1476.
327. Kestler HW III, Ringler DJ, Mori K, et al. Importance of the *nef* gene for maintenance of high virus loads and for development of AIDS. *Cell* 1991;65:651–662.
328. Kewalramani VN, Emerman M. Vpx association with mature core structures of HIV-2. *Virology* 1996;218:159–168.
329. Kiernan RE, Freed EO. Cleavage of the murine leukemia virus transmembrane env protein by human immunodeficiency virus type 1 protease: Transdominant inhibition by matrix mutations. *J Virol* 1998; 72:9621–9627.
330. Kiernan RE, Ono A, Englund G, et al. Role of matrix in an early postentry step in the human immunodeficiency virus type 1 life cycle. *J Virol* 1998;72:4116–4126.
331. Kilby JM, Hopkins S, Venetta TM, et al. Potent suppression of HIV-1 replication in humans by T-20, a peptide inhibitor of gp41-mediated virus entry. *Nat Med* 1998;4:1302–1307.
332. Kim JY, Gonzalez-Scarano F, Zeichner SL, et al. Replication of type 1 human immunodeficiency viruses containing linker substitution mutations in the −201 to −130 region of the long terminal repeat. *J Virol* 1993;67:1658–1662.
333. Kim YH, Chang SH, Kwon JH, et al. HIV-1 Nef plays an essential role in two independent processes in CD4 down-regulation: Dissociation of the CD4-p56(lck) complex and targeting of CD4 to lysosomes. *Virology* 1999;257:208–219.
334. Kino T, Gragerov A, Kopp JB, et al. The HIV-1 virion-associated protein vpr is a coactivator of the human glucocorticoid receptor. *J Exp Med* 1999;189:51–62.
335. Kirchhoff F, Greenough TC, Brettler DB, et al. Brief report: Absence of intact *nef* sequences in a long-term survivor with nonprogressive HIV-1 infection. *N Engl J Med* 1995;332:228–232.
336. Klebe C, Bischoff FR, Ponstingl H, et al. Interaction of the nuclear GTP-binding protein Ran with its regulatory proteins RCC1 and RanGAP1. *Biochemistry* 1995;34:639–647.
337. Kledal TN, Rosenkilde MM, Coulin F, et al. A broad-spectrum chemokine antagonist encoded by Kaposi's sarcoma-associated herpesvirus. *Science* 1997;277:1656–1659.
338. Klimkait T, Strebel K, Hoggan MD, et al. The human immunodeficiency virus type 1-specific protein *vpu* is required for efficient virus maturation and release. *J Virol* 1990;64:621–629.
339. Koga Y, Nakamura K, Sasaki M, et al. The difference in gp160 and gp120 of HIV type 1 in the induction of CD4 downregulation preceding single-cell killing. *Virology* 1994;201:137–141.
340. Kohlstaedt LA, Wang J, Friedman JM, et al. Crystal structure at 3.5 Å resolution of HIV-1 reverse transcriptase complexed with an inhibitor. *Science* 1992;256:1783–1790.
341. Kolchinsky P, Mirzabekov T, Farzan M, et al. Adaptation of a CCR5-using, primary human immunodeficiency virus type 1 isolate for CD4-independent replication. *J Virol* 1999;73:8120–8126.
342. Kondo E, Mammano F, Cohen EA, et al. The $p6^{gag}$ domain of human immunodeficiency virus type 1 is sufficient for the incorporation of Vpr into heterologous viral particles. *J Virol* 1995;69:2759–2764.
343. Koot M, Vos AH, Keet RP, et al. HIV-1 biological phenotype in long-term infected individuals evaluated with an MT-2 cocultivation assay. *AIDS* 1992;6:49–54.

344. Korber B, Kuiken C, Foley B, et al., eds. *Human Retroviruses and AIDS 1998*. Los Alamos, NM: Los Alamos National Laboratory, 1998.
345. Korin YD, Zack JA. Progression to the $G_1{}^b$ phase of the cell cycle is required for completion of human immunodeficiency virus type 1 reverse transcription in T cells. *J Virol* 1998;72:3161–3168.
346. Kostrikis LG, Huang Y, Moore JP, et al. A chemokine receptor CCR2 allele delays HIV-1 disease progression and is associated with a CCR5 promoter mutation. *Nat Med* 1998;4:350–353.
347. Kotler M, Simm M, Zhao YS, et al. Human immunodeficiency virus type 1 (HIV-1) protein Vif inhibits the activity of HIV-1 protease in bacteria and in vitro. *J Virol* 1997;71:5774–5781.
348. Kotov A, Zhou J, Flicker P, et al. Association of Nef with the human immunodeficiency virus type 1 core. *J Virol* 1999;73:8824–8830.
349. Kräusslich H-G. Human immunodeficiency virus proteinase dimer as component of the viral polyprotein prevents particle assembly and viral infectivity. *Proc Natl Acad Sci U S A* 1991;88:3213–3217.
350. Kwong PD, Wyatt R, Robinson J, et al. Structure of an HIV gp120 envelope glycoprotein in complex with the CD4 receptor and a neutralizing human antibody. *Nature* 1998;393:648–659.
351. LaBranche CC, Sauter MM, Haggarty BS, et al. A single amino acid change in the cytoplasmic domain of the simian immunodeficiency virus transmembrane molecule increases envelope glycoprotein expression on infected cells. *J Virol* 1995;69:5217–5227.
352. Lapatto R, Blundell T, Hemmings A, et al. X-ray analysis of HIV-1 proteinase at 2.7 Å resolution confirms structural homology among retroviral enzymes. *Nature* 1989;342:299–302.
353. Lapham CK, Ouyang J, Chandrasekhar B, et al. Evidence for cell-surface association between fusin and the CD4-gp120 complex in human cell lines. *Science* 1996;274:602–605.
354. Lapham CK, Zaitseva MB, Lee S, et al. Fusion of monocytes and macrophages with HIV-1 correlates with biochemical properties of CXCR4 and CCR5. *Nat Med* 1999;5:303–308.
355. Laspia MF, Rice AP, Mathews MB. HIV-1 Tat protein increases transcriptional initiation and stabilizes elongation. *Cell* 1989;59:283–292.
356. Le Gall S, Erdtmann L, Benichou S, et al. Nef interacts with the μ subunit of clathrin adaptor complexes and reveals a cryptic sorting signal in MHC I molecules. *Immunity* 1998;8:483–495.
357. Lee CH, Saksela K, Mirza UA, et al. Crystal structure of the conserved core of HIV-1 Nef complexed with a Src family SH3 domain. *Cell* 1996;85:931–942.
358. Lee MS, Craigie R. A previously unidentified host protein protects retroviral DNA from autointegration. *Proc Natl Acad Sci U S A* 1998;95:1528–1533.
359. Lee S, Lapham CK, Chen H, et al. Coreceptor competition for association with CD4 may change the susceptibility of human cells to infection with T-tropic and macrophagetropic isolates of human immunodeficiency virus type 1. *J Virol* 2000;74:5016–5023.
360. Lee YM, Yu XF. Identification and characterization of virus assembly intermediate complexes in HIV-1-infected CD4+ T cells. *Virology* 1998;243:78–93.
361. Leiden JM, Wang CY, Petryniak B, et al. A novel Ets-related transcription factor, Elf-1, binds to human immunodeficiency virus type 2 regulatory elements that are required for inducible trans activation in T cells. *J Virol* 1992;66:5890–5897.
362. Leitner T. Genetic subtypes of HIV-1. In: Myers G, Foley B, Mellors JW, et al., eds. *Human Retroviruses and AIDS 1996*. Los Alamos, NM: Los Alamos National Laboratory, 1996:III-29–III-40.
363. Lenburg ME, Landau NR. Vpu-induced degradation of CD4: Requirement for specific amino acid residues in the cytoplasmic domain of CD4. *J Virol* 1993;67:7238–7245.
364. Leonard CK, Spellman MW, Riddle L, et al. Assignment of intrachain disulfide bonds and characterization of potential glycosylation sites of the type 1 recombinant human immunodeficiency virus envelope glycoprotein (gp120) expressed in Chinese hamster ovary cells. *J Biol Chem* 1990;265:10373–10382.
365. Leonard J, Khillan JS, Gendelman HE, et al. The human immunodeficiency virus long terminal repeat is preferentially expressed in Langerhans cells in transgenic mice. *AIDS Res Hum Retroviruses* 1989;5:421–430.
366. Leonard J, Parrott C, Buckler-White AJ, et al. The NF-κB binding sites in the human immunodeficiency virus type 1 long terminal repeat are not required for virus infectivity. *J Virol* 1989;63:4919–4924.
367. Leonard JM, Abramczuk JW, Pezen DS, et al. Development of disease and virus recovery in transgenic mice containing HIV proviral DNA. *Science* 1988;242:1665–1670.
368. Letvin NL, Daniel MD, Sehgal PK, et al. Induction of AIDS-like disease in macaque monkeys with T-cell tropic retrovirus STLV-III. *Science* 1985;230:71–73.
369. Levy DN, Fernandes LS, Williams WV, et al. Induction of cell differentiation by human immunodeficiency virus 1 vpr. *Cell* 1993;72:541–550.
370. Levy DN, Refaeli Y, MacGregor RR, et al. Serum Vpr regulates productive infection and latency of human immunodeficiency virus type 1. *Proc Natl Acad Sci U S A* 1994;91:10873–10877.
371. Levy JA, Hoffman AD, Kramer SM, et al. Isolation of lymphocytopathic retroviruses from San Francisco patients with AIDS. *Science* 1984;225:840–842.
372. Li J, Lord CI, Haseltine W, et al. Infection of cynomolgus monkeys with a chimeric HIV-1/SIVmac virus that expresses the HIV-1 envelope glycoproteins. *J Acquir Immune Defic Syndr* 1992;5:639–646.
373. Li Y, Flanagan PM, Tschochner H, et al. RNA polymerase II initiation factor interactions and transcription start site selection. *Science* 1994;263:805–807.
374. Liang C, Li X, Rong L, et al. The importance of the A-rich loop in human immunodeficiency virus type 1 reverse transcription and infectivity. *J Virol* 1997;71:5750–5757.
375. Lindemann D, Wilhelm R, Renard P, et al. Severe immunodeficiency associated with a human immunodeficiency virus 1 NEF/3′-long terminal repeat transgene. *J Exp Med* 1994;179:797–807.
376. Liu B, Dai R, Tian CJ, et al. Interaction of the human immunodeficiency virus type 1 nucleocapsid with actin. *J Virol* 1999;73:2901–2908.
377. Liu H, Chao D, Nakayama EE, et al. Polymorphism in RANTES chemokine promoter affects HIV-1 disease progression. *Proc Natl Acad Sci U S A* 1999;96:4581–4585.
378. Liu H, Wu X, Newman M, et al. The Vif protein of human and simian immunodeficiency viruses is packaged into virions and associates with viral core structures. *J Virol* 1995;69:7630–7638.
379. Liu R, Paxton WA, Choe S, et al. Homozygous defect in HIV-1 coreceptor accounts for resistance of some multiply-exposed individuals to HIV-1 infection. *Cell* 1996;86:367–377.
380. Lodge R, Gottlinger H, Gabuzda D, et al. The intracytoplasmic domain of gp41 mediates polarized budding of human immunodeficiency virus type 1 in MDCK cells. *J Virol* 1994;68:4857–4861.
381. Lodi PJ, Ernst JA, Kuszewski J, et al. Solution structure of the DNA binding domain of HIV-1 integrase. *Biochemistry* 1995;34:9826–9833.
382. Lori F, di Marzo Veronese F, de Vico AL, et al. Viral DNA carried by human immunodeficiency virus type 1 virions. *J Virol* 1992;66:5067–5074.
383. Louwagie J, Janssens W, Mascola J, et al. Genetic diversity of the envelope glycoprotein from human immunodeficiency virus type 1 isolates of African origin. *J Virol* 1995;69:263–271.
384. Louwagie J, McCutchan FE, Peeters M, et al. Phylogenetic analysis of *gag* genes from 70 international HIV-1 isolates provides evidence for multiple genotypes. *AIDS* 1993;7:769–780.
385. Lu H, Zawel L, Fisher L, et al. Human general transcription factor IIH phosphorylates the C-terminal domain of RNA polymerase II. *Nature* 1992;358:641–645.
386. Lu X, Yu H, Liu S-H, et al. Interactions between HIV1 Nef and vacuolar ATPase facilitate the internalization of CD4. *Immunity* 1998;8:647–656.
387. Lu YL, Bennett RP, Wills JW, et al. A leucine triplet repeat sequence $(LXX)_4$ in $p6^{gag}$ is important for Vpr incorporation into human immunodeficiency virus type 1 particles. *J Virol* 1995;69:6873–6879.
388. Lu YL, Spearman P, Ratner L. Human immunodeficiency virus type 1 viral protein R localization in infected cells and virions. *J Virol* 1993;67:6542–6550.
389. Luban J, Bossolt KL, Franke EK, et al. Human immunodeficiency virus type 1 Gag protein binds to cyclophilins A and B. *Cell* 1993;73:1067–1078.
390. Luciw PA, Cheng-Mayer C, Levy JA. Mutational analysis of the human immunodeficiency virus: The *orf*-B region down-regulates virus replication. *Proc Natl Acad Sci U S A* 1987;84:1434–1438.
391. Luo W, Peterlin BM. Activation of the T-cell receptor signaling pathway by Nef from an aggressive strain of simian immunodeficiency virus. *J Virol* 1997;71:9531–9537.
392. Luo Y, Madore SJ, Parslow TG, et al. Functional analysis of interac-

tions between Tat and the trans-activation response element of human immunodeficiency virus type 1 in cells. *J Virol* 1993;67:5617–5622.
393. Macreadie IG, Castelli LA, Hewish DR, et al. A domain of human immunodeficiency virus type 1 Vpr containing repeated H(S/F)RIG amino acid motifs causes cell growth arrest and structural defects. *Proc Natl Acad Sci U S A* 1995;92:2770–2774.
394. Madani N, Kabat D. An endogenous inhibitor of human immunodeficiency virus in human lymphocytes is overcome by the viral Vif protein. *J Virol* 1998;72:10251–10255.
395. Maddon PJ, Dalgleish AG, McDougal JS, et al. The T4 gene encodes the AIDS virus receptor and is expressed in the immune system and the brain. *Cell* 1986;47:333–348.
396. Maddon PJ, McDougal JS, Clapham PR, et al. HIV infection does not require endocytosis of its receptor, CD4. *Cell* 1988;54:865–874.
397. Maddon PJ, Molineaux SM, Maddon DE, et al. Structure and expression of the human and mouse T4 genes. *Proc Natl Acad Sci U S A* 1987;84:9155–9159.
398. Madore SJ, Cullen BR. Genetic analysis of the cofactor requirement for human immunodeficiency virus type 1 Tat function. *J Virol* 1993; 67:3703–3711.
399. Madore SJ, Tiley LS, Malim MH, et al. Sequence requirements for Rev multimerization in vivo. *Virology* 1994;202:186–194.
400. Mahalingam S, Ayyavoo V, Patel M, et al. Nuclear import, virion incorporation, and cell cycle arrest/differentiation are mediated by distinct functional domains of human immunodeficiency virus type 1 Vpr. *J Virol* 1997;71:6339–6347.
401. Mahalingam S, Ayyavoo V, Patel M, et al. HIV-1 Vpr interacts with a human 34-kDa mov34 homologue, a cellular factor linked to the G2/M phase transition of the mammalian cell cycle. *Proc Natl Acad Sci U S A* 1998;95:3419–3424.
402. Maldarelli F, Chen M-Y, Willey RL, et al. Human immunodeficiency virus type 1 Vpu protein is an oligomeric type I integral membrane protein. *J Virol* 1993;67:5056–5061.
403. Maldarelli F, Martin MA, Strebel K. Identification of posttranscriptionally active inhibitory sequences in human immunodeficiency virus type 1 RNA: Novel level of gene regulation. *J Virol* 1991;65: 5732–5743.
404. Malim MH, Böhnlein S, Hauber J, et al. Functional dissection of the HIV-1 Rev *trans*-activator—Derivation of a trans-dominant repressor of Rev function. *Cell* 1989;58:205–214.
405. Malim MH, Hauber J, Le S-Y, et al. The HIV-1 *rev trans*-activator acts through a structured target sequence to activate nuclear export of unspliced viral mRNA. *Nature* 1989;338:254–257.
406. Malim MH, McCarn DF, Tiley LS, et al. Mutational definition of the human immunodeficiency virus type 1 Rev activation domain. *J Virol* 1991;65:4248–4254.
407. Malim MH, Tiley LS, McCarn DF, et al. HIV-1 structural gene expression requires binding of the Rev trans-activator to its RNA target sequence. *Cell* 1990;60:675–683.
408. Mammano F, Kondo E, Sodroski J, et al. Rescue of human immunodeficiency virus type 1 matrix protein mutants by envelope glycoproteins with short cytoplasmic domains. *J Virol* 1995;69:3824–3830.
409. Mancebo HS, Lee G, Flygare J, et al. P-TEFb kinase is required for HIV Tat transcriptional activation in vivo and in vitro. *Genes Dev* 1997;11:2633–2644.
410. Mann DA, Mikaelian I, Zemmel RW, et al. A molecular rheostat. Cooperative rev binding to stem I of the rev-response element modulates human immunodeficiency virus type-1 late gene expression. *J Mol Biol* 1994;241:193–207.
411. Mansky LM. The mutation rate of human immunodeficiency virus type 1 is influenced by the *vpr* gene. *Virology* 1996;222:391–400.
412. Mansky LM. Retrovirus mutation rates and their role in genetic variation. *J Gen Virol* 1998;79:1337–1345.
413. Mansky LM, Temin HM. Lower in vivo mutation rate of human immunodeficiency virus type 1 than that predicted from the fidelity of purified reverse transcriptase. *J Virol* 1995;69:5087–5094.
414. Margottin F, Bour SP, Durand H, et al. A novel human WD protein, h-βTrCP, that interacts with HIV-1 Vpu connects CD4 to the ER degradation pathway through an F-box motif. *Mol Cell* 1998;1:565–574.
415. Markovitz DM, Smith MJ, Hilfinger J, et al. Activation of the human immunodeficiency virus type 2 enhancer is dependent on purine box and kappa B regulatory elements. *J Virol* 1992;66:5479–5484.
416. Marsh JW. The numerous effector functions of Nef. *Arch Biochem Biophys* 1999;365:192–198.
417. Marshall NF, Peng J, Xie Z, et al. Control of RNA polymerase II elongation potential by a novel carboxyl-terminal domain kinase. *J Biol Chem* 1996;271:27176–27183.
418. Marshall NF, Price DH. Purification of P-TEFb, a transcription factor required for the transition into productive elongation. *J Biol Chem* 1995;270:12335–12338.
419. Martin KA, Wyatt R, Farzan M, et al. CD4-independent binding of SIV gp120 to rhesus CCR5. *Science* 1997;278:1470–1473.
420. Martin MP, Dean M, Smith MW, et al. Genetic acceleration of AIDS progression by a promoter variant of CCR5. *Science* 1998;282:1907–1911.
421. Martinez MA, Vartanian JP, Wain-Hobson S. Hypermutagenesis of RNA using human immunodeficiency virus type 1 reverse transcriptase and biased dNTP concentrations. *Proc Natl Acad Sci U S A* 1994; 91:11787–11791.
422. Massiah MA, Starich MR, Paschall C, et al. Three-dimensional structure of the human immunodeficiency virus type 1 matrix protein. *J Mol Biol* 1994;244:198–223.
423. Mattaj IW, Englmeier L. Nucleocytoplasmic transport: The soluble phase. *Annu Rev Biochem* 1998;67:265–306.
424. Mauclere P, Loussert-Ajaka I, Damond F, et al. Serological and virological characterization of HIV-1 group O infection in Cameroon. *AIDS* 1997;11:445–453.
425. McBride MS, Panganiban AT. The human immunodeficiency virus type 1 encapsidation site is a multipartite RNA element composed of functional hairpin structures [published erratum appears in *J Virol* 1997;71:858]. *J Virol* 1996;70:2963–2973.
426. McCune JM. SCID mice as immune system models. *Curr Opin Immunol* 1991;3:224–228.
427. McCune JM, Rabin LB, Feinberg MB, et al. Endoproteolytic cleavage of gp160 is required for the activation of human immunodeficiency virus. *Cell* 1988;53:55–67.
428. McDermott DH, Zimmerman PA, Guignard F, et al. CCR5 promoter polymorphism and HIV-1 disease progression. *Lancet* 1998;352: 866–870.
429. McDougal JS, Cort SP, Kennedy MS, et al. Immunoassay for the detection and quantitation of infectious human retrovirus, lymphadenopathy-associated virus (LAV). *J Immunol Methods* 1985;76:171–183.
430. McDougal JS, Mawle A, Cort SP, et al. Cellular tropism of the human retrovirus HTLV-III/LAV. I. Role of T cell activation and expression of the T4 antigen. *J Immunol* 1985;135:3151–3162.
431. McKeating JA, Shotton C, Cordell J, et al. Characterization of neutralizing monoclonal antibodies to linear and conformation-dependent epitopes within the first and second variable domains of human immunodeficiency virus type 1 gp120. *J Virol* 1993;67:4932–4944.
432. McKnight A, Wilkinson D, Simmons G, et al. Inhibition of human immunodeficiency virus fusion by a monoclonal antibody to a coreceptor (CXCR4) is both cell type and virus strain dependent. *J Virol* 1997;71:1692–1696.
433. McNally LM, McNally MT. SR protein splicing factors interact with the Rous sarcoma virus negative regulator of splicing element. *J Virol* 1996;70:1163–1172.
434. Meyer BE, Malim MH. The HIV-1 Rev trans-activator shuttles between the nucleus and the cytoplasm. *Genes Dev* 1994;8:1538–1547.
435. Meyerhans A, Cheynier R, Albert J, et al. Temporal fluctuations in HIV quasispecies in vivo are not reflected by sequential HIV isolations. *Cell* 1989;58:901–910.
436. Miller MD, Wang B, Bushman FD. Human immunodeficiency virus type 1 preintegration complexes containing discontinuous plus strands are competent to integrate in vitro. *J Virol* 1995;69:3938–3944.
437. Miller MD, Warmerdam MT, Ferrell SS, et al. Intravirion generation of the C-terminal core domain of HIV-1 Nef by the HIV-1 protease is insufficient to enhance viral infectivity. *Virology* 1997;234:215–225.
438. Miller MD, Warmerdam MT, Gaston I, et al. The human immunodeficiency virus-1 *nef* gene product: A positive factor for viral infection and replication in primary lymphocytes and macrophages. *J Exp Med* 1994;179:101–113.
439. Molla A, Korneyeva M, Gao Q, et al. Ordered accumulation of mutations in HIV protease confers resistance to ritonavir. *Nat Med* 1996; 2:760–766.
440. Momany C, Kovari LC, Prongay AJ, et al. Crystal structure of dimeric HIV-1 capsid protein. *Nat Struct Biol* 1996;3:763–770.
441. Montagnier L, Chermann JC, Barré-Sinoussi F, et al. A new human T-lymphotropic retrovirus: Characterization and possible role in lymphadenopathy and acquired immune deficiency syndromes. In: Gallo RC, Essex ME, Gross L, eds. *Human T-Cell Leukemia/Lymphoma Virus. The Family of Human T-Lymphotropic Retroviruses: Their Role*

in Malignancies and Association with AIDS. Cold Spring Harbor, NY: Cold Spring Harbor Laboratory, 1984:363–379.
442. Moore JP, McKeating JA, Weiss RA, et al. Dissociation of gp120 from HIV-1 virions induced by soluble CD4. *Science* 1990;250:1139–1142.
443. Morellet N, Jullian N, De Rocquigny H, et al. Determination of the structure of the nucleocapsid protein NCp7 from the human immunodeficiency virus type 1 by 1H NMR. *EMBO J* 1992;11:3059–3065.
444. Moriuchi H, Moriuchi M, Combadiere C, et al. CD8+ T-cell-derived soluble factor(s), but not β-chemokines RANTES, MIP-1α, and MIP-1β, suppress HIV-1 replication in monocyte/macrophages. *Proc Natl Acad Sci U S A* 1996;93:15341–15345.
445. Mosier DE, Gulizia RJ, Baird SM, et al. Human immunodeficiency virus infection of human-PBL-SCID mice. *Science* 1991;251:791–794.
446. Mosier DE, Gulizia RJ, MacIsaac PD, et al. Rapid loss of CD4+ T cells in human-PBL-SCID mice by noncytopathic HIV isolates. *Science* 1993;260:689–692.
447. Muller MC, Saksena NK, Nerrienet E, et al. Simian immunodeficiency viruses from Central and Western Africa: Evidence for a new species-specific lentivirus in tantalus monkeys. *J Virol* 1993;67:1227–1235.
448. Murakami T, Freed EO. Genetic evidence for an interaction between human immunodeficiency virus type 1 matrix and α-helix 2 of the gp41 cytoplasmic tail. *J Virol* 2000;74:3548–3554.
449. Murakami T, Freed EO. The long cytoplasmic tail of gp41 is required in a cell type-dependent manner for HIV-1 envelope glycoprotein incorporation into virions. *Proc Natl Acad Sci U S A* 2000;97:343–348.
450. Murakami T, Nakajima T, Koyanagi Y, et al. A small molecule CXCR4 inhibitor that blocks T cell line-tropic HIV-1 infection. *J Exp Med* 1997;186:1389–1393.
451. Muro-Cacho CA, Pantaleo G, Fauci AS. Analysis of apoptosis in lymph nodes of HIV-infected persons. Intensity of apoptosis correlates with the general state of activation of the lymphoid tissue and not with stage of disease or viral burden. *J Immunol* 1995;154:5555–5566.
452. Mwaengo DM, Novembre FJ. Molecular cloning and characterization of viruses isolated from chimpanzees with pathogenic human immunodeficiency virus type 1 infections. *J Virol* 1998;72:8976–8987.
453. Myers G. Tenth anniversary perspectives on AIDS. HIV: Between past and future. *AIDS Res Hum Retroviruses* 1994;10:1317–1324.
454. Myers G, Pavlakis GN. Evolution potential of complex retroviruses. In: Levy JA, ed. *The Retroviridae.* New York: Plenum Press, 1992:51–105.
455. Nabel G, Baltimore D. An inducible transcription factor activates expression of human immunodeficiency virus in T cells [published erratum appears in *Nature* 1990;344:178]. *Nature* 1987;326:711–713.
456. Nakielny S, Fischer U, Michael WM, et al. RNA transport. *Annu Rev Neurosci* 1997;20:269–301.
457. Namikawa R, Kaneshima H, Lieberman M, et al. Infection of the SCID-hu mouse by HIV-1. *Science* 1988;242:1684–1686.
458. Navia MA, Fitzgerald PMD, McKeever BM, et al. Three-dimensional structure of aspartyl protease from human immunodeficiency virus HIV-1. *Nature* 1989;337:615–620.
459. Negroni M, Buc H. Recombination during reverse transcription: An evaluation of the role of the nucleocapsid protein. *J Mol Biol* 1999;286:15–31.
460. Nelson JA, Ghazal P, Wiley CA. Role of opportunistic viral infections in AIDS. *AIDS* 1990;4:1–10.
461. Neville M, Stutz F, Lee L, et al. The importin-β family member Crm1p bridges the interaction between Rev and the nuclear pore complex during nuclear export. *Curr Biol* 1997;7:767–775.
462. Nigg EA. Nucleocytoplasmic transport: Signals, mechanisms and regulation. *Nature* 1997;386:779–787.
463. Nishi K, Yoshida M, Fujiwara D, et al. Leptomycin B targets a regulatory cascade of crm1, a fission yeast nuclear protein, involved in control of higher order chromosome structure and gene expression. *J Biol Chem* 1994;269:6320–6324.
464. Novembre FJ, Saucier M, Anderson DC, et al. Development of AIDS in a chimpanzee infected with human immunodeficiency virus type 1. *J Virol* 1997;71:4086–4091.
465. Novitsky VA, Montano MA, McLane MF, et al. Molecular cloning and phylogenetic analysis of human immunodeficiency virus type 1 subtype C: A set of 23 full-length clones from Botswana. *J Virol* 1999;73:4427–4432.
466. O'Brien T, Hardin S, Greenleaf A, et al. Phosphorylation of RNA polymerase II C-terminal domain and transcriptional elongation. *Nature* 1994;370:75–77.
467. O'Brien WA, Namazi A, Kalhor H, et al. Kinetics of human immunodeficiency virus type 1 reverse transcription in blood mononuclear phagocytes are slowed by limitations of nucleotide precursors. *J Virol* 1994;68:1258–1263.
468. Ochsenbauer C, Wilk T, Bosch V. Analysis of vif-defective human immunodeficiency virus type 1 (HIV-1) virions synthesized in 'non-permissive' T lymphoid cells stably infected with selectable HIV-1. *J Gen Virol* 1997;78:627–635.
469. Ogert RA, Lee LH, Beemon KL. Avian retroviral RNA element promotes unspliced RNA accumulation in the cytoplasm. *J Virol* 1996;70:3834–3843.
470. Ohkuma Y, Roeder RG. Regulation of TFIIH ATPase and kinase activities by TFIIE during active initiation complex formation. *Nature* 1994;368:160–163.
471. Ohno H, Aguilar RC, Fournier MC, et al. Interaction of endocytic signals from the HIV-1 envelope glycoprotein complex with members of the adaptor medium chain family. *Virology* 1997;238:305–315.
472. Ohno H, Stewart J, Fournier MC, et al. Interaction of tyrosine-based sorting signals with clathrin-associated proteins. *Science* 1995;269:1872–1875.
473. Ono A, Demirov D, Freed EO. Relationship between human immunodeficiency virus type 1 Gag multimerization and membrane binding. *J Virol* 2000;74:5142–5150.
474. Ono A, Freed EO. Binding of human immunodeficiency virus type 1 Gag to membrane: Role of the matrix amino terminus. *J Virol* 1999;73:4136–4144.
475. Ono A, Huang M, Freed EO. Characterization of human immunodeficiency virus type 1 matrix revertants: Effects on virus assembly, Gag processing, and Env incorporation into virions. *J Virol* 1997;71:4409–4418.
476. Ono A, Orenstein JM, Freed EO. Role of the Gag matrix domain in targeting human immunodeficiency virus type 1 assembly. *J Virol* 2000;74:2855–2866.
477. Orenstein JM, Meltzer MS, Phipps T, et al. Cytoplasmic assembly and accumulation of human immunodeficiency virus types 1 and 2 in recombinant human colony-stimulating factor-1-treated human monocytes: An ultrastructural study. *J Virol* 1988;62:2578–2586.
478. Ostrowski MA, Chun TW, Justement SJ, et al. Both memory and $CD45RA^+/CD62L^+$ naive $CD4^+$ T cells are infected in human immunodeficiency virus type 1-infected individuals. *J Virol* 1999;73:6430–6435.
479. Ott DE. Cellular proteins in HIV virions. *Rev Med Virol* 1997;7:167–180.
480. Ott DE, Hewes SM, Alvord WG, et al. Inhibition of Friend virus replication by a compound that reacts with the nucleocapsid zinc finger: Anti-retroviral effect demonstrated in vivo. *Virology* 1998;243:283–292.
481. Owens RJ, Dubay JW, Hunter E, et al. Human immunodeficiency virus envelope protein determines the site of virus release in polarized epithelial cells. *Proc Natl Acad Sci U S A* 1991;88:3987–3991.
482. Page KA, Stearns SM, Littman DR. Analysis of mutations in the V3 domain of gp160 that affect fusion and infectivity. *J Virol* 1992;66:524–533.
483. Paillart JC, Gottlinger HG. Opposing effects of human immunodeficiency virus type 1 matrix mutations support a myristyl switch model of gag membrane targeting. *J Virol* 1999;73:2604–2612.
484. Paillart JC, Skripkin E, Ehresmann B, et al. A loop-loop "kissing" complex is the essential part of the dimer linkage of genomic HIV-1 RNA. *Proc Natl Acad Sci U S A* 1996;93:5572–5577.
485. Palombella VJ, Rando OJ, Goldberg AL, et al. The ubiquitin-proteasome pathway is required for processing the NF-κB1 precursor protein and the activation of NF-κB. *Cell* 1994;78:773–785.
486. Pandori MW, Fitch NJ, Craig HM, et al. Producer-cell modification of human immunodeficiency virus type 1: Nef is a virion protein. *J Virol* 1996;70:4283–4290.
487. Parada CA, Roeder RG. Enhanced processivity of RNA polymerase II triggered by Tat-induced phosphorylation of its carboxy-terminal domain. *Nature* 1996;384:375–378.
488. Parent LJ, Bennett RP, Craven RC, et al. Positionally independent and exchangeable late budding functions of the Rous sarcoma virus and human immunodeficiency virus Gag proteins. *J Virol* 1995;69:5455–5460.

489. Parren PW, Ditzel HJ, Gulizia RJ, et al. Protection against HIV-1 infection in hu-PBL-SCID mice by passive immunization with a neutralizing human monoclonal antibody against the gp120 CD4-binding site. *AIDS* 1995;9:F1–6.
490. Pasquinelli AE, Ernst RK, Lund E, et al. The constitutive transport element (CTE) of Mason-Pfizer monkey virus (MPMV) accesses a cellular mRNA export pathway. *EMBO J* 1997;16:7500–7510.
491. Pathak VK, Hu W-S. "Might as well jump!" Template switching by retroviral reverse transcriptase, defective genome formation, and recombination. *Semin Virol* 1997;8:141–150.
492. Pathak VK, Temin HM. Broad spectrum of in vivo forward mutations, hypermutations, and mutational hotspots in a retroviral shuttle vector after a single replication cycle: Substitutions, frameshifts, and hypermutations. *Proc Natl Acad Sci U S A* 1990;87:6019–6023.
493. Pathak VK, Temin HM. Broad spectrum of in vivo forward mutations, hypermutations, and mutational hotspots in a retroviral shuttle vector after a single replication cycle: Deletions and deletions with insertions. *Proc Natl Acad Sci U S A* 1990;87:6024–6028.
494. Paxton W, Connor RI, Landau NR. Incorporation of Vpr into human immunodeficiency virus type 1 virions: Requirement for the p6 region of gag and mutational analysis. *J Virol* 1993;67:7229–7237.
495. Paxton WA, Martin SR, Tse D, et al. Relative resistance to HIV-1 infection of CD4 lymphocytes from persons who remain uninfected despite multiple high-risk sexual exposures. *Nat Med* 1996;2:412–417.
496. Peeters M, Liegeois F, Torimiro N, et al. Characterization of a highly replicative intergroup M/O human immunodeficiency virus type 1 recombinant isolated from a Cameroonian patient. *J Virol* 1999;73:7368–7375.
497. Peng J, Marshall NF, Price DH. Identification of a cyclin subunit required for the function of *Drosophila* P-TEFb. *J Biol Chem* 1998;273:13855–13860.
498. Peng J, Zhu Y, Milton JT, et al. Identification of multiple cyclin subunits of human P-TEFb. *Genes Dev* 1998;12:755–762.
499. Perkins ND, Edwards NL, Duckett CS, et al. A cooperative interaction between NF-kappa B and Sp1 is required for HIV-1 enhancer activation. *EMBO J* 1993;12:3551–3558.
500. Piguet V, Chen YL, Mangasarian A, et al. Mechanism of Nef-induced CD4 endocytosis: Nef connects CD4 with the μ chain of adaptor complexes. *EMBO J* 1998;17:2472–2481.
501. Piguet V, Gu F, Foti M, et al. Nef-induced CD4 degradation: A diacidic-based motif in Nef functions as a lysosomal targeting signal through the binding of β-COP in endosomes. *Cell* 1999;97:63–73.
502. Piller SC, Jans P, Gage PW, et al. Extracellular HIV-1 virus protein R causes a large inward current and cell death in cultured hippocampal neurons: Implications for AIDS pathology. *Proc Natl Acad Sci U S A* 1998;95:4595–4600.
503. Platt EJ, Haffar OK. Characterization of human immunodeficiency virus type 1 $Pr55^{gag}$ membrane association in a cell-free system: Requirement for a C-terminal domain. *Proc Natl Acad Sci U S A* 1994;91:4594–4598.
504. Poon B, Grovit-Ferbas K, Stewart SA, et al. Cell cycle arrest by Vpr in HIV-1 virions and insensitivity to antiretroviral agents. *Science* 1998;281:266–269.
505. Popov S, Rexach M, Ratner L, et al. Viral protein R regulates docking of the HIV-1 preintegration complex to the nuclear pore complex. *J Biol Chem* 1998;273:13347–13352.
506. Popov S, Rexach M, Zybarth G, et al. Viral protein R regulates nuclear import of the HIV-1 pre-integration complex. *EMBO J* 1998;17:909–917.
507. Popovic M, Sarngadharan MG, Read E, et al. Detection, isolation, and continuous production of cytopathic retroviruses (HTLV-III) from patients with AIDS and pre-AIDS. *Science* 1984;224:497–500.
508. Potempa S, Picard L, Reeves JD, et al. CD4-independent infection by human immunodeficiency virus type 2 strain ROD/B: The role of the N-terminal domain of CXCR-4 in fusion and entry. *J Virol* 1997;71:4419–4424.
509. Preston BD, Dougherty JP. Mechanisms of retroviral mutation. *Trends Microbiol* 1996;4:16–21.
510. Preston BD, Poiesz BJ, Loeb LA. Fidelity of HIV-1 reverse transcriptase. *Science* 1988;242:1168–1171.
511. Puffer BA, Parent LJ, Wills JW, et al. Equine infectious anemia virus utilizes a YXXL motif within the late assembly domain of the Gag p9 protein. *J Virol* 1997;71:6541–6546.
512. Puffer BA, Watkins SC, Montelaro RC. Equine infectious anemia virus Gag polyprotein late domain specifically recruits cellular AP-2 adapter protein complexes during virion assembly. *J Virol* 1998;72:10218–10221.
513. Purcell DF, Martin MA. Alternative splicing of human immunodeficiency virus type 1 mRNA modulates viral protein expression, replication, and infectivity. *J Virol* 1993;67:6365–6378.
514. Quinnan GV Jr, Masur H, Rook AH, et al. Herpesvirus infections in the acquired immune deficiency syndrome. *JAMA* 1984;252:72–77.
515. Ragheb JA, Anderson WF. pH-independent murine leukemia virus ecotropic envelope-mediated cell fusion: Implications for the role of the R peptide and p12E TM in viral entry. *J Virol* 1994;68:3220–3231.
516. Rao Z, Belyaev AS, Fry E, et al. Crystal structure of SIV matrix antigen and implications for virus assembly. *Nature* 1995;378:743–747.
517. Ratner L, Haseltine W, Patarca R, et al. Complete nucleotide sequence of the AIDS virus, HTLV-III. *Nature* 1985;313:277–284.
518. Re F, Braaten D, Franke EK, et al. Human immunodeficiency virus type 1 Vpr arrests the cell cycle in G2 by inhibiting the activation of p34cdc2-cyclin B. *J Virol* 1995;69:6859–6864.
519. Refaeli Y, Levy DN, Weiner DB. The glucocorticoid receptor type II complex is a target of the HIV-1 vpr gene product. *Proc Natl Acad Sci U S A* 1995;92:3621–3625.
520. Reil H, Bukovsky AA, Gelderblom HR, et al. Efficient HIV-1 replication can occur in the absence of the viral matrix protein. *EMBO J* 1998;17:2699–2708.
521. Reimann KA, Li JT, Veazey R, et al. A chimeric simian/human immunodeficiency virus expressing a primary patient human immunodeficiency virus type 1 isolate *env* causes an AIDS-like disease after in vivo passage in rhesus monkeys. *J Virol* 1996;70:6922–6928.
522. Rein A, Henderson LE, Levin JG. Nucleic-acid-chaperone activity of retroviral nucleocapsid proteins: Significance for viral replication. *Trends Biochem Sci* 1998;23:297–301.
523. Rein A, Mirro J, Haynes JG, et al. Function of the cytoplasmic domain of a retroviral transmembrane protein: P15E-p2E cleavage activates the membrane fusion capability of the murine leukemia virus Env protein. *J Virol* 1994;68:1773–1781.
524. Rey O, Canon J, Krogstad P. HIV-1 Gag protein associates with F-actin present in microfilaments. *Virology* 1996;220:530–534.
525. Rice P, Mizuuchi K. Structure of the bacteriophage Mu transposase core: A common structural motif for DNA transposition and retroviral integration. *Cell* 1995;82:209–220.
526. Rice WG, Schaeffer CA, Harten B, et al. Inhibition of HIV-1 infectivity by zinc-ejecting aromatic C-nitroso compounds. *Nature* 1993;361:473–475.
527. Rice WG, Supko JG, Malspeis L, et al. Inhibitors of HIV nucleocapsid protein zinc fingers as candidates for the treatment of AIDS. *Science* 1995;270:1194–1197.
528. Riley JL, Levine BL, Craighead N, et al. Naïve and memory CD4 T cells differ in their susceptibilities to human immunodeficiency virus type 1 infection following CD28 costimulation: Implications for transmission and pathogenesis. *J Virol* 1998;72:8273–8280.
529. Rizzuto CD, Wyatt R, Hernandez-Ramos N, et al. A conserved HIV gp120 glycoprotein structure involved in chemokine receptor binding. *Science* 1998;280:1949–1953.
530. Roberts JD, Bebenek K, Kunkel TA. The accuracy of reverse transcriptase from HIV-1. *Science* 1988;242:1171–1173.
531. Robertson DL, Sharp PM, McCutchan FE, et al. Recombination in HIV-1 [letter]. *Nature* 1995;374:124–126.
532. Rodgers DW, Gamblin SJ, Harris BA, et al. The structure of unliganded reverse transcriptase from the human immunodeficiency virus type 1. *Proc Natl Acad Sci U S A* 1995;92:1222–1226.
533. Roos MT, Lange JM, de Goede RE, et al. Viral phenotype and immune response in primary human immunodeficiency virus type 1 infection. *J Infect Dis* 1992;165:427–432.
534. Rosen CA, Sodroski JG, Haseltine WA. The location of *cis*-acting regulatory sequences in the human T cell lymphotropic virus type III (HTLV-III/LAV) long terminal repeat. *Cell* 1985;41:813–823.
535. Rosen CA, Terwilliger E, Dayton A, et al. Intragenic cis-acting *art* gene-responsive sequences of the human immunodeficiency virus. *Proc Natl Acad Sci U S A* 1988;85:2071–2075.
536. Ross EK, Buckler-White AJ, Rabson AB, et al. Contribution of NF-κB and Sp1 binding motifs to the replicative capacity of human immunodeficiency virus type 1: Distinct patterns of viral growth are determined by T-cell types. *J Virol* 1991;65:4350–4358.
537. Ross TM, Cullen BR. The ability of HIV type 1 to use CCR-3 as a coreceptor is controlled by envelope V1/V2 sequences acting in con-

junction with a CCR-5 tropic V3 loop. *Proc Natl Acad Sci U S A* 1998;95:7682–7686.
538. Rossio JL, Esser MT, Suryanarayana K, et al. Inactivation of human immunodeficiency virus type 1 infectivity with preservation of conformational and functional integrity of virion surface proteins. *J Virol* 1998;72:7992–8001.
539. Roth MJ, Schwartzberg PL, Goff SP. Structure of the termini of DNA intermediates in the integration of retroviral DNA: Dependence on IN function and terminal DNA sequence. *Cell* 1989;58:47–54.
540. Rothe M, Sarma V, Dixit VM, et al. TRAF2-mediated activation of NF-κ B by TNF receptor 2 and CD40. *Science* 1995;269:1424–1427.
541. Rowell JF, Stanhope PE, Siliciano RF. Endocytosis of endogenously synthesized HIV-1 envelope protein. Mechanism and role in processing for association with class II MHC. *J Immunol* 1995;155:473–488.
542. Roy S, Delling U, Chen C-H, et al. A bulge structure in HIV-1 TAR RNA is required for Tat binding and Tat-mediated *trans*-activation. *Genes Dev* 1990;4:1365–1373.
543. Ruben S, Perkins A, Purcell R, et al. Structural and functional characterization of human immunodeficiency virus tat protein. *J Virol* 1989;63:1–8.
544. Rubin H. A virus in chick embryos which induces resistance in vitro to infection with Rous sarcoma virus. *Proc Natl Acad Sci U S A* 1960; 46:1105–1119.
545. Saag MS, Hahn BH, Gibbons J, et al. Extensive variation of human immunodeficiency virus type-1 in vivo. *Nature* 1988;334:440–444.
546. Sadaie MR, Rappaport J, Benter T, et al. Missense mutations in an infectious human immunodeficiency viral genome: Functional mapping of *tat* and identification of the *rev* splice acceptor. *Proc Natl Acad Sci U S A* 1988;85:9224–9228.
547. Sakaida H, Hori T, Yonezawa A, et al. T-tropic human immunodeficiency virus type 1 (HIV-1)-derived V3 loop peptides directly bind to CXCR-4 and inhibit T-tropic HIV-1 infection. *J Virol* 1998;72: 9763–9770.
548. Saksela K, Cheng G, Baltimore D. Proline-rich (PxxP) motifs in HIV-1 Nef bind to SH3 domains of a subset of Src kinases and are required for the enhanced growth of Nef+ viruses but not for down-regulation of CD4. *EMBO J* 1995;14:484–491.
549. Samson M, Libert F, Doranz BJ, et al. Resistance to HIV-1 infection in caucasian individuals bearing mutant alleles of the CCR-5 chemokine receptor gene. *Nature* 1996;382:722–725.
550. Sandefur S, Varthakavi V, Spearman P. The I domain is required for efficient plasma membrane binding of human immunodeficiency virus type 1 $Pr55^{Gag}$. *J Virol* 1998;72:2723–2732.
551. Sarngadharan MG, Popovic M, Bruch L, et al. Antibodies reactive with human T-lymphotropic retroviruses (HTLV-III) in the serum of patients with AIDS. *Science* 1984;224:506–508.
552. Sattentau QJ, Moore JP. Conformational changes induced in the human immunodeficiency virus envelope glycoprotein by soluble CD4 binding. *J Exp Med* 1991;174:407–415.
553. Sattentau QJ, Moore JP, Vignaux F, et al. Conformational changes induced in the envelope glycoproteins of the human and simian immunodeficiency viruses by soluble receptor binding. *J Virol* 1993; 67:7383–7393.
554. Sawaya BE, Khalili K, Mercer WE, et al. Cooperative actions of HIV-1 Vpr and p53 modulate viral gene transcription. *J Biol Chem* 1998;273:20052–20057.
555. Schmidtmayerova H, Alfano M, Nuovo G, et al. Human immunodeficiency virus type 1 T-lymphotropic strains enter macrophages via a CD4- and CXCR4-mediated pathway: Replication is restricted at a postentry level. *J Virol* 1998;72:4633–4642.
556. Schmidtmayerova H, Sherry B, Bukrinsky M. Chemokines and HIV replication. *Nature* 1996;382:767.
557. Schnittman SM, Lane HC, Greenhouse J, et al. Preferential infection of CD4+ memory T cells by human immunodeficiency virus type 1: Evidence for a role in the selective T-cell functional defects observed in infected individuals. *Proc Natl Acad Sci U S A* 1990;87:6058–6062.
558. Schubert U, Bour S, Ferrer-Montiel AV, et al. The two biological activities of human immunodeficiency virus type 1 Vpu protein involve two separable structural domains. *J Virol* 1996;70:809–819.
559. Schubert U, Ferrer-Montiel AV, Oblatt-Montal M, et al. Identification of an ion channel activity of the Vpu transmembrane domain and its involvement in the regulation of virus release from HIV-1-infected cells. *FEBS Lett* 1996;398:12–18.
560. Schubert U, Henklein P, Boldyreff B, et al. The human immunodeficiency virus type 1 encoded Vpu protein is phosphorylated by casein kinase-2 (CK-2) at positions Ser52 and Ser56 within a predicted α-helix-turn-α-helix-motif. *J Mol Biol* 1994;236:16–25.
561. Schubert U, Strebel K. Differential activities of the human immunodeficiency virus type 1-encoded Vpu protein are regulated by phosphorylation and occur in different cellular compartments. *J Virol* 1994;68:2260–2271.
562. Schuitemaker H, Kootstra NA, Koppelman MH, et al. Proliferation-dependent HIV-1 infection of monocytes occurs during differentiation into macrophages. *J Clin Invest* 1992;89:1154–1160.
563. Schuler W, Wecker K, de Rocquigny H, et al. NMR structure of the (52-96) C-terminal domain of the HIV-1 regulatory protein Vpr: Molecular insights into its biological functions. *J Mol Biol* 1999;285: 2105–2117.
564. Schwartz O, Marechal V, Danos O, et al. Human immunodeficiency virus type 1 Nef increases the efficiency of reverse transcription in the infected cell. *J Virol* 1995;69:4053–4059.
565. Schwartz O, Marechal V, Le Gall S, et al. Endocytosis of major histocompatibility complex class I molecules is induced by the HIV-1 Nef protein. *Nat Med* 1996;2:338–342.
566. Schwartz S, Felber BK, Benko DM, et al. Cloning and functional analysis of multiply spliced mRNA species of human immunodeficiency virus type 1. *J Virol* 1990;64:2519–2529.
567. Schwartz S, Felber BK, Fenyö E-M, et al. Env and Vpu proteins of human immunodeficiency virus type 1 are produced from multiple bicistronic mRNAs. *J Virol* 1990;64:5448–5456.
568. Schwartzberg P, Colicelli J, Goff SP. Construction and analysis of deletion mutations in the *pol* gene of Moloney murine leukemia virus: A new viral function required for productive infection. *Cell* 1984;37: 1043–1052.
569. Selby MJ, Peterlin BM. *Trans*-activation by HIV-1 Tat via a heterologous RNA binding protein. *Cell* 1990;62:769–776.
570. Sharp PM, Bailes E, Stevenson M, et al. Gene acquisition in HIV and SIV. *Nature* 1996;383:586–587.
571. Shen H, Cheng T, Preffer FI, et al. Intrinsic human immunodeficiency virus type 1 resistance of hematopoietic stem cells despite coreceptor expression. *J Virol* 1999;73:728–737.
572. Sheridan PL, Sheline CT, Cannon K, et al. Activation of the HIV-1 enhancer by the LEF-1 HMG protein on nucleosome-assembled DNA in vitro. *Genes Dev* 1995;9:2090–2104.
573. Shibata R, Kawamura M, Sakai H, et al. Generation of a chimeric human and simian immunodeficiency virus infectious to monkey peripheral blood mononuclear cells. *J Virol* 1991;65:3514–3520.
574. Siekevitz M, Josephs SF, Dukovich M, et al. Activation of the HIV-1 LTR by T cell mitogens and the trans-activator protein of HTLV-I [published erratum appears in *Science* 1988;239:451]. *Science* 1987; 238:1575–1578.
575. Sieweke MH, Tekotte H, Jarosch U, et al. Cooperative interaction of Ets-1 with USF-1 required for HIV-1 enhancer activity in T cells. *EMBO J* 1998;17:1728–1739.
576. Simm M, Shahabuddin M, Chao W, et al. Aberrant Gag protein composition of a human immunodeficiency virus type 1 vif mutant produced in primary lymphocytes. *J Virol* 1995;69:4582–4586.
577. Simmons G, Clapham PR, Picard L, et al. Potent inhibition of HIV-1 infectivity in macrophages and lymphocytes by a novel CCR5 antagonist. *Science* 1997;276:276–279.
578. Simmons G, Reeves JD, McKnight A, et al. CXCR4 as a functional coreceptor for human immunodeficiency virus type 1 infection of primary macrophages. *J Virol* 1998;72:8453–8457.
579. Simmons G, Wilkinson D, Reeves JD, et al. Primary, syncytium-inducing human immunodeficiency virus type 1 isolates are dual-tropic and most can use either Lestr or CCR5 as coreceptors for virus entry. *J Virol* 1996;70:8355–8360.
580. Simon F, Mauclere P, Roques P, et al. Identification of a new human immunodeficiency virus type 1 distinct from group M and group O. *Nat Med* 1998;4:1032–1037.
581. Simon JH, Gaddis NC, Fouchier RA, et al. Evidence for a newly discovered cellular anti-HIV-1 phenotype. *Nat Med* 1998;4:1397–1400.
582. Simon JH, Malim MH. The human immunodeficiency virus type 1 Vif protein modulates the postpenetration stability of viral nucleoprotein complexes. *J Virol* 1996;70:5297–5305.
583. Simon JH, Miller DL, Fouchier RA, et al. Virion incorporation of human immunodeficiency virus type-1 Vif is determined by intracellular expression level and may not be necessary for function. *Virology* 1998;248:182–187.
584. Simon JHM, Miller DL, Fouchier RAM, et al. The regulation of pri-

mate immunodeficiency virus infectivity by Vif is cell species restricted: A role for Vif in determining virus host range and cross-species transmission. *EMBO J* 1998;17:1259–1267.
585. Simpson SB, Zhang L, Craven RC, et al. Rous sarcoma virus direct repeat *cis* elements exert effects at several points in the virus life cycle. *J Virol* 1997;71:9150–9156.
586. Skowronski J, Parks D, Mariani R. Altered T cell activation and development in transgenic mice expressing the HIV-1 *nef* gene. *EMBO J* 1993;12:703–713.
587. Smith MW, Dean M, Carrington M, et al. Contrasting genetic influence of *CCR2* and *CCR5* variants on HIV-1 infection and disease progression. *Science* 1997;277:959–965.
588. Sodroski J, Goh WC, Rosen C, et al. A second post-transcriptional *trans*-activator gene required for HTLV-III replication. *Nature* 1986; 321:412–417.
589. Sodroski J, Goh WC, Rosen C, et al. Replicative and cytopathic potential of HTLV-III/LAV with *sor* gene deletions. *Science* 1986;231: 1549–1553.
590. Sommerfelt MA, Petteway SR Jr, Dreyer GB, et al. Effect of retroviral proteinase inhibitors on Mason-Pfizer monkey virus maturation and transmembrane glycoprotein cleavage. *J Virol* 1992;66: 4220–4227.
591. South TL, Blake PR, Sowder RC III, et al. The nucleocapsid protein isolated from HIV-1 particles binds zinc and forms retroviral-type zinc fingers. *Biochemistry* 1990;29:7786–7789.
592. Sova P, Volsky DJ. Efficiency of viral DNA synthesis during infection of permissive and nonpermissive cells with vif-negative human immunodeficiency virus type 1. *J Virol* 1993;67:6322–6326.
593. Spearman P, Horton R, Ratner L, et al. Membrane binding of human immunodeficiency virus type 1 matrix protein in vivo supports a conformational myristyl switch mechanism. *J Virol* 1997;71:6582–6592.
594. Spina CA, Kwoh TJ, Chowers MY, et al. The importance of nef in the induction of human immunodeficiency virus type 1 replication from primary quiescent CD4 lymphocytes. *J Exp Med* 1994;179:115–123.
595. Stade K, Ford CS, Guthrie C, et al. Exportin 1 (Crm1p) is an essential nuclear export factor. *Cell* 1997;90:1041–1050.
596. Starcich BR, Hahn BH, Shaw GM, et al. Identification and characterization of conserved and variable regions in the envelope gene of HTLV-III/LAV, the retrovirus of AIDS. *Cell* 1986;45:637–648.
597. Stevenson M, Meier C, Mann AM, et al. Envelope glycoprotein of HIV induces interference and cytolysis resistance in CD4+ cells: Mechanism for persistence in AIDS. *Cell* 1988;53:483–496.
598. Stevenson M, Stanwick TL, Dempsey MP, et al. HIV-1 replication is controlled at the level of T cell activation and proviral integration. *EMBO J* 1990;9:1551–1560.
599. Stewart SA, Poon B, Jowett JB, et al. Human immunodeficiency virus type 1 Vpr induces apoptosis following cell cycle arrest. *J Virol* 1997;71:5579–5592.
600. Strebel K, Daugherty D, Clouse K, et al. The HIV "A" (*sor*) gene product is essential for virus infectivity. *Nature* 1987;328:728–730.
601. Strebel K, Klimkait T, Maldarelli F, et al. Molecular and biochemical analyses of human immunodeficiency virus type 1 vpu protein. *J Virol* 1989;63:3784–3791.
602. Strebel K, Klimkait T, Martin MA. A novel gene of HIV-1, *vpu*, and its 16-kilodalton product. *Science* 1988;241:1221–1223.
603. Stutz F, Rosbash M. Nuclear RNA export. *Genes Dev* 1998;12: 3303–3319.
604. Subbarao S, Schochetman G. Genetic variability of HIV-1. *AIDS* 1996;10:S13–23.
605. Sullenger BA, Gallardo HF, Ungers GE, et al. Analysis of trans-acting response decoy RNA-mediated inhibition of human immunodeficiency virus type 1 transactivation. *J Virol* 1991;65:6811–6816.
606. Sullivan N, Sun Y, Li J, et al. Replicative function and neutralization sensitivity of envelope glycoproteins from primary and T-cell line-passaged human immunodeficiency virus type 1 isolates. *J Virol* 1995; 69:4413–4422.
607. Sullivan N, Thali M, Furman C, et al. Effect of amino acid changes in the V1/V2 region of the human immunodeficiency virus type 1 gp120 glycoprotein on subunit association, syncytium formation, and recognition by a neutralizing antibody. *J Virol* 1993;67:3674–3679.
608. Summers MF, Henderson LE, Chance MR, et al. Nucleocapsid zinc fingers detected in retroviruses: EXAFS studies of intact viruses and the solution-state structure of the nucleocapsid protein from HIV-1. *Protein Sci* 1992;1:563–574.
609. Swingler S, Mann A, Jacque J, et al. HIV-1 Nef mediates lymphocyte chemotaxis and activation by infected macrophages. *Nat Med* 1999; 5:997–103.
610. Tachibana K, Hirota S, Iizasa H, et al. The chemokine receptor CXCR4 is essential for vascularization of the gastrointestinal tract. *Nature* 1998;393:591–594.
611. Tan K, Liu J, Wang J, et al. Atomic structure of a thermostable subdomain of HIV-1 gp41. *Proc Natl Acad Sci U S A* 1997;94: 12303–12308.
612. Tanchou V, Decimo D, Pechoux C, et al. Role of the N-terminal zinc finger of human immunodeficiency virus type 1 nucleocapsid protein in virus structure and replication. *J Virol* 1998;72:4442–4447.
613. Telesnitsky A, Goff SP. Reverse transcription and the generation of retroviral DNA. In: Coffin JM, Hughes SH, Varmus HE, eds. *Retroviruses*. Cold Spring Harbor, NY: Cold Spring Harbor Laboratory Press, 1997:121–160.
614. Temin HM. Retrovirus variation and reverse transcription: Abnormal strand transfers result in retrovirus genetic variation. *Proc Natl Acad Sci U S A* 1993;90:6900–6903.
615. Temin HM, Mizutani S. RNA-dependent DNA polymerase in virions of Rous sarcoma virus. *Nature* 1970;226:1211–1213.
616. Tersmette M, Gruters RA, de Wolf F, et al. Evidence for a role of virulent human immunodeficiency virus (HIV) variants in the pathogenesis of acquired immunodeficiency syndrome: Studies on sequential HIV isolates. *J Virol* 1989;63:2118–2125.
617. Terwilliger EF, Cohen EA, Lu Y, et al. Functional role of human immunodeficiency virus type 1 *vpu*. *Proc Natl Acad Sci U S A* 1989; 86:5163–5167.
618. Thali M, Bukovsky A, Kondo E, et al. Functional association of cyclophilin A with HIV-1 virions. *Nature* 1994;372:363–365.
619. Thali M, Moore JP, Furman C, et al. Characterization of conserved human immunodeficiency virus type 1 gp120 neutralization epitopes exposed upon gp120-CD4 binding. *J Virol* 1993;67:3978–3988.
620. Tiley LS, Madore SJ, Malim MH, et al. The VP16 transcription activation domain is functional when targeted to a promoter-proximal RNA sequence. *Genes Dev* 1992;6:2077–2087.
621. Toggas SM, Masliah E, Rockenstein EM, et al. Central nervous system damage produced by expression of the HIV-1 coat protein gp120 in transgenic mice. *Nature* 1994;367:188–193.
622. Toohey MG, Jones KA. In vitro formation of short RNA polymerase II transcripts that terminate within the HIV-1 and HIV-2 promoter-proximal downstream regions. *Genes Dev* 1989;3:265–282.
623. Tristem M, Marshall C, Karpas A, et al. Origin of vpx in lentiviruses. *Nature* 1990;347:341–342.
624. Tristem M, Purvis A, Quicke DL. Complex evolutionary history of primate lentiviral vpr genes. *Virology* 1998;240:232–237.
625. Trkola A, Dragic T, Arthos J, et al. CD4-dependent, antibody-sensitive interactions between HIV-1 and its co-receptor CCR-5. *Nature* 1996;384:184–187.
626. Trono D. Partial reverse transcripts in virions from human immunodeficiency and murine leukemia viruses. *J Virol* 1992;66:4893–4900.
627. Tsunetsugu-Yokota Y, Yasuda S, Sugimoto A, et al. Efficient virus transmission from dendritic cells to $CD4^+$ T cells in response to antigen depends on close contact through adhesion molecules. *Virology* 1997;239:259–268.
628. Turner BG, Summers MF. Structural biology of HIV. *J Mol Biol* 1999;285:1–32.
629. Uchida N, Sutton RE, Friera AM, et al. HIV, but not murine leukemia virus, vectors mediate high efficiency gene transfer into freshly isolated G_0/G_1 human hematopoietic stem cells. *Proc Natl Acad Sci U S A* 1998;95:11939–11944.
630. Unutmaz D, KewalRamani VN, Marmon S, et al. Cytokine signals are sufficient for HIV-1 infection of resting human T lymphocytes. *J Exp Med* 1999;189:1735–1746.
631. Valsamakis A, Schek N, Alwine JC. Elements upstream of the AAUAAA within the human immunodeficiency virus polyadenylation signal are required for efficient polyadenylation in vitro. *Mol Cell Biol* 1992;12:3699–3705.
632. van Kuyk R, Torbett BE, Gulizia RJ, et al. Cloned human CD8+ cytotoxic T lymphocytes protect human peripheral blood leukocyte–severe combined immunodeficient mice from HIV-1 infection by an HLA-unrestricted mechanism. *J Immunol* 1994;153:4826–4833.
633. Van Lint C, Amella CA, Emiliani S, et al. Transcription factor binding sites downstream of the human immunodeficiency virus type 1 transcription start site are important for virus infectivity. *J Virol* 1997; 71:6113–6127.

634. Vartanian JP, Meyerhans A, Sala M, et al. G→A hypermutation of the human immunodeficiency virus type 1 genome: Evidence for dCTP pool imbalance during reverse transcription. *Proc Natl Acad Sci U S A* 1994;91:3092–3096.
635. Verdin E. DNase I–hypersensitive sites are associated with both long terminal repeats and with the intragenic enhancer of integrated human immunodeficiency virus type 1. *J Virol* 1991;65:6790–6799.
636. Verdin E, Paras P Jr, Van Lint C. Chromatin disruption in the promoter of human immunodeficiency virus type 1 during transcriptional activation [published erratum appears in *EMBO J* 1993;12:4900]. *EMBO J* 1993;12:3249–3259.
637. Vicenzi E, Dimitrov DS, Engelman A, et al. An integration-defective U5 deletion mutant of human immunodeficiency virus type 1 reverts by eliminating additional long terminal repeat sequences. *J Virol* 1994;68:7879–7890.
638. Vincent MJ, Raja NU, Jabbar MA. Human immunodeficiency virus type 1 Vpu protein induces degradation of chimeric envelope glycoproteins bearing the cytoplasmic and anchor domains of CD4: Role of the cytoplasmic domain in Vpu-induced degradation in the endoplasmic reticulum. *J Virol* 1993;67:5538–5549.
639. Viscidi RP, Mayur K, Lederman HM, et al. Inhibition of antigen-induced lymphocyte proliferation by Tat protein from HIV-1. *Science* 1989;246:1606–1608.
640. Vodicka MA, Koepp DM, Silver PA, et al. HIV-1 Vpr interacts with the nuclear transport pathway to promote macrophage infection. *Genes Dev* 1998;12:175–185.
641. Vogel J, Hinrichs SH, Reynolds RK, et al. The HIV tat gene induces dermal lesions resembling Kaposi's sarcoma in transgenic mice. *Nature* 1988;335:606–611.
642. Vogt VM. Proteolytic processing and particle maturation. *Curr Top Microbiol Immunol* 1996;214:95–131.
642a. Vogt VM. Ubiquitin in retrovirus assembly: actor or bystander? *Proc Natl Acad Sci USA* 2000;97:12945–12947.
643. Vogt VM, Eisenman R. Identification of a large polypeptide precursor of avian oncornavirus proteins. *Proc Natl Acad Sci U S A* 1973;70: 1734–1738.
644. Vogt VM, Eisenman R, Diggelmann H. Generation of avian myeloblastosis virus structural proteins by proteolytic cleavage of a precursor polypeptide. *J Mol Biol* 1975;96:471–493.
645. von Schwedler U, Kornbluth RS, Trono D. The nuclear localization signal of the matrix protein of human immunodeficiency virus type 1 allows the establishment of infection in macrophages and quiescent T lymphocytes. *Proc Natl Acad Sci U S A* 1994;91:6992–6996.
646. von Schwedler U, Song J, Aiken C, et al. Vif is crucial for human immunodeficiency virus type 1 proviral DNA synthesis in infected cells. *J Virol* 1993;67:4945–4955.
647. von Schwedler UK, Stemmler TL, Klishko VY, et al. Proteolytic refolding of the HIV-1 capsid protein amino-terminus facilitates viral core assembly. *EMBO J* 1998;17:1555–1568.
648. Wain-Hobson S, Sonigo P, Danos O, et al. Nucleotide sequence of the AIDS virus, LAV. *Cell* 1985;40:9–17.
649. Wang L, Mukherjee S, Jia F, et al. Interaction of virion protein Vpr of human immunodeficiency virus type 1 with cellular transcription factor Sp1 and trans-activation of viral long terminal repeat. *J Biol Chem* 1995;270:25564–25569.
650. Weeks KM, Ampe C, Schultz SC, et al. Fragments of the HIV-1 Tat protein specifically bind TAR RNA. *Science* 1990;249:1281–1285.
651. Wei P, Garber ME, Fang SM, et al. A novel CDK9-associated C-type cyclin interacts directly with HIV-1 Tat and mediates its high-affinity, loop-specific binding to TAR RNA. *Cell* 1998;92:451–462.
652. Wei SQ, Mizuuchi K, Craigie R. A large nucleoprotein assembly at the ends of the viral DNA mediates retroviral DNA integration. *EMBO J* 1997;16:7511–7520.
653. Weissenhorn W, Dessen A, Harrison SC, et al. Atomic structure of the ectodomain from HIV-1 gp41. *Nature* 1997;387:426–430.
654. Welker R, Harris M, Cardel B, et al. Virion incorporation of human immunodeficiency virus type 1 Nef is mediated by a bipartite membrane-targeting signal: Analysis of its role in enhancement of viral infectivity. *J Virol* 1998;72:8833–8840.
655. Welker R, Kottler H, Kalbitzer HR, et al. Human immunodeficiency virus type 1 Nef protein is incorporated into virus particles and specifically cleaved by the viral proteinase. *Virology* 1996;219:228–236.
656. Wen W, Meinkoth JL, Tsien RY, et al. Identification of a signal for rapid export of proteins from the nucleus. *Cell* 1995;82:463–473.
657. White JM. Membrane fusion. *Science* 1992;258:917–924.
658. Wiegers K, Rutter G, Schubert U, et al. Cyclophilin A incorporation is not required for human immunodeficiency virus type 1 particle maturation and does not destabilize the mature capsid. *Virology* 1999; 257:261–274.
659. Wild C, Oas T, McDanal C, et al. A synthetic peptide inhibitor of human immunodeficiency virus replication: Correlation between solution structure and viral inhibition. *Proc Natl Acad Sci U S A* 1992; 89:10537–10541.
660. Wilk T, Gowen B, Fuller SD. Actin associates with the nucleocapsid domain of the human immunodeficiency virus Gag polyprotein. *J Virol* 1999;73:1931–1940.
661. Willett BJ, Picard L, Hosie MJ, et al. Shared usage of the chemokine receptor CXCR4 by the feline and human immunodeficiency viruses. *J Virol* 1997;71:6407–6415.
662. Willey RL, Bonifacino JS, Potts BJ, et al. Biosynthesis, cleavage, and degradation of the human immunodeficiency virus 1 envelope glycoprotein gp160. *Proc Natl Acad Sci U S A* 1988;85:9580–9584.
663. Willey RL, Buckler-White A, Strebel K. Sequences present in the cytoplasmic domain of CD4 are necessary and sufficient to confer sensitivity to the human immunodeficiency virus type 1 Vpu protein. *J Virol* 1994;68:1207–1212.
664. Willey RL, Maldarelli F, Martin MA, et al. Human immunodeficiency virus type 1 Vpu protein induces rapid degradation of CD4. *J Virol* 1992;66:7193–7200.
665. Willey RL, Maldarelli F, Martin MA, et al. Human immunodeficiency virus type 1 Vpu protein regulates the formation of intracellular gp160-CD4 complexes. *J Virol* 1992;66:226–234.
666. Willey RL, Rutledge RA, Dias S, et al. Identification of conserved and divergent domains within the envelope gene of the acquired immunodeficiency syndrome retrovirus. *Proc Natl Acad Sci U S A* 1986;83:5038–5042.
667. Wills JW, Cameron CE, Wilson CB, et al. An assembly domain of the Rous sarcoma virus Gag protein required late in budding. *J Virol* 1994;68:6605–6618.
668. Wills JW, Craven RC. Form, function, and use of retroviral gag proteins [editorial]. *AIDS* 1991;5:639–654.
669. Winkler C, Modi W, Smith MW, et al. Genetic restriction of AIDS pathogenesis by an SDF-1 chemokine gene variant. *Science* 1998;279: 389–393.
670. Wlodawer A, Erickson JW. Structure-based inhibitors of HIV-1 protease. *Annu Rev Biochem* 1993;62:543–585.
671. Wlodawer A, Miller M, Jaskólski M, et al. Conserved folding in retroviral proteases: Crystal structure of a synthetic HIV-1 protease. *Science* 1989;245:616–621.
672. Wolff B, Sanglier JJ, Wang Y. Leptomycin B is an inhibitor of nuclear export: Inhibition of nucleo-cytoplasmic translocation of the human immunodeficiency virus type 1 (HIV-1) Rev protein and Rev-dependent mRNA. *Chem Biol* 1997;4:139–147.
673. WHO Network for HIV Isolation and Characterization. HIV type 1 variation in World Health Organization–sponsored vaccine evaluation sites: Genetic screening, sequence analysis, and preliminary biological characterization of selected viral strains. *AIDS Res Hum Retroviruses* 1994;10:1327–1343.
674. Worthylake DK, Wang H, Yoo S, et al. Structures of the HIV-1 capsid protein dimerization domain at 2.6 Å resolution. *Acta Crystallogr D Biol Crystallogr* 1999;55:85–92.
675. Wray V, Kinder R, Federau T, et al. Solution structure and orientation of the transmembrane anchor domain of the HIV-1–encoded virus protein U by high-resolution and solid-state NMR spectroscopy. *Biochemistry* 1999;38:5272–5282.
676. Wu L, Gerard NP, Wyatt R, et al. CD4-induced interaction of primary HIV-1 gp120 glycoproteins with the chemokine receptor CCR-5. *Nature* 1996;384:179–183.
677. Wu L, LaRosa G, Kassam N, et al. Interaction of chemokine receptor CCR5 with its ligands: Multiple domains for HIV-1 gp120 binding and a single domain for chemokine binding. *J Exp Med* 1997;186:1373–1381.
678. Wu X, Conway JA, Kim J, et al. Localization of the Vpx packaging signal within the C terminus of the human immunodeficiency virus type 2 Gag precursor protein. *J Virol* 1994;68:6161–6169.
679. Wyatt R, Kwong PD, Desjardins E, et al. The antigenic structure of the HIV gp120 envelope glycoprotein. *Nature* 1998;393:705–711.
680. Xiao X, Wu L, Stantchev TS, et al. Constitutive cell surface association between CD4 and CCR5. *Proc Natl Acad Sci U S A* 1999;96:7496–7501.

681. Yang X, Gold MO, Tang DN, et al. TAK, an HIV Tat-associated kinase, is a member of the cyclin-dependent family of protein kinases and is induced by activation of peripheral blood lymphocytes and differentiation of promonocytic cell lines. *Proc Natl Acad Sci U S A* 1997;94:12331–12336.
682. Yang X, Herrmann CH, Rice AP. The human immunodeficiency virus Tat proteins specifically associate with TAK in vivo and require the carboxyl-terminal domain of RNA polymerase II for function. *J Virol* 1996;70:4576–4584.
683. Yang ZN, Mueser TC, Bushman FD, et al. Crystal structure of an active two-domain derivative of Rous sarcoma virus integrase. *J Mol Biol* 2000;296:535–548.
684. Yao XJ, Gottlinger H, Haseltine WA, et al. Envelope glycoprotein and CD4 independence of vpu-facilitated human immunodeficiency virus type 1 capsid export. *J Virol* 1992;66:5119–5126.
685. Yasuda J, Hunter E. A proline-rich motif (PPPY) in the Gag polyprotein of Mason-Pfizer monkey virus plays a maturation-independent role in virion release. *J Virol* 1998;72:4095–4103.
686. Yeager M, Wilson-Kubalek EM, Weiner SG, et al. Supramolecular organization of immature and mature murine leukemia virus revealed by electron cryo-microscopy: Implications for retroviral assembly mechanisms. *Proc Natl Acad Sci U S A* 1998;95:7299–7304.
687. Yi Y, Isaacs SN, Williams DA, et al. Role of CXCR4 in cell-cell fusion and infection of monocyte-derived macrophages by primary human immunodeficiency virus type 1 (HIV-1) strains: Two distinct mechanisms of HIV-1 dual tropism. *J Virol* 1999;73:7117–7125.
688. Yi Y, Rana S, Turner JD, et al. CXCR-4 is expressed by primary macrophages and supports CCR5-independent infection by dual-tropic but not T-tropic isolates of human immunodeficiency virus type 1. *J Virol* 1998;72:772–777.
689. Yokoyama WM. Natural killer cell receptors. *Curr Opin Immunol* 1998;10:298–305.
690. Yu X, Yu QC, Lee TH, et al. The C terminus of human immunodeficiency virus type 1 matrix protein is involved in early steps of the virus life cycle. *J Virol* 1992;66:5667–5670.
691. Yu X, Yuan X, Matsuda Z, et al. The matrix protein of human immunodeficiency virus type 1 is required for incorporation of viral envelope protein into mature virions. *J Virol* 1992;66:4966–4971.
692. Yu XF, Yu QC, Essex M, et al. The vpx gene of simian immunodeficiency virus facilitates efficient viral replication in fresh lymphocytes and macrophage. *J Virol* 1991;65:5088–5091.
693. Yuan B, Li X, Goff SP. Mutations altering the Moloney murine leukemia virus p12 Gag protein affect virion production and early events of the virus life cycle. *EMBO J* 1999;18:4700–4710.
694. Yuan X, Matsuda Z, Matsuda M, et al. Human immunodeficiency virus *vpr* gene encodes a virion-associated protein. *AIDS Res Hum Retroviruses* 1990;6:1265–1271.
695. Yuan X, Yu X, Lee TH, et al. Mutations in the N-terminal region of human immunodeficiency virus type 1 matrix protein block intracellular transport of the Gag precursor. *J Virol* 1993;67:6387–6394.
696. Zack JA, Arrigo SJ, Weitsman SR, et al. HIV-1 entry into quiescent primary lymphocytes: Molecular analysis reveals a labile, latent viral structure. *Cell* 1990;61:213–222.
697. Zagury D, Lachgar A, Chams V, et al. C-C chemokines, pivotal in protection against HIV type 1 infection. *Proc Natl Acad Sci U S A* 1998; 95:3857–3861.
698. Zapp ML, Hope TJ, Parslow TG, et al. Oligomerization and RNA binding domains of the type 1 human immunodeficiency virus Rev protein: A dual function for an arginine-rich binding motif. *Proc Natl Acad Sci U S A* 1991;88:7734–7738.
699. Zapp ML, Stern S, Green MR. Small molecules that selectively block RNA binding of HIV-1 Rev protein inhibit Rev function and viral production. *Cell* 1993;74:969–978.
700. Zemmel RW, Kelley AC, Karn J, et al. Flexible regions of RNA structure facilitate co-operative Rev assembly on the Rev-response element. *J Mol Biol* 1996;258:763–777.
701. Zennou V, Petit C, Guetard D, et al. HIV-1 genome nuclear import is mediated by a central DNA flap. *Cell* 2000;101:173–185.
702. Zhang L, He T, Huang Y, et al. Chemokine coreceptor usage by diverse primary isolates of human immunodeficiency virus type 1. *J Virol* 1998;72:9307–9312.
703. Zhang YJ, Dragic T, Cao Y, et al. Use of coreceptors other than CCR5 by non-syncytium-inducing adult and pediatric isolates of human immunodeficiency virus type 1 is rare in vitro. *J Virol* 1998;72:9337–9344.
704. Zhao LJ, Wang L, Mukherjee S, et al. Biochemical mechanism of HIV-1 Vpr function. Oligomerization mediated by the N-terminal domain. *J Biol Chem* 1994;269:32131–32137.
705. Zheng R, Jenkins TM, Craigie R. Zinc folds the N-terminal domain of HIV-1 integrase, promotes multimerization, and enhances catalytic activity. *Proc Natl Acad Sci U S A* 1996;93:13659–13664.
706. Zhou Q, Chen D, Pierstorff E, et al. Transcription elongation factor P-TEFb mediates Tat activation of HIV-1 transcription at multiple stages. *EMBO J* 1998;17:3681–3691.
707. Zhou W, Parent LJ, Wills JW, et al. Identification of a membrane-binding domain within the amino-terminal region of human immunodeficiency virus type 1 Gag protein which interacts with acidic phospholipids. *J Virol* 1994;68:2556–2569.
708. Zhou W, Resh MD. Differential membrane binding of the human immunodeficiency virus type 1 matrix protein. *J Virol* 1996;70:8540–8548.
709. Zhu K, Cordeiro ML, Atienza J, et al. Irreversible inhibition of human immunodeficiency virus type 1 integrase by dicaffeoylquinic acids. *J Virol* 1999;73:3309–3316.
710. Zhu Y, Pe'ery T, Peng J, et al. Transcription elongation factor P-TEFb is required for HIV-1 tat transactivation in vitro. *Genes Dev* 1997; 11:2622–2632.
711. Zolla-Pazner S, Gorny MK, Nyambi PN, et al. Immunotyping of human immunodeficiency virus type 1 (HIV): An approach to immunologic classification of HIV. *J Virol* 1999;73:4042–4051.
712. Zolotukhin AS, Valentin A, Pavlakis GN, et al. Continuous propagation of RRE(−) and Rev(−)RRE(−) human immunodeficiency virus type 1 molecular clones containing a cis-acting element of simian retrovirus type 1 in human peripheral blood lymphocytes. *J Virol* 1994;68:7944–7952.
713. Zou YR, Kottmann AH, Kuroda M, et al. Function of the chemokine receptor CXCR4 in haematopoiesis and in cerebellar development. *Nature* 1998;393:595–599.

CHAPTER 29

Polyomaviridae: The Viruses and Their Replication

Charles N. Cole and Suzanne D. Conzen

DISCOVERY AND CLASSIFICATION

The *Polyomaviridae* were previously considered a subfamily of the *Papovaviridae,* a name derived from the names of three prototypical members: rabbit papilloma virus (pa), mouse polyomavirus (po), and simian virus 40 (SV40), originally called vacuolating virus (va). Their genomes are single molecules of covalently closed, superhelical double-stranded DNA that are replicated in the nucleus. Thorough investigations since the 1980s indicate that SV40 and mouse polyomavirus differ from the papillomaviruses in having smaller capsids (diameters of 45 nm versus 55 nm), smaller genomes (about 5,000 base pairs versus about 8,000 base pairs), and a different genomic organization. The *Polyomaviridae* are now considered an independent family of viruses. In this chapter, the term *polyoma* is used to refer to mouse polyomavirus, whereas the family of viruses is referred to as *polyomaviruses.*

Thirteen members of the *Polyomaviridae* family have now been identified. All have capsids that are the same size and are constructed from three viral capsid proteins. All have genomes of about 5,000 base pairs and display a similar genomic organization. Many regions of their genomes are highly conserved, demonstrating that the *Polyomaviridae* are descended from a common ancestor. Different family members infect several species of mammals, including humans, other primates, rodents, rabbits, as well as birds. Table 1 lists the members of the *Polyomaviridae* and their natural hosts. Most of these viruses display a narrow host range and do not productively infect other species. However, infection of cultured cells in which these viruses cannot grow productively often leads to the malignant transformation of these cells. Some of these viruses also induce tumor formation in newborn hamsters.

These small DNA tumor viruses, particularly SV40 and polyoma, have been subjects of intensive studies by virologists and molecular biologists since their discovery in 1953 (143). Polyoma was the first family member to be discovered. In his studies on the transmission of murine leukemia, Ludwig Gross noted that

TABLE 1. *The polyomaviruses*

Virus	Host species
Polyomavirus (PyV)	Mouse
Simian virus 40 (SV40)	Rhesus monkey
BK virus (BKV)	Human
JC virus (JCV)	Human
K papovavirus (KPV)	Mouse
Hamster papovavirus (HaPV)	Hamster
Lymphotropic papovavirus (LPV)	African green monkey
Simian agent 12 (SA12)	Baboon
Rabbit kidney vacuolating virus (RKV)	Rabbit
Stump-tailed macaque virus (STMV)	Stump-tailed macaque
Budgerigar fledgling disease virus	Bird

extracts from infected animals could be used to transmit leukemia (143). However, some inoculated animals developed salivary gland tumors rather than leukemia. Gross's further studies showed that the two agents could be separated on the basis of differences in sedimentation or filtration (the murine leukemia virus [MLV] was larger) as well as heat inactivation (the agent that induced salivary gland tumors was insensitive to treatment at 65°C, whereas MLV was completely inac tivated). The virus that caused the salivary gland tumors was subsequently named *mouse polyomavirus* because of its ability to cause a variety of different types of tumors in newborn mice (329). Infection of adult mice with polyomavirus does not usually result in tumorigenesis.

SV40 is one of several viruses identified by screening for viruses in the secondary rhesus monkey kidney cell cultures used for production of poliovirus vaccines. Although SV40 does not induce a visible cytopathic effect in rhesus monkey kidney cells, Sweet and Hilleman (338) noted a pronounced cytopathic effect when African green monkey kidney cells were infected with extracts from the rhesus kidney cell cultures. Soon afterward, it was discovered that tumors were induced by injection of SV40 into newborn hamsters (102,133). Many lots of poliovirus vaccine were contaminated with live SV40 virus, raising the concern that this virus, which is oncogenic for newborn hamsters, might also be oncogenic for humans. Fortunately, studies to determine the risk for cancer in those individuals inadvertently inoculated with SV40 during poliovirus vaccination indicate that exposure to the vaccine is not associated with significantly increased rates of ependymomas and other brain cancers, osteosarcomas, or mesotheliomas (244,332). However, SV40 T-antigen sequences have recently been detected in these cancers in the general population, leading to renewed interest in the role of SV40 infection in contributing to the development of some human tumors (reviewed in 39).

Two polyomaviruses of humans have been described. JC virus (JCV) was isolated in 1971 (254) by inoculating human fetal brain cells with extracts of diseased brain tissue from patients with progressive multifocal leukoencephalopathy (PML). BK virus (BKV) was isolated in the same year from the urine of an immunosuppressed renal transplant recipient (123). The genomes of both of these human viruses show closest homology to SV40. Most people worldwide become infected with and acquire antibodies to these viruses during childhood, with no apparent disease manifestations. These viruses are then thought to lie dormant in cells of a subset of infected people. Once extremely rare, the incidence of PML has increased dramatically in recent years as a consequence of the immunosuppression associated with infection by human immunodeficiency virus (HIV). A related simian papovavirus has been isolated from cynomolgus monkeys under immune suppression (363).

Although most polyomaviruses replicate primarily in epithelial or fibroblastic cells, zur Hausen and Gissmann (402) discovered a B-lymphotropic virus antigenically related to SV40 in a B-lymphoblastoid cell line derived from an African green monkey. Because this virus grows only in B-lymphoblastoid cells, it has been named *lymphotropic papovavirus* (LPV). Serologic studies suggest that humans and most other primates harbor viruses antigenically related to LPV. This virus does not induce tumors in newborn hamsters but will transform cultured hamster and mouse cells.

Hamster polyomavirus (HaPV) was isolated originally from a spontaneously occurring hair follicle epithelioma of a Syrian hamster (139). These tumors resemble papillomavirus-induced tumors in being highly keratinized and having virus particles exclusively in the differentiated cell layer. When injected into newborn hamsters, this virus causes leukemias and lymphomas, a tumor spectrum quite distinct in the polyomavirus subfamily. On the basis of nucleic acid sequence homology and genome organization (83,138), this virus is more closely related to polyoma than to SV40 or the human polyomaviruses. Other mammalian polyomaviruses include bovine polyomavirus (ByPV) (293), which is sometimes found in fetal calf serum, a rabbit polyomavirus (RKV) (152), a rat polyomavirus (RPV) (370), and Kilham virus, an additional polyomavirus of mice (231).

The first avian polyomavirus (APV) was identified in 1986 (207). Budgerigar fledgling disease virus (BFDV) is classified as a polyomavirus on the basis of nucleic acid homology to other polyomaviruses as well as on morphologic and serologic criteria. It appears to be more similar to SV40 than to mouse polyomavirus because it lacks a middle T antigen. Several additional APV isolates from a variety of avian species have now been characterized; so far, all belong to one genotype and one serotype within the proposed subgenus *Avipolyomavirus* of the family *Papovaviridae* (258).

POLYOMAVIRUSES AS PARADIGMS

The initial impetus for studies of these viruses was their oncogenic potential. However, these viruses are easy to cultivate in tissue culture and to purify, making them suitable model systems for diverse studies in molecular biology. Because of the small size of their genomes, physical maps of their genomes were generated as soon as restriction endonucleases became available in the 1970s, and they were among the first DNA genomes to be completely sequenced (109,271,310,311). Since the 1970s, these viruses have been used to examine many fundamental questions in eukaryotic molecular biology.

Among the major discoveries resulting from work on these viruses are the structure of supercoiled DNA, the identification of eukaryotic origins of DNA replication, the discovery of enhancers and elucidation of the organization of promoters involved in transcriptional regulation, the discovery of alternative splicing, and detailed understanding of the mechanisms of negative and positive regulation of gene expression. Because viral DNA is organized into chromatin, and because replication of viral DNA involves only a single viral gene product and uses almost all of the proteins used for cellular DNA replication, replication of SV40 origin-containing DNA *in vitro* has served as a model for understanding eukaryotic chromosomal DNA replication. Studies to understand the oncogenic potential of these viruses have provided fundamental insights into cell cycle regulation, oncogenes, and tumor suppressor genes. Much of our understanding of the polyomaviruses derives from studies of SV40 and polyoma, and this chapter focuses primarily on these two viruses.

VIRION STRUCTURE

The capsids of the polyomaviruses contain three virus-encoded proteins, VP1, VP2, and VP3, surrounding a single molecule of viral DNA (Fig. 1A) complexed with cellular histones H2A, H2B, H3, and H4 in the form of chromatin (see Fig. 1B). The sizes of the capsid proteins of SV40 and polyoma are shown in Table 2. These proteins are arranged to form a T=7 icosahedral capsid (see Fig. 1C) containing 360 molecules of the major capsid protein, VP1, organized into 72 pentamers. A single VP2 or VP3 molecule associates with each pentamer. The virus particle is 88% protein and 12% DNA and has a sedimentation coefficient of 240S in sucrose density gradients. Because they lack envelopes, the virus particles are resistant to lipid solvents. They are also relatively resistant to heat inactivation. Virions have a density of 1.34 g/mL in cesium chloride (CsCl) equilibrium density gradients, whereas empty capsids have a density of 1.29 g/mL.

Although originally thought to contain 60 hexameric (hexons) and 12 pentameric (pentons) capsomeres, it is now clear that these viruses contain 72 pentameric capsomers, which each contain five molecules of VP1 (209,269). In fact, polyoma VP1 produced in *Escherichia coli* will self-assemble into pentameric capsomeres, and under appropriate conditions, these molecules will further assemble into virus-like empty capsids and other structures (280). The same is true of SV40 VP1 synthesized *in vitro* (126). Icosahedral viruses have both sixfold and fivefold axes of symmetry, and the structure of the polyoma capsids presents a puzzle because these capsids contain capsomeres that have only fivefold axes of symmetry. The high-resolution structure of the SV40 capsid (209,324,383) indicates that the C-terminal arm of VP1 does not form part of the capsomere structure itself but instead makes contacts with neighboring pentamers (see Fig. 1D). It is the flexible geometry of these contacts that appears to allow the pentamers to fit together in such a way that an icosahedral capsid is formed. Calcium ions are required for virion stability (32,52) and are thought to stabilize pentamer–pentamer interactions (209). There are no disulfide bonds within the SV40 pentamer subunits, but disulfide bonds may exist between adjacent pentamers because reducing agents are required to disassemble virus particles.

The sequences of the minor capsid proteins, VP2 and VP3, are overlapping; VP2 contains the entire VP3 sequence at its C-terminus and an additional sequence of about 115 amino acids at its N-terminus. The N-terminus of SV40 and polyoma VP2 is myristoylated (331). The VP2 and VP3 proteins of all polyomaviruses are most highly conserved near their C-termini, and it is this region that interacts with VP1 through its N-terminal region (13,50). The disorder seen for VP2/3 in earlier virion structures reflects the fact that VP2/3 interacts differently with different VP1 molecules within each capsomere, but has an equal probability of interacting most directly with any of the five VP1 molecules (50). Only VP1 molecules are exposed on the outside of the virion. VP1 contains a small groove that interacts with specific carbohydrate residues on the cell surface (325–327). Oligosaccharide chains that terminate with sialic acid serve as the receptor for mouse polyomavirus (327). Some strains bind only straight-chain oligosaccharides, whereas others bind both straight and branched chains. There are wide variations in the response of mice to polyomavirus infection, ranging from persistent infection to tumorigenesis to death. This can be explained on the basis of the differences in receptor–virion interactions (16,17).

Preparations of polyomaviruses contain three kinds of virus particles. Infectious virus particles contain a single molecule of viral DNA in association with four cellular histones. The DNA and histones are arranged as chromatin, and the histone–viral DNA complex is often referred to as the *viral minichromosome.* This minichromosome has been used as a model system to study the

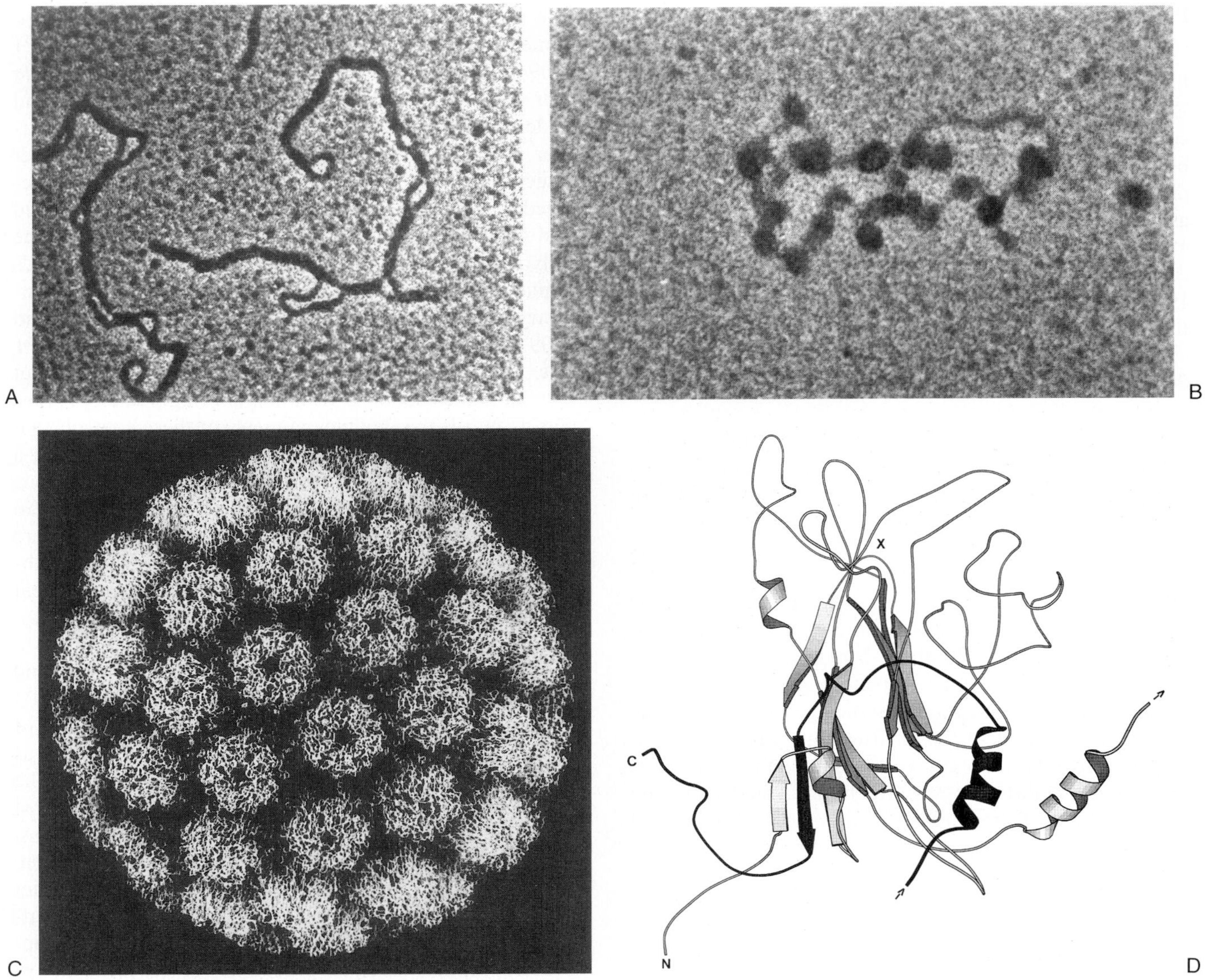

FIG. 1. Viral DNA, minichromosomes, and virions. **A:** Electron micrograph of supercoiled SV40 DNA molecules. **B:** Electron micrograph of an SV40 minichromosome. Note that this particular minichromosome displays a nucleosome-free region. About 20% of minichromosomes have a nucleosome-free region surrounding the regulatory region at the origin of DNA replication. **C:** Computer graphic representation of the structure of the SV40 virion. Note that the shell is made up of 72 pentamers of VP1. Twelve of these lie on icosahedral fivefold axes and are surrounded by five other pentamers. The remaining 60 pentamers, such as the ones near the center of this diagram, are surrounded by six other pentamers. The pentamers are linked together by extended C-terminal arms of VP1 molecules of the subunits. **D:** A ribbon diagram of a VP1 subunit of the mouse polyomavirus virion. *N* refers to the location of residue 15 of the VP1 polypeptide; the first 14 residues are thought to be disordered. *C* is the C-terminus of an invading arm (*darkly shaded*) of another VP1 molecule. At the right of the figure is an *arrow* showing that this VP1 molecule goes off to the right, where it interacts with another VP1 molecule. The interactions of the C-terminal arms of VP1 molecules can be pair-wise with each of two VP1 molecules interacting with the C-terminal arm of the other (as in this figure), or the incoming C-terminal arm of VP1 can come from a third VP1 subunit. (see Chapter 3 for more details on protein–protein interactions in the capsids of the polyomaviruses). *X* is the site of the mouse polyomavirus receptor-binding pocket. (**A** and **B** courtesy of Dr. Jack Griffith, University of North Carolina; **C** and **D** courtesy of Dr. Steven Harrison, Harvard University.)

TABLE 2. *Capsid proteins of the polyomaviruses*

	SV40		Polyoma		JC virus		BK virus	
	Mol. wt.	Amino Acids	Mol. wt.	Amino acids	Mol. Wt.	Amino Acids	Mol. Wt.	Amino Acids
VP1	39,903	362		385	39,606	354	40,106	362
VP2	38,525	352		319	37,366	344	38,345	351
VP3	26,961	234		204	25,743	225	26,718	232

effects of chromatin structure on DNA replication and transcription. Most viral DNA molecules contain a full complement of nucleosomes, but some lack nucleosomes over viral regulatory sequences. Virion minichromosomes lack histone H1, whereas the form of the minichromosome found within infected cells contains it (364). Virion preparations also contain empty capsids as well as pseudovirions, capsids containing cellular rather than viral DNA. Passage of polyomaviruses at high multiplicities of infection leads to the generation of defective viral genomes containing deletions, duplications, and rearrangements of viral genetic information, often with duplications of the viral origin of DNA replication. If within appropriate size limits, these defective viral genomes can be encapsidated.

GENOME ORGANIZATION

The genomes of all polyomaviruses are divided into early and late regions (Fig. 2). The early region is, by definition, that portion of the genome transcribed and expressed early after the virus enters the cells, and it continues to be expressed at late times after infection, after the onset of viral DNA replication. The late region of the genome is expressed efficiently only after viral DNA replication begins, although low levels of transcription of the late region occur early after infection as well. The first maps of the polyoma and SV40 genomes were divided into 100 map units, with the unique Eco RI site in both the SV40 and polyoma genomes defined as 0/100 map units. Because the complete nucleotide sequences of these genomes have been determined, use of nucleotide positions rather than map units permits more precise description of specific sites within the genome. Nucleotide position 1/5243 for SV40 is the center of a 27–base pair palindrome located at the origin of viral DNA replication (*ORI* in Fig. 3). The numbering system used for SV40 is that of Buchman and colleagues (36). The numbering system used for polyomavirus is that of Griffin and associates (141). For polyoma, nucleotide position 1/5295 corresponds to the center of the Hpa II cleavage site at the junction of the fifth and third largest of eight fragments of polyoma DNA produced by cleavage with Hpa II. This site is also close to the polyoma origin of DNA replication.

Two lines of evidence indicate that polyomavirus genomes contain a single unique origin of DNA replication. In one of the earliest uses of restriction endonucleases as tools to address important problems in molecular biology, Danna and Nathans (77) exposed SV40-infected BSC-1 monkey cells to pulses of ^{3}H-thymidine and, at various subsequent times, isolated viral DNA molecules that had completed replication. They then hybridized this labeled DNA to fragments of SV40 DNA generated with restriction endonucleases Hind II + III. In mature viral DNA molecules, label should first appear at sites near the terminus for DNA replication, whereas the origin region should become labeled later because molecules just initiating DNA replication at the time of addition of label require a longer time to be completed. The region of the genome around map position 17 (nucleotide 2622) became labeled first, whereas that near position 67 (nucleotide 0/5243) was labeled last and designated as the origin region.

This location for the origin was also revealed by electron microscopy. Replicating SV40 DNA molecules were cleaved with Eco RI, which cuts SV40 DNA once (nucleotide 1782), and examined by electron microscopy. The unique cleavage site allows mapping of the sites at which replication bubbles are initiated; these studies indicated that replication began one third of the way around the genome from the Eco RI site. By performing similar analyses with viral DNA molecules lacking portions of the early or late region, it was shown that there is no unique site for the termination of DNA replication. Rather, bidirectional replication proceeds away from the origin, with the replication forks meeting at a site about 180 degrees from the initiation site. Detailed mutational analyses to define the origin more precisely are discussed later.

The promoters and enhancers for transcription are located close to the origin of replication (see Figs. 2 and 3). Together, the promoters, enhancers, and origin are referred to as the *viral regulatory region.* Transcription extends bidirectionally from initiation sites near the origin, with early and late messenger RNAs (mRNAs) being transcribed from opposite strands of the viral genome. Thus, the early region extends from the origin to a site about halfway around the genome. The early region encodes the viral regulatory proteins, the tumor, or T, antigens, so called because they can be detected with antisera derived from animals bearing tumors induced by these viruses or by injection of cells transformed by these viruses. SV40 and the other primate polyomaviruses

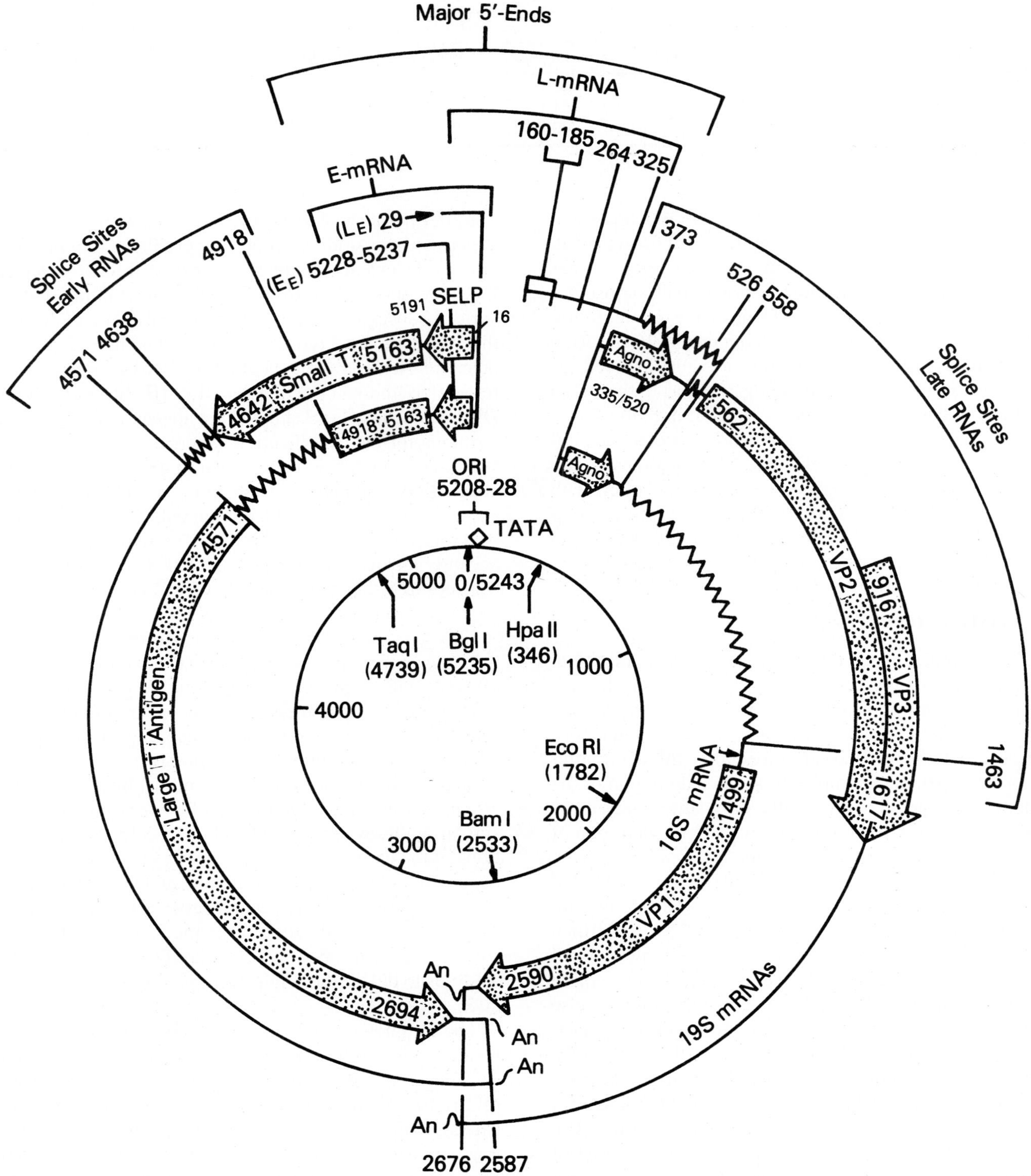

A

FIG. 2. Genomic organization of SV40 and mouse polyoma virus. **A:** SV40. The origin of replication and transcriptional regulatory region is at the top. The early region extends counterclockwise and the late region clockwise from the top. The regions encoding viral proteins are shaded. Also shown are the nucleotide positions for the 5′ and 3′ ends of viral mRNAs and the positions of introns. (From ref. 26, with permission).

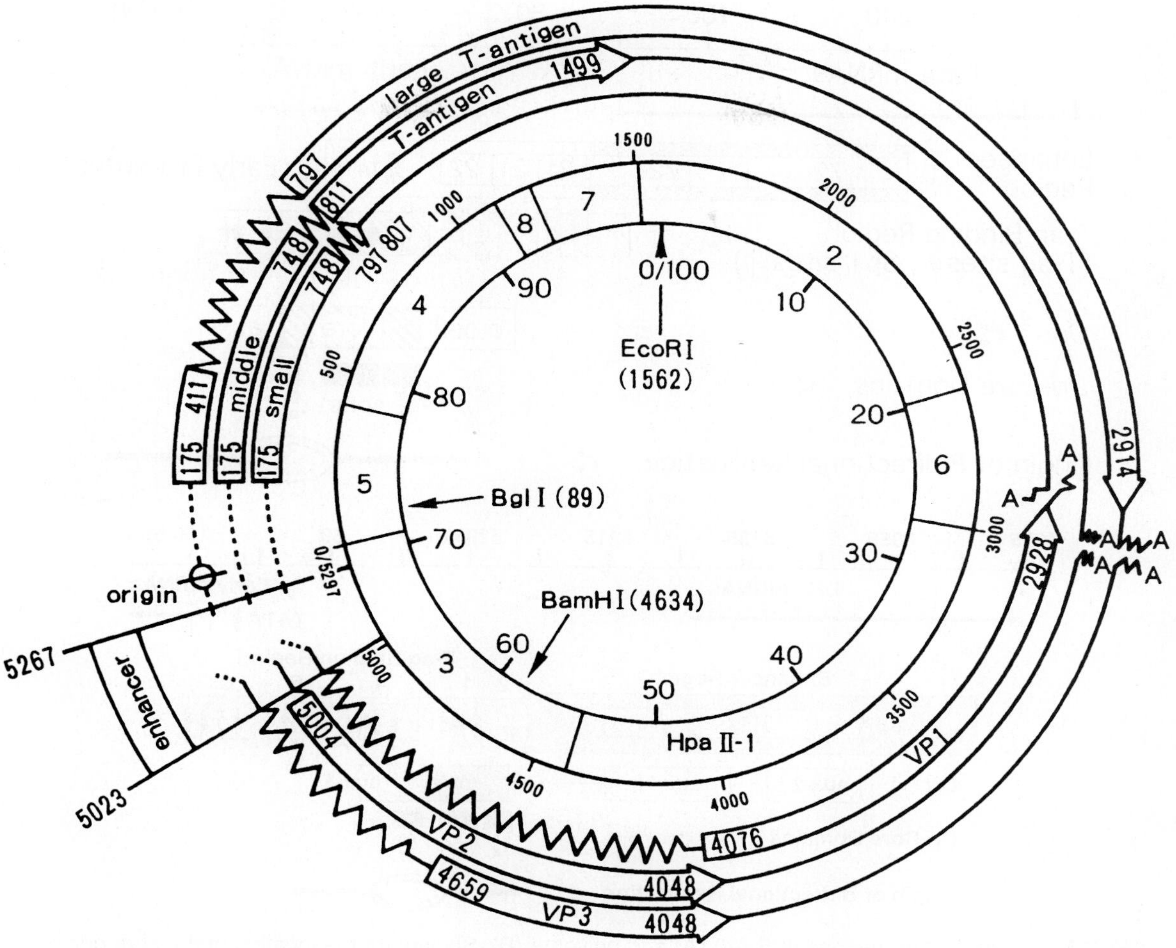

B

FIG. 2. *Continued.* **B:** Mouse polyoma virus. The 0/100 map unit position is at the top and corresponds to the unique Eco RI site. The origin is located counterclockwise about one third the way around the circle. The early region is located in the top half of the figure and the late region in the bottom half. Also shown are the positions where each of the viral gene products are encoded, the nucleotide numbers of the 5′ and 3′ ends of the viral mRNAs, and the nucleotide positions of the introns. (From ref. 350, with permission.)

encode two T antigens—designated large T and small t antigens on the basis of size. Polyoma and closely related viruses encode three T antigens—large T, middle (or medium) T, and small t. All of the T antigens of each virus share N-terminal sequences and contain different C-terminal regions. The mRNAs encoding them are produced by alternative splicing from a common pre-mRNA. Figure 2 shows the common and unique regions of SV40 and polyoma T antigens.

The late regions of these viral genomes encode the three capsid proteins, VP1, VP2, and VP3. As with the early mRNAs, late mRNAs are generated from a common pre-mRNA by alternative splicing. The coding regions of VP2 and VP3 overlap, with VP3 sequences being a subset of VP2 sequences. The coding region for the N-terminus of VP1 overlaps that for the C-termini of VP2 and VP3, with translation of VP1 being from a different reading frame than VP2 and VP3. SV40 and the human polyomaviruses encode a fourth late protein, called the *agnoprotein* (see Table 2). This 62– to 71–amino acid protein is encoded by the leader region of some species of late viral mRNA and accumulates in the perinuclear region during the late phase of the infection cycle (167,253). It was originally named agnoprotein because its function was unknown. It appears to facilitate the localization of the major capsid protein to the nucleus and may also enhance the efficiency with which virus spreads from cell to cell (43,273). Mutants that do not produce the agnoprotein yield fewer progeny virions and produce small plaques (11,238). Pseudorevertants of these mutants map to the major capsid protein, VP1, suggesting a possible interaction between the agnoprotein and VP1. Additional

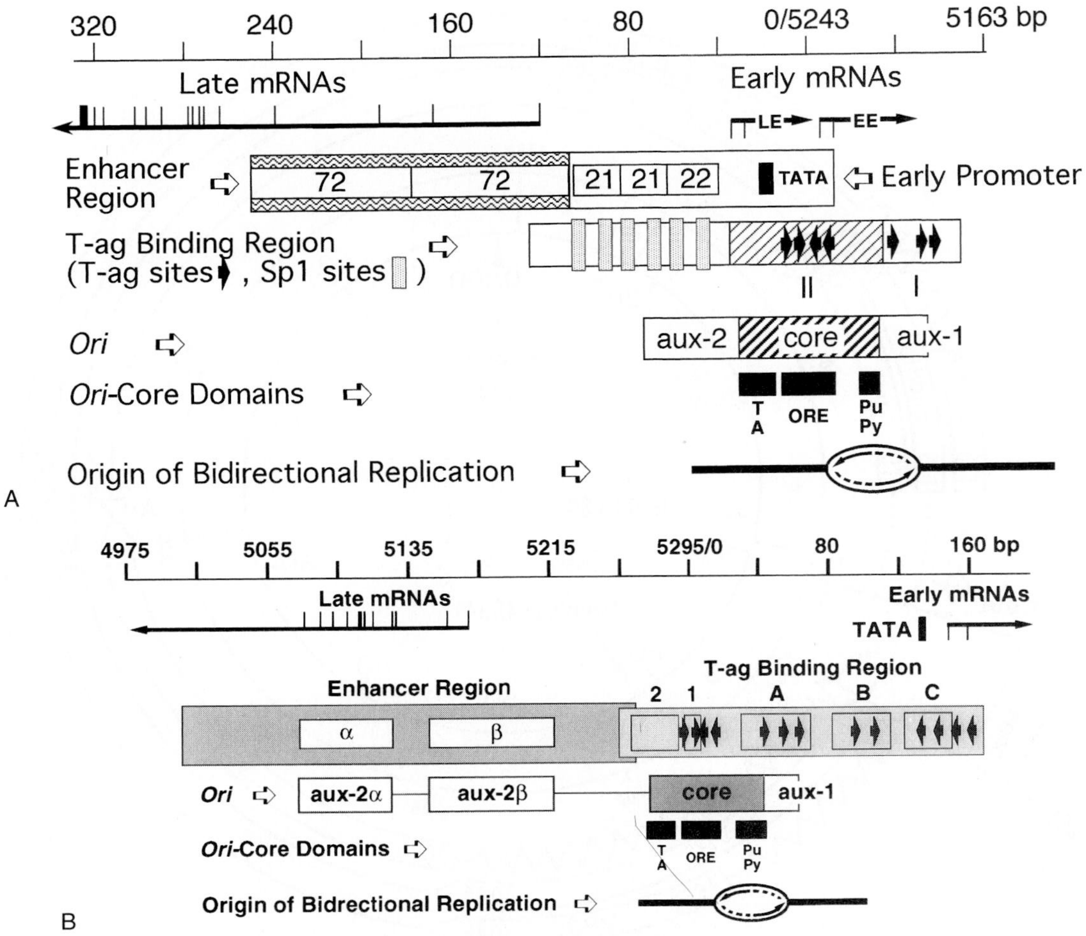

FIG. 3. The regulatory regions of SV40 (**A**) and polyoma (**B**). Shown are the location of the core origin of viral DNA replication and the location of auxiliary sequences (*aux*), which enhance viral DNA replication. Replication of polyoma requires either aux-2α or aux-2β. Within each core origin region are located a TA tract, with a strand bias for Ts and As, the palindromic region that serves as an origin-recognition element (*ORE*), and a region with a purine (*PU*) and pyrimidine (*PY*) strand bias, within which bidirectional DNA replication is initiated. Also shown are sites at which large T antigen binds to viral DNA; pentanucleotides involved directly in binding are indicated by *arrowheads,* which point in the direction of the pentanucleotide, 5′GAGGC3′. Several additional 5′GAGGC3′ pentanucleotides are located in the vicinity of the Sp1 sites, to the left of binding site II, but these bind T antigen very weakly and are not thought to play a role in SV40 replication. Sites within this region at which transcription is initiated for production of viral early and late mRNAs are also indicated. The sites marked *EE* for SV40 are those used early after infection; those marked *LE* are used to produce early mRNAs after the onset of viral DNA replication. Additional sites for production of both SV40 and polyoma late mRNAs are located further downstream for both SV40 and Py. For SV40, the locations of the two 72–base pair repeats, which serve as enhancers, and of the 3 nearly perfect 21–base pair GC-rich repeats are also shown. Within these repeats are six sites to which transcription factor Sp1 can bind. (Courtesy of Dr. Mel DePamphilis, National Institutes of Health, Bethesda, MD.)

small open reading frames that could encode other proteins are found in other species of late mRNA as well as in some species of early-stranded mRNA present late after infection (186). Thus, many SV40 late mRNA species are bi-cistronic.

VIRAL GENETICS

Genetic analyses have played a central role in our understanding of the biology and replication cycle of the polyomaviruses (reviewed in 351). The first mutants to be isolated were host range mutants of polyoma whose growth was restricted to certain mouse cell lines, and temperature-sensitive (ts) mutants of SV40 and polyoma. The availability of restriction endonucleases led to the construction of a wide variety of deletion and substitution mutants during the 1970s and 1980s. Site-directed mutagenesis and polymerase chain reaction–based approaches have also been used to produce mutants of the polyomaviruses. Today, it is relatively easy to construct any desired point, deletion, or substitution mutant of these viruses.

For SV40, ts mutants were divided into five complementation groups, A, B, C, BC, and D, based on their ability to complement one another to produce plaques at the nonpermissive temperature. We now know that the product of the A gene is large T antigen. VP2 and VP3 are both altered by mutations in gene D, whereas mutants in groups B, BC, and C produce altered VP1. Intracistronic complementation is often seen in genes that encode proteins that assemble into multimers or in multifunctional proteins in which separate domains perform distinct roles. Intracistronic complementation is observed between VP1 mutants in groups B and C but not between those in the BC group and either group B or group C. It has also been observed between mutants of large T antigen that affect the host range of the virus and mutants that affect replicative activities of the protein (352). The ts mutants of polyomavirus have been sorted into similar complementation groups.

By infecting cells at the permissive temperature and shifting them to the nonpermissive temperature at various times after infection, it was shown that the products of genes A and D were required early after infection, whereas the products of genes B and C were required only at late stages of infection. It is not surprising that large T antigen is required early after infection because it is required for viral DNA replication. Studies that suggest a role for VP2 and VP3 in adsorption or uncoating of the virus explain the finding that the D gene product is also required for early events of the infection cycle.

The sites of mutation of representative members of each complementation group were mapped by marker rescue using restriction endonuclease fragments of viral DNA (197). This involved producing partial heteroduplexes containing a circular strand of a particular ts mutant and a linear restriction endonuclease fragment. Successful marker rescue depends on the wild-type restriction endonuclease fragment containing the information that is mutated in the mutant genome. In this way, the SV40 A gene was mapped to the early region and the SV40 B, C, BC, and D groups to the late region of the genome. Similar mutants of polyoma were mapped to analogous regions of the polyoma genome.

Although these studies were able to identify viral genes and their positions on the physical map of the viral genome, they did not indicate which of the viral gene products were encoded by each gene. Deletion mutants were constructed using restriction endonucleases, and this permitted assignment of some viral proteins to viral genes because it was easy to determine which viral gene product had been shortened by the deletion mutation. Many of these mutants could be propagated only in the presence of wild-type helper virus. Mutants of SV40 with deletions at the unique Eco RI or BamH I sites produce internally deleted or truncated VP1 polypeptides, indicating that the gene for VP1 spans the Eco RI and Bam HI sites (59). This is the region of the genome where marker rescue studies placed mutations in the B, BC, and C complementation groups.

Mutants with deletions at the unique Hae II site affected only VP2 (59). These mutants were able to form very small plaques and hence could be propagated without helper virus. Because these slow-growing mutants could complement tsD mutants at the nonpermissive temperature, they were assigned to a new complementation group E, with VP3 assigned to complementation group D. SV40 mutants with deletions in the early region were also constructed and found to produce large T antigens of reduced size, thus proving that the large T antigen was the product of the A gene rather than a cellular protein induced by SV40 infection (198).

A set of viable mutants with small deletions located randomly around the SV40 genome was produced. Three regions of the viral genome were identified that could accommodate deletions without impairing the plaque-forming ability of the virus (301). These sites are located in the agnogene region, in the region encoding the 3′-untranslated regions of the early and late mRNAs, and in the early region between map positions 54 and 59 (nucleotides 4900 to 4600, approximately).

Normal-sized plaques were produced by the 54/59 region deletion mutants, but these viruses were unable to transform nonpermissive cells as efficiently as wild-type SV40, suggesting that a gene product needed for transformation was encoded in this region. No tsA mutants (affecting large T antigen) had been mapped to this region. Analysis of T antigens encoded by mutants with deletions in the 54/59 region showed that the deletions did not affect large T antigen, although size measurements of large T suggested that most or all of the early region was required to encode it. Studies by a number of investigators subsequently showed that the SV40 early region encodes both small and large T antigens (22,71,256) and that small t antigen was reduced in size by mutations in the 54/59 region. Alternative splicing allows the production of mRNAs that encode these two early gene products; there is not sufficient genetic information in the SV40 early region to encode distinct polypeptides of 84 and 17 kd.

Viable deletion mutants of polyomavirus have also been isolated and characterized. Host range mutants of polyoma were selected that grew poorly or not at all in mouse 3T3 cells but replicated efficiently in primary cells or in cells transformed by retroviruses or by polyoma itself (18). Because these mutants display this host range phenotype and are also defective for transformation, they are called *hrt* mutants. Marker rescue experiments indicated that the hrt mutants map to the analogous region of the polyoma genome as the SV40 54/59 deletion mutants. Complementation is observed between polyoma tsA and hrt mutants to permit cell transformation at a temperature restrictive for tsA mutants. The hrt mutants are known to encode truncated forms of both small and middle T antigens. The role of these proteins in transformation is discussed later.

BIOLOGIC PROPERTIES OF THE POLYOMAVIRUSES

Although SV40 and polyoma are able to infect a wide range of mammalian cell lines and cultures, the response to infection can be productive or nonproductive. In some types of cells, viral DNA replication occurs, followed by the assembly of progeny virions and, ultimately, the death of the cell. This is called a *productive infection,* and cells in which infection is productive are said to be *permissive* for growth of the virus. Monkey cells are permissive for growth of SV40 and mouse cells for growth of polyoma. Some polyomaviruses show an extremely narrow host range for productive infection. For example, JCV replicates only in human fetal glial cells.

Nonproductive infections result when viral DNA replication cannot take place in the infected cell. For viral DNA replication to occur, SV40 or polyoma must produce adequate levels of large T antigen, the only viral protein needed directly for replication, and this protein must interact with cellular replication factors and the viral origin of DNA replication. An inability of SV40 large T antigen to interact productively with host replication factors in rodent cells is the reason that SV40 infection of rodent cells is unproductive. A similar inability of the polyoma large T antigen to interact productively with simian or human host cell factors is responsible for the inability of polyoma to replicate in primate cells.

In nonproductively infected cells, the infection cycle begins normally. The viral early mRNAs are produced, and the viral T antigens can be detected. The early proteins exert a variety of effects on the host cell. Because the polyomaviruses require the host cell DNA replication machinery, they replicate only during S phase, and T antigen stimulates cells to move through the cell cycle into S phase. When expressed in cells that are nonpermissive for viral replication, the viral T antigens also cause cells to acquire the properties of transformed cells. Such cells proliferate in semisolid media or in the absence of a high concentration of fetal calf serum. Usually, these transformed properties are manifested for only a few days. Usually, the viral genome, which does not replicate, is lost from the cells, and they return to normal growth. Such cells are said to have been "abortively" transformed. At a low frequency, the viral DNA becomes integrated into the host cell genome and is subsequently inherited as if it were a cellular gene. Integration appears to occur randomly with respect to sites in both the viral and host cell genomes. If the arrangement of viral DNA sequences after integration permits continued expression of SV40 large T antigen or polyoma middle T antigen, the transformed phenotype is expressed permanently, and the cell is said to have been *transformed* by the virus.

Most studies of transformation by SV40 have been conducted in mouse, rat, and hamster cells, but primate cells can be transformed by SV40 if replication is prevented by mutation of the viral origin of replication or the viral T antigen gene. The Cos-1 and Cos-7 monkey kidney cell lines express wild-type SV40 large T antigen and contain an integrated copy of SV40 DNA carrying a deletion of sequences within the origin of DNA replication that are essential for DNA replication (135). For polyoma, rat cells are normally used to study viral transformation. Although permissive for replication of polyomavirus, mouse cells can also be transformed by polyoma if the virus carries a mutation affecting large T antigen or its origin of replication or if viral DNA becomes integrated into the mouse cell genome in a way that interrupts the early coding region and prevents continued synthesis of full-length large T antigen. Although multiple regions spanning most of the SV40 large T antigen are required for transformation, the critical protein for transformation by polyoma is the middle T antigen. Although these viral gene products must be present continuously to maintain the transformed phenotype, mutation of cellular genes can eliminate the need for maintenance of the viral transforming region (266,267).

In addition to being able to cause malignant transformation of cultured cells, these viruses can efficiently immortalize primary rodent cells that would normally undergo a limited number of cell doublings. Immortalization is a function of the large T antigens of SV40 and polyoma. Studies of immortalization of primary mouse embryo fibroblasts by mutants of SV40 T antigen suggest that some mutants that can neither immortalize primary cells nor transform established cell lines have the ability to extend the normal lifespan of the primary mouse fibroblasts (64,345). Although the lifespan of human fibroblasts and epithelial cells can also be extended by wild-type SV40 T antigen, their immortalization is a rare event and requires mutations of one or more cellular genes (122,300,362).

THE REPLICATION CYCLES OF SV40 AND POLYOMA

Productive infection of cells by polyomaviruses can be divided into early and late stages. The early stage begins with attachment of virus to cells (Fig. 4) and continues until the beginning of viral DNA replication. Thus, the early stage is marked by adsorption and penetration of the virion and its migration to the nucleus, where the viral genome is uncoated and made available for transcription. During the early phase of infection, the viral early proteins, the T antigens, are produced, and they affect the host cell by stimulating the production of enzymes required for cellular DNA replication, thereby preparing the cell for replication of viral DNA. These viral early proteins also stimulate resting cells to reenter the cell cycle. The late stage of infection extends from the onset of viral DNA replication to the end of the infection cycle and involves the replication of viral DNA, expression of the viral late genes encoding the capsid proteins, assembly of progeny virus particles in the nucleus of the infected cells, and release of virus, possibly at the time of the death of the cell.

The time course of infection by SV40 and polyoma depends primarily on two parameters. Infection proceeds more rapidly at higher multiplicities of infection than at lower multiplicities. This most likely reflects the fact that critical levels of the viral early proteins are attained earlier when more viral genomes are available for transcription to produce the viral early mRNAs. The other critical parameter is the growth state of the host cell. At the same multiplicity of infection, viral DNA replication begins sooner, and the production of progeny virions is completed more rapidly when cells are growing exponentially than when cells are confluent and in a G_0 state at the time of infection. Figure 5 illustrates the time course for the expression of polyoma T antigen, induction of cellular

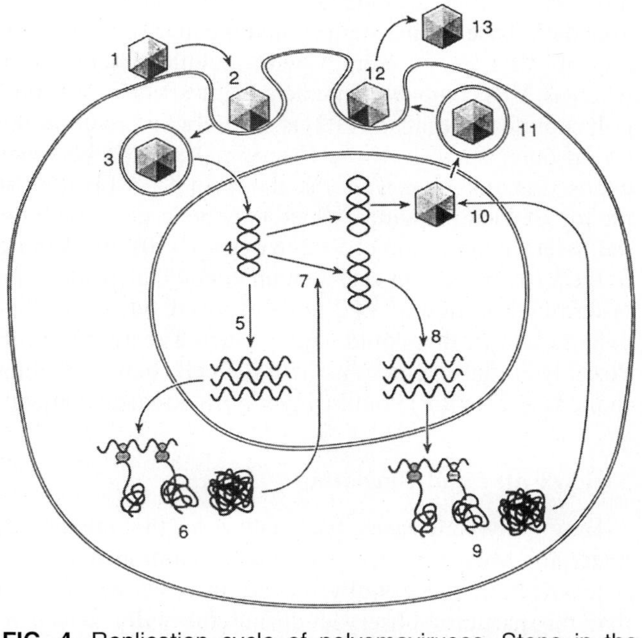

FIG. 4. Replication cycle of polyomaviruses. Steps in the replication cycle are indicated by numbers as follows: *1,* adsorption of virions to the cell surface; *2,* entry by endocytosis; *3,* transport to the cell nucleus (route and mechanism not yet known); *4,* uncoating; *5,* transcription to produce early region mRNAs; *6,* translation to produce early proteins (T antigens); *7,* viral DNA replication; *8,* transcription to produce late region mRNAs; *9,* translation to produce late proteins (capsid proteins); *10,* assembly of progeny virions in the nucleus; *11,* entry of virions into cytoplasmic vesicles (mechanism unknown); *12,* release of virions from the cell by fusion of membrane vesicles with the plasma membrane; *13,* released virion. Virions are most likely also released from cells at cell death when virions have an opportunity to leak out of the nucleus. In nonpermissive cells, the first six steps occur normally, but viral DNA replication cannot occur and subsequent events do not take place.

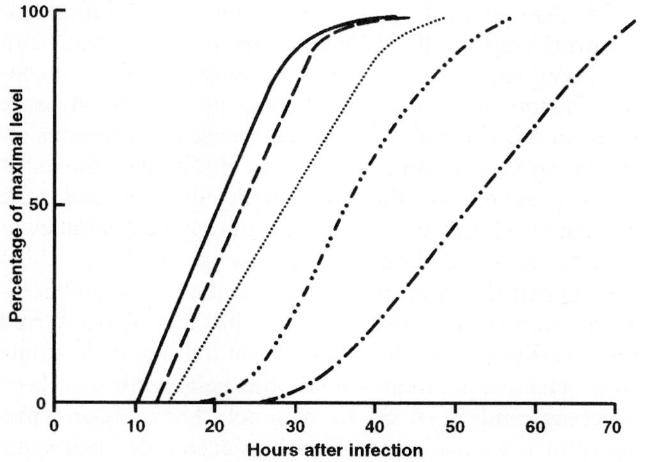

FIG. 5. Idealized time course of central events during productive infection of mouse cells by mouse polyoma virus. Events after infection of monkey cells by simian virus 40 follow a similar course. Parameters shown are expressed as a percentage of maximal level reached. T antigen (———) was measured by percentage of cells showing positive immunofluorescence; the actual rate of accumulation of T antigen may be slower because T-antigen–positive cells continued to synthesize T antigen over a long period. Cellular enzyme production (-----) is expressed as stimulation of enzyme activities compared with activity levels present in uninfected cells. Cellular DNA synthesis (··········), viral DNA and RNA (-··-·), and infectious virus (-·-·-) are expressed as the percentage of the total final yields of these macromolecules attained at particular times, not the rate of production at any particular time. (From ref. 350, with permission.)

enzymes, replication of viral DNA, and production of progeny virions.

Adsorption and Receptors

Early studies of the initial events of polyomavirus infection were complicated by the fact that virus preparations used contained not only infectious virus particles but also empty capsids and pseudovirions. Less ambiguous results have been obtained using purified virion preparations. Norkin and coworkers found that binding of SV40 virions to LLC-MK2 rhesus monkey kidney cells was inhibited by antibodies to class I major histocompatibility complex (MHC) antigens but not by antibodies to other cell surface proteins (34). Little binding was observed to two human lymphoblastoid cell lines that do not express MHC class I molecules owing to failure to express either β_2-microglobulin or HLA class I molecules. Binding occurred when class I expression was restored by transfection of cells with plasmids encoding β_2-microglobulin or HLA class I molecules. Different results were obtained by Basak and colleagues, who studied the binding of SV40 virions to polarized monkey kidney cells (Vero C1008) (14). Binding was restricted to the apical surface of these polarized cells, whereas HLA expression was detected at both the apical and basolateral surfaces.

Perhaps class I MHC molecules are required for adsorption of SV40 virions but are not sufficient, with other cell surface molecules also being part of the receptor. In nonpolarized cells, binding sites for SV40 were distributed uniformly over the cell surface. Different subclones of C1008 Vero cells bound different numbers of virions, and the abundance of binding sites was cell cycle regulated. Those cells that bound the greatest number of virions contained about 10^5 receptors per cell.

Competition experiments indicate that SV40 and polyoma receptors are distinct (14). This was also inferred from earlier studies that showed that binding of polyoma was sensitive to treatment of the cells with sialidase, whereas binding of SV40 was not. The polyomavirus receptor is known to contain oligosaccharide chains terminating with sialic acid. Antibodies to VP1 block adsorption of polyoma virions (25). Small and large plaque strains of polyoma produce different VP1 molecules, suggesting that plaque morphology may reflect different efficiencies of interaction of the virus particles with their receptors. When examined by isoelectric focusing (25), polyoma virions are seen to contain six distinct isoforms of VP1 (A to F), which differ in posttranslational modifications. Empty capsids lack one of these species (E) and do not compete with virions for binding to mouse kidney cells, suggesting that species E plays a central role in specific virus adsorption (26). Empty capsids can still bind to guinea pig erythrocytes and are internalized and degraded in lysosomes, rather than being transported to the nucleus for productive infection. Additional evidence for a role for VP1 in virus binding comes from binding studies with capsid-like structures that self-assemble from polyoma VP1 expressed in and purified from bacteria. The fact that the binding of these "capsids" to quiescent cells stimulates modest induction of *c-fos* and *c-myc* (399) suggests that these capsids may be interacting with a growth factor receptor or related protein.

The VP2 polypeptide of polyoma and SV40 is myristoylated at its N-terminus (331), and this modification plays a role in the early events of infection. Deletion mutants of SV40 that produce no VP2 are weakly viable. Plaques formed by these mutants are extremely slow to appear and enlarge slowly, suggesting that these mutants produce a dramatically reduced yield of infectious progeny (59). However, the yield of physical virus particles is nearly normal, suggesting that these progeny are defective in some early event of the infection cycle, perhaps adsorption. Mutation of polyoma VP2 so that it can no longer be myristoylated still permits its incorporation into virions, but infectivity is reduced 15- to 20-fold, and the infection cycle is prolonged by several hours (196,279). Together, these results suggest that the myristic acid moiety of VP2 may interact with cellular membranes, whereas VP1 probably interacts with specific receptor polypeptides. Because VP2 is entirely internal to the virion outer shell, how the N-terminal portion becomes exposed is unknown. There is about a 12.5 Å opening at the top of each pentamer, which may be large enough for the N-terminal portion of VP2 to emerge (50). Weakening of the VP1 contacts in each pentamer could also allow the N-terminal portion of VP2 to be exposed, but no mechanism is known that could explain such a rearrangement. Possibly, initial interactions with the cell (before binding to the true receptor) could trigger such a rearrangement.

Virion Entry and Uncoating

How polyomaviruses gain entry to the nucleus is uncertain. Most particles in a virus preparation do not initiate infection successfully; hence, there is the problem that the particles observed during the early stages of infection are likely to be primarily those that do not initiate an infectious cycle. After binding to the cell surface, SV40 virions appear to transmit an intracellular signal that in turn facilitates viral entry into caveolae. Class I MHC molecules do not enter cells, indicating that although these molecules mediate binding of virions to cells, they are not required for viral enclosure within the preformed caveolae (2,51). Soon after infection, virus particles can be detected by electron microscopy in small vesicles within the cytoplasm (162,229). These vesicles may ferry virus particles to the nucleus, and the fusion of these vesicles with the nuclear envelope has been observed by electron microscopy (142,250). Virus particles have also been observed within the endoplasmic reticulum (ER) (176); thus, the ER may also provide a pathway to the nuclear envelope.

The nuclear pore complex could serve as an entry portal for virus particles because SV40 virions injected into the cytoplasm enter the nucleus and begin production of SV40 early mRNA (55). This process is blocked by wheat germ agglutinin or by monoclonal antibodies to nuclear pore complex proteins (382), treatments known to block the movement of karyophilic proteins through the nuclear pore complex. Large T antigen is normally not detected until 10 to 12 hours after infection but can be detected within 3 to 4 hours after microinjection of virus particles into the cytoplasm. This time differential may reflect slow steps in penetration and the escape of virions from membrane vesicles into the cytoplasm before entry through the nuclear pore complex. Alternatively, it may mean that the nuclear pore complex is not generally a route of entry into the nucleus for SV40 or polyoma virions, with the pathway to the nucleus involving movement of virus particles within the ER or other membrane-bound structures. Because virus capsid proteins contain nuclear localization signals used to direct the proteins to the nucleus before virion assembly, these same nuclear localization signals may be able to mediate the entry of microinjected virions into the nucleus, even if this route is not normally used.

Most studies indicate that virions are uncoated within the nucleus because intact virions can be detected within the nucleus before expression of the viral T antigen (8,162,219). However, in some studies, partially disassembled virus structures were seen in the cytoplasm and were presumed to be uncoating intermediates (118). Whatever the route of entry, the viral minichromosome is transcribed, replicated, and subsequently encapsidated within the nucleus.

Transcription and Processing of Early Viral Messenger RNAs

Once virions have been uncoated, the viral minichromosome can be used as a template for transcription by RNA polymerase II to produce early viral mRNAs, derived from the early region of the viral genome. Production of mRNAs derived from the late strand of viral DNA is inefficient early after infection. Maximal production of the viral late mRNAs requires both an activity of large T antigen and the onset of viral DNA replication. Viral late mRNAs are discussed later.

For many years, studies on patterns of transcription of polyomavirus genomes were hampered by the very low levels of the viral early mRNAs, which make up only 0.01% to 0.02% of the total cellular RNA synthesized before viral DNA replication. During the initial 10 to 15 hours of an SV40 or polyoma infection, the total production of early mRNA likely represents not more than a few hundred molecules, in comparison to the 300,000 molecules of total mRNA found in a eukaryotic cell (reviewed in 351). From the application of more sophisticated and sensitive mapping techniques, it is now known that transcription initiates within the viral regulatory region and extends at least 180 degrees around the viral genome (188), and may extend further. Functional viral early mRNAs are produced by alternative splicing of this pre-mRNA (22). For SV40, alternative splicing generates two species of early mRNA. Messenger RNAs encoding large T antigen result from excision of an intron that extends from nucleotide 4918 to nucleotide 4571, whereas excision of an intron extending from nucleotide 4638 to the same splice acceptor at 4571 yields mRNAs encoding small t antigen. Thus, the SV40 early pre-mRNA contains two splice donor sites and a common splice acceptor. All of these mRNAs are polyadenylated at the same site at nucleotide 2694. Infected cells may also contain a third alternatively spliced early SV40 mRNA (391).

For polyoma, a similar early pre-mRNA is spliced to generate three polyoma early mRNAs (174,175). These mRNAs share 5′ ends located in the viral origin region and 3′ ends located at nucleotide 2930, and they differ with respect to sequences excised by splicing. The introns for the mRNAs for the polyoma large, middle, and small T antigens extend from nucleotides 409 to 794, 746 to 808, and 746 to 794, respectively. Thus, there are two splice donors and two splices acceptors. Low levels of polyoma early mRNAs that use a weak polyadenylation site at nucleotide 1525 have also been detected (156,354).

Other polyomaviruses show similar patterns of early transcription. For those that produce two T antigens, including JCV and BKV, two early mRNAs are generated by alternative splicing; for those that produce large, middle, and small T antigens, the three mRNAs are produced by alternative splicing from a common precursor, analogous to the situation with polyoma.

Early Promoters and Enhancers

The sites at which SV40 early mRNAs are initiated have been mapped in three ways—by nuclease S1 protection using end-labeled DNA probes, by primer extension of short labeled oligonucleotides, and by analysis of the nucleotide sequences attached to 5′-capped oligonucleotides produced after enzymatic digestion of purified labeled viral early mRNAs. All three approaches can produce artifactual results, particularly if the RNAs to be analyzed are inabundant (as viral early mRNAs are) or if they have significant secondary structure. Taken together, these experiments suggest that there are multiple clustered start sites for the SV40 early mRNAs, positioned around nucleotides 5237 and 5231 (127,146,348) (see Fig. 3).

Additional species of SV40 early mRNA are also detected that contain 5′ ends at nucleotides 34 through 28 (127). Molecules using these upstream starts can be detected relatively early after infection, but these sites become the primary initiation sites after viral DNA replication begins (117). This shift from early-early to late-early start sites requires both T-antigen and viral DNA replication. When all T-antigen–binding sites in the origin region are mutated and a second origin is introduced at another site, the shift from early-early to late-early sites still occurs (37). These 5′-extended early mRNAs have the potential to encode an additional viral polypeptide of 23 amino acids (186) (see Fig. 2), although deletion mutants unable to produce this protein behave like wild-type viruses. Translation from these longer early mRNAs, in which the initiation codon for the T antigens is not the first one, is inefficient (37).

The promoters that govern the production of the SV40 early mRNAs were among the first to be studied in detail and dissected by exhaustive mutagenesis. The critical features of the SV40 regulatory region are shown in Figure 3. Three sites (I, II, and III) for binding of SV40 large T antigen are located in this region. Upstream from the start sites for transcription is located an AT-rich region that contains a TATA box–like element, TATTTAT. Analysis of deletion and point mutants affecting the SV40 early TATA box and sequences between it and the normal transcriptional start sites demonstrated for the first time that TATA boxes function to direct transcription initiation to a site about 30 nucleotides downstream (65). Detailed point mutagenesis of this region indicates that it actually contains two TATA boxes, which specify initiation at the two clusters, around nucleotides 5237 and 5231 (257).

Upstream from the AT-rich region is a GC-rich cluster that contains two repeats of a 21–base pair sequence and a homologous 22–base pair sequence (often referred to as the *three 21–base pair repeats*). Altogether, this region contains six copies of a GC-rich sequence (CCGCCC) present 40 to 103 nucleotides upstream of the RNA initiation sites. Lying further upstream are two copies of a 72–base pair repeat. A variety of *in vivo* and *in vitro* studies have been performed in many laboratories to determine the importance to viral early transcription of these various regulatory region elements. Together, they indicate that the 21–base pair elements are important promoter elements but are not absolutely essential for early transcription (21,105,117,153). Studies of the SV40 promoter indicate that transcription factor Sp1 binds to these sites *in vitro* and is absolutely required for transcription *in vitro* from the SV40 early promoter (95,96).

The 72–base pair repeat elements function as enhancers for the SV40 early promoter. In fact, it was the study of these repeats that led to the discovery of eukaryotic transcriptional enhancers. These elements act to increase transcription initiation in an orientation-independent mechanism when located either upstream or downstream from transcriptional start sites, with little dependence on distance for their enhancing effects. Many different transcription factor–binding sites are located within the SV40 and polyoma enhancers, but it has not yet been possible to identify which factors actually interact with them *in vivo* (reviewed in 168). The SV40 enhancer is quite strong and functions well in cells of a variety of species and types; it has been widely used as an enhancer to drive expression of heterologous genes. The BKV enhancer consists of three repeats of a 68–base pair sequence, with the middle copy containing an internal 18–base pair deletion, and also includes another sequence element located adjacent to the repeat element closest to the BKV late genes (88). JCV contains two copies of a 98–base pair sequence that functions as an enhancer and that, like SV40 and BKV enhancers, is located on the late side of the origin or replication (183).

The organization of the regulatory region of polyomavirus is similar to that of SV40 (see Fig. 3) but has some important differences. Similar approaches were used to map the major sites of transcription initiation to sequences between nucleotides 147 and 158 (67,173). As in the case of SV40, 5′ sites mapping further upstream were detected during the late phase of polyoma infection (67,108,173). In contrast to their production by transcription initiation during SV40 infection, these 5′-extended polyomavirus transcripts appear to arise by processing of long viral pre-mRNAs, which themselves arise by transcription that continues more than once around the complete polyomavirus genome (1). Also in contrast to the late-early SV40 transcripts, these polyoma transcripts are uncapped and primarily nuclear.

The polyomavirus regulatory region contains an enhancer element that has a more complex organization than does the SV40 enhancer. The polyoma enhancer contains a single copy of two different adjacent enhancers, called A and B, or α and β (160), which can function independently and which confer different cell-type specificities. Extensive studies have been conducted of polyomavirus variants selected for efficient growth on either differentiated or undifferentiated embryonal carcinoma cells; these viral variants contain point mutations within the enhancers (76,235,236). Because enhancers contain multiple sites to which transcription factors can bind productively (168), these genetic studies suggest that there has been a selection for mutants that acquire binding sites for transcription factors present in embryonal carcinoma cells.

Regulation of Early Transcription

The early promoters of all polyomaviruses are autoregulated by their large T antigens. This was shown first for SV40 (189,272,344). In cells infected with tsA mutants affecting the large T antigen, early mRNAs are overproduced, and the rate of synthesis of large T antigen is elevated in parallel. A similar result has been obtained for polyoma (57). Autoregulation of viral early transcription has been reproduced *in vitro* and shown to be dependent on T-antigen–binding sites (150,276,277), indicating that large T antigen autoregulates synthesis of its own mRNA. The binding of large T antigen to viral DNA blocks the assembly of a functional transcription complex, thereby repressing early transcription (248). The location of the binding sites that are the target for this repression is different for SV40 and polyoma. The SV40 binding sites I and II (see Fig. 3A) are located downstream of, or overlap, the early mRNA start sites used early after infection, respectively (277), whereas the binding sites critical for autoregulation by polyoma T antigen (see Fig. 3B) are located upstream of the early transcription initiation sites (68,107).

Most studies on autoregulation by large T antigen were performed under conditions in which T-antigen levels were relatively high. Early after infection, when T-antigen levels are much lower, T-antigen–binding sites are unoccupied. Under these conditions, large T antigen stimulates transcription from its own promoter by a mechanism that does not require direct binding of T antigen to viral DNA (375).

Processing of Viral Early Pre-messenger RNAs

Alternative splicing is used to generate multiple species of early mRNA from a single class of mRNA precursor (see Fig. 2). Because of the advantages of working with viral systems, alternative splicing of SV40 pre-mRNA has been extensively analyzed both *in vivo* and *in vitro* as a model system for alternative splicing. The very small size of the intron excised to produce the SV40 small t mRNA (66 nucleotides) helped to define the relationship between minimum intron size and efficiency of excision (119). Splicing to produce large T mRNA uses multiple alternative branch-point sites, whereas splicing to produced small t mRNA uses only the most distal of these sites (251). The use of alternative lariat branch sites is probably central to alternative splicing in other systems. The ratio of small t to large T mRNA produced varies from cell line to cell line and is 10- to 20-fold higher in human 293 cells than in many other mammalian cell lines (119). Because the ratio of large T to small t splicing *in vitro* in HeLa cell extracts is 100:1 (252), extracts supplemented with fractions from a human 293 cell extract were used to identify and purify a factor from 293 cells that promoted use of the small t intron. This resulted in the discovery of ASF, a protein factor that controls alternative splicing for SV40 (124) and that appears to play an important role in alternative splicing in many cellular gene systems.

For polyoma, the 48-nucleotide intron excised to produce small t mRNA is the smallest known mammalian intron and is below the minimum size thought to be required for excision. Excision of this intron involves two branch-point sites, one only 4 nucleotides upstream of the small t 3′ splice acceptor site, and also requires an intact 3′ splice site for middle T antigen, located 14 nucleotides downstream of the small t 3′ splice acceptor site (125). This indicates that the two 3′ splice sites somehow cooperate to permit excision of the tiny small t intron. Such splice-site cooperation could be important for alternative splicing of cellular pre-mRNAs as well.

Synthesis and Functions of the Viral T Antigens

Large T Antigen

The large T antigens of the polyomaviruses are complex multifunctional proteins that have multiple enzymatic activities, interact with several cellular proteins, and perform several different roles during infection. The organization and activities of different large T antigens have been compared and reviewed (260). Considerably more is known about SV40 large T antigen than about the other large T antigens. Although this portion of this chapter focuses on SV40 large T antigen, key differences between SV40 and polyoma are highlighted.

The sizes of the T antigens of several polyomaviridae are listed in Table 2. The functional organization of SV40 and polyoma large T antigens is shown in Figure 6. All of the large T proteins are closely related and contain identical or similar sequences over most of their lengths. Polyoma large T contains a region of 154 amino acids following amino acid 82 with no homology to SV40 large T sequences; the viral DNA encoding this portion of large T is the portion of the polyoma genome that also encodes, in a different reading frame, the unique portion of middle T antigen. Conversely, SV40, JCV, and BKV large T antigen contain about 70 amino acids at their carboxyl termini that have no homology with any sequences in polyoma large T. This carboxyl-terminal domain of large T is involved in host range and adenovirus helper function (see later).

The SV40 large T protein is modified posttranslationally in several ways. It contains two clusters of phosphorylation sites (285,343) (see Fig. 6) and is also modified by *O*-glycosylation (165,289), acylation (192), adenylation (30), poly(ADP)-ribosylation (137), and amino-terminal acetylation (237). Little is known about the functions of most of these modifications. However, phosphorylation is known to play a major role in controlling the activities and functions of the protein, and acylation often permits a modified protein to associate with cellular membranes. More than 95% of SV40 large T antigen is located in the nucleus, although a small percentage is found at the plasma membrane. Nuclear T antigen exists both free in the nucleoplasm and associated with chromatin and nuclear matrix (323). It is estimated that lytically infected cells contain between 5×10^5 and 5×10^6 molecules of large T antigen.

Detailed studies of the sequences of SV40 large T antigen required for nuclear localization led to the definition

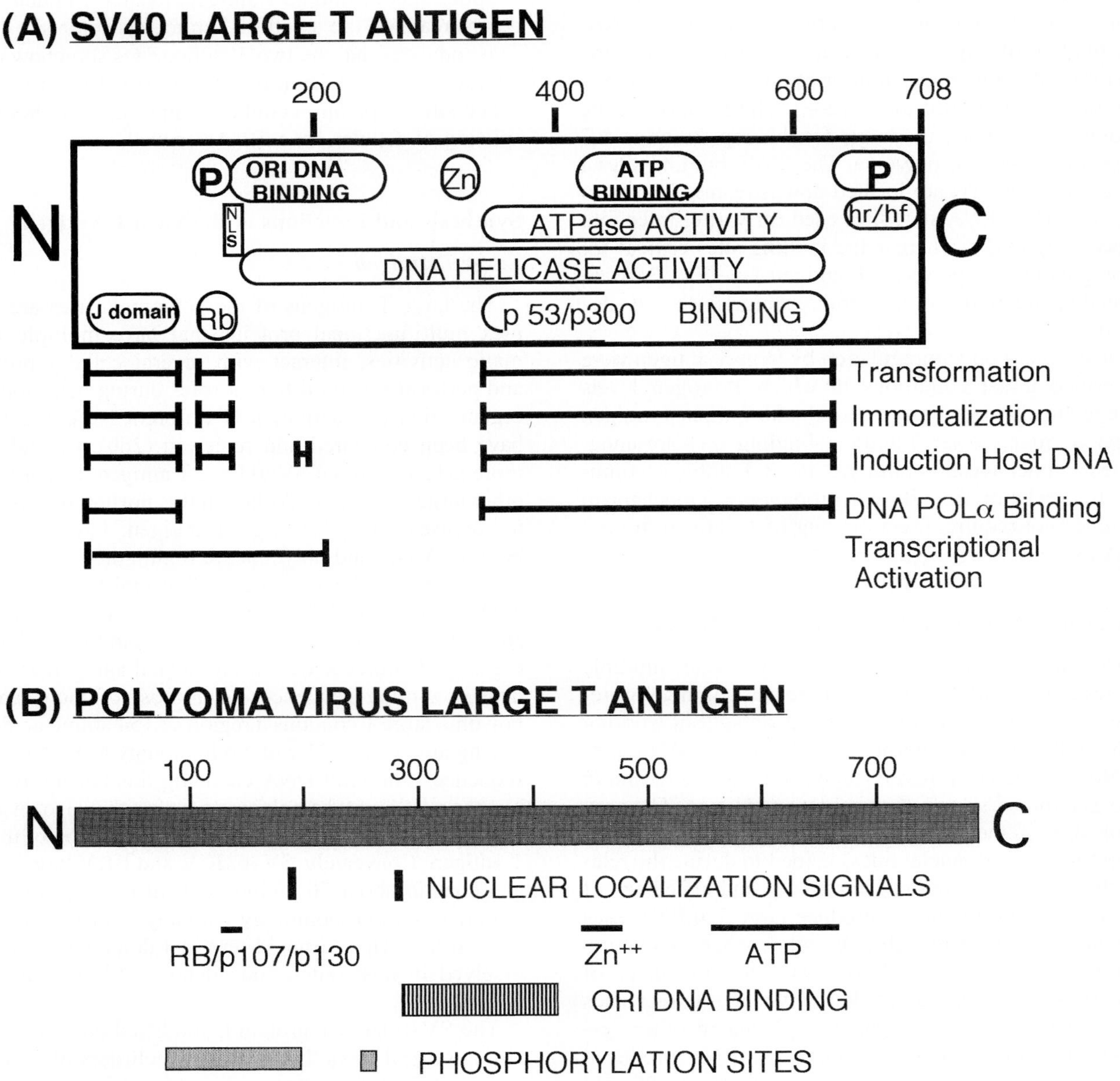

FIG. 6. The domain structures of SV40 large T and mouse polyomavirus large and medium T antigens. **A:** SV40. Shown are the domains of large T antigen required for nuclear localization (*NLS*) and for binding ATP and Zn^{2+} and for binding to the viral origin of DNA replication. The regions of T antigen required for ATPase activity, helicase activity, host range and helper function activity (*hr-hf*), as binding to $p105^{Rb}$/p107/p130 (indicated by *Rb*) and to p53 are shown. The DNA J domain functions like the J domain found in *Escherichia coli* DNA J/hsp40 molecular chaperone proteins and is involved in protein–protein interactions between T antigen and members of the $p105^{Rb}$ family. Also shown are the regions required for transformation of most rodent cell lines, for immortalization of primary mouse fibroblasts, for binding to DNA polymerase α, for induction of host DNA synthesis, and for transcriptional activation of the SV40 late promoter and many simple modular promoters by SV40 large T antigen. **B:** Mouse polyoma virus. Shown are the sequences that serve as nuclear localization signals (*NLS*) and sequences required for binding ATP and Zn^{2+} and for binding to the polyomavirus origin of DNA replication and to $p105^{Rb}$/p107/p130. Sites of phosphorylation are also shown. (**B** courtesy of Dr. Brian Schaffhausen, Tufts University Medical School, Boston, MA.)

of amino acids 127 to 133 (KKKRKVD) as the first identified nuclear localization signal (170,200). Polyoma large T antigen contains two nuclear localization signals, one at a place analogous to the site of the SV40 nuclear localization signal, the other in a region without homology to SV40 T antigen (275). Phosphorylation sites are located near these nuclear localization signals and may be used to regulate the location of T antigen. For both polyoma and SV40, some of the phosphorylation sites are substrates for cell cycle–dependent kinases or for isoforms of casein kinase I.

SV40 large T antigen is a DNA-binding protein that interacts specifically with several pentameric sequences (GAGGC) at the SV40 origin of DNA replication. It also binds, but with considerably lower affinity, to both single- and double-stranded DNA in a sequence-independent manner. The organization of these T-antigen–binding sites is shown in Figure 3. Binding of T antigen to site I permits T antigen to autoregulate production of SV40 early mRNAs (91,150,276). Binding at site II plays a central role in initiation of viral DNA replication. Binding site II is the preferred site for binding of SV40 large T antigen in the presence of physiologic levels of adenosine triphosphate (ATP) (27,80), which induces the formation of double hexamers of T antigen bound to site II (225). Individual pentanucleotides within site I are sufficient to direct hexamer formation, whereas certain pairs of these pentanucleotides can direct formation of T-antigen double hexamers (169). These double hexamers are fully able to initiate the structural changes that occur at the origin of replication after T-antigen binding. Because more pentanucleotides than two in site I are required, the others most likely play a role subsequent to the initial formation of double hexamers. In the presence of ATP, binding of polyoma T antigen to the polyoma regulatory region is also stimulated, and binding occurs over an extended portion of the origin (217). Some mutations of phosphorylation sites affect the DNA replication activities of T antigen, and this appears to affect interactions between T antigen hexamers critical for replication (373).

A second activity of large T antigen is DNA helicase activity (78,321). SV40 large T antigen can bind and hydrolyze ATP, and this activity is stimulated by single-stranded DNA (130,350). Helicase activity is crucial for viral DNA replication and requires functional ATPase activity and the ability to bind to SV40 DNA. *In vitro,* T antigen displays helicase activity with substrates lacking specific T-antigen–binding sites. T antigen also possesses RNA helicase activity (284), but the importance of this activity is unknown. There have also been reports that T antigen has (or is tightly associated with) topoisomerase I activity and that T antigen is able to promote strand reannealing and DNA looping (221,224,287). Formation of double hexamers stimulates the helicase activity of T antigen (308,309).

More recently, the N-termini of all known polyomavirus large T antigens have been noted to have sequence homology with the J domain of the DnaJ (Hsp40) family of molecular chaperones (181,261). The T-antigen J domain contains the Hsp70/DnaK family domain histidine-proline-aspartate (HPD) that is conserved within the J domain of all DnaJ homologs (358). T antigen retains its functions when its J domain is replaced by the J domain of two human J-domain proteins (40). *In vitro* studies indicate that this portion of T antigen can stimulate the ATPase activity of hsc70 and also enhance release of an unfolded polypeptide from hsc70 (317). Furthermore, this region has been shown to function as a molecular chaperone mediating phosphorylation of the T-antigen–associated proteins p107 and p130 (333). The domains of T antigen required for these enzymatic activities are shown in Figure 6.

Based on its primary sequence and structural modeling, the DNA-binding domain of large T antigen does not resemble a known DNA-binding domain, and this is confirmed in the solution structure of the DNA-binding domain of SV40 large T antigen, determined using nuclear magnetic resonance spectroscopy (218). Two nearby loops define a continuous surface of T antigen that is altered in the presence of added GAGGC-containing oligonucleotides, suggesting that this surface is the one that directly contacts DNA. The ATP-binding/ATPase domain of large T shows substantial similarity to many known ATP-binding and hydrolyzing proteins. Located between the DNA-binding domain and the ATP binding/ATPase domain is a zinc finger domain important for the overall structure and function of large T antigen (215). Attempts to crystallize T antigen have so far been unsuccessful, perhaps owing to heterogeneity resulting from nonuniform posttranslational modification. High-resolution electron microscopy, image processing, and three-dimensional reconstruction suggest that each T-antigen hexamer at the origin has a propeller-like shape organized around a central channel, similar to what has been seen in other DNA helicases (282).

T antigen forms complexes with several cellular proteins important for DNA replication, including at least two subunits of DNA polymerase α-primase and the single-stranded DNA-binding protein, replication protein A (RPA) (33,63,93,94,161,234,372). T antigen also binds DNA topoisomerase I, and this interaction serves to stimulate initiation of replication at the origin and to prevent the unwinding of nonorigin sites by T antigen (147,303–305,357).

Complexes are also formed between T antigen and several proteins important for regulation of cell growth. Through conserved sequences located between amino acids 102 and 115, T antigen interacts with the tumor suppressor protein, $p105^{Rb}$, as well as with related cellular proteins, p107 and p130 (82,97,106,149). A sequence very similar to T-antigen amino acids 102 to 115 is found in the adenovirus E1A and the human papillomavirus E7 proteins, which also interact with $p105^{Rb}$ and related proteins. In fact, the adenovirus E1A gene remains functional when its $p105^{Rb}$-binding domain is replaced with the $p105^{Rb}$-binding region of SV40 large T antigen (242). The Dna J domain, in conjunction with an intact $p105^{Rb}$-binding domain, has been shown to perturb p130 and p107 phosphorylation and to target p130 for rapid degradation (334). The mechanism of this effect is thought to require an association between the T-antigen J domain and mammalian hsc70, resulting in activation of the intrinsic ATPase activity associated with hsc70 and alteration of the folding of associated p107 or p130 (81). Small t antigen also contains the J domain and is also able to stimulate the ATPase activity of hsc70 (317).

The tumor suppressor protein p53 forms complexes with SV40 large T antigen (199,213) through portions of a large conformationally sensitive domain located in the carboxyl-terminal half of the protein (190,288,394). Although p53 also interacts with the JCV and BKV T antigens, it does not form complexes with the polyoma large T antigen, and this is one of the most important differences between SV40 and polyoma large T antigens. However, both SV40 (101) and polyoma large T-antigen (249) oncoproteins bind to members of the cap-binding protein (CBP) family of transcriptional adapter proteins (p300 and p400) that contain high histone acetyltransferase activity. The p300 protein, a transcriptional coactivator related to CREB, also binds to the adenovirus E1A protein (374,381), although T antigen and p300 appear to bind to distinct p300 isoforms (5). Furthermore, p300 can also bind directly to and modulate p53 (210), implying the existence of a complex transcriptional regulatory mechanism resulting from the tripartite interaction of large T antigen, p300, and p53.

Small t Antigen

The small t antigens of most polyomaviruses are cysteine-rich proteins of 172 to 195 amino acids (see Table 2) whose amino-terminal 82 amino acids are shared with large T antigen. For those polyomaviruses that encode middle T antigens, almost all of the sequence of small t antigen is contained within the middle T antigen of the same virus. Small t antigen is located in both the nucleus and the cytoplasm (104,398). Studies with mutants of SV40 and polyoma that contain deletions within the region of small t not shared with large T antigen indicate that small t antigen is dispensable for the lytic cycle of these viruses in cultured cells (301,322). SV40 small t antigen promotes G_1 phase progression and increases the efficiency of SV40 transformation of mammalian cells through activation of growth factor–stimulated signaling pathways. Small t antigens (and polyoma middle t antigen) associate with the catalytic (C) and structural (S) subunits of protein phosphatase 2A (PP2A) (255). This interaction displaces the B subunit of PP2A, resulting in inhibition of phosphatase activity (385). Inactivation of PP2A in turn results in the activation of the mitogen-activated protein kinase (314) and stress-activated protein kinase (371) pathways as well as pathways that use nuclear factor-κB (NF-κB), protein kinase C, and phosphatidylinositol-3 kinase (PI-3 kinase) (315). Small t-antigen expression has also been shown to be required to decrease p27 (KIP1) levels during cell cycle reentry of human diploid fibroblasts, perhaps explaining the requirement for small t in cell cycle activation of density-arrested human fibroblasts (263).

In some studies, SV40 small t antigen expressed from plasmids has been shown to be capable of activating transcription from the SV40 late and other viral promoters (23,216). However, when small t was expressed during a viral infection, transcriptional activation was not observed (264), making it uncertain whether small t antigens play a role in regulation of transcription. SV40 small t antigen has been reported to bind zinc ions through its cysteine clusters (361), but the function and importance of this interaction is uncertain because the small t antigens of the bovine and parakeet viruses contain only a single cysteine and would therefore be unable to bind zinc ions. Although the conserved cysteine appears to be required for PP2A binding, interaction with zinc is not required for binding PP2A (226).

There is evidence for yet another t antigen encoded in the SV40 genome, expressed from a third species of SV40 early mRNA that is spliced between nucleotides 4425 and 3679 (391). This alternatively spliced mRNA encodes a 17 kd small t antigen containing the first 131 amino acids of large T antigen and 4 amino acids encoded downstream of the splice junction in an alternate reading frame from that used to produce large T antigen. Whether a similar mRNA and small t antigen is produced by other polyomaviruses is not known.

Middle T Antigen

T antigens of medium size (middle T) are encoded by polyoma and closely related viruses, but not by SV40 or other primate polyomaviruses. The middle T protein is located primarily at the plasma membrane (164,297), where it associates with several cellular proteins important in the signal transduction pathways regulating growth. These include c-src, the cellular homolog of the transforming protein v-src of Rous sarcoma virus (66), and related src family kinase members. This association leads to the activation of the tyrosine kinase activity of c-src. Also complexed with middle T antigen and c-src is PI-3 kinase (4), which in turn leads to activation of the Ser/Thr kinase c-Akt, the cellular homolog of the viral oncogene v-Akt 2A (335). Shc, a two-protein complex that lies upstream of Ras in the signal transduction pathway (41,90) and the A and C subunits of protein phosphatase 2A (255,369), also form complexes with middle T antigen. PP2A binding appears to be required for middle T–src complex formation (134). Mutants of polyomavirus unable to produce middle T antigen are defective for replication, persistence, transformation, and tumor induction in mice (114).

Although formation of complexes with src family kinases and activation of PI-3 kinase signaling pathways are important events for cellular transformation, a role for middle T antigen during lytic infection is not known. Because polyoma large T antigen does not interact with p53, and because the interaction of SV40 large T with p53 is thought to be central to its ability to stimulate cellular S-phase entry and in turn create an optimal environment for viral DNA replication, an interesting possibility is that the polyoma middle T antigen–cellular protein interactions perform a related function for polyoma infection. In this view, middle T antigen plays the role of an activated growth factor receptor through its activation of src family members, PI-3 kinase, and other proteins that mediate signal transduction pathways leading to cell cycle progression and cell division.

Preparation for Viral DNA Replication and Modulation of Cellular Gene Expression

Soon after T antigen is detected within cells, the levels of many cellular enzymes increase (see Fig. 5), and this requires T antigen (reviewed in 351). This probably reflects the ability of T antigen to stimulate expression from a variety of viral and cellular promoters (131,145, 274). Diverse mechanisms underlie the ability of T antigen to alter host cell gene expression. For example, when T antigen forms complexes with $p105^{Rb}$ and related proteins, other host cell proteins, including transcription factors of the E2F family, are released and can reach their promoter targets (6,7,48). Many genes involved in growth regulation and cell cycle progression, including *c-fos* and *c-myc*, contain E2F-binding sites.

The regulation of cellular genes is also affected by binding of p53 to T antigen because p53 is a transcription factor (9,184) with both activating (178,390) and repressing activities (132). Binding of p53 to DNA is inhibited by T antigen (10), abrogating the ability of p53 to stimulate gene expression. Among the targets of p53 transcriptional activation is *WAF1/CIP1,* a potent inhibitor of the cell cycle owing to its ability to block the kinase activity of some cyclin dependent kinase (CDK)–cyclin complexes. It is reasonable that *WAF1/CIP1* expression is reduced in the presence of T antigen because this stimulates cell cycle progression by permitting cyclin-dependent kinase–cyclin complexes to function (103,151,380).

Several studies indicate that T antigen can play the role of a TFIID-associated factor (TAF) in transcription initiation by all three RNA polymerases (73–75,393). T antigen forms a complex with TATA-box binding protein (TBP) and stabilizes the TBP–TFIIA complex on the promoter (74). Direct interactions also occur between T antigen and other cellular transcription factors. Some of these interactions activate, and others repress, transcription of various cellular genes. T antigen also transactivates transcription by RNA polymerases I and III. Because TBP is involved in transcription by all RNA polymerases, the T antigen–TBP interaction may play a role in activation of multiple classes of genes. In addition, T antigen stimulates the phosphorylation of RNA polymerase I transcription factor, UBF, most likely by recruiting a kinase (392).

T antigen stimulates resting cells to enter the cell cycle and replicate their DNA and, by so doing, creates an optimal environment for viral DNA replication. Multiple distinct subregions of large T are independently able to stimulate cellular DNA replication and probably cooperate to provide maximal stimulation and to activate a broad spectrum of cellular genes (92,316,349). These regions are the Rb-binding domain, the DNA-binding domain, and sequences near the carboxyl terminus of large T (92). Polyoma middle T antigen was also able to stimulate cellular DNA replication. Mutants defective for binding to either SHC or PI-3 kinase were able to stimulate cellular replication, whereas a double mutant (Y250F/Y315F), unable to bind either, was not (245). In some cases, SV40 (226,263) and polyoma small t antigens (292) are required for the support of S-phase induction in concert with the respective T antigens, likely through their ability to stimulate growth factor–signaling pathways. However, in other cases, polyoma small t antigen alone can stimulate cell cycle progression, dependent on its ability to interact with PP2A (245). Because the middle T-antigen double mutant (Y250F/Y315F) retains PP2A binding, yet cannot stimulate cellular DNA replication, middle T and small t appear to modulate cellular signaling differently when each binds PP2A.

Viral DNA Replication

Replication of viral DNA within infected cells requires a functional origin of DNA replication, large T antigen with its DNA binding and helicase activities intact, and most of cellular proteins involved in replicative DNA synthesis. Viral DNA is in the form of a minichromosome, and its replication occurs in the nucleus during S phase, like cellular DNA replication. By other parameters, including the enzymes used and the geometry of the replication fork, replication of SV40 and polyoma DNA is sufficiently similar to cellular DNA replication that the viral systems have been exploited as powerful tools to understand cellular DNA replication. Excellent *in vitro* systems have been developed (208,330,368,377) that permit accurate and efficient replication of viral DNA using 10 purified cellular proteins, viral DNA containing a functional origin, and purified large T antigen. Viral DNA replication differs from cellular DNA replication in that the SV40 DNA origin can fire multiple times during

S phase, whereas cellular DNA replication is tightly controlled to prevent any region of the genome from being replicated more than once in a single cell cycle. This difference reflects the use of the cellular origin-recognition complex (ORC) at cellular origins. T antigen performs ORC's origin-recognition function and is not subject to the cellular mechanism that prevents additional rounds of DNA replication within one cell cycle.

Viral Origin of DNA Replication

The region of DNA required in cis for initiation of viral DNA replication (ORI) has been defined genetically for each of the polyomaviruses by the construction and analysis of detailed sets of deletion and point substitution mutations and by the analysis of evolutionary variants of these viruses, which carry deletions of sequences not required for replication (reviewed in 85 and 86). These studies indicate that both SV40 and polyoma contain a core of sequences absolutely required for viral DNA replication and that auxiliary sequences on either side of the core act to enhance initiation of DNA replication within the viral core (see Fig. 3). For SV40, the core origin of 64 base pairs extends from nucleotides 5209 to 29, whereas the auxiliary sequences extend from nucleotides 5164 to 5208 and 30 to 72.

The major difference between SV40 and polyoma in the organization of their ORI regions is that polyoma replication requires promoter and enhancer sequences on the late side of the ORI core, whereas SV40 replication does not. Critical sequences, shown in Figure 3, include the core, auxiliary sequences on the early side of ORI (aux-1), and enhancer sequences. Replication of DNA-containing polyoma sequences requires core and either aux-2α or aux-2β. The polyoma core covers 66 base pairs. Although quite different in sequence, the auxiliary sequences of polyoma can substitute for those of SV40, and the SV40 72–base pair enhancer can be used in place of the polyoma α and β enhancers. The SV40 21–base pair repeats, which play a role as auxiliary origin elements, cannot substitute for the polyoma enhancer elements. Replication of SV40 in monkey cells and polyomavirus in mouse cells absolutely requires the presence of the appropriate core and large T antigen (19). Interestingly, the SV40 core ORI contains start sites for early mRNA, whereas polyoma early mRNAs are initiated at sites that lie outside of the polyoma core ORI.

The features shared by all polyomaviridae ORI regions are an inverted repeat of 14 base pairs on the early gene side of ORI (see *PU/PY* in Fig. 3), a GC-rich palindrome of 23 to 34 base pairs in the center (see *ORE* in Fig. 3), and an AT sequence of 15 to 20 base pairs on the late side (see *TA* in Fig. 3). That all polyomavirus core origins contain these elements suggests that common structures play a role in binding proteins and in initiation of viral DNA replication. SV40, BKV, and JCV contain a second nearby palindrome of differing size, but it is not required for viral DNA replication and is absent from the polyoma genome.

Initiation of Viral DNA Replication

In the absence of ATP, T antigen binds as a tetramer to binding site II in the origin region and protects about 35 base pairs of DNA from DNAse (278). In the presence of ATP, T antigen undergoes a conformational shift, permitting the assembly of a bi-lobed double hexamer of T antigen at the origin of DNA replication (27,79,80,161,225). Although a single monomer of T antigen can bind to a GAGGC pentanucleotide (see *dark arrowheads* in Fig. 3), clearly not all 12 molecules of T antigen will be bound to a pentanucleotide in the assembled dodecamer–DNA structure. Some of the T antigen subunits can be thought of as playing an allosteric role, modifying the conformation of other subunits to permit proper binding and assembly of the double hexamer (29). Studies of T-antigen mutants indicate that each of the two hexamers interacts with the other. ATP hydrolysis is not required for the assembly of this structure on the DNA.

A variety of physical and chemical analyses indicate that the bound T-antigen double hexamer catalyzes the local unwinding of part of the early palindrome (see *PU/PY* in Fig. 3) and the distortion or untwisting of the TA element (27,299). Once this initial unwinding has occurred, T antigen no longer binds specifically to viral DNA because the ORI region is no longer double stranded (3). T antigen then associates with RPA, a three-subunit single-stranded DNA-binding protein that keeps unwound regions single stranded, and this permits more extensive unwinding of the DNA using the helicase activity of T antigen (78,378). In its ability to unwind double-stranded DNA from an internal site, T antigen is unusual among DNA helicases (227,321).

The association of the viral ORI, the T-antigen double hexamer, and RPA, is referred to as the *preinitiation complex*. Recruitment of DNA polymerase α-primase into this complex converts it to an initiation complex. It is this step in viral DNA replication that defines the very limited host range for members of the *Polyomaviridae* family. SV40 DNA can be replicated in extracts prepared from murine cells if these are supplemented with DNA polymerase α-primase from monkey cells (247,320). Specific protein contacts form between T antigen, RPA, and DNA polymerase α-primase (62,93,94,121,307), and the nature of these interactions at the viral origin of replication limits productive complex formation with SV40 and polyomavirus T antigens to primate and murine DNA polymerase α-primases, respectively (290). Polymerase α-primase synthesizes short RNA primers, which it then extends into short DNA fragments (38,155,228).

Processive extension of DNA in eukaryotes requires three factors to coordinate their actions. First, DNA polymerase α-primase synthesizes the primed site. Then, replication factor C loads a proliferating cell nuclear antigen (PCNA) clamp onto the primer. Following this, DNA polymerase δ assembles with PCNA for processive extension. These proteins each bind the primed site tightly and trade places in a highly coordinated fashion such that the primer terminus is never left free of protein. RPA, the single-stranded DNA-binding protein, forms a common touchpoint for each of these proteins, and they compete with one another for it. Thus, these protein exchanges are driven by competition-based protein switches in which two proteins vie for contact with RPA.

DNA Synthesis at the Replication Fork

After initiation, DNA synthesis moves bidirectionally away from the ORI. Replication fork movement is facilitated by the helicase activity of T antigen, which translocates along the DNA. The cellular replication factor C (RFC) binds the 3′ end of elongating DNA strands, displaces polymerase α-primase, and coordinates the switch to DNA polymerase δ. RFC, PCNA, and DNA polymerase δ can each interact with RFA bound to the growing strand. Multiple subunits of RFC coordinate the assembly of the PCNA sliding clamp and then remain associated with the complex through an RFC–RPA interaction. DNA polymerase δ interacts with this complex through its ability to bind to RPA and actually competes with RFC for RPA binding (388). RFC is displaced from the 3′ end of the growing strand but remains associated with this complex, which synthesizes both the continuous leading strand (359,360) and the Okazaki fragments on the lagging strand (368). The actions of RNase H, a 5′to 3′; exonuclease (MFI), and DNA ligase I are required for removal of primers and ligation of Okazaki fragments, yielding covalently closed circular form I DNA (367).

Termination of Replication and Separation of Daughter Molecules

Replicative intermediates have been isolated by sucrose gradient centrifugation and analyzed biochemically, electrophoretically, and electron microscopically. Preparations of replicative intermediates are enriched in molecules that are almost completely replicated. Replication moves bidirectionally around the circular chromosome, with both replication forks advancing at about the same rate. These replication intermediates contain three DNA loops—two daughter loops and the unreplicated parental DNA. Molecules that are 85% to 95% complete are enriched in replicative intermediate pools, suggesting that separation of daughter molecules is a slow step in DNA replication (336,337,341). Topoisomerase II is required for this separation (384). There is no specific termination site for viral DNA replication. Deletion analysis indicates that termination can occur within any sequence located about 180 degrees from the origin.

Regulation of Viral DNA Replication by Phosphorylation

The activity of T antigen in viral DNA replication is regulated by phosphorylation of the protein. Both SV40 and polyoma large T antigens carry phosphorylation sites near their DNA-binding domains in the amino-terminal half of each protein. An underphosphorylated population of T antigen isolated from infected cells, or T antigen that is dephosphorylated enzymatically, is more active in DNA binding and viral DNA replication *in vitro* (240). Although phosphorylation of threonine-124 of SV40 T antigen is essential for unwinding of viral origin DNA and replication (239,373), dephosphorylation (240,365, 366) or substitution (291) of adjacent serine residues enhances origin unwinding and replication. Interestingly, the phosphorylation site at threonine-124 is a substrate for the cyclin-dependent kinases (233), whereas protein phosphatase 2A is active in dephosphorylation of the nearby serines, whose phosphorylation inhibits viral DNA replication *in vitro* (286). This suggests that the replication activity of T antigen may be regulated during the cell cycle so that T is maximally active for replication during S phase and inactive for replication at earlier stages of the viral infection.

Viral Late Gene Expression

The onset of viral DNA replication brings about a shift in the pattern of viral transcription. The start sites for production of the viral early mRNAs shift to upstream positions (see *LE* in Fig. 3A), and there is a dramatic increase in transcription to produce the viral late mRNAs. Early after infection, late transcription is repressed owing to occupancy of the late promoter by a steroid receptor family heterodimer between RXRα and TRα1, a thyroid hormone receptor (376,400,401).

Infected cells contain up to 200,000 molecules of viral DNA, and more than half of this may be encapsidated into progeny virions. With 360 molecules of VP1 per virus particle, a minimum of 3.6×10^8 molecules of VP1 must be produced. Assuming a normal loading of ribosomes on viral late mRNA and a normal rate of translation to produce VP1, each molecule of mRNA encoding VP1 could generate 5,000 to 10,000 molecules of VP1 in an infected cell. Thus, more than 30,000 molecules of message encoding VP1 are required. This is several hundred times greater than the abundance of viral early mRNA, making studies of the synthesis and structure of viral late mRNAs relatively easy.

Late transcription of SV40 and polyoma has been studied in the greatest detail. In both systems, two sets of late mRNAs are produced, originally referred to as 16S and 19S late RNAs based on velocity sedimentation in sucrose gradients. The 16S late mRNAs are considerably more abundant than the 19S late mRNAs. These late mRNAs are all derived by transcription, which begins near the origin and extends around the opposite strand from that transcribed to produce the early mRNAs (see Fig. 2). The start sites for SV40 late mRNAs are heterogeneous and map to many positions (see Fig. 3A) between nucleotides 120 and 482, although the start at nucleotide 325 is the most abundant (128,129,270). All viral late 16S mRNAs contain a leader sequence spliced to a second exon that extends from nucleotide 1464 to a polyadenylation site at nucleotide 2674 (see Fig. 2A). All lack sequences between 527 and 1464. Thus, the 16S late mRNAs differ in the structure of their leader regions, with some containing an additional splice, and a rare group containing a duplication of sequences in the leader region. The 19S late mRNAs are also heterogeneous at both their 5′ ends and in the structure of their leader regions. A minor class is unspliced. All of the others contain a leader spliced to sequences extending from nucleotide 558 to the same polyadenylation site used for 16S late mRNAs at nucleotide 2674. All SV40 late mRNAs are derived by processing of precursors that begin at heterogeneous initiation sites and extend most of the way around the viral genome.

Polyomavirus late transcription differs from SV40 in that most viral late pre-mRNAs are extremely large, resulting from transcription completely around the viral genome multiple times (1,206). The mRNAs produced from these giant transcripts contain a single copy of the coding region for late proteins spliced to multiple copies of the leader region by leader-to-leader splicing (172). As with SV40, the start sites for late transcription are heterogeneous (see Fig. 3B); they extend from nucleotides 5075 to 5170, with about 90% of them lying in the region from nucleotides 5077 to 5101 (69,70,110,355). The late promoters of SV40 and polyoma lack TATA boxes, which likely explains the heterogeneity of initiation sites for viral late transcription. Maximal rates of SV40 late transcription depend on sequences within the 21–base pair GC repeats as well as within the 72–base pair enhancers (180,230).

At least three mechanisms are involved in the production of high levels of the viral late mRNAs: amplification of templates for late transcription by viral DNA replication, relief of repression of the viral late promoter, and T-antigen–mediated activation of transcription from the viral late promoter. Studies with origin-defective viral DNA molecules indicate that genome amplification is not required for activation of the late promoter by large T antigen (31,179). The region of large T antigen involved in activation of the late promoter maps to the amino-terminal half of the protein (395). Transcriptional activation of the late promoter by T antigen requires sequences within the 72–base pair enhancer region, including a unique sequence element located at the junction of the two 72–base pair repeats (144). One factor able to bind to these sequences is TEF-1, which is able to form a complex with large T antigen (145,182). Interactions between T antigen and TBP likely also contribute to activation of the late promoter. One mechanism of T-antigen stimulation of transcription involves T antigen functioning as a TAF. In fact, T antigen can complement the ts defect in TAF_{250} in the ts13 cells (73), a baby hamster kidney with a cell cycle defect (340). As a TAF, T antigen acts to stabilize the complex between TBP and TFIIA (74). T antigen appears to be a promiscuous activator, enhancing transcription of both viral and cellular genes in multiple ways. The structure of replicated minichromosomes likely also plays a key role in activation of late transcription (339). Although transcription factors are thought to stimulate DNA replication, complex formation between T antigen and TBP (and perhaps also with other transcription factors) actually inhibits DNA replication *in vitro,* most likely by occupying a binding surface of T antigen required for viral DNA replication (159). SV40 T antigen also interacts with TAF_{110} (232). Overall, T antigen interacts with many cellular proteins as well as with DNA and possibly RNA. This suggests that competition for T-antigen binding can be used to regulate the course of infection.

Synthesis of Late Proteins and Assembly and Release of Progeny Virions

Within the cytoplasm of infected cells, viral 16S late mRNAs are translated to produce VP1, whereas viral 19S late mRNAs are translated to produce VP2 and VP3. Because the sequence of VP3 is contained entirely within that of VP2, VP3 could be derived from VP2 by proteolytic processing. However, deletion mutants lacking the initiation codon for VP2 still produce VP3, indicating that VP3 can be synthesized independently of synthesis of VP2 (59). Because all of the SV40 late mRNAs are polycistronic and contain open reading frames upstream from the capsid protein genes, leaky scanning permits synthesis of capsid proteins from these mRNAs. For some late mRNAs, the upstream ORF encodes the agnoprotein. Studies of translation of SV40 late mRNAs (294–296) have dramatically increased our understanding of how leaky scanning permits internal AUGs to function efficiently as initiation codons (194,195).

Virion proteins VP1, VP2 and VP3 are synthesized in the cytoplasm of infected cells and transported to the nucleus for assembly into virions. When all three capsid proteins are produced, all three enter the nucleus efficiently. Detailed studies of these proteins indicate that sequences near the amino terminus of VP1 and near the carboxyl termini of VP2 and VP3 are essential for this nuclear accumulation. Within the N-terminus of both SV40 and polyoma VP1 are nuclear localization signals (46,243,379). Sequences required for localization of VP2 and VP3 to the nucleus have also been identified. VP1 is able to cotransport VP2 or VP3, and VP2 or VP3 can cotransport VP1, indicating that these proteins may be imported as a complex as well as separately (13,84,112, 163,177). Within the nucleus, these proteins are found in the same ratio as within the viral capsid (212).

Viral chromatin is not required for the assembly of capsids or capsid-like structures. Purified polyoma VP1 self-assembles into pentamers and capsid-like structures (126,280), whereas coexpression of polyoma or SV40 VP1, VP2, and VP3 in insect cells from baculovirus vectors results in the assembly of capsid-like structures containing all three capsid proteins in about the same relative ratio as is found in mature virions (112,283). Sequences within the regulatory region of SV40 have also been shown to facilitate encapsidation (72).

The precise mechanism of encapsidation in polyoma-infected cells remains uncertain. Available data are consistent with two possibilities. Empty capsids can be purified from infected cells and could be precursors to virions. Alternatively, capsomers may condense on viral chromatin to assemble a virus capsid (387). The 75S to 90S chromatin structures containing viral DNA are detected, as are 200S previrions and 240S virions. Although intracellular chromatin contains histone H1, virion chromatin does not, but the precise time or mechanism of removal of histone H1 is not known. Analysis of immunoprecipitates of insect cells expressing one or more polyomavirus capsid proteins indicates that cellular histones associate with capsid proteins and suggest that VP2 or VP3 may be the direct mediator of capsid protein–histone interactions (112). Polyoma VP1 and SV40 VP2 and VP3 have been shown to bind to DNA in a sequence-independent manner (45,54). The importance of these interactions for virion assembly or stability is uncertain because capsid protein–histone interactions could serve the same roles in assembly or stability as would capsid protein–DNA interactions.

SV40 and other polyomaviruses do not encode a lysozyme that causes cell lysis. It was previously suggested that exit of SV40 virions from infected cells occurs when cells disintegrate or rupture as part of their dying. However, studies of virus-infected epithelial cells lines indicated that SV40 can be released from the cell surface, primarily from the apical surface of polarized epithelial cells and uniformly from the surface of nonpolarized epithelial cells (53). By electron microscopy, SV40 was seen in cytoplasmic smooth membrane vesicles, and release of SV40 was inhibited by monensin, an inhibitor of intracellular vesicular transport. How and where these vesicles form and the fraction of total infectious progeny released in this manner or by leakage from dying cells are not known.

The Host Range and Helper Function of SV40 Large T Antigens

Most monkey cell lines infected by human adenoviruses produce low yields of viral progeny, with the block to productive infection occurring very late in the adenovirus infection cycle (reviewed in 191 and 351). This block can be overcome by the extreme carboxyl terminus of SV40 large T antigen (58,262), which is unrelated to any portions of polyoma large T antigen. Mutants of SV40 whose T antigens lack a normal carboxyl terminus are defective in this helper function and also show a restricted growth range among different African green monkey kidney cell lines (60,61,222,259). Human adenoviruses and host range mutants of SV40 both grow well in some monkey kidney cells lines (e.g., Vero) and poorly in others (e.g., CV-1). This activity of large T antigen is referred to as the *host range and helper function* (hr/hf). It is a distinct and separable activity of large T because a VP1 fusion protein containing the normal carboxyl terminus of large T can provide hr/hf activity (353).

Mutants lacking the hr/hf domain of large T show defects that affect late gene expression. The levels of viral late mRNA and capsid protein are reduced to about one third of their normal levels, but virion production is reduced much more dramatically (319). Agnoprotein is not produced (187,319) because the 5′ ends of late viral mRNAs in mutant-infected cells map to normally used minor sites downstream of the agnoprotein initiation codon (319). Provision of agnoprotein in trans permits hr/hf mutants to form plaques but does not increase late mRNA or VP1 production. This suggests that agnoprotein permits more efficient use of the capsid proteins available in mutant-infected cells. This is consistent with studies that suggested a role for the agnoprotein either in transport of VP1 to the nucleus or in assembly of progeny virions (12,43,273).

Evolutionary Variants and Defective Viral Genomes

As with most animal viruses, passage of polyomaviruses at high multiplicities of infection leads to the generation of defective viral genomes and the accumulation of those that have selective growth advantages. These evolutionary variants contain deletions, inversions, and rearrangements, and they often contain multiple origins of DNA replication (140,203). The only sequence retained by all defective viruses is the viral origin region, indicating that it is the only cis-acting sequence required for propagation of the origin-containing DNA. This has led to the development of many eukaryotic expression vectors containing an SV40 origin of replication. These molecules will replicate in monkey kidney cells that provide the SV40 T antigen constitutively (e.g., Cos cells) owing to the integration into the cellular genome of an origin-defective SV40 genome encoding wild-type T antigen.

Those variants with more than one origin replicate more efficiently than wild-type virus and become enriched. Defective viruses require the presence of wild-type virus for their propagation because they often contain no intact viral genes, but nondefective variants have been constructed that contain two functional origins (220). Virus stocks maintained by high multiplicity passage can become contaminated with these evolutionary variants, but this can be prevented by frequent reisolation of wild-type virus through plaque purification.

TRANSFORMATION AND IMMORTALIZATION BY SV40

The polyomaviruses are also known as small DNA tumor viruses. The ability of these viruses to transform established cell lines, to immortalize primary cell cultures, and to induce tumors in animals resulted in the widespread study of these viruses as a window into understanding the molecular basis of oncogenesis and growth regulation. Transformed cells grow readily into tumors when injected into syngeneic or immunocompromised hosts. Transgenic expression of polyomavirus antigens has provided a useful model for studying the development of cell type–specific tumors.

Early studies indicated that genetic information in the viral early region was necessary and sufficient for transformation (reviewed in 116 and 351). One of the first experiments performed after the development of Southern hybridization was an analysis of the patterns of integration of viral DNA in SV40 transformed cells. Although these studies demonstrated that there were no unique or preferred sites of integration in either the viral or host genomes, a functional viral early region were present in all transformed lines analyzed (28,185,281). For SV40, studies using tsA mutants readily demonstrated that T antigen was required for both the initiation and maintenance of the transformed state (35,223,342).

For polyoma, large T antigen is required for transformation (89,99,115), but subsequent studies indicated that T-antigen expression is needed only for initiation but not for the maintenance of the transformed state. The viral DNA in transformed cells is usually integrated to interrupt the early region, blocking continued expression of large T antigen but permitting continued synthesis of both small and middle T antigens (15,201). Studies of polyoma hrt mutants (18), which encode a wild-type large T antigen, demonstrated that other early region gene products besides large T antigen were required for transformation by polyomavirus (100,111). It is now known that a cyclic DNA encoding just middle T antigen is sufficient to transform established cell lines (265,356). The requirement for polyoma large T antigen to initiate transformation after viral infection may reflect modest amplification of the genome by replication. Subsequent integration of the viral DNA often interrupts the large T-antigen–coding region, thereby eliminating the replicative activities of polyoma large T antigen while leaving the middle T-antigen–coding region intact. Levels of middle T antigen sufficient for transformation may be achieved by transfection, thus eliminating the need for large T antigen. In transformation, polyomavirus middle T antigen activity requires association with the plasma membrane. Here, interaction with many of the same cellular signal transduction proteins mediating growth factor receptor signaling leads to constitutive activation of the cell cycle. Although the interaction between middle T and pp60c-src cannot be essential because middle T antigen can transform cells that contain a disruption of the *c-src* gene, middle T continues to interact with other src family kinases and PI-3 kinase in cells lacking *c-src* (346).

Mutational analyses of transformation by SV40 large T antigen demonstrate that only the amino-terminal portion of large T (amino acids 1 to 121) is required to transform mouse C3H 10T1/2 cells, whereas sequences extending over much of large T antigen are required to transform REF-52 rat embryo fibroblasts and many other established rodent cell lines (318). Transformation by T antigen can be separated from its role in viral DNA replication (136,171) and does not require any of the activities involved in viral DNA replication (e.g., DNA binding, ATP binding, ATPase activity, helicase activity) or host range and helper function. SV40 mutants defective in transformation of REF-52 cells map to three regions of large T antigen: the amino terminus containing the conserved DNA J domain (amino acids 1 to 82), the domain that binds $p105^{Rb}$ and the associated proteins p107 and p130 (amino acids 102 to 114), and the p53/p300 binding domain of the carboxyl half (49,171,396). SV40 small t antigen is clearly required for transformation under many conditions (301,306), but sufficiently high levels of large T antigen (24), growth conditions of the infected cells (298), or contributions to transformation from the cellular genetic background probably account for the lack of a uniform requirement for small t antigen for transformation by SV40. Under circumstances in which SV40 small t antigen is required for transformation, mutants of small t defective for interaction with and inhibition of PP2A are defective for transformation, suggesting that this interaction is central to the effect of small t antigen on cellular growth properties (246).

The requirement for the SV40 large T antigen amino terminus in cellular transformation reflects its DNA J domain activity as a molecular chaperone whereby it disrupts DNA-binding complexes between Rb family proteins and E2F (389). Mutants that express only amino acids 83 to 708 are defective for transformation, as are several deletion, insertion, and point mutations within the first 82 amino acids. Mutants of SV40 that express a T antigen lacking residues 1 to 82 can be complemented for transformation by SV40 small t antigen (241), consistent with the small t-antigen J domain functioning as a molecular chaperone (317). Results of experiments using double knockout mouse embryo fibroblasty (MEFs) (p107–/– and p130–/–) have revealed that the J domain is dispensable for transformation of these cells. This implies that the J domain plays an essential role in SV40 transformation by inactivating p107 and p130 functions (81), even though these proteins do not appear to have tumor suppressor activity.

Binding of T antigen to p105^{Rb}, an important tumor suppressor gene product, and the related cellular proteins p107 and p130, contributes to the disruption of the function of these cellular proteins (389). A clue to the mechanism of p105^{Rb} function in cellular growth control suppression is its interaction with the E2F family of transcription factors (6,47). E2F family members bind as heterodimers to sequence-specific sites present in the promoter-enhancer regions of genes known to have important roles in cellular growth control, including *c-myc* and *c-fos* (158). Different E2F family members are thought to associate with different p105^{Rb}-related proteins at unique points in the cell cycle (98,205). For example, in G_0 phase, hypophosphorylated p105^{Rb} interacts with E2F, preventing E2F from interacting with target genes (47,157). By binding to the hypophosphorylated form of p105^{Rb}, T antigen causes the release of E2F, and this activates E2F-regulated genes, leading to cell cycle progression (48). The related proteins, p107 and p130, complex with different members of the E2F family. The p130 complexes are found predominantly at the G_0–G_1 phase border (56), whereas the p107 complexes are most abundant at the G_1–S phase boundary (98). The concomitant binding of T antigen to p107 and p130 and the amino terminal J domain perturbation of their phosphorylation state result in the release of free and active E2F. Subsequently, genes encoding proteins required for the initiation of DNA synthesis are activated by E2F-dependent mechanisms.

Yet another p105^{Rb}, p107, and p130 ("pocket proteins") mechanism for cell cycle control was identified by the discovery that these proteins, in association with E2Fs, can bind to the cyclins and cdks. The association of pocket protein–E2F complexes with cyclin/cdks appears to be cell cycle regulated and specific for particular cyclin/cdks complexes (42,56,87,204,302). Expression of SV40 large T antigen inhibits the activation of cyclins by cdks, thereby interfering with multiples stages of cell cycle progression (193).

SV40 large T antigen also binds p300 and CBP (5,101) through a common region of T antigen that is required for binding to the tumor suppressor protein p53 (211). The coactivators p300 and CBP form a transcriptional activation complex and can function to promote histone acetylation; binding of p300 and CBP to T antigen disrupts p300-dependent growth control and is likely to contribute to T antigen–induced cell transformation (210). The viral oncoprotein E1A has been shown to repress the normal functions of p300 and CBP by both displacing them from transcriptional coactivating complexes and directly repressing their histone acetyltransferase activity (44). This repression, in turn, leads to p53 deacetylation, thereby disrupting p53 tumor suppressor activities. Whether SV40 large T antigen uses a similar mechanism for direct inhibition of p300 and CBP family histone acetyltransferase activity is not yet known; however, the ability of T antigen to bind directly to p53 (199) is yet another important mechanism through which SV40 can disrupt an important cellular growth checkpoint control protein.

Transgenic mice have been used to study SV40-induced oncogenesis in a broad range of tissues, including mammary gland, salivary gland, pancreas, prostate, liver, lung, kidney, intestine, brain, choroid plexus, lens of the eye, bone, smooth muscle, and cartilage (reviewed in 120). Interestingly, transgenic experiments have suggested that the p300- and p53-binding region may not be required for tumor cell formation in animals. For example, hepatic tumors can be induced by the N-terminal fragment of T antigen (amino acids 1 to 121) encoded by dl1137. This truncated protein retains the ability to bind and inhibit pRb function but cannot bind p53. Surprisingly, these tumors grow significantly faster than those induced by wild-type T antigen (20).

The ability to immortalize primary rodent cells is another property of the large T antigens of polyoma and SV40 that has also been studied in detail. Analysis of the domains of polyoma and SV40 large T antigens required for immortalization have also been performed, but with conflicting results. Some studies demonstrated that the ability of SV40 large T antigen to bind p53 is required for immortalization of primary mouse cells (347,394), whereas others indicated that the amino-terminal 147 amino acids of large T can immortalize primary mouse or rat cells (312,313). Studies with a ts mutant of SV40 T antigen indicated, however, that T antigen is required continuously to maintain immortalization because cultures shifted to the nonpermissive temperature ceased proliferation (166).

Critical to evaluation of the immortalization potential of these viruses and their individual T antigens are the assays used to measure immortalization. If immortalization of primary cultures requires multiple genetic or epigenetic alterations (e.g., the formation of a complex between SV40 T antigen and p53), mutant viral T antigens may provide some or most of the required functions, and a single additional cellular mutation could result in the full spectrum of genetic changes leading to immortalization. In some assays, no attempts were made to distinguish between extension of normal lifespan, with eventual senescence, and true immortalization. In other assays, populations of cells still proliferating at a time when control cells had senesced were serially subcultured and considered to be immortal if the culture survived for several months. However, the probability is high that cellular mutations will occur that contribute to immortalization of cells expressing mutant T antigens, particularly if mutation of one cellular gene in one cell in the population is sufficient to cause its immortalization and eventual predominance in the culture.

There is solid evidence that mutation of p53 plays a central role in immortalization. Mutation of the p53 gene was seen in all spontaneously immortalized mouse embryo fibroblast cell lines examined (154). It is easy to see that mutation of p53 or its functional inactivation by complex formation with SV40 large T antigen could increase the frequency of cellular mutations because p53 loss of function is known to be associated with gene amplification and genomic instability (214,386). In fact, inactivation of p53 by complex formation with SV40 T antigen is likely to be at least partially responsible for the known genomic instability associated with expression of SV40 T antigen (268,328).

Careful analysis of immortalization by mutant SV40 large T antigens suggests that all three domains required for transformation (J domain, binding region for pRb family proteins, and binding region for p53) are required for immortalization of primary mouse embryo fibroblasts. Substantial lifespan extension was seen in cultures expressing mutant T antigens defective for the amino-terminal transformation function or unable to bind $p105^{Rb}$, but a minority of colonies expressing these mutant T antigens became immortalized after continued subculturing. In contrast, neither lifespan extension nor immortalization was achieved with mutants of T antigen unable to bind p53 and p300. Similar results were shown using amino-terminal (amino acids T1 to T147) or carboxyl-terminal (T251 to T708) fragments of large T antigen: these two regions of T antigen appear to function in the same way as in wild-type T antigen to extend cell lifespan, and together they cooperate to immortalize primary B6MEF cells (345). The fact that immortalization of human cells by SV40 is such an exceedingly rare event may reflect a differential requirement for telomerase activity in human versus rodent cell immortalization because recent evidence demonstrates that introduction of the telomerase catalytic subunit hTRT allows human cells expressing SV40 large T antigen to escape crisis and divide indefinitely (148,397).

Fewer studies have been performed to understand immortalization by polyoma large T antigen, which does not bind p53. An essential role in immortalization for the $p105^{Rb}$-binding activity of polyoma large T antigen has been demonstrated (113,202), and it is likely that additional activities are also required.

REFERENCES

1. Acheson NH. Polyoma giant RNAs contain tandem repeats of the nucleotide sequence of the entire viral genome. *Proc Natl Acad Sci U S A* 1978;75:4754–4758.
2. Anderson HA, Chen Y, Norkin LC. Bound simian virus 40 translocates to caveolin-enriched membrane domains, and its entry is inhibited by drugs that selectively disrupt caveolae. *Mol Biol Cell* 1996;7: 1825–1834.
3. Auborn KJ, Markowitz RB, Wang E, et al. Simian virus 40 (SV40) T antigen binds specifically to double-stranded DNA but not to single-stranded DNA or DNA/RNA hybrids containing the SV40 regulatory sequences. *J Virol* 1988;62:2204–2208.
4. Auger KR, Carpenter CL, Shoelson SE, et al. Polyoma virus middle T antigen-pp60c-src complex associates with purified phosphatidylinositol 3-kinase *in vitro*. *J Biol Chem* 1992;267:5408–5415.
5. Avantaggiati ML, Carbone M, Graessmann A, et al. The SV40 large T antigen and adenovirus E1a oncoproteins interact with distinct isoforms of the transcriptional co-activator, p300. *EMBO J* 1996;15: 2236–2248.
6. Bagchi S, Weinmann R, Raychaudhuri P. The retinoblastoma protein copurifies with E2F-1, an E1A-regulated inhibitor of the transcription factor E2F. *Cell* 1991;65:1063–1072.
7. Bandara LR, Adamczewski JP, Hunt T, La Thangue NB. Cyclin A and the retinoblastoma gene product complex with a common transcription factor. *Nature* 1991;352:249–251.
8. Barbanti-Brodano G, Swetly P, Koprowski H. Early events in the infection of permissive cells with simian virus 40: Adsorption, penetration, and uncoating. *J Virol* 1970;6:78–86.
9. Bargonetti J, Friedman PN, Kern SE, et al. Wild-type but not mutant p53 immunopurified proteins bind to sequences adjacent to the SV40 origin of replication. *Cell* 1991;65:1083–1091.
10. Bargonetti J, Reynisdóttir I, Friedman PN, Prives C. Site-specific binding of wild-type p53 to cellular DNA is inhibited by SV40 T antigen and mutant p53. *Genes Dev* 1992;6:1886–1898.
11. Barkan A, Mertz JE. DNA sequence analysis of simian virus 40 mutants with deletions mapping in the leader region of the late mRNAs: Mutants with deletions similar in size and position exhibit varied phenotypes. *J Virol* 1981;37:730–737.
12. Barkan A, Welch RC, Mertz JE. Missense mutations in the VP1 gene of simian virus 40 that compensate for defects caused by deletions in the viral genome. *J Virol* 1987;61:3190–3198.
13. Barouch DH, Harrison SC. Interactions among the major and minor coat proteins of polyomavirus. *J Virol* 1994;68:3982–3989.
14. Basak S, Turner H, Compans RW. Expression of SV40 receptors on apical surfaces of polarized epithelial cells. *Virology* 1992;190: 393–402.
15. Basilico C, Zouzias D, Della-Valle G, et al. Integration and excision of polyoma virus genomes. *Cold Spring Harbor Symp Quant Biol* 1979;44:611-620.
16. Bauer PH, Bronson RT, Fung SC, et al. Genetic and structural analysis of a virulence determinant in polyomavirus VP1. *J Virol* 1995;69: 7925–7931.
17. Bauer PH, Cui C, Stehle T, et al. Discrimination between sialic acid-containing receptors and pseudoreceptors regulates polyomavirus spread in the mouse. *J Virol* 1999;73:5826–5832.
18. Benjamin TL. Host-range mutants of polyoma virus. *Proc Natl Acad Sci U S A* 1970;67:394–401.
19. Bennett ER, Naujokas M, Hassell JA. Requirements for species-specific papovavirus DNA replication. *J Virol* 1989;63:5371–5385.
20. Bennoun M, Grimber G, Couton D, et al. The amino-terminal region of SV40 large T antigen is sufficient to induce hepatic tumours in mice. *Oncogene* 1998;17:1253–1259.
21. Benoist C, Chambon P. *In vivo* sequence requirements of the SV40 early promoter region. *Nature* 1981;290:304–310.
22. Berk, AJ and Sharp, PA. Spliced early mRNAs of simian virus 40. *Proc Natl Acad Sci U S A* 1978;75:1274–1278.
23. Bikel I, Loeken MR. Involvement of simian virus 40 (SV40) small t antigen in transactivation of SV40 early and late promoters. *J Virol* 1992;66:1489–1494.
24. Bikel I, Montano X, Agha M, et al. SV40 small-t antigen enhances the transformation activity of limiting concentrations of SV40 large T antigen. *Cell* 1987;48:321–330.
25. Bolen JB, Anders DG, Trempy J, Consigli RA. Difference in the subpopulatons of the structural proteins of polyoma virions and capsids: Biological functions of the VP1 species. *J Virol* 1981;37:80–91.
26. Bolen JB, Consigli RA. Differential adsorption of polyoma virions and capsids to mouse kidney cells and guinea pig erythrocytes. *J Virol* 1979;32:679–683.
27. Borowiec JA, Hurwitz J. ATP stimulates the binding of simian virus 40 (SV40) large tumor antigen to the SV40 origin of replication. *Proc Natl Acad Sci U S A* 1988;85:64–68.
28. Botchan M, Topp WC, Sambrook J. The arrangement of simian virus 40 sequences in the DNA of transformed cells. *Cell* 1976;9:269–287.

29. Bradley MK. Activation of ATPase activity of simian virus 40 large T antigen by the covalent affinity analog of ATP, fluorosulfonylbenzoyl 5′-adenosine. *J Virol* 1990;64:4939–4947.
30. Bradley MK, Hudson J, Villanueva MS, Livingston DM. Specific *in vitro* adenylation of simian virus 40 large tumor antigen. *Proc Natl Acad Sci U S A* 1984;81:6574–6578.
31. Brady JN, Bolen JB, Radonovich M, et al. Stimulation of simian virus 40 late gene expression by simian virus 40 tumor antigen. *Proc Natl Acad Sci U S A* 1984;81:2040–2044.
32. Brady JN, Wihnston VD, Consigli RA. Dissociation of polyoma virus by chelation of calcium ions found associated with purified virions. *J Virol* 1977;23:717–724.
33. Braun KA, Lao Y, He Z, et al. Role of protein-protein interactions in the function of replication protein A (RPA): RPA modulates the activity of DNA polymerase alpha by multiple mechanisms. *Biochemistry* 1997;36:8443–8454.
34. Breau WC, Atwood WJ, Norkin, LC. Class I major histocompatibility proteins are an essential component of the simian virus 40 receptor. *J Virol* 1992;66:2037–2045.
35. Brugge JS, Butel JS. Involvement of the simian virus 40 gene: A function in maintenance of transformation. *J Virol* 1975;15:619–635.
36. Buchman AR, Burnett L, Berg P. The SV40 nucleotide sequence. In: Tooze J, ed. *DNA tumor viruses*. Cold Spring Harbor, NY: Cold Spring Harbor Laboratory, 1981:799–841.
37. Buchman AR, Fromm M, Berg P. Complex regulation of SV40 early-region transcription from different overlapping promoters. *Mol Cell Biol* 1984;4:1900–1914.
38. Bullock PA, Seo YS, Hurwitz J. Initiation of simian virus 40 DNA synthesis *in vitro*. *Mol Cell Biol* 1991;11:2350–2361.
39. Butel JS, Lednicky JA. Cell and molecular biology of simian virus 40: Implications for human infections and disease. *J Natl Cancer Inst* 1999;91:119–134.
40. Campbell KS, Mullane KP, Aksoy IA, et al. DnaJ/hsp40 chaperone domain of SV40 large T antigen promotes efficient viral DNA replication. *Genes Dev* 1997;11:1098–110.
41. Campbell KS, Ogris E, Burke B, et al. Polyoma middle T antigen interacts with SHC via the NPTY motif in middle T. *Proc Natl Acad Sci U S A* 1994;91:6344–6348.
42. Cao L, Faha B, Dembski M, et al. Independent binding of the retinoblastoma protein and p107 to the transcription factor E2F. *Nature* 1992;355:176–179.
43. Carswell S, Alwine JC. Simian virus 40 agnoprotein facilitates perinuclear-nuclear localization of VP1, the major capsid protein. *J Virol* 1986;60:1055–1061.
44. Chakravarti D, Ogryzko V, Hung-Ying Kao1 AN, et al. A viral mechanism for inhibition of p300 and PCAF acetyltransferase activity. *Cell* 1999;96:393–403.
45. Chang D, Cai X, Consigli RA. Characterization of the DNA binding properties of polyomavirus capsid protein. *J Virol* 1993;67:6327–6331.
46. Chang D, Hayes DI, Brady JN, Consigli RA. The use of additive and subtractive approaches to examine the nuclear localization sequence of the polyomavirus major capsid protein VP1. *Virology* 1992;189: 821–827.
47. Chellappan S, Heibert S, Mudryj M, et al. The E2F cellular transcription factor is a target for the RB protein. Cell 1991;89:4549–4553.
48. Chellappan S, Kraus VB, Kroger B, et al. Adenovirus E1A, simian virus 40 tumor antigen, and human papillomavirus E7 protein share the capacity to disrupt the interaction between transcription factor E2F and the retinoblastoma gene product. *Proc Natl Acad Sci U S A* 1992;89:4549–4553.
49. Chen S, Paucha E. Identification of a region of simian virus 40 large T antigen required for cell transformation. *J Virol* 1990;64:3350–3357.
50. Chen XS, Stehle T, Harrison SC. Interaction of polyomavirus internal protein VP2 with the major capsid protein VP1 and implications for participation ofVP2 in viral entry. *EMBO J* 1998;17:3233–3240.
51. Chen Y, Norkin LC. Extracellular simian virus 40 transmits a signal that promotes virus enclosure within caveolae. *Exp Cell Res* 1999; 246:83–90.
52. Christiansen G, Landers T, Griffith J, Berg P. Characterization of components released by alkali disruption of simian virus 40. *J Virol* 1977; 21:1079–1084.
53. Clayson ET, Brando LV, Compans RW. Release of simian virus 40 virions from epithelial cells is polarized and occurs without cell lysis. *J Virol* 1989;63:2278–2288.
54. Clever J, Dean DA, Kasamatsu H. Identification of a DNA binding domain in simian virus 40 capsid proteins VP2 and VP3. *J Biol Chem* 1993;268:20877–20883.
55. Clever J, Yamada M, Kasamatsu H. Import of simian virus 40 virions through nuclear pore complexes. *Proc Natl Acad Sci U S A* 1991;88: 7333–7337.
56. Cobrinik D, Whyte P, Peeper D, et al. Cell cycle-specific association of E2F with the p130 E1A-binding protein. *Genes Dev* 1993;7: 2392–2404.
57. Cogen B. Virus-specific early RNA in 3T6 cells infected by a tsA mutant of polyoma virus. *Virology* 1978;85:222–230.
58. Cole CN, Crawford LV, Berg P. Simian virus 40 mutants with deletions at the 3′ end of the early region are defective in adenovirus helper function. *J Virol* 1979;30:683–691.
59. Cole CN, Landers T, Goff SP, et al. Physical and genetic characterization of deletion mutants of simian virus 40 constructed *in vitro*. *J Virol* 1977;24:277–294.
60. Cole CN, Stacy TP. Biological properties of simian virus 40 host range mutants lacking the COOH-terminus of large T antigen. *Virology* 1987;161:170–180.
61. Cole CN, Tornow J, Clark R, Tjian R. Properties of the simian virus 40 (SV40) large T antigens encoded by SV40 mutants with deletions in gene A. *J Virol* 1986;57:539–546.
62. Collins KL, Kelly TJ. Effects of T antigen and replication protein A on the initiation of DNA synthesis by DNA polymerase α-primase. *Mol Cell Biol* 1991;11:2108–2115.
63. Collins KL, Russo AA, Tseng BY, Kelly TJ. The role of the 70 kda subunit of human DNA polymerase alpha in DNA replication. *EMBO J* 1993;12:4555–4566.
64. Conzen SD, Cole CN. The three transforming regions of SV40 T antigen are required for immortalization of primary mouse embryo fibroblasts. *Oncogene* 1995;11:2295–2302.
65. Corden J, Wasylyk B, Buchwalder A, et al. Promoter sequences of eukaryotic promoters. *Science* 1980;209:1406–1414.
66. Courtneidge SA, Smith AE. Polyoma virus transforming protein associates with the product of the *c-src* cellular gene. *Nature* 1983;303:435–439.
67. Cowie A, Jat P, Kamen R. Determination of sequences at the capped 5′-ends of polyomavirus early region transcripts synthesized *in vivo* and *in vitro* demonstrates an unusual microheterogeneity. *J Mol Biol* 1982;159:225–255.
68. Cowie A, Kamen R. Multiple binding sites for polyomavirus large T antigen within regulatory sequences of polyomavirus DNA. *J Virol* 1984;52:750–760.
69. Cowie A, Tyndall C, Kamen R. Determination of sequences at the capped 5′-ends of polyomavirus early region transcripts synthesized *in vivo* and *in vitro* demonstrates an unusual microheterogeneity. *J Mol Biol* 1981;159:225–255.
70. Cowie A, Tyndall C, Kamen R. Sequences at the capped 5′-ends of polyomavirus late region mRNAs: An example of extreme heterogeneity. *Nucleic Acids Res* 1981;9:6305–6322.
71. Crawford L, Cole CN, Smith AE, et al. The organization and expression of simian virus 40's early genes. *Proc Natl Acad Sci U S A* 1978;75:117–122.
72. Dalyot-Herman N, Ben-nun-Shaul O, Gordon-Shaag A, Oppenheim A. The simian virus 40 packaging signal ses is composed of redundant DNA elements which are partly interchangeable. *J Mol Biol* 1996;259:69–80.
73. Damania B, Alwine JC. TAF-like function of SV40 large T antigen. *Genes Dev* 1996;10:1369–1381.
74. Damania B, Lieberman P, Alwine JC. Simian virus 40 large T antigen stabilizes the TATA-binding protein-TFIIA complex on the TATA element. *Mol Cell Biol* 1998;18:3926–3935.
75. Damania B, Mital R, Alwine JC. Simian virus 40 large T antigen interacts with human TFIIB-related factor and small nuclear RNA-activating protein complex for transcriptional activation of TATA-containing polymerase III promoters. *Mol Cell Biol* 1998;18:1331–1338.
76. Dandolo L, Blangy D, Kamen R. Regulation of polyoma virus transcription in murine embryonal carcinoma cells. *J Virol* 1983;47:55–64.
77. Danna K, Nathans D. Bidirectional replication of simian virus 40 DNA. *Proc Nat Acad Sci U S A* 1972;69:2391–2395.
78. Dean FB, Bullock P, Murakami Y, et al. Simian virus 40 (SV40) DNA replication: SV40 large T antigen unwinds DNA containing an SV40 origin of DNA replication. *Proc Natl Acad Sci U S A* 1987;84:16–20.

79. Dean FB, Dodson M, Echols H, Hurwitz J. ATP-dependent formation of a specialized nucleoprotein structure by simian virus 40 (SV40) large tumor antigen at the SV40 replication origin. *Proc Natl Acad Sci U S A* 1987;84:8981–8985.
80. Deb SP, Tegtmeyer P. ATP enhances the binding of simian virus 40 large T antigen to the origin of replication. *J Virol* 1987;61: 3649–3654.
81. DeCaprio JA. The role of the J domain of SV40 large T in cellular transformation. *Biologicals* 1999;27:23–28.
82. DeCaprio JA, Ludlow JW, Figge J, et al. SV40 large tumor antigen forms a specific complex with the product of the retinoblastoma susceptibility gene. *Cell* 1988;54:275–283.
83. Delmas V, Bastien C, Scherneck S, Feunteun J. A new member of the polyomavirus family: The hamster papovavirus. Complete nucleotide sequence and transformation properties. *EMBO J* 1985;4:1279–1286.
84. Delos SE, Montross L, Moreland RB, Garcea RL. Expression of the polyomavirus VP2 and VP3 proteins in insect cells: Coexpression with the major capsid protein VP1 alters VP2/3 localization. *Virology* 1993;194:393–398.
85. DePamphilis M. Eukaryotic DNA replication: Anatomy of an origin. *Annu Rev Biochem* 1993;62:29–63.
86. DePamphilis ML, Bradley MK. Replication of SV40 and polyoma virus chromosomes. In: Salzman N, ed. *The papovaviridae*. New York: Plenum Press, 1986:99–246.
87. Devoto S, Mudryj M, Pines J, et al. A cyclin A-protein kinase complex possesses sequence-specific DNA binding-activity: p33 cdk2 is a component of the E2F-cyclin A complex. *Cell* 1992;68:167–176.
88. Deyerle KD, Cassill JA, Subramani S. Analysis of the early regulatory region of the human papovavirus BK. *Virology* 1987;158:181–193.
89. Di Mayorca G, Callender J, Marin G, Giordano R. Temperature-sensitive mutants of polyoma virus. *Virology* 1969;38:126–133.
90. Dilworth SM, Brewster CEP, Jones MD, et al. Transformation by polyoma virus middle T-antigen involves the binding and tyrosine phosphorylation of Shc. *Nature* 1994;367:87–90.
91. DiMaio D, Nathans D. Regulatory mutants of simian virus 40: Effect of mutations at a T antigen binding site on DNA replication and expression of viral genes. *J Mol Biol* 1982;156:531–548.
92. Dobbelstein M, Arthur AK, Dehde S, et al. Intracistronic complementation reveals a new function of SV40 T antigen that co-operates with Rb and p53 binding to stimulate DNA synthesis in quiescent cells. *Oncogene* 1992;7:837–847.
93. Dornreiter I, Erdile LF, Gilbert IU, et al. Interaction of DNA polymerase alpha-primase with cellular replication protein A and SV40 T antigen. *EMBO J* 1992;11:769–776.
94. Dornreiter I, Höss A, Arthur AK, Fanning E. SV40 T antigen binds directly to the large subunit of purified DNA polymerase alpha. *EMBO J* 1990;9:3329–3336.
95. Dynan WS, Tjian R. Isolation of transcription factors that discriminate between different promoters recognized by RNA polymerase II. *Cell* 1983;32:669–680.
96. Dynan WS, Tjian R. The promoter-specific transcription factor Sp1 binds to upstream sequence in the SV40 early promoter. *Cell* 1983;35:79–87.
97. Dyson N, Buchkovich K, Whyte P, Harlow E. The cellular 107K protein that binds to adenovirus E1A also associates with the large T antigens of SV40 and JC virus. *Cell* 1989;58:249–255.
98. Dyson N, Dembski A, Fattaey A, et al. Analysis of the p107-associated proteins: p107 Associates with a form of E2F that differs from pRb-associated E2F-1. *J Virol* 1993;67:7641–7647.
99. Eckhart W. Complementation and transformation by temperature-sensitive mutants of polyoma virus. *Virology* 1969;38:120–125.
100. Eckhart W. Complementation between temperature-sensitive and host range nontransforming mutants of polyoma virus. *Virology* 1977;77: 589–597.
101. Eckner R, Ludlow JW, Lill NL, et al. Association of p300 and CBP with simian virus 40 large T antigen. *Mol Cell Biol* 1996;16: 3454–3464.
102. Eddy BE, Borman GS, Grubbs GE, Young RD. Identification of the oncogenic substance in rhesus monkey kidney cell cultures as simian virus 40. *Virology* 1962;17:65–75.
103. El-Deiry WS, Tokino T, Velculescu VE, et al. WAF1, a potential mediator of p53 tumor suppression. *Cell* 1993;75:817–825.
104. Ellman M, Bikel I, Figge J, et al. Localization of the simian virus 40 small t antigen in the nucleus and cytoplasm of monkey and mouse cells. *J Virol* 1984;50:623–628.
105. Everett RD, Baty D, Chambon P. The repeated GC-rich motifs upstream from the TATA box are important elements of the SV40 early promoter. *Nucleic Acids Res* 1983;11:2447–2464.
106. Ewen ME, Ludlow JW, Marsilio E, et al. An N-terminal transformation-governing sequence of SV40 large T antigen contributes to the binding of both p110Rb and a second cellular protein, p120. *Cell* 1989;58:257–267.
107. Farmerie WG, Folk WR. Regulation of polyoma virus transcription by large T antigen. *Proc Natl Acad Sci U S A* 1984;81:6919–6923.
108. Fenton RG, Basilico C. Changes in the topography of early region transcription during polyoma virus lytic infection. *Proc Natl Acad Sci U S A* 1982;79:7142–7146.
109. Fiers W, Contreras R, Haegeman G, et al. The complete nucleotide sequence of SV40 DNA. *Nature* 1978;273:113–120.
110. Flavell AJ, Cowie A, Arrand JR, Kamen R. Localization of three major capped 5′ ends of polyoma late mRNAs within a single tetranucleotide sequence in the viral genome. *J Virol* 1980;33: 902–908.
111. Fluck MM, Staneloni RJ, Benjamin TL. Hr-t and ts-a: Two early gene functions in polyoma virus DNA. *Virology* 1977;77:610–624.
112. Forstova J, Krauzewica N, Wallace S, et al. Cooperation of structural proteins during late events in the life cycle of polyomavirus. *J Virol* 1993;67:1405–1413.
113. Freund R, Bronson RT, Benjamin TL. Separation of immortalization from tumor induction with polyoma large T mutants that fail to bind the retinoblastoma gene product. *Oncogene* 1992;7:1979–1987.
114. Freund R, Sotnikov A, Bronson RT, Benjamin TL. Polyoma virus middle T is essential for virus replication and persistence as well as for tumor induction in mice. *Virology* 1992;191:716–723.
115. Fried M. Cell-transforming ability of a temperature-sensitive mutant of polyoma virus. *Proc Natl Acad Sci U S A* 1965;53:486–491.
116. Fried M, Prives C. The biology of simian virus 40 and polyomavirus. In Botchan M, Grodzicker T, Sharp P, eds. *Cancer cells 4. DNA tumor viruses: Control of gene expression and replication*. Cold Spring Harbor, NY: Cold Spring Harbor Laboratory, 1986:1–16.
117. Fromm M, Berg P. Deletion mapping of DNA regions required for SV40 early region promoter function *in vivo*. *J Mol Appl Genet* 1982;1:457–481.
118. Frost E, Borgaux P. Decapsidation of polyoma virus: Identification of subviral species. *Virology* 1975;68:245–255.
119. Fu X-Y, Manley JL. Factors influencing alternative splice site utilization *in vivo*. *Mol Cell Biol* 1987;7:738–748.
120. Furth P. SV40 rodent tumour models as paradigms of human disease: transgenic mouse models. *Dev Biol Stand* 1998;94:281–287.
121. Gannon JV, Lane DP. Interactions between SV40 T antigen and DNA polymerase α. *New Biol* 1990;2:84–92.
122. Garbe J, Wong M, Wigington D, et al. Viral oncogenes accelerate conversion to immortality of cultured conditionally immortal human mammary epithelial cells. *Oncogene* 1999;18:2169–2180.
123. Gardner SD, Field AM, Coleman DV, Hulme B. New human papovavirus (B.K.) isolated from urine after renal transplantation. *Lancet* 1971;1:1253–1257.
124. Ge H, Manley JL. A protein factor, ASF, controls cell-specific alternative splicing of SV40 early pre-mRNA *in vitro*. *Cell* 1990;62:25–34.
125. Ge H, Noble J, Colgan J, Manley JL. Polyoma virus small tumor antigen pre-mRNA splicing requires cooperation between 3′ splice sites. *Proc Natl Acad Sci U S A* 1990;87:3338–3342.
126. Gharakhanian E, Sajo AK, Weidman MK. SV40 VP1 assembles into disulfide-linked postpentameric complexes in cell-free lysates. *Virology* 1995;207:251–254.
127. Ghosh PK, Lebowitz P. Simian virus 40 early mRNAs contain multiple 5′-termini upstream and downstream from a Hogness-Goldberg sequence: A shift in 5′-termini during the lytic cycle is mediated by large T antigen. *J Virol* 1981;40:224–240.
128. Ghosh PK, Reddy VB, Swinscoe J, et al. The 5′ terminal leader sequence of late 16S mRNA from cells infected with simian virus 40. *J Biol Chem* 1978;253:3643–3647.
129. Ghosh PK, Reddy VB, Swinscoe J, et al. The heterogeneity and 5′ terminal structures of the late RNAs of simian virus 40. *J Mol Biol* 1978;126:813–846.
130. Giacherio D, Hager LP. A poly(dT) stimulated ATPase activity associated with simian virus 40 large T antigen. *J Biol Chem* 1979;254: 8113–8120.
131. Gilinger G, Alwine JC. Transcriptional activation by simian virus 40 large T antigen: Requirements for simple promoter structures contain-

ing either TATA or initiator elements with variable upstream factor binding sites. *J Virol* 1993;11:6682–6688.
132. Ginsberg D, Mechta F, Yaniv M, Oren M. Wild-type p53 can down-modulate the activity of various promoters. *Proc Natl Acad Sci U S A* 1991;88:9979–9983.
133. Girardi AJ, Sweet BH, Slotnick VB, Hilleman MR. Development of tumors in hamsters inoculated in the neo-natal period with vacuolating virus, SV40. *Proc Soc Exp Biol Med* 1962;109:649–660.
134. Glover HR, Brewster CE, Dilworth SM. Association between src-kinases and the polyoma virus oncogene middle T- antigen requires PP2A and a specific sequence motif. *Oncogene* 1999;18:4364–4370.
135. Gluzman Y. SV40 transformed cells support the replication of early SV40 mutants. *Cell* 1981;23:175–182.
136. Gluzman Y, Ahrens B. SV40 early mutants that are defective for viral synthesis but competent for transformation of cultured rat and simian cells. *Virology* 1982;123:78–92.
137. Goldman ND, Brown M, Khoury G. Modification of SV40 T-antigen by poly ADP-ribosylation. *Cell* 1981;24:567–572.
138. Goutebroze L, Feunteun J. Transformation by hamster polyomavirus: Identification and functional analysis of the early genes. *J Virol* 1992;66:2495–2504.
139. Graffi A, Schramm T, Graffi I, et al. Virus-associated skin tumors of the Syrian hamster: Preliminary note. J Natl Cancer Inst 1968;40:867–873.
140. Griffin B, Fried M. Amplification of a specific region of the polyoma virus genome. *Nature* 1975;256:175–179.
141. Griffin BE, Soeda E, Barrell BG, Staden R. Sequence and analysis of polyoma virus DNA. In: Tooze J, ed. *DNA tumor viruses*. Cold Spring Harbor, NY: Cold Spring Harbor Laboratory, 1981:843–910.
142. Griffith GR, Marriott SJ, Rintoul DA, Consigli RA. Early events in polyomavirus infection: Fusion of mono-pinocytotic vesicles containing virions with mouse kidney cell nuclei. *Virus Res* 1988;10:41–52.
143. Gross L. A filterable agent, recovered from Ak leukemic extracts, causing salivary gland carcinomas in C3H mice. *Proc Soc Exp Biol Med* 1953;83:414–421.
144. Gruda MC, Alwine JC. Simian virus 40 (SV40) T antigen transcriptional activation mediated through the Oct/SPH region of the SV40 late promoter. *J Virol* 1991;65:3553–3558.
145. Gruda MC, Zabolotny JM, Xiao JH, et al. Transcriptional activation by simian virus 40 large T antigen: Interactions with multiple components of the transcription complex. *Mol Cell Biol* 1993;13:961–969.
146. Haegeman G, Fiers W. Characterization of the 5′-terminal cap structures of early simian virus-40 RNA. *J Virol* 1980;35:955–961.
147. Halmer L, Vestner B, Gruss C. Involvement of topoisomerases in the initiation of simian virus 40 minichromosome replication. *J Biol Chem* 1998;273:34792–34798.
148. Halvorsen TL, Leibowitz G, Levine F. Telomerase activity is sufficient to allow transformed cells to escape from crisis. *Mol Cell Biol* 1999; 19:1864–1870.
149. Hannon GJ, Demetrick D, Beach D. Isolation of the RB-related p130 through its interaction with CDK2 and cyclins. *Genes Dev* 1993;7: 2378–2391.
150. Hansen U, Tenen DG, Livingston DM, Sharp PA. T antigen repression of SV40 early transcription from two promoters. *Cell* 1981;27:603–612.
151. Harper JW, Adami GR, Wei N, et al. The p21 Cdk-interacting protein Cip1 is a potent inhibitor of G1 cyclin-dependent kinases. *Cell* 1993; 75:805–816.
152. Hartley JW, Rowe WP. New papovavirus contaminating Shope papillomata. *Science* 1964;143:258–260.
153. Hartzell SW, Yamaguchi J, Subramanian KN. SV40 deletion mutants lacking the 21-bp repeated sequences are viable, but have non-complementable deficiencies. *Nucleic Acids Res* 1983;11:1601–1616.
154. Harvey DM, Levine AJ. p53 Alteration is a common event in the spontaneous immortalization of primary Balb/c murine embryo fibroblasts. *Genes Dev* 5:2375–2385.
155. Hay RT, DePamphilis ML. Initiation of simian virus 40 DNA replication *in vivo:* Location and structure of 5′-ends of DNA synthesized in the ori region. *Cell* 1982;28:767–779.
156. Heiser WC, Eckhart W. Polyoma virus early and late mRNAs in productively infected mouse 3T6 cells. *J Virol* 1982;44:175–188.
157. Helin K, Lees J, Vidal M, et al. A cDNA encoding a pRb-binding protein with properties of the transcription factor E2F. *Cell* 1992;70: 337–350.
158. Helin K, Wu C, Fattaey A, et al. Heterodimerization of the transcription factors E2F and DP-1 leads to cooperative transactivation. *Genes Dev* 1993;7:1850–1861.
159. Herbig U, Weisshart K, Taneja P, Fanning E. Interaction of transcription factor TFIID with simian virus 40 (SV40) large T antigen interferes with replication of SV40 DNA *in vitro. J Virol* 1999;73: 1099–1107.
160. Herbomel P, Bourachot B, Yaniv M. Two distinct enhancers with different cell specificities coexist in the regulatory region of polyoma. *Cell* 1984;39:653–662.
161. Huang SG, Weisshart K, Gilbert I, Fanning E. Stoichiometry and mechanism of assembly of SV40 T antigen complexes with the viral origin of DNA replication and DNA polymerase alpha-primase. *Biochemistry* 1998;37:15345–15352.
162. Hummeler K, Tomassini N, Sokol F. Morphological aspects of the uptake of simian virus 40 by permissive cells. *J Virol* 1970;6:87–93.
163. Ishii N, Nakanishi A, Yamada M, et al. Functional complementation of nuclear targeting-defective mutants of simian virus 40 structural proteins. *J Virol* 1994;68:8209–8216.
164. Ito Y, Brocklehurst JR, Dulbecco R. Virus-specific proteins in the plasma membrane of cells lytically infected or transformed by polyoma virus. *Proc Natl Acad Sci U S A* 1977;74:4666–4670.
165. Jarvis DL, Butel JS. Modification of simian virus 40 large tumor antigen by glycosylation. *Virology* 1985;141:173–189.
166. Jat PS, Sharp PA. Cell lines established by a temperature-sensitive simian virus 40 large-T-antigen gene are growth restricted at the non-permissive temperature. *Mol Cell Biol* 1989;9:1672–1681.
167. Jay G, Nomura S, Anderson CW, Khoury G. Identification of the SV40 agnogene product: a DNA binding protein. *Nature* 1981;291: 346–349.
168. Jones NC, Rigby PWJ, Ziff EB. Trans-acting protein factors and the regulation of eukaryotic transcription: Lessons from studies on DNA tumor viruses. *Genes Dev* 1988;2:267–281.
169. Joo WS, Kim HY, Purviance JD, et al. Assembly of T-antigen double hexamers on the simian virus 40 core origin requires only a subset of the available binding sites. *Mol Cell Biol* 1998;18:2677–2687.
170. Kalderon D, Roberts B, Richardson WD, Smith AE. A short amino acid sequence able to specify nuclear localization. *Cell* 1984;39:499–509.
171. Kalderon D, Smith AE. *In vitro* mutagenesis of a putative DNA binding domain of SV40 large-T antigen. *Virology* 1984;139:109–137.
172. Kamen R, Favaloro J, Parker J. Topography of the three late mRNAs of polyomavirus which encode the virion proteins. *J Virol* 1980;33: 637–651.
173. Kamen R, Jat P, Treisman R, Favaloro J. Termini of polyoma virus early region transcripts synthesized *in vivo* by wild-type virus and viable deletion mutants. *J Mol Biol* 1982;159:189–224.
174. Kamen R, Lindstrom DM, Shure H, Old RW. Virus-specific RNA in cells productively infected or transformed by polyoma virus. *Cold Spring Harbor Symp Quant Biol* 1975;39:187–198.
175. Kamen R, Shure H. Topography of polyoma virus messenger RNA molecules. *Cell* 1976;7:361–371.
176. Kartenbeck J, Stukenbrok H, Helenius A. Endocytosis of simian virus 40 into the endoplasmic reticulum. *J Cell Biol* 1989;109:2721–2729.
177. Kasamatsu H, Nehorayan A. VP1 affects the intracellular localization of VP3 polypeptide during simian virus 40 infection. *Proc Natl Acad Sci U S A* 1979;76:2808–2812.
178. Kastan MB, Onyekwere O, Sidransky D, et al. Participation of p53 protein in the cellular response to DNA damage. *Cancer Res* 1991;51: 6304–6311.
179. Keller JM, Alwine JC. Activation of the SV40 late promoter: Direct effects of T antigen in the absence of viral DNA replication. *Cell* 1984;36:381–389.
180. Keller JM, Alwine JC. Analysis of an activatable promoter: Sequences in the simian virus 40 late promoter required for T-antigen–mediated *trans* activation. *Mol Cell Biol* 1985;5:1859–1869.
181. Kelley WL, Georgopoulos C. The T/t common exon of simian virus 40, JC, and BK polyomavirus T antigens can functionally replace the J-domain of the *Escherichia coli* DnaJ molecular chaperone. *Proc Natl Acad Sci U S A* 1997;94:3679–3684.
182. Kelly JJ, Wildeman AG. Role of the SV40 enhancer in the early to late shift in viral transcription. *Nucleic Acids Res* 1991;19:6799–6804.
183. Kenney S, Natarajan V, Strike D, et al. JC virus enhancer-promoter active in human brain cells. *Science* 1984;226:1337–1339.
184. Kern SE, Kinzler KW, Bruskin A, et al. Identification of p53 as a sequence-specific DNA-binding protein. *Science* 1991;252:1708–1711.
185. Ketner G, Kelly TJ. Integrated simian virus 40 sequences in transformed cell DNA: Analysis using restriction endonucleases. *Proc Natl Acad Sci U S A* 1976;73:1102–1106.

186. Khalili K, Brady J, Khoury G. Translational regulation of SV40 early mRNA defines a new viral protein. *Cell* 1987;48:639–645.
187. Khalili K, Brady J, Pipas JM, et al. Carboxyl-terminal mutants of the large tumor antigen of simian virus 40: A role for the early protein late in the lytic cycle. *Proc Natl Acad Sci U S A* 1988;85:354–358.
188. Khoury G, Howley P, Nathans D, Martin M. Posttranscriptional selection of simian virus 40-specific RNA. *J Virol* 1975;15:433–437.
189. Khoury G, May E. Regulation of early and late simian virus 40 transcription: Overproduction of early viral RNA in the absence of a functional T antigen. *J Virol* 1977;23:167–176.
190. Kierstead TD, Tevethia MJ. Association of p53 binding and immortalization of primary C57BL/6 mouse embryo fibroblasts by using simian virus 40 T-antigen mutants bearing internal overlapping deletion mutations. *J Virol* 1993;67:1817–1829.
191. Klessig DF. Adenovirus–simian virus 40 interactions. In: Ginsberg H, ed. *The adenoviruses*. New York: Plenum, 1984:399–449.
192. Klockmann U, Deppert W. Acylated simian virus 40 large T-antigen: A new subclass associated with a detergent resistant lamina of the plasma membrane. *EMBO J* 1983;2:1151–1157.
193. Knudsen E, Buckmaster C, Chen T-T, et al. Inhibition of DNA synthesis by RB: Effects on G1/S transition and S-phase progression. *Genes Dev* 1998;12:2278–2292.
194. Kozak M. Mechanism of mRNA recognition by eukaryotic ribosomes during initiation of protein synthesis. *Curr Top Microbiol Immunol* 1981;93:81–123.
195. Kozak M. Point mutations define a sequence flanking the AUG initiator codon that modulates translation by eukaryotic ribosomes. *Cell* 1986;44:283–292.
196. Krauzewicz N, Streuli CH, Stuart-Smith N, et al. Myristoylated polyomavirus VP2: Role in the life cycle of the virus. *J Virol* 1990;64:4414–4420.
197. Lai C, Nathans D. A map of temperature-sensitive mutants of simian virus 40. *Virology* 1975;66:70.
198. Lai C-J, Nathans D. Deletion mutants of simian virus 40 generated by enzymatic excision of DNA segments from the viral genome. *J Mol Biol* 1974;89:179–193.
199. Lane DP, Crawford LV. T antigen is bound to a host protein in SV40-transformed cells. *Nature* 1979;278:261–263.
200. Lanford RE, Butel JS. Construction and characterization of an SV40 mutant defective in nuclear transport of T antigen. *Cell* 1984;37:801–813.
201. Lania L, Hayday A, Bjursell G, et al. Organization and expression of integrated polyoma virus DNA in transformed rodent cells. *Cold Spring Harbor Symp Quant Biol* 1979;44:597–603.
202. Larose A, Dyson N, Sullivan M, et al. Polyomavirus large T mutants affected in retinoblastoma protein binding are defective in immortalization. *J Virol* 1991;65:2308–2313.
203. Lee TNH, Brockman WW, Nathans D. Evolutionary variants of SV40: Cloned substituted variants containing multiple initiation sites for DNA replication. *Virology* 1975;66:53–69.
204. Lees E, Faha B, Dulic V, et al. Cyclin E/cdk 2 and cyclin A/cdk2 kinases associate with p107 and E2F in a temporally distinct manner. *Genes Dev* 1992;6:1874–1885.
205. Lees JA, Saito M, Vidal M, et al. The retinoblastoma protein binds to a family of E2F transcription factors. *Mol Cell Biol* 1993;13:7813–7825.
206. Legon S, Flavell A, Cowie A, Kamen R. Amplification of the leader sequences of "late" polyomavirus mRNAs. *Cell* 1979;16:373–388.
207. Lehn H, Müller H. Cloning and characterization of budgerigar fledgling disease virus, an avian polyomavirus. *Virology* 1986;151:362–370.
208. Li JJ, Kelly TJ. Simian virus 40 DNA replication *in vitro*. *Proc Natl Acad Sci U S A* 1984;81:6973–6977.
209. Liddington RC, Yan Y, Moulai J, et al. Structure of simian virus 40 at 3.8-A resolution. *Nature* 1991;354:278–294.
210. Lill NL, Grossman SR, Ginsberg D, et al. Binding and modulation of p53 by p300/CBP coactivators. *Nature* 1997;387:823–827.
211. Lill NL, Tevethia MJ, Eckner R, et al. p300 Family members associate with the carboxyl terminus of simian virus 40 large tumor antigen. *J Virol* 1997;71:129–137.
212. Lin W, Hata T, Kasamatsu H. Subcellular distribution of viral structural proteins during simian virus 40 infection. *J Virol* 1984;50:363–371.
213. Linzer DIH, Levine AJ. Characterization of a 54K dalton cellular SV40 tumor antigen present in SV40 transformed cells and uninfected embryonal carcinoma cells. *Cell* 1979;17:43–52.
214. Livingstone LR, White A, Sprouse J, et al. Altered cell cycle arrest and gene amplification potential accompany loss of wild-type p53. *Cell* 1992;70:923–935.
215. Loeber G, Parsons R, Tegtmeyer P. A genetic analysis of the zinc finger of SV40 large T antigen. *Curr Top Microbiol Immunol* 1989;144:21–29.
216. Loeken MR, Bikel I, Livingston DM, Brady J. Trans-activation of RNA polymerase II and III promoters by SV40 small t antigen. *Cell* 1988;55:1171–1177.
217. Lorimer HE, Wang EH, Prives C. The DNA-binding properties of polyomavirus large T antigen are altered by ATP and other nucleotides. *J Virol* 1991;65:687–699.
218. Luo X, Sanford DG, Bullock PA, Bachovchin WW. Solution structure of the origin DNA-binding domain of SV40 T-antigen. *Nature Struct Biol* 1996;3:1034–1039.
219. Mackay RL, Consigli RA. Early events in polyoma virus infection: Attachment, penetration, and nuclear entry. *J Virol* 1976;19:620–636.
220. Magnusson TG, Nilsson M-G. Viable polyoma virus variant with two origins of DNA replication. *Virology* 1982;119:12–21.
221. Mann K. Topoisomerase activity is associated with purified SV40 T antigen. *Nucleic Acids Res* 1993;21:1697–1704.
222. Manos MM, Gluzman Y. Genetic and biochemical analysis of transformation-competent, replication-defective simian virus 40 large T antigen mutants. *J Virol* 1985;53:120–127.
223. Martin RG, Chou JY. Simian virus 40 functions required for the establishment and maintenance of malignant transformation. *J Virol* 1975;15:599–612.
224. Marton A, Jean D, Delbecchi L, et al. Topoisomerase activity associated with SV40 large tumor antigen. *Nucleic Acids Res* 1990;21:1689–1695.
225. Mastrangelo IA, Hough PVC, Wall JS, et al. ATP-dependent assembly of double hexamers of SV40 T antigen at the viral origin of DNA replication. *Nature* 1989;338:658–662.
226. Mateer CA. Executive function disorders: Rehabilitation challenges and strategies. *Semin Clin Neuropsychiatry* 1999;4:50–59.
227. Matson SW, Kaiser-Rogers KA. DNA helicases. *Annu Rev Biochem* 1990;59:289–329.
228. Matsumoto T, Eki T, Hurwitz J. Studies on the initiation and elongation reactions in the simian virus 40 DNA replication system. *Proc Natl Acad Sci U S A* 1990;87:9712–9716.
229. Mattern CF, Takemoto KK, Daniel WA. Replication of polyoma virus in mouse embryo cells: Electron microscopic observations. *Virology* 1966;30:242–256.
230. May E, Omilli F, Ernoult-Lange E, et al. The sequence motifs that are involved in SV40 enhancer function also control SV40 late promoter activity. *Nucleic Acids Res* 1987;15:2445–2461.
231. Mayer M, Dorries K. Nucleotide sequence and genome organization of the murine polyomavirus, Kilham strain. *Virology* 1991;181:469–480.
232. Mazzarelli JM, Atkins GB, Geisberg JV, Ricciardi RP. T antigen (and other oncoproteins) bind TAF-110. *Oncogene* 1995;11:1859–1864.
233. McVey D, Brizuela L, Mohr I, et al. Phosphorylation of large tumour antigen by cdc2 stimulates SV40 DNA replication. *Nature* 1989;341:503–507.
234. Melendy T, Stillman B. An interaction between replication protein A and SV40 T antigen appears essential for primasome assembly during SV40 DNA replication. *J Biol Chem* 1993;268:3389–3395.
235. Melin F, Pinon H, Kress C, Blangy D. Isolation of polyomavirus mutants multiadapted to murine embryonal carcinoma cells. *J Virol* 1985;28:992–996.
236. Melin F, Pinon H, Reiss C, et al. Common features of polyomavirus mutants selected on PCC4 embryonal carcinoma cells. *EMBO J* 1985;4:1799–1803.
237. Mellor A, Smith AE. Characterization of the amino terminal tryptic peptide of simian virus 40 small-t and large-T antigens. *J Virol* 1978;28:992–996.
238. Mertz JE, Berg P. Viable deletion mutants of simian virus 40: Selective isolation by means of a restriction endonuclease from *Haemophilus parainfluenzae*. *Proc Natl Acad Sci U S A* 1974;71:4879–4883.
239. Moarefi IF, Small D, Gilbert I, et al. Mutation of the cyclin-dependent kinase phosphorylation site in simian virus 40 (SV40) large T antigen specifically blocks SV40 origin DNA unwinding. *J Virol* 1993;67:4992–5002.

240. Mohr IJ, Stillman B, Gluzman Y. Regulation of SV40 DNA replication by phosphorylation of T antigen. *EMBO J* 1987;6:153–160.
241. Montano X, Millikan R, Milhaven JM, et al. Simian virus 40 small tumor antigen and an amino-terminal domain of large tumor antigen share a common transforming function. *Proc Nat Acad Sci U S A* 1990;97:7448–7452.
242. Moran E. A region of SV40 large T antigen can substitute for a transforming domain of the adenovirus E1A products. *Nature* 1988;334: 168–170.
243. Moreland RB, Garcea RL. Characterization of a nuclear localization sequence in the polyomavirus capsid protein VP1. *Virology* 1991;185: 513–518.
244. Mortimer EA, Lepow ML, Gold E, et al. Long-term follow-up of persons inadvertently inoculated with SV40 as neonates. *N Engl J Med* 1981;305:1517–1518.
245. Mullane KP, Ratnofsky M, Cullere X, Schaffhausen B. Signaling from polyomavirus middle T and small T defines different roles for protein phosphatase 2A. *Mol* Cell *Biol* 1998;18:7556–7564.
246. Mungre S, Enderle K, Turk B, et al. Mutations which affect the inhibition of protein phosphatase 2A by simian virus 40 small-t antigen *in vitro* decrease viral transformation. *J Virol* 1994;68:1675–1681.
247. Murakami Y, Wobbe CR, Weissbach L, et al. Role of DNA polymerase α and DNA primase in simian virus 40 DNA replication *in vitro. Proc Natl Acad Sci U S A* 1986;83:2869–2873.
248. Myers RM, Rio DC, Robbins AK, Tjian R. SV40 gene expression is modulated by the cooperative binding of T antigen to DNA. *Cell* 1981;25:373–384.
249. Nemethova M, Wintersberger E. Polyomavirus large T antigen binds the transcriptional coactivator protein p300. *J Virol* 1999;73:1734–1739.
250. Nishimura T, Kawai N, Kawai M, et al. Fusion of SV40-induced endocytic vacuoles with the nuclear membrane. *Cell Struct Funct* 1986;11: 135–141.
251. Noble JCS, Pan Z-Q, Prives C, Manley JL. Splicing of SV40 early pre-mRNA to large T and small t mRNAs utilizes different patterns of lariat branch sites. *Cell* 1987;50:227–236.
252. Noble JCS, Prives C, Manley JL. *In vitro* splicing of simian virus 40 early pre-mRNA. *Nucleic Acids Res* 1986;14:1219–1235.
253. Nomura S, Khoury G, Jay G. Subcellular localization of the simina virus 40 agnoprotein. *J Virol* 1983;45:428–433.
254. Padgett BL, Walker DL, ZuRhein GM, et al. Cultivation of a papovalike virus from human brain with progressive multifocal leukoencephalopathy. *Lancet* 1971;1:1257–1260.
255. Pallas DC, Shahrink LK, Martin BL, et al. Polyoma small and middle T antigens and SV40 small t antigen form stable complexes with protein phosphatase 2A. *Cell* 1990;60:167–176.
256. Paucha E, Mellor A, Harvey R, et al. Large and small tumor antigens from SV40 have identical amino termini mapping at 0.65 map units. *Proc Natl Acad Sci U S A* 1978;75:2165–2169.
257. Pauly M, Treger M, Westhof E, Chambon P. The initiation accuracy of SV40 early transcription is determined by the functional domains of two TATA elements. *Nucleic Acids Res* 1992;20:975–982.
258. Phalen DN, Wilson VG, Gaskin JM, et al. Genetic diversity in twenty variants of the avian polyomavirus. *Avian Dis* 1999;43: 207–218.
259. Pipas JM. Mutations near the carboxyl terminus of the simian virus 40 large T antigen alter viral host range. *J Virol* 1985;54:569–575.
260. Pipas JM. Common and unique features of the T antigens encoded by the polyomavirus group. *J Virol* 1992;66:3979–3985.
261. Pipas JM. Molecular chaperone function of the SV40 large T antigen. *Dev Biol Stand* 1998;94:313–319.
262. Polvino-Bodnar M, Cole CN. Construction and characterization of viable deletion mutants of simian virus 40 lacking sequences near the 3′ end of the early region. *J Virol* 1982;43:489–502.
263. Porras A, Gaillard S, Rundell K. The simian virus 40 small-t and large-T antigens jointly regulate cell cycle reentry in human fibroblasts. *J Virol* 1999;73:3102–3107.
264. Rajan P, Dhamankar V, Rundell K, Thimmapaya B. Simian virus 40 small-t does not transactivate polymerase II promoters in virus infections. *J Virol* 1991;65:6553–6561.
265. Rassoulzadegan M, Cowie A, Carr A, et al. The role of individual polyoma virus early proteins in oncogenic transformation. *Nature* 1982;300:713–718.
266. Rassoulzadegan M, Perbal B, Cuzin F. Growth control in simian virus 40-transformed rat cells-temperature independent expression of transformed phenotype in tsA transformants derived by agar selection. *J Virol* 1978;28:1–5.
267. Rassoulzadegan M, Seif R, Cuzin F. Conditions leading to establishment of N (A gene dependent) and A (A gene independent) transformed states after polyoma virus infection of rat fibroblasts. *J Virol* 1978;28:421–426.
268. Ray FA, Peabody DS, Cooper JL, et al. SV40 T antigen alone drives karyotype instability that precedes neoplastic transformation of human diploid fibroblasts. *J* Cell *Biochem* 1990;42:13–31.
269. Rayment I, Baker TS, Caspar DL, Murakami WT. Polyoma virus capsid structure at 22.5 Å resolution. *Nature* 1982;295:110–115.
270. Reddy VB, Ghosh PK, Lebowitz P, Weissman SM. Gaps and duplicated sequence in the leaders of SV40 16S RNA. *Nucleic Acids Res* 1978;5:4195–4213.
271. Reddy VB, Thimmapaya B, Dhar R, et al. The genome of simian virus 40. *Science* 1978;200:494–502.
272. Reed SI, Stark GR, Alwine JC. Autoregulation of SV40 gene A by T antigen. *Proc Natl Acad Sci U S A* 1976;73:3083–3088.
273. Resnick J, Shenk T. Simian virus 40 agnoprotein facilitates normal nuclear location of the major capsid polypeptide and cell-to-cell spread of virus. *J Virol* 1986;60:1098–1106.
274. Rice PW, Cole CN. Efficient transcriptional activation of many simple modular promoters by simian virus 40 large T antigen. *J Virol* 1993; 67:6689–6697.
275. Richardson WD, Roberts BL, Smith AE. Nuclear location signals in polyoma virus large-T. *Cell* 1986;44:77–85.
276. Rio DC, Robbins A, Myers R, Tjian R. Regulation of SV40 early transcription *in vitro* by a purified tumor antigen. *Proc Natl Acad Sci U S A* 1980;77:5706–5710.
277. Rio DC, Tjian R. SV40 T antigen binding site mutations that affect autoregulation. *Cell* 1983;32:1227–1240.
278. Ryder K, Vakalopoulou E, Mertz R, et al. Seventeen base pairs of region I encode a novel tripartite binding signal for SV40 T antigen. *Cell* 1985;42:539–548.
279. Sahli R, Freund R, Dubensky T, et al. Defect in entry and altered pathogenicity of a polyoma virus mutant blocked in VP2 myristylation. *Virology* 1993;192:142–153.
280. Salunke DM, Caspar DLD, Garcea RL. Self-assembly of purified polyomavirus capsid protein VP1. *Cell* 1986;46:895–904.
281. Sambrook J, Westphal H, Srinivasan PR, Dulbecco R. The integrated state of viral DNA in SV40-transformed cells. *Proc Natl Acad Sci U S A* 1968;60:1288–1295.
282. San Martin MC, Gruss C, Carazo JM. Six molecules of SV40 large T antigen assemble in a propeller-shaped particle around a channel. *J Mol Biol* 1997;268:15–20.
283. Sandalon Z, Oppenheim A. Self-assembly and protein-protein interactions between the SV40 capsid proteins produced in insect cells. *Virology* 1997;237:414–421.
284. Scheffner M, Knippers R, Stahl H. RNA unwinding activity of SV40 large T antigen. *Cell* 1989;57:955–963.
285. Scheidtmann K-H, Echle B, Walter G. Simian virus 40 large T antigen is phosphorylated at multiple sites clustered in two separate regions. *J Virol* 1982;44:116–133.
286. Scheidtmann KH, Virshup DM, Kelly TJ. Protein phosphatase 2A dephosphorylates simian virus 40 large T antigen specifically at residues involved in regulation of DNA-binding activity. *J Virol* 1991; 65:2098–2101.
287. Schiedner G, Wessel R, Scheffner M, Stahl H. Renaturation and DNA looping promoted by SV40 large tumour antigen. *EMBO J* 1990;9: 2937–2943.
288. Schmieg FI, Simmons DT. Characterization of the *in vitro* interaction between SV40 T antigen and p53: Mapping the p53 binding site. *Virology* 1988;164:132–140.
289. Schmitt MK, Mann K. Glycosylation of simian virus 40 T antigen and localization of glycosylated T antigen in the nuclear matrix. *Virology* 1987;156:268–281.
290. Schneider C, Weisshart K, Guarino LA, et al. Species-specific functional interactions of DNA polymerase α-primase with simian virus 40 (SV40) T antigen require SV40 origin DNA. *Mol Cell Biol* 1994; 14:3176–3185.
291. Schneider J, Fanning E. Mutations in the phosphorylation sites of simian virus 40 (SV40) T antigen alter its origin DNA-binding specificity for sites I or II and affect SV40 DNA replication activity. *J Virol* 1988;62:1598–1605.

292. Schuchner S, Wintersberger E. Binding of polyomavirus small T antigen to protein phosphatase 2A is required for elimination of p27 and support of S-phase induction in concert with large T antigen. *J Virol* 1999;73:9266–9273.
293. Schuurman R, Sol C, van der Noordaa J. The complete nucleotide sequence of bovine polyomavirus. *J Gen Virol* 1990;71:1723–1735.
294. Sedman S, Gelembiuk GW, Mertz JE. Translation initiation at a downstream AGU occurs with increased efficiency when the upstream AUG is located very close to the 5′ cap. *J Virol* 1990;64:453–457.
295. Sedman S, Good PJ, Mertz JE. Leader-encoded open reading frames modulate both the absolute and relative rates of synthesis of the virion proteins of simian virus 40. *J Virol* 1989;63:3884–3993.
296. Sedman SA, Mertz JE. Mechanisms of synthesis of virion proteins from the functionally bigenic late mRNAs of simian virus 40. *J Virol* 1988;62:954–961.
297. Segawa K, Ito Y. Differential subcellular localization of *in vivo*-phosphorylated and non-phosphorylated middle-sized tumor antigen of polyma virus and its relationship to middle-sized tumor antigen phosphorylating activity *in vitro. Proc Natl Acad Sci U S A* 1982;79:6812–6816.
298. Seif R, Martin RG. Simian virus 40 small t antigen is not required for the maintenance of transformation but may act as a promoter (cocarcinogen) during establishment of transformation in resting rat cells. *J Virol* 1979;32:979–988.
299. SenGupta DJ, Borowiec JA. Strand and face: The topography of interactions between the SV40 origin of replication and T-antigen during the initiation of replication. *EMBO J* 1994;12:982–992.
300. Shay JW, Wright WE. Quantitation of the frequency of immortalization of normal human diploid fibroblasts by SV40 large T-antigen. *Exp Cell Res* 1989;184:109–118.
301. Shenk TE, Carbon J, Berg P. Construction and analysis of viable deletion mutants of simian virus 40. *J Virol* 1976;18:664–672.
302. Shirodkar S, Ewen M, DeCaprio J, et al. The transcription factor E2F interacts with retinoblastoma product and a p107-cyclin A complex in a cell cycle-regulated manner. *Cell* 1992;68:157–166.
303. Simmons DT, Melendy T, Usher D, Stillman B. Simian virus 40 large T antigen binds to topoisomerase I. *Virology* 1996;222:365–374.
304. Simmons DT, Roy R, Chen L, et al. The activity of topoisomerase I is modulated by large T antigen during unwinding of the SV40 origin. *J Biol Chem* 1998;273:20390–20396.
305. Simmons DT, Trowbridge PW, Roy R. Topoisomerase I stimulates SV40 T antigen-mediated DNA replication and inhibits T antigen's ability to unwind DNA at nonorigin sites. *Virology* 1998;242:435–443.
306. Sleigh MJ, Topp WC, Hanich R, Sambrook JF. Mutants of SV40 with an altered small t protein are reduced in their ability to transform cells. *Cell* 1978;14:79–88.
307. Smale ST, Tjian R. T-antigen-DNA polymerase α complex implicated in simian virus 40 DNA replication. *Mol* Cell *Biol* 1986;6:4077–4087.
308. Smelkova NV, Borowiec JA. Dimerization of simian virus 40 T-antigen hexamers activates T-antigen DNA helicase activity. *J Virol* 1997;71:8766–8773.
309. Smelkova NV, Borowiec JA. Synthetic DNA replication bubbles bound and unwound with twofold symmetry by a simian virus 40 T-antigen double hexamer. *J Virol* 1998;72:8676–8681.
310. Soeda E, Arrand JR, Smolar N, Griffin BE. Sequences from the early region of polyoma virus DNA containing the viral replication origin and encoding small, middle and (part of) large T-antigens. *Cell* 1979;17:357–370.
311. Soeda E, Arrand JR, Smolar N, et al. Coding potential and regulatory signals of the polyoma virus genome. *Nature* 1980;283:445–453.
312. Sompayrac L, Danna KJ. The SV40 sequences between 0.169 and 0.423 map units are not essential to immortalize early passage rat embryo cells. *Mol Cell Biol* 1985;5:1191–1194.
313. Sompayrac L, Danna KJ. The amino-terminal 147 amino acids of SV40 large T antigen transform secondary rat embryo fibroblasts. *Virology* 1991;181:412–415.
314. Sontag E, Federov S, Kamibayashi C, et al. The interaction of SV40 small tumor antigen with protein phosphatase 2A stimulates the map kinase pathway and induces cell proliferation. *Cell* 1993;75:887–897.
315. Sontag E, Sontag JM, Garcia A. Protein phosphatase 2A is a critical regulator of protein kinase C zeta signaling targeted by SV40 small t to promote cell growth and NF-kappaB activation. *EMBO J* 1997;16:5662–5671.
316. Soprano KJ, Galanti N, Jonak GK, et al. Mutational analysis of simian virus 40 T antigen: stimulation of cellular DNA synthesis and activation of rRNA genes by mutants with deletions in the T-antigen gene. *Mol Cell Biol* 1983;3:214–219.
317. Srinivasan A, McClellan AJ, Vartikar J, et al. The amino-terminal transforming region of simian virus 40 large T and small t antigens functions as a J domain. *Mol Cell Biol* 1997;17:4761–4773.
318. Srinivasan A, Peden KW, Pipas JM. The large tumor antigen of simian virus 40 encodes at least two distinct transforming functions. *J Virol* 1989;63:5459–5463.
319. Stacy T, Chamberlain M, Cole CN. Simian virus 40 host range/helper function mutations cause multiple defects in viral late gene expression. *J Virol* 1989;63:5280–5215.
320. Stadlbauer F, Voitenleitner C, Bruckner A, et al. Species-specific replication of simian virus 40 DNA *in vitro* requires the p180 subunit of human DNA polymerase alpha-primase. *Mol Cell Biol* 1996;16:94–104.
321. Stahl H, Dröge P, Knippers R. DNA helicase activity of SV40 large tumor antigen. *EMBO J* 1986;5:1939–1944.
322. Staneloni RJ, Fluck MM, Benjamin TL. Host range selection of transformation-defective hr-t mutants of polyoma virus. *Virology* 1977;77:598–609.
323. Staufenbiel M, Deppert W. Different structural systems of the nucleus are targets for SV40 large T antigen. *Cell* 1983;33:173–181.
324. Stehle T, Gamblin SJ, Yan Y, Harrison SC. The structure of simian virus 40 refined at 3.1 A resolution. *Structure* 1996;4:165–182.
325. Stehle T, Harrison SC. Crystal structure of murine polyomavirus in complex with straight-chain and branched-chain sialyloligosaccharide receptor fragments. *Structure* 1996;4:183–194.
326. Stehle T, Harrison SC. High-resolution structure of a polyomavirus VP1-oligosaccharide complex: Implications for assembly and receptor binding. *EMBO J* 1997;16:5139–5148.
327. Stehle T, Yan Y, Benjamin TL, Harrison SC. Structure of murine polyomavirus complexed with an oligosaccharide receptor fragment. *Nature* 1994;369:160–163.
328. Stewart N, Bacchetti S. Expression of SV40 large T antigen, but not small t antigen, is required for the induction of chromosomal alterations in transformed human cells. *Virology* 1991;180:49–57.
329. Stewart SE, Eddy BE, Borgese NG. Neoplasms in mice inoculated with a tumor agent carried in tissue culture. *J Natl Cancer Inst* 1958;20:1223–1243.
330. Stillman BW, Gluzman Y. Replication and supercoiling of simian virus 40 DNA in cell extracts from human cells. *Mol Cell Biol* 1985;5:2051–2060.
331. Streuli CH, Griffin BE. Myristic acid is coupled to a structural protein of polyoma virus and SV40. *Nature* 1987;326:619–622.
332. Strickler HD, Rosenberg PS, Devesa SS, et al. Contamination of poliovirus vaccines with simian virus 40 (1955–1963) and subsequent cancer rates. *JAMA* 1998;279:292–295.
333. Stubdal H, Zalvide J, Campbell KS, et al. Inactivation of pRB-related proteins p130 and p107 mediated by the J domain of simian virus 40 large T antigen. *Mol Cell Biol* 1997;17:4979–4990.
334. Stubdal H, Zalvide J, DeCaprio JA. Simian virus 40 large T antigen alters the phosphorylation state of the RB-related proteins p130 and p107. *J Virol* 1996;70:2781–2788.
335. Summers SA, Lipfert L, Birnbaum MJ. Polyoma middle T antigen activates the Ser/Thr kinase Akt in a PI3-kinase-dependent manner. *Biochem Biophys Res Commun* 1998;246:76–81.
336. Sundin O, Varshavsky A. Terminal stages of SV40 DNA replication proceed via multiple intertwined catenated dimers. *Cell* 1980;21:103–114.
337. Sundin O, Varshavsky A. Arrest of segregation leads to accumulation of highly intertwined catenated dimers: Dissection of the final stages of SV40 DNA replication. *Cell* 1981;25:659–669.
338. Sweet BH, Hilleman MR. The vacuolating virus, SV40. *Proc Soc Exp Biol Med* 1960;105:420–427.
339. Tack LC, Beard P. Both trans-acting factors and chromatin structure are involved in regulation of transcription from the early and late promoters in simian virus 40 chromosomes. *J Virol* 1985;54:207–218.
340. Talavera A, Basilico C. Temperature sensitive mutants of BHK cells affected in cell cycle progression. *J Cell Physiol* 1977;92:425–436.
341. Tapper DP, DePamphilis ML. Discontinuous DNA replication: Accumulation of simian virus 40 DNA at specific stages in its replication. *J Mol Biol* 1978;120:401–422.
342. Tegtmeyer P. Function of simian virus 40 gene A in transforming infection. *J Virol* 1975;15:613–618.

343. Tegtmeyer P, Rundell K, Collins JK. Modification of simian virus 40 protein A. *J Virol* 1977;21:647–657.
344. Tegtmeyer P, Schwartz M, Collins JK, Rundell K. Regulation of tumor antigen synthesis by simian virus 40 gene A. *J Virol* 1975;16:168–178.
345. Tevethia MJ, Lacko HA, Conn A. Two regions of simian virus 40 large T-antigen independently extend the life span of primary C57BL/6 mouse embryo fibroblasts and cooperate in immortalization. *Virology* 1998;243:303–312.
346. Thomas JE, Aguzzi A, Soriano P, et al. Induction of tumor formation and cell transformation by polyoma middle T antigen in the absence of src. *Oncogene* 1993;8:2521–2529.
347. Thompson DL, Kalderon D, Smith A, Tevethia M. Dissociation of Rb-binding and anchorage-independent growth from immortalization and tumorigenicity using SV40 mutants producing N-terminally truncated large T antigens. *Virology* 1990;178:15–34.
348. Thompson JA, Radonovich MF, Salzman NP. Characterization of the 5′ terminal structure of SV40 early mRNAs. *J Virol* 1979;31:437–446.
349. Tjian R, Fey G, Graessmann A. Biological activity of purified SV40 T-antigen proteins. *Proc Natl Acad Sci U S A* 1978;75:1279–1283.
350. Tjian R, Robbins A. Enzymatic activities associated with a purified SV40 T-antigen related protein. *Proc Natl Acad Sci U S A* 1979;76:610–615.
351. Tooze J. DNA tumor viruses. In: *Molecular biology of tumor viruses,* vol, part 2. Cold Spring Harbor, NY: Cold Spring Harbor Laboratories, 1981.
352. Tornow J, Cole CN. Intracistronic complementation in the simian virus 40 A gene. *Proc Natl Acad Sci U S A* 1983;80:6312–6316.
353. Tornow J, Polvino-Bodnar M, Santangelo G, Cole CN. Two separable functional domains of simian virus 40 large T antigen: Carboxyl-terminal region of simian virus 40 large T antigen is required for efficient capsid protein synthesis. *J Virol* 1985;53:415–424.
354. Treisman R, Cowie A, Favaloro J, et al. The structure of the spliced mRNAs encoding polyoma virus early region proteins. *J Mol Appl Genet* 1981;1:83–92.
355. Treisman R, Kamen R. Structure of polyoma virus late nuclear RNA. *J Mol Biol* 1981;148:273–301.
356. Treisman RH, Novack V, Favaloro J, Kamen R. Transformation of rat cells by an altered polyoma virus genome expressing only the middle T protein. *Nature* 1981;292:595–600.
357. Trowbridge PW, Roy R, Simmons DT. Human topoisomerase I promotes initiation of simian virus 40 DNA replication *in vitro. Mol Cell Biol* 1999;19:1686–1694.
358. Tsai J, Douglas MG. A conserved HPD sequence of the J-domain is necessary for YDJ1 stimulation of Hsp70 ATPase activity at a site distinct from substrate binding. *J Biol Chem* 1996;271:9347–9354.
359. Tsurimoto T, Melendy T, Stillman B. Sequential initiation of lagging and leading strand synthesis by two different polymerase complexes at the SV40 DNA replication origin. *Nature* 1990;346:534–539.
360. Tsurimoto T, Stillman B. Replication factors required for SV40 DNA replication *in vitro.* I. DNA structure-specific recognition of a primer-template junction by eukaryotic DNA polymerases and their accessory proteins. *J Biol Chem* 1991;266:1950–1960.
361. Turk B, Porras A, Mumby MC, Rundell K. Simian virus 40 small-t antigen binds two zinc ions. *J Virol* 1993;67:3671–3673.
362. van der Haegen BA, Shay JW. Immortalization of human mammary epithelial cells by SV40 large T-antigen involves a two-step mechanism. *In Vitro Cell Dev Biol* 1993;29:180–182.
363. van Gorder MA, Della Pelle P, Henson JW, et al. Cynomolgus polyoma virus infection: A new member of the polyoma virus family causes interstitial nephritis, ureteritis, and enteritis in immunosuppressed cynomolgus monkeys. *Am J Pathol* 1999;154:1273–1284.
364. Varshavsky AJ, Bakayev VV, Chumackov PM, Georgiev GP. Minichromosome of simian virus 40: Presence of H1. *Nucleic Acids Res* 1976;3:2101–2113.
365. Virshup DM, Kauffman MG, Kelly TJ. Activation of SV40 DNA replication *in vitro* by cellular protein phosphatase 2A. *EMBO J* 1989;8:3891–3898.
366. Virshup DM, Russo A, Kelly TJ. Mechanism of activation of simian virus 40 DNA replication by protein phosphatase 2A. *Mol Cell Biol* 1992;12:4883–4895.
367. Waga S, Bauer G, Stillman B. Reconstitution of complete SV40 DNA replication with purified replication factors. *J Biol Chem* 1994;269: 10923–10934.
368. Waga S, Stillman B. Anatomy of a DNA replication fork revealed by reconstitution of SV40 DNA replication *in vitro. Nature* 1994;369: 207–212.
369. Walter G, Ruediger R, Slaughter C, Mumby M. Association of protein phosphatase 2A with polyoma virus medium tumor antigen. *Proc Natl Acad Sci U S A* 1990;87:2521–2525.
370. Ward JM, Lock A, Collins J, et al. Papovaviral sialoadenitis in athymic nude rats. *Lab Anim* 1984;18:84–89.
371. Watanabe G, Howe A, Lee RJ, et al. Induction of cyclin D1 by simian virus 40 small tumor antigen. *Proc Natl Acad Sci U S A* 1996;93: 12861–12866.
372. Weisshart K, Taneja P, Fanning E. The replication protein A binding site in simian virus 40 (SV40) T antigen and its role in the initial steps of SV40 DNA replication. *J Virol* 1998;72:9771–9781.
373. Weisshart K, Taneja P, Jenne A, et al. Two regions of simian virus 40 T antigen determine cooperativity of double-hexamer assembly on the viral origin of DNA replication and promote hexamer interactions during bidirectional origin DNA unwinding. *J Virol* 1999;73: 2201–2211.
374. Whyte P, Williamson NM, Harlow E. Cellular targets for transformation by the adenovirus E1A proteins. *Cell* 1989;56:67–75.
375. Wildeman AG. Transactivation of both early and late simian virus 40 promoters by large tumor antigen does not require nuclear localization of the protein. *Proc Natl Acad Sci U S A* 1989;86:2123–2127.
376. Wiley SR, Kraus RJ, Zuo F, et al. SV40 early-to-late switch involves titration of cellular transcriptional repressors. *Genes Dev* 1993;7: 2206–2219.
377. Wobbe CR, Dean F, Weissbach L, Hurwitz J. *In vitro* replication of duplex circular DNA containing the simian virus 40 DNA origin site. *Proc Natl Acad Sci U S A* 1985;82:5710–5714.
378. Wold M, Li J, Kelly T. Initiation of simian virus 40 DNA replication *in vitro:* Large-tumor-antigen- and origin-dependent unwinding of the template. *Proc Natl Acad Sci U S A* 1987;84:3643–3647.
379. Wychowski C, Benichou D, Girard M. A domain of SV40 capsid polypeptide VP1 that specifies migration into the cell nucleus. *EMBO J* 1986;5:2569–2576.
380. Xiong Y, Hannon GJ, Zhang H, et al. p21 Is a universal inhibitor of cyclin kinases. *Nature* 1993;366:701–704.
381. Yaciuk P, Carter MC, Pipas JM, Moran E. Simian virus 40 large T antigen expresses a biological activity complementary to the p300-associated transforming function of the adenovirus E1A gene products. *Mol* Cell *Biol* 1991;11:2116–2124.
382. Yamada M, Kasamatsu H. Role of nuclear pore complex in simian virus 40 nuclear targeting. *J Virol* 1993;67:119–130.
383. Yan Y, Stehle T, Liddington RC, et al. Structure determination of simian virus 40 and murine polyomavirus by a combination of 30-fold and 5-fold electron-density averaging. *Structure* 1996;4:157–164.
384. Yang L, Wold MS, Li JJ, et al. Roles of DNA topoisomerases in simian virus 40 DNA replication *in vitro. Proc Natl Acad Sci U S A* 1987; 84:950–954.
385. Yang S-I, Lickteig RL, Estes RC, et al. Control of protein phosphatase 2A by simian virus 40 small-t antigen. *Mol Cell Biol* 1991;64: 1988–1995.
386. Yin Y, Tainsky MA, Bischoff FZ, et al. Wild-type p53 restores cell cycle control and inhibits gene amplification in cells with mutant p53 alleles. *Cell* 1992;70:937–948.
387. Yuen LKC, Consigli RA. Identification and protein analysis of polyomavirus assembly intermediates from infected primary mouse embryo cells. *Virology* 1985;144:127–138.
388. Yuzhakov A, Kelman Z, Hurwitz J, O'Donnell M. Multiple competition reactions for RPA order the assembly of the DNA polymerase delta holoenzyme. *EMBO J* 1999;18:6189–6199.
389. Zalvide J, Stubdal H, DeCaprio JA. The J domain of simian virus 40 large T antigen is required to functionally inactivate RB family proteins. *Mol Cell Biol* 1998;18:1408–1415.
390. Zambetti GP, Bargonetti J, Walker K, et al. Wild-type p53 mediates positive regulation of gene expression through a specific DNA sequence element. *Genes Dev* 1992;6:1143–1152.
391. Zerrahn J, Knippschild U, Winkler T, Deppert W. Independent expression of the transforming amino-terminal domain of SV40 large T an alternatively spliced third SV40 early mRNA. *EMBO J* 1993;12:4739–4746.
392. Zhai W, Comai L. A kinase activity associated with simian virus 40 large T antigen phosphorylates upstream binding factor (UBF) and promotes formation of a stable initiation complex between UBF and SL1. *Mol Cell Biol* 1999;19:2791–2802.

393. Zhai W, Tuan JA, Comai L. SV40 large T antigen binds to the TBP-TAF(I) complex SL1 and coactivates ribosomal RNA transcription. *Genes Dev* 1997;11:1605–1617.
394. Zhu J, Rice PW, Abate M, Cole CN. The ability of SV40 large T antigen to immortalize primary mouse embryo fibroblasts co-segregates with its ability to bind p53. *J Virol* 1991;65:6872–6880.
395. Zhu J, Rice PW, Chamberlain M, Cole CN. Mapping the transcriptional transactivation function of SV40 large T antigen. *J Virol* 1991; 65:2778–2790.
396. Zhu J, Rice PW, Gorsch L, et al. Transformation of a continuous rat embryo fibroblast cell line requires three separate domains of simian virus 40 large T antigen. *J Virol* 1992;66:2780–2791.
397. Zhu J, Wang H, Bishop JM, Blackburn EH. Telomerase extends the lifespan of virus-transformed human cells without net telomere lengthening. *Proc Natl Acad Sci U S A* 1999;96:3723–3728.
398. Zhu Z, Veldman GM, Cowie A, et al. Construction and functional characterization of polyomavirus genomes that separately encode the three early proteins. *J Virol* 1984;51:170–180.
399. Zullo J, Stiles CD, Garcea RL. Regulation of c-myc and c-fos mRNA levels by polyomavirus: Distinct roles for the capsid protein VP1 and the viral early proteins. *Proc Natl Acad Sci U S A* 1987;84:1210–1214.
400. Zuo F, Kraus RJ, Gulick T, et al. Direct modulation of simian virus 40 late gene expression by thyroid hormone and its receptor. *J Virol* 1997;71:427–436.
401. Zuo F, Mertz JE. Simian virus 40 late gene expression is regulated by members of the steroid/thyroid hormone receptor superfamily. *Proc Natl Acad Sci U S A* 1995;92:8586–8590.
402. zur Hausen H, Gissmann L. Lymphotropic papovaviruses isolated from African green monkey and human cells. *Med Microbiol Immunol* 1979;167:137–153.

CHAPTER 30

Papillomaviruses and Their Replication

Peter M. Howley and Douglas R. Lowy

GENERAL DEFINITION AND PROPERTIES

The papillomaviruses are a group of small DNA viruses that induce warts (or papillomas) in a variety of higher vertebrates, including humans. Some papillomaviruses also have malignant potential for animals and people. A number of human papillomaviruses (HPVs) have been implicated as the etologic agents for cervical cancer and other epithelial tumors.

The viral nature of human warts was first indicated more than 90 years ago by Ciuffo, who demonstrated transmission of common warts using cell-free filtrates (48). The first papillomavirus was described in 1933 when Richard Shope recognized the cottontail rabbit papillomavirus (CRPV) as the etiologic agent responsible for cutaneous papillomatosis in the cottontail rabbit (269). This group of viruses remained refractory to standard virologic study for many years because tissue culture systems for the propagation of any of the papillomaviruses in the laboratory did not exist. It was not until the late 1970s, when the first papillomavirus genome was successfully cloned in bacteria, that investigators had reagents that were sufficiently standardized to begin a detailed analysis of the molecular biology of this group of viruses. In addition to standardizing reagents, the molecular cloning of the papillomavirus genomes provided adequate viral genetic material to permit the sequencing of the genomes of a number of papillomaviruses and to initiate a systematic mutational analysis and definition of the genes encoded by this group of viruses. The study of the papillomaviruses was spurred during the 1980s by the development of *in vitro* transformation assays that permitted the analysis of the viral functions involved in the induction of cellular proliferation. The bovine papillomavirus type 1 (BPV-1) initially served as the prototype for studies on various aspects of the molecular biology of the papillomaviruses; therefore, a major focus of this chapter will be on BPV-1. The recognition that specific HPVs are closely linked with cervical cancer, as well as other human tumors, has focused interest on the subgroup of HPVs that are associated with genital tract lesions. Consequently, information on the molecular biology of these HPVs will also be highlighted in this chapter.

CLASSIFICATION

Historically, the papillomaviruses were grouped together with the polyomaviruses to form the papovavirus family. The term papovavirus is derived from the first two letters of the virus first grouped together to form this family of viruses: rabbit papillomavirus, mouse polyomavirus, and simian vacuolating virus (SV40). The properties shared by these viruses include small size, a nonenveloped virion, an icosahedral capsid, a double-stranded circular DNA genome, and the nucleus as the site of viral DNA replication and virion assembly. The papillomavirus particles are about 55 nm in diameter, whereas those of polyomavirus and SV40 are slightly smaller, measuring about 45 nm. Based on this difference in size, the papovavirus family was initially divided into two genera: the polyomaviruses (which include polyomavirus and SV40) and the papillomaviruses. However, comparative molecular biologic studies made possible by the molecular cloning of papillomavirus genomes indicated there were fundamental differences in the genomic organization of the papillomaviruses and the polyomaviruses. Recognition of these differences, as well as others, has led to the papillomaviruses and polyomaviruses now being considered distinct virus families. The genomes of papillomaviruses are larger than are those of polyomaviruses (8,000 base pairs [bp] versus 5,000 bp). Papillomaviruses have more open reading frames (ORFs) than polyomaviruses and encode a different number of structural and nonstructural proteins. The genes of papillomaviruses are all transcribed from the same DNA strand, whereas some polyomavirus genes are transcribed from one strand but others are transcribed from the opposite strand. The two families can also be distinguished by the presence of conserved family-specific epitopes in their major capsid protein (139).

The papillomaviruses are widespread in nature and have been recognized primarily in higher vertebrates. Viruses have been characterized from humans, cattle, rabbits, horses, dogs, sheep, elk, deer, nonhuman primates, the harvest mouse, and the multimammate mouse (*Mastomys natalensis*). Papillomavirus antigens have been identified in a variety of other mammals, including other nonhuman primates (290). Papillomaviruses have also been described in some avian species, namely the parrot and the chafinch. In general, the papillomaviruses are highly species specific, and there are no examples of a papillomavirus from one species causing a productive infection in a second species. Most papillomaviruses have a specific cellular tropism because squamous epithelial cells are associated with purely squamous epithelial proliferative lesions (warts, papillomas). The lesions can be cutaneous or can involve the mucosal squamous epithelium from the oral pharynx, the esophagus, or the genital tract. Expression of the productive functions necessary for virion replication appears to be limited to the terminally differentiating cells of the squamous epithelium.

There is a distinct group of papillomaviruses, found in ungulates, that induce benign fibropapillomas in which there is a proliferative dermal fibroblastic component in addition to the typical proliferative squamous epithelial component. The best studied papillomavirus of this group is BPV-1. Other papillomaviruses that also induce fibropapillomas include BPV-2, the European elk papillomavirus, the deer papillomavirus, and the reindeer papillomavirus. Interest in this subgroup of papillomaviruses stemmed initially from the fact that, in addition to their ability to induce fibropapillomas in their natural host, they have the ability to induce fibroblastic tumors in other species, such as hamsters (90). Members of this group of papillomaviruses can also readily transform a variety of rodent cells in culture. The capacity of BPV-1 to induce morphologic transformation of tissue culture cells was first demonstrated in the early 1960s (23,25,302). Quantitative transformation focus assays were developed for BPV-1 in the late 1970s, which provided a biologic assay to define and study the viral functions involved in the induction of cell proliferation (79). Although most studies have been carried out with BPV-1, it is notable that the European elk papillomavirus and the deer papillomavirus have also been demonstrated to have these transformation properties.

To date, more than 100 different human papillomaviruses have been characterized, and it is estimated that there may be many additional viral types that have not yet been described (64). Because serologic reagents are not generally available to distinguish each of the known HPV types, they are not referred to as serotypes. The classification of viral types is based on the species of origin and the extent and degree of relatedness of the viral genomes. Hence, the HPV types are often referred to as *genotypes.* For most animal species, only a single papillomavirus type has been described, but this is likely because extensive comparative studies have not yet been carried out for most animal species at a molecular level.

The papillomavirus DNA isolates from one species are classified according to their sequence homology. As noted previously, more than 100 HPV types are now recognized. The initial classification of a specific type was based on the extent of homology of the DNA genomes using liquid hybridization techniques under stringent reassociation conditions (51). Classification of types is now carried out by comparison of the nucleotide sequence of specific regions of the genome. Based on criteria adopted by the Papillomavirus Nomenclature Committee, the nucleotide sequences of the *E6, E7,* and *L1* ORFs of a new type should not exceed 90% of the corresponding sequences of the genomes of known HPV types (63). A closer relationship is considered a subtype or variant of the type with the highest degree of homology.

VIRION STRUCTURE

Papillomaviruses are small, nonenveloped, icosahedral DNA viruses that replicate in the nucleus of squamous epithelial cells. The papillomavirus particles have a sedimentation coefficient (S_{20},W) of 300. The papillomavirus particles are 52 to 55 nm in diameter (Fig. 1). The virion

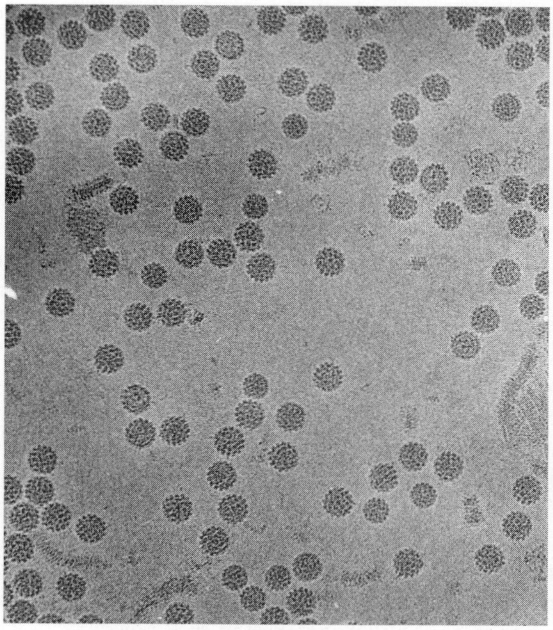

FIG. 1. Electron micrograph of BPV-1 virion particles (55 nm in diameter). (From ref. 10, with permission.)

particles consist of a single molecule of double-stranded circular DNA about 8,000 bp in size, contained within a spherical protein coat, or capsid, composed of 72 capsomers. The virus particles have a density in cesium chloride of 1.34 g/mL (54). Fine structural analysis by cryoelectron microscopy on three-dimensional image reconstruction techniques have revealed that the viruses consist of 72 pentameric capsomers arranged on a T=7 surface lattice (10). Like the polyomavirus capsids, the capsomers exist in two states: one capable of making contact with six neighbors, as observed in the 60 hexavalent capsomers, and the other with 5 neighbors in the 12 pentavalent capsomers (Fig. 2).

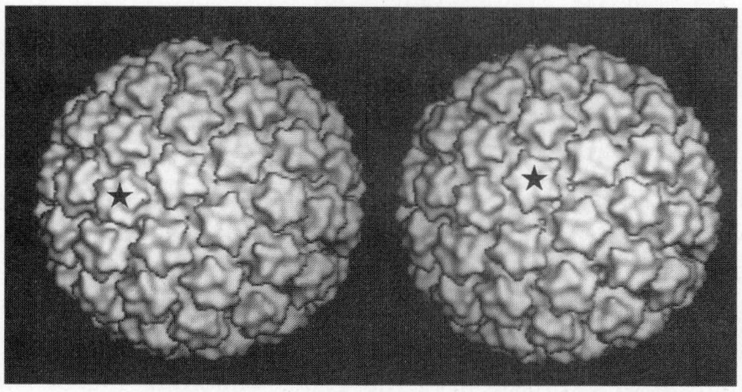

FIG. 2. Surface-shaded displays of papillomavirus three-dimensional image reconstructions of a cryoelectron microscopic analysis of virion particle structures. The individual capsomers exist in either a pentavalent (*starred on left*) or hexavalent (*starred on right*) state. (From ref. 10, with permission.)

The capsid consists of two structural proteins. The major capsid protein (L1) is about 55 kd in size (86,100,222) and represents about 80% of the total viral protein. A minor protein (L2) has a molecular size of about 70 kd. Both of these proteins are virally encoded. In addition, analysis of proteins in the virus particle has shown that the viral DNA is associated with cellular histones to form a chromatin-like complex (86,222). Virus-like particles (VLPs) can be produced from different papillomaviruses by expressing L1 alone or the combination of L1 and L2 using mammalian or nonmammalian expression systems (108,150,243,339). Although not required for assembly, L2 is incorporated into VLPs when coexpressed with L1. The morphology of VLPs containing only L1 appears identical to intact virus particles by cryoelectron microscopy (107). L2 plays a role in the selective encapsidation of papillomavirus DNA in viral capsids and therefore increases the infectivity of papillomavirus virions (338). It colocalizes with the viral E2 transcription and replication factor in PML oncogenic domains (PODs) within the nucleus (60), where it probably fosters virion assembly and perhaps antagonizes some of the activities of E2 (118).

Full papillomavirus particles contain a double-stranded circular DNA viral genome of about 8,000 bp. The guanosine cytosine content of most papillomavirus genomes is about 42%. The DNA constitutes about 12% of the virion by weight, accounting for the density in cesium chloride of about 1.34 g/mL (54).

GENOME STRUCTURE AND ORGANIZATION

The genomes of many of the animal papillomaviruses and human papillomaviruses have been sequenced in their entirety. The genomic organization of each of the papillomaviruses is remarkably similar. The genomic map of BPV-1 DNA is shown in Figure 3. One characteristic of the genomic organization of all of the other papillomaviruses is that all of the ORFs are located on one strand of the viral DNA, indicating that all of the viral genes are located on one strand. Transcriptional studies of the RNAs encoded by the papillomaviruses indicate that only one strand serves as a template for transcription.

The coding strand for each of the papillomaviruses contains about 10 designated translational ORFs that are classified as either early (E) or late (L) ORFs, based on their location in the genome. The early ORFs of the BPV-1 genome are located within the fragment of the BPV-1 genome, which was sufficient for inducing cellular transformation (177). The early region of the viral genome is expressed in nonproductively infected cells and in transformed cells (117). The early region of the papillomavirus genomes encodes viral regulatory proteins, including those viral proteins that are necessary for initiating viral DNA replication. The *L1* and *L2* ORFs encode the viral capsid proteins and are expressed only in pro-

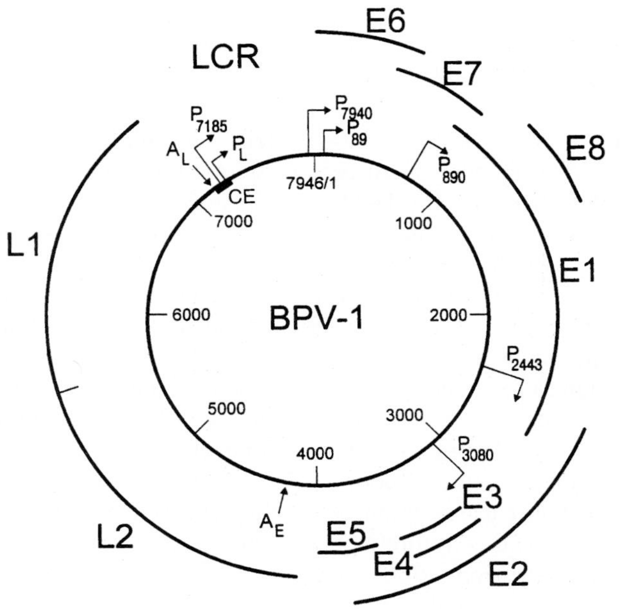

FIG. 3. BPV-1 genomic map. The numbers inside the circle indicate the nucleotide positions. The individual open reading frames of the early (*E*) and late (*L*) regions are depicted as areas outside the double-stranded circular genome. Only one strand is transcribed, and transcription occurs in the clockwise direction. Early promoters are indicated by an arrow labeled P_n, where *n* is the approximate nucleotide position of the RNA initiation site. P_L is the late promoter whose initiation sites map between nucleotides 7214 and 7256. *LCR* designates the long control region, which contains the origin of DNA replication (nucleotides 7911 to 22) (310,328) and the constitutive (*CE*) transcriptional enhancer (nucleotides 7162 to 7275) (312). The early (A_E) and late (A_L) poly(A) sites are located at nucleotides 4203 and 7175, respectively.

ductively infected cells (9). The position, size, and function of many of the ORFs are well conserved among the various papillomaviruses that have been sequenced and studied in detail thus far (7,37). The individual ORFs whose functions have been well characterized are described in more detail in the appropriate sections of this chapter.

There is a region in each of the papillomavirus genomes in which there are no ORFs. The region varies slightly in size among the different papillomavirus genomes; in the BPV-1 genome, it is about 1 kb in size. This region has been referred to by several terms, including the *long control region* (LCR), the *upstream regulatory region*, and the *noncoding region*.

VIRUS REPLICATION

As noted earlier, the papillomaviruses are highly species specific, induce squamous epithelial tumors and fibroepithelial tumors in their natural hosts, and have a specific tropism for squamous epithelial cells. The productive infection of cells by the papillomaviruses can be divided into early and late stages. These stages are linked to the differentiation state of the epithelial cell. Histologically, the lesions induced by papillomaviruses share a number of features. For papillomavirus infections of cutaneous (keratinized) epithelia, there is thickening of the epidermis (acanthosis), usually with some degree of papillomatosis. Keratohyalin granules are often prominent in the granular layer of a keratinized epithelium, and occasionally, basophilic intranuclear inclusions can be detected in the cells of the upper layer of the epidermis. These histologic features reflect the biologic properties of the papillomaviruses; most likely, these morphologic changes are induced by specific viral gene products. The specific tropism of the papillomaviruses for squamous epithelial cells is evidenced by the restriction of the viral replication functions, such as vegetative viral DNA synthesis, the production of viral capsid proteins, and the assembly of virions, to keratinocytes in the process of terminal differentiation. The close link of the papillomavirus life cycle with the differentiation program of the squamous epithelium is depicted in Figure 4.

Because the basal cell is the only cell in the squamous epithelium capable of dividing, the virus must infect the basal cell to induce a lesion that can persist. By *in situ* hybridization, it has been demonstrated that the viral DNA is indeed present within the basal cells and the parabasal cells of a papilloma (263). Furthermore, using probes to the early gene regions of the papillomaviruses, viral transcripts have been detected in the basal cells of the epidermis (283), and at least some early viral protein is found in basal cells (33).

Late gene expression, synthesis of capsid proteins, vegetative viral DNA synthesis, and assembly of virions occur only in terminally differentiating squamous epithelial cells. The link of viral DNA replication to the state of differentiation of the squamous epithelial cell is illustrated in Figure 5B, which shows an *in situ* hybridization of a BPV-1–induced fibropapilloma. Using a BPV-1 DNA probe, which can hybridize to denatured viral DNA, positive hybridization can readily be detected in the nuclei of cells in the middle and upper layers of the squamous epithelium, but not within the cells of the lower portion of the epithelium or within the fibroblasts in the dermis. This represents a relatively short exposure and is only sensitive enough to detect viral DNA in those cells in which there has been significant amplification of the viral DNA (i.e., vegetative viral DNA replication). Thus, vegetative viral DNA synthesis occurs only in differentiating keratinocytes and is therefore linked to the differentiation program of the squamous epithelial cell. The regulation of expression of the genes encoding the capsid protein is at the level of RNA, as demonstrated in the *in situ* hybridization analysis depicted in Figure 5C, in which a probe complementary to the late viral mRNAs localizes the transcripts to the more terminally differentiated keratinocytes within the wart. Conversely, the major

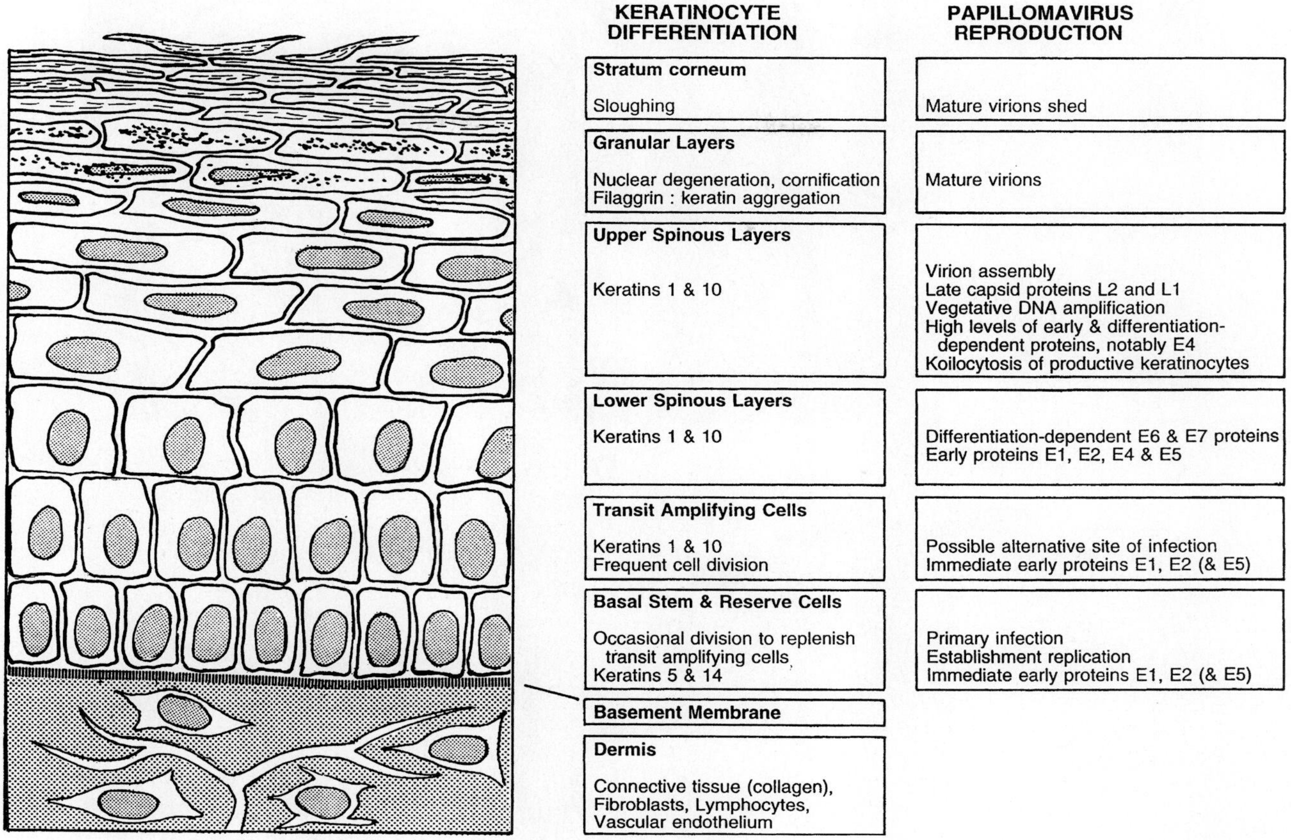

FIG. 4. Differentiation of normal cutaneous squamous epithelium and papillomaviral activities in productively infected benign lesions. The various epithelial strata and the host-differentiation, stage-specific, gene-expression profile are indicated in the *left* and *center* panels. In nonkeratinized squamous epithelia such as cervical or laryngeal, keratins 4 and 13 are expressed in the place of keratins 1 and 10 in the differentiated cells. Although profilaggrin is expressed, there is no granular layer or stratum corneum in nonkeratinized squamous epithelia. The viral activities in the corresponding strata during productive infection shown on the *right* have been determined or inferred from *in situ* hybridization studies. (From ref. 46, with permission.)

capsid protein (L1) can only be detected in the more superficial cells of the wart (139). The replication cycle for the papillomavirus is depicted in Figure 6 and is discussed in detail below in the appropriate sections.

Attachment, Entry, and Uncoating

The first step in viral infection is the binding of the virion to the cell. Binding studies with radiolabeled virions have revealed that the papillomaviruses can bind a wide variety of cell types in addition to the normal host cell, the squamous epithelial cell (197,237). Therefore, the specific tropism of these viruses for keratinocytes does not appear to be due to a cell-type–specific receptor. This observation is consistent with studies with the BPV-1, which have shown that this virus can infect and transform a wide variety of cells, including rodent fibroblasts.

The receptors by which papillomaviruses bind and enter cells have not been unequivocally identified. The α_6 integrin was first identified as a candidate receptor for the papillomaviruses based on studies showing that papillomavirus VLPs bound a protein that was identified as α6 and that antibodies to α6 could block binding of VLPs to cells (85). Recent studies have established that the expression of the α6 integrin in a receptor-negative cell line is sufficient to confer papillomavirus binding to the cell, providing functional evidence for the role of α6 as the receptor (189). The α6 integrin partners with a β integrin subunit, either β1 or β4, on the cell surface. The α6β1 integrin is expressed on a wide range of cells, including platelets, lymphocytes, endothelial cells, and so forth, whereas α6β4 is on relatively restricted epithelial cells, mesenchymal cells, and some neuronal cells (189). Papillomaviruses can bind cells expressing either the α6β1 or the α6β4 complex, although the cells with the highest degree of papillomavirus binding match the α6β4 expression profile. The expression of α_6 is widespread, and it is well conserved among species, consistent with the criteria identified for the papillomavirus

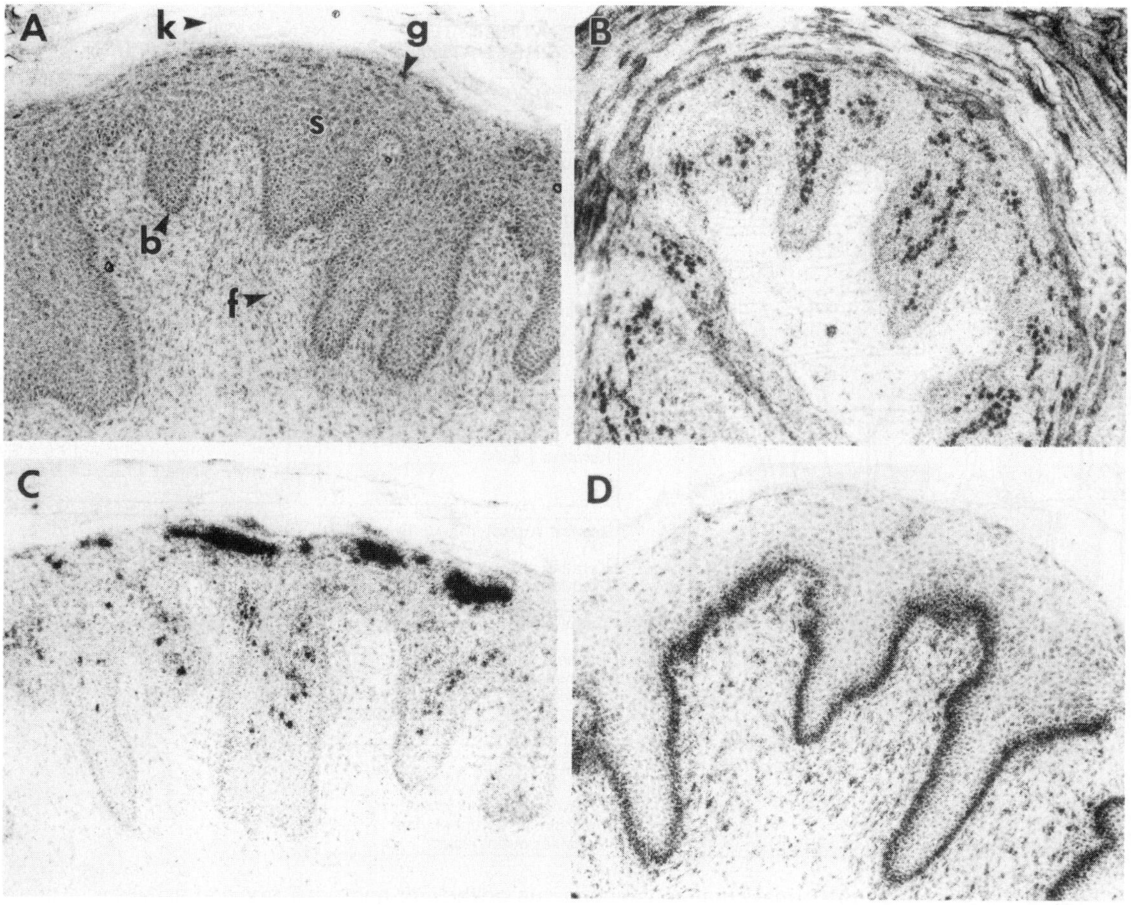

FIG. 5. *In situ* hybridization of a bovine fibropapilloma induced by BPV-1 revealing the linkage of the papillomavirus replication cycle to the squamous epithelial cell differentiation program. **A**: Control section with a sense probe and no denaturation: keratinized horn (*k*), granular layer (*g*), basal layer (*b*), and dermal fibroma (*f*). **B:** Hybridization of a sense probe to a denatured section revealing cells with a high copy number of viral DNA molecules owing to vegetative viral DNA replication. **C:** Hybridization with a probe complementary to the L1 open reading frame indicating late gene expression in the more differentiated epithelial cells of the epithelium. **D:** Hybridization with a probe complementary to a spliced message specific for the E5 transcript revealing maximal expression in the basal cells and some expression in the dermal fibroblasts. (From ref. 14, with permission.)

receptor from the previous binding studies (237). Although evidence suggests that the α6β4 complex is an attractive candidate receptor for papillomaviruses, it is apparently not obligatory because at least some papillomaviruses can infect cells that lack this complex (270). Papillomavirus virions can also bind to heparin and cell surface glycosaminoglycans on human keratinocytes, which may provide an initial binding event that could be followed by receptor binding and internalization (142).

There have been few published studies on the mechanisms by which the papillomavirus enters the cell, gains entry to the nucleus, or uncoats its DNA. It is presumed that these steps proceed similarly to the mechanisms used by the polyomaviruses. In one study using BPV-1, the uptake of the virions was complete by 90 minutes, with most of the capsid antigen localized in the nucleus (337). The virus particles were transported in phagosomes, and their uptake and transport could be inhibited by cytochalasin B and paclitaxel (Taxol), suggesting the possible involvement of microfilaments and microtubules in these processes. Although binding to the plasma membrane and uptake of virions into large cytoplasmic vesicles could be monitored by electron microscopy, no complete virions were observed in the nucleus of infected cells despite a very strong nuclear fluorescent staining for both L1 and L2 proteins (337). This observation suggests that disintegration of the virion occurs in the cytoplasm and that the L1 and L2 proteins may migrate to the nucleus through their nuclear localization signals.

Transcription

The replicative phase of the papillomavirus life cycle has been difficult to study because of its link to the ter-

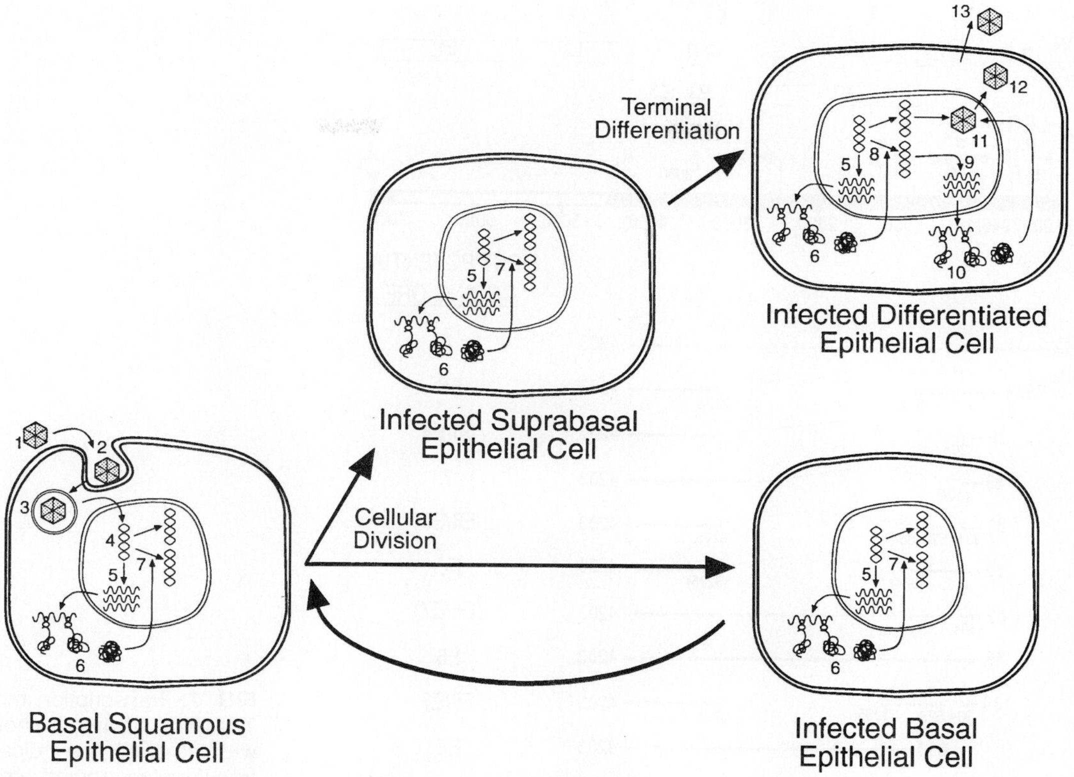

FIG. 6. Replication cycle of a papillomavirus. To establish a wart or papilloma, the virus must infect a basal epithelial cell. Our knowledge is limited about the initial steps in the replication cycle such as attachment (1), uptake (2), endocytosis (3), and transport to the nucleus and uncoating of the viral DNA (4). Early-region transcription (5), translation of the early proteins (6), and steady-state viral DNA replication (7) all occur in the basal cell and in the infected suprabasal epithelial cell. Events in the viral life cycle leading to the production of virion particles occur in the differentiated keratinocyte: vegetative viral DNA replication (8), transcription of the late region (9), production of the capsid proteins L1 and L2 (10), assembly of the virion particles (11), nuclear breakdown (12), and release of virus (13).

minal differentiation program of the epithelium. Historically, BPV-1 has served as the prototype for analyzing the papillomavirus transcription program. The studies have been carried out in a variety of systems, including viral RNAs from rodent cells transformed by BPV-1 as well as those from infected wart tissues. Viral transcription studies have been extended to some of the HPVs associated with genital tract lesions, such as HPV-11, HPV-16, HPV-18, and HPV-31, by using HPV-positive clinical lesions, xenograft tissue in nude mice, cervical carcinoma cell lines, and, more recently, organotypic cultures. This section focuses on BPV-1 and on HPV-31, both of which have been extensively analyzed by *in vitro* culture techniques (192).

Viral RNAs and Promoters

Papillomavirus transcription is complex owing to the presence of multiple promoters, to alternate and multiple splice patterns, and to the differential production of messenger RNA (mRNA) species in different cells. Transcription has been most extensively analyzed for BPV-1, for which seven different transcriptional promoters have been identified (1,9,43,281). Their locations are indicated on the circular genomic map of BPV-1 (see Fig. 3). More than 20 different mRNA species have been identified in BPV-1 transformed cells and in the productively infected cells of fibropapillomas (6). The various RNA species and the genes products they might possibly encode are depicted in Figure 7. The known viral RNA species are often present in very low abundance, making it likely that additional RNA species exist. Most RNA species in warts use a polyadenylation site (A_e) at nucleotide 4180, downstream of the early genes. It is the only polyadenylation site used in transformed rodent cells. The mRNAs in transformed cells principally encode viral factors involved in viral plasmid replication, in the regulation of viral transcription, and in cellular transformation. A second set of RNAs, which are expressed in productively infected cells, use the polyadenylation signal (A_l) at nucleotide 7156, positioned downstream of the *L1* and *L2* ORFs. RNAs that use this late polyadenylation site are

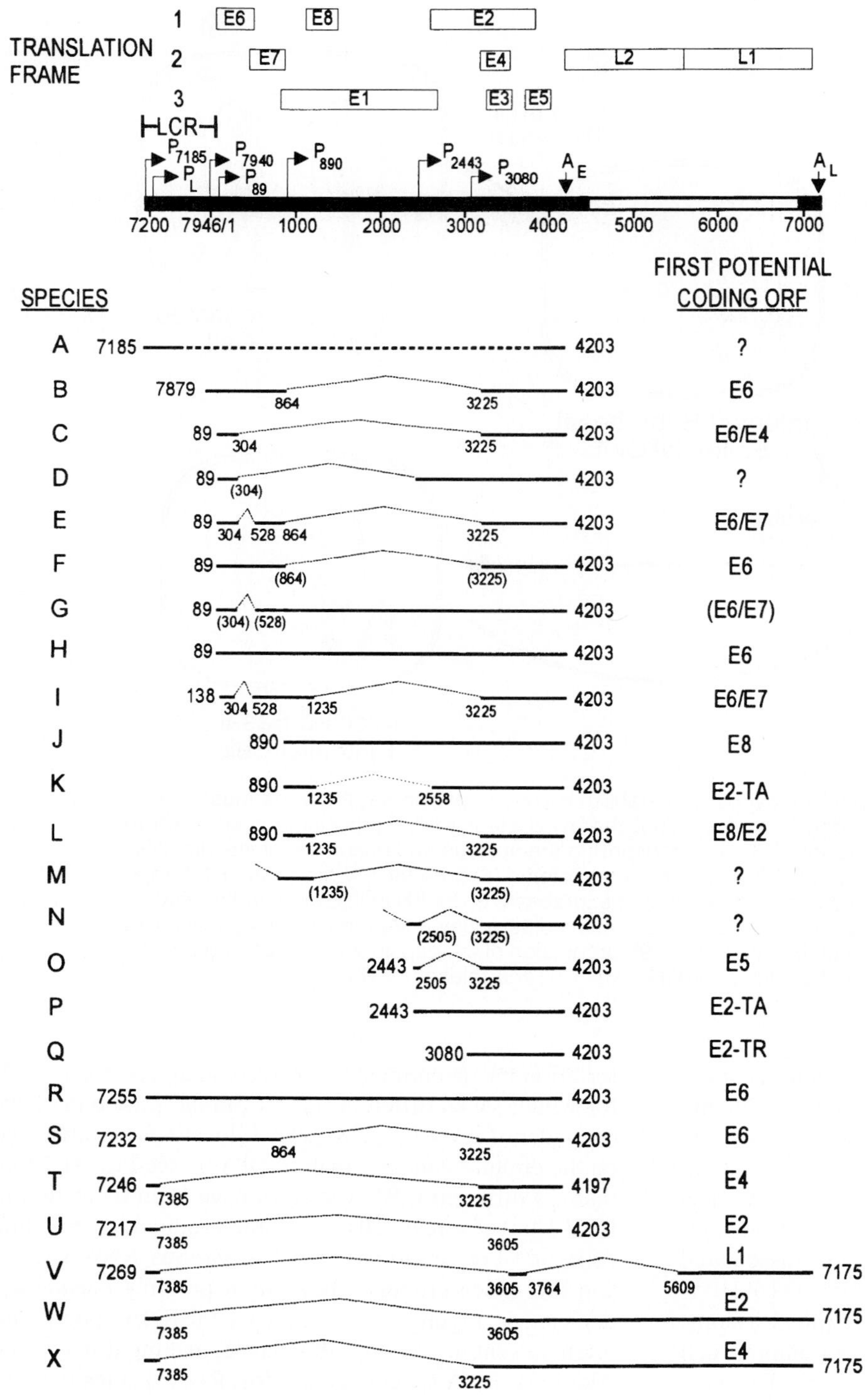

FIG. 7. Transcription map of BPV-1. The genomic map is shown at the *top,* with the *black line* indicating the 69% transforming region containing the long control region (LCR) and the early-region open reading frames (ORFs). The known promoters and poly(A) sites are indicated. The structures of the species A to Q were determined from RNA species in BPV-1 transformed mouse C127 cells by cyclic DNA (cDNA) cloning, electron microscopy, nuclease protection, polymerase chain reaction (PCR), and primer extension. The 5′-most ORF, which is likely to be encoded by the messenger RNA (mRNA) species, is indicated to the *right.* Structures of additional mRNAs that appear to be unique for productively infected BPV-1 fibropapillomas (species R to X) were determined by reverse transcription–PCR and cDNA cloning. Although E2 and E4 are the first significant ORFs for the W and X species, these mRNAs could also encode the L2 capsid protein. (From ref. 6, with permission.)

found only in the terminally differentiating keratinocytes of fibropapillomas and are absent in transformed cells and in the nonproductively infected cells of BPV-1 fibropapillomas. The control of late transcription is complex and involves at least three regulatory mechanisms, as discussed later.

Six of the transcriptional promoters for BPV-1 are active in transformed cells. These promoters are also active in productively infected fibropapillomas (9). The nomenclature that has been generally adopted for use in the papillomavirus field designates the promoters (P) with a subscript indicating the nucleotide position of the 5′ end of the most abundant RNA species expressed from the designated promoter. Thus, for BPV-1, P_{89} is the promoter that has its major transcription start at nucleotide 89. Another promoter, P_{2443}, gives rise to RNA species with 5′ ends heterogeneously mapping in the vicinity of nucleotide 2443. The six promoters active in transformed cells that have been mapped to date are P_{89}, P_{890}, P_{2443}, P_{3080}, P_{7185}, and P_{7940} (1,9,43,281,282). One additional promoter, P_{7250}, is referred to as the *major late promoter* (P_L) and is principally active in productively infected keratinocytes, giving rise to the late mRNA species containing the *E4* and *L1* ORFs (9).

A variety of mRNA and promoter mapping studies have also been carried out with the genital tract–associated papillomaviruses, most notably HPV-11, HPV-16, HPV-18, and HPV-31. A transcription map of HPV-31 is shown in Figure 8. As with BPV-1, multiple promoters are involved in generating the various mRNA species for the genital tract HPVs. For HPV-31, P_{97} is the major promoter active in nonterminally differentiated cells. This promoter, which directs the expression of E6 and E7 as well as several other early gene products, is analogous to P_{97} of HPV-16 and P_{105} of HPV-18. Upon differentiation of immortalized keratinocytes harboring episomal HPV-31 DNA, there is activation of the differentiation-dependent late promoter P_{742}, which directs the expression of the late gene products, including E4, L1, and L2, as well as an increase in the level of the E1 mRNA (153,244).

An important difference in the structures of the E6 and E7 mRNAs and in the manner by which they are expressed distinguishes the high-risk and low-risk HPV types. As discussed in detail in Chapter 66 in *Fields Virology*, 4th ed., the HPVs associated with the genital tract lesions can be divided into high-risk (e.g., HPV types 16 and 18) and low-risk (e.g., HPV types 6 and 11) categories based on the risk for malignant progression of the lesions they induce in the cervix. For the high-risk HPVs, such as HPV-16 and HPV-18, a single promoter (P_{97} for HPV-16 and HPV-31, or P_{105} for HPV-18) directs the synthesis of mRNAs with *E6* and *E7* intact or with splices in the *E6* gene (see Fig. 8). The species with *E6* intact could be translated into E6 but not E7 because there is insufficient spacing for translation reinitiation. The mRNAs with the spliced *E6* splice the 5′ end of the *E6* ORF (referred to as E6*) to a translation frame with stop codons that provides sufficient spacing for translation reinitiation of the *E7* ORF and are therefore likely to represent the E7 mRNAs. In contrast, the *E6* and *E7* genes of the low-risk HPVs, such as HPV-6 and HPV-11, are expressed from two independent promoters (46).

Regulation of Transcription (cis Elements)

Papillomavirus transcription is tightly regulated by the differentiation state of the infected squamous epithelial cell. This is evident in part through the analysis of the differential expression of viral RNAs in the cells in the different levels of the epithelium in warts (14,47). It is also evident *in vitro* through the analysis of infected keratinocytes using organotypic and suspension tissue culture systems that permit epithelial cell differentiation (72,153,191). Cells transformed by bovine papillomavirus have provided a useful model for examining transcriptional regulation in the nonproductively infected cell, in which transcription is also tightly regulated. The genomes of the papillomaviruses contain multiple cis regulatory elements and encode several transcriptional factors that modulate viral gene expression.

The LCR region of papillomavirus contains enhancer elements that are responsive to cellular factors as well as to virally encoded transcriptional regulatory factors. All of the viral LCRs that have been studied in detail have been found to contain constitutive enhancer elements that have some tissue or cell-type specificity (245). This was first established for HPV-16 and HPV-18 (55,297) and has also been shown for HPV-11 (42) as well as for BPV-1 (312,313). It is thought that these constitutive enhancer elements are essential for the initial expression of the viral genes after virus infection and that they may also be important in the maintenance of viral latency. A number of transcription factor–binding sites have been identified in the LCRs of the various papillomaviruses that have been carefully studied. Included among them are sites that bind AP1, SP1, Oct-1, and YY1, among others (17,36,44,45,123,210,299). The HPV-16 LCR has also recently been shown to contain nuclear matrix attachment sites that may be important for controlling viral gene expression (295).

In addition to the binding sites for cellular transcription factors, the LCR contains binding sites for the virally encoded E2 regulatory proteins and the origin of DNA replication that binds the E1 replication factor, discussed in some detail later.

E2 Regulatory Proteins

The papillomavirus *E2* gene products are important regulators of viral transcription and replication. The *E2* gene product of BPV-1 was first described as a transcriptional activator (278) capable of activating viral transcription through E2-responsive elements located within the viral genome (276). The E2 proteins are relatively well conserved among the papillomaviruses in two domains: a sequence-specific DNA-binding and dimerization domain located in the carboxyl-terminal region of the protein, and a transactivating domain that is located within the amino-terminal half of the protein (99,187). These two domains are separated by an internal hinge region, which is not well conserved in size nor in amino acid composition among different papillomaviruses. The E2 proteins bind the consensus sequence, $ACCN_6GGT$ (2,174), and can regulate transcription from promoters containing E2-binding sites (112,122,275). E2 binds $ACCN_6GGT$ motifs as a dimer; the DNA-binding dimerization domain localizes to the carboxyl terminus of E2 (188).

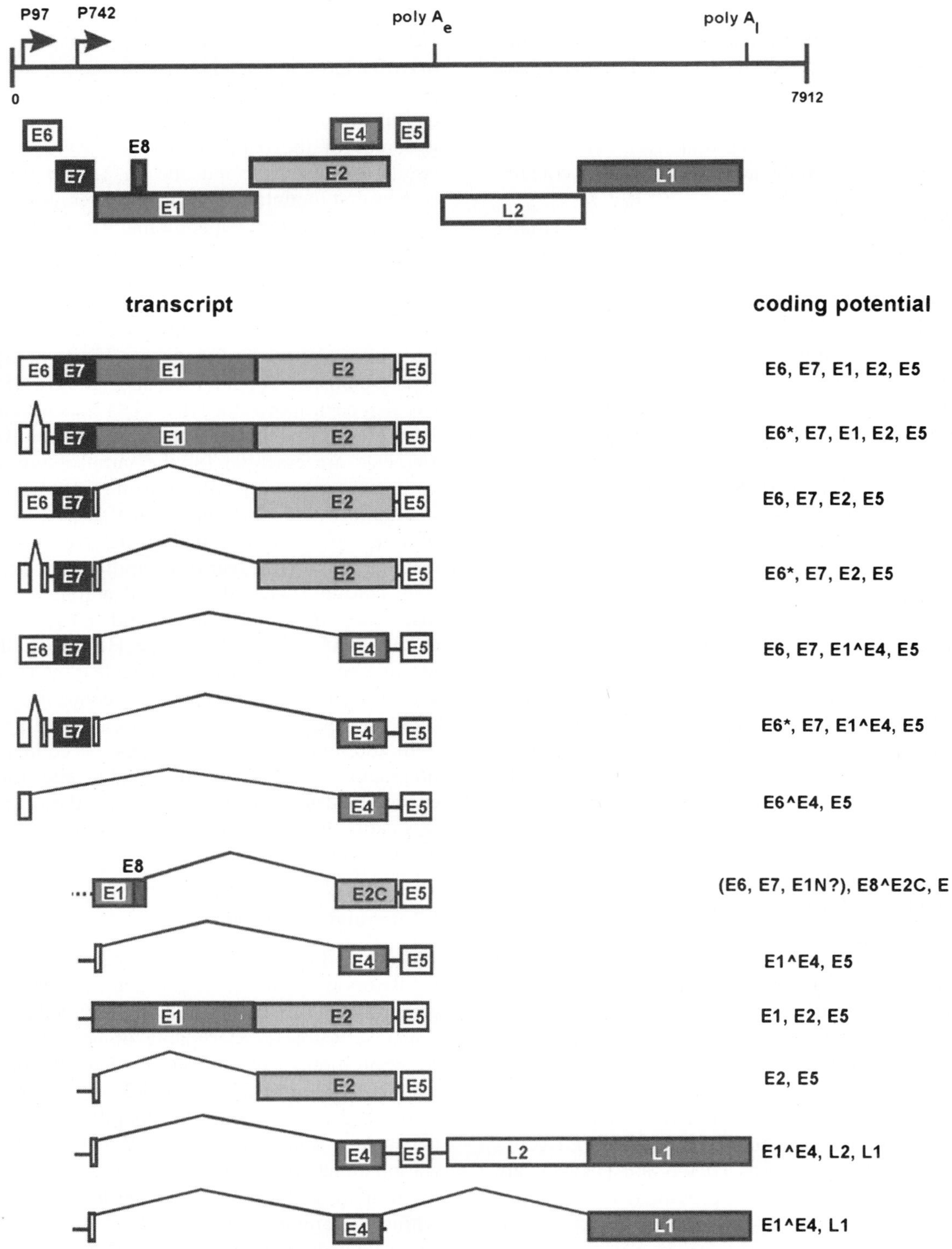

FIG. 8. Transcription map of HPV 31 (134,135,153,213). A linearized version of the genomic map is shown at the *top.* Transcripts initiated at the early viral promoter, designated P_{97}, are expressed in the nonterminally differentiated cells in the lower portion of the epithelium, whereas those initiating at the late promoter (P_{742}) are expressed upon differentiation in the cells committed to the replication of the progeny virions. (From ref. 289, with permission.)

.e E2 proteins have been best studied in the BPV system, where three species have been identified (Fig. 9). The full-length protein (E2TA) can function as a transactivator or a repressor, depending on the location of the E2-binding sites within the enhancer or promoter region (Fig. 10). The two shorter forms of E2, called E2TR and E8/E2, have been described as repressors because they can inhibit the transactivation function of the full-length E2TA (161,162). The shorter E2 proteins contain the DNA-binding and dimerization domains of the C-terminus but lack the transactivation domain. E2TR and E8/E2 can inhibit the transcriptional transactivating function of the full-length polypeptide by competing for its cognate DNA-binding sites and by forming inactive heterodimers with the full-length transactivator protein. The crystal structure of the dimeric DNA-binding domain of BPV-1 E2 revealed a previously unobserved structure for a DNA-binding protein, which is a dimeric antiparallel β-barrel (116). The crystal structure of the N-terminal transactivation domain has also been resolved for HPV-16 and HPV-18 (5,110). The structural studies of the E2 N-terminal domain indicated that it could form a dimer both in the crystal and in solution. Because amino acids that are necessary for transactivation are located at the dimer interface, the dimer structure may be important in the interactions of E2 with viral and cellular transcription factors. The dimer formation may contribute to the stabilization of DNA loops, which may serve to relocate distal DNA-binding transcription factors to the site of human papillomavirus transcription initiation (5).

Mutations in the BPV-1 *E2* ORF have pleiotropic effects on the virus, disrupting transformation, replication, and transcriptional regulation functions. Studies have shown that expression of the early region viral genes is under the control of the viral *E2* gene product through E2-responsive elements located within the viral LCR. The BPV-1 genome contains 17 E2-binding sites (ATTN$_6$GGT), of which 12 are located in the LCR (174). Pairs of the E2-binding sites are sufficient to function as an E2-dependent enhancer (2,113,275). The major E2-dependent enhancer in the LCR, E2RE1, contains four high-affinity E2-binding sites (276) and is located upstream of the P_{89} promoter complex. In addition to activating the P_{89} promoter, E2 can also activate each of the early region promoters (P_{890}, P_{2443}, and P_{3080}) through the E2-dependent enhancer elements in the LCR. Despite

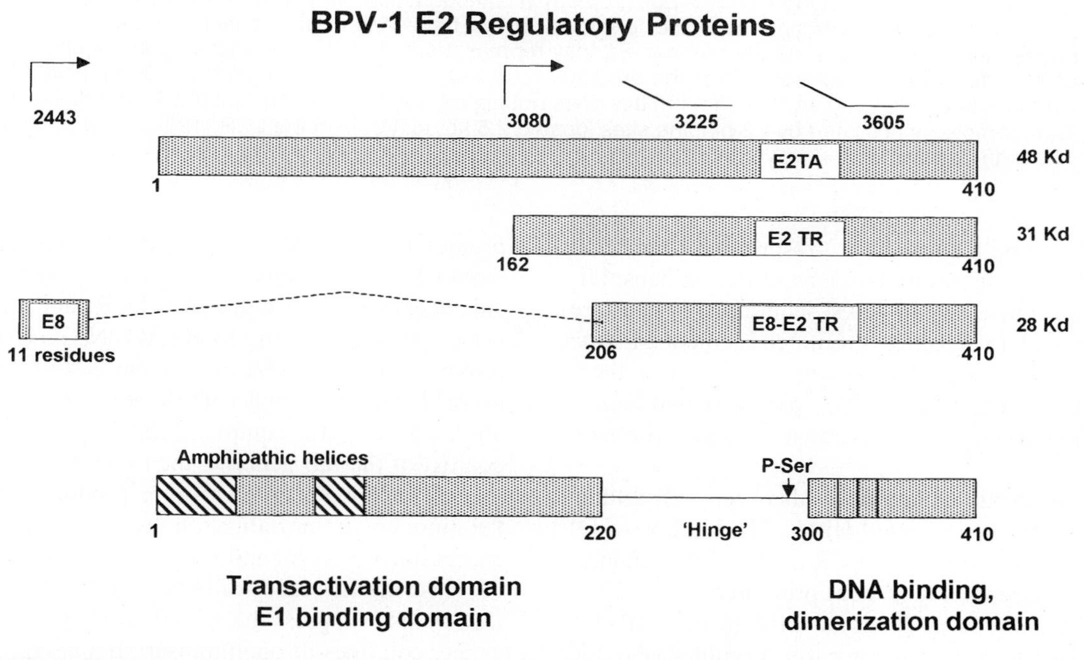

FIG. 9. Structure of the BPV-1 *E2* gene products. The structures of the three known proteins encoded by the BPV-1 *E2* open reading frame are indicated. The 48-kd full-length E2 transactivator can be expressed from an unspliced message from P_{2443} or from a spliced messenger RNA (mRNA) from upstream promoters by using a splice acceptor at nucleotide 2558. The 31-kd and 28-kd forms of the repressor are expressed from P_{3080} and as an E8:E2 fusion by a spliced mRNA as shown, respectively. The transactivation domain consists of a region of about 200 amino acids at the N-terminal region of the full-length E2 protein that is relatively well conserved among papillomaviruses. This region, which is acidic and is predicted to contain amphipathic helices, is only present in the full-length form of E2. The N-terminus of E2 contains the site for binding E1. The 110 C-terminal amino acids are also conserved and make up the DNA-binding and dimerization domain. (Modified from ref. 188, with permission.)

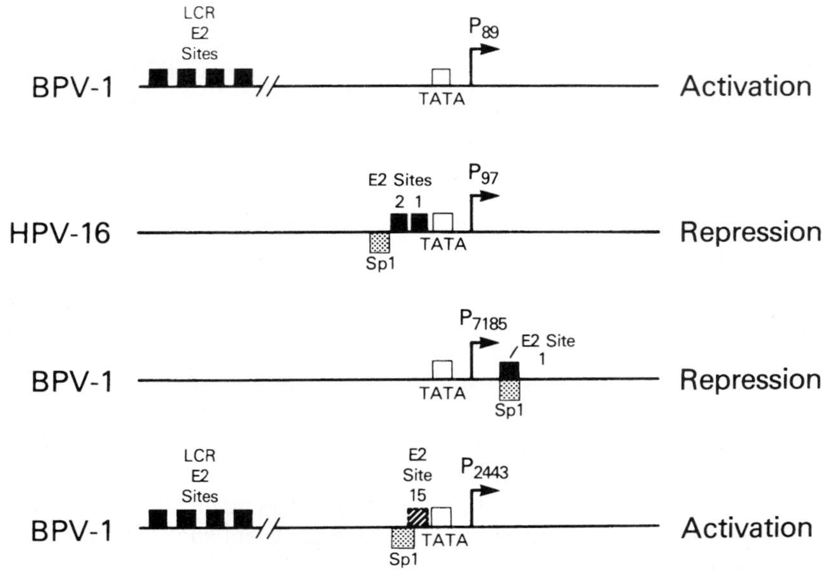

FIG. 10. Papillomavirus E2 transcriptional regulation. Transcriptional activation or repression by E2 depends on the position and proximity of the E2-binding sites in the promoter with respect to the promoter. In this figure, only the E2-binding sites in close proximity to the promoters are indicated. Several E2-binding sites in the BPV-1 long control region (*LCR*) are positioned several hundred base pairs upstream of P_{89}, which is activated by E2 (111,276). The HPV-16 P_{97} promoter (and the analogous P_{105} and P_{97} promoters in HPV-18 and HPV-31, respectively), which directs the synthesis of the E6 and E7 viral oncoproteins, is repressed by E2 through occupancy of E2-binding sites, which overlap an SP1 site and are in close proximity to the TATA box (22,298). It is thought that through displacement of SP1 from the promoter and interference with the formation of the transcription preinitiation complex, E2 may repress transcription. In a similar manner, E2 may repress the BPV-1 P_{7185} promoter by interfering with SP1 binding to a site downstream of the promoter (280,312). The P_{2443} promoter has a low-affinity E2-binding site overlapping an SP1 site, but this does not appear to play an important role in its regulation. The promoter is activated by E2-binding sites located 2.5 kb upstream in the LCR (120,277). (From ref. 188, with permission.)

this dependence on a common E2-responsive element in the LCR, the various promoters have different sensitivities to the E2 transactivator (293). These differences are most likely due to specific promoter elements in the vicinities of the individual promoters. For instance, there is an SP1 site upstream of the P_{2443} promoter that is necessary for both its basal and E2-transactivated expression (277).

E2 transcriptional regulation has also been well studied for the genital tract–associated HPVs. The binding of E2 to its cognate sites within the LCR of the HPV genomes results in the modulation of viral promoter activity. The *E6* and *E7* transforming genes of HPV-16 and HPV-18 are transcribed from the major early promoter (P_{97} and P_{105}, respectively) contained within the LCR of their respective genomes (272,300). Analyses of promoter activity in human epithelial cells have shown that the P_{97} promoter of HPV-16 and the P_{105} promoter of HPV-18 possess a basal activity that can be repressed by full-length *E2* gene products (22,241,298,300). There are four E2-binding sites within the LCRs of the HPV-16 and HPV-18 genomes. Two E2-binding sites are located immediately adjacent to the TATA box of the P_{97} and P_{105} promoters of HPV-16 and HPV-18, respectively. The basal activity is dependent on the keratinocyte-dependent enhancer contained within the LCR, and E2 repression occurs through binding to the $ACCN_6GGT$ sites in close proximity to the TATA box of the early promoter, most probably by interfering with the assembly of the preinitiation transcription complex (22,55,241,291,300). In the context of the full genome, the modulation of HPV gene expression by *E2* is even more pronounced. In human keratinocyte immortalization assays dependent on the expression of the *E6* and *E7* genes, an intact *E2* gene can decrease the efficiency of HPV-16 immortalization (240). E2 can also suppress the growth of HPV-positive cervical cancer cell lines through transcriptional repression of the viral *E6* and *E7* genes (76,89,136,208,300). These results are consistent with the model that at certain concentrations, E2 can repress the viral P97 promoter through binding to the E2 DNA-binding sites in the proximity of the promoter. In contrast to the repression mediated by E2 on the expression of the high-risk HPVs, in BPV-1, the full-length E2TA stimulates the expression of a number of viral genes, including *E2* itself and *E5* (120,229). This finding has raised the question of whether the transcrip-

TABLE 1. *Cellular targets and functions of the papillomavirus E2 oncoproteins*

Associated cellular proteins	Functional consequences	References
TATA-binding protein (TBP)		233
TFIIB		20, 233
AMF-1/Gps2	Enhance transcriptional activation	30
	Enhance E2 interaction with p300	217
YY1		166

tional activation function of E2 is essential for the high-risk HPVs. Indeed, it was recently shown that an HPV-31 genome that carried a mutant *E2* gene, which was defective for transactivation but competent for DNA replication, could still be established as a stable episome and could induce differentiation-dependent late functions (288). Thus, the specific role of E2 as a transcriptional regulator may vary among different papillomavirus types.

E2 is a multifunctional protein. Its functions as a transcriptional activator and repressor are likely mediated by interactions with specific cellular factors, some of which have now been identified (Table 1). In addition to its role as a transcriptional regulator, E2 has critical roles in viral DNA replication and in plasmid maintenance. E2TA, together with the viral E1 protein, is essential for viral DNA replication (41,62,309). E2 may serve as an auxiliary protein in viral DNA replication. This aspect has been best studied in the BPV system, in which E2 was first shown to complex with E1 and to strengthen the affinity of E1 for binding to the origin of DNA replication (195,309). Long-term maintenance of plasmids containing a papillomavirus origin of DNA replication, however, also requires a minichromosome maintenance element, a cis element consisting of multiple E2-binding sites (226). The role of E2TA in plasmid maintenance appears to be due to its role in linking the viral plasmids to the cellular mitotic chromosomes, thereby ensuring that the viral genomes are enclosed within the nuclear envelope for when it reforms during telophase (16,170,271).

Late Gene Expression

The viral late functions, such as vegetative viral DNA synthesis, capsid protein synthesis, and virion assembly, occur exclusively in differentiated keratinocytes. Transcriptional regulation of the late genes has been most extensively studied for BPV-1, HPV-11, HPV-16, and HPV-31. For each of these viruses, there is a specific promoter, which becomes active only in terminally differentiated keratinocytes. For BPV-1, the late RNAs are transcribed from a wart-specific or late promoter (P_L) at nucleotide 7250 that is located in the 5′ end of the LCR (9) (see Fig. 7). Both the *L1* and *L2* genes are expressed from mRNAs transcribed from P_L (14). In addition to the L1 and L2 mRNA species, this promoter also gives rise to other viral mRNAs that are specific for terminally differentiated cells. For instance, one abundant mRNA from P_L gives rise to the message that appears to encode the E4 protein (9), an abundant cytoplasmic protein found predominantly in the differentiated keratinocytes of the wart (73). Thus, although E4 is located in the early region of the viral genomes (see Figs. 3 and 4), it is a late protein by virtue of the promoter from which it is expressed. Interestingly, the late promoters for the human papillomaviruses that have been analyzed do not map to the LCR. Instead, a differentiation-specific promoter has been identified within the E7 coding region of the HPV-31 genome that gives rise to mRNA species whose 5′ ends map to nucleotide 742 (134) (see Fig. 8). The late promoter in HPV-11 also maps to the E7-coding region (46).

Polyadenylation of the BPV-1 L1- and L2-specific mRNAs occurs 3′ to the *L1* ORF at nucleotide 7175, a site not used in transformed cells and therefore considered the late poly(A) site (A_L) (9) (see Fig. 7). In the HPVs that have been analyzed, polyadenylation occurs in a similar region of the genome, 3′ to the *L1* ORF (see Fig. 8).

Papillomavirus *L1* and *L2* gene expression is also regulated at a posttranscriptional level. There are cis-acting elements that have been described for BPV-1, HPV-16, and HPV-1, which serve important roles in regulating late gene expression for these viruses at a posttranscriptional level. In the 3′-untranslated regions (3′-UTRs) of the late RNAs of each of these viruses, there are negative regulatory elements that can inhibit the generation of stable late mRNAs. In the BPV-1 late 3′-UTR, there is an unused 5′ splice element that binds the U1 small nuclear ribonuclear protein and inhibits late polyadenylation, thereby favoring use of the early polyadenylation site (93,94). A negative regulatory element in the HPV-16 3′-UTR contains multiple 5′ splice-like sequences, as well as an inhibitory GU-rich region that reduces mRNA stability, that bind to (65,147,154) three different cellular factors (the U2 auxiliary splicing factor 65-kd subunit, the cleavage stimulation factor 64-kd subunit, and the Elav-like HuR protein) (154). In HPV-1, an AU-rich inhibitory region has been identified in the 3′ UTR that also binds the Elav-like HuR protein (273). The model emerges that these, and perhaps additional cellular factors, are responsible for the nuclear retention or cytoplasmic instability of the nuclear retention element (NRE)–containing late transcripts. Keratinocyte differentiation would then lead to changes in these cell-encoded factors, thus relieving the inhibition of late mRNA processing.

E4 Proteins

The *E4* ORF of the papillomaviruses is located in the early region (see Figs. 3, 7, and 8), yet it is expressed as a late gene with a role in productive infection. It overlaps the *E2* ORF in a different reading frame and therefore encodes a protein with an entirely different amino acid sequence. In general, the *E4* gene is not highly conserved among the papillomaviruses. Transcripts that could encode E4 proteins have been described both for BPV-1 and the HPVs (see Figs. 7 and 8). A viral transcript formed by splicing a few codons from the beginning of E1 to E4 appears to be the major RNA in HPV-induced lesions for the viruses that have been studied. In papillomas, the E4 proteins are expressed primarily in the differentiating layers of the epithelium, and the E4 proteins are expressed in cells in which vegetative viral DNA replication is ongoing (75). The expression of E4 is not coincident with the expression of the capsid proteins (75), and E4 expression precedes the expression of L1 (56). Although the E4 proteins are expressed at high levels in infected tissues, their precise role in the viral life cycle is unclear. E4 proteins are not found in the virion particles. Mutational analysis of the *E4* gene in BPV-1 showed that E4 was not essential for viral transformation or viral DNA replication (119,204).

In cultured epithelial cells, the E4 proteins are associated with the keratin cytoskeleton (74,236,239). The HPV-16 E4 protein has been shown to induce the collapse of the cytokeratin network (74,236), suggesting that it may function to aid the virus in its egress from the cell. A dramatic collapse of the keratin intermediate filaments has not, however, been observed with cells expressing HPV-1 E4, raising some question as to the generality of this effect (236,239). The available data are compatible with the possibility that E4 may contribute to vegetative DNA replication or to altering the cellular environment in a manner that may favor virus synthesis or perhaps virus release.

Virus Assembly and Release

Little is known about the papillomavirus assembly or release. Virus particles are observed in the granular layer of the epithelium and not at lower levels. The virus is not believed to be cytolytic, and the release of the virion particles does not occur before the cornified layers of a keratinized epithelium (see Figs. 4 and 5).

VIRAL DNA REPLICATION

The papillomaviruses have three modes of viral DNA replication. The first occurs during the initial infection of a basal keratinocyte by the virus, when there is an amplification of the viral genome to about 50 to 100 copies. Little is known of this process. The next phase is one of genome maintenance, which occurs in dividing basal cells of the lower portion of the epidermis as well as in the dermal fibroblasts in fibropapillomas such as those induced by BPV-1. In these cells, the viral DNA is maintained as a stable multicopy plasmid. The viral genomes replicate an average of once per cell cycle during S phase in synchrony with the host cell chromosome (98) and may be faithfully partitioned to the daughter cells. This type of DNA replication ensures a persistent and latent infection in the stem cells of the epidermis. The third type of DNA replication is vegetative DNA replication, which occurs in the more differentiated epithelial cells of the papilloma. In these cells, which no longer undergo cellular DNA synthesis, one observes a burst of viral DNA synthesis, generating the genomes to be packaged into progeny virions.

Plasmid Maintenance

Plasmid maintenance has been examined in greatest detail in BPV-1 transformed mouse cells, in which the viral genome exists as a stable multicopy plasmid (163). This system has provided a model for studying nonvegetative viral DNA replication, and it has been assumed that viral DNA replication in these mouse cells may be analogous to the stable plasmid replication seen in the dermal fibroblasts of a fibropapilloma and in the basal keratinocytes of a papillomavirus–associated lesion. During the maintenance phase, the viral genome copy number remains relatively constant for many cell generations.

Origin of DNA Replication

The origin of BPV-1 DNA replication was initially localized to the LCR by electron microscopic analysis of replicative intermediates isolated from BPV-1 transformed rodent cells harboring extrachromosomal viral DNA (317). Papillomavirus DNA replication requires the origin of DNA replication in cis and the viral E1 and E2 proteins in trans. *In vivo,* the minimal origin of replication (nucleotides 7911 to 7927) contains an A+T-rich region (ATR), the E1-binding site that includes a region of dyad symmetry (DSR), and an E2-binding site (310) (Fig. 11). The origins of DNA replication have been mapped for a number of the HPVs and contain similar ATR and DSR domains adjacent to E2-binding sites (41,62). Furthermore, in transient replication assays, the viral E1 and E2 proteins can function in trans on replication origins from heterologous papillomavirus genomes (41). Origin-dependent DNA replication of BPV-1 can be achieved *in vitro* with cell extracts containing high levels of E1 alone in the absence of E2 (267,328).

E1 Protein

Genetic studies have revealed that stable BPV-1 plasmid replication requires the expression of the viral *E1* and *E2* genes. Initial studies of mutated BPV-1 genomes implicated both E1 and E2 as essential for stable viral DNA replication (70,230) and for transient viral DNA replication (309).

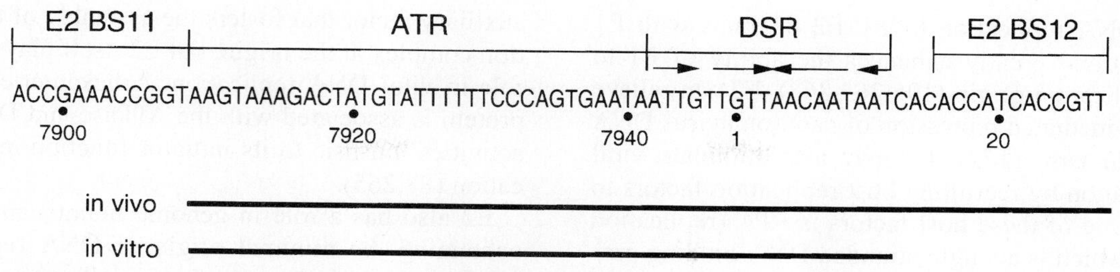

FIG. 11. The BPV-1 origin of DNA replication. The minimal origin for *in vivo* DNA replication (nucleotides 7911 to 7927) requires the A+T-rich region (ATR), the dyad symmetry repeats (DSR), and a binding site for the E2 protein. For *in vitro* DNA replication, there is a requirement only for the ATR and DSR.

However, E1 is the only viral factor that is directly involved in plasmid replication; E2 has auxiliary roles in DNA replication and in plasmid maintenance as discussed below. The *E1* ORF is the largest ORF in the papillomavirus genome and is relatively well conserved among all of the papillomaviruses (Fig. 12). The E1 proteins share structural similarities with portions of the SV40 large tumor antigen (TAg), which is an essential replication protein of that virus. The similarity includes regions of TAg with ATPase, helicase, and nucleotide-binding activities (49,267). The BPV-1 E1 protein is a 68-kd nuclear phosphoprotein that binds specifically to the origin of replication (304,310,324). By itself, E1 binds the origin with weak affinity. However, the binding of E1 to the origin is stabilized through its interaction with E2 and the binding of E2 to its cognate sites adjacent to the origin (195,310).

The papillomavirus E1 protein has DNA-dependent ATPase and DNA helicase activities (28,267,329). E1 is required for both the initiation and elongation of viral DNA synthesis (175). In addition to its interaction with E2, E1 has been shown to bind a number of cellular proteins. E1 interacts with the p180 subunit of the cellular DNA polymerase α-primase and presumably thereby recruits the cellular DNA replication initiation machinery to the viral replication origin (26,215). Several additional host cellular proteins have been found to bind E1, including histone H1 (292), SW1/SNF5 (165), cyclin E/Cdk2 (58,181), Hsp40/Hsp70 (176), and Ubc9 (231,332). Although the physiologic significance of some of these interactions remains to be determined, several appear to be quite interesting. In particular, the efficient cell cycle–regulated replication of papillomavirus genomes is dependent on the association of E1 with the S-phase–specific cyclin E–Cdk2 complex (58). In addition, the interaction of E1 with Ubc9 is required for efficient origin-dependent replication (332). E1 is SUMO-1 modified by Ubc-9, and this modification is required for the intranuclear accumulation of E1 (232).

In addition to the 68-kd protein encoded by the entire gene, the 5′ end of BPV-1 E1 encodes a protein with an apparent molecular weight of 23,000 (303). Although the protein has been detected by BPV-1 transformed cells, no function has yet been ascribed to this N-terminal E1 protein (129).

Role of the E2 Proteins

As noted previously, papillomavirus DNA replication also requires the viral E2 protein (309,328). A requirement for E2 in origin-dependent DNA replication has been shown for the HPVs as well as BPV-1 in transient assays. Although not essential for origin-dependent DNA replication *in vitro,* E2 greatly stimulates the ability of E1

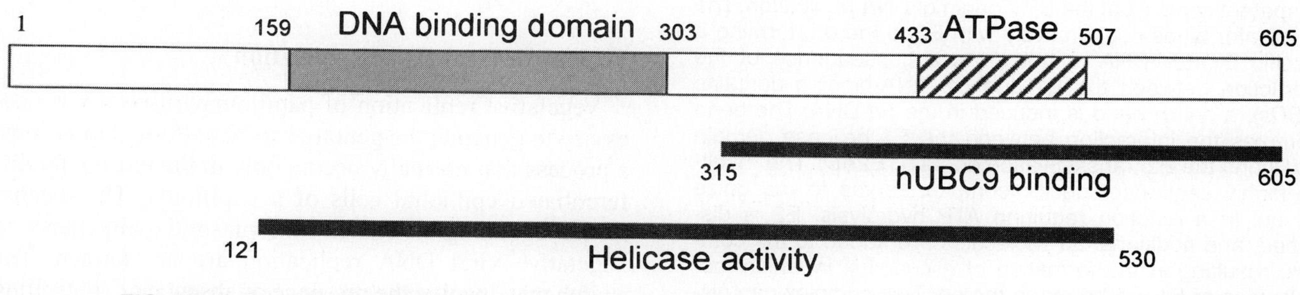

FIG. 12. Schematic representation of the BPV-1 E1 replication protein. The DNA-binding domain of E1 has been mapped to amino acid residues 159 to 303 for BPV-1. The crystal structure of the DNA-binding domain of BPV-1 E1 has recently been determined and shown to resemble (despite an amino acid sequence identity of only 6%) the DNA-binding domain of SV40 tumor antigen (84). The E2-binding domain maps to the C-terminal 266 amino acids.

to initiate DNA replication (328). E2 interacts with E1 (24,179,195) and greatly enhances the ability of E1 to bind the replication origin (195,264,268). E2 can relieve nucleosome-mediated repression of papillomavirus DNA replication *in vitro* (172). E2 may also stimulate viral DNA replication by recruiting host replication factors to the origin. One of these host factors is RPA (replication protein A), which is a single-stranded DNA-binding protein that can bind to acidic transactivation domains such as the one found in E2 (173). The E1:E2 complex is a precursor to a larger multimeric E1 complex, which after the removal of E2 can distort the replication origin and ultimately unwind the DNA (180) (Fig. 13). E2 serves as an auxiliary factor that fosters the assembly of the preinitiation complex at the origin, but E2 itself plays no intrinsic role in viral DNA replication. A hexameric form of E1 protein is associated with the ATPase and DNA helicase activities intrinsic to its initiator function in DNA replication (88,265).

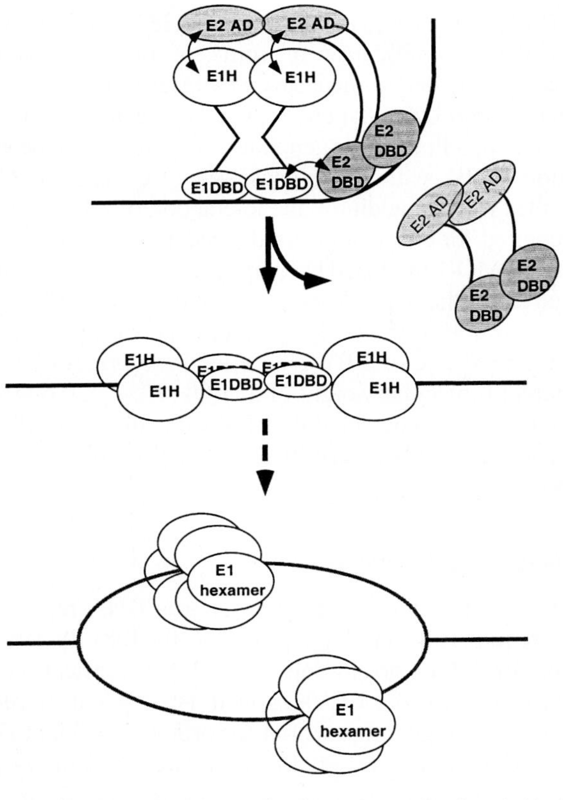

FIG. 13. Proposed pathway for the assembly of an initiation-competent complex at the BPV origin of DNA replication. The E1 initiator binds cooperatively with E2 to the ori, forming a specific $E1_2E2_2$–DNA complex. As a consequence of the interaction between the E1 and E2 DNA-binding domains (*DBDs*), a sharp bend is induced in the ori DNA. The bend promotes the interaction between the E1 helicase domain (*E1H*) and the E2 transactivation domain (*E2AD*). The resulting highly sequence-specific complex serves to recognize the ori. In a reaction requiring ATP hydrolysis, E2 is displaced, and additional E1 molecules are added to the complex, resulting in the formation of a complex in which four molecules of E1 are bound to the ori. This complex can distort the DNA duplex and give rise to partially single-stranded regions. Subsequently, additional molecules are added. In a final step, E1 is assembled onto the exposed single strands, forming a hexameric ringlike structure that constitutes the replicative helicase. (Modified from ref. 84, with permission.)

E2 also has a role in genome maintenance. Plasmids containing the minimal origin of DNA replication are capable of transient replication in cells expressing E1 and E2. With time, however, the plasmids are lost. Long-term, stable plasmid maintenance requires a cis minichromosome maintenance element, which consists of multiple E2-binding sites (226). This, together with the observation that E2TA and the viral genomes are associated with the mitotic chromosomes (137,170,271), suggests that viral E2 protein–mediated attachment of the viral genomes to the host cell chromatin could provide a mechanism for the coupling of viral genome multiplication and partitioning to the host cell cycle during viral latent infection. This association would ensure the localization of the viral genomes within the nuclear envelope when it is reformed during telophase.

Model for Plasmid Replication

In the initial intracellular stages of a papillomavirus infection, the viral genome may undergo amplification for a short period of time. There is then a transition to a maintenance stage in which the plasmids replicate an average of once per cell cycle, in a manner analogous to chromosomal DNA replication. It was initially thought that stable plasmid DNA replication might involve the "marking" of the daughter viral genomes so that they did not return to the replicating pool until the next cell cycle, and that each viral plasmid molecule replicated only once per cell cycle. However, the evidence currently favors an alternative model, in which the plasmid replication is not restricted to once per cell cycle but occurs an average of once per cell cycle and does not rely on plasmid marking (98,202). However, precise mechanisms involved in regulating plasmid maintenance, as well as vegetative DNA replication, have not yet been elucidated.

Vegetative Viral DNA Replication

Vegetative replication of papillomavirus DNA is necessary to generate the genomes to be packaged in virions, a process that normally occurs only in the terminally differentiated epithelial cells of a papilloma. The mechanisms regulating the switch from plasmid maintenance to vegetative viral DNA replication are not known. The switch may involve the presence or absence of controlling cellular factors in differentiating keratinocytes. In addition or alternatively, the relative levels of viral factors such as E1 or E2 (or their modification) may change in terminally differentiating keratinocytes. A high level of

BPV-1 DNA amplification occurs in transformed cells after growth arrest, in a process in which both E1 and E2 have been implicated (34,35). There have been few studies that have examined the mode of vegetative viral DNA replication in differentiated cells. One might anticipate that, as with the polyomaviruses, vegetative DNA replication occurs bi-directionally through theta structure intermediates, as it does in the maintenance replication phase. One intriguing study, however, suggests that there may be a switch from a bi-directional mode of replication to what could be a rolling circle mode (87). Additional studies on the mechanism of vegetative replication would appear to be warranted.

VIRAL TRANSFORMATION

BPV-1 Transformation

Certain papillomaviruses are capable of inducing cellular transformation in tissue culture. The most completely studied of the transforming papillomaviruses has been BPV-1. Morphologic transformation in tissue culture was first described for BPV in the early 1960s (23,25,302). In the late 1970s, a focus assay was developed using established cell lines to study BPV-1 transformation (79). In general, investigators have relied on mouse C127 cells and NIH-3T3 cells for these transformation studies, although a variety of other rodent cells, including hamster and rat cells, are susceptible to BPV-1–mediated transformation. Transformation of mouse C127 cells by BPV-1 causes alterations in morphology, loss of contact inhibition, anchorage independence, and tumorigenicity in nude mice (79).

One interesting characteristic of BPV-1 transformed rodent cells is that the viral DNA is maintained as a stable multicopy plasmid (163). Integration of the viral genome is not required for either the initiation or maintenance of the transformed state. However, transformation is dependent on the continued expression of viral DNA, as evidenced by the loss of the transformed phenotype in mouse cells which have been "cured" of the viral DNA by treatment with interferon (308). The extrachromosomal state of the viral genome, however, is not a prerequisite for this transformation because replication defective viruses are capable of transforming cells (250). In cells in which the extrachromosomal DNA is maintained, it is likely that a high gene dosage resulting from the viral plasmid replication is necessary for efficient transformation by the wild-type genome. Cells harboring BPV-1 mutants, which maintain a low copy number of extrachromosomal DNA, do not have a transformed phenotype (21).

The initial studies with cloned BPV-1 DNA indicated that the entire viral genome was not required for transformation of rodent cells (177). A specific 69% subgenomic fragment was sufficient for inducing cellular transformation; hybrid plasmids containing this 69% fragment could be maintained as stable plasmids within transformed cells. Genetic studies have mapped the BPV-1 transforming genes to the *E5, E6,* and *E7* ORFs, as discussed later. The initial studies establishing that the BPV-1 genome could be maintained as a stable plasmid in rodent cells led to the development of BPV-1–based plasmid vectors for mammalian cells (71,248,249).

BPV-1 has three independent transforming proteins, encoded by the *E6* (258,331), *E7,* and *E5* ORFs (104,259,330). Each of these genes is contained within the 69% transforming fragment, and each is expressed in transformed cells. The *E5* gene is the major transforming gene of BPV-1 in transformed cells. This gene is highly conserved among the group of papillomaviruses that induce fibropapillomas in their natural host and have the capacity to induce fibroblastic tumors in hamsters. The *E5* gene is believed to be responsible for the proliferation of dermal fibroblasts in fibropapillomas.

In addition to the *E5, E6,* and *E7* genes that are directly involved in BPV-1 transformation, the early region also encodes genes that are indirectly involved in transformation. The products of the *E1* and *E2* ORFs that are involved in the transcriptional regulation and replication of the virus regulate the expression of the transforming genes. Initial studies with BPV-1 E2 mutants suggested they were defective for transformation (68,104,230). This defect, however, is not due to the loss of a direct transforming activity of E2 but rather occurs because E2 is necessary for sufficient expression of the E5 viral oncoprotein. Mutations in the *E1* ORF may result in a higher transforming activity as a result of an increase in the transcriptional activity of the mutant viral genome (160,257). BPV-1 E1 can repress the E2 transactivated expression of the virus (246).

BPV-1 E5 Oncoprotein

The BPV-1 *E5* ORF encodes a 44–amino acid protein (262) and is sufficient for the transformation of certain established rodent cells in culture (66,104,230,259). The amino acid sequence of E5 and its predicted structure are shown in Figure 14. Structurally, E5 is composed of two protein domains: a very hydrophobic segment at its amino terminus, which is responsible for localization of E5 in membrane fractions (262), and a carboxyl-terminal hydrophilic domain. The E5 protein is associated with intracellular membranes and is thought to be an integral membrane protein (31). In transformed cells, the E5 protein exists largely as a homodimer and is localized primarily in the Golgi apparatus and in the endoplasmic reticulum (32,33). E5 is not secreted, and the hydrophilic C-terminus extends into the lumen of the Golgi (32). The E5 protein contains two cysteine residues involved in dimer formation that are required for transformation (31,124).

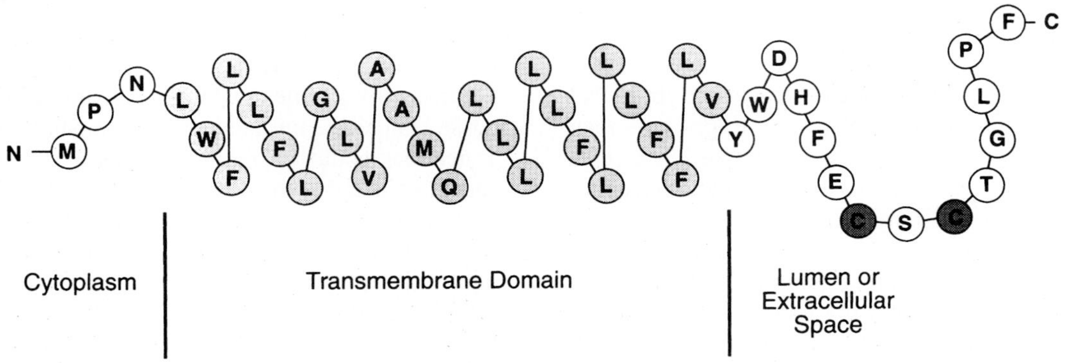

FIG. 14. Amino acid sequence and predicted secondary structure of the BPV-1 E5 oncoprotein. The 27 hydrophobic amino acids composing the first two thirds of the 44–amino acid protein (*shaded lightly*) are predicted to be in α-helical conformation. The 14 carboxyl-terminal residues are predicted to be in a nonhelical configuration. The cysteine residues, which are highly conserved among the E5 proteins of the transforming ungulate papillomaviruses, are *shaded darkly.* These cysteines mediate dimer formation (31,124).

The E5 protein does not possess intrinsic enzymatic activity and functions by altering the activity of cellular membrane proteins involved in proliferation. The first direct evidence that BPV-1 E5 can affect the activity and metabolism of growth factor receptors came from experiments that showed that E5 can cooperate with exogenously introduced epidermal growth factor (EGF) receptor or colony-stimulating factor 1 receptor in the transformation of NIH-3T3 cells (183). Subsequently, it was established that the primary endogenous target for the BPV-1 E5 protein in fibroblasts is the β-receptor for the platelet-derived growth factor (PDGF) (220). There is an increase in the level of tyrosine phosphorylation of the endogenous PDGF receptor in the E5-transformed rodent cells and bovine fibroblasts (218,220), and a prominent form of the tyrosine phosphorylated PDGF receptor in the transformed cells is an intracellular, membrane-associated, premature form of the receptor. Similarly, gene transfer experiments in heterologous cell types demonstrate that BPV-1 E5 transformation can be mediated by the PDGF β-receptor but not by a variety of other growth factor receptors (102,206). E5 activates the receptor and transforms cells in a ligand-independent manner (218, 219). The mechanism of E5 activation of the PDGF β-receptor involves complex formation with the receptor, thereby inducing receptor dimerization, trans-phosphorylation of tyrosine residues in the cytoplasmic domain of the receptor, and recruitment of cellular SH2 domain–containing proteins into a signal transduction complex (67). This is depicted in Figure 15, which shows a model suggesting that the individual subunits of the E5 dimer each bind to two different molecules of the PDGF β-receptor, resulting in receptor dimerization and activation (69). This model is supported by mutational analyses of the E5 protein–PDGF β-receptor interaction, which have identified in E5 the cysteines 37 and 39, glutamine 17, and aspartic acid 33 as essential for receptor binding (124,190,207). Similarly, mutations in the PDGF β-receptor at the transmembrane threonine 513 and juxtamembrane lysine 499 prevent complex formation and transformation (221).

BPV-1 E5 has also been shown to form a complex with the 16-kd transmembrane channel–forming subunit of the vacuolar H^+-ATPase (101,103), an abundant cellular protein located in the membranes of intracytoplasmic membranes and plasma membranes. Golgi acidification has been found to be impaired in cells transformed by the BPV-1 E5 protein, owing to the inhibition of the vacuolar H^+-ATPase (252). It has not yet been shown directly that Golgi alkalinization plays a role in cellular transformation, but there is a good genetic correlation between the ability of specific E5 mutants to transform cells and Golgi alkalization (252). Because many important growth regulatory proteins, including the PDGF β-receptor, transit through the Golgi apparatus, it is possible that the ability of E5 to perturb the pH of intracellular organelles might affect the activity of some of these proteins and, in so doing, contribute to the transformed phenotype. It is additionally possible that the BPV-1–mediated Golgi alkalinization may affect cellular functions unrelated to transformation that are important in the life cycle of the virus.

BPV-1 E6 and E7 Oncoproteins

The BPV-1 *E6* and *E7* genes also encode proteins with transforming activities. In mouse cells, the full transformed phenotype requires the expression of the *E6* and *E7* genes as well as *E5* (203,250). Furthermore, BPV-1 E6 expressed from a strong heterologous promoter is sufficient for transformation of C127 cells (258). The E6 and E7 proteins are themselves structurally related and

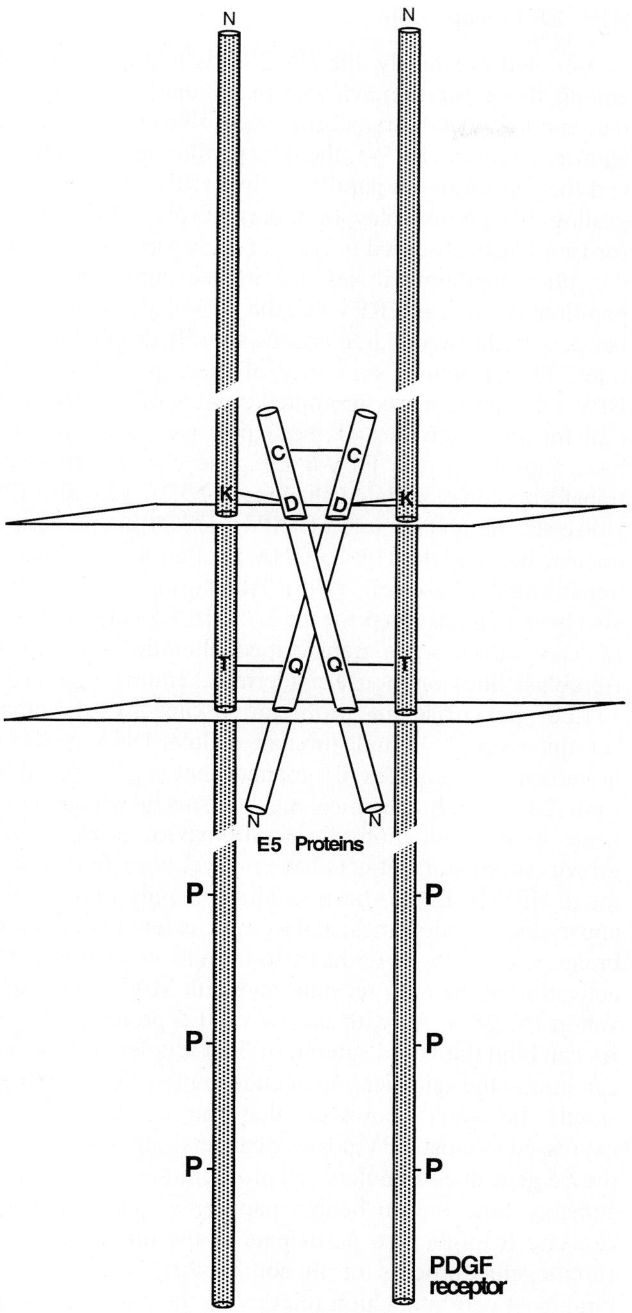

FIG. 15. Schematic model of the E5 protein–platelet-derived growth factor (PDGF) β-receptor complex. The *open rods* represent the E5 dimer, and the *shaded rods* represent two molecules of the PDGF β-receptor. The amino termini of the proteins are designated *N.* The *planes* represent the two faces of the cell membrane. The figure also shows the postulated glutamine-threonine (*Q-T*) hydrogen bond and aspartic acid–lysine (*D-K*) salt bridge linking these two proteins as well as the disulfide bond between the cysteine residues that stabilize the E5 dimer. *P* represents the phosphotyrosines in the cytoplasmic domain of the activated PDGF β-receptor. Not depicted in this figure is the 16-kd transmembrane channel-forming subunit of the vacuolar H^+-ATPase, which also binds E5 (101). (Modified from ref. 67, with permission.)

are conserved, at least in part, among all of the papillomaviruses. In BPV-1 transformed cells, cyclic DNA (cDNA) has been isolated and characterized, which could encode the full-length E6 protein, the full-length E7 protein, as well as the E6 fusion protein in which the amino-terminal half of E6 could be fused to portions of downstream genes (331) (see Fig. 7). To date, no studies have been done on these potential BPV-1 *E6* spliced genes. The *E6* and *E7* genes of all the papillomaviruses encode proteins with conserved structural motifs. They contain domains of almost identically spaced CYS-X-X-CYS motifs (four in *E6* and two in the carboxyl-terminal portion of *E7*). It has been postulated that the *E6* and *E7* genes may have arisen from duplication events involving a 39-codon core sequence containing one of these motifs (52). The CYS-X-X-CYS motifs found in a number of nucleic acid–binding proteins are characteristic of zinc-binding proteins. The papillomavirus E6 and E7 proteins bind zinc through these cysteine residues (13,105).

The E6 protein of BPV-1 is present at low levels in stably transformed cells. Cell fractionation experiments have localized the BPV-1 E6 protein to the nucleus and to nonnuclear membranes of transformed cells (3). No intrinsic enzymatic activities have been identified for BPV-1 E6, and like the oncogenic HPV E6 proteins, it is believed to function through binding cellular targets. Four different cellular proteins have been found to interact with BPV-1 E6: the ubiquitin protein ligase E6AP (see later), E6BP (also known as ERC55), the γ subunit of the AP1 clatherin adaptor complex, and the focal adhesion protein paxillin (38,305,306,311). Unlike the oncogenic HPV E6 proteins (see later), the BPV-1 E6 interaction with E6AP does not result in the binding and degradation of p53. It is not yet known whether the interaction of BPV-1 E6 with E6AP has physiologic consequences for the cell. Similarly, no *in vivo* consequences of the interaction of BPV-1 E6 with either ERC55 or the γ subunit of the AP1 on the cell have yet been determined. Analysis of a series of BPV-1 E6 mutants has shown a good correlation between the binding to paxillin and cellular transformation (59,306,311). This binding has also been shown to correlate with the disruption of the cellular actin cytoskeleton, a characteristic of transformed cells (306). E6 binds to charged leucine motifs in paxillin known as LD motifs and, in doing so, competes with the ability of paxillin to bind to vinculin and the focal adhesion kinase (307,311). Nonetheless, a detailed understanding of the mechanisms by which BPV-1 E6 transforms cells remains to be determined.

The product of the *E7* ORF has been detected in BPV-1 transformed cells (138). Although the *E7* gene by itself is not able to induce foci in transformation assays, its integrity is necessary for the fully transformed phenotype as assayed by anchorage independence and by tumorigenicity (203). BPV-1 E6 and E7 are under the negative regulatory control of the viral *E1* and *E2* genes, and in the absence of these gene products, *E6* and *E7* together are potent oncogenes that are sufficient for the full transformation of C127 cells (314). To date, there have been no functional studies of the BPV-1 E7 protein. Unlike the HPV E7 proteins, BPV-1 E7 does not contain an LXCXE motif for binding the retinoblastoma tumor suppressor gene product (pRB), suggesting that it does not share the property of pRB binding and inactivation with the HPV E7 proteins (see later).

HPV Transformation and Immortalization

Transformation studies with the papillomaviruses have not been limited to BPV-1. Assays have also been developed for the transformation and immortalization functions encoded by those HPVs associated with anogenital cancers in humans. The HPV-16 and HPV-18 genomes are not as efficient as BPV-1 at inducing transformation of established rodent cells; however, alternative assays have been developed. DNA cotransfection with a second dominant selective marker, such as the neomycin resistance gene, and biochemical selection for the transfected cells permit HPV-16 and HPV-18 to transform established rodent cells (333). Assays employing primary rodent cells and primary human fibroblast and keratinocyte cultures have proved even more informative (78,143,185,224,228,261,318). In these assays, the high-risk HPVs, such as HPV-16 and HPV-18, are transformation positive, whereas the low-risk viruses, such as HPV-6 and HPV-11, are not (261,285). These assays have permitted the mapping of the viral genes directly involved in cellular transformation to the *E6* and *E7* ORFs of the high-risk HPV types, which are discussed in detail later.

In established rodent cells, such as the NIH-3T3 cells, the *E7* ORF scores as the major HPV transforming gene (224,296,316,319,334). HPV-16 and HPV-18 by themselves are not able to transform primary rat fibroblasts or baby rat kidney cells (159,224). However, the *E7* gene can cooperate with an activated *ras* oncogene to transform primary rat cells completely (18,174,209,224,285).

The DNA of the high-risk HPVs can also be distinguished from the DNA of the low-risk HPVs by the ability of the high-risk types to immortalize primary cultures of human fibroblasts, human foreskin keratinocytes, and human cervical epithelial cells (78,228,261,318,325). The resulting cell lines are neither anchorage dependent nor tumorigenic in nude mice, but they do display altered growth properties and are resistant in the response to signals for terminal differentiation (78,146,228,261). All of the genital tract HPV types (i.e., HPV-6, HPV-11, HPV-16, and HPV-18) are capable of transiently inducing cellular proliferation. Only the high-risk HPVs, however, are able to extend the life span and give rise to immortalized cell lines that are refractory to differentiation signals (261).

HPV E5 Oncoprotein

As noted previously, the *E5* ORF is highly conserved among those papillomaviruses that induce fibropapillomas and that readily transform rodent fibroblasts in tissue culture, including BPV-1, the deer papillomavirus (DPV), and the European elk papillomavirus (EEPV) (156), suggesting that E5 may play an important role in the tropism for fibroblasts observed *in vivo* for these viruses. Many of the other papillomaviruses that induce purely epithelial papillomas (such as CRPV and the HPVs) also contain *E5* genes with the potential to encode short hydrophobic peptides. The structural similarity of these peptides to the BPV-1 E5 protein has prompted studies of the potential transforming activities of these putative genes. Studies have shown that the HPV-6 *E5* gene can induce some transformation-associated changes of NIH-3T3 cells (39). However, the precise role of HPV-6 E5 in this process is unclear because the HPV-6 DNA is often not retained in transformed mouse cells (196). Transforming activity has also been demonstrated for the HPV-16 *E5* gene. HPV-16 E5 can induce some transformed alterations in mouse fibroblast lines or mouse epidermal keratinocytes (169, 171,287), increase the proliferative capacity of human keratinocytes (284), and stimulate cellular DNA synthesis in human keratinocytes in a manner that is potentiated by EGF (287). The biochemical mechanisms by which the *E5* genes of the epitheliotropic papillomaviruses exert their growth stimulatory effects have not yet been fully elaborated. HPV-16 E5 has been localized mainly to the Golgi apparatus, to endosomes, and to some extent to cell membranes (53). HPV-16 E5 has also been associated with the activation of the EGF receptor and with MAP kinase activation (57,287). As with the BPV-1 E5 protein, HPV-16 E5 can bind the 16-kd subunit of the vacuolar ATPase and can inhibit the acidification of endosomes (53,238,286). It should be noted, however, that the *E5* gene is not expressed in most HPV-positive cancers, suggesting that if the *E5* gene does stimulate cell proliferation *in vivo,* it presumably functions in benign papillomas and not in the cancers. It might also participate in the initiation of the carcinogenic process or in some other aspects of the viral–host cell interaction relevant to the pathogenesis of the HPV infection.

HPV E6 Oncoprotein

Although HPV-16 E7 is sufficient for the transformation of established rodent cells such as NIH-3T3 cells and for cooperation with *ras* in the transformation of baby rat kidney cells, the combination of E6 and E7 is required for the efficient immortalization of primary human fibroblasts or keratinocytes (114,198,318). E6 and E7 together can extend the life span of human keratinocytes and lead to the outgrowth of immortalized clones that are resistant to terminal differentiation. This property is dependent on the full-length *E6* gene; mutational analysis has shown that the putative HPV-16 *E6** gene, encoding a truncated form of E6, cannot provide this function (198). Indeed, it appears that the *E6**, if it is actually made *in vivo,* might function in a dominant negative manner to inhibit some of the activities of the full-length E6 oncoprotein of the cancer associated HPV types (227).

The HPV E6 proteins are about 150 amino acids in size and contain four Cys-X-X-Cys motifs, which are believed to be involved in binding zinc (13,105,106). The E6 proteins from the low-risk and high-risk HPVs appear to have similar transcriptional activation properties, as has been shown using "minimal" promoters containing a TATA box element only (266). Because the E6 proteins of the low-risk HPVs have little or no transformation activity in any of the assays tested, this transactivation property of the E6 proteins may not be linked mechanistically to the transforming functions of the E6 proteins of the high-risk HPVs.

The small DNA tumor viruses have evolved mechanisms to complex and functionally inactivate the tumor suppressor gene product p53 (see Chapter 10). Like the SV40 TAg and the Ad5 E1B 55K proteins, the E6 proteins encoded by the high-risk HPVs can complex with p53; however, a functional *in vivo* interaction between the low-risk HPV E6 proteins and p53 has not been detected (320). Although p53 is not required for normal cellular proliferation, it plays a fundamental role in directing the cellular response to genotoxic and cytotoxic stresses that threaten genomic stability. The function of p53 as a sequence-specific transcriptional activator (92,148) is necessary for its activity in regulating cell growth and in tumor growth suppression. The first downstream target of p53 to be identified was the p21 cyclin-dependent kinase inhibitor, encoded by the *WAF1* or *CIP1* gene (83,109, 327). Thus, the p53-mediated suppression of cell growth is due in part to the transcriptional activation of p21 leading to the inhibition of the cyclin-dependent kinases critical for G_1 progression and cell growth. The p53 protein directly regulates the transcription of additional genes involved in the cellular response to genotoxic and cytotoxic stress, apoptosis and cell cycle control, including *Bax, GADD45, IGF-BP3, cyclin G,* and *14-3-3*γ (315). The viral oncoproteins SV40 TAg, AdE1B 55K, and the high-risk E6 proteins can each efficiently abrogate the transcriptional transactivation activity of p53 (193,335). Thus, as with SV40 TAg and Ad E1B, HPV E6 has anti-apoptotic activities and can interfere with the negative cell cycle regulatory functions of p53.

Although SV40 TAg, the Ad5 E1B 55-kd protein, and the high-risk HPV E6 proteins can all complex p53, the consequence of these interactions are different with respect to the stability of the p53 protein. In SV40 and adenovirus-transformed cells, levels of p53 are usually quite high, and the half-life of p53 is increased (212,234). In contrast, the levels of p53 in HPV-infected cells are low compared with uninfected primary host cells (128, 254). Unlike TAg and the E1B 55-kd protein, which inactivate p53 in part by sequestering it into stable inactive complexes, the E6 proteins of the high-risk HPVs counter p53 by inducing its proteolysis. This was first demonstrated by *in vitro* studies that showed that the high-risk HPV E6 proteins facilitate the rapid degradation of p53 through ubiquitin-dependent proteolysis (256). Under the same conditions, the low-risk HPV E6 proteins, which do not bind detectable amounts of p53, have no detectable effect on p53 stability *in vitro* (256). HPV-16 E6 induces p53 degradation by forming a complex with the cellular ubiquitin–protein ligase E6AP (131,132), which is then able to bind and ubiquitinate p53 (253). E6AP is a component of the ubiquitin-proteasome pathway, which targets proteins for degradation by covalently linking them to multimeric chains of the 76–amino acid protein ubiquitin. In this pathway (shown in Fig. 16), ubiquitin is first activated in an ATP-dependent reaction and then passed from the ubiquitin-activating enzyme (E1) to a ubiquitin-conjugating enzyme (E2). Ubiquitin is then transferred to lysine residues of the target protein with the aid of a ubiquitin–protein ligase (E3). Multi-ubiquitinated proteins are subsequently recognized and degraded by the 26S proteasome (121). Although some classes of E3 proteins, such as the SCF complexes, function as adapters that bring E2 enzymes into complex with their substrates, E6AP belongs to a class of ubiquitin–protein ligases called HECT E3 proteins, which directly transfer ubiquitin to

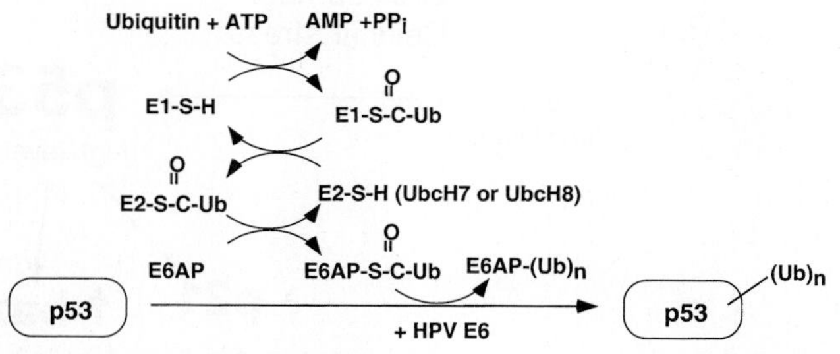

FIG. 16. A ubiquitin thiolester cascade model for the HPV E6–dependent ubiquitination of p53. The E6 protein binds to the cellular protein E6-AP, and the complex together functions as an E3 (ubiquitin protein ligase) in facilitating the ubiquitination of p53 (253). The ubiquitination of a protein involves three cellular activities: E1 (ubiquitin-activating enzyme), E2 (ubiquitin-conjugating enzyme), and E3 (ubiquitin protein ligase). Ubiquitin is activated in an ATP-dependent manner and forms a high-energy thiolester with E1, which can then be transferred to E2 through a thiolester linkage. Ubiquitin can then be transferred to a cysteine within the Hect domain of E6AP, again as a thiolester linkage (255), through the direct binding of E6AP with UbcH7 or UbcH8 (157). In conjunction with HPV-16 E6, E6AP then recognizes p53 and catalyses the formation of an isopeptide bond between the carboxyl-terminal glycine of ubiquitin and a lysine side chain of p53. In catalyzing the ubiquitination of p53, HPV-16 E6 also induces the self-ubiquitination and proteolysis of E6AP (144).

their substrates (255). The catalytic domain of HECT proteins is a conserved 350–amino acid region defined by its *h*omology to the *E*6AP *c*arboxyl *t*erminus (i.e., HECT) (130). The HECT domain binds to specific E2 enzymes (157) and contains an active-site cysteine residue that forms a thiolester bond with ubiquitin (130,255). X-ray crystallography studies have determined that the HECT domain is a bilobed structure, with a larger N-terminal lobe that interacts with the ubiquitin-conjugating enzyme, and a smaller C-terminal lobe containing the catalytic cysteine residue (126). Both E6 and E6-AP are necessary to detect complex formation with p53, and it has not yet been determined whether E6, E6-AP, or both actually contact p53.

In addition to the *in vitro* evidence that the high-risk HPV E6 proteins accelerate the degradation of p53, E6 also affects the stability of intracellular p53 *in vivo* (11,128,164,254). Levels of p53 in E6 immortalized cells or in HPV-positive cervical carcinoma cells are, on average, twofold to threefold lower compared with primary cells (254). The half-life of p53 is reduced from several hours to 20 minutes in human keratinocytes expressing E6 (128). In uninfected cells, intracellular p53 levels increase significantly in response to DNA damage or genotoxic agents (145). The higher levels of p53 result in either a G_1 growth arrest or apoptosis as part of a cell defense mechanism that allows for either the DNA damage to be repaired before the initiation of a new round of DNA replication or removal of the cell. E6-expressing cells, however, do not manifest a p53-mediated cellular response to DNA damage (149), indicating the ability of E6 to promote the degradation of p53 and prevent the steady level of p53 to rise above a certain threshold level (Fig. 17). Under DNA-damaging conditions, the E6-stimulated degradation of p53 abrogates the negative growth regulatory effect of p53 and as such contributes to genomic instability (321). *In vivo* studies have confirmed the role of E6AP in mediating the E6-dependent ubiquitination of p53 and have established that E6AP in the absence of E6AP is not involved in the regulation of p53 stability (19,294). Instead, mdm2 functions as the ubiquitin protein ligase for p53 in normal cells (315).

The HPV-16 E6 protein binds to E6AP within the N-terminal substrate recognition domain, directing E6AP to ubiquitinate p53 (133). Several potential E6-independent substrates of E6AP have now been identified, including the human homolog of the yeast RAD23 protein involved in nucleotide excision repair (HHR23A), the src-family kinase Blk, and the MCM7 subunit of replication licensing factor (155,158,211). In addition, E6 induces self-

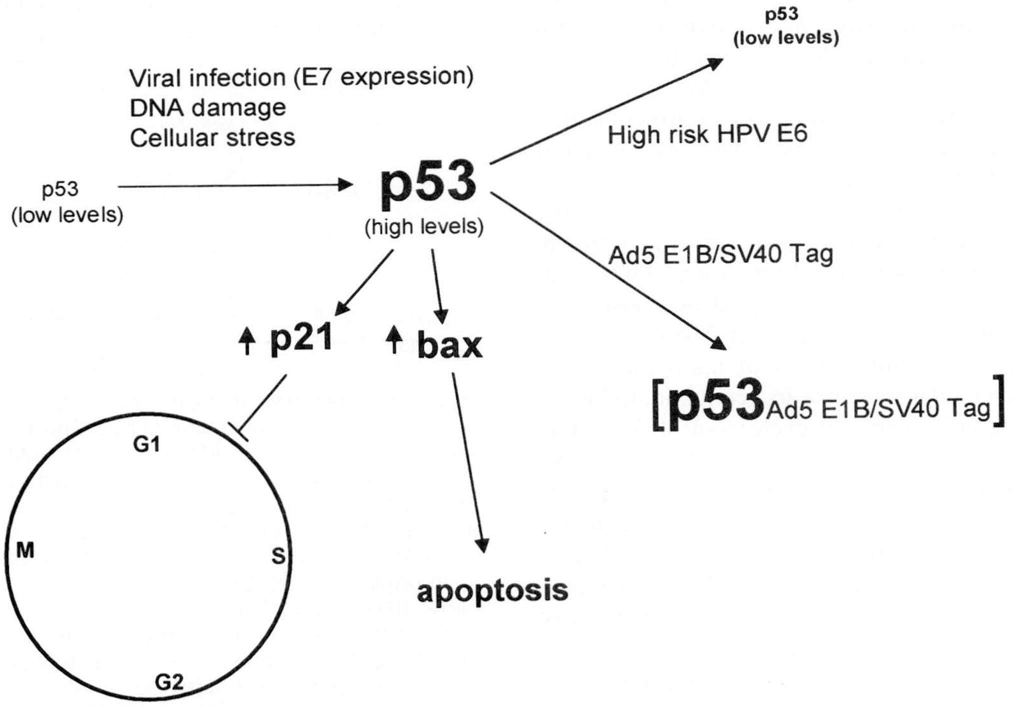

FIG. 17. The level of p53 in primary cells is generally low. DNA damaging agents, viral infection, and expression of E7 increase the level of p53. Elevated levels of p53 can lead to either apoptosis or a cell cycle checkpoint arrest in G_1 phase through the transcriptional activation of *bax* or p21[cip1]. Viral oncoproteins may interfere with this negative growth-regulatory function of p53, either by sequestering p53 into a stable but nonfunctional complex (such as with SV40 TAg or the Ad5 55-kd E1B protein) or by ubiquitination and enhanced proteolysis, as observed with the high-risk HPV E6 proteins.

ubiquitination of E6AP (144). It is conceivable that the redirection of E6AP activity toward p53 by E6 might affect (either enhance or inhibit) the targeting of the normal substrates of E6AP and that such an alteration of E6AP activity could account for some of the transforming activity of E6. Indeed, recent studies suggest that E6 has p53-independent transformation activities. For example, transgenic mice expressing E6 from the epithelial-specific K14 promoter developed epidermal hyperplasia even in a p53-null background (274). Other experiments have shown that an E6 mutant that is unable to bind or degrade p53 can still promote colony formation and growth on soft agar as well as induce cell cycle reentry in cells even when p53 transactivation activity is inhibited (279). Another p53-independent activity of HPV-16 E6 is its ability to activate telomerase, a characteristic of many different types of cancer (152).

A number of additional cellular targets have now been identified for the high-risk E6 proteins in an attempt to define additional p53-independent cellular targets (Table 2). As discussed previously, paxillin, which appears to be a relevant target for the BPV-1 E6 transformation function, can also bind HPV-16 E6, at least *in vitro* (306,311). Interestingly, the high-risk E6 oncoproteins contain a X-(S/T)-X-(V/I/L)-COOH motif at the extreme C-terminus that can mediate the binding of cellular PDZ domain–containing proteins. This motif is unique to high-risk HPV E6 proteins and is not present in the E6 proteins of the low-risk HPV types. The high-risk HPV E6 proteins have been shown to bind a number of cellular PDZ domain–containing proteins, including hDlg (the human homolog of the *Drosophila melanogaster* tumor suppressor disk's large protein), MUPP1 (the multi-PDZ domain protein) and hScrib (the human homolog of *Drosophila scribble*) (151,167,168,201). E6 binding to these PDZ-containing proteins results in their E6AP-mediated ubiquitination and proteolysis (97,201). These PDZ-containing proteins have been shown to be involved in negatively regulating cellular proliferation. At least some of the p53-independent transforming activities of the high-risk E6 oncoproteins may be linked to their ability to bind and degrade some of these PDZ motif–containing proteins. E6 has also been reported to bind the transcriptional coactivator p300/CBP, a target also of adenovirus (Ad) E1A and SV40 large TAg (216,340). The physiologic relevance to the transformation functions of the other E6 cellular targets listed in Table 2 have not yet been elucidated. It is possible that the binding of E6 to some of these targets could contribute to the viral pathogenic functions unrelated to cellular transformation.

HPV E7 Oncoprotein

The E7 protein encoded by the high-risk HPVs is a small nuclear protein of about 100 amino acids, has been shown to bind zinc, and is phosphorylated by casein kinase II (CK II) (199). Insight into its mechanism of action came initially from the recognition that E7 has functional similarities with the Ad 12S E1A product (224). Like Ad E1A, E7 can transactivate the Ad E2 promoter (224), induce DNA synthesis in quiescent cells (251), and cooperate with an activated *ras* oncogene to transform primary rodent cells (185,224).

In addition to these functional similarities, the HPV-16 E7 shares important amino acid sequence similarity with portions of the Ad E1A proteins and the SV40 large TAg (Fig. 18). These conserved regions are critical for the transforming activities in all three viral oncoproteins and have been shown to participate in the binding of a number of important cellular regulatory proteins, including the product of the retinoblastoma tumor suppressor gene *pRB,* and the related pocket proteins, p107 and p130 (61,81,322). Complex formation with pRB involves conserved region 2 of the Ad E1A protein and the corresponding region in the E7 protein and in SV40 large TAg (61,323).

The retinoblastoma protein is a member of a family of cellular proteins that also includes p107 and p130, which are homologous in their binding "pockets" for E7, Ad E1A, and SV40 TAg. The retinoblastoma protein is the most extensively studied member of this family of proteins. Its phosphorylation state is regulated through the

TABLE 2. *Cellular targets of the papillomavirus E6 oncoproteins*

Associated cellular proteins	Functional consequences	References
p53	E6AP-dependent ubiquitination and proteolysis	256, 320
E6-associated protein (E6AP)	Ubiquitination and proteolysis of associated proteins	253
	Enhanced auto-ubiqitination of E6AP	144
E6BP (Erc55)	Unknown	38
Paxillin	Disruption of the actin cytoskeleton	306, 311
HD1g, MUPP1, and hScrib	E6AP-dependent ubiquitination and proteolysis	97, 167, 201
IRF-3	Inhibition of interferon-β induction	242
Clatherin adaptor complex AP-1	Unknown	305
Unknown	Activation of cellular telomerase	152
E6TP1	E6-induced degradation	96
Bak	Inhibition of Bak-induced apoptosis	301
CBP/p300	Inhibition of p53 transcriptional activity	216, 340

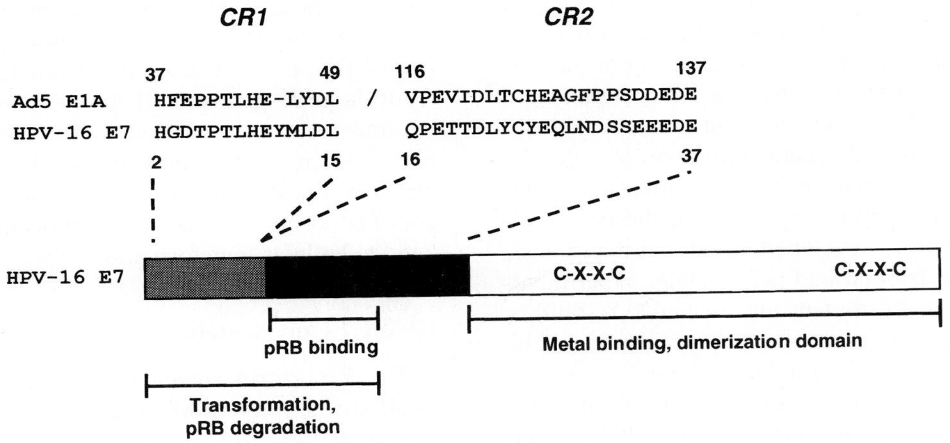

FIG. 18. Amino acid sequence similarity between portions of conserved regions 1 and 2 (*CR1, CR2*) of the Ad5 E1A proteins and the amino-terminal 38 amino acids of HPV-16 E7. CR2 contains the pRB binding site and the casein kinase II (*CKII*) phosphorylation site of HPV-16 E7.

cell cycle, being hypophosphorylated in G_0 and G_1 phase and phosphorylated during S, G_2, and M phase. The pRB protein becomes phosphorylated at multiple serine residues by cyclin-dependent kinases at the G_1-to-S phase boundary and remains phosphorylated until late M phase, when it becomes hypophosphorylated again through the action of a specific phosphatase (Fig. 19). The hypophosphorylated form represents the active form with respect to its ability to inhibit cell cycle progression. HPV-16 E7, like SV40 TAg, binds preferentially to the hypophosphorylated form of pRB, consistent with the model that this interaction results in the functional inactivation of pRB and permits progression of the cell into S phase of the cell cycle (50). This property of the viral oncoproteins to complex pRB would appear to account, at least in part, for their ability to induce DNA synthesis and cellular proliferation.

Members of the E2F family of transcription factors are involved in mediating the functions of the pocket proteins (see Chapter 10). The transcriptional activity of E2F is modulated by pRB; when bound to the G_0- and G_1-specific hypophosphorylated form of pRB, E2F functions as a transcriptional repressor. When pRB is phosphorylated by cyclin-dependent kinase complexes near the G_1-to-S phase boundary, the pRB–E2F complex dissociates, and E2F can act as a transcriptional activator (see Fig. 19). The regulated conversion of the transcriptional activity of E2F between repressor and activator contributes to the regulation of G_1-to-S phase progression. The high-risk HPV E7 proteins, like Ad E1A and SV40 TAg, contribute to carcinogenic progression, therefore, at least in part, by disrupting this regulatory network (205). In the case of the E7–pRB interaction, E7 destabilizes pRB, promoting its proteolysis (27).

The E7 proteins of the HPV high-risk and low-risk types differ in a number of biochemical and biologic properties. The E7 proteins from the low-risk HPV types 6 and 11 bind pRB with about a 10-fold lower efficiency than the E7 proteins of HPV types 16 and 18 (95,200). Furthermore, the E7 proteins of the low-risk HPVs function inefficiently in cellular transformation assays with an activated *ras* oncogene and are phosphorylated by CK II at a lower rate (12). Studies with chimeric E7 proteins containing domains of high-risk and low-risk HPV E7 proteins showed that the difference in transformation efficiency in rodent cells was due to the pRB-binding site (115). Sequence comparison of the pRB-binding sites revealed a single consistent amino acid sequence difference between the high-risk and the low-risk E7 proteins: an aspartic acid residue (Asp 21 in HPV-16 E7) corresponding to a glycine residue in the low-risk E7 sequence (Gly 22 in HPV-6 E7). Substitution of this residue in the respective *E7* genes revealed that this single amino acid residue was the principal determinant responsible for the difference in pRB-binding affinity and in the transforming capacity of the low-risk and the high-risk E7 proteins (115,247).

Mutations in the carboxyl-terminal half of E7 that interfere with E7 function have also generally affected the intracellular stability of the protein (82,223). Nevertheless, several studies have suggested some specific contributions of the carboxyl terminus to E7 functions. E7 can exist as a dimer, and the C-terminal half is important in mediating dimerization (159). The ability of E7 to disrupt the complex between the cellular transcription factor E2F and pRB also involves sequences in the carboxyl terminus of E7, in addition to the pRB-binding site (127,326). Although the ability of E7 to transform rodent cells requires an intact pRB-binding domain, a mutant of HPV-16 E7 that is defective for pRB binding was reported to be competent to cooperate with E6 for the immortalization of primary human genital keratinocytes, indicating that other properties of E7 may also be involved in this function.

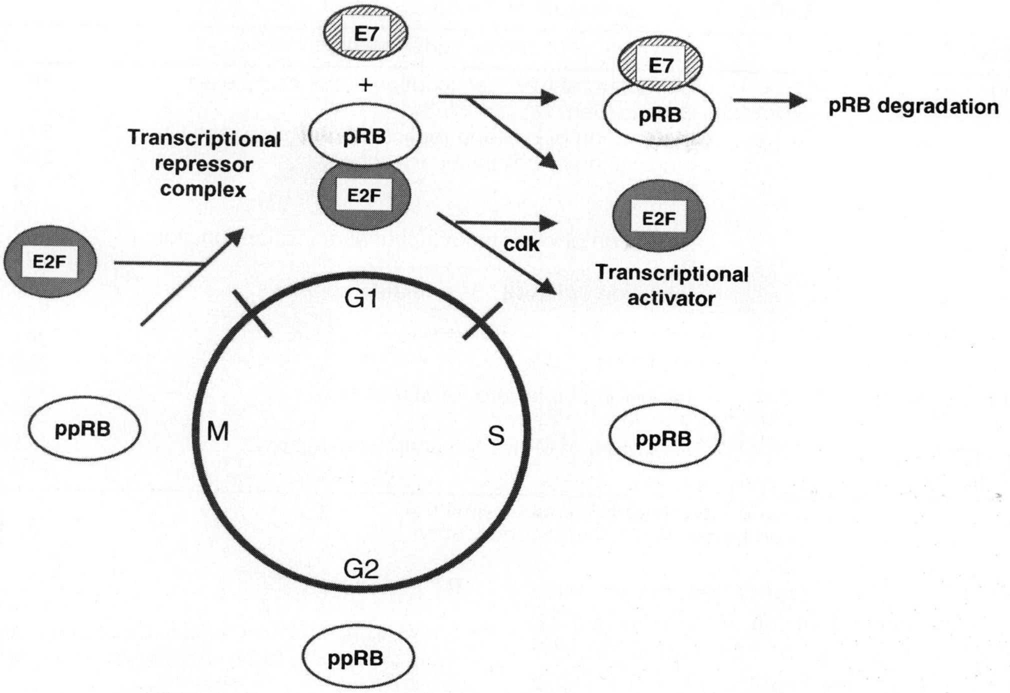

FIG. 19. E7 abrogates the cell cycle regulation mediated by pRB (as well as the related proteins p107 and p130) by complex formation. During the cell cycle, pRB is differentially phosphorylated, and the underphosphorylated form is detected only in the G_0/G_1 phase. This underphosphorylated form is the active form of pRB, acting as a negative regulator of the cell cycle. During the transition to S phase, pRB is phosphorylated by cyclin-dependent kinases (*cdk*), resulting in the inactivation of its cell cycle regulatory functions. Members of the E2F family of cellular transcription factors are preferentially bound to the underphosphorylated form of pRB, and in complex with pRB, they cannot activate transcription. Phosphorylation of pRB or complex formation with E7 results in the release of the E2F factors, allowing them to function as transcriptional activators of cellular genes involved in cellular DNA synthesis and progression into S phase of the cell cycle.

Genetic studies indicate that complex formation between E7 and the pocket proteins, including pRB, is not sufficient to account for its immortalization and transforming functions, suggesting that there are likely to be additional cellular targets of E7 that are relevant to cellular transformation (140). Table 3 provides a list of various cellular targets with which E7 has been shown to bind. The physiologic relevance of many of these interactions is unclear. It is possible that some of the interactions may reflect artifacts of the biochemical or yeast two-hybrid approaches used in their identification. It is also possible that some of the interactions may be of physiologic importance to functions of the E7 protein that are not involved in cellular transformation.

Of particular interest are the reports that E7 can interact with cyclin-dependent kinase inhibitors. As with E1A, HPV-16 E7 interacts with and abrogates the inhibitory activity of $p27^{kip1}$ (336). Because $p27^{kip1}$ is involved in mediating the cellular growth inhibition by transforming growth factor-β (TGF-β) in keratinocytes, this activity may contribute to the ability of E7 to override TGF-β–associated growth arrest (225). HPV-16 E7 can also associate with $p21^{cip1}$ and abrogate its inhibition of cyclin dependent kinases as well as its inhibition of PCNA-dependent DNA replication (91,141). The $p21^{cip1}$ is normally induced during keratinocyte differentiation (194), and presumably its inhibition by E7 may be critical to allowing the replication of papillomavirus DNA in differentiated squamous epithelial cells (40).

HPV-16 E7 has also recently been shown to induce abnormal centrosome duplication (77). Although E6 can potentiate this effect, E7 plays a major role in inducing these centrosome-related mitotic disturbances. The mechanism by which E7 affects these centrosome abnormalities are not yet known. Abnormal centrosome duplication rapidly results in genomic instability and aneuploidy, one of the hallmarks of a cancer cell. This activity is therefore likely to be functionally relevant to the contribution of high-risk HPV to malignant progression.

What are the roles of the E6 and E7 oncoproteins in the normal life cycle of an HPV infection? It is likely that they contribute critical functions by providing a cellular environment that fosters the replication of the viral DNA. The viral E1 and E2 proteins are necessary

TABLE 3. *Cellular targets of the human papillomavirus E7*

Associated cellular proteins	Functional consequences	References
pRB, p107, p130	Disruption of E2F transcription factor complexes	80, 81
	Degradation	27
p21[cip1]	Inactivation of *cdk* and replication inhibitory activity	91, 141
p27[kip1]	Inactivation of *cdk* inhibitory activity	336
TBP	?	184
TAF110	?	186
AP-1	Activation of *c-jun* transcriptional activation function	4
Mi2β (HDAC)	?	29
IGFBP-3	Inhibition of IGFBP-3–mediated apoptosis	182
M2 Pyruvate kinase	?	342
α-Glucosidase	?	341
hTid-1	?	260
p48 component of ISGF3	Inhibition of interferon-α stimulation	15
F-actin	?	235
Forkhead transcription factor MPP2	Activation of MPP2 transcriptional activity	178
S4 subunit of proteasome	?	20a

for the initiation of viral DNA replication, but the virus is otherwise totally dependent on host cell factors, including DNA polymerase α, thymidine kinase, PCNA, and so forth, for the replication of its DNA. These are proteins that are normally only expressed in S phase during cellular DNA replication in cycling cells. Vegetative DNA replication for the papillomaviruses, however, occurs only in the more differentiated cells of the epithelium that are no longer cycling (see Figs. 4 and 5). Thus, the papillomaviruses have evolved a mechanism similar to that of the polyomaviruses and the adenoviruses, to activate the cellular genes necessary for the replication of their own DNA in otherwise quiescent cells. These viruses may do so through the E7 proteins and their ability to release the E2F transcription factors by binding the pocket proteins, including pRB (see Fig. 19). In addition, E7 binds and inhibits the cdk inhibitor p21[cip1] that is normally induced during keratinocyte differentiation, again presumably for the purpose of permitting viral DNA replication in a differentiated cell. Why, then, does E6 target p53 for proteolysis? The high-risk HPV E7 proteins, when expressed in the absence of E6, result in increased levels of p53, resulting in either a G_1-mediated cell cycle arrest or apoptosis, depending on the cell type (125,214). The mechanistic link between the pRB and p53 pathways is discussed in Chapter 10. The proposed model, for which there is some evidence, involves the deregulation of pRB by E7, resulting in the induction of E2F-1, which in turn activates p19[arf], which interferes with the ability of mdm2 to regulate p53 stability. Thus, E7 creates a signal that increases p53 levels. E6, by promoting the degradation of p53, resulting in a lower steady-state level in the cell, counters this activity of E7 and permits the E7-dependent activation of the cellular DNA replication genes required for viral DNA replication.

REFERENCES

1. Ahola H, Stenlund A, Moreno-Lopez J, et al. Promoters and processing sites within the transforming region of bovine papillomavirus type 1. *J Virol* 1987;61:2240–2244.
2. Androphy EJ, Lowy DR, Schiller JT. Bovine papillomavirus E2 trans-activating gene product binds to specific sites in papillomavirus DNA. *Nature* 1987;325:70–73.
3. Androphy EJ, Schiller JT, Lowy DR. Identification of the protein encoded by the E6 transforming gene of bovine papillomavirus. *Science* 1985;230:442–445.
4. Antinore MJ, Birrer MJ, Patel D, et al. The human papillomavirus type 16 E7 gene product interacts with and trans-activates the AP1 family of transcription factors. *EMBO J* 1996;15:1950–1960.
5. Antson AA, Burns JE, Moroz OV, et al. Structure of the intact trans-activation domain of the human papillomavirus E2 protein. *Nature* 2000;403:805–809.
6. Baker CC. The genomes of the papillomaviruses. In: O'Brien SJ eds. *Genetic maps: Locus maps of complex genomes,* 6th ed, vol 1. Cold Spring Harbor, NY: Cold Spring Harbor Laboratory Press, 1993: 134–146.
7. Baker CC. Sequence analysis of papillomavirus genomes. In: Salzman NP, Howley PM eds. *The papillomaviruses, 2.* New York: Plenum Press, 1987;321–385.
8. Deleted in page proofs.
9. Baker CC, Howley PM. Differential promoter utilization by the papillomavirus in transformed cells and productively infected wart tissues. *EMBO J* 1987;6:1027–1035.
10. Baker TS, Newcomb WW, Olson NH, et al. Structures of bovine and human papillomaviruses: Analysis by cryoelectron microscopy and three-dimensional image reconstruction. *Biophys J* 1991;60: 1445–1456.
11. Band V, DeCaprio JA, Delmolino L, et al. Loss of p53 protein in human papillomavirus type 16 E6-immortalized human mammary epithelial cells. *J Virol* 1991;65:6671–6676.
12. Barbosa MS, Edmonds C, Fisher C, et al. The region of the HPV E7 oncoprotein homologous to adenovirus E1a and SV40 large T antigen contains separate domains for RB binding and casein kinase II. *EMBO J* 1990;9:153–160.
13. Barbosa MS, Lowy DR, Schiller JT. Papillomavirus polypeptides E6 and E7 are zinc binding proteins. *J Virol* 1989;63:1404–1407.
14. Barksdale SK, Baker CC. Differentiation-specific expression from the bovine papillomavirus type 1 P_{2443} and late promoters. *J Virol* 1993;67:5605–5616.
15. Barnard P, McMillan NA. The human papillomavirus E7 oncoprotein abrogates signaling mediated by interferon-alpha. *Virology* 1999;259: 305–313.
16. Bastien N, McBride AA. Interaction of the papillomavirus E2 protein with mitotic chromosomes. *Virology* 2000;270:124–34.

17. Bauknecht T, Angel P, Royer HD, et al. Identification of a negative regulatory domain in the human papillomavirus type 18 promoter: Interaction with the transcriptional repressor YY1. *EMBO J* 1992;11: 4607–4617.
18. Beaudenon S, Kremsdorf D, Obalek S, et al. Plurality of genital human papillomaviruses: Characterization of two new types with distinct biological properties. *Virology* 1987;161:374–384.
19. Beer-Romano P, Glass S, Rolfe M. Antisense targeting of E6AP elevates p53 in HPV-infected cells but not in normal cells. *Oncogene* 1997;14:595–602.
20. Benson JD, Lawanda R, Howley PM. Conserved interaction of the papillomavirus E2 transcriptional activator proteins with human and yeast TFIIB proteins. *J Virol* 1997;71:8041–8047.
20a. Berezutskaya E, Bagche S. The human papillomavirus E7 oncoprotein functionally interacts with the S4 subunit of the 26S proteasome. *J Biol Chem* 1997;272:30135–30140.
21. Berg LJ, Singh K, Botchan M. Complementation of a bovine papilloma virus low-copy-number mutant: Evidence for a temporal requirement of the complementing gene. *Mol Cell Biol* 1986;6:859–869.
22. Bernard BA, Bailly C, Lenoir MC, et al. The human papillomavirus type 18 (HPV18) E2 gene product is a repressor of the HPV18 regulatory region in human keratinocytes. *J Virol* 1989;63:4317–4324.
23. Black PH, Hartley JW, Rowe WP, et al. Transformation of bovine tissue culture cells by bovine papilloma virus. *Nature* 1963;199:1016–1018.
24. Blitz IL, Laimins LA. The 68-kilodalton E1 protein of bovine papillomavirus is a DNA-binding phosphoprotein which associates with the E2 transcriptional activator *in vitro*. *J Virol* 1991;65:649–656.
25. Boiron M, Levy JP, Thomas M, et al. Some properties of bovine papilloma virus. *Nature* 1964;201:423–424.
26. Bonne-Andrea C, Santucci S, Clertant P, et al. Bovine papillomavirus E1 protein binds specifically DNA polymerase alpha but not replication protein A. *J Virol* 1995;69:2341–2350.
27. Boyer SN, Wazer DE, Band V. E7 protein of human papilloma virus-16 induces degradation of retinoblastoma protein through the ubiquitin-proteasome pathway. *Cancer Res* 1996;56:4620–4624.
28. Bream GL, Ohmstede C-A, Phelps WC. Characterization of human papillomavirus type 11 E1 and E2 proteins expressed in insect cells. *J Virol* 1993;67:2655–2663.
29. Brehm A, Nielsen SJ, Miska EA, et al. The E7 oncoprotein associates with Mi2 and histone deacetylase activity to promote cell growth. *EMBO J* 1999;18:2449–2458.
30. Breiding DE, Sverdrup F, Grossel MJ, et al. Functional interaction of a novel cellular protein with the papillomavirus E2 transactivation domain. *Mol Cell Biol* 1997;17:7208–7219.
31. Burkhardt A, DiMaio D, Schlegel R. Genetic and biochemical definition of the bovine papillomavirus E5 transforming protein. *EMBO J* 1987;6:2381–2385.
32. Burkhardt A, Willingham M, Gay C, et al. The E5 oncoprotein of bovine papillomavirus is oriented asymmetrically in Golgi and plasma membranes. *Virology* 1989;170:334–339.
33. Burnett S, Jareborg N, DiMaio D. Localization of bovine papillomavirus type 1 E5 protein to transformed keratinocytes and permissive differentiated cells in fibropapilloma tissue. *Proc Natl Acad Sci U S A* 1992;89:5665–5669.
34. Burnett S, Kiessling U, Pettersson U. Loss of bovine papillomavirus DNA replication control in growth-arrested transformed cells. *J Virol* 1989;63:2215–2225.
35. Burnett S, Strom AC, Jareborg N, et al. Induction of bovine papillomavirus E2 gene expression and early region transcription by cell growth arrest: Correlation with viral DNA amplification and evidence for differential promoter induction. *J Virol* 1990;64:5529–5541.
36. Butz K, Hoppe-Seyler F. Transcriptional control of human papillomavirus (HPV) oncogene expression: Composition of the HPV type 18 upstream regulatory region. *J Virol* 1993;67:6476–6486.
37. Chan SY, Delius H, Halpern AL, et al. Analysis of genomic sequences of 95 papillomavirus types: Uniting typing, phylogeny, and taxonomy. *J Virol* 1995;69:3074–3083.
38. Chen JJ, Reid CE, Band V, et al. Interaction of papillomavirus E6 oncoproteins with a putative calcium-binding protein. *Science* 1995;269:529–531.
39. Chen S-L, Mounts P. Transforming activity of E5a protein of human papillomavirus type 6 in NIH3T3 and C127 cells. *J Virol* 1990;64: 3226–3233.
40. Cheng S, Schmidt-Grimminger DC, Murant T, et al. Differentiation-dependent up-regulation of the human papillomavirus E7 gene reactivates cellular DNA replication in suprabasal differentiated keratinocytes. *Genes Dev* 1995;9:2335–2349.
41. Chiang C-M, Ustav M, Stenlund A, et al. Viral E1 and E2 proteins support replication of homologous and heterologous papillomavirus origins. *Proc Nat Acad Sci U S A* 1992;89:5799–5803.
42. Chin MT, Broker TR, Chow LT. Identification of a novel constitutive enhancer element and an associated binding protein: Implications for human papillomavirus type 11 enhancer regulation. *J Virol* 1989;63: 2967–2976.
43. Choe J, Vaillancourt P, Stenlund A, et al. Bovine papillomavirus type 1 encodes two forms of a transcriptional repressor: Structural and functional analysis of new viral cDNAs. *J Virol* 1989;63:1743–1755.
44. Chong T, Apt D, Gloss B, et al. The enhancer of human papillomavirus type 16: Binding sites for the ubiquitous transcription factors oct-1, NFA, TEF-2, NF1, and AP-1 participate in epithelial cell-specific transcription. *J Virol* 1991;65:5933–5943.
45. Chong T, Chan WK, Bernard HU. Transcriptional activation of human papillomavirus 16 by nuclear factor I, AP1, steroid receptors and a possibly novel transcription factor, PVF: A model for the composition of genital papillomavirus enhancers. *Nucleic Acids Res* 1990;18: 465–470.
46. Chow LT, Broker TR. Small DNA tumor viruses. In: Nathanson N eds. *Viral pathogenesis*. Philadelphia: Lippincott-Raven, 1997:267–301.
47. Chow LT, Hirochika H, Nasseri M, et al. Human papilloma virus gene expression. In: Steinberg BM, Brandsma JL, Taichman LB, eds. *Papillomaviruses, 5*. Cold Spring Harbor, NY: Cold Spring Harbor Laboratory Press, 1987:55–72.
48. Ciuffo G. Innesto positivo con filtrato di verruca volgare. *Giorn Ital Mal Venereol* 1907;48:12–17.
49. Clertant P, Seif I. A common function for polyoma virus large-T and papillomavirus E1 proteins. *Nature* 1984;311:276–279.
50. Cobrinik D, Dowdy SF, Hinds PW, et al. The retinoblastoma protein and the regulation of cell cycling. *Trends Biochem Sci* 1992;17: 312–315.
51. Coggin JR, zur Hausen H. Workshop on papillomaviruses and cancer. *Cancer Res* 1979;39:545–546.
52. Cole ST, Danos O. Nucleotide sequence and comparative analysis of the human papillomavirus type 18 genome: Phylogeny of papillomaviruses and repeated structure of the E6 and E7 gene products. *J Mol Biol* 1987;193:599–608.
53. Conrad M, Bubb VJ, Schlegel R. The human papillomavirus type 6 and 16 E5 proteins are membrane-associated proteins which associate with the 16-kilodalton pore-forming protein. *J Virol* 1993;67:6170–6178.
54. Crawford LV, Crawford EM. A comparative study of polyoma and papilloma viruses. *Virology* 1963;21:258–263.
55. Cripe TP, Haugen TH, Turk JP, et al. Transcriptional regulation of the human papillomavirus-16 E6-E7 promoter by a keratinocyte-dependent enhancer, and by viral E2 trans-activator and repressor gene products: Implications for cervical carcinogenesis. *EMBO J* 1987;6: 3745–3753.
56. Crum CP, Barber S, Symbula M, et al. Coexpression of the human papillomavirus type 16 E4 and L1 open reading frames in early cervical neoplasia. *Virology* 1990;178:238–246.
57. Crusius K, Auvinen E, Alonso A. Enhancement of EGF- and PMA-mediated MAP kinase activation in cells expressing the human papillomavirus type 16 E5 protein. *Oncogene* 1997;15:1437–1444.
58. Cueille N, Nougarede R, Mechali F, et al. Functional interaction between the bovine papillomavirus virus type 1 replicative helicase E1 and cyclin E-Cdk2. *J Virol* 1998;72:7255–7262.
59. Das K, Bohl J, Vande Pol SB. Identification of a second transforming function in bovine papillomavirus type 1 E6 and the role of E6 interactions with paxillin, E6BP, and E6AP. *J Virol* 2000;74:812–816.
60. Day PM, Roden RB, Lowy DR, et al. The papillomavirus minor capsid protein, L2, induces localization of the major capsid protein, L1, and the viral transcription/replication protein, E2, to PML oncogenic domains. *J Virol* 1998;72:142–150.
61. DeCaprio JA, Ludlow JW, Figge J, et al. SV40 large tumor antigen forms a specific complex with the product of the retinoblastoma susceptibility gene. *Cell* 1988;54:275–283.
62. Del Vecchio AM, Romanczuk H, Howley PM, et al. Transient replication of human papillomavirus DNAs. *J Virol* 1992;66:5949–5958.
63. Delius H, Hofmann B. Primer-directed sequencing of human papillomavirus types. *Curr Top Microbiol Immunol* 1994;186:13–32.

64. DeVilliers EM. Papillomavirus and HPV typing. *Clin Dermatol* 1997;15:199–206.
65. Dietrich-Goetz W, Kennedy IM, Levins B, et al. A cellular 65-kDa protein recognizes the negative regulatory element of human papillomavirus late mRNA. *Proc Natl Acad Sci U S A* 1997;94:163–168.
66. DiMaio D, Guralski D, Schiller JT. Translation of open reading frame E5 of bovine papillomavirus is required for its transforming activity. *Proc Natl Acad Sci U S A* 1986;83:1797–1801.
67. DiMaio D, Lai C-C, Mattoon D. The platelet-derived growth factor b receptor as a target of the bovine papillomavirus E5 protein. *Cytokine Growth Factor Rev* 2000;11:283–293.
68. DiMaio D, Metherall J, Neary K, et al. Nonsense mutation in open reading frame E2 of bovine papillomavirus DNA. *J Virol* 1986;57:475–480.
69. DiMaio D, Petti L, Hwang E-S. The E5 transforming proteins of the papillomaviruses. *Semin Virol* 1994;5:369–379.
70. DiMaio D, Settleman J. Bovine papillomavirus mutant temperature defective for transformation, replication and transactivation. *EMBO J* 1988;7:1197–1204.
71. DiMaio D, Treisman RH, Maniatis T. Bovine papillomavirus vector that propagates as a plasmid in both mouse and bacterial cells. *Proc Natl Acad Sci U S A* 1982;77:4030–4034.
72. Dollard SC, Wilson JL, Demeter LM, et al. Production of human papillomavirus and modulation of the infectious program in epithelial raft cultures. *Genes Dev* 1992;6:1131–1142.
73. Doorbar J, Campbell D, Grand RJA, et al. Identification of the human papillomavirus-1a E4 gene products. *EMBO J* 1986;5:355–362.
74. Doorbar J, Ely S, Sterling J, et al. Specific interaction between HPV-16 E1-E4 and cytokeratins results in collapse of the epithelial cell intermediate filament network. *Nature* 1991;352:824–827.
75. Doorbar J, Foo C, Coleman N, et al. Characterization of events during the late stages of HPV16 infection *in vivo* using high-affinity synthetic Fabs to E4. *Virology* 1997;238:40–52.
76. Dowhanick JJ, McBride AA, Howley PM. Suppression of cellular proliferation by the papillomavirus E2 protein. *J Virol* 1995;69:7791–7799.
77. Duensing S, Lee LY, Duensing A, et al. The human papillomavirus type 16 E6 and E7 oncoproteins cooperate to induce mitotic defects and genomic instability by uncoupling centrosome duplication from the cell division cycle. *Proc Natl Acad Sci U S A* 2000;97:10002–10007.
78. Durst M, Dzarlieva PR, Boukamp P, et al. Molecular and cytogenetic analysis of immortalized human primary keratinocytes obtained after transfection with human papillomavirus type 16 DNA. *Oncogene* 1987;1:251–256.
79. Dvoretzky I, Shober R, Chattopadhyay SK, et al. A quantitative *in vitro* focus assay for bovine papilloma virus. *Virology* 1980;103:369–375.
80. Dyson N, Guida P, Munger K, et al. Homologous sequences in adenovirus E1A and human papillomavirus E7 proteins mediate interaction with the same set of cellular proteins. *J Virol* 1992;66:6893–6902.
81. Dyson N, Howley PM, Munger K, et al. The human papillomavirus-16 E7 oncoprotein is able to bind the retinoblastoma gene product. *Science* 1989;243:934–937.
82. Edmonds C, Vousden KH. A point mutational analysis of human papillomavirus type 16 E7 protein. *J Virol* 1989;63:2650–2656.
83. El-Diery WS, Tokino T, Velculescu VE, et al. WAF1, a potential mediator of p53 tumor suppression. *Cell* 1993;75:817–825.
84. Enemark EJ, Chen G, Vaughn DE, et al. Crystal structure of the DNA binding domain of the replication initiation protein E1 from papillomavirus. *Mol Cell* 2000;6:149–158.
85. Evander M, Frazer IH, Payne E, et al. Identification of the alpha6 integrin as a candidate receptor for papillomaviruses. *J Virol* 1997;71:2449–2456.
86. Favre M, Breitburd F, Croissant O, et al. Structural polypeptides of rabbit, bovine, and human papilloma viruses. *J Virol* 1975;15:1239–1247.
87. Flores ER, Lambert PF. Evidence for a switch in the mode of human papillomavirus DNA replication during the viral life cycle. *J Virol* 1997;71:7167–7179.
88. Fouts ET, Yu X, Egelman EH, et al. Biochemical and electron microscopic image analysis of the hexameric E1 helicase. *J Biol Chem* 1999;274:4447–4458.
89. Francis DA, Schmid SI, Howley PM. Repression of the integrated papillomavirus E6/E7 promoter is required for growth suppression of cervical cancer cells. *J Virol* 2000;74:2679–2686.
90. Friedman JC, Levy JP, Lasneret J, et al. Induction de fibromes souscutanes chez le hamster dore par inoculation d'extraits acellulaires de papillomes bovins. *C R Acad Sci* 1963;257:2328–2331.
91. Funk JO, Waga S, Harry JB, et al. Inhibition of CDK activity and PCNA-dependent DNA replication by p21 is blocked by interaction with the HPV-16 E7 oncoprotein. *Genes Dev* 1997;11:2090–2100.
92. Funk WD, Pak DT, Karas RH, et al. A transcriptionally active DNA-binding site for human p53 protein complexes. *Mol Cell Biol* 1992;12:2866–2871.
93. Furth PA, Baker CC. An element in the bovine papillomavirus late 3′ untranslated region reduces polyadenylated cytoplasmic RNA levels. *J Virol* 1991;65:5806–5812.
94. Furth PA, Choe W-T, Rex JH, et al. Sequences homologous to 5′ splice sites are required for the inhibitory activity of papillomavirus late 3′ untranslated regions. *Mol Cell Biol* 1994;14:5278–5289.
95. Gage JR, Meyers C, Wettstein FO. The E7 proteins of the nononcogenic human papillomavirus type 6b (HPV-6b) and of the oncogenic HPV-16 differ in retinoblastoma protein binding and other properties. *J Virol* 1990;64:723–730.
96. Gao Q, Srinivasan S, Boyer SN, et al. The E6 oncoproteins of high-risk papillomaviruses bind to a novel putative GAP protein, E6TP1, and target it for degradation. *Mol Cell Biol* 1999;19:733–744.
97. Gardiol D, Kuhne C, Glaunsinger B, et al. Oncogenic human papillomavirus E6 proteins target the discs large tumour suppressor for proteasome-mediated degradation. *Oncogene* 1999;18:5487–5496.
98. Gilbert DM, Cohen SN. Bovine papilloma virus plasmids replicate randomly in mouse fibroblasts throughout S phase of the cell cycle. *Cell* 1987;50:59–68.
99. Giri I, Yaniv M. Study of the E2 gene product of the cottontail rabbit papillomavirus reveals a common mechanism of transactivation among the papillomaviruses. *J Virol* 1988;62:1573–1581.
100. Gissmann L, Pfister H, zur Hausen H. Human papilloma virus (HPV): Characterization of 4 different isolates. *Virology* 1977;76:569–580.
101. Goldstein DJ, Finbow ME, Andersson T, et al. Bovine papillomavirus E5 oncoprotein binds to the 16K component of the vacuolar H+-ATPase. *Nature* 1991;352:347–349.
102. Goldstein DJ, Li W, Wang L-M, et al. The bovine papillomavirus type 1 E5 transforming protein specifically binds and activates the b-type receptor for the platelet-derived growth factor but not other related tyrosine kinase-containing receptors to induce cellular transformation. *J Virol* 1994;68:4432–4441.
103. Goldstein DJ, Schlegel R. The E5 oncoprotein of bovine papillomavirus binds to a 16 kd cellular protein. *EMBO J* 1990;9:137–146.
104. Groff DE, Lancaster WD. Genetic analysis of the 3′ early region transformation and replication functions of bovine papillomavirus type 1. *Virology* 1986;150:221–230.
105. Grossman SR, Laimins LA. E6 protein of human papillomavirus type 18 binds zinc. *Oncogene* 1989;4:1089–1093.
106. Grossman SR, Mora R, Laimins LA. Intracellular localization and DNA-binding properties of human papillomavirus type 18 E6 protein expressed with a baculovirus vector. *J Virol* 1989;63:366–374.
107. Hagensee ME, Olson NH, Baker TS, et al. Three-dimensional structure of vaccinia virus-produced human papillomavirus type 1 capsids. *J Virol* 1994;68:4503–4505.
108. Hagensee ME, Yaegashi N, Galloway DA. Self-assembly of human papillomavirus type 1 capsids by expression of the L1 protein alone or by coexpression of the L1 and L2 capsid proteins. *J Virol* 1993;67:315–322.
109. Harper JW, Adami GR, Wei N, et al. The p21 cdk-interacting protein Cip1 is a potent inhibitor of G1 cyclin dependent kinases. *Cell* 1993;75:805–816.
110. Harris SF, Botchan MR. Crystal structure of the human papillomavirus type 18 E2 activation domain. *Science* 1999;284:1673–1677.
111. Haugen TH, Cripe TP, Ginder GD, et al. Trans-activation of an upstream early gene promoter of bovine papilloma virus-1 by a product of the viral E2 gene. *EMBO J* 1987;6:145–152.
112. Haugen TH, Turek LP, Mercurio FM, et al. Sequence specific and general transactivation by the BPV-1 E2 transactivator require an N-terminal amphipathic helix-containing E2 domain. *EMBO J* 1988;7:4245–4253.
113. Hawley-Nelson P, Androphy EJ, Lowy DR, et al. The specific DNA recognition sequence of the bovine papillomavirus E2 protein is an E2-dependent enhancer. *EMBO J* 1988;7:525–531.

114. Hawley-Nelson P, Vousden KH, Hubbert NL, et al. HPV16 E6 and E7 proteins cooperate to immortalize human foreskin keratinocytes. *EMBO J* 1989;8:3905–3910.
115. Heck DV, Yee CL, Howley PM, et al. Efficiency of binding the retinoblastoma protein correlates with the transforming capacity of the E7 oncoproteins of the human papillomaviruses. *Proc Natl Acad Sci U S A* 1992;89:4442–4446.
116. Hedge RS, Rossman SR, Laimins LA, et al. Crystal structure at 1.7A of the bovine papillomavirus-1 E2 DNA-binding domain bound to its DNA target. *Nature* 1992;359:505–512.
117. Heilman CA, Engel L, Lowy DR, et al. Virus-specific transcription in bovine papillomavirus-transformed mouse cells. *Virology* 1982;119: 22–34.
118. Heino P, Zhou J, Lambert PF. Interaction of the papillomavirus transcription/replication factor, E2, and the viral capsid protein, L2. *Virology* 2000;276:304–314.
119. Hermonat PL, Howley PM. Mutational analysis of the 3′ open reading frames and the splice junction at nucleotide 3225 of bovine papillomavirus type 1. *J Virol* 1987;61:3889–3895.
120. Hermonat PL, Spalholz BA, Howley PM. The bovine papillomavirus P2443 promoter is E2 trans-responsive: Evidence for E2 autoregulation. *EMBO J* 1988;7:2815–2822.
121. Hershko A, Ciechanover A. The ubiquitin system. *Annu Rev Biochem* 1998;67:425–479.
122. Hirochika H, Hirochika R, Broker TR, et al. Functional mapping of the human papillomavirus type 11 transcriptional enhancer and its interaction with the trans-acting E2 proteins. *Genes Dev* 1988;2: 54–67.
123. Hoppe-Seyler F, Butz K, zur Hausen H. Repression of the human papillomavirus type 18 enhancer by the cellular transcription factor Oct-1. *J Virol* 1991;65:5613–5618.
124. Horwitz BH, Burkhardt AL, Schlegel R, et al. The 44 amino acid E5 transforming protein of bovine papillomavirus requires a hydrophobic core and specific carboxyl-terminal amino acids. *Mol Cell Biol* 1988;8:4071–4078.
125. Howes KA, Ransom N, Papermaster DF, et al. Apoptosis or retinoblastoma: Alternative fates of photoreceptors expressing the HPV-16 E7 gene in the presence or absence of p53. *Genes Dev* 1994;8: 1300–1310.
126. Huang L, Kinnucan E, Wang G, et al. Structure of an E6AP-UbcH7 complex: Insights into ubiquitination by the E2-E3 enzyme cascade. *Science* 1999;286:1321–1326.
127. Huang PS, Patrick DR, Edwards G, et al. Protein domains governing interactions between E2F, the retinoblastoma gene product, and human papillomavirus type 16 E7 protein. *Mol Cell Biol* 1993;13: 953–960.
128. Hubbert NL, Sedman SA, Schiller JT. Human papillomavirus type 16 E6 increases the degradation rate of p53 in human keratinocytes. *J Virol* 1992;66:6237–6241.
129. Hubert WG, Lambert PF. The 23-kilodalton phosphoprotein of bovine papillomavirus type 1 is non-essential for stable plasmid replication in murine C127 cells. *J Virol* 1993;67:2932–2937.
130. Huibregtse JM, Scheffner M, Beaudenon S, et al. A family of proteins structurally and functionally related to the E6-AP ubiquitin-protein ligase. *Proc Natl Acad Sci U S A* 1995;92:2563–2567.
131. Huibregtse JM, Scheffner M, Howley PM. A cellular protein mediates association of p53 with the E6 oncoprotein of human papillomavirus types 16 or 18. *EMBO J* 1991;10:4129–4135.
132. Huibregtse JM, Scheffner M, Howley PM. Cloning and expression of the cDNA for E6-AP: A protein that mediates the interaction of the human papillomavirus E6 oncoprotein with p53. *Mol Cell Biol* 1993;13:775–784.
133. Huibregtse JM, Scheffner M, Howley PM. Localization of the E6-AP regions that direct HPV E6 binding, association with p53, and ubiquintination of associated proteins. *Mol Cell Biol* 1993;13:4918–4927.
134. Hummel M, Hudson JB, Laimins LA. Differentiation-induced and constitutive transcription of human papillomavirus type 31b in cell lines containing viral episomes. *J Virol* 1992;66:6070–6080.
135. Hummel M, Lim HB, Laimins LA. Human papillomavirus type 31b late gene expression is regulated through protein kinase C-mediated changes in RNA processing. *J Virol* 1995;69:3381–3388.
136. Hwang ES, Riese DJ, Settleman J, et al. Inhibition of cervical carcinoma cell line proliferation by the introduction of a bovine papillomavirus regulatory gene. *J Virol* 1993;67:3720–3729.
137. Ilves I, Kivi S, Ustav M. Long-term episomal maintenance of bovine papillomavirus type 1 plasmids is determined by attachment to host chromosomes, which is mediated by the viral E2 protein and its binding sites. *J Virol* 1999;73:4404–4412.
138. Jareborg N, Alderborn A, Burnett S. Identification and genetic definition of a bovine papillomavirus type 1 E7 protein and absence of a low-copy-number phenotype exhibited by E5, E6, or E7 viral mutants. *J Virol* 1992;66:4957–4965.
139. Jenson AB, Rosenthal JD, Olson C, et al. Immunologic relatedness of papillomaviruses from different species. *J Natl Cancer Inst* 1980;64: 495–500.
140. Jewers RJ, Hildebrandt P, Ludlow JW, et al. Regions of human papillomavirus type 16 E7 oncoprotein required for immortalization of human keratinocytes. *J Virol* 1992;66:1329–1335.
141. Jones DL, Alani RM, Münger K. The human papillomavirus E7 oncoprotein can uncouple cellular differentiation and proliferation in human keratinocytes by abrogating $p21^{cip1}$-mediated inhibition of cdk2. *Genes Dev* 1997;11:2101–2111.
142. Joyce JG, Tung JS, Przysiecki CT, et al. The L1 major capsid protein of human papillomavirus type 11 recombinant virus-like particles interacts with heparin and cell-surface glycosaminoglycans on human keratinocytes. *J Biol Chem* 1999;274:5810–5822.
143. Kanda T, Watanabe S, Yoshiike K. Immortalization of primary rat cells by human papillomavirus type 16 subgenomic DNA fragments controlled by the SV40 promoter. *Virology* 1988;165:321–325.
144. Kao WH, Beaudenon SL, Talis AL, et al. Human papillomavirus type 16 E6 induces self-ubiquitination of the E6AP ubiquitin-protein ligase. *J Virol* 2000;74:6408–6417.
145. Kastan MB, Zhan Q, El Deiry W-S, et al. A mammalian cell cycle checkpoint pathway utilizing p53 and GADD 45 is defective in ataxia-telangiectasia. *Cell* 1992;71:587–597.
146. Kaur P, McDougall JK. Characterization of primary human keratinocytes transformed by human papillomavirus type 18. *J Virol* 1988;62:1917–1924.
147. Kennedy IM, Haddow JK, Clements JB. A negative regulatory element in the human papillomavirus type 16 genome acts at the level of late mRNA stability. *J Virol* 1991;65:2093–2097.
148. Kern SE, Pietenpol JA, Thiagalingam S, et al. Oncogenic forms of p53 inhibit p53-regulated gene expression. *Science* 1992;256:827–830.
149. Kessis TD, Slebos RJ, Nelson WG, et al. Human papillomavirus 16 E6 expression disrupts the p53-mediated cellular response to DNA damage. *Proc Natl Acad Sci U S A* 1993;90:3988–3992.
150. Kirnbauer R, Booy F, Cheng N, et al. Papillomavirus L1 major capsid protein self-assembles into virus-like particles that are highly immunogenic. *Proc Natl Acad Sci U S A* 1992;89:12180–12184.
151. Kiyono T, Hiraiwa A, Fujita M, et al. Binding of high-risk human papillomavirus E6 oncoproteins to the human homologue of the *Drosophila* discs large tumor suppressor protein. *Proc Nat Acad Sci U S A* 1997;94:11612–11616.
152. Klingelhutz AJ, Foster SA, McDougall JK. Telomerase activation by the E6 gene product of human papillomavirus type 16. *Nature* 1996; 380:79–81.
153. Klumpp DJ, Laimins LA. Differentiation-induced changes in promoter usage for transcripts encoding the human papillomavirus type 31 replication protein E1. *Virology* 1999;257:239–246.
154. Koffa MD, Graham SV, Takagaki Y, et al. The human papillomavirus type 16 negative regulatory RNA element interacts with three proteins that act at different posttranscriptional levels. *Proc Natl Acad Sci U S A* 2000;97:4677–4682.
155. Kuhne C, Banks L. E3-Ubiquitin Ligase/E6-AP links multicopy maintenance protein 7 to the ubiquitination pathway by a novel motif, the L2G Box. *J Biol Chem* 1998;273:34302–34309.
156. Kulke R, DiMaio D. Biological activities of the E5 protein of the deer papillomavirus in mouse C127 cells: Morphologic transformation, induction of cellular DNA synthesis and activation of the PDGF receptor. *J Virol* 1991;65:4943–4949.
157. Kumar S, Kao WH, Howley PM. Physical interaction between specific E2 and Hect E3 enzymes determines functional cooperativity. *J Biol Chem* 1997;272:13548–13554.
158. Kumar S, Talis AL, Howley PM. Identification of HHR23A as a substrate for E6-associated protein-mediated ubiquitination. *J Biol Chem* 1999;274:18785–18792.
159. Laimins LA, Bedell MA, Jones KH, et al. Transformation of NIH-3T3 and primary rat embryo fibroblasts by human papillomavirus type 16

and type 18. In: Steinberg BM, Brandsma JL, Taichman LB, eds. *Papillomaviruses, 5.* Cold Spring Harbor, NY: Cold Spring Harbor Laboratory Press, 1987;201–207.
160. Lambert PF, Howley PM. Bovine papillomavirus type 1 E1 replication-defective mutants are altered in their transcriptional regulation. *J Virol* 1988;62:4009–4015.
161. Lambert PF, Hubbert NL, Howley PM, et al. Genetic assignment of the multiple E2 gene products in bovine papillomavirus transformed cells. *J Virol* 1989;63:3151–3154.
162. Lambert PF, Spalholz BA, Howley PM. A transcriptional repressor encoded by BPV-1 shares a common carboxy terminal domain with the E2 transactivator. *Cell* 1987;50:68–78.
163. Law M-F, Lowy DR, Dvoretzky I, et al. Mouse cells transformed by bovine papillomavirus contain only extrachromosomal viral DNA sequences. *Proc Natl Acad Sci U S A* 1981;78:2727–2731.
164. Lechner MS, Mack DH, Finicle AB, et al. Human papillomavirus E6 proteins bind p53 *in vivo* and abrogate p53-mediated repression of transcription. *EMBO J* 1992;11:3045–3052.
165. Lee D, Sohn H, Kalpana GV, et al. Interaction of E1 and hSNF5 proteins stimulates replication of human papillomavirus DNA. *Nature* 1999;399:487–491.
166. Lee KY, Broker TR, Chow LT. Transcription factor YY1 represses cell-free replication from human papillomavirus origins. *J Virol* 1998; 72:4911–4917.
167. Lee SS, Glaunsinger B, Mantovani F, et al. Multi-PDZ domain protein MUPP1 is a cellular target for both adenovirus E4-ORF1 and high-risk papillomavirus type 18 E6 oncoproteins. *J Virol* 2000;74: 9680–9693.
168. Lee SS, Weiss RS, Javier RT. Binding of human virus oncoproteins to hDlg/SAP97, a mammalian homolog of the *Drosophila* discs large tumor suppressor protein. *Proc Natl Acad Sci U S A* 1997;94: 6670–6675.
169. Leechanachai P, Banks L, Moreau F, et al. The E5 gene from human papillomavirus type 16 is an oncogene which enhances growth factor-mediated signal transduction to the nucleus. *Oncogene* 1992;7:17–25.
170. Lehman CW, Botchan MR. Segregation of viral plasmids depends on tethering to chromosomes and is regulated by phosphorylation. *Proc Natl Acad Sci U S A* 1998;95:4338–4343.
171. Leptak C, Ramon y Cajal S, Kulke R, et al. Tumorigenic transformation of mouse keratinocytes by the E5 genes of human papillomavirus type 16 and bovine papillomavirus type 1. *J Virol* 1991;65:7078–7083.
172. Li R, Botchan MR. Acidic transcription factors alleviate nucleosome-mediated repression of BPV-1 DNA replication. *Proc Natl Acad Sci U S A* 1994;91:7051–7055.
173. Li R, Botchan MR. The acidic transcriptional activation domains of VP16 and p53 bind the cellular replication protein A and stimulate *in vitro* BPV-1 DNA replication. *Cell* 1993;73:1207–1221.
174. Li R, Knight J, Bream G, et al. Specific recognition nucleotides and their context determine the affinity of E2 protein for 17 binding sites in the BPV-1 genome. *Genes Dev* 1989;3:510–526.
175. Liu J-S, Kuo S-R, Broker TR, et al. The functions of human papillomavirus type 11 E1, E2, and E2C proteins in cell-free DNA replication. *J Biol Chem* 1995;270:27283–27291.
176. Liu JS, Kuo SR, Makhov AM, et al. Human Hsp70 and Hsp40 chaperone proteins facilitate human papillomavirus-11 E1 protein binding to the origin and stimulate cell-free DNA replication. *J Biol Chem* 1998;273:30704–30712.
177. Lowy DR, Dvoretzky I, Shober R, et al. *In vitro* tumorigenic transformation by a defined subgenomic fragment of bovine papillomavirus DNA. *Nature* 1980;287:72–74.
178. Luscher-Firzlaff JM, Westendorf JM, Zwicker J, et al. Interaction of the fork head domain transcription factor MPP2 with the human papilloma virus 16 E7 protein: enhancement of transformation and transactivation. *Oncogene* 1999;18:5620–5630.
179. Lusky M, Fontane E. Formation of the complex of bovine papillomavirus E1 and E2 proteins is modulated by E2 phosphorylation and depends upon sequences within the carboxyl terminus of E1. *Proc Natl Acad Sci U S A* 1991;88:6363–6367.
180. Lusky M, Hurwitz J, Seo YS. The bovine papillomavirus E2 protein modulates the assembly of but is not stably maintained in a replication-competent multimeric E1-replication origin complex. *Proc Natl Acad Sci U S A* 1994;91:8895–8899.
181. Ma T, Zou N, Lin BY, et al. Interaction between cyclin-dependent kinases and human papillomavirus replication-initiation protein E1 is required for efficient viral replication. *Proc Natl Acad Sci U S A* 1999; 96:382–387.
182. Mannhardt B, Weinzimer SA, Wagner M, et al. Human papillomavirus type 16 E7 oncoprotein binds and inactivates growth-inhibitory insulin-like growth factor binding protein 3. *Mol Cell Biol* 2000;20: 6483–6495.
183. Martin P, Vass W, Schiller JT, et al. The bovine papillomavirus E5 transforming protein can stimulate the transforming activity of EGF and CSF-1 receptors. *Cell* 1989;59:21–23.
184. Massimi P, Pim D, Storey A, et al. HPV-16 E7 and adenovirus E1a complex formation with TATA box binding protein is enhanced by casein kinase II phosphorylation. *Oncogene* 1996;12:2325–2330.
185. Matlashewski G, Schneider J, Banks L, et al. Human papillomavirus type 16 DNA cooperates with activated ras in transforming primary cells. *EMBO J* 1987;6:1741–1746.
186. Mazzarelli JM, Atkins GB, Geisberg JV, et al. The viral oncoproteins Ad5 E1A, HPV16 E7 and SV40 TAg bind a common region of the TBP-associated factor-110. *Oncogene* 1995;11:1859–1864.
187. McBride AA, Byrne JC, Howley PM. E2 polypeptides encoded by bovine papillomavirus I form dimers through the carboxyl-terminal DNA binding domain: Transactivation is mediated through the conserved amino-terminal domain. *Proc Natl Acad Sci U S A* 1989;86: 510–514.
188. McBride AA, Romanczuk H, Howley PM. The papillomavirus E2 regulatory proteins. *J Biol Chem* 1991;266:18411–18414.
189. McMillan NA, Payne E, Frazer IH, et al. Expression of the alpha6 integrin confers papillomavirus binding upon receptor-negative B-cells. *Virology* 1999;261:271–279.
190. Meyer AN, Xu YF, Webster MK, et al. Cellular transformation by a transmembrane peptide: Structural requirements for the bovine papillomavirus E5 oncoprotein. *Proc Natl Acad Sci U S A* 1994;91: 4634–4638.
191. Meyers C, Frattini MG, Hudson JB, et al. Biosynthesis of human papillomavirus from a continuous cell line upon epithelial differentiation. *Science* 1992;257:971–973.
192. Meyers C, Laimins LA. *In vitro* systems for the study and propagation of human papillomaviruses. *Curr Top Microbiol Immunol* 1994;186: 199–215.
193. Mietz JA, Unger T, Huibregtse JM, et al. The transcriptional transactivation function of wild-type p53 is inhibited by SV40 large T-antigen and by HPV-16 oncoprotein. *EMBO J* 1992;11:5013–5020.
194. Missero C, Calautti E, Eckner R, et al. Involvement of the cell-cycle inhibitor Cip1/WAF1 and the E1A-associated p300 protein in terminal differentiation. *Proc Nat Acad Sci U S A* 1995;92:5451–5455.
195. Mohr IJ, Clark R, Sun S, et al. Targeting the E1 replication protein to the papillomavirus origin of replication by complex formation with the E2 transactivator. *Science* 1990;250:1694–1699.
196. Morgan D, Pecoraro G, Rosenberg I, et al. Human papillomavirus type 6b DNA required for initiation but not maintenance of transformation of C127 mouse cells. *J Virol* 1990;64:969–976.
197. Muller M, Gissmann L, Cristiano RJ, et al. Papillomavirus capsid binding and uptake by cells from different tissues and species. *J Virol* 1995;69:948–954.
198. Münger K, Phelps WC, Bubb V, et al. The E6 and E7 genes of the human papillomavirus type 16 together are necessary and sufficient for transformation of primary human keratinocytes. *J Virol* 1989;63: 4417–4421.
199. Münger K, Scheffner M, Huibregtse JM, et al. Interactions of HPV E6 and E7 with tumor suppressor gene products. *Cancer Surv* 1992;12: 197–217.
200. Münger K, Werness BA, Dyson N, et al. Complex formation of human papillomavirus E7 proteins with the retinoblastoma tumor suppressor gene product. *EMBO J* 1989;8:4099–4105.
201. Nakagawa S, Huibregtse JM. Human scribble (vartul) is targeted for ubiquitin-mediated degradation by the high-risk papillomavirus E6 proteins and the E6AP ubiquitin-protein ligase. *Mol Cell Biol* 2000; 20:8244–8253.
202. Nallaseth FS, DePamphilis ML. Papillomavirus contains cis-acting sequences that can suppress but not replicate origins of DNA replication. *J Virol* 1994;68:3051–3064.
203. Neary K, DiMaio D. Open reading frames E6 and E7 of bovine papillomavirus type 1 are both required for full transformation of mouse C127 cells. *J Virol* 1989;63:259–266.
204. Neary K, Horwitz BH, DiMaio D. Mutational analysis of open read-

ing frame E4 of bovine papillomavirus type 1. *J Virol* 1987;61: 1248–1252.
205. Nevins JR. A link between the Rb tumor suppressor protein and viral oncoproteins. *Science* 1992;258:424–429.
206. Nilson LA, DiMaio D. Platelet-derived growth factor receptor can mediate tumorigenic transformation by the bovine papillomavirus E5 protein. *Mol Cell Biol* 1993;13:4137–4145.
207. Nilson LA, Gottlieb RL, Polack GW, et al. Mutational analysis of the interaction between the bovine papillomavirus E5 transforming protein and the endogenous beta receptor for platelet-derived growth factor in mouse C127 cells. *J Virol* 1995;69:5869–5874.
208. Nishimura A, Ono T, Ishimoto A, et al. Mechanisms of human papillomavirus E2-mediated repression of viral oncogene expression and cervical cancer cell growth inhibition. *J Virol* 2000;74:3752–3760.
209. Nuovo GJ, Crum CP, de Villiers E-M, et al. Isolation of a novel human papillomavirus (type 15) from a cervical condyloma. *J Virol* 1988; 62:1452–1455.
210. O'Connor M, Bernard HU. Oct-1 activates the epithelial-specific enhancer of human papillomavirus type 16 via a synergistic interaction with NFI at a conserved composite regulatory element. *Virology* 1995;207:77–88.
211. Oda H, Kumar S, Howley PM. Regulation of the Src family tyrosine kinase Blk through E6AP-mediated ubiquitination. *Proc Natl Acad Sci U S A* 1999;96:9557–9562.
212. Oren M, Maltzman W, Levine AJ. Post-translational regulation of the 54K cellular tumor antigen in normal and transformed cells. *Mol Cell Biol* 1981;1:101–110.
213. Ozbun MA, Meyers C. Human papillomavirus type 31b E1 and E2 transcript expression correlates with vegetative viral genome amplification. *Virology* 1998;248:218–230.
214. Pan H, Griep AE. Altered cell cycle regulation in the lens of HPV-16 E6 and E7 transgenic mice: Implications for tumor suppressor gene function in development. *Genes Dev* 1994;8:1285–1299.
215. Park P, Copeland W, Yang L, et al. The cellular DNA polymerase a-primase is required for papillomavirus DNA replication and associates with the viral E1 helicase. *Proc Natl Acad Sci U S A* 1994;91: 8700–8704.
216. Patel D, Huang SM, Baglia LA, et al. The E6 protein of human papillomavirus type 16 binds to and inhibits co-activation by CBP and p300. *EMBO J* 1999;18:5061–5072.
217. Peng YC, Breiding DE, Sverdrup F, et al. AMF-1/Gps2 binds p300 and enhances its interaction with papillomavirus E2 proteins. *J Virol* 2000;74:5872–5879.
218. Petti L, DiMaio D. Specific interaction between the bovine papillomavirus E5 transforming protein and the b receptor for platelet-derived growth factor in stably transformed and acutely transfected cells. *J Virol* 1994;68:3582–3592.
219. Petti L, DiMaio D. Stable association between the bovine papillomavirus E5 transforming protein and activated platelet-derived growth factor receptor in transformed mouse cells. *Proc Natl Acad Sci U S A* 1992;89:6736–6740.
220. Petti L, Nilson L, DiMaio D. Activation of the platelet-derived growth factor receptor by the bovine papillomavirus E5 protein. *EMBO J* 1991;10:845–855.
221. Petti LM, Reddy V, Smith SO, et al. Identification of amino acids in the transmembrane and juxtamembrane domains of the platelet-derived growth factor receptor required for productive interaction with the bovine papillomavirus E5 protein. *J Virol* 1997;71:7318–7327.
222. Pfister H, Gissman L, zur Hausen H. Partial characterization of proteins of human papilloma viruses (HPV) 1–3. *Virology* 1977;83: 131–137.
223. Phelps WC, Münger K, Yee CL, et al. Structure-function analysis of the human papillomavirus type 16 E7 oncoprotein. *J Virol* 1992;66: 2418–2427.
224. Phelps WC, Yee CL, Münger K, et al. The human papillomavirus type 16 E7 gene encodes transactivation and transformation functions similar to those of adenovirus E1A. *Cell* 1988;53:539–547.
225. Pietenpol JA, Stein RW, Moran E, et al. TGFb1 inhibition of c-myc transcription and growth in keratinocytes is abrogated by viral transforming proteins with pRB binding domains. *Cell* 1990;61:777–785.
226. Piirsoo M, Ustav E, Mandel T, et al. Cis and trans requirements for stable episomal maintenance of the BPV-1 replicator. *EMBO J* 1996; 15:1–11.
227. Pim D, Massimi P, Banks L. Alternatively spliced HPV-18 E6* protein inhibits E6 mediated degradation of p53 and suppresses transformed cell growth. *Oncogene* 1997;15:257–264.
228. Pirisi L, Yasumoto S, Feller M, et al. Transformation of human fibroblasts and keratinocytes with human papillomavirus type 16 DNA. *J Virol* 1987;61:1061–1066.
229. Prakash SS, Horwitz BH, Zibello T, et al. Bovine papillomavirus E2 gene regulates expression of the viral E5 transforming gene. *J Virol* 1988;62:3608–3613.
230. Rabson MS, Yee C, Yang Y-C, et al. Bovine papillomavirus type 1 3′ early region transformation and plasmid maintenance functions. *J Virol* 1986;60:626–634.
231. Rangasamy D, Wilson VG. Bovine papillomavirus E1 protein is sumoylated by the host cell Ubc9 protein. *J Biol Chem* 2000;275: 30487–30495.
232. Rangasamy D, Woytek K, Khan SA, et al. SUMO-1 modification of bovine papillomavirus E1 protein is required for intranuclear accumulation. *J Biol Chem* 2000;275:37999–38004.
233. Rank NM, Lambert PF. Bovine papillomavirus type 1 E2 transcriptional regulators directly bind two cellular transcription factors, TFIID and TFIIB. *J Virol* 1995;69:6323–6334.
234. Reich NC, Oren M, Levine AJ. Two distinct mechanisms regulate the levels of a cellular tumor antigen. *Mol Cell Biol* 1983;3:2134–2150.
235. Rey O, Lee S, Baluda MA, et al. The E7 oncoprotein of human papillomavirus type 16 interacts with F-actin *in vitro* and *in vivo*. *Virology* 2000;268:372–381.
236. Roberts S, Ashmole I, Johnson GD, et al. Cutaneous and mucosal human papillomavirus E4 proteins form intermediate filament-like structures in epithelial cells. *Virology* 1993;197:176–187.
237. Roden RBS, Kirnbauer R, Jenson AB, et al. Interaction of papillomaviruses with the cell surface. *J Virol* 1994;68:7260–7266.
238. Rodriguez MI, Finbow ME, Alonso A. Binding of human papillomavirus 16 E5 to the 16 kDa subunit c (proteolipid) of the vacuolar H+-ATPase can be dissociated from the E5-mediated epidermal growth factor receptor overactivation. *Oncogene* 2000;19:3727–3732.
239. Rogel-Gaillard C, Pehau-Arnaudet G, Breitburd F, et al. Cytopathic effect in human papillomavirus type 1-induced inclusion warts: *In vitro* analysis of the contribution of two forms of the viral E4 protein. *J Invest Dermatol* 1993;101:843–851.
240. Romanczuk H, Howley PM. Disruption of either the E1 or the E2 regulatory gene of human papillomavirus type 16 increases viral immortalization capacity. *Proc Natl Acad Sci U S A* 1992;89:3159–3163.
241. Romanczuk H, Thierry F, Howley PM. Mutational analysis of cis-elements involved in E2 modulation of human papillomavirus type 16 P97 and type 18 P105 promoters. *J Virol* 1990;64:2849–2859.
242. Ronco LV, Karpova AY, Vidal M, et al. The human papillomavirus 16 E6 oncoprotein binds to interferon regulatory factor-3 and inhibits its transcriptional activity. *Genes Dev* 1998;12:2061–2072.
243. Rose RC, Bonnez W, Reichman RC, et al. Expression of human papillomavirus type 11 L1 protein in insect cells: *in vivo* and *in vitro* assembly of virus like particles. *J Virol* 1993;67:1936–1944.
244. Ruesch MN, Stubenrauch F, Laimins LA. Activation of papillomavirus late gene transcription and genome amplification upon differentiation in semisolid medium is coincident with expression of involucrin and transglutaminase but not keratin-10. *J Virol* 1998;72: 5016–5024.
245. Sailaja G, Watts RM, Bernard HU. Many different papillomaviruses have low transcriptional activity in spite of strong epithelial specific enhancers. *J Gen Virol* 1999;80:1715–1724.
246. Sandler AB, Vande Pol SB, Spalholz BA. Repression of the bovine papillomavirus type 1 transcription by the E1 replication protein. *J Virol* 1993;67:5079–5087.
247. Sang B-C, Barbosa MS. Single amino acid substitutions in "low risk" human papillomavirus (HPV) type 6 E7 protein enhance features characteristic of the "high risk" HPV E7 oncoproteins. *Proc Natl Acad Sci U S A* 1992;89:8063–8067.
248. Sarver N, Byrne JC, Howley PM. Transformation and replication in mouse cells of a bovine papillomavirus-pML2 plasmid vector that can be rescued in bacteria. *Proc Natl Acad Sci U S A* 1982;79:7147–7151.
249. Sarver N, Gruss P, Law M-F, et al. Bovine papilloma virus deoxyribonucleic acid: A novel eucaryotic cloning vector. *Mol Cell Biol* 1981; 1:486–496.
250. Sarver N, Rabson MS, Yang YC, et al. Localization and analysis of bovine papillomavirus type 1 transforming functions. *J Virol* 1984; 52:377–388.

251. Sato H, Furuno A, Yoshiike K. Expression of human papillomavirus type 16 E7 gene induces DNA synthesis of rat 3Y1 cells. *Virology* 1989;168:195–199.
252. Schapiro F, Sparkowski J, Adduci A, et al. Golgi alkalinization by the papillomavirus E5 oncoprotein. *J Cell Biol* 2000;148:305–315.
253. Scheffner M, Huibregtse JM, Vierstra RD, et al. The HPV-16 E6 and E6-AP complex functions as a ubiquitin-protein ligase in the ubiquintination of p53. *Cell* 1993;75:495–505.
254. Scheffner M, Munger K, Byrne JC, et al. The state of the p53 and retinoblastoma genes in human cervical carcinoma cell lines. *Proc Natl Acad Sci U S A* 1991;88:5523–5527.
255. Scheffner M, Nuber U, Huibregtse J. Protein ubiquitination involving an E1-E2-E3 enzyme ubiquitin thioester cascade. *Nature* 1995;373: 81–83.
256. Scheffner M, Werness BA, Huibregtse JM, et al. The E6 oncoprotein encoded by human papillomavirus types 16 and 18 promotes the degradation of p53. *Cell* 1990;63:1129–1136.
257. Schiller JT, Kleiner E, Androphy EJ, et al. Identification of bovine papillomavirus E1 mutants with increased transforming and transcriptional activity. *J Virol* 1989;63:1775–1782.
258. Schiller JT, Vass WC, Lowy DR. Identification of a second transforming region in bovine papillomavirus DNA. *Proc Natl Acad Sci U S A* 1984;81:7880–7884.
259. Schiller JT, Vass WC, Vousden KH, et al. The E5 open reading frame of bovine papillomavirus type 1 encodes a transforming gene. *J Virol* 1986;57:1–6.
260. Schilling B, De-Medina T, Syken J, et al. A novel human DnaJ protein, hTid-1, a homolog of the Drosophila tumor suppressor protein Tid56, can interact with the human papillomavirus type 16 E7 oncoprotein. *Virology* 1998;247:74–85.
261. Schlegel R, Phelps WC, Zhang YL, et al. Quantitative keratinocyte assay detects two biological activities of human papillomavirus DNA and identifies viral types associated with cervical carcinoma. *EMBO J* 1988;7:3181–3187.
262. Schlegel R, Wade-Glass M, Rabson M, et al. The E5 transforming gene of bovine papillomavirus encodes a small, hydrophobic polypeptide. *Science* 1986;233:464–467.
263. Schneider A, Oltersdorf T, Schneider V, et al. Distribution of human papillomavirus 16 genome in cervical neoplasia by molecular *in situ* hybridization of tissue sections. *Int J Cancer* 1987;39:717–721.
264. Sedman J, Stenlund A. Cooperative interaction between the initiator E1 and the transcriptional activator E2 is required for replication of bovine papillomavirus *in vivo* and *in vitro*. *EMBO J* 1995;14: 6218–6228.
265. Sedman J, Stenlund A. The papillomavirus E1 protein forms a DNA-dependent hexameric complex with ATPase and DNA helicase activities. *J Virol* 1998;72:6893–6897.
266. Sedman SA, Barbosa MS, Vass WC, et al. The full-length E6 protein of human papillomavirus type 16 has transforming and trans-activating activities and cooperates with E7 to immortalize keratinocytes in culture. *J Virol* 1991;65:4860–4866.
267. Seo Y, Muller F, Lusky M, et al. Bovine papilloma virus (BPV)-encoded E1 protein contains multiple activities required for BPV DNA replication. *Proc Natl Acad Sci U S A* 1993;90:702–706.
268. Seo Y-S, Muller F, Lusky M, et al. Bovine papillomavirus (BPV)-encoded E2 protein enhances binding of E1 protein to the BPV replication origin. *Proc Natl Acad Sci U S A* 1993;90:2865–2869.
269. Shope RE, Hurst EW. Infectious papillomatosis of rabbits; with a note on the histopathology. *J Exp Med* 1933;58:607–624.
270. Sibbet G, Romero-Graillet C, Meneguzzi G, et al. alpha6 Integrin is not the obligatory cell receptor for bovine papillomavirus type 4. *J Gen Virol* 2000;81:327–334.
271. Skiadopoulos MH, McBride AA. Bovine papillomavirus type 1 genomes and the E2 transactivator protein are closely associated with mitotic chromatin. *J Virol* 1998;72:2079–2088.
272. Smotkin D, Wettstein FO. Transcription of human papillomavirus type 16 early genes in cervical cancer and a cervical cancer derived cell line and identification of the E7 protein. *Proc Natl Acad Sci U S A* 1986;83:4680–4684.
273. Sokolowski M, Furneaux H, Schwartz S. The inhibitory activity of the AU-rich RNA element in the human papillomavirus type 1 late 3′ untranslated region correlates with its affinity for the elav-like HuR protein. *J Virol* 1999;73:1080–1091.
274. Song S, Pitot HC, Lambert PF. The human papillomavirus type 16 E6 gene alone is sufficient to induce carcinomas in transgenic animals. *J Virol* 1999;73:5887–5893.
275. Spalholz BA, Byrne JC, Howley PM. Evidence for cooperativity between E2 binding sites in E2 trans-regulation of bovine papillomavirus type 1. *J Virol* 1988;62:3143–3150.
276. Spalholz BA, Lambert PF, Yee CL, et al. Bovine papillomavirus transcriptional regulation: Localization of the E2-responsive elements of the long control region. *J Virol* 1987;61:2128–2137.
277. Spalholz BA, Vande Pol SB, Howley PM. Characterization of the cis elements involved in the basal and E2 transactivated expression of the bovine papillomavirus P2443 promoter. *J Virol* 1991;65:743–753.
278. Spalholz BA, Yang Y-C, Howley PM. Transactivation of a bovine papillomavirus transcriptional regulatory element by the E2 gene product. *Cell* 1985;42:183–191.
279. Spitkovsky D, Aengeneyndt F, Braspenning J, et al. p53-Independent growth regulation of cervical cancer cells by the papillomavirus E6 oncogene. *Oncogene* 1996;13:1027–1035.
280. Stenlund A, Botchan MR. The E2 trans-activator can act as a repressor by interfering with a cellular transcription factor. *Genes Dev* 1990;4:123–136.
281. Stenlund A, Bream GL, Botchan MR. A promoter with an internal regulatory domain is part of the origin of replication in BPV-1. *Science* 1987;236:1666–1671.
282. Stenlund A, Zabielski J, Ahola H, et al. Messenger RNAs from the transforming region of bovine papilloma virus type 1. *J Mol Biol* 1985;182:541–554.
283. Stoler MH, Broker TR. *In situ* hybridization detection of human papilloma virus DNA and messenger RNA in genital condylomas and a cervical carcinoma. *Hum Pathol* 1986;17:1250–1258.
284. Storey A, Greenfield I, Banks L, et al. Lack of immortalizing activity of a human papillomavirus type 16 variant DNA with a mutation in the E2 gene isolated from normal human cervical keratinocytes. *Oncogene* 1992;7:459–465.
285. Storey A, Pim D, Murray A, et al. Comparison of the *in vitro* transforming activities of human papillomavirus types. *EMBO J* 1988;6: 1815–1820.
286. Straight SW, Herman B, McCance DJ. The E5 oncoprotein of human papillomavirus type 16 inhibits acidification of endosomes in human keratinocytes. *J Virol* 1995;69:3185–3192.
287. Straight SW, Hinkle PM, Jewers RJ, et al. The E5 oncoprotein of human papillomavirus type 16 transforms fibroblasts and effects downregulation of the epidermal growth factor receptor in keratinocytes. *J Virol* 1993;67:4521–4532.
288. Stubenrauch F, Colbert AM, Laimins LA. Transactivation by the E2 protein of oncogenic human papillomavirus type 31 is not essential for early and late viral functions. *J Virol* 1998;72:8115–8123.
289. Stubenrauch F, Laimins LA. Human papillomavirus life cycle: Active and latent phases. *Semin Cancer Biol* 1999;9:379–386.
290. Sundberg JP. Papillomavirus infections in animals. In: Syrjanen K, Gissmann L, Koss LG, eds. *Papillomaviruses and human disease*. Berlin: Springer-Verlag, 1987:40–103.
291. Swift FV, Bhat K, Younghusband HB, et al. Characterization of a cell type-specific enhancer found in the human papilloma virus type 18 genome. *EMBO J* 1987;6:1339–1344.
292. Swindle CS, Engler JA. Association of the human papillomavirus type 11 E1 protein with histone H1. *J Virol* 1998;72:1994–2001.
293. Szymanski P, Stenlund A. Regulation of early gene expression from the bovine papillomavirus genome in transiently transfected C127 cells. *J Virol* 1991;65:5710–5720.
294. Talis AL, Huibregtse JM, Howley PM. The role of E6AP in the regulation of p53 protein levels in human papillomavirus (HPV) positive and HPV negative cells. *J Biol Chem* 1998;273:6439–6445.
295. Tan SH, Bartsch D, Schwarz E, et al. Nuclear matrix attachment regions of human papillomavirus type 16 point toward conservation of these genomic elements in all genital papillomaviruses. *J Virol* 1998; 72:3610–3622.
296. Tanaka A, Noda T, Yajima H, et al. Identification of a transforming gene of human papillomavirus type 16. *J Virol* 1989;63:1465–1469.
297. Thierry F, Garcia-Carranca A, Yaniv M. Elements that control the transcription of genital papillomavirus type 18. *Cancer Cells* 1987;5: 23–32.
298. Thierry F, Howley PM. Functional analysis of E2 mediated repression of the HPV-18 P105 promoter. *New Biologist* 1991;3:90–100.
299. Thierry F, Spyrou G, Yaniv M, et al. Two AP1 sites binding JunB are

essential for HPV18 transcription in keratinocytes. *J Virol* 1992;66: 3740–3748.
300. Thierry F, Yaniv M. The BPV1 E2 trans-acting protein can be either an activator or a repressor of the HPV18 regulatory region. *EMBO J* 1987;6:3391–3397.
301. Thomas M, Banks L. Inhibition of Bak-induced apoptosis by HPV-18 E6. *Oncogene* 1998;17:2943–2954.
302. Thomas M, Boiron M, Tanzer J, et al. *In vitro* transformation of mice by bovine papillomavirus. *Nature* 1964;202:709–710.
303. Thorner L, Bucay N, Choe J, et al. The product of the bovine papillomavirus type 1 modulator gene (M) is a phosphoprotein. *J Virol* 1988;62:2474–2482.
304. Thorner LK, Lim DA, Botchan MR. DNA-binding domain of bovine papillomavirus type 1 E1 helicase: Structural and functional aspects. *J Virol* 1993;67:6000–6014.
305. Tong X, Boll W, Kirschhausen T, et al. Interaction of the bovine papillomavirus E6 protein with the clatherin adaptor complex AP-1. *J Virol* 1998;72:476–482.
306. Tong X, Howley PM. The bovine papillomavirus E6 oncoprotein interacts with paxillin and disrupts the actin cytoskeleton. *Proc Natl Acad Sci U S A* 1997;94:4412–4417.
307. Tong X, Salgia R, Li J-L, et al. The bovine papillomavirus E6 protein binds to the LD motif repeats of paxillin and blocks its interaction with vinculin and the focal adhesion kinase. *J Biol Chem* 1997;272: 33373–33376.
308. Turek LP, Byrne JC, Lowy DR, et al. Interferon induces morphologic reversion with elimination of extrachromosomal viral genomes in bovine papillomavirus-transformed mouse cells. *Proc Natl Acad Sci U S A* 1982;79:7914–7918.
309. Ustav M, Stenlund A. Transient replication of BPV-1 requires two viral polypeptides encoded by the E1 and E2 open reading frames. *EMBO J* 1991;10:449–457.
310. Ustav M, Ustav E, Szymanski P, et al. Identification of the origin of replication of bovine papillomavirus and characterization of the viral origin recognition factor E1. *EMBO J* 1991;10:4321–4329.
311. Vande Pol SB, Brown MC, Turner CE. Association of bovine papillomavirus type 1 E6 oncoprotein with the focal adhesion protein paxillin through a conserved protein interaction motif. *Oncogene* 1998;16:43–52.
312. Vande Pol SB, Howley PM. A bovine papilloma virus constitutive enhancer is negatively regulated by the E2 repressor through competitive binding. *J Virol* 1990;64:5420–5429.
313. Vande Pol SB, Howley PM. The bovine papillomavirus constitutive enhancer is essential for viral transformation, DNA replication, and the maintenance of latency. *J Virol* 1992;66:2346–2358.
314. Vande Pol SB, Howley PM. Negative regulation of the bovine papillomavirus E5, E6, and E7 oncogenes by the viral E1 and E2 genes. *J Virol* 1995;69:395–402.
315. Vogelstein B, Lane D, Levine AJ. Surfing the p53 network. *Nature* 2000;408:307–310.
316. Vousden KH, Doniger J, DiPaolo JA, et al. The E7 open reading frame of human papillomavirus type 16 encodes a transforming gene. *Oncogene Res* 1988;3:167–175.
317. Waldeck S, Rosl F, Zentgraf H. Origin of replication in episomal bovine papilloma virus type 1 DNA isolated from transformed cells. *EMBO J* 1984;3:2173–2178.
318. Watanabe S, Kanda T, Yoshiike K. Human papillomavirus type 16 transformation of primary human embryonic fibroblasts requires expression of open reading frames E6 and E7. *J Virol* 1989;63: 965–969.
319. Watanabe S, Yoshiike K. Transformation of rat 3Y1 cells by human papillomavirus type 18 DNA. *Int J Cancer* 1988;41:896–900.
320. Werness BA, Levine AJ, Howley PM. Association of human papillomavirus types 16 and 18 E6 proteins with p53. *Science* 1990;248: 76–79.
321. White A, Livanos EM, Tlsty TD. Differential disruption of genomic integrity and cell cycle regulation in normal human fibroblasts by the HPV oncoproteins. *Genes Dev* 1994;8:666–677.
322. Whyte P, Buchkovich KJ, Horowitz JM, et al. Association between an oncogene and an anti-oncogene: The adenovirus E1A proteins bind to the retinoblastoma gene product. *Nature* 1988;334:124–129.
323. Whyte P, Williamson NM, Harlow E. Cellular targets for transformation by the adenovirus E1A proteins. *Cell* 1989;56:67–75.
324. Wilson VG, Ludes-Meyers J. A bovine papillomavirus E1-related protein binds specifically to bovine papillomavirus DNA. *J Virol* 1991; 65:5314–5322.
325. Woodworth CD, Bowden PE, Doninger J, et al. Characterization of normal human exocervical epithelial cells immortalized *in vitro* by papillomavirus types 16 and 18 DNA. *Cancer Res* 1988;48: 4620–4628.
326. Wu EW, Clemens KE, Heck DV, et al. The human papillomavirus E7 oncoprotein and the cellular transcription factor E2F bind to separate sites on the retinoblastoma tumor suppressor protein. *J Virol* 1993;67: 2402–2407.
327. Xiong Y, Hannon GJ, Zhang H, et al. p21 Is a universal inhibitor of cyclin kinases. *Nature* 1993;366:701–704.
328. Yang L, Li R, Mohr IJ, et al. Activation of BPV-1 replication *in vitro* by the transcription factor E2. *Nature* 1991;353:628–632.
329. Yang L, Mohr I, Fouts E, et al. The E1 protein of bovine papilloma virus 1 is an ATP-dependent DNA helicase. *Proc Natl Acad Sci U S A* 1993;90:5086–5090.
330. Yang Y-C, Spalholz BA, Rabson MS, et al. Dissociation of transforming and transactivating functions for bovine papillomavirus type 1. *Nature* 1985;318:575–577.
331. Yang YC, Okayama H, Howley PM. Bovine papillomavirus contains multiple transforming genes. *Proc Natl Acad Sci U S A* 1985;82: 1030–1034.
332. Yasugi T, Vidal M, Sakai H, et al. Two classes of human papillomavirus type 16 E1 mutants suggest pleiotropic conformational constraints affecting multimerization, E2 interaction, and interaction with cellular proteins. *J Virol* 1997;71:5942–5951.
333. Yasumoto S, Burkhardt AL, Doninger J, et al. Human papillomavirus type 16-induced malignant transformation of NIH 3T3 cells. *J Virol* 1986;57:572–577.
334. Yatsudo M, Okamoto Y, Hakura A. Functional dissociation of transforming genes of human papillomavirus type 16. *Virology* 1988;166: 594–597.
335. Yew PR, Berk A. Inhibition of p53 transactivation required for transformation by adenovirus early 1B protein. *Nature* 1992;357:82–85.
336. Zerfass-Thome K, Zwerschke W, Mannhardt B, et al. Inactivation of the cdk inhibitor p27KIP1 by the human papillomavirus type 16 E7 oncoprotein. *Oncogene* 1996;13:2323–2330.
337. Zhou J, Gissmann L, Zentgraf H, et al. Early phase in the infection of cultured cells with papillomavirus virions. *Virology* 1995;214:167–176.
338. Zhou J, Stenzel DJ, Sun XY, et al. Synthesis and assembly of infectious bovine papillomavirus particles *in vitro*. *J Gen Virol* 1993;74: 763–768.
339. Zhou J, Sun XY, Stenzel DJ, et al. Expression of vaccinia recombinant HPV 16 L1 and L2 ORF proteins in epithelial cells is sufficient for assembly of HPV virion-like particles. *Virology* 1991;185:251–257.
340. Zimmermann H, Degenkolbe R, Bernard HU, et al. The human papillomavirus type 16 E6 oncoprotein can down-regulate p53 activity by targeting the transcriptional coactivator CBP/p300. *J Virol* 1999;73: 6209–6219.
341. Zwerschke W, Mannhardt B, Massimi P, et al. Allosteric activation of acid alpha-glucosidase by the human papillomavirus E7 protein. *J Biol Chem* 2000;275:9534–9541.
342. Zwerschke W, Mazurek S, Massimi P, et al. Modulation of type M2 pyruvate kinase activity by the human papillomavirus type 16 E7 oncoprotein. *Proc Natl Acad Sci U S A* 1999;96:1291–1296.

CHAPTER 31

Adenoviridae: The Viruses and Their Replication

Thomas E. Shenk

Adenoviruses were first isolated and characterized as distinct viral agents by two groups who were searching for the etiologic agents of acute respiratory infections. In 1953, Rowe and colleagues (333) observed the spontaneous degeneration of primary cell cultures derived from human adenoids. The pathogenic changes proved to result from the replication of previously unidentified viruses present in the adenoid tissues. In 1954, Hilleman and Werner (172) were studying an epidemic of respiratory disease in army recruits, and they isolated agents from respiratory secretions that induced cytopathic changes in cultures of human cells. The viruses discovered by the two groups were soon shown to be related (188), and, in 1956, the agents were named *adenoviruses,* after the original tissue (adenoid) in which the prototype viral strain was discovered (99). Epidemiologic studies confirmed that adenoviruses are the cause of acute febrile respiratory disease among military recruits (90,122). It soon became clear, however, that adenoviruses are not the etiologic agents of the common cold; they are responsible for only a small portion of acute respiratory morbidity in the general population and for about 5% to 10% of respiratory illness in children. Besides respiratory disease, adenoviruses cause epidemic conjunctivitis (196), and they have been associated with a variety of additional clinical syndromes—perhaps most notably, infantile gastroenteritis (450). Today, more than 100 members of the adenovirus group have been identified that infect a wide range of mammalian and avian hosts. All of these viruses contain a linear, double-stranded DNA genome encapsidated in an icosahedral protein shell.

In 1962, Trentin and colleagues (398) made a seminal discovery: human adenovirus type 12 induces malignant tumors after inoculation into newborn hamsters. This was the first time that a human virus was shown to sponsor oncogenesis. No epidemiologic evidence has been reported linking adenoviruses with malignant disease in humans; extensive searches have generally failed to find adenovirus nucleic acids in human tumors (144,254). Nevertheless, the ability to induce tumors in animals and to transform cultured cells has established adenovirus as an important model system for probing the mysteries of oncogenesis.

As the interest in adenoviruses as tumor viruses intensified, their virtues as an experimental system became evident. The prototype human adenoviruses are easily propagated to produce high-titer stocks, and they initiate synchronous infections of established cell lines. Further, the viral genome is readily manipulated, facilitating the study of adenovirus gene functions by mutational analysis. Studies of adenovirus-infected cells have made numerous contributions to our understanding of viral and cellular gene expression and regulation, DNA replication, cell cycle control, and cellular growth regulation.

Perhaps the signal contribution to modern biology of the adenovirus system has been to host the discovery of messenger RNA (mRNA) splicing. Studies on the biogenesis of viral mRNA first demonstrated that many mRNAs are produced from a large nuclear transcript (17,421), and subsequent analysis of the structure of adenovirus mRNAs revealed the existence of introns (30,65). Today, the utility of adenovirus as a vector for gene therapy is the subject of intense exploration. This chapter overviews the structure of the adenovirus particle, the adenovirus replication cycle in human cells, its ability to oncogenically transform cells, and its interactions with host cells and host organisms. Details of adenovirus transformation are also considered in Chapter 10, and a discussion of the pathogenesis, clinical syndromes, epidemiology, techniques for diagnosis, modes of treatment, and utility of adenoviruses as vectors follows in Chapter 68 in *Fields Virology*, 4th ed.

CLASSIFICATION

The adenoviruses constitute the *Adenoviridae* family of viruses, which is divided into two genera, *Mastadenovirus* and *Aviadenovirus* (297). Whereas the *Aviadenovirus* genus is limited to viruses of birds, the *Mastadenovirus* genus includes human, simian, murine, bovine, equine, porcine, ovine, canine, and opossum viruses. Although there is antigenic cross-reactivity among members within each genera owing to conserved epitopes located on the hexon protein of the virion (296), there is no known antigen common to all adenoviruses.

Forty-nine human adenovirus serotypes (Table 1) have been distinguished on the basis of their resistance to neutralization by antisera to other known adenovirus serotypes. Type-specific neutralization results predominantly from antibody binding to epitopes on the virion hexon protein and the terminal knob portion of the fiber protein (296). Hypervariable regions have been identified on the hexon that make up serotype-specific loops on the surface of the protein (75). The various serotypes are classified into six subgroups (see Table 1) based on their ability to agglutinate red blood cells (330). The central shaft of the viral fiber protein is responsible for binding to erythrocytes, and the hemagglutination reaction of an adenovirus is inhibited by antisera specific for viruses of the same type but not by antisera to viruses of different types. A variety of additional classification schemes have been explored, including subgroupings based on oncogenicity in rodents, relatedness of tumor antigens, electrophoretic mobility of virion proteins, or genome homologies. The various schemes produce reasonably concordant groupings (see Table 1), suggesting that the widely used classification based on hemagglutination is a reasonable standard.

VIRION STRUCTURE

Adenoviruses are icosahedral particles measuring 70 to 100 nm in diameter (177) (Fig. 1). The particles (virions) contain DNA (13% of mass), protein (87% of mass), no membrane or lipid, and trace amounts of carbohydrate because the virion fiber protein is modified by addition of glucosamine (143,191). Virions consist of a protein shell surrounding a DNA-containing core. The protein shell (capsid) is composed of 252 subunits (capsomeres), of which 240 are hexons and 12 are pentons (125). As suggested by their names, penton and hexon subunits are surrounded by five and six neighbors, respectively. Each penton contains a base, which forms part of the surface of the capsid, and a projecting fiber whose length varies among different serotypes (295).

Virion Polypeptides and DNA

Most of the structural studies of adenoviruses have focused on the closely related adenoviruses type 2 and 5

TABLE 1. *Classification schemes for human adenoviruses (mastadenovirus H)*

Subgroup	Hemagglutination groups	Serotypes	Oncogenic potential: Tumors in animals	Oncogenic potential: Transformation in tissue culture	Percentage of G-C in DNA
A	IV (little or no agglutination)	12, 18, 31	High	+	48–49
B	I (complete agglutination of monkey erythrocytes)	3, 7, 11, 14, 16, 21, 34, 35	Moderate	+	50–52
C	III (partial agglutination of rat erythrocytes)	1, 2, 5, 6	Low or none	+	57–59
D	II (complete agglutination of rat erythrocytes)	8, 9, 10, 13, 15, 17, 19, 20, 22–30, 32, 33, 36–39, 42–49	Low or none (mammary tumors)	+	57–61
E	III	4	Low or none	+	57–59
F	III	40,41	Unknown		

Modified from refs. 23 and 249, with permission.

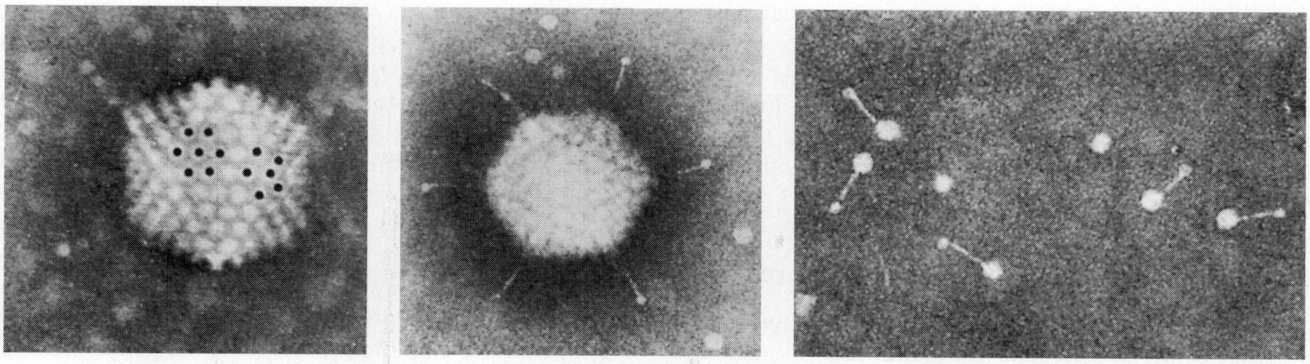

A,B C

FIG. 1. Adenovirus type 5. **A:** The virion is an icosahedron. One of the 240 hexon capsomeres surrounded by 6 hexons and one of the 12 penton capsomeres surrounded by 5 hexons are marked (*dots*). **B:** Six of the 12 fibers that are present on each virus particle are shown projecting from penton capsomeres located at the vertices of the icosahedral capsid. **C:** Free penton capsomeres containing penton base and fiber (×285,000). (From ref. 401, with permission.)

(Ad2 and Ad5). Electrophoretic analyses of purified virions disrupted with sodium dodecylsulfate was employed initially to identify structural polypeptides (191,407). Comparison of electrophoretic results with genomic open reading frames (ORFs) suggests there are probably 11 virion proteins. These proteins are numbered by convention (255), with no polypeptide I because the moiety originally designated I proved to be a mixture of aggregated molecules.

The outer shell or capsid of the virion is composed of seven known polypeptides. Polypeptide II (967 amino acids) is the most abundant virion constituent. The hexon protein is composed of three tightly associated molecules of polypeptide II (179), and this trimeric protein is referred to as the *hexon capsomere.* Polypeptides VI (217 amino acids), VIII (134 amino acids), and IX (139 amino acids) are associated with the hexon protein after various isolation procedures (107). All three polypeptides likely stabilize the hexon capsomere lattice, and polypeptides VI and VIII probably bridge between the capsid and core components of the virion. Five copies of polypeptide III (571 amino acids) associate to form the penton base protein (407), which is found at each vertex of the icosahedral particle. Polypeptide IIIa (566 amino acids) is associated with hexon units that surround the penton after pyridine dissociation of virions, and it appears to link adjacent facets of the capsid and bridge between hexons and polypeptide VII of the core (106). Polypeptide IV (582 amino acids) forms the trimeric fiber protein (407), which projects from the penton base at each vertex of the icosahedron. The combination of penton base plus fiber is called the *penton capsomere.* All human adenoviruses examined to date encode a single fiber protein with the exception of Ad40 and Ad41, which encode two fiber proteins and incorporate both polypeptides into their virions (205). Because the fiber interacts with a cellular receptor protein, the incorporation of two fiber proteins might extend the range of cell types to which these viruses can bind. Hexon and penton capsomeres are the major components on the surface of the virion, and their constituents, polypeptides II, III, and IV, contain tyrosine residues that are exposed on the virion surface and can be labeled by iodination of intact particles (106).

The core of the virion contains four known proteins and the viral genome. Polypeptides V (368 amino acids), VII (174 amino acids), and mu (19 amino acids) are basic, arginine-rich proteins (181,335) that contact the viral DNA (6,56). The function of the mu protein is unknown (181). Polypeptide VII is the major core protein, and it serves as a histone-like center around which the viral DNA is wrapped (56,272). Polypeptide V can bind to a penton base (106), and it might bridge between the core and capsid, positioning one relative to the other. The fourth protein in the core is the *terminal protein* (671 amino acids), which is covalently attached to the ends of the viral DNA. It was first identified indirectly by its ability to mediate circularization of the viral DNA through a protease-sensitive, noncovalent interaction (327). The circularizing agent was shown to be a 55-kd protein covalently attached to each 5′ end of the viral DNA (324), and the protein was subsequently visualized on viral DNA by avidin-biotin labeling (110a). The linkage between DNA and protein is a phosphodiester bond formed between the β-hydroxyl group of a serine (residue 562 of terminal protein) and the 5′ hydroxyl of the terminal deoxycytosine residue (83,360). The protein is not evident in electrophoretic analyses of virion proteins because it is present in only two copies per particle. The terminal protein serves as a primer for DNA replication (49,52,236,382), and it mediates attachment of the viral genome to the nuclear matrix (36,115,342).

Ad2 DNA was the first adenovirus genome to be completely sequenced (326), and it includes a total of 35,937 base pairs (bp). Ad5 (67), Ad12 (365), murine adenovirus (268), canine adenovirus (279), and avian adenovirus genomes (62,312) have also been sequenced. The DNAs of different adenoviruses have inverted terminal repeat sequences ranging in size from about 40 to 160 bp (12,119,396). The inverted repeats enable single strands of viral DNA to circularize by base-pairing of their terminal sequences, and the resulting base-paired panhandles are thought to be important for replication of the viral DNA.

Capsid and Core Three-Dimensional Structure

X-ray crystallography, electron microscopy, and combinations of the two methods have been used to generate a fairly refined picture of the adenovirus capsid (reviewed in 372). The x-ray structure of the major capsid protein, the hexon, has been determined to a resolution of 2.9 Å (13,325). The hexon protein, which is also referred to as the hexon capsomere, is a trimer composed of three interwoven hexon polypeptides. As described first for the picornaviruses, a β-structure stabilizes the association of the three subunits into a larger structure consisting of two domains: a triangular top facing the outside of the capsid and a hexagonal base with a central cavity. Group-of-nine hexons ("ninemers"), which can be isolated from each triangular face of the virion by treatment with 10% pyridine (313), provided insight to how interactions between hexons are stabilized. The structure of these ninemers was examined by subtracting an array of nine projected x-ray–determined hexons from scanning transmission electron microscopic images (116). The resulting two-dimensional difference image revealed density from a minor protein component extending along the hexon–hexon interfaces. Biochemical analysis had previously identified this component as polypeptide IX (407), a minor capsid constituent involved in stabilization of the capsid (69). Its carboxy-terminal domain is exposed on the surface of the capsid (3).

The three-dimensional structure of the complete adenovirus particle was determined to 21 Å resolution by image reconstruction from cryoelectron micrographs (63,371,372). A density map of the virion was generated from multiple images of the particle in different orientations. The reconstruction process relied on the known icosahedral symmetry of the virion to align the individual images. This work provided the first detailed visualization of the vertex proteins, including the penton base and its protruding fiber; it confirmed the earlier placement of protein IX; and it located minor capsid polypeptides at the edges of triangular facets, bridging hexons in adjacent facets. The three-dimensional structure of the virion has been refined by subtracting 240 copies of the crystallographic hexon from the cryoelectron microscopic image reconstruction (372). The difference map revealed more precisely the positions of several capsid proteins (Fig. 2). A less abundant stabilizing protein is located at each specialized position in the hexon assemblage. The penton complex fills the large gaps at the vertices, polypeptide IX stabilizes hexon–hexon contacts within a facet, polypeptide IIIa joins hexons of adjacent facets, and polypeptide VI anchors the ring of peripentonal hexons on the inside surface of the capsid and connects the capsid to the core. The structure of the particle has been further refined by employing constrained maximum entropy tomography (359).

The fiber protein that projects from each vertex of the particle is composed of three copies of polypeptide IV (334,407). The amino-terminal 40 residues of each sub-

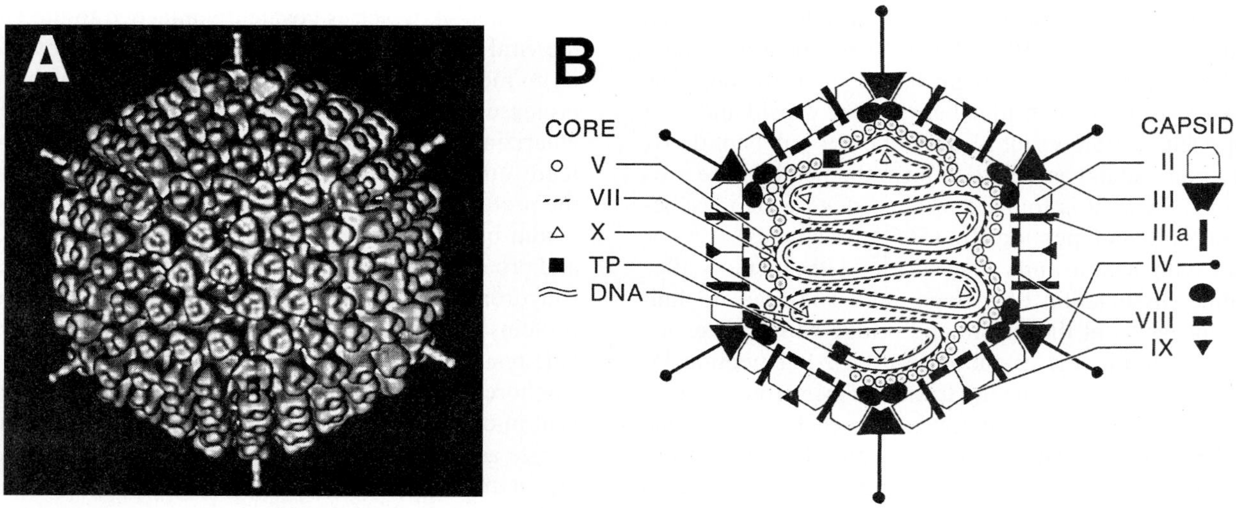

FIG. 2. Models of the adenovirus virion. **A:** Three-dimensional image reconstruction of the intact adenovirus particle viewed along an icosahedral threefold axis. **B:** Stylized section of the adenovirus particle based on current understanding of its polypeptide components and DNA. No real section of the icosahedral virion would contain all components. Virion constituents are designated by their polypeptide numbers with the exception of the terminal protein (*TP*). A from ref. 371, with permission; B from ref. 370, with permission.)

unit are embedded in the penton base (84,423). A central extended shaft is composed of repeating motifs about 15 amino acids in length, and the number of repeat units differs among adenovirus serotypes (145). The carboxy-terminal 180-residue segment of each subunit composing the fiber protein contributes to formation of a terminal bulb (84). The structure of the terminal bulb has been determined at 1.7 Å resolution (442), and a three-dimensional model of the fiber shaft has been proposed (375), predicting that its constituent polypeptide chains form a left-handed, triple helical structure composed of short β-strands interspersed with extended loops that follow the overall helical path. This model fits reasonably well with the cryoelectron microscopic results (372) and mutational studies (173).

The adenovirus core is composed of the linear, double-stranded DNA and four virus-coded proteins. Unlike cellular chromatin, which yields discrete mononucleosomal DNA fragments of about 146 bp on digestion with micrococcal nuclease, the adenovirus core yields a heterogeneous population of DNA fragments ranging from about 50 to 300 bp in length (74,272,410,411). These fragments are associated with polypeptide VII (272,410). Although the reason for the variability in DNA length is not understood, it nevertheless seems clear that adenovirus chromatin is organized into unit particles composed of DNA and polypeptide VII (272,410). The notion that adenovirus chromatin is arranged in a repeating unit is consistent with electron microscopic visualization of particles within the adenovirus core (41,411) and with x-ray scattering patterns obtained with cores (85). Digestion of cores with limiting amounts of nuclease fails to produce a ladder-like series of DNA fragments on electrophoresis, as would be predicted for an oligomeric structure, and this might be due to the fragile and unstable nature of the core after release from virions (411).

The higher-level organization of the core remains obscure. Psoralen cross-linking of viral DNA within partially disassembled virions indicates that the linear molecule is organized into eight supercoiled domains (440), in agreement with earlier electron microscopic studies suggesting that the core is organized into 8 to 12 domains (41). It is intriguing to note that the eight-domain organization places most of the viral transcription units into independent supercoiled domains (440).

GENOME ORGANIZATION

All human adenovirus genomes that have been examined to date have the same general organization; that is, the genes encoding specific functions are located at the same position on the viral chromosome. Avian adenoviruses differ in that they lack several of the early genes identified in the human viruses and contain ORFs of unrelated sequence in their place (62,312). The linear genome contains two origins for DNA replication. The two origins are identical, and one is present in each terminal repeat. The genome also includes a cis-acting packaging sequence (135,155,166,168) that must be located within several hundred base pairs of an end of the chromosome to direct the interaction of the viral DNA with its encapsidating proteins (165).

The viral chromosome carries five early transcription units (E1A, E1B, E2, E3, and E4), two delayed early units (IX and IVa2), and one late unit (major late) that is processed to generate five families of late mRNAs (L1 to L5), all of which are transcribed by RNA polymerase II (reviewed in 308) (Fig. 3). Families of mRNAs were initially localized on the adenovirus map by hybridization to restriction enzyme–generated fragments of the viral DNA (351), and transcription units were defined by ultraviolet light–mapping experiments (32,439). The chromosome also carries one or two (depending on the serotype) virus-associated (VA) genes transcribed by RNA polymerase III. By convention, the map is drawn with the E1A gene at the left end. Both strands of the viral DNA are transcribed with the so-called rightward reading strand on the conventional map coding for the E1A, E1B, IX, major late, VA RNA, and E3 units and the leftward reading strand coding the E4, E2, and IVa2 units.

Little is known about the functional and evolutionary considerations that have led to the current organization of the transcription units on the viral chromosome. Their arrangement might serve a timing function. Viral cores have an organized structure (41,440), and they are converted from a more compact to a more open structure as

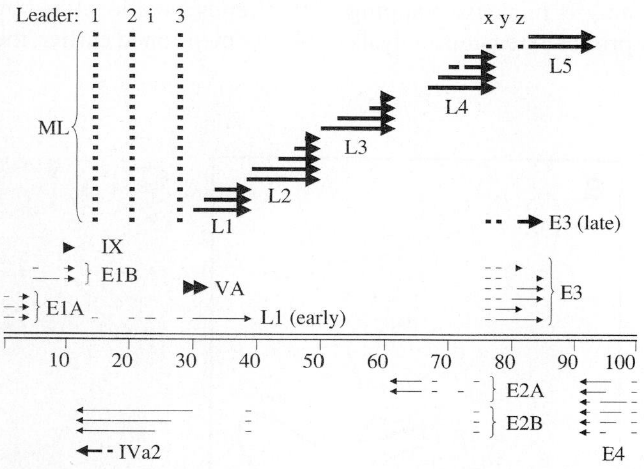

FIG. 3. Transcription map of adenovirus type 2. The early mRNAs are diagrammed with their exons represented by *thin arrows,* late mRNAs are drawn with *heavy arrows,* and delayed early mRNAs (*1Va2* and *IX*) are designated with *arrows of intermediate thickness.* Most late mRNAs originate at 16.3 map units and contain the tripartite leader whose components are labeled *1, 2,* and *3.* Some of the late mRNAs also contain leader segments *i, y,* or *z* polypeptide. Introns are indicated by gaps in the lines comprising the *arrows.*

the early phase of infection progresses (41,440). Perhaps RNA polymerase initially interacts with promoters exposed at the ends of the chromosome, and transcription of the terminal units drives further opening of the core structure. This proposal predicts that the terminal E1A and E4 transcription units would be the first to be expressed, and this is the case. Thus, the location of a transcription unit on the chromosome could influence the order in which it is expressed relative to other units during the early phase of the infectious cycle.

The activation of transcription units can also be influenced by their location relative to other units on the chromosome. Insertion of a strong transcriptional termination sequence between the E1A and E1B units inhibits activation of the E1B unit, suggesting that transcriptional readthrough from E1A to E1B contributes to the activation of E1B (108). One might also imagine that transcription units embedded within the major late unit would be influenced in cis by its very active expression late after infection. However, different viral molecules could serve as templates for early and late transcription units, avoiding complications that might arise from overlapping transcription units. Further, initiation is rate limiting; hence, even if opposing and overlapping units were transcribed from the same template, transcription complexes would seldom meet on the chromosome.

Each of the adenovirus genes transcribed by RNA polymerase II gives rise to multiple mRNAs that are differentiated by alternative splicing and in some cases by the use of different poly(A) sites. The structures of mRNAs were defined by a variety of procedures, including electron microscopic heteroduplex analysis (64,66) and S1 nuclease mapping (32); 5′ ends were localized by primer extension analysis (464). As mentioned earlier, the analysis of adenovirus mRNA structure led to the discovery of splicing (30,65) (Fig. 4).

Some of the protein products generated from the same transcription unit are partially related in their sequence (e.g., the two major polypeptides encoded by the E1A unit); others have no sequence in common (e.g., the two major E1B-coded polypeptides). Unfortunately, no consistent terminology has been adopted for naming viral proteins: the E1A proteins are named for the sedimentation coefficient of the mRNAs that encode them; E1B and E3 proteins are designated by their molecular mass; E2 proteins are named for their functions; E4 proteins are named for ORFs; and the structural proteins encoded by the late transcription unit are termed II to IX. The various historical names of viral polypeptides are used in this chapter, generally preceded by the name of the transcription unit or family of late mRNAs that encodes them (e.g., E1A 13S, E4orf6, L5-IV).

Many of the individual adenovirus transcription units encode a series of polypeptides with related functions. As discussed later, the E1A unit encodes two proteins that activate transcription and induce the host cell to enter the S phase of the cell cycle; E1B encodes two proteins that block apoptosis; E2 encodes three proteins that function directly in DNA replication; E3 encodes products that modulate the response of the host to infection; and the late family of mRNAs is concerned with the production and assembly of capsid components. Only the E4 unit encodes an apparently disparate set of functions. E4 products mediate transcriptional regulation and mRNA transport and modulate DNA replication and apoptosis. One might speculate that an ancestral adenovirus encoding fewer gene products evolved to generate a modern virus in which many of the ancestral genes have given

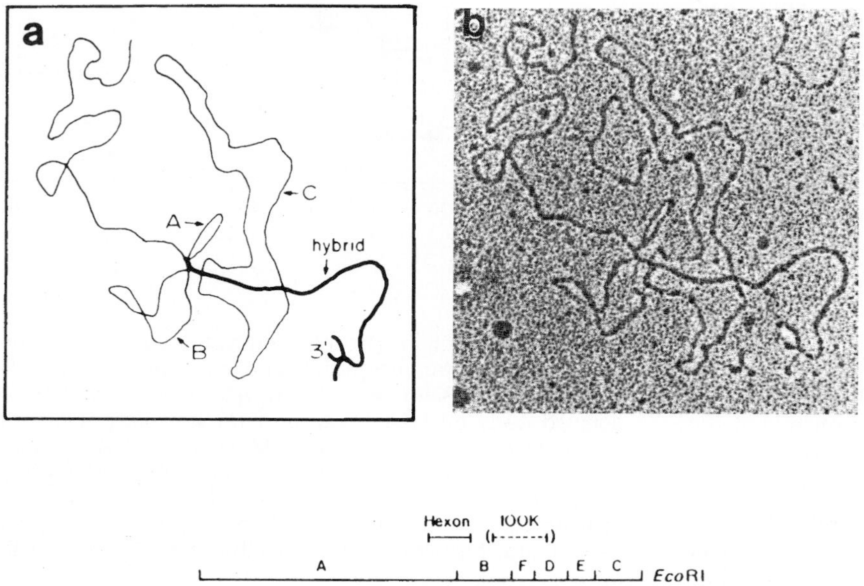

FIG. 4. Detection of adenovirus hexon transcripts processed by splicing near their 5′ ends. When hexon mRNA was hybridized to viral DNA, it formed a duplex structure with three short DNA loops (labeled *A, B,* and *C*), which correspond to introns removed from the mRNA by splicing. **A:** Diagram of duplex molecules. **B:** Electron micrograph of the RNA:DNA hybrid. The position of the hexon and L4 100-kd protein coding regions are displayed on the EcoR1 cleavage map of adenovirus type 2 (*bottom*). (From ref. 30, with permission.)

rise to groups of more specialized products that remain functionally related. The grouping might also be driven in part by the advantage of using a single transcriptional control element to regulate the expression of multiple polypeptides that are needed simultaneously to execute a function such as DNA replication. Further, it might be useful to group closely the coding regions for products that interact physically or functionally to reduce the frequency with which they can be separated by recombination. Otherwise, recombinant variants, which could be defective because they encode products unable to function well together, might be generated at high frequency.

GENETIC SYSTEM AND RECOMBINATION

Adenovirus mutants have proved invaluable as reagents for the study of viral physiologic processes. Most genetic studies have used Ad2 or Ad5. Initially, physical and chemical mutagens were employed to generate variants that could be recognized on the basis of their growth phenotype. Subsequently, mutants have been produced by the targeted manipulation of viral DNA. The ability to propagate mutant viruses is currently the only limitation to their production. Many variants have proved viable, often growing more poorly than their wild-type parent, but growing sufficiently well for the production of useful virus stocks. Other mutants have been selected for conditional growth. These include temperature-sensitive as well as host range variants. Host range mutants have played an especially important role in adenovirus genetics. E1A and E1B mutants can be propagated in 293 cells, a human embryonic kidney cell line that contains and expresses the Ad5 E1A and E1B genes (136); the physiologic consequences of the mutations can then be analyzed in standard laboratory host cells such as HeLa cells. Similarly, complementing cell lines have been developed for propagation of viruses with mutations in the E2, E4, and L5 genes (5,212,221,415,425).

Recombination between adenoviruses contributes to the evolution and diversity of viral serotypes. It is well established that recombination occurs among adenoviruses of the same subgroup. Homologous recombination occurs with high efficiency during growth in co-infected cultured cells (127,437), and comparison of field strains with disparate neutralization (hexon) and hemagglutination (fiber) serology (170) indicates that such exchanges also occur in nature. Recombination between viruses of different subgroups appears to have given rise to Ad4, the sole member of subgroup E adenoviruses. Ad4 exhibits sequence similarity in its E1A (0 to 5 map units) and E2 regions (62 to 66 map units) to group B adenoviruses (209,392), and its hexon gene (51 to 61 map units) is immunologically related to group B viruses (298), whereas the Ad4 fiber gene sequence (146) and immunologic characteristics (296) are most similar to group C viruses. Thus, the simplest model for the origination of Ad4 posits a single recombinatorial crossover event somewhere between the E2 coding region of a group B virus and the fiber coding region of a group C virus (146).

Efficient adenovirus recombination requires viral DNA replication (453), but the virus does not appear to encode any gene products that function specifically to facilitate recombination (103). Rather, it appears that single strands of DNA produced during the viral replication process, which can pair with each other or invade duplex DNAs, are the driving force behind recombination (111).

Although adenoviruses have never unambiguously been shown to integrate into the chromosomes of permissive host cells, integration does occur during the process of transformation. No specific motifs have been identified in the cellular DNA sequences at adenovirus integration sites.

REPLICATIVE CYCLE

Studies of the human adenovirus replication cycle have focused primarily on the closely related Ad2 and Ad5 viruses. These serotypes have been favored because they are easily grown in the laboratory, and an extensive collection of Ad2 and Ad5 mutant viruses have been developed. When other human serotypes have been studied, their growth strategies have proved similar to the paradigm established for the prototypes. Most studies of adenovirus growth have been performed by infection of HeLa or KB cells at fairly high multiplicities of infection (more than 10 plaque-forming units per cell). High multiplicities of infection have been used so that all cells in the culture are synchronously infected, allowing the ordered series of biochemical events during the infectious cycle to be observed in a time-wise fashion. HeLa and KB cells have been favored as hosts because they are easily propagated in large quantities, and the viruses grow in them rapidly and to high yield. These tumor cells support more rapid viral growth than human diploid fibroblasts, in which the replication cycle is substantially prolonged.

The replication cycle is divided by convention into two phases that are separated by the onset of viral DNA replication (Fig. 5). Early events commence as soon as the infecting virus interacts with the host cell. These include adsorption, penetration, movement of the viral DNA to the nucleus, and expression of an early set of genes. Early viral gene products mediate further viral gene expression and DNA replication, induce cell cycle progression, block apoptosis, and antagonize a variety of host antiviral measures. In HeLa cells infected at a multiplicity of 10 plaque-forming units per cell, the early phase lasts for 5 to 6 hours, after which viral DNA replication is first detected. Concomitant with the onset of viral DNA replication, the late phase of the cycle begins with expression of late viral genes and assembly of progeny virions. The infectious cycle is completed after 20 to 24 hours in HeLa cells. At the end of the cycle, about 10^4 progeny virus particles per

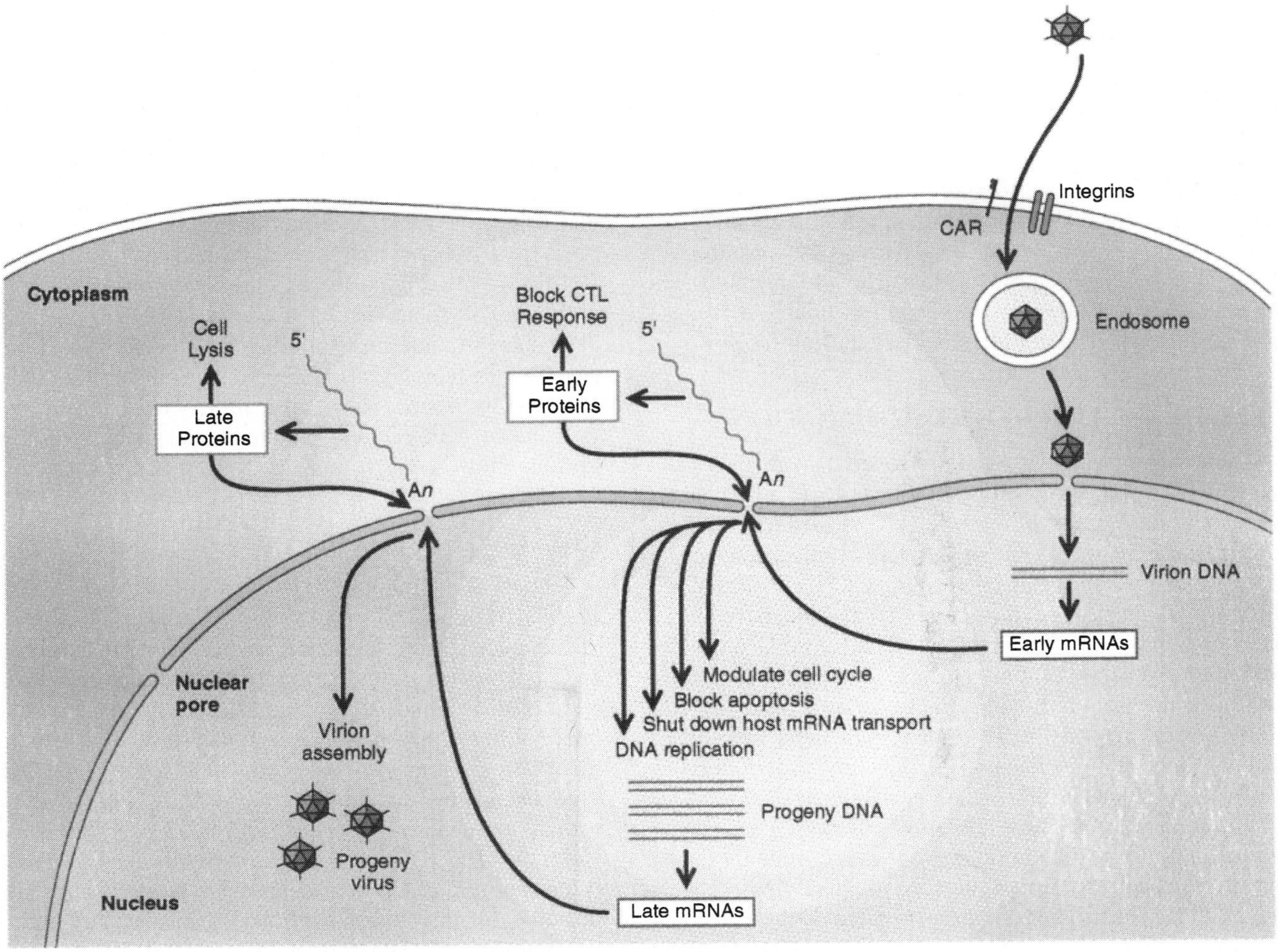

FIG. 5. Cartoon of the adenovirus life cycle.

cell have been produced, along with the synthesis of a substantial excess of virion proteins and DNA that are not assembled into virions (141). Cells infected at high multiplicity seldom divide; hence, at the completion of the replication cycle, the DNA and protein content of the infected cell has increased by a factor of about two.

Although *early* and *late* are convenient terms for description of events that occur during the replication cycle, the functional distinction between early and late events is often blurred. Early genes continue to be expressed at late times after infection, and the promoter controlling expression of the major late transcription unit directs a low level of transcription early after infection. The viral genes encoding proteins IVa2 and IX begin to be expressed at an intermediate time (308) and thus form a *delayed-early* category.

Adsorption and Entry

Attachment of Ad2 to cells is mediated by its fiber protein (246). The distal, carboxy-terminal domain of the fiber protein terminates in a knob that binds to the cellular receptor (84). The CAR (coxsackievirus and adenovirus receptor) protein, which belongs to the immunoglobulin superfamily, is an adenovirus receptor (29,395). It serves as a high-affinity receptor for human adenoviruses from subgroups A, C, D, E, and F, but not subgroup B (329). The class I major histocompatibility complex (MHC) α_2 domain has also been reported to serve as a receptor for Ad5 (174).

The observation that Ad2 binds to some cells but does not efficiently enter them (357) raised the possibility that a second protein–protein recognition event might be needed for internalization, and a second interaction has been identified. The penton base protein binds to members of a family of heterodimeric cell surface receptors, termed *integrins* (436). The $\alpha_v\beta_3$- and $\alpha_v\beta_5$-integrins and perhaps other integrin family members interact with the viral protein. The interaction occurs through an arg-gly-asp (RGD) sequence present in each of the five polypeptide III molecules that compose the penton base, the same sequence motif present in a number of extracellular adhesion molecules that bind to integrins. RGD-containing peptides can block internalization of Ad2 (436), and Ad5 variants with mutations that alter the RGD sequence in polypeptide III exhibit a delay in the onset of viral DNA synthesis under certain conditions, consistent with a reduced efficiency of internalization (20). The structure of $\alpha_V\beta_5$-integrin bound to virions has been determined at 21 Å resolution by cryoelectron microscopy (63).

It seems likely that the fiber–receptor interaction serves to bring the virion to the cell surface, facilitating the critical integrin–receptor interaction. Consistent with this view, insertion of an RGD motif into the Ad5 hexon partially overcomes the need for a fiber–receptor interaction (414).

The tropism of adenoviruses is influenced by the availability of cellular receptors for fiber and penton. Airway epithelial cells lack both receptors (128,455). This deficiency might reflect evolutionary pressure to block a port of entry for respiratory adenoviruses, and it has frustrated efforts to use adenovirus as a vector to introduce therapeutic genes to the lungs.

After adsorption, Ad2–receptor complexes diffuse into coated pits, and they are internalized by receptor-mediated endocytosis (54,55,110,409). The process is triggered by the penton–integrin interaction because purified penton but not fiber protein is rapidly internalized by cultured cells (436). The process requires dynamin (419), a protein that specifically regulates clathrin-mediated endocytosis; and it requires activation of the lipid kinase phosphotidylinositol-3-OH kinase (230), which induces reorganization of actin filaments. The internalization of adsorbed virus is remarkably efficient (140). Eighty to 85% of virus that binds to the surface of a susceptible cell is internalized, and penetration occurs rapidly, with half of the adsorbed virus moving to endosomes within 10 minutes. About 90% of the virus within endosomes successfully moves to the cytosol with a half time of about 5 minutes. The movement to the cytosol is triggered by the acidic pH of the endosome (349,379), and the penton base is believed to play an essential role in the process. The rapidity of the movement to the cytosol suggests that the virus escapes from the endosomal unit, known as the *early endosome,* before formation of a lysosome (270). The endosome appears to be substantially disrupted because DNA–protein complexes that enter the endosome together with virus particles—but not physically attached to virions—also escape to the cytosol with high efficiency (451). Virus particles are transported across the cytoplasm to the nucleus by a process that involves microtubules (76,378). *In vitro* studies have shown that virions can attach to microtubules through the hexon, and some drugs that interact with microtubules can inhibit adenovirus infection (76). About 40 minutes after penetration, virus particles are seen at nuclear pore complexes by electron microscopy. After 120 minutes, about 40% of internalized particles have released their DNA free from hexon proteins, although it is not known what portion of this released DNA is localized to the nucleus (140). Inhibitors of nuclear import block the accumulation of adenovirus DNA in the nucleus, indicating that it enters through the nuclear pore (138).

During the internalization process, there is a sequential disassembly of the virion (140). The disassembly occurs by selective dissociation and proteolytic degradation of virion constituents. First, the proteins at the vertices of the particle are lost. Polypeptide IV that trimerizes to form the fiber, polypeptide IIIa located near the peripentonal hexons linking adjacent facets of the capsid, and polypeptide III that forms the pentameric penton base are substantially lost by 15 minutes after penetration of the cell. Polypeptides IV and IIIa dissociate somewhat more rapidly than III, and this could reflect a need to free the penton base for a role in escape from the endosome. Polypeptide VIII dissociates from the particle as the penton capsomeres are lost, and, shortly after entry of the particle to the cytosol, polypeptide VI is degraded by the virus-coded protease (139). Both polypeptides VI and VIII bridge from the DNA core to the capsid, and their loss prepares the particle for release of its DNA. Somewhat later, polypeptide IX, which stabilizes hexon facets, exits from the infecting particle; finally, the DNA-containing core is freed from hexons. Thus, the virion, which is very stable outside the cell, is dismantled by an ordered elimination of structural proteins on entry to the cell so that it can deliver its DNA to the nucleus.

The events that signal disassembly are mostly unknown. Acidification induces exit of the infecting particle from the endosome to the cytosol, but disassembly of the vertex constituents can occur in the absence of acidification (140). It seems likely that the signal for the initial dissociation of the fiber from the penton is a determining event that initiates a cascade in which each sequential disassembly event is driven by changes in the structure of the virion that result from previous events.

A DNA–protein VII complex reaches the nucleus (138). The viral DNA has been reported to convert into a structure that can be digested with a low concentration of DNase I to generate DNA fragments that form a ladder pattern similar to that of cellular chromatin on electrophoresis (384), suggesting that cellular histone proteins might replace polypeptide VII, the major core constituent, before the infecting DNA is transcribed. However, using sensitive assays, others have been unable to detect nucleosomal particles composed of viral DNA and cellular histones (410). It is possible that the viral genome is expressed as a chromosomal structure containing protein VII rather than cellular histones. When the viral DNA reaches the nucleus, it associates with the nuclear matrix through its terminal protein (36,115,342). DNAs from mutant Ad5 variants with lesions in their terminal protein genes fail to become tightly associated with the nuclear matrix, and they also fail to be efficiently transcribed (342). This correlation between nuclear matrix association and activation of transcription suggests the two events are functionally interrelated. Apparently, the terminal protein, which arrives with the infecting genome, is the first viral gene product that functions within the nucleus to initiate the program of viral gene expression.

Activation of Early Viral Genes

There are three main goals of early adenovirus gene expression. The first is to induce the host cell to enter the S phase of the cell cycle, providing an optimal environment for viral replication. As discussed later (see Interactions with the Host), E1A, E1B, and E4 gene products play roles in this process. The second is to set up viral systems that protect the infected cell from various antiviral defenses of the host organism. The E3 and VA RNA genes contribute to these defenses, and these are also discussed later (see Interactions with the Host). The third is to synthesize viral gene products needed for viral DNA replication. All three of these goals depend on the transcriptional activation of the viral genome, and the principal activating proteins of adenovirus are encoded by the E1A gene.

E1A is the first transcription unit to be expressed after the viral chromosome reaches the nucleus. Transcription of the E1A unit is controlled by a constitutively active promoter, and it encodes two mRNAs during the early phase of infection (Fig. 6). Three additional E1A mRNA species accumulate later in the infectious cycle (369), but no distinct function has been described for their products. The two early mRNAs contain identical 5′ and 3′ ends, differ internally owing to differential splicing, and encode proteins that are identical except for an additional 46 amino acid segment that is present in the larger polypeptide. The two polypeptides are commonly referred to as the 12S and 13S E1A proteins. The primary E1A translation products undergo extensive phosphorylation that is mediated, at least in part, by cyclin-dependent kinases (256) and mitogen-activated protein kinase (430).

When the amino acid sequences of the E1A proteins encoded by a variety of human serotypes are compared, the E1A products prove to be constructed of three conserved regions (CR1, CR2, and CR3) (see Fig. 6) separated by less highly conserved domains (278,290,408). The E1A proteins do not exhibit sequence-specific DNA binding; rather, they bind to cellular proteins and modulate their function. The three conserved regions in the E1A proteins mark domains that play major roles in protein–protein interactions.

The ability of E1A proteins to activate expression of the other adenovirus transcription units was discovered when viral mutants were examined that carried either a single base-pair substitution (31) or a deletion (198,353) within the E1A coding region. These mutant viruses, which could be grown in transformed human cells expressing the E1A and E1B genes (293 cells) (136), failed to accumulate early viral mRNAs with normal kinetics when grown in HeLa cells that were unable to

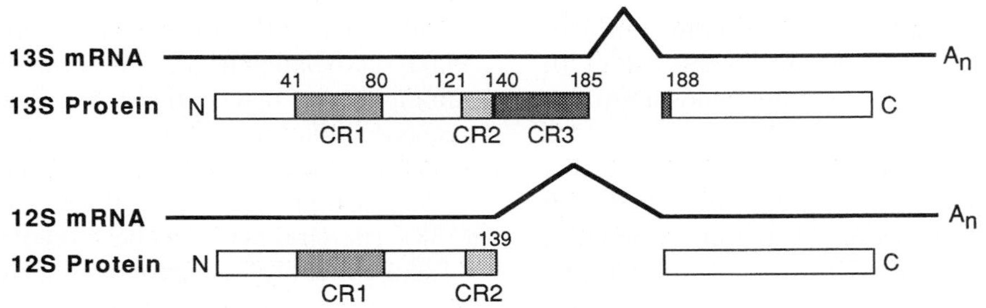

CR1
41-PTLHELYDLDVTAPEDPNEEAVSQIFPDSVMLAVQEGIDL-80

CR2
121-DLTCHEAGFPPSDDEDEEG-139

CR3
140-EEFVLDYVEHPGHG**C**RS**C**HYHRRNTGDPDIM**C**SL**C**YMRTCGMFVYSPVS-188

FIG. 6. Diagram of E1A mRNAs, the polypeptides they encode, and the amino acid sequence of conserved domains. 13S and 12S mRNA exons are represented (*lines*), as are introns (*carets*) and poly(A) sequences (A_n) The polypeptides encoded by the 13S and 12S mRNAs are designated (*rectangles*). Domains in the proteins that are conserved among adenovirus serotypes are identified as conserved regions 1 to 3 (CR1, CR2, CR3), and the amino acids at the boundaries of conserved regions are indicated (*above rectangles*). The amino acid sequences of the conserved domains are displayed at the bottom of the figure, and the cysteines composing the zinc finger motif in CR3 are marked (*enlarged bold letters*).

complement the defect. Compared to wild-type virus, they accumulated reduced quantities of early mRNAs only after a long delay. Subsequent analysis demonstrated that E1A proteins acted to increase the rate of transcription (289). Since the E1A proteins can activate other genes in trans, they are often referred to as *trans-activators*.

Initially, attempts to identify a promoter element that is responsive to the E1A proteins proved frustrating. In a number of studies, it was possible to mutate any specific DNA element without blocking the ability of E1A to activate test promoters, provided that basal transcription was not eliminated. The reason for the promiscuous activation is now clear. The E1A proteins activate transcription by binding to a variety of cellular transcription factors and regulatory proteins (Table 2). The E1A proteins can interact directly with auxiliary factors that mediate basal transcription, with activating proteins that bind to upstream promoter and enhancer elements, and with regulatory subunits that influence the activity of DNA-binding factors. All three conserved domains of E1A mediate protein–protein interactions that activate transcription.

E1A proteins activate transcription through the TATA motif (142,441), an element found 25 to 30 bp upstream of transcriptional initiation sites in many viral and cellular genes. The activation is believed to result in part from the ability of the 13S E1A protein to bind directly to the TATA-binding protein (TBP) (175,226), which is the DNA-binding subunit of the auxiliary transcription factor IID (TFIID), the first auxiliary transcription factor to interact with TATA-containing promoters. The interaction between TBP and E1A is mediated by the 13S-specific CR3 domain of the E1A protein (226), and this helps to explain why the 13S E1A protein activates transcription through TATA motifs more efficiently than the 12S protein. Part of the mechanism by which the 13S E1A protein activates transcription as a result of binding to TBP appears to involve the cellular tumor suppressor protein, p53, which can bind to TFIID (244,350) and repress transcription (350). The two proteins bind to overlapping domains on TBP, and the E1A protein can displace p53 from TBP and relieve p53-mediated repression (176). The 12S E1A protein can also activate through a TATA motif (219), but more weakly than the 13S protein. This activation event involves Dr1, a factor that can bind to TBP and inhibit transcription (190). The 12S and 13S proteins bind directly to Dr1, preventing it from associating with TBP (218). Thus, both 12S and 13S proteins can activate transcription through TATA motifs by binding to cellular factors and relieving transcriptional repression. E1A also has been reported to bind to several TAF subunits of TFIID (121,265) and to the rap30 subunit of TFIIF (242).

Recently, the 13S-specific CR3 domain of E1A has been shown to bind to the human SUR-2 protein (38). This interaction is very likely to be functionally significant because point mutations in CR3 that block transcriptional activation also block the interaction with SUR-2. SUR-2 is a constituent of a large protein complex known as *Srb/Mediator* or *TRAP*. The complex contains about 30 polypeptides and functions as a transcriptional coactivator or corepressor. The herpesvirus VP16 and p53 activation domains also interact with this complex, but through a different subunit (38,192).

In addition to interactions with the basal transcriptional machinery, E1A proteins can activate transcription through the binding sites for factors that bind well upstream of the basal promoter. The best-studied activation event occurs through E2F-binding sites. This transcription factor is named for the first promoter where it

TABLE 2. *Cellular E1A binding partners*

E1A-binding protein	Binds to 12S E1A	13S E1A	Other proteins in complex
pRB	+	+	Unknown
p107	+	+	Cyclin A, cdk2/cyclin E
p130	+	+	Cyclin A, cdk2/cyclin E
p300	+	+	Unknown
TBP	−	+	Unknown
hTAF(II)135	−	+	Unknown
SUR-2	−	+	Unknown
Dr1	+	+	Unknown
ATF-2	−	+	Unknown
YY1	+	+	Unknown
Sp1	?	+	Unknown
MAZ	?	+	Unknown
STAT1	+	+	Unknown

Note: This listing contains only those cellular proteins that have been shown to bind directly to E1A proteins, and it is limited to binding partners for which there is evidence that the interaction is biologically relevant.

pRB, retinoblastoma susceptibility protein; cdk2, cyclin-dependent kinase 2; TBP, TATA-binding protein; TAFs, TBP-associated factors.

was found to bind, the adenovirus E2 promoter (214). E2F forms a complex with the cellular retinoblastoma tumor suppressor protein, pRB, and pRB inhibits transcriptional activation by E2F. The 12S and 13S E1A proteins activate transcription through E2F-binding sites (215,445,456), and both E1A proteins bind to pRB (435) through CR1 and CR2 (96,189), dissociating it from E2F (18,19,21). The strong correlation between the dissociation of the E2F–pRB complex and transcriptional activation by E1A proteins argues that E1A activates transcription by dissociating pRB from E2F. The activation of E2F by E1A not only affects the expression of viral genes but also influences the expression of cellular genes, dramatically affecting cell cycle progression (see Activation of the Host Cell).

E1A activates transcription by binding directly to several additional cellular factors. All of the early adenovirus promoters, with the exception of the E1B promoter, contain binding sites for the ATF (also termed *CREB*) family of transcription factors. E1A activates transcription through ATF-binding sites (243), presumably in part because the 13S E1A protein can bind to ATF-2 (1,239, 243). The interaction occurs between the DNA binding domain of ATF-2 and CR3 of E1A. Different subdomains of CR3 mediate E1A binding to ATF-2 and TBP, raising the possibility that E1A functions as an adapter, bridging between ATF-2 bound at an upstream site and TBP (226). The SUR-2–containing complex, discussed previously, might also participate in the bridging. Such a bridging function might stabilize the initiation complex at the promoter.

E1A proteins can also activate through YY1 recognition sites (354). YY1 represses transcription when bound upstream of a transcriptional initiation site. The E1A proteins bind to YY1 through an amino-terminal sequence of E1A, and, in the case of the 13S E1A protein, the interaction is stabilized by CR3 (229). This binding correlates with the relief of repression mediated by YY1. The murine *c-fos* promoter provides a specific example of YY1-mediated repression that is relieved by E1A (462). This promoter contains both YY1- and ATF/CREB-binding sites, and YY1 binds to ATF/CREB, inhibiting its ability to activate transcription. E1A binds to YY1, blocking its interaction with ATF/CREB and relieving the repression. YY1 also interacts with p300 (see Activation of the Host Cell), and E1A potentially influences the activity of the YY1–p300 complex through its ability to bind to p300 (224).

E1A proteins have been reported to both activate and repress through the transcription factor AP1. These activities involve an amino-terminal domain and the CR1 domain of E1A (101,299). E1A can repress the action of AP1 through its consensus binding sites in the collagenase and stromelysin genes (299) and enhance the ability of AP1 to activate through the ATF sites (to which AP1 can bind) of adenovirus early genes (100,157). The AP1 transcription factor is a dimeric molecule that is generally composed of *c-fos* and *c-jun* family members, although *jun* family members can also heterodimerize with members of the ATF family (27). E1A repression appears to result from a block to DNA binding by *c-fos/c-jun* heterodimers (151), and activation by E1A through AP1 occurs, at least in part, by an indirect mechanism. E1A proteins cooperate with cyclic adenosine monophosphate (cAMP) to induce the level of AP1, which activates transcription of viral genes (284). The E1A-mediated induction of AP1 activity results from transcriptional activation of the *c-fos* and *junB* genes through their TATA motifs (211), and the *c-jun* gene has been shown to be induced through an ATF-like element in its promoter, which probably responds to a *c-jun*/ATF-2 heterodimer (402). Hence, E1A can activate transcription indirectly through AP1-binding sites by inducing AP1 activity, and E1A can activate through ATF-binding sites either directly by binding to ATF-2 or indirectly by inducing AP1 activity. A second adenovirus protein contributes to the induction of AP1 activity. The E1B 19-kd protein activates the *c-jun* N-terminal kinase (JNK) (347), which strongly induces *c-jun*–dependent transcription.

Expression of the adenovirus VA RNA genes is induced by the E1A proteins (358,452). These genes are transcribed by RNA polymerase III, and it appears that the amount of the 110-kd subunit of transcription factor IIIC2a is increased by the E1A proteins (358). RNA polymerase III–sponsored transcription is repressed by pRB (434); hence, E1A might act through pRB to induce the synthesis of the 110-kd subunit.

Besides the E1A proteins, two additional early gene products have been shown to activate adenovirus promoters. The E4orf6/7 polypeptide binds to the cellular transcription factor E2F, with two molecules of the E4 protein apparently bridging between a pair of E2F molecules and causing them to bind cooperatively to the pair of E2F-binding sites within the E2 promoter (156,187,318). The E2 DNA-binding protein can activate a variety of early adenovirus promoters as well as the major late promoter (53), but the mechanism by which it stimulates transcription is unclear.

Individual adenovirus early promoters are activated by multiple mechanisms. For example, the E2 promoter can be activated by E1A through its TATA motif, ATF site, or E2F sites. In addition, the E4orf6/7 protein contributes to activation at the E2F sites, and the E2 promoter can also be induced by the E2 DNA-binding protein. Perhaps the activation pathways function with different efficiencies within various cell types, and these apparently redundant activation mechanisms have evolved to ensure that early viral promoters will be efficiently activated in a variety of different cell types as the virus spreads within its infected host.

Generally, adenovirus early genes remain active throughout the viral replication cycle, although the rate at which they are transcribed slowly declines. In part, the decline results from cell death. However, there are three known down-regulatory events, and in each case, it appears that a viral protein, which accumulates in response to an activation event, subsequently acts to inhibit continued transcriptional stimulation mediated by one or more early promoter elements. First, the E1A proteins can repress the activity of a variety of known enhancers, including the enhancer residing upstream of the E1A gene itself. This down-regulatory function correlates with the ability of the E1A protein to bind to a cellular protein, p300 (368), and the consequences of this protein–protein interaction are considered later (see Activation of the Host Cell). Second, whereas the E2 DNA-binding protein activates some promoters (53), it inhibits transcription from the E4 promoter (293) by an unknown mechanism. Third, the induction of AP1 activity by E1A and cAMP is transient (284). It is antagonized by the E4orf4 polypeptide, which accumulates in response to the E1A-mediated activation of the E4 gene (283). Mutant viruses unable to produce E4orf4 protein are viable but are more cytopathic than the wild-type virus, a counter-intuitive result because expression of E4orf4 in the absence of infection induces apoptosis (222,356). E4orf4 binds to protein phosphatase 2A, and phosphatase activity is essential for the down-regulatory event (211).

Once early mRNAs have been synthesized, they are translated on polysomes together with cellular mRNAs. Initially, they do not appear to enjoy a competitive advantage, but as the infection enters the late phase, cellular mRNAs are excluded from polysomes (see Activation of Late Gene Expression and Host Cell Shutoff).

Activation of the Host Cell

Adenovirus infection has long been known to induce quiescent cells to enter the S phase of the cell cycle, creating an environment optimally conducive to viral replication. Modulation of the cell cycle is primarily a function of the E1A proteins, and the modulation is mediated by their CR1, CR2, and nonconserved amino-terminal domains. The key to understanding how E1A proteins manipulate cell cycle regulation came from the observation that a set of cellular proteins can be co-immunoprecipitated with the E1A proteins (158,446). The most abundant coprecipitating cellular polypeptides have molecular weights of about 33, 60, 80, 90, 105, 107, 130, 300, and 400 kd (Fig. 7); several of these polypeptides have been shown to interact directly with E1A proteins (see Table 2). The 105-kd moiety was the first to be identified (435). It is the retinoblastoma tumor suppressor protein, pRB, which, as discussed earlier (see Activation of Early Viral Genes), regulates the ability of the E2F cellular transcription factor to activate transcription. The human papillomavirus E7 protein and the large T antigens of papovaviruses also bind to pRB, underscoring its

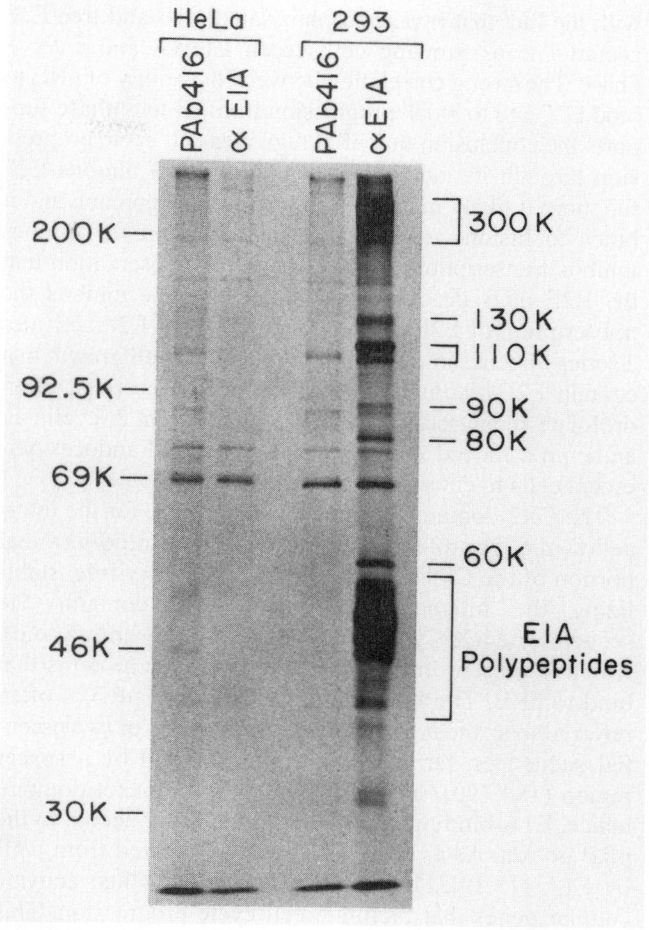

FIG. 7. Co-immunoprecipitation of cellular polypeptides with E1A proteins. Radioactively labeled polypeptides were immunoprecipitated from lysates of HeLa or 293 cells with a monoclonal antibody specific for SV40 T antigen (PAb416) or a mixture of antibodies specific for E1A proteins (αE1A), and immune complexes were analyzed by electrophoresis. The size (kd) of marker proteins is indicated (*left*), and the size of polypeptides coimmunoprecipitated with E1A proteins, as well as the location of E1A polypeptides, is indicated (*right of autoradiogram*). (From ref. 158, with permission.)

importance as a target of oncoproteins encoded by DNA tumor viruses. Although E2F sites are present in the adenovirus E1A and E2 promoters and contribute to their activation, neither papovaviruses nor papillomaviruses have E2F binding sites in their genome. Therefore, tumor virus oncoproteins must target pRB for reasons other than to influence E2F function at their own promoters.

Overexpression of pRB inhibits cell cycle progression, causing cells to arrest in middle to late G_1 phase, and growth arrest correlates with the ability of pRB to bind to E2F and block E2F-dependent transcriptional activation. pRB activity is regulated by cyclin-dependent kinases. Hyperphosphorylation of pRB inhibits the formation of the pRB–E2F complex, and it reverses the ability of pRB to arrest cell growth. These observations are consistent with the fact that hyperphosphorylated pRB and free E2F accumulate as growing cells reach late G_1 and enter S phase. The strong correlation between the ability of pRB to bind E2F and to block progression from G_1 to S phase supports the conclusion that pRB regulates cell cycle progression through its interactions with E2F. pRB inhibits E2F function: it likely masks the E2F activation domain, and it binds to histone deacetylase. Deacetylation of histones inhibits transcription, consistent with the observation that the E2F–pRB–deacetylase complex actively inhibits the transcription of E2F-responsive genes. Free E2F activates a series of genes important for S phase and cell growth that contain E2F-binding sites in their promoters (e.g., dihydrofolate reductase, DNA polymerase α, *cdc2,* cyclin E, and *c-myc.* Indeed, ectopic expression of E2F induces quiescent cells to enter the S phase of the cell cycle.

The CR2 domain is primarily responsible for the interaction of E1A proteins with pRB, and the amino-terminal portion of the CR1 domain plays an auxiliary role, stabilizing the interaction (96,189). CR2 contains the sequence Leu-X-Cys-X-Glu (where X is any amino acid), which is present in other viral and cellular proteins that bind to pRB. The E1A-binding domain on pRB is often referred to as the *pocket,* and it is composed of two essential sequences, termed A and B, separated by a spacer region (184,199). E2F also binds to the pocket domain; hence, E1A binding competes with E2F for access to the pRB pocket. As a result, E2F can be liberated from pRB by E1A (18,19,21), and the free E2F can then activate cellular genes that facilitate cell cycle progression. This accomplishes what appears to be a common goal of DNA tumor viruses: to move the infected cell into the S phase, creating an environment favorable for efficient viral DNA replication. Mutant E1A proteins that fail to bind pRB are unable to activate transcription through E2F or modulate cellular growth.

Two additional cellular pRB family members have been identified that interact with E2F—p107 and p130—and E1A can bind to them (see Fig. 7), dissociating E2F. As is the case for pRB, the interaction is mediated by the E1A CR2 domain, and E1A–p107 binding is stabilized by interactions within the CR1 domain (418). The proteins p107 and p130 associate with cyclins and cyclin-dependent kinases. E1A can be found in complexes that include kinase activities (169,210), and the phosphorylation state of p107 and p130 in these complexes is substantially elevated (22). Whether these complexes represent nonfunctional byproducts of the release of E2F or whether the complexes that include E1A, p107 or p130, cyclin and cyclin-dependent kinase (p60 and p33) (see Fig. 7) perform an active, E1A-modulated function is unknown. Not only are there multiple pRB family members present in E2F complexes, but there are also multiple E2Fs. The E2F transcription factor is a heterodimer composed of one of six known E2F family members and one of three DP family members. In summary, the E1A proteins disrupt a series of complexes that contain different pRB family members and multiple E2F subunits, forcing quiescent cells to begin DNA synthesis.

In addition to disrupting pRB–E2F complexes, E1A blocks the action of a cyclin-dependent kinase inhibitory protein. Cyclin-dependent kinases target pRB family members and regulate their activities. Hyperphosphorylated pRB does not bind E2F, allowing the transcription factor to stimulate S-phase entry. Cyclin-dependent kinases are themselves regulated by several mechanisms, including association with cyclin-dependent kinase inhibitory proteins, such as $p27_{kip1}$. Overexpression of $p27_{kip1}$ blocks cell cycle progression in the G_1 compartment. E1A antagonizes the inhibitory activity of $p27_{kip1}$ (4,257), preventing G_1 arrest and favoring progression to the S phase.

The E1A proteins facilitate cell cycle progression through a second pathway by binding to the closely related p300 and CBP proteins (see Fig. 7). Their binding site on E1A includes the poorly conserved amino-terminus and the carboxy-terminal half of CR1 (418). E1A mutants lacking CR2 and unable to bind pRB family members can nevertheless stimulate cellular DNA synthesis, provided their p300/CBP-binding site remains intact. Thus, the E1A proteins contain two independent domains, either of which can stimulate cells to progress from G_1 to S phase (183,240,459). The p300/CBP proteins serve as coactivaters for a number of transcription factors, including CREB, STATs, and nuclear receptors. The coactivaters are brought to the promoter through their interaction with DNA-binding factors. The p300/CBP proteins exhibit intrinsic histone acetylase activity, and they interact with a factor termed *P/CAF* that is also a histone acetyltransferase. Acetylation of histones is believed to weaken their interaction with DNA, producing a chromatin structure that is more conducive to transcription. Thus, p300/CBP is thought to function, at least in part, by modifying chromatin structure. When E1A binds to p300 or CBP, it simultaneously displaces P/CAF and inhibits the intrinsic acetyltransferase activity of the coactivator (48,154,307,444). The inhibition of p300/CBP acetyltransferase activity can explain the earlier observation that E1A inhibits the function of some enhancer elements (328,368,418).

S-phase entry is facilitated by the ability of E1A to inhibit p300/CBP function. The p53 tumor suppressor protein is one target of this activity. The *p53* gene is the most commonly mutated gene in human tumors, and the loss of p53 function or its alteration by mutation can contribute to tumor progression. Consistent with its frequent loss in tumor cells, high-level expression of p53 promotes cell cycle arrest or apoptosis. The p53 protein is a DNA-binding transcription factor, and p300/CBP serves as a coactivator for p53. By inhibiting p300/CBP activity, E1A proteins antagonize p53 function (238,362). Although inhibition of p53 will relieve a block to cell cycle progression, it does not by itself stimulate progression into S phase. It is likely that there are unidentified genes whose expression is modulated by the interaction of E1A with p300/CBP, inducing the cell to synthesize DNA. Alternatively, the domain on E1A that mediates its interaction with p300/CBP might interact with another unidentified target. Indeed, this domain binds to p400, the largest protein known to interact with E1A. Although p400 and p300/CBP are related in their amino acid sequences (22), the function of p400 is unknown.

Two separate regions of the E1A proteins can induce cells to move from G_1 to S phase through two independent mechanisms: binding to pRB family members and binding to p300/CBP. Presumably, E1A proteins employ two mechanisms because together they function more effectively than either alone or because there may be cells in which one pathway works more efficiently than the other. Further, although the E1A domains mediating binding to either pRB family members or p300/CBP can induce DNA synthesis in quiescent cells, both regions are required to pass the G_2- to M-phase checkpoint and progress to mitosis (182,183,417,459). This could be an important function in animal hosts, in which infections are likely to proceed much more slowly than in cultured cells. Without the ability to divide, cells that pass completely through S phase would be stuck in G_2; if the cells can divide, they can continue cycling and return to S phase, during which viral replication is most efficient. Possibly, the simultaneous inhibition of both the pRB family and p300/CBP by E1A binding somehow enables the infected cell to pass through the G_2- to M-phase checkpoint. Alternatively, E1A proteins might alter the function of these regulatory proteins rather than simply inhibit them. E1A has been reported to bind simultaneously to a pRB family member and p300/CBP (22), and this new complex might influence passage through mitosis. It is also possible that E1A proteins bind to additional, as yet unidentified, proteins to antagonize this checkpoint.

The level and activity of p53 are induced in response to a variety of stresses, including the presence of E1A proteins (79,248,337). E1A activates p53 through a pathway that includes the p19^{ARF} tumor suppressor protein (78). This protein can associate with p53 to alter its level and activity. E1A induces p19^{ARF} through the same domains required for the induction of p53, and E1A fails to induce p53 in cells lacking p19^{ARF}. Although E1A inhibits the p53 transcriptional coactivator p300/CBP, p53 nevertheless acts to limit its oncogenic potential. As noted previously, high-level expression of p53 promotes cell cycle arrest at the G_1- to S-phase boundary or apoptosis. Although the transcriptional activation function of p53 mediates its block to cell cycle progression and apoptosis, p53 can induce apoptosis through a second pathway that does not depend on its ability to stimulate transcription. This helps to explain why adenoviruses have evolved additional mechanisms to counter p53 function.

The Ad5 E1B 55-kd protein binds to p53 within infected cells (339), and it can block transcriptional activation by p53. Analysis of mutant E1B 55-kd proteins has revealed a strict correlation between the ability of E1B to block p53-mediated transcriptional activation and its ability to cooperate with E1A in the oncogenic transformation of cells (447). The E1A and E1B proteins of adenovirus are oncoproteins (see Oncogenesis), and they cooperate to transform cultured cells. Oncogenic transformation is a manifestation of the ability of these proteins to interfere with the normal function of tumor suppressor proteins. Thus, the correlation between a block to transcriptional activation and transforming activity of the viral protein suggests that the E1B 55-kd protein antagonizes the ability of p53 to block cell cycle progression and induce apoptosis by inhibiting its activation function. The E1B 55-kd protein binds to the amino-terminal, acidic transcriptional activation domain of p53 (200), and this suggests that the viral protein might simply mask the activation domain. Steric hindrance might contribute to the ability of the E1B 55-kd protein to block activation by p53, but it is not the entire mechanism. The E1B 55-kd protein can inhibit transcription if it is artificially anchored to a promoter, indicating that it can actively repress transcription (448). Not only does the interaction of the E1B 55-kd protein with p53 serve to bring the viral protein to the promoter, but also the E1B 55-kd protein increases the affinity of p53 for its DNA-binding site (261). In conjunction with an as yet unidentified corepressor (261), the E1B 55-kd protein not only blocks the activation function of p53 but also actively represses transcription. Thus, like E1A, the E1B 55-kd protein binds to a tumor suppressor protein, antagonizes its normal activity, and helps to deregulate cell cycle progression.

In contrast to E1A, expression of the E1B 55-kd protein alone is not sufficient to stimulate quiescent cells to enter the S phase of the cell cycle. This is consistent with the observation that deletion of both p53 alleles does not directly lead to the loss of regulated cell division (93). Nevertheless, p53 is targeted by a variety of tumor virus oncoproteins: SV40 large T antigen binds to p53, blocks its DNA-binding activity, and interferes with its ability to activate transcription; and human papillomavirus type 16 E6 protein complexes with p53 and cooperates with cellular proteins to promote its degradation. Presumably, then, the E1B 55-kd protein collaborates with E1A to activate quiescent cells more effectively. Further, because E1A causes p53 to accumulate, E1B must contribute to the activation of quiescent cells by preventing the implementation of a cell cycle block or apoptosis by elevated levels of p53.

The E1B 55-kd protein also enables the virus to overcome a restriction to its replication imposed by the cell cycle (131) independently of the presence of wild-type p53 (132). Mutant viruses unable to express the E1B 55-kd protein fail to produce progeny efficiently unless cells are infected in the S phase of the cell cycle. The mechanism by which the E1B 55-kd protein mediates this intriguing function is uncertain. Mutant viruses that fail to express E4orf6 protein exhibit a similar cell cycle phenotype as E1B mutants (133). A complex of the E1B and E4 proteins controls the transport of viral and host mRNAs from nucleus to cyto plasm (see Activation of Late Gene Expression and Host Cell Shutoff), but this function does not appear to underlie the effect of the E1B 55-kd and E4orf6 proteins on the cell cycle restriction.

It is noteworthy that the Ad12 homolog of the Ad5 E1B 55-kd protein can inhibit p53-mediated transcriptional activation and cooperate with E1A to transform cells (447), even though it shows no indication of p53 binding (137,458). Also, the Ad5 E1B protein can sequester a substantial portion of the cell's p53 in a discrete cytoplasmic structure outside of the nucleus (457), whereas the Ad12 protein cannot (458). This has been taken as further evidence that the Ad12 protein does not bind to p53. The Ad12 E1B protein might bind weakly to p53, and the resulting complex might not be sufficiently stable to be detected by the assays that have been employed. The p53 protein is stabilized in Ad12 transformed cells, and the stabilization is dependent on expression of the E1B protein (403). Stabilization is often observed for mutant p53, but the p53 present in the Ad12 transformed cells is wild type. Further, although the Ad5 E1B protein inhibited transformation by *myc* plus *ras,* the Ad12 E1B protein, like mutant p53, enhanced the number of foci produced by *myc* plus *ras.* If there is no direct interaction between the Ad12 E1B protein and p53, these observations suggest that the Ad12 protein somehow causes wild-type p53 to be modified, perhaps by association with another cellular protein, so that it behaves in some respects like mutant p53.

In addition to the E1B 55-kd protein, the E4orf6 protein can bind to p53 and block its transcriptional activation function (92). Like the E1B 55-kd protein, E4orf6 inhibits the interaction of p53 with the TAF31 subunit of TFIID; however, unlike the E1B 55-kd protein, which binds to the amino-terminal activation domain of p53, E4orf6 binds within its carboxy-terminal region. The E1B and E4 proteins cooperate to shorten markedly the half life of p53 (276,287,331,366). Given its ability to antagonize p53, it is not surprising that E4orf6 can cooperate with E1A in cell transformation assays (see Oncogenesis).

E4or6, but not the E1B 55-kd protein, can bind to p73 and inhibit its function (171,367). The p73 protein is a member of the p53 family that is able to activate transcription through p53 response elements. Thus, E4orf6 antagonizes the function of both p53 and p73, blocking their potential inhibitory effects on viral replication.

Inhibition of Apoptosis

E1A proteins trigger apoptosis through both p53-dependent and p53-independent mechanisms (386). The p53-independent apoptosis is an indirect effect of E1A. It results from the E1A-mediated expression of the E4orf4 protein (222,356). E4orf4 might induce apoptosis as a consequence of its ability to bind to protein phosphatase 2A and inhibit its activity (211). This phosphatase targets Bcl-2 and caspase 3, which are known to regulate and mediate apoptosis, respectively. Apoptosis is not observed when E4orf4 functions in the context of an infected cell.

As has been found for other viruses, adenoviruses encode proteins (E1B 55-kd, E1B 19-kd, and E4orf6) that block apoptosis. As discussed previously, the E1B 55-kd and E4orf6 proteins bind to p53 and inhibit its function, blocking p53-dependent apoptosis. The E1B 19-kd protein is a member of the Bcl-2 family of proteins and can block p53-dependent or p53-independent apoptosis (316). In this respect, it is similar to Bcl-2, which resides in the outer mitochondrial membrane and inhibits the translocation of cytochrome c from mitochondria to the cytoplasm. When cytochrome c enters the cytoplasm, it facilitates activation of caspase-9, provoking an apoptotic response.

Adenovirus mutants that fail to produce a functional E1B 19-kd protein induce extensive degradation of host cell and viral DNA, enhanced cytopathic effect, and reduced virus yield when grown in cultured cells (310,380,433). Presumably, the inhibitory effects of premature cell death on viral propagation would be even more severe in natural infections, in which the viral growth cycle is slower than in cultured HeLa cells. Thus, apoptosis is an example of a cellular response to infection that has the potential to inhibit viral growth and block its spread within the infected organism.

Adenoviruses encode additional proteins (E3 gp19-kd, E3 14.7-kd, E3 14.5-kd, and E3 10.4-kd) that block the induction of apoptosis by cytotoxic T lymphocytes (CTLs) and macrophages, and their mode of action is discussed later (see Viral Antagonists of Cytotoxic T Lymphocytes and Tumor Necrosis Factor-α).

Viral DNA Replication

As E2 gene products accumulate, the stage is set for viral DNA replication. Ad2 or Ad5 DNA replication begins between 5 to 8 hours after infection of HeLa cells at a multiplicity of 10 plaque-forming units per cell, and it continues until the host cell dies.

The inverted terminal repeats of the viral chromosome serve as replication origins. *In vivo* studies support a model in which adenovirus DNA replication takes place in two stages (223) (Fig. 8). First, synthesis is initiated at either terminus of the linear DNA and proceeds in a continuous fashion to the other end of the genome. Only one of the two DNA strands serves as a template for the synthesis; thus, the products of the replication are a duplex consisting of a daughter and parental strand plus a displaced single strand of DNA. In the second stage of the

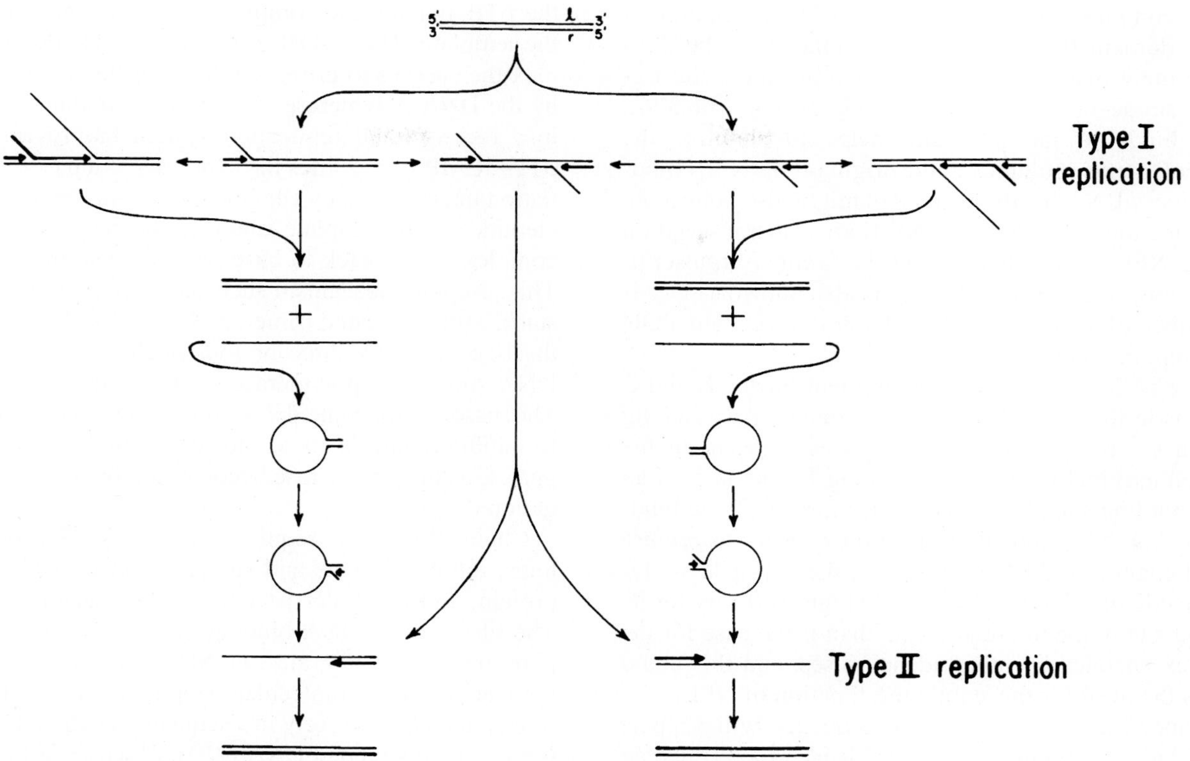

FIG. 8. A model for adenovirus DNA replication. Replication begins at either end of the duplex adenovirus DNA molecule, displacing one of the parental strands and subsequently replicating the displaced strand. Type I replication refers to replication on duplex templates, and type II replication refers to replication initiated on a single-stranded molecule. (From ref. 223, with permission.)

replication process, a complement to the displaced single strand is synthesized. The single-stranded template circularizes through annealing of its self-complementary termini, and the resulting duplex "panhandle" has the same structure as the termini of the duplex viral genome. This structure allows it to be recognized by the same initiation machinery that operates in the first stage of replication, and complementary strand synthesis generates a second completed duplex consisting of one parental and one daughter strand. Adenovirus DNA was the first eukaryotic template to be replicated *in vitro* (50), and increasingly, defined cell-free systems have allowed the analysis of replication in considerable detail.

The cis-Acting sequences composing the replication origins are located within the inverted terminal repeats of the viral chromosome. Three functional domains have been defined within the terminal 51 bp of the repeats. Domain A consists of the first 18 bp of the viral DNA, and it functions as a minimal origin of replication. This domain is required for replication but supports only limited replication on its own. The sequence between base pairs 9 to 18 (5′ATAATATACC-3′) is conserved among different human adenovirus serotypes, and a complex of two viral proteins binds here (59,281,385): the preterminal protein (pTP) and the DNA polymerase. The E2-coded terminal protein (TP) is synthesized as an 80-kd polypeptide (pTP) that is active in initiation of DNA replication (49,373) and, as discussed previously, is found covalently attached to the 5′ ends of the viral chromosome. It is subsequently processed by proteolysis during assembly of virions to generate a 55-kd fragment (TP) that is covalently attached to the genome (51), but it appears that the entire protein with cleaved peptide bonds remains associated with the genomic termini (342). The E2-coded polymerase is a 140-kd protein with biochemical properties distinct from other known DNA polymerases (102,109). It contains both 5′-to-3′ polymerase activity and 3′-to-5′ exonuclease activity, which probably serves a proofreading function during polymerization (109). The pTP and the polymerase form a heterodimeric complex in solution (102,235,374,385) and thus would be expected to bind to the origin as a unit.

Domain B consists of base pairs 19 to 39, and domain C includes base pairs 40 to 51. These two elements are not absolutely required for adenovirus DNA replication, but they substantially enhance the efficiency of the initiation reaction. Cellular factors bind to these elements: nuclear factor I (NFI) binds as a dimer in domain B, and nuclear factor III (NFIII) binds in domain C. NFI interacts with the DNA polymerase, stabilizing the pTP–polymerase complex at the origin (37,59,282). The binding of NFI at domain B appears to be stimulated by the third viral protein that functions in DNA replication, the E2-coded single-stranded DNA-binding protein (68,376). NFIII binds to the pTP and helps to stabilize the pTP–polymerase complex at the origin (406). NFIII binding induces DNA bending, and this might also contribute to its function (413). NFI and NFIII are also transcription factors. NFI is a member of the CTF family of transcriptional activators (197), and NFIII is also known as Oct 1, a member of the family of proteins that contain POU DNA-binding domains (302,315).

There is flexibility in the requirement for the B and C domains in the replication origin. A mutant Ad5 lacking domain C grows well, with sequences adjacent to the inverted terminal repeat compensating for the lack of an NFIII-binding site (162). Ad4 lacks domain B, the binding site for NFI, and its replication appears to require only domain A (159,163). Possibly, the Ad4 pTP–polymerase complex has an intrinsically higher affinity for its binding site in the minimal origin than is the case for the complex encoded by other adenoviruses, and this could bypass the need for the stabilizing function of NFI.

A cloned adenovirus terminal sequence will support the initiation of replication if it is cleaved to produce an end near the normal terminus (382). However, a natural template with a molecule of TP attached at its 5′ end is replicated at much higher efficiency. The activity of the cloned template can be substantially increased if it is treated with a 5′-to-3′ exonuclease. Thus, the production of a single-stranded 3′-terminus can compensate for the absence of an attached molecule at the 5′-terminus, and this suggests that TP bound to the template DNA normally helps to open the terminal duplex. The pTP–polymerase complex can bind in a sequence-specific fashion to the double-stranded form of the A domain of the replication origin (385), and it also can bind to single-stranded DNA (59,204). A sequential interaction of the pTP–polymerase complex, first with the duplex terminus and subsequently with a single strand, could help to unwind the terminal duplex DNA.

The pTP interacts with the nuclear matrix (36,115,342) and serves as a primer for DNA replication. Within the nuclear matrix, pTP appears to contact CAD, a multifunctional pyrimidine biosynthesis enzyme (9). This interaction might anchor adenovirus replication complexes in the vicinity of useful cellular factors.

As a primer, pTP preserves the integrity of the viral chromosome's terminal sequence during multiple rounds of DNA replication. The priming reaction begins with the formation of an ester bond between the β-OH of a serine residue in pTP and the α-phosphoryl group of deoxycytidine monophosphate (dCMP), the first residue at the 5′ end of the DNA chain (49,236). The pTP–dCMP interaction requires the presence of polymerase and is template dependent (52,236,382), suggesting that it occurs after the pTP–polymerase complex is properly positioned on the template. The 3′-OH group of the pTP–dCMP complex then serves to prime synthesis of the nascent strand by the DNA polymerase. The study of mutant templates in a reconstituted replication system has revealed that pTP–dCMP first primes the synthesis of a pTP–CAT initiation intermediate by copying the second three mononucleotides of the template, and then the newly synthesized complex jumps back to base pair at the terminus (207). This jumping mechanism succeeds because the sequence starts with a repeated trimer: 3′-GTAGTA. After the synthesis of the first three or four nucleotides of the new DNA strand, the polymerase separates from pTP (206). The dissociation coincides with a change in its sensitivity to inhibitors and in its K_m for deoxynucleoside triphosphates, as the polymerase becomes a more efficient elongation enzyme.

Chain elongation requires two virus E2-coded proteins, the polymerase and single-stranded DNA-binding protein, and a cellular protein, nuclear factor II (NFII). The virus-coded DNA-binding protein is a 59-kd phosphoprotein that migrates in SDS-polyacrylamide gels with an apparent molecular weight of 72 kd. It binds tightly and cooperatively in a sequence-independent fashion to single-stranded DNA (404). The role of the DNA-binding protein in DNA replication was first revealed by analysis of an adenovirus temperature-sensitive variant carrying a mutation within the E2 gene; its ability to replicate DNA is exquisitely temperature dependent (405). The three-dimensional structure of the DNA-binding protein has been determined (400), and it contains a terminal extension that hooks onto an adjacent DNA-binding protein monomer. This drives the formation of long, multimeric protein chains bound to single-stranded DNA. If the carboxy-terminal extension is removed from the DNA-binding protein, strand displacement on a double-stranded template no longer occurs (81). This indicates that the polymerization of the DNA-binding protein on single-stranded DNA drives strand separation, consistent with the lack of a requirement for a DNA helicase to unwind the double-stranded template in reconstituted adenovirus DNA replication reactions. In the presence of the DNA-binding protein, the polymerase is highly processive (109,241) and can travel the entire length of the chromosome after it has separated from pTP. NFII copurifies with a cellular DNA topoisomerase activity (285), and mammalian topoisomerase I will substitute for it in an *in vitro* replication reaction. NFII does not significantly enhance the synthesis of nascent chains up to 9,000 nucleotides in length; hence, it must be needed to overcome a DNA structural problem that arises only after extensive replication.

In summary, a set of proteins has been identified that mediates the initiation of adenovirus DNA replication (pTP, polymerase, NFI, and NFIII) and chain elongation (polymerase, DNA-binding protein, and NFII). These polypeptides, together with a template containing an adenovirus replication origin, are sufficient to reconstitute the complete viral DNA replication reaction *in vitro*. The adenovirus E4 gene encodes one or more products required for efficient DNA replication (39,153,426), but their role in the process is almost certainly indirect (266).

Activation of Late Gene Expression and Host Cell Shutoff

Adenovirus late genes begin to be expressed efficiently at the onset of viral DNA replication. The adenovirus late coding regions are organized into a single large transcription unit whose primary transcript is about 29,000 nucleotides in length (105,291). This transcript is processed by differential poly(A) site utilization and splicing to generate multiple distinct mRNAs (see Fig. 3). These mRNAs have been grouped into five families, termed L1 to L5, based on the use of common poly(A) addition sites (66,291,463). Expression of this large family of late mRNAs is controlled by the major late promoter. This promoter exhibits a low level of activity early after infection, and it becomes several hundred-fold more active on a per DNA molecule basis at late times (352). It is strongly activated by the E1A proteins through its TATA motif and Sp1/MAZ binding sites (E1A binds to the Sp1 and MAZ transcription factors) (306), but this does not account for the delayed kinetics of the activation event. There appear to be at least two distinct components that contribute to the delayed activation of the major late promoter: a cis-acting change in the viral chromosome, and induction of at least one virus-coded transacting factor.

The time-dependent cis-acting modification of the adenovirus chromosome was revealed by the sequential infection of cells with two closely related adenovirus strains whose late products could be distinguished (389). Although the first virus to reach the nucleus was actively expressing its late products, the second viral chromosome did not express late gene products until it had completed the early phase and had begun DNA replication. Thus, gene products from the first virus did not act in trans to initiate late expression from the second virus.

There are several possible explanations for this observation. It might be necessary to alter the constituents of the viral chromatin during the process of DNA replication to activate the major late promoter. Unreplicated viral chromatin appears to be associated with a different set of proteins than replicated chromatin (56,82). Viral DNA might remain associated with virus-coded core proteins until cellular histones bind during replication. Such an exchange could be required to activate the major late promoter. However, this proposal seems unlikely. Adenovirus DNA does not appear to be associated with histones (410), and papovaviruses exhibit a DNA replication–coupled early-to-late switch even though they package their DNA in cellular histones. Perhaps the replication process allows transcription factors to gain access to the promoter. Histones or histone-like proteins are displaced and then reassemble on DNA during replication, and this could provide an opportunity for transcription factors to compete for binding to the DNA. Alternatively, a newly arriving viral core might simply require a period of time to decondense and become available to the transcription machinery. Chromosomal domains could become accessible to the transcriptional machinery in a defined order, and the promoter responsible for most late gene expression might become accessible only after a delay. The major late promoter is active at a low level early after infection, but this might reflect early activation by a relatively minor subset of the total infecting population of viral chromosomes. It is also possible that the viral chromosome might establish a compartmentalized environment in the nucleus, and it might take a period of time to recruit cellular factors to its defined environment that are needed for late gene expression. Discrete viral centers at which replication and transcription occur have been observed in the infected nucleus by electron microscopy (262,280).

Whatever the underlying mechanism, *in vivo* footprint analysis has revealed that a transcription factor, termed *USF* or *MLTF* (45,273,341), binds to its upstream site in the major late promoter after the onset of DNA replication but not before (397). This factor activates transcription when it is bound to its recognition sequence in the major late promoter. However, a point mutation that blocks binding of USF/MLTF does not prevent the normal activation of the major late promoter (319,320). Hence, if it normally plays an important role in the late activation process, there must be redundant activators that can work in its absence, or USF/MLTF might be brought to the promoter through a protein–protein interaction in the absence of its binding site. Nevertheless, the demonstration that a factor gains access to the major late promoter only after the onset of DNA replication suggests that the time-dependent cis-acting modification to viral chromatin likely involves changes that permit access of transcription factors to the template.

The second component that contributes to activation of the major late promoter is a virus-coded transcription factor. In addition to the upstream region with USF/MLTF-, CAAT-, Sp1/MAZ-, and TATA-binding motifs, the region between +85 and +120, downstream of the initiation site, contributes to activation of the promoter (227,259). This downstream domain contains binding sites for at least two factors that can cooperate with the upstream USF/MLTF element to activate transcription (274,275). One of these factors is coded by the adenovirus *IVa2* gene (399). The *IVa2* gene has been classified as a delayed early gene because it is activated somewhat later than the standard early genes. Its promoter also contains important downstream elements (43,201), and these elements include the binding site for a factor that represses *IVa2* transcription (58). The mechanism by which repression is relieved is not yet known, but it seems likely that an early gene product plays a role. One can build a model in which a cascade of events leads to activation of the major late promoter: early transcription is activated; an early gene product relieves repression of the IVa2 promoter; and the IVa2 protein binds downstream of the major late start site and contributes to its induction. This model is attractive because the sequential nature of these events can serve as a timer, and this clock, together with the requirement for DNA replication, delays the synthesis of the late mRNAs until their products are needed for virus assembly. The IVa2 protein might work in concert with the L1 52/55-kd protein to activate the major late promoter because the two proteins have been reported to interact (149).

Adenovirus encodes a second delayed early gene product, protein IX. It activates transcription in transfection assays but does not exhibit specificity for the major late promoter (250).

Accumulation of late mRNA not only requires activation of the major late promoter but also depends on the alleviation of premature termination by RNA polymerase as it traverses the 29,000-bp late unit. Premature termination occurs at two positions within the unit. The first termination occurs close to the start site. During the late phase of infection, 80% of the RNA chains initiated at the major late promoter terminate before elongation has proceeded 500 nucleotides (104,114,348). This termination primarily mitigates against late mRNA accumulation because prematurely terminated transcripts with 3′ ends in this region are not detected early after infection (114). The second termination event occurs early after infection when molecules of polymerase fail to transcribe beyond the end of the L2 coding region (292); later, the polymerase transcribes through all of the late coding regions to the end of the genome (113). The molecular basis for the termination at early but not late times remains a mystery. Among other possibilities, it could result from cis-acting changes in the structure of adenovirus chromatin.

When DNA replication begins and all the late mRNAs are synthesized, the cytoplasmic accumulation of cellular mRNAs is blocked (26). Synthesis and processing of cellular transcripts continue, but the mRNAs fail to accumulate in the cytoplasm, suggesting that their transport is blocked. The block to cellular mRNA accumulation is mediated by the E1B 55-kd polypeptide (15,311) and by the E4 34-kd polypeptide (153,426), which exist in a complex (338). The same E1B and E4 proteins are required for efficient cytoplasmic accumulation of viral mRNAs late after infection (16,153,311,426). Thus, a complex that includes two viral proteins inhibits accumulation of cellular mRNAs and facilitates cytoplasmic accumulation of viral mRNAs. Analysis of late viral mRNA metabolism in cells infected with a mutant virus unable to synthesize the E1B 55-kd protein indicated that a block occurred immediately before movement of the mRNA from the nucleus to the cytoplasm (228). As discussed previously, the E1B 55-kd protein also binds to p53, but there is no evidence that p53 plays a role in the mRNA transport function mediated by the complex formed between the E1B and E4 proteins.

How does the E1B–E4 complex move mRNAs from the site of synthesis? The E4orf6 protein shuttles between the nucleus and cytoplasm (91,134). E4orf6 contains a nuclear export sequence, a motif first identified in the human immunodeficiency virus (HIV) rev protein, that would be expected to mediate its interaction with the cellular nucleocytoplasmic shuttling apparatus. How does the E1B–E4 complex interact with RNAs to be transported? The E1B 55-kd protein has been reported to exhibit intrinsic RNA-binding activity (178), and the viral protein interacts with a cellular protein termed *E1B-AP5* (117). E1B-AP5 is a member of the heterogeneous nuclear ribonucleoprotein family of RNA-binding proteins, it contains an RNA-binding motif, and its overexpression overcomes the block to host cell mRNA cytoplasmic accumulation in adenovirus-infected cells. A complex of the E1B and E4 proteins with their cellular partners transports newly synthesized viral mRNAs to the cytoplasm.

The discrimination between host and viral mRNAs for transport to the cytoplasm within virus-infected cells is not based on the identity of individual mRNAs. Cellular genes expressed from recombinant viral chromosomes accumulate in the cytoplasm late after infection as if they were viral mRNAs (120,167). Further, mRNAs are transported to the cytoplasm when encoded by cellular genes, such as the *hsp70* gene, that are transcriptionally induced within infected cells (277,443). Immunoelectron microscopy revealed that the E1B–E4 protein complex is localized within and surrounding intranuclear inclusions believed to represent viral transcription and replication centers (304). Together, these observations suggest a model in which the E1B–E4 complex relocalizes to viral transcription centers a cellular factor required for transport of mRNAs (304). This proposal can explain the simultaneous inhibition of host and activation of viral mRNA transport because a transport factor would be moved from the many sites of host transcription and processing to the viral centers.

In addition to their facilitated transport from the nucleus, viral mRNAs are preferentially translated when they reach the cytoplasm late after infection (461). During this period, when viral mRNAs constitute about 20% of the total cytoplasmic pool (381), they are translated to the exclusion of host mRNAs (14,449). Host mRNAs are not degraded; if they are extracted from the infected cell, they can be translated with normal efficiency in a cell-free extract (387). The translational block is not dependent on the inhibition of host cell mRNA accumulation in the cytoplasm. In contrast to most host mRNAs, β-tubulin mRNA continues to accumulate in the cytoplasm, but it is not translated (277). Also, 2-aminopurine can prevent the inhibition of translation without relieving the block to accumulation of host mRNAs (185).

Several regulatory components cooperate to facilitate selective translation of viral mRNAs late after infection. The first involves the cellular protein kinase R (PKR), which is activated by double-stranded RNA that accumulates within adenovirus-infected cells (260,301). After activation, it can phosphorylate the eukaryotic initiation factor-2α (eIF-2α), inactivating the initiation factor and blocking translation. Translation of host cell mRNAs is not inhibited after infection of cells deficient in PKR activity (185,300), suggesting that the kinase, and presumably inactivation of eIF-2α, are key components of the block to host cell translation. The adenovirus-coded VA RNAs (see Viral Antagonists of Interferon-α and -β) inhibit activation of the cellular PKR. These small RNAs have been shown to copurify with viral mRNAs (263); as a result, they might protect viral but not cellular protein synthesis, providing a functional compartmentalization.

Inactivation of eIF-4F also contributes to selective translation in adenovirus-infected cells (186). This initiation factor binds to the cap of mRNAs and facilitates scanning of the 40S ribosome from the cap to the AUG through its intrinsic helicase activity. eIF-4F is normally activated by phosphorylation, and it becomes substantially inactivated by dephosphorylation late after adenovirus infection when cellular mRNAs are not translated. The five families of mRNAs encoded by the adenovirus major late transcription unit all contain the same 200-nucleotide 5′-noncoding region, which has been termed the *tripartite leader sequence* (30). This 5′-noncoding region is important for translation of mRNAs late but not early after infection (33,245). Tripartite leader–containing adenovirus mRNAs continue to be translated late after infection because the 40S ribosome can scan from cap to AUG by a process termed *ribosome jumping* (454), without the need for a helicase as eIF-4F activity becomes limiting. In contrast, most cellular mRNAs are no longer translated in the absence of eIF-4F because they require the helicase to permit scanning through the more extensive secondary structure at their 5′ ends.

Finally, there is a selective activation of late viral protein synthesis by the 100-kd protein encoded by the L4 family of late mRNAs (164). A mutant virus expressing defective L4 100-kd protein fails to translate its late mRNAs efficiently, but it is nevertheless able to block host cell translation. The L4 100-kd protein can bind to mRNA (2), suggesting it may function at the polysome to facilitate translation.

Virus Assembly and Release from the Cell

The replication of viral DNA, coupled with the production of large quantities of the adenovirus structural polypeptides, sets the stage for virus assembly. Trimeric hexon capsomeres are rapidly assembled from monomers after their synthesis in the cytoplasm (180). Assembly of the hexon requires the participation of a second late viral protein (the L4 100-kd protein), the same protein that stimulates late viral translation. Biochemical experiments indicate that a multimeric complex of the L4 100-kd protein binds to hexon monomers (47), and genetic analyses have demonstrated that mutations in the L4 100-kd protein can block assembly of the hexon capsomere (237, 303). Apparently, the L4-coded protein acts as a scaffold to facilitate assembly of trimers, but the mechanism underlying the process is unknown. Penton capsomeres consisting of a pentameric penton base and trimeric fiber assemble somewhat more slowly in the cytoplasm (180). Pulse-chase experiments indicate that the penton base and fiber assemble independently and subsequently join to form a complete penton capsomere (180,412). After their production, hexon and penton capsomeres accumulate in the nucleus, where assembly of the virion occurs.

Mutations within a variety of viral genes can interfere with the assembly process. As would be expected, alterations in structural polypeptides that comprise the hexon or penton base can prevent accumulation of mature virions as well as subassemblies, such as empty capsids (87, 97,336). Alterations in the polypeptide forming the fiber, polypeptide IIIa, or in the L1 52/55-kd protein can prevent assembly of virions and lead to the accumulation of incomplete capsid-like particles (57,86,87,97,336). Finally, a mutant virus with a defective L3-coded protease accumulates noninfectious virion-like particles with a set of unprocessed polypeptides (420).

Studies of mutant viruses, combined with analysis of the kinetics with which polypeptides are incorporated into capsids and mature virions, have provided a rough outline of the adenovirus assembly process. Assembly appears to begin with the formation of an empty capsid (309,377). Subsequently, a viral DNA molecule enters the capsid. The DNA–capsid recognition event is mediated by the packaging sequence, a cis-acting DNA element that is centered about 260 bp from the left end of the viral chromosome (135,155,165,390). Several cellular proteins have been reported to bind at the packaging sequence (343), but their role in the interaction between DNA and capsid is unclear. The packaging element can function only when it is positioned near an end of the viral chromosome, raising the possibility that proteins interacting at the terminal replication origin might contribute to its function. This could explain the ability of mutations in the virus-coded DNA polymerase to interfere with assembly (87). No empty capsids accumulate in cells infected with a mutant adenovirus containing a partially defective packaging sequence, even though all of the known constituents of the capsid accumulate (160, 166). This suggests that capsid assembly does not occur spontaneously in the absence of an interacting DNA;

rather, it is probably initiated in association with a viral DNA, an association mediated by the viral packaging sequence. Encapsidation of the chromosome is polar, beginning with the left end of the viral DNA (390), as one might anticipate given the location of the packaging sequence. The mechanism by which the viral DNA enters the capsid is controversial (87,160,422). Some experiments favor the possibility that viral DNA replication and encapsidation are coupled; that is, that the viral DNA enters the capsid as it is replicated. Other work suggests that ongoing viral DNA replication is not required and that replication and encapsidation occur in separate nuclear compartments. The L1 52/55-kd protein, which is composed of two differentially phosphorylated forms of a 48-kd precursor polypeptide, facilitates the encapsidation process (148,160,161). The L3-coded proteinase, a cysteine proteinase that requires DNA and a fragment of another viral polypeptide as cofactors (89,258,391,424), functions late in the assembly process. It cleaves at least four virion constituents, generating the mature VI, VII, and VIII and terminal protein moieties. These cleavages stabilize the particle and render it infectious.

There appear to be at least two viral systems that facilitate the escape and spread of progeny virus. The first involves disruption of intermediate filaments, which are components of the cytoskeleton. Vimentin is cleaved rapidly after infection, reportedly both by a reaction initiated by the adsorption process that does not require viral gene expression (24) and in response to the E1B 19-kd protein (431,432). As a result, the extended vimentin system collapses into the perinuclear region (80,460). Late in the infectious cycle, the L3 proteinase cleaves the cellular cytokeratin K18 (61). The cleavage event occurs at amino acid 74 of the cytokeratin, creating a "headless" protein that is not able to polymerize and form filaments; rather, it accumulates in cytoplasmic clumps. A normal intermediate filament system helps to maintain the mechanical integrity of cells, and perturbations to the network would be expected to make the infected cell more susceptible to lysis. The second system that facilitates the release of progeny virions involves the E3 11.6-kd protein. This protein, which is also referred to as the *adenovirus death protein,* kills cells as it accumulates during the late stage of infection (394). The mechanism by which it kills is not known.

INTERACTIONS WITH THE HOST

Adenovirus can maintain a long-term association with its human host, persisting for years after an initial infection. Adenovirus DNA has been identified by *in situ* hybridization in 1 in 10^4 to 10^6 peripheral lymphocytes of healthy individuals (123), and lymphocytes could be the source of virus in the original isolations of adenoviruses from adenoid tissue. Thus, adenovirus probably persists in lymphocytes. The virus encodes three gene products that should facilitate persistence by antagonizing antiviral responses of the host: E1A proteins and VA RNAs, which inhibit the cellular response to interferon-α and -β; and E3-coded products that protect infected cells from killing by CTLs and tumor necrosis factor (TNF). It is intriguing to note that these protective viral products are expressed from the three adenovirus genes most likely to be expressed in lymphocytes in the absence of active viral replication. The E1A promoter and the polymerase III–transcribed VA RNAs are constitutively expressed in all cells that have been tested, and the E3 promoter is unique among adenovirus control elements in that it contains several binding sites for the lymphoid-specific NFκB transcription factor, facilitating constitutive expression in lymphoid cells (438). Additionally, it appears that these protective viral genes might be further induced in response to the production of interleukin-6 (IL-6), a cytokine that is induced at the site of adenovirus infection in experimental animals (124), as a host antiviral measure. Transcription of the E2 gene is strongly activated by IL-6 through the cellular transcription factor NF–IL-6 (364); the resulting E2-coded DNA-binding protein, in turn, can activate the E1A and E3 promoters (53). Thus, the production of a cytokine by the host as a protective response likely induces a viral countermeasure.

Viral Antagonists of Interferon-α and -β

The adenovirus E1A protein and virus-associated (VA) RNAs both afford protection from interferon-α and -β. E1A proteins inhibit the antiviral affect of interferon (7) by blocking the activation of interferon response genes (150,321). At least part of this effect results from the ability of E1A to bind to STAT1 (247) and its coactivator p300/CPB (see Activation of the Host Cell) and inhibit their activity. STAT1 is a transcription factor that mediates activation of interferon-responsive genes.

The small, abundant VA RNAs were named when their viral origin was still uncertain (322). Different adenovirus serotypes have been reported to encode one or two VA RNAs; Ad2 and Ad5 encode two species, termed VA RNA_I and VA RNA_{II}. The RNAs are each about 160 nucleotides in length, are GC rich, adopt stable secondary structures that are important for their function, and are transcribed by RNA polymerase III (112,147,427). VA RNA synthesis begins during the early phase of the infectious cycle and dramatically accelerates during the late phase. VA RNA_I accumulates to about 10^8 molecules per infected HeLa cell, roughly the abundance of ribosomes, and VA RNA_{II} reaches about 10^7 molecules per cell.

The first hint to the function of VA RNAs came from analysis of a mutant Ad5 virus in which the VA RNA_I gene was deleted (387). The virus grew poorly, and its defect was traced to inefficient protein synthesis during the late phase of infection. Additional work identified a defect in polypeptide chain initiation (323,345) resulting from phosphorylation of the eukaryotic initiation factor-2 (eIF-2) (323,344).

The eIF-2, which includes three subunits (α, β, and γ), is central to one of the best-studied pathways of translational control. Early in the initiation process, eIF-2 binds to guanosine triphosphate (GTP) and the initiator transfer RNA (tRNA) to form a ternary complex, which then interacts with the 40S ribosomal subunit. Subsequent steps in the initiation process involving additional factors result in the binding of mRNA and the 60S ribosomal subunit. As the round of initiation is completed, eIF-2 leaves the ribosome, lacking the initiator tRNA and complexed with guanosine diphosphate (GDP) instead of GTP. For eIF-2–GDP to participate in another round of initiation, its GDP must be replaced with GTP in a reaction catalyzed by eIF-2B (also termed *guanosine nucleotide exchange factor*). The exchange reaction is inhibited by phosphorylation of the α subunit of eIF-2. The eIF-2α(P) forms a tight complex with eIF-2B, preventing it from cycling and catalyzing the exchange reaction. As a result, initiation is brought to a halt when about one third to one half of eIF-2 is phosphorylated, trapping all available eIF-2B. The degree of eIF-2α phosphorylation is greatly increased during the late phase of infection with the VA RNA_I–negative mutant (301), and protein synthesis in extracts of these infected cells can be restored to normal levels by addition of eIF-2 or eIF-2B (323,344). Further, the mutant phenotype is abrogated in cells that contain mutant forms of the eIF-2α subunit (77) or lack the eIF-2α kinase (301,344). Thus, the reduction in late translation results from the phosphorylation and inactivation of eIF-2.

Phosphorylation of eIF-2 is mediated by PKR. Synthesis of an inactive form of PKR is induced by interferon, and the latent enzyme is activated by double-stranded RNA. PKR is activated by autophosphorylation, which appears to require that two molecules of the enzyme interact with a molecule of double-stranded RNA (213). Activated PKR can phosphorylate the eIF-2α subunit; this leads to sequestration of eIF-2B and the cessation of translation. VA RNA_I can bind to PKR (203,269) and block its activation (208,300). The current structural model for VA RNA_I (Fig. 9A) suggests that it consists of two extended duplex domains bracketing a central domain that is composed of several stem-loop structures. The central domain includes two complementary tetranucleotides that are conserved in VA RNAs encoded by a variety of adenovirus serotypes (251,253), and mutational analysis indicates that the conserved tetranucleotide pair is essential for VA RNA_I structure and function (252).

In an adenovirus-infected cell, PKR is probably activated by double-stranded RNA produced as a result of the symmetric transcription of the viral chromosome (260, 301). Activation of endogenous latent kinase is likely responsible for the inhibition of translation observed in cells infected with VA RNA_I–negative mutants (264). The level of latent PKR is induced by a factor of 5 to 10 in response to interferon. Thus, one might anticipate that VA RNA_I antagonizes the antiviral effect of interferon by blocking activation of PKR, and this has proved to be the case (208). Whereas interferon-α inhibits the growth of VA RNA_I–negative virus, it has no effect on wild-type Ad5 (see Fig. 9B). In summary, VA RNA_I blocks activation of latent PKR, and this function would seem critical for optimal viral growth in an infected host capable of responding to viral infection by the production of interferon.

In contrast to VA RNA_I, VA RNA_{II} exhibits limited ability to block PKR activation. VA RNA_{II} binds to RNA helicase A and NF90, a component of the nuclear factor of activated T cells (234). It is not yet understood how these interactions might promote viral replication.

Viral Antagonists of Cytotoxic T Lymphocytes and Tumor Necrosis Factor-α

Upon intranasal inoculation of cotton rats (*Sigmodon hispidus*) or mice with Ad5, viral gene expression is detected in the epithelial cells of the bronchi and bronchioles of the lung and nasal mucosa. The pulmonary histopathology is similar to that observed in humans (126), and disease proceeds in two stages (314). The earlier stage consists of a mild-to-moderate damage to bronchiolar epithelial cells and a diffuse cellular infiltration of peribronchiolar and alveolar regions. At this time, TNF-α, IL-1, and IL-6 appear in infected lung tissue (124). The later stage of the disease consists almost entirely of an infiltration of lymphocytes. A normal early phase ensues, but little late response is observed when athymic nude mice are infected (124), consistent with the interpretation that the late phase results from infiltration of virus-specific CTLs. Thus, the two stages of pathogenesis appear to result from an initial nonspecific host response to viral infection that includes synthesis of cytokines followed by an immunologically specific CTL response. Adenovirus E3-coded proteins, which are not needed for efficient viral growth in cultured cells, combat at least a portion of these host antiviral measures, inhibiting cytolysis of infected cells by CTLs or TNF-α.

Recognition and lysis of a virus-infected cell by CTLs requires that viral peptide antigens be displayed on the infected cell's surface in a complex with a class I MHC antigen. Ad2- or Ad5-infected cells expressing the E3-coded 19-kd glycoprotein (E3 gp19-kd) are considerably less sensitive to CTL-mediated lysis than cells infected with mutant viruses unable to express the E3 protein (8,42). E3gp 19-kd is a transmembrane protein of 142 amino acids, after removal of its amino-terminal signal sequence. It resides in the membrane of the endoplasmic reticulum, where it is held through the action of a retention signal that has been mapped to its C-terminal domain (305). The luminal domain of E3gp 19-kd binds directly

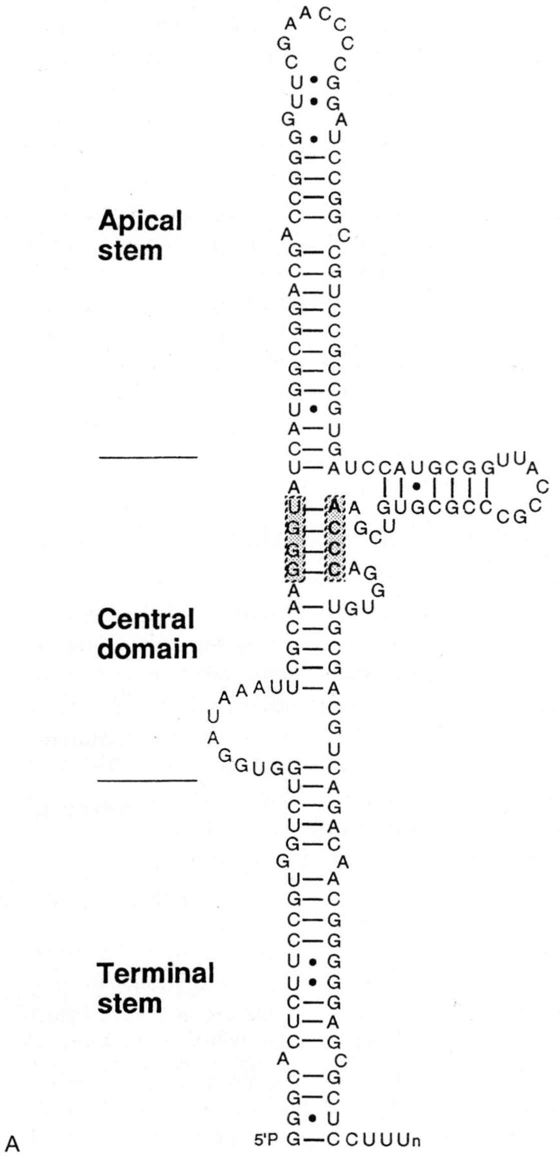

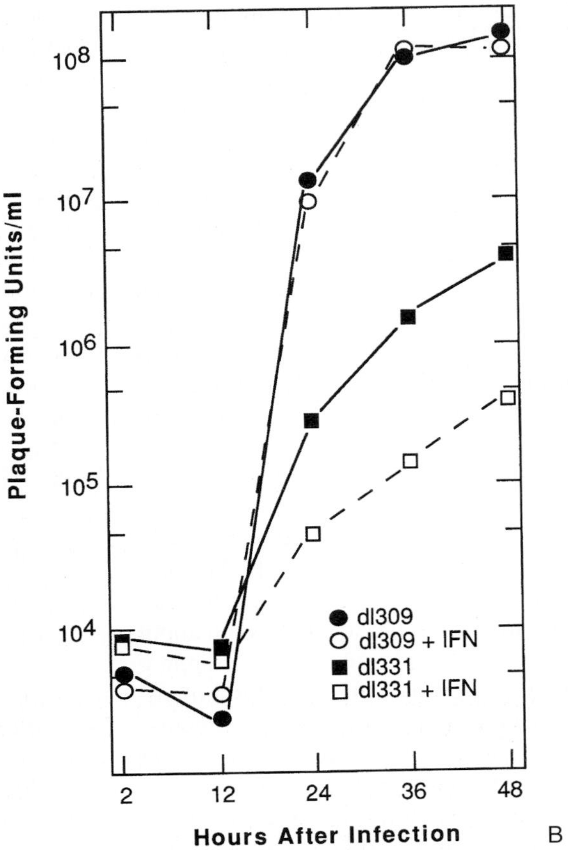

FIG. 9. Adenovirus VA RNA structure and function. **A:** Current model for the secondary structure of Ad2 VA RNA_1. The molecule is divided into three domains by convention: apical stem, central domain, and terminal stem. The two tetranucleotides in the central domain that are conserved among different adenovirus serotypes are identified (*shading*). **B:** VA RNA_1 antagonizes the antiviral effects of α-interferon. *Cell*s were infected with a virus that contained a wild-type VA RNA_1 gene (*d1309, circles*) or a mutant with a deletion blocking expression of VA RNA_1 (*d1331, squares*), and either treated (*open symbols*) or not treated (*solid symbols*) with α-interferon. The adenovirus with the wild-type VA RNA_1 gene was resistant to α-interferon, whereas the mutant virus was inhibited. (**A** modified from ref. 252, with permission; **B** from ref. 208, with permission.)

to the peptide-binding domain of class I MHC antigens (42,220), and this interaction retains class I antigen in the endoplasmic reticulum through the di-lysine retention signal in the E3 protein. E3 gp19-kd also binds to TAP (28) and prevents it from transferring peptides processed in the cytosol to class I antigen in the endoplasmic reticulum. A reduced level of class I antigen on the cell surface and a block to TAP-mediated loading of class I antigen should protect against premature lysis of the infected cell by CTLs. Such protection can be inferred from experiments with cotton rats (126), but not mice (363). Pulmonary infection of cotton rats with a mutant virus, unable to express E3gp 19-kd, induced a markedly enhanced late phase inflammatory response (126). Thus, the E3 protein apparently ameliorates the late-phase response in cotton rats by protecting against lysis by CTLs.

CTLs carry the Fas ligand on their cell surface and induce apoptosis when the Fas ligand interacts with the Fas receptor (CD95) on a target cell. Products of the E3 region block Fas-mediated apoptosis. The membrane-bound E3 14.4-kd–E3 10.4-kd protein complex mediates internalization and degradation of the Fas receptor (98, 355,393). Further, the E3 14.7-kd protein interacts with FLICE, a caspase acting downstream of the Fas receptor, and inhibits Fas ligand-induced apoptosis (60).

TNF-α is a cytokine that is secreted by activated macrophages and lymphocytes. It exerts cytotoxic or cytostatic effects on many tumor cells, and it can induce apoptosis and the subsequent lysis of cells infected with some viruses. Whereas uninfected cells or cells infected with wild-type adenovirus are not affected, cells infected with mutant adenoviruses lacking the E3 coding region are lysed by TNF-α (129). The CR1 domain of the E1A proteins is responsible for inducing susceptibility to TNF-α (95). This is the same E1A domain that has been reported to antagonize the activation of interferon-responsive genes, and the mapping does not precisely correlate with the binding requirements for any known E1A target. Either the E3 14.7-kd protein (129) or the E3 14.5-kd–E3 10.4-kd protein complex can prevent cytolysis by TNF-α (130). Both inhibit the activation of cytosolic phospholipase A2, which acts downstream of the TNF-α receptor (88,216,465). As noted previously, the E3 14.7-kd protein interacts with FLICE (caspase 8) (60). FLICE acts downstream of both the FAS and TNF receptors, and this interaction likely accounts for part of the mechanism by which the E3 14.7-kd protein blocks the induction of apoptosis by both receptors. The E3 14.7-kd protein also binds to a set of proteins termed FIP-1, -2, and -3 (231–233). When overexpressed, FIP-3 appears to activate a cell death pathway and to block an NFκB-mediated survival pathway (231). The interaction of the E3 14.7-kd protein with FIP-3 presumably blocks both of these pro-apoptotic activities.

In addition to its effect on the Fas receptor and the response to TNF-α, the E3 14.5-kd–E3 10.4-kd protein complex reduces the level of epidermal growth factor receptor on the surface of infected cells by inducing its internalization (44,393). It is not yet clear whether the internalization stimulates an epidermal growth factor–like response or abrogates function of the receptor.

ONCOGENESIS

All human adenoviruses that have been tested are able to transform cultured rodent cells to an oncogenic phenotype. The transformants undergo morphologic changes, and they tend to grow as dense, multilayered colonies. They can display various phenotypic hallmarks of oncogenic transformation, including growth in reduced serum, anchorage-independent growth, and growth to higher densities than normal. Only a subset of adenovirus serotypes can directly induce the formation of tumors within rats and hamsters (see Table 1). Group A adenoviruses (e.g., Ad12, Ad18) are highly oncogenic, producing tumors in most animals within 4 months; group B viruses (e.g., Ad3, Ad7) are weakly oncogenic, inducing tumors within 4 to 18 months; at least one group D virus (Ad9) is oncogenic, efficiently inducing mammary tumors within 3 to 5 months; and group C and E viruses are not known to be tumorigenic.

Adenoviruses transform rodent cells much more efficiently than human cells, and the oncogenic adenoviruses induce tumors in rodents, whereas extensive screens have failed to correlate the presence of adenoviruses with human cancer. Initially, it seemed that the more efficient oncogenic transformation of rodent than human cells might result from the fact that rodent cells are generally less permissive for growth of human adenoviruses, and, as a result, they could more readily survive an infection and yield transformants. However, cloned E1A and E1B genes exhibit the same host cell preferences for transformation as does whole virus, arguing that differences in permissivity to viral growth are not a primary determining factor in transformation efficiency. There is a fundamental difference in the biology of rodent and human somatic cells that likely influences their response to adenovirus oncoproteins. Murine cells express telomerase and have longer telomeres than their human counterparts, which lack telomerase activity. It has recently been shown that the catalytic subunit of telomerase can cooperate with SV40 T antigen plus an oncogenic H-ras protein to transform efficiently human fibroblasts to a tumorigenic phenotype (152). T antigen plus oncogenic H-ras do not transform human cells in the absence of telomerase. This experiment suggests that the lack of telomerase expression in somatic cells is, at least in part, responsible for the block to adenovirus oncogenicity in humans. It is also possible that the immune response to adenovirus transformants (see Tumorigenesis) is fundamentally different in rodents and humans.

Transformation

Three lines of evidence initially demonstrated that the E1A and E1B genes mediate transformation. First, virus-transformed cells always contain and express these genes; second, transfection of cultured cells with cloned E1A and E1B genes leads to transformation; and, third, mutant viruses with alterations to these genes can be defective for transformation. As discussed previously, the E1A and E1B proteins manipulate cellular growth regulation. In a lytically infected human cell, E1A proteins induce quiescent cells to enter the S phase of the cell cycle, and E1B proteins prevent p53-mediated G_1 phase arrest and block the onset of apoptosis, creating an environment optimally conducive to viral replication. In the context of a rodent cell, these same events lead to oncogenic transformation.

One can construct a model for how the E1A and E1B 55-kd oncoproteins deregulate the G_0- to G_1- to S-phase cell cycle checkpoint through their interactions with pRB family members, p300 and p53. However, although E1A proteins have been shown to drive cells past the G_2- to M-phase checkpoint into mitosis, the mechanism by which this checkpoint is antagonized remains a mystery. Mutations in the E1A proteins that interfere with the binding of p300 or pRB family members can block the ability of E1A proteins to induce mitosis (182). Perhaps these cellular proteins, either in their normal complexes or as a result of their interaction with E1A proteins, influence both the G_0- to G_1- to S-phase and the G_2- to M-phase cell cycle checkpoints. Alternatively, the E1A proteins interact with additional, as yet unidentified proteins that control the G_2- to M-phase checkpoint.

Either the E4orf6 (276,286) or the E4orf3 protein (288) can substitute for E1B and cooperate with E1A to transform cells. Further, both of these proteins can enhance the tumorigenic potential of cells transformed with the E1A plus E1B oncogenes. E4orf6 inhibits p53 function and cooperates with the E1B 55-kd protein to reduce the half life of p53 (see Activation of the Host Cell). The ability to neutralize p53 probably accounts for the oncogenic activity of E4orf6. E4orf3 and E1A localize to and cause a morphologic rearrangement of POD/ND10 structures (46,94). The function of these intranuclear structures and their possible relationship to the oncogenic activity of E4orf3 are unknown.

Tumorigenesis

Rat cells transformed by the highly oncogenic Ad12 generally produce tumors in newborn syngeneic rats, whereas most cells transformed by the nononcogenic adenoviruses, such as Ad2 or Ad5, are not tumorigenic. However, some Ad2-transformed rat cell lines can induce tumors in immunosuppressed rats (118), suggesting that cells transformed by nononcogenic adenoviruses are rejected by the host's immune system. Newborn hamsters, which have not yet developed a thymus-dependent immune response, are also susceptible to tumor production by Ad2-transformed cells. Although thymectomized hamsters remain susceptible, normal animals become resistant to tumor challenge at the age of about 3 weeks when their thymic response has developed (71), suggesting that the thymus-dependent cellular immune system plays a key role in the rejection.

The thymus-dependent CTL response leads to lysis of transformed cells. As mentioned earlier, CTLs target tumor cells by recognizing foreign antigens displayed on their cell surface in the context of class I MHC antigens. In the case of Ad5 transformed cells, the E1A protein itself serves as a cell surface target (25), and several specific E1A-encoded epitopes have been identified that serve as targets of class I–restricted CTLs (202,332).

The Ad12 E1A proteins inhibit the CTL response that blocks tumor formation by cells transformed with nononcogenic adenoviruses (35). Ad12-transformed cells contain reduced quantities of class I MHC antigen on their surface (346), and, after introduction of a class I gene MHC that cannot be down-regulated by the Ad12 E1A proteins, Ad12 transformants are unable to induce tumors (383). Thus, the Ad12 E1A proteins repress expression of the class I antigen, and this prevents recognition by CTLs. The repression occurs at the level of transcription, and it appears that the activity of at least two factors that interact with the class I gene control region are altered (217,267,294).

Not all Ad12 transformants have proved resistant to CTL lysis (271), and some Ad12 transformed lines have become more tumorigenic (i.e., fewer cells can induce a tumor) when they were modified to express higher levels of class I antigen (361). Thus, although Ad12 E1A proteins reduce class I MHC levels in some transformed cells, facilitating escape from class I–restricted CTL-mediated destruction, the correlation is not reliable. This indicates that there are additional immune mechanisms that govern adenovirus tumor formation.

Many Ad2 transformed cells are markedly less efficient than Ad12 transformants in the formation of tumors in athymic nude mice that lack class I–restricted CTLs. Nude mice possess natural killer (NK) cells, a class of immunologically nonspecific cytotoxic lymphocytes. Ad2 transformants are more susceptible to NK cell–mediated lysis than their Ad12 counterparts (70,317). Susceptibility to NK killing is governed by the E1A gene (72,73,340); addition of the Ad5 E1A gene to a highly tumorigenic sarcoma cell line induced susceptibility to lysis by NK cells, blocking its ability to form tumors (416).

Non-E1A–mediated mechanisms can also influence tumorigenesis. The E3 19-kd glycoprotein can influence class I MHC levels (see Viral Antagonists of Cytotoxic T Lymphocytes and Tumor Necrosis Factor-α). Thus, the E3 gene might also contribute to the differential CTL sensitivity of Ad12 versus Ad2 or Ad5 transformants. Although the E3 gene is often present in Ad12 transformants, it is generally not present in Ad2 or Ad5 transformed cells. Although there are exceptions, most rodent cells transformed with Ad2 or Ad5 contain only portions of the viral genome; only the E1A and E1B genes are consistently present. In a similar vein, additional E3-coded proteins, if present, might afford protection from TNF-α. The notion that additional genes play auxiliary roles in tumorigenesis is consistent with the observation that substitution of the Ad12 E1A or E1B genes into the corresponding Ad5 domain did not equip the resulting hybrid viruses to induce tumors in newborn rats or hamsters (34,340).

In contrast to group A adenoviruses such as Ad12, which induces tumors at the site of injection, Ad9, a group D virus, induces mammary tumors, irrespective of the site of injection. Subcutaneous injection of newborn Wistar-Furth rats produces mammary tumors in females but not males (11). The tumors are predominantly benign fibroadenomas, but phyllodes-like tumors and malignant sarcomas are also produced; all of the tumors are estrogen dependent (10,193). When hybrid viruses were constructed between Ad9 and a closely related group D virus that fails to induce mammary tumors, the Ad9 E4 gene was found to be required for mammary tumorigenesis (194). Remarkably, the E1A and E1B genes are dispensable for tumor induction (388). The Ad9 E4orf1 protein is responsible for Ad9 tumorigenesis. It is able to transform cultured cells efficiently to an oncogenic phenotype (195), and E4orf1 from group A and C adenoviruses can also transform cells if overexpressed (428). The 12.5-kd E4orf1 protein is localized predominantly to the cytoplasm (429), and it binds to a PDZ domain–containing protein, hDlg/SAP97 (225), a human homolog of the *Drosophila* discs large tumor suppressor protein. The carboxy-terminal domain of E4orf1 that is required for oncogenesis is also required for hDlg/SAP97 binding, suggesting that E4orf1 might act through this protein to mediate its oncogenic activity.

PERSPECTIVES

Much is known about the adenovirus growth cycle; indeed, the advances in our understanding during the 5 years since I first wrote this chapter are remarkable. An adenovirus host cell receptor has been identified, the protective (from the virus's point of view) roles of E3 proteins have been clarified, and the oncogenic potential of E4 proteins has been discovered. Yet, much remains a mystery, including the structure of the viral core both within the virion and as viral DNA is transcribed, the mechanism by which viral DNA is encapsidated, and the basis for host restrictions and tissue tropisms in infected organisms. There is no doubt that these and many other questions will be resolved in the near future.

Adenoviruses have brought much more to the table than a system of viral replication; they have also contributed to a molecular understanding of many fundamental cellular processes. For example, studies of adenoviruses have yielded important insights to the complex mechanisms by which cells express and process mRNAs and control their growth. Early adenovirus gene products have helped to identify many important cell cycle regulatory proteins, and they continue to serve as probes with which to manipulate these cellular factors and reveal their normal functions.

Adenoviruses no longer serve simply as systems for study. As discussed in Chapter 68 in *Fields Virology*, 4th ed., they are now being developed as vectors for gene therapy. Indeed, adenovirus vectors have been created that carry no viral genes, and it is becoming possible to modify the tropism of vectors by directing the virus to proteins on the cell surface other than its natural receptor. If the virus can be tamed so that it delivers and expresses therapeutic genes without attendant pathology, we will undoubtedly find ourselves "sleeping with the enemy" in the near future.

REFERENCES

1. Abdel-Hafiz HA, Chen CY, Marcell T, et al. Structural determinants outside of the leucine zipper influence the interactions of CREB and ATF-2: Interaction of CREB with ATF-2 blocks E1a-ATF-2 complex formation. *Oncogene* 1993;8:1161–1174.
2. Adam SA, Dreyfuss G. Adenovirus proteins associated with mRNA and hnRNA in infected HeLa cells. *J Virol* 1987;61:3276–3283.
3. Akalu A, Liebermann H, Bauer U, et al. The subgenus-specific C-terminal region of protein IX is located on the surface of the adenovirus capsid. *J Virol* 1999;73:6182–6187.
4. Alevizopoulos K, Catarin B, Vlach J, Amati B. A novel function of adenovirus E1A is required to overcome growth arrest by the CDK2 inhibitor p27(Kip1). *EMBO J* 1998;17:5987–5997.
5. Amalfitano A, Begy CR, Chamberlain JS. Improved adenovirus packaging cell lines to support the growth of replication-defective gene-delivery vectors. *Proc Natl Acad Sci U S A* 1996;93:3352–3356.
6. Anderson CW, Young ME, Flint SJ. Characterization of the adenovirus 2 virion protein, mu. *Virology* 1989;172:506–512.
7. Anderson KP, Fennie EH. Adenovirus early region 1A modulation of interferon antiviral activity. *J Virol* 1987;61:787–795.
8. Andersson M, McMichael A, Peterson PA. Reduced allorecognition of adenovirus 2 infected cells. *J Immunol* 1987;138:3960–3966.
9. Angeletti PC, Engler JA. Adenovirus preterminal protein binds to the CAD enzyme at active sites of viral DNA replication on the nuclear matrix. *J Virol* 1998;72:2896–2904.
10. Ankerst J, Jonsson N. Adenovirus type 9-induced tumorigenesis in the rat mammary gland related to sex hormonal state. *J Natl Cancer Inst* 1989;81:294–298.
11. Ankerst J, Jonsson N, Kjellen L, et al. Induction of mammary fibroadenomas in rats by adenovirus type 9. *Int J Cancer* 1974;13:286–290.
12. Arrand JR, Roberts RJ. The nucleotide sequences at the termini of adenovirus-2 DNA. *J Mol Biol* 1979;128:577–594.
13. Athappilly FK, Murali R, Rux JJ, et al. The refined crystal structure of hexon, the major coat protein of adenovirus type 2, at 2.9 Å resolution. *J Mol Biol* 1994;242:430–455.
14. Babich A, Feldman LT, Nevins JR, et al. Effect of adenovirus on metabolism of specific host mRNAs: transport control and specific translational discrimination. *Mol Cell Biol* 1983;3:1212–1221.
15. Babiss LE, Ginsberg HS. Adenovirus type 5 early region 1b gene product is required for efficient shutoff of host protein synthesis. *J Virol* 1984;50:202–212.
16. Babiss LE, Ginsberg HS, Darnell JE Jr. Adenovirus E1B proteins are required for accumulation of late viral mRNA and for effects on cellular mRNA translation and transport. *Mol Cell Biol* 1985;5:2552–2558.
17. Bachenheimer S, Darnell JE. Adenovirus-2 mRNA is transcribed as part of a high-molecular-weight precursor RNA. *Proc Natl Acad Sci U S A* 1975;72:4445–4449.
18. Bagchi S, Raychaudhuri P, Nevins JR. Adenovirus E1A proteins can dissociate heteromeric complexes involving the E2F transcription factor: A novel mechanism for E1A trans-activation. *Cell* 1990;62:659–669.
19. Bagchi S, Weinmann R, Raychaudhuri P. The retinoblastoma protein copurifies with E2F-I, an E1A-regulated inhibitor of the transcription factor E2F. *Cell* 1991;65:1063–1072.
20. Bai M, Harfe B, Freimuth P. Mutations that alter an Arg-Gly-Asp (RGD) sequence in the adenovirus type 2 penton base protein abolish its cell-rounding activity and delay virus reproduction in flat cells. *J Virol* 1993;67:5198–5205.
21. Bandara LR, La Thangue NB. Adenovirus E1A prevents the retinoblastoma gene product from complexing with a cellular transcription factor. *Nature* 1991;351:494–497.
22. Barbeau D, Charbonneau R, Whalen SG, et al. Functional interactions within adenovirus E1A protein complexes. *Oncogene* 1994;9:359–373.
23. Baum SG. Adenoviridae. In: Mandel GL, Douglas RG, Bennet JE, eds. *Principals and practice of infectious diseases.* 2nd ed. New York: John Wiley and Sons, 1984:1353–1361.
24. Belin MT, Boulanger P. Processing of vimentin occurs during the early stages of adenovirus infection. *J Virol* 1987;61:2559–2566.
25. Bellgrau D, Walker TA, Cook JL. Recognition of adenovirus E1A gene products on immortalized cell surfaces by cytotoxic T lymphocytes. *J Virol* 1988;62:1513–1519.
26. Beltz GA, Flint SJ. Inhibition of HeLa cell protein synthesis during adenovirus infection: Restriction of cellular messenger RNA sequences to the nucleus. *J Mol Biol* 1979;131:353–373.
27. Benbrook DM, Jones NC. Heterodimer formation between CREB and JUN proteins. *Oncogene* 1990;5:295–302.
28. Bennett EM, Bennink JR, Yewdell JW, Brodsky FM. Cutting edge: Adenovirus E19 has two mechanisms for affecting class I MHC expression. *J Immunol* 1999;162:5049–5052.
29. Bergelson JM, Cunningham JA, Droguett G, et al. Isolation of a common receptor for coxsackie B viruses and adenoviruses 2 and 5. *Science* 1997;275:1320–1323.
30. Berget SM, Moore C, Sharp PA. Spliced segments at the 5′ terminus of adenovirus 2 late mRNA. *Proc Natl Acad Sci U S A* 1977;74:3171–3175.

31. Berk AJ, Lee F, Harrison T, et al. Pre-early adenovirus 5 gene product regulates synthesis of early viral messenger RNAs. *Cell* 1979;17:935–944.
32. Berk AJ, Sharp PA. Sizing and mapping of early adenovirus mRNAs by gel electrophoresis of S1 endonuclease-digested hybrids. *Cell* 1977;12:721–732.
33. Berkner KL, Sharp PA. Effect of the tripartite leader on synthesis of a non-viral protein in an adenovirus 5 recombinant. *Nucleic Acids Res* 1985;13:841–857.
34. Bernards R, de Leeuw MG, Vaessen MJ, et al. Oncogenicity by adenovirus is not determined by the transforming region only. *J Virol* 1984;50:847–853.
35. Bernards R, Schrier PI, Houweling A, et al. Tumorigenicity of cells transformed by adenovirus type 12 by evasion of T-cell immunity. *Nature* 1983;305:776–779.
36. Bodnar JW, Hanson PI, Polvino-Bodnar M, et al. The terminal regions of adenovirus and minute virus of mice DNAs are preferentially associated with the nuclear matrix in infected cells. *J Virol* 1989;63:4344–4353.
37. Bosher J, Robinson EC, Hay RT. Interactions between the adenovirus type 2 DNA polymerase and the DNA binding domain of nuclear factor I. *New Biol* 1990;2:1083–1090.
38. Boyer TG, Martin ME, Lees E, et al. Mammalian Srb/mediator complex is targeted by adenovirus E1A protein. *Nature* 1999;399:276–279.
39. Bridge E, Medghalchi S, Ubol S, et al. Adenovirus early region 4 and viral DNA synthesis. *Virology* 1993;193:794–801.
40. Deleted in page proofs.
41. Brown DT, Westphal M, Burlingham BT, et al. Structure and composition of the adenovirus type 2 core. *J Virol* 1975;16:366–387.
42. Burget HG, Kvist S. The E3/19K protein of adenovirus type 2 binds to the domains of histocompatibility antigens required for CTL recognition. *EMBO J* 1987;6:2019–2026.
43. Carcamo J, Maldonado E, Cortes P, et al. A TATA-like sequence located downstream of the transcription initiation site is required for expression of an RNA polymerase II transcribed gene. *Genes Dev* 1990;4:1611–1622.
44. Carlin CR, Tollefson AE, Brady HA, et al. Epidermal growth factor receptor is down-regulated by a 10,400 MW protein encoded by the E3 region of adenovirus. *Cell* 1989;57:135–144.
45. Carthew RW, Chodosh LA, Sharp PA. An RNA polymerase II transcription factor binds to an upstream element in the adenovirus major late promoter. *Cell* 1985;43:439–448.
46. Carvalho T, Seeler JS, Ohman K, et al. Targeting of adenovirus E1A and E4-ORF3 proteins to nuclear matrix-associated PML bodies. *J Cell Biol* 1995;131:45–56.
47. Cepko CL, Sharp PA. Assembly of adenovirus major capsid protein is mediated by a nonvirion protein. *Cell* 1982;31:407–415.
48. Chakravarti D, Ogryzko V, Kao HY, et al. A viral mechanism for inhibition of p300 and PCAF acetyltransferase activity. *Cell* 1999;96:393–403.
49. Challberg MD, Desiderio SV, Kelly TJ Jr. Adenovirus DNA replication in vitro: Characterization of a protein covalently linked to nascent DNA strands. *Proc Natl Acad Sci U S A* 1980;77:5105–5109.
50. Challberg MD, Kelly TJ Jr. Adenovirus DNA replication in vitro. *Proc Natl Acad Sci U S A* 1979;76:655–659.
51. Challberg MD, Kelly TJ Jr. Processing of the adenovirus terminal protein. *J Virol* 1981;38:272–277.
52. Challberg MD, Ostrove JM, Kelly TJ Jr. Initiation of adenovirus DNA replication: Detection of covalent complexes between nucleotide and the 80-kilodalton terminal protein. *J Virol* 1982;41:265–270.
53. Chang LS, Shenk T. The adenovirus DNA-binding protein stimulates the rate of transcription directed by adenovirus and adeno-associated virus promoters. *J Virol* 1990;64:2103–2109.
54. Chardonnet Y, Dales S. Early events in the interaction of adenoviruses with HeLa cells. I. Penetration of type 5 and intracellular release of the DNA genome. *Virology* 1970;40:462–477.
55. Chardonnet Y, Dales S. Early events in the interaction of adenoviruses with HeLa cells. II. Comparative observations on the penetration of types 1, 5, 7 and 12. *Virology* 1970;40:478–485.
56. Chatterjee PK, Vayda ME, Flint SJ. Identification of proteins and protein domains that contact DNA within adenovirus nucleoprotein cores by ultraviolet light crosslinking of oligonucleotides 32P-labelled in vivo. *J Mol Biol* 1986;188:23–37.
57. Chee-Sheung CC, Ginsberg HS. Characterization of a temperature-sensitive fiber mutant of type 5 adenovirus and effect of the mutation on virion assembly. *J Virol* 1982;42:932–950.
58. Chen H, Vinnakota R, Flint SJ. Intragenic activating and repressing elements control transcription from the adenovirus IVa2 initiator. *Mol Cell Biol* 1994;14:676–685.
59. Chen M, Mermod N, Horwitz MS. Protein-protein interactions between adenovirus DNA polymerase and nuclear factor I mediate formation of the DNA replication preinitiation complex. *J Biol Chem* 1990;265:18634–18642.
60. Chen P, Tian J, Kovesdi I, Bruder JT. Interaction of the adenovirus 14.7-kDa protein with FLICE inhibits Fas ligand-induced apoptosis. *J Biol Chem* 1998;273:5815–5820.
61. Chen PH, Ornelles DA, Shenk T. The adenovirus L3 23-kilodalton proteinase cleaves the amino-terminal head domain from cytokeratin 18 and disrupts the cytokeratin network of HeLa cells. *J Virol* 1993;67:3507–3514.
62. Chiocca S, Kurzbauer R, Schaffner G, et al. The complete DNA sequence and genomic organization of the avian adenovirus CELO. *J Virol* 1996;70:2939–2949.
63. Chiu CY, Mathias P, Nemerow GR, Stewart PL. Structure of adenovirus complexed with its internalization receptor, alphavbeta5 integrin. *J Virol* 1999;73:6759–6768.
64. Chow LT, Broker TR, Lewis JB. Complex splicing patterns of RNAs from the early regions of adenovirus 2. *J Mol Biol* 1979;134:265–303.
65. Chow LT, Gelinas RE, Broker TR, Roberts RJ. An amazing sequence arrangement at the 5′ ends of adenovirus 2 messenger RNA. *Cell* 1977;12:1–8.
66. Chow LT, Roberts JM, Lewis JB, Broker TR. A map of cytoplasmic RNA transcripts from lytic adenovirus type 2, determined by electron microscopy of RNA:DNA hybrids. *Cell* 1977;11:819–836.
67. Chroboczek J, Bieber F, Jacrot B. The sequence of the genome of adenovirus type 5 and its comparison with the genome of adenovirus type 2. *Virology* 1992;186:280–285.
68. Cleat PH, Hay RT. Co-operative interactions between NFI and the adenovirus DNA binding protein at the adenovirus origin of replication. *EMBO J* 1989;8:1841–1848.
69. Colby WW, Shenk T. Adenovirus type 5 virions can be assembled in vivo in the absence of detectable polypeptide IX. *J Virol* 1981;39:977–980.
70. Cook JL, Hibbs JB Jr, Lewis AM Jr. DNA virus-transformed hamster cell-host effector cell interactions: Level of resistance to cytolysis correlated with tumorigenicity. *Int J Cancer* 1982;30:795–803.
71. Cook JL, Lewis AM Jr. Host response to adenovirus 2-transformed hamster embryo cells. *Cancer Res* 1979;39:1455–1461.
72. Cook JL, May DL, Lewis AM Jr, Walker TA. Adenovirus E1A gene induction of susceptibility to lysis by natural killer cells and activated macrophages in infected rodent cells. *J Virol* 1987;61:3510–3520.
73. Cook JL, Walker TA, Lewis AM Jr, et al. Expression of the adenovirus E1A oncogene during cell transformation is sufficient to induce susceptibility to lysis by host inflammatory cells. *Proc Natl Acad Sci U S A* 1986;83:6965–6969.
74. Corden J, Engelking HM, Pearson GD. Chromatin-like organization of the adenovirus chromosome. *Proc Natl Acad Sci U S A* 1976;73:401–404.
75. Crawford-Miksza L, Schnurr DP. Analysis of 15 adenovirus hexon proteins reveals the location and structure of seven hypervariable regions containing serotype-specific residues. *J Virol* 1996;70:1836–1844.
76. Dales S, Chardonnet Y. Early events in the interaction of adenoviruses with HeLa cells. IV. Association with microtubules and the nuclear pore complex during vectorial movement of the inoculum. *Virology* 1973;56:465–483.
77. Davies MV, Furtado M, Hershey JW, et al. Complementation of adenovirus-associated RNA I gene deletion by expression of a mutant eukaryotic translation initiation factor. *Proc Natl Acad Sci U S A* 1989;86:9163–9167.
78. de Stanchina E, McCurrach ME, Zindy F, et al. E1A signaling to p53 involves the p19(ARF) tumor suppressor. *Genes Dev* 1998;12:2434–2442.
79. Debbas M, White E. Wild-type p53 mediates apoptosis by E1A, which is inhibited by E1B. *Genes Dev* 1993;7:546–554.
80. Defer C, Belin MT, Caillet-Boudin ML, Boulanger P. Human adenovirus-host cell interactions: Comparative study with members of subgroups B and C. *J Virol* 1990;64:3661–3673.

81. Dekker J, Kanellopoulos PN, Loonstra AK, et al. Multimerization of the adenovirus DNA-binding protein is the driving force for ATP-independent DNA unwinding during strand displacement synthesis. *EMBO J* 1997;16:1455–1463.
82. Dery CV, Toth M, Brown M, et al. The structure of adenovirus chromatin in infected cells. *J Gen Virol* 1985;66:2671–2684.
83. Desiderio SV, Kelly TJ Jr. Structure of the linkage between adenovirus DNA and the 55,000 molecular weight terminal protein. *J Mol Biol* 1981;145:319–337.
84. Devaux C, Caillet-Boudin ML, Jacrot B, Boulanger P. Crystallization, enzymatic cleavage, and the polarity of the adenovirus type 2 fiber. *Virology* 1987;161:121–128.
85. Devaux C, Timmins PA, Berthet-Colominas C. Structural studies of adenovirus type 2 by neutron and X-ray scattering. *J Mol Biol* 1983;167:119–132.
86. D'Halluin JC, Milleville M, Boulanger PA, Martin GR. Temperature-sensitive mutant of adenovirus type 2 blocked in virion assembly: Accumulation of light intermediate particles. *J Virol* 1978;26:344–356.
87. D'Halluin JC, Milleville M, Martin GR, Boulanger P. Morphogenesis of human adenovirus type 2 studied with fiber- and fiber and penton base-defective temperature-sensitive mutants. *J Virol* 1980;33:88–99.
88. Dimitrov T, Krajcsi P, Hermiston TW, et al. Adenovirus E3-10.4K/14.5K protein complex inhibits tumor necrosis factor-induced translocation of cytosolic phospholipase A2 to membranes. *J Virol* 1997;71:2830–2837.
89. Ding J, McGrath WJ, Sweet RM, Mangel WF. Crystal structure of the human adenovirus proteinase with its 11 amino acid cofactor. *EMBO J* 1996;15:1778–1783.
90. Dingle JH, Langmuir AD. Epidemiology of acute, respiratory disease in military recruits. *Am Rev Respir Dis* 1968;97[Suppl]:1–65.
91. Dobbelstein M, Roth J, Kimberly WT, et al. Nuclear export of the E1B 55-kDa and E4 34-kDa adenoviral oncoproteins mediated by a rev-like signal sequence. *EMBO J* 1997;16:4276–4284.
92. Dobner T, Horikoshi N, Rubenwolf S, Shenk T. Blockage by adenovirus E4orf6 of transcriptional activation by the p53 tumor suppressor. *Science* 1996;272:1470–1473.
93. Donehower LA, Harvey M, Slagle BL, et al. Mice deficient for p53 are developmentally normal but susceptible to spontaneous tumours. *Nature* 1992;356:215–221.
94. Doucas V, Ishov AM, Romo A, et al. Adenovirus replication is coupled with the dynamic properties of the PML nuclear structure. *Genes Dev* 1996;10:196–207.
95. Duerksen-Hughes PJ, Hermiston TW, Wold WS, Gooding LR. The amino-terminal portion of CD1 of the adenovirus E1A proteins is required to induce susceptibility to tumor necrosis factor cytolysis in adenovirus-infected mouse cells. *J Virol* 1991;65:1236–1244.
96. Dyson N, Guida P, McCall C, Harlow E. Adenovirus E1A makes two distinct contacts with the retinoblastoma protein. *J Virol* 1992;66:4606–4611.
97. Edvardsson B, Ustacelebi S, Williams J, Philipson L. Assembly intermediates among adenovirus type 5 temperature-sensitive mutants. *J Virol* 1978;25:641–651.
98. Elsing A, Burgert HG. The adenovirus E3/10.4K-14.5K proteins down-modulate the apoptosis receptor Fas/Apo-1 by inducing its internalization. *Proc Natl Acad Sci U S A* 1998;95:10072–10077.
99. Enders JF, Bell JA, Dingle JH, et al. "Adenoviruses": Group name proposed for new respiratory-tract viruses. *Science* 1956;124:119–120.
100. Engel DA, Hardy S, Shenk T. cAMP acts in synergy with E1A protein to activate transcription of the adenovirus early genes E4 and E1A. *Genes Dev* 1988;2:1517–1528.
101. Engel DA, Muller U, Gedrich RW, et al. Induction of c-fos mRNA and AP-1 DNA-binding activity by cAMP in cooperation with either the adenovirus 243- or the adenovirus 289-amino acid E1A protein. *Proc Natl Acad Sci U S A* 1991;88:3957–3961.
102. Enomoto T, Lichy JH, Ikeda JE, Hurwitz J. Adenovirus DNA replication in vitro: Purification of the terminal protein in a functional form. *Proc Natl Acad Sci U S A* 1981;78:6779–6783.
103. Epstein LH, Young CS. Adenovirus homologous recombination does not require expression of the immediate-early E1A gene. *J Virol* 1991;65:4475–4479.
104. Evans R, Weber J, Ziff E, Darnell JE. Premature termination during adenovirus transcription. *Nature* 1979;278:367–370.
105. Evans RM, Fraser N, Ziff E, et al. The initiation sites for RNA transcription in Ad2 DNA. *Cell* 1977;12:733–739.
106. Everitt E, Lutter L, Philipson L. Structural proteins of adenoviruses. XII. Location and neighbor relationship among proteins of adenovirion type 2 as revealed by enzymatic iodination, immunoprecipitation and chemical cross-linking. *Virology* 1975;67:197–208.
107. Everitt E, Sundquist B, Pettersson U, Philipson L. Structural proteins of adenoviruses. X. Isolation and topography of low molecular weight antigens from the virion of adenovirus type 2. *Virology* 1973;52:130–147.
108. Falck-Pedersen E, Logan J, Shenk T, Darnell JE Jr. Transcription termination within the E1A gene of adenovirus induced by insertion of the mouse beta-major globin terminator element. *Cell* 1985;40:897–905.
109. Field J, Gronostajski RM, Hurwitz J. Properties of the adenovirus DNA polymerase. *J Biol Chem* 1984;259:9487–9495.
110. FitzGerald DJ, Padmanabhan R, Pastan I, Willingham MC. Adenovirus-induced release of epidermal growth factor and pseudomonas toxin into the cytosol of KB cells during receptor-mediated endocytosis. *Cell* 1983;32:607–617.
110a. Flint SJ. Structure and genome organization of adenoviruses. In: Tooze J, ed. *DNA tumor viruses: Molecular biology of DNA tumor viruses.* Cold Spring Harbor, NY: Cold Spring Harbor Laboratory. 1981:408–409.
111. Flint SJ, Berget SM, Sharp PA. Characterization of single-stranded viral DNA sequences present during replication of adenovirus types 2 and 5. *Cell* 1976;9:559–571.
112. Fowlkes DM, Shenk T. Transcriptional control regions of the adenovirus VAI RNA gene. *Cell* 1980;22:405–413.
113. Fraser NW, Nevins JR, Ziff E, Darnell JE Jr. The major late adenovirus type-2 transcription unit: Termination is downstream from the last poly(A) site. *J Mol Biol* 1979;129:643–656.
114. Fraser NW, Sehgal PB, Darnell JE Jr. Multiple discrete sites for premature RNA chain termination late in adenovirus-2 infection: Enhancement by 5,6-dichloro-1-beta-D-ribofuranosylbenzimidazole. *Proc Natl Acad Sci U S A* 1979;76:2571–2575.
115. Fredman JN, Engler JA. Adenovirus precursor to terminal protein interacts with the nuclear matrix in vivo and in vitro. *J Virol* 1993;67:3384–3395.
116. Furcinitti PS, van Oostrum J, Burnett RM. Adenovirus polypeptide IX revealed as capsid cement by difference images from electron microscopy and crystallography. *EMBO J* 1989;8:3563–3570.
117. Gabler S, Schutt H, Groitl P, et al. E1B 55-kilodalton-associated protein: A cellular protein with RNA-binding activity implicated in nucleocytoplasmic transport of adenovirus and cellular mRNAs. *J Virol* 1998;72:7960–7971.
118. Gallimore PH. Tumour production in immunosuppressed rats with cells transformed in vitro by adenovirus type 2. *J Gen Virol* 1972;16:99–102.
119. Garon CF, Berry KW, Rose JA. A unique form of terminal redundancy in adenovirus DNA molecules. *Proc Natl Acad Sci U S A* 1972;69:2391–2395.
120. Gaynor RB, Hillman D, Berk AJ. Adenovirus early region 1A protein activates transcription of a nonviral gene introduced into mammalian cells by infection or transfection. *Proc Natl Acad Sci U S A* 1984;81:1193–1197.
121. Geisberg JV, Chen JL, Ricciardi RP. Subregions of the adenovirus E1A transactivation domain target multiple components of the TFIID complex. *Mol Cell Biol* 1995;15:6283–6290.
122. Ginsberg HS, Gold E, Jordan WS Jr. Relation of the new respiratory agents to acute respiratory diseases. *Am J Publ Health* 1955;45:915–922.
123. Ginsberg HS, Lundholm-Beauchamp U, Prince G. Adenovirus as a model of disease. In: Russell W, Almond J, eds. *Molecular basis of virus disease.* New York: Cambridge University Press, 1987:245–258.
124. Ginsberg HS, Moldawer LL, Sehgal PB, et al. A mouse model for investigating the molecular pathogenesis of adenovirus pneumonia. *Proc Natl Acad Sci U S A* 1991;88:1651–1655.
125. Ginsberg HS, Pereira HG, Valentine RC, Wilcox WC. A proposed terminology for the adenovirus antigens and virion morphological subunits. *Virology* 1966;28:782–783.
126. Ginsberg HS, Prince G. Gene functions directing adenovirus pathogenesis. In: Notkins A, Oldstone M, eds. *Concepts in viral pathogenesis III.* New York: Springer-Verlag, 1989:275–281.
127. Ginsberg HS, Young CSH. The genetics of adenoviruses. In: Fraenkel-Conrat H, Wagner RR, eds. *Comprehensive virology.* Vol. 9. New York: Plenum Press, 1977.
128. Goldman MJ, Wilson JM. Expression of alpha v beta 5 integrin is nec-

essary for efficient adenovirus-mediated gene transfer in the human airway. *J Virol* 1995;69:5951–5958.

129. Gooding LR, Elmore LW, Tollefson AE, et al. A 14,700 MW protein from the E3 region of adenovirus inhibits cytolysis by tumor necrosis factor. *Cell* 1988;53:341–346.
130. Gooding LR, Ranheim TS, Tollefson AE, et al. The 10,400- and 14,500-dalton proteins encoded by region E3 of adenovirus function together to protect many but not all mouse cell lines against lysis by tumor necrosis factor. *J Virol* 1991;65:4114–4123.
131. Goodrum FD, Ornelles DA. The early region 1B 55-kilodalton oncoprotein of adenovirus relieves growth restrictions imposed on viral replication by the cell cycle. *J Virol* 1997;71:548–561.
132. Goodrum FD, Ornelles DA. p53 Status does not determine outcome of E1B 55-kilodalton mutant adenovirus lytic infection. *J Virol* 1998; 72:9479–9490.
133. Goodrum FD, Ornelles DA. Roles for the E4 orf6, orf3, and E1B 55-kilodalton proteins in cell cycle-independent adenovirus replication. *J Virol* 1999;73:7474–7488.
134. Goodrum FD, Shenk T, Ornelles D. Adenovirus early region 4 34-kilodalton protein directs the nuclear localization of the early region 1B 55-kilodalton protein in primate cells. *J Virol* 1996;70:6323–6335.
135. Grable M, Hearing P. cis And trans requirements for the selective packaging of adenovirus type 5 DNA. *J Virol* 1992;66:723–731.
136. Graham FL, Smiley J, Russell WC, Nairn R. Characteristics of a human cell line transformed by DNA from human adenovirus type 5. *J Gen Virol* 1977;36:59–74.
137. Grand RJ, Lecane PS, Roberts S, et al. Overexpression of wild-type p53 and c-Myc in human fetal cells transformed with adenovirus early region 1. *Virology* 1993;193:579–591.
138. Greber UF, Suomalainen M, Stidwill RP, et al. The role of the nuclear pore complex in adenovirus DNA entry. *EMBO J* 1997;16:5998–6007.
139. Greber UF, Webster P, Weber J, Helenius A. The role of the adenovirus protease on virus entry into cells. *EMBO J* 1996;15:1766–1777.
140. Greber UF, Willetts M, Webster P, Helenius A. Stepwise dismantling of adenovirus 2 during entry into cells. *Cell* 1993;75:477–486.
141. Green M. Biochemical studies on adenovirus multiplication. I. Kinetics of nucleic acid and protein synthesis in suspension cultures. *Virology* 1961;13:169–176.
142. Green M. Transcriptional activation of cloned human β-globin genes by viral immediate-early gene products. *Cell* 1983;35:137–148.
143. Green M, Pina M. Biochemical studies on adenovirus multiplication. IV. Isolation, purification, and chemical analysis of adenovirus. *Virology* 1963;20:199–207.
144. Green M, Wold WSM, Brackmann KH, et al. Human adenovirus transforming genes: Group relationships, integration, expression in transformed cells and analysis of human cancers and tonsils. In: Essex M, Todaro G, zurHausen H, eds. *Seventh Cold Spring Harbor Conference on Cell Proliferation Viruses in Naturally Occurring Tumors.* Cold Spring Harbor, NY: Cold Spring Harbor Laboratory, 1980: 373–397.
145. Green NM, Wrigley NG, Russel WC, et al. Evidence for a repeating β-sheet structure in the adenovirus fibre. *EMBO J* 1983;8:1357–1365.
146. Gruber WC, Russell DJ, Tibbetts C. Fiber gene and genomic origin of human adenovirus type 4. *Virology* 1993;196:603–611.
147. Guilfoyle R, Weinmann R. Control region for adenovirus VA RNA transcription. *Proc Natl Acad Sci U S A* 1981;78:3378–3382.
148. Gustin KE, Imperiale MJ. Encapsidation of viral DNA requires the adenovirus L1 52/55-kilodalton protein. *J Virol* 1998;72:7860–7870.
149. Gustin KE, Lutz P, Imperiale MJ. Interaction of the adenovirus L1 52/55-kilodalton protein with the IVa2 gene product during infection. *J Virol* 1996;70:6463–6470.
150. Gutch MJ, Reich NC. Repression of the interferon signal transduction pathway by the adenovirus E1A oncogene. *Proc Natl Acad Sci U S A* 1991;88:7913–7917.
151. Hagmeyer BM, Konig H, Herr I, et al. Adenovirus E1A negatively and positively modulates transcription of AP-1 dependent genes by dimer-specific regulation of the DNA binding and transactivation activities of Jun. *EMBO J* 1993;12:3559–3572.
152. Hahn W, Counter C, Lundberg A, et al. Creation of human tumor cells with defined genetic elements. *Nature* 1999;400:464–468.
153. Halbert DN, Cutt JR, Shenk T. Adenovirus early region 4 encodes functions required for efficient DNA replication, late gene expression, and host cell shutoff. *J Virol* 1985;56:250–257.
154. Hamamori Y, Sartorelli V, Ogryzko V, et al. Regulation of histone acetyltransferases p300 and PCAF by the bHLH protein twist and adenoviral oncoprotein E1A. *Cell* 1999;96:405–413.
155. Hammarskjold ML, Winberg G. Encapsidation of adenovirus 16 DNA is directed by a small DNA sequence at the left end of the genome. *Cell* 1980;20:787–795.
156. Hardy S, Engel DA, Shenk T. An adenovirus early region 4 gene product is required for induction of the infection-specific form of cellular E2F activity. *Genes Dev* 1989;3:1062–1074.
157. Hardy S, Shenk T. Adenoviral control regions activated by E1A and the cAMP response element bind to the same factor. *Proc Natl Acad Sci U S A* 1988;85:4171–4175.
158. Harlow E, Whyte P, Franza BR Jr, Schley C. Association of adenovirus early-region 1A proteins with cellular polypeptides. *Mol Cell Biol* 1986; 6:1579–1589.
159. Harris MP, Hay RT. DNA sequences required for the initiation of adenovirus type 4 DNA replication in vitro. *J Mol Biol* 1988;201:57–67.
160. Hasson TB, Ornelles DA, Shenk T. Adenovirus L1 52- and 55-kilodalton proteins are present within assembling virions and colocalize with nuclear structures distinct from replication centers. *J Virol* 1992; 66:6133–6142.
161. Hasson TB, Soloway PD, Ornelles DA, et al. Adenovirus L1 52- and 55-kilodalton proteins are required for assembly of virions. *J Virol* 1989;63:3612–3621.
162. Hatfield L, Hearing P. The NFIII/OCT-1 binding site stimulates adenovirus DNA replication in vivo and is functionally redundant with adjacent sequences. *J Virol* 1993;67:3931–3939.
163. Hay RT. The origin of adenovirus DNA replication: Minimal DNA sequence requirement in vivo. *EMBO J* 1985;4:421–426.
164. Hayes BW, Telling GC, Myat MM, et al. The adenovirus L4 100-kilodalton protein is necessary for efficient translation of viral late mRNA species. *J Virol* 1990;64:2732–2742.
165. Hearing P, Samulski RJ, Wishart WL, Shenk T. Identification of a repeated sequence element required for efficient encapsidation of the adenovirus type 5 chromosome. *J Virol* 1987;61:2555–2558.
166. Hearing P, Shenk T. The adenovirus type 5 E1A transcriptional control region contains a duplicated enhancer element. *Cell* 1983;33:695–703.
167. Hearing P, Shenk T. Sequence-independent autoregulation of the adenovirus type 5 E1A transcription unit. *Mol Cell Biol* 1985;5: 3214–3221.
168. Hearing P, Shenk T. The adenovirus type 5 E1A enhancer contains two functionally distinct domains: One is specific for E1A and the other modulates all early units in cis. *Cell* 1986;45:229–236.
169. Hermann CH, Su L-K, Harlow E. Adenovirus E1A is associated with a serine/threonine protein kinase. *J Virol* 1991;65
170. Hierholzer JC, Wigand R, Anderson LJ, et al. Adenoviruses from patients with AIDS: A plethora of serotypes and a description of five new serotypes of subgenus D (types 43-47). *J Infect Dis* 1988;158: 804–813.
171. Higashino F, Pipas JM, Shenk T. Adenovirus E4orf6 oncoprotein modulates the function of the p53-related protein, p73. *Proc Natl Acad Sci U S A* 1998;95:15683–15687.
172. Hilleman MR, Werner JH. Recovery of new agents from patients with acute respiratory illness. *Proc Soc Exp Biol Med* 1954;85:183–188.
173. Hong JS, Engler JA. Domains required for assembly of adenovirus type 2 fiber trimers. *J Virol* 1996;70:7071–7078.
174. Hong SS, Karayan L, Tournier J, et al. Adenovirus type 5 fiber knob binds to MHC class I alpha2 domain at the surface of human epithelial and B lymphoblastoid cells. *EMBO J* 1997;16:2294–2306.
175. Horikoshi N, Maguire K, Kralli A, et al. Direct interaction between adenovirus E1A protein and the TATA box binding transcription factor IID. *Proc Natl Acad Sci U S A* 1991;88:5124–5128.
176. Horikoshi N, Usheva A, Chen J, et al. Two domains of p53 interact with the TATA-binding protein, and the adenovirus 13S E1A protein disrupts the association, relieving p53-mediated transcriptional repression. *Mol Cell Biol* 1995;15:227–234.
177. Horne RW, Bonner S, Waterson AP, Wildy P. The icosahedral form of an adenovirus. *J Mol Biol* 1959;1:84–86.
178. Horridge JJ, Leppard KN. RNA-binding activity of the E1B 55-kilodalton protein from human adenovirus type 5. *J Virol* 1998;72:9374–9379.
179. Horwitz MS, Maizel JV Jr, Scharff MD. Molecular weight of adenovirus type 2 hexon polypeptide. *J Virol* 1970;6:569–571.
180. Horwitz MS, Scharff MD, Maizel JV Jr. Synthesis and assembly of adenovirus 2. I. Polypeptide synthesis, assembly of capsomeres, and morphogenesis of the virion. *Virology* 1969;39:682–694.

181. Hosakawa K, Sung MT. Isolation and characterization of an extremely basic protein from adenovirus type 5. *J Virol* 1976;17:924–934.
182. Howe JA, Bayley ST. Effects of Ad5 E1A mutant viruses on the cell cycle in relation to the binding of cellular proteins including the retinoblastoma protein and cyclin A. *Virology* 1992;186:15–24.
183. Howe JA, Mymryk JS, Egan C, et al. Retinoblastoma growth suppressor and a 300-kDa protein appear to regulate cellular DNA synthesis. *Proc Natl Acad Sci U S A* 1990;87:5883–5887.
184. Hu QJ, Dyson N, Harlow E. The regions of the retinoblastoma protein needed for binding to adenovirus E1A or SV40 large T antigen are common sites for mutations. *EMBO J* 1990;9:1147–1155.
185. Huang JT, Schneider RJ. Adenovirus inhibition of cellular protein synthesis is prevented by the drug 2-aminopurine. *Proc Natl Acad Sci U S A* 1990;87:7115–7119.
186. Huang JT, Schneider RJ. Adenovirus inhibition of cellular protein synthesis involves inactivation of cap-binding protein. *Cell* 1991;65: 271–280.
187. Huang M-M, Hearing P. The adenovirus early region 4 open reading frame 6/7 protein regulates the DNA binding activity of the cellular transcription factor, E2F, through a direct complex. *Genes Dev* 1989; 3:1699–1710.
188. Huebner RJ, Rowe WP, Ward TG, et al. Adenoidal-pharyngeal conjunctival agents. *N Engl J Med* 1954;251:1077–1086.
189. Ikeda MA, Nevins JR. Identification of distinct roles for separate E1A domains in disruption of E2F complexes. *Mol Cell Biol* 1993;13: 7029–7035.
190. Inostroza JA, Mermelstein FH, Ha I, et al. Dr1, a TATA-binding protein-associated phosphoprotein and inhibitor of class II gene transcription. *Cell* 1992;70:477–489.
191. Ishibashi M, Maizel JV Jr. The polypeptides of adenovirus. VI. Early and late glycopolypeptides. *Virology* 1974;58:345–361.
192. Ito M, Yuan CX, Malik S, et al. Identity between TRAP and SMCC complexes indicates novel pathways for the function of nuclear receptors and diverse mammalian activators. *Mol Cell* 1999;3:361–370.
193. Javier R, Raska K Jr, Macdonald GJ, Shenk T. Human adenovirus type 9-induced rat mammary tumors. *J Virol* 1991;65:3192–3202.
194. Javier R, Raska K Jr, Shenk T. Requirement for the adenovirus type 9 E4 region in production of mammary tumors. *Science* 1992;257: 1267–1271.
195. Javier RT. Adenovirus type 9 E4 open reading frame 1 encodes a transforming protein required for the production of mammary tumors in rats. *J Virol* 1994;68:3917–3924.
196. Jawetz E. The story of shipyard eye. *Br Med J* 1959;1:873–878.
197. Jones KA, Kadonaga JT, Rosenfeld PJ, et al. A cellular DNA-binding protein that activates eukaryotic transcription and DNA replication. *Cell* 1987;48:79–89.
198. Jones N, Shenk T. An adenovirus type 5 early gene function regulates expression of other early viral genes. *Proc Natl Acad Sci U S A* 1979; 76:3665–3669.
199. Kaelin WG Jr, Ewen ME, Livingston DM. Definition of the minimal simian virus 40 large T antigen- and adenovirus E1A-binding domain in the retinoblastoma gene product. *Mol Cell Biol* 1990;10:3761–3769.
200. Kao CC, Yew PR, Berk AJ. Domains required for in vitro association between the cellular p53 and the adenovirus 2 E1B 55K proteins. *Virology* 1990;179:806–814.
201. Kasai Y, Chen H, Flint SJ. Anatomy of an unusual RNA polymerase II promoter containing a downstream TATA element. *Mol Cell Biol* 1992;12:2884–2897.
202. Kast WM, Offringa R, Peters PJ, et al. Eradication of adenovirus E1-induced tumors by E1A-specific cytotoxic T lymphocytes. *Cell* 1989; 59:603–614.
203. Katze MG, DeCorato D, Safer B, et al. Adenovirus VAI RNA complexes with the 68 000 Mr protein kinase to regulate its autophosphorylation and activity. *EMBO J* 1987;6:689–697.
204. Kenny MK, Hurwitz J. Initiation of adenovirus DNA replication. II. Structural requirements using synthetic oligonucleotide adenovirus templates. *J Biol Chem* 1988;263:9809–9817.
205. Kidd AH, Chroboczek J, Cusack S, Ruigrok RW. Adenovirus type 40 virions contain two distinct fibers. *Virology* 1993;192:73–84.
206. King AJ, Teertstra WR, van der Vliet PC. Dissociation of the protein primer and DNA polymerase after initiation of adenovirus DNA replication. *J Biol Chem* 1997;272:24617–24623.
207. King AJ, van der Vliet PC. A precursor terminal protein-trinucleotide intermediate during initiation of adenovirus DNA replication: Regeneration of molecular ends in vitro by a jumping back mechanism. *EMBO J* 1994;13:5786–5792.
208. Kitajewski J, Schneider RJ, Safer B, et al. Adenovirus VAI RNA antagonizes the antiviral action of interferon by preventing activation of the interferon-induced eIF-2 alpha kinase. *Cell* 1986;45:195–200.
209. Kitchingman GR. Sequence of the DNA-binding protein of a human subgroup E adenovirus (type 4): Comparisons with subgroup A (type 12), subgroup B (type 7), and subgroup C (type 5). *Virology* 1985; 146:90–101.
210. Kleinberger T, Shenk T. A protein kinase is present in a complex with adenovirus E1A proteins. *Proc Natl Acad Sci U S A* 1991;88:11143–11147.
211. Kleinberger T, Shenk T. Adenovirus E4orf4 protein binds to protein phosphatase 2A, and the complex down regulates E1A-enhanced junB transcription. *J Virol* 1993;67:7556–7560.
212. Klessig DF, Brough DE, Cleghon V. Introduction, stable integration, and controlled expression of a chimeric adenovirus gene whose product is toxic to the recipient human cell. *Mol Cell Biol* 1984;4: 1354–1362.
213. Kostura M, Mathews MB. Purification and activation of the double-stranded RNA-dependent eIF-2 kinase DAI. *Mol Cell Biol* 1989;9: 1576–1586.
214. Kovesdi I, Reichel R, Nevins JR. Identification of a cellular transcription factor involved in E1A trans-activation. *Cell* 1986;45:219–228.
215. Kovesdi I, Reichel R, Nevins JR. Role of an adenovirus E2 promoter binding factor in E1A-mediated coordinate gene control. *Proc Natl Acad Sci U S A* 1987;84:2180–2184.
216. Krajcsi P, Dimitrov T, Hermiston TW, et al. The adenovirus E3-14.7K protein and the E3-10.4K/14.K complex of proteins, which independently inhibit tumor necrosis factor (TNF)-induced apoptosis, also independently inhibit TNF-induced release of arachidonic acid. *J Virol* 1996;70:4904–4913.
217. Kralli A, Ge R, Graeven U, et al. Negative regulation of the major histocompatibility complex class I enhancer in adenovirus type 12-transformed cells via a retinoic acid response element. *J Virol* 1992;66: 6979–6988.
218. Kraus VB, Inostroza JA, Yeung K, et al. Interaction of the Dr1 inhibitory factor with the TATA binding protein is disrupted by adenovirus E1A. *Proc Natl Acad Sci U S A* 1994;91:6279–6282.
219. Kraus VB, Moran E, Nevins JR. Promoter-specific trans-activation by the adenovirus E1A12S product involves separate E1A domains. *Mol Cell Biol* 1992;12:4391–4399.
220. Kvist S, Ostberg L, Persson H, et al. Molecular association between transplantation antigens and cell surface antigen in adenovirus-transformed cell line. *Proc Natl Acad Sci U S A* 1978;75:5674–5678.
221. Langer SJ, Schaack J. 293 Cell lines that inducibly express high levels of adenovirus type 5 precursor terminal protein. *Virology* 1996;221: 172–179.
222. Lavoie JN, Nguyen M, Marcellus RC, et al. E4orf4, a novel adenovirus death factor that induces p53-independent apoptosis by a pathway that is not inhibited by zVAD-fmk. *J Cell Biol* 1998;140:637–645.
223. Lechner RL, Kelly TJ Jr. The structure of replicating adenovirus 2 DNA molecules. *Cell* 1977;12:1007–1020.
224. Lee JS, Galvin KM, See RH, et al. Relief of YY1 transcriptional repression by adenovirus E1A is mediated by E1A-associated protein p300 [published erratum appears in *Genes Dev* 1995;9:1948–1949]. *Genes Dev* 1995;9:1188–1198.
225. Lee SS, Weiss RS, Javier RT. Binding of human virus oncoproteins to hDlg/SAP97, a mammalian homolog of the Drosophila discs large tumor suppressor protein. *Proc Natl Acad Sci U S A* 1997;94:6670–6675.
226. Lee WS, Kao CC, Bryant GO, et al. Adenovirus E1A activation domain binds the basic repeat in the TATA box transcription factor. *Cell* 1991;67:365–376.
227. Leong K, Lee W, Berk AJ. High-level transcription from the adenovirus major late promoter requires downstream binding sites for late-phase-specific factors. *J Virol* 1990;64:51–60.
228. Leppard KN, Shenk T. The adenovirus E1B 55 kd protein influences mRNA transport via an intranuclear effect on RNA metabolism. *EMBO J* 1989;8:2329–2336.
229. Lewis BA, Tullis G, Seto E, et al. Adenovirus E1A proteins interact with the cellular YY1 transcription factor. *J Virol* 1995;69:1628–1636.
230. Li E, Stupack D, Bokoch GM, Nemerow GR. Adenovirus endocytosis requires actin cytoskeleton reorganization mediated by Rho family GTPases. *J Virol* 1998;72:8806–8812.

231. Li Y, Kang J, Friedman J, et al. Identification of a cell protein (FIP-3) as a modulator of NF-kappaB activity and as a target of an adenovirus inhibitor of tumor necrosis factor alpha-induced apoptosis. *Proc Natl Acad Sci U S A* 1999;96:1042–1047.
232. Li Y, Kang J, Horwitz MS. Interaction of an adenovirus 14.7-kilodalton protein inhibitor of tumor necrosis factor alpha cytolysis with a new member of the GTPase superfamily of signal transducers. *J Virol* 1997;71:1576–1582.
233. Li Y, Kang J, Horwitz MS. Interaction of an adenovirus E3 14.7-kilodalton protein with a novel tumor necrosis factor alpha-inducible cellular protein containing leucine zipper domains. *Mol Cell Biol* 1998; 18:1601–1610.
234. Liao HJ, Kobayashi R, Mathews MB. Activities of adenovirus-associated RNAs: Purification and characterization of RNA binding proteins. *Proc Natl Acad Sci U S A* 1998;95:8514–8519.
235. Lichy JH, Field J, Horwitz MS, Hurwitz J. Separation of the adenovirus terminal protein precursor from its associated DNA polymerase: Role of both proteins in the initiation of adenovirus DNA replication. *Proc Natl Acad Sci U S A* 1982;79:5225–5229.
236. Lichy JH, Horwitz MS, Hurwitz J. Formation of a covalent complex between the 80,000-dalton adenovirus terminal protein and 5′-dCMP in vitro. *Proc Natl Acad Sci U S A* 1981;78:2678–2682.
237. Liebowitz J, Horwitz MS. Synthesis and assembly of adenovirus polypeptides. III. Reversible inhibition of hexon assembly in adenovirus type 5 temperature-sensitive mutants. *Virology* 1975;66:10–24.
238. Lill NL, Grossman SR, Ginsberg D, et al. Binding and modulation of p53 by p300/CBP coactivators. *Nature* 1997;387:823–827.
239. Lillie JW, Green MR. Transcription activation by the adenovirus E1a protein. *Nature* 1989;338:39–44.
240. Lillie JW, Loewenstein PM, Green MR, Green M. Functional domains of adenovirus type 5 E1a proteins. *Cell* 1987;50:1091–1100.
241. Lindenbaum JO, Field J, Hurwitz J. The adenovirus DNA binding protein and adenovirus DNA polymerase interact to catalyze elongation of primed DNA templates. *J Biol Chem* 1986;261:10218–10227.
242. Lipinski KS, Esche H, Brockmann D. Amino acids 1-29 of the adenovirus serotypes 12 and 2 E1A proteins interact with rap30 (TF(II)F) and TBP in vitro. *Virus Res* 1998;54:99–106.
243. Liu F, Green MR. A specific member of the ATF transcription factor family can mediate transcription activation by the adenovirus E1A protein. *Cell* 1990;61:1217–1224.
244. Liu X, Miller CW, Koeffler PH, Berk AJ. The p53 activation domain binds the TATA box-binding polypeptide in Holo-TFIID, and a neighboring p53 domain inhibits transcription. *Mol Cell Biol* 1993;13: 3291–3300.
245. Logan J, Shenk T. Adenovirus tripartite leader sequence enhances translation of mRNAs late after infection. *Proc Natl Acad Sci U S A* 1984;81:3655–3659.
246. Londberg-Holm K, Philipson L. Early events of virus-cell interactions in an adenovirus system. *J Virol* 1969;4:323–338.
247. Look DC, Roswit WT, Frick AG, et al. Direct suppression of Stat1 function during adenoviral infection. *Immunity* 1998;9:871–880.
248. Lowe SW, Ruley HE. Stabilization of the p53 tumor suppressor is induced by adenovirus 5 E1A and accompanies apoptosis. *Genes Dev* 1993;7:535–545.
249. Lukashok SA, Horwitz MS. New perspectives in adenoviruses. *Curr Clin Top Infect Dis* 1998;18:286–305.
250. Lutz P, Rosa-Calatrava M, Kedinger C. The product of the adenovirus intermediate gene IX is a transcriptional activator. *J Virol* 1997;71: 5102–5109.
251. Ma Y, Mathews MB. Comparative analysis of the structure and function of adenovirus virus-associated RNAs. *J Virol* 1993;67: 6605–6617.
252. Ma Y, Mathews MB. Secondary and tertiary structure in the central domain of adenovirus type 2 VA RNA I. *RNA* 1996;2:937–951.
253. Ma Y, Mathews MB. Structure, function and evolution of adenovirus-associated RNA: A phylogenetic approach. *J Virol* 1996;70:5083–5099.
254. Mackey JK, Rigden PM, Green M. Do highly oncogenic group A human adenoviruses cause human cancer? Analysis of human tumors for adenovirus 12 transforming DNA sequences. *Proc Natl Acad Sci U S A* 1976;73:4657–4661.
255. Maizel JV Jr, White DO, Scharff MD. The polypeptides of adenovirus. II. Soluble proteins, cores, top components and the structure of the virion. *Virology* 1968;36:126–136.
256. Mal A, Piotrkowski A, Harter ML. Cyclin-dependent kinases phosphorylate the adenovirus E1A protein, enhancing its ability to bind pRb and disrupt pRb-E2F complexes. *J Virol* 1996;70:2911–2921.
257. Mal A, Poon RY, Howe PH, et al. Inactivation of p27Kip1 by the viral E1A oncoprotein in TGFbeta-treated cells. *Nature* 1996;380:262–265.
258. Mangel WF, McGrath WJ, Toledo DL, Anderson CW. Viral DNA and a viral peptide can act as cofactors of adenovirus virion proteinase activity. *Nature* 1993;361:274–275.
259. Mansour SL, Grodzicker T, Tjian R. Downstream sequences affect transcription initiation from the adenovirus major late promoter. *Mol Cell Biol* 1986;6:2684–2694.
260. Maran A, Mathews MB. Characterization of the double-stranded RNA implicated in the inhibition of protein synthesis in cells infected with a mutant adenovirus defective for VA RNA. *Virology* 1988;164: 106–113.
261. Martin ME, Berk AJ. Adenovirus E1B 55K represses p53 activation in vitro. *J Virol* 1998;72:3146–3154.
262. Martinez-Palomo A, Granboulan N. Electron microscopy of adenovirus 12 replication. II. High-resolution autoradiography of infected KB cells labeled with tritiated thymidine. *J Virol* 1967;1:1010–1018.
263. Mathews MB. Binding of adenovirus VA RNA to mRNA: A possible role in splicing? *Nature* 1980;285:575–577.
264. Mathews MB, Shenk T. Adenovirus virus-associated RNA and translation control. *J Virol* 1991;65:5657–5662.
265. Mazzarelli JM, Mengus G, Davidson I, Ricciardi RP. The transactivation domain of adenovirus E1A interacts with the C terminus of human TAF(II)135. *J Virol* 1997;71:7978–7983.
266. Medghalchi S, Padmanabhan R, Ketner G. Early region 4 modulates adenovirus DNA replication by two genetically separable mechanisms. *Virology* 1997;236:8–17.
267. Meijer I, Boot AJ, Mahabir G, et al. Reduced binding activity of transcription factor NF-kappa B accounts for MHC class I repression in adenovirus type 12 E 1-transformed cells. *Cell Immunol* 1992;145:56–65.
268. Meissner JD, Hirsch GN, LaRue EA, et al. Completion of the DNA sequence of mouse adenovirus type 1: Sequence of E2B, L1, and L2 (18-51 map units). *Virus Res* 1997;51:53–64.
269. Mellits KH, Mathews MB. Effects of mutations in stem and loop regions on the structure and function of adenovirus VA RNAI. *EMBO J* 1988;7:2849–2859.
270. Mellman I. The importance of being acid: The role of acidification in intracellular membrane traffic. *J Exp Biol* 1992;172:39–45.
271. Mellow GH, Fohring B, Dougherty J, et al. Tumorigenicity of adenovirus-transformed rat cells and expression of class I major histocompatibility antigen. *Virology* 1984;134:460–465.
272. Mirza MA, Weber J. Structure of adenovirus chromatin. *Biochem Biophys Acta* 1982;696:76–86.
273. Miyamoto NG, Moncollin V, Egly JM, Chambon P. Specific interaction between a transcription factor and the upstream element of the adenovirus-2 major late promoter. *EMBO J* 1985;4:3563–3570.
274. Mondesert G, Kedinger C. Cooperation between upstream and downstream elements of the adenovirus major late promoter for maximal late phase-specific transcription. *Nucleic Acids Res* 1991;19:3221–3228.
275. Mondesert G, Tribouley C, Kedinger C. Identification of a novel downstream binding protein implicated in late-phase-specific activation of the adenovirus major late promotor. *Nucleic Acids Res* 1992; 20:3881–3889.
276. Moore M, Horikoshi N, Shenk T. Oncogenic potential of the adenovirus E4orf6 protein. *Proc Natl Acad Sci U S A* 1996;93:11295–11301.
277. Moore M, Schaack J, Baim SB, et al. Induced heat shock mRNAs escape the nucleocytoplasmic transport block in adenovirus-infected HeLa cells. *Mol Cell Biol* 1987;7:4505–4512.
278. Moran E, Mathews MB. Multiple functional domains in the adenovirus E1A gene. *Cell* 1987;48:177–178.
279. Morrison MD, Onions DE, Nicolson L. Complete DNA sequence of canine adenovirus type 1. *J Gen Virol* 1997;78:873–878.
280. Moyne G, Pichard E, Bernhard W. Localization of simian adenovirus 7 (SA 7) transcription and replication in lytic infection: An ultracytochemical and autoradiographical study. *J Gen Virol* 1978;40:77–92.
281. Mul YM, Van der Vliet PC. Nuclear factor I enhances adenovirus DNA replication by increasing the stability of a preinitiation complex. *EMBO J* 1992;11:751–760.
282. Mul YM, Verrijzer CP, van der Vliet PC. Transcription factors NFI and NFIII/oct-1 function independently, employing different mechanisms to enhance adenovirus DNA replication. *J Virol* 1990;64: 5510–5518.

283. Muller U, Kleinberger T, Shenk T. Adenovirus E4orf4 protein reduces phosphorylation of c-Fos and E1A proteins while simultaneously reducing the level of AP-1. *J Virol* 1992;66:5867–5878.
284. Muller U, Roberts MP, Engel DA, et al. Induction of transcription factor AP-1 by adenovirus E1A protein and cAMP. *Genes Dev* 1989;3: 1991–2002.
285. Nagata K, Guggenheimer RA, Hurwitz J. Adenovirus DNA replication in vitro: Synthesis of full-length DNA with purified proteins. *Proc Natl Acad Sci U S A* 1983;80:4266–4270.
286. Nevels M, Rubenwolf S, Spruss T, et al. The adenovirus E4orf6 protein can promote E1A/E1B-induced focus formation by interfering with p53 tumor suppressor function. *Proc Natl Acad Sci U S A* 1997; 94:1206–1211.
287. Nevels M, Spruss T, Wolf H, Dobner T. The adenovirus E4orf6 protein contributes to malignant transformation by antagonizing E1A-induced accumulation of the tumor suppressor protein p53. *Oncogene* 1999;18:9–17.
288. Nevels M, Tauber B, Kremmer E, et al. Transforming potential of the adenovirus type 5 E4orf3 protein. *J Virol* 1999;73:1591–1600.
289. Nevins JR. Mechanism of activation of early viral transcription by the adenovirus E1A gene product. *Cell* 1981;26:213–220.
290. Nevins JR. E2F: A link between the Rb tumor suppressor protein and viral oncoproteins. *Science* 1992;258:424–429.
291. Nevins JR, Darnell JE. Groups of adenovirus type 2 mRNAs derived from a large primary transcript: Probable nuclear origin and possible common 3′ ends. *J Virol* 1978;25:811–823.
292. Nevins JR, Wilson MC. Regulation of adenovirus-2 gene expression at the level of transcriptional termination and RNA processing. *Nature* 1981;290:113–118.
293. Nevins JR, Winkler JJ. Regulation of early adenovirus transcription: A protein product of early region 2 specifically represses region 4 transcription. *Proc Natl Acad Sci U S A* 1980;77:1893–1897.
294. Nielsch U, Zimmer SG, Babiss LE. Changes in NF-kappa B and ISGF3 DNA-binding activities are responsible for differences in MHC and beta-IFN gene expression in Ad5-versus Ad12-transformed cells. *EMBO J* 1991;10:4169–4175.
295. Norrby E. The relationship between soluble antigens and the virion of adenovirus type 3. I. Morphological characteristics. *Virology* 1966;28: 236–248.
296. Norrby E. The structural and functional diversity of Adenovirus capsid components. *J Gen Virol* 1969;5:221–236.
297. Norrby E, Bartha A, Boulanger P, et al. Adenoviridae. *Intervirology* 1976;7:117–125.
298. Norrby E, Wadell G. Immunological relationships between hexons of certain human adenoviruses. *J Virol* 1969;4:663–670.
299. Offringa R, Gebel S, van Dam H, et al. A novel function of the transforming domain of E1A: Repression of AP-1 activity. *Cell* 1990;62: 527–538.
300. O'Malley RP, Duncan RF, Hershey JW, Mathews MB. Modification of protein synthesis initiation factors and the shut-off of host protein synthesis in adenovirus-infected cells. *Virology* 1989;168:112–118.
301. O'Malley RP, Mariano TM, Siekierka J, Mathews MB. A mechanism for the control of protein synthesis by adenovirus VA RNAI. *Cell* 1986;44:391–400.
302. O'Neill EA, Fletcher C, Burrow CR, et al. Transcription factor OTF-1 is functionally identical to the DNA replication factor NF-III. *Science* 1988;241:1210–1213.
303. Oosterom-Dragon EA, Ginsberg HS. Characterization of two temperature-sensitive mutants of type 5 adenovirus with mutations in the 100,000-dalton protein gene. *J Virol* 1981;40:491–500.
304. Ornelles DA, Shenk T. Localization of the adenovirus early region 1B 55-kilodalton protein during lytic infection: Association with nuclear viral inclusions requires the early region 4 34-kilodalton protein. *J Virol* 1991;65:424–429.
305. Paabo S, Bhat BM, Wold WS, Peterson PA. A short sequence in the COOH-terminus makes an adenovirus membrane glycoprotein a resident of the endoplasmic reticulum. *Cell* 1987;50:311–317.
306. Parks CL, Shenk T. Activation of the adenovirus major late promoter by transcription factors MAZ and Sp1. *J Virol* 1997;71:9600–9607.
307. Perissi V, Dasen JS, Kurokawa R, et al. Factor-specific modulation of CREB-binding protein acetyltransferase activity. *Proc Natl Acad Sci U S A* 1999;96:3652–3657.
308. Pettersson U, Roberts RJ. Adenovirus gene expression and replication: A historical review. *Cancer Cells* 1986;4:37–57.
309. Philipson L. Adenovirus assembly. In: Ginsberg H, ed. *The adenoviruses*. New York: Plenum Press, 1984:309–337.
310. Pilder S, Logan J, Shenk T. Deletion of the gene encoding the adenovirus 5 early region 1b 21,000- molecular-weight polypeptide leads to degradation of viral and host cell DNA. *J Virol* 1984;52:664–671.
311. Pilder S, Moore M, Logan J, Shenk T. The adenovirus E1B-55K transforming polypeptide modulates transport or cytoplasmic stabilization of viral and host cell mRNAs. *Mol Cell Biol* 1986;6:470–476.
312. Pitcovski J, Mualem M, Rei-Koren Z, et al. The complete DNA sequence and genome organization of the avian adenovirus, hemorrhagic enteritis virus. *Virology* 1998;249:307–315.
313. Prage L, Pettersson U, Hoglund S, et al. Structural proteins of adenoviruses. IV. Sequential degradation of the adenovirus type 2 virion. *Virology* 1970;42:341–358.
314. Prince GA, Porter DD, Jenson AB, et al. Pathogenesis of adenovirus type 5 pneumonia in cotton rats (Sigmodon hispidus). *J Virol* 1993;67: 101–111.
315. Pruijn JM, van der Vliet PC, Dathan NA, Mattaj IW. Anti-OTF-1 antibodies inhibit NFIII stimulation of in vitro adenovirus DNA replication. *Nucleic Acids Res* 1989;17:1845–1863.
316. Rao L, Debbas M, Sabbatini P, et al. The adenovirus E1A proteins induce apoptosis, which is inhibited by the E1B 19-kDa and Bcl-2 proteins [published erratum appears in *Proc Natl Acad Sci U S A* 1992;89:9974]. *Proc Natl Acad Sci U S A* 1992;89:7742–7746.
317. Raska K Jr, Gallimore PH. An inverse relation of the oncogenic potential of adenovirus-transformed cells and their sensitivity to killing by syngeneic natural killer cells. *Virology* 1982;123:8–18.
318. Raychaudhuri P, Bagchi S, Neill SD, Nevins JR. Activation of the E2F transcription factor in adenovirus-infected cells involves E1A-dependent stimulation of DNA-binding activity and induction of cooperative binding mediated by an E4 gene product. *J Virol* 1990;64: 2702–2710.
319. Reach M, Babiss LE, Young CS. The upstream factor-binding site is not essential for activation of transcription from the adenovirus major late promoter. *J Virol* 1990;64:5851–5860.
320. Reach M, Xu LX, Young CS. Transcription from the adenovirus major late promoter uses redundant activating elements. *EMBO J* 1991;10: 3439–3446.
321. Reich N, Pine R, Levy D, Darnell JE Jr. Transcription of interferon-stimulated genes is induced by adenovirus particles but is suppressed by E1A gene products. *J Virol* 1988;62:114–119.
322. Reich PR, Rose J, Forget B, Weissman SM. RNA of low molecular weight in KB cells infected with Ad2. *J Mol Biol* 1966;17:428–439.
323. Reichel PA, Merrick WC, Siekierka J, Mathews MB. Regulation of a protein synthesis initiation factor by adenovirus virus-associated RNA. *Nature* 1985;313:196–200.
324. Rekosh DM, Russell WC, Bellet AJ, Robinson AJ. Identification of a protein linked to the ends of adenovirus DNA. *Cell* 1977;11:283–295.
325. Roberts MM, White JL, Grutter MG, Burnett RM. Three-dimensional structure of the adenovirus major coat protein hexon. *Science* 1986; 232:1148–1151.
326. Roberts RJ, O'Neill KE, Yen CT. DNA sequences from the adenovirus 2 genome. *J Biol Chem* 1984;259:13968–13975.
327. Robinson AJ, Younghusband HB, Bellett AJ. A circular DNA-protein complex from adenoviruses. *Virology* 1973;56:54–69.
328. Rochette-Egly C, Fromental C, Chambon P. General repression of enhanson activity by the adenovirus-2 E1A proteins. *Genes Dev* 1990; 4:137–150.
329. Roelvink PW, Lizonova A, Lee JG, et al. The coxsackievirus-adenovirus receptor protein can function as a cellular attachment protein for adenovirus serotypes from subgroups A, C, D, E, and F. *J Virol* 1998;72:7909–7915.
330. Rosen I. A hemagglutination-inhibitor technique for typing adenoviruses. *Am J Hyg* 1960;71:120–128.
331. Roth J, Konig C, Wienzek S, et al. Inactivation of p53 but not p73 by adenovirus type 5 E1B 55-kilodalton and E4 34-kilodalton oncoproteins. *J Virol* 1998;72:8510–8516.
332. Routes JM, Bellgrau D, McGrory WJ, et al. Anti-adenovirus type 5 cytotoxic T lymphocytes: Immunodominant epitopes are encoded by the E1A gene. *J Virol* 1991;65:1450–1457.
333. Rowe WP, Huebner RJ, Gilmore LK, et al. Isolation of a cytopathogenic agent from human adenoids undergoing spontaneous degeneration in tissue culture. *Proc Soc Exp Biol Med* 1953;84:570–573.
334. Ruigrok RW, Barge A, Albiges-Rizo C, Dayan S. Structure of aden-

ovirus fibre. II. Morphology of single fibres. *J Mol Biol* 1990;215: 589–596.

335. Russell WC, Laver WG, Sanderson PJ. Internal components of adenovirus. *Nature* 1968;219:1127–1130.
336. Russell WC, Newman C, Williams JF. Characterization of temperature-sensitive mutants of adenovirus type 5-serology. *J Gen Virol* 1972; 17:265–279.
337. Samuelson AV, Lowe SW. Selective induction of p53 and chemosensitivity in RB-deficient cells by E1A mutants unable to bind the RB-related proteins. *Proc Natl Acad Sci U S A* 1997;94:12094–12099.
338. Sarnow P, Hearing P, Anderson CW, et al. Adenovirus early region 1B 58,000-dalton tumor antigen is physically associated with an early region 4 25,000-dalton protein in productively infected cells. *J Virol* 1984;49:692–700.
339. Sarnow P, Ho YS, Williams J, Levine AJ. Adenovirus E1b-58kd tumor antigen and SV40 large tumor antigen are physically associated with the same 54 kd cellular protein in transformed cells. *Cell* 1982;28: 387–394.
340. Sawada Y, Fohring B, Shenk TE, Raska K Jr. Tumorigenicity of adenovirus-transformed cells: Region E1A of adenovirus 12 confers resistance to natural killer cells. *Virology* 1985;147:413–421.
341. Sawadogo M, Roeder RG. Interaction of a gene-specific transcription factor with the adenovirus major late promoter upstream of the TATA box region. *Cell* 1985;43:165–175.
342. Schaack J, Ho WY, Freimuth P, Shenk T. Adenovirus terminal protein mediates both nuclear matrix association and efficient transcription of adenovirus DNA. *Genes Dev* 1990;4:1197–1208.
343. Schmid SI, Hearing P. Cellular components interact with adenovirus type 5 minimal DNA packaging domains. *J Virol* 1998;72:6339–6347.
344. Schneider RJ, Safer B, Munemitsu SM, et al. Adenovirus VAI RNA prevents phosphorylation of the eukaryotic initiation factor 2 alpha subunit subsequent to infection. *Proc Natl Acad Sci U S A* 1985;82: 4321–4325.
345. Schneider RJ, Weinberger C, Shenk T. Adenovirus VAI RNA facilitates the initiation of translation in virus-infected cells. *Cell* 1984;37: 291–298.
346. Schrier PI, Bernards R, Vaessen RT, et al. Expression of class I major histocompatibility antigens switched off by highly oncogenic adenovirus 12 in transformed rat cells. *Nature* 1983;305:771–775.
347. See RH, Shi Y. Adenovirus E1B 19,000-molecular-weight protein activates c-Jun N-terminal kinase and c-Jun-mediated transcription. *Mol Cell Biol* 1998;18:4012–4022.
348. Seiberg M, Kessler M, Levine AJ, Aloni Y. Human RNA polymerase II can prematurely terminate transcription of the adenovirus type 2 late transcription unit at a precise site that resembles a prokaryotic termination signal. *Virus Genes* 1987;1:97–116.
349. Seth P, Fitzgerald DJ, Willingham MC, Pastan I. Role of a low-pH environment in adenovirus enhancement of the toxicity of a Pseudomonas exotoxin-epidermal growth factor conjugate. *J Virol* 1984;51:650–655.
350. Seto E, Usheva A, Zambetti GP, et al. Wild-type p53 binds to the TATA-binding protein and represses transcription. *Proc Natl Acad Sci U S A* 1992;89:12028–12032.
351. Sharp PA, Gallimore PH, Flint SJ. Mapping of adenovirus 2 RNA sequences in lytically infected cells and transformed cell lines. *Cold Spring Harb Symp Quant Biol* 1975;39:457–474.
352. Shaw AR, Ziff EB. Transcripts from the adenovirus-2 major late promoter yield a single early family of 3′ coterminal mRNAs and five late families. *Cell* 1980;22:905–916.
353. Shenk T, Jones N, Colby W, Fowlkes D. Functional analysis of adenovirus type 5 host-range deletion mutants defective for transformation of rat embryo cells. *Cold Spring Harbor Symp Quant Biol* 1979;44: 367–375.
354. Shi Y, Seto E, Chang LS, Shenk T. Transcriptional repression by YY1, a human GLI-Kruppel-related protein, and relief of repression by adenovirus E1A protein. *Cell* 1991;67:377–388.
355. Shisler J, Yang C, Walter B, et al. The adenovirus E3-10.4K/14.5K complex mediates loss of cell surface Fas (CD95) and resistance to Fas-induced apoptosis. *J Virol* 1997;71:8299–8306.
356. Shtrichman R, Kleinberger T. Adenovirus type 5 E4 open reading frame 4 protein induces apoptosis in transformed cells. *J Virol* 1998; 72:2975–2982.
357. Silver L, Anderson CW. Interaction of human adenovirus serotype 2 with human lymphoid cells. *Virology* 1988;165:377–387.
358. Sinn E, Wang Z, Kovelman R, Roeder RG. Cloning and characterization of a TFIIIC2 subunit (TFIIIC beta) whose presence correlates with activation of RNA polymerase III-mediated transcription by adenovirus E1A expression and serum factors. *Genes Dev* 1995;9: 675–685.
359. Skoglund U, Ofverstedt LG, Burnett RM, Bricogne G. Maximum-entropy three-dimensional reconstruction with deconvolution of the contrast transfer function: A test application with adenovirus. *J Struct Biol* 1996;117:173–188.
360. Smart JE, Stillman BW. Adenovirus terminal protein precursor: Partial amino acid sequence and the site of covalent linkage to virus DNA. *J Biol Chem* 1982;257:13499–13506.
361. Soddu S, Lewis AM Jr. Driving adenovirus type 12-transformed BALB/c mouse cells to express high levels of class I major histocompatibility complex proteins enhances, rather than abrogates, their tumorigenicity. *J Virol* 1992;66:2875–2884.
362. Somasundaram K, El-Deiry WS. Inhibition of p53-mediated transactivation and cell cycle arrest by E1A through its p300/CBP-interacting region. *Oncogene* 1997;14:1047–1057.
363. Sparer TE, Tripp RA, Dillehay DL, Hermiston TW. The role of human adenovirus early region 3 proteins (gp19K, 10.4K, 14.5K, and 14.7K) in a murine pneumonia model. *J Virol* 1996;70:2431–2439.
364. Spergel JM, Hsu W, Akira S, et al. NF-IL6, a member of the C/EBP family, regulates E1A-responsive promoters in the absence of E1A. *J Virol* 1992;66:1021–1030.
365. Sprengel J, Schmitz B, Heuss-Neitzel D, Doerfler W. The complete nucleotide sequence of the DNA of human adenovirus type 12. *Curr Top Microbiol Immunol* 1995;199:189–274.
366. Steegenga WT, Riteco N, Jochemsen AG, et al. The large E1B protein together with the E4orf6 protein target p53 for active degradation in adenovirus infected cells. *Oncogene* 1998;16:349–357.
367. Steegenga WT, Shvarts A, Riteco N, et al. Distinct regulation of p53 and p73 activity by adenovirus E1A, E1B, and E4orf6 proteins. *Mol Cell Biol* 1999;19:3885–3894.
368. Stein RW, Corrigan M, Yaciuk P, et al. Analysis of E1A-mediated growth regulation functions: Binding of the 300-kilodalton cellular product correlates with E1A enhancer repression function and DNA synthesis-inducing activity. *J Virol* 1990;64:4421–4427.
369. Stephens C, Harlow E. Differential splicing yields novel adenovirus 5 E1A mRNAs that encode 30 kd and 35 kd proteins. *EMBO J* 1987;6: 2027–2035.
370. Stewart P, Burnett RM. Adenovirus structure as revealed by x-ray crystallography, electron microscopy, and difference imaging. *Jpn J Appl Phys* 1993;32:1342–1347.
371. Stewart PL, Burnett RM, Cyrklaff M, Fuller SD. Image reconstruction reveals the complex molecular organization of adenovirus. *Cell* 1991; 67:145–154.
372. Stewart PL, Fuller SD, Burnett RM. Difference imaging of adenovirus: Bridging the resolution gap between X-ray crystallography and electron microscopy. *EMBO J* 1993;12:2589–2599.
373. Stillman BW, Lewis JB, Chow LT, et al. Identification of the gene and mRNA for the adenovirus terminal protein precursor. *Cell* 1981;23: 497–508.
374. Stillman BW, Tamanoi F, Mathews MB. Purification of an adenovirus-coded DNA polymerase that is required for initiation of DNA replication. *Cell* 1982;31:613–623.
375. Stouten PF, Sander C, Ruigrok RW, Cusack S. New triple-helical model for the shaft of the adenovirus fibre. *J Mol Biol* 1992;226: 1073–1084.
376. Stuiver MH, van der Vliet PC. The adenovirus DNA binding protein forms a multimeric protein complex with double-stranded DNA and enhances binding of nuclear factor I. *J Virol* 1990;64:379–386.
377. Sundquist B, Everitt E, Philipson L, Hoglund S. Assembly of adenoviruses. *J Virol* 1973;11:449–459.
378. Suomalainen M, Nakano MY, Keller S, et al. Microtubule-dependent plus- and minus end-directed motilities are competing processes for nuclear targeting of adenovirus. *J Cell Biol* 1999;144:657–672.
379. Svensson U. Role of vesicles during adenovirus 2 internalization into HeLa cells. *J Virol* 1985;55:442–449.
380. Takemori N, Cladaras C, Bhat B, et al. cyt Gene of adenoviruses 2 and 5 is an oncogene for transforming function in early region E1B and encodes the E1B 19,000-molecular-weight polypeptide. *J Virol* 1984; 52:793–805.
381. Tal J, Craig EA, Raskas HJ. Sequence relationships between aden-

ovirus 2 early RNA and viral RNA size classes synthesized at 18 hours after infection. *J Virol* 1975;15:137–144.

382. Tamanoi F, Stillman BW. Function of adenovirus terminal protein in the initiation of DNA replication. *Proc Natl Acad Sci U S A* 1982;79: 2221–2225.
383. Tanaka K, Isselbacher KJ, Khoury G, Jay G. Reversal of oncogenesis by the expression of a major histocompatibility complex class I gene. *Science* 1985;228:26–30.
384. Tate VE, Philipson L. Parental adenovirus DNA accumulates in nucleosome-like structures in infected cells. *Nucleic Acids Res* 1979;6: 2769–2785.
385. Temperley SM, Hay RT. Recognition of the adenovirus type 2 origin of DNA replication by the virally encoded DNA polymerase and preterminal proteins. *EMBO J* 1992;11:761–768.
386. Teodoro JG, Shore GC, Branton PE. Adenovirus E1A proteins induce apoptosis by both p53-dependent and p53-independent mechanisms. *Oncogene* 1995;11:467–474.
387. Thimmappaya B, Weinberger C, Schneider RJ, Shenk T. Adenovirus VAI RNA is required for efficient translation of viral mRNAs at late times after infection. *Cell* 1982;31:543–551.
388. Thomas DL, Shin S, Jiang BH, et al. Early region 1 transforming functions are dispensable for mammary tumorigenesis by human adenovirus type 9. *J Virol* 1999;73:3071–3079.
389. Thomas GP, Mathews MB. DNA replication and the early to late transition in adenovirus infection. *Cell* 1980;22:523–533.
390. Tibbetts C. Viral DNA sequences from incomplete particles of human adenovirus type 7. *Cell* 1977;12:243–249.
391. Tihanyi K, Bourbonniere M, Houde A, et al. Isolation and properties of adenovirus type 2 proteinase. *J Biol Chem* 1993;268:1780–1785.
392. Tokunaga O, Yaegashi T, Lowe J, et al. Sequence analysis in the E1 region of adenovirus type 4 DNA. *Virology* 1986;155:418–433.
393. Tollefson AE, Hermiston TW, Lichtenstein DL, et al. Forced degradation of Fas inhibits apoptosis in adenovirus-infected cells. *Nature* 1998;392:726–730.
394. Tollefson AE, Scaria A, Hermiston TW, et al. The adenovirus death protein (E3-11.6K) is required at very late stages of infection for efficient cell lysis and release of adenovirus from infected cells. *J Virol* 1996;70:2296–2306.
395. Tomko RP, Xu R, Philipson L. HCAR and MCAR: The human and mouse cellular receptors for subgroup C adenoviruses and group b Coxsackieviruses. *Proc Natl Acad Sci U S A* 1997;94:3352–3356.
396. Tooze J. DNA tumor viruses. In: *Molecular biology of tumor viruses.* 2nd ed. Cold Spring Harbor, NY: Cold Spring Harbor Laboratory, 1981.
397. Toth M, Doerfler W, Shenk T. Adenovirus DNA replication facilitates binding of the MLTF/USF transcription factor to the viral major late promoter within infected cells. *Nucleic Acids Res* 1992;20:5143–5148.
398. Trentin JJ, Yabe Y, Taylor G. The quest for human cancer viruses. *Science* 1962;137:835–849.
399. Tribouley C, Lutz P, Staub A, Kedinger C. The product of the adenovirus intermediate gene IVa2 is a transcriptional activator of the major late promoter. *J Virol* 1994;68:4450–4457.
400. Tucker PA, Tsernoglou D, Tucker AD, et al. Crystal structure of the adenovirus DNA binding protein reveals a hook-on model for cooperative DNA binding. *EMBO J* 1994;13:2994–3002.
401. Valentine RC, Pereira HG. Antigens and structure of the adenovirus. *J Mol Biol* 1965;13:13–20.
402. van Dam H, Duyndam M, Rottier R, et al. Heterodimer formation of cJun and ATF-2 is responsible for induction of C-jun by the 243 amino acid adenovirus E1A protein. *EMBO J* 1993;12:479–487.
403. van den Heuvel SJ, van Laar T, The I, van der Eb AJ. Large E1B proteins of adenovirus types 5 and 12 have different effects on p53 and distinct roles in cell transformation. *J Virol* 1993;67:5226–5234.
404. van der Vliet PC, Levine AJ. DNA-binding proteins specific for cells infected by adenovirus. *Nature* 1973;246:170–174.
405. van Der Vliet PC, Levine AJ, Ensinger MJ, Ginsberg HS. Thermolabile DNA binding proteins from cells infected with a temperature-sensitive mutant of adenovirus defective in viral DNA synthesis. *J Virol* 1975;15:348–354.
406. van Leeuwen HC, Rensen M, van der Vliet PC. The Oct-1 POU homeodomain stabilizes the adenovirus preinitiation complex via a direct interaction with the priming protein and is displaced when the replication fork passes. *J Biol Chem* 1997;272:3398–3405.
407. van Oostrum J, Burnett RM. Molecular composition of the adenovirus type 2 virion. *J Virol* 1985;56:439–448.
408. van Ormondt H, Maat J, Dijkema R. Comparison of nucleotide sequences of the early E1a regions for subgroups A, B and C of human adenoviruses. *Gene* 1980;12:63–76.
409. Varga MJ, Weibull C, Everitt E. Infectious entry pathway of adenovirus type 2. *J Virol* 1991;65:6061–6070.
410. Vayda ME, Flint SJ. Isolation and characterization of adenovirus core nucleoprotein subunits. *J Virol* 1987;61:3335–3339.
411. Vayda ME, Rogers AE, Flint SJ. The structure of nucleoprotein cores released from adenovirions. *Nucleic Acids Res* 1983;11:441–460.
412. Velicer LF, Ginsberg HS. Synthesis, transport, and morphogenesis of type adenovirus capsid proteins. *J Virol* 1970;5:338–352.
413. Verrijzer CP, van Oosterhout JA, van Weperen WW, van der Vliet PC. POU proteins bend DNA via the POU-specific domain. *EMBO J* 1991;10:3007–3014.
414. Vigne E, Mahfouz I, Dedieu JF, et al. RGD inclusion in the hexon monomer provides adenovirus type 5-based vectors with a fiber knob-independent pathway for infection. *J Virol* 1999;73:5156–5161.
415. Von Seggern DJ, Kehler J, Endo RI, Nemerow GR. Complementation of a fibre mutant adenovirus by packaging cell lines stably expressing the adenovirus type 5 fibre protein. *J Gen Virol* 1998;79:1461–1468.
416. Walker TA, Wilson BA, Lewis AM Jr, Cook JL. E1A oncogene induction of cytolytic susceptibility eliminates sarcoma cell tumorigenicity. *Proc Natl Acad Sci U S A* 1991;88:6491–6495.
417. Wang HG, Draetta G, Moran E. E1A induces phosphorylation of the retinoblastoma protein independently of direct physical association between the E1A and retinoblastoma products. *Mol Cell Biol* 1991;11: 4253–4265.
418. Wang HG, Rikitake Y, Carter MC, et al. Identification of specific adenovirus E1A N-terminal residues critical to the binding of cellular proteins and to the control of cell growth. *J Virol* 1993;67:476–488.
419. Wang K, Huang S, Kapoor-Munshi A, Nemerow G. Adenovirus internalization and infection require dynamin. *J Virol* 1998;72:3455–3458.
420. Weber J. Genetic analysis of adenovirus type 2. III. Temperature sensitivity of processing of viral proteins. *J Virol* 1976;17:462–471.
421. Weber J, Jelinek W, Darnell JE Jr. The definition of a large viral transcription unit late in Ad2 infection of HeLa cells: Mapping of nascent RNA molecules labeled in isolated nuclei. *Cell* 1977;10:611–616.
422. Weber JM, Dery CV, Mirza MA, Horvath J. Adenovirus DNA synthesis is coupled to virus assembly. *Virology* 1985;140:351–359.
423. Weber JM, Talbot BG, Delorme L. The orientation of the adenovirus fiber and its anchor domain identified through molecular mimicry. *Virology* 1989;168:180–182.
424. Webster A, Hay RT, Kemp G. The adenovirus protease is activated by a virus-coded disulphide-linked peptide. *Cell* 1993;72:97–104.
425. Weinberg DH, Ketner G. A cell line that supports the growth of a defective early region 4 deletion mutant of human adenovirus type 2. *Proc Natl Acad Sci U S A* 1983;80:5383–5386.
426. Weinberg DH, Ketner G. Adenoviral early region 4 is required for efficient viral DNA replication and for late gene expression. *J Virol* 1986; 57:833–838.
427. Weinmann R, Raskas HJ, Roeder RG. Role of DNA-dependent RNA polymerases II and III in transcription of the adenovirus genome late in productive infection. *Proc Natl Acad Sci U S A* 1974;71:3426–3430.
428. Weiss RS, Lee SS, Prasad BV, Javier RT. Human adenovirus early region 4 open reading frame 1 genes encode growth-transforming proteins that may be distantly related to dUTP pyrophosphatase enzymes. *J Virol* 1997;71:1857–1870.
429. Weiss RS, McArthur MJ, Javier RT. Human adenovirus type 9 E4 open reading frame 1 encodes a cytoplasmic transforming protein capable of increasing the oncogenicity of CREF cells. *J Virol* 1996;70: 862–872.
430. Whalen SG, Marcellus RC, Whalen A, et al. Phosphorylation within the transactivation domain of adenovirus E1A protein by mitogen-activated protein kinase regulates expression of early region 4. *J Virol* 1997;71:3545–3553.
431. White E, Cipriani R. Specific disruption of intermediate filaments and the nuclear lamina by the 19-kDa product of the adenovirus E1B oncogene. *Mol Cell Biol* 1989;10:120–130.
432. White E, Cipriani R. Role of adenovirus E1B proteins in transformation: Altered organization of intermediate filaments in transformed cells that express the 19-kilodalton protein. *Mol Cell Biol* 1990;10:120–130.
433. White E, Grodzicker T, Stillman BW. Mutations in the gene encoding the adenovirus early region 1B 19,000-molecular-weight tumor antigen cause the degradation of chromosomal DNA. *J Virol* 1984;52:410–419.

434. White RJ, Trouche D, Martin K, et al. Repression of RNA polymerase III transcription by the retinoblastoma protein. *Nature* 1996;382:88–90.
435. Whyte P, Buchkovich KJ, Horowitz JM, et al. Association between an oncogene and an anti-oncogene: The adenovirus E1A proteins bind to the retinoblastoma gene product. *Nature* 1988;334:124–129.
436. Wickham TJ, Mathias P, Cheresh DA, Nemerow GR. Integrins alpha v beta 3 and alpha v beta 5 promote adenovirus internalization but not virus attachment. *Cell* 1993;73:309–319.
437. Williams J, Grodzicker T, Sharp P, Sambrook J. Adenovirus recombination: Physical mapping of crossover events. *Cell* 1975;4:113–119.
438. Williams JL, Garcia J, Harrich D, et al. Lymphoid specific gene expression of the adenovirus early region 3 promoter is mediated by NF-kappa B binding motifs. *EMBO J* 1990;9:4435–4442.
439. Wilson MC, Fraser NW, Darnell JE Jr. Mapping of RNA initiation sites by high doses of uv irradiation: Evidence for three independent promoters within the left 11% of the Ad-2 genome. *Virology* 1979;94:175–184.
440. Wong ML, Hsu MT. Linear adenovirus DNA is organized into supercoiled domains in virus particles. *Nucleic Acids Res* 1989;17:3535–3550.
441. Wu L, Rosser DS, Schmidt MC, Berk A. A TATA box implicated in E1A transcriptional activation of a simple adenovirus 2 promoter. *Nature* 1987;326:512–515.
442. Xia D, Henry LJ, Gerard RD, Deisenhofer J. Crystal structure of the receptor-binding domain of adenovirus type 5 fiber protein at 1.7 A resolution. *Structure* 1994;2:1259–1270.
443. Yang UC, Huang W, Flint SJ. mRNA export correlates with activation of transcription in human subgroup C adenovirus-infected cells. *J Virol* 1996;70:4071–4080.
444. Yang XJ, Ogryzko VV, Nishikawa J, et al. A p300/CBP-associated factor that competes with the adenoviral oncoprotein E1A. *Nature* 1996;382:319–324.
445. Yee AS, Raychaudhuri P, Jakoi L, Nevins JR. The adenovirus-inducible factor E2F stimulates transcription after specific DNA binding. *Mol Cell Biol* 1989;9:578–585.
446. Yee SP, Branton PE. Detection of cellular proteins associated with human adenovirus type 5 early region 1A polypeptides. *Virology* 1985;147:142–153.
447. Yew PR, Berk AJ. Inhibition of p53 transactivation required for transformation by adenovirus early 1B protein. *Nature* 1992;357:82–85.
448. Yew PR, Liu X, Berk AJ. Adenovirus E1B oncoprotein tethers a transcriptional repression domain to p53. *Genes Dev* 1994;8:190–202.
449. Yoder SS, Robberson BL, Leys EJ, et al. Control of cellular gene expression during adenovirus infection: Induction and shut-off of dihydrofolate reductase gene expression by adenovirus type 2. *Mol Cell Biol* 1983;3:819–828.
450. Yolken RH, Lawrence F, Leister F, et al. Gastroenteritis associated with enteric type adenovirus in hospitalized infants. *J Pediatr* 1982;101:21–26.
451. Yoshimura K, Rosenfeld MA, Seth P, Crystal RG. Adenovirus-mediated augmentation of cell transfection with unmodified plasmid vectors. *J Biol Chem* 1993;268:2300–2303.
452. Yoshinaga S, Dean N, Han M, Berk AJ. Adenovirus stimulation of transcription by RNA polymerase III: Evidence for an E1A-dependent increase in transcription factor IIIC concentration. *EMBO J* 1986;5:343–354.
453. Young CS, Cachianes G, Munz P, Silverstein S. Replication and recombination in adenovirus-infected cells are temporally and functionally related. *J Virol* 1984;51:571–577.
454. Yueh A, Schneider RJ. Selective translation initiation by ribosome jumping in adenovirus-infected and heat-shocked cells. *Genes Dev* 1996;10:1557–1567.
455. Zabner J, Freimuth P, Puga A, et al. Lack of high affinity fiber receptor activity explains the resistance of ciliated airway epithelia to adenovirus infection. *J Clin Invest* 1997;100:1144–1149.
456. Zamanian M, La Thangue NB. Adenovirus E1A prevents the retinoblastoma gene product from repressing the activity of a cellular transcription factor. *EMBO J* 1992;11:2603–2610.
457. Zantema A, Fransen JAM, Davis-Olivier A, et al. Localization of the E1B proteins of adenovirus 5 in transformed cells is revealed by interaction with monoclonal antibodies. *Virology* 1985;142:44–58.
458. Zantema A, Schrier PO, Davis-Olivier A, et al. Adenovirus serotype determines association and localization of the large E1B tumor antigen with cellular tumor antigen p53 in transformed cells. *Mol Cell Biol* 1985;5:3084–3091.
459. Zerler B, Roberts RJ, Mathews MB, Moran E. Different functional domains of the adenovirus E1A gene are involved in regulation of host cell cycle products. *Mol Cell Biol* 1987;7:821–829.
460. Zhai ZH, Wang X, Qian XY. Nuclear matrix-intermediate filament system and its alteration in adenovirus infected HeLa cell. *Cell Biol Int Rep* 1988;12:99–108.
461. Zhang Y, Schneider R. Adenovirus inhibition of cellular protein synthesis and the specific translation of late viral mRNAs. *Semin Virol* 1993;4:229–236.
462. Zhou Q, Engel DA. Adenovirus E1A243 disrupts the ATF/CREB-YY1 complex at the mouse c-fos promoter. *J Virol* 1995;69:7402–7409.
463. Ziff E, Fraser N. Adenovirus type 2 late mRNA's: Structural evidence for 3′-coterminal species. *J Virol* 1978;25:897–906.
464. Ziff EB, Evans RM. Coincidence of the promoter and capped 5′ terminus of RNA from the adenovirus 2 major late transcription unit. *Cell* 1978;15:1463–1476.
465. Zilli D, Voelkel-Johnson C, Skinner T, Laster SM. The adenovirus E3 region 14.7 kDa protein, heat and sodium arsenite inhibit the TNF-induced release of arachidonic acid. *Biochem Biophys Res Commun* 1992;188:177–183.

CHAPTER 32

Parvoviridae: The Viruses and Their Replication

Nicholas Muzyczka and Kenneth I. Berns

The parvoviruses are among the smallest of the DNA animal viruses. The virion has a diameter of 18 to 26 nm and is composed entirely of protein and DNA. The family *Parvoviridae* (21) contains two subfamilies: the *Parvovirinae*, which infect vertebrates, and the *Densovirinae*, which infect insects. Each of the subfamilies contains three genera (Table 1). Because the host range of the *Densovirinae* lies outside the scope of this volume, the replication of these viruses is not reviewed. The interested reader is referred to several recent articles (14,29,151). The *Parvovirinae* have a wide distribution among warm-blooded animals, ranging from domestic fowl to humans (see Table 1). Dependoviruses, also known as adeno-associated viruses (AAV), are unique among animal viruses in that, except under special conditions, they require co-infection with an unrelated helper virus, either an adenovirus (Ad) or a herpesvirus, for productive infection in cell culture (11,38). In spite of this distinction, there are many similarities between AAV and the members of the *Parvovirus* and *Erythrovirus* genera in genome structure, organization, and expression. It is the intent of this chapter to compare and contrast the replication of these three genera at the molecular and biologic levels.

THE VIRION

The parvovirus virion has a relatively simple structure composed of a mixture of VP1, VP2, and VP3, which encapsidates a linear, single-strand DNA molecule. The particle has icosahedral symmetry (277). The crystal structures of canine parvovirus (CPV), feline panleukopenia parvovirus (FPV), minute virus of mice (MVM), human parvovirus B19, and wax moth densovirus have been determined and their basic capsid organizations are similar (2,3,277, and refs. therein). The 60 protein subunits that make up the capsid have a common structure, arranged with T=1 icosahedral symmetry. The main structural motif is an eight-stranded, antiparallel β-barrel, which also has been found in most other viral capsid structures. The β-barrel motif contains only approximately one third of the amino acid composition of VP2, the major structural protein in most parvoviruses that comprises about 90% of the capsid. The remaining two thirds is present as large loops connecting the strands of the β-barrel. The loops form much of the capsid surface, onto which a number of biologic features, such as host species and tissue tropism, receptor binding, and antigenic properties have been structurally and genetically mapped. The insertions between the

TABLE 1. *Parvoviridae*

- Subfamily *Parvovirinae*
  - Genus *Parvovirus*
    - Members
      - Aleutian mink disease virus (ADV) (M20036; NC_001662; GI:10580)
      - Barbarie duck parvovirus (U22967.1; GI:1113784)
      - Bovine parvovirus (BPV) (M14363; NC_001540; GI:10358)
      - Canine parvovirus (M19296; NC_001539; GI:10357)
      - Feline panleukopenia (M75728; M38246.1; GI:333471)
      - Goose parvovirus (GPV) (NC_001701; GI:10689)
      - H1 parvovirus (XO1457; NC_001358; GI:10057)
      - Hamster parvovirus (HaPV)
      - HB parvovirus
      - Lapine parvovirus (LPV)
      - LuIII (M81888, M81888.1; GI:333487)
      - Minute virus of mice (MVM or MMV) (J02275; NC_001510; GI:10316)
      - Mink enteritis virus (MEV)
      - Minute virus of canine (MVC)
      - Mouse parvovirus 1 (NC_001630; GI:10516)
      - Muscovy duck parvovirus (MDPV) (X75093.1; GI:609091; U22967)
      - Porcine parvovirus (PPV) (DO0623; NC_001718; GI:10886)
      - RA1
      - Raccoon parvovirus (RPV) (M24005)
      - Rat parvovirus (RV-1a) (AF036710)
      - Rat virus (also Kilham rat virus or H3) (RV or KRV or H3) U79033
      - RT parvovirus (RTV)
      - Tumor virus X
  - Genus *Erythrovirus*
    - Members
      - B19 virus (M13178, M24682; NC_000883; GI:9632996)
      - Chipmunk parvovirus (U86868.1; GI:2584818)
      - Pig-tailed macaque parvovirus
      - Rhesus macaque parvovirus
      - Simian parvovirus (U26342.1; GI:968937)
      - Manchurian chipmunk parvovirus
  - Genus *Dependovirus*
    - Members
      - Adeno-associated type 1 (AAV1) (NC_002077; GI:9632547)
      - Adeno-associated type 2 (AAV2) (J01901; NC_001401; GI:9626146)
      - Adeno-associated type 3 (AAV3) (NC_001729; GI:9628918)
      - Adeno-associated type 4 (AAV4) (NC_001829; GI:9629641)
      - Adeno-associated type 5 (AAV5) (AF085716.1; GI:4249656)
      - Adeno-associated type 6 (AAV6) (NC_001862; GI:9629894)
      - Avian adeno-associated
      - Bovine adeno-associated
      - Canine adeno-associated
      - Equine adeno-associated
      - Ovine adeno-associated
- Subfamily *Densovirinae*
  - Genus *Densovirus*
    - Members
      - *Acheta domestica* densovirus (AdDNV)
      - *Agraulis vanillae* densovirus (AvDNV)
      - *Culex pipiens* (DNV)
      - *Diatraea saccharalis* densovirus (NC_001899; GI:9630378)
      - *Junonia coenia* densovirus (JcDNV) (S47266.1; GI:257675)
      - *Galleria mellonella* densovirus (GmDNV) (L32896.1; GI:556172)
  - Genus *Iteravirus*
    - Members
      - *Bombyx mori* densovirus (Bombyx DNV) (M15123, M60583, M60584; AB042597.1; GI:7959360)
      - *Casphalia extranea densovirus*
  - Genus *Contravirus*
    - Members
      - *Aedes aegypti* densovirus (AaDNV)
      - *Aedes albopictus* densovirus (AaPV or AlDNV) (X74945.1; GI:510569)
      - *Aedes* densonucleosis virus (AeDNV) (M37899.1; GI:209745)
      - Hepatopancreatic parvo-like virus of shrimps
    - Tentative species in the genus
      - *Aedes pseudoscutellaris* densovirus
      - *Euxoa auxiliaris* densovirus
      - *Leucorrhinia dubia* densovirus
      - *Lymantria dubia* densovirus
      - *Periplanata fuliginosa* densovirus (NC_000936; GI:9633605)
      - *Pieris rapae* densovirus
      - *Pseudaletia includens* densovirus
      - *Sibine fusca* densovirus
      - *Simulium vittatum* densovirus
  - Tentative species in the subfamily
    - Parvo-like virus of crabs

DNA sequence accession numbers and common abbreviations for each virus are shown in parentheses. The table is derived from ref. 21, and from the NCBI Taxonomy browser at *www.nlm.nih.gov/htbin-post/Taxonomy/wgetorg,* with permission. The parvovirus taxonomy continues to evolve as additional sequence information is obtained and new serotypes are isolated or reclassified. The reader should not assume that Table 1 represents a definitive list.

βD and βE strands of the β-barrel form an antiparallel β-ribbon, which together with similar insertions in four other fivefold related polypeptides form a cylinder about the fivefold icosahedral axes, with an opening to the exterior surface of the capsid in CPV, FPV, and MVM, but not in B19. VP2 is thought to be externalized for maturation cleavage to VP3 via this opening in the latter viruses. Other characteristic features of the parvoviral capsid (Fig. 1) include spikelike protrusions at the icosahedral threefold axes, a 15-Å canyon-like depression about the fivefold axes, and a dimple-like depression at the icosahedral twofold axes. Antigenic regions have been mapped to the threefold protrusions (2), and the twofold depression has been implicated in the attachment of host cell factors (3).

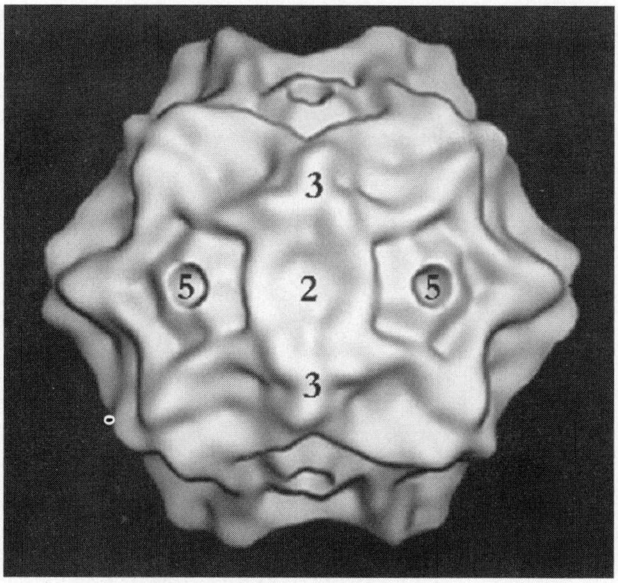

FIG. 1. *Parvovirus* structure. Cryoelectron micrograph of canine parvovirus showing some of the surface features around the two-, three-, and fivefold axes of symmetry.

The particle has a molecular weight (MW) of 5.5 to 6.2 $\times 10^6$ daltons. Approximately 50% of the mass is protein, and the remainder is DNA. Because of the relatively high DNA-to-protein ratio, the buoyant density of the intact virion in cesium chloride (CsCl) is 1.39 to 1.42 g/cm^3 (21). The heavy buoyant density in CsCl permits the ready separation of AAV from helper Ad in co-infections. Both heavier and lighter forms of the virion occur (22,84). The latter are particles containing DNA molecules with significant deletions, and these particles can function as defective interfering (DI) particles. The exact role of the heavier-than-normal particles in infections is unknown. The encapsidated DNA molecules are indistinguishable from those of normal-density particles and so, presumably, some of the coat protein molecules are missing. Whether the missing proteins constitute a specific set is unknown. Finally, the sedimentation coefficient of the virion in neutral sucrose gradients is 110 to 122 (300).

Possibly as a consequence of its structural simplicity, the virion is extremely resistant to inactivation. It is stable between pH 3 and 9 and at 56°C for 60 min. The virus can be inactivated by formalin, β-propriolactone, hydroxylamine, and oxidizing agents (21).

The Genome

The genome is a linear, single-stranded polydeoxynucleotide chain (80,237). Several parvovirus DNAs have been completely sequenced (see Table 1) and the genome size is typically about 5 kilobases (kb). MVM DNA (the prototype autonomous parvovirus) contains 5,084 bases; AAV2 DNA (the prototype dependovirus) contains 4,679 bases (10,264). In general, autonomous parvoviruses encapsidate primarily strands of one polarity, the strand that is complementary to mRNA (i.e., the minus strand), whereas AAV encapsidates strands of both polarities with equal frequency (80,237). However, this distinction is not absolute. In the case of bovine parvovirus (BPV), only approximately 20% to 30% of the encapsidated strands are of the same polarity as mRNA, and in some hosts, LuIII (another autonomous parvovirus) encapsidates equal numbers of strands of both polarities (17).

All autonomous parvovirus genomes have palindromic sequences at both the 5′ and the 3′ termini of the virion (antimessenger) strand (Fig. 2). The palindromic sequence at the 3′ end of the virion strand (also commonly referred to as the left end) of most murine autonomous parvovirus DNAs is approximately 115 bases long (8). In the human parvovirus B19, this sequence is more than 300 nucleotides in length (86). Because of its palindromic nature, the 3′ end can fold back on itself to form a hairpin structure stabilized by hydrogen bonding between self-complementary sequences. This hairpin structure (see Fig. 2) is believed to be shaped like either a Y or a T, but its exact three-dimensional structure is not known. There is also a conserved GAA/GA mismatch bubble in the stem of the hairpin.

The 5′ end (or right end) of autonomous parvoviruses is also palindromic and can form a hairpin, but the sequence is completely unrelated to that at the 3′ end of the virion strand (see Fig. 2). An exception is the 5′ end of the human B19 genome, in which the two ends are identical (86). The MVM 5′ palindrome is 207 bases long (10). Like the 3′ terminal sequence, the 5′ terminal sequence of MVM is not a perfect palindrome (see Fig. 2); again there are short, self-contained internal palindromic sequences (not shown) and an AGA bubble. The 5′ terminal sequence is also not unique. Two sequences that represent an inversion of the terminal segment of the genome are found with equal frequency and are called flip and flop. The two orientations are a consequence of the fact that an inversion of the 5′ sequence occurs during DNA replication (see later). Because the 5′ hairpin is not perfectly symmetric, the two forms can be distinguished by restriction analysis.

In contrast to the sequence at the 5′ end of the virion strand, which can exist in either of two orientations, the 3′ terminal sequence is usually unique; only one orientation is found. (The relevance of this organization to the process of DNA replication is discussed later.) The exception is BPV, in which about 10% of the 3′ end of the genome is, like its 5′ end, inverted (255).

Unlike autonomous parvovirus DNA, the AAV genome has an inverted terminal repetition of 145 nucleotides (181). The first 125 bases form a palindromic sequence that, when folded to maximize base-pairing, forms a T-shaped structure almost identical to that formed by the 3′ terminal sequence of the virion strand of

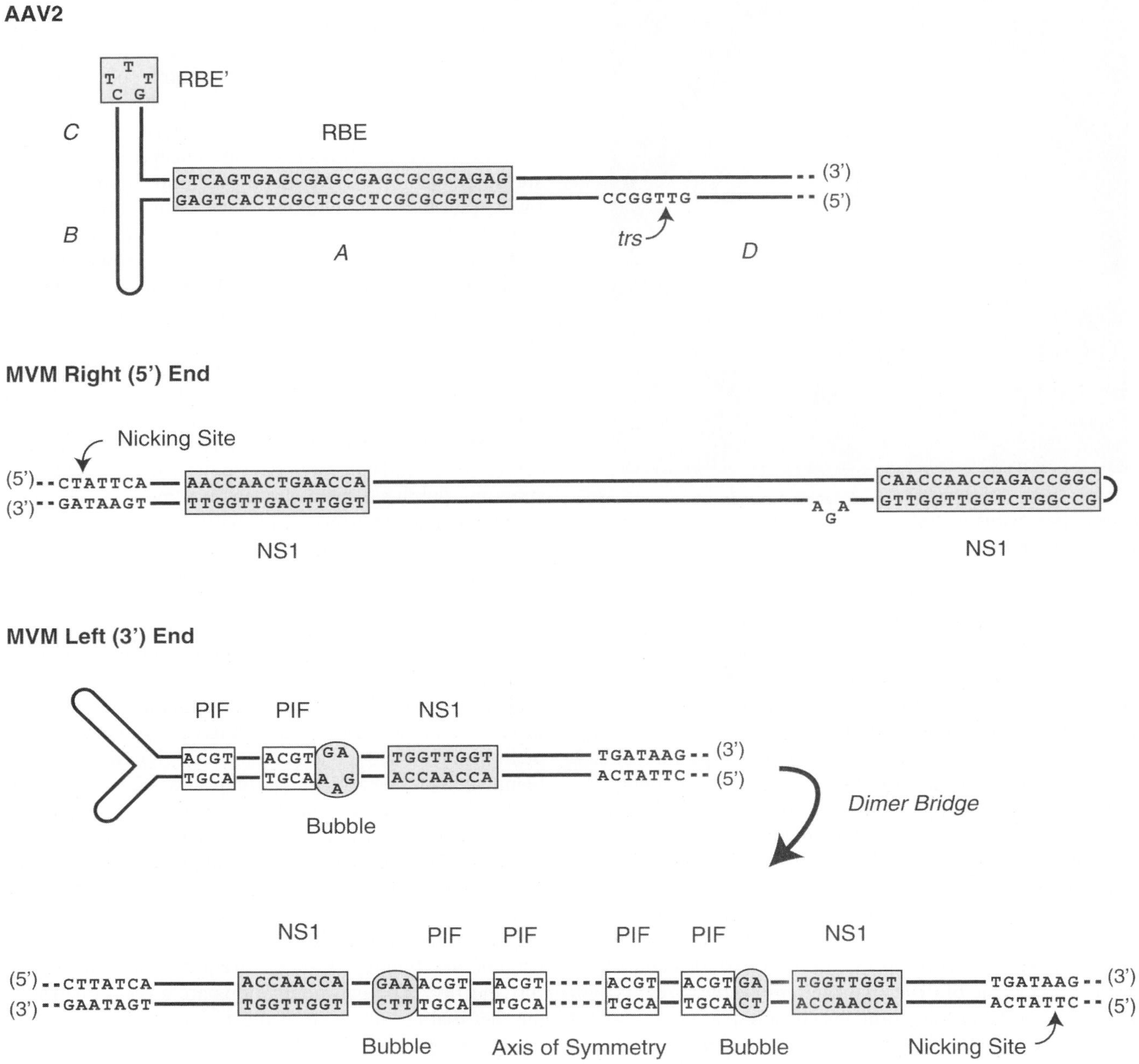

FIG. 2. Comparison of the 3′ and 5′ terminal palindromic structures of MVM DNA with the AAV2 terminal repeat, which is identical at both ends. Also shown is the 3′ dimer bridge that is formed in a dimer replicative intermediate during MVM DNA replication. In each case, the key sequence elements are indicated that are required for AAV Rep nicking at the *trs*, or MVM NS1 nicking at the 5′ (right end) hairpin or in the 3′ (left end) dimer bridge. The hairpin sequences are shown in their most stable secondary structure. In the AAV hairpin, B and C by convention are the small internal palindromes flanked by the A palindrome that forms the stem of the first 125 bases. The D sequence comprises the remaining 20 bases of the TR that are inboard of the *trs*. See text for details.

autonomous parvoviruses (see Fig. 2). As with the sequence in autonomous parvovirus DNA, the palindromic terminal sequence in AAV DNA may be characterized more accurately as two internal palindromes (nucleotides 42 to 84) flanked by a more extensive palindrome (nucleotides 1 to 41 and 85 to 125). In the folded configuration, only seven of 125 bases remain unpaired. Six are required to allow the internal palindromes to fold over, and the seventh separates the two internal palindromes. Both ends of AAV exist in two orientations, flip and flop, which are essentially inversions of the terminal 125 bases. In this respect, the AAV terminal repeats

(...) are similar to the autonomous parvovirus 5′ (right end) palindromic sequence. Again, the two orientations can be detected because the two internal palindromes are not identical. In the flip orientation, the B palindrome (see Fig. 2) is closer to the end of the genome than the C palindrome, whereas in the flop orientation, the C palindrome is closer to the end. Furthermore, there is an additional heterogeneity in the extreme terminal bases. The canonical 5′ terminal sequence in AAV2 DNA is 5′ TTG. However, 50% of the molecules isolated from virions lack the first T, and a further 15% lack both Ts.

Because mature virion DNA is the end product of DNA replication, any model proposed must be able to account for the nucleotide sequence arrangements found in virion DNA. The terminal sequence organization has offered valuable clues to the mechanism of DNA replication. Thus, the similarities and differences between the terminal sequence arrangements of autonomous parvovirus DNA and those of AAV DNA have led to similar models of DNA replication for the two genera that differ in several key steps (see later).

There are additional similarities in the internal organization of the genomes of the vertebrate viruses (Fig. 3).

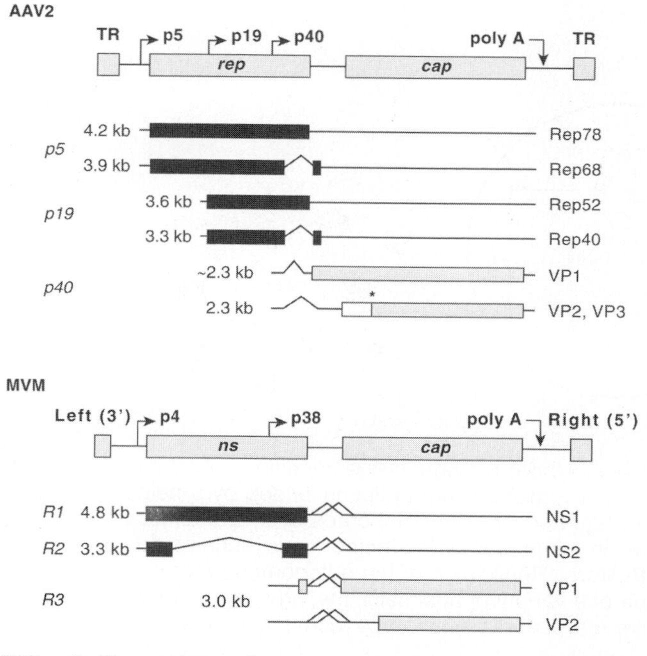

FIG. 3. Transcriptional maps of MVM, the prototype autonomous parvovirus, and AAV2, the prototype dependovirus. Terminal palindromes and ORFs are represented by *boxes.* The approximate positions of the promoters and polyadenylation sites in each genome are indicated by *arrows.* AAV has three promoters, at map positions 5, 19, and 40; MVM has two promoters, at mps 4 and 38. All AAV and MVM transcripts are co-terminal at a polyadenylation signal near the right end of the genome. Below each genome are the major mRNAs synthesized by each virus along with (on the left) their common names and their sizes in kilobases. At the right of each message is (or are) the viral protein(s) translated from each mRNA.

All have two large open reading frames (ORFs) that do not overlap (10,228,264). One extends approximately from map position (mp) 5 to 40, whereas the second extends approximately from mp 50 to 90. As is discussed later, the ORF in the right half of the genome codes for all the caspsid proteins, and that in the left half codes for nonstructural proteins.

Coat Proteins

Both autonomous parvovirus and AAV virions contain three capsid proteins [with the exception of Aleutian disease virus (ADV), B19, and simian parvovirus, which contain only two coat proteins] (21). For different species of autonomous parvoviruses, the proteins have approximate MWs of 80,000 to 86,000 (VP1), 64,000 to 75,000 (VP2), and 60,000 to 62,000 (VP3). Those of lapine parvovirus are significantly larger: 96,000 (VP1), 85,000 (VP2), and 75,000 (VP3). Except for ADV, VP3 is the major coat protein, representing 80% to 90% of the total mass. Some virus preparations are lacking in VP3, and its abundance appears to depend on the time during infection when the virions are isolated. LuIII preparations, for example, may contain only VP3 in detectable quantities. All AAV preparations characterized to date have three coat proteins: VP1, 87,000; VP2, 73,000; and VP3, 62,000 (143). In neither genus is there any evidence for glycosylation of any of the coat proteins; however, all parvovirus proteins appear to be phosphorylated. The N terminus is blocked in the case of the AAV VP3 protein (19,143).

In addition to the fact that all three parvovirus coat proteins appear to be coded for by overlapping in-frame DNA sequences, a further complexity has been reported. In the cases of both AAV1 and AAV2, the coat proteins VP1 and VP3 can be further subdivided by polyacrylamide gel electrophoresis into several subspecies (191). The molecular basis for the difference in mobility is unknown.

PARVOVIRUS INFECTION

Host Range

Parvoviruses replicate in the nuclei of infected cells. Of all the DNA viruses, they seem to be among the most dependent on cellular function. The autonomous parvoviruses require the cell to go through S phase to replicate (269). Unlike the polyomaviruses and Ad, the parvoviruses do not have the ability to stimulate or turn on host DNA synthesis in resting cells. The autonomous parvoviruses simply wait for S phase in the host they infect. AAV relies on a helper virus, adeno- or herpesvirus, to induce S phase or its equivalent (11,38) (Fig. 4). (The nature of the helper factors is described later.) There are also cell lines that can be made semipermissive for AAV

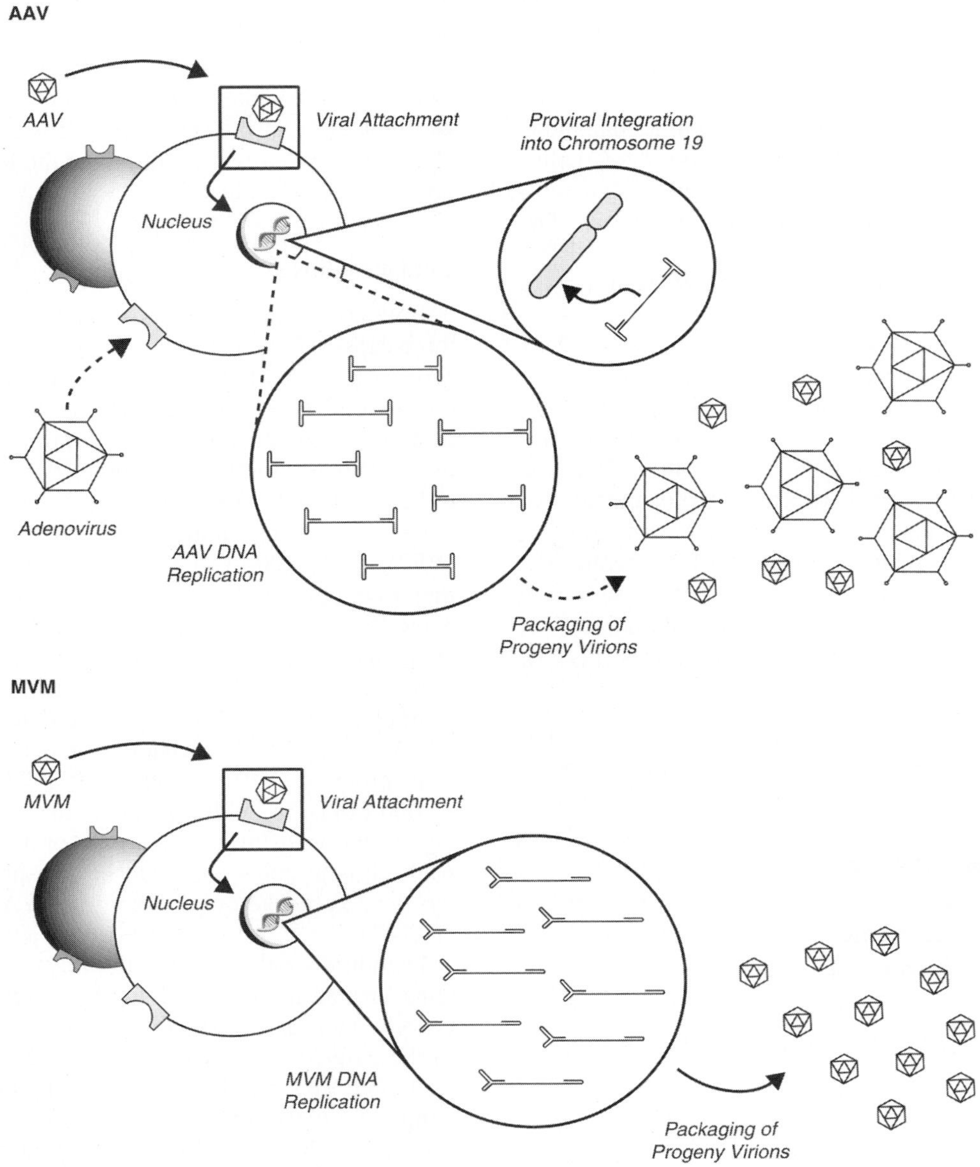

FIG. 4. Top: Replication of adeno-associated virus (AAV). Under nonpermissive conditions, AAV integrates into the q arm of human chromosome 19, where it remains silent until challenged by a helper virus (e.g., an adenovirus). This leads to rescue of the integrated virus from the chromosome and induction of the lytic cycle. Under permissive conditions (i.e., in the presence of a helper virus, such as adenovirus), AAV replicates, resulting in host cell lysis. **Bottom:** Replication of the autonomous *Parvoviridae.* After adsorption of the virus at the cell membrane of a variety of host cells, the virus enters and is transported to the nucleus. During S phase, the cellular replication machinery is recruited for viral replication, leading to virus production and cell lysis.

infection, without helper co-infection, by various chemical or physical treatments, described in the section on helper functions. The autonomous parvoviruses are relatively species specific, although some hamster viruses were first isolated as apparent contaminants from human tumor cells grown in the laboratory, and MVM will grow in both mouse and human transformed cell lines (73). In the case of MVM, tissue specificity has been observed for differentiated cells (262). The prototype strain MVM(p) replicates in murine fibroblasts but not in T lymphocytes. A second strain has been discovered, MVM(i), that displays the opposite phenotype.

Genetic analysis of parvoviruses has been greatly facilitated by the discovery that clones of complete parvovirus genomes in bacterial plasmids are infectious when transfected into mammalian cells. This fact, together with the complete sequence of several prototype strains, notably MVM and AAV2, has made it possible to construct and propagate any mutant in a bacterial plasmid vector, and then to transfect the intact plasmid clone into cell culture. If the cells are permissive or (in the case of AAV) infected by helper virus, the parvoviral genes are expressed, the inserted genome is rescued from the plasmid and replicated, and infectious virions are produced. In this way, it has been possible to correlate specific phenotypes with specific mutations at fixed points along the genome, and thus it has been possible to develop meaningful genetic maps (125,244). The infectivity of parvovirus plasmids has also been the key to their development as mammalian transduction vectors (126).

Tissue Specificity, Viral Entry, and Cryptic Infection

Although dividing cells are required for the replication of autonomous parvoviruses, not all dividing cells are susceptible to, or permissive for, viral infection. In the case of MVM, susceptible cells have large numbers of surface receptors (10^5 or more). The nature of these receptors has not been defined; however, the receptors appear to contain sialic acid, as pretreatment of cells with neuraminidase prevents viral attachment (73). The surface receptors are missing from B lymphocytes. Additionally, MVM(p) is restricted in T lymphocytes at the level of gene expression even though the virus can enter the cell; in contrast, the related variant MVM(i) is permissive in T cells (262). The host range restriction is caused by several mutations in the capsid (13). In other cells, transcription can occur but DNA replication is inhibited. The loss of permissiveness seen at the level of cell culture is reflected in the general resistance of older animals to infection in spite of the presence of rapidly dividing tissues.

The narrow host range of B19 virus (primarily erythrocyte precursors) is partly the result of the distribution of its receptor. The human B19 virus receptor is globoside, the blood group P antigen, which is found on only a few cell types (35). Some of the narrow host-range specificity can also be attributed to tissue-specific gene expression (162). Both nonstructural (NS) and capsid genes have been implicated in the porcine parvovirus host range (281). In the case of MVM, NS2 has been specifically implicated in tissue specificity (198).

Parvoviruses frequently cause semipermissive (sometimes called restrictive) infections, which can imply a low level of viral multiplication in the intact host (73). At the level of cell culture, this seems best illustrated by the establishment of carrier cultures in which viral multiplication also occurs at a low level. The situation is the result of a low fraction of cells that are permissive, and it is plastic in that viral variants frequently arise that can infect the majority of cells in the culture (236). The reciprocal situation has also been observed, in which resistant cells arise from clones of susceptible cells. The frequency of semipermissive infection raises the question of whether the autonomous parvoviruses can cause latent infections by integration of the viral genome into cellular DNA as a provirus, as is seen with AAV. To date, no evidence for integration of autonomous parvoviral DNA during viral replication can be detected, nor has integration been observed during abortive infections.

Several receptors used by AAV2 for viral entry have been identified. These include heparin sulfate proteoglycan (267), the fibroblast growth factor receptor 1 (222), and the integrin $\alpha_v\beta_5$ (266). Uptake of AAV by susceptible cells occurs rapidly (half-life, 10 min) through a standard receptor-mediated endocytosis from clathrin-coated pits (16). When the virus escapes from endosomes is not clear, but within 30 minutes the virus accumulates perinuclearly and within 2 hours virus particles are detected within the nucleus. It is still not clear whether uncoating occurs in the nucleus or at the nuclear pore.

DEPENDOVIRUSES

Overview

One of the outstanding features of AAV replication in cell culture has been the requirement for co-infection of the cell by an unrelated helper virus (see Fig. 4). Either an Ad or a herpesvirus can supply complete helper functions for fully permissive AAV infection (11,38). In the absence of helper virus, AAV can establish a latent infection in cell culture that involves integration of the viral genome into a unique site on human chromosome 19 (48, 155,248). Superinfection of cell lines carrying a provirus with Ad or herpes will rescue the integrated genome and initiate a fully productive infection (48,169,190). In light of this, it has been assumed that AAV uses latency in chromosome 19 as a strategy to survive in the absence of a helper.

The situation during natural infections is not as clear. *In vivo* (i.e., in human infections), AAV has typically been found as a contaminant of Ad isolates (24). It is generally assumed, therefore, that natural AAV infections occur via the respiratory or gastrointestinal route as is the case for Ad. However, as yet, it is not clear what tissue or organ is a preferred site of latency in humans. Efforts by several groups to demonstrate latency in human lung samples have failed to detect AAV. AAV has been recovered from a small percentage (1% to 5%) of hematopoietic cells and from the genital tract of female patients suspected of herpes infections (106,117). One report (273) suggested that AAV was present in some first-trimester abortion material, but this has not been confirmed (106). However, AAV has been found at a surprisingly high frequency (20%) in muscle biopsies (Xiao, personal communication, 2000). Recently, Dutheil et al. (97) demonstrated that the chromosome 19 integration site that is preferred by AAV is linked to the slow skeletal muscle–specific gene troponin T1 (TNNT1), and the cardiac troponin I gene (TNNI3). Several proviral cell lines established *in vitro* were shown to contain rearrangements of the TNNT1 gene due to integration. Additionally, Samulski and his colleagues (Samulski, personal communication, 2000) have demonstrated that recombinant AAV preferentially transduces slow skeletal muscle fibers in rodent models. Together, these observations have led to the hypothesis that the natural site of AAV latency in humans might be skeletal muscle. Skeletal muscle is known to be resistant to Ad and herpes infection when these viruses are administered intravascularly, thus muscle could be a reservoir that is protected from rescue by AAV helper viruses. Because muscle fibers are multinucleated, integration of AAV and the possible disruption of the TNNT1 locus would produce minimal effects on the host. However, as yet, no one has demonstrated that AAV is integrated into the chromosome 19 target in human samples.

As discussed later, the role of the Ad helper functions seems in part to be the induction of the appropriate cellular milieu required for AAV DNA replication. The notion that AAV replication is possible once the appropriate cellular genes have been induced suggests that the appropriate cellular milieu could be established in the absence of helper virus. Indeed, several groups have reported that pretreatment of transformed or tumor cell lines with a variety of genotoxic agents can render the cells semipermissive for AAV replication in the absence of helper virus co-infection (307, and refs. therein). Agents that have been successfully used include ultraviolet (UV) irradiation, cycloheximide, hydroxyurea, aphidicolin, topoisomerase inhibitors, and several chemical carcinogens. Recently, Hermonat and colleagues (personal communication, 2000) have demonstrated that keratinocyte cultures can support AAV replication, albeit poorly, in the absence of a helper virus. In this system, basal cells are nonpermissive for replication but become semipermissive as the cells differentiate. The value of these semipermissive systems is that they may help identify cellular functions that are normally induced by the helper virus.

Helper Functions

Adenoviruses, herpes simplex virus (HSV) types I and II, cytomegalovirus, and pseudorabies virus all serve as complete helpers for AAV replication (11,38,197). The AAV host range is identical to the normal host range for the helper virus. Genetic analysis of helper functions has been most extensive for Ad. Many of the identified Ad early functions serve as helper functions for AAV replication, but no Ad late functions have been found to be necessary. Four Ad proteins have been shown to be required for complete helper function: the early region IA (EIA) transactivator protein, the EIB 55-kd protein, the E4 34-kd protein, and the E2A DNA-binding protein. Additionally, synthesis of the Ad virus-associated (VA) RNAs is required. Ad EIA function is required for the other Ad early regions to be transcribed (197). Similarly, an EIA function is required for AAV transcripts to be detected by Northern blotting (140,170,232). Two EIA proteins with overlapping sequences of 289 and 243 amino acids, respectively, have been identified. The former can both activate and inhibit gene expression in trans, whereas the latter primarily inhibits gene expression. The 289-amino-acid EIA protein is responsible for transactivation of AAV gene expression (46). EIA, in concert with other Ad early genes, also induces a variety of changes in cellular gene expression. The most important may be that EIA induces cells to enter S phase and to synthesize cellular DNA replication proteins that are likely to be needed for AAV DNA replication (197).

E4 was originally identified as encoding a helper function specifically required for AAV DNA replication. The E4 product involved is a 34-kd protein that is the product of the E4 ORF 6 gene and it can form a complex with the 55-kd EIB protein during a productive Ad infection (135). Both the 55-kd and the 34-kd proteins have been shown to regulate the expression of AAV genes, possibly at the level of transport of mRNA to the cytoplasm (246). In a general sense, EIB has also been identified as being required for AAV DNA replication to occur, but it does not seem to have a consistent effect on AAV transcript accumulation (140,170,232,246). More recently, studies of transduction mediated by recombinant AAVs (rAAVs) that carry marker genes have suggested that the E4 ORF 6 protein enhances the conversion of single-stranded input viral genomes to a duplex form by promoting second-strand synthesis (101,102). Grifman et al. (115) have shown that the ORF 6 gene product promotes degradation of cyclin A and inhibits the kinase activity of cdc2. The net effect of these changes would be to stop the cell cycle in late S or G2. Because cellular DNA replication enzymes are induced during this phase of the cell cycle, this could in part explain the effect of ORF 6 on AAV DNA replication.

E2A encodes a 72-kd single-strand DNA binding protein (DBP) that is required for Ad DNA synthesis but that does not appear to be required for AAV DNA replication (39), although particle formation is greatly inhibited by certain E2A gene mutations (141). DBP stimulates transcription from AAV promoters (39,45) and may be involved in mRNA transport and stability. In spite of the absence of genetic evidence that Ad DBP is required for AAV DNA replication, recent *in vitro* studies of AAV DNA replication using cell-free extracts suggest that Ad DBP is preferentially used for AAV DNA replication in place of the human single-strand DBP, replication protein A (RPA) (290). In contrast, the E2B region, which produces the Ad terminal protein, and the Ad DNA polymerase, both of which are directly involved in the process of Ad DNA replication, is not required for AAV replication. Finally, Ad VAI RNA has been reported to facilitate the initiation of AAV protein synthesis (139) by preventing the interferon-induced host-cell shutoff of translation.

Two detailed studies on the HSV-1 genes required for productive AAV infection have been reported. Unfortunately, the conclusions were somewhat different. The first study (193) identified the following HSV proteins as providing helper functions for AAV: ICP4 transactivator, DNA polymerase, ICP8 single-strand DBP, the origin-binding protein, and two of the three subunits of the helicase–primase complex (UL5, UL8). The second study (294) identified ICP8 and all three components of the helicase–primase complex as helper functions. It should be noted that the latter study used a heterologous promoter; normally, ICP4 function is required for expression of HSV replication genes. The former study found that maximal AAV replication required all the genes identified but that only ICP4 was essential for AAV replication per se. It is not clear why with Ad, most of the viral DNA replication genes are not required, but with herpes, most of the helper functions are replication enzymes.

Genetic Map

The AAV genetic map (see Fig. 3) has been derived primarily from studies of AAV2 (125,190,247,252,274) but is highly conserved among all of the AAV serotypes. There is a large ORF (cap) on the right side of the genome (mp 50 to 90), which encodes the three coat proteins of the virus. Frameshift and deletion mutants within this region do not block DNA replication, but the accumulation of progeny single strands is inhibited, presumably because this requires encapsidation (126,274). Mutations in the N-terminal region of the cap ORF, which affect VP1 exclusively, package DNA but produce virus particles that have lower infectivity. There is also a large ORF in the left half of the genome (mp 5 to 40), which has been called the rep region because any frameshift mutation or significant deletion within the region blocks DNA replication (126,274). At least four proteins have been detected (Rep78, Rep68, Rep52, and Rep40), which correspond to the four mRNAs that have been mapped to this region (see Fig. 3) (192). It is possible to selectively eliminate Rep78 and 68 (from the p5 transcripts), and this type of mutation completely blocks all AAV-directed transcript accumulation that can be detected by Northern analysis, and it completely eliminates DNA replication (126,168).

The larger Rep proteins play a critical regulatory role in every phase of the AAV life cycle. Under nonpermissive conditions (no helper virus) Rep68/78 negatively regulates AAV gene expression and DNA replication and is required for site-specific integration in the host cell genome to establish a latent infection (148,164,253,275). In the presence of helper, Rep68/78 is a transactivator of AAV gene expression (168) and is essential for DNA replication and rescue of the viral genome from the integrated state (125). Mutants that are defective for the synthesis of the two smaller Rep proteins (Rep52 and 40 from the p19 promoter) have been made by changing the initiator AUG for these proteins to GGG (47). The resulting mutant is able to replicate DNA, but no mature single-stranded DNA is encapsidated. The phenotype is thus similar to a coat protein mutant. Other smaller ORFs exist near the middle of the genome, but the production of proteins corresponding to these regions is less clear.

Mutations in either the rep or cap ORFs can be complemented in trans. In contrast, the inverted TRs of 145 bases are required in cis for both DNA replication and transcription (18,252). In addition to these functions, the TR is required for encapsidation (190), integration of the genome during the establishment of a latent infection (309), and rescue of the genome from the integrated state (247). All of these functions are detailed later.

Transcription

In a productive infection, six polyadenylated, capped RNAs are detectable by Northern blotting (see Fig. 3) (171). In decreasing size, the mRNAs have apparent lengths of 4.2 kb, 3.9 kb, 3.6 kb, 3.3 kb, 2.6 kb, and 2.3 kb. These are synthesized from three conventional RNA polymerase II promoters at mp 5, 19, and 40 (114,182). All of the RNAs are 3′ co-terminal and are polyadenylated downstream from an AATAAA signal at mp 96 (264). The two largest transcripts (4.2 and 3.9 kb) are synthesized from the promoter at mp 5 (p5), the next two (3.6 and 3.3 kb) are from the promoter at mp 19 (p19), and the two smallest RNAs (2.6 and 2.3 kb) are from the promoter at mp 40 (p40). There is an intron at mp 42 to 46, and there are both spliced and unspliced mRNAs produced from all three promoters, hence the three pairs of transcripts. The smallest RNA (2.3 kb) is the major species and is produced from the p40 promoter. It is used to translate all three capsid proteins. The 2.3-kb species actually consists of two alternatively spliced mRNAs (196). The major spliced species directs the synthesis of the major capsid protein, VP3, from a conventional AUG codon, and the minor capsid protein, VP2, from an upstream in-frame ACG codon. The minor spliced 2.3-kb message includes an upstream AUG codon that allows the translation of the entire cap ORF to produce the minor capsid protein VP1. No clear role has been established for the unspliced 2.6-kb message. The p5 and p19 promoters generate two mRNA species each (spliced and unspliced), which code for the four AAV nonstructural proteins, Rep78 and 68 from p5, and Rep52 and 40 from p19 (182,192). In the case of the p5 and p19 RNAs, the unspliced species is the major one, but the reverse is true of the p40 RNAs. During the course of infection, the unspliced p5 transcript, and the Rep78 protein coded by it, appear first (192). This is followed shortly by the synthesis of the p19 and p40 transcripts and the proteins they encode. Additionally, the spliced p5 and p19 RNA species accumulate later in infection than the unspliced species. This is apparently the result of a change in splicing that is caused by either Ad infection or Rep78 expression (276).

Several groups have mapped the regulatory signals that control AAV transcription (Fig. 5). Chang et al. (46) mapped two regulatory sequences in the p5 promoter. The first corresponded to a sequence in the Ad major late promoter activated by EIA (Ad MLP). The second was a sequence that binds the cellular transcription factor YYI. Two YYI sites were found, one upstream of the TATA box and one overlapping the p5 message start site. McCarty et al. (188) subsequently mapped a Rep binding element (RBE) between the TATA box and the downstream YYI site. There are four additional RBEs, two in each of the two TRs. Together, these elements seem to be responsible for controlling AAV p5 transcription (164,212). Regulatory sequences upstream of the p19 and p40 promoters have also been identified (see Fig. 5). In the p19 pro-

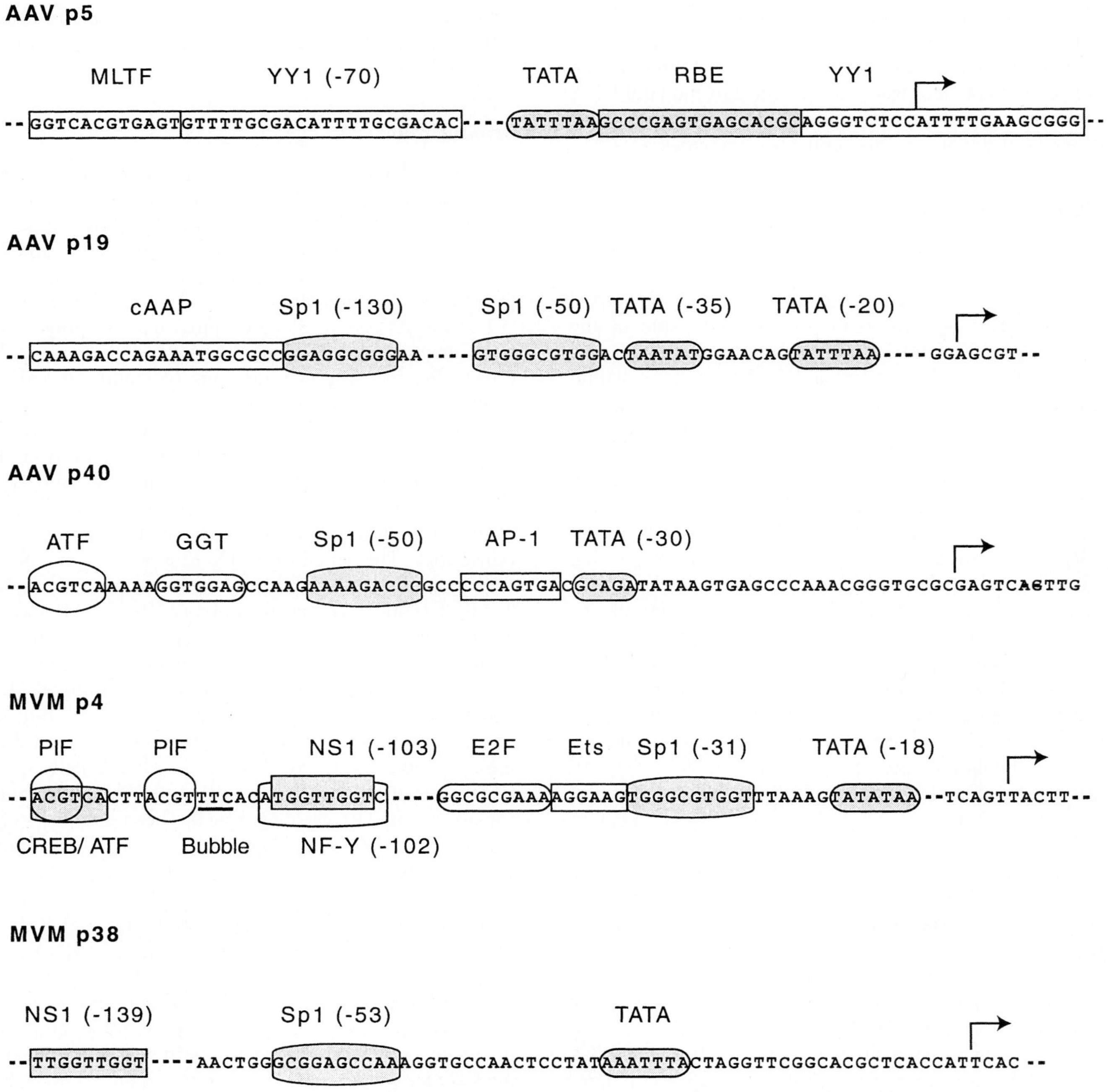

FIG. 5. Approximate position of promoter elements within the AAV2 and MVM promoters. *Arrow* indicates the start of the major mRNA from each promoter. See text for details.

moter, the proximal TATA box, two Sp1 sites, and a novel sequence that binds an as yet unidentified cellular factor, cellular AAV activating protein (cAAP), were found to be sufficient by mutation analysis for p19 transcription (214). In the p40 promoter, an Sp1 site and the TATA box were essential, and ATF and AP1 sites also may play a role (213). The regulation of AAV transcription is complex. This is apparently because following infection, the virus can choose one of two paths for persistence: It can either establish a latent infection or proceed through a productive viral infection. The switch for these two paths appears to be controlled primarily by the Ad EIA gene and the AAV *rep* gene, as discussed later.

In the absence of helper virus, only a small amount of Rep78 is synthesized from the p5 promoter. This is sufficient to bind to the p5 RBE and completely repress further p5 transcription (164,212). Mutation of the p5 RBE can lead to higher p5 expression and a virus that is partially permissive for DNA replication in some cell lines (288). Repression is tight, so that generally it is not possible to detect p5 transcripts or Rep protein. However, it is possible to detect *rep* gene function biologically because Rep inhibits expression from a number of heterologous promoters (122,128,134,167). Although the domain of Rep78/68 that binds to the RBE has been mapped to the region of Rep78 that is not present in Rep52 and 40 (210), the p19 Rep proteins are also capable of repressing the p5 promoter (163). Furthermore, although there is no strong RBE within the p19 promoter, Rep52 is capable of repressing p19 transcription (134, 163). This suggests that binding to the RBE at p5 is not the sole mechanism by which Rep proteins can repress transcription. Indeed, studies of the papilloma virus transcription control region and the human immunodeficiency virus (HIV) long terminal repeat (LTR) suggest that Rep can repress transcription from these heterologous promoters, which have no RBE, by interacting with a variety of transcription factors (134). Although there is active repression of p5 and p19 promoter activity by the Rep proteins, repression of p40 has been difficult to demonstrate. Yet there is little accumulation of p40 transcripts or capsid protein in the absence of Ad infection (169,186).

In the presence of Ad co-infection, a cascade of transcriptional regulation seems to rapidly induce the synthesis of all AAV genes. First, the Ad EIA transactivator protein induces transcription from the p5 promoter and synthesis of Rep78/68. The mechanism of EIA transactivation of p5 is not clear, but it may involve interaction with YYI, which can function as a transactivator or a repressor (254). Additionally, Rep may interact with the TATA binding protein (TBP) or Rep may be displaced from the p5 RBE by YY1, thereby derepressing the p5 promoter (127,164). Rep78/68 in turn now behaves like a transactivator protein rather than a repressor and induces transcription from the p5 and p19 promoters (168,212, 293). To accomplish this, Rep apparently needs to be bound to the RBE that is present either in the TR or at the p5 promoter, as the absence of both elements reduces transactivation of p19 and p40. Curiously, mutations in the p5 RBE continue to derepress p5 transcription (212), suggesting that Rep bound to the p5 RBE continues to repress p5 even while it transactivates p19 and p40. The absence of the RBE within the TR, however, leads to lower p5 activity, suggesting that Rep bound to the TR transactivates the p5 promoter as well as the p19 and p40 promoters (18,212). Finally, transactivation of the p19 and p40 promoters and repression of p5 appears to be coordinately regulated by the p5 RBE and Rep protein (186,212–214). Deletion of the p5 RBE element (and the TR) simultaneously increases p5 transcription and decreases p19 and p40 transcription. The elements in p5, p19, and p40 required for this coordination have been partially mapped (see Fig. 5). p19 Transcription requires the p5 or TR RBE, as well as the −50 p19 Sp1 site and the cAAP site upstream of p19 (214). Transactivation of p40 requires the same elements required for p19 transactivation and the proximal −50 Sp1 site upstream of the p40 start (213). How this is accomplished is not clear, but Rep has been shown to bind to Sp1 (214), TBP (127), and PC4 (292), a general transactivation protein for pol II transcription. Presumably, some or all of these Rep interactions are involved.

Several other regulatory circuits have been uncovered: (a) Rep52/40, which represses p5 in the absence of Ad, derepresses p5 in the presence of Ad, possibly by interacting with the larger Rep proteins (212). (b) Overexpression of Rep78/68 reduces the level of capsid protein by a posttranscriptional mechanism, possibly by reducing translation of the capsid message (276). (c) At least one cis-active negative regulatory sequence has been mapped to a region between mp 28 and 37 (168). Deletion of the sequence leads to higher levels of the upstream transcripts, and insertion of the sequence downstream of the p40 promoter reduces p40 transcript levels. Whether this cis-active negative regulatory sequence inhibits transcript elongation or adversely affects transcript stability is not known.

The net effect of these positive and negative feedback loops appears to be the maintenance of a constant ratio of Rep78/68, Rep52/40, and the three capsid proteins during productive infection. Why it is critical to maintain this ratio so tightly is not entirely clear. One possibility is that overexpression of capsid proteins might prematurely deplete the pool of replicative intermediates required to sustain a productive infection. On the other hand, overexpression of the Rep proteins might increase the replicative pool of DNA at the expense of packaging.

DNA Replication

AAV DNA replication occurs via a single-strand displacement mechanism (Fig. 6) (120,265). No evidence

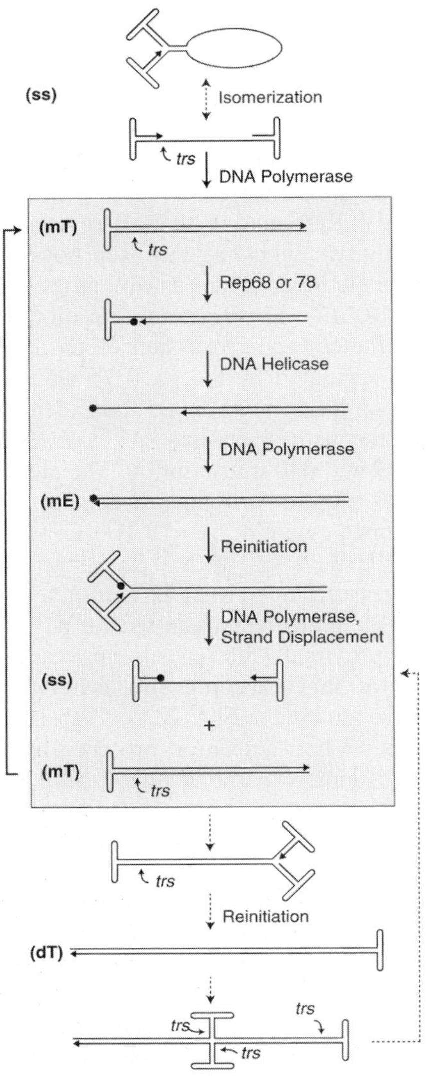

FIG. 6. Model for AAV DNA replication. *Gray box* highlights the reactions essential for generating single-stranded progeny DNA. mT, monomer turnaround RF; dt, dimer turnaround RF; ss, single-stranded viral DNA; mE, monomer extended RF. See text for details.

has been found for RNA primers or for the equivalent of Okazaki fragments (the presence of which would be indicative of lagging strand synthesis). Because all known DNA polymerases have a requirement for a primer with an available 3′ OH, in addition to a template, linear DNA genomes have had to evolve specialized terminal sequences to allow them to maintain the 5′ terminal sequences intact when the primer structure is resolved during replication. The basic model for parvovirus DNA replication (often called the rolling hairpin model) was first described by Straus et al. (265) and Tattersall and Ward (272). As noted earlier, the two ends of AAV are identical in sequence and palindromic. The palindromic inverted TR at the 3′ end of either strand can form a hairpin to serve as a primer to initiate synthesis of the complementary strand (181). This produces a linear duplex molecule in which the original 3′ end is covalently closed in the hairpin configuration, also called a monomer turnaround form (see Fig. 6, mT). The hairpin is nicked at a site near the end of the terminal palindrome (nucleotide 124 of the AAV sequence), and this produces a new 3′-hydroxyl primer that allows repair synthesis of the hairpin. This process is called terminal resolution (or strand transfer) and the site-specific and strand-specific nicking site is called the terminal resolution site (trs). The net result of terminal resolution is the first complete duplex molecule in which both ends are extended, the monomer extended form (see Fig. 6, mE). Either end can then denature and reanneal to form a double hairpinned structure, or rabbit ears (a process sometimes called reinitiation), and the newly hairpinned 3′ end initiates leading-strand displacement synthesis to generate a single-stranded genome (which is packaged) and a duplex genome covalently closed at one end. The process of terminal resolution and reinitiation is then repeated (see Fig. 6, gray box). Each time the cycle is completed, a new single-stranded progeny strand (see Fig. 6, ss) is generated, and the strand transfer process that occurs during terminal resolution inverts the TR. If a molecule covalently closed at one end is not resolved before completion of strand displacement from the other end, then a dimer molecule can be formed in which two genomes are present in an inverted orientation (head to head or tail to tail) with a single TR at their junction (see Fig. 6, dimer turnaround or dT).

A large amount of evidence now supports this mechanism. All of the predicted replicative intermediates have been found *in vivo* (201,265) and can also be generated with *in vitro* replication systems (201). These include monomers and dimers, with both ends extended or with one end covalently closed (201,265). Two orientations of the TR (flip and flop) are seen in replicative intermediates and in packaged DNA as predicted (180,244). Biochemical analysis of the Rep protein carried out by several groups *in vitro* also supports this mechanism. This has shown that Rep78/68 protein carries out the site-specific nicking reaction necessary for terminal resolution and has a DNA-DNA (and DNA-RNA) helicase activity and an ATPase activity, that is essential for nicking and probably for strand displacement (138,260,302).

The outstanding feature of the TR is the T- or Y-shaped structure that is formed when the terminal 125 bases are folded on themselves to optimize base-pairing (181). This structure is quite stable and appears to exist predominantly as B form DNA. Recent thermal melting and UV spectra analysis suggests a ΔH_{cal} of 614 kcal mol^{-1} (226). Thus, the T-shaped structure is likely to need the active intervention of a DNA helicase to unwind during terminal resolution and to re-form during the reinitiation step following resolution. Another issue is that the nicking site (*trs*) is present in both the hairpinned and linear extended forms of the TR, as well as in the linear junction between two genomes within a dimer molecule. Thus, some method for discriminating between these three forms must exist that allows nicking preferentially on the hairpinned substrate and the dimer, rather than on the linear extended TR, in which nicking appears to be minimal (50,188).

Mutational analyses of both the Rep coding sequence and the TR, as well as the development of a number of *in vitro* biochemical assays, have led to a good preliminary understanding of the terminal resolution reaction (see Fig. 2). The TR contains at least three specific sequences that direct the Rep-mediated *trs* endonuclease reaction. A 20- to 22-bp linear sequence, the RBE (also called RRS or RBS), within the stem of the T structure is sufficient to bind a Rep78 or 68 complex that consists of two to six Rep molecules (50,188,241,259,295). Most of the RBE sequence consists of a tandem $(GAGC)_4$ repeat. As few as two GAGC repeats are sufficient to bind Rep, and considerable heterogeneity in the RBE is tolerated (51,188,303). One of the functions of the RBE is apparently to assemble the Rep complex in a particular orientation that is subsequently required for *trs* endonuclease activity. Substrates that contain inversions of the RBE, for example, will bind Rep but are poorly nicked (32). The enzyme also makes contact with a GTTTC motif that is present in the small internal palindrome that is furthest away from the *trs*. This sequence motif, called the RBE′ (or RRS′), is present in both the flip and the flop orientations in the same position with respect to the *trs* (see Fig. 2) (32,241). Contacts with this motif as well as with several other bases within the small internal palindromes apparently account for the difference in binding affinity between the hairpinned and linear forms of the TR, which has been estimated to be as much as 100-fold (189,259), and the fact that the linear form of the TR is nicked with a lower efficiency than the hairpin (32,50,188,259,304). DNase protection and chemical interference assays suggest that the enzyme complex bound to the RBE in the absence of ATP does not actually make contact with the *trs* site (137,241).

Once bound to the TR, Rep carries out two sequential reactions. First, the DNA helicase activity of Rep unwinds the stem of the TR in a reaction that requires ATP hydrolysis and generates a single-stranded *trs* site (31,83,259); this explains why the *trs* endonuclease reaction is ATP dependent (138). A highly conserved inverted repeat sequence that flanks the nick site is probably used to form a cruciform structure, which brings the *trs* closer to the Rep complex that is still bound to the RBE (31,32). Evidence that Rep does not let go of the RBE prior to nicking comes from mutants in which the spacing between the RBE and the *trs* is increased; insertion of even three bases significantly reduces nicking activity (32). In the second step of the reaction, the endonuclease active site carries out a transesterification reaction, in which the tyrosine at amino acid position 156 of Rep is covalently joined to the 5′ phosphate end of the nick at the *trs* (83,138,257). This reaction is ATP independent. Y156 is part of a rolling circle replication (RCR) protein motif that is common to all parvovirus NS proteins and is similar to motifs found in many enzymes of bacterial and eukaryotic origin that nick the origin of plasmids that undergo rolling circle DNA replication (136).

The *trs* is also a specific sequence recognized by Rep. It consists of a seven-base sequence (3′CCGGT/TG5′) that is recognized only on the correct strand (31). Nicking occurs between the two Ts (138), and mutation of any of the seven bases on the nicked strand reduces nicking (31). Changes in the sequence of the complementary strand, however, have no effect on nicking. Thus, the AAV origin for DNA replication is a tripartite sequence that consists of the RBE, the RBE′, and the *trs*.

Several groups have clearly demonstrated that the transesterification reaction does not require ATP. The best evidence is that Rep will nick a variety of substrates in an ATP-independent reaction, provided that the RBE is duplex but the *trs* is single stranded (259). Generally, these substrates lose some specificity in the nicking site. However, recently Brister and Muzyczka (31) have constructed what appears to be the actual intermediate for nicking by deleting the *trs* sequences on the complementary strand, thus artificially extruding the *trs* into a stem-loop structure that contains the *trs* in a single-stranded loop. This substrate is cleaved in an ATP-independent fashion only at the correct nicking site; moreover, the substrate is nicked more efficiently than the conventional hairpin. Most recently, Rep also has been shown to nick a completely single-stranded substrate that contains only one strand of the RBE and the *trs* (257).

Additional evidence for the two-step *trs* endonuclease reaction comes from mutagenic analysis of the Rep coding sequence. Rep contains two domains that can be functionally separated. The C-terminal end that is present in Rep52 and 40 contains the Rep-associated DNA helicase activity (256). Rep52, like Rep78 and 68, has full DNA helicase activity when tested on primed single-stranded DNA substrates and behaves like a conventional 3′ to 5′ DNA helicase (256,316). In contrast, C-terminal truncations of Rep78, which retain the N-terminal sequences that are not present in Rep52, have no helicase or ATPase activity, but they are capable of binding to the RBE and they nick substrates that contain a single-stranded *trs*—that is, substrates in which the DNA helicase activity is not necessary to generate a single-stranded *trs* (83). Thus, the N-terminus of Rep78/68 contains most of the amino acid residues that are required for specific binding to the RBE and nicking the *trs*.

Unlike conventional RCR proteins, there does not appear to be an unlinking step for the Rep tyrosine phosphate bond with DNA. The Rep protein continues to be joined to the 5′ end of the nick through subsequent steps of DNA replication, and it apparently remains attached during packaging of the progeny strand (96,161,219,300). Mature, highly purified virus particles, however, do not appear to have significant quantities of Rep protein (161,317); thus, some mechanism exists for hydrolyzing the tyrosine phosphate linkage that has not yet been discovered.

Once the terminal hairpin is nicked, it is believed that the Rep helicase unwinds the hairpin and a cellular DNA polymerase copies the TR to form an extended terminal sequence. Evidence for this comes primarily from *in vitro* reactions in which Rep is the only helicase available (138). The possibility that a cellular helicase or a viral-encoded helicase (in the case of herpesvirus) participates in the reaction has not been excluded. Rep helicase is then most likely responsible for unwinding and refolding the duplex end to form the double-hairpin TR that is needed for further DNA synthesis. Evidence for this comes from *in vitro* assays in which cell-free extracts are used (289). By themselves, the extracts replicate linear AAV templates poorly. When purified Rep is added, these extracts become competent for AAV DNA replication. This suggests that Rep78/68 can induce the formation of the double-hairpin substrate required to initiate strand displacement synthesis. That Rep is capable of initiating the double-hairpin intermediate is also supported by characterization of its DNA helicase activity using defined substrates. Simple linear oligonucleotides appear to be poor substrates for Rep helicase, but oligonucleotides that contain an RBE can be unwound efficiently (316). Thus, the extended duplex TR, which contains two RBEs, is an efficient substrate for Rep helicase activity.

Both uninfected and Ad infected cell-free extracts have been used to replicate AAV DNA *in vitro* in a Rep and AAV ori-dependent manner. Typically, these extracts are supplemented with Rep78 or 68 purified from baculovirus, vaccinia, or bacterial clones, and study of these *in vitro* systems has provided additional information about AAV DNA replication. In general, Ad-infected extracts are significantly more active for *in vitro* AAV DNA synthesis (131,202,289). The block in DNA synthesis when uninfected extracts are used is not in the terminal resolution reaction but rather in the elongation reaction during strand displacement synthesis (202,289). Ward et al. (290) have presented evidence that the Ad-encoded DBP increases the processivity of AAV replication *in vivo*, allowing more efficient strand elongation. In spite of the fact that deletions of DBP are apparently viable for AAV DNA replication *in vivo* (39), DBP is preferentially used in place of the host single-strand binding complex, RPA, in the *in vitro* reaction. However, adding Ad DBP to uninfected extracts does not raise the level of DNA replication to the same level seen with an Ad-infected extract, suggesting that there are additional factors in an Ad-infected extract that are needed.

Ni et al. (201) have also examined AAV DNA replication in uninfected extracts. This group found conditions for stressing cells that apparently produced cell extracts that were permissive in the absence of Ad infection. Such conditions might be a model for the semipermissive *in vivo* AAV replication that has been demonstrated by several groups. As expected, Ni et al. (201) found that AAV DNA replication did not depend on DNA polymerase alpha–primase but was dependent on the presence of RPA, proliferating cell nuclear antigen (PCNA), and replication factor C (RFC). PCNA is a processivity factor that is essential for DNA polymerase delta and epsilon, both of which are believed to be involved in replication of cellular DNA. Epsilon was originally identified as a DNA repair enzyme. Both polymerases are essentially leading-strand DNA synthesis enzymes, and either would be appropriate for AAV DNA replication. RFC is a 3′ primer recognition enzyme that assembles PCNA at a 3′ hydroxyl. Reconstitution of the *in vitro* reaction with one or both purified polymerases, however, did not restore AAV DNA replication, suggesting again that there is an additional unidentified cellular factor necessary for AAV DNA replication.

At least two other cellular factors have been implicated in AAV DNA replication. The first is high mobility group protein 1 (HMG1), a protein that binds cruciform DNA (65). This protein has been shown to bind AAV hairpins and Rep. HMG1 stimulates Rep nicking of the TR, Rep ATPase activity and Rep repression of the p5 promoter. It is, therefore, likely to be directly involved in DNA replication. The second factor is a protein that binds specifically to one strand of the D sequence within the AAV TR (see Fig. 2), hence the name single-stranded D binding protein (ssD-BP) (183,223). This protein exists in two phosphorylation states. When bound by the phosphorylated form, the input single-stranded AAV genome is unable to synthesize the second strand to form the first replicative intermediate. The protein, which appears to be the 52-kd FK506 binding protein, FKBP52, binds to the 10 bases of D sequences (see Fig. 2) proximal to the *trs* and prevents DNA replication. When the nonphosphorylated form of the protein binds, second-strand synthesis proceeds normally. Phosphorylation of the protein appears to be controlled by the epidermal growth factor receptor protein (EGF-R) tyrosine kinase and correlates well with the ability of cells to be transduced by recombinant AAV vectors in the absence of helper virus. This is because the input vector single-stranded DNA must synthesize the second strand to produce a substrate for RNA polymerase II transcription. The role of this protein in productive infections (i.e., when helper virus is present) has not been reported.

Three types of substrates have been used for *in vitro* DNA replication. The first is a linear AAV duplex molecule, which is covalently cross-linked at both ends by the hairpinned form of the TR, a substrate called NE (no end) DNA. In this assay, Rep 68/78 protein is required, as is an extract from cells infected by Ad (202). The major product is linear duplex AAV DNA containing one newly synthesized strand and extended ends. Extracts of uninfected HeLa cells do not support replication, even if supplemented with Rep68. A second assay has been described (49,131,132,291) in which the substrate is either linear duplex AAV DNA or the same DNA contained in a bacterial plasmid vector. Again, Rep68/78 is required and an extract from uninfected HeLa cells does support replication. When the template is the plasmid construct, replication leads to rescue of the AAV insert from pBR322 and, in some instances, pBR322 gets replicated in addition to AAV. Whether the vector sequences are preferentially replicated as opposed to the AAV sequences appears to depend on the presence of Ad DBP.

An important observation is that rescue of the AAV insert from bacterial plasmids *in vitro* can be separated from the initiation of DNA replication in terms of template sequence requirement. Deletion of the terminal 55 bases from both TRs in the plasmid construct prevents rescue of the AAV insert but allows the entire construct to be replicated. The implications of this are that ori function does not require the entire TR and that a hairpin per se is not required for DNA replication (131). The minimal requirements for this reaction are an RBE and a *trs*. Replication in this case appears to be similar to the *in vitro* replication seen with plasmids that contain a copy of the chromosome 19 integration sequence (280). These plasmids have been shown to undergo a rolling circle type of replication in the presence of Rep and cell-free extracts, and a nick at the *trs*-like site within chromosome 19 apparently initiates replication. In both cases, nicking by Rep appears to occur because of the presence of an RBE and a nearby *trs* without an RBE′ or significant secondary structure. *In vitro* assays using such substrates have demonstrated that Rep can both bind and nick substrates that do not have an RBE′ or the cross-arms of the AAV hairpin (50,188). This reaction proceeds 20- to 100-fold less efficiently than nicking of the complete hairpin and may be an important aspect of the mechanism for AAV integration or rescue from human chromosome 19. There is evidence as well that rescue of AAV does not require Rep or DNA replication. One group identified a cellular enzyme, endo R, that recognizes potential triple-stranded DNA in the TR and excises AAV from recombinant plasmids (113). Another group has shown that a plasmid containing a single TR with two D sequences, analogous to an internal TR junction from a dimer replicative form (RF) molecule (see Fig. 6), can be converted rapidly to linear molecules when transfected into cells in the absence of Rep expression (306).

Single-stranded AAV DNA can form circles that are hydrogen bonded through the 20-bp D sequence (see Fig. 6). This type of structure is believed to be responsible for the ability of AAV TR deletions to be repaired to the wild-type sequence (247). As described earlier, the cloned duplex form of the genome is infectious when transfected into Ad-infected cells. Clones with deletions of up to 113 bases at one end are still infectious, and the resulting progeny contain genomes with wild-type termini at both ends (247). The repair process is thought to involve (a) base-pairing between the remaining complementary bases (32 base pairs in this case) and (b) use of the shorter 3′-terminal strand as a primer for repair synthesis, using the intact 5′ TR strand as the template. Mutants with deletions that extend beyond the bounds of the TR cannot be rescued. Thus, not only does the TR help to resolve the problem inherent to linear genomes of maintaining the integrity of the 5′-terminal sequences during the process of DNA replication, but it also confers the ability to repair terminal deletions of the type described earlier.

Deletion of an 11-base symmetrical sequence (at nucleotides 50 to 60) from both TRs, thus effectively removing one of the cross-arms of the T, abolishes the ability of a cloned genome to be rescued and replicated (247). Substitution of an alternative 8- or 12-base symmetrical sequence restores viability to the cloned genome (172). No differences can be detected in either the rate or the extent of DNA replication that occurs after viral infection under permissive conditions. Substitution of an asymmetric 12-base sequence does not significantly restore viability (28). This observation has been interpreted to mean that, at least in the region of the cross-arms, the conformation of the TR, when folded on itself, takes precedence over the actual sequence in terms of rescue and replication of the genome from the cloned state in a plasmid. However, it is now known that the sequence deleted in these constructs was the RBE′ motif that makes specific contacts with Rep. The RBE′ has a specific three-dimensional location with respect to the RBE and *trs* in the hairpinned TR and this, in addition to the sequence of the RBE′, may play a role in TR recognition by Rep. Thus far, it has been difficult to separate the role of the hairpin secondary structure from the RBE′ sequence for Rep binding, helicase, and nicking activity. Recent experiments in which the RBE′ sequence has been mutated without changing the overall structure of the TR suggest that the RBE′ contacts are important primarily for initiating DNA helicase activity on the hairpin and are essentially dispensable for the transesterification reaction (32).

The viability of the symmetrical substitutions offers the possibility of testing whether or not the ability of the TRs to perfectly base-pair and form a single-stranded circle is a requirement for normal AAV DNA replication. Constructs in which a viable TR substitution is inserted in one end and not the other are found to be capable of being packaged. Under some conditions, the chimeras were able to undergo many rounds of replication and encapsidation without the occurrence of gene conversion (27). Similarly, packaged genomes derived from wild-type AAV are equally divided between those whose TRs at both ends are in the same orientation (flip or flop) and those with TRs in the opposite orientation (180). Thus, although the termini definitely can interact during the process of replication, TR interaction or gene conversion does not appear to be essential for replication.

As with many DNA viruses, AAV DNA replication generates defective genomes. These structures contain internal deletions flanked by TRs. In some cases, the defective genomes contained inverted duplications of sequences from either end of the genome (84,121).

Protein Synthesis

Four nonstructural proteins, Rep78, 68, 52, and 40, have been identified immunologically and purified from bacterial or eukaryotic expression vectors. They have been named according to their apparent MWs on sodium dodecyl sulfate (SDS) acrylamide gels, but their actual MWs are 72, 62, 46, and 34 kd, respectively. The amounts of the individual proteins correspond reasonably well to the relative accumulations of the individual transcripts. The two larger species are predominantly nuclear proteins, whereas the smaller ones, Rep52 and 40, are also found in the cytoplasm (192).

Various functions ascribed to the Rep proteins have been mapped along the primary structure. As noted earlier, Rep52 (amino acids 225 to 621 of the rep ORF) retains full helicase activity (256). The region unique to Rep78/68 plus a few amino acids shared with Rep52/40 (amino acids 3 to 251) are sufficient for nicking a single-stranded *trs* substrate (83), and a slightly smaller N-terminal region is sufficient for RBE binding (210). Efficient TR binding, however, requires sequences within the C-terminal region as well (187). A number of specific amino acids involved in TR binding have been mapped (82,110,187,279). The N-terminal region contains several motifs common to RCR proteins (amino acids 9 to 14, 89 to 94, and 146 to 156) (136) that are believed to be involved in nicking activity, and mutations in these motifs are defective in both *trs* endonuclease activity and integration at chromosome 19 (279). This includes the tyrosine residue at amino acid 156 that makes a covalent linkage with the *trs* site (83,257). C-terminal deletions (amino acids 490 to 621) appear to retain most Rep functions *in vivo* and *in vitro* (134,154). This includes the region of Rep52 and 78 that is spliced out in Rep40 and 68 (amino acids 529 to 621). However, repression of the p5 promoter and a heterologous promoter, the HPV18 upstream regulatory region, was most pronounced with Rep78, followed by Rep68 and Rep52. Rep40 repression was undetectable (134). Transactivation of the p40 promoter appears to be exclusively caused by either Rep78 or 68, with Rep68 having a more pronounced effect (293). A zinc-binding domain in the C-terminal region that is spliced out in Rep68 and 40 has been mutated; the mutant Rep78 protein no longer binds Zn *in vitro*, but the mutation does not change the ability of Rep78 to inhibit transcription from AAV or heterologous promoters *in vivo* (134). Rep is phosphorylated primarily on threonine residues, but these have not been mapped (62). As yet there is no clear evidence that Rep phosphorylation has an effect on any of its biochemical activities. A canonical ATP binding site is located at amino acids 334 to 349. Mutations in this region are defective for ATPase and helicase activity, DNA replication, and transactivation and repression of the p5 promoter *in vivo*; however, they retain some ability to repress the p19 and heterologous promoters. Curiously, virtually all mutants that are defective for helicase or DNA replication activity are also defective for transactivation; this has led to the suggestion that the helicase activity may be involved in transactivation (187). Mutants in other putative helicase motifs conserved among parvovirus nonstructural proteins eliminated helicase activity (187,284). A divalent cation binding site, apparently the one used for DNA helicase activity, has been mapped at amino acid 421 (110). Another divalent cation binding site in the N-terminus that is used for nuclease activity (presumably one of the conserved RCR motifs discussed earlier) remains to be definitively mapped. A nuclear localization region has been mapped to amino acids 483 to 519 (313). Rep 68/78 inhibits oncogenesis induced by a variety of carcinogens; mutants involving amino acids 25 to 56, 73 to 74, 164 to 165, and 257 to 346 had a significantly reduced capacity to inhibit EIA + *ras* transformation (312). Rep interacts with a variety of cellular proteins, but most of the interaction domains have not been completely mapped. Most of the N-terminal region (amino acids 1 to 174) is dispensable for interaction with PC4 (a transcription activator), as well as for inhibition of herpes virus replication (154,292). Rep–Rep interaction domains have been mapped to several specific regions (82,83,96,258), and Rep–capsid protein interaction has been mapped to amino acids 322 to 482 (96).

As mentioned earlier, all of the coat proteins, VP1 to VP3, are translated from two alternatively spliced p40 mRNAs (196). The most abundant of these messages is used to translate VP2 from a nonconventional ACG codon, and VP3 from a downstream AUG. VP1 is translated from the low-abundance spliced p40 message. All three proteins share the same ORF. Amino acid numbers below begin with amino acid 1 of VP1; VP2 begins at amino acid 138, and VP3 at 203. Why the first AUG in the predominant mRNA should be so far downstream is uncertain. However, evidence has been presented that *rep* activity can inhibit gene expression from the p40 promoter at the level of protein translation when a vector with a reporter gene under control of the p40 promoter is co-transfected with a plasmid containing *rep* into Ad-infected cells (275). Thus, it is possible that the long leader sequence in the major p40 spliced RNA from which VP2 and VP3 are translated serves to protect against this type of inhibition.

Expression of the structural proteins in insect cells leads to spontaneous particle self-assembly. VP2 was specifically required for self-assembly; either VP1 or VP3 could be omitted, but all three were required for infectivity (239). VP3, however, lacks a nuclear localization signal (NLS) (299); if a heterologous NLS is fused to VP3, it also becomes capable of self-assembly into empty particles (133). At least one NLS has been mapped to the N-terminus of VP2, amino acids 167 to 172 (133), but there appear to be redundant NLS sequences (305). As mentioned earlier, AAV2 uses heparin sulfate proteoglycans as a primary cell surface receptor (267). The heparin sulfate binding region of the AAV2 capsid protein has been mapped to two clusters, amino acids 509 to 522 and 561 to 591 (305). Several substitution and insertion mutants have been characterized in a preliminary way (305, and refs. therein). In general, insertions into putative loop regions are on the surface of the capsid and at least partially viable. The N-terminus of VP2 and a portion of the N-terminus of VP1 are also on the capsid surface. The N-terminus of VP3 and the C-terminus are internal to the capsid and essential for capsid structural integrity. One mutant (R432A) makes only empty capsids. Nonviable mutants tend to map to alpha-helix or beta-sheet regions, which are known to be necessary for capsid integrity.

Latent Infection

In the absence of a helper virus co-infection, the AAV genome is often integrated into cellular DNA to establish a latent infection that can be activated by a subsequent helper virus infection. AAV latent infection was discovered by Hoggan et al. (130) in the course of a federal project to screen primary cell lots intended for vaccine production. Although there was no immunologic evidence for AAV, upon challenge by Ad infection, 20% of the lots of African green monkey kidney cells and 1% to 2% of the lots of human embryonic kidney cells tested produced AAV. Thus, AAV latent infection *in vivo* appeared to be common. Although most human transmission of AAV appears to be horizontal, evidence for vertical germline transmission of avian AAV has been reported in chickens (23). Human cells in culture can be latently infected simply by infecting with a high multiplicity of AAV (multiplicity of infection of 10 to 1,000) in the absence of helper virus (126,169). The frequency of positive clones (estimated either by isolation of single-cell colonies or by selection with recombinant vectors carrying a *rep* gene and a selectable marker) suggests that up to 10% of the infected cells become latently infected (126,169). These figures exceed those seen with other DNA animal viruses and approach the efficiency of lambda bacteriophage lysogeny and rescue.

Characterization of AAV DNA in latently infected clones shows that the viral genome is in most cases integrated into cellular DNA (48,169). The junction with cellular sequences is usually within the TR, but the site of integration within the viral TR is not unique. Recombination junctions occur throughout the TR sequences and the p5 promoter region (155,309), and portions of the TR are deleted. The viral DNA in most latently infected cell lines is integrated as a tandem (head-to-tail) array of several genome equivalents (48,169,190). Inverted (tail-to-tail or head-to-head) arrays have also been seen but occur at a much lower frequency (155). The presence of TR deletions raises the question of how the AAV provirus is rescued. Presumably this occurs by excision of an internal tandemly repeated genome that is intact. Indeed, the junctions between tandem repeats appear to be intact, consist of a single TR flanked by two D sequences, and correlate with rescue (94,190,306).

It is not known whether deletions of the TR occur during integration or during subsequent passage of the cells. In one clone of latently infected cells that was followed for over 100 passages, the restriction patterns obtained, using enzymes that cut in the unique sequences, were unchanged, but significant changes were noted using a restriction enzyme that cuts exclusively in the TR (48). This raises the possibility that the TR is an unstable sequence. This notion was supported by the observation that after 100 passages, free copies of the AAV genome were present, even though all of the detectable sequences had been integrated into high-MW DNA in earlier passages.

Initially, it was concluded that integration was random with respect to cellular sequences because restriction analysis found that junction fragments of viral and cellular DNA differed in size in every independently derived clone carrying a provirus. It is now clear that integration occurs at a specific site on human chromosome 19q13.3-qter (157,158,248). Integration is by nonhomologous recombination, although there are four to five base homologies at the site of recombination, and integration is often associated with rearrangements and inversions of both viral DNA and cellular sequences (156,309). Although integration is site specific, it is not specific at the individual nucleotide level but occurs within a region of several hundred nucleotides (156,248,309). Additionally, only about 70% of the integration events appear to occur on chromosome 19.

The preintegration site has been isolated as an 8-kb fragment, of which the first 4 kb have been sequenced (156). The sequenced region, called AAVS1, contains all of the known sites of recombination. The average base composition is 82% GC in the first 900 bases, which are near the recombination sites. Toward the 3′ end of the AAVS1 sequence, there is a tandem repeat of 10 copies of a 35-mer minisatellite, which occurs at 60 places in the human genome, all of which are on 19q. There are also a large number of direct repeats in which there is an 11/12 base match. The first 900 bases fulfill the criteria for a

CpG island, which could serve as a promoter for expression of the ORF found in the middle of the sequenced region. As noted earlier, Dutheil et al. (97) have recently identified two of the coding regions within this region. A gene proximal to the integration site codes for the slow skeletal muscle troponin T gene, TNNT1, previously mapped to 19q13.4. This gene is located approximately 15 kb to the telomere side of AAVS1, and integration into AAVS1 has been shown to cause rearrangements of TNNT1 in some proviral clones.

The most interesting feature of the preintegration site is that it contains an RBE and an abbreviated version of the *trs*. The sequences within the AAVS1 site necessary for site-specific recombination have been identified by the use of an extrachromosomal Epstein-Barr virus shuttle vector carrying the preintegration sequence. When human cells carrying the shuttle vector are infected with wild-type AAV virions, the viral genome preferentially integrates into the chromosome 19 target site. The critical region has been mapped to a 500-base fragment, which contains the RBE and a *trs*-like element (111). It was possible to dissociate the RBE from the sequences at which recombination occur in the latently infected cell lines. Thus, it appears as though the critical factor is a recognition site, and the actual recombination takes place several hundred bases distal to the recognition site. Additionally, any higher-order chromatin structure specific to chromosome 19q does not appear to be essential for site-specific integration. Site-specific mutagenesis has been used to further define the critical elements. Mutation of either the RBE or the putative *trs* site dramatically reduces site-specific integration (176), and these two elements appear to be the only essential elements required for integration.

Several groups have shown that Rep expression is essential for site-specific integration. Recombinant AAV (rAAV) vectors carrying a selectable marker flanked by two TRs, but deleted for the *rep* gene, do not integrate into chromosome 19 (148), whereas those that contain the *rep* gene integrate site specifically. Plasmids carrying an rAAV genome, when co-transfected with a Rep-expressing plasmid (or Rep protein) into human cells, will excise the rAAV genome and integrate it into chromosome 19 (253). The same occurs when human cells are infected with herpes, Ad, or baculovirus vectors carrying an rAAV genome, provided Rep is expressed (225, and references therein). Most recently, site-specific integration has been demonstrated in nonhuman cells. Mice do not have the AAVS1 preintegration sequence. However, when cells from transgenic mice carrying the AAVS1 locus are infected with *rep*$^+$ AAV, integration occurs in the transgenic S1 locus (233).

Biochemical evidence also supports a role for Rep in site-specific integration. Weitzman et al. (295) have demonstrated that Rep68 can bind to a plasmid containing a fragment of the preintegration site and can also serve as a bridge between the AAV TR and the chromosome 19 RBE. Thus, *in vitro*, Rep can bring the chromosome 19 target site and the AAV genome together through Rep-Rep contacts. As noted earlier, Urcelay et al. (280) have shown that plasmids containing the AAVS1 site can be nicked by Rep, which in turn initiates DNA replication. Recently, Smith and Kotin (257) have shown that Rep can both nick a *trs* and ligate the nicked DNA to another sequence in a second transesterification reaction *in vitro*. Dyall et al. (99) have also provided evidence for nicking and joining *in vitro*.

Integration in the absence of Rep generates proviral structures in cell culture that are essentially the same as those seen in the presence of Rep, with the exception that the site of integration is not chromosome 19 (93,190,240, 309). (This includes the formation of head-to-tail repeats, deletions within the TR, rearrangements of cellular DNA, and microhomologies at junctions between cellular and viral DNA.) The efficiency of Rep-minus integration is variable and seems to depend on the cell line under study, but it can be as high as 80% (190). This suggests that cellular enzymes are largely responsible for recombination, and Rep is essential only for site specificity. The only AAV related sequence that is necessary for integration seems to be the TR, which is recognized by the cellular machinery as a recombination or amplification signal (309).

No clear consensus model has emerged thus far for integration. The key elements to explain are the tandem (head-to-tail) repeats, the high rescue frequency implying that at least one intact copy is always integrated, the role of Rep, the ability of Rep to rearrange the host target site even in the absence of an input AAV genome, and the lack of site specificity at the sequence level for either viral or host DNA. The existence of head-to-tail repeats prompted some to suggest that the integration intermediate is a circular AAV genome that undergoes RCR (169,190). Both AAV and chromosome 19 could be nicked at their respective *trs*s, exposing a TR end for illegitimate recombination to a random cellular sequence in the S1 site. This would explain the frequent occurrence of tandem repeats with intact internal TRs. Giraud et al. (112) have suggested that copy-choice replication mechanisms during RCR could account for the rearrangements and inversions that have been found in some proviruses. Dyall et al. (98) have suggested a deletion substitution method of recombination.

The need for *trs* nicking on the input genome apparently has been eliminated by Young and Samulski (314), who demonstrated that site-specific integration occurs even when plasmids carrying AAV with mutant *trs*s are transfected into human cells. The mutant *trs* is defective for Rep-mediated nicking or DNA replication, but it integrates into chromosome 19 at about the same frequency as wild-type DNA.

Evidence for the formation of circular intermediates comes from recent studies of rAAV transduction in cell culture and muscle tissue (94). These experiments are done in the absence of Rep expression but, as noted earlier, this produces similar proviral structures in cell culture. Persistent transduction appeared to correlate with the formation of circular rAAV intermediates, which could be recovered by subsequent transfection into bacteria. Previous studies had shown that the expression of the Ad E4 ORF 6 gene product or a variety of genotoxic agents would increase transduction or reduce the time required for expression of a transgene in cell culture and *in vivo* (101,102). This was interpreted to mean that a variety of agents could promote second-strand synthesis, which was required for transcription. More recent experiments suggest that either linear duplex or circular duplex intermediates are formed, depending on the type of stimulus—for example, UV light versus ORF 6 gene expression (249). The significance of this is not clear.

Perhaps the most surprising development in rAAV integration has been the realization that recombinant AAV genomes persist *in vivo* for extended periods of time (up to a year) as episomes. These are converted slowly from linear or circular monomer genomes to high-MW concatemers, and this may or may not be accompanied by integration (1,105,148,184,282). In addition, it is now clear that two different rAAV genomes will recombine to form circular or linear concatemers. Several groups have shown that this occurs frequently and can be used to reconstruct split genes that are infected into cells in two different vectors (95,268,308).

AAV as a Vector

AAV has received a significant amount of interest as a potential vector for gene therapy (41,126,245). There are a number of characteristics that contribute to the potential utility of the virus for this purpose. Recombinant AAV vectors can efficiently transduce a variety of nondividing, terminally differentiated tissues *in vivo*. These include cells of the eye, central nervous system, muscle, liver, and lung. Significantly, the vector genome persists for extended periods (up to 2 years in muscle, brain, and eye of rodents) with no apparent decrease in expression. In part, this is because essentially no pathogenicity or inflammatory response is generated by *in vivo* injections of vector. The cytotoxic T-lymphocyte (CTL) response also appears to be lower than that seen with most other viral vectors (20,52,129). This may be due in part to the absence of genes (other than the transgene) in the vector, or to the observation that AAV does not efficiently infect antigen-presenting cells (145). Long-lived expression is due also to the fact that foreign promoters appear to behave as expected in the context of an AAV vector. Tissue-specific and inducible promoters are expressed only in the appropriate cell types or in the presence of inducer and do not appear to be shut off by mechanisms that affect other types of vectors. Although the AAV TR is itself a TATA-less promoter (104), its basal level of expression is low and detectable only in some cell types. Expression from an rAAV vector typically takes 3 to 6 weeks to reach a maximum level (149,261). The slow onset is generally believed to result from the slow synthesis of the second strand (101,102).

Ex vivo gene therapy has also been investigated, particularly in hematopoietic cells. One group has successfully transplanted ablated mice with transduced hematopoietic stem cells and achieved long-term expression in recipients. However, it is clear that the efficiency of transduction is variable, and that it depends on several factors that have so far been poorly defined but may include the genotype of the donor cells (218), the phosphorylation state of ssD-BP (221), the ability of virus to traffic to the nucleus, or the presence of the appropriate cell surface receptors (222,266,267).

Permanent transduction in cell culture was first shown by Hermonat and Muzyczka (126). The vectors used in these studies deleted the capsid gene and substituted foreign DNA. This type of vector retains the *rep* gene and can integrate with high frequency into chromosome 19. The second type of vector, which simply puts an AAV TR on both ends of the foreign DNA (190), has received the most attention because it contains more room for the transgene, about 4.5 kb. This type of vector was the first to be used *in vivo* (103), and it is currently being used in two human trials for the treatment of cystic fibrosis and factor IX deficiency. Preliminary results from both trials have been encouraging (147,283).

The rAAV vector system has suffered from several disadvantages, some of which have now been addressed or eliminated. The small packaging size has been a problem for some transgene–promoter combinations. Two groups have recently showed that this problem can be overcome by the use of split genes that are cloned into two separate vectors (95,268,308). These are expressed *in vivo* from head-to-tail concatemers of the vector with the use of appropriate splice signals. Another problem has been the lack of effective methods for purification of rAAV virus, and this also has been addressed. There are now several new methods for virus production and purification that produce virus with low particle-to-infectivity ratios and low wild-type AAV and helper contamination (59,116,317). Scalable production methods have also been developed (59,63,108). Several problems remain, however. The slow onset of transgene expression eliminates rAAV as a vector for acute clinical applications. It is still not clear from biodistribution experiments whether rAAV permanently transduces germline cells *in vivo*. Finally, because rAAV integrates into some primary cells, the potential long-term risk from insertional mutagenesis needs to be assessed.

Inhibition of Helper Virus Replication and Heterologous Gene Expression

In addition to AAV gene expression and replication being affected by Ad or herpes co-infection, the course of

Ad infection is also significantly affected by AAV co-infection (40,42,43). There is also evidence that Rep can directly or indirectly interfere with replication of other viral genomes, specifically SV40, papilloma, and herpes, as well as with replication of cellular DNA (123,154,166, 310,311). In the case of Ad, the net effect is enhanced AAV gene expression and replication, with greatly reduced Ad gene expression and replication. These effects depend on the ratio of the multiplicities of infection of the two viruses and the temporal order of addition. AAV is effectively autoinhibitory because, if the ratio of AAV to Ad becomes too great, the inhibition of Ad gene expression is sufficient that it no longer provides the helper functions needed for AAV replication. By the same token, if AAV infection is delayed until Ad DNA synthesis has begun, AAV replication occurs but that of Ad is not inhibited. The inhibition appears to require *rep* gene expression because DI particles of AAV, which have very large internal deletions but intact TRs, cannot inhibit Ad replication (84). Whether the inhibition of Ad includes direct effects on DNA replication or simply a lack of early regulatory proteins is not known. This type of inhibition is not usually seen with herpesvirus co-infections (15), probably because the herpesvirus infection is so rapid, but it is seen when the *rep* gene is over-expressed (154).

Initially, infection by AAV in the absence of helper virus was not noted to affect the cell phenotype. More detailed studies of latently infected cells have indicated several phenotypic changes. These include decreased plating efficiency, evidence of cell cycle arrest, and increased sensitivity to a variety of genotoxic agents [e.g., UV, chemical carcinogens (286,287)]. Latent infection can also inhibit DNA amplification after exposure to genotoxic agents (298). AAV infection of the human leukemic cell line HL60 and immortalized keratinocyte lines led to reduced cell growth and reduced levels of detectable differentiation-associated antigens, plus altered expression of c-*myc*, c-*myb*, and c-*fos* (153). In the case of c-*myc* and c-*fos*, this appears to result from Rep repression of the cellular promoters (124). This may also account for the observation of Yang et al. (311), who have shown that the *rep* gene is cytostatic. Cells carrying an inducible *rep* gene were arrested for growth when the *rep* gene was induced and returned to normal growth in the absence of inducer. Even low constitutive levels of *rep* expression increased cell doubling time.

AAV has also been reported to inhibit permanent cellular transformation by selectable markers under the control of the SV40 early promoter, the HSV type 11 thymidine kinase promoter, and the inducible murine metallothionein promoter. The level of inhibition was greater than 95% and depended on an intact *rep* gene. Under the conditions employed, the cells were not killed by *rep* gene expression, nor was the ability of plasmid DNA to integrate into cellular DNA decreased. Thus, it appeared as though the inhibition was caused by repression of gene expression. This notion was supported by the observation that in co-transfections, the AAV *rep* gene was able to inhibit chloramphenical acetyl transferase (CAT) expression under control of the SV40 early promoter. These types of inhibitory effects have been observed in both murine and human cells (167,276), but the extent of inhibition was very dependent on the specific cells used.

Inhibition of Adenovirus, Herpesvirus, and Papillomavirus Oncogenicity

Oncogenic serotypes of Ad induce tumors in newborn Syrian hamsters. Co-infection of AAV with oncogenic Ad reduces the frequency of tumors and lengthens the induction time of those that do occur (152,185). AAV co-infection also inhibits the ability of Ad to transform cells. Ad-transformed hamster cells are also oncogenic in the newborn, and this oncogenicity was reduced by infection of the cells with AAV, although the growth rate in culture was unaltered (209). The primary effect appeared to be on the level of E1B expression in the transformed cells. de la Maza and Carter (85) reported that DI particles of AAV and DI genomes could inhibit Ad induction of tumors in hamsters. Because some of the preparations of defective particles contained only the termini of the AAV genome, it was suggested that the termini may be sufficient for inhibiting Ad oncogenicity. AAV has also been reported to inhibit the oncogenicity of HSV-II-transformed cells after infection (81). Not only was the incidence of tumor induction decreased after cells were injected into hamsters, but the induction period was lengthened. Possibly the most interesting result was that even in those animals that did develop tumors there was no evidence of metastasis. AAV has also been shown to inhibit transformation by bovine papilloma virus and human papilloma virus 16 (HPV16), and this inhibition is attributable to Rep (123,285). Rep-mediated inhibition appears to involve binding of Rep to an HPV16 promoter and direct interaction between Rep and the HPV E7 oncoprotein (128). Similarly, Rep inhibits cell transformation by the combined action of the E1A and human *ras* oncogenes (150).

The reports of AAV inhibition of oncogenicity have raised the question of whether AAV might inhibit oncogenicity in humans. More than 90% of adults are seropositive for AAV, suggesting that many carry AAV as a latent infection. According to the model hypothesized, latent virus might be activated by oncogenic virus infection and, once activated, inhibit oncogenesis. Several retrospective epidemiologic studies have been done, studying patients suffering from cervical carcinoma. Interestingly, in each study the patients were markedly deficient in antibodies to AAV compared to a group of matched controls (263, and references therein). These results raise the unusual possibility that a viral infection might, for once, be beneficial to the host.

AUTONOMOUS PARVOVIRUSES

Genetic Map

Like that of AAV, the autonomous parvovirus genome contains two large ORFs (see Fig. 3). The first covers much of the left half of the genome (approximately mps 6 to 42) and encodes two NS proteins, NS1 and NS2, from alternately spliced mRNAs that are initiated at mp 4 (see Fig. 3). Mutations within NS1 block viral replication and gene expression (229,230). Only NS1 is absolutely required for DNA replication. NS2-specific mutants are defective for capsid synthesis, gene expression, and DNA replication in murine cells but show variable phenotypes in human cells (36,68,174,198,199). The second large ORF occupies much of the right half of the genome (mp 45 to 90) and encodes the coat proteins (228,255). Up to three coat proteins have been detected in the virion. In the case of MVM, the smallest capsid protein, VP3, is generated in the intact capsid by proteolytic cleavage of VP2 (271). The amino acid sequences of VP1 and VP2 are identical except for additional amino acids at the N terminus of VP1, and they are synthesized from two alternatively spliced messages initiated at mp 38 (see Fig. 3). The VP1 message contains a second (smaller) ORF at the 5′ end of the major right-hand ORF (165,194). Mutants altered in either the NS or coat protein ORFs can be complemented in trans. However, the palindromic sequences at both termini are required in cis for DNA replication and packaging.

Transcription

For most autonomous parvoviruses, three major size classes of polyadenylated transcripts have been identified (see Fig. 3). Two of these (R1 and R2) are initiated downstream of a promoter (TATA box) at mp 4 and extend to a point near the right end of the genome near mps 95 to 96, where a polyadenylation signal (AATAAA) is located. Both of these transcripts have an intron removed between mps 44 and 46, and one has a large intron removed between mps 10 and 39 (144,194,217). These two transcripts are translated to yield NS proteins NS1 and NS2, respectively (72,228). The other major size class (R3) is initiated downstream from a promoter at mp 38 and alternatively spliced between mps 44 and 46 to produce the coat proteins VP1 and VP2 (165,194). The region between mps 44 and 46 is unusual in that two pairs of donor and acceptor splice sites occur in a very small region. In all, three of the four possible splicing combinations that could occur in this region are observed in each of the three major mRNA size classes, R1, R2, and R3 (see Fig. 3), to produce a total of nine mRNA species that are made at detectable steady-state levels (144,194). Unspliced mRNA species are also a major portion of nuclear RNA found in infected cells. In the case of MVM, excision of the large intron and the ratio of the R1 and R2 messages depend on sequences within the small intron (mps 44 to 46). The role of the small intron in this process has been hypothesized to involve initial entry of the spliceasome (315). Improvement of the polypyrimidine tract of the large intron relieves the requirement for the small intron and makes prior excision of the small intron unnecessary for large intron excision. As an added factor, any mutations that insert stop codons in either exon will block splicing (200).

Significant variations of this general scheme occur. All transcripts of the autonomous human parvovirus B19 have been reported to initiate from the promoter at mp 6 (25,90,211). Potential internal polyadenylation signals (AATAAA) exist near the middle of several parvovirus genomes, and these sequences are used for polyadenylation in the case of ADV and B19 virus (6,211). An additional NS protein, NS3, has been identified in ADV, which is coded by an alternatively spliced left-side ORF transcript (58).

Both MVM NS1 and H1 NS1 (a closely related parovirus) are necessary for transactivation of their respective p38 promoters (92,230). In the absence of functional NS1, p38 mRNA is difficult to detect by most RNA detection methods. The transactivation domain in NS1 has been mapped to the C-terminal 129 amino acid residues (173). Three sequences are essential for transactivation. The first is the tar element (transactivation response element, sensitive to NS1) or an alternative NS1 binding site–containing sequence (178,179,231). NS1 binds to the tar region in an ATP-dependent manner (53). However, because there are many NS1 binding sequences upstream of the p38 promoter (more than 100), mutations of the NS1 binding site within the tar region have not always shown a decrease in p38 transcription, presumably because of redundant NS1 binding sequences. Two other sequences are essential for transactivation, an SP1 site and the TATA box (5,179) (see Fig. 5). NS1 can bind to Sp1, and the general transcription proteins TBP and TFIIA in the absence of DNA (159,179), and, presumably, these interactions are involved in transactivation. However, the mechanism of transactivation is not yet clear.

Activation of p4 transcription by NS1 has been seen in LuIII, B19, and MVM (91,119), and it depends in part on sequences within the upstream terminal palindrome, presumably because they contain NS1 binding sites (see Fig. 5). Transactivation of p4 by NS1 essentially creates a positive feedback loop for p4 transcription, thereby creating a switch that commits the virus to lytic infection.

Several other elements necessary for p4 transcription have also been mapped in MVM (4,87,88,107,118,215). A TATA box and an Sp1 site at –29 and –45 bases relative to the p4 mRNA start (see Fig. 5) are essential for promoter activity (4). Additionally, because MVM requires cellular proteins that are expressed in S phase for productive infection, some mechanism must exist for sensing when S phase begins, because unregulated expression of NS1 is cytotoxic

(235). This is apparently supplied by an E2F site (see Fig. 5) at –60 relative to the message start (87,88). Mutation of this site abolishes NS1 induction in S phase and produces a replication-negative phenotype that can be rescued only if NS1 is supplied in trans. The E2F transcription factor consists of a heterodimeric factor composed of E2F and DP family members. Their transcriptional activity is controlled during the cell cycle by binding to members of the pocket protein family (pRb, p130, and p107). Free E2F heterodimers are active for transactivation and are released at the G1–S transition as a result of phosphorylation of the pocket proteins by cell-cycle-regulated cyclin-dependent kinases. A second transcription factor family also is involved in sensing and responding to the cell cycle. Two cyclic AMP response elements (see Fig. 5, CREs), which are present within the left palindrome (at –130 and –160), and which bind the ATF/CREB family of transcription factors, activate the p4 promoter in growing and serum-starved cells but repress the p4 promoter in contact-inhibited cells (87,215). Promoter silencing in contact-inhibited cells is apparently mediated by the cyclin-dependent kinase inhibitor (CKI) p27, as overexpression of p27 reduces p4 transcription in growing cells. Thus, control of NS1 expression by the E2F and CREB families of transcription factors effectively couples MVM p4 transcription (and DNA replication) to the cell cycle.

Two other transcription factors participate in p4 control, NF-Y and Ets (see Fig. 5). NF-Y binds to an atypical site, CCAAC, which is present in the left TR (–100 upstream of p4) as well as at the internal dimer junction of MVM. Its mutation reduces p4 transcription approximately twofold (118). The Ets transcription factor binding site is located at approximately–50, just upstream of the Sp1 site, and it also increases p4 transcription (about threefold) (107). The Ets site appears to cooperate with the nearby Sp1 site in activating p4. Interestingly, both the Ets site and the CRE sites increase transcription from the p4 promoter in a *ras*-transformed cell (107,215). The increased NS1 levels in *ras*-transformed cells may account in part for the well established sensitivity of some tumor cells to MVM killing (235).

Negative regulation of p38 has also been observed (109,160), which can be caused by a cellular repressor. Evidence for regulation by RNA processing and protein stability has also been found (251). Another form of regulation that apparently occurs involves attenuation of transcription of the p4 promoter via an RNA polymerase pause site (*att*) between nucleotides 259 and 383. The *att* site contains a sequence that can form a cruciform in the DNA template (216, and refs. therein). Temporal regulation of gene expression has been reported for MVM (61), which is consistent with transactivation of the p38 transcript by the NS1 protein.

Regulation of gene expression is also a major factor in tissue specificity. The parvovirus HI NS2 gene regulates gene expression in a manner dependent on cell type; it does so by virtue of sequences in the 3′ untranslated region (175). As noted earlier, a different type of host-range mutant is observed for MVM. Wild-type MVM(p) productively infects murine fibroblasts but not T lymphocytes. A mutant MVM(i) has the reverse phenotype. Both strains are replicated for one round after transfection. The genetic difference is in the middle of the capsid gene and represents several amino changes on the surface of the virion. However, simple binding to the cells is not affected. Thus, the physiologic lesion is somewhere between entry and uncoating (13).

DNA Replication

Like AAV, autonomous parvovirus DNA replication takes place in the nucleus. The location of replication, combined with the fact that the cell is required to go through S phase for replication to occur (227,269,301), suggests a very close relationship between viral and cellular DNA replication. Sequence analysis of the termini of virion and replicative forms of MVM DNA suggests a modified rolling hairpin model for autonomous parvovirus DNA replication (7,272). However, there are some important differences between the model for autonomous parvoviruses and the mechanism described for AAV. Like AAV, the autonomous parvovirus genome has palindromic ends. Unlike AAV, the two ends are not identical in size or primary sequence (9,228). Furthermore, unlike in AAV, only one of the two strands (the minus or noncoding strand) is packaged in most rodent autonomous parvoviruses. This places significant constraints on the model of autonomous parvovirus DNA replication (Fig. 7) as compared with the AAV model described earlier (see Fig. 6). The following is currently the consensus model for rodent autonomous parvovirus DNA replication, and it is drawn primarily from work done with MVM. However, there are still some significant steps that are not clearly supported with experimental evidence, so the model should be considered one example of how MVM might replicate its DNA to generate the species of replicative intermediates and packaged viral DNA that are seen in cell culture.

FIG. 7. Model for MVM DNA replication. See text for details. ABa, 3′ terminal palindrome of virion strand; FGf, 5′ terminal palindrome of virion strand; e, 18- to 26-nucleotide sequence present in replicative intermediates but not in DNA of nuclease-treated virions; V, virion strand; V^{par}, parental virion strand; V^{prog}, progeny virion strand; C, complementary strand; *heavy arrows*, new DNA synthesis; *solid circle*, site of nicks and NS1 covalent attachment in right end and dimer bridge. (The model was developed from the discussion in ref. 78, with permission.)

It is assumed that the 3′ terminus (by convention the left end) of the virion strand folds back on itself to serve as the primer to initiate DNA synthesis of the complementary strand (see Fig. 7). When DNA synthesis reaches

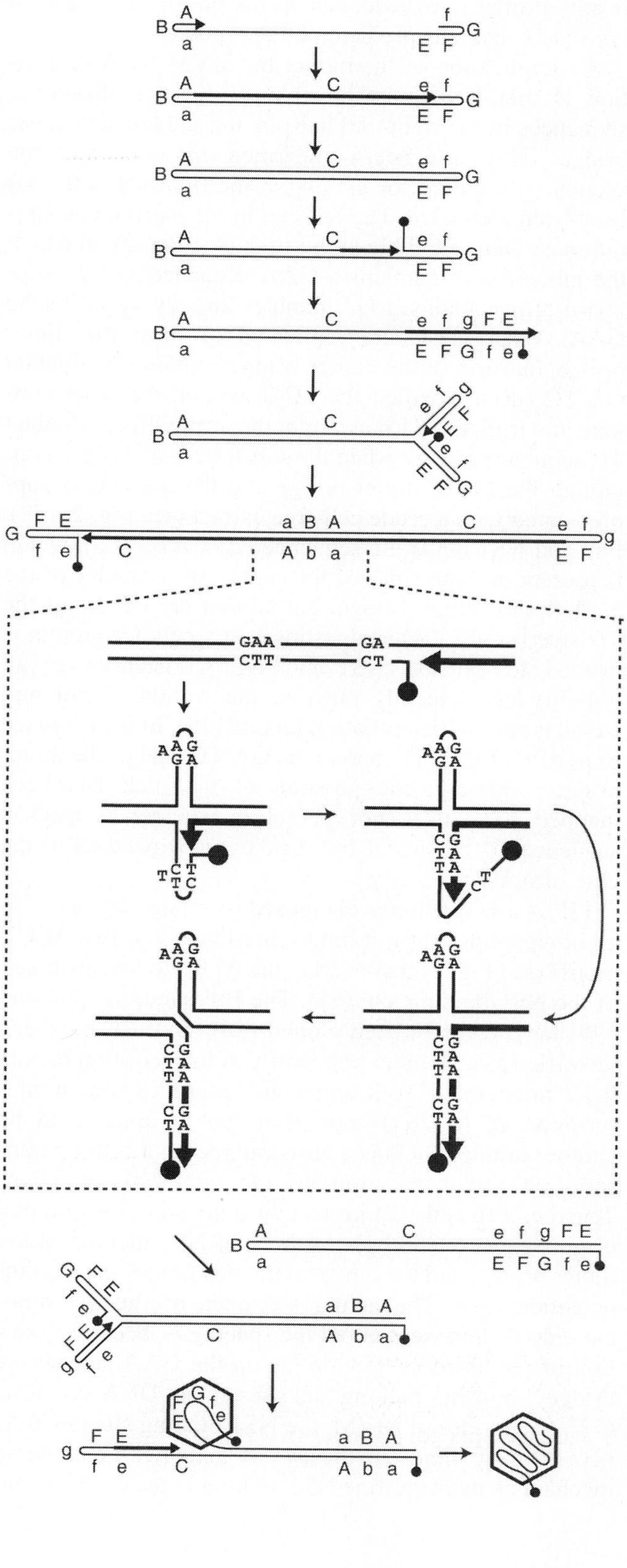

the hairpinned 5′ end, it is believed that a ligation occurs to produce a linear molecule in which both ends are covalently joined—that is, there are no free 5′ or 3′ ends. Such molecules have been found *in vivo* (69). (They can be thought of as single-stranded dimer circles that have collapsed via base pairing to duplex linear molecules.) The 5′ end (by convention the right end) is then nicked at a site that is inboard of the original 5′ end of the parental molecule by NS1, which forms a covalent linkage with the 5′ end of the nick. This generates a 3′ OH that is used to repair the right end to a duplex extended form (see Fig. 7, steps 4 and 5). In the process, the right end undergoes a strand-transfer event, which inverts its sequence and results in the two orientations seen at the right end, flip and flop. Subsequently, the newly repaired extended right end forms a double hairpinned intermediate in which the 3′ strand at the right end of the genome serves as a primer for further DNA synthesis (see Fig. 7, steps 6 and 7). Synthesis proceeds through the left end to form a duplex dimer molecule in which the left end (the original 3′ end) is now in the form of a linear junction between two copies of the MVM genome that are inverted with respect to each other. The viral right ends, which flank the dimer, can continue to undergo terminal resolution and strand transfer, generating flip and flop orientations. The junction in the middle of the dimer is often called the left-left junction, the dimer bridge, or the 3′ junction. Unlike the right end that exists in two orientations (flip and flop), the left end is found in only one orientation, called flip. Thus, a mechanism exists to maintain only one orientation of the left end and to generate only one strand of the viral genome for packaging. This is accomplished by asymmetric nicking at the internal left-left junction in a process called junction resolution (see Fig. 7, steps 8 to 12), which generates 3′ termini in only one orientation (7,78). Thus, one of the key replicative species in MVM DNA replication appears to be an obligatory dimer intermediate containing a left end–left end junction. The products of bridge resolution have been shown *in vitro* (71) to be a monomer intermediate that is covalently joined at the left end and a monomer intermediate in which both ends are extended (see Fig. 7, step 13). The latter can undergo DNA replication from the right end (the 5′ end) of MVM to generate the minus strand of the virus with the correct orientation at its 3′ end (and either orientation at its 5′ end) for packaging into mature virions. (This process could be repeated multiple times.) The former intermediate can also undergo DNA replication from its right end to regenerate a dimer intermediate with a left end–left end bridge.

The details of this model have not been completely settled but several lines of evidence support the keys steps outlined. Concatemers of dimer and tetramer length, as well as molecules covalently closed at both ends, have been detected in parvovirus-infected cells (69,270) as predicted by the model. Additionally, the expected bias toward left-left bridges has been seen *in vivo* (278). Biochemical characterization of NS1 also supports the model. In addition to having endonuclease activity, NS1, like the AAV Rep protein, is a DNA helicase and an ATPase (57,297). Whenever NS1 nicks, it forms a covalent linkage with the 5′ end of the cut (12,74). Linkage is through a tyrosine residue at amino acid 210 of NS1 (204), which is part of the RCR motif (136). NS1 cuts the 5′ (right end) at a position some 18 bases upstream of the sequence that is found in viral DNA (7), and it remains attached to the DNA during packaging. Mature MVM virus particles initially contain NS1 still attached to the DNA on the outside of the viral capsid (75). The protein is subsequently removed along with some of the 5′-end DNA, by nucleases in the culture medium or during cell entry. Recovery of the 18 bases missing from the right end presumably occurs when NS1 nicks the initial RF form (12,69), which is made *in vivo* and is covalently closed at both ends.

In vitro DNA replication studies using viral single-stranded DNA (or duplex RF) and cell-free crude extracts supplemented with purified NS1, have also confirmed key elements of the model (12,296). First, there is an apparent preference for formation of the linear duplex covalently closed at both ends from viral DNA, which is apparently the first RF intermediate made (12). Second, the left end is relatively insensitive to NS1 resolution when it is in the hairpin configuration (12); NS1 cuts the left end only when it is in the linear dimer bridge form. This is important because it accounts for why only one orientation of the left end (flip) is seen. Third, NS1 helicase activity is apparently responsible for unwinding and refolding the linear extended right end into the double hairpin that is used for initiation of DNA replication at several steps in the model (296). Unwinding is ATP dependent and NS1 mutants that have mutations in the canonical ATP binding site are inactive for the refolding reaction. Additionally, the TR isomerization occurs more efficiently at the right extended TR than at the left end in the extended configuration (12). This means that initiation of strand-displacement DNA synthesis is initiated preferentially at right ends. Coupled with the absence of left-end hairpin resolution, this would explain the preferential formation of dimer molecules with left-end bridges and the predominant synthesis of only minus strands.

Resolution of left-left and right-right end junctions also has been demonstrated *in vitro* and *in vivo* using plasmids that contain these junctions. In both cases nicking requires MVM NS1 protein and NS1 becomes covalently attached to the 5′ end of the nick (70,71,76,77, 177). Resolution of the left-left dimer bridge *in vitro* and *in vivo* is asymmetric as predicted, producing predominantly extended forms from one arm of the bridge and predominantly hairpinned (also called turn-around) forms from the other arm (71,76). Precisely how one of the products winds up having a covalently closed end is still not clear. The model illustrated in Figure 7 is just one possible mechanism. Cleavage of the right-right junctions, on the other hand, produces predominantly extended structures in both the flip and flop orientations with covalently associated copies of NS1 (70,76). NS1 also cuts the right end hairpin conformation, which results primarily in extended forms both *in vivo* and *in vitro* (12), again as predicted by the model.

An implication of the model for MVM DNA replication is that NS1 must be able to cut two dissimilar sequences in the right-end hairpin and the left-left dimer bridge. This has been confirmed *in vitro* and the sequences required for nicking at the right and left ends have been identified. The left end in the hairpin configuration contains a bubble in the stem (see Fig. 2), in which the inboard arm contains a GAA sequence and the outboard arm contains a GA doublet directly opposite the GAA. When these are replicated to form the dimer bridge, one arm of the duplex bridge contains the doublet GA/TC (usually called the TC arm) and the other contains the triplet. NS1 nicks only the arm with the doublet TC sequence *in vitro* when the substrate is a plasmid containing the MVM dimer bridge and the reaction is supplemented with a crude cell-free extract (see Fig. 2) (77). Purified NS1 binds the sequence $(ACCA)_{2\text{-}3}$ (66), which is present on both sides of the center of symmetry of the 3′ (left end) dimer bridge, but neither the GAA nor the TC side is cut (204), suggesting that a cellular protein is needed to activate NS1 nicking. Christensen et al. (54–56) have recently purified the cellular factor and called it parvovirus initiation factor (PIF). In the presence of purified PIF, NS1 cleaves the GA/TC side of the dimer bridge. Although the position of the nick has been mapped (77), it is not yet clear whether a specific sequence at the site of the nick is recognized as in the case of AAV.

PIF is a heterodimer composed of related 96- and 79-kd polypeptides (56); it binds coordinately to two ACGT motifs (see Fig. 2) that overlap the ATF site just upstream of the NS1 binding site (55). The PIF subunits (p96 and p79) have recently been cloned (56), and PIF has been identified as a member of a family of transcription factors that contain the KDWK amino acid motif. Its role in transcription of MVM is not clear, but it appears to be another example of how a virus can recruit a cellular transcription factor to promote the synthesis of DNA. Together, PIF and NS1 protect virtually all of the minimal origin sequence (50 bp) required for NS1 nicking of the dimer bridge, and they meet at the position of the TC dinucleotide (55). The actual sequence of the TC dinucleotide is not essential but the spacing is, because insertion of any third nucleotide (as on the GAA side of the bridge) abolishes nicking and subsequent DNA synthesis (77). In the case of MVM, the NS1 binding site (ACCA) occurs many times in the MVM genome. Thus, some mechanism must confine NS1 nicking to the right hairpin and the left-end dimer bridge, and prevent nicking within the 3′ hairpin or at other locations within the MVM genome. PIF (and the spacing between the PIF site and the NS1 site) apparently serves this function by stimulating nicking on only one side, the TC side, of the 3′ bridge. Presumably, the same mechanism inhibits nicking of the same 3′ origin sequence when it is in the hairpin configuration.

Cotmore et al. (67,79) have identified the sequences and cellular protein required for nicking at the right (5′) end of MVM (see Fig. 2). In this case, NS1 must nick and resolve a covalently closed hairpinned species to continue DNA synthesis. The cellular cofactor required to activate NS1 in an *in vitro* reaction is either HMG1 or HMG2 (HMG1/2) (79). In the absence of either protein, NS1 does not nick the hairpin. HMG1/2 preferentially binds bent DNA, cruciform DNA, or four-way junctions (i.e., Holliday intermediates). Three sequence elements are essential for nicking the 5′ hairpin (see Fig. 2): (a) an NS1 binding site at the very end of the hairpinned 5′ end, just beyond the AGA bubble, (b) an NS1 binding site near the nick site, approximately 110 bp upstream of the first NS1 site, and (c) a specific sequence at the nick site just inboard of the second NS1 site (67). In the presence of HMG protein, the NS1 sites appear to form a higher-order nucleoprotein complex, in which the intervening sequence is distorted in a way that suggests the formation of a double helical loop. Thus, NS1 carries out a similar reaction at the left-left dimer junction and the hairpinned right end, two distinct sequences, by interacting with two different cellular proteins.

Although the two NS1 sites and the nicking site appear to be the essential sequences required for endonuclease activity in the right hairpin, Costello et al. (64) showed that *in vivo* the presence of the unpaired AGA triplet within the left hairpin was important for efficient DNA replication. Absence of the bubble significantly reduced replication of the mutant MVM genome, but replacement of the bubble with a different sequence restored DNA replication, suggesting that the sequence of the bubble was not important but the actual presence of unpaired bases was. Additionally, in both 3′ dimer bridge nicking and 5′ hairpin nicking, ATP is required for the reaction to proceed. This may simply reflect the fact that NS1 binding requires ATP, unlike AAV Rep. Alternatively, it may mean that the DNA helicase activity of MVM must modify the DNA substrate prior to nicking. The nature of the modification, however, is not clear. In the 5′ hairpin, a potential cruciform structure could form that would include the NS1 site at the tip of the hairpin. Mutation analysis of this cruciform structure, as well as the companion NS1 site that is present just inboard of the right end hairpin (not shown in Fig. 2), indicated that neither was essential for nicking the 5′ hairpin (67).

In addition to the sequences within the 5′ palindrome, two other sequences at the right end of the genome but inboard of the palindrome have been shown to have an effect on DNA replication. One of these is a 65-bp repeat between nucleotides (nts) 4,760 and 4,850 of MVM, each of which contains multiple copies of a CC(C/A) repeat (243). Deletion of this sequence reduces DNA replication in some cell lines by as much as 100-fold, and a similar sequence has been mapped in H1. The second sequence is located between nts 4,489 and 4,695 (37). This region has been referred to as an internal replication sequence (IRS). Mutation of this region has identified two sequence blocks that reduce DNA replication about five-fold, and several cellular proteins that bind specifically to this region of the genome have been detected. It is not clear what role these internal sequences play in DNA replication, but some groups have suggested that they may act as internal origins that initiate DNA replication via a cellular primase (37, and refs. therein). Initiation of DNA replication close to the 5′ end has been postulated to be a possible alternative mechanism for unwinding and refolding the right-end palindromic sequence, a step that is normally energetically unfavorable (37).

Christensen et al. (54) have identified some of the other cellular factors that are required *in vitro* for replication when a 3′ dimer bridge origin is used. In addition to PIF, DNA synthesis required PCNA, RPA (the cellular single-strand DBP), and a partially purified fraction that contains DNA polymerases. PCNA is an accessory protein for DNA polymerases δ and ε, suggesting that one of these two polymerases is involved in MVM DNA replication. *In vitro* studies using purified DNA polymerases or polymerase inhibitors have not definitively identified the cellular DNA polymerase used *in vivo*, but they do show that the viral single-stranded DNA can be converted into a double-stranded RF *in vitro* using a variety of DNA polymerases (73).

Any model of DNA replication must be able to account for the particular features found in mature virion DNA, as well as for intracellular structures (73). In particular, the model in Figure 7 is somewhat more complex than that illustrated earlier for AAV, because the rodent parvoviruses, which have been studied in most detail, have terminal sequence arrangements in which the 5′ terminal sequence of the virion is inverted during replication but the 3′ terminal sequence is not. Additionally, the rodent viruses tend to package only one of the two strands. There are some exceptions to these features among the other autonomous parvoviruses, and presumably this means that alternative mechanisms for parvovirus DNA replication will be uncovered. BPV DNA, for example, shows evidence that both terminal sequences are inverted during replication, although the majority of the virion strands have the 3′-terminal sequence in the same orientation (255). An additional complexity of replication is the generation of variant genomes similar to those seen with AAV (73). The first represents internal deletions of varying extents, and the second is a duplex hairpin molecule representing segments from either the left or the right end of the molecule. Virions containing the incomplete genomes can function as DI particles.

Protein Synthesis

Synthesis of the NS proteins appears to occur first, because the NS protein transcripts appear earlier in the course of infection than the transcripts for the structural proteins, and because one or both of the NS proteins regulate gene expression (91,175,231). Both NS1 and NS2 are phosphorylated subsequent to translation (73). NS1 binds poorly to its recognition site, but binding can be detected in the presence of ATP (53). Binding, ATPase, and DNA helicase activity are modulated by phosphorylation of NS1 (89,203,205). Phosphorylation is on serine and threonine residues by the lambda isoform of protein kinase C and possibly other PKC family members. Dephosphorylated protein has lower nickase and helicase activity but enhanced binding activity, and it retains its ability to regulate transcription. Thus, the phosphorylation state of the NS1 protein seems to determine whether it will be used for transcriptional control or DNA replication. The ATPase binding site and several helicase motifs have been mapped with specific mutations (142), as has a metal coordination site (204). NS1 self-associates prior to nuclear localization (206), and at least one interaction domain has been mapped between amino acids 261 and 280 (220). MVM NS2 is required for efficient virus growth in a host-range-dependent manner. Although not required in hamster, transformed rat, monkey, or human cell lines, it is essential for growth in mouse cell lines and in the whole animal (36,44,198,199). An earlier report suggested that NS2 is required for efficient translation of MVM mRNA (199), but subsequent studies suggested that it was more likely to be involved in particle assembly (68). NS2 also has been shown to interact with 14-3-3 proteins and CRM1 (26,33,207).

The capsid proteins are thought to be acetylated at the N termini (143). VP2 has also been reported to be phosphorylated (250). Synthesis of coat proteins is marked by two unusual phenomena. The first is that the major coat protein, VP2, is proteolytically cleaved to produce VP3 during entry into the cell, and it can be cleaved *in vitro*, but only in the context of full virions (271). The ratio of VP2 to VP3 depends on the time course of the infection. The second is that, as in the case of the AAV capsid proteins VP2 and VP3, the initiator AUG for MVM VP1 is several hundred bases (the whole of the NS2 second exon) downstream from the cap site. The AUG codon for VP2 is another several hundred nucleotides farther downstream. The reason for this is not clear. When expressed in insect cells, the coat proteins can self-assemble to form particles (34,60,146). In the case of B19, the unique region of VP1 (the N terminus) appears to project from the surface of the particle (238).

Oncolysis

Autonomous parvoviruses are normally species restricted. However, transformation of nonpermissive cells, including human cells, with a variety of viral and cellular oncogenes or chemical carcinogens can render the cells permissive for productive infection by rodent parvoviruses such as MVM (reviewed in refs. 234 and 235). In cell culture experiments, infection of transformed cells with MVM or H1 leads to lytic death of the culture; in animal experiments, infection of tumor cells inhibits tumor formation or progression and leads to improved animal survival. A variety of experiments have led to the conclusion that the cytotoxic effect of MVM (or H1) on tumor cells is the result of expression of NS1. Notably, Mousset et al. (195) isolated a Fisher rat fibroblast cell line (FR3T3) that expressed NS1 under the control of an inducible mouse mammary tumor virus (MMTV) promoter. When NS1 was induced in this cell line, no cell death was seen. However, when the same cell was transformed with c-Ha-*ras* or the polyoma oncogenes, the cells died within a few days after induction of NS1. Many but not all oncogenes produced similar NS-induced cytotoxicity. For example, in one study (242), FR3T3 cells transformed with SV40, v-*myc*, and v-*src* were susceptible to MVM killing, but cells transformed by BPV1 were not. If the BPV-transformed cells were supertransformed with Ha-*ras*, they became susceptible to the MVM cytotoxic effect. Although NS1 expression appears to be sufficient for tumor cell killing, NS2 expression had a synergistic effect in some cell types (30).

NS1 expression in nontransformed and transformed cells leads to cell accumulation in the G2 phase of the cell cycle, suggesting that at least part of the cytotoxic phenotype has to do with alteration of the cell cycle (208), but the essential trigger for tumor cell killing is not yet clear. In this respect, Rayet et al. (224) have recently shown that H1 infection of human U937 tumor cells downregulates c-*myc* and activates the CPP322 ICE-like protease (believed to be involved in apoptosis). This is similar to what happens when these cells undergo killing due to tumor necrosis factor (TNF)-α, and it suggests that the TNF pathway may be one of the signaling pathways involved in tumor cell cytotoxicity. It is worth noting that the oncosuppressive effect of parvovirus infection is potentially of clinical value. For example, Faisst et al. (100) have demonstrated that mice with severe combined immunodeficiency disease (SCID), injected with human tumor cells and then infected with H1, showed a dose-dependent regression of the tumors.

SUMMARY AND CONCLUSION

In terms of physical structure, genetic map, autoregulation, and close dependence on the state of the intracellular milieu, the autonomous parvoviruses are closely related to the dependoviruses. There are significant stretches of homology at the amino acid sequence level in both structural and NS proteins of viruses of both genera, and the details of the biochemical reactions involved in DNA synthesis illustrate how the same RCR reaction can be modified to produce quite different overall outcomes. This produces a continuous spectrum of properties among the viruses of both genera—for example, LuIII and BPV encapsidate both strands, the 3′ terminal palindrome of the BPV shows evidence of inversion during replication, and B19 contains TRs. However, there remain several major differences at the biologic level. It seems certain that latent infection plays a major role in the replication cycle of AAV, whereas this is not the case with the autonomous parvoviruses. They do frequently cause cryptic infections, and perhaps these are the biologic equivalent of the AAV latent infection. Another major difference, of course, is that all of the autonomous viruses are serious pathogens in their normal hosts, whereas AAV has yet to be associated with disease. The key difference between the genera seems to be that autonomous viruses simply wait for the cell to enter S phase, relying entirely on their ability to infect dividing cells or tumor cells. In contrast, AAV relies on a helper virus, which can induce S phase in a variety of terminally differentiated, nondividing cells, to expand its host range; but this comes at a price—the helper virus is not always available.

REFERENCES

1. Afione SA, Conrad CK, Kearns WG, et al. *In vivo* model of adeno-associated virus vector persistence and rescue. *J Virol* 1996;70:3235.
2. Agbandje M, Parrish CR, Rossmann MG. The structure of parvoviruses. *Semin Virol* 1995;6:299.
3. Agbandje-McKenna M, Llamas-Saiz AL, Wang F, et al. Functional implications of the structure of the murine parvovirus, minute virus of mice. *Structure* 1998;6:1369.
4. Ahn JK, Gavin BJ, Kumar G, Ward DC. Transcriptional analysis of minute virus of mice P4 promoter mutants. *J Virol* 1989;63:5425.
5. Ahn JK, Pitluk ZW, Ward DC. The GC box and TATA transcription control elements in the P38 promoter of the minute virus of mice are necessary and sufficient for transactivation by the nonstructural protein NS1. *J Virol* 1992;66:3776.
6. Alexandersen S, Bloom ME, Perryman S. Detailed transcription map of Aleutian mink disease parvovirus. *J Virol* 1988;62:3684.
7. Astell CR, Chow MB, Ward DC. Sequence analysis of the termini of virion and replicative forms of minute virus of mice DNA suggests a modified rolling hairpin model for autonomous parvovirus DNA replication. *J Virol* 1985;54:171.
8. Astell CR, Smith M, Chow MB, Ward DC. Structure of the 3′ hairpin termini of four rodent parvovirus genomes: Nucleotide sequence homology at origins of DNA replication. *Cell* 1979;17:691.
9. Astell CR, Thomson M, Chow MB, Ward DC. Structure and replication of minute virus of mice DNA. *Cold Spring Harb Symp Quant Biol* 1983;47:751.
10. Astell CR, Thomson M, Merchlinsky M, Ward DC. The complete DNA sequence of minute virus of mice, an autonomous parvovirus. *Nucleic Acids Res* 1983;11:999.
11. Atchison RW, Casto BC, Hammon W. Adenovirus-associated defective virus particles. *Science* 1965;149:754.
12. Baldauf AQ, Willwand K, Mumtsidu E, et al. Specific initiation of replication at the right-end telomere of the closed species of minute virus of mice replicative-form DNA. *J Virol* 1997;71:971.
13. Ball-Goodrich LJ, Tattersall P. Two amino acid substitutions within the capsid are coordinately required for acquisition of fibrotropism by the lymphotropic strain of minute virus of mice. *J Virol* 1992;66:3415.
14. Bando H, Kusuda J, Gojobori T, et al. Organization and nucleotide sequence of a densovirus genome imply a host-dependent evolution of the parvoviruses. *J Virol* 1987;61:553.
15. Bantel Schaal U, zur Hausen H. Adeno-associated viruses inhibit SV40 DNA amplification and replication of herpes simplex virus in SV40-transformed hamster cells. *Virology* 1988;164:64.
16. Bartlett JS, Wilcher R, Samulski RJ. Infectious entry pathway of adeno-associated virus and adeno-associated virus vectors. *J Virol* 2000;74:2777.
17. Bates RC, Snyder CE, Banerjee PT, Mitra S. Autonomous parvovirus LuIII encapsidates equal amounts of plus and minus DNA strands. *J Virol* 1984;49:319.
18. Beaton A, Palumbo P, Berns KI. Expression from the adeno-associated virus p5 and p19 promoters is negatively regulated in trans by the rep protein. *J Virol* 1989;63:4450.
19. Becerra SP, Rose JA, Hardy M, et al. Direct mapping of adeno-associated virus capsid proteins B and C: A possible ACG initiation codon. *Proc Natl Acad Sci U S A* 1985;82:7919.
20. Beck SE, Jones LA, Chesnut K, et al. Repeated delivery of adeno-associated virus vectors to the rabbit airway. *J Virol* 1999;73:9446.
21. Berns KI, Bergoin M, Bloom M, et al. *Parvoviridae*. VIth report of International Committee on Taxonomy of Viruses. In: Murphy FA, Fauquet CM, Bishop DHL, et al., eds. *Virus Taxonomy*. Vienna: Springer-Verlag, 1994:166.
22. Berns KI, Hauswirth WW. Adeno-associated viruses. *Adv Virus Res* 1979;25:407.
23. Berns KI, Hauswirth WW, Fife KH, Lusby E. Adeno-associated virus DNA replication. *Cold Spring Harb Symp Quant Biol* 1979;43:781.
24. Blacklow NR, Hoggan MD, Sereno MS, et al. A seroepidemiologic study of adenovirus-associated virus infection in infants and children. *Am J Epidemiol* 1971;94:359.
25. Blundell MC, Beard C, Astell CR. *In vitro* identification of a B19 parvovirus promoter. *Virology* 1987;157:534.
26. Bodendorf U, Cziepluch C, Jauniaux JC, et al. Nuclear export factor CRM1 interacts with nonstructural proteins NS2 from parvovirus minute virus of mice. *J Virol* 1999;73:7769.
27. Bohenzky RA, Berns KI. Interactions between the termini of adeno-associated virus DNA. *J Mol Biol* 1989;206:91.
28. Bohenzky RA, LeFebvre RB, Berns KI. Sequence and symmetry requirements within the internal palindromic sequences of the adeno-associated virus terminal repeat. *Virology* 1988;166:316.
29. Boublik Y, Jousset FX, Bergoin M. Complete nucleotide sequence and genomic organization of the *Aedes albopictus* parvovirus (AaPV) pathogenic for *Aedes aegypti* larvae. *Virology* 1994;200:752.
30. Brandenburger A, Legendre D, Avalosse B, Rommelaere J. NS-1 and NS-2 proteins may act synergistically in the cytopathogenicity of parvovirus MVMp. *Virology* 1990;174:576.
31. Brister JR, Muzyczka N. Rep-mediated nicking of the adeno-associated virus origin requires two biochemical activities, DNA helicase activity and transesterification. *J Virol* 1999;73:9325.
32. Brister JR, Muzyczka N. Mechanism of Rep-mediated adeno-associated virus origin nicking. *J Virol* 2000;74:7762.
33. Brockhaus K, Plaza S, Pintel DJ, et al. Nonstructural proteins NS2 of minute virus of mice associate *in vivo* with 14-3-3 protein family members. *J Virol* 1996;70:7527.
34. Brown CS, Van Lent JW, Vlak JM, Spaan WJ. Assembly of empty capsids by using baculovirus recombinants expressing human parvovirus B19 structural proteins. *J Virol* 1991;65:2702.
35. Brown KE, Hibbs JR, Gallinella G, et al. Resistance to parvovirus B19 infection due to lack of virus receptor (erythrocyte P antigen). *N Engl J Med* 1994;330:1192.
36. Brownstein DG, Smith AL, Johnson EA, et al. The pathogenesis of infection with minute virus of mice depends on expression of the small nonstructural protein NS2 and on the genotype of the allotropic determinants VP1 and VP2. *J Virol* 1992;66:3118.
37. Brunstein J, Astell CR. Analysis of the internal replication sequence indicates that there are three elements required for efficient replication of minute virus of mice minigenomes. *J Virol* 1997;71:9087.
38. Buller RM, Janik JE, Sebring ED, Rose JA. Herpes simplex virus types 1 and 2 completely help adenovirus-associated virus replication. *J Virol* 1981;40:241.

39. Carter BJ, Antoni BA, Klessig DF. Adenovirus containing a deletion of the early region 2A gene allows growth of adeno-associated virus with decreased efficiency. *Virology* 1992;191:473.
40. Carter BJ, Laughlin CA, de la Maza LM, Myers M. Adeno-associated virus autointerference. *Virology* 1979;92:449.
41. Carter PJ, Samulski RJ. Adeno-associated viral vectors as gene delivery vehicles (review). *Int J Mol Med* 2000;6:17.
42. Casto BC, Atchison RW, Hammon WM. Studies on the relationship between adeno-associated virus type I (AAV-1) and adenoviruses. I. Replication of AAV-1 in certain cell cultures and its effect on helper adenovirus. *Virology* 1967;32:52.
43. Casto BC, Goodheart CR. Inhibition of adenovirus transformation *in vitro* by AAV-1. *Proc Soc Exp Biol Med* 1972;140:72.
44. Cater JE, Pintel DJ. The small non-structural protein NS2 of the autonomous parvovirus minute virus of mice is required for virus growth in murine cells. *J Gen Virol* 1992;73:1839.
45. Chang LS, Shenk T. The adenovirus DNA-binding protein stimulates the rate of transcription directed by adenovirus and adeno-associated virus promoters. *J Virol* 1990;64:2103.
46. Chang LS, Shi Y, Shenk T. Adeno-associated virus P5 promoter contains an adenovirus E1A-inducible element and a binding site for the major late transcription factor. *J Virol* 1989;63:3479.
47. Chejanovsky N, Carter BJ. Mutagenesis of an AUG codon in the adeno-associated virus *rep* gene: Effects on viral DNA replication. *Virology* 1989;173:120.
48. Cheung AK, Hoggan MD, Hauswirth WW, Berns KI. Integration of the adeno-associated virus genome into cellular DNA in latently infected human Detroit 6 cells. *J Virol* 1980;33:739.
49. Chiorini JA, Weitzman MD, Owens RA, et al. Biologically active Rep proteins of adeno-associated virus type 2 produced as fusion proteins in *Escherichia coli*. *J Virol* 1994;68:797.
50. Chiorini JA, Wiener SM, Owens RA, et al. Sequence requirements for stable binding and function of Rep68 on the adeno-associated virus type 2 inverted terminal repeats. *J Virol* 1994;68:7448.
51. Chiorini JA, Yang L, Safer B, Kotin RM. Determination of adeno-associated virus Rep68 and Rep78 binding sites by random sequence oligonucleotide selection. *J Virol* 1995;69:7334.
52. Chirmule N, Xiao W, Truneh A, et al. Humoral immunity to adeno-associated virus type 2 vectors following administration to murine and nonhuman primate muscle. *J Virol* 2000;74:2420.
53. Christensen J, Cotmore SF, Tattersall P. Minute virus of mice transcriptional activator protein NS1 binds directly to the transactivation region of the viral P38 promoter in a strictly ATP-dependent manner. *J Virol* 1995;69:5422.
54. Christensen J, Cotmore SF, Tattersall P. A novel cellular site-specific DNA-binding protein cooperates with the viral NS1 polypeptide to initiate parvovirus DNA replication. *J Virol* 1997;71:1405.
55. Christensen J, Cotmore SF, Tattersall P. Parvovirus initiation factor PIF: A novel human DNA-binding factor which coordinately recognizes two ACGT motifs. *J Virol* 1997;71:5733.
56. Christensen J, Cotmore SF, Tattersall P. Two new members of the emerging KDWK family of combinatorial transcription modulators bind as a heterodimer to flexibly spaced PuCGPy half-sites. *Mol Cell Biol* 1999;19:7741.
57. Christensen J, Pedersen M, Aasted B, Alexandersen S. Purification and characterization of the major nonstructural protein (NS-1) of Aleutian mink disease parvovirus. *J Virol* 1995;69:1802.
58. Christensen J, Storgaard T, Bloch B, et al. Expression of Aleutian mink disease parvovirus proteins in a baculovirus vector system. *J Virol* 1993;67:229.
59. Clark KR, Liu X, McGrath JP, Johnson PR. Highly purified recombinant adeno-associated virus vectors are biologically active and free of detectable helper and wild-type viruses. *Hum Gene Ther* 1999;10:1031.
60. Clemens DL, Wolfinbarger JB, Mori S, et al. Expression of Aleutian mink disease parvovirus capsid proteins by a recombinant vaccinia virus: Self-assembly of capsid proteins into particles. *J Virol* 1992;66:3077.
61. Clemens KE, Pintel DJ. The two transcription units of the autonomous parvovirus minute virus of mice are transcribed in a temporal order. *J Virol* 1988;62:1448.
62. Collaco R, Prasad KM, Trempe JP. Phosphorylation of the adeno-associated virus replication proteins. *Virology* 1997;232:332.
63. Conway JE, Ap Rhys CMJ, Zolotukhin I, et al. High titer recombinant adeno-associated virus production utilizing a recombinant herpes simplex virus type 1 vector expressing AAV-2 rep and cap. *Gene Ther* 1999;6:986.
64. Costello E, Sahli R, Hirt B, Beard P. The mismatched nucleotides in the 5′-terminal hairpin of minute virus of mice are required for efficient viral DNA replication. *J Virol* 1995;69:7489.
65. Costello E, Saudan P, Winocour E, et al. High mobility group chromosomal protein 1 binds to the adeno-associated virus replication protein (Rep) and promotes Rep-mediated site-specific cleavage of DNA, ATPase activity and transcriptional repression. *EMBO J* 1997; 16:5943.
66. Cotmore SF, Christensen J, Nuesch JP, Tattersall P. The NS1 polypeptide of the murine parvovirus minute virus of mice binds to DNA sequences containing the motif $[ACCA]_{2-3}$. *J Virol* 1995;69:1652.
67. Cotmore SF, Christensen J, Tattersall P. Two widely spaced initiator binding sites create an HMG1-dependent parvovirus rolling-hairpin replication origin. *J Virol* 2000;74:1332.
68. Cotmore SF, D'Abramo AM Jr, Carbonell LF, et al. The NS2 polypeptide of parvovirus MVM is required for capsid assembly in murine cells. *Virology* 1997;231:267.
69. Cotmore SF, Gunther M, Tattersall P. Evidence for a ligation step in the DNA replication of the autonomous parvovirus minute virus of mice. *J Virol* 1989;63:1002.
70. Cotmore SF, Nuesch JP, Tattersall P. *In vitro* excision and replication of 5′ telomeres of minute virus of mice DNA from cloned palindromic concatemer junctions. *Virology* 1992;190:365.
71. Cotmore SF, Nuesch JP, Tattersall P. Asymmetric resolution of a parvovirus palindrome *in vitro*. *J Virol* 1993;67:1579.
72. Cotmore SF, Sturzenbecker LJ, Tattersall P. The autonomous parvovirus MVM encodes two nonstructural proteins in addition to its capsid polypeptides. *Virology* 1983;129:333.
73. Cotmore SF, Tattersall P. The autonomously replicating parvoviruses of vertebrates. *Adv Virus Res* 1987;33:91.
74. Cotmore SF, Tattersall P. The NS-1 polypeptide of minute virus of mice is covalently attached to the 5′ termini of duplex replicative-form DNA and progeny single strands. *J Virol* 1988;62:851.
75. Cotmore SF, Tattersall P. A genome-linked copy of the NS-1 polypeptide is located on the outside of infectious parvovirus particles. *J Virol* 1989;63:3902.
76. Cotmore SF, Tattersall P. *In vivo* resolution of circular plasmids containing concatemer junction fragments from minute virus of mice DNA and their subsequent replication as linear molecules. *J Virol* 1992;66:420.
77. Cotmore SF, Tattersall P. An asymmetric nucleotide in the parvoviral 3′ hairpin directs segregation of a single active origin of DNA replication. *EMBO J* 1994;13:4145.
78. Cotmore SF, Tattersall P. Parvovirus DNA replication. In: DePamphilis ML, ed. *DNA Replication in Eukaryotic Cells.* Cold Spring Harbor, NY: Cold Spring Harbor Laboratory Press, 1996:799.
79. Cotmore SF, Tattersall P. High-mobility group 1/2 proteins are essential for initiating rolling-circle-type DNA replication at a parvovirus hairpin origin. *J Virol* 1998;72:8477.
80. Crawford LV, Follett EA, Burdon MG, McGeoch DJ. The DNA of a minute virus of mice. *J Gen Virol* 1969;4:37.
81. Cukor G, Blacklow NR, Kibrick S, Swan IC. Effect of adeno-associated virus on cancer expression by herpesvirus-transformed hamster cells. *J Natl Cancer Inst* 1975;55:957.
82. Davis MD, Wonderling RS, Walker SL, Owens RA. Analysis of the effects of charge cluster mutations in adeno-associated virus Rep68 protein *in vitro*. *J Virol* 1999;73:2084.
83. Davis MD, Wu J, Owens RA. Mutational analysis of adeno-associated virus type 2 rep68 protein endonuclease activity on partially single-stranded substrates. *J Virol* 2000;74:2936.
84. de la Maza LM, Carter BJ. Molecular structure of adeno-associated virus variant DNA. *J Biol Chem* 1980;255:3194.
85. de la Maza LM, Carter BJ. Inhibition of adenovirus oncogenicity in hamsters by adeno-associated virus DNA. *J Natl Cancer Inst* 1981;67: 1323.
86. Deiss V, Tratschin JD, Weitz M, Siegl G. Cloning of the human parvovirus B19 genome and structural analysis of its palindromic termini. *Virology* 1990;175:247.
87. Deleu L, Fuks F, Spitkovsky D, et al. Opposite transcriptional effects of cyclic AMP-responsive elements in confluent or p27KIP-overexpressing cells versus serum-starved or growing cells. *Mol Cell Biol* 1998;18:409.

88. Deleu L, Pujol A, Faisst S, Rommelaere J. Activation of promoter P4 of the autonomous parvovirus minute virus of mice at early S phase is required for productive infection. *J Virol* 1999;73:3877.
89. Dettwiler S, Rommelaere J, Nuesch JP. DNA unwinding functions of minute virus of mice NS1 protein are modulated specifically by the lambda isoform of protein kinase C. *J Virol* 1999;73:7410.
90. Doerig C, Beard P, Hirt B. A transcriptional promoter of the human parvovirus B19 active *in vitro* and *in vivo*. *Virology* 1987;157:539.
91. Doerig C, Hirt B, Antonietti JP, Beard P. Nonstructural protein of parvoviruses B19 and minute virus of mice controls transcription. *J Virol* 1990;64:387.
92. Doerig C, Hirt B, Beard P, Antonietti JP. Minute virus of mice non-structural protein NS-1 is necessary and sufficient for trans-activation of the viral P39 promoter. *J Gen Virol* 1988;69:2563.
93. Duan D, Fisher KJ, Burda JF, Engelhardt JF. Structural and functional heterogeneity of integrated recombinant AAV genomes. *Virus Res* 1997;48:41.
94. Duan D, Yan Z, Yue Y, Engelhardt JF. Structural analysis of adeno-associated virus transduction circular intermediates. *Virology* 1999; 261:8.
95. Duan D, Yue Y, Yan Z, Engelhardt JF. A new dual-vector approach to enhance recombinant adeno-associated virus-mediated gene expression through intermolecular cis activation. *Nat Med* 2000;6:595.
96. Dubielzig R, King JA, Weger S, et al. Adeno-associated virus type 2 protein interactions: Formation of pre-encapsidation complexes. *J Virol* 1999;73:8989.
97. Dutheil N, Shi F, Dupressoir T, Linden RM. Adeno-associated virus site-specifically integrates into a muscle-specific DNA region. *Proc Natl Acad Sci U S A* 2000;97:4862.
98. Dyall J, Berns KI. Site-specific integration of adeno-associated virus into an episome with the target locus via a deletion-substitution mechanism. *J Virol* 1998;72:6195.
99. Dyall J, Szabo P, Berns KI. Adeno-associated virus (AAV) site-specific integration: Formation of AAV-AAVS1 junctions in an *in vitro* system. *Proc Natl Acad Sci U S A* 1999;96:12849.
100. Faisst S, Guittard D, Benner A, et al. Dose-dependent regression of HeLa cell-derived tumours in SCID mice after parvovirus H-1 infection. *Int J Cancer* 1998;75:584.
101. Ferrari FK, Samulski T, Shenk T, Samulski RJ. Second-strand synthesis is a rate-limiting step for efficient transduction by recombinant adeno-associated virus vectors. *J Virol* 1996;70:3227.
102. Fisher KJ, Gao GP, Weitzman MD, et al. Transduction with recombinant adeno-associated virus for gene therapy is limited by leading-strand synthesis. *J Virol* 1996;70:520.
103. Flotte TR, Afione SA, Conrad C, et al. Stable *in vivo* expression of the cystic fibrosis transmembrane conductance regulator with an adeno-associated virus vector. *Proc Natl Acad Sci U S A* 1993;90: 10613.
104. Flotte TR, Afione SA, Solow R, et al. Expression of the cystic fibrosis transmembrane conductance regulator from a novel adeno-associated virus promoter. *J Biol Chem* 1993;268:3781.
105. Flotte TR, Afione SA, Zeitlin PL. Adeno-associated virus vector gene expression occurs in nondividing cells in the absence of vector DNA integration. *Am J Respir Cell Mol Biol* 1994;11:517.
106. Friedman-Einat M, Grossman Z, Mileguir F, et al. Detection of adeno-associated virus type 2 sequences in the human genital tract. *J Clin Microbiol* 1997;35:71.
107. Fuks F, Deleu L, Dinsart C, et al. *ras* oncogene-dependent activation of the P4 promoter of minute virus of mice through a proximal P4 element interacting with the Ets family of transcription factors. *J Virol* 1996;70:1331.
108. Gao GP, Qu G, Faust LZ, et al. High-titer adeno-associated viral vectors from a Rep/Cap cell line and hybrid shuttle virus. *Hum Gene Ther* 1998;9:2353.
109. Gavin BJ, Ward DC. Positive and negative regulation of the minute virus of mice P38 promoter. *J Virol* 1990;64:2057.
110. Gavin DK, Young SM Jr, Xiao W, et al. Charge-to-alanine mutagenesis of the adeno-associated virus type 2 Rep78/68 proteins yields temperature-sensitive and magnesium-dependent variants [published erratum appears in *J Virol* 2000;74:591]. *J Virol* 1999;73:9433.
111. Giraud C, Winocour E, Berns KI. Site-specific integration by adeno-associated virus is directed by a cellular DNA sequence. *Proc Natl Acad Sci U S A* 1994;91:10039.
112. Giraud C, Winocour E, Berns KI. Recombinant junctions formed by site-specific integration of adeno-associated virus into an episome. *J Virol* 1995;69:6917.
113. Gottlieb J, Muzyczka N. Substrate specificity of HeLa endonuclease R. A G-specific mammalian endonuclease. *J Biol Chem* 1990;265: 10842.
114. Green MR, Roeder RG. Definition of a novel promoter for the major adenovirus-associated virus mRNA. *Cell* 1980;22:231.
115. Grifman M, Chen NN, Gao GP, et al. Overexpression of cyclin A inhibits augmentation of recombinant adeno-associated virus transduction by the adenovirus E4orf6 protein. *J Virol* 1999;73:10010.
116. Grimm D, Kleinschmidt JA. Progress in adeno-associated virus type 2 vector production: Promises and prospects for clinical use. *Hum Gene Ther* 1999;10:2445.
117. Grossman Z, Mendelson E, Brok Simoni F, et al. Detection of adeno-associated virus type 2 in human peripheral blood cells. *J Gen Virol* 1992;73:961.
118. Gu Z, Plaza S, Perros M, et al. NF-Y controls transcription of the minute virus of mice P4 promoter through interaction with an unusual binding site. *J Virol* 1995;69:239.
119. Hanson ND, Rhode SL. Parvovirus NS1 stimulates P4 expression by interaction with the terminal repeats and through DNA amplification. *J Virol* 1991;65:4325.
120. Hauswirth WW, Berns KI. Origin and termination of adeno-associated virus DNA replication. *Virology* 1977;78:488.
121. Hauswirth WW, Berns KI. Adeno-associated virus DNA replication: Nonunit-length molecules. *Virology* 1979;93:57.
122. Hermonat PL. Inhibition of H-*ras* expression by the adeno-associated virus Rep78 transformation suppressor gene product. *Cancer Res* 1991;51:3373.
123. Hermonat PL. Inhibition of bovine papillomavirus plasmid DNA replication by adeno-associated virus. *Virology* 1992;189:329.
124. Hermonat PL. Down-regulation of the human c-*fos* and c-*myc* proto-oncogene promoters by adeno-associated virus Rep78. *Cancer Lett* 1994;81:129.
125. Hermonat PL, Labow MA, Wright R, et al. Genetics of adeno-associated virus: Isolation and preliminary characterization of adeno-associated virus type 2 mutants. *J Virol* 1984;51:329.
126. Hermonat PL, Muzyczka N. Use of adeno-associated virus as a mammalian DNA cloning vector: Transduction of neomycin resistance into mammalian tissue culture cells. *Proc Natl Acad Sci U S A* 1984;81: 6466.
127. Hermonat PL, Santin AD, Batchu RB, Zhan D. The adeno-associated virus Rep78 major regulatory protein binds the cellular TATA-binding protein *in vitro* and *in vivo*. *Virology* 1998;245:120.
128. Hermonat PL, Santin AD, Zhan D. Binding of the human papillomavirus type 16 E7 oncoprotein and the adeno-associated virus Rep78 major regulatory protein *in vitro* and in yeast and the potential for downstream effects. *J Hum Virol* 2000;3:113.
129. Hernandez YJ, Wang J, Kearns WG, et al. Latent adeno-associated virus infection elicits humoral but not cell-mediated immune responses in a nonhuman primate model. *J Virol* 1999;73:8549.
130. Hoggan MD, Thomas GF, Thomas FB, Johnson FB. Continuous "carriage" of adenovirus associated virus genome in cell cultures in the absence of helper adenoviruses. In: Hoggan MD, Thomas GF, Thomas FB, Johnson FB, eds. *Proceedings of the Fourth Lepetit Colloquium, Cocoyac, Mexico.* Amsterdam: North Holland, 1972.
131. Hong G, Ward P, Berns KI. *In vitro* replication of adeno-associated virus DNA. *Proc Natl Acad Sci U S A* 1992;89:4673.
132. Hong G, Ward P, Berns KI. Intermediates of adeno-associated virus DNA replication *in vitro*. *J Virol* 1994;68:2011.
133. Hoque M, Ishizu K, Matsumoto A, et al. Nuclear transport of the major capsid protein is essential for adeno-associated virus capsid formation. *J Virol* 1999;73:7912.
134. Horer M, Weger S, Butz K, et al. Mutational analysis of adeno-associated virus Rep protein-mediated inhibition of heterologous and homologous promoters. *J Virol* 1995;69:5485.
135. Huang MM, Hearing P. Adenovirus early region 4 encodes two gene products with redundant effects in lytic infection. *J Virol* 1989;63:2605.
136. Ilyina TV, Koonin EV. Conserved sequence motifs in the initiator proteins for rolling circle DNA replication encoded by diverse replicons from eubacteria, eucaryotes and archaebacteria. *Nucleic Acids Res* 1992;20:3279.
137. Im DS, Muzyczka N. Factors that bind to adeno-associated virus terminal repeats. *J Virol* 1989;63:3095.

138. Im DS, Muzyczka N. The AAV origin binding protein Rep68 is an ATP-dependent site-specific endonuclease with DNA helicase activity. *Cell* 1990;61:447.
139. Janik JE, Huston MM, Cho K, Rose JA. Requirement of adenovirus DNA binding protein and VA-1 RNA for production of adeno-associated virus polypeptides. *J Cell Biochem (Suppl)* 1982;6:209.
140. Janik JE, Huston MM, Rose JA. Locations of adenovirus genes required for the replication of adenovirus-associated virus. *Proc Natl Acad Sci U S A* 1981;78:1925.
141. Jay FT, Laughlin CA, Carter BJ. Eukaryotic translational control: Adeno-associated virus protein synthesis is affected by a mutation in the adenovirus DNA-binding protein. *Proc Natl Acad Sci U S A* 1981; 78:2927.
142. Jindal HK, Yong CB, Wilson GM, et al. Mutations in the NTP-binding motif of minute virus of mice (MVM) NS-1 protein uncouple ATPase and DNA helicase functions. *J Biol Chem* 1994;269:3283.
143. Johnson FB. Parvovirus proteins. In: Berns KI, ed. *The Parvoviruses.* New York: Plenum Press, 1983:329.
144. Jongeneel CV, Sahli R, McMaster GK, Hirt B. A precise map of splice junctions in the mRNAs of minute virus of mice, an autonomous parvovirus. *J Virol* 1986;59:564.
145. Jooss K, Yang Y, Fisher KJ, Wilson JM. Transduction of dendritic cells by DNA viral vectors directs the immune response to transgene products in muscle fibers. *J Virol* 1998;72:4212.
146. Kajigaya S, Fujii H, Field A, et al. Self-assembled B19 parvovirus capsids, produced in a baculovirus system, are antigenically and immunogenically similar to native virions. *Proc Natl Acad Sci U S A* 1991;88:4646.
147. Kay MA, Manno CS, Ragni MV, et al. Evidence for gene transfer and expression of factor IX in haemophilia B patients treated with an AAV vector [see comments]. *Nat Genet* 2000;24:257.
148. Kearns WG, Afione SA, Fulmer SB, et al. Recombinant adeno-associated virus (AAV-CFTR) vectors do not integrate in a site-specific fashion in an immortalized epithelial cell line. *Gene Ther* 1996;3:748.
149. Kessler PD, Podsakoff GM, Chen X, et al. Gene delivery to skeletal muscle results in sustained expression and systemic delivery of a therapeutic protein. *Proc Natl Acad Sci U S A* 1996;93:14082.
150. Khleif SN, Myers T, Carter BJ, Trempe JP. Inhibition of cellular transformation by the adeno-associated virus *rep* gene. *Virology* 1991;181:738.
151. Kimmick MW, Afanasiev BN, Beaty BJ, Carlson JO. Gene expression and regulation from the p7 promoter of *Aedes densonucleosis* virus. *J Virol* 1998;72:4364.
152. Kirschstein RL, Smith KO, Peters EA. Inhibition of adenovirus 12 oncogenicity by adeno-associated virus. *Proc Soc Exp Biol Med* 1968; 128:670.
153. Klein Bauernschmitt P, zur Hausen H, Schlehofer JR. Induction of differentiation-associated changes in established human cells by infection with adeno-associated virus type 2. *J Virol* 1992;66:4191.
154. Kleinschmidt JA, Mohler M, Weindler FW, Heilbronn R. Sequence elements of the adeno-associated virus *rep* gene required for suppression of herpes-simplex-virus-induced DNA amplification. *Virology* 1995;206:254.
155. Kotin RM, Berns KI. Organization of adeno-associated virus DNA in latently infected Detroit 6 cells. *Virology* 1989;170:460.
156. Kotin RM, Linden RM, Berns KI. Characterization of a preferred site on human chromosome 19q for integration of adeno-associated virus DNA by non-homologous recombination. *EMBO J* 1992;11:5071.
157. Kotin RM, Menninger JC, Ward DC, Berns KI. Mapping and direct visualization of a region-specific viral DNA integration site on chromosome 19q13-qter. *Genomics* 1991;10:831.
158. Kotin RM, Siniscalco M, Samulski RJ, et al. Site-specific integration by adeno-associated virus. *Proc Natl Acad Sci U S A* 1990;87:2211.
159. Krady JK, Ward DC. Transcriptional activation by the parvoviral nonstructural protein NS-1 is mediated via a direct interaction with Sp1. *Mol Cell Biol* 1995;15:524.
160. Krauskopf A, Aloni Y. A cellular repressor regulates transcription initiation from the minute virus of mice P38 promoter. *Nucleic Acids Res* 1994;22:828.
161. Kube DM, Ponnazhagan S, Srivastava A. Encapsidation of adeno-associated virus type 2 Rep proteins in wild-type and recombinant progeny virions: Rep-mediated growth inhibition of primary human cells. *J Virol* 1997;71:7361.
162. Kurpad C, Mukherjee P, Wang XS, et al. Adeno-associated virus 2-mediated transduction and erythroid lineage-restricted expression from parvovirus B19p6 promoter in primary human hematopoietic progenitor cells. *J Hematother Stem Cell Res* 1999;8:585.
163. Kyostio SR, Owens RA, Weitzman MD, et al. Analysis of adeno-associated virus (AAV) wild-type and mutant Rep proteins for their abilities to negatively regulate AAV p5 and p19 mRNA levels. *J Virol* 1994;68:2947.
164. Kyostio SR, Wonderling RS, Owens RA. Negative regulation of the adeno-associated virus (AAV) P5 promoter involves both the P5 rep binding site and the consensus ATP-binding motif of the AAV Rep68 protein. *J Virol* 1995;69:6787.
165. Labieniec-Pintel L, Pintel D. The minute virus of mice P39 transcription unit can encode both capsid proteins. *J Virol* 1986;57:1163.
166. Labow MA, Berns KI. The adeno-associated virus *rep* gene inhibits replication of an adeno-associated virus/simian virus 40 hybrid genome in cos-7 cells. *J Virol* 1988;62:1705.
167. Labow MA, Graf LH Jr, Berns KI. Adeno-associated virus gene expression inhibits cellular transformation by heterologous genes. *Mol Cell Biol* 1987;7:1320.
168. Labow MA, Hermonat PL, Berns KI. Positive and negative autoregulation of the adeno-associated virus type 2 genome. *J Virol* 1986;60: 251.
169. Laughlin CA, Cardellichio CB, Coon HC. Latent infection of KB cells with adeno-associated virus type 2. *J Virol* 1986;60:515.
170. Laughlin CA, Jones N, Carter BJ. Effect of deletions in adenovirus early region 1 genes upon replication of adeno-associated virus. *J Virol* 1982;41:868.
171. Laughlin CA, Westphal H, Carter BJ. Spliced adenovirus-associated virus RNA. *Proc Natl Acad Sci U S A* 1979;76:5567.
172. LeFebvre RB, Riva S, Berns KI. Conformation takes precedence over sequence in adeno-associated virus DNA replication. *Mol Cell Biol* 1984;4:1416.
173. Legendre D, Rommelaere J. Targeting of promoters for trans activation by a carboxy-terminal domain of the NS-1 protein of the parvovirus minute virus of mice. *J Virol* 1994;68:7974.
174. Li X, Rhode SL. Nonstructural protein NS2 of parvovirus H-1 is required for efficient viral protein synthesis and virus production in rat cells *in vivo* and *in vitro*. *Virology* 1991;184:117.
175. Li X, Rhode SL. The parvovirus H-1 NS2 protein affects viral gene expression through sequences in the 3′ untranslated region. *Virology* 1993;194:10.
176. Linden RM, Winocour E, Berns KI. The recombination signals for adeno-associated virus site-specific integration. *Proc Natl Acad Sci U S A* 1996;93:7966.
177. Liu Q, Yong CB, Astell CR. *In vitro* resolution of the dimer bridge of the minute virus of mice (MVM) genome supports the modified rolling hairpin model for MVM replication. *Virology* 1994;201:251.
178. Lorson C, Burger LR, Mouw M, Pintel DJ. Efficient transactivation of the minute virus of mice P38 promoter requires upstream binding of NS1. *J Virol* 1996;70:834.
179. Lorson C, Pearson J, Burger L, Pintel DJ. An Sp1-binding site and TATA element are sufficient to support full transactivation by proximally bound NS1 protein of minute virus of mice. *Virology* 1998;240:326.
180. Lusby E, Bohenzky R, Berns KI. Inverted terminal repetition in adeno-associated virus DNA: Independence of the orientation at either end of the genome. *J Virol* 1981;37:1083.
181. Lusby E, Fife KH, Berns KI. Nucleotide sequence of the inverted terminal repetition in adeno-associated virus DNA. *J Virol* 1980;34:402.
182. Lusby EW, Berns KI. Mapping of the 5′ termini of two adeno-associated virus 2 RNAs in the left half of the genome. *J Virol* 1982;41:518.
183. Mah C, Qing K, Khuntirat B, et al. Adeno-associated virus type 2-mediated gene transfer: Role of epidermal growth factor receptor protein tyrosine kinase in transgene expression. *J Virol* 1998;72:9835.
184. Malik AK, Monahan PE, Allen DL, et al. Kinetics of recombinant adeno-associated virus-mediated gene transfer. *J Virol* 2000;74:3555.
185. Mayor HD, Houlditch GS, Mumford DM. Influence of adeno-associated satellite virus on adenovirus-induced tumours in hamsters. *Nature New Biol* 1973;241:44.
186. McCarty DM, Christensen M, Muzyczka N. Sequences required for coordinate induction of adeno-associated virus p19 and p40 promoters by Rep protein. *J Virol* 1991;65:2936.
187. McCarty DM, Ni TH, Muzyczka N. Analysis of mutations in adeno-associated virus Rep protein *in vivo* and *in vitro*. *J Virol* 1992;66:4050.
188. McCarty DM, Pereira DJ, Zolotukhin I, et al. Identification of linear

DNA sequences that specifically bind the adeno-associated virus Rep protein. *J Virol* 1994;68:4988.
189. McCarty DM, Ryan JH, Zolotukhin S, et al. Interaction of the adeno-associated virus Rep protein with a sequence within the A palindrome of the viral terminal repeat. *J Virol* 1994;68:4998.
190. McLaughlin SK, Collis P, Hermonat PL, Muzyczka N. Adeno-associated virus general transduction vectors: Analysis of proviral structures. *J Virol* 1988;62:1963.
191. McPherson RA, Rose JA. Structural proteins of adenovirus-associated virus: Subspecies and their relatedness. *J Virol* 1983;46:523.
192. Mendelson E, Trempe JP, Carter BJ. Identification of the trans-acting Rep proteins of adeno-associated virus by antibodies to a synthetic oligopeptide. *J Virol* 1986;60:823.
193. Mishra L, Rose JA. Adeno-associated virus DNA replication is induced by genes that are essential for HSV-1 DNA synthesis. *Virology* 1990;179:632.
194. Morgan WR, Ward DC. Three splicing patterns are used to excise the small intron common to all minute virus of mice RNAs. *J Virol* 1986; 60:1170.
195. Mousset S, Ouadrhiri Y, Caillet-Fauquet P, Rommelaere J. The cytotoxicity of the autonomous parvovirus minute virus of mice nonstructural proteins in FR3T3 rat cells depends on oncogene expression. *J Virol* 1994;68:6446.
196. Muralidhar S, Becerra SP, Rose JA. Site-directed mutagenesis of adeno-associated virus type 2 structural protein initiation codons: Effects on regulation of synthesis and biological activity. *J Virol* 1994; 68:170.
197. Muzyczka N. Use of adeno-associated virus as a general transduction vector for mammalian cells. *Curr Top Microbiol Immunol* 1992;158: 97.
198. Naeger LK, Cater J, Pintel DJ. The small nonstructural protein (NS2) of the parvovirus minute virus of mice is required for efficient DNA replication and infectious virus production in a cell-type-specific manner. *J Virol* 1990;64:6166.
199. Naeger LK, Salome N, Pintel DJ. NS2 is required for efficient translation of viral mRNA in minute virus of mice-infected murine cells. *J Virol* 1993;67:1034.
200. Naeger LK, Schoborg RV, Zhao Q, et al. Nonsense mutations inhibit splicing of MVM RNA in cis when they interrupt the reading frame of either exon of the final spliced product. *Genes Dev* 1992;6:1107.
201. Ni TH, McDonald WF, Zolotukhin I, et al. Cellular proteins required for adeno-associated virus DNA replication in the absence of adenovirus coinfection. *J Virol* 1998;72:2777.
202. Ni TH, Zhou X, McCarty DM, et al. *In vitro* replication of adeno-associated virus DNA. *J Virol* 1994;68:1128.
203. Nuesch JP, Corbau R, Tattersall P, Rommelaere J. Biochemical activities of minute virus of mice nonstructural protein NS1 are modulated *in vitro* by the phosphorylation state of the polypeptide. *J Virol* 1998; 72:8002.
204. Nuesch JP, Cotmore SF, Tattersall P. Sequence motifs in the replicator protein of parvovirus MVM essential for nicking and covalent attachment to the viral origin: Identification of the linking tyrosine. *Virology* 1995;209:122.
205. Nuesch JP, Dettwiler S, Corbau R, Rommelaere J. Replicative functions of minute virus of mice NS1 protein are regulated *in vitro* by phosphorylation through protein kinase C. *J Virol* 1998;72:9966.
206. Nuesch JP, Tattersall P. Nuclear targeting of the parvoviral replicator molecule NS1: Evidence for self-association prior to nuclear transport. *Virology* 1993;196:637.
207. Ohshima T, Nakajima T, Oishi T, et al. CRM1 mediates nuclear export of nonstructural protein 2 from parvovirus minute virus of mice. *Biochem Biophys Res Commun* 1999;264:144.
208. Op De Beeck A, Anouja F, Mousset S, et al. The nonstructural proteins of the autonomous parvovirus minute virus of mice interfere with the cell cycle, inducing accumulation in G2. *Cell Growth Differ* 1995;6: 781.
209. Ostrove JM, Duckworth DH, Berns KI. Inhibition of adenovirus-transformed cell oncogenicity by adeno-associated virus. *Virology* 1981;113:521.
210. Owens RA, Weitzman MD, Kyostio SR, Carter BJ. Identification of a DNA-binding domain in the amino terminus of adeno-associated virus Rep proteins. *J Virol* 1993;67:997.
211. Ozawa K, Ayub J, Hao YS, et al. Novel transcription map for the B19 (human) pathogenic parvovirus. *J Virol* 1987;61:2395.
212. Pereira DJ, McCarty DM, Muzyczka N. The adeno-associated virus (AAV) Rep protein acts as both a repressor and an activator to regulate AAV transcription during a productive infection. *J Virol* 1997;71: 1079.
213. Pereira DJ, Muzyczka N. The adeno-associated virus type 2 p40 promoter requires a proximal Sp1 interaction and a p19 CArG-like element to facilitate Rep transactivation. *J Virol* 1997;71:4300.
214. Pereira DJ, Muzyczka N. The cellular transcription factor SP1 and an unknown cellular protein are required to mediate Rep protein activation of the adeno-associated virus p19 promoter. *J Virol* 1997;71: 1747.
215. Perros M, Deleu L, Vanacker JM, et al. Upstream CREs participate in the basal activity of minute virus of mice promoter P4 and in its stimulation in *ras*-transformed cells. *J Virol* 1995;69:5506.
216. Perros M, Spegelaere P, Dupont F, et al. Cruciform structure of a DNA motif of parvovirus minute virus of mice (prototype strain) involved in the attenuation of gene expression. *J Gen Virol* 1994;75:2645.
217. Pintel D, Dadachanji D, Astell CR, Ward DC. The genome of minute virus of mice, an autonomous parvovirus, encodes two overlapping transcription units. *Nucleic Acids Res* 1983;11:1019.
218. Ponnazhagan S, Mukherjee P, Wang XS, et al. Adeno-associated virus type 2-mediated transduction in primary human bone marrow-derived CD34+ hematopoietic progenitor cells: Donor variation and correlation of transgene expression with cellular differentiation. *J Virol* 1997; 71:8262.
219. Prasad KM, Zhou C, Trempe JP. Characterization of the Rep78/adeno-associated virus complex. *Virology* 1997;229:183.
220. Pujol A, Deleu L, Nuesch JP, et al. Inhibition of parvovirus minute virus of mice replication by a peptide involved in the oligomerization of nonstructural protein NS1. *J Virol* 1997;71:7393.
221. Qing K, Khuntirat B, Mah C, et al. Adeno-associated virus type 2-mediated gene transfer: Correlation of tyrosine phosphorylation of the cellular single-stranded D sequence-binding protein with transgene expression in human cells *in vitro* and murine tissues *in vivo*. *J Virol* 1998;72:1593.
222. Qing K, Mah C, Hansen J, et al. Human fibroblast growth factor receptor 1 is a co-receptor for infection by adeno-associated virus 2 [see comments]. *Nat Med* 1999;5:71.
223. Qing K, Wang XS, Kube DM, et al. Role of tyrosine phosphorylation of a cellular protein in adeno-associated virus 2-mediated transgene expression. *Proc Natl Acad Sci U S A* 1997;94:10879.
224. Rayet B, Lopez-Guerrero JA, Rommelaere J, Dinsart C. Induction of programmed cell death by parvovirus H-1 in U937 cells: Connection with the tumor necrosis factor alpha signalling pathway. *J Virol* 1998; 72:8893.
225. Recchia A, Parks RJ, Lamartina S, et al. Site-specific integration mediated by a hybrid adenovirus/adeno-associated virus vector. *Proc Natl Acad Sci U S A* 1999;96:2615.
226. Ren J, Qu X, Chaires JB, et al. Spectral and physical characterization of the inverted terminal repeat DNA structure from adenoassociated virus 2. *Nucleic Acids Res* 1999;27:1985.
227. Rhode SL. Replication process of the parvovirus H-1. I. Kinetics in a parasynchronous cell system. *J Virol* 1973;11:856.
228. Rhode SL, Paradiso PR. Parvovirus genome: Nucleotide sequence of H-1 and mapping of its genes by hybrid-arrested translation. *J Virol* 1983;45:173.
229. Rhode SL. Complementation for replicative form DNA replication of a deletion mutant of H-1 by various parvoviruses. *J Virol* 1982;42:1118.
230. Rhode SL. trans-Activation of parvovirus P38 promoter by the 76K noncapsid protein. *J Virol* 1985;55:886.
231. Rhode SL, Richard SM. Characterization of the trans-activation-responsive element of the parvovirus H-1 P38 promoter. *J Virol* 1987;61:2807.
232. Richardson WD, Westphal H. Requirement for either early region 1a or early region 1b adenovirus gene products in the helper effect for adeno-associated virus. *J Virol* 1984;51:404.
233. Rizzuto G, Gorgoni B, Cappelletti M, et al. Development of animal models for adeno-associated virus site-specific integration. *J Virol* 1999;73:2517.
234. Rommelaere J, Cornelis JJ. Antineoplastic activity of parvoviruses. *J Virol Methods* 1991;33:233.
235. Rommelaere J, Tattersall P. Oncosuppression by parvoviruses. In: Tijssen P, ed. *Handbook of Parvoviruses.* Boca Raton, FL: CRC Press, 1990:41.
236. Ron D, Tal J. Coevolution of cells and virus as a mechanism for the

persistence of lymphotropic minute virus of mice in L-cells. *J Virol* 1985;55:424.
237. Rose JA, Berns KI, Hoggan MD, Koczot FJ. Evidence for a single-stranded adenovirus-associated virus genome: Formation of a DNA density hybrid on release of viral DNA. *Proc Natl Acad Sci U S A* 1969;64:863.
238. Rosenfeld SJ, Yoshimoto K, Kajigaya S, et al. Unique region of the minor capsid protein of human parvovirus B19 is exposed on the virion surface [published erratum appears in *J Clin Invest* 1992;90:2609]. *J Clin Invest* 1992;89:2023.
239. Ruffing M, Zentgraf H, Kleinschmidt JA. Assembly of viruslike particles by recombinant structural proteins of adeno-associated virus type 2 in insect cells. *J Virol* 1992;66:6922.
240. Rutledge EA, Russell DW. Adeno-associated virus vector integration junctions. *J Virol* 1997;71:8429.
241. Ryan JH, Zolotukhin S, Muzyczka N. Sequence requirements for binding of Rep68 to the adeno-associated virus terminal repeats. *J Virol* 1996;70:1542.
242. Salome N, van Hille B, Duponchel N, et al. Sensitization of transformed rat cells to parvovirus MVMp is restricted to specific oncogenes. *Oncogene* 1990;5:123.
243. Salvino R, Skiadopoulos M, Faust EA, et al. Two spatially distinct genetic elements constitute a bipartite DNA replication origin in the minute virus of mice genome. *J Virol* 1991;65:1352.
244. Samulski RJ, Berns KI, Tan M, Muzyczka N. Cloning of adeno-associated virus into pBR322: Rescue of intact virus from the recombinant plasmid in human cells. *Proc Natl Acad Sci U S A* 1982;79:2077.
245. Samulski RJ, Sally M, Muzyczka N. *Adeno-Associated Viral Vectors.* Cold Spring Harbor, NY: Cold Spring Harbor Laboratory Press, 1998.
246. Samulski RJ, Shenk T. Adenovirus E1B 55-Mr polypeptide facilitates timely cytoplasmic accumulation of adeno-associated virus mRNAs. *J Virol* 1988;62:206.
247. Samulski RJ, Srivastava A, Berns KI, Muzyczka N. Rescue of adeno-associated virus from recombinant plasmids: Gene correction within the terminal repeats of AAV. *Cell* 1983;33:135.
248. Samulski RJ, Zhu X, Xiao X, et al. Targeted integration of adeno-associated virus (AAV) into human chromosome 19 [published erratum appears in *EMBO J* 1992;11:1228]. *EMBO J* 1991;10:3941.
249. Sanlioglu S, Duan D, Engelhardt JF. Two independent molecular pathways for recombinant adeno-associated virus genome conversion occur after UV-C and E4orf6 augmentation of transduction. *Hum Gene Ther* 1999;10:591.
250. Santaren JF, Ramirez JC, Almendral JM. Protein species of the parvovirus minute virus of mice strain MVMp: Involvement of phosphorylated VP-2 subtypes in viral morphogenesis. *J Virol* 1993;67:5126.
251. Schoborg RV, Pintel DJ. Accumulation of MVM gene products is differentially regulated by transcription initiation, RNA processing and protein stability. *Virology* 1991;181:22.
252. Senapathy P, Tratschin JD, Carter BJ. Replication of adeno-associated virus DNA. Complementation of naturally occurring *rep*-mutants by a wild-type genome or an *ori*-mutant and correction of terminal palindrome deletions. *J Mol Biol* 1984;179:1.
253. Shelling AN, Smith MG. Targeted integration of transfected and infected adeno-associated virus vectors containing the neomycin resistance gene. *Gene Ther* 1994;1:165.
254. Shi Y, Seto E, Chang LS, Shenk T. Transcriptional repression by YY1, a human GLI-Kruppel-related protein, and relief of repression by adenovirus E1A protein. *Cell* 1991;67:377.
255. Shull BC, Chen KC, Lederman M, et al. Genomic clones of bovine parvovirus: Construction and effect of deletions and terminal sequence inversions on infectivity. *J Virol* 1988;62:417.
256. Smith RH, Kotin RM. The Rep52 gene product of adeno-associated virus is a DNA helicase with 3′-to-5′ polarity. *J Virol* 1998;72:4874.
257. Smith RH, Kotin RM. An adeno-associated virus (AAV) initiator protein, Rep78, catalyzes the cleavage and ligation of single-stranded AAV ori DNA. *J Virol* 2000;74:3122.
258. Smith RH, Spano AJ, Kotin RM. The Rep78 gene product of adeno-associated virus (AAV) self-associates to form a hexameric complex in the presence of AAV ori sequences. *J Virol* 1997;71:4461.
259. Snyder RO, Im DS, Ni T, et al. Features of the adeno-associated virus origin involved in substrate recognition by the viral Rep protein. *J Virol* 1993;67:6096.
260. Snyder RO, Samulski RJ, Muzyczka N. *In vitro* resolution of covalently joined AAV chromosome ends. *Cell* 1990;60:105.
261. Song S, Morgan M, Ellis T, et al. Sustained secretion of human alpha-1-antitrypsin from murine muscle transduced with adeno-associated virus vectors. *Proc Natl Acad Sci U S A* 1998;95:14384.
262. Spalholz BA, Tattersall P. Interaction of minute virus of mice with differentiated cells: Strain-dependent target cell specificity is mediated by intracellular factors. *J Virol* 1983;46:937.
263. Sprecher Goldberger S, Thiry L, Lefebvre N, et al. Complement-fixation antibodies to adenovirus-associated viruses, cytomegaloviruses and herpes simplex viruses in patients with tumors and in control individuals. *Am J Epidemiol* 1971;94:351.
264. Srivastava A, Lusby EW, Berns KI. Nucleotide sequence and organization of the adeno-associated virus 2 genome. *J Virol* 1983;45:555.
265. Straus SE, Sebring ED, Rose JA. Concatemers of alternating plus and minus strands are intermediates in adenovirus-associated virus DNA synthesis. *Proc Natl Acad Sci U S A* 1976;73:742.
266. Summerford C, Bartlett JS, Samulski RJ. AlphaVbeta5 integrin: A co-receptor for adeno-associated virus type 2 infection [see comments]. *Nat Med* 1999;5:78.
267. Summerford C, Samulski RJ. Membrane-associated heparan sulfate proteoglycan is a receptor for adeno-associated virus type 2 virions. *J Virol* 1998;72:1438.
268. Sun L, Li J, Xiao X. Overcoming adeno-associated virus vector size limitation through viral DNA heterodimerization. *Nat Med* 2000;6:599.
269. Tattersall P. Replication of the parvovirus MVM. I. Dependence of virus multiplication and plaque formation on cell growth. *J Virol* 1972;10:586.
270. Tattersall P, Crawford LV, Shatkin AJ. Replication of the parvovirus MVM. II. Isolation and characterization of intermediates in the replication of the viral deoxyribonucleic acid. *J Virol* 1973;12:1446.
271. Tattersall P, Shatkin AJ, Ward DC. Sequence homology between the structural polypeptides of minute virus of mice. *J Mol Biol* 1977; 111:375.
272. Tattersall P, Ward DC. Rolling hairpin model for replication of parvovirus and linear chromosomal DNA. *Nature* 1976;263:106.
273. Tobiasch E, Rabreau M, Geletneky K, et al. Detection of adeno-associated virus DNA in human genital tissue and in material from spontaneous abortion. *J Med Virol* 1994;44:215.
274. Tratschin JD, Miller IL, Carter BJ. Genetic analysis of adeno-associated virus: Properties of deletion mutants constructed *in vitro* and evidence for an adeno-associated virus replication function. *J Virol* 1984; 51:611.
275. Tratschin JD, Tal J, Carter BJ. Negative and positive regulation in trans of gene expression from adeno-associated virus vectors in mammalian cells by a viral *rep* gene product. *Mol Cell Biol* 1986;6:2884.
276. Trempe JP, Carter BJ. Regulation of adeno-associated virus gene expression in 293 cells: Control of mRNA abundance and translation. *J Virol* 1988;62:68.
277. Tsao J, Chapman MS, Agbandje M, et al. The three-dimensional structure of canine parvovirus and its functional implications. *Science* 1991;251:1456.
278. Tullis G, Schoborg RV, Pintel DJ. Characterization of the temporal accumulation of minute virus of mice replicative intermediates. *J Gen Virol* 1994;75:1633.
279. Urabe M, Hasumi Y, Kume A, et al. Charged-to-alanine scanning mutagenesis of the N-terminal half of adeno-associated virus type 2 Rep78 protein. *J Virol* 1999;73:2682.
280. Urcelay E, Ward P, Wiener SM, et al. Asymmetric replication *in vitro* from a human sequence element is dependent on adeno-associated virus Rep protein. *J Virol* 1995;69:2038.
281. Vasudevacharya J, Compans RW. The NS and capsid genes determine the host range of porcine parvovirus. *Virology* 1992;187:515.
282. Vincent-Lacaze N, Snyder RO, Gluzman R, et al. Structure of adeno-associated virus vector DNA following transduction of the skeletal muscle. *J Virol* 1999;73:1949.
283. Wagner JA, Reynolds T, Moran ML, et al. Efficient and persistent gene transfer of AAV-CFTR in maxillary sinus [letter]. *Lancet* 1998; 351:1702.
284. Walker SL, Wonderling RS, Owens RA. Mutational analysis of the adeno-associated virus type 2 Rep68 protein helicase motifs. *J Virol* 1997;71:6996.
285. Walz C, Deprez A, Dupressoir T, et al. Interaction of human papillomavirus type 16 and adeno-associated virus type 2 co-infecting human cervical epithelium. *J Gen Virol* 1997;78:1441.

286. Walz C, Schlehofer JR. Modification of some biological properties of HeLa cells containing adeno-associated virus DNA integrated into chromosome 17. *J Virol* 1992;66:2990.
287. Walz C, Schlehofer JR, Flentje M, et al. Adeno-associated virus sensitizes HeLa cell tumors to gamma rays. *J Virol* 1992;66:5651.
288. Wang XS, Srivastava A. Rescue and autonomous replication of adeno-associated virus type 2 genomes containing Rep-binding site mutations in the viral p5 promoter. *J Virol* 1998;72:4811.
289. Ward P, Berns KI. *In vitro* replication of adeno-associated virus DNA: Enhancement by extracts from adenovirus-infected HeLa cells. *J Virol* 1996;70:4495.
290. Ward P, Dean FB, O'Donnell ME, Berns KI. Role of the adenovirus DNA-binding protein in *in vitro* adeno-associated virus DNA replication. *J Virol* 1998;72:420.
291. Ward P, Urcelay E, Kotin R, et al. Adeno-associated virus DNA replication *in vitro*: Activation by a maltose binding protein/Rep 68 fusion protein. *J Virol* 1994;68:6029.
292. Weger S, Wendland M, Kleinschmidt JA, Heilbronn R. The adeno-associated virus type 2 regulatory proteins rep78 and rep68 interact with the transcriptional coactivator PC4. *J Virol* 1999;73:260.
293. Weger S, Wistuba A, Grimm D, Kleinschmidt JA. Control of adeno-associated virus type 2 cap gene expression: Relative influence of helper virus, terminal repeats, and Rep proteins. *J Virol* 1997;71:8437.
294. Weindler FW, Heilbronn R. A subset of herpes simplex virus replication genes provides helper functions for productive adeno-associated virus replication. *J Virol* 1991;65:2476.
295. Weitzman MD, Kyostio SR, Kotin RM, Owens RA. Adeno-associated virus (AAV) Rep proteins mediate complex formation between AAV DNA and its integration site in human DNA. *Proc Natl Acad Sci U S A* 1994;91:5808.
296. Willwand K, Mumtsidu E, Kuntz-Simon G, Rommelaere J. Initiation of DNA replication at palindromic telomeres is mediated by a duplex-to-hairpin transition induced by the minute virus of mice nonstructural protein NS1. *J Biol Chem* 1998;273:1165.
297. Wilson GM, Jindal HK, Yeung DE, et al. Expression of minute virus of mice major nonstructural protein in insect cells: Purification and identification of ATPase and helicase activities. *Virology* 1991;185:90.
298. Winocour E, Puzis L, Etkin S, et al. Modulation of the cellular phenotype by integrated adeno-associated virus. *Virology* 1992;190:316.
299. Wistuba A, Kern A, Weger S, et al. Subcellular compartmentalization of adeno-associated virus type 2 assembly. *J Virol* 1997;71:1341.
300. Wistuba A, Weger S, Kern A, Kleinschmidt JA. Intermediates of adeno-associated virus type 2 assembly: Identification of soluble complexes containing Rep and Cap proteins. *J Virol* 1995;69:5311.
301. Wolter S, Richards R, Armentrout RW. Cell cycle-dependent replication of the DNA of minute virus of mice, a parvovirus. *Biochim Biophys Acta* 1980;607:420.
302. Wonderling RS, Kyostio SR, Owens RA. A maltose-binding protein/adeno-associated virus Rep68 fusion protein has DNA-RNA helicase and ATPase activities. *J Virol* 1995;69:3542.
303. Wonderling RS, Owens RA. Binding sites for adeno-associated virus Rep proteins within the human genome. *J Virol* 1997;71:2528.
304. Wu J, Davis MD, Owens RA. Factors affecting the terminal resolution site endonuclease, helicase, and ATPase activities of adeno-associated virus type 2 Rep proteins. *J Virol* 1999;73:8235.
305. Wu P, Xiao W, Conlon T, et al. Mutational analysis of the Adeno-associated virus type 2(AAV2) capsid gene and construction of AAV2 vectors with altered tropism. *J Virol* 2000;74:8635.
306. Xiao X, Xiao W, Li J, Samulski RJ. A novel 165-base-pair terminal repeat sequence is the sole cis requirement for the adeno-associated virus life cycle. *J Virol* 1997;71:941.
307. Yakobson B, Koch T, Winocour E. Replication of adeno-associated virus in synchronized cells without the addition of a helper virus. *J Virol* 1987;61:972.
308. Yan Z, Zhang Y, Duan D, Engelhardt JF. Trans-splicing vectors expand the utility of adeno-associated virus for gene therapy. *Proc Natl Acad Sci U S A* 2000;97:6716.
309. Yang CC, Xiao X, Zhu X, et al. Cellular recombination pathways and viral terminal repeat hairpin structures are sufficient for adeno-associated virus integration *in vivo* and *in vitro*. *J Virol* 1997;71:9231.
310. Yang Q, Chen F, Ross J, Trempe JP. Inhibition of cellular and SV40 DNA replication by the adeno-associated virus Rep proteins. *Virology* 1995;207:246.
311. Yang Q, Chen F, Trempe JP. Characterization of cell lines that inducibly express the adeno-associated virus Rep proteins. *J Virol* 1994;68:4847.
312. Yang Q, Kadam A, Trempe JP. Mutational analysis of the adeno-associated virus *rep* gene. *J Virol* 1992;66:6058.
313. Yang Q, Trempe JP. Analysis of the terminal repeat binding abilities of mutant adeno-associated virus replication proteins. *J Virol* 1993;67:4442.
314. Young SM, Samulski RJ. AAV chromosome 19 site specific recombination soes not require a Rep dependent origin of replication on the AAV inverted terminal repeat sequence. In: Young SM, Samulski RJ, eds. *VIII Parvovirus Workshop,* Mont-Tremblant, Quebec, Canada, 2000.
315. Zhao Q, Gersappe A, Pintel DJ. Efficient excision of the upstream large intron from P4-generated pre-mRNA of the parvovirus minute virus of mice requires at least one donor and the 3′ splice site of the small downstream intron. *J Virol* 1995;69:6170.
316. Zhou X, Zolotukhin I, Im DS, Muzyczka N. Biochemical characterization of adeno-associated virus rep68 DNA helicase and ATPase activities. *J Virol* 1999;73:1580.
317. Zolotukhin S, Byrne BJ, Mason E, et al. Recombinant adeno-associated virus purification using novel methods improves infectious titer and yield. *Gene Ther* 1999;6:973.

CHAPTER 33

Herpes Simplex Viruses and Their Replication

Bernard Roizman and David M. Knipe

> Dans l'ignorance ou nous vivons du processus exact de l'herpes, nous voyons chaque generation medicale creer une theorie adaptee aux idees, aux decovertes du moment.
> Castel DU, Herpes P *Pratique dermatologique,* vol. II. Paris: Masson, 1901:814, 815.

Herpes simplex viruses (HSVs) were the first of the human herpesviruses to be discovered and are among the most intensively investigated of all viruses. Their attractions are their biologic properties, particularly their abilities to cause a variety of infections, to remain latent in their host for life, and to be reactivated to cause lesions at or near the site of initial infection. They serve as models and tools for the study of translocation of proteins, synaptic connections in the nervous system, membrane structure, gene regulation, gene therapy, and a myriad of other biologic problems, both general to viruses and specific to HSV. For years, their size and complexity served as formidable obstacles to intensive research. More than 40 years passed from the time of their isolation (341) until Schneweiss (542) demonstrated that there were in fact two serotypes of HSV, HSV-1 and HSV-2, whose formal designations under International Committee on Taxonomy of Viruses (ICTV) rules are now human herpesviruses 1 and 2 (508). Not until 1961 were practical plaque assays published (513), and only much later were the genome sizes and the extent of homology between these two viruses reported. This chapter recounts well established facts, but its main emphasis is on burning issues, the problems whose time has come.

To the preface to the third edition of this book, which we affirm but do not repeat here, we add an additional comment. The field has grown enormously since the dawn of studies on the molecular biology of HSV more than 40 years ago. Studies on HSV are entering, at last, a most exciting period for two reasons. First, the words *structure* and *function* are beginning to have an operational meaning. Second, HSV gene products have become powerful probes for the study of cellular metabolic pathways. Host factors crucial to virus multiplication and, potentially, to latency are being identified. The armamentarium for a major assault on the mysteries underlying the biology of these viruses is in place and reflects the contributions of many laboratories over many, many years.

At the same time, the field and the literature have grown enormously. The task before us was far greater for not having followed Ludwig Wittgenstein's dictum that "Whereof one cannot speak, thereof one must be silent," but chapters of citations bereft of commentary are dull. The decision to avoid assembling an annotated bibliography was in large part dictated by the space available to us.

VIRION STRUCTURE

The HSV virion (Fig. 1) consists of 4 elements: (a) an electron-opaque core, (b) an icosadeltahedral capsid surrounding the core, (c) an amorphous tegument surrounding the capsid, and (d) an outer envelope exhibiting spikes on its surface (509). The core contains the double-stranded DNA (dsDNA) genome wrapped as a toroid (171) or spool (702) and possibly in a liquid crystalline state (42). The tegument is largely unstructured, except for some icosahedral structure around the pentons (702). The capsid is composed of 162 capsomers (676) arranged in a T=16 icosahedral symmetry. Finally, the envelope consists of a lipid bilayer with about 12 different viral glycoproteins embedded in it.

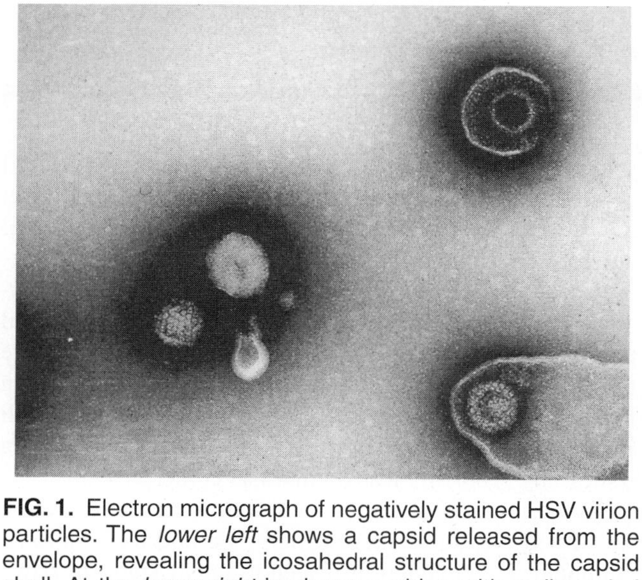

FIG. 1. Electron micrograph of negatively stained HSV virion particles. The *lower left* shows a capsid released from the envelope, revealing the icosahedral structure of the capsid shell. At the *lower right* is shown a virion with a distended envelope. The *upper right* shows a more intact particle, in which stain has penetrated to the core of the particle revealing the multiple layers of the virion, including the envelope as the outer layer, then the dark tegument layer, the capsid shell, and the dark core.

The dry masses of herpes simplex virions, full nucleocapsids, empty nucleocapsids, and cores were calculated from permeability of virions to electrons to be $13.33 \pm 2.56 \times 10^{-16}$ g, $7.55 \pm 1.11 \times 10^{-16}$ g, $5.22 \pm 1.10 \times 10^{-16}$ g, and $2.07 \pm 0.95 \times 10^{-16}$ g, respectively. The average mass ratios of the virion, full capsid, and core to DNA are 8.1, 4.6, and 1.25, respectively. The experimentally derived ratio of virus mass to DNA is 10.73 ± 0.96, from which it has been calculated that the virion contains 19.4×10^{-16} g of protein (216). A similar value was derived from counts of virions in purified virus preparations (R. W. Honess and B. Roizman, unpublished data), although the error in these determinations was higher. This ratio was used in the calculation of the polypeptide content of HSV virions by Heine and colleagues (216).

Virion Polypeptides

Early studies on purified HSV-1 virions suggested that they contain more than 30 distinct proteins, which were designated as virion polypeptides (VP) and given serial numbers (216,589). All of the virion proteins were made after infection, and no host proteins could be detected in purified virion preparations. Of the about 30 known and another 10 suspected virion proteins (Table 1), at least 11 are on the surface of the virion (accessible to antibody), and at least 10 are glycosylated. The glycoproteins are gB (VP7 and VP8.5), gC (VP8), gD (VP17 and VP18) and gE (VP12.3 and VP12.6), gG, gH, gI, gK, gL, and gM. The presence of gJ (U_S5) and gN (U_L49.5) in virions has not been demonstrated. Virion envelopes also contain at least two (U_L20 and U_S9) and possibly more (U_L24, U_L43, and U_L34) nonglycosylated intrinsic membrane proteins. Stannard and associates (599) reported that spikes projecting from envelopes are, as was expected, the viral glycoproteins, and that the latter were nonrandomly distributed.

Gibson and Roizman (188,189) described three kinds of capsids: those that lack DNA and were never enveloped (type A), those that contain DNA and were never enveloped (type B), and those that contain DNA and were obtained by deenveloping intact virions (type C). In the current nomenclature, the term *A capsid* refers to capsids without an internal toroidal structure; those with internal scaffolding proteins but without DNA are designated as *B capsids*; and those with DNA have been designated as the C capsids. The A capsids are a defective byproduct (558) rather than precursors of the B capsids. A short-lived assembly intermediate termed the *procapsid* has recently been described (636).

The empty (A) capsids consist of four proteins: VP5 (U_L19), VP19C (U_L38), VP23 (U_L38), and a smaller Mr 12,000 protein described subsequently (95) and often referred to as VP26 (U_L35) (110,439). VP5 was estimated to be present in ratios of 850 to 1,000 per virion, that is, about six per hexameric capsomere (216,509,647), but Schrag and co-investigators (543) suggested that VP5 is a

TABLE 1. *HSV genes and their functions*

Gene	Protein	Essential or nonessential	Kinetic class	Comments
$\gamma_1$34.5	ICP34.5	N	γ_1	Multifunctional protein; carboxyl-terminal domain homologous to the corresponding domain of GADD34 and acts as a phosphatase accessory factor; it binds and redirects protein phosphatase 1 to dephosphorylate the α subunit of the translation initation factor 2 (eIF-2α) and thereby preclude the shutoff of protein synthesis caused by activated protein kinase R. Aminoterminal domain binds U_S11 through an RNase-sensitive bond.
ORF P	ORF P	N	pre-α	Open reading frame (ORF) is antisense to the $\gamma_1$34.5 gene normally repressed by ICP4. ORF P protein is pulled down by antibody to splicing factor SC35. Derepression of ORF P results in retardation of the expression of α proteins made from spliced mRNAs (e.g., ICPO, ICP22).
ORF O	ORF O	N	pre-α	ORF is antisense to the $\gamma_1$34.5 gene normally repressed by ICPO. Protein synthesis is initiated from ORF P initiator methionine but shifts to another reading frame before codon 35. ORF P binds ICP4 and precludes the latter from binding to cognate sites on DNA.
α0	ICPO	N	α	A multifunctional protein characterized best as a promiscuous transactivator of genes introduced by transfection or infection; optimal activity requires presence of ICP4. Deletion mutants debilitated at low multiplicities of infection. ICPO is nucleotidylylated by casein kinase II and extensively phosphorylated by HSV U_L13 and U_s3 and by cellular kinase. ICPO accumulates in nuclei early in infection and in the cytoplasm at later times. ICPO binds numerous cellular proteins.
U_L1	gL	E	γ	Complex with gH required for transport of both proteins to plasma membrane and for entry mediated by gH. Required for fusion of membranes. Contains *syn* locus.
U_L2		N	β	Uracil DNA glycosylase.
U_L3		N	Unknown	Initiates predominantly from second methionine in ORF and is highly processed by U_L13 and cellular kinases. Colocalizes in small dense nuclear bodies with ICP22. mRNA corresponding to U_L3 protein is conspicuously absent.
U_L4		N	γ_2	M_r 60-Kd species is found in virions and light particles. Colocalizes with U_L3.
U_L5		E	β	Component of helicase-primase complex with U_L8 and U_L52 proteins.
U_L6		E	Unknown	Capsid protein; required for DNA cleavage and packaging.
U_L7		E	Unknown	Unknown.
U_L8		E	β	Component of helicase-primase complex with U_L5 and U_L52.
U_L8.5		E	γ_1	ORF encodes the carboxyl-terminal domain of U_L9.
U_L9		E	β	DNA origins binding protein; carries out helicase and ATPase activities.
U_L9.5		N	γ_2	Antisense to U_L10 ORF
U_L10		N	γ	Glycoprotein present in virions and plasma membranes; interacts with gB.
U_L10.5	?	?	Unknown	Unknown.
U_L11	gM	N	γ	Myristoylated protein; necessary for efficient capsid envelopment and exocytosis.
U_L12		N	β	Alkaline exonuclease (DNAse); required for processing of DNA replication intermediates.
U_L13		N	γ	Virion protein kinase; substrates include viral [ICPO, ICP22, U_S1.5, vhs (U_L41), gE, U_L49] and cellular (e.g., EF-1δ) proteins. Complexes with gE.
U_L14		N	γ_2	Virion tegument; aids in spread from cell to cell. Null mutants debilitated.
U_L15		E	γ	Required for packaging of DNA. Associated with B but not C capsids; ORF in two exons.
U_L16		N	Unknown	Capsid-associated protein required for cleavage-packaging of DNA. ORF located within intron of *U_L15*.
U_L17		E	γ	Tegument protein required for cleavage packaging of DNA and transport within nuclei. ORF located within intron of *U_L15*.
U_L15.5		E	γ	Corresponds to exon II of *U_L15*; function not known.
U_L18	VP23	E	γ_1	Together with VP19C forms triplexes which connect adjacent hexons and pentons in C capsids. Required for capsid formation and cleavage-packaging of replicated viral DNA.
U_L19	VP5; ICP5	E	γ_1	Major capsid protein. Interacts with ICP35.

(Continues)

TABLE 1. Continued

Gene	Protein	Essential or nonessential	Kinetic class	Comments
U_L20		N	γ	Intrinsic membrane protein associated with nuclear membranes and Golgi stacks but not with extracellular virions. Necessary for viral exocytosis, particularly in cells in which the Golgi apparatus is fragmented and dispersed.
$U_L20.5$		N	γ_2	Unknown function; colocalizes with U_L3 but does not interact with U_L3 or ICP22. Not present in HSV-2
U_L21		N	γ_1	Nucleotidylylated phosphoprotein; unknown function.
U_L22	gH	E	γ	Forms complex with gL (see above). Appears to play a role in entry, egress, and cell-to-cell spread.
U_L23	ICP36	N	β	Nucleoside kinase, known as thymidine kinase.
U_L24		N	Unknown	*Syn* locus; membrane-associated protein
U_L25		E	γ_2	Capsid protein required for penetration into cells and for DNA packaging.
U_L26		E	γ	A polyprotein self-cleaved to yield a serine protease (amino-terminal, also known as VP24) and one of its substrates (carboxyl-terminal of U_L36 protein, also known as VP21).
$U_L26.5$	ICP35	E	γ	Protein (ICP35c, d) made from a transcript initiated in the coding domain of U_L26; cleaved by protease to ICPe,f. ICP35 forms the scaffolding for DNA packaging in B capsids. During packaging of DNA, it is extruded and is absent from the mature, C capsids.
U_L27	gB, VP7	E	γ	Glycoprotein required for viral entry; forms a dimer and induces neutralizing antibody. A *syn*⁻ locus maps to the carboxyl terminus.
$U_L27.5$		?	γ_2	ORF antisense to U_L27. Cytoplasmic protein; shares epitope with gJ.
U_L28	ICP18.5	E	γ	Required for DNA cleavage-packaging. Associated with B but not C capsids.
U_L29	ICP8	E	β_1	Binds single-stranded DNA cooperatively, required for viral DNA replication: forms complex with DNA polymerase and U_L42. Mutants are DNA negative; hence, expression of early and late genes may be affected positively or negatively by the function of ICP8. Because ICP8 denatures DNA, it affects renaturation of complementary strands of DNA and affects homologous pairing and strand transfer.
U_L30		E	γ	DNA polymerase; forms complex with U_L42 protein and with ICP8.
U_L31		E	γ_2	Nucleotidylylated phosphoprotein, associates with nuclear lamina and cofractionates with nuclear matrix and interacts with U_L34. Required for envelopment.
U_L32		E	γ_2	Required for DNA packaging but not associated with capsids.
U_L33		E	Unknown	Required for DNA packaging but not associated with capsids.
U_L34		E	γ_1	Abundant nonglycosylated, membrane-associated, virion protein phosphorylated by protein kinase U_S3; required for localization of U_L31 protein in nuclei.
U_L35	VP26	E	γ_2	Basic phosphorylated capsid protein.
U_L36	ICP1-2	E	γ	Tegument phosphoprotein. In cells infected with temperature-sensitive mutant at nonpermissive temperature DNA is not released from capsids at nuclear pores. Reported to form complex with a 140-Kd protein that binds *a*-sequence DNA. May be involved in cleavage and/or packaging of newly synthesized viral DNA.
U_L37		E	γ_1	Cytoplasmic phosphoprotein; transported to nucleus in the presence of ICP8. Minor tegument component.
U_L38	ICP32/VP19C	E	γ_2	Capsid assembly protein, binds DNA and may be involved in anchoring DNA in the capsid. Efficient synthesis of U_L38 protein requires functional ICP22/$U_S1.5$ and U_L13 proteins.
U_L39	ICP6	N	β_1	Large subunit of ribonucleotide reductase. Autophosphorylates via unique amino terminus but does not trans-phosphorylate. HSV-2 homolog can be trans-phosphorylated.
U_L40		N	β_1	Small subunit of ribonucleotide reductase.
U_L41	vhs	N	γ_1	Tegument phosphoprotein causes nonspecific degradation of mRNA and shutoff of macro-molecular synthesis after infection. Efficient synthesis of U_L41 protein requires functional ICP22/$U_S1.5$ and U_L13 proteins.
U_L42		E	β	Double-stranded DNA-binding protein, binds to and increases processivity of DNA polymerase.
U_L43		N	γ	Amino acid sequence predicts membrane-associated protein.

(Continues)

TABLE 1. Continued

Gene	Protein	Essential or nonessential	Kinetic class	Comments
U_L43.5		N	γ	ORF antisense to U_L43. Low-abundance nuclear protein accumulates in assemblons.
U_L44	gC, VP7.5	N	γ_2	Glycoprotein involved in cell attachment; required for attachment to the apical surface of polarized MDCK cells and may play a role in blocking host response to infection.
U_L45		N	γ	Intrinsic, type 2 membrane protein; may play a role in cell fusion.
U_L46	VP11/12	N	γ	Tegument phosphoprotein reported to modulate the activity of U_L48 (αTIF) protein.
U_L47	VP13/14	N	γ_1	Tegument phosphoprotein; 0-glycosylated, phosphorylated by U_L13, nucleotidylylated. Reported to modulate the activity of U_L48 (αTIF) protein, associate with the nuclear matrix, and bind DNA.
U_L48	VP16; ICP25, αTIF	E	γ	Tegument protein, induces α genes by interacting with host proteins Oct-I and HCF The complex binds to specific sequences with the consensus GyATGnTAATGArATTCyTTGnGGG-NC.
U_L49	VP22	E	γ	Tegument protein, O-linked glycosylated, nucleotidylylated mono(ADP-ribosyl)ated tegument phosphoprotein. It is transported from infected to uninfected cells by direct extension; in dividing cells, it associates with chromatin.
U_L49.5		E	γ_2	Sequence predicts a M_r 12,000 membrane-associated protein.
U_L50		N	β	dUTPase.
U_L51		N	γ	Unknown
U_L52		E	β	Component of the helicase/primase complex with U_L5 and U_L8.
U_L53	gK	N	γ	Glycoprotein required for efficient viral exocytosis; contains *syn*$^-$ locus but not found in plasma membrane.
U_L54	α27; ICP27	E	α	Nucleotidylylated regulatory protein required for some early and all late gene expression. Early ICP27 redistributes snRNPs and inhibits splicing. Late ICP27 in replication compartments and shuttles to cytoplasm.
U_L55		N	γ_1	Nuclear protein associated with nuclear matrix (?) and assemblons.
U_L56			γ_2	Nuclear, virion-associated protein of unknown function; reduces virulence.
α4	ICP4	E	α	Nucleotidylylated, poly(ADP-ribosyl)ated phosphoprotein required for expression of most β and γ genes. ICP4 represses itself, ORF P, and ORF O by binding to DNA in sequence-specific fashion.
α22	U_S1, ICP22	N	α	Nucleotidylylated regulatory protein, phosphorylated by U_L13 protein kinase, required for optimal expression of ICPO and of a subset of γ proteins.
U_S1.5		N	α	Regulatory protein phosphorylated by U_L13 and by U_S3; colinear with carboxyl terminal of ICP22.
U_S2		N	γ_2	Nuclear, tegument protein.
U_S3		N	γ	Protein kinase; major substrates are α22 and U_L34. Exhibits anti-apoptotic activity.
U_S4	gG	N	γ	Glycoprotein required for entry into polarized cells; plays a role in egress and cell-to-cell spread.
U_S5	gJ	N	γ	Minor glycoprotein reported to block apoptosis.
U_S6	gD, VP17/18	E	γ	Glycoprotein required for postattachment entry of virus into cells.
U_S7	gI	N	γ	gI and gE glycoproteins form complex for transport to plasma membrane and also to constitute a high affinity Fc receptor. gI is required for basolateral spread of virus in polarized cells. Phosphorylated by U_L13.
U_S8	gE	N	γ_1	Fc receptor; involved in basolateral spread of virus in polarized cells. Affinity for and phosphorylated by U_L13.
U_S8.5		N	γ_1	Unknown.
U_S9		N	γ	Tegument protein.
U_S10		N	γ_1	Tegument protein.
U_S11		N	γ_2	Abundant virion tegument protein binds to U_L34 mRNA in sequence- and conformation-specific fashion and acts as an antiattenuation factor; binds to the 60S ribosomal subunit, and localizes in the nucleolus; if expressed early in infection, it blocks PKR from shutting off protein synthesis.
U_S12	α47; ICP47	N	α	Reported to block antigen presentation to CD8+ cells.
Ori_STU	Ori_S RNA	N	Unknown	RNA transcribed across S component origins of DNA synthesis. Most probably not translated and function is not known.
LATU	LATs (RNAs)	N	Unknown	Transcripts, some spliced, from the inverted repeat sequences flanking U_L sequences. The function of these transcripts is not known.

component of both pentameric and hexameric capsomeres. VP19C and VP5 appear to be linked by disulfide bonds (706) and are present in about similar ratios per virion (216). Braun and associates (45) showed that VP19C, identified as the infected cell protein (ICP) 32, bound to DNA and may be involved in anchoring the viral DNA in the capsid. The HSV-2 counterpart has also been mapped (694). VP26 is located at the hexon tips. B-type capsids differ from the A type in that they contain three proteins: VP21, VP22a, and VP24. VP22a corresponds to ICP35e-f, the product of the open reading frame (ORF) U_L26.5 cleaved at the carboxyl terminus by the protease resident in VP24 (333,334). VP21 corresponds to ICP35b (amino acids 248 to 610) of the protease Pra, the nascent U_L26 gene product. VP24 corresponds to the N-terminal domain (codons 1 through 247) of Pra designated as Prn, the smallest form of the protease encoded by the ORF U_L26. Pra is cleaved by the autologous protease between ala247 and ser248 and between ala610 and ser611 (126,331). The ICP35 family of proteins described by Braun and colleagues (45) plays a vital role in capsid assembly and encapsidation of viral DNA (178,462,493,558). Gibson and Roizman (189) suggested that VP21 is an internal capsid protein. Newcomb and Brown (404,405) demonstrated that VP19C and VP23 are on the surface of the capsid and form triplex structures that link the hexon capsomers and that VP22a is in the interior of the capsid and forms a ringlike structure that is quantitatively removed by 2.0 molar (M) guanidine hydrochloride.

Type C capsids were reported to contain a smaller protein—VP22—but not VP22a, and it has been suggested that the proteins are related (189). Sherman and Bachenheimer (558) and Rixon and colleagues (493) suggested that the VP22 found in the C-type capsids may not be related to VP22a. Depending on the procedure for stripping the envelope, the C-type capsids may contain variable amounts of tegument proteins. C capsids retain VP24 (the protease).

Cryoelectron microscopy has provided moderately high-resolution models of the HSV nucleocapsid and virion (42,543,702). These studies have shown that the HSV nucleocapsid is composed of three layers: the outer layer arranged in a T=16 symmetry, an intermediate layer organized in a T=4 lattice, and an inner layer consisting of genomic DNA (543). The same study concluded that the outer and intermediate layers are organized so that channels along their icosahedral twofold axes coincide, forming a direct pathway and potential channel between the DNA layer and the exterior of the virion (543). Another study of intact virions has shown that the channel is plugged, possibly with tegument proteins (702). These authors suggested that the VP1-3 tegument proteins regulate the transport of DNA through the channel.

In the interval between 1965 and 1974, a large number of articles dealt with the structure and morphogenesis of herpesvirus capsids; a list of citations and review of that literature was published by Roizman and Furlong (509). On the basis of the electron microscopic appearance of the capsid and the core, as many as eight distinct capsid forms were identified (509). Although the various forms probably reflect different stages of capsid assembly, the reagents necessary to relate the various forms to specific proteins are only now becoming available. The use of specific antibody reagents, viral assembly mutants, cryoelectron microscopy, and methods for *in vitro* as well as *in vivo* assembly hold out the prospect of relating specific proteins, protein assemblies, and capsid forms in a comprehensive view of capsid morphogenesis.

The space between the undersurface of the envelope and the surface of the capsid was designated as the tegument (509); thus, it contains the rest of the virion proteins (see Table 1). The most notable of the proteins associated with the space between the underside of the envelope and the capsid are the α-trans-inducing factor (αTIF; ICP25; VP16), VP11-12 (U_L46), VP13-14 (U_L47), the virion host shutoff (vhs) protein (U_L41); the product of the U_S11 gene; and a very large protein (VP1-2) associated with a complex that binds to the terminal *a* sequence of the viral genome (22,79,483,521,522). Extensive discussion of the various types of capsids and virions can be found elsewhere (227,509,604).

Several publications have reported on the production of "light particles" that are devoid of DNA. These particles consist of enveloped tegument-like structures (371,492,616). They appear to contain, in addition, other nonstructural proteins previously associated with virions (e.g., ICP4) (690). Little is known of their synthesis beyond the facts that they do not appear to be uniform in size and that the capsid is not an essential trigger for envelopment or egress.

Viral DNA

Like other herpesvirus DNAs, the bulk of packaged HSV DNA is linear and double stranded (24,272,444). In the virion, HSV DNA is packaged in the form of a toroid (171) or a spool (702). The ends of the genome are probably held together or are in close proximity inasmuch as a small fraction of the packaged DNA appears to be circular and the bulk of the linear DNA circularizes rapidly in the absence of protein synthesis after it enters the nuclei of infected cells (445). DNA extracted from virions contains ribonucleotides, nicks, and gaps (26,169,677).

Based on physical characterization studies, the HSV genome was originally estimated to be about 150 kilobase pairs (kbp), with a G+C content of 68% for HSV-1 and 69% HSV-2 (24,272). Complete sequencing of the HSV-1 strain 17 genome described the genome as 152,260 base pairs (bp) (accession number X14112) (363); minor updates altered this sequence to 152,261 bp (132). Complete sequencing of the HSV-2 strain HG52 genome defined it as 154,746 bp (accession number 286099) (132). However, these numbers include only single copies of the *a* sequence at the ends of the L component and do not take into account the variation in the size of the *a* sequences (200 to 500 bp each) or the variable number of direct repeats present throughout the genome but especially in the inverted repeats flanking the L and S components.

The HSV genome can be viewed as consisting of two covalently linked components, designated as L (long) and S (short) (Fig. 2). Each component consists of unique sequences bracketed by inverted repeats (650). The repeats of the L component are designated *ab* and *b′a′*, whereas those of the S component are *a′c′* and *ca* (see Fig. 2). The number of *a* sequence repeats at the L-S junction and at the L terminus is variable; thus, the HSV genome can then be represented as follows:

$$a_La_nb\text{-}U_L\text{-}b'a'_mc'\text{-}U_S\text{-}ca_S$$

where a_L and a_S are terminal sequences with unique properties (described later), and a_n and a_m are terminal *a* sequences directly repeated 0 or more times (n) or present in one to many copies (m) (335,503,505,650,655). The structure of the *a* sequence is highly conserved, but it consists of a variable number of repeat elements. In the HSV-1 (F) strain, the *a* sequence consists of a 20-bp direct repeat (DR1), a 65-bp unique sequence (U_b), a 12-bp direct repeat (DR2) present in 19 to 23 copies per *a* sequence, a 37-bp direct repeat (DR4) present in 2 to 3 copies, a 58-bp unique sequence (U_c), and a final copy of DR1 (388,389). The size of the *a* sequence varies from strain to strain, reflecting in part the number of copies of DR2 and DR4. The structure of the HSV-1 (F) *a* sequence can be represented as follows:

$$DR1—U_b—DR2_n—DR4_m—U_c—DR1$$

with the adjacent *a* sequences sharing the intervening DR1. Linear virion DNA contains asymmetric terminal *a* sequence ends. The terminal *a* sequence of the L component (a_L) contains a truncated DR1 with 18 bp and one 3′ nucleotide extension, whereas the terminal *a* sequence of the S component (a_S) ends with a DR1 containing only 1 bp and one 3′-overhanging nucleotide (390). The two truncated DR1 sequences form one complete DR1 upon circularization.

The L and S components of HSV are found inverted relative to one another, to yield four linear isomers. Populations of unit-length DNA from wild-type virus-infected cells consist of equimolar concentrations of the four predicted isomers (see Fig. 2) (120,211). The iso-

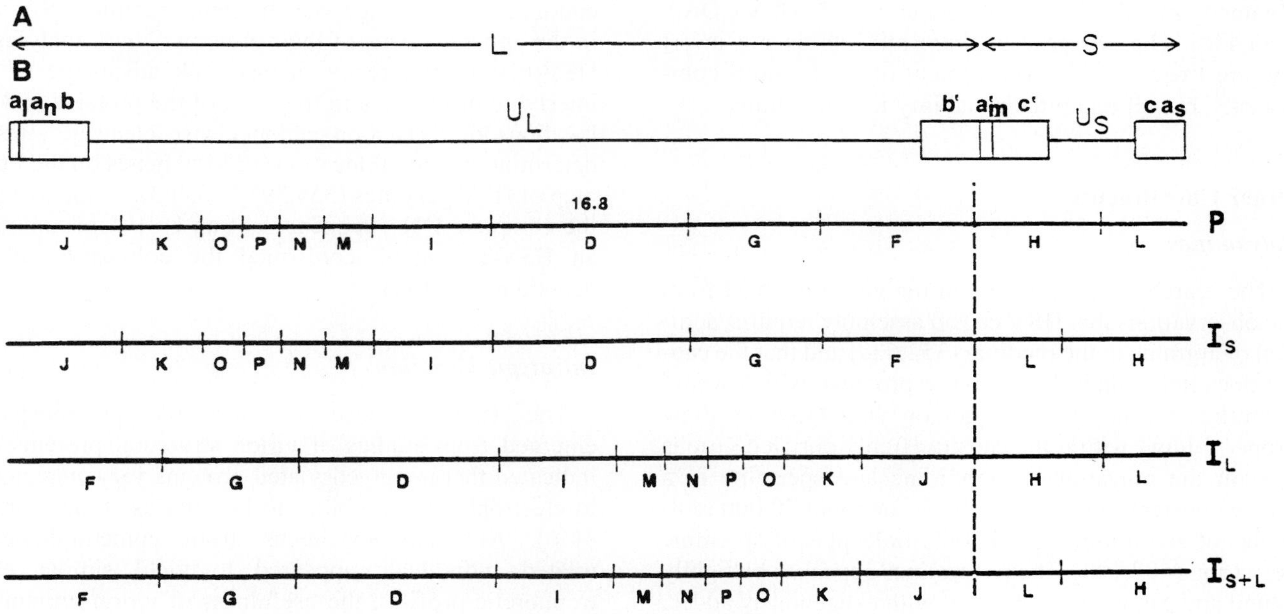

FIG. 2. Schematic representation of the arrangement of DNA sequences in the HSV genome. **A:** The domains of the L and S components are denoted by the *arrows.* The second line shows the unique sequences (*thin lines*) flanked by the inverted repeats (*boxes*). The letters above the second line designate the terminal *a* sequence of the L component (a_L), a variable (*n*) number of additional *a* sequences, the *b* sequence, the unique sequence of the L component (U_L), the repetitions of the *b* sequence and of a variable (*m*) number of sequences (a_m), the inverted *c* sequence, the unique sequence of the S component (U_S), and finally the terminal *a* sequence (a_S) of the S component. **B:** The HindIII restriction endonuclease map of HSV-1 (F) strain for the P, I_S, I_L, and I_{SL} isomers of the DNA. Note that, because HindIII does not cleave within the inverted repeat sequences, there are four terminal fragments and four fragments spanning the internal inverted repeats in concentrations of 0.5 and 0.25 M, respectively, relative to the concentration of the viral DNA.

mers have been designated as P (prototype), I_L (inversion of the L component), I_S (inversion of the S component), and I_{SL} (inversion of both S and L components) (211,395, 396). The first evidence for the existence of repetition of terminal sequences in inverted orientation was based on electron microscopic studies of denatured HSV-1 DNA allowed to self-anneal (554). Electron microscopic analyses of denatured molecules allowed to self-anneal and of partial denaturation profiles of HSV DNA revealed that the terminal repeats are also repeated internally and that the repeats flanking the L component differ from those of the S component in size and sequence arrangement (650). The demonstration that restriction endonucleases that cleave outside the inverted repeats yield four terminal fragments, each present in half of the molecules (also called half molar or 0.5M fragments), and 4 L-S component junction fragments that are each present in one fourth of the molecules (also called *quarter molar* or 0.25M fragments) (211) (see Fig. 2), as well as analyses of the partial denaturation profiles of Wadsworth and coauthors (650), supported the conclusion that the L and S components can invert relative to each other.

The internal inverted repeat sequences are not essential for growth of the virus in cell culture; thus, mutants from which portions of unique sequences and most of the internal inverted repeats have been deleted have been obtained in all four arrangements of HSV DNA (253,446). The genomes of these mutants do not invert and are frozen in one arrangement of the L and S components, but all retain their viability in cell culture.

Other Constituents

Polyamines

The search for polyamines in the virion evolved from the observations that HSV capsid assembly requires addition of arginine to the medium (352,620) and that the capsid does not contain highly basic proteins, which would neutralize the negative charges on viral DNA to allow proper folding within the capsid. Highly purified virions contain the polyamines spermidine and spermine in a nearly constant ratio of $1.6 \pm 0.2{:}1$, or about 70,000 molecules of spermidine and 40,000 molecules of spermine per virion (187,190). The polyamines appear to be tightly bound and cannot be exchanged with exogenously added, labeled polyamines. Disruption of the envelope with nonionic detergents and urea removed the spermidine but not the spermine. The spermine contained in the virion is sufficient to neutralize about 40% of the DNA phosphate (190). Parenthetically, proteins have been noted in association with the toroidal structure (171) in the capsid, and a capsid protein has been reported to bind DNA (45).

The compartmentalization of spermine and spermidine may reflect the distribution of polyamines in the infected cell. It is of interest to note that after infection, the conversion of ornithine to putrescine appears to be blocked, but the synthesis of spermine and spermidine does not appear to be affected (190).

Lipids

It has been assumed that HSV acquires the envelope lipids from its host. The hypothesis that the lipid composition of the viral envelope is determined by the host was supported by the observation that the buoyant density of the virus was host cell dependent on serial passage of HSV-1 alternately in HEp-2 and chick embryo cells (588). More recent studies (642) suggest that the virion lipids are similar to those of cytoplasmic membranes and different from those of nuclear membranes of uninfected cells. This conclusion assumes that the lipid content of nuclear membranes remains unchanged during infection notwithstanding the change in the overall surface area of nuclear membranes and lack of *de novo* synthesis of cellular proteins in infected cells.

Herpes Simplex Virus Polymorphism

Intertypic Variation

Although the genetic maps of HSV-1 and HSV-2 are largely colinear, they differ in the locations of restriction endonuclease cleavage sites in their genomic DNAs and in the apparent sizes of their proteins. Thus, analyses of HSV-1 × HSV-2 recombinants took advantage of the intertypic differences in the sizes of the proteins and the locations of restriction endonuclease cleavage sites to determine the initial locations of viral genes on the linear map of HSV genomes (354,395,396,463). Comparison of the complete DNA sequences of an HSV-1 genome and an HSV-2 genome confirmed the colinearity of the genetic maps (132).

Intratypic Variation

The first evidence of intratypic polymorphism emerged from studies of virion structural proteins and indicated that nonglycosylated proteins vary sufficiently in electrophoretic mobility to be used as strain markers (436). Although specimens from epidemiologically related individuals appeared to yield similar electrophoretic profiles, the usefulness of virion proteins as markers for molecular epidemiologic studies was limited by the effort required to purify virions for such analyses.

At the DNA level, differences between HSV-1 strains appear to result from (a) base substitutions, which may add or eliminate a restriction endonuclease cleavage site, and on occasion change an amino acid; and (b) variability in the number of repeated sequences present in a number of regions of the genome (e.g., $\gamma_1 34.5$, $U_S 11$) (82,494). The restriction endonuclease cleavage patterns of a given strain are relatively stable, whereas the number of repeats is not (53,210,507,632). Thus, no changes in restriction endonuclease patterns were noted in isolates from the same individual over an interval of 13 years or in genomes of an HSV-1 strain passaged serially numerous times in cell culture. However, restriction endonuclease site polymorphism was readily noted in isolates from epidemiologically unrelated individuals (202,520). On the basis of these properties, restriction endonuclease site polymorphism was used in several epidemiologic studies of HSV transmission in the human population (53,507, 520), and blind restriction endonuclease analysis of virus isolates has been used to trace the spread of infection from patients to hospital personnel (51), from patient to patient (328), and from hospital personnel to patient (3,52). Sakaoka and associates (529) reported on clustering of divergent sites along geographically and racially distinct areas. Although these authors concluded that the evolution of HSV-1 may be host dependent, it seems more likely that random mutations were conserved and dispersed in different populations.

GENOME STRUCTURE AND ORGANIZATION

Viral Genes: Pattern of Organization and Expression

Distribution and Organization of Transcriptional Units

The HSV DNA encodes by current count about 90 unique transcriptional units (see Table 1). The HSV-1 sequence and gene map can be found at website http://www.stdgene.lanl.gov/. At least 84 of these transcriptional units encode proteins. As described in more detail later, these genes are classified into at least three general kinetic classes: α, or immediate early; β, or early; and γ, or late. The key elements of genome organization are as follows:

1. With three known exceptions, each viral transcript encodes a single protein. In the first exception, a single transcript serves as the template for both ORF P and ORF 0 proteins. Protein synthesis is initiated from a single methionine but diverges between the 1st and 35th codons to yield different polypeptides (480). Second, the *U_L26* gene encodes a polypeptide that cleaves itself to form two proteins. The amino-terminal product functions as a protease. The carboxyl-terminal product, ICP35a,b, is a component of the capsid scaffolding. The third exception is the messenger RNA (mRNA) that encodes the U_L3 protein. This RNA, 2.9 kb in size, contains the ORFs of U_L1, U_L2, and U_L3, but U_L1 and U_L2 proteins are encoded by distinct mRNAs (569). The mechanism of expression of U_L3 protein is unknown.
2. Many clusters of transcriptional units are 3′ co-terminal. In addition, these clusters may be arranged either head-to-head, head-to-tail, or tail-to-tail. The precise transcription initiation sites are not known for all transcriptional units. In many instances, but especially late in infection, transcription termination sites are ignored, with the consequence that run-on transcripts of giant size are present along with the properly terminated transcripts. Some of the 3′ co-terminal mRNAs initiate within the body of an expressed ORF and encode only the carboxyl-terminal portion of the protein encoded by the ORF. For example, the mRNA encoding U_S1.5 initiates within the ORF expressing ICP22, and the amino acid sequence of U_S1.5 is identical to that of the carboxyl-terminal domain of ICP22. The same situation exists for U_L26 and U_L26.5.
3. Some of the expressed ORFs are antisense to each other. These include *ICP34.5* and *ORF P*, *U_L43* and *U_L43.5*, and *gB* and *U_L27.5*. The existence of additional antisense ORFs cannot be excluded.
4. Few of the transcripts accumulating in infected cells arise as a consequence of splicing of RNA. In only two cases, those encoding ICP0 and U_L15, are the introns within coding domains. The intron of U_L15 is transcribed antisense to U_L15 and encodes two ORFs, U_L16 and U_L17 (363). The intron of ICP0 mRNA is stable and transported into the cytoplasm but appears to play no role in productive infection because substitution of the wild-type *ICP0* gene with an intronless *ICP0* gene has no effect on its known functions (147). In all other cases (genes encoding ICP22, ICP47, and gC), the introns are in the 5′-noncoding domains. In one instance, that of the gene encoding ICP34.5, an intron is present in the coding domain of HSV-2 but not that of HSV-1 (362,482).
5. Several transcripts appear not to encode expressed ORFs. Those best known are the latency-associated transcripts (LATs) described in the section dealing with latency and the *Ori_S* mRNA that is expressed late in infection and is 3′ co-terminal with the mRNA encoding ICP4. The functions of these RNAs in productive infection are not known.

Functional Organization of Herpes Simplex Virus Genomes

α genes map near the termini of the L and S components (9,258,259,347,396,400,463,661,662). The *α0* and *α4* genes map within the inverted repeats of the L and S components, respectively, and are therefore each present in two copies per wild-type genome. However, a single copy of each is sufficient inasmuch as mutants lacking the internal inverted repeats are viable but are attenuated for growth in animals (446).

With few exceptions, β and γ genes are scattered in the unique sequences of both the L and S components. The exceptions are the *$\gamma_1$34.5* and *ORF P* genes located in the reiterated sequences flanking the L component between the terminal *a* sequence and the *α0* gene (2,84,307). At present, only two functional gene clusters are strikingly apparent, but their significance is uncertain: The β genes specifying the DNA polymerase and the ICP8 single-stranded DNA (ssDNA)-binding protein flank the L component origin of DNA synthesis (Ori_L) (98,226,478), and the γ genes specifying membrane glycoproteins D, E, G, I, and J map next to each other within the unique sequences of the S component (2,165,311,490,510,526, 584,662).

Application of Genetic Techniques to the Identification of Gene Product Function: Genes Essential and Nonessential for Growth in Cell Cultures

Key to the identification of viral functions and mapping of viral genes encoding these functions are temperature sensitive (ts) and null mutants. Earlier studies identified about 30 complementation groups (668)—an extraordinary accomplishment in itself given the difficulties inherent in the selection and testing of the numerous mutants produced by many laboratories. The ts mutants have been enormously helpful in mapping genes. Nevertheless, this approach to identification and mapping of viral functions suffers from several problems: (a) the phenotypes of viruses containing mutations in nonessential genes cannot be readily differentiated from that of the wild type parent; (b) conditional lethal (e.g., ts) mutants produced by general mutagenesis of the viral genome may contain a large number of silent nonlethal mutations in both essential and nonessential genes; (c) the phenotypes of mutations introduced into domains shared by more than one gene cannot be readily attributed to the malfunction of a specific gene product; and (d) although the usefulness of ts mutants is in part dependent on their efficiency of plating at permissive and nonpermissive temperatures, tight mutants with high permissive-to-nonpermissive ratios may well contain more than one point mutation. Although the presence of multiple mutations in a single gene should not affect the mapping or identification of the gene function, it does present a problem in mapping the functional domains of the gene.

An alternative to the random or fragment-specific substitution of bases in DNA is localized mutagenesis of the viral genome. Much of the HSV genetic work thus far has used a co-transfection procedure involving the introduction of infectious viral DNA with a viral DNA fragment that contains a marker or mutation to be introduced into the viral genome by a double crossover event (279,526, 611). This has been used for marker rescue mapping of viral ts mutants, introduction of markers into a viral genome (marker transfer) (279,526), and introduction of mutations into a viral genome (86,98).

A protocol for site-specific insertion and deletion of viral genes was reported by Post and Roizman (454). It was based on selection of recombinants generated by double recombination through homologous flanking sequences between an intact viral DNA molecule and a DNA fragment containing an insertion or deletion and a selectable marker. The selectable marker used in these studies was the viral thymidine kinase (*tk*) gene because (a) it can be deleted from the HSV genome without affecting the growth of virus in cell culture, (b) a plasmid-borne *tk* gene can be altered so that it cannot recombine by double crossover to repair the deletion in the genomic *tk* gene; (c) viruses carrying a functional *tk* gene can be selected against by plating viral progeny in the presence of nucleoside analogs phosphorylated by the viral thymidine kinase (TK) (e.g., Ara T), and (d) viruses expressing the TK gene can be selected for by plating the virus on TK-negative cells in medium containing methotrexate or aminopterin, which blocks the conversion of thymidine monophosphate (TMP) from deoxyuridine monophosphate (dUMP) by thymidylate synthetase and precludes the *de novo* pathway of TMP synthesis. This procedure permits the selection of viable mutants with deletions or insertions in genes that appear to be nonessential for growth in cells in culture.

A second popular approach for mutagenesis of a specific gene is to replace the gene with *Escherichia coli lac*Z coding sequences so that the β-galactosidase enzyme is expressed by the recombinant virus. The recombinant virus can be identified by the formation of blue plaques in the presence of chromogenic substrates such as X-GAL (194). If the recombinant virus can be isolated and propagated on normal cells, such as Vero cells, the mutated gene is considered to be nonessential. If the viral gene is essential for growth in that cell line, stable complementing cell lines have often been used to propagate these null mutant viruses (122). In this protocol, the gene to be mutated is transfected into and stably maintained in a cell line that serves as the complementing cell line. The complementing cell line is then transfected with intact viral DNA and the mutated DNA fragment. The progeny of transfection are screened for mutants that form blue plaques or multiply only in the complementing cells (122,326,424).

In recent years, several other techniques have come into vogue that promise to simplify greatly the construction of mutants. The first involves the use of overlapping cosmids that contain viral DNA sequences that encompass the entire genome. After transfection into cells, viral gene expression from the overlapping cosmids enables recombination at the overlapping ends to reconstitute the intact genome (104). The second technique is based on the use of bacterial artificial chromosomes to propagate the viral genome in bacterial cells. Mutations can be introduced into the HSV sequences, and introduction of the recombinant bacterial artificial chromosome into mammalian cells yields infectious virus (235). Both techniques enable construction of multiple mutants. The genomes cloned as bacterial accessory chromosomes are amenable to random insertional mutagenesis by transposons. Finally, an adjunct to all methods designed to inactivate viral genes is the use of baculoviruses carrying the target gene under a viral promoter. Such genes are expressed only in infected cells and enable selection of mutants lacking essential genes (691).

The genes known to be dispensable for viral replication in cells in culture are listed in Table 1. Of importance, most of the dispensable genes are required for replication in experimental animal systems, and in no instance has a virus lacking a dispensable gene been isolated from human lesions (although viruses that fail to react with a specific monoclonal antibody are readily isolated).

Genes dispensable for viral replication in cells in culture fall into several groups whose products are involved in entry of HSV into cells, regulation of gene expression, posttranslational modification of proteins, exocytosis, inhibition of host response to infection, and spread of virus from cell to cell.

In a special category are deletion mutants, whose ability to multiply in cells is species dependent. One example of such mutants is the $\alpha22^-$ virus, which grows well in Vero and HEp-2 cell lines but not in human fibroblast strains or in rodent cell lines (547). In the nonpermissive cells, the virus fails to express $\gamma2$ genes efficiently. Another example of a cell-specific gene is $\gamma_1 34.5$, which enables HSV to multiply in human cells but is dispensable in Vero, baby hamster kidney cells, and so forth. In the absence of the gene, there is total shutoff of protein synthesis before significant amounts of virus are synthesized (78,80,81).

It could be predicted that viral genes that specify products whose functions are identical and interchangeable with those of cellular genes would be dispensable, at least in cells that express these functions. In this category are the *tk* gene and the genes specifying ribonucleotide reductase. The observation that some virion proteins are dispensable for infection and replication of virus at least in cell culture presented was puzzling for many years. Although we cannot exclude the possibility that cells express proteins with similar functions that complement the deletion mutants, a more likely scenario is that cells in culture express many more genes than cells *in situ* in animal organs. The exceptions to date are polarized epithelial cells and neuroblastoma cells, in which the gene products are sorted differently or which differ from other cells in culture with respect to the nature of the genes that are expressed. HSV may carry a set of genes that enables the virus to enter (e.g., the dispensable glycoproteins), multiply (e.g., $\gamma_1 34.5$) or egress (e.g., $U_L 20$) from a wide variety of human cells. Because these genes are not required for replication in all cells, there exists the formal possibility that functional analogs of the viral gene are encoded and may be expressed by cells. The obvious examples are the *tk,* ribonucleotide reductase, and so forth. The less obvious homologs are the cellular protein kinases that substitute for some of the viral enzymes and the homolog of $U_L 20$, which enables virus to egress from a variety of cell lines other than Vero cells. The complexity involved in defining the function of the numerous genes whose products are dispensable for viral replication in at least some cells in culture is offset by the fact that these genes are excellent probes of cellular functions that, at least in some instances, complement the missing viral function.

VIRAL REPLICATION

Overview of Replication

It is convenient to begin this section on viral replication with a bird's eye view of the major events of HSV replication (Fig. 3).

To initiate infection, the virus must attach to cell surface receptors. Fusion of the envelope with the plasma membrane rapidly follows the initial attachment. The deenveloped tegument–capsid structure is then transported to the nuclear pores, where DNA is released into the nucleus.

Transcription of the viral genome, replication of viral DNA, and assembly of new capsids take place in the nucleus. Viral DNA is transcribed throughout productive infection by host RNA polymerase II, but with the participation of viral factors at all stages of infection. The synthesis of viral gene products is tightly regulated: Viral gene expression is coordinately regulated and sequentially ordered in a cascade fashion. The gene products studied to date form at least five groups as a result of both transcriptional and posttranscriptional regulation.

Several of the gene products are enzymes and DNA-binding proteins involved in viral DNA replication. The bulk of viral DNA is synthesized by a rolling-circle mechanism, yielding concatemers, which are cleaved into monomers during the process of nucleocapsid assembly.

Assembly occurs in several stages. After packaging of DNA into preassembled capsids, the virus matures and acquires infectivity by budding through the inner lamella of the nuclear membrane. The transit of virions from the space between the inner and outer nuclear membranes to the subcellular space is less well defined. It has been suggested that the virion envelope is processed by transit through Golgi stacks or by being deenveloped and then reenveloped at the trans-Golgi network. In fully permissive tissue culture cells, the entire process takes about 18 to 20 hours.

Virus Attachment and Entry

Entry of HSV into cells is effected in three stages (Fig. 4). The first involves the attachment of the virion to the surface of the cell. The second step involves the interaction of gD with one of several cellular receptors. In the last step, the viral envelope and the plasma membrane fuse to

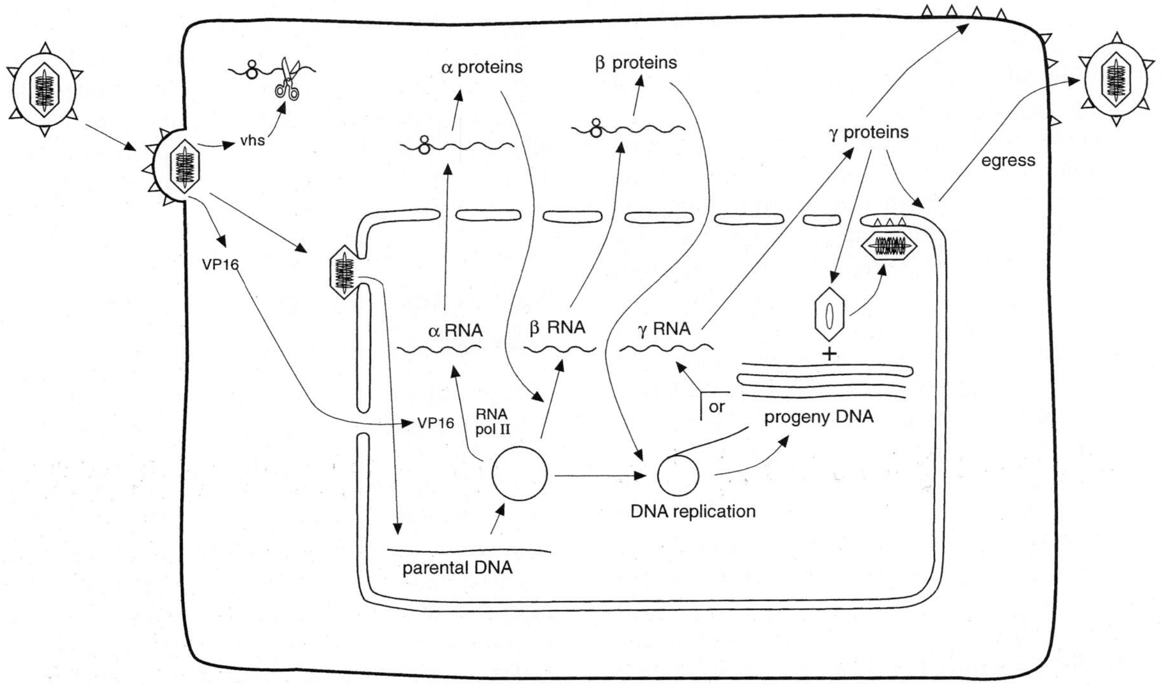

FIG. 3. Diagram of the replication cycle of HSV. At the *upper left,* the virion binds to the cell plasma membrane, and the virion envelope fuses with the plasma membrane, releasing the capsid and tegument proteins into the cytoplasm. The vhs protein acts to cause degradation of mRNAs. The capsid is transported to the nuclear pore, where the viral DNA is released into the nucleus. The viral DNA circularizes and is transcribed by host RNA polymerase II to give first the IE or α mRNAs. IE gene transcription is stimulated by the VP16 tegument protein. Five of the six IE proteins act to regulate viral gene expression in the nucleus. They transactivate E or β gene transcription. The E proteins are involved in replicating the viral DNA molecule. Viral DNA synthesis stimulates L or γ gene expression. The L proteins are involved in assembling the capsid in the nucleus and modifying the membranes for virion formation. The filled capsid buds through the inner membrane to form an enveloped virion, and the virion exits from the cell by mechanisms described in the section on Virion Assembly and Egress.

release the capsid–tegument structure into the cytoplasm. Most of the information on this process is based on studies of nonpolarized cells in which the membrane proteins interacting with envelope proteins are most likely randomly distributed. Attachment and entry of viruses into polarized cells—most epithelial cells in the human body—may differ in detail.

The initial attachment to nonpolarized cells involves the interaction of the viral envelope gC, and, to a lesser extent gB, with the glycosaminoglycan moieties of cell surface heparan sulfate (560,686). Although gC confers the greatest efficiency for attachment in these systems, it is not essential for either entry or viral replication (216).

Attachment to heparan sulfate enhances infection but is not an absolute requirement for HSV infection of cells because cells devoid of heparan sulfate but expressing other glycosaminoglycans (e.g., chondroitin sulfate) can be infected. Cells devoid of both of these types of glycosaminoglycans can also be infected, although at a reduced efficiency (19). The second, sequential step, designated here as binding to a coreceptor, involves the interaction of gD with one of several cellular molecules that belong to three structurally unrelated molecular families. As is often the case, they have been given different designations based on their cellular function or their function in viral infection.

The first of these coreceptors is a member of the tumor necrosis factor (TNF) receptor family originally called *herpes virus entry mediator* (HVEM) (392) but renamed HveA after other receptors were discovered (659). HveA is present primarily in lymphoid cells, and thus it is unlikely to function as the major mediator of HSV entry into human cells. It serves as a receptor for entry of some selected HSV-1 strains, HSV-2, but not for the related alphaherpesvirus, pseudorabies (PRV) virus (392,670).

The second family of coreceptors belongs to the immunoglobulin superfamily and is related to the poliovirus receptors (183). The first identified members of this family were named HveB (659) and HveC (183) and herpesvirus immunoglobulin-like receptor (HIgR) (92). This family includes several isoforms present in

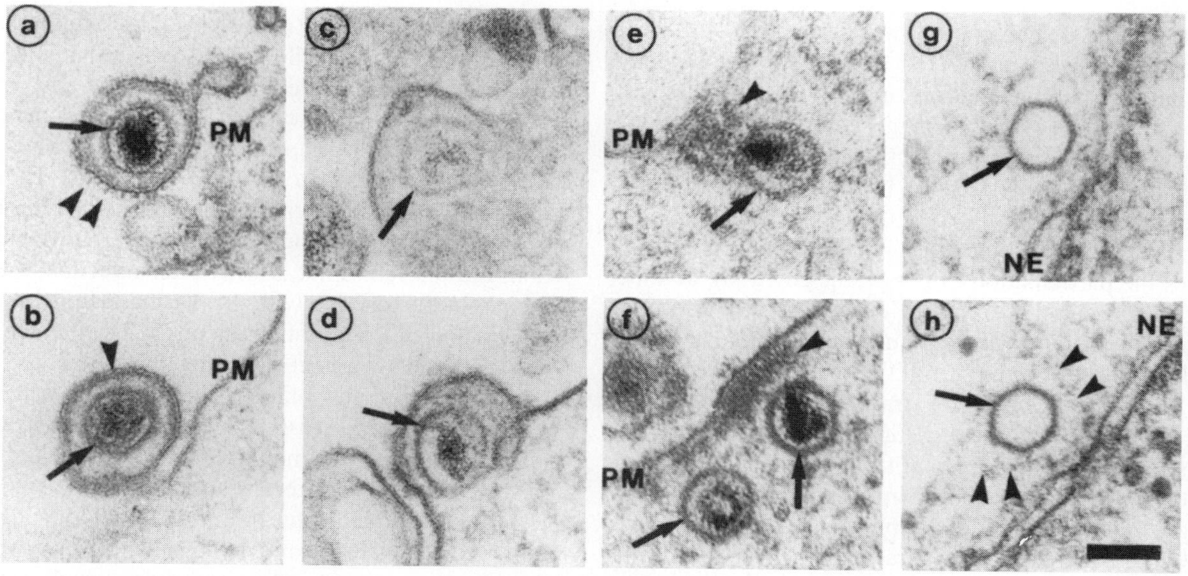

FIG. 4. Entry and uncoating of HSV-1. Shown are ultrathin Epon sections of Vero cells infected with HSV-1 at an MOI of 500 in the presence of cycloheximide (*CH*). After 2 hours of virus binding at 4°C, the cells were either fixed immediately (***a*** and ***b***), or warmed up for 30 (***c*** to ***f***) or 60 (***g*** and ***h***) minutes. Binding (***a*** and ***b***). The main morphologic features of the intact virus bound to the plasma membrane (*PM*) are the viral envelope (***b,*** *arrowhead*) with the viral spikes (***a,*** *arrowhead*), the viral capsid (*arrow*), and the electron-dense viral DNA genome within the capsid. Fusion (***c*** and ***d***). Upon warming up, the viral envelope fuses with the plasma membrane, and the capsid (*arrow*) and the tegument proteins are released into the cytosol. Release of the capsid (***e*** and ***f***). Preparations, which display a prominent contrast of the tegument, show that the tegument (*arrowheads*) stays behind at the PM. Binding to the nuclear pore (***g*** and ***h***). At later time points, the capsids (*arrows*) have arrived at the nuclear envelope (*NE*), where they are exclusively located in close apposition to the nuclear pore complexes. Occasionally, fibers emanating from the pores (*arrowheads*) are visible, to which the capsids appear to bind. Almost all of the capsids at the nuclear pores appear empty and have lost the electron-dense DNA core. Bar, 100 nm. (From ref. 578, with permission).

both human and nonhuman cells that are encoded by mRNAs generated by alternative mRNA splicing. More recently, these cellular proteins have been shown to act as intercellular adhesion molecules and to be localized at adhesion junctions where their C-terminal domains bind to L-afadin, a PDZ-binding protein that anchors these molecules to cytoskeleton and adherens junctions. On the basis of their cellular function, they have been named *nectins* (617); therefore, the designations that appear now in the literature are nectin-1α (HveC, Prr1), nectin-1β (HIgR), nectin-2α (HveB, Prr2), and nectin-2δ (91,340, 586). Nectin-1α and nectin-1β, two splice variants with a common ectodomain, are broadly expressed in cells of epithelial, fibroblastic, neural, and hematopoietic origin; in keratinocytes; and in human tissues that are targets of HSV infection, including skin, brain, and spinal ganglia (92,183). They mediate entry of all HSV-1 strains tested, HSV-2, PRV, and bovine herpes virus 1 (183). They also mediate cell-to-cell spread of HSV (91). Nectin-2α (HveB) and nectin-2δ, also splice variant isoforms, mediate the entry of HSV-2, PRV, and certain viable mutants of HSV-1, but not of wild-type HSV-1 (340,659). The distribution of this general class (immunoglobulin superfamily) of receptors in human tissues reflects the susceptibility of cells to infection and is likely to account for both entry and spread of virus from cell to cell.

Homologs of human nectins have been found in a wide variety of species. The murine homolog of human nectin-1 also mediates entry of HSV-1 and HSV-2 into murine cells (382). This raises the possibility that the ability to use the animal homologs of the nectin-type proteins can account for the broad host range of HSV in cell cultures and animals of different species. Interestingly, this receptor activity was reported to function independently of gD binding (382).

The third family has to date only one member: 3-*O*-sulfated heparan sulfate (563). The 3-*O*-sulfated heparan sulfates are broadly distributed on human cells and tissues and mediate efficient HSV-1 but not HSV-2 entry (563). Whether they can mediate entry into human cells remains to be determined. It is interesting that either protein molecules or specific sites on heparan sulfate can serve as receptors for HSV entry.

The last step in entry is the fusion of the viral envelope with the plasma membrane of the host cell. There is overwhelming acceptance of the hypothesis that productive infection results from the entry of virus mediated by fusion of the envelope and plasma membranes (394). Key evidence is the demonstration that gI and gE—the viral Fc receptors—can be detected on the surface of cells immediately after penetration of the virus (430). Conversely, a body of evidence suggests that entry by endocytosis does not result in productive infection. Thus, cells expressing gD internalize virus by endocytosis, but viral replication does not ensue (58,703).

Current evidence indicates that virus–cell fusion requires the participation of gD (326), gB (536), and the gH-gL heterodimer (164). The exact role of these proteins in the fusion process is unknown, but one could speculate that the binding of gD to the cellular receptors leads to a rearrangement of viral proteins on the virion surface, a conformational change in their structure, or both, so that gB, gH/gL, or both can promote fusion. An additional observation underlying the hypotheses is that cells are infected with wild-type virus aggregate (*syn*$^+$ phenotype), whereas certain viral mutants cause the cells to fuse (called either *syn*$^-$ or *syn* phenotype). *Syn*$^-$ mutations map in the genes encoding gB, gH, and gK and in the U_L24 membrane protein (526). The data suggest that these proteins may form a complex and that mutations in any one of the syn proteins cause a rearrangement or a conformational change in the complex, resulting in cell fusion (526). For detailed reviews on this topic, see references 57 and 585.

Studies on viral entry into polarized cells have progressed to a much lesser extent. Current data are based on studies of viral entry into a few polarized cell lines in culture and on corneal cells *in vivo*. These data indicate that attachment to the apical surface is gC dependent, whereas entry through the basolateral surface is gC independent (548), and that gG, a viral glycoprotein with no other known function, plays a key role in the postattachment entry on the apical surface but is not essential for basolateral entry (633).

The transition from attached to penetrated virus, as measured by the loss of susceptibility to neutralization, inactivation by acidic pH, or proteases, is very rapid and occurs within minutes (121,236).

Transport to the Cell Nucleus

After fusion of the envelope to the plasma membrane, some tegument proteins remain in the cytoplasm (e.g., vhs, U_S11) whereas others are either transported to the nucleus (VP16) or may remain associated with the capsid (e.g., VP1-2), as discussed later in the text. The capsid with associated tegument structures is then transported through the microtubular network to the nuclear pore. The extent of our knowledge of virus transport is limited but can be described as follows:

HSV capsids have been observed bound to microtubules in neurons (343,344,433). In cultured cells, antibodies specific for capsid proteins co-localize with microtubules after viral entry (578). Microtubule depolymerizing agents such as colchicine and nocodazole block the transport of nucleocapsids to the cell nucleus, and antibody labeling of dynein, the microtubule-dependent motor, showed that it was attached to HSV capsids (578). These authors proposed that incoming capsids bind to microtubules and use dynein to propel them to the cell nucleus. The precise mechanism of loading capsid–tegument structures onto the cytoplasmic dynein motors is unknown, but two observations are relevant. First, shortly after infection, the microtubules at the junction with the plasma membrane become disrupted (657), suggesting the possibility that the loading of the capsid–tegument structures may affect the interaction of microtubules or associated proteins with cognate structures in the plasma membrane. More extensive rearrangements of the microtubular network take place late in infection. Second, recent studies have shown that the U_L34 protein binds the amino-terminal domain of the intermediate chain 1α of cytoplasmic neuronal dynein and that, in the presence of nocodazole, which causes the depolymerization of dynein, U_L34 protein is not transported to the nucleus (692). Finally, because the normal dynein motor terminus is at the microtubule-organizing center, it is not clear how the nucleocapsids ultimately come in apposition with the nuclear pore complex.

After intracytoplasmic transport, the nucleocapsids accumulate at the nuclear envelope and associate with the nuclear pore complexes (21,578) (see Fig. 4). At the pore, the nucleocapsid releases its DNA into the nucleus, leaving an empty capsid at the cytoplasmic side of the complex. Little is known about the mechanisms of HSV DNA release and transport through the nuclear pore into the nucleus. The HSV-1 ts mutant *ts*B7 is completely blocked for viral gene expression at the nonpermissive temperature (NPT) (278) because it is defective for the release of DNA from capsids at the NPT (21). The ts mutation in *ts*B7 maps in the *VP1/2* gene (21), suggesting that this large tegument protein plays a role in DNA release at the nuclear pores. These results also suggest that the VP1/2 tegument protein is transported to the nuclear pore with the capsid; nevertheless, it is still conceivable that the defective protein is unable to be released in the cytoplasm and thus is kept artifactually with the nucleocapsid during transport through the cytoplasm and blocks uncoating at the nuclear pore. Recent *in vitro* results have shown that binding of the capsid to the nuclear pores is blocked by wheat germ agglutinin, antinuclear pore complex antibodies, or antibodies against importin β (422). Thus, the available data suggest that the interaction of capsid–tegument structures with the nuclear pore proteins causes a structural change in the former, with the consequence that viral DNA is extruded from the capsids into the nucleus; however, the molecular details remain to be defined. The presence of intact, empty capsids for at least 2 hours after exposure of cells to the virus suggests that the extrusion of the DNA does not coincide with complete dissociation of the capsid.

Some of the functions of viral tegument proteins and of genes expressed after infection suggest that the environment inside the host cell is decidedly hostile to the incoming virus. The tegument proteins are introduced into the cell concurrently with the capsid, and some play a key role in creating an environment that allows efficient viral replication. Although the functions of many tegument proteins remain elusive, it seems clear that their distribution varies early in infection. For example, two of these proteins, VP16 and U_L41, are described in detail in later sections, but they promote α gene transcription in the nucleus and shutoff of host protein synthesis in the cytoplasm, respectively. These two virion proteins play a clear role in preparing the host cell for efficient viral replication.

Table 1 lists a large number of viral proteins reported to be components of the viral tegument. With the two exceptions listed previously, the functions of the tegument proteins are not readily discernible, largely because many are either dispensable for viral replication or their function as tegument proteins is different from that expressed in the course of productive infection after *de novo* synthesis. For example, U_S11, genetically engineered to be expressed early in infection, blocks the shutoff of protein synthesis induced by activated protein kinase R (PKR) (66). Virions carry about 2,000 copies of U_S11 protein; after infection, these are associated with polyribosomes and 60S ribosomal subunits and do not block the shutoff of protein synthesis caused by activated PKR in cells infected with $\gamma_1 34.5$-negative mutants. Similarly, ICP22 and other α proteins are posttranslationally modified by both the U_L13 and U_S3 viral protein kinases. However, there is no evidence that ICP22 is modified by the viral kinases introduced into the infected cell as tegument proteins (421,471,472). Thus, the functions of many of the tegument proteins remain to be identified. Nevertheless, the process of entry and release of tegument proteins can be harmful to the cell because cells arrested at the stage of release of tegument proteins can undergo apoptosis (176,700).

The Fate of Viral DNA upon Entry into the Nucleus

The bulk of the incoming viral DNA circularizes rapidly after infection and in the absence of viral protein synthesis (179,445), suggesting that under these conditions, circularization of the genome is promoted by cellular proteins or viral proteins brought into the infected cell in the virion. It has been suggested that the viral DNA ends are held together in the virion and are rapidly ligated by cellular enzymes (445). Because viral DNA is nicked and contains ribonucleotides (see Genome Structure and Organization), repair, circularization, and conversion to the appropriate conformation must then take place. These events may explain the involvement of the RCC1 (regulator of chromosome condensation) gene product in early events in viral infection reported by Umene and Nishimoto (638), but this remains to be verified. It has also been suggested that circularization may result from recombination between direct repeats in the terminal *a* sequences (37), consistent with the hypothesis that fluctuation in the number of *a* sequences could be the consequence of recombination between free ends (390). Such recombination events undoubtedly take place because the number of such repeats varies within the DNA populations arising from a single plaque. It is likely, however, that such recombination events also occur during viral DNA synthesis and packaging.

Leinbach and Summers (317) reported that HSV DNA remains in a nonnucleosomal form during the course of productive infection of cells.

Overview of Productive Infection Gene Expression

During productive infection, more than 80 HSV proteins are expressed in a highly regulated cascade fashion (Fig. 5) in a number of coordinately expressed groups of gene products (230), and several viral proteins play a role in regulation of viral gene expression. Transcription of viral DNA takes place in the nucleus, and as would be expected, all viral proteins are synthesized in the cytoplasm. The host RNA polymerase II is responsible for transcription of all viral genes on the viral DNA during infection (8,102), although viral gene products may modify its activity and structure. Very soon after infection,

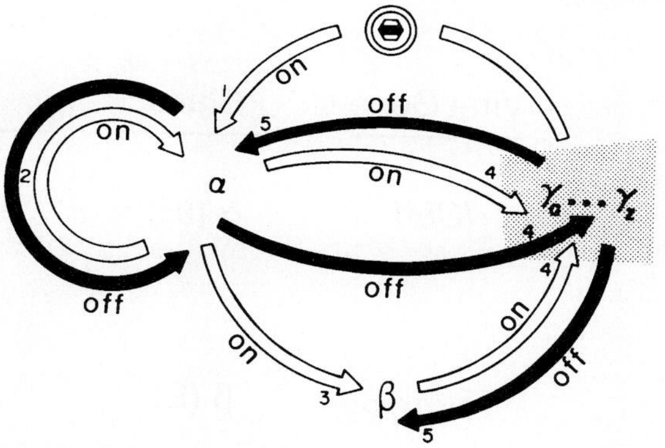

FIG. 5. Schematic representation of the regulation of HSV gene expression. *Open* and *filled arrows* represent events in the reproductive cycle that turn gene expression "on" and "off," respectively. 1. Turning on of α gene transcription by α-TIF, a γ protein packaged in the virion. 2. Autoregulation of α gene expression. 3. Turning on of β gene transcription. 4. Turning on of γ gene transcription by α and β gene products through transactivation of γ genes, release of γ genes from repression, and replication of viral DNA. Note that γ genes differ with respect to the stringency of the requirement for DNA synthesis. The heterogeneity is shown as a continuum in which inhibitors of viral DNA synthesis are shown to have minimal effect on γ_a gene expression but totally preclude the expression of γ_z genes. 5. Turning off of α and β gene expression by the products of γ genes late in infection.

about 2 to 4 hours postinfection (hpi) at a multiplicity of infection (MOI) of 10 to 20 or in the absence of other *de novo* synthesized viral proteins, the viral α or immediate-early (IE) genes are expressed. These consist of six proteins designated as ICP0, ICP4, ICP22, ICP27, ICP47, and Us1.5. Although transcription of α genes requires no prior viral protein synthesis, an HSV protein brought in with the virion tegument, VP16 (also called αTIF and Vmw65), stimulates the transcription of the α genes, as described later. Five of the six α gene products, including ICP4, ICP0, ICP27, ICP22, and Us1.5, stimulate E gene expression in at least some types of cells. As described later, HSV infection inhibits host transcription, RNA splicing and transport, and protein synthesis to facilitate the transition from cellular to viral gene expression.

Expression of the next set of HSV genes, the β or early genes, requires at least the presence of functional ICP4 but not the onset of viral DNA synthesis. Between about 4 to 8 hpi, the β proteins are expressed at peak rates. Among these are proteins involved in replication of the viral DNA and nucleotide metabolism. These viral proteins promote viral DNA replication, and expression of γ, or late, genes is then stimulated. Two general groups of β proteins have been identified, although rigid criteria for classification into the two groups have not been defined. The β1 genes are expressed within a short time after or almost concurrently with the onset of synthesis of α proteins and are exemplified by *UL29* encoding ICP8, the single-stranded protein, and *UL39* encoding ICP6, the large subunit of ribonucleotide reductase. The β_2 genes are expressed with more delay after α protein expression and are exemplified by *UL23* encoding thymidine kinase. Some of the β genes require ICP27 for their expression, and this may correlate with the later kinetics characteristic of β_2 genes.

The γ, or late, genes are expressed at peak times after viral DNA synthesis has commenced, and their expression is enhanced by viral DNA synthesis. They have been lumped for convenience into two groups, one called γ_1, early-late, or leaky-late, and one called γ_2, late, or true-late, although in reality, they form a continuum differing in their timing and dependence on viral DNA synthesis for expression (98,101,259,565,651). The typical γ_1 gene (e.g., the genes encoding ICP5, gB, gD, and ICP34.5) is expressed relatively early in infection and is stimulated a few fold by viral DNA synthesis. The relatively abundant major capsid protein ICP5 is made both early and late in infection. In contrast, typical γ_2 genes (e.g., *UL44*, the gene encoding gC, *UL41, UL36, UL38*, and *Us11*) are expressed late in infection and are not expressed in the presence of effective concentrations of inhibitors of viral DNA synthesis.

Based on our limited knowledge of the structure of the promoter and regulatory regions of HSV genes at this time, there appear to be differences in the general organization of the promoter and regulatory sequences of typical genes in each class (Fig. 6). In general, the α gene promoters contain numerous binding sites for cellular transcription factors (see Fig. 6, *ICP4* gene) upstream of a TATA box. The β gene promoters thus far studied contain binding sites for two or three cellular transcription factors upstream of the transcriptional start site (see Fig. 6, *TK* gene). The γ_1 gene promoters contain only one or

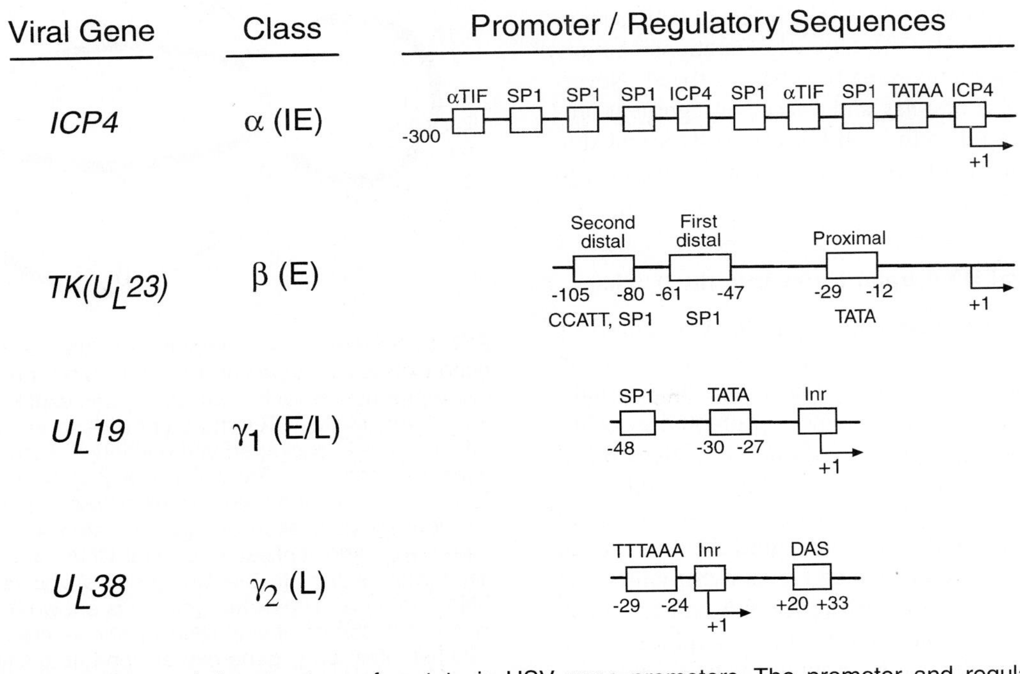

FIG. 6. Diagram of the structure of prototypic HSV gene promoters. The promoter and regulatory sequences of prototypic genes of α, β, γ_1, and γ_2 kinetic classes are diagrammed.

two upstream binding sites (see Fig. 6, *ICP5* gene), whereas the γ_2 promoters consist of a TATA box, an initiator element, and a downstream activator element, each of which may vary considerably from cellular homologs (see Fig. 6, *gC* or *U_L44* gene). The level of transcription of viral genes increases in general for the later kinetic classes of genes (699), likely because large amounts of late proteins are needed for virion assembly. This increased level of transcription is apparently due to increased template number and virus-induced modification of the transcription apparatus that is operating on the viral DNA molecule.

We would like to emphasize that although there are prototype genes that allow the definition of four post-α classes of genes, there is likely to be a continuum of genes from β_2 to γ_1 genes, in terms of their kinetics and requirements for viral gene expression. First, β and γ gene expression in the context of the viral genome requires the participation of five of the six α proteins: ICP0 (528), ICP4 (279,456), ICP27 (527), ICP22 (454, 547), and US1.5 (421). Only a few viral genes have been completely characterized with regard to their requirement for these α proteins; thus, we do not know how the requirement for these genes correlates with the kinetic classes already defined. Second, the differences between β and γ_1 genes are difficult to quantify and are not perfectly delineated. In principle, the expression of β genes is not augmented by the onset of DNA synthesis, whereas the expression of γ_1 genes is reduced in the presence of inhibitors of DNA synthesis. However, expression of some of the β genes is inhibited slightly by inhibitors of viral DNA synthesis (639), whereas some γ_1 genes are expressed early and are affected only minimally by inhibitors of DNA synthesis (e.g., *gB*) (478). Nevertheless, it is useful to consider β and γ gene expression separately while discussing events in the course of productive infection.

The *ORF O* and *ORF P* genes present a special case. These genes are repressed by ICP4 and therefore are not expressed during productive infection or in the presence of functional ICP4. These genes have been designated as pre-α genes in recognition of the special requirements for their expression (307).

Expression of α Genes

Upon entry into the cell nucleus, the HSV genome, presumably in a circular form, localizes to intranuclear sites near the cellular ND10 structures where transcription of α genes is thought to take place (358). The α gene promoters contain numerous binding sites for cellular transcriptional factors. The major characteristic that differentiates α genes from other viral genes is the presence of the consensus sequence 5′-GyATGnTAATGArATTCyTTGnGGG-3′ in one to several copies within several hundred base pairs upstream of the cap site (173,346–348). This sequence binds Oct-1 but acts as a response element to a complex of the viral protein VP16, host cell factor (HCF) or C1, cellular Oct-1, and other transcriptional factors to promote the expression of the α genes (185,292,293,295,418,459,634).

VP16

VP16 was first described as a virion protein number 16 (VP16) by Spear and Roizman (589) and as ICP25 during the enumeration of proteins accumulating in cells after infection (230). The first evidence that HSV encodes a function that transactivates α genes after infection was reported by Post and co-investigators (453). Subsequently, this virion factor, named α gene transactivating factor (α-TIF) was shown to be a component of the tegument capable of inducing genes carrying the cognate promoter response element, even in the absence of the release of viral DNA into the nucleus (22). VP16 was identified as the virion protein responsible for the transactivation of α genes by Campbell and colleagues (61), and the gene was sequenced by Pellett and associates (432). Upon release from the tegument, VP16 binds to a cellular protein called host cell factor (HCF) or C1 (265,297,603,688). It has been reported that HCF carries VP16 into the nucleus (302), where the VP16–HCF complex binds to Oct-1 bound to viral DNA, forming the activator complex.

The functional organization of VP16 involves several domains of the protein: Residues 378 to 389 are required for interaction with the POU domain of Oct-1 (197,198, 297,603), residues 173 to 241 are required for binding of the complex to DNA (603), and the acidic carboxyl-terminal residues 411 to 490 are required for transactivation (634). The C-terminal region likely activates transcription by interaction with host transcription factors, possibly the TFII-B (327) and TFII-D general transcription factors (612). Little is known about the portions of VP16 needed for assembly into virions other than the observation that the amino-terminal 389 residues are sufficient for interaction with the vhs protein, another tegument component (570).

As illustrated in the case of the gene encoding ICP4 (see Fig. 6), α promoters also contain binding sites for other cellular transcriptional activators (e.g., Sp1) in addition to Oct-1. The precise mix of cellular and viral response elements varies between different α gene promoter and regulatory sequences, and their relative contribution to the abundance and duration of transcription has been investigated in only a few instances. In rapidly dividing cells, VP16 increases the accumulation of transcripts by about fourfold and is not a critical factor in viral gene expression (592). Presumably, Oct-1, Sp1, and other cellular transactivating factors account for the basal level of α gene expression. The requirement for VP16 may be different in resting cells or differentiated cells in which these transcriptional factors are unavailable or tightly regulated.

Shutoff of α *Gene Expression*

The mechanism of the shutoff of α gene transcription is not entirely clear, but three mechanisms are thought to play a role:

1. ICP4 represses its own gene by binding to its cognate DNA binding site located across the transcription initiation site (see Fig. 6). The original consensus sequence of the binding site reported by Faber and Wilcox (154) was ATCGTCNNNNYCGRC, but binding sites vary considerably with respect to degeneracy and affinity for ICP4. The strongest binding sites are those located across the transcription initiation sites of the *ICP4* and the *ORF P* and *ORF O* genes (154,296,399). The effectiveness of the binding site in repressing transcription in the context of the viral genome varies depending on the distance from the transcriptional initiation site. The further downstream it is, the less the repression. Also, displacement by half of a helical turn is more effective in minimizing repression than that by a full helical turn (320). In addition, whereas mutagenesis of the ICP4-binding site across the transcription initiation site resulted in a 10-fold increase in accumulation of transcripts, the added mutagenesis of the upstream and more distant binding site had barely a twofold effect on transcript accumulation (320). It is less clear whether ICP4 represses the expression of the other α genes. ICP4 binds upstream of the *ICP0* gene transcriptional initiation site (294), and ICP4 represses the *ICP0* promoter in transfected cells (181). Nevertheless, the specific effect of ICP4 on *ICP0* gene expression in infected cells has not been defined by construction of a mutant virus with the binding site in the *ICP0* gene mutated. Consensus ICP4-binding sites are not evident in or near the promoters of the other α genes.
2. During productive infection, β gene products downregulate α gene expression (230). One β protein identified as a candidate is ICP8, the ssDNA-binding protein encoded by the β_1 gene U_L29. ICP8 decreases the expression of all genes from the parental viral DNA molecules (191,192), in particular transcription of the gene encoding ICP4 (193). The mechanism of this effect of ICP8 is not known, but it may involve the sequestration of viral DNA molecules in replication complexes, changes in the conformation of viral DNA, or displacement of DNA to sites of DNA synthesis away from those required for transcription.
3. In cells infected with *vhs* mutants, the transition from α to β and subsequently to γ protein synthesis lags behind that observed in wild-type virus-infected cells. One function of *vhs* is to synchronize sequential viral gene expression. Underlying this process is the expectation that the α transcripts would overwhelm and outcompete the β mRNAs with respect to translation initiation.

Activation of β Gene Expression

The β_1 and β_2 groups of polypeptides reach peak rates of synthesis about 5 to 7 hours after infection (230). The β_1 proteins, exemplified by polypeptides ICP6 (the large component of the viral ribonucleotide reductase (239) and ICP8 (the major DNA binding protein (98), appear very early after infection and in the past have been mistaken for α proteins (90). They are differentiated from the latter by their requirement for functional ICP4 protein for their synthesis (230,231). The β_2 polypeptides include the viral TK and DNA polymerase. The appearance of β gene products signals the onset of viral DNA synthesis, and most viral genes involved in viral nucleic acid metabolism appear to be in the β group. The β genes are heterogeneous with respect to time of peak synthesis, although those defined as β_2 are generally made later in infection.

Unlike α genes, β or γ genes do not share common promoter elements that instantly predict the timing, duration, or abundance of gene expression. Rather, the overall impression is that they appear to be made up of a diversity of elements, and both the organization and the context in which these elements are placed determine the expression of the gene.

ICP4

ICP4 is required for all post-α gene expression (90,130,279,456,660), and the effect of ICP4 is exerted at the transcriptional level, as demonstrated by nuclear runoff assays (193). Despite the extensive studies of ICP4 through transfection studies, viral genetic studies, and biochemical studies, the mechanism by which ICP4 transactivates post-α genes remains elusive; however, three lines of investigation are noteworthy.

The first centers on the DNA-binding activity of ICP4. As noted earlier in the text, ICP4 binds to both consensus and nonconsensus sites as measured by gel shift assays (294,384,385). Binding of ICP4 to specific DNA sites seems unlikely to explain its transactivation activity because the strongest affinity of ICP4 is for sites known to repress rather than activate transcription (e.g., at the transcription initiation sites of the *ICP4* or *ORF P* genes), and destruction of the sole sequence-specific binding site of ICP4 upstream of the transcription initiation site of the *ICP4* gene attenuated repression in the context of the viral genome (320). With regard to the role of DNA-binding in the transactivation function of ICP4, early mutational analysis studies showed that the sequence-specific binding activity of ICP4 correlated extensively with its ability to activate β gene expression in infected cells (556). In addition, insertion of ICP4 binding sites was reported to render reporter genes responsive to ICP4, albeit in transfected cells (622). However, at least one viral mutant has been obtained in which the DNA-binding activity of ICP4 was greatly reduced but the ability to activate β genes in infected cells was nearly unchanged (555). Furthermore, most post-α genes do not have recognizable consensus binding sites for ICP4, and mutation of consensus sites has not affected the level of expression of the surrounding genes in the viral genome (572). Thus, the bulk of the data from studies of infected cells have failed to correlate ICP4 DNA binding with transactivation of β genes.

As noted earlier, gel shift studies have shown that ICP4 binds to several nonconsensus β and γ gene sequences (241,384,385,427,428). It was postulated that, by binding to DNA sequences near promoters, ICP4 might stabilize the binding of cellular transcription factors to the β gene promoters (427,428).

The second line of studies has centered on the interaction of ICP4 with transcriptional factors. ICP4 has been shown to form complexes *in vitro* with TATA-binding protein, TFII-B, and TAF250 (63,573), and most current models for ICP4 transactivation involve interactions with cellular transcription factors to stimulate transcription. Again, given the ability of ICP4 to both activate and repress gene expression, it is not clear whether the binding of cellular transcriptional factors represents the transactivation or repressive function of ICP4.

The mechanism of activation of β genes has also been approached in studies attempting to map the cis-acting sequences needed for activation by virus infection or ICP4. The most extensively studied β gene promoter is that of the *UL23* or *tk* gene. Extensive mutagenic analysis of the promoter showed that the sequences needed for basal level transcription (369) or activated transcription (94) were the same (see Fig. 6): (1) a proximal signal from nt −12 to −29 containing a TATA box and (2) two distal signals from nt −47 to −61 and −80 to −105 containing an SP1 transcription factor–binding site, an SP1 site, and a CCAAT transcription factor (CTF) site, respectively. These studies also supported the hypothesis that ICP4 transactivates β gene promoters through interactions with cellular basal transcription factors.

Considerable work has been devoted to defining the functional organization of the ICP4 molecule. Residues 143 to 210 and 800 to 1298 are required for transactivation (431,556); residues 263 to 487 are required for DNA-binding (556,683); residues 723 to 732 are required for nuclear localization (123,398); residues 309 to 489, including the DNA-binding domain, are required for dimerization (557,682); and residues 171 to 251, including the serine-rich domain from residues 175 to 198, are required for phosphorylation (123,687).

ICP4 is modified extensively by phosphorylation, poly(ADP-ribosyl)ation *in vitro* (461) and *in vivo* (27), and nucleotidylylation (30). The latter modification, carried out by casein kinase II (386), is signaled by the sequence RPRA/S-R shared with the nucleotidylylated proteins ICP0, ICP22, ICP27, and the products of the *UL21*, *UL31*, *UL47*, and *UL49* genes (28). The available evidence suggests that nucleotidylylation of some α proteins requires the presence of proteins made later in infection (27).

Posttranslational processing of ICP4 is associated with translocation into the nucleus. ICP4 forms numerous spots in two-dimensional gels (1) and at least three bands named ICP4a, b, and c in one-dimensional SDS-PAGE gels (437). The slower one-dimensional electrophoretic forms are due to posttranslational modifications. They appear at about the time when ICP4 associates with the nucleus (158), and they do not form with ts mutant ICP4 molecules that are unable to localize into the nucleus (279,456). ICP4 is probably phosphorylated at multiple sites, as suggested by the complex pattern of phosphopeptides generated from it (687). The serine-rich region from residues 142 to 210 contains many potential sites for phosphorylation, and this region has been shown to be phosphorylated. The serine-rich region or its phosphorylation is essential for efficient phosphorylation of the rest of the molecule (687).

Residues 515 to 520 of ICP4, gly-tyr-gly-ala-ala-gly, match an adenosine triphosphate (ATP)-binding motif, gly-X-gly-X-X-gly, characteristic of the catalytic domain of certain protein kinases (687). ICP4 has a tightly associated protein kinase activity (687), but it is not known if this activity is intrinsic to ICP4.

There is considerable indirect evidence that the various isoforms of ICP4 may have different properties and functions. The isoforms of ICP4 differ in their affinities for different DNA-binding sites (385). A later study reported that dephosphorylated forms of ICP4 bound to α promoters, whereas phosphorylated forms bound to β and γ promoters (429). The transition from one isoform to another may well be dependent on the function of other α proteins inasmuch as ICP27 causes a shift of ICP4 to a faster migrating form (485,613) and stimulates the transactivation of γ genes by ICP4. Some of the ICP4 isoforms cycle phosphate on and off (675), an activity that may be related to the protein kinase activity tightly associated with the protein (687).

In summary, ICP4 performs the functions of a transcriptional activator but, except for its repressive functions, does not behave like a classic transcriptional regulator. The many isoforms accumulating in the infected cells suggest that its different functions may be dependent on the posttranscriptional modification and the context of the cognate DNA-binding site. A perhaps simplistic view summarizing the current models of ICP4 action is that it represses transcription by binding to consensus sequences near sites of transcriptional initiation but activates transcription by binding to transcription factors and perhaps nonspecifically to DNA.

ICP27

ICP27 is an essential (360,527), multifunctional α protein that is required for expression of several classes of post-α genes (360,489,527,639), viral inhibition of RNA splicing (206,208), and inhibition of transcription of many host genes (593). ICP27 localizes into the nucleus independently of other viral proteins and, at early times, has been reported to be distributed diffusely in the nucleus or with small nuclear ribonucleoprotein particles (snRNPs) (441,534) and in replication compartments at later times of infection (114).

Functional domains mapped on the 512-residue ICP27 molecule include an amino-terminal acidic region essential for viral replication from residues 12 to 63 (487), an N-terminal nuclear localization signal from residues 110 to 137 (375), an N-terminal leucine-rich nuclear export signal from residues 7 to 15 (532), a methylated internal RGG box required for RNA-binding (378), a C-terminal transactivator region from residues 262 to 512 and a transrepressor region from 434 to 512 (533), and a zinc finger motif from 483 to 508 (646).

Early studies on viral gene expression concluded that ICP27 is required only for viral DNA replication and late gene expression (485,527), but recent results have shown that ICP27 is also needed for efficient expression of certain β genes (365,530,639), in particular the less abundant viral DNA replication proteins (639). Thus, ICP27 is required indirectly for viral DNA replication to promote the expression of viral gene products that are essential for viral DNA synthesis. These studies have shown that ICP27 increases the mRNA levels for these β genes, but it has not been determined whether this effect is transcriptional or posttranscriptional. Further discussion of the mechanisms by which ICP27 stimulates γ gene expression and inhibits RNA splicing and host transcription is presented in the sections that follow.

ICP0

ICP0 is not essential for viral replication but promotes viral infection and viral gene expression, especially at low multiplicities of infection (MOI) (528,610). At low MOIs, cells infected with ICP0 deletion mutants yield about 10- to 100-fold less virus than cells infected with wild-type virus. ICP0 null mutant viruses are able to enter cells and express α proteins but are defective for progression through the productive cycle. Therefore, the particle-to-plaque-forming unit (PFU) ratios of ICP0 null mutant virus stocks are significantly higher than those of wild-type virus stocks (610). The phenotype of ICP0 null mutants is MOI dependent because at MOIs of 5 and higher, ICP0 null mutants give viral yields similar to those of wild-type virus.

The early literature on ICP0 clearly established that it is a nonspecific (sometimes called promiscuous) transactivator because in transfected cells, it induces the expression of HSV α, β, and γ promoters (148,182,419,476) as well as heterologous promoters (401). ICP0 null mutants are defective for expression of α, β, and γ mRNAs (74), a defect manifest at the level of RNA synthesis (260). Because ICP0 does not bind DNA directly (153), it appears to be affecting transcription indirectly. Functional analysis of mutant proteins has defined an N-terminal C3HC4 zinc-binding domain or RING finger motif (146). ICP0 is phosphorylated by both viral (U_L13) and cellular kinases in infected cells (420) and is nucleotidylylated (29).

The mechanisms by which ICP0 stimulates viral gene transcription in infected cells have not been defined, but a number of interactions of ICP0 with cellular proteins and organelles have been observed, and these may ultimately lead to an understanding of the mechanism of action of ICP0.

1. Early in infection, ICP0 localizes in the nucleus. Beginning 3 hours after infection, ICP0 is translocated to the cytoplasm (primary human embryonic lung fibroblasts). The translocation is nearly complete by 7 to 9 hours, depending on multiplicity of infection. Translocation is blocked by inhibitors of DNA synthesis, suggesting that the translocation required γ_2 proteins (644).
2. During the nuclear phase, ICP0 localizes at or near nuclear structures known as *nuclear domain 10* (ND10) structures and causes the loss of the ND10 component PML and the disorganization of the ND10 structures (151,356,357). The function of these cellular structures is not known, but several viral DNA genomes are believed to target to these structures early in infection (243,244). A key component of ND10 is PML, named after promyelocytic leukemia, in which an aberrant form consisting of PML fused to rectinoic acid receptor-α accumulates. Certain forms of PML are lost after HSV infection. A simple model for this viral effect on the host cell is that the ND10 structures are part of a host cell repression system that the virus evades by causing disruption of the structure.
3. ICP0 interacts with components of the protein degradation machinery (150,152). ICP0 binds to a ubiquitin-specific protease named HAUSP and increases its localization to ND10 sites (152). ICP0 and HSV infection causes a loss of PML isoforms that are known to be conjugated to SUMO-1 or PIC1 (150). Thus, it has been hypothesized that ICP0 binds to HAUSP and stimulates the cleavage of SUMO-1 from PML and possibly other proteins, allowing their ubiquitination and subsequent degradation (150). ICP0 is also required for the loss of the regulatory subunit of the cellular DNA-dependent protein kinase (313), which may be a result of this same activity.
4. In dividing cells, ICP0 associates with kinetochores and causes the degradation of centomeric protein C

(CENP-C) (149). This protein plays a key role in the assembly of the kinetochore, and non–virus-induced degradation of this protein results in delayed transit ion of metaphase to anaphase. The zinc finger is required to bind to the kinetochore, but the actual structure to which it binds is unknown; thus, the mutation that abolishes the degradation overlaps the site required for binding of the ubiquitin-specific protease and may be a manifestation of the interaction of ICP0 with the latter protein.

5. ICP0 also binds several other proteins. These include cyclin D3, BMAL-1, elongation factor-1δ (eF-1δ), and a protein currently known as p60. In cells infected with wild-type virus, the levels of cyclin D3 and D1 decrease with time after infection (136,269,581). However, the rate of decay in cyclin D3 levels in cells infected with wild-type virus is slower than in cells infected with ICP0-negative mutant or a mutant whose ICP0 (D199A) does not bind cyclin D3. In addition, in cells infected with wild-type viruses, cdk4, the partner of D cyclins, is activated because p21, the cdk4 inhibitor, is degraded; whereas in cells infected with the D199A mutant, cdk4 is not activated, and p21 levels remain unchanged. The D199A mutant showed reduced capacity to replicate in stationary contact-inhibited cells and reduced neurotoxicity in mice infected by a peripheral route (643). The D199A co-localizes with PML and causes the disaggregation of ND10, but unlike the wild-type virus, it is not transported out of the nucleus into the cytoplasm. Neither wild-type nor the D199A mutant activates cdk2. Analyses of the interaction of cyclin D3 with ICP0 led to two significant observations. First, cyclin D3 co-localizes with wild-type ICP0 but not with the D199A mutant during the nuclear phase of ICP0. Second, overexpression of cyclin D3 accelerates the transport of ICP0 to the cytoplasm (644). The picture that emerges is that by stabilizing cyclin D3, ICP0 also stabilizes the cyclin-dependent kinase cdk4 and cyclin D1, another partner of cdk4. The function of cdk4–cyclin D complexes is not known. By analogy with the apparent function of activated cdc2, the activated function of cdk4–cyclin D complexes may lead to more rapid activation of viral DNA synthesis, synthesis of late proteins, and translocation of ICP0 into the cytoplasm. The apparent preoccupation of HSV with D cyclins is underscored by the observation that members of other herpesvirus subfamilies either induce a D-type cyclin (568) or encode a cyclin D homolog (70,261,324,411).
6. ICP0 has been shown to interact with eF-1δ (267). The interaction of ICP0 with eF-1δ, an elongation factor responsible for adenosine diphosphate (ADP)-ATP exchange, appears to be significant inasmuch as a truncated ICP0 polypeptide containing the binding site interfered with *in vitro* synthesis of a reporter protein. The significance that HSV places on eF-1δ is underscored by the observations that U_L13 phosphorylates eF-1δ and that this protein is also phosphorylated in cells infected with representative betaherpesviruses and gammaherpesviruses. The protein p60 binds ICP0 and ICP22 and is discussed in conjunction with the latter protein. ICP0 appears to have other functions, which are dealt with in the section on cell death.
7. ICP0 has also been postulated to have an effect similar to that of a histone deacetylase inhibitor (224), potentially resulting in increased acetylation of histones and increased gene expression from DNA condensed in nucleosomes. It seems more likely that alterations of histone acetylation would affect transfected genes or viral reactivation as compared with HSV productive infection because the former forms of DNA are wrapped in nucleosomes whereas HSV DNA during productive infection is not.

In summary, ICP0 is emerging as a multifunctional protein directed primarily toward modification of cellular functions to promote viral gene expression and viral productive infection. Precisely how the sum total of all of these modifications account for the function of ICP0 remains to be ascertained.

ICP22 and $U_S1.5$

As noted previously, the $U_S1.5$ transcription unit resides within the coding sequence of the gene encoding ICP22, and the amino acid sequence of the corresponding protein is identical to the carboxyl-terminal two thirds of the amino acid sequence of ICP22 (64). Like ICP22, $U_S1.5$ is expressed as an α protein.

Viral mutants that fail to express the carboxyl-terminal half of ICP22 (454) have been studied extensively and exhibit several phenotypes, such as (a) restricted growth in primary human fibroblasts, rabbit, mouse, and rat cells (549); (b) attenuated virulence by intracerebral inoculation in mouse; (c) reduced expression of some (e.g., U_S11, U_L38, U_L41) but not all γ_2 (e.g., gC) proteins; (d) abolished posttranslational modification of the C-terminal domain of the large subunit of RNA polymerase II, which takes place in some but not all cell lines (338); (e) reduced stability of ICP0 mRNA (64); and (f) increased stability of several cell cycle proteins (e.g. cyclins A and B) (4). The same phenotype is exhibited by a mutant defective for the U_L13 protein kinase (471,472). ICP22 also interacts with p60, a protein that also binds ICP0, and with p78, a cell cycle protein of unknown function (50).

ICP22 and $U_S1.5$ are phosphorylated by the U_L13 and U_S3 viral protein kinases, and ICP22 is nucleotidylylated by casein kinase II. Sequential deletions have established a relatively detailed functional map of ICP22 (421) and made apparent three significant features of its structure and organization. First, a mutant lacking the sequences unique to ICP22 (i.e., not shared with $U_S1.5$) behaved like the wild-type parent with respect to expression of γ_2 genes but was avirulent on intracerebral inoculation of mice. Second, two sets of sequences are required for the phosphorylation of ICP22 by U_L13 and U_S3. One is within the carboxyl-terminal domain shared with $U_S1.5$; whereas the other highly homologous sequence is within the amino-terminal portion of ICP22 that is not shared with $U_S1.5$. Alteration of either sequence abolishes the phosphorylation of ICP22. Mutagenesis of the amino-terminal domain enables wild-type expression of γ_2 proteins, but alteration of the carboxyl-terminal sequence caused a reduction in the expression of the selected γ_2 proteins, similar to that seen in cells infected with deletion mutants in ICP22 (452). These studies indicate that U_L13 and ICP22 and $U_S1.5$ proteins act independently and either jointly or sequentially to regulate several aspects of HSV gene expression.

Synthesis and Processing of Viral Proteins

Viral proteins appear to be made on both free and bound polyribosomes. Many HSV proteins are posttranslationally modified, and these modifications include cleavage, phosphorylation, sulfation, *N*-linked and *O*-linked glycosylation, myristoylation, ADP-ribosylation, and nucleotidylylation (514). With the exception of some glycoproteins, the extent to which processing is a requirement of virus growth rather than the consequence of an encounter between cellular or viral enzymes and molecules resembling natural substrates remains uncertain. Much of this processing is by cellular enzymes and pathways (reviewed in 514), but some enzymes are virus encoded. The HSV-encoded protease is discussed later in the section on capsid assembly.

Herpes Simplex Virus Protein Kinases

HSV specifies at least three protein kinases, the large subunit of the ribonucleotide reductase (RR1), U_L13, and U_S3.

RR1

A protein kinase activity was first reported to be associated with the large subunit of the ribonucleotide reductase (ICP6) of HSV-2 but not of HSV-1 (87). Later studies showed autophosphorylation activity with the HSV-1 RR1 protein as well (99). Whereas the ribonucleotide reductase activity is associated with the conserved carboxyl-terminal domain, the protein kinase activity maps near the amino terminus (7,99). The large subunit of ribonucleotide reductase is therefore a multifunctional protein. The substrate of this protein kinase activity is not known.

U_S3

McGeoch and Davison (364) predicted that U_S3 encodes a protein kinase on the basis of its sequence, a prediction borne out by biochemical (166) and genetic studies (470). A major substrate of this enzyme is an intrinsic membrane protein exposed on the surface of infected cells and encoded by *U_L34*. The U_L34 protein contains the amino acid motif recognized by the U_S3 protein kinase; thus, substitution of the serine or threonine residues within this motif with alanine resulted in a loss of phosphorylation, but the virus grew poorly and revertants were readily detected. It is noteworthy that four prominent phosphoproteins unrelated to the U_L34 protein appear in lysates of baby hamster kidney cells infected with the U_L3-negative mutant or with mutants in the amino acid motif recognized in U_L34 by the U_S3 kinase. The anti-U_L34 serum copreciptates the four phosphoproteins along with the U_L34 protein. It would appear that the four phosphoproteins compensate in some fashion for the absence of phosphorylation by U_S3 kinase. U_S3 also phosphorylates the U_L3 protein and ICP22 (353,421, 452). The major targets of U_S3, however, may well be host proteins, as discussed in the section on apoptosis.

U_L13

Smith and Smith (577) and Chee and coauthors (73) reported that the sequence of the *U_L13* ORF contains the signature amino acid motif common to other protein kinases and is shared among alphaherpesviruses, betaherpesviruses, and gammaherpesviruses. Cunningham and colleagues (105) reported on the properties of a new kinase very similar to the protein kinase activity demonstrated in tegument–capsid structures described by Lemaster and Roizman (319) and ascribed the new kinase to the product of the *U_L13* gene. Studies of U_L13- and U_L13-U_S3-negative mutants led to the conclusion that the U_L13 protein kinase affects the phosphorylation and processing of the gene products of ICP22 and $U_S1.5$, ICP0, and U_L47 and affects the accumulation of the $\alpha0$, U_L26 and $U_L26.5$ (protease and its substrate), U_L38 encoding the VP19C capsid protein, U_L41, and U_S11 gene products (471,472).

Although the U_L13 protein kinase is associated with structural proteins, the enzyme brought into the infected cell by the virion does not phosphorylate the newly synthesized ICP22. The phenotype of the U_L13-negative virus is similar to that described for the $\alpha22$-negative mutant by Sears and coauthors (6,471,547). As noted earlier in the text, U_L13 protein kinase phosphorylates EF-1δ. This function appears to be highly conserved among herpesvirus subfamilies.

A large number of other proteins (e.g., ICP4, gE; see Table 1 for a more detailed list) are phosphorylated in the course of the reproductive cycle. The kinases responsible for the phosphorylation and the role of phosphorylation in the functions of these gene products have not been elucidated.

Adenosine Diphosphate Ribosylation

Preston and Notarianni (461) reported that ICP4 and VP23 are poly(ADP-ribosyl)ated in isolated nuclei, a significant finding that nevertheless left unanswered the question of whether this reaction actually takes place in the infected cell. Blaho and coworkers (27) reported that antibody specific for poly(ADP-ribose) reacts with ICP4 extracted from cells late in infection, in effect answering the question in the affirmative. However, the poly(ADP-ribose) added to ICP4 was digested by poly(ADP-ribose) glycohydrolase, but only after denaturation of the protein. In contrast, poly(ADP-ribose) added to ICP4 in isolated nuclei was readily removed from the native protein by the glycohydrolase. The results indicate that ICP4 is poly(ADP-ribosyl)ated and suggest that, in the isolated nuclei, the poly(ADP-ribose) is added either by elongation of existing chains or to novel sites.

Nucleotidylylation of Viral Proteins

An initial report by Blaho and Roizman (30) showed that ICP4 is both guanylated and adenylated. The label transferred by α^{32}P-ATP or α^{32}P-guanosine triphosphate (GTP) is associated with the slowly migrating forms of the protein. Conclusive evidence for the nucleotidylylation emerged from transfer of a ^{3}H-labeled purine ring from ATP to ICP4. Subsequent studies revealed that ICP0, ICP22, ICP27, and the proteins encoded by U_L21, U_L31, U_L47, and U_L49 are also nucleotidylylated and that all these proteins share the sequence R/PRAPS/R (27, 28). Nucleotidylylation is carried out by casein kinase II. U_L21 is dispensable for growth in cultured cells (15), U_L31 cofractionates with the nuclear matrix (71) and appears to be an important component of the nuclear membrane of the infected cell (Baines, personal communication), and U_L47 may interact with VP16 (368). U_L49 is a virion protein (VP22/3?) that is labeled in cells with [^{32}P]orthophosphate and also is (ADP-ribosyl)ated.

Modification of Membrane-associated Proteins

Of the 11 predicted glycoproteins, at least 10 have been studied in sufficient detail to demonstrate the presence of oligosaccharide chains. The 11th, gJ, remains elusive, although recent studies indicating that gJ plays a role in blocking apoptosis are likely to lead to more extensive studies of this protein (254,700). In addition, it has been reported recently that the products of the U_L47 gene, VP13-14, contain *O*-linked polysaccharide chains and are phosphorylated (383).

At least one protein, the product of the U_L11 gene, has been shown to be myristoylated (349). Deletion mutants in the U_L11 gene show an impairment in egress from infected cells (17).

Viral DNA Replication

Once the β proteins are expressed, several of these proteins localize into the nucleus and assemble onto the parental viral DNA molecules in punctate structures called *prereplicative sites* located near ND10 structures (243,639) (Fig. 7A), where viral DNA synthesis initiates on the circular molecule, probably to give theta replicative forms. As viral DNA synthesis progresses, the progeny DNA molecules and replication complexes accumulate in the nucleus in globular structures called *replication compartments* (475) (see Fig. 7B). Viral DNA synthesis proceeds within these areas of the nucleus. At some point, presumably relatively early after its initiation, viral DNA synthesis switches from a theta replication mechanism to a rolling-circle mechanism, the latter producing concatemeric molecules. Thus, most of the viral progeny DNA molecules that accumulate in the infected cell nucleus are "head-to-tail" concatemers containing the four sequence isomers described previously (245).

Seven viral proteins are required for viral DNA replication. Phenotypic analysis of viral ts mutants first identified two virus-encoded gene products required for viral DNA synthesis, the viral DNA polymerase (469) and the

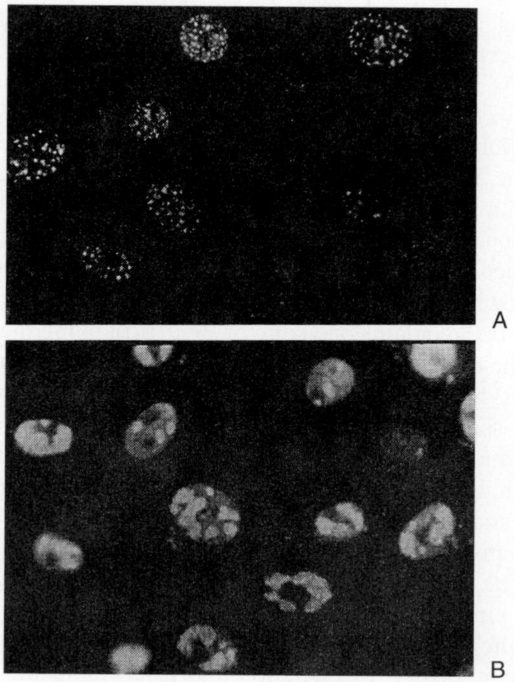

FIG. 7. Prereplicative sites and replication compartments. Immunofluorescence micrographs showing the localization of the ICP8 to prereplicative sites (**A**) when viral DNA synthesis is inhibited and to replication compartments, and (**B**) when viral DNA replication is proceeding. (Micrographs courtesy of E. McNamee.)

ICP8 ssDNA-binding protein (98), and transfection studies showed that seven viral genes are sufficient to replicate a viral origin sequence co-transfected into cells (69,681). The gene products of the other five genes were identified through biochemical purification and genetic studies. The seven gene products are the viral DNA polymerase (U_L30) and its accessory protein or processivity factor (U_L42), an origin-binding protein (U_L9), the ICP8 ssDNA-binding protein (SSB; U_L29), and the helicase–primase or primeosome complex of three proteins, U_L5, U_L8, and U_L52. Host cell factors are presumably also involved in viral DNA synthesis, but these have not been identified, in large part because HSV DNA replication involving origin-dependent initiation and synthesis has not been achieved *in vitro.* Nevertheless, host enzymes, including the DNA polymerase α-primase, DNA ligase, and topoisomerase II, are probably also required.

The origins of viral DNA synthesis were identified through mapping of sequences found in defective viral genomes (168,336) and sequences needed for plasmid DNA amplification in transfection studies (390,648,669). The origins include *oriS,* a sequence located in the *c* sequences bounding the S component and therefore present in two copies in the viral genome, and *oriL,* a sequence located between the divergent transcription units of the genes for two viral DNA replication proteins, ICP8 and DNA polymerase.

Both *oriS* and *oriL* are palindromic structures, *oriL* being a 144-bp palindrome (281,337,477,669) and *oriS* being a shorter palindrome of 45bp (116,390,607,608) that center around AT-rich regions of 18 and 20 bp, respectively. Inverted repeats that contain binding sites for the U_L9 protein, called Box I, are located on either side of the AT-rich region of *oriL.* The *oriS* contains a Box I sequence to the 5′ side of the AT-rich region and a similar sequence with a 10-fold lower binding affinity for U_L9, called Box II, located 3′ to the AT-rich region. In *oriL,* the Box I sequences are flanked by another homologous sequence, called Box III, which has greatly reduced affinity for U_L9. The *oriS* contains one copy of Box III flanking the 5′ Box I. The *oriL* is notoriously unstable when cloned into plasmids; hence, little genetic analysis has been performed on this sequence. Box I is required for *oriS* function, and mutations in Box II greatly reduce DNA replication. Although Box III shows weak binding to U_L9 *in vitro,* mutations in Box III reduce replication by about fivefold in transfection assays.

The reasons for three potential origins of replication in the viral genome are not apparent at this time. Neither origin is specifically required for viral replication. A mutant virus with a deletion in *oriL* is viable and showed normal burst size and latent infection (450). In addition, mutant viruses with both *oriS* sequences deleted showed at most a fourfold reduction in viral yields and only slightly delayed viral DNA synthesis (240). It has been suggested that one of these origins may represent vestigial origins from the L and S components of the viral genome (514) and that one of these origins, *oriL,* may function in reactivation from latent infection (207).

Viral DNA Replication Proteins

The properties and functions of the seven essential HSV DNA replication proteins are summarized here but reviewed in detail elsewhere (37).

Origin-binding Protein, U_L9, OBP

The U_L9 origin-binding protein forms a homodimer and binds specifically to the sequence CGTTCGCACTT (139,140,283,284). U_L9 also has ATP-binding and DNA helicase motifs that are essential for viral replication. Binding of U_L9 to origin sequences induces a bend in the DNA and formation of a single-stranded stem-loop structure. The addition of the HSV ssDNA-binding protein, ICP8 (see later), allows U_L9 to unwind Box I of *oriS* if an 18-nucleotide single strand tail is present 3′ to Box I. Thus, ICP8 may provide a ssDNA region in the AT-rich region, from which U_L9 can separate the strands. As an origin-binding protein, U_L9 would play a role in origin-dependent synthesis originating from the circular molecules, but once synthesis has converted to a rolling-circle mode, U_L9 would presumably not be needed as an origin-binding protein.

Single-Stranded DNA-Binding Protein, ICP8, U_L29.

ICP8 is an abundant protein in HSV-infected cells and was first identified as the major DNA-binding protein in HSV-infected cells (23). ICP8 binds preferentially to ssDNA (310,525), and this ssDNA-binding (SSB) function is essential for viral DNA replication. ICP8 also exhibits a helix-destabilizing activity but can also catalyze the renaturation of complementary single strands (134). Probably as a consequence of the latter two activities, ICP8 can promote strand transfer (43), and this may contribute to the high frequency of homologous recombination observed in infected cells. In addition to its SSB function, ICP8 interacts with several other viral DNA replication proteins, as evidenced by its physical interaction and stimulation of U_L9 helicase activity (36, 38,162), stimulation of the $U_L5/8/52$ helicase activity (155,201,619), functional interaction with DNA polymerase (77,218), and coimmunoprecipitation with U_L9, U_L8, and pol proteins (639). Consistent with these numerous interactions, ICP8 is required for localization of other viral proteins and cellular proteins to prereplicative sites in infected cell nuclei (54,112,329,342). As a result of its size and numerous protein interactions, ICP8 is likely to play a scaffold role in assembly of HSV DNA replication complexes (112). ICP8 also exerts a repressive effect on IE and E gene expression under certain conditions (191–193), possibly as a consequence of promoting the formation of DNA replication complexes on viral DNA.

DNA Helicase–Primase Complex

This complex, which contains the protein products of the U_L5, U_L8, and U_L52 genes, was first identified as a helicase activity from infected cells (103). The complex unwinds short oligonucleotides annealed to single-stranded M13 DNA in the 5′ to 3′ direction. U_L5 has ATP-binding and DNA helicase motifs, and these are essential for DNA replication (704). U_L52 has a proposed divalent metal-binding motif that is conserved in DNA polymerases and primases, and this motif is required for DNA replication. A complex of U_L5 and U_L52 has DNA-dependent ATPase, helicase, and primase activities; hence, this constitutes the core enzyme. U_L8 promotes the nuclear localization of this complex and, in concert with ICP8, stimulates optimal activities of the core enzyme. Thus, the holoenzyme can unwind a 2.3-kbp nicked plasmid in the presence of ICP8. The primase activity produces oligoribonucleotides 6 to 13 bases in length, and the preferred template sequence is 3′AGCC-CTCCCA, with synthesis initiating at the first C.

DNA Polymerase

The HSV DNA polymerase has been studied extensively, partly as a result of its potential as a target for antiviral drugs. A new DNA polymerase activity was detected in HSV-infected cells in the 1960s (270), but formal genetic proof that it was virus encoded was not provided until the late 1970s when temperature-sensitive and drug-resistant mutations affecting the properties of the polymerase were isolated and mapped to the viral genome (469). The HSV DNA polymerase holoenzyme is a heterodimer of the 136-kd U_L30 protein complexed with the 65-kd U_L42 protein. The U_L30 protein contains the polymerase activity, and it contains three sequence motifs that are homologous and align with sequence motifs I, II, and III of other DNA polymerases (186). The U_L30 protein also has an intrinsic 3′-5′-exonuclease activity, which can serve as a proofreading activity. U_L42 increases the processivity of the U_L30 DNA polymerase. The interaction between U_L30 and U_L42 is essential for viral DNA replication *in vivo,* and these interaction sites are being investigated as possible targets for antiviral compounds.

The HSV DNA polymerase has a broader substrate specificity than cellular polymerases, and this has allowed the development of compounds that specifically inhibit the viral DNA polymerase. These compounds are discussed in Chapters 15 and 73 in *Fields Virology*, 4th ed.

Based on the available information, a model for HSV DNA replication (Fig. 8) has been formulated (reviewed in 37). The first steps in HSV DNA replication involve the binding of the U_L9 protein to the origin sequences and the looping and distortion of the origin sequences by U_L9. ICP8 then binds to U_L9 or ssDNA regions, and the U_L9 helicase activity unwinds the DNA. The helicase–primase complex is then recruited to the origin by interactions with U_L9 or ICP8. Leading-strand synthesis involves the unwinding of the DNA and synthesis of a primer by the

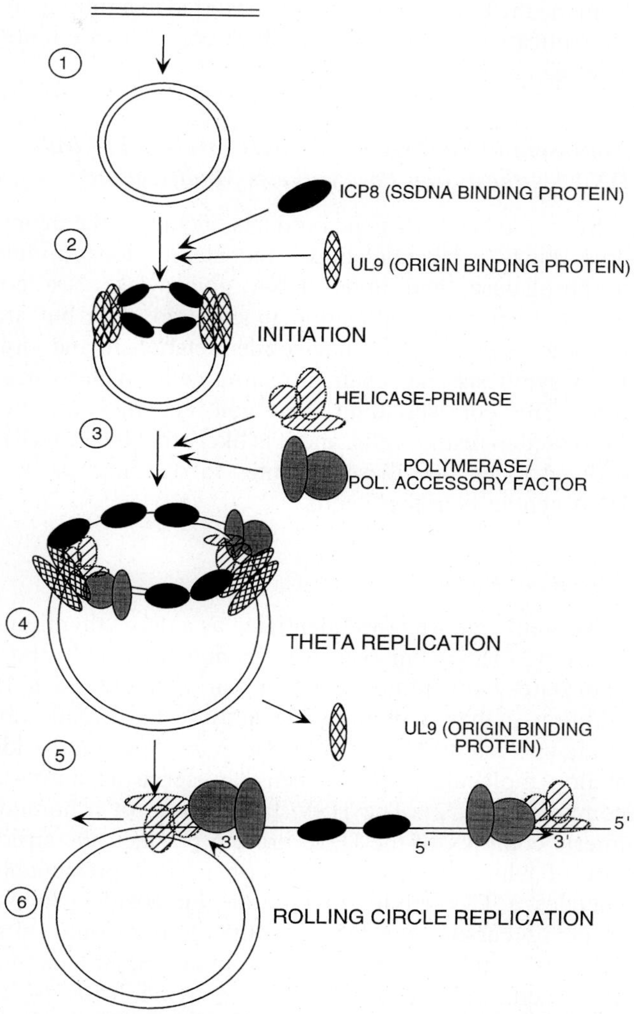

FIG. 8. Diagram of a model of HSV DNA replication, with the following steps: 1. Input DNA is circularized upon entry into the nucleus. 2. U_L9 (the origin-binding protein) initially binds to specific elements in the origin (either *ori*$_L$ or *ori*$_S$) and begins to unwind the DNA. U_L9 then recruits ICP8 (the single-stranded DNA-binding protein) to the unwound single-stranded DNA. 3. U_L9 and ICP8 recruit the five remaining viral DNA replication proteins to the replication forks. 4. The helicase–primase proteins and the viral polymerase complex assemble at each replication fork for initial rounds of theta-form replication. 5. Replication switches from theta to rolling-circle mode by an unknown mechanism. U_L9 is not necessary for rolling-circle replication because it is not origin dependent. 6. Rolling-circle DNA replication produces long head-to-tail concatamers of viral DNA, which are cleaved into monomeric molecules during packaging. (Diagram courtesy of E. McNamee.)

HSV helicase–primase complex, from which leading-strand synthesis can be accomplished by the HSV pol-U_L42 holoenzyme. Alternatively, primers may be synthesized by the cellular polymerase α-primase. Lagging-strand synthesis is then accomplished by primer synthesis and pol-U_L42 extension of the DNA strand. Because the progeny DNA is largely head-to-tail concatemers (245), it is believed that although synthesis initiates from the theta form, it is rapidly converted to a rolling-circle replicative mechanism, by which concatemeric molecules can be synthesized.

Nonessential Viral Gene Products Involved in Viral DNA Synthesis and Postsynthesis Modification

Several other HSV gene products, including the thymidine kinase, ribonucleotide reductase, deoxyuridine triphosphatase, and uracil DNA glycosylase, are not essential for viral replication in cultured cells but are likely to be essential for nucleotide metabolism and viral DNA synthesis and repair in resting cells, such as neurons. The corresponding host cell enzymes are not expressed in resting cells, and it is likely that the virus has evolved to encode these enzymes to optimize its own DNA synthesis in these cells.

Thymidine Kinase

This enzyme was first identified as a deoxythymidine kinase (273), giving rise to its name. In fact, it phosphorylates pyrimidines and even purine nucleosides. In addition, it has a thymidylate activity. Its broad substrate specificity allows it to phosphorylate nucleoside analog molecules, which then can serve as antiviral compounds (172). The HSV TK consists of a homodimeric complex of the U_L23 protein product, the structure of which has been solved (47). HSV presumably encodes a TK activity to provide nucleoside triphosphate precursors for DNA synthesis in resting cells, such as neurons, where the cellular enzyme is not expressed (see later). The viral enzyme leads to an increase in deoxythymidine triphosphate (dTTP) pools relative to that seen in uninfected cells or early in infection. This complicates the use of radioactive thymidine for labeling of viral DNA synthesis in infected cells because the specific activity of the labeled DNA will be lower at later times of infection.

Deoxyuridine Triphosphatase

Deoxyuridine triphosphatase (dUTPase) hydrolyzes dUTP to dUMP and pyrophosphate, preventing the incorporation of uracil into DNA and generating dUMP, the precursor of dTTP. The HSV enzyme is a monomer of the U_L50 protein product (464) and appears to be most essential for viral replication in the nervous system (473).

Ribonucleotide Reductase

Ribonucleotide reductase catalyzes the reduction of ribonucleoside diphosphates to the corresponding deoxyribonucleoside diphosphate. The HSV enzyme consists of a complex of the U_L39 and U_L40 proteins as an $\alpha_2\beta_2$ tetramer (14). The HSV ribonucleotide reductase is not subject to the same allosteric controls as the cellular enzyme; thus, the HSV enzyme is not inhibited by the increased dTTP pools in HSV-infected cells. The HSV ribonucleotide reductase is required for viral replication in nondividing cells (194). The large subunit has an intrinsic serine-threonine kinase activity that is separable from the ribonucleotide reductase activity. The role of the protein kinase activity is not known, although there has been one report that the HSV-2 protein kinase activity is required for IE gene expression and virus growth (574).

Uracil N-Glycosylase

This enzyme removes uracil bases from DNA, bases that arise in DNA by the deamination of cytosine to form uracil, by the cleavage of the *N*-glycosidic bond linking uracil to the deoxyribose sugar. The site is then repaired so that a mutagenic event converting a G-C base pair to an A-T base pair does not occur. The HSV enzyme is encoded by the *U_L2* gene (62). This gene product is not essential for replication in growing cells in culture, but it plays a role in viral pathogenicity and reactivation from latent infection (474).

Alkaline Nuclease

This enzyme is a phosphoprotein encoded by the *U_{L12}* gene (20,458), has endonuclease and exonuclease activities, and is active at pH 9.0 to 10.0 (270,271,625). As described later, this nuclease plays a role in DNA maturation and encapsidation. It is believed to interact with the ICP8 (625), possibly to allow the nuclease to act directly on viral replication intermediates or products. The HSV nuclease may be required to resolve concatenated viral DNA for packaging (553).

Viral DNA Recombination

Homologous recombination is very efficient in HSV-infected cells, and multiple crossover events between co-infecting viral genomes are apparent in progeny viruses, even between HSV-1 and HSV-2 genomes (396). Viral DNA replication is required for this high level of homologous recombination, and the time courses of DNA replication and recombination are parallel in cells transfected with viral *oriS* plasmids (133). The mechanism by which replication of the DNA promotes recombination is not known, but the single-stranded regions or the concatemeric molecules might be targets for cellular or viral recombination machinery. In addition, ICP8 is known to promote strand transfer; hence, it might play a role in recombination in infected cells.

Inversion of the genomic L and S segments also involves recombination between the terminal repeats and the internal inverted repeats. As described previously, HSV virion DNA contains four populations of molecules bearing the four orientations of the L and S components of the genome. This novel feature of the genome of HSV and certain other, but not all, herpesviruses (see Chapter 71 in *Fields Virology*, 4th ed.) has long intrigued the field, and interest has been further piqued by the observation that viruses without internal repeats are viable, indicating that inversion is not essential for viral replication (253,446). These mutant viruses are less virulent, but the role of the internal repeats as protein-coding sequences versus their structural role as repeated sequences has not been separated. The L–S junction sequences and, in particular, the *a* sequences promote high-efficiency inversion in that insertion of a copy of these sequences at other sites in the genome leads to inversion of these sequences (83,387–389). Duplication of certain other viral sequences at a second site in the viral genome can lead to additional inversion events (448,663), but these events appear to be less efficient than *a* sequence–mediated inversion. The 95-bp Uc-DR1 sequence is specifically required for inversion at the *a* sequence (133), but it remains to be determined if this event involves site-specific recombination or a hot spot for recombination. This may be resolved by the further purification of the activity needed for inversion (49).

Activation of Late Viral Transcription

Once viral DNA replication has initiated, expression of γ genes is increased (232), largely as a result of increases in their transcription (193,666,699). For some genes called γ_1, early-late, or leaky-late genes, this represents an increase in expression that was already occurring under early conditions. These include the genes encoding ICP5 (*U_L19*), gB (*U_L27*), and gD (*U_S6*). Other genes, called γ_2, late, or true-late genes, are transcribed at significant levels only after viral DNA synthesis. These include *U_L38*, *gC* (*U_L44*), *U_S11*, *U_S9*, and *U_L49.5*. Whereas γ_2 genes are unambiguously defined as requiring the onset of viral DNA synthesis for their expression, the γ_1 group lumps together all genes whose expression is enhanced by the onset of viral DNA synthesis but in reality contains a continuum of genes that either resemble γ genes but are expressed late in infection or are partially expressed in the absence of DNA synthesis but kinetically are not different from the γ_2 genes.

Late transcription takes place in replication compartments within the infected cell nucleus, as evidenced by (a) the localization of ICP4 (280,481), pol II (323,488), and ICP22 (323) to replication compartments at late times; and (b) RNA-pulse labeling of replication compartments at late times (443). Thus, the transition from β to γ gene transcription involves a change in the nuclear location of transcription from sites near ND10 domains to replication compartments. This is likely to play a significant role in this change in viral gene transcription.

Although the complete mechanism for stimulation of late viral gene expression has not been defined, it is known that transcription of late genes increases upon viral DNA synthesis (193), that the alteration in the viral DNA template is cis-acting (359), and that the viral proteins ICP4, ICP27, and ICP8 are required. The cis-acting effect on the template could be due to changes in the viral DNA molecules themselves by exposure of single-stranded regions or by conversion from a circular form to a linear form. Alternatively, the cis-acting effect could be due to proteins tightly bound to the viral parental DNA that do not exchange to other DNA molecules in the infected cell.

As a general rule, while sequences upstream of transcription initiation are sufficient to endow a reporter gene with the kinetics of β gene expression both in transfected cells and in the context of the viral genome (94,666), this is not generally true of γ genes (359,565). In the context of the viral genome, expression of reporter genes as γ_2 genes also requires regulatory elements present in the 5′-transcribed noncoding domains (229). Even then, such chimeras are expressed as β genes in cells transfected with the chimera and then superinfected with the virus (565).

The HSV γ_1 promoters have not been studied as extensively as some of the other viral promoters, but the *ICP5* (*U_L19*) gene promoter elements have been defined (see Fig. 6). The essential elements of the minimal *ICP5* promoter are an SP1-binding site at –48, a TATA box at –30, and and an essential cis-acting element between –2 and +10 whose sequence resembles the human immunodeficiency virus (HIV) initiator element (238). A cellular factor that binds at the cap site has been identified (237). The γ_1 gene promoters are heterogeneous in that the minimal *VP16* gene promoter from base pair –90 to +6 contains an E Box (CACGTG) at –85, a CAAT box at –77, and an SP1 site at –48 as well as a different initiator element (325).

Analyses of the γ_2 viral gene promoters have shown that the upstream sequences consist of a TATA box with few other upstream transcription factor–binding sites (163,228,229,257) and with additional sequences needed for activation within the 5′-untranslated region (200,229, 359,601,667). For example, the γ_2 *U_L38* gene promoter (see Fig. 6) contains three elements: (a) an unusual TATA element with the sequence TTTAAA at –31, (b) a consensus initiator element at the transcriptional start site, and (c) a downstream activation sequence (DAS) from base pair +20 to +33 that is required for normal levels of gene expression (200). The DAS appears to increase transcriptional initiation (199), and several other HSV γ genes, including *U_S11*, *gC* (*U_L44*), *gB* (*U_L27*), *L/ST*, and *U_L49.5*, have similar downstream control elements in their promoter (reviewed in 199). In addition, the *gC* gene DAS can partially substitute for the U_L38 DAS (199), suggesting that common mechanisms may act on the different DAS sequences. One cellular protein purified on the basis of binding to the DAS has been identified as the DNA-binding subunit of the DNA-dependent protein kinase (440). Given that HSV infection leads to the degradation of the catalytic subunit of DNA-PK and loss of kinase activity (313), this effect may free up the DNA-binding subunit for interaction with viral DNA.

In addition to ICP4, γ gene expression requires ICP27 (489,527). As described previously, ICP27 stimulates expression of viral DNA replication proteins and thereby viral DNA synthesis (639), but it is also specifically required for γ gene expression (489). The mechanism by which ICP27 stimulates γ gene expression has not been completely defined because there is evidence that its effects may be both transcriptional and posttranscriptional. Posttranscriptional effects of ICP27 were initially inferred from its stimulation of reporter gene expression in transfected cells in which the stimulation appeared to be dependent on sequences in the 3′-untranslated region of the reporter gene (72,535). Similarly, a late polyadenylation factor (LPF) was reported to be dependent on ICP27 (370). In infected cells, γ viral transcription was not inhibited when cells infected with the ICP27 ts mutant *ts*LG4 were shifted to the nonpermissive temperature (575). Based on this result, it was concluded that ICP27 stimulated late gene expression by posttranscriptional mechanisms. Nevertheless, the *ts*LG4 ICP27 may not be thermolabile for transcriptional functions upon shift to the NPT.

In addition, ICP27 was shown to bind to RNA (46, 242,377), and one report indicated sequence specificity in this binding activity (46), whereas others failed to observe this specificity (242,377). A portion of the nuclear ICP27 can shuttle from the nucleus to the cytoplasm in infected cells (376,442,579). This activity requires an RNA-binding sequence, an export sequence, and an export control sequence on ICP27 (580). A correlation has been reported between the ability of ICP27 to shuttle from the nucleus to the cytoplasm and its ability to stimulate gene expression, suggesting that ICP27 stimulates gene expression by shuttling late mRNAs from the nucleus to the cytoplasm (579).

Not all studies, however, support the hypothesis that the effect of ICP27 on viral gene expression is solely a consequence of posttranscriptional effects. ICP27 has been shown to bind to ICP4 (426), to alter the phosphorylation of ICP4 (485,613,687), and to localize to replication compartments (115). These properties are all consistent with effects on transcription of late HSV genes.

The ability of ICP27 to promote γ viral gene expression is likely a distinct function derived from its ability to stimulate viral DNA synthesis because at least one mutant virus, *n*504, separates these two functions. This mutant is defective for γ gene expression, in particular γ_2 proteins, while maintaining normal levels of viral DNA synthesis (486). This unique mutant virus has been used further to demonstrate that ICP27 stimulates transcription of γ genes independently of its role in stimulating β gene expression and viral DNA replication (252). This study found that ICP27 promotes transcription of at least two γ_2 genes, U_L44 and U_L47, in infected cells, as assayed by *in vivo* pulse labeling of RNA, without any apparent effects on transport or stability of these transcripts.

ICP27 has also been reported to stimulate the use of weak polyadenylation sites (365) and downstream polyadenylation sites (203). Thus, ICP27 appears to have roles in transcription, processing, and transport of late mRNAs in infected cells, a multifunctional role similar to the HIV Rev protein. Interestingly, ICP27 has been reported to interact with the hnRNP K protein, which also plays a role in both transcriptional and RNA processing and transport events, and with casein kinase 2 (649). ICP27 may stimulate late transcription or RNA processing by binding to nascent RNA transcripts and promoting transcriptional elongation like HIV Tat protein or by altering the phosphorylation of viral and cellular proteins involved in transcription and RNA processing and transport.

ICP8 has also been found to stimulate γ gene expression from progeny DNA templates (76,177). This ability to stimulate late gene expression correlates with the ability of the virus to form large replication compartments in infected cells (374). Thus, transcription of γ_2 genes such as *gC* may require the movement of viral progeny DNA to new sites in the nucleus in a process promoted by ICP8.

Finally, the accumulation of a subset of γ_2 proteins exemplified by U_S11, U_L41, and U_L38 is significantly reduced in the absence of the carboxyl-terminal portion of ICP22 or $U_S1.5$, or U_L13 proteins (421,452,471). The same two proteins, $U_S1.5$ and U_L13, are required for degradation of cyclins A and B and for the activation of cdc2. The connection may be a requirement for cdc2 for the expression of U_S11, and so forth, inasmuch as in cells transfected with dominant negative cdc2 and infected with wild-type virus, α, β and γ_1 proteins are expressed, but U_S11 is not (6).

The ultimate goal of viral late gene expression is to express large amounts of viral structural proteins for assembly of progeny viral particles.

Viral Capsid Assembly

After synthesis of the γ capsid proteins, they are localized into the infected cell nucleus, where capsid assembly occurs. Empty shells containing an internal scaffolding are assembled first, and the scaffolding is lost upon DNA encapsidation or insertion of viral DNA into the capsid. Our knowledge about the mechanisms of assembly of the HSV capsid has come from several lines of experimentation: (a) study of infected cell complexes and structures,

(b) assembly of capsid structures from extracts of insect cells infected with baculoviruses expressing HSV scaffolding proteins, (c) study of protein localization using immunofluorescence, and (d) genetic analysis of the functions of capsid and scaffolding proteins. Each of these approaches has contributed important information to our understanding of this process (reviewed in 227 and 604).

Immunofluorescence studies have shown that the initial stages of assembly of at least some capsid proteins occur in the cytoplasm (412,491). VP5, the major capsid protein, VP26, the outer tip of hexons, and VP23, a triplex protein are incapable of nuclear localization on their own, but VP5 can be carried into the nucleus by VP19C, a capsid triplex protein, or pre-VP22a, a scaffolding protein. VP23 localizes into the nucleus with VP19C, consistent with their interaction in triplexes, and VP26 localizes into the nucleus only when it is expressed with both VP5 and VP19C or pre-VP22.

Electron microscopic studies have shown that the final assembly of capsids occurs in the nucleus. Three types of capsids, called *A-, B-,* and *C-capsids,* have been identified from infected cell nuclear extracts by sucrose density gradient ultracentrifugation (189). All three types of capsids are about 120 nm in diameter, with an outer shell consisting of hexons and pentons made up of VP5, the major capsid protein. The capsomers are linked by triplex structures composed of the two minor capsid proteins VP19C (U$_L$38) and VP23 (U$_L$18), each complex consisting of one molecule of VP19C and two molecules of VP23 (409). C-capsids contain viral DNA and can mature into infectious virions by budding through the nuclear membrane (434). A- and B-capsids lack DNA, but B-capsid cavities are filled with VP22a and VP21, the cleaved forms of the scaffolding protein, and a viral protease, VP24 (189,404). The internal proteins, including the scaffolding proteins and protease, are removed upon encapsidation of DNA (111,189). A-capsids are not filled with DNA or scaffolding protein and are believed to be abortive forms that result from failed attempts to package DNA.

In the nucleus, the VP5–pre-VP22a complexes come together as a result of self-interactions of pre-VP22a molecules. The triplex proteins are then added to form a partial capsid. As hexons and pentons are added, the partial capsid assembles into a round procapsid (406). The procapsid structures undergo a structural transformation and become angular and polyhedral (88,630,636). It is controversial whether the round or the polyhedral B capsids are the structure into which viral DNA is encapsidated (312,435,636). Much of our knowledge of the capsid assembly process has come from analysis of structures formed in insect cells infected with baculoviruses expressing HSV capsid or scaffolding proteins (621,631) and in extracts from these infected cells (408). In these studies, a series of baculovirus recombinants were constructed that each express one capsid or scaffolding protein, and B-capsids with normal structure were formed when insect cells were co-infected with viruses encoding VP5, VP19C, VP23, and U_L26 or $U_L26.5$ gene products. When the U_L26 and $U_L26.5$ gene products were left out, no intact capsids were formed, indicating that these gene products are needed to form a scaffold structure around which the shell proteins could form a closed capsid. Similar phenotypes were observed with HSV strains in which the U_L26 and $U_L26.5$ genes were mutated (124). In the baculovirus studies, when the U_L26 gene was omitted, large cored B-capsids were observed because in the absence of the maturational protease, the U$_L$26.5 protein is not cleaved. Thus, cleavage of the U$_L$26.5 scaffolding protein leads to condensation of the core. When the $U_L26.5$ gene was omitted, intact capsids were observed, but no core structure was apparent. Viruses mutated for U$_L$26.5 can still produce infectious virus, but progeny virus yields are reduced by 10^2- to 10^3-fold relative to wild-type virus (178). These data indicate that the U$_L$26 gene products can serve as scaffolding proteins, but they form a different core and one that is not as effective as cores containing U$_L$26.5 gene products.

In vitro assembly of B-capsids can occur in extracts when the insect cell extracts from cells individually infected with baculoviruses expressing VP5, VP19, VP23, U_L26, and $U_L26.5$ gene products are mixed and incubated (406). *In vitro* assembly of procapsids requires only the purified viral components VP5, VP19C, VP23, and a scaffolding protein; hence, assembly of procapsids does not require any cellular proteins (407). It has been hypothesized that procapsids may be involved in the early stages of viral DNA packaging, much like the prohead structures of bacteriophages (227).

Although the other capsid proteins are encoded in separate transcriptional units (see Table 1), the scaffolding proteins and maturational protease are encoded by the overlapping U_L26 and $U_L26.5$ genes, which encode a complex set of gene products involved in formation of a core for capsid assembly and for capsid maturation (331, 333,334,462). The U_L26 gene encodes a 635–amino acid residue precursor protein with an intrinsic protease activity that cleaves either autoproteolytically or in trans after residues 247, the R site, and 610, the M site, in the precursor molecule. The amino-terminal 247-residue fragment is VP24, which retains protease activity. The fragment from residues 248 to 610 is VP21, which can serve as a scaffolding for capsid assembly. The $U_L26.5$ gene mRNA initiates within the U_L26 gene and encodes a protein that is read in the same reading frame as U$_L$26. The U$_L$26.5 protein, pre-VP22a, is equivalent to the C-terminal 329 residues of U$_L$26 and is also subject to cleavage by the U$_L$26 protease at the M site near its C-terminus to give a 304-residue protein, which is known as VP22a. The pre-VP22a protein functions as the major scaffolding protein for capsid assembly. The carboxyl-terminal 14 residues of pre-VP22a (and VP21) are recognized by VP5 during capsid assembly (233).

The protease activity encoded by the $U_{L}26$ gene is a serine protease (332) whose activity is required for virus assembly (178). Cleavage at the R site is required for viral infectivity (496), and cleavage at the M site is believed to be involved in release of the scaffolding protein from the capsid interior. Mutagenesis studies have identified two histidines and two glutamic acid residues essential for proteolytic activity, but a conserved cysteine was dispensable in the 247–amino acid polypeptide (331,332). Proteases have been targets for drug development in many biologic systems, and considerable effort has been devoted to identifying specific inhibitors of the HSV protease as possible antiviral compounds. The crystal structures of the HSV-1 and HSV-2 proteases have been solved (234).

Assembly of capsids may take place within specialized infected cell nuclear structures called *assemblons* (403, 658), or they may be assembled within replication compartments at sites near the sites of viral DNA replication (85,88,114,309,373). However, there is more general agreement that the next step in viral replication, encapsidation, occurs in replication compartments (15,309,658).

Encapsidation of Viral DNA

Encapsidation of HSV DNA involves a process in which cleavage of HSV progeny DNA concatemers into unit-length monomers and packaging of the monomers is linked, as originally shown for pseudorabies virus (304, 305). This process is not well defined, but the concatemeric progeny molecules are likely fed into the capsid concomitant with displacement of the scaffolding molecules, VP21 and VP22a, from the capsid. The viral DNA concatemer is believed to be cleaved upon encapsidation of a length of DNA that fills the capsid or when a "headful" (a term that originated with bacteriophage head assembly) of DNA has been inserted. Varmuza and Smiley (645) first mapped signals for cleavage and packaging within the U_b and U_c domains of the *a* sequences, and Deiss and colleagues (118) mapped these precisely and designated the two DNA packaging elements as *pac1* and *pac2,* respectively.

Concatemers are cleaved into unit-length molecules during packaging (118,262,335,445,559,582,608,609, 645). Cleavage occurs site specifically within the DR1 sequences of the *a* sequences (388) and involves two site-specific breaks at defined distances from the *pac1* and *pac2* packaging signals (118,571,645). The maturational process duplicates the sequences between these two cleavage sites, so that cleavage at sites bearing only one *a* sequence leads to two molecules with terminal *a* sequences (119,571,645). Several models have been proposed to explain the cleavage and metabolism of viral DNA during encapsidation (118,645). In general, these

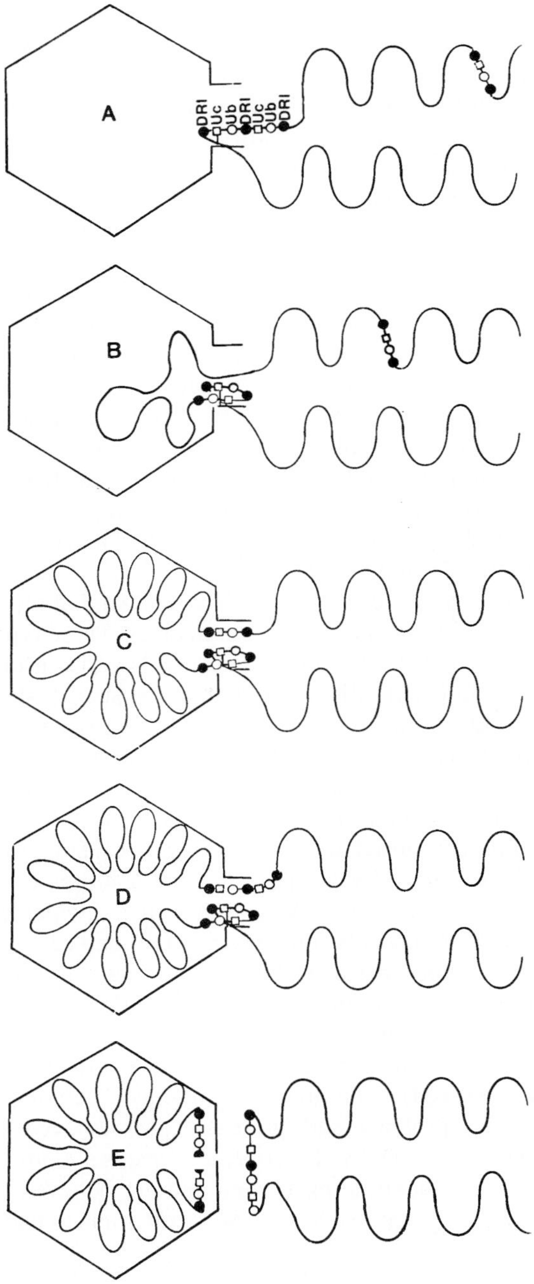

FIG. 9. Packaging of HSV-1 DNA. This general model predicts that (a) proteins attach to components of the *a* sequence, probably U_c; (b) empty capsids scan concatemeric DNA until contact is made in a specific orientation with the first protein-U_c sequence (capsid A); (c) the DNA is then taken into the capsid B until a "headful" or contact is made with a sequence whose nucleotide arrangement is in the same orientation (i.e., one genome equivalent in length away) is encountered (capsid C); (d) the packaging signal requires nicking of both strands from signals on opposite sites of a DR1 sequence. In the absence of two adjacent *a* sequences (capsid D), the juxtaposition of the *a* sequences would result in duplication of the *a* sequence (capsid E). (Model based on refs. 118 and 645.)

models propose that a packaging complex binds to the DNA and scans for a U_c sequence (Fig. 9). Cleavage occurs at a DR1 element proximal to the U_c sequence, and then the packaging complex scans the DNA as it is packaged until a directly repeated junction is encountered. Alternatively, two cleavages at L- and S-termini produce a monomer molecule. The amplification of the *a* sequence may occur by staggered nick-repair or gene conversion. The terminal *a* sequence generated by the cleavage may be recombinogenic in either a single-stranded or double-stranded form and promote inversions or *a* sequence amplification. In any event, the process must yield the virion form of the genome with an L-terminus containing one or more *a* sequences and a 3′ single-base overhang, a unit-length genome with an L and S component, and an S-terminus containing a single *a* sequence and a 3′ single-base overhang.

Encapsidation of viral DNA requires several viral gene products, including the U_L6, U_L15, U_L25, U_L28, U_L32, U_L33, U_L36, and U_L37 gene products, but the mechanisms of this process remain to be defined. Several biochemical activities that may be involved in this process have been identified, including virus-encoded proteins that bind to the *pac2* site (79) and a virus-encoded endonuclease that introduces double-stranded cuts in the U_c domain of the *a* sequence (135,679).

Virion Assembly and Egress

After encapsidation of full-length viral genomic DNA molecules, the nucleocapsids are capable of budding through the inner nuclear membrane (648). Interactions between capsid and tegument proteins and between tegument proteins and viral glycoproteins in the inner nuclear membrane promote this budding process. It is clear that nucleocapsids acquire a tegument layer upon budding through the inner nuclear membrane, although the tegument of virions in the internuclear membrane space appears less dense than that of extracellular virions (184,596). This apparent change in the tegument during egress of the virions may be due to maturation or exchange of tegument layers, as discussed later. Some tegument proteins play essential roles in the assembly process. VP16 has been reported to be required for envelopment at the inner nuclear membrane (665) or for another step downstream of nuclear envelopment (397). In addition, the U_L11 gene product increases the efficiency of envelopment (17,349).

Knowledge of the localization patterns of the tegument proteins could be informative as to the site of tegument assembly, but thus far, the results on tegument protein localization are complex. VP16 has been reported to localize to the cytoplasm and the nucleus (141) and at early times to the nucleus in diffuse patterns or replication compartments and later times also to a perinuclear distribution (303). Thus, VP16 could be available for nuclear or cytoplasmic assembly of tegument structures. The potential role for VP16 in replication compartments remains to be explored. The localization patterns of the VP22 tegument protein also show complex results, but this protein has displayed some novel properties. In some studies VP22, was shown to localize primarily to the cytoplasm in a perinuclear pattern in infected cells (141), whereas others have observed significant accumulations of VP22 in nuclei (451). The latter study found that nuclear VP22 is phosphorylated. Thus, VP22 could also assemble into tegument structures in either the nucleus or cytoplasm. Interestingly, VP22 has the property of intercellular transport in transfected and infected cells (142). VP22 is found in the cytoplasm of the cell where it is synthesized, but it is localized to the nucleus of the surrounding cells where it traffics. Intercellular trafficking occurs by a nonclassic, Golgi-independent mechanism apparently involving microfilaments. The function of this unique property in viral infection is not known, but applications of this property to delivery of proteins and other molecules inside of cells are being actively sought (127).

The route for egress of the virion particle from the space between the inner and outer nuclear membranes to the exterior of the infected cell is controversial. Two general pathways have been hypothesized for virion egress (Fig. 10), originally based on electron microscopic evidence. In pathway A, often called the *reenvelopment pathway,* the enveloped particle fuses with the outer nuclear membrane, resulting in deenvelopment of the nucleocapsid and its entry into the cytoplasm. The nucleocapsid then buds into the trans-Golgi network, and the enveloped particle is then released through secretory vesicles. The early electron microscopic evidence for this pathway came from observations of naked nucleocapsids in the cytoplasm of cells infected with HSV or a frog herpesvirus (566,596). In pathway B, called the *lumenal pathway* by Enquist and associates (144), the enveloped particle moves through the cytoplasm in the lumen of the endoplasmic reticulum (ER) or in vesicles either to the trans-Golgi network or Golgi vesicles where final maturation of the virion glycoproteins occurs. The early electron microscopic evidence for this pathway was that cytoplasmic viral particles largely showed enveloped particles in vesicles (109) or in tubular membrane structures (545). Further evidence interpreted in favor of this pathway came from studies involving monensin treatment of HSV-infected cells (256). Monensin, an ionophore that inhibits the secretory pathway, blocked viral egress and caused accumulation of virions in cytoplasmic vesicles. Thus, it appeared that egress involved the secretory pathway. Studies on the lipid content of virions have shown that virions are similar to cytoplasmic membranes rather than nuclear membranes, supporting the reenvelopment model (642); however, as noted earlier, the comparison is between virion envelopes and nuclear membranes of

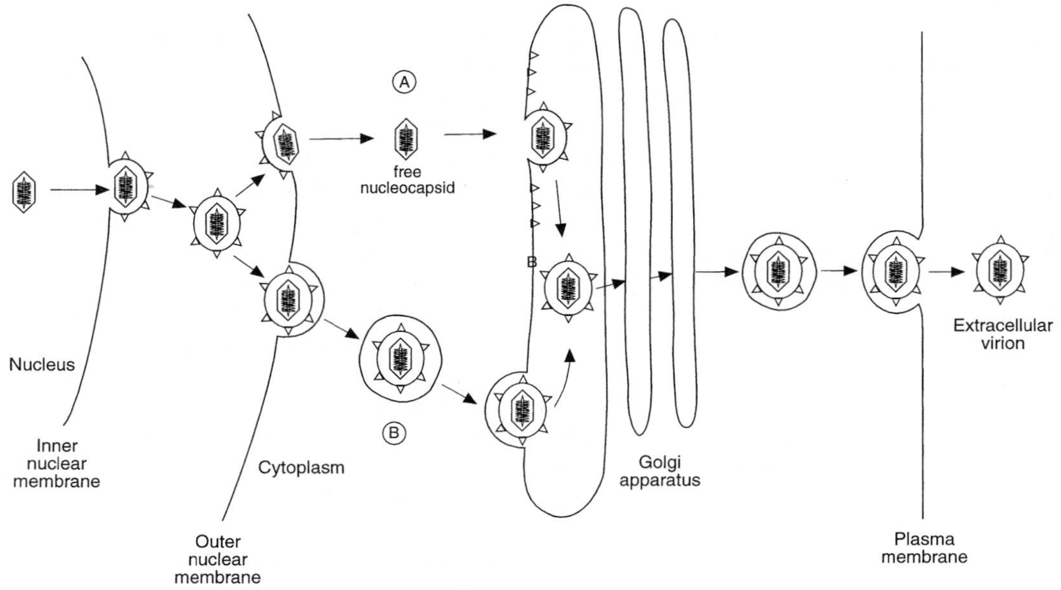

FIG. 10. Diagram of pathways of egress. HSV capsids bud through the inner nuclear membrane, forming an enveloped virion particle. Egress of the virions from the host cell may occur by either of two general pathways. **A:** The envelope fuses with the outer nuclear membrane, de-enveloping the capsid and releasing it into the cytoplasm. The capsid then buds into the Golgi apparatus, forming an enveloped virion, which is transported to the surface by vesicular transport. **B:** The virion particle buds through the outer nuclear membrane and is transported by vesicular movement through the Golgi apparatus to the exterior of the cell.

uninfected cells. The assumption underlying this comparison may not be tenable in light of the many modifications known to take place in the nuclear membrane.

The major new type of evidence favoring the reenvelopment model comes from genetic studies of virus release in cells infected with viruses expressing viral glycoproteins with novel targeting signals. A virus encoding a mutant glycoprotein H with an ER retention signal released normal numbers of extracellular particles that contained no gH and that were not infectious (48). Similarly, viruses encoding gD molecules with ER retention or ER-retrieval signals produced 10- to 100-fold less extracellular virus, whereas viruses encoding gD molecules with Golgi-retention or Golgi-retrieval signals formed normal amounts of extracellular infectious virus (671). Preliminary results with a viral mutant encoding an ER-retained gD indicate that viral particles within the nuclear membranes contain gD, whereas extracellular virions do not (A. Minson, personal communication). These studies argue that virus acquires its final membrane in a compartment that contains Golgi-targeted gD but from which ER-retrieved gD is excluded. However, the published data have not shown that gD or gH reach the nuclear membranes.

Whatever scheme is eventually shown to be correct, it must take into account two additional observations. First, in many cell types, the Golgi apparatus is fragmented and dispersed, a phenomenon that may be related to rearrangement of the cytoskeleton (59,657). Curiously, the Golgi apparatus is not fragmented in cells infected with *syn*$^-$ mutants. The second observation is that the U_L20 gene product plays an important role in viral egress from the infected cell. In cells in which the Golgi apparatus is fragmented, virions accumulate in the space between the inner and outer nuclear membrane, whereas the glycoproteins are transported to the trans-Golgi network (18).

In addition to spreading from one cell to the next through the extracellular space, HSV can spread directly from cell to cell, likely through cell junctions. The gE and gI glycoproteins are required for this mode of spread (128), possibly because the gE–gI complex can target to cell junctions and mediate movement of virions through these junctions (129).

THE FATE OF THE INFECTED CELL

Viruses require living cells for their replication. The longer the infected cells remain alive, the more progeny viruses are made, and ultimately the more the virus spreads. From an anthropomorphic viewpoint, viruses, unlike most bacteria, benefit from maintaining the cell alive. Cells productively infected with herpesviruses do not survive. Cell death is the result of not only irreparable injury caused by viral replication but also cellular responses to infection. This section deals with changes induced by the virus. Almost from the beginning of the reproductive cycle, the infected cells undergo major structural and biochemical alterations that ultimately result in their destruction.

Structural Alterations

Changes in Host Chromatin

As described in detail elsewhere (509), one of the earliest manifestations of productive infection is in the nucleolus. In infected cells, the nucleolus becomes enlarged, is displaced toward the nuclear membrane, and ultimately disaggregates or fragments. Concurrently, host chromosomes become marginated, and later in infection, the nucleus becomes distorted and multilobed. The numerous protrusions and distortions have in the past been mistaken for amitotic division (263,546). Margination of the chromosomes may or may not be linked with the chromosome breakage reported by numerous investigators (reviewed in 509).

Virus-induced Alteration of Cellular Membranes

Duplication and Folding of Intracellular Membranes

Changes in the appearance of cellular membranes and, in particular, of nuclear membranes are characteristic of cells late in infection. Deposition of material (tegument proteins?) on the inner surface facing the nucleoplasm or cytoplasm, but not in the space between inner and outer lamella or in the cisternae of the ER, results in the formation of thickened patches along the membranes. Ultimately, the patches in the nuclear membrane coalesce and fold upon themselves to give the impression of reduplicated membranes (100,145,314,361,393,413,455,544,562, 680).

Fragmentation and Dispersal of Golgi Stacks. HSV also causes a cell-type–dependent fragmentation and dispersal of Golgi vesicles. In cells in which this occurs, the Golgi vesicles fragment into myriad small vesicles that become dispersed throughout the cytoplasm (59). Disruption of microtubules is essential but not sufficient to induce the fragmentation of the Golgi apparatus. (13). In cells in which the Golgi apparatus is fragmented and dispersed, transport of virions from the nuclear membrane to the extracellular space requires the U_L20 gene product (18). In cells in which the Golgi stacks remain intact (e.g., in 143 TK-negative cells and in cells undergoing polykaryocytosis), the U_L20 protein plays a less prominent role in virion transport. In these cells, the Golgi stacks aggregate in what appears to be a central location. The distribution of viral glycoprotein D matches the distribution of the Golgi stacks, suggesting that the aggregated Golgi stacks funnel viral glycoproteins and viral particles to a limited region of the plasma membrane of the polykaryocytes rather than directing exocytic flow in a more dispersed fashion as seen in *syn*$^+$ (wild-type) virus-infected cells exhibiting fragmented and dispersed Golgi (657).

Insertion of Viral Proteins into Cellular Membranes. The first inkling that herpesviruses modify cellular membranes was based on the observation that mutant strains can differ from wild-type strains with respect to their effects on cells. For example, although wild-type viruses usually cause cells to round up and clump together, some mutant viruses cause cells to fuse into polykaryocytes (137,504). These observations led to the prediction that herpesviruses alter the structure and antigenicity of cellular membranes—a prediction fulfilled by the demonstration of altered structure and antigenic specificity (495,512,513,519) and the presence of viral glycoproteins in the cytoplasmic and plasma membranes of infected cells (217,517,518,587).

Polykaryocytosis. Both HSV-1 and HSV-2 cause infected cells to round up and adhere to each other. Some viral mutants cause cells to fuse into polykaryocytes, and this fusion may be cell-type specific or cell-type independent (137,225,526). Polykaryocytosis has been studied for several reasons: (a) as a probe of the structure and function of cellular membranes reflected in the "social behavior of cells," (b) as a tool for analyses of the functions of viral membrane proteins, and (c) as a model of the initial interaction between HSV and susceptible cells that results in the fusion of the viral envelope and the plasma membrane (60,504,583,584). Cell fusion induced by HSV also requires conditions that favor processing of high mannose glycans to complex glycans, but in this regard, it is not clear whether complex glycans must be present only on viral glycoproteins present on the surface of the infected recruiter cells, or on both the recruiter cells and on the uninfected cells being recruited into polykaryocytes (60,583,584).

Polykaryocytosis can be viewed as an aberrant manifestation of the interaction of altered membrane domains of infected cells and unaltered membranes of juxtaposed cells (504). Genetic analyses have shown that syncytial (*syn*) mutations that confer the capacity to fuse cells map in at least five and possibly more loci within the viral genome (16,41,117,330,350,447,449,523,526,689). These loci map within the domains of the *gB, gK, gL,* U_L24, and U_L20. One interpretation of these observations is that the membrane proteins form complexes whose structure and conformation become altered by mutations in any of the component polypeptides, and that the changes in the conformation are similar to those that occur in the envelopes of virions interacting with the plasma membrane (526).

Rearrangement of the Microtubular Network

Changes in the microtubular network are apparent very early in infection. Thus, the microtubules at the junction of the network with the plasma membrane appear to be disrupted in cells exposed to either *syn*$^+$ (wild-type) or *syn*$^-$ virus either in the presence or absence of cycloheximide. The overall arrangement of microtubules, however, is similar to that of uninfected cells. Late in infection, microtubules rearrange to form parallel bundles surrounding the nucleus. In polykaryocytes induced by the virus, microtubules form parallel bundles extending along the axis of recruitment of new cells (657).

Formation of Intranuclear Inclusion Bodies

Electron microscopy of herpesvirus-infected cells showed electron-translucent intranuclear inclusions surrounded by marginated and compacted cell chromatin (108,545) (see Fig. 9 in Chapter 7). Light microscopic observation of nuclear inclusions shows an hourglass appearance of the inclusions at early times and an eosinophilic staining at later times (402,576). Immunofluorescence experiments using antibodies specific for HSV DNA replication proteins have shown that viral DNA replication proteins accumulate in intranuclear foci by 3 hours after infection and that these foci enlarge into globular nuclear structures called *replication compartments* (112,475). The replication compartments are likely to be equivalent to (a) the translucent nuclear inclusions seen by EM and (b) the early nuclear inclusions seen by light microscopy.

These replication compartments are located in the interior of the nucleus as shown by EM (108,545) and by confocal microscopy (113). Viral DNA synthesis, late gene transcription, capsid assembly, and DNA encapsidation may all occur within these nuclear factories. Thus, the accumulation of replication proteins, progeny viral DNA, and nucleocapsid components within these replication compartments may cause the nuclear cytopathic effect described as *nuclear inclusion bodies*.

Host Macromolecular Metabolism

Background

It has been known for many years that HSV shuts off host RNA, DNA, and protein synthesis rapidly after infection (511). Thus, host DNA synthesis is shut off (511), host protein synthesis declines rapidly (506,614, 615), and glycosylation of host proteins ceases (572). Host macromolecular metabolism is altered in infected cells in at least four different ways: (a) mRNA present in infected cells at the time of infection is degraded, and this degradation continues for at least several hours; (b) transcription appears to be turned off; (c) cellular proteins are selectively degraded or stabilized; and (d) cellular proteins are redirected to perform novel tasks.

Shutoff of the Synthesis of Cellular Products

HSV host shutoff occurs in two stages: degradation of host mRNA and inhibition of further synthesis and processing of host mRNAs.

Virion Host Shutoff and Degradation of RNA

The existence and properties of a virion lost shutoff (*vhs*) function were documented in several stages. The first stage, documented initially by Fenwick and Walker (160) and by Nishioka and Silverstein (414–416), involves structural proteins of the virus and does not require *de novo* protein synthesis. Thus, HSV shutoff of host protein synthesis occurs in physically or chemically enucleated cells (158). Furthermore, the shutoff was effected by density gradient purified virus but not by purified virus inactivated by heating or neutralization with antibody. The shutoff is faster and more effective in HSV-2– than in HSV-1–infected cells, and this observation permitted the initial mapping of the genetic locus that confers upon HSV-1 × HSV-2 recombinants the accelerated shutoff characteristic of HSV-2 (157).

The second stage began with the isolation of *vhs*$^-$ mutants that failed to shut off host polypeptide synthesis in HSV-infected cells (483). Viral mutants of HSV-1 that were defective for shutoff of host cell protein synthesis were identified. The *vhs* function was initially mapped to 0.52 to 0.59 map units (157). Isolation of a mutant defective in this function (483) allowed further mapping of the gene responsible. Mapping studies by Oroskar and Read (425) and Kwong and colleagues (301) have identified sequences mapping from 0.604 to 0.606 map units on the viral genome (U_L41 ORF) as being responsible for the *vhs*$^-$ phenotype of the mutants. U_L41 RNA is expressed as a γ_1 gene (170). The products of U_L41 are an abundant phosphoprotein of Mr 58,000 and a less abundant, more extensively phosphorylated protein of apparent Mr 59,500. Only the faster, migrating protein is found in virions (484). Conclusive evidence that vhs acts in the absence of other viral proteins emerged from studies of Zelus and associates (698), but the question of whether it acts directly as a ribonuclease or indirectly to activate a cellular nuclease remains unresolved. Virions have a ribonuclease activity that is inactivated by anti-vhs antiserum (698). The observation that vhs has weak sequence similarity to the fen-1 family of nucleases suggested that it has intrinsic nuclease activity. Consistent with this view, Elgadi and associates (138) reported that the vhs protein induces endoribonucleolytic cleavage of mRNAs *in vitro,* whereas Karr and Read (264) noted that vhs causes the degradation of the 5′ end of mRNAs before that of the 3′ end. Recently, it has been reported that vhs interacts with the translation factor eIF-4H and that this interaction is essential for the RNase activity and perhaps for targeting of vhs to polyribosomes for selective degradation of mRNAs (S. Read, personal communication; J.

Smiley, personal communication). The complex appears to cause the decapping of cellular mRNAs from the 5′ terminus.

In cells infected with a *vhs*⁻ mutant, host protein synthesis is not shut off, at least early in infection, and the duration of α and β protein synthesis is prolonged compared to wild type. Both of these effects have been shown to be due to a stabilization of host and viral mRNAs in cells infected by *vhs*⁻ mutants; thus, vhs protein accelerates the degradation of both cellular and viral mRNAs (300,425) and serves to inhibit translation of cellular mRNA. Combined with the viral effects of inhibition of host transcription and RNA splicing, the cellular mRNA pools are not replenished, and as viral mRNA accumulates, it is preferentially translated. It has been suggested that vhs serves to facilitate the transitions from α to β to γ protein synthesis by shortening the life of viral mRNA (300,425). As infection progresses, the degradation of RNA by vhs appears to be reduced or blocked altogether. The most direct observation in support of this conclusion is that the half-lives of viral mRNAs increase with time after infection (159). A compelling rationale for the turnoff of vhs function is that the vhs protein accumulates in appreciable amounts late in infection. If the nascent protein were functional, it would be expected that it would totally degrade viral mRNA concurrent with its accumulation in the infected cell. VP16 and vhs interact (570), and this interaction blocks the degradation of RNA by vhs (308). Thus, assembly of vhs into tegument complexes not only allows the virion to bring vhs into the cell and inhibit host translation but also serves to modulate the activity of vhs at later times of infection when mostly viral mRNA is present in the cell. The conditions required for the dissociation of vhs and VP16 proteins at the outset of infection remain to be defined.

Shutoff of Transcription

To facilitate the transition from cellular to viral gene transcription, HSV infection causes a rapid decrease in host RNA synthesis (209,654). Transcription by all three cellular RNA polymerases declines to less than 50% of uninfected cell levels by 4 hours postinfection (460). Repression of host cell poll II transcription requires multiple HSV genes, the specific gene dependence varying with the cellular gene (593). HSV infection causes changes in the phosphorylation of RNA pol II (593) in some cell lines, and this effect on the host cell requires ICP22 and U_L13 protein kinase. However, the relationship of this change in pol II to inhibition of host gene transcription and promotion of viral gene transcription remains to be defined.

Inhibition of Splicing of Messenger RNA

Early in infection, some of the intranuclear ICP27 localizes to spliceosomes, causing a redistribution of host snRNPs (441,534). Two cellular snRNP proteins, U1 and a 70-kd protein, coprecipitate with ICP27, and ICP27 causes an increase in their phosphorylation (533). Phosphorylation of U1 protein impairs its ability to stimulate RNA splicing. Thus, this effect of ICP27 may contribute to its ability to inhibit RNA splicing. This effect on splicing has little or no effect on viral RNA synthesis because three of the genes encoding spliced RNAs are α genes ($\alpha 0$, $\alpha 22$, and $\alpha 47$). Late in infection, ICP27 is localized to replication compartments and shuttles to the cytoplasm, and at this stage, it may no longer repress RNA splicing, allowing U_L15 RNA to be spliced.

Selective Degradation of Cellular Proteins

Destruction or posttranslational modification of cellular protein is implied by the changes in microtubular network, nucleoli, mitochondria, Golgi apparatus, ND10 structures, and so forth. Recent studies have shown that HSV causes both accelerated destruction and stabilization of cellular proteins.

Accelerated destruction of specific proteins in infected cells was described earlier. These included PML, the kinetochore protein CENP-C (149), and cyclins A and B (4). The destruction of CENP-C is mediated by ICP0, whereas the destruction of cyclins A and B requires two functions, that of ICP22 and of U_L13 protein kinase (5). Additional evidence for selective destruction of cellular proteins is likely to emerge given the increasing prominence of viral–cellular protein interactions in current research. What differentiates normal turnover of cellular proteins from selective degradation is evidence that specific viral proteins mediate this degradation.

Selective Stabilization and Activation of Cellular Proteins

As noted earlier, ICP0 stabilizes cyclin D1 and D3 and activates cdc2 cell cycle kinase. The stabilization of cyclins D1 and D3 is mediated by ICP0 (269,644). Thus, wild-type ICP0 binds cyclin D3 and stabilizes it. Mutants lacking ICP0 or carrying an alanine substitution in place of aspartic acid 199 fail to bind cyclin D3 and are less pathogenic when administered to mice at a peripheral site (643). The D199A mutation is pleiotropic in the sense that both cyclin D3 and cyclin D1 are destabilized and degraded within a few hours after infection (643). Moreover, the D199A mutant is not transported from the nucleus into the cytoplasm (644). The stabilization of cyclin D3 and D1 is surprising in light of the observation that cdk2 is inactive (136). The pRB protein is hypophosphorylated, E2F-pRB and E2F-p107 complexes accumulate, E2F-dependent gene expression decreases, and E2F proteins are posttranslationally modified and inactive (5,6,136,223,423,581), all suggesting that S-phase genes are unlikely to be activated.

The hypothesis that HSV uses cyclins D1 and D3 for purposes other than to induce S phase is supported indirectly by another observation. Thus, 5 to 9 hours after infection, cyclins A and B are destroyed, but their catalytic partner, cdc2, is activated (5), prompting the question of how catalytic subunit regulation occurs in the absence of the normal cyclin subunit. In addition, cdc2 is required for the expression of a subset of γ_2 genes exemplified by U_S11 (6). More recent studies indicate that cdc2 can phosphorylate ICP0 and ICP22 *in vitro* and in the context of infected cells (S. J. Advani and B. Roizman, manuscript in preparation). Activation of cdc2 is mediated by ICP22 and the U_L13 protein kinase.

The conscription of cdc2 to phosphorylate viral proteins is not an isolated phenomenon. As noted elsewhere in this chapter, the $\gamma_1 34.5$ protein binds and redirects protein phosphatase 1 to dephosphorylate eIF-2α (215). As analyses of viral–cellular protein interactions progress, many more examples of diversion of cellular proteins to meet viral needs will emerge. Equally significant, posttranslational modifications of cellular proteins are also likely to be commonplace as more and more cellular proteins are studied in depth in the context of infected cells. The distinction between specific and nonspecific modification will depend on the viral genes that are involved in the process and evidence that they play a role in viral gene expression. A case in point is the phosphorylation of translation factor EF-1δ in infected cells by the U_L13 protein kinase. The specificity of this reaction was reinforced by the observation that EF-1δ is hyperphosphorylated in cells infected with representative alphaherpesviruses, betaherpesviruses, and gammaherpesviruses and that in cytomegalovirus (CMV)-infected cells, the phosphorylation of EF-1δ is mediated by the U_L97 protein, the CMV homolog of U_L13 protein kinase (268). An additional example of the activation of cellular kinases is the activation of p38 and JNK stress-activated kinases, which augments viral yield (372,697).

Effects of Herpes Simplex Virus Infection on the Cell Cycle Machinery

HSV infection causes several changes in the cell cycle machinery. First, it causes a block in the cell cycle in either the G_2 (96) or the G_1 (112) phase of the cell cycle. The G_1 phase block is distinct from the viral inhibition of cell DNA synthesis because early to mid G_1 phase events are blocked, including pRB protein phosphorylation and induction of cyclins and cyclin-dependent kinases (136, 581). The net effect of HSV infection on cells is to lower the level of G_1 phase–specific functions, including cyclin D3 protein levels (581) and cdk2 kinase activity (136). This is interesting in light of several reports indicating that HSV infection requires cyclin-dependent kinases (539–541). Clearly, we have much more to learn about the interactions of HSV with the cell cycle machinery.

VIRULENCE

Background

During infection of humans, viral disease includes primary and recurrent epithelial lesions as well as disseminated disease and encephalitis. In studies on the molecular basis of disease induced by HSV, the end point of the research objective—disease—is often taken to be synonymous with the destruction of central nervous system (CNS) tissue. In healthy, immunocompetent humans, encephalitis occurs rarely but with catastrophic results (672). In experimental animals, it is frequently a major component of the disease. Neurogrowth, the ability to grow in nervous system tissue, as measured solely by intracerebral inoculation of virus, is the most commonly measured aspect of virulence. Direct injection of virus into the CNS measures the capacity of the virus to destroy an amount of CNS tissue that will result in death before the immune system blocks further virus spread. Because in most instances destruction of the CNS and death are related to virus multiplication, in quantitative terms, the growth of the virus in the CNS is measured in terms of the amount of virus required to reach a specific level of mortality (50% of inoculated animals).

A second attribute of virulence is invasiveness—the capacity to reach a target organ from the portal of entry. To disseminate to the target organ, it is necessary for the virus to multiply at peripheral sites. In experimental systems, virulence is composed of (a) peripheral multiplication, (b) invasion of the CNS, and (c) growth in the CNS. Peripheral growth and invasiveness into the CNS can be quantified by measuring the amount of virus recovered at the peripheral site and in the CNS as a function of the quantity of virus inoculated at a peripheral site (e.g., footpad, eye, ear).

The sum total of events defined under the heading "virulence" reflects two distinct sets of viral functions. The first comprises viral genes responsible for access to and injury of the cells whose destruction is responsible for the disease. The second, less well appreciated, are viral genes and gene functions that turn off host responses to infection.

Viral Functions that Contribute to Viral Invasiveness and Replication

Several types of studies have been done to define genes required for neurovirulence or neuroinvasiveness. They may be summarized as follows:

1. An important question is whether the virus that causes adult encephalitis is different from that which establishes recurrent labial infections. Viral isolates taken either from CNS tissues of encephalitis patients, from facial or genital isolates of the same patients, or from normal individuals have been com-

pared in mice inoculated intracranially or through peripheral routes with respect to neurogrowth. Although the encephalitis isolates appear to have slightly lower average PFU/LD_{50} values as compared with nonencephalitis strains, no correlation was apparent between encephalitis in humans and neurogrowth or neuroinvasiveness in experimental animals (R. J. Whitley, personal communication). However, as a variant of this approach, infection of neurons in culture has indicated that virus isolates from encephalitis cases are better able to infect and be transported to the cell body than isolates from peripheral lesions (25).

2. Numerous studies have been undertaken to assess the relative abilities of various viral mutants to grow in the CNS after direct intracerebral inoculation. What has emerged from the accumulated data is that so-called neurovirulence factors are not the exception, but the rule. Almost all virus mutants tested to date, including a number of HSV-1 × HSV-2 recombinants, many ts viruses, a variety of spontaneous mutants, and myriad recombinant viruses with deletions in one or more genes, exhibit LD_{50} values following intracerebral inoculation ranging from 100- to 100,000-fold higher than those of the parental strains. Experiments using nongenetically engineered viruses mapped loci implicated in "neurovirulence" to a number of regions, including the *tk* gene and sequences around the right terminus of the L component (68,161,249–251,282,465,524,598,626,627). Recombinant viruses with elevated intracerebral LD_{50} values include those with deletions in the genes encoding ICP22, U_S2, U_S3 protein kinase, U_L13, U_L16, U_L24, gG, gJ, gE, gI, ribonucleotide reductase, thymidine kinase, $\gamma_1 34.5$, U_L55, and U_L56 (56,379,380,547,664, 673; E. Kern, B. Meignier, J. Baines, R. J. Whitley, A. Sears, and B. Roizman, unpublished results). Most of the attenuated deletion mutants listed previously also exhibit impaired growth in peripheral tissues (e.g., cornea) as assayed either by the occurrence of epithelial lesions or by quantitation of infectious virus in the tissues, indicating that the genes deleted are required generally for growth in differentiated or polarized cells, not specifically for growth in neurons or in CNS tissues (44,246,247; A. Sears, B. Meignier, and B. Roizman, unpublished results). In fact, the only genes that have to date been shown *not* to be required for neurovirulence in the murine model are *gC, U_S9, U_S10, U_S11,* and *α47* (417; R. J. Roller, B. Roizman, unpublished data). Because the function of *α47* appears to be human cell specific (695), it is conceivable that if the *U_S9* to *U_S11* genes share in this property, their function will be inapparent in the mouse.

The conclusion that emerges is that all HSV genes are important in enabling optimal viral replication and viral spread in the CNS. The special importance of some genes is nevertheless obvious. Mutations in *gD* that restrict or expand the host range are likely to have a significant impact on viral pathogenicity. Another, as yet not fully defined function that plays a significant role in viral pathogenesis is that which enables capsid–tegument structures to be transported retrograde in axons leading to sensory neurons or the CNS.

Viral Functions that Block Host Responses to Infection

Of the 84 ORFs identified to date, more than half are dispensable for replication in cells in culture. Some (e.g., thymidine kinase) are not essential in dividing cells but must be present in nondividing cells to enable viral replication. A large number of the "dispensable" genes as well as some "essential" genes, however, appear to target host responses to infection. These genes may be divided into two groups: (a) those that block *de novo* synthesis of cellular gene proteins that may adversely affect viral replication, and (b) those that block the function of preexisting proteins residing in cells after infection. Examples of the former are vhs, the product of *U_L41* gene, and ICP27. The former causes degradation of mRNA present in infected cells, whereas the latter mediates an inhibition of transcription and splicing during the initial stages of infection. Included in this list are the other viral gene functions that block transcription of cellular genes discussed earlier in the text. This section concerns viral gene functions that block the activation of proteins preexisting in the cell at the time of infection.

ICP34.5, U_S11 protein, and the RNA-dependent Protein Kinase (PKR)

One of the principal but easily defeated host defenses is PKR. This enzyme resides in small amounts in uninfected cells but its expression is induced by interferon. PKR is activated by some forms of dsRNA. Activated PKR causes the phosphorylation of the α subunit of eIF-2. Phosphorylated eIF-2α causes total shutoff of protein synthesis. In cells infected with a $\gamma_1 34.5$-negative mutant, protein synthesis is shut off after the onset of viral DNA synthesis concomitant with the phosphorylation of eIF-2α and the appearance of complementary viral RNA capable of self-annealing to form dsRNA (80,248,288). All viruses that cause the synthesis of RNA with extensive secondary structure must block PKR from shutting off protein synthesis. The manner in which HSV does this is quite different from that of other viruses: ICP34.5 binds protein phosphatase 1α and redirects it to dephosphorylate eIF-2α (215). The virus totally ignores the activated PKR. The domain of ICP34.5 responsible for this function resides in the carboxyl terminus of ICP34.5 and exhibits two attributes. First, it contains the motif of the protein phosphatase accessory protein necessary to direct the phosphatase to specific targets. Mutagenesis of two key amino acids within this motif precludes ICP34.5 from causing the dephosphorylation of eIF-2α (214). Second, the carboxyl-terminal domain of ICP34.5 is highly homologous to the corresponding domain of a conserved mammalian protein known as growth arrest and DNA damage 34 (GADD34) protein. The GADD34 domain substitutes for the corresponding ICP34.5 domain in blocking the effects of PKR (213).

Mohr and Gluzman (391) serially passaged a $\gamma_1$34.5-negative mutant and obtained a phenotypic revertant. The revertant showed a spontaneous deletion of the coding sequence of *α47* and the adjacent promoter of U_L11 gene such that the α promoter of *α47* became juxtaposed to the U_L11 gene. The net consequence was that U_L11 was expressed earlier in infection (212). Subsequent studies showed that PKR interacted physically with U_L11 *in vitro* and that the capacity of U_S11 protein to block activation of PKR was dependent on the time and order of additional U_S11 protein. Exposure of PKR to U_S11 protein before its activation was effective in precluding the phosphorylation of eIF-2δ, whereas activated PKR responded poorly to added U_S11 protein (67).

As noted in Chapter 71 in *Fields Virology*, 4th ed., the *$\gamma_1$34.5* gene is conserved only in HSV-1, HSV-2, and simian B virus, the implication being that *$\gamma_1$34.5* gene is a late acquisition by these herpesviruses. Therefore, the HSV progenitor may have dealt with PKR differently, perhaps by U_S11 protein expressed earlier in infection.

Apoptosis

Several HSV-1 deletion mutants have now been shown to induce classic apoptosis, characterized by chromatin condensation, release of cytochrome C from mitochondria, fragmentation of cellular DNA, vacuolization, and blebbing of the cytoplasm. The mutants shown to cause programmed cell death in at least one cell line include *α4*⁻, *α27*⁻, *ts*B7 carrying a ts lesion in the U_L36 protein and maintained at the nonpermissive temperature, and *(gD, gJ)*⁻ mutant viruses. Conversely, wild-type HSV-1 blocks apoptosis induced by osmotic shock, thermal shock, Fas ligand, and TNF-α (11,12,176,255,287,321, 564). The salient features of the available data may be summarized as follows:

1. Apoptosis is cell-type dependent. For example, the *d*120 mutant lacking the *α4* gene induces apoptosis in all continuous cell lines (175,176) tested but not in human embryonic lung cells (175,701). *ts*B7 at the nonpermissive temperature induces programmed cell death in Vero cells but not in the human SK-N-SH cells derived from a malignant glioma (176).
   The pathway leading to programmed cell death is also cell-type dependent. For example, the *d*120 mutant induced caspase 3–independent apoptosis in SK-N-SH cells but caspase 3–dependent apoptosis in HEp-2 cells. Recently, a novel caspase-independent pathway mediated by a mitochondrial protein designated *apoptosis-inducing factor* (AIF) was described. In induced cells, AIF is translocated from mitochondria into the nucleus. In induced human embryonic cells, AIF is translocated into the nucleus, but apoptosis does not ensue.
   These observations suggest that different cells react differently to the same stimulus, that mutants differ in the stimuli they induce, and that wild-type virus blocks all viral activators of programmed cell death to achieve its optimal replication.
2. Little is known of the mechanism by which HSV mutants induce apoptosis. It has been reported that HSV degrades Bcl2 (355), and indeed overexpression of Bcl2 in HEp-2 cells blocks apoptosis induced by the *d*120 mutant (174). The delay in the cytopathic effects induced by wild-type HSV-1 suggests that the cytopathic effects observed in cells undergoing productive infection may at least in part be due to apoptosis. Consistent with this view is the observation that the cytopathic effect of *d*120 virus was more extensive than that caused by wild-type virus, whereas mutants lacking both *α0* and *α4* genes were far less cytopathic (531,684).
3. There is also a paucity of data on the mechanism by which HSV blocks apoptosis. One observation of particular interest was that in SK-N-SH cells treated with sorbitol, (osmotic shock) HSV blocked fragmentation of DNA but not activation of caspase 3 or release of cytochrome C (175,176). Viral genes shown to date to block apoptosis are *gD, gJ,* and the protein kinase *U_S3* (254,322,700). ICP4 and ICP27 deleted from respective viruses most likely block apoptosis by enabling the synthesis of proteins made late in infection. The *gD* and *gJ* genes were able to block apoptosis only in cells infected with a mutant lacking both genes but not in cells exposed to TNF-α or Fas ligand (703); therefore, they may be necessary and sufficient in some circumstances but not in all systems studied to date.

In essence, cell death appears to be a complex phenomenon resulting in part from injury to the cell and in part from the cell response to infection. A major cause of cell death even in wild-type virus-infected cells may result from exhaustion of mitochondria and ultimately necrosis, if the levels of ATP have been totally exhausted, or apoptosis, if the cell can still react to the injury caused by viral gene products.

Herpes Simplex Virus and the Immune System

York and colleagues (695) were the first to report that HSV blocks the presentation of antigenic peptides by class I major histocompatibility complex (MHC) proteins. As the story unfolded, it became clear that ICP47, a small protein encoded by the *α47* (*Us12*) gene binds to the transporter associated with antigen processing (TAP) and blocks the transport of peptides into the ER. ICP47 appears to have a high affinity for human and porcine TAP but not for murine homologs of the transport proteins. It may explain why the anti-HSV response in mice is so much more effective than in humans.

There is no current evidence that HSV blocks presentation by class II MHC proteins.

LATENCY

The ability of HSV to establish a lifelong latent infection in the human host is the most intellectually challenging aspect of HSV biology. The available data support the following sequence of events: The virus enters nerve endings and is transported retrograde to the nucleus of sensory nerves innervating mucosal epithelium (Fig. 11). In latently infected neurons, viral genomes acquire the characteristics of endless or circular DNA (167,381,497,498), and no replicating virus can be detected in the sensory ganglia innervating the site of inoculation. In a fraction of neurons harboring latent HSV, the virus is periodically reactivated. Infectious virus is carried anterogradely to peripheral tissues by axonal transport (97), usually to cells at or near the site of initial infection (65,106,195,502). Depending on several factors, including the host immune status, the reactivation may be asymptomatic or lead to a recurrent lesion, which may vary considerably in severity from punctate lesions that are invisible to the naked eye to severe, debilitating lesions in immunosuppressed individuals.

Viral DNA fragments have been detected in CNS and other tissues; thus, to differentiate between presence of defective genomes and latent infections, the operational definition of latent infections has historically embodied the requirement that wild-type virus must be able to reactivate from latent state under appropriate experimental conditions. Operationally, this meant that virus could be detected after incubation of intact ganglionic tissue with suitable susceptible cells, but not by inoculation of the susceptible cells with homogenized ganglia (597). This definition obviously also included the ability to reactivate and replicate to detectable levels in the ganglia. Because virus has been reactivated from sensory and autonomic ganglia only, this definition restricts viral latency to only these tissues. More recently, the definition of latency was

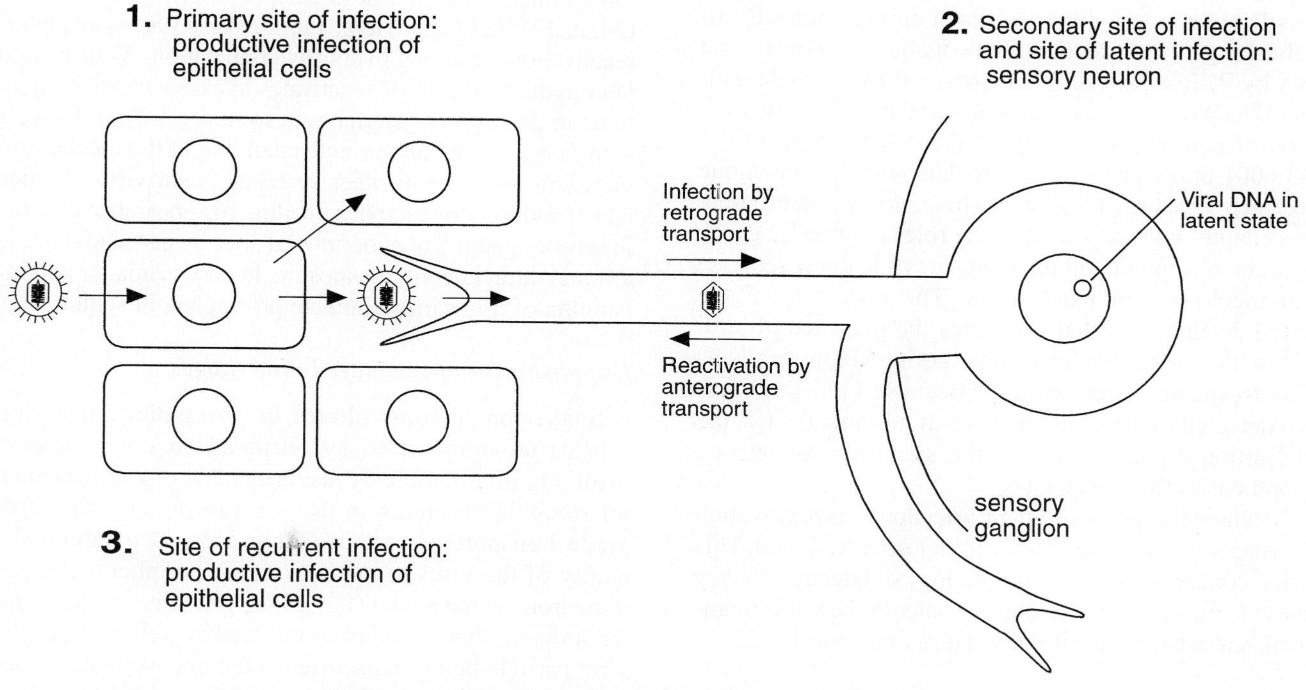

FIG. 11. Stages of HSV infection of the host. 1. HSV is introduced onto a mucosal surface or a break in the skin; it replicates productively in epithelial cells at the site of inoculation and spreads through the tissue. Virus enters sensory neuron axons and is transported to the cell body in a ganglion. 2. Virus either replicates productively or establishes a latent infection in the neuronal cell nucleus. Viral DNA is circular and in a nucleosomal form. Upon neuronal damage or activation, the virus reactivates and undergoes at least a limited productive cycle. Capsids are transported by anterograde transport to the axonal termini and virions are released. 3. Reactivated virus causes a recurrent infection of the mucosal tissue, causing the shedding of virus.

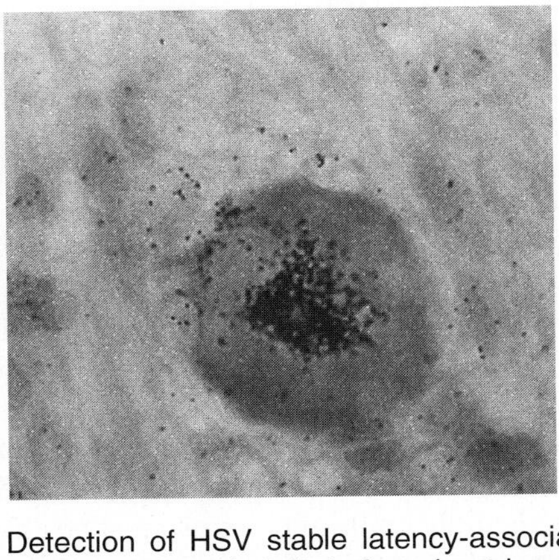

FIG. 12. Detection of HSV stable latency-associated transcript (LAT) RNA in latently infected murine trigeminal ganglion neurons by *in situ* hybridization. Mice were infected with HSV-1 after corneal scarification. At 30 days postinfection, the mice were sacrificed, and trigeminal ganglia were frozen and sectioned. The sections were hybridized with a ^{3}H-labeled DNA probe detecting the LAT RNA as described (93). (Micrograph courtesy of Magdalena Kosz-Vnenchak.)

extended to include viruses that can be detected in sensory ganglia several weeks after infection by *in situ* hybridization (Fig. 12) with probes for latency-associated transcripts (described later) or by assays of viral DNA in ganglia (93,266,316,318,345,623). At the present time, the only technique for proving that a virus is incapable of establishing latent infections is the inability to detect viral DNA by PCR assays of DNA extracted from whole ganglia (378a,478a). A possible new standard is the identification of neurons containing viral DNA by *in situ* PCR (143,600), although the results to date with this technique have been variable (378,478a). This redefinition of latent virus enables an assessment of the roles of specific genes in the establishment and maintenance of latency, separate from their roles in reactivation. The downside of the revised definition is that it equates the presence of viral DNA with a *bona fide* latent state defined biologically as at least capable of reactivation. Because viral DNA has been detected in the CNS and even at peripheral sites, the redefinition arguably extends the sites of viral latency beyond currently proven sites.

The clinical aspects of latent infection and reactivation are discussed in Chapter 73 in *Fields Virology*, 4th ed. This section concerns the molecular biology of latency. The key issues are how the virus establishes latency, how it is maintained, and what makes it reactivate spontaneously.

Herpes Simplex Virus Latency in Experimental Systems

The Experimental Models

The most useful animal model systems are mice, guinea pigs, and rabbits. In all three species, inoculation of wild-type virus results in viral replication at the peripheral site, retrograde transport of virus to the nucleus of dorsal root neuron, followed ultimately by establishment of latency. In all three systems, a fraction of sensory neurons replicate the virus after entry into the neuron (274–277,366, 367,466,467,637,656,678). It is not known whether acute viral replication also occurs in humans or whether this replication reflects the animal system, route of inoculation, induction of host transactivating factors, or the large amount of virus used in the inoculum to attain a high percentage of latently infected ganglia.

Explantation of dorsal root ganglia causes the latent virus to replicate and spread from cell to cell. There are several key differences in the animal models. In rabbits, both HSV-1 and HSV-2 reactivate spontaneously. The rabbit eye model is particularly useful for studies of spontaneous reactivation because the virus is readily detected in lacrimal secretions. The guinea pig is a useful model of HSV-2 genital infections. The virus reactivates spontaneously, causing lesions containing small amounts of virus, although the acute and recurrent phases are somewhat artificially defined. The virtues of the mouse model are twofold. First, highly inbred strains differ with respect to their susceptibility to infection, and knock-out mice have been particularly useful in studies of immune responses to infection (339). Second, spontaneous reactivations of virus resulting in the appearance of infectious virus either in ganglia or at peripheral sites are very rare (34,35,221,222,605). Here, the key issue is spontaneous reactivations resulting in abortive replication. As discussed later in the text, if HSV reactivates to cause abortive infections in dorsal root ganglia ever so rarely, it would have a significant impact on our understanding of the mechanism of reactivation. As in other systems, latent virus in mice can be induced to reactivate, leading to appearance of virus in sensory ganglia or at peripheral sites by peripheral tissue trauma, ultraviolet light exposure, hyperthermia, or administration of drugs that stimulate prostaglandin synthesis.

Establishment of Latency: Initial Stages

Studies on neurons cultured *in vitro* indicate that viral capsids are transported by retrograde axonal transport involving microtubules; thus, drugs that disrupt neuronal microtubule structures, or that are known to inhibit retrograde transport of certain compounds, also inhibit the ability of the virus to move from the peripheral endings of neurons to the nuclei (291). Electron microscopic studies indicate that in neurons infected in cell culture, the viral particle being transported is the unenveloped nucleocapsid or nucleocapsid–tegument structure (344,433).

Several important facets of latent infections relate to the role of virus multiplication, both at the portal of entry and in the neurons harboring the virus.

1. As noted previously, HSV must have access to the nerve endings to establish latency; therefore, it could be expected that the greater the number of peripheral

cells that become infected and support virus multiplication, the larger the number of neurons that will harbor latent virus. The relevant phenomenon in humans is that the frequency of reactivations resulting in recrudescences of lesions is related to the severity of lesions caused by the first infection. In the model discussed subsequently, the frequency of recurrences would be determined in part by the number of neurons harboring virus.

2. Because wild-type viruses multiply in sensory neurons during the first 7 to 10 days after peripheral inoculation, most of the information available to date on the establishment of the latent state is based on studies done 2 weeks or more after infection and therefore adequately reflects maintenance rather than establishment. Studies with mutants lacking essential genes have been very revealing in several respects.

First, viruses lacking the essential *α4* and *α27* genes, totally unable to replicate in cultured cells in the absence of complementing viral genes, were shown to be able to establish and maintain latent infections but were unable to reactivate (266,552). The fact that no deletion mutant totally failed to establish latency raises the question of whether any viral gene is essential for this process and suggests that no viral function is absolutely required for the establishment of latency. Nevertheless, viral gene products may affect the levels of DNA persisting in latent viral ganglia. For example, recent studies have shown that an HSV-2 U_L5-negative, U_L29-negative mutant virus is defective for stable maintenance of viral DNA in trigeminal ganglia (107).

Second, either viral latency is determined by cellular functions or virion proteins and no viral gene function expressed *de novo* is required to establish latency, or viral DNA entering neurons is retained in an episomal form irrespective of its ability to express any function, and therefore at least some of the deletion mutants may not be truly latent but merely retained in dorsal root neurons. Differentiation between these two alternatives requires an analysis of dorsal root ganglia during the first few hours after infection. Alas, the small number of neurons harboring these mutants makes effective analyses of the early events in the establishment of latency very difficult. In essence, no gene has been identified as essential for establishment of latency based on analyses of latent virus present during the maintenance phase, although certain viral functions, such as the LATs and the missing functions in the *dl*5-29 mutant, appear to increase the efficiency of latent infection.

Function(s) of Latency-associated Transcripts

The major viral gene products expressed during latent infection are the LATs (606). This transcriptional unit is expressed from the *b* repeat sequences of the L component (Fig. 13), and the more than 8-kb transcript is antisense to ICP0 mRNA and possibly ICP4 mRNA. The viral promoter driving expression of this transcriptional unit functions efficiently in sensory neurons, and expression of LAT ensues rapidly after viral infection of sensory neurons (285,595). Latent infection is favored in certain subsets of murine trigeminal ganglion sensory neurons, as evidenced by expression of LATs, whereas productive infection is favored in other types of the sensory neurons, as evidenced by expressing of lytic antigens (351). LAT-negative mutant viruses exhibit increased acute expression of viral α, β, and γ genes in sensory neurons as compared with rescued or wild-type viruses (180), suggesting that LATs in some way down-regulate lytic gene expression in neurons. The threefold increase in neurons expressing lytic genes with LAT-negative viruses correlates with the similar decrease in latently infected neurons with LAT-negative viruses (628). Thus, LAT may play a role in promoting latent infection by down-regulation of lytic gene expression. The mechanism of this effect could include antisense down-regulation of ICP0 or ICP4 mRNA, structural effects of the transcript on the viral genome, or expression of a protein product.

A promising observation that did not live up to its expectation is that ORF P and ORF O were encoded in the domain transcribed by the 8.3-kb LAT. The transcript was detected late in infection and in nuclear runoff experiments, but not in cells treated with cycloheximide from the time of infection (40,693). The transcript or the protein it encodes has been detected early in infection in cells infected with *α4*-negative virus (693) or at 39°C, the temperature at which ICP4 of a wild-type virus is nonfunctional (306). Although attempts to detect the transcript in latently infected neurons have been unsuccessful (693), the results remain inconclusive because both the transcript and the protein are made in very small amounts. In addition, Yeh and Schaffer (693) failed to detect the 8.3-kbp LAT, which contains the sequences contained in the *ORF P* transcript. The transcription initiation site contains a high-affinity binding site for ICP4, and the genes are expressed only in the absence of functional ICP0 (480). Both ORF O and ORF P proteins are expressed from a single mRNA; thus, they share the amino-terminal 1 to 35 codons but diverge thereafter owing to RNA editing or undetected splicing. Overexpressed ORF P protein co-localized with spliceosomes and reduced the accumulation of ICP22 and ICP0, whereas the ORF O protein bound ICP4 and interfered with its binding to cognate sites on HSV DNA. Notwithstanding these attributes, mutagenesis of the initiator methionine, which abrogated the synthesis of ORF P and ORF O, had no effect on the ability of the virus to replicate in experimental animal systems and only a slight effect on the amount of virus recovered

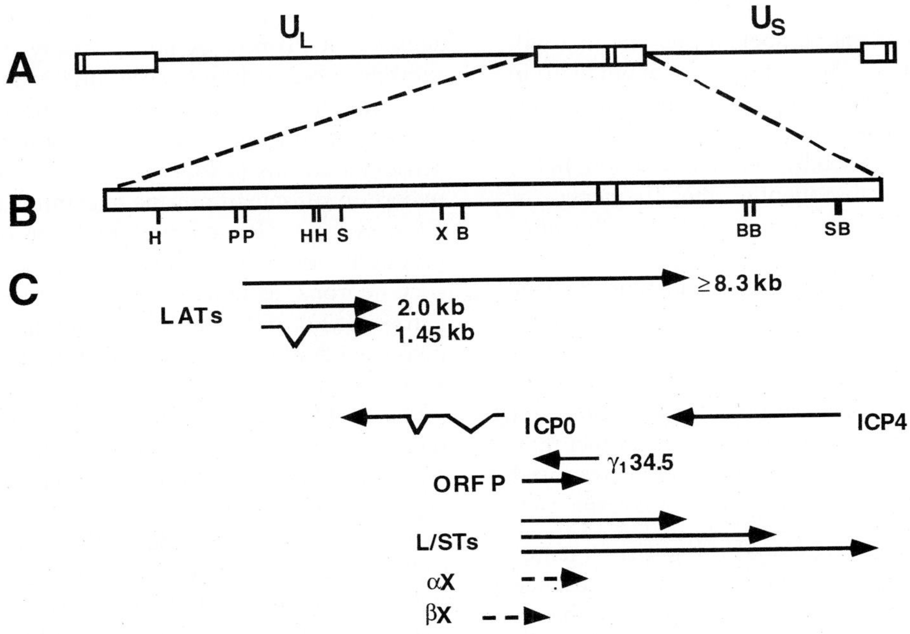

FIG. 13. Map of the latency-associated transcript (LAT) transcriptional unit. Map of the HSV-1 genome showing the LAT transcriptional unit. **A:** HSV-1 genome in the prototype orientation; U_L and U_S denote the unique sequences of the long (L) and short (S) components of the genome, respectively, and the *open boxes* denote repeat sequences. **B:** Expanded view of the L-S junction region with restriction endonuclease cleavage sites: B, BamHI; H, HpaI; P, PstI; S, SalI; X, XhoI. **C:** Locations and orientations of transcripts of the L-S junction region are denoted by *solid arrows* and include the LATs, ICP0, ICP4, $\gamma_1$34.5 (78,82), ORF P (306), L/STs (693), and partially mapped transcripts (*dashed arrows*) αX and βX (39,40).

from latently infected ganglia (479). *ORF P* and *O* gene products may contribute to the establishment but are not key determinants of latency.

In the absence of detailed analyses of the events occurring during the first few hours after entry of viral DNA into dorsal root ganglia, one key hypothesis regarding the establishment of latency remains unchallenged. In essence, the hypothesis predicts that latency is established by default in the absence of initial sustained expression of α genes. The lack of α gene expression is likely explained by several mechanisms acting in combination: (a) lack of nuclear forms of host factors necessary for α gene transcription (298,640), (b) hormonally regulated repression of viral gene expression (674), and (c) LAT-mediated repression of α gene expression (180). The hypothesis that lack of α gene expression is central to latency is further supported by two sets of observations.

The first set stems from attempts to establish latency in cultured cells *in vitro.* Initial attempts were based on suppression of viral multiplication by high temperatures or antiviral drugs. Although these early attempts used nonphysiologic means and lacked the power of modern analytic tools, they did show that the HSV resident in these cells could be reactivated by superinfection with unrelated human CMV. More recent studies in so-called quiescent systems have yielded similar information, but in this instance, the power of the analytic tools applied to the system indicate that HSV does remain quiescent (nonreplicating) if α gene expression immediately after entry of the virus into the cell is repressed. The mechanism of repression after the initial stages of infection is unknown.

The second set of supporting data comes from two series of experiments. In chronologic order, the first was based on the hypothesis that the tegument protein αTIF or VP16 does not reach the neuronal nucleus. This possibility was tested using a recombinant virus that contained an insertion of a second copy of the *αTIF* gene under the control of the mouse metallothionein (MT) promoter (548). Despite expression of the chimeric *αTIF* gene in latently infected sensory neurons, latent infection continued. Furthermore, expression of the same chimeric gene in transgenic mice also failed to prevent establishment or maintenance of latency. *In situ* hybridization with probes specific for Oct-1 demonstrated detectable levels of Oct-1 mRNA in the sensory neurons of the MT–αTIF transgenics (V. Hukkannen and B. Roizman, unpublished data), indicating that the presence of both αTIF and Oct-1 was insufficient to prevent latent infection. A formal explanation as to why MT–αTIF failed to induce viral multiplication emerged from studies of Kristie and co-investigators (298), who showed that HCF or C1, the cellular cofactor required for enhancement of α gene expression, along with Oct-1 and αTIF, resides in the cytoplasm and is translocated into the nucleus only under conditions of reactivation, such as explantation of ganglia in culture.

Maintenance Phase of Latency: The Latency-associated Transcripts

Extensive studies on ganglia harboring latent HSV have been rewarded by an extreme paucity of evidence for viral gene expression. The only transcripts regularly detected in a large fraction of latently infected neurons have been designated as the LATs (606). They constitute a family of transcripts mapping to the inverted repeats flanking the U_L sequence (see Fig. 13). The full-length 8.3-kb transcript accumulates at low levels in latently infected neurons, whereas the 2.0- and 1.5-kb introns processed from a full-length transcript are abundant and accumulate in the nucleus (125,290,499,594,606,652, 653,705). These introns are highly stable as a result of unusual lariat structures (156,500,685,696). The literature on LATs is enormous but fortuitously does lend itself to a brief summation. Viruses deleted in various domains of LATs have been reported to establish latency at normal levels (250,315,602) or at threefold reduced levels (628). Several studies have shown reduced explant reactivation of virus from ganglia latently infected with LAT-negative mutant viruses (31, 220,250,315,551,602), although in many instances, LAT-negative mutant viruses show reduced replicative ability (31; Garber et al., manuscript in preparation; Lagunoff and Roizman, unpublished studies). The region of the LATs associated with decreased reactivation has been mapped to a 348-bp sequence in the 5′ end of LAT (33,219).

Notwithstanding several reports (131,624), the stable 2.0- and 1.5-kb LATs have not been shown unambiguously to express ORFs. The functions attributed to LATs have been numerous and varied. Thus LATs, have been reported to (a) block productive infection gene expression by blocking the transcription of the gene encoding ICP0 located antisense or by other mechanisms (75,180), (b) enable reactivation of virus from latent state, and (c) maintain virus in latent state. Each of these putative mechanisms has been disputed (32,75,89,180,196,221, 315,316,628,635). The most recent function attributed to LATs is that they protect neurons from apoptosis. Thus, a virus deleted for LAT was reported to induce apoptosis in rabbit trigeminal ganglia at slightly higher levels than the wild-type virus (438). The substance of the report is that LATs do spare the neurons from destruction but not the mechanism by which this takes place. This report requires confirmation. If LATs do protect neurons from apoptosis, the question arises as to how RNA does this, and whether reactivation is the cause or consequence of failure of LAT to protect neurons from programmed cell death. Irrespective of the final determination of the functions of LATs, current data suggest that LATs exert a quantitative effect on latency rather than an absolute role.

Copy Number of Viral DNA in Latently Infected Neurons

In a different category from LATs is the observation that in trigeminal ganglia harboring latent virus, there are between 0.1 and 1 viral genome equivalents per cell genome (55,468,497,498). This datum posed an intriguing question. Heretofore, the number of neurons harboring virus was thought to be about 3% of total neurons. Rodahl and Stevens (501) indicated that under some circumstances, the number can be higher; however, neurons account for only about 10% of the total cells in a sensory ganglion. Unless viral genomes are contained in every single cell in a ganglion, including glial cells, it is obvious that, as was first calculated a number of years ago (516), each latently infected neuron must contain more than one viral genome.

Two series of experiments indicate that, as was predicted earlier (516), replication of viral DNA by viral enzymes is not necessary for the establishment of latent infection and is not responsible for the attainment of the high copy number. In these experiments (567,590,591), mice were infected by the footpad route, and assays of LAT, lytic antigens, and DNA copy number were done. Although there was a correlation between levels of lytic replication and the level of viral DNA per LAT-positive neuron, even those ganglia that showed little or no sign of viral antigen expression still had DNA copy numbers of greater than 20 viral genomes per LAT-positive neuron. To account for the high number of viral genomes per cell harboring latent virus, it is then necessary to postulate that (a) more than one viral genome can enter a single neuron during the establishment of latency, or (b) viral genomes are amplified by the cellular machinery during latency (516). In support of the second of these hypotheses, at least one host-dependent origin of DNA replication embedded within the viral genome has been identified (550). A second, symmetrically arranged copy was also found (A. E. Sears, personal communication). As discussed later, one hypothesis governing these studies is that one of the cellular polymerases amplifies resident viral genomes at a low rate. The dogma, however, has been that there is no DNA replication machinery in neurons.

On the other hand, evidence in favor of the high copy number being due to viral DNA replication functions includes (a) the constant level of viral DNA during latent infection by viruses incapable of viral DNA replication in neurons as determined by quantitative PCR (289,641) and (b) the general correlation between ganglionic replication and latent DNA load (629).

Reactivation of Virus from Latent State

The issues central to understanding viral reactivation from latent state are fivefold: (a) Do the events surrounding viral recrudescences in humans provide a clue to the events leading to reactivation? (b) Is there a specific viral gene whose function is unambiguously required for viral reactivation? (c) What is the order of expression of viral genes in the course of reactivation? (d) What is the significance of the observation that not all neurons harboring virus reactivate all at once? and (e) What is the fate of the neuron in which virus reactivated? It is convenient to consider these questions in the order stated.

a. In humans, latent virus is reactivated after local stimuli, such as injury to tissues innervated by neurons harboring latent virus, or by systemic stimuli, such as physical or emotional stress, hyperthermia, exposure to ultraviolet light, menstruation, hormonal imbalance, and so forth, which may reactivate virus simultaneously in neurons of diverse ganglia (e.g., trigeminal and sacral). In experimental systems, multiplication of latent virus has been induced by physical trauma to tissues innervated by the neurons harboring virus (10,204), by iontophoresis of epinephrine (299) or other chemicals or drugs (204,205,561), by transient hyperthermia (537,538), or by corneal scarification (640). The most plausible common denominator is that injury or stimulation of cells innervated by dorsal root neurons harboring latent virus is a common trigger of recrudescence of lesions caused by reactivated virus. The nature of the transduced signal is unknown.
b. It is a common practice to test deletion mutants for ability to establish latent infections and to reactivate. Not surprisingly, a large number of deletion mutants either failed to reactivate or reactivated poorly. Included in this list are virtually all of the genes essential for viral replication in cell culture but also mutants lacking thymidine kinase, ICP0, ribonucleotide reductase, $\gamma_1 34.5$, and so forth. A central problem with these claims is that neuronal cells harboring virus are relatively nonpermissive and devoid of enzymes necessary for viral nucleic acid metabolism. In the context of experimental tools based on explantation of sensory ganglia, it is virtually impossible to differentiate between genes required for optimal replication in tissues *in vivo* and those dedicated to reactivation of virus from latent state.
c. For years, the prevailing hypothesis concerning the regulation and order of gene expression during acute infection and reactivation was that it matched the program of viral gene expression taking place in infected cells in culture, that is, α genes are expressed first, followed by β and γ genes. Recent evidence supporting the idea that α genes are expressed first is the rapid translocation (within minutes) of the HCF or C1 transcription factor from the cytoplasm to nucleus upon explantation of trigeminal ganglia (298). Nevertheless, theoretical arguments and experimental observations have suggested that viral gene expression may be regulated differently in neurons. Theoretical considerations have argued that HSV depends to a large extent on cellular factors for its gene expression, that the order of viral gene expression depends on available factors, and that in neuronal cells, the available factors differ from those of run-of-the-mill cultured cells (457). The experimental observations are of two kinds. First, Kosz-Vnenchak and associates (286) reported that high-level expression of α and β genes depended on viral DNA synthesis during acute ganglionic infection and in explanted ganglia. It was postulated that, in neurons, low levels of α and β gene expression preceded viral DNA synthesis and γ gene expression, which then further activated α and β gene expression. The latter hypothesis was supported using reverse transcription PCR (RT-PCR) and PCR methods to detect viral RNA and DNA levels, respectively (289). Nevertheless, it has been argued that viral gene expression may not be detectable in the initial infected neuron and that viral spread amplifies the signal so that high-level α and β gene expression can be detected. By this hypothesis, viral DNA synthesis is needed for progeny virus formation and spread and not direct induction of α and β gene expression. The currently available experimental data cannot rule out this alternative explanation for the *in vivo* data. However, one study of infections of sensory neurons in culture has supported the idea that viral gene expression is regulated differently in neurons. Nichol and colleagues (410) observed that, in HSV-infected sensory neurons in culture, viral DNA synthesis stimulates α and β gene expression. These results support the hypothesis of Kosz-Vnenchak and associates (286) that viral DNA synthesis stimulates α and β gene expression in neurons, but further studies are needed to rule out the possibility that viral spread accounts for the results *in vivo* and in explanted tissue. Second, Tal-Singer and colleagues (618) reported that they could detect β gene expression before α gene expression during explant reactivation. In this study, they used RT-PCR to detect viral transcripts, but they did not show that the assays for each of the transcripts was equally sensitive; therefore, it is conceivable that the differences in kinetics of appearance reflected sensitivity of the detection assay rather than the true order of appearance. The order

of expression of HSV genes may be different during reactivation, but additional studies are needed to adequately document this.

d. Unlike the reactivation of varicella-zoster virus, not all neurons harboring latent HSV reactivate at once. The current consensus is that the recurrent lesions caused by reactivated virus are the reservoir for transmission of virus from person to person. Because transmission depends on physical contact between infected and uninfected individuals, frequent protracted recurrences would enhance transmission far more than a single synchronous transmission. One hypothetical model detailed elsewhere (45,515) that could explain asynchronous reactivation takes into account the DNA copy number per latently infected neurons. Briefly, the model is that each stimulus leading to reactivation causes an increase in the copy number of viral DNA. The stimulus may be local or systemic. At a certain point when the viral DNA copy number becomes very high, the virus reactivates either by diluting a repressor (copy number effect) or by competing more effectively for a scarce host factor necessary for basal level of viral gene expression (multiplicity effect). This model predicts that the decrease in recurrence rate reflects exhaustion of neurons that are stimulated to increase viral DNA copy number and, therefore, the larger the initial burden of latent virus, the more frequent or longer lasting interval of recurrences. This DNA level threshold could be achieved by host replicative mechanisms (516) or by viral replicative mechanisms (286).

e. The fate of the neurons after viral reactivation is a hotly debated topic. The proponents of the notion that neurons survive to reactivate again and again base their arguments on two observations. The first is that local anesthesia is not a sequelae in patients suffering from frequent recurrences at the same site. A formal rebuttal of this argument is that nerve endings from adjacent unaffected neurons grow into the healed area and reestablish a network. The second and more weighty observation is that women with recurrent genital lesions shed virus in the interim between clinically manifest lesions. The shed virus appears to originate from punctate, microscopic lesions that arise frequently and for long intervals. If each microscopic lesion arose from a reactivated neuron, there would not be enough neurons to support viral reactivation over many years if the neurons perished as a consequence of this process. The questions that have not been resolved yet is whether each lesion is the consequence of reactivation and whether chronic infections of mucosal tissues characterized by the observed microscopic lesions can be ruled out.

The studies on the molecular biology of viral replication and especially the effects of viral gene products on cellular structures and gene products detailed in this chapter do not support the hypothesis that neurons expressing viral gene products necessary for productive infection can survive and continue to function. A strange and unsupported model that satisfies the requirement that the neuron survive reactivation is that the neuron transport anterograde to peripheral sites not virions but viral DNA replicated by cellular enzymes.

CONCLUSIONS

There is an apocryphal story of three blind people asked to deduce the nature of an elephant. Each touched a different part and the identity became elusive. This probably was the case with herpesvirus research 50 years ago. In the interim, thousands of investigators explored every facet of HSV biology. We know what it consists of and the end result of infection: thousands of replicas and a very dead cell. The mass of data has produced a giant mosaic with huge gaps, but the designer's intent and general strategy of HSV design emerges. What is apparent is the following:

1. The overall strategy is total control of its own replication and of the cellular environment in which replication takes place.
2. A large fraction of viral coding sequence is devoted to changing the environment of the cell. The objectives of viral functions are the shutoff of *de novo* cellular gene expression, scavenging existing cellular proteins to redirect them to either block the host or to assist in viral replication, and complete dedication to the task of producing lots of viral progeny.
3. Many functions overlap. For example, several viral genes independently target *de novo* synthesis of cellular gene products. Many viral objectives are reached by accretion rather than by a single function of a viral gene.
4. Many, if not most, HSV proteins are multifunctional. In some instances, the functions can be mapped to blocks of amino acids. There is sufficient evidence to postulate that the function performed by individual proteins is determined by posttranslational modifications. Indeed, viral proteins are extensively posttranslationally modified.
5. Other members of the herpesvirus family with a much more restricted host range encode homologs of cellular genes. HSV encodes instead sequences that interact with and stabilize or redirect cellular proteins. The net effect is that whereas a homolog basically performs a single function, viral proteins containing amino acids blocks that redirect cellular proteins can perform multiple functions. This design presents a curious problem: It is much easier to identify a homolog than to detect the intent or function of an amino acid block that interacts with a similar cellular protein.

6. Latent infection of sensory neurons by HSV is likely to be a complex process in which numerous factors, including missing host cell factors, cellular repressor molecules, and viral functions, may each play a role in this alternative infection pathway.

Notwithstanding the many problems, the virus is no match to the effort, modern technology, and ingenuity of the blind investigators.

REFERENCES

1. Ackermann M, Braun DK, Pereira L, Roizman B. Characterization of herpes simplex virus 1 alpha proteins 0, 4, and 27 with monoclonal antibodies. *J Virol* 1984;52:108–118.
2. Ackermann M, Longnecker R, Roizman B, Pereira L. Identification, properties, and gene location of a novel glycoprotein specified by herpes simplex virus 1. *Virology* 1986;150:207–220.
3. Adams G, Stover BH, Keenlyside RA, et al. Nosocomial herpetic infections in a pediatric intensive care unit. *Am J Epidemiol* 1981;113:126–132.
4. Advani SJ, Brandimarti R, Weichselbaum RR, Roizman B. The disappearance of cyclins A and B and the increase in the activity of the G2/M phase cellular kinase cdc2 in herpes simplex virus 1-infected cells requires the expression of alpha 22/US1.5 and UL viral genes. *J Virol* 2000;74:8–15.
5. Advani SJ, Weichselbaum RR, Roizman B. E2F proteins are postranslationally modified concomitantly with a reduction in nuclear binding activity in cells infected with herpes simplex virus 1. *J Virol* 2000;74:7842–7850.
6. Advani SJ, Weichselbaum RR, Roizman B. The role of cdc2 in the expression of herpes simplex virus genes. *Proc Natl Acad Sci U S A* 2000;97:10996–11001.
7. Ali MA, Prakash SS, Jariwalla RJ. Localization of the antigenic sites and intrinsic protein kinase domain within a 300 amino acid segment of the ribonucleotide reductase large subunit from herpes simplex virus type 2. *Virology* 1992;187:360–367.
8. Alwine JC, Steinhart WL, Hill CW. Transcription of herpes simplex type 1 DNA in nuclei isolated from infected HEp-2 and KB cells. *Virology* 1974;60:302–307.
9. Anderson KP, Costa RH, Holland LE, Wagner EK. Characterization of herpes simplex virus type 1 RNA present in the absence of *de novo* protein synthesis. *J Virol* 1980;34:9–27.
10. Anderson WA, Magruder B, Kilbourne ED. Induced reactivation of herpes simplex virus in healed rabbit corneal leasions. *Proc Soc Exp Biol Med* 1961;107:628–632.
11. Aubert M, Blaho JA. The herpes simplex virus type 1 regulatory protein ICP27 is required for the prevention of apoptosis in infected human cells. *J Virol* 1999;73:2803–1813.
12. Aubert M, O'Toole J, Blaho JA. Induction and prevention of apoptosis in human HEp-2 cells by herpes simplex virus type 1. *J Virol* 1999;73:10359–10370.
13. Avitabile E, Di Gaeta S, Torrisi MR, et al. Redistribution of microtubules and Golgi apparatus in herpes simplex virus-infected cells and their role in viral exocytosis. *J Virol* 1995;69:7472–7482.
14. Bacchetti S, Evelegh MJ, Muirhead B. Identification and separation of the two subunits of the herpes simplex virus ribonucleotide reductase. *J Virol* 1986;57:1177–1181.
15. Baines JD, Koyama AH, Huang T, Roizman B. The UL21 gene products of herpes simplex virus 1 are dispensable for growth in cultured cells. *J Virol* 1994;68:2929–2936.
16. Baines JD, Roizman B. The open reading frames UL3, UL4, UL10, and UL16 are dispensable for the replication of herpes simplex virus 1 in cell culture. *J Virol* 1991;65:938–944.
17. Baines JD, Roizman B. The UL11 gene of herpes simplex virus 1 encodes a function that facilitates nucleocapsid envelopment and egress from cells. *J Virol* 1992;66:5168–5174.
18. Baines JD, Ward PL, Campadelli-Fiume G, Roizman B. The UL20 gene of herpes simplex virus 1 encodes a function necessary for viral egress. *J Virol* 1991;65:6414–6424.
19. Banfield BW, Leduc Y, Esford L, et al. Evidence for an interaction of herpes simplex virus with chondroitin sulfate proteoglycans during infection. *Virology* 1995;208:531–539.
20. Banks LM, Halliburton IW, Purifoy DJ, et al. Studies on the herpes simplex virus alkaline nuclease: Detection of type-common and type-specific epitopes on the enzyme. *J Gen Virol* 1985;66:1–14.
21. Batterson W, Furlong D, Roizman B. Molecular genetics of herpes simplex virus. VIII. Further characterization of a temperature-sensitive mutant defective in release of viral DNA and in other stages of the viral reproductive cycle. *J Virol* 1983;45:397–407.
22. Batterson W, Roizman B. Characterization of the herpes simplex virion-associated factor responsible for the induction of alpha genes. *J Virol* 1983;46:371–377.
23. Bayliss GJ, Marsden HS, Hay J. Herpes simplex virus proteins: DNA-binding proteins in infected cells and in the virus structure. *Virology* 1975;68:124–134.
24. Becker Y, Dym H, Sarov I. Herpes simplex virus DNA. *Virology* 1968;36:184–192.
25. Bergstrom T, Lycke E. Neuroinvasion by herpes simplex virus: An in vitro model for characterization of neurovirulent strains. *J Gen Virol* 1990;71:405–410.
26. Biswal N, Murray BK, Benyesh-Melnick M. Ribonucleotides in newly synthesized DNA of herpes simplex virus. *Virology* 1974;61:87–99.
27. Blaho JA, Michael N, Kang V, et al. Differences in the poly(ADP-ribosyl)ation patterns of ICP4, the herpes simplex virus major regulatory protein, in infected cells and in isolated nuclei. *J Virol* 1992;66:6398–6407.
28. Blaho JA, Mitchell C, Roizman B. An amino acid sequence shared by the herpes simplex virus 1 alpha regulatory proteins 0, 4, 22, and 27 predicts the nucleotidylylation of the UL21, UL31, UL47, and UL49 gene products. *J Biol Chem* 1994;269:17401–17410.
29. Blaho JA, Mitchell C, Roizman B. Guanylylation and adenylylation of the alpha regulatory proteins of herpes simplex virus require a viral beta or gamma function. *J Virol* 1993;67:3891–3900.
30. Blaho JA, Roizman B. ICP4, the major regulatory protein of herpes simplex virus, shares features common to GTP-binding proteins and is adenylated and guanylated. *J Virol* 1991;65:3759–3769.
31. Block TM, Deshmane SL, Masonis J, et al. An HSV LAT null mutant reactivates slowly from latent infection and makes small plaques on CV-1 monolayers. *Virology* 1993;192:618–630.
32. Block TM, Spivack JG, Steiner I, et al. A herpes simplex virus type 1 latency-associated transcript mutant reactivates with normal kinetics from latent infection [published erratum appears in *J Virol* 1990 Sep;64(9):4603]. *J Virol* 1990;64:3417–3426.
33. Bloom DC, Hill JM, Devi-Rao G, et al. A 348-base-pair region in the latency-associated transcript facilitates herpes simplex virus type 1 reactivation. *J Virol* 1996;70:2449–2459.
34. Blue WT, Winland RD, Stobbs DG, et al. Effects of adenosine monophosphate on the reactivation of latent herpes simplex virus type 1 infections of mice. *Antimicrob Agents Chemother* 1981;20:547–548.
35. Blyth WA, Hill TJ, Field HJ, Harbour DA. Reactivation of herpes simplex virus infection by ultraviolet light and possible involvement of prostaglandins. *J Gen Virol* 1976;33:547–550.
36. Boehmer PE, Dodson MS, Lehman IR. The herpes simplex virus type-1 origin binding protein: DNA helicase activity. *J Biol Chem* 1993;268:1220–1225.
37. Boehmer PE, Lehman IR. Herpes simplex virus DNA replication. *Annu Rev Biochem* 1997;66:347–384.
38. Boehmer PE, Lehman IR. Physical interaction between the herpes simplex virus 1 origin-binding protein and single-stranded DNA-binding protein ICP8. *Proc Natl Acad Sci U S A* 1993;90:8444–8448.
39. Bohenzky RA, Lagunoff M, Roizman B, et al. Two overlapping transcription units which extend across the L-S junction of herpes simplex virus type 1. *J Virol* 1995;69:2889–2897.
40. Bohenzky RA, Papavassiliou AG, Gelman IH, Silverstein S. Identification of a promoter mapping within the reiterated sequences that flank the herpes simplex virus type 1 UL region. *J Virol* 1993;67:632–642.
41. Bond VC, Person S. Fine structure physical map locations of alterations that affect cell fusion in herpes simplex virus type 1. *Virology* 1984;132:368–376.
42. Booy FP, Newcomb WW, Trus BL, et al. Liquid-crystalline, phage-like packing of encapsidated DNA in herpes simplex virus. *Cell* 1991;64:1007–1015.

43. Bortner C, Hernandez TR, Lehman IR, Griffith J. Herpes simplex virus 1 single-strand DNA-binding protein (ICP8) will promote homologous pairing and strand transfer. *J Mol Biol* 1993;231: 241–250.
44. Brandt CR, Kintner RL, Pumfery AM, et al. The herpes simplex virus ribonucleotide reductase is required for ocular virulence. *J Gen Virol* 1991;72:2043–2049.
45. Braun DK, Batterson W, Roizman B. Identification and genetic mapping of a herpes simplex virus capsid protein that binds DNA. *J Virol* 1984;50:645–648.
46. Brown CR, Nakamura MS, Mosca JD, et al. Herpes simplex virus trans-regulatory protein ICP27 stabilizes and binds to 3′ ends of labile mRNA. *J Virol* 1995;69:7187–7195.
47. Brown DG, Visse R, Sandhu G, et al. Crystal structures of the thymidine kinase from herpes simplex virus type-1 in complex with deoxythymidine and ganciclovir. *Nat Struct Biol* 1995;2:876–881.
48. Browne H, Bell S, Minson T, Wilson DW. An endoplasmic reticulum-retained herpes simplex virus glycoprotein H is absent from secreted virions: Evidence for reenvelopment during egress. *J Virol* 1996;70: 4311–4316.
49. Bruckner RC, Dutch RE, Zemelman BV, et al. Recombination *in vitro* between herpes simplex virus type 1 a sequences. *Proc Natl Acad Sci U S A* 1992;89:10950–10954.
50. Bruni R, Roizman B. Open reading frame P: A herpes simplex virus gene repressed during productive infection encodes a protein that binds a splicing factor and reduces synthesis of viral proteins made from spliced mRNA. *Proc Natl Acad Sci U S A* 1996;93: 10423–10427.
51. Buchman TG, Roizman B, Adams G, Stover BH. Restriction endonuclease fingerprinting of herpes simplex virus DNA: A novel epidemiological tool applied to a nosocomial outbreak. *J Infect Dis* 1978;138: 488–498.
52. Buchman TG, Roizman B, Nahmias AJ. Demonstration of exogenous genital reinfection with herpes simplex virus type 2 by restriction endonuclease fingerprinting of viral DNA. *J Infect Dis* 1979;140: 295–304.
53. Buchman TG, Simpson T, Nosal C, et al. The structure of herpes simplex virus DNA and its application to molecular epidemiology. *Ann N Y Acad Sci* 1980;354:279–290.
54. Bush M, Yager DR, Gao M, et al. Correct intranuclear localization of herpes simplex virus DNA polymerase requires the viral ICP8 DNA-binding protein. *J Virol* 1991;65:1082–1089.
55. Cabrera CV, Wohlenberg C, Openshaw H, et al. Herpes simplex virus DNA sequences in the CNS of latently infected mice. *Nature* 1980; 288:288–290.
56. Cameron JM, McDougall I, Marsden HS, et al. Ribonucleotide reductase encoded by herpes simplex virus is a determinant of the pathogenicity of the virus in mice and a valid antiviral target. *J Gen Virol* 1988;69:2607–2612.
57. Campadelli-Fiume G. Virus receptor arrays, CD46 and human herpesvirus 6. *Trends Microbiol* 2000;10:436–438.
58. Campadelli-Fiume G, Arsenakis M, Farabegoli F, Roizman B. Entry of herpes simplex virus 1 in BJ cells that constitutively express viral glycoprotein D is by endocytosis and results in degradation of the virus. *J Virol* 1988;62:159–167.
59. Campadelli-Fiume G, Brandimarti R, Di Lazzaro C, et al. Fragmentation and dispersal of Golgi proteins and redistribution of glycoproteins and glycolipids processed through Golgi following infection with herpes simplex virus 1. *Proc Natl Acad Sci U S A* 1993;90: 2798–2802.
60. Campadelli-Fiume G, Serafini-Cessi F. Processing of the oligosaccharide chains of herpes simplex virus type 1 glycoproteins. In: Roizman B, ed. *The herpesviruses,* vol. 3. New York: Plenum, 1985: 357–382.
61. Campbell MEM, Palfreyman JW, Preston CM. Identification of herpes simplex virus DNA sequences which encode a trans-acting polypeptide responsible for stimulation of immediate early transcription. *J Mol Biol* 1984;180:1–19.
62. Caradonna S, Worrad D, Lirette R. Isolation of a herpes simplex virus cDNA encoding the DNA repair enzyme uracil-DNA glycosylase. *J Virol* 1987;61:3040–3047.
63. Carrozza M, DeLuca N. Interactions of the viral activator protein ICP4 with TFIID through TAF250. *Mol Cell Biol* 1996;16: 3085–3093.
64. Carter KL, Roizman B. Alternatively spliced mRNAs predicted to yield frame-shift proteins and stable intron 1 RNAs of the herpes simplex virus 1 regulatory gene alpha 0 accumulate in the cytoplasm of infected cells. *Proc Natl Acad Sci U S A* 1996;93:12535–12540.
65. Carton CA, Kilbourne ED. Activation of latent herpes simplex by trigeminal sensory-root section. *N Engl J Med* 1952;246:172–176.
66. Cassady KA, Gross M, Roizman B. The herpes simplex virus US11 protein effectively compensates for the gamma1(34.5) gene if present before activation of protein kinase R by precluding its phosphorylation and that of the alpha subunit of eukaryotic translation initiation factor 2. *J Virol* 1998;72:8620–8626.
67. Cassady KA, Gross M, Roizman B. The second-site mutation in the herpes simplex virus recombinants lacking the gamma 134.5 genes precludes shutoff of protein synthesis by blocking the phosphorylation of eIF-2 alpha. *J Virol* 1998;72:7005–7011.
68. Centifanto-Fitzgerald YM, Varnell ED, Kaufman HE. Initial herpes simplex virus type 1 infection prevents ganglionic superinfection by other strains. *Infect Immun* 1982;35:1125–1132.
69. Challberg MD. A method for identifying the viral genes required for herpesvirus DNA replication. *Proc Natl Acad Sci U S A* 1986;83: 9094–9098.
70. Chang Y, Cesarman E, Pessin MS, et al. Identification of herpesvirus-like DNA sequences in AIDs-associated kaposis sarcoma. *Science* 1994;266:1865–1869.
71. Chang YE, Roizman B. The product of the UL31 gene of herpes simplex virus 1 is a nuclear phosphoprotein which partitions with the nuclear matrix. *J Virol* 1993;67:6348–6356.
72. Chapman CJ, Harris JD, Hardwicke MA, et al. Promoter-independent activation of heterologous virus gene expression by the herpes simplex virus immediate-early protein ICP27. *Virology* 1992;186:573–578.
73. Chee M, Rudolph SA, Plachter B, et al. Identification of the major capsid protein gene of human cytomegalovirus. *J Virol* 1989;63: 1345–1353.
74. Chen J, Silverstein S. Herpes simplex viruses with mutations in the gene encoding ICP0 are defective in gene expression. *J Virol* 1992;66: 2916–2927.
75. Chen SH, Kramer MF, Schaffer PA, Coen DM. A viral function represses accumulation of transcripts from productive-cycle genes in mouse ganglia latently infected with herpes simplex virus. *J Virol* 1997;71:5878–5884.
76. Chen YM, Knipe DM. A dominant mutant form of the herpes simplex virus ICP8 protein decreases viral late gene transcription. *Virology* 1996;221:281–290.
77. Chiou HC, Weller SK, Coen DM. Mutations in the herpes simplex virus major DNA-binding protein gene leading to altered sensitivity to DNA polymerase inhibitors. *Virology* 1985;145:213–226.
78. Chou J, Kern ER, Whitley RJ, Roizman B. Mapping of herpes simplex virus-1 neurovirulence to gamma 134.5, a gene nonessential for growth in culture. *Science* 1990;250:1262–1266.
79. Chou J, Roizman B. Characterization of DNA sequence-common and sequence-specific proteins binding to cis-acting sites for cleavage of the terminal a sequence of the herpes simplex virus 1 genome. *J Virol* 1989;63:1059–1068.
80. Chou J, Roizman B. The gamma 1(34.5) gene of herpes simplex virus 1 precludes neuroblastoma cells from triggering total shutoff of protein synthesis characteristic of programed cell death in neuronal cells. *Proc Natl Acad Sci U S A* 1992;89:3266–3270.
81. Chou J, Roizman B. Herpes simplex virus 1 gamma(1)34.5 gene function, which blocks the host response to infection, maps in the homologous domain of the genes expressed during growth arrest and DNA damage. *Proc Natl Acad Sci U S A* 1994;91:5247–5251.
82. Chou J, Roizman B. The herpes simplex virus 1 gene for ICP34.5, which maps in inverted repeats, is conserved in several limited-passage isolates but not in strain 17syn+. *J Virol* 1990;64:1014–1020.
83. Chou J, Roizman B. Isomerization of herpes simplex virus 1 genome: Identification of the cis-acting and recombination sites within the domain of the a sequence. *Cell* 1985;41:803–811.
84. Chou J, Roizman B. The terminal a sequence of the herpes simplex virus genome contains the promoter of a gene located in the repeat sequences of the L component. *J Virol* 1986;57:629–637.
85. Chowdhury SI, Batterson W. Transinhibition of herpes simplex virus replication by an inducible cell-resident gene encoding a dysfunctional VP19C capsid protein. *Virus Res* 1994;33:67–87.
86. Chu CT, Parris DS, Dixon RA, et al. Hydroxylamine mutagenesis of

HSV DNA and DNA fragments: Introductin of mutations into selected regions of the viral genome. *Virology* 1979;98:168–181.
87. Chung TD, Wymer JP, Smith CC, et al. Protein kinase activity associated with the large subunit of herpes simplex virus type 2 ribonucleotide reductase (ICP10). *J Virol* 1989;63:3389–3398.
88. Church GA, Wilson DW. Study of herpes simplex virus maturation during a synchronous wave of assembly. *J Virol* 1997;71:3603–3612.
89. Clements GB, Stow ND. A herpes simplex virus type 1 mutant containing a deletion within immediate early gene 1 is latency-competent in mice. *J Gen Virol* 1989;70:2501–2506.
90. Clements JB, Watson RJ, Wilkie NM. Temporal regulation of herpes simplex virus type 1 transcription: Location of transcripts on the viral genome. *Cell* 1977;12:275–285.
91. Cocchi F, Menotti L, Dubreuil P, et al. Cell-to-cell spread of wild-type herpes simplex virus type 1, but not of syncytial strains, is mediated by the immunoglobulin-like receptors that mediate virion entry, nectin 1 (PRR1/HveC/HIgR) and nectin 2 (PRR2/HveB). *J Virol* 2000;74: 3909–3917.
92. Cocchi F, Menotti L, Mirandola P, et al. The ectodomain of a novel member of the immunoglobulin subfamily related to the poliovirus receptor has the attributes of a bona fide receptor for herpes simplex virus types 1 and 2 in human cells. *J Virol* 1998;72:9992–10002.
93. Coen DM, Kosz-Vnenchak M, Jacobson JG, et al. Thymidine kinase-negative herpes simplex virus mutants establish latency in mouse trigeminal ganglia but do not reactivate. *Proc Natl Acad Sci U S A* 1989;86:4736–4740.
94. Coen DM, Weinheimer SP, McKnight SL. A genetic approach to promoter recognition during trans induction of viral gene expression. *Science* 1986;234:53–59.
95. Cohen GH, Ponce de Leon M, Diggelmann H, et al. Structural analysis of the capsid polypeptides of herpes simplex virus types 1 and 2. *J Virol* 1980;34:521–531.
96. Cohen GH, Vaughan RK, Lawrence WC. Deoxyribonucleic acid synthesis in synchronized mammalian KB cells infected with herpes simplex virus. *J Virol* 1971;7:783–791.
97. Colberg-Poley AM, Isom HC, Rapp F. Involvement of an early human cytomegalovirus function in reactivation of quiescent herpes simplex virus type 2. *J Virol* 1981;37:1051–1059.
98. Conley AJ, Knipe DM, Jones PC, Roizman B. Molecular genetics of herpes simplex virus. VII. Characterization of a temperature-sensitive mutant produced by in vitro mutagenesis and defective in DNA synthesis and accumulation of gamma polypeptides. *J Virol* 1981;37: 191–206.
99. Conner J, Macfarlane J, Lankinen H, Marsden H. The unique N terminus of the herpes simplex virus type 1 large subunit is not required for ribonucleotide reductase activity. *J Gen Virol* 1992;73:103–112.
100. Cook ML, Stevens JG. Replication of varicella-zoster virus in cell cultures: An ultrastructural study. *J Ultrastruct Res* 1970;32:334–350.
101. Costa RH, Devi BG, Anderson KP, et al. Characterization of a major late herpes simplex virus type 1 mRNA. *J Virol* 1981;38:483–496.
102. Costanzo F, Campadelli-Fiume G, Foa-Tomasi L, Cassai E. Evidence that herpes simplex virus DNA is transcribed by cellular RNA polymerase B. *J Virol* 1977;21:996–1001.
103. Crute JJ, Mocarski ES, Lehman IR. A DNA helicase induced by herpes simplex virus type 1. *Nucleic Acids Res* 1988;16:6585–6596.
104. Cunningham C, Davison AJ. A cosmid-based system for constructing mutants of herpes simplex virus type 1. *Virology* 1993;197:116–124.
105. Cunningham C, Davison AJ, Dolan A, et al. The UL13 virion protein of herpes simplex virus type 1 is phosphorylated by a novel virus-induced protein kinase. *J Gen Virol* 1992;73:303–311.
106. Cushing H. Surgical aspects of major neuralgia of trigeminal nerve: Report of 20 cases of operation upon the gasserian ganglion with anatomic and physiologic notes on the consequences of its removal. *JAMA* 1905;4:1002–1008.
107. Da Costa XJ, Jones CA, Knipe DM. Immunization against genital herpes with a vaccine virus that has defects in productive and latent infection. *Proc Natl Acad Sci U S A* 1999;96:6994–6998.
108. Darlington RW, James C. Biological and morphological aspects of the growth of equine abortion virus. *J Bacteriol* 1966;92:250–257.
109. Darlington RW, Moss LH. The envelope of herpesvirus. *Prog Med Virol* 1969;11:16–45.
110. Davison AJ, Wilkie NM. Nucleotide sequences of the joint between the L and S segments of herpes simplex virus types 1 and 2. *J Gen Virol* 1981;55:315–331.
111. Davison MD, Rixon FJ, Davison AJ. Identification of genes encoding two capsid proteins (VP24 and VP26) of herpes simplex virus type 1. *J Gen Virol* 1992;73:2709–2713.
112. de Bruyn Kops A, Knipe DM. Formation of DNA replication structures in herpes virus-infected cells requires a viral DNA binding protein. *Cell* 1988;55:857–868.
113. de Bruyn Kops A, Knipe DM. Preexisting nuclear architecture defines the intranuclear location of herpesvirus DNA replication structures. *J Virol* 1994;68:3512–3526.
114. de Bruyn Kops A, Uprichard SL, Chen M, Knipe DM. Comparison of the intranuclear distributions of herpes simplex virus proteins involved in different viral functions. *Virology* 1998;252:162–178.
115. De Bruyne T, Pieters L, Witvrouw M, et al. Biological evaluation of proanthocyanidin dimers and related polyphenols. *J Nat Prod* 1999; 62:954–8.
116. Deb S, Doelberg M. A 67-base-pair segment from the Ori-S region of herpes simplex virus type 1 encodes origin function. *J Virol* 1988;62: 2516–2519.
117. Debroy C, Pederson N, Person S. Nucleotide sequence of a herpes simplex virus type 1 gene that causes cell fusion. *Virology* 1985;145: 36–48.
118. Deiss LP, Chou J, Frenkel N. Functional domains within the a sequence involved in the cleavage-packaging of herpes simplex virus DNA. *J Virol* 1986;59:605–618.
119. Deiss LP, Frenkel N. Herpes simplex virus amplicon: Cleavage of concatemeric DNA is linked to packaging and involves amplification of the terminally reiterated a sequence. *J Virol* 1986;57:933–941.
120. Delius H, Clements JB. A partial denaturation map of herpes simplex virus type 1 DNA: Evidence for inversions of the unique DNA regions. *J Gen Virol* 1976;33:125–133.
121. DeLuca N, Bzik D, Person S, Snipes W. Early events in herpes simplex virus type 1 infection: photosensitivity of fluorescein isothiocyanate-treated virions. *Proc Natl Acad Sci U S A* 1981;78:912–916.
122. DeLuca NA, McCarthy AM, Schaffer PA. Isolation and characterization of deletion mutants of herpes simplex virus type 1 in the gene encoding immediate-early regulatory protein ICP4. *J Virol* 1985;56: 558–570.
123. DeLuca NA, Schaffer PA. Physical and functional domains of the herpes simplex virus transcriptional regulatory protein ICP4. *J Virol* 1988;62:732–743.
124. Desai P, Watkins SC, Person S. The size and symmetry of B capsids of herpes simplex virus type 1 are determined by the gene products of the UL26 open reading frame. *J Virol* 1994;68:5365–5374.
125. Devi-Rao GB, Goodart SA, Hecht LM, et al. Relationship between polyadenylated and nonpolyadenylated herpes simplex virus type 1 latency-associated transcripts. *J Virol* 1991;65:2179–2190.
126. DiIanni CL, Drier DA, Deckman IC, et al. Identification of the herpes simplex virus-1 protease cleavage sites by direct sequence analysis of autoproteolytic cleavage products. *J Biol Chem* 1993;268: 2048–2051.
127. Dilber MS, Phelan A, Aints A, et al. Intracellular delivery of thymidine kinase prodrug activating enzyme by the herpes simplex virus protein, VP22. *Gene Ther* 1999;6:12–21.
128. Dingwell KS, Brunetti CR, Hendricks RL, et al. Herpes simplex virus glycoproteins E and I facilitate cell-to-cell spread in vivo and across junctions of cultured cells. *J Virol* 1994;68:834–845.
129. Dingwell KS, Johnson DC. The herpes simplex virus gE-gI complex facilitates cell-to-cell spread and binds to components of cell junctions. *J Virol* 1998;72:8933–8942.
130. Dixon RA, Schaffer PA. Fine-structure mapping and functional analysis of temperature-sensitive mutants in the gene encoding the herpes simplex virus type 1 immediate early protein VP175. *J Virol* 1980; 36:189–203.
131. Doerig C, Pizer LI, Wilcox CL. An antigen encoded by the latency-associated transcript in neuronal cell cultures latently infected with herpes simplex virus type 1. *J Virol* 1991;65:2724–2727.
132. Dolan A, Jamieson FE, Cunnigham C, et al. The genome sequence of herpes simplex virus type 2. *J Virol* 1998;72:2010–2021.
133. Dutch RE, Bruckner RC, Mocarski ES, Lehman IR. Herpes simplex virus type 1 recombination: Role of DNA replication and viral a sequences. *J Virol* 1992;66:277–285.
134. Dutch RE, Lehman IR. Renaturation of complementary DNA strands by herpes simplex virus type 1 ICP8. *J Virol* 1993;67:6945–6949.
135. Dutch RE, Zemelman BV, Lehman IR. Herpes simplex virus type 1

recombination: The Uc-DR1 region is required for high-level a-sequence-mediated recombination. *J Virol* 1994;68:3733–3741.

136. Ehmann GL, McLean TI, Bachenheimer SL. Herpes simplex virus type 1 infection imposes a G(1)/S block in asynchronously growing cells and prevents G(1) entry in quiescent cells. *Virology* 2000;267:335–349.
137. Ejercito PM, Kieff ED, Roizman B. Characterization of herpes simplex virus strains differing in their effect on social behavior of infected cells. *J Gen Virol* 1968;2:357–364.
138. Elgadi MM, Smiley JR. Picornavirus internal ribosome entry site elements target RNA cleavage events induced by the herpes simplex virus virion host shutoff protein. *J Virol* 1999;73:9222–9231.
139. Elias P, Lehman IR. Interaction of origin binding protein with an origin of replication of herpes simplex virus 1. *Proc Natl Acad Sci U S A* 1988;85:2959–2963.
140. Elias P, O'Donnell ME, Mocarski ES, Lehman IR. A DNA binding protein specific for an origin of replication of herpes simplex virus type 1. *Proc Natl Acad Sci U S A* 1986;83:6322–6326.
141. Elliott G, Mouzakitis G, O'Hare P. VP16 interacts via its activation domain with VP22, a tegument protein of herpes simplex virus, and is relocated to a novel macromolecular assembly in coexpressing cells. *J Virol* 1995;69:7932–7941.
142. Elliott G, O'Hare P. Intercellular trafficking and protein delivery by a herpesvirus structural protein. *Cell* 1997;88:223–233.
143. Embretson J, Zupanicic M, Beneke J, et al. Analysis of human immunodeficiency virus-infected tissues by amplification and in situ hybridization reveals latent and permissive infections at single-cell resolution. *Proc Natl Acad Sci U S A* 1993;90(1):357–361.
144. Enquist LW, Husak PJ, Banfield BW, Smith GA. Infection and spread of alphaviruses in the nervous system. *Adv Virus Res* 1999;51: 237–347.
145. Epstein MA. 1962. Observations on the mode of release of herpes virus from infected HeLa cells. *J Cell Biol* 1962;12:589–597.
146. Everett R, O'Hare P, O'Rourke D, et al. Point mutations in the herpes simplex virus type 1 Vmw110 RING finger helix affect activation of gene expression, viral growth, and interaction with PML-containing nuclear structures. *J Virol* 1995;69:7339–7344.
147. Everett RD. Construction and characterization of herpes simplex type 1 viruses without introns in immediate early gene 1. *J Gen Virol* 1991; 72:651–659.
148. Everett RD. Transactivation of transcription by herpes virus products: Requirement for two HSV-1 immediate-early polypeptides for maximum activity. *EMBO J* 1984;3:3135–3141.
149. Everett RD, Earnshaw WC, Findlay J, Lomonte P. Specific destruction of kinetochore protein CENP-C and disruption of cell division by herpes simplex virus immediate-early protein Vmw110. *EMBO J* 1999; 18:1526–1538.
150. Everett RD, Freemont P, Saitoh H, et al. The disruption of ND10 during herpes simplex virus infection correlates with the Vmw110- and proteasome-dependent loss of several PML isoforms. *J Virol* 1998;72: 6581–6591.
151. Everett RD, Maul GG. HSV-1 IE protein VMW 110 causes redistribution of PML. *EMBO J* 1994;13:5062–5069.
152. Everett RD, Meredith M, Orr A, et al. A novel ubiquitin-specific protease is dynamically associated with the PML nuclear domain and binds to a herpesvirus regulatory protein. *EMBO J* 1997;16:566–577.
153. Everett RD, Orr A, Elliott M. High level expression and purification of herpes simplex virus type 1 immediate early polypeptide Vmw110. *Nucleic Acids Res* 1991;19:6155–6161.
154. Faber SW, Wilcox KW. Association of the herpes simplex virus regulatory protein ICP4 with specific nucleotide sequences in DNA. *Nucleic Acids Res* 1986;14:6067–6083.
155. Falkenberg M, Bushnell DA, Elias P, Lehman IR. The UL8 subunit of the heterotrimeric herpes simplex virus type 1 helicase-primase is required for the unwinding of single strand DNA-binding protein (ICP8)-coated DNA substrates. *J Biol Chem* 1997;272:22766–22770.
156. Farrell MJ, Dobson AT, Feldman LT. Herpes simplex virus latency-associated transcript is a stable intron. *Proc Natl Acad Sci U S A* 1991;88:790–794.
157. Fenwick M, Morse LS, Roizman B. Anatomy of herpes simplex virus DNA. XI. Apparent clustering of functions effecting rapid inhibition of host DNA and protein synthesis. *J Virol* 1979;29:825–827.
158. Fenwick M, Roizman B. Regulation of herpesvirus macromolecular synthesis. VI. Synthesis and modification of viral polypeptides in enucleated cells. *J Virol* 1977;22:720–725.
159. Fenwick ML, Owen SA. On the control of immediate early (alpha) mRNA survival in cells infected with herpes simplex virus. *J Gen Virol* 1988;69:2869–2877.
160. Fenwick ML, Walker MJ. Suppression of the synthesis of cellular macromolecules by herpes simplex virus. *J Gen Virol* 1978;41:37–51.
161. Field HJ, Darby G. Pathogenicity in mice of strains of herpes simplex virus which are resistant to acyclovir in vitro and in vivo. *Antimicrob Agents Chemother* 1980;17:209–216.
162. Fierer DS, Challberg MD. Purification and characterization of UL9, the herpes simplex virus type 1 origin-binding protein. *J Virol* 1992; 66:3986–3995.
163. Flanagan WM, Papavassiliou AG, Rice M, et al. Analysis of the herpes simplex virus type 1 promoter controlling the expression of UL38, a true late gene involved in capsid assembly. *J Virol* 1991;65:769–786.
164. Forrester A, Farrell H, Wilkinson G, et al. Construction and properties of a mutant of herpes simplex virus type 1 with glycoprotein H coding sequences deleted. *J Virol* 1992;66:341–348.
165. Frame MC, Marsden HS, Dutia BM. The ribonucleotide reductase induced by herpes simplex virus type 1 involves minimally a complex of two polypeptides (136K and 38K). *J Gen Virol* 1985;66:1581–1587.
166. Frame MC, Purves FC, McGeoch DJ, et al. Identification of the herpes simplex virus protein kinase as the product of viral gene US3. *J Gen Virol* 1987;68:2699–2704.
167. Fraser JW, Deatly AM, Mellerick MI, et al. Molecular biology of latent HSV-1. In: Lopez C, Roizman B, eds. *Human herpesvirus infections: Pathogenesis, diagnosis, and treatment.* New York: Raven, 1986:39–54.
168. Frenkel N, Locker H, Batterson W, et al. Anatomy of herpes simplex virus DNA. VI. Defective DNA originates from the S component. *J Virol* 1976;20:527–531.
169. Frenkel N, Roizman B. Separation of the herpesvirus deoxyribonucleic acid on sedimentation in alkaline gradients. *J Virol* 1972;10: 565–572.
170. Frink RJ, Anderson KP, Wagner EK. Herpes simplex virus type 1 HindIII fragment L encodes spliced and complementary mRNA species. *J Virol* 1981;39:559–572.
171. Furlong D, Swift H, Roizman B. Arrangement of herpesvirus deoxyribonucleic acid in the core. *J Virol* 1972;10:1071–1074.
172. Fyfe JA, Keller PM, Furman PA, et al. Thymidine kinase from herpes simplex virus phosphorylates the new antiviral compound, 9-(2-hydroxyethoxymethyl)guanine. *J Biol Chem* 1978;253:8721–8727.
173. Gaffney DF, McLauchlan J, Whitton JL, Clements JB. A modular system for the assay of transcription regulatory signals: The sequence TAATGARAT is required for herpes simplex virus immediate early gene activation. *Nucleic Acids Res* 1985;13:7847–7863.
174. Galvan V, Brandimarti R, Munger J, Roizman B. Bcl-2 blocks a capase-dependent pathway of apoptosis activated by herpes simplex virus 1 infection in HEp-2 cells. *J Virol* 2000;74:1931–1938.
175. Galvan V, Brandimarti R, Roizman B. Herpes simplex virus 1 blocks caspase-3-independent and caspase-dependent pathways to cell death. *J Virol* 1999;73:3219–3226.
176. Galvan V, Roizman B. Herpes simplex virus 1 induces and blocks apoptosis at multiple steps during infection and protects cells from exogenous inducers in a cell-type-dependent manner. *Proc Natl Acad Sci U S A* 1998;95:3931–3936.
177. Gao M, Knipe DM. Potential role for herpes simplex virus ICP8 DNA replication protein in stimulation of late gene expression. *J Virol* 1991; 65:2666–2675.
178. Gao M, Matusick-Kumar L, Hurlburt W, et al. The protease of herpes simplex virus type 1 is essential for functional capsid formation and viral growth. *J Virol* 1994;68:3702–3712.
179. Garber DA, Beverley SM, Coen DM. Demonstration of circularization of herpes simplex virus DNA following infection using pulsed field gel electrophoresis. *Virology* 1993;197:459–462.
180. Garber DA, Schaffer PA, Knipe DM. A LAT-associated function reduces productive-cycle gene expression during acute infection of murine sensory neurons with herpes simplex virus type 1. *J Virol* 1997;71:5885–5893.
181. Gelman IH, Silverstein S. Herpes simplex virus immediate-early promoters are responsive to virus and cell trans-acting factors. *J Virol* 1987;61:2286–2296.
182. Gelman IH, Silverstein S. Identification of immediate early genes from herpes simplex virus that transactivate the virus thymidine kinase gene. *Proc Natl Acad Sci U S A* 1985;82:5265–5269.

183. Geraghty RJ, Krummenacher C, Cohen GH, et al. Entry of alphaherpesviruses mediated by poliovirus receptor-related protein 1 and poliovirus recptor. *Science* 1998;280:1618–1620.
184. Gershon AA, Sherman DL, Zhu Z, et al. Intracellular transport of newly synthesized varicella-zoster virus: Final envelopment in the trans-Golgi network. *J Virol* 1994;68:6372–6390.
185. Gerster T, Roeder RG. A herpesvirus trans-activating protein interacts with transcription factor OTF-1 and other cellular proteins. *Proc Natl Acad Sci U S A* 1988;85:6347–6351.
186. Gibbs JS, Chiou HC, Bastow KF, et al. Identification of amino acids in herpes simplex virus DNA polymerase involved in substrate and drug recognition. *Proc Natl Acad Sci U S A* 1988;85:6672–6676.
187. Gibson W, Roizman B. Compartmentalization of spermine and spermidine in the herpes simplex virion. *Proc Natl Acad Sci U S A* 1971; 68:2818–2821.
188. Gibson W, Roizman B. Proteins specified by herpes simplex virus. X. Staining and radiolabeling properties of B capsid and virion proteins in polyacrylamide gels. *J Virol* 1974;113:155–165.
189. Gibson W, Roizman B. Proteins specified by herpes simplex virus. VIII. Characterization and composition of multiple capsid forms of subtypes 1 and 2. *J Virol* 1972;10:1044–1052.
190. Gibson W, Roizman B. The structural and metabolic involvement of polyamines with herpes simplex virus. In: Russell DH, ed. *Polyamines in normal and neoplastic growth.* New York: Raven, 1973:123–135.
191. Godowski PJ, Knipe DM. Identification of a herpes simplex virus function that represses late gene expression from parental viral genomes. *J Virol* 1985;55:357–365.
192. Godowski PJ, Knipe DM. Mutations in the major DNA-binding protein gene of herpes simplex virus type 1 result in increased levels of viral gene expression. *J Virol* 1983;47:478–486.
193. Godowski PJ, Knipe DM. Transcriptional control of herpesvirus gene expression: Gene functions required for positive and negative regulation. *Proc Natl Acad Sci U S A* 1986;83:256–260.
194. Goldstein DJ, Weller SK. Herpes simplex virus type 1-induced ribonucleotide reductase activity is dispensable for virus growth and DNA synthesis: Isolation and characterization of an ICP6 lacZ insertion mutant. *J Virol* 1988;62:196–205.
195. Goodpasture EW. Herpectic infections with special reference to involvement of the nervous system. *Medicine* (Baltimore) 1929;8: 223–243.
196. Gordon YJ, McKnigt JLC, Ostrove JM, et al. Host species and strain differences affect the ability of an HSV-1 ICP0 deletion mutant to establish latency and spontaneously reactivate in vivo. *Virology* 1990; 178:469–477.
197. Greaves R, O'Hare P. Separation of requirements for protein-DNA complex assembly from those for functional activity in the herpes simplex virus regulatory protein Vmw65. *J Virol* 1989;63:1641–1650.
198. Greaves RF, O'Hare P. Structural requirements in the herpes simplex virus type 1 transactivator Vmw65 for interaction with the cellular octamer-binding protein and target TAATGARAT sequences. *J Virol* 1990;64:2716–2724.
199. Guzowski JF, Singh J, Wagner EK. Transcriptional activation of the herpes virus type 1 UL38 promoter conferred by the cis-acting downstream activation sequence is mediated by a cellular transcription factor. *J Virol* 1994;68:7774–7789.
200. Guzowski JF, Wagner EK. Mutational analysis of the herpes simplex virus type 1 strict late UL38 promoter/leader reveals two regions critical in transcriptional regulation. *J Virol* 1993;67:5098–5108.
201. Hamatake RK, Bifano M, Hurlburt WW, Tenney DJ. 1997. A functional interaction of ICP8, the herpes simplex virus single-stranded DNA-binding protein, and the helicase-primase complex that is dependent on the presence of the UL8 subunit. *J Gen Virol* 1997;78:857–865.
202. Hammer SM, Buchman TG, D'Angelo LJ, et al. Temporal cluster of herpes simplex encephalitis: Investigation by restriction endonuclease cleavage of viral DNA. *J Infect Dis* 1980;141:436–440.
203. Hann LE, Cook WJ, Uprichard SL, et al. The role of herpes simplex virus ICP27 in the regulation of UL24 gene expression by differential polyadenylation. *J Virol* 1998;72:7709–7714.
204. Harbour DA, Hill TJ, Blyth WA. Recurrent herpes simplex in the mouse: Inflammation in the skin and activation of virus in the ganglia following peripheral stimulation. *J Gen Virol* 1983;64:1491–1498.
205. Hardwick J, Romanowski E, Araullo-Cruz T, Gordon YJ. Timolol promotes reactivation of latent HSV-1 in the mouse iontophoresis model. *Invest Ophthalmol Vis Sci* 1987;28:580–584.
206. Hardwicke MA, Sandri-Goldin RM. The herpes simplex virus regulatory protein ICP27 contributes to the decrease in cellular mRNA levels during infection. *J Virol* 1994;68:4797–4810.
207. Hardwicke MA, Schaffer PA. Differential effects of nerve growth factor and dexamethasone on herpes simplex virus type 1 oriL- and oriS-dependent DNA replication in PC12 cells. *J Virol* 1997;71: 3580–2587.
208. Hardy WR, Sandri-Goldin RM. Herpes simplex virus inhibits host cell splicing, and regulatory protein ICP27 is required for this effect. *J Virol* 1994;68:7790–7799.
209. Hay J, Koteles GJ, Keir HM, Subak-Sharpe H. Herpes virus specified ribonucleic acids. *Nature* 1966;210:387–390.
210. Hayward GS, Frenkel N, Roizman B. Anatomy of herpes simplex virus DNA: Strain differences and heterogeneity in the locations of restriction endonuclease cleavage sites. *Proc Natl Acad Sci U S A* 1975;72:1768–1772.
211. Hayward GS, Jacob RJ, Wadsworth SC, Roizman B. Anatomy of herpes simplex virus DNA: Evidence for four populations of molecules that differ in the relative orientations of their long and short components. *Proc Natl Acad Sci U S A* 1975;72:4243–4247.
212. He B, Chou J, Brandimarti R, et al. Suppression of the phenotype of gamma(1)34.5-herpes simplex virus 1: Failure of activated RNA-dependent protein kinase to shut off protein synthesis is associated with a deletion in the domain of the alpha47 gene. *J Virol* 1997;71: 6049–6054.
213. He B, Chou J, Liebermann DA, et al. The carboxyl terminus of the murine MyD116 gene substitutes for the corresponding domain of the gamma(1)34.5 gene of herpes simplex virus to preclude the premature shutoff of total protein synthesis in infected human cells. *J Virol* 1996; 70:84–90.
214. He B, Gross M, Roizman B. The gamma134.5 protein of herpes simplex virus 1 has the structural and functional attributes of a protein phosphatase 1 regulatory subunit and is present in a high molecular weight complex with the enzyme in infected cells. *J Biol Chem* 1998; 273:20737–20743.
215. He B, Gross M, Roizman B. The gamma (1)34.5 protein of herpes simplex virus 1 complexes with protein phosphatase 1 alpha to dephosphorylate the alpha subunit of the eukaryotic translation initiation factor 2 and preclude the shutoff of protein synthesis by double-stranded RNA-activated protein kinase. *Proc Natl Acad Sci U S A* 1997;94:843–848.
216. Heine JW, Honess RW, Cassai E, Roizman B. Proteins specified by herpes simplex virus. XII. The virion polypeptides of type 1 strains. *J Virol* 1974;14:640–651.
217. Heine UI. 1974. Intranuclear viruses. In: Busch H, ed. *The cell nucleus.* New York: Academic Press, 1974:489.
218. Hernandez TR, Lehman IR. Functional interaction between the herpes simplex-1 DNA polymerase and UL42 protein. *J Biol Chem* 1990; 265:11227–11232.
219. Hill JM, Gebhardt BM, Wen R, et al. Quantitation of herpes simplex virus type 1 DNA and latency-associated transcripts in rabbit trigeminal ganglia demonstrates a stable reservoir of viral nucleic acids during latency. *J Virol* 1996;70:3137–3141.
220. Hill JM, Sedarati F, Javier RT, et al. Herpes simplex virus latent phase transcription facilitates in vivo reactivation. *Virology* 1990;174: 117–125.
221. Hill TJ, Blyth WA, Harbour DA. Recurrent herpes simplex in mice: Topical treatment with acyclovir cream. *Antiviral Res* 1982;2:135–146.
222. Hill TJ, Blyth WA, Harbour DA. Trauma to the skin causes recurrence of herpes simplex in the mouse. *J Gen Virol* 1978;39:21–28.
223. Hilton MJ, Mounghane D, McLean T, et al. Induction by herpes simplex virus of free and heteromeric forms of E2F transcription factor. *Virology* 1995;213:624–638.
224. Hobbs WE II, DeLuca NA. Perturbation of cell cycle progression and cellular gene expression as a function of herpes simplex virus ICP0. *J Virol* 1999;73:8245–8255.
225. Hoggan MD, Roizman B. The isolation and properties of a variant of herpes simplex producing multinucleated giant cells in monolayer cultures in the prescence of antibody. *Am J Hyg* 1959;70:208–219.
226. Holland LE, Sandri-Goldin RM, Goldin AL, et al. Transcriptional and genetic analyses of the herpes simplex virus type 1 genome: Coordinates 0.29 to 0.45. *J Virol* 1984;49:947–959.
227. Homa FL, Brown JC. Capsid assembly and DNA packaging in herpes simplex virus. *Rev Med Virol* 1997;7:107–122.

228. Homa FL, Glorioso JC, Levine M. A specific 15-bp TATA box promoter element is required for expression of a herpes simplex virus type 1 late gene. *Genes Dev* 1988;2:40–53.
229. Homa FL, Otal TM, Glorioso JC, Levine M. Transcriptional control signals of a herpes simplex virus type 1 late (gamma 2) gene lie within bases −34 to +124 relative to the 5′ terminus of the mRNA. *Mol Cell Biol* 1986;6:3652–3666.
230. Honess RW, Roizman B. Regulation of herpesvirus macro-molecular synthesis. I. Cascade regulation of the synthesis of three groups of viral proteins. *J Virol* 1974;14:8–19.
231. Honess RW, Roizman B. 1975. Regulation of herpesvirus macromolecular synthesis: Sequential transition of polypeptide synthesis requires functional viral polypeptides. *Proc Natl Acad Sci U S A* 1975; 72:1276–1280.
232. Honess RW, Watson DH. Herpes simplex virus-specific polypeptides studied by polyacrylamide gel electrophoresis of immune precipitates. *J Gen Virol* 1974;22:171–185.
233. Hong Z, Beaudet-Miller M, Durkin J, et al. Identification of a minimal hydrophobic domain in the herpes simplex virus type 1 scaffolding protein which is required for interaction with the major capsid protein. *J Virol* 1996;70:533–540.
234. Hoog SS, Smith WW, Qiu X, et al. Active site cavity of herpesvirus protesase revealed by the crystal structure of herpes simplex virus protease/inhibitor complex. *Biochemistry* 1997;36:14023–14029.
235. Horsburgh BC, Hubinette MM, Tufaro F. Genetic manipulation of herpes simplex virus using bacterial artificial chromosomes. *Methods Enzymol* 1999;306:337–352.
236. Huang AS, Wagner RR. Penetration of herpes simplex virus into human epidermoid cells. *Proc Social Exp Biol Med* 1964;116:863–869.
237. Huang CJ, Petroski MD, Pande NT, et al. The herpes simplex virus type 1 VP5 promoter contains a cis-acting element near the cap site which interacts with a cellular protein. *J Virol* 1996;70:1898–1904.
238. Huang CJ, Wagner EK. The herpes simplex virus type 1 major capsid protein (VP5-UL19) promoter contains two cis-acting elements influencing late expression. *J Virol* 1994;68:5738–5747.
239. Huszar D, Bacchetti S. Partial purification and characterization of the ribonucleotide reductase induced by herpes simplex virus infection of mammalian cells. *J Virol* 1981;37:580–588.
240. Igarashi K, Fawl R, Roller RJ, Roizman B. Construction and properties of a recombinant herpes simplex virus 1 lacking both S-component origins of DNA synthesis. *J Virol* 1993;67:2123–2132.
241. Imbalzano AN, Shepard AA, DeLuca NA. Functional relevance of specific interactions between herpes simplex virus type 1 ICP4 and sequences from the promoter-regulatory domain of the viral thymidine kinase gene. *J Virol* 1990;64:2620–2631.
242. Ingram A, Phelan A, Dunlop J, Clements JB. Immediate early protein IE63 of herpes simplex virus type 1 binds RNA directly. *J Gen Virol* 1996;77:1847–1851.
243. Ishov AM, Maul GG. The periphery of nuclear domain 10 (ND10) as site of DNA virus deposition. *J Cell Biol* 1996;134:815–826.
244. Ishov AM, Stenberg RM, Maul GG. Human cytomegalovirus immediate early interaction with host nuclear structures: Definition of an immediate transcript environment. *Cell Biol* 1997;138:5–16.
245. Jacob RJ, Morse LS, Roizman B. Anatomy of herpes simplex virus DNA. XII. Accumulation of head-to-tail concatemers in nuclei of infected cells and their role in the generation of the four isomeric arrangements of viral DNA. *J Virol* 1979;29:448–457.
246. Jacobson JG, Leib DA, Goldstein DJ, et al. A herpes simplex virus ribonucleotide reductase deletion mutant is defective for productive acute and reactivatable latent infections of mice and for replication in mouse cells. *Virology* 1989;173:276–283.
247. Jacobson JG, Martin SL, Coen DM. A conserved open reading frame that overlaps the herpes simplex virus thymidine kinase gene is important for viral growth in cell culture. *J Virol* 1989;63:1839–1843.
248. Jacquemont B, Roizman B. RNA synthesis in cells infected with herpes simplex virus. X. Properties of viral symmetric transcripts and of double-stranded RNA prepared from them. *J Virol* 1975;15:707–713.
249. Javier RT, Izumi KM, Stevens JG. Localization of a herpes simplex virus neurovirulence gene dissociated from high-titer virus replication in the brain. *J Virol* 1988;62:1381–1387.
250. Javier RT, Stevens JG, Dissette VB, Wagner EK. A herpes simplex virus transcript abundant in latently infected neurons is dispensable for establishment of the latent state. *Virology* 1988;166:254–257.
251. Javier RT, Thompson RL, Stevens JG. Genetic and biological analyses of a herpes simplex virus intertypic recombinant reduced specifically for neurovirulence. *J Virol* 1987;61:1978–1984.
252. Jean S, LeVan KM, Song B, Levine M, Knipe DM. HSV-1 ICP27 is required for transcription of two viral late (γ_2) genes in infected cells. *Virology* 2001. In press.
253. Jenkins FJ, Roizman B. Herpes simplex virus 1 recombinants with noninverting genomes frozen in different isomeric arrangements are capable of independent replication. *J Virol* 1986;59:494–499.
254. Jerome KR, Fox R, Chen Z, et al. Herpes simplex virus inhibits apoptosis through the action of two genes, Us5 and Us3. *J Virol* 1999;73: 8950–8957.
255. Jerome KR, Tait JF, Koelle DM, Corey L. Herpes simplex virus type 1 renders infected cells resistant to cytotoxic T-lymphocyte-induced apoptosis. *J Virol* 1998;72:436–441.
256. Johnson DC, Spear PG. Monensin inhibits the processing of herpes simplex virus glycoproteins, their transport to the cell surface, and the egress of virions from infected cells. *J Virol* 1982;43:1102–1112.
257. Johnson PA, Everett RD. The control of herpes simplex virus type-1 late gene transcription: A 'TATA-box'/cap site region is sufficient for fully efficient regulated activity. *Nucleic Acids Res* 1986;14:8247–8264.
258. Jones PC, Hayward GS, Roizman B. Anatomy of herpes simplex virus DNA. VII. alpha-RNA is homologous to noncontiguous sites in both the L and S components of viral DNA. *J Virol* 1977;21:268–276.
259. Jones PC, Roizman B. Regulation of herpesvirus macromolecular synthesis. VIII. The transcription program consists of three phases during which both extent of transcription and accumulation of RNA in the cytoplasm are regulated. *J Virol* 1979;31:299–314.
260. Jordan R, Schaffer PA. Activation of gene expression by herpes simplex virus type 1 ICP0 occurs at the level of mRNA synthesis. *J Virol* 1997;71:6850–6862.
261. Jung JU, Stager M, Desrosiers RC. Virus-encoded cyclin. *Mol Cell Biol* 1994;14:7235–7244.
262. Kaerner HC, Maichle IB, Ott A, Schroder CH. Origin of two different classes of defective HSV-1 Angelotti DNA. *Nucleic Acids Res* 1979;6: 1467–1478.
263. Kaplan AS, Ben-Porat T. The effect of pseudorabies virus on the nucleic acid metabolism and on the nuclei of rabbit kidney cells. *Virology* 1959;8:352–366.
264. Karr BM, Read GS. The virion host shutoff function of herpes simplex virus degrades the 5′ end of a target mRNA before the 3′ end. *Virology* 1999;264:195–204.
265. Katan M, Haigh A, Verrijzer CP, et al. Characterization of a cellular factor which interacts functionally with Oct-1 in the assembly of a multicomponent transcription complex. *Nucleic Acids Res* 1990;18: 6871–6880.
266. Katz JP, Bodin ET, Coen DM. Quantitative polymerase chain reaction analysis of herpes simplex virus DNA in ganglia of mice infected with replication-incompetent mutants. *J Virol* 1990;64:4288–4295.
267. Kawaguchi Y, Bruni R, Roizman B. Interaction of herpes simplex virus 1 alpha regulatory protein ICP0 with elongation factor 1d: ICP0 affects translational machinery. *J Virol* 1997;71:1019–1024.
268. Kawaguchi Y, Matsumura T, Roizman B, Hirai K. Cellular elongation factor 1delta is modified in cells infected with representative alpha-, beta-, or gammaherpesviruses. *J Virol* 1999;73:4456–4460.
269. Kawaguchi Y, Van Sant C, Roizman B. Herpes simplex virus 1 alpha regulatory protein ICP0 interacts with and stabilizes the cell cycle regulator cyclin D3. *J Virol* 1997;71:7328–7336.
270. Keir HM, Gold E. Deoxyribonucleotidyl transferase and deoxyribonuclease from cultured cells infected with herpes simplex virus. *Biochem Biophys Acta Rev* 1963;72:263–276.
271. Keir HM, Hay J, Morrison JM, Subak-Sharpe H. Altered properties of deoxyribonucleic acid nucleotidyltransferase after infection of mammalian cells with herpes simplex virus. *Nature* 1966;210:369–371.
272. Kieff ED, Bachenheimer SL, Roizman B. Size, composition, and structure of the deoxyribonucleic acid of herpes simplex virus subtypes 1 and 2. *J Virol* 1971;8:125–132.
273. Kit S, Dubbs DR. Properties of deoxythymidine kinase partially purified from noninfected and virus-infected mouse fibroblast cells. *Virology* 1965;26:16–27.
274. Klein RJ. Effect of immune serum on the establishment of herpes simplex virus infection in trigeminal ganglia of hairless mice. *J Gen Virol* 1980;49:401–405.
275. Klein RJ. Pathogenetic mechansims of recurrent herpes simplex virus infections. *Arch Virol* 1976;51:1–13.

276. Klein RJ, Friedman-Kien AE, Brady E. Latent herpes simplex virus in ganglia of mice after primary infection and reinoculation at a distant site. *Arch Virol* 1978;57:161–166.
277. Klein RJ, Friedman-Kien AE, Yellin PB. Orofacial herpes simplex virus infection in hairless mice: Latent virus in trigeminal ganglia after topical antiviral treatment. *Infect Immun* 1978;20:130–135.
278. Knipe DM, Ruyechan WT, Roizman B. Molecular genetics of herpes simplex virus. III. Fine mapping of a genetic locus determining resistance to phosphonoacetate by two methods of marker transfer. *J Virol* 1979;29:698–704.
279. Knipe DM, Ruyechan WT, Roizman B, Halliburton IW. Molecular genetics of herpes simplex virus: Demonstration of regions of obligatory and nonobligatory identity within diploid regions of the genome by sequence replacement and insertion. *Proc Natl Acad Sci U S A* 1978; 75:3896–3900.
280. Knipe DM, Senechek D, Rice SA, Smith JL. Stages in the nuclear association of the herpes simplex virus transcriptional activator protein ICP4. *J Virol* 1987;61:276–284.
281. Knopf CW. Nucleotide sequence of the DNA polymerase gene of herpes simplex virus type 1 strain Angelotti. *Nucleic Acids Res* 1986;14: 8225–8226.
282. Koch HG, Rosen A, Ernst F, et al. Determination of the nucleotide sequence flanking the deletion (0.762 to 0.789 map units) in the genome of an intraperitoneally avirulent HSV-1 strain HFEM. *Virus Res* 1987;7:105–115.
283. Koff A, Schwedes JF, Tegtmeyer P. Herpes simplex virus origin-binding protein (UL9) loops and distorts the viral replication origin. *J Virol* 1991;65:3284–3292.
284. Koff A, Tegtmeyer P. Characterization of major recognition sequences for a herpes simplex virus type 1 origin-binding protein. *J Virol* 1988; 62:4096–4103.
285. Kosz-Vnenchak M, Coen DM, Knipe DM. Restricted expression of herpes simplex virus lytic genes during establishment of latent infection by thymidine kinase-negative mutant viruses. *J Virol* 1990;64: 5396–5402.
286. Kosz-Vnenchak M, Jacobson J, Coen DM, Knipe DM. Evidence for a novel regulatory pathway for herpes simplex virus gene expression in trigeminal ganglion neurons. *J Virol* 1993;67:5383–5393.
287. Koyama AH, Miwa Y. Suppression of apoptotic DNA fragmentation in herpes simplex virus type 1-infected cells. *J Virol* 1997;71: 2567–2571.
288. Kozak M, Roizman B. RNA synthesis in cells infected with herpes simplex virus. IX. Evidence for accumulation of abundant symmetric transcripts in nuclei. *J Virol* 1975;15:36–40.
289. Kramer MF, Chen SH, Knipe DM, Coen DM. Accumulation of viral transcripts and DNA during establishment of latency by herpes simplex virus. *J Virol* 1998;72:1177–1185.
290. Krause PR, Croen KD, Straus SE, Ostrove JM. Detection and preliminary characterization of herpes simplex virus type 1 transcripts in latently infected human trigeminal ganglia. *J Virol* 1988;62: 4819–4823.
291. Kristensson K, Lycke E, Roytta M, et al. Neuritic transport of herpes simplex virus in rat sensory neurons *in vitro*: Effects of substances interacting with microtubular function and axonal flow [nocodazole, Taxol and erythro-9-3-(2-hydroxynonyl)adenine]. *J Gen Virol* 1986; 67:2023–2028.
292. Kristie TM, LeBowitz JH, Sharp PA. The octamer-binding proteins form multi-protein–DNA complexes with the HSV alpha TIF regulatory protein. *EMBO J* 1989;8:4229–4238.
293. Kristie TM, Roizman B. Differentiation and DNA contact points of host proteins binding at the cis site for virion-mediated induction of alpha genes of herpes simplex virus 1. *J Virol* 1988;62:1145–1157.
294. Kristie TM, Roizman B. DNA-binding site of major regulatory protein alpha 4 specifically associated with promoter-regulatory domains of alpha genes of herpes simplex virus type 1. *Proce Natl Acad Sci U S A* 1986;83:4700–4704.
295. Kristie TM, Roizman B. Host cell proteins bind to the cis-acting site required for virion-mediated induction of herpes simplex virus 1 alpha genes. *Proc Natl Acad Sci U S A* 1987;84:71–75.
296. Kristie TM, Roizman B. Separation of sequences defining basal expression from those conferring alpha gene recognition within the regulatory domains of herpes simplex virus 1 alpha genes. *Proc Natl Acad Sci U S A* 1984;81:4065–4069.
297. Kristie TM, Sharp PA. Interactions of the Oct-1 POU subdomains with specific DNA sequences and with the HSV alpha-trans-activator protein. *Genes Dev* 1990;4:2383–2396.
298. Kristie TM, Vogel JL, Sears AE. Nuclear localization of the C1 factor (host cell factor) in sensory neurons correlates with reactivation of herpes simplex virus from latency. *Proc Natl Acad Sci U S A* 1999;96: 1229–1233.
299. Kwon BS, Gangarosa LP, Burch KD, et al. Induction of ocular herpes simplex virus shedding by iontophoresis of epinephrine into rabbit cornea. *Invest Ophthalmol Visual Sci* 1981;21:442–449.
300. Kwong AD, Frenkel N. Herpes simplex virus-infected cells contain a function(s) that destabilizes both host and viral mRNAs. *Proc Natl Acad Sci U S A* 1987;84:1926–1930.
301. Kwong AD, Kruper JA, Frenkel N. Herpes simplex virus virion host shutoff function. *J Virol* 1988;62:912–921.
302. La Boissiere S, Hughes T, O'Hare P. HCF-dependent nucear import of VP16. *EMBO J* 1999;18:480–489.
303. La Boissiere S, O'Hare P. Analysis of HCF, the cellular cofactor of VP16, in herpes simplex virus-infected cells. *J Virol* 2000;74:99–109.
304. Ladin BF, Blankenship ML, Ben-Porat T. Replication of herpesvirus DNA II: The maturation of concatemeric DNA of pseudo rabies virus to genome length is related to capsid formation. *J Virol* 1980;33: 1151–1164.
305. Ladin BF, Ihara S, Hampl H, Ben-Porat T. Pathway of assembly of herpesvirus capsids: An analysis using DNA temperature sensitive mutants of pseudorabies virus. *Virology* 1982;116:544–561.
306. Lagunoff M, Roizman B. Expression of a herpes simplex virus 1 open reading frame antisense to the gamma(1)34.5 gene and transcribed by an RNA 3′ coterminal with the unspliced latency-associated transcript. *J Virol* 1994;68:6021–6028.
307. Lagunoff M, Roizman B. The regulation of synthesis and properties of the protein product of open reading frame P of the herpes simplex virus 1 genome. *J Virol* 1995;69:3615–3623.
308. Lam Q, Smibert CA, Koop KE, et al. Herpes simplex virus VP16 rescues viral mRNA from destruction by the virion host shutoff function. *EMBO J* 1996;15:2575–2581.
309. Lamberti C, Weller SK. The herpes simplex virus type 1 cleavage/packaging protein, UL32, is involved in efficient localization of capsids to replication compartments. *J Virol* 1998;72: 2463–2473.
310. Lee CK, Knipe DM. An immunoassay for the study of DNA-binding activities of herpes simplex virus protein ICP8. *J Virol* 1985;54: 731–738.
311. Lee GT, Para MF, Spear PG. Location of the structural genes for glycoproteins gD and gE and for other polypeptides in the S component of herpes simplex virus type 1 DNA. *J Virol* 1982;43:41–49.
312. Lee JY, Irmiere A, Gibson W. Primate cytomegalovirus assembly: Evidence that DNA packaging occurs subsequent to B capsid assembly. *Virology* 1988;167:87–96.
313. Lees-Miller SP, Long MC, Kilvert MA, et al. Attenuation of DNA-dependent protein kinase activity and its catalytic subunit by the herpes simpelx virus type 1 transactivator ICP0. *J Virol* 1996;70: 7471–7477.
314. Leestma JE, Bornstein MB, Sheppard RD, Feldman LA. 1969. Ultrastructural aspects of herpes simplex virus infection in organized cultures of mammalian nervous tissue. *Lab Invest* 1969;20:70–78.
315. Leib DA, Bogard CL, Kosz-Vnenchak M, et al. A deletion mutant of the latency-associated transcript of herpes simplex virus type 1 reactivates from the latent state with reduced frequency. *J Virol* 1989; 63:2893–2900.
316. Leib DA, Coen DM, Bogard CL, et al. Immediate-early regulatory gene mutants define different stages in the establishment and reactivation of herpes simplex virus latency. *J Virol* 1989;63:759–768.
317. Leinbach SS, Summers WC. The structure of herpes simplex virus type 1 DNA as probed by micrococcal nuclease digestion. *J Gen Virol* 1980;51:45–59.
318. Leist TP, Sandri-Goldin RM, Stevens JG. Latent infections in spinal ganglia with thymidine kinase-deficient herpes simplex virus. *J Virol* 1989;63:4976–4978.
319. Lemaster S, Roizman B. Herpes simplex virus phosphoproteins. II. Characterization of the virion protein kinase and of the polypeptides phosphorylated in the virion. *J Virol* 1980;35:798–811.
320. Leopardi R, Michael N, Roizman B. Repression of the herpes simplex virus 1 alpha 4 gene by its gene product (ICP4) within the context of the viral genome is conditioned by the distance and stereoaxial align-

ment of the ICP4 DNA binding site relative to the TATA box. *J Virol* 1995;69:3042–3048.

321. Leopardi R, Roizman B. The herpes simplex virus major regulatory protein ICP4 blocks apoptosis induced by the virus or by hyperthermia. *Proc Natl Acad Sci U S A* 1996;93:9583–9587.
322. Leopardi R, Van Sant C, Roizman B. The herpes simplex virus 1 protein kinase US3 is required for protection from apoptosis induced by the virus. *Proc Natl Acad Sci U S A* 1997;94:7891–7896.
323. Leopardi R, Ward PL, Ogle WO, Roizman B. Association of herpes simplex virus regulatory protein ICP22 with transcriptional complexes containing EAP, ICP4, RNA polymerase II, and viral DNA requires posttranslational modification by the U(L)13 protein kinase. *J Virol* 1997;71:1133–1139.
324. Li M, Lee H, Yoon DW, et al. Kaposi's sarcoma-associated herpesvirus encodes a functional cyclin. *J Virol* 1997;71:1984–1991.
325. Lieu PT, Wagner EK. Two leaky-late HSV-1 promoters differ significantly in structural architecture. *Virology* 2000;272:191–203.
326. Ligas MW, Johnson DC. A herpes simplex virus mutant in which glycoprotein D sequences are replaced by beta-galactosidase sequences binds to but is unable to penetrate into cells. *J Virol* 1988;62: 1486–1494.
327. Lin Y, Green MR. Mechanism of action of an acidic transcriptional activator *in vitro*. *Cell* 1991;64:971–981.
328. Linnemann CC Jr, Buchman TG, Light IJ, Ballard JL. Transmission of herpes-simplex virus type 1 in a nursery for the newborn. Identification of viral isolates by D.N.A. "fingerprinting." *Lancet* 1978;1: 964–966.
329. Liptak L, Uprichard SL, Knipe DM. Functional order of assembly of herpes simplex virus DNA replication proteins into prereplicative site structures. *J Virol* 1996;70:1759–1767.
330. Little SP, Schaffer PA. Expression of the syncytial (syn) phenotype in HSV-12, strain KOS: Genetic and phenotypic studies of mutants in two syn loci. *Virology* 1981;112:686–702.
331. Liu F, Roizman B. Characterization of the protease and other products of amino-terminus-proximal cleavage of the herpes simplex virus 1 UL26 protein. *J Virol* 1993;67:1441–1452.
332. Liu F, Roizman B. Differentiation of multiple domains in the herpes simplex virus 1 protease encoded by the UL26 gene. *Proc Natl Acad Sci U S A* 1992;89:2076–2080.
333. Liu FY, Roizman B. The herpes simplex virus 1 gene encoding a protease also contains within its coding domain the gene encoding the more abundant substrate. *J Virol* 1991;65:5149–5156.
334. Liu FY, Roizman B. The promoter, transcriptional unit, and coding sequence of herpes simplex virus 1 family 35 proteins are contained within and in frame with the UL26 open reading frame. *J Virol* 1991; 65:206–212.
335. Locker H, Frenkel N. BamI, KpnI, and SalI restriction enzyme maps of the DNAs of herpes simplex virus strains Justin and F: Occurrence of heterogeneities in defined regions of the viral DNA. *J Virol* 1979; 32:429–441.
336. Locker H, Frenkel N, Halliburton I. Structure and expression of class II defective herpes simplex virus genomes encoding infected cell polypeptide number 8. *J Virol* 1982;43:574–593.
337. Lockshon D, Galloway DA. Cloning and characterization of oriL2, a large palindromic DNA replication origin of herpes simplex virus type 2. *J Virol* 1986;58:513–521.
338. Long MC, Leong V, Schaffer PA, et al. ICP22 and the UL13 protein kinase are both required for herpes simplex virus-induced modification of the large subunit of RNA polymerase II. *J Virol* 1999;73: 5593–5604.
339. Lopez C. Genetics of natural resistance to herpesvirus infections in mice. *Nature* 1975;258:152–153.
340. Lopez M, Cocchi F, Menotti L, et al. Nectin 2 alpha (PRR2 alpha or HveB) and nectin 2 gamma are low-efficiency mediators for entry of herpes simplex virus mutants carrying the Leu25Pro subsitution in glycoprotein D. *J Virol* 2000;74:1267–1274.
341. Lowenstein A. Aetiologische untersuchungen uber den fieberhaften, herpes. *Munch Med Wochenschr* 1919;66:769–770.
342. Lukonis CJ, Weller SK. Characterization of nuclear structures in cells infected with herpes simplex virus type 1 in the absence of viral DNA replication. *J Virol* 1996;70:1751–1758.
343. Lycke E, Hamark B, Johansson M, et al. Herpes simplex virus infection of the human sensory neuron. An electron microscopy study. *Arch Virol* 1988;101:87–104.
344. Lycke E, Kristensson K, Svennerholm B, et al. Uptake and transport of herpes simplex virus in neurites of rat dorsal root ganglia cells in culture. *J Gen Virol* 1984;65:55–64.
345. Lynas C, Laycock KA, Cook SD, et al. Detection of herpes simplex virus type 1 gene expression in latently and productively infected mouse ganglia using the polymerase chain reaction. *J Gen Virol* 1989; 70:2345–2355.
346. Mackem S, Roizman B. Differentiation between alpha promoter and regulator regions of herpes simplex virus 1: The functional domains and sequence of a movable alpha regulator. *Proc Natl Acad Sci U S A* 1982;79:4917–4921.
347. Mackem S, Roizman B. 1980. Regulation of herpesvirus macromolecular synthesis: Transcription-initiation sites and domains of alpha genes. *Proc Natl Acad Sci U S A* 1980;77:7122–7126.
348. Mackem S, Roizman B. Structural features of the herpes simplex virus alpha gene 4, 0, and 27 promoter-regulatory sequences which confer alpha regulation on chimeric thymidine kinase genes. *J Virol* 1982;44:939–949.
349. MacLean CA, Dolan A, Jamieson FE, McGeoch DJ. The myristylated virion proteins of herpes simplex virus type 1: Investigation of their role in the virus life cycle. *J Gen Virol* 1992;73:539–547.
350. Manservigi R, Spear PG, Buchan A. Cell fusion induced by herpes simplex virus is promoted and suppressed by different viral glycoproteins. *Proc Natl Acad Sci U S A* 1977;74:3913–3917.
351. Margolis TP, Dawson CR, LaVail JH. Herpes simplex viral infection of the mouse trigeminal ganglion: Immunohistochemical analysis of cell populations. *Invest Ophthalmol Visual Sci* 1992;33:259–267.
352. Mark GE, Kaplan AS. Synthesis of protein in cells infected with herpesvirus. VII. Lack of migration of structural viral proteins to the nucleus of arginine-deprived cells. *Virology* 1971;45:53–60.
353. Markovitz N, Filatov F, Roizman B. The UL3 protein of herpes simplex virus 1 is translated predominantly from the second in-frame methionine codon and is subject to at least two postranslational modifications. *J Virol* 1999;73:8010–8013.
354. Marsden HS, Stow ND, Preston VG, et al. Physical mapping of herpes simplex virus-induced polypeptides. *J Virol* 1978;28:624–642.
355. Mastino A, Sciortino MT, Medici MA, et al. Herpes simplex virus 2 causes apoptotic infection in monocytoid cells. *Cell Death Differen* 1997;4:629–638.
356. Maul GG, Everett RD. The nuclear location of PML, a cellular member of the C3HC4 zinc-binding domain protein family, is rearranged during herpes simplex virus infection by the C3HC4 viral protein ICPO. *J Gen Virol* 1994;75:1223–1233.
357. Maul GG, Guldner HH, Spivack JG. Modification of discrete nuclear domains induced by herpes simplex virus type 1 immediate early gene 1 product (ICP0). *J Gen Virol* 1993;74:2679–2690.
358. Maul GG, Ishov AM, Everett RD. Nuclear domain 10 as preexisting potential replication start sites of herpes simplex virus type 1. *Virology* 1996;217:67–75.
359. Mavromara-Nazos P, Roizman B. Activation of herpes simplex virus 1 gamma 2 genes by viral DNA replication. *Virology* 1987;161: 593–598.
360. McCarthy AM, McMahan L, Schaffer PA. Herpes simplex virus type 1 ICP27 deletion mutants exhibit altered patterns of transcription and are DNA deficient. *J Virol* 1989;63:18–27.
361. McCracken RM, Clarke JK. A thin section study of the morphogenesis of Aujeszky's disease virus in synchronously infected cell culutres. *Arch Ges Virusforsch* 1971;34:189–201.
362. McGeoch DJ, Cunningham C, McIntyre G, Dolan A. Comparative sequence analysis of the long repeat regions and adjoining parts of the long unique regions in the genomes of herpes simplex viruses types 1 and 2. *J Gen Virol* 1991;72:3057–3075.
363. McGeoch DJ, Dalrymple MA, Davison AJ, et al. The complete DNA sequence of the long unique region in the genome of herpes simplex virus type 1. *J Gen Virol* 1988;69:1531–1574.
364. McGeoch DJ, Davison AJ. 1986. Alphaherpesviruses possess a gene homologous to the protein kinase gene family of eukaryotes and retroviruses. *Nucleic Acids Res* 1986;14:1765–1777.
365. McGregor F, Phelan A, Dunlop J, Clements JB. Regulation of herpes simplex virus poly(A) site usage and the action of immediate-early protein IE63 in the early-late switch. *J Virol* 1996;70:1931–1940.
366. McKendall RR. Efficacy of herpes simplex virus type 1 immunization in protecting against acute and latent infection by herpes simplex virus type 2 in mice. *Infect Immun* 1977;16:717–719.

367. McKendall RR, Klassen T, Baringer JR. Host defenses in herpes simplex infections of the nervous system: Effect of antibody on disease and viral spread. *Infect Immun* 1979;23:305–311.
368. McKnight JL, Pellett PE, Jenkins FJ, Roizman B. Characterization and nucleotide sequence of two herpes simplex virus 1 genes whose products modulate alpha-trans-inducing factor-dependent activation of alpha genes. *J Virol* 1987;61:992–1001.
369. McKnight SL, Kingsbury RC. Transcriptional control signals of a eukaryotic protein-coding gene. *Science* 1982;217:316–324.
370. McLauchlan J, Phelan A, Loney C, et al. Herpes simplex virus IE63 acts at the posttranscriptional level to stimulate viral mRNA 3′ processing. *J Virol* 1992;66:6939–6945.
371. McLauchlan J, Rixon FJ. Characterization of enveloped tegument structures (L particles) produced by alphaherpesviruses: Integrity of the tegument does not depend on the presence of capsid or envelope. *J Gen Virol* 1992;73:269–276.
372. McLean TI, Bachenheimer SL. Activation of cJUN N-terminal kinase by herpes simplex virus type 1 enhances viral replication. *Virology* 1999;73:8415–8426.
373. McNabb DS, Courtney RJ. Posttranslational modification and subcellular localization of the p12 capsid protein of herpes simplex virus type 1. *J Virol* 1992;66:4839–4847.
374. McNamee EE, Taylor TJ, Knipe DM. A dominant-negative herpesvirus protein inhibits intranuclear targeting of viral proteins: Effects on DNA replication and late gene expression. *J Virol* 2000;74:10122–10131.
375. Mears WE, Lam V, Rice SA. Identification of nuclear and nucleolar localization signals in the herpes simplex virus regulatory protein ICP27. *J Virol* 1995;69:935–947.
376. Mears WE, Rice SA. The herpes simplex virus immediate-early protein ICP27 shuttles between nucleus and cytoplasm. *Virology* 1998;242:128–137.
377. Mears WE, Rice SA. 1996. The RGG box motif of the herpes simplex virus ICP27 protein mediates an RNA-binding activity and determines in vivo methylation. *J Virol* 1996;70:7445–7453.
378. Mehta A, Maggioncalda J, Bagasra O, et al. In situ DNA PCR and RNA hybridization detection of herpes simplex virus sequences in trigeminal ganglia of latently infected mice. *Virology* 1995;206(1):633–640.
379. Meignier B, Longnecker R, Mavromara-Nazos P, et al. Virulence of and establishment of latency by genetically engineered deletion mutants of herpes simplex virus 1. *Virology* 1988;162:251–254.
380. Meignier B, Longnecker R, Roizman B. *In vivo* behavior of genetically engineered herpes simplex viruses R7017 and R7020: Construction and evaluation in rodents. *Journal of Infectious Diseases* 1988;158:602–614.
381. Mellerick DM, Fraser NW. Physical state of the latent herpes simplex virus genome in a mouse model system: Evidence suggesting an episomal state. *Virology* 1987;158:265–275.
382. Menotti L, Lopez M, Avitabile E, et al. The murine homolog of human nectin1delta serves as a species nonspecific mediator for entry of human and animal alpha herpesviruses in a pathway independent of a detectable binding to gD. *Proc Natl Acad Sci U S A* 2000;97:4867–4872.
383. Meredith DM, Lindsay JA, Halliburton IW, Whittaker GR. Post-translational modification of the tegument proteins (VP13 and VP14) of herpes simplex virus type 1 by glycosylation and phosphorylation. *J Gen Virol* 1991;72:2771–2775.
384. Michael N, Roizman B. Binding of the herpes simplex virus major regulatory protein to viral DNA. *Proc Natl Acad Sci U S A* 1989;86:9808–9812.
385. Michael N, Spector D, Mavromara-Nazos P, et al. The DNA-binding properties of the major regulatory protein alpha 4 of herpes simplex viruses. *Science* 1988;239:1531–1534.
386. Mitchell C, Blaho JA, McCormick AL, Roizman B. The nucleotidylylation of herpes simplex virus 1 regulatory protein alpha 22 by human casein kinase II. *J Biol Chem* 1997;272:25394–25400.
387. Mocarski ES, Post LE, Roizman B. Molecular engineering of the herpes simplex virus genome: Insertion of a second L-S junction into the genome causes additional genome inversions. *Cell* 1980;22:243–255.
388. Mocarski ES, Roizman B. Herpesvirus-dependent amplification and inversion of cell-associated viral thymidine kinase gene flanked by viral a sequences and linked to an origin of viral DNA replication. *Proc Natl Acad Sci U S A* 1982;79:5626–5630.
389. Mocarski ES, Roizman B. Site-specific inversion sequence of the herpes simplex virus genome: Domain and structural features. *Proc Natl Acad Sci U S A* 1981;78:7047–7051.
390. Mocarski ES, Roizman B. Structure and role of the herpes simplex virus DNA termini in inversion, circularization and generation of virion DNA. *Cell* 1982;31:89–97.
391. Mohr I, Gluzman Y. A herpesvirus genetic element which affects translation in the absence of the viral GADD34 function. *EMBO J* 1996;15:4759–4766.
392. Montgomery RI, Warner MS, Lum BJ, Spear PG. Herpes simplex virus-1 entry into cells mediated by a novel member of the TNF/NGF receptor family. *Cell* 1996;87:427–436.
393. Morgan C, Holden M, Jones EP. Electron microscopic observations on the development of herpes simplex virus. *J Exp Med* 1959;110:643–656.
394. Morgan C, Rose HM, Mednis B. Electron microscopy of herpes simplex virus. I. Entry. *J Virol* 1968;2:507–516.
395. Morse LS, Buchman TG, Roizman B, Schaffer PA. Anatomy of herpes simplex virus DNA. IX. Apparent exclusion of some parental DNA arrangements in the generation of intertypic (HSV-1 X HSV-2) recombinants. *J Virol* 1977;24:231–248.
396. Morse LS, Pereira L, Roizman B, Schaffer PA. Anatomy of herpes simplex virus (HSV) DNA. X. Mapping of viral genes by analysis of polypeptides and functions specified by HSV-1 X HSV-2 recombinants. *J Virol* 1978;26:389–410.
397. Mossman KL, Sherburne R, Lavery C, et al. Evidence that herpes simplex virus VP16 is required for viral egress downstream of the initial envelopment event. *J Virol* 2000;74:6287–6299.
398. Mullen MA, Ciufo DM, Hayward GS. Mapping of intracellular localization domains and evidence for colocalization interactions between the IE110 and IE175 nuclear transactivator proteins of herpes simplex virus. *J Virol* 1994;68:3250–3266.
399. Muller MT. Binding of the herpes simplex virus immediate-early gene product ICP4 to its own transcription start site. *J Virol* 1987;61:858–865.
400. Murchie MJ, McGeoch DJ. DNA sequence analysis of an immediate-early gene region of the herpes simplex virus type 1 genome (map coordinates 0.950 to 0.978). *J Gen Virol* 1982;62:1–15.
401. Nabel GJ, Rice SA, Knipe DM, Baltimore D. Alternative mechanisms for activation of human immunodeficiency virus enhancer in T cells. *Science* 1988;239:1299–1302.
402. Naib ZM, Clepper AS, Elliott SR. Exfoliative cytology as an aid in diagnosis of ophthalmic lesions. *Acta Cytol* 1967;11:295–303.
403. Nalwanga D, Rempel S, Roizman B, Baines JD. The UL16 gene product of herpes simplex virus 1 is a virion protein that colocalizes with intranuclear capsid proteins. *Virology* 1996;226:236–242.
404. Newcomb WW, Brown JC. Structure of the herpes simplex virus capsid: Effects of extraction with guanidine hydrochloride and partial reconstitution of extracted capsids. *J Virol* 1991;65:613–620.
405. Newcomb WW, Brown JC. Use of Ar+ plasma etching to localize structural proteins in the capsid of herpes simplex virus type 1. *J Virol* 1989;63:4697–4702.
406. Newcomb WW, Homa FL, Thomsen DR, et al. Assembly of the herpes simplex virus capsid: Characterization of intermediates observed during cell-free capsid formation. *J Mol Biol* 1996;263:432–446.
407. Newcomb WW, Homa FL, Thomsen DR, et al. Assembly of the herpes simplex virus procapsid from purified components and identification of small complexes containing the major capsid and scaffolding proteins. *J Virol* 1999;73:4239–4250.
408. Newcomb WW, Homa FL, Thomsen DR, et al. Cell-free assembly of the herpes simplex virus capsid. *J Virol* 1994;68:6059–6063.
409. Newcomb WW, Trus BL, Booy FP, et al. Structure of the herpes simplex virus capsid: Molecular composition of the pentons and the triplexes. *J Mol Biol* 1993;232:499–511.
410. Nichol PF, Chang JY, Johnson EM Jr, Olivo PD. Herpes simplex virus gene expression in neurons: Viral DNA synthesis is a critical regulatory event in the branch point between the lytic and latent pathways. *J Virol* 1996;70:5476–5486.
411. Nicholas J, Cameron KR, Honess RW. Herpesvirus saimiri encodes homologues of G protein-coupled receptor and cyclins. *Nature* 1992;355:362–365.
412. Nicholson P, Addison C, Cross AM, et al. Localization of the herpes simplex virus type 1 major capsid protein VP5 to the cell nucleus requires the abundant scaffolding protein VP22a. *J Gen Virol* 1994;75:1091–1099.

413. Nii S, Morgan C, Rose HM, Hsu KC. Electron microscopy of herpes simplex virus. IV. Studies with ferritin-conjugated antibodies. *J Virol* 1968;2:1172–1184.
414. Nishioka Y, Silverstein S. Alterations in the protein synthetic apparatus of Friend erythroleukemia cells infected with vesicular stomatitis virus or herpes simplex virus. *J Virol* 1978;25:422–426.
415. Nishioka Y, Silverstein S. Degradation of cellular mRNA during infection by herpes simplex virus. *Proc Natl Acad Sci U S A* 1977;74: 2370–2374.
416. Nishioka Y, Silverstein S. Requirement of protein synthesis for the degradation of host mRNA in Friend erythroleukemia cells infected with HSV-1. *J Virol* 1978;27:619–627.
417. Nishiyama Y, Kurachi R, Daikoku T, Umene K. The US 9, 10, 11, and 12 genes of herpes simplex virus type 1 are of no importance for its neurovirulence and latency in mice. *Virology* 1993;194:419–423.
418. O'Hare P, Goding CR. Herpes simplex virus regulatory elements and the immunoglobulin octamer domain bind a common factor and are both targets for virion transactivation. *Cell* 1988;52:435–445.
419. O'Hare P, Hayward GS. Evidence for a direct role for both the 175,000- and 110,000-molecular-weight immediate-early proteins of herpes simplex virus in the transactivation of delayed-early promoters. *J Virol* 1985;53:751–760.
420. Ogle WO, Ng TI, Carter KL, Roizman B. The UL13 protein kinase and the infected cell type are determinants of posttranslational modification of ICP0. *Virology* 1997;235:406–413.
421. Ogle WO, Roizman B. Functional anatomy of herpes simplex virus 1 overlapping genes encoding infected-cell protein 22 and US1.5 protein. *J Virol* 1999;73:4305–4315.
422. Ojala PM, Sodeik B, Ebersold MW, et al. Herpes simplex virus type 1 entry into host cells: Reconstitution of capsid binding and uncoating at the nuclear pore complex in vitro. *Mol Cell Biol* 2000;20:4922–4931.
423. Olgiate J, Ehmann GL, Vidyarthi S, et al. Herpes simplex virus induces intracellular redistribution of E2F4 and accumulation of E2F pocket protein complexes. *Virology* 1999;258:257–270.
424. Orberg PK, Schaffer PA. Expression of herpes simplex virus type 1 major DNA-binding protein, ICP8, in transformed cell lines: Complementation of deletion mutants and inhibition of wild-type virus. *J Virol* 1987;61:1136–1146.
425. Oroskar AA, Read GS. A mutant of herpes simplex virus type 1 exhibits increased stability of immediate early (alpha) mRNAs. *J Virol* 1987;61:604–606.
426. Panagiotidis CA, Lium EK, Silverstein SJ. 1997. Physical and functional interactions between herpes simplex virus immediate-early proteins ICP4 and ICP27. *J Virol* 1997;71:1547–1557.
427. Papavassiliou AG, Silverstein SJ. Characterization of DNA-protein complex formation in nuclear extracts with a sequence from the herpes simplex virus thymidine kinase gene. *J Biol Chem* 1990;265: 1648–1657.
428. Papavassiliou AG, Silverstein SJ. Interaction of cell and virus proteins with DNA sequences encompassing the promoter/regulatory and leader regions of the herpes simplex virus thymidine kinase gene. *J Biol Chem* 1990;265:9402–9412.
429. Papavassiliou AG, Wilcox KW, Silverstein SJ. The interaction of ICP4 with cell/infected-cell factors and its state of phosphorylation modulate differential recognition of leader sequences in herpes simplex virus DNA. *EMBO J* 1991;10:397–406.
430. Para MF, Baucke RB, Spear PG. Immunoglobulin G(Fc)-binding receptors on virions of herpes simplex virus type 1 and transfer of these receptors to the cell surface by infection. *J Virol* 1980;34:512–520.
431. Paterson T, Everett RD. Mutational dissection of the HSV-1 immediate-early protein Vmw175 involved in transcriptional transactivation and repression. *Virology* 1988;166:186–196.
432. Pellett PE, McKnight JL, Jenkins FJ, Roizman B. Nucleotide sequence and predicted amino acid sequence of a protein encoded in a small herpes simplex virus DNA fragment capable of trans-inducing alpha genes. *Proc Natl Acad Sci U S A* 1985;82:5870–5874.
433. Penfold ME, Armati P, Cunningham AL. Axonal transport of herpes simplex virions to epidermal cells: Evidence for a specialized mode of virus transport and assembly. *Proc Natl Acad Sci U S A* 1994;91: 6529–6533.
434. Perdue ML, Cohen JC, Randall CC, O'Callaghan DJ. Biochemical studies of the maturation of herpesvirus nucleocapsid species. *Virology* 1976;1.
435. Perdue ML, Kemp MC, Randall CC, O'Callaghan DJ. Studies of the molecular anatomy of the L-M cell strain of equine herpes virus type 1: Proteins of the nucleocapsid and intact virion. *Virology* 1974;59: 201–216.
436. Pereira L, Cassai E, Honess RW, et al. Variability in the structural polypeptides of herpes simplex virus 1 strains: Potential application in molecular epidemiology. *Infect Immun* 1976;13:211–220.
437. Pereira L, Wolff MH, Fenwick M, Roizman B. Regulation of herpes virus macromolecular synthesis. V. Properties of a polypeptides made in HSV-1 and HSV-2 infected cells. *Virology* 1977;77:733–749.
438. Perng GC, Jones C, Ciacci-Zanella J, et al. Virus-induced neuronal apoptosis blocked by the herpes simplex virus latency-associated transcript. *Science* 2000;287:1500–1503.
439. Person S, Laquerre S, Desai P, Hempel J. Herpes simplex virus type 1 capsid protein, VP21, originates within the UL26 open reading frame. *J Gen Virol* 1993;74:2269–2273.
440. Petroski MD, Wagner EK. Purification and characterization of a cellular protein that binds to the downstream activation sequence of the strict late UL38 promoter of herpes simplex virus type 1. *J Virol* 1998;72:8181–8190.
441. Phelan A, Carmo-Fonseca M, McLaughlan J, et al. A herpes simplex virus type 1 immediate-early gene product, IE63, regulates small nuclear ribonucleoprotein distribution. *Proc Natl Acad Sci U S A* 1993;90:9056–9060.
442. Phelan A, Clements JB. Herpes simplex virus type 1 immediate early protein IE63 shuttles between nuclear compartments and the cytoplasm. *J Gen Virol* 1997;78:3327–3331.
443. Phelan A, Dunlop J, Patel AH, et al. Nuclear sites of herpes simplex virus type 1 DNA replication and transcription colocalize at early times postinfection and are largely distinct from RNA processing factors. *J Virol* 1997;71:1124–1132.
444. Plummer G, Goodheart CR, Henson D, Bowling CP. A comparative study of the DNA density and behavior in tissue cultures of fourteen different herpesviruses. *Virology* 1969;39:134–137.
445. Poffenberger KL, Roizman B. Studies on non-inverting genome of a viable herpes simplex virus 1: Presence of head-to-tail linkages in packaged genomes and requirements for circularization after infection. *J Virol* 1985;53:589–595.
446. Poffenberger KL, Tabares E, Roizman B. Characterization of a viable, noninverting herpes simplex virus 1 genome derived by insertion and deletion of sequences at the junction of components L and S. *Proc Natl Acad Sci U S A* 1983;80:2690–2694.
447. Pogue-Geile KL, Lee GT, Shapira SK, Spear PG. Fine mapping of mutations in the fusion-inducing MP strain of herpes simplex virus type 1. *Virology* 1984;136:100–109.
448. Pogue-Geile KL, Lee GT, Spear PG. Novel rearrangements of herpes simplex virus DNA sequences resulting from duplication of a sequence within the unique region of the L component. *J Virol* 1985; 53:456–461.
449. Pogue-Geile KL, Spear PG. The single base pair substitution responsible for the Syn phenotype of herpes simplex virus type 1, strain MP. *Virology* 1987;157:67–74.
450. Polvino-Bodnar M, Orberg PK, Schaffer PA. Herpes simplex virus type 1 oriL is not required for virus replication or for the establishment and reactivation of latent infection in mice. *J Virol* 1987;61: 3528–3535.
451. Pomeranz LE, Blaho JA. Modified VP22 localizes to the cell nucleus during synchronized herpes simplex virus type 1 infection. *J Virol* 1999;73:6769–6781.
452. Poon APW, Ogle WO, Roizman B. The posttranslational processing of infected cell protein 22 mediated by viral protein kinases is sensitive to amino acid substitution at distant sites and can be cell-type specific. *J Virol* 2000;71:11210–11214.
453. Post LE, Mackem S, Roizman B. Regulation of alpha genes of herpes simplex virus: Expression of chimeric genes produced by fusion of thymidine kinase with alpha gene promoters. *Cell* 1981;24:555–565.
454. Post LE, Roizman B. A generalized technique for deletion of specific genes in large genomes: Alpha Gene 22 of herpes simplex virus 1 is not essential for growth. *Cell* 1981;25:227–232.
455. Powell KL, Purifoy DJ. Nonstructural proteins of herpes simplex virus. I. Purification of the induced DNA polymerase. *J Virol* 1977;24: 618–626.
456. Preston CM. Control of herpes simplex virus type 1 mRNA synthesis in cells infected with wild-type virus or the temperature-sensitive mutant tsK. *J Virol* 1979;29:275–284.

457. Preston CM. Repression of viral transcription during herpes simplex virus latency. *J Gen Virol* 2000;81:1–19.
458. Preston CM, Cordingley MG. mRNA- and DNA-directed synthesis of herpes simplex virus-coded exonuclease in *Xenopus laevis* oocytes. *J Virol* 1982;43:386–394.
459. Preston CM, Frame MC, Campbell MEM. A complex formed between cell components and an HSV structural polypeptide binds to a viral immediate early gene regulatory DNA sequence. *Cell* 1988;52: 425–434.
460. Preston CM, Newton AA. The effects of herpes simplex virus type 1 on cellular DNA-dependent RNA polymerase activities. *J Gen Virol* 1976;33:471–482.
461. Preston CM, Notarianni EL. Poly(ADP-ribosyl)ation of a herpes simplex virus immediate early polypeptide. *Virology* 1983;131: 492–501.
462. Preston VG, Coates JA, Rixon FJ. Identification and characterization of a herpes simplex virus gene product required for encapsidation of virus DNA. *J Virol* 1983;45:1056–1064.
463. Preston VG, Davison AJ, Marsden HS, et al. Recombinants between herpes simplex virus types 1 and 2: Analyses of genome structures and expression of immediate early polypeptides. *J Virol* 1978;28: 499–517.
464. Preston VG, Fisher FB. Identification of the herpes simplex virus type 1 gene encoding the dUTPase. *Virology* 1984;138:58–68.
465. Price RW, Khan A. Resistance of peripheral autonomic neurons to in vivo productive infection by herpes simplex virus mutants deficient in thymidine kinase activity. *Infect Immun* 1981;34:571–580.
466. Price RW, Schmitz J. Route of infection, systemic host resistance, and integrity of ganglionic axons influence acute and latent herpes simplex virus infection of the superior cervical ganglion. *Infect Immun* 1979;23:373–383.
467. Price RW, Walz MA, Wohlenberg C, Notkins AL. Latent infection of sensory ganglia with herpes simplex virus: Efficacy of immunization. *Science* 1975;188:938–940.
468. Puga A, Rosenthal JD, Openshaw H, Notkins AL. Herpes simplex virus DNA and mRNA sequences in acutely and chronically infected trigeminal ganglia of mice. *Virology* 1978;89:102–111.
469. Purifoy DJ, Lewis RB, Powell KL. Identification of the herpes simplex virus DNA polymerase gene. *Nature* 1977;269:621–623.
470. Purves FC, Longnecker RM, Leader DP, Roizman B. Herpes simplex virus 1 protein kinase is encoded by open reading frame US3 which is not essential for virus growth in cell culture. *J Virol* 1987;61: 2896–2901.
471. Purves FC, Ogle WO, Roizman B. Processing of the herpes simplex virus regulatory protein alpha 22 mediated by the UL13 protein kinase determines the accumulation of a subset of alpha and gamma mRNAs and proteins in infected cells. *Proc Natl Acad Sci U S A* 1993;90: 6701–6705.
472. Purves FC, Roizman B. The UL13 gene of herpes simplex virus 1 encodes the functions for posttranslational processing associated with phosphorylation of the regulatory protein alpha 22. *Proc Natl Acad Sci U S A* 1992;89:7310–7314.
473. Pyles RB, Sawtell NM, Thompson RL. Herpes simplex virus type 1 dUTPase mutants are attenuated for neurovirulence, neuroinvasiveness, and reactivation from latency. *J Virol* 1992;66:6706–6713.
474. Pyles RB, Thompson RL. Evidence that the herpes simplex virus type 1 uracil DNA glycosylase is required for efficient viral replication and latency in the murine nervous system. *J Virol* 1994;68: 4963–4972.
475. Quinlan MP, Chen LB, Knipe DM. The intranuclear location of a herpes simplex virus DNA-binding protein is determined by the status of viral DNA replication. *Cell* 1984;36:857–868.
476. Quinlan MP, Knipe DM. Stimulation of expression of a herpes simplex virus DNA-binding protein by two viral functions. *Mol Cell Biol* 1985;5:957–963.
477. Quinn JP, McGeoch DJ. DNA sequence of the region in the genome of herpes simplex virus type 1 containing the genes for DNA polymerase and the major DNA binding protein. *Nucleic Acids Res* 1985; 13:8143–8163.
478. Rafield LF, Knipe DM. Characterization of the major mRNAs transcribed from the genes for glycoprotein B and DNA-binding protein ICP8 of herpes simplex virus type 1. *J Virol* 1984;49:960–969.
478a. Ramakrishnen R, Levine M, Fink DJ. PCR-based analysis of herpes simplex virus type 1 latency in the rat trigeminal ganglion established with a ribonucleotide reductase-deficient mutant. *J Virol* 1994;68: 7083–7091.
479. Randall G, Lagunoff M, Roizman B. Herpes simplex virus 1 open reading frames O and P are not necessary for establishment of latent infection in mice. *J Virol* 2000;74:9019–9027.
480. Randall G, Lagunoff M, Roizman B. The product of ORF O located within the domain of herpes simplex virus 1 genome transcribed during latent infection binds to and inhibits in vitro binding of infected cell protein 4 to its cognate DNA site. *Proc Natl Acad Sci U S A* 1997;94:10379–10384.
481. Randall RE, Dinwoodie N. Intranuclear localization of herpes simplex virus immediate-early and delayed-early proteins: Evidence that ICP 4 is associated with progeny virus DNA. *J Gen Virol* 1986;67:2163–2177.
482. Ravi V, Kennedy PG, MacLean AR. Functinal analysis of the herpes simplex virus type 2 strain HG52 RL1 gene: The intron plays no role in virulence. *J Gen Virol* 1998;79:1613–1617.
483. Read GS, Frenkel N. Herpes simplex virus mutants defective in the virion-associated shutoff of host polypeptide synthesis and exhibiting abnormal synthesis of alpha (immediate early) viral polypeptides. *J Virol* 1983;46:498–512.
484. Read GS, Karr BM, Knight K. Isolation of a herpes simplex virus type 1 mutant with a deletion in the virion host shutoff gene and identification of multiple forms of the vhs (UL41) polypeptide. *J Virol* 1993; 67:7149–7160.
485. Rice SA, Knipe DM. Gene-specific transactivation by herpes simplex virus type 1 alpha protein ICP27. *J Virol* 1988;62:3814–3823.
486. Rice SA, Knipe DM. Genetic evidence for two distinct transactivation functions of the herpes simplex virus alpha protein ICP27. *J Virol* 1990;64:1704–1715.
487. Rice SA, Lam V, Knipe DM. The acidic amino-terminal region of herpes simplex virus type 1 alpha protein ICP27 is required for an essential lytic function. *J Virol* 1993;67:1778–1787.
488. Rice SA, Long MC, Lam V, Spencer CA. RNA polymerase II is aberrantly phosphorylated and localized to viral replication compartments following herpes simplex virus infection. *J Virol* 1994;68:988–1001.
489. Rice SA, Su LS, Knipe DM. Herpes simplex virus alpha protein ICP27 possesses separable positive and negative regulatory activities. *J Virol* 1989;63:3399–3407.
490. Richman DD, Buckmaster A, Bell S, et al. Identification of a new glycoprotein of herpes simplex virus type 1 and genetic mapping of the gene that codes for it. *J Virol* 1986;57:647–655.
491. Rixon FJ, Addison C, McGregor A, et al. Multiple interactions control the intracellular localization of the herpes simplex virus type 1 capsid proteins. *J Gen Virol* 1996;77:2251–2260.
492. Rixon FJ, Addison C, McLauchlan J. Assembly of enveloped tegument structures (L particles) can occur independently of virion maturation in herpes simplex virus type 1-infected cells. *J Gen Virol* 1992;73: 277–284.
493. Rixon FJ, Cross AM, Addison C, Preston VG. The products of herpes simplex virus type 1 gene UL26 which are involved in DNA packaging are strongly associated with empty but not with full capsids. *J Gen Virol* 1988;69:2879–2891.
494. Rixon FJ, McGeoch DJ. A 3′ co-terminal family of mRNAs from the herpes simplex virus type 1 short region: Two overlapping reading frames encode unrelated polypeptide one of which has highly reiterated amino acid sequence. *Nucleic Acids Res* 1984;12:2473–2487.
495. Roane PRJ, Roizman B. Studies of the determinant antigens of viable cells. II. Demonstration of altered antigenic reactivity of HEp-2 cells infected with herpes simplex virus. *Virology* 1964;22:1–8.
496. Robertson BJ, McCann PJ 3rd, Matusick-Kumar L, et al. Separate functional domains of the herpes simplex virus type 1 protease: Evidence for cleavage inside capsids. *J Virol* 1996;70:4317–4328.
497. Rock DL, Fraser NW. Detection of HSV-1 genome in central nervous system of latently infected mice. *Nature* 1983;302:523–525.
498. Rock DL, Fraser NW. Latent herpes simplex virus type 1 DNA contains two copies of the virion DNA joint region. *J Virol* 1985;55: 849–852.
499. Rock DL, Nesburn AB, Ghiasi H, et al. Detection of latency-related viral RNAs in trigeminal ganglia of rabbits latently infected with herpes simplex virus type 1. *J Virol* 1987;61:3820–3826.
500. Rodahl E, Haarr L. Analysis of the 2-kilobase latency-associated transcript expressed in PC12 cells productively infected with herpes simplex virus type 1: Evidence for a stable, nonlinear structure. *J Virol* 1997;71:1703–1707.

501. Rodahl E, Stevens JG. Differential accumulation of herpes simplex virus type 1 latency-associated transcripts in sensory and autonomic ganglia. *Virology* 1992;189:385–388.
502. Roizman B. An inquiry into the mechanisms of recurrent herpes infection of man, p. 283–304. In: Pollard M, ed. *Perspectives in virology,* vol. IV. New York: Harper-Row, 1966:283–304.
503. Roizman B. The organization of the herpes simplex virus genomes. *Annu Rev Genet* 1979;13:25–57.
504. Roizman B. Polykaryocytosis. *Cold Spring Harbor Symp Quant Biol* 1962;27:327–340.
505. Roizman B. The structure and isomerization of herpes simplex virus genomes. *Cell* 1979;16:481–494.
506. Roizman B, Borman GS, Kamali-Rousta M. Macromolecular synthesis in cells infected with herpes simplex virus. *Nature* 1965;206:1374–1375.
507. Roizman B, Buchman T. The molecular epidemiology of herpes simplex viruses. *Hosp Pract* 1979;14:95–104.
508. Roizman B, Carmichael LE, Deinhardt F, et al. Herpesviridae: Definition, provisional nomenclature and taxonomy. *Intervirology* 1981;16: 201–217.
509. Roizman B, Furlong D. The replication of herpesviruses. In: Fraenkel-Conrat H, Wagner RR, eds. *Comprehensive virology*. New York: Plenum, 1974:229–403.
510. Roizman B, Norrild B, Chan C, Pereira L. Identification and preliminary mapping with monoclonal antibodies of a herpes simplex virus 2 glycoprotein lacking a known type 1 counterpart. *Virology* 1984;133: 242–247.
511. Roizman B, Roane PRJ. The multiplication of HSV II. The relation between protein synthesis and the duplication of viral DNA in infected HEp-2 cells. *Virology* 1964;22:262–269.
512. Roizman B, Roane PRJ. A physical difference between two strains of herpes simplex virus apparent on sedimenation in cesium chloride. *Virology* 1961;15:75–79.
513. Roizman B, Roane PRJ. 1961. Studies on the determinant antigens of viable cells. I. A method, and its application in tissue culture studies, for enumeration of killed cells, based on the failure of virus multiplication following injury by cytotoxic antibody and complement. *J Immunol* 1961;87:714–727.
514. Roizman B, Sears A. Herpes simplex viruses and their replication. In: Fields BN, Knipe DM, Howley PM, eds. *Fields virology,* 3rd ed. Philadelphia: Lippincott-Raven, 1996:2231–2296.
515. Roizman B, Sears AE. Herpes simplex viruses and their replication. In: Fields BN, Knipe DM, Chanock RM, et al, eds. *Virology,* 2nd ed. New York: Raven, 1990:1795–1841.
516. Roizman B, Sears AE. An inquiry into the mechanisms of herpes simplex virus latency. *Annu Rev Microbiol* 1987;41:543–571.
517. Roizman B, Spear PG. Herpesvirus antigens on cell membranes detected by centrifugation of membrane-antibody complexes. *Science* 1971;171:298–300.
518. Roizman B, Spear PG. The role of herpes virus glycoproteins in the modification of membranes of infected cells. Proceedings of the Miami Winter Symposia, January 18–22, 1971, pp. 435–455. In: Ribbons DW, Woessner JF, Schulz J, eds. *Nucleic acid-protein interactions and nucleic acid synthesis in viral infection,* vol. 2. Amsterdam: North Holland Publishing, 1971.
519. Roizman B, Spring SB. Alteration in immunologic specificity of cells infected with cytolytic viruses. In: Trentin JJ, ed. *Proceedings of the Conference on Cross Reacting Antigens.* Baltimore: Williams & Wilkins, 1967:85–96.
520. Roizman B, Tognon M. Restriction endonuclease patterns of herpes simplex virus DNA: Application to diagnosis and molecular epidemiology. *Curr Top Microbiol Immunol* 1983;104:273–286.
521. Roller RJ, Roizman B. The herpes simplex virus 1 RNA binding protein US11 is a virion component and associates with ribosomal 60S subunits. *J Virol* 1992;66:3624–3632.
522. Roller RJ, Roizman B. Herpes simplex virus 1 RNA-binding protein US11 negatively regulates the accumulation of a truncated viral mRNA. *J Virol* 1991;65:5873–5879.
523. Romanelli MG, Cattozzo EM, Faggioli L, Tognon M. Fine mapping and characterization of the Syn 6 locus in the herpes simplex virus type 1 genome. *J Gen Virol* 1991;72:1991–1995.
524. Rosen A, Ernst F, Koch HG, et al. Replacement of the deletion in the genome (0.762–0.789) of avirulent HSV-1 HFEM using cloned MluI DNA fragment (0.7615–0.796) of virulent HSV-1 F leads to generation of virulent intratypic recombinant. *Virus Res* 1986;5:157–175.
525. Ruyechan WT. The major herpes simplex virus DNA-binding protein holds single-stranded DNA in an extended configuration. *J Virol* 1983;46:661–666.
526. Ruyechan WT, Morse LS, Knipe DM, Roizman B. Molecular genetics of herpes simplex virus. II. Mapping of the major viral glycoproteins and of the genetic loci specifying the social behavior of infected cells. *J Virol* 1979;29:677–697.
527. Sacks WR, Greene CC, Aschman DP, Schaffer PA. Herpes simplex virus type 1 ICP27 is an essential regulatory protein. *J Virol* 1985;55:796–805.
528. Sacks WR, Schaffer PA. Deletion mutants in the gene encoding the herpes simplex virus type 1 immediate-early protein ICP0 exhibit impaired growth in cell culture. *J Virol* 1987;61:829–839.
529. Sakaoka H, Kurita K, Iida Y, et al. Quantitative analysis of genomic polymorphism of herpes simples virus type 1 from six countries: Studies of molecular evolution and molecular epidemiology of the virus. *J Gen Virol* 1994;74:513–527.
530. Samaniego LA, Webb AL, DeLuca NA. Functional interactions between herpes simplex virus immediate early proteins during infection: Gene expression as a consequence of ICP27 and different domains of ICP4. *J Virol* 1995;69:5705–5715.
531. Samaniego LA, Wu N, DeLuca NA. The herpes simplex virus immediate-early protein ICP0 affects transcription from the viral genome and infected-cell survival in the absence of ICP4 and ICP27. *J Virol* 1997;71:4614–4625.
532. Sandri-Goldin RM. Interactions between a herpes simplex virus regulatory protein and cellular mRNA processing pathways. *Methods* 1998;16:95–104.
533. Sandri-Goldin RM, Hibbard MK. The herpes simplex virus type 1 regulatory protein ICP27 coimmunoprecipitates with anti-Sm antiserum, and the the C terminus appears to be required for this interaction. *J Virol* 1996;70:108–118.
534. Sandri-Goldin RM, Hibbard MK, Hardwicke MA. The C-terminal repressor region of herpes simplex virus type 1 ICP27 is required for the redistribution of small nuclear ribonucleoprotein particles and splicing factor SC35; however, these alterations are not sufficient to inhibit host cell splicing. *J Virol* 1995;69:6063–6076.
535. Sandri-Goldin RM, Mendoza GE. A herpesvirus regulatory protein appears to act post-transcriptionally by affecting mRNA processing. *Genes Dev* 1992;6:848–863.
536. Sarmiento M, Haffey M, Spear PG. Membrane proteins specified by herpes simplex viruses. III. Role of glycoprotein VP7(B2) in virion infectivity. *J Virol* 1979;29:1149–1158.
537. Sawtell NM, Thompson RL. Herpes simplex virus type 1 latency-associated transcription unit promotes anatomical site-dependent establishment and reactivation from latency. *J Virol* 1992;66: 2157–2169.
538. Sawtell NM, Thompson RL. Rapid *in vivo* reactivation of herpes simplex virus in latently infected murine ganglionic neurons after transient hyperthermia. *J Virol* 1992;66:2150–2156.
539. Schang LM, Hwang GJ, Dynlacht BD, et al. Human PC4 is a substrate-specific inhibitor of RNA polymerase II phosphorylation. *J Biol Chem* 2000;275:6071–6074.
540. Schang LM, Phillips J, Schaffer PA. Requirement for cellular cyclin-dependent kinases in herpes simplex virus replication and transcription. *J Virol* 1998;72:5626–5637.
541. Schang LM, Rosenberg A, Schaffer PA. Transcription of herpes simplex virus immediate-early and early genes is inhibited by roscovitine, an inhibitor specific for cellular cyclin-dependent kinases. *J Virol* 1999;73:2161–2172.
542. Schneweiss KE. Untersuchungen zur typendifferenzierung des herpesvirus hominis. *Z Immuno-Forsch* 1962;124:24–28.
543. Schrag JD, Prasad BVV, Rixon RJ, Chiu W. Three dimensional structure of the HSV-1 nucleocapsid. *Cell* 1989;56:651–660.
544. Schwartz J, Roizman B. Concerning the egress of herpes simplex virus from infected cells: electron and light microscope observations. *Virology* 1969;38:42–49.
545. Schwartz J, Roizman B. Similarities and differences in the development of laboratory strains and freshly isolated strains of herpes simplex virus in HEp-2 cells: Electron microscopy. *J Virol* 1969;4: 879–889.
546. Scott TF, Burgoon CF, Coriell LL, Blank H. The growth curve of the virus of herpes simplex in rabbit corneal cells grown in tissue culture with parallel observations on the development of the intranuclear inclusion body. *J Immunol* 1953;71:385–396.

547. Sears AE, Halliburton IW, Meignier B, et al. Herpes simplex virus 1 mutant deleted in the alpha 22 gene: Growth and gene expression in permissive and restrictive cells and establishment of latency in mice. *J Virol* 1985;55:338–346.
548. Sears AE, McGwire BS, Roizman B. Infection of polarized MDCK cells with herpes simplex virus 1: Two asymmetrically distributed cell receptors interact with different viral proteins. *Proc Natl Acad Sci U S A* 1991;88:5087–5091.
549. Sears AE, Meignier B, Roizman B. Establishment of latency in mice by herpes simplex virus 1 recombinants that carry insertions affecting regulation of the thymidine kinase gene. *J Virol* 1985;55: 410–416.
550. Sears AE, Roizman B. Amplification by host cell factors of a sequence contained within the herpes simplex virus 1 genome. *Proc Natl Acad Sci U S A* 1990;87:9441–9444.
551. Sedarati F, Izumi KM, Wagner EK, Stevens JG. Herpes simplex virus type 1 latency-associated transcription plays no role in establishment or maintenance of a latent infection in murine sensory neurons. *J Virol* 1989;63:4455–4458.
552. Sedarati F, Margolis TP, Stevens JG. Latent infection can be established with drastically restricted transcription and replication of the HSV-1 genome. *Virology* 1993;192:687–691.
553. Shao L, Rapp LM, Weller SK. Herpes simplex virus 1 alkaline nuclease is required for efficient egress of capsids from the nucleus. *Virology* 1993;196:146–162.
554. Sheldrick P, Berthelot N. Inverted repetitions in the chromosome of herpes simplex virus. *Cold Spring Harbor Symp Quant Biol* 1975;39: 667–678.
555. Shepard AA, DeLuca NA. A second-site revertant of a defective herpes simplex virus ICP4 protein with restored regulatory activities and impaired DNA-binding properties. *J Virol* 1991;65:787–795.
556. Shepard AA, Imbalzano AN, DeLuca NA. Separation of primary structural components conferring autoregulation, transactivation, and DNA-binding properties to the herpes simplex virus transcriptional regulatory protein ICP4. *J Virol* 1989;63:3714–3728.
557. Shepard AA, Tolentino P, DeLuca NA. Trans-dominant inhibition of herpes simplex virus transcriptional regulatory protein ICP4 by heterodimer formation. *J Virol* 1990;64:3916–3926.
558. Sherman G, Bachenheimer SL. Characterization of intranuclear capsids made by ts morphogenic mutants of HSV-1. *Virology* 1988;163: 471–480.
559. Sherman G, Bachenheimer SL. DNA processing in temperature-sensitive morphogenic mutants of HSV-1. *Virology* 1987;158:427–430.
560. Shieh MT, WuDunn D, Montgomery RI, et al. Cell surface receptors for herpes simplex virus are heparan sulfate proteoglycans. *J Cell Biol* 1992;116:1273–1281.
561. Shimomura Y, Gangarosa LP Sr, Kataoka M, Hill JM. HSV-1 shedding by Iontophoresis of 6-hydroxydopamine followed by topical epinephrine. *Invest Ophthalmol Visual Sci* 1983;24:1588–1594.
562. Shipkey FH, Erlandson RA, Bailey RB, et al. Virus biographies. II. Growth of herpes simplex virus in tissue culture. *Exp Mol Pathol* 1967;6:39–67.
563. Shukla D, Liu J, Blaiklock P, et al. A novel role for 3-O-sulfated heparan sulfate in herpes simplex virus 1 entry. *Cell* 1999;99:13–22.
564. Sieg S, Yildirim Z, Smith D, et al. Herpes simplex virus type 2 inhibition of Fas ligand expression. *J Virol* 1966;70:8747–8751.
565. Silver S, Roizman B. gamma 2-Thymidine kinase chimeras are identically transcribed but regulated a gamma 2 genes in herpes simplex virus genomes and as beta genes in cell genomes. *Mol Cell Biol* 1985; 5:518–528.
566. Siminoff P, Menefee MG. Normal and 5-bromodeoxyuridine-inhibited development of herpes simplex virus: An electron microscope study. *Exp Cell Res* 1966;44:241–255.
567. Simmons A, Slobedman B, Speck P, et al. Two patterns of persistence of herpes simplex virus DNA sequences in the nervous systems of latently infected mice. *J Gen Virol* 1992;73:1287–1291.
568. Sinclair MC, McLauchlan J, Marsden H, Brown SM. Characterization of a herpes simplex virus type 1 deletion variant (1703) which underproduces Vmw63 during immediate early conditions of infection. *J Gen Virol* 1994;75:1083–1089.
569. Singh J, Wagner EK. Transcriptional analysis of the herpes simplex virus type 1 region containing the TRL/UL junction. *Virology* 1993; 196:220–231.
570. Smibert CA, Popova B, Xiao P, et al. Herpes simplex virus VP16 forms a complex with the virion host shutoff protein vhs. *J Virol* 1994; 68:2339–2346.
571. Smiley JR, Duncan J, Howes M. Sequence requirements for DNA rearrangements induced by the terminal repeat of herpes simplex virus type 1 KOS DNA. *J Virol* 1990;64:5036–5050.
572. Smiley JR, Johnson DC, Pizer LI, Everett RD. The ICP4 binding sites in the herpes simplex virus type 1 glycoprotein D (gD) promoter are not essential for efficient gD transcription during virus infection. *J Virol* 1992;66:623–631.
573. Smith CA, Bates P, Rivera-Gonzalez R, et al. ICP4, the major transcriptional regulatory protein of herpes simplex virus type 1, forms a tripartite complex with TATA-binding protein and TFIIB. *J Virol* 1993;67:4676–4687.
574. Smith CC, Peng T, Kulka M, Aurelian L. The PK domain of the large subunit of herpes simplex virus type 2 ribonucleotide reductase (ICP10) is required for immediate-early gene expression and virus growth. *J Virol* 1998;72:9131–9141.
575. Smith IL, Hardwicke MA, Sandri-Goldin RM. Evidence that the herpes simplex virus immediate early protein ICP27 acts post-transcriptionally during infection to regulate gene expression. *Virology* 1992; 186:74–86.
576. Smith RD, Sutherland K. The cytopathology of virus infections. In: Spector S, Lancz GJ, ed. *Clinical virology manual.* New York: Elsevier Science, 1986:53–69.
577. Smith RF, Smith TF. Identification of new protein kinase-related genes in three herpesviruses, herpes simplex virus, varicella-zoster virus, and Epstein-Barr virus. *J Virol* 1989;63:450–455.
578. Sodeik B, Ebersold M, Helenius A. Dynein mediated transport of incoming herpes simplex virus 1 capsids to the nucleus. *J Cell Biol* 1997;136:1007–1021.
579. Soliman TM, Sandri-Goldin RM, Silverstein SJ. Shuttling of the herpes simplex virus type 1 regulatory protein ICP27 between the nucleus and cytoplasm mediates the expression of late proteins. *J Virol* 1997;71:9188–9197.
580. Soliman TM, Silverstein SJ. Identification of an export control sequence and a requirement for the KH domains in ICP27 from herpes simplex virus type 1. *J Virol* 2000;74:7600–7609.
581. Song B, Liu JJ, Yeh KC, et al. Herpes simplex virus infection blocks events in the G1 phase of the cell cycle. *Virology* 2000;267:326–334.
582. Spaete RR, Frenkel N. The herpes simplex virus amplicon: Analyses of cis-acting replication functions. *Proc Natl Acad Sci U S A* 1985;82: 694–698.
583. Spear PG. Antigenic structure of herpes simplex viruses. In: van Regenmortel MHV, Neurath AR, ed. *Immunochemistry of viruses: The basis for serodiagnosis and vaccines.* Amsterdam: Elsevier Science, 1985:425–446.
584. Spear PG. Glycoproteins specified by herpes simplex viruses. In: Roizman B, ed. *The herpesviruses,* vol. 3. New York: Plenum, 1985: 315–356.
585. Spear PG. Membrane fusion induced by herpes simplex virus. In: Bentz J, ed. *Viral fusion mechanisms.* Boca Raton, FL: CRC Press, 1993:201–232.
586. Spear PG, Eisenberg RJ, Cohen GH. Three classes of cell surface receptors for alphaherpesvirus entry. *Virology* 2000;275:1–8.
587. Spear PG, Kellejmroian B. Proteins spcified by herpes simplex virus. II. Viral glycoprotins associated with cellular membranes. *J Virol* 1970;5:123–131.
588. Spear PG, Roizman B. Buoyant density of herpes simplex virus in solutions of caesium chloride. *Nature* 1967;214:713–714.
589. Spear PG, Roizman B. Proteins specified by herpes simplex virus. V. Purification and structural proteins of the herpesvirion. *J Virol* 1972; 9:143–159.
590. Speck PG, Simmons A. Divergent molecular pathways of productive and latent infection with a virulent strain of herpes simplex virus type 1. *J Virol* 1991;65:4001–4005.
591. Speck PG, Simmons A. Synchronous appearance of antigen-positive and latently infected neurons in spinal ganglia of mice infected with a virulent strain of herpes simplex virus. *J Gen Virol* 1992;73:1281–1285.
592. Spector D, Purves F, Roizman B. Role of alpha-transinducing factor (VP16) in the induction of alpha genes within the context of viral genomes. *J Virol* 1991;65:3504–3513.
593. Spencer CA, Dahmus ME, Rice SA. Repression of host RNA polymerase II transcription by herpes simplex virus type 1. *J Virol* 1997; 71:2031–2040.

594. Spivack JG, Fraser NW. Detection of herpes simplex virus type 1 transcripts during latent infection in mice [published erratum appears in *J Virol* 1988 Feb;62(2):663]. *J Virol* 1987;61:3841–3847.
595. Spivack JG, Fraser NW. Expression of herpes simplex virus type 1 latency-associated transcripts in the trigeminal ganglia of mice during acute infection and reactivation of latent infection. *J Virol* 1988;62: 1479–1485.
596. Stackpole CW. Herpes-type virus of the frog renal adenocarcinoma. I. Virus development in tumor transplants maintained at low temperature. *J Virol* 1969;4:75–93.
597. Stanberry LR, Kern ER, Richards JT, et al. Genital herpes in guinea pigs: Pathogenesis of the primary infection and description of recurrent disease. *J Infect Dis* 1982;146:397–404.
598. Stanberry LR, Kit S, Myers MG. Thymidine kinase-deficient herpes simplex virus type 2 genital infection in guinea pigs. *J Virol* 1985;55: 322–328.
599. Stannard LM, Fuller AO, Spear PG. Herpes simplex virus glycoproteins associated with different morphological entities projecting from the virion envelope. *J Gen Virol* 1987;68:715–725.
600. Staskus KA, Couch L, Bitterman P, et al. *In situ* amplification of visna virus DNA in tissue sections reveals a reservoir of latently infected cells. *Microb Pathog* 1991;11:67–76.
601. Steffy KR, Weir JP. Mutational analysis of two herpes simplex virus type 1 late promoters. *J Virol* 1991;65:6454–6460.
602. Steiner I, Spivack JG, Lirette RP, et al. Herpes simplex virus type 1 latency-associated transcripts are evidently not essential for latent infection. *EMBO J* 1989;8:505–511.
603. Stern S, Herr W. The herpes simplex virus trans-activator VP16 recognizes the Oct-1 homeo domain: Evidence for a homeo domain recognition subdomain. *Genes Dev* 1991;5:2555–2566.
604. Steven AC, Spear PG. Herpesvirus capsid assembly and envelopment. In: Burnett R, Chiu W, Garcea R, eds. *Structural biology of viruses.* New York: Oxford University Press, 1997:312–391.
605. Stevens JG, Cook ML. Latent herpes simplex virus in spinal ganglia of mice. *Science* 1971;173:843–845.
606. Stevens JG, Wagner EK, Devi-Rao GB, et al. RNA complementary to a herpesvirus alpha gene mRNA is prominent in latently infected neurons. *Science* 1987;235:1056–1059.
607. Stow ND. Localization of an origin of DNA replication within the TRS/IRS repeated region of the herpes simplex virus type 1 genome. *EMBO J* 1982;1:863–867.
608. Stow ND, McMonagle EC. Characterization of the TRS/IRS origin of DNA replication of herpes simplex virus type 1. *Virology* 1983;130: 427–438.
609. Stow ND, McMonagle EC, Davison AJ. Fragments from both termini of the herpes simplex virus type 1 genome contain signals required for the encapsidation of viral DNA. *Nucleic Acids Res* 1983;11: 8205–8220.
610. Stow ND, Stow EC. Isolation and characterization of a herpes simplex virus type 1 mutant containing a deletion within the gene encoding the immediate early polypeptide Vmw110. *J Gen Virol* 1986;67: 2571–2585.
611. Stow ND, Subak-Sharpe JH, Wilkie NM. Physical mapping of herpes simplex virus type 1 mutations by marker rescue. *J Virol* 1978;28: 182–192.
612. Stringer KF, Ingles CJ, Greenblatt J. Direct and selective binding of an acidic transcriptional activation domain to the TATA-box factor TFIID. *Nature* 1990;345:783–786.
613. Su L, Knipe DM. Herpes simplex virus alpha protein ICP27 can inhibit or augment viral gene transactivation. *Virology* 1989;170: 496–504.
614. Summers WP, Wagner M, Summers WC. Possible peptide chain termination mutants in thymide kinase gene of a mammalian virus, herpes simplex virus. *Proc Natl Acad Sci U S A* 1975;72:4081–4084.
615. Sydiskis RJ, Roizman B. The disaggregation of host polyribosomes in productive and abortive infection with herpes simplex virus. *Virology* 1966;32:678–686.
616. Szilagyi JF, Cunningham C. Identification and characterization of a novel non-infectious herpes simplex virus-related particle. *J Gen Virol* 1991;72:661–668.
617. Takahashi K, Nakanishi H, Miyahara M, et al. Nection/PRR: An immunoglobulin-like cell adhesion molecule recruited to cadherin-based adherens junctions through interaction with afadin, a PDZ domain-containing protein. *J Cell Biol* 1999;145:539–549.
618. Tal-Singer R, Lasner TM, Podrzucki W, et al. Gene expression during reactivation of herpes simplex virus type 1 from latency in the peripheral nervous system is different from that during lytic infection of tissue cultures. *J Virol* 1997;71:5268–5276.
619. Tanguy LeGac N, Villani G, Boehmer PE. Herpes simplex virus type-1 single-stranded DNA-binding protein (ICP8) enhances the ability of the viral DNA helicase-primase to unwind cisplatin-modified DNA. *J Biol Chem* 1998;273:13801–13807.
620. Tankersley RW. Amino acid requirements of herpes simplex virus in human cells. *J Bacteriol* 1964;87:609–613.
621. Tatman JD, Preston VG, Nicholson P, et al. Assembly of herpes simplex virus type 1 capsids using a panel of recombinant baculoviruses. *J Gen Virol* 1994;75:1101–1113.
622. Tedder DG, Everett RD, Wilcox KW, et al. ICP4-binding sites in the promoter and coding regions of the herpes simplex virus gD gene contribute to activation of in vitro transcription by ICP4. *J Virol* 1989; 63:2510–2520.
623. Tenser RB, Hay KA, Edris WA. Latency-associated transcript but not reactivatable virus is present in sensory ganglion neurons after inoculation of thymidine kinase-negative mutants of herpes simplex virus type 1. *J Virol* 1989;63:2861–2865.
624. Thomas HC, Torok ME, Foster GR. Hepatitis C virus dynamics *in vivo* and the antiviral efficacy of interferon alfa therapy. *Hepatology* 1999;29:1333–1334.
625. Thomas MS, Gao M, Knipe DM, Powell KL. Association between the herpes simplex virus major DNA-binding protein and alkaline nuclease. *J Virol* 1992;66:1152–1161.
626. Thompson RL, Cook ML, Devi-Rao GB, et al. Functional and molecular analyses of the avirulent wild-type herpes simplex virus type 1 strain KOS. *J Virol* 1986;58:203–211.
627. Thompson RL, Devi-Rao GV, Stevens JG, Wagner EK. Rescue of a herpes simplex virus type 1 neurovirulence function with a cloned DNA fragment. *J Virol* 1985;55:504–508.
628. Thompson RL, Sawtell NM. The herpes simplex virus type 1 latency-associated transcript gene regulates the establishment of latency. *J Virol* 1997;71:5432–5440.
629. Thompson RL, Sawtell NM. Replication of herpes simplex virus type 1 within trigeminal ganglia is required for high frequency but not high viral genome copy number latency. *J Virol* 2000;74:965–974.
630. Thomsen DR, Newcomb WW, Brown JC, Homa FL. Assembly of the herpes simplex virus capsid: Requirement for the carboxyl-terminal twenty-five amino acids of the proteins encoded by the UL26 and UL26.5 genes. *J Virol* 1995;69:3690–3703.
631. Thomsen DR, Roof LL, Homa FL. Assembly of herpes simplex virus (HSV) intermediate capsids in insect cells infected with recombinant baculoviruses expressing HSV capsid proteins. *J Virol* 1994;68: 2442–2457.
632. Tognon M, Furlong D, Conley AJ, Roizman B. Molecular genetics of herpes simplex virus. V. Characterization of a mutant defective in ability to form plaques at low temperatures and in a viral fraction which prevents accumulation of coreless capsids at nuclear pores late in infection. *J Virol* 1981;40:870–880.
633. Tran LC, Kissner JM, Westerman LE, Sears AE. A herpes simplex virus 1 recombinant lacking the glycoprotein G coding sequences is defective in entry through apical surfaces of polarized epithelial cells in culture and in vivo. *Proc Natl Acad Sci U S A* 2000;97:1818–1822.
634. Triezenberg SJ, Kingsbury RC, McKnight SL. Functional dissection of VP16, the trans-activator of herpes simplex virus immediate early gene expression. *Genes Dev* 1988;2:718–729.
635. Trousdale MD, Steiner I, Spivack JG, et al. *In vivo* and *in vitro* reactivation impairment of a herpes simplex virus type 1 latency-associated transcript variant in a rabbit eye model. *J Virol* 1991;65: 6989–6993.
636. Trus BL, Booy FP, Newcomb WW, et al. The herpes simplex procapsid: Structure, conformational changes upon maturation, and roles of the triplex proteins VP19C and VP23 in assembly. *J Mol Biol* 1996; 263:447–462.
637. Tullo AB, Shimeld C, Blyth WA, et al. Spread of virus and distribution of latent infection following ocular herpes simplex in the non-immune and immune mouse. *J Gen Virol* 1982;63:95–101.
638. Umene K, Nishimoto T. Replication of herpes simplex virus type 1 DNA is inhibited in a temperature-sensitive mutant of BHK-21 cells lacking RCC1 (regulator of chromosome condensation) and virus DNA remains linear. *J Gen Virol* 1996;77:2261–2270.

639. Uprichard SL, Knipe DM. Herpes simplex virus ICP27 mutant viruses exhibit reduced expression of specific DNA replication genes. *J Virol* 1996;70:1969–1980.
640. Valyi-Nagy T, Deshmane SL, Dillner A, Fraser NW. Induction of cellular transcription factors in trigeminal ganglia of mice by corneal scarification, herpes simplex virus type 1 infection, and explantation of trigeminal ganglia. *J Virol* 1991;65:4142–4152.
641. Valyi-Nagy T, Gesser RM, Raengsakulrach B, et al. A thymidine kinase-negative HSV-1 strain establishes a persistent infection in SCID mice that features uncontrolled peripheral replication but only marginal nervous system involvement. *Virology* 1994;199:484–490.
642. van Genderen IL, Brandimarti R, Torrisi MR, et al. The phospholipid composition of extracellular herpes simplex virions differs from that of host cell nuclei. *Virology* 1994;200:831–836.
643. Van Sant C, Kawaguchi Y, Roizman B. A single amino acid substitution in the cyclin D binding domain of the infected cell protein no. 0 abrogates the neuroinvasivesness of herpes simplex virus without affecting its ability to replicate. *Proc Natl Acad Sci U S A* 1999;96:8184–8189.
644. Van Sant C, Lopez P, Advani SJ, Roizman B. The role of cyclin D3 in the biology of the infected cell protein No. 0 of herpes simplex virus 1. *J Virol* 2001;75:1888–1898.
645. Varmuza SL, Smiley JR. Signals for site-specific cleavage of HSV DNA: Maturation involves two separate cleavage events at sites distal to the recognition sequences. *Cell* 1985;41:793–802.
646. Vaughan PJ, Thibault KJ, Hardwicke MA, Sandri-Goldin RM. The herpes simplex virus immediate early protein ICP27 encodes a potential metal binding domain and binds zinc in vitro. *Virology* 1992;189:377–384.
647. Vernon SK, Ponce de Leon M, Cohen GH, et al. Morphological components of herpesvirus. III. Localization of herpes simplex virus type 1 nucleocapsid polypeptides by immune electron microscopy. *J Gen Virol* 1981;54:39–46.
648. Vlazny DA, Kwong A, Frenkel N. Site-specific cleavage/packaging of herpes simplex virus DNA and the selective maturation of nucleocapsids containing full-length viral DNA. *Proc Natl Acad Sci U S A* 1982;79:1423–1427.
649. Wadd S, Bryant H, Filhol O, et al. The multifunctional herpes simplex virus IE63 protein interacts with heterogeneous ribonucleoprotein K and with casein kinase 2. *J Biol Chem* 1999;274:28991–28998.
650. Wadsworth S, Jacob RJ, Roizman B. Anatomy of herpes simplex virus DNA. II. Size, composition, and arrangement of inverted terminal repetitions. *J Virol* 1975;15:1487–1497.
651. Wagner EK. Individual HSV transcripts: Characterisation of specific genes. In: Roizman B, ed. *The herpesviruses.* New York: Plenum, 1985:45–104.
652. Wagner EK, Devi-Rao G, Feldman LT, et al. Physical characterization of the herpes simplex virus latency-associated transcript in neurons. *J Virol* 1988;62:1194–1202.
653. Wagner EK, Flanagan WM, Devi-Rao G, et al. The herpes simplex virus latency-associated transcript is spliced during the latent phase of infection. *J Virol* 1988;62:4577–4585.
654. Wagner EK, Roizman B. RNA synthesis in cells infected with herpes simplex virus. II. Evidence that a class of viral mRNA is derived from a high molecular weight precursor synthesized in the nucleus. *Proc Natl Acad Sci U S A* 1969;64:626–633.
655. Wagner MJ, Summers WC. Structure of the joint region and the termini of the DNA of herpes simplex virus type 1. *J Virol* 1978;27:374–387.
656. Walz MA, Yamamoto H, Notkins AL. Immunological response restricts number of cells in sensory ganglia infected with herpes simplex virus. *Nature* 1976;264:554–556.
657. Ward PL, Avitabile E, Campadelli-Fiume G, Roizman B. Conservation of the architecture of the Golgi apparatus related to a differential organization of microtubules in polykaryocytes induced by syn–mutants of herpes simplex virus 1. *Virology* 1998;241:189–199.
658. Ward PL, Barker DE, Roizman B. A novel herpes simplex virus 1 gene, UL43.5, maps antisense to the UL43 gene and encodes a protein which colocalizes in nuclear structures with capsid proteins. *J Virol* 1996;70:2684–2690.
659. Warner MS, Geraghty RJ, Martinez WM, et al. A cell surface protein with herpesvirus entry activity (HveB) confers susceptibility to infection by mutants of herpes simplex virus type 1, herpes simplex virus type 2 and pseudorabies virus. *Virology* 1998;246:179–189.
660. Watson RJ, Clements JB. A herpes simplex virus type 1 function continuously required for early and late virus RNA synthesis. *Nature* 1980;285:329–330.
661. Watson RJ, Sullivan M, Vande Woude GF. Structures of two spliced herpes simplex virus type 1 immediate-early mRNAs which map at the junctions of the unique and reiterated regions of the virus DNA S component. *J Virol* 1981;37:431–444.
662. Watson RJ, Weis JH, Salstrom JS, Enquist LW. Herpes simplex virus type-1 glycoprotein D gene: Nucleotide sequence and expression in *Escherichia coli. Science* 1982;218:381–384.
663. Weber PC, Challberg MD, Nelson NJ, et al. Inversion events in the HSV-1 genome are directly mediated by the viral DNA replication machinery and lack sequence specificity. *Cell* 1988;54:369–381.
664. Weber PC, Levine M, Glorioso JC. Rapid identification of nonessential genes of herpes simplex virus type 1 by Tn5 mutagenesis. *Science* 1987;236:576–579.
665. Weinheimer SP, Boyd BA, Durham SK, et al. Deletion of the VP16 open reading frame of herpes simplex virus type 1. *J Virol* 1992;66:258–269.
666. Weinheimer SP, McKnight SL. 1987. Transcriptional and post-transcriptional controls establish the cascade of herpes simplex virus protein synthesis. *J Mol Biol* 1987;195:819–833.
667. Weir JP, Narayanan PR. The use of beta-galactosidase as a marker gene to define the regulatory sequences of the herpes simplex virus type 1 glycoprotein C gene in recombinant herpesviruses [published erratum appears in *Nucleic Acids Res* 1989;17(5):2157]. *Nucleic Acids Res* 1988;16:10267–10282.
668. Weller SK, Lee KJ, Sabourin DJ, Schaffer PA. Genetic analysis of temperature-sensitive mutants which define the gene for the major herpes simplex virus type 1 DNA-binding protein. *J Virol* 1983;45:354–366.
669. Weller SK, Spadaro A, Schaffer JE, et al. Cloning, sequencing, and functional analysis of oriL, a herpes simplex virus type 1 origin of DNA synthesis. *Mol Cell Biol* 1985;5:930–942.
670. Whitbeck JC, Peng C, Lou H, et al. Glycoprotein D of herpes simplex virus (HSV) binds directly to HVEM, a member of the tumor necrosis factor receptor superfamily and a mediator of HSV entry. *J Virol* 1997;71:6083–6093.
671. Whiteley A, Bruun B, Minson T, Browne H. Effects of targeting herpes simplex virus type 1 gD to the endoplasmic reticulum and trans-golgi network. *J Virol* 1999;73:9515–9520.
672. Whitley RJ. Epidemiology of herpes simplex viruses. In: Roizman B, ed. *The herpesviruses.* New York: Plenum, 1985:1–44.
673. Whitley RJ, Kern ER, Chatterjee S, et al. Replication, establishment of latency, and induced reactivation of herpes simplex virus gamma 1 34.5 deletion mutants in rodent models. *J Clin Invest* 1993;91:2837–2843.
674. Wilcox CL, Johnson EM Jr. Nerve growth factor deprivation results in the reactivation of latent herpes simplex virus *in vitro. J Virol* 1987;61:2311–2315.
675. Wilcox KW, Kohn A, Sklyanskaya E, Roizman B. Herpes simplex virus phosphoproteins. I. Phosphate cycles on and off some viral polypeptides and can alter their affinity for DNA. *J Virol* 1980;33:167–182.
676. Wildy P, Russell WC, Horne RW. The morphology of herpes virus. *Virology* 1960;12:204–222.
677. Wilkie NM. The synthesis and substructure of herpesvirus DNA: The distribution of alkali labile strand interruptions in HSV-1 DNA. *J Gen Virol* 1973;21:453–467.
678. Wohlenberg CR, Walz MA, Notkins AL. Efficacy of phosphonoacetic acid on herpes simplex virus infection of sensory ganglia. *Infect Immun* 1976;13:1519–1521.
679. Wohlrab F, Chatterjee S, Wells RD. The herpes simplex virus 1 segment inversion site is specifically cleaved by a virus-induced nuclear endonuclease. *Proc Natl Acad Sci U S A* 1991;88:6432–6436.
680. Wolf K, Darlington RW. Channel catfish virus: A new herpesvirus of ictalurid fish. *J Virol* 1971;8:525–533.
681. Wu CA, Nelson NJ, McGeoch DJ, Challberg MD. Identification of herpes simplex virus type 1 genes required for origin-dependent DNA synthesis. *J Virol* 1988;62:435–443.
682. Wu CL, Wilcox KW. Codons 262 to 490 from the herpes simplex virus ICP4 gene are sufficient to encode a sequence-specific DNA binding protein. *Nucleic Acids Res* 1990;18:531–538.
683. Wu CL, Wilcox KW. The conserved DNA-binding domains encoded by the herpes simplex virus type 1 ICP4, pseudorabies virus IE180,

and varicella-zoster virus ORF62 genes recognize similar sites in the corresponding promoters. *J Virol* 1991;65:1149–1159.
684. Wu N, Watkins SC, Schaffer PA, DeLuca NA. Prolonged gene expression and cell survival after infection by a herpes simplex virus mutant defective in the immediate-early genes encoding ICP4, ICP27, and ICP22. *J Virol* 1996;70:6358–6369.
685. Wu TT, Su YH, Block TM, Taylor JM. Evidence that two latency-associated transcripts of herpes simplex virus type 1 are nonlinear. *J Virol* 1996;70:5962–5967.
686. WuDunn D, Spear PG. Initial interaction of herpes simplex virus with cells is binding to heparan sulfate. *J Virol* 1989;63:52–58.
687. Xia K, DeLuca NA, Knipe DM. Analysis of phosphorylation sites of the herpes simplex virus 1 infected cell protein 4 (ICP4). *J Virol* 1996; 70:1061–1071.
688. Xiao P, Capone JP. A cellular factor binds to the herpes simplex virus type 1 transactivator Vmw65 and is required for Vmw65-dependent protein-DNA complex assembly with Oct-1. *Mol Cell Biol* 1990;10: 4974–4977.
689. Yamamoto S, Kabuta H. Genetic analysis of polykaryocytosis by herpes simplex virus. III. Complementation and recombination between non-fusing mutants and construction of a linkage map with regard to the fusion function. *Kurume Med J* 1977;24:163.
690. Yao F, Courtney RJ. Association of ICP0 but not ICP27 with purified virions of herpes simplex virus type 1. *J Virol* 1992;66:2709–2716.
691. Ye GJ, Roizman B. The essential protein encoded by the UL31 gene of herpes simplex virus 1 depends for its stability on the presence of UL34 protein. *Proc Natl Acad Sci U S A* 2000;97:11002–11007.
692. Ye GJ, Vaughan KT, Vallee RB, Roizman B. The herpes simplex virus 1 U(L)34 protein interacts with a cytoplasmic dynein intermediate chain and targets nuclear membrane. *J Virol* 2000;74:1355–1363.
693. Yeh L, Schaffer PA. A novel class of transcripts expressed with late kinetics in the absence of ICP4 spans the junction between the long and short segments of the herpes simplex virus type 1 genome. *J Virol* 1993;67:7373–7382.
694. Yei SP, Chowdhury SI, Bhat BM, et al. Identification and characterization of the herpes simplex virus type 2 gene encoding the essential capsid protein ICP32/VP19c. *J Virol* 1990;64:1124–1134.
695. York IA, Roop C, Andrews DW, et al. A cytosolic herpes simplex virus protein inhibits antigen presentation to CD8+ T lymphocytes. *Cell* 1994;77:525–535.
696. Zabolotny JM, Krummenacher C, Fraser NW. The herpes simplex virus type 1 2.0-kilobase latency-associated transcript is a stable intron which branches at a guanosine. *J Virol* 1997;71:4199–4208.
697. Zachos G, Clements B, Conner J. Herpes simplex virus type 1 infection stimulates p38/c-Jun N-terminal mitogen-activated protein kinase pathways and activates transcription factor AP-1. *J Biol Chem* 1999; 274:5097–5103.
698. Zelus BD, Stewart RS, Ross J. The virion host shutoff protein of herpes simplex virus type 1: Messenger ribonucleolytic activity in vitro. *J Virol* 1996;70:2411–2419.
699. Zhang YF, Devi-Rao GB, Rice M, et al. The effect of elevated levels of herpes simplex virus alpha-gene products on the expression of model early and late genes in vivo. *Virology* 1987;157:99–106.
700. Zhou G, Galvan V, Campadelli-Fiume G, Roizman B. Glycoprotein D or J delivered in trans blocks apoptosis in SK-N-SH cells induced by a herpes simplex virus 1 mutant lacking intact genes expressing both glycoproteins. *J Virol* 2000;74:11782–11791.
701. Zhou G, Roizman B. Wild-type herpes simplex virus 1 blocks programmed cell death and release of cytochrome c but not the translocation of mitochondrial apoptosis-inducing factorto the nuclei of human embryonic lung fibroblasts. *J Virol* 2000;74:9048–9053.
702. Zhou ZH, Chen DH, Jakana J, et al. Visualization of tegument-capsid interactions and DNA in intact herpes simplex virus type 1 virions. *J Virol* 1999;73:3210–3218.
703. Zhou ZH, Dougherty M, Jakana J, et al. Seeing the herpesvirus capsid at 8.5 Å. *Science* 2000;288:877–880.
704. Zhu LA, Weller SK. The six conserved helicase motifs of the UL5 gene product, a component of the herpes simplex virus type 1 helicase-primase, are essential for its function. *J Virol* 1992;66:469–479.
705. Zwaagstra JC, Ghiasi H, Slanina SM, et al. Activity of herpes simplex virus type 1 latency-associated transcript (LAT) promoter in neuron-derived cells: Evidence for neuron specificity and for a large LAT transcript. *J Virol* 1990;64:5019–5028.
706. Zweig M, Heilman CJ Jr, Hampar B. Identification of disulfide-linked protein complexes in the nucleocapsids of herpes simplex virus type 2. *Virology* 1979;94:442–450.

CHAPTER 34

Epstein-Barr Virus and Its Replication

Elliott Kieff and Alan B. Rickinson

CLASSIFICATION

Epstein-Barr virus (EBV) was discovered in 1964 (192). Beginning in the 1940s, Denis Burkitt, a British missionary surgeon, observed and treated children with previously undescribed extranodal lymphomas. He noted that the lymphomas were frequent in regions of equatorial Africa with holoendemic malaria and rarely occurred elsewhere. Burkitt wrote and spoke widely about the unusual epidemiologic and clinical features of this lymphoma, raising the specter of an infectious etiology (81). After hearing Burkitt speak about this new disease at Bristol University, Tony Epstein arranged collaborations to obtain tumor biopsies and succeeded in culturing the lymphoma cells. Epstein, Achong, and Barr identified a herpesvirus in electron micrographs of the tumor cells growing in culture. They showed that the virus differed from the known human herpesviruses in being unable to replicate in other cultured cells and in being nonreactive with antibodies to other known human herpesviruses. EBV became the first candidate human tumor virus.

EBV is now the prototype of the gamma subfamily of potentially oncogenic herpesviruses. The gamma herpesvirus subfamily includes both the gamma 1, or *Lymphocryptovirus* (LCV), and gamma 2, or *Rhadinovirus* (RDV), genera. EBV is the only human LCV, and the recently discovered Kaposi's sarcoma–associated herpesvirus (KSHV) is the only human RDV (93). Herpesvirus saimiri (HVS), an RDV that was discovered in New World primates and found to cause lymphomas in experimental infection, was the previous prototype RDV (10). Many Old World primate species have their own endemic LCV, and recent evidence suggests that some New World primate species also have endemic LCVs (61,207,244,246,313,457,474,676). In contrast, RDVs have been identified not only in many primate species but also in many subprimate mammalian species (9,11,188, 858). At this stage of accumulation of LCV and RDV DNA sequences, RDV DNAs are more diverse than LCV DNAs. The endemicity of RDVs in a broader range of mammalian species and their greater genome divergence are evidence that RDVs evolved earlier than the LCVs. Given the many similarities of the LCV and RDV genomes and the restriction of LCVs to primates, LCVs are likely to have evolved from an early primate RDV. This would explain the presence of LCVs only in primates.

The LCV genomes are very similar to each other in structure and gene organization. In general, their DNAs are composed of colinearly homologous sequences. The EBV genome organization is shown in Figure 1 and compared to that of KSHV. The schematic diagram is based on the published analyses of KSHV DNA sequences. The LCVs share structural features such as similar 0.5-kbp

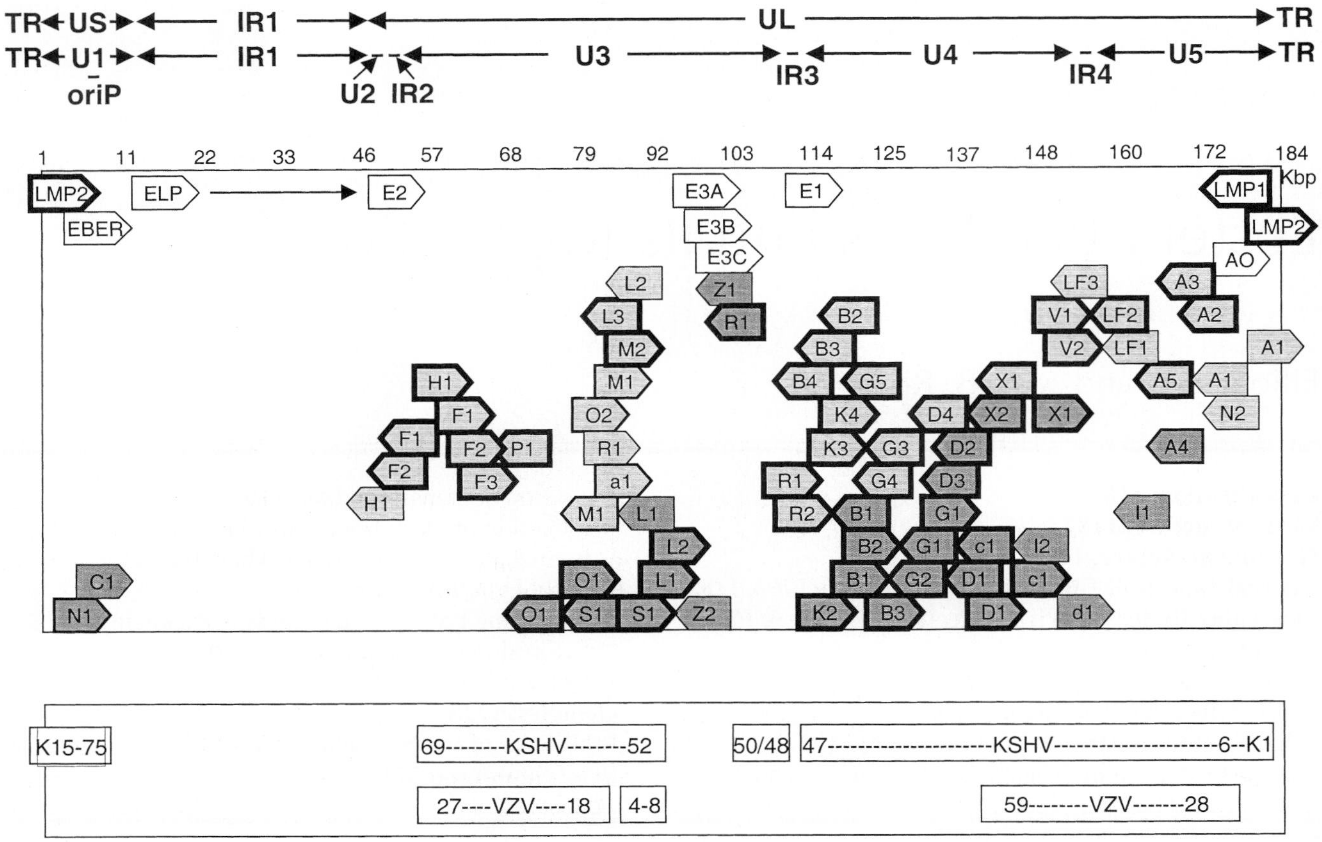

FIG. 1. Schematic depiction of the linear EBV genome, and comparison with the genomes of KSHV (712) and VZV (154,155). At the *top* of the figure, the terminal repeat (TR), internal repeat (IR1-4), and the largely unique sequence domains (U1-U5) of the EBV genome are depicted in proportion to their overall size. The position of the cis-acting element for episome maintenance and replication in latent infection, oriP, is indicated. The origins for EBV DNA replication in lytic infection are in U3 and U5 just to the right of IR2 and IR4. The P3HR-1 EBV strain is deleted for DNA between 45 and 52 kbp in the indicated map. EBV open reading frames (*ORFs*) are indicated based on the size of the encoding *Bam*HI fragment (A, B, C, etc., in decreasing size), using the convention of Barrell et al. (36,209). The origins and direction of the reading frames are indicated in the *large panel* according to scale. However, the size of the text box and end of the ORFs are not to scale. ORFs expressed in EBV latent infection are in *clear text boxes*, immediate-early in *dark gray*, early in *light gray*, and late in *medium gray*. ORFs that are conserved in KSHV are indicated by *thick outline* and by blocks shown in the *lower panel*. The numbers in the lower panel refer to homologous ORFs of KSHV (712) or VZV (154), which are displayed by their corresponding EBV map location.

terminal (TR), 3-kbp internal (IR1), and short internal (IR2, IR4) tandem direct repeats (142,143,313,314,316, 474,714). The LCV open reading frames (ORFs) also encode colinearly homologous, antigenically related, structural and nonstructural proteins (384,648,690).

LCV genomes include genes that are shared by most herpesviruses, genes that are shared among gamma herpesviruses but not with other herpesviruses, and a number of genes that are characteristic only of LCVs (see Fig. 1). The genes that are shared with most herpesviruses include genes that encode for proteins that are involved in nucleotide metabolism, genes that encode for proteins that replicate viral DNA, genes that encode for proteins that comprise the structural components of the virion, and genes that encode for proteins that package viral DNA, modify the infected cell, and enable the virus envelope to fuse with the cell membrane. Despite base compositions ranging from 43% guanine plus cytosine for varicella-zoster virus (VZV) to 71% guanine plus cytosine for herpes simplex virus (HSV), herpesvirus DNAs have large regions with colinear, distant homology at the predicted protein level (see Fig. 1) (36,154,155,442). For example, one large conserved domain, homologous to VZV ORFs 28 to 59 (see Fig. 1), encodes for the major DNA binding protein, DNA polymerase, glycoprotein (gp) B (gB), thymidine kinase (TK), and gH. Similarities notwithstanding, base-pair conservation even in the homologous domains is inadequate to permit EBV DNA to hybridize to the homologous HSV, VZV, cytomegalovirus (CMV), or even KSHV DNAs. Furthermore, antigenic cross-reactivity between EBV and other human herpesviruses is rare, even among proteins encoded by the most conserved genes. The genes that are shared among the gamma herpesviruses and have more limited or less obvious representation in the genomes of other herpesviruses include genes that encode several immediate-early or early regulators of viral gene expression, an antiapoptotic Bcl-2 homolog, and two integral membrane proteins that in EBV are designated LMP1 and LMP2. LCVs and RDVs also have analogous, but nonhomologous, cis-acting DNA sequences and transacting nuclear proteins that are necessary and sufficient for persistence of the genomes as episomes in dividing cells (41,910). The genes that are well conserved among only LCVs include a set of genes that encode nuclear and integral membrane proteins that are important for latent B-lymphocyte infection and cell growth transformation, genes that encode two small nonpolyadenylated RNAs, genes that encode an interleukin (IL)-10 homolog, and a gene that encodes a glycoprotein that binds to a B-lymphocyte surface protein, CD21.

Overall, the LCV and RDV genomes are much more closely related to each other than to the genomes of the alpha or beta herpesviruses (36,154,155,712). Of the 75 KSHV predicted ORFs, 54 are colinearly homologous to ORFs of EBV (see Fig. 1). Only one of these 54 is out of place relative to its position in EBV. The mean amino acid identity to EBV among the 54 KSHV ORFs is 35%, with only two less than 21%.

Nevertheless, LCV and RDV are clearly distinct genera. The sequence homology between EBV and KSHV is insufficient to detect significant cross-reactive antibody or T-cell responses. Primates including humans can be persistently systemically infected by viruses of both genera. Whereas LCVs are able to efficiently immortalize B lymphocytes of their natural host, RDVs lack similar activity. At the genome level, RDVs have very highly reiterated terminal direct repeats and lack long internal direct repeats. Most RDVs have a common set of cellular genes that include dihydrofolate reductase, interferon regulator factors, G-protein coupled receptors, chemokine analogs, and a cyclin homolog, none of which have been found in LCVs.

The gamma herpesvirus subfamily classification was initially established not on the basis of similarity in genome organization but on the basis of similarity in biologic properties. EBV and KSHV have particularly limited host ranges for *in vitro* infection and are associated with human malignancies. Much of the interest in these viruses is because of their association with cancer. These and other gamma herpesviruses also establish latent infection in lymphocytes, but they are not unique in this regard; beta herpesviruses such as HHV-6, HHV-7, and CMV latently infect lymphocytes. Although the oncogenic properties of LCVs and RDVs were historically important in segregating them into the gamma herpes subfamily, the nucleotide and protein sequence relationships provide a more enduring basis for phylogenetic classification.

Taxonomists have renamed EBV as human herpesvirus 4 (HHV4). Although most authors still use the name EBV, some indexing services have adopted HHV4, so both entries should be used when doing bibliographic searches.

VIRUS STRUCTURE

Like other herpesviruses, EBV has a toroid-shaped protein core that is wrapped with DNA, a nucleocapsid with 162 capsomeres, a protein tegument between the nucleocapsid and the envelope, and an outer envelope with external glycoprotein spikes (172,173,192,659). The major EBV capsid proteins are 160, 47, and 28 kd, similar in size to the major HSV-1 capsid proteins (172,173). EBV has a range of envelope glycoproteins, including several that are homologs of relatively well conserved herpesvirus glycoproteins. These include homologs of HSV gH, gL, gB, gM, and gN, which are also known as EBV gp85 or BXLF2, gp25 or BKRF2, gp110 or BALF4, gp84/113 or BBRF3, and gp15 or BLRF1, respectively. However, the most abundant EBV envelope and tegument proteins are 350/220 and 152 kd, respectively, and these are not homologous to major envelope and tegument proteins of HSV-1 (172,173,597,668,669,820,822).

GENOME STRUCTURE

The EBV genome is a linear, double-stranded, 184-kbp DNA composed of 60 mole percent guanine or cytosine (see Fig. 1) (36,142,253–255,379,405,662,663,673). The characteristic features of EBV and most other LCV genomes include the following (see Fig. 1): (a) a single overall format and gene arrangement (142,147,253–255, 671); (b) tandem, reiterated, 0.5-kbp direct repeats of the same sequence at both termini (TR) (255,304,430); (c) six to 12 tandem reiterations of 3-kbp, internal direct repeats (IR1) (103,104,253,254,305), and (d) short and long, largely unique sequence domains (U_S and U_L) that have almost all of the genome coding capacity. Although largely unique DNA, U_L and U_S include perfect and imperfect tandem DNA repeats, most of which are within ORFs. A duplicated region, D_L, near the left end of U_L, consists of multiple, highly conserved, G-C-rich, tandem 125-bp repeats and 2 kbp of adjacent unique DNA, all of which have extensive homology to the D_R region, near the right end of U_L. D_R consists of multiple, highly conserved, G-C-rich, tandem, 102-bp repeats and 1 kbp of nearby unique DNA (149,311,313,314,316,351,378,463). The D_L and D_R repeats are within ORFs. Because the D_L repeat is 125 bp and not divisible by three, sequential iterations are translated in different reading frames, resulting in an unusual protein. D_L and D_R also include the origins for initiation of viral DNA replication in lytic infection.

The reiteration frequency of the EBV tandem perfect repeats becomes variable during viral DNA replication, with the average number of repeats being identical to the parent genome, and most of the progeny having a number of repeats that is identical or similar to that of the parental genome. When EBV infects a cell, the genome becomes an episome with a characteristic number of TRs, dependent on the number of TRs in the parental genome, with variation introduced during viral DNA replication and the unique cleavage and joining events of the single infecting viral genome. If the infection is nonpermissive for viral replication and permissive for latent infection and continued cell growth, each EBV episome in progeny infected cells will usually have the same number of TRs as the parent cell. Homogeneity or heterogeneity in the number of TRs is therefore useful in determining whether a group of latently infected cells arose from a single common progenitor infected cell or from multiple progenitors (76,674). The number of 3-kbp IR1 repeats also varies among EBVs and among progeny of EBV replication, but this is more difficult to assess as a marker of heterogeneity because of the 18- to 30-kbp size of the total IR1 element. Other, smaller, imperfect or less highly reiterated repeats within ORFs are more stable during replication but differ sufficiently among different virus isolates that the size of the encoded proteins can be used to uniquely identify each isolate.

Because of the limited host range for EBV replication *in vitro* and the difficulty in obtaining large amounts of viral DNA for molecular biologic investigation, EBV was the first herpesvirus whose complete genome fragments were cloned into *Escherichia coli* (33,77,142,216,656, 673). EBV was also the first herpesvirus to be completely sequenced (36,301,632). Since the EBV genome was sequenced from a *Bam*HI fragment library, genes, promoters, ORFs, and polyadenylation sites are frequently referenced to the corresponding *Bam*HI fragment (36). Thus, the EBV DNA polymerase gene is frequently referred to as BALF3 for *Bam*HI A fragment, third leftward ORF. Exons of spliced mRNAs are also frequently designated by the *Bam*HI DNA fragment that encodes the exon.

Two EBV types circulate in most populations. The two types are now usually designated 1 and 2, although A and B were widely used in the past. Type 1 is far more common in most populations. EBV type 2 is nearly as common as type 1 in equatorial Africa and New Guinea, and it is also not infrequent among people infected with human immunodeficiency virus (HIV) (4,30,144,147, 206,288,311,419,426,549,710,725,740,741,761,901,903, 904,920). The only significant differences between the genomes of the two types are in the genes that encode for the EBV nuclear proteins [or antigens (EBNA)] LP, 2, 3A, 3B, and 3C. The type 1 and 2 alleles for EBNA-2, -3A, -3B, and -3C differ in predicted primary amino acid sequence by 47%, 16%, 20%, and 28%, respectively (4,144,723). EBNA-LP differs less overall (144,381). Other than these differences, the genomes of various isolates of type 1 or type 2 EBV strains from widely different geographic areas have single base changes and repeat reiteration frequency differences from prototype genomes, with an overall difference in nucleotide sequence between type 1 and type 2 isolates outside of the EBNA-LP, -2, -3A, -B, or -3C ORFs of less than 4%. Differences among individual type 1 or type 2 isolates are more in the range of 1% (266–269,288,419,549). Similarities in the numbers of DNA repeats at various sites in the EBV genome among EBV isolates from a given geographic area have been used to group isolates into strains and to epidemiologically track EBV infection. Similar strain variations have been noted among both type 1 and type 2 isolates, consistent with the notion that these polymorphisms evolve regularly in nature. Persistent infection with more than one EBV type or strain is not unusual, particularly for more promiscuous and immunocompromised people. Intertypic recombinants have been identified in the oropharynx and lymphocytes of immunocompromised people and less commonly from otherwise healthy people (5,266,269,288,419,549,761,860–863, 901,903).

GENERAL ASPECTS OF EBV INFECTION OF CELLS *IN VITRO*

The *in vitro* host range for efficient EBV infection is restricted to primary human B lymphocytes (323,660). EBV readily infects B lymphocytes derived from peripheral blood, tonsils, or fetal cord blood (29,319,403,697, 883,897,921). B lymphocytes at earlier stages of development from adult or fetal bone marrow or fetal liver, as well as leukemic and non-EBV-infected Burkitt's lymphoma (BL) cell lines, can also be infected, although the efficiency of infection is lower than with peripheral blood (20,35,85,87,175,195,294,435,528,529,815). Fully differentiated plasma cells cannot be infected. The outcome of infection of primary human B lymphocytes with EBV is nonpermissiveness for virus replication and conversion of the infected cells to continuous proliferation into long-term lymphoblastoid cell lines (LCLs) (323,660). The seminal observation that latent EBV infection efficiently causes perpetual B-lymphocyte proliferation was critically important in establishing that EBV has oncogenic potential (323,563,607,608,660).

EBV can also establish latent infection in other cell types, including T or natural killer (NK) cells, although the efficiency is low, even compared to non-EBV-infected BL cells, which are usually 10-fold less susceptible to infection than primary B lymphocytes (397,398,745). Primary epithelial cells (763,918) are also relatively resistant to infection, whereas some epithelial cell lines, including HEK293 (213), gastric carcinoma cell lines (916), and biliary, laryngeal, hepatocellular, colon, and bladder carcinoma cell lines (365), can be infected with efficiencies that approach those of BL cells.

Wild-type virus can be obtained from human saliva or from infected human B lymphocytes growing in culture. Most adults have been infected by EBV and intermittently shed virus in saliva (245,902). They also have EBV in a latent state in approximately 1 in 10^5 to 10^6 of their peripheral blood B lymphocytes (608). When 10^6 to 10^7 peripheral blood B lymphocytes from an EBV-seropositive person are put in culture in the absence of functional T lymphocytes, EBV-infected B lymphocytes are likely to grow out, without adding exogenous virus (608,685,821). These cell lines are then a source of infectious EBV. Interestingly, the recovery of EBV-infected cells from such cultures in the absence of exogenously added virus can be blocked by inhibitors of virus replication or the addition of neutralizing antibody (687,819). Explantation to culture can apparently cause a rare EBV infected cell to become permissive for virus replication. The newly replicated virus can then infect other B cells in the culture, and thereby initiate a latent, immortalizing infection, whereas the *in vivo* latently infected cell cannot spontaneously convert to a transformation type of latent infection. Virtually all cell lines that arise from cultures of normal blood cells are EBV immortalized B LCLs.

EBV infection of primary B cells, *in vitro*, results in about 10% of the cells becoming latently infected and proliferating as immortalized or "transformed" latently infected LCLs (319,783). Virus replication in LCLs is usually minimal or undetectable. The presence of the "latent" virus in each of the infected cells can be readily detected using antibodies to any of the eight different virus proteins that are characteristically expressed in LCLs. The eight viral encoded proteins include six nuclear proteins (the EBNAs) and two integral membrane proteins (the LMPs) (Fig. 2). In this context, the virus genome is hardly inactive and the infection is latent only in the absence of lytic virus infection.

	I	II	III
EBNA-1	Qp	Qp	Wp, Cp
EBNA-2, LP, 3A-C°			+
LMP1, LMP2		+	+
EBERs°	+	+	+
BARTs	+	+	+
Example	EBV-BL	HD, NPC	LCL, EBV-BL

FIG. 2. Types of EBV latent infection observed in Burkitt's lymphoma (*BL*) cells growing in culture (types I or III), or in nasopharyngeal carcinoma or Hodgkin's disease cells *in vivo* (type II). Type III latency is also characteristic of human B lymphocytes that have been infected with EBV and are proliferating as a consequence of latent EBV infection.

The standard conditions for clonal infection of primary B lymphocytes with EBV are to add less than 50 transforming units of EBV to 10^7 T-cell-depleted lymphocytes, and to then plate the infected cells in 96 wells of a microtiter tray in 0.1 to 0.15 mL of a complete growth medium consisting of the defined constituents of RPMI 1640 (Sigma Chemical Company, St. Louis, MO) and 10% to 20% fetal calf serum. Each infectious virus will give rise to a macroscopically visible cell line by 5 weeks of incubation. The virus titer is usually defined by this most sensitive assay of EBV infection. If the purpose is to study the biochemical events of primary infection, lymphocytes are infected with three transforming units of virus per cell and kept in bulk culture. Higher multiplicities are rarely used because of the practical difficulty of obtaining high-titer EBV preparations. For the cloning of virus or latently infected cells, putatively infected cells are fed every 2 weeks, and the assay is scored after 6 to 8 weeks, by which time an infected cell will usually have multiplied into more than 10^5 progeny cells. The cloning efficiency can be modestly improved by culturing the infected lymphocytes on irradiated human diploid fibroblasts, which enriches the culture conditions beyond those provided initially by the 10^5 uninfected lymphocytes, residual macrophages, and complete growth medium.

In latently infected B lymphocytes, EBV expresses not only the six EBNAs and two LMPs but also two small nonpolyadenylated RNAs (or EBERs) and highly spliced *Bam* A rightward transcripts, or BARTs (see Fig. 2). These viral gene products maintain the latent infection and cause the previously resting B lymphocytes to enter cycle and continuously proliferate. The effect on cell growth is immediate, and most infected B cells enter the first round of cell DNA synthesis 48 to 72 hours after EBV infection (12,594–596). The target cell that is most amenable to conversion to an LCL has a resting B-lymphocyte phenotype (22).

Aside from the presence of the EBV genome and its gene products, the EBV-infected proliferating B lymphocytes are similar to lymphocytes proliferating in response to antigen, mitogen, or IL4 and anti-CD40 in their expression of a similar repertoire of "activation"-associated proteins, their secretion of immunoglobulin (Ig), their high level of expression of adhesion molecules, and their adherence to each other (42,67,85–87,363,635,636, 785,826,828,867–869). EBV-infected B lymphocytes may continue to secrete immunoglobulin for months or even years in culture. Some cells can continue to differentiate and undergo class switching in culture when exposed to IL4 (243,373).

Most non-EBV-infected BL cell lines can be infected with EBV *in vitro* (85,87). The growth of non-EBV-infected BL cells *in vitro* is substantially the result of a characteristic reciprocal chromosome translocation involving the c-*myc* and Ig heavy or light chain loci. This results in constitutive c-*myc* expression (141; for review see ref. 531). Other changes are presumed to be necessary for the development of BL *in vivo*, including changes in chromosome 1 (52). Still other genetic changes occur in BL cells during growth *in vitro*. BL cells frequently grow as single cells and can regrow from true single-cell end-point dilution. They are similar to germinal-center B lymphocytes in their expression of surface markers including IgM, and they differ from LCLs in their high-level expression of Bcl-6 and CD10 and low-level expression of activation markers and adhesion molecules. When EBV infects BL cells *in vitro*, the virus usually initially expresses the same program of latency as in LCLs. This type of latency, characteristic of LCLs and marked by the expression of the six EBNAs, two LMPs, two EBERs, and BARTs, is termed latency III (21,271,708) (Figs. 2 and 3). Latency III EBV gene expression causes the cells to grow in tight clumps, express activation markers, down-regulate Bcl-6 and CD10, and otherwise assume the phenotype of LCLs (1,57,133,134,321,453,527,867–869,871,873). Over the ensuing months of culture, however, some of the cells may lose the EBV genome and revert to a germinal center BL phenotype. Some BL cell lines, infected with EBV *in vitro* and maintained in culture for several months, remain EBV infected and continue in a latency III phenotype. Others convert to a latency 1 phenotype and express only EBNA-1, EBERs, and BARTs (see Fig. 3). Some BL cells retain the EBV genome as an episome, whereas in other cells, the EBV genome can be integrated into the cell genome (318,361,467,543). Some BL cells with integrated EBV DNA maintain a latency III phenotype.

As described in Chapter 75 in *Fields Virology*, 4th ed., most EBV-infected BL tumors have a latency I phenotype. When these cells are explanted to culture, they initially maintain latency I and express only EBNA-1, EBERs, and BARTs. Paradoxically, on continued culture, many of the *in vivo*–infected BL cells switch to a latency III phenotype and grow in clumps similar to LCLs. Most *in vivo*–infected BL cells never lose their EBV episomes when the cells are grown *in vitro*, whereas BL cells infected *in vitro* may lose their EBV genomes entirely or may have only integrated EBV DNA (361,527,871). The persistence of EBV episomes in most *in vivo*–infected BL cell lines that have been maintained for years in culture is compatible with the possibility that the episome is important for cell proliferation or survival. Cells of other B- or even T-lymphocyte malignancies that can be grown as continuous cells lines *in vitro*, and that express low levels of EBV receptors, usually express only EBNA-1, EBERs, and BARTs when infected with EBV *in vitro*.

With a frequency characteristic of each EBV-infected B-lymphocyte line, some progeny latently infected proliferating cells growing *in vitro* become spontaneously permissive for virus replication. Primary human B-lymphocyte-derived cell lines (LCLs) vary from zero to a few percent of cells permissive for EBV replication. *In vitro*–infected BL cell lines tend to be even less permissive for virus replication, whereas *in vivo*–infected BL cell lines are frequently substantially more permissive for virus replication than LCLs. The lack of permissivity of *in vitro*–infected BL cells for EBV replication is in part related to the poor persistence of EBV episomes in such cells, as lytic replication probably requires episomal viral DNA.

In all instances, permissively infected cells exhibit the characteristic cytopathic changes associated with herpesvirus replication, including formation of an intranuclear inclusion in the center of the nucleus at the site of lytic infection DNA replication, margination of nuclear chromatin, assembly of capsids within the nucleus near the nuclear membrane, budding of virus through the nuclear membrane, and formation of cytoplasmic vesicles containing enveloped virus (189–193,261,659). As with other herpesviruses, cell macromolecular synthesis is inhibited early in EBV replication (247).

The frequency with which latently infected lymphocytes become permissive for virus replication can sometimes be influenced by specific culture conditions. Transient exposure to drugs that inhibit host macromolecular synthesis, cell starvation, arginine-free media, inhibition of DNA methylation with azacytidine, exposure to butyric acid (which inhibits histone deacetylase), treatment with phorbol ester to stimulate protein kinase C (PKC), exposure to ionophores (which increases intracellular free calcium), or cross-linking of surface Ig can each increase the permissivity of some EBV-infected cells for lytic infection (45,152,350,464,717,802,804,805,896,898,899).

Analyses of cultures of a latently infected BL tumor–derived cell line that is particularly permissive for virus replication led to the identification of defective EBV genomes in these cultures (332,559,678). The defective genomes express an EBV immediate-early protein, BZLF1 or Z (381,383). The expression of Z following heterologous gene transfer is now frequently used to induce lytic EBV replication in latently infected cells (129,130,264,564). Not all cells in which Z is expressed go on to lytic infection (129).

The most sensitive method for recovering EBV from a latently infected cell line that is largely nonpermissive for virus replication is to lethally irradiate 10^4 induced cells and co-cultivate them with 10^5 primary B lymphocytes in 150 μL of complete medium in a microwell (566,567). This allows maximal contact between the rare cell that becomes permissive for lytic EBV infection and uninfected B lymphocytes. Under such conditions, the irradiated cells also provide feeder effects and enhance the growth of the newly infected primary B lymphocytes. In the absence of autologous or heterologous feeder cells, EBV-transformed B lymphocytes do not usually regrow from suspensions of single cells in 100 μL of rich growth medium.

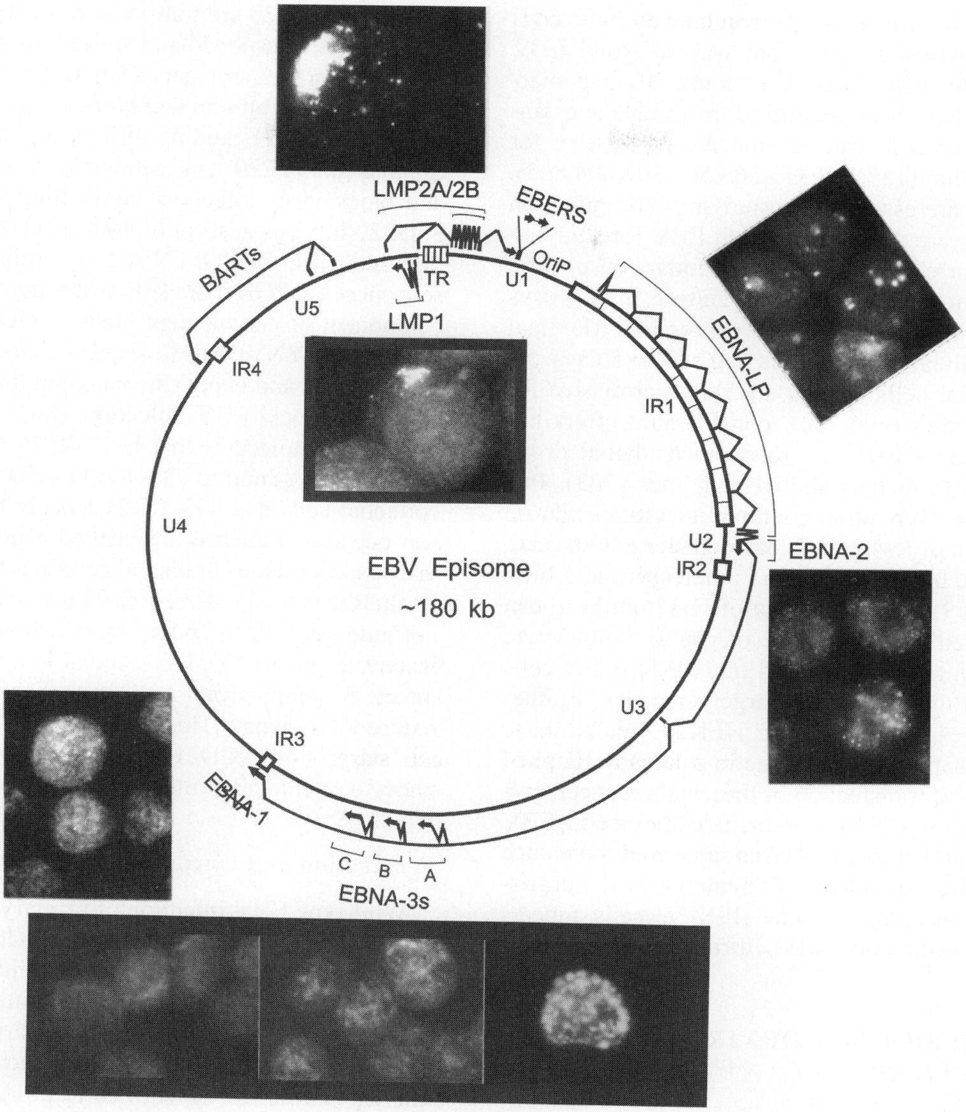

FIG. 3. EBV episome, transcripts, mRNAs, and proteins in type III latent B-lymphocyte infection. Largely unique (U1-U5) and repetitive internal (IR1-4) or terminal (TR) repeat DNA segments are indicated. The origin for latent infection EBV episome replication, oriP, is also indicated. Exons encoding EBV nuclear proteins (EBNA-1, -2, -3A, -3B, -3C, and -LP) and EBV integral membrane proteins (LMP1, -2A, or -2B) are indicated by *vertical lines* radiating from the circular episome map. EBNA transcription is shown as it is first initiated from the IR1 or Wp promoter. In many infected lymphocytes, after expression of EBNA-LP and EBNA-2, the Cp promoter in U1 dominates EBNA transcription. Alternative polyadenylation and splicing lead the various EBNA mRNAs. EBNA-LP is encoded by repeating exons from IR1 and two short unique exons from U2. The EBERs are two small, nonpolyadenylated RNAs transcribed in latent or productive infection. LMP1 is transcribed in the direction opposite to the EBNAs, LMP2A and -B, EBERs, and BARTs. The typical intracellular localizations of the proteins that are known to be expressed in type III latency are shown on the EBV DNA map on the *left.* The proteins are identified by immune fluorescence microscopy using specific antisera. The smaller episome drawing on the *right* shows the terminal exons of the differentially spliced Bam A fragment rightward transcripts that are likely to encode the proteins provisionally designated RPMS1 and BARF0 in all three types of latent infection (234,422,716,766). LMP2A also has an upstream EBNA-2 response element, whereas LMP1 and LMP2B share the same EBNA-2 response element.

The induction of virus replication in latently infected B lymphocytes remains the principal way to study EBV replication. Fortunately, latently infected BL and marmoset cell lines have been identified in which a substantial fraction of the cells can be rendered permissive for lytic virus infection (137,138,333,566,567,802,804,805). These cell lines are essential for studying lytic infection *in vitro*, and they are the best source of EBV for studying virus structure or cell infection. After induction of lytic EBV infection in B lymphocytes in culture, 2 to 3 days are required for maximal late gene expression. Maximal titers of extracellular virus are reached at 4 to 5 days.

Since epithelial cells *in vivo* are fully permissive for lytic EBV infection (606,760), considerable effort has been made to adopt EBV to growth in epithelial organ cultures or transformed epithelial cell lines (763). Primary cultures or even some continuous cultures can be infected, particularly when incubated with cells that are producing virus, but the infection is inefficient and little virus results (759). The efficiency of infection has been slightly improved by expression of the B lymphocyte EBV receptor in an epithelial cell line (481). More cells are infected but the infection is largely abortive. Epithelial cell cultures, especially of HEK293 cells, have recently been useful for EBV genetic studies because of the relative ease of transfection of these adherent cell cultures with plasmid DNAs that include the entire EBV genome. The small amount of virus recovered from such cells can then be expanded in B lymphocytes. Surprisingly, the EBV receptor on some HEK293 cells appears to be the same as the normal B-cell receptor (213).

MOLECULAR BIOLOGY OF VIRAL INFECTION OF CELLS *IN VITRO*

Adsorption

The *in vitro* host range restriction of LCVs to B lymphocytes is partly the result of a restriction in high-level expression of a cell surface protein, CD21, which is an efficient receptor for EBV and for the C3d component of complement (214,456,878,879). Efficient B-lymphocyte infection correlates with the stages of B-lymphocyte development in which CD21 is expressed (364,390). Monoclonal antibodies to CD21 block virus infection (214). Furthermore, purified CD21 binds to EBV and can block infection (604,605). Moreover, CD21 expression on heterologous cells confers the ability to adsorb EBV (6,481). CD21 is an immunoglobulin superfamily glycoprotein, and it consists of 15 or 16 imperfect repeats of a 60-plus amino acid domain, a transmembrane domain, and a short carboxyl-terminal cytoplasmic domain (588,878). EBV binding activity maps to the two aminoterminal domains (537,582,587,604).

The most abundant EBV outer envelope glycoprotein, gp350/220, is the CD21 ligand (602,603,810,811,880). Gp350 and gp220 are translated from abundant late-replication-cycle nonspliced and spliced mRNAs that are transcribed from the same gene (50). CD21 is the only B-lymphocyte surface protein that binds to gp350/220 (810). The gp350/220–CD21 binding affinity is 1.2×10^{-8} M (811). Soluble gp350/220 can saturate B-lymphocyte receptors and block virus infection, confirming a key role for gp 350/220 in virus adsorption (604,811). A gp350/220 peptide sequence EDPGFFNVEI is similar to the peptide sequence EDPGKQLYNVEA through which the C3d component of complement binds to CD21. Peptides containing the LYNVEA C3d sequence block C3d binding to CD21 (456), and peptides containing the EDPGFFNVEA sequence block EBV infection (602), whereas mutant gp350/220 molecules that lack VE in the EDPGFFNVE peptide do not bind to CD21 (811). The EBV receptor on epithelial cells that lack CD21 has not been identified, in part because of the less efficient adsorption of EBV to primary or continuous epithelial cell lines than to B lymphocytes. Recently, the derivation of a virus that has an insertion into gp350/220 codon 79, which should functionally inactivate gp350/220, has resulted in a virus that can still infect B lymphocytes and epithelial cells, albeit with reduced efficiency. This indicates that gp350/220-mediated adsorption to CD21 is not absolutely required for lymphocyte or epithelial infection (375).

Penetration and Uncoating

Wild-type EBV infection of primary B lymphocytes is initiated by gp350/220 adsorption to CD21 on the B-lymphocyte plasma membrane, aggregation of CD21 in the plasma membrane, and internalization of EBV into cytoplasmic vesicles (91,601). CD21 is part of a complex that includes CD19 and associated intracellular tyrosine kinases, similar to the surface Ig (sIg)–associated signal transducing cell surface proteins. EBV aggregation of CD21 probably results in CD21-mediated tyrosine kinase signal transduction, and this may have an activating effect on the B lymphocyte (536,541). Infected cells begin to synthesize RNA, enlarge, express activation and adhesion molecules, clump, and secrete Ig soon after exposure to virus (12,24,363,810). CD21 ligation also increases NF-κB activation and may up-regulate the EBNA Wp promoter at the start of EBV infection (782). The precise role of these effects in initial infection is somewhat uncertain, because inhibitors of cell protein synthesis, of tyrosine kinases, or of PI3 kinase do not block initial EBNA RNA transcription (756).

The EBV gH homolog, gp85, is the second most abundant envelope glycoprotein (177,178,310,779). EBV gp85 is part of two virion glycoprotein complexes: a heterodimeric complex with the EBV gL homolog, gp25, a product of BKRF2, and a heterotrimeric of gp85, gp25, and gp42, the product of BZLF2. EBV gL is all that is necessary for gp85 processing (666,905). Studies with a monoclonal antibody to gp85 that does not affect virus adsorption to B lymphocytes but that blocks EBV envelope fusion with B lymphocyte membranes, provided an initial indication that gp85 is particularly important in envelope fusion with cellular membranes (289,480,568). This role of gp85 is similar to that of HSV-1 gH, which mediates envelope fusion with the cell membrane and thereby enables nucleocapsid exocytosis into the cytoplasm (260).

The heterotrimeric complexes of EBV gH/gL and gp42 (905) have a unique role in mediating a coreceptor interaction in B lymphocyte infection by gp42 engagement of human leukocyte antigen (HLA) class II, D_R, D_P, and a subset of D_Q alleles (286,287,479,581,776,875,876). Epithelial cells do not express HLA class II, and antibody to gp42 blocks B-lymphocyte infection but not epithelial infection (480). The lack of effect of gp42-specific antibody on epithelial infection suggested the possibility that gp42 has an insignificant or different role in epithelial infection. Recent studies with an EBV recombinant that does not express gp42 confirm a key role for gp42 in efficient B-lymphocyte infection and a noncritical role in epithelial cell infection (581,875,876).

EBV gH and the gH/gL heterodimer have still another role in epithelial infection. An EBV recombinant that does not express gp85 adsorbs normally to B lymphocytes and is not only deficient in fusion with B-lymphocyte membranes but is unable to adsorb to epithelial cells (581,623). These latter studies confirm the importance of gp85 in fusion with B-lymphocyte membranes and indicate a unique role for gp85/gp25 dimeric complexes in interaction with a putative epithelial cell receptor or coreceptor.

Early Intracellular Events in Infection

Little is known about EBV capsid dissolution, genome transport to the cell nucleus, or DNA circularization. By analogy with other DNA viruses that replicate in the nucleus, the cytoskeleton is likely to mediate EBV capsid transport to the nucleus or to nuclear pores (140). A protein similar in size to the HSV virion tegumentary protein VMW 65, or VP16, has been detected in purified EBV preparations and remains associated with cells after infection (12). HSV VP16 is a key trans-inducer of immediate-early lytic virus gene expression (see Chapter 73 in *Fields Virology*, 4th ed.). The EBV BPLF1 ORF is colinearly 30% homologous to the HSV VP16 ORF. EBV BPLF1 could therefore be a transactivator of lytic EBV replication in epithelial cells. The role of BPLF1 in lymphocyte infection is even less predictable. The initial latent infection promoter, Wp (12,721,773,855), has high constitutive activity in B lymphocytes (852).

The first evidence that herpesvirus genomes circularize in infected cells arose from the observation that almost all EBV-infected cells contain covalently closed circular EBV episomes (3,496). In primary B lymphocytes, EBV genome circularization precedes or coincides with earliest virus gene expression and may require activation from G0 to G1 (12,363). Whether the putative viral protein that recognizes EBV TR for cleavage and packaging (see later section, Late Gene Expression, Cleavage, Packaging, Envelopment, and Egress) facilitates the joining of the linear virion EBV TRs to produce genome circularization is not known. A cellular protein complex that includes Sp1 has also been identified that can recognize the ends of the DNA and could be involved in genome circularization (790,791). By 16 hours after infection, each infected cell contains one EBV episome. In some experiments, the addition of inhibitors of DNA, RNA, or protein synthesis to cells at the time of infection blocked genome circularization, indicating that active cell macromolecular synthesis is required for circularization. Inhibition of infected cell protein synthesis does not, however, prevent viral gene transcription (756).

Latent Infection in Primary B Lymphocytes and Growth Transformation

Viral Gene Expression in Latent Infection

EBV infection of primary human B lymphocytes *in vitro* results in type III latency (see Fig. 2) and transformation of the infected cell into a proliferating lymphoblast capable of long-term growth as an LCL. In defining the genes expressed in latent infection, it is important to recognize that most latently infected cell cultures have a small number of cells that are spontaneously permissive for virus replication. Since virus gene expression in lytic infection is at a much higher level than in latent infection, lytic-cycle RNAs or proteins are frequently detectable in predominantly latently infected B-cell lines. Proof that an EBV gene is expressed in latent infection requires the demonstration that the specific virus gene product is in most latently infected cells in a culture. This has usually been accomplished by defining an mRNA sequence whose abundance is not affected by the number of permissively infected cells (212,317,427,428,852,853), deriving monospecific antibody to the putative protein product using heterologous antigen expression systems (324–329,511,650–652,870) or peptide synthesis (169–171), and using the antibody to identify the protein in latently infected cells by immune microscopy (324,325,327, 329,511,650,652,870).

The time course of events in *in vitro* primary B-lymphocyte infection varies somewhat, depending on the virus inoculum and the physiologic state of the lymphocytes. The EBV genome circularizes in the infected cell nucleus within 12 to 16 hours of infection (see Fig. 3). At about the same time, the Wp promoter in the 3-kbp, Bam or IR1, long internal direct repeat element initiates rightward transcription (12,16,362,594,595,702). The B-cell specificity of the W promoter derives at least in part from the presence of upstream BSAP/Pax5 sites (830). As is true of the other herpesviruses, EBV does not encode an RNA polymerase, and host cell RNA polymerase II transcribes viral mRNAs. By nuclear run-on or transient transfection analysis, the initial EBNA promoter, Wp, and the more upstream promoter, Cp, which is activated by EBNA-2, are the strongest EBV pol II promoters in latent EBV infection (719,720,852). The promoter in the leftmost repeat appears to dominate, as most of the EBNA cDNAs have multiple exons from downstream copies of the W repeat (62–66,719). The simplest model for the domination of the leftmost W repeat element is a positive transcriptional element in the upstream U1 region (see Fig. 2).

Wp promotes the transcription of the first EBV mRNAs, and these are differentially spliced to encode EBNA-LP and EBNA-2, two proteins that coordinately up-regulate transcription from viral and cellular promoters, including Wp and an activatible upstream surrogate, Cp (66,198,886–888). The initial mRNAs have a 40-base first exon, W0, which ends with an AT (12,721). The W0 exon is spliced to a 66-base W1 exon or to a 5′ 5-base truncated W01 exon. The W01 exon begins with a G, creating a translational start site, whereas the W1 exon has no translational start site. The W1 exons are followed by a 132-base W2 exon, by repeating 66-base and 132-base W1W2 exons derived from successive reiterations of the long internal repeats, by two short exons, Y1 and Y2, and then by one long exon (YH) from the unique DNA (Bam Y and H) downstream of Bam W long internal repeats (see Fig. 3) (12,719,870). The resulting mRNAs translate either EBNA-LP from the W01 translational start site or EBNA-2 from a translational start site near the 5′ end of the YH exons of those alternatively spliced RNAs that lack the W01 translational initiation site. EBNA-LP derives its name from the fact that it is a nuclear protein encoded by the potential 5′ ORF in the leader of the EBNA-2 mRNA.

The efficient translation of EBNA-2 from only those mRNAs that lack the EBNA-LP translational start site and therefore have a long untranslated 5′ leader is surprising, because 40s ribosomal subunits usually associate with mRNAs at the 5′ cap and then move along the untranslated leader without a stabilizing 60s subunit, until either disengaging or encountering a translational initiation codon (444). Translation of the 5′ EBNA-LP ORF would be expected to stabilize mRNA interaction with the ribosome and yield more efficient translation of the 3′ EBNA-2 ORF. Although expected, an independent ribosome entry sequence upstream of the EBNA-2 ORF has not been defined, and this enigma has not been resolved.

EBNA-LP and EBNA-2 reach the level that is maintained in transformed B lymphocytes (LCLs) by 24 to 32 hours after infection (12). EBNA-2 has a well-characterized role in up-regulating virus and cell gene expression, including expression of the virus-encoded EBNAs, LMP1 and LMP2, and the cell-encoded CD23, CD21, c-*fgr*, and c-*myc* proteins (Fig. 4) (1,12,127,199,200,437, 844,865,867,868,870,871,925,930). Up-regulation of CD23, CD21, and c-*fgr* is observed following transient or stable expression of EBNA-2 in non-EBV-infected BL cells. C-*myc* expression is also up-regulated in primary B-lymphocyte infection at the time that EBNA-LP and EBNA-2 are expressed, and c-*myc* expression is continuously dependent on EBNA-2 expression (12,394). EBNA-2 also up-regulates various LMP1 (1,199,388, 764,848,873), LMP2 (460,461,930,931), and Cp (322, 386,498,499,793,895) promoter constructs following transient transfection with an EBNA-2 expression vector into non-EBV-infected B-lymphoma cells.

EBNA-2 has three critical components to its transcriptional up-regulating effects (see Fig. 3) (125,296,842, 894). First, the specificity of EBNA-2 effects on certain virus and cell promoters and not others is caused by an EBNA-2 domain that interacts with cell-sequence-specific DNA binding proteins (125,276,322,388,895). The

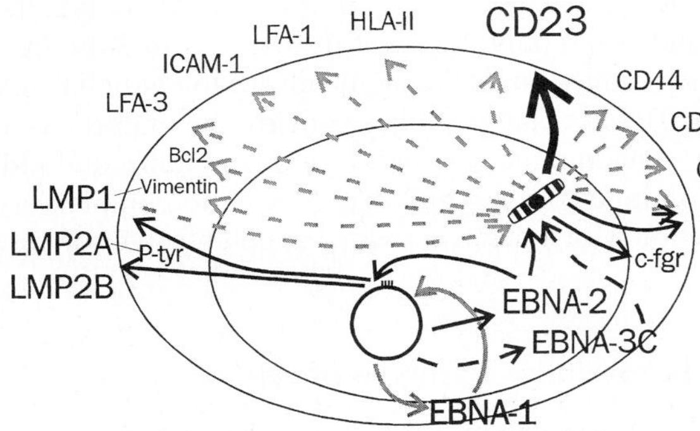

FIG. 4. Expression of EBNAs or LMPs in BL lymphoblasts provides indications of the biochemical mechanisms by which these proteins effect changes in lymphocyte growth or survival. EBNA-1 binds to oriP and to chromosomes and enables the EBV episome to partition to progeny cells. EBNA-2 specifically up-regulates cellular CD23, CD21, c-*myc*, and c-*fgr* expression and viral EBNA, LMP1, and LMP2 expression. EBNA-3C can also up-regulate CD23 expression, although the effects are much less than those of EBNA-2. LMP1 patches in the cell plasma membrane where it is associated with and induces higher level expression of vimentin. LMP1 has dramatic effects on BL cell growth; it functionally activates homotypic adhesion; it up-regulates ICAM 1, LFA 1, and LFA 3; it up-regulates bcl2; it raises the lymphocyte intracellular free calcium; it up-regulates activation markers including transferrin receptor, HLA-II, CD21, CD23, CD39, CD40, and CD44; and it down-regulates CD10 and bcl-6. LMP1 also alters lymphoblast TGF-beta responsiveness. Each of these effects is cell-line dependent, and most effects are not evident in all BL cell lines. LMP2A constitutively activates B-cell receptor tyrosine kinase signalling pathways at a low level and desensitizes B lymphoblasts to further B-cell receptor–type tyrosine kinase signal transduction.

repertoire of cellular transcription factors includes RBP-Jk, a transcription factor expressed in all cells (276,322, 895), and PU.1, a hematopoietic transcription factor that is particularly important in B lymphocytes (388). Second, once it is near promoter sites, EBNA-2 has an acidic activating domain that recruits basal and activation-associated transcription factors, including transcription factor IIB (TFIIB), TAF40, TBP, transcription factor IIH (TFIIH), and CBP/p300 (123,124,839–841,874). Much of the EBNA-2 acidic domain is complexed with a cell nuclear protein, p100, that has coactivating effects with EBNA-2 (840). P100 is a scaffolding protein for the acidic domain, for TFIIE, for c-*myb*, and for PIM-1. Third, efficient assembly of multiple transcription factors at promoter sites appears to require multiple EBNA-2 acidic domains. EBNA-2 has two separate domains in its amino terminus that can mediate homotypic association, thereby enabling EBNA-2 to assemble multiple transcription factors near a promoter that has RBP-Jk or PU.1 sites (894). The ability of EBNA-2 to self-associate may account for the large size of EBNA-2 complexes in cell extracts.

Because EBNA-LP is transcribed along with EBNA-2 at the initiation of EBV infection in primary B lymphocytes and because it is a nuclear protein, it is a prime candidate for cooperation with EBNA-2 in the regulation of virus and cell gene expression (see Fig. 4). Indeed, EBNA-LP substantially enhances EBNA-2 up-regulation of virus and cell gene transcription (295,609). The effect is evident in transient expression assays with artificial LMP1 promoter constructs and with endogenous LMP1 expression in EBV-infected BL cells that are otherwise in latency I and fail to express LMP1 until EBNA-2 and EBNA-LP are coexpressed in these cells following gene transfer. EBNA-LP has no promoter-specific effects alone and stringently requires EBNA-2 for activation of specific promoters. Surprisingly, the EBNA-LP effect requires only the EBNA-2 acidic domain near a promoter site and expression of the repeating domains of EBNA-LP (295). Thus, EBNA-LP is likely to biochemically interact with the EBNA-2 acidic domain or with another factor that binds to the acidic domain.

Probably as a consequence of EBNA-2 effects on a response element in the unique DNA in the EBV Bam C fragment that is upstream of the long internal repeat, EBNA promoter usage in many EBV-infected primary B lymphocytes moves from Wp to the nearby Cp latency promoter (295,386,789,882,885,914). In those cells in which the Cp promoter is turned on and supplants Wp, two short exons downstream of the Cp promoter, C1 and C2, replace the short W0 exon in the EBNA mRNAs (66). As with the W0 exon, the C2 exon ends in an AT that is spliced to either the 66-base or the 61-base internal-repeat-derived exon, W1 or W01, resulting in an mRNA leader incapable or capable, respectively, of translating EBNA-LP. All resulting C- or W-initiated mRNAs have the same repeating 66- and 132-base exons in their leader (62–66,387,653,699,721,773). A potential splice donor near the beginning of the EBNA-2-encoding YH exon but preceding the EBNA-2 initiation codon is now activated in some transcripts, and some RNA molecules are spliced to a far downstream acceptor in Bam U (62,65,66,653, 721,773). The U exon is then spliced to any of four alternative acceptor sites of exons that begin the ORFs that encode for the amino terminus of EBNA-3A, EBNA-3B, or EBNA-3C, or for EBNA-1 (see Fig. 3). As a consequence of alternate 5′ splicing of the Cp- or Wp-initiated RNAs, some mRNAs will still encode EBNA-LP. As a consequence of partial use of the alternative donor site between the beginning of the YH exon and the EBNA-2 initiation codon, some RNAs that do not encode for EBNA-LP or for EBNA-2 are spliced to the U exon and now encode for EBNA-3A, -3B, -3C, or -1 instead of EBNA-2. Alternative acceptor site usage after the U donor site determines the frequency with which transcripts encode EBNA-3A, -3B, -3C, or -1 (see Fig. 2).

The simplest model to explain the turn-on of EBNA-3A, -3B, -3C, and -1 expression is that EBNA-LP and EBNA-2 up-regulation of the EBNA-2 response element upstream of the Cp promoter leads to higher level transcription of the EBNA mRNAs by Cp or by Wp in those cells that do not switch to Cp. In a partial test of this hypothesis, cell lines were derived that were infected with an EBV recombinant that is deleted for the EBNA-2 response element upstream of the Cp promoter. As expected from the model, cells transformed with the response-element-deleted virus were biased toward initial Wp promoter usage relative to cell lines transformed with wild-type virus (915). Not surprisingly, given the need for EBNA-3A, -3C, and -1 for the establishment and maintenance of transformation (469,837), stable EBNA transcripts were not different in cell lines transformed by mutant and wild-type virus. Surprisingly, the mutant virus was not markedly impaired in transformation efficiency (914). A corollary of the model is that Cp dominates over Wp after EBNA-LP and -2 expression, because the EBNA-2 response element is upstream of the Cp promoter and the increased activity of the Cp promoter overrides and interferes with the 3-kb-downstream Wp promoter. In support of this aspect of the model, mutations that down-modulated Cp activity or reversed Cp direction resulted in up-regulation of Wp activity (664).

Whether the net effect of EBNA-LP and -2 is to up-regulate Cp or Wp, increased transcription by either or both promoters probably accounts for transcripts that extend past the polyadenylation site downstream of the EBNA-2 ORF and through the polyadenylation sites downstream of the EBNA-3A, -3B, -3C, or -1 ORFs. Presumably, the efficiency of polyadenylation at each site determines the relative amount of each of these downstream EBNA mRNAs. The subsequent processing of the transcripts is likely to be determined by the characteristics of their polyadenylation sites. The EBNA mRNAs are all at low abundance, with the EBNA-3 or EBNA-1 mRNAs estimated to be several copies per cell.

EBNA-1 expression probably further activates EBNA transcription by enabling EBNA-1 to bind to the EBNA-1-dependent enhancer component of oriP that is 3.5 kb upstream of Cp (241,665,683). The up-regulation of the Cp and Wp promoters first by EBNA-2 and EBNA-LP and then by EBNA-1 would be anticipated to result in unbridled up-regulation of EBNA mRNA transcription were it not for the repressive effect of EBNA-3A, -3B, and -3C expression on transcription mediated by EBNA-2 and EBNA-LP activation of the Cp enhancer (389,534,692,693,864,926). EBNA-3A, -3B, and -3C bind more strongly to RBP-Jk than EBNA-2 and associate with much of the RBP-Jk in the cell. Because the EBNA-3s have no demonstrable positive effects on the Cp enhancer, their net effect is to limit EBNA-2-mediated effects on this element. EBNA-3C has more complicated effects on the LMP1 promoter and can, under certain circumstances, up-regulate LMP1 expression (927).

Concomitant with up-regulation of the Cp and Wp promoters, EBNA-2 and EBNA-LP also up-regulate cell promoters, including c-*myc*, CD23, and the virus LMP1, -2A, and -2B promoters (12). LMP2 transcription is in the same direction as EBNA transcription, and the two LMP2 promoters bracket the LMP1 promoter, with the LMP2A promoter being 3.3 kbp 5′ of the LMP2B promoter (see Fig. 3) (462,465,724). LMP2A and -2B transcription are regulated through EBNA-2 response elements upstream of their promoter (925,930). LMP1 transcription is in the opposite direction, and the LMP1 transcript is entirely within the first intron of, and antisense to, the LMP2A transcript (212). The LMP1 promoter upstream regulatory sequence is also the upstream regulatory sequence of the LMP2B promoter. The LMP1 and -2B promoters regulate transcription in opposite directions and are separated by only 266 bases.

LMP2A and -2B differ only in their first exons. The LMP2A first exon is 419 bases and the LMP2B first exon is 167 bases. The LMP2A exon encodes an amino-terminal 120-amino-acid cytoplasmic signaling domain of LMP2A, whereas the LMP2B first exon is noncoding. The remaining LMP2 exons are common to both LMP2A and -2B and are transcribed from U1. By 32 hours after infection of primary B lymphocytes, all EBNA and LMP mRNAs are expressed (12). Cell DNA synthesis follows the onset of LMP1 expression. By 48 hours after primary human B-lymphocyte infection *in vitro*, all of the EBNAs and LMP1 are near the levels that are maintained consistently through latent infection (12,16,362,594,595,700, 702).

EBER expression lags by approximately 24 hours and does not reach substantial levels until 70 hours after infection (12). The EBER-1 and EBER-2 RNAs are mostly transcribed by cell RNA polymerase III, although polymerase II may also be involved (32,340,342,376,475, 701). The EBERs have typical intragenic control regions common to pol III transcripts and upstream Sp1, ATF, and TATA box elements characteristic of pol II transcriptional sites (342). At steady-state levels in latently infected B lymphocytes, the EBERs are the most heavily transcribed and most abundant EBV RNAs. The EBERs are estimated to accumulate in cell nuclei at about 50,000 copies per cell (32,340,427,428,660,720,842).

The delineation of the highly spliced EBNA and LMP1 transcripts through Northern blot, S1 nuclease mapping, cDNA cloning and sequencing, and nuclear run-on studies explains the observations that latently infected cell nuclei have transcripts from most of the EBV genome, yet cytoplasmic polyadenylated polyribosomal mRNA is much less complex (146,303,306,427,428,628). Nuclear run-on studies indicate that almost the entire rightward or clockwise strand of the genome 3′ to the Wp promoter is transcribed, although the rate of transcription drops off somewhat downstream of EBNA-2 and again downstream of EBNA 1 (see Fig. 3) (719). Transcription, per se, does not regulate EBV gene expression. As indicated previously, the differential use of latent infection polyadenylation sites probably determines upstream splicing and thereby regulates synthesis of the six EBNA mRNAs from the same promoter.

Each EBNA primary transcript has multiple copies of IR1 or Bam W–encoded RNA, and each copy has a 500-base segment that can form an extensively base-paired structure (104). This unusual sequence could have a cis-acting role in processing of EBNA transcripts, but such a role has not as yet been identified. Analysis of a defective EBV DNA indicates that the corresponding DNA sequence can be a site for inversion within the EBV genome (381). This suggests that extensive base-pairing may occur within this nucleotide sequence under physiologic conditions.

Latent Infection Proteins

EBNA-LP

Because the number of copies of the IR1 repeat varies among EBV isolates, and because IR1-derived exons W1 and W2 encode repeating 22- and 44-amino-acid segments of EBNA-LP (Fig. 5), the size of EBNA-LP is frequently different in cells infected by different EBV isolates (169,215,872). The 44-amino-acid repeat domain encoded by W2 exons has two runs of basic amino acids, RRHR or RRVRRR, which are responsible for EBNA-LP nuclear localization (648). Aside from the N-terminal repeat domain, EBNA-LP has a unique 45-amino-acid carboxyl-terminal sequence. EBNA-LP is phosphorylated at multiple sites, probably at least once within each 44-amino-acid repeat, because the number of isoelectric forms varies with the W1W2 exon repeat number (651).

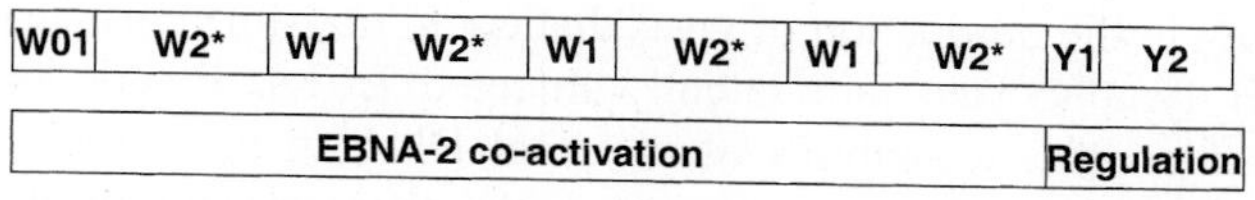

*Composite NLS and p34^{cdc2} site

FIG. 5. Schematic diagram of the repeat and unique exon and domain structure of EBNA-LP. The EBNA-LP repeat domain can coactivate transcription mediated by the EBNA-2 acidic domain. The unique carboxyl terminus of EBNA-LP modulates EBNA-LP effects.

The EBNA-LP 44-amino-acid repeat domain has a near consensus casein kinase II serine phosphorylation site. *In vitro*, p34cdc2 can phosphorylate this serine as well as a C-terminal unique serine. Casein kinase II can also phosphorylate only the unique C-terminal serine (433). EBNA-LP is highly phosphorylated in G2/M, consistent with a role for p34cdc2 in phosphorylation of EBNA-LP *in vivo* (433). At the present time, the effects of phosphorylations on EBNA-LP functionality are uncertain.

EBNA-LP is more associated with the nuclear matrix fraction than the other EBNAs (651). In immune microscopy of LCLs or of non-EBV-infected BL lymphoblasts in which EBNA-LP is expressed alone by gene transfer, EBNA-LP localizes to nuclear dots that correspond to sites of ND10 proteins (800,870). Some EBNA-LP is also diffusely spread through the nucleus. RNA *in situ* cytohybridizations with EBV IR1 DNA reveal similar intranuclear structures (466). These observations suggest the possibility that EBNA-LP could associate with EBNA transcripts and play a role in RNA processing.

EBV recombinant molecular genetic analyses of EBNA-LP have focused on the carboxyl-terminal two exons. Mutations in the repeating exons of EBNA-LP are more difficult to construct. Specific deletion of DNA encoding the carboxyl-terminal two exons, or placement of a nonsense codon at the beginning of the last two exons, has resulted in EBV recombinants that are deficient in primary lymphocyte transformation into LCLs (291,525). In two series of experiments that resulted in many wild-type EBV recombinant LCLs, only two LCLs were obtained that were infected with recombinants that are deleted for the carboxyl-terminal two exons, and these LCLs were deficient for growth. Transfection of one of these LCLs with an expression vector for wild-type EBNA-LP enabled the transfected LCLs expressing wild-type EBNA-LP to grow more rapidly than the LCLs that did not express wild-type EBNA-LP (13). Despite growth of infected primary B lymphocytes on fibroblast feeder layers, the frequency of derivation of nonsense recombinant transformed LCLs was less than 5% of wild-type, and infected cell growth was slower than with wild-type recombinants. One mutant recombinant infected LCL was obtained that had wild-type growth characteristics, and that LCL proved to be infected with a revertant (525). Passage of the deletion or nonsense EBNA-LP recombinants into other primary B lymphocytes further confirmed the reduced transformation phenotype (525). Infection of multiple primary B lymphocytes with higher-titer mutant recombinant virus enabled better outgrowth of LCLs infected with the mutant EBNA-LP EBV recombinants, presumably because of an enabling effect of cross-feeding among the multiple mutant EBV-infected cells (525). The mutant virus–infected LCLs were more highly differentiated toward immunoglobulin secretion, compatible with the possibility that wild-type EBNA-LP inhibits differentiation. In other experiments, transient expression of EBNA-LP and EBNA-2 in primary B lymphocytes co-stimulated with gp 350 resulted in induction of cyclin D2 (755). Thus, overall, these experiments favor the model that EBNA-LP has a key role in up-regulating cell gene expression critical for LCL outgrowth.

The effects of EBNA-LP on cell gene expression are likely to be similar to EBNA-LP effects in strongly coactivating viral promoters with EBNA-2. EBNA-LP coactivates EBNA-2-mediated transcription from the Cp and LMP1 promoters in transient transfection assays with reporter constructs, and it also coactivates EBNA-2 up-regulation of LMP1 expression in latency 1 EBV–infected BL cells (295,609). The EBNA-LP 22- and 44-amino-acid repeat domains have most of the activity of wild-type EBNA-LP, exerting very similar effects on EBNA-2 up-regulation of the Cp and LMP1 promoters or of a simple multimerized RBP-Jk site position near a basal promoter (295). Interactions with DNA sequence-specific transcription factors other than RBP-Jk are not critical for EBNA-LP coactivation with EBNA-2. EBNA-LP coactivation with EBNA-2 does not even require that EBNA-2 interact through RBP-Jk, because EBNA-LP robustly coactivates transcription mediated by the EBNA-2 acidic domain alone fused to the Gal-4 DNA binding domain when cells are co-transfected with a minimal promoter/reporter plasmid that has multiple upstream Gal-4 binding sites (295).

The unique 3′ exons of EBNA-LP encode 11- and 34-amino-acid carboxyl-terminal domains. Whereas the repeating exons are efficient coactivators, addition of 11 or even 35 of the carboxyl-terminal residues results in nearly complete loss of coactivating effects. Addition of the entire 45 carboxyl-terminal amino acids restores wild-type coactivation. These data indicate that the first 35 carboxyl-terminal amino acids have a strong negative regulatory effect on coactivation, and that the last 10 amino acids effectively silence the negative regulatory effect (295). The negative effect of the stop codon mutation that prevented expression of the last 45 amino acids on primary B-lymphocyte transformation (525) is evidence of the importance of this complex regulatory domain for efficient lymphocyte growth transformation. Differential phosphorylation of EBNA-LP by p34cdc2 or casein kinase II may be important in the natural regulatory effects of the carboxyl-terminal domain.

An effect of EBNA-LP on Rb and p53 has been suggested based on *in vitro* biochemical interactions and colocalization of EBNA-LP with Rb as detected with one monoclonal antibody but not with others (385,797). However, EBNA-LP is not associated with Rb family proteins or p53 in cell lysates, and expression of EBNA-LP in transgenic mice had no discernible effect on development or tumor incidence. The EBNA-LP transgenic mice died of heart failure, which was likely to be due to a toxic effect of EBNA-LP expression or to an insertion site effect (355). Immunoprecipitations of EBNA-LP from B lymphoblasts have resulted in the identification of the DNA-PK catalytic subunit, an AKAP 95 homolog HA95, HSP70, and HSP27 as EBNA-LP-associated proteins (434,526,799).

EBNA-2

Early studies identified a transformation-incompetent but replication-competent laboratory strain of EBV, P3HR-1 (565,598). The search for the biochemical basis of the nontransforming phenotype led to the discovery and characterization of EBNA-2 (Fig. 6). P3HR-1 is deleted for the DNA that encodes RNA and protein in latently infected cells, and the principal ORF in the DNA deleted from P3HR-1 encodes EBNA-2 (144,311,327,427,675).

Superinfection of latently infected cells with P3HR-1 induced replication of the endogenous viral genome, resulting in the production of virus that could transform primary B lymphocytes into latently infected LCLs. Restriction endonuclease analyses of the viral DNA in the resultant LCLs for polymorphisms that are characteristic of the P3HR-1 genome indicated that many of the genomes were partly from the P3HR-1 EBV. All of the viral DNAs were wild type at the site of the P3HR-1 deletion, supporting the hypothesis that the EBNA-2-encoding DNA is critical for LCL outgrowth (765).

More precise recombinant EBV molecular genetic experiments done by transfection of cells that are infected with the P3HR-1 EBV with molecularly cloned wild-type EBV DNA fragments that span the deletion resulted in homologous recombination and restoration of the deleted DNA segment in 1 in 10^5 progeny virus (126,290). The recombinant virus could be easily recovered because of its unique ability to transform primary B lymphocytes into LCLs. Transfection with cloned EBV DNA fragments deleted for part of the EBNA-2 ORF, or containing a stop codon one third of the way into the ORF, repeatedly failed to restore transforming ability, whereas wild-type DNA or DNA with a small marker deletion restored transforming ability. Recombinant EBVs with a nontransforming EBNA-2 mutation could also be recovered by infection of EBV-negative BL cells (527). Thus, several different genetic analyses proved that EBNA-2 is essential for primary B-lymphocyte growth transformation.

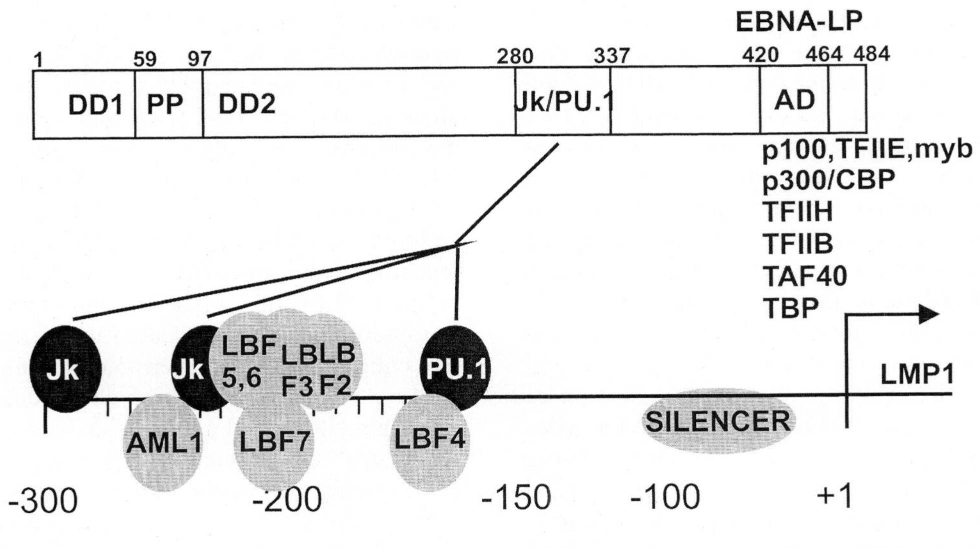

FIG. 6. Schematic depiction of the biochemical mechanisms by which EBNA-2 and EBNA-LP up-regulate transcription by the LMP1 promoter in B lymphocytes. EBNA-2 is an acidic transcriptional transactivator that biochemically interacts with the cellular sequence-specific DNA binding proteins RBP-Jk and PU.1 to bring it to specific promoters, including the LMP1 promoter. The EBNA-2 amino terminus has two domains that can mediate homotypic association with other EBNA-2 molecules. The EBNA-2 acidic domain interacts with TFIIB, TAF40, TFIIH, TBP, p100, P300/CBP, and EBNA-LP in stimulating transcription. The EBNA-2 acidic domain is extensively associated with p100, which is a scaffolding protein for *c-myb* and PIM-1.

EBNA-2 also differs more extensively between EBV types 1 and 2 than any other latent infection–associated protein, and that difference results in a differential ability to cause LCL outgrowth (7,126,144,722,723,835). Infection of primary human B lymphocytes with EBV type 2 rarely gives rise to rapidly growing LCLs (689). Restoration of the P3HR-1 deletion with prototype type 1 or type 2 EBNA-2 genes indicated that EBNA-2 is the principal determinant that enables type 1 EBV to more efficiently transform primary B lymphocytes than type 2 EBV strains (126). Primary B lymphocytes infected with the type 2 P3HR-1 EBV that had its deletion cured with type 1 EBV DNA proliferated into LCLs as rapidly as lymphocytes transformed by type 1 EBV strains. In contrast, recombination of cloned type 2 EBNA-2 DNA into the site of the P3HR-1 deletion resulted in the deficient transformation phenotype characteristic of type 2 EBV strains (126).

Comparison of the nucleotide and predicted amino acid sequence of the EBV type 1 and 2 EBNA-2s, or the corresponding sequences of other LCVs, reveals conserved or divergent domains that in general correspond with sequences that are more or less critical in genetic and biochemical analyses (see Fig. 6) (123–125,144,276, 296,322,498,500,647,840,842,894,895): (a) The amino-terminal 57 amino acids contain a motif like the immunoreceptor tyrosine-based activation motif (ITAM), have an overall negative charge, and are highly conserved between types 1 and 2. (b) The polyproline repeat of type 1 EBNA-2 is usually longer than that of type 2. (c) The 46 amino acids carboxyl-terminal to the polyproline repeat are well conserved between types 1 and 2, with 30 identical amino acids. (d) Only 52 of the next 149 amino acids are identical between types 1 and 2. (e) Carboxyl-terminal to this highly divergent region is a 46-amino-acid domain with 26 type-common amino acids. (f) A 26-amino-acid imperfect Arg-Gly repeat, of which 13 amino acids are Arg or Lys, is highly conserved. (g) In the 121-amino-acid carboxyl terminus, 84 amino acids are identical in types 1 and 2, and 16 are acidic. And (h) near the carboxyl terminus is a Lys-Arg-Pro-Arg sequence that can provide nuclear localization. In EBNA-2, the Arg-Gly repeat region near the carboxyl terminus can provide nuclear localization (125).

EBNA-2 is associated with nucleoplasmic, chromatin, and nuclear matrix fractions and localizes to large nuclear granules (327,651). It is phosphorylated on serine and threonine residues and may undergo significant post-translational modification other than phosphorylation, as the size of the nascent protein is 10 kd smaller than stable intranuclear EBNA-2 (265,870). The basis for this modification is not known. EBNA-2 extracted from lymphoblasts or even from baculovirus-infected sf-9 cells is heterogeneous in velocity sedimentation and gel elusion chromatography. EBNA-2 can form homotypic complexes the size of tetramers or larger, and some of the EBNA-2 complexes in lymphoblasts are larger than 1 MDa (265,850,891,892). The size of EBNA-2 complexes is at least in part due to the ability of EBNA-2 to homotypically self-associate through two separate domains: the amino-terminal 57 amino acids before the polyproline domain and the 120 amino acids after the polyproline domain.

EBNA-2 is a specific transactivator of cell and viral gene expression, a property first described in delineation of the mechanism for up-regulated expression of CD23 (865), a B-lymphocyte-specific surface protein expressed in high abundance on EBV-transformed or antigen-activated primary B lymphocytes (362,429). EBNA-2 transactivates CD23 expression through an EBNA-2 responsive element upstream of the CD23 promoter (867,868). Subsequently, EBNA-2 has been shown to also up-regulate the cellular CD21 (25,127,868), c-*fgr* (437), and c-*myc* mRNAs (394), as well as the viral LMP1 (1,199, 200,248,873), and LMP2A and -B (930) and Bam C promoter mRNAs (386,793). Curiously, EBNA-2 also transactivates the HIV LTR, and the transactivation is dependent on the NF-κB and PU.1 sites in the LTR, despite the absence of NF-κB sites in other EBNA-responsive cis-acting elements (730).

EBNA-2 response elements upstream of the CD23, LMP1, LMP2A, and Bam C promoters have been defined by deletional analyses and by positioning the response elements near a heterologous basal promoter (199,386,461,498,546,848,870,873,930). The LMP1 promoter, EBNA-2 response element, is largely restricted in EBNA-2 responsiveness to human B lymphocytes (200) and was not observed in epithelial cells, probably because of the role of the B-lymphocyte-specific factor, PU.1 in EBNA-2 activation of the LMP1 promoter (388,764).

Analysis of EBNA-2 using recombinant EBV molecular genetics with marker rescue of primary B-lymphocyte transforming activity in the EBNA-2-deleted, nontransforming, P3HR-1 EBV background has identified three essential EBNA-2 domains, and these domains are also critical for LMP1p or Cp promoter up-regulation. The essential domains correspond to a requirement for either of the amino-terminal domains that mediate homotypic association, the domain between 280 and 337 that mediates interaction with cellular DNA binding proteins, or the domain between amino acids 420 and 464 that is an acidic activation domain (123–126,296,840,842,894,895).

The EBNA-2 acidic domain is similar but not identical to the prototype VP16 acidic domain (123–125). Despite little colinear homology, both acidic domains include similarly placed critical hydrophobic residues, a phenylalanine in VP16 and a tryptophan in EBNA-2. A fusion of 28 amino acids of the EBNA-2 acidic domain to the Gal-4 DNA-binding domain is nearly as strong in activation of basal reporter constructs with multiple upstream Gal-4 binding sites as the core VP16 14 amino acids, whereas the corresponding EBNA-2 14 amino acids have only

25% of the VP16 activity. Despite their greater activity in transient assays, the VP16 14 amino acids can substitute for the corresponding EBNA-2 residues when expressed from an EBV recombinant (123). The EBNA-2 acidic domain is more active in BL cells than in Chinese hamster ovary (CHO) cells, and the VP16 acidic domain is more active in CHO cells than in BL cells, evidence of EBNA-2 selectivity for B lymphocytes (124). The EBNA-2 acidic domain shares with VP16 an affinity for TFIIB, TAF40, TFIIH, RPA70, and p300/CBP, but it has much less affinity for TBP (839–841,874). In contrast, the EBNA-2 acidic domain has greater affinity for p100 than does VP16, and the EBNA-2 acidic domain is highly complexed with p100 in LCLs (840). P100 is a scaffolding protein for c-*myb* and PIM-1 (150,476) and also can interact with TFIIE (840). Given the extent of association between the EBNA-2 acidic domain and p100, and the potential for p100 to recruit TFIIE, c-*myb*, and PIM-1, p100 is likely to have an important role in regulating EBNA-2-mediated transcription. Although p300 and CBP are less stably associated with EBNA-2, p300 and CBP are also likely to be critical for EBNA-2-mediated transactivation because of their intrinsic histone acetylase activities, because of their ability to recruit PCAF histone acetylase, and because of their interaction with other transcription factors. Much of the substantial histone acetylase activity that can bind to the EBNA-2 acidic domain is associated with p300/CBP (874). CBP has been specifically implicated in EBNA-2 activation of the c-*myc* promoter, whereas p300 appear to be repressive (377).

The second domain of EBNA-2 that is critical for transformation mediates an interaction and high-level association with a cellular sequence-specific DNA binding protein, RBP-Jk, also known as CBF1 (276,322,389, 895). The EBNA-2 amino acid sequence that binds to RBP-Jk includes amino acids 290 to 337. Although PWWPP is the core sequence that interacts with RBP-Jk, and mutations of the WW to FF or SS are sufficient to ablate binding, deletion of amino acids 292 to 310 also significantly disrupts the ability of EBNA-2 to associate with RBP-Jk (276,296,497,895). The WWP sequence in EBNA-2 closely mimics the WFP sequence in the Notch-receptor intracellular domain that normally mediates tight association of the Notch intracellular domain with RBP-Jk for up-regulating HES1 in tissue development (808). The WW to SS mutation ablates EBNA-2 ability to up-regulate the Cp promoter, reduces the ability to activate the LMP-1 promoter by 50%, and ablates the ability of the specifically mutated EBV recombinant to transform primary B lymphocytes into LCLs (895). These point mutation data are strong evidence for the key role of RBP-Jk association in promoter choice, promoter regulation, and LCL outgrowth; the data also support the hypothesis that RBP-Jk-mediated promoter regulation is linked to the transformation of resting B lymphocytes into LCLs.

RBP-Jk has intrinsic repressive activity that is at least in part mediated by interaction with SKIP, a component of the SMRT, Sin3A, and HDAC 2 corepressor complex (928,929). Notch and EBNA-2 may partly activate transcription from RBP-Jk-responsive promoters by interacting with SKIP and interfering with SMRT interaction with SKIP. The interaction with SKIP may also stabilize Notch and EBNA-2 interaction with RBP-Jk.

RBP-Jk recognizes the nucleotide sequence GTGGGAA (276,322,499). This sequence is part of the EBNA-2 responsive elements that have been implicated in Cp, LMP1, LMP2A, CD23, IL6, and c-*fgr* promoter regulation in LCLs (174,284,386,848,870,931). Although existing data favor the possibility that the PRF site in the c-*myc* promoter is critical in EBNA-2 promoter regulation (377), the first intron of c-*myc* has a GTGGGAA sequence that could also, or alternatively, mediate EBNA-2 up-regulation. The latter possibility might also explain the role of constitutively activated Notch receptors in human T-cell leukemia and in inducing mouse T-cell leukemia (185,640).

EBNA-2 enjoys a high-level continuous association with RBP-Jk in LCLs (389). Further, a multimerized Cp sequence that contains the RBP-Jk binding site or a multimerized minimal synthetic RBP-Jk binding site can convey EBNA-2 responsiveness to minimal promoters (295,499). However, analyses of EBNA-2-mediated activation of those EBNA-2-responsive enhancer elements that have been most extensively studied from the LMP1p and Cp promoters show that responsiveness requires at least one other cellular sequence-specific DNA binding protein, PU.1 for LMP1 (388) and AUF1 for Cp (238). Mutation of the sole RBP-Jk site in the LMP1 EBNA-2-responsive enhancer element, or point mutation of the EBNA-2 WW to SS so that EBNA-2 cannot interact with RBP-Jk, only reduces EBNA-2 responsiveness 50%. In contrast, mutation of the PU.1 binding site ablates EBNA-2 responsiveness (388). The EBNA-2 domain that interacts with PU.1 appears to include the site that interacts with RBP-Jk, and more-carboxyl EBNA-2 amino acids, because bacterial fusion proteins that include these EBNA-2 amino acid sequences can efficiently remove PU.1 from nuclear extracts (388). However, unlike RBP-Jk, which readily coimmunoprecipitates with EBNA-2 from LCL cell lysates, PU.1 does not coimmunoprecipitate with EBNA-2 (388). The targeting of PU.1 by EBNA-2 in transcriptional activation is an important aspect of EBV adaptation to lymphoid cells, because PU.1/Spi1 is a key Ets family regulator of the IgH enhancer (600). The role of AUF1 binding to CBF2 in complementing EBNA-2 interaction with CBF1 also seems to involve a AUF1 functional interaction with EBNA-2 that may be independent of EBNA-2 interaction with CBF1. AUF1 is a component of the cellular DNA binding protein complex that interacts with CBF2, and a highly multimerized CBF2 can be activated by EBNA-2 expression (238). Further, EBNA-2 activation through CBF2 is indirectly enhanced by protein kinase A (PKA) (238), as has been shown in regulation through an AUF1 site in the EBNA-2-responsive CD21 promoter (834). Although direct interaction or association of EBNA-2 with AUF1 has not been demonstrated, EBNA-2 activation of a minimal promoter through a mutimerized CBF2 element is coactivated by AUF1 overexpression and PKA activation (238).

The third EBNA-2 domain that is important for primary B-lymphocyte growth transformation appears to be either of the domains that are amino- or carboxyl-terminal to the polyproline repeat. Either domain, amino-terminal amino acids 1 to 57 or carboxyl-terminal amino acids 97 to 210, or almost all the prolines, can be deleted with only a moderate loss of primary B-lymphocyte growth transformation and Cp promoter activation, but deletion of *all* the prolines is incompatible with the mutant EBV initiating primary B-lymphocyte growth transformation (894). Biochemical studies indicate that either domain can mediate homotypic association. Homotypic association is likely to be critical to the ability of EBNA-2 to form large homotypic and larger heterotypic complexes (265,850,891,892) that can facilitate simultaneous recruitment of multiple transcription factors and enhance transcription. This probably explains the unusual effect of the deletion of both domains.

Although not essential per se for transformation or transcriptional activation, the domain that is carboxyl-terminal to the polyprolines has also been implicated in an interactions with human SNF5/Ini1 and the DEAD box protein DP103. Ini1 and DP103 interact with EBNA-2 amino acids 112 to 344 in yeast two-hybrid screens (281,891). DP103 is a DEAD box protein with imputed RNA helicase activity that appears to have transcription-repressive effects (629). *In vitro*, translated EBNA-2 amino acids 1 to 210 bind to Gst-Ini1, and a small fraction of phosphorylated EBNA-2 coimmunoprecipitates with Ini1 from 1.5- to 2-MDa fractions of cell lysates. Consistent with EBNA-2 recruitment of Ini1 to specific sites, immunoprecipitation of chromatin fragments with Ini1 antibody enriches for promoter DNA sequences downstream of LMP2A-derived enhancer construct or CD23 first-exon DNA in EBNA-2-positive cells (892). Thus, EBNA-2 interaction with Ini1 could be physiologically significant.

Deletion of the EBNA-2 DNA segment encoding the Arg-Gly repeat domain RGQSRGRGRGRGRGRGKG, amino acids 337 to 354, results in EBV recombinants that transform primary B lymphocytes with decreased activity. The transformed cells grow slowly and require maintenance at a high density. The Arg-Gly repeat has an intrinsic ability to bind to histone H1, to many other proteins (including EBNA-1), and to nucleic acids, especially poly(G). The strong interaction of the Arg-Gly domain with histone H1 is consistent with the observed effect of deletion of the Arg-Gly domain on release of a significant fraction of EBNA-2 that is in the 0.4 M salt–extractable chromatin fraction to the isotonic salt–extractable nucleoplasmic fraction in LCLs transformed by the mutant recombinant EBV. EBNA-2 deleted for the Arg-Gly domain is better than wild-type EBNA-2 at transactivating the LMP1 promoter and is as active as EBNA-2 in transactivating the *Bam*HI-C promoter. These data are most compatible with a model in which the Arg-Gly domain of region 3 is a modulator of EBNA-2 interactions with chromatin and activities in up-regulating gene expression.

EBNA-3A, -3B, -3C

The EBNA-3 genes are tandemly placed in the genome (see Fig. 3) and are transcribed from the far-upstream Cp or Wp EBNA promoters. The EBNA-3A, -3B, and -3C ORFs share colinear distant homology and are each encoded in the 3′ terminal short and long exons of their mRNAs (36,62,64,65,325,329,387,395,418,651,653,721). Latently infected cells have only a few copies of each EBNA-3 mRNA. EBNA-3A, -3B, and -3C have repeating polypeptide domains near their carboxyl termini, representing unusual examples of domain amplifications within ORFs of genes that are themselves amplified from a common progenitor. Type 1 EBNA-3A, -3B, and -3C are 944, 938, and 992 amino acids, respectively. The type 2 EBNA-3A, -3B, and -3C proteins are 925, 946, and 1,069 amino acids and are 84%, 80%, and 72% identical to their type 1 counterparts (725).

The EBNA-3 proteins (see Fig. 5) are remarkably hydrophilic, with up to 20% charged amino acids. Each has several localized concentrations of arginines or lysines, which could be responsible for nuclear localization; heptad repeats of leucine, isoleucine, or valine that could facilitate hydrophobic homo- or heterodimerization; and LXLXXL motifs that could enable interaction with nuclear hormone receptors. Despite the very low abundance of the three mRNAs in latently infected cells, EBNA-3A, -3B, and -3C are stable proteins. The EBNA-3s accumulate in intranuclear clumps, sparing the nucleolus (325,651,653). With differential salt extraction, EBNA-3A, -3B, and -3C partition to the nuclear matrix, chromatin, and nucleoplasmic fractions (651).

Although significantly divergent in nucleotide and amino acid sequence, type 1 and type 2 EBNA-3A, -3B, and -3C have similar effects in B-lymphocyte growth transformation (835). EBV recombinants made in a type 2 EBV P3HR-1 background with type 1 EBNA-LP and EBNA-2 have the robust primary B-lymphocyte transformation phenotype characteristic of type 1 EBV strains. Replacement of the P3HR-1 type 2 EBNA-3s with type 1 EBNA-3s does not alter infected B-cell outgrowth into LCLs, or the ability of the recombinant to replicate in response to induction of permissive infection. Thus,

EBNA-3 type specificity does not affect latent or lytic virus infection of B lymphocytes *in vitro*.

EBNA-3B is not critical for latent infection of primary B lymphocytes, for LCL outgrowth, for cell survival, or for lytic virus replication (836). EBV recombinants with a nonsense codon after codon 109 of the 938 type 1 EBNA-3B codons are indistinguishable from wild-type recombinants in latent infection of primary B lymphocytes *in vitro*, in LCL outgrowth, and in lytic infection. The finding that EBNA-3B is not essential for any aspect of lymphocyte infection *in vitro* is surprising because EBNA-3B epitopes are frequently recognized by human immune cytotoxic T lymphocytes (see Chapter 75 in *Fields Virology*, 4th ed.). Immune recognition would be expected to provide strong *in vivo* selection against a nonessential gene. Consistent with the lack of effect of the putative null EBNA-3B mutation on lymphocyte infection and LCL outgrowth *in vitro*, and the expectation that EBV strains with altered or absent EBNA-3B genes would be expected to emerge under immune selection, an EBV mutant with a truncated EBNA-3B ORF was recently discovered in a transplant patient with EBV-associated lymphoproliferative disease who was undergoing therapy with anti-EBNA-3B cytotoxic T lymphocytes. Nevertheless, the consistent presence of EBNA-3B in EBV isolates from normal people is evidence that EBNA-3B is important in natural infection, one aspect of which may be to contribute to immune recognition.

In contrast to the lack of phenotypic association with truncation of the EBNA-3B ORF, a nonsense codon after codon 302 of EBNA-3A or codon 365 of EBNA3C results in EBV recombinants that are unable to transform primary B lymphocytes (835). These experiments indicate that EBNA-3A and -3C are critical for B-lymphocyte growth transformation or survival, and that they differ significantly from EBNA-3B in their roles in EBV infection. Subsequent experiments with EBV recombinants that have a missense mutation beginning at EBNA-3A codon 304 confirm a critical role for EBNA-3A in LCL outgrowth and survival (412). However, two of more than 40 LCLs that were obtained in this latter study eventually grew in culture without wild-type EBNA-3A expression, indicating that EBNA-3A is not absolutely required for continued LCL proliferation or survival. Recombination of rhesus LCV EBNA-3A, -3B, and -3C, or -3B and -3C, into EBV results in recombinants that cannot transform human B lymphocytes into LCLs, consistent with the critical role of EBNA-3A and -3C in LCL outgrowth (384).

Surprisingly, EBNA-3A, -3B, and -3C are similar to EBNA-2 in being able to bind to and stably associate with RBP-Jk (389,446,534,692,693,864,926). In associating with RBP-Jk, the EBNA-3s effectively compete for RBP-Jk with EBNA-2 and Notch and limit EBNA-2 strong up-regulation through RBP-Jk (389,446,468,534,692,693, 864,926). An RBP-Jk domain as small as amino acids 125 to 181 can bind to EBNA-3C, and amino acids 172 to 223 of EBNA-3C, which are relatively well conserved in all three EBNA-3 family members, can interact with RBP-Jk (926). EBNA-3A amino acids 224 to 556 also bind well to RBP-Jk, and amino acids 1 to 138 can bind at a low level (122,693).

Because of their role in LCL outgrowth, more attention has been given to the biochemical properties of EBNA-3A and -3C than to EBNA-3B. When expressed alone in B-lymphoma cells, EBNA-3s effect modest changes in cell gene expression. EBNA-3C up-regulates CD21 expression, but not that of CD23, CD10, CD30, CD39, CD40, CD44, or cellular adhesion molecules in BJAB cells (868), whereas EBNA-3B up-regulates vimentin, CD40, and Bcl-2 expression and down-regulates CD77 in DG75 cells (751,752).

EBNA-3C can increase the levels of LMP1 expression, which fall off normally in RAJI cells that arrest in G1 when they grow to saturation (17). EBNA-3C is unique among the EBNA-3s in its ability to coactivate the LMP1 promoter with EBNA-2 (534,927). This effect can occur independently of the RBP-Jk binding site in the LMP1 promoter and of the RBP-Jk site in EBNA-3C. The effect depends on the LMP1 promoter PU.1 site and appears to be mediated by an interaction of the bZIP domain of EBNA-3C with the Ets domain of PU.1 or Spi-B. When fused to the Gal-4 DNA binding domain, EBNA-3C glutamine- and proline-rich amino acids 724 to 826 can activate transcription from a Gal-4-responsive promoter (534). However, EBNA-3C also has repressive effects. Full-length EBNA-3C fused to the Gal-4 DNA binding domain represses transcription from a variety of promoters in a variety of cell types, and the effect is independent of the presence of RBP-Jk sites on the promoter plasmid (40,71). The repressive effects map to amino acids 280 to 525; the larger proline- and glutamine-rich regions corresponding to amino acids 580 to 992 also have repressive activity (40). EBNA-3C also represses transcription from the Cp promoter. In this instance, the effect depends on interaction with RBP-Jk and on the EBNA-3C repression domain. The repressive effect of EBNA-3C is in part attributable to an interaction and association with HDAC1, but that interaction maps to a region of EBNA-3C that includes the RBP-Jk binding domain (679). EBNA-3C has been reported to cooperate with oncogenic Ras in transforming rat embryo fibroblasts, and a low level of *in vitro* interaction with RB has been detected (633). In NIH3T3 fibroblasts or human U2OS cells compelled to arrest by serum withdrawal, EBNA-3C expression can inhibit the accumulation of p27(K1P1) and can cause bi- and multinucleated cells by abrogating the mitotic spindle checkpoint (634). EBNA-3C amino acids 365 to 509 avidly bind prothymosin-alpha, a 112-amino-acid nuclear protein that can interact with histone (128). Although only about 2% of EBNA-3C coimmunoprecipitated with ProT-α and much less than 1% of ProT-α coimmunoprecipitated with EBNA-3C, EBNA-3C appeared to co-localize with ProT-α in nuclei (128). These data indicate that EBNA-3C could be involved in transcriptional effects through interaction with ProT-α.

EBNA-3A also represses the activity of the Cp promoter in B cells and in epithelial cells, and this activity largely depends on the domain through which EBNA-3A interacts with RBP-Jk (122). Using Gal-4 EBNA-3A fusion proteins and Gal-4-responsive promoters, the EBNA-3A-repressive domain has been mapped to 143 amino acids that do not interact with RBP-Jk and can mediate down-regulation of transcription (71,122). EBNA-3A also has a potential weak activation domain that is evident when EBNA-3A lacking the amino acid 100-to-364 repressive domain are fused to the Gal-4 DNA binding domain and expressed in B lymphoblasts along with a Gal-4-responsive promoter (122). The activation effects appear to be B-cell specific and are not evident in epithelial cells. EBNA-3A used as bait in a yeast two-hybrid search for interacting proteins curiously retrieved the carboxyl part of the epsilon subunit of the chaperonin T-complex protein 1, and the p38 subunit of the aryl hydrocarbon receptor complex (401,402). EBNA-3A binds to p38 and causes p38 to partially localize to the nucleus (401).

EBNA-1

EBNA-1 was initially identified as an EBV nuclear neoantigen that is present in all EBV-infected cells, regardless of the state of EBV infection (682). This was the first evidence that EBV encoded a nuclear protein in latently infected cells, perhaps similar to T antigen in simian virus 40 (SV40)-transformed cells. Soon thereafter, EBNA-1 was shown to associate diffusely with mitotic chromosomes (625). EBNA-1 is unique among the EBNAs in this regard (274,652). The significance of EBNA-1 association with chromosomes emerged later from the discovery that EBV has a cis-acting element, termed oriP, that enables the persistence of episomes in EBV-infected cells or in any human cells in which EBNA-1 is expressed (906,910). EBV and other oriP-containing episomes associate randomly with human chromosomes in cells that express EBNA-1 (159,299, 753). The unique random association of EBNA-1 with chromosomes, the association of EBV or other oriP plasmid DNA with chromosomes in EBNA-1 expressing cells, and the need for EBNA-1 in oriP persistence, position EBNA-1 as the key mediator of EBV DNA binding to chromosomes and episome persistence. Indeed, EBNA-1 is essential for EBV episome maintenance (469).

OriP has at least two components: a family of 20 copies of a 30-bp repeat, FR, that can be an EBNA-1-dependent enhancer, and a dyad symmetry, DS, of four copies of the 30-bp repeat, two in tandem and two in a larger dyad symmetry, that are required for episome maintenance (683,684). A key component of the mechanism by which this system works is that EBNA-1 binds specifically to the 30-bp repeat (most strongly to the 20×30-bp repeat element) and then to the dyad symmetry element, and to another site within the EBNA transcript (681). An EBNA-1 expression vector and oriP can be combined with a cassette for positive selection to make a plasmid into which any gene can be cloned to enable its maintenance as an episome in human cells (784). The EBNA-1 and oriP system has been widely exploited to achieve heterologous gene expression. In one use, oriP enabled plasmids containing 150 to 200 kbp fragments of random human DNA to persist as multicopy episomes in EBNA-1-expressing cells. Two such plasmids could persist in the same cell (792). Although essential for oriP enablement of plasmid persistence, excess EBNA-1 expression does not increase oriP-replicated plasmid copy number. Cellular controls limit DNA replication to one initiation event per DNA molecule per S phase (2,909), and equal numbers of plasmids are distributed to cell progeny (787).

EBNA-1 is encoded by the 2-kb 3′-terminal exon of spliced mRNAs. In type 3 latency, the 3.5-kb EBNA-1 mRNA is initiated at the Cp or Wp promoter and is highly spliced, and the primary transcript is about 100 kb (see Fig. 3) (62–66,317,326,327,719,774,788). Transcription from the Wp promoter is initially regulated by cellular factors. Wp is up-regulated and Cp turned on by EBNA-2 and -LP. EBNA-1 then further up-regulates Wp and Cp. Eventually, high-level expression of EBNA-3s down-modulates the strong up-regulating effects of EBNA-2 and EBNA-LP and prevents runaway EBNA transcription (295,468,665,692,693,788,793,886). In latency type 1 or 2, the EBNA-1-specific 2.4-kb mRNA is primarily initiated at n62423, with secondary sites at 62392 and 62340 in the prototype B95 sequence (36,611–614,733). This latency type 1 and 2 Qp promoter lacks a recognizable TATAA element. Transcription appears to be positively regulated by an unknown factor, LBP-1 (611), by IRF1 and 2 (613,731), and by E2F (612,794), which bind to three distinct sites bracketing the n62423 initiation site. The two EBNA-1 binding sites just 3′ to the transcriptional start site are the principal elements that self-regulate EBNA-1 transcription in latency type 1 and 2 (720,732,794). Similar regulatory sites are conserved in the baboon LCV (711).

EBNA-1 from the prototypical B95 EBV strain consists of 641 amino acids. The protein has a high proline content, is charged, and migrates on denaturing polyacrylamide gels with an apparent size of 76 kd. From amino to carboxyl terminus, EBNA-1 has four components: (a) an amino-terminal 89 amino acids, which include amino acids 32 to 83 and are Arg rich, (b) amino acids 90 to 327, which are an irregular copolymer of Gly and Ala, (c) amino acids 328 to 386, which are Arg rich and include a nuclear localization sequence at amino acids 379 to 386, and (d) carboxyl-terminal amino acids 387 to 641, which include amino acids 459 to 607 that bind DNA and dimerize. The two Arg-rich regions of EBNA-1 amino acids 1 to 379 can each bind to chromosomes and together reconstitute the chromosome association characteristic of EBNA-1 (360,532). Whereas EBNA-1 amino acids 379 to 641 appear to permit initial accumulation of oriP-containing plasmids in cells, the chromosome-associating domains are necessary for long-term plasmid maintenance, presumably because of their role in interacting with chromosomal proteins (349) and partitioning oriP episomes to progeny nuclei. Cellular chromosomal proteins, HMG-I amino acids 1 to 90, or histone H1 can functionally substitute for EBNA-1 amino acids 1 to 378 in enabling long-term episome persistence (360).

Identification of the biochemical interactions of the EBNA-1 carboxyl-terminal domain with oriP is facilitated by the high expression level of the EBNA-1 carboxyl terminus in bacteria- or baculovirus-infected sf9 cells (230,574). EBNA-1 amino acids 450 to 641 or 607 have similar DNA binding and dimerization activity to full-length EBNA-1 (26,27,391,573,681). The core amino acids for DNA interaction are amino acids 459 to 500, particularly 462 to 477, whereas the core residues for dimerization are amino acids 501 to 532 and 554 to 598. A dimer of an EBNA-1 oligopeptide corresponding to amino acids 458 to 478 can bind DNA, albeit nonspecifically (99,100). Surprisingly, amino acids 450 to 641 fused to the pyruvate kinase ORF and the EBNA-1 nuclear localization signal (NLS) are sufficient for wild-type EBNA-1 transcriptional activation through FR upstream of a minimal TK promoter in Vero cells, and the carboxyl-terminal acidic domain is critical for activation (26).

Each 30-bp EBNA-1 dimer-binding site is a partial dyad similar to TAGGATAGCATATGCTACCCA-GATCCAG (27,391,681). Relative to the center of each half of the dyad, nucleotides 3 to 8 are most critical for EBNA-1 binding (27). EBNA-1 has a high affinity for its cognate sequence, and interactions with the cognate sequence can be demonstrated even after protein denaturation and renaturation on cellulose nitrate. EBNA-1 not only dimerizes on 30-bp elements but also forms higher-order oligomers. Oligomerization of EBNA-1 on templates that have EBNA-1 binding sites separated by intervening sequence induces looping-out of the intervening DNA (230,259,548,781). On oriP, EBNA-1 first saturates FR and then binds to DS, looping out the intervening DNA (230). EBNA-1 amino acids 322 to 377 are important for efficient looping of EBNA-1 bound to FR and DS, or for linking multiple oriP DNA molecules to each other in a larger complex (228,518–520). Only DNA-bound EBNA-1 can participate in the large, linked EBNA-1 DNA complexes.

The binding of EBNA-1 to oriP results in two thymine residues, 64 bp apart in the region of dyad symmetry, becoming reactive to potassium permanganate, indicative of a helical distortion. EBNA-1 binding to DS lengthens interstrand H-bonds for three base-pairs centered over the permanganate-sensitive thymine base and three potential intrastrand H-bonds are formed between adjacent bases. Dimethyl sulfate protection studies indicate that EBNA-1 binds on the opposite face of the helix from the reactive thymines (229,307). Analyses on oriP in EBV-infected cells indicate that similar permanganate- and dimethyl sulfate–reactive sites exist *in vivo* (344).

Crystal structures of the EBNA-1 carboxyl-terminal 255-amino-acid dimer have been resolved at 2.5 Å, and of the dimer of cognate DNA at 2.4 and 2.2 Å (58–60). The EBNA-1 DNA binding domain has two structural motifs: a core domain that mediates protein dimerization and is similar to the DNA binding domain of the papillomavirus E2 protein, and a flanking domain that mediates sequence-specific contacts. Genetic and biochemical studies of the EBNA-1 core domain residues, which are structural homologs of the E2 residues that mediate sequence-specific DNA binding, implicate the corresponding EBNA-1 residues in DNA binding. The EBNA-1 core domain, when expressed in the absence of the flanking domain, has sequence-specific DNA binding activity, and the flanking domain residues contribute to the DNA binding. Thus, both the core and the flanking domains of EBNA-1 play direct roles in DNA recognition (132).

Only seven to eight copies of the 30-bp repeats are required for full activity of FR in transcription or episomal DNA replication (893). EBNA-1 binding to FR may effect up-regulation of the Wp and Cp promoters and of the far-upstream LMP1 and LMP2B promoters (241,665). The requirement for FR to enhance transcription and for episomal DNA replication can be partially replaced by a tandem duplication of DS (893). Tandem duplication of DS decreases its ability to serve as an origin (655). FR also arrests and functionally terminates the replication of episomes containing oriP in cells expressing EBNA-1 (167,240).

FR increases the retention and enhances transcription of oriP plasmids in cells, whereas DS is the site of initiation of plasmid DNA replication (300). DS supports EBNA-1-dependent replication in the absence of the FR (908). DNA synthesis begins in DS and proceeds bidirectionally from DS (240). Plasmids containing two copies of DS are not amplified relative to wild-type oriP (431). Two EBNA-1 binding sites in DS appear to be adequate for initial DNA replication (300,908). The ease of unwinding the 65-bp dyad symmetry of two EBNA-1 binding sites in DS, or relative nucleosome sparing in DS (i.e., relative to other sites in oriP) may contribute to the preferential use of DS as an origin (744,882). DS is not stringently required for episome maintenance, and other sequences can substitute for DS in initiation of DNA synthesis (109), including another site in oriP, designated

Rep* (432). DS is also a preferential but not exclusive site for EBV genome replication, and deletion of DS does not prevent EBV episome persistence (501,617).

At least one cellular cofactor that is not conserved in rodent cells is required for DS origin function and not for FR enhancer activity, as EBNA 1 enhances transcription in mouse or human cells, whereas oriP episomes do not replicate in rodent cells (893). Replication in rodent cells can be restored by replacing DS with a rodent DNA origin; such vectors are still dependent on the enhancer function of EBNA-1 and the family of repeats (447). Similarly, human cell DNA that contains a putative origin for DNA replication can functionally substitute for DS in oriP to allow persistence as an episome in human cells (448,542). A human cell cDNA has been identified that encodes a protein that interacts specifically with EBNA-1 cognate DNA, although the relevance of this protein to oriP function in DNA synthesis has not been established (924).

The ability of Rep*, human cell DNA origins, or rodent cell DNA origins to substitute for DS in the context of oriP in an EBNA-1-expressing cell, calls into question the fundamental role of EBNA-1 in DNA replication versus episome persistence (8). Indeed, oriP increases the conversion of transfected plasmid DNA to Dpn1 resistance about 10-fold in the absence of EBNA-1 at 48 hours after transfection and about 20-fold in the presence of EBNA-1. This DNA had gone through two cycles of DNA replication as evidenced by Dpn1 resistance and by bromodeoxyuridine incorporation. The major EBNA-1 effect occurred at 96 hours after transfection, at which point Dpn-resistant DNA disappeared from cells that lack EBNA-1. Further, DS was not specifically required for persistence; FR with a triplicate of Rep* DNA replicates and persists as well as wild-type oriP in cells that express EBNA-1.

EBNA-1 amino acids 90 to 327 are an irregular glycine–alanine repeat domain. The DNA encoding this domain is similar to repeat sequences in cell DNA, and similar polypeptides may be encoded from the cell genome (312). EBV isolates frequently differ in the length of this repeat. This difference has been useful in identifying the EBNA-1 ORF and typing EBV isolates (204,267–269,326). Deletion of the repeat does not affect EBNA-1 stability or function (907). EBNA-1 expressed in murine cells does not engender a specific cytotoxic T-cell response in mice (847). The failure to recognize EBNA-1 as foreign is due to the EBNA-1 Gly-Ala repeat, which inhibits EBNA-1 processing through proteosomes (477). Because proteosome-mediated degradation is necessary for antigen processing into major histocompatibility complex (MHC) class I molecules for presentation at the cell surface, epitopes in EBNA-1 are poor targets for attack by CD8 cytotoxic T cells. Fusion of the Gly-Ala domain to the EBNA-3B ORF down-regulates CD8 recognition of EBNA-3B-expressing cells. Other proteins are also protected from proteosome degradation by fusion to the glycine–alanine repeat (746). The length of the repeat and particularly the alanines are critical for this effect. Primate LCVs have shorter Gly-Ala repeats that do not have a similar effect on proteosome processing, leaving open the possibility that the Gly-Ala repeat domain may have yet another role in EBV infection.

EBNA-1 is very stable and is phosphorylated on serine residues in at least two separable domains in the carboxyl half of the molecule (308,652,658). The role of these phosphorylations in EBNA-1 function has not as yet been established through genetic analyses. Further, EBV DNA in human cells that express EBNA-1 associates with the nuclear matrix. The fragment of EBV DNA that associates with the matrix includes oriP, potentially linking oriP to a site for DNA replication or transcription. EBNA-1 can also interact with diverse nucleic acid substrates *in vitro*, including EBER-1 and HIV-TAR (768).

EBNA-1 is the only EBNA that continues to be transcribed when cells are activated to lytic infection (317,706,873,877). Cp and Wp promoter activities cease in lytic infection, and the downstream Fp promoter is activated (614). The lytic mRNA initiates in an Fp promoter just upstream of the Qp promoter and otherwise has the same sequence as the latent infection RNA.

LMP1

Despite being a weak promoter for the LMP1 gene relative to the Cp and Wp EBNA promoters, as revealed by nuclear run-on assays, LMP1 mRNA is almost 10 times more abundant than the EBNA mRNAs in latently infected B lymphocytes (212,720). In epithelial cells, LMP1 transcription is mediated by an upstream promoter that initiates transcription from multiple TATA-less sites in the nearest copy of TR, resulting in a 3.5-kb transcript with a long, largely untranslated 5′ exon (251,715). The LMP1 transcripts have two short introns (44,212). The EBNA proteins are remarkably stable, whereas a significant fraction of LMP1 has a short half-life. The primary amino acid sequence of LMP1 is that of an integral membrane protein and includes at least three domains: (a) a 20-amino-acid, arginine- and proline-rich, hydrophilic amino terminus lacking the characteristics of a signal peptide; (b) six markedly hydrophobic 20-amino-acid, alpha-helical, transmembrane segments, separated by five reverse turns, each eight to ten amino acids in length; and (c) a 200-amino-acid carboxyl terminus, rich in acidic residues (Fig. 8). LMP1, translated *in vitro*, post-translationally inserts into cell membranes consistent with the expected membrane insertion properties of the three pairs of highly hydrophobic transmembrane segments joined by short reverse turns (490,492,724). Although LMP1 has little primary sequence homology to other proteins, aspects of its three-domain organization are similar to some other integral membrane proteins

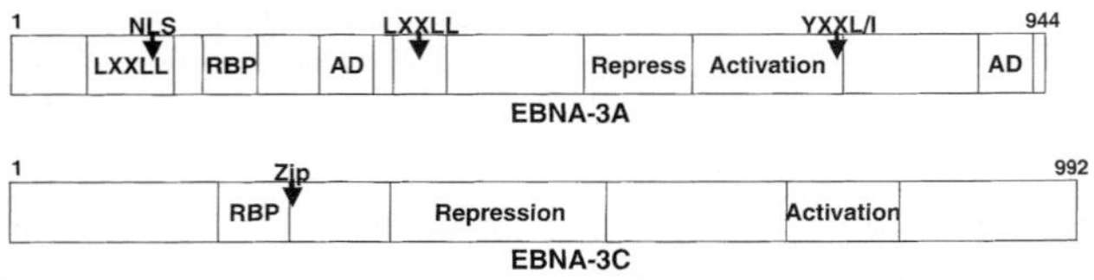

FIG. 7. Schematic diagram of the EBNA-3A and EBNA-3C open reading frames. Indicated are domains that associate with RBP-Jkappa as well as domains that have activating or repressive effects when fused to the Gal-4 DNA binding domains and assayed for transcriptional up- or down-regulating effects in transient transfection assays with a promoter that has multiple upstream Gal-4 binding sites.

such as erythrocyte membrane band three or the *mas* oncogene.

Immunofluorescence microscopy (324,492), membrane fractionation (523), and live-cell protease cleavage studies (492) indicate that about half of the cellular LMP1 is in the plasma membrane. LMP1 is less abundant in other cytoplasmic membranes. Live-cell protease cleavage studies also indicate that both the N- and C-termini are on the cytoplasmic side of the plasma membrane and only three short reverse-turn domains are on the extracellular side of the plasma membrane (492).

LMP1 is phosphorylated on serine and threonine residues, at a ratio of 6:1, and is not phosphorylated on tyrosines (38,490,524,589,591). Half or more of LMP1 is associated with the cytoplasmic cytoskeleton as defined by resistance to extraction with buffers supplemented with nonionic detergents (490,492,524,589,591). The half-life of LMP1 has been measured by determining the time to reach stable levels of ^{35}S-methionine label in LMP1 and by determining the rate of decay of LMP1 in the presence of protein synthesis inhibitors. The data do not precisely agree, possibly because of an effect of the protein synthesis inhibitors in increasing total LMP1 turnover, or differences in the cell lines studied (38,490,524,589,591). Clearly, nascent, nonionic, detergent-soluble LMP1 has a half-life of less than 2 hours and is converted to a more stable cytoskeleton-associated form. Cytoskeletal LMP1 is phosphorylated, and soluble LMP1 is not (490,524,589,591). LMP1 is ultimately cleaved near the beginning of the carboxyl-terminal cytoplasmic domain, resulting in a transiently stable soluble C-terminal domain of about 25 kd (589,591). The principal serine and threonine phosphorylation sites are near each other in the 25-kd cleavage product (591).

LMP1 constitutively forms discrete patches in the plasma membrane, which are often further organized into a single caplike structure, which localizes to the uropod (324,492). LMP1 aggregates in patches in LCLs or other cell plasma membranes in the absence of exogenous growth factors; the aggregation appears to be an intrinsic property of the multiple hydrophobic transmembrane domains (490,492). Vimentin co-localizes with the LMP1 cap in the latently infected B-lymphocyte plasma membranes (490). Vimentin is not ordinarily found in a plasma membrane patch and is drawn into this patch by LMP1. Vimentin relocalizes into perinuclear rings and coils when cells are treated with colcemid, and LMP1 then relocalizes to the vimentin rings (490). Thus, once LMP1 is associated with vimentin, vimentin can further direct LMP1's localization. LMP1 aggregates in patches and caps in the plasma membrane of cells that lack vimentin or other EBV proteins and does not require vimentin for its signal transducing effects (489,491,866). Thus LMP1 interacts with itself or with other cell membrane proteins to form large, noncovalently linked membrane complexes. LMP1 is partially associated with cholesterol-rich membrane microdomains (31).

In single gene transfer experiments under heterologous promoters, LMP1 has transforming effects in continuous rodent fibroblast cell lines (39,865,866,590). In Rat-1 or NIH3T3 cells, LMP1 alters cell morphology and enables cells to grow in medium supplemented with a low concentration of serum. In Rat-1 cells, LMP1 also causes loss of contact inhibition, so that cells heap up in monolayer culture (865). Rat-1 or BALB/c 3T3 cells lose anchorage dependence and grow in soft agar after LMP1 expression (39,866). Rat-1 cells expressing LMP1 are tumorigenic in nude mice, whereas control Rat-1 cells are nontumorigenic (865). The growth of BALB/c 3T3 cells in soft agar correlates quantitatively with the extent of LMP1 expression up to the levels ordinarily expressed in LCLs (866). Expression at higher levels results in toxicity. The hypothesis has been put forward that the toxic effects of LMP1 expressed at high levels may be a useful surrogate marker for LMP1 biologic activity in rodent fibroblasts; LMP1 mutants that have transforming activity when expressed at levels similar to LCLs, are usually toxic when expressed at higher levels (538). Comparison of the transforming properties of LMP1 with those of D1LMP1 indicates that D1LMP1 does not have these effects (37,866). D1LMP1 lacks the amino-terminal cytoplasmic domain and the first four transmembrane domains, inserts into cell membranes, and does not patch; these data indicate that the amino terminus and the first four transmembrane domains are essential for LMP1 transforming effects in BALB/c 3T3 cells. Addition of the 25-amino-acid N-terminal cytoplasmic domain to the amino terminus of D1LMP did not restore the ability to cause anchorage-independent growth of BALB/c 3T3 cells (37,538), indicating that abnormal transforming phenotype of D1LMP is not caused by an absence of the amino-terminal cytoplasmic domain. Carboxyl-terminal cytoplasmic domain truncations have been variable in rodent fibroblast effects but consistently unable to cause loss of contact inhibition in Rat-1 cells (590). These data suggest that the carboxyl-terminal cytoplasmic domain is important for loss of contact inhibition in Rat-1 cells.

LMP1 also dramatically alters the growth of EBV-negative BL lymphoblasts or even primary B lymphocytes when expressed stably or transiently at the appropriate level in such cells following gene transfer (57,321,489, 645,646,649,709,867,868). LMP1 induces many of the changes usually associated with EBV infection of primary B lymphocytes or with antigen activation of primary B lymphocytes, including cell clumping; increased villous projections; increased vimentin expression; increased cell surface expression of CD23, CD39, CD40, CD44, and class II MHC; increased IL10 expression; decreased expression of CD10; and increased expression of the cell adhesion molecules LFA-1, ICAM-1, and LFA-3 (867). Not only does LMP1 increase plasma membrane expression of adhesion molecules, but it also functionally activates adhesion and induces higher levels of LFA-1 mRNA (866,867). D1LMP1 has none of these effects, confirming the importance of the amino terminus and multiple transmembranes for domains for phenotypic effects (491,867). LMP1 has also been shown to protect B lymphocytes from apoptosis (270,321,709). These effects are mediated in part through LMP1 induction of bcl-2 (321,539,707). LMP1 effects in BL cells or rodent fibroblasts vary with the particular cell background and particularly in B lymphoblasts with the basal level of activation molecule expression. LMP1 induction of B-lymphocyte adhesion molecules may be important, as homotypic B-lymphocyte adhesion or adhesion to other cells can facilitate cell growth through autocrine or paracrine growth factors and ligands expressed on other cell surfaces. Also, adhesion is important for the immune elimination of EBV-transformed B lymphocytes *in vivo*, and therefore for continued virus infection. Despite the robust and pleotropic effects of LMP1 expression in human B-lymphoma cells, the effects of deletion mutants that partially affect the membrane-patching properties of LMP1 on each of the phenotypes is intermediate without a clear loss of some effects and the retention of others (491).

LMP1 expression also alters cell growth and gene expression in multipotent hematopoietic stem cells and epithelial cells (156,201,202,346). The effects of LMP1 on epithelial cell growth are evident with transgenic expression of LMP1 in the skin of mice: LMP1 induces epidermal hyperplasia and alters keratin gene expression (885). In monolayer cultures, LMP1 alters keratinocyte morphology and cytokeratin expression (201). In stratified air–liquid interface raft cultures of immortalized epithelial cell lines, LMP1 inhibits cell differentiation (156). In C33 cervical carcinoma cells, LMP1 expression induces matrix metalloproteinase 9 expression; matrix metalloproteinases are believed to be important in tissue invasion (807,917).

The ability of EBV recombinants specifically mutated in LMP1 to transform primary B lymphocytes into LCLs is a definitive assay for EBV transforming effects, because primary human B lymphocytes grow out as LCLs only in response to EBV infection. This assay has proven to be quite useful for defining the critical components of LMP1. As expected from the transforming effects of LMP1 expression in rodent fibroblasts and B-lymphoma cells, LMP1 is essential for primary B-lymphocyte growth transformation (409). EBV recombinants with mutations in LMP1 that result in amino-terminal truncation of the cytoplasmic and first transmembrane domain have a nontransforming phenotype (409). This form of LMP1 is expressed as a stable protein, localizes to the plasma membrane, but does not aggregate in the plasma membrane, indicating the importance of plasma membrane aggregation in LMP1 effects on primary B-lymphocyte transformation into LCLs (409,491). Similarly, expression of the last three transmembrane domains and the carboxyl-terminus resulted in a nontransforming phenotype; this form of LMP1 localizes to all cytoplasmic membrane without evidence of accumulation in the plasma membrane or aggregation (409,491). The effects of these mutations are not caused by specific interactions mediated by the amino-terminal cytoplasmic domain, because deletion of any part of the amino-terminal cytoplasmic domain results in at least 10% residual transforming efficiency, and the LCLs have a normal growth phenotype (368). The most severe effects of mutation in the amino-terminal cytoplasmic domain are associated with deletion of all of the arginines, which appears to interfere with membrane positioning effects of the transmembrane domains. In contrast, expression of the amino-terminal 187 amino acids of LMP1, which includes the amino-terminal cytoplasmic domain and all of the transmembrane domains but not the carboxyl-terminal cytoplasmic 200 amino acids, ablates primary B-lymphocytes transformation (411).

Specifically mutated EBV recombinants that allow expression of the amino-terminal 231 amino acids, which includes only the first 45 of the 200 amino acids of the carboxy-terminal cytoplasmic domain, results in LCL outgrowth that depends on fibroblast feeder layers (409). The LMP1 1 to 231 recombinant EBV is nearly wild type in the initiation of foci of LCL outgrowth, but most of these foci cannot be expanded to LCLs; their growth is unusually dependent on a high cell density (410). In contrast, an EBV recombinant deleted for DNA encoding only the first 15 amino acids of the cytoplasmic carboxyl terminus is unable to transform primary B lymphocytes (367). These data indicate that the first 15 amino acids of the carboxyl-terminal cytoplasmic domain include part of a site whose first 45 amino acids are essential for LCL outgrowth and even sufficient, in the context of the transmembrane domains, for initial B-cell transformation. Further, these data indicate that efficient LCL outgrowth requires the more carboxyl-terminal 155 amino acids. The first mutations of two of the three LMP1 carboxyl-terminal amino acids that were tested in an EBV recombinant defined a second site of up to 35 amino acids that is important for efficient transformation of primary B lymphocytes (370). Despite the fact that multiple sites between the first 45 and last 35 amino acids of the LMP1 carboxyl terminus have been implicated in various biologic or biochemical processes, specific deletion of all of the LMP1 codons for amino acids 232 to 351 results in an EBV recombinant that is indistinguishable from wild-type LMP1 in primary B-lymphocyte growth transformation, LCL outgrowth, LCL growth characteristics, or lytic EBV replication (371). Thus, the nontransforming phenotype resulting from the deletion of the first 15 codons of the cytoplasmic carboxyl terminus, the robust initial transformation phenotype of the LMP1 amino acids 1 to 231, the deficient LCL outgrowth phenotype of the recombinant with two of the last three carboxyl-terminal amino acids mutated, and the wild-type phenotype of the recombinant deleted for codons 232 to 351 indicate that LMP1 carboxyl-terminal residues 187 to 231 and 352 to 386 are the only residues that are critical for LMP1 cytoplasmic signalling effects in the conversion of primary B lymphocytes to LCLs. Therefore, these two domains have been given the acronym TES1 and 2, for transformation effector sites 1 and 2.

Investigations of the biochemical bases of LMP1 effects in up-regulating expression of B-lymphocyte activation markers, adhesion molecules, HIV, or A20 (an antiapoptosis factor) led to the identification of NF-κB activation as one basis for LMP1 signalling effects (292,453). The domains of LMP1 required for NF-κB activation are the multiple transmembrane domains and the carboxyl-terminal 55 amino acids or the carboxyl-terminal 36 amino acids and first 45 amino acids of the cytoplasmic carboxyl terminus; the amino-terminal cytoplasmic amino acids are not specifically required (356, 578). The amino-terminal 45 and carboxyl-terminal 36 amino acids of the cytoplasmic carboxyl terminus are therefore designated C-terminal NF-κB activation regions 1 and 2, or CTAR1 and -2 (356). The need for the LMP1 transmembrane domains could be replaced in various ways, including expression of CD2-CTAR1 and -2, or CD2-CTAR2 chimeric fusions in cells, and adding anti-CD2 antibody to induce aggregation, confirming the important constitutive homoaggregating role of the LMP1 transmembrane domains (226,252).

The biochemical mechanisms that underly the transformation effector sites and NF-κB activating domains were initially united by the yeast two-hybrid-based discovery that LMP1 TES1/CTAR1 interacts with, and in the context of the LMP1 transmembrane domains constitutively associates with, human tumor necrosis factor (TNF)-associated cell cytoplasmic factors hTRAF3 and hTRAF1 (593); the mouse TRAF1 and -2 were described several months before by their interaction with the type 2 TNF-receptor cytoplasmic domains (703). LMP1 TES1 is structurally and functionally homologous to the TNF receptor (TNFR), CD40 (593), which, when activated, induces effects in B lymphocytes that are similar to LMP1 (42,101,585). The structural basis for LMP1 and CD40 engagement with TRAFs and many of the downstream effects are equivalent (74,164,166,180–184,225, 227,302,408,424,572,667,726,798,854,911). LMP1 and CD40 share a PXQXT motif (164,227) that interacts with a shallow canyon on the surface of TRAF trimers (911,912). The biochemical effect is to stabilize TRAF1 and -2 and TRAF3 and -5 homo- and heterodimers on LMP1 TES1/CTAR1 and in the cytoplasm (164,166). TRAF trimers that incorporate TRAF2 and TRAF5 are particularly implicated in forward signalling from TNFRs. One aspect of LMP1 signalling through TRAFs is that the LMP1 PXQXT domain has a higher affinity for TRAF1 and -3 than for TRAF2 and -5 (164,166). TRAF1 is expressed at low levels in B lymphocytes and is then induced by LMP1 expression, whereas in epithelial cells or other cell types expression of TRAF1 may be minimal or not inducible, and this may affect the level of LMP1 signalling through TES1/CTAR1 in these cells.

TES2/CTAR2 also engages TNFR signalling pathways and ultimately signals through TRAFs (369,372). A yeast two-hybrid screen with TES2 bait retrieved the TNFR-I associated death domain protein, TRADD (369). The LMP1 carboxyl-terminal 11 amino acids interact with and constitutively associate with TRADD and RIP (369,372). LMP1 engages a small component of the death domain and does not propagate death domain complex recruitment or induce cell death. Much of the signal that LMP1 transmits through TRADD and RIP appears to then be mediated by TRAFs, which are known to mediate nondeath signalling from TRADD and RIP. Dominant negative mutants of TRAFs block NF-κB activation from both TES1/CTAR1 and TES2/CTAR2 (408). Further, dominant negative mutants of the NF-κB-inducing kinase, NIK, or of the IKK inducing kinases, IKK α or β block TES1/CTAR1 and TES2/CTAR2-mediated NF-κB activation (Fig. 8) (798). However, NIK is probably only one component of the kinases that mediate signalling downstream of the TRAFs. NIK is probably not even the principal kinase that connects TRAFs to the IKKs. Furthermore, signalling downstream of the TRAFs activates not only IKKs and NF-κB, but also JUNK and *jun/fos*, p38 and AP-1, and CDC42 (180,182,184,302,423,667). Thus, while LMP1 signalling through TRAFs mediates most or all of LMP1's effects, aspects of these pathways are as yet incompletely delineated. One incompletely understood aspect of LMP1 signalling is the preferential role of TES1/CTAR1 over TES2/CTAR2 in the activation of EGF receptor expression in epithelial cells, or of TRAF1 expression in B lymphocytes (166,569–572). NF-κB activation is an important component of many of these transcriptional activations and is critical to LCL survival (82). Despite continued high level expression of Bcl-2 and Bcl-XI, inhibition of NF-κB activation results in apoptosis of LCLs.

LMP1 and EBNA-1 are the only latent infection–associated genes that are also transcribed in lytic EBV infec-

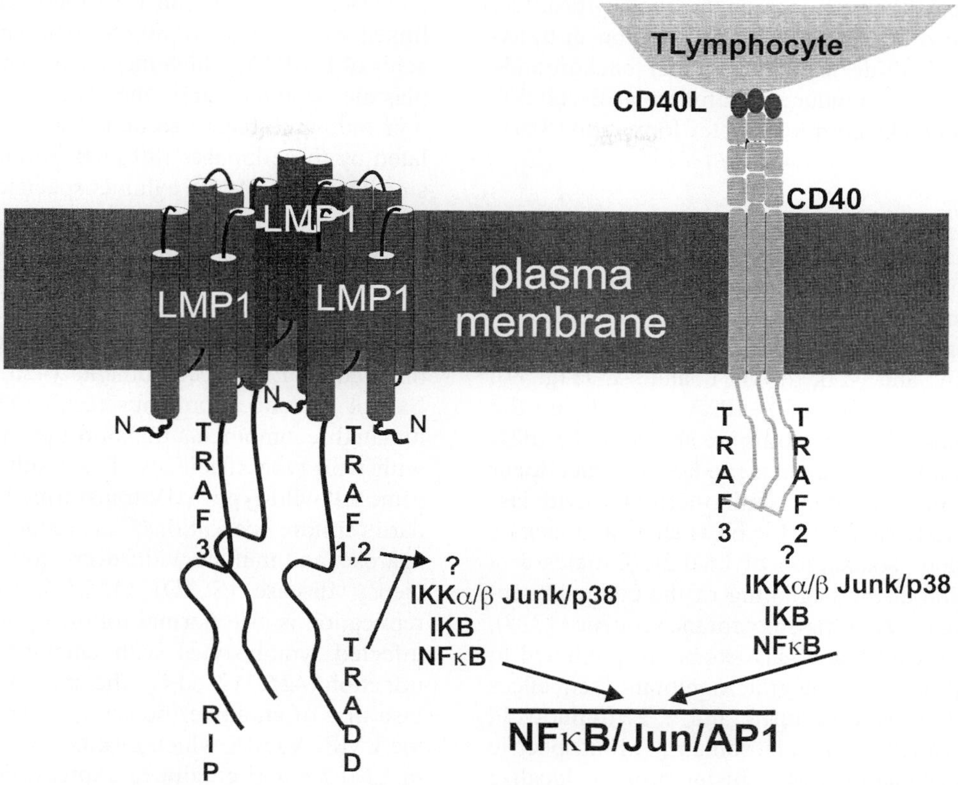

FIG. 8. Schematic diagram of biochemical mechanisms by which LMP1 effects cell growth and survival pathways by constitutively mimicking an activated tumor necrosis factor (TNF) receptor such as CD40. The six hydrophobic transmembrane domains of LMP1 enable LMP1 to aggregate in the plasma membrane. The amino-terminal cytoplasmic domain is fully dispensable for primary B-lymphocyte growth transformation, and its primary function is in tethering the amino terminus of the first transmembrane domain to the cytoplasmic side of the plasma membrane. The transmembrane domains and the carboxyl-terminal cytoplasmic domain are essential for primary B-lymphocyte growth transformation. The carboxyl-terminal cytoplasmic domain is composed of 200 amino acids and it has two essential components: One is the first 44 amino acids, which associate with TNF receptor-associated factors. The second is the carboxyl-terminal 30 amino acids, which associate with the TNFR-associated death domain proteins, TRADD and RIP, without propagating a death signal. Both domains activate the IkB kinases causing phosphorylation of IkB, IkB degradation, and NF-kB activation. Both domains also activate Junk and p38 kinases. The rest of the carboxyl-terminal cytoplasmic domain can be deleted without loss of B-lymphocyte transforming activity.

tion. In some latently infected BL cells such as Raji, LMP1 expression can be increased by treatment with activators of PKC, which increase early lytic cycle promoter activity (68,464,704). The promoter for full-length LMP1 expression in lytic infection has not been characterized. In late lytic infection, a promoter in the third LMP1 exon transcribes the part of the LMP1 ORF that encodes the last two transmembrane domains and the entire LMP1 cytoplasmic domain (353). This smaller integral membrane protein, referred to as D1LMP1, localizes to cytoplasmic membranes and does not have the transforming or cell activating properties of LMP1 and does not associate with vimentin or other cytoskeletal elements (490,491,523). The detection of LMP1 but not D1LMP1 in preparations of purified virus and newly infected cells indicates that LMP1 may be incorporated into virions (194,523). This raises the possibility that virion-associated LMP1 could have an effect on the growth of newly infected cells.

The expression of LMP1 in three lineages of transgenic mice under control of the immunoglobulin heavy-chain promoter and enhancer results in low-level expression in normal lymphoid tissue and an increase in B-cell hyperplasia and lymphomas (449). The incidence of lymphoma increased significantly with age with lymphomas developing in 42% of transgenic mice over 18 months of age. The lymphomas are monoclonal or oligoclonal by IgH rearrangement, and LMP1 is expressed at LCL levels in the lymphomas. These data indicate that LMP1 alone can be oncogenic in B lymphocytes *in vivo*. B cells of transgenic mice expressing LMP1 under the control of immunoglobulin promoter/enhancer–displayed enhanced expression of activation antigens, spontaneously proliferated and produced antibody. LMP1 expression in transgenic mice in CD40-deficient or normal backgrounds mimics CD40 signals to induce extrafollicular B-cell differentiation and blocks germinal center formation (854).

LMP2A and -2B

The cloning and sequencing of cDNAs (462,465,724) to 2.3- and 2.0-kb cytoplasmic polyadenylated RNAs (856) from latently infected cells provided the first evidence for two integral membrane proteins that were designated LMP2A and -2B, or TP1 and -2 (Fig. 9). (231,511). The first exons of LMP2A and -2B are the only unique exons; all other exons are shared by LMP2A and -2B. The first LMP2A exon is predicted to encode for a 119-amino-acid hydrophilic amino-terminal cytoplasmic domain. The first LMP2B exon is short and lacks a methionine codon. Translation of LMP2B initiates at a methionine codon at the beginning of the common second exon, before the first transmembrane sequence (724). The remaining LMP2A and -2B exons are predicted to encode 12 hydrophobic integral membrane sequences separated by short reverse turns and a 27-amino-acid hydrophilic carboxyl-terminal domain. Monospecific antisera generated against LMP2 fusion proteins localize LMP2A to a patch in the plasma membrane of latently infected B lymphocytes, where it co-localizes with LMP1 (510,511). LMP2A localizes to the same site in the plasma membrane of B-lymphoma cells whether or not LMP1 is expressed in the same cell.

LMP2A is a substrate for and is associated with B-lymphocyte src family tyrosine kinases. Antiphosphotyrosine antibodies localize sites of constitutive tyrosine phosphorylation in the plasma membrane of cells that express LMP2A (510). The sites of tyrosine phosphorylation coincide with LMP2A, indicating that LMP2A is one of the few localized stable tyrosine phosphorylated proteins in BL cells or LCLs (510). LMP2A is stably associated with src family tyrosine kinases and with syk, unlike the sIg B-cell receptor complex, which markedly increases its association with these kinases when cross-linked by antigen (78,80,88,510). The first 167 amino acids of LMP2A, which include the amino-terminal cytoplasmic domain and the first two transmembrane domains, are able to associate with and be phosphorylated by these kinases (80,510). Among src family tyrosine kinases, LMP2A exhibits specificity for fyn and lyn in B lymphocytes (80).

Despite the interaction of LMP2A with B-lymphocyte tyrosine kinases, LMP2A and -2B do not effect EBV transformation of primary B lymphocytes into LCLs or LCL survival. LMP2A and -2B have been extensively mutated in EBV recombinants (425,512–514,698,771). Except for one anomalous result (73), the specifically mutated recombinants transform primary B lymphocytes with wild-type efficiency. The resultant LCLs grow the same as wild-type EBV-transformed LCLs under standard culture conditions, in reduced serum, in soft agarose, and in mice with severe combined immunodeficiency disease (SCID) (425,512–514,698,771). Virus replication is also normal following treatment of latently infected lymphocytes with chemical inducers of lytic infection (425,512–514). The specific mutations include insertion of an amber nonsense linker after codon 19 of the LMP2A ORF, which results in ablation of expression of LMP2A and continued expression of LMP2B (512); insertion of an amber nonsense linker after DNA encoding the first five transmembrane domains, which results in ablation of expression in the last seven transmembrane domains and the carboxy-terminus of LMP2A and -2B (513); and deletion of DNA encoding the first five transmembrane domains of LMP2A and -2B, which results in truncation of LMP2A after the amino-terminal cytoplasmic domain and the addition of missense codons (514).

LMP2A expression in BL lymphoblasts constitutively blocks the signal transduction events that would follow the cross-linking of sIgM, CD19, or class II MHC on cells that do not express LMP2A (552,555). This blockade is similar to the desensitization that occurs after sIg signal transduction (78,88). LMP2A effects depend on the LMP2 transmembrane domains that mediate aggrega-

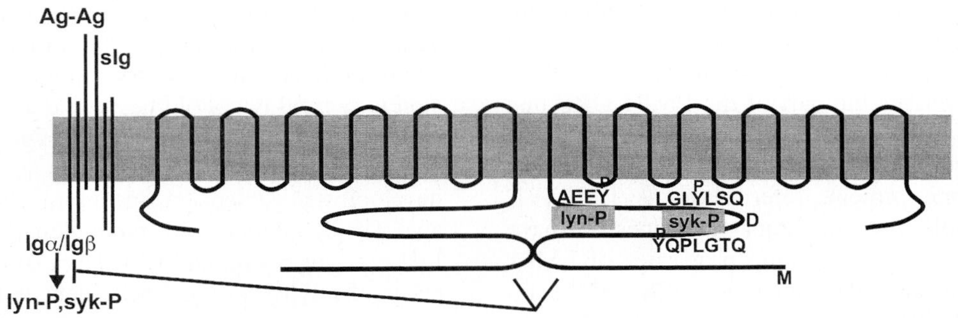

FIG. 9. Schematic diagram of the biochemical mechanisms by which LMP2 constitutively effects tyrosine kinase signalling pathways, inducing low-level activation and high-level global desensitization.

tion in the cell plasma membrane and on the LMP2A amino terminal cytoplasmic domain. The simplest model that would account for this activity is that LMP2 transmembrane domain–mediated aggregation of LMP2A results in phosphorylation of LMP2A, constitutive binding of src and syk, a constitutive low level of forward signaling, and turn-on of a down-regulatory kinase or phosphatase that globally blocks other src family–associated receptor tyrosine kinase–mediated signal transduction. Indeed, the basal tyrosine phosphorylation of many cellular proteins, including lyn, syk, and the p85 subunit of PI3 kinase, are higher in LCLs transformed by EBV recombinants that express wild-type LMP2A than in LCLs transformed by EBV recombinants that do not express LMP2A. Further, cross-linking of sIg on wild-type EBV–transformed LCLs results in abrogation of tyrosine kinase signalling at the first steps of src family and syk phosphorylation, whereas cross-linking of sIg on LMP2 null mutant recombinant–transformed LCLs results in normal sIg protein tyrosine kinase signal transduction, including transient phosphorylation of lyn, fyn, syk, p85, Vav, PLCgamma, SHC, and Grb2 (552). The amino terminus of LMP2A has a $YXXL(N)_7YXXL$ sequence that in the B-cell receptor–associated molecules Ig alpha and Ig beta binds syk, and a YEEI sequence that binds lyn or other src family tyrosine kinases (88). When these LMP2A domains are fused to the CD8 surface and transmembrane domains and CD8 is cross-linked on cells that express the chimeric protein, the LMP2A domains transmit an increase in intracellular free calcium and are then refractory to further stimulation, as is characteristic of sIg cross-linking (49). The key roles for the LMP2 putative src family PTK binding site at Y112 and the putative syk binding site at the ITAM motif have been directly demonstrated by expression of the appropriate mutant proteins in BL cells and by examining sIg signal transduction in LCLs transformed by specifically mutated EBV recombinants (235–237). Both Y112 and the ITAM are stringently required for B-cell receptor desensitization.

The effect of LMP2A expression on LCLs is to block lytic infection that would occur in the absence of LMP2A following cross-linking of sIg on the surface of LCLs. Cross-linking of sIg on primary B lymphocytes transformed by LMP2 null mutant recombinants results in normal sIg-mediated signal transduction and activation of EBV replication (553,554). The LMP2A blockade to lytic activation can be bypassed by activating PKC and raising intracellular free calcium with phorbol ester (TPA) and calcium ionophore treatment. Treatment of wild-type or mutant transformed cells with TPA and calcium ionophore results in similar inductions of lytic infection (554). Because LMP2A is expressed in most latently infected B lymphocytes *in vivo*, one role may be to keep EBV infection latent in these cells when they encounter T lymphocytes or other potentially activating signals; a corollary of this hypothesis is that activation of lytic EBV infection in a latently infected lymphocyte could still be triggered by a cytokine released from an epithelial cell that might trigger a G protein–coupled receptor or JAK kinase signal transduction pathway (758).

A second role for LMP2 may be to provide survival and antidifferentiation signals to B cells that are not in type 3 latency. LMP2A expression in transgenic mice under control of IgH chain promoter and enhancer results sIg-negative B cells escaping from the bone marrow and colonizing peripheral lymphoid organs, bypassing normal B-lymphocyte developmental checkpoints (84). This indicates that LMP2A has sufficient constitutive forward signaling activity to affect the biology of normal B cells. The LMP2A effect is also evident in RAG 1(–/–) mice and is dependent on the LMP2A ITAM (83,547). Thus, LMP2A expression could have a role in latency type 2–infected lymphocytes in enhancing cell survival, in lymphoid organ persistence, or in blocking differentiation. As described in Chapter 75 in *Fields Virology*, 4th ed., LMP2A is also expressed in type 2 latency in Hodgkin's disease and nasopharyngeal carcinoma. Constitutive forward signalling effects of LMP2 could also be important in the pathogenesis of these malignancies. The effects of LMP2 are, however, subtle. No effect on epithelial differentiation or survival is evident with transgenic expression of LMP2A in normal mouse epithelium under control of the keratin 14 promoter (509). Effects on cell survival are evident with LMP2A expression in the human keratinocyte cell line, HaCaT. LMP2A-expressing cells are hyperproliferative in raft cultures, differentiation is inhibited, and cloning efficiency in soft agar is substantially increased (737). Cells that grew in soft agar formed aggressive, poorly differentiated tumors in nude mice. PI3 kinase and AKT were activated in the LMP2A-expressing cells and tumors. Thus, in the appropriate cell type, LMP2A can have survival-enhancing effects.

EBERs

The EBV-encoded, small, nonpolyadenylated RNAs are by far the most abundant EBV RNAs in latently infected cells. Estimates of abundance place the EBERs at 10^4–10^5 copies per cell (32,340,343). EBER-1 is transcribed by RNA polymerases II and III, whereas EBER-2 is solely transcribed by RNA polymerase III (340–342). The EBERs localize to the cell nucleus, where they are complexed with the cellular proteins La and EBER-associated protein (EAP) (475,832,833). The EBER RNAs have stable secondary structures that persist in RNA La protein complexes (256). La protein is associated with the 3′ terminus of the EBER RNAs (256), whereas EAP is associated with the stem-loop 3 structure (832,833). Most of the EBER-1 is precipitable with antibody to EAP. EAP is L22 ribosomal and about half of the EAP in EBER-expressing cells is in EBER-1 ribonucleoprotein (RNP) particles in the nucleoplasm (831). The EBER RNPs are predominantly in the nucleoplasm. L22 is associated with chromosomal translocation in leukemia, raising the possibility L22 association with EBERs could be of functional significance. EBER-1 and -2 have extensive primary sequence similarity to adenovirus VA1 and VA2 and cell U6 small RNAs, both of which also form similar secondary structures and complex with La protein (256).

EBER-1 or -2, adenovirus VA, and U6 cell RNAs may have similar primary sequences, secondary structures, and association with La protein in order to accomplish similar functions. Based on the known functions of VA and U6 RNAs, two alternative roles have been proposed for the EBERs. In adenovirus infection, VA1 RNA acts in the cytoplasm to directly inhibit activation of the interferon-induced protein kinase PKR, which would, in the absence of VAI RNA, phosphorylate protein synthesis initiation factor eIF-2 alpha and block translation (736). EBER-1 and -2, provided by transfection into cells or substituted in to the adenovirus genome, can partially complement the replication of adenovirus with null mutations in VA1 and -2 (53,54). EBER-1 can also inhibit PKR *in vitro*, at levels that are similar to VA1 RNA (116–119,747). Moreover, EBV-mediated growth transformation is sensitive to high levels of interferon, and the EBV Bam W latency 3 EBNA transcript can activate PKR, so a role for the EBERs in inhibiting PKR could be important (179). However, evidence that PKR is inhibited in latency 1, 2, or 3 infected cells has not been obtained.

Small nuclear RNAs have long been suspected to be involved in RNA splicing, partly because of base complementarity to splice sites. U6 RNA has been shown to be base-paired to U4 RNA in particles required for *in vitro* RNA splicing. Six of seven identical nucleotides to those through which U6 binds to U4 are in a single-strand loop in EBER-2 RNA (256).

EBV recombinants specifically deleted for the EBER genes have been compared with wild-type recombinants in primary B-lymphocyte infection (797). EBER-deleted virus was as able to initiate primary B-lymphocyte infection and growth transformation as wild-type virus. No difference could be found in the growth of LCLs infected with EBER-deleted or control virus or in the permissivity of these cells for lytic virus infection following induction.

To further evaluate the hypothesis that the EBERs could have an antiinterferon effect, the effect of the EBERs on the replication of an interferon-sensitive virus in EBV-transformed human B lymphocytes was determined (796). Replication of vesicular stomatitis virus (VSV) in human lymphocytes is sensitive to interferon. However, interferon had a similar inhibitory effect on VSV replication in LCLs infected with EBER-deleted or wild-type virus (796). Further, lytic wild-type EBV replication could not be inhibited by high levels of interferon, and replication in cells infected with EBER-deleted virus was not more sensitive to interferon. Moreover, EBER-deleted virus was not more sensitive to the antitransforming effects of interferon (796). Once established as LCLs, neither EBER-deleted nor wild-type EBV–infected LCLs were sensitive to potential antiproliferative effects of interferon. Thus, the role of the EBERs in EBV infection is not obvious from studies in B lymphocytes *in vitro* and may emerge from testing of the mutants in other cell types or in an *in vivo* model.

Recent data indicate that EBER expression may increase the tumorigenicity of BL cells or non-EBV-infected nasopharyngeal carcinoma cells, in which EBERs have been specifically expressed (440,441,818). Surprisingly, EBER expression in Akata BL cells resulted in increased Bcl-2 levels (440).

Other Viral Gene Products Expressed in Latent EBV Infection: BARF0, RPMS1, A73, and BHRF1

Complementary-strand Bam A rightward transcripts, also known as CSTs, BARTs, or BARF0 RNAs, are differentially spliced RNAs that were identified in the cloning of cDNAs from RNA of latently infected nasopharyngeal carcinoma cells grown in nude mice (98,251,334,399,716, 766). CSTs have also been identified in latently infected BL cells (75,766), latently infected lymphocytes from human peripheral blood or marmoset tumors (97,922), and early primary infection of B cells *in vitro* (75) and LCLs (75,766). These RNAs initiate at n 150645 in the B95 sequence (36,716,766). Transfection of EBV DNA sequences corresponding to n 150199–151283 results in expression of the first exon in HeLa cells (766). Three ORFs in the differentially spliced CSTs may encode protein in latently infected cells, BARF0, RPMS1, and A73. BARF0 is potentially encoded in the most 3′ ORF of the CSTs. Humans have antibody to the 173-amino-acid BARF0 polypeptide, consistent with its expression at some point in EBV infection (251). Two differentially spliced forms of BARF0 are described, BARF0 and the further spliced ORF, RK-BARF0 (234,421). Both are encoded by CST exon 7 (766). RK-BARF0 has a signal peptide sequence and interacts with the Notch4 ligand binding domain in yeast two-hybrid, coimmunoprecipitation, and confocal microscopy assays (452). RK-BARF0 expression can induce translocation of part of Notch4 to the nucleus and can turn on LMP1 expression in latency 1 infected BL cells.

RPMS1 is encoded in an ORF formed by the fourth exon and components of the fifth exon of some CSTs, includes a WWP motif similar to EBNA-2, interacts with RBP-Jk amino acids 310 to 500 in yeast two-hybrid assays, and blocks EBNA-2 transactivation of a promoter with a multimerized upstream RBP-Jk site (766). Expression of RPMS1 alone does not up- or down-regulate promoters. Thus, RK-BARF0 can potentially up-regulate promoters with upstream RBP-Jk sites, and RPMS1 would modulate that activity.

The third potential CST ORF, A73, is formed by components of exons 6 and 7 (766). A73 is expressed as a cytoplasmic protein that can interact with the cell RACK1 protein in yeast two-hybrid assays, and it can associate with a small fraction of RACK1 in 293 cells. A73 could potentially affect RACK1 modulation of PKC or src tyrosine kinase signaling.

Although the CSTs are likely to be important in latent EBV infections, infections of primary B lymphocytes with EBV recombinants that are deleted for the DNA that encodes the CSTs efficiently results in LCLs that can be readily expanded *in vitro* (412,691,694). Thus, at this first level of analysis, CSTs are not critical for EBV transformation of primary B lymphocytes *in vitro* or for LCL outgrowth or survival.

Some EBNA-type Bam W transcripts from various latently infected cells include BHRF1 at their 3′ end (34,721). BHRF1 is expressed at high levels early in lytic infection, it is a bcl-2 homolog, and it has antiapoptotic effects (320,339,641). These antiapoptotic effects are likely to be quite important for efficient lytic infection in most cell types. Expression at even a low level in latent infection could be of significance. However, searches for the protein in latently infected cells using polyclonal or monoclonal antibodies that readily detect the protein in lytically infected cells fail to detect BHRF1 in LCLs or type 3 latently infected BL cells (641). BHRF1 protein has been detected transiently after refeeding growth-arrested Raji cells but not in similarly treated LCLs (G. Pearson, personal communication).

Consistent with the failure to detect BHRF1 protein expression in latently infected LCLs and the abundant expression of antiapoptotic Bcl-2 family proteins in these cells (82,321,775), EBV recombinants with a nonsense mutation or deletion of the BHRF1 ORF are fully competent for the transformation of primary B lymphocytes into actively growing LCLs (471,530). Mutant recombinant virus replicated in LCLs could be recovered from these cells, and it transformed primary B lymphocytes with efficiencies similar to wild-type virus. BHRF1 is therefore not critical for outgrowth or survival of latency 3 infected LCLs or for EBV replication in such cells.

Role of Latency 3 Infection Proteins in LCL Outgrowth and Survival

EBV-transformed primary B lymphocytes are nearly indistinguishable from B lymphocytes proliferating in response to polyvalent antigen and T-cell help or IL4, IL10, and CD40 in their growth and display of molecular markers of adhesion, activation, and differentiation (23, 24,42,85,263,337,363,585,635,661,688,824,825,829,913). The growth and survival of LCLs is highly dependent on autocrine and paracrine signalling mediated by IL5, IL6, IL10, TNF-beta, and transforming growth factor (TGF) (19,48,79,165,168,183,186,197,263,330,345,436,445,544, 584,599,638,639,705,728,729,778,812,829,845,846,859). The major characteristics that distinguish LCLs from B lymphocytes proliferating in response to polyvalent antigen and T-cell help are the expression of EBV latency 3–associated genes, immortality, and autonomy. For heuristic purposes, two hypotheses are considered here and in Chapter 75 in *Fields Virology*, 4th ed. First, the unique set of genes that LCVs use to cause LCL outgrowth evolved to enable these viruses to rapidly expand the number of latently infected B lymphocytes in the course of primary infection and to periodically reexpand that pool to further the persistence of virus infection *in vivo*. Second, the principal constraint in evolution of these genes is that they use normal B-cell growth pathways and leave the cell susceptible to checkpoint controls, external regulatory signals, and immune surveillance, so as to minimally damage the host. LCVs encode EBNAs to constitutively activate and regulate transcription from Notch- and PU.1-responsive promoters in cell DNA, including the c-*myc*, c-*fgr*, CD21, and CD23 promoters. EBV regulation of c-*myc* is significantly more akin to c-*myc* regulation by B-cell growth stimulatory processes. Constitutive c-*myc* expression in an LCL radically alters the cell phenotype (135,508,657). Constitutive c-*myc* expression in LCLs negatively regulates endogenous c-*myc*, alters adhesion and activation molecule expression so that the cells have the characteristics of a BL cell, increases susceptibility to NK cell cytotoxicity, and increases tumorigenesis in nude mice.

EBV has evolved EBNA-2 responsive cis-acting transcriptional regulatory sequences that bind RBP-Jk and PU.1 to autoregulate EBNA and LMP transcription from the viral genome. LMP1 constitutively activates the TNFR/CD40 downstream signalling pathways to costimulate cell growth and survival through NF-κB, junk, and p38 map kinase activation. These two pathways are depicted in Figure 10. *In vivo*, EBV regulation of LCL growth can be overridden by the microenvironment of infected cells: simply resuspension of the dispersed cells in dilute culture medium stops growth for weeks until the medium is adequately conditioned. Some of the mechanism by which the normal cell and the EBV-transformed cell regulate progress through the cell cycle, maintain telomeres through multiple rounds of expansion, and escape programmed cell death are unclear and present substantial future challenges in this area of EBV investigation. A substantial body of genetic and biochemical data described in this chapter and in the references indicate that the EBV latency-associated genes do not inactivate normal cell checkpoint controls such as Rb or p53 (18,89,366). EBNAs and LMPs do have "transforming effects." EBNA-2, expressed under control of the SV40 promoter and enhancer in transgenic mice, caused islands of kidney tubular hyperplasia at 20 weeks in all animals (843). At 50 weeks, multiple foci of microscopic renal tubular adenocarcinomas were evident; eventually, 90% of the transgenic mice has renal tubular adenocarcino-

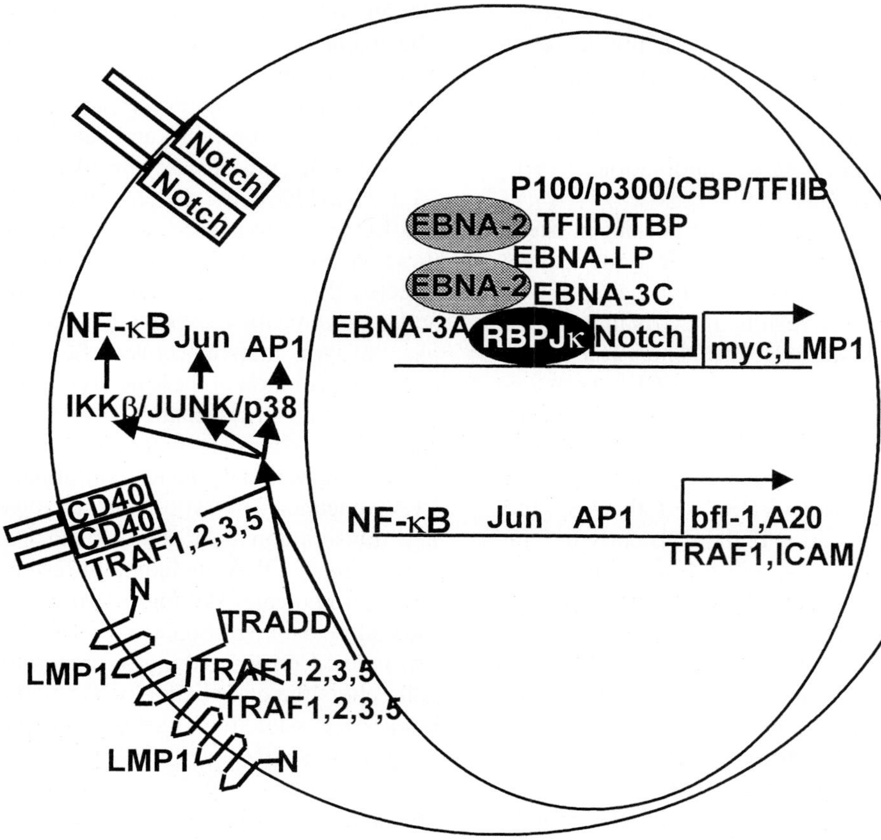

FIG. 10. Schematic diagram of the biochemical mechanisms by which EBNA-2, -LP, -3A, and -3C and LMP1 collaborate to induce primary B-lymphocyte growth transformation and survival. EBNA-2, -LP, -3A, and -3C use the nuclear anchor for Notch signaling and the B-cell Ets family protein PU.1 to constitutively up-regulate cellular and viral promoters including the *c-myc* promoter, the LMP1 promoter, and the EBNA promoter. LMP1 constitutively activates TNFR-associated factor signalling, inducing NF-κB, Jun/Fos, and AP-1.

mas. *In vitro*, EBNA-2 lowers the serum dependence of Rat-1 cells (148). EBNA-2 also exerts strong activating effects on genes that are regulated by Notch: Constitutive Notch activation in T cells induces leukemia (185,640). Moreover, EBNA-2 is involved in up-regulation of c-*myc* in LCLs (394). However, EBNA-2 has not been reported to have SV40 virus–like T antigen, or adenovirus-like E1A effects in collaborating with activated Ras in primary rodent cell immortalization. As described earlier, LMP1 has multiple activated Ras–like effects on immortalized rodent fibroblast cell lines, and transgenic LMP1 expression in mice results in increased incidence of lymphoma. LMP1 is not reported to substitute for activated Ras in complementing T or E1A in primary rodent fibroblast transformation. EBNA-1 has had a c-*myc*-like effect in inducing lymphomas in transgenic mice (884). However, the one lineage with this robust effect on lymphoma incidence did not express EBNA-1 in the transgenic normal lymphocytes. Only one study ascribed an E1A-like effect to one of the EBNAs in primary rat fibroblast immortalization experiments (633). The potential basis for the latter effect has not as yet emerged from intensive investigation of EBNA-3C.

Persistence of EBV DNA in Latently Infected Cells

The circularization of linear input EBV DNA in the nuclei of acutely infected lymphocytes requires 12 to 24 hours (12,362). Cells do not enter S phase until all of the EBNAs and LMPs are expressed. Stable latently infected proliferating lymphocytes characteristically contain multiple copies of EBV episomes (3,400,496,616,786,809). Most LCLs have about 10 episomes per cell. The range of episome copy number in BL cells is greater. Raji cells have 50 episomes per cell and the number has been stable over 30 years in culture (2,26). EBV episomes are replicated early in S phase by cell DNA polymerase (2,283,293). The initial amplification of circular EBV DNA is at the start of latent infection and requires early S phase DNA synthesis, as prior to S phase each infected cell has only one episome (12,786).

Although EBV DNA usually persists in cells as an episome, the EBV genome can also integrate into chromosomal DNA, and both integrated and episomal DNA coexist in some cells (159,282,318,361,393,467,543, 889). In one EBV-infected human Burkitt tumor cell line, EBV DNA has persisted by integrating on chromosome one at IP35 (318,467). The entire EBV genome is integrated into A-T-rich cell DNA through the EBV TR (543). More than 15 kb of cell DNA were deleted by the integration of the 170-kb complete EBV genome. The entire block of cell DNA with the integrated EBV genome has then been duplicated as an inverted DNA domain (467). Another example is a latently infected fetal human LCL that contains an EBV genome integrated at chromosome 4q25 (318,543). In this instance, integration appears to be through a site within U1 (315,318), and there are several EBV genomes integrated in tandem (362). In the first instance, integration through TR favors the hypothesis that integration occurred prior to circularization; however, in the second instance, integration through U1 and the finding of tandem repeats of the EBV genome are more consistent with the hypothesis that integration occurred after initial circularization. Integration occurs frequently when BL cells are infected with EBV *in vitro* and extensively passaged (361). In contrast, infection of BL cells with EBV and selection for cells infected with virus almost always results in cell lines that contain episomal EBV DNA (527–529,869). The genome persists as an episome in such cell lines for at least 1 year. Clearly, integration is not a regular feature of EBV infection or EBV induced cell growth transformation. However, because LMP2 is the only EBV gene that spans the TR, and LMP2 is not required for cell transformation, EBV may be able to transform cells with the genome persisting solely as integrated DNA.

Episomal DNA is likely to be necessary for lytic cycle EBV DNA replication, because lytic herpesvirus DNA replication characteristically proceeds from a circular DNA intermediate (for review, see Chapter 33). Circular EBV DNA copy number increases in lytic infection (747a). Lytic EBV replication has not been observed in cells that contain only integrated EBV DNA, and virus has not been recovered from such cells in response to known inducers of virus replication.

In the establishment of latent infection, the EBV genome undergoes progressive methylation (203,347, 374,429,458,459,478,540,577,615,650,695,718,801,813, 814) and associates with chromosomal proteins so as to give a nucleosomal pattern after micrococcal nuclease digestion (176,654,744,747b). Regulatory domains involved in maintaining latent infection such as oriP tend to be undermethylated in latently infected cells relative to DNA that is expressed only in lytic infection (196,203, 205,347,374,546,575,576,615,695). Extensive methylation of lytic genes and their regulatory elements probably helps to maintain latency by inhibiting lytic gene expression. Treatment of latently infected cells with drugs that reduce DNA methylation increases the frequency of spontaneous activation to lytic infection (51,540,696).

Induction of Lytic Infection

Lytic EBV infection is usually studied by inducing latently infected BL cells to become permissive for lytic virus replication (51,350,516,680,717,933). Various induction strategies give characteristic, although not precisely reproducible, levels of permissivity for each latently infected B cell line. Autocrine TGF-beta may participate in lytic reactivation, as antibody to TGF-beta reduces the responsiveness of cells to lytic induction (168). Phorbol esters are among the most reproducible and most broadly applicable inducers. The effect is probably mediated by PKC activation of *jun-fos* interaction with AP-1 sites upstream of the immediate-early virus genes (28,139,210,211,218,219,221–224,464,473,486, 817). The rapidity of activation of immediate-early EBV genes by phorbol ester is most consistent with the activation of a preexisting transcriptional coactivator of lytic cycle gene expression, or with inactivation of an active repressor of lytic infection. PKC does activate BZLF1 itself, and the effect of PKC could be to increase background activity of the BZLF1 promoter through autostimulation (47). Among latently infected LCLs, marmoset LCLs tend to be more inducible than adult human lymphoblasts, and neonatal human lymphoblasts are least inducible for virus replication (558,561,562,566, 567, and for review see ref. 556). A few cell lines can be consistently induced to permit lytic virus replication in 10% of the cells (333,567,802,803). One cell line, Akata, can be induced to 20% to 50% lytic infection by cross-linking sIg; it is currently the best source for large quantities of EBV (803). SIg cross-linking activates phospholipase-C-gamma. Phospholipase-C-gamma releases IP3 and diacylglycerol, which mobilize calcium from intracellular stores and activate PKC. Treatment of cells with calcium ionophore and phorbol ester induces a rise in intracellular free calcium and activates PKC but is only a partial surrogate for sIg cross-linking, compatible with the possibility that other pathways activated by sIg cross-linking may have a role in the induction of lytic infection in Akata cells (95,136,137,139,257,505,507,748,772). Several elements upstream of the BZLF1 promoter seem to mediate the sIg response: Sp1, Sp3, myocyte enhancer factor 2D, ATF-1, and ATF-2 (505). The ATF-1 and ATF-2 binding sites correspond to a site that is regulated in part by CAM kinase IV (95). The initial activation of Z may be dependent on two 7-bp dyad symmetry elements separated by 27 bp. These sequences are similar to a reversible YY1-dependent silencing element in adeno-associated virus and may contribute to the lack of Z expression during latency (583). Other negative regulatory elements are more upstream from the transcriptional initiation site (739). Changes in the BZLF1 promoter histone acetylation appear to be critical for BZLF1 activation (380).

The responsiveness of Akata cells to sIg cross-linking is due in part to stable latency 1 infection. The absence of LMP2A enables sIg cross-linking induced signal transduction and induction of lytic EBV infection. In latency 3–infected lymphocytes where LMP2A is expressed, calcium ionophore and TPA can be used to induce virus replication (554). An alternative strategy is to use cells infected with EBV recombinants with specific null mutations in the LMP2A gene (551,554).

A second approach to studying virus replication is to induce lytic replication by superinfection of Raji cells with the P3HR-1 EBV (55,597,670). Raji is an EBV-infected Burkitt tumor–derived cell line that has an unusually high EBV episome copy number and is responsive to this type of induction. The endogenous Raji genome has at least two deletions and is defective for EBV DNA replication and late gene expression (301, 656). Thus, EBV late genes are expressed in Raji cells only after superinfection. The P3HR-1 virus is efficient in inducing lytic infection in Raji because of defective virus genomes in most noncloned P3HR-1 cell cultures (129,311,559,564,701). An abundant class of defective virions from noncloned P3HR-1 cells has rearranged EBV DNA molecules in which the Z or R and Z immediate-early transactivator(s) are downstream of the latent infection cycle IR1 EBNA gene promoter and are, therefore, expressed in latently infected cell lines following superinfection (110,311,381–383,564,677,678). The induction of productive infection following high multiplicity superinfection is more rapid and synchronous than following chemical induction. Maximal late virus protein expression and enveloped virus release requires 48 to 96 hours.

Following induction, cells that have become permissive for virus replication undergo cytopathic changes characteristic of herpesviruses, including margination of nuclear chromatin (406), inhibition of host macromolecular synthesis, replication of viral DNA at the center of the nucleus, assembly of nucleocapsids at the nuclear periphery, nucleation of nucleocapsids, and envelopment of virus by budding through the inner nuclear membrane (158,247,261,262,631,727). Virus gene expression follows a temporal and sequential order (for review, see refs. 209 and 803). Some virus mRNAs are expressed early after induction despite the inhibition of new protein synthesis. These RNAs are classified as immediate-early (630). Most early lytic virus genes that are expressed before the onset of virus DNA replication are dependent on the immediate-early BZLF1 or BRLF1 protein transcription factors for their expression. Genes are formally classified as early if their expression is not affected by inhibition of viral DNA synthesis. Late proteins are expressed temporally later but are formally categorized as late based on the marked reduction in their mRNA abundance in the presence of viral DNA synthesis inhibitors.

Immediate-Early Genes and Their Targets

In typical herpesvirus infection, immediate-early genes are defined by their transcription following infection in the presence of inhibitors of protein synthesis (for review, see Chapter 33). Characteristically, a virion tegument protein contributes to the activation of immediate-early gene expression. *In vivo*, EBV replicates in epithelial cells of the oropharynx before infecting B lymphocytes. Infection of epithelial cells lines *in vitro* is not efficient, and studies of the biochemical events of synchronous lytic infection in permissive epithelial cell cultures has not been feasible. Only B lymphocytes can be efficiently infected by EBV, and the outcome of infection is nonpermissivity for virus replication and the expression of the EBNA-2 and EBNA-LP mRNAs. EBNA-2 and -LP are likely to be immediate-early gene products in primary B lymphocytes, given the constitutive activity of the Wp EBNA promoter and the indications that EBNA-LP and -2 are the first EBV mRNAs expressed in these cells, but independence of transcription from new protein synthesis has not been demonstrated. Similarly, the constitutive activity of the Bam Q EBNA-1 promoter in BL cells (718) and the early expression of EBNA-1 mRNA in infected BL cells may be in the mode of an immediate-early gene.

Because synchronous lytic EBV infection *in vitro* can be studied only by induction of permissivity in cells that are already latently infected, the definition of immediate-early lytic infection–associated gene expression must be modified to acknowledge the potential direct or indirect effects of EBV latent infection genes on transcription from the activated EBV genome or the potential effect of the induction strategy on the transcription of specific EBV genes. Moreover, chemical induction may fail to activate an immediate-early gene whose transcription in lymphocytes or primary epithelial cells depends on a virion trans-acting factor. Thus, our current definition of BZLF1 and BRLF1 as the principal immediate-early viral genes may be incomplete.

P3HR-1 superinfection of Raji cells and inhibition of protein synthesis with anisomycin results in accumulation of 1-kb BZLF1, 2.8-kb BRLF1, and 4.1-kb BI′LF4 mRNAs (55). Induction of lytic infection in Akata cells by sIg cross-linking and incubation of the cells in the presence of moderately high concentrations of cycloheximide (50 μg/mL) results in relatively abundant expression of the 1-kb BZLF1 and 2.8-kb BRLF1 mRNAs, confirming that these are immediate-early gene products (803). Cycloheximide resistant 1.6- and 4.1-kb mRNAs from Bam M and A, respectively, are also expressed in induced Akata cells, but these mRNAs are much less abundant in cycloheximide-treated cells than in non-treated cells. In the absence of cycloheximide, the Bam M and A mRNAs are most abundant from 4 to 12 hours after induction, whereas the BZLF1 and BRLF1 mRNAs are expressed earlier. Thus, the M and A mRNAs appear to be early but not immediate-early genes. The Bam A mRNA is encoded by BALF2, which is the EBV homolog of HSV-1 ICP8. ICP8 is also expressed very early in HSV infection and is less sensitive to viral protein synthesis inhibition than other early virus genes. Another immediate-early gene is encoded from the BI′LF4 ORF (533).

The first evidence that BZLF1- and BRLF1-encoded proteins are key transactivators of lytic EBV gene expression (Fig. 11) came from the discovery that highly defective P3HR-1 virus preparations that induce lytic infection in EBV-infected BL cells express BZLF1, or BZLF1 and BRLF1, under control of the Wp promoter (381–383,557, 564). BZLF1 expression from heterologous vectors broadly activates lytic infection (272,381–383). BZLF1 and BRLF1 coordinately up-regulate expression from early EBV promoters (96,105,106). BI′LF4 also has transactivating effects, although these effects are restricted to specific types (533). Consistent with these *in vitro* observations, BZLF1 is expressed in advancing margins of lytic EBV infection in oropharyngeal epithelia (919).

Two key early promoter regulatory elements within D_L and D_R (duplication, left and right) are coordinately up-regulated by the BZLF1- and BRLF1-encoded proteins. D_L and D_R encode abundant early mRNAs (149,232, 351,357,620,621) and include the origins for lytic viral DNA replication within their promoter upstream regulatory domains (291). BZLF1 and BRLF1 synergistically up-regulate the bidirectional BHLF1 and BHRF1 D_L promoters in transient transfection assays (96,105,106,131). Promoter activation has a strong positive effect on DNA

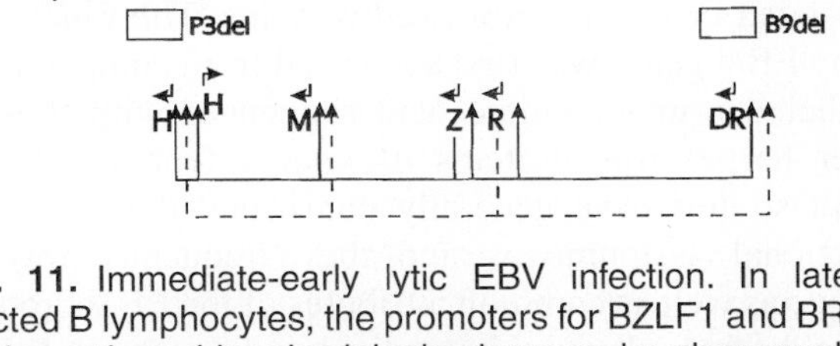

FIG. 11. Immediate-early lytic EBV infection. In latently infected B lymphocytes, the promoters for BZLF1 and BRLF1 can be activated by physiologic changes, by pharmacologic treatment, or by heterologous Z overexpression. In newly infected epithelial cells, the BZLF1 and BRLF1 promoters are presumed to be activated by virion-associated transactivators. BZLF1 and BRLF1 are transcribed, translated, and localized to the nucleus, where they coordinately further up-regulate their promoters and turn early genes, including BHLF1, BHRF1, D_R, BSMLF1, and BALF2 (not shown).

synthesis from the neighboring D_L origin. The cis-acting domains of D_R and D_L have been partially dissected and have many similarities including multiple BZLF1 binding sites (96,105,106,297,486,735). The promoter proximal domain (−79 to −221 bp relative to BHLF1) confers strong promoter activity in HeLa or Vero cells only when BZLF1 is provided in trans (736). ZBP-89 and Sp1 bind synergistically to a site near the promoter, stimulate transcription, and interact with the viral DNA polymerase and processivity factor (46). PKC phosphorylation of BZLF1 S186 increases BZLF1 transactivation and DNA replication effects (47). A DNA segment 639 bp upstream of the BHLF1 cap site is a position- and orientation-independent enhancer composed of one component with constitutive activity in fibroblasts or epithelial lines but not in B lymphocytes, and a second component, TTGTCC-CGTGGACAATGTCC, which is responsive to the BRLF1 transactivator. Although BZLF1 interaction with this site has negligible effects on transcription from the BHRF1 promoter, BRLF1 activates transcription and BZLF1 strongly up-regulates transcription with BRLF1 (131). Regulation of the D_R element appears to be different, in that BZLF1 does not strongly up-regulate the BZRF1 effects on D_R (279).

The BSMLF1 and BMRF1 promoters are also coordinately regulated by BZLF1 and BRLF1 (336,672). Direct BRLF1 binding to the BMRF1 promoter upstream DNA is essential for BMRF1 coordinate up-regulation by the BZLF1 and BRLF1 transactivators (672). BRLF1 transactivation of the BSMLF1 early promoter is also mediated by activation of an upstream sequence CCGTGGA-GAATGTC similar to the activation sequence in BHLF1 (277,413). *In vitro* translated R binds directly to this R response elements by interacting with two sequences cat-GTCCCtctatcatGGCGCagac within the element that are close to an optimal R binding site (277,278,280). The BZLF1 protein interacts with a TPA response element upstream of the BSMLF1 promoter (506).

The BZLF1 protein interacts with NF-κB, p53, and virion proteins (285,338,925). NF-κB interaction inhibits the transactivating effects of BZLF1. Similarly, the BZLF1 coiled-coil dimerization domain interacts with the carboxyl-terminal portion of p53, the two proteins associate *in vivo*, and both proteins are transcriptionally inactivated by the association. BZLF1-mediated inhibition of p53 could be important in preventing p53-induced apoptosis in response to lytic EBV DNA replication. Later in lytic infection, BZLF1 becomes associated with virion structural proteins; BZLF1 has not been detected in virus (404). The interaction of BZLF1 with NF-κB, p53, and virion structural proteins could down-modulate BZLF1 activity late in infection so as to minimize the toxic effects of high-level BZLF1 expression.

A minor immediate-early RNA encodes an unusual spliced product of the BRLF1 and BZLF1 bi-cistronic transcript that could also down-modulate BZLF1 activity

(239,742). This RNA has the beginning of the BRLF1 ORF spliced in-frame to the DNA binding and dimerization domains of BZLF1. Because the BRLF1 activation domain is at the C-terminus and the BZLF1 activation domain is at the N-terminus, the spliced product lacks an activation domain and when dimerized with Z, it represses Z activity (239).

BZLF1 can down-regulate the EBNA Cp promoter, perhaps facilitating the transition from latent to lytic infection (415,754). The action of BZLF1 on Cp appears to be indirect, involving the up-regulation of *fos* by BZLF1 and the down-modulation of the positive effect of a glucocorticoid response element, which maps about 1 kbp upstream of Cp (450,754,757). Glucocorticoid withdrawal from culture media increases permissivity for replication, indicative of a mutual antagonism between Cp function and lytic reactivation. The Cp promoter may antagonize lytic infection, in part because Cp transcription is antisense to BZLF1 and BRLF2 transcription.

BZLF1 probably autoregulates its own promoter and the BRLF1 promoter (218). The Z promoter has several AP1-like upstream elements that mediate activation in the presence of low levels of Z and repression in the presence of high levels of Z. Differential Z binding to the various upstream sites could be mediated by changes in Z abundance during lytic infection.

BZLF1 mRNA is composed from three exons, each encoding a separate functional domain (215,485). The first exon encodes amino acids 1 to 167, which constitute a transactivating domain when fused to a Gal-4 DNA binding domain (107,218,483,560). The activating domain can recruit TAFs and stabilize TFIID association with TATA elements through protein–protein interactions (483,484,488). Replacement of the BZLF1-activating domain with the VP16 acidic domain results in enhanced transactivation of early promoters (48). The second exon encodes amino acids 168 to 202, a sequence that includes a strongly basic domain with homology to a conserved region of the c-*fos* and c-*jun* family of transcriptional modulators (211). This domain confers the ability to interact with AP1-related sites in DNA (94,220, 482,483,485,486) and also targets Z to the nucleus (550). A BZLF1 intron also has homology to the 3′ untranslated c-*fos* sequences, suggesting that BZLF1 relatively recently evolved from c-*fos* (211). The third exon encodes for amino acids 203 to 245, a sequence that includes a near-perfect leucine and isoleucine heptad repeat capable of coiled-coil dimer formation (94,211,219,220,443, 483). Like c-*fos*, BZLF1 is a dimerizing DNA binding protein that binds directly to AP1-related sequences (211, 220,222–224,483,485,486). Dimerization may facilitate high affinity interaction with templates having two or more Z binding sites (92).

BZLF1 is multiply phosphorylated by casein kinase II, PKA, and PKC on serines 173, 186, and 336 (47,136, 439). The phosphorylation regulates DNA binding activity and transcriptional activating effects. Phosphorylation of S186 in response to PKC activation stimulates transcription but decreases affinity for cognate DNA (47).

The R transactivator is also a DNA sequence-specific acidic transactivator and has distant homology to c-*myb* (280,521,522). C-*myb* can interact synergistically with Z in transactivating the BMRF1 promoter in lymphocytes (414). Two domains of R when fused to the Gal-4 DNA binding domain have transactivating activity for Gal-4 response elements upstream of basal promoters (297,298). Amino acids 416 to 519 are weakly activating and are required only for activation in B lymphocytes, whereas the carboxyl-terminal amino acids 520 to 605 are a potent acidic transactivating domain similar to VP16.

Early Lytic Infection

EBV early replicative cycle genes are operationally differentiated from late genes by their persistent transcription in the presence of inhibitors of viral DNA synthesis. By this criterion, at least 30 EBV mRNAs are early mRNAs, and almost 30 EBV mRNAs are late mRNAs (see Fig. 1) (36,43,55,56,209,210,249,250,301, 352–354,358). Early and late mRNAs are intermingled through most of the EBV genome. Frequently, different promoters initiate nested transcripts, which begin with different ORFs and terminate at the same polyadenylation site, so that the longer mRNAs include all of the shorter mRNAs; the primary reading frames of the shorter mRNAs are 3′ to the primary reading frame in the longer mRNAs and are likely to remain untranslated or inefficiently translated in this context. Some early and late genes are spliced, and others are not. Minor spliced mRNA species have frequently been discerned when genes have been studied in detail.

Because of the difficulty of doing genetic studies of EBV, proteins encoded by EBV early or late genes have usually been identified and assigned functions from predictions based on the ORF sequence, from the temporal class and abundance of the RNA or the size of its *in vitro* translation products, or from functional assays of *in vitro* translated or *in vivo* expressed proteins. The function of many EBV genes was first suggested from comparison of predicted primary amino acid sequences with those of other herpesvirus proteins of known function. Subsequent studies have generally confirmed these tentative functional assignments, and they frequently revealed unique as well as common attributes of the EBV proteins.

Aside from the two immediate-early proteins BZLF1 and BRLF1, the EBV early proteins BSMLF1 and BMRF1 may also transactivate expression of other early EBV genes. Both are moderately abundant early nuclear proteins (113,114). BMRF1 activity has been demonstrated only by co-transfection with SV40 promoter driven by chloramphenicol acetyl transferase reporter gene

DNA into BHK cells (624). BSMLF1 is a promiscuous transactivator of gene expression that acts synergistically with BZLF1 or BRLF1 in inducing higher-level expression in transient expression assays (413,415,416,487,624, 890). The level of CAT reporter gene mRNA does not increase in cells co-transfected with BSMLF1-expressing plasmids (417). BSMLF1 does not effect increased transcription in nuclear on assays (72,713). Instead, BSMLF1 increases cytoplasmic transport of unspliced mRNAs, and this accounts for the promiscuity of its effects in transactivation (72,713). Both cytoplasmic transport and promiscuous transactivation depend on BSMLF1 association with CRM1.

Two other EBV early proteins are quite abundant. One encodes the 135-kd BALF2 protein (357). This protein has primary amino acid sequence homology to the major HSV DNA binding protein ICP8, and it is important in DNA replication (217). A second RNA that is less abundant encodes BHRF1 (34,641). BHRF1 encodes an 18-kd protein that consists of a predicted hydrophobic signal peptide, a 135-amino-acid hydrophilic domain that contains two potential N-linked glycosylation sites, a hydrophobic potential transmembrane domain, and a short carboxyl-terminal cytoplasmic domain. BHRF1 has extensive colinear homology with *bcl-2*, a cell gene activated by the chromosome 14/18 translocation in human follicular B-cell lymphomas (120). Immunofluorescent microscopy with specific sera reveals nuclear membrane and cytoplasmic localization compatible with endoplasmic reticulum or mitochondrial residence (641). *Bcl-2* is important in lymphocyte survival because of its role in stabilizing mitochondrial membrane potential and preventing apoptotic death, and BHRF1 appears to have similar effects in preventing apoptotic cell death in lytic EBV infection (320). The effects of BHRF1 are evident with lytic replication of EBV in type 1 latency–infected BL cells, but they are not evident when lytic commences in type III latency–infected LCLs because of their high-level expression of other antiapoptotic proteins (82). EBV recombinants with a stop codon early in BHRF1, or with deletions of the BHRF1 ORF, are fully able to initiate or maintain cell growth transformation, enter lytic cycle, and produce virus even in media with low serum or low cell concentration (471,530). BHRF1 is expected to have a similar role in epithelial infection. EBV BALF1 also has significant homology to *bcl-2* and is likely to have similar antiapoptotic effects (535).

Among the EBV early genes identified by their homology to early genes of other herpesviruses are several that are linked to DNA replication. These include DNA polymerase (BALF5), major DNA binding protein (BALF2), ribonucleotide reductase (BORF2 and BARF1), thymidine kinase (BXLF1), and alkaline exonuclease (BGLF5). These genes are distributed through the long EBV U_L domain (see Fig. 1).

The EBV DNA polymerase has been extensively purified and is 117 kd (396). Partially purified DNA polymerase is associated with several other EBV nuclear proteins, including the 50-kd protein encoded by BMRF1 (420,481). The catalytic subunit expressed in insect cells from a baculovirus vector has 3′-to-5′ proofreading exonuclease activity in addition to DNA polymerase activity (851). Reconstitution of baculovirus-expressed polymerase with a 2:1 molar ratio of baculovirus-expressed BMRF1 enhances the double-strand 3′-to-5′ exonuclease activity fourfold (849) and the DNA polymerase activity tenfold (848). BMRF1 also markedly enhances polymerase processivity and results in full-length products (848). Unlike cellular polymerases, the EBV polymerase is active in 100mM ammonium sulfate or in KCl and is sensitive to inhibition by ethyl maleimide, phosphonoacetic acid, phosphonoformic acid, arabinofuranosylthymine, and acycloguanosine triphosphate (14,102,108, 121,143–149,151–153,275,344–346,348,625–627,786). The EBV DNA polymerase also differs from HSV DNA polymerase in its salt sensitivity and its relative resistance to amphidicolin. The EBV DNA polymerase only weakly distinguishes between 2-amino-purine nucleoside triphosphate and dATP, so that 2-amino-purine is preferentially incorporated into viral as opposed to cell DNA (273).

The EBV, VZV, and HSV ribonucleotide reductases are extensively colinearly homologous. The large HSV subunit is 140 kd, whereas the EBV subunit is 85 kd, and VZV is predicted to be 87 kd (250). The EBV, VZV, and HSV large and small subunits have domains that are common to ribonucleotide reductases from a wide variety of prokaryotic and eukaryotic species (90,606). The HSV-1 large subunit has an amino-terminal domain that is absent from other ribonucleotide reductases. Surprisingly, the EBV ribonucleotide reductase large subunit is confined to multiple discrete regions in the cytoplasm of productively infected cells (258). The large subunit is a delayed early protein that accumulates in cells approximately 4 hours after the MRF1 nuclear early protein (258,641). Acetone fixation of cells destroys the immunologic reactivity of the large subunit, suggesting that it may be a major component of the restricted early antigen complex originally identified by EBV immune human sera from African patients with BL (see Chapter 75 in *Fields Virology*, 4th ed.).

The existence of an EBV-specific deoxypyrimidine kinase was inferred from the co-induction of EBV lytic replication and a new kinase activity in P3HR-1 cells (157,777). An EBV-induced dTK and dCK activity elutes as a single peak on DEAE-cellulose, away from the cellular dTK and dCK activities. Gene transfer of EBV DNA, or of the EBV DNA fragment with homology to HSV TK, into TK-mammalian cells or into TK-*E. coli* restores TK activity mapping the kinase activity to this DNA fragment (502–504). The EBV TK is similar to HSV TK in accepting a broad range of nucleosides or nucleoside analogs as substrates and has some antigenic cross-reactivity with the HSV TK (503).

The D_L and D_R EBV DNA segments (see Fig. 1) that have strong early promoter activity are also origins of lytic infection viral DNA replication (290,730,734). Using transient transfection to activate lytic EBV replication co-transfection of either of these EBV DNA segments on plasmids results in replication of the plasmid DNAs in the lytically infected cells. An essential 1.4-kb core element replicates with considerably reduced efficiency (290). The core 1.4-kb origin has numerous inverted repeat elements that could serve as the definitive origin. Even within the 1.4-kb segment, at least three domains contribute to the replicative activity. One domain can be functionally replaced in part by the CMV immediate-early promoter and enhancer, suggesting that this domain is important for lytic origin function because of transcriptional enhancement (163). Interestingly, when cells containing lytic origin plasmids are induced to lytic EBV infection, plasmid copy number increases slightly and linear concatemers are produced. With induction of lytic EBV replication, episome copy number increases, and labeled thymidine, initially incorporated into circular EBV DNA, chases into very large, presumably linear concatemeric EBV DNA (115,757,762). Other LCVs have D_L and D_R elements; these are anticipated to have similar roles in DNA replication (313,314,316,474). The herpesvirus Papio element has transcriptional activation and DNA replication sites that are similar to those in EBV (714).

Considerable progress has been made in constituting an *in vitro* minimal replication system similar to the Challberg HSV system (217). The components include BALF5, which encodes the core DNA polymerase; BALF2, the single-strand DNA binding protein; BMRF1, the processivity factor; BSLF1 and BBLF4, the primase and helicase complex; BBLF2/3, a spliced primase helicase complex component; and BKRF3, the uracil DNA glycosylase. A surprising aspect of the EBV DNA replication genes is the extent to which they are dependent on expression of the BZLF1, BRLF1, and BSMLF1 transactivators. EBV DNA replication also requires topoisomerase 1 and 2 activity (407). The redistribution of BZLF1 and BMRF1 gene products to the same nuclear site may identify the site at which viral DNA is replicated (806).

Late Gene Expression, Cleavage, Packaging, Envelopment, and Egress

The EBV TR has obvious similarities to the HSV "a" sequence (543,580,767,769,770). Both EBV TR and the HSV "a" sequence are directly repeated at both ends of the DNA. Both sequences are high in G+C composition, with runs of three to five Cs. In both HSV and EBV, there is a short extra oligonucleotide segment (D_R1) where the repeat joins the unique DNA. The EBV D_R1 oligonucleotide GCATGGGGGG brackets the multiple TR copies (543,580). In HSV-1, D_R1 is the site of cleavage of head full-length DNA for packaging into virions (767,769,770). There seems to be little sequence specificity for D_R1, because the nonhomologous oligonucleotides of HSV-1, HSV-2, and CMV are interchangeable (770). HSV or CMV cleavage and packaging appear to occur 33 bases 3′ to a conserved sequence of $C(G)_{6-8}TGT(G/T)(T)_3NG(C/G)(G)_6(G/C)(T/C)$. A similar sequence $C(G)_5TGT(T)_2CCT(G)_5CC$ occurs 25 bases before the EBV D_R1 and is the key cleavage packaging recognition sequence for EBV. The EBV rightmost TR acquires a short unique sequence from the leftmost TR during cleavage and packaging, and that sequence becomes the left end of the DNA (932). Plasmids containing the EBV latent infection episome origin, the EBV lytic origin, and the EBV terminal repeat sequence are stably maintained as an episome in latently infected cells, are replicated into linear concatemers by EBV DNA polymerase when lytic infection is induced, and are cleaved and packaged into infectious virions (291,871). Cell lines have recently been derived that are infected with a TR-negative EBV that cannot itself be packaged, but they are suitable hosts to support the replication and packaging of plasmids that include oriLyt and EBV DNA termini .

The viral glycoprotein genes that have been identified so far are all late genes (50,208,262,310,359,451,454, 455,480,517,610,622,643,644,905). These have been more intensively studied than other late genes because of their potential importance in antibody-mediated immunity to virus infection (70,289,331,472,479,480,568, 581,631,776,875,876). Current knowledge of nonglycoprotein late genes is quite limited. Among the nonglycoprotein late genes, the major nucleocapsid protein is almost certainly encoded by BcLF1 based on homology to the major HSV capsid-protein gene (545). Further, BcLF1 encodes a 4.5-kb late mRNA that, translated *in vitro*, yields a 150-kd protein, identical in size to the major EBV nucleocapsid protein (357). Similarly, BNRF1 probably encodes a major 140-kd virion nonglycoprotein. The NRF1 4.1-kb late mRNA, translated *in vitro*, produces a 140-kd protein, identical in size to the virion component (357). Because the BNRF1 predicted sequence has no major hydrophobic domains or glycosylation sites, it is more likely to encode a tegument protein than an integral membrane protein. Another late RNA includes an ORF BXRF1 homologous to the VZV basic virion core protein gene (154,232).

The known (gp25) EBV glycoprotein genes are BLLF1 (gp350/220), BALF4 (gp110), BXLF2 (gp85), BKRF2, BZLF2 (gp42), BILF2 (gp55/80), BDLF3 (gp150), BLRF1 (gp15), BBRF3 (gp84/113), and BILF1 (gp64) (50,245,262,273,310,359,517,621). Other glycoproteins may be encoded by BFRF1 and BMRF2. BILF2 expressed from a recombinant vaccinia virus is 55 to 80 kd. A 78-kd glycoprotein has been identified in EBV lytically infected cells and in virus using antiserum from recombinant vaccinia virus–infected rabbits or EBV-immunized mice. The BILF2 glycoprotein corresponds to an abundant glycoprotein in purified virus preparations. Antibody to BILF2, however, fails to neutralize virus infectivity (517).

BDLF3 cDNA cloning and sequencing confirm that BDLF3 mRNA is not spliced (245). The predicted amino acid sequence includes a hydrophobic amino terminus, consistent with a signal peptide, a hydrophilic external domain with nine potential N-linked glycosylation sites, and a single hydrophobic transmembrane domain. Translation of the 0.9-kb mRNA *in vitro* yields a 32-kd protein that is processed by dog pancreas microsomes to 60 kd, and the size of the fully processed glycoprotein in EBV infected cell is 150 kd. Disruption of gp150 expression for the context of a specifically mutated EBV indicates that gp150 is not critically important for lymphocyte infection.

Because HSV-1 gB is a major virion and infected cell surface glycoprotein, the homologous EBV BALF4 ORF is of interest (187,262,642). Both BALF4 and HSV-1 gB are predicted from their primary amino acid sequence to have amino-terminal cleavable signal peptides, external domains of 650 amino acids with four potential N-linked glycosylation sites, three potential membrane-spanning domains, and a 150-amino-acid cytoplasmic domain (642). BALF4 encodes two late mRNAs: an abundant 3-kb RNA that is not spliced and a scarce 1.8-kb RNA (262). The BALF4-encoded 3-kb mRNA translates a 93-kd protein that is glycosylated to 110 kd (261,262). Gp110 is one of the most abundant late EBV proteins (187,261,262). The glycosylation is probably both N- and O-linked, because N-glycanase, which cleaves N-linked oligosaccharides, only reduces gp110 to 105 kd (261,262). Endoglycosidase H has a similar effect on almost all of the gp110. Because endoglycosidase H cleaves only N-linked oligosaccharides that have not been modified in the Golgi, this suggests that most of the gp110 is not Golgi processed. A small fraction of gp110 is processed to a form compatible with a size of 120 kd. This 120-kd glycoprotein is not endo-H sensitive and is partially incorporated into virus (Alfieri and Kieff, manuscript in preparation). The intracellular distribution of gp110 closely parallels that of an endoplasmic reticulum resident protein (261,262). Immune light or electron microscopy localizes gp110 to the inner and outer nuclear membranes and to cytoplasmic membranes frequently surrounding enveloped virus, but not to the Golgi or plasma membrane. Further, despite the high abundance of gp110 in the inner nuclear membrane through which nucleocapsids bud to acquire their initial envelope, only small amounts of gp110 are in enveloped extracellular virus, as seen by immune electron microscopy (261,262). Protein and sugar stains of polyacrylamide gel–separated proteins from purified virus confirms that gp110 is not a major virion glycoprotein. Thus, EBV gp110 is a very abundant glycoprotein in the nuclear and endoplasmic reticular membranes and may have a critical role in initial envelopment, but only a small amount of gp110 is in the definitive virion envelope.

In contrast to gp110, gp85 and gp350/220 are processed much more efficiently through the Golgi and are found on the virus and in the plasma membrane of lytically infected cells (50,172,173,261,262,309,310,335, 517,597,618,619,621,622,668–670,780,822,823,827).

Gp85 is encoded by XLF2, which has significant colinear homology to HSV-1 gH (310,622), whereas gp350/220 is encoded by LLF, which has only a small region of distant homology to HSV-1 gC (50). Gp85 is a relatively minor virus component, important in fusion of the virus and cell membranes (568), whereas gp350/220 is the dominant external virus glycoprotein that mediates virus binding to the B-lymphocyte receptor, CD21 (see preceding). Interestingly, gp85 expressed in NIH3T3 cells localizes to the internal cytoplasmic and nuclear membranes, whereas gp350/220 localizes to the Golgi and plasma membrane (262,881). In fact, gp85 requires another virus protein to bring it to the plasma membrane of lytically infected lymphocytes, where it is characteristically found, whereas gp350/220 possesses the necessary signals for efficient Golgi transport, processing, and plasma membrane insertion. Gp85 complexes with the BKRF2-encoded protein, which enables its transport to the plasma membrane (905). Two homologous glycoproteins, gH and gL, heterologomerize and have similar functions in HSV replication: EBV gp85 (gH) has a dual role both in fusion and in coreceptor recognition. A third glycoprotein, gp42 or BZLF2, is a component of gH–gL complexes. BZLF2 binds to several HLA class II complexes and is critical for B cell infection. Overexpression of gp42 results in saturation of gH/gL complexes with gp42, a virus that can infect only B lymphocytes and not epithelial cells. Thus, BZLF2 could have a critical role in directing the virus toward B lymphocytes versus epithelial cells. In B lymphocytes, gp42 may have still another role in down-modulatory class II expression.

Although gp350/220 is the most abundant viral protein in the lytically infected cell plasma membrane and in the virus envelope, only small amounts of gp350/220 accumulate in the lytically infected cell nuclear membrane (261). EBV gp350/220 is extensively N- and O-glycosylated (261,743,822,823,827,881). Gp350 nascent protein has an apparent size of 135 kd, and 37 potential N-linked glycosylation sites, whereas mature glycoprotein has an apparent size of 350 kd. Approximately half of the glycosylation is due to N linkage and half to O linkage. Virtually all of the N-linked oligosaccharides are complex, with tri- and tetra-antennary chains, whereas most O-linked chains are probably di- or tri-N-acetyl lactosamine, consistent with extensive Golgi processing (743).

Early electron microscopic observations of lymphocytes lytically infected with EBV revealed the presence of nucleocapsids in the cytoplasm. Although this could occur as a consequence of nuclear disruption late in infection or as a consequence of reinfection of the infected cell by released virus, an alternative hypothesis is that virus acquires an initial envelope as it buds through the nuclear membrane, that de-envelopment occurs within cytoplasmic vesicles resulting in release of nucleocapsids into the cytoplasm, and that re-envelopment occurs at the plasma membrane, where the virus acquires a definitive envelope rich in gp350/220 and gH/gL. Consistent with this hypothesis, the plasma membrane and virus are both rich in gp350/220, whereas the nuclear membrane is relatively deficient (261). Even if this hypothesis is correct, late in infection, as the cell deteriorates, partially enveloped or initially enveloped virus may be released in substantial quantity. The relative importance of these various pathways in natural infection is difficult to evaluate. A second possible role for high-level plasma membrane gp350/220 expression is in saturation of lymphocyte CD21 and HLA class II, so that virus can be completely released from and not reabsorbed to the lytically infected cells. A price may be paid for such efficiency, however, because antibody to gp350/220 and gH/gL may fix complement and cause lysis of infected cells *in vivo*.

Gp350/220 is not only the most abundant viral protein in the lytically infected cell plasma membrane, it is also one of the most abundant late viral proteins and the most abundant protein on the outer surface of the virus. Surprisingly, disruption of the gp350/220 ORF is not lethal to the virus, and both lymphocytes and epithelial cells can be infected with reduced efficiency. Most EBV neutralizing antibody response is directed to gp350/220 (827). Gp350/220 is therefore an important component of any prospective EBV vaccine that would aim to engender neutralizing antibody (592,618). Significant parts or all of the protein have been expressed in *E. coli*, in *Saccharomyces cerevisiae*, and in mammalian cells, and a recombinant VZV that expresses Gp350/220 under control of the gpI promoter has been constructed (50,604, 738,811,881,923). Gp350 is expressed in large amounts in recombinant VZV-infected cells, and it is incorporated into the infected cell plasma membrane and into the VZV outer envelope (515). Gp350/220 has also been inserted into vaccinia capable of under control of the p8.5 promoter (592). Injection with purified EBV gp350/220, or infection with vaccinia expressing gp350/220, protects cottontop tamarins against a lethal, lymphomagenic EBV challenge (592).

BCRF1 is a close colinear homolog to the human IL10 gene, with nearly 90% colinear identity in amino acid sequence (345,857). BCRF1 is expressed only late in EBV replication despite its location in the middle of the EBNA regulatory domain between oriP and the Cp promoter. IL10 has B-cell growth factor activity (586), and some data have suggested that BCRF1 could be important in latent EBV infection (579). However, nonsense or deletion mutations involving BCRF1 have no effect on the ability of the recombinants to initiate growth transformation, to maintain wild-type latent infection and transformed cell growth, or to lytically infect induced B lymphocytes *in vitro* (795). Thus, the role of BCRF1 is in lytic infection *in vivo*. The principal role of IL10 in mice and humans appears to be as a negative regulator of macrophage and NK cell functions that otherwise positively regulate TH1 cytotoxic T lymphocytes (586). BCRF1 has most of the activities of human IL10 *in vitro*.

Thus, BCRF1 is likely to act to blunt the initial NK and T-cell cytotoxic response to EBV infection in epithelial cells and B lymphocytes. One important aspect of that response is the release of gamma interferon. The initiation of cell growth transformation is quite sensitive to interferon (242,795). A mixture of lytically infected EBV recombinant transformed LCLs with normal peripheral blood mononuclear cells results in low interferon release and efficient transformation of primary B lymphocytes, whereas a mixture of lytically induced BCRF1 null mutant recombinant infected LCLs with peripheral blood mononuclear cells results in high-level gamma interferon release and inefficient transformation of the primary B lymphocytes (795). A second aspect of the NK and CD8 cytotoxic responses is the direct cytotoxic component. Blunting of that component is likely to be important in both primary EBV infection and in reactivation of lytic infection in B lymphocytes. To create an analogous murine model for this possible effect, infection of C57BL/6 mice with vaccinia virus expressing beta galactosidase was compared with infection of C57BL/6 mice with vaccinia virus expressing murine IL10. The NK- and vaccinia-specific CD8 cytotoxic responses were lower in the mice infected with vaccinia virus expressing IL10, although there was no difference in virulence or in antibody response (438). Thus, virally expressed IL10 appears to have an effect on the initial interferon and NK and CD8 cytotoxic responses and may have a local effect on these responses to reactivated virus infection.

Defective Virus

The complete EBV genome is usually maintained as an episome in latently infected lymphocytes, including BL lymphoblasts when there is restricted EBV gene expression. However, in several instances, incomplete genomes have been detected in latently infected BL cells growing in culture or in subclones of such cells. The three best-studied examples are the EBV genomes in the Raji, P3HR-1, and Daudi cell lines (69,110–112,162,301, 311,378,381–383,392,426,675). The Raji cell has 50

EBV episomes, each of which is deleted for EBNA-3C and for BALF2, the 135-kd, major DNA binding protein. As a consequence of the deletion of the BALF2 gene, the EBV genome in Raji cells is not replicated by the Raji DNA polymerase when lytic infection is induced. Thus, no late genes are expressed and the infection is abortive. Expression of BALF2 in Raji cells allows lytic infection to proceed, and virus is produced.

P3HR-1 and Daudi have fewer EBV episomes and are deleted for a single EBV DNA fragment that includes some of the IR1 copies, all of U2 and IR2, and several hundred base pairs of U3. The P3HR-1 EBV deletion appears to have arisen on *in vitro* passage, because the parent cell lines from which P3HR-1 was cloned are not deleted (4,426,677). The EBV genome in P3HR-1 can be induced to full lytic infection and virus is produced. Thus, EBV genes deleted from P3HR-1, including EBNA-LP, EBNA-2, and HLF1, are not necessary for EBV replication in B-lymphoma cells *in vitro*. The resulting P3HR-1 or Daudi virus cannot transform normal B lymphocytes. These cell lines carrying minimally defective EBV genomes are useful for EBV recombinant genetic studies (see later). Interestingly, similar defectives arise during EBV infection in epithelial cells *in vivo* (637,762).

Aside from the minimally defective EBV DNA, some of the EBV DNA in P3HR-1 cells is more highly defective. There are several formats for the more highly defective DNAs and several biologic properties have been delineated (110,112,311,381–383,816). Analysis of P3HR-1 subclones reveals that most cells contain only the minimally defective EBV P3HR-1 genome (332). A rare cell contains both the minimally and the more defective P3HR-1 EBV genomes. The more defective genome is spread by cell-to-cell transmission following spontaneous reactivation of lytic EBV replication (559). Reactivation occurs in cells containing the defective genomes because the defective genomes contain the ZLF1 immediate-early transactivator under control of the IR1 latent infection cycle promoter (381–383). One population of defective genomes appears to be centered about the IR1 palindrome (272,381–383). In the highly defective DNA, the left arm of the palindrome is a complete inverted copy of the right arm. The IR1 sequence to the right of the palindrome now also extends from the palindrome in the opposite direction into a new linkage with the right end of Bam Z. A second new linkage joins the left of Bam Z to Bam S and Bam M. A third new linkage joins Bam M to Bam B1, W1I1 and *Bam*HI A. *Bam*HI A is presumably linked to TR. The lytic ori in *Bam*HI B1 and the TR presumably provide the necessary cis-acting lytic EBV DNA replication origin and packaging signals, respectively, to ensure the perpetuation of the defective virus in the P3HR-1 cell cultures. The specific and selective inclusion of BZLF1, BSMLF1, and BI′LF1 probably arises because of the adjuvant effect of these transactivators on lytic EBV replication.

GENETICS

Attempts at constructing EBV recombinants have been hindered by the limitation in the EBV host range to human B lymphocytes and the nonpermissivity of these cells for EBV replication. The development of strategies for switching latently infected cells into lytic infection has partially alleviated this major experimental barrier. The first attempt at developing an EBV recombinant genetics system was to infect replication-defective Raji cells with P3HR-1 EBV stocks, and to plate the resultant virus onto primary B lymphocytes (111,233). Raji EBV cannot replicate its own genome in lytic infection because of deletion of the major single-strand DNA binding protein BALF2, but it has EBNA-LP and EBNA-2. Raji is also deleted for EBNA-3C, which in later experiments turned out to be a critical gene for B-lymphocyte growth transformation. The P3HR-1 EBV genome is lytic replication competent, but it is transformation incompetent because of the deletion of a DNA segment that encodes EBNA-LP and EBNA-2. Infection of Raji cells with P3HR-1 EBV induced partial permissivity for lytic infection, and replication of both genomes ensued. Because Raji cells contain 50 episome copies of EBV DNA, most of the transforming virus that came out of the infection should have been simply Raji EBV genomes. However, the few transforming viruses that were obtained in transformed primary B-lymphocyte-derived cell lines were in fact recombinants between Raji and P3HR-1 that had restored the deleted EBNA-LP and EBNA-2 encoding fragment, providing initial genetic evidence that EBNA-2 or EBNA-LP is essential for transformation (765). In retrospect, these results also provided an indication that the Raji EBV genome was itself transformation incompetent because of the EBNA-3C deletion. Recent attempts to exploit the EBNA-3C deletion in Raji to assay the ability of wild-type or specifically mutated LBNA-3C genes to marker-rescue a transforming EBV amma from Raji have met with very limited success because of the limited virus from Raji cells even when BALF2 is provided by a heterologous expression vector.

More recently, the entire EBV genome has become amenable to molecular genetic manipulation. In these experiments, specifically mutated recombinant EBV genomes have been obtained by transfecting latently infected lymphocytes with specifically mutated recombinant EBV DNA fragments that had been cloned and amplified in *E. coli*. When virus replication is then induced, the mutant EBV DNA fragment undergoes homologous recombination with replicating viral DNA (125,126,290,368,409,411,470,471,512–514,525,527–530,694,795,797,835–838,871). Parental and recombinant virus can be used to infect primary B lymphocytes or non-EBV-infected BL cells. Because primary B lymphocytes depend on EBV infection for their ability to grow *in vitro*, a mutation in an essential transforming gene will only be recoverable in primary B lymphocytes if the cells are co-infected with a defective EBV that is wild type for the mutated gene. The usual source for defective EBV is P3HR-1 cells, because 10^{7-8} P3HR-1 EBVs can be obtained from 10^7 P3HR-1 cells, and the virus is wild type except for the EBNA-LP and EBNA-2 deletion. BL cells are not dependent on EBV for their growth in culture and therefore are potentially useful for recovery of recombinants with mutations in essential transforming genes (527–530,871). BL cells or primary B lymphocytes can be made dependent on recombinant virus for their growth by including a positive selection marker such as SV40 promoter-driven hygromycin phosphotransferase in the transfected recombinant EBV DNA. Only cells infected with a recombinant virus will then grow out under selective conditions (871). Alternatively, cells infected with the replication-competent but transformation-defective P3HR-1 EBV can be used as the source of a parent virus strain. When these cells are transfected with a wild-type EBV DNA fragment spanning the EBNA-LP and EBNA-2 deletion, a small number of transformation-competent wild-type EBNA-LP and EBNA-2 P3HR-1 EBV recombinants result, and these can be specifically isolated in primary B-lymphocyte-derived cell lines, because only the recombinants will be able to cause LCL outgrowth (125,126,290).

Because transfection with a wild-type EBV cosmid DNA fragment that includes EBNA-LP and EBNA-2 into P3HR-1 EBV-infected cells and induction of lytic infection results in homologous recombination between the transfected DNA and the replicating P3HR-1 EBV with restoration of transforming ability to recombinant P3HR-1 genomes, the effect on transformation of specific EBNA-LP or EBNA-2 mutations or of EBNA-LP or EBNA-2 type-specific differences could be determined (125,126,290,525). Recombination with a wild-type EBV cosmid DNA fragment that spans the deletion uniformly resulted in transforming recombinants. The number of transforming recombinants was sufficiently consistent in a clonal transformation assay that differences in transformation efficiency could be detected. Some deletion mutations within the EBNA-2 ORF or a stop-codon mutation resulted in no transforming recombinants, demonstrating that EBNA-2 is essential for lymphocyte growth transformation. EBNA-2 was also shown to account for the differences between high-transforming type 1 EBV strains and low-transforming type 2 EBV strains (126). Analysis of the phenotype of 11 linker insertion and 15 deletion mutations within the EBNA-2 ORF revealed four separable domains that are essential for transformation of primary B lymphocytes (125). Subsequent experiments with EBV recombinants containing EBNA-LP deletion or stop-codon insertion mutants revealed a markedly reduced B-lymphocyte transformation efficiency.

The use of large cosmid DNA fragment for EBNA-2/EBNA-LP marker rescue of transformation in P3HR-1 cells enables specific mutations to be made in genes mapping near EBNA-LP and EBNA-2 and within the flanking EBV DNA that is common to both the P3HR-1 and transfected EBV DNA fragment. Deletion of the EBER-encoding DNA, or mutation of the BHLF1 or BHRF1 ORFs in the cosmid fragment, resulted in many of the transforming recombinants being also mutant in the adjacent gene (530,797). The resultant mutant EBV recombinants transform cells with wild-type efficiency and replicate following induction.

This led to the observation that almost as high a frequency of incorporation into recombinant EBV genomes occurs with a second, nonlinked, cosmid EBV DNA fragment transfected along with the EBNA-LP and EBNA-2 cosmid DNA into P3HR-1 cells (835–837). Using this strategy of second-site homologous recombination, mutations could be made on any EBV DNA fragment, and, after transfection into P3HR-1 cells, harvest of the resultant virus, and clonal infection of primary B lymphocytes, a substantial fraction of the resultant LCLs are infected with mutant recombinants. The frequency of incorporation of nonlinked second EBV DNA fragments is directly related to transfected fragment size. Fragments of 4 to 5 kb are incorporated with about 20% to 30% of the efficiency of 40-kb fragments, the latter being incorporated into about 10% of the EBV DNAs that recombine with the EBNA-LP/2-positive selection marker.

An alternative strategy for constructing EBV recombinants, which is particularly useful for making deletions in the EBV genome, is to use the P3HR-1 cells as a lytic infection transcomplementing and packaging cell line for cosmid cloned EBV DNA fragments (694,837). Approximately 50% of all transforming recombinants from cells transfected with five overlapping EBV DNA fragments representative of the entire genome consist of the transfected cosmid DNAs without any evidence for recombination with the P3HR-1 EBV genome. For studying the transforming EBV genes, only two and a half cosmid-cloned EBV DNA fragments are necessary, because all of the genome between EBNA-1 and LMP1 is unnecessary and most of the noncoding exons and introns of the EBNA mRNAs can be deleted.

Although positive selection for transformation from the transformation-negative P3HR-1 parent strain is useful for making specifically mutated recombinants in most genes, there are limitations. First, nontransforming mutations in EBNA-LP or EBNA-2 cannot be recovered, and the effect of the mutation can be ascertained only by the failure to generate a transforming recombinant from P3HR-1. Second, nontransforming mutations in other essential or critical transforming genes such as EBNA-3A or -3C or LMP1 can be recovered only when the wild-type EBNA-3A, -3C, or LMP1 is provided to the infected primary B lymphocyte. In many instances, this can be conveniently provided by nonrecombinant P3HR-1 virus, as 10^{7-8} nonrecombinant P3HR-1 EBVs are in each preparation of 50 to 200 recombinant EBVs. Because the virus preparation is used to infect 10^7 primary B lymphocytes, 50% of the primary B lymphocytes are initially infected with nonrecombinant P3HR-1. Any cell infected with a recombinant therefore has a 50% chance of being initially co-infected with a nonrecombinant. Both genomes can stably persist in cells and function, although the nonrecombinant P3HR-1 genome is usually lost over a few months in continuous culture of the resultant LCL if it is not required to maintain cell growth transformation. The characterization of the mutant recombinant genome in co-infected cells is more complicated than in cells infected with a single EBV genome. Furthermore, in some instances, the mutant recombinant can be lost, because the mutant recombinant with its mutated EBNA-3A, EBNA-3C, or LMP1 gene and its wild-type EBNA-2 and EBNA-LP genes undergoes secondary recombination with the co-infecting P3HR-1 EBV, which is wild type for EBNA-3A, EBNA-3C, or LMP1 but deleted for EBNA-2 and EBNA-LP. The secondary recombinant genome could be fully wild type. Third, the efficiency of second-site recombination is about 10%. Many recombinants are obtained that are not mutant at the second site, and these must be identified by polymerase chain reaction for the mutated DNA.

To circumvent some of these problems, non-EBV-infected BL cells or primary B lymphocytes can be used to isolate and recover mutant EBV recombinants carrying a selectable marker (470,471,527–529,871). BL cells can be infected with EBV *in vitro*. The efficiency of infection varies among BL cell lines and is frequently 10% of the efficiency of primary B-lymphocyte infection. Mutant recombinant virus can be recovered from such cells. Because the BL cells are not dependent on EBV for their ability to grow *in vitro*, mutant recombinants deleted for an essential transforming gene can be transferred to non-EBV-infected BL cells and marker-rescue experiments similar to those done in P3HR-1 cells can be carried out. A limitation of this strategy has been alleviated with the derivation of EBV-negative Akata BL cells, which retain EBV episomes and can be induced to become permissive for EBV replication (749).

Recently, several alternative strategies have been developed for making EBV recombinants. One strategy uses targeted homologous recombination to insert mutations, cassettes for expression of positive selection markers, or bacterial replicons into wild-type EBV episomes in cells that can be readily induced to lytic infection, such as Akata or B95 cells (750). The resultant virus can then be harvested and passaged into EBV-negative Akata cells, induced to replicate in these cells, and used for subsequent genetic studies (365,900). EBV recombinants with positive selection markers inserted using this strategy have been used to study the *in vitro* host range for EBV infection, and to show that EBV gp85 is essential for B lymphocyte and epithelial cell infection *in vitro*, that gp42 is critical for B-lymphocyte infection *in vitro*, and that gp150 deletion enhances the efficiency of epithelial cell infection (70,365,581,623,875,900).

A second strategy is a further modification, importing the entire EBV genome into *E. coli* using F plasmids and recombination-deficient cells. Targeted insertional mutations can then be made in cells that have recombination functions. F plasmids containing the entire EBV genome and a positive selection marker for mammalian cells have been recovered from *E. coli* and transferred to human epithelial 293 cells. These plasmids can be induced to replicate in the infected 293 cells and small amounts of virus can be obtained to study the effects of specific mutations on virus infection, replication, or cell growth transformation (160,161). This system should improve the efficiency of EBV genetic studies, assuming that the EBV genome proves to be stable in the recombination-deficient *E. coli*. Initial experiments that demonstrate the utility of the system for investigating the dependence of EBV on gp350 for B-lymphocyte or epithelial cell infection indicate that the system is useful (375).

INHIBITORS OF VIRUS REPLICATION

Lytic EBV infection in B lymphocytes *in vitro* and in EBV infection *in vivo* (see Chapter 75 in *Fields Virology*, 4th ed.) are quite sensitive to acycloguanosine, which is a substrate for the EBV deoxynucleoside kinase (14,15, 494,502) and an inhibitor of EBV DNA polymerase. Other inhibitors of herpesvirus DNA polymerases such as phosphonoacetic acid and phosphonoformic acid are also useful for *in vitro* inhibition of EBV DNA polymerase in B lymphocytes, so as to distinguish early from late gene expression (153,493,495,686). Because of the limited clinical benefit in inhibiting EBV replication with acycloguanosine in patients with acute primary EBV infection (see Chapter 75 in *Fields Virology*, 4th ed.), there has been little effort to develop other specific inhibitors of lytic EBV infection.

BRIEF SUMMARY

In the first decade of EBV research, a great deal was learned about the biology of EBV infection *in vitro* and *in vivo*. The virus was found to cause infectious mononucleosis and to be latent in most adult humans. The tight linkage to BL and NPC, the rare occurrence of lymphoproliferative disease in young children and renal transplant recipients, and the ability of the virus to efficiently immortalize lymphocytes *in vitro* and to induce lymphomas in marmosets provided a biologic framework indicating that EBV can be oncogenic under unusual circumstances. The discovery of cell lines that could be induced to replicate EBV led in the second decade to increasingly sophisticated biochemical analyses. The structure of the genome was determined, the genome cloned, the transcriptional program in latent and lytic infection worked out, and the entire genome sequenced. EBNA became a protein on an acrylamide gel, and then more than one protein. EBV mRNAs in latently infected and growth-transformed B lymphocytes were cloned, sequenced, and expressed in heterologous cells.

By the beginning of the third decade, the genes encoding the EBV latent-infection nuclear and membrane proteins and the proteins themselves were identified in rapid succession. Six EBNAs, two LMPs, and two EBERs were involved in Latency III and cell growth transformation. Studies of the biologic activity of these genes following single-gene transfer revealed EBNA-1 and oriP to be sufficient for plasmid episome maintenance, and LMP1 to have significant transforming activity in rodent fibroblasts. Gene transfer into BL cells and recombinant EBV molecular genetics emerged as important experimental paradigms. Activities of the EBNAs and LMPs were more evident in human B lymphocytes, a natural target of EBV infection.

In the last 5 years, knowledge of the roles of the EBNAs and LMPs in maintaining latent infection and growth transformation and of the various types of latent infection has rapidly advanced. The interaction of EBNAs and LMPs with B-lymphocyte proteins is offering increasing understanding of the mechanisms of EBV-induced and normal B-lymphocyte activation, proliferation, and survival. Molecular targets for inhibition of EBV-mediated growth transformation and cell survival have been identified. Immediate-early and early regulation of lytic EBV infection are better understood. New strategies for manipulating the transition to lytic infection and for genetic analyses have facilitated EBV research. These discoveries and those described in Chapter 75 in *Fields Virology*, 4th ed. on the molecular pathogenesis of EBV infection *in vivo* open new possibilities for understanding, preventing, diagnosing, and treating EBV infection and its associated malignancies.

REFERENCES

1. Abbot SD, Rowe M, Cadwallader K, et al. Epstein-Barr virus nuclear antigen 2 induces expression of the virus-encoded latent membrane protein. *J Virol* 1990;64:2126–2134.
2. Adams A. Replication of latent Epstein-Barr virus genomes in Raji cells. *J Virol* 1987;61:1743–1746.
3. Adams A, Lindahl T. Epstein-Barr virus genomes with properties of circular DNA molecules in carrier cells. *Proc Natl Acad Sci U S A* 1975;72:1477–1481.
4. Adldinger HK, Delius H, Freese UK, et al. A putative transforming gene of Jijoye virus differs from that of Epstein-Barr virus prototypes. *Virology* 1985;141:221–234.
5. Aguirre AJ, Robertson ES. Epstein-Barr virus recombinants from BC-1 and BC-2 can immortalize human primary B lymphocytes with different levels of efficiency and in the absence of coinfection by Kaposi's sarcoma-associated herpesvirus. *J Virol* 2000;74: 735–743.
6. Ahearn JM, Hayward SD, Hickey JC, Fearon DT. Epstein-Barr virus (EBV) infection of murine L cells expressing recombinant human EBV/C3d receptor. *Proc Natl Acad Sci U S A* 1988;85:9307–9311.
7. Aitken C, Sengupta SK, Aedes C, et al. Heterogeneity within the Epstein-Barr virus nuclear antigen 2 gene in different strains of Epstein-Barr virus. *J Gen Virol* 1994;75:95–100.
8. Aiyar A, Tyree C, Sugden B. The plasmid replicon of EBV consists of multiple cis-acting elements that facilitate DNA synthesis by the cell and a viral maintenance element. *EMBO J* 1998;17:6394–6403.
9. Albrecht JC. Primary structure of the Herpesvirus ateles genome. *J Virol* 2000;74:1033–1037.
10. Albrecht JC, Nicholas J, Biller D, et al. Primary structure of the herpesvirus saimiri genome. *J Virol* 1992;66:5047–5058.
11. Alexander L, Denekamp L, Knapp A, et al. The primary sequence of rhesus monkey rhadinovirus isolate 26-95: Sequence similarities to Kaposi's sarcoma-associated herpesvirus and rhesus monkey rhadinovirus isolate 17577. *J Virol* 2000;74:3388–3398.
12. Alfieri C, Birkenbach M, Kieff E. Early events in Epstein-Barr virus infection of human B lymphocytes [published erratum appears in *Virology* 1991;185:946]. *Virology* 1991;181:595–608.
13. Allan GJ, Inman GJ, Parker BD, et al. Cell growth effects of Epstein-Barr virus leader protein. *J Gen Virol* 1992;73:1547–1551.
14. Allaudeen HS. Distinctive properties of DNA polymerases induced by herpes simplex virus type-1 and Epstein-Barr virus. *Antiviral Res* 1985;5:1–12.
15. Allaudeen HS, Descamps J, Sehgal RK. Mode of action of acyclovir triphosphate on herpesviral and cellular DNA polymerases. *Antiviral Res* 1982;2:123–133.
16. Allday MJ, Crawford DH, Griffin BE. Epstein-Barr virus latent gene expression during the initiation of B cell immortalization. *J Gen Virol* 1989;70:1755–1764.
17. Allday MJ, Farrell PJ. Epstein-Barr virus nuclear antigen EBNA3C/6 expression maintains the level of latent membrane protein 1 in G1-arrested cells. *J Virol* 1994;68:3491–3498.
18. Allday MJ, Sinclair A, Parker G, et al. Epstein-Barr virus efficiently immortalizes human B cells without neutralizing the function of p53. *EMBO J* 1995;14:1382–1391.
19. Altiok A, Bejarano MT, Klein E. Effect of TGF-beta on the proliferation of B cell lines and on the immortalisation of B cells by EBV. *Curr Top Microbiol Immunol* 1990;166:375–380.
20. Altiok E, Klein G, Zech L, et al. Epstein-Barr virus-transformed pro-B cells are prone to illegitimate recombination between the switch region of the mu chain gene and other chromosomes [published erratum appears in *Proc Natl Acad Sci U S A* 1990;87:7345]. *Proc Natl Acad Sci U S A* 1989;86:6333–6337.
21. Altiok E, Minarovits J, Hu LF, et al. Host-cell-phenotype-dependent control of the BCR2/BWR1 promoter complex regulates the expression of Epstein-Barr virus nuclear antigens 2-6 [published erratum appears in *Proc Natl Acad Sci U S A* 1992;89:6225]. *Proc Natl Acad Sci U S A* 1992;89:905–909.
22. Aman P, Ehlin-Henriksson B, Klein G. Epstein-Barr virus susceptibility of normal human B lymphocyte populations. *J Exp Med* 1984; 159:208–220.
23. Aman P, Gordon J, Lewin N, et al. Surface marker characterization of EBV target cells in normal blood and tonsil B lymphocyte populations. *J Immunol* 1985;135:2362–2367.
24. Aman P, Lewin N, Nordstrom M, Klein G. EBV-activation of human B-lymphocytes. *Curr Top Microbiol Immunol* 1986;132:266–271.
25. Aman P, Rowe M, Kai C, et al. Effect of the EBNA-2 gene on the surface antigen phenotype of transfected EBV-negative B-lymphoma lines. *Int J Cancer* 1990;45:77–82.
26. Ambinder RF, Mullen MA, Chang YN, et al. Functional domains of Epstein-Barr virus nuclear antigen EBNA-1. *J Virol* 1991;65: 1466–1478.
27. Ambinder RF, Shah WA, Rawlins DR, et al. Definition of the sequence requirements for binding of the EBNA-1 protein to its palindromic target sites in Epstein-Barr virus DNA. *J Virol* 1990;64: 2369–2379.
28. Angel P, Imagawa M, Chiu R, et al. Phorbol ester-inducible genes contain a common cis element recognized by a TPA-modulated trans-acting factor. *Cell* 1987;49:729–739.
29. Anvret M, Miller G. Copy number and location of Epstein-Barr Viral genomes in neonatal human lymphocytes transformed after separation by size and treatment with mitogens. *Virology* 1981;111:47–55.

30. Apolloni A, Sculley TB. Detection of A-type and B-type Epstein-Barr virus in throat washings and lymphocytes. *Virology* 1994;202: 978–981.
31. Ardila-Osorio H, Clausse B, Mishal Z, et al. Evidence of LMP1-TRAF3 interactions in glycosphingolipid-rich complexes of lymphoblastoid and nasopharyngeal carcinoma cells. *Int J Cancer* 1999; 81:645–649.
32. Arrand JR, Rymo L. Characterization of the major Epstein-Barr virus-specific RNA in Burkitt lymphoma-derived cells. *J Virol* 1982;41: 376–389.
33. Arrand JR, Rymo L, Walsh JE, et al. Molecular cloning of the complete Epstein-Barr virus genome as a set of overlapping restriction endonuclease fragments. *Nucleic Acids Res* 1981;9:2999–3014.
34. Austin PJ, Flemington E, Yandava CN, et al. Complex transcription of the Epstein-Barr virus *Bam*HI fragment H rightward open reading frame 1 (BHRF1) in latently and lytically infected B lymphocytes. *Proc Natl Acad Sci U S A* 1988;85:3678–3682.
35. Avila-Carino J, Lewin N, Yamamoto K, et al. EBV infection of B-CLL cells *in vitro* potentiates their allostimulatory capacity if accompanied by acquisition of the activated phenotype. *Int J Cancer* 1994;58: 678–685.
36. Baer R, Bankier AT, Biggin MD, et al. DNA sequence and expression of the B95-8 Epstein-Barr virus genome. *Nature* 1984;310:207–211.
37. Baichwal VR, Sugden B. The multiple membrane-spanning segments of the BNLF-1 oncogene from Epstein-Barr virus are required for transformation. *Oncogene* 1989;4:67–74.
38. Baichwal VR, Sugden B. Posttranslational processing of an Epstein-Barr virus-encoded membrane protein expressed in cells transformed by Epstein-Barr virus. *J Virol* 1987;61:866–875.
39. Baichwal VR, Sugden B. Transformation of Balb 3T3 cells by the BNLF-1 gene of Epstein-Barr virus. *Oncogene* 1988;2:461–467.
40. Bain M, Watson RJ, Farrell PJ, Allday MJ. Epstein-Barr virus nuclear antigen 3C is a powerful repressor of transcription when tethered to DNA. *J Virol* 1996;70:2481–2489.
41. Ballestas ME, Chatis PA, Kaye KM. Efficient persistence of extrachromosomal KSHV DNA mediated by latency-associated nuclear antigen. *Science* 1999;284:641–644.
42. Banchereau J, de Paoli P, Valle A, et al. Long-term human B cell lines dependent on interleukin-4 and antibody to CD40. *Science* 1991;251: 70–72.
43. Bankier AT, Deininger PL, Farrell PJ, Barrell BG. Sequence analysis of the 17,166 base-pair *Eco*RI fragment C of B95-8 Epstein-Barr virus. *Mol Biol Med* 1983;1:21–45.
44. Bankier AT, Deininger PL, Satchwell SC, et al. DNA sequence analysis of the *Eco*RI Dhet fragment of B95-8 Epstein-Barr virus containing the terminal repeat sequences. *Mol Biol Med* 1983;1:425–445.
45. Bauer G, Hofler P, zur Hausen H. Epstein-Barr virus induction by a serum factor. I. Induction and cooperation with additional inducers. *Virology* 1982;121:184–194.
46. Baumann M, Feederle R, Kremmer E, Hammerschmidt W. Cellular transcription factors recruit viral replication proteins to activate the Epstein-Barr virus origin of lytic DNA replication, oriLyt [published erratum appears in *EMBO J* 2000;19:315]. *EMBO J* 1999;18: 6095–6105.
47. Baumann M, Mischak H, Dammeier S, et al. Activation of the Epstein-Barr virus transcription factor BZLF1 by 12-O-tetradecanoylphorbol-13-acetate-induced phosphorylation. *J Virol* 1998;72: 8105–8114.
48. Baumann MA, Paul CC. Interleukin-5 is an autocrine growth factor for Epstein-Barr virus-transformed B lymphocytes. *Blood* 1992;79: 1763–1767.
49. Beaufils P, Choquet D, Mamoun RZ, Malissen B. The (YXXL/I)2 signalling motif found in the cytoplasmic segments of the bovine leukaemia virus envelope protein and Epstein-Barr virus latent membrane protein 2A can elicit early and late lymphocyte activation events. *EMBO J* 1993;12:5105–5112.
50. Beisel C, Tanner J, Matsuo T, et al. Two major outer envelope glycoproteins of Epstein-Barr virus are encoded by the same gene. *J Virol* 1985;54:665–674.
51. Ben-Sasson SA, Klein G. Activation of the Epstein-Barr virus genome by 5-aza-cytidine in latently infected human lymphoid lines. *Int J Cancer* 1981;28:131–135.
52. Berger R, Bernheim A. Cytogenetics of Burkitt's lymphoma-leukaemia: A review. *IARC Sci Publ* 1985;60:65–80.
53. Bhat RA, Thimmappaya B. Construction and analysis of additional adenovirus substitution mutants confirm the complementation of VAI RNA function by two small RNAs encoded by Epstein-Barr virus. *J Virol* 1985;56:750–756.
54. Bhat RA, Thimmappaya B. Two small RNAs encoded by Epstein-Barr virus can functionally substitute for the virus-associated RNAs in the lytic growth of adenovirus 5. *Proc Natl Acad Sci U S A* 1983;80: 4789–4793.
55. Biggin M, Bodescot M, Perricaudet M, Farrell P. Epstein-Barr virus gene expression in P3HR1-superinfected Raji cells. *J Virol* 1987;61: 3120–3132.
56. Biggin M, Farrell PJ, Barrell BG. Transcription and DNA sequence of the *Bam*HI L fragment of B95-8 Epstein-Barr virus. *EMBO J* 1984;3: 1083–1090.
57. Birkenbach M, Liebowitz D, Wang F, et al. Epstein-Barr virus latent infection membrane protein increases vimentin expression in human B-cell lines. *J Virol* 1989;63:4079–4084.
58. Bochkarev A, Barwell JA, Pfuetzner RA, et al. Crystal structure of the DNA-binding domain of the Epstein-Barr virus origin-binding protein, EBNA1, bound to DNA. *Cell* 1996;84:791–800.
59. Bochkarev A, Barwell JA, Pfuetzner RA, et al. Crystal structure of the DNA-binding domain of the Epstein-Barr virus origin-binding protein EBNA 1. *Cell* 1995;83:39–46.
60. Bochkarev A, Bochkareva E, Frappier L, Edwards AM. The 2.2 Å structure of a permanganate-sensitive DNA site bound by the Epstein-Barr virus origin binding protein, EBNA1. *J Mol Biol* 1998;284: 1273–1278.
61. Bocker JF, Tiedemann KH, Bornkamm GW, zur Hausen H. Characterization of an EBV-like virus from African green monkey lymphoblasts. *Virology* 1980;101:291–295.
62. Bodescot M, Brison O, Perricaudet M. An Epstein-Barr virus transcription unit is at least 84 kilobases long. *Nucleic Acids Res* 1986;14:2611–2620.
63. Bodescot M, Chambraud B, Farrell P, Perricaudet M. Spliced RNA from the IR1–U2 region of Epstein-Barr virus: Presence of an open reading frame for a repetitive polypeptide. *EMBO J* 1984;3: 1913–1917.
64. Bodescot M, Perricaudet M. Clustered alternative splice sites in Epstein-Barr virus RNAs. *Nucleic Acids Res* 1987;15:5887.
65. Bodescot M, Perricaudet M. Epstein-Barr virus mRNAs produced by alternative splicing. *Nucleic Acids Res* 1986;14:7103–7114.
66. Bodescot M, Perricaudet M, Farrell PJ. A promoter for the highly spliced EBNA family of RNAs of Epstein-Barr virus. *J Virol* 1987;61: 3424–3430.
67. Bonnefoy JY, Defrance T, Peronne C, et al. Human recombinant interleukin 4 induces normal B cells to produce soluble CD23/IgE-binding factor analogous to that spontaneously released by lymphoblastoid B cell lines. *Eur J Immunol* 1988;18:117–122.
68. Boos H, Berger R, Kuklik-Roos C, et al. Enhancement of Epstein-Barr virus membrane protein (LMP) expression by serum, TPA, or n-butyrate in latently infected Raji cells. *Virology* 1987;159:161–165.
69. Bornkamm GW, Hudewentz J, Freese UK, Zimber U. Deletion of the nontransforming Epstein-Barr virus strain P3HR-1 causes fusion of the large internal repeat to the DSL region. *J Virol* 1982;43:952–968.
70. Borza CM, Hutt-Fletcher LM. Epstein-Barr virus recombinant lacking expression of glycoprotein gp150 infects B cells normally but is enhanced for infection of epithelial cells. *J Virol* 1998;72:7577–7582.
71. Bourillot PY, Waltzer L, Sergeant A, Manet E. Transcriptional repression by the Epstein-Barr virus EBNA3A protein tethered to DNA does not require RBP-Jkappa. *J Gen Virol* 1998;79:363–370.
72. Boyle SM, Ruvolo V, Gupta AK, Swaminathan S. Association with the cellular export receptor CRM 1 mediates function and intracellular localization of Epstein-Barr virus SM protein, a regulator of gene expression. *J Virol* 1999;73:6872–6881.
73. Brielmeier M, Mautner J, Laux G, Hammerschmidt W. The latent membrane protein 2 gene of Epstein-Barr virus is important for efficient B cell immortalization. *J Gen Virol* 1996;77:2807–2818.
74. Brodeur SR, Cheng G, Baltimore D, Thorley-Lawson DA. Localization of the major NF-kappaB-activating site and the sole TRAF3 binding site of LMP-1 defines two distinct signaling motifs. *J Biol Chem* 1997;272:19777–19784.
75. Brooks LA, Lear AL, Young LS, Rickinson AB. Transcripts from the Epstein-Barr virus *Bam*HI A fragment are detectable in all three forms of virus latency. *J Virol* 1993;67:3182–3190.

76. Brown NA, Liu C, Garcia CR, et al. Clonal origins of lymphoproliferative disease induced by Epstein-Barr virus. *J Virol* 1986;58: 975–978.
77. Buell GN, Reisman D, Kintner C, et al. Cloning overlapping DNA fragments from the B95-8 strain of Epstein-Barr virus reveals a site of homology to the internal repetition. *J Virol* 1981;40:977–982.
78. Buhl AM, Cambier JC. Co-receptor and accessory regulation of B-cell antigen receptor signal transduction. *Immunol Rev* 1997;160: 127–138.
79. Burdin N, Peronne C, Banchereau J, Rousset F. Epstein-Barr virus transformation induces B lymphocytes to produce human interleukin 10. *J Exp Med* 1993;177:295–304.
80. Burkhardt AL, Bolen JB, Kieff E, Longnecker R. An Epstein-Barr virus transformation-associated membrane protein interacts with src family tyrosine kinases. *J Virol* 1992;66:5161–5167.
81. Burkitt D, Wright D. Geographical and tribal distribution of the African lymphoma in Uganda. *Br Med J* 1966;5487:569–573.
82. Cahir-McFarland ED, Davidson DM, Schauer SL, et al. NF-kappa B inhibition causes spontaneous apoptosis in Epstein-Barr virus-transformed lymphoblastoid cells. *Proc Natl Acad Sci U S A* 2000;97: 6055–6060.
83. Caldwell RG, Brown RC, Longnecker R. Epstein-Barr virus LMP2A-induced B-cell survival in two unique classes of EmuLMP2A transgenic mice. *J Virol* 2000;74:1101–1113.
84. Caldwell RG, Wilson JB, Anderson SJ, Longnecker R. Epstein-Barr virus LMP2A drives B cell development and survival in the absence of normal B cell receptor signals. *Immunity* 1998;9:405–411.
85. Calender A, Billaud M, Aubry JP, et al. Epstein-Barr virus (EBV) induces expression of B-cell activation markers on *in vitro* infection of EBV-negative B-lymphoma cells. *Proc Natl Acad Sci U S A* 1987;84: 8060–8064.
86. Calender A, Billaud M, Lenoir G. Cooperation between cellular and Epstein-Barr virus genes in the genesis of Burkitt's lymphoma. *IARC Sci Publ* 1988;92:159–164.
87. Calender A, Cordier M, Billaud M, Lenoir GM. Modulation of cellular gene expression in B lymphoma cells following *in vitro* infection by Epstein-Barr virus (EBV). *Int J Cancer* 1990;46:658–663.
88. Cambier JC, Bedzyk W, Campbell K, et al. The B-cell antigen receptor: Structure and function of primary, secondary, tertiary and quaternary components. *Immunol Rev* 1993;132:85–106.
89. Cannell EJ, Farrell PJ, Sinclair AJ. Epstein-Barr virus exploits the normal cell pathway to regulate Rb activity during the immortalisation of primary B-cells. *Oncogene* 1996;13:1413–1421.
90. Caras IW, Levinson BB, Fabry M, et al. Cloned mouse ribonucleotide reductase subunit M1 cDNA reveals amino acid sequence homology with *Escherichia coli* and herpesvirus ribonucleotide reductases. *J Biol Chem* 1985;260:7015–7022.
91. Carel JC, Myones BL, Frazier B, Holers VM. Structural requirements for C3d,g/Epstein-Barr virus receptor (CR2/CD21) ligand binding, internalization, and viral infection. *J Biol Chem* 1990;265: 12293–12299.
92. Carey M, Kolman J, Katz DA, et al. Transcriptional synergy by the Epstein-Barr virus transactivator ZEBRA. *J Virol* 1992;66: 4803–4813.
93. Chang Y, Cesarman E, Pessin MS, et al. Identification of herpesvirus-like DNA sequences in AIDS-associated Kaposi's sarcoma [see comments]. *Science* 1994;266:1865–1869.
94. Chang YN, Dong DL, Hayward GS, Hayward SD. The Epstein-Barr virus Zta transactivator: A member of the bZIP family with unique DNA-binding specificity and a dimerization domain that lacks the characteristic heptad leucine zipper motif. *J Virol* 1990;64: 3358–3369.
95. Chatila T, Ho N, Liu P, et al. The Epstein-Barr virus-induced Ca2+/calmodulin-dependent kinase type IV/Gr promotes a Ca(2+)-dependent switch from latency to viral replication. *J Virol* 1997;71: 6560–6567.
96. Chavrier P, Gruffat H, Chevallier-Greco A, et al. The Epstein-Barr virus (EBV) early promoter DR contains a cis-acting element responsive to the EBV transactivator EB1 and an enhancer with constitutive and inducible activities. *J Virol* 1989;63:607–614.
97. Chen H, Smith P, Ambinder RF, Hayward SD. Expression of Epstein-Barr virus *Bam*HI-A rightward transcripts in latently infected B cells from peripheral blood. *Blood* 1999;93:3026–3032.
98. Chen HL, Lung MM, Sham JS, et al. Transcription of *Bam*HI-A region of the EBV genome in NPC tissues and B cells. *Virology* 1992; 191:193–201.
99. Chen MR, Middeldorp JM, Hayward SD. Separation of the complex DNA binding domain of EBNA-1 into DNA recognition and dimerization subdomains of novel structure. *J Virol* 1993;67:4875–4885.
100. Chen MR, Zong J, Hayward SD. Delineation of a 16 amino acid sequence that forms a core DNA recognition motif in the Epstein-Barr virus EBNA-1 protein. *Virology* 1994;205:486–495.
101. Cheng G, Cleary AM, Ye ZS, et al. Involvement of CRAF1, a relative of TRAF, in CD40 signaling. *Science* 1995;267:1494–1498.
102. Cheng YC, Huang ES, Lin C, et al. Unique spectrum of activity of 9-[(1,3-dihydroxy-2-propoxy)methyl]-guanine against herpesviruses *in vitro* and its mode of action against herpes simplex virus type 1. *Proc Natl Acad Sci U S A* 1983;80:2767–2770.
103. Cheung A, Kieff E. Epstein-Barr virus DNA. X. Direct repeat within the internal direct repeat of Epstein-Barr virus DNA. *J Virol* 1981;40: 501–507.
104. Cheung A, Kieff E. Long internal direct repeat in Epstein-Barr virus DNA. *J Virol* 1982;44:286–294.
105. Chevallier-Greco A, Gruffat H, Manet E, et al. The Epstein-Barr virus (EBV) DR enhancer contains two functionally different domains: Domain A is constitutive and cell specific, domain B is transactivated by the EBV early protein R. *J Virol* 1989;63:615–623.
106. Chevallier-Greco A, Manet E, Chavrier P, et al. Both Epstein-Barr virus (EBV)-encoded trans-acting factors, EB1 and EB2, are required to activate transcription from an EBV early promoter. *EMBO J* 1986; 5:3243–3249.
107. Chi T, Carey M. The ZEBRA activation domain: Modular organization and mechanism of action. *Mol Cell Biol* 1993;13:7045–7055.
108. Chiou JF, Cheng YC. Interaction of Epstein-Barr virus DNA polymerase and 5′-triphosphates of several antiviral nucleoside analogs. *Antimicrob Agents Chemother* 1985;27:416–418.
109. Chittenden T, Lupton S, Levine AJ. Functional limits of oriP, the Epstein-Barr virus plasmid origin of replication. *J Virol* 1989;63: 3016–3025.
110. Cho MS, Bornkamm GW, zur Hausen H. Structure of defective DNA molecules in Epstein-Barr virus preparations from P3HR-1 cells. *J Virol* 1984;51:199–207.
111. Cho MS, Fresen KO, zur Hausen H. Multiplicity-dependent biological and biochemical properties of Epstein-Barr virus (EBV) rescued from non-producer lines after superinfection with P3HR-1 EBV. *Int J Cancer* 1980;26:357–363.
112. Cho MS, Gissmann L, Hayward SD. Epstein-Barr virus (P3HR-1) defective DNA codes for components of both the early antigen and viral capsid antigen complexes. *Virology* 1984;137:9–19.
113. Cho MS, Jeang KT, Hayward SD. Localization of the coding region for an Epstein-Barr virus early antigen and inducible expression of this 60-kilodalton nuclear protein in transfected fibroblast cell lines. *J Virol* 1985;56:852–859.
114. Cho MS, Milman G, Hayward SD. A second Epstein-Barr virus early antigen gene in *Bam*HI fragment M encodes a 48- to 50-kilodalton nuclear protein. *J Virol* 1985;56:860–866.
115. Cho MS, Tran VM. A concatenated form of Epstein-Barr viral DNA in lymphoblastoid cell lines induced by transfection with BZLF1. *Virology* 1993;194:838–842.
116. Clarke PA, Schwemmle M, Schickinger J, et al. Binding of Epstein-Barr virus small RNA EBER-1 to the double-stranded RNA-activated protein kinase DAI. *Nucleic Acids Res* 1991;19:243–248.
117. Clarke PA, Sharp NA, Arrand JR, Clemens MJ. Epstein-Barr virus gene expression in interferon-treated cells. Implications for the regulation of protein synthesis and the antiviral state. *Biochim Biophys Acta* 1990;1050:167–173.
118. Clarke PA, Sharp NA, Clemens MJ. Expression of genes for the Epstein-Barr virus small RNAs EBER-1 and EBER-2 in Daudi Burkitt's lymphoma cells: Effects of interferon treatment. *J Gen Virol* 1992;73:3169–3175.
119. Clarke PA, Sharp NA, Clemens MJ. Translational control by the Epstein-Barr virus small RNA EBER-1. Reversal of the double-stranded RNA-induced inhibition of protein synthesis in reticulocyte lysates. *Eur J Biochem* 1990;193:635–641.
120. Cleary ML, Smith SD, Sklar J. Cloning and structural analysis of cDNAs for bcl-2 and a hybrid bcl-2/immunoglobulin transcript resulting from the t(14;18) translocation. *Cell* 1986;47:19–28.
121. Clough W, McMahon J. Characterization of the Epstein-Barr virion-

associated DNA polymerase as isolated from superinfected and drug-stimulated cells. *Biochim Biophys Acta* 1981;656:76–85.
122. Cludts I, Farrell PJ. Multiple functions within the Epstein-Barr virus EBNA-3A protein. *J Virol* 1998;72:1862–1869.
123. Cohen JI. A region of herpes simplex virus VP16 can substitute for a transforming domain of Epstein-Barr virus nuclear protein 2. *Proc Natl Acad Sci U S A* 1992;89:8030–8034.
124. Cohen JI, Kieff E. An Epstein-Barr virus nuclear protein 2 domain essential for transformation is a direct transcriptional activator. *J Virol* 1991;65:5880–5885.
125. Cohen JI, Wang F, Kieff E. Epstein-Barr virus nuclear protein 2 mutations define essential domains for transformation and transactivation. *J Virol* 1991;65:2545–2554.
126. Cohen JI, Wang F, Mannick J, Kieff E. Epstein-Barr virus nuclear protein 2 is a key determinant of lymphocyte transformation. *Proc Natl Acad Sci U S A* 1989;86:9558–9562.
127. Cordier M, Calender A, Billaud M, et al. Stable transfection of Epstein-Barr virus (EBV) nuclear antigen 2 in lymphoma cells containing the EBV P3HR1 genome induces expression of B-cell activation molecules CD21 and CD23. *J Virol* 1990;64:1002–1013.
128. Cotter MA 2nd, Robertson ES. Modulation of histone acetyltransferase activity through interaction of Epstein-Barr nuclear antigen 3C with prothymosin alpha. *Mol Cell Biol* 2000;20:5722–5735.
129. Countryman J, Jenson H, Seibl R, et al. Polymorphic proteins encoded within BZLF1 of defective and standard Epstein-Barr viruses disrupt latency. *J Virol* 1987;61:3672–3679.
130. Countryman J, Miller G. Activation of expression of latent Epstein-Barr herpesvirus after gene transfer with a small cloned subfragment of heterogeneous viral DNA. *Proc Natl Acad Sci U S A* 1985;82:4085–4089.
131. Cox MA, Leahy J, Hardwick JM. An enhancer within the divergent promoter of Epstein-Barr virus responds synergistically to the R and Z transactivators. *J Virol* 1990;64:313–321.
132. Cruickshank J, Shire K, Davidson AR, et al. Two domains of the Epstein-Barr virus origin DNA-binding protein, EBNA1, orchestrate sequence-specific DNA binding. *J Biol Chem* 2000;275:22273–22277.
133. Cuomo L, Ramquist T, Trivedi P, et al. Expression of the Epstein-Barr virus (EBV)-encoded membrane protein LMP1 impairs the *in vitro* growth, clonability and tumorigenicity of an EBV-negative Burkitt lymphoma line. *Int J Cancer* 1992;51:949–955.
134. Cuomo L, Trivedi P, Wang F, et al. Expression of the Epstein-Barr virus (EBV)-encoded membrane antigen (LMP) increases the stimulatory capacity of EBV-negative B lymphoma lines in allogeneic mixed lymphocyte cultures. *Eur J Immunol* 1990;20:2293–2299.
135. Cuomo L, Zhang QJ, Lombardi L, et al. Over-expression of C-myc increases the sensitivity of Epstein-Barr virus immortalized lymphoblastoid cells to non-MHC-restricted cytotoxicity. *Int J Cancer* 1993;53:1008–1012.
136. Daibata M, Humphreys RE, Sairenji T. Phosphorylation of the Epstein-Barr virus BZLF1 immediate-early gene product ZEBRA. *Virology* 1992;188:916–920.
137. Daibata M, Humphreys RE, Takada K, Sairenji T. Activation of latent EBV via anti-IgG-triggered, second messenger pathways in the Burkitt's lymphoma cell line Akata. *J Immunol* 1990;144:4788–4793.
138. Daibata M, Sairenji T. Epstein-Barr virus (EBV) replication and expressions of EA-D (BMRF1 gene product), virus-specific deoxyribonuclease, and DNA polymerase in EBV-activated Akata cells. *Virology* 1993;196:900–904.
139. Daibata M, Speck SH, Mulder C, Sairenji T. Regulation of the BZLF1 promoter of Epstein-Barr virus by second messengers in anti-immunoglobulin-treated B cells. *Virology* 1994;198:446–454.
140. Dales S, Chardonnet Y. Early events in the interaction of adenoviruses with HeLa cells. IV. Association with microtubules and the nuclear pore complex during vectorial movement of the inoculum. *Virology* 1973;56:465–483.
141. Dalla-Favera R, Martinotti S, Gallo RC, et al. Translocation and rearrangements of the c-*myc* oncogene locus in human undifferentiated B-cell lymphomas. *Science* 1983;219:963–967.
142. Dambaugh T, Beisel C, Hummel M, et al. Epstein-Barr virus (B95-8) DNA VII: Molecular cloning and detailed mapping. *Proc Natl Acad Sci U S A* 1980;77:2999–3003.
143. Dambaugh T, Heller M, Raab-Traub N, et al. DNAs of Epstein-Barr virus and herpes virus Papio. In: *The Human Herpes Viruses.* New York: Elsevier, 1980:85–90.
144. Dambaugh T, Hennessy K, Chamnankit L, Kieff E. U2 region of Epstein-Barr virus DNA may encode Epstein-Barr nuclear antigen 2. *Proc Natl Acad Sci U S A* 1984;81:7632–7636.
145. Dambaugh T, Hennessy K, Fennewald S, Kieff E. The Epstein-Barr virus genome and its expression in latent infection. In: Epstein M, Achong BG, eds. *The Epstein-Barr Virus: Recent Advances.* London: Lilliam Heinemann, 1986:13–45.
146. Dambaugh T, Nkrumah FK, Biggar RJ, Kieff E. Epstein-Barr virus RNA in Burkitt tumor tissue. *Cell* 1979;16:313–322.
147. Dambaugh T, Raab-Traub N, Heller M, et al. Variations among isolates of Epstein-Barr virus. *Ann N Y Acad Sci* 1980;354:309–325.
148. Dambaugh T, Wang F, Hennessy K, et al. Expression of the Epstein-Barr virus nuclear protein 2 in rodent cells. *J Virol* 1986;59:453–462.
149. Dambaugh TR, Kieff E. Identification and nucleotide sequences of two similar tandem direct repeats in Epstein-Barr virus DNA. *J Virol* 1982;44:823–833.
150. Dash AB, Orrico FC, Ness SA. The EVES motif mediates both intermolecular and intramolecular regulation of c-Myb. *Genes Dev* 1996;10:1858–1869.
151. Datta AK, Colby BM, Shaw JE, Pagano JS. Acyclovir inhibition of Epstein-Barr virus replication. *Proc Natl Acad Sci U S A* 1980;77:5163–5166.
152. Datta AK, Feighny RJ, Pagano JS. Induction of Epstein-Barr virus-associated DNA polymerase by 12-O-tetradecanoylphorbol-13-acetate. Purification and characterization. *J Biol Chem* 1980;255:5120–5125.
153. Datta AK, Hood RE. Mechanism of inhibition of Epstein-Barr virus replication by phosphonoformic acid. *Virology* 1981;114:52–59.
154. Davison AJ, Scott JE. The complete DNA sequence of varicella-zoster virus. *J Gen Virol* 1986;67:1759–1816.
155. Davison AJ, Taylor P. Genetic relations between varicella-zoster virus and Epstein-Barr virus. *J Gen Virol* 1987;68:1067–1079.
156. Dawson CW, Rickinson AB, Young LS. Epstein-Barr virus latent membrane protein inhibits human epithelial cell differentiation. *Nature* 1990;344:777–780.
157. de Turenne-Tessier M, Ooka T, de The G, Daillie J. Characterization of an Epstein-Barr virus-induced thymidine kinase. *J Virol* 1986;57:1105–1112.
158. Decaussin G, Leclerc V, Ooka T. The lytic cycle of Epstein-Barr virus in the nonproducer Raji line can be rescued by the expression of a 135-kilodalton protein encoded by the BALF2 open reading frame. *J Virol* 1995;69:7309–7314.
159. Delecluse HJ, Bartnizke S, Hammerschmidt W, et al. Episomal and integrated copies of Epstein-Barr virus coexist in Burkitt lymphoma cell lines. *J Virol* 1993;67:1292–1299.
160. Delecluse HJ, Hilsendegen T, Pich D, et al. Propagation and recovery of intact, infectious Epstein-Barr virus from prokaryotic to human cells. *Proc Natl Acad Sci U S A* 1998;95:8245–8250.
161. Delecluse HJ, Pich D, Hilsendegen T, et al. A first-generation packaging cell line for Epstein-Barr virus-derived vectors. *Proc Natl Acad Sci U S A* 1999;96:5188–5193.
162. Delius H, Bornkamm GW. Heterogeneity of Epstein-Barr virus. III. Comparison of a transforming and a nontransforming virus by partial denaturation mapping of their DNAs. *J Virol* 1978;27:81–89.
163. DePamphilis ML. Transcriptional elements as components of eukaryotic origins of DNA replication. *Cell* 1988;52:635–638.
164. Devergne O, Hatzivassiliou E, Izumi KM, et al. Association of TRAF1, TRAF2, and TRAF3 with an Epstein-Barr virus LMP1 domain important for B-lymphocyte transformation: Role in NF-kappaB activation. *Mol Cell Biol* 1996;16:7098–7108.
165. Devergne O, Hummel M, Koeppen H, et al. A novel interleukin-12 p40-related protein induced by latent Epstein-Barr virus infection in B lymphocytes [published erratum appears in *J Virol* 1996;70:2678]. *J Virol* 1996;70:1143–1153.
166. Devergne O, McFarland EC, Mosialos G, et al. Role of the TRAF binding site and NF-kappaB activation in Epstein-Barr virus latent membrane protein 1-induced cell gene expression. *J Virol* 1998;72:7900–7908.
167. Dhar V, Schildkraut CL. Role of EBNA-1 in arresting replication forks at the Epstein-Barr virus oriP family of tandem repeats. *Mol Cell Biol* 1991;11:6268–6278.
168. di Renzo L, Altiok A, Klein G, Klein E. Endogenous TGF-beta contributes to the induction of the EBV lytic cycle in two Burkitt lymphoma cell lines. *Int J Cancer* 1994;57:914–919.

169. Dillner J, Kallin B, Alexander H, et al. An Epstein-Barr virus (EBV)-determined nuclear antigen (EBNA5) partly encoded by the transformation-associated Bam WYH region of EBV DNA: Preferential expression in lymphoblastoid cell lines. *Proc Natl Acad Sci U S A* 1986;83:6641–6645.
170. Dillner J, Kallin B, Klein G, et al. Antibodies against synthetic peptides react with the second Epstein-Barr virus-associated nuclear antigen. *EMBO J* 1985;4:1813–1818.
171. Dillner J, Sternas L, Kallin B, et al. Antibodies against a synthetic peptide identify the Epstein-Barr virus-determined nuclear antigen. *Proc Natl Acad Sci U S A* 1984;81:4652–4656.
172. Dolyniuk M, Pritchett R, Kieff E. Proteins of Epstein-Barr virus. I. Analysis of the polypeptides of purified enveloped Epstein-Barr virus. *J Virol* 1976;17:935–949.
173. Dolyniuk M, Wolff E, Kieff E. Proteins of Epstein-Barr Virus. II. Electrophoretic analysis of the polypeptides of the nucleocapsid and the glucosamine- and polysaccharide-containing components of enveloped virus. *J Virol* 1976;18:289–297.
174. Dou S, Zeng X, Cortes P, et al. The recombination signal sequence-binding protein RBP-2N functions as a transcriptional repressor. *Mol Cell Biol* 1994;14:3310–3319.
175. Doyle MG, Catovsky D, Crawford DH. Infection of leukaemic B lymphocytes by Epstein Barr virus. *Leukemia* 1993;7:1858–1864.
176. Dyson PJ, Farrell PJ. Chromatin structure of Epstein-Barr virus. *J Gen Virol* 1985;66:1931–1940.
177. Edson CM, Thorley-Lawson DA. Epstein-Barr virus membrane antigens: Characterization, distribution, and strain differences. *J Virol* 1981;39:172–184.
178. Edson CM, Thorley-Lawson DA. Synthesis and processing of the three major envelope glycoproteins of Epstein-Barr virus. *J Virol* 1983;46:547–556.
179. Elia A, Laing KG, Schofield A, et al. Regulation of the double-stranded RNA-dependent protein kinase PKR by RNAs encoded by a repeated sequence in the Epstein-Barr virus genome. *Nucleic Acids Res* 1996;24:4471–4478.
180. Eliopoulos AG, Blake SM, Floettmann JE, et al. Epstein-Barr virus-encoded latent membrane protein 1 activates the JNK pathway through its extreme C terminus via a mechanism involving TRADD and TRAF2. *J Virol* 1999;73:1023–1035.
181. Eliopoulos AG, Dawson CW, Mosialos G, et al. CD40-induced growth inhibition in epithelial cells is mimicked by Epstein-Barr Virus-encoded LMP1: Involvement of TRAF3 as a common mediator. *Oncogene* 1996;13:2243–2254.
182. Eliopoulos AG, Gallagher NJ, Blake SM, et al. Activation of the p38 mitogen-activated protein kinase pathway by Epstein-Barr virus-encoded latent membrane protein 1 coregulates interleukin-6 and interleukin-8 production. *J Biol Chem* 1999;274:16085–16096.
183. Eliopoulos AG, Stack M, Dawson CW, et al. Epstein-Barr virus-encoded LMP1 and CD40 mediate IL-6 production in epithelial cells via an NF-kappaB pathway involving TNF receptor-associated factors. *Oncogene* 1997;14:2899–2916.
184. Eliopoulos AG, Young LS. Activation of the cJun N-terminal kinase (JNK) pathway by the Epstein-Barr virus-encoded latent membrane protein 1 (LMP1). *Oncogene* 1998;16:1731–1742.
185. Ellisen LW, Bird J, West DC, et al. TAN-1, the human homolog of the *Drosophila* notch gene, is broken by chromosomal translocations in T lymphoblastic neoplasms. *Cell* 1991;66:649–661.
186. Emilie D, Touitou R, Raphael M, et al. *In vivo* production of interleukin-10 by malignant cells in AIDS lymphomas. *Eur J Immunol* 1992;22:2937–2942.
187. Emini EA, Luka J, Armstrong ME, et al. Identification of an Epstein-Barr virus glycoprotein which is antigenically homologous to the varicella-zoster virus glycoprotein II and the herpes simplex virus glycoprotein B. *Virology* 1987;157:552–555.
188. Ensser A, Pflanz R, Fleckenstein B. Primary structure of the alcelaphine herpesvirus 1 genome. *J Virol* 1997;71:6517–6525.
189. Epstein M, Achong B. The Epstein-Barr virus. *Ann Rev Microbiol* 1973;27:413–436.
190. Epstein M, Achong B. *The Epstein-Barr Virus.* London: Springer-Verlag, 1979.
191. Epstein M, Achong B. *The Epstein-Barr Virus. Recent Advances.* London: Heinemann, 1986.
192. Epstein M, Achong B, Barr Y. Morphological and biological studies on a virus in cultured lymphoblasts from Burkitt's lymphoma. *J Exp Med* 1965;121:761–770.
193. Epstein M, Achong B, Barr Y. Virus particles in cultured lymphoblasts from Burkitt's lymphoma. *Lancet* 1964;1.
194. Erickson KD, Martin JM. Early detection of the lytic LMP-1 protein in EBV-infected B-cells suggests its presence in the virion. *Virology* 1997;234:1–13.
195. Ernberg I, Falk K, Hansson M. Progenitor and pre-B lymphocytes transformed by Epstein-Barr virus. *Int J Cancer* 1987;39:190–197.
196. Ernberg I, Falk K, Minarovits J, et al. The role of methylation in the phenotype-dependent modulation of Epstein-Barr nuclear antigen 2 and latent membrane protein genes in cells latently infected with Epstein-Barr virus [published erratum appears in *J Gen Virol* 1990;71:499]. *J Gen Virol* 1989;70:2989–3002.
197. Estrov Z, Kurzrock R, Pocsik E, et al. Lymphotoxin is an autocrine growth factor for Epstein-Barr virus-infected B cell lines. *J Exp Med* 1993;177:763–774.
198. Evans TJ, Farrell PJ, Swaminathan S. Molecular genetic analysis of Epstein-Barr virus Cp promoter function. *J Virol* 1996;70:1695–1705.
199. Fahraeus R, Jansson A, Ricksten A, et al. Epstein-Barr virus-encoded nuclear antigen 2 activates the viral latent membrane protein promoter by modulating the activity of a negative regulatory element. *Proc Natl Acad Sci U S A* 1990;87:7390–7394.
200. Fahraeus R, Jansson A, Sjoblom A, et al. Cell phenotype-dependent control of Epstein-Barr virus latent membrane protein 1 gene regulatory sequences. *Virology* 1993;195:71–80.
201. Fahraeus R, Rymo L, Rhim JS, Klein G. Morphological transformation of human keratinocytes expressing the LMP gene of Epstein-Barr virus. *Nature* 1990;345:447–449.
202. Fairbairn LJ, Stewart JP, Hampson IN, et al. Expression of Epstein-Barr virus latent membrane protein influences self-renewal and differentiation in a multipotential murine haemopoietic "stem cell" line. *J Gen Virol* 1993;74:247–254.
203. Falk K, Ernberg I. An origin of DNA replication (oriP) in highly methylated episomal Epstein-Barr virus DNA localizes to a 4.5-kb unmethylated region. *Virology* 1993;195:608–615.
204. Falk K, Gratama JW, Rowe M, et al. The role of repetitive DNA sequences in the size variation of Epstein-Barr virus (EBV) nuclear antigens, and the identification of different EBV isolates using RFLP and PCR analysis. *J Gen Virol* 1995;76:779–790.
205. Falk KI, Szekely L, Aleman A, Ernberg I. Specific methylation patterns in two control regions of Epstein-Barr virus latency: The LMP-1-coding upstream regulatory region and an origin of DNA replication (oriP). *J Virol* 1998;72:2969–2974.
206. Falk KI, Zou JZ, Lucht E, et al. Direct identification by PCR of EBV types and variants in clinical samples. *J Med Virol* 1997;51:355–363.
207. Falk L, Deinhardt F, Nonoyama M, et al. Properties of a baboon lymphotropic herpesvirus related to Epstein-Barr virus. *Int J Cancer* 1976;18:798–807.
208. Farina A, Santarelli R, Gonnella R, et al. The BFRF1 gene of Epstein-Barr virus encodes a novel protein. *J Virol* 2000;74:3235–3244.
209. Farrell PJ. Epstein-Barr virus. In: O'Brien SJ, ed. *Genetic Maps.* New York: Cold Spring Harbor Press, 1992:120–133.
210. Farrell PJ, Bankier A, Seguin C, et al. Latent and lytic cycle promoters of Epstein-Barr virus. *EMBO J* 1983;2:1331–1338.
211. Farrell PJ, Rowe DT, Rooney CM, Kouzarides T. Epstein-Barr virus BZLF1 trans-activator specifically binds to a consensus AP-1 site and is related to c-fos. *EMBO J* 1989;8:127–132.
212. Fennewald S, van Santen V, Kieff E. Nucleotide sequence of an mRNA transcribed in latent growth-transforming virus infection indicates that it may encode a membrane protein. *J Virol* 1984;51:411–419.
213. Fingeroth JD, Diamond ME, Sage DR, et al. CD21-dependent infection of an epithelial cell line, 293, by Epstein-Barr virus. *J Virol* 1999;73:2115–2125.
214. Fingeroth JD, Weis JJ, Tedder TF, et al. Epstein-Barr virus receptor of human B lymphocytes is the C3d receptor CR2. *Proc Natl Acad Sci U S A* 1984;81:4510–4514.
215. Finke J, Rowe M, Kallin B, et al. Monoclonal and polyclonal antibodies against Epstein-Barr virus nuclear antigen 5 (EBNA-5) detect multiple protein species in Burkitt's lymphoma and lymphoblastoid cell lines. *J Virol* 1987;61:3870–3878.
216. Fischer DK, Miller G, Gradoville L, et al. Genome of a mononucleosis Epstein-Barr virus contains DNA fragments previously regarded to be unique to Burkitt's lymphoma isolates. *Cell* 1981;24:543–553.
217. Fixman ED, Hayward GS, Hayward SD. Trans-acting requirements for replication of Epstein-Barr virus ori-Lyt. *J Virol* 1992;66:5030–5039.

218. Flemington E, Speck SH. Autoregulation of Epstein-Barr virus putative lytic switch gene BZLF1. *J Virol* 1990;64:1227–1232.
219. Flemington E, Speck SH. Epstein-Barr virus BZLF1 trans activator induces the promoter of a cellular cognate gene, c-fos. *J Virol* 1990; 64:4549–4552.
220. Flemington E, Speck SH. Evidence for coiled-coil dimer formation by an Epstein-Barr virus transactivator that lacks a heptad repeat of leucine residues. *Proc Natl Acad Sci U S A* 1990;87:9459–9463.
221. Flemington E, Speck SH. Identification of phorbol ester response elements in the promoter of Epstein-Barr virus putative lytic switch gene BZLF1. *J Virol* 1990;64:1217–1226.
222. Flemington EK, Borras AM, Lytle JP, Speck SH. Characterization of the Epstein-Barr virus BZLF1 protein transactivation domain. *J Virol* 1992;66:922–929.
223. Flemington EK, Goldfeld AE, Speck SH. Efficient transcription of the Epstein-Barr virus immediate-early BZLF1 and BRLF1 genes requires protein synthesis. *J Virol* 1991;65:7073–7077.
224. Flemington EK, Lytle JP, Cayrol C, et al. DNA-binding-defective mutants of the Epstein-Barr virus lytic switch activator Zta transactivate with altered specificities. *Mol Cell Biol* 1994;14:3041–3052.
225. Floettmann JE, Eliopoulos AG, Jones M, et al. Epstein-Barr virus latent membrane protein-1 (LMP1) signalling is distinct from CD40 and involves physical cooperation of its two C-terminus functional regions. *Oncogene* 1998;17:2383–2392.
226. Floettmann JE, Rowe M. Epstein-Barr virus latent membrane protein-1 (LMP1) C-terminus activation region 2 (CTAR2) maps to the far C-terminus and requires oligomerisation for NF-kappaB activation. *Oncogene* 1997;15:1851–1858.
227. Franken M, Devergne O, Rosenzweig M, et al. Comparative analysis identifies conserved tumor necrosis factor receptor-associated factor 3 binding sites in the human and simian Epstein-Barr virus oncogene LMP1. *J Virol* 1996;70:7819–7826.
228. Frappier L, Goldsmith K, Bendell L. Stabilization of the EBNA1 protein on the Epstein-Barr virus latent origin of DNA replication by a DNA looping mechanism. *J Biol Chem* 1994;269:1057–1062.
229. Frappier L, O'Donnell M. EBNA1 distorts oriP, the Epstein-Barr virus latent replication origin. *J Virol* 1992;66:1786–1790.
230. Frappier L, O'Donnell M. Epstein-Barr nuclear antigen 1 mediates a DNA loop within the latent replication origin of Epstein-Barr virus. *Proc Natl Acad Sci U S A* 1991;88:10875–10879.
231. Frech B, Zimber-Strobl U, Suentzenich KO, et al. Identification of Epstein-Barr virus terminal protein 1 (TP1) in extracts of four lymphoid cell lines, expression in insect cells, and detection of antibodies in human sera. *J Virol* 1990;64:2759–2767.
232. Freese UK, Laux G, Hudewentz J, et al. Two distant clusters of partially homologous small repeats of Epstein-Barr virus are transcribed upon induction of an abortive or lytic cycle of the virus. *J Virol* 1983; 48:731–743.
233. Fresen KO, Cho MS, Gissmann L, zur Hausen H. NC37-R1 Epstein-Barr virus (EBV): A possible recombinant between intracellular NC37 viral DNA and superinfecting P3HR-1 EBV. *Intervirology* 1980;12:303–310.
234. Fries KL, Sculley TB, Webster-Cyriaque J, et al. Identification of a novel protein encoded by the *Bam*HI A region of the Epstein-Barr virus. *J Virol* 1997;71:2765–2771.
235. Fruehling S, Lee SK, Herrold R, et al. Identification of latent membrane protein 2A (LMP2A) domains essential for the LMP2A dominant-negative effect on B-lymphocyte surface immunoglobulin signal transduction. *J Virol* 1996;70:6216–6226.
236. Fruehling S, Longnecker R. The immunoreceptor tyrosine-based activation motif of Epstein-Barr virus LMP2A is essential for blocking BCR-mediated signal transduction. *Virology* 1997;235:241–251.
237. Fruehling S, Swart R, Dolwick KM, et al. Tyrosine 112 of latent membrane protein 2A is essential for protein tyrosine kinase loading and regulation of Epstein-Barr virus latency. *J Virol* 1998;72:7796–7806.
238. Fuentes-Panana EM, Peng R, Brewer G, et al. Regulation of the Epstein-Barr virus C promoter by AUF1 and the cyclic AMP/protein kinase A signaling pathway. *J Virol* 2000;74:8166–8175.
239. Furnari FB, Zacny V, Quinlivan EB, et al. RAZ, an Epstein-Barr virus transdominant repressor that modulates the viral reactivation mechanism. *J Virol* 1994;68:1827–1836.
240. Gahn TA, Schildkraut CL. The Epstein-Barr virus origin of plasmid replication, oriP, contains both the initiation and termination sites of DNA replication. *Cell* 1989;58:527–535.
241. Gahn TA, Sugden B. An EBNA-1-dependent enhancer acts from a distance of 10 kilobase pairs to increase expression of the Epstein-Barr virus LMP gene. *J Virol* 1995;69:2633–2636.
242. Garner JG, Hirsch MS, Schooley RT. Prevention of Epstein-Barr virus-induced B-cell outgrowth by interferon alpha. *Infect Immun* 1984;43:920–924.
243. Gauchat JF, Gascan H, de Waal Malefyt R, de Vries JE. Regulation of germ-line epsilon transcription and induction of epsilon switching in cloned EBV-transformed and malignant human B cell lines by cytokines and CD4+ T cells. *J Immunol* 1992;148:2291–2299.
244. Gerber P, Birch SM. Complement-fixing antibodies in sera of human and nonhuman primates to viral antigens derived from Burkitt's lymphoma cells. *Proc Natl Acad Sci U S A* 1967;58:478–484.
245. Gerber P, Lucas S, Nonoyama M, et al. Oral excretion of Epstein-Barr virus by healthy subjects and patients with infectious mononucleosis. *Lancet* 1972;2:988–989.
246. Gerber P, Pritchett RF, Kieff ED. Antigens and DNA of a chimpanzee agent related to Epstein-Barr virus. *J Virol* 1976;19:1090–1099.
247. Gergely L, Klein G, Ernberg I. Host cell macromolecular synthesis in cells containing EBV-induced early antigens, studied by combined immunofluorescence and radioautography. *Virology* 1971;45:22–29.
248. Ghosh D, Kieff E. Cis-acting regulatory elements near the Epstein-Barr virus latent-infection membrane protein transcriptional start site. *J Virol* 1990;64:1855–1858.
249. Gibson T, Stockwell P, Ginsburg M, Barrell B. Homology between two EBV early genes and HSV ribonucleotide reductase and 38K genes. *Nucleic Acids Res* 1984;12:5087–5099.
250. Gibson TJ, Barrell BG, Farrell PJ. Coding content and expression of the EBV B95-8 genome in the region from base 62,248 to base 82, 920. *Virology* 1986;152:136–148.
251. Gilligan K, Sato H, Rajadurai P, et al. Novel transcription from the Epstein-Barr virus terminal *Eco*RI fragment, DIJhet, in a nasopharyngeal carcinoma. *J Virol* 1990;64:4948–4956.
252. Gires O, Zimber-Strobl U, Gonnella R, et al. Latent membrane protein 1 of Epstein-Barr virus mimics a constitutively active receptor molecule. *EMBO J* 1997;16:6131–6140.
253. Given D, Kieff E. DNA of Epstein-Barr virus. IV. Linkage map of restriction enzyme fragments of the B95-8 and W91 strains of Epstein-Barr Virus. *J Virol* 1978;28:524–542.
254. Given D, Kieff E. DNA of Epstein-Barr virus. VI. Mapping of the internal tandem reiteration. *J Virol* 1979;31:315–324.
255. Given D, Yee D, Griem K, Kieff E. DNA of Epstein-Barr virus. V. Direct repeats of the ends of Epstein-Barr virus DNA. *J Virol* 1979;30: 852–862.
256. Glickman JN, Howe JG, Steitz JA. Structural analyses of EBER1 and EBER2 ribonucleoprotein particles present in Epstein-Barr virus-infected cells. *J Virol* 1988;62:902–911.
257. Goldfeld AE, Liu P, Liu S, et al. Cyclosporin A and FK506 block induction of the Epstein-Barr virus lytic cycle by anti-immunoglobulin. *Virology* 1995;209:225–229.
258. Goldschmidts W, Luka J, Pearson GR. A restricted component of the Epstein-Barr virus early antigen complex is structurally related to ribonucleotide reductase. *Virology* 1987;157:220–226.
259. Goldsmith K, Bendell L, Frappier L. Identification of EBNA1 amino acid sequences required for the interaction of the functional elements of the Epstein-Barr virus latent origin of DNA replication. *J Virol* 1993;67:3418–3426.
260. Gompels U, Minson A. The properties and sequence of glycoprotein H of herpes simplex virus type 1. *Virology* 1986;153:230–247.
261. Gong M, Kieff E. Intracellular trafficking of two major Epstein-Barr virus glycoproteins, gp350/220 and gp110. *J Virol* 1990;64: 1507–1516.
262. Gong M, Ooka T, Matsuo T, Kieff E. Epstein-Barr virus glycoprotein homologous to herpes simplex virus gB. *J Virol* 1987;61:499–508.
263. Gordon J, Guy G, Walker L. Autocrine models of B-lymphocyte growth. II. Interleukin-1 supports the proliferation of transformed lymphoblasts but not the stimulation of resting B cells triggered through their receptors for antigen. *Immunology* 1986;57:419–423.
264. Gradoville L, Grogan E, Taylor N, Miller G. Differences in the extent of activation of Epstein-Barr virus replicative gene expression among four nonproducer cell lines stably transformed by oriP/BZLF1 plasmids. *Virology* 1990;178:345–354.
265. Grasser FA, Haiss P, Gottel S, Mueller-Lantzsch N. Biochemical characterization of Epstein-Barr virus nuclear antigen 2A. *J Virol* 1991;65: 3779–3788.
266. Gratama JW, Lennette ET, Lonnqvist B, et al. Detection of multiple

Epstein-Barr viral strains in allogeneic bone marrow transplant recipients. *J Med Virol* 1992;37:39–47.
267. Gratama JW, Oosterveer MA, Klein G, Ernberg I. EBNA size polymorphism can be used to trace Epstein-Barr virus spread within families. *J Virol* 1990;64:4703–4708.
268. Gratama JW, Oosterveer MA, Lepoutre JM, et al. Serological and molecular studies of Epstein-Barr virus infection in allogeneic marrow graft recipients [published erratum appears in *Transplantation* 1990;50:910]. *Transplantation* 1990;49:725–730.
269. Gratama JW, Oosterveer MA, Weimar W, et al. Detection of multiple "Ebnotypes" in individual Epstein-Barr virus carriers following lymphocyte transformation by virus derived from peripheral blood and oropharynx. *J Gen Virol* 1994;75:85–94.
270. Gregory CD, Dive C, Henderson S, et al. Activation of Epstein-Barr virus latent genes protects human B cells from death by apoptosis. *Nature* 1991;349:612–614.
271. Gregory CD, Rowe M, Rickinson AB. Different Epstein-Barr virus-B cell interactions in phenotypically distinct clones of a Burkitt's lymphoma cell line. *J Gen Virol* 1990;71:1481–1495.
272. Grogan E, Jenson H, Countryman J, et al. Transfection of a rearranged viral DNA fragment, WZhet, stably converts latent Epstein-Barr viral infection to productive infection in lymphoid cells. *Proc Natl Acad Sci U S A* 1987;84:1332–1336.
273. Grogan E, Miller G, Henle W, et al. Expression of Epstein-Barr viral early antigen in monolayer tissue cultures after transfection with viral DNA and DNA fragments. *J Virol* 1981;40:861–869.
274. Grogan EA, Summers WP, Dowling S, et al. Two Epstein-Barr viral nuclear neoantigens distinguished by gene transfer, serology, and chromosome binding. *Proc Natl Acad Sci U S A* 1983;80:7650–7653.
275. Grossberger D, Clough W. Characterization of purified Epstein-Barr virus induced deoxyribonucleic acid polymerase: Nucleotide turnover, processiveness, and phosphonoacetic acid sensitivity. *Biochemistry* 1981;20:4049–4055.
276. Grossman SR, Johannsen E, Tong X, et al. The Epstein-Barr virus nuclear antigen 2 transactivator is directed to response elements by the J kappa recombination signal binding protein. *Proc Natl Acad Sci U S A* 1994;91:7568–7572.
277. Gruffat H, Duran N, Buisson M, et al. Characterization of an R-binding site mediating the R-induced activation of the Epstein-Barr virus BMLF1 promoter. *J Virol* 1992;66:46–52.
278. Gruffat H, Manet E, Rigolet A, Sergeant A. The enhancer factor R of Epstein-Barr virus (EBV) is a sequence-specific DNA binding protein. *Nucleic Acids Res* 1990;18:6835–6843.
279. Gruffat H, Moreno N, Sergeant A. The Epstein-Barr virus (EBV) ORI1yt enhancer is not B-cell specific and does not respond synergistically to the EBV transcription factors R and Z. *J Virol* 1990;64:2810–2818.
280. Gruffat H, Sergeant A. Characterization of the DNA-binding site repertoire for the Epstein-Barr virus transcription factor R. *Nucleic Acids Res* 1994;22:1172–1178.
281. Grundhoff AT, Kremmer E, Tureci O, et al. Characterization of DP103, a novel DEAD box protein that binds to the Epstein-Barr virus nuclear proteins EBNA2 and EBNA3C. *J Biol Chem* 1999;274:19136–19144.
282. Gulley ML, Raphael M, Lutz CT, et al. Epstein-Barr virus integration in human lymphomas and lymphoid cell lines. *Cancer* 1992;70:185–191.
283. Gussander E, Adams A. Electron microscopic evidence for replication of circular Epstein-Barr virus genomes in latently infected Raji cells. *J Virol* 1984;52:549–556.
284. Gutkind JS, Link DC, Katamine S, et al. A novel c-fgr exon utilized in Epstein-Barr virus-infected B lymphocytes but not in normal monocytes. *Mol Cell Biol* 1991;11:1500–1507.
285. Gutsch DE, Holley-Guthrie EA, Zhang Q, et al. The bZIP transactivator of Epstein-Barr virus, BZLF1, functionally and physically interacts with the p65 subunit of NF-kappa B. *Mol Cell Biol* 1994;14:1939–1948.
286. Haan KM, Kwok WW, Longnecker R, Speck P. Epstein-Barr virus entry utilizing HLA-DP or HLA-DQ as a coreceptor. *J Virol* 2000;74:2451–2454.
287. Haan KM, Longnecker R. Coreceptor restriction within the HLA-DQ locus for Epstein-Barr virus infection. *Proc Natl Acad Sci U S A* 2000;97:9252–9257.
288. Habeshaw G, Yao QY, Bell AI, et al. Epstein-Barr virus nuclear antigen 1 sequences in endemic and sporadic Burkitt's lymphoma reflect virus strains prevalent in different geographic areas. *J Virol* 1999;73:965–975.
289. Haddad RS, Hutt-Fletcher LM. Depletion of glycoprotein gp85 from virosomes made with Epstein-Barr virus proteins abolishes their ability to fuse with virus receptor-bearing cells. *J Virol* 1989;63:4998–5005.
290. Hammerschmidt W, Sugden B. Genetic analysis of immortalizing functions of Epstein-Barr virus in human B lymphocytes. *Nature* 1989;340:393–397.
291. Hammerschmidt W, Sugden B. Identification and characterization of oriLyt, a lytic origin of DNA replication of Epstein-Barr virus. *Cell* 1988;55:427–433.
292. Hammerskjold M, Simurda M. Epstein-Barr virus latent membrane protein transactivates the human immunodeficiency virus type 1 long terminal repeat through induction of NF-kB activity. *J Virol* 1992;66:6496–6501.
293. Hampar B, Tanaka A, Nonoyama M, Derge JG. Replication of the resident repressed Epstein-Barr virus genome during the early S phase (S-1 period) of nonproducer Raji cells. *Proc Natl Acad Sci U S A* 1974;71:631–633.
294. Hansson M, Falk K, Ernberg I. Epstein-Barr virus transformation of human pre-B cells. *J Exp Med* 1983;158:616–622.
295. Harada S, Kieff E. Epstein-Barr virus nuclear protein LP stimulates EBNA-2 acidic domain-mediated transcriptional activation. *J Virol* 1997;71:6611–6618.
296. Harada S, Yalamanchili R, Kieff E. Residues 231 to 280 of the Epstein-Barr virus nuclear protein 2 are not essential for primary B-lymphocyte growth transformation. *J Virol* 1998;72:9948–9954.
297. Hardwick JM, Lieberman PM, Hayward SD. A new Epstein-Barr virus transactivator, R, induces expression of a cytoplasmic early antigen. *J Virol* 1988;62:2274–2284.
298. Hardwick JM, Tse L, Applegren N, et al. The Epstein-Barr virus R transactivator (Rta) contains a complex, potent activation domain with properties different from those of VP16. *J Virol* 1992;66:5500–5508.
299. Harris A, Young BD, Griffin BE. Random association of Epstein-Barr virus genomes with host cell metaphase chromosomes in Burkitt's lymphoma-derived cell lines. *J Virol* 1985;56:328–332.
300. Harrison S, Fisenne K, Hearing J. Sequence requirements of the Epstein-Barr virus latent origin of DNA replication. *J Virol* 1994;68:1913–1925.
301. Hatfull G, Bankier AT, Barrell BG, Farrell PJ. Sequence analysis of Raji Epstein-Barr virus DNA. *Virology* 1988;164:334–340.
302. Hatzivassiliou E, Miller WE, Raab-Traub N, et al. A fusion of the EBV latent membrane protein-1 (LMP1) transmembrane domains to the CD40 cytoplasmic domain is similar to LMP1 in constitutive activation of epidermal growth factor receptor expression, nuclear factor-kappa B, and stress-activated protein kinase. *J Immunol* 1998;160:1116–1121.
303. Hayward D, Pritchett R, Orellana T, et al. The DNA of Epstein-Barr virus fragments produced by restriction enzymes: Homologous DNA and RNA in lymphoblastoid cells. In: Baltimore D, et al., eds. *Animal Virology.* New York: Academic Press, 1976:619–639.
304. Hayward SD, Kieff E. DNA of Epstein-Barr virus. II. Comparison of the molecular weights of restriction endonuclease fragments of the DNA of Epstein-Barr virus strains and identification of end fragments of the B95-8 strain. *J Virol* 1977;23:421–429.
305. Hayward SD, Lazarowitz SG, Hayward GS. Organization of the Epstein-Barr virus DNA molecule. II. Fine mapping of the boundaries of the internal repeat cluster of B95-8 and identification of additional small tandem repeats adjacent to the HR-1 deletion. *J Virol* 1982;43:201–212.
306. Hayward SD, Nogee L, Hayward GS. Organization of repeated regions within the Epstein-Barr virus DNA molecule. *J Virol* 1980;33:507–521.
307. Hearing J, Mulhaupt Y, Harper S. Interaction of Epstein-Barr virus nuclear antigen 1 with the viral latent origin of replication. *J Virol* 1992;66:694–705.
308. Hearing JC, Levine AJ. The Epstein-Barr virus nuclear antigen (*Bam*HI K antigen) is a single-stranded DNA binding phosphoprotein. *Virology* 1985;145:105–116.
309. Heineman T. The University of Chicago, 1988.
310. Heineman T, Gong M, Sample J, Kieff E. Identification of the Epstein-Barr virus gp85 gene. *J Virol* 1988;62:1101–1107.

311. Heller M, Dambaugh T, Kieff E. Epstein-Barr virus DNA. IX. Variation among viral DNAs from producer and nonproducer infected cells. *J Virol* 1981;38:632–648.
312. Heller M, Flemington E, Kieff E, Deininger P. Repeat arrays in cellular DNA related to the Epstein-Barr virus IR3 repeat. *Mol Cell Biol* 1985;5:457–465.
313. Heller M, Gerber P, Kieff E. DNA of herpesvirus pan, a third member of the Epstein-Barr virus-Herpesvirus papio group. *J Virol* 1982;41: 931–939.
314. Heller M, Gerber P, Kieff E. Herpesvirus papio DNA is similar in organization to Epstein-Barr virus DNA. *J Virol* 1981;37:698–709.
315. Heller M, Henderson A, Ripley S, et al. The IR3 repeat in Epstein-Barr virus DNA has homology to cell DNA, encodes part of a messenger RNA in EBV transformed cells but does not mediate integration of Epstein-Barr virus DNA. In: Prasad U, et al., eds. *Nasopharyngeal Carcinoma: Current Concepts*, vol. 6. Kuala Lumpur: University of Malaysia, 1983:177–202.
316. Heller M, Kieff E. Colinearity between the DNAs of Epstein-Barr virus and herpesvirus papio. *J Virol* 1981;37:821–826.
317. Heller M, van Santen V, Kieff E. Simple repeat sequence in Epstein-Barr virus DNA is transcribed in latent and productive infections. *J Virol* 1982;44:311–320.
318. Henderson A, Ripley S, Heller M, Kieff E. Chromosome site for Epstein-Barr virus DNA in a Burkitt tumor cell line and in lymphocytes growth-transformed *in vitro*. *Proc Natl Acad Sci U S A* 1983; 80:1987–1991.
319. Henderson E, Miller G, Robinson J, Heston L. Efficiency of transformation of lymphocytes by Epstein-Barr virus. *Virology* 1977;76: 152–163.
320. Henderson S, Huen D, Rowe M, et al. Epstein-Barr virus-coded BHRF1 protein, a viral homologue of Bcl-2, protects human B cells from programmed cell death. *Proc Natl Acad Sci U S A* 1993;90: 8479–8483.
321. Henderson S, Rowe M, Gregory C, et al. Induction of bcl-2 expression by Epstein-Barr virus latent membrane protein 1 protects infected B cells from programmed cell death. *Cell* 1991;65:1107–1115.
322. Henkel T, Ling PD, Hayward SD, Peterson MG. Mediation of Epstein-Barr virus EBNA2 transactivation by recombination signal-binding protein J kappa. *Science* 1994;265:92–95.
323. Henle W, Diehl V, Kohn G, et al. Herpes-type virus and chromosome marker in normal leukocytes after growth with irradiated Burkitt cells. *Science* 1967;157:1064–1065.
324. Hennessy K, Fennewald S, Hummel M, et al. A membrane protein encoded by Epstein-Barr virus in latent growth-transforming infection. *Proc Natl Acad Sci U S A* 1984;81:7207–7211.
325. Hennessy K, Fennewald S, Kieff E. A third viral nuclear protein in lymphoblasts immortalized by Epstein-Barr virus. *Proc Natl Acad Sci U S A* 1985;82:5944–5948.
326. Hennessy K, Heller M, van Santen V, Kieff E. Simple repeat array in Epstein-Barr virus DNA encodes part of the Epstein-Barr nuclear antigen. *Science* 1983;220:1396–1398.
327. Hennessy K, Kieff E. One of two Epstein-Barr virus nuclear antigens contains a glycine-alanine copolymer domain. *Proc Natl Acad Sci U S A* 1983;80:5665–5669.
328. Hennessy K, Kieff E. A second nuclear protein is encoded by Epstein-Barr virus in latent infection. *Science* 1985;227:1238–1240.
329. Hennessy K, Wang F, Bushman EW, Kieff E. Definitive identification of a member of the Epstein-Barr virus nuclear protein 3 family. *Proc Natl Acad Sci U S A* 1986;83:5693–5697.
330. Herbst H, Foss HD, Samol J, et al. Frequent expression of interleukin-10 by Epstein-Barr virus-harboring tumor cells of Hodgkin's disease. *Blood* 1996;87:2918–2929.
331. Herrold RE, Marchini A, Fruehling S, Longnecker R. Glycoprotein 110, the Epstein-Barr virus homolog of herpes simplex virus glycoprotein B, is essential for Epstein-Barr virus replication *in vivo*. *J Virol* 1996;70:2049–2054.
332. Heston L, Rabson M, Brown N, Miller G. New Epstein-Barr virus variants from cellular subclones of P3J-HR-1 Burkitt lymphoma. *Nature* 1982;295:160–163.
333. Hinuma Y, Konn M, Yamaguchi J, et al. Immunofluorescence and herpes-type virus particles in the P3HR-1 Burkitt lymphoma cell line. *J Virol* 1967;1:1045–1051.
334. Hitt MM, Allday MJ, Hara T, et al. EBV gene expression in an NPC-related tumour. *EMBO J* 1989;8:2639–2651.
335. Hoffman GJ, Lazarowitz SG, Hayward SD. Monoclonal antibody against a 250,000-dalton glycoprotein of Epstein-Barr virus identifies a membrane antigen and a neutralizing antigen. *Proc Natl Acad Sci U S A* 1980;77:2979–2983.
336. Holley-Guthrie EA, Quinlivan EB, Mar EC, Kenney S. The Epstein-Barr virus (EBV) BMRF1 promoter for early antigen (EA-D) is regulated by the EBV transactivators, BRLF1 and BZLF1, in a cell-specific manner. *J Virol* 1990;64:3753–3759.
337. Hollyoake M, Stuhler A, Farrell P, et al. The normal cell cycle activation program is exploited during the infection of quiescent B lymphocytes by Epstein-Barr virus. *Cancer Res* 1995;55:4784–4787.
338. Hong Y, Holley-Guthrie E, Kenney S. The bZip dimerization domain of the Epstein-Barr virus BZLF1 (Z) protein mediates lymphoid-specific negative regulation. *Virology* 1997;229:36–48.
339. Horner D, Lewis M, Farrell PJ. Novel hypotheses for the roles of EBNA-1 and BHRF1 in EBV-related cancers. *Intervirology* 1995;38: 195–205.
340. Howe JG, Shu MD. Epstein-Barr virus small RNA (EBER) genes: Unique transcription units that combine RNA polymerase II and III promoter elements. *Cell* 1989;57:825–834.
341. Howe JG, Shu MD. Isolation and characterization of the genes for two small RNAs of herpesvirus papio and their comparison with Epstein-Barr virus-encoded EBER RNAs. *J Virol* 1988;62:2790–2798.
342. Howe JG, Shu MD. Upstream basal promoter element important for exclusive RNA polymerase III transcription of the EBER 2 gene. *Mol Cell Biol* 1993;13:2655–2665.
343. Howe JG, Steitz JA. Localization of Epstein-Barr virus-encoded small RNAs by in situ hybridization. *Proc Natl Acad Sci U S A* 1986;83: 9006–9010.
344. Hsieh DJ, Camiolo SM, Yates JL. Constitutive binding of EBNA1 protein to the Epstein-Barr virus replication origin, oriP, with distortion of DNA structure during latent infection. *EMBO J* 1993;12: 4933–4944.
345. Hsu DH, de Waal Malefyt R, Fiorentino DF, et al. Expression of interleukin-10 activity by Epstein-Barr virus protein BCRF1. *Science* 1990;250:830–832.
346. Hu LF, Chen F, Zheng X, et al. Clonability and tumorigenicity of human epithelial cells expressing the EBV encoded membrane protein LMP1. *Oncogene* 1993;8:1575–1583.
347. Hu LF, Minarovits J, Cao SL, et al. Variable expression of latent membrane protein in nasopharyngeal carcinoma can be related to methylation status of the Epstein-Barr virus BNLF-1 5′-flanking region. *J Virol* 1991;65:1558–1567.
348. Hu LF, Zabarovsky ER, Chen F, et al. Isolation and sequencing of the Epstein-Barr virus BNLF-1 gene (LMP1) from a Chinese nasopharyngeal carcinoma. *J Gen Virol* 1991;72:2399–2409.
349. Huber MD, Dworet JH, Shire K, et al. The budding yeast homolog of the human EBNA1-binding protein 2 (Ebp2p) is an essential nucleolar protein required for pre-rRNA processing. *J Biol Chem* 2000;275:28764–28773.
350. Hudewentz J, Bornkamm GW, zur Hausen H. Effect of the diterpene ester TPA on Epstein-Barr virus antigen-and DNA synthesis in producer and nonproducer cell lines. *Virology* 1980;100:175–178.
351. Hudewentz J, Delius H, Freese UK, et al. Two distant regions of the Epstein-Barr virus genome with sequence homologies have the same orientation and involve small tandem repeats. *EMBO J* 1982;1:21–26.
352. Hudson GS, Bankier AT, Satchwell SC, Barrell BG. The short unique region of the B95-8 Epstein-Barr virus genome. *Virology* 1985;147: 81–98.
353. Hudson GS, Farrell PJ, Barrell BG. Two related but differentially expressed potential membrane proteins encoded by the *Eco*RI Dhet region of Epstein-Barr virus B95-8. *J Virol* 1985;53:528–535.
354. Hudson GS, Gibson TJ, Barrell BG. The *Bam*HI F region of the B95-8 Epstein-Barr virus genome. *Virology* 1985;147:99–109.
355. Huen DS, Fox A, Kumar P, Searle PF. Dilated heart failure in transgenic mice expressing the Epstein-Barr virus nuclear antigen-leader protein. *J Gen Virol* 1993;74:1381–1391.
356. Huen DS, Henderson SA, Croom-Carter D, Rowe M. The Epstein-Barr virus latent membrane protein-1 (LMP1) mediates activation of NF-kappa B and cell surface phenotype via two effector regions in its carboxy-terminal cytoplasmic domain. *Oncogene* 1995;10:549–560.
357. Hummel, M, Kieff E. 1982. Epstein-Barr virus RNA. VIII. Viral RNA in permissively infected B95-8 cells. *J Virol* 43:262–72.
358. Hummel, M, Kieff E. 1982. Mapping of polypeptides encoded by the

Epstein-Barr virus genome in productive infection. *Proc Natl Acad Sci U S A* 79:5698–702.

359. Hummel, M, D. Thorley-Lawson, Kieff E. 1984. An Epstein-Barr virus DNA fragment encodes messages for the two major envelope glycoproteins (gp350/300 and gp220/200). *J Virol* 49:413–7.
360. Hung, S. C, M. S. Kang, Kieff E. Maintenance of EBV oriP-based episomes requires EBV-encoded nuclear antigen-1 chromosome-binding domains, which can be replaced by high-mobility group-I or histone H1. *Proc Natl Acad Sci U S A* 2001;98:1865–1870.
361. Hurley, E. A, S. Agger, J. A. McNeil, J. B. Lawrence, A. Calendar, G. Lenoir, D. A. Thorley-Lawson. 1991. When Epstein-Barr virus persistently infects B-cell lines, it frequently integrates. *J Virol* 65:1245–54.
362. Hurley, E. A, L. D. Klaman, S. Agger, J. B. Lawrence, D. A. Thorley-Lawson. 1991. The prototypical Epstein-Barr virus-transformed lymphoblastoid cell line IB4 is an unusual variant containing integrated but no episomal viral DNA. *J Virol* 65:3958–63.
363. Hurley, E. A, D. A. Thorley-Lawson. 1988. B cell activation and the establishment of Epstein-Barr virus latency. *J Exp Med* 168:2059–75.
364. Hutt-Fletcher, L. M, E. Fowler, J. D. Lambris, R. J. Feighny, J. G. Simmons, G. D. Ross. 1983. Studies of the Epstein Barr virus receptor found on Raji cells. II. A comparison of lymphocyte binding sites for Epstein Barr virus and C3d. *J Immunol* 130:1309–12.
365. Imai, S, J. Nishikawa, K. Takada. 1998. Cell-to-cell contact as an efficient mode of Epstein-Barr virus infection of diverse human epithelial cells. *J Virol* 72:4371–8.
366. Inman, G. J, Farrell PJ. 1995. Epstein-Barr virus EBNA-LP and transcription regulation properties of pRB, p107 and p53 in transfection assays. *J Gen Virol* 76:2141–9.
367. Izumi, K. M, K. M. Kaye, E. D. Kieff. 1997. The Epstein-Barr virus LMP1 amino acid sequence that engages tumor necrosis factor receptor associated factors is critical for primary B lymphocyte growth transformation. *Proc Natl Acad Sci U S A* 94:1447–52.
368. Izumi, K. M, K. M. Kaye, E. D. Kieff. 1994. Epstein-Barr virus recombinant molecular genetic analysis of the LMP1 amino-terminal cytoplasmic domain reveals a probable structural role, with no component essential for primary B-lymphocyte growth transformation. *J Virol* 68:4369–76.
369. Izumi, K. M, E. D. Kieff. 1997. The Epstein-Barr virus oncogene product latent membrane protein 1 engages the tumor necrosis factor receptor-associated death domain protein to mediate B lymphocyte growth transformation and activate NF-kappaB. *Proc Natl Acad Sci U S A* 94:12592–7.
370. Izumi, K. M, E. D. Kieff. 1997. The Epstein-Barr virus oncogene product latent membrane protein 1 engages the tumor necrosis factor receptor-associated death domain protein to mediate B lymphocyte growth transformation and activate NF-kappaB. *Proc Natl Acad Sci U S A* 94:12592–7.
371. Izumi, K. M, E. C. McFarland, E. A. Riley, D. Rizzo, Y. Chen, Kieff E. 1999. The residues between the two transformation effector sites of Epstein-Barr virus latent membrane protein 1 are not critical for B-lymphocyte growth transformation. *J Virol* 73:9908–16.
372. Izumi, K. M, E. C. McFarland, A. T. Ting, E. A. Riley, B. Seed, E. D. Kieff. 1999. The Epstein-Barr virus oncoprotein latent membrane protein 1 engages the tumor necrosis factor receptor-associated proteins TRADD and receptor-interacting protein (RIP) but does not induce apoptosis or require RIP for NF-kappaB activation. *Mol Cell Biol* 19:5759–67.
373. Jabara, H. H, L. C. Schneider, S. K. Shapira, C. Alfieri, C. T. Moody, Kieff E, R. S. Geha, D. Vercelli. 1990. Induction of germ-line and mature C epsilon transcripts in human B cells stimulated with rIL-4 and EBV. *J Immunol* 145:3468–73.
374. Jansson, A, M. Masucci, L. Rymo. 1992. Methylation of discrete sites within the enhancer region regulates the activity of the Epstein-Barr virus BamHI W promoter in Burkitt lymphoma lines. *J Virol* 66:62–9.
375. Janz, A, M. Oezel, C. Kurzeder, J. Mautner, D. Pich, M. Kost, W. Hammerschmidt, H. J. Delecluse. 2000. Infectious Epstein-Barr virus lacking major glycoprotein BLLF1 (gp350/220) demonstrates the existence of additional viral ligands. *J Virol* 74:10142–52.
376. Jat, P, J. R. Arrand. 1982. *In vitro* transcription of two Epstein-Barr virus specified small RNA molecules. *Nucleic Acids Res* 10:3407–25.
377. Jayachandra, S, K. G. Low, A. E. Thlick, J. Yu, P. D. Ling, Y. Chang, P. S. Moore. 1999. Three unrelated viral transforming proteins (vIRF, EBNA2, and E1A) induce the MYC oncogene through the interferon-responsive PRF element by using different transcription coadaptors. *Proc Natl Acad Sci U S A* 96:11566–71.
378. Jeang, K. T, Hayward SD. 1983. Organization of the Epstein-Barr virus DNA molecule. III. Location of the P3HR-1 deletion junction and characterization of the NotI repeat units that form part of the template for an abundant 12–O-tetradecanoylphorbol-13-acetate-induced mRNA transcript. *J Virol* 48:135–48.
379. Jehn, U, T. Lindahl, C. Klein. 1972. Fate of virus DNA in the abortive infection of human lymphoid cell lines by Epstein-Barr virus. *J Gen Virol* 16:409–12.
380. Jenkins, P. J, U. K. Binne, Farrell PJ. 2000. Histone acetylation and reactivation of Epstein-Barr virus from latency. *J Virol* 74:710–20.
381. Jenson, H. B, Farrell PJ, G. Miller. 1987. Sequences of the Epstein-Barr Virus (EBV) large internal repeat form the center of a 16-kilo-base-pair palindrome of EBV (P3HR-1) heterogeneous DNA [published erratum appears in J Virol 1987 Sep;61(9):2950]. *J Virol* 61: 1495–506.
382. Jenson, H. B, G. Miller. 1988. Polymorphisms of the region of the Epstein-Barr virus genome which disrupts latency. *Virology* 165: 549–64.
383. Jenson, H. B, M. S. Rabson, G. Miller. 1986. Palindromic structure and polypeptide expression of 36 kilobase pairs of heterogeneous Epstein-Barr virus (P3HR-1) DNA. *J Virol* 58:475–86.
384. Jiang, H, Y. G. Cho, F. Wang. 2000. Structural, functional, and genetic comparisons of Epstein-Barr virus nuclear antigen 3A, 3B, and 3C homologues encoded by the rhesus lymphocryptovirus. *J Virol* 74: 5921–32.
385. Jiang, W. Q, L. Szekely, V. Wendel-Hansen, N. Ringertz, Klein G, A. Rosen. 1991. Co-localization of the retinoblastoma protein and the Epstein-Barr virus-encoded nuclear antigen EBNA-5. *Exp Cell Res* 197:314–8.
386. Jin, X. W, S. H. Speck. 1992. Identification of critical cis elements involved in mediating Epstein-Barr virus nuclear antigen 2-dependent activity of an enhancer located upstream of the viral *Bam*HI C promoter. *J Virol* 66:2846–52.
387. Joab, I, D. T. Rowe, M. Bodescot, J. C. Nicolas, Farrell PJ, M. Perricaudet. 1987. Mapping of the gene coding for Epstein-Barr virus-determined nuclear antigen EBNA3 and its transient overexpression in a human cell line by using an adenovirus expression vector. *J Virol* 61:3340–4.
388. Johannsen, E, E. Koh, G. Mosialos, X. Tong, Kieff E, S. R. Grossman. 1995. Epstein-Barr virus nuclear protein 2 transactivation of the latent membrane protein 1 promoter is mediated by J kappa and PU.1. *J Virol* 69:253–62.
389. Johannsen, E, C. L. Miller, S. R. Grossman, Kieff E. 1996. EBNA-2 and EBNA-3C extensively and mutually exclusively associate with RBPJkappa in Epstein-Barr virus-transformed B lymphocytes. *J Virol* 70:4179–83.
390. Jondal, M, Klein G, M. B. Oldstone, V. Bokish, E. Yefenof. 1976. Surface markers on human B and T lymphocytes. VIII. Association between complement and Epstein-Barr virus receptors on human lymphoid cells. *Scand J Immunol* 5:401–10.
391. Jones, C. H, Hayward SD, D. R. Rawlins. 1989. Interaction of the lymphocyte-derived Epstein-Barr virus nuclear antigen EBNA-1 with its DNA-binding sites. *J Virol* 63:101–10.
392. Jones, M. D, L. Foster, T. Sheedy, B. E. Griffin. 1984. The EB virus genome in Daudi Burkitt's lymphoma cells has a deletion similar to that observed in a non-transforming strain (P3HR-1) of the virus. *EMBO J* 3:813–21.
393. Jox, A, C. Rohen, G. Belge, S. Bartnitzke, M. Pawlita, V. Diehl, J. Bullerdiek, J. Wolf. 1997. Integration of Epstein-Barr virus in Burkitt's lymphoma cells leads to a region of enhanced chromosome instability. *Ann Oncol* 8:131–5.
394. Kaiser, C, G. Laux, D. Eick, N. Jochner, G. W. Bornkamm, B. Kempkes. 1999. The proto-oncogene c-*myc* is a direct target gene of Epstein-Barr virus nuclear antigen 2. *J Virol* 73:4481–4.
395. Kallin, B, J. Dillner, I. Ernberg, B. Ehlin-Henriksson, A. Rosen, W. Henle, G. Henle, Klein G. 1986. Four virally determined nuclear antigens are expressed in Epstein-Barr virus-transformed cells. *Proc Natl Acad Sci U S A* 83:1499–503.
396. Kallin, B, L. Sternas, A. K. Saemundssen, J. Luka, H. Jornvall, B. Eriksson, P. Z. Tao, M. T. Nilsson, Klein G. 1985. Purification of Epstein-Barr virus DNA polymerase from P3HR-1 cells. *J Virol* 54:561–8.

397. Kanegane, H, T. Wado, K. Nunogami, H. Seki, N. Taniguchi, G. Tosato. 1996. Chronic persistent Epstein-Barr virus infection of natural killer cells and B cells associated with granular lymphocytes expansion. *Br J Haematol* 95:116–22.
398. Kanegane, H, A. Yachie, T. Miyawaki, G. Tosato. 1998. EBV-NK cells interactions and lymphoproliferative disorders. *Leuk Lymphoma* 29:491–8.
399. Karran, L, Y. Gao, P. R. Smith, B. E. Griffin. 1992. Expression of a family of complementary-strand transcripts in Epstein-Barr virus-infected cells. *Proc Natl Acad Sci U S A* 89:8058–62.
400. Kaschka-Dierich, C, A. Adams, T. Lindahl, G. W. Bornkamm, G. Bjursell, Klein G, B. C. Giovanella, S. Singh. 1976. Intracellular forms of Epstein-Barr virus DNA in human tumour cells *in vivo*. *Nature* 260:302–6.
401. Kashuba, E, V. Kashuba, K. Pokrovskaja, Klein G, L. Szekely. 2000. Epstein-Barr virus encoded nuclear protein EBNA-3 binds XAP-2, a protein associated with Hepatitis B virus X antigen. *Oncogene* 19: 1801–6.
402. Kashuba, E, K. Pokrovskaja, Klein G, L. Szekely. 1999. Epstein-Barr virus-encoded nuclear protein EBNA-3 interacts with the epsilon-subunit of the T-complex protein 1 chaperonin complex. *J Hum Virol* 2: 33–7.
403. Katsuki, T, Y. Hinuma. 1976. A quantitative analysis of the susceptibility of human leukocytes to transformation by Epstein-Barr virus. *Int J Cancer* 18:7–13.
404. Katz, D. A, R. P. Baumann, R. Sun, J. L. Kolman, N. Taylor, G. Miller. 1992. Viral proteins associated with the Epstein-Barr virus transactivator, ZEBRA. *Proc Natl Acad Sci U S A* 89:378–82.
405. Kawai, Y, M. Nonoyama, J. S. Pagano. 1973. Reassociation kinetics for Epstein-Barr virus DNA: Nonhomology to mammalian DNA and homology of viral DNA in various diseases. *J Virol* 12:1006–12.
406. Kawanishi, M. 1993. Epstein-Barr virus induces fragmentation of chromosomal DNA during lytic infection. *J Virol* 67:7654–8.
407. Kawanishi, M. 1993. Topoisomerase I and II activities are required for Epstein-Barr virus replication. *J Gen Virol* 74:2263–8.
408. Kaye, K. M, O. Devergne, J. N. Harada, K. M. Izumi, R. Yalamanchili, Kieff E, G. Mosialos. 1996. Tumor necrosis factor receptor associated factor 2 is a mediator of NF-kappa B activation by latent infection membrane protein 1, the Epstein-Barr virus transforming protein. *Proc Natl Acad Sci U S A* 93:11085–90.
409. Kaye, K. M, K. M. Izumi, Kieff E. 1993. Epstein-Barr virus latent membrane protein 1 is essential for B-lymphocyte growth transformation. *Proc Natl Acad Sci U S A* 90:9150–4.
410. Kaye, K. M, K. M. Izumi, H. Li, E. Johannsen, D. Davidson, Longnecker R, Kieff E. 1999. An Epstein-Barr virus that expresses only the first 231 LMP1 amino acids efficiently initiates primary B-lymphocyte growth transformation. *J Virol* 73:10525–30.
411. Kaye, K. M, K. M. Izumi, G. Mosialos, Kieff E. 1995. The Epstein-Barr virus LMP1 cytoplasmic carboxy terminus is essential for B-lymphocyte transformation; fibroblast cocultivation complements a critical function within the terminal 155 residues. *J Virol* 69:675–83.
412. Kempkes, B, D. Pich, R. Zeidler, B. Sugden, W. Hammerschmidt. 1995. Immortalization of human B lymphocytes by a plasmid containing 71 kilobase pairs of Epstein-Barr virus DNA. *J Virol* 69:231–8.
413. Kenney, S, E. Holley-Guthrie, E. C. Mar, M. Smith. 1989. The Epstein-Barr virus BMLF1 promoter contains an enhancer element that is responsive to the BZLF1 and BRLF1 transactivators. *J Virol* 63: 3878–83.
414. Kenney, S, J. Kamine, E. Holley-Guthrie, J. C. Lin, E. C. Mar, J. Pagano. 1989. The Epstein-Barr virus (EBV) BZLF1 immediate-early gene product differentially affects latent versus productive EBV promoters. *J Virol* 63:1729–36.
415. Kenney, S, J. Kamine, E. Holley-Guthrie, E. C. Mar, J. C. Lin, D. Markovitz, J. Pagano. 1989. The Epstein-Barr virus immediate-early gene product, BMLF1, acts in trans by a posttranscriptional mechanism which is reporter gene dependent. *J Virol* 63:3870–7.
416. Kenney, S, J. Kamine, D. Markovitz, R. Fenrick, J. Pagano. 1988. An Epstein-Barr virus immediate-early gene product trans-activates gene expression from the human immunodeficiency virus long terminal repeat. *Proc Natl Acad Sci U S A* 85:1652–6.
417. Kenney, S. C, E. Holley-Guthrie, E. B. Quinlivan, D. Gutsch, Q. Zhang, T. Bender, J. F. Giot, A. Sergeant. 1992. The cellular oncogene c-myb can interact synergistically with the Epstein-Barr virus BZLF1 transactivator in lymphoid cells. *Mol Cell Biol* 12:136–46.
418. Kerdiles, B, D. Walls, H. Triki, M. Perricaudet, I. Joab. 1990. cDNA cloning and transient expression of the Epstein-Barr virus-determined nuclear antigen EBNA3B in human cells and identification of novel transcripts from its coding region. *J Virol* 64:1812–6.
419. Khanim, F, Q. Y. Yao, G. Niedobitek, S. Sihota, A. B. Rickinson, L. S. Young. 1996. Analysis of Epstein-Barr virus gene polymorphisms in normal donors and in virus-associated tumors from different geographic locations. *Blood* 88:3491–501.
420. Kiehl, A, D. I. Dorsky. 1991. Cooperation of EBV DNA polymerase and EA-D(BMRF1) *in vitro* and colocalization in nuclei of infected cells. *Virology* 184:330–40.
421. Kienzle, N, M. Buck, S. Greco, K. Krauer, T. B. Sculley. 1999. Epstein-barr virus-encoded RK-BARF0 protein expression. *J Virol* 73:8902–6.
422. Kienzle, N, T. B. Sculley, L. Poulsen, M. Buck, S. Cross, N. Raab-Traub, R. Khanna. 1998. Identification of a cytotoxic T-lymphocyte response to the novel BARF0 protein of Epstein-Barr virus: A critical role for antigen expression. *J Virol* 72:6614–20.
423. Kieser, A, E. Kilger, O. Gires, M. Ueffing, W. Kolch, W. Hammerschmidt. 1997. Epstein-Barr virus latent membrane protein-1 triggers AP-1 activity via the c-Jun N-terminal kinase cascade. *EMBO J* 16: 6478–85.
424. Kilger, E, A. Kieser, M. Baumann, W. Hammerschmidt. 1998. Epstein-Barr virus-mediated B-cell proliferation is dependent upon latent membrane protein 1, which simulates an activated CD40 receptor. *EMBO J* 17:1700–9.
425. Kim, O. J, J. L. Yates. 1993. Mutants of Epstein-Barr virus with a selective marker disrupting the TP gene transform B cells and replicate normally in culture. *J Virol* 67:7634–40.
426. King, W, T. Dambaugh, M. Heller, J. Dowling, Kieff E. 1982. Epstein-Barr virus DNA XII. A variable region of the Epstein-Barr virus genome is included in the P3HR-1 deletion. *J Virol* 43:979–86.
427. King, W, A. L. Thomas-Powell, N. Raab-Traub, M. Hawke, Kieff E. 1980. Epstein-Barr virus RNA. V. Viral RNA in a restringently infected, growth-transformed cell line. *J Virol* 36:506–18.
428. King, W, V. Van Santen, Kieff E. 1981. Epstein-Barr virus RNA. VI. Viral RNA in restringently and abortively infected Raji cells. *J Virol* 38:649–60.
429. Kintner, C, B. Sugden. 1981. Conservation and progressive methylation of Epstein-Barr viral DNA sequences in transformed cells. *J Virol* 38:305–16.
430. Kintner, C. R, B. Sugden. 1979. The structure of the termini of the DNA of Epstein-Barr virus. *Cell* 17:661–71.
431. Kirchmaier, A. L, B. Sugden. 1995. Plasmid maintenance of derivatives of oriP of Epstein-Barr virus. *J Virol* 69:1280–3.
432. Kirchmaier, A. L, B. Sugden. 1998. Rep*: A viral element that can partially replace the origin of plasmid DNA synthesis of Epstein-Barr virus. *J Virol* 72:4657–66.
433. Kitay, M. K, D. T. Rowe. 1996. Cell cycle stage-specific phosphorylation of the Epstein-Barr virus immortalization protein EBNA-LP. *J Virol* 70:7885–93.
434. Kitay, M. K, D. T. Rowe. 1996. Protein-protein interactions between Epstein-Barr virus nuclear antigen-LP and cellular gene products: Binding of 70-kilodalton heat shock proteins. *Virology* 220:91–9.
435. Klein, G, B. Sugden, W. Leibold, J. Menezes. 1974. Infection of EBV-genome-negative and –positive human lymphoblastoid cell lines with biologically different preparations of EBV. *Intervirology* 3:232–44.
436. Klein, S. C, D. Kube, H. Abts, V. Diehl, H. Tesch. 1996. Promotion of IL8, IL10, TNF alpha and TNF beta production by EBV infection. *Leuk Res* 20:633–6.
437. Knutson, J. C. 1990. The level of c-fgr RNA is increased by EBNA-2, an Epstein-Barr virus gene required for B-cell immortalization. *J Virol* 64:2530–6.
438. Koizumi, S, X. K. Zhang, S. Imai, M. Sugiura, N. Usui, T. Osato. 1992. Infection of the HTLV-I-harbouring T-lymphoblastoid line MT-2 by Epstein-Barr virus. *Virology* 188:859–63.
439. Kolman, J. L, N. Taylor, D. R. Marshak, G. Miller. 1993. Serine-173 of the Epstein-Barr virus ZEBRA protein is required for DNA binding and is a target for casein kinase II phosphorylation. *Proc Natl Acad Sci U S A* 90:10115–9.
440. Komano, J, S. Maruo, K. Kurozumi, T. Oda, K. Takada. 1999. Oncogenic role of Epstein-Barr virus-encoded RNAs in Burkitt's lymphoma cell line Akata. *J Virol* 73:9827–31.
441. Komano, J, M. Sugiura, K. Takada. 1998. Epstein-Barr virus con-

tributes to the malignant phenotype and to apoptosis resistance in Burkitt's lymphoma cell line Akata. *J Virol* 72:9150–6.
442. Kouzarides, T, A. T. Bankier, S. C. Satchwell, K. Weston, P. Tomlinson, B. G. Barrell. 1987. Large-scale rearrangement of homologous regions in the genomes of HCMV and EBV. *Virology* 157:397–413.
443. Kouzarides, T, G. Packham, A. Cook, Farrell PJ. 1991. The BZLF1 protein of EBV has a coiled coil dimerisation domain without a heptad leucine repeat but with homology to the C/EBP leucine zipper. *Oncogene* 6:195–204.
444. Kozak, M. 1989. The scanning model for translation: An update. *J Cell Biol* 108:229–41.
445. Krauer, K. G, D. K. Belzer, D. Liaskou, M. Buck, S. Cross, T. Honjo, T. Sculley. 1998. Regulation of interleukin-1beta transcription by Epstein-Barr virus involves a number of latent proteins via their interaction with RBP. *Virology* 252:418–30.
446. Krauer, K. G, N. Kienzle, D. B. Young, T. B. Sculley. 1996. Epstein-Barr nuclear antigen-3 and -4 interact with RBP-2N, a major isoform of RBP-J kappa in B lymphocytes. *Virology* 226:346–53.
447. Krysan, P. J, M. P. Calos. 1993. Epstein-Barr virus-based vectors that replicate in rodent cells. Gene. 136:137–43.
448. Krysan, P. J, S. B. Haase, M. P. Calos. 1989. Isolation of human sequences that replicate autonomously in human cells. *Mol Cell Biol* 9:1026–33.
449. Kulwichit, W, R. H. Edwards, E. M. Davenport, J. F. Baskar, V. Godfrey, N. Raab-Traub. 1998. Expression of the Epstein-Barr virus latent membrane protein 1 induces B cell lymphoma in transgenic mice. *Proc Natl Acad Sci U S A* 95:11963–8.
450. Kupfer, S. R, W. C. Summers. 1990. Identification of a glucocorticoid-responsive element in Epstein-Barr virus. *J Virol* 64:1984–90.
451. Kurilla, M. G, T. Heineman, L. C. Davenport, Kieff E, L. M. Hutt-Fletcher. 1995. A novel Epstein-Barr virus glycoprotein gp150 expressed from the BDLF3 open reading frame. *Virology* 209:108–21.
452. Kusano, S, N. Raab-Traub. 2001. An Epstein-Barr virus protein interacts with notch [In Process Citation]. *J Virol* 75:384–95.
453. Laherty, C. D, H. M. Hu, A. W. Opipari, F. Wang, V. M. Dixit. 1992. The Epstein-Barr virus LMP1 gene product induces A20 zinc finger protein expression by activating nuclear factor kappa B. *J Biol Chem* 267:24157–60.
454. Lake, C. M, L. M. Hutt-Fletcher. 2000. Epstein-barr virus that lacks glycoprotein gN is impaired in assembly and infection. *J Virol* 74:11162–72.
455. Lake, C. M, S. J. Molesworth, L. M. Hutt-Fletcher. 1998. The Epstein-Barr virus (EBV) gN homolog BLRF1 encodes a 15-kilodalton glycoprotein that cannot be authentically processed unless it is coexpressed with the EBV gM homolog BBRF3. *J Virol* 72:5559–64.
456. Lambris, J. D, V. S. Ganu, S. Hirani, H. J. Muller-Eberhard. 1985. Mapping of the C3d receptor (CR2)-binding site and a neoantigenic site in the C3d domain of the third component of complement. *Proc Natl Acad Sci U S A* 82:4235–9.
457. Landon, J. C, L. B. Ellis, V. H. Zeve, D. P. Fabrizio. 1968. Herpes-type virus in cultured leukocytes from chimpanzees. *J Natl Cancer Inst* 40:181–92.
458. Larocca, D, W. Clough. 1982. Hypomethylation of Epstein-Barr virus DNA in the nonproducer B-cell line EBR. *J Virol* 43:1129–31.
459. Larocca, D, D. Homisak, W. Clough. 1981. Synthesis of hypomethylated Epstein-Barr viral DNA is stimulated by dimethylsulfoxide treatment of lymphoblastoid cells. *Biochem Biophys Res Commun* 100:559–65.
460. Laux, G, B. Adam, L. J. Strobl, F. Moreau-Gachelin. 1994. The Spi-1/PU.1 and Spi-B Ets family transcription factors and the recombination signal binding protein RBP-J kappa interact with an Epstein-Barr virus nuclear antigen 2 responsive cis-element. *EMBO J* 13:5624–32.
461. Laux, G, F. Dugrillon, C. Eckert, B. Adam, U. Zimber-Strobl, G. W. Bornkamm. 1994. Identification and characterization of an Epstein-Barr virus nuclear antigen 2-responsive cis element in the bidirectional promoter region of latent membrane protein and terminal protein 2 genes. *J Virol* 68:6947–58.
462. Laux, G, A. Economou, Farrell PJ. 1989. The terminal protein gene 2 of Epstein-Barr virus is transcribed from a bidirectional latent promoter region. *J Gen Virol* 70:3079–84.
463. Laux, G, U. K. Freese, G. W. Bornkamm. 1985. Structure and evolution of two related transcription units of Epstein-Barr virus carrying small tandem repeats. *J Virol* 56:987–95.
464. Laux, G, U. K. Freese, R. Fischer, A. Polack, E. Kofler, G. W. Bornkamm. 1988. TPA-inducible Epstein-Barr virus genes in Raji cells and their regulation. *Virology* 162:503–7.
465. Laux, G, M. Perricaudet, Farrell PJ. 1988. A spliced Epstein-Barr virus gene expressed in immortalized lymphocytes is created by circularization of the linear viral genome. *EMBO J* 7:769–74.
466. Lawrence, J. B, R. H. Singer, L. M. Marselle. 1989. Highly localized tracks of specific transcripts within interphase nuclei visualized by in situ hybridization. *Cell* 57:493–502.
467. Lawrence, J. B, C. A. Villnave, R. H. Singer. 1988. Sensitive, high-resolution chromatin and chromosome mapping in situ: Presence and orientation of two closely integrated copies of EBV in a lymphoma line. *Cell* 52:51–61.
468. Le Roux, A, B. Kerdiles, D. Walls, J. F. Dedieu, M. Perricaudet. 1994. The Epstein-Barr virus determined nuclear antigens EBNA-3A, -3B, and -3C repress EBNA-2-mediated transactivation of the viral terminal protein 1 gene promoter. *Virology* 205:596–602.
469. Lee, M. A, M. E. Diamond, J. L. Yates. 1999. Genetic evidence that EBNA-1 is needed for efficient, stable latent infection by Epstein-Barr virus. *J Virol* 73:2974–82.
470. Lee, M. A, O. J. Kim, J. L. Yates. 1992. Targeted gene disruption in Epstein-Barr virus. *Virology* 189:253–65.
471. Lee, M. A, J. L. Yates. 1992. BHRF1 of Epstein-Barr virus, which is homologous to human proto-oncogene bcl2, is not essential for transformation of B cells or for virus replication *in vitro*. *J Virol* 66: 1899–906.
472. Lee, S. K, Longnecker R. 1997. The Epstein-Barr virus glycoprotein 110 carboxy-terminal tail domain is essential for lytic virus replication. *J Virol* 71:4092–7.
473. Lee, W, P. Mitchell, R. Tjian. 1987. Purified transcription factor AP-1 interacts with TPA-inducible enhancer elements. *Cell* 49:741–52.
474. Lee, Y. S, A. Tanaka, R. Y. Lau, M. Nonoyama, H. Rabin. 1981. Linkage map of the fragments of herpesvirus papio DNA. *J Virol* 37: 710–20.
475. Lerner, M. R, N. C. Andrews, G. Miller, J. A. Steitz. 1981. Two small RNAs encoded by Epstein-Barr virus and complexed with protein are precipitated by antibodies from patients with systemic lupus erythematosus. *Proc Natl Acad Sci U S A* 78:805–9.
476. Leverson, J. D, P. J. Koskinen, F. C. Orrico, E. M. Rainio, K. J. Jalkanen, A. B. Dash, R. N. Eisenman, S. A. Ness. 1998. Pim-1 kinase and p100 cooperate to enhance c-Myb activity. Mol *Cell* 2:417–25.
477. Levitskaya, J, A. Sharipo, A. Leonchiks, A. Ciechanover, M. G. Masucci. 1997. Inhibition of ubiquitin/proteasome-dependent protein degradation by the Gly-Ala repeat domain of the Epstein-Barr virus nuclear antigen 1. *Proc Natl Acad Sci U S A* 94:12616–21.
478. Lewin, N, J. Minarovits, G. Weber, B. Ehlin-Henriksson, T. Wen, H. Mellstedt, Klein G, Klein E. 1991. Clonality and methylation status of the Epstein-Barr virus (EBV) genomes in *in vivo*-infected EBV-carrying chronic lymphocytic leukemia (CLL) cell lines. *Int J Cancer* 48:62–6.
479. Li, Q, M. K. Spriggs, S. Kovats, S. M. Turk, M. R. Comeau, B. Nepom, L. M. Hutt-Fletcher. 1997. Epstein-Barr virus uses HLA class II as a cofactor for infection of B lymphocytes. *J Virol* 71:4657–62.
480. Li, Q, S. M. Turk, L. M. Hutt-Fletcher. 1995. The Epstein-Barr virus (EBV) BZLF2 gene product associates with the gH and gL homologs of EBV and carries an epitope critical to infection of B cells but not of epithelial cells. *J Virol* 69:3987–94.
481. Li, Q. X, L. S. Young, G. Niedobitek, C. W. Dawson, M. Birkenbach, F. Wang, A. B. Rickinson. 1992. Epstein-Barr virus infection and replication in a human epithelial cell system. *Nature* 356:347–50.
482. Lieberman, P. 1994. Identification of functional targets of the Zta transcriptional activator by formation of stable preinitiation complex intermediates. *Mol Cell Biol* 14:8365–75.
483. Lieberman, P. M, A. J. Berk. 1990. *In vitro* transcriptional activation, dimerization, and DNA-binding specificity of the Epstein-Barr virus Zta protein. *J Virol* 64:2560–8.
484. Lieberman, P. M, A. J. Berk. 1994. A mechanism for TAFs in transcriptional activation: Activation domain enhancement of TFIID-TFIIA–promoter DNA complex formation. *Genes Dev* 8:995–1006.
485. Lieberman, P. M, A. J. Berk. 1991. The Zta trans-activator protein stabilizes TFIID association with promoter DNA by direct protein-protein interaction. *Genes Dev* 5:2441–54.
486. Lieberman, P. M, J. M. Hardwick, J. Sample, G. S. Hayward, Hayward SD. 1990. The zta transactivator involved in induction of lytic cycle gene expression in Epstein-Barr virus-infected lymphocytes binds to

both AP-1 and ZRE sites in target promoter and enhancer regions. *J Virol* 64:1143–55.
487. Lieberman, P. M, P. O'Hare, G. S. Hayward, Hayward SD. 1986. Promiscuous trans activation of gene expression by an Epstein-Barr virus-encoded early nuclear protein. *J Virol* 60:140–8.
488. Lieberman, P. M, J. Ozer, D. B. Gursel. 1997. Requirement for transcription factor IIA (TFIIA)-TFIID recruitment by an activator depends on promoter structure and template competition. *Mol Cell Biol* 17:6624–32.
489. Liebowitz, D, Kieff E. 1989. Epstein-Barr virus latent membrane protein: Induction of B-cell activation antigens and membrane patch formation does not require vimentin. *J Virol* 63:4051–4.
490. Liebowitz, D, R. Kopan, E. Fuchs, J. Sample, Kieff E. 1987. An Epstein-Barr virus transforming protein associates with vimentin in lymphocytes. *Mol Cell Biol* 7:2299–308.
491. Liebowitz, D, J. Mannick, K. Takada, Kieff E. 1992. Phenotypes of Epstein-Barr virus LMP1 deletion mutants indicate transmembrane and amino-terminal cytoplasmic domains necessary for effects in B-lymphoma cells. *J Virol* 66:4612–6.
492. Liebowitz, D, D. Wang, Kieff E. 1986. Orientation and patching of the latent infection membrane protein encoded by Epstein-Barr virus. *J Virol* 58:233–7.
493. Lin, J. C, E. DeClercq, J. S. Pagano. 1987. Novel acyclic adenosine analogs inhibit Epstein-Barr virus replication. *Antimicrob Agents Chemother* 31:1431–3.
494. Lin, J. C, H. Machida. 1988. Comparison of two bromovinyl nucleoside analogs, 1-beta-D-arabinofuranosyl-E-5-(2-bromovinyl)uracil and E-5-(2-bromovinyl)-2′-deoxyuridine, with acyclovir in inhibition of Epstein-Barr virus replication. *Antimicrob Agents Chemother* 32: 1068–72.
495. Lin, J. C, Z. X. Zhang, M. C. Smith, K. Biron, J. S. Pagano. 1988. Anti-human immunodeficiency virus agent 3′-azido-3′-deoxythymidine inhibits replication of Epstein-Barr virus. *Antimicrob Agents Chemother* 32:265–7.
496. Lindahl, T, A. Adams, G. Bjursell, G. W. Bornkamm, C. Kaschka-Dierich, U. Jehn. 1976. Covalently closed circular duplex DNA of Epstein-Barr virus in a human lymphoid cell line. *J Mol Biol* 102: 511–30.
497. Ling, P. D, Hayward SD. 1995. Contribution of conserved amino acids in mediating the interaction between EBNA2 and CBF1/RBPJk. *J Virol* 69:1944–50.
498. Ling, P. D, J. J. Hsieh, I. K. Ruf, D. R. Rawlins, Hayward SD. 1994. EBNA-2 upregulation of Epstein-Barr virus latency promoters and the cellular CD23 promoter utilizes a common targeting intermediate, CBF1. *J Virol* 68:5375–83.
499. Ling, P. D, D. R. Rawlins, Hayward SD. 1993. The Epstein-Barr virus immortalizing protein EBNA-2 is targeted to DNA by a cellular enhancer-binding protein. *Proc Natl Acad Sci U S A* 90:9237–41.
500. Ling, P. D, J. J. Ryon, Hayward SD. 1993. EBNA-2 of herpesvirus papio diverges significantly from the type A and type B EBNA-2 proteins of Epstein-Barr virus but retains an efficient transactivation domain with a conserved hydrophobic motif. *J Virol* 67:2990–3003.
501. Little, R. D, C. L. Schildkraut. 1995. Initiation of latent DNA replication in the Epstein-Barr virus genome can occur at sites other than the genetically defined origin. *Mol Cell Biol* 15:2893–903.
502. Littler, E, J. R. Arrand. 1988. Characterization of the Epstein-Barr virus-encoded thymidine kinase expressed in heterologous eucaryotic and procaryotic systems. *J Virol* 62:3892–5.
503. Littler, E, I. W. Halliburton, K. L. Powell, B. W. Snowden, J. R. Arrand. 1988. Immunological conservation between Epstein-Barr virus and herpes simplex virus. *J Gen Virol* 69:2021–31.
504. Littler, E, J. Zeuthen, A. A. McBride, E. Trost Sorensen, K. L. Powell, J. E. Walsh-Arrand, J. R. Arrand. 1986. Identification of an Epstein-Barr virus-coded thymidine kinase. *EMBO J* 5:1959–66.
505. Liu, P, S. Liu, S. H. Speck. 1998. Identification of a negative cis element within the ZII domain of the Epstein-Barr virus lytic switch BZLF1 gene promoter. *J Virol* 72:8230–9.
506. Liu, Q, W. C. Summers. 1992. Identification of the 12–O-tetradecanoylphorbol-13-acetate-responsive enhancer of the MS gene of the Epstein-Barr virus. *J Biol Chem* 267:12049–54.
507. Liu, S, P. Liu, A. Borras, T. Chatila, S. H. Speck. 1997. Cyclosporin A-sensitive induction of the Epstein-Barr virus lytic switch is mediated via a novel pathway involving a MEF2 family member. *EMBO J* 16:143–53.
508. Lombardi, L, E. W. Newcomb, R. Dalla-Favera. 1987. Pathogenesis of Burkitt lymphoma: Expression of an activated c-*myc* oncogene causes the tumorigenic conversion of EBV-infected human B lymphoblasts. *Cell* 49:161–70.
509. Longan, L, Longnecker R. 2000. Epstein-barr virus latent membrane protein 2A has no growth-altering effects when expressed in differentiating epithelia. *J Gen Virol* 81 Pt 9:2245–52.
510. Longnecker, R, B. Druker, T. M. Roberts, Kieff E. 1991. An Epstein-Barr virus protein associated with cell growth transformation interacts with a tyrosine kinase. *J Virol* 65:3681–92.
511. Longnecker, R, Kieff E. 1990. A second Epstein-Barr virus membrane protein (LMP2) is expressed in latent infection and colocalizes with LMP1. *J Virol* 64:2319–26.
512. Longnecker, R, C. L. Miller, X. Q. Miao, A. Marchini, Kieff E. 1992. The only domain which distinguishes Epstein-Barr virus latent membrane protein 2A (LMP2A) from LMP2B is dispensable for lymphocyte infection and growth transformation *in vitro*; LMP2A is therefore nonessential. *J Virol* 66:6461–9.
513. Longnecker, R, C. L. Miller, X. Q. Miao, B. Tomkinson, Kieff E. 1993. The last seven transmembrane and carboxy-terminal cytoplasmic domains of Epstein-Barr virus latent membrane protein 2 (LMP2) are dispensable for lymphocyte infection and growth transformation *in vitro*. *J Virol* 67:2006–13.
514. Longnecker, R, C. L. Miller, B. Tomkinson, X. Q. Miao, Kieff E. 1993. Deletion of DNA encoding the first five transmembrane domains of Epstein-Barr virus latent membrane proteins 2A and 2B. *J Virol* 67:5068–74.
515. Lowe, R. S, P. M. Keller, B. J. Keech, A. J. Davison, Y. Whang, A. J. Morgan, Kieff E, R. W. Ellis. 1987. Varicella-zoster virus as a live vector for the expression of foreign genes. *Proc Natl Acad Sci U S A* 84:3896–900.
516. Luka, J, B. Kallin, Klein G. 1979. Induction of the Epstein-Barr virus (EBV) cycle in latently infected cells by n-butyrate. *Virology* 94: 228–31.
517. Mackett, M, M. J. Conway, J. R. Arrand, R. S. Haddad, L. M. Hutt-Fletcher. 1990. Characterization and expression of a glycoprotein encoded by the Epstein-Barr virus *Bam*HI I fragment. *J Virol* 64: 2545–52.
518. Mackey, D, T. Middleton, B. Sugden. 1995. Multiple regions within EBNA1 can link DNAs. *J Virol* 69:6199–208.
519. Mackey, D, B. Sugden. 1999. The linking regions of EBNA1 are essential for its support of replication and transcription. *Mol Cell Biol* 19:3349–59.
520. Mackey, D, B. Sugden. 1997. Studies on the mechanism of DNA linking by Epstein-Barr virus nuclear antigen 1. *J Biol Chem* 272: 29873–9.
521. Manet, E, C. Allera, H. Gruffat, I. Mikaelian, A. Rigolet, A. Sergeant. 1993. The acidic activation domain of the Epstein-Barr virus transcription factor R interacts *in vitro* with both TBP and TFIIB and is cell-specifically potentiated by a proline-rich region. *Gene Expr* 3:49–59.
522. Manet, E, A. Rigolet, H. Gruffat, J. F. Giot, A. Sergeant. 1991. Domains of the Epstein-Barr virus (EBV) transcription factor R required for dimerization, DNA binding and activation. *Nucleic Acids Res* 19:2661–7.
523. Mann, K. P, D. Staunton, D. A. Thorley-Lawson. 1985. Epstein-Barr virus-encoded protein found in plasma membranes of transformed cells. *J Virol* 55:710–20.
524. Mann, K. P, D. Thorley-Lawson. 1987. Posttranslational processing of the Epstein-Barr virus-encoded p63/LMP protein. *J Virol* 61:2100–8.
525. Mannick, J. B, Cohen JI, M. Birkenbach, A. Marchini, Kieff E. 1991. The Epstein-Barr virus nuclear protein encoded by the leader of the EBNA RNAs is important in B-lymphocyte transformation. *J Virol* 65:6826–37.
526. Mannick, J. B, X. Tong, A. Hemnes, Kieff E. 1995. The Epstein-Barr virus nuclear antigen leader protein associates with hsp72/hsc73. *J Virol* 69:8169–72.
527. Marchini, A, Cohen JI, F. Wang, Kieff E. 1992. A selectable marker allows investigation of a nontransforming Epstein-Barr virus mutant. *J Virol* 66:3214–9.
528. Marchini, A, Kieff E, Longnecker R. 1993. Marker rescue of a transformation-negative Epstein-Barr virus recombinant from an infected Burkitt lymphoma cell line: A method useful for analysis of genes essential for transformation. *J Virol* 67:606–9.

529. Marchini, A, Longnecker R, Kieff E. 1992. Epstein-Barr virus (EBV)-negative B-lymphoma cell lines for clonal isolation and replication of EBV recombinants. *J Virol* 66:4972–81.
530. Marchini, A, B. Tomkinson, Cohen JI, Kieff E. 1991. BHRF1, the Epstein-Barr virus gene with homology to Bc12, is dispensable for B-lymphocyte transformation and virus replication. *J Virol* 65: 5991–6000.
531. Marcu, K. B, S. A. Bossone, A. J. Patel. 1992. myc function and regulation. *Annu Rev Biochem* 61:809–60.
532. Marechal, V, A. Dehee, R. Chikhi-Brachet, T. Piolot, M. Coppey-Moisan, J. C. Nicolas. 1999. Mapping EBNA-1 domains involved in binding to metaphase chromosomes. *J Virol* 73:4385–92.
533. Marschall, M, F. Schwarzmann, U. Leser, B. Oker, P. Alliger, H. Mairhofer, H. Wolf. 1991. The BI'LF4 trans-activator of Epstein-Barr virus is modulated by type and differentiation of the host cell. *Virology* 181:172–9.
534. Marshall, D, C. Sample. 1995. Epstein-Barr virus nuclear antigen 3C is a transcriptional regulator. *J Virol* 69:3624–30.
535. Marshall, W. L, C. Yim, E. Gustafson, T. Graf, D. R. Sage, K. Hanify, L. Williams, J. Fingeroth, R. W. Finberg. 1999. Epstein-Barr virus encodes a novel homolog of the bcl-2 oncogene that inhibits apoptosis and associates with Bax and Bak. *J Virol* 73:5181–5.
536. Martin, D. R, R. L. Marlowe, J. M. Ahearn. 1994. Determination of the role for CD21 during Epstein-Barr virus infection of B-lymphoblastoid cells. *J Virol* 68:4716–26.
537. Martin, D. R, A. Yuryev, K. R. Kalli, D. T. Fearon, J. M. Ahearn. 1991. Determination of the structural basis for selective binding of Epstein-Barr virus to human complement receptor type 2. *J Exp Med* 174: 1299–311.
538. Martin, J, B. Sugden. 1991. Transformation by the oncogenic latent membrane protein correlates with its rapid turnover, membrane localization, and cytoskeletal association. *J Virol* 65:3246–58.
539. Martin, J. M, D. Veis, S. J. Korsmeyer, B. Sugden. 1993. Latent membrane protein of Epstein-Barr virus induces cellular phenotypes independently of expression of Bcl-2. *J Virol* 67:5269–78.
540. Masucci, M. G, B. Contreras-Salazar, E. Ragnar, K. Falk, J. Minarovits, I. Ernberg, Klein G. 1989. 5–Azacytidine up regulates the expression of Epstein-Barr virus nuclear antigen 2 (EBNA-2) through EBNA-6 and latent membrane protein in the Burkitt's lymphoma line rael. *J Virol* 63:3135–41.
541. Masucci, M. G, R. Szigeti, I. Ernberg, C. P. Hu, S. Torsteinsdottir, R. Frade, Klein E. 1987. Activation of B lymphocytes by Epstein-Barr virus/CR2 receptor interaction. *Eur J Immunol* 17:815–20.
542. Masukata, H, H. Satoh, C. Obuse, T. Okazaki. 1993. Autonomous replication of human chromosomal DNA fragments in human cells. *Mol Biol Cell* 4:1121–32.
543. Matsuo, T, M. Heller, L. Petti, E. O'Shiro, Kieff E. 1984. Persistence of the entire Epstein-Barr virus genome integrated into human lymphocyte DNA. *Science* 226:1322–5.
544. Matsushima, K, G. Tosato, D. Benjamin, J. J. Oppenheim. 1985. B-cell-derived interleukin-1 (IL-1)-like factor. II. Sources, effects, and biochemical properties. *Cell Immunol* 94:418–26.
545. McGeoch, D. J, M. A. Dalrymple, A. J. Davison, A. Dolan, M. C. Frame, D. McNab, L. J. Perry, J. E. Scott, P. Taylor. 1988. The complete DNA sequence of the long unique region in the genome of herpes simplex virus type 1. *J Gen Virol* 69:1531–74.
546. Meitinger, C, L. J. Strobl, G. Marschall, G. W. Bornkamm, U. Zimber-Strobl. 1994. Crucial sequences within the Epstein-Barr virus TP1 promoter for EBNA2-mediated transactivation and interaction of EBNA2 with its responsive element. *J Virol* 68:7497–506.
547. Merchant, M, R. G. Caldwell, Longnecker R. 2000. The LMP2A ITAM is essential for providing B cells with development and survival signals *in vivo*. *J Virol* 74:9115–24.
548. Middleton, T, B. Sugden. 1992. EBNA1 can link the enhancer element to the initiator element of the Epstein-Barr virus plasmid origin of DNA replication. *J Virol* 66:489–95.
549. Midgley, R. S, N. W. Blake, Q. Y. Yao, D. Croom-Carter, S. T. Cheung, S. F. Leung, A. T. Chan, P. J. Johnson, D. Huang, A. B. Rickinson, S. P. Lee. 2000. Novel intertypic recombinants of Epstein-Barr virus in the chinese population. *J Virol* 74:1544–8.
550. Mikaelian, I, E. Drouet, V. Marechal, G. Denoyel, J. C. Nicolas, A. Sergeant. 1993. The DNA-binding domain of two bZIP transcription factors, the Epstein-Barr virus switch gene product EB1 and Jun, is a bipartite nuclear targeting sequence. *J Virol* 67:734–42.
551. Miller, C. L, A. L. Burkhardt, J. H. Lee, B. Stealey, Longnecker R, J. B. Bolen, Kieff E. 1995. Integral membrane protein 2 of Epstein-Barr virus regulates reactivation from latency through dominant negative effects on protein-tyrosine kinases. *Immunity* 2:155–66.
552. Miller, C. L, A. L. Burkhardt, J. H. Lee, B. Stealey, Longnecker R, J. B. Bolen, Kieff E. 1995. Integral membrane protein 2 of Epstein-Barr virus regulates reactivation from latency through dominant negative effects on protein-tyrosine kinases. *Immunity* 2:155–66.
553. Miller, C. L, J. H. Lee, Kieff E, A. L. Burkhardt, J. B. Bolen, Longnecker R. 1994. Epstein-Barr virus protein LMP2A regulates reactivation from latency by negatively regulating tyrosine kinases involved in sIg-mediated signal transduction. *Infect Agents Dis* 3:128–36.
554. Miller, C. L, J. H. Lee, Kieff E, Longnecker R. 1994. An integral membrane protein (LMP2) blocks reactivation of Epstein-Barr virus from latency following surface immunoglobulin crosslinking. *Proc Natl Acad Sci U S A* 91:772–6.
555. Miller, C. L, Longnecker R, Kieff E. 1993. Epstein-Barr virus latent membrane protein 2A blocks calcium mobilization in B lymphocytes. *J Virol* 67:3087–94.
556. Miller, G. 1989. The Epstein-Barr virus. In B. Fields and D. Knipe (ed.), *Fields Virology*. Raven, New York.
557. Miller, G. 1989. The switch between EBV latency and replication. *Yale J Biol Med* 62:205–13.
558. Miller, G. 1990. The switch between latency and replication of Epstein-Barr virus. *J Infect Dis* 161:833–44.
559. Miller, G, L. Heston, J. Countryman. 1985. P3HR-1 Epstein-Barr virus with heterogeneous DNA is an independent replicon maintained by cell-to-cell spread. *J Virol* 54:45–52.
560. Miller, G, H. Himmelfarb, L. Heston, J. Countryman, L. Gradoville, R. Baumann, T. Chi, M. Carey. 1993. Comparing regions of the Epstein-Barr virus ZEBRA protein which function as transcriptional activating sequences in Saccharomyces cerevisiae and in B cells. *J Virol* 67:7472–81.
561. Miller, G, M. Lipman. 1973. Comparison of the yield of infectious virus from clones of human and simian lymphoblastoid lines transformed by Epstein-Barr virus. *J Exp Med* 138:1398–412.
562. Miller, G, M. Lipman. 1973. Release of infectious Epstein-Barr virus by transformed marmoset leukocytes. *Proc Natl Acad Sci U S A* 70:190–4.
563. Miller, G, H. Lisco, H. I. Kohn, D. Stitt, J. F. Enders. 1971. Establishment of cell lines from normal adult human blood leukocytes by exposure to Epstein-Barr virus and neutralization by human sera with Epstein-Barr virus antibody. *Proc Soc Exp Biol Med* 137:1459–65.
564. Miller, G, M. Rabson, L. Heston. 1984. Epstein-Barr virus with heterogeneous DNA disrupts latency. *J Virol* 50:174–82.
565. Miller, G, J. Robinson, L. Heston, M. Lipman. 1975. Differences between laboratory strains of Epstein-Barr virus based on immortalization, abortive infection and interference. *IARC Sci Publ* 11:395–408.
566. Miller, G, J. Robinson, L. Heston, M. Lipman. 1974. Differences between laboratory strains of Epstein-Barr virus based on immortalization, abortive infection, and interference. *Proc Natl Acad Sci U S A* 71:4006–10.
567. Miller, G, T. Shope, H. Lisco, D. Stitt, M. Lipman. 1972. Epstein-Barr virus: Transformation, cytopathic changes, and viral antigens in squirrel monkey and marmoset leukocytes. *Proc Natl Acad Sci U S A* 69:383–7.
568. Miller, N, L. M. Hutt-Fletcher. 1988. A monoclonal antibody to glycoprotein gp85 inhibits fusion but not attachment of Epstein-Barr virus. *J Virol* 62:2366–72.
569. Miller, W. E, J. L. Cheshire, A. S. Baldwin, Jr, N. Raab-Traub. 1998. The NPC derived C15 LMP1 protein confers enhanced activation of NF-kappa B and induction of the EGFR in epithelial cells. *Oncogene* 16:1869–77.
570. Miller, W. E, J. L. Cheshire, N. Raab-Traub. 1998. Interaction of tumor necrosis factor receptor-associated factor signaling proteins with the latent membrane protein 1 PXQXT motif is essential for induction of epidermal growth factor receptor expression. *Mol Cell Biol* 18:2835–44.
571. Miller, W. E, H. S. Earp, N. Raab-Traub. 1995. The Epstein-Barr virus latent membrane protein 1 induces expression of the epidermal growth factor receptor. *J Virol* 69:4390–8.
572. Miller, W. E, G. Mosialos, Kieff E, N. Raab-Traub. 1997. Epstein-Barr virus LMP1 induction of the epidermal growth factor receptor is

mediated through a TRAF signaling pathway distinct from NF-kappaB activation. *J Virol* 71:586–94.
573. Milman, G, E. S. Hwang. 1987. Epstein-Barr virus nuclear antigen forms a complex that binds with high concentration dependence to a single DNA-binding site. *J Virol* 61:465–71.
574. Milman, G, A. L. Scott, Cho MS, S. C. Hartman, D. K. Ades, G. S. Hayward, P. F. Ki, J. T. August, Hayward SD. 1985. Carboxyl-terminal domain of the Epstein-Barr virus nuclear antigen is highly immunogenic in man. *Proc Natl Acad Sci U S A* 82:6300–4.
575. Minarovits, J, L. F. Hu, Z. Marcsek, S. Minarovits-Kormuta, Klein G, I. Ernberg. 1992. RNA polymerase III-transcribed EBER 1 and 2 transcription units are expressed and hypomethylated in the major Epstein-Barr virus-carrying cell types. *J Gen Virol* 73:1687–92.
576. Minarovits, J, L. F. Hu, S. Minarovits-Kormuta, Klein G, I. Ernberg. 1994. Sequence-specific methylation inhibits the activity of the Epstein-Barr virus LMP 1 and BCR2 enhancer-promoter regions. *Virology* 200:661–7.
577. Minarovits, J, S. Minarovits-Kormuta, B. Ehlin-Henriksson, K. Falk, Klein G, I. Ernberg. 1991. Host cell phenotype-dependent methylation patterns of Epstein-Barr virus DNA. *J Gen Virol* 72:1591–9.
578. Mitchell, T, B. Sugden. 1995. Stimulation of NF-kappa B-mediated transcription by mutant derivatives of the latent membrane protein of Epstein-Barr virus. *J Virol* 69:2968–76.
579. Miyazaki, I, R. K. Cheung, H. M. Dosch. 1993. Viral interleukin 10 is critical for the induction of B cell growth transformation by Epstein-Barr virus. *J Exp Med* 178:439–47.
580. Mocarski, E. S, B. Roizman. 1982. Structure and role of the herpes simplex virus DNA termini in inversion, circularization and generation of virion DNA. *Cell* 31:89–97.
581. Molesworth, S. J, C. M. Lake, C. M. Borza, S. M. Turk, L. M. Hutt-Fletcher. 2000. Epstein-Barr virus gH is essential for penetration of B cells but also plays a role in attachment of virus to epithelial cells. *J Virol* 74:6324–32.
582. Molina, H, C. Brenner, S. Jacobi, J. Gorka, J. C. Carel, T. Kinoshita, V. M. Holers. 1991. Analysis of Epstein-Barr virus-binding sites on complement receptor 2 (CR2/CD21) using human-mouse chimeras and peptides. At least two distinct sites are necessary for ligand-receptor interaction. *J Biol Chem* 266:12173–9.
583. Montalvo, E. A, Y. Shi, T. E. Shenk, A. J. Levine. 1991. Negative regulation of the BZLF1 promoter of Epstein-Barr virus. *J Virol* 65: 3647–55.
584. Moore, K. W, A. O'Garra, R. de Waal Malefyt, P. Vieira, T. R. Mosmann. 1993. Interleukin-10. *Annu Rev Immunol* 11:165–90.
585. Moore, K. W, F. Rousset, J. Banchereau. 1991. Evolving principles in immunopathology: Interleukin 10 and its relationship to Epstein-Barr virus protein BCRF1. *Springer Semin Immunopathol* 13:157–66.
586. Moore, K. W, P. Vieira, D. F. Fiorentino, M. L. Trounstine, T. A. Khan, T. R. Mosmann. 1990. Homology of cytokine synthesis inhibitory factor (IL-10) to the Epstein-Barr virus gene BCRFI [published erratum appears in Science 1990 Oct 26;250(4980):494]. *Science* 248:1230–4.
587. Moore, M. D, M. J. Cannon, A. Sewall, M. Finlayson, M. Okimoto, G. R. Nemerow. 1991. Inhibition of Epstein-Barr virus infection *in vitro* and *in vivo* by soluble CR2 (CD21) containing two short consensus repeats. *J Virol* 65:3559–65.
588. Moore, M. D, N. R. Cooper, B. F. Tack, G. R. Nemerow. 1987. Molecular cloning of the cDNA encoding the Epstein-Barr virus/C3d receptor (complement receptor type 2) of human B lymphocytes. *Proc Natl Acad Sci U S A* 84:9194–8.
589. Moorthy, R, D. A. Thorley-Lawson. 1990. Processing of the Epstein-Barr virus-encoded latent membrane protein p63/LMP. *J Virol* 64: 829–37.
590. Moorthy, R. K, D. A. Thorley-Lawson. 1993. All three domains of the Epstein-Barr virus-encoded latent membrane protein LMP-1 are required for transformation of rat-1 fibroblasts. *J Virol* 67:1638–46.
591. Moorthy, R. K, D. A. Thorley-Lawson. 1993. Biochemical, genetic, and functional analyses of the phosphorylation sites on the Epstein-Barr virus-encoded oncogenic latent membrane protein LMP-1. *J Virol* 67:2637–45.
592. Morgan, A. J, M. Mackett, S. Finerty, J. R. Arrand, F. T. Scullion, M. A. Epstein. 1988. Recombinant vaccinia virus expressing Epstein-Barr virus glycoprotein gp340 protects cottontop tamarins against EB virus-induced malignant lymphomas. *J Med Virol* 25:189–95.
593. Mosialos, G, M. Birkenbach, R. Yalamanchili, T. VanArsdale, C. Ware, Kieff E. 1995. The Epstein-Barr virus transforming protein LMP1 engages signaling proteins for the tumor necrosis factor receptor family. *Cell* 80:389–99.
594. Moss, D. J, S. R. Burrows, P. G. Parsons. 1984. Calcium concentration defines two stages in transformation of lymphocytes by Epstein-Barr virus. *Int J Cancer* 33:587–90.
595. Moss, D. J, A. B. Rickinson, L. E. Wallace, M. A. Epstein. 1981. Sequential appearance of Epstein-Barr virus nuclear and lymphocyte-detected membrane antigens in B cell transformation. *Nature* 291: 664–6.
596. Moss, D. J, T. B. Sculley, J. H. Pope. 1986. Induction of Epstein-Barr virus nuclear antigens. *J Virol* 58:988–90.
597. Mueller-Lantzsch, N, B. Georg, N. Yamamoto, H. zur Hausen. 1980. Epstein-Barr virus-induced proteins. III. Analysis of polypeptides from P3HR-1–EBV-superinfected NC37 cells by immunoprecipitation. *Virology* 102:231–3.
598. Nagoya, T, Y. Hinuma. 1972. Production of infective Epstein-Barr virus in a Burkitt lymphoma cell line, P3HR-1. *Gann* 63:87–93.
599. Nakagomi, H, R. Dolcetti, M. T. Bejarano, P. Pisa, R. Kiessling, M. G. Masucci. 1994. The Epstein-Barr virus latent membrane protein-1 (LMP1) induces interleukin-10 production in Burkitt lymphoma lines. *Int J Cancer* 57:240–4.
600. Nelsen, B, G. Tian, B. Erman, J. Gregoire, R. Maki, B. Graves, R. Sen. 1993. Regulation of lymphoid-specific immunoglobulin mu heavy chain gene enhancer by ETS-domain proteins. *Science* 261:82–6.
601. Nemerow, G. R, N. R. Cooper. 1984. Early events in the infection of human B lymphocytes by Epstein-Barr virus: The internalization process. *Virology* 132:186–98.
602. Nemerow, G. R, R. A. Houghten, M. D. Moore, N. R. Cooper. 1989. Identification of an epitope in the major envelope protein of Epstein-Barr virus that mediates viral binding to the B lymphocyte EBV receptor (CR2). *Cell* 56:369–77.
603. Nemerow, G. R, C. Mold, V. K. Schwend, V. Tollefson, N. R. Cooper. 1987. Identification of gp350 as the viral glycoprotein mediating attachment of Epstein-Barr virus (EBV) to the EBV/C3d receptor of B cells: Sequence homology of gp350 and C3 complement fragment C3d. *J Virol* 61:1416–20.
604. Nemerow, G. R, J. J. d. Mullen, P. W. Dickson, N. R. Cooper. 1990. Soluble recombinant CR2 (CD21) inhibits Epstein-Barr virus infection. *J Virol* 64:1348–52.
605. Nemerow, G. R, M. F. Siaw, N. R. Cooper. 1986. Purification of the Epstein-Barr virus/C3d complement receptor of human B lymphocytes: Antigenic and functional properties of the purified protein. *J Virol* 58:709–12.
606. Niedobitek, G, L. S. Young, R. Lau, L. Brooks, D. Greenspan, J. S. Greenspan, A. B. Rickinson. 1991. Epstein-Barr virus infection in oral hairy leukoplakia: Virus replication in the absence of a detectable latent phase. *J Gen Virol* 72:3035–46.
607. Nilsson, K. 1971. High-frequency establishment of human immunoglobulin-producing lymphoblastoid lines from normal and malignant lymphoid tissue and peripheral blood. *Int J Cancer* 8:432–42.
608. Nilsson, K, Klein G, W. Henle, G. Henle. 1971. The establishment of lymphoblastoid lines from adult and fetal human lymphoid tissue and its dependence on EBV. *Int J Cancer* 8:443–50.
609. Nitsche, F, A. Bell, A. Rickinson. 1997. Epstein-Barr virus leader protein enhances EBNA-2-mediated transactivation of latent membrane protein 1 expression: A role for the W1W2 repeat domain. *J Virol* 71:6619–28.
610. Nolan, L. A, A. J. Morgan. 1995. The Epstein-Barr virus open reading frame BDLF3 codes for a 100–150 kDa glycoprotein. *J Gen Virol* 76: 1381–92.
611. Nonkwelo, C, E. B. Henson, J. Sample. 1995. Characterization of the Epstein-Barr virus Fp promoter. *Virology* 206:183–95.
612. Nonkwelo, C, I. K. Ruf, J. Sample. 1997. The Epstein-Barr virus EBNA-1 promoter Qp requires an initiator-like element. *J Virol* 71:354–61.
613. Nonkwelo, C, I. K. Ruf, J. Sample. 1997. Interferon-independent and -induced regulation of Epstein-Barr virus EBNA-1 gene transcription in Burkitt lymphoma. *J Virol* 71:6887–97.
614. Nonkwelo, C, J. Skinner, A. Bell, A. Rickinson, J. Sample. 1996. Transcription start sites downstream of the Epstein-Barr virus (EBV) Fp promoter in early-passage Burkitt lymphoma cells define a fourth promoter for expression of the EBV EBNA-1 protein. *J Virol* 70:623–7.
615. Nonkwelo, C. B, W. K. Long. 1993. Regulation of Epstein-Barr virus *Bam*HI-H divergent promoter by DNA methylation. *Virology* 197: 205–15.

616. Nonoyama, M, A. Tanaka. 1975. Plasmid DNA as a possible state of Epstein-Barr virus genomes in nonproductive cells. *Cold Spring Harb Symp Quant Biol* 39:807–10.
617. Norio, P, C. L. Schildkraut, J. L. Yates. 2000. Initiation of DNA replication within oriP is dispensable for stable replication of the latent Epstein-Barr virus chromosome after infection of established cell lines. *J Virol* 74:8563–74.
618. North, J. R, A. J. Morgan, M. A. Epstein. 1980. Observations on the EB virus envelope and virus-determined membrane antigen (MA) polypeptides. *Int J Cancer* 26:231–40.
619. Nucifora, G, C. R. Begy, P. Erickson, H. A. Drabkin, J. D. Rowley. 1993. The 3;21 translocation in myelodysplasia results in a fusion transcript between the AML1 gene and the gene for EAP, a highly conserved protein associated with the Epstein-Barr virus small RNA EBER 1. *Proc Natl Acad Sci U S A* 90:7784–8.
620. Nuebling, C. M, N. Mueller-Lantzsch. 1989. Identification and characterization of an Epstein-Barr virus early antigen that is encoded by the NotI repeats. *J Virol* 63:4609–15.
621. Nuebling, C. M, N. Mueller-Lantzsch. 1991. Identification of the gene product encoded by the PstI repeats (IR4) of the Epstein-Barr virus genome. *Virology* 185:519–23.
622. Oba, D. E, L. M. Hutt-Fletcher. 1988. Induction of antibodies to the Epstein-Barr virus glycoprotein gp85 with a synthetic peptide corresponding to a sequence in the BXLF2 open reading frame. *J Virol* 62: 1108–14.
623. Oda, T, S. Imai, S. Chiba, K. Takada. 2000. Epstein-barr virus lacking glycoprotein gp85 cannot infect B cells and epithelial cells. *Virology* 276:52–8.
624. Oguro, M. O, N. Shimizu, Y. Ono, K. Takada. 1987. Both the rightward and the leftward open reading frames within the *Bam*HI M DNA fragment of Epstein-Barr virus act as trans-activators of gene expression. *J Virol* 61:3310–3.
625. Ohno, S, J. Luka, T. Lindahl, Klein G. 1977. Identification of a purified complement-fixing antigen as the Epstein-Barr-virus determined nuclear antigen (EBNA) by its binding to metaphase chromosomes. *Proc Natl Acad Sci U S A* 74:1605–9.
626. Ooka, T, A. Calender. 1980. Effects of arabinofuranosylthymine on Epstein-Barr virus replication. *Virology* 104:219–23.
627. Ooka, T, M. De Turenne, G. De The, J. Daillie. 1984. Epstein-Barr virus-specific DNase activity in nonproducer Raji cells after treatment with 12-o-tetradecanoylphorbol-13-acetate and sodium butyrate. *J Virol* 49:626–8.
628. Orellana, T, Kieff E. 1977. Epstein-barr virus-specific RNA. II. Analysis of polyadenylated viral RNA in restringent, abortive, and productive infections. *J Virol* 22:321–30.
629. Ou, Q, J. F. Mouillet, X. Yan, C. Dorn, P. A. Crawford, Y. Sadovsky. 2001. The DEAD Box Protein DP103 Is a Regulator of Steroidogenic Factor-1. *Mol Endocrinol* 15:69–79.
630. Packham, G, M. Brimmell, D. Cook, A. J. Sinclair, Farrell PJ. 1993. Strain variation in Epstein-Barr virus immediate early genes. *Virology* 192:541–50.
631. Papworth, M. A, A. A. Van Dijk, G. R. Benyon, T. D. Allen, J. R. Arrand, M. Mackett. 1997. The processing, transport and heterologous expression of Epstein-Barr virus gp110. *J Gen Virol* 78:2179–89.
632. Parker, B. D, A. Bankier, S. Satchwell, B. Barrell, Farrell PJ. 1990. Sequence and transcription of Raji Epstein-Barr virus DNA spanning the B95-8 deletion region. *Virology* 179:339–46.
633. Parker, G. A, T. Crook, M. Bain, E. A. Sara, Farrell PJ, M. J. Allday. 1996. Epstein-Barr virus nuclear antigen (EBNA)3C is an immortalizing oncoprotein with similar properties to adenovirus E1A and papillomavirus E7. *Oncogene* 13:2541–9.
634. Parker, G. A, R. Touitou, M. J. Allday. 2000. Epstein-Barr virus EBNA3C can disrupt multiple cell cycle checkpoints and induce nuclear division divorced from cytokinesis. *Oncogene* 19:700–9.
635. Patarroyo, M, E. A. Clark, J. Prieto, C. Kantor, C. G. Gahmberg. 1987. Identification of a novel adhesion molecule in human leukocytes by monoclonal antibody LB-2. *FEBS Lett* 210:127–31.
636. Patarroyo, M, J. Prieto, I. Ernberg, C. G. Gahmberg. 1988. Absence, or low expression, of leukocyte adhesion molecules CD11 and CD18 on Burkitt lymphoma cells. *Int J Cancer* 41:901–7.
637. Patton, D. F, P. Shirley, N. Raab-Traub, L. Resnick, J. W. Sixbey. 1990. Defective viral DNA in Epstein-Barr virus-associated oral hairy leukoplakia. *J Virol* 64:397–400.
638. Paul, C. C, M. A. Baumann. 1990. Modulation of spontaneous outgrowth of Epstein-Barr virus immortalized B-cell clones by granulocyte-macrophage colony-stimulating factor and interleukin-3. *Blood* 75:54–8.
639. Paul, C. C, J. R. Keller, J. M. Armpriester, M. A. Baumann. 1990. Epstein-Barr virus transformed B lymphocytes produce interleukin-5. *Blood* 75:1400–3.
640. Pear, W. S, J. C. Aster, M. L. Scott, R. P. Hasserjian, B. Soffer, J. Sklar, D. Baltimore. 1996. Exclusive development of T cell neoplasms in mice transplanted with bone marrow expressing activated Notch alleles. *J Exp Med* 183:2283–91.
641. Pearson, G. R, J. Luka, L. Petti, J. Sample, M. Birkenbach, D. Braun, Kieff E. 1987. Identification of an Epstein-Barr virus early gene encoding a second component of the restricted early antigen complex. *Virology* 160:151–61.
642. Pearson, G. R, B. Vroman, B. Chase, T. Sculley, M. Hummel, Kieff E. 1983. Identification of polypeptide components of the Epstein-Barr virus early antigen complex with monoclonal antibodies. *J Virol* 47: 193–201.
643. Pellett, P. E, M. D. Biggin, B. Barrell, B. Roizman. 1985. Epstein-Barr virus genome may encode a protein showing significant amino acid and predicted secondary structure homology with glycoprotein B of herpes simplex virus 1. *J Virol* 56:807–13.
644. Penaranda, M. E, L. A. Lagenaur, L. T. Pierik, J. W. Berline, L. A. MacPhail, D. Greenspan, J. S. Greenspan, J. M. Palefsky. 1997. Expression of Epstein-Barr virus BMRF-2 and BDLF-3 genes in hairy leukoplakia [published erratum appears in *J Gen Virol* 1998; 79:1321]. *J Gen Virol* 78:3361–70.
645. Peng, M, E. Lundgren. 1993. Transient expression of the Epstein-Barr virus LMP1 gene in B-cell chronic lymphocytic leukemia cells, T cells, and hematopoietic cell lines: Cell-type-independent-induction of CD23, CD21, and ICAM-1. *Leukemia* 7:104–12.
646. Peng, M, E. Lundgren. 1992. Transient expression of the Epstein-Barr virus LMP1 gene in human primary B cells induces cellular activation and DNA synthesis. *Oncogene* 7:1775–82.
647. Peng, R, A. V. Gordadze, E. M. Fuentes Panana, F. Wang, J. Zong, G. S. Hayward, J. Tan, P. D. Ling. 2000. Sequence and functional analysis of EBNA-LP and EBNA2 proteins from nonhuman primate lymphocryptoviruses. *J Virol* 74:379–89.
648. Peng, R, J. Tan, P. D. Ling. 2000. Conserved regions in the Epstein-Barr virus leader protein define distinct domains required for nuclear localization and transcriptional cooperation with EBNA2. *J Virol* 74:9953–63.
649. Peng-Pilon, M, K. Ruuth, E. Lundgren, P. Brodin. 1995. The cytoplasmic C-terminal domain but not the N-terminal domain of latent membrane protein 1 of Epstein-Barr virus is essential for B cell activation. *J Gen Virol* 76:767–77.
650. Perlmann, C, A. K. Saemundsen, Klein G. 1982. A fraction of Epstein—Barr virus virion DNA is methylated in and around the *Eco*RI-J fragment. *Virology* 123:217–21.
651. Petti, L, Kieff E. 1988. A sixth Epstein-Barr virus nuclear protein (EBNA3B) is expressed in latently infected growth-transformed lymphocytes. *J Virol* 62:2173–8.
652. Petti, L, C. Sample, Kieff E. 1990. Subnuclear localization and phosphorylation of Epstein-Barr virus latent infection nuclear proteins. *Virology* 176:563–74.
653. Petti, L, J. Sample, F. Wang, Kieff E. 1988. A fifth Epstein-Barr virus nuclear protein (EBNA3C) is expressed in latently infected growth-transformed lymphocytes. *J Virol* 62:1330–8.
654. Pfuller, R, W. Hammerschmidt. 1996. Plasmid-like replicative intermediates of the Epstein-Barr virus lytic origin of DNA replication. *J Virol* 70:3423–31.
655. Platt, T. H, I. Y. Tcherepanova, C. L. Schildkraut. 1993. Effect of number and position of EBNA-1 binding sites in Epstein-Barr virus oriP on the sites of initiation, barrier formation, and termination of replication. *J Virol* 67:1739–45.
656. Polack, A, H. Delius, U. Zimber, G. W. Bornkamm. 1984. Two deletions in the Epstein-Barr virus genome of the Burkitt lymphoma nonproducer line Raji. *Virology* 133:146–57.
657. Polack, A, K. Hortnagel, A. Pajic, B. Christoph, B. Baier, M. Falk, J. Mautner, C. Geltinger, G. W. Bornkamm, B. Kempkes. 1996. c-*myc* activation renders proliferation of Epstein-Barr virus (EBV)-transformed cells independent of EBV nuclear antigen 2 and latent membrane protein 1. *Proc Natl Acad Sci U S A* 93:10411–6.
658. Polvino-Bodnar, M, J. Kiso, P. A. Schaffer. 1988. Mutational analysis

of Epstein-Barr virus nuclear antigen 1 (EBNA 1). *Nucleic Acids Res* 16:3415–35.

659. Pope, J. H, B. G. Achong, M. A. Epstein. 1968. Cultivation and fine structure of virus-bearing lymphoblasts from a second New Guinea Burkitt lymphoma: Establishment of sublines with unusual cultural properties. *Int J Cancer* 3:171–82.
660. Pope, J. H, M. K. Horne, W. Scott. 1968. Transformation of foetal human keukocytes *in vitro* by filtrates of a human leukaemic cell line containing herpes-like virus. *Int J Cancer* 3:857–66.
661. Prieto, J, P. G. Beatty, E. A. Clark, M. Patarroyo. 1988. Molecules mediating adhesion of T and B cells, monocytes and granulocytes to vascular endothelial cells. *Immunology* 63:631–7.
662. Pritchett, R, M. Pendersen, Kieff E. 1976. Complexity of EBV homologous DNA in continous lymphoblastoid cell lines. *Virology* 74: 227–31.
663. Pritchett RF, Hayward SD, Kieff ED. 1975. DNA of Epstein-Barr virus. I. Comparative studies of the DNA of Epstein-Barr virus from HR-1 and B95-8 cells: Size, structure, and relatedness. *J Virol* 15: 556–9.
664. Puglielli, M. T, N. Desai, S. H. Speck. 1997. Regulation of EBNA gene transcription in lymphoblastoid cell lines: Characterization of sequences downstream of BCR2 (Cp). *J Virol* 71:120–8.
665. Puglielli, M. T, M. Woisetschlaeger, S. H. Speck. 1996. oriP is essential for EBNA gene promoter activity in Epstein-Barr virus-immortalized lymphoblastoid cell lines. *J Virol* 70:5758–68.
666. Pulford, D. J, P. Lowrey, A. J. Morgan. 1995. Co-expression of the Epstein-Barr virus BXLF2 and BKRF2 genes with a recombinant baculovirus produces gp85 on the cell surface with antigenic similarity to the native protein. *J Gen Virol* 76:3145–52.
667. Puls, A, A. G. Eliopoulos, C. D. Nobes, T. Bridges, L. S. Young, A. Hall. 1999. Activation of the small GTPase cdc42 by the inflammatory cytokines TNFα and IL-1, and by the Epstein-Barr virus transforming protein LMP1. *J Cell Sci* 112:2983–92.
668. Qualtiere, L. F, J. F. Decoteau, M. Hassan Nasr-el-Din. 1987. Epitope mapping of the major Epstein-Barr virus outer envelope glycoprotein gp350/220. *J Gen Virol* 68:535–43.
669. Qualtiere, L. F, G. R. Pearson. 1979. Epstein-Barr virus-induced membrane antigens: Immunochemical characterization of Triton X-100 solubilized viral membrane antigens from EBV-superinfected Raji cells. *Int J Cancer* 23:808–17.
670. Qualtiere, L. F, G. R. Pearson. 1980. Radioimmune precipitation study comparing the Epstein-Barr virus membrane antigens expressed on P3HR-1 virus-superinfected Raji cells to those expressed on cells in a B-95 virus-transformed producer culture activated with tumor-promoting agent (TPA). *Virology* 102:360–9.
671. Quinlivan, E. B, E. Holley-Guthrie, E. C. Mar, M. S. Smith, S. Kenney. 1990. The Epstein-Barr virus BRLF1 immediate-early gene product transactivates the human immunodeficiency virus type 1 long terminal repeat by a mechanism which is enhancer independent. *J Virol* 64:1817–20.
672. Quinlivan, E. B, E. A. Holley-Guthrie, M. Norris, D. Gutsch, S. L. Bachenheimer, S. C. Kenney. 1993. Direct BRLF1 binding is required for cooperative BZLF1/BRLF1 activation of the Epstein-Barr virus early promoter, BMRF1 [corrected and republished with original paging, article originally printed in Nucleic Acids Res 1993 Apr 25;21(8):1999–2007]. *Nucleic Acids Res* 21:1999–2007.
673. Raab-Traub, N, T. Dambaugh, Kieff E. 1980. DNA of Epstein-Barr virus VIII: B95-8, the previous prototype, is an unusual deletion derivative. *Cell* 22:257–67.
674. Raab-Traub, N, K. Flynn. 1986. The structure of the termini of the Epstein-Barr virus as a marker of clonal cellular proliferation. *Cell* 47:883–9.
675. Raab-Traub, N, R. Pritchett, Kieff E. 1978. DNA of Epstein-Barr virus. III. Identification of restriction enzyme fragments that contain DNA sequences which differ among strains of Epstein-Barr virus. *J Virol* 27:388–98.
676. Rabin, H, R. H. Neubauer, R. F. d. Hopkins, M. Nonoyama. 1978. Further characterization of a herpesvirus-positive orang-utan cell line and comparative aspects of *in vitro* transformation with lymphotropic old world primate herpesviruses. *Int J Cancer* 21:762–7.
677. Rabson, M, L. Gradoville, L. Heston, G. Miller. 1982. Non-immortalizing P3J-HR-1 Epstein-Barr virus: A deletion mutant of its transforming parent, Jijoye. *J Virol* 44:834–44.
678. Rabson, M, L. Heston, G. Miller. 1983. Identification of a rare Epstein-Barr virus variant that enhances early antigen expression in Raji cells. *Proc Natl Acad Sci U S A* 80:2762–6.
679. Radkov, S. A, R. Touitou, A. Brehm, M. Rowe, M. West, T. Kouzarides, M. J. Allday. 1999. Epstein-Barr virus nuclear antigen 3C interacts with histone deacetylase to repress transcription. *J Virol* 73: 5688–97.
680. Ragona, G, I. Ernberg, Klein G. 1980. Induction and biological characterization of the Epstein-Barr virus (EBV) carried by the Jijoye lymphoma line. *Virology* 101:553–7.
681. Rawlins, D. R, G. Milman, Hayward SD, G. S. Hayward. 1985. Sequence-specific DNA binding of the Epstein-Barr virus nuclear antigen (EBNA-1) to clustered sites in the plasmid maintenance region. *Cell* 42:859–68.
682. Reedman, B. M, Klein G. 1973. Cellular localization of an Epstein-Barr virus (EBV)-associated complement-fixing antigen in producer and non-producer lymphoblastoid cell lines. *Int J Cancer* 11:499–520.
683. Reisman, D, B. Sugden. 1986. trans activation of an Epstein-Barr viral transcriptional enhancer by the Epstein-Barr viral nuclear antigen 1. *Mol Cell Biol* 6:3838–46.
684. Reisman, D, J. Yates, B. Sugden. 1985. A putative origin of replication of plasmids derived from Epstein-Barr virus is composed of two cis-acting components. *Mol Cell Biol* 5:1822–32.
685. Rickinson, A. B, D. Crawford, M. A. Epstein. 1977. Inhibition of the *in vitro* outgrowth of Epstein-Barr virus-transformed lymphocytes by thymus-dependent lymphocytes from infectious mononucleosis patients. *Clin Exp Immunol* 28:72–9.
686. Rickinson, A. B, M. A. Epstein. 1978. Sensitivity of the transforming and replicative functions of Epstein—Barr virus to inhibition by phosphonoacetate. *J Gen Virol* 40:409–20.
687. Rickinson, A. B, S. Finerty, M. A. Epstein. 1978. Inhibition by phosphonoacetate of the *in vitro* outgrowth of Epstein-Barr virus genome-containing cell lines from the blood of infectious mononucleosis patients. *IARC Sci Publ* 24:721–8.
688. Rickinson, A. B, J. E. Jarvis, D. H. Crawford, M. A. Epstein. 1975. Observations on the nature of Epstein-Barr virus infection of peripheral lymphoid cells in infectious mononucleosis. *IARC Sci Publ* 11: 169–77.
689. Rickinson, A. B, L. S. Young, M. Rowe. 1987. Influence of the Epstein-Barr virus nuclear antigen EBNA 2 on the growth phenotype of virus-transformed B cells. *J Virol* 61:1310–7.
690. Rivailler, P, C. Quink, F. Wang. 1999. Strong selective pressure for evolution of an Epstein-Barr virus LMP2B homologue in the rhesus lymphocryptovirus. *J Virol* 73:8867–72.
691. Robertson, E, Kieff E. 1995. Reducing the complexity of the transforming Epstein-Barr virus genome to 64 kilobase pairs. *J Virol* 69: 983–93.
692. Robertson, E. S, S. Grossman, E. Johannsen, C. Miller, J. Lin, B. Tomkinson, Kieff E. 1995. Epstein-Barr virus nuclear protein 3C modulates transcription through interaction with the sequence-specific DNA-binding protein J kappa. *J Virol* 69:3108–16.
693. Robertson, E. S, J. Lin, Kieff E. 1996. The amino-terminal domains of Epstein-Barr virus nuclear proteins 3A, 3B, and 3C interact with RBPJ(kappa). *J Virol* 70:3068–74.
694. Robertson, E. S, B. Tomkinson, Kieff E. 1994. An Epstein-Barr virus with a 58-kilobase-pair deletion that includes BARF0 transforms B lymphocytes *in vitro*. *J Virol* 68:1449–58.
695. Robertson, K. D, R. F. Ambinder. 1997. Methylation of the Epstein-Barr virus genome in normal lymphocytes. *Blood* 90:4480–4.
696. Robertson, K. D, Hayward SD, P. D. Ling, D. Samid, R. F. Ambinder. 1995. Transcriptional activation of the Epstein-Barr virus latency C promoter after 5-azacytidine treatment: Evidence that demethylation at a single CpG site is crucial. *Mol Cell Biol* 15:6150–9.
697. Robinson, J, A. Frank, E. Henderson, J. Schweitzer, G. Miller. 1979. Surface markers and size of lymphocytes in human umbilical cord blood stimulated into deoxyribonucleic acid synthesis by Epstein-Barr virus. *Infect Immun* 26:225–31.
698. Rochford, R, C. L. Miller, M. J. Cannon, K. M. Izumi, Kieff E, Longnecker R. 1997. *In vivo* growth of Epstein-Barr virus transformed B cells with mutations in latent membrane protein 2 (LMP2). *Arch Virol* 142:707–20.
699. Rogers, R. P, J. L. Strominger, S. H. Speck. 1992. Epstein-Barr virus in B lymphocytes: Viral gene expression and function in latency. *Adv Cancer Res* 58:1–26.
700. Rogers, R. P, M. Woisetschlaeger, S. H. Speck. 1990. Alternative

splicing dictates translational start in Epstein-Barr virus transcripts. *EMBO J* 9:2273–7.
701. Rooney, C, N. Taylor, J. Countryman, H. Jenson, J. Kolman, G. Miller. 1988. Genome rearrangements activate the Epstein-Barr virus gene whose product disrupts latency. *Proc Natl Acad Sci U S A* 85:9801–5.
702. Rooney, C. M, M. Brimmell, M. Buschle, G. Allan, Farrell PJ, J. L. Kolman. 1992. Host cell and EBNA-2 regulation of Epstein-Barr virus latent-cycle promoter activity in B lymphocytes. *J Virol* 66: 496–504.
703. Rothe, M, S. C. Wong, W. J. Henzel, D. V. Goeddel. 1994. A novel family of putative signal transducers associated with the cytoplasmic domain of the 75 kDa tumor necrosis factor receptor. *Cell* 78:681–92.
704. Roubal, J, B. Kallin, J. Luka, Klein G. 1981. Early DNA-binding polypeptides of Epstein-Barr virus. *Virology* 113:285–92.
705. Rousset, F, E. Garcia, T. Defrance, C. Peronne, N. Vezzio, D. H. Hsu, R. Kastelein, K. W. Moore, J. Banchereau. 1992. Interleukin 10 is a potent growth and differentiation factor for activated human B lymphocytes. *Proc Natl Acad Sci U S A* 89:1890–3.
706. Rowe, D. T, L. Hall, I. Joab, G. Laux. 1990. Identification of the Epstein-Barr virus terminal protein gene products in latently infected lymphocytes. *J Virol* 64:2866–75.
707. Rowe, M, H. S. Evans, L. S. Young, K. Hennessy, Kieff E, A. B. Rickinson. 1987. Monoclonal antibodies to the latent membrane protein of Epstein-Barr virus reveal heterogeneity of the protein and inducible expression in virus-transformed cells. *J Gen Virol* 68:1575–86.
708. Rowe, M, A. L. Lear, D. Croom-Carter, A. H. Davies, A. B. Rickinson. 1992. Three pathways of Epstein-Barr virus gene activation from EBNA1–positive latency in B lymphocytes. *J Virol* 66:122–31.
709. Rowe, M, M. Peng-Pilon, D. S. Huen, R. Hardy, D. Croom-Carter, E. Lundgren, A. B. Rickinson. 1994. Upregulation of bcl-2 by the Epstein-Barr virus latent membrane protein LMP1: A B-cell-specific response that is delayed relative to NF-kappa B activation and to induction of cell surface markers. *J Virol* 68:5602–12.
710. Rowe, M, L. S. Young, K. Cadwallader, L. Petti, Kieff E, A. B. Rickinson. 1989. Distinction between Epstein-Barr virus type A (EBNA 2A) and type B (EBNA 2B) isolates extends to the EBNA 3 family of nuclear proteins. *J Virol* 63:1031–9.
711. Ruf, I. K, A. Moghaddam, F. Wang, J. Sample. 1999. Mechanisms that regulate Epstein-Barr virus EBNA-1 gene transcription during restricted latency are conserved among lymphocryptoviruses of Old World primates. *J Virol* 73:1980–9.
712. Russo, J. J, R. A. Bohenzky, M. C. Chien, J. Chen, M. Yan, D. Maddalena, J. P. Parry, D. Peruzzi, I. S. Edelman, Y. Chang, P. S. Moore. 1996. Nucleotide sequence of the Kaposi sarcoma-associated herpesvirus (HHV8). *Proc Natl Acad Sci U S A* 93:14862–7.
713. Ruvolo, V, E. Wang, S. Boyle, S. Swaminathan. 1998. The Epstein-Barr virus nuclear protein SM is both a post-transcriptional inhibitor and activator of gene expression. *Proc Natl Acad Sci U S A* 95:8852–7.
714. Rymo, L, T. Lindahl, A. Adams. 1979. Sites of sequence variability in Epstein-Barr virus DNA from different sources. *Proc Natl Acad Sci U S A* 76:2794–8.
715. Sadler, R. H, N. Raab-Traub. 1995. The Epstein-Barr virus 3.5-kilobase latent membrane protein 1 mRNA initiates from a TATA-less promoter within the first terminal repeat. *J Virol* 69:4577–81.
716. Sadler, R. H, N. Raab-Traub. 1995. Structural analyses of the Epstein-Barr virus *Bam*HI A transcripts. *J Virol* 69:1132–41.
717. Saemundsen, A. K, B. Kallin, Klein G. 1980. Effect of n-butyrate on cellular and viral DNA synthesis in cells latently infected with Epstein-Barr virus. *Virology* 107:557–61.
718. Saemundsen, A. K, C. Perlmann, Klein G. 1983. Intracellular Epstein-Barr virus DNA is methylated in and around the *Eco*RI-J fragment in both producer and nonproducer cell lines. *Virology* 126:701–6.
719. Sample, J, L. Brooks, C. Sample, L. Young, M. Rowe, C. Gregory, A. Rickinson, Kieff E. 1991. Restricted Epstein-Barr virus protein expression in Burkitt lymphoma is due to a different Epstein-Barr nuclear antigen 1 transcriptional initiation site. *Proc Natl Acad Sci U S A* 88:6343–7.
720. Sample, J, E. B. Henson, C. Sample. 1992. The Epstein-Barr virus nuclear protein 1 promoter active in type I latency is autoregulated. *J Virol* 66:4654–61.
721. Sample, J, M. Hummel, D. Braun, M. Birkenbach, Kieff E. 1986. Nucleotide sequences of mRNAs encoding Epstein-Barr virus nuclear proteins: A probable transcriptional initiation site. *Proc Natl Acad Sci U S A* 83:5096–100.
722. Sample, J, E. F. Kieff, E. D. Kieff. 1994. Epstein-Barr virus types 1 and 2 have nearly identical LMP-1 transforming genes. *J Gen Virol* 75:2741–6.
723. Sample, J, G. Lancz, M. Nonoyama. 1986. Mapping of genes in *Bam*HI fragment M of Epstein-Barr virus DNA that may determine the fate of viral infection. *J Virol* 57:145–54.
724. Sample, J, D. Liebowitz, Kieff E. 1989. Two related Epstein-Barr virus membrane proteins are encoded by separate genes. *J Virol* 63:933–7.
725. Sample, J, L. Young, B. Martin, T. Chatman, Kieff E, A. Rickinson. 1990. Epstein-Barr virus types 1 and 2 differ in their EBNA-3A, EBNA-3B, and EBNA-3C genes. *J Virol* 64:4084–92.
726. Sandberg, M, W. Hammerschmidt, B. Sugden. 1997. Characterization of LMP-1's association with TRAF1, TRAF2, and TRAF3. *J Virol* 71: 4649–56.
727. Savard, M, C. Belanger, M. Tardif, P. Gourde, L. Flamand, J. Gosselin. 2000. Infection of primary human monocytes by Epstein-Barr virus. *J Virol* 74:2612–9.
728. Scala, G, Y. D. Kuang, R. E. Hall, A. V. Muchmore, J. J. Oppenheim. 1984. Accessory cell function of human B cells. I. Production of both interleukin 1-like activity and an interleukin 1 inhibitory factor by an EBV-transformed human B cell line. *J Exp Med* 159:1637–52.
729. Scala, G, I. Quinto, M. R. Ruocco, A. Arcucci, M. Mallardo, P. Caretto, G. Forni, S. Venuta. 1990. Expression of an exogenous interleukin 6 gene in human Epstein Barr virus B cells confers growth advantage and *in vivo* tumorigenicity. *J Exp Med* 172:61–8.
730. Scala, G, I. Quinto, M. R. Ruocco, M. Mallardo, C. Ambrosino, B. Squitieri, P. Tassone, S. Venuta. 1993. Epstein-Barr virus nuclear antigen 2 transactivates the long terminal repeat of human immunodeficiency virus type 1. *J Virol* 67:2853–61.
731. Schaefer, B. C, E. Paulson, J. L. Strominger, S. H. Speck. 1997. Constitutive activation of Epstein-Barr virus (EBV) nuclear antigen 1 gene transcription by IRF1 and IRF2 during restricted EBV latency. *Mol Cell Biol* 17:873–86.
732. Schaefer, B. C, J. L. Strominger, S. H. Speck. 1995. Redefining the Epstein-Barr virus-encoded nuclear antigen EBNA-1 gene promoter and transcription initiation site in group I Burkitt lymphoma cell lines. *Proc Natl Acad Sci U S A* 92:10565–9.
733. Schaefer, B. C, J. L. Strominger, S. H. Speck. 1997. Host-cell-determined methylation of specific Epstein-Barr virus promoters regulates the choice between distinct viral latency programs. *Mol Cell Biol* 17:364–77.
734. Schaefer, B. C, M. Woisetschlaeger, J. L. Strominger, S. H. Speck. 1991. Exclusive expression of Epstein-Barr virus nuclear antigen 1 in Burkitt lymphoma arises from a third promoter, distinct from the promoters used in latently infected lymphocytes. *Proc Natl Acad Sci U S A* 88:6550–4.
735. Schepers, A, D. Pich, W. Hammerschmidt. 1996. Activation of oriLyt, the lytic origin of DNA replication of Epstein-Barr virus, by BZLF1. *Virology* 220:367–76.
736. Schepers, A, D. Pich, W. Hammerschmidt. 1993. A transcription factor with homology to the AP-1 family links RNA transcription and DNA replication in the lytic cycle of Epstein-Barr virus. *EMBO J* 12: 3921–9.
737. Scholle, F, K. M. Bendt, N. Raab-Traub. 2000. Epstein-barr virus LMP2A transforms epithelial cells, inhibits cell differentiation, and activates Akt. *J Virol* 74:10681–9.
738. Schultz, L. D, J. Tanner, K. J. Hofmann, E. A. Emini, J. H. Condra, R. E. Jones, Kieff E, R. W. Ellis. 1987. Expression and secretion in yeast of a 400-kDa envelope glycoprotein derived from Epstein-Barr virus. *Gene* 54:113–23.
739. Schwarzmann, F, N. Prang, B. Reichelt, B. Rinkes, S. Haist, M. Marschall, H. Wolf. 1994. Negatively cis-acting elements in the distal part of the promoter of Epstein-Barr virus trans-activator gene BZLF1. *J Gen Virol* 75:1999–2006.
740. Sculley, T. B, A. Apolloni, L. Hurren, D. J. Moss, D. A. Cooper. 1990. Coinfection with A- and B-type Epstein-Barr virus in human immunodeficiency virus-positive subjects. *J Infect Dis* 162:643–8.
741. Sculley, T. B, D. G. Sculley, J. H. Pope, G. W. Bornkamm, G. M. Lenoir, A. B. Rickinson. 1988. Epstein-Barr virus nuclear antigens 1 and 2 in Burkitt lymphoma cell lines containing either `A'- or `B'-type virus. *Intervirology* 29:77–85.
742. Segouffin, C, H. Gruffat, A. Sergeant. 1996. Repression by RAZ of Epstein-Barr virus bZIP transcription factor EB1 is dimerization independent. *J Gen Virol* 77:1529–36.

743. Serafini-Cessi, F, N. Malagolini, M. Nanni, F. Dall'Olio, G. Campadelli-Fiume, J. Tanner, Kieff E. 1989. Characterization of N- and O-linked oligosaccharides of glycoprotein 350 from Epstein-Barr virus. *Virology* 170:1–10.
744. Sexton, C. J, J. S. Pagano. 1989. Analysis of the Epstein-Barr virus origin of plasmid replication (oriP) reveals an area of nucleosome sparing that spans the 3′ dyad. *J Virol* 63:5505–8.
745. Shapiro, I. M, D. J. Volsky, A. K. Saemundsen, E. Anisimova, Klein G. 1982. Infection of the human T-cell-derived leukemia line Molt-4 by Epstein-Barr virus (EBV): Induction of EBV-determined antigens and virus reproduction. *Virology* 120:171–81.
746. Sharipo, A, M. Imreh, A. Leonchiks, S. Imreh, M. G. Masucci. 1998. A minimal glycine-alanine repeat prevents the interaction of ubiquitinated I kappaB alpha with the proteasome: A new mechanism for selective inhibition of proteolysis [see comments]. Nat Med. 4:939–44.
747. Sharp, T. V, M. Schwemmle, I. Jeffrey, K. Laing, H. Mellor, C. G. Proud, K. Hilse, M. J. Clemens. 1993. Comparative analysis of the regulation of the interferon-inducible protein kinase PKR by Epstein-Barr virus RNAs EBER-1 and EBER-2 and adenovirus VAI RNA. *Nucleic Acids Res* 21:4483–90.
747a. Shaw JE. The circular intracellular vorm of Epstein-Barr virus DNA is amplified by the virus-associated DNA polymerase. *J Virol* 1985 53:1012–1015.
747b. Shaw JE, Levinger, Carter CW. Nucleosomal structure of Epstein-Barr virus DNA in transformed cell lines. *J Virol* 1979;29:657–665.
748. Shimizu, N, K. Takada. 1993. Analysis of the BZLF1 promoter of Epstein-Barr virus: Identification of an anti-immunoglobulin response sequence. *J Virol* 67:3240–5.
749. Shimizu, N, A. Tanabe-Tochikura, Y. Kuroiwa, K. Takada. 1994. Isolation of Epstein-Barr virus (EBV)-negative cell clones from the EBV-positive Burkitt's lymphoma (BL) line Akata: Malignant phenotypes of BL cells are dependent on EBV. *J Virol* 68:6069–73.
750. Shimizu, N, H. Yoshiyama, K. Takada. 1996. Clonal propagation of Epstein-Barr virus (EBV) recombinants in EBV-negative Akata cells. *J Virol* 70:7260–3.
751. Silins, S. L, T. B. Sculley. 1995. Burkitt's lymphoma cells are resistant to programmed cell death in the presence of the Epstein-Barr virus latent antigen EBNA-4. *Int J Cancer* 60:65–72.
752. Silins, S. L, T. B. Sculley. 1994. Modulation of vimentin, the CD40 activation antigen and Burkitt's lymphoma antigen (CD77) by the Epstein-Barr virus nuclear antigen EBNA-4. *Virology* 202:16–24.
753. Simpson, K, A. McGuigan, C. Huxley. 1996. Stable episomal maintenance of yeast artificial chromosomes in human cells. *Mol Cell Biol* 16:5117–26.
754. Sinclair, A. J, M. Brimmell, Farrell PJ. 1992. Reciprocal antagonism of steroid hormones and BZLF1 in switch between Epstein-Barr virus latent and productive cycle gene expression. *J Virol* 66:70–7.
755. Sinclair, A. J, M. Brimmell, F. Shanahan, Farrell PJ. 1991. Pathways of activation of the Epstein-Barr virus productive cycle. *J Virol* 65:2237–44.
756. Sinclair, A. J, Farrell PJ. 1995. Host cell requirements for efficient infection of quiescent primary B lymphocytes by Epstein-Barr virus. *J Virol* 69:5461–8.
757. Sinclair, A. J, M. G. Jacquemin, L. Brooks, F. Shanahan, M. Brimmell, M. Rowe, Farrell PJ. 1994. Reduced signal transduction through glucocorticoid receptor in Burkitt's lymphoma cell lines. *Virology* 199: 339–53.
758. Sinha, S. K, S. C. Todd, J. A. Hedrick, C. L. Speiser, J. D. Lambris, C. D. Tsoukas. 1993. Characterization of the EBV/C3d receptor on the human Jurkat T cell line: Evidence for a novel transcript. *J Immunol* 150:5311–20.
759. Sixbey, J. W, D. S. Davis, L. S. Young, L. Hutt-Fletcher, T. F. Tedder, A. B. Rickinson. 1987. Human epithelial cell expression of an Epstein-Barr virus receptor. *J Gen Virol* 68:805–11.
760. Sixbey, J. W, J. G. Nedrud, N. Raab-Traub, R. A. Hanes, J. S. Pagano. 1984. Epstein-Barr virus replication in oropharyngeal epithelial cells. *N Engl J Med* 310:1225–30.
761. Sixbey, J. W, P. Shirley, P. J. Chesney, D. M. Buntin, L. Resnick. 1989. Detection of a second widespread strain of Epstein-Barr virus. *Lancet* 2:761–5.
762. Sixbey, J. W, P. Shirley, M. Sloas, N. Raab-Traub, V. Israele. 1991. A transformation-incompetent, nuclear antigen 2-deleted Epstein-Barr virus associated with replicative infection. *J Infect Dis* 163:1008–15.
763. Sixbey, J. W, E. H. Vesterinen, J. G. Nedrud, N. Raab-Traub, L. A. Walton, J. S. Pagano. 1983. Replication of Epstein-Barr virus in human epithelial cells infected *in vitro*. *Nature* 306:480–3.
764. Sjoblom, A, A. Jansson, W. Yang, S. Lain, T. Nilsson, L. Rymo. 1995. PU box-binding transcription factors and a POU domain protein cooperate in the Epstein-Barr virus (EBV) nuclear antigen 2-induced transactivation of the EBV latent membrane protein 1 promoter. *J Gen Virol* 76:2679–92.
765. Skare, J, J. Farley, J. L. Strominger, K. O. Fresen, Cho MS, H. zur Hausen. 1985. Transformation by Epstein-Barr virus requires DNA sequences in the region of *Bam*HI fragments Y and H. *J Virol* 55:286–97.
766. Smith, P. R, O. de Jesus, D. Turner, M. Hollyoake, C. E. Karstegl, B. E. Griffin, L. Karran, Y. Wang, Hayward SD, Farrell PJ. 2000. Structure and coding content of CST (BART) family RNAs of Epstein-Barr virus. *J Virol* 74:3082–92.
767. Smith, P. R, B. E. Griffin. 1992. Transcription of the Epstein-Barr virus gene EBNA-1 from different promoters in nasopharyngeal carcinoma and B-lymphoblastoid cells. *J Virol* 66:706–14.
768. Snudden, D. K, J. Hearing, P. R. Smith, F. A. Grasser, B. E. Griffin. 1994. EBNA-1, the major nuclear antigen of Epstein-Barr virus, resembles `RGG' RNA binding proteins. *EMBO J* 13:4840–7.
769. Songyang, Z, S. E. Shoelson, M. Chaudhuri, G. Gish, T. Pawson, W. G. Haser, F. King, T. Roberts, S. Ratnofsky, R. J. Lechleider, et al. 1993. SH2 domains recognize specific phosphopeptide sequences. *Cell* 72:767–78.
770. Spaete, R. R, N. Frenkel. 1985. The herpes simplex virus amplicon: Analyses of cis-acting replication functions. *Proc Natl Acad Sci U S A* 82:694–8.
771. Speck, P, K. A. Kline, P. Cheresh, Longnecker R. 1999. Epstein-Barr virus lacking latent membrane protein 2 immortalizes B cells with efficiency indistinguishable from that of wild-type virus. *J Gen Virol* 80:2193–203.
772. Speck, S. H, T. Chatila, E. Flemington. 1997. Reactivation of Epstein-Barr virus: Regulation and function of the BZLF1 gene. *Trends Microbiol* 5:399–405.
773. Speck, S. H, A. Pfitzner, J. L. Strominger. 1986. An Epstein-Barr virus transcript from a latently infected, growth-transformed B-cell line encodes a highly repetitive polypeptide. *Proc Natl Acad Sci U S A* 83:9298–302.
774. Speck, S. H, J. L. Strominger. 1985. Analysis of the transcript encoding the latent Epstein-Barr virus nuclear antigen I: A potentially polycistronic message generated by long-range splicing of several exons. *Proc Natl Acad Sci U S A* 82:8305–9.
775. Spender, L. C, E. J. Cannell, M. Hollyoake, B. Wensing, J. M. Gawn, M. Brimmell, G. Packham, Farrell PJ. 1999. Control of cell cycle entry and apoptosis in B lymphocytes infected by Epstein-Barr virus. *J Virol* 73:4678–88.
776. Spriggs, M. K, R. J. Armitage, M. R. Comeau, L. Strockbine, T. Farrah, B. Macduff, D. Ulrich, M. R. Alderson, J. Mullberg, Cohen JI. 1996. The extracellular domain of the Epstein-Barr virus BZLF2 protein binds the HLA-DR beta chain and inhibits antigen presentation. *J Virol* 70:5557–63.
777. Sternas, L, T. Middleton, B. Sugden. 1990. The average number of molecules of Epstein-Barr nuclear antigen 1 per cell does not correlate with the average number of Epstein-Barr virus (EBV) DNA molecules per cell among different clones of EBV-immortalized cells. *J Virol* 64:2407–10.
778. Stewart, J. P, F. G. Behm, J. R. Arrand, C. M. Rooney. 1994. Differential expression of viral and human interleukin-10 (IL-10) by primary B cell tumors and B cell lines. *Virology* 200:724–32.
779. Strnad, B. C, M. R. Adams, H. Rabin. 1983. Glycosylation pathways of two major Epstein-Barr virus membrane antigens. *Virology* 127: 168–76.
780. Strnad, B. C, R. H. Neubauer, H. Rabin, R. A. Mazur. 1979. Correlation between Epstein-Barr virus membrane antigen and three large cell surface glycoproteins. *J Virol* 32:885–94.
781. Su, W, T. Middleton, B. Sugden, H. Echols. 1991. DNA looping between the origin of replication of Epstein-Barr virus and its enhancer site: Stabilization of an origin complex with Epstein-Barr nuclear antigen 1. *Proc Natl Acad Sci U S A* 88:10870–4.
782. Sugano, N, W. Chen, M. L. Roberts, N. R. Cooper. 1997. Epstein-Barr virus binding to CD21 activates the initial viral promoter via NF-kappaB induction. *J Exp Med* 186:731–7.
783. Sugden, B, W. Mark. 1977. Clonal transformation of adult human leukocytes by Epstein-Barr virus. *J Virol* 23:503–8.

784. Sugden, B, K. Marsh, J. Yates. 1985. A vector that replicates as a plasmid and can be efficiently selected in B-lymphoblasts transformed by Epstein-Barr virus. *Mol Cell Biol* 5:410–3.
785. Sugden, B, S. Metzenberg. 1983. Characterization of an antigen whose cell surface expression is induced by infection with Epstein-Barr virus. *J Virol* 46:800–7.
786. Sugden, B, M. Phelps, J. Domoradzki. 1979. Epstein-Barr virus DNA is amplified in transformed lymphocytes. *J Virol* 31:590–5.
787. Sugden, B, N. Warren. 1988. Plasmid origin of replication of Epstein-Barr virus, oriP, does not limit replication in cis. *Mol Biol Med* 5:85–94.
788. Sugden, B, N. Warren. 1989. A promoter of Epstein-Barr virus that can function during latent infection can be transactivated by EBNA-1, a viral protein required for viral DNA replication during latent infection. *J Virol* 63:2644–9.
789. Summers, W. C, Klein G. 1976. Inhibition of Epstein-Barr virus DNA synthesis and late gene expression by phosphonoacetic acid. *J Virol* 18:151–5.
790. Sun, R, T. A. Spain, S. F. Lin, G. Miller. 1994. Autoantigenic proteins that bind recombinogenic sequences in Epstein-Barr virus and cellular DNA. *Proc Natl Acad Sci U S A* 91:8646–50.
791. Sun, R, T. A. Spain, S. F. Lin, G. Miller. 1997. Sp1 binds to the precise locus of end processing within the terminal repeats of Epstein-Barr virus DNA. *J Virol* 71:6136–43.
792. Sun, T, D. A. Fenstermacher, J. H. Vos. 1994. Human artificial episomal chromosomes for cloning large DNA fragments in human cells. *Nature Genetics* 8:33–41.
793. Sung, N. S, S. Kenney, D. Gutsch, J. S. Pagano. 1991. EBNA-2 transactivates a lymphoid-specific enhancer in the *Bam*HI C promoter of Epstein-Barr virus. *J Virol* 65:2164–9.
794. Sung, N. S, J. Wilson, M. Davenport, N. D. Sista, J. S. Pagano. 1994. Reciprocal regulation of the Epstein-Barr virus *Bam*HI-F promoter by EBNA-1 and an E2F transcription factor. *Mol Cell Biol* 14:7144–52.
795. Swaminathan, S, R. Hesselton, J. Sullivan, Kieff E. 1993. Epstein-Barr virus recombinants with specifically mutated BCRF1 genes. *J Virol* 67:7406–13.
796. Swaminathan, S, B. S. Huneycutt, C. S. Reiss, Kieff E. 1992. Epstein-Barr virus-encoded small RNAs (EBERs) do not modulate interferon effects in infected lymphocytes. *J Virol* 66:5133–6.
797. Swaminathan, S, B. Tomkinson, Kieff E. 1991. Recombinant Epstein-Barr virus with small RNA (EBER) genes deleted transforms lymphocytes and replicates *in vitro*. *Proc Natl Acad Sci U S A* 88:1546–50.
798. Sylla, B. S, S. C. Hung, D. M. Davidson, E. Hatzivassiliou, N. L. Malinin, D. Wallach, T. D. Gilmore, Kieff E, G. Mosialos. 1998. Epstein-Barr virus-transforming protein latent infection membrane protein 1 activates transcription factor NF-kappaB through a pathway that includes the NF-kappaB-inducing kinase and the IkappaB kinases IKKalpha and IKKbeta. *Proc Natl Acad Sci U S A* 95:10106–11.
799. Szekely, L, W. Q. Jiang, K. Pokrovskaja, K. G. Wiman, Klein G, N. Ringertz. 1995. Reversible nucleolar translocation of Epstein-Barr virus-encoded EBNA-5 and hsp70 proteins after exposure to heat shock or cell density congestion. *J Gen Virol* 76:2423–32.
800. Szekely, L, K. Pokrovskaja, W. Q. Jiang, H. de The, N. Ringertz, Klein G. 1996. The Epstein-Barr virus-encoded nuclear antigen EBNA-5 accumulates in PML-containing bodies. *J Virol* 70:2562–8.
801. Szyf, M, L. Eliasson, V. Mann, Klein G, A. Razin. 1985. Cellular and viral DNA hypomethylation associated with induction of Epstein-Barr virus lytic cycle. *Proc Natl Acad Sci U S A* 82:8090–4.
802. Takada, K. 1984. Cross-linking of cell surface immunoglobulins induces Epstein-Barr virus in Burkitt lymphoma lines. *Int J Cancer* 33:27–32.
803. Takada, K, Y. Ono. 1989. Synchronous and sequential activation of latently infected Epstein-Barr virus genomes. *J Virol* 63:445–9.
804. Takada, K, N. Shimizu, S. Sakuma, Y. Ono. 1986. trans activation of the latent Epstein-Barr virus (EBV) genome after transfection of the EBV DNA fragment. *J Virol* 57:1016–22.
805. Takada, K, H. zur Hausen. 1984. Induction of Epstein-Barr virus antigens by tumor promoters for epidermal and nonepidermal tissues. *Int J Cancer* 33:491–6.
806. Takaki, K, A. Polack, G. W. Bornkamm. 1984. Expression of a nuclear and a cytoplasmic Epstein-Barr virus early antigen after DNA transfer: Cooperation of two distant parts of the genome for expression of the cytoplasmic antigen. *Proc Natl Acad Sci U S A* 81:4568–72.
807. Takeshita, H, T. Yoshizaki, W. E. Miller, H. Sato, M. Furukawa, J. S. Pagano, N. Raab-Traub. 1999. Matrix metalloproteinase 9 expression is induced by Epstein-Barr virus latent membrane protein 1 C-terminal activation regions 1 and 2. *J Virol* 73:5548–55.
808. Tamura, K, Y. Taniguchi, S. Minoguchi, T. Sakai, T. Tun, T. Furukawa, T. Honjo. 1995. Physical interaction between a novel domain of the receptor Notch and the transcription factor RBP-J kappa/Su(H). *Curr Biol* 5:1416–23.
809. Tanaka, A, M. Nonoyama. 1975. Latent genomes of Epstein-Barr virus. *IARC Sci Publ* 11:133–7.
810. Tanner, J, J. Weis, D. Fearon, Y. Whang, Kieff E. 1987. Epstein-Barr virus gp350/220 binding to the B lymphocyte C3d receptor mediates adsorption, capping, and endocytosis. *Cell* 50:203–13.
811. Tanner, J, Y. Whang, J. Sample, A. Sears, Kieff E. 1988. Soluble gp350/220 and deletion mutant glycoproteins block Epstein-Barr virus adsorption to lymphocytes. *J Virol* 62:4452–64.
812. Tanner, J. E, G. Tosato. 1992. Regulation of B-cell growth and immunoglobulin gene transcription by interleukin-6. *Blood* 79:452–9.
813. Tao, Q, K. D. Robertson, A. Manns, A. Hildesheim, R. F. Ambinder. 1998. The Epstein-Barr virus major latent promoter Qp is constitutively active, hypomethylated, and methylation sensitive. *J Virol* 72:7 075–83.
814. Tao, Q, L. J. Swinnen, J. Yang, G. Srivastava, K. D. Robertson, R. F. Ambinder. 1999. Methylation status of the Epstein-Barr virus major latent promoter C in iatrogenic B cell lymphoproliferative disease. Application of PCR-based analysis. *Am J Pathol* 155:619–25.
815. Tatsumi, E, S. Harada, T. Bechtold, H. Lipscomb, J. Davis, C. Kuszynski, D. J. Volsky, T. Han, J. Armitage, D. T. Purtilo. 1986. In-vitro infection of chronic lymphocytic leukemia cells by Epstein-Barr virus (EBV). *Leuk Res* 10:167–77.
816. Taylor, N, J. Countryman, C. Rooney, D. Katz, G. Miller. 1989. Expression of the BZLF1 latency-disrupting gene differs in standard and defective Epstein-Barr viruses. *J Virol* 63:1721–8.
817. Taylor, N, E. Flemington, J. L. Kolman, R. P. Baumann, S. H. Speck, G. Miller. 1991. ZEBRA and a Fos-GCN4 chimeric protein differ in their DNA-binding specificities for sites in the Epstein-Barr virus BZLF1 promoter. *J Virol* 65:4033–41.
818. Teramoto, N, A. Maeda, K. Kobayashi, K. Hayashi, T. Oka, K. Takahashi, K. Takada, Klein G, T. Akagi. 2000. Epstein-Barr virus infection to Epstein-Barr virus-negative nasopharyngeal carcinoma cell line TW03 enhances its tumorigenicity. *Lab Invest* 80:303–12.
819. Thorley-Lawson, D, J. L. Strominger. 1976. Transformation of human lymphocytes by Epstein-Barr virus is inhibited by phosphonoacetic acid. *Nature* 263:332–4.
820. Thorley-Lawson, D. A. 1979. Characterization of cross-reacting antigens on the Epstein-Barr virus envelope and plasma membranes of producer cells. *Cell* 16:33–42.
821. Thorley-Lawson, D. A, L. Chess, J. L. Strominger. 1977. Suppression of *in vitro* Epstein-Barr virus infection. A new role for adult human T lymphocytes. *J Exp Med* 146:495–08.
822. Thorley-Lawson, D. A, C. M. Edson. 1979. Polypeptides of the Epstein-Barr virus membrane antigen complex. *J Virol* 32:458–67.
823. Thorley-Lawson, D. A, K. Geilinger. 1980. Monoclonal antibodies against the major glycoprotein (gp350/220) of Epstein-Barr virus neutralize infectivity. *Proc Natl Acad Sci U S A* 77:5307–11.
824. Thorley-Lawson, D. A, K. P. Mann. 1985. Early events in Epstein-Barr virus infection provide a model for B cell activation. *J Exp Med* 162:45–59.
825. Thorley-Lawson, D. A, E. M. Miyashita, G. Khan. 1996. Epstein-Barr virus and the B cell: That's all it takes. *Trends Microbiol* 4:204–8.
826. Thorley-Lawson, D. A, L. M. Nadler, A. K. Bhan, R. T. Schooley. 1985. BLAST-2 [EBVCS], an early cell surface marker of human B cell activation, is superinduced by Epstein Barr virus. *J Immunol* 134:3007–12.
827. Thorley-Lawson, D. A, C. A. Poodry. 1982. Identification and isolation of the main component (gp350–gp220) of Epstein-Barr virus responsible for generating neutralizing antibodies *in vivo*. *J Virol* 43: 730–6.
828. Thorley-Lawson, D. A, R. T. Schooley, A. K. Bhan, L. M. Nadler. 1982. Epstein-Barr virus superinduces a new human B cell differentiation antigen (B-LAST 1) expressed on transformed lymphoblasts. *Cell* 30:415–25.
829. Thyphronitis, G, J. Banchereau, C. Heusser, G. C. Tsokos, A. D. Levine, F. D. Finkelman. 1991. Kinetics of interleukin-4 induction and interferon-gamma inhibition of IgE secretion by Epstein-Barr virus-infected human peripheral blood B cells. Cell Immunol. 133:408–19.

830. Tierney, R, H. Kirby, J. Nagra, A. Rickinson, A. Bell. 2000. The Epstein-Barr virus promoter initiating B-cell transformation is activated by RFX proteins and the B-cell-specific activator protein BSAP/Pax5. *J Virol* 74:10458–67.
831. Toczyski, D. P, A. G. Matera, D. C. Ward, J. A. Steitz. 1994. The Epstein-Barr virus (EBV) small RNA EBER1 binds and relocalizes ribosomal protein L22 in EBV-infected human B lymphocytes. *Proc Natl Acad Sci U S A* 91:3463–7.
832. Toczyski, D. P, J. A. Steitz. 1993. The cellular RNA-binding protein EAP recognizes a conserved stem-loop in the Epstein-Barr virus small RNA EBER 1. *Mol Cell Biol* 13:703–10.
833. Toczyski, D. P, J. A. Steitz. 1991. EAP, a highly conserved cellular protein associated with Epstein-Barr virus small RNAs (EBERs). *EMBO J* 10:459–66.
834. Tolnay, M, J. D. Lambris, G. C. Tsokos. 1997. Transcriptional regulation of the complement receptor 2 gene: Role of a heterogeneous nuclear ribonucleoprotein. *J Immunol* 159:5492–501.
835. Tomkinson, B, Kieff E. 1992. Second-site homologous recombination in Epstein-Barr virus: Insertion of type 1 EBNA 3 genes in place of type 2 has no effect on *in vitro* infection. *J Virol* 66:780–9.
836. Tomkinson, B, Kieff E. 1992. Use of second-site homologous recombination to demonstrate that Epstein-Barr virus nuclear protein 3B is not important for lymphocyte infection or growth transformation *in vitro*. *J Virol* 66:2893–903.
837. Tomkinson, B, E. Robertson, Kieff E. 1993. Epstein-Barr virus nuclear proteins EBNA-3A and EBNA-3C are essential for B-lymphocyte growth transformation. *J Virol* 67:2014–25.
838. Tomkinson, B, E. Robertson, R. Yalamanchili, Longnecker R, Kieff E. 1993. Epstein-Barr virus recombinants from overlapping cosmid fragments. *J Virol* 67:7298–306.
839. Tong, X, R. Drapkin, D. Reinberg, Kieff E. 1995. The 62– and 80-kDa subunits of transcription factor IIH mediate the interaction with Epstein-Barr virus nuclear protein 2. *Proc Natl Acad Sci U S A* 92:3259–63.
840. Tong, X, R. Drapkin, R. Yalamanchili, G. Mosialos, Kieff E. 1995. The Epstein-Barr virus nuclear protein 2 acidic domain forms a complex with a novel cellular coactivator that can interact with TFIIE. *Mol Cell Biol* 15:4735–44.
841. Tong, X, F. Wang, C. J. Thut, Kieff E. 1995. The Epstein-Barr virus nuclear protein 2 acidic domain can interact with TFIIB, TAF40, and RPA70 but not with TATA-binding protein. *J Virol* 69:585–8.
842. Tong, X, R. Yalamanchili, S. Harada, Kieff E. 1994. The EBNA-2 arginine-glycine domain is critical but not essential for B-lymphocyte growth transformation; the rest of region 3 lacks essential interactive domains. *J Virol* 68:6188–97.
843. Tornell, J, S. Farzad, A. Espander-Jansson, G. Matejka, O. Isaksson, L. Rymo. 1996. Expression of Epstein-Barr nuclear antigen 2 in kidney tubule cells induce tumors in transgenic mice. *Oncogene* 12:1521–8.
844. Tosato, G, R. M. Blaese. 1985. Epstein-Barr virus infection and immunoregulation in man. *Adv Immunol* 37:99–149.
845. Tosato, G, K. B. Seamon, N. D. Goldman, P. B. Sehgal, L. T. May, G. C. Washington, K. D. Jones, S. E. Pike. 1988. Monocyte-derived human B-cell growth factor identified as interferon-beta 2 (BSF-2, IL-6). *Science* 239:502–4.
846. Tosato, G, J. Tanner, K. D. Jones, M. Revel, S. E. Pike. 1990. Identification of interleukin-6 as an autocrine growth factor for Epstein-Barr virus-immortalized B cells. *J Virol* 64:3033–41.
847. Trivedi, P, M. G. Masucci, G. Winberg, Klein G. 1991. The epstein-Barr-virus-encoded membrane protein LMP but not the nuclear antigen EBNA-1 induces rejection of transfected murine mammary carcinoma cells. *Int J Cancer* 48:794–800.
848. Tsang, S. F, F. Wang, K. M. Izumi, Kieff E. 1991. Delineation of the cis-acting element mediating EBNA-2 transactivation of latent infection membrane protein expression. *J Virol* 65:6765–71.
849. Tsoukas, C. D, J. D. Lambris. 1993. Expression of EBV/C3d receptors on T cells: Biological significance. *Immunol Today* 14:56–9.
850. Tsui, S, W. H. Schubach. 1994. Epstein-Barr virus nuclear protein 2A forms oligomers *in vitro* and *in vivo* through a region required for B-cell transformation. *J Virol* 68:4287–94.
851. Tsurumi, T, T. Daikoku, R. Kurachi, Y. Nishiyama. 1993. Functional interaction between Epstein-Barr virus DNA polymerase catalytic subunit and its accessory subunit *in vitro*. *J Virol* 67:7648–53.
852. Tugwood, J. D, W. H. Lau, S. K. O, S. Y. Tsao, W. M. Martin, W. Shiu, C. Desgranges, P. H. Jones, J. R. Arrand. 1987. Epstein-Barr virus-specific transcription in normal and malignant nasopharyngeal biopsies and in lymphocytes from healthy donors and infectious mononucleosis patients. *J Gen Virol* 68:1081–91.
853. Uchibayashi, N, H. Kikutani, E. L. Barsumian, R. Hauptmann, F. J. Schneider, R. Schwendenwein, W. Sommergruber, W. Spevak, I. Maurer-Fogy, M. Suemura, et al. 1989. Recombinant soluble Fc epsilon receptor II (Fc epsilon RII/CD23) has IgE binding activity but no B cell growth promoting activity. *J Immunol* 142:3901–8.
854. Uchida, J, T. Yasui, Y. Takaoka-Shichijo, M. Muraoka, W. Kulwichit, N. Raab-Traub, H. Kikutani. 1999. Mimicry of CD40 signals by Epstein-Barr virus LMP1 in B lymphocyte responses. *Science* 286: 300–3.
855. van Santen, V, A. Cheung, M. Hummel, Kieff E. 1983. RNA encoded by the IR1–U2 region of Epstein-Barr virus DNA in latently infected, growth-transformed cells. *J Virol* 46:424–33.
856. van Santen, V, A. Cheung, Kieff E. 1981. Epstein-Barr virus RNA VII: Size and direction of transcription of virus-specified cytoplasmic RNAs in a transformed cell line. *Proc Natl Acad Sci U S A* 78:1930–4.
857. Vieira, P, R. de Waal-Malefyt, M. N. Dang, K. E. Johnson, R. Kastelein, D. F. Fiorentino, J. E. deVries, M. G. Roncarolo, T. R. Mosmann, K. W. Moore. 1991. Isolation and expression of human cytokine synthesis inhibitory factor cDNA clones: Homology to Epstein-Barr virus open reading frame BCRFI. *Proc Natl Acad Sci U S A* 88:1172–6.
858. Virgin, H. W. 4th, P. Latreille, P. Wamsley, K. Hallsworth, K. E. Weck, A. J. Dal Canto, S. H. Speck. 1997. Complete sequence and genomic analysis of murine gammaherpesvirus 68. *J Virol* 71:5894–904.
859. Wakasugi, H, L. Rimsky, Y. Mahe, A. M. Kamel, D. Fradelizi, T. Tursz, J. Bertoglio. 1987. Epstein-Barr virus-containing B-cell line produces an interleukin 1 that it uses as a growth factor. *Proc Natl Acad Sci U S A* 84:804–8.
860. Walling, D. M, N. M. Clark, D. M. Markovitz, T. S. Frank, D. K. Braun, E. Eisenberg, D. J. Krutchkoff, D. H. Felix, N. Raab-Traub. 1995. Epstein-Barr virus coinfection and recombination in non-human immunodeficiency virus-associated oral hairy leukoplakia [see comments]. *J Infect Dis* 171:1122–30.
861. Walling, D. M, S. N. Edmiston, J. W. Sixbey, M. Abdel-Hamid, L. Resnick, N. Raab-Traub. 1992. Coinfection with multiple strains of the Epstein-Barr virus in human immunodeficiency virus-associated hairy leukoplakia. *Proc Natl Acad Sci U S A* 89:6560–4.
862. Walling, D. M, A. G. Perkins, J. Webster-Cyriaque, L. Resnick, N. Raab-Traub. 1994. The Epstein-Barr virus EBNA-2 gene in oral hairy leukoplakia: Strain variation, genetic recombination, and transcriptional expression. *J Virol* 68:7918–26.
863. Walling, D. M, N. Raab-Traub. 1994. Epstein-Barr virus intrastrain recombination in oral hairy leukoplakia. *J Virol* 68:7909–17.
864. Waltzer, L, M. Perricaudet, A. Sergeant, E. Manet. 1996. Epstein-Barr virus EBNA3A and EBNA3C proteins both repress RBP-J kappa-EBNA2-activated transcription by inhibiting the binding of RBP-J kappa to DNA. *J Virol* 70:5909–15.
865. Wang, D, D. Liebowitz, Kieff E. 1985. An EBV membrane protein expressed in immortalized lymphocytes transforms established rodent cells. *Cell* 43:831–40.
866. Wang, D, D. Liebowitz, Kieff E. 1988. The truncated form of the Epstein-Barr virus latent-infection membrane protein expressed in virus replication does not transform rodent fibroblasts. *J Virol* 62:2337–46.
867. Wang, D, D. Liebowitz, F. Wang, C. Gregory, A. Rickinson, R. Larson, T. Springer, Kieff E. 1988. Epstein-Barr virus latent infection membrane protein alters the human B-lymphocyte phenotype: Deletion of the amino terminus abolishes activity. *J Virol* 62:4173–84.
868. Wang, F, C. Gregory, C. Sample, M. Rowe, D. Liebowitz, R. Murray, A. Rickinson, Kieff E. 1990. Epstein-Barr virus latent membrane protein (LMP1) and nuclear proteins 2 and 3C are effectors of phenotypic changes in B lymphocytes: EBNA-2 and LMP1 cooperatively induce CD23. *J Virol* 64:2309–18.
869. Wang, F, C. D. Gregory, M. Rowe, A. B. Rickinson, D. Wang, M. Birkenbach, H. Kikutani, T. Kishimoto, Kieff E. 1987. Epstein-Barr virus nuclear antigen 2 specifically induces expression of the B-cell activation antigen CD23. *Proc Natl Acad Sci U S A* 84:3452–6.
870. Wang, F, H. Kikutani, S. F. Tsang, T. Kishimoto, Kieff E. 1991. Epstein-Barr virus nuclear protein 2 transactivates a cis-acting CD23 DNA element. *J Virol* 65:4101–6.
871. Wang, F, A. Marchini, Kieff E. 1991. Epstein-Barr virus (EBV) recombinants: Use of positive selection markers to rescue mutants in EBV-negative B-lymphoma cells. *J Virol* 65:1701–9.

872. Wang, F, L. Petti, D. Braun, S. Seung, Kieff E. 1987. A bicistronic Epstein-Barr virus mRNA encodes two nuclear proteins in latently infected, growth-transformed lymphocytes. *J Virol* 61:945–54.
873. Wang, F, S. F. Tsang, M. G. Kurilla, Cohen JI, Kieff E. 1990. Epstein-Barr virus nuclear antigen 2 transactivates latent membrane protein LMP1. *J Virol* 64:3407–16.
874. Wang, L, S. R. Grossman, Kieff E. 2000. Epstein-Barr virus nuclear protein 2 interacts with p300, CBP, and PCAF histone acetyltransferases in activation of the LMP1 promoter. *Proc Natl Acad Sci U S A* 97:430–5.
875. Wang, X, L. M. Hutt-Fletcher. 1998. Epstein-Barr virus lacking glycoprotein gp42 can bind to B cells but is not able to infect. *J Virol* 72:158–63.
876. Wang, X, W. J. Kenyon, Q. Li, J. Mullberg, L. M. Hutt-Fletcher. 1998. Epstein-Barr virus uses different complexes of glycoproteins gH and gL to infect B lymphocytes and epithelial cells. *J Virol* 72:5552–8.
877. Weigel, R, D. K. Fischer, L. Heston, G. Miller. 1985. Constitutive expression of Epstein-Barr virus-encoded RNAs and nuclear antigen during latency and after induction of Epstein-Barr virus replication. *J Virol* 53:254–9.
878. Weis, J. J, D. T. Fearon, L. B. Klickstein, W. W. Wong, S. A. Richards, A. de Bruyn Kops, J. A. Smith, J. H. Weis. 1986. Identification of a partial cDNA clone for the C3d/Epstein-Barr virus receptor of human B lymphocytes: Homology with the receptor for fragments C3b and C4b of the third and fourth components of complement. *Proc Natl Acad Sci U S A* 83:5639–43.
879. Weis, J. J, T. F. Tedder, D. T. Fearon. 1984. Identification of a 145,000 Mr membrane protein as the C3d receptor (CR2) of human B lymphocytes. *Proc Natl Acad Sci U S A* 81:881–5.
880. Wells, A, N. Koide, Klein G. 1982. Two large virion envelope glycoproteins mediate Epstein-Barr virus binding to receptor-positive cells. *J Virol* 41:286–97.
881. Whang, Y, M. Silberklang, A. Morgan, S. Munshi, A. B. Lenny, R. W. Ellis, Kieff E. 1987. Expression of the Epstein-Barr virus gp350/220 gene in rodent and primate cells. *J Virol* 61:1796–807.
882. Williams, D. L, D. Kowalski. 1993. Easily unwound DNA sequences and hairpin structures in the Epstein-Barr virus origin of plasmid replication. *J Virol* 67:2707–15.
883. Wilson, G, G. Miller. 1979. Recovery of Epstein-Barr virus from non-producer neonatal human lymphoid cell transformants. *Virology* 95: 351–8.
884. Wilson, J. B, J. L. Bell, A. J. Levine. 1996. Expression of Epstein-Barr virus nuclear antigen-1 induces B cell neoplasia in transgenic mice. *EMBO J* 15:3117–26.
885. Wilson, J. B, W. Weinberg, R. Johnson, S. Yuspa, A. J. Levine. 1990. Expression of the BNLF-1 oncogene of Epstein-Barr virus in the skin of transgenic mice induces hyperplasia and aberrant expression of keratin 6. *Cell* 61:1315–27.
886. Woisetschlaeger, M, X. W. Jin, C. N. Yandava, L. A. Furmanski, J. L. Strominger, S. H. Speck. 1991. Role for the Epstein-Barr virus nuclear antigen 2 in viral promoter switching during initial stages of infection. *Proc Natl Acad Sci U S A* 88:3942–6.
887. Woisetschlaeger, M, J. L. Strominger, S. H. Speck. 1989. Mutually exclusive use of viral promoters in Epstein-Barr virus latently infected lymphocytes. *Proc Natl Acad Sci U S A* 86:6498–502.
888. Woisetschlaeger, M, C. N. Yandava, L. A. Furmanski, J. L. Strominger, S. H. Speck. 1990. Promoter switching in Epstein-Barr virus during the initial stages of infection of B lymphocytes. *Proc Natl Acad Sci U S A* 87:1725–9.
889. Wolf, J, M. Pawlita, A. Jox, S. Kohls, S. Bartnitzke, V. Diehl, J. Bullerdiek. 1993. Integration of Epstein Barr virus near the breakpoint of a translocation 11;19 in a Burkitt's lymphoma cell line. *Cancer Genet Cytogenet* 67:90–4.
890. Wong, K. M, A. J. Levine. 1986. Identification and mapping of Epstein-Barr virus early antigens and demonstration of a viral gene activator that functions in trans. *J Virol* 60:149–56.
891. Wu, D. Y, G. V. Kalpana, S. P. Goff, W. H. Schubach. 1996. Epstein-Barr virus nuclear protein 2 (EBNA2) binds to a component of the human SNF-SWI complex, hSNF5/Ini1. *J Virol* 70:6020–8.
892. Wu, D. Y, A. Krumm, W. H. Schubach. 2000. Promoter-specific targeting of human SWI-SNF complex by Epstein-Barr virus nuclear protein 2. *J Virol* 74:8893–903.
893. Wysokenski, D. A, J. L. Yates. 1989. Multiple EBNA1-binding sites are required to form an EBNA1-dependent enhancer and to activate a minimal replicative origin within oriP of Epstein-Barr virus. *J Virol* 63:2657–66.
894. Yalamanchili, R, S. Harada, Kieff E. 1996. The N-terminal half of EBNA2, except for seven prolines, is not essential for primary B-lymphocyte growth transformation. *J Virol* 70:2468–73.
895. Yalamanchili, R, X. Tong, S. Grossman, E. Johannsen, G. Mosialos, Kieff E. 1994. Genetic and biochemical evidence that EBNA 2 interaction with a 63-kDa cellular GTG-binding protein is essential for B lymphocyte growth transformation by EBV. *Virology* 204:634–41.
896. Yamamoto, H, T. Katsuki, Y. Hinuma, H. Hoshino, M. Miwa, H. Fujiki, T. Sugimura. 1981. Induction of Epstein-Barr virus by an new tumor promoter, teleocidin, compared to induction by TPA. *Int J Cancer* 28:125–9.
897. Yamamoto, N, T. Katsuki, Y. Hinuma. 1976. Transformation of tonsil lymphocytes by Epstein-Barr virus. *J Natl Cancer Inst* 56:1105–7.
898. Yamamoto, N, N. Mueller-Lantzsch, H. zur Hausen. 1980. Effect of actinomycin D and cycloheximide on Epstein-Barr virus early antigen induction in lymphoblastoid cells. *J Gen Virol* 51:255–61.
899. Yamamoto, N, H. zur Hausen. 1981. Induction of Epstein-Barr virus early antigens by intercalating chemicals in B95-8 cells. *Virology* 115:390–4.
900. Yanai, H, K. Takada, N. Shimizu, Y. Mizugaki, M. Tada, K. Okita. 1997. Epstein-Barr virus infection in non-carcinomatous gastric epithelium. *J Pathol* 183:293–8.
901. Yao, Q. Y, D. S. Croom-Carter, R. J. Tierney, G. Habeshaw, J. T. Wilde, F. G. Hill, C. Conlon, A. B. Rickinson. 1998. Epidemiology of infection with Epstein-Barr virus types 1 and 2: Lessons from the study of a T-cell-immunocompromised hemophilic cohort. *J Virol* 72:4352–63.
902. Yao, Q. Y, A. B. Rickinson, M. A. Epstein. 1985. Oropharyngeal shedding of infectious Epstein-Barr virus in healthy virus-immune donors. A prospective study. *Chin Med J (Engl)* 98:191–6.
903. Yao, Q. Y, R. J. Tierney, D. Croom-Carter, G. M. Cooper, C. J. Ellis, M. Rowe, A. B. Rickinson. 1996. Isolation of intertypic recombinants of Epstein-Barr virus from T-cell-immunocompromised individuals. *J Virol* 70:4895–903.
904. Yao, Q. Y, R. J. Tierney, D. Croom-Carter, D. Dukers, G. M. Cooper, C. J. Ellis, M. Rowe, A. B. Rickinson. 1996. Frequency of multiple Epstein-Barr virus infections in T-cell-immunocompromised individuals. *J Virol* 70:4884–94.
905. Yaswen, L. R, E. B. Stephens, L. C. Davenport, L. M. Hutt-Fletcher. 1993. Epstein-Barr virus glycoprotein gp85 associates with the BKRF2 gene product and is incompletely processed as a recombinant protein. *Virology* 195:387–96.
906. Yates, J, N. Warren, D. Reisman, B. Sugden. 1984. A cis-acting element from the Epstein-Barr viral genome that permits stable replication of recombinant plasmids in latently infected cells. *Proc Natl Acad Sci U S A* 81:3806–10.
907. Yates, J. L, S. M. Camiolo. 1988. Dissection of DNA replication and enhancer activation function of Epstein-Barr virus nuclear antigen 1. *Cancer Cells* 6:197–205.
908. Yates, J. L, S. M. Camiolo, J. M. Bashaw. 2000. The minimal replicator of Epstein-Barr virus oriP. *J Virol* 74:4512–22.
909. Yates, J. L, N. Guan. 1991. Epstein-Barr virus-derived plasmids replicate only once per cell cycle and are not amplified after entry into cells. *J Virol* 65:483–8.
910. Yates, J. L, N. Warren, B. Sugden. 1985. Stable replication of plasmids derived from Epstein-Barr virus in various mammalian cells. *Nature* 313:812–5.
911. Ye, H, Y. C. Park, M. Kreishman, Kieff E, H. Wu. 1999. The structural basis for the recognition of diverse receptor sequences by TRAF2. *Mol Cell* 4:321–30.
912. Ye, H, H. Wu. 2000. Thermodynamic characterization of the interaction between TRAF2 and tumor necrosis factor receptor peptides by isothermal titration calorimetry. *Proc Natl Acad Sci U S A* 97:8961–6.
913. Yokochi, T, R. D. Holly, E. A. Clark. 1982. B lymphoblast antigen (BB-1) expressed on Epstein-Barr virus-activated B cell blasts, B lymphoblastoid cell lines, and Burkitt's lymphomas. *J Immunol* 128: 823–7.
914. Yoo, L, S. H. Speck. 2000. Determining the role of the Epstein-Barr virus Cp EBNA2-dependent enhancer during the establishment of latency by using mutant and wild-type viruses recovered from cotton-top marmoset lymphoblastoid cell lines. *J Virol* 74:11115–20.

915. Yoo, L. I, M. Mooney, M. T. Puglielli, S. H. Speck. 1997. B-cell lines immortalized with an Epstein-Barr virus mutant lacking the Cp EBNA2 enhancer are biased toward utilization of the oriP-proximal EBNA gene promoter Wp1. *J Virol* 71:9134–42.
916. Yoshiyama, H, S. Imai, N. Shimizu, K. Takada. 1997. Epstein-Barr virus infection of human gastric carcinoma cells: Implication of the existence of a new virus receptor different from CD21. *J Virol* 71:5688–91.
917. Yoshizaki, T, H. Sato, M. Furukawa, J. S. Pagano. 1998. The expression of matrix metalloproteinase 9 is enhanced by Epstein-Barr virus latent membrane protein 1. *Proc Natl Acad Sci U S A* 95:3621–6.
918. Young, L. S, D. Clark, J. W. Sixbey, A. B. Rickinson. 1986. Epstein-Barr virus receptors on human pharyngeal epithelia. *Lancet* 1:240–2.
919. Young, L. S, R. Lau, M. Rowe, G. Niedobitek, G. Packham, F. Shanahan, D. T. Rowe, D. Greenspan, J. S. Greenspan, A. B. Rickinson, et al. 1991. Differentiation-associated expression of the Epstein-Barr virus BZLF1 transactivator protein in oral hairy leukoplakia. *J Virol* 65:2868–74.
920. Young, L. S, Q. Y. Yao, C. M. Rooney, T. B. Sculley, D. J. Moss, H. Rupani, G. Laux, G. W. Bornkamm, A. B. Rickinson. 1987. New type B isolates of Epstein-Barr virus from Burkitt's lymphoma and from normal individuals in endemic areas. *J Gen Virol* 68:2853–62.
921. Zerbini, M, I. Ernberg. 1983. Can Epstein-Barr virus infect and transform all the B-lymphocytes of human cord blood? *J Gen Virol* 64 Pt 3:539–47.
922. Zhang, C. X, P. Lowrey, S. Finerty, A. J. Morgan. 1993. Analysis of Epstein-Barr virus gene transcription in lymphoma induced by the virus in the cottontop tamarin by construction of a cDNA library with RNA extracted from a tumour biopsy. *J Gen Virol* 74:509–14.
923. Zhang, P. F, C. J. Marcus-Sekura. 1993. Conformation-dependent recognition of baculovirus-expressed Epstein-Barr virus gp350 by a panel of monoclonal antibodies. *J Gen Virol* 74:2171–9.
924. Zhang, Q, L. Brooks, P. Busson, F. Wang, D. Charron, Kieff E, A. B. Rickinson, T. Tursz. 1994. Epstein-Barr virus (EBV) latent membrane protein 1 increases HLA class II expression in an EBV-negative B cell line. *Eur J Immunol* 24:1467–70.
925. Zhang, Q, D. Gutsch, S. Kenney. 1994. Functional and physical interaction between p53 and BZLF1: Implications for Epstein-Barr virus latency. *Mol Cell Biol* 14:1929–38.
926. Zhao, B, D. R. Marshall, C. E. Sample. 1996. A conserved domain of the Epstein-Barr virus nuclear antigens 3A and 3C binds to a discrete domain of Jkappa. *J Virol* 70:4228–36.
927. Zhao, B, C. E. Sample. 2000. Epstein-barr virus nuclear antigen 3C activates the latent membrane protein 1 promoter in the presence of Epstein-Barr virus nuclear antigen 2 through sequences encompassing an spi-1/Spi-B binding site. *J Virol* 74:5151–60.
928. Zhou, S, M. Fujimuro, J. J. Hsieh, L. Chen, Hayward SD. 2000. A role for SKIP in EBNA2 activation of CBF1-repressed promoters. *J Virol* 74:1939–47.
929. Zhou, S, M. Fujimuro, J. J. Hsieh, L. Chen, A. Miyamoto, G. Weinmaster, Hayward SD. 2000. SKIP, a CBF1-associated protein, interacts with the ankyrin repeat domain of NotchIC To facilitate NotchIC function. *Mol Cell Biol* 20:2400–10.
930. Zimber-Strobl, U, E. Kremmer, F. Grasser, G. Marschall, G. Laux, G. W. Bornkamm. 1993. The Epstein-Barr virus nuclear antigen 2 interacts with an EBNA2 responsive cis-element of the terminal protein 1 gene promoter. *EMBO J* 12:167–75.
931. Zimber-Strobl, U, K. O. Suentzenich, G. Laux, D. Eick, M. Cordier, A. Calender, M. Billaud, G. M. Lenoir, G. W. Bornkamm. 1991. Epstein-Barr virus nuclear antigen 2 activates transcription of the terminal protein gene. *J Virol* 65:415–23.
932. Zimmermann, J, W. Hammerschmidt. 1995. Structure and role of the terminal repeats of Epstein-Barr virus in processing and packaging of virion DNA. *J Virol* 69:3147–55.
933. zur Hausen, H, G. W. Bornkamm, R. Schmidt, E. Hecker. 1979. Tumor initiators and promoters in the induction of Epstein-Barr virus. *Proc Natl Acad Sci U S A* 76:782–5.

CHAPTER 35

Poxviridae: The Viruses and Their Replication

Bernard Moss

The *Poxviridae* comprise a family of complex DNA viruses that replicate in the cytoplasm of vertebrate or invertebrate cells. These viruses are of special interest because of their unique biologic properties and impact on human health. Two members of the family—variola virus and molluscum contagiosum virus—are obligate human pathogens, and many others can be transmitted to humans from other animal hosts (see Chapter 85 in *Fields Virology*, 4th ed.). Variola virus can cause smallpox, a once common and devastating disease that altered human history. Smallpox was eradicated in 1977, nearly two centuries after the introduction of prophylactic inoculations with cowpox and vaccinia virus, through a dedicated effort spearheaded by the World Health Organization. Vaccination contributed to present concepts of infectious disease and immunity. Moreover, vaccinia virus was the first animal virus seen microscopically, grown in tissue culture, accurately titered, physically purified, and chemically analyzed. A once prevalent view of virus particles as packets of nucleic acid was revised after the discovery of RNA synthetic activity in purified vaccinia virions. This finding stimulated investigations that led to the discovery of transcriptase and reverse transcriptase activities in RNA viruses and to the elucidation of structural features of viral and eukaryotic messenger RNA (mRNA), including the 5′ cap and 3′ poly(A) tail. Recombinant DNA technology eliminated obstacles to working with these large viruses, and considerable progress has been made in elucidating the cycle of virus replication (Fig. 1). Discoveries of virus-encoded proteins that affect cell growth and modulate immune defense mechanisms provided new insights into virus–host relationships. In addition, the development of vaccinia virus as a live recombinant expression vector provided a powerful tool for immunologists and biochemists as well as an alternative approach to the development of vaccines against a variety of infectious agents.

CLASSIFICATION

The general properties of *Poxviridae* include: a large complex virion containing enzymes that synthesize mRNA; a genome composed of a single linear double-stranded DNA molecule of 130 to 300 kilobase pairs (kbp) with a hairpin loop at each end; and a cytoplasmic site of replication. The *Poxviridae* are divided into two subfamilies, *Chordopoxvirinae* and *Entomopoxvirinae*, based on vertebrate and insect host range (Table 1). DNA sequencing has confirmed the genetic relationship

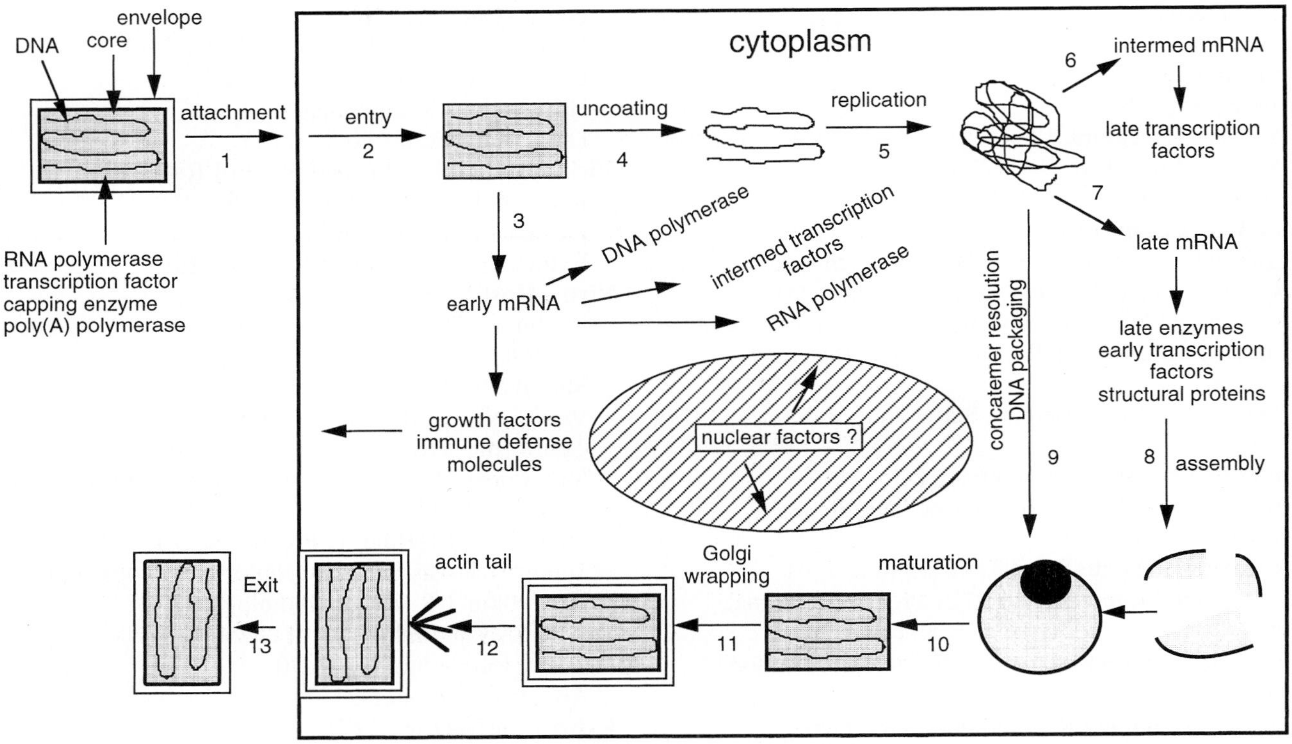

FIG. 1. The replication cycle of vaccinia virus. Virions, containing a double-stranded DNA genome, enzymes, and transcription factors, attach to cells (*1*) and penetrate the cell membrane, releasing cores into the cytoplasm (*2*). The cores synthesize early mRNAs that are translated into a variety of proteins, including growth factors, immune defense molecules, enzymes, and factors for DNA replication and intermediate transcription (*3*). Uncoating occurs (*4*), and the DNA is replicated to form concatemeric molecules (*5*). Intermediate genes in the progeny DNA are transcribed, and the mRNAs are translated to form late transcription factors (*6*). The late genes are transcribed, and the mRNAs are translated to form virion structural proteins, enzymes, and early transcription factors (*7*). Assembly begins with the formation of discrete membrane structures (*8*). The concatemeric DNA intermediates are resolved into unit genomes and packaged in immature virions (*9*). Maturation proceeds to the formation of infectious intracellular mature virions (*10*). The virions are wrapped by modified Golgi membranes, are transported to the periphery of the cell (*11*), and acquire actin tails (*12*). Fusion of the wrapped virions with the plasma membrane results in release of extracellular enveloped virus (*13*). Although replication occurs entirely in the cytoplasm, nuclear factors may be involved in transcription and assembly.

TABLE 1. *Family* Poxviridae

Subfamilies	Genera	Member viruses	Features
Chordopoxvirinae	*Orthopoxvirus*	Camelpox, cowpox, ectromelia, monkeypox, raccoonpox, skunkpox, [a]Uasin Gishu, [b,c]vaccinia, [c]variola, volepox	Brick-shaped virion, DNA ~200 kbp, G + C ~36%, wide to narrow host range, variola (smallpox), vaccinia (smallpox vaccine)
	Parapoxvirus	[a]Auzduk disease, [a]chamois contagious ecthyma, [b]orf, pseudocowpox, parapox of deer, [a]sealpox	Ovoid virion, DNA ~140 kbp, G + C ~64%
	Avipoxvirus	Canarypox, [b,c]fowlpox, juncopox, mynahpox, pigeonpox, psittacinepox, quailpox, [a]peacockpox, [a]penguinpox, sparrowpox, starlingpox, turkeypox	Brick shaped, DNA ~260 kbp, G + C ~35%, birds, arthropod transmission
	Capripoxvirus	Goatpox, lumpy skin disease, [b]sheeppox	Brick-shaped, DNA ~150 kbp, ungulates, arthropod transmission
	Leporipoxvirus	Hare fibroma, [b,c]myxoma, [c]rabbit fibroma, squirrel fibroma	Brick-shaped, DNA ~160 kbp, G + C ~40%, leporids and squirrels
	Suipoxvirus	Swinepox	Brick-shaped, DNA ~170 kbp, narrow host range
	Molluscipoxvirus	[c]Molluscum contagiosum	Brick-shaped, DNA ~180 kbp, G + C ~60%, human host, localized tumors, contact spread
	Yatapoxvirus	Tanapox, [b]Yaba monkey tumor	Brick-shaped, DNA ~145 kbp, G + C ~33%, primates and ? rodents
Entomopoxvirinae	*Entomopoxvirus* A	[b]*Melontha melontha*	Ovoid virion, DNA ~260–370 kbp, Coleoptera
	Entomopoxvirus B	[b,c]*Amsacta moorei*, [c]*Melanoplus sanguinipes*	Ovoid, DNA ~236 kbp, G + C ~18%, Lepidoptera and Orthoptera
	Entomopoxvirus C	[b]*Chrionimus luridus*	Brick-shaped, DNA ~250–380 kbp, Diptera

[a]Probable member of genus.
[b]Prototypal member.
[c]Completely sequenced.

between the two subfamilies. African swine fever virus shares some properties with poxviruses but is morphologically and genetically distinct and separately classified.

The *Chordopoxvirinae* consist of eight genera: *Orthopoxvirus, Parapoxvirus, Avipoxvirus, Capripoxvirus, Leporipoxvirus, Suipoxvirus, Molluscipoxvirus,* and *Yatapoxvirus* (see Table 1). Members of the same genus are genetically and antigenically related and have a similar morphology and host range. The orthopoxviruses have been studied most intensively. The prototypal member, vaccinia virus, has an unknown origin (41) and no known natural host, although it has been isolated from buffalo that probably contracted it from humans (149). DNA sequencing revealed that the genes common to vaccinia, variola, and cowpox viruses are greater than 90% identical (186,311,456,457), whereas limited data on orthopoxviruses indigenous to the Americas (e.g., raccoonpox virus and volepox virus) indicate that they are more genetically divergent (263). There are much less comparative data for individual members of the other poxvirus genera.

The *Entomopoxvirinae* have been divided into three genera based on the insect host of isolation (20). The prototypal members are listed in Table 1. The recent complete sequence analysis of the *Melanoplus sanguinipes* and *Amsacta moorei* viruses suggest that the Orthopteran and Lepidopteran members of genus B should be split into separate genera (1,40).

VIRION STRUCTURE

Morphology

Poxvirus virions are larger than those of other animal viruses and are discernible by light microscopy. The ultrastructural appearances of the particles varies according to the preparation methods. Vaccinia virions are visualized as smooth, rounded rectangles of about 350×270 nm by cryoelectron microscopy of unfixed and unstained vitrified samples (148) (Fig. 2). A 30-nm, membrane-delimited surface layer surrounds a homogenous core. Using the same technique, cores produced by treating virions with a detergent, reducing

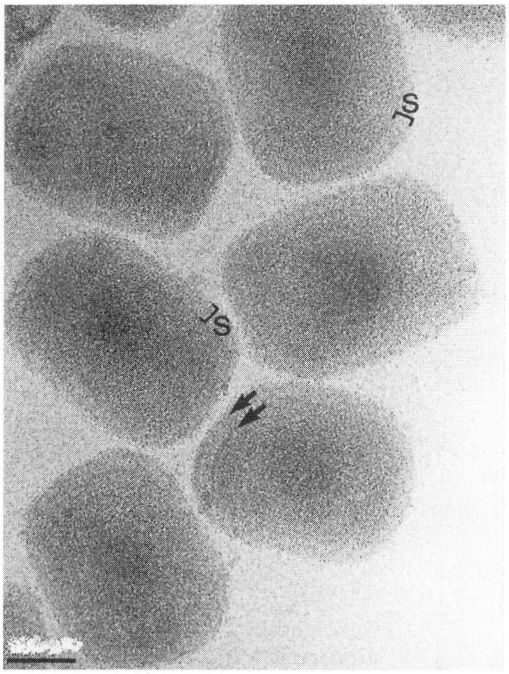

FIG. 2. Vitrified suspension of intracellular mature vaccinia virus particles observed by cryoelectron microscopy. The 30-nm thick surface domain (*S*) is delimited by arrows. (From ref. 148, with permission.)

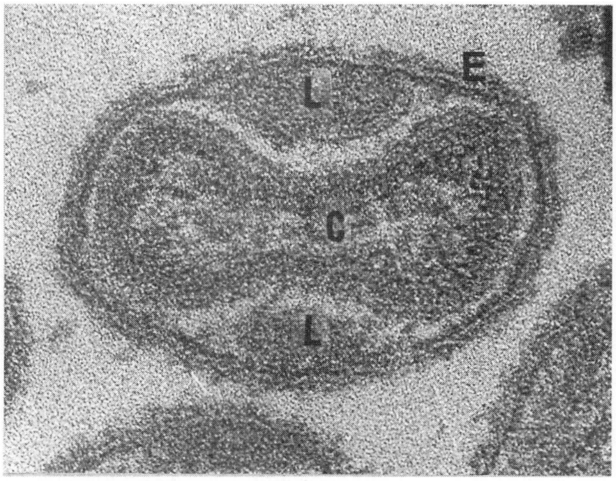

FIG. 3. Electron-microscopic image of a thin-sectioned intracellular mature vaccinia virus particle showing core (*C*), lateral bodies (*L*), and external membrane (*E*). (From ref. 393, with permission.)

agent, and deoxyribonuclease appear to be studded with 20-nm spikes. Two types of particles, C and M, are seen by negative staining of whole virions (359,546). The C form has a smooth exterior similar to the particles viewed by cryoelectron microscopy, whereas the M form has a beaded or tubular appearance also noted by freeze-etching (321). Incubation of virions with a nonionic detergent converts the M forms to C forms, but otherwise, the morphology appears unchanged (154). Further treatment with a reducing agent leads to removal of the outer coat, suggesting that disulfide-bonded proteins hold the latter together (154,422). Negatively stained images of cores, isolated by treatment with a detergent and reducing agent, have a rectangular shape; the wall of the core appears to be composed of an outer layer of cylindrical subunits 10 nm in length and 5 nm in diameter and an inner 5-nm thick smooth layer (154). Trypsin-sensitive structures called *lateral bodies* remain associated with cores prepared in this manner. In fixed and stained thin sections of virions, the core frequently appears dumbbell-shaped, with the lateral bodies in the concavities (126) (Fig. 3). It has been suggested that the surface tubules and the dumbbell-shaped cores result from nonisotropic drying because they are most clearly seen in dehydrated samples (148). Even so, an underlying structure must contribute to the acquisition of this highly characteristic appearance. Cylindrical elements that may take an S shape, or more complex flower-like structures, presumably representing nucleoprotein, have been visualized within poxvirus cores (227,390).

The preceding descriptions apply to cytoplasmic infectious particles that are called *intracellular mature virions* (IMVs). *Extracellular enveloped virions* (EEVs), isolated from the tissue culture medium, contain an additional somewhat fragile lipoprotein envelope and have a lower buoyant density than IMVs (378,422). Thus far, EEVs from only vaccinia virus have been analyzed.

Chemical Composition

The large size of poxvirus virions facilitated their isolation by low-speed centrifugation and permitted accurate chemical determinations in the early 1940s (483). The principal components of vaccinia virions are protein, lipid, and DNA. These account for 90%, 5%, and 3.2%, respectively, of the dry weight (575), which has been estimated to be about 5×10^{-15} g (484). In contrast, about one-third of fowlpox virions is lipid (298). The lipid components of vaccinia virions are predominantly cholesterol and phospholipids (492,498), whereas fowlpox virions also contain squalene and cholesterol esters (298). Carbohydrate is present in the EEV as a constituent of glycoproteins. Spermine and spermidine (278) and trace amounts of RNA (420) have also been found in vaccinia virions, but their significance has not been established.

Genome

Poxviruses have linear double-stranded DNA genomes that vary from 130 kbp in parapoxviruses to about 230 kbp in avipoxviruses. All poxviruses examined have *inverted terminal repetitions* (ITRs), which are identical but oppositely oriented sequences at the two ends of the genome (176) (Fig. 4). The ITRs include: an A+T-rich, incompletely base-paired, hairpin loop that connects the two DNA strands (36); a highly conserved region of less than 100 bp that contains sequences required for the resolution of replicating concatemeric forms of DNA (136,324); variable-length sets of short, tandemly repeated sequences (557); and up to several open reading frames (ORFs). The ITRs are variable in length owing to deletions, repetitions, and transpositions.

Complete genome sequences have been reported for six chordopoxviruses—vaccinia virus (19,186), variola virus (311,456), molluscum contagiosum virus (450), myxoma virus (89), Shope fibroma virus (552), and fowlpox virus (2)—and for two entomopoxviruses (1,40). There are about 100 ORFs that are represented in all chordopoxviruses and about 50 that are shared by chordopoxviruses and entomopoxviruses. Several generalizations can be made: ORFs are largely nonoverlapping, tend to occur in blocks pointing toward the nearer end of the genome, are usually located in the central region if highly conserved and concerned with essential replication functions, and are usually located in the end regions if variable and concerned with host interactions. The arrangement of the central genes is remarkably similar in all chordopoxviruses. The convention for naming orthopoxvirus ORFs was adopted before obtaining the complete genome sequence and consists of using the HindIII restriction endonuclease DNA fragment letter, followed by the ORF number (from left to right) within the fragment, and L or R, depending on the direction of the ORF. An exception to this rule was made for the HindIII C fragment; the ORFs were numbered from right to left to avoid starting at the left end of the genome, which is highly variable. For reference, the physical order of the 16 HindIII fragments of vaccinia virus is C, N, M, K, F, E, P, O, I, G, L, J, H, D, A, B. With the other poxviruses, the convention has been to number the ORFs continuously starting from one end.

Polypeptides

Consistent with their size and complex structures, poxvirus virions are composed of a large number of polypeptides. About 30 bands are readily resolved by one-dimensional polyacrylamide gel electrophoresis of vaccinia virus virions that have been purified from infected cells and disrupted with sodium dodecyl sulfate and a reducing agent, and considerably more can be detected by two-dimensional analysis (240). Twelve

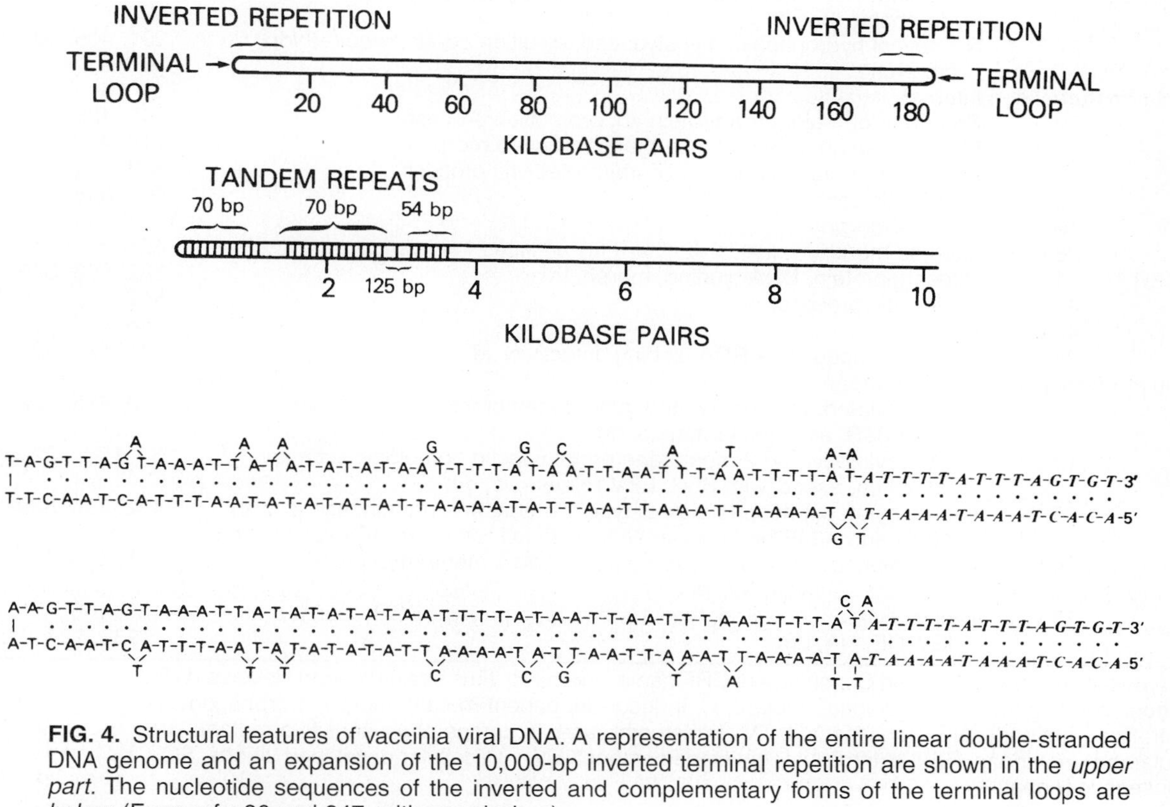

FIG. 4. Structural features of vaccinia viral DNA. A representation of the entire linear double-stranded DNA genome and an expansion of the 10,000-bp inverted terminal repetition are shown in the *upper part.* The nucleotide sequences of the inverted and complementary forms of the terminal loops are *below.* (From refs. 36 and 347, with permission.)

polypeptides have been localized near the exterior of the IMV by one or more of the following procedures: surface-specific labeling, sensitivity to proteases, extraction with nonionic detergents, and reactivity with virus-neutralizing antibodies (Table 2). Some of these proteins may form a disulfide-bonded matrix because both a reducing agent and a nonionic detergent are required for their release (233). There is evidence for physical association of the A17L, A27L, and A14L polypeptides in a complex (418). The L1R polypeptide is myristylated (405), and the A14L and A17L proteins are phosphorylated (55,143). Many of the IMV membrane proteins have unusual topologies: the A17L protein crosses the membrane twice with both the N- and C-terminal ends in the cytoplasm (54). The D8L (434) and the H3L (120) proteins are anchored by N- and C-terminal hydrophobic domains, respectively.

After IMVs are treated with a nonionic detergent and reducing agent, the cores can be recovered by low-speed centrifugation. Disruption of the core with deoxycholate releases a soluble enzyme fraction (described in the next section) from insoluble structural proteins. Four of the latter proteins, encoded by the F17R, L4R, A3L, and A10L ORFs, account for about 70% of the viral core by weight (see Table 2). The F17R 11-kd phosphoprotein and the L4R 25-kd polypeptide bind DNA and may cor-

TABLE 2. *Nonenzymatic vaccinia virion components*

ORF	Size (kda)	Properties	Selected references
Intracellular mature virion membrane associated			
A9L	12.1	Putative signal peptide and TM domain, required for morph, id	572
A13L	7.7	N-terminal hydrophobic	434, 507
A14L	10.0	Phosphorylated, myristylated, assoc. with A17L, required morph, id	55, 418, 419, 520
A14.5	6.2	Largely hydrophobic, NE, dm	56
A17L	23.0	N- and C-terminal processing, TM domains, phosphorylated, assoc. with A14L and A27L, NA, required morph, id	53, 54, 143, 271, 413, 560
A27L	12.6	"Fusion protein," heparin-binding, required for EEV, NA, id	106, 416, 417, 537
D8L	35.3	Binds chondroitin sulfate, dm	218, 491
D13L	61.9	Rifampicin resistance, virus morph, ? virion assoc., id, ts	240, 332, 493, 578
E10R	10.8	N-terminal hydrophobic, redox function, required for morph, id	452, 453
H3L	37.5	C-terminal TM, enhances IMV morph, heparin-binding, NA, dm, id	120, 121, 286
I5L	8.7	Hydrophobic, basic	507
L1R	27.3	N-terminal hydrophobic, myristyolated, disulfide bonds, required for morph, id	231, 405, 406, 561
Intracellular mature virion internal			
A3L	72.6	Precursor of major core protein 4b, proteolytic process	343, 428, 533
[a]A4/5L	30.8	Matrix between core and membrane, required morph, id	118, 412, 545, 553
A10L	102.3	Precursor of major core protein 4a, proteolytic process	343, 536, 556
A12L	20.5	Proteolytic process	507, 548
D2L	16.9	Core, ts morph	151
D3R	28.0	Core, ts morph	151
[a]F17/18R	11.3	Phosphoprotein, DNA binding, morph, id	382, 556, 579
G7L	41.9	Proteolytic process	507
I7L	49.0	ts morph	246
L4R	28.5	Single-stranded DNA/RNA binding, infectivity, id	44, 549, 550
Extracellular enveloped virion-membrane			
A33R		N-glycosylated, phosphorylated, type 2 membrane protein, assoc. with A36R, actin tail formation, dm	423, 425, 562
A34R	19.5	N-glycosylated, type 2 membrane protein, lectin homology, actin tail formation, assoc. with B5R, EEV release, id, dm	62, 150, 432, 559
A36R	25.1	N-glycosylated, phosphorylated, type 1 membrane protein, assoc. with A33R and A34R and cellular Nck, actin tail formation, IEV-specific, dm	432, 436, 529
A56R	34.8	Hemagglutinin, *N*- and *O*-glycosylated, type 1 membrane protein, prevents syncytia, NE, dm	448, 459, 460
B5R	35.1	*N*-glycosylated, acylated, type 1 membrane protein, SCR, required for IEV, NE, NA, dm	155, 156, 173, 203, 237, 294, 312, 543

[a]ORF name in vaccinia virus strain Copenhagen; ORF name in vaccinia virus strain Western Reserve (WR).

ORF, open reading frame; dm, deletion mutant; id, inducer-dependent mutant; morph, morphogenesis; NA, neutralizing antibody; NE, nonessential; TM, transmembrane; ts, temperature-sensitive mutant; IMV, intracellular mature virions; EEV, extracellular enveloped virions; IEV, intracellular enveloped virions; SCR, short consensus repeat.

respond to nucleoprotein constituents (233). The mature G7L, L4R, A3L, A10L, and A12L proteins are processed from larger precursors at Ala-Gly-Ala/Ser motifs during morphogenesis (343,536). Vaccinia virus EEVs have a lower buoyant density than IMVs because of the additional lipid membrane and contain several unique glycosylated proteins with type I or II topologies encoded by the A33R, A34R, A36R, A56R, and B5R ORFs (see Table 2) and by F13L, a nonglycosylated phospholipase (Table 3).

Enzymes

Infectious poxvirus particles contain a transcription system (248,354) that can carry out *in vitro* synthesis of mRNAs that are polyadenylylated (247), capped, and methylated (544). A large number of virus-encoded enzymes and factors are packaged in the virus particle (see Table 3). Many of these, including the RNA polymerase, RNA polymerase-associated protein of 94 kd (RAP94), vaccinia early transcription factor (VETF), capping and methylating enzymes, poly(A) polymerase,

TABLE 3. *Vaccinia virion enzymes and factors*

Enzymes/factors	ORF	Size (kda)	Properties	Selected references
RNA polymerase			Multisubunit	35, 341, 495
RPO 147	J6R	147	Cell RPO homol, ts	78, 514
RPO 132	A24R	132	Cell RPO homol, ts	14, 213
RPO 35	A29R	35		16
RPO 30	E4L	30	Eukaryote TFIIS homol	3, 81
RPO 22	J4R	22	ts, histidine tag mutant	78, 251, 514
RPO 19	A5R	19		8
RPO 18	D7R	18	ts	5, 401
RPO 7	G5.5R	7	Eukaryote homol	15
RNA polymerase-associated protein (RAP94)	H4L	94	Early promoter specificity factor, ts	4, 7, 142, 245
Early transcription factor (VETF)			Binds early promoter, DNA-dependent ATPase	75, 77, 82
Large subunit	A7/8L	82	Binds promoter	96, 180, 222
Small subunit	D6R	74	ts	73, 74, 96, 180, 221, 285
Capping enzyme			RNA triphosphase, guanylyltransferase, guanine-7-methyltransferase, termination factor	295, 307, 469, 538
Large subunit	D1R	97	Covalent GMP, catalytic activities, ts	194, 337, 356, 472, 473
Small subunit	D12L	33	Stimulates guanine-7-methyltransferase, ts	115, 363
Poly(A) polymerase			Primer-depend	177, 344
Large subunit	E1L	55	Poly(A) polymerase catalytic subunit	178, 182, 183
Small subunit	J3R	39	Poly(A) polymerase stimulatory subunit	178, 181
RNA nucleoside-2′-methyltransferase	J3R	39	Methylates capped end of mRNA, stimulates transcription	209, 444, 568
Nucleoside triphosphate phosphohydrolase I (NPH I)	D11L	72	DExH box family, DNA-dependent ATPase RNA helicase, transcription termination factor, ts	79, 105, 141, 372, 415
Nucleoside triphosphate phosphohydrolase II (NPH II)	I8R	77	DExH box family, DNA/RNA-dependent ribonucleoside triphosphatase, RNA helicase, early transcription, ts	43, 167, 190, 372, 467
DNA helicase	A18R		DNA-dependent ATPase, transcript release factor, ts	42, 273, 476, 477
DNA topoisomerase I	H6R	37	Sequence-specific nicking	39, 466, 475
Protein kinase 1	B1R	34	Serine/threonine, ts	32, 47, 288, 410
Protein kinase 2	F10L	52	Serine/threonine, ts	259, 287, 518, 542
Protein phosphatase	H1L		Dual (ser/tyr) specificity	192, 290
Glutaredoxin 1	O2L	12	Thioltransferase, cofactor for viral ribonucleotide reductase, NE	9, 402
Glutaredoxin 2	G4L		Thioltransferase, id	195, 547
Phospholipase	F13L		Phospholipase, EEV membrane, dm	25, 60, 424

ORF, open reading frame; homol, homology; ts, temperature-sensitive mutant; NE, nonessential; id, inducer-dependent mutant; dm, deletion mutant.

and nucleoside triphosphate phosphohydrolase (NPH) I are directly involved in the synthesis and modification of mRNA. Additional enzymes may also be involved in synthesis of RNA or in virus assembly, protein processing, or DNA packaging.

VIRUS ENTRY

Studies of poxvirus entry into cells are complicated by the existence of multiple infectious forms that may use different and still unidentified cellular receptors and viral proteins (381,530). Although IMVs are commonly used by investigators to infect cells, they are only released by cell lysis; EEVs (68,380), and particularly the related *cell-associated enveloped virions* (CEVs) (61), are important for efficient cell-to-cell spread. IMVs are generally thought to enter cells by fusion with the plasma membrane or vesicles formed by surface invaginations (98,124,146,238). The inhibition of IMV entry by cytochalasin B and D suggests a role for actin filaments (381,530). In contrast to IMVs, some data suggest that EEVs enter cells by a mechanism that involves endocytosis followed by low pH disruption of the EEV outer membrane and fusion of the released IMV with endosomal membranes (228,530). The fusion of infected cells to each other, mediated by short exposure to a low pH, may mimic the latter process by disrupting the outer membrane of virus particles on the cell surface (146,187).

Poxvirus Receptors

A virus receptor is usually defined as a component on the cell surface to which a virus specifically binds and that mediates virus internalization. Because vaccinia virus can enter virtually all cell lines tested, there must be either many receptors or one that is ubiquitous. Thus far, however, no receptor has been unequivocally identified for any poxvirus. A virus-binding site, in contrast to a receptor, allows virus attachment but not necessarily entry. Evidence that IMV and EEV have different binding sites includes the efficiency with which the two virus types bind to different cell lines, differential effects of cell surface digestion with proteases, and the specific effect of a monoclonal antibody on binding of IMV (101,532). Heparin sulfate binds to vaccinia IMV and can inhibit infection by IMV of several orthopoxviruses and leporipoxviruses, suggesting that cell surface proteoglycans could serve as general mediators of poxvirus infection (106). It will be important, however, to rule out the possibility that heparin sulfate binding is an adaptation to passage in tissue culture. A candidate cell surface receptor was identified with a monoclonal antibody that blocked binding of IMV to cells (101). A suggestion that the epidermal growth factor (EGF) receptor serves as a portal of entry for vaccinia virus (305) has not been generally accepted (225). An exciting, albeit short-lived, proposal that poxviruses use chemokine receptors was based on studies with Shope fibroma virus (277). However, recent data (G. McFadden, personal communication) does not support this hypothesis.

Poxvirus Entry Proteins

Information about which viral proteins mediate cell entry and penetration is limited. At least four vaccinia IMV proteins—L1R, A27L, D8R, and H3L—have been implicated. Monoclonal antibodies to the L1R (231,561) and A27L (414) proteins neutralize the infectivity of IMV. In addition, the A27L protein plays a critical role in low pH–mediated cell-to-cell fusion, and an N-terminal domain binds heparin sulfate (187,217,537). The H3L protein also binds heparin sulfate, and a deletion mutant was reported to bind less efficiently to cells under some conditions (286), but not others (121). A role for the D8L protein was suggested by its ability to bind to cell surface chondroitin sulfate and by decreased binding of virions with a mutation in the *D8L* gene (218,274). Treatment of vaccinia virions with proteases increases infectivity, apparently by enhancing cell penetration (232).

A difficulty in studying entry of EEV is that purified preparations may contain damaged particles with exposed IMV membranes. In addition, deletion or repression of some genes encoding EEV membrane proteins may affect formation of the membrane, precluding an analysis of their role in entry. Repression of the *A34R* gene, which encodes a glycoprotein with a putative lectin domain, however, leads to increased production of EEV with reduced infectivity (319). Whether this reduction is due to a defect in cell binding or later steps has not been determined. The B5R protein has also been implicated in cell entry because polyclonal antibodies to its extracellular domain neutralize EEV (173). Nevertheless, the extracellular domain does not appear to be essential for infectivity (203,312). Mutations of the hemagglutinin or the K2L glycoprotein result in the fusion of infected cells (448,524). However, neither the mechanism of fusion inhibition nor the roles of these proteins are understood.

Cell-to-cell spread is mediated most efficiently by CEVs, which resemble EEVs except that they are still attached to the plasma membrane of the parental cell (61). Vaccinia virus strains, such as WR, that produce mostly CEV form large, round plaques; whereas those that release large numbers of EEVs, such as IHD, form long comet-like plaques on cell monolayers under a liquid overlay. The different plaque phenotypes were mapped to a single amino acid substitution in the putative lectin domain of the A34R glycoprotein (62). Most orthopoxviruses have the WR-like sequence, suggesting that increased EEV may be an adaptation to spread in tissue culture. The extracellular domain of the B5R protein may also have a role in release of cell-associated virions (312). The efficient spread of CEVs is facilitated by their location at the tips of long microvilli that form by attachment of actin tails to the viral particles (119,499). Deletion of the *A34R, A33R,* or *A36R* gene prevents actin tail and microvillus formation and reduces the efficiency of virus spread (423,437,559,563). Presumably, the CEVs have the same outer membrane as EEVs, and details regarding their entry will be similar. A further discussion of these topics appears in a later section on EEV.

UNCOATING

After entry into the cytoplasm, virus cores are transported to juxtanuclear locations where they synthesize mRNA and undergo a second uncoating step. Electron microscopic images suggest that the nucleoprotein complex passes out through breaches in the core wall (123). Susceptibility of the virion DNA to treatment with deoxyribonuclease has been used as biochemical evidence of uncoating (241). Prevention of the uncoating process by inhibitors of transcription or translation (242) indicates a requirement for either a virus-induced or virus-encoded protein. A putative 23-kd uncoating protein with trypsin-like activity was partially purified from infected cell extracts (383). Viral particles in intermediate stages of disassembly have been isolated, and the polypeptide compositions have been analyzed (382).

GENE EXPRESSION

Programmed Expression of Poxvirus Genes

Studies primarily with vaccinia virus have led to a general understanding of how the DNA genomes of poxviruses are expressed within the cytoplasm of infected cells (see Fig. 1). A complete early transcription system is synthesized late in infection and packaged within the core of an infectious poxvirus particle, providing a mechanism for the initial synthesis of viral mRNAs. These early mRNAs encode enzymes and factors needed for transcription of the intermediate class of genes that in turn encode enzymes and factors for late gene expression (Table 4).

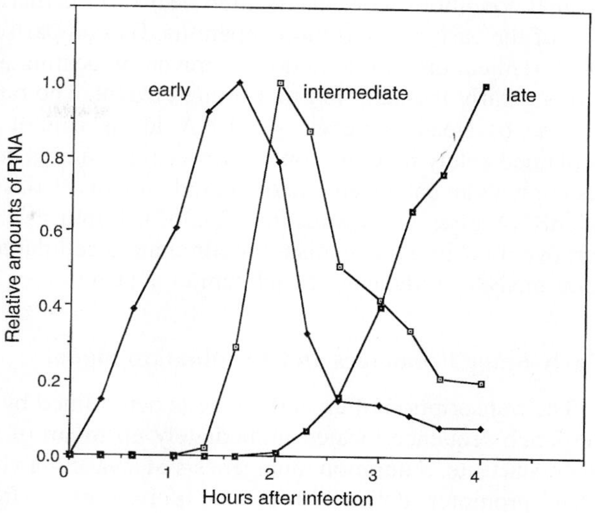

FIG. 5. Steady-state levels of representative early-, intermediate-, and late-stage messenger RNAs (mRNAs) in vaccinia virus–infected cells. Total RNA was isolated from infected HeLa cells at various times after infection and hybridized to antisense RNA probes specific for the 5′ ends of mRNAs encoded by the C11R (early), G8R (intermediate), or F17R (late) open reading frames (ORFs) (28). After ribonuclease digestion, the protected probe fragments were analyzed by polyacrylamide gel electrophoresis and the radioactivity quantified. The numbers were normalized to the peak value in each case.

Regulation of Early-Stage Transcription

Vaccinia virus early mRNA is detected within 20 minutes after infection and accumulates to maximal levels in 1 to 2 hours (28) (Fig. 5). About half of the vaccinia virus genome is transcribed before DNA replication (65,371), including genes encoding proteins involved in host interactions, viral DNA synthesis, and intermediate gene expression. When uncoating of the core is prevented by protein synthesis inhibitors, early mRNA synthesis is increased and prolonged (28,564), suggesting that under

TABLE 4. *Stage-specific transcription factors encoded by vaccinia virus*

Stage	Factor	ORF	Promoter	Properties	Selected references
Early	VETF	A7L, D6R	Late	Heterodimer, DNA binding, ATPase	75, 77, 82, 96 73, 74, 180, 285
	RAP94	H4L	Late	Associated with RNA polymerase	4, 7, 142
Intermediate	VITF 1	E4L	Early	Homology to TFIIS, also RNA polymerase subunit RP030	426
	VITF 3	A8R, A23R	Early	Heterodimer	439, 440
	Capping enzyme	D1R, D12L	Early	Heterodimer, also functions to modify mRNA	202, 540
Late	VLTF 1	G8R	Intermed	Interacts with self and VLTF 2	253, 314, 566, 580
	VLTF 2	A1L	Intermed	Interacts with VLTF 1, zinc binding	92, 253, 255, 314, 565
	VLTF 3	A2L	Intermed	Zinc binding	223, 253, 254, 375
	VLTF 4	H5R	Early	Stimulates transcription	269

ORF, open rending frame.

normal conditions, core disassembly leads to the disruption of the early transcription apparatus. By comparison, DNA replication inhibitors do not prevent uncoating and prolong early transcription to a limited extent. The rapid decline of steady-state early mRNA levels cannot be explained solely by cessation of transcription and is consistent with an enhanced rate of degradation of all classes of mRNA after virus infection (28,366). Rapid mRNA turnover may be a mechanism for eliminating cellular and viral mRNAs at the end of each temporal stage.

Early-Stage Promoters and Termination Signal

The transcription of an early gene is determined by an A+T-rich sequence located immediately upstream of the RNA start site. Saturation mutagenesis of a vaccinia virus early promoter defined a critical core region, from nucleotide −13 to −27, in which many single substitutions have a drastic effect on expression (131) (Fig. 6). A consensus core sequence AAAAAATGAAAAAA/TA is close to the optimal one defined by mutagenesis. Transcription initiation occurs with a purine, predominantly 12 to 17 nucleotides downstream of the core region. The intervening DNA, between the core and RNA start site, appears to have a spacer role, and there are no evident sequence requirements upstream of the core or downstream of the initiation site. Promoter sequences are conserved between poxvirus genera, partially explaining the phenomenon called *nongenetic reactivation,* which consists of rescue of a heat-inactivated poxvirus by co-infection with a second poxvirus (169,200). Thus, the heat-killed poxvirus provides the template and the second poxvirus provides the enzymes for transcription.

The 3′ ends of vaccinia virus early mRNAs occur 20 to 50 bp downstream of the sequence TTTTTNT (574). Such termination sequences are present near the ends of most viral early genes but only rarely in their middle. When absent, the mRNA may extend through the next early gene downstream. *In vivo* studies suggested that the efficiency of termination is about 80% (152), although in some cases, it is much less, probably because of RNA secondary structure (282,296). TTTTTNT sequences have been noted near the ends of putative early genes in other poxvirus genera, suggesting a similar role in termination. As discussed later, the TTTTTNT sequence is actually recognized as UUUUUNU in RNA (474).

VACCINIA VIRUS PROMOTER SEQUENCES

	CORE	INITIATOR
EARLY	AAAA T GAAA TA	A/G
INTER	T TT AAA AA	TAAA
LATE	A/T-rich	TAAATG/A
	−30 −20 −10	+1

FIG. 6. Early-, intermediate-, and late-stage promoter sequences. Nucleotides that have a strong positive effect on transcription are shown. Positions of nucleotides in the nontemplate strand are relative to the RNA start site (+1). (From ref. 340, with permission.)

Enzymes and Factors for Early-Stage Transcription

A complete early transcription system is packaged within the core of an infectious poxvirus particle (248, 354). Soluble extracts of vaccinia virus virions can transcribe an early promoter template *in vitro* to generate properly initiated and terminated mRNAs (421) and therefore provide a source of materials for characterization of the relevant enzymes and factors. The virion RNA polymerase is eukaryotic-like with regard to its size and subunit complexity (35). The subunits, ranging from 7- to 147-kd, are encoded by at least eight viral genes (see Table 3). There is a single copy of each large subunit, but the stoichiometry of the small subunits has not been accurately determined, partly because of polypeptide heterogeneity caused by alternative transcriptional and translational start sites. RPO147 and RPO132 are homologous to the corresponding large subunits of cellular RNA polymerase and resemble those of eukaryotes and archae (20% to 30% amino acid identities over the entire proteins) slightly more than those of bacteria. The vaccinia virus RPO30 subunit is about 23% identical in sequence to eukaryotic transcription elongation factor SII (TFIIS); RPO7, the smallest vaccinia virus RNA polymerase subunit, is about 23% identical in amino acid sequence with the smallest eukaryotic RNA polymerase subunit. Although the functions of the individual viral RNA polymerase subunits have not been investigated, the large ones are likely to catalyze nucleotide addition based on homology with the cellular enzymes. Temperature-sensitive (ts) mutants with defects mapped to RNA polymerase subunits have been isolated (213,514). Mutant virions, propagated at the permissive temperature, generally contain active RNA polymerase, and early gene expression occurs even when cells are infected at the nonpermissive temperature. The phenotype of these mutants is a block in late gene expression, probably caused by aberrant assembly of the multisubunit enzyme.

An additional polypeptide is associated with RNA polymerase molecules in vaccinia virions (4,7,142). This RAP94 is specifically required for transcription of early promoter templates in conjunction with the VETF. RNA polymerase lacking RAP94 can transcribe single-stranded DNA nonspecifically or double-stranded intermediate or late promoter templates with the corresponding transcription factors. It seems likely that RAP94 interacts with VETF, although this has yet to be demonstrated. Synthesis of RAP94 occurs late, at the time of virion assembly, consistent with its exclusive role as a virion-associated early transcription factor. In this regard, RAP94 is distinct from the RNA polymerase subunits that are synthesized throughout the infectious cycle for intermediate and late transcription.

Transcriptional activity can be reconstituted *in vitro* with RNA polymerase and VETF, a heterodimer of 82 and 70 kd subunits (82,180). VETF, like RAP94, is synthesized only at late times after infection. The protein binds to the core region of early promoters and to DNA downstream of the RNA start site, thereby altering the conformation of the DNA (75,96). Single nucleotide substitutions in the core sequence of the promoter that decrease transcription also abrogate specific DNA binding (573). A DNA-dependent adenosine triphosphatase (ATPase) activity associated with the small subunit of VETF is not required for promoter binding but is essential for transcription, possibly through a promoter clearance mechanism (71,77,283). Complexes of VETF and RNA polymerase have been detected, suggesting that VETF may recruit RNA polymerase to the promoter (27,80,251,284). The elongation complex has a 3′ RNase activity that permits resumption of transcription by stalled polymerase (197). A role for RPO30 has been suggested because the latter RNase activity is similar to one exhibited by eukaryotic RNA polymerase II in the presence of TFIIS, an RPO30 homolog.

A physical complex of RNA polymerase, VETF, capping enzyme, and NPH I (a DNA-dependent ATPase) can accurately terminate, as well as initiate, transcription on DNA templates containing an early promoter and TTTTTNT sequence (80,574). Although RNA polymerase and VETF can reconstitute the transcription initiation and elongation activities, capping enzyme and NPH I are needed to release nascent mRNA containing a UUUUUNU sequence from the transcription complex in an adenosine triphosphate (ATP)-dependent reaction (105, 141,469,474). The physical interaction of NPH I with RAP94 may explain the specificity of this termination system for early transcripts (334). NPH I also serves as a polymerase elongation factor to facilitate read-through of intrinsic pause sites (141).

Because early viral transcripts made *in vivo* or *in vitro* are capped (64,544) and polyadenylylated (247), they structurally and functionally resemble eukaryotic mRNAs. RNAs synthesized by virus cores contain a cap I structure that consists of a terminal 7-methylguanosine connected by a triphosphate bridge to a 2′-*O*-methylribonucleoside. The N^7-methylguanosine component of the cap is required for mRNA stability and for binding of vaccinia virus mRNA to ribosomes, whereas the role of ribose methylation is undetermined (355). Capping occurs during transcription when the nascent RNA chains are about 30 nucleotides long (196). The steps in cap formation are: (a) removal of the terminal phosphate of the triphosphate end of the nascent RNA to form a pp(5′)N-terminus, (b) transfer of a guanosine monophosphate (GMP) residue from guanosine triphosphate (GTP) to form G(5′)ppp(5′)N-, (c) transfer of a methyl group from *S*-adenosylmethionine to produce m^7G(5′)ppp(5′)N-, and (d) transfer of a second methyl group to form m^7G(5′)ppp(5′)Nm. The first three reactions are catalyzed by the virus-encoded 127-kd heterodimeric capping enzyme (307,308,538). The fourth step in cap formation, ribose methylation of the penultimate nucleoside, is mediated by a separate viral enzyme (34). The capping enzyme large subunit forms a covalent lysyl-GMP intermediate (114,362,431,472). The RNA triphosphatase and guanylyltransferase activities reside in an N-terminal segment of the large subunit (357,473), whereas a complex of the C-terminal part of the large subunit and the small subunit contains the N^7-methyltransferase activity (205, 304). The nucleoside 2′-methyltransferase is a 39-kd protein that exists as a monomeric species and as a subunit of the poly(A) polymerase (444). High-resolution x-ray crystal structures of the nucleoside 2′-methyltransferase complexed to its methyl donor and mRNA cap have been determined (209,210). Viral mRNAs synthesized *in vivo* have additional base and ribose methylations that are catalyzed by cellular enzymes (64).

The enzyme that catalyzes poly (A) tail formation is a heterodimer of virus-encoded 55- and 39-kd subunits called VP55 and VP39, respectively (178,344). VP55 binds to uridylate sequences near the end of the RNA chain and catalyzes the processive addition of 30 to 35 adenylate residues before changing to a slow and nonprocessive mechanism (140,183). VP39 binds poly(A) and stimulates VP55 to add additional adenylate residues (181). Thus, VP39, which is present in an excess over VP55, serves as a processivity factor for the poly(A) polymerase as well as a methyltransferase. The two activities are independent because mutated forms of VP39 that lack methyltransferase but retain adenylyltransferase stimulatory activity *in vitro* have been produced (445,458). Genetic and biochemical studies indicate an additional role of VP39 as an RNA elongation factor for intermediate and late RNA synthesis (279,568), discussed later. The finding that the capping enzyme and termination factor and the ribose methyltransferase and poly(A) polymerase processivity factor function at the 5′ and 3′ ends of the mRNA is intriguing. Whether the association of such apparently disparate functions in the same enzymes provides a specific advantage or represents an economical use of proteins is unknown.

The minimal components for synthesis of correctly initiated, terminated, capped, and polyadenylylated mRNA were defined by *in vitro* reconstitution assays. However, additional enzymes may be needed within the virus core. One example is NPH II, an enzyme with RNA-dependent RNA nucleoside triphosphatase and RNA helicase (372,468) activities. Permeabilized mutant virions lacking NPH II have diminished transcription activity and produce longer than normal RNAs that remain virion associated, suggesting a role in transcription termination or extrusion (191). Studies with ts mutants suggest that the A18R DNA helicase has a role in early, as well as late, transcription (476,477). Biochemical studies indicate that the A18R protein, along with an unidentified cellular component, acts a transcript release factor (273). Virions deficient in the H1L serine-tyrosine phosphatase have low transcription activity, suggesting a regulatory role along with that of the virion-associated protein kinases (290).

Regulation of Intermediate-Stage Transcription

DNA replication precedes a shift in viral gene expression. Amino acid labeling (346,385) and transcription (28,541) studies indicated the existence of an intermediate class of genes that are expressed after DNA replication but before expression of the late genes (see Fig. 1). After synchronous infection, intermediate mRNAs were detected at 100 minutes, the time of peak early mRNA accumulation (see Fig. 5). Intermediate mRNAs reached their peak values soon after and then declined in quantity. Only seven vaccinia virus genes belonging to the intermediate class have been identified thus far (253,271, 541), although additional ones exist (580). Three of these (*A1L, A2L,* and *G8R*) encode transactivators of late gene expression (253), and one (*I8R*) encodes the RNA helicase NPH II (467). Two have both early and intermediate promoters; of these, I3L is a single-stranded DNA binding protein that interacts with ribonucleotide reductase (130,521), and K2L (also called SPI-3) is a member of the serine protease inhibitor (SERPIN) superfamily with an unknown role (523,524).

The DNA replication requirement for intermediate gene expression may result from the inaccessibility of the genome within the infecting particle to the newly synthesized RNA polymerase and transcription factors. This hypothesis is consistent with transfection experiments showing that the DNA isolated from purified virus particles can serve as a template for intermediate and late transcription in the absence of DNA replication (253). The proposed inaccessibility of the parental DNA could be nonspecific owing to remaining virion proteins or to putative specific repressor proteins.

Intermediate-Stage Promoters

Mutagenesis of intermediate promoters indicated two important regions: a 14-bp core element separated by 10 or 11 bp from a 4-bp initiator element (29). The intermediate core element resembles that of early promoters in A+T richness but differs in specific sequence (see Fig. 6). The tetranucleotide TAAA serves as an initiator element of intermediate promoters. Intermediate-stage RNAs are initiated within the AAA triplet, but as discussed later, they contain additional A residues incorporated by a polymerase slippage mechanism. With a slight adjustment, early and intermediate promoter motifs can be accommodated within a single, dual-function, synthetic early-intermediate promoter (28), raising the possibility that such dual promoters occur naturally.

Analysis of some intermediate mRNAs by agarose gel electrophoresis indicated diffuse bands, equal to and longer than the coding regions, suggesting preferred sites of 3′-end formation that did not correlate with early gene transcriptional termination signals (28).

Enzymes and Factors for Intermediate-Stage Transcription

Intermediate promoter templates can be transcribed by extracts prepared from cells infected with vaccinia virus in the presence of an inhibitor of DNA replication (541). Further studies indicated a role for both viral and cellular proteins. The viral proteins (see Table 4) include capping enzyme, which acts by a cap-independent mechanism (202,539,540); VITF-1, which is encoded by the gene for RPO30, a viral RNA polymerase subunit with homology to eukaryotic transcription elongation factor TFIIS (426); and VITF-3, a heterodimer composed of polypeptides encoded by ORFs *A8R* and *A23R* (439). Unlike the early transcription factor, neither VITF-1 nor VITF-3 has ATPase activity or exhibits sequence-specific DNA binding. It is uncertain which component corresponds to the promoter melting factor (539). The cellular component, VITF-2, was extracted from the nucleus of uninfected HeLa cells but was distributed within the cytoplasmic and nuclear fractions of infected cells (427). Whether vaccinia virus infection induces transit of VITF-2 out of the nucleus, activates a cryptic cytoplasmic factor, or depends on newly synthesized VITF-2 has not yet been determined. A relationship between VITF-2 activity and certain examples of host range restriction has been suggested (503). One intriguing possibility is that VITF-2 provides a gate-keeper role between the prereplicative and postreplicative phases of the virus cycle by signaling whether a quiescent cell has been activated to allow optimal replication.

Genetic studies have provided evidence for positive and negative regulators of intermediate or late transcriptional elongation. Initial experiments pointed to similar effects on RNA metabolism of vaccinia virus mutants that mapped to the *A18R* gene, now known to encode a DNA helicase, and those produced by the antiviral drug isatin-β-thiosemicarbazone (IBT) (369). Subsequent experiments indicated that IBT-resistant mutants of vaccinia virus mapped to the RNA polymerase subunit RPO132 (111), whereas IBT-dependent mutants mapped to G2R, a protein of unknown function (322). The story became more intriguing when it was discovered that mutations in the *A18R* gene increased transcriptional readthrough of downstream gene sequences (571), whereas mutations of the *G2R* gene produced decreased-length mRNAs (57). Remarkably, *G2R* mutants rescued *A18R* mutants (113), and physical interactions between the proteins encoded by *G2R, A18R,* and *H5R* (a late transcription factor) were demonstrated (58,314). Recent biochemical studies suggest that the *A18R* helicase is a transcript release factor and acts in conjunction with an unidentified cellular protein (273). Similar genetic approaches led to the identification of the product of the *J3R* gene, which also serves as the cap 2′-*O*-methyltransferase and as a subunit of the poly(A) polymerase, as an mRNA elongation factor (279,568).

Regulation of Late-Stage Transcription

The transcription of late genes follows that of intermediate genes (see Fig. 1). In HeLa cells, late-stage RNA is detected at 140 minutes after synchronous infection with vaccinia virus and continues for about 48 hours (see Fig. 5). The persistent synthesis of late proteins reflects continued transcription because the half-life of late mRNAs has been estimated to be 30 minutes or less (366). Many late proteins, including the major virion components, accumulate in large amounts during this long period. Other late proteins include the factors that are specifically required for transcription of early genes, such as VETF and RAP94, as well as certain other virion enzymes (see Table 3). Although distributed throughout the genome, the late-stage genes cluster in the central region.

Late-Stage Promoters and RNA Processing Signal

Late-stage promoters may be considered in terms of three regions: a core sequence of about 20 bp with some consecutive T or A residues, separated by a region of about 6 bp from a highly conserved TAAAT element within which transcription initiates (132) (see Fig. 6). A synthetic promoter with exclusively T residues forming the core sequence was stronger than tested natural late promoters. Any mutations of TAAAT severely decreased transcription. G or A usually follows the late promoter TAAAT sequence; in the former case, the TAAATG transcription initiation sequence and the ATG translation initiation codon overlap. The seeming absence of an untranslated RNA leader in this situation was puzzling, until it was found that late mRNAs have a 5′-capped, heterogeneous-length, poly(A) sequence formed by RNA polymerase slippage (6,376,446). Poly(A) leaders are also present on mRNAs of a few early genes that have a TAAAT initiation site (5,235) as well as on intermediate mRNAs (28), suggesting that slippage on an AAA sequence is an intrinsic property of the viral RNA polymerase.

Most late transcripts are long and heterogeneous and lack defined 3′-ends (117,303). The early termination signal is not recognized by the late transcription system; consequently, TTTTTNT is frequently present within the coding region of late genes. Terminal heterogeneity, combined with transcription from both DNA strands, explains the ability of late transcripts to self-anneal or anneal with early transcripts to form ribonuclease-resistant hybrids (66,109). The vaccinia virus–encoded double-stranded RNA-binding protein (100) or RNA helicase (467) may prevent deleterious effects of the double-stranded RNA, although this idea is entirely speculative. Alternatively, the 5′ poly(A) leader could compensate for the complementary RNA by providing a single-stranded binding site for initiation factors and the 40s ribosomal subunit, which would then move unimpeded by antisense RNA to the first AUG codon where ribosome assembly and translation occur.

An exception to the general 3′ heterogeneity of late mRNAs was discovered (18). The cowpox virus late mRNA encoding the A-type inclusion protein has a 3′ end corresponding to a precise site in the DNA template. The DNA sequence at this position encodes an RNA cis-acting signal for RNA 3′-end formation that can function independently of either the nature of the promoter or the RNA polymerase responsible for generating the primary RNA (214). There is evidence for induction or activation of a specific endoribonuclease that cleaves this RNA, which is then polyadenylylated. The number of late mRNAs that are processed in this manner remains to be determined. Therefore, poxviruses employ at least two mechanisms of RNA 3′-end formation. The first, operative at early times in viral replication, terminates transcription downstream of an RNA signal, whereas the second, operative at late times, involves RNA site-specific cleavage.

Enzymes and Factors for Late-Stage Transcription

Templates containing late promoters can be transcribed by extracts prepared from cells at the late stage of vaccinia virus infection (567). Late transcription factors were identified by the systematic screening of cloned DNA fragments: ORFs *A1L, A2L,* and *G8R* were necessary and sufficient for transactivation of a transfected late promoter reporter gene in vaccinia virus–infected cells that were blocked in DNA replication (253). An intermediate promoter regulates each of these late transcription factor genes (see Table 4), which is consistent with a cascade model of regulation. *In vitro* studies confirmed that the products of the *G8R, A1L,* and *A2L* genes are vaccinia virus late transcription factors (223,255,375,565,566), and they have been named VLTF-1, VLTF-2, and VLTF-3, respectively (see Table 4). In addition, ts and repressible mutations of *A1L* and *G8R,* respectively, block late gene expression under nonpermissive conditions (92,580). Both VLTF-2 and VLTF-3 can bind zinc (254), and yeast two-hybrid studies indicate interactions of VLTF-1 with itself and with VLTF-2 (314). *In vitro* studies indicated that the product of the early *H5R* gene, named VLTF-4, stimulated late transcription several-fold (269). Evidence has been obtained for a cell-derived late transcription factor that binds late promoters (193). Other studies demonstrated that the cellular transcription factor YY1 is found in the cytoplasm of infected cells and can bind to at least two late promoters (76), but it remains to be shown that this protein has a role in vaccinia virus transcription. Several studies have been cited as evidence for a role of host RNA polymerase II in late vaccinia virus gene expression (122), but this has not been demonstrated directly.

Posttranscriptional Regulation of Viral Gene Expression

Poxvirus mRNAs are made in the cytoplasm, and no evidence of splicing has been reported. As noted earlier, accelerated mRNA degradation induced by vaccinia virus facilitates rapid changes in viral mRNA populations (see Fig. 5), although the basis for this effect is unknown. The finding that intermediate and late mRNAs contain 5′ poly(A) sequences, whereas such sequences are uncommon on early mRNAs, raises the possibility that this structural feature enhances translation. However, critical experiments to test such a hypothesis have not been reported.

DNA REPLICATION

General Features

Poxvirus DNA replication takes place in the cytoplasm, a characteristic shared only with African swine fever virus, and has been reported to occur in enucleated cells (386,398). Discrete cytoplasmic foci of replication, termed *factory areas,* were discerned by light and electron microscopic autoradiography and microscopic procedures (88,201,249).

Enzymes Involved in DNA Precursor Metabolism

Some poxviruses encode enzymes involved in the synthesis of deoxyribonucleotides, evidently to enhance DNA replication in cells with suboptimal precursor pools; whereas other poxviruses lack some or all of these enzymes and are dependent on the host. In orthopoxviruses, these enzymes include a thymidine kinase (26,216), thymidylate kinase (489), ribonucleotide reductase (478,510), and dUTPase (72). In addition, there is an incomplete guanylate kinase (488), raising the possibility that an intact form might be found in some other poxvirus. Leporipoxviruses are missing genes encoding the large subunit of ribonucleotide reductase, thymidylate kinase, and remnants of the guanylate kinase (89,552); whereas molluscum contagiosum virus has no known enzymes involved in nucleotide precursor formation (450). Fowlpox virus encodes a protein related to human deoxycytidine kinase that is not present in the other poxviruses (266). The completely sequenced genome of the entomopoxvirus *Melanoplus sanguinipes* lacks all of the previously described poxvirus genes involved in nucleotide metabolism but has a thymidylate synthetase homolog (1). However, a homologous thymidine kinase gene is present in *Amsacta moorei* (40) and other entomopoxviruses.

The thymidine kinases encoded by orthopoxviruses, avipoxviruses, suipoxviruses, capripoxviruses, leporipoxviruses, and some entomopoxviruses are 20 to 25 kd and related in sequence to corresponding eukaryotic enzymes (35% to 70% amino acid identity), but not to the pyrimidine kinase of herpesviruses. The thymidine kinase gene is regulated by an early promoter, as befits its role in increasing the precursors for DNA replication. The vaccinia virus enzyme exists as a tetramer, has ATP- and Mg^{2+}-binding domains, and is susceptible to feedback inhibition by dTDP or dTTP (59). Although the thymidine kinase gene is not required for virus growth in tissue culture cells, deletion mutants are attenuated *in vivo* (86).

Thymidylate kinase catalyzes the next step in thymidine monophosphate (TMP) metabolism. The vaccinia virus gene encodes a 23.2-kd protein that can complement *Saccharomyces cerevisiae* mutants deficient in the homologous enzyme (224). The protein is expressed early in infection and is not required for virus replication in tissue culture.

The synthesis of ribonucleotide reductase, an enzyme that converts ribonucleoside diphosphates to deoxyribonucleoside diphosphates, occurs soon after vaccinia virus infection (480). Both the small catalytic subunit and the large regulatory subunit closely resemble their eukaryotic counterparts both structurally (70% to 80% identity) and functionally (215,479). Catalytic activity is inhibited by hydroxyurea, and drug-resistant mutants generate direct tandem repeats of the gene encoding the catalytic subunit (482). Mutation of the large subunit prevented induced ribonucleotide reductase activity in tissue culture cells without affecting replication (104). However, the mutant virus was mildly attenuated in a mouse model.

The hydrolysis of dUTP by the vaccinia virus dUTPase provides dUMP, an intermediate in the biosynthesis of thymidine triphosphate (TTP), and might also minimize dUTP incorporation into DNA (72). The protein is synthesized early in infection (481) and is nonessential for virus replication (388).

DNA Synthesis

The time of onset of DNA synthesis varies with different members of the poxvirus family and to some extent with the multiplicity of infection and cell type. In cells synchronously infected with vaccinia virus, DNA replication begins 1 to 2 hours after infection and results in the generation of about 10,000 genome copies per cell, of which half are ultimately packaged into virions (243,435). Studies depending on thymidine incorporation instead of hybridization for DNA quantification generally underestimate the length of the replication period, probably because of a decline in the activity of the viral thymidine kinase used for incorporation of the radioactive precursor through the salvage pathway.

A plausible model for poxvirus DNA replication begins with the introduction of a nick near one or both of the hairpin termini, followed by nucleotide addition to the free 3′ end, strand displacement, and concatemer resolution. Nicking is supported by changes in the sedimentation of the parental viral DNA (394) (although the cleavage site remains to be defined), and labeling studies suggested that replication begins near the ends of the genome (396). The presence of single-stranded DNA is consistent with a strand-displacement mechanism, and the report of small DNA fragments covalently linked to RNA primers suggests lagging strand synthesis (158–160,395), but this needs further investigation with current methods. The presence of transient concatemeric DNA intermediates were demonstrated by the presence of junction fragments (37,352) and high-molecular-weight DNA (135,329).

Efforts to locate a specific poxvirus origin using a plasmid replication assay in transfected cells led to a surprising conclusion that any supercoiled plasmid replicated in cells infected with Shope fibroma (137) or vaccinia virus (330). The absence of any stimulatory effect of vaccinia virus DNA sequences resulted in speculation that poxviruses, unlike nuclear DNA viruses, do not require specific origin sequences. Recently, however, more specific results were obtained by transfecting a linear DNA molecule containing vaccinia virus hairpin ends (147). With this assay, an enhancing effect was found when the template contained the terminal 200 bp of the viral genome.

Viral Proteins Involved in DNA Replication

Several complementation groups of ts mutants that express vaccinia virus early proteins but are impaired in DNA synthesis have been found (112,317). One group contains mutations in the DNA polymerase, which has a mass of about 110 kd, an associated 3′ exonuclease activity and sequence similarities with other eukaryotic and viral DNA polymerases (97,153,316). Certain codon substitutions confer resistance to inhibitors of DNA synthesis, providing information regarding the active site of the polymerase (134,153,505,506,519).

The second DNA-negative complementation group maps to the *D5R* gene, which encodes a 90-kd protein with a nucleic acid–independent nucleoside triphosphatase activity (163,165,429). An abrupt cessation of DNA synthesis occurred upon a shift to the nonpermissive temperature of cells infected with one of the *D5R* mutants, suggesting a direct but still unknown role in replication (164). The third DNA-negative complementation group was mapped to the *B1R* ORF, which encodes a serine-threonine protein kinase that is expressed early in infection, and is packaged in virions (32,288,410). An early protein encoded by the *H5R* gene has been shown to be a substrate for the B1R kinase (47), and interactions between these proteins was demonstrated by the yeast two-hybrid system (314). Although the H5R protein appears to be involved in late transcription (58,269), it has no known role in DNA replication. Two human homologs of B1R have been identified, but their functions are unknown (361).

Another vaccinia virus ts mutant impaired in DNA replication was mapped to the *D4R* ORF (331). A mutant with a deleted *D4R* gene was also impaired in DNA replication but could be propagated in a transfected cell line stably transfected with *D4R* (212). Both the *D4R* ORF and its Shope fibroma virus homolog encode functional uracil DNA glycosylases (502,528). Because these enzymes remove uracil residues that have been introduced into DNA, either through misincorporation of dUTP or through the deamination of cytosine, a DNA-negative phenotype was surprising.

Additional ts mutants impaired in DNA replication were derived by directed mutagenesis of the *A20R* gene (264). The protein encoded by this gene interacts in the yeast two-hybrid system with the DNA glycosylase and the D5R protein, both of which are involved in DNA replication (314). Traktman (517) cited evidence that the A20R protein is the DNA polymerase processivity factor previously detected in infected cell extracts (315).

Vaccinia virus encodes a functional ATP-dependent DNA ligase that is not essential for viral replication in tissue culture, although it affects virulence as well as sensitivity to DNA-damaging agents (110,256). Whether DNA ligation is unnecessary for replication or this requirement is fulfilled by the cellular homolog is unknown.

Three of the putative replication proteins encoded by orthopoxviruses (the DNA polymerase, nucleoside triphosphatase, and DNA glycosylase) have homologs in all sequenced poxvirus genomes pointing to their central roles. B1R protein kinase homologs are present in all sequenced poxviruses except for molluscum contagiosum virus; putative processivity factor homologs are present in all except entomopoxviruses; an ATP-dependent DNA ligase is encoded by leporipoxviruses but not by either molluscum contagiosum virus or entomopoxviruses. *Melanoplus sanguinipes,* however, encodes a putative NAD^+-dependent DNA ligase (1).

Concatemer Resolution

The replication of the poxvirus genome involves the formation of concatemeric intermediates and their resolution into unit-length molecules. The concatemer junction consists of a precise duplex copy of the hairpin loop present at the ends of mature DNA genomes (see Fig. 4). Studies with ts mutants of vaccinia virus, as well as specific inhibitors, indicate that concatemeric forms of DNA accumulate when late gene expression is prevented (135,329). Resolution occurs upon allowing late proteins to be made, providing evidence that the concatemers are replicative intermediates.

Circular plasmids containing vaccinia virus (328) or Shope fibroma virus (138) concatemer junctions are converted into linear molecules with hairpin termini when transfected into poxvirus-infected cells. Using this assay, the structural and sequence requirements for resolution of concatemer junctions were determined by site-directed mutagenesis (136,318,324,327). The minimal requirement for resolution is two copies of the sequence T_6-N_{7-9}-T/C-A_3-T/A present in an inverted repeat orientation on either side of an extended double-stranded copy of the hairpin loop. Structurally and functionally similar resolution sequences are present in at least four poxvirus genera: *Orthopoxvirus, Leporipoxvirus, Capripoxvirus,* and *Avipoxvirus* (Fig. 7). The sequence of the intervening region, destined to form the hairpin loop, is not highly conserved but must be palindromic and less than 200 bp long. Further studies suggested that resolution is accomplished either by conservative site-specific recombination and oriented branch migration (325) or by nicking and sealing of an extruded cruciform structure (318).

Data showing that all conditional lethal mutants of vaccinia virus that are blocked in late gene expression are also defective in concatemer resolution at the nonpermissive temperature were interpreted as indicating a requirement for a specific viral late protein (135,329). However, the resolution sequence contains a functional late promoter (374,501) (compare Figs. 6 and 7). Therefore, it is unclear whether transcription of the resolution sequence, the translation product of a late transcript, or both are required.

There are at least three viral late proteins that might be components of a resolvase. One is a type 1 topoisomerase that structurally and functionally resembles its eukaryotic counterpart (39,261,470,475), except for a specificity for the sequence C/TCCTT (465). Similar sequence-specific topoisomerases are encoded by orf virus (260), entomopoxvirus (272,391), Shope fibroma virus (370), and molluscum contagiosum virus (226). Despite extensive biochemical analyses and evidence that the gene is essential for virus replication (466,471), its biologic role remains uncertain. The ability of poxvirus topoisomerases to resolve Holliday junctions, a key intermediate in both homologous and site-specific recombination, and generate hairpin ends suggest that this enzyme might be involved either in resolving concatemer junctions or in general recombination (370,449).

A 50-kd homodimeric DNase with nicking and joining activity (275,326,409) was recently identified as the product of the *K4L* ORF (M. Merchlisky, Food and Drug Administration, personal communication) and is present in vaccinia virus cores. The nicking and joining reaction requires no energy cofactor and generates 3′-P- and 5′-OH-termini. When the purified enzyme was incubated with concatemeric junction fragments, cleavage occurred at the apex of the cruciform instead of at the base, which would be necessary for telomere formation (409).

Most recently, a bacterial-type Holliday junction resolvase was found to be encoded by the *A22R* gene of vaccinia virus and homologs are present in all poxviruses (174). *In vitro,* the recombinant A22R protein can resolve synthetic Holliday junctions or cruciform structures extruded by a supercoiled plasmid. Furthermore, a vaccinia virus mutant in which the *A22R* gene was repressed is defective in concatemer resolution (175).

Homologous Recombination

High rates of recombination occur within poxvirus-infected cells (168). Recombination has apparently occurred naturally between two leporipoxviruses—Shope fibroma virus, which produces benign fibromas in rabbits, and myxoma virus, the agent of myxomatosis—to form malignant rabbit fibroma virus (63), and between individual capripoxviruses (179). Recombination between the terminal sequences of poxvirus DNA may explain variations in the number of tandem repeats and translocations. Most extraordinarily, field and vaccine strains of fowlpox virus carry a nearly full-length and apparently infectious integrated avian retrovirus genome (204).

Recombination can also occur between virus-derived genomic DNA and transfected subgenomic DNA fragments, and this has been exploited to map and construct mutations and to insert genes for expression. Viral genomes rapidly eliminate direct repeats with the formation of intramolecular and intermolecular recombination products (31). Single- and double-crossover

VA	TTTTTTTCTAG	ACAC	TAAAT	--hairpin loop--	ATTTA	GTGT	CTAGAAAAAAA
CP	TTTTTTTCTAG	ACAC	TAAAT	--hairpin loop--	ATTTA	GTGT	CTAGAAAAAAA
RP	TTTTTTTCTAG	ACAT	TAAAT	--hairpin loop--	ATTTA	ATGT	CTAGAAAAAAA
SF	TTTTTTTCTAG	GGTTA	TAAAT	--hairpin loop--	ATTTA	TAACC	CTAGAAAAAAA

FIG. 7. Concatemer resolution sequence. The *boxed regions* represent conserved sequences necessary for concatemer resolution. Extended palindromic hairpin loop sequences are indicated. VA, vaccinia; CP, cowpox; RP, rabbitpox; SF, Shope fibroma.

products, resulting from recombination between transfected plasmids and viral genomes (497), and intermolecular and intramolecular plasmid or bacteriophage DNA recombinants (162,373) have been detected in poxvirus-infected cells. Recombination does not require late gene products, and there appears to be a strong connection between recombination and replication (323,551). After phage lambda DNA was transfected into Shope fibroma virus–infected cells, heteroduplex formation coincided with the onset of both replication and recombination, suggesting that poxviruses make no clear biochemical distinction between these processes (170). Evidence for DNA strand exchange catalyzed by proteins from vaccinia virus–infected cells has been reported, and a derivative of the T4-replication–primed recombination model has been suggested (576). The roles in recombination of the poxvirus encoded topoisomerase and Holiday junction endonuclease, discussed in the previous section, remain to be determined.

DNA Replication Model

Although there are large gaps in our understanding of poxvirus DNA replication, the unique terminal structure of the poxvirus genome, evidence that initiation occurs near the ends of the molecule, and the presence of concatemer junctions in replicating DNA suggest a model similar to that proposed for replication of single-stranded parvovirus DNA. As depicted in Figure 8, a hypothetical nick occurring at one or both ends of the genome provides a free 3′ end for priming. The replicated DNA strand then folds back on itself and copies the remainder of the genome. Concatemer junctions form by replication through the hairpin; very large branched concatemers can arise by initiating new rounds of replication before resolution occurs. Recombinational strand invasion may further contribute to the formation of complex multibranched molecules. After the onset of late-stage transcription, unit-length genomes are resolved, and the incompletely base-paired

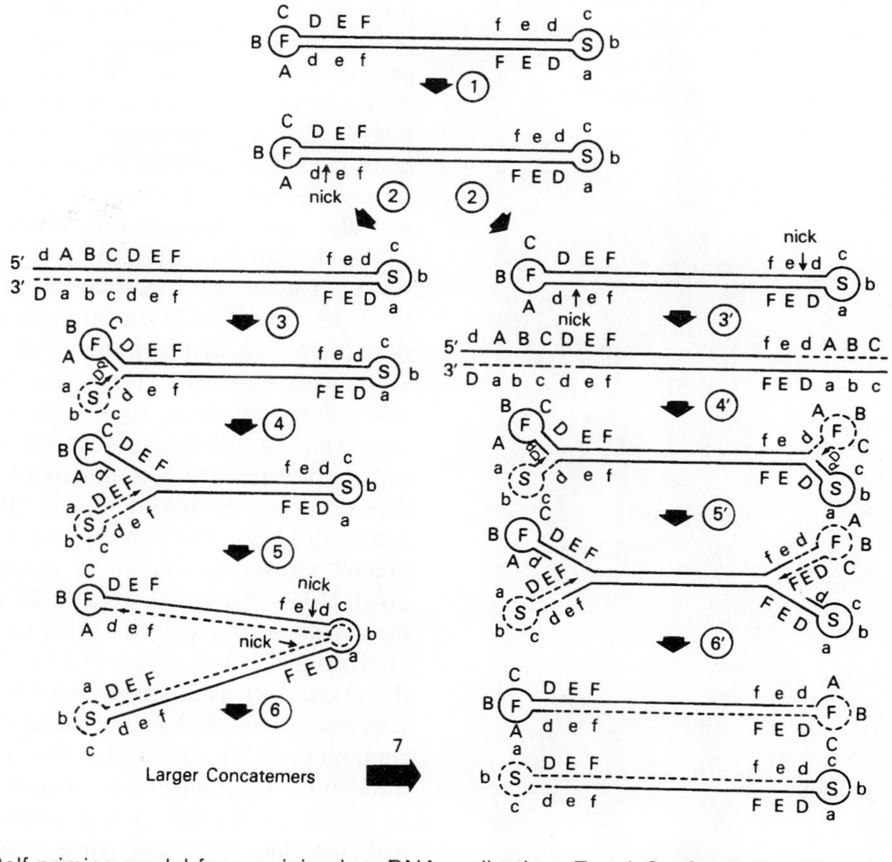

FIG. 8. Self-priming model for vaccinia virus DNA replication. *F* and *S* refer to the difference in electrophoretic mobilities of the two alternative inverted and complementary hairpin sequences present at the ends of the vaccinia virus genome. The scheme *on the left* assumes that the replication of a single DNA molecule is initiated at one end and continues to the other end to form a concatemer, whereas *on the right,* initiation occurs at both ends without concatemer formation. (From ref. 347, with permission.)

terminal loops, with inverted and complementary sequences, are regenerated.

VIRION ASSEMBLY, MATURATION, AND RELEASE

Intracellular Mature Virions

Assembly begins in circumscribed, granular, electron-dense areas of the cytoplasm. The first morphologically distinct structure is a crescent (or cupulae in three dimensions) consisting of a membrane with a brushlike border of spicules on the convex surface and granular material adjacent to the concave side (Fig. 9, *panel 1*). Electron micrographs showing a single bilayer membrane with no apparent continuity with cellular organelles have been published by several groups (125,189,211). How such a membrane could form *de novo,* however, is unclear. One unprecedented and highly speculative possibility is the assembly of a protein lattice or scaffold with hydrophobic domains into which lipids could be deposited. An alternate view, more in line with cell biology, is that the viral membrane is composed of two tightly apposed membranes derived by a wrapping mechanism from the intermediate compartment between the endoplasmic reticulum and Golgi network (434,492). A third scheme, in which vesicles bud from cellular organelles and then coalesce to form the viral membrane, is suggested by the

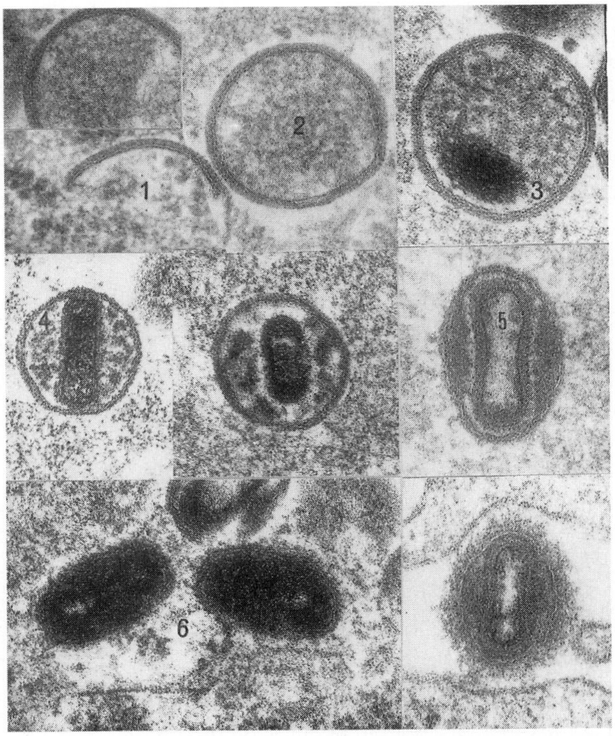

FIG. 9. Electron micrographs of developing and mature virus particles in thin section. (Courtesy of P. Grimley, Uniformed Services University of the Health Sciences.)

accumulation of small vesicles in the viral factory area when morphogenesis is blocked by repression of the *A17L* (418,560) or *A14L* (419,520) genes. In subsequent stages of development, the crescent membranes are transformed into circular (or spherical in three dimensions) immature virions with a dense nucleoprotein mass embedded in a granular matrix (see Fig. 9, *panels 2 and 3*). Occasional electron-microscopic pictures suggest that the nucleoprotein enters the immature envelopes just before they are completely sealed (336). Further steps in maturation are inferred from selected images (see Fig. 9, *panels 4 to 6*).

Studies of the early stages of morphogenesis have been facilitated by the combined use of drugs or conditional lethal mutants to arrest assembly and immunoelectron microscopy to locate viral proteins in the abortive structures. No viral membranes can be detected at their usual time of formation when viral DNA replication is stringently inhibited, consistent with the finding of late promoters on the membrane proteins. The earliest defect in morphogenesis occurs with a ts F10L kinase mutant (518,542). At the nonpermissive temperature, late viral proteins were made, but recognizable viral membranes were not seen. A similar phenotype was also described for a ts mutant in the *H5R* gene (139), which was surprising because other studies had indicated a role for this protein in RNA synthesis. When synthesis of the A17L or A14L proteins, which associate with each other, is repressed, small vesicles accumulate instead of a continuous membrane (418,419,520,560). There is, however, some difference in the locations of the vesicles that form with the two mutants and the block appears to be more stringent with the A17L mutant. Both the A17L and A14L proteins are phosphorylated apparently by the F10L kinase (55,143). In the presence of the antibiotic rifampicin, irregular viral membranes that lack spicules accumulate (345,358) (Fig. 10) Within minutes after removal of the drug, the membranes become spicule coated and assume a regular crescent shape (see Fig. 10), even in the presence of inhibitors of RNA or protein synthesis, suggesting that rifampicin directly interferes with assembly (189). The gene responsible for resistance of mutant viruses to rifampicin has been mapped to the *D13L* ORF, which encodes a 65-kd protein (30,509) that rapidly associates with the rifampicin body membranes after drug removal (332,493,534). When expression of the *D13L* ORF is repressed, morphogenesis of the viral envelope is blocked at the same stage as occurs with rifampicin (578). The 65-kd protein appears to concentrate on the inner side of the membrane, perhaps serving as a scaffold. A block at later stages, in which crescents and circular immature virus particles accumulated, occurred when expression of the A9L (572), L1R (406), or H3L (121,286) membrane protein was repressed.

Several vaccinia virus major core proteins have been detected within the immature particles visualized by

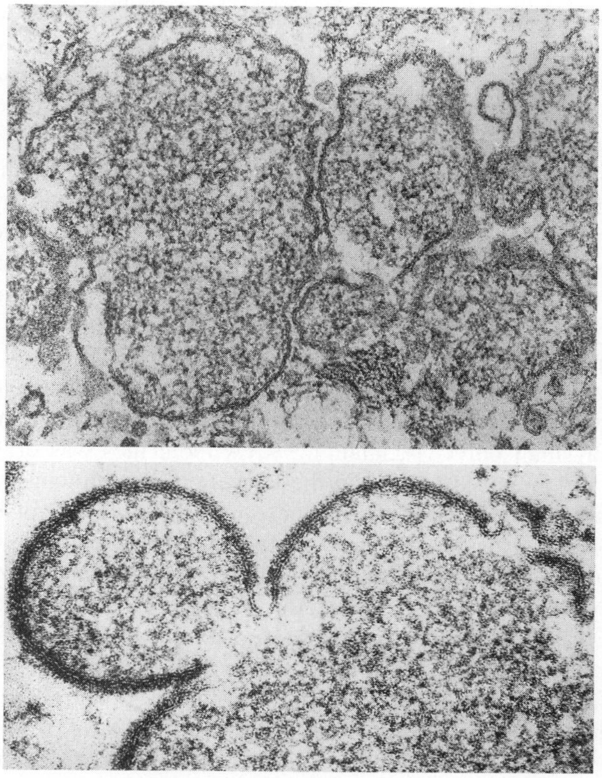

FIG. 10. Electron micrographs of thin sections of cell infected in the presence of rifampicin. **Upper panel:** HeLa cells were fixed and sectioned at 8 hours after infection in the presence of rifampicin. **Lower panel:** Cells were fixed and sectioned at 10 minutes after removal of rifampicin. (From ref. 189, with permission.)

immunoelectron microscopy (412,534) or isolated by sedimentation (442,535). Pulse-chase experiments indicated that several late polypeptides, including major structural proteins of the core, undergo proteolytic processing (343) at Ala-Gly-Ala/Ser motifs (280). Processing of the major structural proteins is coupled to virus assembly because their cleavage is prevented by rifampicin or mutants that interfere with early steps in morphogenesis (252). Repression of synthesis of certain core proteins, such as the F17R phosphoprotein or the I1L DNA-binding protein, halts assembly at an immature particle stage and prevents proteolytic processing (262,579). Under nonpermissive conditions, ts mutants with substitutions in the *I7L* ORF appear to be blocked at a slightly earlier stage, but protein processing was not examined (246). Repression of the *A32L* gene, a predicted ATPase, interfered with the packaging of DNA and led to the formation of aberrant particles (95). The question of how the transcription apparatus becomes enclosed within the core of the assembling virus particle is intriguing. It seems unlikely that each enzyme has its own targeting signal. A clue to possible mechanisms was obtained by examining the noninfectious virus particles that formed when synthesis of RAP94, the RNA polymerase-associated protein that confers specificity for early promoters, was repressed. Such particles contained an apparently complete set of structural proteins as well as the early transcription factor VETF but lacked the viral RNA polymerase, poly(A) polymerase, capping enzyme, topoisomerase, NPH I, and NPH II (577). Such a specific effect could result if these proteins formed a complex that associates with promoter-bound VETF through RAP94. Evidence for an interaction between NPH I and RAP94 has been obtained (334). Reduced amounts of RNA polymerase in virions formed with a ts mutation in VETF (285) is also consistent with the latter model. Repression of synthesis of either subunit of VETF, however, leads to a more severe defect with accumulation of immature virus particles (221,222).

Because disulfide bonds usually form in the endoplasmic reticulum, the presence of intramolecular and intermolecular disulfides in cytoplasmic vaccinia virus core and membrane proteins (229,291,416,561) raise the possibility that poxviruses encode novel thiol oxidoreductases. Proteins with predicted C-X-X-C redox motifs include the vaccinia virus O2L and G4L glutaredoxins, which have been shown to have thiol transferase activities *in vitro* (9,195), and the E10R protein, a member of the eukaryotic ERV1/ALR family (450). Of these, the G4L and E10R proteins are conserved in all poxviruses and are essential for morphogenesis (452,547). Recent data suggest that the E10R and G4L proteins are components of a cytoplasmic disulfide bond pathway (453).

Occluded Virions

The IMV of some *Chordopoxvirinae* (e.g., cowpox, ectromelia, and fowlpox) become occluded in a dense protein matrix referred to as *A-type inclusions* to differentiate them from the sites of virus replication and assembly, which are sometimes called *B-type inclusions* (250). Presumably, the A-type inclusions are released into the environment after degeneration of infected cells. The major A-type inclusion protein of cowpox virus is a 160-kd species that may represent up to 4% of the total cell protein at late times after infection (172,377). Some cowpox virus mutants form inclusions without virions, implicating a role for the IMV-specific protein 4C (461,525). Although vaccinia virus does not form A-type inclusions, a smaller homologous protein is made because of a frameshift mutation (17,133). Both the cowpox and vaccinia virus inclusion proteins are myristylated (306).

The virions of *Entomopoxvirinae* are also occluded to protect them from the environment (51). After ingestion by a new larval host, infectious particles may be released in the alkaline pH of the gut. The sequences of homologous occlusion proteins, called *spheroidin* or *spherulin,* have been deduced from the ORFs of several entomopoxviruses (1,33,198,199,441). These proteins are cysteine-rich, about 100 kd, and lack homology to fusolin, the abundant 50-kd spindle-body protein of entomopoxviruses (127), the A-type inclusion protein of chordopoxviruses, or the polyhedrin protein of baculoviruses.

Extracellular Enveloped Virions

The movement of IMV out of the assembly areas to the cell periphery is microtubule dependent and requires the A27L membrane protein (438). The IMV become wrapped by additional membranes, derived from the trans-Golgi or early endosomal network, that contain viral proteins (206,230,336,443,516). Studies with mutant vaccinia viruses indicate that wrapping requires expression of at least one IMV membrane protein, the A27L 14-kd protein (417), and two EEV membrane proteins: the F13L 37-kd phospholipase (25,60,424) and the B5R 42-kd glycoprotein (156,558). Fusion of the wrapped particles with the plasma membrane results in the externalization of the virus, with loss of the outermost Golgi-derived membrane. Only some of the externalized virions are found in the medium as EEV, whereas the rest adheres to the cell surface (CEVs). The ratio of adherent to released virions varies with different cell hosts and different vaccinia virus strains (379), largely because of a single amino acid difference in the putative lectin-binding domain of the membrane protein encoded by the *A34R* ORF (62). The extracellular virions are important for virus dissemination (68,380). On cell monolayers, the CEVs can mediate efficient cell-to-cell spread and plaque formation, whereas the EEVs provide long-range dissemination (61).

The efficient cell-to-cell spread of CEVs appears to be due to their location at the tip of motile, actin-containing microvilli that have been visualized by fluorescence and electron microscopy (119,207,499). When the *A33R, A34R,* or *A36R* ORFs are not expressed, actin-containing microvilli are not formed, resulting in a small plaque phenotype (423,436,559,563). Nucleation of the actin tails depends on tyrosine phosphorylation of the A36R protein by Src-family kinases: the phosphorylated A36R protein interacts with the adaptor protein Nck, which results in the recruitment of the Ena/VASP family member N-WASP to the site of actin assembly (171).

VIRUS–HOST INTERACTIONS

Inhibitory Effects on Host Macromolecular Synthesis

Infection of tissue culture cells with vaccinia virus or other orthopoxviruses results in profound cytopathic effects (21), changes in membrane permeability (93), and inhibition of DNA, RNA, and protein synthesis. The effects on protein synthesis are dramatic (161,346). It seems likely that several factors may lead to the switch from host to viral protein synthesis and that the relative contribution of each factor may depend on the virus multiplicity, cell type, time of analysis, and use of metabolic inhibitors. Some experiments suggested that inhibition of host protein synthesis could occur in the absence of viral gene expression, thereby implicating a protein in the vaccinia virus particle. Candidate inhibitors are the surface tubules (313), the F17R phosphoprotein (389), and the B1R protein kinase (49). There is indirect evidence that some viral early proteins may allow translation of viral mRNA to continue under conditions that inhibit host protein synthesis (48,342). Other studies suggested that viral transcription is necessary for inhibition of host protein synthesis. For example, high concentration of actinomycin D and cordycepin prevented this inhibition (22). Also, in some cell lines, inhibition of host protein synthesis remains incomplete until after DNA replication. An inhibitory role for small poly(A)-containing RNA molecules was originally proposed to explain the effects on host protein synthesis that occur in the presence of actinomycin D or by ultraviolet-irradiated virus (184,430). Subsequent reports, however, suggested that small poly(A)-containing RNAs may have an inhibitory role during normal virus infection (23,24,87). After several hours, most of the mRNA present in the cytoplasm of infected cells is viral, accounting for the predominance of viral protein synthesis regardless of translational effects (65,116). The shift in mRNA species results from the short half-life of all mRNAs following vaccinia virus infection (50,447), coupled with very active virus transcription and inhibition of host RNA synthesis and transport. Rapid degradation of actin and tubulin mRNAs has been demonstrated (411). Viral inhibitory effects on the synthesis or processing of cellular RNAs have been reported (50,239,447). This inhibition involves all classes of RNA and requires vaccinia virus protein synthesis; heated or ultraviolet irradiated virus was ineffective (384). The inhibition was correlated with the transit of RNA polymerase II activity from the nucleus to the cytoplasm (338,554). However, whole cell extracts of vaccinia virus–infected cells were no longer able to transcribe genes regulated by eukaryotic RNA polymerase II promoters, although they were still able to transcribe a polymerase III promoter (399). Nuclear DNA replication is also inhibited (144,244). Under certain nonpermissive conditions of vaccinia virus infection, the inhibition of host macromolecular synthesis may be accelerated. These situations include the restricted growth of vaccinia virus in Chinese hamster ovary cells, which can be overcome by the cowpox virus gene encoding a 77-kd protein (494); host range mutants of rabbitpox virus (351); and vaccinia virus K1L deletion mutants (185,387,503).

Stimulatory Effects on Cell Growth

Many poxviruses induce hyperplastic responses and even tumors in the skin of infected animals. These effects are pronounced with fowlpox virus (103), Shope fibroma virus (464), Yaba virus (364), and molluscum contagiosum virus (397). In the case of orthopoxviruses, the hyperplasia is due to secretion of a homolog of EGF (83,84,500). Leporipoxviruses have structural and functional homologs of EGF that are nonessential for replication in tissue culture but contribute to virulence (102,289, 368). A gene encoding a mitogenic polypeptide with homology to mammalian vascular endothelial growth factor is present in the orf virus genome (555).

Viral Defense Molecules

Host immune responses can halt the spread of viruses and eliminate them. Immediately after virus invasion, nonspecific mechanisms involving interferons (IFNs), complement, cytokines, and natural killer cells predominate; subsequently, cytotoxic T cells and antibodies assume importance in defense (85). In response to these selective pressures, poxviruses encode multiple proteins that interfere with the induction or activity of complement and the principal cytokines (Table 5). The inhibitory proteins fall into three main classes: virokines, which are secreted from infected cells and resemble host cytokines or soluble immune regulators (268); viroceptors, which are altered cellular receptors that have lost their transmembrane anchor sequences and consequently are secreted from infected cells and sequester ligands (526); and intracellular proteins that interfere with signaling or effector pathways (407).

Complement Regulatory Protein

One of the major secreted proteins of vaccinia virus consists largely of four, tandem, inexact copies of a 60–amino acid sequence known as the *short consensus repeat* (SCR) that is found in complement regulatory proteins (268). This vaccinia viral protein, called VCP, inhibits the classic and alternative pathways of complement activation through its ability to bind and inactivate both C4B and C3B (267,320,433) and contributes to virulence (236). B5R, an EEV membrane protein of vaccinia virus also has SCRs, but there is no evidence that it has complement inhibitory activity. Host proteins incorporated into the EEV membrane could also inhibit complement activation (531).

Inhibitors of Interferon and Interferon Transduction Pathways

Secreted proteins that bind to type I or II IFNs are encoded by poxviruses of several different genera. The IFN-γ–binding proteins of myxoma virus (M-T7) and

TABLE 5. *Poxvirus immune defense molecules*

Viral protein	Role	Virus/Gene	Selected references
Secreted complement binding protein	Binds C4B, C3B; inhibits complement activation	Orthopox (VAC C3L)	236, 267, 268, 320, 433
Soluble IFN-γ receptor	Binds and antagonizes IFN-γ	Orthopox (VAC B8R), Leporipox (MYX M-T7)	12, 349, 350, 527
Soluble IFN-α/β receptor	Binds and antagonizes IFN-α/β	Orthopox (VAC B18R)	108, 504
Soluble TNF receptor	Binds and antagonizes TNF-α	Orthopox (CPV crmA), Leporipoz (MYX M-T2)	219, 293, 301, 485, 486, 526
Soluble IL-1β receptor	Binds and antagonizes IL-1β	Orthopox (VAC B15R)	10, 11, 496
Secreted IL-18–binding protein	Binds and antagonizes IL-18	Molluscipox (MC54), Orthopox (ECT p13/16)	67, 490, 569, 570
Secreted chemokine-binding protein	Binds and antagonizes CC chemokines	Orthopox (VAC 35 kd), Leporipox (M-T1)	13, 91, 188, 487
Secreted chemokine homolog	Binds and antagonizes CCR8	Molluscipox (MC148)	128, 270, 297
dsRNA-binding protein	Prevents activation of protein kinase PKR and 2.5A synthetase	Orthopox (VAC E3L)	45, 99, 100, 455
EIF-2a homolog	Inhibits protein kinase PKR	Orthopox (VAC K3L)	46, 94, 129
Caspase inhibitor	Inhibits caspase 1 to prevent processing of IL-1β and IL-18 precursors and procaspase 8 to block TNF and Fas-induced apoptosis	Orthopox (CPX crmA), Leporipox (MYX SERP2)	257, 265, 392, 407, 511, 581
Serine protease inhibitor	Inhibits serine proteases	Leporipox (MYX SERP1)	302, 360
FLIP (FLICE-like inhibitory protein)	Binds FADD and procaspase 8 to prevent TNF and Fas-induced apoptosis	Molluscipox (MC159)	52, 220, 513
Glutathione peroxidase	Hydrolyzes peroxides from inflammatory cells or UV rays	Molluscipox (MC66)	463
Class I MHC homolog	Binds β_2-microglobulin	Molluscipox (MC80R)	451

IFN, interferon; TNF, tumor necrosis factor; IL, interleukin; dsRNA, double-stranded RNA; EIF, eukaryotic translation initiation factor; FADD, Fas-associated death domain protein; FLICE, FADD-like IL-1β converting enzyme; MHC, major histocompatibility complex.

orthopoxviruses (vaccinia B8R) are similar in sequence to the extracellular domain of the IFN-γ receptor and consequently bind IFN-γ (12,350,527). Deletion of the gene encoding the IFN-γ–binding protein of myxoma virus greatly attenuates disease in European rabbits (349). A protein from the supernatant of cells infected with tanapoxvirus has been reported to bind IFN-γ and also interleukin-2 (IL-2) and IL-5 (157).

A type I IFN inhibitor is present in the supernatants and on the surfaces of cells infected with vaccinia and other orthopoxviruses (108,504). The protein has some sequence similarities with regions of cellular type I IFN receptor and binds IFN-α with high affinity but less species specificity than the receptors. Vaccinia viruses with a deletion of the type I IFN-binding protein gene are attenuated in mice, suggesting that the protein is a virulence factor.

Orthopoxviruses encode a double-stranded RNA-binding protein (e.g. vaccinia virus E3L) that prevents the activation of the IFN response protein kinase (PKR), which inhibits translation initiation (99,100,455). Vaccinia virus E3L deletion mutants show host range restriction and enhanced apoptosis, RNA degradation, and IFN sensitivity (45,258). Orthopoxviruses also encode a homolog of the translation initiation factor eIF-2α (e.g., vaccinia virus K3L) that inhibits eIF-2α phosphorylation by PKR (94,129). Deletion of K3L increases the IFN sensitivity of vaccinia virus (46). Therefore, the E3L and K3L proteins have overlapping roles in blocking IFN action.

Interleukin-18–Binding Proteins

IL-18 induces IFN-γ production, acts in synergy with IL-12 to induces natural killer (NK) cell activation, T-cell activation and helper T-cell type 1 response polarization, and can protect mice from vaccinia virus infection (508). molluscum contagiosum virus (MCV) and orthopoxviruses encode secreted proteins that are homologous to the mammalian IL-18–binding protein and that bind IL-18 and block IFN-γ production (67,490,569,570). An ectromelia deletion mutant induced elevated intraperitoneal NK cell activity and cytokine production and decreased virus replication compared with wild-type virus (67).

Tumor Necrosis Factor Receptor Homologs

Tumor necrosis factor (TNF) binds to its cognate receptors and induces proinflammatory responses or death of virus-infected cells. Leporipoxviruses (301,485,526) and orthopoxviruses (219,293,486) encode one or more soluble type II TNF receptor homologs that can block TNF-α–mediated cytolysis *in vitro* and attenuate virulence.

Interleukin-1 Receptor Homologs

IL-1β mediates a broad response to virus infection by binding to a high-affinity cellular receptor and triggering a signal transduction pathway. Orthopoxviruses encode homologs of the IL-1 receptor that bind IL-1β (11,496). Depending on the route of inoculation, deletion of the gene can reduce or enhance virulence (10,496). Frameshift mutations in the variola homolog preclude synthesis of an active protein.

SERPINS and Inhibitors of Cytokine Processing

IL-1β and IL-18 are produced by caspase-1 cleavage of inactive precursors. CrmA (also called SPI-2), a member of the SERPIN superfamily encoded by cowpox virus, was identified by its antiinflammatory properties and shown to inhibit caspase-1, a cysteine aspartic protease, and activation of IL-1β (265,407). An effect on activation of IL-18 is presumed, although it has not been shown directly. Further studies showed that CrmA protects cells against apoptosis by inactivation of additional caspases (581). Other orthopoxviruses and leporipoxviruses also encode CrmA homologs that inhibit caspase-1 (257,392). Attenuation of cowpox or rabbitpox viruses results from deletion of the *crmA* gene (515).

Orthopoxviruses and LeporIpoxviruses encode additional members of the SERPIN superfamily. SPI-1 and SPI-3 have been shown to complex with certain proteinases *in vitro,* but whether these proteinases are important targets *in vivo* is unknown (335,523). Deletion of SPI-1 causes a host range effect and nuclear changes but not other signs of apoptosis (335,462). Deletion of the *SPI-3* gene induces fusion of infected cells, but this activity does not require the SERPIN active site (523). Another SERPIN (SERP-1), encoded by leporipoxviruses, is secreted from infected cells, interferes with inflammation, and is required for virus-induced disease in rabbits (302). SERP-1 inhibits a number of serine proteases (plasmin, urokinase, tissue plasminogen activator, and a member of the complement cascade) *in vitro*, but whether any or all of these are significant biologic targets *in vivo* is unknown (292).

Chemokine Inhibitors

MCV encodes a CC chemokine homolog (MC148) that is predicted to be an antagonist based on the absence of the conserved N-terminal region (450). MC148 was found to bind specifically to the CCR8 chemokine receptor and to inhibit competitively the binding of I-309, the natural ligand (297). Other reports, based mainly on chemotaxis assays, suggest a broader activity (128,270).

Secreted proteins that bind to CC chemokines but lack sequence similarity to chemokine receptors are encoded by leporipoxviruses (M-T1) and orthopoxviruses (35-kd proteins) (13,91,188,487). These proteins prevent activation and chemotaxis of leukocytes. An influx of inflammatory cells into tissues infected with a rabbitpox virus 35-kd protein deletion mutant was described (188), although no difference in virulence was detected (309).

M-T7, the myxoma virus IFN-γ receptor–binding protein, also interacts with chemokines but with low affinity through the heparin-binding site, suggesting that it could alter their tissue localization (276). The influx of leukocytes into tissues infected with a M-T7 deletion mutant could be due to loss of either the chemokine or IFN-γ–binding activities.

Genes encoding homologs of seven transmembrane receptors have been identified in swinepox and capripox viruses (90,310), although their ligand-binding properties are unknown.

Apoptosis Inhibitors

CrmA was described previously as an inhibitor of caspase-1, the IL-1β–converting enzyme. However, CrmA and other orthopoxvirus homologs also block apoptosis activated through the Fas and TNF receptors (145,333, 512) and potently inhibited caspase-8, the apical caspase in these pathways (581). CrmA also binds granzyme B, a serine protease associated with lytic granules released by cytotoxic T lymphocytes (CTLs) (400). It is difficult to evaluate the specific roles of CrmA during a natural infection. CrmA can protect target cells against Fas-mediated lysis by alloreactive CTLs (300,512), but wild-type cowpox or ectromelia virus–infected target cells are not protected against lysis by class I major histocompatibility complex restricted CTLs (353). Although *crmA* deletion mutants replicate normally in most cell lines without inducing apoptosis, a cowpox *crmA* deletion mutant induced apoptosis in a pig kidney cell line but without affecting the virus yield (299,408). The effect on virulence caused by deletion of *crmA* or *SPI-2* has varied in different animal models (257,515).

MCV encodes two proteins with death effector domains (DEDs) (450). DEDs are also present in FADD and procaspase-8 and mediate their interaction after the binding of TNF or FasL to their receptors. One of these MCV proteins, MC159, binds FADD and protects transfected cells against death effector filament formation and apoptosis induced by Fas and other members of the TNF receptor superfamily (52,220,513,522). The role of the second DED-containing protein, MC160, is uncertain.

MCV encodes a selenocysteine-containing protein, MC66, that is homologous to cellular glutathione peroxidase and that can protect cells against the cytotoxic effects of hydrogen peroxide and ultraviolet (UV) irradiation (450,463). Peroxides may be formed by activated inflammatory cells and by UV light. A putative glutathione peroxidase is also encoded by fowlpox virus (2).

Ectromelia virus encodes a protein called p28 that contains a really interesting new gene (RING) finger motif that is required for virulence in mice (454) and that acts upstream of caspase-3 to block UV-induced apoptosis (69). Overexpression of the Shope fibroma virus RING finger protein N1R can also block apoptosis induced by UV light (70).

Several unrelated myxoma virus proteins prevent apoptosis. The protein encoded by the *M11L* gene localizes in the mitochondrial membrane and is required for virulence, to block myxoma-induced apoptosis of primary rabbit monocytes and staurosporine-induced apoptosis activation of caspase-3 (166,367). The M-T4 protein localizes to the endoplasmic reticulum of infected cells and is required for virulence and to prevent induction of apoptosis in a rabbit CD4+ T-cell line or primary rabbit lymphocytes (38,208). The M-T5 protein has a single ankyrin motif, is related to orthopoxvirus host range genes, and is required to prevent apoptosis in a rabbit CD4+ T-cell line (348).

CHOhr is a host range gene of cowpox virus that is disrupted or deleted from vaccinia virus strains and that is required for vaccinia virus replication in Chinese hamster ovary (CHO) cells (494). In the absence of the host range gene, there is a rapid cessation of host and viral protein synthesis and accelerated apoptosis in vaccinia virus–infected CHO cells (234,365,404). Apoptosis was induced at an unidentified viral postbinding step (403) and could be prevented by expression of the adenovirus *E1B-19K* gene or *Bcl2* gene in RK-13 (107,234).

The *E3L* gene of vaccinia virus was described previously as a double-stranded RNA-binding protein that protects against the action of protein kinase PKR and provides resistance to the action of IFN. *E3L* deletion mutants induced apoptosis in HeLa cells through failure to inhibit PKR (258,281).

EXPRESSION VECTORS

Several attributes of poxviruses have led to their extensive use as expression vectors (339). These include relative ease of formation and isolation of recombinant viruses, capacity for large amounts of DNA, relatively high expression, and wide host range. Expression has been achieved either by using poxvirus promoters or by employing bacteriophage RNA polymerases and cognate promoters. Recombinant viruses have been used for the synthesis of proteins *in vivo* or *in vitro* and as vaccine candidates.

CONCLUSIONS

The poxviruses are among the largest and most genetically complex of all animal viruses. Unlike most other DNA viruses, they replicate in the cytoplasm and encode many proteins that permit transcription and replication to occur outside of the nucleus. Gene expression is stringently regulated by a cascade mechanism, and virion assembly is a complex process that involves the formation of multiple membranes. Viral proteins are used for evasion of the host immune defense system.

REFERENCES

1. Afonso CL, Tulman ER, Lu Z, Oma E, et al. The genome of Melanoplus sanguinipes entomopoxvirus. *J Virol* 1999;73:533–552.
2. Afonso CL, Tulman ER, Lu Z, et al. The genome of fowlpox virus. *J Virol* 2000;74:3815–3831.
3. Ahn BY, Gershon PD, Jones EV, Moss B. Identification of rpo30, a vaccinia virus RNA polymerase gene with structural similarity to a eukaryotic transcription factor. *Mol Cell Biol* 1990;10:5433–5441.
4. Ahn BY, Gershon PD, Moss B. RNA-polymerase associated protein RAP94 confers promoter specificity for initiating transcription of vaccinia virus early stage genes. *J Biol Chem* 1994;269:7552–7557.
5. Ahn BY, Jones EV, Moss B. Identification of the vaccinia virus gene encoding an 18-kilodalton subunit of RNA polymerase and demonstration of a 5′ poly(A) leader on its early transcript. *J Virol* 1990;64:3019–3024.
6. Ahn BY, Moss B. Capped poly(A) leader of variable lengths at the 5′ ends of vaccinia virus late mRNAs. *J Virol* 1989;63:226–232.
7. Ahn BY, Moss B. RNA polymerase-associated transcription specificity factor encoded by vaccinia virus. *Proc Natl Acad Sci U S A* 1992;89:3536–3540.
8. Ahn BY, Rosel J, Cole NB, Moss B. Identification and expression of rpo19, a vaccinia virus gene encoding a 19-kilodalton DNA-dependent RNA polymerase subunit. *J Virol* 1992;66:971–982.
9. Ahn BY, Moss B. Glutaredoxin homolog encoded by vaccinia virus is a virion-associated enzyme with thioltransferase and dehydroascorbate reductase activities. *Proc Natl Acad Sci U S A* 1992;89:7060–7064.
10. Alcami A, Smith GL. A mechanism for inhibition of fever by a virus. *Proc Natl Acad Sci U S A* 1996;93:11029–11034.
11. Alcami A, Smith GL. A soluble receptor for interleukin-1b encoded by vaccinia virus: A novel mechanism of virus modulation of the host response to infection. *Cell* 1992;71:153–167.
12. Alcami A, Smith GL. Vaccinia, cowpox, and camelpox viruses encode soluble gamma interferon receptors with novel broad species specificity. *J Virol* 1995;69:4633–4639.
13. Alcami A, Symons JA, Collins PD, et al. Blockade of chemokine activity by a soluble chemokine binding protein from vaccinia virus. *J Immunol* 1998;160:624–633.
14. Amegadzie B, Holmes M, Cole NB, et al. Identification, sequence, and expression of the gene encoding the second-largest subunit of the vaccinia virus DNA polymerase. *Virology* 1991;180:88–98.
15. Amegadzie BY, Ahn BY, Moss B. Characterization of a 7-kilodalton subunit of vaccinia virus DNA-dependent RNA polymerase with structural similarities to the smallest subunit of eukaryotic RNA polymerase-II. *J Virol* 1992;66:3003–3010.
16. Amegadzie BY, Cole N, Ahn BY, Moss B. Identification, sequence and expression of the gene encoding a Mr 35,000 subunit of the vaccinia virus DNA-dependent RNA polymerase. *J Biol Chem* 1991;266:13712–13718.
17. Amegadzie BY, Sisler JR, Moss B. Frame-shift mutations within the vaccinia virus A-type inclusion protein gene. *Virology* 1992;186:777–782.
18. Antczak JB, Patel DD, Ray CA, et al. Site-specific RNA cleavage generates the 3′ end of a poxvirus late mRNA. *Proc Natl Acad Sci U S A* 1992;89:12033–12037.
19. Antoine G, Scheiflinger F, Dorner F, Falkner FG. The complete genomic sequence of the modified vaccinia Ankara strain: Comparison with other orthopoxviruses. *Virology* 1998;244:365–396.
20. Arif BM. The entomopoxviruses. *Adv Virus Res* 1984;29:195–213.
21. Bablanian R, Baxt B, Sonnabend JA, Esteban M. Studies on the mechanisms of vaccinia virus cytopathic effects. II. Early cell rounding is associated with virus polypeptide synthesis. *J Gen Virol* 1978;39:403–413.
22. Bablanian R, Coppola G, Scribani S, Esteban M. Inhibition of protein synthesis by vaccinia virus. IV. The role of low-molecular-weight viral RNA in the inhibition of protein synthesis. *Virology* 1981;112:13–24.
23. Bablanian R, Goswami SK, Esteban M, et al. Mechanism of selective translation of vaccinia virus mRNAs: Differential role of poly(A) and initiation factors in the translation of viral and cellular mRNAs. *J Virol* 1991;65:4449–4460.
24. Bablanian R, Scribani S, Esteban M. Amplification of polyadenylated nontranslated small RNA sequences (POLADS) during superinfection correlates with the inhibition of viral and cellular protein synthesis. *Cell Mol Biol Res* 1993;39:243–255.
25. Baek SH, Kwak JY, Lee SH, et al. Lipase activities of p37, the major envelope protein of vaccinia virus. *J Biol Chem* 1997;272:32042–32049.
26. Bajszar G, Wittek R, Weir JP, Moss B. Vaccinia virus thymidine kinase and neighboring genes: mRNAs and polypeptides of wild type virus and putative nonsense mutants. *J Virol* 1983;45:62–72.
27. Baldick CJ, Cassetti MC, Harris N, Moss B. Ordered assembly of a functional preinitiation transcription complex, containing vaccinia virus early transcription factor and RNA polymerase, on an immobilized template. *J Virol* 1994;68:6052–6056.
28. Baldick CJ Jr, Moss B. Characterization and temporal regulation of mRNAs encoded by vaccinia virus intermediate stage genes. *J Virol* 1993;67:3515–3527.
29. Baldick CJ, Keck JG, Moss B. Mutational analysis of the core, spacer and initiator regions of vaccinia virus intermediate class promoters. *J Virol* 1992;66:4710–4719.
30. Baldick CJ, Moss B. Resistance of vaccinia virus to rifampicin conferred by a single nucleotide substitution near the predicted NH2 terminus of a gene encoding an Mr 62,000 polypeptide. *Virology* 1987;156:138–145.
31. Ball LA. High frequency recombination in vaccinia virus DNA. *J Virol* 1987;61:1788–1795.
32. Banham A, Smith GL. Vaccinia virus gene B1R encodes a 34-kDa serine/threonine protein kinase that localizes in cytoplasmic factories and is packaged into virions. *Virology* 1992;191:803–812.
33. Banville M, Duma SF, Trifiro S, et al. The predicted amino acid sequence of the spheroidin protein of *Amsacta moorei* entomopoxvirus: Lack of homology between major occlusion body proteins of different poxviruses. *J Gen Virol* 1992;73:559–566.
34. Barbosa E, Moss B. mRNA (nucleoside-2′)-methyltransferase from vaccinia virus: Characteristics and substrate specificity. *J Biol Chem* 1978;253:7698–7702.
35. Baroudy BM, Moss B. Purification and characterization of a DNA-dependent RNA polymerase from vaccinia virions. *J Biol Chem* 1980;255:4372–4380.
36. Baroudy BM, Venkatesan S, Moss B. Incompletely base-paired flip-flop terminal loops link the two DNA strands of the vaccinia virus genome into one uninterrupted polynucleotide chain. *Cell* 1982;28:315–324.
37. Baroudy BM, Venkatesan S, Moss B. Structure and replication of vaccinia virus telomeres. *Cold Spring Harbor Symp Quant Biol* 1982;47:723–729.
38. Barry M, Hnatiuk S, Mossman K, et al. The myxoma virus M-T4 gene encodes a novel RDEL-containing protein that is retained within the endoplasmic reticulum and is important for the productive infection of lymphocytes. *Virology* 1997;239:360–377.
39. Bauer WR, Ressner EC, Kates J, Patzke J. A DNA nicking-closing enzyme encapsidated in vaccinia virus: Partial purification and properties. *Proc Natl Acad Sci U S A* 1977;74:1841–1845.
40. Bawden AL, Glassberg KJ, Diggans J, et al. Complete genomic sequence of the *Amsacta moorei* entomopoxvirus: Analysis and comparison with other poxviruses. *Virology* 2000;274:120–139.
41. Baxby D. *Jenner's smallpox vaccine:* The riddle of vaccinia virus and its origin. London: Heinemann Educational, 1981:1–214.
42. Bayliss CD, Condit RC. The vaccinia virus A18R gene product is a DNA-dependent ATPase. *J Biol Chem* 1995;270:1550–1556.
43. Bayliss CD, Smith GL. A vaccinia virion protein I8R has both DNA and RNA helicase activities: Implications for vaccinia virus transcription. *J Virol* 1996;70:794–800.
44. Bayliss CD, Smith GL. Vaccinia virion protein VP8, the 25 kDa product of the L4R gene, binds single-stranded DNA and RNA with similar affinity. *Nucleic Acids Res* 1997;25:3984–3990.
45. Beattie E, Paoletti E, Tartaglia J. Distinct patterns of IFN sensitivity observed in cells infected with vaccinia K3L- and E3L- mutant viruses. *Virology* 1995;210:254–263.
46. Beattie E, Tartaglia J, Paoletti E. Vaccinia virus encoded eIF-2a homolog abrogates the antiviral effect of interferon. *Virology* 1991;183:419–422.
47. Beaud G, Beaud R, Leader DP. Vaccinia virus gene H5R encodes a protein that is phosphorylated by the multisubstrate vaccinia virus B1R protein kinase. *J Virol* 1995;69:1819–1826.
48. Beaud G, Dru A. Protein synthesis in vaccinia virus-infected cells in

the presence of amino acid analogs: A translational control mechanism. *Virology* 1980;100:10–21.
49. Beaud G, Sharif A, Topamass A, Leader DP. Ribosomal-protein S2/SA kinase purified from HeLa cells infected with vaccinia virus corresponds to the B1R protein-kinase and phosphorylates *in-vitro* the viral ssDNA-bindng protein. *J Gen Virol* 1994;75:283–293.
50. Becker Y, Joklik WK. Messenger RNA in cells infected with vaccinia virus. *Proc Natl Acad Sci U S A* 1964;51:577–584.
51. Bergoin M, Devauchelle G, Vago C. Electron microscopy study of the pox-like virus of *Melolontha melolontha* L (*Coleptera, Scarabeidae*) virus morphogenesis. *Arch Virusforsch* 1969;28:285–302.
52. Bertin J, Armstrong RC, Ottilie S, et al. DED-containing herpesvirus and poxvirus proteins inhibit both Fas- and TNFR1-induced apoptosis. *Proc Natl Acad Sci U S A* 1997;94:1172–1176.
53. Betakova T, Moss B. Disulfide bonds and membrane topology of the vaccinia virus A17L envelope P protein. *J Virol* 2000;74:2438–2442.
54. Betakova T, Wolffe EJ, Moss B. Membrane topology of the vaccinia virus A17L envelope protein. *Virology* 1999;261:347–356.
55. Betakova T, Wolffe EJ, Moss B. Regulation of vaccinia virus morphogenesis: Phosphorylation of the A14L and A17L membrane proteins and C-terminal truncation of the A17L protein are dependent on the F10L protein kinase. *J Virol* 1999;73:3534–3543.
56. Betakova T, Wolffe EJ, Moss B. Vaccinia virus A14.5L gene encodes a hydrophobic 53-amino acid virion membrane protein that enhances virulence in mice and is conserved amongst vertebrate poxviruses. *J Virol* 2000;74:4085–4092.
57. Black EP, Condit RC. Phenotypic characterization of mutants in vaccinia virus gene G2R, a putative transcription elongation factor. *J Virol* 1996;70:47–54.
58. Black EP, Moussatche N, Condit RC. Characterization of the interactions among vaccinia virus transcription factors G2R, A18R, and H5R. *Virology* 1998;245:313–322.
59. Black ME, Hruby DE. A single amino acid substitution abolishes feedback inhibition of vaccinia virus thymidine kinase. *J Biol Chem* 1992;267:9743–9748.
60. Blasco R, Moss B. Extracellular vaccinia virus formation and cell-to-cell virus transmission are prevented by deletion of the gene encoding the 37,000 Dalton outer envelope protein. *J Virol* 1991;65:5910–5920.
61. Blasco R, Moss B. Role of cell-associated enveloped vaccinia virus in cell-to-cell spread. *J Virol* 1992;66:4170–4179.
62. Blasco R, Sisler JR, Moss B. Dissociation of progeny vaccinia virus from the cell membrane is regulated by a viral envelope glycoprotein: Effect of a point mutation in the lectin homology domain of the A34R gene. *J Virol* 1993;67:3319–3325.
63. Block W, Upton C, McFadden G. Tumorigenic poxviruses: Genomic organization of malignant rabbit virus, a recombinant between Shope fibroma virus and myxoma virus. *Virology* 1985;140:113–124.
64. Boone RF, Moss B. Methylated 5′ terminal sequences of vaccinia virus mRNA species made in vivo at early and late times after infection. *Virology* 1977;79:67–80.
65. Boone RF, Moss B. Sequence complexity and relative abundance of vaccinia virus mRNA's synthesized *in vivo* and *in vitro*. *J Virol* 1978;26:554–569.
66. Boone RF, Parr RP, Moss B. Intermolecular duplexes formed from polyadenylated vaccinia virus RNA. *J Virol* 1979;30:365–374.
67. Born TL, Morrison LA, Esteban DJ, et al. A poxvirus protein that binds to and inactivates IL-18, and inhibits NK cell response. *J Immunol* 2000;164:3246–3254.
68. Boulter EA, Appleyard G. Differences between extracellular and intracellular forms of poxvirus and their implications. *Prog Med Virol* 1973;16:86–108.
69. Brick DJ, Burke RD, Minkley AA, Upton C. Ectromelia virus virulence factor p28 acts upstream of caspase-3 in response to UV light-induced apoptosis. *J Gen Virol* 2000;81:1087–1097.
70. Brick DJ, Burke RD, Schiff L, Upton C. Shope fibroma virus RING finger protein N1R binds DNA and inhibits apoptosis. *Virology* 1998;249:42–51.
71. Broyles SS. A role for ATP hydrolysis in vaccinia virus early gene transcription. *J Biol Chem* 1991;266:15545–15548.
72. Broyles SS. Vaccinia virus encodes a functional dUTPase. *Virology* 1993;195:863–865.
73. Broyles SS, Fesler BS. Vaccinia virus gene encoding a component of the viral early transcription factor. *J Virol* 1990;64:1523–1529.
74. Broyles SS, Li J. The small subunit of the vaccinia virus early transcription factor contacts the transcription promoter DNA. *J Virol* 1993;67:5677–5680.
75. Broyles SS, Li J, Moss B. Promoter DNA contacts made by the vaccinia virus early transcription factor. *J Biol Chem* 1991;266:15539–15544.
76. Broyles SS, Liu X, Zhu M, Kremer M. Transcription factor YY1 is a vaccinia virus late promoter activator. *J Biol Chem* 1999;274:35662–35667.
77. Broyles SS, Moss B. DNA-dependent ATPase activity associated with vaccinia virus early transcription factor. *J Biol Chem* 1988;263:10761–10765.
78. Broyles SS, Moss B. Homology between RNA polymerases of poxviruses, prokaryotes, and eukaryotes: Nucleotide sequence and transcriptional analysis of vaccinia virus genes encoding 147-kDa and 22-kDa subunits. *Proc Natl Acad Sci U S A* 1986;83:3141–3145.
79. Broyles SS, Moss B. Identification of the vaccinia virus gene encoding nucleoside triphosphate phosphohydrolase I, a DNA-dependent ATPase. *J Virol* 1987;61:1738–1742.
80. Broyles SS, Moss B. Sedimentation of an RNA polymerase complex from vaccinia virus that specifically initiates and terminates transcription. *Mol Cell Biol* 1987;7:7–14.
81. Broyles SS, Pennington MJ. Vaccinia virus gene encoding a 30-kilodalton subunit of the viral DNA-dependent RNA polymerase. *J Virol* 1990;64:5376–5382.
82. Broyles SS, Yuen L, Shuman S, Moss B. Purification of a factor required for transcription of vaccinia virus early genes. *J Biol Chem* 1988;263:10754–10760.
83. Buller RM, Chakrabarti S, Cooper JA, et al. Deletion of the vaccinia virus growth factor gene reduces virus virulence. *J Virol* 1988;62:866–877.
84. Buller RML, Chakrabarti S, Moss B, Frederickson T. Cell proliferative response to vaccinia virus is mediated by VGF. *Virology* 1988;164:182–192.
85. Buller RML, Palumbo GJ. Poxvirus pathogenesis. *Microbiol Rev* 1991;55:80–122.
86. Buller RML, Smith GL, Cremer K, Notkins AL, Moss B. Decreased virulence of recombinant vaccinia virus expression vectors is associated with a thymidine kinase-negative phenotype. *Nature* 1985;317:813–815.
87. Cacoullos N, Bablanian R. Role of polyadenylated RNA sequences (POLADS) in vaccinia virus infection: Correlation between accumulation of POLADS and extent of shut-off in infected cells. *Cell Mol Biol Res* 1993;39:657–664.
88. Cairns J. The initiation of vaccinia infection. *Virology* 1960;11:603–623.
89. Cameron C, Hota-Mitchell S, Chen L, et al. The complete DNA sequence of myxoma virus. *Virology* 1999;264:298–318.
90. Cao JX, Gershon PD, Black DN. Sequence analysis of HindIII Q2 fragment of capripoxvirus reveals a putative gene encoding a G-protein-coupled chemokine receptor homologue. *Virology* 1995;209:207–212.
91. Carf A, Smith CA, Smolak PJ, et al. Structure of a soluble secreted chemokine inhibitor vCCI (p35) from cowpox virus. *Proc Natl Acad Sci U S A* 1999;96:12379–12383.
92. Carpenter MS, DeLange AM. Identification of a temperature-sensitive mutant of vaccinia virus defective in late but not intermediate gene expression. *Virology* 1992;188:233–244.
93. Carrasco L, Esteban M. Modification of membrane permeability in vaccinia virus-infected cells. *Virology* 1982;117:62–69.
94. Carroll K, Elroy-Stein O, Moss B, Jagus R. Recombinant vaccinia virus K3L gene product prevents activation of double-stranded RNA-dependent, initiation factor 2 alpha-specific protein kinase. *J Biol Chem* 1993;268:12837–12842.
95. Cassetti MC, Merchlinsky M, Wolffe EJ, et al. DNA packaging mutant: Repression of the vaccinia virus A32 gene results in noninfectious, DNA-deficient, spherical, enveloped particles. *J Virol* 1998;72:5769–5780.
96. Cassetti MC, Moss B. Interaction of the 82-kDa subunit of the vaccinia virus early transcription factor heterodimer with the promoter core sequence directs downstream DNA binding of the 70-kDa subunit. *Proc Natl Acad Sci U S A* 1996;93:7540–7545.
97. Challberg MD, Englund PT. Purification and properties of the deoxyribonucleic acid polymerase induced by vaccinia virus. *J Biol Chem* 1979;254:7812–7819.

98. Chang A, Metz DH. Further investigations on the mode of entry of vaccinia virus into cells. *J Gen Virol* 1976;32:275–282.
99. Chang HW, Jacobs BL. Identification of a conserved motif that is necessary for binding of the vaccinia virus E3L gene products to double-stranded RNA. *Virology* 1993;194:537–547.
100. Chang HW, Watson JC, Jacobs BL. The E3L gene of vaccinia virus encodes an inhibitor of the interferon-induced, double-stranded RNA-dependent protein kinase. *Proc Natl Acad Sci U S A* 1992;89: 4825–4829.
101. Chang W, Hsiao JC, Chung CS, Bair CH. Isolation of a monoclonal antibody which blocks vaccinia virus infection. *J Virol* 1995;69: 517–522.
102. Chang W, Macaulay C, Hu SL, et al. Tumorigenic poxviruses: Characterization of the expression of an epidermal growth factor related gene in Shope fibroma virus. *Virology* 1990;179:926–930.
103. Cheevers WP, O'Callaghan DJ, Randall CC. Biosynthesis of host and viral deoxyribonucleic acid during hyperplastic fowlpox-infection *in vivo*. *J Virol* 1968;2:421–429.
104. Child SJ, Palumbo G, Buller RM, Hruby D. Insertional inactivation of the large subunit of ribonucleotide reductase encoded by vaccinia virus is associated with reduced virulence *in vivo*. *Virology* 1990;174: 625–629.
105. Christen LM, Sanders M, Wiler C, Niles EG. Vaccinia virus nucleoside triphosphate phosphohydrolase I is an essential viral early gene transcription termination factor. *Virology* 1998;245:360–371.
106. Chung CS, Hsiao JC, Chang YS, Chang W. A27L protein mediates vaccinia virus interaction with cell surface heparin sulfate. *J Virol* 1998;72:1577–1585.
107. Chung CS, Vasilevskaya IA, Wang SC, et al. Apoptosis and host restriction of vaccinia virus in RK13 cells. *Virus Res* 1997;52: 121–132.
108. Colamonici OR, Domanski P, Sweitzer SM, et al. Vaccinia virus B18R gene encodes a type I interferon-binding protein that blocks interferon alpha transmembrane signaling. *J Biol Chem* 1995;270:15974–15978.
109. Colby C, Jurale C, Kates JR. Mechanism of synthesis of vaccinia virus double-stranded ribonucleic acid *in vivo* and *in vitro*. *J Virol* 1971;7:71–76.
110. Colinas RJ, Goebel SJ, Davis SW, et al. A DNA ligase gene in the Copenhagen strain of vaccinia virus is nonessential for viral replication and recombination. *Virology* 1990;179:267–275.
111. Condit RC, Easterly R, Pacha RF, et al. A vaccinia virus isatin-b-thiosemicarbazone resistance mutation maps in the viral gene encoding the 132-kDa subunit of RNA polymerase. *Virology* 1991;185: 857–861.
112. Condit RC, Motyczka A. Isolation and preliminary characterization of temperature-sensitive mutants of vaccinia virus. *Virology* 1981;113: 224–241.
113. Condit RC, Xiang Y, Lewis JI. Mutation of vaccinia virus gene G2R causes suppression of gene A18R ts mutants: Implication for control of transcription. *Virology* 1996;220:10–19.
114. Cong P, Shuman S. Mutational analysis of mRNA capping enzyme identifies amino acids involved in GTP binding, enzyme-guanylate formation, and GMP transfer to RNA. *Mol Cell Biol* 1995;15: 6222–6231.
115. Cong PJ, Shuman S. Methyltransferase and subunit association domains of vaccinia virus messenger RNA capping enzyme. *J Biol Chem* 1992;267:16424–16429.
116. Cooper JA, Moss B. *In vitro* translation of immediate early, early and late classes of RNA from vaccinia virus infected cells. *Virology* 1979; 96:368–380.
117. Cooper JA, Wittek R, Moss B. Extension of the transcriptional and translational map of the left end of the vaccinia virus genome to 21 kilobase pairs. *J Virol* 1981;39:733–745.
118. Cudmore S, Blasco R, Vincentelli R, et al. A vaccinia virus core protein, p39, is membrane associated. *J Virol* 1996;70:6909–6921.
119. Cudmore S, Cossart P, Griffiths G, Way M. Actin-based motility of vaccinia virus. *Nature* 1995;378:636–638.
120. da Fonseca FG, Weisberg A, Wolffe EJ, Moss B. Characterization of the vaccinia virus H3L envelope protein: Topology and post-translational membrane insertion via the C-terminal hydrophobic tail. *J Virol* 2000;74:7508–7517.
121. da Fonseca FG, Wolffe EJ, Weisberg A, Moss B. Effects of deletion or stringent repression of the H3L envelope gene on vaccinia virus replication. *J Virol* 2000;74:7518–7528.
122. Dales S. Reciprocity in the interactions between the poxviruses and their host cells. *Annu Rev Microbiol* 1990;44:173–192.
123. Dales S. Relation between penetration of vaccinia, release of viral DNA, and initiation of genetic functions. *Perspect Virol* 1965;4: 47–71.
124. Dales S, Kajioka R. The cycle of multiplication of vaccinia virus in Earle's strain L cells. I. Uptake and penetration. *Virology* 1964;24: 278–294.
125. Dales S, Mosbach EH. Vaccinia as a model for membrane biogenesis. *Virology* 1968;35:564–583.
126. Dales S, Siminovitch L. The development of vaccinia virus in Earle's L strain cells as examined by electron microscopy. *J Biophys Biochem Cytol* 1961;10:475–503.
127. Dall D, Sriskantha A, Verra A, et al. A gene encoding a highly expressed spindle body protein of *Heliothis armigera* entomopoxvirus. *J Gen Virol* 1993;74:1811–1818.
128. Damon I, Murphy PM, Moss B. Broad spectrum chemokine antagonist activity of a human poxvirus chemokine homolog. *Proc Natl Acad Sci U S A* 1998;95:6403–6407.
129. Davies MV, Elroy-Stein O, Jagus R, et al. The vaccinia virus K3L gene product potentiates translation by inhibiting double-stranded-RNA-activated protein kinase and phosphorylation of the alpha subunit of eukaryotic initiation factor 2. *J Virol* 1992;66:1943–1950.
130. Davis RE, Mathews CK. Acidic-C terminus of vaccinia virus DNA-Binding protein interacts with ribonucleotide reductase. *Proc Natl Acad Sci U S A* 1993;90:745–749.
131. Davison AJ, Moss B. The structure of vaccinia virus early promoters. *J Mol Biol* 1989;210:749–769.
132. Davison AJ, Moss B. The structure of vaccinia virus late promoters. *J Mol Biol* 1989;210:771–784.
133. De Carlos A, Paez E. Isolation and characterization of mutants of vaccinia virus with a modified 94-kDa inclusion protein. *Virology* 1991;185:768–778.
134. DeFilippes FM. Site of the base change in the vaccinia virus DNA polymerase gene which confers aphidicolin resistance. *J Virol* 1989; 63:4060–4063.
135. DeLange AM. Identification of temperature-sensitive mutants of vaccinia virus that are defective in conversion of concatemeric replicative intermediates to the mature linear DNA genome. *J Virol* 1989;63: 2437–2444.
136. DeLange AM, McFadden G. Efficient resolution of replicated poxvirus telomeres to native hairpin structures requires two inverted symmetrical copies of a core target DNA sequence. *J Virol* 1987;61: 1957–1963.
137. DeLange AM, McFadden G. Sequence-nonspecific replication of transfected plasmid DNA in poxvirus-infected cells. *Proc Natl Acad Sci U S A* 1986;83:614–618.
138. Delange AM, Reddy M, Scraba D, et al. Replication and resolution of cloned poxvirus telomeres *in vivo* generates linear minichromosomes with intact viral hairpin termini. *J Virol* 1986;59:249–259.
139. DeMasi J, Traktman P. Clustered charge-to-alanine mutagenesis of the vaccinia virus H5 gene: Isolation of a dominant, temperature-sensitive mutant with a profound defect in morphogenesis. *J Virol* 2000;74: 2393–2405.
140. Deng L, Beigelman L, Matulic-Adamic J, et al. Specific recognition of an rU2-N15-rU motif by VP55, the vaccinia virus poly(A) polymerase catalytic subunit. *J Biol Chem* 1997;272:31542–31552.
141. Deng L, Shuman S. Vaccinia NPH-I, a DExH-box ATPase, is the energy coupling factor for mRNA transcription termination. *Genes Dev* 1998;12:538–546.
142. Deng S, Shuman S. A role for the H4 subunit of vaccinia RNA polymerase in transcription initiation at a viral early promoter. *J Biol Chem* 1994;269:14323–14329.
143. Derrien M, Punjabi A, Khanna R, et al. Tyrosine phosphorylation of A17 during vaccinia virus infection: Involvement of the H1 phosphatase and the F10 kinase. *J Virol* 1999;73:7287–7296.
144. des Gouttes Olgiati D, Pogo BG, Dales S. Biogenesis of vaccinia: Specific inhibition of rapidly labeled host DNA in vaccinia inoculated cells. *Virology* 1976;71:325–335.
145. Dobbelstein M, Shenk T. Protection against apoptosis by the vaccinia virus SPI-2 (B13R) gene product. *J Virol* 1996;70:6479–6485.
146. Doms RW, Blumenthal R, Moss B. Fusion of intra- and extracellular forms of vaccinia virus with the cell membrane. *J Virol* 1990;64: 4884–4892.

147. Du S, Traktman P. Vaccinia virus DNA replication: Two hundred base pairs of telomeric sequence confer optimal replication efficiency on minichromosome templates. *Proc Natl Acad Sci U S A* 1996;93: 9693–9698.
148. Dubochet J, Adrian M, Richter K, et al. Structure of intracellular mature vaccine virus observed by cryoelectron microscopy. *J Virol* 1994;68:1935–1941.
149. Dumbell K, Richardson M. Virological investigations of specimens from buffaloes affected by buffalopox in Maharashtra State, India between 1985 and 1987. *Arch Virol* 1993;128:257–267.
150. Duncan SA, Smith GL. Identification and characterization of an extracellular envelope glycoprotein affecting vaccinia virus egress. *J Virol* 1992;66:1610–1621.
151. Dyster LM, Niles EG. Genetic and biochemical characterization of vaccinia virus genes D2L and D3R which encode virion structural proteins. *Virology* 1991;182:455–467.
152. Earl PL, Hügin AW, Moss B. Removal of cryptic poxvirus transcription termination signals from the human immunodeficiency virus type 1 envelope gene enhances expression and immunogenicity of a recombinant vaccinia virus. *J Virol* 1990;64:2448–2451.
153. Earl PL, Jones EV, Moss B. Homology between DNA polymerases of poxviruses, herpesviruses, and adenoviruses: Nucleotide sequence of the vaccinia virus DNA polymerase gene. *Proc Natl Acad Sci U S A* 1986;83:3659–3663.
154. Easterbrook KB. Controlled degradation of vaccinia virions in vitro: An electron microscopic study. *J Ultrastruct Res* 1966;14:484–496.
155. Engelstad M, Howard ST, Smith GL. A constitutively expressed vaccinia gene encodes a 42-kDa glycoprotein related to complement control factors that forms part of the extracellular virus envelope. *Virology* 1992;188:801–810.
156. Engelstad M, Smith GL. The vaccinia virus 42-kDa envelope protein is required for the envelopment and egress of extracellular virus and for virus virulence. *Virology* 1993;194:627–637.
157. Essani K, Chalasani S, Eversole R, et al. Multiple anti-cytokine activities secreted from tanapox virus-infected cells. *Microbiol Pathog* 1994;17:347–353.
158. Esteban M, Flores L, Holowczak JA. Model for vaccinia virus DNA replication. *Virology* 1977;83:467–473.
159. Esteban M, Flores L, Holowczak JA. Topography of vaccinia virus DNA. *Virology* 1977;82:163–181.
160. Esteban M, Holowczak JA. Replication of vaccinia DNA in mouse L cells. I. In vivo DNA synthesis. *Virology* 1977;78:57–75.
161. Esteban M, Metz DH. Early virus protein synthesis in vaccinia virus-infected cells. *J Gen Virol* 1973;19:201–216.
162. Evans DH, Stuart D, McFadden G. High levels of genetic recombination among cotransfected plasmid DNAs in poxvirus-infected mammalian cells. *J Virol* 1988;62:367–375.
163. Evans E, Klemperer N, Ghosh R, Traktman P. The vaccinia virus D5 protein, which is required for DNA replication, is a nucleic acid-independent nucleotide triphosphatase. *J Virol* 1995;69:5353–5361.
164. Evans E, Traktman P. Characterization of vaccinia virus DNA replication mutants with lesions in the D5 gene. *Chromosoma* 1992;102: S72–S82.
165. Evans E, Traktman P. Molecular genetic analysis of a vaccinia virus gene with an essential role in DNA replication. *J Virol* 1987;61: 3152–3162.
166. Everett H, Barry M, Lee SF, et al. M11L: A novel mitochondria-localized protein of myxoma virus that blocks apoptosis of infected leukocytes. *J Exp Med* 2000;191:1487–1498.
167. Fathi Z, Condit RC. Phenotypic characterization of a vaccinia virus temperature-sensitive complementation group affecting a virion component. *Virology* 1991;181:272–276.
168. Fenner F, Comben BM. Genetic studies with mammalian poxviruses. I. Demonstration of recombination between two strains of poxviruses. *Virology* 1958;5:530–548.
169. Fenner F, Woodroofe GM. The reactivation of poxviruses. II. The range of reactivating viruses. *Virology* 1960;11:185–201.
170. Fisher C, Parks RJ, Lauzon ML, Evans DH. Heteroduplex DNA formation is associated with replication and recombination in poxvirus-infected cells. *Genetics* 1991;129:7–18.
171. Frischknecht F, Moreau V, Rottger S, et al. Actin-based motility of vaccinia virus mimics receptor tyrosine kinase signalling. *Nature* 1999;401:926–929.
172. Funahashi S, Sato T, Shida H. Cloning and characterization of the gene encoding the major protein of the A-type inclusion body of cowpox virus. *J Gen Virol* 1988;69:35–47.
173. Galmiche MC, Goenaga J, Wittek R, Rindisbacher L. Neutralizing and protective antibodies directed against vaccinia virus envelope antigens. *Virology* 1999;254:71–80.
174. Garcia AD, Aravind L, Koonin EV, Moss B. Bacterial-type DNA Holliday junction resolvases in eukaryotic viruses. *Proc Natl Acad Sci U S A* 2000;97:8926–8931.
175. Garcia AD, Moss B. Repression of vaccinia virus Holliday Junction resolvase inhibits processing of viral DNA into unit-length genones. *J Virol* 2001; in press.
176. Garon CF, Barbosa E, Moss B. Visualization of an inverted terminal repetition in vaccinia virus DNA. *Proc Natl Acad Sci U S A* 1978;75: 4863–4867.
177. Gershon PD. mRNA 3′ end formation by vaccinia virus: Mechanism of action of a heterodimeric poly(A) polymerase. *Semin Virol* 1998;8: 343–350.
178. Gershon PD, Ahn BY, Garfield M, Moss B. Poly(A) polymerase and a dissociable polyadenylation stimulatory factor encoded by vaccinia virus. *Cell* 1991;66:1269–1278.
179. Gershon PD, Kitching RP, Hammond JM, Black DN. Poxvirus genetic recombination during natural virus transmission. *J Gen Virol* 1989;70: 485–489.
180. Gershon PD, Moss B. Early transcription factor subunits are encoded by vaccinia virus late genes. *Proc Natl Acad Sci U S A* 1990;87:4401–4405.
181. Gershon PD, Moss B. Stimulation of poly(A) tail elongation by the VP39 subunit of the vaccinia virus-encoded poly(A) polymerase. *J Biol Chem* 1993;268:2203–2210.
182. Gershon PD, Moss B. Transition from rapid processive to slow nonprocessive polyadenylation by vaccinia virus poly(A) polymerase catalytic subunit is regulated by the net length of the poly(A) tail. *Genes Dev* 1992;6:1575–1586.
183. Gershon PD, Moss B. Uridylate-containing RNA sequences determine specificity for binding and polyadenylation by the catalytic subunit of vaccinia virus poly(A) polymerase. *EMBO J* 1993;12:4705–4714.
184. Gershowitz A, Moss B. Abortive transcription products of vaccinia virus are guanylylated, methylated and polyadenylated. *J Virol* 1979; 31:849–853.
185. Gillard S, Spehner D, Drillien R, Kirn A. Localization and sequence of a vaccinia virus gene required for multiplication in human cells. *Proc Natl Acad Sci U S A* 1986;83:5573–5577.
186. Goebel SJ, Johnson GP, Perkus ME, et al. The complete DNA sequence of vaccinia virus. *Virology* 1990;179:247–266.
187. Gong SC, Lai CF, Esteban M. Vaccinia virus induces cell fusion at acid pH and this activity is mediated by the N-terminus of the 14-kDa virus envelope protein. *Virology* 1990;178:81–91.
188. Graham KA, Lalani AS, Macen JL, et al. The T1/35kDa family of poxvirus-secreted proteins bind chemokines and modulate leukocyte influx into virus-infected tissues. *Virology* 1997;229:12–24.
189. Grimley PM, Rosenblum EN, Mims SJ, Moss B. Interruption by rifampin of an early stage in vaccinia virus morphogenesis: Accumulation of membranes which are precursors of virus envelopes. *J Virol* 1970;6:519–533.
190. Gross CH, Shuman S. The nucleoside triphosphatase and helicase activities of vaccinia virus NPH-II are essential for virus replication. *J Virol* 1998;72:4729–4736.
191. Gross CH, Shuman S. Vaccinia virions lacking the RNA helicase nucleoside triphosphate hydrolase II are defective in early transcription. *J Virol* 1996;70:8549–8570.
192. Guan K, Broyles SS, Dixon JE. A Tyr/Ser protein phosphatase encoded by vaccinia virus. *Nature* 1991;350:359–362.
193. Gunasinghe SK, Hubbs AE, Wright CF. A vaccinia virus late transcription factor with biochemical and molecular identity to a human cellular protein. *J Biol Chem* 1998;273:27524–27530.
194. Guo P, Moss B. Interaction and mutual stabilization of the two subunits of vaccinia virus mRNA capping enzyme coexpressed in *Escherichia coli*. *Proc Natl Acad Sci U S A* 1990;87:4023–4027.
195. Gvakharia BO, Koonin E, Mathews CK. Vaccinia virus G4L gene encodes a second glutaredoxin. *Virology* 1996;226:408–411.
196. Hagler J, Shuman S. A freeze-frame view of eukaryotic transcription during elongation and capping of nascent mRNA. *Science* 1992;255: 983–986.
197. Hagler J, Shuman S. Nascent RNA cleavage by purified ternary complexes of vaccinia RNA polymerase. *J Biol Chem* 1993;268:2166–2173.

198. Hall RL, Moyer RW. Identification, cloning, and sequencing of a fragment of Amsacta moorei entomopoxvirus DNA containing the spheroidin gene and three vaccinia virus-related open reading frames. *J Virol* 1991;65:6516–6527.
199. Hall RL, Moyer RW. Identification of an Amsacta spheroidin-like protein within the occlusion bodies of *Choristoneura entomopox* viruses. *Virology* 1993;192:179–187.
200. Hanafusa H, Hanafusa T, Kamahora J. Transformation phenomena in the pox group viruses. II. Transformation between several members of the pox group. *Biken J* 1959;2:85–91.
201. Harford C, Hamlin A, Riders E. Electron microscopic autoradiography of DNA synthesis in cell infected with vaccinia virus. *Exp Cell Res* 1966;42:50–57.
202. Harris N, Rosales R, Moss B. Transcription initiation factor activity of vaccinia virus capping enzyme is independent of mRNA guanylylation. *Proc Natl Acad Sci U S A* 1993;90:2860–2864.
203. Herrera E, del Mar Lorenzo M, Blasco R, Isaacs SN. Functional analysis of vaccinia virus B5R protein: Essential role in virus envelopment is independent of a large portion of the extracellular domain. *J Virol* 1998;72:294–302.
204. Hertig C, Coupar BEH, Gould AR, Boyle DB. Field and vaccine strains of fowlpox virus carry integrated sequences from the avian retrovirus, reticuloendotheliosis virus. *Virology* 1997;235:367–376.
205. Higman MA, Christen LA, Niles EG. The mRNA (guanine-7-) methyltransferase domain of the vaccinia virus mRNA capping enzyme: Expression in *Escherichia coli* and structural and kinetic comparison to the intact capping enzyme. *J Biol Chem* 1994;269: 14974–14981.
206. Hiller G, Weber K. Golgi-derived membranes that contain an acylated viral polypeptide are used for vaccinia virus envelopment. *J Virol* 1985;55:651–659.
207. Hiller G, Weber K, Schneider L, et al. Interaction of assembled progeny pox viruses with the cellular cytoskeleton. *Virology* 1979;98: 142–153.
208. Hnatiuk S, Barry M, Zeng W, et al. Role of the C-terminal RDEL motif of the myxoma virus M-T4 protein in terms of apoptosis regulation and viral pathogenesis. *Virology* 1999;263:290–306.
209. Hodel AE, Gershon PD, Shi X, Quiocho FA. The 1.8 Å structure of vaccinia protein VP39: A bifunctional enzyme that participates in the modification of both mRNA ends. *Cell* 1996;85:247–256.
210. Hodel AE, Gershon PD, Shi X, et al. Specific protein recognition of an mRNA cap through its alkylated base. *Nat Struct Biol* 1997;4: 350–354.
211. Hollinshead M, Vanderplasschen A, Smith GL, Vaux DJ. Vaccinia virus intracellular mature virions contain only one lipid membrane. *J Virol* 1999;73:1503–1517.
212. Holzer GW, Gritschenberger W, Mayrhofer JA, et al. Dominant host range selection of vaccinia recombinants by rescue of an essential gene. *Virology* 1998;249:160–166.
213. Hooda-Dhingra U, Patel DD, Pickup DJ, Condit RC. Fine structure mapping and phenotypic analysis of five temperature sensitive mutations in the second largest subunit of vaccinia virus DNA-dependent RNA polymerase. *Virology* 1990;174:60–69.
214. Howard ST, Ray CA, Patel DD, et al. A 43-nucleotide RNA cis-acting element governs the site-specific formation of the 3′ end of a poxvirus late mRNA. *Virology* 1999;255:190–204.
215. Howell ML, Sanders-Loehr J, Loehr TM, et al. Cloning of the vaccinia virus ribonucleotide reductase small subunit gene: Characterization of the gene product expressed in *Escherichia coli. J Biol Chem* 1992; 267:1705–1711.
216. Hruby DE, Maki RA, Miller DB, Ball LA. Fine structure analysis and nucleotide sequence of the vaccinia virus thymidine kinase gene. *Proc Natl Acad Sci U S A* 1983;80:3411–3415.
217. Hsiao JC, Chung CS, Chang W. Cell surface proteoglycans are necessary for A27L protein-mediated cell fusion: Identification of the N-terminal region of A27L protein as the glycosaminoglycan-binding domain. *J Virol* 1998;72:8374–8379.
218. Hsiao JC, Chung CS, Chang W. Vaccinia virus envelope D8L protein binds to cell surface chondroitin sulfate and mediates the adsorption of intracellular mature virions to cells. *J Virol* 1999;73:8750–8761.
219. Hu FQ, Smith CA, Pickup DJ. Cowpox virus contains two copies of an early gene encoding a soluble secreted form of the type II TNF receptor. *Virology* 1994;204:343–356.
220. Hu S, Vincenz C, Buller M, Dixit VM. A novel family of viral death effector domain-containing molecules that inhibit both CD-95- and tumor necrosis factor receptor-1-induced apoptosis. *J Biol Chem* 1997;272:9621–9624.
221. Hu X, Carroll LJ, Wolffe EJ, Moss B. *De novo* synthesis of the early transcription factor 70-kDa subunit is required for morphogenesis of vaccinia virions. *J Virol* 1996;70:7669–7677.
222. Hu X, Wolffe EJ, Weisberg AS, et al. Repression of the A8L gene, encoding the early transcription factor 82-kilodalton subunit, inhibits morphogenesis of vaccinia virions. *J Virol* 1998;72:104–112.
223. Hubbs AE, Wright CF. The A2L intermediate gene product is required for *in vitro* transcription from a vaccinia virus late promoter. *J Virol* 1996;70:327–331.
224. Hughes SJ, Johnston LH, Decarlos A, Smith GL. Vaccinia virus encodes an active thymidylate kinase that complements a cdc8 mutant of *Saccharomyces cerevisiae. J Biol Chem* 1991;266:20103–20109.
225. Hugin AW, Hauser C. The epidermal growth factor receptor is not a receptor for vaccinia virus. *J Virol* 1994;68:8409–8412.
226. Hwang Y, Wang B, Bushman FD. Molluscum contagiosum virus topoisomerase: Purification, activities, and response to inhibitors. *J Virol* 1998;72:3401–3406.
227. Hyde JM, Peters D. The organization of nucleoprotein within fowlpox virus. *J Ultrastruct Res* 1971;35:626–641.
228. Ichihashi Y. Extracellular enveloped vaccinia virus escapes neutralization. *Virology* 1996;217:478–485.
229. Ichihashi Y. Unit complex of vaccinia polypeptides linked by disulfide bridges. *Virology* 1981;113:277–284.
230. Ichihashi Y, Matsumoto S, Dales S. Biogenesis of poxviruses: Role of A-type inclusions and host cell membranes in virus dissemination. *Virology* 1971;46:507–532.
231. Ichihashi Y, Oie M. Neutralizing epitopes on penetration protein of vaccinia virus. *Virology* 1996;220:491–494.
232. Ichihashi Y, Oie M. Proteolytic activation of vaccinia virus for penetration phase of infection. *Virology* 1982;116:297–305.
233. Ichihashi Y, Oie M, Tsuruhara T. Location of DNA-binding proteins and disulfide-linked proteins in vaccinia virus structural elements. *J Virol* 1984;50:929–938.
234. Ink BS, Gilbert CS, Evan GI. Delay of vaccinia virus-induced apoptosis in nonpermissive hamster ovary cells by the cowpox virus CHOhr and adenovirus E1B 19K genes. *J Virol* 1995;69:661–668.
235. Ink BS, Pickup DJ. Vaccinia virus directs the synthesis of early mRNAs containing 5′ poly(A) sequences. *Proc Natl Acad Sci U S A* 1990;87:1536–1540.
236. Isaacs SN, Kotwal GJ, Moss B. Vaccinia virus complement-control protein prevents antibody-dependent complement-enhanced neutralization of infectivity and contributes to virulence. *Proc Natl Acad Sci U S A* 1992;89:628–632.
237. Isaacs SN, Wolffe EJ, Payne LG, Moss B. Characterization of a vaccinia virus-encoded 42-kilodalton class I membrane glycoprotein component of the extracellular virus envelope. *J Virol* 1992;66: 7217–7224.
238. Janeczko RA, Rodriguez JF, Esteban M. Studies on the mechanism of entry of vaccinia virus into animal cells. *Arch Virol* 1987;92:135–150.
239. Jefferts ER, Holowczak. RNA synthesis in vaccinia-infected L cells: Inhibition of ribosome formation and maturation. *Virology* 1971;46: 730–744.
240. Jensen ON, Houthaeve T, Shevchenko A, et al. Identification of the major membrane and core proteins of vaccinia virus by two-dimensional electrophoresis. *J Virol* 1996;70:7485–7497.
241. Joklik WK. The intracellular uncoating of poxvirus DNA. I. The fate of radioactively-labeled rabbitpox virus. *J Mol Biol* 1964;8:263–276.
242. Joklik WK. The intracellular uncoating of poxvirus DNA. II. The molecular basis of the uncoating process. *J Mol Biol* 1964;8:277–288.
243. Joklik WK, Becker Y. The replication and coating of vaccinia DNA. *J Mol Biol* 1964;10:452–474.
244. Jungwirth C, Launer J. Effects of poxvirus infection on host cell deoxyribonucleic acid synthesis. *Virology* 1968;2:401–408.
245. Kane EM, Shuman S. Temperature-sensitive mutations in the vaccinia Virus-H4 gene encoding a component of the virion RNA polymerase. *J Virol* 1992;66:5752–5762.
246. Kane EM, Shuman S. Vaccinia virus morphogenesis is blocked by a temperature sensitive mutation in the I7 gene that encodes a virion component. *J Virol* 1993;67:2689–2698.
247. Kates J, Beeson J. Ribonucleic acid synthesis in vaccinia virus. II. Synthesis of polyriboadenylic acid. *J Mol Biol* 1970;50:19–23.

248. Kates JR, McAuslan BR. Poxvirus DNA-dependent RNA polymerase. *Proc Natl Acad Sci U S A* 1967;58:134–141.
249. Kato S, Kameyama S, Kamahora J. Autoradiography with tritium-labeled thymidine of pox virus and human amnion cell system in tissue culture. *Biken J* 1960;3:135–138.
250. Kato S, Takahashi M, Kameyama S, Kamahora J. A study on the morphological and cyto-immunological relationship between the inclusions of variola, cowpox, rabbitpox, vaccinia (variola origin) and vaccinia IHD, and a consideration of the term "Guarnieri body." *Biken J* 1959;2:353–363.
251. Katsafanas GC, Moss B. Histidine codons appended to the gene encoding the RP022 subunit of vaccinia virus RNA polymerase facilitate the isolation and purification of functional enzyme and associated proteins from virus-infected cells. *Virology* 1999;258:469–479.
252. Katz E, Moss B. Formation of a vaccinia virus structural polypeptide from a higher molecular weight precursor: Inhibition by rifampicin. *Proc Natl Acad Sci U S A* 1970;6:677–684.
253. Keck JG, Baldick CJ, Moss B. Role of DNA replication in vaccinia virus gene expression: A naked template is required for transcription of three late transactivator genes. *Cell* 1990;61:801–809.
254. Keck JG, Feigenbaum F, Moss B. Mutational analysis of a predicted zinc binding motif in the 26-kDa protein encoded by the vaccinia virus A2L gene: Correlation of zinc binding with late transcriptional activity. *J Virol* 1993;67:5740–5748.
255. Keck JG, Kovacs GR, Moss B. Overexpression, purification and late transcription factor activity of the 17-kDa protein encoded by the vaccinia virus A1L gene. *J Virol* 1993;67:5740–5748.
256. Kerr SM, Johnston LH, Odell M, et al. Vaccinia DNA ligase complements *Saccharomyces cerevisiae* Cdc9, localizes in cytoplasmic factories and affects virulence and virus sensitivity to DNA damaging agents. *EMBO J* 1991;10:4343–4350.
257. Kettle S, Alcami A, Khanna A, et al. Vaccinia virus serpin B13R (SPI-2) inhibits interleukin-1-b converting enzyme and protects virus-infected cells from TNF- and Fas-mediated apoptosis, but does not prevent IL-1b-induced fever. *J Gen Virol* 1997;78:677–685.
258. Kibler KV, Shors T, Perkins KB, et al. Double-stranded RNA is a trigger for apoptosis in vaccinia virus-infected cells. *J Virol* 1997;71:1992–2003.
259. Kleiman JH, Moss B. Characterization of a protein kinase and two phosphate acceptor proteins from vaccinia virions. *J Biol Chem* 1975;250:2430–2437.
260. Klemperer N, Lyttle DJ, Tauzin D, et al. Identification and characterization of the orf virus type 1 topoisomerase. *Virology* 1995;206:203–215.
261. Klemperer N, Traktman P. Biochemical analysis of mutant alleles of the vaccinia virus topoisomerase I carrying targeted substitutions in a highly conserved domain. *J Biol Chem* 1993;268:15887–15899.
262. Klemperer N, Ward J, Evans E, Traktman P. The vaccinia virus I1 protein is essential for the assembly of mature virions. *J Virol* 1997;71:9285–9294.
263. Knight JC, Goldsmith CS, Tamin A, et al. Further analyses of the orthopoxviruses volepox virus and raccoon poxvirus. *Virology* 1992;190:423–433.
264. Koji I, Moss B. Role of the vaccinia virus A20R protein in DNA replication: Construction and characterization of temperature-sensitive mutants. *J Virol* 2001;75:1656–1663.
265. Komiyama T, Ray CA, Pickup DJ, et al. Inhibition of interleukin-1 beta converting enzyme by the cowpox virus serpin CrmA: An example of cross-class inhibition. *J Biol Chem* 1994;269:19331–19337.
266. Koonin EV, Senkevich TG. Fowlpox virus encodes a protein related to human deoxycytidine kinase: Further evidence for independent acquisition of genes for enzymes of nucleotide metabolism by different viruses. *Virus Genes* 1993;7:289–295.
267. Kotwal GJ, Isaacs SN, Mckenzie R, et al. Inhibition of the complement cascade by the major secretory protein of vaccinia virus. *Science* 1990;250:827–830.
268. Kotwal GJ, Moss B. Vaccinia virus encodes a secretory polypeptide structurally related to complement control proteins. *Nature* 1988;335:176–178.
269. Kovacs GR, Moss B. The vaccinia virus H5R gene encodes late gene transcription factor 4: purification, cloning and overexpression. *J Virol* 1996;70:6796–6802.
270. Krathwohl MD, Hromas R, Brown DR, et al. Functional characterization of the C-C chemokine-like molecules encoded by molluscum contagiosum virus types 1 and 2. *Proc Natl Acad Sci U S A* 1997;94:9875–9880.
271. Krijnse-Locker J, Schleich S, Rodriguez D, et al. The role of a 21-kDa viral membrane protein in the assembly of vaccinia virus from the intermediate compartment. *J Biol Chem* 1996;271:14950–14958.
272. Krogh BO, Cheng CH, Burgin A, Shuman S. *Melanoplus sanguinipes* entomopoxvirus DNA topoisomerase: Site-specific DNA transesterification and effects of 5′-bridging phosphorothiolates. *Virology* 1999;264:441–451.
273. Lackner CA, Condit RC. Vaccinia virus gene A18R DNA helicase is a transcript release factor. *J Biol Chem* 2000;275:1485–1494.
274. Lai C, Gong S, Esteban M. The 32-kilodalton envelope protein of vaccinia virus synthesized in *Escherichia coli* binds with specificity to cell surfaces. *J Virol* 1991;65:499–504.
275. Lakritz N, Fogelsong PD, Reddy M, et al. A vaccinia virus DNase preparation which cross-links superhelical DNA. *J Virol* 1985;53:935–943.
276. Lalani AS, Graham K, Mossman K, et al. The purified myxoma virus gamma interferon receptor homolog M-T7 interacts with the heparin-binding domains of chemokines. *J Virol* 1997;71:4356–4363.
277. Lalani AS, Masters J, Zeng W, et al. Use of chemokine receptors by poxviruses. *Science* 1999;286:1968–1971.
278. Lanzer W, Holowczak JA. Polyamines in vaccinia virions and polypeptides released from viral cores by acid extraction. *J Virol* 1975;16:1254–1264.
279. Latner DR, Xiang Y, Lewis JI, et al. The vaccinia virus bifunctional gene J3 (nucleoside-2′-O-)-methyltransferase and poly(A) polymerase stimulatory factor is implicated as a positive transcription elongation factor by two genetic approaches. *Virology* 2000;269:345–355.
280. Lee P, Hruby DE. Proteolytic cleavage of vaccinia virus virion proteins. Mutational analysis of the specificity determinants. *J Biol Chem* 1994;269:8616–8622.
281. Lee SB, Esteban M. The interferon-induced double-stranded RNA-activated protein kinase induces apoptosis. *Virology* 1994;199:491–496.
282. Lee-Chen GJ, Bourgeois N, Davidson K, et al. Structure of the transcription initiation and termination sequences of seven early genes in the vaccinia virus HindIII D fragment. *Virology* 1988;163:64–79.
283. Li J, Broyles SS. The DNA-dependent ATPase activity of vaccinia virus early gene transcription factor is essential for its transcription activation function. *J Biol Chem* 1993;268:20016–20021.
284. Li J, Broyles SS. Recruitment of vaccinia virus RNA polymerase to an early gene promoter by the viral early transcription factor. *J Biol Chem* 1993;268:2773–2780.
285. Li J, Pennington MJ, Broyles SS. Temperature-sensitive mutations in the gene encoding the small subunit of the vaccinia virus early transcription factor impair promoter binding, transcription activation, and packaging of multiple virion components. *J Virol* 1994;68:2605–2614.
286. Lin CL, Chung CS, Heine HG, Chang W. Vaccinia virus envelope H3L protein binds to cell surface heparan sulfate and is important for intracellular mature virion morphogenesis and virus infection *in vitro* and *in vivo*. *J Virol* 2000;74:3353–3365.
287. Lin S, Broyles SS. Vaccinia protein kinase 2: A second essential serine/threonine protein kinase encoded by vaccinia virus. *Proc Natl Acad Sci U S A* 1994;91:7653–7657.
288. Lin S, Chen W, Broyles SS. The vaccinia virus B1R gene product is a serine/threonine protein kinase. *J Virol* 1992;66:2717–2723.
289. Lin YZ, Ke XH, Tam JP. Synthesis and structure-activity study of myxoma virus growth factor. *Biochemistry* 1991;30:3310–3314.
290. Liu K, Lemon B, Traktman P. The dual-specificity phosphatase encoded by vaccinia virus, VH1, is essential for viral transcription in vivo and in vitro. *J Virol* 1995;69:7823–7834.
291. Locker JK, Griffiths G. An unconventional role for cytoplasmic disulfide bonds in vaccinia virus proteins. *J Cell Biol* 1999;144:267–279.
292. Lomas DA, Evans DL, Upton C, et al. Inhibition of plasmin, urokinase, tissue plasminogen activator, and C1S by a myxoma virus serine proteinase inhibitor. *J Biol Chem* 1993;268:516–521.
293. Loparev VN, Parsons JM, Knight JC, et al. A third distinct tumor necrosis factor receptor of orthopoxviruses. *Proc Natl Acad Sci U S A* 1998;95:3786–3791.
294. Lorenzo MD, Herrera E, Blasco R, Isaacs SN. Functional analysis of vaccinia virus B5R protein: Role of the cytoplasmic tail. *Virology* 1998;252:450–457.

295. Luo Y, Mao X, Deng L, et al. The D1 and D12 subunits are both essential fo the transcription termination factor activity of vaccinia virus capping enzyme. *J Virol* 1995;69:3852–3856.
296. Luo Y, Shuman S. Antitermination of vaccinia virus early transcription: Possible role of RNA secondary structure. *Virology* 1991;185: 432–436.
297. Luttichau HR, Stine J, Boesen TP, et al. A highly selective CC chemokine receptor (CCR)8 antagonist encoded by the poxvirus molluscum contagiosum. *J Exp Med* 2000;191:171–179.
298. Lyles DS, Randall CC, Gafford LG, White HB Jr. Cellular fatty acids during fowlpox virus infection of three different host systems. *Virology* 1976;70:227–229.
299. Macen J, Takahashi A, Moon KB, et al. Activation of caspases in pig kidney cells infected with wild-type and crmA/SPI-2 mutants of cowpox and rabbitpox viruses. *J Virol* 1998;72:3524–3533.
300. Macen JL, Garner R, Musy PY, et al. Differential inhibition of the Fas- and granule-mediated cytolysis pathways by the orthopoxvirus cytokine response modifier A/SPI-2 and SPI-1 protein. *Proc Natl Acad Sci U S A* 1996;93:9108–9113.
301. Macen JL, Graham KA, Lee SF, et al. Expression of the myxoma virus tumor necrosis factor receptor homologue and M11L genes is required to prevent virus-induced apoptosis in infected rabbit T lymphocytes. *Virology* 1996;218:232–237.
302. Macen JL, Upton C, Nation N, McFadden G. SERP1, a serine protease inhibitor encoded by myxoma virus, is a secreted glycoprotein that interferes with inflammation. *Virology* 1993;195:348–363.
303. Mahr A, Roberts BE. Arrangement of late RNAs transcribed from a 7.1 kilobase Eco R1 vaccinia virus DNA fragment. *J Virol* 1984;49: 510–520.
304. Mao X, Shuman S. Intrinsic RNA (guanine-7) methyltransferase activity of the vaccinia virus capping enzyme D1 subunit is stimulated by the D12 subunit. Identification of amino acid residues in the D1 protein required for subunit association and methyl group transfer. *J Biol Chem* 1994;269:24472–24479.
305. Marsh YV, Eppstein DA. Vaccinia virus and the EGF receptor: a portal of entry for infectivity? *J Cell Biochem* 1987;34:239–245.
306. Martin KH, Franke CA, Hruby DE. Novel acylation of poxvirus A-type inclusion proteins. *Virus Res* 1999;60:147–157.
307. Martin SA, Moss B. Modification of RNA by mRNA guanylyltransferase and mRNA (guanine-7-)methyl-transferase from vaccinia virions. *J Biol Chem* 1975;250:9330–9335.
308. Martin SA, Moss B. mRNA guanylyltransferase and mRNA (guanine-7)methyltransferase from vaccinia virions: Donor and acceptor substrate activities. *J Biol Chem* 1976;251:7313–7321.
309. Martinez-Pomares L, Thompson JP, Moyer RW. Mapping and investigation of the role in pathogenesis of the major unique secreted protein of rabbitpox virus. *Virology* 1995;206:591–600.
310. Massung RF, Jayarama V, Moyer RW. DNA sequence analysis of conserved and unique regions of swinepox virus: Identification of genetic elements supporting phenotypic observations including a novel G protein-coupled receptor homologue. *Virology* 1993;197:511–528.
311. Massung RF, Liu LI, Qi J, et al. Analysis of the complete genome of smallpox variola major virus strain Bangladesh-1975. *Virology* 1994; 201:215–240.
312. Mathew E, Sanderson CM, Hollinshead M, Smith GL. The extracellular domain of vaccinia virus protein B5R affects plaque phenotype, extracellular enveloped virus release, and intracellular actin tail formation. *J Virol* 1998;72:2429–2438.
313. Mbuy GN, Morris RE, Bubel HC. Inhibition of cellular protein synthesis by vaccinia virus surface tubules. *Virology* 1982;116:137–147.
314. McCraith S, Holtzman T, Moss B, Fields S. Genome-wide analysis of vaccinia virus protein-protein interactions. *Proc Natl Acad Sci U S A* 2000;97:4879–4884.
315. McDonald WF, Klemperer N, Traktman P. Characterization of a processive form of the vaccinia virus DNA polymerase. *Virology* 1997; 234:168–175.
316. McDonald WF, Traktman P. Vaccinia virus DNA polymerase. *J Biol Chem* 1994;269:1–8.
317. McFadden G, Dales S. Biogenesis of poxviruses: Preliminary characterization of conditional lethal mutants of vaccinia virus defective in DNA synthesis. *Virology* 1980;103:68–79.
318. McFadden G, Stuart D, Upton C, et al. Replication and resolution of poxvirus telomeres. *Cancer Cells* 1988;6:77–85.
319. McIntosh AA, Smith GL. Vaccinia virus glycoprotein A34R is required for infectivity of extracellular enveloped virus. *J Virol* 1996; 70:272–281.
320. McKenzie R, Kotwal GJ, Moss B, et al. Regulation of complement activity by vaccinia virus complement-control protein. *J Infect Dis* 1992;166:1245–1250.
321. Medzon EL, Bauer H. Structural features of vaccinia virus revealed by negative staining. *Virology* 1970;40:860–867.
322. Meis RJ, Condit RC. Genetic and molecular biological characterization of a vaccinia virus gene which renders the virus dependent on isatin-b-thiosemicarbazone (IBT). *Virology* 1991;182:442–454.
323. Merchlinsky M. Intramolecular homologous recombination in cells infected with temperature-sensitive mutants of vaccinia virus. *J Virol* 1989;63:2030–2035.
324. Merchlinsky M. Mutational analysis of the resolution sequence of vaccinia virus DNA: Essential sequence consists of 2 separate AT-rich regions highly conserved among poxviruses. *J Virol* 1990;64: 5029–5035.
325. Merchlinsky M. Resolution of poxvirus telomeres: Processing of vaccinia virus concatemer junctions by conservative strand exchange. *J Virol* 1990;64:3437–3446.
326. Merchlinsky M, Garon C, Moss B. Molecular cloning and sequence of the concatemer junction from vaccinia virus replicative DNA: Viral nuclease cleavage sites in cruciform structures. *J Mol Biol* 1988;199: 399–413.
327. Merchlinsky M, Moss B. Nucleotide sequence required for resolution of the concatemer junction of vaccinia virus DNA. *J Virol* 1989;63: 4354–4361.
328. Merchlinsky M, Moss B. Resolution of linear minichromosomes with hairpin ends from circular plasmids containing vaccinia virus concatemer junctions. *Cell* 1986;45:879–884.
329. Merchlinsky M, Moss B. Resolution of vaccinia virus DNA concatemer junctions requires late gene expression. *J Virol* 1989;63: 1595–1603.
330. Merchlinsky M, Moss B. Sequence-independent replication and sequence-specific resolution of plasmids containing the vaccinia virus concatemer junction: Requirements for early and late trans-acting factors. In: Kelly T, Stillman B, eds. *Cancer cells 6/eukaryotic DNA replication.* Cold Spring Harbor, NY: Cold Spring Harbor Laboratory Press, 1988;87–93.
331. Millns AK, Carpenter MS, DeLange AM. The vaccinia virus-encoded uracil DNA glycosylase has an essential role in viral DNA replication. *Virology* 1994;198:504–513.
332. Miner JN, Hruby DE. Rifampicin prevents virosome localization of L65, an essential vaccinia virus polypeptide. *Virology* 1989;170: 227–237.
333. Miura M, Friedlander RM, Yuan J. Tumor necrosis factor-induced apoptosis is mediated by a CrmA-sensitive cell death pathway. *Proc Natl Acad Sci U S A* 1995;92:8318–8322.
334. Mohamed MR, Niles EG. Interaction between nucleoside triphosphate phosphohydrolase I and the H4L subunit of the viral RNA polymerase is required for vaccinia virus early gene transcript release. *J Biol Chem* 2000;275:25798–25804.
335. Moon KB, Turner PC, Moyer RW. SPI-1-dependent host range of rabbitpox virus and complex formation with cathepsin G is associated with serpin motifs. *J Virol* 1999;73:8999–9010.
336. Morgan C. Vaccinia virus reexamined: Development and release. *Virology* 1976;73:43–58.
337. Morgan JR, Cohen LK, Roberts BE. Identification of the DNA sequences encoding the large subunit of the mRNA capping enzyme of vaccinia virus. *J Virol* 1984;52:206–214.
338. Morrison DK, Moyer RW. Detection of a subunit of cellular pol II within highly purified preparations of RNA polymerase isolated from poxvirus virions. *Cell* 1986;44:587–596.
339. Moss B. Genetically engineered poxviruses for recombinant gene expression, vaccination, and safety. *Proc Natl Acad Sci U S A* 1996; 93:11341–11348.
340. Moss B. Vaccinia virus transcription. In: Conaway R, Conaway J, eds. *Transcription mechanisms and regulation.* New York: Raven, 1994; 185–205.
341. Moss B, Ahn BY, Amegadzie BY, et al. Cytoplasmic transcription system encoded by vaccinia virus. *J Biol Chem* 1991;266:1355–1358.
342. Moss B, Filler R. Irreversible effects of cycloheximide during the early period of vaccinia virus replication. *J Virol* 1970;5:99–108.
343. Moss B, Rosenblum EN. Protein cleavage and poxvirus morphogene-

sis: Tryptic peptide analysis of core precursors accumulated by blocking assembly with rifampicin. *J Mol Biol* 1973;81:267–269.

344. Moss B, Rosenblum EN, Gershowitz A. Characterization of a polyriboadenylate polymerase from vaccinia virions. *J Biol Chem* 1975;250: 4722–4729.
345. Moss B, Rosenblum EN, Katz E, Grimley PM. Rifampicin: A specific inhibitor of vaccinia virus assembly. *Nature* 1969;224:1280–1284.
346. Moss B, Salzman NP. Sequential protein synthesis following vaccinia virus infection. *J Virol* 1968;2:1016–1027.
347. Moss B, Winters E, Jones EV. Replication of vaccinia virus. In: Cozzarelli N, ed. *Mechanics of DNA replication and recombination.* New York: A. Liss, 1983:449–461.
348. Mossman K, Lee SF, Barry M, et al. Disruption of M-T5, a novel myxoma virus gene member of the poxvirus host range superfamily, results in dramatic attenuation of myxomatosis in infected European rabbits. *J Virol* 1996;70:4394–4410.
349. Mossman K, Nation P, Macen J, et al. Myxoma virus M-T7, a secreted homolog of the interferon-γ receptor, is a critical virulence factor for the development of myxomatosis in European rabbits. *Virology* 1996;215:17–30.
350. Mossman K, Upton C, Buller RM, McFadden G. Species specificity of ectromelia virus and vaccinia virus interferon-gamma binding proteins. *Virology* 1995;208:762–769.
351. Moyer RW, Brown GD, Graves RL. The white pock mutants of rabbit poxvirus. II. The early white pock (m) host range (hr) mutants of rabbit poxvirus uncouple transcription and translation in non-permissive cells. *Virology* 1980;106:234–249.
352. Moyer RW, Graves RL. The mechanism of cytoplasmic orthopoxvirus DNA replication. *Cell* 1981;27:391–401.
353. Mullbacher A, Wallich R, Moyer RW, Simon MM. Poxvirus-encoded serpins do not prevent cytolytic T cell-mediated recovery from primary infections. *J Immunol* 1999;162:7315–7321.
354. Munyon WE, Paoletti E, Grace JT Jr. RNA polymerase activity in purified infectious vaccinia virus. *Proc Natl Acad Sci U S A* 1967;58: 2280–2288.
355. Muthukrishnan S, Moss B, Cooper JA, Maxwell ES. Influence of 5′ terminal cap structure on the initiation of translation of vaccinia virus mRNA. *J Biol Chem* 1978;253:1710–1715.
356. Myette JR, Niles EG. Characterization of the vaccinia virus RNA 5′-triphosphatase and nucleotide triphosphate phosphohydrolase activities: Demonstrate that both activities are carried out at the same active site. *J Biol Chem* 1996;271:11945–11952.
357. Myette JR, Niles EG. Domain structure of the vaccinia virus mRNA capping enzyme: Expression in *Escherichia coli* of a subdomain possessing the RNA 5′-triphosphatase and guanylyltransferase activities and a kinetic comparison to the full-size enzyme. *J Biol Chem* 1996; 271:11936–11944.
358. Nagayama A, Pogo BGT, Dales S. Biogenesis of vaccinia: Separation of early stages from maturation by means of rifampicin. *Virology* 1970;40:1039–1051.
359. Nagington J, Horne RW. Morphological studies of orf and vaccinia viruses. *Virology* 1962;16:248–260.
360. Nash P, Whitty A, Handwerker J, et al. Inhibitory specificity of the anti-inflammatory myxoma virus serpin, SERP-1. *J Biol Chem* 1998; 273:20982–20991.
361. Nezu JI, Oku A, Jones MH, Shimane M. Identification of two novel human putative serine/threonine kinases, VRK1 and VRK2, with structural similarity to vaccinia virus B1R kinase. *Genomics* 1997;45: 327–331.
362. Niles EG, Christen L. Identification of the vaccinia virus mRNA guanyltransferase active site lysine. *J Biol Chem* 1993;268: 24986–24989.
363. Niles EG, Lee-Chen GJ, Shuman S, et al. Vaccinia virus gene D12L encodes the small subunit of the viral mRNA capping enzyme. *Virology* 1989;172:513–522.
364. Niven JSF, Armstrong JA, Andrewes CH, et al.. Subcutaneous "growths" in monkeys produced by a poxvirus. *J Pathol Bacteriol* 1961;81:1–10.
365. Njayou M, Drillien R, Kirn A. Characteristics of the inhibition of protein synthesis by vaccinia virus in nonpermissive Chinese hamster ovary cells. *Ann Virol* 1982;133E:393–402.
366. Oda K, Joklik WK. Hybridization and sedimentation studies on "early" and "late" vaccinia messenger RNA. *J Mol Biol* 1967;27: 395–419.
367. Opgenorth A, Graham K, Nation N, et al. Deletion analysis of 2 tandemly arranged virulence genes in myxoma virus, M11L and myxoma growth factor. *J Virol* 1992;66:4720–4731.
368. Opgenorth A, Strayer D, Upton C, Mcfadden G. Deletion of the growth factor gene related to EGF and TGF-alpha reduces virulence of malignant rabbit fibroma virus. *Virology* 1992;186:175–191.
369. Pacha RF, Condit RC. Characterization of a temperature-sensitive mutant of vaccinia virus reveals a novel function that prevents virus-induced breakdown of RNA. *J Virol* 1985;56:395–403.
370. Palaniyar N, Gerasimopoulos E, Evans DH. Shops fibroma virus DNA topoisomerase catalyses Holliday junction resolution and hairpin formation in vitro. *J Mol Biol* 1999;287:9–20.
371. Paoletti E, Grady LJ. Transcriptional complexity of vaccinia virus in vivo and in vitro. *J Virol* 1977;23:608–615.
372. Paoletti E, Moss B. Two nucleic acid-dependent nucleoside triphosphate phosphohydrolases from vaccinia virus: Nucleotide substrate and polynucleotide cofactor specificities. *J Biol Chem* 1974;249: 3281–3286.
373. Parks RJ, Evans DH. Effect of marker distance and orientation on recombinant formation in poxvirus-infected cells. *J Virol* 1991;65: 1263–1272.
374. Parsons BL, Pickup DJ. Transcription of orthopoxvirus telomeres at late times during infection. *Virology* 1990;175:69–80.
375. Passarelli AL, Kovacs GR, Moss B. Transcription of a vaccinia virus late promoter template: Requirement for the product of the A2L intermediate-stage gene. *J Virol* 1996;70:4444–4450.
376. Patel DD, Pickup DJ. Messenger RNAs of a strongly-expressed late gene of cowpox virus contains a 5′-terminal poly(A) leader. *EMBO J* 1987;6:3787–3794.
377. Patel DD, Pickup DJ, Joklik WK. Isolation of cowpox virus A-type inclusions and characterization of their major protein component. *Virology* 1986;149:174–189.
378. Payne L. Polypeptide composition of extracellular enveloped vaccinia virus. *J Virol* 1978;27:28–37.
379. Payne LG. Identification of the vaccinia hemagglutinin polypeptide from a cell system yielding large amounts of extracellular enveloped virus. *J Virol* 1979;31:147–155.
380. Payne LG. Significance of extracellular virus in the *in vitro* and *in vivo* dissemination of vaccinia virus. *J Gen Virol* 1980;50:89–100.
381. Payne LG, Norrby E. Adsorption and penetration of enveloped and naked vaccinia virus particles. *J Virol* 1978;27:19–27.
382. Pedersen K, Snijder EJ, Schleich S, et al. Characterization of vaccinia virus intracellular cores: Implications for viral uncoating and core structure. *J Virol* 2000;74:3525–3536.
383. Pedley CB, Cooper RJ. The assay, purification and properties of vaccinia virus-induced uncoating protein. *J Gen Virol* 1987;68: 1021–1028.
384. Pedley S, Cooper RJ. The inhibition of HeLa cell RNA synthesis following infection with vaccinia virus. *J Gen Virol* 1984;65:1687–1697.
385. Pennington TH. Vaccinia virus polypeptide synthesis: Sequential appearance and stability of pre- and post-replicative polypeptides. *J Gen Virol* 1974;25:433–444.
386. Pennington TH, Follett EA. Vaccinia virus replication in enucleated BSC-1 cells: Particle production and synthesis of viral DNA and proteins. *J Virol* 1974;13:488–493.
387. Perkus ME, Goebel SJ, Davis SW, et al. Vaccinia virus host range genes. *Virology* 1990;179:276–286.
388. Perkus ME, Goebel SJ, Davis SW, et al. Deletion of 55 open reading frames from the termini of vaccinia virus. *Virology* 1991;180:406–410.
389. Person-Fernandez A, Beaud G. Purification and characterization of a protein synthesis inhibitor associated with vaccinia virus. *J Biol Chem* 1986;261:8283–8289.
390. Peters D, Müller G. The fine structure of the DNA containing core of vaccinia virus. *Virology* 1963;21:266–269.
391. Petersen BO, Hall RL, Moyer RW, Shuman S. Characterization of a DNA topoisomerase encoded by Amsacta moorei entomopoxvirus. *Virology* 1997;230:197–206.
392. Petit F, Bertagnoli, Gelfi J, et al. Characterization of a myxoma virus-encoded serpin-like protein with activity against interleukin-1b-converting enzymes. *J Virol* 1996;70:5860–5866.
393. Pogo BGT, Dales S. Two deoxyribonuclease activities within purified vaccinia virus. *Proc Natl Acad Sci U S A* 1969;63:820–827.
394. Pogo BGT, O'Shea M, Freimuth P. Initiation and termination of vaccinia virus DNA replication. *Virology* 1981;108:241–248.

395. Pogo BGT, O'Shea MT. The mode of replication of vaccinia virus DNA. *Virology* 1978;86:1–8.
396. Pogo BGT. Changes in parental vaccinia virus DNA after viral penetration into cells. *Virology* 1980;101:520–524.
397. Postlethwaite R. Molluscum contagiosum: A review. *Arch Environ Health* 1970;21:432–452.
398. Prescott DM, Kates J, Kirkpatrick JB. Replication of vaccinia virus DNA in enucleated L-cells. *J Mol Biol* 1971;59:505–508.
399. Puckett C, Moss B. Selective transcription of vaccinia virus genes in template dependent soluble extracts of infected cells. *Cell* 1983;35: 441–448.
400. Quan LT, Caputo A, Bleackley RC, et al. Granzyme B is inhibited by the cowpox virus serpin cytokine response modifier A. *J Biol Chem* 1995;270:10377–10379.
401. Quick SD, Broyles SS. Vaccinia virus gene D7R encodes a 20,000-Dalton subunit of the viral DNA-dependent RNA polymerase. *Virology* 1990;178:603–605.
402. Rajagopal I, Ahn BY, Moss B, Mathews CK. Roles of vaccinia virus ribonucleotide reductase and glutaredoxin in DNA precursor biosynthesis. *J Biol Chem* 1995;270:27415–27418.
403. Ramsey-Ewing A, Moss B. Apoptosis induced by a postbinding step of vaccinia virus entry into Chinese hamster ovary cells. *Virology* 1998;242:138–149.
404. Ramsey-Ewing A, Moss B. Restriction of vaccinia virus replication in CHO cells occurs at the stage of viral intermediate protein synthesis. *Virology* 1995;206:984–993.
405. Ravanello MP, Hruby DE. Characterization of the vaccinia virus L1R myristylprotein as a component of the intracellular virion envelope. *J Gen Virol* 1994;75:1479–1483.
406. Ravanello MP, Hruby DE. Conditional lethal expression of the vaccinia virus L1R myrstylated protein reveals a role in virus assembly. *J Virol* 1994;68:6401–6410.
407. Ray CA, Black RA, Kronheim SR, et al. Viral inhibition of inflammation: Cowpox virus encodes an inhibitor of the interleukin-1b converting enzyme. *Cell* 1992;69:597–604.
408. Ray CA, Pickup DJ. The mode of death of pig kidney cells infected with cowpox virus is governed by the expression of the crmA gene. *Virology* 1996;217:384–391.
409. Reddy MK, Bauer WR. Activation of the vaccinia virus nicking-joining enzyme by trypsinization. *J Biol Chem* 1989;264:443–449.
410. Rempel RE, Traktman P. Vaccinia virus-B1 kinase: phenotypic analysis of temperature-sensitive mutants and enzymatic characterization of recombinant proteins. *J Virol* 1992;66:4413–4426.
411. Rice AP, Roberts BE. Vaccinia virus induces cellular mRNA degradation. *J Virol* 1983;47:529–539.
412. Risco C, Rodriguez JR, Demkowicz W, et al. The vaccinia virus 39-kDa protein forms a stable complex with the p4a/4a major core protein early in morphogenesis. *Virology* 1999;265:375–386.
413. Rodriguez D, Esteban M, Rodriguez JR. Vaccinia virus A17L gene product is essential for an early step in virion morphogenesis. *J Virol* 1995;69:4640–4648.
414. Rodriguez JF, Janeczko R, Esteban M. Isolation and characterization of neutralizing monoclonal antibodies to vaccinia virus. *J Virol* 1985; 56:482–488.
415. Rodriguez JF, Kahn JS, Esteban M. Molecular cloning, encoding sequence, and expression of vaccinia virus nucleic acid-dependent nucleoside triphosphatase gene. *Proc Natl Acad Sci U S A* 1986;83: 9566–9570.
416. Rodriguez JF, Paez E, Esteban M. A 14,000-Mr envelope protein of vaccinia virus is involved in cell fusion and forms covalently linked trimers. *J Virol* 1987;61:395–404.
417. Rodriguez JF, Smith GL. IPTG-dependent vaccinia virus: Identification of a virus protein enabling virion envelopment by Golgi membrane and egress. *Nucleic Acids Res* 1990;18:5347–5351.
418. Rodriguez JR, Risco C, Carrascosa JL, et al. Characterization of early stages in vaccinia virus membrane biogenesis: implications of the 21-kilodalton protein and a newly identified 15-kilodalton envelope protein. *J Virol* 1997;71:1821–1833.
419. Rodriguez JR, Risco C, Carrascosa JL, et al. Vaccinia virus 15-kilodalton (A14L) protein is essential for assembly and attachment of viral crescents to virosomes. *J Virol* 1998;72:1287–1296.
420. Roening G, Holowczak JA. Evidence for the presence of RNA in the purified virions of vaccinia virus. *J Virol* 1974;14:704–708.
421. Rohrmann G, Yuen L, Moss B. Transcription of vaccinia virus early genes by enzymes isolated from vaccinia virions terminates downstream of a regulatory sequence. *Cell* 1986;46:1029–1035.
422. Roos N, Cyrklaff M, Cudmore S, et al. A novel immunogold cryoelectron microscopic approach to investigate the structure of the intracellular and extracellular forms of vaccinia virus. *EMBO J* 1996;15: 2343–2355.
423. Roper R, Wolffe EJ, Weisberg A, Moss B. The envelope protein encoded by the A33R gene is required for formation of actin-containing microvilli and efficient cell-to-cell spread of vaccinia virus. *J Virol* 1998;72:4192–4204.
424. Roper RL, Moss B. Envelope formation is blocked by mutation of a sequence related to the HKD phospholipid metabolism motif in the vaccinia virus F13L protein. *J Virol* 1999;73:1108–1117.
425. Roper RL, Payne LG, Moss B. Extracellular vaccinia virus envelope glycoprotein encoded by the A33R gene. *J Virol* 1996;70:3753–3762.
426. Rosales R, Harris N, Ahn BY, Moss B. Purification and identification of a vaccinia virus-encoded intermediate stage promoter-specific transcription factor that has homology to eukaryotic transcription factor SII (TFIIS) and an additional role as a viral RNA polymerase subunit. *J Biol Chem* 1994;269:14260–14267.
427. Rosales R, Sutter G, Moss B. A cellular factor is required for transcription of vaccinia viral intermediate stage genes. *Proc Natl Acad Sci U S A* 1994;91:3794–3798.
428. Rosel J, Moss B. Transcriptional and translational mapping and nucleotide sequence analysis of a vaccinia virus gene encoding the precursor of the major core polypeptide 4b. *J Virol* 1985;56:830–838.
429. Roseman NA, Hruby DE. Nucleotide sequence and transcript organization of a region of the vaccinia virus genome which encodes a constitutively expressed gene required for DNA replication. *J Virol* 1987; 61:1398–1406.
430. Rosemond-Hornbeak H, Moss B. Inhibition of host protein synthesis by vaccinia virus: Fate of cell mRNA and synthesis of small poly(A)-rich polyribonucleotides in the presence of actinomycin D. *J Virol* 1975;16:34–42.
431. Roth MJ, Hurwitz J. RNA capping by the vaccinia virus guanylyltransferase: Structure of enzyme-guanylate intermediate. *J Biol Chem* 1984;259:13488–13494.
432. Rottger S, Frischknecht F, Reckmann I, et al. Interactions between vaccinia virus IEV membrane proteins and their roles in IEV assembly and actin tail formation. *J Virol* 1999;73:2863–2875.
433. Sahu A, Isaacs SN, Soulika AM, Lambris JD. Interaction of vaccinia virus complement control protein with human complement proteins: Factor I-mediated degradation of C3b to iC3b1 inactivates the alternative complement pathway. *J Immunol* 1998;160:5596–5604.
434. Salmons T, Kuhn A, Wylie F, et al. Vaccinia virus membrane proteins p8 and p16 are cotranslationally inserted into the rough endoplasmic reticulum and retained in the intermediate compartment. *J Virol* 1997;71:7404–7420.
435. Salzman NP. The rate of formation of vaccinia deoxyribonucleic acid and vaccinia virus. *Virology* 1960;10:150–152.
436. Sanderson CM, Frischknecht F, Way M, et al. Roles of vaccinia virus EEV-specific proteins in intracellular actin tail formation and low pH-induced cell-cell fusion. *J Gen Virol* 1998;79:1415–1425.
437. Sanderson CM, Frischknecht F, Way M, et al. Roles of vaccinia virus EEV-specific proteins in intracellular actin tail formation and low pH-induced cell-cell fusion. *J Gen Virol* 1998;79:1415–1425.
438. Sanderson CM, Hollinshead M, Smith GL. The vaccinia virus A27L protein is needed for the microtubule-dependent transport of intracellular mature virus particles. *J Gen Virol* 2000;81:47–58.
439. Sanz P, Moss B. Identification of a transcription factor, encoded by two vaccinia virus early genes, that regulates the intermediate stage of viral gene expression. *Proc Natl Acad Sci U S A* 1999;96:2692–2697.
440. Sanz P, Moss B. A new vaccinia virus intermediate transcription factor. *J Virol* 1998;72:6880–6883.
441. Sanz P, Veyrunes JC, Cousserans F, Bergoin M. Cloning and sequencing of the Spherulin gene, the occlusion body major polypeptide of the *Melolontha melolontha* entomopoxvirus (MmEPV). *Virology* 1994; 202:449–457.
442. Sarov I, Joklik W. Isolation and characterization of intermediates in vaccina virus morphogenesis. *Virology* 1973;52:223–233.
443. Schmelz M, Sodeik B, Ericsson M, et al. Assembly of vaccinia virus: The second wrapping cisterna is derived from the trans Golgi network. *J Virol* 1994;68:130–147.
444. Schnierle BS, Gershon PD, Moss B. Cap-specific mRNA (nucleoside-

O2′-)-methyltransferase and poly(A) polymerase stimulatory activities of vaccinia virus are mediated by a single protein. *Proc Natl Acad Sci U S A* 1992;89:2897–2901.
445. Schnierle BS, Gershon PD, Moss B. Mutational analysis of a multifunctional protein, with mRNA 5′ cap-specific (nucleoside-2′-O-)-methyltransferase and 3′ adenylyltransferase stimulatory activities, encoded by vaccinia virus. *J Biol Chem* 1994;269:20700–20706.
446. Schwer B, Visca P, Vos JC, Stunnenberg HG. Discontinuous transcription or RNA processing of vaccinia virus late messengers results in a 5′ poly(A) leader. *Cell* 1987;50:163–169.
447. Sebring ED, Salzman NP. Metabolic properties of early and late vaccinia messenger ribonucleic acid. *J Virol* 1967;1:550–575.
448. Seki M, Oie M, Ichihashi Y, Shida H. Hemadsorption and fusion inhibition activities of hemagglutinin analyzed by vaccinia virus mutants. *Virology* 1990;175:372–384.
449. Sekiguchi J, Seeman NC, Shuman S. Resolution of Holliday junctions by eukaryotic DNA topoisomerase I. *Proc Natl Acad Sci U S A* 1996;93:785–789.
450. Senkevich TG, Koonin EV, Bugert JJ, et al. The genome of molluscum contagiosum virus: Analysis and comparison with other poxviruses. *Virology* 1997;233:19–42.
451. Senkevich TG, Moss B. Domain structure, intracellular trafficking, and beta 2-microglobulin binding of a major histocompatibility complex class I homolog encoded by molluscum contagiosum virus. *Virology* 1998;250:397–407.
452. Senkevich TG, Weisberg A, Moss B. Vaccinia virus E10R protein is associated with the membrane of intracellular mature virions and has role in morphogenesis. *Virology* 2000;278:244–252.
453. Senkevich TG, White CL, Koonin EV, Moss B. A viral member of the ERV1/ALR protein family participates in a novel pathway of disulfide bond formation. *Proc Natl Acad Sci U S A* 2000;97:12068–12073.
454. Senkevich TG, Wolffe EJ, Buller MI. Ectromelia virus RING finger protein is localized in virus factories and is required for virus replication in macrophages. *J Virol* 1995;69:4103–4111.
455. Sharp TV, Moonan F, Romashko A, et al. The vaccinia virus E3L gene product interacts with both the regulatory and the substrate binding regions of PKR: Implications for PKR autoregulation. *Virology* 1998;250:302–315.
456. Shchelkunov SN, Massung RF, Esposito JJ. Comparison of the genome DNA sequences of Bangladesh-1975 and India-1967 variola viruses. *Virus Res* 1995;36:107–118.
457. Shchelkunov SN, Safronov PF, Totmenin AV, et al. The genomic sequence analysis of the left and right species-specific terminal region of a cowpox virus strain reveals unique sequences and a cluster of intact orfs for immunomodulatory and host range proteins. *Virology* 1998;243:432–460.
458. Shi X, Yao P, Jose T, Gershon PD. Methyltransferase-specific domains within VP39, a bifunctional protein which participates in the modification of both mRNA ends. *RNA* 1996;2:88–101.
459. Shida H. Nucleotide sequence of the vaccinia virus hemagglutinin gene. *Virology* 1986;150:451–462.
460. Shida H, Dales S. Biogenesis of vaccinia: Carbohydrate of the hemagglutinin molecule. *Virology* 1981;111:56–72.
461. Shida H, Tanabe K, Matsumoto S. Mechanism of virus occlusion into A-type inclusion during poxvirus infection. *Virology* 1977;76:217–233.
462. Shisler JL, Isaacs SN, Moss B. Vaccinia virus serpin-1 deletion mutant exhibits a host range defect characterized by low levels of intermediate and late mRNAs. *Virology* 1999;262:298–311.
463. Shisler JL, Senkevich TG, Berry MJ, Moss B. Ultraviolet-induced cell death blocked by a selenoprotein from a human dermatotropic poxvirus. *Science* 1998;279:102–105.
464. Shope RE. A filtrable virus causing a tumor-like condition in rabbits and its relationship to virus myxomatosum. *J Exp Med* 1932;56: 803–822.
465. Shuman S. Site-specific DNA cleavage by vaccinia virus DNA topoisomerase-I: Role of nucleotide sequence and DNA secondary structure. *J Biol Chem* 1991;266:1796–1803.
466. Shuman S. Vaccinia virus DNA topoisomerase: A model eukaryotic type IB enzyme. *Biochim Biophys Acta* 1998;1400:321–337.
467. Shuman S. Vaccinia virus RNA helicase: An essential enzyme related to the DE-H family of RNA-dependent NTPases. *Proc Natl Acad Sci U S A* 1992;89:10935–10939.
468. Shuman S. Vaccinia virus RNA helicase: Directionality and substrate specificity. *J Biol Chem* 1993;268:11798–11802.
469. Shuman S, Broyles SS, Moss B. Purification and characterization of a transcription termination factor from vaccinia virions. *J Biol Chem* 1987;262:12372–12380.
470. Shuman S, Golder M, Moss B. Characterization of vaccinia virus DNA topoisomerase I expressed in *Escherichia coli. J Biol Chem* 1988;263:16401–16407.
471. Shuman S, Golder M, Moss B. Insertional mutagenesis of the vaccinia virus gene encoding a type I DNA topoisomerase: Evidence that the gene is essential for virus growth. *Virology* 1989;170:302–306.
472. Shuman S, Hurwitz J. Mechanism of mRNA capping by vaccinia virus guanylyltransferase: Characterization of an enzyme-guanylate intermediate. *Proc Natl Acad Sci U S A* 1981;78:187–191.
473. Shuman S, Morham SG. Domain structure of vaccinia virus messenger RNA capping enzyme: Activity of the MR 95,000 subunit expressed in *Escherichia coli. J Biol Chem* 1990;265:11967–11972.
474. Shuman S, Moss B. Bromouridine triphosphate inhibits transcription termination and mRNA release by vaccinia virions. *J Biol Chem* 1989;264:21356–21360.
475. Shuman S, Moss B. Identification of a vaccinia virus gene encoding a type I DNA topoisomerase. *Proc Natl Acad Sci U S A* 1987;84: 7478–7482.
476. Simpson DA, Condit RC. The vaccinia virus A18R protein plays a role in viral transcription during both the early and late phase of infection. *J Virol* 1994;68:3642–3649.
477. Simpson DA, Condit RC. Vaccinia virus gene A18R encodes an essential DNA helicase. *J Virol* 1995;69:6131–6139.
478. Slabaugh M, Roseman N, Davis R, Mathews C. Vaccinia virus-encoded ribonucleotide reductase: Sequence conservation of the gene for the small subunit and its amplification in hydroxyurea-resistant mutants. *J Virol* 1988;62:519–527.
479. Slabaugh MB, Davis RE, Roseman NA, Mathews CK. Vaccinia virus ribonucleotide reductase expression and isolation of the recombinant large subunit. *J Biol Chem* 1993;268:17803–17810.
480. Slabaugh MB, Johnson TL, Mathews CK. Vaccinia virus induces ribonucleotide reductase in primate cells. *J Virol* 1984;52:507–514.
481. Slabaugh MB, Roseman NA. Retroviral protease-like gene in the vaccinia virus genome. *Proc Natl Acad Sci U S A* 1989;86:4152–4155.
482. Slabaugh MB, Roseman NA, Mathews CK. Amplification of the ribonucleotide reductase small subunit gene: Analysis of novel joints and the mechanism of gene duplication in vaccinia virus. *Nucleic Acids Res* 1989;17:7073–7088.
483. Smadel JE, Hoagland CL. Elementary bodies of vaccinia. *Bacteriol Rev* 1942;6:79–110.
484. Smadel Je, Hoagland CL. Estimation of the purity of preparation of elementary bodies of vaccinia. *J Exp Med* 1939;70:379–385.
485. Smith CA, Davis T, Wignall JM, et al. T2 open reading frame from the Shope fibroma virus encodes a soluble form of the TNF receptor. *Biochem Biophys Res Commun* 1991;176:335–342.
486. Smith CA, Hu FQ, Smith TD, et al. Cowpox virus genome encodes a second soluble homologue of cellular TNF receptors, distinct from CrmB, that binds TNF but not LT alpha. *Virology* 1996;223:132–147.
487. Smith CA, Smith TD, Smolak PJ, et al. Poxvirus genomes encode a secreted, soluble protein that preferentially inhibits b chemokine activity yet lacks sequence homology to known chemokine receptors. *Virology* 1997;236:316–327.
488. Smith GL, Chan YS, Howard ST. Nucleotide sequence of 42 kbp of vaccinia virus strain WR from near the right inverted terminal repeat. *J Gen Virol* 1991;72:1349–1376.
489. Smith GL, de Carlos A, Chan YS. Vaccinia virus encodes a thymidylate kinase gene: Sequence and transcriptional mapping. *Nucleic Acids Res* 1989;17:7581–7590.
490. Smith VP, Bryant NA, Alcami A. Ectromelia, vaccinia and cowpox viruses encode secreted interleukin-18-binding proteins. *J Gen Virol* 2000;81:1223–1230.
491. Sodeik B, Cudmore S, Ericsson M, et al. Assembly of vaccinia virus: Incorporation of p14 and p32 into the membrane of the intracellular mature virus. *J Virol* 1995;69:3560–3574.
492. Sodeik B, Doms RW, Ericsson M, et al. Assembly of vaccinia virus: Role of the intermediate compartment between the endoplasmic reticulum and the Golgi stacks. *J Cell Biol* 1993;121:521–541.
493. Sodeik B, Griffiths G, Ericsson M, et al. Assembly of vaccinia virus: Effects of rifampin on the intracellular distribution of viral protein p65. *J Virol* 1994;68:1103–1114.
494. Spehner D, Gillard S, Drillien R, Kirn A. A cowpox virus gene

required for multiplication in Chinese hamster ovary cells. *J Virol* 1988;62:1297–1304.
495. Spencer E, Shuman S, Hurwitz J. Purification and properties of vaccinia virus DNA-dependent RNA polymerase. *J Biol Chem* 1980;255:5388–5395.
496. Spriggs MK, Hruby DE, Maliszewski CR, et al. Vaccinia and cowpox viruses encode a novel secreted interleukin-1-binding protein. *Cell* 1992;71:145–152.
497. Spyropoulos DD, Roberts BE, Panicali DL, Cohen LK. Delineation of the viral products of recombination in vaccinia virus-infected cells. *J Virol* 1988;62:1046–1054.
498. Stern W, Dales S. Biogenesis of vaccinia: Concerning the origin of the envelope phospholipids. *Virology* 1974;62:293–306.
499. Stokes GV. High-voltage electron microscope study of the release of vaccinia virus from whole cells. *J Virol* 1976;18:636–643.
500. Stroobant P, Rice AP, Gullick WJ, et al. Purification and characterization of vaccinia virus growth factor. *Cell* 1985;42:383–393.
501. Stuart D, Graham K, Schreiber M, et al. The target DNA sequence for resolution of poxvirus replicative intermediates is an active late promoter. *J Virol* 1991;65:61–70.
502. Stuart DT, Upton C, Higman MA, et al. A poxvirus-encoded uracil DNA glycosylase is essential for virus viability. *J Virol* 1993;67:2503–2512.
503. Sutter G, Ramsey-Ewing A, Rosales R, Moss B. Stable expression of the vaccinia virus K1L gene in rabbit cells complements the host range defect of a vaccinia virus mutant. *J Virol* 1994;68:4109–4116.
504. Symons JA, Alcami A, Smith GL. Vaccinia virus encodes a soluble type 1 interferon receptor of novel structure and broad species specificity. *Cell* 1995;81:551–560.
505. Taddie JA, Traktman P. Genetic characterization of the vaccinia virus DNA polymerase: Cytosine arabinoside resistance requires a variable lesion conferring phosphonoacetate resistance in conjunction with an invariant mutation localized to the 3′-5′ exonuclease domain. *J Virol* 1993;67:4323–4336.
506. Taddie JA, Traktman P. Genetic characterization of the vaccinia virus DNA polymerase: Identification of point mutations conferring altered drug sensitivities and reduced fidelity. *J Virol* 1991;65:869–879.
507. Takahashi T, Oie M, Ichihashi Y. N-terminal amino acid sequences of vaccinia virus structural proteins. *Virology* 1994;202:844–852.
508. Tanaka-Kataoka M, Kunikata T, Takayama S, et al. *In vivo* antiviral effect of interleukin 18 in a mouse model of vaccinia virus infection. *Cytokine* 1999;11:593–599.
509. Tartaglia J, Piccini A, Paoletti E. Vaccinia virus rifampicin-resistance locus specifies a late 63,000 Da gene product. *Virology* 1986;150:45–54.
510. Tengelsen LA, Slabaugh MB, Bibler JK, Hruby DE. Nucleotide sequence and molecular genetic analysis of the large subunit of ribonucleotide reductase encoded by vaccinia virus. *Virology* 1988;164:121–131.
511. Tewari M, Dixit VM. Fas- and tumor necrosis factor-induced apoptosis is inhibited by the poxvirus crmA gene product. *J Biol Chem* 1995;270:3255–3260.
512. Tewari M, Telford WG, Miller RA, Dixit VM. CrmA, a poxvirus-encoded serpin, inhibits cytotoxic T-lymphocyte-mediated apoptosis. *J Biol Chem* 1995;270:22705–22708.
513. Thome M, Schneider P, Hofmann K, et al. Viral flice-inhibitory proteins (FLIPs) prevent apoptosis induced by death receptors. *Nature* 1997;386:517–521.
514. Thompson CL, Hooda-Dhingra U, Condit RC. Fine structure mapping of five temperature-sensitive mutants in the 22- and 147-kilodalton subunits of vaccinia virus DNA-dependent RNA polymerase. *J Virol* 1989;63:705–713.
515. Thompson JP, Turner PC, Ali AN, et al. The effects of serpin gene mutations on the distinctive pathobiology of cowpox and rabbitpox virus following intranasal inoculation of balb/c mice. *Virology* 1993;197:328–338.
516. Tooze J, Hollinshead M, Reis B, et al. Progeny vaccinia and human cytomegalovirus particles utilize early endosomal cisternae for their envelopes. *Eur J Cell Biol* 1993;60:163–178.
517. Traktman P. Poxvirus DNA replication. In: DePamphilis ML, ed. *DNA replication in eukaryotic cells.* Cold Spring Harbor, NY: Cold Spring Harbor Laboratory Press, 1996;775–793.
518. Traktman P, Caligiuri A, Jesty SA, Sankar U. Temperature-sensitive mutants with lesions in the vaccinia virus F10 kinase undergo arrest at the earliest stage of morphogenesis. *J Virol* 1995;69:6581–6587.
519. Traktman P, Kelvin M, Pacheco S. Molecular genetic analysis of vaccinia virus DNA polymerase mutants. *J Virol* 1989;63:841–846.
520. Traktman P, Liu K, DeMasi J, et al. Elucidating the essential role of the A14 phosphoprotein in vaccinia virus morphogenesis: Construction and characterization of a tetracycline-inducible recombinant. *J Virol* 2000;74:3682–3695.
521. Tseng M, Palaniyar N, Zhang WD, Evans DH. DNA binding and aggregation properties of the vaccinia virus I3L gene product. *J Biol Chem* 1999;274:21637–21644.
522. Tsukumo SI, Yonehara S. Requirement of cooperative functions of two repeated death effector domains in caspase-8 and in MC159 for induction and inhibition of apoptosis, respectively. *Genes Cells* 1999;4:541–549.
523. Turner PC, Baquero MT, Yuan S, et al. The cowpox virus serpin SPI-3 complexes with and inhibits urokinase-type and tissue-type plasminogen activators and plasmin. *Virology* 2000;272:267–280.
524. Turner PC, Moyer RW. Orthpoxvirus fusion inhibitor glycoprotein SPI-3 (open reading frame K2L) contains motifs characteristic of serine protease inhibitors that are not required for control of cell fusion. *J Virol* 1995;69:5978–5987.
525. Ulaeto D, Grosenbach D, Hruby DE. The vaccinia virus 4c and A-type inclusion proteins are specific markers for the intracellular mature virus particle. *J Virol* 1996;70:3372–3375.
526. Upton C, Macen JL, Schreiber M, McFadden G. Myxoma virus expresses a secreted protein with homology to the tumor necrosis factor receptor gene family that contributes to viral virulence. *Virology* 1991;184:370–382.
527. Upton C, Mossman K, McFadden G. Encoding of a homolog of the IFN-γ receptor by myxoma virus. *Science* 1992;258:1369–1373.
528. Upton C, Stuart DT, McFadden G. Identification of a poxvirus gene encoding a uracil DNA glycosylase. *Proc Natl Acad Sci U S A* 1993;90:4518–4522.
529. van Eijl H, Hollinshead M, Smith GL. The vaccinia virus A36R protein Is a type Ib membrane protein present on intracellular but not extracellular enveloped virus particles. *Virology* 2000;271:26–36.
530. Vanderplasschen A, Hollinshead M, Smith GL. Intracellular and extracellular vaccinia virions enter cells by different mechanisms. *J Gen Virol* 1998;79:877–887.
531. Vanderplasschen A, Mathew E, Hollinshead M, et al. Extracellular enveloped vaccinia virus is resistant to complement because of incorporation of host complement control proteins into its envelope. *Proc Natl Acad Sci U S A* 1998;95:7544–7549.
532. Vanderplasschen A, Smith GL. A novel virus binding assay using confocal microscopy: Demonstration that intracellular and extracellular vaccinia virions bind to different cellular receptors. *J Virol* 1997;71:4032–4041.
533. Vanslyke JK, Franke CA, Hruby DE. Proteolytic maturation of vaccinia virus core proteins: Identification of a conserved motif at the N termini of the 4b and 25K virion proteins. *J Gen Virol* 1991;72:411–416.
534. Vanslyke JK, Hruby DE. Immunolocalization of vaccinia virus structural proteins during virion formation. *Virology* 1994;198:624–635.
535. VanSlyke JK, Lee P, Wilson EM, Hruby DE. Isolation and analysis of vaccinia virus previrions. *Virus Genes* 1993;7:311–324.
536. VanSlyke JK, Whitehead SS, Wilson EM, Hruby DE. The multistep proteolytic maturation pathway utilized by vaccinia virus P4a protein: A degenerate conserved cleavage motif within core proteins. *Virology* 1991;183:467–478.
537. Vazquez MI, Esteban M. Identification of functional domains in the 14-kilodalton envelope protein (A27L) of vaccinia virus. *J Virol* 1999;73:9098–9109.
538. Venkatesan S, Gershowitz A, Moss B. Modification of the 5′-end of mRNA: Association of RNA triphosphatase with the RNA guanylyltransferase-RNA (guanine-7)methyltransferase complex from vaccinia virus. *J Biol Chem* 1980;255:903–908.
539. Vos JC, Sasker M, Stunnenberg HG. Promoter melting by a stage-specific vaccinia virus transcription factor is independent of the presence of RNA polymerase. *Cell* 1991;65:105–114.
540. Vos JC, Sasker M, Stunnenberg HG. Vaccinia virus capping enzyme is a transcription initiation factor. *EMBO J* 1991;10:2553–2558.
541. Vos JC, Stunnenberg HG. Derepression of a novel class of vaccinia virus genes upon DNA replication. *EMBO J* 1988;7:3487–3492.

542. Wang S, Shuman S. Vaccinia virus morphogenesis is blocked by temperature-sensitive mutations in the F10 gene, which encodes protein kinase 2. *J Virol* 1995;69:6376–6388.
543. Ward BM, Moss B. Golgi network targeting and plasma membrane internalization signals in vaccinia virus B5R envelope protein. *J Virol* 2000;74:3771–3780.
544. Wei CM, Moss B. Methylated nucleotides block 5′-terminus of vaccinia virus mRNA. *Proc Natl Acad Sci U S A* 1975;72:318–322.
545. Weir JP, Moss B. Use of a bacterial expression vector to identify the gene encoding a major core protein of vaccinia virus. *J Virol* 1985;56:534–540.
546. Westwood JCN, Harris WJ, Zwartouw HT, et al. Studies on the structure of vaccinia virus. *J Gen Microbiol* 1964;34:67–78.
547. White CL, Weisberg AS, Moss B. A glutaredoxin, encoded by the G4L gene of vaccinia virus, is essential for virion morphogenesis. *J Virol* 2000;74:9175–9183.
548. Whitehead WS, Hruby DE. Differential utilization of a conserved motif for the proteolytic maturation of vaccinia virus proteins. *Virology* 1994;200:154–161.
549. Wilcock D, Smith GL. Vaccinia virions lacking core protein VP8 are deficient in early transcription. *J Virol* 1996;70:934–943.
550. Wilcock D, Smith GL. Vaccinia virus core protein VP8 is required for virus infectivity, but not for core protein processing or for INV and EEV formation. *Virology* 1994;202:294–304.
551. Willer DO, Mann MJ, Zhang WD, Evans DH. Vaccinia virus DNA polymerase promotes DNA pairing and strand-transfer reactions. *Virology* 1999;257:511–523.
552. Willer DO, McFadden G, Evans DH. The complete genome sequence of Shope (rabbit) fibroma virus. *Virology* 1999;264:319–343.
553. Williams O, Wolffe EJ, Weisberg AS, Merchlinsky M. Vaccinia virus WR gene A5L is required for morphogenesis of mature virions. *J Virol* 1999;73:4590–4599.
554. Wilton S, Dales S. Relationship between RNA polymerase II and efficiency of vaccinia virus replication. *J Virol* 1989;63:1540–1548.
555. Wise LM, Veikkola T, Mercer AA, et al. Vascular endothelial growth factor (VEGF)-like protein from orf virus NZ2 binds to VEGFR2 and neuropilin-1. *Proc Natl Acad Sci U S A* 1999;96:3071–3076.
556. Wittek R, Hanggi M, Hiller G. Mapping of a gene coding for a major late structural polypeptide on the vaccinia virus genome. *J Virol* 1984;49:371–378.
557. Wittek R, Moss B. Tandem repeats within the inverted terminal repetition of vaccinia virus DNA. *Cell* 1980;21:277–284.
558. Wolffe EJ, Isaacs SN, Moss B. Deletion of the vaccinia virus B5R gene encoding a 42-kilodalton membrane glycoprotein inhibits extracellular virus envelope formation and dissemination. *J Virol* 1993;67:4732–4741.
559. Wolffe EJ, Katz E, Weisberg A, Moss B. The A34R glycoprotein gene is required for induction of specialized actin-containing microvilli and efficient cell-to-cell transmission of vaccinia virus. *J Virol* 1997;71:3904–3915.
560. Wolffe EJ, Moore DM, Peters PJ, Moss B. Vaccinia virus A17L open reading frame encodes an essential component of nascent viral membranes that is required to initiate morphogenesis. *J Virol* 1996;70:2797–2808.
561. Wolffe EJ, Vijaya S, Moss B. A myristylated membrane protein encoded by the vaccinia virus L1R open reading frame is the target of potent neutralizing monoclonal antibodies. *Virology* 1995;211:53–63.
562. Wolffe EJ, Weisberg A, Moss B. The vaccinia virus A33R protein provides a chaperone function for viral membrane localization and tyrosine phosphorylation of the A36R protein. *J Virol* 2000;74:9701–9711.
563. Wolffe EJ, Weisberg AS, Moss B. Role for the vaccinia virus A36R outer envelope protein in the formation of virus-tipped actin-containing microvilli and cell-to-cell virus spread. *Virology* 1998;244:20–26.
564. Woodson B. Vaccinia mRNA synthesis under conditions which prevent uncoating. *Biochem Biophys Res Commun* 1967;27:169–175.
565. Wright CF, Coroneos AM. Purification of the late transcription system of vaccinia virus: Identification of a novel transcription factor. *J Virol* 1993;67:7264–7270.
566. Wright CF, Keck JG, Moss B. A transcription factor for expression of vaccinia virus late genes is encoded by an intermediate gene. *J Virol* 1991;65:3715–3720.
567. Wright CF, Moss B. *In vitro* synthesis of vaccinia virus late mRNA containing a 5′ poly(A) leader sequence. *Proc Natl Acad Sci U S A* 1987;84:8883–8887.
568. Xiang Y, Latner DR, Niles EG, Condit RC. Transcription elongation activity of the vaccinia virus J3 protein *in vivo* is independent of poly(A) polymerase stimulation. *Virology* 2000;269:356–369.
569. Xiang Y, Moss B. Identification of human and mouse homologs of the MC51L-53L-54L family of secreted glycoproteins encoded by the molluscum contagiosum poxvirus. *Virology* 1999;257:297–302.
570. Xiang Y, Moss B. IL-18 binding and inhibition of interferon gamma induction by human poxvirus-encoded proteins. *Proc Natl Acad Sci U S A* 1999;96:11537–11542.
571. Xiang Y, Simpson DA, Spiegel J, et al. The vaccinia virus A18R DNA helicase is a postreplicative negative transcription elongation factor. *J Virol* 1998;72:7012–7023.
572. Yeh WW, Moss B, Wolffe EJ. The vaccinia virus A9 gene encodes a membrane protein required for an early step in virion morphogenesis. *J Virol* 2000;74:9701–9711.
573. Yuen L, Davison AJ, Moss B. Early promoter-binding factor from vaccinia virions. *Proc Natl Acad Sci U S A* 1987;84:6069–6073.
574. Yuen L, Moss B. Oligonucleotide sequence signaling transcriptional termination of vaccinia virus early genes. *Proc Natl Acad Sci U S A* 1987;84:6417–6421.
575. Zartouw HT. The chemical composition of vaccinia virus. *J Gen Microbiol* 1964;34:115–123.
576. Zhang WD, Evans DH. DNA strand exchange catalyzed by proteins from vaccinia virus-infected cells. *J Virol* 1993;67:204–212.
577. Zhang Y, Ahn BY, Moss B. Targeting of a multicomponent transcription apparatus into assembling vaccinia virus particles requires RAP94, an RNA polymerase-associated protein. *J Virol* 1994;68:1360–1370.
578. Zhang Y, Moss B. Immature viral envelope formation is interrupted at the same stage by lac operator-mediated repression of the vaccinia virus D13L gene and by the drug rifampicin. *Virology* 1992;187:643–653.
579. Zhang Y, Moss B. Vaccinia virus morphogenesis is interrupted when expression of the gene encoding an 11-kilodalton phosphorylated protein is prevented by the *Escherichia coli* lac repressor. *J Virol* 1991;65:6101–6110.
580. Zhang YF, Keck JG, Moss B. Transcription of viral late genes is dependent on expression of the viral intermediate gene G8R in cells infected with an inducible conditional-lethal mutant vaccinia virus. *J Virol* 1992;66:6470–6479.
581. Zhou Q, Snipas S, Orth K, et al. Target protease specificity of the viral serpin CrmA: Analysis of five caspases. *J Biol Chem* 1997;272:7797–7800.

CHAPTER 36

Hepadnaviridae: The Viruses and Their Replication

Donald Ganem and Robert J. Schneider

Of the many viral causes of human hepatitis, few are of greater global importance than hepatitis B virus (HBV). More than 300 million people worldwide are persistently infected with HBV, and of these, a significant fraction develop severe pathologic consequences, including chronic hepatitis, cirrhosis, and hepatocellular carcinoma (22,23,289). The epidemiology, natural history, and therapy of HBV infection are reviewed by Hollinger in Chapter 87. Here, we focus on the cellular and molecular mechanisms of the replication of HBV and its related viruses.

For many years, insight into the fundamentals of the HBV life cycle was impeded by severe experimental obstacles posed by (a) the narrow host range of the virus (resulting in the absence of convenient animal models of infection and disease), and (b) the lack of cell lines that support productive HBV replication. However, the molecular cloning of the viral genome (150,334,392, 489,556,558), the development of cell culture–based assays for viral replication (95,151,211,477,516,593), and the discovery of natural animal models of viral infection (335,338,342,514) radically changed this picture. These advances ultimately resulted in the development of recombinant HBV vaccine (344), the first successful recombinant vaccine for a human infectious disease, and the seminal discovery that these viruses replicate their DNA through the reverse transcription of an RNA intermediate (510). The latter finding established HBVs as distant evolutionary relatives of the retroviruses and stimulated the identification of clinically effective drugs based on the inhibition of the viral reverse transcriptase. The more recent development of transgenic mouse models of virus-induced liver injury (86) has led to new ways of thinking about the pathophysiology of viral clearance and persistence, with profound implications for the design of strategies for intervening in the natural history of chronic infection. Virology affords few better examples of the close relationship between research into the molecular aspects of viral replication and advances in clinical diagnosis and therapy.

HEPATITIS B VIRUS BIOLOGY: AN OVERVIEW

Primary HBV infection of susceptible adults results from sexual contact with an infected host or from parenteral exposure to virus-containing blood or blood products (154,217,219,269,289). Primary infection may be asymptomatic or may result in varying degrees of acute liver injury (acute hepatitis). Although such hepatitis can be severe, in most adults, the primary infection resolves (219,233). Host immune responses to viral antigens result in the clearance of infected cells from the liver and the removal of virions from the bloodstream; lasting immunity to clinically evident reinfection typically results (217; but see later section, Viral Pathogenesis and Immunity, for an important caveat). However, in a small proportion of infected adults (generally less than 5%), the primary infection does not resolve (233). These individuals go on to a persistent infection characterized by active viral replication in hepatocytes and variable (but usually substantial) levels of viremia. As in primary infection, the clinical manifestations of the persistent infection vary greatly: many patients are relatively symptom free, whereas others have varying grades of chronic liver injury and inflammation (chronic hepatitis B) (289). Although it is the minority outcome of primary infection, persistence is important for several reasons. First, most of the morbidity and mortality of hepatitis B virus infection results from the persistent infection. Some subsets of symptomatic patients (e.g., those with severe chronic active hepatitis B) have 5-year survival rates of less than 50%, with most deaths resulting from liver failure and its complications (289). Chronic hepatitis B patients who survive 25 to 30 years of viral persistence also have a markedly increased risk for developing heptocellular carcinoma (23), a dreaded malignancy that is usually fatal. Finally, the asymptomatic carriers are the major epidemiologic reservoir of infection: it is principally from them that spread of HBV to susceptible hosts occurs.

The reasons that some individuals resolve HBV infection whereas others do not remain poorly understood. Much correlative clinical evidence suggests that variations in host immune responses are a critical variable. For example, individuals with overt deficits in cell-mediated immunity (e.g., transplant recipients, patients with acquired immunodeficiency syndrome [AIDS]) are more likely to become chronic carriers than are fully immunocompetent hosts. The most biologically important example of this phenomenon is seen in the vertical transmission of HBV from pregnant mother to newborn baby. HBV transmission to babies usually takes place at the time of delivery, when the newborn is exposed to large quantities of viremic maternal blood during passage through the birth canal. The cellular immune system of the neonate is known to be incompletely developed at birth; in this context, 80% to 90% of HBV exposures result in persistent infections (24,294,381,502). Much has been learned in recent years about the immunologic mechanisms governing viral clearance; these are discussed in more detail later (see Viral Pathogenesis and Immunity).

VIRION STRUCTURE

Particle Types

HBV is unusual among animal viruses in that infected cells produce multiple types of virus-related particles (21,103,444). Electron microscopy of partially purified preparations of HBV shows three types of particles: (a) 42- to 47-nm double-shelled particles (known as *Dane particles,* after their discoverer); (b) 20-nm spheres, usually present in a 10,000- to 1,000,000-fold excess over Dane particles; and (c) smaller quantities of filaments of 20 nm diameter and variable length (Fig. 1). All three forms have a common antigen on their surface, termed *hepatitis B surface antigen* (HBsAg). HBsAg is present in enormous quantity in the serum of infected hosts, with concentrations ranging from 50 to 300 μg/mL; most of the circulating pool of HBsAg is composed of 20-nm spheres, which can reach titers as high as 10^{12}/mL. This unprecedented amount of viral antigen in the circulation allows physicians to use direct viral antigen detection as a sensitive diagnostic test for HBV infection.

The Dane particle is the infectious virion of HBV; titers of Dane particles in the blood can range from less than 10^4/mL to greater than 10^9/mL. Its outer shell is a lipoprotein envelope containing the viral surface glycoproteins, originally detected serologically as HBsAg (35). These are the determinants against which neutralizing antibody (anti-HBs) is directed (217). The envelope can be removed by treatment with nonionic detergents, liberating an inner core particle or nucleocapsid of 25 to 27 nm. The major structural protein of the core is the C protein, a 21-kd basic phosphoprotein that was also originally detected serologically (218) and that is still frequently called *hepatitis B core antigen* (HBcAg) (442,511). Within the core is the viral DNA and a polymerase (P) activity (255,443) now known to be centrally involved in viral genomic replication. Purified cores also contain a protein kinase activity detected by its ability to phosphorylate C protein *in vitro* (2,135,165); because recombinant C and P proteins do not possess kinase activity, it is thought that this enzyme is of host origin. Whether it is truly an internal capsid component or merely tightly associated with cores during extract preparation is still uncertain, as is its biologic role (although there is no doubt that C protein is phosphorylated *in vivo*) (328,421,449,602,609).

The 20-nm spheres and filaments are composed exclusively of HBsAg and host-derived lipid (about 30% by weight); their principal lipids include phospholipids, cholesterol, cholesterol esters, and triglycerides (160,405, 406). These particles lack nucleic acid altogether and hence are noninfectious. Nonetheless, in pure form, these particles are highly immunogenic and efficiently induce a neutralizing anti-HBs antibody response. Such 20-nm spheres, as purified from the serum of HBV carriers, in fact served as the initial form of HBV vaccine before the

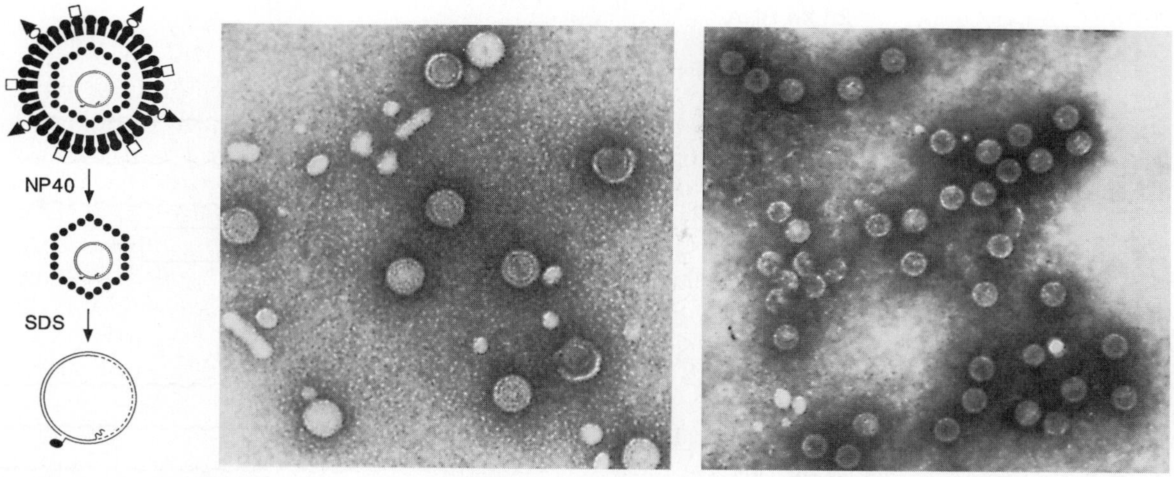

FIG. 1. The structure of hepadnaviral virions and subviral particles. **Left:** Schematic depiction of virion (*top*), core particle (*middle*), and virion DNA (*bottom*). The outer envelope of the virion contains three related surface glycoproteins (*L, M,* and *S*); the inner nucleocapsid contains a single capsid protein (*C*). The viral DNA contains a terminal protein (*oval*) attached to the negative strand and a short RNA (*wavy line*) attached to the positive strand. *Dashes* indicate single-stranded gap region on virion DNA. **Center:** Electron micrograph of hepatitis B virus particles, including virions, 20-nm spheres, and filaments. **Right:** Electron micrograph of virion cores produced by detergent (NP40) treatment of virions. (Experiment by June Almeida, United Medical School, Guy's Hospital, London, U.K.)

development of recombinant HBsAg preparations (269). Natural infection thus presents the seeming paradox of efficient progression despite the accompanying production of highly immunogenic particles that can elicit neutralizing host responses. How this comes about is not known; one school of thought is that the excess HBsAg particles function to adsorb neutralizing antibody and thus help shield virions from host defenses.

The Viral Genome

HBV virion DNA is a relaxed circular, partially duplex species of 3.2 kb whose circularity is maintained by 5′-cohesive ends (442,458,511) (Fig. 2). This molecule has an unusual structure in that its two DNA strands are not perfectly symmetric. The viral negative strand is unit length and has protein covalently linked to its 5′ end (156,166,351). The existence of this terminal protein emerged from the observation that the viral DNA was extracted from the aqueous phase by phenol unless the genome was first treated with proteases. Restriction endonuclease digestion of viral DNA indicated that only terminal DNA fragments bearing the negative strand 5′ end displayed this behavior, indicating linkage of the protein to the 5′ end of negative-stranded DNA. By contrast, the positive strand is less than unit length and bears a capped oligoribonucleotide at its 5′ end (309,472,581). The presence of these terminal structures explains the longstanding observation that neither 5′ end of viral DNA can be phosphorylated by polynucleotide kinase. Importantly, the positions of the 5′ ends of both strands map to the regions of short (11 nucleotides) direct repeats (DRs) in viral DNA. The 5′ end of negative-stranded DNA maps within the repeat termed DR1, whereas positive-stranded DNA begins within DR2 (309,352,472,581) (see Fig. 2). As detailed later, these repeats are importantly involved in priming the synthesis of their respective DNA strands.

Virion DNA thus contains a single-stranded region or gap of fixed polarity but variable length. Early studies showed that cores purified from extracellular virions contain a polymerase activity that can fill in this gap, generating a fully duplex genome (255,443,511). In this so-called endogenous polymerase reaction (EPR), the 3′ hydroxyl of positive-stranded DNA serves as the primer, with synthesis extending along negative-stranded DNA templates. The newly synthesized product is therefore entirely of positive-stranded polarity, an asymmetry that is not simply reconciled with a standard semiconservative DNA replication scheme (see later).

Molecular cloning of HBV DNA extracted from Dane particles reveals a coding organization that is highly compact: every nucleotide in the genome is within a coding region, and more than half of the sequence is translated in more than one frame (150,558). As shown in Figure 2, four open reading frames (ORFs) are present in the DNA. The viral polymerase, the central enzymatic activity in genomic replication, is encoded by the *P* gene; ORF *P* also encodes the terminal protein found on negative-stranded DNA (37) (see later). The C (core) region encodes the structural protein of the nucleocapsid (392), whereas ORF *S*/pre-S encodes the viral surface glycoproteins (556).

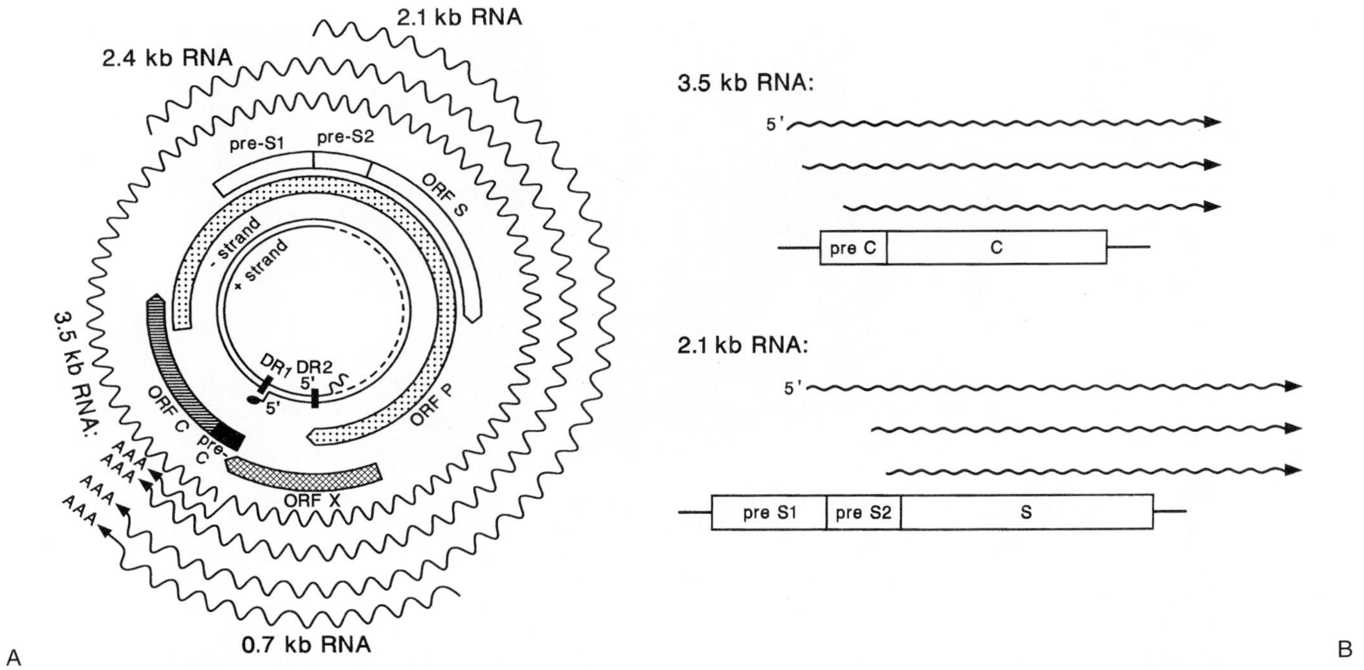

FIG. 2. A: Diagrammatic representation of the hepatitis B virus coding organization. *Inner circle* represents virion DNA, with dashes signifying the single-stranded genomic region; the locations of DR1 and DR2 sequence elements are as indicated. *Boxes* denote viral coding regions, with *arrows* indicating direction of translation. *Outermost wavy lines* depict the viral RNAs identified in infected cells, with arrows indicating direction of transcription. **B:** Fine structure of the 5′ ends of the pre-C/C transcripts (*top*) and pre-S2/S transcripts (*bottom*) relative to their respective open reading frames.

The DNA sequence of HBV revealed a number of surprises not anticipated from earlier biologic studies. Chief among these was the existence of ORF *X,* a coding region whose product had not previously been detected. The product of ORF *X* is a complex regulatory protein that is required for viral infectivity *in vivo* and modulates the expression of heterologous and homologous genes in trans, at least in transient assays performed in cultured cells (451). How it does so is a matter of considerable debate and is considered in a later section.

Moreover, the coding organization of the genes for the known virion structural components (HBsAg and HBcAg) turned out to be more complex than expected. Early studies had suggested that the major component of HBsAg was a protein of 24 kd (30% to 50% of which is glycosylated, appearing as a second species of 27 kd), but small quantities of larger polypeptides often copurified with this material (164). The coding region for HBsAg was identified by aligning the translated HBV DNA sequence with the known N-terminal amino acid sequence of the 24-kd chain (556). This revealed that the reading frame for this antigen was open for about 400 nucleotides 5′ to its AUG (initiation codon) and that this upstream (or pre-S) ORF could be divided into two subregions (pre-S1 and pre-S2) by the presence of two in-frame initiation codons (see Fig. 2). This coding organization provided an explanation for most of the larger polypeptides earlier observed in HBsAg preparations. The largest of these so-called pre-S proteins is the 39-kd L (pre-S1) protein, which is the product of initiation at the first AUG of the ORF (204,585). Initiation at the second AUG generates the 31-kd M (pre-S2) protein (326,327,401,503). Both proteins share the common C-terminal S domain and differ principally by the length and structure of their N-terminal (pre-S) extensions. Classic HBsAg, which contains only the S domain, is now more commonly referred to as the *S protein.*

Both pre-S–encoded polypeptides are quantitatively minor components of the circulating pool of S-related antigens, with the M protein accounting for about 5% to 15% of the total and the L protein typically representing only 1% to 2% or less of the total. Each protein exists in two isomeric forms, differing only by the presence or absence of S-domain glycosylation; in addition, the M protein contains an additional *N*-linked oligosaccharide on its pre-S2–specific domain (204,503). The L protein contains a further posttranslational modification, a myristic acid group in amide linkage to its amino-terminal glycine residue (403). Despite their low abundance, L chains are now thought to play a key role in viral assembly and infectivity (46,235,301,330).

Careful fractionation studies (204) have established that the three envelope glycoproteins are not distributed uniformly among the various HBV particle types. Subviral 20-nm particles are composed predominantly of the S protein, with variable quantities of M polypeptides and few or no L chains. By contrast, Dane particles are substantially enriched for L chains. Because L chains are thought to carry the receptor recognition domain (235,264,411), this enrichment may prevent the more numerous 20-nm particles from competing effectively with virions for cell surface receptors.

The coding organization of the core protein gene revealed a similar surprise: again, two in-frame AUGs were found in the core ORF, with the classic HBcAg being the product of initiation from the more internal start codon (580). Initiation at the upstream AUG gives rise to a C-related protein that is not incorporated into virions but instead is independently secreted from cells, accumulating in serum as an immunologically distinct antigen known as *HBeAg* (159,345,388,448,498). The function of HBeAg remains enigmatic (see later).

CLASSIFICATION

The *Hepadnaviridae* Family

These unusual structural features clearly set HBV apart from the other families of animal DNA viruses. HBV is the prototype member of a family of related viruses known as hepadnaviruses (for hepatotropic DNA viruses). The first of the nonhuman hepadnaviruses to be discovered was the woodchuck hepatitis virus (WHV). In a colony of captive woodchucks (*Marmota monax*), veterinarians noted the frequent presence of chronic active hepatitis and hepatoma at necropsy (515); these features recalled the histopathology of advanced HBV infection. A search for HBV-like particles in serum from these animals ultimately culminated in the identification of WHV (514), a novel virus that is morphologically indistinguishable from HBV and whose genome shares about 60% nucleotide sequence identity with its human counterpart (149,268). A series of similar viruses have now been recovered from a variety of animal species, including the Beechey ground squirrel, *Spermophilis beecheyi* (ground squirrel hepatitis virus [GSHV]) (156,157,337, 338), and the Pekin duck, *Anas domesticus* (duck hepatitis B virus [DHBV]) (336,337,342,497). Less well-characterized viruses have been recovered from arctic ground squirrels, wild herons, several varieties of wild and domestic geese, marsupials, and orangutans (496,527, 530). All of these viruses share the following common properties: (a) enveloped virions bearing 3- to 3.3-kb relaxed circular, partially duplex DNA; (b) virion-associated polymerases that can repair the gap in the virion DNA template; (c) the production of excess subviral lipoprotein particles composed of envelope proteins; (d) narrow host range, growing only in species close to the natural host (14,285,336,422,475,542); and (e) production of persistent infections displaying pronounced (but not absolute) hepatotropism.

Table 1 summarizes the biologic properties of the most intensively studied hepadnaviruses. Although the similarities between these viruses outnumber the differences, there are important distinctions to be made among the individual members of this virus family. In general, the avian viruses are the most divergent: their viral genomes are smaller than those of the mammalian viruses and share little primary nucleotide sequence homology with them (334). Most avian viruses encode only two envelope proteins (L and S) rather than three (423,463) and lack the classic X coding region (although a small ORF beginning with a noncanonical initiator is present in this position and can be expressed in transfected cells (H. Will, personal communication). Although they too display a very narrow host range, their hepatotropism is less marked: viral antigens and replicative intermediates can

TABLE 1. *The hepadnaviridae family*

	HBV	WHV	GSHV	DHBV
Genome	3.2 kb	3.3 kb	3.3 kb	3.0 kb
ORFs	S, C, P, X, S, C, P, X	S, C, P, X	S, C, P	
Hosts	Humans Chimps	Woodchucks	Ground squirrels Woodchucks Chipmunks	Ducks Geese
Replication	Liver Kidney Pancreas WBC	Liver Kidney Pancreas WBC Other	Liver	Liver Kidney Pancreas Spleen Other
Diseases	ACS Hepatitis Cirrhosis HCC	ACS Hepatitis HCC	ACS Hepatitis HCC	ACS Hepatitis

ACS, asymptomatic carrier state; DHBV, duck hepatitis B virus; HBV, hepatitis B virus; GSHV, ground squirrel hepatitis virus; HCC, hepatocellular carcinoma; ORF, open reading frame; WBC, white blood cells; WHV, woodchuck hepatitis virus.

be readily detected in several extrahepatic sites, including the pancreas, kidney, and spleen (193–196,220,247). In animals infected *in ovo,* the yolk sac is a major site of viral replication (520). Extrahepatic infection is also well-documented for HBV (412,447,605) and WHV (274–276,379), but the titers of their extrahepatic viral DNAs are generally much lower than those observed for DHBV. Nonetheless, even in the avian viruses, the liver remains the predominant site of virus production. Most strikingly, DHBV infection, although it can be associated with mild grades of hepatitis, is not strongly linked to the development of HCC. Although some DHBV-infected flocks in China and Japan have noted the occasional occurrence of hepatoma (234,383,606), infected birds in U.S. and European flocks (and laboratory-held animals) virtually never develop this lesion. It seems likely that the Asian flocks have been exposed to environmental cofactors that may accelerate HCC formation; dietary aflatoxin, a potent hepatic carcinogen, is a leading candidate for this cofactor role (100).

VIRAL REPLICATION

Overview of the Life Cycle

The peculiar asymmetries of virion DNA (and of the endogenous polymerase reaction) provided early clues that a mechanism other than semiconservative DNA synthesis is involved in hepadnaviral genomic replication. Examination of intrahepatic replicative intermediates revealed even more striking asymmetries. Infected liver cells harbor large quantities of negative strands of less than unit length, most of which are not associated with positive strands (340,578). In 1982, Summers and Mason (510) reported seminal experiments establishing that viral DNA replication proceeds not by conventional semiconservative DNA synthesis but by reverse transcription of an RNA intermediate. To do this, they first prepared subviral particles from DHBV-infected liver; these particles, unlike mature virions, incorporate labeled deoxyribonucleoside triphosphates (dNTPs) into both positive and negative strands of viral DNA, exactly as would be anticipated for authentic replication intermediates. Electron microscopy of the particles proved them to be immature (unenveloped) cores that were cytoplasmic in location; thus, most viral replication was occurring outside of the nucleus, the principal site of host DNA synthesis. Importantly, the synthesis of negative-stranded DNA was resistant to actinomycin D, implying its template was not DNA, whereas positive-stranded synthesis was sensitive to this compound. In addition, a portion of newly made negative-stranded DNA was found in the form of RNA–DNA hybrids. These observations suggested that negative-stranded DNA was made from an RNA template, whereas the positive strand was copied from a DNA template—by inference the negative-stranded DNA whose RNA template had been removed.

These experiments predicted the existence of a full-length, unspliced RNA that would serve as the template for reverse transcription, and such an RNA was indeed identified soon thereafter (55,123,355). This RNA (sometimes called *pregenomic RNA* [pgRNA] to denote its role in genomic replication) has all the hallmarks of a transcript produced by host RNA polymerase II (pol II). But if pol II, a nuclear enzyme, is the enzyme responsible for genomic RNA synthesis, clearly a subpopulation of nuclear viral DNA molecules must exist to serve as its template. This function is provided by a nuclear pool of viral DNA consisting of 10 to 20 molecules/cell of unit-length, covalently closed circular DNA (cccDNA) (340,578). As the presumed viral transcriptional template, these molecules thus play in the hepadnaviral life cycle the role analogous to that of integrated proviral DNA in retroviral replication; however, in hepadnaviral infection, these molecules remain episomal. Presumably, incoming viral DNA is transported to the nucleus and converted to the cccDNA form. Consistent with this, cccDNA is the first novel virus-specific DNA species to appear after DHBV infection, preceding the accumulation of viral RNA (341).

These observations allow formulation of a model for the overall viral replicative cycle (Fig. 3). After receptor binding, virions deliver their nucleocapsids to the cytoplasm. These then translocate to the nucleus, where their genomic DNA is matured to the cccDNA form. This DNA is then transcribed by host RNA pol II, and the resulting RNAs translated to give rise to the P, C, pre-S/S and (in mammalian viruses) X gene products. Viral pregenomic RNAs are selectively encapsidated within core particles in the cytoplasm (124,510), together with the P gene product. Within this structure, viral DNA synthesis is initiated; after negative-stranded synthesis (and concomitant degradation of the RNA template), positive-stranded DNA synthesis occurs. Upon completion of genomic DNA synthesis, progeny cores bud into intracellular membranes, generally the endoplasmic reticulum (ER) or proximal Golgi (252,446), to acquire their glycoprotein envelope. Enveloped virions are then secreted through the constitutive pathway of vesicular transport.

Many of the events schematized in Figure 3 can now be studied in cell culture. Although there are still no established cell lines that support infection with HBV virions (see later), primary duck hepatocytes freshly explanted directly from liver will support DHBV infection (152,424,546). These are terminally differentiated epithelial cell cultures that engage in little or no cell division and cannot be passaged long-term *in vitro.* Similar preparations of mammalian hepatocytes appear to support mammalian hepadnaviral infections, but much less efficiently (175,176,376). The reasons for this inefficiency are unclear, but HBV infection of primary human hepa-

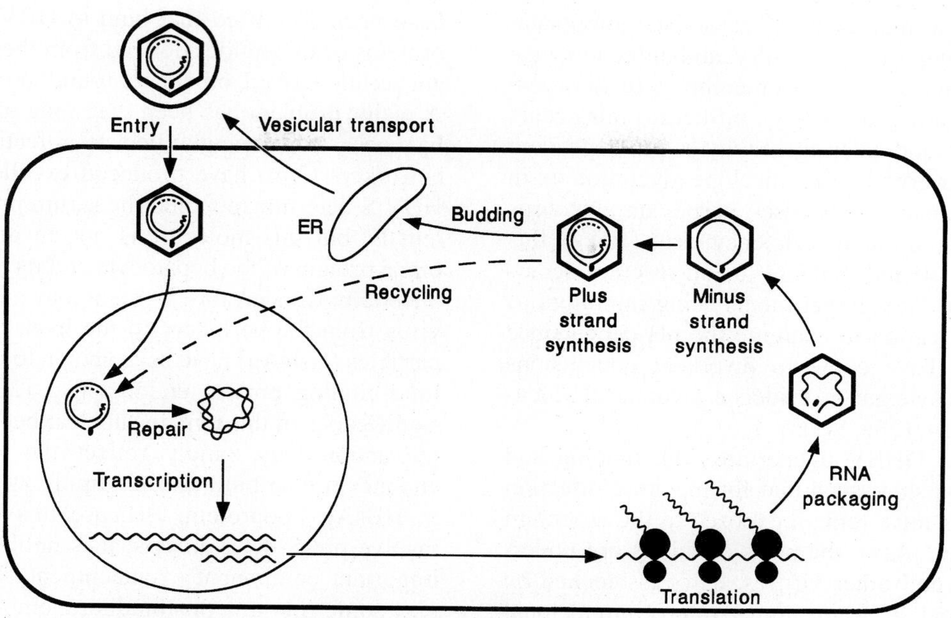

FIG. 3. Schematic depiction of the hepadnaviral life cycle. See text for details.

tocytes can be significantly enhanced by the addition of low concentrations of polyethylene glycol to the medium (175), suggesting that inefficient membrane fusion may be the cause.

Although they will not support virion infection, several well-differentiated and immortalized hepatoma cell lines (e.g., human HepG2 or HuH7, and chick LMH cells) support viral replication and release if cloned viral DNA is delivered by transfection (95,151,425,477,516,593). Presumably, the incoming transfected DNA functionally substitutes for cccDNA upon arrival in the nucleus, allowing the generation of the correct panel of viral transcripts; these can then encode the viral gene products necessary to complete all subsequent stages of the life cycle. Even fibroblasts can support hepadnaviral production after transfection by cloned viral DNA, provided that a heterologous promoter is used to drive expression of pgRNA (470), suggesting that transcription of pgRNA is a major determinant of liver specificity in wild-type hepadnavirus infection. Transfection of hepatocytes can also occur *in vivo* after the direct inoculation of cloned hepadnaviral DNA into the liver of susceptible hosts (471,497,579). In this case, progeny virions elaborated by the transfected cells establish a hepatic and systemic infection exactly as observed after virion inoculation. Similarly, HBV replication can proceed in transgenic mice bearing chromosomal copies of overlength HBV genomes (92,186). In these cases, the integrated transgenes serve the function of transcriptional templates for pgRNA production. Because mouse cells lack the HBV entry pathway, there is no horizontal spread of virus in these animals; however, such spread is not required to maintain viremia because every hepatocyte in the liver harbors a transcriptionally competent integrated viral genome from birth.

The availability of these systems has made possible mutational analysis of virtually all steps in replication. These systems have also revealed an important additional feature of the replication cycle: its noncytocidal nature. Primary cells supporting productive infection generally show no cytopathic effects and are morphologically normal (176,545,546); transfected hepatoma cells bearing viral replicative intermediates display growth rates identical to those of their untransfected parents (516). These facts agree well with clinical observations that many densely infected HBV carriers have minimal or no hepatocellular injury and support the contention that such injury *in vivo* is largely the result of host immune or inflammatory responses (see later). The phenotype of HBV-positive transgenic mice bears further witness to this model: the livers of these mice (which are immunologically tolerant to the viral antigens) harbor high levels of viral replicative intermediates but remain histologically normal throughout life (185,186,354).

Attachment and Entry

Little is known about the earliest events in the viral life cycle. Enveloped virions must first bind to the cell surface, a reaction that has been best studied for DHBV. Binding occurs at 4°C, but at this temperature, no productive infection takes place. The binding reaction appears to have two components: a low-affinity, nonsaturable one and a high-affinity, saturable component (264). On warming to 37°C, entry and infection take place. After binding, a virus–host membrane fusion event must occur. For some viruses (e.g,. influenza) this occurs after endocytosis and is triggered by a pH-dependent fusion reaction governed by an envelope glycoprotein; in other viruses (e.g. paramyxoviruses, herpes simplex virus [HSV], and human immunodeficiency virus [HIV]), this is mediated by a pH-independent fusion reaction occurring at the cell surface. Experiments using inhibitors of endosomal acidification to examine the pH dependence of DHBV entry have come to divergent conclusions (377,441), but the weight of evidence favors a pH-independent mechanism (266,441).

The kinetics of DHBV uptake are odd: binding and entry appear to be slow, such that for maximal infection to occur, the cells must remain exposed to the inoculum for up to 16 hours (424); the basis of this is not understood. As for several other viruses, entry is blocked by suramin (404) and by some antienvelope monoclonal antibodies (MAbs) (80,81,284,286,612).

Much work has been done on the viral envelope components that may be involved in host cell interactions. For HBV and DHBV, several lines of evidence indicate that pre-S proteins participate in cellular receptor binding. Binding of HBV virions to human liver plasma membrane fractions is blocked by MAbs to the HBV pre-S1 domain; antipeptide antibodies to pre-S1 block adherence of HBV particles to HepG2 cells (370,411). Unfortunately, neither experiment is able to relate binding to productive infection. However, using recombinant DHBV envelope proteins, it has been shown that S proteins do not block DHBV infection of primary duck hepatocytes, whereas recombinant preparations containing both pre-S and S proteins do (264).

Another strong inference that pre-S determinants play a key role in receptor interactions comes from genetic studies of viral host range determinants. Hepadnaviruses typically are restricted to species close to that of their natural host, and DNA transfection experiments show that the block to efficient cross-species infection is at the level of virus entry (151,485). For example, the heron hepatitis B virus (HHBV) grows in herons but not in ducks or chicks, despite its substantial sequence homology with DHBV (496). If the normal entry pathway is bypassed by transfecting HHBV DNA into heterologous cells, replication proceeds normally. Consistent with this, pseudotyping experiments show that HHBV can be enveloped by DHBV envelope proteins and that these pseudotyped virions can efficiently infect duck hepatocytes (235). Examination of HHBV and DHBV chimeric envelope proteins in such pseudotyping assays indicates that pre-S determinants play the dominant role in host range determination (235).

Much less is known of the identities of the cellular receptors for hepadnaviruses. A large variety of proteins have been identified that bind to HBV envelope glycoproteins or to peptides derived from them. Some of these are serum derived, others are found in or on hepatocytes. A major problem has been that none of these molecules has been convincingly tied to infectivity. Mehdi and coworkers (346) have produced excellent evidence that HBV S determinants bind the serum protein apolipoprotein H, but this molecule is not an integral transmembrane protein of the hepatocyte and its role in infection is uncertain. Conceivably, it might play a role in delivery of virus from the periphery to the liver. Similarly, HBV S particles (HBsAg) have been shown to bind the phospholipid-binding protein endonexin 2 (207). The biologic significance of this remains unclear because the observed interaction may simply reflect the known ability of endonexin 2 to bind phospholipids, which are abundant in HBsAg lipoprotein. Because this binding does not involve pre-S determinants, it is unlikely to be the sole important component of attachment; it might, however, play some role in a postbinding membrane fusion event. Other studies have suggested possible roles for yet other molecules in viral entry (51,147,272,273,370–372,413), but no evidence that these proteins play a role in permissive infection has yet been forthcoming.

Progress in receptor identification has been greater in the DHBV system. In 1994, Kuroki and associates (278) identified a 180-kd surface glycoprotein (gp180) that binds to DHBV virions. Binding is specific to the pre-S region of the viral L protein (237,278,536,555) and is blocked by neutralizing (but not by nonneutralizing) antiviral MAbs. The species distribution of this protein mirrors the known host range of DHBV. All pre-S mutations that block this binding without affecting viral assembly destroy DHBV infectivity (237). Cloning of the cyclic DNA (cDNA) encoding this molecule revealed it to be a novel member of the carboxypeptidase family (279). The protein, also designated *carboxypeptidase D* (CPD), is enzymatically active, but this activity is separable from the virus-binding activity (125). Antibody to gp180 blocks DHBV infection of primary hepatocytes, as does soluble recombinant gp180 (S. Urban and H. Schaller, personal communication), demonstrating a key role for this molecule in viral entry. However, the protein is expressed on a wide variety of cell types in the animal, including many (e.g. fibroblasts) that are not thought to be susceptible to infection, and cDNA transfection into most nonpermissive cell lines (e.g., LMH cells) does not confer DHBV susceptibility (40,278). Thus, CPD is unlikely to be the sole component of the DHBV entry pathway; as in other virus systems, coreceptor proteins are likely to exist, and their identification constitutes one of the great remaining challenges to the field. Although gp180 is found in small quantities on the cell surface, most of it resides on intracellular (Golgi) membranes (40,279), suggesting that recycling of the protein between the cell surface and Golgi may occur. In accord with this,

DHBV particles bound to CPD-expressing cells can be internalized (40). It is therefore possible that the accessory components of the viral entry pathway may act not at the cell surface but on intracellular vesicles bearing internalized DHBV.

The subsequent, postreceptor steps in hepadnaviral entry are even less well characterized (267). Cytoplasmic cores must be delivered to the nucleus, where their DNA is converted to the superhelical form. Nothing is known of this delivery process. Conceivably, microtubule-based motor systems might play a role in their transport across the cytoplasm to the nuclear envelope. Consistent with this, microtubule assembly inhibitors profoundly depress viral replication (D. Kedes and DG, unpublished observations), but the exact mechanism of this inhibition remains uncertain (especially because these drugs display considerable nonspecific toxicity).

Once cores arrive at the nuclear envelope, they or their DNA contents must translocate across this structure. Some believe that core particles themselves are transported to the nucleus because (a) C protein is known to harbor nuclear localization signals in its C-terminus (120,390,601), and (b) the diameter of viral cores (about 25 to 27 nm) is just at the limit of the functional nuclear pore size as determined by experimental measurements in *Xenopus* species oocytes (136). However, the possibility that cores disassemble in the cytosol (perhaps at the nuclear pore) and deliver their DNA to the nucleus in nonparticulate form, as posited for adenovirus, has not been excluded (254). The exclusively cytosolic location of C protein in HBV transgenic mice (184,185) is sometimes cited as evidence in support of this notion. However, because such mice do not support cccDNA accumulation, it is difficult to know whether their phenotype is relevant to authentic viral infection—it may be that it is precisely their failure to transmit cores across their nuclear pore that underlies the absence of cccDNA in their nuclei. Recently, HBV core particle import into the nucleus has been examined in an *in vitro* system (631). Mature capsids purified from infected cells were presented to digitonin-permeablized cells in the presence of a cytoplasmic extract and adenosine triphosphate (ATP), a system in which soluble proteins competent for nuclear import are properly transported. HBV C protein accumulated efficiently in the target nuclei in particulate form. Interestingly, however, these particles appeared to lack viral DNA, suggesting that capsids might have released their genomes during or after import. Alternatively, cores might have disassembled during or after import, then reassembled within the nucleus once separated from their DNA.

Treatment of primary duck hepatocytes with glucagon has been shown to inhibit DHBV replication at a step occurring after receptor binding but before cccDNA formation—compatible with a block involving the cytoplasmic transport or nuclear translocation of cores (or their DNA) (209). Because glucagon modulates the activity of the cyclic adenosine monophosphate (cAMP)-dependent protein kinase A, it is tempting to speculate that at least one step in this process may be regulated by phosphorylation. However, the target of this phosphorylation remains unknown.

Once in the nucleus, the partially duplex viral DNA is repaired to the cccDNA form. This requires repair of the single-stranded gap, removal of the 5′-terminal structures (RNA and P protein), and covalent ligation of the strands. Several lines of evidence suggest that this process can be carried out largely by host machinery. The cloning of Dane particle DNA in *Escherichia coli* results in the recovery of fully duplex, superhelical plasmid clones in which the terminal structures have been correctly processed; thus, there would appear to be no need for viral machinery to effect these steps. Consistent with this notion, DHBV cccDNA formation in primary hepatocytes is not inhibited by phosphonoformate, a known inhibitor of P protein polymerase activity (267); however, the biochemical mechanisms by which the terminal structures are removed remain largely unknown.

Viral Transcription

Overview

Mammalian and avian hepadnaviruses use the circular 3-kb, cccDNA nuclear form of the genome as the template for viral transcription. Figure 2 shows the transcriptional organization of human HBV, which is similar to other mammalian hepadnaviruses. Avian hepadnaviruses differ from the related mammalian viruses in lacking an *X* gene ORF and an X promoter element. There are two classes of transcripts synthesized from cccDNA, known as the *genomic* and *subgenomic* classes, that have been identified in transfected cells in culture and in virus-infected liver. Both classes contain several transcripts, all are capped, and all are polyadenylated at a common polyadenylation sequence located within the core gene. The subgenomic transcripts function exclusively as messenger RNAs (mRNAs) for translation of the envelope pre-S1, pre-S2, S (also known as L, M, and S proteins) and X protein. The two genomic mRNAs encode the pre-C, C, and P ORFs. The C/P genomic mRNA is bifunctional, serving as the template for reverse transcription of the viral DNA negative strand (therefore known as *pregenomic RNA*), in addition to its role in translation of C and P protein products. The pre-C mRNA is not used for reverse transcription and functions only in translation of pre-C protein. Functional transcripts of the hepadnavirus genome are synthesized from the negative strand of the viral cccDNA template. RNAs transcribed from positive-stranded DNA, although detected in cells transfected in culture with viral genomic DNA, have not been found in infected cells or have not been found to encode viral polypeptides. None of the major hepadnavirus mRNAs contain classic introns. However, spliced viral transcripts have been detected for both avian and mammalian hepadnavirus mRNAs in cells transfected with genomic DNAs and in infected liver (74,508,517,529,586). Moreover, a spliced transcript encoding an alternately transcribed form of the S protein has been identified for the avian DHBV hepadnavirus in cultured hepatocytes and infected liver (375). Elimination of the spliced transcript by site-directed mutagenesis demonstrated that it is essential for viral replication in culture and in ducks. All of the hepadnavirus transcription elements, including promoters, enhancers, and the single polyadenylation signal, reside within viral genes that are actively transcribed and translated. This unusual arrangement reflects the compact organization of the hepadnavirus genome.

cis-Acting Transcription Elements

In HBV, the four overlapping ORFs are controlled by two enhancer elements and four (possibly five) promoters, corresponding to independent transcription from *pre-S1* (L protein), *pre-S2/S* (M and S proteins), *C* (core protein), *X* (X protein), and possibly *pre-C* (precore protein) genes (5,58,190,191,216,333,435,436,448,487,488,540, 553,591,600,619). The fine structure and function of the individual HBV promoters have been very well characterized and shown in Figure 4. Most studies have investigated the activity of individual DNA fragments and used site-directed mutagenesis to then map transcriptional promoters that direct transcription of reporter genes. Several studies have also examined the transcriptional activity of DNA regions in the context of the virus genome. From these studies, it can be concluded that the *pre-C/C, pre-S1, pre-S2/S,* and *X* genes are controlled by independent promoters. Transcription from the pre-C/C promoter (5,216,448,592) is highly restricted to liver (216,431). Studies in transfected cultured cells suggest that transcription of pre-C and C RNAs is controlled by two physically overlapping, but functionally distinct, promoters that are differentially regulated (72,305,610,611). Studies have not yet verified the dual disposition of the pre-C and

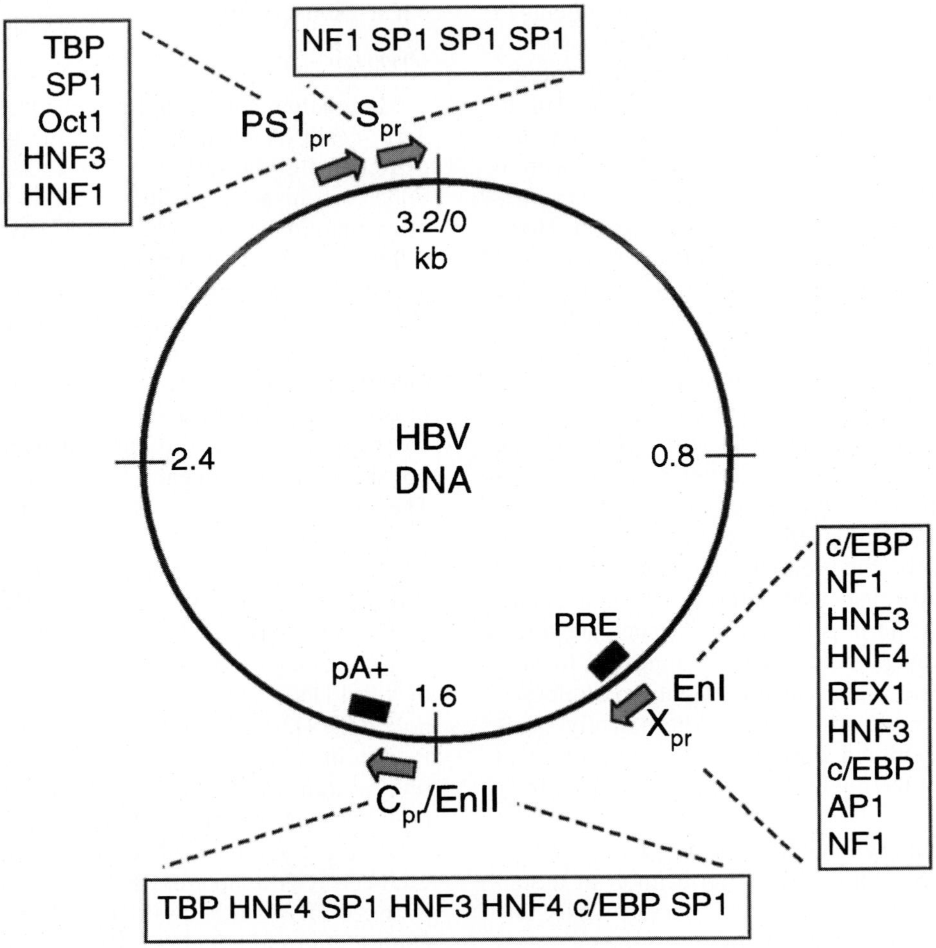

FIG. 4. Fine structure of hepatitis B virus promoter regions.

C promoters in infected cells. However, a frequently arising mutation in the presumptive pre-C promoter region has been documented in HBV-infected individuals, which results in selective down-regulation of pre-C mRNA and protein (50,305,459). These results are fully consistent with the separate regulation of transcription by pre-C and C promoters. The liver-specific expression of *C* gene transcription is thought to result from the combined requirement for multiple liver-enriched transcription factors in the pre-C/C promoter. These include factors c/EBP, HBF1, HNF3, and HNF4 (64,73,112,158,189, 249,321,322,430,437). The C promoter is thought to be controlled by both positive and negative regulation (431,611). Binding by the factor COUP-TF suppresses transcription from both promoters, HNF4 suppresses the presumptive pre-C promoter, and RXRα specifically enhances C promoter activity. Thus, part of the hepatotropism of HBV is likely attributable to liver-specific transcription of the C promoter, which is required for synthesis of pregenomic RNA.

The HBV pre-S1 promoter directs transcription of the 2.4-kb large envelope (pre-S1 or L [large] HBsAg mRNA). It is located immediately upstream of the pre-S1 protein AUG initiation codon (64,65,434,436). The pre-S1 promoter functions weakly within the context of the virus genome, and when tested independently of other viral transcription elements, is consistent with the low level of pre-S1 protein observed during infection (5,434, 436). The liver specificity of the pre-S1 promoter is derived from its dependence on liver-enriched transcription factor HNF1 (98). The S promoter directs transcription of several mRNAs of about 2.1 kb, which are translated to produce the pre-S2 (middle) and the S (small) HBsAg polypeptides (54,64,105,128,432,435,436,482, 487,622). The S promoter is located within the coding region of the *pre-S1* gene and lacks a classic TATA sequence (5,64), likely accounting for the transcriptional stuttering that gives rise to mRNAs that either contain or lack the pre-S2 translation AUG initiation codon. The S promoter is constitutively active in a wide range of cell types, although it is more active in hepatocyte-related cell lines and in the liver of transgenic mice (7,11,64,91,105, 128,132,133,499,501). The increased liver-specific transcription of the S promoter is probably related to the greater activity of enhancer II in hepatocytes (discussed later) (622).

The mammalian virus *X* gene mRNA is generally of low abundance *in vivo,* consistent with the low levels of X protein observed (101,102). When studied in transfected hepatoma cells independently of other viral elements, a region identified as the X promoter is considerably more active than in the context of the virus genome (5,190,434,488,540,543,592). In HBV, the X promoter is located adjacent to and downstream of enhancer I (EnI), which is within the ORF *P.* Based on transfection of cells with subgenomic HBV DNA fragments, the 5′ end of the X mRNA appears to initiate at heterogeneous sites (488,540,543), consistent with the absence of canonical TATA and CAAT elements. X-promoter activity involves binding of both liver-enriched transcription factors (e.g., c/EBP) and ubiquitous factors (e.g., AP-1, ATF/CREB) and is strongly augmented by EnI (5,27,111,112,127,148, 189,190,192,241,321,393,448,483,543).

Two genomic regions identified as EnI and EnII have been shown in HBV to fulfill the classic definition of transcriptional enhancer elements. These DNA fragments provide position- and orientation-independent stimulation of transcription when examined independently of viral genes in transient reporter assays (73,75,483,531, 572,600,614). Regions corresponding to HBV EnI and EnII were also found to display DNase hypersensitivity patterns consistent with transcriptional activity when examined as integrants in transgenic mice (1), consistent with their identification as enhancer elements. Although both EnI and EnII can increase transcription from a variety of heterologous promoters, the activity of EnII is largely restricted to hepatic cells (600,615). HBV EnI functions in both hepatic and nonhepatic cells, although it more strongly activates transcription in hepatocytes (5,148,241,483,559,613,615). Accordingly, EnI has been shown to be activated by the binding of both ubiquitous and liver-enriched transcription factors, including c/EBP, HBF4, and HBLF (27,127,148,158,189,384,386,490, 543). Although EnI is located adjacent to and upstream of the X promoter (and within the ORF *P*), it strongly upregulates all of the major HBV promoters, both in heterologous reporter constructs and in the native context of the viral genome (5,225). WHV probably does not contain a region equivalent to HBV EnI (108). EnII is located within the ORF *X* and is adjacent to the pre-C/C promoter that directs transcription of pregenomic RNAs (600,615). EnII is a bipartite element that contains binding sites for, and is activated by, a constellation of liver-enriched transcription factors, including the c/EBP family of proteins, HBF1, HNF3, HNF4, and possibly a novel factor known as hB1F (189,249,283,307,308,321,322,431,433,625). One factor (E4BP4) has also been identified as a negative regulator of EnII, based on studies using artificial reporter constructs (283). In a similar manner, a negative regulatory element was identified within EnII that suppresses its activity (314). EnII strongly promotes liver-specific transcription of the pregenomic C promoter, and possibly X and S promoters, but not the pre-S1 promoter, for unknown reasons (108,216,308,322,506,572,614, 624). It was also shown by mutagenesis of EnII that within the context of the viral genome, transcription of the viral genome is significantly (more than 10-fold) reduced with EnII impairment (576).

In addition to its role in activating viral transcription in a liver-specific manner, EnII plays an important role in oncogenesis by WHV. Unlike HBV, which integrates apparently at random, woodchuck hepatocellular carcinoma (HCC) tumors usually contain WHV sequences integrated from 2 to 200 kb away from the two *N-myc* gene loci (141,144,222). The genetic arrangement of WHV–cellular gene junctions of genomic integrants implicated WHV EnII in up-regulation of *N-myc* genes (126,574). This is supported by studies using artificial constructs in which EnII was shown to be capable of directly activating *N-myc* genes (553,574).

Transcriptional Regulation of the Hepadnavirus Genome

The congested architecture of hepadnaviral transcriptional elements, with promoter and enhancer elements embedded within coding regions and physically adjacent or overlapping, necessitates complex regulatory controls. Studies have begun to examine transcriptional regulation of the hepadnavirus genome. The ratio of pre-S1 to pre-S2/S transcription appears to be one such form of regulation and is an important control point in the viral life cycle. The pre-S1 L protein product acts as an inhibitor of virus secretion (described later), and therefore its level must be tightly controlled. When assayed in reporter constructs independent of other viral genes, the pre-S1 and pre-S2/S promoters display similar activities, whereas in the context of the viral genome, the pre-S1 promoter is much less active (5). The S promoter down-regulates the pre-S1 promoter in the context of the HBV genome (54,323). Down-regulation is attributed to interference in pre-S1 transcriptional elongation, possibly by a CCAAT/NF-Y–binding element (323,324). Other complex regulatory circuits are emerging as well. In DHBV, an active C promoter appears to impair the usage of downstream pre-S and S promoters (228). The mechanism of promoter occlusion is thought to be involved, in which elongating transcription complexes originating from the C promoter impair pre-S1 and S promoters by passing through. Despite the fact that the pre-S1 promoter is located immediately upstream of the S promoter, there is no evidence for promoter occlusion in this complex arrangement.

Hepadnavirus Posttranscriptional Regulatory Element

RNA splicing in eukaryotes is tightly coupled to 3′ end formation and export of the RNA from the nucleus to the cytoplasm (373). Consequently, intronless RNAs are poorly exported to the cytoplasm. A number of animal viruses encode intronless mRNAs that nevertheless efficiently accumulate in the cytoplasm. To overcome the export restriction to intronless RNAs, hepadnaviruses use a large RNA element known as the *posttranscriptional regulatory element* (PRE) (reviewed in 604). The PRE is located partially within the X promoter and ORF and downstream of the ORF *S,* indicating that it is contained in all viral transcripts (227,230,231,560). The PRE was shown to promote directly the export of unspliced transcripts. The HBV PRE and the HIV Rev response element (RRE), which performs a similar function, are largely but not completely interchangeable (113,231). However, the HBV PRE is not dependent on HBV proteins for export activity, whereas the HIV RRE requires binding by HIV Rev protein (227,230,231). The HBV PRE is conserved in mammalian hepadnaviruses, and a similar element has been described in WHV (114,630). The mechanism by which the PRE functions is not well understood. In contrast to the HIV RRE–Rev complex, the HBV PRE is not inhibited by the antibiotic leptomycin B, which poisons the nuclear export signal (NES) receptor CRM1/exportin-1 (387).

Processing of Viral RNA

The co-terminal nature of the viral transcripts (see Fig. 2) poses an interesting problem in the control of RNA processing. The subgenomic mRNAs are efficiently polyadenylated at a signal within ORF *C.* The genomic RNAs, being terminally redundant, contain two copies of this signal: one at the 5′ end of the transcript and one at the 3′ end. Thus, the transcriptional apparatus, which efficiently polyadenylates at this signal in subgenomic RNAs, must bypass this signal on its first pass in genomic RNA synthesis but use it efficiently on its second pass. (This problem is formally analogous to that encountered in retroviral genomic RNA synthesis, in which polyadenylation signals embedded in the 5′-LTR are ignored, but identical signals in the 3′-LTR are used).

Exactly how this problem is solved is still somewhat unclear, but the elements of the solution have at least been identified. Canonical eukaryotic poly(A) signals include the hexanucleotide AAUAAA, a cleavage site about 30 nucleotides downstream, and a U- or GU-rich element 3′ to the cleavage site. Mammalian hepadnaviruses have polyadenylation signals that resemble these canonical signals, with one exception: the hexanucleotide is UAUAAA, which is known to function inefficiently. To bolster the efficiency of hepadnaviral RNA processing, the virus has evolved additional elements upstream of the hexanucleotide that enhance its use (455). Some of these elements are 5′ to the genomic RNA cap site, such that full processing efficiency is possible only at the 3′ end of the RNA. However, beyond this, it appears the the proximity of the 5′ processing site to the 5′ end of the RNA somehow drastically curtails its use (78,79). The mechanism by which cap-site proximity exerts this effect is unknown, but similar effects have been observed in cellular and retroviral transcripts (238).

X Protein and Its Role in the Virus Life Cycle

X Protein Is Required for Mammalian Hepadnavirus Infection in Animals

The small ORF located between EnI and the single polyadenylation signal of the HBV, WHV, and GSHV genome is referred to as the *X* gene, *HBx* or *pX,* originally reflecting a lack of evidence for gene expression. Subsequently, several groups showed that some infected individuals develop antibodies to X protein during natural infection (208,257,304), and X protein was detected by radioimmunoassay in some infected patients (407). The ORF *X* is contained within all of the mammalian hepadnavirus mRNAs, given its location just upstream of the single polyadenylation signal. However, a 0.7- to 1-kb RNA, corresponding solely to the ORF *X,* has been detected in hepatoma cells transfected with the entire HBV genome (191), and a specific *X* gene promoter was identified in transfected cells (190,509). It is assumed, but not proven, that the X protein is translated from the 0.7- to 1-kb transcript rather than from the core, pre-S1, or S antigen mRNAs through internal ribosome entry. An *X* gene–specific transcript was also detected in the livers of woodchucks chronically infected with WHV (102, 253). In HBV-infected human liver tissue, a putative *X* gene mRNA was indirectly detected by reverse transcription–polymerase chain reaction amplification of X region–specific RNA (109,394). Although X protein has been detected in infected liver tissue (304,407,618), it is often difficult to do so because the protein is poorly immunogenic and has a short half-life (101,460). Consequently, it has been shown that immunohistochemical detection of X protein in infected liver tissue with certain antibodies can represent cross-reaction to cellular polypeptides (416,507). Nevertheless, it has been possible to unambiguously detect X protein in acute and chronically infected woodchuck livers using high-affinity, multiple X protein–specific antibodies (102,240), where it is estimated to accumulate at 10,000 to 50,000 copies per cell (102). HBV X protein has been detected by a similar approach in infected human liver (416,507).

Seminal studies from Zoulim and colleagues (628) and Chen and associates (70) demonstrated that X protein performs an essential (but still unknown) function in WHV infection of woodchucks. Wild-type WHV genomic DNA, which expresses X protein, establishes an infection and an easily detectable viremia when directly injected into the liver of young woodchucks. Mutation of the *X* gene in a manner that does not disrupt the overlying Pol reading frame, either by elimination of the ORF *X* AUG codon or by severely truncating the COOH-terminus of the X protein, fully blocks establishment of infection. It was concluded that X protein performs an essential function in the infectious cycle of the virus, possibly to initiate or maintain viral replication, because there was no detectable level of WHV in serum or in liver tissue (628). This is consistent with a report that X protein expression strongly co-localized with active centers of WHV replication in the liver of chronically infected woodchucks (102). Consequently, HBV X protein is also thought to be essential for human infection. Although a replication function for X protein in viral infection still remains to be described in animal models, the first standard by which to consider various X protein activities is the requirement for viral infection in animals.

X Protein Is a Weak Transcriptional Activator

By comparing the location of the ORF *X* in the HBV genome to the genetic organization of complex retroviruses, it was proposed that the 154–amino acid (17-kd) X protein might possess transcriptional transactivating activity similar to the regulatory proteins Tat of HIV and Tax of human T-cell lymphotropic virus type I (HTLV-I) (350). HBV X protein was subsequently shown to possess a moderate ability (3- to 10-fold) to stimulate transcription of reporter genes (495,549). Subsequently, many reports demonstrated that HBV, WHV, and GSHV X proteins display a weak to moderate ability to stimulate transcription of a wide variety of enhancers and promoters (reviewed in 450 and 603). These include viral elements, such as the SV40 early promoter, the HIV LTR, the HSV tyrosine kinase promoter, and HBV EnI (303,480,486, 488,495,549,584,616). Cellular promoter elements stimulated by X protein include those for interleukin-8, c-fos, c-myc, class I major histocompatibility complex, and tumor necrosis factor-α (TNF-α), among others (9,10,12, 171,288,332,623; an extensive list can be found in 450). X protein also stimulates RNA pol I– and pol III–dependent promoters (adenovirus virion associated (VA) RNA, cellular transfer RNA [tRNA], and U6 elements) (6,8, 282,563–565). RNA pol II transcriptional elements activated by the X protein usually contain a DNA-binding site for either NF-κB, AP-1, AP-2, c-EBP, ATF/CREB, or the calcium-activated factor NF-AT, among others (129, 258,287,303,325,331,332,478,547,548,583). Biochemical evidence for activation of DNA-binding activity of NF-κB, AP-1, ATF/CREB, and NF-AT was also obtained (15,29,83,287,331,367,504,577,583).

The effect of X protein on HBV, WHV, and GSHV transcription elements is consistent with the weak transactivation observed for non-HBV transcriptional elements. When studied within the context of the whole viral genome in transfected hepatoma cells, most studies found that expression of X protein stimulates a modest increase (threefold to eightfold) in accumulation of viral mRNAs (94,263,295,362,594,628), although no effect on transcription was also observed in certain cell lines (34). These results imply that stimulation of transcription may not be a critical function of X protein during infection. Weak up-regulation of viral transcription is also not consistent with the absolute requirement for X protein in WHV infection (628). If the major function of X protein is to stimulate viral transcription slightly, then in its absence, there should be only a concomitant decrease in viremia. In contrast, serum and tissue levels of virus are actually undetectable in the absence of X protein expression (628).

Although it is possible during whole animal infection that X protein might stimulate viral transcription much more strongly than in cultured cells, there is presently no evidence to support this contention. Transgenic mice have been developed to express the HBV X protein specifically in the liver. When crossed with mice that express a reporter gene controlled by the HIV LTR, liver-specific expression of the reporter was increased by only three to six times (13). Therefore, X protein only modestly stimulates transcription of a wide variety of different elements, whether expressed in the context of the whole viral genome, independently in transfected cells, or in the liver of experimental animals. The importance of this weak transactivation activity in establishment of infection and virus replication remains to be determined in relevant animal models.

Mechanism of X Protein Action

Overview

A considerable amount of effort has been directed toward understanding the fundamental molecular activity of X protein. Although there has traditionally been little consensus regarding a common mechanism of action of X protein, several patterns have emerged, which are summarized here and reviewed later.

1. X protein is found largely in the cytoplasm and in small amounts in the nucleus of cells, whether expressed independently of other viral genes in transfected cells, in the context of HBV or WHV genomes, or in infected livers of humans and woodchucks (101,102,115,206,240, 287,380,416,492,507,577). A few studies have described X protein as a predominantly nuclear protein in cell lines (202,214,488). In two of these instances (214,488), the nuclear location of X protein can be explained by the coexpression of SV40 large T antigen, which mediates nuclear accumulation of certain proteins, including X protein (115,479). Cytoplasmic X protein has not been found in association with organelles (115), although there is the possibility of an association with proteasomes (226,492).

2. X protein probably functions by several distinct mechanisms, which include direct interaction with components of the transcriptional machinery and stimulation of cytoplasmic signal transduction pathways.

3. The molecular actions of X protein are not restricted to transcriptional activation. Several studies concur that a fraction of X protein interacts with a probable DNA repair protein, known as UVDDB, which might affect viral replication, pathogenesis, and carcinoma (26,30; for an extensive review, see 56, 296, and 493). Whether X protein interaction with UVDDB alters nucleotide excision repair is presently unresolved. Using essentially similar assay systems to measure excision repair fidelity and frequency, several groups observed a slight to moderate decrease on expression of X protein (26,177,245,420), whereas another report did not (30). X protein has also been widely reported either to induce or sensitize cells to induction of apoptosis by pro-apoptotic cytokines and chemical agents in experimental cell systems and transgenic mice (30,84,261,505,528). However, in some systems, X protein is found to inhibit induction of cellular apoptosis (122,172,571), and the relationship of these observations to viral pathogenesis in animals and humans has not been investigated.

4. X protein is probably only weakly oncogenic at best, perhaps contributing indirectly to development of HCC (for an extensive review, see 4). Although X protein expressed in the liver of transgenic mice was originally reported to strongly promote tumorigenesis (259), this has not been found in subsequent studies, except perhaps at supraphysiologic levels of X protein expression (53,271,297). Moreover, studies implicating X protein interaction with, and impairment of, cellular p53 protein (134,541,570) have not been substantiated in more recent investigations (426, reviewed in 603). However, X protein was found to moderately promote development of HCC in the liver of transgenic mice coexpressing the *c-myc* gene (528) or when animals were exposed to hepatocarcinogens at levels that do not independently promote tumor development (102,494). Thus, it is probably correct to conclude that X protein expression is slightly pro-oncogenic.

X Protein Interacts with Several Components of the Transcriptional Apparatus

Most studies agree that X protein does not act by directly binding DNA (evidence reviewed in 603). Through interaction-cloning techniques using overexpressed proteins, it was shown that X protein associates with several components of the basal transcription machinery, including factors TFIIB and TFIIH, the RPB5 subunit of RNA polymerases, and TATA-binding protein (77,201,203,311,358,427,428). In these studies, coassociation of X protein and components of the basal transcription apparatus was observed in mammalian cells upon overexpression of both X and target proteins. Nevertheless, it is still possible that low levels of X-interacting complexes are sufficient to stimulate transcription but cannot be readily detected. X protein also directly interacts, *in vitro* and in cells upon overexpression, with the cyclic adenosine monophosphate (cAMP) response element–binding protein (CREB), a b-Zip family transcription factor (331,583). Evidence that X protein possesses a nuclear function in transcription, possibly by interaction with transcription components, is derived from three sets of observations:

1. X protein can stimulate transcription if tethered to a DNA-binding domain (202,478), which is consistent

with, but does not prove, a direct mode of transcriptional activation.

2. X protein directly interacts with the basic leucine zipper region of CREB (583), which is involved in DNA-binding activity, and increases CREB affinity for its DNA-binding site by an order of magnitude (15,391,583). Occupation of the HBV EnI ATF/CREB-binding site is strongly enhanced *in vitro* by X protein interaction with CREB and correlates with CREB-dependent transcriptional activation of this element *in vivo* by X protein expression (4,15, 399,583). A similar mechanism of action was described for X protein interaction with another b-Zip transcription factor, cEBPα (90).
3. X protein engineered to contain a nuclear localization signal, and shown to accumulate exclusively in the nucleus, strongly stimulates transcription from an EnI reporter construct in transfected cells, but no longer activates transcription dependent on factors NF-κB and AP-1 (115).

It should now be possible, using experimental approaches such as nuclear-targeted X protein, to determine whether nuclear activation of transcription occurs in the context of viral replication and whether it plays a role in the viral life cycle, pathogenesis, or transformation.

X Protein Stimulates Cytoplasmic Signal Transduction Pathways

Evidence from a number of groups indicates that X protein in the cytoplasm activates several related signal transduction pathways. It was first shown that dominant-inhibiting forms of the kinase Raf, an effector of the Ras-Raf-MAP kinase signal transduction pathway, could block X protein–induced activation of transcription factor AP-1–dependent transcription, as shown in transient transfection studies (99). It was then shown that a dominant-inhibiting form of Ras also blocks X protein activation of AP-1–dependent transcription (28,367,368). X protein increased Ras activity by increasing guanosine triphosphate (GTP) loading onto Ras, not by altering Ras-GAP activity (29). Importantly, the magnitude of Ras activation by X protein is not like that of growth factor stimulation, which strongly but transiently stimulates Ras. Rather, X protein only modestly stimulates Ras, but the activation is sustained or at least periodic (29,206). X protein stimulation of the Ras-Raf-MAP kinase pathway is critical for activation of transcription factor AP-1 in transiently transfected cells (28,29,97,99,115,262,367,368,504). More recently, X protein was found to stimulate Ras-Raf-MAP kinase signal transduction when expressed in the context of replicating HBV or WHV in hepatoma cells in culture (262,263). X protein stimulation of Ras was also found to be essential for its activation of RNA pol I– and pol III–dependent transcription in stably transfected insect cells (563–565). Thus, the ability of X protein to stimulate Ras is observed in a variety of cell types under different conditions. Retargeting X protein to the nucleus, by fusion to a nuclear localization signal, abolished activation of the Ras pathway (115). The activation of cytoplasmic signaling pathways by X protein is consistent with its predominant cytoplasmic location.

X protein was also shown to stimulate the stress-activated protein kinase (SAPK)-NH2-terminal-Jun kinase (JNK) pathway (29). This pathway is primarily activated by the Ras-related G protein Rac (107). Activation of the SAPK-JNK pathway by X protein was shown by several groups working with a variety of different cell lines, under different conditions (29,206,522; O. Andrisani, personal communication). Thus, there is good evidence that X protein stimulates Ras-Raf-MAP kinase and SAPK-JNK signal transduction pathways in the cytoplasm of a variety of different cells, whether expressed independently of other viral genes or from viral genomes during viral replication. It is not known whether these signal transduction pathways are activated by X protein in natural infection of animals and humans.

Although studies uniformly concur that X protein activates transcription factor NF-κB, whether activation of Ras or other signaling pathways is involved is not resolved. One report found an essential requirement for X protein stimulation of protein kinase C in activation of NF-κB (258), whereas others did not (99,325,358,368, 504). Two studies found that Ras signaling is necessary for NF-κB activation (115,504), whereas another did not (83). These discrepancies may result from the fact that NF-κB consists of multiple related proteins that may be activated to different extents in different ways (343,617). Related NF-κB proteins include p65/RelA, c-rel, and p105 (617). In most cells, NF-κB is sequestered in the cytoplasm, bound to inhibiting IκB proteins, which release NF-κB when phosphorylated by the IκB kinase (617). It has been reported that X protein directly binds to the cytoplasmic IκBα protein when both are overexpressed, mediating direct release of NF-κB and becoming transported to the nucleus (577). However, two previous studies did not detect direct interaction of X protein with endogenous NF-κB or IκB (83,504).

Activation of Ras by X protein is indirect because it has not been found in association with Ras, Ras-GAP, the GTP exchange factor Sos, or Ras adapter proteins Grb2 or Shc (29,262). More recent studies demonstrated that X protein activates Ras by activating the nonreceptor tyrosine kinases of the Src family, which are upstream activators of Ras GTPases (262). X protein constitutively activated Src kinases when expressed from WHV or HBV genomes during viral replication in cultured hepatoma cells and when expressed independently of the viral genome. Activation of Src kinases was modest (twofold to fourfold), as observed for X activation of Ras-signaling pathways. Additional evidence consistent with X protein activation of Src kinases includes X protein activation of the JAK-STAT signaling pathway (299), which is directly activated by Src kinases (544,607).

It is possible that some of the complications and contrasting results in the field of X protein research may be related to the finding that expression of the *X* gene in transfected cells can give rise to several related X proteins by alternate ribosome initiation at several in-frame AUG codons by leaky ribosome scanning (256,282,362,369, 621). Although multiple X protein products have not been detected during replication of WHV in cultured cells (101,102), in transfected cells, they can apparently be synthesized from certain constructs and display somewhat different activities (282,362). Thus, expression of different related X proteins (whether biologically relevant or not) could influence different mechanisms of activation.

Possible Function of X Protein in Virus Infection and Replication

The molecular function of X protein in infection of animals and humans has not been investigated. However, studies have examined the function of X protein in WHV and HBV replication in cultured cells. Using cell culture systems, the activation of Src kinases by X protein, but not Ras, was found to stimulate HBV and WHV replication in hepatoma cell lines (263). In this system, ablation of X protein expression by mutation of the *X* gene impairs HBV and WHV replication 5- to 20-fold (94,263,295, 347,362,594,628). Accordingly, inhibition of Src kinases impaired HBV and WHV replication 10- to 15-fold at the levels of reverse transcription of pregenomic core-associated RNA, and second-stranded DNA synthesis (263). Viral-specific transcription and translation were reduced only twofold to fourfold. However, it is not known whether X protein stimulates Src kinases during natural infection, nor whether the molecular function of Src kinases in viral replication is the same as in hepatoma cells. Importantly, activation of Src kinases cannot account for the entire function of X protein in viral replication in cultured cells because a constitutively activated form of Src only partially replaced X protein function (263). The mechanism by which X protein activates Src kinases has not been established, but it appears to involve calcium-dependent activation of the tyrosine kinase Pyk2 (M. Bouchard and R. Schneider, unpublished results), which is an upstream, calcium-dependent entry point into the Src pathway (110,302). Given X protein stimulation of calcium-dependent transcription factor NF-AT (287), it is possible that a fundamental activity of X protein is to release intracellular calcium, which could account for many of the reported activities of X protein.

Translation of Viral Gene Products

Hepadnaviruses have evolved multiple transcriptional and translational strategies to maximize the use of the limited coding capacity of their DNA. As previously noted, they make extensive use of overlapping reading frames (see Fig. 2), and within reading frames, they often employ multiple initiation codons to generate structurally related but functionally distinct proteins. Because of their 5′-scanning mechanism, host ribosomes tend not to initiate internally with high efficiency (277). Thus, to guarantee host ribosomes access to these internal AUG codons, the viral transcriptional program has deployed separate mRNA 5′ ends just 5′ to each AUG. In the case of the envelope proteins, it does this by (a) employing a dedicated promoter for the pre-S1 mRNAs, and (b) having the TATA-less S promoter display microheterogeneity of its start sites, such that some begin 5′ to the pre-S2 AUG and others just 3′ to it (58,499). In this way, both M and S proteins can be translated as the first ORF of a transcript (see Fig. 2).

Heterogeneous start sites also characterize the genomic promoter, whose RNA 5′ ends bracket the pre-C AUG. Those initiating 3′ to this AUG encode the C protein, the structural protein of the nucleocapsid (123,355,581). Those initiating 5′ to this AUG encode the pre-C protein, which enjoys an altogether different biosynthetic fate. The pre-C region encodes a signal sequence that targets this protein to the secretory pathway (159,388,498). After cleavage of the signal in the ER lumen, the protein is transported through the vesicular transport system, undergoing cleavage of its basic C-terminal region in the process (242,243,462,498,569). Ultimately, it is secreted from the cell, accumulating in the extracellular medium (or serum) as the 17-kd protein known serologically as *e antigen* (HBeAg). In a minority of chains, ER translocation is aborted after signal peptide cleavage, and the resulting products are returned to the cytosol (159) or even the nucleus (390). The significance of these unusual events is uncertain. HBeAg immunoreactivity can also be found on the plasma membrane (462,466), although the mechanism of this cell surface localization is not well defined.

The function of HBeAg is still unknown. Clearly, it is dispensable for replication *in vitro* because nonsense or frameshift mutations within pre-C grow relatively well in cultured cells or in experimental animals (62,71,465, 467). However, clinical studies of human HBV carriers show that during persistent infection, mutant viruses with pre-C lesions spontaneously and regularly arise, often coming to prevail over the wild-type virus after years of carriage (41,42,188,382,456,457,538). Transmission of these mutants confirms that they are infectious (198). This implies that there is some selection against HBeAg expression. Such a selection has also been seen in some experimental infections with mixtures of wild-type and pre-C–mutant DHBV isolates, although it is not a uniform occurrence in that setting (620). Because deliberate overexpression of pre-C can interfere with wild-type replication (186), it is conceivable that normal levels of pre-C expression may confer a subtle growth disadvantage on the wild-type genome. Alternatively, host immunologic attack on HBeAg-bearing cells may select against cells infected by viruses expressing pre-C polypeptides. Whatever the mechanism of selection, all this raises a deeper paradox that is as yet unresolved: if there is a selection against pre-C products at the level of the individual host, how has the *pre-C* gene been maintained in the population? No entirely satisfactory answer to this question has yet been forthcoming. One proposal is that HBeAg may serve as a neonatal tolerogen (348); if so, transmission of pre-C–positive viruses could be selected for during vertical transmission because the induction of neonatal immune tolerance to HBV would promote the development of chronic infection in the infected baby. However, experimental studies do not show an important effect of pre-C proteins on immune function (440). Thus, the forces selecting for or against pre-C expression remain deeply enigmatic at present.

The genomic RNA species that initiates downstream of the pre-C AUG is the mRNA not only for C protein but also for P protein. Evidence that this is so comes from several sources: (a) it is the only identified viral transcript bearing the entire P coding region; (b) no viral transcripts have been identified with 5′ ends just upstream of the P AUG, despite vigorous and sensitive searches; and (c) the fact that DHBV pregenomic RNAs are infectious (229) implies that P protein must have been translated from the input RNA. Examination of the coding organization of pgRNA shows that ORF *P* overlaps the 3′ end of the upstream *C* gene; the P frame is +1 relative to the C frame. This organization recalls that of most retroviruses, whose upstream core gene (*gag*) overlaps the downstream polymerase gene (*pol*); there, however, the *pol* reading frame is −1 relative to that of *gag*. In those cases, the retroviral polymerase is expressed as a gag-pol polyprotein by ribosomal frameshifting in the overlap region (239). Early assumptions that this would prove true for hepadnaviruses seemed to be supported by the finding of proteins with both C and P immunoreactivity in HBV-infected liver samples (582). However, genetic studies with DHBV soon established that polymerase is made by *de novo* initiation at the P initiator rather than by C-P frameshifting. These studies showed that (a) mutation of the first P AUG to an ACU codon inactivates DNA synthesis; (b) stop codons in ORF *P* located 3′ but not 5′ to this AUG inactivate polymerase activity; and (c) *C* gene frameshift mutations do not impair the production of P protein (66,68,464). Subsequent experiments in HBV confirmed these findings and indicated that missense mutations in the P AUG could be reverted by construction of a new, in-frame AUG either upstream or downstream of the original mutation (244,454).

The mechanism by which ribosomes gain access to this internal AUG remains incompletely understood. Attempts to identify internal ribosome entry sequences of the type that function in picornavirus translation have failed, and *P* gene translation appears fully sensitive to poliovirus superinfection (66), suggesting that, like most translational events, it is cap dependent. Elaborate genetic studies have led to a model that invokes modified ribosomal scanning from the 5′ end of genomic RNA. In this model, ribosomes scan from the cap site until they reach a small ORF overlapping the *C* gene; translation of this ORF allows bypass of a strong out-of-frame AUG that would otherwise occlude scanning further downstream, thereby allowing ribosomes that originated at the 5′ end of the transcript access to the internal P AUG (140).

Genomic Replication

The Viral Polymerase

Early inferences that ORF *P* encoded the viral polymerase were strongly supported by the recognition of homology between this coding region and those of retroviral reverse transcriptases (532). Since then, many other reverse transcriptases have been identified from numerous sources, and all of them share sequence relatedness to the hepadnaviral enzyme. Sequence alignments between these coding regions reveal the existence of subregions with obvious homology to either other polymerases (including RNA-directed RNA and DNA polymerases) or to *E. coli* RNaseH (67,212,429,468). Mutational analysis of retroviral *pol* genes has confirmed that these regions indeed represent functional domains that control the polymerase and RNaseH activities of the retroviral enzyme (521). In hepadnaviruses, the polymerase homology domain is centrally located, whereas the RNaseH homology region is located near the C-terminus of the chain (Fig. 5).

In retroviruses and many retrotransposons, polymerase genes also encode protease and endonuclease activities, and recognizable homologies also characterize each of these activities. As might have been anticipated from the absence of a known role for integration in the growth of hepadnaviruses, no homology exists between ORF *P* and the integrases of other reverse-transcribing elements. Similarly, no functional protease homologies have been located within ORF *P* (or ORF *C*) (364), consistent with the fact that P protein is not processed from a C-P polyprotein.

The functional significance of these homology-based domain assignments has been validated *in vivo* through the study of mutant viral genomes bearing lesions in these regions. HBV and DHBV mutants bearing point mutations in highly conserved residues within the polymerase homology region are defective for viral DNA synthesis, whereas certain mutations within the RNaseH homology region allow negative-stranded but not positive-stranded DNA synthesis (67,130,429). Just upstream

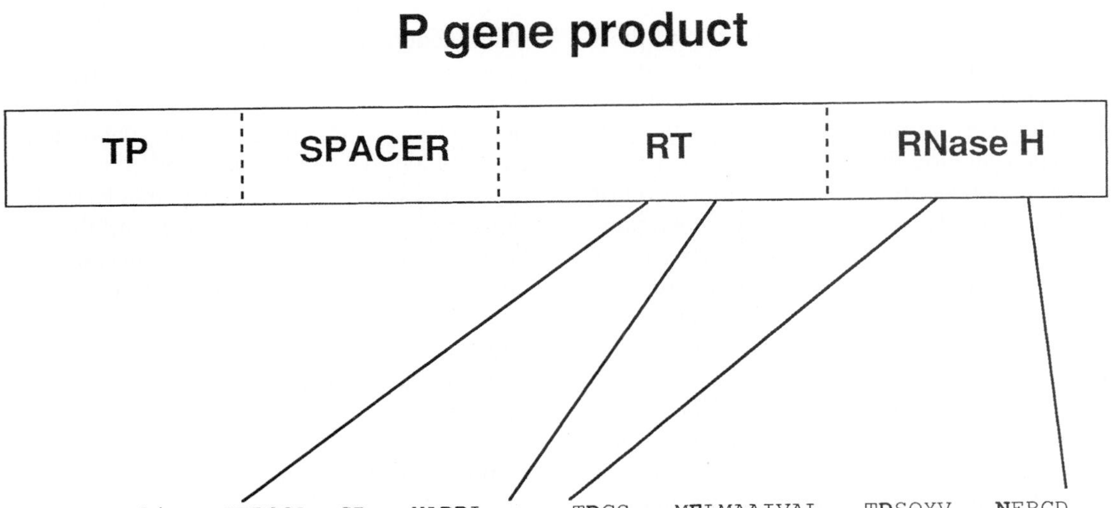


```
E. coli ...LLPQGA--SP...YADDL......TDGS...MELMAAIVAL...TDSQYV...NERCD
Ty1      ...APPPHL--ND...FVDDM......
Copia    ...ALPQGI--NS...YVDDV......
RSV     ...VLPQGM--SP...YMDDL......TDAS...LEARAVAMAL...TDSAFV...NDVAD
MoMLV   ...RLPQGF--SP...YVDDL......TDGS...AELIALTQAL...TDSRYA...NRMAD
BLV     ...VLPQGF--SP...YMDDI......SDGA...GELAGLLAGL...VDSKYL...NNYVD
HIV     ...VLPQGW--SP...YMDDL......VDGA...TELQAIYLAL...TDSQYA...NEQVD
CaMV    ...VVPFGL--AP...YVDDI......TDAS...KETLAVINTI...TDNTHF...NHFAD
HBV      ...KIPMGV--SP...YMDDV......ADAT...AELLAACFAR...TDNSVV...NP AD
DHBV     ...KAPMGV--SP...YMDDF......TDAT...QELIMSCLAK...SDSTFV...NP AD

               Conserved RT                        Conserved RNaseH
```

FIG. 5. Domain structure of the hepadnaviral P protein. **Top:** Schematic depiction of the functional domains of P protein. TP, terminal protein; RT, reverse transcriptase; RNaseH, ribonuclease H. **Bottom:** Amino acid sequence alignments with other RNA-dependent DNA polymerases; these homologies form the basis of the assignment of the RT and RNaseH domains.

of the polymerase homology region, overlapping the pre-S coding domain, is a region of the *P* gene that is apparently unrelated to other polymerases and displays high sequence divergence between different hepadnaviral *P* genes. This region appears to define an unessential portion of the P protein because it tolerates a wide variety of substitution, deletion, and insertion mutations (18,67,306); 5′ to it is the region implicated in the covalent linkage of the P protein to the viral DNA (see later). For this reason, the unessential region is often referred to as a "spacer" or "tether" region connecting the terminal protein (TP) domain to the polymerase and RNaseH domains (see Fig. 5).

Owing to the low abundance of P protein *in vivo,* it has been difficult to visualize P chains in virions. Attempts to do so by immunoblotting (329) or activity gel analysis (20,374) have often revealed species of less than full length, raising the question of posttranslational proteolytic processing. However, by engineering a protein kinase recognition site into the P chain (17), investigators were able to visualize directly encapsidated P chains after their phosphorylation *in vitro;* these studies strongly suggest that cores bear full-length P chains.

RNA Encapsidation

The classic experiments of Summers and Mason (510) indicated that virtually all reverse transcription takes place within subviral core particles, thereby implying that encapsidation of the genomic RNA template must represent the initial step in the genomic replication pathway. As noted previously, hepadnaviral genomic RNAs display microheterogeneities at their 5′ ends (see Fig. 2), with the longer ones encoding pre-C proteins and the smallest one encoding the C and P gene products. Importantly, only the smallest genomic mRNA is encapsidated into the core particle (124), indicating that only this transcript (pgRNA) can serve as a template for reverse transcription; host RNAs, subgenomic RNAs, and even the closely similar longer genomic transcripts are excluded. (The basis of this fine discrimination among such closely related RNAs will be discussed later).

The viral proteins required for encapsidation have been identified by examining the impact of mutations in individual genes on pgRNA packaging. As expected, C protein is required to form the structure into which the RNA is packaged (212,293). Capsid formation is independent of pgRNA packaging: isolated *C* gene expression in heterologous hosts results in the accumulation of morphologically normal capsids devoid of pgRNA (33,93,388, 448,580,626,627). However, such recombinant capsids do contain host and viral RNAs, which are encapsidated by virtue of the sequence-nonspecific nucleic acid–binding properties of the arginine-rich C-terminal domain of the molecule (33,153,199,363). (Deletion of this region still allows capsid formation, but not RNA encapsidation.) Assembly of capsids proceeds through C protein dimer intermediates (627); these dimers form very rapidly, perhaps even while the chains are still nascent (63). Once the dimers have reached a threshold concentration (estimated at 1 μmol), a sharply cooperative assembly reaction takes place to yield intact capsids (476). In general, no higher-order assembly intermediates can be detected *in vivo* between dimers and capsids. As a result, it is not yet known exactly where in this sequence the addition of RNA occurs.

The fine structure of recombinant HBV core particles produced by C protein expression in *E. coli* has been examined by cryoelectron microscopy (38) and x-ray crystallography (588). The individual C monomers have a unique folding pattern, unrelated to the β-barrel structure so often seen in capsid proteins in other viruses. Dimerization of these monomers occurs through association of two amphipathic α-helical hairpins, generating a four-helix bundle that protrudes from the capsid surface as a spike. Surprisingly, two different particle structures form in *E. coli*: T=3 capsids containing 180 C subunits, and T=4 structures containing 240 such subunits (38). Both particle types seem likely to exist *in vivo,* but it is unclear which can support formation of an infectious virion in the presence of pgRNA and the remaining viral proteins (or if both can do so). It is equally unclear what forces govern the assembly of C into these distinct structures.

In addition to the expected requirement for C protein, P gene products are also necessary for RNA packaging (16,212). Null mutations in ORF *P* result in cores with reduced or undetectable levels of pregenomic RNA. The P protein function required for packaging can be dissociated from those involved in DNA synthesis: many missense mutations that ablate polymerase or RNaseH activity are still competent for RNA encapsidation (212,429, 453). This requirement for polymerase gene products in packaging of viral RNA is strikingly different from the retroviral case, in which only gag proteins are required.

How does the encapsidation machinery select the proper RNA? First, a cis-acting packaging signal is present on the encapsidated message. The location of this packaging signal was determined by assaying for the ability of hepadnaviral sequences to confer encapsidation upon heterologous transcripts to which they were fused. In HBV, a small (about 100 nucleotides) region from the 5′ end of pgRNA (termed ε) suffices to allow packaging (82,250,409). In DHBV, the corresponding ε region is necessary but not sufficient; a second, noncontiguous region downstream of ε is also required (57,213). Because of the terminal redundancy in pgRNA, the ε element is present at both ends of the RNA. Interestingly, however, only the 5′ copy is functional for RNA packaging; deletion of the 3′ element has no impact on viral replication (213). How this position dependence comes about is unknown, but it helps to explain the exclusion of subgenomic RNAs from encapsidation (124). Although all viral transcripts harbor ε sequences at their 3′ ends, only the genomic RNAs harbor them in the 5′ (functional) position (see Fig. 2); thus, subgenomic RNAs cannot be encapsidated.

Examination of the nucleotide sequence within ε reveals a series of inverted repeats that can be predicted to fold into an RNA stem-loop structure (Fig. 6). This predicted stem-loop is phylogenetically conserved among all hepadnaviruses despite significant primary sequence variation in this region among the avian viruses (250). Consistent with this finding, direct biochemical analyses confirm that such a structure actually exists in HBV RNA (265,409). Mutational analyses have probed the regions of this structure that are functionally important for encapsidation (265,409,537). The lower stem (but only limited portions of the upper stem) must be base-paired, but primary sequence in this region is not critical; the 6-nucleotide bulge must be present, but again, primary sequence within the bulge can be radically altered without impairment of encapsidation. By contrast, the specific nucleotide sequence in the loop is critical, and base changes there are poorly tolerated by the packaging machinery.

What is the ε recognition apparatus? The simplest model compatible with the genetic analysis of encapsidation is that P protein directly recognizes this element, and *in vitro* evidence for P protein–RNA interactions have been obtained by several groups (223,410). That this binding relates importantly to RNA encapsidation is supported by analysis of ε mutations; all such mutations that block the P-ε interaction *in vitro* block RNA encapsidation *in vivo.* However, there is one important discordance: loop mutations, known to strongly impair packaging *in vivo,* do not abolish P-ε binding (410). This might mean that additional factors, possibly of host origin, may be binding to the loop region; alternatively (or additionally), lesions in the loop may subtly affect ε structure. Searches for host proteins that bind to the apical loop have been unrevealing (400), but evidence for structural changes in ε after P binding has recently been presented (25). Loop mutations that block encapsidation do not display these changes, suggesting that they are functionally significant (25).

The assembly of the P-ε ribonucleoprotein (RNP) has recently been found to require host molecular chaperones and ATP (223,224). Addition of monoclonal antibodies to heat shock protein 90 (hsp90) blocks the ability of P synthesized *in vitro* to bind to ε RNA, as does geldanomycin, a drug that blocks the association of hsp90 with its essential cofactor p23. (Interestingly, p23 also appears to bind

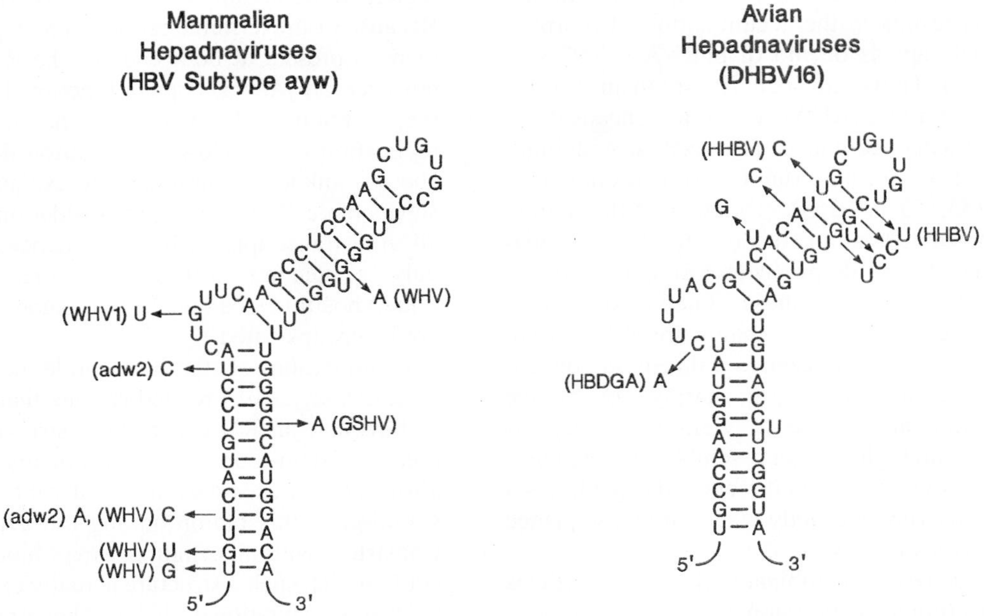

FIG. 6. Phylogenetic conservation of the ε stem-loop structure in mammalian (*left*) and avian (*right*) hepadnaviruses. The positions of base changes in naturally occurring isolates are indicated.

directly to DHBV P protein, in a geldanomycin-resistant fashion.) The proteins p23 (and presumably hsp90) remain associated with the polymerase after encapsidation; this is unlike many other chaperone-assisted reactions, in which the association of chaperone and target is transient. However, clever temperature-shift experiments with a temperature-sensitive DHBV polymerase reveal that, after encapsidation and DNA priming, geldanomycin has no impact on subsequent reverse transcription (224). Thus, hsp90–p23 complexes act primarily to assist in the formation of an RNP competent for encapsidation and DNA priming (see later).

The next step in RNA encapsidation is presumably the association of the P-ε complex with assembling core subunits. Detailed understanding of these events is lacking, but recent evidence indicates that HBV P protein produced in baculovirus-infected cells can interact noncovalently with C protein (R. Lanford, personal communication). Additional information has emerged from the study of structure–function relations within the DHBV P protein. By examining truncation mutants of DHBV P produced by *in vitro* translation, it has been shown that the C-terminus of P protein is dispensable for ε binding; however, this same region is important for RNA encapsidation *in vivo* (212,410). This is compatible with a model in which the N-terminal two thirds of P protein binds pgRNA, leaving the C-terminus free to interact (directly or indirectly) with assembling C polypeptides. A full accounting of the mechanism of the encapsidation reaction will likely require development of an *in vitro* system in which the entire process is faithfully reproduced. The first step in this direction has been achieved: the assembly of "empty" HBV cores from C proteins produced in cell-free translation systems (312). However, no group has yet succeeded in observing P-dependent RNA encapsidation into such structures *in vitro.*

Thus, in hepadnaviruses, the encapsidation of polymerase occurs by a fundamentally different mechanism from that employed by retroviruses. The latter produce pol as a gag-pol polyprotein, which is assembled into capsids by interactions of its gag domain with assembling gag polypeptides. In hepadnaviruses, P protein is bound to the RNA that is destined for encapsidation, and noncovalent interactions, direct or indirect, between C and the P-containing RNP must exist to package the pregenome. Such interactions, however, must depend on a unique property of the P-ε complex not shared by free P because DHBV genomes bearing ε deletions produce cores that lack P protein as well as RNA (19). Perhaps one function of the stably complexed chaperones in the RNP is to maintain P protein in a conformation that is competent for interactions with assembling C subunits; evidence that P undergoes conformational changes after ε binding has in fact been presented (525).

An interesting feature of the encapsidation reaction is the marked preference of the P gene product for its own mRNA during the packaging process. This is most easily demonstrated by cotransfecting a wild-type and P-negative mutant genome (which is differentially marked with a new restriction enzyme site). Examination of either the encapsidated RNA or the subsequently reverse-transcribed viral DNA reveals that the mRNA encoding the wild-type (functional) P gene product is preferentially encapsidated (90% to 95% of the encapsidated genomes are of wild-type origin) (212,293). The mechanistic basis of this cis-preference is unclear. One possibility is that the nascent P polypeptide co-translationally binds to its own mRNA. Alternatively, the levels of functional P gene product might be limiting, so that concentrations of P sufficient for encapsidation are found only in the vicinity of its own mRNA. In the case of HBV, the inefficiency in trans complementation can be at least partially overcome by deleting the encapsidation signal (16).

As noted earlier, the 5′ ends of the genomic RNAs are heterogeneous, but only the shortest of these RNAs is encapsidated (124). Because all these transcripts contain an intact 5′ copy of ε, how is packaging of all but the shortest pregenomic RNA suppressed? Examination of the 5′ termini of these RNAs indicates that all but the shortest transcript (i.e., pgRNA) include the upstream, in-frame pre-C AUG (see Fig. 2). Mutations that inactivate this AUG allow these longer messages to be encapsidated (365). These and other data suggest that translation through this region suppresses recognition of ε. Because the shortest genomic RNA (pgRNA) lacks the pre-C AUG, such ribosome-mediated suppression cannot operate on this RNA.

Viral DNA Synthesis

The complex mechanism by which single-stranded pregenomic RNA is converted to partially duplex virion DNA is now understood in considerable detail. The current view of this reaction is summarized schematically in Figure 7. Pregenomic RNA is terminally redundant; its about 200-nucleotide redundancies (termed R) include the ε stem-loop and a short sequence of 11 to 12 nucleotides termed *DR1*. Another copy of this same sequence is present near the 3′ portion of the unique region of the RNA and is termed *DR2*. The potential importance of the DR sequences in viral DNA synthesis was recognized when the 5′ termini of the viral DNA strands were precisely mapped. This showed that the 5′ end of negative-stranded DNA mapped within DR1, whereas the 5′ end of positive-stranded DNA mapped to DR2 (96,309,352,472,581). The exact roles of these sequences are discussed later.

Negative-Stranded Synthesis

Negative-stranded DNA has protein covalently linked to its 5′ end (156,166,351). This so-called terminal protein was identified as the viral P protein by showing that viral DNA could be immunoprecipitated by anti–P protein antibodies (37). Limited proteolysis suggested that the N-terminal portion of the P polypeptide contained the site of covalent attachment to the DNA (18); this has now been directly confirmed for DHBV, in which the DNA protein joint has been precisely mapped to tyrosine 96 of the P protein (573,629).

Because of the fact that all nascent chains of viral DNA are found linked to P protein (351), virologists have for years suspected that the protein serves as the primer for DNA synthesis, in a fashion formally analogous to that established for the terminal protein of adenovirus DNA (61). This inference has now been directly sustained by a seminal experiment of Wang and Seeger (561). When DHBV P protein was translated *in vitro* (from a mRNA that also contains DR1 and ε sequences) in the presence of ^{32}P- dNTPs, P protein chains become labeled by covalent attachment of nucleotides. Most product consists of P chains bearing about 4 nucleotides; longer products (up to several hundred nucleotides) are present at a very low level. That this reaction reflects authentic viral DNA synthesis is indicated by the following: it is inhibited by mutations in the reverse transcription active site, and the sequence of bases at the DNA protein joint corresponds exactly to the authentic 5′ end of viral DNA. In this reaction, the priming hydroxyl group is supplied not by a 3′OH of DNA or RNA but by the side chain of a tyrosine residue on P protein (573,629).

If P protein is the primer, what is the template for initiation? Because the 5′ ends of viral DNA map to DR1, it was long assumed that the priming of negative-stranded DNA was templated by DR1 sequences. However, analyses of the DHBV priming reaction both *in vitro* (562,629) and in recombinant yeast expressing functional P protein (523,526) indicate that this is not the case. Rather, negative-stranded initiation is templated by sequences within the bulge of the ε stem-loop. The involvement of ε sequences in the reverse transcription reaction had previously gone unrecognized because *in vivo* ε is required for the RNA packaging step that is a necessary precondition for DNA synthesis. Thus, defects in DNA synthesis due to ε mutations could be accounted for entirely by their RNA packaging defect. However, both of the recombinant P protein expression systems mentioned previously were designed to be independent of DHBV packaging functions. Under these conditions, the involvement of ε in reverse transcription rapidly became apparent: deletions of ε (or even of the ε bulge alone) completely ablated all viral reverse transcription. Analysis of large numbers of more subtle ε mutations reveals a close correlation between lesions affecting RNA packaging and those affecting DNA priming, suggesting that the same RNA protein recognition reaction underlies both processes (410). In accord with this, blockade of P-ε RNP formation with anti-hsp90 or geldanomycin also blocks DNA priming (223,224). Taken together, these data all indicate that initiation of viral DNA synthesis occurs within ε, not DR1 as initially supposed.

There is growing evidence that this critical step results in structural changes in both the RNA template and the enzyme that may be required to facilitate the subsequent events in the replication cycle. Beck and Nassal (25) have shown that the fine structure of ε is subtly altered by P protein binding, and analysis of ε mutants indicates that

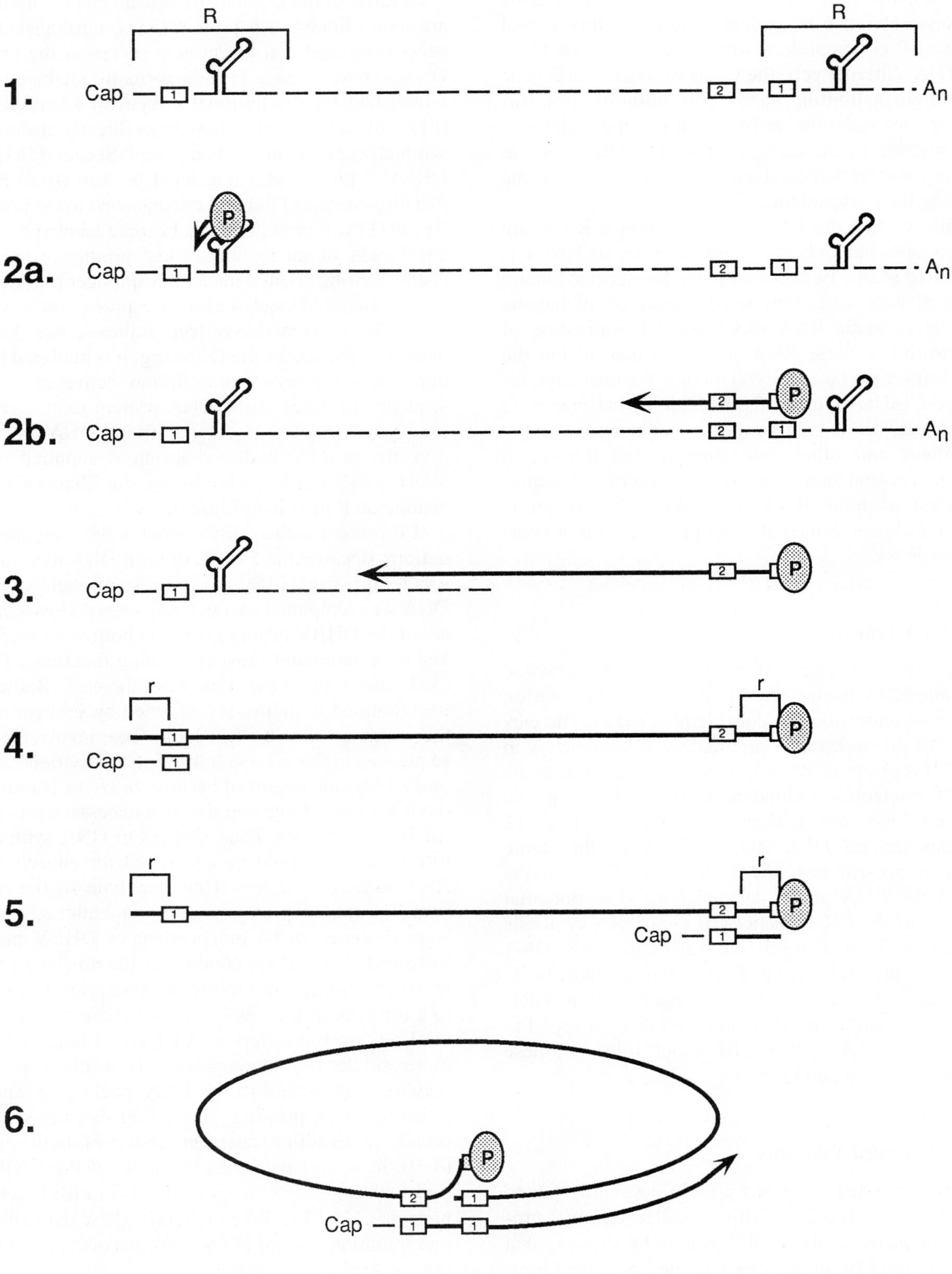
R
R
1.
Cap
1
2
1
An
P
2a.
Cap
1
2
1
An
2b.
Cap
1
2
P
2
1
An
3.
Cap
1
2
P
r
r
4.
1
2
P
Cap
1
r
r
5.
1
2
P
Cap
1
6.
P
2
1
Cap
1
1

this change is correlated with competence for DNA synthesis. Similarly, the P protein may also undergo conformational changes following binding. This was initially revealed by an altered susceptibility of P to proteolytic digestion after contact with ε RNA. All ε mutations that allow DNA priming induce this change, whereas those that do not (including apical loop mutations that can still bind P but do not allow DNA synthesis) fail to induce the change (525). Thus, the ε RNA might serve not only as the template for the polymerase but also as its allosteric effector.

The next events in replication are depicted schematically in Figure 7. After P-ε binding, initiation occurs within the ε bulge, generating an initial P-linked oligonucleotide of about 4 nucleotides. Because the sequences of the ε bulge and DR1 share 4 nucleotides of identity, this DNA product can be transferred and annealed to DR1 sequences; from this position, the DNA can be extended by traditional elongation mechanisms (524,526,562). This strand transfer reaction has been studied in great detail but remains incompletely understood. It is clear that sequence homology between donor and acceptor sites is required for the reaction because disruption of the homology strongly impairs transfer (246,315,524). However, second-site mutations in DR1 that restore complementarity to a mutant ε region do not always restore efficient transfer, indicating that homology, although necessary, is not sufficient for the reaction. Many other factors appear to be involved, including local sequence or structure surrounding the acceptor site, the position of the acceptor site relative to the donor, and the length of the transferred strand (317,524).

Both DR1 and ε are represented twice in the pgRNA template. The fact that the 3′ copy of ε can be deleted from pgRNA without blocking viral replication (473,474) suggests that it is the 5′ copy of ε that is functional in initiation. This inference has been directly validated by genetically marking the 5′ ε with a sequence polymorphism and showing that this sequence marker appears at the 5′ end of negative-stranded DNA after one round of reverse transcription (526,562). Analogous genetic tagging experiments indicate that it is the 3′ copy of DR1 to which the nascent P-linked primer is transferred (473). Once this transfer reaction is complete, elongation can continue to the end of the RNA template. As negative-stranded elongation proceeds, degradation of the newly copied pregenomic RNA template occurs concomitantly (349,510); this is necessary to make negative-stranded DNA available to template positive-stranded synthesis. As in other reverse transcription reactions, this function is attributed to the RNaseH activity of the viral polymerase itself (429). Consistent with this notion, lesions in the RnaseH domain of P inhibit positive-stranded synthesis (67,429). The final product of this elongation reaction is a negative-stranded DNA that is actually terminally redundant by about 8 nucleotides (this shorter redundancy is known as r) (309,472,581).

Positive-Stranded Synthesis

After negative-stranded DNA synthesis is complete, positive-stranded DNA synthesis can begin. Positive strands are initiated at DR2 (309,472,581) (see Fig. 7), in a reaction primed by short (about 15 to 18 nucleotides), capped oligoribonucleotides derived from the 5′ of pregenomic RNA; these include DR1 sequences and the 6-nucleotide 5′ end of DR1. The viral RnaseH activity is also presumed to be responsible for the cleavages that generate these primers. The reaction does not proceed by sequence-specific endonucleolytic cleavage at the border of DR1 because nucleotide changes around the cleavage sites do not perturb either the specificity or efficiency of cleavage (500). However, when insertions or deletions are placed between the 5′ end of pregenome and the 3′ end of DR1 (316), the sites of cleavage remain a constant distance (15 to 18 nucleotides) from the 5′ end of the pregenome. This indicates that the cleavages are somehow positioned by measurement from the end of the template and that the actual scission event is independent of the sequence at the cleavage site. A model for how this distance might be measured has been proposed (316).

FIG. 7. The hepadnaviral reverse transcription pathway. Pregenomic RNA (*dashed line,* step 1) is capped and polyadenylated and has a large terminal redundancy (*R*). The locations of direct repeats 1 and 2 (DR1 and DR2) are shown as correspondingly numbered boxes, and the ε stem-loops are indicated. Pregenomic RNA packaging into cores is initiated by the interaction of P protein with the 5′ copy of ε. P initiates reverse transcription at the 5′ stem-loop and extends negative-stranded DNA (*solid line*) for 3 to 4 nucleotides (step 2a). P and the covalently attached nascent DNA are then transferred to the 3′ copy of DR1 (step 2b), and the DNA is extended. During negative-stranded elongation, pgRNA is degraded by the RNaseH activity of P (step 3). When P reaches the 5′ end of the template, its RNaseH activity leaves an RNA oligomer consisting of r plus DR1 sequences (step 4). This RNA oligomer is translocated and annealed to DR2, where it primes positive-stranded DNA synthesis (*lower solid line,* step 5). Positive-stranded elongation proceeds to the 5′ end of the negative-stranded DNA template, including the sequences denoted as r. Because complementary r sequences are found at the 3′ end of negative-strandeds DNA, a second homology-mediated template transfer can now circularize the genome. The positive strand is then extended for a variable length (step 6) to yield mature viral DNA.

The site of primer generation is many hundreds of bases away from the actual site of positive-stranded DNA synthesis at DR2. Thus, the newly cleaved RNA primer must be translocated to the 5′ end of negative-stranded DNA to base-pair with DR2 for positive-stranded DNA synthesis to begin. Because the primer is being moved from a region (including r and DR1), where it is base-paired for 18 nt to a region (DR2) where it is base-paired for only 12 nt (see Fig. 7); this primer translocation is not thought to occur passively. Most likely, it is actively facilitated by proteins, but how this is accomplished remains a matter of conjecture. It is known that positive-stranded synthesis is very sensitive to mutations not only within the primer but also to lesions in several other regions of the template, including a region in the middle of the genome and others near DR2 and DR1 (200,315,318,319, 357). The two terminal regions have the potential to base-pair with the central region (D. Loeb, personal communication), suggesting that these regions may be important in maintaining a structure in the template that facilitates the transfer, perhaps by juxtaposing the donor and acceptor sites.

Occasionally, primers that are cleaved fail to be translocated. This occurs at a low rate with wild-type virus genomes (about 1% to 5% of primers) but can be greatly increased by cis-acting mutations in and around DR1. Typically, primers that are cleaved but not translocated are instead extended from their original position, a process referred to as *in situ* priming. The result is fully duplex linear viral DNA (500). Such molecules are found in all stocks of hepadnaviral particles. Many of these duplex linear DNAs are dead-end products. However, recent work has shown that some of these species can participate in a variety of illegitimate recombination reactions, with interesting consequences. Although the viral life cycle is maintained by episomal DNA, integration of the genome into host DNA is known to occur at low frequency, an event that in some systems plays a role in hepatocellular carcinogenesis (see later). Analysis of these integrants suggests that a substantial fraction of them likely derive from double-stranded linear DNAs produced by *in situ* priming (168–170; W. Yang and J. Summers, personal communication). Illegitimate recombination can also circularize such linear DNAs, generating cccDNA forms with abnormal circle junctions. Some of these are competent to undergo additional rounds of transcription and reverse transcription, a process that has been termed *illegitimate replication* (597–599).

Once the RNA primer is translocated, synthesis of positive-stranded DNA can begin. Elongation proceeds to the 5′ end of negative-stranded DNA, at which point the template is exhausted and an intramolecular strand transfer is required to complete positive-stranded synthesis (see Fig. 7). This transfer is facilitated by the short redundancy (r) in the negative-stranded DNA template: annealing of the nascent positive strand DNA (by its r homology) to the 3′ end of the negative strand circularizes the genome and allows continuation of positive-stranded synthesis. As for other hepadnaviral strand transfers, sequence complementarity is necessary but not sufficient for this process. Circularization can be affected by other variables, including the sequence and length of the transferred strand and the sequences adjacent to DR1 at the 3′ end of negative-stranded DNA (200,315,318,319). Once accomplished, the strand transfer allows positive-stranded synthesis access to the rest of the negative-stranded DNA template. However, in most cases, synthesis does not proceed to completion (the exception is DHBV, in which 80% of the positive strands complete elongation) (310,352). The result is the characteristic single-stranded gap that is a hallmark of hepadnaviral DNA.

Why positive-stranded synthesis terminates prematurely is not entirely clear but might be related to the process of viral budding. The DNA of cytoplasmic core particles is substantially more immature than that of extracellular virions, suggesting that maturation of viral DNA synthesis is somehow coupled with envelopment and secretion of the Dane particle. In keeping with this, *P* gene mutations affecting viral DNA synthesis can strongly influence envelopment and release (162,576). Presumably, a structural change or posttranslational modification of the core particle occurs concomitant with reaching a certain stage in genome maturation (608), creating a signal for core envelopment. Once budded into the ER, the core particle would presumably no longer have access to cytoplasmic dNTP pools, and further DNA synthesis would be expected to arrest.

Viral Assembly and Release

20-nm Subviral Particle Assembly

As noted previously, 20-nm particles contain predominantly the S protein with variable amounts of M and only trace quantities of L subunits. With the advent of cloned HBV DNA, it became possible to express the surface protein coding regions in heterologous cells, leading to the discovery that cells expressing only the S polypeptide can assemble and secrete morphologically normal 20-nm particles. Thus, all of the viral information necessary for this assembly process resides in the S domain (290,313,401). Because the cellular machinery for particle assembly is present in virtually all vertebrate cells, expression of 20-nm particles is possible in a wide variety of expression systems (116,353,501). This has made possible the development of recombinant HBV vaccine, the first recombinant DNA-based vaccine licensed for any human infectious disease. Interestingly, yeast cells (the source of one widely used recombinant vaccine) do not secrete HBsAg and may not form intracellular particles at all. However, subparticulate lipoprotein aggregates of S subunits likely do form intracellularly and may rearrange during extraction to yield immunogenic particulate antigen (557,560).

How do 20-nm particles form in mammalian cells? Early electron microscopic studies of infected liver revealed that particles accumulated within cisternae of the ER (161), an observation also confirmed by later electron microscopic studies of transfected, HBsAg-positive cells in culture (395). Consistent with this is the fact that intracellular particles contain asparagine-linked high-mannose oligosaccharide chains, a modification specific to the ER (396). Subsequent biochemical studies have more precisely localized the major site of particle assembly to the so-called intermediate compartment between the ER and Golgi (232). Assembled complexes are then transported through the constitutive secretory pathway, traversing the Golgi complex, where their carbohydrates are processed to the complex, endoglycosidase H-resistant form (396). Transport of the complexes through the Golgi appears to be the rate-limiting step in export because all intracellular glycosylated S protein is found in the endoH-sensitive form, whereas all extracellular glycosylated HBsAg is endoH resistant.

S proteins are synthesized in the ER as integral membrane proteins. Their transmembrane topology has been determined in cell-free translation systems supplemented with ER-derived microsomal vesicles (117,119). In these experiments, nascent S protein chains were found to be oriented in the bilayer such that both N- and C-termini are in the vesicle lumen. To do so, the polypeptide must span the bilayer at least twice; many current models, based largely on theoretical considerations, envision up to four transmembrane passages (Fig. 8). (The S coding region contains three hydrophobic domains, encompassing residues 4 to 28, 80 to 100, and 164 to 221. Hydrophobicity and other considerations lead most to assume that all of these regions are located within the bilayer, generating the model of Figure 8. However, the disposition of the C-terminal hydrophobic domain has not been experimentally assessed.) This topology is achieved through the conjoint action of two topogenic signal sequences. Signal I corresponds to the first hydophobic domain and initiates chain translocation across the bilayer. It resembles conventional N-terminal signal sequences except for the fact that it remains uncleaved during translocation. Signal II (corresponding to the second hydrophobic domain) is a complex topogenic element that serves both as a stop-transfer sequence (anchoring the protein in the bilayer with residue 80 facing the cytoplasm and residue 100 facing the ER lumen) and a signal sequence directing the translocation of the distal region of the molecule. Thus, the region between signals I and II is a cytoplasmic loop; downstream of signal II is the major glycosylation site of S as well as its immunodominant surface epitope.

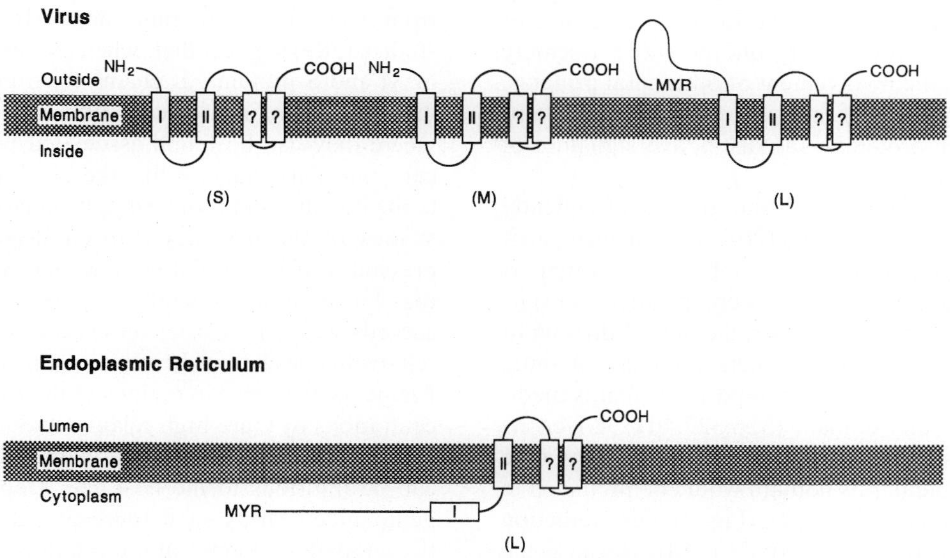

FIG. 8. Top: Proposed transmembrane topologies for the HBV L, M, and S glycoproteins in the virion envelope. *Rectangles* denote S-protein hydrophobic domains. [The transmembrane orientation of domains I and II have been addressed experimentally (87), whereas the disposition of the remaining hydrophobic regions remains speculative.] The *psi* symbol denotes *N*-linked carbohydrate. *Myr* is the myristate group in amide linkage to glycine at the N-terminus of L protein (292). **Bottom:** Transmembrane structure of L protein in endoplasmic reticulum membranes. Virtually all pre-S sequences reside on the cytoplasmic face of the membrane. (The disposition of S hydrophobic region I is here drawn as cytoplasmic, but this has not been directly validated.)

This transmembrane form of S is only a transient intermediate in particle formation; *in vivo,* this form is rapidly converted to a series of defined assembly intermediates (232,491), and *S* gene mutations affecting one or more of these steps have been examined (44,418). After membrane insertion, the transmembrane monomers aggregate and in the process exclude host proteins from the complex. (With one exception, in DHBV, subviral particles also harbor large quantities of the host chaperone hsp70, a known participant in many protein-folding reactions. Because hsp70 is a cytosolic protein, it must be interacting with cytoplasmically disposed regions of the viral envelope proteins. It is not clear, however, why so much hsp70 remains in the final particle because in most other folding reactions, the chaperone is released from its targets once folding is accomplished.) The aggregate then buds or extrudes into the lumen. It is likely that this extrusion event differs from more conventional viral budding reactions in that the "budded" product lacks a typical unit membrane structure. In addition, its lipid content is much lower than that of most cellular membranes, suggesting that that the host lipids may be substantially reorganized in the process.

This pathway shares many features with morphogenetic events postulated for the envelope proteins of other animal viruses: transmembrane insertion, aggregation, and budding. However, in other viruses, envelope glycoproteins remain anchored in the bilayer until interactions with other viral components (e.g., nucleocapsid or matrix proteins) trigger the budding step, thus ensuring that envelope proteins can exit the cell only by enveloping the nucleocapsid. The distinctive feature of the S protein is that it can carry out the entire assembly sequence without the involvement of other viral proteins. The result is the release of the subviral particles containing only envelope proteins—the distinctive signature of hepadnaviral infection.

In authentic viral infection, 20-nm particles frequently contain M as well as S subunits (204,503). In such particles, the pre-S2–encoded domain of the M protein is exposed on the particle surface, as demonstrated by (a) its reactivity with antisera specific for the pre-S2 domain of M, and (b) its ability to bind polymers of human albumin, an activity of uncertain biologic importance that is mediated uniquely by this domain (326,327,401). Given its surface location on the particle, in the transmembrane form of the M protein, this domain would be predicted to be translocated into the ER lumen (Fig. 9); this prediction has been experimentally confirmed (118). Because the pre-S2–encoded domain lacks a definable signal sequence, its transmembrane transport must be mediated by the downstream signals in the S domain.

As noted previously, natural 20-nm particles often lack detectable L protein (204). The reason for the low abundance of L chains on 20-nm particles became clear in experiments in which L chains were deliberately overexpressed in cultured cells. In cells infected with vaccinia vectors that express only the L protein, the L chains themselves are not secreted, despite the presence of an intact S domain that contains all the information required for the export process (76). This suggests that the pre-S1–specific domain of L contains signals that promote intracellular retention of the chain and that can override the secretory elements in the S domain. When L chains are overexpressed in the presence of M and S chains, the ability of the M and S chains to be secreted is inhibited in a dose-dependent fashion (76,88,389,402); all three chains accumulate intracellularly (87). Presumably, this reflects the formation of mixed arrays of L, M, and S subunits, with the inhibitory influence of the pre-S1 domain now being conferred upon the entire aggregate. The inhibitory effect of L overexpression on S particle secretion explains the underrepresentation of L chains on 20-nm spherical particles.

The region of the pre-S1 domain that specifies the intracellular retention of HBsAg has been mapped by deletion mutagenesis to the extreme N-terminus of the molecule (281). The observation that this region of the L protein is myristoylated (403) raised the possibility that ER retention might be mediated by the affinity of this hydrophobic fatty acid for the ER membrane. However, point mutations that ablate myristylation have either no (281) or only incomplete (417) effects on secretion-inhibition, indicating that primary sequences in this region of the chain are important for this activity. The mechanism of the secretion-inhibition by L remains uncertain. Early models proposed that L chains might not be mobilized from their transmembrane state. However, subsequent studies (589) suggest that, when expressed in the absence of M and S proteins, L chains form intraluminal aggregates that remain trapped within the secretory system, where they can be found associated with the chaperone calnexin. This suggests that the block to release is distal to the budding step. Interestingly, in electron microscopic studies of the hepatocytes of transgenic mice overexpressing L chains (relative to M and S), 20-nm filamentous forms were frequently observed in the ER (87). This accords well with earlier observations that filaments are relatively enriched in L subunits (204) and suggests that filaments may arise in regions of the ER where local concentrations of L are high relative to S.

The overaccumulation of retained L-M-S aggregates can be injurious to the host cell. Hepatocytes of transgenic mice bearing such aggregates develop characteristic cytopathic effects (in the relative absence of inflammation) and are very sensitive to killing induced by interferon-α (IFN-α) and TNF (361). Morphologically similar cells, termed *ground-glass hepatocytes* by pathologists, are sometimes seen in biopsy specimens from acute hepatitis B, indicating that deregulation of envelope protein expression may make some contribution to the process of liver cell injury. The magnitude of

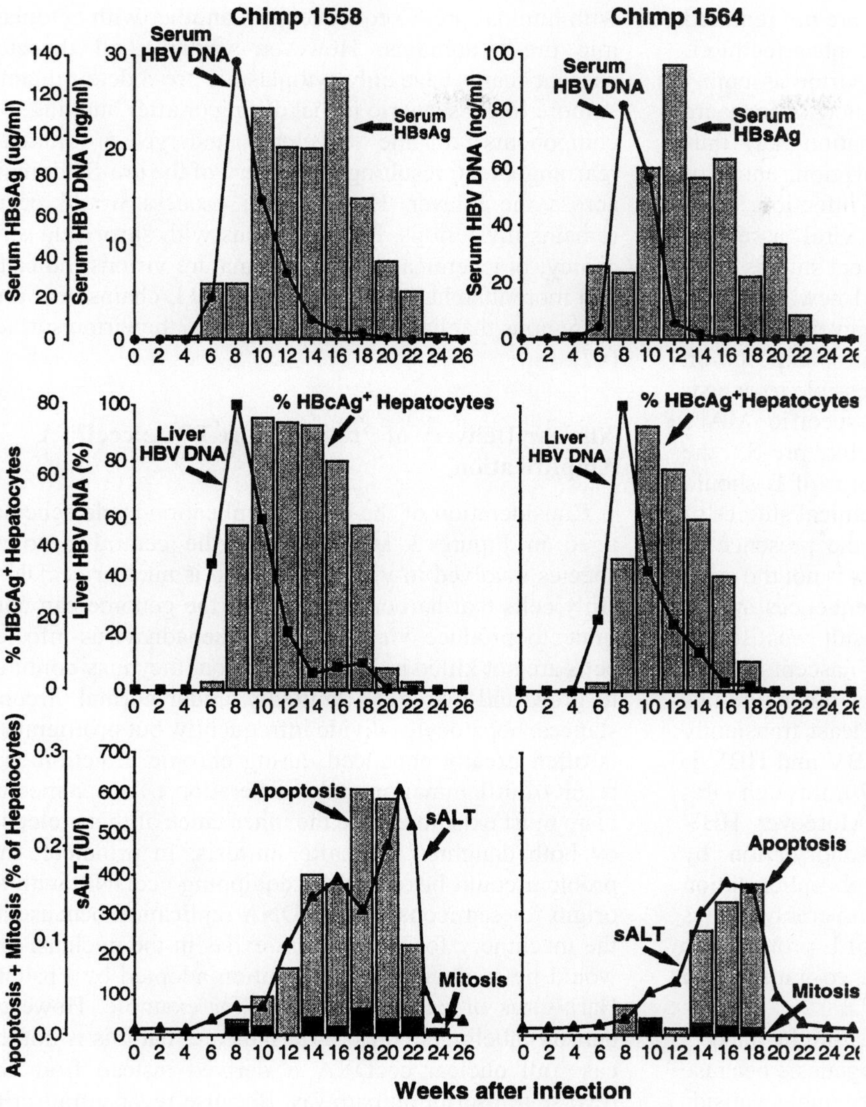

FIG. 9. Natural history of experimental HBV infection of two chimpanzees. **Left:** Chimpanzee, 1558. **Right:** Chimpanzee, 1564. **Top:** serum hepatitis B virus DNA levels and HBsAg levels as a function of time post inoculation. **Center:** Liver HBV DNA levels and the percentage of HBcAg-positive hepatocytes as a function of time after inoculation. **Bottom:** Serum transaminase levels and the percentage of hepatocytes undergoing mitosis (*black bars*) or apoptosis (*gray bars*) as a function of time after inoculation. (From ref. 187, with permission.)

this contribution, however, is uncertain, and is likely to be modest.

Dane Particle Assembly

Conceptual views of Dane particle assembly have been heavily influenced by the emerging understanding of the morphogenesis of subviral particles. Because all three HBV envelope proteins are expressed primarily on intracellular membranes rather than on the cell surface (389), virion formation almost certainly proceeds on intracellular membranes; EM studies consistent with this have been reported (252,446). However, an important distinguishing feature of virions is that they contain relatively large quantities of L proteins; in the best preparations, the ratio of L to M to S subunits was about 1:1:4 (204). Because these preparations are often contaminated to some extent with 20-nm particles, it is possible that the ratio of L to S chains in authentic virions is still higher. It is unlikely that subviral particles bearing this much L protein could be efficiently released; this suggests that distinctive mechanisms are involved in virion assembly and export.

To define the components required for Dane particle production, permissive HepG2 cells have been transfected with missense or nonsense mutants selectively affecting the HBV L, M, or S proteins and the ability of these mutants to support virion release assayed (45). Several conclusions have emerged from these studies: (a) unlike retroviruses, whose nucleocapsids can still bud out of cells in the absence of envelope proteins, no HBV cores are exported if the synthesis of all envelope proteins is aborted by nonsense mutations in S; and (b) both L and S proteins are required for virion formation and release.

Although one report to the contrary has appeared (552), the weight of evidence is that M proteins are not required for assembly (45,137,457). Missense mutants affecting L myristylation also remain competent for virion assembly and secretion, although the unmyristylated virions are noninfectious (45,46,330,513). Myristylation may thus play its most important role in the adsorption, entry, or uncoating of virions on the next cycle of infection.

How the L protein contributes to viral assembly remains incompletely understood, but recent studies of its transmembrane topology have suggested new possibilities. Studies of HBV virion architecture reveal that the L protein–specific, pre-S1–encoded domain is exposed on the virion surface. For example, it is accessible to exogenous proteases as well as to pre-S1–specific MAbs (204,280,385). This would suggest that, like pre-S2, the pre-S1 domain in the transmembrane form of L should reside in the ER lumen. However, biochemical studies of HBV L chains synthesized *in vitro* in the presence of microsomal membranes indicated that this is not the case; rather, most pre-S–encoded L protein sequences are on the cytoplasmic surface (385). This result was subsequently confirmed by similar analysis of nascent HBV L chains *in vivo* (47,419) and is supported by other findings that indicate that pre-S1 regions are at least transiently cytosolic (see Fig. 8). For example, DHBV and HBV L chains can associate with cytosolic hsp70, through sites mapped to the pre-S region (320,518). Moreover, HBV and DHBV pre-S can undergo phosphorylation by cytosolic kinases (173,174,452). This phosphorylation has no impact on viral replication or assembly but is required for yet another known activity of L protein—its ability to up-regulate reporter genes in co-transfection assays (210).

This topology helps to explain how L might make a distinctive contribution to virion morphogenesis because it now can present unique determinants to nucleocapsids on the cytoplasmic face of the ER membrane. In one attractive model, capsid–L protein interactions trigger the budding event that incorporates the mature core into the viral envelope. This notion is supported by mutational studies examining the impact of pre-S topology on virion assembly. If the pre-S region of L is delivered to the ER lumen by an engineered N-terminal signal sequence, no virions can be formed, despite the fact that subviral particles can still be assembled and released (47). Examination of deletions and linker scanning mutations within pre-S confirms that only those mutations whose pre-S domain is cytosolically disposed are competent for virion assembly, and point to a region at the pre-S1–pre-S2 border as critical for virus production (43,48,49). The simplest model is that this region is directly involved in contacting the nucleocapsid.

We are left, however, with an important remaining problem: how does the pre-S1 domain wind up on the surface of the budded virion? One possibility is that nascent L chains exist in two orientations in the ER: one with luminal pre-S sequences and another with cytoplasmic pre-S domains. However, virtually all detected nascent chains have only cytoplasmic pre-S determinants. A more likely scenario is that during or after budding, the components of the envelope undergo a dramatic rearrangement, resulting in delivery of the pre-S1 domain across the bilayer. How such a process would occur remains mysterious, but it happens with surprising efficiency; biochemical analysis of mature virions indicates that more than half of their constituent L chains bear pre-S1 regions that have been transposed to the virion surface (47).

Nuclear Delivery of Progeny Core DNA: cccDNA Amplification

Consideration of the overall replication cycle schematized in Figure 3 indicates that the central genomic species involved in viral persistence is nuclear cccDNA. Only cells that harbor this form of the genome can continue to produce virus. Because hepadnavirus-infected cells are not killed by viral replication, they may continue to grow and divide. (Admittedly, under normal circumstances, hepatocytes divide infrequently, but proliferation is often greatly enhanced during chronic infection as a result of inflammation and regeneration.) Thus, a mechanism must exist to ensure the inheritance of this molecule by both daughter cells after mitosis. In principle, this problem could be solved by equipping cccDNA with an origin for semiconservative DNA replication because all the machinery for this process exists in the nucleus; this would be analogous to the solution adopted by Epstein-Barr virus or papillomaviruses, for example. However, density labeling studies (545) indicate that this is not the case: all nuclear cccDNA is derived instead from the reverse transcription pathway. Because reverse transcription is a cytoplasmic process, this implies that mechanisms exist to deliver cytoplasmic reverse transcription products into the nucleus. For DHBV, such mechanisms operate efficiently early in the establishment of infection in primary duck hepatocytes, leading to the rapid accumulation of 10 to 20 or more copies of cccDNA per nucleus.

One possible way to account for the maintenance of a pool of cccDNA would be to imagine that it was replenished by reinfection of cells by extracellular virus. However, it was soon shown that cccDNA amplification could be observed in the presence of inhibitors of viral entry like suramin or neutralizing antibody; it also can occur after transfection of viral DNA into cells that lack the surface receptor, thereby eliminating the possibility of reinfection by released progeny virus (587). Thus, cytoplasmic cores bearing virion DNA can be shunted to the nucleus by an intracellular pathway. A key step forward was made with the recognition that DHBV mutants lacking the L envelope protein (or bearing certain point mutations in pre-S) (301) displayed greatly enhanced amplification, resulting in the nuclear accumulation of very high levels of cccDNA (512,513). This implies that the subcellular trafficking of cores is regulated: early in infection, when envelope proteins are at low levels, nuclear delivery is favored, allowing accumulation of cccDNA. This ensures that this infected cell will be stably colonized. Late in infection, with rising levels of envelope proteins, export of cores as virions is favored, allowing horizontal spread of infection to surrounding cells. Thus, in this view, nuclear transit is the default pathway; as envelope proteins accumulate, cores are shunted from this pathway to the export pathway.

Examination of DHBV pre-S mutants that up-regulate cccDNA accumulation reveals that these variants are often cytotoxic; presumably, cells do not tolerate high levels of cccDNA or the resulting elevated levels of viral gene products. The mechanisms of this toxicity are unknown but are not immune mediated because this phenomenon is also observed in cultured cells. Infection of animals with DHBV pre-S point mutants that display deregulated cccDNA gives rise to an early phase of liver injury, which subsequently resolves; this resolution is accompanied by the outgrowth of noncytopathic second-site revertants that restore normal cccDNA regulation (300).

VIRAL PATHOGENESIS AND IMMUNITY

Save for the rare pre-S mutants just described, hepadnaviruses are generally agreed to be noncytopathic. If the viral replication cycle is not itself injurious to hepatocytes, how does clinical hepatitis arise? And why do some individuals develop serious liver disease, whereas others escape with only minor pathologic changes? Correlative clinical data suggested early on that host immune attack on infected hepatocytes, a response normally designed for clearance of infection, might also be the prime source of the injury (and that variations in the magnitude or nature of this response might account for the variety of clinical outcomes in different hosts). Here we summarize the growing body of experimental evidence that supports this inference and outline the mechanisms now thought to be involved.

The study of immune responses to HBV has long been bedeviled by a number of experimental obstacles that have only recently been overcome. HBV grows only in humans and higher primates, a fact that has severely constrained immunologic investigation. Apart from the evident ethical constraints involved in human experimentation, all primate hosts are genetically outbred, making many experimental manipulations of immunity (e.g., adoptive transfer of sensitized lymphocytes) impossible. Similar difficulties apply to the study of the other animal hepadnaviruses (e.g., WHV and DHBV), all of which grow poorly or not at all outside of their outbred native hosts. Thus, efforts to understand immune responses to hepadnaviruses in their native hosts have been limited largely to descriptive studies. Nonetheless, such studies have provided a useful starting point for hepadnaviral immunology because any model for immune-mediated liver injury must account for their observations.

As noted at the outset of this chapter, most primary infections of immunocompetent adults result in variable degrees of acute hepatitis, following which viral infection is cleared. Figure 9 depicts the virologic, serologic, and pathologic events seen in a primary HBV infection, here studied in two experimentally inoculated chimpanzees (187). After an incubation period of 4 to 6 weeks, HBsAg and viral DNA become evident in the serum, peaking at about postinoculation week 8, at which time more than 75% of hepatocytes in the liver display HBcAg by immunohistochemical analysis. In DHBV and WHV, virtually 100% of hepatocytes are infected in a typical primary infection (247,248,251). Importantly, at the peak of virus production, there is little evidence of liver injury, either histologically or by measurement of serum transaminases—in keeping with the noncytocidal nature of the viral replicative cycle. However, beginning 1 to 3 weeks thereafter, serum markers of liver injury become dramatically abnormal, along with histologic evidence of inflammatory cell infiltrates and cell destruction—markers of cell-mediated immunity. A particularly important point is that a 10-fold decrease in intrahepatic (and serum) viral DNA is evident even before the onset of liver injury (see Fig. 9; more about this anon). Ultimately, viral DNA and antigens are cleared from liver and blood, inflammatory infiltrates resolve, and serum antibody to HBsAg provides immunity to reinfection.

Given the enormous size of the liver and the huge burden of infection achieved, clearance of HBV and other hepadnaviruses during acute hepatitis is remarkably efficient. However, although this clearance process achieves eradication of clinically detectable infection, there is evidence that a few infected cells may persist in the hosts after successful resolution of acute disease. For example, very sensitive nested polymerase chain reaction assays can detect low quantities of viral DNA in liver and serum of some such hosts years after primary infection (438, 439). Virus-specific cytotoxic T lymphocytes (CTLs) are also detectable at high frequency in most such cases many years later (438,439). In fact, such CTLs may display activation markers, suggesting that a few persistently infected cells remain in the body and serve as ongoing stimuli of such responses. Rare reports that organ donors with serologic profiles compatible with resolved infection can occasionally transmit HBV after liver transplantation are compatible with this notion (69).

What are the determinants of successful clearance? Efforts to answer this question have focused on comparison of HBV-specific immune responses in patients who clear primary infection with those who fail to do so. Particular emphasis has been placed on the role of CTLs in this process (86). In those in whom primary infection resolves, the CTL response to HBV is vigorous, polyclonal, and directed against most or all of the viral gene products (31,85,181,236,397,398). The breadth of these responses may be important in preventing the emergence of CTL escape mutants, although rare escape or antagonist mutations have been observed (32). By contrast, in chronic HBV carriers, CTL responses to viral antigens are weak or undetectable. Such carriers often display weak responses of helper (CD4+) T cells to viral antigens as well. The latter may not be due to deletion of such cells because successful reduction of viral loads with lamivudine can restore significant CD4+ cell proliferative responses to viral antigen (36), although this does not result in clearance of infection.

These correlative clinical data have focused attention on T-cell responses (especially CTL responses) to HBV as the key to understanding viral clearance and immunity. However, meaningful analysis of the biologic roles of antiviral CTLs had to await development of tractable experimental systems for the study of HBV immunity. This became possible with the development by Chisari and coworkers (86) and Moriyama and associates (354) of transgenic mouse models of HBV infection and disease. The models involve inbred mice bearing one of two classes of HBV transgenes: those bearing subgenomic fragments expressing one or more viral antigen, and those bearing intact, replication-competent viral DNA. The latter mice have the full complement of viral replicative intermediates in the liver and release infectious virus into the bloodstream. These mice display two important virologic differences from natural infection: (a) because they lack HBV receptors, there is no horizontal spread of virus between cells; and (b) for unknown reasons, they do not support cccDNA formation. However, their integrated HBV transgenes serve to replace the transcriptional template function of cccDNA. Most HBV transgenic mice do not experience liver disease because replication is noncytopathic and they are immunologically tolerant to the transgene products, which are viewed as self because their genes are present from conception. One exception to this is the case of transgenic mice that overexpress the viral L protein relative to S and M. These mice accumulate viral glycoproteins to pathologic levels in their ER and display cytotoxicity on this basis (87–89).

Although these mice experience no liver disease in the ground state, when sensitized T cells from an immunized syngeneic mouse are adoptively transferred into them, dramatic liver injury results (354). CTLs account for the bulk of this injury, which can be reproduced with individual CTL clones; CD4+ cells can also mediate liver injury, but do so with much lower efficiency and intensity (146,398). CTL-mediated injury is dependent on viral antigen expression in the recipient and is class I major histocompatibility complex restricted. These studies provided the first experimental proof that CTLs could mediate liver injury as well as participate in viral clearance and put notions of HBV immunopathogenesis on a firm experimental footing.

They also permitted a major insight into the role of these cells in viral clearance. In addition to producing liver cell injury, transfer of CTLs to mice bearing replicating HBV resulted in a dramatic decrease in viral replication (178,183). Careful quantitation of direct CTL-mediated killing in the livers of these animals revealed that the reduction in viral load achieved after CTL transfer was much greater than could be accounted for by the number of infected hepatocytes directly killed by CTL contact. In fact, large fields of viable hepatocytes surrounding isolated CTL infiltrates could be shown to have lost HBcAg and viral DNA. This suggested that paracrine, noncytopathic mechanisms might be operating to effect much of the observed viral clearance, an inference sustained by the discovery that this clearance could be blocked by administration of antibodies to TNF-α and IFN-γ. It is now thought that these cytokines, which are released from CTLs after contact with their targets, are major effectors of the antiviral response seen to accompany CTL administration. The molecular basis of this response is now under active study; the cytokines appear able to reduce the accumulation of viral RNA (perhaps by engagement of the 2′,5′oligo(A) synthase–RnaseL pathway) and also, in some settings, to destabilize viral capsid components (59,167,182,205).

If intrahepatic cytokine release is in fact an important determinant of HBV clearance, other stimuli to their release should also produce a similar result. This is supported by the finding that many other infectious agents that replicate in the liver of HBV transgenic mice can suppress HBV replication. For example, LCMV strains that replicate in hepatic macrophages (but not in hepatocytes) dramatically suppressed HBV replication in hepatocytes—a suppression that could be reversed with antibodies to TNF-α and IFN (in this case, IFN-α and -β) (179,180). Induction of the same cytokines was shown to mediate a similar suppression of HBV replication by hepatocyte superinfection with adenovirus or cytomegalovirus (60). Apart from their intrinsic interest, these reports may have direct clinical relevance because it has been observed that superinfection of human HBV carriers with hepatitis A virus or hepatitis C virus has occasionally resulted in the resolution of the underlying HBV infection (60).

Does this form of noncytocidal antiviral mechanism operate during normal viral clearance? The best evidence that it might comes from consideration of the experimental study of acute HBV infection of chimpanzees (see Fig. 9). Recall that a significant decrement in virus production was achieved in the period before histologic evidence of massive cellular infiltration or hepatocyte destruction.

Local production of IFN-γ and TNF is demonstrable during this interval, although the source of these cytokines is not yet clear. Recent experimental evidence indicates that cells from the innate immune system, possibly derived from the natural killer T-cell population normally resident in the liver, may be important sources of these cytokines early in the infectious process, before the development of adaptive CTL responses (J. Baron and D. Ganem, unpublished results).

Could this understanding of clearance during acute hepatitis be parlayed into a strategy for the immunotherapy of chronic hepatitis B? The answer to this is presently unclear because the basis of the absence of HBV-specific CTLs from chronic carriers is not understood. However, if the burden of infected cells could be reduced by long-term administration of antiviral drugs, up-regulation of CTL responses by therapeutic vaccination—or modulation of cytokine production by other means (e.g., gene therapy)—might provide a way to eliminate the remaining reservoir of HBV-positive cells.

HEPADNAVIRUSES AND HEPATOCELLULAR CARCINOMA

Biology and Epidemiology

The first indication that chronic HBV infection might predispose to the development of hepatocellular carcinoma emerged from studies of the global epidemiology of HBV carriage (519). These studies revealed that HBV is not uniformly distributed among human populations. In Western Europe and North America, only about 0.1% to 0.5% of individuals are HBsAg carriers; however, in Southeast Asia and Subsaharan Africa, fully 5% to 15% of all humans are chronically infected with HBV. (The remaining areas of the globe have an intermediate prevalence of HBV carriage.) This pattern of HBV infection strikingly reproduces the known global epidemiology of HCC, a rare tumor in the West but long known as a leading malignancy in Africa and Asia. This remarkable finding prompted deeper investigation of this linkage.

In HBV-endemic countries, most HCCs arise in patients who are HBV carriers (22,154,514); even though carriers may represent 5% to 10% of the population, they represent 50% to 80% of HCC patients in those societies. However, the strongest evidence for an association comes from careful prospective studies done in Taiwan, in which large numbers of carriers and noncarriers were followed prospectively and deaths due to HCC recorded. These classic studies demonstrated that chronic HBV carriage is associated with a 100-fold increase in risk for HCC relative to noncarriers (22,23). This massive increment in cancer risk makes HBV one of the most important environmental risk factors in human cancer epidemiology.

In Taiwan (as in all HBV-endemic areas), most infections are acquired in the first decade of life (154). Thus, in these studies, most of the individuals being followed had been carrying HBV for many decades. From the age distribution of Taiwanese hepatoma cases, it can be inferred that most tumors arise after 30 or more years of persistent infection; relatively few cases occur in children and adolescents. Extrapolation of this estimate of relative cancer risk to Western societies should be done with caution. In the West, most infections are acquired in young adulthood, as a result of sexual transmission or parenteral drug abuse. Although few doubt that such infections present an increase in cancer risk, it is unclear if the magnitude of this risk is as large as in the HBV-endemic zones, if only because those infected as adults have fewer years at risk. Nonetheless, even in the West, the interval between acquisition of infection and HCC development remains at least 30 years (154).

Further support for the oncogenic potential of hepadnavirus infection came with the discovery of the animal hepadnaviruses. Studies of WHV infection showed that this virus is even more potent than HBV as a hepatic carcinogen: nearly 100% of woodchucks infected from birth with WHV develop HCC, starting at about 18 to 24 months of age (163,414,415,469). Uninfected woodchucks housed in similar circumstances do not develop HCC at all. The oncogenic drive accompanying this infection is so strong that many animals develop multiple independent hepatic tumors; even animals who experienced only a transient WHV infection (as judged by the presence of antisurface and anticore antibodies in the absence of surface antigenemia) display an increased prevalence of HCC (163). Ground squirrels infected with GSHV also display an increased prevalence of HCC, although the tumors are less frequent and arise much later in life (339,539). Because WHV and GSHV can both be grown in woodchucks (3,475), it has been possible to compare the oncogenic potential of both infections in a common host. These studies (469) showed that the biology just described is determined largely by the viral genome and not by the host: GSHV-infected woodchucks display HCC later in life and at a lower frequency than WHV-infected woodchucks. As noted earlier, studies of the oncogenic potential of DHBV have not clearly established it as a tumor virus. Although some DHBV-infected flocks in Asia have shown HCC, most laboratory-raised animals or commercial flocks in America and Europe have not exhibited HCC (100), suggesting that environmental factors (or cofactors) may account for a large portion of the oncogenesis in Asia. There is no evidence that Asian DHBV isolates (550) differ from Western isolates in their oncogenicity.

Viral DNA and Hepatocellular Carcinoma

When the tumors themselves are examined, some can be shown to produce one or more viral antigens, but many have extinguished all HBV gene expression.

Nonetheless, most (85% or more) of such tumors harbor integrated viral DNA, often multiple copies per cell (39,481,484). The HBV integrants are usually highly rearranged, with deletions, inversions, and sequence reiterations all commonly observed (121,359); as expected, most of these rearrangements ablate viral gene expression. WHV insertions in woodchuck HCC in general display similar features (378). In addition, alterations of host DNA often accompany these integrations. Described alterations include deletions or repeats at the host–virus junctions (445,484,534,535,590) as well as (more rarely) large chromosomal translocations, some of which harbor HBV sequences at the interchomosomal junctions (533); the latter might have arisen by homologous recombination between viral integrants on two different chromosomes. Importantly, tumors are clonal with respect to these integrants; that is, every cell in the tumor harbors an identical complement of HBV insertions. This implies that the integration events accompanied or preceded the clonal expansion of the cells. Although much has been made of this fact, by itself, it puts HBV DNA at the scene of the crime but does not establish criminality.

How HBV integration is achieved is poorly understood. As opposed to its role in retroviral replication, integration is not an obligatory part of the hepadnaviral replication cycle; it is therefore not surprising that hepadnaviruses have no virus-encoded integration machinery. Presumably, HBV DNA is assimilated into the nucleus by host mechanisms; it is reasonable to suppose that this event proceeds by pathways akin to those operating in the integration of exogenous DNA in transfected mammalian cells in culture. Such mechanisms likely involve topoisomerase I (461,566) and other host enzymes involved in DNA recombination and repair. A major problem that has confounded study of the integration process has been that the integrants characterized in HCC specimens are many years removed from the primary insertion event. During this (about 30-year) interval, there has presumably been strong immunologic selection against viral antigen expression; this is the likely force that has selected the genomic rearrangements described previously. Recently, it has become possible to examine the structure of integrants newly generated in cultured cells permissive for DHBV replication. In acute infection of primary duck hepatocytes, integrated DHBV DNA can be detected as early as six days after infection, although such integration is a rare event (estimated at 1 insertion per 1000 to 10,000 hepatocytes; W. Yang and J. Summers, personal communication). LMH cells stably transfected with overlength DHBV clones similarly accumulate new DHBV insertions during serial passage (168–170). In both systems, many of the resulting integrants have structures compatible with a derivation from the double-stranded liner genomes produced by *in situ* priming; in accord with this, mutant DHBV genomes that display enhanced *in situ* priming display an increased frequency of integration.

Models for Hepatitis B Virus Oncogenesis

The molecular mechanisms by which hepadnaviruses predispose to malignancy remain much debated. Models for how they might act fall into two broad categories, direct and indirect, according to the roles they envision for the viral genome and its products (155).

Direct Models

Direct models posit that viral DNA makes a direct genetic contribution to the lesion, either by providing cis-acting sequences that activate or suppress host growth-regulating genes or by elaborating trans-acting factors that alter the program of cellular growth control. The most straightforward version of such a model is that a viral protein might act as a dominant oncogene, much as src does in Rous sarcoma virus infection. However, hepadnaviruses carry no gene directly transduced from the host cell genome; in addition, hepadnaviral infection does not lead to growth transformation or immortalization of primary cells *in vitro,* although there is one report (215) of further growth deregulation induced by HBV X expression in a cell line already immortalized by SV40 T antigen. These facts, together with the prolonged incubation period between infection and tumor development, make it extremely unlikely that the direct action of a single viral gene product can itself transform a hepatocyte. However, they by no means exclude more subtle roles for viral proteins that might help initiate the loss of growth control, even if they cannot by themselves complete this process.

In this connection, two viral proteins are frequently mentioned. Primary attention has centered on the X protein, for two reasons: (a) it is highly divergent or absent in the avian viruses, the only hepadnaviruses not reliably associated with HCC; and (b) as a known regulator of signal transduction, it is easy to envision models for how such a molecule might affect cellular growth. The debate about X protein's role in oncogenesis has been powerfully influenced by reports that transgenic mice bearing X sequences under the control of the X promoter and EnI develop HCC (260,270). However, this effect has not been observed by other groups using X vectors driven by heterologous promoters (298), nor has comparable oncogenesis been seen in transgenic mice bearing other subgenomic or genomic HBV DNAs containing the X region (11,92,131,133). The reasons for these divergent results are obscure; possibilities include differing levels of X expression or the different genetic backgrounds of the mice used in different laboratories. One thing is certain: if X protein plays a role in oncogenesis, it cannot be necessary for the entire life of the transformed cell because most advanced tumors have extinguished all HBV gene expression. Thus, if X is required early in oncogenesis to promote cell proliferation, this requirement must be obviated at later stages of transformation.

The second viral gene product for which a role in oncogenesis has been postulated is the truncated M protein generated by occasional viral integration events (291,292,366). The roles ascribed to such factors are formally identical to those outlined previously for X protein, but experimental evidence supporting such roles is scant at present: many tumors cannot encode such M variants, and expression of these proteins in cultured cells does not lead to loss of growth control. Finally, rare viral integration events might be able to generate other novel proteins by fusion of viral coding sequences with adjacent cellular genes, analogous to the generation of novel oncogenic proteins by chromosomal translocations in other settings. One potential example of this surfaced in a human HCC, in which integration fused the HBV pre-S region to a retinoic acid receptor locus (104,106). However, such events have been documented extremely rarely and are unlikely to represent a major pathway of oncogenesis.

Most advocates of direct models favor the notion that viral sequences act primarily by contributing cis-acting sequences rather than coding regions. There is unequivocal evidence for this mode of oncogenesis in WHV infection. In this system, about 40% of all HCCs contain an integrated WHV genome within several kilobases of one of two *N-myc* loci; these *N-myc* rearrangements are readily detected by Southern blotting (145,197). *N-myc* genes are normally silent in adult liver but are transcriptionally activated by enhancer elements within WHV DNA (575); recent studies implicate EnII (and, less frequently, EnI) in this effect (138,139,143,551,554). Interestingly, *N-myc* transcription is elevated very early in the oncogenic process, even in premalignant nodules (595), and is observed in virtually 100% of cases. Moreover, among many tumors that lack *N-myc* rearrangements by conventional Southern blotting, integrated WHV DNA can be found in cis to *N-myc2* by pulse-field gel analysis, at distances up to 150 to 180 kb away from the activated locus (142). This raises the possibility that all WHV-associated HCC may be initiated by insertional activation of *N-myc,* with many cases resulting from previously unsuspected long-range activation events. Consistent with this, antisense inhibition of *N-myc* expression in a woodchuck hepatoma cell line reverts its growth phenotype (567), and overexpression of *myc* in the livers of transgenic mice gives rise to HCC (52,221,356). Tumors in such mice require many months to develop, consistent with a requirement for multiple additional genetic hits in the pathogenesis of full malignancy.

N-myc expression may also explain other known features of the biology of woodchuck HCC. For example, it has long been known that such tumors overexpress insulin-like growth factor-2 (IGF-2) (595). Recent studies show that *N-myc2* overexpression often triggers apoptosis, and this effect can be suppressed by exogenous IGF-2 (551,596). It is likely that the up-regulation of IGF-2 naturally observed in HCC is the result of selective pressure exerted by the insertional activation of *N-myc* alleles by WHV.

Efforts to make a similar case for insertional activation by HBV have been largely unsuccessful. Dozens of human hepatomas have been screened for common sites of HBV integration (359,534). This is done by cloning HBV integrants and using the flanking host DNA as a probe to screen Southern blots of DNA from other HCCs for rearrangements of the corresponding host sequences. (This is the same strategy that was employed productively for WHV.) To date, no rearrangements common to many human HCCs have been detected; although a few isolated examples of insertions near interesting loci have been reported (104,106,568), these insertions appear to be unique to the tumors in which they were discovered. Similarly, deliberate screens of human HCCs for rearrangements of known host oncogenes have likewise been largely unrevealing. It should be emphasized, however, that all of these methods can only detect rearrangements within a few kilobases of the locus being probed; if long-range activation events of the type identified for WHV (142) operate in HBV infection, insertional activation might still contribute to the biology of HBV-induced HCC.

Indirect Models

The relative paucity of experimental support for direct models of HBV-induced oncogenesis has led to the growing popularity of indirect models. Here, the term *indirect* means that HBV genes and their products make no direct genetic contribution to the transforming event. Rather, HBV-induced liver injury (itself largely the result of host immune or inflammatory responses to infection) triggers a series of stereotypic host responses that lead to liver cell regeneration. Vertebrate hosts are known to respond to liver cell injury of many types with a brisk regenerative response (although the mechanism of this response is poorly understood). Under conditions of chronic regeneration, the increase in the number of cells undergoing DNA synthesis results in an increased probability of mutation; this in turn increases the probability that one or more of the resulting mutant cells will have a proliferative advantage. As this cell is preferentially expanded, the same logic predicts an increased opportunity for additional mutational lesions in its progeny (and so on, until full growth transformation is achieved). Thus, in indirect models, the role of HBV is to act as an agent of liver injury; everything else—in particular, the growth-deregulating mutations directly responsible for tumorigenesis—is contributed by the host. (The identification of host mutations in HCC is now an active area of inquiry that has turned up numerous candidate loci. Readers interested in this aspect of HCC research are referred to references 52 and 408 for recent review.)

Supporters of indirect models point to several compelling facts, chief among which is that most conditions in human medicine that lead to chronic liver injury are associated to one degree or another with a risk for HCC: alcoholic cirrhosis, α_1-antitrypsin deficiency, Wilson's disease, and so forth. Even hepatitis C virus, an RNA virus with no known DNA intermediate, can predispose to HCC during chronic infection. However, none of these precedents can fully explain why the magnitude of the HCC risk appears to be so much larger in chronic HBV infection. Strong experimental support for this hypothesis is derived from influential experiments in transgenic mice (89). These mice were engineered to overexpress the HBV L protein relative to the M and S proteins. As noted previously, when L is overexpressed, it leads to retention of all the viral envelope glycoproteins in the ER (87,88); this retention is toxic to cells, although the mechanism of this toxicity is unknown. Initially, the mice display only hepatocellular necrosis and accompanying regeneration. Over time, however, malignant HCC arises with great regularity.

Confusion has arisen over the proper interpretation of this experiment, in part because it uses HBV gene products to drive the liver injury. Strictly speaking, the experiment demonstrates that chronic liver injury promotes regeneration and HCC. Although it raises the possibility that viral envelope glycoproteins might contribute to this injury, it does not establish that this form of injury is relevant to clinical hepatitis B. Indeed, it appears unlikely that this would be so; most evidence favors the notion that the bulk of the injury is produced by immune attack on infected hepatocytes (86), and the relative levels of L protein in natural infection are nowhere near those achieved in the HCC-prone transgenic mice. Although hepatocytes with the histologic appearance of cells undergoing damage from deregulated envelope expression can be seen in hepatitis B, in most cases, they are not numerous enough to explain the regenerative drive that accompanies this infection.

A more recent transgenic mouse experiment has affirmed that immune-mediated injury mechanisms can drive hepatic oncogenesis. This study employed mice expressing HBV envelope components at nontoxic levels (akin to those encountered in natural infection) (360). The tolerized immune systems of such animals were ablated by lethal irradiation and replaced with bone marrow and splenocytes from syngeneic mice immunized with a vaccina virus expressing HBsAg. As expected, the recipients developed a chronic hepatitis due to immune attack of the sensitized donor cells on their antigen-expressing hepatocytes. By 17 months after transfer, nearly all such animals had developed HCC, whereas control recipients that received immunocytes from a tolerized (HBV-transgenic) donor developed only minimal liver injury and had a low incidence of HCC. Thus, immune-mediated injury is sufficient to drive hepatic oncogenesis; direct cytotoxicity from deregulated L protein expression is not required.

REFERENCES

1. Akmal M, el-Ghor A, Burk RD. DNase I hypersensitive site maps to the HBV enhancer. *Virology* 1989;172(2):478–488.
2. Albin C, Robinson WS. Protein kinase activity in hepatitis B virus. *J Virol* 1980;34(1):297–302.
3. Aldrich CE, Coates L, Wu TT, et al. *In vitro* infection of woodchuck hepatocytes with woodchuck hepatitis virus and ground squirrel hepatitis virus. *Virology* 1989;172(1):247–252.
4. Andrisani O, Barnabas S. The transcriptional function of the hepatitis B virus X protein and its role in hepatocarcinogenesis [Review]. *Int J Oncol* 1999;15:1–7.
5. Antonucci TK, Rutter WJ. Hepatitis B virus (HBV) promoters are regulated by the HBV enhancers in a tissue-specific manner. *J Virol* 1989;63(2):579–583.
6. Antunovic J, DiCarlo A, Cromlish JA. The novel purification of functional RNA polymerase III VAI transcription preinitiation complexes. *Cell Mol Biol Res* 1993;39:141–158.
7. Araki K, Miyazaki JI, Hino O, et al. Expression and replication of hepatitis B virus genome in transgenic mice. *Proc Natl Acad Sci U S A* 1989;86:207–211.
8. Aufiero B, Schneider RJ. The hepatitis B virus X-gene product trans-activates both RNA polymerase II and III promoters. *EMBO J* 1990; 9:497–504.
9. Avantaggiati ML, Balsano C, Natoli G, et al. The hepatitis B virus X protein transactivation of c-fos and c-myc proto-oncogenes is mediated by multiple transcription factors. *Arch Virol* 1992;4:57–61.
10. Avantaggiati ML, Natoli G, Balsano C, et al. The hepatitis B virus (HBV) pX transactivates the c-fos promoter through multiple cis-acting elements. *Oncogene* 1993;8:1567–1574.
11. Babinet C, Farza H, Morello D, et al. Specific expression of hepatitis B surface antigen (HBsAg) in transgenic mice. *Science* 1985;230 (4730):1160–1163.
12. Balsano C, Avantaggiati ML, Natoli G, et al. Full-length and truncated versions of the hepatitis B virus (HBV) X protein (pX) transactivate the c-myc proto-oncogene at the transcriptional level. *Biochem Biophys Res Commun* 1991;176:985–992.
13. Balsano C, Billet O, Bennoun M, et al. Hepatitis B virus X gene product acts as a transactivator *in vivo*. *J Hepatol* 1994;21:103–109.
14. Barker LF, Chisari FV, McGrath PP, et al. Transmission of type B viral hepatitis to chimpanzees. *J Infect Dis* 1973;127(6):648–662.
15. Barnabas S, Hai T, Andrisani OM. The hepatitis B virus X protein enhances the DNA binding potential and transcription efficacy of bZip transcription factors. *J Biol Chem* 1997;272(33):20684–20690.
16. Bartenschlager R, Junker-Niepmann M, Schaller H. The P gene product of hepatitis B virus is required as a structural component for genomic RNA encapsidation. *J Virol* 1990;64(11):5324–5332.
17. Bartenschlager R, Kuhn C, Schaller H. Expression of the P-protein of the human hepatitis B virus in a vaccinia virus system and detection of the nucleocapsid-associated P-gene product by radiolabelling at newly introduced phosphorylation sites. *Nucleic Acids Res* 1992; 20(2):195–202.
18. Bartenschlager R, Schaller H. The amino-terminal domain of the hepadnaviral P-gene encodes the terminal protein (genome-linked protein) believed to prime reverse transcription. *EMBO J* 1988;7(13): 4185–4192.
19. Bartenschlager R, Schaller H. Hepadnaviral assembly is initiated by polymerase binding to the encapsidation signal in the viral RNA genome. *EMBO J* 1992;11(9):3413–3420.
20. Bavand MR, Laub O. Two proteins with reverse transcriptase activities associated with hepatitis B virus-like particles. *J Virol* 1988;62(2): 626–628.
21. Bayer ME, Blumberg BS, Werner B. Particles associated with Australia antigen in the sera of patients with leukaemia, Down's syndrome and hepatitis. *Nature* 1968;218(146):1057–1059.

22. Beasley RP. Hepatitis B virus: The major etiology of hepatocellular carcinoma. *Cancer* 1988;61(10):1942–1956.
23. Beasley RP, Hwang LY, Lin CC, Chien CS. Hepatocellular carcinoma and hepatitis B virus: A prospective study of 22 707 men in Taiwan. *Lancet* 1981;2(8256):1129–1133.
24. Beasley RP, Trepo C, Stevens CE, Szmuness W. The e antigen and vertical transmission of hepatitis B surface antigen. *Am J Epidemiol* 1977;105(2):94–98.
25. Beck J, Nassal M. Formation of a functional hepatitis B virus replication initiation complex involves a major structural alteration in the RNA template. *Mol Cell Biol* 1998;18(11):6265–6272.
26. Becker SA, Lee T-H, Butel JS, Slagle BL. Hepatitis B virus X protein interferes with cellular DNA repair. *J Virol* 1998;72:266–272.
27. Ben-Levy R, Faktor O, Berger I, Shaul Y. Cellular factors that interact with the hepatitis B virus enhancer. *Mol Cell Biol* 1989;9:1804–1809.
28. Benn J, Schneider RJ. Hepatitis B virus HBx protein activates Ras-GTP complex formation and establishes a Ras, Raf, MAP kinase signalling cascade. *Proc Natl Acad Sci U S A* 1994;91:10350–10354.
29. Benn J, Su F, Doria M, Schneider RJ. Hepatitis B virus HBx protein induces transcription factor AP-1 by activation of extracellular signal-regulated and c-Jun N-terminal mitogen-activated protein kinases. *J Virol* 1996;70:4978–4985.
30. Bergametti F, Prigent S, Luber B, et al. The proapoptotic effect of hepatitis B virus HBx protein correlates with its transactivation activity in stably transfected cell lines. *Oncogene* 1999;18:2860–2871.
31. Bertoletti A, Ferrari C, Fiaccadori F, et al. HLA class I-restricted human cytotoxic T cells recognize endogenously synthesized hepatitis B virus nucleocapsid antigen. *Proc Natl Acad Sci U S A* 1991;88 (23):10445–10449.
32. Bertoletti A, Sette A, Chisari FV, et al. Natural variants of cytotoxic epitopes are T-cell receptor antagonists for antiviral cytotoxic T cells [see Comments]. *Nature* 1994;369(6479):407–410.
33. Birnbaum F, Nassal M. Hepatitis B virus nucleocapsid assembly: Primary structure requirements in the core protein. *J Virol* 1990;64(7): 3319–3330.
34. Blum HE, Zhang Z, Galun E, et al. Hepatitis B virus X protein Is not central to the viral life cycle *in vitro*. *J Virol* 1992;66:1223–1227.
35. Blumberg B, Alter H, Visnich S. A "new" antigen in leukemia sera. *JAMA* 1965;191:541–546.
36. Boni C, Bertoletti A, Penna A, et al. Lamivudine treatment can restore T cell responsiveness in chronic hepatitis B [see Comments]. *J Clin Invest* 1998;102(5):968–975.
37. Bosch V, Bartenschlager R, Radziwill G, Schaller H. The duck hepatitis B virus P-gene codes for protein strongly associated with the 5′-end of the viral DNA minus strand. *Virology* 1988;166(2):475–485.
38. Bottcher B, Wynne SA, Crowther RA. Determination of the fold of the core protein of hepatitis B virus by electron cryomicroscopy [see Comments]. *Nature* 1997;386(6620):88–91.
39. Brechot C, Pourcel C, Louise A, et al. Presence of integrated hepatitis B virus DNA sequences in cellular DNA of human hepatocellular carcinoma. *Nature* 1980;286(5772):533–535.
40. Breiner KM, Urban S, Schaller H. Carboxypeptidase D (gp180), a Golgi-resident protein, functions in the attachment and entry of avian hepatitis B viruses. *J Virol* 1998;72(10):8098–8104.
41. Brunetto MR, Giarin MM, Oliveri F, et al. Wild-type and e antigen-minus hepatitis B viruses and course of chronic hepatitis. *Proc Natl Acad Sci U S A* 1991;88(10):4186–4190.
42. Brunetto MR, Stemmler M, Schodel F, et al. Identification of HBV variants which cannot produce precore-derived HBeAg and may be responsible for severe hepatitis. *Ital J Gastroenterol* 1989;21: 151–154.
43. Bruss V. A short linear sequence in the pre-S domain of the large hepatitis B virus envelope protein required for virion formation. *J Virol* 1997;71(12):9350–9357.
44. Bruss V, Ganem D. Mutational analysis of hepatitis B surface antigen particle assembly and secretion. *J Virol* 1991;65(7):3813–3820.
45. Bruss V, Ganem D. The role of envelope proteins in hepatitis B virus assembly. *Proc Natl Acad Sci U S A* 1991;88(3):1059–1063.
46. Bruss V, Hagelstein J, Gerhardt E, Galle PR. Myristylation of the large surface protein is required for hepatitis B virus *in vitro* infectivity. *Virology* 1996;218(2):396–399.
47. Bruss V, Lu X, Thomssen R, Gerlich WH. Post-translational alterations in transmembrane topology of the hepatitis B virus large envelope protein. *EMBO J* 1994;13(10):2273–2279.
48. Bruss V, Thomssen R. Mapping a region of the large envelope protein required for hepatitis B virion maturation. *J Virol* 1994;68(3): 1643–1650.
49. Bruss V, Vieluf K. Functions of the internal pre-S domain of the large surface protein in hepatitis B virus particle morphogenesis. *J Virol* 1995;69(11):6652–6657.
50. Buckwold VE, Xu Z, Chen M, et al. Effects of a naturally occurring mutation in the hepatitis B virus basal core promoter on precore gene expression and viral replication. *J Virol* 1996;70(9):5845–5851.
51. Budkowska A, Quan C, Groh F, et al. Hepatitis B virus (HBV) binding factor in human serum: Candidate for a soluble form of hepatocyte HBV receptor. *J Virol* 1993;67(7):4316–4322.
52. Buendia MA. Hepatitis B viruses and cancerogenesis. *Biomed Pharmacother* 1998;52(1):34–43.
53. Buendia MA. Hepatitis B viruses and carcinogenesis. *Biomed Pharmacother* 1998;52:34–43.
54. Bulla G, Siddiqui A. The hepatitis B virus enhancer modulates transcription of the hepatitis B virus surface antigen gene from an internal location. *J Virol* 1988;62:1437–1441.
55. Buscher M, Reiser W, Will H, Schaller H. Transcripts and the putative RNA pregenome of duck hepatitis B virus: Implications for reverse transcription. *Cell* 1985;40(3):717–724.
56. Butel JS, Lee T-H, Slagle BL. Is the DNA repair system involved in hepatitis B virus mediated hepatocellular carcinogenesis? *Trends Microbiol* 1996;4:119–124.
57. Calvert J, Summers J. Two regions of an avian hepadnavirus RNA pregenome are required in cis for encapsidation. *J Virol* 1994;68(4): 2084–2090.
58. Cattaneo R, Will H, Hernandez N, Schaller H. Signals regulating hepatitis B surface antigen transcription. *Nature* 1983;305(5932): 336–338.
59. Cavanaugh VJ, Guidotti LG, Chisari FV. Interleukin-12 inhibits hepatitis B virus replication in transgenic mice. *J Virol* 1997;71(4): 3236–3243.
60. Cavanaugh VJ, Guidotti LG, Chisari FV. Inhibition of hepatitis B virus replication during adenovirus and cytomegalovirus infections in transgenic mice. *J Virol* 1998;72(4):2630–2637.
61. Challberg MD, Kelly TJ. Animal virus DNA replication. *Annu Rev Biochem* 1989;58:671–717.
62. Chang C, Enders G, Sprengel R, et al. Expression of the precore region of an avian hepatitis B virus is not required for viral replication. *J Virol* 1987;61(10):3322–3325.
63. Chang C, Zhou S, Ganem D, Standring DN. Phenotypic mixing between different hepadnavirus nucleocapsid proteins reveals C protein dimerization to be cis preferential. *J Virol* 1994;68(8):5225–5231.
64. Chang HK, Ting LP. The surface gene promoter of the human hepatitis B virus displays a preference for differentiated hepatocytes. *Virology* 1989;170(1):176–183.
65. Chang HK, Wang BY, Yuh CH, et al. A liver-specific nuclear factor interacts with the promoter region of the large surface protein gene of human hepatitis B virus. *Mol Cell Biol* 1989;9(11):5189–5197.
66. Chang LJ, Ganem D, Varmus HE. Mechanism of translation of the hepadnaviral polymerase (P) gene. *Proc Natl Acad Sci U S A* 1990;87 (13):5158–5162.
67. Chang LJ, Hirsch RC, Ganem D, Varmus HE. Effects of insertional and point mutations on the functions of the duck hepatitis B virus polymerase. *J Virol* 1990;64(11):5553–5558.
68. Chang LJ, Pryciak P, Ganem D, Varmus HE. Biosynthesis of the reverse transcriptase of hepatitis B viruses involves *de novo* translational initiation not ribosomal frameshifting. *Nature* 1989;337(6205): 364–368.
69. Chazouilleres O, Mamish D, Kim M, et al. "Occult" hepatitis B virus as source of infection in liver transplant recipients [see Comments]. *Lancet* 1994;343(8890):142–146.
70. Chen H, Kaneko S, Girones R, et al. The woodchuck hepatitis virus X gene is important for establishment of virus infection in woodchucks. *J Virol* 1993;67:1218–1226.
71. Chen HS, Kew MC, Hornbuckle WE, et al. The precore gene of the woodchuck hepatitis virus genome is not essential for viral replication in the natural host. *J Virol* 1992;66(9):5682–5684.
72. Chen IH, Huang CJ, Ting LP. Overlapping initiator and TATA box functions in the basal core promoter of hepatitis B virus. *J Virol* 1995;69(6):3647–3657.
73. Chen M, Hieng S, Qian X, et al. Regulation of hepatitis B virus ENI

enhancer activity by hepatocyte-enriched transcription factor HNF3. *Virology* 1994;205(1):127–132.
74. Chen PJ, Chen CR, Sung JL, Chen DS. Identification of a doubly spliced viral transcript joining the separated domains for putative protease and reverse transcriptase of hepatitis B virus. *J Virol* 1989;63 (10):4165–4171.
75. Chen ST, La Porte P, Yee JK. Mutational analysis of hepatitis B virus enhancer 2. *Virology* 1993;196:652–659.
76. Cheng KC, Smith GL, Moss B. Hepatitis B virus large surface protein is not secreted but is immunogenic when selectively expressed by recombinant vaccinia virus. *J Virol* 1986;60(2):337–344.
77. Cheong J-H, Yi M-K, Lin Y, Murakami S. Human RPB5, a subunit shared by eukaryotic nuclear polymerases, binds human hepatitis B virus X protein and may play a role in X transactivation. *EMBO J* 1995;14:143–150.
78. Cherrington J, Ganem D. Regulation of polyadenylation in human immunodeficiency virus (HIV): Contributions of promoter proximity and upstream sequences. *EMBO J* 1992;11(4):1513–1524.
79. Cherrington J, Russnak R, Ganem D. Upstream sequences and cap proximity in the regulation of polyadenylation in ground squirrel hepatitis virus. *J Virol* 1992;66(12):7589–7596.
80. Cheung RC, Robinson WS, Marion PL, Greenberg HB. Epitope mapping of neutralizing monoclonal antibodies against duck hepatitis B virus. *J Virol* 1989;63(6):2445–2451.
81. Cheung RC, Trujillo DE, Robinson WS, et al. Epitope-specific antibody response to the surface antigen of duck hepatitis B virus in infected ducks. *Virology* 1990;176(2):546–552.
82. Chiang PW, Jeng KS, Hu CP, Chang CM. Characterization of a cis element required for packaging and replication of the human hepatitis B virus. *Virology* 1992;186(2):701–711.
83. Chirillo P, Falco M, Puri PL, et al. Hepatitis B virus pX activates NF-kB-dependent transcription through a Raf-independent pathway. *J Virol* 1996;70:641–646.
84. Chirillo P, Pagano S, Natoli G, et al. The hepatitis B virus X gene induces p53-mediated programmed cell death. *Proc Natl Acad Sci U S A* 1997;94:8162–8167.
85. Chisari FV. Cytotoxic T cells and viral hepatitis. *J Clin Invest* 1997;99 (7):1472–1477.
86. Chisari FV, Ferrari C. Hepatitis B virus immunopathogenesis. *Annu Rev Immunol* 1995;13:29–60.
87. Chisari FV, Filippi P, Buras J, et al. Structural and pathological effects of synthesis of hepatitis B virus large envelope polypeptide in transgenic mice. *Proc Natl Acad Sci U S A* 1987;84(19):6909–6913.
88. Chisari FV, Filippi P, McLachlan A, et al. Expression of hepatitis B virus large envelope polypeptide inhibits hepatitis B surface antigen secretion in transgenic mice. *J Virol* 1986;60(3):880–887.
89. Chisari FV, Klopchin K, Moriyama T, et al. Molecular pathogenesis of hepatocellular carcinoma in hepatitis B virus transgenic mice. *Cell* 1989;59(6):1145–1156.
90. Choi BH, Park GT, Rho HM. Interaction of hepatitis B viral X protein and CCAAT/enhancer-binding protein alpha synergistically activates the hepatitis B viral enhancer II/pregenomic promoter. *J Biol Chem* 1999;274:2858–2865.
91. Choo KB, Liew LN, Chong KY, et al. Transgenome transcription and replication in the liver and extrahepatic tissues of a human hepatitis B virus transgenic mouse. *Virology* 1991;182:785–792.
92. Choo KB, Liew LN, Chong KY, et al. Transgenome transcription and replication in the liver and extrahepatic tissues of a human hepatitis B virus transgenic mouse. *Virology* 1991;182(2):785–792.
93. Cohen BJ, Richmond JE. Electron microscopy of hepatitis B core antigen synthesized in *E. coli. Nature* 1982;296(5858):677–679.
94. Colgrove R, Simon G, Ganem D. Transcriptional activation of homologous and heterologous genes by the hepatitis B virus X gene product in cells permissive for viral replication. *J Virol* 1989;63:4019–4026.
95. Condreay LD, Aldrich CE, Coates L, et al. Efficient duck hepatitis B virus production by an avian liver tumor cell line. *J Virol* 1990;64(7): 3249–3258.
96. Condreay LD, Wu TT, Aldrich CE, et al. Replication of DHBV genomes with mutations at the sites of initiation of minus- and plus-strand DNA synthesis. *Virology* 1992;188(1):208–216.
97. Cong YS, Yao YL, Yang WM, et al. The hepatitis B virus X-associated protein, XAP3, is a protein kinase C-binding protein. *J Biol Chem* 1997;272:16482–16489.
98. Courtois G, Baumhueter S, Crabtree GR. Purified hepatocyte nuclear factor 1 interacts with a family of hepatocyte-specific promoters. *Proc Natl Acad Sci U S A* 1988;85(21):7937–7941.
99. Cross JC, Wen P, Rutter WJ. Transactivation by hepatitis B virus X protein is promiscuous and dependent on mitogen activated cellular serine/threonine kinases. *Proc Natl Acad Sci U S A* 1993;90: 8078–8082.
100. Cullen JM, Marion PL, Sherman GJ, et al. Hepatic neoplasms in aflotoxin B1-treated congenitally DHBV-infected and virus-free. In: Hollinger FB, Lemon SM, Margolis H, eds. *Viral hepatitis and liver disease.* Proceedings of the 1990 International Symposium on Viral Hepatitis and Liver Disease: Contemporary Issues and Future Prospects. Baltimore: Williams & Wilkins, 1990:601–604.
101. Dandri M, Petersen J, Stockert RJ, et al. Metabolic labeling of woodchuck hepatitis B virus X protein in naturally infected hepatocytes reveals a bimodal half-life and association with the nuclear framework. *J Virol* 1998;72(11):9359–9364.
102. Dandri M, Schirmacher P, Rogler CE. Woodchuck hepatitis virus X protein is present in chronically infected woodchuck liver and woodchuck hepatocellular carcinomas which are permissive for viral replication. *J Virol* 1996;70:5246–5254.
103. Dane DS, Cameron CH, Briggs M. Virus-like particles in serum of patients with Australia-antigen-associated hepatitis. *Lancet* 1970;1 (7649):695–698.
104. de The H, Marchio A, Tiollais P, Dejean A. A novel steroid thyroid hormone receptor-related gene inappropriately expressed in human hepatocellular carcinoma. *Nature* 1987;330(6149):667–670.
105. De-Medina T, Faktor O, Shaul Y. The S promoter of hepatitis B virus is regulated by positive and negative elements. *Mol Cell Biol* 1988; 8(6):2449–2455.
106. Dejean A, Bougueleret L, Grzeschik KH, Tiollais P. Hepatitis B virus DNA integration in a sequence homologous to v-erb-A and steroid receptor genes in a hepatocellular carcinoma. *Nature* 1986;322 (6074):70–72.
107. Derijard B, Hibi M, Wu IH, et al. JNK1: A protein kinase stimulated by UV light and Ha-Ras that binds and phosphorylates the c-Jun activation domain. *Cell* 1994;76:1025–1037.
108. Di Q, Summers J, Burch JB, Mason WS. Major differences between WHV and HBV in the regulation of transcription. *Virology* 1997;229: 25–35.
109. Diamantis ID, McGandy CE, Chen TJ, et al. Hepatitis B X-gene expression in hepatocellular carcinoma. *J Hepatol* 1992;1992: 400–403.
110. Dikic I, Tokiwa G, Lev S, et al. A role for Pyk2 and Src in linking G-protein-coupled receptors with MAP kinase activation. *Nature* 1996;383:547–550.
111. Dikstein R, Faktor O, Ben-Levy R, Shaul Y. Functional organization of the hepatitis B virus enhancer. *Mol Cell Biol* 1990;10(7): 3682–3689.
112. Dikstein R, Faktor O, Shaul Y. Hierarchic and cooperative binding of the rat liver nuclear protein C/EBP at the hepatitis B virus enhancer. *Mol Cell Biol* 1990;10(8):4427–4430.
113. Donello JE, Beeche AA, Smith GJ 3rd, et al. The hepatitis B virus posttranscriptional regulatory element is composed of two subelements. *J Virol* 1996;70(7):4345–4351.
114. Donello JE, Loeb JE, Hope TJ. Woodchuck hepatitis virus contains a tripartite posttranscriptional regulatory element. *J Virol* 1998;72(6): 5085–5092.
115. Doria M, Klein N, Lucito R, Schneider RJ. Hepatitis B virus HBx protein is a dual specificity cytoplasmic activator of Ras and nuclear activator of transcription factors. *EMBO J* 1995;14:4747–4757.
116. Dubois MF, Pourcel C, Rousset S, et al. Excretion of hepatitis B surface antigen particles from mouse cells transformed with cloned viral DNA. *Proc Natl Acad Sci U S A* 1980;77(8):4549–4553.
117. Eble BE, Lingappa VR, Ganem D. Hepatitis B surface antigen: An unusual secreted protein initially synthesized as a transmembrane polypeptide. *Mol Cell Biol* 1986;6(5):1454–1463.
118. Eble BE, Lingappa VR, Ganem D. The N-terminal (pre-S2) domain of a hepatitis B virus surface glycoprotein is translocated across membranes by downstream signal sequences. *J Virol* 1990;64(3): 1414–1419.
119. Eble BE, MacRae DR, Lingappa VR, Ganem D. Multiple topogenic sequences determine the transmembrane orientation of the hepatitis B surface antigen. *Mol Cell Biol* 1987;7(10):3591–3601.
120. Eckhardt SG, Milich DR, McLachlan A. Hepatitis B virus core anti-

gen has two nuclear localization sequences in the arginine-rich carboxyl terminus. *J Virol* 1991;65(2):575–582.
121. Edman JC, Gray P, Valenzuela P, et al. Integration of hepatitis B virus sequences and their expression in a human hepatoma cell. *Nature* 1980;286(5772):535–538.
122. Elmore LW, Hancock AR, Chang SF, et al. Hepatitis B virus X protein and p53 tumor suppressor interactions in the modulation of apoptosis. *Proc Natl Acad Sci U S A* 1997;94(26):14707–14712.
123. Enders GH, Ganem D, Varmus H. Mapping the major transcripts of ground squirrel hepatitis virus: The presumptive template for reverse transcriptase is terminally redundant. *Cell* 1985;42(1):297–308.
124. Enders GH, Ganem D, Varmus HE. 5′-Terminal sequences influence the segregation of ground squirrel hepatitis virus RNAs into polyribosomes and viral core particles. *J Virol* 1987;61(1):35–41.
125. Eng FJ, Novikova EG, Kuroki K, et al. gp180, A protein that binds duck hepatitis B virus particles, has metallocarboxypeptidase D-like enzymatic activity. *J Biol Chem* 1998;273(14):8382–8388.
126. Etiemble J, Degott C, Renard CA, et al. Liver specific expression and high oncogenic efficiency of a c-myc transgene activated by woodchuck hepatitis virus insertion. *Oncogene* 1994;9:727–737.
127. Faktor O, Budlovsky S, Ben-Levy R, Shaul Y. A single element within the hepatitis B virus enhancer binds multiple proteins and responds to multiple stimuli. *J Virol* 1990;64:1861–1863.
128. Faktor O, De-Medina T, Shaul Y. Regulation of hepatitis B virus S gene promoter in transfected cell lines. *Virology* 1988;162(2): 362–368.
129. Faktor O, Shaul Y. The identification of hepatitis B virus X gene responsive elements reveals functional similarity of X and HTLV-I tax. *Oncogene* 1990;5:867–872.
130. Faruqi AF, Roychoudhury S, Greenberg R, et al. Replication-defective missense mutations within the terminal protein and spacer/intron regions of the polymerase gene of human hepatitis B virus. *Virology* 1991;183(2):764–768.
131. Farza H, Hadchouel M, Scotto J, et al. Replication and gene expression of hepatitis B virus in a transgenic mouse that contains the complete viral genome. *J Virol* 1988;62(11):4144–4152.
132. Farza H, Hadchovel M, Scotto J, et al. Replication and gene expression of hepatitis B virus in a transgenic mouse that contains the complete viral genome. *J Virol* 1988;62:4144–4152.
133. Farza H, Salmon AM, Hadchouel M, et al. Hepatitis B surface antigen gene expression is regulated by sex steroids and glucocorticoids in transgenic mice. *Proc Natl Acad Sci U S A* 1987;84(5):1187–1191.
134. Feitelson M, Zhu M, Duan LX, London WT. Hepatitis B x antigen and p53 are associated *in vitro* and in liver tissues from patients with primary hepatocellular carcinoma. *Oncogene* 1993;8:1109–1117.
135. Feitelson MA, Marion PL, Robinson WS. Core particles of hepatitis B virus and ground squirrel hepatitis virus. II. Characterization of the protein kinase reaction associated with ground squirrel hepatitis virus and hepatitis B virus. *J Virol* 1982;43(2):741–748.
136. Feldherr CM, Kallenbach E, Schultz N. Movement of a karyophilic protein through the nuclear pores of oocytes. *J Cell Biol* 1984;99(6): 2216–2222.
137. Fernholz D, Wildner G, Will H. Minor envelope proteins of duck hepatitis B virus are initiated at internal pre-S AUG codons but are not essential for infectivity. *Virology* 1993;197(1):64–73.
138. Flajolet M, Gegonne A, Ghysdael J, et al. Cellular and viral trans-acting factors modulate N-myc2 promoter activity in woodchuck liver tumors. *Oncogene* 1997;15(9):1103–1110.
139. Flajolet M, Tiollais P, Buendia MA, Fourel G. Woodchuck hepatitis virus enhancer I and enhancer II are both involved in N-myc2 activation in woodchuck liver tumors. *J Virol* 1998;72(7):6175–6180.
140. Fouillot N, Tlouzeau S, Rossignol JM, Jean-Jean O. Translation of the hepatitis B virus P gene by ribosomal scanning as an alternative to internal initiation. *J Virol* 1993;67(8):4886–4895.
141. Fourel G, Couturier J, Wei Y, et al. Evidence for long-range oncogene activation by hepadnavirus insertion. *EMBO J* 1994;13:2526–2534.
142. Fourel G, Couturier J, Wei Y, et al. Evidence for long-range oncogene activation by hepadnavirus insertion. *EMBO J* 1994;13(11): 2526–2534.
143. Fourel G, Ringeisen F, Flajolet M, et al. The HNF1/HNF4-dependent We2 element of woodchuck hepatitis virus controls viral replication and can activate the N-myc2 promoter. *J Virol* 1996;70(12): 8571–8583.
144. Fourel G, Trepo C, Bougueleret L, et al. Frequent activation of N-myc genes by hepadnavirus insertion in woodchuck liver tumors. *Nature* (London) 1990;347:294–298.
145. Fourel G, Trepo C, Bougueleret L, et al. Frequent activation of N-myc genes by hepadnavirus insertion in woodchuck liver tumours [see comments]. *Nature* 1990;347(6290):294–298.
146. Franco A, Guidotti LG, Hobbs MV, et al. Pathogenetic effector function of CD4-positive T helper 1 cells in hepatitis B virus transgenic mice. *J Immunol* 1997;159(4):2001–2008.
147. Franco A, Paroli M, Testa U, et al. Transferrin receptor mediates uptake and presentation of hepatitis B envelope antigen by T lymphocytes. *J Exp Med* 1992;175(5):1195–1205.
148. Fukai K, Takada S, Yokosuka O, et al. Characterization of a specific region in the hepatitis B virus enhancer I for the efficient expression of X gene in the hepatic cell. *Virology* 1997;236(2):279–287.
149. Galibert F, Chen TN, Mandart E. Nucleotide sequence of a cloned woodchuck hepatitis virus genome: comparison with the hepatitis B virus sequence. *J Virol* 1982;41(1):51–65.
150. Galibert F, Mandart E, Fitoussi F, et al. Nucleotide sequence of the hepatitis B virus genome (subtype ayw) cloned in *E. coli*. *Nature* 1979;281(5733):646–650.
151. Galle PR, Schlicht HJ, Fischer M, Schaller H. Production of infectious duck hepatitis B virus in a human hepatoma cell line. *J Virol* 1988;62(5):1736–1740.
152. Galle PR, Schlicht HJ, Kuhn C, Schaller H. Replication of duck hepatitis B virus in primary duck hepatocytes and its dependence on the state of differentiation of the host cell. *Hepatology* 1989;10(4): 459–465.
153. Gallina A, Bonelli F, Zentilin L, et al. A recombinant hepatitis B core antigen polypeptide with the protamine-like domain deleted self-assembles into capsid particles but fails to bind nucleic acids. *J Virol* 1989;63(11):4645–4652.
154. Ganem D. Persistent infection of humans with hepatitis B virus: Mechanisms and consequences. *Rev Infect Dis* 1982;4(5):1026–1047.
155. Ganem D. Oncogenic viruses. Of marmots and men [News; comment]. *Nature* 1990;347(6290):230–232.
156. Ganem D, Greenbaum L, Varmus HE. Virion DNA of ground squirrel hepatitis virus: Structural analysis and molecular cloning. *J Virol* 1982;44(1):374–383.
157. Ganem D, Weiser B, Barchuk A, et al. Biological characterization of acute infection with ground squirrel hepatitis virus. *J Virol* 1982; 44(1):366–373.
158. Garcia AD, Ostapchuk P, Hearing P. Functional interaction of nuclear factors EF-C, HNF-4, and RXR alpha with hepatitis B virus enhancer I. *J Virol* 1993;67(7):3940–3950.
159. Garcia PD, Ou JH, Rutter WJ, Walter P. Targeting of the hepatitis B virus precore protein to the endoplasmic reticulum membrane: After signal peptide cleavage translocation can be aborted and the product released into the cytoplasm. *J Cell Biol* 1988;106(4):1093–1104.
160. Gavilanes F, Gonzalez-Ros JM, Peterson DL. Structure of hepatitis B surface antigen: Characterization of the lipid components and their association with the viral proteins. *J Biol Chem* 1982;257(13): 7770–7777.
161. Gerber MA, Hadziyannis S, Vissoulis C, et al. Electron microscopy and immunoelectronmicroscopy of cytoplasmic hepatitis B antigen in hepatocytes. *Am J Pathol* 1974;75(3):489–502.
162. Gerelsaikhan T, Tavis JE, Bruss V. Hepatitis B virus nucleocapsid envelopment does not occur without genomic DNA synthesis. *J Virol* 1996;70(7):4269–4274.
163. Gerin JL, Cote PJ, Korba BE, et al. Hepatitis B virus and liver cancer: The woodchuck as an experimental model of hepadnavirus-induced liver cancer. In: Hollinger FB, Lemon SM, Margolis H, eds. *Viral hepatitis and liver disease.* Proceedings of the 1990 International Symposium on Viral Hepatitis and Liver Disease: Contemporary Issues and Future Prospects. Baltimore: Williams & Wilkins, 1990: 556–558.
164. Gerin JL, Purcell RH, Hoggan MD, et al. Biophysical properties of Australia antigen. *J Virol* 1969;4(5):763–768.
165. Gerlich WH, Goldmann U, Muller R, et al. Specificity and localization of the hepatitis B virus-associated protein kinase. *J Virol* 1982; 42(3):761–766.
166. Gerlich WH, Robinson WS. Hepatitis B virus contains protein attached to the 5′ terminus of its complete DNA strand. *Cell* 1980; 21(3):801–809.
167. Gilles PN, Fey G, Chisari FV. Tumor necrosis factor alpha negatively

regulates hepatitis B virus gene expression in transgenic mice. *J Virol* 1992;66(6):3955–3960.
168. Gong SS, Jensen AD, Chang CJ, Rogler CE. Double-stranded linear duck hepatitis B virus (DHBV) stably integrates at a higher frequency than wild-type DHBV in LMH chicken hepatoma cells. *J Virol* 1999; 73(2):1492–1502.
169. Gong SS, Jensen AD, Rogler CE. Loss and acquisition of duck hepatitis B virus integrations in lineages of LMH-D2 chicken hepatoma cells. *J Virol* 1996;70(3):2000–2007.
170. Gong SS, Jensen AD, Wang H, Rogler CE. Duck hepatitis B virus integrations in LMH chicken hepatoma cells: Identification and characterization of new episomally derived integrations. *J Virol* 1995; 69(12):8102–8108.
171. Gonzalez-Amaro R, Garcia-Monzon C, Garcia-Buey L, et al. Induction of tumor necrosis factor α production by human hepatocytes in chronic viral hepatitis. *J Exp Med* 1994;179:841–848.
172. Gottlob K, Fulco M, Levrero M, Graessmann A. The hepatitis B virus HBx protein inhibits caspase 3 activity. *J Biol Chem* 1998;273: 33347–33353.
173. Grgacic EV, Anderson DA. The large surface protein of duck hepatitis B virus is phosphorylated in the pre-S domain. *J Virol* 1994;68(11): 7344–7350.
174. Grgacic EV, Lin B, Gazina EV, et al. Normal phosphorylation of duck hepatitis B virus L protein is dispensable for infectivity. *J Gen Virol* 1998;79(11):2743–2751.
175. Gripon P, Diot C, Guguen-Guillouzo C. Reproducible high level infection of cultured adult human hepatocytes by hepatitis B virus: Effect of polyethylene glycol on adsorption and penetration. *Virology* 1993;192(2):534–540.
176. Gripon P, Diot C, Theze N, et al. Hepatitis B virus infection of adult human hepatocytes cultured in the presence of dimethyl sulfoxide. *J Virol* 1988;62(11):4136–4143.
177. Groisman IJ, Koshy R, Henkler F, et al. Downregulation of DNA excision repair by the hepatitis B virus-x protein occurs in p53-proficient and p53-deficient cells. *Carcinogenesis* 1999;20(3):479–483.
178. Guidotti LG, Ando K, Hobbs MV, et al. Cytotoxic T lymphocytes inhibit hepatitis B virus gene expression by a noncytolytic mechanism in transgenic mice. *Proc Natl Acad Sci U S A* 1994;91(9):3764–3768.
179. Guidotti LG, Borrow P, Brown A, et al. Noncytopathic clearance of lymphocytic choriomeningitis virus from the hepatocyte. *J Exp Med* 1999;189(10):1555–1564.
180. Guidotti LG, Borrow P, Hobbs MV, et al. Viral cross talk: Intracellular inactivation of the hepatitis B virus during an unrelated viral infection of the liver. *Proc Natl Acad Sci U S A* 1996;93(10):4589–4594.
181. Guidotti LG, Chisari FV. To kill or to cure: Options in host defense against viral infection. *Curr Opin Immunol* 1996;8(4):478–483.
182. Guidotti LG, Guilhot S, Chisari FV. Interleukin-2 and alpha/beta interferon down-regulate hepatitis B virus gene expression *in vivo* by tumor necrosis factor-dependent and -independent pathways. *J Virol* 1994;68(3):1265–1270.
183. Guidotti LG, Ishikawa T, Hobbs MV, et al. Intracellular inactivation of the hepatitis B virus by cytotoxic T lymphocytes. *Immunity* 1996;4(1): 25–36.
184. Guidotti LG, Martinez V, Loh YT, et al. Hepatitis B virus nucleocapsid particles do not cross the hepatocyte nuclear membrane in transgenic mice. *J Virol* 1994;68(9):5469–5475.
185. Guidotti LG, Matzke B, Chisari FV. Hepatitis B virus replication is cell cycle independent during liver regeneration in transgenic mice. *J Virol* 1997;71(6):4804–4808.
186. Guidotti LG, Matzke B, Pasquinelli C, et al. The hepatitis B virus (HBV) precore protein inhibits HBV replication in transgenic mice. *J Virol* 1996;70(10):7056–7061.
187. Guidotti LG, Rochford R, Chung J, et al. Viral clearance without destruction of infected cells during acute HBV infection. *Science* 1999;284(5415):825–829.
188. Gunther S, Meisel H, Reip A, et al. Frequent and rapid emergence of mutated pre-C sequences in HBV from e-antigen positive carriers who seroconvert to anti-HBe during interferon treatment. *Virology* 1992; 187(1):271–279.
189. Guo W, Chen M, Yen TS, Ou JH. Hepatocyte-specific expression of the hepatitis B virus core promoter depends on both positive and negative regulation. *Mol Cell Biol* 1993;13(1):443–448.
190. Guo WT, Bell KD, Ou JS. Characterization of the hepatitis B virus EnhI and X promoter complex. *J Virol* 1991;65:6686–6692.
191. Guo WT, Wang J, Tam G, et al. Leaky transcription termination produces larger and smaller than genome size hepatitis B virus X gene transcripts. *Virology* 1991;181:630–636.
192. Gustin K, Shapiro M, Lee W, Burk RD. Characterization of the role of individual protein binding motifs within the hepatitis B virus enhancer I on X promoter activity using linker scanning mutagenesis. *Virology* 1993;193:653–660.
193. Halpern MS, Egan J, McMahon SB, Ewert DL. Duck hepatitis B virus is tropic for exocrine cells of the pancreas. *Virology* 1985;146(1): 157–161.
194. Halpern MS, England JM, Deery DT, et al. Viral nucleic acid synthesis and antigen accumulation in pancreas and kidney of Pekin ducks infected with duck hepatitis B virus. *Proc Natl Acad Sci U S A* 1983; 80(15):4865–4869.
195. Halpern MS, England JM, Flores L, et al. Individual cells in tissues of DHBV-infected ducks express antigens crossreactive with those on virus surface antigen particles and immature viral cores. *Virology* 1984;137(2):408–413.
196. Halpern MS, McMahon SB, Mason WS, O'Connell AP. Viral antigen expression in the pancreas of DHBV-infected embryos and young ducks. *Virology* 1986;150(1):276–282.
197. Hansen LJ, Tennant BC, Seeger C, Ganem D. Differential activation of myc gene family members in hepatic carcinogenesis by closely related hepatitis B viruses. *Mol Cell Biol* 1993;13(1):659–667.
198. Hasegawa K, Huang JK, Wands JR, et al. Association of hepatitis B viral precore mutations with fulminant hepatitis B in Japan. *Virology* 1991;185(1):460–463.
199. Hatton T, Zhou S, Standring DN. RNA- and DNA-binding activities in hepatitis B virus capsid protein: A model for their roles in viral replication. *J Virol* 1992;66(9):5232–5241.
200. Havert MB, Loeb DD. cis-Acting sequences in addition to donor and acceptor sites are required for template switching during synthesis of plus-strand DNA for duck hepatitis B virus. *J Virol* 1997;71(7): 5336–5344.
201. Haviv I, Shamay M, Doitsch G, Shaul Y. Hepatitis B virus pX targets TFIIB in transcription coactivation. *Mol Cell Biol* 1998;18: 1562–1569.
202. Haviv I, Vaizel D, Shaul Y. The X protein of hepatitis B virus coactivates potent activation domains. *Mol Cell Biol* 1995;15: 1079–1085.
203. Haviv I, Vaizel D, Shaul Y. pX, the HBV-encoded coactivator, interacts with components of the transcription machinery and stimulates transcription in a TAF-independent manner. *EMBO J* 1996;15: 3413–3420.
204. Heermann KH, Goldmann U, Schwartz W, et al. Large surface proteins of hepatitis B virus containing the pre-s sequence. *J Virol* 1984; 52(2):396–402.
205. Heise T, Guidotti LG, Cavanaugh VJ, Chisari FV. Hepatitis B virus RNA-binding proteins associated with cytokine-induced clearance of viral RNA from the liver of transgenic mice. *J Virol* 1999;73(1): 474–481.
206. Henkler F, Lopes AR, Jones M, Koshy R. Erk-independent partial activation of AP-1 sites by the hepatitis B virus HBx protein. *J Gen Virol* 1998;79:2737–2742.
207. Hertogs K, Leenders WP, Depla E, et al. Endonexin II, present on human liver plasma membranes, is a specific binding protein of small hepatitis B virus (HBV) envelope protein. *Virology* 1993;197(2): 549–557.
208. Hess J, Stemler M, Will H, et al. Frequent detection of antibodies to hepatitis B virus x-protein in acute, chronic and resolved infections. *Med Microbiol Immunol* 1988;177:195–205.
209. Hild M, Weber O, Schaller H. Glucagon treatment interferes with an early step of duck hepatitis B virus infection. *J Virol* 1998;72(4): 2600–2606.
210. Hildt E, Saher G, Bruss V, Hofschneider PH. The hepatitis B virus large surface protein (LHBs) is a transcriptional activator. *Virology* 1996;225(1):235–239.
211. Hirsch R, Colgrove R, Ganem D. Replication of duck hepatitis B virus in two differentiated human hepatoma cell lines after transfection with cloned viral DNA. *Virology* 1988;167(1):136–142.
212. Hirsch RC, Lavine JE, Chang LJ, et al. Polymerase gene products of hepatitis B viruses are required for genomic RNA packaging as wel as for reverse transcription. *Nature* 1990;344(6266):552–555.
213. Hirsch RC, Loeb DD, Pollack JR, Ganem D. cis-Acting sequences

required for encapsidation of duck hepatitis B virus pregenomic RNA. *J Virol* 1991;65(6):3309–3316.

214. Hohne M, Schaefer S, Seifer M, et al. Malignant transformation of immortalized transgenic hepatocytes after transfection with hepatitis B virus DNA. *EMBO J* 1990;9:1137–1145.
215. Hohne M, Schaefer S, Seifer M, et al. Malignant transformation of immortalized transgenic hepatocytes after transfection with hepatitis B virus DNA. *EMBO J* 1990;9(4):1137–1145.
216. Honigwachs J, Faktor O, Dikstein R, et al. Liver-specific expression of hepatitis B virus is determined by the combined action of the core gene promoter and the enhancer. *J Virol* 1989;63(2):919–924.
217. Hoofnagle JH. Serologic markers of hepatitis B virus infection. *Annu Rev Med* 1981;32:1–11.
218. Hoofnagle JH, Gerety RJ, Barker LF. Antibody to hepatitis-B-virus core in man. *Lancet* 1973;2(7834):869–873.
219. Hoofnagle JH, Seeff LB, Bales ZB, et al. Serologic responses in HB. In: Vyas GN, Cohen SN, Schmid R, eds. *Viral hepatitis: A contemporary assessment of etiology, epidemiology, pathogenesis, and prevention.* Philadelphia: Franklin Institute Press, 1978:219–244.
220. Hosoda K, Omata M, Uchiumi K, et al. Extrahepatic replication of duck hepatitis B virus: More than expected. *Hepatology* 1990;11(1):44–48.
221. Hsu T, Moroy T, Etiemble J, et al. Activation of c-myc by woodchuck hepatitis virus insertion in hepatocellular carcinoma. *Cell* 1988;55(4): 627–635.
222. Hsu TY, Moroy T, Etiemble J, et al. Activation of c-myc by woodchuck hepatitis virus insertion in hepatocellular carcinoma. *Cell* 1988;55: 627–635.
223. Hu J, Seeger C. Hsp90 is required for the activity of a hepatitis B virus reverse transcriptase. *Proc Natl Acad Sci U S A* 1996;93(3): 1060–1064.
224. Hu J, Toft DO, Seeger C. Hepadnavirus assembly and reverse transcription require a multi-component chaperone complex which is incorporated into nucleocapsids. *EMBO J* 1997;16(1):59–68.
225. Hu KQ, Siddiqui A. Regulation of the hepatitis B virus gene expression by the enhancer element I. *Virology* 1991;181(2):721–726.
226. Hu Z, Zhang Z, Doo E, et al. Hepatitis B virus X protein is both a substrate and a potential inhibitor of the proteasome complex. *J Virol* 1999;73(9):7231–7240.
227. Huang J, Liang TJ. A novel hepatitis B virus (HBV) genetic element with Rev response element-like properties that is essential for expression of HBV gene products. *Mol Cell Biol* 1993;13(12):7476–7486.
228. Huang M, Summers J. pet, A small sequence distal to the pregenome cap site, is required for expression of the duck hepatitis B virus pregenome. *J Virol* 1994;68(3):1564–1572.
229. Huang MJ, Summers J. Infection initiated by the RNA pregenome of a DNA virus. *J Virol* 1991;65(10):5435–5439.
230. Huang ZM, Yen TS. Hepatitis B virus RNA element that facilitates accumulation of surface gene transcripts in the cytoplasm. *J Virol* 1994;68(5):3193–3199.
231. Huang ZM, Yen TS. Role of the hepatitis B virus posttranscriptional regulatory element in export of intronless transcripts. *Mol Cell Biol* 1995;15(7):3864–3869.
232. Huovila AP, Eder AM, Fuller SD. Hepatitis B surface antigen assembles in a post-ER, pre-Golgi compartment. *J Cell Biol* 1992;118(6): 1305–1320.
233. Hyams KC. Risks of chronicity following acute hepatitis B virus infection: A review. *Clin Infect Dis* 1995;20(4):992–1000.
234. Imazeki F, Yaginuma K, Omata M, et al. Integrated structures of duck hepatitis B virus DNA in hepatocellular carcinoma. *J Virol* 1988; 62(3):861–865.
235. Ishikawa T, Ganem D. The pre-S domain of the large viral envelope protein determines host range in avian hepatitis B viruses. *Proc Natl Acad Sci U S A* 1995;92(14):6259–6263.
236. Ishikawa T, Kono D, Chung J, et al. Polyclonality and multispecificity of the CTL response to a single viral epitope. *J Immunol* 1998;161 (11):5842–5850.
237. Ishikawa T,Kuroki K, Lenhoff R, et al. Analysis of the binding of a host cell surface glycoprotein to the preS protein of duck hepatitis B virus. *Virology* 1994;202(2):1061–1064.
238. Iwasaki K, Temin HM. The efficiency of RNA 3′-end formation is determined by the distance between the cap site and the poly(A) site in spleen necrosis virus. *Genes Dev* 1990;4(12B):2299–2307.
239. Jacks T, Varmus HE. Expression of the Rous sarcoma virus pol gene by ribosomal frameshifting. *Science* 1985;230(4731):1237–1242.
240. Jacob JR, Ascenzi MA, Roneker CA, et al. Hepatic expression of the woodchuck hepatitis virus X-antigen during acute and chronic infection and detection of a woodchuck hepatitis virus X-antigen antibody response. *Hepatology* 1997;26:1607–1615.
241. Jameel S, Siddiqui A. The human hepatitis B virus enhancer requires trans-acting cellular factor(s) for activity. *Mol Cell Biol* 1986;6(2): 710–715.
242. Jean-Jean O, Levrero M, Will H, et al. Expression mechanism of the hepatitis B virus (HBV) C gene and biosynthesis of HBe antigen. *Virology* 1989;170(1):99–106.
243. Jean-Jean O, Salhi S, Carlier D, et al. Biosynthesis of hepatitis B virus e antigen: directed mutagenesis of the putative aspartyl protease site. *J Virol* 1989;63(12):5497–5500.
244. Jean-Jean O, Weimer T, de Recondo AM, et al. Internal entry of ribosomes and ribosomal scanning involved in hepatitis B virus P gene expression. *J Virol* 1989;63(12):5451–5454.
245. Jia L, Wang XW, Harris CC. Hepatitis B virus X protein inhibits nucleotide excision repair. *Int J Cancer* 1999;80(6):875–879.
246. Jiang H, Loeb DD. Insertions within epsilon affect synthesis of minus-strand DNA before the template switch for duck hepatitis B virus. *J Virol* 1997;71(7):5345–5354.
247. Jilbert AR, Freiman JS, Gowans EJ, et al. Duck hepatitis B virus DNA in liver, spleen, and pancreas: Analysis by *in situ* and Southern blot hybridization. *Virology* 1987;158(2):330–338.
248. Jilbert AR, Wu TT, England JM, et al. Rapid resolution of duck hepatitis B virus infections occurs after massive hepatocellular involvement. *J Virol* 1992;66(3):1377–1388.
249. Johnson JL, Raney AK, McLachlan A. Characterization of a functional hepatocyte nuclear factor 3 binding site in the hepatitis B virus nucleocapsid promoter. *Virology* 1995;208:147–158.
250. Junker-Niepmann M, Bartenschlager R, Schaller H. A short cis-acting sequence is required for hepatitis B virus pregenome encapsidation and sufficient for packaging of foreign RNA. *EMBO J* 1990;9(10): 3389–3396.
251. Kajino K, Jilbert AR, Saputelli J, et al. Woodchuck hepatitis virus infections: Very rapid recovery after a prolonged viremia and infection of virtually every hepatocyte. *J Virol* 1994;68(9):5792–5803.
252. Kamimura T, Yoshikawa A, Ichida F, Sasaki H. Electron microscopic studies of Dane particles in hepatocytes with special reference to intracellular development of Dane particles and their relation with HBeAg in serum. *Hepatology* 1981;1(5):392–397.
253. Kaneko S, Miller RH. X-region-specific transcript in mammalian hepatitis B virus-infected liver. *J Virol* 1988;62:3979–3984.
254. Kann M, Bischof A, Gerlich WH. *In vitro* model for the nuclear transport of the hepadnavirus genome. *J Virol* 1997;71(2):1310–1316.
255. Kaplan PM, Greenman RL, Gerin JL, et al. DNA polymerase associated with human hepatitis B antigen. *J Virol* 1973;12(5):995–1005.
256. Kay A, Dupont de Dinechin S, Vitvitski-Trepo L, et al. Recognition of the N-terminal, C-terminal, and interior portions of HBx by sera from patients with hepatitis B. *J Med Virol* 1991;33:228–235.
257. Kay A, Mandart E, Trepo C, Galibert F. The HBV HBx gene expressed in *E. coli* is recognized by sera from hepatitis patients. *EMBO J* 1985;4:1287–1292.
258. Kekule AS, Lauer U, Weiss L, et al. Hepatitis B virus transactivator HBx uses a tumor promoter signalling pathway. *Nature* 1993;361: 742–745.
259. Kim CM, Koike K, Saito I, et al. HBx gene of hepatitis B virus induces liver cancer in transgenic mice. *Nature* 1991;353:317–320.
260. Kim CM, Koike K, Saito I, et al. HBx gene of hepatitis B virus induces liver cancer in transgenic mice. *Nature* 1991;351(6324): 317–320.
261. Kim H, Lee H, Yun Y. X-gene product of hepatitis B virus induces apoptosis in liver cells. *J Biol Chem* 1998;273:381–385.
262. Klein N, Schneider RJ. Activation of Src family kinases by HBV HBx protein, and coupled signalling to Ras. *Mol Cell Biol* 1997;17: 6427–6436.
263. Klein N, Schneider RJ. Src kinases involved in hepatitis B virus replication. *EMBO J* 1999;18:5019–5027.
264. Klingmuller U, Schaller H. Hepadnavirus infection requires interaction between the viral pre-S domain and a specific hepatocellular receptor. *J Virol* 1993;67(12):7414–7422.
265. Knaus T, Nassal M. The encapsidation signal on the hepatitis B virus RNA pregenome forms a stem-loop structure that is critical for its function. *Nucleic Acids Res* 1993;21(17):3967–3975.

266. Kock J, Borst EM, Schlicht HJ. Uptake of duck hepatitis B virus into hepatocytes occurs by endocytosis but does not require passage of the virus through an acidic intracellular compartment. *J Virol* 1996;70(9): 5827–5831.
267. Kock J, Schlicht HJ. Analysis of the earliest steps of hepadnavirus replication: Genome repair after infectious entry into hepatocytes does not depend on viral polymerase activity. *J Virol* 1993;67(8): 4867–4874.
268. Kodama K, Ogasawara N, Yoshikawa H, Murakami S. Nucleotide sequence of a cloned woodchuck hepatitis virus genome: Evolutional relationship between hepadnaviruses. *J Virol* 1985;56(3):978–986.
269. Koff RS, Galambos JT. Viral hepatitis. In: Schiff L, Schiff ER, eds. *Diseases of the liver,* 6th ed. Philadelphia: JB Lippincott, 1987: 457–581.
270. Koike K, Moriya K, Iino S, et al. High-level expression of hepatitis B virus HBx gene and hepatocarcinogenesis in transgenic mice. *Hepatology* 1994;19(4):810–819.
271. Koike K, Moriya K, Iino S, et al. High-level expression of hepatitis B virus HBx gene and heptocellular carcinogenesis in transgenic mice. *Hepatology* 1994;19:810–819.
272. Komai K, Kaplan M, Peeples ME. The Vero cell receptor for the hepatitis B virus small S protein is a sialoglycoprotein. *Virology* 1988; 163(2):629–634.
273. Komai K, Peeples ME. Physiology and function of the vero cell receptor for the hepatitis B virus small S protein. *Virology* 1990;177(1): 332–338.
274. Korba BE, Gowans EJ, Wells FV, et al. Systemic distribution of woodchuck hepatitis virus in the tissues of experimentally infected woodchucks. *Virology* 1988;165(1):172–181.
275. Korba BE, Wells F, Tennant BC, et al. Lymphoid cells in the spleens of woodchuck hepatitis virus-infected woodchucks are a site of active viral replication. *J Virol* 1987;61(5):1318–1324.
276. Korba BE, Wells F, Tennant BC, et al. Hepadnavirus infection of peripheral blood lymphocytes *in vivo:* Woodchuck and chimpanzee models of viral hepatitis. *J Virol* 1986;58(1):1–8.
277. Kozak M. The scanning model for translation: An update. *J Cell Biol* 1989;108(2):229–241.
278. Kuroki K, Cheung R, Marion PL, Ganem D. A cell surface protein that binds avian hepatitis B virus particles. *J Virol* 1994;68(4):2091–2096.
279. Kuroki K, Eng F, Ishikawa T, et al. gp180, A host cell glycoprotein that binds duck hepatitis B virus particles, is encoded by a member of the carboxypeptidase gene family. *J Biol Chem* 1995;270(25): 15022–15028.
280. Kuroki K, Floreani M, Mimms LT, Ganem D. Epitope mapping of the PreS1 domain of the hepatitis B virus large surface protein. *Virology* 1990;176(2):620–624.
281. Kuroki K, Russnak R, Ganem D. Novel N-terminal amino acid sequence required for retention of a hepatitis B virus glycoprotein in the endoplasmic reticulum. *Mol Cell Biol* 1989;9(10):4459–4466.
282. Kwee L, Lucito R, Aufiero B, Schneider RJ. Alternate translation initiation on hepatitis B virus X mRNA produces multiple polypeptides that differentially transactivate class II and III promoters. *J Virol* 1992;66:4382–4389.
283. Lai CK, Ting LP. Transcriptional repression of human hepatitis B virus genes by a bZIP family member, E4BP4. *J Virol* 1999;73(4): 3197–3209.
284. Lambert V, Chassot S, Kay A, et al. *In vivo* neutralization of duck hepatitis B virus by antibodies specific to the N-terminal portion of pre-S protein. *Virology* 1991;185(1):446–450.
285. Lambert V, Cova L, Chevallier P, et al. Natural and experimental infection of wild mallard ducks with duck hepatitis B virus. *J Gen Virol* 1991;72(2):417–420.
286. Lambert V, Fernholz D, Sprengel R, et al. Virus-neutralizing monoclonal antibody to a conserved epitope on the duck hepatitis B virus pre-S protein. *J Virol* 1990;64(3):1290–1297.
287. Lara-Pezzi E, Armesilla AL, Majano PL, et al. The hepatitis B virus X protein activates nuclear factor of activated T cells (NF-AT) by a cyclosporin A-sensitive pathway. *EMBO J* 1998;17:7066–7077.
288. Lara-Pezzi E, Majano PL, Gomez-Gonzalo M, et al. The hepatitis B virus X protein up-regulates tumor necrosis factor-α gene expression in hepatocytes. *Hepatology* 1998;28:1013–1021.
289. Lau JY, Wright TL. Molecular virology and pathogenesis of hepatitis B [see Comments]. *Lancet* 1993;342(8883):1335–1340.
290. Laub O, Rall LB, Truett M, et al. Synthesis of hepatitis B surface antigen in mammalian cells: expression of the entire gene and the coding region. *J Virol* 1983;48(1):271–280.
291. Lauer U, Weiss L, Hofschneider PH, Kekule AS. The hepatitis B virus pre-S/S(t) transactivator is generated by 3′ truncations within a defined region of the S gene. *J Virol* 1992;66(9):5284–5289.
292. Lauer U, Weiss L, Lipp M, et al. The hepatitis B virus preS2/St transactivator utilizes AP-1 and other transcription factors for transactivation. *Hepatology* 1994;19(1):23–31.
293. Lavine J, Hirsch R, Ganem D. A system for studying the selective encapsidation of hepadnavirus RNA. *J Virol* 1989;63(10):4257–4263.
294. Lee AK, Ip HM, Wong VC. Mechanisms of maternal-fetal transmission of hepatitis B virus. *J Infect Dis* 1978;138(5):668–671.
295. Lee H, Lee YH, Huh YS, et al. X-gene product antagonizes the p53-mediated inhibition of hepatitis B virus replication through regulation of the pregenomic/core promoter. *J Biol Chem* 1995;270: 31405–31412.
296. Lee TH, Elledge SJ, Butel JS. Hepatitis B virus X protein interacts with a probably cellular DNA repair protein. *J Virol* 1995;69: 1107–1114.
297. Lee TH, Finegold MJ, Shen RF, et al. Hepatitis B virus transactivator X protein is not tumorigenic in transgenic mice. *J Virol* 1990;64: 5939–5947.
298. Lee TH, Finegold MJ, Shen RF, et al. Hepatitis B virus transactivator X protein is not tumorigenic in transgenic mice. *J Virol* 1990;64(12): 5939–5947.
299. Lee YH, Yun Y. HBx protein of hepatitis B virus activates Jak1-STAT signaling. *J Biol Chem* 1998;273(39):25510–25515.
300. Lenhoff RJ, Luscombe CA, Summers J. Acute liver injury following infection with a cytopathic strain of duck hepatitis B virus. *Hepatology* 1999;29(2):563–571.
301. Lenhoff RJ, Summers J. Coordinate regulation of replication and virus assembly by the large envelope protein of an avian hepadnavirus. *J Virol* 1994;68(7):4565–4571.
302. Lev S, Moreno H, Martinez R, et al. Protein tyrosine kinase Pyk2 involved in Ca2+-induced regulation of ion channel and MAP kinase functions. *Nature* 1995;376:737–745.
303. Levrero M, Balsano C, Natoli G, et al. Hepatitis B virus X protein transactivates the long terminal repeats of human immunodeficiency virus types 1 and 2. *J Virol* 1990;64:3082–3086.
304. Levrero M, Jean-Jean O, Balsano C, et al. Hepatitis B vIrus (HBV) X gene expression in human cells and anti-HBx antibodies detection in chronic HBV infection. *Virology* 1990;174:299–304.
305. Li J, Buckwold VE, Hon M-W, Ou J-H. Mechanism of suppression of hepatitis B virus precore RNA transcription by a frequent double mutation. *J Virol* 1999;73:1239–1244.
306. Li JS, Cova L, Buckland R, et al. Duck hepatitis B virus can tolerate insertion, deletion, and partial frameshift mutation in the distal pre-S region. *J Virol* 1989;63(11):4965–4968.
307. Li M, Xie Y, Wu X, et al. HNF3 binds and activates the second enhancer, ENII, of hepatitis B virus. *Virology* 1995;214(2):371–378.
308. Li M, Xie YH, Kong YY, et al. Cloning and characterization of a novel human hepatocyte transcription factor, hB1F, which binds and activates enhancer II of hepatitis B virus. *J Biol Chem* 1998;273(44): 29022–29031.
309. Lien JM, Aldrich CE, Mason WS. Evidence that a capped oligoribonucleotide is the primer for duck hepatitis B virus plus-strand DNA synthesis. *J Virol* 1986;57(1):229–236.
310. Lien JM, Petcu DJ, Aldrich CE, Mason WS. Initiation and termination of duck hepatitis B virus DNA synthesis during virus maturation. *J Virol* 1987;61(12):3832–3840.
311. Lin Y, Nomura T, Cheong J, et al. Hepatitis B virus X protein is a transcriptional modulator that communicates with transcription factor IIB and RNA polymerase II subunit 5. *J Biol Chem* 1997;272:7132–7139.
312. Lingappa JR, Martin RL, Wong ML, et al. A eukaryotic cytosolic chaperonin is associated with a high molecular weight intermediate in the assembly of hepatitis B virus capsid, a multimeric particle. *J Cell Biol* 1994;125(1):99–111.
313. Liu CC, Yansura D, Levinson AD. Direct expression of hepatitis B surface antigen in monkey cells from an SV40 vector. *DNA* 1982;1(3):213–221.
314. Lo WY, Ting LP. Repression of enhancer II activity by a negative regulatory element in the hepatitis B virus genome. *J Virol* 1994;68: 1758–1764.
315. Loeb DD, Gulya KJ, Tian R. Sequence identity of the terminal redun-

dancies on the minus-strand DNA template is necessary but not sufficient for the template switch during hepadnavirus plus-strand DNA synthesis. *J Virol* 1997;71(1):152–160.
316. Loeb DD, Hirsch RC, Ganem D. Sequence-independent RNA cleavages generate the primers for plus strand DNA synthesis in hepatitis B viruses: Implications for other reverse transcribing elements. *EMBO J* 1991;10(11):3533–3540.
317. Loeb DD, Tian R. Transfer of the minus strand of DNA during hepadnavirus replication is not invariable but prefers a specific location. *J Virol* 1995;69(11):6886–6891.
318. Loeb DD, Tian R, Gulya KJ. Mutations within DR2 independently reduce the amount of both minus- and plus-strand DNA synthesized during duck hepatitis B virus replication. *J Virol* 1996;70(12): 8684–8690.
319. Loeb DD, Tian R, Gulya KJ, Qualey AE. Changing the site of initiation of plus-strand DNA synthesis inhibits the subsequent template switch during replication of a hepadnavirus. *J Virol* 1998;72(8): 6565–6573.
320. Loffler-Mary H, Werr M, Prange R. Sequence-specific repression of cotranslational translocation of the hepatitis B virus envelope proteins coincides with binding of heat shock protein Hsc70. *Virology* 1997; 235(1):144–152.
321. Lopez-Cabrera M, Letovsky J, Hu KQ, Siddiqui A. Multiple liver-specific factors bind to the hepatitis B virus core/pregenomic promoter: Trans-activation and repression by CCAAT/enhancer binding protein. *Proc Natl Acad Sci U S A* 1990;87(13):5069–5073.
322. Lopez-Cabrera M, Letovsky J, Hu KQ, Siddiqui A. Transcriptional factor C/EBP binds to and transactivates the enhancer element II of the hepatitis B virus. *Virology* 1991;183(2):825–829.
323. Lu CC, Chen M, Ou JH, Yen TS. Key role of a CCAAT element in regulating hepatitis B virus surface protein expression. *Virology* 1995; 206(2):1155–1158.
324. Lu CC, Yen TS. Activation of the hepatitis B virus S promoter by transcription factor NF-Y via a CCAAT element. *Virology* 1996;225(2): 387–394.
325. Lucito R, Schneider RJ. Hepatitis B virus X protein activates transcription factor NF-kB without a requirement for protein kinase C. *J Virol* 1992;66:983–991.
326. Machida A, Kishimoto S, Ohnuma H, et al. A polypeptide containing 55 amino acid residues coded by the pre-S region of hepatitis B virus deoxyribonucleic acid bears the receptor for polymerized human as well as chimpanzee albumins. *Gastroenterology* 1984;86(5 Pt 1): 910–918.
327. Machida A, Kishimoto S, Ohnuma H, et al. A hepatitis B surface antigen polypeptide (P31) with the receptor for polymerized human as well as chimpanzee albumins. *Gastroenterology* 1983;85(2):268–274.
328. Machida A, Ohnuma H, Tsuda F, et al. Phosphorylation in the carboxyl-terminal domain of the capsid protein of hepatitis B virus: Evaluation with a monoclonal antibody. *J Virol* 1991;65(11):6024–6030.
329. Mack DH, Bloch W, Nath N, Sninsky JJ. Hepatitis B virus particles contain a polypeptide encoded by the largest open reading frame: A putative reverse transcriptase. *J Virol* 1988;62(12):4786–4790.
330. Macrae DR, Bruss V, Ganem D. Myristylation of a duck hepatitis B virus envelope protein is essential for infectivity but not for virus assembly. *Virology* 1991;181(1):359–363.
331. Maguire HF, Hoeffler JP, Siddiqui A. HBV X protein alters the DNA binding specificity of CREB and ATF-2 by protein-protein interactions. *Science* 1991;252:842–844.
332. Mahe Y, Mukaida N, Kuno K, et al. Hepatitis B virus X protein transactivates human interleukin-8 gene through acting on nuclear factor kB and CCAAT/enhancer-binding protein-like cis elements. *J Biol Chem* 1991;266:13759–13763.
333. Malpiece Y, Michel ML, Carloni G, et al. The gene S promoter of hepatitis B virus confers constitutive gene expression. *Nucleic Acids Res* 1983;11(13):4645–4654.
334. Mandart E, Kay A, Galibert F. Nucleotide sequence of a cloned duck hepatitis B virus genome: Comparison with woodchuck and human hepatitis B virus sequences. *J Virol* 1984;49(3):782–792.
335. Marion PL. Use of animal models to study hepatitis B virus. *Prog Med Virol* 1988;35:43–75.
336. Marion PL, Cullen JM, Azcarraga RR, et al. Experimental transmission of duck hepatitis B virus to Pekin ducks and to domestic geese. *Hepatology* 1987;7(4):724–731.
337. Marion PL, Knight SS, Ho BK, et al. Liver disease associated with duck hepatitis B virus infection of domestic ducks. *Proc Natl Acad Sci U S A* 1984;81(3):898–902.
338. Marion PL, Oshiro LS, Regnery DC, et al. A virus in Beechey ground squirrels that is related to hepatitis B virus of humans. *Proc Natl Acad Sci U S A* 1980;77(5):2941–2945.
339. Marion PL, Van Davelaar MJ, Knight SS, et al. Hepatocellular carcinoma in ground squirrels persistently infected with ground squirrel hepatitis virus. *Proc Natl Acad Sci U S A* 1986;83(12):4543–4546.
340. Mason WS, Aldrich C, Summers J, Taylor JM. Asymmetric replication of duck hepatitis B virus DNA in liver cells: Free minus-strand DNA. *Proc Natl Acad Sci U S A* 1982;79(13):3997–4001.
341. Mason WS, Halpern MS, England JM, et al. Experimental transmission of duck hepatitis B virus. *Virology* 1983;131(2):375–384.
342. Mason WS, Seal G, Summers J. Virus of Pekin ducks with structural and biological relatedness to human hepatitis B virus. *J Virol* 1980; 36(3):829–836.
343. May MJ, Ghosh S. Signal transduction through NF-kappa B. *Immunol Today* 1998;19(2):80–88.
344. McAleer WJ, Buynak EB, Maigetter RZ, et al. Human hepatitis B vaccine from recombinant yeast. *Nature* 1984;307(5947):178–180.
345. McLachlan A, Milich DR, Raney AK, et al. Expression of hepatitis B virus surface and core antigens: Influences of pre-S and precore sequences. *J Virol* 1987;61(3):683–692.
346. Mehdi H, Kaplan MJ, Anlar FY, et al. Hepatitis B virus surface antigen binds to apolipoprotein H. *J Virol* 1994;68(4):2415–2424.
347. Melegari M, Scaglioni PP, Wands JR. Cloning and characterization of a novel hepatitis B virus x binding protein that inhibits viral replication. *J Virol* 1998;72(3):1737–1743.
348. Milich DR, Jones JE, Hughes JL, et al. Is a function of the secreted hepatitis B e antigen to induce immunologic tolerance in utero? *Proc Natl Acad Sci U S A* 1990;87(17):6599–6603.
349. Miller RH, Marion PL, Robinson WS. Hepatitis B viral DNA-RNA hybrid molecules in particles from infected liver are converted to viral DNA molecules during an endogenous DNA polymerase reaction. *Virology* 1984;139(1):64–72.
350. Miller RH, Robinson WS. Common evolutionary origin of hepatitis B virus and retroviruses. *Proc Natl Acad Sci U S A* 1986;83:2531–2535.
351. Molnar-Kimber KL, Summers J, Taylor JM, Mason WS. Protein covalently bound to minus-strand DNA intermediates of duck hepatitis B virus. *J Virol* 1983;45(1):165–172.
352. Molnar-Kimber KL, Summers JW, Mason WS. Mapping of the cohesive overlap of duck hepatitis B virus DNA and of the site of initiation of reverse transcription. *J Virol* 1984;51(1):181–191.
353. Moriarty AM, Hoyer BH, Shih JW, et al. Expression of the hepatitis B virus surface antigen gene in cell culture by using a simian virus 40 vector. *Proc Natl Acad Sci U S A* 1981;78(4):2606–2610.
354. Moriyama T, Guilhot S, Klopchin K, et al. Immunobiology and pathogenesis of hepatocellular injury in hepatitis B virus transgenic mice. *Science* 1990;248(4953):361–364.
355. Moroy T, Etiemble J, Trepo C, et al. Transcription of woodchuck hepatitis virus in the chronically infected liver. *EMBO J* 1985;4(6): 1507–1514.
356. Moroy T, Marchio A, Etiemble J, et al. Rearrangement and enhanced expression of c-myc in hepatocellular carcinoma of hepatitis virus infected woodchucks. *Nature* 1986;324(6094):276–279.
357. Mueller-Hill K, Loeb DD. Previously unsuspected cis-acting sequences for DNA replication revealed by characterization of a chimeric heron/duck hepatitis B virus. *J Virol* 1996;70(12): 8310–8317.
358. Murakami S, Cheong J-H, Ohno S, et al. Transactivation of human hepatitis B virus X protein, HBx, operates through a mechanism distinct from protein kinase C and okadaic acid activation pathways. *Virology* 1994;199:243–246.
359. Nagaya T, Nakamura T, Tokino T, et al. The mode of hepatitis B virus DNA integration in chromosomes of human hepatocellular carcinoma. *Genes Dev* 1987;1(8):773–782.
360. Nakamoto Y, Guidotti LG, Kuhlen CV, et al. Immune pathogenesis of hepatocellular carcinoma. *J Exp Med* 1998;188(2):341–350.
361. Nakamoto Y, Guidotti LG, Pasquetto V, et al. Differential target cell sensitivity to CTL-activated death pathways in hepatitis B virus transgenic mice. *J Immunol* 1997;158(12):5692–5697.
362. Nakatake H, Chisaka O, Yamamoto S, et al. Effect of X protein on transactivation of hepatitis B virus promoters and on viral replication. *Virology* 1993;195:305–314.

363. Nassal M. The arginine-rich domain of the hepatitis B virus core protein is required for pregenome encapsidation and productive viral positive-strand DNA synthesis but not for virus assembly. *J Virol* 1992; 66(7):4107–4116.
364. Nassal M, Galle PR, Schaller H. Proteaselike sequence in hepatitis B virus core antigen is not required for e antigen generation and may not be part of an aspartic acid-type protease. *J Virol* 1989;63(6): 2598–2604.
365. Nassal M, Junker-Niepmann M, Schaller H. Translational inactivation of RNA function: Discrimination against a subset of genomic transcripts during HBV nucleocapsid assembly. *Cell* 1990;63(6): 1357–1363.
366. Natoli G, Avantaggiati ML, Balsano C, et al. Characterization of the hepatitis B virus preS/S region encoded transcriptional transactivator. *Virology* 1992;187(2):663–670.
367. Natoli G, Avantaggiati ML, Chirillo P, et al. Induction of the DNA-binding activity of c-Jun/c-Fos heterodimers by the hepatitis B virus transactivator pX. *Mol Cell Biol* 1994;14:989–998.
368. Natoli G, Avantaggiati ML, Chirillo P, et al. Ras- and raf- dependent activation of c-jun transcriptional activity by the hepatitis B virus transactivator pX. *Oncogene* 1994;9:2837–2843.
369. Naumann H, Schaefer S, Yoshida CFT, et al. Identification of a new hepatitis B virus (HBV) genotype from Brazil that expresses HBV surface antigen subtype adw4. *J Gen Virol* 1993;74:1627–1632.
370. Neurath AR, Kent SB, Strick N, Parker K. Identification and chemical synthesis of a host cell receptor binding site on hepatitis B virus. *Cell* 1986;46(3):429–436.
371. Neurath AR, Strick N, Li YY. Cells transfected with human interleukin 6 cDNA acquire binding sites for the hepatitis B virus envelope protein. *J Exp Med* 1992;176(6):1561–1569.
372. Neurath AR, Strick N, Sproul P, et al. Detection of receptors for hepatitis B virus on cells of extrahepatic origin. *Virology* 1990;176(2): 448–457.
373. Nigg EA. Nucleocytoplasmic transport: Signals, mechanisms and regulation. *Nature* 1997;386(6627):779–787.
374. Oberhaus SM, Newbold JE. Detection of DNA polymerase activities associated with purified duck hepatitis B virus core particles by using an activity gel assay. *J Virol* 1993;67(11):6558–6566.
375. Obert S, Zachmann-Brand B, Deindl E, et al. A spliced hepadnavirus RNA that is essential for virus replication. *EMBO J* 1996;15: 2565–2574.
376. Ochiya T, Tsurimoto T, Ueda K, et al. An *in vitro* system for infection with hepatitis B virus that uses primary human fetal hepatocytes. *Proc Natl Acad Sci U S A* 1989;86(6):1875–1879.
377. Offensperger WB, Offensperger S, Walter E, et al. Inhibition of duck hepatitis B virus infection by lysosomotropic agents. *Virology* 1991; 183(1):415–418.
378. Ogston CW, Jonak GJ, Rogler CE, et al. Cloning and structural analysis of integrated woodchuck hepatitis virus sequences from hepatocellular carcinomas of woodchucks. *Cell* 1982;29(2):385–394.
379. Ogston CW, Schechter EM, Humes CA, Pranikoff MB. Extrahepatic replication of woodchuck hepatitis virus in chronic infection. *Virology* 1989;169(1):9–14.
380. Oguey D, Dumenco LL, Pierce RH, Fausto N. Analysis of the tumorigenicity of the X gene of hepatitis B virus in a nontransformed hepatocyte cell line and the effects of cotransfection with a murine p53 mutant equivalent to human codon 249. *Hepatology* 1996;24: 1024–1033.
381. Okada K, Kamiyama I, Inomata M, et al. e Antigen and anti-e in the serum of asymptomatic carrier mothers as indicators of positive and negative transmission of hepatitis B virus to their infants. *N Engl J Med* 1976;294(14):746–749.
382. Okamoto H, Yotsumoto S, Akahane Y, et al. Hepatitis B viruses with precore region defects prevail in persistently infected hosts along with seroconversion to the antibody against e antigen. *J Virol* 1990;64(3): 1298–1303.
383. Omata M, Uchiumi K, Ito Y, et al. Duck hepatitis B virus and liver diseases. *Gastroenterology* 1983;85(2):260–267.
384. Ori A, Shaul Y. Hepatitis B virus enhancer binds and is activated by the hepatocyte nuclear factor 3. *Virology* 1995;207(1):98–106.
385. Ostapchuk P, Hearing P, Ganem D. A dramatic shift in the transmembrane topology of a viral envelope glycoprotein accompanies hepatitis B viral morphogenesis. *EMBO J* 1994;13(5):1048–1057.
386. Ostapchuk P, Scheirle G, Hearing P. Binding of nuclear factor EF-C to a functional domain of the hepatitis B virus enhancer region. *Mol Cell Biol* 1989;9:2787–2797.
387. Otero GC, Harris ME, Donello JE, Hope TJ. Leptomycin B inhibits equine infectious anemia virus rev and feline immunodeficiency virus rev function but not the function of the hepatitis B virus posttranscriptional regulatory element. *J Virol* 1998;72(9):7593–7597.
388. Ou JH, Laub O, Rutter WJ. Hepatitis B virus gene function: The precore region targets the core antigen to cellular membranes and causes the secretion of the e antigen. *Proc Natl Acad Sci U S A* 1986;83(6): 1578–1582.
389. Ou JH, Rutter WJ. Regulation of secretion of the hepatitis B virus major surface antigen by the preS-1 protein. *J Virol* 1987;61(3): 782–786.
390. Ou JH, Yeh CT, Yen TS. Transport of hepatitis B virus precore protein into the nucleus after cleavage of its signal peptide. *J Virol* 1989; 63(12):5238–5243.
391. Palmer CR, Gegnas L, Schepartz A. Mechanism of DNA binding enhancement by hepatitis B virus protein X. *Biochemistry* 1997;36: 15349–15355.
392. Pasek M, Goto T, Gilbert W, et al. Hepatitis B virus genes and their expression in *E. coli. Nature* 1979;282(5739):575–579.
393. Patel NU, Jameel S, Isom H, Siddiqui A. Interactions between nuclear factors and the hepatitis B virus enhancer. *J Virol* 1989;63(12): 5293–5301.
394. Paterlini P, Poussin K, Kew M, et al. Selective accumulation of the X transcript of hepatitis B virus in patients negative for hepatitis B surface antigen with hepatocellular carcinoma. *Hepatology* 1995;21: 313–321.
395. Patzer EJ, Nakamura GR, Simonsen CC, et al. Intracellular assembly and packaging of hepatitis B surface antigen particles occur in the endoplasmic reticulum. *J Virol* 1986;58(3):884–892.
396. Patzer EJ, Nakamura GR, Yaffe A. Intracellular transport and secretion of hepatitis B surface antigen in mammalian cells. *J Virol* 1984;51(2): 346–353.
397. Penna A, Chisari FV, Bertoletti A, et al. Cytotoxic T lymphocytes recognize an HLA-A2-restricted epitope within the hepatitis B virus nucleocapsid antigen. *J Exp Med* 1991;174(6):1565–1570.
398. Penna A, Fowler P, Bertoletti A, et al. Hepatitis B virus (HBV)-specific cytotoxic T-cell (CTL) response in humans: Characterization of HLA class II-restricted CTLs that recognize endogenously synthesized HBV envelope antigens. *J Virol* 1992;66(2):1193–1198.
399. Perini G, Oetjen E, Green MR. The hepatitis B pX protein promotes dimerization and DNA binding of cellular basic region/leucine zipper proteins by targeting the conserved basic region. *J Biol Chem* 1999; 274(20):13970–13977.
400. Perri S, Ganem D. A host factor that binds near the termini of hepatitis B virus pregenomic RNA. *J Virol* 1996;70(10):6803–6809.
401. Persing DH, Varmus HE, Ganem D. A frameshift mutation in the pre-S region of the human hepatitis B virus genome allows production of surface antigen particles but eliminates binding to polymerized albumin. *Proc Natl Acad Sci U S A* 1985;82(10):3440–3444.
402. Persing DH, Varmus HE, Ganem D. Inhibition of secretion of hepatitis B surface antigen by a related presurface polypeptide. *Science* 1986;234(4782):1388–1391.
403. Persing DH, Varmus HE, Ganem D. The preS1 protein of hepatitis B virus is acylated at its amino terminus with myristic acid. *J Virol* 1987;61(5):1672–1677.
404. Petcu DJ, Aldrich CE, Coates L, et al. Suramin inhibits *in vitro* infection by duck hepatitis B virus, Rous sarcoma virus, and hepatitis delta virus. *Virology* 1988;167(2):385–392.
405. Peterson DL. Isolation and characterization of the major protein and glycoprotein of hepatitis B surface antigen. *J Biol Chem* 1981; 256(13):6975–6983.
406. Peterson DL. The structure of hepatitis B surface antigen and its antigenic sites. *Bioessays* 1987;6(6):258–262.
407. Pfaff E, Salfeld J, Gmelin K, et al. Synthesis of the X-protein of hepatitis B virus *in vitro* and detection of anti-X antibodies in human sera. *Virology* 1987;158:456–460.
408. Pineau P, Nagai H, Prigent S, et al. Identification of three distinct regions of allelic deletions on the short arm of chromosome 8 in hepatocellular carcinoma. *Oncogene* 1999;18(20):3127–3134.
409. Pollack JR, Ganem D. An RNA stem-loop structure directs hepatitis B virus genomic RNA encapsidation. *J Virol* 1993;67(6):3254–3263.
410. Pollack JR, Ganem D. Site-specific RNA binding by a hepatitis B

virus reverse transcriptase initiates two distinct reactions: RNA packaging and DNA synthesis. *J Virol* 1994;68(9):5579–5587.

411. Pontisso P, Petit MA, Bankowski MJ, Peeples ME. Human liver plasma membranes contain receptors for the hepatitis B virus pre-S1 region and, via polymerized human serum albumin, for the pre-S2 region. *J Virol* 1989;63(5):1981–1988.
412. Pontisso P, Poon MC, Tiollais P, Brechot C. Detection of hepatitis B virus DNA in mononuclear blood cells. *Br Med J* (*Clin Res Ed*) 1984; 288(6430):1563–1566.
413. Pontisso P, Ruvoletto MG, Tiribelli C, et al. The preS1 domain of hepatitis B virus and IgA cross-react in their binding to the hepatocyte surface. *J Gen Virol* 1992;73(8):2041–2045.
414. Popper H, Roth L, Purcell RH, et al. Hepatocarcinogenicity of the woodchuck hepatitis virus. *Proc Natl Acad Sci U S A* 1987;84(3): 866–870.
415. Popper H, Shih JW, Gerin JL, et al. Woodchuck hepatitis and hepatocellular carcinoma: Correlation of histologic with virologic observations. *Hepatology* 1981;1(2):91–98.
416. Poussin K, Dienes H, Sirma H, et al. Expression of mutated hepatitis B virus X genes in human hepatocellular carcinomas. *Int J Cancer* 1999;80(4):497–505.
417. Prange R, Clemen A, Streeck RE. Myristylation is involved in intracellular retention of hepatitis B virus envelope proteins. *J Virol* 1991; 65(7):3919–3923.
418. Prange R, Nagel R, Streeck RE. Deletions in the hepatitis B virus small envelope protein: effect on assembly and secretion of surface antigen particles. *J Virol* 1992;66(10):5832–5841.
419. Prange R, Streeck RE. Novel transmembrane topology of the hepatitis B virus envelope proteins. *EMBO J* 1995;14(2):247–256.
420. Prost S, Ford JM, Taylor C, et al. Hepatitis B x protein inhibits p53-dependent DNA repair in primary mouse hepatocytes. *J Biol Chem* 1998;273:33327–33332.
421. Pugh J, Zweidler A, Summers J. Characterization of the major duck hepatitis B virus core particle protein. *J Virol* 1989;63(3):1371–1376.
422. Pugh JC, Simmons H. Duck hepatitis B virus infection of Muscovy duck hepatocytes and nature of virus resistance *in vivo. J Virol* 1994; 68(4):2487–2494.
423. Pugh JC, Sninsky JJ, Summers JW, Schaeffer E. Characterization of a pre-S polypeptide on the surfaces of infectious avian hepadnavirus particles. *J Virol* 1987;61(5):1384–1390.
424. Pugh JC, Summers JW. Infection and uptake of duck hepatitis B virus by duck hepatocytes maintained in the presence of dimethyl sulfoxide. *Virology* 1989;172(2):564–572.
425. Pugh JC, Yaginuma K, Koike K, Summers J. Duck hepatitis B virus (DHBV) particles produced by transient expression of DHBV DNA in a human hepatoma cell line are infectious *in vitro. J Virol* 1988;62(9): 3513–3516.
426. Puisieux A, Ji J, Guillot C, et al. p53-Mediated cellular response to DNA damage in cells with replicative hepatitis B virus. *Proc Natl Acad Sci U S A* 1995;92:1342–1346.
427. Qadri I, Conaway JW, Conaway RC, et al. Hepatitis B virus transactivator protein, HBx, associates with the components of TFIIH and stimulates the DNA helicase activity of TFIIH. *Proc Natl Acad Sci U S A* 1996;93:10578–10583.
428. Qadri I, Maguire HF, Siddiqui A. Hepatitis B virus transactivator protein X interacts with the TATA-binding protein. *Proc Natl Acad Sci U S A* 1995;92:1003–1007.
429. Radziwill G, Tucker W, Schaller H. Mutational analysis of the hepatitis B virus P gene product: Domain structure and RNase H activity. *J Virol* 1990;64(2):613–620.
430. Raney AK, Easton AJ, Milich DR, McLachlan A. Promoter-specific transactivation of hepatitis B virus transcription by a glutamine- and proline-rich domain of hepatocyte nuclear factor 1. *J Virol* 1991; 65(11):5774–5781.
431. Raney AK, Johnson JL, Palmer CN, McLachlan A. Members of the nuclear receptor superfamily regulate transcription from the hepatitis B virus nucleocapsid promoter. *J Virol* 1997;71(2):1058–1071.
432. Raney AK, Le HB, McLachlan A. Regulation of transcription from the hepatitis B virus major surface antigen promoter by the Sp1 transcription factor. *J Virol* 1992;66(12):6912–6921.
433. Raney AK, McLachlan A. Characterization of the hepatitis B virus major surface antigen promoter hepatocyte nuclear factor 3 binding site. *J Gen Virol* 1997;78(11):3029–3038.
434. Raney AK, Milich DR, Easton AJ, McLachlan A. Differentiation-specific transcriptional regulation of the hepatitis B virus large surface antigen gene in human hepatoma cell lines. *J Virol* 1990;64(5): 2360–2368.
435. Raney AK, Milich DR, McLachlan A. Characterization of hepatitis B virus major surface antigen gene transcriptional regulatory elements in differentiated hepatoma cell lines. *J Virol* 1989;63(9):3919–3925.
436. Raney AK, Milich DR, McLachlan A. Complex regulation of transcription from the hepatitis B virus major surface antigen promoter in human hepatoma cell lines. *J Virol* 1991;65(9):4805–4811.
437. Raney AK, Zhang P, McLachlan A. Regulation of transcription from the hepatitis B virus large surface antigen promoter by hepatocyte nuclear factor 3. *J Virol* 1995;69(6):3265–3272.
438. Rehermann B, Ferrari C, Pasquinelli C, Chisari FV. The hepatitis B virus persists for decades after patients' recovery from acute viral hepatitis despite active maintenance of a cytotoxic T- lymphocyte response. *Nat Med* 1996;2(10):1104–1108.
439. Rehermann B, Lau D, Hoofnagle JH, Chisari FV. Cytotoxic T lymphocyte responsiveness after resolution of chronic hepatitis B virus infection. *J Clin Invest* 1996;97(7):1655–1665.
440. Reifenberg K, Deutschle T, Wild J, et al. The hepatitis B virus e antigen cannot pass the murine placenta efficiently and does not induce CTL immune tolerance in H-2b mice in utero. *Virology* 1998;243(1): 45–53.
441. Rigg RJ, Schaller H. Duck hepatitis B virus infection of hepatocytes is not dependent on low pH. *J Virol* 1992;66(5):2829–2836.
442. Robinson WS, Clayton DA, Greenman RL. DNA of a human hepatitis B virus candidate. *J Virol* 1974;14(2):384–391.
443. Robinson WS, Greenman RL. DNA polymerase in the core of the human hepatitis B virus candidate. *J Virol* 1974;13(6):1231–1236.
444. Robinson WS, Lutwick LI. The virus of hepatitis, type B (first of two parts). *N Engl J Med* 1976;295(21):1168–1175.
445. Rogler CE, Sherman M, Su CY, et al. Deletion in chromosome 11p associated with a hepatitis B integration site in hepatocellular carcinoma. *Science* 1985;230(4723):319–322.
446. Roingeard P, Lu SL, Sureau C, et al. Immunocytochemical and electron microscopic study of hepatitis B virus antigen and complete particle production in hepatitis B virus DNA transfected HepG2 cells. *Hepatology* 1990;11(2):277–285.
447. Romet-Lemonne JL, McLane MF, Elfassi E, et al. Hepatitis B virus infection in cultured human lymphoblastoid cells. *Science* 1983; 221(4611):667–669.
448. Roossinck MJ, Jameel S, Loukin SH, Siddiqui A. Expression of hepatitis B viral core region in mammalian cells. *Mol Cell Biol* 1986;6(5):1393–1400.
449. Roossinck MJ, Siddiqui A. *In vivo* phosphorylation and protein analysis of hepatitis B virus core antigen. *J Virol* 1987;61(4):955–961.
450. Rossner MT. Hepatitis B virus X-gene product: A promiscuous transcriptional activator. *J Med Virol* 1992;36:101–117.
451. Rossner MT. Hepatitis B virus X-gene product: A promiscuous transcriptional activator [Review]. *J Med Virol* 1992;36(2):101–117.
452. Rothmann K, Schnolzer M, Radziwill G, et al. Host cell-virus cross talk: Phosphorylation of a hepatitis B virus envelope protein mediates intracellular signaling. *J Virol* 1998;72(12):10138–10147.
453. Roychoudhury S, Faruqi AF, Shih C. Pregenomic RNA encapsidation analysis of eleven missense and nonsense polymerase mutants of human hepatitis B virus. *J Virol* 1991;65(7):3617–3624.
454. Roychoudhury S, Shih C. cis Rescue of a mutated reverse transcriptase gene of human hepatitis B virus by creation of an internal ATG. *J Virol* 1990;64(3):1063–1069.
455. Russnak R, Ganem D. Sequences 5′ to the polyadenylation signal mediate differential poly(A) site use in hepatitis B viruses. *Genes Dev* 1990;4(5):764–776.
456. Santantonio T, Jung MC, Miska S, et al. Prevalence and type of pre-C HBV mutants in anti-HBe positive carriers with chronic liver disease in a highly endemic area. *Virology* 1991;183(2):840–844.
457. Santantonio T, Jung MC, Schneider R, et al. Hepatitis B virus genomes that cannot synthesize pre-S2 proteins occur frequently and as dominant virus populations in chronic carriers in Italy. *Virology* 1992;188(2):948–952.
458. Sattler F, Robinson WS. Hepatitis B viral DNA molecules have cohesive ends. *J Virol* 1979;32(1):226–233.
459. Scaglioni PP, Melegari M, Wands JR. Biologic properties of hepatitis B viral genomes with mutations in the precore promoter and precore open reading frame. *Virology* 1997;233(2):374–381.

460. Schek N, Bartenschlager R, Kuhn C, Schaller H. Phosphorylation and rapid turnover of hepatitis B virus X protein expressed in HepG2 cells from a recombinant vaccinia virus. *Oncogene* 1991;6: 1735–1744.
461. Schirmacher P, Wang H, Stahnke G, et al. Sequences and structures at hepadnaviral integration: Recombination sites implicate topoisomerase I in hepadnaviral DNA rearrangements and integration. *J Hepatol* 1995;22(1):21–33.
462. Schlicht HJ. Biosynthesis of the secretory core protein of duck hepatitis B virus: Intracellular transport, proteolytic processing, and membrane expression of the precore protein. *J Virol* 1991;65(7): 3489–3495.
463. Schlicht HJ, Kuhn C, Guhr B, et al. Biochemical and immunological characterization of the duck hepatitis B virus envelope proteins. *J Virol* 1987;61(7):2280–2285.
464. Schlicht HJ, Radziwill G, Schaller H. Synthesis and encapsidation of duck hepatitis B virus reverse transcriptase do not require formation of core-polymerase fusion proteins. *Cell* 1989;56(1):85–92.
465. Schlicht HJ, Salfeld J, Schaller H. The duck hepatitis B virus pre-C region encodes a signal sequence which is essential for synthesis and secretion of processed core proteins but not for virus formation. *J Virol* 1987;61(12):3701–3709.
466. Schlicht HJ, Schaller H. The secretory core protein of human hepatitis B virus is expressed on the cell surface. *J Virol* 1989;63(12): 5399–5404.
467. Schneider R, Fernholz D, Wildner G, Will H. Mechanism, kinetics, and role of duck hepatitis B virus e-antigen expression *in vivo. Virology* 1991;182(2):503–512.
468. Schodel F, Weimer T, Will H, Sprengel R. Amino acid sequence similarity between retroviral and *E. coli* RNase H and hepadnaviral gene products [Letter]. *AIDS Res Hum Retroviruses* 1988;4(6):ix–xi.
469. Seeger C, Baldwin B, Hornbuckle WE, et al. Woodchuck hepatitis virus is a more efficient oncogenic agent than ground squirrel hepatitis virus in a common host. *J Virol* 1991;65(4):1673–1679.
470. Seeger C, Baldwin B, Tennant BC. Expression of infectious woodchuck hepatitis virus in murine and avian fibroblasts. *J Virol* 1989; 63(11):4665–4669.
471. Seeger C, Ganem D, Varmus HE. Nucleotide sequence of an infectious molecularly cloned genome of ground squirrel hepatitis virus. *J Virol* 1984;51(2):367–375.
472. Seeger C, Ganem D, Varmus HE. Biochemical and genetic evidence for the hepatitis B virus replication strategy. *Science* 1986;232(4749): 477–484.
473. Seeger C, Maragos J. Identification and characterization of the woodchuck hepatitis virus origin of DNA replication. *J Virol* 1990;64(1): 16–23.
474. Seeger C, Maragos J. Identification of a signal necessary for initiation of reverse transcription of the hepadnavirus genome. *J Virol* 1991; 65(10):5190–5195.
475. Seeger C, Marion PL, Ganem D, Varmus HE. *In vitro* recombinants of ground squirrel and woodchuck hepatitis viral DNAs produce infectious virus in squirrels. *J Virol* 1987;61(10):3241–3247.
476. Seifer M, Zhou S, Standring DN. A micromolar pool of antigenically distinct precursors is required to initiate cooperative assembly of hepatitis B virus capsids in *Xenopus* oocytes. *J Virol* 1993;67(1): 249–257.
477. Sells MA, Chen ML, Acs G. Production of hepatitis B virus particles in Hep G2 cells transfected with cloned hepatitis B virus DNA. *Proc Natl Acad Sci U S A* 1987;84(4):1005–1009.
478. Seto E, Mitchell PJ, Yen TSB. Transactivation by the hepatitis B virus X protein depends on AP-2 and other transcription factors. *Nature* 1990;344:72–74.
479. Seto E, Yen TSB. Mutual functional antagonism of the simian virus 40 T antigen and the hepatitis B virus trans activator. *J Virol* 1991;65: 2351–2356.
480. Seto E, Yen TSB, Peterlin BM, Ou J-H. Trans-activation of the human immunodeficiency virus long terminal repeat by the hepatitis B virus X protein. *Proc Natl Acad Sci U S A* 1988;85:8290–8286.
481. Shafritz DA, Shouval D, Sherman HI, et al. Integration of hepatitis B virus DNA into the genome of liver cells in chronic liver disease and hepatocellular carcinoma: Studies in percutaneous liver biopsies and post-mortem tissue specimens. *N Engl J Med* 1981;305(18): 1067–1073.
482. Shaul Y, Ben-Levy R, De-Medina T. High affinity binding site for nuclear factor I next to the hepatitis B virus S gene promoter. *EMBO J* 1986;5(8):1967–1971.
483. Shaul Y, Rutter WJ, Laub O. A human hepatitis B virus enhancer element. *EMBO J* 1985;4:427–430.
484. Shih C, Burke K, Chou MJ, et al. Tight clustering of human hepatitis B virus integration sites in hepatomas near a triple-stranded region. *J Virol* 1987;61(11):3491–3498.
485. Shih CH, Li LS, Roychoudhury S, Ho MH. *In vitro* propagation of human hepatitis B virus in a rat hepatoma cell line. *Proc Natl Acad Sci U S A* 1989;86(16):6323–6327.
486. Siddiqui A, Gaynor R, Srinivasan A, et al. Trans-activation of viral enhancers including long terminal repeat of the human immunodeficiency virus by the hepatitis B virus X protein. *Virology* 1989;169: 479–484.
487. Siddiqui A, Jameel S, Mapoles J. Transcriptional control elements of hepatitis B surface antigen gene. *Proc Natl Acad Sci U S A* 1986; 83(3):566–570.
488. Siddiqui A, Jameel S, Mapoles J. Expression of the hepatitis B virus X gene in mammalian cells. *Proc Natl Acad Sci U S A* 1987;84: 2513–2517.
489. Siddiqui A, Sattler F, Robinson WS. Restriction endonuclease cleavage map and location of unique features of the DNA of hepatitis B virus, subtype adw2. *Proc Natl Acad Sci U S A* 1979;76(9): 4664–4668.
490. Siegrist CA, Durand B, Emery P, et al. RFX1 is identical to enhancer factor C and functions as a transactivator of the hepatitis B virus enhancer. *Mol Cell Biol* 1993;13(10):6375–6384.
491. Simon K, Lingappa VR, Ganem D. Secreted hepatitis B surface antigen polypeptides are derived from a transmembrane precursor. *J Cell Biol* 1988;107(6 Pt 1):2163–2168.
492. Sirma H, Weil R, Rosmorduc O, et al. Cytosol is the prime compartment of hepatitis B virus X protein where it colocalizes with the proteasome. *Oncogene* 1998;16(16):2051–2063.
493. Sitterlin D, Lee T-H, Prigent S, et al. Interaction of the UV-damaged DNA-binding protein with hepatitis B virus X protein is conserved among mammalian hepadnaviruses and restricted to transactivation-proficient X-insertion mutants. *J Virol* 1997;71:6194–6199.
494. Slagle BL, Lee TH, Medina D, et al. Increased sensitivity to the hepatocarcinogen diethylnitrosamine in transgenic mice carrying the hepatitis B virus X gene. *Mol Carcinog* 1996;15:261–269.
495. Spandau DF, Lee CH. Trans-activation of viral enhancers by the hepatitis B virus X protein. *J Virol* 1988;62:427–434.
496. Sprengel R, Kaleta EF, Will H. Isolation and characterization of a hepatitis B virus endemic in herons. *J Virol* 1988;62(10):3832–3839.
497. Sprengel R, Kuhn C, Manso C, Will H. Cloned duck hepatitis B virus DNA is infectious in Pekin ducks. *J Virol* 1984;52(3):932–937.
498. Standring DN, Ou JH, Masiarz FR, Rutter WJ. A signal peptide encoded within the precore region of hepatitis B virus directs the secretion of a heterogeneous population of e antigens in *Xenopus* oocytes. *Proc Natl Acad Sci U S A* 1988;85(22):8405–8409.
499. Standring DN, Rutter WJ, Varmus HE, Ganem D. Transcription of the hepatitis B surface antigen gene in cultured murine cells initiates within the presurface region. *J Virol* 1984;50(2):563–571.
500. Staprans S, Loeb DD, Ganem D. Mutations affecting hepadnavirus plus-strand DNA synthesis dissociate primer cleavage from translocation and reveal the origin of linear viral DNA. *J Virol* 1991;65(3): 1255–1262.
501. Stenlund A, Lamy D, Moreno-Lopez J, et al. Secretion of the hepatitis B virus surface antigen from mouse cells using an extra-chromosomal eucaryotic vector. *EMBO J* 1983;2(5):669–673.
502. Stevens CE, Beasley RP, Tsui J, Lee WC. Vertical transmission of hepatitis B antigen in Taiwan. *N Engl J Med* 1975;292(15):771–774.
503. Stibbe W, Gerlich WH. Structural relationships between minor and major proteins of hepatitis B surface antigen. *J Virol* 1983;46(2): 626–628.
504. Su F, Schneider RJ. HBV HBx protein activates transcription factor NF-kB by acting on multiple cytoplasmic inhibitors of rel-related proteins. *J Virol* 1996;70:4558–4566.
505. Su F, Schneider RJ. Hepatitis B virus HBx protein sensitizes cells to apoptotic killing by TNFα. *Proc Natl Acad Sci U S A* 1997;94: 8744–8749.
506. Su H, Yee JK. Regulation of hepatitis B virus gene expression by its two enhancers. *Proc Natl Acad Sci U S A* 1992;89(7):2708–2712.
507. Su Q, Schroder CH, Hofman WJ, et al. Expression of hepatitis B virus

X protein in HBV-infected human livers and hepatocellular carcinomas. *Hepatology* 1998;27:1109–1120.
508. Su TS, Lai CJ, Huang JL, et al. Hepatitis B virus transcript produced by RNA splicing. *J Virol* 1989;63(9):4011–4018.
509. Sugata F, Chen HS, Kaneko S, et al. Analysis of the X gene promoter of woodchuck hepatitis virus. *Virology* 1994;205:314–320.
510. Summers J, Mason WS. Replication of the genome of a hepatitis B–like virus by reverse transcription of an RNA intermediate. *Cell* 1982;29(2):403–415.
511. Summers J, O'Connell A, Millman I. Genome of hepatitis B virus: Restriction enzyme cleavage and structure of DNA extracted from Dane particles. *Proc Natl Acad Sci U S A* 1975;72(11):4597–4601.
512. Summers J, Smith PM, Horwich AL. Hepadnavirus envelope proteins regulate covalently closed circular DNA amplification. *J Virol* 1990;64(6):2819–2824.
513. Summers J, Smith PM, Huang MJ, Yu MS. Morphogenetic and regulatory effects of mutations in the envelope proteins of an avian hepadnavirus. *J Virol* 1991;65(3):1310–1317.
514. Summers J, Smolec JM, Snyder R. A virus similar to human hepatitis B virus associated with hepatitis and hepatoma in woodchucks. *Proc Natl Acad Sci U S A* 1978;75(9):4533–4537.
515. Summers J, Smolec JM, Werner BG. Hepatitis B virus and woodchuck hepatitis virus are members of a novel class of DNA viruses. In: Essex M, Todaro G, zur Hausen H, eds. *Viruses in naturally occurring tumors*. Cold Spring Harbor conference on cell proliferation VII. Cold Spring Harbor, NY: Cold Spring Harbor Press, 1979:459–470.
516. Sureau C, Romet-Lemonne JL, Mullins JI, Essex M. Production of hepatitis B virus by a differentiated human hepatoma cell line after transfection with cloned circular HBV DNA. *Cell* 1986;47(1):37–47.
517. Suzuki T, Masui N, Kajino K, et al. Detection and mapping of spliced RNA from a human hepatoma cell line transfected with the hepatitis B virus genome. *Proc Natl Acad Sci U S A* 1989;86(21):8422–8426.
518. Swameye I, Schaller H. Dual topology of the large envelope protein of duck hepatitis B virus: Determinants preventing pre-S translocation and glycosylation. *J Virol* 1997;71(12):9434–9441.
519. Szmuness W. Hepatocellular carcinoma and the hepatitis B virus: Evidence for a causal association. *Prog Med Virol* 1978;24:40–69.
520. Tagawa M, Robinson WS, Marion PL. Duck hepatitis B virus replicates in the yolk sac of developing embryos. *J Virol* 1987;61(7): 2273–2279.
521. Tanese N, Goff SP. Domain structure of the Moloney murine leukemia virus reverse transcriptase: Mutational analysis and separate expression of the DNA polymerase and RNase H activities. *Proc Natl Acad Sci U S A* 1988;85(6):1777–1781.
522. Tarn C, Bilodeau ML, Hullinger RL, Andrisani OM. Differential immediate early gene expression in conditional hepatitis B virus pX-transforming versus nontransforming hepatocyte cell lines. *J Biol Chem* 1999;274(4):2327–2336.
523. Tavis JE, Ganem D. Expression of functional hepatitis B virus polymerase in yeast reveals it to be the sole viral protein required for correct initiation of reverse transcription. *Proc Natl Acad Sci U S A* 1993; 90(9):4107–4111.
524. Tavis JE, Ganem D. RNA sequences controlling the initiation and transfer of duck hepatitis B virus minus-strand DNA. *J Virol* 1995; 69(7):4283–4291.
525. Tavis JE, Ganem D. Evidence for activation of the hepatitis B virus polymerase by binding of its RNA template. *J Virol* 1996;70(9): 5741–5750.
526. Tavis JE, Perri S, Ganem D. Hepadnavirus reverse transcription initiates within the stem-loop of the RNA packaging signal and employs a novel strand transfer. *J Virol* 1994;68(6):3536–3543.
527. Tennant BC, Mrosovsky N, McLean K, et al. Hepatocellular carcinoma in Richardson's ground squirrels (*Spermophilus richardsonii*): Evidence for association with hepatitis B-like virus infection. *Hepatology* 1991;13(6):1215–1221.
528. Terradillos O, Billet O, Rnard CA, et al. The hepatitis B virus X gene potentiates c-myc-induced liver oncogenesis in transgenic mice. *Oncogene* 1997;14:395–404.
529. Terre S, Petit MA, Brechot C. Defective hepatitis B virus particles are generated by packaging and reverse transcription of spliced viral RNAs *in vivo*. *J Virol* 1991;65(10):5539–5543.
530. Testut P, Renard CA, Terradillos O, et al. A new hepadnavirus endemic in arctic ground squirrels in Alaska. *J Virol* 1996;70(7):4210–4219.
531. Tognoni A, Cattaneo R, Serfling E, Schaffner W. A novel expression selection approach allows precise mapping of the hepatitis B virus enhancer. *Nucleic Acids Res* 1985;13:7457–7472.
532. Toh H, Hayashida H, Miyata T. Sequence homology between retroviral reverse transcriptase and putative polymerases of hepatitis B virus and cauliflower mosaic virus. *Nature* 1983;305(5937):827–829.
533. Tokino T, Fukushige S, Nakamura T, et al. Chromosomal translocation and inverted duplication associated with integrated hepatitis B virus in hepatocellular carcinomas. *J Virol* 1987;61(12):3848–3854.
534. Tokino T, Matsubara K. Chromosomal sites for hepatitis B virus integration in human hepatocellular carcinoma. *J Virol* 1991;65(12): 6761–6764.
535. Tokino T, Tamura H, Hori N, Matsubara K. Chromosome deletions associated with hepatitis B virus integration. *Virology* 1991;185(2): 879–882.
536. Tong S, Li J, Wands JR. Interaction between duck hepatitis B virus and a 170-kilodalton cellular protein is mediated through a neutralizing epitope of the pre-S region and occurs during viral infection. *J Virol* 1995;69(11):7106–7112.
537. Tong SP, Li JS, Vitvitski L, et al. Evidence for a base-paired region of hepatitis B virus pregenome encapsidation signal which influences the patterns of precore mutations abolishing HBe protein expression. *J Virol* 1993;67(9):5651–5655.
538. Tran A, Kremsdorf D, Capel F, et al. Emergence of and takeover by hepatitis B virus (HBV) with rearrangements in the pre-S/S and pre-C/C genes during chronic HBV infection. *J Virol* 1991;65(7): 3566–3574.
539. Transy C, Fourel G, Robinson WS, et al. Frequent amplification of c-myc in ground squirrel liver tumors associated with past or ongoing infection with a hepadnavirus. *Proc Natl Acad Sci U S A* 1992;89(9): 3874–3878.
540. Treinin M, Laub O. Identification of a promoter element located upstream from the hepatitis B virus X gene. *Mol Cell Biol* 1987;7: 545–548.
541. Truant R, Antunovic J, Greenblatt J, et al. Direct interaction of the hepatitis B virus HBx protein with p53 leads to inhibition by HBx of p53 response element-directed transcativation. *J Virol* 1995;69: 1851–1859.
542. Trueba D, Phelan M, Nelson J, et al. Transmission of ground squirrel hepatitis virus to homologous and heterologous hosts. *Hepatology* 1985;5(3):435–439.
543. Trujillo MA, Letovsky J, Maguire HF, et al. Functional analysis of a liver-specific enhancer of the hepatitis B virus. *Proc Natl Acad Sci U S A* 1991;88(9):3797–3801.
544. Turkson J, Bowman T, Garcia R, et al. Stat3 activation by Src induces specific gene regulation and is required for cell transformation. *Mol Cell Biol* 1998;18(5):2545–2552.
545. Tuttleman JS, Pourcel C, Summers J. Formation of the pool of covalently closed circular viral DNA in hepadnavirus-infected cells. *Cell* 1986;47(3):451–460.
546. Tuttleman JS, Pugh JC, Summers JW. *In vitro* experimental infection of primary duck hepatocyte cultures with duck hepatitis B virus. *J Virol* 1986;58(1):17–25.
547. Twu JS, Lai MY, Chen DS, Robinson WS. Activation of protooncogene c-jun by the X protein of hepatitis B virus. *Virology* 1993;192: 346–350.
548. Twu JS, Robinson WS. Hepatitis B virus X gene can transactivate heterologous viral sequences. *Proc Natl Acad Sci U S A* 1989;86: 2046–2050.
549. Twu JS, Schloemer RH. Transcriptional trans-activating function of hepatitis B virus. *J Virol* 1987;61:3448–3453.
550. Uchida M, Esumi M, Shikata T. Molecular cloning and sequence analysis of duck hepatitis B virus genomes of a new variant isolated from Shanghai ducks. *Virology* 1989;173(2):600–606.
551. Ueda K, Ganem D. Apoptosis is induced by N-myc expression in hepatocytes, a frequent event in hepadnavirus oncogenesis, and is blocked by insulin-like growth factor II. *J Virol* 1996;70(3): 1375–1383.
552. Ueda K, Tsurimoto T, Matsubara K. Three envelope proteins of hepatitis B virus: Large S, middle S, and major S proteins needed for the formation of Dane particles. *J Virol* 1991;65(7):3521–3529.
553. Ueda K, Wei Y, Ganem D. Activation of N-myc2 gene expression by cis-acting elements of oncogenic hepadnaviral genomes: Key role of enhancer II. *Virology* 1996;217:413–417.
554. Ueda K, Wei Y, Ganem D. Activation of N-myc2 gene expression by

cis-acting elements of oncogenic hepadnaviral genomes: Key role of enhancer II. *Virology* 1996;217(1):413–417.
555. Urban S, Breiner KM, Fehler F, et al. Avian hepatitis B virus infection is initiated by the interaction of a distinct pre-S subdomain with the cellular receptor gp180. *J Virol* 1998;72(10):8089–8097.
556. Valenzuela P, Gray P, Quiroga M, et al. Nucleotide sequence of the gene coding for the major protein of hepatitis B virus surface antigen. *Nature* 1979;280(5725):815–819.
557. Valenzuela P, Medina A, Rutter WJ, et al. Synthesis and assembly of hepatitis B virus surface antigen particles in yeast. *Nature* 1982; 298(5872):347–350.
558. Valenzuela P, Quiroga M, Zaldivar J, et al. The nucleotide sequence of the hepatitis B viral genome and the identification of the major viral genes. In: Fields BN, Jaenisch R, eds. *Animal virus genetics.* Proceedings of the 1980 ICN/UCLA Symposia on Animal Virus Genetics. New York: Academic Press, 1980:57–70.
559. Vannice JL, Levinson AD. Properties of the human hepatitis B virus enhancer: Position effects and cell-type nonspecificity. *J Virol* 1988; 62(4):1305–1313.
560. Wampler DE, Lehman ED, Boger J, et al. Multiple chemical forms of hepatitis B surface antigen produced in yeast. *Proc Natl Acad Sci U S A* 1985;82(20):6830–6834.
561. Wang GH, Seeger C. The reverse transcriptase of hepatitis B virus acts as a protein primer for viral DNA synthesis. *Cell* 1992;71(4):663–670.
562. Wang GH, Seeger C. Novel mechanism for reverse transcription in hepatitis B viruses. *J Virol* 1993;67(11):6507–6512.
563. Wang H-D, Trivedi A, Johnson DL. Hepatitis B virus X protein induces RNA polymerase III-dependent gene transcription and increases cellulae TATA-binding protein by activating the Ras signaling pathway. *Mol Cell Biol* 1997;17:6838–6846.
564. Wang HD, Yuh CH, Dang CV, Johnson DL. The hepatitis B virus X protein increases the cellular level of TATA-binding protein which mediates transactivation of RNA polymerase III genes. *Mol Cell Biol* 1995;15:6720–6728.
565. Wang HD, Trivedi A, Johnson DL. Regulation of RNA polymerase I-dependent promoters by the hepatitis B virus X protein via activated Ras and TATA-binding protein. *Mol Cell Biol* 1998;18(12): 7086–7094.
566. Wang HP, Rogler CE. Topoisomerase I-mediated integration of hepadnavirus DNA *in vitro. J Virol* 1991;65(5):2381–2392.
567. Wang HP, Zhang L, Dandri M, Rogler CE. Antisense downregulation of N-myc1 in woodchuck hepatoma cells reverses the malignant phenotype. *J Virol* 1998;72(3):2192–2198.
568. Wang J, Chenivesse X, Henglein B, Brechot C. Hepatitis B virus integration in a cyclin A gene in a hepatocellular carcinoma. *Nature* 1990;343(6258):555–557.
569. Wang J, Lee AS, Ou JH. Proteolytic conversion of hepatitis B virus e antigen precursor to end product occurs in a postendoplasmic reticulum compartment. *J Virol* 1991;65(9):5080–5083.
570. Wang XW, Forrester K, Yeh H, et al. Hepatitis B virus X protein inhibits p53 sequence-specific DNA binding, transcriptional activity, and association with transcription factor ERCC3. *Proc Natl Acad Sci U S A* 1994;91:2230–2234.
571. Wang XW, Gibson MK, Vermeulen W, et al. Abrogation of p-53-induced apoptosis by the hepatitis B virus X gene. *Cancer Res* 1995; 55:6012–6016.
572. Wang Y, Chen P, Wu X, et al. A new enhancer element, ENII, identified in the X gene of hepatitis B virus. *J Virol* 1990;64(8):3977–3981.
573. Weber M, Bronsema V, Bartos H, et al. Hepadnavirus P protein utilizes a tyrosine residue in the TP domain to prime reverse transcription. *J Virol* 1994;68(5):2994–2999.
574. Wei Y, Fourel G, Ponzetto A, et al. Hepadnavirus integration: Mechanisms of activation of the N-myc2 retrotransposon in woodchuck liver tumors. *J Virol* 1992;66:5265–5276.
575. Wei Y, Fourel G, Ponzetto A, et al. Hepadnavirus integration: Mechanisms of activation of the N-myc2 retrotransposon in woodchuck liver tumors. *J Virol* 1992;66(9):5265–5276.
576. Wei Y, Tavis JE, Ganem D. Relationship between viral DNA synthesis and virion envelopment in hepatitis B viruses. *J Virol* 1996;70(9): 6455–6458.
577. Weil R, Sirma H, Giannini C, et al. Direct association and nuclear import of the hepatitis B virus X protein with the NF-kB inhibitor IkBa. *Mol Cell Biol* 1999;19:6345–6354.
578. Weiser B, Ganem D, Seeger C, Varmus HE. Closed circular viral DNA and asymmetrical heterogeneous forms in livers from animals infected with ground squirrel hepatitis virus. *J Virol* 1983;48(1):1–9.
579. Will H, Cattaneo R, Koch HG, et al. Cloned HBV DNA causes hepatitis in chimpanzees. *Nature* 1982;299(5885):740–742.
580. Will H, Cattaneo R, Pfaff E, et al. Expression of hepatitis B antigens with a simian virus 40 vector. *J Virol* 1984;50(2):335–342.
581. Will H, Reiser W, Weimer T, et al. Replication strategy of human hepatitis B virus. *J Virol* 1987;61(3):904–911.
582. Will H, Salfeld J, Pfaff E, et al. Putative reverse transcriptase intermediates of human hepatitis B virus in primary liver carcinomas. *Science* 1986;231(4738):594–596.
583. Williams JS, Andrisani OM. The hepatitis B virus X protein targets the basic region-leucine zipper domain of CREB. *Proc Natl Acad Sci U S A* 1995;92:3819–3823.
584. Wollersheim M, Debelka U, Hofschneider PH. A transactivating function encoded in the hepatitis B virus X gene is conserved in the integrated state. *Oncogene* 1988;3:545–552.
585. Wong DT, Nath N, Sninsky JJ. Identification of hepatitis B virus polypeptides encoded by the entire pre-s open reading frame. *J Virol* 1985;55(1):223–231.
586. Wu HL, Chen PJ, Tu SJ, et al. Characterization and genetic analysis of alternatively spliced transcripts of hepatitis B virus in infected human liver tissues and transfected HepG2 cells. *J Virol* 1991;65(4): 1680–1686.
587. Wu TT, Coates L, Aldrich CE, et al. In hepatocytes infected with duck hepatitis B virus, the template for viral RNA synthesis is amplified by an intracellular pathway. *Virology* 1990;175(1):255–261.
588. Wynne SA, Crowther RA, Leslie AG. The crystal structure of the human hepatitis B virus capsid. *Mol Cell* 1999;3(6):771–780.
589. Xu Z, Bruss V, Yen TS. Formation of intracellular particles by hepatitis B virus large surface protein. *J Virol* 1997;71(7):5487–5494.
590. Yaginuma K, Kobayashi M, Yoshida E, Koike K. Hepatitis B virus integration in hepatocellular carcinoma DNA: Duplication of cellular flanking sequences at the integration site. *Proc Natl Acad Sci U S A* 1985;82(13):4458–4462.
591. Yaginuma K, Koike K. Identification of a promoter region for 3.6-kilobase mRNA of hepatitis B virus and specific cellular binding protein. *J Virol* 1989;63(7):2914–2920.
592. Yaginuma K, Nakamura I, Takada S, Koike K. A transcription initiation site for the hepatitis B virus X gene is directed by the promoter-binding protein. *J Virol* 1993;67(5):2559–2565.
593. Yaginuma K, Shirakata Y, Kobayashi M, Koike K. Hepatitis B virus (HBV) particles are produced in a cell culture system by transient expression of transfected HBV DNA. *Proc Natl Acad Sci U S A* 1987; 84(9):2678–2682.
594. Yaginuma K, Shirakata Y, Kobayashi M, Koike K. Hepatitis B virus (HBV) particles are produced in a cell culture system by transient expression of transfected HBV DNA. *Proc Natl Acad Sci U S A* 1987; 84:2678–2682.
595. Yang D, Alt E, Rogler CE. Coordinate expression of N-myc 2 and insulin-like growth factor II in precancerous altered hepatic foci in woodchuck hepatitis virus carriers. *Cancer Res* 1993;53(9): 2020–2027.
596. Yang D, Faris R, Hixson D, et al. Insulin-like growth factor II blocks apoptosis of N-myc2-expressing woodchuck liver epithelial cells. *J Virol* 1996;70(9):6260–6268.
597. Yang W, Mason WS, Summers J. Covalently closed circular viral DNA formed from two types of linear DNA in woodchuck hepatitis virus-infected liver. *J Virol* 1996;70(7):4567–4575.
598. Yang W, Summers J. Illegitimate replication of linear hepadnavirus DNA through nonhomologous recombination. *J Virol* 1995;69(7): 4029–4036.
599. Yang W, Summers J. Infection of ducklings with virus particles containing linear double-stranded duck hepatitis B virus DNA: Illegitimate replication and reversion. *J Virol* 1998;72(11):8710–8717.
600. Yee J. A liver specific enhancer in the core promoter region of human hepatitis B virus. *Science* 1989;246:658–661.
601. Yeh CT, Liaw YF, Ou JH. The arginine-rich domain of hepatitis B virus precore and core proteins contains a signal for nuclear transport. *J Virol* 1990;64(12):6141–6147.
602. Yeh CT, Ou JH. Phosphorylation of hepatitis B virus precore and core proteins. *J Virol* 1991;65(5):2327–2331.
603. Yen TSB. Hepadnaviral X protein: Review of recent progress. *J Biomed Sci* 1996;3:20–30.

604. Yen TSB. Posttranscriptional regulation of gene expression in hepadnaviruses. *Semin Virol* 1998;8:319–326.
605. Yoffe B, Noonan CA, Melnick JL, Hollinger FB. Hepatitis B virus DNA in mononuclear cells and analysis of cell subsets for the presence of replicative intermediates of viral DNA. *J Infect Dis* 1986; 153(3):471–477.
606. Yokosuka O, Omata M, Zhou YZ, et al. Duck hepatitis B virus DNA in liver and serum of Chinese ducks: Integration of viral DNA in a hepatocellular carcinoma. *Proc Natl Acad Sci U S A* 1985;82(15): 5180–5184.
607. Yu CL, Meyer DJ, Campbell GS, et al. Enhanced DNA-binding activity of a Stat3-related protein in cells transformed by the Src oncoprotein. *Science* 1995;269(5220):81–83.
608. Yu M, Summers J. A domain of the hepadnavirus capsid protein is specifically required for DNA maturation and virus assembly. *J Virol* 1991;65(5):2511–2517.
609. Yu M, Summers J. Phosphorylation of the duck hepatitis B virus capsid protein associated with conformational changes in the C terminus. *J Virol* 1994;68(5):2965–2969.
610. Yu X, Mertz JE. Promoters for synthesis of the pre-C and pregenomic mRNAs of human hepatitis B virus are genetically distinct and differentially regulated. *J Virol* 1996;70(12):8719–8726.
611. Yu X, Mertz JE. Differential regulation of the pre-C and pregenomic promoters of human hepatitis B virus by members of the nuclear receptor superfamily. *J Virol* 1997;71(12):9366–9374.
612. Yuasa S, Cheung RC, Pham Q, et al. Peptide mapping of neutralizing and nonneutralizing epitopes of duck hepatitis B virus pre-S polypeptide. *Virology* 1991;181(1):14–21.
613. Yuh CH, Chang YL, Ting LP. Transcriptional regulation of precore and pregenomic RNAs of hepatitis B virus. *J Virol* 1992;66(7): 4073–4084.
614. Yuh CH, Ting LP. The genome of hepatitis B virus contains a second enhancer: Cooperation of two elements within this enhancer is required for its function. *J Virol* 1990;64(9):4281–4287.
615. Yuh CH, Ting LP. Differentiated liver cell specificity of the second enhancer of hepatitis B virus. *J Virol* 1993;67(1):142–149.
616. Zahm P, Hofschneider PH, Koshy R. The HBV X-ORF encodes a transactivator: a potential factor in viral hepatocarcinogenesis. *Oncogene* 1988;3:169–177.
617. Zandi E, Karin M. Bridging the gap: Composition, regulation, and physiological function of the IkappaB kinase complex. *Mol Cell Biol* 1999;19(7):4547–4551.
618. Zentgraf H, Herrmann G, Klein R, et al. Mouse monoclonal antibody against hepatitis B virus X protein synthesized in *Escherichia coli:* Detection of reactive antigen in liver cell carcinoma and chronic hepatitis. *Oncology* 1990;47:143–148.
619. Zhang P, Raney AK, McLachlan A. Characterization of the hepatitis B virus X- and nucleocapsid gene transcriptional regulatory elements. *Virology* 1992;191(1):31–41.
620. Zhang YY, Summers J. Enrichment of a precore-minus mutant of duck hepatitis B virus in experimental mixed infections. *J Virol* 1999;73(5): 3616–3622.
621. Zheng Y-X, Riegler J, Wu J, Yen TSB. Novel short transcripts of hepatis B virus X gene derived from intragenic promoter. *J Biol* Chem 1994;269:22593–22598.
622. Zhou D, Yen TSB. Differential regulation of the hepatitis B virus surface gene promoters by a second viral enhancer. *J Biol Chem* 1990;265(34):20732–20734.
623. Zhou DX, Taraboulous A, Ou JH, Yen TSB. Activation of class I major histocompatability complex gene expression by hepatitis B virus. *J Virol* 1990;64:4025–4028.
624. Zhou DX, Yen TS. The hepatitis B virus S promoter comprises A CCAAT motif and two initiation regions. *J Biol Chem* 1991;266(34): 23416–23421.
625. Zhou DX, Yen TS. The ubiquitous transcription factor Oct-1 and the liver-specific factor HNF-1 are both required to activate transcription of a hepatitis B virus promoter. *Mol Cell Biol* 1991;11(3):1353–1359.
626. Zhou S, Standring DN. Cys residues of the hepatitis B virus capsid protein are not essential for the assembly of viral core particles but can influence their stability. *J Virol* 1992;66(9):5393–5398.
627. Zhou S, Yang SQ, Standring DN. Characterization of hepatitis B virus capsid particle assembly in *Xenopus* oocytes. *J Virol* 1992;66(5): 3086–3092.
628. Zoulim F, Saputelli J, Seeger C. Woodchuck hepatitis virus X protein is required for viral infection *in vivo. J Virol* 1994;68:2026–2030.
629. Zoulim F, Seeger C. Reverse transcription in hepatitis B viruses is primed by a tyrosine residue of the polymerase. *J Virol* 1994;68(1): 6–13.
630. Zufferey R, Donello JE, Trono D, Hope TJ. Woodchuck hepatitis virus posttranscriptional regulatory element enhances expression of transgenes delivered by retroviral vectors. *J Virol* 1999;73(4):2886–2892.
631. Kann M, Sodeik B, Vlachou A, et al. Phosphorylation-dependent binding of hepatitis B virus core particles to the nuclear pore complex. *J Cell Biol* 1999;145:45–55.

CHAPTER 37

Prions

Stanley B. Prusiner

Prions are infectious proteins that cause fatal neurodegeneration in humans and animals (156). The prion diseases, also referred to as the transmissible spongiform encephalopathies, are uniquely manifest as sporadic, genetic, and infectious illnesses. The only known component of the prion is a protein designated PrP^{Sc}. The prion protein (PrP) gene found on the short arm of chromosome 20 of humans encodes a protein of 253 amino acids termed PrP^{C}. Both PrP^{C} and PrP^{Sc} have the same covalent structure, but through a poorly understood process, PrP^{C} is refolded into PrP^{Sc}. The accumulation of PrP^{Sc} in the central nervous system (CNS) causes neurologic disease, and the refolding of PrP^{C} is stimulated by the product of the reaction PrP^{Sc}.

For many years, investigators classified scrapie, the prototypic prion disease of sheep, as a slow viral illness. Many aspects of scrapie in sheep and goats mimic viral diseases (Table 1). The term *slow viruses* was introduced by Bjorn Sigurdsson in 1954 to characterize the sheep diseases called visna and scrapie (184). He suggested that the long latency periods between inoculation and the onset of disease was a special feature of slow- or delayed-acting viruses. Eventually, the visna agent was shown to be a lentivirus, the same family to which the human immunodeficiency virus (HIV) belongs.

TABLE 1. *Features of scrapie suggesting that it might be caused by a virus*

Scrapie is a transmissible disease.
Infectious pathogen is small and filterable.
Accumulation of the scrapie pathogen causes disease.
Distinct strains of the scrapie agent cause different patterns of disease, as measured by the length of the incubation time and the neuropathologic lesion profile.

As early as 1967, several experimental findings by Tikvah Alper and her colleagues suggested that the infectious pathogen causing scrapie might be unusual (1,2). Most notable were the results of radiation inactivation studies suggesting that the scrapie might not contain a nucleic acid and that the infectious particle might be extremely small. On one hand, those conclusions were vigorously challenged (165–168), and on the other, they prompted a myriad of hypotheses (Table 2). The most prescient of these speculations were those suggesting that the scrapie agent might be a protein. I. Pattison (143) proposed that the scrapie agent was a basic protein, and J. S. Griffith (72) published three hypotheses: that it was (a) a protein that induces its own gene transcription, (b) an antibody-like molecule stimulating more of itself, and (c) a protein that acquires a disease-inducing conformation. Although the first two hypotheses proved to be incorrect, the last resembles what was eventually discovered. Interestingly, the conformational proposal violated considerable data arguing that each protein has only one biologically active conformation (5,6).

The tortuous path of the scientific investigation that led to an understanding of familial Creutzfeldt-Jakob disease (CJD) chronicles a remarkable scientific odyssey. By 1930, the high incidence of familial (f) CJD in some families was known (127,189). Almost 60 years were to pass before the significance of this finding could be appreciated (84,120,152). CJD remained a curious, rare neurodegenerative disease of unknown etiology throughout this period of threescore years (102). Only with the transmission of disease to apes after inoculation of brain extracts prepared from patients who died of CJD did the story begin to unfold (67).

TABLE 2. *Hypothetical structures proposed for the scrapie agent*

Sarcosporidia-like parasite
"Filterable" virus
Small DNA virus
Replicating protein
Replicating abnormal polysaccharide with membrane
DNA subvirus controlled by a transmissible linkage substance
Provirus consisting of recessive genes generating RNA particles
Naked nucleic acid similar to plant viroids
Unconventional virus
Aggregated conventional virus with unusual properties
Replicating polysaccharide
Nucleoprotein complex
Nucleic acid surrounded by a polysaccharide coat
Spiroplasma-like microorganism
Multicomponent system with one component quite small
Membrane-bound DNA
Virino (viroid-like DNA complexed with host proteins)
Filamentous animal virus [scrapie-associated fibrils (SAF)]
Aluminum-silicate amyloid complex
Amyloid-inducing virus
Complex of apo- and co-prions (unified theory)
Nemavirus (SAF surrounded by DNA)
Retrovirus
Soil bacterium

Source: Adapted from Prusiner SB. Development of the prion concept. In: *Prion Biology and Diseases.* Cold Spring Harbor, N.Y.: Cold Spring Harbor Press, 1999, with permission.

Once CJD was shown to be an infectious disease, relatively little attention was paid to the familial form of the disease, as most cases were not found in families. It is interesting to speculate how the course of scientific investigation might have proceeded had transmission studies not been performed until after the molecular genetic lesion had been identified. Had that sequence of events transpired, then the prion concept, which readily explains how a single disease can have a genetic or infectious etiology, might have been greeted with much less skepticism (154).

Epidemiologic studies designed to identify the source of the CJD infection were unable to identify any predisposing risk factors, although some geographic clusters were found (19,45,74,117). Libyan Jews living in Israel developed CJD about 30 times more frequently than other Israelis (94). This finding prompted some investigators to propose that the Libyan Jews had contracted CJD by eating lightly cooked brain from scrapie-infected sheep when they lived in Tripoli prior to emigration. Subsequently, the Libyan Jewish patients were all found to carry a mutation at codon 200 in their PrP gene (61,70,85).

Although the brains of patients appear grossly normal upon postmortem examination, they usually show spongiform degeneration and astrocytic gliosis under the light microscope (Fig. 1). In all cases of Gerstmann-Sträussler-Scheinker disease (GSS) and variant (v) CJD, PrP amyloid plaques are found (213). Before PrP immunostaining was available, histochemical staining was used to examine brains from patients with kuru, and 70% of cases were thought to have amyloid plaques (103). The presence or absence of PrP amyloid plaques in sporadic and inherited CJD is quite variable (50).

Human prion disease should be considered in any patient who develops a progressive subacute or chronic decline in cognitive or motor function. Typically, adults between 40 and 80 years of age are affected (169). The young age of more than 100 people who have died of vCJD in Britain and France has raised the possibility that these individuals were infected with bovine prions that contaminated beef products (34,46,213). Over 100 young adults have also been diagnosed with iatrogenic CJD from 4 to 30 years after receiving human growth hormone (HGH) or gonadotrophin derived from cadaveric pituitaries (105,148). The longest incubation periods (20 to 30 years) are similar to those associated with more recent cases of kuru (65,104).

In scrapie, kuru, CJD, and all the other disorders now referred to as prion diseases (Table 3), spongiform degeneration and astrocytic gliosis are found on microscopic

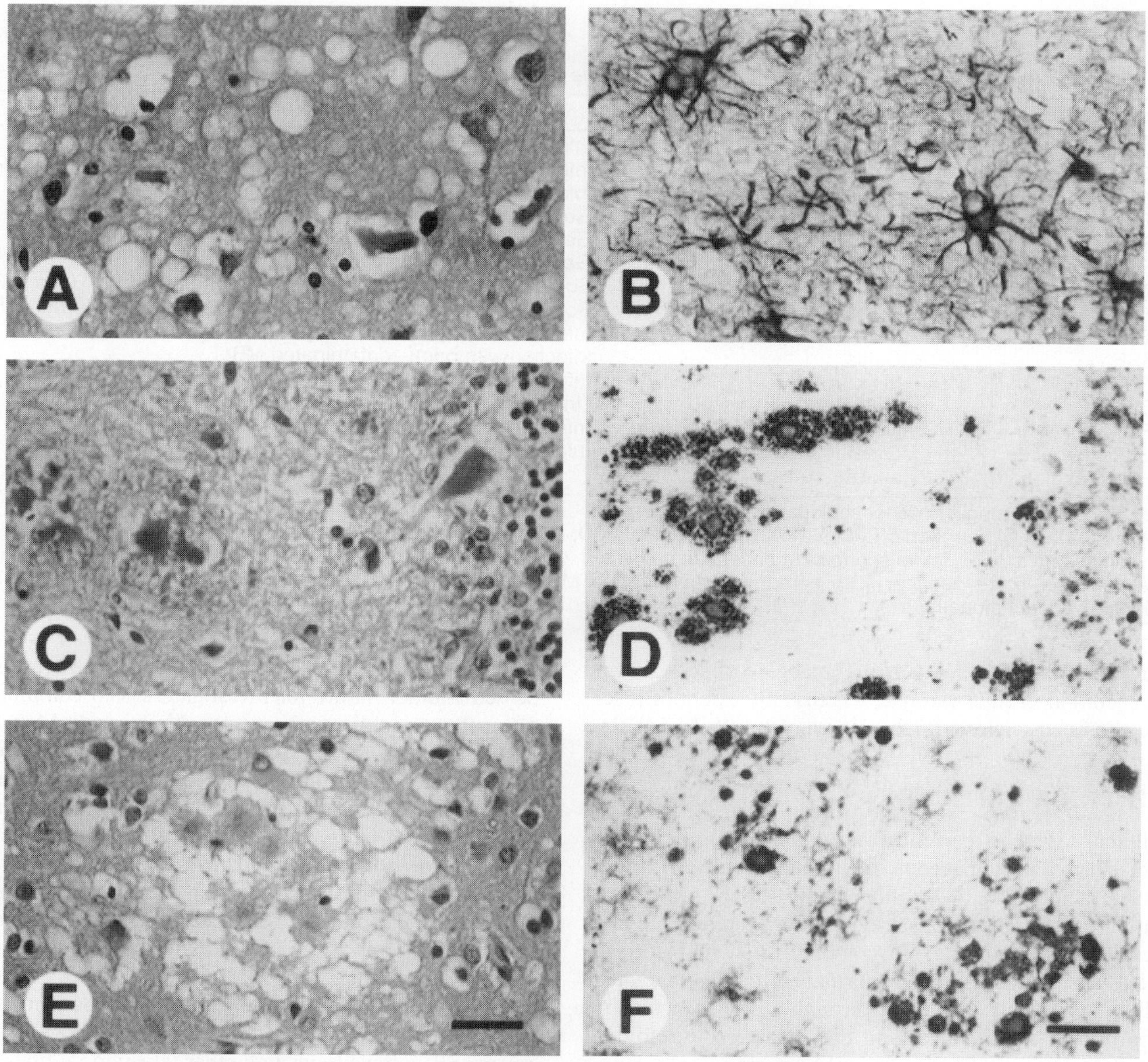

FIG. 1. Neuropathology of human prion diseases. Sporadic Creutzfeldt-Jakob disease (CJD) is characterized by vacuolation of the neuropil of the gray matter, by exuberant reactive astrocytic gliosis, the intensity of which is proportional to the degree of nerve cell loss, and rarely by PrP amyloid plaque formation (not shown). The neuropathology of familial CJD is similar. GSS(P102L), as well as other inherited forms of Gerstmann-Sträussler-Scheinker disease (GSS) (not shown), is characterized by numerous deposits of PrP amyloid throughout the CNS. New variant CJD (nvCJD) has clinical and epidemiologic features that suggest it was acquired by infection with prions. The neuropathologic features of nvCJD are unique among CJD cases because of the abundance of PrP amyloid plaques that are often surrounded by a halo of intense vacuolation. **A:** Sporadic CJD. Cerebral cortex demonstrates widespread spongiform degeneration (H&E). **B:** Sporadic CJD. Cerebral cortex immunostained with anti-GFAP (glial fibrillary acidic protein) antibodies demonstrates the widespread reactive gliosis. **C:** GSS. Cerebellum with most of the GSS plaques in the molecular layer (left 80% of micrograph); many but not all are periodic acid Schiff (PAS)–reaction positive. Granule cells and a single Purkinje cell are seen in the right 20% of the panel. **D:** GSS. Cerebellum at the same location as (C). PrP immunohistochemistry after hydrolytic autoclaving reveals more PrP plaques than seen with the PAS reaction. **E:** Variant CJD. Cerebral cortex, showing the plaque deposits uniquely located within vacuoles (H&E). With this histology, these amyloid deposits have been referred to as florid plaques. **F:** Variant CJD. Cerebral cortex stained with PrP immunohistochemistry after hydrolytic autoclaving reveals numerous PrP plaques, often occurring in clusters as well as minute PrP deposits surrounding many cortical neurons and their proximal processes. *Bar* in (E) = 50 μm, and scale applies also to (A), (B), and (C). *Bar* in F = 100 μm, and scale applies also to (D). (Photomicrographs prepared by Stephen DeArmond.)

TABLE 3. *The prion diseases*

Disease	Host	Mechanism of pathogenesis
A. Kuru	Fore people	Infection through ritualistic cannibalism
iCJD	Humans	Infection from prion-contaminated HGH, dura mater grafts, etc.
vCJD	Humans	Infections from bovine prions?
fCJD	Humans	Germline mutations in PrP gene
GSS	Humans	Germline mutations in PrP gene
FFI	Humans	Germline mutation in PrP gene (D178N, M129)
sCJD	Humans	Somatic mutation or spontaneous conversion of PrP^{C} into PrP^{Sc}?
sFI	Humans	Somatic mutation or spontaneous conversion of PrP^{C} into PrP^{Sc}?
B. Scrapie	Sheep	Infection in genetically susceptible sheep
BSE	Cattle	Infection with prion-contaminated MBM
TME	Mink	Infection with prions from sheep or cattle
CWD	Mule deer, elk	Unknown
FSE	Cats	Infection with prion-contaminated beef
Exotic ungulate encephalopathy	Greater kudu, nyala, oryx	Infection with prion-contaminated MBM

BSE, bovine spongiform encephalopathy; CJD, Creutzfeldt-Jakob disease; sCJD, sporadic CJD; fCJD, familial CJD; iCJD, iatrogenic CJD; vCJD, (new) variant CJD; CWD, chronic wasting disease; FFI, fatal familial insomnia; FSE, feline spongiform encephalopathy; sFI, sporadic fatal insomnia; GSS, Gerstmann-Sträussler-Scheinker disease; HGH, human growth hormone; MBM, meat and bone meal; TME, transmissible mink encephalopathy.

examination of the CNS (215). The degree of spongiform degeneration is quite variable, whereas the extent of reactive gliosis correlates with the degree of neuron loss (121).

THE PRION PARTICLE

Perhaps the best current working definition of a prion is that it is a proteinaceous infectious particle that lacks nucleic acid (155). A wealth of data supports the contention that scrapie prions are devoid of nucleic acid and seem to be composed exclusively of a modified isoform of PrP, designated PrP^{Sc}. The normal cellular PrP, denoted PrP^{C}, is converted into PrP^{Sc} through a process whereby a portion of its α-helical and coil structure is refolded into β-sheet (139). This structural transition is accompanied by profound changes in the physicochemical properties of the PrP. Whereas PrP^{C} is soluble in nondenaturing detergents, PrP^{Sc} is not. PrP^{C} is readily digested by proteases, whereas PrP^{Sc} is partially resistant (137). Because prions appear to be composed entirely of a protein that adopts an abnormal conformation, it is not unreasonable to think of prions as infectious proteins (139,198). But we hasten to add that we still cannot eliminate the possibility of a small ligand bound to PrP^{Sc} as an essential component of the infectious prion particle.

In a broader view, prions are elements that impart and propagate variability through multiple conformers of a normal cellular protein. The species of a particular prion is encoded by the sequence of the chromosomal PrP gene of the mammal in which it last replicated. In contrast to pathogens with a nucleic acid genome that encode strain-specific properties in genes, prions seem to encipher these properties in the tertiary structure of PrP^{Sc} (12,155,198).

The discovery that mutations of the PrP gene caused dominantly inherited prion diseases in humans linked the genetic and infectious forms of prion diseases and presented another hurdle for investigators who continued to argue that prion diseases are caused by viruses. More than 20 mutations of the PrP gene are now known to cause the inherited human prion diseases, and significant genetic linkage has been established for five of these mutations (84, and reviewed in ref. 155). The prion concept readily explains how a disease can manifest as a heritable as well as an infectious illness. Moreover, the hallmark common to all of the prion diseases, whether sporadic, dominantly inherited, or acquired by infection, is that they involve the aberrant metabolism of the PrP (153).

Although PrP^{Sc} is the only known component of the infectious prion particles, these unique pathogens share several phenotypic traits with other infectious entities such as viruses. Because some features of the diseases caused by prions and viruses are similar, some scientists have difficulty accepting the existence of prions despite a wealth of scientific data supporting this concept (37,38,112,119).

MOLECULAR GENETICS OF PRION DISEASES

Once a PrP cDNA probe became available, molecular genetic studies were undertaken to determine whether the PrP gene controls scrapie incubation times in mice. Independent of the enriching of brain fractions for scrapie infectivity that led to the discovery of PrP^{Sc}, the PrP gene was shown to be genetically linked to a locus controlling the incubation time (28). Subsequently, mutation of the PrP gene was shown to be genetically linked to the development of familial prion disease (84). At the same time, expression of a Syrian hamster (SHa) PrP transgene in mice was shown to render the animals highly susceptible to SHa prions, which demonstrated that expression of a foreign PrP gene could abrogate the species barrier (176).

Later, PrP-deficient (*Prnp*$^{0/0}$) mice were found to be resistant to prion infection and failed to replicate prions, as expected (23,157). The results of these studies indicated that PrP must play a central role in the transmission and pathogenesis of prion disease, but equally important, they established that the abnormal isoform is an essential component of the prion particle (153).

PrP Gene Dosage Controls Length of Incubation Time

Scrapie incubation times in mice were used to distinguish prion strains and to identify a gene controlling incubation length (53,177). This gene was initially called *Sinc*, based on genetic crosses between C57Bl and VM mice that exhibited short and long incubation times, respectively (53). Because the distribution of VM mice was restricted, we searched for another mouse with long incubation times. I/Ln mice proved to be a suitable substitute for VM mice; eventually, I/Ln and VM mice were found to be derived from a common ancestor. Subsequently, the PrP gene was shown to control the length of the scrapie incubation time in mice (27,131).

Overexpression of wt PrP Transgenes

Mice were constructed expressing different levels of the wild-type (wt) SHaPrP transgene (Tg) (176). Inoculation of these Tg(SHaPrP) mice with SHa prions demonstrated abrogation of the species barrier, resulting in abbreviated incubation times as a result of a nonstochastic process (159). The length of the incubation time after inoculation with SHa prions was inversely proportional to the level of SHaPrP^{C} in the brains of Tg(SHaPrP) mice (159). Bioassays of brain extracts from clinically ill Tg(SHaPrP) mice inoculated with mouse (Mo) prions revealed that only Mo prions but no SHa prions were produced. Conversely, inoculation of Tg(SHaPrP) mice with SHa prions led only to the synthesis of SHa prions. Thus, the rate of PrP^{Sc} synthesis appears to be a function of the level of PrP^{C} expression in Tg mice; however, the level to which PrP^{Sc} accumulates appears to be independent of PrP^{C} concentration (159).

PrP-Deficient Mice

The development and life span of two lines of *Prnp*$^{0/0}$ mice denoted Zrch and Npu were indistinguishable from controls (24,118), whereas another line (Ngsk) exhibited ataxia and Purkinje cell degeneration at about 70 weeks of age (172). In the former two lines, with normal development, altered sleep–wake cycles (201) and synaptic behavior in brain slices have been reported (44), but the synaptic changes could not be confirmed by others (78,116). The lack of severe defects in these two lines of *Prnp*$^{0/0}$ mice were ascribed to adaptation, because PrP was absent throughout embryogenesis. However, bigenic mice expressing inducible PrP transgenes that were rendered PrP deficient as adults by the administration of doxycycline have remained healthy for more than 1.5 years (202). This argues against the adaptation hypothesis and raises the likelihood of surrogate proteins with functions overlapping that of PrP^{C}.

Prnp$^{0/0}$ mice are resistant to prions (23,157). *Prnp*$^{0/0}$ mice were sacrificed 5, 60, 120, and 315 days after inoculation with Rocky Mountain Laboratory (RML) prions, and brain extracts were bioassayed in CD-1 Swiss mice (Table 4). Except for residual infectivity from the inoculum detected at 5 days after inoculation, no infectivity was detected in the brains of the *Prnp*$^{0/0}$ mice (157). One group of investigators found that *Prnp*$^{0/0}$ mice inoculated

TABLE 4. *Prion titers in brains of Prnp*$^{0/0}$ *and Prnp*$^{+/0}$ *mice*

Mouse	Time of sacrifice after inoculation with RML scrapie prions: 5 days	60 days	120 days	315 days	500 days
	Log scrapie prion titers (ID_{50} units/mL ± SE)[a]				
Prnp$^{+/+}$	<1	3.9 ± 0.4	6.4 ± 0.3		
	<1	4.8 ± 0.3	7.1 ± 0.1		
	<1	4.6 ± 0.2	6.6 ± 0.2		
Prnp$^{+/0}$	<1	<1	5.1 ± 0.2		
	0.6 ± 0.7	<1	5.2 ± 0.6		
	1.2 ± 0.1[b]	3.4 ± 0.2	2.8 ± 0.1		
Prnp$^{0/0}$	<1[c]	<1	<1	<1	<1
	<1[d]	<1	<1	<1	<1
		<1			<1
					<1

[a]Titers are for 10% (w/v) brain homogenates. Log titers of <1 reflect no signs of CNS dysfunction in CD-1 mice for >250 days after inoculation, except as noted.
[b]3/9 mice developed scrapie between 208 and 210 days after inoculation.
[c]2/9 mice developed scrapie between 208 and 225 days after inoculation.
[d]2/10 mice developed scrapie between 208 and 225 days after inoculation.
RML, Rocky Mountain Laboratory.

with RML prions and sacrificed 20 weeks later had $10^{3.6}$ ID_{50} units/mL of homogenate by bioassay (23). Others have used this report to argue that prion infectivity replicates in the absence of PrP (38,112). Neither we nor the authors of the initial report could confirm the finding of prion replication in *Prnp*$^{0/0}$ mice (157,171).

Doppel Up-regulation in *Prnp*$^{0/0}$ Mice

Since a common approach to determining the function of a gene is the analysis of related genes, we searched for PrP-related genes by hybridization; however, these studies were uninformative (208). Vertebrate genomes contain a number of protein families sharing sequence homology and showing overlapping function (77), and because a number of them have been shown to be organized in clusters, we undertook sequencing of large cosmid clones containing the PrP gene (113). Studies of regions flanking the human, sheep, and mouse PrP genes in cosmid clones failed to reveal additional open reading frames (ORFs) (113). Only when the sequencing of a cosmid clone isolated from a *Prnp*$^{b/b}$ mouse (I/LnJ-4) was extended downstream of PrP was a novel PrP-like gene found.

The locus *Prnd* is 16-kb downstream of the PrP gene, *Prnp*, and it encodes a 179-residue PrP-like protein designated doppel (Dpl) (132). *Prnd* generates major transcripts of 1.7 and 2.7 kb, as well as some unusual chimeric transcripts generated by intergenic splicing with *Prnp*. Like PrP, Dpl mRNA is expressed during embryogenesis, but in contrast to PrP, it is expressed minimally in the CNS. Unexpectedly, Dpl is up-regulated in the CNS of two *Prnp*$^{0/0}$ lines of mice (Ngsk and Rcm0), both of which develop a late-onset ataxia, raising the possibility that Dpl may provoke neurodegeneration (130,172). It has been suggested that PrP may have a role in the long-term survival of Purkinje neurons; however, it was puzzling that Ngsk and Rcm0 *Prnp*$^{0/0}$ mice should develop a fatal ataxia, whereas two other lines (Zrch and Npu) of *Prnp*$^{0/0}$ mice did not exhibit CNS dysfunction. In an effort to determine the role of PrP in this phenotype, Ngsk *Prnp*$^{0/0}$ mice were crossed with transgenic (Tg) mice overexpressing wild-type mouse PrP. This rescued the phenotype in Ngsk *Prnp*$^{0/0}$ offspring expressing PrP (135).

Our findings suggest that Dpl may provoke neurodegeneration in PrP-deficient mice—an observation that may explain why some lines of *Prnp*$^{0/0}$ mice develop cerebellar dysfunction and Purkinje cell death while others do not. The homology between Dpl and PrP suggests that these two proteins may share some biologic properties, and as such, Dpl may open new avenues of investigation in prion biology.

Our findings suggesting that Dpl may provoke degeneration in Purkinje cells force a reevaluation of Tg mice generated using the I/LnJ-4 cosmid. One explanation for spontaneous neurodegeneration reported in Tg(MoPrP-B) mice with high copy-number arrays of the I/LnJ-4 cosmid transgene is the overexpression of *Prnd* (206). In the case of the Tg(MoPrP,P101L) mice constructed with the I/LnJ-4 cosmid transgene (86,87), *Prnd* overexpression is an unlikely explanation, because similar results were obtained with Tg(MoPrP,P101L) mice constructed using the SHa Cos.Tet vector, which does not contain the *Prnd* gene (178,197,200).

Whether cerebellar degeneration in Zrch *Prnp*$^{0/0}$ mice expressing N-terminally truncated PrP transgenes is explained by Dpl overexpression remains to be established. The expression of N-terminally truncated PrPs carrying either codon 32–121 or 32–134 deletions caused degeneration of granule cells in the cerebellum of neonates, but the smaller 32–106 deletion did not (183). Interestingly, this granule cell dysfunction was mitigated by expression of wild-type MoPrP^{C}. One interpretation of these studies is that PrP carrying either the 32–121 or 32–134 deletion assumes a Dpl-like conformation that is neurotoxic and results in the killing of granule cells because the transgene construct used in those Tg mice is expressed in granule cells but not Purkinje cells (57).

Dpl is the first PrP-like protein to be described in mammals, and because Dpl seems to be similar to PrP in causing neurodegeneration, the linked expression of the *Prnp* and *Prnd* genes may play a previously unrecognized role in the pathogenesis of prion diseases or other illnesses.

PRION PROTEIN STRUCTURE

Once cDNA probes for PrP became available, the PrP gene was found to be constitutively expressed in adult, uninfected brain (39,137). This finding eliminated the possibility that PrP^{Sc} stimulated production of more of itself by initiating transcription of the PrP gene, as proposed nearly two decades earlier (72). Determination of the structure of the PrP gene eliminated a second possible mechanism that might explain the appearance of PrP^{Sc} in brains already synthesizing PrP^{C}. As the entire protein coding region was contained within a single exon, there was no possibility that the two PrP isoforms were the products of alternatively spliced mRNAs (8). Next, a posttranslational chemical modification that distinguishes PrP^{Sc} from PrP^{C} was considered but none was found in an exhaustive study (187), and we considered it likely that PrP^{C} and PrP^{Sc} differed only in their conformations, a hypothesis also proposed earlier (72).

When the secondary structures of the PrP isoforms were compared by optical spectroscopy, they were found to be markedly different (139). Fourier transform infrared (FTIR) and circular dichroism (CD) spectroscopy studies showed that PrP^{C} contains about 40% α-helix and little β-sheet, whereas PrP^{Sc} is composed of about 30% α-helix and 45% β-sheet (139). That the two PrP isoforms have the same amino acid sequence runs counter to the widely accepted view that the amino acid sequence specifies only one biologically active conformation of a protein (5).

Prior to comparative studies on the structures of PrP^C and PrP^{Sc}, metabolic labeling studies showed that the acquisition of PrP^{Sc} protease resistance is a posttranslational process (15). In a search for chemical differences that would distinguish PrP^{Sc} from PrP^C, we identified ethanolamine in hydrolysates of PrP 27–30, which signalled the possibility that PrP might contain a glycosylphosphatidyl inositol (GPI) anchor (188). Both PrP isoforms were found to carry GPI anchors, and PrP^C was found on the surface of cells where it could be released by cleavage of the anchor. Subsequent studies showed that PrP^{Sc} formation occurs after PrP^C reaches the cell surface (31) and is localized to caveolae-like domains (71,195).

Computational Models and Optical Spectroscopy

Modeling studies and subsequent nuclear magnetic resonance (NMR) investigations of a synthetic PrP peptide containing residues 90 to 145 suggested that PrP^C might contain an α-helix within this region (Fig. 2) (88). This peptide contains the residues 113 to 128, which are most highly conserved among all species studied (see Fig. 2A) and correspond to a transmembrane region of PrP that was delineated in cell-free translation studies. A transmembrane form of PrP was found in brains of patients with GSS caused by the A117V mutation and in Tg mice overexpressing either the mutant or wt PrP (76). That no evidence for an α-helix in this region has been found in NMR studies of recombinant PrP in an aqueous environment (54,93,162) suggests that these recombinant PrPs correspond to the secreted form of PrP that was also identified in the cell-free translation studies. This contention is supported by studies with recombinant antibody fragments (Fabs) showing that GPI-anchored PrP^C on the surface of cells exhibits an immunoreactivity similar to that of recombinant PrP prepared with an α-helical conformation (146).

Models of PrP^{Sc} suggest that formation of the disease-causing isoform involves refolding of a region corresponding roughly to residues 108 to 144 into β-sheets (89); the single disulfide bond joining the COOH-terminal helices would remain intact, as the disulfide is required for PrP^{Sc} formation (Fig. 3D) (134). Deletion of each of several regions of putative secondary structure in PrP, except for the NH_2-terminal 66 amino acids (residues 23 to 88) and a 36-amino-acid stretch (Mo residues 141 to 176), prevented formation of PrP^{Sc} as measured in scrapie-infected cultured neuroblastoma cells (134). With α-PrP Fabs selected from phage display libraries and two monoclonal antibodies (MAb) derived from hybridomas, a major conformational change that occurs during conversion of PrP^C into PrP^{Sc} has been localized to residues 90 to 112 (146). Studies with an α-PrP IgM MAb, which was reported to immunoprecipitate PrP^{Sc} selectively (107), support this conclusion. Although these results indicate that PrP^{Sc} formation involves a conformational change at the NH_2-terminus, mutations causing inherited prion diseases have been found throughout the protein (see Fig. 2B). Interestingly, all of the known point mutations in PrP with biologic significance occur either within or adjacent to regions of secondary structure in PrP and as such could destabilize the structure of PrP^C or stabilize a transition state between PrP^C and PrP^{Sc} (42,88,162,163).

NMR Structure of Recombinant PrP

The NMR structure of recombinant (r) SHaPrP(90–231) was determined after the protein was purified and refolded (see Fig. 3A). Residues 90 to 112 are not shown in the figure, because marked conformational heterogeneity was found in this region, whereas residues 113 to 126 constitute the conserved hydrophobic region that also displays some structural plasticity (93,115). Although some features of the structure of rPrP(90–231) are similar to those reported earlier for the smaller recombinant MoPrP(121–231) fragment (162), substantial differences were found. For example, the loop at the NH_2-terminus of helix B is defined in rPrP(90—231) but is disordered in MoPrP(121–231); in addition, helix C is composed of residues 200 to 227 in rPrP(90–231) but extends only from 200 to 217 in MoPrP(121–231). The loop and the COOH-terminal portion of helix C are particularly important, as described later (see Fig. 3B). Whether the differences between the two recombinant PrP fragments are the result of (a) their different lengths, (b) species-specific differences in sequences, or (c) the conditions used for solving the structures remains to be determined.

Recent NMR studies of full-length MoPrP(23–231) and SHaPrP(29–231) have shown that the NH_2-termini are highly flexible and lack identifiable secondary structure under the experimental conditions employed (see Fig. 3C) (54). Studies of SHaPrP(29–231) indicate transient interactions between the COOH-terminal end of helix B and the highly flexible, NH_2-terminal random-coil containing the octarepeats (residues 29 to 125) (54).

PrP Appears to Bind Copper

The highly flexible NH_2-terminus of recombinant PrP may be more structured in the presence of copper. Each SHaPrP(29–231) molecule was found to bind two Cu^{2+} ions at pH 6.5; peptide studies suggest that four Cu^{2+} ions will bind at pH 7.4 (17,203). Using tryptophan fluorescence assay, only Cu^{2+} was found to bind recombinant SHaPrP(29–231); other divalent cations including Ca^{2+}, Co^{2+}, Mg^{2+}, Mn^{2+}, Ni^{2+}, and Zn^{2+} did not bind to PrP (190). Earlier studies with synthetic peptides corresponding to the octarepeat sequence demonstrated the binding of Cu^{2+} ions (81,82), and optical spectroscopy showed that Cu^{2+} induced an α-helix formation in these peptides (128). More recently, PrP-deficient (*$Prnp^{0/0}$*) mice were found to have lower levels of Zn/Cu superoxide dismu-

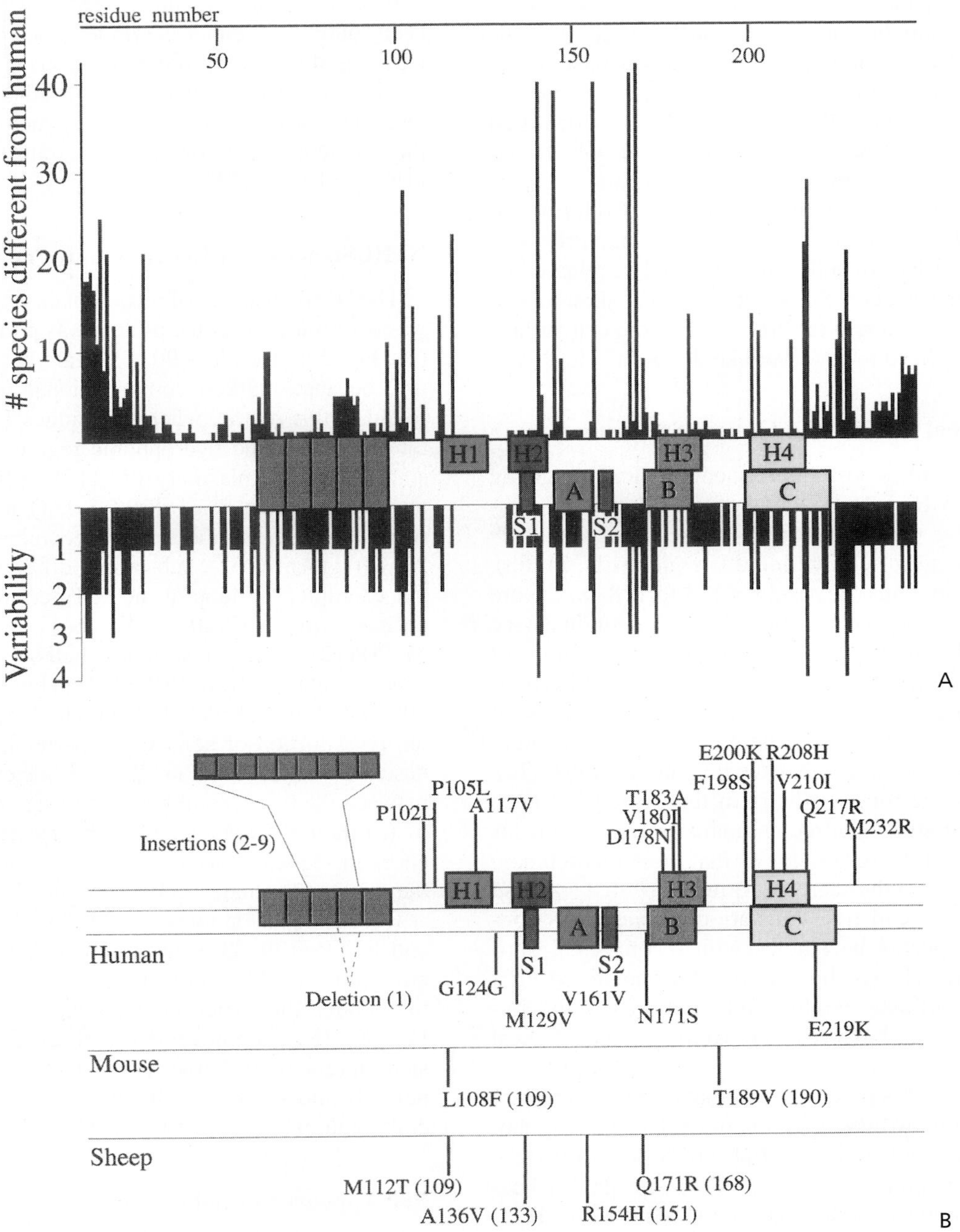

FIG. 2. Species variations and mutations of the prion protein gene. **A:** Species variations. The x-axis represents the human PrP sequence, with the five octarepeats and H1–H4 regions of putative secondary structure shown, as well as the three α-helices A, B, and C and the two β-strands S1 and S2. *Vertical bars* above the axis indicate the number of species that differ from the human sequence at each position. Below the axis, the length of the *bars* indicates the number of alternative amino acids at each position in the alignment. **B:** Mutations causing inherited human prion disease and polymorphisms in human, mouse, and sheep. Above the line of the human sequence are mutations that cause prion disease. Below the lines are polymorphisms, some but not all of which are known to influence the onset as well as the phenotype of disease. (Data compiled by Paul Bamborough and Fred E. Cohen.)

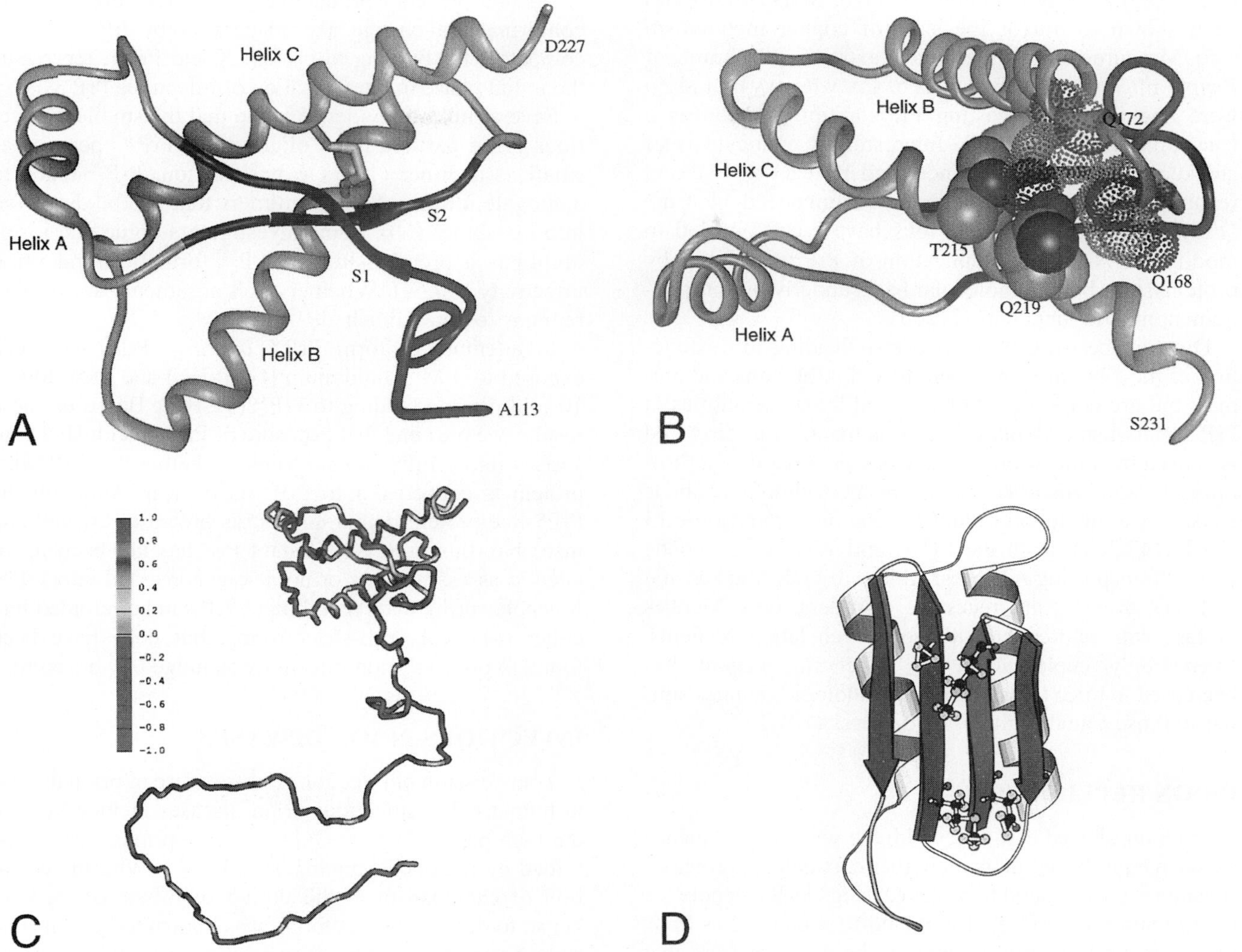

FIG. 3. Structures of prion proteins. **A:** NMR structure of Syrian hamster (SHa) recombinant (r) PrP(90–231). Presumably, the structure of the α-helical form of rPrP(90–231) resembles that of PrP^{C}. rPrP(90–231) is viewed from the interface where PrP^{Sc} is thought to bind to PrP^{C}. The color scheme is as follows: α-helices A (residues 144–157), B (172–193), and C (200–227) in *pink*; disulfide between Cys-179 and Cys-214 in *yellow*; conserved hydrophobic region composed of residues 113–126 in *red*; loops in *gray*; residues 129–134 in *green* encompassing strand S1, and residues 159–165 in *blue* encompassing strand S2. The *arrows* span residues 129–131 and 161–163, as these show a closer resemblance to the β-sheet (93). **B:** NMR structure of rPrP(90–231) is viewed from the interface where protein X is thought to bind to PrP^{C}. Protein X appears to bind to the side chains of residues that form a discontinuous epitope. Some amino acids are in the loop composed of residues 165–171 and at the end of helix B (Gln-168 and Gln-172 with a low-density van der Waals rendering), and others are on the surface of helix C (Thr-215 and Gln-219 with a high-density van der Waals rendering) (96). **C:** Schematic diagram showing the flexibility of the polypeptide chain for PrP(29–231) (54). The structure of the portion of the protein representing residues 90–231 was taken from the coordinates of PrP(90–231) (93). The remainder of the sequence was hand-built for illustration purposes only. The color scale corresponds to the heteronuclear ^{1}H–^{15}N NOE data: *red* for the lowest (most negative) values, where the polypeptide is most flexible, to *blue* for the highest (most positive) values in the most structured and rigid regions of the protein. **D:** Plausible model for the tertiary structure of human PrP^{Sc} (89). Color scheme is as follows: S1 β-strands are 108–113 and 116–122 in *red*; S2 β-strands are 128–135 and 138–144 in *green*; α-helices H3 (residues 178–191) and H4 (residues 202–218) in *gray*; loop (residues 142–177) in *yellow*. Four residues implicated in the species barrier are shown in ball-and-stick form (Asn-108, Met-112, Met-129, Ala-133).

tase (SOD) activity than controls (18); SOD activity has been shown to mirror the state of copper metabolism (75). Measurements of membrane extracts from brains of *Prnp*$^{0/0}$ mice showed low levels of Cu, whereas Fe and Zn were unchanged, suggesting PrP^{C} might function as a Cu^{2+} binding protein (17). Interestingly, endocytosis of chicken PrP seems to be increased by Cu^{2+} (144), and renaturation of PrP^{Sc} appears to be enhanced by Cu^{2+} (125). Both Cu^{2+} and Zn^{2+} ions have been reported to modify the N-terminal truncation of PrP^{Sc} catalyzed by proteinase K, but the molecular basis underlying this phenomenon is not understood (205).

Disturbances in Cu^{2+} homeostasis leading to dysfunction of the CNS are well documented in humans and animals but are not known to be caused by abnormalities in PrP metabolism; Menkes disease is manifest at birth and is caused by a mutation of the MNK gene on the X chromosome, and Wilson's disease appears in childhood and is caused by a mutation of the WD gene on chromosome 13 (26,35,147,204). Both the MNK and WD genes encode copper transporting ATPases. Although both Menkes and Wilson's diseases are recessive disorders, only Menkes disease can be treated with copper chelating reagents. Interestingly, cuprizone, a Cu^{2+} chelating reagent, has been used in mice to induce neuropathologic changes similar to those found in the prion diseases (101,142).

PRION REPLICATION

In an uninfected cell, PrP^{C} with the wild-type sequence exists in equilibrium in its monomeric, α-helical, protease-sensitive state or bound to protein X (Fig. 4). We denote the conformation of PrP^{C} that is bound to protein X as PrP* (41); this conformation is likely to be different from that determined under aqueous conditions for monomeric recombinant PrP. The PrP*–protein X complex will bind PrP^{Sc}, thereby creating a replication-competent assembly. Additional experiments demonstrate that for PrP^{C}, protein X binding precedes productive PrP^{Sc} interactions (96). A conformational change takes place whereby PrP, in a shape competent for binding to protein X and PrP^{Sc}, represents the initial phase in the formation of infectious PrP^{Sc}.

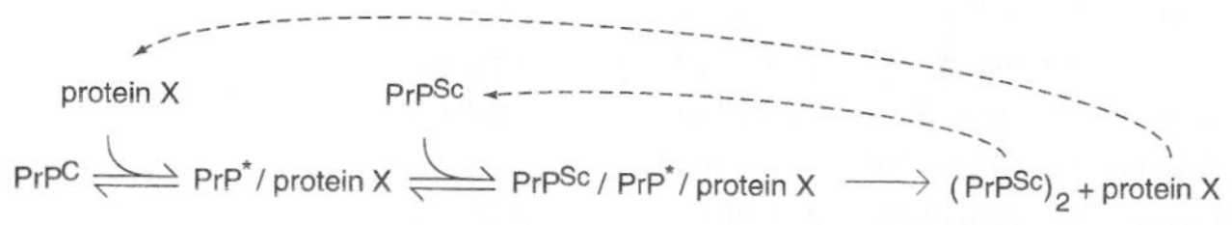

FIG. 4. Schematic diagram showing template-assisted PrP^{Sc} formation. In the initial step, PrP^{C} binds to protein X to form the PrP*–protein X complex. Next, PrP^{Sc} binds to PrP* that has already formed a complex with protein X. When PrP* is transformed into a nascent molecule of PrP^{Sc}, protein X is released and a dimer of PrP^{Sc} remains. The inactivation target size of an infectious prion suggests that it is composed of a dimer of PrP^{Sc} (10). In the model depicted here, a fraction of infectious PrP^{Sc} dimers dissociate into uninfectious monomers as the replication cycle proceeds, whereas most of the dimers accumulate in accordance with the increase in prion titer that occurs during the incubation period. The precise stoichiometry of the replication process remains uncertain.

Several lines of evidence argue that the smallest infectious prion particle is an oligomer of PrP^{Sc}, perhaps as small as a dimer (10). On purification, PrP^{Sc} tends to aggregate into insoluble multimers that can be dispersed into liposomes (60). Some investigators argue that insolubility is a prerequisite for PrP^{Sc} formation and prion infectivity (30,64). Whether such arguments are correct remains to be established.

In attempts to form PrP^{Sc} *in vitro*, PrP^{C} has been exposed to 3 M guanidinium (Gdn) HCl and then diluted 10-fold prior to binding to PrP^{Sc} (95,106). Based on these results, we presume that exposure of PrP^{C} to GdnHCl converts it into a PrP*-like molecule. Whether this PrP*-like protein is converted into PrP^{Sc} is unclear. Although the PrP*-like protein bound to PrP^{Sc} is protease resistant and insoluble, this protease-resistant PrP has not been reisolated to assess whether or not it was converted into PrP^{Sc}. It is noteworthy that recombinant PrP can be refolded into either α-helical or β-sheet forms, but none have been found to possess prion infectivity as judged by bioassay.

INFECTIOUS PRION DISEASES

Transmission of infection is a rare cause of prion disease in humans. The infectious prion diseases include kuru of the Fore people in New Guinea, where prions were transmitted by ritualistic cannibalism (3,4,63). With the cessation of cannibalism at the urging of missionaries, kuru began to decline long before it was known to be transmissible. Sources of prions causing infectious CJD on several different continents include improperly sterilized depth electrodes, transplanted corneas, HGH, gonadotrophin derived from cadaveric pituitaries, and dura mater grafts (20). Over 90 young adults have developed CJD after treatment with cadaveric HGH; the incubation periods range from 3 to more than 20 years (13,148). Dura mater grafts implanted during neurosurgical procedures seem to have caused more than 60 cases of CJD; these incubation periods range from 1 to more than 14 years (33,56,110).

New Variant Creutzfeldt-Jakob Disease

In 1994, the first cases of CJD in teenagers and young adults that were eventually labeled new variant (nv) CJD occurred in Britain (212,213). The young age of these patients was unusual (9,16), and their brains showed numerous PrP amyloid plaques surrounded by a halo of intense spongiform degeneration (92). One French patient meeting these criteria later followed (34). These unusual neuropathologic changes have not been seen in CJD cases in the United States, Australia, or Japan (32). Both macaque monkeys and marmosets developed neurologic disease several years after inoculation with bovine prions (7), but only the macaques exhibited numerous PrP plaques similar to those found in nvCJD (111).

Have Bovine Prions Been Transmitted to Humans?

The restricted geographical occurrence and chronology of vCJD have raised the possibility that bovine spongiform encephalopathy (BSE) prions have been transmitted to humans. From 1994 until the last quarter of 1998, the incidence of vCJD seemed to be constant at about eight cases per year. This now seems to have changed with the report of 27 new cases in 2000 (212). This dramatic change in the incidence of vCJD raises the possibility that we are beginning to see a substantial increase in the number of patients dying of vCJD. Still, epidemiologic studies have not identified a set of dietary habits that distinguishes vCJD patients from apparently healthy people. Moreover, there is no explanation for the predilection of vCJD for teenagers and young adults. Why have older individuals not developed vCJD-based neuropathologic criteria? It is noteworthy that epidemiologic studies over the past three decades have failed to find evidence for transmission of sheep prions to humans (45). Attempts to predict the future number of cases of vCJD, assuming exposure to bovine prions prior to the offal ban, have been uninformative because so few cases of vCJD have occurred (46).

Strain of BSE Prions

Was a particular conformation of bovine (Bo) PrP^{Sc} selected for heat resistance during the rendering process and then reselected multiple times as cattle, infected by ingesting prion-contaminated meat and bone meal (MBM), were slaughtered and their offal rendered into more MBM? Recent studies of PrP^{Sc} from brains of patients who died of vCJD show a pattern of PrP glycoforms different from those found for sporadic (s) or iatrogenic (i) CJD (43,80). But the utility of measuring PrP glycoforms is questionable in trying to relate BSE to vCJD (185), because PrP^{Sc} is formed after the protein is glycosylated (15,31) and enzymatic deglycosylation of PrP^{Sc} requires denaturation. Alternatively, it may be possible to establish a relationship between the conformations of PrP^{Sc} from cattle with BSE and those from humans with vCJD by using Tg mice, as was done for strains generated in the brains of patients with the familial form of fatal insomnia (FFI) or fCJD (179,198). A relationship between vCJD and BSE has been suggested by finding similar incubation times in non-Tg RIII mice 310 days after inoculation with Hu or Bo prions (22).

Transgenetic Studies of BSE Prions

When Tg(BoPrP)*Prnp*$^{0/0}$ mice are inoculated with either nvCJD prions from humans or BSE prions previously passaged once through these same Tg(BoPrP)*Prnp*$^{0/0}$ mice (179), the resulting lesion profiles as measured by neuronal vacuolation, PrP^{Sc} distribution on histoblots, and PrP amyloid deposition as well as the incubation times were all indistinguishable (179a). Interestingly, Tg(BoPrP)*Prnp*$^{0/0}$ mice are also highly susceptible to natural and experimental sheep scrapie. Although the incubation times are similar, the neuronal vacuolation, PrP^{Sc} distribution on histoblots, and PrP amyloid deposition are extremely different.

We believe these data provide the first rational experimental studies that establish a clear link between BSE and nvCJD. Indeed, there is an eerie symmetry about these experimental results, where the one passage of BSE prions from humans is equivalent to the first passage from cattle through Tg(BoPrP)*Prnp*$^{0/0}$ mice.

Inherited and Sporadic Prion Diseases

For inherited and sporadic prion diseases, the major question is how the first PrP^{Sc} molecules are formed. Once these are formed, replication presumably follows the mechanism outlined for infectious disease. Several lines of evidence suggest that PrP^{Sc} is more stable than PrP^{C}, and a kinetic barrier precludes the formation of PrP^{Sc} under normal conditions. In the case of the initiation of inherited prion diseases, the barrier to PrP^{Sc} formation must be lower for the mutant (ΔPrP^{C}) than the wild-type, and thus ΔPrP^{*} can spontaneously rearrange to form ΔPrP^{Sc}. Although the known mutations would appear to be destabilizing to the structure of PrP^{C}, we lack useful information about the structure of the transition state for either the mutant or wild-type sequences. Studies of PrP in the brains of patients who were heterozygous for the E200K mutation revealed ΔPrP^{Sc}(E200K) molecules that were both detergent insoluble and resistant to limited proteolysis, whereas most wild-type PrP was detergent insoluble but protease sensitive (62). These results suggest that in familial (f) CJD(E200K), insoluble wt PrP might represent a form of PrP* (62). In studies with Chinese hamster ovary (CHO) cells, expression of ΔPrP(E200K) was found to be accompanied by the posttranslational acquisition of resistance to limited proteolysis (114), but whether such cell lines expressing ΔPrP(E200K) produce infectious prions is unknown. It is noteworthy that levels of proteinase K used in the studies where ΔPrP(E200K) was expressed in CHO cells were lower by a factor of 10 to 100 compared to digestions of PrP^{Sc} derived from brain or scrapie-infected neuroblastoma (ScN2a) cells. Whether these alterations in the properties of ΔPrP(E200K) in CHO cells provide evidence for ΔPrP*, or such changes lie outside the pathway of ΔPrP^{Sc}(E200K) formation, remains to be determined.

Initiation of sporadic disease may follow from a somatic mutation and thus follows a path similar to that for germline mutations in inherited disease. In this situation, the mutant PrP^{Sc} must be capable of co-opting wt PrP^{C}, a process known to be possible for some mutations (e.g., E200K, D178N) but less likely for others (e.g., P102L) (198,200). Alternatively, the activation barrier separating wt PrP^{C} from PrP^{Sc} could be crossed on rare occasions when viewed in the context of a population. Most individuals would be spared, although presentations in the elderly with an incidence of about one per million would be seen.

Transgenic Mice Expressing Mutant PrP

With the identification of mutant genes causing familial forms of neurodegeneration, it became possible to model this process in Tg mice. The first mice expressing a mutant gene that developed CNS degeneration were those expressing the P102L mutation of GSS disease in a mutant PrP transgene (87). The age of onset of CNS dysfunction was found to depend on the level of expression of the mutant PrP transgene in Tg(MoPrP,P101L) mice. The higher the level of expression of the mutant PrP transgene, the earlier the age of onset (197). Additionally, Tg(MoPrP,P101L)*Prnp*$^{0/0}$ mice that were deficient for wild-type MoPrP exhibit a relatively uniform age onset of disease. Not only did the Tg(MoPrP,P101L) mice develop neurodegeneration spontaneously but they also transmitted disease to inoculated recipients that express the same transgene at a much lower level (86,197). These recipient mice, designated Tg(MoPrP,P101L)196/*Prnp*$^{0/0}$ (or Tg196), infrequently develop spontaneous neurodegeneration. Recently, a 55-residue synthetic peptide carrying the P102L mutation in a β-sheet conformation has been shown to induce disease in Tg196 mice (96a). This mutant 55-mer polypeptide can be refolded into at least two distinct conformations. When inoculated intracerebrally into Tg196 mice, 20 of 20 mice receiving the β-form of this peptide developed signs of CNS dysfunction at about 360 days, with neurohistologic changes that are pathognomonic of GSS. By contrast, 8 of 8 mice receiving a non-β-form of the peptide failed to develop any neuropathologic changes more than 600 days after peptide injections. We conclude that a chemically synthesized peptide refolded into the appropriate conformation can accelerate or possibly initiate prion disease. Also noteworthy is the production of neurodegeneration in Tg mice expressing mutant PrP with an expanded octarepeat region (40). This mutation is known to produce inherited prion disease in humans (138,150).

Mechanism of Prion Propagation?

From the foregoing formalism, we can ask, What is the rate-limiting step in prion formation? First, we must consider the impact of the concentration of PrP^{Sc} in the inoculum, which is inversely proportional to the length of the incubation time. Second, we must consider the sequence of PrP^{Sc} that forms an interface with PrP^{C}. When the sequences of the two isoforms are identical, the shortest incubation times are observed. Third, we must consider the strain-specific conformation of PrP^{Sc}. Some prion strains exhibit longer incubation times than others; interestingly, the levels of protease-sensitive PrP^{Sc} increase with prolongation of the incubation time, as described later (170). From these considerations, there exists a set of conditions under which initial PrP^{Sc} concentrations can be rate limiting. These effects presumably relate to the stability of the PrP^{Sc}, its targeting to the correct cells and subcellular compartments, and its ability to be cleared. Once infection in a cell is initiated and endogenous PrP^{Sc} production is operative, then the following discussion of PrP^{Sc} formation seems most applicable. If the assembly of PrP^{Sc} into a specific dimeric or multimeric arrangement was difficult, then a nucleation-polymerization (NP) formalism would be relevant. In NP processes, nucleation is the rate-limiting step and elongation or polymerization is facile. These conditions are frequently observed in peptide models of aggregation phenomena (30); however, studies with Tg mice expressing foreign PrP genes suggest that a different process is occurring. From investigations with mice expressing both the SHaPrP transgene and the endogenous MoPrP gene, it is clear that PrP^{Sc} provides a template for directing prion replication, where we define a template as a catalyst that leaves its imprint on the product of the reaction (159). Inoculation of these mice with $SHaPrP^{Sc}$ leads to the production of nascent $SHaPrP^{Sc}$ and not $MoPrP^{Sc}$. Conversely, inoculation of the Tg(SHaPrP) mice with $MoPrP^{Sc}$ results in $MoPrP^{Sc}$ formation and not $SHaPrP^{Sc}$. Even stronger evidence for templating has emerged from studies of prion strains passaged in Tg(MHu2M)*Prnp*$^{0/0}$ mice expressing a chimeric Hu/MoPrP gene as described in more detail later (155,198). Even though the conformational templates were initially generated with PrP^{Sc} molecules having different sequences in patients with inherited prion diseases, these templates are sufficient to direct replication of distinct PrP^{Sc} molecules when the amino acid sequences of the substrate PrPs are identical. If the formation of this template were rate limiting, then an NP model could apply. However, studies of PrP^{Sc} formation in ScN2a cells point to a distinct rate-limiting step.

Cell biologic and transgenetic investigations argue for the existence of a chaperone-like molecule referred to as protein X that is required for PrP^{Sc} formation (200). As described later, mutagenesis experiments have created dominant negative forms of ΔPrP^{C} that inhibit the formation of wt PrP^{Sc} by binding protein X (96). This implies that the rate-limiting step *in vivo* in prion replication, under conditions where PrP^{Sc} is sufficient, must be the conversion of PrP^{C} to PrP* because a dominant negative derived from a single point mutation could gate only a kinetically critical step in a cellular process. In the template-directed model, the conversion of PrP^{C} to PrP* is a first-order process. By contrast, NP processes follow higher-order kinetics [$(\text{monomer})^{m}$, where m is the number of monomers in the nucleus]. The experimental implications of these rate relationships are apparent in transgenic studies; if first-order kinetics operate, halving the gene dose (hemizygotes) should double the incubation time, whereas doubling the dose of a transgene array should halve the time to disease. This quantitative behavior has been observed in several studies in mice with altered levels of PrP expression (25,27,157,159). The existence of prion strains that are conformational isoforms of PrP^{Sc} with distinct structures, incubation times, and neurohistopathology must also be considered in an analysis of the kinetics of PrP^{Sc} accumulation. Because the rate-limiting step in PrP^{Sc} formation cannot involve the unique template provided by a strain, differential rates of intercellular spread, cellular uptake, and clearance seem most likely to account for the variation in incubation times. This is consistent with results described later for eight prion strains in which the levels of protease-sensitive PrP^{Sc} correlate with the length of the incubation times (170). We have suggested that protease-sensitive PrP^{Sc} might serve as a surrogate marker for PrP^{Sc} clearance. In addition to these findings, different patterns of protease sensitivity and glycosylation for distinct prion strains support the proposal of clearance of PrP^{Sc} features in determining the length of the incubation time (12,43,185,198).

However, we hasten to add that NP models can provide a useful description of other biologic phenomena. Under conditions when the monomer is relatively rare and/or the conformational change is facile (e.g., short peptides), the NP model will dominate. However, when the monomer is sufficiently abundant and/or the conformational conversion is difficult to accomplish, the template assistance formalism provides a more likely description of the process.

Evidence for Protein X

Protein X was postulated to explain the results on the transmission of human (Hu) prions to Tg mice (Table 5) (199,200). Mice expressing both Mo and HuPrP were resistant to Hu prions, whereas those expressing only HuPrP were susceptible. These results argue that $MoPrP^{C}$ inhibited transmission of Hu prions—that is, the formation of nascent $HuPrP^{Sc}$. In contrast to the foregoing studies, mice expressing both MoPrP and chimeric MHu2M PrP were susceptible to Hu prions, and mice expressing MHu2M PrP alone were only slightly more susceptible. These findings contend that $MoPrP^{C}$ has only a minimal effect on the formation of chimeric $MHu2MPrP^{Sc}$.

When the data on Hu prion transmission to Tg mice were considered together, they suggested that $MoPrP^{C}$ prevented the conversion of $HuPrP^{C}$ into PrP^{Sc} by binding to another Mo protein but that it had little effect on the conversion of MHu2M into PrP^{Sc}. We interpreted these results in terms of $MoPrP^{C}$ binding to this Mo protein with a higher affinity than does $HuPrP^{C}$. We postulated that $MoPrP^{C}$ had little effect on the formation of PrP^{Sc} from MHu2M (see Table 5) because MoPrP and MHu2M share the same amino acid sequence at the COOH-terminus. This also suggested that $MoPrP^{C}$ only weakly inhibited transmission of SHa prions to Tg(SHaPrP) mice because SHaPrP is more closely related to MoPrP than is HuPrP.

Using scrapie-infected mouse neuroblastoma cells transfected with chimeric Hu/Mo PrP genes, we extended our studies of protein X. Substitution of a Hu residue at position 214 or 218 prevented PrP^{Sc} formation (see Fig. 3B) (96). The side chains of these residues protrude from the same surface of the COOH-terminal α-helix, forming a discontinuous epitope with residues 167 and 171 in an adjacent loop. Substitution of a basic residue at positions 167, 171, or 218 prevented PrP^{Sc} formation; these mutant PrPs appear to act as "dominant negatives" by binding protein X and rendering it unavailable for prion propagation. Our findings seem to explain the protective effects of basic polymorphic residues in PrP of humans and sheep (90,181,209).

Is Protein X a Molecular Chaperone?

Because PrP undergoes a profound structural transition during prion propagation, it seems likely that other proteins such as chaperones participate in this process. Whether protein X functions as a classical molecular chaperone or participates in PrP binding as part of its normal function, but can also facilitate pathogenic aspects of PrP biology, is unknown. Interestingly, scrapie-infected cells in culture display marked differences in the induction of heat-shock proteins (Hsp) (196), and Hsp70 mRNA has been reported to increase in scrapie of mice (99). Although attempts to isolate specific proteins that bind to PrP have been disappointing (136), PrP has been shown to interact

TABLE 5. *Evidence for protein X from transmission studies of human prions*

Inoculum	Host	MoPrP gene	Incubation time (days ± SEM) (n/n_0)
sCJD	Tg(HuPrP)	*Prnp*$^{+/+}$	721 (1/10)
sCJD	Tg(HuPrP)*Prnp*$^{0/0}$	*Prnp*$^{0/0}$	263 ± 2 (6/6)
sCJD	Tg(MHu2M)	*Prnp*$^{+/+}$	238 ± 3 (8/8)
sCJD	Tg(MHu2M)*Prnp*$^{0/0}$	*Prnp*$^{0/0}$	191 ± 3 (10/10)

Source: Data with inoculum RG from ref. 200, with permission.
n, number of sick mice; n_0, number of inoculated mice.

with Bcl-2, Hsp60, and the laminin receptor protein by two-hybrid analysis in yeast (108,161). Although these studies are suggestive, no molecular chaperone involved in prion formation in mammalian cells has been identified.

MINIPRIONS

Using the four-helix-bundle model of PrP^C (88), each region of proposed secondary structure was systematically deleted and the mutant constructs expressed in ScN2a cells and Tg mice (133,134). Deletion of any of the four putative helical regions prevented PrP^{Sc} formation, whereas deletion of the NH_2-terminal region containing residues 23 to 89 did not affect the yield of PrP^{Sc}. In addition to the 67 residues at the NH_2-terminus, 36 residues from position 141 to 176 could be deleted without altering PrP^{Sc} formation. The resulting PrP molecule of 106 amino acids was designated PrP106. In this mutant PrP, helix A as well as the S2 β-strand were removed. Whether the structure of PrP^{Sc}106 can be more readily determined than that of full-length PrP^{Sc} remains uncertain.

Transgene-Specified Susceptibility

Tg(MHM2PrP106)*Prnp*$^{0/0}$ mice that expressed PrP106 developed neurologic dysfunction about 300 days after inoculation with RML prions previously passaged in CD-1 Swiss mice (191). The resulting prions containing PrP^{Sc}106 produced CNS disease in about 66 days on subsequent passage in Tg(MHM2PrP106)*Prnp*$^{0/0}$ mice. Besides widespread spongiform degeneration and PrP deposits, the pyramidal cells of the hippocampus comprising the CA-1, CA-2, and CA-3 fields disappeared in Tg(MHM2PrP106)*Prnp*$^{0/0}$ mice inoculated with prions containing PrP^{Sc}106. In no previous study of Tg mice have we seen similar neuropathologic lesions. The Tg(MoPrP-A) mice overexpressing MoPrP are resistant to RML106 miniprions but are highly susceptible to RML prions. These mice require more than 180 days to produce illness after inoculation with miniprions but develop disease in about 50 days when inoculated with RML prions containing full-length $MoPrP^{Sc}$.

Smaller Prions and Mythical Viruses

The unique incubation times and neuropathology in Tg mice caused by miniprions are difficult to reconcile with the notion that scrapie is caused by an as-yet-unidentified virus. When the mutant or wild-type PrP^C of the host matched PrP^{Sc} in the inoculum, the mice were highly susceptible. However, when there was a mismatch between PrP^C and PrP^{Sc}, the mice were resistant to the prions. This principle of homologous PrP interactions—which underlies the species barrier—is recapitulated in studies of PrP106 in which the amino acid sequence has been drastically changed by deleting nearly 50% of the residues. Indeed, the unique properties of the miniprions provide another persuasive argument supporting the contention that prions are infectious proteins.

Strains of Prions

The existence of prion strains raises the question of how heritable biologic information can be enciphered in any molecule other than nucleic acid (53). Strains or varieties of prions have been defined by incubation times and the distribution of neuronal vacuolation (53,59). Subsequently, the patterns of PrP^{Sc} deposition were found to correlate with vacuolation profiles, and these patterns were also used to characterize strains of prions (21,49,51).

The typing of prion strains in C57Bl, VM, and F1(C57Bl × VM) inbred mice began with isolates from sheep with scrapie. The prototypic strains called Me7 and 22A gave incubation times of about 150 and about 400 days in C57Bl mice, respectively (53). The PrPs of C57Bl and I/Ln (and later VM) mice differ at two residues and control incubation times (27,131).

Until recently, support for the hypothesis that the tertiary structure of PrP^{Sc} enciphers strain-specific information (153) was minimal except for the DY strain isolated from mink with transmissible encephalopathy (12). PrP^{Sc} in DY prions showed diminished resistance to proteinase K digestion as well as an anomalous site of cleavage. The DY strain presented a puzzling anomaly because other prion strains exhibiting similar incubation times did not show this altered susceptibility to proteinase K digestion of PrP^{Sc} (177). Also notable was the generation of new strains during passage of prions through animals with different PrP genes (177).

PrP^{Sc} Conformation Enciphers Variation in Prions

Persuasive evidence that strain-specific information is enciphered in the tertiary structure of PrP^{Sc} comes from transmission of two different inherited human prion diseases to mice expressing a chimeric MHu2M PrP transgene (198). In FFI, the protease-resistant fragment of PrP^{Sc} after deglycosylation has an M_r of 19 kd, whereas in fCJD(E200K) and most sporadic prion diseases, it is 21 kd (Table 6) (129). This difference in molecular size was shown to be the result of different sites of proteolytic cleavage at the NH_2-termini of the two human PrP^{Sc} molecules, reflecting different tertiary structures (129). These distinct conformations were not unexpected, because the amino acid sequences of the PrPs differ.

Extracts from the brains of FFI patients transmitted disease into mice expressing a chimeric MHu2M PrP gene about 200 days after inoculation and induced formation of the 19-kd PrP^{Sc}, whereas fCJD(E200K) and sCJD produced the 21-kd PrP^{Sc} in mice expressing the same transgene (198). On second passage, Tg(MHu2M) mice inoculated with FFI prions showed an incubation time of about 136 days and a 19-kd PrP^{Sc}, whereas those

TABLE 6. *Distinct prion strains generated in humans with inherited, infectious, and sporadic prion diseases and transmitted to transgenic mice*

Inoculum	Host species	Host PrP genotype	Incubation time (days ± SEM) (n/n_0)	PrP^{Sc} (kd)
Inherited prion diseases—mutant PrP^{Sc}				
None	Human	FFI(D178N,M129)		19
FFI	Mouse	Tg(MHu2M)	191 ± 4 (10/10)	19
FFI → Tg(MHu2M)	Mouse	Tg(MHu2M)	136 ± 1 (6/6)	19
None	Human	fCJD(E200K)		21
fCJD	Mouse	Tg(MHu2M)	170 ± 2 (10/10)	21
fCJD → Tg(MHu2M)	Mouse	Tg(MHu2M)	167 ± 4 (13/13)	21
Infectious and sporadic prion diseases—wild-type PrP^{Sc}				
BSE	Human	wt(M/M129)		19
nvCJD	Mouse	Tg(MHu2M)	483 ± 44 (8/8)	19
nvCJD → Tg(MHu2M)	Mouse	Tg(MHu2M)	169 ± 3 (6/6)	19
None	Human	wt(M/M129)		21
sCJD	Mouse	Tg(MHu2M)	191 ± 3 (9/9)	21
sCJD → Tg(MHu2M)	Mouse	Tg(MHu2M)	177 ± 3 (10/10)	21

Data from ref. 198.

inoculated with fCJD(E200K) prions exhibited an incubation time of about 170 days and a 21-kd PrP^{Sc} (155). The experimental data demonstrate that $MHu2MPrP^{Sc}$ can exist in two different conformations based on the sizes of the protease-resistant fragments; yet, the amino acid sequence of $MHu2MPrP^{Sc}$ is invariant.

The results of our studies argue that PrP^{Sc} acts as a template for the conversion of PrP^C into nascent PrP^{Sc}. Imparting the size of the protease-resistant fragment of PrP^{Sc} through conformational templating provides a mechanism for both the generation and the propagation of prion strains.

Interestingly, the protease-resistant fragment of PrP^{Sc} after deglycosylation, with an M_r of 19 kd, has been found in patients who died after developing a clinical disease similar to FFI (66,124,140). Since both PrP alleles encoded the wild-type sequence and a Met at position 129, these cases were designated sporadic fatal insomnia (sFI). At autopsy, the spongiform degeneration, reactive astrogliosis, and PrP^{Sc} deposition were confined to the thalamus as found in FFI (123,124,126). Extracts from the thalamus of an sFI patient transmitted disease to Tg(MHu2M)*Prnp$^{0/0}$* mice. PrP^{Sc} accumulated primarily in the thalamus of these Tg mice and after deglycosylation, a 19-kd protease-resistant fragment was identified (124). These findings are similar to those noted earlier for FFI transmission to Tg mice (198). The results of FFI and sFI studies argue persuasively that the clinicopathologic phenotype is determined by the conformation of PrP^{Sc} and not the amino acid sequence (124).

Evidence for Different Conformations of PrP^{Sc} in Eight Prion Strains

Using a highly sensitive conformation-dependent immunoassay for measurement of PrP^{Sc} in tissue homogenates, eight different prion strains passaged in SHas were examined (170). Brains from SHas were collected when the animals displayed signs of neurologic dysfunction; the incubation times for the prion strains varied from 70 to 320 days. Most of the PrP in the brains of SHas with signs of neurologic disease was PrP^{Sc}, as defined by the β-sheet conformation. The level of PrP^{Sc} in the brains of these clinically ill animals exceeded that of PrP^C by 3- to 10-fold (Fig. 5A). The highest levels of PrP^{Sc} were found in the brains of SHas infected with the Me7-H strain; in contrast, the lowest levels were found in the brains of SHas inoculated with the SHa(Me7) strain (see Fig. 5A). Interestingly, the Me7-H and SHa(Me7) strains, both derived from Me7 passaged in mice (177), possessed similar denatured-to-native PrP ratios, but they accumulated PrP^{Sc} at quite different levels (see Fig. 5A and B). The highest denatured-to-native PrP ratio of all tested strains was SHa(RML).

The apparent independence of the ratio of denatured-to-native PrP from the concentration of PrP^{Sc} became apparent after plotting both parameters in a single graph (see Fig. 5B). Each strain occupied a unique position, indicating differences in the conformation of accumulated PrP^{Sc}. Because the PrP^C concentration in each strain was less than or equal to 5 μg/mL and the PrP ratio for PrP^C was less than or equal to 1.8, the expected impact of the presence of PrP^C on the final PrP ratio was less than or equal to 15%.

Because only the most tightly folded conformers of PrP^{Sc} are likely to be protease resistant, we digested each of the brain homogenates with proteinase K prior to measuring the ratio of denatured-to-native PrP (see Fig. 5C). As shown, the positions of many strains changed when the protease-sensitive conformers of PrP^{Sc} were enzymatically hydrolyzed (see Fig. 5C). Most notable was the DY

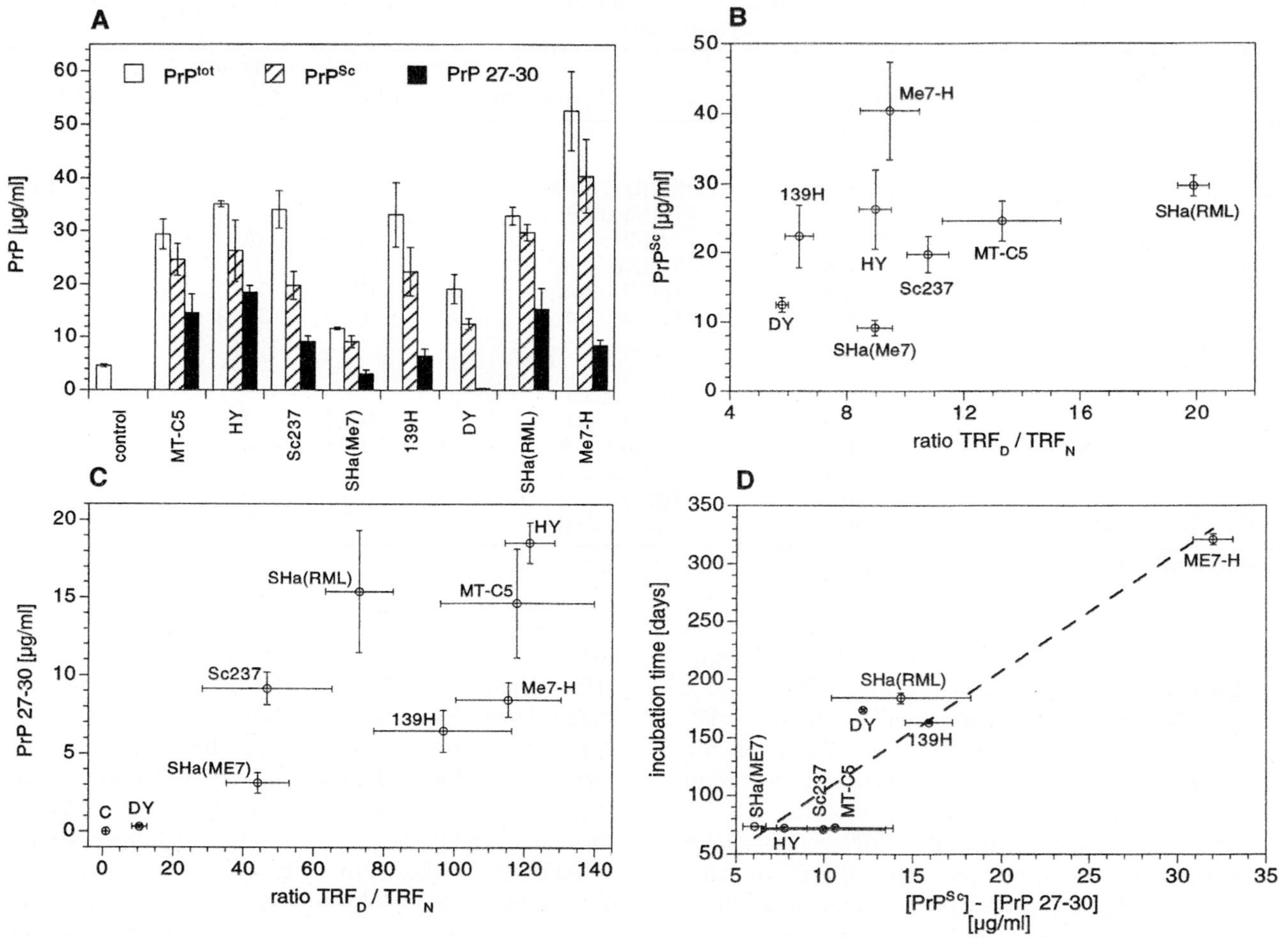

FIG. 5. Eight prion strains distinguished by the conformation-dependent immunoassay. **A:** Concentration of PrP^{Sc} and PrP 27–30. The *columns* and *bars* represent the average ±SEM obtained from three different brains of LVG/LAK Syrian hamsters infected with different prion strains and measured in three independent experiments. **B:** Ratio of antibody binding to denatured/native PrP and a function of concentration of PrP^{Sc} in the brains of Syrian hamsters (SHa) infected with different prion strains. Concentration of PrP^{Sc} and the ratio of antibody binding to denatured/native PrP were measured by the conformation-dependent immunoassay. **C:** Brain homogenates of SHa inoculated with different scrapie strains and uninoculated controls, denoted *C*, were digested with 50 µg/mL of proteinase K for 2 hours at 37°C prior to the conformation-dependent immunoassay. **D:** Incubation time plotted as a function of the concentration of the proteinase K–sensitive fraction of PrP^{Sc} ([PrP^{Sc}]-[PrP 27–30]).

strain, which was readily detectable before limited proteolysis by immunoassay (see Fig. 5B) but became almost undetectable after digestion (see Fig. 5C), in accordance with earlier Western blot studies (11,12). Equally important, strains such as Sc237 and HY were marginally separated prior to proteinase K digestion (see Fig. 5B) but became quite distinct afterwards (see Fig. 5C).

These findings argue that Sc237 and HY are distinct strains although they exhibit similar incubation times of about 70 days when passaged in SHas (177). It is noteworthy that limited proteolysis of PrP^{Sc} from Sc237- and HY-infected brains produced PrP 27–30 proteins that were indistinguishable by migration in sodium dodecyl sulfate–polyacrylamide gel electrophoresis (SDS-PAGE) as detected by Western immunoblotting (177).

When the incubation times of these eight strains were plotted as a function of the concentration of either PrP^{Sc} or PrP 27–30, no relationship could be discerned. Incubation times were also plotted as a function of the ratio of denatured-to-native PrP, and again no correlation could be found.

To assess the fraction of PrP^{Sc} that is sensitive to proteolysis during limited digestion with proteinase K, we subtracted the protease-resistant PrP 27–30 fraction (see Fig. 5C) from the total PrP^{Sc} (see Fig. 5B) for each of the eight prion strains. We asked whether the proteinase K-sensitive fraction of PrP^{Sc} ([PrP^{Sc}]–[PrP 27–30]) might reflect those PrP^{Sc} molecules that are most readily cleared by cellular proteases. The clearance of PrP^{Sc} is of considerable interest with respect to control of the length of the incubation time and other phenotypic features of prion strains (160). When the [PrP^{Sc}]–[PrP 27–30] fraction was plotted as a function of the incubation time, a linear relationship was found with an excellent correlation coefficient ($r = 0.94$) (see Fig. 5D).

The preceding results demonstrate that eight different strains possess at least eight different conformations (see Fig. 5B and C). Additional data argue that each strain is composed of a spectrum of conformations as revealed by limited protease digestion and GdnHCl denaturation studies (170). These findings contrast with the until-recently held notion that the primary structure of a protein determines a single tertiary structure (5).

How many distinct tertiary and quaternary structures can PrP^{Sc} adopt? The conformation-dependent immunoassay described here provides a rapid tool capable of discriminating the secondary, tertiary, and perhaps quaternary structures of a substantial number of PrP^{Sc} molecules.

As noted, for studies of strains passaged from humans with fCJD(E200K) and FFI, PrP^{Sc} must act as a template in the replication of nascent PrP^{Sc} molecules. Also as discussed, it appears likely that the binding of PrP^{C} or a metastable intermediate PrP* to protein X is the initial step in PrP^{Sc} formation, and that this is the rate-limiting step in prion replication (42,96,160). PrP^{Sc} interacts with PrP^{C} but not protein X in the PrP^{C}–protein X complex. When PrP^{C} or PrP* is converted into a nascent PrP^{Sc} molecule, protein X is released.

It also follows from these observations that the different incubation times of various prion strains should arise predominantly from distinct rates of PrP^{Sc} clearance rather than from the different rates of PrP^{Sc} formation (160). Thus, prion strains that are readily cleared should have prolonged incubation times, whereas those that are poorly cleared should display abbreviated incubation periods. We investigated this hypothesis by relying on the difference in brain PrP^{Sc} concentrations before and after proteinase K treatment as a surrogate for *in vivo* clearance of each prion strain. When clearance, as approximated by [PrP^{Sc}]–[PrP 27–30], was plotted as a function of the incubation time for eight strains, a linear relationship was found (see Fig. 5D). It is important to recognize that proteinase K sensitivity is an imperfect model for *in vivo* clearance and that only one strain with a long incubation time (exceeding 300 days) has been studied.

Although it has been suggested that asparagine (Asn)-linked carbohydrates (CHOs) specify prion strains (43), this proposal is difficult to reconcile with the addition of high-mannose oligosaccharides to Asn-linked consensus sites on PrP in the endoplasmic reticulum (ER) and with the subsequent remodeling of the sugar chains in the Golgi (55). Modification of the complex CHOs attached to PrP^{C} is clearly completed prior to PrP^{C} trafficking to the cell surface (15,31), which indicates that the Asn-linked CHOs of PrP^{Sc} do not instruct the addition of such complex-type sugars to PrP^{C}. It remains a formal possibility that specific prion strains preferentially recognize subsets of PrP^{C} glycoforms generated during protein maturation in the Golgi and then facilitate the conformational conversion of these glycoforms into nascent PrP^{Sc}.

Recently, evidence against the proposal that variations in the glycoform ratio encrypt prion strain properties has emerged. Patients with FFI have symptoms and neuropathologic profiles indistinguishable from patients with sFI (124,140). Although PrP^{Sc} from FFI patients shows relatively large amounts of the diglycosylated glycoform because of the D178N mutation adjacent to one of the consensus Asn-linked glycosylation sites (129), $wtPrP^{Sc}$ from sFI patients shows substantially less of the diglycosylated form (124,140). Following transmission to Tg(MHu2M) mice, FFI prions produced an identical pattern of neuropathology to that found in Tg mice infected with sFI prions, arguing that the same prion strain is responsible for the two forms of the disease (124,198). Furthermore, deglycosylated PrP 27–30 migrated at 19 kd whether it was obtained from patients with FFI or sFI, as well as from Tg mice inoculated with FFI or sFI prions (124). These findings with FFI and sFI also argue that the conformation of PrP^{Sc}, not the amino acid sequence, determines the strain-specified disease phenotype. Further evidence arguing against any involvement of the pattern of glycosylation in specifying strain properties has emerged through the discovery that the PrP^{Sc} glycoform ratios found in tonsil tissue differed markedly from those found in the brain of the same patient with nvCJD (79).

Mutagenesis of the complex-type sugar attachment sites (NXT → NXA) seemed to increase the rate of PrP^{Sc} formation in cultured cells (194) but resulted in prolonged incubation times in Tg mice and differences in the patterns of PrP^{C} distribution and PrP^{Sc} deposition in mice expressing mutant PrPs (51). These studies suggest that Asn-linked glycosylation might alter the stability of PrP, and, in the case of PrP^{Sc}, that it results in various patterns of PrP^{Sc} deposition. Thus, different clearance rates of PrP^{Sc} may be important in determining not only strain-specific neuropathology but also the length of the incubation time (160).

Mechanism of Selective Neuronal Targeting?

In addition to incubation times, neuropathologic profiles of spongiform change have been used to characterize prion strains (59). However, recent studies with PrP transgenes argue that such profiles are not an intrinsic feature of strains (29,51). The mechanism by which prion strains modify the pattern of spongiform degeneration was perplexing because earlier investigations had shown that PrP^{Sc} deposition precedes neuronal vacuolation and reactive gliosis (49). When FFI prions were inoculated into Tg(MHu2M) mice, PrP^{Sc} was confined largely to the thalamus (Fig. 6A), as is the case for FFI in humans (198). In contrast, fCJD(E200K) prions inoculated into Tg(MHu2M) mice produced widespread deposition of PrP^{Sc} throughout the cortical mantel and many of the deep structures of the CNS (see Fig. 6B), as is seen in fCJD(E200K) of humans. To examine whether the diverse patterns of PrP^{Sc} deposition are influenced by Asn-linked glycosylation of PrP^{C}, we constructed Tg mice expressing PrPs mutated at one or both of the Asn-linked glycosylation consensus sites (51). These mutations resulted in aberrant neuroanatomic topologies of PrP^{C} within the CNS, whereas pathologic point mutations adjacent to the consensus sites did not alter the distribution of PrP^{C}. Tg mice with a mutation of the second PrP glycosylation site exhibited prion incubation times of more than 500 days and unusual patterns of PrP^{Sc} deposition. These findings raise the possibility that glycosylation can modify the conformation of PrP and affect either the turnover of PrP^{C} or the clearance of PrP^{Sc}. Regional differences in the rate of deposition or clearance would result in specific patterns of PrP^{Sc} accumulation.

A

B

C

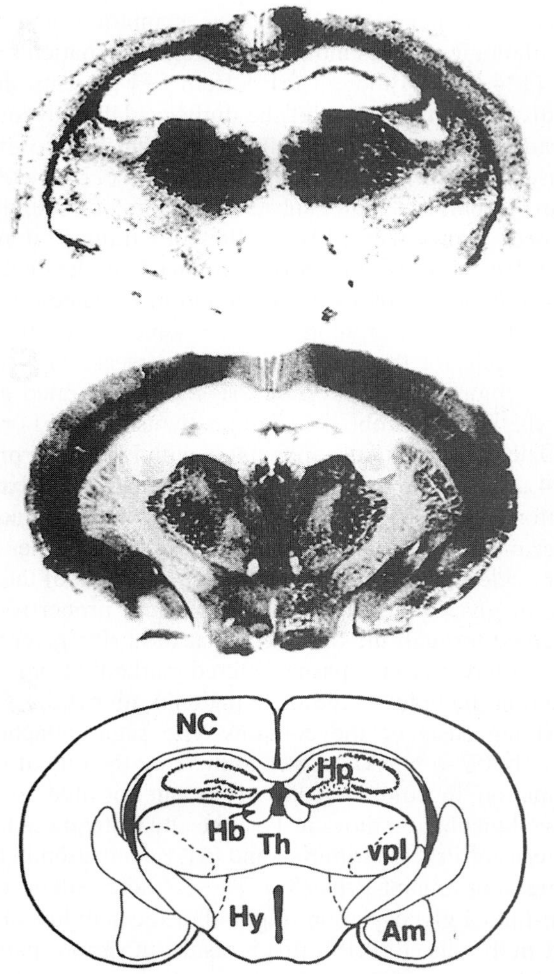

FIG. 6. Regional distribution of PrP^{Sc} deposition in Tg(MHu2M)*Prnp$^{0/0}$* mice inoculated with prions from humans who died of inherited prion diseases. Histoblot of PrP^{Sc} deposition in a coronal section of a Tg(MHu2M)*Prnp$^{0/0}$* mouse through the hippocampus and thalamus (198). **A:** The Tg mouse was inoculated with brain extract prepared from a patient who died of familial fatal insomnia (FFI). **B:** The Tg mouse was inoculated with extract from a patient with fCJD(E200K). Cryostat sections were mounted on nitrocellulose and treated with proteinase K to eliminate PrP^{C} (193). To enhance the antigenicity of PrP^{Sc}, the histoblots were exposed to 3-guanidinium isothiocyanate before immunostaining using α-PrP 3F4 monoclonal antibody (98). **C:** Labelled diagram of a coronal section of the hippocampus/thalamus region. NC, neocortex; Hp, hippocampus; Hb, habenula; Th, thalamus; vpl, ventral posterior lateral thalamic nucleus; Hy, hypothalamus; Am, amygdala.

FUNGAL PRIONS

Although prions were originally defined in the context of an infectious mammalian pathogen (151), it is now becoming widely accepted that prions are elements that impart and propagate variability through multiple conformers of a normal cellular protein. Such a mechanism must surely not be restricted to a single class of transmissible pathogens. Indeed, it is likely that the original definition will need to be extended to encompass other situations in which a similar mechanism of information transfer occurs.

Two notable prion-like determinants, [URE3] and [PSI], have already been described in yeast, and one in another fungus denoted [Het-s*] has been reported (36,47,210). Studies of candidate PrPs in yeast may prove particularly helpful in the dissection of some of the events that feature in PrP^{Sc} formation. Interestingly, different strains of yeast prions have been identified (52). Conversion to the prion-like [PSI] state in yeast requires the molecular chaperone Hsp104; however, no homolog of Hsp104 has been found in mammals (36). The NH_2-terminal prion domains of Ure2p and Sup35 that are responsible for the [URE3] and [PSI] phenotypes in yeast have been identified. In contrast to PrP, which is a GPI-anchored membrane protein, both Ure2p and Sup35 are cytosolic proteins (211). When the prion domains of these yeast proteins were expressed in *Escherichia coli*, the proteins were found to polymerize into fibrils with properties similar to those of proteolytically trimmed PrP and other amyloids (83,145).

Whether prions explain some other examples of acquired inheritance in lower organisms is unclear (109). For example, studies on the inheritance of positional order and cellular handedness on the surface of small organisms have demonstrated the epigenetic nature of these phenomena, but the mechanism remains unclear (58).

THERAPEUTIC APPROACHES TO PRION DISEASES

It seems likely that it will be possible to design effective therapeutics for prion diseases as our understanding of prion propagation increases. Because people at risk for inherited prion diseases can now be identified decades before neurologic dysfunction is evident, the development of an effective therapy for these fully penetrant disorders is imperative. Although we have no way of predicting the number of individuals who may develop neurologic dysfunction from bovine prions in the future, seeking an effective therapy now seems most prudent (155). Interfering with the conversion of PrP^C to PrP^{Sc} seems to be the most attractive therapeutic target. Both stabilizing the structure of PrP^C via the formation of a PrP^C-drug complex, and modifying the action of protein X, which might function as a molecular chaperone (see Fig. 3B), are reasonable strategies. Whether it is more efficacious to design a drug that binds to PrP^C at the protein X binding site or one that mimics the structure of PrP^C with basic polymorphic residues that seem to prevent scrapie and CJD remains to be determined (96,181). As PrP^{Sc} formation seems limited to caveolae-like domains (71,195), drugs designed to inhibit this process need not penetrate the cytosol of cells, but they do need to be able to enter the CNS. Alternatively, drugs that destabilize the structure of PrP^{Sc} might also prove useful.

The production of domestic animals that do not replicate prions may also be important with respect to preventing prion disease. Sheep encoding the R/R polymorphism at position 171 seem to be resistant to scrapie (90,209); presumably, this was the genetic basis of James Parry's scrapie eradication program in Great Britain 30 years ago (141). A more effective approach, using dominant negatives for producing prion-resistant domestic animals, including sheep and cattle, is probably the expression of PrP transgenes encoding R171 or basic residues at the protein X binding site (see Fig. 3B) (96). Such an approach can be readily evaluated in Tg mice and, once shown to be effective, could be instituted by artificial insemination of sperm from males homozygous for the transgene. Less practical is the production of PrP-deficient cattle and sheep. Although such animals would not be susceptible to prion disease (23,157), they might suffer some deleterious effects from ablation of the PrP gene (44,116,172,201).

Whether gene therapy for the human prion diseases will prove feasible using the dominant negative approach described earlier for prion-resistant animals depends on the availability of efficient vectors for delivery of the transgene to the CNS.

CONCLUDING REMARKS

Although the study of prions has taken several unexpected directions over the past three decades, a novel and fascinating story of prion biology is emerging. Investigations of prions have elucidated a previously unknown mechanism of disease in humans and animals. Although learning the details of the structures of PrPs and deciphering the mechanism of PrP^C transformation into PrP^{Sc} will be important, the fundamental principles of prion biology have become reasonably clear. Although some investigators prefer to view the composition of the infectious prion particle as unresolved (37,112,119), such a perspective denies an enlarging body of data, none of which refutes the prion concept. Moreover, the discovery of prion-like phenomena mediated by proteins unrelated to PrP in yeast and other fungi serves not only to strengthen the prion concept but also to widen it.

The discovery that prion diseases in humans are uniquely both genetic and infectious greatly extended the prion concept. To date, 20 different mutations in the human PrP gene, all resulting in nonconservative substitutions, have been found either to be genetically linked to or to segregate with the inherited prion diseases (see Fig. 2B). Yet, the transmissible prion particle is composed largely, if not exclusively, of an abnormal isoform of the PrP designated PrP^{Sc} (153).

Aberrant PrP Metabolism

The hallmark of all prion diseases—whether sporadic, dominantly inherited, or acquired by infection—is that they involve the aberrant metabolism and resulting accumulation of the PrP (see Table 3) (153). The conversion of PrP^C into PrP^{Sc} involves a conformation change whereby the α-helical content diminishes and the amount of β-sheet increases (139). These findings provide a reasonable mechanism to explain the conundrum presented by the three different manifestations of prion disease.

Understanding how PrP^C unfolds and refolds into PrP^{Sc} will be of paramount importance in transferring advances in the prion diseases to studies of other degenerative illnesses. The mechanism by which PrP^{Sc} is formed must involve a templating process whereby existing PrP^{Sc} directs the refolding of PrP^C into a nascent PrP^{Sc} with the same conformation. Not only will knowledge of PrP^{Sc} formation help in the rational design of drugs that interrupt the pathogenesis of prion diseases, but it may also open new approaches to deciphering the causes of and to developing effective therapies for the more common neurodegenerative diseases, including Alzheimer's disease, Parkinson's disease, and amyotrophic lateral sclerosis (ALS). Indeed, the expanding list of prion diseases and their novel modes of transmission and pathogenesis (Table 3), as well as the unprecedented mechanisms of prion propagation and information transfer, indicate that much more attention to these fatal disorders of protein conformation is urgently needed.

Over the past two decades, advances in our understanding of the prion diseases have helped refine our definition of neurodegenerative diseases. In addition to the more common neurodegenerative diseases just men-

TABLE 7. *Neurodegenerative diseases*

Neurodegenerative disease	CNS protein deposits	Mutant genes in familial disorders
Prion diseases	PrP^{Sc}, PrP amyloid plaques	PrP
Alzheimer's disease (AD)	Aβ, Aβ amyloid plaques Tau, neurofibrillary tangles	APP, PS1, PS2, ApoE[a]
Parkinson's disease	α-Synuclein, Lewy bodies	α-Synuclein, Parkin
Amyotrophic lateral sclerosis (ALS)		Superoxide dismutase
Frontotemporal dementia (FTD)	Tau, fibrils and pickbodies	Tau
Huntington's disease (HD)	HD, nuclear HD aggregates	HD

[a]ApoE genotype modulates the age of onset of both familial and sporadic AD.

tioned, there are less prevalent maladies, including frontotemporal dementia, Huntington's disease, and the prion diseases (Table 7). With the exception of Huntington's disease, a minority of all of these neurodegenerative disorders exhibit an autosomal dominant pattern of inheritance, and the majority are sporadic. In all of these illnesses, including Huntington's disease, the onset of CNS dysfunction is usually seen in adults and the neurologic deterioration is progressive.

Abnormal protein deposits are found in all these diseases and the pathogenic process seems to evade immune surveillance. In Alzheimer's disease and the prion diseases, amyloid plaques are found, but the proteins in these plaques are different (68,122,158). In Alzheimer's disease, the plaques contain a peptide called Aβ, which is derived from a large protein designated the amyloid precursor protein, or APP (97). In the prion diseases, the plaques are a nonobligatory feature of the illness (159); the plaques contain substantial amounts of PrP fragments (48,158,192). Mutations in the genes encoding these proteins are found in inherited forms of the disease (69,84). In familial Alzheimer's disease, mutations in the presenilin genes have also been implicated and are thought by some investigators to operate by modifying the processing of APP into Aβ (14,164,180,214).

The time of onset of the prion diseases in experimental animals is determined by the level of PrP^C expression, the sequence of PrP, and the strain of prions (53,159,207). In Alzheimer's disease, the haplotype of apolipoprotein E (ApoE) greatly influences the age of onset of both the familial and sporadic forms of the illness (174). In Huntington's disease, the age of onset is governed by the size of the triplet repeat expansion encoding the polyglutamine segment (100).

Protein aggregates in the nuclei of some neurons can be observed in Huntington's disease (173,175), whereas in Parkinson's disease, intraneuronal inclusions called Lewy bodies are often found (186). Similarly, mutations in the genes encoding these proteins are found in inherited forms of the disease (73,149). In the inherited frontotemporal dementias and Pick's disease, mutations in the tau gene are the cause (91). In all of these diseases, astrocytic gliosis is seen. In some of these diseases, vacuolation in the neuropil is seen, but the most prominent vacuolation can be seen in the prion diseases where vacuoles may coalesce to create spongiform change. The degree of spongiform change is quite variable, whereas the extent of reactive gliosis correlates with the degree of neuron loss in CJD (121).

But prions may have even wider implications than those noted for the common neurodegenerative diseases. If we think of prion diseases as disorders of protein conformation and do not require the diseases to be transmissible, then what we have learned from the study of prions may reach far beyond these common illnesses.

Conformational Diversity

The discovery that proteins may have multiple biologically active conformations may prove no less important than the implications of prions for diseases. How many different tertiary structures can PrP^{Sc} adopt? This query not only addresses the issue of the limits of prion diversity but also applies to proteins as they normally function within the cell or act to affect homeostasis in multicellular organisms. The expanding list of chaperones that assist in the folding and unfolding of proteins promises much new knowledge about this process. For example, it is now clear that pro-proteases can carry their own chaperone activity where the *pro* portion of the protein functions as a chaperone in cis to guide the folding of the proteolytically active portion before it is cleaved (182). Such a mechanism might well feature in the maturation of polypeptide hormones. Interestingly, mutation of the chaperone portion of prosubtilisin resulted in the folding of a subtilisin protease with different properties from the one folded by the wild-type chaperone. Such chaperones have also been shown to work in trans (182). Besides transient metabolic regulation within the cell and hormonal regulation of multicellular organisms, it is not unreasonable to suggest that assembly of proteins into multimeric structures such as intermediate filaments might be controlled, at least in part, by alternative conformations of proteins. Such regulation of multimeric protein assemblies might occur either in the proteins that form the multimers or in the proteins that function to facilitate the assembly process. Additionally, apoptosis during development and throughout adult life might also be regulated, at least in part, by alternative tertiary structures of proteins.

Future Studies

The wealth of data establishing the essential role of PrP in the transmission of prions and the pathogenesis of prion diseases has provoked consideration of how many biologic processes are controlled by changes in protein conformation. The extreme radiation resistance of the scrapie infectivity suggested that the pathogen causing this disease and related illnesses would be different from viruses, viroids, and bacteria (1). Indeed, an unprecedented mechanism of disease has been revealed whereby an aberrant conformational change in a protein is propagated. The future of this emerging area of biology should prove even more interesting and productive as many new discoveries emerge.

REFERENCES

1. Alper T, Cramp WA, Haig DA, Clarke MC. Does the agent of scrapie replicate without nucleic acid? *Nature* 1967;214:764–766.
2. Alper T, Haig DA, Clarke MC. The exceptionally small size of the scrapie agent. *Biochem Biophys Res Commun* 1966;22:278–284.
3. Alpers M. Epidemiology and clinical aspects of kuru. In: Prusiner SB, McKinley MP, eds. *Prions—Novel Infectious Pathogens Causing Scrapie and Creutzfeldt-Jakob Disease.* Orlando: Academic Press, 1987:451–465.
4. Alpers MP. Kuru: Implications of its transmissibility for the interpretation of its changing epidemiological pattern. In: Bailey OT, Smith DE, eds. *The Central Nervous System: Some Experimental Models of Neurological Diseases.* Baltimore: Williams & Wilkins, 1968:234–251.
5. Anfinsen CB. Principles that govern the folding of protein chains. *Science* 1973;181:223–230.
6. Anfinsen CB, Haber E, Sela M, White FH. The kinetics of formation of native ribonuclease during oxidation of the reduced polypeptide chain. *Proc Natl Acad Sci U S A* 1961;47:1309–1313.
7. Baker HF, Ridley RM, Wells GAH. Experimental transmission of BSE and scrapie to the common marmoset. *Vet Rec* 1993;132:403–406.
8. Basler K, Oesch B, Scott M, et al. Scrapie and cellular PrP isoforms are encoded by the same chromosomal gene. *Cell* 1986;46:417–428.
9. Bateman D, Hilton D, Love S, et al. Sporadic Creutzfeldt-Jakob disease in a 18-year-old in the UK [Letter]. *Lancet* 1995;346:1155–1156.
10. Bellinger-Kawahara CG, Kempner E, Groth DF, et al. Scrapie prion liposomes and rods exhibit target sizes of 55,000 Da. *Virology* 1988; 164:537–541.
11. Bessen RA, Marsh RF. Biochemical and physical properties of the prion protein from two strains of the transmissible mink encephalopathy agent. *J Virol* 1992;66:2096–2101.
12. Bessen RA, Marsh RF. Distinct PrP properties suggest the molecular basis of strain variation in transmissible mink encephalopathy. *J Virol* 1994;68:7859–7868.
13. Billette de Villemeur T, Deslys J-P, Pradel A, et al. Creutzfeldt-Jakob disease from contaminated growth hormone extracts in France. *Neurology* 1996;47:690–695.
14. Borchelt DR, Ratovitski T, van Lare J, et al. Accelerated amyloid deposition in the brains of transgenic mice coexpressing mutant presenilin 1 and amyloid precursor proteins. *Neuron* 1997;19:939–945.
15. Borchelt DR, Scott M, Taraboulos A, et al. Scrapie and cellular prion proteins differ in their kinetics of synthesis and topology in cultured cells. *J Cell Biol* 1990;110:743–752.
16. Britton TC, Al-Sarraj S, Shaw C, et al. Sporadic Creutzfeldt-Jakob disease in a 16-year-old in the UK [Letter]. *Lancet* 1995;346:1155.
17. Brown DR, Qin K, Herms JW, et al. The cellular prion protein binds copper *in vivo. Nature* 1997;390:684–687.
18. Brown DR, Schulz-Schaeffer WJ, Schmidt B, Kretzschmar HA. Prion protein-deficient cells show altered response to oxidative stress due to decreased SOD-1 activity. *Exp Neurol* 1997;146:104–112.
19. Brown P, Cathala F, Raubertas RF, et al. The epidemiology of Creutzfeldt-Jakob disease: Conclusion of a 15-year investigation in France and review of the world literature. *Neurology* 1987;37: 895–904.
20. Brown P, Preece MA, Will RG. "Friendly fire" in medicine: Hormones, homografts, and Creutzfeldt-Jakob disease. *Lancet* 1992;340:24–27.
21. Bruce ME, McBride PA, Farquhar CF. Precise targeting of the pathology of the sialoglycoprotein, PrP, and vacuolar degeneration in mouse scrapie. *Neurosci Lett* 1989;102:1–6.
22. Bruce ME, Will RG, Ironside JW, et al. Transmissions to mice indicate that "new variant" CJD is caused by the BSE agent. *Nature* 1997;389: 498–501.
23. Büeler H, Aguzzi A, Sailer A, et al. Mice devoid of PrP are resistant to scrapie. *Cell* 1993;73:1339–1347.
24. Büeler H, Fischer M, Lang Y, et al. Normal development and behaviour of mice lacking the neuronal cell-surface PrP protein. *Nature* 1992;356:577–582.
25. Büeler H, Raeber A, Sailer A, et al. High prion and PrP^{Sc} levels but delayed onset of disease in scrapie-inoculated mice heterozygous for a disrupted PrP gene. *Mol Med* 1994;1:19–30.
26. Bull PC, Thomas GR, Rommens JM, et al. The Wilson disease gene is a putative copper transporting P-type ATPase similar to the Menkes gene. *Nat Genet* 1993;5:327–337.
27. Carlson GA, Ebeling C, Yang S-L, et al. Prion isolate specified allotypic interactions between the cellular and scrapie prion proteins in congenic and transgenic mice. *Proc Natl Acad Sci U S A* 1994;91: 5690–5694.
28. Carlson GA, Kingsbury DT, Goodman PA, et al. Linkage of prion protein and scrapie incubation time genes. *Cell* 1986;46:503–511.
29. Carp RI, Meeker H, Sersen E. Scrapie strains retain their distinctive characteristics following passages of homogenates from different brain regions and spleen. *J Gen Virol* 1997;78:283–290.
30. Caughey B, Kocisko DA, Raymond GJ, Lansbury PT Jr. Aggregates of scrapie-associated prion protein induce the cell-free conversion of protease-sensitive prion protein to the protease-resistant state. *Chem Biol* 1995;2:807–817.
31. Caughey B, Raymond GJ. The scrapie-associated form of PrP is made from a cell surface precursor that is both protease- and phospholipase-sensitive. *J Biol Chem* 1991;266:18217–18223.
32. Centers for Disease Control. Surveillance for Creutzfeldt-Jakob Disease—United States. *MMWR Morb Mortal Wkly Rep* 1996;45:665–668.
33. Centers for Disease Control. Creutzfeldt-Jakob disease associated with cadaveric dura mater grafts—Japan, January 1979–May 1996. *MMWR Morb Mortal Wkly Rep* 1997;46:1066–1069.
34. Chazot G, Broussolle E, Lapras CI, et al. New variant of Creutzfeldt-Jakob disease in a 26-year-old French man. *Lancet* 1996;347:1181.
35. Chelly J, Tümer Z, Tønnesen T, et al. Isolation of a candidate gene for Menkes disease that encodes a potential heavy metal binding protein. *Nat Genet* 1993;3:14–19.
36. Chernoff YO, Lindquist SL, Ono B, et al. Role of the chaperone protein Hsp104 in propagation of the yeast prion-like factor [psi+]. *Science* 1995;268:880–884.
37. Chesebro B. Prion diseases: BSE and prions: Uncertainties about the agent. *Science* 1998;279:42–43.
38. Chesebro B, Caughey B. Scrapie agent replication without the prion protein? *Curr Biol* 1993;3:696–698.
39. Chesebro B, Race R, Wehrly K, et al. Identification of scrapie prion protein-specific mRNA in scrapie-infected and uninfected brain. *Nature* 1985;315:331–333.
40. Chiesa R, Piccardo P, Ghetti B, Harris DA. Neurological illness in transgenic mice expressing a prion protein with an insertional mutation. *Neuron* 1998;21:1339–1351.
41. Cohen FE, Pan K-M, Huang Z, et al. Structural clues to prion replication. *Science* 1994;264:530–531.
42. Cohen FE, Prusiner SB. Pathologic conformations of prion proteins. *Annu Rev Biochem* 1998;67:793–819.
43. Collinge J, Sidle KCL, Meads J, et al. Molecular analysis of prion strain variation and the aetiology of "new variant" CJD. *Nature* 1996; 383:685–690.
44. Collinge J, Whittington MA, Sidle KC, et al. Prion protein is necessary for normal synaptic function. *Nature* 1994;370:295–297.
45. Cousens SN, Harries-Jones R, Knight R, et al. Geographical distribu-

tion of cases of Creutzfeldt-Jakob disease in England and Wales 1970–84. *J Neurol Neurosurg Psychiatry* 1990;53:459–465.
46. Cousens SN, Vynnycky E, Zeidler M, et al. Predicting the CJD epidemic in humans. *Nature* 1997;385:197–198.
47. Coustou V, Deleu C, Saupe S, Begueret J. The protein product of the het-s heterokaryon incompatibility gene of the fungus *Podospora anserina* behaves as a prion analog. *Proc Natl Acad Sci U S A* 1997; 94:9773–9778.
48. DeArmond SJ, McKinley MP, Barry RA, et al. Identification of prion amyloid filaments in scrapie-infected brain. *Cell* 1985;41:221–235.
49. DeArmond SJ, Mobley WC, DeMott DL, et al. Changes in the localization of brain prion proteins during scrapie infection. *Neurology* 1987;37:1271–1280.
50. DeArmond SJ, Prusiner SB. Prion diseases. In: Lantos P, Graham D, eds. *Greenfield's Neuropathology*, 6th ed. London: Edward Arnold, 1997:235–280.
51. DeArmond SJ, Sánchez H, Yehiely F, et al. Selective neuronal targeting in prion disease. *Neuron* 1997;19:1337–1348.
52. Derkatch IL, Chernoff YO, Kushnirov VV, et al. Genesis and variability of [PSI] prion factors in *Saccharomyces cerevisiae. Genetics* 1996; 144:1375–1386.
53. Dickinson AG, Meikle VMH, Fraser H. Identification of a gene which controls the incubation period of some strains of scrapie agent in mice. *J Comp Pathol* 1968;78:293–299.
54. Donne DG, Viles JH, Groth D, et al. Structure of the recombinant full-length hamster prion protein PrP(29–231): The N terminus is highly flexible. *Proc Natl Acad Sci U S A* 1997;94:13452–13457.
55. Endo T, Groth D, Prusiner SB, Kobata A. Diversity of oligosaccharide structures linked to asparagines of the scrapie prion protein. *Biochemistry* 1989;28:8380–8388.
56. Esmonde T, Lueck CJ, Symon L, et al. Creutzfeldt-Jakob disease and lyophilised dura mater grafts: Report of two cases. *J Neurol Neurosurg Psychiatry* 1993;56:999–1000.
57. Fischer M, Rülicke T, Raeber A, et al. Prion protein (PrP) with amino-proximal deletions restoring susceptibility of PrP knockout mice to scrapie. *EMBO J* 1996;15:1255–1264.
58. Frankel J. Positional order and cellular handedness. *J Cell Sci* 1990; 97:205–211.
59. Fraser H, Dickinson AG. The sequential development of the brain lesions of scrapie in three strains of mice. *J Comp Pathol* 1968;78: 301–311.
60. Gabizon R, McKinley MP, Groth D, Prusiner SB. Immunoaffinity purification and neutralization of scrapie prion infectivity. *Proc Natl Acad Sci U S A* 1988;85:6617–6621.
61. Gabizon R, Rosenmann H, Meiner Z, et al. Mutation and polymorphism of the prion protein gene in Libyan Jews with Creutzfeldt-Jakob disease (CJD). *Am J Hum Genet* 1993;53:828–835.
62. Gabizon R, Telling G, Meiner Z, et al. Insoluble wild-type and protease-resistant mutant prion protein in brains of patients with inherited prion disease. *Nat Med* 1996;2:59–64.
63. Gajdusek DC. Unconventional viruses and the origin and disappearance of kuru. *Science* 1977;197:943–960.
64. Gajdusek DC. Transmissible and non-transmissible amyloidoses: Autocatalytic post-translational conversion of host precursor proteins to β-pleated sheet configurations. *J Neuroimmunol* 1988;20:95–110.
65. Gajdusek DC, Gibbs CJ Jr, Asher DM, et al. Precautions in medical care of, and in handling materials from, patients with transmissible virus dementia (Creutzfeldt-Jakob disease). *N Engl J Med* 1977;297: 1253–1258.
66. Gambetti P, Parchi P. Insomnia in prion diseases: Sporadic and familial. *N Engl J Med* 1999;340:1675–1677.
67. Gibbs CJ Jr, Gajdusek DC, Asher DM, et al. Creutzfeldt-Jakob disease (spongiform encephalopathy): Transmission to the chimpanzee. *Science* 1968;161:388–389.
68. Glenner GG, Wong CW. Alzheimer's disease: Initial report of the purification and characterization of a novel cerebrovascular amyloid protein. *Biochem Biophys Res Commun* 1984;120:885–890.
69. Goate A, Chartier-Harlin M-C, Mullan M, et al. Segregation of a missense mutation in the amyloid precursor protein gene with familial Alzheimer's disease. *Nature* 1991;349:704–706.
70. Goldfarb L, Korczyn A, Brown P, et al. Mutation in codon 200 of scrapie amyloid precursor gene linked to Creutzfeldt-Jakob disease in Sephardic Jews of Libyan and non-Libyan origin. *Lancet* 1990;336: 637–638.
71. Gorodinsky A, Harris DA. Glycolipid-anchored proteins in neuroblastoma cells form detergent-resistant complexes without caveolin. *J Cell Biol* 1995;129:619–627.
72. Griffith JS. Self-replication and scrapie. *Nature* 1967;215:1043–1044.
73. Group THsDCR. A novel gene containing a trinucleotide repeat that is expanded and unstable on Huntington's disease chromosomes. *Cell* 1993;72:971–983.
74. Harries-Jones R, Knight R, Will RG, et al. Creutzfeldt-Jakob disease in England and Wales, 1980–1984: A case-control study of potential risk factors. *J Neurol Neurosurg Psychiatry* 1988;51:1113–1119.
75. Harris ED. Copper as a cofactor and regulator of copper, zinc superoxide dismutase. *J Nutr* 1992;122:636–640.
76. Hegde RS, Mastrianni JA, Scott MR, et al. A transmembrane form of the prion protein in neurodegenerative disease. *Science* 1998;279: 827–834.
77. Henikoff S, Greene EA, Pietrokovski S, et al. Gene families: The taxonomy of protein paralogs and chimeras. *Science* 1997;278:609–614.
78. Herms JW, Kretzschmar HA, Titz S, Keller BU. Patch-clamp analysis of synaptic transmission to cerebellar purkinje cells of prion protein knockout mice. *Eur J Neurosci* 1995;7:2508–2512.
79. Hill AF, Butterworth RJ, Joiner S, et al. Investigation of variant Creutzfeldt-Jakob disease and other human prion diseases with tonsil biopsy samples. *Lancet* 1999;353:183–189.
80. Hill AF, Desbruslais M, Joiner S, et al. The same prion strain causes vCJD and BSE. *Nature* 1997;389:448–450.
81. Hornshaw MP, McDermott JR, Candy JM. Copper binding to the N-terminal tandem repeat regions of mammalian and avian prion protein. *Biochem Biophys Res Commun* 1995;207:621–629.
82. Hornshaw MP, McDermott JR, Candy JM, Lakey JH. Copper binding to the N-terminal tandem repeat region of mammalian and avian prion protein: Structural studies using synthetic peptides. *Biochem Biophys Res Commun* 1995;214:993–999.
83. Horwich AL, Weissman JS. Deadly conformations—Protein misfolding in prion disease. *Cell* 1997;89:499–510.
84. Hsiao K, Baker HF, Crow TJ, et al. Linkage of a prion protein missense variant to Gerstmann-Sträussler syndrome. *Nature* 1989;338: 342–345.
85. Hsiao K, Meiner Z, Kahana E, et al. Mutation of the prion protein in Libyan Jews with Creutzfeldt-Jakob disease. *N Engl J Med* 1991;324: 1091–1097.
86. Hsiao KK, Groth D, Scott M, et al. Serial transmission in rodents of neurodegeneration from transgenic mice expressing mutant prion protein. *Proc Natl Acad Sci U S A* 1994;91:9126–9130.
87. Hsiao KK, Scott M, Foster D, et al. Spontaneous neurodegeneration in transgenic mice with mutant prion protein. *Science* 1990;250: 1587–1590.
88. Huang Z, Gabriel J-M, Baldwin MA, et al. Proposed three-dimensional structure for the cellular prion protein. *Proc Natl Acad Sci U S A* 1994;91:7139–7143.
89. Huang Z, Prusiner SB, Cohen FE. Scrapie prions: A three-dimensional model of an infectious fragment. *Folding Design* 1995;1:13–19.
90. Hunter N, Goldmann W, Benson G, et al. Swaledale sheep affected by natural scrapie differ significantly in PrP genotype frequencies from healthy sheep and those selected for reduced incidence of scrapie. *J Gen Virol* 1993;74:1025–1031.
91. Hutton M, Lendon CL, Rizzu P, et al. Association of missense and 5′-splice-site mutations in tau with the inherited dementia FTDP-17. *Nature* 1998;393:702–705.
92. Ironside JW. The new variant form of Creutzfeldt-Jakob disease: A novel prion protein amyloid disorder [Editorial]. *Int J Exp Clin Invest* 1997;4:66–69.
93. James TL, Liu H, Ulyanov NB, et al. Solution structure of a 142-residue recombinant prion protein corresponding to the infectious fragment of the scrapie isoform. *Proc Natl Acad Sci U S A* 1997;94: 10086–10091.
94. Kahana E, Milton A, Braham J, Sofer D. Creutzfeldt-Jakob disease: Focus among Libyan Jews in Israel. *Science* 1974;183:90–91.
95. Kaneko K, Wille H, Mehlhorn I, et al. Molecular properties of complexes formed between the prion protein and synthetic peptides. *J Mol Biol* 1997;270:574–586.
96. Kaneko K, Zulianello L, Scott M, et al. Evidence for protein X binding to a discontinuous epitope on the cellular prion protein during scrapie prion propagation. *Proc Natl Acad Sci U S A* 1997;94:10069–10074.
96a. Kaneko K, Ball H, Wille H, et al. A synthetic peptide initiates "Gerst-

mann-Sträussler-Scheinker (G55) disease in transgenic mice. *J Mol Biol* 2000;295:997–1007.
97. Kang J, Lemaire H-G, Unterbeck A, et al. The precursor of Alzheimer's disease amyloid A4 protein resembles a cell-surface receptor. *Nature* 1987;325:733–736.
98. Kascsak RJ, Rubenstein R, Merz PA, et al. Mouse polyclonal and monoclonal antibody to scrapie-associated fibril proteins. *J Virol* 1987;61:3688–3693.
99. Kenward N, Hope J, Landon M, Mayer RJ. Expression of polyubiquitin and heat-shock protein 70 genes increases in the later stages of disease progression in scrapie-infected mouse brain. *J Neurochem* 1994;62:1870–1877.
100. Kieburtz K, MacDonald M, Shih C, et al. Trinucleotide repeat length and progression of illness in Huntington's disease. *J Med Genet* 1994; 31:872–874.
101. Kimberlin RH, Millson GC, Bountiff L, Collis SC. A comparison of the biochemical changes induced in mouse brain by cuprizone toxicity and by scrapie infection. *J Comp Pathol* 1974;84:263–270.
102. Kirschbaum WR. *Jakob-Creutzfeldt Disease.* Amsterdam: Elsevier, 1968.
103. Klatzo I, Gajdusek DC, Zigas V. Pathology of kuru. *Lab Invest* 1959; 8:799–847.
104. Klitzman RL, Alpers MP, Gajdusek DC. The natural incubation period of kuru and the episodes of transmission in three clusters of patients. *Neuroepidemiology* 1984;3:3–20.
105. Koch TK, Berg BO, DeArmond SJ, Gravina RF. Creutzfeldt-Jakob disease in a young adult with idiopathic hypopituitarism. Possible relation to the administration of cadaveric human growth hormone. *N Engl J Med* 1985;313:731–733.
106. Kocisko DA, Come JH, Priola SA, et al. Cell-free formation of protease-resistant prion protein. *Nature* 1994;370:471–474.
107. Korth C, Stierli B, Streit P, et al. Prion (PrP^{Sc})-specific epitope defined by a monoclonal antibody. *Nature* 1997;389:74–77.
108. Kurschner C, Morgan JI. Analysis of interaction sites in homo- and heteromeric complexes containing Bcl-2 family members and the cellular prion protein. *Mol Brain Res* 1996;37:249–258.
109. Landman OE. The inheritance of acquired characteristics. *Annu Rev Genet* 1991;25:1–20.
110. Lane KL, Brown P, Howell DN, et al. Creutzfeldt-Jakob disease in a pregnant woman with an implanted dura mater graft. *Neurosurgery* 1994;34:737–740.
111. Lasmézas CI, Deslys J-P, Demaimay R, et al. BSE transmission to macaques. *Nature* 1996;381:743–744.
112. Lasmézas CI, Deslys J-P, Robain O, et al. Transmission of the BSE agent to mice in the absence of detectable abnormal prion protein. *Science* 1997;275:402–405.
113. Lee IY, Westaway D, Smit AFA, et al. Complete genomic sequence and analysis of the prion protein gene region from three mammalian species. *Genome Res* 1998;8:1022–1037.
114. Lehmann S, Harris DA. Two mutant prion proteins expressed in cultured cells acquire biochemical properties reminiscent of the scrapie isoform. *Proc Natl Acad Sci U S A* 1996;93:5610–5614.
115. Liu H, Farr-Jones S, Ulyanov NB, et al. Solution structure of Syrian hamster prion protein rPrP(90-231). *Biochemistry* 1999;38: 5362–5377.
116. Lledo P-M, Tremblay P, DeArmond SJ, et al. Mice deficient for prion protein exhibit normal neuronal excitability and synaptic transmission in the hippocampus. *Proc Natl Acad Sci U S A* 1996; 93:2403–2407.
117. Malmgren R, Kurland L, Mokri B, Kurtzke J. The epidemiology of Creutzfeldt-Jakob disease. In: Prusiner SB, Hadlow WJ, eds. *Slow Transmissible Diseases of the Nervous System*, vol. 1. New York: Academic Press, 1979:93–112.
118. Manson JC, Clarke AR, Hooper ML, et al. 129/Ola mice carrying a null mutation in PrP that abolishes mRNA production are developmentally normal. *Mol Neurobiol* 1994;8:121–127.
119. Manuelidis L, Fritch W. Infectivity and host responses in Creutzfeldt-Jakob disease. *Virology* 1996;216:46–59.
120. Masters CL, Gajdusek DC, Gibbs CJ Jr. Creutzfeldt-Jakob disease virus isolations from the Gerstmann-Sträussler syndrome. *Brain* 1981; 104:559–588.
121. Masters CL, Richardson EP Jr. Subacute spongiform encephalopathy Creutzfeldt-Jakob disease—The nature and progression of spongiform change. *Brain* 1978;101:333–344.
122. Masters CL, Simms G, Weinman NA, et al. Amyloid plaque core protein in Alzheimer disease and Down syndrome. *Proc Natl Acad Sci U S A* 1985;82:4245–4249.
123. Mastrianni J, Nixon F, Layzer R, et al. Fatal sporadic insomnia: Fatal familial insomnia phenotype without a mutation of the prion protein gene. *Neurology* 1997;48(suppl):A296.
124. Mastrianni JA, Nixon R, Layzer R, et al. Prion protein conformation in a patient with sporadic fatal insomnia. *N Engl J Med* 1999;340: 1630–1638.
125. McKenzie D, Bartz J, Mirwald J, et al. Reversibility of scrapie inactivation is enhanced by copper. *J Biol Chem* 1998;273:25545–25547.
126. Medori R, Tritschler H-J, LeBlanc A, et al. Fatal familial insomnia, a prion disease with a mutation at codon 178 of the prion protein gene. *N Engl J Med* 1992;326:444–449.
127. Meggendorfer F. Klinische und genealogische Beobachtungen bei einem Fall von spastischer Pseudosklerose Jakobs. *Z Gesamte Neurol Psychiatr* 1930;128:337–341.
128. Miura T, Hori-i A, Takeuchi H. Metal-dependent α-helix formation promoted by the glycine-rich octapeptide region of prion protein. *FEBS Lett* 1996;396:248–252.
129. Monari L, Chen SG, Brown P, et al. Fatal familial insomnia and familial Creutzfeldt-Jakob disease: Different prion proteins determined by a DNA polymorphism. *Proc Natl Acad Sci U S A* 1994;91:2839–2842.
130. Moore R. Gene targeting studies at the mouse prion protein locus. Dissertation, University of Edinburgh, 1997.
131. Moore RC, Hope J, McBride PA, et al. Mice with gene targetted prion protein alterations show that *Prn-p*, *Sinc* and *Prni* are congruent. *Nat Genet* 1998;18:118–125.
132. Moore RC, Lee IY, Silverman GL, et al. Ataxia in prion protein (PrP) deficient mice is associated with upregulation of the novel PrP-like protein doppel. *J Mol Biol* 1999;292:797–817.
133. Muramoto T, DeArmond SJ, Scott M, et al. Heritable disorder resembling neuronal storage disease in mice expressing prion protein with deletion of an α-helix. *Nat Med* 1997;3:750–755.
134. Muramoto T, Scott M, Cohen FE, Prusiner SB. Recombinant scrapie-like prion protein of 106 amino acids is soluble. *Proc Natl Acad Sci U S A* 1996;93:15457–15462.
135. Nishida N, Tremblay P, Sugimoto T, et al. A mouse prion protein transgene rescues mice deficient for the prion protein gene from purkinje cell degeneration and demyelination. *Lab Invest* 1999;79:689–697.
136. Oesch B, Teplow DB, Stahl N, et al. Identification of cellular proteins binding to the scrapie prion protein. *Biochemistry* 1990;29:5848–5855.
137. Oesch B, Westaway D, Wälchli M, et al. A cellular gene encodes scrapie PrP 27-30 protein. *Cell* 1985;40:735–746.
138. Owen F, Poulter M, Lofthouse R, et al. Insertion in prion protein gene in familial Creutzfeldt-Jakob disease. *Lancet* 1989;1:51–52.
139. Pan K-M, Baldwin M, Nguyen J, et al. Conversion of α-helices into β-sheets features in the formation of the scrapie prion proteins. *Proc Natl Acad Sci U S A* 1993;90:10962–10966.
140. Parchi P, Capellari S, Chin S, et al. A subtype of sporadic prion disease mimicking fatal familial insomnia. *Neurology* 1999;52:1757–1763.
141. Parry HB. Scrapie: A transmissible and hereditary disease of sheep. *Heredity* 1962;17:75–105.
142. Pattison IH, Jebbett JN. Clinical and histological observations on cuprizone toxicity and scrapie in mice. *Res Vet Sci* 1971;12:378–380.
143. Pattison IH, Jones KM. The possible nature of the transmissible agent of scrapie. *Vet Rec* 1967;80:1–8.
144. Pauly PC, Harris DA. Copper stimulates endocytosis of the prion protein. *J Biol Chem* 1998;273:33107–33110.
145. Paushkin SV, Kushnirov VV, Smirnov VN, Ter-Avanesyan MD. *In vitro* propagation of the prion-like state of yeast Sup35 protein. *Science* 1997;277:381–383.
146. Peretz D, Williamson RA, Matsunaga Y, et al. A conformational transition at the N terminus of the prion protein features in formation of the scrapie isoform. *J Mol Biol* 1997;273:614–622.
147. Petrukhin K, Fischer SG, Pirastu M, et al. Mapping, cloning and genetic characterization of the region containing the Wilson disease gene. *Nat Genet* 1993;5:338–343.
148. PHS: Public Health Service Interagency Coordinating Committee. Report on human growth hormone and Creutzfeldt-Jakob disease. 1997.
149. Polymeropoulos MH, Lavedan C, Leroy E, et al. Mutation in the α-synuclein gene identified in families with Parkinson's disease. *Science* 1997;276:2045–2047.
150. Poulter M, Baker HF, Frith CD, et al. Inherited prion disease with 144

base pair gene insertion. 1. Genealogical and molecular studies. *Brain* 1992;115:675–685.
151. Prusiner SB. Novel proteinaceous infectious particles cause scrapie. *Science* 1982;216:136–144.
152. Prusiner SB. Scrapie prions. *Annu Rev Microbiol* 1989;43:345–374.
153. Prusiner SB. Molecular biology of prion diseases. *Science* 1991;252: 1515–1522.
154. Prusiner SB. The prion diseases. *Sci Am* 1995;272:48–51, 54–57.
155. Prusiner SB. Prion diseases and the BSE crisis. *Science* 1997;278: 245–251.
156. Prusiner SB. Prions. *Proc Natl Acad Sci U S A* 1998;95:13363–13383.
157. Prusiner SB, Groth D, Serban A, et al. Ablation of the prion protein (PrP) gene in mice prevents scrapie and facilitates production of anti-PrP antibodies. *Proc Natl Acad Sci U S A* 1993;90:10608–10612.
158. Prusiner SB, McKinley MP, Bowman KA, et al. Scrapie prions aggregate to form amyloid-like birefringent rods. *Cell* 1983;35:349–358.
159. Prusiner SB, Scott M, Foster D, et al. Transgenetic studies implicate interactions between homologous PrP isoforms in scrapie prion replication. *Cell* 1990;63:673–686.
160. Prusiner SB, Scott MR, DeArmond SJ, Cohen FE. Prion protein biology. *Cell* 1998;93:337–348.
161. Rieger R, Edenhofer F, Lasmézas CI, Weiss S. The human 37-kDa laminin receptor precursor interacts with the prion protein in eukaryotic cells. *Nat Med* 1997;3:1383–1388.
162. Riek R, Hornemann S, Wider G, et al. NMR structure of the mouse prion protein domain PrP(121-231). *Nature* 1996;382:180–182.
163. Riek R, Wider G, Billeter M, et al. Prion protein NMR structure and familial human spongiform encephalopathies. *Proc Natl Acad Sci U S A* 1998;95:11667–11672.
164. Rogaev EI, Sherrington R, Rogaeva EA, et al. Familial Alzheimer's disease in kindreds with missense mutations in a gene on chromosome 1 related to the Alzheimer's disease type 3 gene. *Nature* 1995;376: 775–778.
165. Rohwer RG. Scrapie infectious agent is virus-like in size and susceptibility to inactivation. *Nature* 1984;308:658–662.
166. Rohwer RG. Virus-like sensitivity of the scrapie agent to heat inactivation. *Science* 1984;223:600–602.
167. Rohwer RG. Estimation of scrapie nucleic acid molecular weight from standard curves for virus sensitivity to ionizing radiation. *Nature* 1986;320:381.
168. Rohwer RG. The scrapie agent: "A virus by any other name." *Curr Top Microbiol Immunol* 1991;172:195–232.
169. Roos R, Gajdusek DC, Gibbs CJ Jr. The clinical characteristics of transmissible Creutzfeldt-Jakob disease. *Brain* 1973;96:1–20.
170. Safar J, Wille H, Itri V, et al. Eight prion strains have PrP^{Sc} molecules with different conformations. *Nat Med* 1998;4:1157–1165.
171. Sailer A, Büeler H, Fischer M, et al. No propagation of prions in mice devoid of PrP. *Cell* 1994;77:967–968.
172. Sakaguchi S, Katamine S, Nishida N, et al. Loss of cerebellar Purkinje cells in aged mice homozygous for a disrupted PrP gene. *Nature* 1996;380:528–531.
173. Sandou F, Finkbeiner S, Devys D, Greenberg ME. Huntingtin acts in the nucleus to induce apoptosis but death does not correlate with the formation of intranuclear inclusions. *Cell* 1998;95:55–66.
174. Saunders AM, Strittmatter WJ, Schmechel D, et al. Association of apolipoprotein E allele ε4 with late-onset familial and sporadic Alzheimer's disease. *Neurology* 1993;43:1467–1472.
175. Scherzinger E, Sittler A, Schweiger K, et al. Self-assembly of polyglutamine-containing huntingtin fragments into amyloid-like fibrils: Implications for Huntington's disease pathology. *Proc Natl Acad Sci U S A* 1999;96:4604–4609.
176. Scott M, Foster D, Mirenda C, et al. Transgenic mice expressing hamster prion protein produce species-specific scrapie infectivity and amyloid plaques. *Cell* 1989;59:847–857.
177. Scott MR, Groth D, Tatzelt J, et al. Propagation of prion strains through specific conformers of the prion protein. *J Virol* 1997;71: 9032–9044.
178. Scott MR, Köhler R, Foster D, Prusiner SB. Chimeric prion protein expression in cultured cells and transgenic mice. *Protein Sci* 1992;1: 986–997.
179. Scott MR, Safar J, Telling G, et al. Identification of a prion protein epitope modulating transmission of bovine spongiform encephalopathy prions to transgenic mice. *Proc Natl Acad Sci U S A* 1997;94: 14279–14284.
179a. Scott MR, Will R, Ironside J, et al. Compelling transgenetic evidence for transmission of bovine spongiform encephalopathy prions to humans. *Proc Natl Acad Sci* 1999;96:15137–15142.
180. Sherrington R, Rogaev EI, Liang Y, et al. Cloning of a gene bearing missense mutations in early-onset familial Alzheimer's disease. *Nature* 1995;375:754–760.
181. Shibuya S, Higuchi J, Shin R-W, et al. Protective prion protein polymorphisms against sporadic Creutzfeldt-Jakob disease. *Lancet* 1998; 351:419.
182. Shinde UP, Liu JJ, Inouye M. Protein memory through altered folding mediated by intramolecular chaperones. *Nature* 1997;389:520–522.
183. Shmerling D, Hegyi I, Fischer M, et al. Expression of amino-terminally truncated PrP in the mouse leading to ataxia and specific cerebellar lesions. *Cell* 1998;93:203–214.
184. Sigurdsson B. Rida, a chronic encephalitis of sheep with general remarks on infections which develop slowly and some of their special characteristics. *Br Vet J* 1954;110:341–354.
185. Somerville RA, Chong A, Mulqueen OU, et al. Biochemical typing of scrapie strains. *Nature* 1997;386:564.
186. Spillantini MG, Crowther RA, Jakes R, et al. α-Synuclein in filamentous inclusions of Lewy bodies from Parkinson's disease and dementia with Lewy bodies. *Proc Natl Acad Sci U S A* 1998;95:6469–6473.
187. Stahl N, Baldwin MA, Teplow DB, et al. Structural analysis of the scrapie prion protein using mass spectrometry and amino acid sequencing. *Biochemistry* 1993;32:1991–2002.
188. Stahl N, Borchelt DR, Hsiao K, Prusiner SB. Scrapie prion protein contains a phosphatidylinositol glycolipid. *Cell* 1987;51:229–240.
189. Stender A. Weitere Beiträge zum Kapitel "Spastische Pseudosklerose Jakobs." *Z Gesamte Neurol Psychiatr* 1930;128:528–543.
190. Stöckel J, Safar J, Wallace AC, et al. Prion protein selectively binds copper (II) ions. *Biochemistry* 1998;37:7185–7193.
191. Supattapone S, Bosque P, Muramoto T, et al. Prion protein of 106 residues creates an artificial transmission barrier for prion replication in transgenic mice. *Cell* 1999;96:869–878.
192. Tagliavini F, Prelli F, Ghiso J, et al. Amyloid protein of Gerstmann-Sträussler-Scheinker disease (Indiana kindred) is an 11 kd fragment of prion protein with an N-terminal glycine at codon 58. *EMBO J* 1991; 10:513–519.
193. Taraboulos A, Jendroska K, Serban D, et al. Regional mapping of prion proteins in brains. *Proc Natl Acad Sci U S A* 1992;89:7620–7624.
194. Taraboulos A, Rogers M, Borchelt DR, et al. Acquisition of protease resistance by prion proteins in scrapie-infected cells does not require asparagine-linked glycosylation. *Proc Natl Acad Sci U S A* 1990;87: 8262–8266.
195. Taraboulos A, Scott M, Semenov A, et al. Cholesterol depletion and modification of COOH-terminal targeting sequence of the prion protein inhibits formation of the scrapie isoform. *J Cell Biol* 1995;129:121–132.
196. Tatzelt J, Zuo J, Voellmy R, et al. Scrapie prions selectively modify the stress response in neuroblastoma cells. *Proc Natl Acad Sci U S A* 1995;92:2944–2948.
197. Telling GC, Haga T, Torchia M, et al. Interactions between wild-type and mutant prion proteins modulate neurodegeneration in transgenic mice. *Genes Dev* 1996;10:1736–1750.
198. Telling GC, Parchi P, DeArmond SJ, et al. Evidence for the conformation of the pathologic isoform of the prion protein enciphering and propagating prion diversity. *Science* 1996;274:2079–2082.
199. Telling GC, Scott M, Hsiao KK, et al. Transmission of Creutzfeldt-Jakob disease from humans to transgenic mice expressing chimeric human-mouse prion protein. *Proc Natl Acad Sci U S A* 1994;91: 9936–9940.
200. Telling GC, Scott M, Mastrianni J, et al. Prion propagation in mice expressing human and chimeric PrP transgenes implicates the interaction of cellular PrP with another protein. *Cell* 1995;83:79–90.
201. Tobler I, Gaus SE, Deboer T, et al. Altered circadian activity rhythms and sleep in mice devoid of prion protein. *Nature* 1996;380:639–642.
202. Tremblay P, Meiner Z, Galou M, et al. Doxycyline control of prion protein transgene expression modulates prion disease in mice. *Proc Natl Acad Sci U S A* 1998;95:12580–12585.
203. Viles JH, Cohen FE, Prusiner SB, et al. Copper binding to the prion protein: Structural implications of four identical cooperative binding sites. *Proc Natl Acad Sci U S A* 1999;96:2042–2047.
204. Vulpe C, Levinson B, Whitney S, et al. Isolation of a candidate gene for Menkes disease and evidence that it encodes a copper-transporting ATPase. *Nat Genet* 1993;3:7–13.

205. Wadsworth JDF, Hill AF, Joiner S, et al. Strain-specific prion-protein conformation determined by metal ions. *Nat Cell Biol* 1999;1:55–59.
206. Westaway D, DeArmond SJ, Cayetano-Canlas J, et al. Degeneration of skeletal muscle, peripheral nerves, and the central nervous system in transgenic mice overexpressing wild-type prion proteins. *Cell* 1994; 76:117–129.
207. Westaway D, Goodman PA, Mirenda CA, et al. Distinct prion proteins in short and long scrapie incubation period mice. *Cell* 1987;51:651–662.
208. Westaway D, Prusiner SB. Conservation of the cellular gene encoding the scrapie prion protein. *Nucleic Acids Res* 1986;14:2035–2044.
209. Westaway D, Zuliani V, Cooper CM, et al. Homozygosity for prion protein alleles encoding glutamine-171 renders sheep susceptible to natural scrapie. *Genes Dev* 1994;8:959–969.
210. Wickner RB. [URE3] as an altered URE2 protein: Evidence for a prion analog in *Saccharomyces cerevisiae. Science* 1994;264:566–569.
211. Wickner RB. A new prion controls fungal cell fusion incompatibility [Commentary]. *Proc Natl Acad Sci U S A* 1997;94:10012–10014.
212. Will RG, Cousens SN, Farrington CP, et al. Deaths from variant Creutzfeldt-Jakob disease. *Lancet* 1999;353:979.
213. Will RG, Ironside JW, Zeidler M, et al. A new variant of Creutzfeldt-Jakob disease in the UK. *Lancet* 1996;347:921–925.
214. Wolfe MS, Xia W, Ostaszewski BL, et al. Two transmembrane aspartates in presenilin-1 required for presenilin endoproteolysis and γ-secretase activity. *Nature* 1999;398:513–517.
215. Zlotnik I, Stamp JL. Scrapie disease of sheep. *World Neurol* 1961;2: 895–907.

Subject Index

An *f* after a page number indicates a figure. A *t* indicates a table.

C